# Free personal online access
# for 5 years

The copy of *New Oxford Textbook of Psychiatry* you have purchased entitles you to free personal online access for 5 years.

Customers outside North and South America, please visit:
**https://subscriberservices.sams.oup.com/token to set up access.**
Customers in North and South America, please visit:
[**https://ams.oup.com/order/OTPSYCHSCRIP**] to set up access.
<u>Please note</u>: the URL is case-sensitive.

To register, enter the code on this page. Please keep the number for future reference as, in the event of a query, you may be asked for it. Please note that as part of the registration process you will be informed of our terms and conditions, and will be asked to accept these to confirm your online access.

| Unique code: | JE19991635396913 |
|---|---|

The online access provided free with this book is for individuals who have purchased a personal copy only, and this will be verified as part of the access process. Users of library copies should ask their librarian about access in their institution.

**CUSTOMER SUPPORT**

Customers outside North & South America
Tel: +44 (0) 1865 353705
Email: accesstokens@oup.com

**Customers in North & South America**

Tel: 1-800-334-4249 ext. 6484
Email: oxfordonline@oup.com

New Oxford Textbook of

# Psychiatry

# New Oxford Textbook of

# Psychiatry

## THIRD EDITION

EDITED BY

## John R. Geddes

*Professor of Epidemiological Psychiatry*
*Head of the Department of Psychiatry*
*Warneford Hospital*
*University of Oxford*
*Oxford, UK*

## Nancy C. Andreasen

*Professor of Psychiatry*
*Andrew H. Woods Chair of Psychiatry*
*Department of Psychiatry*
*University of Iowa Carver College of Medicine*
*Iowa City, USA*

## Guy M. Goodwin

*Senior Research Fellow*
*Department of Psychiatry*
*Warneford Hospital*
*University of Oxford*
*Oxford, UK*

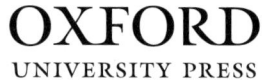

OXFORD
UNIVERSITY PRESS

# OXFORD
### UNIVERSITY PRESS

Great Clarendon Street, Oxford, OX2 6DP,
United Kingdom

Oxford University Press is a department of the University of Oxford.
It furthers the University's objective of excellence in research, scholarship,
and education by publishing worldwide. Oxford is a registered trade mark of
Oxford University Press in the UK and in certain other countries

First Edition published 2000
Second Edition published 2009
Third Edition published 2020

Impression: 1

Published in the United States of America by Oxford University Press
198 Madison Avenue, New York, NY 10016, United States of America

British Library Cataloguing in Publication Data
Data available

Library of Congress Control Number: 2019931646

ISBN 978-0-19-871300-5

Printed in Great Britain by
Bell & Bain Ltd., Glasgow

# Preface

This is the third edition of the textbook. We decided to rethink the size and content completely when planning this edition. Our sense was that a larger and larger archive of accumulated knowledge is no longer feasible or desirable in the digital age. We wanted to produce a single volume with a more defined point of view, that better reflects the challenge of the future.

Psychiatry is a medical specialty. Medicine took its origins in simple observation and classification and the serendipitous discovery of palliative treatments. The application of science has transformed much of medicine by providing an understanding of mechanisms of pathology. The scientific method provides the only way to reliable knowledge, and medical science is slowly developing rational treatments that are potentially curative. However, aside from treatable infections, we have a long way to go. The trajectory of medical advance in the practice of psychiatry has been slower than for other disease areas in recent years, but neuroscience is difficult. What underwrites our confidence in what is sometimes disparagingly described as the medical model is the fact that psychiatric disorders, especially severe disorders, have a genetic basis. Genetic risks are largely unidirectional and they are biological. They guarantee some kind of future biological explanation for the phenomena they describe. So if you decide that schizophrenia is a myth, a social construct, or a plot by psychiatrists to enhance their social status, you have to explain why its inheritance is what it is.

If, like us, you find the genetic data compelling, then you accept the grand challenge of working out the neurobiology of psychiatric disorder. We cannot know how quickly it will translate into improved treatments, but we think there are already promising developments from molecular biology and neuroimaging. Imaging has been particularly important because it has stimulated the development of a completely brain-based cognitive neuroscience. This is a major intellectual shift. Forty years ago, an experimental psychologist would have said that the brain was unimportant for the study of mental mechanisms and even less important for the development of psychological treatments. As this view changes, so the advances of neuroscience can be translated into patient benefit as scientifically guided psychotherapy.

Our authors are drawn from all over the world, and they illustrate the simple truth that science is universal. We thank them most sincerely for their efforts in bringing the project to completion.

## The layout of the book

The content of chapters was not highly pre-specified, and the chapters themselves have not been edited for conformity with the editors' views. They can be read as free-standing contributions. Accordingly, there is both overlap and divergence in how topics are covered, which will reflect the writers' priorities and interests.

In the previous edition of the textbook, the editors identified convergence as an important theme of the book. We are not convinced further convergence has occurred since 2001. Instead we have seen a surprising amount of divergence in the claims made about psychiatry. Our section on approaches to psychiatry reflects some of the key issues relating to the patient's perspective, stigma, the global challenge of mental disorder, practical ethics, and the foundations of psychiatry as phenomenology and a medical discipline. It further sets the scene for current controversies around diagnosis, psychopathology, evidence, and drug terminology.

The chapters in the section on the scientific basis of psychiatric aetiology and treatment provide simple introductions to the relevant disciplines that underpin our scientific understanding.

Individual disorders are covered in sections that follow the structure of the *Diagnostic and Statistical Manual of Mental Disorders*, fifth edition (DSM-5). DSM-5 was published in 2013. It had been envisaged that it would be possible to make major changes to the approach of DSM-IV. Thus, major advances in genetics, imaging, and neurobiology were widely expected to transform psychiatry, following the success of the human genome project and the decade of the brain. This transformation has not yet happened. Hence, DSM-5 (and the International Classification of Diseases, eleventh revision) follow a much more conventional, clinically led summary of how patients present with psychiatric disorder. We see no reason to deny the utility of symptom-based diagnoses and the consensus that created the current categories. However, the project of applying neuroscience to psychiatry has not failed, as has sometimes been implied by criticism of DSM-5. For these reasons, we have included chapters on genetics, neurobiological targets, and imaging in the sections of the book focused on specific disorders.

We have also included sections on service provision and forensic psychiatry because these are critical to the context in which psychiatric disorder is managed.

We thank the staff of OUP for their support and encouragement and Andy Richford who has been our project manager sans pareil.

John R. Geddes
Nancy C. Andreasen
Guy M. Goodwin

## Professor Michael Gelder (1929–2018)

*Michael Gelder, one of the founding editors of the* New Oxford Textbook of Psychiatry, *sadly died in 2018. We dedicate this new edition of the book to Michael's memory.*

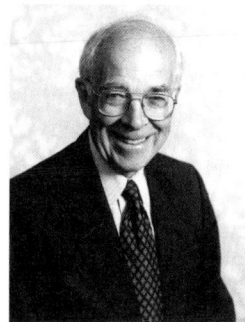

Michael was the first WA Handley Professor of Psychiatry at the University of Oxford and founded the Department of Psychiatry in 1969. He led the Department for 27 years until he retired in 1996. Before arriving in Oxford, at the Institute of Psychiatry, Michael developed a treatment for anxiety based on desensitization, in which gradual exposure to the feared stimulus was coupled with physical relaxation. He described the first controlled trial of this psychological therapy in patients with severe agoraphobia in his seminal 1966 publication with Isaac Marks.

Michael possessed remarkable organizational abilities and leadership skills and he built a thriving Department of Psychiatry in Oxford with a particular focus on developing both psychological and physical treatments. This departmental focus continues into the present. When JRG interviewed him in 2018, very shortly before he died, Michael admitted to being particularly proud of the Department's development of cognitive behaviour therapy (CBT) under his leadership. These treatments include highly effective forms of CBT for anxiety disorders, post-traumatic stress disorder, chronic fatigue syndrome, and eating disorders. All have been widely adopted in clinical practice and have benefited enormous numbers of people worldwide. Michael also developed a psychopharmacology research unit based on powerful cross-departmental collaboration within the University. The unit has a strong track record of investigating the mechanisms of action of antidepressants and anxiolytics and its work has fundamentally shaped our understanding of the biology underlying psychiatric disorder.

Michael was also a committed and inspirational teacher and the driving force behind a successful series of psychiatry textbooks. The first, in 1983, was the *Oxford Textbook of Psychiatry* (now in its seventh edition). Translated into six languages, this became the standard textbook for psychiatric trainees. Then came the *Concise Textbook* (aimed at medical students and now in its fifth edition) and the current *New Oxford Textbook of Psychiatry* (targeted at postgraduates—this is the third edition).

As he passed the age of 80, Michael had finally retired from editing textbooks (although he was delighted that his colleagues continue to revise them!), but he closely followed the development of the Department. He will be greatly missed. Michael was a truly remarkable clinical academic, inspirational in his ability to combine research with clinical practice, teaching, and leadership.

# Contents

# Abbreviations

| | |
|---|---|
| α-MSH | alpha-melanocyte-stimulating hormone |
| G × E | gene and environment |
| μg | microgram |
| AA | arachidonic acid |
| AAO | age at onset |
| AAS | ascending arousal system |
| AASM | American Academy of Sleep Medicine |
| ABA | applied behavioural analysis; activity-based anorexia |
| Abeta | amyloid beta |
| AC | adenylyl cyclase |
| ACC | anterior cingulate cortex |
| ACE | angiotensin-converting enzyme; adverse childhood experience |
| ACE(R) | Addenbrooke Cognitive Examination (Revised) |
| aCGH | array-comparative genomic hybridization |
| ACh | acetylcholine |
| ACMG | American College of Medical Genetics and Genomics |
| ACQ | Agoraphobia Cognition Questionnaire |
| ACT | acceptance and commitment therapy; assertive community treatment |
| ACTH | adrenocorticotrophic hormone |
| AD | axial diffusivity; Alzheimer's disease; Alzheimer's dementia; adjustment disorder |
| ADAMHA | US Alcohol, Drug Abuse, and Mental Health Administration |
| ADAPT | Adaption and Development After Persecution and Trauma (model) |
| ADAS-cog | Alzheimer's Disease Assessment Scale-cognitive subscale |
| ADD | attention deficit disorder |
| ADDUCE | Attention Deficit Hyperactivity Disorder Drugs Use Chronic Effects |
| ADH | alcohol dehydrogenase; antidiuretic hormone |
| ADHD | attention-deficit/hyperactivity disorder |
| ADP | adenosine diphosphate |
| A&E | accident and emergency |
| aFTLD-U | atypical fronto-temporal lobar degeneration with ubiquitinated inclusions |
| AGD | argyrophilic grain disease |
| AgRP | agouti-related protein |
| AHI | apnoea–hypopnea index |
| aHR | adjusted hazard ratio |
| AICD | APP intracellular domain |
| AIDS | acquired immune deficiency syndrome |

| | |
|---|---|
| AIMS | Abnormal Involuntary Movement Scale |
| AL | allostatic load |
| ALDH | acetaldehyde dehydrogenase |
| ALIC | anterior limb of the internal capsule |
| ALFF | amplitude of low-frequency fluctuations |
| ALS | amyotrophic lateral sclerosis |
| AMBIT | adolescent mentalization-based integrative therapy |
| AMDP | Association for Methodology and Documentation in Psychiatry; alternative DSM-5 model for personality disorders |
| AMP | adenosine monophosphate-activated protein; amphetamine |
| AMPA | α-amino-3-hydroxy-5-methyl-4-isoxazolepropionic acid |
| AMTS | Abbreviated Mental Test Score |
| AN | anorexia nervosa |
| ANA | antinuclear antibody |
| ANP | atrial natriuretic peptide |
| AN-R | restrictive subtype of anorexia nervosa |
| AO | assertive outreach |
| aOR | adjusted odds ratio |
| AOS | apraxia of speech |
| AP | agoraphobia; area postrema |
| APA | American Psychiatric Association |
| APD | antisocial personality disorder |
| APOE | apolipoprotein E |
| APP | amyloid β precursor protein |
| APS | attenuated psychotic symptoms |
| ARFID | avoidant restrictive food intake disorder |
| ARID | autosomal recessive forms of intellectual disability |
| ARMS | at-risk mental state |
| ARP | aripiprazole |
| AS | anxiety sensitivity |
| ASCOT | Adult Social Care Outcome Toolkit |
| ASD | autism spectrum disorder; acute stress disorder |
| ASI | Anxiety Sensitivity Index |
| ASIC | acid-sensing ion channel |
| ASL | arterial spin labelling |
| ASN | asenapine |
| AsPD | antisocial personality disorder |
| ASPD | antisocial personality disorder |
| ASPS | advanced sleep phase syndrome |
| ASWPD | advanced sleep–wake phase disorder |
| ATC | Anatomical Therapeutic Chemical |
| ATF6 | activating transcription factor 6 |

| | | | |
|---|---|---|---|
| ATL | anterior temporal lobe | CADASIL | cerebral autosomal dominant arteriopathy with subcortical infarcts and leukoencephalopathy |
| ATP | adenosine triphosphate | CAM | Confusion Assessment Method |
| ATPD | acute and transient psychotic disorder | CAMCOG(R) | Cambridge Cognitive Assessment (Revised) |
| ATX | atomoxetine | CAMHS | child and adolescent mental health services |
| AUC | area under the curve | cAMP | cyclic adenosine monophosphate |
| AUD | alcohol use disorder | CAPA | Child and Adolescent Psychiatric Assessment |
| AUDADIS-IV | Alcohol Use Disorder and Associated Disabilities Interview Schedule-IV | CAPP | Comprehensive Assessment of Psychopathic Personality Disorder |
| AVP | vasopressin | CART | cocaine- and amphetamine-related transcript |
| AvPD | avoidant personality disorder | CAS9 | CRISPR-associated protein 9 |
| AVPD | avoidant personality disorder | CAT | cognitive analytic therapy |
| BBB | blood–brain barrier | CATCH-IT | Competent Adulthood Transition with Cognitive Behavioural and Interpersonal Training |
| BBV | blood-borne virus | CATIE | Clinical Antipsychotic Trial of Intervention Effectiveness (study) |
| BD | bipolar disorder | CBA | cost-benefit analysis |
| BDD | body dysmorphic disorder | CBC | complete blood count |
| BDI | Beck Depression Inventory | CBCL | Child Behavior Problems Checklist |
| BDNF | brain-derived neurotrophic factor | CBCM | cognitive behavioural case management |
| BDSM | bondage, dominance and submission, sadism, and masochism | CBD | cortico-basal degeneration; cannabidiol |
| BED | binge eating disorder | CBF | cerebral blood flow |
| BET | brief eclectic therapy | CBG | cortico-basal ganglia |
| BF | basal forebrain | CBG-GSH | guided self-help cognitive behavioural therapy |
| BI | behavioural inhibition | CBI | classroom-based intervention |
| BIA | budget impact analysis | CBIT | Comprehensive Behavioral Intervention for Tics |
| BIBD | basophilic inclusion body disease | CBO | community-based organization |
| BIPS | Brief Intermittent Psychotic Symptoms | CBS | cortico-basal syndrome |
| BIT | behavioural intervention team | CBT | cognitive behavioural therapy |
| BLA | basolateral amygdala | CBT-E | enhanced cognitive behavioural treatment |
| BLIPS | Brief Limited Intermittent Psychotic Symptoms | CBTi | cognitive behavioural therapy for insomnia |
| BMI | body mass index | CBT-PD | cognitive behavioural therapy for personality disorder |
| BMP | bone morphogenetic protein | CC | collaborative care |
| BN | bulimia nervosa | CCA | cost-consequences analysis |
| BNM | biophysical network model | CCK | cholecystokinin |
| B/NRT | bupropion/nicotine replacement therapy | CCK-4 | cholecystokinin tetrapeptide |
| BOLD | blood oxygen level-dependent | CCL | conventional consultation liaison |
| BOTMP | Bruininks–Oseretsky Test of Motor Proficiency | CCM | collaborative care management |
| BP | blood pressure | CD | coeliac disease |
| BPD | borderline personality disorder; bipolar disorder | CDC | Center for Disease Control and Prevention |
| BPI | bipolar disorder type I | CDDG | *Clinical Descriptions and Diagnostic Guidelines* (from *ICD-10 Classification of Mental and Behavioral Disorders*) |
| BPII | bipolar disorder type II | | |
| bpm | beats per minute | | |
| BPRS | Brief Psychiatric Rating Scale | | |
| BPSD | behavioural and psychological symptoms of dementia | CEA | cost-effectiveness analysis |
| BS | basic symptoms | CEST | chemical exchange saturation transfer |
| BSE | bovine spongiform encephalopathy | CET | cue-exposure treatment |
| BTSAS | Behavioural Treatment for Substance Abuse in Severe and Persistent Mental Illness | CETA | Common Elements Treatment Approach |
| bvFTD | behavioural-variant fronto-temporal dementia | CFIR | Consolidated Framework for Implementation Research |
| BWLT | behavioural weight loss therapy | CFS | chronic fatigue syndrome |
| BZD | benzodiazepine | CGAS | Child Global Assessment Scale |
| C&A | children and adolescents | CGE | caudal ganglionic eminence |
| Ca²⁺ | calcium | CGI-I | Clinical Global Impression of Improvement |
| CAA | cerebral amyloid angiopathy | cGMP | cyclic guanosine monophosphate |
| CAARMS | Comprehensive Assessment of At-Risk Mental State | CGMV | cortical grey matter volume |
| CAC | Clinical Assessment of Confusion | CH | congenital hypothyroidism |
| CAD | coronary artery disease | | |

| | | | |
|---|---|---|---|
| CHARGE | Cohorts for Heart and Aging Research in Genomic Epidemiology | CRISPR | clustered regularly interspaced short palindromic repeat |
| CHAT | Comprehensive Health Assessment Tool | CRN | correct related negativity |
| CHMP | Committee for Medicinal Products for Human Use | CRP | C-reactive protein |
| CHMP2B | charged multivesicular body protein 2b | CrPR | Criminal Procedure Rules |
| CHOICE | CHOosing Interventions that are Cost-Effective (project) | CRSWD | circadian rhythm sleep–wake disorder |
| | | CS | conditioned stimulus; compulsive shopping |
| CHOP | Children's Hospital of Philadelphia | CSA | child sexual abuse |
| CHR | clinical high-risk | CSB | compulsive sexual behaviour |
| CI | confidence interval | CSF | cerebrospinal fluid |
| CIDI | Composite International Diagnostic Instrument | CSS | chromosomal substitution strain |
| CIR | Clutter Image Rating | CSTC | cortico-striato-thalamo-cortical |
| CJD | Creutzfeldt–Jakob disease | CT | computed tomography |
| CLiPS | Collaborative Longitudinal Personality Disorders Study | CTD | chronic tic disorder |
| | | CTE | chronic traumatic encephalopathy |
| CLP | consultation-liaison psychiatry | CTO | community treatment order |
| CLPDS | Collaborative Longitudinal Personality Disorders Study | CU | callous-unemotional |
| | | CUA | cost-utility analysis |
| CLPS | Collaborative Longitudinal Personality Study | CUtLASS | Cost Utility of the Latest Antipsychotic drugs in Schizophrenia Study |
| cm | centimetre | |
| CM | contingency management; crisis management | CVD | cardiovascular disease |
| CMA | chromosomal microarray analysis; chaperone-mediated autophagy; cost-minimization analysis | CVO | circumventricular organ |
| | | CWMV | cerebral white matter volume |
| | | CY-BOCS | Children's Yale-Brown Obsessive Compulsive Scale |
| CMAT | Changes to the Matrix Council | DA | dopamine |
| CMD | common mental disorder | dACC | dorsal anterior cingulate cortex |
| CMHD | common mental health disorder | DACCP | Dundee ADHD Clinical Care Pathway |
| CMHT | community mental health team | DAG | diacylglycerol |
| CMP | comprehensive metabolic panel | DAGK | diacylglycerol kinase |
| CMS-R | Comorbidity Survey-Replication | DALY | disability-adjusted life year |
| CNGC | cyclic nucleotide-gated channel | DAMP | damage-associated molecular pattern |
| CNS | central nervous system | DAPP | Differential Assessment of Personality Pathology |
| CNV | copy number variant | |
| COG | centre of gravity | DARI | dopamine reuptake inhibitor |
| COGA | Collaborative Studies on Genetics of Alcoholism | DAT | dopamine; dopamine transporter |
| COGEND | Collaborative Genetic Study of Nicotine Dependence | DAWS | dopamine agonist withdrawal syndrome |
| COMT | catechol-O-methyltransferase | DBH | dopamine-beta-hydroxylase |
| CONSORT | Consolidated Standards of Reporting Trial | DBS | deep brain stimulation |
| CONVERGE | China, Oxford, and Virginia Commonwealth University Experimental Research on Genetic Epidemiology | DBT | dialectical behaviour therapy |
| | | DCD | developmental co-ordination disorder |
| | | DCM | dynamic causal model |
| COPC | chronic overlapping pain condition | DCR | Diagnostic Criteria for Research (from *ICD-10 Classification of Mental and Behavioral Disorders*) |
| C9ORF72 | chromosome 9 open reading frame 72 | |
| CoSA | Circles of Support and Accountability | DCS | d-cycloserine |
| COX-2 | cyclo-oxygenase-2 | DD | delay discounting |
| CP | choroid plexus | DDA | direct detection assay |
| CPA | Care Programme Approach | DDP | dynamic deconstructive psychotherapy |
| CPES | Collaborative Psychiatric Epidemiological Studies | DEX | dextroamphetamine |
| CPR | Civil Procedure Rules | DFC | dorsolateral prefrontal cortex |
| CPT | cognitive processing therapy | 2-DG | 2-deoxyglucose |
| Cr | creatine | DHA | docosahexaenoic acid |
| CR | cognitive rehabilitation; conditioned response | DHPG | dihydroxyphenylethylene glycol |
| CRA | community reinforcement approach | DIAN | Dominantly Inherited Alzheimer Network |
| CREB | cAMP response element binding protein | DIRT | Danger ideation reduction therapy |
| CRF | corticotropin-releasing factor | DIRUM | Database of Instruments for Resource Use Measurement |
| CRF1 | corticotropin-releasing factor 1 | |
| CRH | corticotropin-releasing hormone | DIS | Diagnostic Interview Schedule |
| CR/HT | crisis resolution/home treatment | DISC | Diagnostic Interview Schedule for Children |
| | | DISC1 | Disrupted in Schizophrenia 1 |

| | | | | |
|---|---|---|---|---|
| DLB | dementia with Lewy bodies | | ED | elimination disorder; emergency department; eating disorder; erectile disorder |
| DLMO | dim light melatonin onset | | EDNOS | eating disorder not otherwise specified |
| dlPFC | dorsolateral prefrontal cortex | | EDSP | Early Developmental Stages of Psychopathology (study) |
| DLPFC | dorsolateral prefrontal cortex | | EEG | electroencephalogram |
| DM | diabetes mellitus | | EFFEKTE-E | *Entwicklungsförderung in Familien: Eltern- und Kinder-Training in emotional belasteten Familien* |
| DMH | dorsomedial nucleus of the hypothalamus | | EGF | epidermal growth factor |
| DM-ID | Diagnostic Manual-Intellectual Disabilities | | EHS | essential hypersomnia syndrome |
| DMN | default mode network | | EI | early intervention |
| DMT | dimethyltryptamine | | EMA | European Medicines Agency; ecological momentary assessment |
| DNA | deoxyribonucleic acid | | EMDR | eye movement desensitization and reprocessing |
| DNIC | diffuse noxious inhibitory control | | EMG | electromyography |
| DOMINO | Donepezil and Memantine in Moderate to Severe Alzheimer's Disease (study) | | ENCODE | Encyclopedia of DNA Elements |
| DOMS | delayed onset of muscular soreness | | ENIGMA | Enhancing NeuroImaging Genetics through Meta-Analysis (Consortium) |
| DOR | delta opioid receptor | | EOG | electro-oculography |
| DOSS | Delirium Observation Screening Scale | | EOS | endogenous opioid system |
| DPD | dependent personality disorder | | EP | explaining pain |
| DPMS | descending pain modulatory system | | EPA | eicosapentanoic acid |
| DR | dorsal raphe | | EPAD | European Prevention of Alzheimer's Dementia Consortium |
| DRD4 | dopamine receptor type 4 | | EPDS | Edinburgh Postnatal Depression scale |
| DRG | diagnosis-related group | | EPI | echo planar imaging |
| DRN | dorsal raphe nuclei | | ePREP | Prevention and Relationship Enhancement Programme |
| DRPLA | dentatorubropallidoluysian atrophy | | EPS | extra-pyramidal side effect |
| DRS-R-98 | Delirium Rating Scale-Revised-98 | | EPSE | extra-pyramidal side effect |
| DS | dorsal striatum | | ER | endoplasmic reticulum |
| DSED | disinhibited social engagement disorder | | ERF | event-related field |
| DSM | *Diagnostic and Statistical Manual of Mental Disorders* | | ERK | extracellular regulated kinase |
| DSM-III | Third revision of the Diagnostic and Statistical Manual of Mental Disorders | | ERN | error-related negativity |
| DSM-III-R | DSM-III-Revised | | ERP | event-related potential; exposure and response prevention |
| DSM-IV-TR | DSM-IV 'Text Revision' | | ES | effect size |
| DSM-5 | 5th edition of the Diagnostic and Statistical Manual of Mental Disorders | | ESDM | Early Start Denver Model |
| DST | daylight saving times; dexamethasone suppression test | | ESR | erythrocyte sedimentation rate |
| DSWPD | delayed sleep–wake phase disorder | | ESS | Epworth Sleepiness Scale |
| DTC | democratic therapeutic community | | ESSENCE | Early Symptomatic Syndromes Eliciting Neurodevelopmental Clinical Examination |
| DTI | diffusion tensor imaging | | EU | European Union |
| DTS | diffusion tensor spectroscopy | | EUFEST | European First Episode Schizophrenia Trial |
| DUB | deubiquitinating enzyme | | EULAR | European League Against Rheumatism |
| DUD | drug use disorders | | EUnetHTA | European Network for Health Technology Assessment |
| DUI | daytime urinary incontinence; duration of untreated illness | | FA | fractional anisotropy |
| DUP | duration of untreated psychosis | | FACT | functional assertive community treatment |
| DURG | Drug Utilisation Research Group | | fAD | familial Alzheimer's disease |
| DVA | domestic violence and abuse | | FASD | fetal alcohol spectrum disorders |
| DWI | diffusion-weighted imaging | | fcMRI | functional connectivity magnetic resonance imaging |
| DXA | dual-energy X-ray absorptiometry | | FDA | US Food and Drug Administration |
| DY-BOCS | Dimensional Yale-Brown Obsessive Compulsive Scale | | FDG | fluorodeoxyglucose |
| DZ | dizygotic | | FDOPA | 18F-fluorodopa |
| EAGG | European ADHD Guideline Group | | FEP | first-episode psychosis |
| EAS | euthanasia or assisted suicide | | FFI | fatal familial insomnia |
| EC | enhanced care | | FFM | five-factor model of personality |
| ECA | Epidemiologic Catchment Area (study) | | | |
| ECG | electrocardiography | | | |
| ECNP | European College of Neuropsychopharmacology | | | |
| ECT | electroconvulsive therapy | | | |

| | | | |
|---|---|---|---|
| FFT | family-focused therapy; functional family therapy | GI | gyrification index; gender incongruence |
| FGA | first-generation antipsychotic | GID | gender identity disorder |
| FGCB | Family Group Cognitive-Behavioural | GIDC | gender identity disorder of childhood |
| FGF | fibroblast growth factor | GIDYQ-AA | Gender Identity/Gender Dysphoria Questionnaire for Adolescents and Adults |
| FI | faecal incontinence | | |
| FINGER | Finnish Geriatric Intervention Study to Prevent Cognitive Impairment and Disability (study) | GIP | G protein-coupled receptor-interacting protein |
| | | GJ | gap junction |
| FLAIR | fluid-attenuated inversion recovery | GLM | general linear model |
| FL-APM | first-line dopamine antagonist medication | GM | grey matter |
| FM | fibromyalgia | GMV | grey matter volume |
| fMRI | functional magnetic resonance imaging | GnIH | gonadotrophin-inhibitory hormone |
| FMRP | fragile X mental retardation protein | GnRH | gonadotrophin-releasing hormone |
| FMT | 6-18F-fluoro-l-m-tyrosine | GnRHa | gonadotrophin-releasing hormone analogue |
| FNSD | functional neurological symptom disorder | GO | Gene Ontology |
| FOCUS | Families OverComing Under Stress | GORD | gastro-oesophageal reflux disease |
| FPN | frontal-parietal network | GPCR | G protein-coupled receptor |
| FPR | Family Procedure Rules | GPPPD | genito-pelvic pain/penetration disorder |
| FSCD | Family Study of Cocaine Dependence | GR | glucocorticoid receptor |
| FSIAD | female sexual interest/arousal disorder | GRADE | Grading of Recommendations, Assessment, Development, and Evaluations |
| fT | femtotesla | | |
| FTD | fronto-temporal dementia | GRDS | genetic risk and deterioration syndrome |
| FTDC | International Behavior-variant FTD Criteria Consortium | GRE | gradient echo |
| | | GREML | genomic-relatedness-matrix restricted maximum likelihood |
| FTE | full-time equivalent | | |
| FTI | family therapeutic intervention | GRK | G protein-coupled receptor kinase |
| FTLD | fronto-temporal lobar degeneration | GRML | genomic relationship–matrix restricted maximum likelihood |
| FTLD-ni | fronto-temporal lobar degeneration without inclusions | | |
| | | GRN | granulin |
| FTLD-tau | fronto-temporal lobar degeneration with tau-positive inclusions | GRS | genetic risk scoring |
| | | GSK-3β | glycogen synthase kinase-3β |
| FTLD-UPS | fronto-temporal lobar degeneration with immunohistochemistry against proteins of the ubiquitin proteosomal system | GSS | Gerstmann–Sträussler syndrome |
| | | GTP | guanosine triphosphate |
| | | GWA | genome-wide association |
| FUS | fused in sarcoma (protein) | GWAS | genome-wide association studies |
| FXS | fragile X syndrome | GWES | genome-wide exome sequencing |
| g | gram; effect size | HAI | health care-associated infection |
| GA | Gamblers Anonymous | HAROLD | Hemispheric Asymmetry Reduction in Old Adults (model) |
| GABA | gamma aminobutyric acid | | |
| GAD | generalized anxiety disorder | HbA1c | glycated haemoglobin |
| GAF | Global Assessment of Functioning (scale) | HBV | hepatitis B virus |
| GAPD | General Assessment of Personality Disorder | HCR-20 | Historical, Clinical Risk Management-20 |
| GAR | Global Attentiveness Rating | HCV | hepatitis C virus |
| GBA | glucocerebrosidase | HD | Huntington's disease; hoarding disorder |
| GBD | Global Burden of Disease (studies) | HDAC | histone deacetylation |
| GBL | gamma butyrolactone | HD-D | Hoarding Disorder Dimensional Scale |
| GCAN | Genetic Consortium for Anorexia Nervosa | HDE | humanitarian device exemption |
| GCase | β-glucocerebrosidase 1 | HDL | high-density lipoprotein |
| GCMS | gas chromatography–mass spectrometry | HDRS | Hamilton Depression Rating Scale |
| GCS | Glasgow Coma Scale | HF | high frequency |
| GCT | gender-confirming treatment | HFS | high-frequency stimulation |
| GCTA | genome-wide complex trait analysis | 5-HIAA | 5-hydroxyindoleacetic acid |
| GD | gender dysphoria; gambling disorder | HIC | high-income country |
| GDNF | glial cell-derived neurotrophic factor | HiTOP | Hierarchical Taxonomy of Psychopathology |
| GDP | guanosine diphosphate; gross domestic product | HIV | human immunodeficiency virus |
| | | HKD | hyperkinetic disorder |
| GET | graded exercise therapy | HLA | human leucocyte antigen |
| GF | germ-free | HoNOS | Health of the Nation Outcome Scales |
| GHB | gamma hydroxybutyrate | HOT | hyperbaric oxygen therapy |
| GHRF | growth-hormone releasing factor | | |

| | | | | |
|---|---|---|---|---|
| HPA | hypothalamus–pituitary–adrenal | | IM | intramuscular |
| HPD | histrionic personality disorder | | ImPACT | Immediate Post-Concussion Assessment and Cognitive Testing |
| HPLC | high-performance liquid chromatography | | IMPase | inositol-1-monophosphatase |
| HPPD | hallucinogen persisting perceptual disorder | | IMPC | International Mouse Phenotyping Consortium |
| HPRD | human protein reference database | | INAHTA | International Network of Agencies for Health Technology Assessment |
| HR | heart rate; hazard ratio | | INN | international non-proprietary name |
| HRI | high risk index | | iNOS | inducible nitric oxide synthase |
| HR-QoL | health-related quality of life | | IOCDF-GC | International OCD Foundation Genetics Collaborative |
| HRS-I | Hoarding Rating Scale-Interview | | IOM | Institute of Medicine |
| HRS-SR | Hoarding Rating Scale-Self Report | | $IP_3$ | inositol 1,4,5-triphosphate |
| HRT | habit reversal training; hormone replacement therapy | | IPDE | International Personality Disorders Examination |
| HSP90 | heat shock protein 90 | | IPL | inferior parietal lobe |
| 5-HT | 5-hydroxytryptamine | | iPSC | induced pluripotent stem cell |
| HTA | health technology appraisal; health technology assessment | | IPSRT | interpersonal and social rhythm therapy |
| | | | IPT | interpersonal psychotherapy |
| HTAi | Health Technology Assessment international | | IPV | intimate partner violence |
| HTT | huntingtin | | IQ | intelligence quotient |
| HVA | homovanillic acid | | IR | immediate release; insulin resistance |
| HYE | health year equivalent | | IRE1 | inositol-requiring enzyme 1 |
| Hz | hertz | | IRGC | intermediate radial glia cell |
| IADL | instrumental activity of daily living | | IRLSS | International Restless Legs Syndrome Study Group |
| IAPT | Improving Access to Psychological Therapies | | IRT | item response theory; individual resilience training; imagery relief therapy |
| IBD | inflammatory bowel disease | | | |
| IBMPFD | inclusion body myopathy with Paget's disease of bone and fronto-temporal dementia | | ISBD | International Society for Bipolar Disorders |
| | | | ISC | International Schizophrenia Consortium |
| IBS | irritable bowel syndrome | | ISoS | International Study of Schizophrenia |
| ICA | independent component analysis | | isvz | inner subventricular zone |
| ICCS | International Children's Continence Society | | ISWRD | irregular sleep–wake rhythm disorder |
| ICD | impulse-control disorder | | ITP | inferior thalamic peduncle |
| ICD | International Classification of Diseases | | IUPHAR | International Union of Basic and Clinical Pharmacology |
| ICD-10 | International Classification of Diseases, tenth revision | | | |
| | | | IVF | *in vitro* fertilization |
| ICD-11 | International Classification of Diseases, eleventh revision | | JASPER | Joint Attention, Symbolic Play, Engagement and Regulation |
| ICECAP | ICEpop CAPability | | K | kelvin |
| ICER | incremental cost-effectiveness ratio | | $K^+$ | potassium |
| ICF | International Classification of Functioning and Disability | | kb | kilobase |
| | | | kDa | kilodalton |
| ICOCS | International College of Obsessive–Compulsive Spectrum Disorders | | KEGG | *Kyoto Encyclopaedia of Genes and Genomes* |
| | | | KFS | Keeping Families Strong |
| ICSD-3 | International Classification of Sleep Disorder, third edition | | kg | kilogram |
| | | | KO | knockout |
| ICU | intensive care unit | | KOR | kappa opioid receptor |
| ID | intellectual disabilities; insomnia disorder | | K-SADS | Schedule for Affective Disorders and Schizophrenia for School Age Children |
| IDD | intellectual developmental disorder | | | |
| IDO | indoleamine 2,3-dioxygenase | | L | litre |
| IED | intermittent explosive disorder | | LAI | long-acting injected |
| IFC | inferior frontal cortex | | LB | Lewy body |
| IFG | inferior frontal gyrus | | LBD | Lewy body dementia |
| IFN | interferon | | LC | locus caeruleus |
| IGF | insulin-like growth factor | | LD | linkage disequilibrium; learning disability |
| IGF-1 | insulin-like growth factor 1 | | L/D | light/dark |
| IgG | immunoglobulin G | | LDL | low-density lipoprotein |
| IHSC | interhemispheric spectral coherence | | L-dopa | levodopa |
| IL | interleukin | | LDX | lisdexamfetamine |
| IL-2 | interleukin 2 | | | |
| IL-6 | interleukin 6 | | | |

| | | | |
|---|---|---|---|
| LF | low frequency | MDA | methylenedioxyamphetamine |
| LFP | local field potential | MDAS | Memorial Delirium Assessment Scale |
| LGD | likely gene disrupting | MDD | major depressive disorder |
| LGE | lateral ganglionic eminence | MDI | manic–depressive illness |
| lGI | local gyrification index | MDMA | 3,4-methylenedioxymethamphetamine |
| LH | lateral hypothalamic | MDMA-AP | MDMA-assisted psychotherapy |
| LHA | lateral hypothalamus | MDT | mode deactivation therapy |
| LHb | lateral habenula | ME | myalgic encephalomyelitis |
| LHRH | luteinizing hormone-releasing hormone | M/EEG | MEG and EEG |
| LMIC | low- and middle-income country | MEG | magnetoencephalography |
| lncRNA | long non-coding ribonucleic acid | MET | motivational enhancement therapy |
| LOC | loss of consciousness | MFB | medial forebrain bundle |
| LOD | logarithm of the odds | MFC | medial frontal cortical (regions) |
| LoF | loss of function | MFG | medial frontal gyrus |
| LOS | length of stay | MGB | microbiota–gut–brain (axis) |
| LPFS | Level of Personality Functioning Scale | MGD | Mouse Genome Database |
| LPS | lipopolysaccharide | MGE | medial ganglionic eminence |
| LSD | lysergic acid diethylamide | mGluR | metabotropic glutamatergic receptor |
| LTC | long-term care | MGMH | Movement for Global Mental Health |
| LTD | long-term depression | MHC | major histocompatibility complex |
| LTG | lamotrigine | mhGAP | Mental Health Gap Action Programme |
| LTP | long-term potentiation | MHIN | Mental Health Innovation Network |
| LUR | lurasidone | MHP | mental health professional |
| LUTS | lower urinary tract symptoms | MHPG | 3-methoxy-4-hydroxyphenylglycol |
| MABC | Movement Assessment Battery for Children | MHRA | Medicines and Healthcare products Regulatory Agency |
| MADRS | Montgomery-Åsberg Depression Rating Scale | MHS | mental health services |
| MAM | mitochondria-associated membrane | MI | motivational interviewing |
| MANTRA | Maudsley Model of Anorexia Nervosa Treatment for Adults | MIBG | $^{123}$I-metaiodobenzylguanidine |
| MAO | monoamine oxidase | MID | monetary incentive delay |
| MAOA | monoamine oxidase A | MIPS | myo-inositol-3-phosphate synthase |
| MAOA-H | monoamine oxidase-high (allele) | miRNA | microribonucleic acid |
| MAOA-L | monoamine oxidase-low (allele) | mm | millimetre |
| MAOI | monoamine oxidase inhibitor | MMN | mismatch negativity |
| MAP | mitogen-activated protein; microtubule-associated protein | MMPI | Minnesota Multiphasic Personality Inventory |
| MAPK | mitogen-activated protein kinase | MMSE | Mini-Mental State Examination |
| MAPS | Multidisciplinary Association for Psychedelic Studies (project) | MND | motor neuron disease; Malingered Neurocognitive Dysfunction |
| MAPT | microtubule-associated protein tau | MOA | mechanism of action |
| MARAC | multi-agency risk assessment conference | MoCA | Montreal Cognitive Assessment |
| MAYSI-2 | Massachusetts Youth Screening Instrument-Version 2 | mOFC | medial orbitofrontal cortex |
| | | MOR | mu-opioid receptor |
| MBCT | mindfulness-based cognitive therapy | mPFC | medial prefrontal cortex |
| MBP | myelin basic protein | MPH | methylphenidate |
| MBSR | mindfulness-based stress reduction | MPP+ | 1-methyl-4-phenylpyridinium |
| MBT | mentalization-based treatment | MPTP | methyl-4-phenyl-1,2,3,6-tetrahydropyridine |
| MBT-A | mentalization-based treatment for adolescents | MR | mineralocorticoid receptor; magnetic resonance |
| MBU | mother and baby unit | mRASS | modified Richmond Agitation and Sedation Scale |
| MCA | middle cerebral artery | MRF | modifiable risk factor |
| MCC | mid cingulate cortex | MRI | magnetic resonance imaging |
| MCDA | multi-criteria decision analysis | MRN | medial raphe nuclei |
| MC4R | melanocortin-4 receptor | mRNA | messenger ribonucleic acid |
| MCH | melatonin-concentrating hormone | MRS | magnetic resonance spectroscopy |
| MCI | mild cognitive impairment | MSA | multiple system atrophy |
| MCMI-III | Millon Clinical Multiaxial Inventory-III | MSAD | McLean Study of Adult Development |
| MCTQ | Munich ChronoType Questionnaire | MSF | mid-sleep on free day |
| MD | mean diffusivity | MSH | melanocyte-stimulating hormone |
| | | MSI-2 | Multiphasic Sex Inventory-2 |

| | |
|---|---|
| MSLT | multiple sleep latency test |
| MSR | magnetically shielded room |
| MST | multi-systemic therapy |
| MSW | mid-sleep on workdays |
| MT | magnetization transfer |
| mTBI | mild traumatic brain injury |
| mtDNA | mitochondrial DNA |
| MTFC | multi-dimensional treatment foster care |
| mTOR | mammalian target of rapamycin |
| MTR | magnetization transfer ratio |
| MVPC | multivariate pattern classification |
| MZ | monozygotic |
| Na$^+$ | sodium |
| NA | noradrenaline |
| NAA | *N*-acetyl aspartate |
| NAC | nucleus accumbens; *N*-acetylcysteine |
| NAcc | nucleus accumbens |
| nAChR | nicotinic acetylcholine receptor |
| NAM | negative allosteric modulation |
| NAMHC | National Advisory Mental Health Council |
| NaSSA | noradrenergic and specific serotonergic antidepressant |
| Natsal-3 | third National Surveys of Sexual Attitudes and Lifestyles |
| NB | net benefit |
| NbN | Neuroscience-based Nomenclature |
| NcAcc | nucleus accumbens |
| NCD | neurocognitive disorder |
| NCDLB | neurocognitive disorder with Lewy bodies |
| NCGS | non-coeliac gluten sensitivity |
| ncRNA | non-coding RNA |
| NCS | National Comorbidity Survey |
| NCS-A | National Comorbidity Survey Adolescent Supplement |
| NCS-R | National Comorbidity Survey-Replication |
| NDA | National Institute of Mental Health Data Archive; new drug approval |
| NDD | neurodegenerative disease |
| NDRI | noradrenaline/dopamine reuptake inhibitor |
| NE | nocturnal enuresis |
| NEAT | non-exercise activity thermogenesis |
| NES | night eating syndrome |
| NESARC | National Epidemiological Survey on Alcohol and Related Conditions |
| NET | noradrenaline (norepinephrine) transporter; narrative exposure therapy |
| NF-κB | nuclear factor κB |
| nfvPPA | non-fluent-variant primary progressive aphasia |
| NGF | nerve growth factor |
| NGO | non-governmental organization |
| NGS | next-generation sequencing |
| NHMRC | National Health and Medical Research Council |
| NICE | National Institute for Health and Care Excellence |
| NIDA | National Institute of Drug Abuse |
| NIFID | neuronal intermediate filament inclusion disease |
| NIH | National Institutes of Health |
| NIMH | National Institute of Mental Health |
| NIMH-RGR | NIMH Repository and Genomics Resource |

| | |
|---|---|
| NJRE | Not Just Right Experience |
| NK-1 | neurokinin 1 |
| NMDA | *N*-methyl-*D*-aspartate |
| NMDAR | *N*-methyl-*D*-aspartate receptor |
| NMR | nuclear magnetic resonance |
| NMS | neuroleptic malignant syndrome |
| NND | number needed to detain |
| NNI | NMDAR-neuromodulator interaction |
| NNP | number needed to prevent |
| NNT | number needed to treat |
| NO | nitric oxide |
| NOS | not otherwise specified; nitric oxide synthase |
| NPC | neural progenitor cell |
| NPD | narcissistic personality disorder |
| NPI | neuropsychiatric inventory |
| NPS | novel psychoactive substance; neuropeptide S |
| NPY | neuropeptide Y |
| NREM | non-rapid eye movement |
| NRI | selective noradrenergic reuptake inhibitor |
| NRT | nicotine replacement therapy |
| NSAID | non-steroidal anti-inflammatory drug |
| NSS | neurological soft sign |
| NSSI | non-suicidal self-injury |
| NSSID | non-suicidal self-injury disorder |
| N24SWD | non-24-hour sleep–wake disorder |
| NTD | neurofibrillary tangle dementia |
| Nu-DESC | Nursing Delirium Screening Scale |
| NVAWS | National Violence Against Women Survey |
| OAB | overactive bladder |
| OC | obsessive–compulsive |
| OCD | obsessive–compulsive disorder |
| OCDUS | Obsessive Compulsive Drug Use Scale |
| OCGAS | OCD Collaborative Genetic Association Study |
| OCPD | obsessive–compulsive personality disorder |
| OCRD | obsessive–compulsive and related disorder |
| OCSD | obsessive–compulsive spectrum disorder |
| ODD | oppositional defiant disorder |
| OECD | Organisation for Economic Co-operation and Development |
| OED | other eating disorder |
| OFC | orbitofrontal cortex |
| OLZ | olanzapine |
| ONS | Office of National Statistics |
| OPD | operational psychodynamic diagnostics |
| OPM | optically pumped magnetometer |
| OPRI | octapeptide repeat insertion |
| OR | odds ratio |
| OSA | obstructive sleep apnoea |
| OSE | other stressor event |
| OSFED | other specified feeding and eating disorders |
| OST | opiate substitution therapy |
| osvz | outer subventricular zone |
| OxCAP-MH | Oxford CAPabilities questionnaire-Mental Health |
| OXTR | oxytocin receptor |
| PA | periaqueductal |
| PACAP | pituitary adenylyl cyclase-activating polypeptide |
| PACT | Preschool Autism Communication Trial |
| PAF | population-attributable fraction |

| | | | |
|---|---|---|---|
| PAG | periaqueductal grey | PM+ | Problem Management Plus |
| PAI | Personality Assessment Inventory | PMA | paramethoxyamphetamine |
| PAL | paliperidone | PMDD | premenstrual dysphoric disorder |
| PAM | positive allosteric inhibitor; positive allosteric modulation | PMMA | paramethoxymethamphetamine |
| | | PND | postnatal depression |
| PAMP | pathogen-associated molecular pattern | PoA | preoptic area |
| PANDAS | Paediatric autoimmune neuropsychiatric disorder associated with streptococcal infections | POMC | pro-opiomelanocortin |
| | | PP | post-partum (puerperal) psychosis |
| PANESS | Physical and Neurological Examination for Soft Signs | PPAR | peroxisome proliferator-activated receptor |
| | | PPD | paranoid personality disorder |
| PaPA | Perceptions and Practicalities Approach | P&PD | DSM-5 Personality and Personality Disorders Work Group |
| PAR | population-attributable risk | | |
| PATS | Preschoolers with ADHD Treatment Study | PPG | penile plethysmography |
| PBMC | peripheral blood mononuclear cell | PPI | protein–protein interaction |
| PBP | Parent-Based Prevention | PPV | positive predictive value |
| PCBD | persistent complex bereavement disorder | pRGC | photosensitive retinal ganglion cell |
| PCC | posterior cingulate cortex | PRIME | Programme for Improving Mental Health Care (study) |
| PCL | paracentral lobule | | |
| PCL-R | Psychopathy Checklist Revised | PROM | patient-reported outcome measure |
| PCL-YV | Psychopathy Checklist: Youth Version | PrP | prion protein; Penn Resilience Program |
| PCP | primary care physician | $PrP^C$ | cellular prion protein |
| PCPA | para-chlorophenylalanine | $PrP^{Sc}$ | scrapie form of prion protein |
| PCS | post-concussion syndrome | PRS | polygenic risk scoring |
| PD | panic disorder; proton density; Parkinson's disease; personality disorder | PSA | prostate-specific antigen |
| | | PSD | post-synaptic density; post-stroke depression |
| PDAQ | Penn Daily Activities Questionnaire | PSE | Present State Examination |
| PD-CFRS | PD-Cognitive Function Rating Scale | PSG | polysomnography |
| PDD | pervasive developmental disorder; Parkinson's disease dementia | PSP | progressive supranuclear palsy |
| | | PSQI | Pittsburgh Sleep Quality Index |
| PDE | phosphodiesterase | PST | problem-solving therapy |
| PDE-5 | phosphodiesterase type 5 | PTA | post-traumatic amnesia; Positive Thoughts and Action Program |
| PD-MCI | Parkinson's disease with mild cognitive impairment | | |
| PD-TS | personality disorder–trait specified | p-tau | phosphorylated tau |
| PE | prolonged exposure; premature ejaculation | PTE | potentially traumatic event |
| PEG | polyethyleneglycol | PTSD | post-traumatic stress disorder |
| PEPS | psychoeducation with problem-solving | PU | premonitory urge |
| PERK | protein kinase RNA-like endoplasmic reticulum kinase | PUFA | polyunsaturated fatty acid |
| | | PVE | partial volume effect |
| PET | positron emission tomography | PVFS | post-viral fatigue syndrome |
| PET-MR | positron emission tomography–magnetic resonance | PVN | paraventricular hypothalamic nucleus |
| PFA | psychological first aid | QALY | quality-adjusted life year |
| PFC | prefrontal cortex | QOF | quality and outcomes framework |
| PGAD | persistent genital arousal disorder | QoL | quality of life |
| PGC | Psychiatric Genetics Consortium | QTL | quantitative trait locus |
| PGC-ED | Eating Disorders Working Group of the Psychiatric Genomics Consortium | QTP | quetiapine |
| | | rACC | rostral anterior cingulate cortex |
| $PGE_2$ | prostaglandin $E_2$ | RAD | reactive attachment disorder; Reynolds Adolescent Depression |
| PGRS | polygenic risk score | | |
| PI | phosphoinositide/phosphoinositol; polarity index | RAID | Rapid Assessment, Interface, and Discharge (model) |
| PiB | Pittsburgh compound B | RANZP | Royal Australian and New Zealand College of Psychiatrists |
| PIGD | postural instability gait disorder | | |
| $PIP_2$ | phosphotidyl inositol 4,5-biphosphate | RAP | Resourceful Adolescent Program |
| piRNA | piwi-interacting ribonucleic acid | RAR | retinoic acid receptor |
| PKA | protein kinase A | RBANS | Repeatable Battery for the Assessment of Neuropsychological Status |
| PKC | protein kinase C | | |
| PKU | phenylketonuria | RBD | rapid eye movement sleep behaviour disorder |
| PLC | phospholipase C | rCBF | regional cerebral blood flow |
| PLE | psychotic-like experience | rCMRglu | regional cerebral metabolic rate for glucose |

| | | | |
|---|---|---|---|
| RCT | randomized controlled trial | SCZ | schizophrenia |
| RCV | rare coding variant | SD | sleep deprivation |
| RD | radial diffusivity | SDQ | Strengths and Difficulties Questionnaire |
| RDC | Research Diagnostic Criteria | SDS | standard deviation score |
| RDoC | Research Domain Criteria | SEID | systemic exertion intolerance disease |
| RdoCdb | Research Domain Criteria Database | SERCA | sarco(endo)plasmic reticulum calcium ATPase |
| REE | resting energy expenditure | SERT | serotonin; serotonin transporter |
| REM | rapid eye movement | SES | socio-economic status |
| REMS | risk evaluation and mitigation strategies | SF-36 | Short Form Health Survey 36 |
| RESH | Repeated Episodes of Self-Harm (score) | SFO | subfornical organ |
| REST | RE1-silencing transcription factor | SFT | schema-focused therapy |
| RF | radiofrequency | SG | somatosensory gating |
| RFLP | restriction fragment length polymorphism | SGA | second-generation antipsychotic |
| RGS | G-protein signalling protein | sgACC | subgenual anterior cingulate cortex |
| RHT | retinohypothalamic tract | sgp130 | soluble glycoprotein 130 |
| RLE | real life experience | sgRNA | single-guide ribonucleic acid |
| RLS | restless legs syndrome | SHA | System of Health Accounts |
| RNA | ribonucleic acid | SHORT IQ-CODE | short form of the Informant Questionnaire on Cognitive Decline in the Elderly |
| RNP | ribonucleoprotein | | |
| ROADMAP | Real world Outcomes across the Alzheimer's Disease spectrum for better care: Multi-modal data Access Platform | SHQ | Clarke Sex History Questionnaire |
| | | SIADH | syndrome of inappropriate antidiuretic hormone |
| | | SIDP-IV | Structured Interview for DSM-IV Personality Disorders |
| ROI | region of interest | SIH | stress-induced hyperthermia |
| ROM | routine outcome measure | SIHD | Structured Interview for Hoarding Disorder |
| ROS | reactive oxygen species | SIPP | Severity Indices of Personality Problems |
| ROSE | Reach Out, Stand Strong, Essentials for new mothers (programme) | SIPS | Structured Interview for Prodromal Syndromes; Structured Interview for Psychosis-Risk Syndromes |
| RPS | risk profile scoring | SI-R | Saving Inventory-Revised |
| RR | relative risk | siRNA | short interfering ribonucleic acid |
| RRBI | restricted and repetitive behaviours and interests | SIT | stress inoculation training |
| RRT | rapid response team | SLC | solute carrier |
| RS | rumination syndrome | slMFB | superolateral branch of the medial forebrain bundle |
| rsfMRI | resting-state functional magnetic resonance imaging | SMA | supplementary motor area |
| RSN | resting state network | SMD | standardized mean difference |
| rTMS | repetitive transcranial magnetic stimulation | SMG | supramarginal gyrus |
| RT-QuIC | real-time quaking-induced conversion | SMI | severe mental illness |
| RVM | rostral ventromedial medulla | SMIT 1 | sodium/$myo$-inositol transporter 1 |
| RYGB | Roux-En-Y gastric bypass | SMOC | second messenger-operated channel |
| sAD | sporadic Alzheimer's disease | SMR | standard mortality ratio; standardized mortality rate |
| SAD | social anxiety disorder; seasonal affective disorder | SN | substantia nigra |
| SANS | Scale for the Assessment of Negative Symptoms | SNAP | Swanson, Nolan, and Pelham (scale); Schedule for Nonadaptive and Adaptive Personality |
| SAPS | Scale for the Assessment of Positive Symptoms | SNP | single-nucleotide polymorphism |
| SAPS-PD | Scale for Assessment of Positive Symptoms in Parkinson's Disease | SNR | signal-to-noise ratio |
| | | SNRI | serotonin/noradrenaline reuptake inhibitor |
| SARI | serotonin antagonist and reuptake inhibitor | SNV | single nucleotide variant |
| SAVRY | Structured Assessment of Violence Risk in Youth | SOC | store-operated channel |
| SCAN | Schedule for Clinical Assessment in Neuropsychiatry | SOC-7 | Standards of Care for the Health of Transsexual, Transgender, and Gender-Non-conforming People, Version 7 |
| SCC | subcallosal cingulate cortex | | |
| SCD | social (pragmatic) communication disorder | SOD | superoxide dismutase |
| SCFA | short-chain fatty acid | SOFAS | Social and Occupational Functioning Assessment Scale |
| SCID-II | Structured Clinical Interview for DSM-IV Axis II personality disorders | | |
| | | SORAG | Sex Offender Risk Appraisal Guide |
| sCJD | sporadic Creuztfeldt–Jakob disease | SOREMP | sleep-onset REM period |
| SCL-90 | Symptom Checklist-90 | SP | specific phobia; subplate (zone) |
| SCM | structured clinical management | SPD | schizotypal personality disorder |
| SCN | suprachiasmatic nucleus | | |
| SCO | subcommissural organ | | |
| SCRD | sleep and circadian rhythm disruption | | |

| | | | |
|---|---|---|---|
| SPECT | single-photon emission computed tomography | TMF | Trzepacz, Meagher, and Franco (research diagnostic criteria) |
| SPZ | subparaventricular zone | TMN | tuberomammillary nucleus |
| SQUID | superconducting quantum interference device | TMS | transcranial magnetic stimulation |
| SRAI | structured risk assessment instrument | TNF | tumour necrosis factor |
| SRI | serotonin reuptake inhibitor | TOR | target of rapamycin |
| SRS | sex reassignment surgery | TPD | Tobacco Products Directive |
| SRT | sleep restriction therapy | TPJ | temporo-parietal junction |
| SSCM | specialist supportive clinical management | TR | repetition time |
| SSRI | selective serotonin reuptake inhibitor | TRD | treatment-resistant depression |
| STAT3 | signal transducer and activator of transcription 3 | TRH | thyrotropin-releasing hormone |
| STEP-BD | Systematic Treatment Enhancement Program for Bipolar Disorder | TRN | thalamic reticular nucleus |
| | | TRP | transient receptor potential |
| STEPPS | Systems Training for Emotional Predictability and Problem Solving | TS | Tourette's syndrome |
| | | TSC | tuberous sclerosis complex |
| STL | superior temporal lobe | TSF | 12-step facilitation |
| STN | subthalamic nucleus | TSH | thyroid-stimulating hormone |
| StPD | schizotypal personality disorder | TSO | total sexual outlet |
| STPD | schizotypal personality disorder | TSPO | translocator protein |
| STPP | short-term psychodynamic psychotherapy | TSST | Trier Social Stress Test |
| SUD | substance use disorder | t-tau | total tau |
| SUVr | regional standard uptake value | TTFL | transcriptional–translational feedback loop |
| svPPA | semantic-variant primary progressive aphasia | UA | uric acid |
| SVT | symptom validity test | UDS | urinary drug screen |
| SWAN | Strengths and Weaknesses of ADHD-symptoms and Normal-behavior (scale) | UGDS | Utrecht Gender Dysphoria Scale |
| | | UHR | ultra-high-risk |
| SWI | susceptibility-weighted imaging | UHSS | UCLA Hoarding Severity Scale |
| SWS | slow-wave sleep | UI | uncertainty interval |
| T | tesla; testosterone | UK | United Kingdom cHECK 1-4!!! |
| tACS | transcranial alternating current stimulation | UN | United Nations |
| TADS | Treatment for Adolescents with Depression Study | UP | Unified Protocol for Transdiagnostic Treatment of Emotional Disorders |
| TAP-MS | tandem affinity purification and mass spectrometry | | |
| TAU | treatment as usual | UPD | uniparental disomy |
| TBARS | thiobarbituric acid reactive substances | UPR | unfolded protein response |
| TBI | traumatic brain injury | UPS | unspecified prodromal symptoms |
| TBK1 | TANK-binding kinase 1 | US | unconditioned stimulus; United States |
| TBSS | tract-based spatial statistics | USD | United States dollar |
| TCA | tricarboxylic acid; tricyclic antidepressant | USI-model | Universal, Selected and Indicated preventive model |
| TCI | Temperament and Character Inventory | uVNTR | upstream variable number of tandem repeats |
| TD | typically developing; tardive dyskinesia | VaD | vascular dementia |
| tDCS | transcranial direct current stimulation | VasD | vascular dementia |
| T2DM | type 2 diabetes mellitus | VBM | voxel-based morphometry |
| TDP | TAR-DNA binding protein | VCFS | velo-cardio-facial syndrome |
| TDP43 | TAR-DNA binding protein 43 | VCI | vascular cognitive impairment |
| tds | three times daily | vCJD | variant Creuztfeldt–Jakob disease |
| TEMPS | Temperament Evaluation scale from Memphis, Pisa, and San Diego | VCP | valosin-containing protein |
| | | VC/VS | ventral capsule/ventral striatum |
| TENS | transcutaneous electrical nerve stimulation | VEGF | vascular endothelial growth factor |
| TFBS | transcription factor binding site | VIAAT | vesicular inhibitory amino acid transporter |
| TF-CBT | trauma-focused cognitive behavioural therapy | VIP | vasoactive intestinal peptide |
| TFP | transference-focused psychotherapy | VLPO | ventrolateral preoptic |
| TGA | transient global amnesia | VMAT2 | vesicular monoamine transporter-2 |
| TGMD | Test for Gross Motor Development, second edition | VMHC | voxel-mirrored homotopic connectivity |
| Th2 | T helper 2 | vmPFC | ventromedial prefrontal cortex |
| THC | tetrahydrocannabinol | VNS | vagal nerve stimulation |
| TIA | transient ischaemic attack | VNTR | variable numbers of tandem repeat |
| TIPS | Treatment and Intervention in Psychosis Study | VNUT | vesicular nucleotide transporter |
| TJ | tight junction | VPA | valproate |
| TLR | Toll-like receptor | | |

| | |
|---|---|
| VPAG | ventral periaqueductal grey |
| VR | virtual reality |
| VRAG | Violence Risk Appraisal Guide |
| VRAG-R | Violence Risk Appraisal Guide-Revised |
| VRET | virtual reality exposure therapy |
| VS/NcAcc | ventral striatum/nucleus accumbens |
| VTA | ventral tegmental area |
| WASO | wake after sleep onset |
| WCST | Wisconsin Card Sorting Task |
| WFSBP | World Federation of Societies of Biological Psychiatry |
| WHO | World Health Organization |
| WHO-DAS | World Health Organization Disability Assessment Schedule |
| WM | white matter |
| WMH | World Mental Health; white matter hyperintensity |
| WPA | World Psychiatric Association |
| WTCCC3 | Wellcome Trust Case-Control Consortium 3 |
| XMRV | xenotropic murine leukaemia virus-related virus |
| Y-BOCS | Yale-Brown Obsessive Compulsive Scale |
| YFAS | Yale Food Addiction Scale |
| Y2H | Yeast 2 Hybrid |
| YLD | year of life lived with disability |
| YLL | year of life lost |
| YSR | Youth Self-Report |
| ZIP | ziprasidone |

# Contributors

**Dag Aarsland**, Department of Old Age Psychiatry, Institute of Psychiatry, Psychology, and Neuroscience, King's College London, London, UK; Mental Health of Older Adults and Dementia Clinical Academic Group, South London and Maudsley NHS Foundation Trust, London, UK

**Kwangmi Ahn**, Child Psychiatry Branch, NIMH, Bethesda, MD, USA

**Renato D. Alarcón**, Mayo Clinic College of Medicine, Rochester, MN, USA; Cayetano Heredia University, Lima, Peru

**Kirstie N. Anderson**, Institute of Neuroscience, Newcastle University, UK; Regional Sleep Service, Newcastle upon Tyne Hospitals NHS Foundation Trust, UK

**Erik M. Andersson**, Department of Clinical Neuroscience, Karolinska Institutet, Stockholm, Sweden

**Nancy C. Andreasen**, Department of Psychiatry, University of Iowa Carver College of Medicine, Iowa City, IA, USA

**Roberto Andreatini**, Department of Pharmacology, Federal University of Paraná, Curitiba, Brazil

**Jochen Antel**, Department of Child and Adolescent Psychiatry, Psychosomatics and Psychotherapy, University Hospital Essen, University of Essen-Duisburg, Essen, Germany

**Filip K. Arnberg**, National Centre for Disaster Psychiatry, Department of Neuroscience, Psychiatry, Uppsala, Sweden; Stress Research Institute, Stockholm University, Sweden

**Nerys M. Astbury**, Nuffield Department of Primary Care Health Sciences, University of Oxford, Oxford, UK

**Kammarauche Asuzu**, Department of Psychiatry and Behavioral Sciences, Duke University Health System, Durham, NC, USA

**José L. Ayuso-Mateos**, Department of Psychiatry, Faculty of Medicine, Autonomous University of Madrid, La Princesa University Hospital, CIBERSAM, Spain

**Fahd Baig**, Nuffield Department of Clinical Neurosciences, John Radcliffe Hospital, Oxford, UK

**Sue Bailey**, Chair of Centre for Mental Health, London, UK

**David S. Baldwin**, Department of Psychiatry, University of Southampton, Southampton, UK

**John Bancroft**, Oxford, UK

**Judy Bass**, Department of Mental Health, Johns Hopkins Bloomberg School of Public Health, Baltimore, MD, USA

**Matthew L. Baum**, Harvard Medical School, Harvard-MIT Division of Health Sciences and Technology, Boston, MA, USA

**Katja Beesdo-Baum**, Behavioral Epidemiology, Institute of Clinical Psychology and Psychotherapy, Technical University Dresden, Dresden, Germany

**Dörte Bemme**, Department of Anthropology, University of North Carolina at Chapel Hill, USA

**Oded Ben-Arush**, Israeli Center for the Treatment of Obsessive-Compulsive Related Disorders, Mesilat Zion, Israel

**Chantal Berna**, Pain Center, Division of Anesthesiology, Lausanne University Hospital, Lausanne, Switzerland

**Laura A. Berner**, UCSD Eating Disorders Center for Treatment and Research, San Diego, CA, USA

**Michael J. Berridge**, Laboratory of Molecular Signalling, The Babraham Institute, Babraham Research Campus, Cambridge, UK

**Ravi S. Bhat**, Rural Health Centre, University of Melbourne, Melbourne, VIC, Australia

**Donald W. Black**, Department of Psychiatry, University of Iowa Carver College of Medicine, Iowa City, IA, USA

**William V. Bobo**, Department of Psychiatry and Psychology, Mayo Clinic College of Medicine, Rochester, MN, USA

**Emre Bora**, Melbourne Neuropsychiatry Centre, Department of Psychiatry, The University of Melbourne and Melbourne Health; Carlton South, VIC, Australia; DokuzEylül University, Faculty of Medicine, Department of Psychiatry, Izmir, Turkey

**Daniel W. Bradford**, Department of Psychiatry and Behavioral Sciences, Duke University Medical Center, Durham, NC, USA

**Maria Bragesjö**, Department of Clinical Neuroscience, Karolinska Institutet, Stockholm, Sweden

**Courtney Breen**, National Drug and Alcohol Research Centre, University of New South Wales, Sydney, NSW, Australia

**Gerome Breen**, MRC Social Genetic and Developmental Psychiatry Centre, Institute of Psychiatry, Psychology and Neuroscience, King's College London, London, UK

**Michael Browning**, Department of Psychiatry, Warneford Hospital, Oxford, UK

**Alec Buchanan**, Department of Psychiatry, Yale School of Medicine, Division of Law and Psychiatry, New Haven, CT, USA

**Noel J. Buckley**, Department of Psychiatry, Warneford Hospital, University of Oxford, Oxford, UK

**Jan K. Buitelaar**, Department of Cognitive Neuroscience, Donders Institute for Brain, Cognition and Behaviour, Radboud University Medical Center, Nijmegen, The Netherlands

**Cynthia M. Bulik**, Department of Medical Epidemiology and Biostatistics, Karolinska Institutet, Stockholm, Sweden; Department of Nutrition, University of North Carolina at Chapel Hill, Chapel Hill, NC, USA

**Eric Burguière**, ICM Brain and Spine Institute, Pitié-Salpêtrière Hospital, Paris, France

**Tom Burns**, University of Oxford, Department of Psychiatry, Warneford Hospital, Oxford, UK

**Joanne A. Byars**, Department of Psychiatry and Behavioral Sciences, Baylor College of Medicine, TIRR Memorial Hermann, Houston, TX, USA

**Lior Carmi**, Post Trauma Center, Chaim Sheba Medical Center, and Tel Aviv University, Israel

**Sara Carucci**, Child and Adolescent Neuropsychiatric Unit, Department of Biomedical Sciences, University of Cagliari & 'G. Brotzu' Hospital Trust, Cagliari, Italy

**Javier R. Caso**, Department of Pharmacology, Faculty of Medicine, Complutense University of Madrid; CIBERSAM, Imas12, IUIN, Madrid, Spain

**David J. Castle**, St. Vincent's Hospital, The University of Melbourne, Fitzroy, VIC, Australia

**Amy Chan**, Centre for Behavioural Medicine, Department of Practice and Policy, UCL School of Pharmacy, London, UK

**Prathiba Chitsabesan**, Pennine Care NHS Foundation Trust, Manchester, UK; Department of Health Psychology, Manchester Metropolitan University, Manchester, UK

**Helen Christensen**, University of New South Wales, Prince of Wales Hospital, Randwick, NSW, Australia

**Grant C. Churchill**, Department of Pharmacology, University of Oxford, Oxford, UK

**Eduardo Cinosi**, NHS East of England Highly Specialised Service (HSS) for Treatment Resistant OCD/BDD, Obsessive Compulsive and Related Spectrum Disorders and Applied Neuroscience Department, Hertfordshire Partnership University NHS Foundation Trust and University of Hertfordshire, Hatfield, UK

**Andrea Cipriani**, Department of Psychiatry, University of Oxford, Warneford Hospital; Oxford Health NHS Foundation Trust, Warneford Hospital, Oxford, UK

**C. Robert Cloninger**, Center for Psychobiology of Personality, Washington University School of Medicine, St. Louis, MO, USA

**Michael J. Coleman**, Psychiatry Neuroimaging Laboratory, Brigham and Women's Hospital, Boston, MA, USA

**John Collinge**, National Hospital for Neurology and Neurosurgery, UCL Institute of Neurology, London, UK

**Sally-Ann Cooper**, Institute of Health and Wellbeing, University of Glasgow, Gartnavel Royal Hospital, Glasgow, UK

**Philip J. Cowen**, University Department of Psychiatry, Warneford Hospital, Oxford, UK

**Andrea Crowell**, Department of Psychiatry, Emory University, Atlanta, GA, USA

**Dianne Currier**, Melbourne School of Population and Global Health, University of Melbourne, Melbourne, VIC, Australia

**Bruce N. Cuthbert**, National Institute of Mental Health, Bethesda, MD, USA

**Thien Thanh Dang-Vu**, Center for Studies in Behavioral Neurobiology and Department of Health, Kinesiology and Applied Physiology, Concordia University, Montreal, QC, Canada; PERFORM Centre, Concordia University, Montreal, QC, Canada; Centre de recherche de l'institut universitaire de gériatrie de Montréal (CRIUGM), Montreal, QC, Canada; Department of Neurosciences, University of Montreal, Montreal, QC, Canada

**Deborah Davis**, Department of Social Psychology, University of Nevada, Reno, Reno, NV, USA

**Liliana Dell'Osso**, Psychiatric Unit I, Department of Clinical and Experimental Medicine, University of Pisa, Pisa, Italy

**Sevilla Detera-Wadlieigh**, Human Genetics Branch, National Institute of Mental Health, Intramural Research Program, Bethesda, MD, USA

**Arianna Di Florio**, Cardiff University, School of Medicine, Division of Psychological Medicine and Clinical Neurosciences, Cardiff, UK

**Andreea O. Diaconescu**, Translational Neuromodeling Unit (TNU), Institute for Biomedical Engineering, University of Zurich and Swiss Federal Institute of Technology (ETH Zurich), Zurich; Department of Psychiatry, University of Basel, Basel, Switzerland

**Katharina Domschke**, Department of Psychiatry and Psychotherapy, Medical Center – University of Freiburg, and Center for Basics in NeuroModulation (NeuroModulBasics), Medical Center – University of Freiburg, Faculty of Medicine, University of Freiburg, Freiburg, Germany

**Julianne Dorset**, Yale School of Medicine, Department of Psychiatry, New Haven, CT, USA

**Wayne C. Drevets**, Neuroscience, Janssen Research and Development, LLC, of Johnson and Johnson, Titusville, PA, USA

**Lynne M. Drummond**, NHS England Highly Specialised Service (HSS) for Treatment Resistant OCD/BDD, South West London and St. Georges Mental Health Trust and St. George's, University of London, London, UK

**Julie Dunsmore**, Trauma Recovery, RNS Community Health Centre, St. Leonards, NSW, Australia

**Klaus P. Ebmeier**, Department of Psychiatry, Warneford Hospital, University of Oxford, Oxford, UK

**Christine Ecker**, Department of Child and Adolescent Psychiatry, Psychosomatics and Psychotherapy, University Hospital, Goethe University Frankfurt am Main, Frankfurt, Germany

**Els Elaut**, Department of Sexology and Gender, Ghent University Hospital, Ghent, Belgium

**Annette Erlangsen**, Danish Research Institute for Suicide Prevention, Mental Health Center Copenhagen, University of Copenhagen, Copenhagen, Denmark

**Colin A. Espie**, Sleep and Circadian Neuroscience Institute, Nuffield Department of Clinical Neurosciences, University of Oxford, Oxford, UK

**Barry J. Everitt**, Department of Psychology, Behavioural and Clinical Neuroscience Institute, University of Cambridge, Cambridge, UK

**Christopher G. Fairburn**, Department of Psychiatry, University of Oxford, Warneford Hospital, Oxford, UK

**Stephen V. Faraone**, SUNY Upstate Medical University, Syracuse, NY, USA

**Michael Farrell**, National Drug and Alcohol Research Centre, University of New South Wales, Sydney, NSW, Australia

**Mina Fazel**, Department of Psychiatry, Medical Sciences Division, University of Oxford, Warneford Hospital, Oxford, UK

**Seena Fazel**, Department of Psychiatry, University of Oxford, Warneford Hospital, Oxford, UK

**Thomas V. Fernandez**, Yale Child Study Center, Yale School of Medicine, New Haven, CT, USA

**Lorena Fernández de la Cruz**, Department of Clinical Neuroscience, Karolinska Institutet, Stockholm, Sweden

**Naomi A. Fineberg**, NHS East of England Highly Specialised Service (HSS) for Treatment Resistant OCD/BDD, Obsessive Compulsive and Related Spectrum Disorders and Applied Neuroscience Department, Hertfordshire Partnership University NHS Foundation Trust and University of Hertfordshire, Hatfield, UK

**Angus S. Fisk**, Sleep and Circadian Neuroscience Institute (SCNi), Nuffield Department of Clinical Neurosciences, University of Oxford, Oxford, UK

**Remy Flechais**, Marina House, London, UK

**Russell G. Foster**, Sleep and Circadian Neuroscience Institute (SCNi), Nuffield Department of Clinical Neurosciences, University of Oxford, Oxford, UK

**Barbara Franke**, Department of Human Genetics and Department of Psychiatry, Donders Institute for Brain, Cognition and Behaviour, Radboud University Medical Center, Nijmegen, The Netherlands

**Oliver Freudenreich**, Department of Psychiatry, Massachusetts General Hospital Schizophrenia Clinical and Research Program, Harvard Medical School, Boston, MA, USA

**Matthew J. Friedman**, National Center for PTSD, Dartmouth Medical School, Hanover, NH, USA

**John Gallacher**, Department of Psychiatry, Medical Sciences Division, University of Oxford, Oxford, UK

**Borja García-Bueno**, Department of Pharmacology, Faculty of Medicine, Complutense University of Madrid; CIBERSAM, Imas12, IUIN, Madrid, Spain

**John R. Geddes**, Department of Psychiatry, Warneford Hospital, University of Oxford, Oxford, UK

**Philip R. Gehrman**, University of Pennsylvania, Perelman School of Medicine, Philadelphia, PA, USA

**S. Nassir Ghaemi**, Department of Psychiatry, Tufts University, Tufts Medical Center; Department of Psychiatry, Harvard Medical School, Boston, MA, USA

**Amanda K. Gilmore**, Department of Psychiatry and Behavioral Science, National Crime Victims Research and Treatment Center, Medical University of South Carolina, Charleston, SC, USA

**David P. Goldberg**, Institute of Psychiatry, Psychology and Neuroscience, King's College London, London, UK

**Wayne K. Goodman**, Menninger Department of Psychiatry and Behavioral Sciences, Baylor College of Medicine, Houston, TX, USA

**Guy M. Goodwin**, Department of Psychiatry, Warneford Hospital, University of Oxford, Oxford, UK

**Philip Gorwood**, Saint-Anne Hospital, Paris Descartes University, Paris, France

**Michael G. Gottschalk**, Department of Psychiatry and Psychotherapy, Medical Center – University of Freiburg, Faculty of Medicine, University of Freiburg, Freiburg, Germany; Department of Psychiatry, Psychosomatics and Psychotherapy, Center of Mental Health, University of Würzburg, Würzburg, Germany

**Meryem Grabski**, Clinical Psychopharmacology Unit, Research Department of Clinical, Educational and Health Psychology, University College London, London, UK

**Cynthia A. Graham**, Department of Psychology, Faculty of Environmental and Life Sciences, University of Southampton, Southampton, UK

Anna I. Guerdjikova, Linder Center of HOPE, Mason, OH, USA; Department of Psychiatry and Behavioral Neuroscience, University of Cincinnati College of Medicine, Cincinnati, OH, USA

Abha R. Gupta, Department of Pediatrics, Yale University School of Medicine, New Haven, CT, USA

Katherine A. Halmi, Weill Cornell Medical College, White Plains, NY, USA

Jamie Hartmann-Boyce, Nuffield Department of Primary Care Health Sciences, University of Oxford, Oxford, UK

Keith Hawton, Centre for Suicide Research, University of Oxford, Department of Psychiatry, Warneford Hospital, Oxford, UK

Johannes Hebebrand, Department of Child and Adolescent Psychiatry, Psychosomatics and Psychotherapy, University Hospital Essen, University of Essen-Duisburg, Essen, Germany

Verena Heise, Warneford Hospital, Department of Psychiatry, University of Oxford, Oxford, UK

Alasdair L. Henry, Big Health Ltd, London, UK/ San Francisco, USA; Sleep and Circadian Neuroscience Institute, Nuffield Department of Clinical Neurosciences, University of Oxford, Oxford, UK

Beate Herpertz-Dahlmann, Department of Child and Adolescent Psychiatry, Psychosomatics and Psychotherapy, University Hospital Aachen, Technical University of Aachen, Aachen, Germany

Leigh van den Heuvel, Department of Psychiatry, Faculty of Medicine and Health Sciences, Stellenbosch University, Cape Town, South Africa

Gunter Heylens, Department of Psychiatry, Ghent University Hospital, Ghent, Belgium

Cecilia A. Hinojosa, School of Arts and Sciences, Department of Psychology, Tufts University, Medford, MA, USA

Ellen J. Hoffman, Yale Child Study Center, Yale School of Medicine, New Haven, CT, USA

Anthony J. Holland, Cambridge Neuroscience, University of Cambridge, Cambridge, UK

Emily A. Holmes, Department of Psychology, Uppsala University, Sweden; Department of Clinical Neuroscience, Karolinska Institutet, Stockholm, Sweden; Department of Psychiatry, University of Oxford, Oxford, UK

Rob Horne, Centre for Behavioural Medicine, Department of Practice and Policy, UCL School of Pharmacy, London, UK

Paul L. Houser, Linder Center of HOPE, Mason, OH, USA; Department of Psychiatry and Behavioral Neuroscience, University of Cincinnati College of Medicine, Cincinnati, OH, USA

Louise M. Howard, Institute of Psychiatry, King's College London, London, UK

Michele Hu, Nuffield Department of Clinical Neurosciences, John Radcliffe Hospital, Oxford, UK

Christopher Hübel, MRC Social Genetic and Developmental Psychiatry Centre, Institute of Psychiatry, Psychology and Neuroscience, King's College London, London, UK

Stephen J. Hucker, Division of Forensic Psychiatry, University of Toronto, Toronto, ON, Canada

Jennifer L. Hudson, Centre for Emotional Health, Department of Psychology, Macquarie University, Sydney, NSW, Australia

Nathan T. M. Huneke, Clinical and Experimental Sciences, Faculty of Medicine, University of Southampton, Southampton, UK

Sandra Iglesias, Translational Neuromodeling Unit (TNU), Institute for Biomedical Engineering, University of Zurich and Swiss Federal Institute of Technology (ETH Zurich), Zurich, Switzerland

Assen Jablensky, Royal Perth Hospital, The University of Western Australia, Crawley, WA, Australia

Scott L. J. Jackson, Office of Assessment and Analytics, Southern Connecticut State University, New Haven, CT, USA; Child Study Center, Yale University School of Medicine, New Haven, CT, USA

Kay Redfield Jamison, Department of Psychiatry, The Johns Hopkins University School of Medicine, Johns Hopkins Hospital, Baltimore, MD, USA

Mahesh Jayaram, Melbourne Neuropsychiatry Centre, Department of Psychiatry, The University of Melbourne and Melbourne Health; Carlton South, VIC, Australia; NorthWestern Mental Health, Melbourne Health, Parkville, VIC, Australia

Susan A. Jebb, Nuffield Department of Primary Care Health Sciences, University of Oxford, Oxford, UK

Mark Jenkinson, Nuffield Department of Clinical Neurosciences, John Radcliffe Hospital, Oxford, UK

Emily J. H. Jones, Centre for Brain and Cognitive Development, School of Psychology, Birkbeck College, London, UK

Ian Jones, Cardiff University, School of Medicine, Division of Psychological Medicine and Clinical Neurosciences, Cardiff, UK

Ricardo E. Jorge, Department of Psychiatry and Behavioral Sciences, Baylor College of Medicine, TIRR Memorial Hermann, Houston, TX, USA; Michael E. DeBakey Veterans Affairs Medical Center, Houston, TX, USA

Adam Ian Kaplin, Departments of Psychiatry and Neurology, Johns Hopkins University School of Medicine, Johns Hopkins Hospital, Baltimore, MD, USA

Nav Kapur, Centre for Suicide Prevention, Centre for Mental Health and Safety, University of Manchester, Manchester, UK; Greater Manchester Mental Health NHS Foundation Trust, Manchester, UK

Martien J. Kas, Groningen Institute for Evolutionary Life Sciences (GELIFES), University of Groningen, Groningen, The Netherlands

Navneet Kaur, School of Arts and Sciences, Department of Psychology, Tufts University, Medford, MA, USA

Walter H. Kaye, UCSD Eating Disorders Center for Treatment and Research, San Diego, CA, USA

Paul E. Keck, Jr., Linder Center of HOPE, Mason, OH, USA; Department of Psychiatry and Behavioral Neuroscience, University of Cincinnati College of Medicine, Cincinnati, OH, USA

Lena Katharina Keller, Institute for Medical Psychology, Medical Faculty, Ludwig-Maximilian-University, Munich, Germany; Department of Child and Adolescent Psychiatry, Psychosomatics and Psychotherapy, University Hospital Munich, Munich, Germany

Megan M. Kelly, Edith Nourse Rogers Memorial Veterans Hospital, Bedford, MA, USA; Department of Psychiatry, University of Massachusetts Medical School, Worcester, MA, USA

Kimberley M. Kendall, MRC Centre for Neuropsychiatric Genetics and Genomics, School of Medicine, Cardiff University, Cardiff, UK

Tony Kendrick, Primary Care and Population Sciences, University of Southampton, Aldermoor Health Centre, Southampton, UK

Lars Vedel Kessing, Psychiatric Center Copenhagen and University of Copenhagen, Faculty of Health and Medical Sciences, Copenhagen, Denmark

Falk Kiefer, Central Institute for Mental Health, Mannheim, Germany

Dean G. Kilpatrick, Department of Psychiatry, Medical University of South Carolina, Charleston, SC, USA

Martin Knapp, Care Policy and Evaluation Centre, London School of Economics and Political Science; and NIHR School for Social Care Research, London, UK

Nastassja Koen, Department of Psychiatry and Mental Health, University of Cape Town, South Africa; South African Medical Research Council (SAMRC) Unit on Risk and Resilience in Mental Disorders, Cape Town, South Africa

Inga K. Koerte, Psychiatry Neuroimaging Laboratory, Department of Psychiatry, Brigham and Women's Hospital, Harvard Medical School, Boston, MA, USA; and Department of Child and Adolescent Psychiatry, Psychosomatic, and Psychotherapy, Ludwig-Maximilian-University, Munich, Germany

Cary S. Kogan, School of Psychology, Faculty of Social Sciences, University of Ottawa, Ottawa, ON, Canada

Mirja Koschorke, Institute of Psychiatry, Psychology and Neuroscience, King's College London, London, UK

Ivan Koychev, Department of Psychiatry, Medical Sciences Division, University of Oxford, Oxford, UK

David J. Kupfer, Department of Psychiatry, University of Pittsburgh, Pittsburgh, PA, USA

**Natalie Kurniadi**, UCSD Eating Disorders Center for Treatment and Research, San Diego, CA, USA

**Simon D. Kyle**, Sleep and Circadian Neuroscience Institute, Nuffield Department of Clinical Neurosciences, University of Oxford, Oxford, UK

**Kate Langley**, School of Psychology, Cardiff University, Cardiff, UK; MRC Centre for Psychiatric Genetics and Genomics, Cardiff University, Cardiff, UK

**Briony Larance**, National Drug and Alcohol Research Centre, University of New South Wales, Sydney, NSW, Australia

**Matthew Large**, School of Psychiatry, University of New South Wales, Sydney, NSW, Australia

**Yann Le Strat**, Hospital Louis Mourrier, Department of Psychiatry, Colombes, France

**Gregor Leicht**, University Medical Center Hamburg-Eppendorf, Department of Psychiatry and Psychotherapy, Psychiatry Neuroimaging Branch, Hamburg, Germany

**Christian Lepage**, Psychiatry Neuroimaging Laboratory, Department of Psychiatry, Brigham and Women's Hospital, Harvard Medical School, Boston, MA, USA

**Stefan Leucht**, Department of Psychiatry and Psychotherapy, Klinikum rechts der Isar, School of Medicine, Technical University of Munich, Munich, Germany

**Juan C. Leza**, Department of Pharmacology, Faculty of Medicine, Complutense University of Madrid; CIBERSAM, Imas12, IUIN, Madrid, Spain

**Anne Lingford-Hughes**, Centre for Psychiatry, Department of Medicine, Imperial College London, London, UK

**Elizabeth F. Loftus**, School of Social Ecology, University of California, Irvine, CA, USA

**Crick Lund**, Alan J. Flisher Centre for Public Mental Health, Department of Psychiatry and Mental Health, University of Cape Town, Cape Town, South Africa; Centre for Global Mental Health, King's Global Health Institute, Health Service and Population Research Department, Institute of Psychiatry, Psychology and Neuroscience, King's College London, London, UK

**Antonella Macerollo**, Department of Neurology, The Walton Centre NHS Foundation Trust, Liverpool; School of Psychology, Faculty of Health and Life Sciences, University of Liverpool, Liverpool, UK

**Clare Mackay**, University of Oxford, Department of Psychiatry, Warneford Hospital, Oxford, UK

**Deirdre MacManus**, Institute of Psychiatry, King's College London, London, UK

**Trine Madsen**, Danish Research Institute for Suicide Prevention, Mental Health Center Copenhagen, University of Copenhagen, Copenhagen, Denmark

**Gin S. Malhi**, Discipline of Psychiatry, Sydney Medical School, Faculty of Medicine and Health, The University of Sydney, Australia

**Luc Mallet**, Personalized Neurology and Psychiatry University Department, University Hospital of Henri-Mondor, Créteil, France

**J. John Mann**, Department of Psychiatry, Columbia University/New York State Psychiatric Institute, New York, NY, USA

**Russell L. Margolis**, Division of Neurobiology, Department of Psychiatry, Johns Hopkins University School of Medicine, Baltimore, MD, USA

**Andreas Marneros**, Clinic for Psychiatry and Psychotherapy, Martin Luther University of Halle-Wittenberg, Halle, Germany

**Davide Martino**, Department of Clinical Neurosciences, Cumming School of Medicine, University of Calgary and Hotchkiss Brain Institute, Calgary, AB, Canada

**David Mataix-Cols**, Department of Clinical Neuroscience, Karolinska Institutet, Stockholm, Sweden

**Sivan Mauer**, Department of Psychiatry, Tufts University,, Tufts Medical Center, Boston, MA, USA

**Helen S. Mayberg**, Center for Advanced Circuit Therapeutics, Mount Sinai Icahn School of Medicine, New York, NY, USA

**Diego R. Mazzotti**, Center for Applied Genomics, The Children's Hospital of Philadelphia, Philadelphia, PA, USA

**Susan L. McElroy**, Linder Center of HOPE, Mason, OH, USA; Department of Psychiatry and Behavioral Neuroscience, University of Cincinnati College of Medicine, Cincinnati, OH, USA

**Joseph P. McEvoy**, Department of Psychiatry and Health Behavior, Medical College of Georgia, Augusta University, Augusta, GA,, USA

**Bruce S. McEwen**, Laboratory of Neuroendocrinology, The Rockefeller University, New York, NY, USA

**Francis J. McMahon**, Human Genetics Branch, National Institute of Mental Health, Intramural Research Program, Bethesda, MD, USA

**Herbert Y. Meltzer**, Northwestern University Feinberg School of Medicine, Chicago, IL, USA

**Harald Merckelbach**, Forensic Psychology Section, Maastricht University, Maastricht, The Netherlands

**Alison K. Merikangas**, Department of Psychiatry, Perelman School of Medicine, University of Pennsylvania, Philadelphia, PA, USA

**Kathleen R. Merikangas**, Intramural Research Program, National Institute of Mental Health, Bethesda, MD, USA

**Thomas Merten**, Department of Neurology, Vivantes Friedrichshain Hospital, Berlin, Germany

**David J. Miklowitz**, Department of Psychiatry, University of California, Los Angeles School of Medicine, Los Angeles, CA, USA

**Bruce Miller**, Memory and Aging Center, Department of Neurology, University of California, San Francisco, CA, USA

**TzeHow Mok**, National Hospital for Neurology and Neurosurgery, UCL Institute of Neurology, London, UK

**Hans-Jürgen Möller**, Department of Psychiatry, Ludwig Maximilian University, Munich, Germany

**Adam Moreton**, Centre for Suicide Prevention, Centre for Mental Health and Safety, University of Manchester, Manchester, UK; Greater Manchester Mental Health NHS Foundation Trust, Manchester, UK

**Umberto Moretto**, Center for Studies in Behavioral Neurobiology and Department of Exercise Science, Concordia University, Montreal, QC, Canada; PERFORM Centre, Concordia University, Montreal, QC, Canada; Research Center, Institute of Geriatrics, University of Montreal, Montreal, QC, Canada; Psychiatric Unit I, Department of Clinical and Experimental Medicine, University of Pisa, Pisa, Italy

**Leslie C. Morey**, Department of Psychology, Texas A&M University, College Station, TX, USA

**Nicole Mori**, Linder Center of HOPE, Mason, OH, USA; Department of Psychiatry and Behavioral Neuroscience, University of Cincinnati College of Medicine, Cincinnati, OH, USA

**Sarah E. Morris**, National Institute of Mental Health, Bethesda, MD, USA

**Katherine H. Moyer**, Central Alabama Veterans Administration Health Care System, Tuskegee AL, USA

**Davis N. Mpavaenda**, NHS East of England Highly Specialised Service (HSS) for Treatment Resistant OCD/BDD, Obsessive Compulsive and Related Spectrum Disorders and Applied Neuroscience Department, Hertfordshire Partnership University NHS Foundation Trust and University of Hertfordshire, Hatfield, UK

**Roger Mulder**, University of Otago, Newtown, Wellington, New Zealand

**Christoph Mulert**, Centre for Psychiatry and Psychotherapy, Justus-Liebig-University, Giessen, Germany

**Paul E. Mullen**, Centre for Forensic Behavioural Sciences, Swinburne University, Hawthorn, VIC, Australia

**Marcus Munafò**, School of Experimental Psychology, University of Bristol, Bristol, UK

**Declan Murphy**, Department of Forensic and Neurodevelopmental Sciences, and the Sackler Institute for Translational Neurodevelopmental Sciences, Institute of Psychiatry, Psychology and Neuroscience, King's College London, London, UK

**Rebecca Murphy**, Department of Psychiatry, University of Oxford, Warneford Hospital, Oxford, UK

**Gerald Nestadt**, Department of Psychiatry and Behavioral Sciences, The Johns Hopkins University School of Medicine, Baltimore, MD, USA

**Charles R. Newton**, Department of Psychiatry, Warneford Hospital, Oxford, UK

**Giles Newton-Howes**, University of Otago, Newtown, Wellington, New Zealand

Olav Nielssen, School of Psychiatry, University of New South Wales, Sydney, NSW, Australia

Akin Nihat, National Hospital for Neurology and Neurosurgery, UCL Institute of Neurology, London, UK

Anna Christina Nobre, Oxford Centre for Human Brain Activity, Department of Psychiatry, Department of Experimental Psychology, and Wellcome Centre for Integrative Neuroimaging, University of Oxford, Oxford, UK

Merete Nordentoft, Mental Health Centre, Copenhagen University, Copenhagen, Denmark

Michael C. O'Donovan, MRC Centre for Neuropsychiatric Genetics and Genomics, School of Medicine, Cardiff University, Cardiff, UK

John O'Grady, Eardisley, Herefordshire, UK

Berend Olivier, Groningen Institute for Evolutionary Life Sciences (GELIFES), University of Groningen, Groningen, The Netherlands; Division of Pharmacology, Utrecht Institute for Pharmaceutical Sciences and Brain Centre Rudolf Magnus, Utrecht University, The Netherlands; Department of Psychiatry, Yale University School of Medicine, New Haven, CT, USA

Isabella Pacchiarotti, Hospital Clinic, Institute of Neuroscience, University of Barcelona, IDIBAPS, CIBERSAM, Barcelona, Spain

Jennifer Pacheco, National Institute of Mental Health, Bethesda, MD, USA

Allan I. Pack, Center for Sleep and Circadian Neurobiology, Division of Sleep Medicine/Department of Medicine, University of Pennsylvania, Perelman School of Medicine, Philadelphia, PA, USA

Brian A. Palmer, Mercy Hospital, Coon Rapids, MN, USA; formerly Department of Psychiatry, Mayo Clinic College of Medicine, Rochester, MN, USA

Melanie Palmer, Institute of Psychiatry, Psychology and Neuroscience, King's College London, London, UK

Nicola Palomero-Gallagher, Institute of Neuroscience and Medicine (INM-1), Research Centre Jülich, Jülich, Germany; Department of Psychiatry, Psychotherapy and Psychosomatics, Medical Faculty, RWTH Aachen, Aachen, Germany

Christos Pantelis, Melbourne Neuropsychiatry Centre, Department of Psychiatry, The University of Melbourne and Melbourne Health; Carlton South, VIC, Australia; NorthWestern Mental Health, Melbourne Health, Parkville, VIC, Australia; Adult Mental Health Rehabilitation Unit, Sunshine Hospital; St Albans, VIC, Australia

Christian Paret, Department of Psychosomatic Medicine, Central Institute of Mental Health Mannheim, Medical Faculty Mannheim, Heidelberg University, Heidelberg, Germany

Steve Pearce, Department of Psychiatry, Medical Sciences Division, University of Oxford, Oxford, UK

Stuart N. Peirson, Sleep and Circadian Neuroscience Institute (SCNi), Nuffield Department of Clinical Neurosciences, University of Oxford, Oxford, UK

Marcela Pereira, Section of Translational Neuropharmacology, Department of Clinical Neuroscience, Center of Molecular Medicine, Karolinska Institute, Stockholm, Sweden

Katharine A. Phillips, Rhode Island Hospital, Providence, RI, USA; Department of Psychiatry and Human Behavior, The Warren Alpert Medical School of Brown University, Providence, RI, USA

Mary L. Phillips, Department of Psychiatry, University of Pittsburgh, Western Psychiatric Institute and Clinic, Pittsburgh PA, USA

Pierre Pichot, National Academy of Medicine, Paris, France

Alexandra Pitman, Division of Psychiatry, University College London, London, UK

Guilherme V. Polanczyk, Department of Psychiatry, University of São Paulo Medical School, São Paulo, Brazil

Jonathan Price, Department of Psychiatry, Medical Sciences Division, University of Oxford, Oxford, UK

David Pritchett, Sleep and Circadian Neuroscience Institute (SCNi), Nuffield Department of Clinical Neurosciences, University of Oxford, Oxford, UK

Rosemary Purcell, Orygen, The National Centre of Excellence in Youth Mental Health and the Centre for Youth Mental Health, The University of Melbourne, Melbourne, VIC, Australia

Anto P. Rajkumar, Institute of Mental Health, University of Nottingham, Nottingham, UK; Department of Old Age Psychiatry, Institute of Psychiatry, Psychology, and Neuroscience, King's College London, London, UK

Nicolas Ramoz, INSERM, Center of Psychiatry and Neuroscience, Paris, France

Beverley Raphael[†], Academic Unit of Psychiatry and Addiction Medicine, ANU Medical School, The Canberra Hospital, Garran, ACT, Australia

Judith L. Rapoport, Child Psychiatry Branch, NIMH, Bethesda, MD, USA

Geoffrey M. Reed, Department of Mental Health and Substance Abuse, World Health Organization, Geneva, Switzerland; Department of Psychiatry, Columbia University Vagelos College of Physicians and Surgeons, New York, NY, USA

Susan Rees, Psychiatry Research and Teaching Unit, University of New South Wales, Mental Health Unit, The Liverpool Hospital, Liverpool, NSW, Australia

Darrel A. Regier, Center for the Study of Traumatic Stress (CSTS), Department of Psychiatry, Uniformed Services University (USUHS), Bethesda, MD, USA

Jemma Reid, NHS East of England Highly Specialised Service (HSS) for Treatment Resistant OCD/BDD, Obsessive Compulsive and Related Spectrum Disorders and Applied Neuroscience Department, Hertfordshire Partnership University NHS Foundation Trust and University of Hertfordshire, Hatfield, UK

Patricio Riva-Posse, Department of Psychiatry, Emory University, Atlanta, GA, USA

Trevor W. Robbins, Department of Psychology, Behavioural and Clinical Neuroscience Institute, University of Cambridge, Cambridge, UK

Kenneth Rockwood, Dalhousie University, Halifax, NS, Canada

Till Roenneberg, Institute for Medical Psychology, Medical Faculty, Ludwig-Maximilian-University, Munich, Germany

James Rucker, The Institute of Psychiatry, Psychology and Neuroscience, King's College London, London, UK

Julia Russell, School of Arts and Sciences, Department of Psychology, Tufts University, Medford, MA, USA

Jack Samuels, Department of Psychiatry and Behavioral Sciences, The Johns Hopkins University School of Medicine, Baltimore, MD, USA

Charles A. Sanislow, Department of Psychology and Program in Neuroscience and Behavior, Wesleyan University, Middletown, CT, USA

Kate E. A. Saunders, Department of Psychiatry, Medical Sciences Division, University of Oxford, Oxford, UK

Julian Savulescu, Oxford Uehiro Centre for Practical Ethics, Faculty of Philosophy, University of Oxford; Wellcome Centre for Ethics and Humanities, University of Oxford, Oxford, UK; Murdoch Children's Research Institute; Melbourne Law School, University of Melbourne, Melbourne, Australia

Christian Schmahl, Department of Psychosomatic Medicine, Central Institute of Mental Health Mannheim, Medical Faculty Mannheim, Heidelberg University, Heidelberg, Germany

Sophie C. Schneider, Menninger Department of Psychiatry and Behavioral Sciences, Baylor College of Medicine, Houston, TX, USA

Vivian Schultz, Psychiatry Neuroimaging Laboratory, Department of Psychiatry, Brigham and Women's Hospital, Boston, MA, USA; and Department of Child and Adolescent Psychiatry, Psychosomatic, and Psychotherapy, Ludwig-Maximilian-University, Munich, Germany

Stephen Scott, Institute of Psychiatry, Psychology and Neuroscience, King's College London, London, UK

Soraya Seedat, Stellenbosch University, Stellenbosch, South Africa

Rebbia Shahab, Department of Psychiatry, New York University School of Medicine, New York, NY, USA; Nathan Kline Institute for Psychiatric Research, Orangeburg, NY, USA

Trevor Sharp, Department of Pharmacology, University of Oxford, Oxford, UK

Michael Sharpe, Department of Psychiatry, University of Oxford, Oxford, UK

Philip Shaw, Child Psychiatry Branch, National Institute of Mental Health, Bethesda, MD, USA

Martha E. Shenton, Psychiatry Neuroimaging Laboratory, Department of Psychiatry and Radiology, Brigham and Women's Hospital, Harvard Medical School, Boston; and VA Boston Healthcare System, Brockton, MA, USA

Lisa M. Shin, School of Arts and Sciences, Department of Psychology, Tufts University, Medford, MA, USA

Derrick Silove, School of Psychiatry, University of New South Wales, NSW, Australia

Judit Simon, Department of Health Economics, Center for Public Health, Medical University of Vienna, Vienna, Austria; Department of Psychiatry, Nuffield Department of Public Health, University of Oxford, Oxford, UK

Emily Simonoff, Department of Child and Adolescent Psychiatry, Institute of Psychiatry, Psychology and Neuroscience, King's College London, London, UK

Julia M. A. Sinclair, Clinical and Experimental Sciences, Faculty of Medicine, University of Southampton, Southampton, UK

Ilina Singh, Department of Psychiatry, Wellcome Centre for Ethics and Humanities, University of Oxford, Oxford, UK

Nisha Singh, Centre for Neuroimaging Sciences, Institute of Psychiatry, Psychology and Neuroscience, London, UK

Andrew E. Skodol, Department of Psychiatry, University of Arizona College of Medicine, Tucson, AZ, USA

William H. Sledge, Yale School of Medicine, Department of Psychiatry, New Haven, CT, USA

Dylan Smith, Center for Studies in Behavioral Neurobiology and Department of Exercise Science, Concordia University, Montreal, QC, Canada; PERFORM Centre, Concordia University, Montreal, QC, Canada

Olaf Sporns, Department of Psychological and Brain Sciences, Indiana University, Bloomington, IN, USA

Sarah Steeg, Centre for Suicide Prevention, Centre for Mental Health and Safety, University of Manchester, Manchester, UK

Dan J. Stein, Department of Psychiatry and Mental Health, University of Cape Town, Cape Town, South Africa; South African Medical Research Council (SAMRC) Unit on Risk and Resilience in Mental Disorders, Cape Town, South Africa

Klaas E. Stephan, Translational Neuromodeling Unit (TNU), Institute for Biomedical Engineering, University of Zurich and Swiss Federal Institute of Technology (ETH Zurich), Zurich, Switzerland; Wellcome Trust Centre for Neuroimaging, University College London, London, UK

Emily R. Stern, Department of Psychiatry, New York University School of Medicine, New York, NY, USA; Nathan Kline Institute for Psychiatric Research, Orangeburg, NY, USA

Jon Stone, Department of Clinical Neurosciences, Centre for Clinical Brain Sciences, University of Edinburgh, Western General Hospital, Edinburgh, UK

William S. Stone, Department of Psychiatry, Beth Israel Deaconess Medical Center, Boston, MA, USA

Eric A. Storch, Menninger Department of Psychiatry and Behavioral Sciences, Baylor College of Medicine, Houston, TX, USA

Per Svenningsson, Section of Translational Neuropharmacology, Department of Clinical Neuroscience, Center of Molecular Medicine, Karolinska Institute, Stockholm, Sweden

Eszter Szekely, Section on Neurobehavioral Clinical Research, Social and Behavioral Research Branch, National Human Genome Research Institute, National Institute of Mental Health, Intramural Program, Bethesda, MD, USA

Akitoshi Takeda, Memory and Aging Center, Department of Neurology, University of California, San Francisco, CA, USA; Department of Neurology, Osaka City University Graduate School of Medicine, Osaka, Japan

Eric Taylor, Department of Child and Adolescent Psychiatry, Institute of Psychiatry, Psychology and Neuroscience, King's College London, London, UK

Anita Thapar, Division of Psychological Medicine and Clinical Neurosciences, School of Medicine, Cardiff University, Cardiff, UK; MRC Centre for Psychiatric Genetics and Genomics, Cardiff University, Cardiff, UK

Graham Thornicroft, Institute of Psychiatry, Psychology and Neuroscience, King's College London, London, UK

George K. Tofaris, Nuffield Department of Clinical Neurosciences, John Radcliffe Hospital, University of Oxford, Oxford, UK

Mark Toynbee, Department of Psychiatry, University of Oxford, Warneford Hospital, Oxford, UK

Irene Tracey, Nuffield Department of Clinical Neurosciences, University of Oxford, Oxford, UK

Ming T. Tsuang, Department of Psychiatry, Institute for Genomic Medicine, UC San Diego, La Jolla, CA, USA

Bedirhan T. Üstün, Department of Psychiatry, Koc University, Istanbul, Turkey

Wim van den Brink, Academic Medical Center, Department of Psychiatry, University of Amsterdam, Amsterdam, The Netherlands

Michael B. VanElzakker, School of Arts and Sciences, Department of Psychology, Tufts University, Medford, MA, USA

Eduard Vieta, Hospital Clinic, Institute of Neuroscience, University of Barcelona, IDIBAPS, CIBERSAM, Barcelona, Spain

Fred R. Volkmar, Department of Psychiatry, Child Study Center, Yale University, New Haven, CT, USA

Alexander von Gontard, Department of Child and Adolescent Psychiatry, Saarland University Hospital, Homburg, Germany

Nicole Votruba, Centre for Global Mental Health, Institute of Psychiatry, Psychology and Neuroscience, King's College London, London, UK

Jane Walker, Department of Psychiatry, University of Oxford, Oxford, UK

James T. R. Walters, MRC Centre for Neuropsychiatric Genetics and Genomics, School of Medicine, Cardiff University, Cardiff, UK

Caleb Webber, Department of Physiology, Anatomy and Genetics, University of Oxford, Oxford, UK

Aliza Werner-Seidler, Black Dog Institute, University of New South Wales, Randwick, Sydney, NSW, Australia

Christina E. Wierenga, UCSD Eating Disorders Center for Treatment and Research, San Diego, CA, USA

Eva C. Winnebeck, Institute for Medical Psychology, Medical Faculty, Ludwig-Maximilian-University, Munich, Germany

Adam Winstock, Institute of Epidemiology and Health Care, University College London London, UK

Hans-Ulrich Wittchen, Clinical Psychology and Psychotherapy RG, Department of Psychiatry and Psychotherapy, Ludwig-Maximilian-University, Munich, Germany

Sally Wooding, Mental Health Branch, NSW Health Department, Sydney, NSW, Australia

Mark Woolrich, Oxford Centre for Human Brain Activity (OHBA), University Department of Psychiatry, Warneford Hospital, Oxford, UK

Dale Zhou, Child Psychiatry Branch, NIMH, Bethesda, MD, USA

Karl Zilles, Institute of Neuroscience and Medicine (INM-1), Research Centre Jülich, Jülich, Germany; Department of Psychiatry, Psychotherapy and Psychosomatics, Medical Faculty, RWTH Aachen, Aachen, Germany; JARA-BRAIN, Jülich-Aachen Research Alliance, Jülich, Germany

Joseph Zohar, Post Trauma Center, Chaim Sheba Medical Center, and Tel Aviv University, Israel

Enikő Zsoldos, Warneford Hospital, Department of Psychiatry, University of Oxford, Oxford, UK

Alessandro Zuddas, Child and Adolescent Neuropsychiatric Unit, Department of Biomedical Sciences, University of Cagliari and 'G. Brotzu' Hospital Trust, Cagliari, Italy

# Free personal online access for five years

Individual purchasers of this book are also entitled to free personal access to the online edition for five years on *Oxford Medicine Online* (www.oxfordmedicine.com). Please refer to the access token card for instructions on token redemption and access.

*Oxford Medicine Online* allows you to print, save, cite, email, and share content; download high-resolution figures as PowerPoint® slides; save often-used books, chapters, or searches; annotate; and quickly jump to other chapters or related material on a mobile-optimized platform.

# SECTION 1

# The subject matter and approach to psychiatry

# Section 1

# The subject matter and approach to psychiatry

# The patient's perspective

*Kay Redfield Jamison and Adam Ian Kaplin*

## Introduction

It is difficult to be a psychiatric patient, but a good doctor can make it less so. Confusion and fear can be overcome by knowledge and compassion, and resistance to treatment is often, although by no means always, amenable to change by intelligent persuasion that leads to better healing. The devil, as the fiery melancholic Byron knew, is in the details.

## Delivering the diagnosis, prognosis, and plan

Patients, when first given a psychiatric diagnosis, are commonly both relieved and frightened—relieved because often they have been overwhelmed by pain, anxiety, and hopelessness for a considerable period of time, and frightened because they do not know what the diagnosis means, what the treatment will entail, and their likelihood of obtaining a meaningful response. They do not know if they will return to the way they once were, whether the treatment they have been prescribed will or will not work, and, even if it does work, at what cost it will be to them in terms of their notions of themselves, potentially unpleasant side effects, and the reactions of their family members, friends, colleagues, and employers. Perhaps most disturbing, they do not know if their depression, psychosis, anxieties, or compulsions will return to become a permanent part of their lives. Caught in a state often characterized by personal anguish, social isolation, and confusion, newly diagnosed patients find themselves on a quest to regain a sense of mastery of themselves and their surroundings. One of the main goals of therapies of all types is to empower the patient and give them some control back over their world and rechart the meaning and purpose of their lives under altered circumstances.

The specifics of what the doctor says and the manner in which he or she says it are critically important from the start and will colour the patient's ongoing treatment course for years to come. Most patients who complain about receiving poor psychiatric care do so on several grounds—their doctors, they feel, spend too little time explaining the nature of their illnesses and treatment; they are reluctant to consult with, or actively involve, family members; they are patronizing and do not adequately listen to what the patient has to say; they do not encourage questions or sufficiently address the concerns of the patient; they do not discuss alternative treatments, the risks of treatment, and the risks of no treatment; and they do not thoroughly forewarn about side effects of medications.

Most of these complaints are avoidable. Time, although difficult to come by, is well spent early on in the course of treatment when the manifestations of confusion and hopelessness are greatest, the risk of non-adherence is highest, and the possibility of suicide substantially increased. Hope can be realistically extended to patients and family members, and its explicit extension is vital to those whose illnesses have robbed them not only of hope, but also of belief in themselves, their future, and the very meaning of their lives. The hope provided needs to be tempered, however, by an honest and realistic explication of possible difficulties yet to be encountered: unpleasant side effects from medications; a rocky time course to meaningful recovery which will often consist of many discouraging cycles of feeling the progress of marching towards wellness, only to stumble and slide temporarily backwards towards illness again; and the probable personal, professional, and financial repercussions that come in the wake of having a psychiatric illness.

## Importance of doctor–patient communication

It is terrifying to lose one's sanity or to be seized by a paralysing depression. No medication alone can substitute for a good doctor's clinical expertise and the kindness of a doctor who understands both the medical and psychological sides of mental illness. Nor can any medication alone substitute for a good doctor's capacity to listen to the fears and despair of patients trying to come to terms with what has happened to them. A good doctor is a therapeutic optimist who is able to instil hope and confidence to combat bewilderment and despair. Great doctors are able to provide the unwavering care to their patients that they would want a member of their own family to receive, blending empathy and compassion with expertise and confidence.

Doctors need to be direct in answering questions, to acknowledge the limits of their understanding, and to encourage specialist consultations when the clinical situation warrants it. They also need to create a therapeutic climate in which patients and their families feel free, when necessary, to express their concerns about treatment or to request a second opinion. There must also be a willingness by doctors to collaborate across medical disciplines in the care of their psychiatric patients because of the influence and, likewise, the impact of somatic diseases on mental illness—for example, there is evidence that depression predisposes people to conditions such as myocardial infarction, diabetes, and multiple sclerosis, all of which conversely increase the likelihood of depression. Moreover, persons with major depression and schizophrenia have a 40–60% greater chance of dying prematurely than the general population, due to physical health problems that are often left unattended or exacerbated by the side effects of psychotropic medications. Doctors are also frequently called upon to advocate for their psychiatric patients who are frequently stigmatized and therefore at great risk of being discriminated against by being deprived of their professional, economic, social, and cultural rights. Particular care must be taken by doctors to prevent their patients from receiving substandard care by refusing to share, against their patient's better judgement, important aspects of their mental illness with non-mental health medical practitioners.

Treatment non-adherence, one of the major causes of unnecessary suffering, relapse, hospitalization, and suicide must be addressed head-on. Unfortunately, doctors are variable in their ability to assess, predict, and facilitate adherence in their patients [1]. Asking directly and often about medication concerns and side effects, scheduling frequent follow-up visits after the initial diagnostic evaluation and treatment recommendation, and encouraging adjunctive psychotherapy or involvement in patient support groups can make a crucial difference in whether or not a patient takes medication in a way that is most effective. Aggressive treatment of unpleasant or intolerable side effects, minimizing the dosage and number of doses, and providing ongoing, frequently repetitive education about the illness and its treatment are likewise essential, if common-sense, ways to avert or minimize non-adherence.

## Communication in the digital age

The ever-expanding availability of health information technology, ranging from assistive devices (that permit regular tracking of symptoms and reminders to facilitate treatment adherence such as automated texting and telemedicine) to therapeutic tools (that provide interventions such as online cognitive behavioural therapy), will continue to improve the ease with which care can be delivered. But in the end, it is the therapeutic alliance between patient and clinician, honed and proven over two and a half millennia since the time of Hippocrates, that will and must remain central to the healing process. Technology can assist and enhance, but not replace, the doctor–patient relationship.

## Doctor as teacher

Education is, of course, integral to the good treatment of any illness, but this is especially true when the illnesses are chronic and shrouded in the secrecy that is caused by both social and personal stigma. The term 'doctor' derives originally from the Latin word for teacher, and it is in their roles as teachers that doctors provide patients with the knowledge and understanding to combat

the confusion and unpredictability that surround mental illness. Patients and their family members should be encouraged to write down any questions they may have, as many individuals are intimidated once they find themselves in a doctor's office. Any information that is given orally to patients should be repeated as often as necessary (due to the cognitive difficulties experienced by many psychiatric patients, especially when acutely ill or recovering from an acute episode) and, whenever feasible, provided in written form as well. Additional information is available to patients and family members in books and pamphlets obtainable from libraries, bookstores, and patient support groups, but, ever more commonly, information is accessible through the Internet as videos, websites, and online support groups [2, 3]. Visual aids, such as charts portraying the natural course of the treated and untreated illness or the causes and results of sleep deprivation and medication cessation, are also helpful to many [4–6]. Finally, providing the patients with self-report scales to monitor their daily progress, such as mood charts in affective disorder, not only provides invaluable clinical data, but also teaches patients and their physicians to better understand the patient's illnesses and their response to therapeutic interventions and exacerbating stressors. Family members and significant others can, and usually do, play key roles as outside sources of information which can be critically important in ensuring that the proper diagnosis is made at the outset. Patients, when they are well, also often benefit from a meeting with their family members and their doctor that focuses upon drawing up contingency plans in case their illness should recur. These meetings also provide an opportunity to shore up the support system the patient has by educating their caregivers about the nature, cause, manifestations, and treatment of their loved one's mental illness. Such meetings may also include what is to be done in the event that a psychiatric emergency arises and hospitalization is required, a discussion of early warning signs of impending psychotic or depressive episodes, methods for regularizing sleep and activity patterns, techniques to protect patients financially, and ways to manage suicidal behaviour should it occur. Suicide, globally the second leading cause of death in 15- to 29-year olds, is the major cause of premature death in severe psychiatric illnesses [7, 8], and its prevention is of first concern. Those illnesses most likely to result in suicide (mood disorders, comorbid alcohol and drug abuse, and schizophrenia) need to be treated early, aggressively, and often for an indefinite period of time [2, 10]. Lithium, which has demonstrated significant efficacy in preventing suicide, should be considered when appropriate [11]. The increasing evidence that treatment early in psychiatric illness may improve the long-term course needs to be considered in light of the reluctance of many patients to stay in treatment [10, 12, 14].

## Conclusions

The ancient proverb *medice, cura te ipsum* (physician, heal thyself) applies most pressingly to mental illness, because the rates of burnout, depression, and suicide among doctors are deeply concerning. A willingness to change the culture of medicine, so that more time, attention, and education is given to the critically important aspects of mental health, routine screening, and treatment of depression to encourage, rather than punish, seeking help.

No one who has treated or suffered from mental illness would minimize the difficulties involved in successful treatment. Modern medicine gives options that did not exist even 10 years ago, and there is every reason to expect that improvements in psychopharmacology, psychotherapy, and diagnostic techniques will continue to develop at a galloping pace. Still, the relationship between the patient and doctor will remain central to the treatment, as Morag Coate wrote more than 40 years ago in *Beyond All Reason* [13]:

'Because the doctors cared, and because one of them still believed in me when I believed in nothing, I have survived to tell the tale. It is not only the doctors who perform hazardous operations or give life-saving drugs in obvious emergencies who hold the scales at times between life and death. To sit quietly in a consulting room and talk to someone would not appear to the general public as a heroic or dramatic thing to do. In medicine there are many different ways of saving lives. This is one of them.'

## FURTHER INFORMATION

Non-governmental mental health websites: USA
http://www.nami.org/
http://www.dbsalliance.org/site/PageServer?pagename=home
Governmental mental health websites: USA
http://www.nimh.nih.gov/
https://www.samhsa.gov/treatment
Non-governmental mental health websites: UK
http://www.mentalhealth.org.uk/
http://www.mind.org.uk
Governmental mental health websites: UK
https://www.nice.org.uk/guidance/conditions-and-diseases/
    mental-health-and-behavioural-conditions
http://mentalhealthcare-uk.com

## REFERENCES

1. Osterberg, L. and Blaschke, T. (2005). Adherence to medication. *New England Journal of Medicine*, 353, 487–97.
2. Goodwin, F.K. and Jamison, K.R. (2007). *Manic-depressive illness* (2nd edn). Oxford University Press, New York, NY.
3. Wyatt, R.J. and Chew, R.H. (2005). *Practical psychiatric practice. Forms and protocols for clinical use* (3rd edn). American Psychiatric Association, Washington, D.C.
4. Post, R.M., Rubinow, D.R., and Ballenger, J.C. (1986). Conditioning and sensitisation in the longitudinal course of affective illness. *British Journal of Psychiatry*, 149, 191–201.
5. Wehr, T.A., Sack, D.A., and Rosenthal, N.E. (1987). Sleep reduction as a final common pathway in the genesis of mania. *American Journal of Psychiatry*, 144, 201–4.
6. Baldessarini, R.J., Tondo, L., and Hennen, J. (2003). Lithium treatment and suicide risk in major affective disorders: update and new findings. *Journal of Clinical Psychiatry*, 64(Suppl 5), 44–52.
7. World Health Organization. (2014). *Preventing suicide: a global imperative*. http://www.who.int/mental_health/suicide-prevention/world_report_2014/en/
8. Institute of Medicine (IoM). (2002). *Reducing suicide: a national imperative*. National Academy Press, Washington, D.C.
10. Wyatt, R.J. (1995). Early intervention for schizophrenia: can the course of the illness be altered? *Biological Psychiatry*, 38, 1–3.
11. Cipriani A, Hawton K, Stockton S, Geddes JR. (2013). Lithium in the prevention of suicide in mood disorders: updated systematic review and meta-analysis. *BMJ*, 346, f3646.
12. Berger, G., Dell'Olio, M., Amminger, P., *et al.* (2007). Neuroprotection in emerging psychotic disorders. *Early Intervention in Psychiatry*, 1, 114–27.
13. Coate, M. (1964). *Beyond all reason*. Constable, London.
14. Jamison, K.R., Gerner, R.H., and Goodwin, F.K. (1979). Patient and physician attitudes toward lithium: relationship to compliance. *Archives of General Psychiatry*, 36, 866–9.

# Public attitudes and the challenge of stigma

*Nicole Votruba, Mirja Koschorke, and Graham Thornicroft*

## Introduction

Stigma can be considered as an overarching term that includes challenges faced by people with mental illness related to knowledge, attitudes, and behaviour [1]. The knowledge domain includes low levels of mental health literacy, for example among the general population (ignorance); the attitudinal domain relates to almost entirely negative affect towards people with experience of mental illness (prejudice), while the behavioural aspects reflect predominantly forces for the social exclusion and diminished citizenship for people with mental illness (discrimination). This chapter considers the evidence of the implications of these elements and also summarizes the literature on what can be done to effectively reduce stigma and discrimination.

## The practical implications of stigma and discrimination

The consequences of stigma and discrimination are wide-reaching and severe, and affect people with mental disorders, their family members, mental health staff, institutions, and treatments, as well as society as a whole.

Discrimination, the behavioural consequence of stigma, adds to the disability of persons with mental illness and leads to disadvantages in many aspects of life, including personal relationships, education, and work [1, 2]. It limits the life opportunities of those affected, through loss of income, prolonged unemployment, reduced access to housing or health care, for example, and therefore reduced access to important means of recovery [3]. Commonly, people with mental disorders experience unequal treatment for physical health conditions, leading to rates of morbidity and mortality much beyond what is attributable to their primary mental disorder [4]. Discrimination because of mental illness is pervasive and universal—international studies of mental illness discrimination have shown that rates of both anticipated and experienced discrimination are consistently high across countries among people with mental disorders [5–8].

Yet another form of devaluation takes place when individuals affected by mental illness stigma accept the negative beliefs held against them and lose self-esteem, resulting in self-stigma (or 'internalized stigma') [9–11]. Internal consequences of stigma and discrimination have been the subject of a number of studies and include feelings of shame, a loss of emotional well-being, poor self-efficacy, and negative recovery outcomes [12–19].

What self-stigma can mean is vividly described in a quote by Gallo [20, pp. 407–8] quoted in Angell *et al.* (2005) [21]—a statement from a person with mental illness on how stigma and discrimination have changed the way she feels about herself:

> 'I perceive myself, quite accurately, unfortunately, as having a serious mental illness and therefore as having been relegated to what I called "the social garbage heap", I tortured myself with the persistent and repetitive thought that I would encounter, even total strangers, did not like me and wished that mentally ill people like me did not exist. Thus I would do things such as standing away from others at bus stops and hiding and cringing in the far corners of subway cars. Thinking of myself as garbage, I would even leave the side walk in what I thought of as exhibiting the proper difference to those above me in social class. The latter group, of course, included all other human beings.' [20][1]

Internal consequences of stigma and discrimination can further lead to hopelessness and depression, social withdrawal, and reduced participation in treatment programmes [3] and act as a stressor that perpetuates ill health and makes recovery more difficult [22, 23]. Coping responses, such as secrecy about the condition and avoidance of others, further feed into the cycle of isolation and alienation [3].

In addition to experiences of direct discrimination from others, persons suffering from mental illness face several forms of structural discrimination, for example manifest in the lack of resources allocated to the care of mental disorders, the location and quality of some treatment facilities, and inadequate attention to the physical health needs of people with mental disorders [24, 25].

Paradoxically, stigmatizing practices and even human rights violations are found within mental health services worldwide [26–28]. Undesirable conditions in mental health institutions, as well as the shame and fear of disclosure associated with attending them, act as a barrier for help-seeking and the effective treatment of mental health conditions [29]. For example, people with mental disorders may delay seeking treatment or terminate treatment prematurely for fear of being labelled and discriminated against [3, 30].

A statement from Diana on restrained treatment by health-care professionals in a psychiatric hospital:

'There were between six and eight staff members, I am not sure, I can't remember too much. I didn't have a very clear vision. I saw people surrounding me, holding me by the hand, holding me by the legs. I don't think it was something they had to do. There was no talking. They would have helped better if they would have been more understanding and more talking… more respect. I felt really bad. While I was in hospital I tried to complain but I don't know if anybody was listening. It was a nightmare.' [1, p. 87]²

Another very commonly cited source of stigma is family members. Even although many people experience great support from their families, it is family members too who often hold negative attitudes towards people with mental illness and even within their families treat them in a discriminatory way.

'There I was, the eldest son suffering a sudden deep depression, crying and unable to work. Often threatened by my confused Dad as being "weak", "a fuck-up", and a "nutter". No-one else in the family going back generations had gone "mad like that". I was told not to tell any of the neighbours what was happening – to stop the gossip. (Paul)' [1, p. 2]³

In many societies where services are scarce and support systems inadequate, families feel forced to resort to chaining and other practices to restrain relatives with mental illness [28, 31].

Research has shown that mental health professionals themselves hold negative stereotypes and attitudes similar to the general population and even more pessimistic views in the domain of recovery, possibly due to their disproportionate contact with those with poorer outcomes [32]. Service users commonly report lack of empathy and interest from health professionals, diagnoses being given with negative prognosis, and lack of information and involvement in decision-making [33].

'Some of the worst experiences I have had have been in psychiatric hospitals. I recognise the need to be kept safe but often I have felt that my rights and dignity have been stripped away. Being intimately searched again and again and constantly followed whilst under "close observation" just leaves me feeling singled out and perceived as little more than a nuisance ("there's to be no trouble on my shift") [ … ] I have heard many comments along the lines of "Oh, she's cut again. Why doesn't she do it properly and kill herself". (Sandra) [1], p. 94]⁴

Stigma and discrimination do not only affect persons suffering from mental illness, but also families [34–36]. The effect of negative attitudes towards the family members of people with mental illness has been described as 'stigma by association' and may lead to

experiences of direct discrimination, as well as feelings of shame and self-blame [1]. In societies where the cohesion of family networks is strong, the impact of stigma by association may be severe and can include economic consequences, as well as impact on work or marital prospects [37].

## Contextual factors relevant to stigma and discrimination

The manifestations of stigma and discrimination are subject to the influence of a range of cultural and contextual factors [38]. Key domains through which culture shapes the manifestations of stigma include: (1) notions of 'mental illness' and explanatory models (for example, in many settings, psychiatric symptoms may not be seen as indicative of an 'illness'); (2) cultural meanings of the impairments and manifestations caused by the disorder and its stigma (for example, the impact of stigma on marital prospects may have more severe implications in cultural contexts where marriage is central); and (3) notions of self and personhood (for example, higher levels of family cohesion may offer more support but also go along with a more widespread impact of stigma across family members and generations).

Also socio-economic factors, such as poverty and access to health care, determine the context in which stigma is enacted and experienced [7, 9, 39, 40]. In low- and middle-income countries (LMICs) and other settings where most people with mental illness do not have access to social welfare benefits, the negative economic consequences of stigma, for example, through discrimination in work, may be so severe as to threaten the economic survival of entire families [41].

## Global patterns of stigma and discrimination

There are few studies comparing the frequency of experiences of stigma and discrimination in different contexts, and recent research has sought to address this gap in the literature. International surveys of experienced and anticipated discrimination among people with schizophrenia (27 countries) and among people with depression (39 countries), for example, found rates of both outcomes to be consistently high across cultures [5, 7, 8]. Significant between-country variation was found for experienced discrimination, but not for anticipated discrimination reported by people with schizophrenia [7]. A report on the qualitative data collected as part of the same study, however, found few transnational differences [6]. Another study looking at public attitudes across 16 countries identified a 'backbone' of certain prejudices that were held across all settings, even where overall stigma was relatively low [42].

On the other hand, some smaller studies suggest stark differences between high-income country (HIC) and LMIC settings, for example, studies from China [43] and India [41], with rates of experienced discrimination much lower than those commonly reported from HIC studies, and qualitative differences in the meaning and appraisal of the experiences made. At first sight, this appears to support the findings of early cross-cultural research on stigma, suggesting that the stigma of mental illness may be less marked in non-industrialized societies due to a more supportive environment with more social cohesion, and

---

² Reproduced from Thornicroft G, *Shunned: Discrimination against people with mental illness*, p. 87, Copyright (2006), with permission from Oxford University Press.

³ Reproduced from Thornicroft G, *Shunned: Discrimination against people with mental illness*, p. 2, Copyright (2006), with permission from Oxford University Press.

⁴ Reproduced from Thornicroft G, *Shunned: Discrimination against people with mental illness*, p. 94, Copyright (2006), with permission from Oxford University Press.

therefore less risk of prolonged rejection, isolation, segregation, and institutionalization [44, 45; 46, 47 cited in 48]. The better prognosis of schizophrenia found in international studies by the World Health Organization (WHO) [49–52] has therefore commonly been attributed to less stigmatization in LMICs [53].

Yet, in contradiction to this, there is now a considerable body of evidence documenting that in many LMIC settings, experiences of stigma, discrimination, and human rights abuses due to mental illness are common and severe [5, 11, 27, 37, 54–62]. One international study using population-wide data from 16 countries found even higher rates of reported stigma among people with mental disorders in developing (31.2%) than in developed (20%) countries [55].

In conclusion, our understanding of global patterns of stigma and discrimination is still rather limited to date, and further high-quality cross-cultural research is needed to throw light on the forces that drive intercultural differences in the manifestation of stigma. Understanding the factors that shape stigma distinctly in different contexts will serve to inform the development of context-specific anti-stigma interventions.

## How to measure stigma

Alongside the development of research into stigma, the creation and validation of instruments to measure stigma and discrimination took their beginnings in the 1960s. Early scales focused largely on the measurement of stigmatizing attitudes among the general population. Since, numerous scales have been developed, incorporating a wider range of perspectives on stigma and discrimination, notably the inclusion of the perspectives and experiences of service users and carers [63]. Nevertheless, there continues to be a distinct lack of measures developed or validated in LMIC settings and/or non-Western cultures [64]. Several methods have been put forward which seek to achieve cultural validity of measures of stigma and discrimination, including an approach by Yang *et al.* which proposes to focus on 'what matters most' in a given culture [65, 66]. A recent review concluded that future efforts in the domain of measuring stigma and discrimination should focus on: (i) procedures for achieving cultural validity of measurement tools, (ii) indicators for structural stigma and stigmatizing behaviour (underrepresented in current scales), and (iii) targeted or tailored measures for specific subgroups, all with a particular focus on LMIC countries where literature is sparse [63]. This is important as the appropriate measurement of stigma and discrimination is critical to understanding whether and how anti-stigma interventions are effective [63].

## How to tackle stigma

The critical question to tackle stigma in mental health is: what interventions work? In the past years, research on anti-stigma interventions to change knowledge, attitudes, and behaviour towards people with mental illness has increased. Most interventions aim at changing one or several of these aspects through education, social contact, or behavioural interventions.

A recent narrative review concluded with the following main findings on the evidence of anti-stigma interventions [64]:

(1) 'at the population level there is a fairly consistent pattern of short-term benefits for positive attitude change, and some lesser evidence for knowledge improvement;

(2) for people with mental illness, some group-level anti-stigma inventions show promise and merit further assessment;

(3) for specific target groups, such as students, social-contact-based interventions usually achieve short-term (but less clearly long-term) attitudinal improvements, and less often produce knowledge gains;

(4) this is a heterogeneous field of study with few strong study designs with large sample sizes;

(5) research from low-income and middle-income countries is conspicuous by its relative absence;

(6) caution needs to be exercised in not overgeneralising lessons from one target group to another;

(7) there is a clear need for studies with longer-term follow-up to assess whether initial gains are sustained or attenuated, and whether booster doses of the intervention are needed to maintain progress;

(8) few studies in any part of the world have focused on either the service user's perspective of stigma and discrimination or on the behaviour domain of behavioural change, either by people with or without mental illness in the complex processes of stigmatisation.'[5]

It has been found that generally the effectiveness of the interventions depends much on the target group and the time frame of the intervention. However, most studies are short-term effectiveness studies looking at attitudes of the general public towards people with mental disorders in HICs. The most widely evaluated interventions are education/information and social contact [63].

Overall there remains a large knowledge gap for medium- to long-term anti-stigma interventions, and particularly for interventions in low-income countries where evidence is almost absent [63]. There is also a need for: (i) more high-quality interventions based on robust methods and validated measures, (ii) more systematic reviews on long-term effectiveness, (iii) more randomized controlled trials, and (iv) more evidence from LMICs [67].

## Social contact-based interventions

Interventions using social contact as a key element have been found to be the most effective type of interventions [68]. At the same time, social contact is also the best evidence-based intervention, particularly in short-term outcomes. Evidence from systematic reviews suggests that social contact is the most effective intervention in terms of achieving short-term improvements in knowledge and attitudes among adults.

An account by a young man who participated in the German school project 'Crazy? So what!':

'Eight years ago I became ill: I developed schizophrenia [ … ]. I've been feeling better now for two years. But I do have to take good care of myself. But hiding because of that? These times are over. I finally want to live now! Talking to the students is exhausting but also really great [ … ] they discover that there are a lot more commonalities than differences between us, that their images of the 'crazy ones' are

---

[5] Reproduced from *The Lancet*, 387(10023), Thornicroft G, Mehta N, Clement S, *et al.*, Evidence for effective interventions to reduce mental-health-related stigma and discrimination, pp. 1123–1132, Copyright (2015), with permission from Elsevier.

not true. It feels really good to contribute to achieving that we finally can talk openly about mental illness, and that nobody has to hide because of a mental health problem.' [69][6]

Social contact is the most effective type of intervention in the short term, but it is not clear whether effectiveness is sustained in the medium to longer term [67]. While social contact has been reported to be the most effective intervention in adults, these evaluations are mostly based on intervention studies from HICs. There is a great need for more evidence from LMICs to assess whether social contact is as effective there and how to implement it to suit local requirements. In addition, more research is needed to investigate the long-term effectiveness of social contact interventions.

## Educational interventions

'The [ … ] practical way to stop stigma and discrimination is by better education of schoolchildren at an early age and to reinforce this message through lifelong learning. Each course or class should not only start with "household" messages about fire escapes, etc., but that bullying or discrimination will not be tolerated whilst on the course.' (Paul) [1]

(Thornicroft, 2006)

While direct social contact interventions have been found to be the most effective intervention in adults, systematic reviews have found that in students, educational interventions are more effective in reducing stigma in students' knowledge and attitudes in the short term. However, the evidence base for effectiveness in the medium to longer term is weak [64]. A meta-analysis found both social contact as well as educational interventions reduce stigma significantly and, importantly, irrespectively if these interventions are delivered face-to-face or via Internet programmes [70]. Moreover, Thornicroft et al. have found evidence that education and information seem to be the most effective interventions in the medium and long terms [64]. Evaluations in HICs have found that stigma and discrimination against people with mental illness can be reduced through focused, long-term information campaigns like Time to Change in the United Kingdom (UK) [71]. High-quality effectiveness evaluations for educational interventions are scarce for LMICs. Several national and regional campaigns from LMICs report qualitative changes in attitudes and behaviour; however, these effects lack high-quality evaluation for quantitative efficiency [72].

## Behavioural domain

Overall the effect of behavioural therapy and psychotherapy has not been sufficiently researched. In persons with mental illness, psychoeducational therapy, including elements of cognitive behavioural therapy (CBT), seem to be effective in reducing self-stigma

[73]. Yet, CBT has been found not to be effective in reducing stigma in other groups.

For medium- or long-term outcomes, systematic reviews have found there was not sufficient research to believe psychotherapy or entertainment/arts interventions can help to reduce stigma [64].

## Conclusions

From this discussion, the authors draw the following conclusions. Stigma and discrimination appear to be universal in their presence and impact, although there are clear local and regional variations in their content and manifestations. Lay stigma by the general public constitutes a powerful force for social exclusion, and in addition there is also strong evidence that stigma among health-care professionals is a powerful barrier to the mental and physical health care needed by people with mental illness. There is now increasingly strong evidence that personal and social contact methods, including filmed/virtual contact, is the most strongly evidence-based method to reduce stigma and discrimination. This evidence is now accumulating at inter-personal, organizational, and national levels. But as yet, there are few longer-term studies to know if such gains are sustainable in the long term. Nearly all the research evidence is from HICs, with a distinct evidence gap from LMICs. For the future, it is clear that service users are the central pioneers/key active ingredients in anti-stigma programmes and that interventions specifically locally and culturally adapted for use in LMICs are a pressing priority.

## REFERENCES

1. Thornicroft, G. (2006). *Shunned: discrimination against people with mental illness*. Oxford University Press, New York, NY.
2. Corrigan, P.W. (2005). *On the stigma of mental illness: practical strategies for research and social change*. American Psychological Association, Washington, D.C.
3. Yang, L., Cho, S.H., and Kleinman, A. (2010). Stigma of mental illness. In: Patel, V., Woodward, A., Feigin, V., Quah S.R., Heggenhougen, K. (eds.) *Mental and neurological public health: a global perspective*. Elsevier, San Diego, CA. pp. 219–30.
4. Thornicroft, G. (2011). Physical health disparities and mental illness: the scandal of premature mortality. *British Journal of Psychiatry*, 199, 441–2.
5. Lasalvia, A., Zoppei, S., Van Bortel, T., et al. (2013). Global pattern of experienced and anticipated discrimination reported by people with major depressive disorder: a cross-sectional survey. *The Lancet*, 381, 55–62.
6. Rose, D., Willis, R., Brohan, E., et al. 2011. Reported stigma and discrimination by people with a diagnosis of schizophrenia. *Epidemiology and Psychiatric Sciences*, 20, 193–204.
7. Thornicroft, G., Brohan, E., Rose, D., Sartorius, N., and Leese, M.; INDIGO Study Group. (2009). Global pattern of experienced and anticipated discrimination against people with schizophrenia: a cross-sectional survey. *The Lancet*, 373, 408–15.
8. Ucok, A., Brohan, E., Rose, D., et al. (2012). Anticipated discrimination among people with schizophrenia. *Acta Psychiatrica Scandinavica*, 125, 77–83.
9. Livingston, J.D. and Boyd J.E. (2010). Correlates and consequences of internalized stigma for people living with mental illness: a systematic review and meta-analysis. *Social Science and Medicine*, 71, 2150–61.

---

[6] Reproduced from *Informationsbroschuere; (Information brochure), Stark, wenn sich einer traut ueber seelische Probleme zu reden! Verrueckt? Na und! Das Schulprojekt von Irrsinnig Menschlich e.V.; (Cool when someone dares to speak about mental health problems! Crazy? So what! The School Project of the Association Irrsinnig Menschlich e.V.*, Copyright (2002), with permission from Irrsinnig Menschlich e.V.

10. Ritsher, J.B., Otilingam, P.G., and Grajales, M. (2003). Internalized stigma of mental illness: psychometric properties of a new measure. *Psychiatry Research*, 121, 31–49.

11. Sorsdahl, K.R., Kakuma, R., Wilson, Z., and Stein, D.J. (2012). The internalized stigma experienced by members of a mental health advocacy group in South Africa. *International Journal of Social Psychiatry*, 58, 55–61.

12. Fung, K.M., Tsang, H.W., Corrigan, P.W., Lam, C.S., and Cheung, W.M. (2007). Measuring self-stigma of mental illness in China and its implications for recovery. *International Journal of Social Psychiatry*, 53, 408–18.

13. Ritsher, J.B. and Phelan, J.C. (2004). Internalized stigma predicts erosion of morale among psychiatric outpatients. *Psychiatry Research*, 129, 257–65.

14. Vauth, R., Kleim, B., Wirtz, M., and Corrigan, P.W. (2007). Self-efficacy and empowerment as outcomes of self-stigmatizing and coping in schizophrenia. *Psychiatry Research*, 150, 71–80.

15. Watson, A.C., Corrigan, P., Larson, J.E., and Sells, M. (2007). Self-stigma in people with mental illness. *Schizophrenia Bulletin*, 33, 1312–18.

16. Yanos, P.T., Roe, D., Markus, K., and Lysaker, P.H. (2008). Pathways between internalized stigma and outcomes related to recovery in schizophrenia spectrum disorders. *Psychiatric Services*, 59, 1437–42.

17. Link, B.G., Struening, E.L., Neese-Todd, S., Asmussen, S., and Phelan, J.C. (2001). Stigma as a barrier to recovery: The consequences of stigma for the self-esteem of people with mental illnesses. *Psychiatric Services*, 52, 1621–6.

18. Link, B.G., Struening, E.L., Rahav, M., Phelan, J.C., and Nuttbrock, L. (1997). On stigma and its consequences: evidence from a longitudinal study of men with dual diagnoses of mental illness and substance abuse. *Journal of Health and Social Behaviour*, 38, 177–90.

19. Lysaker, P.H., Davis, L.W., Warman, D.M., Strasburger, A., and Beattie, N. (2007). Stigma, social function and symptoms in schizophrenia and schizoaffective disorder: Associations across 6 months. *Psychiatry Research*, 149, 89–95.

20. Gallo, K.M. (1994). First person account: self-stigmatization. *Schizophrenia Bulletin*, 20, 407–10.

21. Angell, B., Cooke, A., and Kovac, K. (2005). First-person accounts of stigma. In: Corrigan, P. (ed.) *On the stigma of mental illness. Practical strategies for research and social change.* American Psychological Association, Washington, D.C. pp. 69–98.

22. Mak, W.W., Poon, C.Y., Pun, L.Y., and Cheung, S.F. (2007). Meta-analysis of stigma and mental health. *Social Science and Medicine*, 65, 245–61.

23. Sirey, J.A., Bruce, M.L., Alexopoulos, G.S., Perlick, D.A., Friedman, S.J., and Meyers, B.S. (2001). Stigma as a barrier to recovery: perceived stigma and patient-rated severity of illness as predictors of antidepressant drug adherence [see comment]. *Psychiatric Services*, 52, 1615–20.

24. Link, B.G. and Phelan, J.C. (2001). On stigma and its public health implications. Paper presented at *Stigma and Global Health: Developing a Research Agenda*, 5–7 September, 2001. Bethesda, MD.

25. Corrigan, P.W., Markowitz, F.E., and Watson, A.C. (2004). Structural levels of mental illness stigma and discrimination. *Schizophrenia Bulletin*, 30, 481–91.

26. Hunt, P. (2006). The human right to the highest attainable standard of health: new opportunities and challenges. *Transactions of the Royal Society of Tropical Medicine and Hygiene*, 100, 603–7.

27. Drew, N., Funk, M., Tang, S., et al. (2011). Human rights violations of people with mental and psychosocial disabilities: an unresolved global crisis. *The Lancet*, 378, 1664–75.

28. Patel, V., Saraceno, B., and Kleinman, A. (2006). Beyond evidence: the moral case for international mental health. *American Journal of Psychiatry*, 163, 1312–15.

29. Clement, S., Schauman, O., Graham, T., *et al.* (2014). What is the impact of mental health-related stigma on help-seeking? A systematic review of quantitative and qualitative studies. *Psychological Medicine*, 1–17.

30. Schomerus, G. and Angermeyer, M.C. (2008). Stigma and its impact on help-seeking for mental disorders: What do we know? *Epidemiologia e Psichiatria Sociale*, 17, 31–7.

31. Minas, H. and Diatri, H. (2008). Pasung: physical restraint and confinement of the mentally ill in the community. *International Journal of Mental Health Systems*, 2, 8.

32. Thornicroft, G., Rose, D., and Mehta, N. (2010). Discrimination against people with mental illness: what can psychiatrists do? *Advances in Psychiatric Treatment*, 16, 53–9.

33. Henderson, C., Noblett, J., Parke, H., *et al.* (2014). Mental health-related stigma in health care and mental health-care settings. *The Lancet Psychiatry*, 1, 467–82.

34. Sartorius, N. (2007). Stigma and mental health. *The Lancet*, 370, 810–11.

35. Larson, J. and Corrigan, P. (2008). The stigma of families with mental illness. *Academic Psychiatry*, 32, 87–91.

36. Phelan, J.C., Bromet, E.J., and Link, B.G. (1998). Psychiatric illness and family stigma. *Schizophrenia Bulletin*, 24, 115–26.

37. Phillips, M.R., Pearson, V., Li, F., Xu, M., and Yang, L. (2002). Stigma and expressed emotion: a study of people with schizophrenia and their family members in China. *British Journal of Psychiatry*, 181, 488–93.

38. Murthy, R.S. (2002). Stigma is universal but experiences are local. *World Psychiatry*, 1, 28.

39. Switaj, P., Wciorka, J., Smolarska-Switaj, J., and Grygiel, P. (2009). Extent and predictors of stigma experienced by patients with schizophrenia. *European Psychiatry*, 24, 513–20.

40. Evans-Lacko, S., Knapp, M., Mccrone, P., Thornicroft, G., and Mojtabai, R. (2013). The mental health consequences of the recession: economic hardship and employment of people with mental health problems in 27 European countries. *PLoS One*, 8, e69792.

41. Koschorke, M., Padmavati, R., Kumar, S., *et al.* 2014. Experiences of stigma and discrimination of people with schizophrenia in India. *Social Science and Medicine*, 123, 149–59.

42. Pescosolido, B.A., Medina, T.R., Martin, J.K., and Long, J.S. (2013). The 'backbone' of stigma: identifying the global core of public prejudice associated with mental illness. *American Journal of Public Health*, 103, 853–60.

43. Chung, K. and Wong, M. (2004). Experience of stigma among Chinese mental health patients in Hong Kong. *Psychiatric Bulletin*, 28, 451–54.

44. Cooper, J. and Sartorius, N. (1977). Cultural and temporal variations in schizophrenia: a speculation on the importance of industrialization. *British Journal of Psychiatry*, 130, 50–5.

45. Waxler, N. (1979). Is outcome of schizophrenia better in non-industrial societies? The case of Sri Lanka. *Jounal of Nervous and Mental Diseases*, 167, 144–58.

46. El-Islam, E.F. (1979). A better outlook for schizophrenics living in extended families. *British Journal of Psychiatry*, 135, 343–7.

47. Askenasy, A. and Zavalloni, M. (1974). *Attitudes toward mental patients: a study across cultures.* Mouton and Co, The Hague.

48. Littlewood, R. (1998). Cultural variation in the stigmatisation of mental illness. *The Lancet*, 352, 1056–7.

49. World Health Organization. (1979). *Schizophrenia: an international follow-up study*. John Wiley and Sons, Chichester.

50. Jablensky, A., Sartorius, N., Ernberg, G., *et al.* 1992. Schizophrenia: manifestations, incidence and course in different cultures. A World Health Organization ten-country study. *Psychological Medicine Monograph Supplement*, 20, 1–97.

51. Harrison, G., Hopper, K., Craig, T., *et al.* 2001. Recovery from psychotic illness: a 15- and 25-year international follow-up study. *British Journal of Psychiatry*, 178, 506–17.

52. Hopper, K., Harrison, G., and Wanderling, J.A. (2007). An overview of course and outcome in ISoS [References]. In: Hopper, K., Harrison, G., Janca, A., and Sartorius, N. (eds.) *Recovery from schizophrenia: an international perspective. A report from the WHO Collaborative Project, the international study of schizophrenia*. Oxford University Press, New York, NY.

53. Rosen, A. (2003). What developed countries can learn from developing countries in challenging psychiatric stigma. *Australasian Psychiatry*, 11, S89–95.

54. Alonso, J., Buron, A., Rojas-Farreras, S., *et al.* (2009). Perceived stigma among individuals with common mental disorders. *Journal of Affective Disorders*, 118, 180–6.

55. Alonso, J., Buron, A., Bruffaerts, R., *et al.* 2008. Association of perceived stigma and mood and anxiety disorders: results from the World Mental Health Surveys. *Acta Psychiatrica Scandinavica*, 118, 305–14.

56. Barke, A., Nyarko, S., and Klecha, D. (2011). The stigma of mental illness in Southern Ghana: attitudes of the urban population and patients' views. *Social Psychiatry and Psychiatric Epidemiology*, 46, 1191–202.

57. Botha, U.A., Koen, L., and Niehaus, D.J. (2006). Perceptions of a South African schizophrenia population with regards to community attitudes towards their illness. *Social Psychiatry and Psychiatric Epidemiology*, 41, 619–23.

58. Lauber, C. and Rossler, W. (2007). Stigma towards people with mental illness in developing countries in Asia. *International Review of Psychiatry*, 19, 157–78.

59. Lee, S., Chiu, M.Y., Tsang, A., Chui, H., and Kleinman, A. (2006). Stigmatizing experience and structural discrimination associated with the treatment of schizophrenia in Hong Kong. *Social Science and Medicine*, 62, 1685–96.

60. Lee, S., Lee, M.T., Chiu, M.Y., and Kleinman, A. (2005). Experience of social stigma by people with schizophrenia in Hong Kong. *British Journal of Psychiatry*, 186, 153–7.

61. Murthy R.S. (2002). Stigma is universal but experiences are local. *World Psychiatry*, 1, 28.

62. Thara, R., Kamath, S., and Kumar, S. (2003). Women with schizophrenia and broken marriages--doubly disadvantaged? Part I: patient perspective. *International Journal of Social Psychiatry*, 49, 225–32.

63. Semrau, M., Evans-Lacko, S., Koschorke, M., Ashenafi, L., and Thornicroft, G. (2015). Stigma and discrimination related to mental illness in low- and middle-income countries. *Epidemiology and Psychiatric Sciences*, 24, 382–94.

64. Thornicroft, G., Mehta, N., Clement, S., *et al.* 2015. Evidence for effective interventions to reduce mental-health-related stigma and discrimination. *The Lancet*, 387, 1123–32.

65. Yang, L.H., Chen, F.P., Sia, K.J., *et al.* (2014). 'What matters most:' a cultural mechanism moderating structural vulnerability and moral experience of mental illness stigma. *Social Science and Medicine*, 103, 84–93.

66. Yang, L.H., Thornicroft, G., Alvarado, R., Vega, E., and Link, B.G. (2014). Recent advances in cross-cultural measurement in psychiatric epidemiology: utilizing 'what matters most' to identify culture-specific aspects of stigma. *International Journal of Epidemiology*, 43, 494–510.

67. Mehta, N., Clement, S., Marcus, E., *et al.* (2015). Evidence for effective interventions to reduce mental health-related stigma and discrimination in the medium and long term: systematic review. *British Journal of Psychiatry*, 207, 377–84.

68. Corrigan, P.W., Morris, S.B., Michaels, P.J., Rafacz, J.D., and Rüsch, N. (2012). Challenging the public stigma of mental illness: a meta-analysis of outcome studies. *Psychiatric Services*, 63, 963–73.

69. Irrsinig Menschlich, E.V. (2002). *'Stark, wenn sich einer traut ueber seelische Probleme zu reden!' Verrueckt? Na und! Das Schulprojekt von Irrsinnig Menschlich e.V.*; (*'Cool when someone dares to speak about mental health problems!' Crazy? So what! The School Project of the Association 'Irrsinnig Menschlich e.V.'*. Information brochure. Informationsbroschuere. Leipzig.

70. Griffiths, K.M., Carron-Arthur, B., Parsons, A., and Reid, R. (2014). Effectiveness of programs for reducing the stigma associated with mental disorders. A meta-analysis of randomized controlled trials. *World Psychiatry*, 13, 161–75.

71. Henderson, C. and Thornicroft, G. (2013). Evaluation of the Time to Change programme in England 2008–2011. *British Journal of Psychiatry*, 202, S45–8.

72. Khairy, N., Hamdi, E., Sidrak, A., *et al.* 2012. Impact of the first national campaign against the stigma of mental illness. *Egyptian Journal of Psychiatry*, 33, 35.

73. Mittal, D., Sullivan, G., Chekuri, L., Allee, E., and Corrigan, P.W. (2012). Empirical studies of self-stigma reduction strategies: a critical review of the literature. *Psychiatric Services*, 63, 974–81.

# 3

# Global mental health

*Crick Lund, Dörte Bemme, and Judy Bass*

## Introduction

Global health has been defined as 'an area for study, research and practice that places a priority on improving health and achieving equity in health for all people worldwide' [1]. In a similar vein, global mental health has emerged in recent years as a field of research, advocacy, and practice that is focused on improving the mental health of populations and reducing inequity in the global burden of mental illness. Because these challenges are multi-faceted, global mental health has been marked from its inception as a multi-disciplinary field, incorporating disciplines of psychiatry, psychology, epidemiology, health economics, anthropology, and implementation science. Although much of the work of global mental health has been focused on the needs of women and men living in low- and middle-income countries (LMICs), there is increasing awareness that many of the mental health challenges faced by populations in LMICs are also encountered in high-income countries (HICs).

Why then is it important to think about mental health in global terms? Firstly, despite the massive and growing global burden of mental illness, mental health has been neglected in global health and international development policy [2]. For example, mental health was excluded from the 2000–2015 Millenium Development Goals, and much of the focus and funding of agencies like the Global Fund and the Bill and Melinda Gates Foundation has been on communicable diseases. Secondly, emerging evidence from the WHO Atlas surveys informs us that the world's mental health resources are largely concentrated in HICs and in wealthier, largely urban settings of LMICs—in short, there is a global maldistribution of mental health resources [3]. Thirdly, human rights abuses and stigma, especially against people with severe mental illness, are global problems that pervade all cultures of the world [4]. Fourthly, there is strong emerging evidence regarding the links between the global challenge of poverty and mental health—poverty is a key social determinant of population mental health, and mental illness leads to individual and household impoverishment [5]. Finally, there are important links between mental health and many other global development challenges, including gender inequity, violence, forced migration, and climate change. As several have argued, there is no sustainable development without mental health [6].

This chapter sets out to provide an overview of the emerging and dynamic field of global mental health. It starts with a brief history

of the field, noting landmark publications and events. The chapter then introduces key areas of enquiry and action in global mental health, including epidemiology, mental health policy and services, intervention research, implementation science, humanitarian settings, qualitative research, instrument development, and economic evaluation. Finally, it concludes with reflections on critiques of the field and future directions.

## Global mental health: a brief history

The emergence of global mental health marks a departure from, but also continuity with, earlier efforts to conceptualize and address mental health problems around the world. While historical accounts have traced the evolution and proliferation of psychiatric knowledge back to antiquity, the rise of institutional care in Europe, and the spread of the psychiatric asylum to many countries during the colonial era [7], global mental health as a specific institutional and programmatic assemblage has emerged out of a more recent post-Second World War history. During this period, mental health became the subject of international public health and psychiatric epidemiology, which rendered mental disorders comparable across regions and other diseases, and allowed for mental health to become visible as a 'global' problem.

### Post-war History

Initially, after the founding of WHO in 1948, mental health promotion followed a pacifist agenda and conceived of mental health as a vehicle to further 'harmonious relationships between men' and ultimately 'world peace' [8]. WHO's initial focus was not on distinct mental illnesses, but on mental health as a positive state of well-being in the tradition of the 'mental hygiene' movement, which had advocated for the prevention of mental illness through education since the 1920s [9]. The dual goal of building harmonious 'world citizenship' and mental health education also informed the founding of the World Mental Health Federation in 1948, the first non-governmental organization (NGO) with which WHO collaborated on matters of mental health policy [10].

A stronger focus on mental disorders came about with the rise of psychiatric epidemiology in international mental health in the 1970s, which sought to assess the prevalence, distribution, and determinants of mental illness. One key challenge to the epidemiological approach was the lack of standardization in the classification and interpretation of mental disorders. While the early versions of the WHO International Classification of Diseases (ICD-6) (1948) and ICD-7 (1955) contained sections on mental illness, they were not widely accepted internationally. Comparative studies on diagnostic practice had also shown large differences in the clinical interpretation of disease categories [11]. Comparable data on mental disorders thus depended on the development of standardized instruments and classifications. In 1966, WHO initiated what would become a series of cross-cultural proof-of-concept studies on schizophrenia that demonstrated that the disorder existed around the world, that it could be measured with standardized instruments, and that it had greatly varying outcomes across developed and developing settings [12]. Greater standardization of psychiatric classification and practice was achieved through the publication of the *Diagnostic and Statistical Manual of Mental Disorders*, version 3 (DSM III) in 1980, which abandoned the psychodynamic aetiological model in favour of a symptom-based approach with no aetiological underpinning. The DSM classification subsequently increased its harmonization with WHO's ICD system, and a number of instruments were developed to facilitate the collection of comparable data, including the Present State Examination (PSE), the Schedule for Clinical Assessment in Neuropsychiatry (SCAN), and the Composite International Diagnostic Instrument (CIDI).

### Disability and disability-adjusted life years

Another important factor lending mental health increasing importance within international health was the development of disability frameworks beginning in the 1980s and leading up to the creation of a new statistical measure that combined morbidity and mortality into the assessment of the global burden of disease through the disability-adjusted life years (DALYs) measure, as part of the *World Development Report* in 1993. This marked the World Bank's increasing investment in health, based on a 'human capital' logic, and its entrance into 'Global Health' [13]. DALYs laid the foundation for the influential 'Global Burden of Disease (GBD)' studies [14], which fundamentally changed how health was measured on a global scale. For the mental health agenda, this shift towards morbidity had a significant impact as mental and neurological disorders became visible as one of the largest contributors to the GBD [15]. Subsequently, medical anthropologists, including Robert Desjarlais, Leon Eisenberg, Byron Good, and Arthur Kleinman, drew further attention to this enormous burden and formulated a call for international action on mental health in the landmark *World Mental Health Report* [16], which combined global data with local case studies. The report was launched at the United Nations in 1995, and in response, WHO initiated the *Nations for Mental Health* programme a year later, which promoted mental health service delivery for underserved populations [17]. These efforts marked a shift towards service delivery rather than pure epidemiology in international mental health.

### World Health Report 2001

The year 2001 was a significant year for global mental health when, with the support of the new WHO Director General Gro Harlem Brundtland, the World Health Day and World Health Report were dedicated in their entirety to mental health. The theme of the day 'Stop exclusion—Dare to care' speaks of this shift towards care

delivery and the human rights agenda. In conjunction, the first WHO *Mental Health Atlas* provided a global overview over the existing mental health care resources [18], marking another important step towards the quantification of the global 'treatment gap'. Parallel to these developments, the wider field of global health consolidated in the early 2000s [13] and mental health advocates sought to emulate its achievements and strategies, especially the enormous success of the HIV/AIDS advocacy movement.

## Global mental health

Global mental health as a distinct global health community and programme was officially inaugurated in 2007 when *The Lancet* published a special series on global mental health, edited by Patel and colleagues. This series documented the links between mental health and other health conditions [19], presented a systematic review of the evidence for cost-effective prevention and treatment interventions in LMICs [20], and called for the scaling up of evidence-based mental health care in LMICs [21]. The field of global mental health has since grown significantly, with the creation of a distinct assemblage of institutions and training programmes, including Masters and doctoral programmes and short courses; online networks [the Movement for Global Mental Health (MGMH) and the Mental Health Innovation Network (MHIN)]; specialty journals such as *Journal of Global Mental Health* and *International Journal of Mental Health Systems*; funding streams, for example United States National Institute of Mental Health's Office on Disparity and Global Mental Health, Grand Challenges Canada, United Kingdom's Department for International Development, European Commission, and Wellcome Trust; international agencies (in particular, the WHO Department of Mental Health and Substance Abuse); and international NGOs such as Transcultural Psychosocial Organization and BasicNeeds.

What distinguishes global mental health from earlier international mental health efforts are five particular features—firstly, the strengthened emphasis on the development of research-driven *evidence-based* interventions. Commitment to the production of evidence-based interventions favours randomized controlled trial (RCT) research designs to test innovative interventions, with the subsequent goal of implementation and scaling-up. Evidence-based practice guidelines, such as the WHO's *mhGAP Intervention Guide* that outlines the treatment of eight priority disorders [22] and the Inter-Agency Standing Committee's *Guideline for Mental Health and Psychosocial Support in Emergency Settings* [23], have thus become central tools in organizing this new field of practice.

A second distinguishing feature is the consideration of care *delivery* in low-resource settings, for example through the training and supervision of non-specialist health providers—a strategy referred to as task shifting or task sharing [24]. Global mental health pays particular attention to the modalities and limitations of service delivery in low-resource settings by using task-sharing models and simplified and adapted treatment protocols, with an increasing focus on implementation science [25].

Thirdly, global mental health is characterized by multidisciplinarity and multi-stakeholder involvement. For example, the landmark research agenda-setting article *Grand challenges in global mental health* was based on an extensive international Delphi stakeholder consultation process [26]. This commitment to multidisciplinary engagement has built a novel knowledge base, adjacent to academic psychiatry, combining the expertise of public health, psychology, health economics, development studies, anthropology, and the experience of NGOs.

Fourthly, global mental health is characterized by a strong emphasis on human rights and the need to strengthen legislation and regulatory environments to protect and promote the rights of people living with psychosocial disabilities [27]. This has been exemplified in the WHO QualityRights initiative, which has developed a tool to assess human rights protection in the provision of mental health care and campaigned for the reduction of human rights violations, particularly against people living with severe mental illness, whether in communities or in psychiatric institutions [28].

Fifthly, despite efforts to raise the profile of mental health as a specific global health priority, global mental health is working towards the *integration* of mental health into other agendas, including sustainable development, non-communicable diseases, and maternal and child health. This includes efforts towards the integration of mental health care into primary care [29]. In particular, recent global mental health advocacy and research have highlighted its links with the development agenda by demonstrating the link between mental health and poverty [30] and the economically promising 'return on investment' of mental health care [31], and by successfully advocating for the inclusion of mental health into the sustainable development goals.

In 2016, the World Bank Group and WHO hosted a high-level meeting entitled *Out of the shadows: making mental health a global development priority* in Washington DC, which was attended by over 500 delegates from the research, business, clinical, policy, and donor communities. At this meeting, the president of the World Bank Dr Jim Kim and the Director General of WHO Dr Margaret Chan committed themselves and their organizations to giving greater priority to global mental health [32].

## Epidemiology

### Global burden of mental illness

A major breakthrough in the measurement of the global burden of mental disorders came with the development of the DALY measure, first published in the 1993 World Development Report [33]. The DALY combines a measure of mortality [years of life lost (YLLs)] with a measure of morbidity [years of life lived with disability (YLDs)], to assess the burden of all diseases and injuries using the metric of time. This allows for comparison of a wide variety of conditions, from human immunodeficiency virus (HIV)/acquired immune deficiency syndrome (AIDS) to cancers and to depression, with the latest 2015 GBD study covering over 300 diseases and injuries. Further details of the assumptions and methods in the latest 2015 GBD study can be found elsewhere [34]. From a health policy perspective, this has been transformative for the field of mental health, because it has moved to the foreground the substantial contribution of mental disorders to the global burden of disease.

Data from the latest available 2015 GBD study show that the total proportion of the global burden of disease attributable to mental, neurological, and substance use disorders has increased substantially from approximately 6.5% in 1990 to over 10% in 2015. For mental and substance use disorders alone, there was a 14.9% increase between 2005 and 2015 [34]. These increases have been largely driven by demographic factors, chiefly population growth and ageing, with age-standardized DALYs per 100,000 population for mental and substance use disorders showing a 0.3% decrease between 2005 and 2015.

There are important gender differences in the burden of mental and substance use disorders, with women accounting for more DALYs in all disorders, except for childhood mental disorders, substance use disorders, epilepsy, and Parkinson's disease, which are more prevalent among boys and men. There are also important age variations, with the burden of mental, neurological, and substance use disorders peaking in young adult years (Fig. 3.1). Fig. 3.1 also visually depicts the relative contribution of specific mental and substance use disorders to the total burden of all mental and substance use disorders.

### Social determinants of mental health

Along with the growing awareness of the burden of mental illness, social epidemiology in the last 30 years has generated new knowledge on the social determinants of mental health [35]. Social determinants are a wide range of social and economic risk and protective factors that influence population mental health across the life course. These social determinants include five broad domains: demographic, social, economic, neighbourhood, and environmental events [36]. The *demographic domain* includes the effects of age, gender, and ethnicity on mental health. In addition to age and gender differences in the burden mental illness, members of minority ethnic groups have been found to have an increased risk for psychosis and depression, particularly in the context of migration or as a result of experiences of discrimination or exclusion [37]. In relation to the *social domain*, social capital, particularly cognitive social capital, has been shown to offer protection against common mental disorders such as depression and anxiety disorders [38]. Education is important for adolescent well-being, is highly protective against later-life depression, and improves cognitive reserve that may be protective against dementia [39]. In relation to the *economic domain*, there is robust evidence showing a strong association between poverty, unemployment, and adverse mental health outcomes, including common mental disorders and schizophrenia [5, 40]. The relationship between poverty and mental illness is bidirectional, characterized by social causation and social drift/selection [30, 40]. In relation to the *neighbourhood domain*, the characteristics of a local area or neighbourhood have an important bearing on population mental health, over and above the effects of individual level socio-economic deprivation [41]. Finally, *environmental events*, such as natural disasters, industrial disasters, war, civil conflict, forced migration, and the effects of climate change, have been shown to have a range of negative mental health consequences. These include post-traumatic stress disorder (PTSD), depression, and anxiety among adults [42], and emotional and behavioural disturbances, sleep difficulties, and disturbed play in children [43].

## Mental health policy and services

Given the major global burden of mental disorders and the powerful social determinants that influence the mental health of populations, what can governments and civil society do? A key area of global mental health research and advocacy since the World Health Report 2001 has been mental health policy and service development.

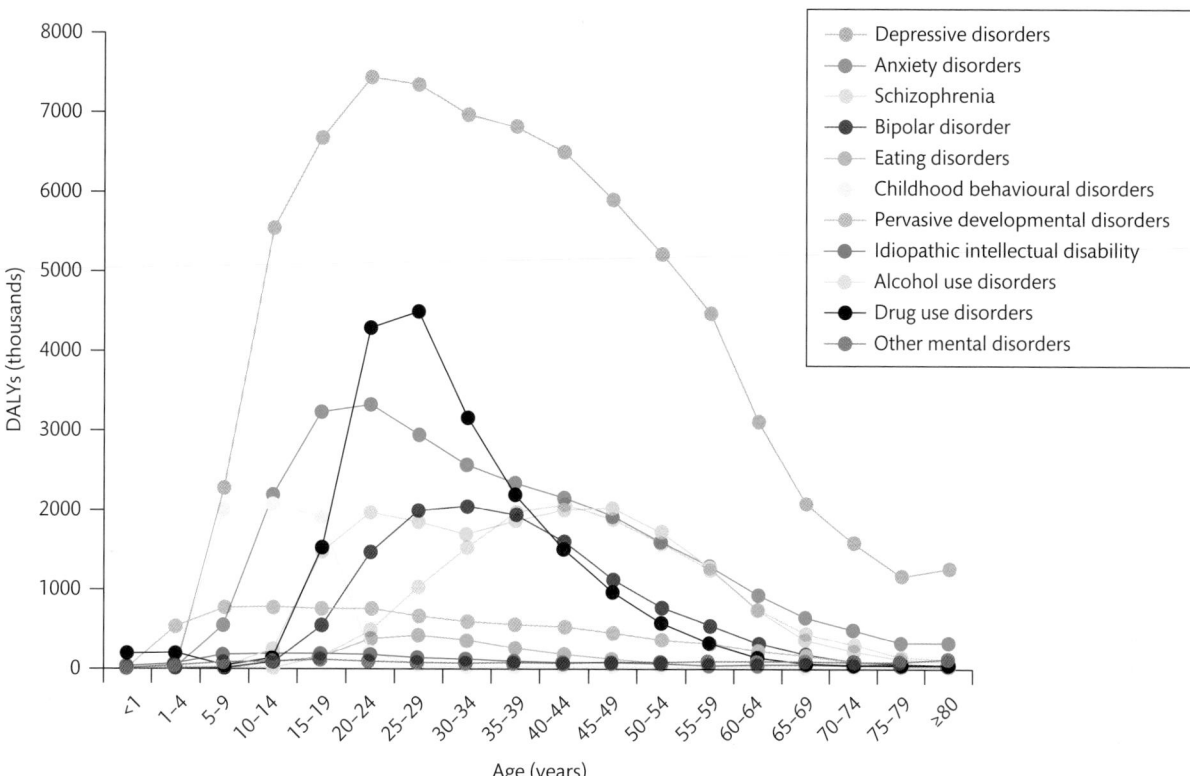

**Fig. 3.1** (see Colour Plate section) Disability-adjusted life years (DALYs) for each mental and substance use disorder in 2010, by age.
Reproduced from *The Lancet*, 382(9904), Whiteford HA, Degenhardt L, Rehm J, *et al.*, Global burden of disease attributable to mental and substance use disorders: findings from the Global Burden of Disease Study 2010, pp. 1575–86, Copyright (2013), with permission from Elsevier Ltd.

One of the major WHO recommendations from that report was that countries should develop national mental health policies and plans, and make the most efficient use of their available resources by implementing these policies and plans using cost-effective interventions. From 2001 to 2005, the WHO developed guidelines to assist countries (particularly LMICs) to develop national mental health policies, plans, and programmes. These practical step-by-step guidelines are set out in the WHO Mental Health Policy and Service Guidance Package [44]. Policies and plans are vital for several reasons—a policy provides a roadmap to guide a ministry of health and other relevant ministries; without such a policy, governments do not have a clear mandate or a mechanism to allocate much needed resources; the process of developing a national policy and plan is also an important means of developing consensus among a range of stakeholders; and a clearly articulated policy and plan with the appropriate targets and indicators can facilitate evaluation of the extent to which the mental health needs of populations are being met.

At a global level, these aspirations were subsequently developed and adopted in the WHO Global Mental Health Action Plan (2013–2020), endorsed by all United Nations member states. The objectives of this plan are to: (1) strengthen effective leadership and governance for mental health; (2) provide comprehensive, integrated, and responsive mental health and social care services in community-based settings; (3) implement strategies for promotion and prevention in mental health; and (4) strengthen information systems, evidence, and research for mental health [45].

In relation to the delivery of mental health services, the WHO has recommended an optimal mix of services, which can be depicted in a pyramid (Fig. 3.2) [46]. This emphasizes the promotion of self-care, the development of primary care and community-based services, the integration of mental health into general health care services, and the provision of a small number of specialist mental health services. Within this overall framework, the Disease Control Priorities initiative has provided a detailed review of the most cost-effective interventions, to be delivered through service platforms, targeting mental health promotion and prevention, treatment, and rehabilitation of mental, neurological, and substance use disorders [47].

## Intervention research, trials, and innovations

Much of the intervention research in LMIC settings at the beginning of the twenty-first century has focused on treatments for common mental disorders, specifically depression, anxiety, and trauma-based syndromes. This focus was, in part, due to the high prevalence of these disorders in LMIC populations, as well as a growing recognition of the large treatment gap for accessing any type of mental health services outside of urban psychiatric centres [3]. The predominant model of service provision has used task-sharing models. Evidence is growing that task sharing can be an effective strategy for providing mental health services where few mental health professionals exist [48], though Padmanathan and De Silva [49] identified important barriers to the acceptability and feasibility of task-sharing models if sufficient financial resources are not provided to support these programmes.

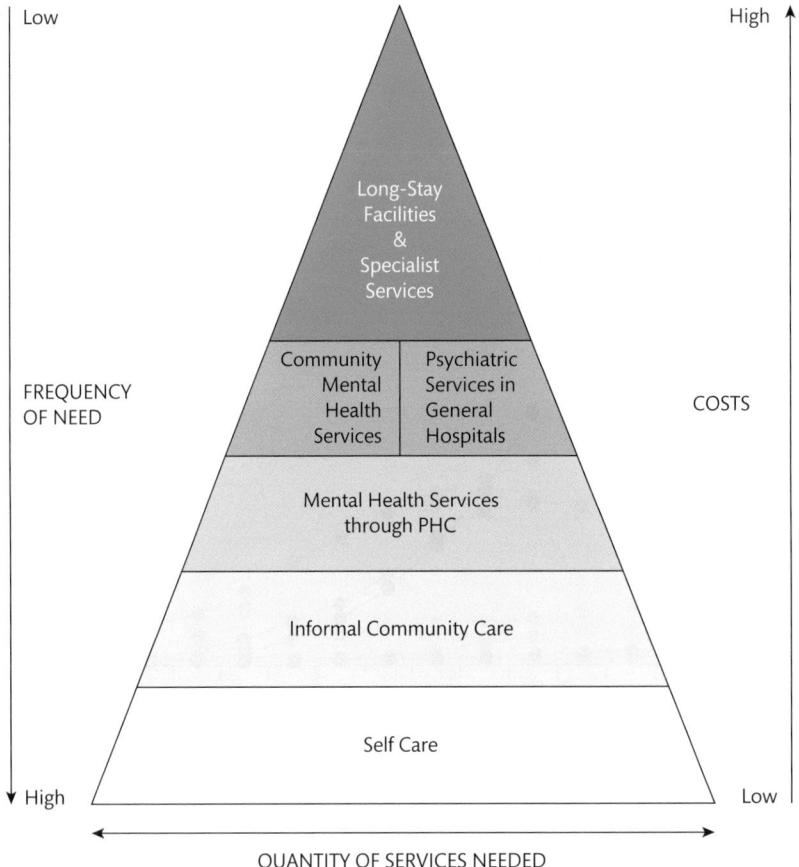

**Fig. 3.2** Optimal mix of mental health services.
Reproduced from *Mental Health Policy and Service Guidance Package*, Copyright (2003) with permission from the World Health Organisation. Available from http://www.who.int/mental_health/policy/services/essentialpackage1v2/en/

Numerous randomized trials in LMIC settings across multiple continents have demonstrated the effectiveness of evidence-based psychotherapies, including cognitive behavioural, interpersonal, and cognitive processing therapies, in reducing the burden of common mental disorders [48]. Research has also identified the utility of using these approaches to improve non-mental health outcomes among high-risk populations, with a growing evidence base of the feasibility and impact of treating mental health problems among HIV-infected populations on HIV treatment adherence [50].

Building on task-sharing approaches, intervention research in LMIC settings has also investigated collaborative care and stepped care models, which integrate task-sharing treatment into primary care systems [51].

An area of current innovation in intervention research is the development of cross-diagnostic and trans-diagnostic treatment models. These models are designed to treat multiple common disorders, rather than being disorder-specific (for example, treatments for depression alone). This is an important consideration, as disorder comorbidity is common and being able to train providers in a single treatment, rather than different treatments for each disorder, can improve treatment fidelity, coverage, and quality, particularly for lay providers. Some of these approaches, such as Problem Management Plus (PM+), have a unified treatment protocol that can be applied to individuals with a range of common mental health problems [52].

Current evidence for PM+ indicates that it is acceptable and feasible to implement [53]; impact results are forthcoming. An alternative to a unified treatment approach is the model developed by Murray and colleagues—Common Elements Treatment Approach (CETA)—that includes a set of treatment components that can be delivered in varying combinations to address a range of common mental health problems and comorbidities that present within a population [54]. Two randomized trials of CETA have shown that this model is acceptable, feasible, and effective for reducing the burden of common mental health problems, such as depression, anxiety, and post-traumatic stress, in LMIC populations [55, 56].

## Implementation science

A critical finding from existing global implementation research is that, regardless of positive reports of acceptability and feasibility by providers and consumers, evidence-based mental health programming is still not being scaled up or sustained [57]. The field of implementation science is needed to provide evidence for how these interventions can be effectively integrated and sustained into existing care systems through identifying and addressing barriers at the organizational and policy levels that are impeding implementation efforts.

In LMICs, like in many HICs, a range of organizations provide mental health services, including hospitals and primary care clinics, NGOs, educational settings, and social service agencies. Primary care settings provide an important opportunity for integrating mental health care with care for other health conditions under a single system. One large research project that has investigated the integrating and scaling up of mental health care packages in primary and maternal health care contexts in five LMIC settings is the Programme for Improving Mental Health Care (PRIME) study [58]. One of the first steps taken in PRIME was to develop and implement district-level mental health care integration plans in all five country sites at four service levels: health service organization, specialist mental health services, primary care facilities, and the community [59]. While the integration goals, to improve quality and access to mental health services, were common across sites, the system approaches required to achieve these goals were variable, for example in the types of providers used to deliver mental health care (lay and community providers vs more highly qualified and specialist mental health workers). The identified variations mean that different systems approaches will be needed to ensure quality mental health services are provided and sustained over time.

While primary care settings are important for integrating mental health care with other health conditions, for many LMIC populations, accessing mental health services in primary health care settings is neither feasible (because of stigma or logistical barriers) nor preferred (because mental health problems may not be considered to be in the domain of what doctors or health providers treat). NGOs and community-based organizations (CBOs) frequently are direct providers of mental health services, with some at the forefront of investigating how to scale up services through non-health care systems. One example is the international NGO Strong Minds which has been working to scale up interpersonal psychotherapy (IPT), an evidence-based treatment for depression in Uganda [60], through local organizations and community groups [61].

In addition, it is recognized that the health sector often needs to interact with other sectors to improve mental health outcomes—what the WHO defines as 'intersectoral action for health' [62]. A qualitative study in South Africa that investigated the challenges and possibilities for intersectoral care for mental health services noted several challenges in this regard, including the lack of systematic strategies for delineating care roles and the lack of communication and referral systems. These limited the success of the multi-system strategies of care, despite the recognition among stakeholders that providing care across multiple systems is necessary [63].

## Qualitative research

Global mental health's emphasis on multi-stakeholder engagement and the recognition that mental health interventions and instruments need to be culturally and linguistically adapted have made qualitative research an important aspect of piloting, implementing, and evaluating mental health interventions. *Ethnographic approaches* have had a strong influence on global mental health, largely due to the anthropologist Arthur Kleinman's seminal work on the expression of mental distress and somatization in China and Asia [64]. While such long-term, in-depth ethnographic engagement is rare nowadays, global mental health draws extensively on qualitative

health research to tailor interventions and research tools to local contexts and to ensure linguistic and cultural appropriateness [65]. A large body of literature has emerged on '*local idioms of distress*' [66] describing local concepts for mental suffering such as 'heart–mind' problems in Nepal [67] and 'thinking too much' in Haiti ('Reflechi twop') [68] and Zimbabwe ('Kufungisisa') [69], which are similar, but not identical, to the category of 'depression'.

Another area in which qualitative research has been integrated into the design of global mental health interventions are studies investigating the *acceptability and feasibility* of mental health interventions or barriers to their implementation within specific populations. For example, task-sharing approaches have been assessed through qualitative research in a great number of contexts [70], while other research has explored the barriers to collaboration with traditional healers [71].

Qualitative research has also become increasingly important for *implementation science* [25]. Multi-country consortia like PRIME routinely collect qualitative interview data on the implementation process of their interventions to assess health system bottlenecks, as well as service user and stakeholder perceptions of the service. Qualitative case studies have also been identified as an important tool for *evaluation*, as they allow for the documentation and dissemination of the specific lessons that are learnt on the ground, including processes of delivering interventions [72].

## Instrument development

In the measurement of mental health problems globally, it is important to consider the validity, reliability, and utility of measurement tools. In general, a valid instrument is one that measures the construct it is intended to measure and a reliable instrument is one that can consistently measure the construct of interest over time (test–retest reliability) and ensure that this consistency does not vary, based on who administers the instrument (inter-rater reliability). Utility refers to how practical and useful the instrument is for a given problem in a given context.

The development of valid and reliable tools to assess mental health problems across different cultures and contexts has been an area of research for some time. One reason for the importance of focusing on instrument development is that the nature and meaning of mental health symptoms can differ by culture and context [73]. For example, in a review of the qualitative literature on the expression of depression globally, Haroz and colleagues found that many symptoms of depression in non-Western populations are not captured in standard measurement tools based on Western diagnostic criteria and that some of the symptoms that frequently appear in standard depression measures, such as psychomotor agitation or slowing, were infrequently mentioned in non-Western populations [74].

To reconcile local characterization of mental health problems with the desire to use standard instruments that can allow for cross-population comparisons, researchers are now using mixed methods approaches that include qualitative methods to identify symptoms relevant to local populations. For example, Wilk and Bolton's qualitative study of depressive disorders among HIV-affected Ugandan adults found many of the standard symptoms related to depressive disorders, while also identifying symptoms such as 'hating the world', 'bad, criminal or reckless behavior', and 'unappreciative of assistance' as relevant manifestations of locally defined depression [75]. These locally relevant symptoms were added to an existing depression measure to create a more locally valid measure that could still be used to compare the burden of illness with other populations [76]. Similar methods have been used, for example, to develop valid and reliable measures of post-partum depression among women in the Democratic Republic of Congo [77], post-traumatic stress problems among youth in Zambia [78], and disruptive behaviour problems among youth in Nepal [79].

While global mental health researchers have increasingly focused on improving reliability and validity of mental health instruments across contexts, developing tools that are practical and useful for screening and ongoing treatment monitoring and evaluation has been more difficult. And as mental health services are integrated in other care systems and scaled up for delivery, having useful measures becomes increasingly important. In considering utility, two important factors are the length of the measure and the usefulness of individual items to assess different mental disorders, as well as the severity of the disorders. One analytic approach that is currently being used to generate useful measures is item response theory (IRT). IRT is a type of latent variable modelling approach that models the probability of a given response as a function of a respondent's underlying level of a latent trait. IRT can help to refine scales by identifying well-performing items at varying levels of a latent trait, assisting in shortening of a scale for screening or monitoring purposes, preventing floor and ceiling effects [80], and identifying where, along a latent trait, a scale is underperforming and additional items are needed in order to better assess individuals with those levels [81]. Tang and colleagues have used this approach to develop a brief depression measure for older adults in Hong Kong [82], and Haroz and colleagues have used IRT analyses to develop a depression measure that more accurately captures the presentation of depression across cultures [83].

## Economic evaluation

Given the severely resource-constrained environment facing mental health systems in most countries, particularly LMICs, it is vital that the available resources are used efficiently. Policymakers face several difficult economic questions in relation to mental health care, namely: (1) what goods and services should a health system produce—for example, should these provide care for infectious diseases, non-communicable diseases, or mental health, and how should these priorities be set?; (2) what is the most efficient and effective way of delivering mental health interventions (for example, through community-based care, primary care services, or hospitals), and who should the key delivery agents be?; and (3) which population groups should be given special attention, for example women, children, older adults, or the economically vulnerable?

A key area of enquiry in global mental health is therefore the economic evaluation of mental health interventions. Economic evaluation has been defined as 'the comparative analysis of alternative courses of action in terms of both their cost and consequences' [84]. Economic evaluations are essential to assist policymakers to set priorities among competing health needs [85]. One of the major concerns of economic evaluation is the relationship between allocated inputs (resources) and outcomes (health benefits). An intervention

is considered technically inefficient if the same, or a greater, health benefit could be obtained with less resources.

The three major methods of conducting economic evaluations are cost-effectiveness analysis, cost–utility analysis, and cost–benefit analysis. All three methods are interested in measuring costs but differ in their measurement of outcomes. In the case of cost-effectiveness analysis, the outcome is measured in the appropriate (usually clinical) measure to assess the effect of the intervention, for example reduction in clinical symptoms or improvement in functioning. In the case of cost–utility analysis, the outcome is measured using a standardized comparable measure of utility such as a combination of life years with the quality of life [quality-adjusted life years (QALYs)] or DALYs, allowing for comparison of the health impacts across a range of interventions and health conditions. In the case of a cost–benefit analysis, the outcome is measured in monetary terms. This latter approach allows policymakers to assess the economic gains from a particular set of service costs or the return on investment.

Some examples of economic evaluations in global mental health research have been Patel and colleagues' cost-effectiveness analysis of primary care for common mental disorders in Goa in India [86] and a task-shifting cognitive behavioural therapy delivered by paraprofessionals for alcohol use in Kenya [87].

In a recent publication, to coincide with the historic World Bank/WHO 'Out of the Shadows' meeting in April 2016, Dan Chisholm and colleagues conducted a global return-on-investment analysis for scaling up care for depression and anxiety disorders between 2015 and 2030. They estimated that for every dollar invested, there would be a $2.3 to $3 return on investment when economic benefits alone were considered, and a $3.3 to $5.7 return on investment when the value of health returns were also included [31].

## Gaps in the field and critiques

In the years following *The Lancet* series on global mental health in 2007, the field attracted some critical attention from transcultural psychiatrists and social scientists who questioned the agenda of this emerging field. These criticisms have focused on a number of key issues.

*Weak evidence.* Critics have drawn attention to the long-standing controversies surrounding the DSM classification system, especially the cross-cultural validity of psychiatric disease models and the efficacy of psychotropic drugs that Western psychiatry promotes [88]. These critics have argued that the evidence base of psychiatry is too weak to be exported to low-resource settings. Existing evidence, they argued, has been predominantly collected in HICs and may not be applicable to other communities. Instead, local idioms of distress and cultural systems of healing should be included in the evidence base and outcome measures of global mental health [89]. Furthermore, scholars have argued that the production of evidence itself is an uneven playing field because RCTs are costly and complex, and require a high degree of technical expertise, which excludes poor countries from the production of formalized evidence [90].

*Too medical.* Global mental health's focus on evidence-based interventions led some scholars to caution that the distribution of medication may, in practice, be prioritized over the development of complex and context-sensitive psychosocial interventions [89].

*Too individualized.* Other scholars critiqued that the Western psychiatric disease model only focuses on the individual, based on the assumption of an underlying, universal brain disorder [91]. Instead, they argued human emotions and behaviour cannot be understood without social context and a meaningful engagement of the community [92] and more attention should be paid to the social determinants of mental health [93].

*Social determinants of health.* Some have argued that the root causes of mental suffering, such as poverty, structural violence, and globalization [93], need to be addressed by tackling the upstream structural determinants of mental health, such as poverty and violence, rather than dedicating most resources to narrower downstream interventions such as mental health treatments [94].

*Limitations of economic arguments for investing in mental health care.* The economic argument for mental health care has also been challenged for its potential to undermine calls for care, based on equity, justice, and the right to social participation [95]. A sole focus on 'return on investment' may prioritize the treatment of common mental disorders at the expense of severe spectrum disorders, which require more care and resources [94].

*Neo-colonial.* Some scholars have gone so far as to describe global mental health as a neo-colonial imposition of Western psychiatric knowledge onto populations in LMICs, driven by the pharmaceutical industry, powerful international institutions, and Western psychiatry [96]. Such an imposition of the biomedical model, they argue, risks the replacement of religious, spiritual, and communal systems of meaning, which may themselves be protective for mental health and offer effective strategies of care [91].

*Insufficient attention to substance abuse.* Much of the focus of global mental health innovations has been on mental illness, and substance abuse has been relatively neglected, despite the evidence for the major burden associated with substance use disorders and cost-effectiveness interventions.

*Critique of the critique.* In the aftermath of some of these vociferous critiques, a set of counter-arguments have emerged, including an analysis of the assumptions underlying the polarized debates between 'global' vs 'local' conceptions of mental health and highlighting the need and potential avenues of integrating both perspectives [97].

Although the above critiques present an important challenge to the field of global mental health, many who work in the field are acutely aware of these issues. For example, the issue of cross-cultural validity is an ongoing challenge and many of the leaders in global mental health have focused their research attention on trying to understand local idioms of distress and develop culturally valid and reliable instruments [69]. Similarly, global mental health as a field has focused a good deal of its attention on understanding the social determinants of mental health and developing interventions that can address these determinants [30].

## Future directions

As a young, rapidly expanding, and dynamic field, global mental health can be said to have 'come of age' [98]. Nevertheless, many challenges remain. In addition to the above critiques, there are ongoing challenges of inadequate policy priority and resources for mental health, particularly in LMICs. There is also a challenging geopolitical environment, with rising income inequality, ongoing violence, and forced migration in the Middle East and sub-Saharan Africa, and the growing reality of climate change—all of which carry major implications for global mental health.

These challenges require the field of global mental health to expand its focus from the earlier calls to scale up mental health care [21] towards interventions that promote population mental heath and prevent mental illness. Given the powerful effects of the social determinants of mental health, it is unlikely that the global burden of mental disorders can be addressed through treatment alone. This requires a more refined understanding of the mechanisms of the social determinants of mental health, for example through larger longitudinal studies, particularly in LMICs. It also requires a greater integration of mental health and well-being into the broader sustainable development agenda of 2015–2030 [6].

The field also requires a greater convergence of approaches, bringing together the fields of genetics and epigenetics with those of social epidemiology and anthropology, to gain a greater understanding of gene–environment interactions and opportunities for interventions across the life course. This implies the need for a more nuanced understanding of the local and the global, and which interventions work for whom, under what circumstances. In this process, greater partnerships are required between people with lived experience of mental illness, their families, clinicians, and researchers.

Finally, the field needs to move away from categorical classifications of mental disorders towards a more dimensional understanding of mental health, on a continuum from disability to well-being. This requires a staged approach to detection and treatment using trans-diagnostic intervention models, with health systems having the capacity to detect problems early and provide care and support in an empowering and collaborative manner. These challenges remain compelling and have managed to galvanize a significant level of international collaboration, funding, and advocacy, to constitute global mental health as a vibrant, dynamic, and growing field.

## REFERENCES

1. Koplan, J.P., Bond, T.C., Merson, M.H., *et al.*; Consortium of Universities for Global Health Executive Board. (2009). Towards a common definition of global health. *The Lancet*, 373, 1993–5.
2. Tomlinson, M. and Lund, C. (2012). Why does mental health not get the attention it deserves? An application of the Shiffman and Smith Framework. *PLoS Medicine*, 9, e1001178.
3. World Health Organization. (2015). *Mental Health Atlas 2014*. World Health Organization, Geneva.
4. Thornicroft, G. (2006). *Shunned: Discrimination against people with mental illness*. Oxford University Press, Oxford.
5. Lund, C., Breen, A., Flisher, A.J., *et al.* (2010). Poverty and common mental disorders in low and middle income countries: a systematic review. *Social Science and Medicine*, 71, 517–28.
6. Thornicroft, G. and Votruba, N. (2016). Does the United Nations care about mental health? *The Lancet Psychiatry*, 3, 599–600.
7. Cohen, A., Patel, V., Minas, H. (2014). A brief history of global mental health. In: Patel, V., Minas, H., Cohen, A., and Prince, M.J. (eds.). *Global mental health: principles and practice*. Oxford University Press, Oxford. pp. 3–26.
8. Lovell, A.M. (2014). The World Health Organization and the contested beginnings of psychiatric epidemiology as an internationaldiscipline: one rope, many strands. *International Journal of Epidemiology*, 43, 16–18.

9. Okpaku, S.O. and Biswas, S. (2014). History of global mental health. *Essentials of Global Mental Health*, 1–10.

10. Brody, E.B. (2004). The World Federation for Mental Health: its origins and contemporary relevance to WHO and WPA policies. *World Psychiatry*, 3, 54–5.

11. Cooper, J.E. (1972). *Psychiatric diagnosis in New York and London: a comparative study of mental hospital admissions.* Oxford University Press, Oxford.

12. Padma, T. (2014). Developing countries: the outcomes paradox. *Nature*, 508, S14–15.

13. Brown, T.M., Cueto, M., and Fee, E. (2006). The World Health Organization and the transition from 'international' to 'global' public health. *American Journal of Public Health*, 96, 62–72.

14. Murray, C.J., Lopez, A.D., World Health Organization, World Bank, and Harvard School of Public Health. (1996). *The global burden of disease: a comprehensive assessment of mortality and disability from diseases, injuries, and risk factors in 1990 and projected to 2020: summary.* http://www.who.int/iris/handle/10665/41864

15. Whiteford, H.A., Degenhardt, L., Rehm, J., *et al.* 2013. Global burden of disease attributable to mental and substance use disorders: findings from the Global Burden of Disease Study 2010. *The Lancet*, 382, 1575–86.

16. Desjarlais, R., Eisenberg, L., Good, B., and Kleinman, A. (eds.). (1995). *World mental health: problems and priorities in low-income countries*: Oxford University Press, New York, NY.

17. Jenkins, R. (1997). Nations for mental health. *Social Psychiatry and Psychiatric Epidemiology*, 32, 309–11.

18. World Health Organization. (2001). *Atlas of mental health resources in the world 2001.* World Health Organization, Geneva.

19. Prince, M., Patel, V., Saxena, S., *et al.* (2007). No health without mental health. *The Lancet*, 370, 859–77.

20. Patel, V., Araya, R., Chatterjee, S., *et al.* (2007). Treatment and prevention of mental disorders in low-income and middle-income countries. *The Lancet*, 370, 991–1005.

21. Lancet Global Mental Health Group. (2007). Scale up services for mental disorders: a call for action. *The Lancet*, 370, 1241–52.

22. World Health Organization. (2010). *mhGAP intervention guide for mental, neurological and substance use disorders in non-specialized health settings: mental health Gap Action Programme (mhGAP).* World Health Organization, Geneva.

23. Inter-Agency Standing Committee (IASC) (2007). *IASC guidelines on mental health and psychosocial support in emergency settings.* IASC, Geneva.

24. Kakuma, R., Minas, H., Van Ginneken, N., *et al.* (2011). Human resources for mental health care: current situation and strategies for action. *The Lancet*, 378, 1654–63.

25. De Silva, M.J. and Ryan, G. (2016). Global mental health in 2015: 95% implementation. *The Lancet Psychiatry*, 3, 15–17.

26. Collins, P.Y., Patel, V., Joestl, S., March, D., Insel, T.R., and Daar, A.S. (2011). Grand challenges in global mental health. *Nature*, 475, 27–30.

27. Dudley, M., Silove, D., and Gale, F. (2012). *Mental health and human rights: vision, praxis and courage.* Oxford University Press, Oxford.

28. World Health Organization. (2012). *WHO QualityRights tool kit: assessing and improving quality and human rights in mental health and social care facilities.* World Health Organization, Geneva.

29. World Health Organization and World Organization of Family Doctors. (2008). *Integrating mental health into primary care: a global perspective.* World Health Organization, Geneva.

30. Lund, C., De Silva, M., Plagerson, S., *et al.* (2011). Poverty and mental disorders: breaking the cycle in low-income and middle-income countries. *The Lancet*, 378, 1502–14.

31. Chisholm, D., Sweeny, K., Sheehan, P., *et al.* (2016). Scaling up treatment of depression and anxiety: a global return on investment analysis. *The Lancet Psychiatry*, 3, 415–24.

32. World Health Organization and World Bank. (2016). *Out of the shadows: making mental health a global development priority.* World Bank, Washington D.C.

33. World Bank. (1993). *World development report 1993: investing in health.* Oxford University Press, New York, NY.

34. GBD 2015 DALYs and HALE Collaborators. (2016). Global, regional, and national disability-adjusted life-years (DALYs) for 315 diseases and injuries and healthy life expectancy (HALE), 1990-2015: a systematic analysis for the Global Burden of Disease Study 2015. *The Lancet*, 388, 1603–58.

35. World Health Organization and Calouste Gulbenkian Foundation. (2014). *Social determinants of mental health.* World Health Organization, Geneva.

36. Lund, C., Stansfeld, S., and De Silva, M.J. (2014). Social determinants of mental health. In: Patel, V., Minas, H., Cohen, A., and Prince, M. (eds.) *Global mental health: principles and practice.* Oxford University Press, Oxford. pp. 116–36.

37. Veling, W. (2013). Ethnic minority position and risk for psychotic disorders. *Current Opinion in Psychiatry*, 26, 166–71.

38. Ehsan, A.M. and De Silva, M.J. (2015). Social capital and common mental disorder: a systematic review. *Journal of Epidemiology and Community Health*, 69, 1021–8.

39. Beydoun, M.A., Beydoun, H.A., Gamaldo, A.A., Teel, A., Zonderman, A.B., and Wang, Y. (2014). Epidemiologic studies of modifiable factors associated with cognition and dementia: systematic review and meta-analysis. *BMC Public Health*, 14, 643.

40. Dohrenwend, B.P., Levav, I., Shrout, P.E., *et al.* (1992). Socioeconomic status and psychiatric disorders: the causation-selection issue. *Science*, 255, 946–52.

41. Truong, K.D. and Ma, S. (2006). A systematic review of relations between neighborhoods and mental health. *Journal of Mental Health Policy and Economics*, 9, 137–54.

42. Goldmann, E. and Galea, S. (2014). Mental health consequences of disasters. *Annual Review of Public Health*, 35, 169–83.

43. Attanayake, V., McKay, R., Joffres, M., Singh, S., Burkle, F., Jr., and Mills, E. (2009). Prevalence of mental disorders among children exposed to war: a systematic review of 7,920 children. *Medicine, Conflict, and Survival*, 25, 4–19.

44. World Health Organization. (2005). *Mental health policy, plans and programmes. WHO mental health policy and service guidance package.* World Health Organization, Geneva.

45. World Health Organization. (2013). *Mental health action plan 2013–2020.* World Health Organization, Geneva.

46. World Health Organization. (2003). *Organization of services for mental health. WHO mental health policy and service guidance package.* World Health Organization, Geneva.

47. Patel, V., Chisholm, D., Dua, T., Laxminarayan, R., and Medine Mora, M.E. (2016). *Mental, neurological and substance use disorders. Disease control priorities* (3rd edn). World Bank Group, Washington D.C.

48. Singla, D.R., Kohrt, B.A., Murray, L.K., Anand, A., Chorpita, B.F., and Patel, V. (2017). Psychological treatments for the world: lessons from low- and middle-income countries. *Annual Review of Clinical Psychology*, 13, 149–81.

49. Padmanathan, P. and De Silva, M.J. (2013). The acceptability and feasibility of task-sharing for mental healthcare in low and

middle income countries: a systematic review. *Social Science and Medicine*, 97, 82–6.

50. Abas, M., Nyamayaro, P., Bere, T., *et al.* (2018). Feasibility and acceptability of a task-shifted intervention to Enhance Adherence to HIV Medication and Improve Depression in People Living with HIV in Zimbabwe, a Low Income Country in Sub-Saharan Africa. *AIDS and Behavior*, 22, 86–101.

51. Araya, R., Rojas, G., Fritsch, R., *et al.* (2003). Treating depression in primary care in low-income women in Santiago, Chile: a randomised controlled trial. *The Lancet*, 361, 995–1000.

52. Dawson, K.S., Bryant, R.A., Harper, M., *et al.* (2015). Problem Management Plus (PM+): a WHO transdiagnostic psychological intervention for common mental health problems. *World Psychiatry*, 14, 354–7.

53. Rahman, A., Riaz, N., Dawson, K.S., *et al.* (2016). Problem Management Plus (PM+): pilot trial of a WHO transdiagnostic psychological intervention in conflict-affected Pakistan. *World Psychiatry*, 15, 182–3.

54. Murray, L.K., Dorsey, S., Haroz, E., *et al.* (2014). A common elements treatment approach for adult mental health problems in low- and middle-income countries. *Cognitive and Behavioral Practice*, 21, 111–23.

55. Bolton, P., Lee, C., Haroz, E.E., *et al.* (2014). A transdiagnostic community-based mental health treatment for comorbid disorders: development and outcomes of a randomized controlled trial among Burmese refugees in Thailand. *PLoS Medicine*, 11, e1001757.

56. Weiss, W.M., Murray, L.K., Zangana, G.A., *et al.* (2015). Community-based mental health treatments for survivors of torture and militant attacks in Southern Iraq: a randomized control trial. *BMC Psychiatry*, 15, 249.

57. World Health Organization. (2008). *Mental Health Gap Action Programme: scaling up care for mental, neurological and substance use disorders*. World Health Organization, Geneva.

58. Lund, C., Tomlinson, M., De Silva, M., *et al.* (2012). PRIME: a programme to reduce the treatment gap for mental disorders in five low- and middle-income countries. *PLoS Medicine*, 9, e1001359.

59. Hanlon, C., Fekadu, A., Jordans, M., *et al.* (2016). District mental healthcare plans for five low- and middle-income countries: commonalities, variations and evidence gaps. *British Journal of Psychiatry*, 208(Suppl 56), s47–54.

60. Bolton, P., Bass, J., Neugebauer, R., *et al.* (2003). Group interpersonal psychotherapy for depression in rural Uganda: a randomized controlled trial. *JAMA*, 289, 3117–24.

61. Peterson, K. (2015). *Impact evaluation: end of phase two impact evaluation for the treating of depression at scale in Africa program in Uganda*. StrongMinds. https://strongminds.org/wp-content/uploads/2013/07/StrongMinds-Phase-Two-Impact-Evaluation-Report-July-2015-FINAL.pdf

62. World Health Organization. (1997). *Report of a conference on intersectoral action for health: a cornerstone for health-for-all in the twenty-first century, 20–23 April 1997, Halifax, Nova Scotia, Canada*. World Health Organization, Geneva.

63. Brooke-Sumner, C., Lund, C., and Petersen, I. (2016). Bridging the gap: investigating challenges and way forward for intersectoral provision of psychosocial rehabilitation in South Africa. *International Journal of Mental Health Systems*, 10, 21.

64. Kleinman, A. (1986). *Social origins of distress and disease: depression, neurasthenia, and pain in modern China*. Yale University Press, New Haven, CT.

65. Kohrt, B.A. and Mendenhall, E. (2016). *Global mental health: anthropological perspectives*. Routledge, Abingdon.

66. Nichter, M. (2010). Idioms of distress revisited. *Culture, Medicine, and Psychiatry*, 34, 401–16.

67. Kohrt, B.A. and Harper, I. (2008). Navigating diagnoses: understanding mind–body relations, mental health, and stigma in Nepal. *Culture, Medicine, and Psychiatry*, 32, 462.

68. Kaiser, B.N., McLean, K.E., Kohrt, B.A., *et al.* (2014). Reflechi twòp—Thinking Too Much: Description of a Cultural Syndrome in Haiti's Central Plateau. *Culture, Medicine, and Psychiatry*, 38, 448–72.

69. Patel, V. (1995). Explanatory models of mental illness in sub-Saharan Africa. *Social Science and Medicine*, 40, 1291–8.

70. Mendenhall, E., De Silva, M.J., Hanlon, C., *et al.* (2014). Acceptability and feasibility of using non-specialist health workers to deliver mental health care: Stakeholder perceptions from the PRIME district sites in Ethiopia, India, Nepal, South Africa, and Uganda. *Social Science and Medicine*, 118, 33–42.

71. Ae-Ngibise, K., Cooper, S., Adiibokah, E., Akpalu, B., Lund, C., Doku, V., Mhapp Research Programme Consortium. (2010). 'Whether you like it or not people with mental problems are going to go to them': a qualitative exploration into the widespread use of traditional and faith healers in the provision of mental health care in Ghana. *International Review of Psychiatry*, 22, 558–67.

72. Cohen, A., Eaton, J., Radtke, B., *et al.* (2011). Three models of community mental health services in low-income countries. *International Journal of Mental Health Systems*, 5, 3.

73. Bass, J.K., Bolton, P.A., and Murray, L.K. (2007). Do not forget culture when studying mental health. *The Lancet*, 370, 918–19.

74. Haroz, E.E., Ritchey, M., Bass, J.K., *et al.* (2017). How is depression experienced around the world? A systematic review of qualitative literature. *Social Science and Medicine*, 183, 151–62.

75. Wilk, C.M. and Bolton, P. (2002). Local perceptions of the mental health effects of the Uganda acquired immunodeficiency syndrome epidemic. *Journal of Nervous and Mental Disease*, 190, 394–7.

76. Bolton, P., Wilk, C.M., and Ndogoni, L. (2004). Assessment of depression prevalence in rural Uganda using symptom and function criteria. *Social Psychiatry and Psychiatric Epidemiology*, 39, 442–7.

77. Bass, J.K., Ryder, R.W., Lammers, M.C., Mukaba, T.N., and Bolton, P.A. (2008). Post-partum depression in Kinshasa, Democratic Republic of Congo: validation of a concept using a mixed-methods cross-cultural approach. *Tropical Medicine and International Health*, 13, 1534–42.

78. Murray, L.K., Bass, J., Chomba, E., *et al.* (2011). Validation of the UCLA Child Post traumatic stress disorder-reaction index in Zambia. *International Journal of Mental Health Systems*, 5, 24.

79. Burkey, M.D., Ghimire, L., Adhikari, R.P., *et al.* (2016). Development process of an assessment tool for disruptive behavior problems in cross-cultural settings: the Disruptive Behavior International Scale—Nepal version (DBIS-N). *International Journal of Culture and Mental Health*, 9, 387–98.

80. Edelen, M.O. and Reeve, B.B. (2007). Applying item response theory (IRT) modeling to questionnaire development, evaluation, and refinement. *Quality of Life Research*, 16(Suppl 1), 5–18.

81. Hays, R.D., Morales, L.S., and Reise, S.P. (2000). Item response theory and health outcomes measurement in the 21st century. *Medical Care*, 38(9 Suppl), Ii28–42.

82. Tang, W.K., Wong, E., Chiu, H.F., Lum, C.M., and Ungvari, G.S. (2005). The Geriatric Depression Scale should be shortened: results of Rasch analysis. *International Journal of Geriatric Psychiatry*, 20, 783–9.

83. Haroz, E.E., Bolton, P., Gross, A., Chan, K.S., Michalopoulos, L., and Bass, J. (2016). Depression symptoms across cultures: an IRT analysis of standard depression symptoms using data from eight countries. *Social Psychiatry and Psychiatric Epidemiology*, 51, 981–91.

84. Drummond, M.F., Sculpher, M.J., Torrance, G.W., O'Brien, B.J., and Stoddart, G.L. (2005). *Methods for the economic evaluation of health care programmes* (3rd edn). Oxford University Press, Oxford.

85. Knapp, M. (1995). *The economic evaluation of mental health care.* Aldershot, Arena.

86. Patel, V., Chisholm, D., Rabe-Hesketh, S., Dias-Saxena, F., Andrew, G., and Mann, A. (2003). Efficacy and cost-effectiveness of a drug and psychological treatment for common mental disorders in general health care in Goa, India: a randomised controlled trial. *The Lancet*, 361, 33–9.

87. Galarraga, O., Gao, B., Gakinya, B.N., *et al.* (2017). Task-shifting alcohol interventions for HIV+ persons in Kenya: a cost-benefit analysis. *BMC Health Services Research*, 17, 239.

88. Summerfield, D. (2008). How scientifically valid is the knowledge base of global mental health? *BMJ*, 336, 992–4.

89. Kirmayer, L.J. and Swartz, L. (2014). Culture and global mental health. In: Patel, V., Minas, H., Cohen, A., and Prince, M.J. (eds.). *Global mental health: principles and practice.* Oxford University Press, Oxford. pp. 41–62.

90. Hickling, F.W., Gibson, R.C., and Hutchinson, G. (2013). Current research on transcultural psychiatry in the Anglophone Caribbean: epistemological, public policy, and epidemiological challenges. *Transcultural Psychiatry*, 50, 858–75.

91. Bracken, P., Giller, J., and Summerfield, D. (2016). Primum non nocere. The case for a critical approach to global mental health. *Epidemiology and Psychiatric Sciences*, 1–5.

92. Campbell, C. and Burgess, R. (2012). The role of communities in advancing the goals of the Movement for Global Mental Health. *Transcultural Psychiatry*, 49 (3–4), 379–95.

93. Kirmayer, L.J. and Pedersen, D. (2014). Toward a new architecture for global mental health. *Transcultural Psychiatry*, 51, 759–76.

94. Freeman, M. (2016). Global mental health in low and middle income, especially African countries. *Epidemiology and Psychiatric Sciences*, 25, 503–5.

95. Das, A. and Rao, M. (2012). Universal mental health: re-evaluating the call for global mental health. *Critical Public Health*, 23, 1–7.

96. Mills, C. (2014). Decolonizing global mental health: the psychiatrization of the majority world. Routledge, Hove and New York, NY.

97. Bemme, D. and D'Souza, N.A. (2014). Global mental health and its discontents: an inquiry into the making of global and local scale. *Transcultural Psychiatry*, 51, 850–74.

98. Patel, V. and Prince, M. (2010). Global mental health: a new global health field comes of age. *JAMA*, 303, 1976–7.

# 4

# The history of psychiatry as a medical specialty[1]

*Pierre Pichot and Guy M. Goodwin*

## Introduction

In 1918, Emil Kraepelin wrote [2]:

> 'A hundred years ago, there were practically no alienists. The care of the mental patients was nearly everywhere in the hands of head supervisors, attendants and administrators of the houses for the mentally ill and the role of the physicians was limited to the treatment of the physical illnesses of the patients.[2]

He pointed out that, in the first decades of the nineteenth century, many of the books dealing with psychiatric themes were still written by medical doctors, such as Reil (who coined the word psychiatry), who had few contacts with mental patients or even by philosophers and theologians, and that only in the great scientific centres had specialists appeared 'who had decided to spend their life in the study and treatment of mental diseases'.

The history of psychiatry as a medical specialty has to be distinguished from the history of psychiatric medical knowledge which began in ancient Greece with the birth of medicine as a science. For more than 2000 years, only physicians observed and treated mental illnesses, and institutions were created in which the 'lunatics' and the 'insane' were received. But, as rightly pointed out by Kraepelin, the truth is that psychiatry was not really a medical specialty. One can argue about the precise date of the appearance of psychiatry as a specific field of medicine and of the psychiatrist as a specialist, devoting his professional competence exclusively to the care of the mentally ill. Denis Leigh recognizes that 'some degree of specialization occurred [in England] among respectable physicians' in the middle of the eighteenth century when the monopoly of Bethlem was broken and new 'lunatic hospitals', such as St Luke's, were opened [2]. On the other hand, the American historian Jan Goldstein stresses that in

France the language, as an exact reflection of the underlying reality, began to use expressions such as *homme spécial* to describe a physician specializing in a branch of medicine such as psychiatry only around 1830 [3].

## Pinel and the birth of psychiatry as a branch of medicine

Despite those divergences, it is generally accepted that the work of Philippe Pinel constitutes a turning point. His role has several aspects. He is known worldwide as the physician who 'liberated the insane from their chains' in a dramatic initiative he started in 1793, at the height of the French revolution, at the Bicêtre asylum and completed 3 years later at the Salpêtrière asylum. However, the reality is more complex.

Pinel, who was born in 1745, had studied medicine, translated Cullen's books into French, and published scientific papers on various subjects. He acted as a physician in a small Parisian 'madhouse'—the Pension Belhomme, in which wealthy lunatics were confined at the request of their families. At that time, most of the Parisian insanes were confined for a few weeks in the general hospital—the Hôtel Dieu. If their state did not rapidly improve, they were considered as incurable and sent to Bicêtre or the Salpêtrière, built a century before, which also received other social deviants like beggars and prostitutes. Pinel, who was known by his politically influential friends for his progressive scientific ideas, was appointed physician to Bicêtre. The division for the insane was under the direction of an overseer (*surveillant*)—Pussin, who had already introduced humanitarian reforms in the care of the patients. Pinel's merit was to approve and systematically develop Pussin's empirical measures and to propose an explicit scientific theory for their mode of action. Inspired by Crichton's views about the nature of the 'passions' by Condillac's psychology and by the ideas of Jean-Jacques Rousseau, he created the *traitement moral*, which he claimed to be effective with patients previously considered as incurably ill.

The improvement of the conditions in which the insane were cared for, supported and expanded by Pinel, was not an isolated

---

French phenomenon. In Tuscany, Chiarugi in 1789 had already asserted that the basis of the extensive reforms he had introduced in the local asylum for the insane was that 'it is a supreme moral duty and a medical obligation to respect the mental patient as a person'. In England, where the public had been shocked by the inhumane treatment to which King George III had been submitted during his mental illness, and where a pious Quaker—William Tuke—deeply affected by the conditions in which the wife of a member of the Society of Friends had died in York lunatic asylum, decided to set up a special institution under the government of the Friends 'for the care and accommodation of their own members'. At the Retreat, opened in 1796 near York, physical restraints were largely abolished, and religious and moral values were emphasized in relations with the patients.

Chiarugi's reforms did not survive the upheavals caused by subsequent wars and the political divisions of Italy, and Tuke's creation of the Retreat had not been prompted by medical considerations but was the expression of religious humanitarian purposes. The role played by Pinel was decisive, not so much because of the changes he promoted in the conditions of the patients, although they had a profound influence, but because he made the study and treatment of mental disorders a branch of medicine.

In 1801, Pinel published the *Medico-philosophical Treatise on Mental Alienation*. In it, he presented the various clinical manifestations he had observed, proposed a simple nosological system largely borrowed from older authors, examined possible aetiological factors, and described his 'moral treatment' in detail. The book has remained a landmark in the history of psychiatry, even being considered by the philosopher Hegel as a 'moment of capital importance in the history of humanity'. For Pinel, insanity was a disease, and the patient affected by it remained, despite the loss of his reason, a human being. Its study, like the rest of medicine, had to be 'a science which consists of carefully observed facts'. Goldstein [3] has shown that Pinel's main preoccupation was to prove this scientific nature of the new medical specialty by repudiating the previous practices of the 'empirics' and 'charlatans'--the two terms being practically synonymous. He had accepted the method Pussin had developed empirically and transformed it in his moral treatment by providing a scientific theory of its mode of action. A curiously premonitory aspect of his emphasis on the necessity of a scientific methodology is to be found in his *Tables to Determine How Probable is the Curability of Alienation*, published in 1808. He provided statistical data on the efficacy of his therapeutic method according to the types of mental disorders and in comparison with spontaneous evolution, and concluded that medicine can only be a true science through the use of the calculus of probability!

## Psychiatry as a profession: Esquirol and the clinical approach

If, because of the international influence of the ideas expressed in his book, Pinel is the founder of psychiatry as a medical discipline, he was not a psychiatric specialist in the strict meaning of the term. Although he retained his position at the Salpêtrière until his death in 1826 and is known today for his contributions to mental medicine, he had many other medical interests which gave him, in his time,

a leading position among the Paris physicians; his *Philosophical Nosology*, published in 1796 and a classical reference for several decades, deals with general pathology. The case of his pupil and successor Esquirol, who became the prototype of the psychiatric specialist, was very different. At the Salpêtrière, he was only in charge of the 'section of the insane'. He was later appointed medical director of the Charenton psychiatric asylum near Paris and owned, in addition, a small clinic, in which he treated his private patients. All his activities were exclusively dedicated to the study and treatment of mental disorders and the teaching of psychiatry. His book *On Mental Diseases*, published in 1838, in which he collected his previous publications, acquired fame as great as Pinel's *Treatise*. In 1913, Karl Jaspers recognized that the later great representatives of German psychiatry, such as Griesinger and Kraepelin, were strongly indebted to Esquirol. He, and the school he founded, effectively developed one of the basic tenets of the new medical specialty. For Esquirol, careful objective observation and analysis of the symptoms and behaviour of the patients were fundamental. He originated the descriptive clinical approach expanded by his pupils. Even more than Pinel, he was suspicious of unproved theories, and when he eventually suggested relations between pathogenic factors and syndromes, he remained extremely cautious in his interpretations. Zilboorg, the psychoanalytically oriented historian of psychiatry, has accused this predominantly descriptive approach of creating 'psychiatry without psychology' because, lacking psychodynamic concepts, its attempted objectivity remained at an allegedly superficial level [4]. The truth is that it laid the foundations of the present description of the mental disorders. The 'atheoretical' descriptive approach adopted in the present nosological systems—both the American *Diagnostic and Statistical Manual* and the *International Classification of Diseases*—of which the proclaimed purpose is to emphasize the medical character of psychiatry is, in this respect, a return to Esquirol's principles.

## The social aspects of psychiatry and the asylum system

By the end of the eighteenth century it was recognized that the study of mental alienation was part of medicine. However, mental diseases were of such a nature that it was not possible to treat the insane in the same conditions as patients affected by other diseases. Their most obvious manifestations had social consequences. According to the prevailing philosophical view, the mentally ill were deprived of free will by their illness. In practice, they were unable to participate in the normal life of society and were often considered as potentially dangerous. Because of this, they had generally been confined in madhouses of various kinds. One of the aspects of the reforms initiated by Pinel had been to make more explicit the difference in nature between the socially deviant behaviour of the insane, which, being the consequence of an illness, belonged exclusively to medicine, and the other deviations which society had to control and eventually to repress. The implementation of this fundamental distinction during the first half of the nineteenth century helped to give psychiatry its specific shape as a profession by being at the origin of forensic psychiatry and by leading to the formulation of precise rules concerning the commitment of the insane to institutions of a strictly medical character.

The legal code promulgated by Napoleon in 1810 stipulated that 'no crime or delict exists if committed in a state of dementia', with the old term dementia being used as a synonym of Pinel's mental alienation. This legal provision, introduced in similar forms in other countries, opened an important domain of activity to the medical profession of the psychiatrist. Because of their now recognized specialized knowledge, the alienists were to help the judges in determining whether the mental state of an individual convicted of a 'crime or delict' was normal or pathological, with decisive consequences on the subsequent decision. The title of Esquirol's *Treatise* mentions explicitly that it describes mental diseases 'in their medical, hygienic and medico-legal aspects'. The conflict (which still exists) between the judges, usually supported by public opinion, who took a restrictive view of the concept of mental disease, and the psychiatrists, who tended to expand it to include new types of deviant behaviour, is illustrated by the violent controversies provoked by Esquirol's description of 'homicidal monomania'. They had an even more famous counterpart in England. J.C. Pritchard, an admirer of Esquirol, had isolated 'moral insanity' as a specific mental disorder in two books published in 1837 and 1842; in the second, he examined its 'relations to jurisprudence'. Half a century later, in 1897, Henry Maudsley, who was in favour of the use of this diagnosis, recognized that this category, although internationally accepted by the psychiatrists, corresponded to:

> ' … a form of mental alienation which has so much the look of vice and crime that may persons regard it as an unfounded medical invention. Judges have repeatedly denounced it from the bench as a "most dangerous medical doctrine", "a dangerous innovation" which, in the interest of society, should be reprobated.'
>
> Henry Maudsley, 1897.

The general acceptance of the new medical concept of mental alienation implied the existence of adequate facilities for the treatment of the patients. The creation of new asylums—the term was retained—and the reorganization of the old ones were the answers. The French law of 1838 that fixed the detailed rules for the expansion of the new system to the whole country and for its functioning and financial support had a model character. Similar results were obtained in, for example, England with the Asylum Act 1828 and the Lunacy Act 1845. Outwardly, the new system was an extension, under more humane conditions, of the previous institutional practices. However, it had radically original features. While recognizing the necessity of protecting society, it stressed the fact that the insane had a fundamental right to be protected and medically treated in a competent way. The deprivation of liberty for the patients, which it still implied, was strictly controlled to prevent possible misuse and was anyway justified, according to Esquirol and most contemporary psychiatrists, not only by the loss of free will, which was a consequence of the illness, but also by the therapeutic value of separation from a pathogenic milieu.

The asylum system became the central element of psychiatric care and was both the consequence and the determining factor of the emergence of psychiatry as a medical specialty to which it gave, until the end of the nineteenth century and even beyond, an original character. The asylums acquired quasi-monopoly in the care of the mentally ill. The few private institutions reserved for the wealthier members of the population, which often belonged to alienists in charge of the asylum, were generally submitted to the same legal rules. Private practice with ambulatory patients, as existing today, was exceptional or dealt with cases which were not then considered to belong to mental alienation. As a result, the study of mental illness was predominantly restricted to the more severe forms of disorder. Another consequence was that the alienists in charge of patients committed to the asylums had a dual function, a fact that differentiated them from other hospital physicians. In addition to their medical duties, they were involved in legal procedures which determined the conditions of admission, stay, and eventually release of the mentally ill. As superintendents, they also often had economic and financial responsibilities, being in charge of the material, as well as the medical aspects of the functioning of their institutions.

Despite the fact that the laws now strictly differentiated the nature of the limitations of liberty in asylums and in prisons, the participation of the alienist in a form of social control was eventually perceived negatively by the public, and often by other physicians, and contributed to accentuating the specificity of psychiatry inside medicine. During the third and fourth decades of the nineteenth century, which saw the birth of the asylum system, psychiatrists became really conscious of their identity as a professional group. In England, France, Germany, and the United States, they founded societies and began to publish journals with specialized scientific goals. Such a description oversimplifies an evolution which was progressive and, in some cases, took different directions. The creation and extension of the asylum system took many years; it did not reach its classical form until the last part of the century, as testified by the famous campaign conducted in the United States during the 1840s by Dorothea Dix who complained that many of the mentally ill were still incarcerated in almshouses and prisons. The moral treatment practised in the institutions was eventually used to justify brutal measures, alleged to be therapeutic, and the behaviour of the attendants, who were not usually medically trained (significantly, they were known as *surveillants* in France), was too often of a purely repressive character. It was a long time before the proposals made in 1856 by the British psychiatrist John Conolly in his book *The Treatment of the Insane Without Mechanical Restraints* were put into practice everywhere.

## The biological and the psychological model

The clinical orientation of Pinel, Esquirol, and their followers was basically empirical. By concentrating on describing observable symptoms and abnormal behaviours, it avoided theoretical controversies. However, many believed that if psychiatry was to become a branch of the medical sciences and to progress, it had to adopt models similar to those accepted by the rest of medicine. According to the anatomoclinical perspective, which was now dominant, diseases were distinct entities. Each disease was defined by a characteristic pattern of symptoms provoked by a lesion or eventually a dysfunction of an organ to be discovered at autopsy. In 1821, Bayle, following this scheme, described the typical clinical symptoms and lesions of the brain in the general paralysis of the insane. Despite the disappointing results of further anatomopathological studies (brain lesions were observed in only a small proportion of cases), there was increasing conviction that, with better investigation methods, mental disorders, like other diseases, could be explained by somatic causes. The degeneration theory, proposed in 1857 by Morel, which attributed many forms of insanity to the hereditary transmission of dysfunction of the nervous system produced by the noxious effects of environmental factors, and whose influence lasted until Kraepelin, is another expression of this biological orientation, the aim of which was to give psychiatry an undisputed medical status.

The biological and the purely clinical approaches were concerned with different conceptual levels—the discovery of the causes of insanity and the description of its manifestations, respectively. Therefore, they could easily coexist. Even when the followers of Pinel and Esquirol expressed reservations about the applicability of the biological model to every type of mental disorder, they still believed in the medical nature of psychiatry. The situation created in the German-speaking countries by the school of the 'mentalists' (the term *Psychiker* by which they were known means 'psychologically oriented'), who were predominant during the first half of the nineteenth century, was very different. Influenced by philosophical, religious, and romantic trends, these psychiatrists took a radical dualistic position, postulating the absolute difference between the physical body and the spiritual soul. The soul was the source of the whole psychic life and hence eventually of its abnormal aspect—insanity. A term such as disease, appropriate for the somatic illness, could only be used metaphorically in psychiatry. The sins of the patients were the origin of the mental disorders, and psychiatry belonged more to moral philosophy than to medicine. These ideas were developed in various related forms by the majority of the German psychiatrists of the period (Heinroth, Ideler, Langerman, and many others). Their ideological position had two consequences—scientific relations with other schools, such as the French and the English who saw in the publications of the mentalists obscure philosophical theories devoid of medical character, were largely cut off; and they provoked a violent reaction in Germany itself. The most extreme representatives of the contending group of 'somatists' (*Somatiker*), such as Jakobi and Friedreich, saw the mental disorders as symptoms of somatic diseases, not necessarily of the brain. In fact, for them, mental diseases as such did not exist. They defended aggressively their biological and sometimes bizarre hypotheses, such as the aetiological role of intestinal worms, against the mentalists. Finally, around 1850, they gained the upper hand. The publication in 1845 of *Pathology and Therapy of the Nervous Diseases* by Wilhelm Griesinger, an heir to their school who was also influenced by the French alienists, is a landmark in the history of German psychiatry. With his appointment in 1865 as professor of psychiatry in Berlin, where he succeeded the mentalist Ideler, medical psychiatry was definitely established in Germany as a branch of the natural sciences.

## The rise of neuropsychiatry

Romberg's *Lehrbuch der Nervenkrankheiten* symbolizes the birth of neurology as an autonomous medical specialty studying and treating the diseases of the nervous system. It was published 5 years after Griesinger's *Textbook* in which, adopting and expanding Bayle's anatomoclinical model, he had affirmed: 'Mental diseases are diseases of the brain'. If both psychiatric and neurological symptoms originated in the nervous system, some form of association between the two specialties was a logical step, at least at the conceptual level. One aspect of their complex relationship was the creation of neuropsychiatry which developed its most characteristic aspects in the German-speaking countries.

Universities acquired considerable power and influence in the second half of the nineteenth century. From the 1850s on, chairs were created for the teaching of the new common discipline, and special institutions—university clinics—were built with hospital beds for psychiatric patients (if their disorders became chronic, they were sent to the nearest asylum), and laboratories for research on neurophysiology and neuroanatomy and special wards for neurological cases were developed. Griesinger's first move when he took over the chair of psychiatry at Berlin was the creation of neurological wards at the Charité. The leading neuropsychiatrists in charge of these institutions often performed research in both fields with equal competence, as shown by the work of Wernicke and Westphal, and later of Kleist and Bonhöffer in Germany and of Meynert in Austria.

The concept of neuropsychiatry, appearing at a period during which the German school was progressively gaining influence, had a deep impact on psychiatric thought and the psychiatric profession, even if its institutional driving force—the university clinic system—was not developed everywhere to the same extent as in Germany. For example, it was conspicuously absent in England, despite the fact that the theoretical position taken by the most important psychiatrist of the time Henry Maudsley was very close to that of Griesinger. The National Hospital in Queen's Square, London, founded in 1860, retained a virtual monopoly on the teaching of neurology for many decades, and psychiatry, taught essentially in hospitals, was not represented at university level until the 1930s. However, in most countries, neuropsychiatric institutions coexisted with asylums where the alienists had the unenviable task of caring for chronic mental patients, often with inadequate means. The concept of neuropsychiatry reflected a basically biological perspective on the aetiology of the mental illnesses, expressed in the creation of a new specialty associating competence in the two previously separated domains of medicine. However, it provoked ideological and professional tension between the 'pure' psychiatrists, mainly those in charge of asylums, and the neuropsychiatrists, predominantly involved in teaching and research. In the long term, this conflict was one of the factors which finally led, in the 1960s, to the almost complete administrative and institutional separation of the two specialties in countries such as France where they had been, at least formally, associated. But many traces of the old situation remain. The most influential scientific journal published in German *Nervenarzt* still deals equally with neurology and psychiatry, and the term 'neuropsychiatric' survives in the titles of many teaching and research institutions.

## The neuroses and birth of the psychotherapies

The study of the neuroses, in which the relation between psychiatry and neurology was also involved, resulted in completely different, but equally important, changes to psychiatry as a medical specialty. The term neurosis had been coined in 1769 by Cullen to describe a class of diseases he attributed to a dysfunction of the nervous system. In this very heterogenous group, two entities of very ancient origin—hysteria and hypochondriasis—had predominantly psychological manifestations. Since the affected patients were not usually commited to asylums, they were not normally studied by alienists, but by specialists in internal medicine such as Briquet, who, in 1859, wrote the classical *Treatise on Hysteria*. Because of the assumed nature of the neuroses, the new discipline of neurology rapidly took an interest in them.

Charcot, the founder of the French neurological school, was responsible for the internal medicine wards at the Salpêtrière—they were not associated with the 'divisions of the insane' at the same hospital, the domain of the alienists. In about 1880, he became interested in hysterical patients who, because of their seizures, were admitted to the same ward as the epileptics. He developed a purely neurological theory of the disease, which he described and studied using hypnosis. This was the former 'animal magnetism', long fallen into disrepute, but to which he gave a new scientific status. Charcot's descriptions of the *grande hystérie*, which he demonstrated on selected patients in his famous public lectures, were justly criticized later, but his international fame attracted students from all over the world. One of them was a young lecturer in neuropathology at the University of Vienna—Sigmund Freud, who, impressed by Charcot's lectures, decided to devote all his energies to the study and treatment of the neuroses. Another was a French professor of philosophy (psychology was then a branch of philosophy)—Pierre Janet, who had become interested in the psychological aspects of the neuroses. He was later to develop, in parallel with Freud, a psychopathological theory which, despite the traces it has left (the concepts of psychasthenia and the dissociative processes in hysteria), was not to be as internationally successful as Freud's psychoanalysis. Charcot's ideas were opposed by Bernheim, the professor of internal medicine at the Nancy Medical School and also an adept of hypnosis. He attacked the neurological interpretations of the Salpêtrière and claimed that suggestion played a central role in the phenomena described by Charcot.

The general interest in the neuroses, which extended beyond medicine to *fin de siècle* literature, was an international phenomenon. In 1880, Beard, an American neurologist, described a new neurosis—neurasthenia, which soon aroused even more interest than Charcot's hysteria. Psychiatry had played almost no part in this evolution, but this was to change under the influence of three related developments: the changes which took place within the concept of neurosis, the birth of the psychotherapies, and the incorporation in the field of psychiatry of psychopathological manifestations, even if they were of minor intensity.

The transformation of the concept of neurosis is apparent in the position taken by Kraepelin in the 1904 edition of his *Textbook*. He introduced a chapter called 'The psychogenic neuroses', on the grounds that 'among the neuroses, to which belong epilepsy and chorea, one must isolate a sub-group characterized by the purely psychological cause of the apparition of the symptoms'. The disintegration of the old concept left to neurology, which, from now on, abandoned the generic term, diseases (such as epilepsy and chorea) whose somatic manifestations could be shown to express a dysfunction of a precise part of the nervous system. Psychiatry took charge of hysteria, hypochondriasis, neurasthenia, and the related phobic, obsessional, and anxious disorders, which constituted the new neuroses. This concept was justified by the psychological nature of the symptoms and the causes recognized even by a biologically oriented psychiatrist such as Kraepelin. This redrawing of the frontier between the neurological and psychiatric specialties also testified to the extension of the limits of psychiatry. Pinel's insanity, until then defined by the necessity of commitment to special institutions, was replaced by a broader concept. A new class corresponding to our present personality disorders had already appeared in the 1894 edition of Kraepelin's *Textbook*. It had been isolated for the first time in 1872–1874 by the psychiatrist Koch. Like the neuroses, the cases were rarely observed in asylums, but nevertheless, they were now considered as belonging to the psychiatric field of study.

This field was further modified by the birth of the psychotherapies. In fact, they had a long history. In 1803, one of the first German mentalists Reil had described, under the name of 'psychic therapy' (*psychische Curmethode*), a number of procedures, including very violent somatic ones, which could influence the 'perturbed passions of the soul', and Pinel's moral therapy contained psychotherapeutic elements. However, psychotherapies, as techniques of which the formal rules were based on an explicit theory about their psychological mechanisms of action, derived mainly from Mesmer's animal magnetism, as rehabilitated by Charcot. The emergence of the psychotherapies, characteristic of the last decades of the nineteenth century, was intimately related to the renewed study of the neuroses. After he had abandoned hypnosis, Freud developed psychoanalysis, but many other techniques evolved during the same period, which were as well, or even better, known at the time, although they were to have a less lasting success. One of these was the method of Janet, who still occasionally used hypnosis. In 1904, Dubois, a Swiss neuropathologist from Bern, introduced a technique influenced by Bernheim's theory of suggestion in *The Psychoneuroses and their Moral Treatment*, and claimed to produce 'psychological re-education' by a combination of rational and persuasive elements. His international reputation brought him patients from all over the world. The 'rest cure', proposed in 1877 by the American neurologist S. Weir Mitchell for the treatment of hysteria and later of neurasthenia, was combined with Dubois' method by Dejerine, Charcot's successor as professor of neurology in Paris.

This very incomplete summary illustrates the striking fact that, because of their intimate connections with the neuroses, psychotherapies originated inside neurology. When the study and treatment of the neuroses were incorporated into psychiatry, psychiatrists considered that they were an integral part of their activity and tried to retain the monopoly of their practice. They never completely succeeded. Already Freud had, according to his biographer Jones, 'warmly welcomed the incursion in the therapeutic field of suitable people from another walk of life than medicine'. The problem of 'lay analysts', a source of conflict within the psychoanalytic movement, is only an aspect of a broader question which was later to involve the relations of the medical specialty of psychiatry with the new professional group of clinical psychologists.

## From the beginning of the twentieth century to the Second World War

During the first half of the twentieth century, psychiatry developed in many directions. Kraepelin's monumental synthesis [5] established in around 1900 a nosological system which, in its broad outlines, has remained valid until today. Without being radically altered, it was completed to mention only a few contributions, in 1911, by Bleuler's description of schizophrenia and in 1913, by Jaspers' psychopathological perspective, developed by the Heidelberg school and Kurt Schneider and by other psychiatrists working in academic institutions. However, the old conflict between the 'mentalists' and the 'somatists' reappeared in a modified form. The mainstream of psychiatry had abandoned the extreme positions of the 'brain pathologists' of the Meynert–Wernicke type but, while recognizing a limited influence of psychological factors, admitted in a general way the biological origin of the more severe mental disorders—the psychoses. The empirical discoveries of biological treatments—of general paralysis by malaria therapy (Wagner von Jauregg in 1917), of schizophrenia by insulin coma (Sakel in 1933) or by chemically induced seizures (von Meduna in 1935), and of depression by electroconvulsive therapy (Cerletti in 1938)—not only helped to dispel the prevailing therapeutic pessimism, but also provided supporting arguments. However, an opposing ideological current represented by psychoanalysis had arisen from the study of the neuroses. Its attention was concentrated on the study of complex psychopathological mechanisms postulated to be at the origin of the neurotic, and later also of the psychotic, symptoms, favoured psychogenetic aetiological theories, and advocated psychotherapy as the fundamental form of treatment. Psychoanalysis expanded steadily during this period and gained enthusiastic adherents in many countries. However, partly because of the suspicion, and even hostility, of many members of the psychiatric establishment, they remained isolated in close-knit groups, with their own teaching system independent of the official medical curriculum, and the use of their therapeutic technique was restricted to a small number of mostly neurotic patients seen in outpatient clinics or, more often, in private practice.

The great majority of patients suffering from mental disorders were still confined in asylums, and the enormous increase in their number, mainly related to the social changes accompanying industrialization and urbanization, although other factors have been invoked, was striking. In Great Britain, it grew from 16,000 in 1860 to 98,000 in 1910, three times more rapidly than the population. A similar phenomenon was observed in all countries and persisted until the end of the 1940s, despite the introduction of the first biological therapies. In the United States, there were already 188,000 patients in mental hospitals in 1910, and by the end of the Second World War, 850,000 were lodged in huge institutions which were overpopulated and understaffed, and could only provide custodial care. This obvious degeneracy of the asylum system, contrasting with the progresses in the scientific field, stimulated efforts to improve the practice of psychiatry and its institutional framework. Most of these improvements took place after 1920 and, although their results remained relatively limited, they were the forerunners of later more drastic changes.

The education of psychiatric specialists, which had varied widely from country to country, was improved and systematized. A convergence of evolution is apparent during this period which can be said, to some extent, to have seen the formal administrative recognition of psychiatry as a medical specialty. Educational programmes and controls of the level of competence were introduced, which extended beyond psychiatrists in academic positions. Limited teaching of psychiatry became compulsory, even in the general medical curriculum. In France, psychiatrists for public asylums and, in some cases, residents in psychiatry were selected by a competitive examination system. In England, the Board of Control recommended in 1918 that a leading position in a psychiatric institution could only be occupied by a physician who had obtained a Diploma in Psychological Medicine awarded by the Royal College of Physicians and by five

universities. In the United States, the moving force behind the reforms was Adolf Meyer, the Director of Henry Phipps Clinic at Johns Hopkins University from 1913 to 1939, who organized a systematic residency system and promoted the creation of the Board of Neurology and Psychiatry. This Board was established in 1936 and awarded a diploma ,which it became necessary to hold, to be recognized as a specialist.

The changes were reflected in the vocabulary. The term psychiatry, originating in the German-speaking countries and mostly used there, was adopted everywhere at the beginning of the century. In France, the health authorities officially substituted '*hôpital psychiatrique*' for '*asile d'aliénés*' and '*psychiatre*' for '*aliéniste*' in the 1930s. In England, a Royal Commission used the words 'hospital', 'nurse', and 'patient', instead of 'asylum', 'attendant', and 'lunatic', for the first time between 1924 and 1926. However, efforts were also made to dissociate, when possible, the social protection function of the institutions from their medical role by allowing them to admit patients under the same conditions as the general hospitals. In 1923, a special section was created in the Paris Sainte-Anne asylum which provided treatment to voluntary patients and had both hospital beds and a large outpatient department. In England, the Mental Health Act of 1930 made voluntary admissions to psychiatric hospitals possible; by 1938, they already constituted 35% of all admissions.

Social considerations had always been evident in psychiatry, but their traditional expressions had mainly been of a negative nature, that is the confinement of patients in asylums. The new possibility of free admissions reflected an increase in tolerance towards the disturbing character of mental illness. At the same time, a differently oriented and broader social perspective appeared. The concept of mental hygiene originated in the United States in 1919 with the creation by a former patient Clifford Beers of an organization whose internationally growing influence was manifested by well-attended congresses held in Washington in 1930 and in Paris in 1937. From its beginning, the movement was not purely medical and was influenced by various humanitarian philosophical trends. It emphasized the role of social factors, such as living conditions or educational practices, in the origin of mental disturbances and promoted their prevention and treatment by the close co-operation of psychiatrists and nurses with non-medical groups in the community. One of the institutional consequences of these ideas was the creation of the profession of social worker. They began their activity in Adolf Meyer's clinic (Adolf Meyer had been an early supporter of the mental hygiene movement whose principles converged with his own ideas) at the Sainte-Anne Hospital in Paris, in England where the London School of Economics opened a special training course in 1929, and elsewhere.

Contemporary with the emergence of psychiatric social work was the expansion of clinical psychology. The Binet–Simon scale for the measurement of intelligence, developed in 1905, was the first application to psychiatry of the new discipline of experimental psychology which had originated at the end of the previous century. This initial contribution led to the creation of a professional class of clinical psychologists who were initially concerned with the development and use of psychological assessment instruments and with theoretical research in a few psychiatric centres. Their number initially remained low; in 1945, the United States, where they were the most numerous, had only 200 clinical psychologists.

## The expansion of psychiatry after 1945

The Second World War coincided with a major transformation of the psychiatric specialty. The war had vividly demonstrated the frequency of mental disorders in the United States; they had proved to be the leading cause of medical discharges from the military service and the primary cause of almost 40% of selective service rejections. The previously prevailing view that psychiatry was a minor and often somewhat despised medical discipline, concerned primarily with the custodial care of psychologically deviant and potentially troublesome individuals, was progressively dispelled. The preservation and restoration of mental health—an expression from now on often used by national and international institutions—began to be considered by governments as an important task. The fundamental changes which took place after 1945 and shaped psychiatry as we know it today were the result of this new atmosphere and of the emergence of new perspectives in the three traditional domains—the psychological, the social, and the biological. Some appeared in slightly different forms at different times; their relative influence was submitted to variations, and eventually they came into conflict. The result has been an impressive expansion and increase of the efficacy of psychiatry, profound institutional transformations, and successive ideological waves which have had a major impact on the professional position of the psychiatrist.

The demographic data reflect the new importance of psychiatry in medicine. In the United States, the proportion of psychiatrists in the medical profession was 0.7% in 1920, 1.4% in 1940, and 5.5% in 1970, the rate of growth having doubled after the Second World War. In France, at present, there are 18 psychiatrists for 100,000 inhabitants; they constitute 6% of all physicians. Similar levels were reached during the post-war decades in developed countries and remain relatively stable today. Even before this spectacular increase in numbers, psychiatrists had been becoming conscious of the necessity to affirm the identity of their discipline. The First World Congress of Psychiatry, held in Paris in 1950, has been followed by periodic meetings and by the creation of the World Psychiatric Association to which almost every national society of psychiatry belongs. The health authorities of various countries have become conscious of the necessity to provide adequate financial means to support research and training in the discipline. In 1946, the United States government created the National Institutes of Mental Health for such a purpose, and similar efforts were made in many countries, although the structures of the organizations formed were different. To promote the same goals at an international level, the WHO, created immediately after the Second World War, had a Section (later Division) of Mental Health which, among other co-ordinating activities, tried to overcome the difficulties of communication between the national schools by establishing a common nosological language.

While the changes affected almost all countries, they were the most spectacular in the United States. From the end of the nineteenth century until the 1930s, the concepts developed in German-speaking countries had been the most influential. This disappeared with the advent of the National Socialist regime which, under the cover of racist theories, expelled many of the leading psychiatrists from Germany and Austria, introduced compulsory sterilization for several varieties of mental illnesses, and promoted the voluntary killing in psychiatric hospitals of mentally retarded children and chronic patients. The United States, which had emerged from the Second World War as the most powerful country in the world, began to exert a widespread influence in psychiatry as in the rest of medicine. Because of the prestige of its research and teaching institutions and the worldwide influence of its scientific publications, reinforced by the progressive adoption of English as the language of international scientific communication, American psychiatry became a model in many countries, even though many of the theoretical trends and technical advances it adopted and developed had originated in Europe. However, in the United States, with a local colouring, they took on a special intensity.

### The psychodynamic wave

An important factor in the spread of the doctrine of psychoanalysis was the emigration of a relatively large number of German and Austrian psychoanalysts to the United States from 1933 onwards. They had been compelled to leave their home countries for racial reasons—psychoanalysis had been condemned by the National Socialist regime, as Jewish and Freud's books had been publicly burnt. Many of the young psychiatrists trained in large numbers to answer the demands of the armed forces adopted psychoanalysis under the influence of some of those in charge of the programmes. For a generation, until the end of the 1960s, psychoanalysis became the dominant ideology in American psychiatry.

The American form of psychodynamism often deviated from Freudian orthodoxy, but it emphasized the role of psychogenetic factors, the value of the study of intrapsychic mechanisms, and the basic importance of psychotherapy, while giving little consideration to the traditional clinical approach and to nosology. The domination of this essentially psychological orientation, sometimes compared with the success of the German mentalist school during the first half of the nineteenth century, had important consequences. Although the disorders of hospitalized psychotics were eventually interpreted according to the psychoanalytic theory, psychotherapy was mostly used, as it has been since its beginning, for ambulatory neurotic patients. As early as 1951–1952, three out of every seven American psychiatrists identified private practice as their main activity, and in 1954, the number of private psychiatrists exceeded that of their salaried colleagues for the first time, with a quarter of the former devoted exclusively to psychotherapy. However, with the initial encouragement of official institutions such as the Veterans Administration, clinical psychologists began to engage in psychotherapeutic activities. The number of members of the Clinical Psychology Section of the American Psychological Association reached 20,000 in 1980, at a time when they were 26,000 psychiatrists in the United States. In public opinion, and to a certain extent in general medical opinion also, psychiatry was assumed to consist only of psychotherapy and psychology.

In most other countries, the developments that occurred in the United States were not as intense, generally appeared later, and were modified by local traditions and influences. In German-speaking countries, they were delayed by the still powerful neuropsychiatric perspective and the temporary vogue for existential phenomenology. In the United Kingdom, the eclectic current fostered by the influential Institute of Psychiatry in London during the decades following the war restricted the advance of psychodynamism; in 1956, *Time Magazine* could affirm, as a conclusion of a survey, that 'all of Great Britain [had] half as many analysts as New York City'. In

France, the psychoanalyst Jacques Lacan gave the doctrine a special colouring. On the whole, however, the rise of psychodynamism was a general phenomenon, except in communist countries where Freud's doctrine had been condemned on ideological grounds.

A reaction began in the 1960s with the successes of the new pharmacotherapies. Clinical psychologists had developed alternative radically different psychotherapeutic methods based on learning theories, especially the behaviour therapy introduced in 1958 by Wolpe, supported in the United Kingdom by Eysenck, and the cognitive therapy often associated with it. These methods competed successfully with the psychodynamic techniques and conquered a large part of the field. Psychodynamism did not disappear; many of its concepts retained their place in psychiatry, and psychotherapeutic methods continued to be practised, but it lost its predominant ideological position. In addition to its theoretical contributions, when its influence on the professional aspect of psychiatry is considered from a historical perspective, it has been an important factor in the further expansion of the activity of psychiatrists in the treatment of relatively minor disorders and has also encouraged clinical psychologists to play an active and independent role in this field.

### The social wave

At the end of the Second World War, there was a great desire for social change; one of its aspects was the belief that everyone had a 'right to health' or at least the right to receive adequate medical care, regardless of the ability to pay. This resulted in the creation of the National Health Service in the United Kingdom in 1948 and the Social Security system in France, together with similar developments in other countries. The social perspective, which was one of the basic principles underlying these developments, initiated major institutional changes in psychiatry. They were the result of a number of factors—the necessity to give to the whole population easy access to psychiatric care, and also the belief that social elements played an important role in the aetiology of mental disorders and that they could greatly contribute to the healing process, with the aim of progressively reintegrating the patient in the community.

The most spectacular aspect of the new policy was the decline of the asylum system, still in a dominant position in psychiatry; in fact, the number of patients in psychiatric hospitals in developed countries reached its peak in 1955. The criticisms of the 'degeneration' of the functioning of psychiatric hospitals and the segregation of patients in institutions, often located far from their homes and families, were not new. However, the previous partial improvements, such as the decrease in the number of compulsory commitments or the creation of outpatient departments, were replaced by the creation of completely new structures. Ideally, the country would be divided into geographical zones or sectors with a population of about 100,000, and each zone would have a multi-disciplinary team of psychiatrists, nurses, clinical psychologists, social workers, and occupational therapists responsible for mental health. Visits and therapeutic interventions in the patient's home and easily accessible outpatient departments were to play an increasingly important role. If hospitalization was necessary, it should be, as far as possible, in small units located in a general hospital where the time of stay was to be reduced to the absolute minimum. Special institutions, such as day hospitals, night hospitals, and specially adapted workshops, would contribute to the progressive readaptation of the patient to life in the community. The introduction of this 'community

care', which was expected to work in close co-operation with general practitioners and various public and private institutions, would result in the disappearance of the traditional psychiatric hospital and 'deinstitutionalizing' psychiatry. The new system was introduced in various forms in most countries after 1969. In the United States, the Community Mental Health Center Act was promulgated in 1967. In the United Kingdom, which had strong traditions of social psychiatry, plans for the implementation of community care were discussed in the 1960s, and in 1975, the Government White Paper *Better Services for the Mentally Ill* encouraged the formation of multi-disciplinary 'primary care teams', which also included general practitioners. In France, an official directive in 1960 created the *psychiatrie de secteur*, which was expected to result in the progressive elimination of *hospitalocentrisme*. The WHO encouraged all its member countries to adopt similar practices.

Although, in the last 40 years, community care has become the official doctrine everywhere, except in Japan where the rate of hospitalization in mostly private hospitals has grown continuously, its implementation has not been easy despite the major therapeutic improvements brought about by pharmacotherapy. In some parts of the United States, the sudden closure of public psychiatric hospitals, combined with the inadequacies of the community mental health centers, was for a time at the origin of an appalling lack of care for a number of mentally ill people. The expected 'fading out' of hospitalization has been slow. According to the WHO, in 1976, the number of mental health beds (including beds for the mentally retarded) per 100 population was 6.5 in Sweden, 5.5 in the United Kingdom, 3 in France, and 2 in Germany. These figures have since decreased, and the types of hospitalization have changed. In 1955, 77% of 'psychiatric care episodes' in the United States occurred in public psychiatric hospitals, compared with 20% in 1990. In 1994, 1.4 million mental patients were hospitalized, but only 35% in public psychiatric hospitals, compared with 43% in general hospitals and 11% in private psychiatric hospitals, which increased in number from 150 in 1970 to 444 in 1988. In France, where the total number of psychiatric patients treated in public institutions (including children) is now about a million, 60% are seen exclusively on an ambulatory basis, but the number of hospital beds has only been reduced by half.

Reflecting the increasing influence of social perspectives, the organizational changes modified psychiatry as a profession. The increase in the number of psychiatrists in private practice was paralleled, in general to a lesser extent, by an increase in the public sector where their role was modified. In the traditional asylum, the authority of the psychiatrist was unchallenged and limited only by the legal provisions related to the procedures of commitment. Nurses, and later clinical psychologists, social workers, and occupational therapists, were 'paramedical auxiliaries' in a subordinate position. The creation of multi-disciplinary teams, working in various settings, gave the psychiatrist a function of co-ordination, made increasingly complex by the claims of professional autonomy made by the former auxiliaries. In some cases, such as in American mental health centres, psychiatrists, who were a small minority in the team and had less and less control over its functioning, resented what they considered to be the loss of their medical status.

The importance given to social factors was not limited to the system by which care was delivered. Sometimes, combined with radical ideological and political attitudes, it took more extreme forms.

The criticisms, which first centred on the inadequacies of the existing institutions, extended to the concept of mental disease itself. The antipsychiatry movement claimed that mental diseases were artificial constructs which were not related to diseases in the medical meaning of the term. The allegedly pathological behaviours, such as those conceptualized as schizophrenia, were in fact normal reactions to an inadequate social system. The so-called treatments were techniques used by the ruling classes to preserve the social order of which they were the beneficiaries. The only solution was a drastic reform of society. Such theses varied in their content and in the arguments used. They were developed by authors such as Szasz, Laing, and Cooper in the English-speaking world, the philosopher Foucault in France, and the psychiatrist Basaglia in Italy. They reached their greatest influence in the 1960s, and a few attempts were made to put their ideological principles into practice. Although they attracted much attention at the time, they were very limited and short-lived. One of the few countries where this movement had a practical impact was Italy. Basaglia's strongly politically oriented theories were influential in the later legal reform of the antiquated asylum system, but, despite the apparently revolutionary character of some of the new administrative provisions, the changes made (notably the closure of large institutions) were very similar to those taking place in other countries.

## The biological wave

Psychotropic drugs, such as opium, had been used since the origin of medical treatment of psychiatric patients. During the nineteenth century and the first half of the twentieth century, synthetic drugs such as the bromides, the barbiturates, and the amphetamines were developed. Some of them, especially the sedatives and hypnotics, had a real, but in practice marginal, value in alleviating some symptoms. They had never constituted an effective treatment of mental disorders. Modern psychopharmacology not only initiated what has been rightly called a therapeutic revolution in psychiatry, but also gave a powerful new impulse to the biological perspective. Its date of birth is usually considered to be 1952, when the remarkable activity of chlorpromazine on the symptoms of schizophrenia and mania was discovered. This had been preceded in 1949 by the demonstration of the value of lithium salts in manic states. A few years later, it was shown that the continuous administration of lithium salts prevented the recurrence of manic and depressive phases in the mood disorders. This was followed by the introduction of drugs acting on depressive manifestations (imipramine and monoamine oxidase inhibitors in 1957) and on anxiety (including chlordiazepoxide, the prototype of benzodiazepines, in 1960). In one decade, clinicians had empirically discovered the fields of application of the main classes of psychoactive drugs—the neuroleptics, the antidepressants, the anxiolytics, and the mood stabilizers—which had been synthesized by biochemists and previously tested by pharmacologists on animal models. The scale and rapidity of the spread of their use had major repercussions.

The first was a modification of the image of psychiatry. The layman generally expected a physician to prescribe drugs to treat the disease from which he suffered. In part, because it did not conform to the expected therapeutic behaviour, psychiatry had been seen as an atypical and almost non-medical specialty. In addition to the specificity of the institutions in which it was generally practised, psychological techniques were unknown in the rest of medicine, and even

the recently introduced biological techniques (the shock therapies and the lobotomy) had a somewhat strange and frightening character. The establishment of pharmacotherapy contributed strongly to modifying this perception, even if it did not completely remove the traditional prejudices.

The second consequence was even more important. There were, at least initially, controversies about the roles of pharmacotherapy and of the new social perspectives in the restructuring of the mental health care system. In fact, the number of inpatients in psychiatric hospitals began to decrease from 1955 on, and it seems obvious that the main cause was the therapeutic efficacy of the drugs. They reduced the mean length of hospitalization and eventually even made it unnecessary. Although some types of patients did not benefit from them and the mental state of others was only improved, many who had previously been condemned to long stays in the hospital were able to return to the community, with their treatment eventually being continued in rehabilitation settings and often on an ambulatory basis. Pharmacotherapy had made possible the practical implementation of social trends. In addition to this basic contribution to the 'deinstitutionalization' movement, pharmacotherapy was an essential factor in the growth of private practice. The success of psychotherapy had been one contribution to this, but the complexity of its techniques, the length of the treatment, its applicability to only a few types of disorders, and the uncertainty of the results limited its use to a relatively small number of selected patients, even in the United States during the period of the greatest popularity of psychodynamism. Pharmacotherapy could be used much more easily, on a much larger number of patients, and did not require long and complex training. Some of the drugs, such as the anxiolytics, had an immediate symptomatic effect, and others (the antidepressants and the neuroleptics) could attenuate or suppress the pathological manifestations in a few weeks and, outside the acute phase requiring hospitalization, could be used on an ambulatory basis. It was not only private psychiatrists who were able to treat many of their patients successfully; general practitioners also began to prescribe psychotropic drugs on a large scale.

The third consequence was the explosive development of biological research in psychiatry. The first therapeutic discoveries were largely empirical, but new biochemical techniques allowed some of the modes of action of the drugs to be elucidated. From 1960 on, studies of the influence of these drugs on various aspects of neurotransmission in the brain stimulated hypotheses about the abnormal biochemical mechanisms considered to be the physical substrate of the mental disorders. Meanwhile new methods had been introduced for the examination of morphological modifications of the living brain and even of the nature and localization of the biochemical processes taking place in its different parts. The discovery by Watson and Crick in 1953 of the chemical basis of heredity and the subsequent spectacular advances in molecular biology gave a fresh impulse to psychiatric genetics, which had been partly discredited by their misuse by the National Socialist regime. Under the name of neurosciences, these new fields of enquiry progressively acquired a dominant role in psychiatric research at the same time as the introduction of an ever increasing number of drugs, eventually more potent, usually with less inconvenient side effects, and sometimes with new therapeutic indications.

## 'Remedicalization' of psychiatry

In 1983, Melvin Sabshin, the director of the American Psychiatric Association, summarized the overlapping chronologies of the psychodynamic, biological, and social waves as follows [6]:

'Psychoanalysis surged through the United States during the 1940s and the 1950s. During the 1950s, a new psychopharmacological approach emerged which had great impact on psychiatric practice generally … The 1960s saw the dawning of a community psychiatric approach which attempted to accomplish a massive desinstitutionalization of patients from public psychiatric hospitals.'

Although less radical and not strictly identical, the general picture was similar in other countries. The 1960s saw an often uneasy coexistence of three schools. 'During that decade', wrote Sabshin, 'American psychiatry enlarged its boundaries and its practices so broadly that many critics grew increasingly concerned with the 'bottomless pit' of the field'. The extension of the practice of psychotherapy, frequently to cases with no clear pathological character, tended to blur the limits of the mental disease concept and to neglect the traditional diagnostic approach. Social work was also tempted to concern itself with problems with no obvious medical nature, such as those still described in 1978 in the United States by the President's Commission of Mental Health, which asserted that 'American mental health cannot be defined only in terms of disabling mental illness and identified mental disorders' and identified as a domain of concern for workers in the field 'unrelenting poverty and unemployment and the institutionalized discrimination that occurs on the basis of race, sex, class, age … ' In sharp contrast, the new biological psychiatry recognized only a strictly medical model, stressing the necessity of an accurate diagnosis for the prescription of drugs and for the testing of their efficacy, and advocated restrictive limits in the definition of mental diseases.

In around 1970, a profound change took place. Although the institutional modifications of the care system favoured by the generalization of drug therapy continued and expanded under its various forms everywhere, the influence of psychodynamism began to decline within the psychiatric profession. According to the director of the National Institutes for Mental Health, 'it was nearly impossible in 1945 for a non-psychoanalyst to become Chairman of a Department of Psychiatry (in the United States)', but by the mid 1970s, the situation was reversed. The publication by the American Psychiatric Association of the Third Revision of the *Diagnostic and Statistical Manual of Mental Disorders* (DSM-III) is often considered as the symbolic expression of the change. This took place in 1980, but its origins were more than a decade previously, and it was significantly presented by its apologists, such as Klerman, as 'a decisive turning point in the history of American psychiatry … an affirmation of its medical identity'. The new nosology, which was categorical in nature and introduced diagnostic criteria borrowed from experimental psychology in the delimitation of the categories, did not allow any reference to 'unproven' aetiological factors or pathogenic mechanisms, unless 'scientifically demonstrated'. It claimed to be purely descriptive and therefore acceptable as a means of communication by all psychiatrists, whatever their individual orientation may be. It was, in fact, perceived, not only in its country of origin as a reaction against the extreme socio-psychological positions—the deletion of the term neurosis because of its usual association with the psychoanalytic theory of intrapsychic conflicts raised violent controversies—but, despite its proclaimed 'a-theorism', also as favouring the biological medical model. Although initially exclusively devised for the use of American psychiatrists, to the surprise of its authors, it was rapidly accepted in all countries, and the WHO adopted finally its principles in its own nosological system—the International Classification of Diseases. Originally, the result of a brutal reversal of trends in American psychiatry, it expressed a general change of direction in the psychiatric way of thinking towards affirmation, against the forces believed to threaten it of the medical character of psychiatry.

## Crisis in psychiatry?

At first glance, the new status of psychiatry seems to have taken firm root in the last four decades. It rests on the general acceptance of the medical definition of the concept of mental disease and of the progressive realization of a diversified, but co-ordinated, institutional system of mental health care. The biological perspective, even if it has taken a prominent place in research and therapy, is now combined with psychological and social approaches in the bio-psychosocial model. The psychiatrist, in accordance with his medical professional responsibilities, occupies a central position in a multi-disciplinary team whose members contribute their special competences to the common goal.

This idyllic picture is far from a reflection of reality, even in developed countries, and the existence of a crisis in psychiatry is evoked with increasing frequency. Under the pressure of economic constraints, efforts are made everywhere to control the rising burden of medical care. They have taken different forms according to the country—from the managed care system in the United States to the *numerus clausus* system in France, in which the number of internships available is determined by the government—but their common aim is to limit the number of psychiatrists and the cost of their activities. In the United Kingdom, the most socialized top–down health care system in the world, managers are now responsible for clinical governance, rather than doctors themselves. This has already resulted in a complete system failure at one general hospital. Psychiatry has proved particularly vulnerable to management edict, and recruitment of competent consultant psychiatrists has become increasingly difficult. Paradoxically, the recognition of the frequency of mental disorders and the growing demand for psychiatric treatments has been associated with a reduction in the domain of action of psychiatrists, who are now often vastly outnumbered by clinical psychologists and social workers. In the United States, by 1990, 80,000 'clinical' social workers were active in the psychiatric socio-psychological domain, a quarter of them in part- or full-time private practice. The claims of these powerful professional groups are not limited to a completely autonomous status but, in the case of clinical psychologists, extend to the demand for a legal recognition of such typical 'medical privileges' as the right to hospitalize patients and to prescribe drugs. The most impressive change has been in the proportion of mental disorders being now treated by general practitioners as a result of the availability of psychotropic drugs with fewer side effects; in France, 60% of antidepressants are now prescribed by general practitioners. Professional jealousies also wax and wane but undoubtedly affect the attractiveness of psychiatry as a profession.

These examples may not be a fair representation of the global picture, but there is undoubtedly a movement towards a limitation of the psychiatric specialty to the care of the most severe cases—in practice, the psychotic cases. This reached its most extreme expression in the United Kingdom with the development of the National Service Framework in 1997. This, in effect, refocused secondary care on 'psychosis'. Some neuroscientists raise doubts about the usefulness of maintaining psychiatry as a specialty, even in this field. Influential, biologically oriented psychiatrists have recently proposed, on theoretical and practical grounds, that psychiatry should be absorbed into a new medical discipline, akin to former neuropsychiatry, and all or most of its socio-psychological aspects should be left to non-medical professions.

In the last decade, medicine in general, but psychiatry in particular, has been accused of selling out to the pharmaceutical industry. This has been based on the high profitability of patented drugs prescribed for psychiatric problems and the fact that large marketing budgets were devoted to the education and entertainment of prescribers. Individual doctors undoubtedly profited from their involvement with companies, and companies obviously influenced how information about new treatments was delivered. However, companies are highly regulated, and indeed off-label promotion, to take one example, has been heavily penalized. The idea that anyone with a so-called conflict of interest (that is, has been paid for professional work by a company) forfeits the right to make a scientific judgement about a treatment is too extreme to be useful. For most doctors, it is their time that is for sale, not their integrity. Suspicion about relationships with big pharma is, however, set to decline with the virtual withdrawal of companies from neuroscience research in the last 10 years.

## Conclusions

Since psychiatry has emerged as a specialty, it has been submitted to conflicting forces. The demands of society, changes in the concept of mental disorder and of its limits, variations in the role played by different theoretical perspectives, and successive scientific discoveries have been responsible for an evolution reflected in the professional status and role of the psychiatrist. Displacements of the centre of gravity of a complex structure in which biological, psychological, and social factors interact have modified the image of psychiatry. The threat of being incorporated in other medical specialties or of being deprived of its medical character is but another transitory episode in its history.

## FURTHER INFORMATION

Hunter, R. and Macalpine, I. (1963). *Three hundred years of psychiatry 1535–1860*. Oxford University Press, Oxford.
Pichot, P. (1996). *Un siècle de psychiatrie*. Synthélabo, Le Plessis-Robinson.
Postel, J. and Questel, U. (eds.). (1994). *Nouvelle histoire de la psychiatrie*. Dunod, Paris.
Shorter, E.A. (1997). *History of psychiatry: from the era of the asylum to the age of Prozac*. Wiley, New York, NY.

## REFERENCES

1. Kraepelin, E. (1918). Hundert Jahre Psychiatrie. *Zeitschrift für die gesamte Neurologie und Psychiatrie*, 38, 161–275.
2. Leigh, D. (1961). *The historical development of British psychiatry*. Vol. I, *Eighteenth and nineteenth centuries*. Pergamon Press, Oxford.
3. Goldstein, J. (1987). *Console and classify: the French psychiatric profession in the nineteenth century*. Cambridge University Press, Cambridge.
4. Zilboorg, G. (1941). *A history of medical psychology*. Norton, New York, NY.
5. Kraepelin, E. (1904). *Psychiatrie* (7th edn). Barth, Leipzig.
6. Sabshin, M. (1983). Preface. In: Spitzer, R.L., Williams, J.B.W., and Skodol, A.E. (eds.) *International perspectives on DSM-III*. American Psychiatric Press, Washington D.C.

# 5

# New ethics for twenty-first-century psychiatry

*Matthew L. Baum, Julian Savulescu, and Ilina Singh*

## Introduction

We need new ethics for twenty-first-century psychiatry. Twenty-first-century psychiatry will not be grounded in categorical diagnosis, office-based therapy, medicalization, and use of drugs. It will be oriented around a view of mental health as a continuum; it will bring novel therapeutics, alternative sites of clinical practice, and new targets of intervention (for example, not patients, but the prodrome; not the individual, but the family). In some ways, it may be a return to the bio-psychosocial formulation of the patient as an agent in an embedded social context, with interventions aimed at promoting well-being, rather than the treatment of psychiatric disorder.

In this chapter, we consider a set of innovations in psychiatry that either raise new ethical questions for psychiatrists and for the psychiatric profession or require a revision of prior understanding of what constitutes ethical behaviour in a psychiatric context. We examine two novel neurointerventions at opposite poles—as an example of neuroengineering efforts for increasingly specific interventions at the level of neural circuits, we highlight deep brain stimulation (DBS), and perhaps as an example of an intervention at the other end of the 'specificity' spectrum, we highlight the therapeutic use of placebos. We spend the remainder of the chapter discussing ethical and philosophical issues spurred by endeavours to enable a future in which psychiatry is increasingly preventative. The discussion is intended to be exemplary, rather than comprehensive; we hope to prompt sustained reflection and debate on these topics in the profession and, in particular, as part of psychiatric training.

## Novel neurointerventions in psychiatry

### The case of deep brain stimulation for the treatment of anorexia nervosa

Perhaps the greatest challenges for psychiatric ethics have arrived in the form of technologies that allow for strategic interventions directly into neural circuits and mental processes. Examples include gamma knife surgery and invasive and non-invasive brain stimulation, including optogenetics. As a case study of this trend

in neurointerventions, we consider the use of DBS to treat anorexia nervosa.

DBS is a non-ablative neurosurgical procedure that has been used with great success to ameliorate motor symptoms in treatment-refractory patients suffering from Parkinson's disease. While the use of the procedure in this context was supported by the UK's National Institute for Health and Care Excellence (NICE) in 2003, DBS is being increasingly considered as an experimental therapy for a wide range of neurological and psychiatric conditions, including (among others) chronic pain, depression, epilepsy, and anorexia nervosa. Preliminary evidence from the experimental use of DBS in these contexts suggests that the procedure may be used to achieve highly beneficial treatment outcomes for treatment-refractory patients suffering from these conditions [1, 2]. Furthermore, DBS has advantages over existing treatment methods since levels of stimulation can be tailored to the needs of the individual patient and it is reversible—treatment can be stopped and electrodes even removed at the request of the patient [3, 4].

The ethically challenging properties of DBS emerge from the technology's ability to specifically interfere with neural activity in the brain and modify brain states. Of course, it is true that any intervention affecting feeling, experience, motivation, and behaviour ultimately modifies neural activity. This is true of indirect psychological interventions such as psychotherapy, as well as direct interventions such as drugs, surgery, or DBS; in some sense, they all involve the modification of brain states, so ethical issues raised by one potentially apply to others. That said, the 'holy grail' of neurointervention is *precise* control of the activation of neurons in specific circuits to produce targeted effects. Perhaps the most controversial application of this kind of precision in neurointervention would be to bring desire under close cognitive control. Choosing what to desire to do, and being able to do that, is an enormous power with implications for freedom, autonomy, and well-being. Although we are not yet at the stage where agents are enabled to simply will a desire into existence, such that it motivates them sufficiently to act, DBS moves us much closer to this than we have ever been before.

In the context of anorexia nervosa (AN), DBS could be used to impose a motivating desire to eat or to give patients the cognitive control required to resist compulsive motivation to engage in dangerous weight loss behaviour. However, other mechanisms, such as the use of this technology to alter first-order motivating desires or the patient's emotional traits, may confer significant harms as well as potential benefits. For example, amplification of first-order desires to eat without higher-level endorsement may undermine, rather than promote, autonomy [5]. The various ways in which different mechanisms are likely to affect AN patients' experiences of themselves and their ability to be self-governing must be borne in mind in research and clinical development protocols for DBS treatment. Furthermore, practitioners should be wary of the new ways in which the use (and indeed, mere prospect) of DBS treatment could introduce new avenues of perceived coercion and new problems regarding the authenticity of AN patients' desires regarding their continued treatment and eating behaviours [5].

### The case of placebo for the treatment of depression

In 2008, Irving Kirsch published the results of a meta-analysis that, for the first time, included unpublished trials of modern antidepressant drugs that were logged with the Food and Drug Administration. Across 47 clinical trials, these antidepressants failed to perform significantly better than placebo in mildly depressed patients and performed only somewhat better than placebo in severely depressed patients. Furthermore, while antidepressants did perform better than placebo for severely depressed patients, the data suggested that as patients became more severely depressed, the group who were given the drug did not fare any better; rather, the control group who were taking placebo fared worse [6, 7]. If these findings are correct, it would seem that severely depressed patients do not respond as strongly to the placebo effect. Consequently, although there is a larger difference between the drug group and the placebo group among severely depressed patients, the drug is no more effective.

Such studies raise the important issue of the extent of the placebo effect in psychiatric treatment and the moral status of such an effect. Since depression, like pain, is a subjective experience, what matters is subjective improvement, and not how it is brought about. That is, two challenges facing psychiatry are to properly ascertain the treatment effect, excluding publication bias, and to better utilize the placebo effect in modern psychiatric practice. Many doctors are forbidden by law or by professional codes of ethics from prescribing placebos without revealing them to their patients [7, 8] , but the moral status quo is under pressure as evidence mounts showing that placebos have substantial subjective benefits and that they may even form a larger component of existing popular therapies than was previously thought [9, 10, 11].

## Early intervention and prevention in psychiatry

### Efforts in predictive biomarker development

'A young man presents to a clinic concerned that people are talking about him on the public bus on his way to school. He knows that they are probably not, but he is troubled by the disconcerting feeling and it is starting to make him dread the idea of taking public transport. He takes a clinical assessment designed in part to detect other sorts of "attenuated" psychotic symptoms; approximately one third of the individuals who scored as highly as he does go on to have a full psychotic break within two years, one third maintain the current level of troubling attenuated symptoms, one third get better. What should the clinician do with this information? Does the young man have a disorder or is he "merely" at risk of a disorder?'

[Case adapted from Baum 2016]

In the revision of DSM-IV-TR to DSM-5, a vigorous debate surfaced about whether to include a disorder characterized chiefly by the risk of first psychosis [12]. Clinical tools designed to assay attenuated psychotic symptoms had been shown in multiple clinical sites to be able to delineate a group of help-seeking young people, 20–40% of whom would go on to have a psychotic break in the next 2 years. The main opposition to creating such a category in the DSM-5 was that it was inappropriate to have disorders 'based on risk' and that telling someone like the young man in this case that he is at high risk of psychosis could be needlessly traumatic, as a large portion of individuals did not, in fact, go on to develop the psychosis. Proponents responded by sidestepping the concern about risk—that even those who did not develop psychosis still had troubling symptoms that were deserving of care. In the end, this category was not included in DSM-V [13], but the debate about the proper role of risk in psychiatry should be far from over.

At the laboratory bench and super-computing clusters, neuroscientists and bioinformaticians are hard at work to uncover biomarkers in blood, saliva, brain images, and cerebrospinal fluid for diverse phenotypes in psychiatry from psychosis, suicide, and abuse to PTSD and dementia. Efforts do not stop at individual biomarkers, however, as current thinking suggests that an assemblage of multiple biomarkers, demographics, and patient history into actuarial risk predictor tools could yield more predictive power, as does the fracture risk score (FRAX) for all-cause risk of hip fracture, or the Reynolds risk score for 10-year cardiovascular event. The quest for a better classification is increasingly aided by advances in machine learning and has even spilled beyond the medical world into social media where Facebook is currently developing and deploying machine-learning classifiers to identify posts that may indicate the author is at risk of suicide [14]. What makes matters more complex is that this work is beginning to reveal a risk landscape where biomarkers do not map cleanly onto existing disorders but sometimes indicate cross-disorder risk or risk of *events* like suicide, rather than disorders themselves. As this research progresses, the current lines between disordered and well will be blurred and replaced by differential magnitudes of risk of different harmful symptoms and events. Psychiatry as a field will have an increasing number of debates similar to that about young individuals with a clinical high risk of psychosis, and it will have to grapple with the question of how to incorporate risk into its nosology and, more broadly, how risk should change physicians', patients', and society's obligations to each other (for an extended discussion of the neuroethics of biomarkers, see [15]).

### The role of risk in the concept of disorder

So what role should quantitative risk play in psychiatric nosology? Should we have disorders based on risk or on categories of risk of disorders? Interestingly, if one delves into the (seldom read) first few pages of DSM where it discussed what, broadly, should be thought of as a disorder, one can see a telling evolution of a response to these questions. In DSM-IV-TR, risk is explicitly highlighted in a 'risk clause' [16]:

> '[A disorder is a dysfunction in the individual] "Associated with present distress (e.g. a painful symptom) or disability (i.e. impairment in one or more important areas of functioning) *or with a significantly increased risk of suffering death, pain, disability, or an important loss of freedom*'.
>
>                                        (American Psychiatric Association [APA] 2000) [Our emphasis].

But faced with the prospect of throngs of predictive biomarkers, a proposal was put forward to drop the risk clause entirely, with an explanation that the purpose of doing so was to 'differentiate more clearly between disorders and risk factors' [17]. One of us has argued that elevated risk of harmful symptoms or of harmful events is precisely why we care about a disorder [15] and that it is really the combination of an unhelpful idea that human existence is neatly cleaved into two conditions, healthy or sick, with disagreements over the *magnitude* of risk and whether the symptoms/events are indeed *harmful* that undergirds disagreements about whether a risk state should be a disorder or not. To see this intuitively, note that we can have highly painful, but quickly resolving, conditions like cramp, which we are unlikely to think of as a disorder (or at least a serious one) *unless we think it is highly likely to happen again or repeatedly in the future*; similarly, people who have a single, unprovoked seizure, though often harmed during the seizure itself (if only by loss of bodily autonomy), are monitored for biomarkers of future seizure risk [for example, epileptiform activity on an encephalogram (EEG)] that could be suggestive of a disorder of sustained predisposition to seizures, e.g. epilepsy. On the other hand, a predictive biomarker like profoundly thickened heart walls indicates a high risk of sudden cardiac death and is relatively uncontroversially thought of as the disorder of hypertrophic cardiomyopathy.

What *should* be controversial and debated openly is the proper course of action indicated by a particular risk and the *types of risks we should care about*. If the 'other risk factors' are indeed of very very low predictive value, this is what matters, not that they are 'risk factors'; indeed, machine-learning classifiers based on the profile of risk factors may soon have higher predictive value of harms we care about than currently accepted clinical standards; for example, in a recent meta-analysis, all of the currently accepted ways of estimating who is at risk of suicidal ideation and attempt, including the oft held idea that those with disorders such as depression and bipolar disorder are at elevated risk, were found to perform only marginally better than chance [18]; several recent machine-learning classifiers, however, performed astronomically better, with one metric of prediction accuracy—the area under the curve (AUC)—of 0.7–0.9 where AUCs of 1 represent perfect prediction and 0.5 represent chance level [for comparison, an elevated score on a prostate-specific antigen (PSA) test has an AUC of 0.68–0.83 for detecting cancer, depending on the PSA cut-off value and the grade of cancer] [19]. Though these algorithms require validation on independent datasets, presumably if part of the reason we care about some psychiatric disorders is the risk of suicide, should we not be even more concerned for the welfare of those identified by an algorithm to be high risk, even if the individual does not map to a currently named disorder?

One of the benefits of being challenged by the development of predictive biomarkers is that it forces us to recognize, more than is currently the case, that the hard conceptual work in psychiatric nosology should be deciding whether a risk is clinically (or morally) significant, whether something is harmful, and whether harms are due primarily to an unjust organization of society [15]. Because the field of psychiatry is unlikely to abandon current nosology entirely, perhaps an interim solution is to retain traditional psychiatric categories but to think of them as useful heuristics for estimating the likelihood of important point outcomes like suicide, future decreases in well-being, or conversely, resolution of symptoms, which can be supplemented with algorithmic and machine learning—similarly to the way a diagnosis of lung cancer is now supplemented by a range of biomarkers from clinical and anatomical pathology to create a better estimate of prognosis.

### The role of welfare in the concept of disorder

A complementary approach has also been put forward—treatment should be primarily about improving well-being, and therefore, disorder categories are useful only in so far as they help us to that end [20, 21]. The debate in psychiatry should be less about whether an individual has a disorder, but how best to improve that individual's quality of life. Thus, a more fruitful question than 'does this child have attention-deficit/hyperactivity disorder' is 'would stimulants improve this child's quality of life (with a whole-life view)?'. Coming back to risk, if awareness, medical, environmental, or other intervention to alter that risk can improve the individual's well-being, then that course of action should be considered. Of course, this sentence should provoke the question 'under what conditions would a reduction of risk improve well-being?'.

To answer this question, it is helpful to frame it within a welfarist account of disability [20, 21]. According to this account, a person has a disability if they have some stable psychological or biological state that makes it likely that their life will get worse, in terms of their own well-being, in the social and environmental context they inhabit. This conception of disability has several morally relevant properties. Firstly, it makes no reference to normality; as such, it does not invite a distinction between treatments that count as therapy and those that count as enhancement. Secondly, it makes no recommendation about the best way to treat disability. The biological, psychological, social, cultural, and other factors that contribute to a person having a disability are relevant only in so far as they negatively impact that person's well-being. The disability may be treated by addressing any one or more of these factors. While it may be appropriate to treat disability by addressing the biological factors that contribute to it—by prescribing medication or surgery, for example—it may also be appropriate, instead, to address non-biological factors. Imagine someone whose leg has been amputated and who qualifies by the welfarist account as disabled because the amputation makes it difficult for her to negotiate the stairs to the second-floor flat where she lives. This combination of factors reduces her well-being. (For simplicity, imagine that no other factors combine with her amputation to reduce her well-being.) Her well-being will improve if she is fitted with a prosthetic limb; alternatively, it will also improve if a lift is installed in the building where she lives. The medical route to treating disability, then, is not the only route, nor even the most obvious or appropriate.

We believe that the current approach to mental health and illness would benefit from considering a welfarist approach [22]. Such an approach to the goals of psychiatry requires an account of welfare or well-being. Measures of well-being have not been widely used in psychiatry until very recently, largely because the criterion of 'impairment' has not been framed in alliance with such epidemiological measures. There is some suggestion that this is changing and that, as quality of life measures enter psychiatry, they may need to be re-normed to take account of the various cognitive, behavioural, and other differences entailed in living life with mental health challenges [22].

In philosophy, three broad theories of well-being have been described: hedonistic, desire fulfilment, and objective list. According to hedonistic theory, what makes someone's life go well are positive experiences such as pleasure. According to desire fulfilment theory, what is good is satisfaction of one's desires, even if one does not gain pleasure from that satisfaction. According to objective theory, certain things are good for people, irrespective of whether they desire them or gain pleasure from them [23].

Psychiatrists routinely encounter cases where these three accounts of well-being come into conflict. A patient may enjoy something he desires not to enjoy or *should not* enjoy, even if he does, e.g. sadistic pleasure. Hedonistic and desire fulfilment theories are both subjective theories of the good or value. In this sense, 'beauty is in the eye of the beholder'. The quality of a life is relative to that individual's own valuation.

This is the kind of view that is often put forward by some disability activists and patient advocacy groups; they claim that because the disabled are as satisfied with the quality of their lives as the non-disabled, the quality of their lives is just as good. In a well-cited study, becoming paraplegic has very negative effects on a person in the short term—it causes a significant decrement in subjective life satisfaction. However, over time, the quality of life returns to nearly normal. Many people with paraplegia adapt to their state [24]. Yet, it could be argued that the loss of independence and mobility are serious disadvantages (though clearly ones whose badness depends on the built environment), even if people are equally satisfied.

There are good reasons to include at least an objective element within an account of well-being, especially within psychiatry. In psychiatry, the subjective perspective is often fundamentally affected by the disorder, and it is important to tether treatment to some objective perspective. It is important to recognize that even within a subjectivist framework, however, a person can be mistaken about what is of value. People can be wrong about the facts, for example believing that they are receiving medical care that is beneficial to them when it is not. Or people could be wrong about whether a particular state of affairs instantiates what they value [25]. For example, suppose someone values empathy but mistakenly applies the value of empathy to support a 'tough love' approach. Anorexia might be one psychiatric condition that involves both factual and evaluative errors about body image and shape. However, the problem with subjectivist accounts of well-being—and more generally of value or reasons—is that such accounts are, at base, unfettered—one can literally desire anything.

Each of the three accounts of well-being—hedonistic, desire fulfilment, and objective list theories—has some plausibility. Parfit concludes that an adequate account of well-being must accord weight to all of valuable mental states, desire satisfaction, and objectively valuable activity [26]. It may be best not only to engage in activities that possess objective value, but to also *want* to engage in such activities and to derive pleasure from them. Thus, a welfarist account

would posit that any changes to features of our genetics or biology that make it more conducive to possessing, desiring, and enjoying the things that are objectively good for us should be furthered as a goal of medicine. And in our utilization of biological or algorithmic technology, it is perhaps equally important to seek better estimations of the likelihood that things will go better for an individual as it is that things will go worse.

## Personalized medicine, predictive psychiatry, and enhanced clinician responsibilities

Consider the following hypothetical case.

A young woman with florid first-episode psychosis and cognitive impairment was put on antipsychotic medication and consequently developed neuroleptic malignant syndrome (NMS). A case of negligence was brought against the prescribing psychiatrist; one piece of evidence brought forward by the prosecution was that the physician considered, but did not test the woman for, anti-*N*-methyl-*D*-aspartate (NMDA) receptor autoantibodies, which would have provided some probabilistic information on NMS risk (for example, see [27]). If the physician had ordered this serological test, he would have found that the woman had high titres of anti-NMDA antibodies. The prosecution claimed that since this test would have yielded relevant information, the physician should have ordered it; because he did not, his prescription was negligent.

Are liability cases like this one poised to proliferate in psychiatry? A psychiatrist might be expected to ensure that a patient does not carry significant risks of a bad reaction to psychopharmaceuticals. How will the responsibilities of the clinician adapt when the ability to detect risks of bad reactions and to perform other risk assessments greatly expand with the development of other predictive biomarkers and algorithms?

Aristotle posited that for someone to be properly held responsible for a state of affairs, she had to have acted voluntarily and with knowledge of what she was doing [28]. If I were not in control of my actions, or if I were not know what I did (or failed to do) was wrong, I would be excused from blame. If a patient deliberately overdosed on a tricyclic antidepressant, but the psychiatrist did not know that the patient was suicidal, this ignorance might excuse the psychiatrist from blame. Yet the technical ability to foresee, to some extent, clinically significant events in psychiatry is poised to drastically shrink the number of cases where one could validly appeal to the excuse of ignorance.

All the way back to Aristotle, theories of moral responsibility have incorporated something similar to a risk clause that permits an individual to be blamed for harm, even if they were in no control or did not know what they were doing at the time the harm came about. Aristotle considers the case of someone who chooses to drink and because of his drunkenness does wrong; that person is still blameworthy for the wrong, even though he had no control over his actions during the highly drunken state, Aristotle argues, because the person could foresee entering such a state when he decided to drink (those who have had training in the treatment of alcohol and substance abuse disorders may have a more nuanced version of these arguments).

In the case of the young woman, even though the clinician had no meaningful control over the harmful reaction at the time that the woman developed NMS, it might be argued that he did have some sort of control at an earlier time point in so far as he made a choice about whether to prescribe antipsychotics or another course of therapy and could have foreseen the possibility that she would develop NMS as a result of antipsychotic treatment. The prosecution is arguing that the psychiatrist is therefore blameworthy for the harm to the patient. It is certainly true, however, that there is *always a possibility* that a patient given antipsychotics will develop NMS, and it is hardly true that the prescribing psychiatrist would properly be blameworthy for *every case of NMS*. The validity of the prosecution's claim therefore lies in arguing that the psychiatrist becomes blameworthy because the likelihood of NMS would be elevated if the person had anti-NMDA antibodies, that is, the *magnitude of the probability* makes all the difference between NMS being unfortunate or culpable.

One of us has pointed out, however, that philosophical theories of responsibility and legal structures offer little guidance as to the magnitudes of probabilities necessary for a psychiatrist to be culpable; those theories of moral responsibility that mention risk often do so in a binary fashion (for example, it was foreseen or not foreseen, significant risk or insignificant risk) or even posit that the necessary magnitude of risk is a 'non-zero probability' [15]; indeed by ordering whole-exome sequencing, which is quickly becoming cheaper than ordering several individual genetic tests (and thus being considered for genomic screening of newborns in some countries), a clinician instantly gains knowledge of thousands of foreseeable non-zero probabilities.

Discussion of which risks create liability and which risks can be justifiably ignored is all the more pressing because risk assessments in psychiatry are far from being restricted to estimating bad reactions to pharmaceuticals. Here we consider two further cases: risk of relapse and risk of harm to third parties.

The miniaturization of biosensors has enabled them to be integrated into medications where they can wirelessly report ingestion events [29]. This is designed to aid monitoring of patient compliance with a prescribed drug therapy. In psychiatry, however, one could easily see how such a technology could create new obligations for the psychiatrist. It is common for discontinuation of antipsychotic medication (aka non-compliance) to precede an acute phase of psychosis that sometimes results in traumatic, forced hospitalization. What would be the responsibility of the prescribing psychiatrist who would be notified by the biosensor that a patient might be discontinuing medication? One practical solution might be to involve the patient through an extension of a so-called 'Ulysses Contract' (for example, reference [30]). In Homer's Odyssey, Ulysses ordered his men to lash him to the mast so that he could not throw himself into the sea upon hearing the sirens' song, the watery plunge being a foreseeable side effect of carrying out his desire to hear their voices. So too, patients might, when well and in full possession of mental faculties of judgement, pre-emptively give their treatment team permission to intervene and hospitalize early when medication discontinuation is detected, even though the patient at the time of discontinuation would not meet the criteria for involuntary hospitalization.

Overall, the role of patient participation in decision-making may increase as prognostic ability grows through the use of biomarkers and big data algorithms. For example, there have been some cases where people with anorexia in the UK have been allowed to die after a long and protracted course with multiple relapses [31]), while it is more normal to force-feed people with anorexia who have a dangerously low body weight [32]. Greater prognostication may allow high-risk people with anorexia to be identified, and targeted in-depth discussions undertaken during periods of competence to elicit preferences for what should be done when life-threatening anorexia is reached. In this way, better definition of potential patient pathways makes it possible for patients to better and more empathetically engage with their possible futures, and for clinicians to elicit their values in relation to those futures. In this way, patient autonomy can be enhanced as part of a framing of mental health and illness as continuous and dimensional.

Risk assessment in psychiatry also can include risk of harm to third parties. Already, over 200 different actuarial tools are being used in forensic psychiatry to estimate the risk of violent behaviour [33]. There are also individual behavioural biomarkers that may be informative of the risk of violent behaviour, with one of the most discussed in the bioethics literature being the monoamine oxidase A (MAOA) gene × environment interaction (reviewed in [34, 35]). Briefly, MAOA, involved in the metabolism of monoamine neurotransmitters, is present in two common genetic alleles, MAOA-low (*MAOA-L*) and MAOA-high (*MAOA-H*), named according to their metabolic activity *in vitro*. When raised in an environment where they experienced maltreatment, boys with *MAOA-L* were found to be at elevated risk of future violent behaviour, while boys with *MAOA-H* were found to be resilient. There are nuances and remaining controversies about this gene × environment interaction, but for the purposes of this chapter, we wish to highlight the cross-cutting moral implications of such a biological risk of harm to others. Specifically, we might ask if knowledge of differential susceptibility to the violence-predisposing effects of maltreatment should change how public health programmes and social workers prioritize the use of limited social supports (if there is not enough support for all children, should programmes prioritize aiding boys at highest risk of expressing violent behaviour, even if the differential risk is small), or change how courts should evaluate the blameworthiness of individuals who do commit violence. In regard to the latter, one of us previously argued that such a predisposition would affect culpability only if the risk of violence was increased through a legally relevant mechanism; while most jurisdictions would offer no excuse or mitigation for a predisposition that resulted from decreased impulse control, some would allow a partial defence of provocation if an individual were more likely to react with violence due to an increased perceived gravity of a threat to the individual, a possibility supported by some evidence in the case of the *MAOA-L* gene × environment interaction.

One further challenge may arise for the child/adolescent psychiatrist who suspects that a boy in their clinical care may be at high risk of maltreatment [34]. Should the threshold for intervention in the family be lowered if the boy has the *MAOA-L* variant? Conversely, since disruption of family units is itself not without risk to a young person, should the threshold for intervention be raised if the boy's biomarker profile suggests he might be more resistant to one of the negative effects of possible maltreatment?

We will conclude this section by highlighting that the increased ability to gain probabilistic information about the risks patients pose to themselves or pose to others, and that others pose to the patients begs the question of when an individual *should have* known something; for example, they could have learnt more about the risk of suicide, the risk of bleeding, and the risk of violent behaviour but did not and, because of that ignorance, did wrong. For example, if I said I did not know that the person was drunk (and therefore at high risk of driving dangerously), someone may rightly counter that perhaps I *should have known*. Being blameworthy for not knowing something is referred to, in the legal-philosophy literature, as 'culpable ignorance'.

A useful concept from the literature of culpable ignorance is the 'benighting act':

> 'An initial act, in which the agent fails to improve (or positively impairs) his cognitive position, [followed by] a subsequent act in which he does wrong because of his resulting ignorance.'
>
> (Smith 1983, p. 547).

Smith uses the example of a clinician who fails to do relevant continuing education to keep up with standards in the field and, because of that benighting act, wrongs a patient. We can update the case to consider a physician who fails to use predictive technology and, because they lack that knowledge, wrongs a patient; though we discussed the case where the absence of action by the psychiatrist might harm the patient (by failing to intervene to minimize the risk of suicide), it may be the case that the clinician would actually overestimate the risk of suicide (by relying on traditional risk factors; see [18]) and thus wrong the patient by acting, for example, to deprive them of their liberty, if only for a night, under the supervision of a psychiatric nurse.

Smith (1983) [36] highlights that theorists differ in how they respond to culpable ignorance. Some (for example, see [37]), including Aristotle, hold the person equally blameworthy for the wrong, as if they did it without ignorance. Liberal theorists evaluate the blameworthiness of the individual on the benighting act itself, modulating blame according to the likelihood that the act would lead to a wrong. Regardless of which stance one takes, the proliferation of predictive technologies renders the necessity of taking a stance increasingly likely for psychiatrists in training and practice.

## Prediction and distributive justice

Distributive justice permeates every facet of psychiatry. There is a global shortage of psychiatrists (and indeed all mental health workers), for example, with only one psychiatrist per 1,000,000 people in low-income countries (vs. one psychiatrist per 472 people in the UK), and even in countries with larger psychiatric workforces, there is a paucity of psychiatrists per capita in rural, compared to urban, areas [38]. So in this sense, psychiatrists themselves are a limited resource that the academies and governing bodies have some concern about how to fairly distribute. Individual psychiatrists must decide: do I accept only private clients? Do I take public insurance? Do I spend time only with the patients I think will benefit the most from my clinical skills, or do I also take on 'tough cases' where the chances of my benefiting the person are lower but the person is more deeply affected by the psychiatric disorder?

If we have a limited supply of goods—time, personnel, funding, etc.—with which to benefit people, how should we go about distributing those goods? What counts as fair, or just, distribution can take many shapes. We might think we should distribute all goods equally among the eligible beneficiaries. But sometimes this strategy can make no one better off and some worse off; if one man had an overcoat on a cold winter day, it would do no one good to distribute the cloth equally among a throng of cold individuals—no one would receive a large enough piece of cloth to warm themselves, and now the man who used to have the coat would also freeze. To counter such an objection to increasing equality by 'levelling down', many theories incorporate some element of distributing in order to do good, to benefit people. However, if one posits that it is better to benefit those who are currently worse off over those who are better off, one endorses some version of the priority principle—that one should give priority to benefiting the worse off, even if this means there is less benefit overall.

If it is important to benefit those who are worse off, however, one must have ways of knowing who is worse off. It would be at best callous and at worst a miscarriage of justice to benefit those who are better off over those who are worse off. Historically in psychiatry, diagnostic categories, clinical interviews, and demographics have been used to identify those who are worse off. This information determines who is given priority on waiting lists for mental health services or publicly supported social supports, who is given the 'direct line' to a psychiatrist's pager or office and who will need to speak with a receptionist for triage, who is directly monitored for suicide risk and who is not, or, in forensic psychiatry, who is let out on parole and who stays incarcerated.

If those at higher risk of harm are actually worse off, not 'merely at risk of being worse off' [15], then as they develop, predictive biomarkers and algorithms will increasingly be able to inform us about who is at elevated risk of harm, and thus worse off and deserving of distributive priority. Since many of the goods discussed would benefit someone, regardless of whether their risk is detectable through traditional or novel means, then it could be argued that the utilization of predictive bioinformatics could support fair distribution, regardless of whether the test would change clinical management in the narrower sense. This sort of 'moral utility' of predictive testing should be considered, in addition to a test's 'clinical utility'. When we consider this in conjunction with the concept of 'culpable ignorance' raised earlier in this chapter, it is possible that psychiatric practices could encounter scenarios where it is no longer permissible to allocate certain resources considering traditional clinical information only, without utilizing novel bioinformatics methods.

Just as the development of bioprediction may change what is considered as ethical behaviour of psychiatrists, so too may developments in e-health. Many academies and public health systems have incentives for psychiatrists to practise in underserved areas. Often, such programmes come at considerable monetary cost; the Headspace programme for youth mental health in Australia came under the critical spotlight for the variance in the cost of services in remote communities vs. urban communities, for example [39]. However, it is generally viewed as permissible for psychiatrists to choose to practise in big cities where the population's access to psychiatric services is much better; the justice claims in these cases might have been judged to have been outweighed by the magnitude of the costs to the psychiatrist of satisfying those claims (perhaps their family or research is in the city).

But does the advent of better telepsychiatry and online-mediated treatments change this calculus? One might argue that access to modern outpatient psychiatric services can largely be accomplished online; indeed, emerging evidence suggests that there is little, if any, enhanced therapeutic value of having bodies in the same room, especially in the treatment of anxiety and depression [40]. If this is true, psychiatrists living in cities may no longer have the same costs in serving rural or foreign populations. Conversely, academies and public health systems may have less justification in continuing to offer incentives for psychiatrists to physically locate their practices in underserved areas. Extending this line of reasoning, should national health insurance move to save costs (and thus be able to re-allocate funds) by eliminating office space for outpatient visits and replacing with a telepsychiatry studio altogether?

Against this possibility, one might raise two objections: (1) even if it does not substantively change outpatient experience, having psychiatric services with a presence in hospitals is important in establishing and maintaining parity between mental health care and the rest of health care; (2) as neurotechnologies and biomarkers improve, psychiatrists will increasingly avail themselves of a hospital's other services, such as molecular pathology, imaging suites, etc., that are currently under-utilized in psychiatric practice. If we accept these objections, psychiatrists will regrettably have to continue to grapple with concerns of geography when evaluating justice regarding access to mental health care.

Another justice-based issue arises in e-health with the rapid expansion of peer-support apps and apps designed to aid in unmediated psychiatric treatment. While there is justified concern that peer-support apps are under-regulated, leading to suboptimal support for those who use it (for example, one peer-support app advises listeners to immediately end the chat if a user mentions suicide or suicidal ideation), it is reasonable to think that this family of apps may soon be able to provide some mental health services currently provided by mental health professionals. Because the time of mental health professionals is a limited resource, should mental health professionals strive to maximally use these unmediated tools, thereby freeing up the time they themselves currently spend providing those services and enabling them to provide to more people the services that are not outsourceable? Such a scenario would be supported by desires to do the most good and increase access to care for more people.

## Generalizing the new ethics

The pace of change in therapeutics, diagnostics, and prediction in psychiatry is poised to enter an inflection point. This change raises new ethical challenges for the practice of psychiatry, whether from the precision of neuroengineering-based therapies or the embraced imprecision of placebos, but also challenges the field's ethical frameworks as our ability to gain probabilistic insight into the mental vulnerabilities of ourselves and others. There is much of moral relevance under way that we have not discussed—the Do-It-Yourself movement in brain stimulation and the rapid progress of brain–computer interfaces, to name two examples. We hope, however, to have chosen cases that raise transferrable ethical challenges and, hopefully, places to start in thinking about, and discussing, how the practice of psychiatry *should* change in this rising tide of technology.

### REFERENCES

1. Holtzheimer, P.E. and Mayberg, H.S. (2011). Deep brain stimulation for psychiatric disorders. *Annual Review of Neuroscience*, 34, 289–307.

2. Mayberg, H.S., Riva-Posse, P., and Crowell, A.L. (2016). Deep brain stimulation for depression: keeping an eye on a moving target. *JAMA Psychiatry*, 73, 439–40.

3. Park, R.J., Godier, L.R., and Cowdrey, F.A. (2014). Hungry for reward: how can neuroscience inform the development of treatment for anorexia nervosa? *Behaviour Research and Therapy*, 62, 47–59.

4. Kocabicak, E., Temel, Y., Höllig, A., Falkenburger, B., and Tan, S.K. (2015). Current perspectives on deep brain stimulation for severe neurological and psychiatric disorders. *Neuropsychiatric Disease and Treatment*, 11, 1051–66.

5. Maslen, H., Pugh, J., and Savulescu, J. (2015). The ethics of deep brain stimulation for the treatment of anorexia nervosa. *Neuroethics*, 8, 215–30.

6. Kirsch, I., Deacon, B.J., Huedo-Medina, T.B., Scoboria, A., Moore, T.J., and Johnson, B.T. (2008). Initial severity and antidepressant benefits: a meta-analysis of data submitted to the Food and Drug Administration. *PLoS Medicine*, 5, e45.

7. Foddy, B., Kahane, G., and Savulescu, J. (2013). Practical neuropsychiatric ethics. In: Fulford, K.W.M., Davies, M., Gipps, R., *et al.* (eds.) *The Oxford handbook of philosophy and psychiatry*. Oxford University Press, Oxford. pp. 1185–201.

8. Shah, K.R. and Goold, S.D. (2009). The primacy of autonomy, honesty, and disclosure--Council on Ethical and Judicial Affairs' placebo opinions. *American Journal of Bioethics*, 9, 15–17.

9. Bingel, U. (2014). Avoiding nocebo effects to optimize treatment outcome. *JAMA*, 312, 693–4.

10. Enck, P., Bingel, U., Schedlowski, M., and Rief, W. (2013). The placebo response in medicine: minimize, maximize or personalize? *Nature Reviews Drug Discovery*, 12, 191–204.

11. Schedlowski, M., Enck, P., Rief, W., and Bingel, U. (2015). Neuro-bio-behavioral mechanisms of placebo and nocebo responses: implications for clinical trials and clinical practice. *Pharmacological Reviews*, 67, 697–730.

12. Nelson, B. and Yung, A.R. (2011). Should a risk syndrome for first episode psychosis be included in the DSM-5? *Current Opinion in Psychiatry*, 24, 128–33.

13. American Psychiatric Association. (2013). *Diagnostic and statistical manual of mental disorders (DSM-5)* (5th edn). American Psychiatric Association, Arlington, VA.

14. Kwon, D. 2017, march 8,-last update, *Can Facebook's Machine-Learning Algorithms Accurately Predict Suicide?*. Available: https://www-scientificamerican-com.ezp-prod1.hul.harvard.edu/article/can-facebooks-machine-learning-algorithms-accurately-predict-suicide/ [2017, Jul 24,].

15. Baum, M. (2016). *The neuroethics of biomarkers: what the development of bioprediction means for moral responsibility, justice, and the nature of mental disorder* (1st edn). Oxford University Press, Oxford and New York, NY.

16. American Psychiatric Association. (2000). *Diagnostic and statistical manual of mental disorders: DSM-IV-TR* (4th edn, text revision edn). American Psychiatric Association, Washington DC.

17. Stein, D.J., Phillips, K.A., Bolton, D., Fulford, K.W.M., Sadler, J.Z., and Kendler, K.S. (2010). What is a mental/psychiatric disorder? from DSM-IV to DSM-V. *Psychological Medicine*, 40, 1759–65.

18. Franklin, J.C., Ribeiro, J.D., Fox, K.R., *et al.* (2017). Risk factors for suicidal thoughts and behaviors: a meta-analysis of 50 years of research. *Psychological Bulletin*, 143, 187–232.

19. Thompson, I.M., Ankerst, D.P., Chi, C., *et al.* (2005). Operating characteristics of prostate-specific antigen in men with an initial PSA level of 3.0 ng/ml or lower. *JAMA*, 294, 66–70.

20. Savulescu, J. and Kahane, G. (2011). Disability: a welfarist approach. *Clinical Ethics*, 6, 45–51.

21. Savulescu, J. and Kahane, G. (2009). The welfarist account of disability. In: Cureton, A. and Brownlee, K. (eds.) *Disability and disadvantage*. Oxford University Press, Oxford. pp. 14–53.

22. Jonsson, U., Alaie, I., Löfgren W., *et al.* (2017). Annual Research Review: quality of life and childhood mental and behavioural disorders—a critical review of the research. *Journal of Child Psychology and Psychiatry*, 58, 439–69.

23. Savulescu, J. and Kahane, G. (2017) Understanding procreative beneficence: the nature and extent of the moral obligation to have the best child. In: Francis, L. (ed.) *The Oxford Handbook of Reproductive Ethics*. Oxford University Press, Oxford. pp. 592–622.

24. Kahneman, D. and Varey, C. (1991). Notes on the psychology of utility. In: Elster, J. and Roemer, J.E. (eds.) *Interpersonal comparisons of well-being*. Cambridge University Press, New York, NY. pp. 127–63.

25. Savulescu, J. and Momeyer, R.W. (1997). Should informed consent be based on rational beliefs? *Journal of Medical Ethics*, 23, 282–8.

26. Parfit, D. (1984). *Reasons and persons*. Oxford University Press, Oxford.

27. Lejuste, F., Thomas, L., Picard, G., *et al.* (2016). Neuroleptic intolerance in patients with anti-NMDAR encephalitis. *Neurology Neuroimmunology and Neuroinflammation*, 3, e280.

28. Aristotle. (1999). *Nicomachean ethics* (2nd edn), translated by Irwin, T. Hackett Publishing Company, Indianapolis, IN.

29. Chai, P.R., Castillo-Mancilla, J., Buffkin, E., *et al.* (2015). Utilizing an ingestible biosensor to assess real-time medication adherence. *Journal of Medical Toxicology*, 11, 439–44.

30. Dresser, R.S. (1982). Ulysses and the psychiatrists: a legal and policy analysis of the voluntary commitment contract. *Harvard Civil Rights-Civil Liberties Law Review*, 16, 777–854.

31. EWHC 2741 (COP). (2012). *The NHS Trust v L and Others*. http://www.39essex.com/cop_cases/the-nhs-trust-v-l-and-others/ (accessed 6 February 2018).

32. EWHC 1639 (COP). (2012). *A Local Authority v E and Others*. http://www.39essex.com/cop_cases/a-local-authority-v-e-and-others/ (accessed 6 February 2018).

33. Douglas, T., Pugh, J., Singh, I., Savulescu, J., and Fazel, S. (2017). Risk assessment tools in criminal justice and forensic psychiatry: the need for better data. *European Psychiatry*, 42, 134–7.

34. Baum, M.L. and Savulescu, J. (2013). Behavioural biomarkers: what are they good for? In: Singh, I., Sinott-Armstrong, W., and Savulescu, J. (eds) *Bioprediction of bad behavior: scientific, legal, and ethical challenges*. Oxford University Press, New York, NY. pp. 12–41.

35. Baum, M.L. (2013). The monoamine oxidase A (MAOA) genetic predisposition to impulsive violence: is it relevant to criminal trials? *Neuroethics*, 6, 287–306.

36. Smith, H. (1983). Culpable ignorance. *The Philosophical Review*, 92, 543–71.

37. Glannon, W. (1998). Moral responsibility and personal identity. *American Philosophical Quarterly*, 35, 249.

38. World Health Organization. (2015). *Mental health atlas 2014*. World Health Organization, Geneva.

39. Hilferty, F., Cassells, R., Muir, K., *et al.* (2015). *Is headspace making a difference to young people's lives? Final Report of the independent evaluation of the headspace program*. Social Policy Research Centre, University of New South Wales, Sydney.

40. Andersson, G., Cuijpers, P., Carlbring, P., Riper, H., and Hedman, E. (2014). Guided Internet-based vs. face-to-face cognitive behavior therapy for psychiatric and somatic disorders: a systematic review and meta-analysis. *World Psychiatry*, 13, 288–95.

# 6

# Foundations of phenomenology/ descriptive psychopathology

*Hans-Jürgen Möller*

## Introduction

Phenomenology or descriptive psychopathology, that is the knowledge of psychopathological phenomena or symptoms, has a long tradition in psychiatry and is much older than the diagnostic systems commonly used today. Correctly applied, it forms the basis for clinical psychiatry as an empirical science [1]. Because the term phenomenology also has a broader, philosophical meaning, the term 'descriptive psychopathology' is much more commonly used nowadays.

In psychiatry the term phenomenology is sometimes used in a wider sense to refer to a method of describing, holistically and hermeneutically, all that is characteristic for a person and his situation, a notion which is used in anthropological or 'daseins'-analytical psychiatry [2]. This methodological approach, which is not very common in modern psychiatry, is based, among other things, on the philosophical tradition of the philosophers Husserl and, in particular, Heidegger (with components such as 'essences', 'interpretation of senses', 'existential interpretation of an individual rational world', 'study of structures', etc.). The approach is characterized by intuitive holistic perception and understanding of the world and the person [3–5]. However, this chapter will not cover this extension of phenomenology but rather review descriptive psychopathology in the stricter sense.

## Principles and limitations of descriptive psychopathology

In this context, 'descriptive' means that symptoms are recorded as far as possible without any theoretical assumptions, for example with respect to certain disease diagnoses or hypotheses of causes, and as far as possible objectively. In clinical diagnostics, the descriptive psychopathological assessment and the creation of a disease/ disorder diagnosis or formulation are ideally performed in two independent stages. Nevertheless, it may be useful later in the further course of diagnosing a particular patient, once a presumed diagnosis has been established, to explore more closely particular symptoms that may or may not be relevant for a specific diagnosis.

Descriptive psychopathology is based on an assessment of symptoms that is as objective as possible, that is, the abnormalities found in the experience and behaviour of the patient should preferably not depend on the individual examiner, the adherence to a particular psychiatric school, the methodology of exploration, the general theoretical attitude (for example, more neurobiological or more psychological), positive and negative expectations, the psychological interaction with the examinee, etc. Moreover, the assessment should be determined in generally the same way by other professionally competent examiners. For various reasons, for example different definitions of symptoms, the completely independent psychopathological diagnostic assessment is in danger of failing to achieve this ideal. To increase the validity and reliability of the assessment, examiners use aids such as symptom lists with exact symptom definitions or even fully structured interviews, especially in research contexts. The clinical psychopathological diagnostic assessment then moves increasingly towards being a fully standardized diagnostic approach, usually involving the use of scales that no longer only make qualitative, but also quantitative, statements. When applying these standardized assessment methods, the diagnostic concordance of the examiners is often additionally improved by 'rater training'. This use of scales is a modern variant of descriptive psychopathology [6] that does not have the width and subtle differentiation of classical descriptive psychopathology.

Regardless of efforts to improve inter-observer reliability, every psychopathological diagnostic assessment—the classical clinical one, as well as the standardized one—is threatened by various biases, as described in the field of empirical social psychology. These cannot be completely excluded, but rather limited by careful conscious control of the interview process [7, 8].

Systematic distortion of the assessor's observations can result from the following factors in particular:

- Rosenthal effect: the assessors expectations influence the result of the assessment; tendency on the side of the assessor to systematically over- or under-rate the degree of disturbance.

- Halo effect: the results of the assessment of one characteristic are influenced by the assessors knowledge of the patient's other characteristics or by the overall impression made by the patient.
- Logical errors: the result of the assessment is influenced by assessors reporting only those detailed observations that make sense to them in the context of their theoretical and logical preconceptions.

Another limiting factor of a diagnostic assessment is the patient him- or herself. The patient may show only limited openness to describing psychopathological changes or may have a distorted perception of them. Besides these main types of self-report distortions, one must consider the following:

- Conscious or unconscious tendencies to exaggerate or conceal symptoms.
- Positive response bias and social desirability effects.

There are several others causes of discrepancy between observer views and patient self-reports. In the field of standardized rating scales, examples of the quality and quantity of such discrepancies can be found by comparing the results of observer rating scales and self-rating scales [7, 8]. The risk of discrepant findings can be reduced by having as optimal an interaction with the patient as possible and using a competent and sensitive interview technique.

Descriptive psychopathology is understood as the description of observable phenomena or those experienced and reported by the patient. It does not mean the phenomena developed under psychodynamic/psychoanalytic reconstruction.

It is a general rule of assessment in the context of descriptive psychopathology that an empathic, understanding attitude based on respect is the essential basis for a careful and patient-oriented assessment of psychopathological findings. To guarantee as objective an assessment as possible, it is also important to find the right balance between empathy-related closeness and objectivity-related distance.

## Objective 'description' of psychopathological phenomena as an ideal standard

If we designate a psychopathological procedure as 'descriptive', we require that the symptoms be recorded and named as simply as possible in a way that is verifiable and clearly organized, without letting aetiological assumptions, pathogenetic hypotheses, or interpretative elements about the individual or social 'meaning' of certain symptoms (or their meaning as would be typical for the reference group) be included in this phase of the diagnostic process.

Some experts claim that less attention should be paid to symptoms whose presence cannot be 'determined' but only inferred. This is an echo of the distinction between 'signs' and 'symptoms', which is well established in the English-speaking world, but less known elsewhere. Thus, DSM-IV defines a sign as 'an objective manifestation of a pathological condition' that is 'observed by the examiner rather than reported by the affected individual', and the symptom as 'a subjective manifestation of a pathological condition' that is 'reported by the affected individual rather than observed by the examiner'.

In practice, descriptive psychopathological diagnostic assessment no longer so clearly preserves this distinction, and it is no longer found in this strict version in DSM-5. This is demonstrated in particular by psychomotor symptoms, which refer to the inseparable binding of subjective experience that relates to mood with objective, directly observable motor behaviour [9].

Without question, the impartial assessment of mental phenomena, that is of what a patient describes and experiences, what they remember, what they plan, and the way they act, is a crucial prerequisite for all careful psychiatric practice and research. However, it would be premature to consider this objective fully achievable by choosing a descriptive approach.

Incidentally, this approach can be applied in the same way at the nosological level. DSM-III, published in 1980, was the first standardized diagnostic manual that placed the focus on the independence of the descriptive from the aetiological level and referred to this approach with the rather prematurely chosen term 'atheoretical'. Since then, a process of differentiation has taken place, which highlights more clearly that freedom from *any* theoretical presupposition—which is basically impossible—was and is not meant. Rather, freedom is sought from implicit assumptions about the cause of each symptom or of the respective disorder. In order to prevent the emergence or strengthening of scientific prejudices during the diagnostic process, recognition of implicit assumptions is of crucial importance, be it on the symptom, syndrome, or nosological level [9]. 'Description' can be easily understood as a sober, factual portrayal of something 'objectively' present, similar to the function of a photographic apparatus used by the examiner. The description of psychopathological symptoms, however, is a communication between the patient and the examiner, that is an interpersonal process [4]. This has a different meaning for different symptoms—a symptom such as 'disoriented to place' can be more clearly and 'objectively' determined than the presence of 'thought broadcasting', for example. However, this does not change the fundamental nature of psychopathological description as a process that is characterized through a relationship, among other things.

In general terms, this means that the description is highly dependent on the nature of the symptom, because observable behaviour can be more easily described than internal experiences. Karl Jaspers attached great importance to the finding that 'mental phenomena' never show themselves directly (and consequently also cannot be directly observed), but only indirectly through language, writing, gestures, facial expressions, artistic expression, or behaviour. Therefore, it is all the more important always to be clear about what is actually being 'described' in the descriptive approach [9], that is about:

- The externally recognizable behaviour of the patient.
- His own statements about the current experience.
- Assumptions about the current subjective experience of the patient that the examiner makes on the basis of certain perceptions and ratings (What? Why this one?), although the patient himself perhaps explains them quite differently or even not at all.
- Information from a third party about the patient's behaviour and experiences.

These examples illustrate that in psychopathology, 'description' refers to a complex field of activity. Besides the recording of psychopathological information, it also includes the critical consideration of the respective sources of the things being described and the respective relational context. The procedure is complicated, among other things, by the fact that the effort to achieve a descriptive recording of the 'phenomenon' cannot, in principle, be entirely separated from a basic understanding of psychopathology and the associated view of human beings. The examiner should be aware that every psychopathological 'description' moves necessarily between the poles of the subjective experience of the patient and examiner, their relationship, and the objectifying determination of facts.

## Pioneers of descriptive psychopathology

### Karl Jaspers

Jaspers' work *General Psychopathology* [10–12] is still regarded as the standard work of descriptive psychopathology. In it, he not only gave an excellent description of psychopathological phenomena, but also additionally discussed fundamental questions about assessing mental phenomena and, going far beyond a mere description of symptoms, discussed aspects of the relationship and backgrounds of psychopathological phenomena. His distinction between 'explaining' and 'understanding' has meaning still today.

Thus, Jaspers made a strong distinction between scientific explanation, which is based on causality, and understanding, which aims to recreate the mental thoughts of another person. He also spoke in this context of the 'phenomenological direction' in psychopathology, with which he mainly meant the respectful and careful engaging of the examiner with the patient's self-portrayal; he warned about prematurely following the supposed obligation to objectify and standardize the findings. He would not have favoured check-box approaches to the identification of symptoms in structured interviews.

Jaspers was fully aware of the importance of a clear terminology for psychopathology. His response to the inherent tension, present in each diagnostic assessment, between subjective experience and standardization, was: 'The envisioning of mental experiences and states, their differentiation and determination, so that one can always mean the same with the terms, is the task of phenomenology' [12, p. 22 ff]. As the first, indispensable step, however, such a phenomenological approach provides the examiner only with 'a number of fragments of the real mental experience', and he envisions 'individual qualities, individual states viewed as dormant' and thus practises 'static understanding'.

'Genetic understanding' appeared to be more important to him in the psychopathological assessment. This 'understanding' deals with the relationship between individual psychological states—in Jaspers' words, with the understanding of 'how mental processes emerge with evidence from mental processes' [12].

An important aspect for Jaspers was the 'genetic understanding of biographical contexts' with psychopathological phenomena. This may seem reminiscent of psychodynamic approaches, but the theoretical context is completely different and makes no psychoanalytic assumptions. It is instead based on a 'common sense psychology' of the relevant own life experiences of the examiner. Jaspers described not only clinical–psychopathological phenomena (which he did with impressive conciseness and often supplemented with case reports), but also the basics of a healthy psyche. One could only approach assessing the entirety of the mentally healthy or disturbed person—this is one of the core ideas—via the uniqueness of each patient, which is based on the patient's biography. However, this entirety is never fully accessible by scientific means.

This brief description will have made clear that he was concerned with far more than describing the specific mental/psychopathological phenomenon, with the holistic assessment of the inner connection of mental phenomena and their relationship to personal experiences.

## Kurt Schneider

Like Jaspers, Kurt Schneider is another important representative of the descriptive approach in psychiatry. Unlike Jaspers, he represents a descriptive approach in the narrower sense, and accordingly his remarks are less extensive. In continuation of Jaspers' perspective, however, he did not split the mental state into unconnected adjoining single elements but preserved an understanding of the overall context. He called this process 'descriptive-analytic'. Even more so than Jaspers, Schneider was interested in carefully clinically justified and, if possible, highly selective psychopathological terminology that should be the guiding principle for the diagnostic process. He was also interested, among other things, in the question of whether characteristic, or possibly even pathognomonic, symptoms exist for certain diseases. Representative of this approach are his remarks about 'first-rank symptoms' and 'second-rank symptoms', with which he paved the way for modern operationalized diagnostics. His most famous work *Clinical Psychopathology* was continually developed in individual contributions from the 1920s; the book appeared under this title for the first time in 1950; the fifteenth edition appeared in 2007 [13, 14].

Recently, efforts have been made to assess descriptively and operationally even more theoretically fraught and not directly observable psychopathological conditions, such as aspects of psychodynamic relationships and defensive strategies [15]. They represent attempts supplementary to operational psychodynamic diagnostics (OPD) [16] but go beyond traditional classical descriptive phenomenology.

## Descriptive assessment of psychopathological symptoms

The descriptive assessment of psychopathological symptoms which follows is based on the most recent version of the manual by the Association for Methodology and Documentation in Psychiatry (AMDP) [17, 18]. Earlier editions of the AMDP manual, which was originally published in German, have been translated into several languages, including English [19].

The AMDP system was chosen because it reflects most comprehensively the continental European psychopathological tradition. Also, despite all its differentiation, it covers the whole spectrum of psychopathology, with a special focus on productive-psychotic and affective symptoms, and is easy to use both clinically and scientifically. In the recent past, enhancements were made in certain areas that were previously assessed only somewhat or not at all in the AMDP system, such as psychomotor function, basic schizophrenic disorders, personality traits, and some symptoms common in 'neurotic' disorders. In order to address these shortcomings, in particular with a view to their use in psychiatric research, additional 'modules' for the AMDP system were also developed [20].

## Disturbances of consciousness

'Disturbance of consciousness' is the generic term for any changes in the level of consciousness. A distinction is made between quantitative changes in consciousness (reduced awareness in the sense of the sleep–wake scale) and qualitative changes (reduced, limited, and shifted consciousness).

A quantitative disturbance of consciousness (reduction of vigilance) is assumed if a patient appears dazed or drowsy and a reduced perception of external stimuli can be detected. The degrees of impaired consciousness can be described as follows:

- Decreased clarity: the patient is very contemplative, slowed down, and restricted in acquiring and processing information.
- Somnolence: the patient is abnormally drowsy but is easily woken up.
- Stupor: the patient is asleep, and only strong stimuli can wake him.
- Coma: the patient is unconscious and cannot be woken up. In a deep coma, the pupillary, corneal, and tendon reflexes are absent.

### Qualitative disturbances of consciousness

- Clouded consciousness: lack of clarity of awareness of oneself or the environment. The associations of experience are lost, and consciousness is as if fragmented. Thinking and acting are confused. Clouding of consciousness is easily recognizable for anyone who has seen this state.
- Narrowed consciousness: narrowing of field of consciousness, for example by focusing on a specific experience (intra-personal or in the environment), mostly combined with reduced response to stimuli (for example, the epileptic semi-conscious state). The experience is changed in a dream-like way. Complicated and outwardly organized actions, such as travel, are nevertheless still possible. The assessment of narrowed consciousness can be problematic precisely because of the ability to perform outwardly organized actions.
- Changed consciousness: change in consciousness, compared with the usual daily consciousness. There is a feeling of increased intensity and brightness and of increased awareness regarding alertness and perception of happenings inside or in the outside world and/or a feeling of magnification of the space or depth that can be consciously recognized (expansion of consciousness). This condition is difficult to detect and only possible on the basis of subjective information provided by the person being examined.

### Disturbances of orientation

Lack of knowledge about temporal, spatial, situational, and/or personal circumstances. Depending on the intensity of the disturbance, one can differentiate between restricted orientation or loss of orientation.

The following forms are distinguished:

- Time: patients do not know the date, day, year, or season.
- Place: patients do not know where they are.
- Situation: patients are not aware of the situation in which they currently find themselves (for example, examination in the hospital).
- Self: patients lack knowledge about their own name, date of birth, and other important personal biographical circumstances.

## Disorders of attention and concentration

Disorders of attention and concentration are defined as an impairment in the ability to fully direct the perception mediated by the sensations or perceptions to focus on a particular subject.

- Attention disorders: scope and intensity of the assimilation of perceptions, ideas, or thoughts are impaired.
- Concentration disorders: ability to maintain attention on a specific activity or a particular object or situation is impaired.

The course of the interview will provide indications of whether patients are restricted in their ability to fully focus their perception on the information mediated by their sensations or in their ability to concentrate on a particular object or situation. Abnormalities in writing, such as omissions or duplication of letters, may also provide clues.

### Perception disorders

Perception disorders are defined as an impairment of the ability to understand the relevance of perceptual experiences and to interconnect them. Perception may be wrong, slowed or completely missing.

### Retention and memory disorders

These disorders are defined as a reduced ability to recall new and old experiences. Traditional psychopathology differentiates between retention and memory disorders. Modern psychological theories of memory differentiate between ultra-short (seconds), short-term (minutes), and long-term memory.

Disorders of memory functions can be generally assessed during the evaluation interview. Can the patient remember the examiner's questions? Do they know what was discussed in an earlier part of the conversation? They may report spontaneously about subjectively perceived forgetfulness. Perhaps they now have to use written reminders to help with shopping or in other life situations, whereas they previously did not make any such notes. The description of the life history and current life situation often provides clear indications of memory gaps, which are then sometimes filled by confabulations. Time lattice defects, that is the inability to report biographical facts in the correct temporal order, also provide information on memory disorders.

Besides the question of subjectively perceived disorders of retention and memory, such disorders are assessed by a preliminary clinical evaluation. Objectively observable behavioural traits are of greater importance than the patient's self-assessment, which can be marked by affect-related feelings of insufficiency.

- *Retention disorders* refer to a recall period of up to about 10 minutes.
- *Memory disorders* refer to a recall period of longer than about 10 minutes. A distinction is made between recent and remote memory disorders:
  - *Short-term memory disorder*: the reduction or loss of the ability to retain impressions or experiences for up to 60 minutes.
  - *Long-term memory disorder*: the reduction or loss of the ability to retain impressions or experiences that took place longer than 60 minutes ago or even further in the past, including biographical events, for example.

Memory disorders also include amnesia.

*Amnesia*: memory gaps limited to a particular event or time. With respect to a traumatic event (for example, brain damage), a distinction is made between retrograde amnesia, in which a certain period of time before the event is affected, and anterograde amnesia, in which a certain period of time after the event is affected. In anterograde amnesia, the duration of the memory gap is usually longer than the duration of unconsciousness. With regard to the period affected by the memory gap, one can distinguish between total and lacunar (episodic) amnesia.

- *Confabulations*: memory gaps are filled with ideas that patients themselves view as memories.
- *Paramnesias (delusional memories)*: memory disorders with fantasy memories. These also include the so-called false recognition, for example the feeling of having experienced certain situations previously ('déjà vu') or never having experienced them ('jamais vu').
- *Transient global amnesia (TGA)*: acute, transient episode of retention and memory disorders of unclear aetiology. Routine actions are possible. Amnesia exists for the duration of the episode.

## Disorders of intelligence

Intelligence is a complex ability of people to find their way in unfamiliar situations, to capture meaning and relationship contexts, and to meet new requirements through logical functions. Intellectual impairment disorders can be congenital or acquired later in life.

The main indications of the patient's intellectual level are already apparent from their *life story*, for example the type of school education, being held back a year in school, school-leaving qualification, professional status achieved, recreational interests. Also the style of speaking and thought processes (abstract level) during the interview allow orientating conclusions to be drawn. A decrease in professional standing and a reduction in the intellectual level of leisure activities, compared to the past, may also indicate an acquired mental retardation, after other factors have been excluded.

## Formal thought disorders

Formal thought disorders are disorders of thought sequence. They are subjectively perceived by the patient or express themselves in verbal utterances.

The following forms are distinguished:

- *Retarded thinking*: the thought process is slow and delayed, appears to be tedious for the patient and is often experienced subjectively by the patient as inhibited thinking.
- *Circumstantial thinking*: thinking is circuitous; irrelevant thoughts are not separated from relevant ones. The main point is lost in the portrayal of insignificant details.
- *Restricted thinking*: restriction of the substantive scope of thinking, attached to an issue or a few topics.
- *Perseveration*: repetition of the same thought contents and adherence to previous words or information that were used but now no longer make sense.
- *Rumination*: constantly busy with certain, usually unpleasant, thoughts that are not experienced by the patient as foreign and usually are related to the current life situation.

- *Pressured thinking*: the patient feels under excessive pressure from many ideas and also constantly recurring thoughts.
- *Flight of ideas*: excessive imaginative thought. Thinking no longer follows a strict direction but changes or loses the goal because of interruptive associations.
- *Tangential thinking*: the patient does not respond to the question and talks around or past the point, although it is apparent from the response and/or situation that they have understood the question.
- *Thought blocking*: sudden interruption of an otherwise fluent train of thought for no apparent reason.
- *Paralogia*: the sentence structure is grammatically still intact, but the consequence of the intellectual context and/or the level of detail of what is said is reduced.
- *Incoherence*: erratic, dissociated thought process, in which the logical and associative dimensions are missing. In severe forms, the grammatical sentence structure is lacking (paragrammatism), all the way to an incomprehensible mix of words and syllables ('word salad', schizophasia).
- *Neologisms*: building of new phrases or words that do not meet the usual language conventions and often are not easily understood.

## Delusions

A delusion is an *uncorrectable* false assessment of reality that occurs independently of experience and which the patient holds onto with *subjective certainty*. The conviction is therefore contrary to reality and to the conviction of others. Delusional phenomena can occur in different forms and with different content.

Delusions belong to the group of *content thought disorders*. They are often hidden and, if suspected, need to be specifically explored and differentiated from *overvalued ideas*. In the latter, strongly emotional thoughts about experiences dominate thinking in a non-objective and one-sided way, but such ideas are not absolutely incorrigible.

Depending on the type of delusion formation, the following forms are distinguished:

- *Sudden delusional thoughts*: sudden occurrence of delusional beliefs.
- *Delusional perceptions*: a normal perception gives rise to an interpretation of delusional and abnormal importance.
- *Explanatory delusions*: delusional conviction for the explanation of psychotic symptoms (for example, hallucinations).

The following terms are useful for the further characterization of the delusional experience:

- *Delusional mood*: sense of the uncanny, the ambiguous, from which delusional ideas arise. General, unclear feeling that something is wrong and is in the air, and that everything concerns the person. The events in the surroundings seem strange and unusual to the person. Because they do not know what is happening to them and what is going on, they become anxious, perplexed, and bewildered. A delusional mood frequently precedes delusional perception.
- *Delusional dynamics*: affective participation in the delusion; the driving force and strength of the emotions in the delusion.
- *Systematic delusions*: delusional ideas are embellished with logical or paralogical associations to a delusional building.

Depending on the content of the delusion, the following can be distinguished:

- *Delusions of reference*: random events are ascribed particular importance for the self.
- *Delusions of persecution*: patients have delusions of being the target of persecution.
- *Delusions of jealousy*: delusional conviction of being cheated on or deceived by one's partner.
- *Delusions of love*: delusional conviction of being loved by another.
- *Delusions of guilt*: delusional conviction to have defied, for example, God's commandments or a higher moral instance.
- *Delusions of impoverishment*: delusional conviction that the financial basis of life is threatened or lost.
- *Hypochondriacal delusions*: delusional conviction that health is threatened or lost or that one has a specific physical illness.
- *Nihilistic delusions*: delusional conviction that all is lost, everything is forlorn, everything is hopeless.
- *Delusions of grandiosity*: delusional overestimation of self all the way to identification with famous personalities from the past or present.
- *Delusions of memory*: delusional falsification of memories.
- *Doppelgänger delusions*: delusional notion that there is a doppelgänger.

### Hallucinations

Hallucinations are perceptual experiences without an appropriate external stimulus, but which are still considered to be real sensations. They are also referred to as false perceptions and can occur in all sensory domains. The degree to which they are convincingly real may differ.

If the unreality of the hallucination is recognized, one refers to *pseudohallucinations*. These are to be differentiated from *illusions*, in which something that really exists is believed to be something else than it actually is (misreading of sensations).

Depending on the sensory area, one differentiates between the following:

- *Auditory hallucinations*: they can range from unformed, elementary acoustic perceptions (acoasma) to hallucinatory experiences of complicated acoustic phenomena (for example, hearing voices).
- *Optical hallucinations*: they can range from unformed, elementary optical illusions (photomes) to the hallucinatory experience of crafted scenes.
- *Olfactory and gustatory hallucinations*: patients with a delusional fear of poisoning claim, for example, to smell gas.
- *Bodily hallucinations*: bodily perceptions are not perceived as being due to external stimulation.

### Hypnagogic hallucinations

These are optical and acoustic hallucinations that occur when people are half asleep, that is when waking up or falling asleep. They can also occur in healthy people without mental illness, as can any hallucinations in various borderline situations (for example, in case of sensory deprivation and meditation).

### Other disorders of perception

Unlike hallucinations, these changes in perception are usually much easier to assess because they do not appear to patients as being so far from normal mental experience.

- *Change in the intensity of perceptions*: sensory impressions are more colourful, lively, colourless, or hazy.
- *Micro-/macropsia*: objects are perceived to be smaller, or further away, or closer.
- *Metamorphopsia (dysmorphopsia)*: the colour or shape of objects is perceived to be changed or distorted.

## Disorders of ego

Disorders in which the egocentricity of experience is altered (derealization, depersonalization) or the boundary between self and the environment appears to be porous.

One differentiates between the following:

- *Depersonalization*: the own ego or bodily parts are perceived as being foreign, unreal, or changed.
- *Derealization*: the environment appears to patients as unreal, strange, or spatially altered.
- *Thought broadcasting*: the patient complains that their thoughts no longer belong to them alone and that others are sharing them and know what they think.
- *Thought withdrawal*: patients have the feeling that thoughts are being taken away from them.
- *Thought insertion*: patients are of the opinion that their thoughts and ideas are externally inserted, influenced, guided, and controlled.
- *Other feelings of alien influence*: patients are of the opinion that their feelings, aspirations, will, and actions are externally made, directed, and controlled.

## Disorders of affect

The realm of affect includes the usually only brief *emotions* ('waves of emotion', for example, anger, rage, hate, joy) and the longer-lasting *moods* (for example, depression).

- *Affective lability/mood lability*: rapid change in affect or mood.
- *Affective incontinence*: lack of control of expressed emotions.
- *Blunted affect*: state of low affect and emotional responsivity. Patients appear indifferent, emotionally restrained, listless, and disinterested.
- *Feelings of loss of feeling*: painfully experienced lack or loss of affective emotion.
- *Affective rigidity*: reduction in the ability to modulate affect. Patients remain in certain moods or affects, regardless of the external situation.
- *Inner restlessness*: patients complain that they are emotionally moved and are agitated or tense.
- *Dysphoria*: sullen mood.
- *Irritability*: tendency for aggressive emotional outbursts.

- *Ambivalence*: contradictory feelings towards a particular person, idea, or action exist side-by-side and lead to a tense state.
- *Euphoria*: state of excessive well-being and of pleasure, joy, confidence, and increased vitality.
- *Foolish affect*: silly, empty cheerfulness with a touch of simple-mindedness, foolishness, and immaturity.
- *Depressed mood*: depressed, rather negative state in the sense of dejection, sadness, listlessness, and hopelessness.
- *Loss of vitality*: reduced general feelings of energy and vitality, of physical and mental freshness, and of being unimpaired.
- *Feelings of inadequacy*: feeling of having no value and of being inept and incapable.
- *Exaggerated self-esteem*: the feeling of being particularly valuable and particularly competent.
- *Parathymia*: inappropriate mood; expressions of emotion and experiences do not match.

The prevailing mood and emotions can be evaluated in the course of the interview, as long as the interview is sufficiently long and gives patients the opportunity to talk about their emotions. Through targeted exploration, one can try to obtain a differentiated description from patients about their affective state.

## Compulsions, phobias, anxiety, and hypochondriasis

- *Fear*: feeling of threat and danger, usually accompanied by vegetative symptoms such as palpitations, sweating, shortness of breath, tremor, dry mouth, or gastric pressure.
- *Phobias*: fear of an object or situation.
- *Suspiciousness*: fear that one is the object of someone's scheming.
- *Hypochondriasis*: concern about one's own health that cannot be objectively explained but that is tenaciously held on to.
- *Obsessive thoughts*: thoughts that cannot be suppressed and that are either senseless or whose persistence and penetrance are perceived to be meaningless and mostly distressing.
- *Compulsive actions*: actions perceived as meaningless and mostly distressing that usually cannot be suppressed; mostly due to compulsive impulses or compulsive fears.

## Disturbances of drive and psychomotility

This term summarizes all disorders that affect the energy, initiative, and activity of a person (*drive*) and the overall movements affected by mental processes (*psychomotility*). These disorders are usually diagnosed by observing the patient.

The following types are distinguished:

- *Lack of drive*: lack of energy and initiative, can be recognized by the scarcity of spontaneous motor activity and lack of activity.
- *Inhibition of drive*: in contrast to lack of drive, patients with inhibited drive do not experience their initiative and energy as reduced, but rather as inhibited. 'Everything is a little harder than usual; it's as if I'm inhibited, but so far hardly anyone has noticed.'
- *Stuporous*: motor immobility and lack of reactions despite normal neurological findings (in contrast to coma).
- *Mutism*: ranges from taciturnity to not speaking, even though organs of speech and the ability to speak are intact.
- *Logorrhoea*: excessive talkativeness. Because of an insatiable urge to speak, no meaningful communication is possible with the patient. Patients ignore or reject attempts to interrupt them.
- *Increased drive*: increased activity and initiative during organized (targeted) activity. Patients express numerous wishes and plans, which are only partially put into action. They are constantly active, are not impressed by counterarguments and ignore or do not care about personal consequences.
- *Motor restlessness*: aimless and undirected motor activity that can increase up to a frenzy. Patients are constantly moving and can therefore have hardly any or no normal social contacts. During the evaluation they cannot stay sitting on the chair and have to get up and walk up and down.
- *Automatisms*: patients perform automatic actions which they describe as not being intentional. These include negativisms (in response to a request, they automatically perform the opposite or nothing at all), automatic obedience (automatic following of instructions), and echolalia/echopraxia (everything a patient hears or sees is repeated or imitated).
- *Indecisiveness*: simultaneous, contradictory impulses make decisive actions impossible.
- *Stereotypy*: language and motor expressions that are repeated in the same way and seem to be meaningless.
- *Tics*: uniformly recurring, rapid, and involuntary muscle twitches, possibly with expressive content.
- *Paramimia*: Mimicking behaviour and affective experience do not concur.
- *Mannerisms*: strange, unnatural, contrived, posing behavioural traits.
- *Histrionics*: patients give the impression that they are presenting themselves in a way that dramatizes their situation or symptoms.
- *Aggressiveness*: tendency to act violently.
- *Social withdrawal*: reduction in social contacts.
- *Social activity*: expansion of social contacts. Patients approach many people, frequently cling indiscriminately to people, lack distance and are always on the go and querulous. They constantly talk to strangers and do not notice when they annoy others. The environment reacts negatively.

Some of these symptoms are traditionally regarded as *catatonic symptoms*. These symptoms are particularly common in the context of the catatonic subtype of schizophrenia and are divided into:

- *Psychomotor hyperphenomena*: psychomotor agitation, movement and speech stereotypes, automatic obedience (echopraxia, echolalia).
- *Psychomotor hypophenomena*: blocking, stupor and mutism, negativism, catalepsy (remaining in a position with passive bodily posture), stereotypical positions, and flexibilitas cerea (wax-like flexibility when moved passively).

## Summarizing psychopathological findings: the psychopathological state (mental state examination)

At the end of the exploration, the symptomatology is summarized as a *psychopathological evaluation*. One tries to create a picture of the patient's current psychopathological condition in an abstract, and yet still concrete enough, manner.

One usually starts with the appearance (habitus, external presentation, physiognomy, and also psychomotility and drive), because this is the easiest to assess. Then the specific behaviour and speech (way of speaking, sound of the voice, modulation, spontaneity) during the interview are described. Thereafter (if applicable!), details are given on changes in consciousness, attention, attitude, orientation, memory, affect, and drive (affective contact, intensity and modulation of affective reactions, basic mood, mood swings, compulsive needs, will control, etc.). This is followed by a discussion of disorders of perception (including hallucinations), disturbances of formal thought and thought content (delusions, obsessive thoughts), and disorders of ego.

One should note that the summary is not just a list of psychopathological terms with a note on whether they are not at all present or mild, moderate, or severe. Rather, one must create a true picture of the *current mental state* of the patient.

One should also go beyond these areas and provide information on possible demonstrative traits or simulation/dissimulation tendencies, malaise and illness insight, and special risks.

## Conclusions

Descriptive psychopathology, or the knowledge of psychopathological symptoms and abnormal experiences and behaviours, is the basis for clinical diagnosis in psychiatry. The symptoms or syndromes recorded within the descriptive psychopathological assessment can be used in the clinical or scientific context, for example in the sense of a syndrome diagnosis [21]. They can also serve to make a diagnosis at a higher level of diagnostics by using certain traditional nosological entities or modern operationalized disease/disorder concepts such as those defined in ICD-10 or DSM-5, for example. While the criteria for the different diseases/disorders can change with each revision of the classification systems, as happened, for example, in the transition from DSM-IV to DSM-5 [22, 23], the description of the symptoms almost always remains stable. Thus, descriptive psychopathology represents the basis of our practice as clinical psychiatrists, and we should use it in everyday clinical practice, as well as in clinical research. Although knowledge of, and competency in, traditional descriptive psychopathology have tended continuously to decrease as part of the development of the operational diagnosis systems such as ICD-10 and especially DSM-IV and DSM-5 [24], descriptive psychopathology is still an important tool for clinical psychiatry [25].

The Research Domain Criteria (RDoC), developed by the National Institute of Mental Health (NIMH), tend to greatly limit the importance of classical descriptive psychopathology and clinical findings for research approaches [26] (see Chapter 8). The reason is that the RDoC focus more on reductionist dimensions detectable at a neuropsychological level as the target of neurobiological research, rather than on complex psychopathological syndromes. This approach may make it easier to achieve research results, but the transformation of these results into the more complex constructs (syndromes) of clinical psychopathology is difficult; for example, a 'depressive syndrome' is more than just a score on a 'negative valence system'.

Psychopathological findings represent the core of psychiatric diagnosis. This statement, which, at first glance, appears obvious, is nowadays no longer a general consensus. In particular, other diagnostic procedures, such as neuropsychological, neurophysiological, biochemical, genetic, and imaging procedures, have greatly increased in relevance and authority through the scientific developments of the last decades. We stand at an important historical juncture where these diagnostic methods have increased in importance but have not come close to replacing the psychopathological assessment. Whether they ever will is an intriguing question for the future.

## REFERENCES

1. Möller, H.-J. (1976). *Methodische Grundprobleme der Psychiatrie*. Kohlhammer, Stuttgart.
2. Blankenburg, W. (1983). Phänomenologie der Lebenswelt—Bezogenheit des Menschen und Psychopathologie. In: Grathoff, R. and Waldenfels, B. (eds.) *Sozialität und Intersubjektivität*. Fink Verlag, Munich.
3. Doerr-Zegers, O. (2000). Existential and phenomenological approach to psychiatry. In: Gelder, M.G., López-Ibor, J.J., and Andreasen, N.C. (eds.) *New Oxford Textbook of Psychiatry*, Vol. 1. Oxford University Press, Oxford. pp. 357–62.
4. Fuchs, T. (2000). *Leib, Raum, Person. Entwurf einer phänomenologischen Anthropologie*. Klett-Cotta Verlag, Stuttgart.
5. Doerr-Zegers, O. (2016). Present and future of Lopez-Ibor's concept of thymopathy. In: Gutierrez-Fentes, M.A., Lopez-Ibor, A., and Sacristan, J.A. (eds.) *Psiquiatría: Situación actual y perspectivas de futuro*. Union Editorial, Madrid. pp. 197–220.
6. Moller, H.J. (2009). Standardised rating scales in psychiatry: methodological basis, their possibilities and limitations and descriptions of important rating scales. *World Journal of Biological Psychiatry*, 10, 6–26.
7. Moller, H.J. (2014). Observer rating scales. In: Alexopoulos, G., Kasper, S., Möller, H.J., and Moreno, C. (eds.) *Guide to assessment scales in major depressive disorder*. Springer Heidelberg: New York, NY and London. pp. 7–22.
8. Möller, H.J. (2014). Self-rating scales. In: Alexopoulos, G., Kasper, S., Möller, H.J., and Moreno, C. (eds.) *Guide to assessment scales in major depressive disorder*. Springer Heidelberg: New York, NY and London. pp. 23–34.
9. Saß, H. and P. Hoff. (2017). Deskriptiv-psychopathologische Befunderhebung in der Psychiatrie. In: Möller, H.-J, Laux, G., and Kapfhammer, H.-P. (eds.) *Psychiatrie, Psychosomatik, Psychotherapie*, Vol 1 (5th edn). Springer Heidelberg, New York, NY and Berlin. pp. 559–76.
10. Jaspers, K. (1913). *Allgemeine Psychopathologie*. Springer, Berlin.
11. Jaspers, K. (1997). *General psychopathology*, Vols 1 and 2 (translated by Hoenig, J. and Hamilton, M.W.). Johns Hopkins University Press, Baltimore, MD.
12. Jaspers, K. (1973). *Allgemeine Psychopathologie* (9th edn). Springer-Verlag, Berlin Heidelberg.
13. Schneider, K. (2007). *Klinische Psychopathologie* (15th edn). Georg Thieme Verlag, Stuttgart.
14. Schneider, K. (1959). *Clinical psychopathology* (translated by Hamilton, M.W.). Grune and Stratton, New York, NY.

15. Möller, H.J. (1978). *Psychoanalyse—Erklärende Wissenschaft oder Deutungskunst?* Fink, Munich.

16. Schneider, W., Klauer, T., and Freyberger, H.J. (2008). Operationalized psychodynamic diagnosis in planning and evaluating the psychotherapeutic process. *European Archives of Psychiatry and Clinical Neuroscience*, 258(Suppl 5), 86–91.

17. Arbeitsgemeinschaft für Methodik und Dokumentation in der Psychiatrie. (2016). *Das AMDP-System. Manual zur Dokumentation psychiatrischer Befunde. 9., überarbeitete und erweiterte Auflage.* Hogrefe, Göttingen.

18. Fähndrich, E. and Stieglitz, R.-D. (2016). *Leitfaden zur Erfassung des psychopathologischen Befundes. Halbstrukturiertes Interview anhand des AMDP-Systems. 4, überarbeitete und erweiterte Auflage.* Hogrefe, Göttingen.

19. Ban, T.A. and Guy, W.E. (1982). *The manual for the assessment and documentation of psychopathology (AMDP system)*. Springer, Berlin.

20. Freyberger, H.J. and Möller, H.J. (2004). *Die AMDP-Module.* Hogrefe, Göttingen.

21. Moller, H.J. (2005). Problems associated with the classification and diagnosis of psychiatric disorders. *World Journal of Biological Psychiatry*, 6, 45–56.

22. Moller, H.J., Bandelow, B., Bauer, M., *et al.* (2015). DSM-5 reviewed from different angles: goal attainment, rationality, use of evidence, consequences-part 2: bipolar disorders, schizophrenia spectrum disorders, anxiety disorders, obsessive-compulsive disorders, trauma- and stressor-related disorders, personality disorders, substance-related and addictive disorders, neurocognitive disorders. *European Archives of Psychiatry and Clinical Neuroscience*, 265, 87–106.

23. Moller, H.J., Bandelow, B., Bauer, M., *et al.* (2015). DSM-5 reviewed from different angles: goal attainment, rationality, use of evidence, consequences—part 1: general aspects and paradigmatic discussion of depressive disorders. *European Archives of Psychiatry and Clinical Neuroscience*, 265, 5–18.

24. Andreasen, N.C. (2007). DSM and the death of phenomenology in America: an example of unintended consequences. *Schizophrenia Bulletin*, 33, 108–12.

25. Hoff, P. (2008). Do social psychiatry and neurosciences need psychopathology—and if yes, what for? *International Review of Psychiatry*, 20, 515–20.

26. Insel, T., Cuthbert, B., Garvey, M., *et al.* (2010). Research domain criteria (RDoC): toward a new classification framework for research on mental disorders. *American Journal of Psychiatry*, 167h, 748–51.

# 7

# DSM-5 and ICD-11 classifications

*Darrel A. Regier, David P. Goldberg, Bedirhan T. Üstün, and Geoffrey M. Reed*

## Brief history of mental disorder classification

The classification of medical conditions has historically included the naming (nomenclature) and description (nosology) of recognized illnesses, and the placement of all such conditions into an organizational structure (taxonomy—classifications) that recognizes similarities and boundaries among these conditions. Similar efforts have been useful for other scientific areas such as chemistry, with the periodic table of elements, and biology, with the recognition and organization of genera and species in the classification of Linnaeus.

With the establishment of asylums for the mentally ill in the eighteenth and nineteenth centuries, there was an opportunity to systematically observe the course of psychiatric illnesses, conduct medical autopsies, and advance new classification structures. Alzheimer's recognition of pathological changes in brains of patients with dementia at autopsy became a biological standard, but Emil Kraepelin was unable to identify parallel changes for dementia praecox. However, Kraepelin's descriptive classification, based on symptom expression and the course of illness, enabled an important separation of schizophrenia and affective psychoses, and his textbooks were widely influential. For asylum directors in the nineteenth century, there was a need to collect statistical information on the types of disorders affecting their patients, and these rudimentary classifications were then used to collect prevalence data by census takers. However, the earliest nineteenth-century international medical statistical classifications focused primarily on listing causes of death (and later diseases) that could aid in standardizing vital statistics reporting for public health monitoring.

At the end of World War II, the United Nations (UN) was established, including the World Health Organization (WHO) as its specialized agency in health. All member states of the UN, which then became signatories to the WHO, agreed to collect common mortality statistics on the causes of death, and morbidity statistics of known medical and mental disorders to develop comparable national and international health statistics. The sixth revision of the *Manual of International Statistical Classification of Diseases, Injuries, and Causes of Death* (ICD-6) was approved by the World Health Assembly, the WHO's governing body, in 1948. Relatively minor revisions were made in the Seventh Revision in 1955, followed by a more extensive Eighth Revision completed in 1965. The increased use of the classification for medical records resulted in individual countries, such as the United States, making 'clinical modifications', which involved additional codes for both outpatient and inpatient hospital use. This continued for the ninth edition in 1977 and the tenth edition in 1992 [1].

## DSM-I to DSM-IV and ICD-10 mental disorder classification links

Although the American Psychiatric Association (APA) contributed to the ICD-6 mental disorders chapter, it also published a separate *Diagnostic and Statistical Manual of Mental Disorders* (DSM-I) in 1952 that more closely reflected Adolf Meyer's view of mental disorders as psychobiological reactions to critical life and developmental events. In preparation for ICD-8 in 1965, the WHO recognized the wide disparity in different national nomenclatures and lists of mental disorders used throughout the world. The WHO commissioned a British psychiatrist—Erwin Stengel—to survey all the major national and academic classifications available at the time as the basis for proposing a feasible international mental disorder classification in future editions of the ICD. Because of the lack of knowledge and differing opinions regarding the pathology and aetiology, he suggested using 'operationalized definitions' of mental disorders, based on observable syndrome criteria that could be reliably reported. In bypassing disagreements about the aetiology of these syndromes, he suggested that such an approach could lead to a greater measure of agreement about the value of specific treatments and facilitate a broad epidemiological approach to psychiatric research [2].

Unfortunately, the recommendations of Stengel were not followed for ICD-8 in 1965 or the parallel second edition of the DSM published by the APA in 1968. Nonetheless, there were several factors which led to the eventual adoption of Stengel's recommendations. The statistical classification of mental hospital admission diagnoses in the United States and the UK demonstrated marked differences in the prevalence rates of schizophrenia and manic depressive disorder. A study to evaluate the basis for this discrepancy showed that the use of common 'operationalized definitions' of these two disorders and a structured psychiatric interview greatly increased the comparability of prevalence rates for these mental disorders [3]. After this study, the WHO realized that additional guidance was needed to improve comparable clinical applications of ICD-8 diagnoses and published a glossary of terms in 1974—a glossary that was fully incorporated into ICD-9 in 1977. At about the same time, psychiatrists at Washington University, St Louis embarked on an effort to 'operationalize' diagnostic criteria for 16 mental disorders (the Feighner criteria) in what was referred to as a neo-Kraepelinian or descriptive approach to psychiatric diagnosis. The approach was recognized as useful for a proposed NIMH longitudinal study of depressive disorders and was modified to become the Research Diagnostic Criteria (RDC) [4]. When Spitzer was also selected to be Chair of the DSM-III Task Force to prepare an edition comparable to the ninth edition of the ICD, the Task Force decided to go beyond the ICD-9 glossary of terms and introduce explicit symptom criteria for each psychiatric disorder—using the RDC as the model for the entire DSM-III [5].

Following the DSM-III publication in 1980, the WHO Division of Mental Health was contacted by the US Alcohol, Drug Abuse, and Mental Health Administration (ADAMHA) to develop a joint effort to bring greater international agreement on definitions and 'operationalized criteria' for mental disorders. A series of international conferences was supported, as was a major international conference of psychiatric leaders from 37 countries held in Copenhagen in 1982 [6]. An agreement was reached at this meeting for these countries to work jointly with the WHO on the development of the Mental and Behavioural Disorders chapter of ICD-10 that would also follow the recommendations of Stengel and the model most fully realized at that time by DSM-III. Subsequently, a co-operative agreement was reached with the WHO and NIMH to support collaboration with the DSM-IV Task Force and the development of three research instruments that would facilitate assessments of both DSM-IV and the newly 'operationalized' ICD-10 diagnoses [7]. These included the Composite International Diagnostic Interview (CIDI) for epidemiological studies that was based on the Diagnostic Interview Schedule (DIS) used in the NIMH Epidemiological Catchment Area Study—the first study to realize the epidemiological research potential of operationalized diagnostic criteria (in DSM-III) anticipated by Stengel [8]. The other two instruments included the Schedule for Clinical Assessment in Neuropsychiatry (SCAN), based on the Present State Examination (PSE) used in the United States/UK study, and the International Personality Disorders Examination (IPDE), based on Loranger's Personality Disorder Examination. The most widely used of these instruments has been the CIDI, which, with some modifications, became the assessment instrument for the extensive World Mental Health Surveys [9]. This work substantially influenced guidance published by the WHO for ICD-10 Mental and Behavioural Disorders, including the *Clinical Descriptions and Diagnostic Guidelines* [10], intended for use in clinical settings, and the *Diagnostic Criteria for Research* [11].

When the co-operative agreement between the NIMH and the WHO for ICD-10 diagnostic instruments was completed in 1992—it was extended to 2001 to develop the WHO Disability Assessment Schedule (WHO-DAS) [12]—an assessment instrument that would support the International Classification of Functioning and Disability (ICF) [13].

## DSM-5 and ICD-11 classification development

In 1999, the APA initiated a review of DSM-IV [14] and ICD-10 [1, 10, 11] approaches to mental disorder diagnosis and invited the WHO, the World Psychiatric Association, and the National Institutes of Health (NIH) to join in this effort. Although the exercise resulted in a monograph entitled *A Research Agenda for DSM-V* [15], it also served as the basis for a co-operative agreement application from the APA and the WHO to three NIH institutes entitled *Developing the Research Base for DSM-V and ICD-11* [16]. From 2004 to 2008, there were 13 conferences, involving about 400 clinicians and scientists from around the world to review the evidence base for major groups of mental disorders and a review of the public health implications of changes in psychiatric classification [17]. The conferences, a list of conference series publications, on 'developing a research agenda for DSM-5', are available on the web at http://www.dsm5.org.

The DSM-5 Task Force Chair and Vice-Chair were appointed in 2006, with the Task Force that included work group chairs and consultants in 2007, and the 13 diagnostic work groups involving a total of about 160 multi-disciplinary and international members were all vetted for conflict of interest issues by the APA Board of Trustees and fully functioning by 2008. Three drafts of proposed diagnostic criteria were posted on the http://www.dsm5.org website in 2010, 2011, and 2012. There were over 13,000 recommendations from clinicians, research investigators, and the general public received on the http://www.dsm5.org website in response to these postings. In addition, there was a remarkable level of international media interest in the process, and thousands of petitions, e-mails, and letters were received about proposed changes for selected disorders. Field trials to assess the reliability of diagnoses and dimensional measures were conducted in 11 academic settings [18–20] and in over 600 routine clinical practice settings to assess the clinical utility of the revisions [21]. A multi-level review process was established by the APA Board of Trustees, and DSM-5 was approved by the Board of Trustees in December 2012 and published for release in May 2013 [22].

As with previous editions of the DSM and ICD, it was expected that there would be extensive consultation between the two classifications and that they would be published at about the same time. The ICD-11 revision process was launched in 2007, and a DSM–ICD harmonization co-ordinating group was organized to use the jointly developed research base from the conferences to enhance the consistency of DSM and ICD revisions for clinical guidance. A DSM-5 Task Force initiative to develop a more useful and evidence-based organizational structure of the mental disorder classification was converted into a joint DSM–ICD effort to examine the degree to which individual disorders and groups of disorders had been 'validated' in research studies. An expanded set of 'validity criteria' from the one proposed in 1970 by Robins and Guze was applied in a series of analyses and papers published in 2009 [23].

It was readily apparent that the alignment of multiple validators was much more meaningful for larger groups or disorder spectra than for individual categorical diagnoses. As a result, there was agreement that both DSM-5 and ICD-11 would—to the extent possible given the different conventions and constituencies of the two systems—share a common organizational structure or 'metastructure' that would be reflective of the evidence base accumulated in this exercise. However, since the ICD-11 process continued for more than 6 years after publication of DSM-5, several significant additional structural changes in the mental disorders chapter have been made in the context of the larger ICD-11 revisions.

## DSM-5

In the three decades between the publication of DSM-III and DSM-5, there was a remarkable increase in the amount of epidemiologic, clinical, and basic neuroscience research on mental disorders. This research has demonstrated the high levels of mental disorder comorbidity, similarities in pharmacologic and psychosocial treatment effectiveness across diagnostic boundaries, and an increasingly complex set of genetic and pathophysiological correlates with a spectrum of clinical syndromes defined in DSM-III to DSM-IV as separate and distinct disorders. The cumulative effect of this research was to support a reconceptualization of the approach to classifying mental disorders that emphasized developmental similarities, common neurobiological correlates, and common phenomenological features that emerged from factor analyses of clinical symptoms and 'personality' traits in both general and clinical populations.

This revised approach appears to be supportive of conceptualizing clinical disorders as central tendencies in more continuous syndromes with multi-causal aetiologies. It acknowledges the heterogenous nature of current categorical mental disorder diagnoses, such as major depressive disorder, which requires any five out of nine diagnostic criteria for diagnosis and allows up to 256 different combinations with 3–4 different levels of severity. In addition, there are now specifiers for anxiety symptoms and contextual factors such as peri-partum status in females that add to the heterogeneity of this disorder. The inclusion of a 'clinically significant distress or disability' threshold criterion for almost all DSM-IV and DSM-5 disorders results in adding mood and anxiety symptoms for virtually all disorders. The overlap of mood and anxiety disorder symptoms with stress-induced disorder criteria for a condition like PTSD further reduces the ability of strict categorical diagnostic criteria boundaries to identify homogenous clinical populations.

### Conceptual approach to linking categorical and dimensional diagnostic assessments

The emergence of a new understanding of mental disorders conceptualizes them as the likely result of multiple genetic and environmental exposure factors, rather than discrete causes such as single genes (for example, Down's syndrome—due to trisomy 21), nutritional or toxic exposures (for example, pellagra—due to niacin deficiency), or single infectious agents [for example, central nervous system (CNS) lues—due to syphilis spirochaete]. This provides an entirely different approach to assessing the validity and reliability of psychiatric diagnoses. It affects how we should conduct field trials of diagnostic criteria and interpret statistical measures of diagnostic reliability such as Kappa—a measure that is greatly affected by the comorbidity of the clinical population from which subjects are recruited and the use of exhaustive research vs usual clinical interviews [19, 24]. If there are perhaps as many as a thousand different genes that contribute some degree of vulnerability to the diagnosis of schizophrenia, and some of these are shared with vulnerability genes for autism spectrum disorders (ASD), attention-deficit/hyperactivity disorder, bipolar disorder, and major depressive disorder [25], the potential for overlapping symptoms and comorbidity

becomes apparent. The emerging appreciation of the influence of psychosocial or physical environmental exposures to the epigenetic switching on or off of any of the vulnerable genes for mental disorders only adds to the aetiological complexity and interpretation of biological 'validators'.

The tension between the psychoanalytic concept of all mental disorders being on a single continuum from normal to psychosis and that of the neo-Kraepelinians that all disorders are discontinuous, discrete disease entities can now be reinterpreted with a better understanding of aetiological factors and statistical analyses of psychopathological symptoms, traits, and clinical course of illness. From a clinician's perspective, there is clearly something different about the core clinical expression and clinical course of patients with autism spectrum, schizophrenic spectrum, and bipolar and major depressive disorder diagnoses—even if some of the same vulnerability genes are shared. Although a strict dimensional scoring of all biological and symptomatic domains as continuous variables would undoubtedly provide a more precise description of psychopathology, a hybrid model that contains both categorical diagnoses and dimensional variations is much more useful for clinical practice. As a result, DSM-5 has recommended the following modifications in clinical diagnosis:

1. The assessment of cross-cutting symptom domains for adults that include depression, anger, hypomania, anxiety, somatic, suicide risk, hallucinations, sleep, cognition, obsessive–compulsive, dissociation, personality, substance use, attention, and irritability—the last two for children and adolescents. A Level 1 screening and a Level 2 confirmation of higher symptom levels are recommended, regardless of diagnosis.

2. An assessment of disability using the WHO-DAS that replaces the previous DSM-IV Axis V Global Assessment of Function (GAF) scale.

3. Revised syndrome-based categorical diagnoses with porous boundaries that are organized into larger spectrum groups to facilitate assessments of common comorbidity.

4. Explicit threshold criteria are retained for research and clinical communication about the characteristics of the diagnostic syndrome.

5. Diagnostic severity measures that are freely available for downloading online in English and with select translation editions.

6. Use of 'Other specified' and 'Unspecified' categorical diagnoses, instead of the 'Not otherwise specified (NOS)' convention of previous DSM editions.

7. Associated text on diagnostic features, prevalence, development and course, risk and prognostic factors, culture-related diagnostic issues, suicide risk, functional consequences, gender-related issues, differential diagnosis, and comorbidity.

8. Recommended comprehensive case formulations for clinical assessments.

9. Use of a Cultural Formulation Interview to facilitate understanding of cultural expressions that may be misunderstood as evidence of psychopathology—particularly where there are cultural differences between the clinician and the individual patient.

**Table 7.1** Proposed overall 'metastructure' or groupings of DSM-5 and ICD-11 mental, behavioural, and neurodevelopmental disorders

| DSM-5 | ICD-11 |
| --- | --- |
| Neurodevelopmental disorders | Neurodevelopmental disorders |
| Schizophrenia spectrum and other psychotic disorders | Schizophrenia spectrum and other primary psychotic disorders |
| (No 'General mood disorders' grouping) | Mood disorders |
| Bipolar and related disorders | Bipolar and related disorders |
| Depressive disorders | Depressive disorders |
| Anxiety disorders | Anxiety and fear-related disorders |
| Obsessive–compulsive and related disorders | Obsessive–compulsive and related disorders |
| Trauma- and stressor-related disorders | Disorders specifically associated with stress |
| Dissociative disorders | Dissociative disorders |
| Somatic symptom and related disorders | Bodily distress disorders |
| Feeding and eating disorders | Feeding and eating disorders |
| Elimination disorders | Elimination disorders |
| Sleep–wake disorders | (Separate ICD-11 chapter on 'Sleep–wake disorders') |
| Sexual dysfunctions | (In separate ICD-11 chapter on 'Conditions related to sexual health') |
| Gender dysphoria | (In separate ICD-11 chapter on 'Conditions related to sexual health') |
| Disruptive, impulse-control, and conduct disorders | Impulse-control disorders (separate grouping from 'Disruptive behaviour and dissocial disorders'; different order: appears after 'Disorders due to substance use and addictive behaviours') |
| | Disruptive behaviour and dissocial disorders (separate grouping from 'Impulse-control disorders'; different order: appears after 'Disorders due to substance use and addictive behaviours') |
| Substance-related and addictive disorders | Disorders due to substance use and addictive behaviours |
| Paraphilic disorders | Paraphilic disorders |
| (Included under 'Somatic symptom disorders') | Factitious disorders |
| Neurocognitive disorders | Neurocognitive disorders (different order; appears after 'Personality disorders') |
| Personality disorders | Personality disorders |
| Other mental disordersz | (Residual categories for each grouping are included by ICD-11 convention) |
| (Not a grouping in DSM-5) | Mental and behavioural disorders associated with pregnancy, childbirth, and the puerperium, not elsewhere classified |
| (DSM-5 divides these up into the section that corresponds to the expressed symptoms. For example, 'Depressive disorder associated with another medical condition' is listed under 'Depressive disorders') | Secondary mental and behavioural disorders syndromes |
| Medication-induced movement disorders and other adverse effects of medication | (In ICD-11 chapter on 'Diseases of the nervous system' or chapter on 'External causes of morbidity or mortality') |
| Other conditions that may be a focus of clinical attention | (Separate ICD-11 chapter on 'Factors influencing health status and encounters with health services') |

Source: data from American Psychiatric Association, *Diagnostic and statistical manual of mental disorders*, 5th edition (DSM-5), Copyright (2013) American Psychiatric Association; World Health Organization, *The ICD-11 Classification of Mental and Behavioural Disorders*, Copyright (2018), World Health Organization.

## The metastructure of DSM-5 classification of diagnostic categories

The anticipated reorganization of the entire ICD statistical coding system from the ICD-9 numeric (000.00–999.99) and ICD-10 alphanumeric (A00.00–Z99.99) system to an ICD-11 numeric-alphanumeric (01A00–99Z99) system opened the possibility for reconceptualizing the grouping and specifiers for individual diagnoses. The previous hierarchy of 'organic dementia', followed by substance-induced disorders and psychoses, could be replaced by a more developmental concept of psychopathology that begins with neurodevelopmental disorders, and place acquired neurocognitive disorders far later in the organizational structure. This structure has

been largely adopted in both DSM-5 and ICD-11 and is shown in Table 7.1.

DSM-5 includes an introductory Section 1 that provides operational definitions and guidance regarding the use of the manual. Section 2 contains the diagnostic criteria and relevant ICD statistical codes within the organizational structure shown in Table 7.1. There is also a very substantive Section 3 that includes the previously mentioned dimensional assessment measures, guidance related to cultural formulation, an alternative 'hybrid model' for personality disorders, and conditions for further study.

Embedded within this new organizational arrangement is a much greater appreciation of more continuous diagnostic spectra containing previously described separate and discrete disorders.

Examples of the compression of previous separate disorders into single disorder spectra include ASD, specific learning disorder, several sleep disorders, somatic symptom disorder, and substance use disorders. Altogether, 50 separate disorders in DSM-IV were reduced to 22 spectrum disorders—with the greatest number contributed by merging abuse and dependence disorders for ten substances into mild, moderate, and severe forms of substance use disorders. Several new disorders were added, including social (pragmatic) communication disorder (SCD) and hoarding disorder, that contained more limited symptom domains than were present in other disorders in the related disorder spectra. For example, ASD required deficits in both social communication and restricted, repetitive behaviours and interest domains, whereas some patients who demonstrated deficits only in social communication required a separate SCD diagnosis.

Major changes in the grouping of disorders include the movement of attention-deficit/hyperactivity disorder into the 'Neurodevelopmental disorder' chapter, and gambling disorder into the 'Substance-related and addictive disorders' chapter. There are also new placements of disorders that were previously in other sections of the mental disorder classifications; for example, body dysmorphic disorder from the DSM-IV 'Somatoform disorders' group and trichotillomania (hair pulling disorder) from the DSM-IV 'Impulse-control disorders' group were moved into the DSM-5 'Obsessive–compulsive and related disorders' group, which also added new hoarding disorder and excoriation (skin picking) disorder conditions.

For a more complete description of individual diagnoses in DSM-5, the reader is referred to Section II of DSM-5 (pp. 31–727). Highlights of changes in individual diagnoses from DSM-IV to DSM-5 are contained in the full DSM-5 (pp. 809–16).

## Mental and behavioural disorders in ICD-11

### ICD-10: the current global standard

The WHO member states agree to use the ICD as the basis for reporting health statistics on mortality and morbidity. The ICD-10 (Tenth Revision) was approved in 1990 and included a listing of all of the health conditions in alphanumeric order, ranging from A00 to Z99, with each chapter corresponding to a major area (for example, neoplasms, diseases of the circulatory system). The 'Mental and behavioural disorders' chapter of ICD-10 was the only chapter to include glossary definitions for each condition. However, the WHO has specifically indicated that these definitions did not provide sufficient information for clinical implementation by mental health professionals. Rather, the statistical version of ICD-10 was intended for use by 'coders or clerical workers and also serves as a reference point for compatibility with other classifications' [1].

For implementation of ICD-10 in mental health service settings, the WHO developed the *ICD-10 Classification of Mental and Behavioral Disorders: Clinical Descriptions and Diagnostic Guidelines* (CDDG) [10], which provided a description of the main clinical and associated features of the disorder, together with diagnostic guidelines designed to assist mental health clinicians in making a confident diagnosis. The diagnostic guidelines in the CDDG differed from DSM diagnostic criteria in offering more flexible, prototypic guidance intended to allow for clinical judgement and global variation, rather than strict criteria.

The WHO also published the *ICD-10 Classification of Mental and Behavioral Disorders: Diagnostic Criteria for Research* (DCR) [11], containing fully operationalized diagnostic criteria. The differences between the CDDG and the DCR reflected their different purposes. The diagnostic guidelines contained in the CDDG were intended to help the clinician identify the category that is most likely to offer relevant information for treatment and management. In this context, false negatives based on arbitrary or overly specified criteria, such as precise duration requirements and symptom counts, were problematic because they offered no guidance to the clinician [26]. In contrast, the DCR were intended primarily for identifying more homogenous research populations such as for clinical trials or epidemiological studies.

Therefore, while the ICD-10 CDDG were substantively quite different from DSM-IV, the ICD-10 DCR were intentionally highly similar to DSM-IV's diagnostic criteria—a similarity that was explicitly permitted by a joint agreement between the WHO and the APA. Still, there were important differences. Of the 176 diagnostic categories the two systems had in common, there were some differences in all but one category (transient tic disorder), with differences judged to be conceptual or substantive in the case of 39 disorders [27].

The largest single source of differences between the ICD-10 DCR and DSM-IV was DSM-IV's 'clinical significance' criterion, which effectively required the presence of distress and/or functional impairment as a part of DSM-IV criteria sets. This difference reflected the WHO's view of distress (other than the specific forms of distress that constitute the symptoms of particular disorders) and changes in functional status—the main components of DSM-IV's clinical significance criterion—as consequences or outcomes of health conditions, rather than their inherent features [28]. The inclusion of these features as a part of specific ICD-10 disorder guidelines or RDC criteria sets was therefore restricted to those conditions in which they were considered necessary for distinguishing disorder from normality. These issues are further discussed in the section on the WHO's ICF.

Finally, the WHO published a version of ICD-10 mental and behavioural disorders intended for use in global primary care settings [29]. The primary care version (ICD-10 PHC) contains only 26 disorder categories and was the predecessor for a similar ICD-11 version.

### Development of ICD-11 mental and behavioural disorders

Because the ICD plays such a crucial role in the international health community, it is critical that it is based on the best available scientific knowledge and that it keeps pace with significant advances in health care that have the potential to improve its reliability, validity, and utility. Increasingly, in most countries, the ICD must also be compatible with electronic information infrastructure. ICD-10 was approved by the World Health Assembly in 1990 and published in 1992, prior to the current digital age, making the current period the longest in the history of the ICD without a major revision.

The development of ICD-11 was a huge undertaking that involved a review of necessary changes in the classification of all health conditions, of which mental and behavioural disorders represent only a small part. It was made even more complex by the requirement that ICD-11 must be suitable for a range of different uses by all WHO member states. Responsibility for co-ordinating the development of the ICD-11 chapter on mental and behavioural disorders was assigned to the WHO Department of Mental Health and Substance Abuse. That department appointed an International Advisory Group in 2007 to provide advice and consultation throughout the process.

The public health focus of the WHO Department of Mental Health and Substance Abuse substantially influenced the priorities and methods for developing diagnostic guidelines for ICD-11. Mental and substance use disorders account for a greater proportion of global disease burden than any other category of non-communicable diseases and are the leading cause of disability worldwide [30]. Yet, they are dramatically undertreated, with up to half of individuals with severe mental disorders in HICs and more than three-quarters in LMICs receiving no treatment at all [31]. Moreover, people with serious mental disorders experience a much higher prevalence of other health conditions, such as cardiovascular, metabolic, and respiratory diseases [32, 33], and disproportionately higher rates of mortality, resulting in a substantial reduction in life expectancy [34].

The WHO therefore saw the development of the ICD-11 as an opportunity to provide WHO member states with a better tool to help them reduce the disease burden of mental, behavioural, and neurodevelopmental disorders and to provide health professionals at various levels of care with better tools for identifying people in need of mental health services and which treatments are most likely to be effective. With very limited exceptions, substantial gains in clinical, neuroscience, and genetic research has not produced validity information on which to base major changes in diagnostic classification [35, 36]. However, current knowledge is amply sufficient to provide vastly more effective and more accessible mental health services than are currently provided at a global level, and the WHO provided a set of specific strategies for doing so in its Comprehensive Mental Health Action Plan 2013–2020 [37]. These considerations have led the WHO to focus particularly on improving the classification's clinical utility and global applicability in developing diagnostic guidelines for ICD-11 mental, behavioural, and neurodevelopmental disorders [38].

The International Advisory Group and all Working Groups for ICD-11 Mental, Behavioural, and Neurodevelopmental disorders included representation from all WHO global regions. Professional surveys [39, 40] and formative studies [41, 42] intended to inform early decisions about the structure of the classification were conducted in multiple languages and with international groups of participants. Diagnostic guidelines for the ICD-11 CDDG include a specific section on cultural issues related to the clinical presentation and diagnosis of each condition.

Clinical utility and global applicability are critical, in part, because the ICD-11 CDDG and primary care versions are intended to function as important interfaces between health encounters and health information [41]. A classification that does not provide clinically and locally useful information to health professionals has little hope of being implemented consistently at the encounter level. In that case, diagnostic data that are aggregated from health encounters at the facility, system, national, and global levels will be unable to provide an optimal basis for global health data or for decision-making such as resource allocation.

To achieve its goal for ICD-11, the WHO took a highly systematic approach to the development of ICD-11 diagnostic guidelines by multi-disciplinary and broadly international expert Working Groups, particularly including substantial representation of experts from LMICs where 80% of the world's population lives. Substantial

improvements, as compared to ICD-10, included the adoption of a lifespan approach and the incorporation of dimensional approaches, particularly for personality disorders and primary psychotic disorders, that are more consistent with current evidence, more compatible with recovery-based approaches, eliminate artificial comorbidity, and more effectively capture changes over time. New categories were added, including bipolar type II disorder, complex post-traumatic stress disorder, prolonged grief disorder, body dysmorphic disorder, olfactory reference disorder, hoarding disorder, binge eating disorder, and compulsive sexual behaviour disorder [43]. In addition, the WHO implemented a systematic global programme of field studies using innovative methodologies specifically intended to examine the clinical utility and global applicability of the ICD-11 diagnostic guidelines [44].

In June 2018 the WHO released a pre-final version of the 1CD-11 for mortality and morbidity statistics to its 194 member states, for review and preparation for implementation, including considering how the ICD-11 will be incorporated in policies, laws, health systems, translations, and training of health professionals. The World Health Assembly, comprising the ministers of health of all member states, formally approved the ICD-11 in May 2019. Member states are now beginning a process of transition from the ICD-10 to the ICD-11, with reporting of health statistics to the WHO using the ICD-11 to begin on 1 January 2022. The WHO Department of Mental Health and Substance Abuse will publish Clinical Descriptions and Diagnostic Guidelines (CDDG) and separate guidance for the identification of mental health conditions in primary care settings.

### Structure of ICD-11 mental and behavioural disorders and compatibility with DSM-5

The ICD-11 was also developed in the context of full knowledge of DSM-5, both in its formative stages and in its 2013 published version. Working Groups were specifically instructed to consider DSM-5 formulations and their suitability for global application but were not prohibited from departing from them when indicated. Therefore, differences between ICD-11 and DSM-5 are intentional.

The proposed groupings for the ICD-11 chapter on mental and behavioural disorders are listed in Table 7.1, which also includes a comparison with the structure of DSM-5. Generally, the comparability of the structure of the two classifications can be counted as a success of harmonization efforts between the WHO and the APA. Some structural differences reflect ICD-wide conventions related to residual categories and mental disorders associated with other underlying disease. Others are the result of deliberations involving the WHO, the Advisory Group, and the various Working Groups, such as in the diagnostic treatment of chronic irritability and anger in children [45] and somatoform disorders [46]. Another difference is related to the integration of the classifications of 'organic' and 'non-organic' aspects of sleep–wake disorders and conditions related to sexual health and gender identity [47] in new ICD-11 chapters in ways that are more consistent with current evidence and clinical practice.

### Structure and content of ICD-11 clinical descriptions and diagnostic guidelines

The structure and information contained for each category of the ICD-11 CDDG are expected to enhance the clinical utility of the manual by providing clearly organized, consistent information across disorders that is flexible enough to allow for cultural variation and the exercise of clinical judgement. The categories of information to be provided for each category in the CDDG are: Category Name, Brief Description (100–125 words), Essential (Required) Features, Boundary with Normality (Threshold), Boundary with Other Disorders (Differential Diagnosis), Coded Qualifiers/Subtypes, Course Features, Associated Clinical Presentations, Culture-Related Features, Developmental Presentations, and Gender-Related Features.

As noted previously, the utility and effectiveness of this format in producing more consistent clinical judgements in ICD-11, as compared to ICD-10, has been tested in a series of international field studies [48, 49].

## ICD-11 mental disorders for primary care

The first version of the ICD classification of mental disorders specifically designed for use in primary care settings (ICD-10 PHC) [29] was produced by the WHO in 1996 and included 26 mental disorders that were either very common in these settings or quite important for primary care professionals to recognize. It had several features that distinguished it from the parent version of ICD-10—for each disorder, common presentations in primary care, distinguishing features, and relevant differential diagnoses were described. Also included was information for the patient and family, response to both psychological and pharmacological treatment, and indications for specialist referral [50].

The most compelling rationale for a version of the ICD designed for primary care is that the spectrum of psychological disorders seen in general medical settings is very different from that seen in specialist mental health settings. These patients in primary care settings commonly present with untidy combinations of somatic, anxious, and depressive symptoms, rather than the more elaborated diagnostic entities that are seen as more prototypic by clinicians working in specialist settings. Many of these patients do not see themselves as psychologically disordered, despite having all the symptoms required for various mental disorders—they are worried about their somatic symptoms and hope that the primary care clinician will exclude a physical cause for their symptoms and offer relief from the pain and distress associated with them.

In specialist mental health settings, the diagnostic task of the mental health professional can be characterized as asking systematically about the full range of known disorders. In contrast, the task of a clinician in primary care is to recognize a range of common mental disorders (CMDs), as well as some other severe mental disorders, and a range of problems associated with sleep, eating, alcohol, and drugs. The boundaries of the various overlapping syndromes of CMDs are of less importance than the existence of psychological distress accompanying any presenting physical disorder. The subtle distinctions between many of the individual disorders separately described by the main classifications are of limited value in primary care where clinicians work with the full range of general medical, behavioural, and social problems. A smaller set of disorders, broadly comparable to the main ICD, reflecting the most common conditions seen in this setting, is required for primary care.

### Conceptual developments for the new version of the primary care version of ICD-11

Since ICD-10 PHC was released, there have been a number of developments in knowledge and conceptualizations regarding common psychological disorders occurring in primary care settings. These are related to the relationship between anxious and depressive symptoms, the importance of recognizing depressive symptoms that commonly accompany chronic physical disorders, and the management of multiple somatic symptoms without any accompanying physical disease.

Both major international classifications recognize that depression and generalized anxiety disorder (GAD) commonly accompany each other, but the diagnostic requirements for depression include a duration of only 2 weeks, while the requirement for GAD is several months. Yet many patients develop anxious symptoms around the time they develop depressive symptoms, so that states of both anxiety and depressive symptoms are very much more common than 'comorbidity' between depression and GAD.

If the same duration of illness is used to define both depression and anxiety, those with both sets of symptoms have a much worse course, are more resistant to treatment, and are more likely to commit suicide [51]. The depressive symptoms in episodes of depression accompanied by significant anxiety are more severe than in depressive episodes not accompanied by anxiety [52, 53]. Individuals with episodes of such 'anxious depression' are more likely to have harm-avoidant symptoms and to also present with a wide range of family members with other anxiety disorders [54]. Focus groups of primary care physicians (PCPs) and nurses were held in eight countries in order to assess the views of PCPs towards the introduction of a category for anxious depression into ICD-11 PHC—they were uniformly enthusiastic [55].

It is true that both anxious and depressive symptoms can and do occur on their own, and therefore, they must both retain their different names, but anxious depression deserves recognition in its own right [56]. Finally, states of mixed anxiety and depressive symptoms that fall just short of the threshold requirements for either are very common in community settings and indeed account for more sickness absence in the UK than either depression or anxiety [57]. These mild disorders tend either to become formally diagnosable or to resolve within the next few months [58].

These various studies encouraged the Primary Care Consultation Group of the WHO to recommend that when the diagnostic requirements for both anxiety and depression are satisfied, although using a shorter duration requirement for anxiety that matches that of depression, patients are diagnosed as 'anxious depression', but when one is at 'case' level and the other well short of it, these conditions are diagnosed as 'depression (non-anxious)' or 'current anxiety'. When symptoms of both are present, but both just fail to reach the required severity, the individual may be diagnosed with 'subclinical anxious depression'.

### The use of screening instruments for psychological problems

Even in HICs, primary care professionals have difficulty remembering and implementing the complex diagnostic algorithms used by mental health professionals [59], there is considerable pressure on time and resources, and options for specialist referral for CMDs may be limited. Available written screening questionnaires may be of limited usefulness for reasons of language or literacy, not only in low-resource settings, but also in primary care settings in HICs which serve increasingly diverse populations.

The ICD-11 Primary Care Consultation Group therefore evaluated two brief screening scales for anxiety and depression to assist PCPs in deciding whether a diagnosable psychological problem was likely to be present. These screening questions were derived from an earlier WHO international study, in which it had been possible to compute sensitivity and specificity values for both sets of questions [60]. Given time and resource pressures and linguistic and literacy issues, these screening scales may be of considerable value, especially in LMICs, but also in HICs, and will be published along with the ICD-11 PHC.

## International classification of functioning disability and health

### Mental disorders and disability: assessment and classification

Mental disorders are strongly associated with disability—detriments in functioning of the brain, the body, and the person in general. People with mental disorders experience impairments in their body and brain functions, limitations in their personal daily activities, and restrictions in their social lives. These disabilities are part and parcel of the clinical picture of persons with mental disorders. The association between a mental disorder and disability may be causal, consequential, or difficult to disentangle. Disability is usually a key determinant for individuals seeking care and a significant factor for providers in making a clinical case formulation. Yet the form, frequency, and outcome of disabilities in mental disorders are not well defined or studied scientifically. Moreover, their use in formulating diagnoses of mental disorders has been unclear and inconsistent.

The WHO and the APA have used the construct of disability differently in their classification systems until recently. The WHO ICD definitions have, as far as possible, kept disability outside the diagnostic classification, as per the model articulated in the WHO's *International Classification of Functioning, Disability and Health* (ICF) [61]. DSM has kept disability as part of the functional impairment component of the clinical significance criteria. However, in the creation of DSM-5, the clinical significance criteria have been aligned to match the operational disability definition in the ICF. This has been an important step to scientifically disentangle disability from the disease process as much as possible in the formulation of mental disorder diagnoses in both ICD and DSM systems.

Ideally, the scientific definitions of a disease or disorder should be based on the aetiology and the pathological process that takes place in bodily systems. Such definitions do not require any sort of disability such as detriments in work capacity. While the consequences of disease are important clinical factors that trigger the recognition of a case by providers and often determine the types of health services and level of care required, they are not always a part of the diagnostic definition of the disease process itself. For example, people with different levels of general intellectual functioning and education may have similar levels of neuronal loss as a result of a brain injury but display different patterns of limitations in their activities. However, poor self-care and social performance are included as negative symptoms in schizophrenia diagnoses. Hence, although most mental disorders do not have known aetiology and specific pathophysiology, the potential benefits of more explicitly defining disability separately from the other signs and symptoms of mental disorders are similar to those of other diseases and disorders. A common disability metric for GBD estimates associated with all diseases and disorders will be helpful [30].

DSM-IV and DSM-5, contrary to the ICD system, make *clinical significance* an explicit part of the criteria for establishing a diagnosis.

The addition of this criterion to almost all disorders occurred after the National Institute of Mental Health Epidemiologic Catchment Area Program (ECA) study demonstrated that use of the DSM-III diagnostic criteria alone in community population studies led to relatively high prevalence rates of disorders—with some subjects having no evidence of distress or impairment [62]. Clinical significance has two main components: *distress* and *functional impairment*. Distress is expressed by the individual in the form of worry and concern about the condition. It has been operationally defined for epidemiological studies (for example, with the K-6 instrument) as including a combination of anxiety and depressive symptoms [63]. Sometimes it may not be expressed or may be explicitly denied. Functional impairment refers to limitations due to the illness, particularly in the social and occupational spheres of life, given that people with a disease or a disorder may not carry out certain functions in their daily lives. As part of the clinical significance criterion, distress and functional impairment help to establish the threshold for the diagnosis of a disorder. No guidance is given for determining the level of disability that would constitute the threshold for a diagnosis; this is left open to the clinical judgement of the clinician.

Operationally, functional impairment as used in the construct of clinical significance is roughly equivalent to the concept of 'disability' in WHO's ICF. The ICF does not use the term functional impairment. In the ICF, the term *functioning* is a neutral one, encompassing all body functions, activities, and involvement in life situations. The term *disability* means the decrements to these functions, which are known at the body level as impairments, at the person level as activity limitations, and at the societal level as participation restriction.

During the development of DSM-5, an attempt was made to align DSM's use of functional impairment more explicitly with ICF's concept of disability. The DSM's concept of social functioning would include the ICF's interpersonal interactions and relationships but might also include some of the items concerning participation in community, social, and civic life. The DSM's occupational functioning would include the activities listed under the ICF's categories of work and employment.

DSM-5 and ICD-11 now use ICF as an anchor to define and quantify disability. The WHO's Disability Assessment Schedule (WHO-DAS 2.0) has been officially recognized to assess the level of disability in DSM-5 Section 3. In this way, it will be easier to measure and identify levels of disability in terms of activity limitations and participation restrictions.

### Disability and severity concepts in classifying mental disorders

Traditionally, both in DSM and ICD systems, the disability and functioning concepts have often been used to determine the level of severity of the diagnosed disorder. Three levels of severity are frequently specified (mild, moderate, and severe), which include either the number or the intensity of symptoms and impairments in social and occupational functioning. Determining the level of severity is a clinical judgement. For example, DSM-5's guidance for 'mild' and 'severe' includes either 'few' or 'many' symptoms over the required number and either 'minor' or 'marked' impairments in social or occupational functioning. 'Moderate' is in between.

The criteria for neurodevelopmental disorders such as ASD are somewhat more explicit. Anchors are provided in DSM-5 for mild, moderate, and severe impairment in specific symptomatic domains for intellectual disability (disorders of intellectual development in ICD-11) and ASD. These domains include conceptual, social, and practical (occupational) areas of intellectual disability, and social communication and restricted, repetitive behaviours in ASD. In both of these disorders, the ability to engage in social activities and the need for supervision are assessed where the amount of supervision required provides an anchor for severity.

In ICD-11, *functioning properties* are being integrated into the information that is being developed to describe health conditions [64]. These are listings of specific functional domains that are specifically relevant to a given disease or disorder, including mental, behavioural, and neurodevelopmental disorders, and may be important foci of assessment. The explicit identification of functioning properties related to specific health conditions is intended to provide a broader and more meaningful picture of an individual's overall health in order to guide clinical decision-making.

Domains of functioning and disability in ICF and WHODAS 2.0 include the following: (1) understanding and communicating with the world (cognition); (2) moving and getting around (mobility); (3) self-care; (4) getting along with people (interpersonal relationships); (5) domestic life, occupation, school, and leisure; and (6) participation in society [65]. The more explicit descriptions of these six domains are intended to facilitate a clinical focus on reducing specific limitations separately, but in conjunction with reducing the symptoms of mental disorders.

## Future of mental disorder classification

At the beginning of the DSM-5 and ICD-11 developmental process, there was a nicely articulated summary of the challenges and obstacles to developing a fully explicated aetiological and pathophysiologically based classification system for mental disorders [66]. An overreliance on DSM-IV and ICD-10 symptom clusters as phenotypes for genetic markers and targets for medication development was noted. Findings such as common genetic markers for multiple disorders and pharmacological and psychosocial treatment effectiveness that did not correspond with DSM or ICD diagnostic boundaries called for new research strategies. Out of this background, the NIMH launched the RDoC strategy to facilitate greater attention to the relationships among multiple biological and phenomenological domains—including negative valence systems, positive valence systems, cognitive systems, systems for social processes, and arousal/modulatory systems—as a basis for future breakthroughs in understanding and treating mental disorders [67]. Although it was fully understood in the field that it would be years, if not decades, before such a fully articulated system could be completed, there was an unfortunate initial juxtaposition of the DSM-5 and RDoC systems as competitive, rather than collaborative, efforts to advance our understanding of these disorders. It is now clear that when genes, molecules, cells, circuits, and physiology emerge that correlate with behavioural and symptomatic syndromes and can be assessed in routine clinical settings, they can be incorporated into future versions of clinical classification systems [68, 69]. Such biological measures must be able to demonstrate the level of sensitivity and specificity needed for clinical decision-making.

From a clinical practice perspective, the increasing concern about the quality of care will require more 'measurement-based outcome' approaches for clinicians, as well as for reassuring health care

administrators of the value received for their organizations and funding. The increasing standardization of medical terminology and the use of dimensional measures of symptomatic and disability domains will be fully operational only in the context of electronic health records. By providing more detailed information about clinical status, these measures will have a major impact on risk adjustment for severely ill patients and on outcome assessment for value-based reimbursement to clinicians. In primary care and low-resource settings, use of simple screening methods to identify mental disorders and to monitor treatment response will be important next steps. With the current DSM-5 and ICD-11 classification structures in place, it is expected that more iterative revisions that can be integrated more seamlessly into health statistics and clinical practice will emerge over the next few decades, rather than large-scale, more disruptive edition changes.

## REFERENCES

1. World Health Organization. (1992). *Manual of the international statistical classification of diseases, injuries, and causes of death. Tenth revision of the international classification of diseases.* World Health Organization, Geneva.
2. Stengel, E. (1959). Classification of mental disorders. *Bulletin of the World Health Organization*, 21, 601–63.
3. Cooper, J.E., Kendell, R.E., Gurland, B.J., Sharpe, L., Copeland, J.R.M., and Simon, R. (1972). *Psychiatric diagnosis in New York and London: a comparative study of mental hospital admissions.* Oxford University Press, Oxford.
4. Spitzer, R.L., Endicott, J., and Robins, E. (1978). Research diagnostic criteria. Rationale and reliability. *Archives of General Psychiatry*, 35, 773–82.
5. American Psychiatric Association. (1980). *Diagnostic and statistical manual of mental disorders, third edition (DSM-III).* American Psychiatric Association, Washington D.C.
6. Jablensky, A., Sartorius, N., Hirschfeld, R., *et al.* (1983). Diagnosis and classification of mental disorders and alcohol- and drug-related problems: a research agenda for the 1980s. *Psychological Medicine*, 13, 907–21.
7. Sartorius, N. Principal Investigator. *The WHO/Alcohol, Drug Abuse, and Mental Health Administration Joint Project on Diagnosis and Classification.* Cooperative agreement U01MH035883, from the National Institute of Mental Health to the World Health Organization, 1983–2001.
8. Regier, D.A., Narrow, W.E., Rae, D.S., Manderscheid, R.W., Locke, B.Z., Goodwin, F.K. (1993). The de facto US mental and addictive disorders service system: epidemiologic catchment area prospective 1-year prevalence rates of disorders and services. *Archives of General Psychiatry*, 50, 85–94.
9. Kessler, R.C. and Üstün, T.B. (2004). The world mental health (WMH) survey initiative version of the World Health Organization (WHO) Composite International Diagnostic Interview (CIDI). *International Journal of Methods in Psychiatric Research*, 13, 93–121.
10. World Health Organization. (1992). *ICD-10 classification of mental and behavioural disorders. Clinical descriptions and diagnostic guidelines.* World Health Organization, Geneva.
11. World Health Organization. (1993). *The ICD-10 classification of mental and behavioral disorders: diagnostic criteria for research.* World Health Organization, Geneva.
12. Üstün, T.B., Chatterji, S., Kostanjsek, N., *et al.*; WHO/NIH Joint Project. (2010). Developing the World Health Organization

Disability Assessment Schedule 2.0. *Bulletin of the World Health Organization*, 88, 815–23.

13. Üstün, T.B., Chatterji, S., Bickenbach, J., Kostanjsek, N., and Schneider, M. (2003). The international classification of functioning, disability and health: a new tool for understanding disability and health. *Disability and Rehabilitation*, 25, 565–71.

14. American Psychiatric Association. (1994). *Diagnostic and statistical manual of mental disorders, fourth edition (DSM-IV)*. American Psychiatric Association, Washington DC.

15. Kupfer, D.J., First, M.B., and Regier, D.A. (eds.). (2002). *A research agenda for DSM-V*. American Psychiatric Association, Washington D.C.

16. Regier DA. Principal Investigator. *Developing the Research Base for DSM-V and ICD-11*. Cooperative agreement U13MH067855 from the National Institute of Mental Health, National Institute on Drug Abuse, and National Institute on Alcohol Abuse and Alcoholism to American Psychiatric Institute for Research and Education, 2003–2008.

17. Saxena, S., Esparza, P., Regier, D.A., Saraceno, B., and Sartorius, N. (eds.). (2012). *Public health aspects of diagnosis and classification of mental and behavioral disorders—refining the research agenda for DSM-5 and ICD-11*. World Health Organization, Geneva and American Psychiatric Publishing, Arlington, VA.

18. Clarke, D.E., Narrow, W.E., Regier, D.A., *et al.* (2013). DSM-5 field trials in the United States and Canada, part I: study design, sampling strategy, implementation, and analytic approaches. *American Journal of Psychiatry*, 170, 43–58.

19. Regier, D.A., Narrow, W.E., Clarke, D.E., *et al.* (2013). DSM-5 field trials in the United States and Canada, part II: test-retest reliability of selected categorical diagnoses. *American Journal of Psychiatry*, 170, 59–70.

20. Narrow, W.E., Clarke, D.E., Kuramoto, S.J., *et al.* (2013). DSM-5 field trials in the United States and Canada, part III: development and reliability testing of a cross-cutting symptom assessment for DSM-5. *American Journal of Psychiatry*, 170 71–82.

21. Moscicki, E.K., Clarke, D.E., Kuramoto, S.J., *et al.* (2013). Testing DSM-5 in routine clinical practice settings: feasibility and clinical utility. *Psychiatric Services*, 64, 952–60.

22. American Psychiatric Association. (2013). *Diagnostic and statistical manual of mental disorders, fifth edition (DSM-5)*. American Psychiatric Association, Arlington, VA.

23. Andrews, G., Goldberg, D.P., Krueger, R.F., *et al.* (2009). Exploring the feasibility of a meta-structure for DSM-V and ICD-11: could it improve utility and validity? *Psychological Medicine*, 39, 1993–2000.

24. Kraemer, H.C., Kupfer, D.J., Clarke, D.E., Narrow, W.E., and Regier, D.A. (2012). DSM-5: how reliable is reliable enough? *American Journal of Psychiatry*, 169, 13–15.

25. Cross-Disorder Group of the Psychiatric Genomics Consortium. (2013). Identification of risk loci with shared effects on five major psychiatric disorders: a genome-wide analysis. *The Lancet*, 381, 1371–9.

26. First, M.B., Reed, G.M., Hyman, S.E., and Saxena, S. (2015). The development of the ICD-11 Clinical Descriptions and Diagnostic Guidelines for Mental and Behavioral Disorders. *World Psychiatry*, 14, 82–90.

27. First, M.B. (2009). Harmonization of ICD-11 and DSM-V: opportunities and challenges. *British Journal of Psychiatry*, 19, 382–90.

28. International Advisory Group for the Revision of ICD-10 Mental and Behavioral Disorders. (2011). A conceptual framework for the revision of the ICD-10 classification of mental and behavioral disorders. *World Psychiatry*, 10, 86–92.

29. World Health Organization. (1996). *Diagnostic and management guidelines for mental disorders in primary care: ICD-10 Chapter V Primary Care Version*. Hogrefe and Huber, Göttingen.

30. Whiteford, H.A., Degenhardt, L., Rehm, J., *et al.* (2013). Global burden of disease attributable to mental and substance use disorders: findings from the Global Burden of Disease Study 2010. *The Lancet*, 382, 1575–86.

31. World Health Organization World Mental Health Survey Consortium. (2004). Prevalence, severity, and unmet need for treatment of mental disorders in the World Health Organization World Mental Health Surveys. *JAMA*, 291, 2581–90.

32. De Hert, M., Correll, C.U., Bobes, J., *et al.* (2011). Physical illness in patients with severe mental disorders. I. Prevalence, impact of medications and disparities in health care. *World Psychiatry*, 10, 52–77.

33. Svendsen, D., Singer, P., Foti, M.E., and Mauer, B. (2006). *Morbidity and mortality in people with serious mental illness*. Alexandria, VA, USA: National Association of State Mental Health Program Directors (NASMHPD) Medical Directors Council, 2006.

34. Walker, E.R., McGee, R.E., and Druss, B.G. (2015). Mortality in mental disorders and global disease burden implications: a systematic review and meta-analysis. *JAMA Psychiatry*, 72, 334–41.

35. Hyman, S.E. (2007). Can neuroscience be integrated into the DSM-V? *Nature Reviews Neuroscience*, 8, 725–32.

36. Insel, T. (2013). *Transforming diagnosis*. Director's Blog, National Institute of Mental Health. http://www.nimh.nih.gov/about/director/2013/transforming-diagnosis.shtml.

37. Saxena, S., Funk, M., and Chisholm, D. (2013). World Health Assembly adopts Comprehensive Mental Health Action Plan 2013–2020. *The Lancet*, 381, 1970–1.

38. Reed, G.M. (2010). Toward ICD-11: improving the clinical utility of WHO's international classification of mental disorders. *Professional Psychology: Research and Practice*, 41, 457–64.

39. Reed, G.M., Correia, J., Esparza, P., Saxena, S., and Maj, M. (2011). The WPA-WHO global survey of psychiatrists' attitudes towards mental disorders classification. *World Psychiatry*, 10, 118–31.

40. Evans, S.C., Reed, G.M., Roberts, M.C., *et al.* (2013). Psychologists' perspectives on the diagnostic classification of mental disorders: results from the WHO-IUPsyS Global Survey. *International Journal of Psychology*, 48, 177–93.

41. Reed, G.M., Roberts, M.C., Keeley, J., *et al.* (2013). Mental health professionals' natural taxonomies of mental disorders: implications for clinical utility of ICD-11 and DSM-5. *Journal of Clinical Psychology*, 69, 1191–212.

42. Roberts, M.C., Reed, G.M., Medina-Mora, M.E., *et al.* (2012). A global clinicians' map of mental disorders to improve ICD-11. *International Review of Psychiatry*, 24, 578–90.

43. Reed, G.M., First, M.B., Kogan, C.S., *et al.* (2019). Innovations and changes in the ICD-11 classification of mental, behavioural and neurodevelopmental disorders. *World Psychiatry*, 18, 3–19.

44. Keeley, J.W., Reed, G.M., Roberts, M.C., *et al.* (2016). Developing a science of clinical utility in diagnostic classification systems: field study strategies for ICD-11 Mental and Behavioural Disorders. *American Psychologist*, 71, 3–16.

45. Evans, S.C., Burke, J.D., Roberts, M.C., *et al.* (2017). Irritability in child and adolescent psychopathology: an integrative review for ICD-11. *Clinical Psychology Review*, 53, 29–45.

46. Gureje, O. and Reed, G.M. (2016). Bodily distress disorder in ICD-11: problems and prospects. *World Psychiatry*, 15, 291–322.

47. Reed, G.M., Drescher, J., Krueger, R.B., *et al.* (2016). Disorders related to sexuality and gender identity in the ICD-11: revising the ICD-10 classification based on current scientific evidence, best clinical practices, and human rights considerations. *World Psychiatry*, 15, 205–21.

48. Reed, G.M., Sharan, P., Rebello, T.J., *et al.* (2018). The ICD-11 developmental field study of reliability of diagnoses of high-burden mental disorders: Results among adult patients in mental health settings of 13 countries. *World Psychiatry*, 17, 174–86.

49. Reed, G.M., Sharan, P., Rebello, T.J., *et al.* (2018). Clinical utility of ICD-11 diagnostic guidelines for high-burden mental disorders: Results from mental health settings in 13 countries. *World Psychiatry*, 17, 306–15.

50. Üstün, T.B., Goldberg, D.P., Cooper, J., and Sartorius, N. (1995). A new classification for mental disorders with management guidelines for use in primary care: ICD-10 PHC chapter five. *British Journal of General Practice*, 45, 211–15.

51. Goldberg, D.P. and Fawcett, J. (2012). The importance of anxiety in both major depression and bipolar disorder. *Depression and Anxiety*, 29, 471–8.

52. Fava, M., Alpert, J.E., Carmin, C.N., *et al.* (2004). Clinical correlates and symptom patterns of anxious depression among patients with major depression in STAR*D. *Psychological Medicine*, 34, 1299–308.

53. Fava, M., Rush, A.J., and Alpert, J.E. (2008). Difference in treatment outcome in patients with anxious versus non-anxious depression: a STAR*D report. *American Journal of Psychiatry*, 165, 342–51.

54. Goldberg, D.P, Wittchen, H.-U., Zimmermann, P., Pfister, H., and Beesdo-Baum, K. (2014). Anxious and non-anxious forms of major depression: familial, personality and symptom characteristics. *Psychological Medicine*, 44, 1223–34.

55. Lam, T.P., Goldberg, D.P., Dowell, A.C., *et al.* Proposed new diagnoses of anxious depression and bodily stress syndrome in ICD-11-PHC: an international focus group study. *Family Practice*, 30, 76–87.

56. Goldberg, D.P. (2014). Anxious forms of depression. *Depression and Anxiety*, 31, 344–51.

57. Das-Munshi, J., Goldberg, D.P., Bebbington, P.E., Bhugra, D., Dewey, M., and Brugha, T.S. (2008). Public health significance of mixed anxiety and depression: beyond current classification. *British Journal of Psychiatry*, 192, 171–7.

58. Barkow, K., Heuna, R., Wittchen, H.-U., Üstün, B., Gansickea, M., and Maier, W. (2004). Mixed anxiety–depression in a 1 year follow-up study: shift to other diagnoses or remission? *Journal of Affective Disorders*, 75, 235–9.

59. Krupinski, J. and Tiller, J.W. (2001). The identification and treatment of depression by general practitioners. *Australian and New Zealand Journal of Psychiatry*, 35, 827–32.

60. Goldberg, D.P., Prisciandaro, J.J., and Williams, P. (2012). The primary health care version of ICD-11: the detection of common mental disorders in general medical settings. *General Hospital Psychiatry*, 34, 665–70.

61. World Health Organization. (2001). *International classification of functioning, disability and health*. World Health Organization, Geneva.

62. Narrow, W.E., Rae, D.S., Robins, L.E., and Regier, D.A. (2002). Revised prevalence estimates of mental disorders in the United States: Using a clinical significance criterion to reconcile 2 survey's estimates. *Archives of General Psychiatry*, 59, 115–23.

63. Kessler, R.C., Barker, P.R., Colpe, L.J., *et al.* (2003). Screening for serious mental illness in the general population. *Archives of General Psychiatry*, 60, 184–9.

64. Selb, M. (2015). ICD-11: a comprehensive picture of health, an update on the ICD-ICF joint use initiative. *Journal of Rehabilitation Medicine*, 47, 2–8.

65. Üstün, B., Kostanjsek, N., Chatterji, S., and Rehm, J. (eds.). (2010). *Measuring health and disability: manual for WHO Disability Assessment Schedule WHODAS 2.0*. World Health Organization, Geneva.

66. Charney, D.S., Barlow, D.H., Botteron, K., *et al.* (2002). Neuroscience research agenda to guide development of a pathophysiologically based classification system. In: Kupfer, D.J., First, M.B., and Regier, D.A. (eds) *A research agenda for DSM-V*. American Psychiatric Association, Washington D.C. pp. 31–83.

67. Cuthbert, B.N. (2014). The RDoC framework: facilitating transition from ICD/DSM to dimensional approaches that integrate neuroscience and psychopathology. *World Psychiatry*, 13, 28–35.

68. Regier DA. (2015). Potential DSM-5 and RDoC synergy for mental health research, treatment, and health policy advances. *Psychological Inquiry*, 26, 288–71.

69. Clark, L.A., Cuthbert, B., Lewis-Fernández, R., Narrow, W., Reed, G.M. (2017). ICD-11, DSM-5, and RDoC: three approaches to understanding and classifying mental disorder. *Psychological Science in the Public Interest*, 18, 72–145.

# 8

# The National Institute of Mental Health Research Domain Criteria

## An alternative framework to guide psychopathology research

*Charles A. Sanislow, Sarah E. Morris, Jennifer Pacheco, and Bruce N. Cuthbert*

## Introduction

The National Institute of Mental Health (NIMH) launched the Research Domain Criteria (RDoC) in 2009, in response to the 2008 NIMH Strategic Plan, call for new ways of classifying mental illnesses that are based on dimensions of observable behavioural and neurobiological measures. The RDoC initiative was motivated by the need to address the scientific concern that the field had equated psychiatric illness with syndromes based on clinically observed diagnostic criteria, which were not well connected with neural and psychological mechanisms. The RDoC was also motivated because progress in treatment development had been slowed by a disproportionately narrow focus on disorders as defined by mainstream diagnostic criteria. Specifically, psychiatric research strategies have been limited by explanations of disorders that have been organized around clinical presentation.

At the outset, we wish to be clear that DSM-5 and ICD-11 (and their predecessors) have been vital for informing the treatment of human distress and dysfunction, and continue to serve an important clinical role. Despite limitations (detailed in the forthcoming), these diagnostic manuals have been critical for the development of innovative theories of mental disorders (for example, anxiety, depression, bipolar disorder, schizophrenia), which, in turn. have facilitated empirical advances to develop a number of effective treatments. That said, a counterpoint consensus that progress could be accelerated has existed for some time, such that gains in understanding and treating mental illness are modest, relative to the more recent advances in integrative neuroscience. This view holds that research aimed at clarifying mechanisms of psychiatric illness (for example, disrupted neural circuits and mental processes) of clinically described syndromes has reached the asymptote of progress. As a result, research into new and potentially more effective treatments has waned. We argue that a change in the conceptualizations of mental disorders is needed to improve diagnostic validity, to open new avenues of research, and to expedite progress in the development of new and more effective treatments.

## Background and rationale for the RDoC

How did psychiatry research reach the paradoxical state of being constrained by a diagnostic system of its own creation? The answer is a story about reliability and validity. In the late 1960s and early 1970s, Washington University became the centre of psychiatric research in the United States, so much so that influential academic leaders of the time became known in some circles as 'The St Louis Group'. For that era, this was a radical collection of psychiatrists. Researchers leading this charge eschewed aetiological theories (mainly psychoanalytic) on the promissory note (mistaken, as it turns out) that if reliable diagnoses were developed, then laboratory studies to elucidate the biological and genetic underpinnings would follow. The motivation was to bring respect to the field by establishing psychiatry as science, in part because one consequence of the psychoanalytic zeitgeist that had prevailed up until that time was that clinicians frequently disagreed about a patient's diagnosis (that is, reliability was poor). Some psychiatrists were concerned that physicians in other specialties espoused the view that psychiatry was not 'real medicine'. The St Louis Group wanted to change this impression and led the charge for psychiatry researchers to focus squarely on improving reliability, with the expectation that the discovery of biological substrates would eventually follow.

Drawing from the heritage of Emil Kraepelin's work (as well as incorporating efforts by Kurt Schneider), clinically observable diagnostic criteria for psychiatric research were developed—earning the researchers the label 'neo-Kraepelinianians' [1]. The new diagnostic criteria were first colloquially referred to as the 'Feighner Criteria' [2], and later became the Research Diagnostic Criteria, or 'RDC' (not to be confused with RDoC). This was a major advance for psychiatry. The new criteria were largely descriptive, freeing researchers from the constraint of psychoanalytic theory. Importantly, psychiatric researchers could now be confident that they were studying the same symptom sets in patients. Working from these clinical syndromes, it was assumed that valid diagnoses could be established. In this vein, Robins and Guze (1970) [3] proclaimed five criteria for the validity of psychiatric diagnoses: (1) clinical description; (2) laboratory tests; (3) delimitation from other disorders; (4) follow-up studies and course; and (5) family studies. These criteria became the bedrock principles guiding the development of psychiatric nosology for the next five decades [4].

The field was at a crossroads on the clinical side too. The development of a radically changed DSM was on the horizon, and the psychiatrist Robert Spitzer was appointed to revise the manual. Among clinicians, there was resistance for overly rapid change, but the RDC were ready-made to be transposed to clinical diagnoses for the 'new' DSM diagnostic manual. As the research criteria were translated to the clinical realm, much of the resulting formulations were based on 'expert consensus', and this led to some notable changes. In the process, however, some duration criteria were relaxed for clinical translation in ways that, while stringent for research purposes, would be less inclusive for clinical purposes; for instance, in the case of major depressive disorder, depressed mood was tightened from 1 month to 2 weeks [5].

DSM-III [6] was both embraced and disparaged by the field. Clinicians could finally agree on a diagnosis with confidence. This was an improvement for developing coherent treatment plans. When used in research, the uniformity of patient groups was all but guaranteed. However, it gave false assurance that psychiatrists were treating 'real' diseases, giving the impression that these new diagnoses were 'natural kinds', and this led to a problem of reification and overconfidence that corresponding mental and neural mechanisms could be unearthed for each disorder [7]. It also unleashed political fury, consequent to the incorporation of symptom criteria that were criticized for being chosen on the arbitrary basis of clinical consensus and for being value-laden with stereotypical cultural beliefs.

Just over a decade after DSM-III was introduced, Jerome Wakefield (1992) [8] addressed these issues by articulating a definition of mental disorder that he termed 'harmful dysfunction'. His definition held two central tenets for a mental illness—firstly, that an 'internal mechanism' was not functioning, and secondly, that the dysfunction caused harm either to the individual, in the form of subjective distress, or to society by the inability for the afflicted person to fulfil his or her roles according to accepted cultural expectations. In psychology, Wakefield's model became the textbook definition of mental disorder; in psychiatry, the influence of the 'harmful' part of his definition was embraced and its influence persists throughout DSM-5, which relies, in many instances, on functional deficits to determine the clinical threshold. It is the second component of Wakefield's definition—the dysfunction of an 'internal mechanism'—that has yet to be elaborated for DSM-based diagnoses (post-1980 through the present), and it is now widely acknowledged that DSM sacrificed validity for reliability.

## Manifest problems of the descriptive approach

The standardized criteria provided by the prevailing DSM diagnostic systems (DSM-III [6] going forward through the current fifth

edition) and the more recent iterations of the WHO's ICD (through the current eleventh version) have made possible the reliable diagnosis of patients for both clinical and research purposes. This has been essential to an important developmental phase of psychiatric science. The diagnostic manuals also improved the conception of mental disorders, as aspects of many disorders were refined, mainly on the basis of Robins and Guze (1970) [3] criteria of course and outcome, and some by delineation from other disorders. However, validation has come up short, particularly for biologically related systems. Moreover, with accumulated knowledge emerging from research using the tools of modern behavioural neuroscience, it became increasingly clear that the nature of psychopathology mechanisms did not align with the descriptively derived categorical diagnoses [9].

The problems evident from poor validity include polythetic criteria sets, high rates of diagnostic co-occurrence ('comorbidity'), heterogeneity within diagnoses, overspecification, arbitrary or subjective cut points, and a binary classification that excludes a dimensional gradience of symptoms. Phenotypes codified in DSM-III (and subsequently aligned in the ICDs) have yet to be validated with laboratory studies. Mental disorder syndromes based on descriptive diagnosis, it seems, have been lost in translational research. The early commentaries that the fundamental tenets of clinical syndromes for DSM-III, carried forward through DSM-5, were flawed for research purposes had been realized (for example, [10]).

By definition, DSM symptoms are imperfect indicators of the diagnosis to which they refer. No single symptom is required for a diagnosis; rather, collectively, a subgroup of symptoms represents the essence of a construct. This is termed 'polythetic' and means there are sundry ways to 'get' a DSM diagnosis. For instance, there are 256 combinations of symptoms for borderline personality disorder (BPD) [11]; two people can meet criteria for major depressive disorder (MDD) and not share a single symptom in common (if weight loss and weight gain are considered as separate symptoms) (APA, DSM-5). DSM also implies that many symptoms are equally important when actually they may be differentially related to functioning and the threshold number of symptoms required for a diagnosis is not empirically determined [12]. At the same time, clinicians demonstrate a proclivity to overweigh certain symptoms that steer them to a diagnosis, for instance, self-harm behaviour for BPD [13, 14, 15].

The exclusion of 'comorbid' diagnoses can artificially restrict the range of pathological mechanisms in psychiatric research [16]. Moreover, it has been argued that the term 'co-occurrence' is preferred over 'comorbidity' by many, precisely because associated neural and mental mechanisms have not been elaborated and it is unclear if two 'comorbid' psychiatric diagnoses have interrelated psychopathology or are merely different sets of descriptors for the same psychopathological processes (see [17]). Individuals who are diagnosed with more than one disorder are often excluded from research, so that confounding by co-occurring disorders is avoided. This approach may increase the specificity of claims resulting from significant between-groups differences, but the result is a predominant focus on reified patient groups and 'super-normal' comparison groups, neither of which are representative of the general patient and non-patient populations.

Another problem with research focusing on clinically described syndromes is the imposition of categories. By focusing research efforts primarily on comparing individuals who meet diagnostic criteria with those who do not experience psychiatric symptoms, potentially meaningful variance in symptoms and neurobehavioural processes may be excluded. Arguments in favour of diagnostic categories include the idea that these extended phenotypes do not reflect a true continuum in symptoms due to varying degrees of disruption of a common symptom-related mechanism, but rather may be the result of distinct processes that distinguish latent clusters of individuals and result in variable symptom presentations which may relate to the likelihood that an individual will seek treatment [18, 19]. However, dimensionality in neurobehavioural processes is consistent with other disease-relevant biological processes. More generally, in internal medicine, hypertension provides an example. Blood pressure levels fall along a gradient, but a threshold—informed by research and subject to change in response to new information—defines the presence of disease and dictates the type of treatment.

With the DSM approach, many individuals experience psychiatric symptoms such as anxiety, depression, or disruptions in thinking that are not sufficient in number, duration, or severity to meet diagnostic criteria. Some of these cases are handled with the 'Unspecified' (formerly 'Not otherwise specified') categories. When the DSM is used for research purposes, however, these incomplete diagnoses are typically excluded from study design, eliminating a potentially significant range of psychopathology. Epidemiological studies find that sub-syndromal psychiatric symptoms are not unusual in the general population. Thus, using the DSM for research potentially excludes a large segment of the population from a study. When DSM disorders are considered dimensionally, it has been shown for some disorders that those who are sub-diagnostic-threshold suffer similar degrees of functional impairment and distress as those who meet the full criteria for the disorder (for example, [20]). Indeed, there is a solid base of evidence and growing consensus for dimensional approaches to diagnosis [21]. When dimensional approaches are applied to DSM symptom sets, considerable improvement in reliability and validity has been demonstrated [22]. However, to connect clinical symptoms to neurobiological mechanisms, more than a simple dimensionalization DSM category is needed (for example, [23]; see also [24]).

## A new approach

These problems illustrate how dividing the lines between psychological health and mental illness can be clinically subjective and suggest that there may be useful discontinuities or thresholds with implications for treatment decisions or the illness course. However, narrowing the definition of a positive diagnosis for clinical purposes can create problems when applied to research design by focusing only on the extremes of a hypothetical health–illness spectrum, excluding the full variation of symptom expression and associated mechanisms. The reasoning implicit in the current diagnostic frameworks is consistent with an infectious disease model in which an individual is either infected with the disease-causing agent or is not, prompting a dichotomous diagnostic decision for each disorder—are diagnostic criteria met or not? This approach provides an acceptably reliable method for sorting research participants into patient and non-patient groups for the purposes of looking for group differences but may have the unintended consequence

of distorting our understanding of the true nature of the landscape of mental disorders. In an ironic twist, other areas of medicine are confronting similar issues and trying to align their diagnostic systems with a new understanding of systems biology. For instance, the National Academies of Sciences issued in 2011 a call for all disease taxonomies to be revised to align more closely with the new understanding of molecular biological processes [25].

In sum, psychiatric diagnosis achieved good reliability, essential for clinical practice and research, but this came at the expense of validity. Definitions of disorders have evolved over centuries and rely heavily on patient self-report of internal experiences. The diagnoses identify common clinical presentations of syndromes, but the foundations for these frameworks precede modern behavioural neuroscience and do not incorporate an understanding of the ways in which the brain develops and functions. Although neuroscience has yielded important insights about mental disorders, these methods are failing to bring about the revolution in understanding and treatment that was anticipated when they were developed [26].

Finally, a persistent myth that has stymied novel solutions to these problems should not go unmentioned: Over the past several decades, the hope was held that mental disorders would be better understood once better tools were developed. That hope is gradually fading. The brain's complexity is daunting, consisting of millions of neurons and other types of cells, with connections and patterns of activity continually changing according to developmental trajectories and in response to experiences and exposures. Technology for visualizing and quantifying the structure and function of the brain has yielded an ever expanding corpus of published studies, and the tools of genetics, molecular biology, and neuroimaging continue to improve; yet no method has emerged that has detected a specific neuropathological process that accounts for a psychiatric disorder and would determine the classification of individuals into diagnostic groups.

The futility of mapping syndromal phenotypes (that is, DSM-based diagnoses) onto dysfunctional internal mechanisms has also been recognized by those developing pharmaceutical agents [27]. Over the past decade, research driven by pharmaceutical companies waned, in large part due to problems that symptom-based phenotypes were not the right targets for drug development (see [28]). Thus, both scientific concerns about psychiatry's approach to diagnosis, along with practical matters obviating treatment development, were motivations for the development of the RDoC. Indeed, others articulated this problem and argued for approaches that would embrace intermediate phenotypes [29, 30].

Despite widespread recognition of these problems, funding for the bulk of psychopathology research in the United States has curiously remained harnessed to the DSM categories. The DSM classifications had become the de facto standards for psychiatric research, such that the entire scientific cycle, from grant applications, review and funding decisions, to publication, was dominated by DSM-based disorders, and little space was left for psychopathology research conducted outside this framework. Some investigators have reported to their programme officers a reluctance to submit non-DSM-based research for funding applications because of concerns such research would not fare well in review for scientific merit, even for proposals in response to specific requests for funding. Other investigators have complained of arbitrary constraints for how to handle co-occurring diagnoses in the culture of grant review committees, as well as favoritisms for certain DSM disorders [31]. The RDoC was introduced to provide an alternative path for researchers to study psychopathology mechanisms, in part so that these impositions could be circumvented.

Van Praag and colleagues (1990) [32] alerted the field to the risks of 'nosological tunnel vision', noting that 'exclusive adherence to nosology has not served biological psychiatry well [but] has been a factor stunting its growth' ([32], p. 507); a decade later, van Praag diagnosed psychiatry with 'nosologomania' [33]. Psychiatry departments have generally been organized according to DSM disorders, and this might also be seen as an impediment to progress, encouraging both research and training in 'silos' and cordoning off knowledge that ideally would be integrated. As recognition of these impediments has become clearer, the field is responding. The journal *Schizophrenia Bulletin* recently added the subtitle '*The Journal of Psychoses and Related Disorders*' to reflect the changing nature of the field. The NIMH is presently addressing the inherent limitations of extramural research largely programmatically organized around disorders by encouraging a focus on trans-diagnostic diagnoses, cross-cutting features, and the RDoC.

## Development of the RDoC framework

In March 2009, the then NIMH director Thomas Insel formed an Internal Working Group to address the 2008 NIMH Strategic Objective to develop new ways to classify mental illnesses based on dimensions of observable behavioural and neurobiological measures (see [34] for a brief summary of the process, including the original working group members). The initial development of the RDoC was influenced by non-DSM-based models of psychopathology research, including the earlier mentioned intermediate phenotype approach [29, 30], as well as pre-DSM-III [6] experimental psychopathology approaches, including work from experimental psychopathology (for example, [35, 36]) and research in developmental psychology (for example, [37]). Facing a *tabula rasa*, and drawing from these approaches, five domains were initially proposed as a starting point: 'Negative valence systems', 'Positive valence systems', 'Cognitive systems', 'Social processes', and 'Regulatory and arousal systems'. Within each of these five domains were grouped a number of potential constructs (and subconstructs), each with evidence for a valid psychological construct, including evidence for a neural circuit associated with a psychological function relevant to psychopathology.

To integrate basic neural and psychological mechanisms with observable behaviour relevant to palpable psychopathology, the Internal Working Group proposed 'units of analyses'. These included *genes, molecules, neural circuits, physiology, behaviour*, and *self-report* (the latter including patient verbal reports). The framework took shape as a matrix, with the original five domains grouping relevant constructs in the rows of the matrix, and 'units of analysis' forming the columns. An additional column—*paradigms*—was added to the matrix to include tasks and assessments to measure the constructs.

The next step in the development of the RDoC matrix was the collaborative effort of leading scientists across multiple workshops to review the evidence and articulate and define each of the domains. Each of the workshops was focused on evaluating evidence for potential constructs and elaborating specific definitions for each

construct, including differentiating them from related constructs. One workshop was convened for each domain, except for cognitive systems, for which there were two because the first RDoC workshop piloted the Cognitive Construct 'Working Memory'. Proceedings from the workshops can be found on the RDoC website (https://www.nimh.nih.gov/research-priorities/rdoc/development-of-the-rdoc-framework.shtml). Prior to each workshop, surveys were sent to NIMH awardees and psychiatry and psychology department chairs across the United States. Survey feedback was presented at the start of each workshop. Workshop participants (invited by the NIMH, based on expertise in the relevant research domain, as evidenced by published work and funding history) were organized into breakout groups to consider and refine the constructs or to discard them and propose new constructs. The groups examined what was known about the units of analysis for each construct and considered what questions remained unanswered, as well as potential avenues of research that might answer these questions. These considerations were then reported out to each full domain group where construct definitions were minted. The end result included an annotated listing of the elements that would populate the RDoC matrix with respect to the genes, molecules, cells, circuits, physiology, and self-reports comprising each defined construct, as well as the nomination of promising and reliable behavioural tasks (paradigms) that could be used to assess function within a construct. The listings from all six independent meetings, when combined, comprised the first version of the RDoC matrix (see https://www.nimh.nih.gov/research-priorities/rdoc/rdoc-snapshot-version-1-saved-3-7-2016.shtml).

## Structure of the RDoC matrix

The RDoC matrix provides a research framework to specify fundamental processes of mental illness in biological and behavioural units of analyses. The rows of the matrix represent specific dimensions of function (domains and constructs), and columns represent different kinds of observations for study (units of analysis). The constructs embody specified functional dimensions of behaviour and are characterized in the aggregate by the genes, molecules, circuits, etc. that correspond to certain behaviours. Constructs are, in turn, grouped into higher-level domains of functioning, reflecting contemporary knowledge about major systems of cognition, motivation, and social behaviour. In its present form, there are six domains in the RDoC matrix: 'Negative valence systems', 'Positive valence systems', 'Cognitive systems', 'Systems for social processes', and 'Arousal/regulatory systems', and 'Sensorimotor systems', the latter domain incorporated in 2018 (Table 8.1). The matrix columns specify units of analysis used to study the constructs and include genes, molecules, cells, circuits, physiology (for example, heart rate or event-related potentials), behaviour, and self-reports. In the cells of the matrix are specific elements that serve as exemplars which are empirically associated with the construct and the corresponding unit of analysis.

The RDoC domains were selected to be purposefully broad, to link directly to psychopathological mechanisms, and for their potential for theoretical integration. The framework is directed towards constructs most relevant to mental disorders and is not intended to span the entire scope of functional behaviour [38–41]. The domains are 'superordinate', and each one includes

**Table 8.1** RDoC domains, domain definitions, and corresponding constructs and subconstructs

| Domains | Definition | Constructs and subconstructs |
| --- | --- | --- |
| Negative valence systems | Activation of the brain's defensive motivational system to promote behaviours that protect the organism from perceived danger. Normal fear involves a pattern of adaptive responses to conditioned or unconditioned threat stimuli (exteroceptive or interoceptive). Fear can involve internal representations and cognitive processing and can be modulated by a variety of factors | Acute threat ('fear')<br>Potential threat ('anxiety')<br>Sustained threat<br>Loss<br>Frustrative non-reward |
| Positive valence systems | Systems primarily responsible for responses to positive motivational situations or contexts such as reward seeking, consummatory behaviour, and reward/habit learning | Reward responsiveness<br>    Reward anticipation;<br>    Initial response to reward;<br>    Reward satiation<br>Reward learning<br>    Probabilistic and reinforcement learning;<br>    Reward prediction error;<br>    Habit – PVS<br>Reward valuation<br>    Reward (probability);<br>    Delay;<br>    Effort |
| Cognitive systems | Systems are responsible for various cognitive processes | Attention<br>Perception<br>    Visual perception;<br>    Auditory perception;<br>    Olfactory/somatosensory/multimodal perception<br>Declarative memory<br>Language<br>Cognitive control<br>    Goal selection; updating, representation, maintenance<br>    Response selection; inhibition/suppression<br>    Performance monitoring |
| Social processes | Systems that mediate responses to interpersonal settings of various types, including perception and interpretation of others' actions | Affiliation and attachment<br>Social communication<br>    Reception of facial communication;<br>    Production of facial communication;<br>    Reception of non-facial communication;<br>    Production of non-facial communication<br>Working memory<br>    Active maintenance;<br>    Flexible updating;<br>    Limited capacity;<br>    Interference control |
| Arousal and regulatory systems | Systems responsible for generating activation of neural systems as appropriate for various contexts, and providing appropriate homeostatic regulation of such systems as energy balance and sleep | Arousal<br>Circadian rhythms<br>Sleep–wakefulness |
| Sensorimotor systems | Sensorimotor systems are primarily responsible for the control and execution of motor behaviours and their refinement during learning and development | Motor actions<br>    Action, planning and selection;<br>    Sensorimotor dynamics;<br>    Initiation;<br>    Execution;<br>    Inhibition and termination<br>Agency and ownership<br>Habit – sensorimotor<br>Innate motor patterns |

Reproduced from https://www.nimh.nih.gov/research-priorities/rdoc/constructs/rdoc-matrix.shtml

multiple, more specific constructs and subconstructs (indented in the third column of Table 8.1). In devising and defining the constructs that would comprise each domain, workshop members were asked to consider three criteria when evaluating the merits of a construct: (1) sufficient evidence for the validity of the construct as a functional unit of behaviour or cognitive process; (2) sufficient evidence for a neural circuit or system that played a primary role in implementing the construct's function; and (3) sufficient relevance for understanding some aspects of psychopathology [38].

The current set of constructs is focused on, and constrained by, circuit definitions to avoid overspecification and proliferation of constructs. The intent is not to arbitrarily exclude constructs, but rather to foster thinking about how constructs are related across observations of different systems (that is, units of analysis). Acknowledged are the complexities of the brain and behaviour, such that circuits and constructs will necessarily overlap and interrelate, such that, to some degree, arbitrary separations are unavoidable. The spelling out of interrelations among constructs and across units of analysis will help to refine or otherwise clarify the constructs in a bootstrapping fashion. In fact, the framework is meant to foster, not discourage, research that explicates mechanisms within and across the constructs as listed. As such, RDoC research design is likely to foster interdisciplinary research collaborations.

The RDoC matrix is best viewed as a work in progress, and not as fait accompli. The matrix is not a finite determination of the field of psychopathology, and by no means is—or was it ever—meant to be a comprehensive framework of psychopathology to be cast in stone. In other words, constructs (and subconstructs), as well as the tasks that are listed in the matrix, are best viewed as exemplars. From its inception, we have indicated that the matrix is expected to undergo revision and updates with accumulating data, and the understanding of psychopathological systems and symptoms is recognized. Because the RDoC was initiated by the NIMH, the National Advisory Mental Health Council (NAMHC) oversees revisions. The NAMHC has covened a committee—the 'Changes to the Matrix Council' (CMAT) Workgroup—to evaluate alterations, updates, and additions to the matrix. Recent revisions include the addition of the earlier mentioned 'Sensorimotor systems' domain. There have also been revisions motivated by the accumulation of new scientific evidence, as well as for purposes of clarity, for instance an update to the 'Positive valence systems' domain. The CMAT Workgroup is provided with resources to consult with experts in the field and to convene meetings as appropriate. All revisions are detailed and available on the RDoC website (see https://www.nimh.nih.gov/about/advisory-boards-and-groups/namhc/reports/rdoc-changes-to-the-matrix-cmat-workgroup-update-addition-of-the-sensorimotor-domain.shtml and https://www.nimh.nih.gov/about/advisory-boards-and-groups/namhc/reports/cmat-pvs-report-508_157003.pdf, respectively, for these changes).

Some have questioned whether the number of constructs is too sparse. In framing the RDoC, the goal was to include relatively high-level constructs to avoid overspecification of functions that could become unwieldy and thereby necessitate unnecessarily frequent revisions to the list or otherwise constrain investigators as research progresses. As one obvious example, a single 'Perception' construct is listed that includes visual, auditory, and other sensory modalities. Defined in this way, the constructs are more easily subject to refinement as new research emerges. Potential constructs not specified in the matrix can be studied with the RDoC framework. As new constructs are considered, the three criteria outlined should be used to evaluate their merits in order to achieve the goals of the RDoC initiative [38].

## Units of analysis

The columns of the matrix represent the units of analysis typically employed in psychopathology research. The term 'units' was deliberately chosen over the term 'levels' of analyses, so as not to privilege any one type of observation or to imply a reductionist ideology (see [42] for a detailed discussion of these issues). As the RDoC

intends to promote integration of knowledge across multiple disciplines, the framework emphasizes the integration of knowledge about genes, cells, and circuits, with knowledge about cognition, emotion, and behaviour. The 'Circuit' unit of analysis refers to measurements of particular neural circuits, as studied by neuroimaging techniques or other measures, such as event-related potentials with established source localization, that have been validated by animal models or functional neuroimaging. The 'Physiology' unit of analysis refers to measures, such as heart rate and cortisol levels, that are well-established indices of certain constructs but that are not direct measures of neural circuits. The 'Behaviour' unit of analysis can refer variously to behavioural tasks (for example, a working memory task) or to systematic behavioural observations (for example, a toddler behavioural assessment). The 'Self-report' unit of analysis refers to interview-based scales, self-report questionnaires, or other instruments that may encompass normal-range and/or abnormal aspects of the dimension of interest.

When initially constructed, the units of analyses for the 'genes' column included candidate genes relevant to psychopathology. The idea was that connecting certain gene products to physiology would help to clarify specific aberrations in psychopathology. However, some researchers have raised questions about statistical power issues and the replicability of candidate gene studies (see [43]; see also [44]), and ' … the current state of the field emphasizes the need for robust evidence of association, generally resulting from adequately powered genome wide association studies, as opposed to candidate gene approaches' [45]. Interestingly, during the original RDoC workshops, questions about how to distinguish genes from molecules (that is, gene products) were raised on multiple occasions. As evidence and various approaches to genetic studies are further evaluated, this column of the matrix will be updated accordingly.

## Paradigms (tasks)

The matrix includes a separate column to specify well-validated, reliable tasks and measures, or 'paradigms', used in studying each construct. These paradigms may be relevant for more than one unit of analysis, and rather than list them in separate columns, they are included under the 'Paradigms' heading. A National Advisory Mental Health Council (NAMHC) workgroup was assembled and charged with developing recommendations for paradigms for each construct, according to several critical considerations. Their work considered the development of exemplar tasks and led to revisions in the matrix (the full report can be found at: https://www.nimh.nih.gov/about/advisory-boards-and-groups/namhc/reports/rdoc_council_workgroup_report_153440.pdf).

## Development and environment

Since its inception, the RDoC has held that developmental processes and environmental influences are inseparable from the consideration of psychopathology [46]. However, a logistical problem is created if one assumes the two-dimensional RDoC matrix to be a complete model, rather than an organizational framework, in which case the absence of explicitly representing development and environment in the matrix would indeed be problematic. For research purposes, empirical aspects of the matrix may be incorporated into the developmental theory. In this way, the RDoC additionally provides a platform to organize the connections of research findings, or the development of a nomological network, conducted from various theoretical paradigms. Investigators are demonstrating the utility of the RDoC for developmental psychopathology research, as evidenced by the substantial proportion (approximately half, to date) of NIMH-funded RDoC grants that focus on the role of developmental processes and/or environmental factors in psychopathology.

Understanding developmental trajectories across various phases of the lifespan represents a critical consideration that is implicit for the RDoC and might be thought of as a third dimension in the overall framework. To fully explore the contributions of development to RDoC constructs, investigators must bear in mind the complexities of development. Not all capacities develop in a linear manner, and understanding the interaction between constructs as they appear, mature, and differentiate is important. Characterizing these developmental trajectories will help inform how development occurs, which systems come online before or after others, and how they interact differentially across development. It will likewise be important for investigators to explore the continuities (and discontinuities) that exist across development itself, with some behaviours being normal at certain developmental stages, but a sign of mental illness at others. Relatedly, the concept of sensitive periods, when the effects of particular experiences have a strong influence on brain and behaviour, is key to understanding how the timing of events can impact the risk for atypical development [46, 47].

The types of constructs typically found in the literature on human neurodevelopment are similar to several RDoC domains, and many areas of the child psychopathology literature (for example, reward sensitivity, cognitive and emotional dysregulation, behavioural inhibition) serve as a more compatible model for a dimensionally based approach, compared to the highly specified categories of adult psychopathology. The goal is to place these constructs in the context of theories of development (for example, [48]). A more comprehensive understanding of the trajectories that lead to disorders, particularly in the context of quantified measures that can validly identify pre-symptomatic dysfunction, will aid early prevention efforts. In addition, the RDoC's focus on integrative methodologies may lead to earlier detection of psychopathology. By not relying on self-report as the 'gold standard', deviations in developmental processes may be detectable before they are observable as overt clinical symptoms.

The importance of environmental influences on psychiatric illnesses is incontrovertible, and RDoC-based research promotes a systematic focus on development and the environment—as well as with their mutual interactions—and their individual and interacting relationships to specific circuits and functions [38]. One way to approach the environment is to equate it with the variable of time, typically represented in science as 'the fourth dimension'. Just as empirical and theoretical interrelations are expected to be specified across units of analyses and constructs, environmental factors, including those reciprocating with developmental changes, can be theoretically spelt out—and empirically tested—with changes in the elements across time.

Older ideas about environmental influences have given way to advances in neuroscience that articulate how stress and deprivation can have a negative impact, including epigenetic factors. Abnormalities in stress responses can result from maladaptive maturation of the nervous system, including its interaction with the wide variety of external influences beginning at conception. The social and physical environment comprises sources of both risk and protection for many different disorders occurring at all points along the lifespan, and methods for studying phenomena such as gene expression, neural plasticity, and various types of learning are rapidly advancing. As with developmental aspects, environmental influences may thus be considered as another critical element of the RDoC matrix. Particular environmental stressors, such as early child abuse, may increase risk for a wide variety of disorders. Environmental effects are most ideally studied bidirectionally; for example, an individual's behaviour affects his/her social environment (for example, family or friends), which, in turn, affects the nature of others' behaviour towards the individual. Research organized around the relevant circuit-based dimensions that are affected, independent of a particular disorder, may thereby accelerate knowledge regarding environmental influences across multiple units of analysis.

## RDoC research design

What does RDoC research look like? Early in our formulations of how one might conduct RDoC research, we emphasized the idea of choosing a 'sampling frame' or a study group of participants that varied widely enough across a spectrum of symptoms or clinical problems that no relevant mechanisms would be excluded. For instance, a researcher interested in studying fear mechanisms might take 'all comers' at an anxiety disorders treatment clinic (regardless of DSM-5 diagnosis) and then use results from a task or paradigm to determine different study groups or dimensions, for instance, the degree to which a fear response could be extinguished through an extinction paradigm. Even though the dimensions being studied would not involve DSM-5 diagnoses per se, those diagnoses could be adjunctively tracked and used to draw trans-diagnostic connections. The latter would assist in future versions of clinical diagnostic manuals.

A sometimes mistaken notion drawn by investigators is that the RDoC necessitates the complete exclusion of DSM diagnoses. This is not the case. For example, investigators might select participants on the basis of a single DSM diagnosis to clarify component dimensions of that diagnosis, for instance, affective dysregulation among patients diagnosed with BPD. For the RDoC, the caveats of this approach would be that inclusion criteria should not be overly restrictive. For example, in this case, high rates of diagnostic co-occurrence would be expected and co-occurring diagnoses should not be used as a basis of exclusion, lest important variation in systems relevant to the regulation of affect be eliminated. Also, understanding of affective dysregulation would be expected to generalize—and might be studied in follow-up—to those suffering similar problems, but not necessarily diagnosable with BPD.

Research that examines features that cross-cut traditional diagnostic categories or trans-diagnostic research are consistent with the RDoC approach. Several groups of researchers have reported findings using trans-diagnostic approaches that have identified trans-diagnostic features for psychotic disorders (for example, Sabharwal *et al.*, 2017 [49]), obsessive–compulsive disorders (for example, [50]), and attention-deficit/hyperactivity disorder (for example, [52]), and depression (for example, [52]). Similarly, for depression, Liston and colleagues have identified four biotypes of depression using computational approaches [53]. Researchers have been making advances in precision medicine by clarifying such cross-cutting dimensions to serve as treatment targets (for example, [54]). With an RDoC approach, these dimensions provide a new beginning and can serve as a starting point for defining participant groups or dimensions to serve as independent variables for study, in lieu of traditional diagnostic categories or dimensions (see [55]). Tamminga and colleagues identified biotypes from a collective sample across bipolar disorder, schizoaffective disorder, and schizophrenia and found that the biotypes were more predictive of functional impairment [56]. Their approach exemplifies the RDoC approach.

## Change is afoot

Collectively, the field of psychiatry, particularly the area of diagnosis, is in a state of unrest that historically characterizes the conditions under which a paradigm change is afoot [57]. Motivations for NIMH efforts with the RDoC are evident in other quarters. The authors of DSM-5 had strived for the ambitious goal of a paradigm change [58]. For a number of reasons, some logistical and some based on the inherent structure, as discussed in earlier parts of this chapter, this goal was not achieved. However, the cross-cutting symptom checklists for DSM-5 are currently being developed, with evidence of good reliability [59], including dimensional characteristics of severity, number, and duration of symptoms (for example, [60, 61]). The alternative model of personality disorders provides another example where the DSM-approach is progressing [62].

Decades of work on structural approaches to psychopathology have now been codified in the Hierarchical Taxonomy of Psychopathology (HiTOP) [63]. As is the case with the RDoC, the HiTOP approach reorganizes clinical symptoms found throughout the DSM agnostic to the original diagnostic categories; however, links to cross-validate these constructs with internal mechanisms (biological or psychological) are limited [64]. Early efforts on this front are promising, especially the psychoneurometric approach developed by Patrick and colleagues [65, 66]. Observations from computational neuroscience working from the 'bottom up' may be particularly informative to help spell out a theoretical understanding of these connections [67, 68]. Finally, an international effort has been undertaken with the Neuroscience-based Nomenclature (NbN) [69] (see also Chapter 9). The NbN offers a template for clinicians to prescribe, based on common symptom sets of familiar mental disorders, but by aggregating symptoms on the basis of how they connect to neurobiological systems.

## Going forward with the RDoC

The RDoC was developed out of the recognition by NIMH leadership that something radically different was needed to effect change in research, so that advances in integrative neuroscience could inform the understanding of biological and psychological processes involved with human suffering and dysfunction. From its inception, the NIMH has emphasized that the RDoC depends on input from the field and on strong empirical support for both its structure and research executed with the RDoC framework. The degree to which

the RDoC will be embraced by the field—or perhaps, more importantly, the ways that the field will take hold of the RDoC and use it to move research forward—will ultimately be determined by scientific peer review of funding applications and journal publications. To this end, the NIMH/RDoC have relied on the NAMHC to evaluate the future development of the RDoC. New generations of clinical scientists will also determine the future of the RDoC, and early indications suggest that the RDoC offers a viable means to teach translational neuroscience [70].

A second way in which the RDoC approach relates to the field concerns data sharing. The NIMH Data Archive (NDA) (see https://data-archive.nimh.nih.gov/) houses and shares with qualified researchers harmonized, item-level data of all types and concerning all levels of biological and behavioural organization. The NDA is made up of several repositories, including the RDoC Database (RDoCdb) (see https://data-archive.nimh.nih.gov/rdocdb). The RDoCdb provides an infrastructure for sharing subject-level data and serves as a resource for hypothesis testing and exploration. The NIMH encourages the use of these resources to achieve rapid scientific progress. Sharing data, associated tools, and methodologies, rather than just their summaries or interpretations, accelerates research progress by allowing re-analysis of data, as well as re-aggregation, integration, and rigorous comparison with other data, tools, and methods. Data from more than 16,000 research participants have already been received.

To facilitate data sharing and the combination of large data sets, in order to fully understand the mechanisms underlying the psychopathology, it is important to develop a set of paradigms and measures that are generally accepted by the field and can ensure that constructs are being measured using systematic and reliable means. As mentioned earlier, the NAMHC workgroup that was formed to look critically at the 'Paradigms' column of the RDoC matrix offered recommendations for currently existing tasks that adequately measure each construct. An incentive was to have a set of common data elements to be used widely to allow for future aggregation of RDoC data. The resulting report includes an abundance of information from domain area experts, including the items they considered when discussing each task, the overall organization of each domain, and recommendations of tasks that are useable, that need more work, and that should not be used for each construct.

In contrast to clinical diagnostic manuals, as a research framework, the RDoC has the luxury to be more nimble, building on recent findings to test new hypotheses. In contrast, changes in clinical diagnostic manuals have immediate implications for patients in terms of treatment prescriptions or reimbursement, as well as disability services or accommodations. Even with the aspiration to update changes in the present DSM-5 more expeditiously, processes described so far (for example, [71]) still rely on consensus vetting procedures and will need to address the implications of change for patient groups. The RDoC, in contrast, can advance new research ideas that, once fully formed, may be utilized to inform clinical diagnostic manuals. One limitation of RDoC research that will need to be addressed for treatment research will be the way that RDoC constructs will be handled by regulatory bodies.

As the RDoC matrix became established and understood by the field, changes to the matrix have become possible. Recently, some 'cosmetic' changes to the matrix have been made, taking advantage of web-based tools to link constructs and elements of the matrix for a more fluid and intuitive design, allowing for ease of future growth and expansion, along with providing a space to elaborate on certain elements and constructs as data emerged. The CMAT and other appointed workgroups overseen by the NAMHC will continue to be tasked with evaluating matrix updates and revisions, including the evaluation of new domains and constructs. The hope is that the RDoC matrix will reflect the needs and growth of the field, with transparent input from the scientists who use it most. With the 10-year anniversary of the RDoC, the RDoC Unit and working groups have their ears open to the field and their eyes on new and innovative ways to help the RDoC grow and adapt, as psychopathology researchers work to build systematic ties to advances in neuroscience.

## Disclaimer

Charles A. Sanislow, Department of Psychology and Program in Neuroscience and Behavior, Wesleyan University, Middletown, CT; Bruce N. Cuthbert, Sarah E. Morris, and Jennifer Pacheco, NIMH, Bethesda, MD. The authors have no financial conflicts to disclose. The opinions expressed in this piece are those of the authors, and not necessarily those of the NIMH, the National Institutes of Health, or the United States government. Many of the ideas expressed in this chapter reflect work by NIMH RDoC Internal Working Group members, past and present. Current RDoC Internal Working Group members are: Bruce Cuthbert (Chair), Ishmael Amarreh, William Carpenter, Mindy Chai, Rebecca Garcia, Marjorie Garvey, Dede Greenstein, Arina Kadam, Sarah Morris, Gretchen Navidi, Jenni Pacheco, Daniel Pine, Syed Rizvi, Matthew Rudorfer, Charles Sanislow, Janine Simmons, and Uma Vaidyanathan. Deana Barch and Michael First serve as external consultants.

## REFERENCES

1. Blashfield, R.K. (2015). Neo-Kraepelinians. *The Encyclopedia of Clinical Psychology*. pp. 1–3.
2. Feighner, J.P., Robins, E., Guze, S.B., Woodruff, R.A., Winokur, G., and Munoz, R. (1972). Diagnostic criteria for use in psychiatric research. *Archives of General Psychiatry*, 26, 57–63.
3. Robins, E. and Guze, S.B. (1970). Establishment of diagnostic validity in psychiatric illness: its application to schizophrenia. *American Journal of Psychiatry*, 126, 983–7.
4. Kendler, K.S., Muñoz, R.A., and Murphy, G.M.D. (2010). The development of the Feighner Criteria: a historical perspective. *American Journal of Psychiatry*, 167, 134–42.
5. Rudorfer, M. (2016). Personal communication, 12 March 2016.
6. American Psychiatric Association. (1980). *Diagnostic and statistical manual for mental disorders*, 3rd edition. American Psychiatric Association: Washington, DC.
7. Hyman, S.E. (2010). The diagnosis of mental disorders: the problem of reification. *Annual Review of Clinical Psychology*, 6, 155–79.
8. Wakefield J.C. (1992). Disorder as harmful dysfunction: a conceptual critique of DSM-III-R's definition of mental disorder. *Psychological Review*, 99, 232–47.
9. Prata, D., Mechelli, A., and Kapur, S. (2014). Clinically meaningful biomarkers for psychosis: a systematic and quantitative review. *Neuroscience and Biobehavioral Reviews*, 45, 134–41.
10. Follette, W.C. and Houts, A.C. (1996). Models of scientific progress and the role of theory in taxonomy development: a case study of the DSM. *Journal of Consulting and Clinical Psychology*, 64, 1120–32.
11. Sanislow, C.A., Grilo, C.M., Morey, L.C., *et al.* (2002). Confirmatory factor analysis of the DSM-IV criteria for borderline personality disorder: findings from the Collaborative Longitudinal Personality Disorders Study. *American Journal of Psychiatry*, 159, 284–90.
12. Sakashita, C., Slade, T., and Andrews, G. (2007). Empirical investigation of two assumptions in the diagnosis of DSM-IV major depressive episode. *Australian and New Zealand Journal of Psychiatry*, 41, 17–23.
13. Blashfield, R.K. and Herkov, R.J. (1996). Investigating clinician adherence to diagnosis by criteria: a replication of Morey and Ochoa (1989). *Journal of Personality Disorders*, 10, 219–28.
14. Morey, L.C. and Benson, K.T. (2016). An investigation of adherence to diagnostic criteria, revisited: clinical diagnosis of the DSM-IV/DSM-5 Section II Personality Disorders. *Journal of Personality Disorders*, 30, 130–44.
15. Morey, L.C. and Ochoa, E.S. (1989). An investigation of adherence to diagnostic criteria: clinical diagnosis of the DSM-III personality disorders. *Journal of Personality Disorders*, 3, 180–92.
16. Maj, M. (2005). Psychiatric comorbidity: an artefact of current diagnostic systems? *British Journal of Psychiatry*, 186, 182–4.
17. Lilienfeld, S.O., Waldman, I.D., and Israel, A.C. (1994). A critical examination of the use of the term and concept of comorbidity in psychopathology research. *Clinical Psychology: Science and Practice*, 1, 71–83.
18. Howes, O.D. and Kapur, S. (2009). The dopamine hypothesis of schizophrenia: version III—the final common pathway. *Schizophrenia Bulletin*, 35, 549–62.
19. Kaymaz, N. and van Os, J. (2010). Extended psychosis phenotype—yes: single continuum—unlikely. *Psychological Medicine*, 40, 1963–6.
20. Clifton, A., and Pilkonis, P.A. (2007). Evidence for a single latent class of DSM borderline personality pathology. *Comprehensive Psychiatry*, 48, 70–8.
21. Widiger, T.A. and Clark, L.A. (2000). Toward DSM-V and the classification of psychopathology. *Psychological Bulletin*, 126, 946–63.
22. Markon, K.E., Chmielewski, M., and Miller, C.J. (2011). The reliability and validity of discrete and continuous measures of psychopathology: a quantitative review. *Psychological Bulletin*, 137, 856–79.
23. London, E.B. (2014). Categorical diagnosis: a fatal flaw for autism research? *Cell Press*, 37, 683–6.
24. Yee, C.M., Javitt, D.C., and Miller, G.A. (2015). Replacing DSM categorical analyses with dimensional analyses in psychiatry research: the Research Domain Criteria initiative. *JAMA: Psychiatry*, 72, 1159–560.
25. National Research Council (US) Committee on A Framework for Developing a New Taxonomy of Disease. (2011). *Toward precision medicine: building a knowledge network for biomedical research and a new taxonomy of disease*. National Academies Press, Washington DC.
26. Kapur, S., Phillips, A.G., and Insel, T.R. (2012). Why has it taken so long for biological psychiatry to develop clinical tests and what to do about it. *Molecular Psychiatry*, 17, 1174–9.
27. Hyman, S.E. and Fenton, W.S. (2003). What are the right targets for psychopharmacology? *Science*, 299, 350–1.

28. Pankevich, D.E., Altevogt, B.M., Dunlop, J., Gage, F.H., and Hyman, S.E. (2009). Improving and accelerating drug development for nervous system disorders. *Neuron*, 84, 546–53.

29. Insel, T.R. and Cuthbert, B.N. (2009). Endophenotypes: bridging genomic complexity and disorder heterogeneity. *Biological Psychiatry*, 66, 988–9.

30. Meyer-Lindenberg, A. and Weinberger, D.R. (2006). Intermediate phenotypes and genetic mechanisms of psychiatric disorders. *Nature Reviews Neuroscience*, 7, 818–27.

31. Zanarini, M.C., Stanley, B., Black, D.W., *et al.* (2010). Methodological considerations for treatment trials for persons with borderline personality disorder. *Annals of Clinical Psychiatry*, 22, 75–83.

32. van Praag, H.M., Asnis, G.M., Kahn, R.S., *et al.* (1990). Nosological tunnel vision in biological psychiatry. *Annals of the New York Academy of Sciences*, 600, 501–10.

33. van Praag, H.M. (2000). Nosologomania: a disorder of psychiatry. *World Journal of Biological Psychiatry*, 1, 151–8.

34. Sanislow, C.A. (2016). Updating the Research Domain Criteria. *World Psychiatry*, 15, 222–3.

35. Lang, P.J., Bradley, M.M., and Cuthbert, B.N (1998). Emotion, motivation, and anxiety: brain mechanisms and psychophysiology. *Biological Psychiatry*, 44, 1248–63.

36. Maher, B.A. (1966). *Principles of psychopathology*. McGraw Hill, New York, NY.

37. Cicchetti, D. and Rogosch, F.A. (1996). Equifinality and multifinality in developmental psychopathology. *Developmental Psychopathology*, 8, 597–600.

38. Cuthbert, B.N. (2015). Research Domain Criteria: toward future psychiatric nosologies. *Dialogues in Clinical Neuroscience*, 17, 89–97.

39. Cuthbert, B.N. and Kozak, M.J. (2013). Constructing constructs for psychopathology: the NIMH Research Domain Criteria. *Journal of Abnormal Psychology*, 122, 928–37.

40. Insel, T., Cuthbert, B., Garvey, M., *et al.* (2010). Research Domain Criteria (RDoC): developing a valid diagnostic framework for research on mental disorders. *American Journal of Psychiatry*, 167, 748–51.

41. Sanislow, C.A., Pine, D.S., Quinn, K.J., *et al.* (2010). Developing constructs for psychopathology research: Research Domain Criteria. *Journal of Abnormal Psychology*, 119, 631–3.

42. Kozak M.J. and Cuthbert, B.N. (2016). The NIMH Research Domain Criteria Initiative: background, issues, and pragmatics. *Psychophysiology*, 53, 286–97.

43. Duncan, L.E. and Keller, M.C. (2011). A critical review of the first 10 years of candidate gene-by-environment interaction research in psychiatry. *American Journal of Psychiatry*, 168, 1041–9.

44. Risch, N., Herrell, R., Lehner, T., *et al.* (2009). Interaction between the serotonin transporter gene (5–HTTLPR), stressful life events, and risk of depression: a meta-analysis. *JAMA*, 301, 2462–71.

45. National Institute of Mental Health. (2017). *Updates on genes in the RDoC matrix*. https://www.nimh.nih.gov/research-priorities/rdoc/update-on-genes-in-the-rdoc-matrix.shtml

46. Garvey, M., Avenevoli, S., and Anderson, K. (2016). The National Institute of Mental Health Research Domain Criteria and clinical research in child and adolescent psychiatry. *Journal of the American Academy of Child and Adolescent Psychiatry*, 55, 93–8.

47. Casey, B.J., Oliveri, M.E., and Insel, T.A. (2014). Neurodevelopmental perspective on the Research Domain Criteria (RDoC) framework. *Biological Psychiatry*, 76, 350–3.

48. Franklin, J.C., Jamieson, J.P., Glenn, C.R., and Nock, M.K. (2015). How developmental psychopathology theory and research can inform the Research Domain Criteria (RDoC) project. *Journal of Clinical Child and Adolescent Psychology*, 44, 280–90.

49. Sabharwal, A., Szekely, A., Kotov, R., *et al.* (2017). Transdiagnostic neural markers of emotion–cognition interaction in psychotic disorders. *Journal of Abnormal Psychology*, 126, 663–78.

50. Gillan, C.M., Fineberg, N.A., and Robbins, T.W. (2017). A transdiagnostic perspective on obsessive-compulsive disorder. *Psychological Medicine*, 47, 1528–48.

51. Fair, D.A., Nigg, J.T., Iyer, S., *et al.* (2013). Distinct neural signatures detected for ADHD subtypes after controlling for micromovements in resting state functional connectivity MRI data. *Frontiers in Systems Neuroscience*, 6, 80.

52. Hägele, C., Schlagenhauf, F., Rapp, M., *et al.* (2015). Dimensional psychiatry: reward dysfunction and depressive mood across psychiatric disorders. *Psychopharmacology*, 232, 331–41.

53. Drysdale, A.T., Grosenick, L., Downar, J., *et al.* (2017). Resting-state connectivity biomarkers define neurophysiological subtypes of depression. *Nature Medicine*, 23, 28–38.

54. Williams, L.M. (2016). Precision psychiatry: a neural circuit taxonomy for depression and anxiety. *The Lancet Psychiatry*, 3, 472–80.

55. Insel, T.R. and Cuthbert, B.N. (2015). Brain disorders? Precisely. *Science*, 348, 499–500.

56. Clementz, B.A., Sweeney, J.A., Hamm, J.P., *et al.* (2016). Identification of distinct psychosis biotypes using brain-based biomarkers. *American Journal of Psychiatry*, 173, 373–84.

57. Maj, M. (2016). Narrowing the gap between ICD/DSM and RDoC constructs: possible steps and caveats. *World Psychiatry*, 15, 193–4.

58. Kupfer, D.J. and Regier, D.A. (2011). Neuroscience, clinical evidence, and the future of psychiatric classification. *American Journal of Psychiatry*, 168, 672–4.

59. Narrow, W.E., Clarke, D.E. Kuramoto, S.J., *et al.* (2013). DSM-5 field trials in the United States and Canada, Part III: development and reliability testing of a cross-cutting symptom assessment for DSM-5. *American Journal of Psychiatry*, 170, 71–82.

60. Barch, D.M., Bustillo, J., Gaebel, W., *et al.* (2013). Logic and justification for dimensional assessment of symptoms and related clinical phenomena in psychosis: relevance to DSM-5. *Schizophrenia Research*, 150, 15–20.

61. Tandon, R., Gaebel W., Barch, D.M., *et al.* (2013). Definition and description of schizophrenia in the DSM-5. *Schizophrenia Research*, 150, 3–10.

62. Skodol, A.E. (2012). Personality disorders in DSM-5. *Annual Review of Clinical Psychology*, 8, 317–44.

63. Kotov, R., Krueger, R.F., Watson, D., *et al.* (2017). The Hierarchical Taxonomy of Psychopathology (HiTOP): a dimensional alternative to traditional nosologies. *Journal of Abnormal Psychology*, 126, 454–77.

64. Sanislow, C.A. (2016). Connecting psychopathology metastructure and mechanisms. *Journal of Abnormal Psychology*, 125, 1158–65.

65. Yancey, J.R., Venables, N.C., and Patrick, C.J. (2016). Psychoneurometric operationalization of threat sensitivity: relations with clinical symptom and physiological response criteria. *Psychophysiology*, 53, 393–405.

66. Vaidyanathan, U., Patrick, C.J., and Cuthbert, B.N. (2009). Linking dimensional models of internalizing psychopathology to neurobiological systems: affect-modulated startle as an indicator of fear and distress disorders and affiliated traits. *Psychological Bulletin*, 135, 909–42.

67. Huys, Q.J.M., Maia, T.V., and Frank, M.J. (2016). Computational psychiatry as a bridge from neuroscience to clinical applications. *Nature Neuroscience*, 19, 404–13.

68. Marquand, A.F., Wolfers, T., Mennes, M., Buitelaar, J., and Beckmann, C.F. (2016). Beyond lumping and splitting: a review of computational approaches for stratifying psychiatric disorders. *Biological Psychiatry: Cognitive Neuroscience and Neuroimaging*, 1, 433–47.

69. Zohar, J. Nutt, D.J., Kupfer, D.J., and Oller, H.H. (2014). A proposal for an updated neuropsychological nomenclature. *European Neuropsychopharmacology*, 24, 1005–14.

70. Etkin, A. and Cuthbert, B.N. (2014). Beyond the DSM: Development of a transdiagnostic psychiatric neuroscience course. *Academic Psychiatry*, 38, 145–50.

71. First, M.B. (2016). Adopting a continuous improvement model for future DSM revisions. *World Psychiatry*, 15, 223–4.

# 9

# Application of research evidence in clinical practice

*Andrea Cipriani, Stefan Leucht, and John R. Geddes*

## Introduction

More than 20 years ago, evidence-based medicine was defined as 'the conscientious, explicit, and judicious use of current best evidence in making decisions about the care of individual patients, and the integration of clinical expertise and patient values' [1]. Three components are essential: (1) the current best research evidence, which is found in methodologically sound and clinically relevant research reports; (2) clinical expertise, which relates to a clinician's cumulative experience, education, and clinical skills; (3) patients, who bring their own personal preferences, unique concerns, and values to the clinical encounter. The full integration of these three components improves clinical outcomes and quality of life. Evidence-based medicine aimed at closing the gap between research and practice by incorporating the advances in clinical epidemiology and medical knowledge into clinical activities [2]. The reason why evidence-based medicine was developed and adopted worldwide is for clinicians to keep abreast of the latest therapeutic advances, cope with rapidly changing policies, and face increasing public expectations and demands [3]. The best course of action is to use an evidence-based approach, because it optimizes clinical decisions (making practice more standardized and more efficient) and also justifies them [4]. This applies to all fields in medicine, including psychiatry.

The idea that clinical practice should be based on good evidence is not new [5, 6]. Over the years, evidence-based medicine has been criticized because its 'quality mark' has been misappropriated by vested interests and the volume of evidence, especially clinical guidelines, has become unmanageable [7]. However, by providing clinicians with a set of skills which allow them to base clinical decisions on the best available and most up-to-date evidence, evidence-based medicine is not only a useful tool for clinical practice, but also an efficient method of self-directed, career-long learning [8].

Evidence-based medicine has been listed among the most important 15 medical advances since 1840 [9] (Kamath 2016), and nowadays mental health professionals are encouraged to use an evidence-based approach in their daily activities [10]. However, it is known that one of the major challenges for clinicians is to move from the theory of evidence-based medicine to the practice of it.

A study, now over 30 years old, estimated that, on average, five clinical questions are raised at each bedside encounter with a patient [11]. In 1998, it was estimated that only 4% of health care decisions were based on sound evidence, 45% on strong consensus among physicians, and 51% in neither [4]. Evidence-based practice requires new skills of the clinician, including efficient literature searching and the application of formal rules of evidence in evaluating the clinical literature. The implementation of evidence-based practice involves four steps [12]:

- To frame a clear question, based on a clinical problem (which arises from the care of one patient).
- To search for the relevant best available evidence in the literature (selecting the appropriate resource).
- To critically appraise the validity (closeness to the truth) and applicability (usefulness in clinical practice) of the retrieved evidence.
- To apply the findings to clinical decision-making and routine practice (integrating the evidence with clinical expertise and patient's preferences and values).

These steps are referred in some textbooks as the 5 As: *Assess* (the patient), *Ask* (the question), *Acquire* and *Appraise* (the evidence), and *Apply* (talk with the patient), with the fifth step being the all-important evaluation of the clinician's own performance in consultation with the patient (the so-called self-evaluation).

In this chapter, we will explore how research evidence should be used to inform real-world practice, taking into account the perspective of both the practising clinician and the clinical researcher.

## What is evidence and why does it matter?

Decision-making processes are enhanced through the use of valid and reliable evidence. Evidence is the information we gather on which to base, or support, our decisions. It is therefore important to be able to determine which evidence is 'the best evidence', that is, the most valid and reliable. This term is used quite frequently in medical journals and international meetings, and it basically refers to the methodological quality of the study design that produces the information we are looking for, in relation to the clinical question. Studies from the scientific literature can be broadly categorized either as *experimental* (when the investigators assign the exposures) or *observational* (when investigators observe usual clinical practice) [13]. Experimental studies become randomized trials only when the exposures are assigned by a random technique and the allocation of the upcoming assignment is concealed. Experimental and observational studies are placed into a hierarchy which may vary, depending on the specific clinical question to address, but only the study designs at the top are considered 'the best evidence'. For example, in the case of assessing the efficacy of interventions, randomized controlled trials are at the top of the ranking [14]. Randomization approximates the controlled experiment of basic science, and it is the only known way to avoid selection and confounding biases in clinical research. Bias (that is, systematic error) can confound the outcome of a study, such that the study may overestimate or underestimate what the true treatment effect is. Within a sample population, a properly conducted randomization is able to reduce the risk of selection bias by not only controlling for *known*, but also (and possibly more importantly) controlling for *unknown* prognostic variables. This bias-controlling measure helps attain a more accurate estimation of the truth.

Randomized controlled trials have drawbacks too. For instance, a methodologically sound randomized controlled trial can have good *internal validity* (that is, the study measures what it sets out to measure), but it might not have 'good enough' *external validity* (that is, the extent to which results from the individual study can be generalized to the broader community of patients outside the trial). Internal validity relates to whether the study answers its research question *correctly*, that is, in a manner which is free from bias (and researchers and clinicians should learn how to appraise the validity of such studies). By contrast, external validity is closely connected with the applicability of a study's findings, and its assessment depends on the purpose for which the study is to be used. Trials are usually conducted by industry on single patented compounds and are designed to meet the requirements of the regulatory agencies. In order not to delay the introduction of drugs onto the market, the majority of such trials are short term, highly controlled, highly monitored, and typically designed to separate between a new drug and placebo as efficiently as possible. This approach to clinical trial design has been described as *explanatory*, in which the aim is to determine if the treatment *can* work [15]. Patients in these trials are characteristically highly selected, and outcomes are essentially sensitive proxies of clinically relevant outcomes. Even for pharmaceutical companies, the risk of mounting a very large expensive clinical trial on a promising compound has to be offset against the risk that such a trial will demonstrate that the investigational compound is either of limited or no efficacy or causes serious adverse effects. Pharmaceutical companies are therefore under pressure to do everything they can to design the trial to show their product in the optimal light and to ensure that any positive results have maximum impact, leading to as rapid uptake of the new drug as possible following market authorization. Because the design of these trials is based on a negotiation between regulators and the industry, these trials often have substantial limitations for answering clinical questions in the real world, and hence limited clinical external validity. The results of the available evidence often need to

be extrapolated—to an unknown degree—when they are applied to the target clinical question.

Finally, randomized controlled trials are usually very expensive, take many years to be conducted (from conception to publication), and cannot be used in some instances (for example, in special populations such as pregnant women who should not be exposed to potentially harmful substances, as this would be unethical).

It has been recognized that much larger trials are required, and trial procedures should be very simple and efficient, allowing widespread recruitment by practising clinicians [16]. If representative samples of patients are enrolled in the trial, the results will be of widespread applicability to future patients. Inclusion criteria are broad and as unrestrictive as possible. The key entry criterion is that both the patient and the investigator are substantially uncertain which of the trial treatments would be most appropriate. This 'uncertainty principle' is ethical because it effectively excludes patients for whom a specific treatment is known to be the most appropriate. All trial procedures are radically simplified. Keeping the trial procedures and data collection to an absolute minimum is essential to achieve widespread participation, and hence the required sample size for realizing the key objectives of the trial. Such trials are termed *pragmatic* [17] and, in contrast to the question of '*Can* the treatment work?' answered by the explanatory trial?', they ask: '*Does* the intervention work?' [18] Pragmatic trials should not be seen as a research design that should replace explanatory trials. There is a continuum between explanatory and pragmatic trials and, ideally, pragmatic trials should be conducted after the results of explanatory trials allowed a new medicine to enter the market. Important examples of pragmatic trials in psychopharmacology include the Bipolar Affective disorder: Lithium/ANticonvulsant Evaluation [19], the European First Episode Schizophrenia Trial [20], the Clinical Antipsychotic Trials of Intervention Effectiveness [21], the Cost Utility of the Latest Antipsychotic Drugs in Schizophrenia Study [22], and Clozapine plus Haloperidol or Aripiprazole Trial [23].

## How to collect the best available evidence

The number of randomized studies is growing, so too does the science of reviewing trials [24]. The history of synthesizing research is inextricably bound up in the history of evidence-based medicine, but it actually goes back centuries. The pioneer in the field was James Lind, a Scottish naval surgeon, who is credited not only with having produced one of the early records of a scientific trial, but also with having written one of the first systematic reviews of evidence. In 1747, Lind took 12 patients with scurvy, whose cases 'were as similar as I could have them' and divided them into six groups of two [25]. According to his planned intervention, Lind administered six different treatments to each pair of sufferers: (1) cider; (2) elixir vitriol; (3) vinegar; (4) seawater; (5) a combination of oranges and lemons; and (6) a mixture of garlic, mustard seed, and balsam of Peru. A week later, Lind's findings were clear: 'The result of all my experiments was that oranges and lemons were the most effectual remedies for this distemper at sea' (http://www.jameslindlibrary.org). The results of this study were published a few years later, and interestingly, Lind wrote: 'As it is no easy matter to root out prejudices ... it became requisite to exhibit a full and impartial view of what had hitherto been published on the scurvy ... by which the sources of these mistakes may be detected. Indeed, before the subject could be set in a clear and proper light, it was necessary to remove a great deal of rubbish.' To gather the available research, get rid of the 'rubbish', and summarize the best of what remains are essentially the science of a properly conducted systematic review. It took a while to understand the value and the methodological implications of Lind's attitude; however, in the past century, there were eminent figures, like Archie Cochrane, a British epidemiologist, who persuasively advocated the scientific evaluation of commonly used medical therapies through objective sources of information [26]. Even though the importance of evidence synthesis in medicine was recognized since the 1970s, the widespread use of these systematic reviews and meta-analyses did not occur until 1990s, when it became clear that the judgements and opinions of experts were often biased [27].

There are two main approaches to reviewing literature: *narrative reviews* and *systematic reviews* [28].

Narrative reviews are the old, traditional approach. They are broad in scope and qualitative and do not include a method section (where the authors describe how they retrieved the relevant information); therefore, they are mainly based on the experience and subjectivity of the authors, who are often experts in the area. The absence of an objective method section, together with the lack of clear and replicable criteria, leads to a number of methodological flaws (for instance, the bias in selecting the scientific literature), which can materially affect the author's conclusions. The results from narrative reviews must be viewed with suspicion, as they are likely to be misleading (and one of the major problems is that the extent to which they are unreliable is almost impossible to judge).

By contrast, systematic reviews (or sometimes called 'overviews') are syntheses of primary research studies and are qualitative and focused around clinical questions. They describe and use specific, explicit, and therefore reproducible, methodological strategies to identify, assemble, and critically appraise all relevant issues on a specific topic [29]. Systematic reviews should be designed to answer only a narrow and specific question, because, if the question is too broad or too generic, it will be impossible for the researchers to collate and assess all the relevant information. The nature of the question determines the optimal primary study design, and hence the a priori inclusion and exclusion criteria.

If the question concerns efficacy and safety of an intervention (*Which treatment is better? Which dose is better tolerated?*), the most reliable study design would be a randomized controlled trial—randomization avoids any systematic tendency to produce an unequal distribution of prognostic factors between the experimental and control treatments, influencing the outcome [30]. However, randomized controlled trials are certainly not the most appropriate research design for all questions [31]. For example, for aetiological questions, it would be neither possible nor ethical to randomize subjects to many harmful exposures—systematic reviews would therefore need to include cohort and case-control studies. Likewise, a diagnostic question such as '*How well can a screening tool identify patients with a psychiatric disorder?*' would be best answered by a cross-sectional study of patients at risk of being ill [32]. Systematic reviews of these other study designs have their own methodological problems—guidelines exist for undertaking reviews (and meta-analyses) of diagnostic tests [33] and the observational epidemiological designs used in aetiological research [34]. The review protocol is where these criteria are reported and defined before the review starts, and they should be followed by the researchers to select the relevant studies.

There is a further difference between narrative reviews and systematic reviews. New research data emerge continuously, and reviews are useful if they are up-to-date. This tends not to be the case with conventionally published reviews, but the systematic reviews of the Cochrane Library, for instance, are published electronically and periodically updated to take into account the emergence of new evidence (http://www.cochranelibrary.com/). There is evidence that systematic reviews improve the reliability and accuracy of conclusions; however, the results are rarely unequivocal and require careful assessment and interpretation [35]. Evidence-based practice is not cookbook medicine [36], also because clinicians need to integrate the results from systematic reviews with the clinical situation, their own expertise, and patients' preferences.

Despite their potential to avoid bias, a number of factors can adversely affect the conclusions of a systematic review. When conducting a primary study, it is important to ensure that the sample recruited is representative of the target population; otherwise, the results may be misleading (*selection bias*). The most significant form of bias in systematic reviews is analogous to selection bias in primary studies but applies to the selection of primary studies, rather than participants. There are various forms of selection bias, including *publication bias, language of publication bias,* and *biases introduced by an overreliance on electronic databases.*

Publication bias is the tendency of investigators, peer reviewers, and also journal editors to differentially submit or accept manuscripts for publication, based on the direction or strength of the study findings. The conclusions of systematic reviews can be significantly affected by publication bias. The potential pitfalls of publication bias are obvious—if only studies which demonstrate a treatment benefit are published, the conclusions may be misleading if the true effect is neutral or even harmful. As early as 1959 it was noted that 97.3% of articles published in four major journals had statistically significant results, although it is likely that many studies were conducted which produced non-significant results—but these were less likely to be published [37]. Various strategies have been proposed to counter publication bias. These include methods aimed at detecting its presence and preventing its occurrence. It is generally accepted that prevention is likely to be the most effective strategy, and therefore, prospective registries of all clinical studies were established. This means that nowadays a record of a trial exists, regardless of whether or not the study is published, and it reduces the risk of *negative* studies disappearing. Registries of ongoing research have been slow to establish—perhaps because it is not clear who should take a lead or fund them—although some of them are working efficiently (for example, http://www.controlled-trials.com or http://www.clinicaltrials.gov). While such registries are useful for newer or relatively new trials, they do not solve the problem of retrospectively identifying unpublished primary studies. A number of methods for estimating the likelihood of the presence of publication bias in a sample of studies have been developed. One commonly used way of investigating publication bias is the funnel plot [38]. In a funnel plot, the study-specific odds ratios are plotted against a measure of the study's precision—such as the inverse of the standard error or the number of cases in each study. There will be more variation in the results of small studies because of their greater susceptibility to random error, and hence, the results of the larger studies, with less random error, should cluster more closely around the *true value*. If publication bias is not present, the graphical distribution of odds ratios should resemble an inverted funnel. If there is a gap in the region of the funnel where the results of small negative studies would be expected, then this would imply that the results of these studies are missing. This could be due to publication bias or mean that the search failed to find small negative studies.

Restricting a search to one language—for example, searching only for English language papers—can be hazardous. It has been shown that studies which find a treatment effect are more likely to be published in English language journals, while opposing studies may be published in non-English language journals. *Language of publication bias* has also been called the *Tower of Babel* bias [39].

With the increasing availability of convenient electronic bibliographic databases, there is a danger that reviewers may rely on them unduly. This can cause bias because electronic databases do not offer comprehensive or unbiased coverage of the relevant primary literature. For instance, on investigating the adequacy of Medline searches for randomized controlled trials in mental health care, it has been shown that the optimal Medline search had a sensitivity of only 52% [40]. Sensitivity can be improved by searching other databases, in addition to Medline, for example Embase, PsycLIT, PSYNDEX, CINAHL, and Lilacs. To avoid the limitations of relying on electronic databases—or any other resource—for the identification of primary studies, reviews seek to use optimally sensitive, over-inclusive searches to identify as many studies as possible with a combination of electronic searching, hand searching, reference checking, and personal communications. Unpublished data refer to studies that are not published at all, but they may also refer to information that are not included in study reports published in scientific journals. Each study has a unique ID number. Trial registration is requested for study approval by local ethics committees and as a precondition for publication in many journals, so a full report of the study protocol, and sometimes of study results, can be found using the Internet. Clinical trial registries and websites of regulatory agencies are one option, but the most informative sources of unpublished data are pharmaceutical industries' websites. Not all companies have study registries, and not all the companies that have study registries report results in an easy-to-use and comprehensive format. Having access to this information may be useful also when the published paper is available, because it can help retrieve some missing information or, in case of discrepancies or inaccuracies, clarify the exact figures (for instance, when changes in rating scales are reported only in figures or graphs).

As a research tool, a systematic review of the literature can be applied to any form of research question. Results of systematic reviews can reliably and efficiently provide the information needed for rational clinical decision-making. However, the main conclusion of a systematic review may often be that there is little or even no good-quality information in the literature. Even this conclusion may be useful in that it highlights areas in need of further primary research.

## How to synthesize the best available evidence

The terms 'systematic review' and 'meta-analysis' are often used interchangeably, but actually they refer to different things. Systematic reviews are reviews of primary research studies, in which specific methodological strategies that limit bias are used and clearly described in the protocol. By contrast, a meta-analysis is a statistical method to combine and summarize the results of several studies retrieved by a systematic review into one single estimate. This method of pooling research data from more than one study provides an estimate of effect size, which has greater power than any of the constituent studies. This has obvious advantages for clinical research and practice, because it minimizes *random error* and produces more precise, and potentially more generalizable, results. However, meta-analyses are not an essential part of a systematic review because sometimes it may be inappropriate to proceed to a statistical summary of the individual studies (for instance, when studies are not similar enough to be lumped together). Meta-analyses make the assumptions that clinically important differences between treated and untreated groups are not so large as to be intuitively obvious and that, although the treatment's effect varies in size among different patient populations, the effect's direction is consistently either beneficial or harmful [41]. A meta-analysis can estimate the degree of random error by presenting the quantitative results of individual studies and the 'pooled' weighted average result, with a confidence interval that provides a good indication of the precision of the estimate (it shows the extent to which the results are likely to differ from the 'true result' because of chance alone).

The technique of meta-analysis has been controversial, and this is perhaps because it is potentially so powerful, but it is also particularly susceptible to abuse [42]. A number of key issues should be borne in mind when assessing or carrying out a meta-analysis:

* A meta-analysis is a tool that can increase the sample size, and consequently the statistical power by pooling the results of individual trials (in psychiatry, many trials are small because of the difficulties in recruiting patients). Increasing the sample size also allows for more precision, that is, a pooled estimate with narrower confidence intervals [43]. Combining studies, however attractive, may not always be appropriate. The inappropriate pooling of disparate studies can make the final results meaningless. To avoid this, it is necessary to ensure that the individual studies are really looking at the same clinical or research question. Individual studies might vary with respect to study participants, intervention, duration of follow-up, and outcome measures. Such a decision will usually require a measure of judgement, and for this reason, a reviewer should always pre-specify the main criteria for including primary studies in the review protocol. Having decided that the primary studies are investigating a close enough question, an important role of the meta-analysis is to investigate variations between the results of individual studies (the so-called heterogeneity). When such variation exists, it is useful to estimate if more heterogeneity exists than can be reasonably explained by the play of chance alone [44]. If so, attempts should be made to identify the reasons for such heterogeneity, and it may then be decided that it is not reasonable to combine the studies, or that it is, but that the overall pooled estimate needs to take the variation into account.

* Individual studies vary in their methodological quality. Randomization, allocation concealment, blinding, and the type of analysis (for instance, whether or not the study participants are considered in the groups to which they were randomly allocated, that is intention-to-treat analysis) can all affect the direction of the results. In general, studies with poor methodology tend to

overestimate the effect of the intervention [45]. Rating scales and standardized tools have been developed to assess the quality (or risk of bias) of randomized trials. The quality scores can be incorporated into the meta-analysis, with a *quality weight* applied to the study-specific effect estimate. Although there are a large number of scales available, the current consensus is that their use is problematic because of uncertain validity, as it has been shown that using different scales leads to substantial differences in the pooled estimate [46]. The optimal approach at present is to assess the risk of bias of individual studies, focusing on the aspects of trial design that affect its internal validity. Nowadays, one of the most frequently used tools for assessing study quality is the Cochrane risk of bias tool. It is a domain-based evaluation, in which different domains are assessed individually, assigning a judgement of 'low', 'high', or 'unclear' risk of bias: sequence generation, allocation concealment, blinding of participants and personnel, blinding of outcome assessment, incomplete outcome data, selective outcome reporting, and other issues. More recently, a new systematic and explicit approach to making judgements about the quality of evidence and the strength of recommendations has been developed by a group of researchers—the Grading of Recommendations, Assessment, Development, and Evaluations (GRADE) Working Group (http://www.gradeworkinggroup.org/). When using GRADE, researchers rate evidence not study by study, but across studies for specific clinical outcomes. So the GRADE approach can specifically assess methodological flaws within the component studies, the consistency of results across different studies, the generalizability of the results to the wider patient base, and ultimately how effective the treatments have been shown to be.

- It is also possible to investigate and quantify the effect of poor-quality trials on the overall treatment outcome, by conducting pre-planned sensitivity analyses which exclude them from the pooled estimate. The main treatment effect of a trial gives an indication of the average response for an average patient meeting the inclusion criteria. Individual patients in real-life clinical practice deviate from the average to greater or lesser degrees. To tailor the results of a trial to an individual patient, it is tempting to perform a sub-analysis of the trial participants with a specific characteristic or a set of characteristics. Estimates of the treatment in subgroups of patients are more susceptible to random error—and therefore imprecision—than the estimate of the average effect for all patients' overall effect, because subgroups reduce the sample size and statistical power of the results. Furthermore, unless randomization was initially stratified according to the important subgroups, protection from confounding afforded by randomization may not be valid anymore and any observed subgroup difference in treatment effect may be due to type I error (that is, the incorrect rejection of a true null hypothesis, or a false positive). As a take-home message for clinicians, subgroup analyses should always be viewed cautiously.

By synthesizing evidence from studies with a similar design which address the same research question within the frame of a systematic review, standard meta-analyses can compare only two alternative treatments at a time [47]. For most clinical conditions where many treatment regimens already exist, standard meta-analysis approaches result into a plethora of pair-wise comparisons and do not inform on the comparative efficacy of all treatments simultaneously.

Moreover, if no trials exist which directly compare two interventions, it is not possible to estimate their relative efficacy, and thus, this specific information is missing from the overall picture. All this has led to the development of meta-analytical techniques that allow the incorporation of evidence from both direct and indirect comparisons in a network of trials and different interventions to estimate summary treatment effects as comprehensively and precisely as possible [48]. This meta-analytical technique is called *network meta-analysis*, also known as multiple treatments meta-analysis or *mixed-treatment comparison*. The combination of direct and indirect estimates into a single-effect size not only can provide information on missing comparisons, but also can increase the precision of treatment estimates of already existing direct comparisons, reducing confidence intervals and strengthening inferences concerning the relative efficacy of two treatments [49].

Another fruitful role of the network meta-analysis technique is to facilitate simultaneous inference regarding all treatments, in order to rank them according to any outcome of interest, for instance efficacy and acceptability [50]. Using network meta-analyses within the frame of a more complex statistical procedure, it is possible to calculate the probability of each treatment to be the most effective (first-best) regimen, the second-best, the third-best, and so on, and thus to rank treatments according to this hierarchical order. This is a very easy-to-understand and straightforward way to present network meta-analysis results, most of all for clinicians who want to know which the best treatment to be prescribed to patients is, on average [51].

Recently, network meta-analyses have become more widely employed and demanded, with the increased complexity of analyses that underpin clinical guidelines and health technology appraisals [52]. Expert statistical support, as well as subject expertise, is required for carrying out and interpreting network meta-analysis results. Several applications of the methodology have depicted the benefits of a joint analysis, but network meta-analysis approaches are far from being an established practice in the medical literature. Concerns have been expressed about the validity of network meta-analysis methods, as they rely on assumptions that are difficult to test [51]. Although network meta-analysis techniques preserve randomization, indirect evidence is not randomized evidence, as treatments have originally been compared *within*, but *not across*, studies. Therefore, indirect evidence may suffer the biases of observational studies (that is, confounding or selection bias). In this respect, direct evidence remains more robust, and in situations where both direct and indirect comparisons are available in a review, any use of network meta-analyses should be to supplement, rather than to replace, the direct comparisons. Several techniques exist, which can account for, but not eliminate, the impact of effect modifiers across studies involving different interventions [53]. However, recent empirical evidence suggests that direct and indirect evidence are in agreement in the majority of cases and that network meta-analyses can address biases that cannot be addressed in a standard meta-analysis such as sponsorship bias and optimism bias [54].

Meta-analyses can give an indication of the average response for an average patient meeting the inclusion criteria, but individual patients in real-life clinical practice deviate from the average to greater or lesser degrees. A potentially useful approach is to carry out meta-analyses of raw data from the included trials, the so-called 'individual patient data meta-analysis' [55]. In an individual patient data analysis, it is possible to investigate important predictors (that is, baseline clinical and demographic characteristics) that might affect treatment response or prognosis, for example gender, age, ethnicity, family history, dose, severity of illness, age of onset, and number of previous episodes. The individual patient data methodology has been used in large-scale collaborative overviews, in which data from many randomized trials in a particular disease area were brought together [56]. Individual patient data meta-analyses usually require more time, resources, and expertise than other forms of review; however, the process brings with it a number of advantages [57]. The main difference between a standard meta-analysis and an individual patient data meta-analysis is that while the former is based on information that refers to each included study, the latter is based on information that refers to each subject included in the study. Individual patient data meta-analyses allow to describe the effects of competitive treatments over time [58]. In fact, information that refers to the outcome of each included subject is usually collected not only at endpoint, but also at various time intervals after random allocation.

## Conclusions

As new evidence emerges, health care workers are constantly required to update their knowledge. In the scientific literature, a lot of information (sometimes too much and too often misleading) is continuously available and many websites or other sources keep updating, almost in real time, on the newest articles. In 1999, clinicians spoke of surviving an 'information flood', as trends demonstrated that the number of new journals doubled every 10–15 years [59]. In 2014, there were about 28,100 active scholarly peer-reviewed English language journals, collectively publishing 2.5 million articles a year, of which 30% were biomedical [60]. Even restricting reading to high-impact journals in a single field of interest, the number of articles is in the thousands. For this reason, health care workers chose to read so-called 'secondary journals', those which aim to highlight and summarize the recent evidence, methodological advances, and possible clinical implications of research [61]. Things may change in the near future, but at the moment, there are three secondary journals in the field of mental health with large readerships: *Current Opinion in Psychiatry, Harvard Review of Psychiatry*, and *Evidence-Based Mental Health*, established in 1988, 1993, and 1998, respectively. Even though there are differences between them, each adopts a systematic, comprehensive strategy to identify the best and most relevant new evidence for mental health workers and incorporates a rigorous peer review process for their articles [61].

## REFERENCES

1. Sackett, D.L., Rosenberg, W.M., Gray, J.A., Haynes, R.B., and Richardson, W.S. (1996). Evidence based medicine: what it is and what it isn't. *BMJ*, 312, 71–2.
2. Guyatt, G., Cairns, J.U., Churchill, D., *et al.* (1992). Evidence-based medicine. A new approach to teaching the practice of medicine. *JAMA*, 268, 2420–5.
3. Djulbegovic, B. and Guyatt, G.H. (2017). Progress in evidence-based medicine: a quarter century on. *The Lancet*, 390, 415–23.
4. Trivedi, J.K. (2000). Evidence based medicine in psychiatry. *Indian Journal of Psychiatry*, 42, 1–2.
5. Lewis, A. (1958a). Between guesswork and certainty in psychiatry. *The Lancet*, 1, 171–5.
6. Lewis, A. (1958b). Between guesswork and certainty in psychiatry. *The Lancet*, 1, 227–30.
7. Greenhalgh, T., Howick, J., and Maskrey, N. (2014). Evidence based medicine: a movement in crisis? *BMJ*, 348, g3725.
8. Geddes, J.R. and Harrison, P.J. (1997). Closing the gap between research and practice. *British Journal of Psychiatry*, 171, 220–5.
9. Kamath, S. and Guyatt, G. (2016). Importance of evidence-based medicine on research and practice. *Indian Journal of Anaesthesia*, 60, 622–5.
10. Cipriani, A. and Furukawa, T.A. (2014). Advancing evidence-based practice to improve patient care. *Evidence-Based Mental Health*, 17, 1–2.
11. Covell, D.G., Uman, G.C. and Manning, P.R. (1985). Information needs in office practice: are they being met? *Annals of Internal Medicine*, 103, 596–9.
12. Weng, Y.H., Kuo, K.N., Yang, C.Y., Lo, H.L., Chen, C., and Chiu, Y.W. (2013). Implementation of evidence-based practice across medical, nursing, pharmacological and allied healthcare professionals: a questionnaire survey in nationwide hospital settings. *Implementation Science*, 8, 112.
13. Grimes, D.A. and Schulz, K.F. (2002). An overview of clinical research: the lay of the land. *The Lancet*, 359, 57–61.
14. Murad, M.H., Asi, N., Alsawas, M., and Alahdab F. (2016). New evidence pyramid. *Evidence Based Medicine*, 21, 25–7.
15. Schwartz, D. and Lellouch, J. (2009). Explanatory and pragmatic attitudes in therapeutical trials. *Journal of Clinical Epidemiology*, 62, 499–505.
16. Geddes, J.R. (2005). Large simple trials in psychiatry: providing reliable answers to important clinical questions. *Epidemiology and Psychiatric Sciences*, 14, 122–6.
17. Hotopf, M., Churchill, R., and Lewis, G. (1999). Pragmatic randomised controlled trials in psychiatry. *British Journal of Psychiatry*, 175, 217–23.
18. Haynes, B. (1999). Can it work? Does it work? Is it worth it? The testing of healthcare interventions is evolving. *BMJ*, 319, 652–3.
19. Geddes, J.R., Goodwin, G.M., Rendell, J., *et al.* (2010). Lithium plus valproate combination therapy versus monotherapy for relapse prevention in bipolar I disorder (BALANCE): a randomised open-label trial. *The Lancet*, 375, 385–95.
20. Kahn, R.S., Fleischhacker, W.W., Boter, H., *et al.*; EUFEST study group. (2008). Effectiveness of antipsychotic drugs in first-episode schizophrenia and schizophreniform disorder: an open randomised clinical trial. *The Lancet*, 371, 1085–97.
21. Lieberman, J.A., Stroup, T.S., McEvoy, J.P., *et al.*; Clinical Antipsychotic Trials of Intervention Effectiveness (CATIE) Investigators. (2005). Effectiveness of antipsychotic drugs in patients with chronic schizophrenia. *New England Journal of Medicine*, 353, 1209–23.
22. Jones, P.B., Barnes, T.R., Davies, L., *et al.* (2006). Randomized controlled trial of the effect on quality of life of second- vs first-generation antipsychotic drugs in schizophrenia: Cost Utility of the Latest Antipsychotic Drugs in Schizophrenia Study. *Archives of General Psychiatry*, 63, 1079–87.
23. Barbui, C., Accordini, S., Nosè, M., *et al.* (2011). Aripiprazole versus haloperidol in combination with clozapine for treatment-resistant schizophrenia in routine clinical care: a randomized,

controlled trial. *Journal of Clinical Psychopharmacology*, 31, 266–73.

24. Bastian, H., Glasziou, P., and Chalmers, I. (2010). Seventy-five trials and eleven systematic reviews a day: how will we ever keep up? *PLoS Medicine*, 7, e1000326.

25. Lind, J. (1753). *A treatise of the scurvy in three parts. Containing an inquiry into the nature, causes and cure of that disease, together with a critical and chronological view of what has been published on the subject.* A. Millar, London.

26. Cochrane, A.L. (1972). *Effectiveness and efficiency. Random reflections on health services.* Royal Society of Medicine Press, London.

27. Cipriani, A. (2013). Time to abandon evidence based medicine? *Evidence-Based Mental Health*, 16, 91–2.

28. Cook, D.J., Mulrow, C.D., and Haynes, R.B. (1997). Systematic reviews: synthesis of best evidence for clinical decisions. *Annals of Internal Medicine*, 126, 376–80.

29. Carney, S.M. and Geddes, J.R. (2002). *Systematic reviews and meta-analyses. Evidence in mental health care.* Brunner Routledge, Hove.

30. Altman, D.G. and Bland, J.M. (1999). Statistics notes. Treatment allocation in controlled trials: why randomise? *BMJ*, 318, 1209.

31. Sackett, D.L. and Wennberg, J.E. (1997). Choosing the best research design for each question. *BMJ*, 315, 1636.

32. Mulrow, C.D. (1994). Rationale for systematic reviews. *BMJ*, 309, 597–9.

33. Irwig, L., Tosteson, A.N., Gatsonis, C., *et al.* (1994). Guidelines for meta-analyses evaluating diagnostic tests. *Annals of Internal Medicine*, 120, 667–76.

34. Stroup, D.F., Berlin, J.A., Morton, S.C., *et al.* (2000). Meta-analysis of observational studies in epidemiology: a proposal for reporting. Meta-analysis Of Observational Studies in Epidemiology (MOOSE) group. *JAMA*, 283, 2008–12.

35. Hopayian, K. (2001). The need for caution in interpreting high quality systematic reviews. *BMJ*, 323, 681–4.

36. Cipriani, A. and Geddes, J.R. (2014). Placebo for depression: we need to improve the quality of scientific information but also reject too simplistic approaches or ideological nihilism. *BMC Medicine*, 12, 105.

37. Sterling, T.D. (1959). Publication decisions and their possible effects on inferences drawn from tests of significance—or vice-versa. *Journal of American Statistical Association*, 54, 30–4.

38. Egger, M., Davey Smith, G., Schneider, M., and Minder, C. (1997). Bias in meta-analysis detected by a simple, graphical test. *BMJ*, 315, 629–34.

39. Grégoire, G., Derderian, F., and Le Lorier, J. (1995). Selecting the language of the publications included in a meta-analysis: is there a Tower of Babel bias? *Journal of Clinical Epidemiology*, 48, 159–63.

40. Montori, V.M., Wilczynski, N.L., Morgan, D., Haynes, R.B.; Hedges Team. (2005). Optimal search strategies for retrieving systematic reviews from Medline: analytical survey. *BMJ*, 330, 68.

41. Peto, R., Collins, R., and Gray, R. (1995). Large-scale randomized evidence: large simple trials and overviews of trials. *Journal of Clinical Epidemiology*, 48, 23–40.

42. Tyrer, P. (2008). So careless of the single trial. *Evidence-Based Mental Health*, 11, 65–6.

43. Peto, R., Collins, R., and Gray, R. (1993). Large-scale randomized evidence: large, simple trials and overviews of trials. *Annals of the New York Academy of Sciences*, 703, 314–40.

44. Higgins, J.P., Thompson, S.G., Deeks, J.J., and Altman, D.G. (2003). Measuring inconsistency in meta-analyses. *BMJ*, 327, 557–60.

45. Higgins, J.P.T. and Green, S. (eds.). (2011). *Cochrane handbook for systematic reviews of interventions*, version 5.1.0 (updated March 2011). The Cochrane Collaboration, 2011. http://handbook-5-1.cochrane.org/

46. Juni, P., Witschi, A., and Bloch, R. (1999). The hazards of scoring the quality of clinical trials for meta-analysis. *JAMA*, 282, 1054–60.

47. Leucht, S., Chaimani, A., Cipriani, A., Davis, J.M., Furukawa, T.A., and Salanti, G. (2016). Network meta-analyses should be the highest level of evidence in treatment guidelines. *European Archives of Psychiatry and Neurological Sciences*, 266, 477–80.

48. Mavridis, D., Giannatsi, M., Cipriani, A., and Salanti, G. (2015). A primer on network meta-analysis with emphasis on mental health. *Evidence-Based Mental Health*, 18, 40–6.

49. Salanti, G., Higgins, J.P., Ades, A.E., and Ioannidis J.P. (2008). Evaluation of networks of randomized trials. *Statistical Methods in Medical Research*, 17, 279–301.

50. Cipriani, A., Higgins, J.P., Geddes, J.R., and Salanti, G. (2013). Conceptual and technical challenges in network meta-analysis. *Annals of Internal Medicine*, 159, 130–7.

51. Salanti, G., Marinho, V., and Higgins J.P. (2009). A case study of multiple-treatments meta-analysis demonstrates that covariates should be considered. *Journal of Clinical Epidemiology*, 62, 857–64.

52. McLaren, R. and Cipriani, A. (2016). Clinical guidelines for mood disorders: the roads travelled, the road ahead. *Australian and New Zealand Journal of Psychiatry*, 50, 1123–4.

53. Zarin, W., Veroniki, A.A., Nincic, V., *et al.* (2017). Characteristics and knowledge synthesis approach for 456 network meta-analyses: a scoping review. *BMC Medicine*, 15, 3.

54. Salanti, G., Dias, S., and Welton, N.J. (2010). Evaluating novel agent effects in multiple-treatments meta-regression. *Statistics in Medicine*, 29, 2369–83.

55. Tierney, J.F., Vale, C., Riley, R., *et al.* (2015). Individual participant data (IPD) meta-analyses of randomised controlled trials: guidance on their use. *PLoS Medicine*, 12, e1001855.

56. Furukawa, T.A., Levine, S.Z., Tanaka, S., *et al.* (2015). Initial severity of schizophrenia and efficacy of anti-psychotics: participant-level meta-analysis of 6 placebo-controlled studies. *JAMA Psychiatry*, 72, 14–21.

57. Veroniki, A.A., Straus, S.E., Ashoor, H., Stewart, L.A., Clarke, M., and Tricco, A.C. (2016). Contacting authors to retrieve individual patient data: study protocol for a randomized controlled trial. *Trials*, 17, 138.

58. Jeng, G.T., Scott, J.R., and Burmeister, L.F. (1995). A comparison of meta-analytic results using literature vs individual patient data: paternal cell immunization for recurrent miscarriage. *JAMA*, 274, 830–6.

59. Höök, O. (1999). Scientific communications. History, electronic journals and impact factors. *Scandinavian Journal of Rehabilitation Medicine*, 31, 3–7.

60. Ware, M. and Mabe, M. (2015). *The STM Report.* International Association of Scientific, Technical and Medical Publishers, Oxford.

61. Barber, S., Corsi, M., Furukawa, T.A., and Cipriani, A. (2016). Quality and impact of secondary information in promoting evidence-based clinical practice: a cross-sectional study about EBMH. *Evidence-Based Mental Health*, 19, 82–5.

# 10

# A neuroscience-based nomenclature for psychotropic drugs

*Guy M. Goodwin, Joseph Zohar, and David J. Kupfer*

## Introduction

A nomenclature can be defined as the devising or choosing of names for things. It sounds innocent enough, but in science, it is closely linked to the idea of classification or the creation of categories of like things. Such categories can also be the basis for a nomenclature. Since the words we use carry meanings, they influence how we think and communicate. If we need to make distinctions between objects, we need appropriate categories—not too many, not too few. Moreover, we need classifications which assist creative thought and do not retard it.

For many years, there has been dissatisfaction with the nomenclature widely employed to classify the medicines used in the treatment of psychiatric disorder. It has lurched between the obscure, the inconsistent, and the incomprehensible. To start with the obscure, a WHO symposium in Oslo in 1969 agreed a consensus that an international system of drug classification was needed, and the Drug Utilisation Research Group (DURG) was established. It created the WHO ATC (Anatomical Therapeutic Chemical) classification system, first published in 1976 and in use to this day, to present drug utilization data and so make national and international comparisons of drug utilization, evaluate long-term trends in drug use, assess the impact of external events on drug use, and provide denominator data in investigations of drug safety.

The ATC system sorts drugs initially into a target organ system (the nervous system, for psychotropics obviously) and then permits an ad hoc further subdivision broadly by therapeutic indication. Fig. 10.1 illustrates the actual first-stage terminology for drugs targeting the nervous system: anaesthetics, analgesics, anti-epileptics, anti-parkinsonians, psycholeptics, psychoanaleptics, and 'other' (which includes drugs used to treat 'addictive disorders'). The very words 'psycholeptic' and 'psychoanaleptic' are strikingly unfamiliar to most prescribers, even though they fit logically with the therapeutic principle of the classification's structure.

Thus, as further illustrated in Fig. 10.1, 'psychoanaleptics' include anti-dementia, antidepressant, psychostimulant, and psycholeptics and psychoanaleptics in combination. The term psychoanaleptic means 'to exert a stimulating effect on the mind'. It reflects an antique

way of thinking about drug action and now conjures up a property that is too vague to be useful. The further grouping is, in part, a classification by indication (anti-dementia, antidepressant) and, in part, by imprecise drug action (psychostimulation).

## Classification by indication: the overlap in primary indications

Naming drugs by primary indication has an obvious superficial attraction. It means we can remember how to use them easily, the classes automatically give us alternatives, and we can communicate our intention to treat with patients and their families. So, while the terms psycholeptic and psychoanaleptic are unfamiliar, we use the next-level terms routinely. The psycholeptics carve into antipsychotics, anxiolytics, and hypnotics, with corresponding indications of psychosis, anxiety, and insomnia. Moving to the psychoanaleptics, antidepressants are effective in treating depression. This terminology currently covers most of what many non-specialist prescribers probably know about psychotropic drugs.

The immediate difficulty is that these primary indications are not unique to the drugs assigned to the relevant classes. In the case of antipsychotics, a number are effective in resistant depression, quite independently of any antipsychotic action. Moreover, lithium is classified as an antipsychotic but has no primary antipsychotic action. In the case of anxiolytics and hypnotics, many are benzodiazepine derivatives with both anxiolytic and hypnotic actions. Indeed, the most important differences are pharmacokinetic, with shorter-acting drugs being the most suitable to hypnotic actions, but such differences cannot be represented explicitly in the classification.

In the case of antidepressants, many of them are commonly prescribed as monotherapy for anxiety disorders. While a drug like paroxetine has multiple licensed indications for anxiety, other drugs with essentially identical mechanisms of action (selective serotonin reuptake inhibitors—the so-called SSRIs) do not necessarily have evidence to support actions on anxiety. However, they are used by extrapolation to treat anxiety disorders. In addition, SSRIs may be useful to treat a variety of pain states [1]. Nevertheless, SSRIs are all

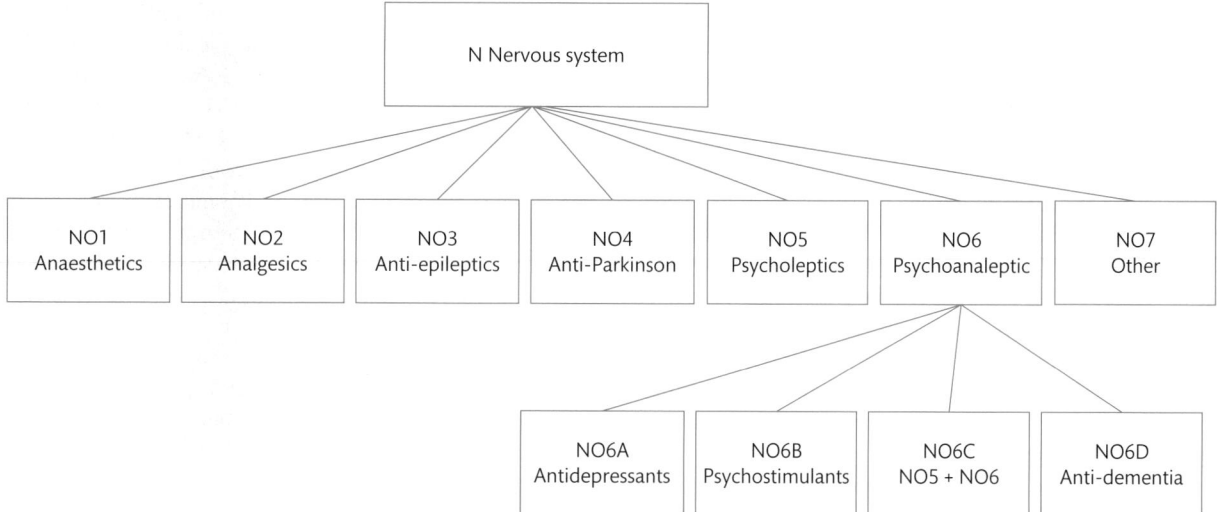

**Fig. 10.1** First-stage terminology for drugs targeting the nervous system.
Source: data from ATC/DDD Index 2017, N NERVOUS SYSTEM, © WHO Collaborating Centre for Drug Statistics Methodology, Oslo, Norway. Available at https://www.whocc.no/atc_ddd_index/?code=N

classified as antidepressants. This inexactitude has a negative effect on public and patient perception of our clinical practice.

Thus, the strident argument has been made that increasing numbers of prescription of SSRIs imply that doctors are overdiagnosing 'depression' and overprescribing 'antidepressants' [2]. It has made for unnecessary controversy and has devalued the evidence that prescribing an SSRI can be both evidence-based and useful to patients [3]. Together with this negative public discourse, the current nomenclature clouds direct personal communication with patients. It must be confusing to find that your anxiety disorder is being treated with an antidepressant. The use of an antipsychotic to augment the treatment for your depression (added to an SSRI or a similar medication) means having to cope with the thought that you have developed psychosis. Psychosis implies both severity of illness and stigma. Finally, anti-epileptic drugs (valproate, carbamazepine, lamotrigine) are used to treat bipolar disorder, but the package inserts for common formulations of these drugs may only reflect their use in epilepsy. The present classification certainly has the potential to confuse patients. Sophisticated prescribers may be well able to tolerate these inconsistencies, but it fails their needs in even more important ways, as will be illustrated later.

Finally, the emphasis on indication has served the purposes of marketing by the makers of drugs perhaps too well. It lends itself to the addition of soothing adjectives. Therefore, we have words like 'atypical', 'second generation', and 'novel' entered in the marketing pitch for new business. It has been almost entirely designed to persuade, Madison Avenue style. Who would want an old smart phone if the next-generation phone were on offer? But the analogy suggested by 'second-generation' antipsychotic drugs is entirely specious. Even specialists appear to have been taken in by this terminology. To take an important example, the CUtLASS trial compared 'first-' with 'second-'generation drugs for psychosis. However many patients in the study received sulpiride as a 'first-generation drug' and amisulpride as a 'second-generation drug'. These drugs are very similar molecules both chemically and pharmacologically, so to compare them is very unlikely to reveal an important difference.

Nevertheless, despite also being underpowered, the CUtLASS study is widely cited as evidence that new drugs for psychosis have no advantage over what went before [4, 5].

In summary, the ATC principle may be adequate for its given limited purposes in pharmacoepidemiology. It probably makes little difference how licensed drugs are actually grouped, since groups may be recombined to answer specific epidemiological questions. Indeed, the home website of the WHO Collaborating Centre for drug statistics methodology carries an important disclaimer: 'the classification of a substance in the ATC/DDD system is not a recommendation for use, nor does it imply any judgements about efficacy or relative efficacy of drugs and groups of drugs' (https://www.whocc.no/atc_ddd_methodology/purpose_of_the_atc_ddd_system/). However, as a classification that is used in everyday practice, it is both confused and confusing. Moreover, it poses a significant barrier to understanding drug action, and hence to rational prescribing. This is a problem psychiatrists need to solve, and the incentive to do so resides in our current practice. We need to change, and this chapter will explain why.

## Classification and the therapeutic challenge

### When chemical classification does not help

The guiding principle of the ATC recognizes 'chemistry' as a key classificatory level. This may sometimes mean pharmacology, but just as often, it is simply a classification on the basis of the organic chemistry of drugs. In the case of anti-epileptics, for example, pharmacology is not considered at all—it is just chemical structures of drugs. This means that the mechanisms of action of anti-epileptics may not be commonly known to prescribers at all. As an example, carbamazepine is an antagonist at the calcium channel [6]. It may be highly relevant that genome-wide association studies implicate variation in the encoding and expression of calcium channels in the aetiology of bipolar disorder and schizophrenia [7]. To describe carbamazepine as an anti-epileptic makes it seem surprising that it is an effective anti-manic drug; to describe it as a calcium channel antagonist at least provokes the thought that its actions might extend beyond the epilepsy indication.

There are many other examples within the existing terminology of psycholeptics and psychoanaleptics that also refer to chemistry. This has the virtue of neutrality, but the vice for most of us of conveying no useful information whatsoever. The case of antipsychotics is particularly instructive. See https://www.whocc.no/atc_ddd_index/?code=N05A for an example of how antipsychotics may be sub-classified. Fig. 10.2 shows how antipsychotics are sub-classified entirely on the basis of chemistry. As trainees, some of us may have attempted to remember the names, if not the chemical structures (for example, phenothiazines, butyrophenones, thioxanthines). All were antagonists at the dopamine D2 receptor, and this monocular perspective on their mode of action was probably encouraged by the pointless nomenclature. This only changed with the commercial effort to produce drugs with a low propensity for producing extrapyramidal side effects (EPS) in the 1980s and 1990s. The so-called atypical drugs fall into three new categories (Fig. 10.2): NO5AE (indole derivatives), NO5AH (diazepines, oxazepines, thiazepines, and oxepines—the '-pines'), and NO5AL (benzamides). However, what is important about indole derivatives and the '-pines' is the addition of affinity for neurotransmitter receptors other than dopamine into their pharmacology. This pharmacology is complex [8]. In the case of the '-pines' from NO5AH, the affinity for 5-HT2A receptors is much higher than for D2 receptors. It is widely believed that this is key to the reduced risk of EPS; moreover, reduced function at 5-HT2A receptors may be intrinsically 'antipsychotic'. Indeed, pimavanserin is a completely novel antipsychotic (developed for the treatment of psychosis in Parkinson's disease), with no dopamine receptor antagonism at all; its mechanism appears to be via an inverse agonist action at the 5-HT2A receptor. So in treating and combining drugs for psychosis, one needs to know that a drug like clozapine will have a small impact on D2 blockade and a large impact on 5-HT2A receptor function, while a drug like amisulpride will block D2/D3 receptors quite selectively (and effectively). If a patient fails to respond fully to clozapine, the addition of amisulpride as augmentation would be more logical than to add olanzapine (which simply mimics a range of the actions of clozapine) [9].

Finally, side effects are an important limitation of most antipsychotic medications. There is a high affinity for histamine

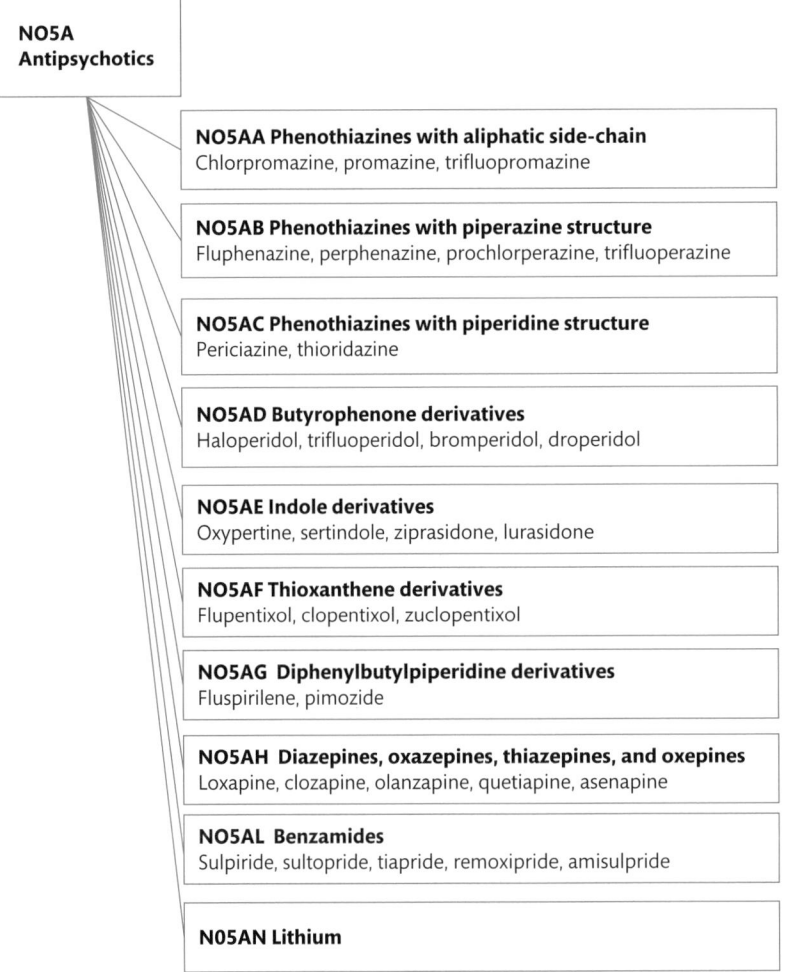

**Fig. 10.2** Current antipsychotic nomenclature under the WHO system.

Source: data from ATC/DDD Index 2017, N05A ANTIPSYCHOTICS, © WHO Collaborating Centre for Drug Statistics Methodology, Oslo, Norway. Available at https://www.whocc.no/atc_ddd_index/?code=N05A

receptors, which may result in weight gain and metabolic disturbance with clozapine, olanzapine, and quetiapine (but not asenapine). For other drugs, there may be a higher affinity for muscarinic receptors, which might be expected to produce a dry mouth, accommodation difficulties, etc. In general, to classify by indication fails to draw the prescriber's attention to the properties of drugs which will be important for treating individual patients.

## Why is pharmacology so important to psychiatry?

Obviously, most doctors take some pride in knowing how drugs work and how to use them. But pharmacological investigation of the mode of action has had a special place in psychiatry, because effective medicines were discovered before their pharmacology was understood. Investigation of the mode of action was, and arguably remains, a cutting-edge theme in neuroscience. Axelrod, Carlsson, von Euler, and Greengard won Nobel prizes for working out how the monoamine systems and the drugs acting on them function in the brain. Completely new fields of cognitive and computational neuroscience have opened up, because we know that dopamine neurons are involved in motor function and decision-making. This scientific development was recognized by the award of the Brain Prize in 2017 for multi-disciplinary analysis of brain mechanisms that link learning to reward (http://www.thebrainprize.org).

Psychopharmacology also provided, and still provides, one of the few starting points for mechanistic understanding of psychiatric disorder. By contrast, diagnosis (the indication) remains quite arbitrary and essentially provisional, based as it is on symptoms, rather than mechanisms of disease (see Chapters 7 and 8). So pharmacology provides a very appropriate space in which to name, describe, summarize, and classify psychotropic medicines. Obviously, some sub-classes of drugs are already described in this way. We have selective monoamine oxidase inhibitors (MAOIs) and SSRIs. The WHO classification of antidepressants (that is, those drugs with evidence for efficacy as monotherapy in unipolar depression) is another case in point (see https://www.whocc.no/atc_ddd_index/?code=N06A). The classification of antidepressants (that is, those drugs with evidence for efficacy as monotherapy in unipolar depression) is shown in Fig. 10.3. Monoamine reuptake inhibitors (non-selective and selective for serotonin) and MAOIs (non-selective and type A-specific) comprise the first four reasonable categories. However, the fifth group N06AX is 'other'. It includes currently 26 chemical entities and seven mechanisms of action (Fig. 10.3). It automatically includes all new drugs with novel mechanisms of action.

Unfortunately, we have even lacked a systematic approach to describing the pharmacological properties of those medicines we do classify by mode of action. The use of the term SSRI was promoted by companies marketing novel antidepressants in the 'Prozac' era. It is a fair summary of the key property of such drugs. However, the term SNRI does not stand for selective *noradrenaline* reuptake inhibitors,

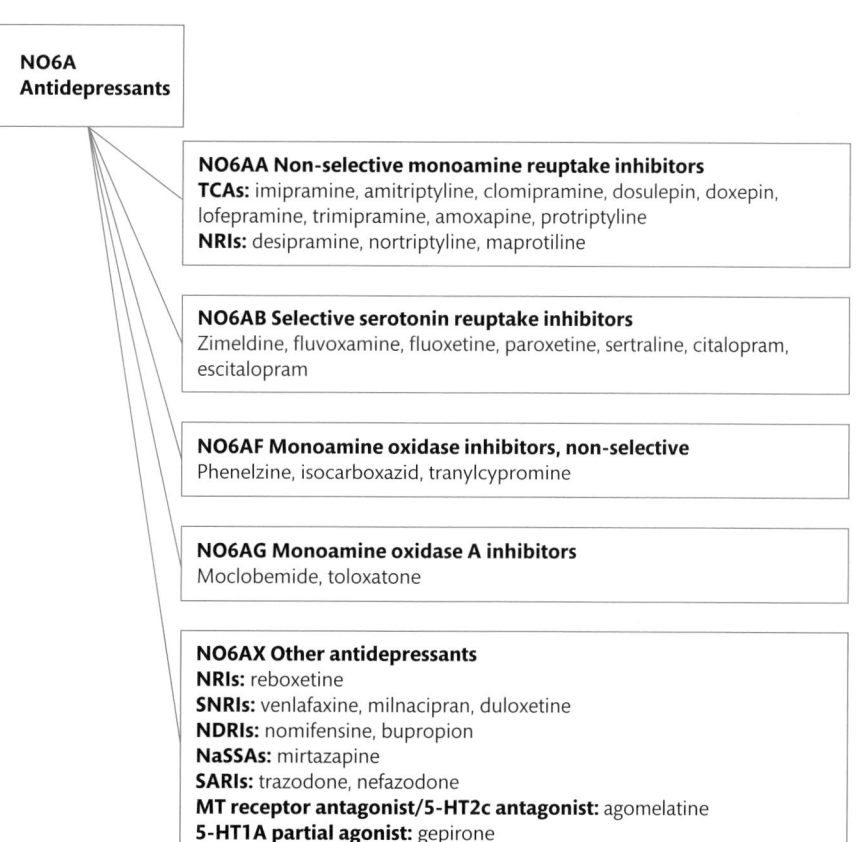

**Fig. 10.3** Current antidepressant nomenclature under the WHO system.

Source: data from ATC/DDD Index 2017, N06A ANTIDEPRESSANTS, © WHO Collaborating Centre for Drug Statistics Methodology, Oslo, Norway. Available at https://www.whocc.no/atc_ddd_index/?code=N06A

as you might expect. Instead, 'SNRI' stands for serotonin/noradrenaline reuptake inhibitor (Fig. 10.2). Selective noradrenergic reuptake inhibitors are instead abbreviated NRIs. More consistently, noradrenaline/dopamine reuptake inhibitors are NDRIs. In the case of serotonin antagonist and reuptake inhibitors, the preferred abbreviation is SARIs. Individual drugs like mirtazapine, agomelatine, and gepirone are single examples of particularly quite complex mechanisms of action.

## Conclusions

So in summary, we have antipsychotics and anti-epileptics used to treat patients with bipolar disorder who are neither psychotic nor epileptic. We have SSRIs and SNRIs, although SNRIs are *not* selective noradrenaline reuptake inhibitors, but instead serotonin/noradrenaline reuptake inhibitors, and finally we have a growing majority of antidepressants classed simply as 'other'. It is undeniably a mess. Does it matter? It has been tolerated for a long time, without serious efforts to change. Our desire to make changes now should be fuelled by embarrassment. However, there are more serious reasons to change too. With Lewis Carroll, we often do not know what we think until we speak. Defining our treatments by diagnoses of limited validity limits our capacity to speak. Our failure to use pharmacological criteria and define drug actions limts our capacity to think. An emphasis on mechanism should stimulate clinicians to think what they are doing when they prescribe for patients. It will be a continuing nudge to stay on top of the science that underpins our understanding. Moreover, a more nuanced system for describing medicines can grow flexibly—it can accommodate a mechanistic understanding at any number of levels, from molecules, to systems, to cognition. There is also the potential to harness the shift in emphasis from operational diagnosis to dimensional neurobiology, as currently enshrined in the RDoC project (see Chapter 8).

## Neuroscience-based nomenclature

The NbN initiative represents the efforts of colleagues from the five major international neuropsychopharmacological scientific organizations to reform the nomenclature of drugs used by psychiatrists. The taskforce was formed in 2008 (Box 10.1).

All expenses related to the project were covered by the European College of Neuropsychopharmacology (ECNP). Throughout the entire process, there was no direct or indirect support from any pharmacological company or other organization.

It was agreed that the guiding criteria were to:

1. Be based on contemporary knowledge.
2. Assist clinicians to make informed choices while prescribing.
3. Provide a system that does not conflict with the use of medications.
4. Be future-proof and accommodate new types of compounds.
5. Decrease stigma attached to a classification by indication (and enhance adherence).

The methodology was expert consensus informed by prescriber feedback [10, 11].

---

**Box 10.1** Organizations contributing to the NbN initiative

*ECNP*—European College of Neuropsychopharmacology
*ACNP*—American College of Neuropsychopharmacology
*AsCNP*—Asian College of Neuropsychopharmacology
*CINP*—International College of Neuropsychopharmacology
*IUPHAR*—International Union of Basic and Clinical Pharmacology

---

## The future of naming by indication

If our existing terminology is misleading and constrains creative thought, we should try to give up this approach completely. This recommendation of the taskforce has been broadly accepted by the editors of many major cognate journals (Box 10.2)

This means trying to use less often the words antipsychotics, antidepressants, anxiolytics, and hypnotics when what we could say is simply 'drugs for psychosis', 'drugs for depression', 'drugs for anxiety', and 'drugs for insomnia'. Simply changing the stress to the indication, rather than the class of drug, is often an easy adjustment to make.

Where an author wants to use the words antipsychotics, antidepressants, anxiolytics, and hypnotics, then s/he should define exactly what is meant. If one is actually wanting to say dopamine antagonists/partial agonists, then that is preferable to 'antipsychotics'. In the case of 'antidepressants' and 'anxiolytics', it is much more difficult to substitute a single word based on the mode of action. However, defining in advance exactly what drugs are subsumed within one's meaning of 'antidepressant' is a good discipline. The British Association for Psychopharmacology guidelines for the treatment of bipolar disorder were written from this perspective and proved acceptable to the consensus group involved [12].

---

**Box 10.2** Journals that have accepted the recommendations of the NbN initiative

*American Journal of Psychiatry*
*The Lancet* Group
*Biological Psychiatry*
*Neuropsychopharmacology*
*Psychological Medicine*
*International Journal of Neuropsychopharmacology*
*European Neuropsychopharmacology*
*World Journal of Biological Psychiatry*
*European Psychiatry*
*Journal of Psychopharmacology*
*CNS Spectrums*
*European Archives of Psychiatry and Clinical Neuroscience*
*Current Psychiatry*
*Japanese Journal of Neuropsychopharmacology* (official journal of Japanese Society of Neuropsychopharmacology)
*Clinical Psychopharmacology and Neuroscience—Korean College of Neuropsychopharmacology* (official journal of AsCNP)
*Chinese Journal of Psychiatry*
*British Journal of Clinical Pharmacology*
*Journal of Clinical Psychopharmacology*
*Pharmacology International* (IUPHAR journal)
*Pharmacopsychiatry*
*Pharmakopsychiatrie* (in German)

## The NbN nomenclature

The NbN nomenclature classifies drug action by domain (the neurotransmitter target) and mechanism of drug action. As shown in Table 10.1, domains range from dopamine or orexin (with quite a restricted anatomy based on small groups of neurons and their projections) to 'ion channels' or GABA (gamma aminobutyric acid) which implies a much more diffuse whole brain anatomy. We currently identify ten domains, but they are very likely to increase over time with the discovery of new drug targets. Some drugs (the SSRIs are an example) have been developed to be highly specific, so we already think of them as working in one domain exclusively. Many other drugs may act on more than one domain. Thus, drugs for psychosis will often be dopamine/serotonin drugs, as described previously. However, the reality is even more complicated, and we believe a dimensional approach is a better way to capture this adequately.

Along with a domain, drugs have different modes of action or functions. Table 10.1 shows the current proposals. Characterization as agonist, antagonist, partial agonist, or partial allosteric modulator defines drug action at the level of the neurotransmitter receptor. Reuptake inhibitor or releaser addresses the functional consequences of drug action. Enzyme inhibitor or modulator, or ion channel blocker, identifies functional targets potentially outside the conceptual synapse. These categories are based on familiarity, rather than a strict understanding of molecular mechanism. It is an open question of whether they will stand the test of time; however, the NbN is equipped to accommodate new insights.

Most of the current pharmacopoeia can be mapped into this nomenclature. For drugs working in a single domain with a single action, like the SRIs, there is little change. Drugs for psychosis pose a different challenge. The '-pines' illustrated previously can be described as dopamine/serotonin receptor inhibitors. Other examples (like aripiprazole and brexpiprazole) produce functional inhibition via partial agonist properties at dopamine receptors and have weaker antagonist properties at 5-HT2A receptors. The NbN approach pushes the prescriber to employ more words to describe their treatments and hopefully think more accurately about what they do. However, this increased complexity is potentially problematic. It exemplifies that medicine is entering a new era, in which

it is being transformed by the explosion of knowledge and access to knowledge. We have deliberately invested in developing an app which will provide the prescribing information we think doctors and patients need. The founding version of the NbN was launched at the ECNP congress in Berlin in 2014 as a booklet and app. The app format allows medicines to be searched under the old categories and new ones. It will allow translation into many languages. It will soon be linked to another specialist database [International Union of Basic and Clinical Pharmacology (IUPHAR)]. It can expand or extend through linking, almost without limit. This would be part of a broader movement to make more informed choices and to practise a more precise pharmacological strategy.

## Use of the NbN app

The NbN app can be searched and downloaded for use on Android (https://play.google.com/store/apps/details?id=il.co.inmanage. nbnomenclature&hl=en_GB)andiOSplatforms(https://itunes.apple. com/gb/app/nbn-neuroscience-based-nomenclature/id927272449? mt=8). Use of the app is explained by a brief tutorial, but it is best appreciated by downloading it and using it. However, Fig. 10.4 shows the opening screen/search page (left) and the result from typing 'olanzapine' (right). Further information (practical notes and neurobiology) can be obtained by scrolling down. The domains are dopamine and serotonin, and the mode of action is receptor antagonism.

The app also shows a brief summary of the approved indications, the spectrum of efficacy, and the adverse reactions commonly associated with olanzapine. The user can scroll down and see practical notes (which describe the availability of depot and the use in combination with fluoxetine for bipolar depression), former terminology (antpsychotic), and a link to a summary of the neurobiology. There are currently 130 drugs in the second edition of NbN (NbN-2) and 40 drugs in the child and adolescent version of NbN (NbN-ca).

## The NbN as a multi-dimensional classificatory system

The searchable fields of the NbN app can also be thought of as a pragmatic multi-axial classificatory system. It recognizes DSM-5 as a system for providing (mostly) familiar diagnoses, which we will continue to use to communicate with ourselves and our patients and estimate societal morbidity. However, the multi-dimensional system of NbN has some parallels with the approach of the RDoC initiative (see Chapter 8). Both highlight heterogeneity, challenge disease-based existing systems, detect subtypes, and provide a better match between research findings and clinical decision-making (Table 10.2).

If the RDoC can create a reliable and valid alternative system for classifying disorders, the NbN may be able to align how it represents drug action. For example, the RDoC proposes the constructs, negative valence, and positive valence, within which different levels of analysis are possible. These RDoC domains have something in common with NbN domains (serotonin and dopamine, for example), and the different levels of analysis in the RDoC (for example, fear, anxiety, loss, frustrated non-reward) provide targets for defining different drug actions. The key property of the

**Table 10.1** The NbN nomenclature classifying drug action by domain (the neurotransmitter target) and mechanism of drug action

| Pharmacological domains | | Modes/mechanisms of actions | |
|---|---|---|---|
| 1 | Acetylcholine | 1 | Receptor agonist |
| 2 | Dopamine | 2 | Receptor partial agonist |
| 3 | GABA | 3 | Receptor antagonist |
| 4 | Glutamate | 4 | Reuptake inhibitor |
| 5 | Histamine | 5 | Releaser |
| 6 | Orexin | 6 | Enzyme inhibitor |
| 7 | Melatonin | 7 | Ion channel blocker |
| 8 | Noradrenaline | 8 | Positive allosteric modulator (PAM) |
| 9 | Opioid | 9 | Enzyme modulator |
| 10 | Serotonin | | |

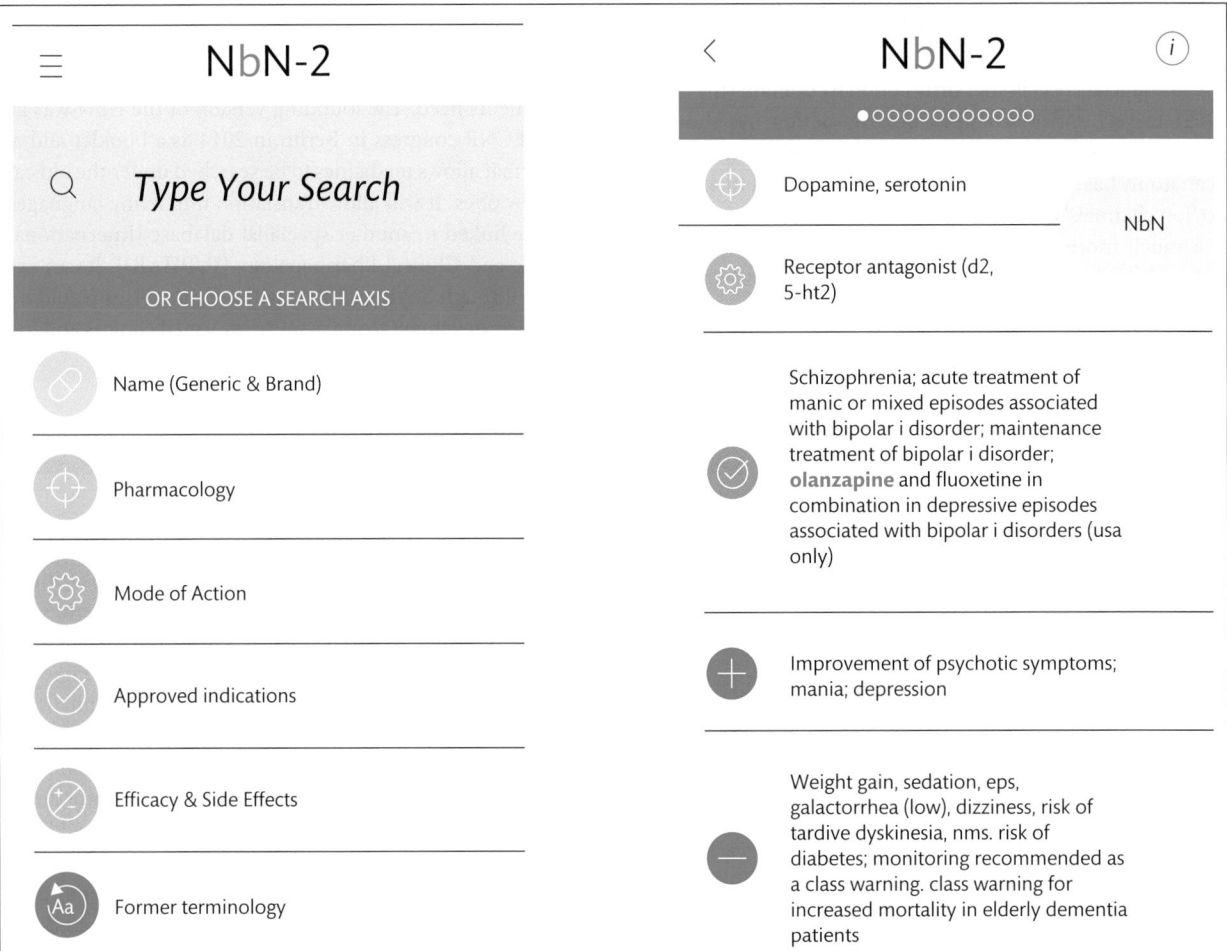

**Fig. 10.4** The NbN app.
Reproduced from the NbN Working Group.

**Table 10.2** Similarities between the RDoC and NbN classifications

|  | RDoC | NbN |
|---|---|---|
| Neuroscience-driven | ✓ | ✓ |
| Highlighting heterogeneity | ✓ | ✓ |
| Using updated medicine tools | ✓ | ✓ |
| Challenging artificial grouping of heterogenous (a) syndromes with different pathophysiological mechanisms and (b) drugs with different pharmacology and/or mode of action | a | b |
| Challenging disease-based existing systems ('horizontal') | ✓ | ✓ |
| Detecting subtypes | ✓ | ✓ |
| Aiming to address individual differences | ✓ | ✓ |
| Paving the way to precise medicine | ✓ | ✓ |
| Building a long-term framework that can accommodate future discoveries in neuroscience | ✓ | ✓ |
| Providing a better match between research findings and clinical decision-making | ✓ | ✓ |
| Focusing on diagnosis | ✓ | - |
| Focusig on drugs | - | ✓ |

NbN is that it is not bound by the limits of a two-dimensional table. Its creation as a digital device builds in a flexibility we have never enjoyed before. Moreover, being on a mobile platform makes it a widely accessible tool for use across the developed and developing world.

As it has developed, the point of the NbN has grown more obvious to more and more people. The major journals have accepted our critique of existing practice and have published editorials recommending change [13–24]. However, it is a work in progress. The hope is that the NbN encourages us to use different words, but crucially more words and concepts when describing our treatments. We may thereby be better informed when we take our initial 'pharmacological step' or later when we combine treatments after a first monotherapy fails. We can also improve how prescribers communicate among themselves and with their patients.

## REFERENCES

1. Patetsos, E. and Horjales-Araujo, E. (2016). Treating chronic pain with SSRIs: what do we know? *Pain Research and Management*, 2016, 2020915.
2. Godlee, F. (2013). Don't keep taking the tablets. *BMJ*, 347, F7438.
3. Reid, I.C. (2013). Are antidepressants overprescribed? *BMJ*, 346, f190.
4. Lewis, S. and Lieberman, J. (2008). CATIE and CUtLASS: can we handle the truth? *British Journal of Psychiatry*, 192, 161–3.
5. Lewis, S. (2009). Second-generation antipsychotics: a therapeutic downturn? *Psychology Medicine*, 39, 1603–6.
6. Cipriani, A., Saunders, K., Attenburrow, M.J., *et al.* (2016). A systematic review of calcium channel antagonists in bipolar disorder and some considerations for their future development. *Molecular Psychiatry*, 21, 1324–32.
7. Harrison, P.J., Cipriani, A., Harmer, C.J., *et al.* (2016). Innovative approaches to bipolar disorder and its treatment. *Annals of the New York Academy of Sciences*, 1366, 76–89.
8. Stahl, S.M. (2013). *Stahl's essential psychopharmacology: neuroscientific basis and practical applications* (4th edn). Cambridge University Press, Cambridge.
9. Goodwin, G., Fleischhacker, W., Arango, C., *et al.* (2009). Advantages and disadvantages of combination treatment with antipsychotics ECNP Consensus Meeting, March 2008, Nice. *European Neuropsychopharmacology*, 19, 520–32.
10. Zohar, J., Nutt, D.J., Kupfer, D.J., *et al.* (2014). A proposal for an updated neuropsychopharmacological nomenclature. *European Neuropsychopharmacology*, 24, 1005–14.
11. Zohar, J., Stahl, S., Moller, H.J., *et al.* (2015). A review of the current nomenclature for psychotropic agents and an introduction to the Neuroscience-based Nomenclature. *European Neuropsychopharmacology*, 25, 2318–25.
12. Goodwin, G.M., Haddad, P.M., Ferrier, I.N., *et al.* (2016). Evidence-based guidelines for treating bipolar disorder: revised third edition recommendations from the British Association for Psychopharmacology. *Journal of Psychopharmacology*. 30, 495–553.
13. Andrade, C. and Sathyanarayana Rao, T.S. (2016). Neuroscience-based nomenclature and medicolegal significance: response. *Indian Journal of Psychiatry*, 58, 346–7.
14. Blier, P., Oquendo, M.A., and Kupfer, D.J. (2017). Progress on the Neuroscience-Based Nomenclature (NbN) for psychotropic medications. *Neuropsychopharmacology*, 42, 1927–8.
15. Bruhl, A.B. and Sahakian, B.J. (2017). Neuroscience-based Nomenclature: improving clinical and scientific terminology in research and clinical psychopharmacology. *Psychology Medicine*, 47, 1339–41.
16. Frazer, A. and Blier, P. (2016). A Neuroscience-Based Nomenclature (NbN) for psychotropic agents. *International Journal of Neuropsychopharmacology*, 19, pyw066.
17. Gorwood, P., Frangou, S., and Heun, R.; Editors-in-chief of European, P. (2017). Editorial: Neuroscience-based Nomenclature (NbN) replaces the current label of psychotropic medications in European psychiatry. *European Psychiatry*, 40, 123.
18. Krystal, J.H., Abi-Dargham, A., Barch, D.M., *et al.* (2016). Biological psychiatry and biological psychiatry: cognitive neuroscience and neuroimaging adopt Neuroscience-Based Nomenclature. *Biological Psychiatry*, 80, 2–3.
19. Moller, H.J., Schmitt, A., and Falkai, P. (2016). Neuroscience-based nomenclature (jNbN) to replace traditional terminology of psychotropic medications. *European Archives of Psychiatry and Clinical Neuroscience*, 266, 385–6.
20. Nutt, D.J. and Blier, P. (2016). Neuroscience-based Nomenclature (NbN) for Journal of Psychopharmacology. *Journal of Psychopharmacology*, 30, 413–15.
21. Uchida, H. and Yamawaki, S. (2016). [Newly developed nomenclature (Neuroscience-based Nomenclature)]. *Nihon Shinkei Seishin Yakurigaku Zasshi* (*Japanese Journal of Psychopharmacology*), 36, 69–71.
22. Uchida, H., Yamawaki, S., Bahk, W.M., and Jon, D.I. (2016). Neuroscience-based Nomenclature (NbN) for clinical psychopharmacology and neuroscience. *Clinical Psychopharmacology and Neuroscience*, 14, 115–16.
23. Worley, L. (2017). Neuroscience-based nomenclature (NbN). *The Lancet Psychiatry*, 4, 272–3.
24. Zohar, J. and Kasper, S. (2016). Neuroscience-based Nomenclature (NbN): a call for action. *World Journal of Biological Psychiatry*, 17, 318–20.

# SECTION 2
# The scientific basis of psychiatric aetiology and treatment

# 11

# Neurodevelopment

*Karl Zilles and Nicola Palomero-Gallagher*

## Neural induction

The central nervous system originates from the midline region of the embryo as a specialized area of the ectoderm—the *neuroectoderm* or *neural plate* (Fig. 11.1a). Fibroblast growth factor (FGF) signalling and bone morphogenetic protein (BMP), as well as *Wnt* (wingless gene) inhibition, are required as steps for neural induction [1]. As the neuroectodermal cells proliferate, the neural plate is transformed into an indentation—the *neural groove* (Fig. 11.1b). The lateral parts of this groove approach each other and join in the midline, forming the *neural tube* (Fig. 11.1c–f). This fusion of the groove to a tube by a folding process starts in the middle portion of the groove and proceeds in rostral and caudal directions like a zipper. The most rostral and caudal parts close only later, initially leaving rostral and caudal neuropores. A small transitional zone between the neural plate and the surrounding ectoderm provides the cells of the *neural crest* (Fig. 11.1a), which develop into post-ganglionic cells of the sympathetic and parasympathetic nervous system, sensory neurons of the spinal ganglia and ganglia of cranial nerves, Schwann cells, and chromaffin cells of the suprarenal glands (Fig. 11.1f).

Neural tube formation requires a controlled expression of cell adhesion molecules in the lateral folds of the neural groove. If the rostral neuropore fails to close, the development of the forebrain is impaired, leading to *anencephaly*. If the caudal neuropore fails to close, the most severe result is *rachischisis*, a malformation with a dorsally exposed neural groove. The mildest outcome is *spina bifida occulta*, which is a cleft of a vertebral arch covered by the epidermis.

As development continues, the neural tube and crest are found between the ectoderm and the notochord. The rostral part of the neural tube differentiates into the brain; the caudal part (behind the fifth somite) differentiates into the spinal cord.

## Organogenesis of the central nervous system

The embryonic brain has three vesicular enlargements: the forebrain (telencephalon plus diencephalon), the midbrain (mesencephalon), and the hindbrain (rhombencephalon, including the cerebellum). At this early stage of brain development, a principal organization of the wall of the neural tube and its derivatives is still recognizable. There is a concentric organization around the central canal, with the ventricular zone most interior, the intermediate zone surrounding the ventricular zone, and an outer cell-sparse marginal zone (Fig. 11.2e). The ventricular zone contains neuroblasts. Sections orthogonal to the longitudinal axis of the neural tube allow the stratification of its wall into four zones in a dorsal to ventral direction: roof plate, alar lamina, basal lamina, and floor plate (Fig. 11.2e). The alar and basal laminae are separated by a shallow sulcus in the ventricular surface, that is the *sulcus limitans* (double arrow in Fig. 11.2e). This sulcus demarcates a principal functional subdivision, since the alar lamina is the source for sensory neurons in the spinal cord and brainstem, whereas motor neurons originate in the basal lamina. Local expression of homeobox genes leads to the formation of the pallium and the ganglionic hill in the forebrain. Because the brain grows much faster than the rest of the embryo, it becomes deflected ventrally. A dorsally convex cephalic flexure marks the border between the hindbrain and the midbrain, and a cervical flexure marks the border between the spinal cord and the hindbrain (Fig. 11.2a–c). The ventrally convex pontine flexure is found at the central level of the hindbrain (Fig. 11.2b). During week 5, the forebrain differentiates further into the rostral telencephalon and the more caudal diencephalon. The telencephalon consists of two hemispheric vesicles connected by a thin lamina terminalis. A part of the lamina terminalis develops into the commissural plate—the *anlage* of the later corpus callosum (Fig. 11.2d). The ventral part of the lamina terminalis differentiates into the anterior commissure. The hemispheric vesicles show a spatially directed growth around the future insular lobe, which leads to a backward-directed elongation towards the occipital lobe and a backward- and ventrally directed growth, forming the temporal lobe (Fig. 11.2f). Further enlargement of the frontal, parietal, and temporal lobes, together with a slower growth rate of the insular lobe, leads to a gradual covering of the latter brain region, a process called *opercularization* (Fig. 11.2g, h). This process is associated with the appearance of the lateral fissure (Fig. 11.2h).

Extensive growth of the parieto-occipito-temporal association cortex leads to a bend in the temporal lobe around the lateral fissure, and the temporal pole is pushed rostrally. This direction of growth (Fig. 11.2f) also affects the structures situated dorsomedially, that is, the archicortex with the hippocampus, corpus striatum, and lateral ventricles. The corpus striatum is split by the ingrowing fibres of the internal capsule into the caudate nucleus and putamen. The head of

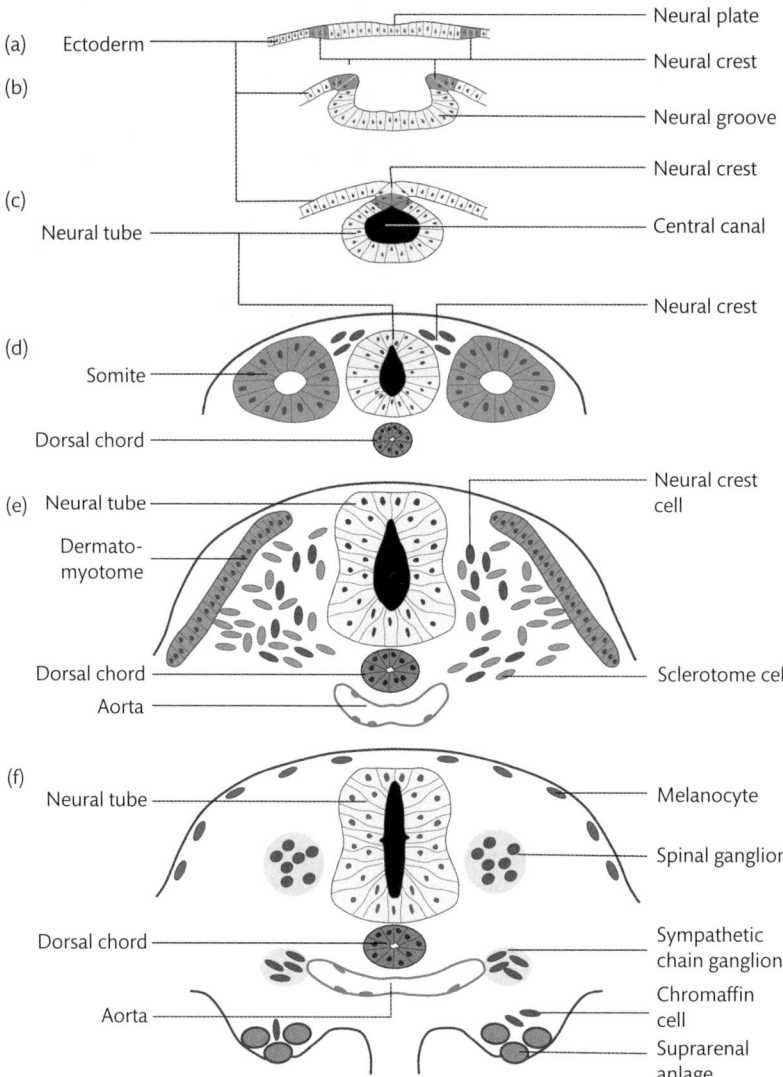

**Fig. 11.1** Early developmental stages of the nervous system in schematic drawings of cross-sections through embryos.

the caudate is situated ventrolateral to the corpus callosum in the frontal lobe, and the tail of the caudate is located dorsal to the inferior horn of the lateral ventricle. The hippocampus forms its largest extension (the retrocommissural part) in the temporal lobe, bends around the posterior end (splenium) of the corpus callosum, and reaches a position on top of the corpus callosum (the supracommissural part). The precommissural part of the hippocampus ends in front of the genu of the corpus callosum. Finally, the first primary sulci appear, for example, the central sulcus (Fig. 11.2h).

The central cavity of the diencephalon (the third ventricle) is connected with the cavities of the hemispheric vesicles (the lateral ventricles) by the interventricular foramen (Fig. 11.2d). The diencephalon forms bilateral evaginations—the eye vesicles—which differentiate into the retina and the optic nerve.

The tectum with the superior and inferior colliculi evolves from midbrain enlargement. Gradients in the expression of *Gbx2* and *Otx2* determine the midbrain–hindbrain boundary [2]. This region is enriched in *Engrailed-1, Engrailed-2, Pax-2, Pax-5,* and *mbx* genes, which are important for the development of the tectum [3, 4].

Meanwhile, the hindbrain becomes subdivided into a rostral part (that is, the metencephalon) and a caudal part (that is, the myelencephalon). The cerebellum starts to develop from the rostral part of the metencephalon during week 6. At first, the enlarged central cavity of the neural tube (the future fourth ventricle) has a thin roof plate, bordered by two thickenings of the neural tube—the *rhombic lips*—which merge in the midline (Fig. 11.2d, f). These thickenings are the source of the later cerebellar hemispheres, while its midline develops into the cerebellar vermis.

The hindbrain is temporarily divided into eight rhombomeres [5], the borders of which are specified by combinations of transcription factors (for example, *Hox, Krox, Wnt* genes). It develops in close association with the visceral arches, which appear during week 4. It innervates these arches and the organs derived from them by a group of branchial nerves, which later become the trigeminal (V), facial (VII), glossopharyngeal (IX), vagal (X), and accessory (XI) cranial nerves. Other cranial nerves develop connections between the hindbrain and peripheral organs not derived from the visceral arches. They are the oculomotor (III), trochlear (IV), abducens (VI),

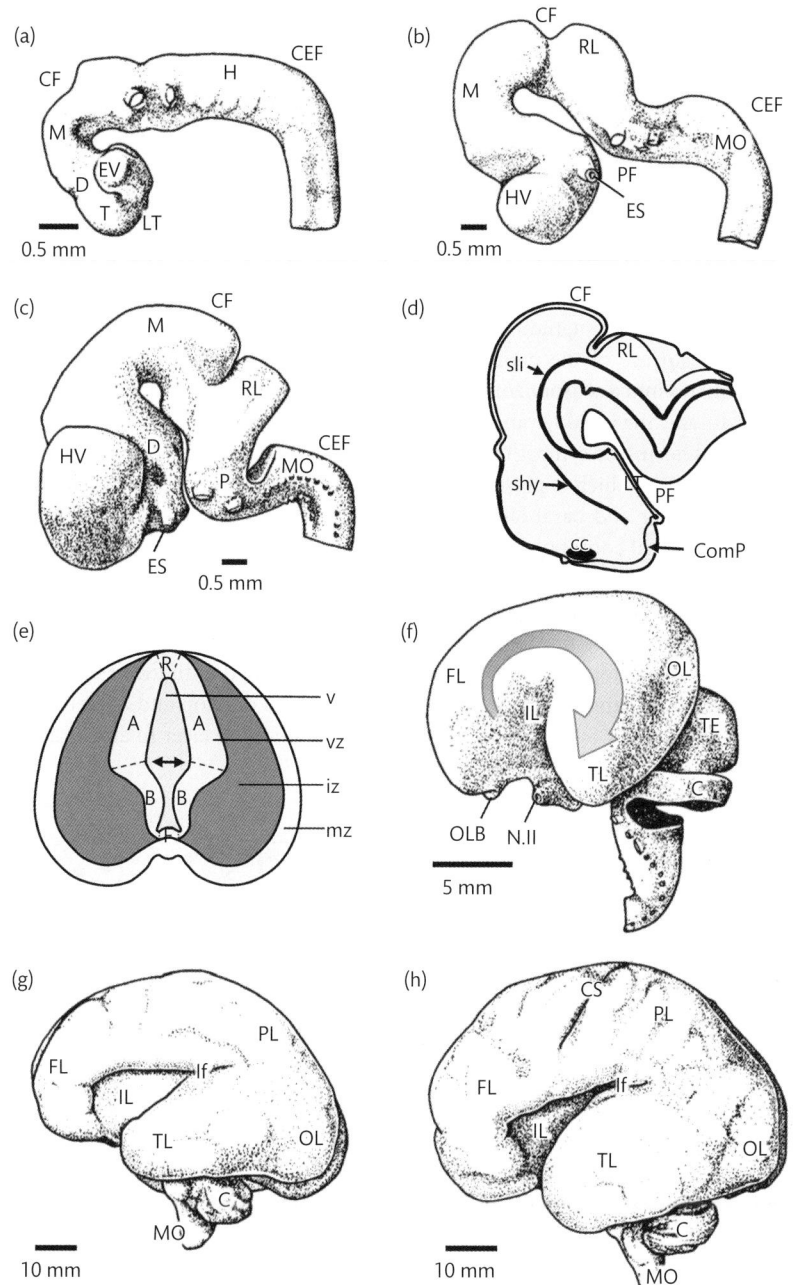

**Fig. 11.2** Development of the human brain. Brains of (a) 4-mm, (b) 10.4-mm (c), 13.8-mm, and (d) 53-mm human embryos, and (e) 21-week and (f) 24-week fetuses. A, alar plate; b, basal plate; c, cerebellum or cerebellar *anlage*; cc, corpus callosum; CEF, cervical flexure; CF, cephalic flexure; ComP, commissural plate; cs, central sulcus; D, diencephalon; ES, eye stalk; EV, eye vesicle; F, floor plate; FL, frontal lobe; H, hindbrain; HV, hemispheric vesicle; IL, insular lobe; iz, intermediate zone; lf, lateral fissure; LT, lamina terminalis; M, mesencephalon; MO, medulla oblongata; mz, mantle zone; N.II, optic nerve; OL, occipital lobe; OLB, olfactory bulb; P, pons; PF, pontine flexure; PL, parietal lobe; R, roof plate; RL, rhombic lip; sli, sulcus limitans; shy, sulcus hypothalamicus; T, telencephalon; TE, tectum; TL, temporal lobe; v, ventricle; vz, ventricular zone.

vestibulocochlear (VIII), and hypoglossal (XII) nerves. The olfactory (I) and optic (II) nerves arise separately as evaginations of the forebrain.

## Histogenesis of the spinal cord

The neural tube initially consists of a single layer of neuroepithelial cells surrounding a central canal filled with cerebrospinal fluid

(Fig. 11.1c–f). The outer surface of the future spinal cord has an external limiting membrane, and the inner surface bordering the central canal has an inner limiting membrane. The entire wall of the early neural tube is called the ventricular zone [6].

The cells of the ventricular zone proliferate, and the surface of the spinal cord enlarges. The cord then thickens, as cells divide further to produce a multi-layered epithelium. The daughter cells have different potentialities; one type of cell (the neuroblast) retains the capability for mitosis, whereas another type (the proneuron) is post-mitotic and represents an immature neuron. Proliferation of neurons is almost complete around birth.

Some neuroepithelial cells develop into precursors of glial cells, that is, glioblasts, which differentiate into astroglial, oligodendroglial, and microglial cells. The first glioblasts differentiate into radially extended cells, spanning the entire width of the wall of the spinal cord (the same occurs in the cerebral hemispheres and the cerebellar cortex, as described here). During later development, these radially extended cells are transformed into ependymal cells and astroglia.

Histogenesis of the spinal cord starts at the cervical level and progresses in a caudal direction. After week 3, the longitudinal sulcus limitans is recognizable on the inner surface of the neural tube (Fig. 11.2e). The alar lamina differentiates into a sensory zone—the dorsal horn of the adult spinal cord—and the basal lamina differentiates into a motor zone—the ventral horn. The sympathetic preganglionic neurons form in the lateral horn, which is present only at thoracic levels. The subdivision into alar and basal laminae is functionally important not only in the spinal cord, but also in the brainstem.

Proneurons leave the ventricular zone and migrate along radial glial cells into the intermediate zone where they become organized into cell groups. The motor neurons develop the axons of the ventral root, and the processes from spinal ganglionic cells grow into the spinal cord to form the dorsal roots. Synapses develop first in the motor zone, and later in the sensory zone, during weeks 10 to 13.

During the third month, the ventricular zone is reduced to a small rim surrounding the central canal and is finally transformed into the ependymal cell layer. The intermediate zone becomes organized into dorsal, ventral, and (at thoracic levels) lateral horns. The ascending and descending fibre tracts of the spinal cord are increased in size in the marginal zone. During weeks 14 and 15, oligodendrocytes begin to myelinate these fibre tracts. The corticospinal, or pyramidal, tract becomes visible for the first time during week 14 and reaches its target neurons, mainly motor neurons of the ventral horn, between weeks 17 and 29. Myelination of the pyramidal tract is completed between the the first and second post-natal years. This late myelination explains the presence of the Babinski reflex in newborns and its disappearance during the first 2 years of life.

## Histogenesis of the brainstem and cerebellum

At the level of the fourth ventricle, the various zones of the hindbrain are arranged in a lateral-to-medial sequence (somatosensory–viscerosensory–visceromotor–somatomotor). In the hindbrain, proneurons not only migrate radially, as in the spinal cord, but also tangentially and longitudinally. This complex migration course and the growth of fibre tracts lead to further changes of the lateral-to-medial and dorsal-to-ventral 'displacements' of cranial nerve nuclei (for example, the facial nucleus) in the adult.

At the level of the cerebellar anlage, the undifferentiated matrix cells form two major zones—a larger ventricular matrix zone and a smaller, most dorsally positioned upper rhombic lip zone. From the upper rhombic lip zone, a first wave of progenitor cells migrate between weeks 10 and 11, which sequentially express *Pax6*, *TBR2*, and *TBR1*, and form a transitory peripheral zone before migrating

down to a position where the adult cerebellar nuclei with their glutamatergic neurons are found (Fig. 11.3a, b). A second wave from the upper rhombic lip zone leads to the formation of an external granular layer (dotted arrow in Fig. 11.3a). Cells in this layer remain mitotically active long after birth. Thus, the external granular layer is a major source of cells for the adult cerebellum. From this layer, cells migrate to form the internal granular layer of the adult cerebellum, with its small and abundant granular cells and the somewhat larger and less abundant Golgi cells. Proneurons from the external granular layer also give rise to the basket and star cells of the adult molecular layer (Fig. 11.3a, b).

A second source of progenitor cells is located around the ventricle, that is, the ventricular matrix zone. The progenitor cells begin to migrate during weeks 12 and 13 along radially extended glial cells—Bergmann glia—into a region below the external granular layer (Fig. 11.3a) where they mature into GABA (gamma aminobutyric acid)-ergic Purkinje cells of the ganglionic layer of the adult cerebellar cortex (Fig. 11.3b). Therefore, the cerebellum originates out of two major migration streams, one starting in the ventricular matrix zone and the upper rhombic lip zone and the other one originating in the external granular layer. Migration of cerebellar proneurons is not completed until the first postnatal year. During weeks 16 and 26, synapses develop and afferent fibre systems begin to form. The external granular layer finally disappears during the first 2 years of

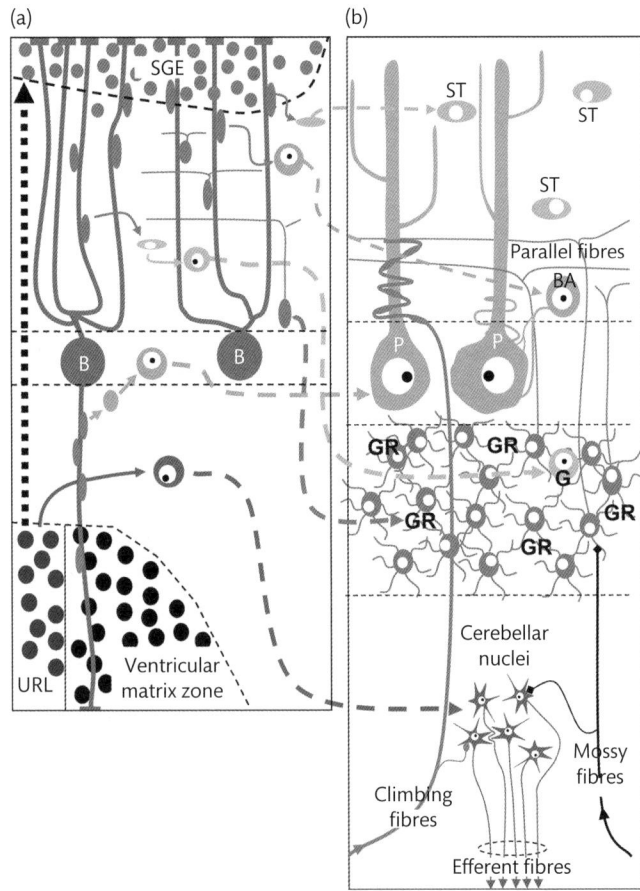

**Fig. 11.3** (see Colour Plate section) Development of the cerebellar cortex and nuclei. (a) Fetal development. (b) Adult stage. B, Bergmann glia; BA, basket cell; G, Golgi cell; GR, granular cell; P, Purkinje cell; SGE, stratum granulosum externum; ST, stellate cell; URL, upper rhombic lip.

life, leaving the three-layered structure (molecular, ganglionic, and internal granular layers) of the adult cerebellar cortex.

## Histogenesis of the cerebral cortex, basal ganglia, amygdala, and basal forebrain

Initially, the entire wall of the hemispheric vesicle consists of very densely packed mitotic cells. These cells undergo more than 28 mitotic rounds in the human brain [7]. In week 5, an inner cell-dense *periventricular zone* and an outer cell-poor *marginal zone* can be recognized. During week 6, the first post-mitotic proneurons leave the inner periventricular zone and form an *intermediate (mantle) zone* between the marginal and periventricular zones. By the end of week 6, the periventricular zone is further subdivided into a cell-dense *ventricular zone* and a less cell-dense *subventricular zone*.

During week 8, the *cortical plate* between the marginal and intermediate zones is formed by proneurons which have migrated along *radial glial cells* from the ventricular and subventricular zones through the intermediate zone (Fig. 11.4a) [6–10]. A single radial glial cell can span the entire distance between the ventricular and pial surfaces. As the proneurons 'climb' to the *cortical plate* along the processes of the radial glial cell, they produce a vertically oriented cortical cell column. This *radial migration* of immature neurons ultimately leads to the formation of cortical layers II to VI, and these proneurons differentiate into the various types of glutamatergic pyramidal neurons in the adult cerebral cortex. A prototype of the structural segregation of the cerebral cortex into numerous areas in the adult brain is already preformed during this migration [11]. A further feature of migration is the *inside-to-outside layering* of the immature, radially migrating neurons. The earliest-born neurons are found in the deepest layers, and the latest in the most superficial layers of the cortical plate. Thus, adult layers V and VI of the cerebral cortex are generated before layer IV, and layer IV is generated before layers III and II (Fig. 11.4b). The inside-out layering process is controlled by the extracellular matrix glycoprotein *reelin*, expressed in the Cajal-Retzius cells of the marginal zone. When cortical proneurons are migrating radially, *reelin* stops the approaching cells as they approach the marginal zone. The next wave of migrating cells moves through the first already 'immobilized' wave and is brought to halt again near the marginal zone. This process continues until the production of proneurons is exhausted, and thus migration is terminated. Therefore, *reelin* is important for the control of the inside-to-outside layering of the cortex [7]. Loss of *reelin* leads to severe disturbances of the normal layering of the cerebral cortex. In addition to reelin, the microtubule regulator protein LIS1, the neuronal migration protein doublecortin DCX, and the tumour suppressor protein p73 are also crucial factors for the normal migration of proneurons.

At the same time, tangential migration of immature cells born in the ganglionic eminence and the preoptic area (PoA) in the subpallium takes place. The ganglionic eminence can be subdivided into a medial (MGE) and a lateral ganglionic eminence (LGE) at more rostral levels, which merge to the caudal ganglionic eminence (CGE) caudally. These immature cells migrate from the MGE, CGE, and PoA through the marginal and intermediate zones into the cortical plate (Fig. 11.5) and develop into the inhibitory interneurons of the adult cerebral cortex [7, 12]. The cells stemming from the dorsal part of the MGE represent 60% of the later cortical interneurons, that is, the parvalbumin-positive basket and chandelier cells, whereas the ventral part of the MGE generates the somatostatin-positive

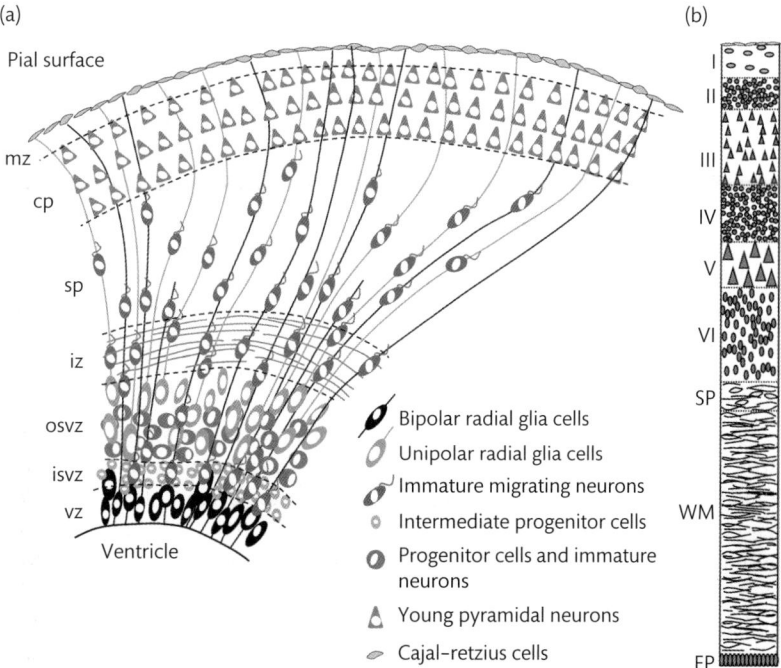

**Fig. 11.4** (see Colour Plate section) Histogenesis and radial migration in the cerebral cortex. (a) Development in the fetal hemispheric wall based on recent data [48, 54–56, 62, 63]. (b) Adult cortical layering in the human neopallium. I–VI, cortical layers; EP, ependymal layer; cp, cortical plate; isvz, inner subventricular zone; iz, intermediate zone with the first arriving nerve fibres establishing connection with immature neurons; mz, marginal zone; sp, subplate; osvz, outer subventricular zone; vz, ventricular zone; WM, white matter.

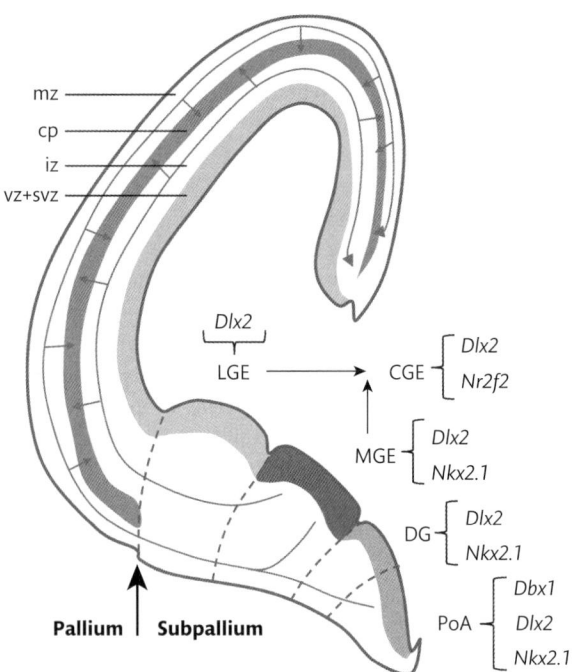

**Fig. 11.5** (see Colour Plate section) Schematic drawing of the precursor regions of inhibitory neurons later found in the cerebral cortex, basal ganglia, amygdala, and basal forebrain [64]. Precursor regions: CGE, caudal ganglionic eminence; DG, diagonal area; LGE, lateral ganglionic eminence; MGE, medial ganglionic eminence; PoA, preoptic area. Transcription factors: Dbx1, developing brain homeobox protein 1; Dlx2, Distal-less protein 2; Nkx2.1, thyroid transcription factor 1; Nr2f2, ligand-activated transcription factor Nr2f2. Cp, cortical plate; iz, intermediate zone; mz, mantle zone; vz + svz, ventricular + subventricular zone.
Source: data from Nieuwenhuys R, Puelles L, *Towards a new neural morphology*, Copyright (2016), Springer International Publishing Switzerland.

interneurons, mainly Martinotti cells [13–16]. The CGE gives rise to about 30% of the later cortical interneurons, which include calretinin and vasoactive inhibitory polypeptide-expressing bipolar and double bouquet cells, as well as reelin-expressing neurogliaform and multipolar cells [17–19]. The cells originating in the PoA contribute to 10% of the cortical interneurons and are represented in all groups of GABAergic interneurons. They all are derived from progenitor cells expressing the developing brain homeobox protein 1 (Dbx1) [16, 20]. Additionally, oligodendrocyte precursor cells migrate from the PoA to the pallium and subpallial target regions [21]. Therefore, the cells of the cerebral cortex have, like those of the cerebellar cortex, two different sources. In the case of the cerebral cortex, the sources are the ventricular and subventricular zones for the glutamatergic pyramidal neurons, and the MGE and CGE, as well as the PoA, for the inhibitory interneurons.

Although interneurons are mainly born in the ganglionic eminence and have completed their tangential migration by the end of fetal development [7, 12], a small number of perinatally born neurons which express doublecortin DCX and markers of interneurons are found during the first 2–5 months of life in the subventricular zone of the lateral ventricles [22]. Some of these young neurons migrate tangentially along the ventricular wall, while others move radially through the developing white matter into the overlying cortex where they develop into GABAergic interneurons, which are thought to contribute to developmental plasticity [22].

The LGE is the precursor region of GABAergic projection neurons of the striatum and pallidum [23, 24], and the MGE of those of the striatum and pallidum [25, 26]. The CGE develops into the larger subpallial part of the amygdala, although the MGE, LGE, CGE, and PoA also contribute precursor cells to the amygdala [23, 27–29]. The progenitor cells from the diagonal area (Fig. 11.5) migrate into the subcortical regions and develop into the adult cholinergic neurons of the basal forebrain and striatum [25, 27].

Regional differences in the development of the cortical plate subdivide the hemisphere into segments. The lateral segment, with a well-developed cortical plate and *presubplate*, develops into the *neocortex*. The mediodorsal segment, with a wide marginal zone and a thin, folded cortical plate, develops into the *archicortex*, including the hippocampus. The mediobasal segment, with its inconspicuously developed cortical plate, is the precursor of the *palaeocortex*. The basolateral segment, that is, the ganglionic eminence, generates cortical interneurons and develops into the corpus striatum, amygdala, and septum.

During weeks 10 and 12, the axons of serotoninergic and noradrenergic neurons contribute to the first synapses in the marginal and presubplate zones where neurotrophin receptors are expressed. During the following 3 weeks, the subplate zone develops, as axons grow in from the basal forebrain and thalamus, dendrites enlarge, and synapses form. From weeks 16–24, the cortical *anlage* has a small marginal zone, a wide cell-dense cortical plate, and a very wide and less cell-dense *subplate*.

Transformation into the adult neocortical pattern starts between weeks 25 and 34, as migration and proliferation of proneurons diminish. Dendrites begin to differentiate, and synapses begin to develop in the deepest cortical layers, progressing to the most superficial layer. Before birth, six cortical layers can be recognized in all regions of the neocortex. In the region of the motor cortex, layer IV (inner granular layer) is invaded by pyramidal cells during the postnatal period, to such a degree that this layer becomes inconspicuous. Therefore, the motor cortex has been classified as five-layered, agranular neocortex [30], although the typical granular cells of layer IV could be demonstrated between the pyramidal cells [31, 32]. Shortly before birth, the subplate, the subventricular zone, and most of the ventricular zone disappear; neuronal proliferation ceases, and the intermediate zone is transformed into the white matter of the pallium. The rest of the ventricular zone contributes to the ependymal layer of the ventricular surface.

Dendritic and axonal differentiation continue after birth and into adult life, and their time courses differ across brain regions. Myelination of the cortical–vestibular system is finished shortly before birth; that of the somatosensory, visual, auditory, pyramidal, and extra-pyramidal fibre tracts is nearly complete by the end of the third postnatal year, and that of the associative fibre tracts in the cerebral hemispheres is continued until the second decade [33, 34]. Although synaptic density in neonatal brains is comparable to that found in adults, synaptogenesis continues after birth, reaches a maximum during the first postnatal year, and proceeds at a lower rate during childhood. The peak period of synapse formation in the primary visual cortex is reached between 3 and 4 months, whereas in the prefrontal cortex, it occurs at around 8 months of age [35, 36]. The key change in synapses after birth, however, is pruning, that is, the process of selective elimination of excess synapses, which is essential for the balance between excitatory and inhibitory synapses and for the normal development of functional neural circuits. Developmental pruning is initiated during late fetal stages; it increases considerably shortly after birth and continues into puberty, when synaptic density stabilizes at adult levels. Pruning occurs earlier in sensorimotor areas than in association cortices.

Microglia play a role in the pruning process, and their activity is modulated by the initiating protein of the classical complement cascade (C1q) and the complement cascade components 3 and 4 (C3 and C4, respectively), as well as the microglial complement receptor 3 (CR3) [37–40]. Early loss of hippocampal synapses, as a result of an abnormally high C1q expression during development, was reported in a mouse model of Alzheimer's disease [40], and the low synapse density found in the brain of schizophrenics has been associated with excessive C4 activity during development [41–43], highlighting the importance of normal pruning process for correct neurodevelopment.

## Cortical folding

After the appearance of the lateral fissure, the neocortical surface develops many additional sulci and gyri during the fetal period (Fig. 11.6). The central, collateral, cingulate, parieto-occipital, superior temporal, and calcarine sulci appear between weeks 16 and 21, followed by the pre- and post-central, frontal, temporal, and intraparietal sulci. Highly variable secondary and tertiary sulci develop between week 29 and birth, when all sulci have been formed [44, 45]. Although all gyri and sulci are present at birth, the depth of the sulci increases until two-thirds of the cortical surface is hidden in them in the adult stage [44]. Measurements of the intensity of cortical folding show that gyrification is greatest in the regions where association cortices are found, particularly in the posterior

prefrontal, parietal, lateral temporal, and occipito-temporal cortices and the cuneus and precuneus (Fig. 11.7b) [44, 46].

The reasons for the formation of gyri in many mammalian brains, including the human brain, are not completely understood. Since the vertical cell columns positioned side by side represent a basic organizational principle of the cerebral cortex, growth of the cortex inevitably leads to a considerable enlargement of the cortical surface. A large unfolded cortical surface would have two major disadvantages: (1) the volume of the skull would increase to such a degree during fetal development that a normal delivery would be impossible; and (2) the distance between cortical regions interconnected by intrahemispheric projection fibres would increase and, with it, the information transmission time. Cortical folding therefore allows a maximal cortical surface in a minimal volume, and an optimization of the speed of neural transmission between cortical areas. This has led to speculations about the relationship between the growing brain surface and the skull size at birth. A large brain surface must be folded in order to minimize the brain diameter and thus enable a minimal skull diameter at the time of birth. In fact, a comparison between the growth of brain weight and cortical folding during human lifespan shows that the increase in cortical folding clearly precedes that of brain weight before and after birth (Fig. 11.7a). This, however, does not explain the mechanisms of cortical folding. Presently, the two most widely discussed hypotheses are the *mechanical tension hypothesis* [47] and the *grey matter hypothesis* [48].

The biophysical basis of the *mechanical tension hypothesis* are the three-dimensional courses and the viscoelastic properties of fibre tracts [47, 49, 50]. The first fibre tracts between cortical and other brain regions are already visible during subplate development and maintained during migration. More tangentially organized cortico-cortical than radially organized cortico-subcortical connections are found in the human brain. Therefore, the tension hypothesis predicts

(a)          (b)          (c)

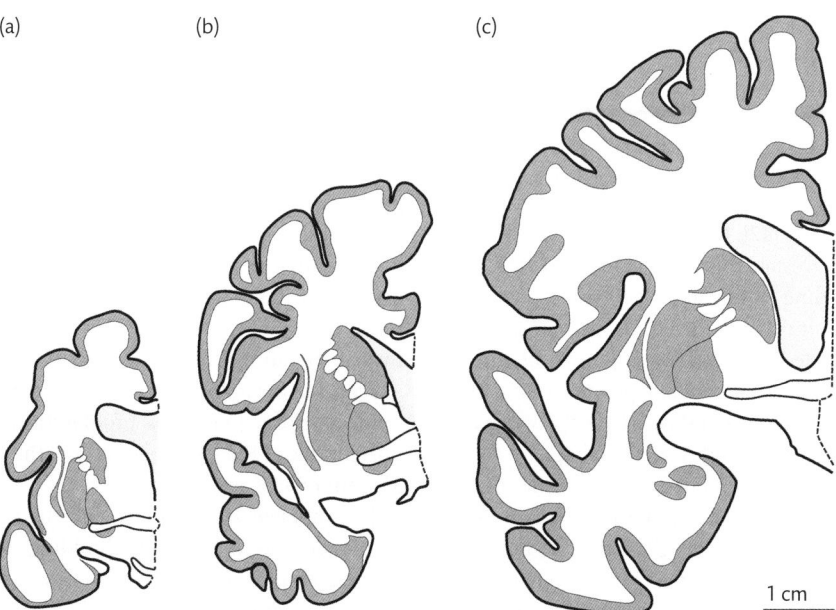

1 cm

**Fig. 11.6** Drawings of coronal sections through a fetal brain during the 30th week of gestation. (a) A newborn brain and (b) an adult brain, (c) showing the increase in cortical folding.

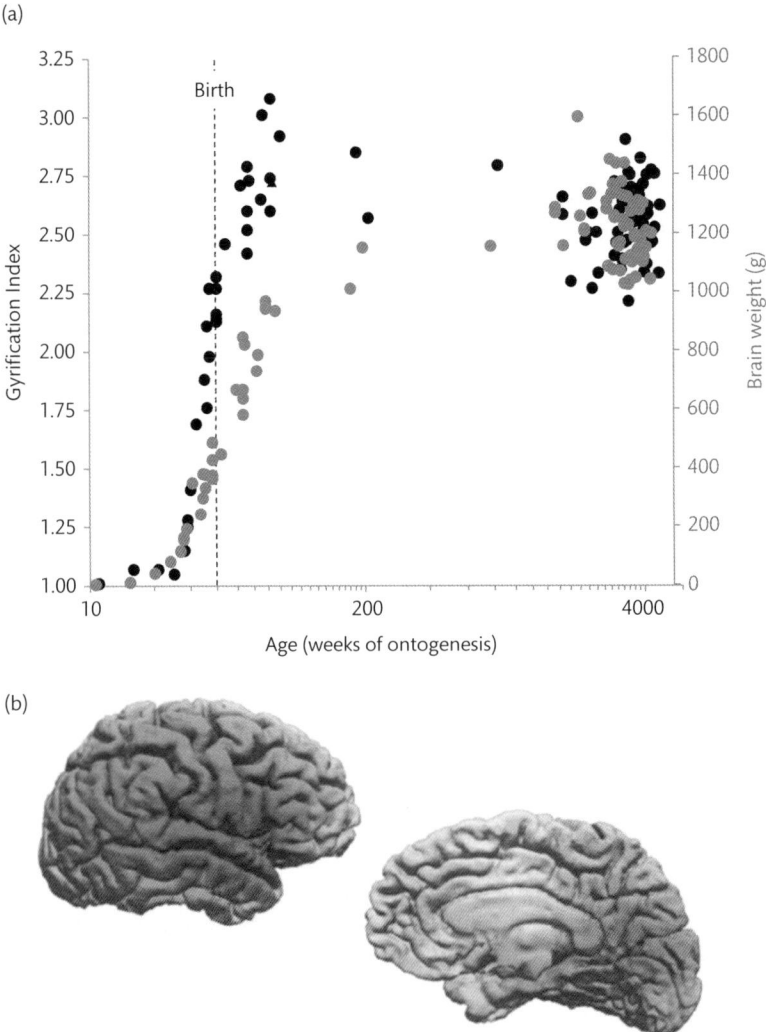

(a)

(b)

**Fig. 11.7** (see Colour Plate section) (a) Development of brain weight and gyrification index (GI) as a measure of the intensity of cortical folding during human lifespan. Data from Zilles *et al.* [44] and Armstrong *et al.* [45]. (b) Distribution of the local degree of cortical folding throughout the adult human brain, after Jockwitz *et al.* [46]. Red (dark grey in the printed version) indicates highest, yellow (pale grey in the printed version) lowest degrees of cortical folding.

an outward folding caused by strong cortico-cortical and weak cortico-subcortical connections [47]. However, tension is not found across developing gyri [51]. Despite this finding, regional variations in tension can shape the folding pattern and its correlation with the spatial organization of the connectome [52, 53]. Using computational modelling, it was demonstrated that differential growth of cortical sites drives folding, consistent with the folding geometry and stress distribution [51]. In summary, the tension-based hypothesis explains a major factor of the mechanisms behind cortical folding.

The *grey matter hypothesis* is founded on the role of the subventricular zone as a precursor domain of a new type of radial glia cells, that is, the intermediate radial glia cells (IRGCs). The subventricular zone of the fetal hemisphere (Fig. 11.4a) consists of an inner (isvz) and an outer (osvz) subventricular zone in human brains [54, 55]. The osvz contains neural stem and intermediate progenitor cells, becomes the predominant proliferative zone in the developing human brain, and expands considerably between

gestational weeks 11–16 in humans [56], just before the beginning of cortical folding. Additionally, a self-amplifying progenitor cell has recently been found in the osvz. This IRGC generates a radially oriented scaffold, in addition to that formed by the classical bipolar radial glia cells (Fig. 11.4b). This way, the osvz can modify the trajectory of migrating proneurons. An experimentally induced reduction of proliferation in the osvz causes a reduced cortical surface area and reduced folding [55]. Thus, proliferation of IRGCs could play an important role in the folding process of the fetal cortex [48, 55, 57] (for a recent review, see [58]).

The subplate zone (SP) reaches its largest extension in the region of the late-maturing and folding association cortices. During fetal development, transient cortico-cortical and callosal connections are found in the SP zone, before they enter the cortical plate [59]. The long, enduring growth of the SP zone and the entire brain (Fig. 11.7a), the regional heterochronicity of cortical folding [45], and particularly the early connections in the SP zone may contribute to mechanical tensions, resulting in the late-appearing, numerous gyri in multimodal association regions. The differential growth of cortical layers may also contribute to cortical folding [60]. Since the growth of the supragranular layers exceeds that of the infragranular layers, folding could be a result of this differential growth process, but the regionally different proportions between supra- and infragranular layers have not been comprehensively studied and precisely related to regions of high or low cortical folding. Finally, previous reports do not support a simple relationship between gyrification and the total number of cortical neurons or the cortical volume. Instead, a recent study demonstrates a universal scaling between cortical folding as a function of the product of the cortical surface area and the square root of cortical thickness in a large sample of mammalian gyrencephalic, as well as lissencephalic, brains [61].

## REFERENCES

1. Ladher, R. and Schoenwolf, G.V. (2005). Making neural tube: neural induction and neurulation. In: Rao, M.S. and Jacobson, M. (eds.) *Developmental neurobiology*. Kluwer Academic/Plenum Publishers, New York, NY. pp. 1–20.
2. Wurst, W. and Bally-Cuif, L. (2001). Neural plate patterning: upstream and downstream of the isthmic organizer. *Nature Reviews Neuroscience*, 2, 99–108.
3. Wurst, W., Auerbach, A.B., and Joyner, A.L. (1994). Multiple developmental defects in *Engrailed-1* mutant mice: an early mid-hindbrain deletion and patterning defects in forelimbs and sternum. *Development*, 120, 2065–75.
4. Kawahara, A., Chien, C.B., and Dawid, I.B. (2002). The homeobox gene *mbx* is involved in eye and tectum development. *Developmental Biology*, 248, 107–17.
5. Lumsden, A. and Krumlauf, R. (1996). Patterning the vertebrate neuraxis. *Science*, 274, 1109–15.
6. Kostovic, I. (1990). Zentralnervensystem. In: Hinrichsen, K.V. (ed.) *Humanembryologie*. Springer-Verlag, Berlin. pp. 381–448.
7. Meyer, G. (2007). Genetic control of neuronal migrations in human cortical development. *Advances in Anatomy, Embryology, and Cell Biology*, 189, 1–111.
8. Levitt, P. and Rakic, P. (1980). Immunoperoxidase localization of glial fibrillary acidic protein in radial glial cells and astrocytes of the developing rhesus monkey brain. *Journal of Comparative Neurology*, 193, 815–40.
9. Rakic, P. (1985). Limits of neurogenesis in primates. *Science*, 227, 1054–6.
10. Supèr, H., Soriano, E., and Uylings, H.B. (1998). The functions of the preplate in development and evolution of the neocortex and hippocampus. *Brain Research. Brain Research Reviews*, 27, 40–64.
11. Rakic, P. (1988). Specification of cerebral cortical areas. *Science*, 241, 170–6.
12. Rakic, P. (1995). Radial versus tangential migration of neuronal clones in the developing cerebral cortex. *Proceedings of the National Academy of Sciences fo the United States of America*, 92, 11323–7.
13. Flames, N., Pla, R., Gelman, D.M., Rubenstein, J.L., Puelles, L., and Marin, O. (2007). Delineation of multiple subpallial progenitor domains by the combinatorial expression of transcriptional codes. *Journal of Neuroscience*, 27, 9682–95.
14. Wonders, C.P., Taylor, L., Welagen, J., Mbata, I.C., Xiang, J.Z., and Anderson, S.A. (2008). A spatial bias for the origins of interneuron subgroups within the medial ganglionic eminence. *Developmental Biology*, 314, 127–36.
15. Wonders, C.P. and Anderson, S.A. (2006). The origin and specification of cortical interneurons. *Nature Reviews Neuroscience*, 7, 687–96.
16. Gelman, D.M. and Marin, O. (2010). Generation of interneuron diversity in the mouse cerebral cortex. *European Journal of Neuroscience*, 31, 2136–41.
17. Miyoshi, G., Hjerling-Leffler, J., Karayannis, T., *et al.* (2010). Genetic fate mapping reveals that the caudal ganglionic eminence produces a large and diverse population of superficial cortical interneurons. *Journal of Neuroscience*, 30, 1582–94.
18. Lee, S., Hjerling-Leffler, J., Zagha, E., Fishell, G., and Rudy, B. (2010). The largest group of superficial neocortical GABAergic interneurons expresses ionotropic serotonin receptors. *Journal of Neuroscience*, 30, 16796–808.
19. Ma, T., Wang, C., Wang, L., *et al.* (2013). Subcortical origins of human and monkey neocortical interneurons. *Nature Neuroscience*, 16, 1588–97.
20. Gelman, D., Griveau, A., Dehorter, N., *et al.* (2011). A wide diversity of cortical GABAergic interneurons derives from the embryonic preoptic area. *Journal of Neuroscience*, 31, 16570–80.
21. Tekki-Kessaris, N., Woodruff, R., Hall, A.C., *et al.* (2001). Hedgehog-dependent oligodendrocyte lineage specification in the telencephalon. *Development*, 128, 2545–54.
22. Paredes, J.A., James, D., Gil-Perotin, S., *et al.* (2016). Extensive migration of young neurons into the infant human frontal lobe. *Science*, 354, pii: aaf7073.
23. Bupesh, M., Legaz, I., Abellan, A., and Medina, L. (2011). Multiple telencephalic and extratelencephalic embryonic domains contribute neurons to the medial extended amygdala. *Journal of Comparative Neurology*, 519, 1505–25.
24. Yun, K., Garel, S., Fischman, S., and Rubenstein, J.L. (2003). Patterning of the lateral ganglionic eminence by the *Gsh1* and *Gsh2* homeobox genes regulates striatal and olfactory bulb histogenesis and the growth of axons through the basal ganglia. *Journal of Comparative Neurology*, 461, 151–65.
25. Marin, O., Anderson, S.A., and Rubenstein, J.L. (2000). Origin and molecular specification of striatal interneurons. *Journal of Neuroscience*, 20, 6063–76.
26. Pauly, M.C., Döbrössy, M.D., Nikkhah, G., Winkler, C., and Piroth, T. (2014). Organization of the human fetal subpallium. *Frontiers in Neuroanatomy*, 7, 54.
27. Garcia-Lopez, M., Abellan, A., Legaz, I., Rubenstein, J.L., Puelles, L., and Medina, L. (2008). Histogenetic compartments of the mouse centromedial and extended amygdala based on gene expression patterns during development. *Journal of Comparative Neurology*, 506, 46–74.
28. Morales-Delgado, N., Merchan, P., Bardet, S.M., Ferran, J.L., Puelles, L., and Diaz, C. (2011). Topography of *somatostatin* gene expression relative to molecular progenitor domains during ontogeny of the mouse hypothalamus. *Frontiers in Neuroanatomy*, 5, 10.
29. Medina, L., Abellan, A., Vicario, A., and Desfilis, E. (2014). Evolutionary and developmental contributions for understanding the organization of the basal ganglia. *Brain, Behavior and Evolution*, 83, 112–25.
30. Brodmann, K. (1909). *Vergleichende Lokalisationslehre der Großhirnrinde in ihren Prinzipien dargestellt auf Grund des Zellbaues*. Barth, Leipzig.
31. Barbas, H. and Garcia-Cabezas, M.A. (2015). Motor cortex layer 4: less is more. *Trends in Neuroscience*, 38, 259–61.
32. Garcia-Cabezas, M.A. and Barbas, H. (2014). Area 4 has layer IV in adult primates. *European Journal of Neuroscience*, 39, 1824–34.

33. Yakolev, P.I. and Lecours, A.R. (1967). The myelogenetic cycles of regional maturation of the brain. In: Minkowski, A. (ed.) *Regional development of the brain in early life*. Blackwell Science, Oxford. pp. 3–70.

34. Miller, D.J., Duka, T., Stimpson, C.D., *et al.* (2012). Prolonged myelination in human neocortical evolution. *Proceedings of the National Academy of Sciences of the United States*, 109, 16480–5.

35. Huttenlocher, P.R. (1979). Synaptic density in human frontal cortex—developmental changes and effects of aging. *Brain Research*, 163, 195–205.

36. Huttenlocher, P.R. (1990). Morphometric study of human cerebral cortex development. *Neuropsychologia*, 28, 517–27.

37. Schafer, D.P., Lehrman, E.K., Kautzman, A.G., *et al.* (2012). Microglia sculpt postnatal neural circuits in an activity and complement-dependent manner. *Neuron*, 74, 691–705.

38. Bialas, A.R. and Stevens, B. (2013). TGF-b signaling regulates neuronal C1q expression and developmental synaptic refinement. *Nature Neuroscience*, 16, 1773–82.

39. Fourgeaud, L. and Boulanger, L.M. (2007). Synapse remodeling, compliments of the complement system. *Cell*, 131, 1034–6.

40. Hong, S., Beja-Glasser, V.F., Nfonoyim, B.M., *et al.* (2016). Complement and microglia mediate early synapse loss in Alzheimer mouse models. *Science*, 352, 712–16.

41. Glantz, L.A. and Lewis, D.A. (2000). Decreased dendritic spine density on prefrontal cortical pyramidal neurons in schizophrenia. *Archives of General Psychiatry*, 57, 65–73.

42. Garey, L.J., Ong, W.Y., Patel, T.S., *et al.* (1998). Reduced dendritic spine density on cerebral cortical pyramidal neurons in schizophrenia. *Journal of Neurology, Neurosurgery, and Psychiatry*, 65, 446–53.

43. Sekar, A., Bialas, A.R., de, R.H., *et al.* (2016). Schizophrenia risk from complex variation of complement component 4. *Nature*, 530, 177–83.

44. Zilles, K., Armstrong, E., Schleicher, A., and Kretschmann, H.-J. (1988). The human pattern of gyrification in the cerebral cortex. *Anatomy and Embryology*, 179, 173–9.

45. Armstrong, E., Schleicher, A., Omram, H., Curtis, M., and Zilles, K. (1995). The ontogeny of human gyrification. *Cerebral Cortex*, 5, 56–63.

46. Jockwitz, C., Caspers, S., Lux, S., *et al.* (2017). Age- and function-related regional changes in cortical folding of the default mode network in older adults. *Brain Structure Function*, 222, 83–99.

47. van Essen, D.C. (1997). A tension-based theory of morphogenesis and compact wiring in the central nervous system. *Nature*, 385, 313–18.

48. Kriegstein, A., Noctor, S., Martinez-Cerdeno, V. (2006). Patterns of neural stem and progenitor cell division may underlie evolutionary cortical expansion. *Nature Reviews Neuroscience*. 7, 883–90.

49. Dennerll, T.J., Lamoureux, P., Buxbaum, R.E., and Heidemann, S.R. (1989). The cytomechanics of axonal elongation and retraction. *Journal of Cell Biology*, 109(6 Pt 1), 3073–83.

50. van Essen, D.C. (2007). Cerebral cortical folding patterns in primates: why they vary and what they signify. In: Kaas, J.H. (ed.) *Evolution of nervous systems*. Elsevier, Amsterdam. pp. 267–76.

51. Xu, G., Knutsen, A.K., Dikranian, K., Kroenke, C.D., Bayly, P.V., and Taber, L.A. (2010). Axons pull on the brain, but tension does not drive cortical folding. *Journal of Biomechanical Engineering*, 132, 071013.

52. Hilgetag, C.C. and Barbas, H. (2006). Role of mechanical factors in the morphology of the primate cerebral cortex. *PLoS Computational Biology*, 2, e22.

53. Toro, R., Perron, M., Pike, B., *et al.* (2008). Brain size and folding of the human cerebral cortex. *Cerebral Cortex*, 18, 2352–7.

54. Fietz, S.A., Kelava, I., Vogt, J., *et al.* (2010). OSVZ progenitors of human and ferret neocortex are epithelial-like and expand by integrin signaling. *Nature Neuroscience*, 13, 690–9.

55. Reillo, I., de Juan, R.C., Garcia-Cabezas, M.A., Borrell, V. (2011). A role for intermediate radial glia in the tangential expansion of the mammalian cerebral cortex. *Cerebral Cortex*, 21, 1674–94.

56. Lui, J.H., Hansen, D.V., and Kriegstein, A.R. (2011). Development and evolution of the human neocortex. *Cell*, 146, 18–36.

57. Molnár, Z. and Clowry, G. (2012). Cerebral cortical development in rodents and primates. *Progress in Brain Research*, 195, 45–70.

58. Zilles, K., Palomero-Gallagher, N., and Amunts, K. (2013). Development of cortical folding during evolution and ontogeny. *Trends in Neuroscience*, 36, 275–84.

59. Kostovic, I. and Judas, M. (2010). The development of the subplate and thalamocortical connections in the human foetal brain. *Acta Paediatrica*, 99, 1119–27.

60. Richman, D.P., Stewart, R.M., Hutchinson, J.W., and Caviness, V. (1975). Mechanical model of brain convolutional development. *Science*, 189, 18–21.

61. Mota, B. and Herculano-Houzel, S. (2015). Cortical folding scales universally with surface area and thickness, not number of neurons. *Science*, 349, 74–7.

62. Hansen, D.V., Lui, J.H., Parker, P.R., and Kriegstein, A.R. (2010). Neurogenic radial glia in the outer subventricular zone of human neocortex. *Nature*, 464, 554–61.

63. Rakic, P. (2009). Evolution of the neocortex: a perspective from developmental biology. *Nature Reviews Neuroscience*, 10, 724–35.

64. Nieuwenhuys, R. and Puelles, L. (2016). *Towards a new neural morphology*. Springer, Cham.

# 12

# Neuroimaging technologies

*Mark Woolrich, Mark Jenkinson, and Clare Mackay*

## Introduction

Brain imaging provides a window into the living brain and is an increasingly essential tool for experimental medicine in psychiatry. The inaccessibility of central nervous system tissues to biopsy and the need to study the 'system', and not just the cell, make advanced brain imaging central to uncovering the pathophysiology, discovering and evaluating new targets, developing and testing the efficacy of drugs, and developing biomarkers for diagnosis, patient stratification, and therapeutic monitoring. Here, we introduce the three technical domains by which we can assay brain structure and function: magnetic resonance imaging (MRI), molecular imaging (positron emission tomography (PET), and single-photon emission computed tomography (SPECT); electrophysiology [electroencephalography (EEG)]; and magnetoencephalograpy (MEG). Each of the imaging modalities has its own strengths and limitations, and the modalities should be regarded as complementary, rather than competing. Typically, the signal that is detected is an average of tens of thousands of cells. Nevertheless, imaging techniques are sensitive to everything, from molecular concentrations up to whole system dynamics, making the essential link between the cell and the system. Table 12.1 gives an overview of the sensitivity of each imaging modality to aspects of neurophysiology.

## Magnetic resonance imaging

One of the most widely used and flexible tools for neuroimaging studies is MRI. This imaging method is non-invasive, causes no tissue damage, and can provide high-quality images of brain anatomy, with excellent soft tissue contrast (structural MRI), or for measuring properties of axonal architecture in the white matter (diffusion MRI), or for detecting neuronal activity (functional MRI). Spatial resolution for MRI is in the order of a millimetre, and MRI scanners are readily available in both clinical and research settings.

### Principles of MRI

MRI is based on magnetic interactions with specific nuclei, using the principle of nuclear magnetic resonance (NMR). Although NMR relies on properties of the nuclei within the atoms, it interacts in a way that does not harm tissue.

Two types of magnetic fields are important in MRI: (1) strong static $B_0$ field; and (2) radiofrequency (RF) fields. The $B_0$ field is created by the large, superconducting coil that defines the strength of the scanner; for instance, a 3T scanner has a $B_0$ field of 3 tesla (T). Both 1.5T and 3T scanners are common in clinical environments, while 3T and 7T scanners are more common for research. Higher-field scanners are advantageous, as they can reduce noise and improve spatial resolution.

RF fields are used to manipulate the magnetization of molecules in the brain. The magnetization can then be detected and measured by the MRI scanner to produce images. For most neuroimaging MRI applications, the RF is tuned to manipulate hydrogen nuclei in water molecules because of their high abundance in all biological tissues. Structural, functional, and diffusion MRI work by manipulating the magnetization in different ways to make it sensitive to particular microscopic properties of water and its environment.

### Overview of acquisition and analysis

MRI acquisitions can be optimized for studies by varying options, for example, the type (modality) of image (for example, functional, diffusion, etc.) and various parameters (for example, echo time). However, some noise and artefacts are common in MRI, caused by scanner imperfections or the physics/physiology of subjects such as head motion. Most MRI artefacts are rare, but some are common (for example, head motion, bias field), and analysis strategies are needed to reduce their effects.

Almost all neuroimaging research studies involve groups of subjects, to infer results about the wider population, accounting for between-subject variation. Statistical analysis is usually conducted separately on each voxel (three-dimensional pixel), with corrections needed for the multiple statistical tests this requires, and results are generated in the form of statistical maps that are displayed as coloured overlays on brain images. These analyses require that all subjects are spatially aligned (registered) together, for anatomical consistency.

### Structural MRI

The most common MRI modality is structural imaging, which is routinely used in both clinical practice and research studies. It provides images of brain anatomy, with excellent soft tissue contrast,

**Table 12.1** The sensitivity of various imaging modalities in aspects of neurophysiology

| Scale | Imaging modality | Examples |
| --- | --- | --- |
| Neurotransmitters | PET, MRS | Radiotracers can probe dopamine and serotonin systems, including labels for synthesis capacity, receptors, and transporters. The glutamate system also has PET ligands. Both GABA and glutamate can be indirectly assayed with high-field MRS |
| Protein aggregates | PET | In ageing and dementia, tracers for amyloid plaques are now commercially available and novel tracers are in development for tau and alpha-synuclein |
| Action potentials | MEG/EEG | Synaptic potentials in the brain give rise to measurable changes in electrical and magnetic fields that are measurable outside the surface of the head |
| Metabolism | PET, MRI | PET radiotracers provide relatively direct measurement of blood flow, blood volume, and oxygen/glucose metabolism. MRI techniques, such as arterial spin labelling, can produce similar measures non-invasively |
| Individual brain structures | MRI | Structural MRI typically has a resolution of 1 mm³ and good tissue contrast for examining individual brain structures |
| Tissue integrity | MRI | MRI provides contrast mechanisms to explore tissue integrity, including relaxometry and susceptibility mapping |
| White matter connectivity | MRI | Diffusion-weighted or diffusion tensor imaging provides indirect estimates of white matter pathways |
| Regional brain function | MRI, PET, M/EEG | PET has largely been replaced by fMRI for studying brain function. fMRI provides good spatial detail, but at low temporal resolution (seconds). This is complemented well by the high temporal resolution (milliseconds) of M/EEG |
| Brain networks | MRI, M/EEG | Brain connectomics is a new and growing field, enabling the use of neuroimaging data to model brain network dynamics |

typical spatial resolution of 1 mm, and typical acquisition times of 3–15 minutes. In clinical practice, radiologists examine these images for signs of pathology for disease diagnosis. In neuroimaging research, images are either analysed directly to extract quantitative measures from them (for example, hippocampal volume) or used as part of other analysis pipelines (for example, for alignment in functional studies).

### Measurement principles

Most structural images are based on three basic properties: proton density (PD), and $T_1$ and $T_2$ relaxation times. Each of these influences the signal that is received from the hydrogen nuclei in water molecules. Proton density is effectively the density of water in tissues, and the received signal is proportional to this, although this alone creates weak tissue contrast for grey and white matter.

The relaxation times $T_1$ and $T_2$ are related to different processes that affect magnetization within water molecules. Many factors affect $T_1$ and $T_2$ relaxation times such as molecular tumbling, chemical environment, geometry of nearby cells/structures, etc. Hence

relaxation times are a complicated function of tissue properties but depend on tissue composition (for example, proportion of neuronal bodies vs axons). These differences in relaxation time provide superior tissue contrast for grey and white matter.

### Acquisitions

Many types of structural MRI acquisition exist, with PD, $T_1$-weighted, $T_2$-weighted, and fluid-attenuated inversion recovery (FLAIR) being the most common (Fig. 12.1). This variety is possible because of the detailed timings of fields applied by the scanner, specified by an MRI pulse sequence. These settings enable the influence of the $T_1$ and $T_2$ relaxation processes on the intensity to be separately adjusted.

For example, for a PD image, the sequence is set such that $T_1$ and $T_2$ relaxation times have minimal effect and the primary contrast (intensity difference between tissues) is driven by the PD. For a $T_1$-weighted image (which is the most commonly acquired structural MRI scan), the sequence is set to enhance the effect of $T_1$ relaxation, while minimizing the effect of $T_2$ relaxation, although

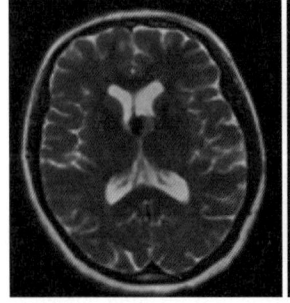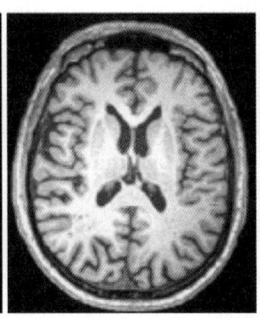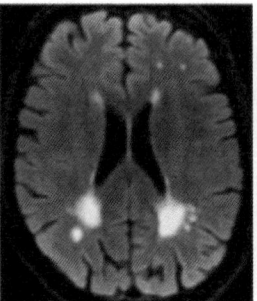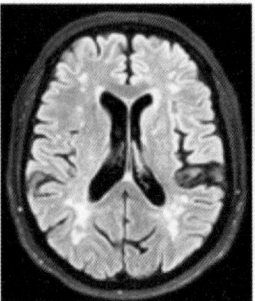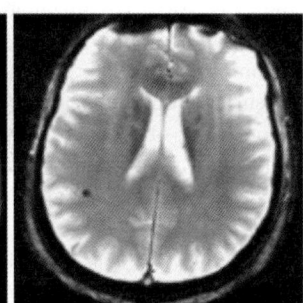

**Fig. 12.1** Examples of the variety of structural images that can be acquired with MRI. From left: $T_1$-weighted, $T_2$-weighted, fluid-attenuated inversion recovery (FLAIR), FLAIR again, susceptibility-weighted gradient echo (SWI). Different types are sensitive to different tissue characteristics, particularly pathological lesions and tissues, and so it is common to get a range of structural images for each subject.

PD weighting remains. Another commonly acquired structural image is FLAIR, which attenuates signal from the cerebrospinal fluid (CSF), to reduce CSF contamination and highlight pathological lesions.

## Limitations and artefacts

Noise is common across all MRI modalities, and this constrains the accuracy of quantitative results and limits statistical power. Consequently, research studies typically require groups of 20 subjects or more.

Another common limitation is the partial volume effect (PVE) due to the finite spatial resolution in MRI—typically between 0.5 and 1mm for structural images. At this scale, a voxel often contains several tissues (for example, in the cortical folds, voxels often contain grey matter and some CSF or white matter). The voxel intensity is then a mixture of tissue intensities, weighted according to the proportion of the voxel volume they occupy. This results in the borders of structures appearing blurry, limiting the precision of boundary localization and volume calculations.

Magnetic resonance intensity values are arbitrarily scaled, and not quantitative. Thus, image analysis techniques are necessary to estimate quantitative information, for example, the volume of grey matter.

It is essential to check for artefacts in MRI studies and keep in mind existing artefacts when interpreting results. One common artefact is bias field, caused by inhomogeneities in the RF fields, and results in large areas of the image being artificially brighter or darker than they should be. This artefact, unless extremely strong, is compensated for very well by analysis methods.

## Analysis

Several different types of analysis are done with structural MRI, some specific for studying anatomical changes and some useful for other experiments such as diffusion MRI, functional MRI, or other modalities like PET, MEG, and EEG.

Registration is a fundamental analysis tool and involves aligning one image with another (for example, two images of the same subject or different subjects). Although modern registration methods work well generally, they cannot overcome some fundamental biological ambiguities such as aligning disparate folding patterns (for example, single vs double gyri, as is common in the cingulate).

Segmentation is another fundamental analysis tool, which involves determining the location of anatomical tissues or structures in the image. The two main types of segmentation are tissue-type segmentation and structural segmentation. Tissue-type segmentation aims to determine where the main 'tissues' (grey matter, white matter, and CSF) are in the image. The result of tissue-type segmentation is typically an image (or a map) where each voxel is assigned a tissue label.

Structural segmentation can identify specific anatomical structures (for example, hippocampus) or the grey matter cortex. Cortical segmentation, or modelling, usually outputs a surface, rather than a voxel-based, image, as this more accurately captures cortical folding and provides clearer ways of displaying the anatomy (Fig. 12.2). Notably, surface-based analysis of functional data is a powerful and growing alternative to voxel-based methods.

Anatomical analysis usually measures differences in structural shape or volume. Cortical thickness is one quantitative measure, and analysing thickness differences is done between groups or with

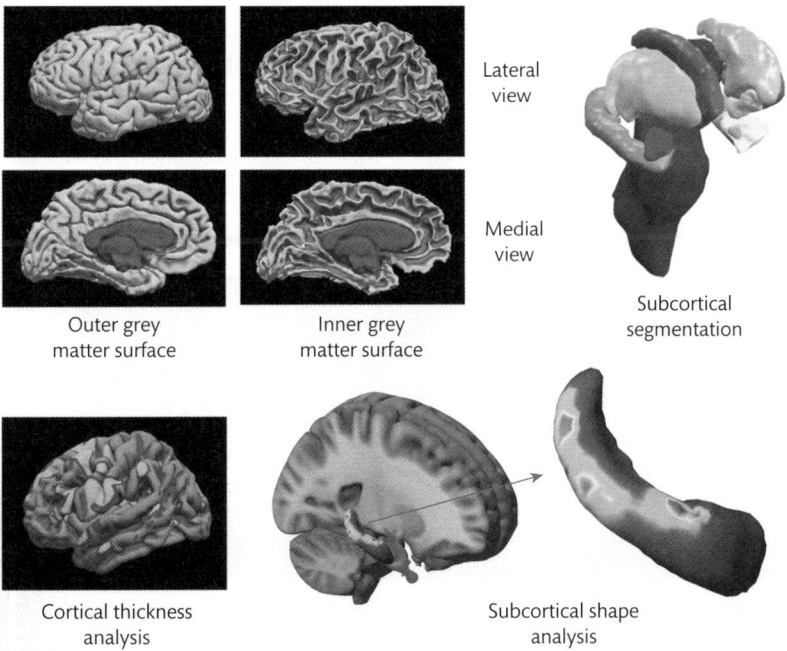

**Fig. 12.2** (see Colour Plate section) Examples of structural segmentation and analysis. Top left shows cortical segmentation (left hemisphere) where the inner and outer surfaces of the cortical grey matter are modelled, and from this, the cortical thickness can be calculated and analysed to show areas of differing thickness between groups (bottom left). Top right shows a set of subcortical structures (for example, caudate, hippocampus, brainstem, etc.), and bottom right shows an example of a shape analysis (hippocampus) displaying localized areas of difference in the shape between a patient and control group.

Adapted from Jenkinson M, Chappell M, *Introduction to Neuroimaging Analysis*, Copyright (2017), with permission from Oxford University Press.

respect to a covariate of interest (for example, disability score). Such analyses use statistical methods to produce a map of significant results—normally displayed as a colour overlay (Fig. 12.2).

Deep grey matter structure segmentations are typically summarized by volume measures or shape characteristics. In shape analysis, each localized region of the boundary is examined to find changes in position that relate to group differences or covariates of interest. This results in a map of significant results at the boundary of the structure (Fig. 12.2).

Whole brain voxel-wise analysis can be used to find anatomical differences at any location, for example, voxel-based morphometry (VBM) [1]. This combines tissue-type segmentation and registration to quantify the amount of 'local' grey matter volume for voxelwise analysis (Fig. 12.3).

### Diffusion MRI

White matter appears fairly uniform in structural MR images, whereas diffusion MRI provides richer information about microstructure and anatomical connectivity.

#### Measurement principles

Axonal fibre bundles restrict how water molecules can diffuse, and this forms the basis of diffusion MRI. Both intracellular and extracellular water in a fibre bundle is less likely to encounter barriers when moving along the direction of the axons, as opposed to moving in other directions. Thus, maximum diffusion occurs along the direction of the axons.

To obtain a measurable signal, it is necessary for a large number of water molecules to behave in the same way, as a voxel is much bigger than an axon diameter. Therefore, only sizeable fibre bundles produce detectable signals. The amount of diffusion, in all directions, is also affected by axon diameter, packing density, and myelination, and diffusion MRI is a sensitive marker of changes in these microstructural properties.

#### Acquisition

Diffusion MRI uses special *diffusion-encoding gradients* (magnetic fields that change in strength along a particular direction) in order to measure the diffusion of water molecules. These gradients lead to a reduction in the signal from water that is diffusing in this encoding direction, and the amount of intensity reduction depends on the amount of diffusion.

A single diffusion magnetic resonance image only provides information about diffusion in one direction. Therefore, many images, with many different encoding directions, are required to build up a full picture of the diffusion. Acquiring many images in a short time requires fast imaging sequences such as *echo planar imaging (EPI)*. Using EPI acquisitions and other accelerations, such as parallel imaging methods [for example, sensitivity encoding (SENSE) or generalized autocalibrating partial parallel acquisition (GRAPPA)] and/or simultaneous multi-slice methods, enables whole brain images to be acquired in a few seconds or less. In neuroimaging research, the number of encoding directions acquired can be up to 200, with acquisition times of around 5–15 minutes. Having a large number of encoding directions is required for tracing anatomical connections; however, this is not often used in clinical practice where a small number of directions (for example, 3–5) is often used for very short acquisitions.

#### Limitations and artefacts

Fast imaging sequences and diffusion encoding come with some drawbacks: lower spatial resolution (around 2–3 mm) and increased artefacts. Diffusion MRI artefacts include eddy current distortions and $B_0$ inhomogeneity distortions and motion, on top of artefacts that also occur in structural MRI. Many artefacts induce geometric distortions that require specialized pre-processing correction tools.

#### Analysis

Pre-processing steps are applied to correct for geometric distortions, though correcting for $B_0$ inhomogeneities requires separate scans (field maps or blip-up–blip-down pairs) to be acquired. After pre-processing, models of the diffusion process are fit to the intensities, to extract information about the physical diffusion of water molecules. One common model is the tensor model (as in *diffusion tensor imaging* or *DTI*), which assumes that the diffusion in different

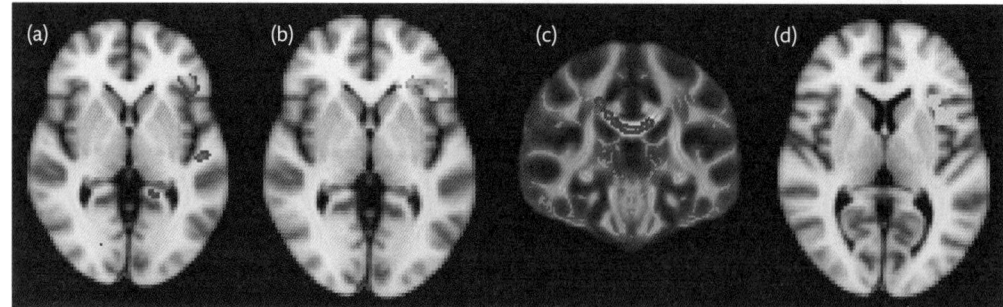

**Fig. 12.3** (see Colour Plate section) Example of standard analysis techniques in patients with schizophrenia (a–c) and carriers of the VAL and MET alleles of the *COMT* gene (d). (a) VBM analysis with areas of significant grey matter reduction in schizophrenia relative to controls shown in red-yellow. (b) fMRI using a letter fluency task showing significant areas of reduced activity in schizophrenia, relative to controls. (c) Diffusion MRI-based TBSS (tract-based spatial statistics) analysis of the same patients with schizophrenia, relative to controls, showing reduced fractional anisotropy in the corpus callosum and forceps major. (d) Resting fMRI analysis of healthy VAL and MET allele homozygotes of the *COMT* gene, showing greater functional connectivity in VAL carriers, relative to METs.

directions can be modelled using a spatial Gaussian probability, often visualized by an ellipsoid. Each voxel is fit separately, resulting in a set of tensor parameters per voxel, that is, a separate map/image of each parameter is obtained. However, this model is not very accurate for voxels containing two or more fibre bundles running in different directions (for example, crossing fibres).

From the tensor parameters, several key values are calculated such as mean diffusivity (MD) (average diffusion in all directions) and fractional anisotropy (FA), a measure of how diffusion varies with direction. The MD can be broken down into axial diffusivity (AD) and radial diffusivity (RD), which quantify the diffusion along the direction of the fibre bundle (AD) and perpendicular to it (RD). All of these quantities are surrogates of biological properties such as axon size, density, and myelination, but independent of direction. Changes in these quantities can help support or refute hypotheses relating to underlying biological changes, but they need to be interpreted carefully.

Analysing changes in DTI measures requires spatial alignment, but structural images are featureless within white matter, and therefore, registrations are based on diffusion information (for example, using original diffusion or FA images). A widely used method for such analyses is tract-based spatial statistics (TBSS), which aligns the centre of major white matter tracts, providing results only in tract centres (the skeleton) where alignment is the most reliable (Fig. 12.3) [2].

Tractography is an alternative analysis tool that traces out the pathways of the major axonal fibre bundles. Pre-processing is the same, but other models are sometimes used that can provide more precise estimates of the direction of the fibre bundle(s) and explicitly account for multiple fibres within a voxel. Information about the direction of fibre bundles is then used to trace out pathways; starting at a seed point and then moving, in small steps, along the locally estimated direction of fibre bundles, allowing entire pathways to be mapped out (Fig. 12.4).

Two main varieties of tractography algorithm exist: deterministic and probabilistic. Deterministic tractography uses a single estimate of direction (for each fibre) at each step. By using multiple seed points, a set of individual pathways, or streamlines, can be constructed, which are often displayed as an entire fibre tract. In probabilistic tractography, a probability distribution of directions is estimated at each voxel (for each fibre), in order to take into account noise and uncertainty.

Tractography outputs can be used to estimate anatomical connectivity matrices (the connectivity between a set of grey matter areas) or to map out the spatial location of tracts (used in presurgical planning) or as a way of parcellating other structures. The latter case—connectivity-based segmentation—is able to parcellate areas of the brain on the basis of where they are most 'strongly' connected, for example, segmenting thalamic nuclei based on connections to the cortex.

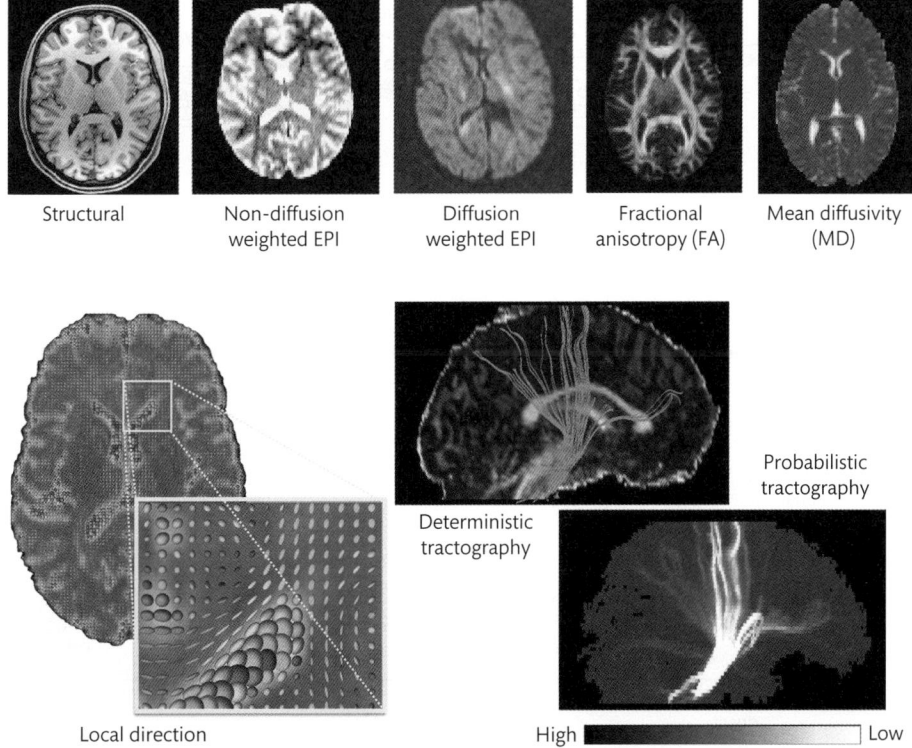

Structural | Non-diffusion weighted EPI | Diffusion weighted EPI | Fractional anisotropy (FA) | Mean diffusivity (MD)

Local direction | Deterministic tractography | Probabilistic tractography | High — Low

**Fig. 12.4** (see Colour Plate section) Examples of diffusion MRI and analysis results. Top row shows a structural image (left) for comparison, along with a non-diffusion-weighted image and a single diffusion-weighted image. Many of these EPI-based images need to be acquired in a diffusion MRI study. The two images on the right of the top row show DTI-based measures calculated from the diffusion-weighted acquisitions, which are often used as surrogate measures of white matter microstructure. The bottom row shows an example of estimated white matter tract directions on the left (colour coding based on direction: red = left–right, green = anterior–posterior, blue = inferior–superior), and the tractography results based on these (right) using either deterministic or probabilistic methods for tracing major fibre pathways.

Adapted from Jenkinson M, Chappell M, *Introduction to Neuroimaging Analysis*, Copyright (2017), with permission from Oxford University Press.

## Functional MRI

Functional MRI (or fMRI) is sensitive to neuronal activity and has two main modes of use: task and resting state. In task fMRI, the participant performs a task in the scanner (for example, sensory, motor, cognitive), in order to determine the location and strength of brain activity related to the task. In resting state fMRI, no task is performed and the objective is to measure intrinsic characteristics of spontaneous brain activity such as functional connectivity between brain regions.

### Measurement principles

fMRI measures neuronal activity indirectly via the BOLD (blood–oxygen level-dependent) effect, based on how activity changes the local concentration of deoxygenated haemoglobin. This is measurable because deoxygenated haemoglobin disturbs the magnetic field around it, reducing the signal from nearby water molecules. Notably, the haemodynamics lag considerably behind the electrical activity of neurons, with the signal peaking approximately 6 seconds after the electrical activity and taking approximately 20–30 seconds to return to the initial baseline level (Fig. 12.5).

### Acquisitions

Measuring neuronal activity indirectly through the slow haemodynamics means that acquiring an image every few seconds is sufficient. This is typically achieved using gradient-echo EPI magnetic resonance images, tuned to detect signal changes caused by local magnetic field disturbances (which changes $T_2^*$ relaxation). A typical fMRI acquisition will have a spatial resolution of 2–3 mm and a temporal resolution [also repetition time (TR), the time taken to acquire one image] of 1–3 seconds.

### Limitations and artefacts

The signal in fMRI is a surrogate haemodynamic measure of neuronal activity, and precise timings in neuronal activity cannot be measured, making causality measurements extremely difficult. Furthermore, changes in fMRI signal between experimental or clinical conditions can be confounded by changes in the vasculature.

The artefacts in fMRI and diffusion are similar because they both use EPI. However, fMRI uses gradient-echo EPI (spin-echo used in diffusion), which causes signal loss in the inferior frontal and temporal areas, due to the proximity of air-filled sinuses and air cells.

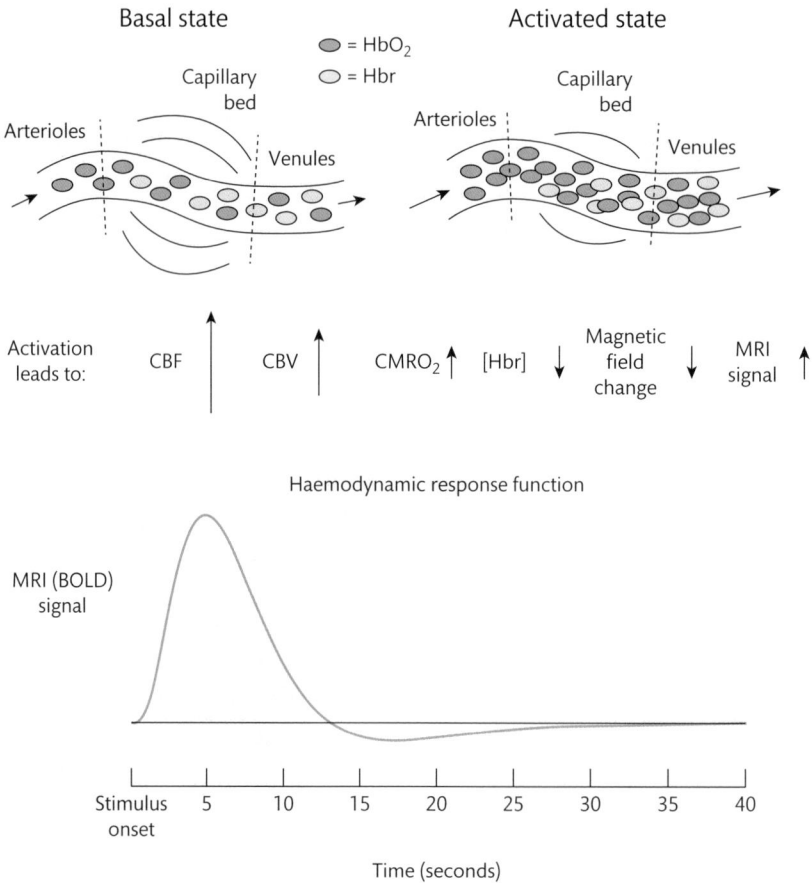

**Fig. 12.5** Illustration of the BOLD (blood oxygenation level-dependent) signal used in fMRI. The top panel shows blood in a capillary within neuronal tissue that is in the basal (left) or activated state (right). Activity of the neurons increases both the cerebral blood flow (CBF) and the cerebral blood volume (CBV) in the tissue more than the oxygen extraction (CMRO₂), resulting in a net decrease in the concentration of deoxygenated haemoglobin (Hbr). Decreased Hbr leads to a greater MRI signal, as it disturbs the local magnetic fields less. The bottom panel demonstrates the typical dynamics of this signal (the haemodynamic response function or HRF) in response to a very short stimulus at time zero.

Adapted from Jenkinson M, Chappell M, *Introduction to Neuroimaging Analysis,* Copyright (2017), with permission from Oxford University Press.

Head motion effects are also a major confound in fMRI, requiring the use of specialized analysis strategies.

### Analysis

Pipelines for fMRI analysis start with pre-processing steps for reducing artefacts or improving the signal-to-noise ratio (SNR). Many pipeline versions exist but share common elements, for example $B_0$ distortion correction, motion correction, slice-timing correction, spatial smoothing, and temporal filtering. Corrections for $B_0$ distortion and motion are broadly the same as for diffusion and still require an additional field map acquisition.

Slice-timing correction is needed in fMRI, since the images are acquired a slice at a time (or several slices at a time for multiband acquisitions), and timing of the analysis and acquisition must match. Spatial smoothing aims to improve the SNR but reduces the effective spatial resolution, and is sometimes avoided in high-quality data to maintain resolution. Temporal filtering removes signals that do not match the characteristics of neuronal signals such as very slow drifts caused by physical or physiological artefacts.

For task fMRI, a model is constructed that incorporates stimulus timings and the known haemodynamic properties to create a predicted response. These predicted responses to tasks are used in a multiple regression that is carried out separately in each voxel. The result is a spatial map showing brain areas that are significantly active (after correction for multiple statistical tests over many voxels) in response to particular tasks. The same framework can also be used to investigate how activation strength compares across differences in stimuli/tasks, groups, covariates, or experimental manipulations.

For resting state fMRI, the two common forms of analysis are: network matrix analysis and independent component analysis (ICA). In network matrix analysis, *functional connectivity*, defined as any measure of statistical dependency, is computed between all pairs of time series (brain activity over time) extracted from all brain regions of interest to build up a network matrix or graph. In fMRI, the most commonly used metric of functional connectivity is correlation. These matrices can then be analysed in various ways, including using graph theory. The analysis of network matrices is of great interest and an active neuroimaging research area.

In ICA, the data set is decomposed into a set of components (similar to principal component analysis), and each one contains a spatial map and time series (Fig. 12.6). Components may relate to neuronal signals, physiological noise, or artefacts. Each neuronally related component represents a set of brain regions that share, at least partially, a common time series. Importantly, certain components are reliably reproduced with recognizable spatial maps, often referred to (misleadingly) as 'networks' with specific names (for example, default mode network, dorsal attention network, etc.), and correspond well with the networks produced using a network matrix analysis approach.

Network analyses can also be used to ask how networks change with task. In general, analysis and interpretation of networks are a relatively new field, and much remains to be understood about functional connectivity. Nonetheless, many applications already exist, including the use of network features as disease biomarkers.

### Other MRI modalities

The three main MRI research modalities have been described in detail, but the versatility of MRI goes beyond these. For example,

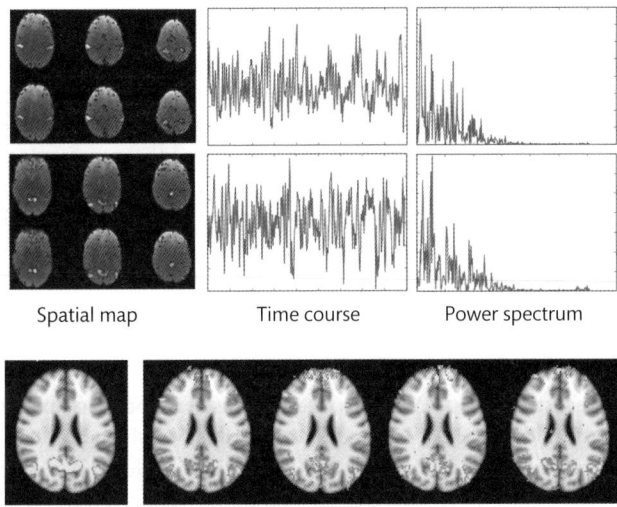

**Fig. 12.6** (see Colour Plate section) Illustration of resting state networks. Top panel shows ICA components corresponding to two networks (motor and default mode in the first and second rows, respectively). These have spatial maps (left) that show the brain areas involved in each network (red-yellow), and time courses (middle) of fMRI signal fluctuations that are common across all parts of that network. The power spectra of the time courses (right) show low frequency fluctuations, characteristic of slow neuronally induced haemodynamic changes. Bottom panel shows an example of the spatial map of a resting state network (default mode network) estimated from a group of subjects (left) and from individual subjects (right). Features from these intrinsic networks can be analysed for differences across clinical populations or experimental conditions.

Adapted from Jenkinson M, Chappell M, *Introduction to Neuroimaging Analysis*, Copyright (2017), with permission from Oxford University Press; Bijsterbosch J, Smith SM, Beckmann CF, *Introduction to Resting State fMRI Functional Connectivity*, Copyright (2017), with permission from Oxford University Press.

magnetization transfer (MT) can be used to detect white matter lesions; susceptibility-weighted imaging (SWI) is used to detect microbleeds or iron deposition; and arterial spin labelling (ASL) magnetically tags blood as an intrinsic contrast agent, providing quantitative measures of perfusion and cerebral blood flow and volume.

An MRI scanner can also be used to acquire information about molecular concentrations. Magnetic resonance spectroscopy (MRS) acquires signals from nuclei in molecules other than water, but their lower concentrations require reduced spatial resolution (several *centimetres*) to obtain sufficient signal, normally from one preselected region. Only signals from certain molecules can be separated by MRS [for example, GABA, *N*-acetyl aspartate (NAA)], which is a limitation, although higher-field scanners (for example, 7T) have greater specificity.

## Molecular imaging

The vast majority of MRI-based research is based on contrasts that can be gleaned from manipulating the proton. The number of molecules that can be probed by emission tomography is far greater, limited only by the creativity of radiochemists and the substantial resources required to develop new tracers.

## How does it work?

PET and SPECT both work on the same principle. A radiotracer is synthesized by adding a radioactive isotope to a molecule of interest. The tracer is injected into a participant who is then placed inside a PET or SPECT camera, and an image is formed that represents the rate of emission of positrons (PET) or gamma rays (SPECT) from a region of interest in the body. The number of PET isotopes is far greater than for SPECT, but SPECT technology is cheaper and more readily available (Fig. 12.7).

### Radioisotopes

The radioisotopes most commonly used for SPECT are iodine-123 and technetium. For PET, the commonly used isotopes are oxygen-15 ($^{15}$O), carbon-11 ($^{11}$C), and fluorine-18 ($^{18}$F), which are manufactured in a particle accelerator (cyclotron). To develop a tracer, the radioisotope must be inserted into the molecule of interest in a way that does not impact the biology of the molecule and in small enough quantities that it does not become pharmacologically active in its own right. In biological compounds, it is relatively easy to insert (or exchange) an oxygen or carbon atom. However, the isotopes for $^{15}$O and $^{11}$C have very short half-lives (2 minutes and 20 minutes, respectively), meaning that for $^{11}$C, the cyclotron must be proximal to the scanner, and for $^{15}$O, the isotope must be piped directly from the cyclotron to radiochemistry and into the participant who is already lying in the scanner, with no delay. With its longer half-life, $^{18}$F (half-life of 110 minutes) might be considered as the most convenient PET isotope, but the radiochemistry can be complex.

### Image acquisition and analysis

Compared with the complex physics involved in MRI acquisition, PET and SPECT image acquisition are relatively straightforward. PET and SPECT 'scanners' are gamma cameras, with detectors arranged in a ring around the object of interest. PET radioisotopes all have unstable nuclei that will emit protons that rapidly collide with an electron, causing an annihilation that generates two gamma rays (photons) with a separation angle of 180°. Two photons will be detected, and a 'line of response' used to localize the source of the annihilation (Fig. 12.7). Data are assimilated from tens of thousands of events, and an image of the relative distribution of the radiotracer in the sample is built up.

Analysis of SPECT images in clinical settings is either qualitative (radiologist's report) or semi-quantitative whereby a signal intensity is obtained from the region of interest and compared with a reference region where the signal is assumed to be unaffected by the experimental manipulation. PET data are amenable to more sophisticated analysis techniques. The unit of analysis is the 'binding potential', which is typically turned into a regional standard uptake value (SUVr) and can be mapped as either a static quantity obtained at a fixed time post-injection or a dynamic quantity with multiple image acquisitions showing both wash-in and washout of the tracer (Fig. 12.8).

PET can be fully quantitative if acquired with an arterial line *in situ*. The arterial input function, combined with metabolite measurement, can be used to produce a full arterial model. However, PET data do not contain any anatomical information, requiring the PET signal to be registered to, or acquired with, a structural scan. Modern PET cameras are usually combined with computed tomography (CT) scanners (PET/CT), and recently it has become possible to combine PET with MRI (PET-MR). PET-MR has advantages relating to the superior tissue contrast of magnetic resonance relative to CT, but there are also methodological hurdles to overcome. In particular, the signal from the annihilation event is attenuated by passing through the skull, and this can be relatively easily mapped using CT (which is, in essence, a 3-dimensional X-ray). MRI is insensitive to bone, so attenuation correction requires a more complex solution.

### Radiotracers

The main innovations in PET come from the development of robust radiotracers by creating a ligand from a radioisotope and a

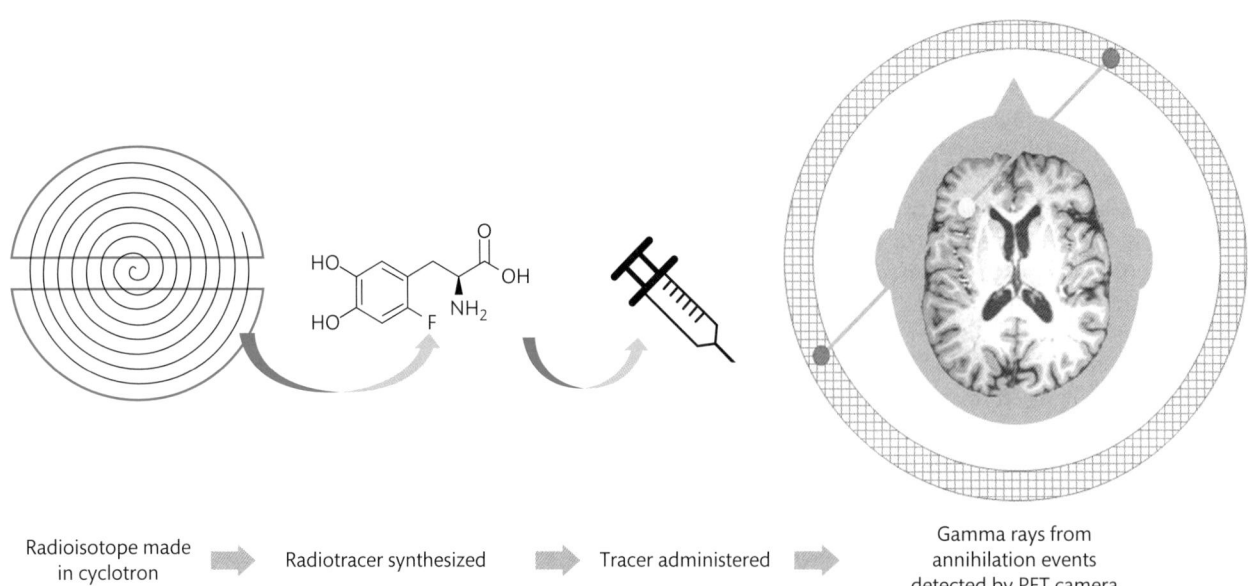

Radioisotope made in cyclotron ⟹ Radiotracer synthesized ⟹ Tracer administered ⟹ Gamma rays from annihilation events detected by PET camera

**Fig. 12.7** How PET imaging works (similar for SPECT). The radioisotope is manufactured in a cyclotron and rapidly combined with the molecule of interest to create the tracer, which is injected into the patient. The patient is then positioned inside the PET scanner (gamma camera), which accumulates the data required to create the image.

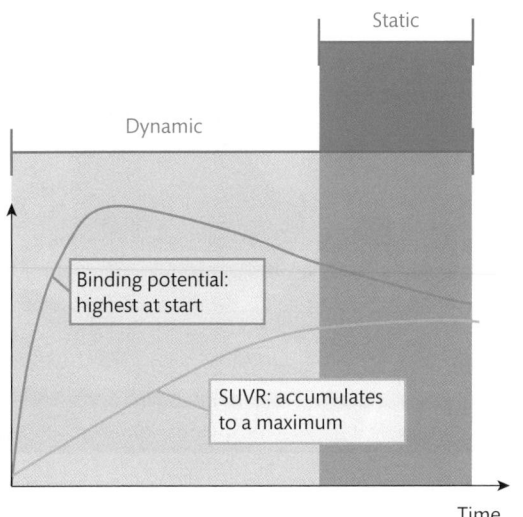

**Fig. 12.8** Signals obtained from semi-quantitative PET. Relative standard uptake units (SUVR) can be acquired from static data acquired at the optimal time post-injection (usually 40–90 minutes, depending on the tracer). Dynamic imaging requires long acquisition times but provides quantification of the pharmacokinetics of the tracer.

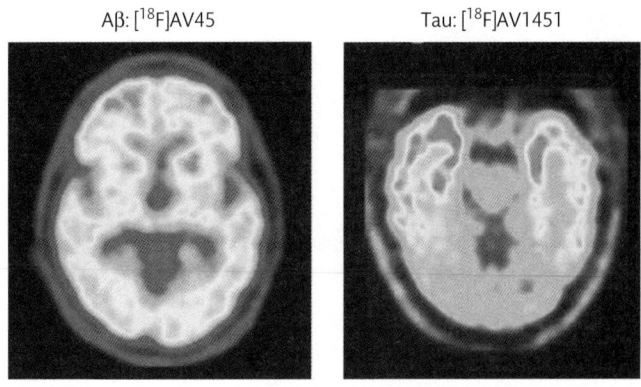

**Fig. 12.9** (see Colour Plate section) Examples of protein aggregate tracers for Alzheimer's disease.
Reproduced courtesy of Roger Gunn and Azadeh Firouzian.

molecule of interest. The most commonly used PET radiotracer is fluorodeoxyglucose (FDG), a glucose analogue, labelled with $^{18}$F, which is readily taken up by metabolically active cells. The resulting FDG-PET images represent regional glucose consumption (and thus metabolic activity), which is widely used in oncology because tumours are typically highly metabolically active. Both FDG and $H_2^{15}O$ have been used as indirect measures of cerebral blood flow changes induced by neuronal activity in cognitive tasks. However, with fMRI being non-invasive, cheaper, and logistically simpler to implement, task-related PET has largely been consigned to history. FDG continues to be a useful tracer for assessment of metabolism, with particular application in dementia and neurodegeneration.

### Neurotransmitter/receptor tracers

Tracers have also been developed for investigating neurotransmitter systems. Two good examples relevant to psychiatric research are the dopamine system in schizophrenia and the serotonin system in mood disorders. For dopamine, the best established PET tracers (for example, $^{11}$C-raclopride and $^{18}$F-fallypride) bind to D2 receptors and are sensitive to changes in the concentration of dopamine through competitive interaction. These tracers are important both for mechanistic studies (for example, reduced D2 receptors in schizophrenia [3]) and to investigate the pharmacokinetic effects of antipsychotic drugs (for example, receptor occupancy studies [4]). Tracers for the serotonin system include $^{11}$C-MDL-1009 for 5-HT2A receptors and $^{11}$C-DASB for the 5-HT transporter and are helping to elucidate mechanisms of response to antidepressants [5].

### Protein aggregate tracers

Pathological aggregated proteins are hallmarks of several neurodegenerative diseases, including Alzheimer's disease and dementia with Lewy bodies (DLB). By developing tracers sensitive to these aggregated proteins, it becomes possible to perform *in vivo* histology and vastly improve stratification for clinical trials [6].

Beta-amyloid plaques and tau tangles are the hallmarks of Alzheimer's disease (see Plate 6). PET with amyloid ligands is part of the leading edge in Alzheimer's disease research [7] and is fast becoming the 'standard' in clinical trials for disease modification. Hot on the heels of amyloid PET are the tau tracers, several of which are now in development [8]. Much international effort is also being spent on developing tracers for alpha-synuclein (the aggregated protein in Lewy bodies) and TDP-43 (hallmark of both fronto-temporal dementia and motor neuron disease) [6] (Fig. 12.9).

## Non-invasive electrophysiology: EEG and MEG

MEG and EEG provide direct measures of neuronal activity, by recording the magnetic or electric fields that propagate outside of the head at millisecond-temporal resolution. As with fMRI, there are two main modes of use—task-based and resting state, both providing a non-invasive window on the brain, at the kind of fast subsecond timescales associated with typical cognition.

### How it works

The different technologies used in MEG and EEG, and their relationship with the underlying electrophysiology, result in contrasting benefits between the two approaches (summarized in Table 12.1).

### EEG

In EEG, the electric currents emanating from brain activity are measured by electrodes in contact with the scalp surface, with arrays of up to 256 electrodes typically housed within a fabric cap (Fig. 12.4). However, the currents measured at the scalp are limited by the distortive effects of the intervening structures in the head, which severely hamper efforts to localize the signal sources precisely. This forms one of the chief motivations for using the alternative technique of MEG, since magnetic fields pass through the dura, the skull, and the scalp relatively unaltered.

### MEG

The magnetic fields produced by the brain are tiny, with field strengths of approximately 10 fT. The highly sensitive superconducting quantum interference device (SQUID) allows for detection of these tiny fields. Sensor arrays provide whole head coverage via a helmet containing up

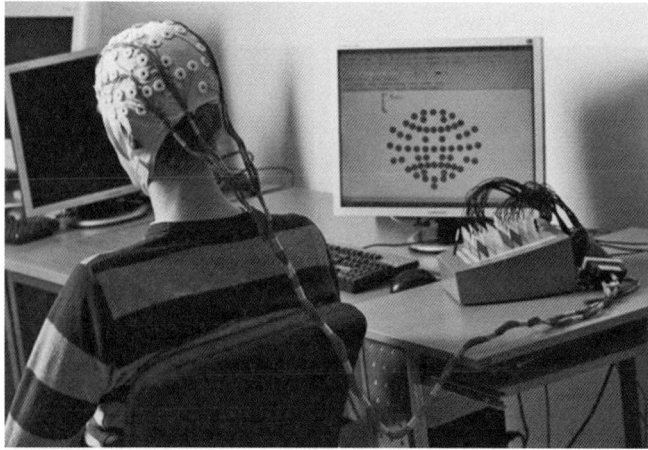 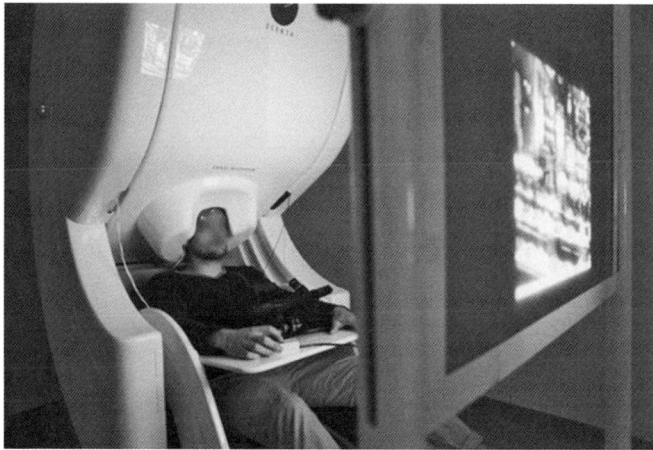

**Fig. 12.10**  Left: subject wearing a 64-channel (electrode) EEG cap. Right: subject doing a visual stimulation study in an MEG scanner housing 306 sensors.

Adapted from Jenkinson M, Chappell M, *Introduction to Neuroimaging Analysis*, Copyright (2017), with permission from Oxford University Press.

to 306 sensors, enveloped in cooling liquid helium. The subject's head is positioned underneath the helmet (Fig. 12.10).

### What are we measuring?

In both MEG and EEG, the measured fields come from neuronal activity at the 'inputs' of neurons—the membrane potentials (also known as the post-synaptic, or local, field potentials), rather than at the 'outputs'—the action potentials. Furthermore, the activity produced by a single neuron is far too small to be detectable; instead signals must sum up over tens of thousands of neurons. This requires a population of neurons to be both temporally synchronous and spatially aligned, with their dendrites pointing in the same directions, such that their individual membrane potentials add up, rather than cancel out. Fortunately, within the cortex, populations of pyramidal neurons tend to fire synchronously and are arranged with their dendrites tending to extend in the same direction, perpendicular to the cortical surface.

### Acquiring data

For EEG to work successfully, care needs to be taken to ensure good conductance between the electrodes and the scalp. This is often achieved by either soaking electrodes in a conducting fluid prior to fitting the cap (a 'wet' cap) or using conducting gels placed on each electrode.

MEG does not require contact between the sensors and the scalp; instead the subject's head is placed as close as comfort allows to the inner surface of the helmet of the scanner. The magnetic field generated by the brain is several orders of magnitude weaker than that of ambient electromagnetic noise, requiring scanners to be placed in magnetically shielded rooms (MSRs).

With both EEG and MEG, it is important that the location of the sensors with respect to subject's head is known, as this aids with mapping activity in the brain (source reconstruction) or with comparing results across subjects. In EEG, the locations of the electrodes are measured, for example by using a stylus pen, the position of which can be triangulated in space, with respect to some anatomical landmarks (for example, the ears and nose). In MEG, the scanner detects small magnetic coils placed at known locations on the subject's head. These can also be used to correct for head motion.

### Data analysis

Both MEG and EEG analyses involve large amounts of data that often need substantial computing power to extract interpretable information from them.

### Artefact cleaning

MEG and EEG recordings typically contain electromagnetic artefacts due to movement of the head or eyes (including saccades and blinking) and skeletal and cardiac muscle electromagnetic activity. To help with identifying artefacts, a combination of surface electro-oculography (EOG), infrared eye tracking, and electrocardiography (ECG) is often used. These recordings can be used in conjunction with techniques like ICA to identify and remove artefactual components in sensor recordings.

### Source reconstruction

Recorded EEG and MEG data at each sensor location represent different weighted summations of the underlying brain activity. In many cases, this sensor–space description of neuronal activity may be sufficient to answer a particular neuroscientific question. Indeed, a large number of studies operate exclusively at this level (see Plate 7a).

Mapping the sources of neuronal activity in the brain (source reconstruction) is often desirable though and requires modelling the relationship between activity and measurable fields in the sensors. This model uses information about the location and geometry of different head structures (for example, scalp, skull, brain tissue) through which the fields pass and is inverted to estimate brain activity. However, the inversion is ill-posed, requiring additional constraints such as assuming the brain activity is sparse or smooth. The resulting spatial maps of brain activity typically have lower spatial resolution than fMRI, in the order of several millimetres (Fig. 12.11).

### Experimental analysis

As with fMRI, M/EEG data analysis comes in two main flavours: task-based and resting state. In task-based M/EEG, the experiments typically consist of many repeats of trials. Data are extracted from each trial and time-locked to a common experimental event of interest

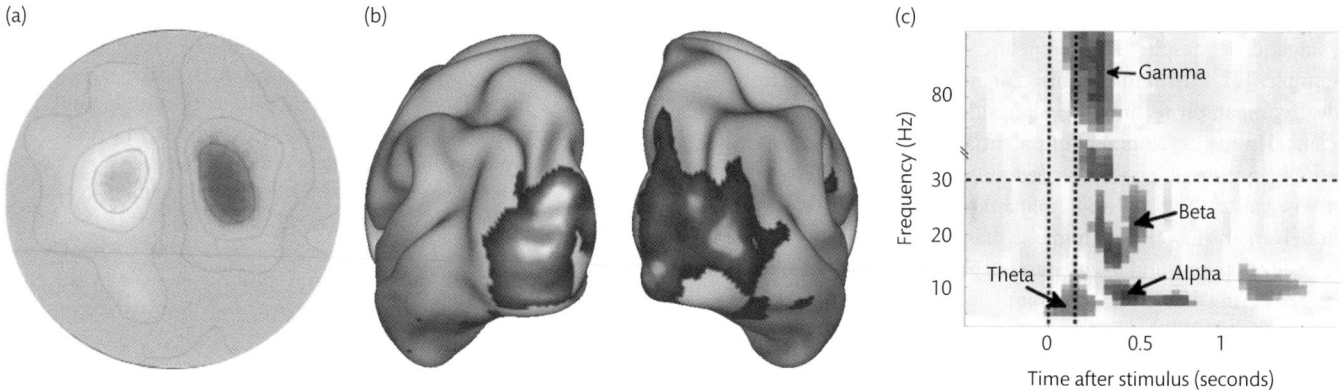

**Fig. 12.11** (see Colour Plate section) (a) Sensor space MEG data presented as a two-dimensional (2D) topographic sensor map of contrasted oscillatory power (between 8 and 12 Hz) in a visual attention task. Power is lower in the contralateral (attending) hemisphere. (b) The same MEG data shown reconstructed into the source (brain) space and presented on a three-dimensional cortical map. (c) Time–frequency plot of oscillatory power in MEG sensors above the visual cortex following presentation of a visual stimulus. Changes in power can be resolved at sub-second resolution, with increases (synchronization) occurring in some frequencies and reductions (desynchronization) occurring in others. Vertical lines denote stimulus onset/offset.

Reproduced from *Practical Neurology*, 14(5), Proudfoot M, Woolrich MW, Nobre AC, *et al.*, Magnetoencephalography, pp. 285–285, Copyright (2014), with permission from *British Medical Journal*.

(for example, the presentation of a visual stimulus; see Plate 1c), and then an average response to the event can be computed over trials. The average response of raw signals is referred to as an event-related field (ERF) in MEG, or an event-related potential (ERP) in EEG.

An alternative to working with raw signals, and a particular strength of M/EEG, is to work with oscillatory brain activity using time-varying frequency representations of the data. This describes task-locked responses in terms of the amount of oscillatory power or phase locking that is present in different frequency bands (see Plate 1c). It is thought that oscillatory power indicates the level of synchrony in the underlying neuronal populations [9].

Resting state M/EEG network matrix analysis, or ICA, often proceeds in a similar manner to fMRI [10, 11]. However, more sophisticated estimates of functional connectivity are needed to account for M/EEG being direct measures of neuronal activity. These are often based on frequency representations (for example, by looking at correlation in oscillatory power) or the phase locking of oscillatory cycles (for example, coherence) between brain areas. As with fMRI, functional connectivity analysis can also be carried out in task data.

### Example applications

MEG and EEG are fundamental tools in both basic and clinical neuroscience research. They can be used to complement the spatial information available from fMRI, with exquisite temporal information.

Basic neuroscience research with M/EEG has often corresponded to the same kind of exploratory brain mapping often carried out with fMRI, albeit extended to also include exploration of the time and frequency domains. Arguably, the most constructive use of M/EEG, and arguably functional neuroimaging in general, comes from more hypothesis-driven work. For example, one approach is to collapse over the spatial dimension and make full use of the temporal information, by asking when in time particular task-related variables can be decoded from the M/EEG data (for example, [12]).

Clinically, EEG and MEG have found important roles in sleep disorders and epilepsy. In sleep research, EEG is used routinely in sleep laboratories to diagnose sleep disorders [13]. In epilepsy, EEG and MEG are used for epileptic source localization, in particular for the planning of subsequent surgery. MEG is particularly promising in this regard, owing to the increased spatial information it has to offer, and shows close correlation to invasive studies of cortical activity [14].

### How imaging is used in psychiatry research

Neuroimaging is now a mainstay of neuroscience research and experimental medicine for mental health diseases and disorders. Examples of its use in specific areas are to be found elsewhere in this book and will include the following.

### Pathophysiology

The pathophysiology of most psychiatric diseases and disorders remains to be fully elucidated, and imaging plays an important role in discovering mechanisms and potential targets. For example, schizophrenia is characterized structurally by increased ventricular volume and subtle grey matter reductions (for example, [15]), and fMRI reveals reduced brain activity in frontal areas (for example, [16]), although the latter is now regarded to be an oversimplification (for example, [17]). Structural MRI abnormalities, albeit more subtle, have also been found in mood disorders (for example, [18]). fMRI has also been employed to produce signatures of brain activity associated with specific clinical phenomena such as auditory hallucinations [19] and PTSD-like flashbacks (for example, [20]).

### Drug action and drug development

Functional imaging, in particular PET and fMRI, has an important role to play in investigations of therapeutic drug action and target engagement. D2 receptor PET has long been used in receptor occupancy studies to estimate the optimal dose of antipsychotics, so that they hit the sweet spot between maximum antipsychotic effect with minimal motor side effects (for example, [4]). In addition to molecular imaging studies, the mechanism of action of antidepressant drugs has been investigated using fMRI, demonstrating that the neural effects of serotonin reuptake inhibitors are detectable after a single dose, despite the therapeutic effect taking 2–4 weeks (for example, [21]). In future, molecular imaging is expected to be an ideal companion technology, alongside cellular/molecular neuroscience, in the development of potential drug targets. In particular, radioligands can be co-developed alongside drug targets to act as *in vivo* validation tools and companion biomarkers. This work, in model organisms and in humans, has the potential to accelerate drug development and to enhance the portfolio of evidence required for partnering on a given compound or target.

## Imaging biomarkers

A common goal of many neuroimaging studies in the context of psychiatric research is to develop novel biomarkers that will be useful for diagnosis, prognosis, stratification of participants for clinical trials, and surrogate endpoints for trials. Neuroimaging biomarkers, including amyloid PET and structural MRI, are now standard in trials for Alzheimer's disease drugs, and hippocampal volumetry is on the verge of being used as standard in memory clinics to aid with both earlier diagnosis and differential diagnosis for patients with cognitive decline. Neuroimaging is further from being ready for standard clinical use in other psychiatric diseases and disorders, but inclusion in trials of novel therapeutics for, for example, mood disorders is ever more common.

## The future of neuroimaging

Each of the imaging modalities described in this chapter are active areas of research, and new ways of acquiring and analysing data are so frequent that a 'state-of-the-art' description would be rapidly out-of-date. For PET, the main areas of innovation are in developing new radiotracers, as well as adapting to new combined PET-MR acquisitions. For MEG, the analysis methodology is rapidly improving and becoming more standardized. The future might involve the use of atomic sensors [for example, optically pumped magnetometers (OPMs)], which could allow the sensors to be placed much nearer to the surface of the head, giving an estimated 5-fold increase in sensitivity. For MRI acquisition, the innovations include acquiring data more quickly, with greater spatial resolution and with an ever greater number of contrast mechanisms that improve sensitivity to specific pathologies. Some of the most exciting innovations come from combining data across modalities (within and beyond neuroimaging) and from 'big data' applications, including scanning much larger populations than ever before (for example, [22] and developing systems and analysis tools for sharing imaging data across cohorts and studies.

## REFERENCES

1. Good, C.D., Johnsrude, I.S., Ashburner, J., Henson, R.N., Friston, K.J., and Frackowiak, R.S. (2001). A voxel-based morphometric study of ageing in 465 normal adult human brains. *NeuroImage*, 14(1 Pt 1), 21–36.
2. Smith, S.M., Jenkinson, M., Johansen-Berg, H., *et al.* (2006). Tract-based spatial statistics: voxelwise analysis of multi-subject diffusion data. *Neuroimage*, 31, 1487–505.
3. Weinstein, J.J., Chohan, M.O., Slifstein, M., Kegeles, L.S., Moore, H., and Abi-Dargham. A. (2017). Pathway-specific dopamine abnormalities in schizophrenia. *Biological Psychiatry*, 81, 31–42.
4. Lako, I.M., van den Heuvel, E.R., Knegtering, H., Bruggeman, R., and Taxis, K. (2013). Estimating dopamine D2 receptor occupancy for doses of 8 antipsychotics: a meta-analysis. *Journal of Clinical Psychopharmacology*, 33, 675–81.
5. Spies, M., Knudsen, G.M., Lanzenberger, R., and Kasper, S. (2015). The serotonin transporter in psychiatric disorders: insights from PET imaging. *The Lancet Psychiatry*, 2, 743–55.
6. Jovalekic, A., Koglin, N., Mueller, A., and Stephens, A.W. (2016). New protein deposition tracers in the pipeline. *EJNMMI Radiopharmacy and Chemistry*, 1, 11.
7. Mathis, C.A., Bacskai, B.J., Kajdasz, S.T., *et al.* (2002). A lipophilic thioflavin-T derivative for positron emission tomography (PET) imaging of amyloid in brain. *Bioorganic and Medicinal Chemistry Letters*, 12, 295–8.
8. James, O.G., Murali Doraiswamy, P., and Borges-Neto, S. (2015). PET imaging of tau pathology in Alzheimer's disease and tauopathies. *Frontiers in Neurology*, 6, 38.
9. Lopes da Silva, F. (2013). EEG and MEG: relevance to neuroscience. *Neuron*, 80, 1112–28.
10. Brookes, M.J., Woolrich, M., Luckhoo, H., *et al.* (2011). Investigating the electrophysiological basis of resting state networks using magnetoencephalography. *Proceedings of the National Academy of Sciences of the United States of America*, 108, 16783–8.
11. Baker, A.P., Brookes, M.J., Rezek, I.A., *et al.* (2014). Fast transient networks in spontaneous human brain activity. *eLife*, 3, e01867.
12. Cichy, R.M., Pantazis, D., and Oliva, A. (2014). Resolving human object recognition in space and time. *Nature Neuroscience*, 17, 455–62.
13. Abad, V.C. and Guilleminault, C. (2003). Diagnosis and treatment of sleep disorders: a brief review for clinicians. *Dialogues in Clinical Neuroscience*, 5, 371–88.
14. Stufflebeam SM. (2011). Clinical magnetoencephalography for neurosurgery. *Neurosurgery Clinics in North America*, 22, 153–67.
15. Honea, R., Crow, T.J,. Passingham, D., and Mackay, C.E. (2005). Regional deficits in brain volume in schizophrenia: a meta-analysis of voxel-based morphometry studies. *American Journal of Psychiatry*, 162, 2233–45.
16. Andreasen, N.C., Rezai, K., Alliger, R., and Swayze, V.W. (1992). Hypofrontality in neuroleptic-naive patients and in patients with chronic schizophrenia: assessment with xenon 133 single-photon emission computed tomography and the Tower of London. *Archives of General Psychiatry*, 49, 943–58.
17. Glahn, D.C., Ragland, J.D., Abramoff, A., *et al.* (2005). Beyond hypofrontality: a quantitative meta-analysis of functional neuroimaging studies of working memory in schizophrenia. *Human Brain Mapping*, 25, 60–9.
18. Hibar, D.P., Westlye, L.T., van Erp, T.G., *et al.* (2016). Subcortical volumetric abnormalities in bipolar disorder. *Molecular Psychiatry*, 21, 1710–16.
19. Dierks, T., Linden, D.E., Jandl, M., *et al.* (1999). Activation of Heschl's gyrus during auditory hallucinations. *Neuron*, 22, 615–21.
20. Clark, I.A., Holmes, E.A., Woolrich, M.W., and Mackay, C.E. (2016). Intrusive memories to traumatic footage: the neural basis of their encoding and involuntary recall. *Psychological Medicine*, 46, 505–18.
21. Harmer, C.J., Mackay, C.E., Reid, C.B., Cowen, P.J., and Goodwin, G.M. (2006). Antidepressant drug treatment modifies the neural processing of nonconscious threat cues. *Biological Psychiatry*, 59, 816–20.
22. Miller, K.L., Alfaro-Almagro, F., Bangerter, N.K., *et al.* (2016). Multimodal population brain imaging in the UK Biobank prospective epidemiological study. *Nature Neuroscience*, 19, 1523–36.

# 13

# The connectome

*Olaf Sporns*

## Introduction

The project of linking anatomical features of the brain to distinct psychological and cognitive processes has been a core objective of cognitive and systems neuroscience for well over a century. A central goal has been the creation of brain maps that chart the localization of function across brain areas and systems [1]. The emphasis on building a cognitive anatomy largely defined by 'place' (topography) is increasingly supplemented by the recognition that cognitive processes are distributed and involve overlapping sets of often remote anatomical regions [2–4]. This complementary view emphasizes the need to map 'relations' (topology) or connectivity across the brain. The idea that connectivity is essential to understand how brain architecture supports cognitive processing underpins the emerging science of brain networks, or connectomics [5–8]. As originally defined [5], the connectome is a comprehensive map of the structural connections linking different elements of the nervous system. These elements may correspond to individual (micro-scale) neurons or entire (macro-scale) brain areas. This structural map is fundamental for a mechanistic account of functional brain activity and connectivity, with structural connections shaping and constraining the response patterns of neurons and brain regions. The study of the structural and functional networks of the human brain comprises the emerging field of 'human connectomics'.

This chapter offers an overview of the core concept of the connectome. After a brief outline of the concept's historical roots and origins, the chapter proceeds to define and contrast the two major modes of structural and functional brain connectivity. This is followed by a survey of the principal findings to date on the network architecture of the connectome, its role in shaping brain dynamics and functional networks, and applications in studies of development and brain disorders.

## Background and origin

Mapping the connections linking neurons and brain regions has been a central goal of neuroscience for many decades—indeed compelling arguments for the importance of connectivity in brain function extend back centuries [9, 10]. The fundamental role of neuroanatomy in neurobiological accounts of brain function and dysfunction was recognized by many nineteenth-century neurologists and anatomists, among whom were Carl Wernicke and Theodor Meynert. Meynert was among the first to clearly articulate that anatomical connectivity establishes physical links among otherwise remote parts of the brain. Distinguishing tracts of 'projection systems' and 'association systems' as major constituents of the cerebral white matter, he wrote that 'the wealth of such fibres, and their variation in length, connecting as they do near and remote parts of the cortex, will suffice, without formulating an anatomical hypothesis, to unite any one part of the cortex to any other' (page 150, ref [11]). In Meynert's theoretical framework, disorganized fibre architecture was an important factor contributing to brain and mental disorders.

Modern studies of brain connectivity at first proceeded in model organisms such as the macaque monkey [12, 13] and other mammalian species. Invasive, but highly sensitive, methods for tracing the trajectories and terminations of axonal pathways were deployed to chart projections between anatomically distinct and functionally specialized brain areas. Comprehensive repositories of individual reports on projection patterns were created for monkey [13, 14] and cat cortex [15] and were studied extensively in search of anatomical substrates that could account for, or predict, functional specialization [16]. The lack of connectivity data for humans triggered calls for developing new methods to map the connectivity of the human brain [17] and eventually led to a proposal for mapping human brain connectivity in its entirety—the human connectome [5]. Over the past decade, these calls have been answered through the creation of multi-site projects aimed at mapping human brain connectivity in large cohorts of human subjects [18], including subject samples across the lifespan and from clinical populations. The connectome has emerged as a core concept in modern systems and cognitive neuroscience, providing a conceptual framework for characterizing structure–function relationships in the healthy and dysfunctional brain.

## Structural and functional networks

Most complex systems in the natural, social, and technological world are composed of large numbers of interacting elements whose collective dynamics gives rise to global system states and determines the evolution of these states through time. To understand the structure or function of a complex system, it is often advantageous to decompose the system into a set of nodes and edges, which can then be studied with the mathematical toolset of graph theory. This is the main idea behind mapping and analysing brain networks, or connectomes. There are two main modes of brain networks, derived from observations on anatomy (structural connectivity) or physiology (functional connectivity). The networks derived from measuring structural and functional connectivity share a set of common attributes. Both comprise collections of nodes (elements such as neurons or areas) and edges (their interrelations or connections). The arrangement of these nodes and edges relative to one another defines the network's topology, which is formally described as a graph. Defining nodes and edges is absolutely fundamental for the creation of any brain network, and a necessary step for any subsequent quantitative analysis of the structure of the graph. At the level of whole-brain human connectome networks, nodes correspond to the basic elements of parcellation of the cortical and subcortical grey matter into a set of areas. Parcellation schemes can be derived, based on a number of anatomical or functional criteria such as cytoarchitectonics, myelination patterns, gene expression profiles, or patterns of anatomical or functional connectivity [19]. The edges linking the nodes record their anatomical or physiological relations and, depending on the nature of the specific measure and how it is recorded, may be binary (0/1) or weighted, symmetric or directed.

Structural connectivity defines networks that record the presence/absence, as well as the strength or density, of physical links between neurons, neuronal populations, or brain areas. The totality of structural connections constitutes the connectome, as originally defined [5]. Human connectome networks derived from non-invasive imaging methodology comprise interregional projections that traverse the brain's white matter and connect cortical and subcortical regions. Because of fundamental limitations, these imaging approaches cannot resolve the directionality of projections and instead deliver measures of undirected connectivity. While most current accounts of human connectomes express connection weights solely in terms of the density or number of streamlines, it should be noted that the relationship of such simple measures to the true anatomical magnitude of a pathway is unclear [20] and that other indices that express connectional microstructure should be taken into account. White matter architecture can show signs of neuroplasticity on timescales of days to weeks [21] and exhibits characteristic changes in the course of development and ageing.

Functional connectivity differs from structural connectivity in several important respects. Firstly, functional connectivity is generally derived from neuronal or haemodynamic time series data and expresses patterns of statistical dependence among these time series [22]. Neuronal time series can be recorded with a broad array of techniques, from invasive multi-electrode recordings to whole brain electrophysiology or fMRI. Analytic techniques for extracting statistical dependence include information theoretic measures (such as mutual information or transfer entropy), spectral coherence, phase locking, and simple Pearson cross-correlation. The latter is currently widely used in human studies carried out with fMRI that track fluctuations in haemodynamic signals, either in response to specific task conditions or in a task-free 'resting state'. Unlike structural connectivity, patterns of functional connectivity can exhibit significant reorganizations over short timescales, as interactions among neurons

and brain areas are continually modulated, reflecting changes in sensory inputs and tasks. Measurement of functional connectivity, especially with fMRI, is prone to numerous sources of physiological noise, including involuntary head motion which can introduce systematic biases into functional connectivity estimates.

Once nodes and edges have been defined and pairwise relations among all system elements have been summarized in a graph or network, a large range of analysis and modelling tools from graph theory can be deployed to characterize or compare network architectures [23–25] (Fig. 13.1). Broadly, these measures can be divided into several classes that capture aspects of segregation, integration, and influence. Measures of segregation capture the extent to which the network is clustered and can be subdivided into separate network communities or modules. Examples are the clustering coefficient, network motifs, and methods for detecting network modules. The latter are particularly important, as they deliver putative structural and/or functional building blocks that have been the focus of much interest and research in cognitive neuroscience [26]. Measures of integration express the degree to which the network is globally interactive. A fundamental concept is that of path length, generally defined as the minimal distance (in terms of topology, that is the number of steps in a network, which may be unrelated to metric separation) between network nodes. In structural networks, the shorter the path length, the more directly two nodes can communicate and exchange information. Across an entire network, this capacity for direct communication is expressed as the network's

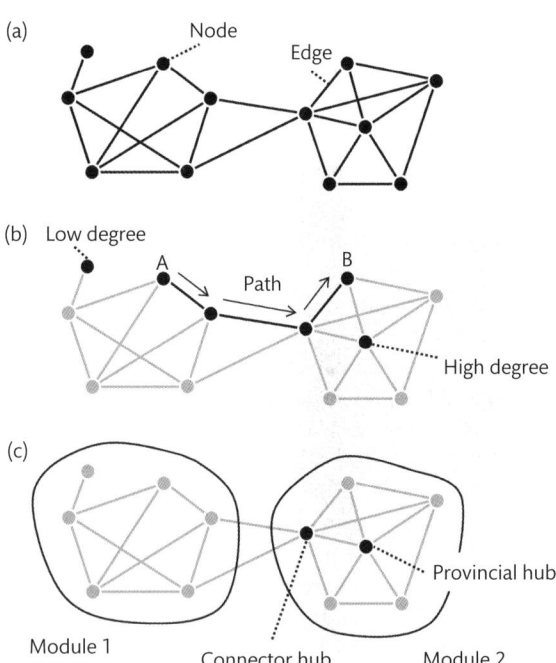

**Fig. 13.1** Elementary graph concepts and measures, illustrated on a schematic illustration of a simple network. (a) The network shown here consists of 12 nodes linked by undirected and unweighted (binary) edges. (b) A low-degree node (maintaining a single edge) and a high-degree node (maintaining five edges) are indicated. Nodes A and B are linked by a minimally short path comprising three edges or steps. (c) The network is shown with a partition into two modules. The node labelled 'connector hub' maintains edges with its own module, as well as across module boundaries. The node labelled 'provincial hub', while highly connected, only links to nodes in its own community.

global efficiency. Measures of influence are useful for detecting those network elements that occupy central positions in the topology and may therefore be particularly important for the functioning of the system. Important nodes are, somewhat informally, designated as network hubs. Some measures of influence rely on local features of a network element (such as the node degree, that is the total number of distinct connections that each node maintains), while others take into account the global web of communication paths across the network (such as betweenness, that is the fraction of optimally short communication paths to which each network elements contributes). Another way to define influence and detect hubs is by evaluating the position of a node or edge relative to network modules. For example, highly connected nodes whose connections span multiple modules (and thus form bridges between them) are considered connector hubs that cross-link different communities. In contrast, highly connected nodes whose connections remain predominantly within one module are considered provincial hubs, with potentially important roles in linking members of a single community to each other.

## The network architecture of the connectome

Connectome data can be assembled from a very broad range of techniques and from virtually any species with a nervous system. Important achievements to date have included the complete reconstruction of the synaptic network of the brain of *Caenorhabditis elegans* [27] as well as the creation of network maps of large portions of the central nervous system of the mouse [28] and rat [29].

Most studies of the structural connectome of the human brain have utilized non-invasive imaging methodology and computational reconstruction to infer the spatial arrangement and trajectories of white matter interregional projections [30, 31]. These trajectories are represented as 'streamlines' that comprise putative white matter tracts. The complete set of these tracts, in combination with parcellation of the grey matter, forms a network of nodes and edges that can be quantitatively analysed with measures and tools from graph theory (Fig. 13.2). While current diffusion imaging and tractography approaches have significant limitations and pitfalls [32], continual refinements are made to better capture complex fibre architecture [33] and develop more principled methods for model-based connectome inference [34]. Despite these ongoing developments, several core findings on human connectome topology have proven to be both robust and reproducible. These include unique 'connectivity fingerprints' of brain areas, a broad distribution of node degrees indicating the presence of network hubs, dense connectivity among hubs linking them into a connective core or 'rich club', and distinct network communities or modules.

Connectivity fingerprints refer to the patterns of inputs and outputs (indistinguishable with diffusion imaging) maintained by each network node [35]. It is thought that these fingerprints are important for defining the functional specialization of nodes, as they determine the neuronal information to which each node has access, as well as the downstream targets to which its output signals are distributed. In all connectome studies carried out so far, anatomically distinct areas have been found to maintain a characteristic and unique connectivity fingerprint. Connectivity fingerprints are more similar among brain regions that contribute to similar functional domains

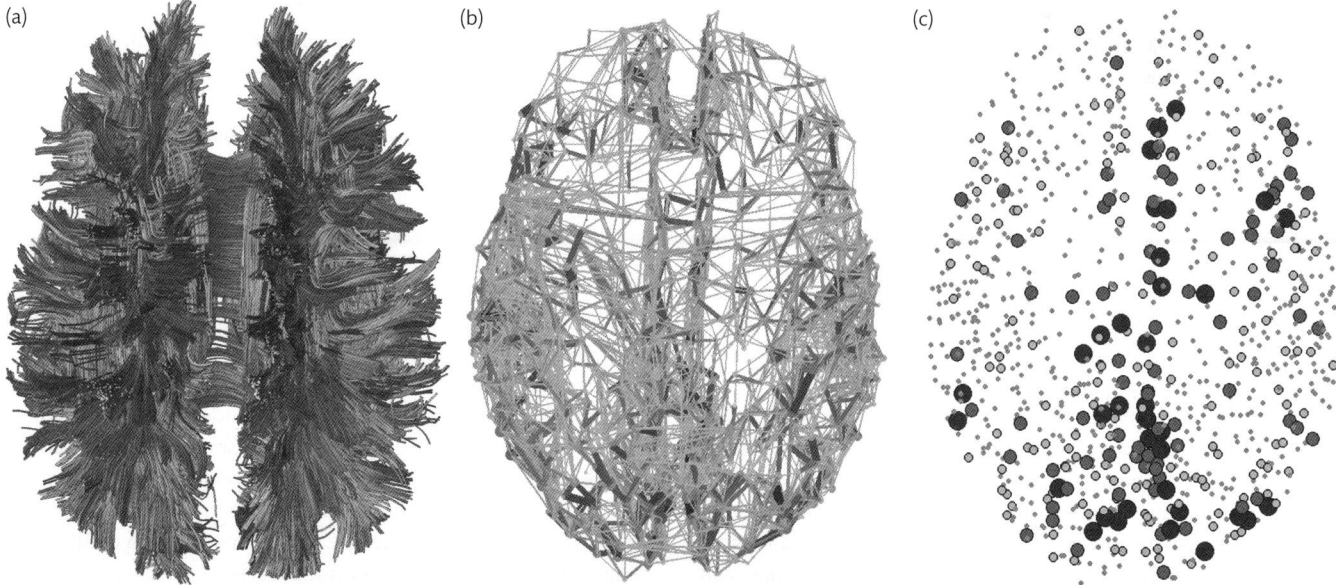

(a)          (b)          (c)

**Fig. 13.2** (see Colour Plate section) Different representations of the connectome. (a) A set of streamlines, derived from diffusion imaging and computational tractography. Red, green, and blue lines indicate putative white matter tracts running along the medial–lateral, anterior–posterior, and dorsal–ventral directions, respectively. (b) Nodes derived from a cortical parcellation are shown as red dots, connected by edges (blue lines) that correspond to the density of streamlines linking each pair of nodes. For clarity, the diagram shows the strongest edges only. (c) Nodes are arranged in the same anatomical positions as in panel (b), with blue-coloured nodes indicating high betweenness centrality, a measure of influence that is computed as the number of optimally short communication paths to which each node contributes. Node diameter is proportional to the number of subjects (0–5), for which a given node received high betweenness scores.

Adapted from *PLOS Biol.*, 6, Hagmann P, Cammoun L, Gigandet X, *et al.*, Mapping the structural core of human cerebral cortex, e159, Copyright (2008), PLOS Biology. Reproduced under the Creative Commons Attribution License CC BY 4.0.

or cognitive processes; conversely, distinct fingerprints can be taken as indications of functional specialization [36]. Connectivity fingerprints can be used for the purpose of parcellation, defining the boundaries between distinct brain areas that maintain distinct patterns of connectivity [19].

Network hubs may be identified on the basis of node degree (that is, the number of connections per node) or other measures of influence. The distribution of node degrees in human connectome studies has invariably been reported as heavy-tailed, that is, strongly skewed towards nodes with low degree. Put differently, a larger number of nodes have relatively few distinct pathways, while a smaller number of nodes maintain a larger set of distinct projections. Broad degree distributions, assuming a log-normal shape, have also been described in tract tracing studies in non-human primates [37]. In the human brain, hub regions have been identified in parts of the orbitofrontal, lateral prefrontal, superior frontal, cingulate, and medial parietal cortex [38], with most of these regions previously classified as multimodal or transmodal, based on their diverse functional responses.

A number of human connectome studies have shown that highly connected hubs are also densely connected to each other, more so than expected by chance. This aspect of network topology, called a 'connective core' or a 'rich club' [39], suggests that hubs are preferentially connected to allow direct communication and sharing of information. Indeed, graph analysis demonstrates that a very large proportion of all short communication paths across the human connectome access some portion of the brain's rich club and that damage to rich club nodes or edges has the potential to disproportionately disrupt patterns of interregional information transfer [40]. An attractive hypothesis suggests that rich club organization offers a structural substrate for integrative processes that may underpin high-level conscious processing. In support of this notion, rich club connectivity has been found to interlink the set of widely distributed resting state networks that form the basic building blocks of functional connectivity [41]. Connections among rich club members may thus play important roles in the exchange of neuronal information across different sensory and task domains.

Human connectome networks exhibit high clustering, with dense structural connections that define local communities or modules. These modules comprise nodes that tend to share not only dense interconnections, but also common sets of inputs and outputs, as well as common physiological responses and co-activation patterns. The concept of modularity has been especially important in studies of human functional networks. A large body of work has examined the topography and specialization of modules corresponding to resting state or intrinsic functional networks [42, 43]. These modules can be derived with a variety of decomposition or clustering techniques. Network-based detection of modules often utilizes an approach known as 'modularity optimization' [26], which attempts to maximize a quality metric that is designed to optimally partition a network into blocks that are internally densely and externally weakly connected. Partitioning of human resting state functional connectivity has resulted in maps of components/modules that are both highly reproducible across different subject cohorts and imaging parameters [44, 45], as well as sensitive to individual variations, including developmental stages and clinical status [46]. Importantly, network modules derived from fMRI time series recorded in the resting state are highly similar to the spatial patterns of

co-activation networks derived from task-evoked activations across large numbers of imaging studies [47, 48]. Hence, it appears that the architecture of functional networks at rest recapitulates or rehearses spatial patterns of co-activation that are engaged as the brain is challenged in different task contexts.

## From the connectome to brain dynamics

The stability and reproducibility of resting state functional networks strongly suggest that these networks have an anatomical origin. Three lines of experimental evidence suggest that this is indeed the case. Firstly, systematic comparison of patterns of structural and functional connectivity recorded in non-human primates [49, 50], as well as in the human brain [51, 52], has shown that they are statistically strongly related. For example, among anatomically directly connected node pairs, the strength of the anatomical projection is partly predictive of the strength of the corresponding functional connection [50, 51]. Secondly, studies of specific resting state functional networks have shown that their constituent components are interconnected by anatomical projections. For example, the anterior and posterior divisions of the default mode network are directly linked by white matter projections running along the cortical midline, and variations in these anatomical projections are correlated with variations in functional connectivity [53]. Thirdly, in rare instances, it has been possible to observe changes in functional networks immediately after experimentally induced disturbances of anatomical connections. For example, transection of interhemispheric cortical pathways in a human patient undergoing surgery for epilepsy resulted in functional disconnection of the two cortical hemispheres [54].

Important insights into the relationship between structural and functional connectivity have come from computational studies of connectome networks (Fig. 13.3). Simulations of neural mass models using a structural coupling matrix, based on the macro-scale connectome of the macaque cerebral cortex, generated functional connectivity that was significantly correlated with the structure of empirical functional networks [50, 55]. Similar results were obtained in simulations of the human connectome [51, 56], including the topography of resting state networks. Additionally, computational studies have demonstrated a number of important dynamic properties of functional connectivity, including temporal fluctuations in network topology [55, 57], as well as the important roles of conduction delays and noise in shaping resting brain functional connectivity [56, 58]. While some research agendas aim to create more realistic and complex neuronal simulations of functional brain dynamics, other studies have attempted to model functional connectivity on the basis of simple dynamic processes such as diffusion [59] and spreading [60]. One example of this approach utilized a measure of 'searchability', derived from studies of network navigability and search, to successfully predict the strength and pattern of functional connectivity in the human brain [61]. What virtually all computational studies have shown is that functional connectivity results (at least in large part) from a complex combination of many (direct and indirect) communication events and dynamic influences that travel across the structural connectome.

While most fMRI studies of functional connectivity in the resting state have examined the structure of functional networks that were estimated over relatively long recording sessions (lasting in the order of 5–10 minutes), recent work has focused on fluctuations

(a)

(b)

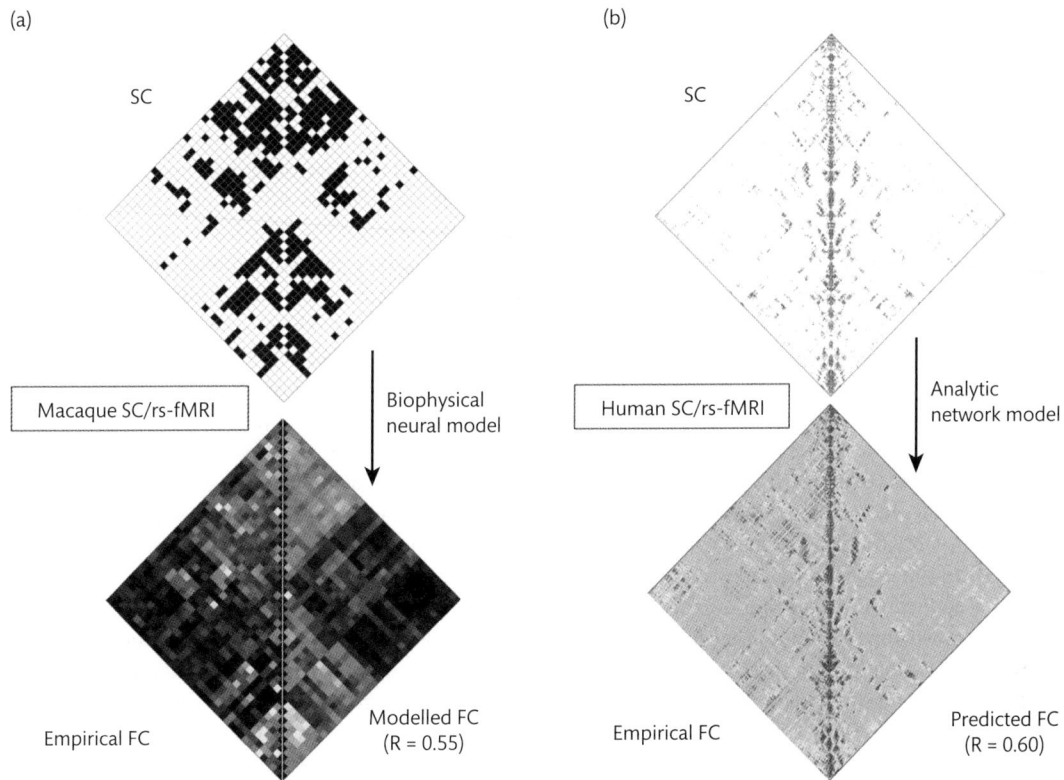

**Fig. 13.3** (see Colour Plate section) Connectome-based computational models of functional connectivity. (a) The matrix at the top shows structural connectivity (SC) of directed projections among a set of macaque cortical areas. This connectome formed the coupling structure for a simulation of neural mass dynamics that generated synthetic fMRI time courses and a 'modelled FC' (functional connectivity) matrix (lower plot, right half). This computational analogue of macaque FC can be compared to empirical recordings of resting-state fMRI. The correlation between the empirical and modelled FC patterns is R = 0.55 [54]. (b) Human SC matrix (from [30]) and empirical FC (from [30]), as well as predicted FC (from [61]). The predicted FC was computed from an analytic model based on measures of communication in the structural graph SC. The correlation between the empirical and predicted FC patterns is R = 0.60 [61].

in functional connectivity that occur on shorter timescales (in the order of tens of seconds) [62]. These fluctuations can be detected by tracking individual functional connections over time [63] or by extracting and clustering network states [64]. Both approaches require the formulation of appropriate statistical null models to exclude spurious detection of fluctuations that are due to measurement artefact or noise. While much of the work in this area is still ongoing, a convergent set of findings suggests that resting brain dynamics seems to reflect ongoing transitions of functional networks between states of high segregation and high integration [65]. Statistically significant fluctuations coalesce into consistent network patterns with high modularity, characterized by a de-coupling of task-positive from task-negative (default mode) networks [66]. Much of the efforts to characterize dynamic changes in functional connectivity are motivated by the possibility that such changes may offer a novel biomarker for clinical disorders.

Another important emerging area is the study of functional connectivity in relation to task and cognitive function [43, 67]. Several studies have shown that functional networks are rapidly reconfigured as the brain engages in different tasks, including in continuous sensorimotor tasks [68] or in switching between continuous mental operation such as working memory, arithmetic, or navigation [69]. A comparison of resting state and task-evoked functional connectivity estimated across a battery of different tasks [70] has shown

the presence of an intrinsic functional connectivity state that persists across tasks and that is highly similar to functional connectivity emerging in the resting state. Task-evoked networks emerge on top of this intrinsic state and are associated with specific patterns of modulated functional connections. A different study showed that transitions between different cognitive tasks were accompanied by transitions between distinct functional connectivity states [71]. Using machine-learning approaches, these functional connectivity states could be used to infer cognitive operations in individual subjects.

## Development and clinical disorders

Important applications of the connectome include the characterization of changes in connectome topology across developmental stages and in clinical populations. These studies pose a number of methodological and analytic challenges. While many study designs rely on comparison of group-averaged connectivity data sets, the heterogeneity of brain structure and function across individuals may be more appropriately captured by looking at longitudinal changes in individuals across development or by employing dimensional designs that can associate continuous variation in behavioural and/or cognitive phenotypes with network markers. In addition to issues of study design, developmental or clinical subject cohorts can present issues related to differential head motion and the associated measurement artefacts.

Numerous studies have shown that structural and functional networks exhibit characteristic changes across the human lifespan. For example, an early study carried out on participants ranging between the ages of 2 and 18 years old showed that human connectome networks increase in density and become more efficient in terms of communication paths and progressively less modular (less highly segregated) with age [72]. These trends mirror similar tendencies in functional networks that were observed across a similar age range [73], with functional modules becoming less determined by spatial clustering and more coherent and integrated across remote regions of the brain. Looking across the human lifespan [74], several structural connectome metrics related to network density and efficiency exhibit inverted U-shaped time courses, with early increases followed by decreases later in life. Rich club organization was present across the entire lifespan, with the most pronounced expression in early adulthood [75]. In parallel with these evolving structural network features, resting state functional networks exhibit developmental trajectories of their own, for example, by becoming internally less strongly coupled, while developing stronger functional links between networks, especially among components of the somatomotor network, the dorsal attention network, and the saliency/ventral attention network [76]. Ongoing lifespan connectomics efforts are extending the range of these observations to neonates and the elderly population.

The fundamental rationale behind connectomics-based approaches to brain disorders is 2-fold. Firstly, most of these conditions cannot be traced to highly localized pathologies but are instead associated with disturbances of network organization across extended parts of the brain [77, 78]. Secondly, connectomics offers an intermediate phenotype, based on structural and functional circuits and connectivity that is interspersed between the domains of genetics and molecular interactions at the lower end and human behaviour and social networks at the upper end of the scale [79] (Fig. 13.4). Structural brain networks not only allow information to become shared and integrated in the course of healthy brain function, but they also promote the spreading of disease processes. Examples are distributed functional changes resulting from brain damage due to an ischaemic attack [80], the progressive spread of degenerative conditions such as Alzheimer's disease along anatomical pathways [81], or the global effects such as generalized seizures that are triggered by focal epileptogenic activity [82]. Several classic clinical concepts, among them diaschisis and cognitive reserve, may be reconceptualized in the context of brain networks and the connectome. Diaschisis [83], which implies functional disruption that occurs at a distance, for example after a stroke, may reflect the brain's response to acute disturbances of connectome topology. For example, network approaches predict that the loss of a set of nodes and edges may be accompanied by altered functional connectivity among remote (including contralateral) brain regions and systems [84]. The extent of this reorganization would likely depend on the topological status of the damaged nodes, with damage to more central nodes (network hubs) causing more severe and widespread disruption. Cognitive reserve [85], or the capacity of the brain to counter impairment with compensatory strategies, may depend on the network's ability to provide alternative functional configurations or paths to counter the loss of nodes and edges. This ability would allow the brain to configure alternative sets of nodes and edges to carry out equivalent ('degenerate' [86, 87]) cognitive or behavioural processes.

A common theme in many clinical and translational applications of the connectome has been the role of important network elements in the origin and progression of brain disorders. Network hubs

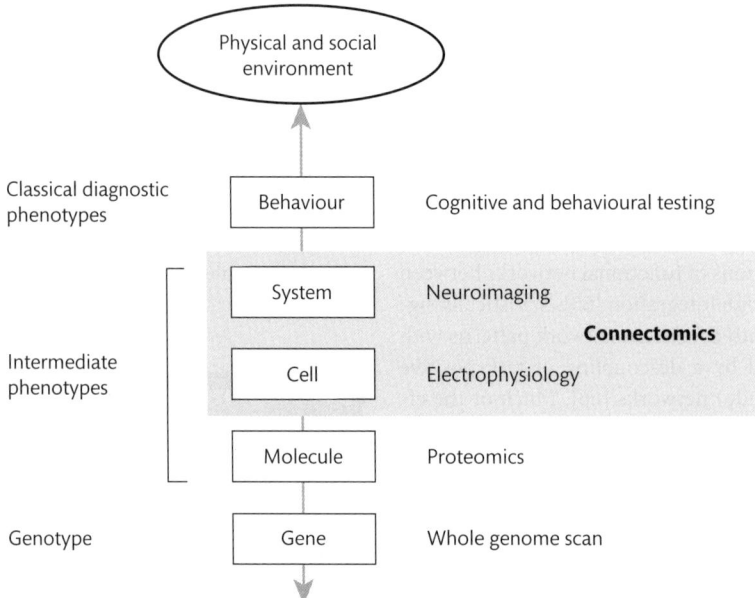

**Fig. 13.4** Brain phenotypes are arranged in a hierarchy spanning several levels of organization, ranging from molecular processes to behaviour and social environment. Genetic and environmental factors contributing to brain disorders converge onto the connectome which occupies the position of an intermediate phenotype that bridges molecular and behavioural scales.

Adapted from *Br J Psychiatry*, 194(4), Bullmore ET, Fletcher P, Jones PB, Why psychiatry can't afford to be neurophobic, pp. 293–295, Copyright (2009), with permission from Royal College of Psychiatrists.

have caught significant attention, as they appear to play a causal role across a wide range of brain disorders. A meta-analysis of data from more than 20,000 subjects and 26 different disorders [88] has shown that many of these disorders were associated with hub-centric neuropathology, that is with lesions that predominantly involved topologically central elements of the hum an connectome. For example, hubs in the medial temporal lobe are among the first brain regions to exhibit pathological changes in Alzheimer's disease [89], while frontal and temporal cortical hubs are implicated in a number of studies of schizophrenia [90]. It appears that the existence of network hubs in the connectome offers unique functional advantages, while also creating points of vulnerability—the benefits of hubs in information integration turn into risk factors, as their disruption has disproportionate effects on the individual's cognitive and behavioural capacities.

## Summary

The connectome refers to a comprehensive map of connections among elements of a neural system. In studies of the human brain, connectomics has so far largely focused on the macro-scale projections among distinct brain areas and their role in shaping functional connectivity during both rest and task-evoked activity. Computational models of the connectome have been instrumental in elucidating potential network mechanisms that create functional connectivity from communication events in structural networks. Numerous applications of the connectome in developmental and clinical studies have shown patterns of change in connectome topology across the lifespan, as well as the network basis of brain disorders. Future work will likely further illuminate the role of the connectome in the functioning of the healthy and diseased brain.

## Acknowledgement

The author's research has been generously supported by the J.S. McDonnell Foundation, the National Science Foundation, and the National Institutes of Health.

## REFERENCES

1. Sporns, O. (2015). Cerebral cartography and connectomics. *Philosophical Transactions of the Royal Society B*, 370, 20140173.
2. Mesulam, M. (1990). Large-scale neurocognitive networks and distributed processing for attention, language, and memory. *Annals of Neurology*, 28, 597–613.
3. McIntosh, A.R. (2000). Towards a network theory of cognition. *Neural Networks*, 13, 861–70.
4. Sporns, O. (2011). *Networks of the brain*. MIT Press, Cambridge, MA.
5. Sporns, O., Tononi, G., Kötter, R. (2005). The human connectome: a structural description of the human brain. *PLoS Computational Biology*, 1, 245–51.
6. Sporns, O. (2012). From simple graphs to the connectome: networks in neuroimaging. *Neuroimage*, 62, 881–6.
7. Sporns, O. (2013). The human connectome: origins and challenges. *Neuroimage*, 80, 53–61.
8. Sporns, O. (2014). Contributions and challenges for network models in cognitive neuroscience. *Nature Neuroscience*, 17, 652–60.
9. Schmahmann, J.D. and Pandya, D.N. (2007). Cerebral white matter—historical evolution of facts and notions concerning the organization of the fiber pathways of the brain. *Journal of the History of the Neurosciences*, 16, 237–67.
10. Catani, M., de Schotten, M.T., Slater, D., and Dell'Acqua, F. (2013). Connectomic approaches before the connectome. *Neuroimage*, 80, 2–13.
11. Meynert, T. (1885). *Psychiatry: a clinical treatise on diseases of the fore-brain*. Putnam's, New York, NY.
12. Zeki, S. and Shipp, S. (1988). The functional logic of cortical connections. *Nature*. 335, 311–17.
13. Felleman, D.J. and Van Essen, D.C. (1991). Distributed hierarchical processing in the primate cerebral cortex. *Cerebral Cortex*, 1, 1–47.
14. Stephan, K.E., Kamper, L., Bozkurt, A., Burns, G.A., Young, M.P., and Kötter, R. (2001). Advanced database methodology for the Collation of Connectivity data on the Macaque brain (CoCoMac). *Philosophical Transactions of the Royal Society London B*, 356, 1159–86.
15. Scannell, J.W., Blakemore, C., and Young, M.P. (1995). Analysis of connectivity in the cat cerebral cortex. *Journal of Neuroscience*, 15, 1463–83.
16. Hilgetag, C.C., Burns, G.A., O'Neill, M.A., Scannell, J.W., and Young, M.P. (2000). Anatomical connectivity defines the organization of clusters of cortical areas in the macaque and the cat. *Philosophical Transactions of the Royal Society London B*, 355, 91–110.
17. Crick, F. and Jones, E. (1993). Backwardness of human neuroanatomy. *Nature*, 361, 109–10.
18. Van Essen, D.C., Smith, S.M., Barch, D.M., *et al.*; WU-Minn HCP Consortium. (2013). The WU-Minn Human Connectome Project: an overview. *Neuroimage*, 80, 62–79.
19. Wig, G.S., Schlaggar, B.L., and Petersen, S.E. (2011). Concepts and principles in the analysis of brain networks. *Annals of the New York Academy of Sciences*, 1224, 126–46.
20. Jones, D.K., Knösche, T.R., and Turner, R. (2013). White matter integrity, fiber count, and other fallacies: the do's and don'ts of diffusion MRI. *Neuroimage*. 73, 239–54.
21. Scholz, J., Klein, M.C., Behrens, T.E., and Johansen-Berg, H. (2009). Training induces changes in white-matter architecture. *Nature Neuroscience*, 12, 1370–1.
22. Friston, K.J. (2011). Functional and effective connectivity: a review. *Brain Connectivity*, 1, 13–36.
23. Rubinov, M. and Sporns, O. (2010). Complex network measures of brain connectivity: uses and interpretations. *Neuroimage*, 52, 1059–69.
24. Bullmore, E. and Sporns, O. (2009). Complex brain networks: graph theoretical analysis of structural and functional systems. *Nature Reviews Neuroscience*, 10, 186–98.
25. Fornito, A., Zalesky, A., and Breakspear, M. (2013). Graph analysis of the human connectome: promise, progress, and pitfalls. *Neuroimage*, 80, 426–44.
26. Sporns, O. and Betzel, R.F. (2016). Modular brain networks. *Annual Review of Psychology*, 67, 613–40.
27. White, J.G., Southgate, E., Thomson, J.N., and Brenner, S. (1986). The structure of the nervous system of the nematode Caenorhabditis elegans. *Philosophical Transactions of the Royal Society London B*, 314, 1–340.

28. Oh, S.W., Harris, J.A., Ng, L., *et al.* (2014). A mesoscale connectome of the mouse brain. *Nature*, 508, 207–14.

29. Bota, M., Sporns, O., and Swanson, L.W. (2015). Architecture of the cerebral cortical association connectome underlying cognition. *Proceedings of the National Academy of Sciences of the United States of America*, 112, E2093–101.

30. Hagmann, P., Cammoun, L., Gigandet, X., *et al.* (2008). Mapping the structural core of human cerebral cortex. *PLoS Biology*, 6, e159.

31. Cammoun, L., Gigandet, X., Meskaldji, D., *et al.* (2012). Mapping the human connectome at multiple scales with diffusion spectrum MRI. *Journal of Neuroscience Methods*, 203, 386–97.

32. Thomas, C., Frank, Q.Y., Irfanoglu, M.O., *et al.* (2014). Anatomical accuracy of brain connections derived from diffusion MRI tractography is inherently limited. *Proceedings of the National Academy of Sciences of the United States of America*, 111, 16574–9.

33. Tuch, D.S., Reese, T.G., Wiegell, M.R., and Wedeen, V.J. (2003). Diffusion MRI of complex neural architecture. *Neuron*, 40, 885–95.

34. Pestilli, F., Yeatman, J.D., Rokem, A., Kay, K.N., and Wandell, B.A. (2014). Evaluation and statistical inference for human connectomes. *Nature Methods*, 11, 1058–63.

35. Passingham, R.E., Stephan, K.E., and Kötter, R. (2002). The anatomical basis of functional localization in the cortex. *Nature Reviews Neuroscience*, 3, 606–16.

36. Markov, N.T., Ercsey-Ravasz, M., Lamy, C., *et al.* (2013). The role of long-range connections on the specificity of the macaque interareal cortical network. *Proceedings of the National Academy of Sciences of the United States of America*, 110, 5187–92.

37. Markov, N.T., Misery, P., Falchier, A., *et al.* (2011). Weight consistency specifies regularities of macaque cortical networks. *Cerebral Cortex*, 21, 1254–72.

38. Van den Heuvel, M.P. and Sporns, O. (2013). Network hubs in the human brain. *Trends in Cognitive Sciences*, 17, 683–96.

39. Van den Heuvel, M.P. and Sporns, O. (2011). Rich-club organization of the human connectome. *Journal of Neuroscience*, 31, 15775–86.

40. van den Heuvel, M.P., Kahn, R.S., Goñi, J., and Sporns, O. (2012). High-cost, high-capacity backbone for global brain communication. *Proceedings of the National Academy of Sciences of the United States of America*, 109, 11372–7.

41. van den Heuvel, M.P. and Sporns, O. (2013). An anatomical substrate for integration among functional networks in human cortex. *Journal of Neuroscience*, 33, 14489–500.

42. Buckner, R.L., Krienen, F.M., and Yeo, B.T. (2013). Opportunities and limitations of intrinsic functional connectivity MRI. *Nature Neuroscience*, 16, 832–7.

43. Petersen, S.E. and Sporns, O. (2015). Brain networks and cognitive architectures. *Neuron*, 88, 207–19.

44. Yeo, B.T.T., Krienen, F.M., Sepulchre, J., *et al.* (2011). The organization of the human cerebral cortex estimated by functional connectivity. *Journal of Neurophysiology*, 106, 1125–65.

45. Power, J.D., Cohen, A.L., Nelson, S.M., *et al.* (2011). Functional network organization of the human brain. *Neuron*, 72, 665–78.

46. Fox, M.D. and Greicius, M. (2010). Clinical applications of resting state functional connectivity. *Frontiers in Systems Neuroscience*, 4, 19.

47. Smith, S.M., Fox, P.T., Miller, K.L., *et al.* (2009). Correspondence of the brain's functional architecture during activation and rest. *Proceedings of the National Academy of Sciences of the United States of America*, 106, 13040–5.

48. Crossley, N.A., Mechelli, A., Vértes, P.E., *et al.* (2013). Cognitive relevance of the community structure of the human brain functional coactivation network. *Proceedings of the National Academy of Sciences of the United States of America*, 110, 11583–8.

49. Vincent, J.L., Patel, G.H., Fox, M.D., *et al.* (2007). Intrinsic functional architecture in the anaesthetized monkey brain. *Nature*, 447, 83–6.

50. Adachi, Y., Osada, T., Sporns, O., *et al.* (2012). Functional connectivity between anatomically unconnected areas is shaped by collective network-level effects in the macaque cortex. *Cerebral Cortex*, 22, 1586–92.

51. Honey, C.J., Sporns, O., Cammoun, L., *et al.* (2009). Predicting human resting-state functional connectivity from structural connectivity. *Proceedings of the National Academy of Sciences of the United States of America*, 106, 2035–40.

52. Hermundstad, A.M., Bassett, D.S., Brown, K.S., *et al.* (2013). Structural foundations of resting-state and task-based functional connectivity in the human brain. *Proceedings of the National Academy of Sciences of the United States of America*, 110, 6169–74.

53. van den Heuvel, M., Mandl, R., Luigjes, J., and Pol, H.H. (2008). Microstructural organization of the cingulum tract and the level of default mode functional connectivity. *Journal of Neuroscience*, 28, 10844–51.

54. Johnston, J.M., Vaishnavi, S.N., Smyth, M.D., *et al.* (2008). Loss of resting interhemispheric functional connectivity after complete section of the corpus callosum. *Journal of Neuroscience*, 28, 6453–8.

55. Honey, C.J., Kötter, R., Breakspear, M., and Sporns, O. (2007). Network structure of cerebral cortex shapes functional connectivity on multiple time scales. *Proceedings of the National Academy of Sciences of the United States of America*, 104, 10240–5.

56. Deco, G., Jirsa, V., McIntosh, A.R., Sporns, O., and Kötter, R. (2009). Key role of coupling, delay, and noise in resting brain fluctuations. *Proceedings of the National Academy of Sciences of the United States of America*, 106, 10302–7.

57. Hansen, E.C., Battaglia, D., Spiegler, A., Deco, G., and Jirsa, V.K. (2015). Functional connectivity dynamics: modeling the switching behavior of the resting state. *Neuroimage*, 105, 525–35.

58. Deco, G., Jirsa, V.K., and McIntosh, A.R. (2011). Emerging concepts for the dynamical organization of resting-state activity in the brain. *Nature Reviews Neuroscience*, 12, 43–56.

59. Abdelnour, F., Voss, H.U., and Raj, A. (2014). Network diffusion accurately models the relationship between structural and functional brain connectivity networks. *Neuroimage*, 90, 335–47.

60. Mišić, B., Betzel, R.F., Nematzadeh, A., *et al.* (2015). Cooperative and competitive spreading dynamics on the human connectome. *Neuron*, 86, 1518–29.

61. Goñi, J., van den Heuvel, M.P., Avena-Koenigsberger, A., *et al.* (2014). Resting-brain functional connectivity predicted by analytic measures of network communication. *Proceedings of the National Academy of Sciences of the United States of America*, 111, 833–8.

62. Hutchison, R.M., Womelsdorf, T., Allen, E.A., *et al.* (2013). Dynamic functional connectivity: promise, issues, and interpretations. *Neuroimage*, 80, 360–78.

63. Zalesky, A., Fornito, A., Cocchi, L., Gollo, L.L., and Breakspear, M. (2014). Time-resolved resting-state brain networks. *Proceedings of the National Academy of Sciences of the United States of America*, 111, 10341–6.

64. Allen, E.A., Damaraju, E., Plis, S.M., Erhardt, E.B., Eichele, T., and Calhoun, V.D. (2014). Tracking whole-brain connectivity dynamics in the resting state. *Cerebral Cortex*, 24, 663–76.

65. Sporns, O. (2013). Network attributes for segregation and integration in the human brain. *Current Opinion in Neurobiology*, 23, 162–71.

66. Betzel, R.F., Fukushima, M., He, Y., Zuo, X.N., and Sporns, O. (2016). Dynamic fluctuations coincide with periods of high and low modularity in resting-state functional brain networks. *NeuroImage*, 127, 287–97.

67. Medaglia, J.D., Lynall, M.E., and Bassett, D.S. (2015). Cognitive network neuroscience. *Journal of Cognitive Neuroscience*, 27, 1471–91.

68. Bassett, D.S., Wymbs, N.F., Rombach, M.P., Porter, M.A., Mucha, P.J., and Grafton, S.T. (2013). Task-based core-periphery organization of human brain dynamics. *PLoS Computational Biology*, 9, e1003171.

69. Cole, M.W., Reynolds, J.R., Power, J.D., Repovs, G., Anticevic, A., and Braver, T.S. (2013). Multi-task connectivity reveals flexible hubs for adaptive task control. *Nature Neuroscience*, 16, 1348–55.

70. Cole, M.W., Bassett, D.S., Power, J.D., Braver, T.S., and Petersen, S.E. (2014). Intrinsic and task-evoked network architectures of the human brain. *Neuron*, 83, 238–51.

71. Gonzalez-Castillo, J., Hoy, C.W., Handwerker, D.A., *et al.* (2015). Tracking ongoing cognition in individuals using brief, whole-brain functional connectivity patterns. *Proceedings of the National Academy of Sciences of the United States of America*, 112, 8762–7.

72. Hagmann, P., Sporns, O., Madan, N., *et al.* (2010). White matter maturation reshapes structural connectivity in the late developing human brain. *Proceedings of the National Academy of Sciences of the United States of America*, 107, 19067–72.

73. Fair, D.A., Cohen, A.L., Power, J.D., *et al.* (2009). Functional brain networks develop from a 'local to distributed' organization. *PLoS Computational Biology*, 5, e1000381.

74. Cao, M., Wang, J.H., Dai, Z.J., *et al.* (2014). Topological organization of the human brain functional connectome across the lifespan. *Developmental Cognitive Neuroscience*, 7, 76–93.

75. Zhao, T., Cao, M., Niu, H., *et al.* (2015). Age-related changes in the topological organization of the white matter structural connectome across the human lifespan. *Human Brain Mapping*, 36, 3777–92.

76. Betzel, R.F., Byrge, L., He, Y., Goñi, J., Zuo, X.N., and Sporns, O. (2014). Changes in structural and functional connectivity among resting-state networks across the human lifespan. *Neuroimage*, 102, 345–57.

77. Fornito, A., Zalesky, A., and Breakspear, M. (2015). The connectomics of brain disorders. *Nature Reviews Neuroscience*, 16, 159–72.

78. Stam, C.J. (2014). Modern network science of neurological disorders. *Nature Reviews Neuroscience*, 15, 683–95.

79. Bullmore, E.T., Fletcher, P., and Jones, P.B. (2009). Why psychiatry can't afford to be neurophobic. *British Journal of Psychiatry*, 194, 293–5.

80. Rehme, A.K. and Grefkes, C. (2013). Cerebral network disorders after stroke: evidence from imaging-based connectivity analyses of active and resting brain states in humans. *Journal of Physiology*, 591, 17–31.

81. Tijms, B.M., Wink, A.M., de Haan, W., *et al.* (2013). Alzheimer's disease: connecting findings from graph theoretical studies of brain networks. *Neurobiology of Aging*, 34, 2023–36.

82. Diessen, E., Diederen, S.J., Braun, K.P., Jansen, F.E., and Stam, C.J. (2013). Functional and structural brain networks in epilepsy: what have we learned? *Epilepsia*, 54, 1855–65.

83. von Monakow, C. (1969). Diaschisis. In: Pribram, K.H. (ed.) *Brain and behaviour Vol.I: mood, states and mind*. Penguin Books, Baltimore, MD. pp. 27–36.

84. Croft, J.J., Higham, D.J., Bosnell, R., *et al.* (2011). Network analysis detects changes in the contralesional hemisphere following stroke. *Neuroimage*, 54, 161–9.

85. Stern, Y. (2002). What is cognitive reserve? Theory and research application of the reserve concept. *Journal of the International Neuropsychological Society*, 8, 448–60.

86. Tononi, G., Sporns, O., and Edelman, G.M. (1999). Measures of degeneracy and redundancy in biological networks. *Proceedings of the National Academy of Sciences of the United States of America*, 96, 3257–62.

87. Price, C.J. and Friston, K.J. (2002). Degeneracy and cognitive anatomy. *Trends in Cognitive Sciences*, 6, 416–21.

88. Crossley, N.A., Mechelli, A., Scott, J., *et al.* (2014). The hubs of the human connectome are generally implicated in the anatomy of brain disorders. *Brain*, 137, 2382–95.

89. Zhou, J. and Seeley, W.W. (2014). Network dysfunction in Alzheimer's disease and frontotemporal dementia: implications for psychiatry. *Biological Psychiatry*, 75, 565–73.

90. Fornito, A. and Bullmore, E.T. (2015). Reconciling abnormalities of brain network structure and function in schizophrenia. *Current Opinion in Neurobiology*, 30, 44–50.

# 14

# Neurotransmitters and signalling

*Trevor Sharp*

## Introduction

The concept of signalling from one neuron to another began to form by the end of the nineteenth century when it was recognized from the histological work of Golgi and Ramon y Cajal that nerve cells were discrete entities and linked by specialized contacts, for which Sherrington coined the term 'synapse'. It took another half century for scientists to finally agree that information passes between neurons principally through the movement across synapses of chemicals, and not electrical current. Today changes in chemical transmission at brain synapses are accepted as being key to both successful drug treatment and the cause of many forms of psychiatric illness. This chapter focuses on fundamental aspects of chemical transmission and describes some recent advances relevant to psychiatry that may indicate the direction of future research.

Seminal work on the autonomic nervous system and glandular secretions around the turn of the twentieth century was conducted by pioneering physiologists like John Langley and his student Thomas Elliott. It culminated in studies in the 1920s by Otto Loewi and then Henry Dale who identified what is often cited as the first neurotransmitter—acetylcholine—the chemical that was released on stimulation of the vagus nerve to inhibit the heart. Subsequently, in 1946, Ulf von Euler reported the identification of the monoamine noradrenaline as the other key autonomic transmitter [1, 2]. Today evidence suggests that, in the brain (and peripheral nervous system), there are many tens, if not hundreds, of molecules that are involved in chemical transmission at synapses. These molecules include acetylcholine and monoamines [noradrenaline, dopamine, and 5-hydroxytryptamine (5-HT; serotonin)], certain amino acids (especially glutamate and GABA), and peptides, as well as specific purines, trophic factors, inflammatory mediators (chemokines and cytokines), lipid-like agents (endocannabinoids), and even gases [nitric oxide (NO)]. Examples of molecules that serve neurotransmitter functions in the brain are listed in Table 14.1. This list is not exhaustive, and more are likely to be discovered.

## Basic principles of chemical transmission

Typically, a molecule is classified as a neurotransmitter if it is localized in neurons, released from nerve terminals (and often soma and dendrites as well) on membrane depolarization, and exerts physiological and molecular effects through acting on postsynaptic receptors. However, the degree to which a particular molecule satisfies these criteria may vary. For example, the term 'neurotransmitter' was once commonly used to define those molecules that exert fast synaptic effects (glutamate, GABA), whereas molecules that exerted slower synaptic effects were often termed 'neuromodulators' (for example, monoamines and peptides). These distinctions are less useful today (and will not be used here) because it is recognized that many transmitter molecules are capable of exerting both fast and slow synaptic effects. For example, both glutamate and

**Table 14.1** Examples of neurotransmitters in the brain

| Chemical class | Example |
| --- | --- |
| Amines | Dopamine<br>Noradrenaline<br>5-hydroxytryptamine (5-HT)<br>Histamine<br>Melatonin<br>Acetylcholine |
| Amino acids | γ-aminobutyric acid (GABA)<br>Glutamate<br>Glycine |
| Neuropeptides | Substance P<br>Leu- and met-enkephalin<br>Galanin<br>Orexin |
| Purines | Adenosine<br>Adenosine triphosphate (ATP) |
| Neurotrophic factors[#] | Neurotrophins (for example, BDNF, NGF)<br>Insulin-like growth factor (IGF)<br>Vascular endothelial growth factor (VEGF) |
| Cytokines[*] | Interleukin-1 (IL-1)<br>Tumour necrosis factor α (TNFα) |
| Chemokines[*] | CC chemokines [for example, interleukin-8 (IL-8)]<br>CXC chemokines |
| Endocannabinoids[#] | Anandamide<br>2-arachidonyl-glycerol (2-AG) |
| Gases[#] | Nitric oxide (NO)<br>Carbon monoxide (CO) |

[*] Putative class of neurotransmitters.
[#] Retrograde messengers.

GABA exert fast and slow synaptic effects, depending on which of their receptors they interact with. Moreover, in contrast to the classical view of neurotransmission in which information passes from the presynaptic to the postsynaptic neuron in an 'anterograde' direction, it is now recognized that certain molecules transfer information at a synapse in a 'retrograde' direction. In this case, the molecules are located in the postsynaptic neuron, and, when their synthesis is activated, the molecules diffuse back across the synapse to act presynaptically.

The general principles of chemical transmission at central synapses are similar for most neurotransmitter molecules. The differences in the detail will be illustrated by transmission mechanisms for small neurotransmitters such as monoamines and amino acids, compared to larger neurotransmitters such as peptides (Fig. 14.1) [3].

## Small neurotransmitters

Typically, small neurotransmitter molecules are synthesized at the nerve terminal by one or a few enzymatic steps, and then packaged in small membrane-bound vesicles via vesicular transporters (proton-coupled), prior to release into the synapse. The latter is triggered via a calcium-dependent mechanism on the arrival of a depolarizing action potential; this release process, referred to as

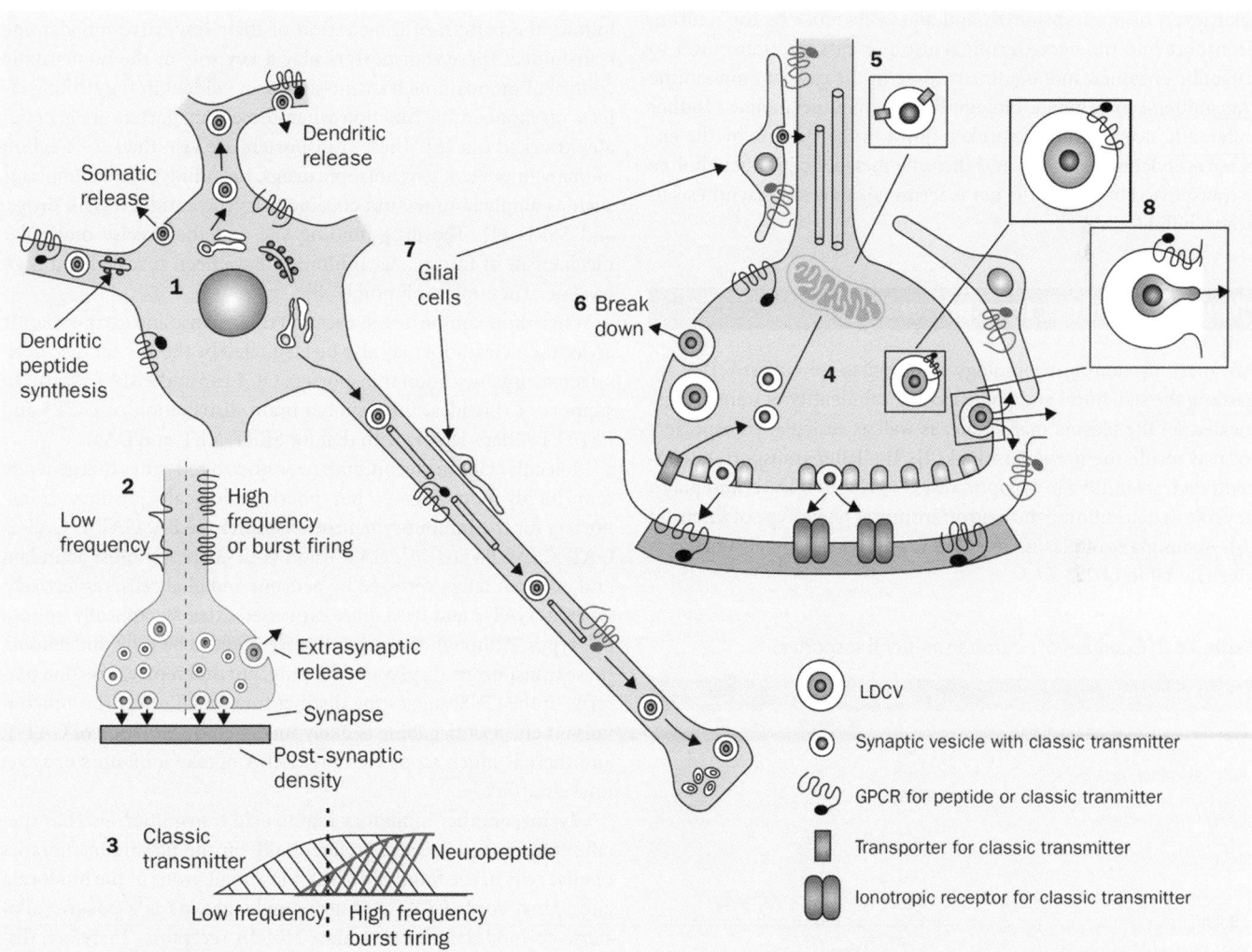

**Fig. 14.1** Summary of the principal steps involved in chemical neurotransmission at CNS synapses. Neuropeptides are synthesized in the cell body and then packaged in large, dense core vesicles (LDCVs) that are transported into axons and dendrites (1). Small 'classic' neurotransmitters (for example, monoamines and amino acids) are synthesized at the nerve terminal and stored in synaptic vesicles, and released into the synaptic cleft. Evidence for the co-release of small transmitters is now clear (2). LDCVs contain proteolytic enzymes (convertases) that generate the active neuropeptide from the precursor. Neurotransmitter receptors are either of the G protein-coupled (metabotropic) or ligand-gated ion channel (ionotropic) type and are present on cell soma, dendrites, axons, and nerve endings (1, 4). The small neurotransmitters are released during low- and high-frequency firing, whereas neuropeptides are preferentially released under burst or high-frequency firing (2–4). Small transmitters have reuptake mechanisms (transporters) at both the plasma membrane and the vesicle membrane (5), which terminate neurotransmitter action and allow recycling (4). In contrast, neuropeptides are broken down by extracellular peptidases (6), and replacement occurs via axonal transport. Glial cells can express neurotransmitter receptors and transporters (7). Receptors are trafficked to and from the cell membrane by G protein-interacting proteins (8).

exocytosis, involves a complex machinery of 20–30 presynaptic proteins. After release, the neurotransmitter diffuses across the synapse to interact with specific receptors localized on the membrane of the postsynaptic neuron to trigger electrical and/or biochemical changes. Small neurotransmitters are also released from the soma and dendrites of neurons, one purpose being to interact with presynaptic receptors that signal negative feedback to the neuron; these receptors are often referred to as autoreceptors, and they are usually also located on the nerve terminals.

Typically, once released, the small neurotransmitters are selectively taken up by another type of transporter (sodium-coupled) located in the plasma membrane of the nerve terminal or neighbouring cells (neurons or glial cells). This transport helps terminate transmission at the postsynaptic receptor, maintains low extracellular levels of the transmitter, and allows its reuse by the neuron. Transport into the nerve terminal also presents the transmitter to catabolic enzymes, monoamine oxidase in the case of monoamine transmitters, to generate biologically inactive metabolites. Rather differently, acetylcholine is broken down in the synapse by the enzyme acetylcholinesterase, and then the metabolic product choline is transported back into the nerve terminal, allowing resynthesis to acetylcholine.

## Neurotransmitter transporters

Advances in cloning technology have led to new discoveries regarding the structural and pharmacological identity of transporters located on the plasma membrane, as well as vesicular transporters located inside the nerve terminal [4]. The latter transporters concentrate transmitters in synaptic vesicles prior to release, and play a key role in determining the neurotransmitter phenotype of a neuron [5]. A summary of plasma membrane and vesicular transporters is given in Table 14.2.

**Table 14.2** Examples of neurotransmitter transporters

| Neurotransmitter | Transporter |
| --- | --- |
| *Plasma membrane transporters* | |
| Dopamine | DAT |
| Noradrenaline | NET |
| 5-HT | SERT |
| GABA | |
| | GAT-1 |
| | GAT-2 |
| | GAT-3 |
| | BGT-1 (primarily in kidney) |
| Glutamate | EAAT-1 (GLAST1) |
| | EAAT-2 (GLT-1) |
| | EAAT-3 (EAAC1) |
| | EAAT-4 |
| | EAAT-5 |
| Glycine | GLYT-1 |
| | GLYT-2 |
| Acetylcholine (choline) | CHT |
| *Vesicular transporters* | |
| Monoamines (dopamine, | VMAT1 |
| noradrenaline, 5-HT, histamine) | VMAT2 |
| GABA | VGAT |
| Glutamate | VGLUT1 |
| | VGLUT2 |
| | VGLUT3 |
| Acetylcholine | VAchT |

### Plasma membrane transporters

The solute carrier (SLC) superfamily of transporters is the second largest family of membrane proteins in the human genome (approximately 52 families, around 400 individual members), after G protein-coupled receptors (GPCRs). These transporters selectively transport into and out of cells a large diversity of solutes, ranging from inorganic ions to amino acids and more complex molecules like haem.

The SLC6 family comprises four subfamilies that form high-affinity and selective transporters for GABA, glycine, and neutral amino acids, as well as the monoamines dopamine (DAT), noradrenaline (NET), and 5-HT (SERT). The latter three transporters have been identified and sequenced, and investigated in detail at the molecular level. Their distribution within the brain closely follows the pattern of innervation of their respective monoamine transmitter. These transporters play a key role in the homeostatic control of monoamine transmission, as is evident in the striking effects on monoamine function when these transporters are genetically knocked out [6]. These transporters are also the site of action of many important psychotropic drugs, including psychostimulants such as amphetamines and cocaine, tricyclic antidepressant drugs, and SSRIs [4]. The drug-binding site and the precise molecular mechanism of transporter inhibition have been revealed at a high level of structural resolution [7, 8].

When monoamines are in excess at the synapse and extra-synaptic areas, their clearance may also be facilitated by the low-affinity, non-selective organic cation transporters OCT1–3 and PMAT [9, 10]. In support of this idea, the regional brain distribution of OCT3 and PMAT overlaps largely with that for SERT, NET, and DAT.

Molecular cloning techniques have uncovered genes that generate four highly homologous, but pharmacologically distinct, transporters for the inhibitory neurotransmitter GABA: GAT-1, GAT-2, GAT-3, and BTG-1 [6]. GAT-1 and GAT-3 are the most abundant and preferentially expressed by neurons and glial cells, respectively, whereas GAT-2 and BTG-1 are expressed extra-synaptically by both cell types. Although their significance is yet to be fully understood, these transporters display overlapping, but different, expression patterns in the CNS, suggesting distinct functional roles. The anticonvulsant effect of tiagabine is likely mediated by blockade of GAT-1, and there is much scope for new GABA uptake inhibitors of as yet unclear utility.

Glycine, another inhibitory amino acid transmitter, also has specific transporters located preferentially on the plasma membranes of glial cells in the forebrain (GLYT1) and neurons of the hindbrain and spinal cord (GLYT2). Interestingly, glycine is a positive allosteric co-modulator of glutamate NMDA receptors. Therefore, disruption of GLYT1 glycine transport blockade may offer a means to facilitate the functioning of the NMDA receptor without incurring excitotoxic effects [4]. The antipsychotic potential of glycine transport inhibitors has been under investigation, because this action is associated with procognitive effects and the symptoms of schizophrenia appear linked to low NMDA receptor function [11]. GLYT2 is expressed by glycinergic neurons and thought to be important for the delivery of glycine into nerve terminals for loading into synaptic vesicles.

Four transporters for the excitatory amino acid neurotransmitter glutamate have been cloned: EAAT1 (excitatory amino acid transporter 1; synonym GLAST), EAAT2 (GLT1), EAAT3 (EAAC1), EAAT4, and EAAT5 [5]. These transporters are located on both neurons (predominantly EAAT3/4/5) and glial cells (predominantly EAAT1/2) and serve to maintain low extracellular concentrations of glutamate, as well as provide a source of intracellular glutamate for metabolism. Pharmacological blockade of glutamate transport may lead to cognition enhancement and other potentially useful therapeutic effects but holds the risk of excitotoxicity, whereas pharmacologically enhanced EAAT expression appears to be neuroprotective [12]. EAAT inhibitors are currently in development, but few brain penetrant or selective agents have been identified thus far.

### Vesicular transporters

Vesicular transporters facilitate the movement of neurotransmitters from the cytoplasm to be concentrated within synaptic vesicles. This transport is often driven by a proton gradient established by an adenosine triphosphate (ATP)-dependent proton pump that acidifies the secretory vesicles. There are two homologous vesicular monoamine transporters—VMAT2 is present in central and peripheral neurons and transports dopamine, noradrenaline, and 5-HT, as well as histamine, into vesicles, whereas VMAT1 is an integral protein in the membrane of secretory vesicles of peripheral neuroendocrine and endocrine cells. Reserpine is a blocker of VMAT and causes depletion of monoamines, and the drug's tranquillizer effects are directly linked to this action. Acetylcholine is loaded into synaptic vesicles by a distinct transporter, VAchT.

Three homologous vesicular transporters for glutamate VGLUT1, VGLUT2, and VGLUT3 have been identified and characterized. While all possess similar molecular properties, they have differential expression patterns, with VGLUT1 arising predominantly from cortical neurons, VGLUT2 from subcortical neurons, and VGLUT3 largely from midbrain neurons [5]. The vesicular GABA transporter is VGAT (also termed vesicular inhibitory amino acid transporter, VIAAT), and this transports GABA or glycine into synaptic vesicles. Loss of VGAT causes a drastic reduction in the release of not only GABA, but also glycine, indicating that glycinergic neurons do not express a separate vesicular transporter for glycine. The vesicular nucleotide transporter (VNUT) is a recent member of this transporter family and functions to load synaptic vesicles with ATP.

There is long-standing evidence that the release of one or more neuropeptides accompanies the release of classical small-molecule neurotransmitters (Fig. 14.1). Interestingly, recent studies based on the localization of vesicular transporters suggest that classical small-molecule neurotransmitters are also co-released. For instance, findings that VGLUT3 is localized in 5-HT-containing neurons and appears to be functional [13] raises the possibility that the release of glutamate contributes to the actions of 5-HT neurons that were previously attributed to 5-HT itself. This is not an isolated case. Neurons previously thought to release only glutamate, acetylcholine, dopamine, or histamine have been found to also release the major inhibitory neurotransmitter GABA [14]. Such evidence supports the emerging view that neuronal communication based on using more than one classical neurotransmitter is prevalent throughout the CNS.

## Neuropeptides

Following the chemical identification of the neuropeptide substance P in 1971, evidence has accumulated that numerous peptides play neurotransmitter roles in the brain [3]. Some examples are shown in Table 14.3. The properties of peptidergic synapses are in many ways different from those of synapses that utilize small neurotransmitters. The neuropeptides comprise 3–100 amino acids and, together with other putative signalling peptides, such as growth factors and cytokines, are synthesized in the nucleus by deoxyribonucleic acid (DNA) transcription, followed by translation from messenger ribonucleic acid (mRNA) into precursor polypeptides (Fig. 14.1). These precursors typically undergo extensive post-translational processing that includes cleavage into smaller peptides by endopeptidases, as well as other enzymatic modifications. The precursor peptides usually contain an N-terminal signal sequence that directs the transport of newly synthesized protein to the lumen of the endoplasmic reticulum, and then the Golgi complex where it is packaged into vesicles (termed 'large, dense core vesicles' due to their appearance under the electron microscope) that are transported along the axon to the synapse. This obviates the need for neuropeptide vesicular transporters.

Proteolytic processing of a single precursor peptide often generates not one, but a family of biologically active peptides, although the proteolytic steps may be tissue-specific. The opioid peptides provide one of the best worked-out examples of this form of processing. Pro-opiomelanocortin (POMC) is a hypothalamic precursor opioid peptide whose structure contains sequences for adrenocorticotropic hormone (ACTH), α-melanocyte-stimulating hormone (α-MSH), and β-endorphin. In the anterior lobe of the pituitary gland, POMC is processed to form ACTH, while in the intermediate lobe, POMC is processed to form α-MSH and β-endorphin. On the other

**Table 14.3** Examples of families of neuropeptides

| | |
|---|---|
| Opioid peptides | Leu-enkephalin
Met-enkephalin
Dynorphin
β-endorphin
Nociceptin |
| Tachykinins | Substance P
Neurokinin A
Neurokinin B |
| Hypothalamic-releasing factors | Thyrotrophin-releasing factor (TRH)
Corticotrophin-releasing factor (CRF)
Growth hormone-releasing hormone (GHRH)
Somatostatin |
| Gut–brain peptides | Cholecystokinin (CCK)
Galanin
Insulin
Neurotensin
Neuropeptide Y (NPY)
Vasointestinal polypeptide (VIP) |
| Other peptides | Bradykinin
Calcitonin gene-related peptide
Melanin-concentrating hormone (MCH)
Melanocortin
Orexin
Oxytocin
Vasopressin |

hand, post-translational processing of the opioid precursor peptide proenkephalin gives rise to multiple copies of the pentapeptide met-enkephalin, as well as a copy of leu-enkephalin, while a third opioid precursor prodynorphin gives rise to dynorphin. In total, the three separate opioid peptide genes give rise to at least 18 endogenous peptides with opiate-like activity.

Many proteolytic enzymes involved in the processing of neuropeptides have been cloned and characterized, including prohormone convertases that produce striking phenotypic effects when genetically manipulated in mutant mouse models [15]. The therapeutic utility of pharmacological manipulation of neuropeptide synthesis and degradation in the brain has yet to be fully realized. However, the success of inhibitors of the prohormone convertase that synthezises angiotensin in the periphery [angiotensin-converting enzyme (ACE) inhibitors], for the treatment of hypertension, sets an important precedent.

In addition to enzymic processing, another mechanism to generate neuropeptide diversity is through alternative ribonucleic acid (RNA) splicing of a single gene. For example, in the case of tachykinins, alternative splicing of preprotachykinin gene A mRNA results in three splice variants which, after translation and post-translational processing, collectively generate the five biologically active peptides of the tachykinin family (including substance P).

To date, there is little evidence that neuropeptides are cleared from the synapse by transporters in the plasma membrane, indicating that they are not recycled after release. Rather, evidence suggests that their action is terminated by peptidases located on extracellular membranes. Thus, replenishment of neuropeptides during high levels of synaptic activity is dependent on the proteolytic enzymes that generate the active peptides in the neurons.

As noted, a feature of most, if not all, neuropeptides is their co-localization with classic neurotransmitters. Some of the best examples include GABA/dynorphin co-localization in movement control pathways (striatonigral neurons), cholecystokinin (CCK)/dopamine in reward pathways (mesoaccumbens neurons), and glutamate/substance P in pain pathways (dorsal root ganglion neurons). The functional significance of this co-localization is not fully clear, but evidence suggests that peptide release requires higher frequencies of neuronal discharge than classical transmitters, and once released, the neuropeptide either facilitates or opposes the function of the co-localized transmitter [3]. In a recent example, co-localization between 5-HT and galanin in midbrain raphe neurons was investigated to reveal an action of the peptide on 5-HT feedback mechanisms. This knowledge has been exploited to develop galanin ligands that are under development as novel antidepressant strategies [16].

## Neurotrophic factors

Neurotrophic factors are brain peptides that were originally recognized for their role in supporting growth, differentiation, and survival of neurons but today these molecules are thought to possess many of the properties of neurotransmitters, including neuronal localization and release and an ability to modulate synaptic function. In addition, there is evidence that neurotrophic factors signal in a retrograde fashion (see later). Neurotrophic factors are currently named according to the action with which they were originally characterized [brain-derived neurotrophic factor (BDNF), nerve growth factor (NGF)], and they comprise many families [17].

Certain features distinguish neurotrophic factors from neuropeptides. In particular, neurotrophic factors are larger molecules; for example, BDNF has a molecular size of 14 kDa, whereas neuropeptides are typically much smaller peptides. Also, while neuropeptides signal via GPCRs, neurotrophic factors signal via direct activation of a class of transmembrane-spanning proteins called protein tyrosine kinases (Trk receptors), of which four types have been identified so far (TrkA, TrkB, TrkC, and p75). In some cases, the neurotrophic factor receptor and protein tyrosine kinase reside in the same protein, while in other cases, the receptor recruits an intracellular protein tyrosine kinase. Specific neurotrophic factors signal via specific protein kinases (for example, NGF–TrkA, BDNF–TrkB). Activation of the protein tyrosine kinase leads to the phosphorylation of proteins via their tyrosine residues and the triggering of signalling cascades that produce not only trophic effects, but also changes in synaptic transmission.

Much recent interest in neurotrophic factors derives from findings that they regulate synaptic transmission in the adult brain and that neurotrophic factor expression can be modulated through interactions with monoamine and amino acid neurotransmitters. For example, repeated administration with monoamine-targeted antidepressants increases BDNF expression in animal models and depressed patients, whereas decreases in BDNF have been linked to depression. These findings have informed a popular hypothesis that changes in neural plasticity at many levels (both BDNF-dependent and non-dependent) are important to the symptoms of depression, as well as the relief of these symptoms by antidepressant drug treatment [18, 19]. A more advanced version of this hypothesis combines with neuropsychological theories to suggest that increased neural plasticity at the molecular and cellular levels arms key neural circuits with the capacity to process emotional information and re-establish positive emotional associations that result in improved mood [20].

## Chemokines and cytokines

Chemokines and cytokines comprise large families of homologous small proteins (6–10 kDa) and differ from neuropeptides and neurotrophic factors in that they are key signalling molecules of the immune system. However, these molecules and some of their receptors are also present in the brain in both glial cells and neurons, raising the possibility that they might also have neurotransmitter-like functions. Although the evidence is incomplete, data show that chemokine and cytokine molecules are synthesized in the brain and have several of the characteristics that define neurotransmitters, including interaction with receptors and modulation of release of other neurotransmitters or neuropeptides [21]. This suggests that chemokine and cytokine signalling may have a role in neuronal and glial cell signalling that is distinct from their role in inflammatory processes. On the other hand, it is quite clear that inflammatory and immunologic changes can trigger responses that play a role in CNS protection, but also a role in CNS injury.

This local presence of chemokine and cytokine signalling provides a route of communication between the immune system and the CNS, but there are many others, including several pathways through which peripheral inflammatory signals can be transmitted to the brain [22]. For example, cytokines may pass directly into the brain via leaky regions in the blood–brain barrier and also bind to peripheral autonomic nerves such as the vagus nerve, resulting in modulation of afferent CNS inputs. A dysfunctional interaction between the immune system and the peripheral inflammatory response, in particular, is presently considered an important contributor to the pathophysiology of a number of psychiatric disorders, including major depression. Moreover, the irrefutable evidence of immunological and CNS interactions has challenged the previously held belief of CNS immune privilege, such that autoimmune mechanisms are emerging as a pathophysiology disease mechanism, as evidenced in recent discoveries of circulating NMDA receptor antibodies in some patients with schizophrenia. The development of drug tools and biologics (for example, antibodies) to target cytokine and chemokine mechanisms is an intense area of current neuroscience research.

## Retrograde messengers

Whereas classical neurotransmitters and neuropeptides are generally considered to signal in an 'anterograde' direction (that is, presynaptic to postsynaptic), it is now recognized that certain brain molecules signal information at a synapse in a 'retrograde' direction. They are released from the postsynaptic neuron to act on the presynaptic neuron. Molecules falling into this category include certain neurotrophic factors, gaseous molecules, and lipid messengers.

## Nitric oxide

One example of a retrograde messenger is the gaseous molecule NO that is produced in neurons from the amino acid *L*-arginine by a neuron-specific isoform of NO synthase (NOS). Some of the first evidence that NO might function as a chemical messenger in the brain came from findings that activation of glutamate NMDA receptors in the cerebellum caused the release of a diffusible messenger, which was subsequently identified as NO [23]. The current thinking is that increased activity at glutamatergic synapses triggers in postsynaptic neurons an NMDA-mediated, calcium-dependent activation of NOS. The resulting NO then diffuses back across the synapse to enhance presynaptic transmission. The latter occurs, at least in part, through NO acting on guanylate cyclase to increase the production of the second messenger cyclic guanosine monophosphate (cGMP). In postsynaptic neurons, NO also regulates certain protein kinase pathways and gene transcription factors, and changes cell signalling events by *S*-nitrosylation.

Since NOS is abundant and widely distributed in the CNS, NO signalling is likely to contribute to many brain functions. Indeed, on the basis of studies on the effects of NO donors and the pharmacological and genetic modulation of NOS, increased NO production is associated with a range of CNS functions, including improved cognition and an associated induction and maintenance of synaptic plasticity, and NO may be neuroprotective under some conditions [24]. However, because excess NO has neurotoxic potential, and because of the difficulty of delivering NO to the CNS without inducing side effects through the many actions of NO on peripheral tissues, the development of NO-based therapies for the treatment of CNS disorders has yet to reach fruition.

## Endocannabinoids

Another example of retrograde signalling is by endocannabinoids [25]. These are a recently discovered family of naturally occurring lipids (including anandamide and 2-arachidonoylglycerol) that interact with cell surface receptors targeted by the psychotropic agent $\Delta^9$-tetrahydrocannabinol (THC). The latter is the principal biologically active constituent of the cannabis plant [26]. In essence, endocannabinoids appear to be to THC and cannabinoid receptors what opioid peptides are to morphine and opiate receptors.

The current thinking is that endocannabinoids are synthesized enzymatically on demand within the postsynaptic neuron and, once produced, diffuse across the synapse in a retrograde direction. Endocannabinoids then suppress neurotransmitter release through activation of a presynaptic $CB_1$ receptor, which is the main type of cannabinoid receptor in the brain (analogous in terms of structure and function to opiate receptors, but quite distinct pharmacologically).

The central actions of THC, including its psychotropic effects, nociception, increased appetite, and anti-emetic effects, are thought to be principally mediated by $CB_1$ receptors. Since $CB_1$ receptors have a powerful influence on synaptic transmission in the brain and have limited distribution in the periphery (although $CB_2$ receptors are abundant in the immune system), drugs targeting these receptors and/or the enzymes involved in endocannabinoid synthesis and metabolism have interesting therapeutic possibilities. Indeed, $CB_1$ receptor agonist preparations are currently prescribed as analgesic and anti-emetic agents.

## Neurotransmitter receptors

Neurotransmitter receptors are located on the cell surface of both pre- and postsynaptic neurons and, as a general rule, can be divided into two main types; one activates an ion channel that is intrinsic to the receptor (ligand-gated ion channel—sometimes called an ionotropic receptor), and the other activates a guanosine triphosphate (GTP)-binding protein which acts as a transducer between the receptor and the effector system (GPCR—sometimes called a metabotropic receptor). As an exception to this general rule, certain trophic factors and cytokines directly activate protein tyrosine kinases, as noted above. In addition, steroid hormones signal in the brain by crossing the plasma membrane and activating receptors in the neuronal cytoplasm that translocate to the nucleus where they bind DNA and function as transcription factors.

Ligand-gated ion channels typically comprise a multimeric plasma membrane receptor complex (4–5 subunits, each with four transmembrane-spanning domains) that gate the influx of ions to evoke fast changes in synaptic signalling. For instance, nicotinic, $5-HT_3$, $GABA_A$, and glycine receptors are pentameric in their subunit composition; these receptors are often termed 'Cys-loop' receptors due to a loop of amino acid residues formed by a disulfide bond in the extracellular domain. GPCRs comprise a superfamily of single proteins (seven transmembrane-spanning domains) that evoke slower changes in synaptic signalling through the generation of second messengers and interactions with intracellular signalling pathways.

A remarkable advance in molecular neuropharmacology in the last 20 years has been the discovery of huge diversity in neurotransmitter receptors. This complexity takes the form of not only several hundred of GPCRs [27], but also considerable heterogeneity in ligand-gated ion channels produced through the assembly of multiple receptor subunits [28, 29]. Receptors were once classified according to their pharmacological properties, but today receptor classification is based on a combination of pharmacological, functional, and structural properties. It is now evident that most, and probably all, neurotransmitters have more than one receptor type. As a consequence of their receptor diversity, individual neurotransmitters are conferred multiple downstream signalling properties. Typically, as soon as neurotransmitter receptors are identified, their distribution within the brain (and other organs and tissues) is established, and then a combination of pharmacological and genetic approaches are used to obtain an understanding of their function, which can then aid the development of novel drug therapies. Some examples are shown in Table 14.4, and more detailed information is available elsewhere [30].

## Ligand-gated ion channels

The amino acids glutamate and GABA are, respectively, the principal excitatory and inhibitory transmitters in the brain and exert their fast synaptic effects via ligand-gated ion channels. Acetylcholine (nicotinic receptors) and ATP ($P_{2X}$ receptors) transmitters also signal fast transmission via ligand-gated ion channels. The 5-$HT_3$ receptor is the only ligand-gated ion channel among the many monoamine receptors, and none exists for neuropeptides.

## Ligand-gated ion channels for glutamate

Glutamate elicits fast excitatory effects by activating ligand-gated ion channels, and there are three types: α-amino-3-hydroxy-5-methyl-4-isoxazolepropionic acid (AMPA) receptors, NMDA receptors, and less abundant kainate receptors. These receptors are named according to their preferred synthetic agonist, and gate cations (sodium, potassium, and calcium) with varying degrees of selectivity. Each receptor is assembled as a tetramer, which can comprise a combination of subunits, and this generates additional heterogeneity. For instance, AMPA receptors are formed from a combination of four subunits (GluA1–4), and NMDA receptors from two subunits (GluN1–2). There are a large number of naturally occurring variants of both AMPA and NMDA subunits generated through RNA editing and alternative splicing (Table 14.4).

The pharmacological and functional significance of this complexity is not yet fully clear, although evidence suggests that different receptor assemblies may confer distinct pharmacological and biophysical properties on the receptor [30]. For example, recent data suggest that changes in AMPA receptor subunit composition cause differences in calcium ion permeability and change synaptic efficacy [29].

In addition to a glutamate-binding site, both AMPA and NMDA receptors demonstrate allosteric modulatory sites, a feature common to many ligand-gated ion channels. Thus, in addition to glutamate, AMPA receptors are sensitive to 'AMPAkines', which comprise a chemically diverse group of exogenous agents that act at separate chemically sensitive site on the receptor. The result is potentiated AMPA receptor ion channel function and associated procognitive effects *in vivo* [31]. Non-glutamate sites on the NMDA receptor include a site for magnesium ions that is the source of a voltage-dependent NMDA receptor block, which requires membrane depolarization to open. In addition, the NMDA receptor has a positive allosteric modulatory site for glycine and *D*-serine, and another for polyamines such as spermidine. While glutamate is released from presynaptic terminals in a phasic, activity-dependent fashion, endogenous glycine, *D*-serine, and polyamines (likely arising from non-neuronal sources) are thought to act as extracellular modulators that are present at more constant levels. These allosteric sites are under investigation as possible sources of NMDA receptor modulatory agents that do not suffer the excitotoxic effects of agonists acting directly at the glutamate site [32]. Such agents include inhibitors of glycine reuptake and *D*-serine metabolism.

## Ligand-gated ion channels for GABA

GABA elicits fast inhibitory effects by activating the $GABA_A$ receptor, which is a ligand-gated ion channel that is selectively permeable to chloride ions. $GABA_A$ receptors are formed from five subunits, of which there are at least 19 types (α1–6, β1–3, γ1–3, ρ1–3, δ, ε, π, θ). Studies co-expressing different $GABA_A$ receptor subunits in simple cells, such as frog oocytes, indicate the potential for several hundreds, if not thousands, of functional $GABA_A$ receptor subunit combinations. However, findings on the distribution and abundance of $GABA_A$ receptor subunits in brain tissue indicate the likely presence of α, β, and γ subunits in the vast majority of receptors, and that the number of naturally occurring types of $GABA_A$ receptors is of the order of ten or fewer [33]. As with the glutamate ionotropic receptors, $GABA_A$ receptors have a number of allosteric modulatory sites, and such sites are sensitive to a variety of pharmacological agents, including benzodiazepines, certain endogenous steroids, steroidal anaesthetic agents such as propofol, and alcohol (ethanol).

$GABA_A$ receptors are influenced by the binding of benzodiazepines, such as diazepam, and 'Z drugs', like zolpidem, which produce their anxiolytic and sedative effects via the benzodiazepine-binding site. Given the high chemical specificity of the benzodiazepine-binding site, there has been an extensive search for an endogenous ligand. This has led to the discovery of the 'endozepine', a diazepam-binding inhibitor, which is a peptide with many of the properties that would be predicted of an endogenous ligand at the benzodiazepine-binding site. This includes secretion (possibly from glial cells) and modulation of the $GABA_A$ receptor, although both positive and negative modulatory effects have been detected [34].

Genetic and pharmacological approaches have been used to identify the pharmacological significance of multiple $GABA_A$ receptor subtypes, and specifically to determine the functional significance of six variants of the α subunit, which is critical to the binding of benzodiazepines [28]. In particular, studies with point-mutated mice have revealed that the sedative effect of diazepam is mediated by α1-containing $GABA_A$ receptors, whereas the anxiolytic action is mediated by α2/α3-containing $GABA_A$ receptors. Moreover, findings that ligands with selective actions at α2- and/or α3-containing $GABA_A$ receptors display anxiolytic activity at doses lower than those that cause sedation [35]. This raises the possibility of interesting future drug therapies, for example drug treatments for anxiety disorder that have the anxiolytic effect of benzodiazepines, such as diazepam, but lack their unwanted adverse effects [36]. Interestingly, $\alpha 5$-containing $GABA_A$ receptors may be an important site of action of alcohol. The $GABA_A$ receptor subunit(s) targeted by steroids to produce CNS inhibitory effects of these agents are currently under investigation.

## G protein-coupled receptors

Almost all neurotransmitters, including glutamate and GABA, signal effects via GPCRs, and most neurotransmitters signal via more than one type of GPCRs. For example, the monoamine 5-HT possesses 14 receptor subtypes (comprising seven receptor families $5\text{-HT}_{1-7}$), 13 of which are GPCRs and one is a ligand-gated ion channel ($5\text{-HT}_3$). Each 5-HT GPCR has high affinity and selectivity for 5-HT, but individually the receptors are pharmacologically distinct, arise from different (but homologous) genes, and are formed from different protein sequences with different distributions and signalling effects [37]. Since several 5-HT GPCRs can co-localize at a single synapse, the signal received by a postsynaptic neuron may be quite complicated. This complexity for 5-HT can be seen in many other transmitters, including dopamine ($D_{1-5}$), glutamate ($mGluR_{1-8}$), noradrenaline ($\alpha_{1A,B,D}$, $\alpha_{2A,B,C}$, $\beta_{1-3}$), endocannabinoids ($CB_{1-2}$), and neuropeptides (Table 14.4).

Typically, GPCRs comprise a single membrane protein with seven transmembrane-spanning domains, an *N*-terminus facing the extracellular space, a *C*-terminus facing the cytoplasm, and several intracellular transmembrane domain linking loops. The *N*-terminus of some GPCRs ($mGluR_{1-8}$, $GABA_B$) contains the ligand-binding site, while for most GPCRs, the predicted ligand-binding site lies within the transmembrane domains. Both the *C*-terminus and the third transmembrane intracellular loops are phosphorylated by protein kinases, which can result in altered GPCR function, as well as trafficking to the plasma membrane. The third intracellular loop is the main site of G protein interaction.

## G proteins

Each G protein is a heterotrimer comprising $\alpha$, $\beta$, and $\gamma$ subunits that dissociate on binding of the ligand to the GPCR. On dissociation, the $\alpha$ subunit binds GTP and, through intrinsic GTPase activity, directly regulates a number of specific downstream effector enzymes and ion channels. The $\beta/\gamma$ subunits are also biologically active and regulate some of the same effector proteins.

There are four major types of G proteins—$G_s$, $G_i$, $G_q$, and $G_0$—that produce the following 'canonical' signalling effects, respectively: activation of adenylyl cyclase, inhibition of adenylyl cyclase, activation of phospholipase C (PLC), and interaction with calcium ion and potassium ion channels. Changes in the activity of adenylyl cyclase result in altered intracellular levels of the 'second messenger' cyclic adenosine monophosphate (cAMP). Similarly, PLC alters intracellular levels of inositol triphosphate ($IP_3$) and diacylglycerol (DAG). Altered levels of these second messengers trigger changes in the activity of specific signalling cascades and ultimately changes in physiological responses.

**Table 14.4** Examples of neurotransmitter receptors

| Transmitter | Receptor | Signal transduction |
|---|---|---|
| Dopamine | $D_1$ family (dopamine $D_1$, $D_5$) | Adenylyl cyclase ($G_s$) |
| | $D_2$ family (dopamine $D_2$, $D_3$, $D_4$) | Adenylyl cyclase ($G_{i/o}$) |
| Noradrenaline | $\alpha_1$ family ($\alpha_{1A, B, D}$) | Phospholipase C ($G_q$) |
| | $\alpha_2$ family ($\alpha_{2A, B, C}$) | Adenylyl cyclase ($G_{i/o}$) |
| | $\beta$ family ($\beta_{1, 2, 3}$) | Adenylyl cyclase ($G_s$) |
| 5-HT | $5\text{-HT}_1$ family ($5\text{-HT}_{1A, B, D, E, F}$) | Adenylyl cyclase ($G_{i/o}$) |
| | $5\text{-HT}_2$ family ($5\text{-HT}_{2A, B, C}$) | Phospholipase C ($G_q$) |
| | $5\text{-HT}_3$ | Cation channel |
| | $5\text{-HT}_4$ | Adenylyl cyclase ($G_s$) |
| | $5\text{-HT}_5$ family ($5\text{-HT}_{5A, B}$) | Not certain |
| | $5\text{-HT}_6$ | Adenylyl cyclase ($G_s$) |
| | $5\text{-HT}_7$ | Adenylyl cyclase ($G_s$) |
| Acetylcholine | $M_1$ (muscarinic) | Phospholipase C ($G_q$) |
| | $M_2$ | Adenylyl cyclase ($G_{i/o}$) |
| | $M_3$ | Phospholipase C ($G_q$) |
| | $M_4$ | Adenylyl cyclase ($G_{i/o}$) |
| | $M_5$ | Phospholipase C ($G_q$) |
| | Nicotinic ($\alpha 1$–10, $\beta 1$–4, $\delta$, $\epsilon$, $\gamma$) | Cation channel |
| GABA | $GABA_A$ ($\alpha 1$–6, $\beta 1$–3, $\gamma 1$–3, $\sigma 1$–3, $\delta$, $\epsilon$, $\pi$, $o$) | Chloride channel |
| | $GABA_B$ | Adenylyl cyclase ($G_{i/o}$) |
| Glutamate | AMPA (GluA1–4) | Cation channel |
| | NMDA (GluN1, GluN2A–D, GluN3A–B) | Cation channel |
| | | Cation channel |
| | Kainate (GluK1–5) | Phospholipase C ($G_q$) |
| | Group I family ($mGluR_{1/5}$) | Adenylyl cyclase ($G_{i/o}$) |
| | Group II family ($mGluR_{2-3}$) | Adenylyl cyclase ($G_{i/o}$) |
| | Group III family ($mGluR_{4, 6, 7, 8}$) | |
| Tachykinin (including substance P) | $NK_1$ | Phospholipase C ($G_q$) |
| | $NK_2$ | Phospholipase C ($G_q$) |
| | $NK_3$ | Phospholipase C ($G_q$) |
| Opioid | $\delta$ | Adenylyl cyclase ($G_{i/o}$) |
| | $\kappa$ | Adenylyl cyclase ($G_{i/o}$) |
| | $\mu$ | Adenylyl cyclase ($G_{i/o}$) |
| Galanin | GAL1 | Adenylyl cyclase ($G_{i/o}$) |
| | GAL2 | Adenylyl cyclase ($G_{i/o}$) |
| | GAL3 | Adenylyl cyclase ($G_{i/o}$) |
| Adenosine | $A_1$ | Adenylyl cyclase ($G_{i/o}$) |
| | $A_2$ family ($A_{2A, B}$) | Adenylyl cyclase ($G_s$) |
| | $A_3$ | Adenylyl cyclase ($G_{i/o}$) |
| ATP | P2X family ($P2X_{1-7}$) | Cation channel |
| | $P2Y_1$ | Phospholipase C ($G_q$) |
| | $P2Y_2$ | Phospholipase C ($G_q$) |
| | $P2Y_4$ | Phospholipase C ($G_q$) |
| | $P2Y_6$ | Phospholipase C ($G_q$) |
| | $P2Y_{11}$ | Phospholipase C ($G_q$) |
| | $P2Y_{12}$ | Adenylyl cyclase ($G_{i/o}$) |
| | $P2Y_{13}$ | Adenylyl cyclase ($G_{i/o}$) |
| | $P2Y_{14}$ | Phospholipase C ($G_q$) |
| Cannabinoid | CB1 | Adenylyl cyclase ($G_{i/o}$) |
| | CB2 | Adenylyl cyclase ($G_{i/o}$) |

The indirect opening of ion channels in response to neurotransmitter-induced GPCR activation leads to direct effects (excitatory or inhibitory) on the electrical properties of neurons, albeit on a longer timescale than effects produced by ligand-gated ion channels. Almost all neurotransmitter classes are able to evoke changes in ion channel opening via GPCRs, and some may be clinically important. For example, the $\alpha_2$-adrenoceptor-induced opening of potassium ion channels on noradrenaline neurons causes a fall in noradrenergic activity and release, which may contribute to the anxiolytic and sedative properties of $\alpha_2$-adrenoceptor agonists such as clonidine. On the other hand, the 5-HT$_{2A}$ receptor-induced closing of potassium ion channels on cortical neurons causes an increase in cortical neuron activity and may underlie the psychotropic effects of lysergic acid diethylamide (LSD) and related hallucinogens [37].

## GPCR regulation

Recent discoveries of interactions between GPCRs and other intracellular proteins have led to a new understanding of how the receptors are regulated and trafficked to and from the plasma membrane. Studies commencing on the $\beta$-adrenoceptor have identified two families of regulatory proteins called $\beta$-arrestins and GPCR kinases (GRKs). Within seconds of being activated by an agonist, the GPCR is phosphorylated by a GRK on the C-terminal cytoplasmic tail and other intracellular domains. This phosphorylation promotes the interaction of $\beta$-arrestins with the GPCR, which limits the signal duration, and causes loss of sensitivity to agonist activation and then receptor internalization from the cell surface [38].

In addition to $\beta$-arrestins, the C-termini of GPCRs associate with a large variety of transmembrane or soluble proteins, termed 'GPCR-interacting proteins' (GIPs). Some GIPs are themselves

GPCRs that form homo- or heterodimers, while other GIPs are ionic channels, ionotropic receptors, and proteins that control GPCR trafficking [39]. One interesting example of a GIP is the molecule p11, which reportedly functions to traffic a 5-HT GPCR (5-HT$_{1B}$) to the plasma membrane. Evidence suggests that p11 expression is reduced in the post-mortem brain of patients committing suicide and that mice with a genetic deletion of p11 have a depressive-like phenotype [40].

## Second messengers

The generation of the second messengers cAMP and DAG by adenylyl cyclase and PLC, respectively, leads to activation of protein kinases that add phosphate groups to specific protein targets to change their activity and ultimately trigger diverse physiological responses (Fig. 14.2). Enzymes called phosphatases, which remove phosphate groups, oppose these signalling effects. Guanylate cyclase is a cytosolic enzyme which also generates a second messenger cGMP. As noted, guanylate cyclase is activated by NO to produce effects on presynaptic function.

Based on molecular cloning studies, nine forms of adenylyl cyclase have been identified (I–IX), and each exhibits a distinct distribution in brain and peripheral tissues [41]. The full implication of this complexity is not yet understood, but it suggests that regulation of

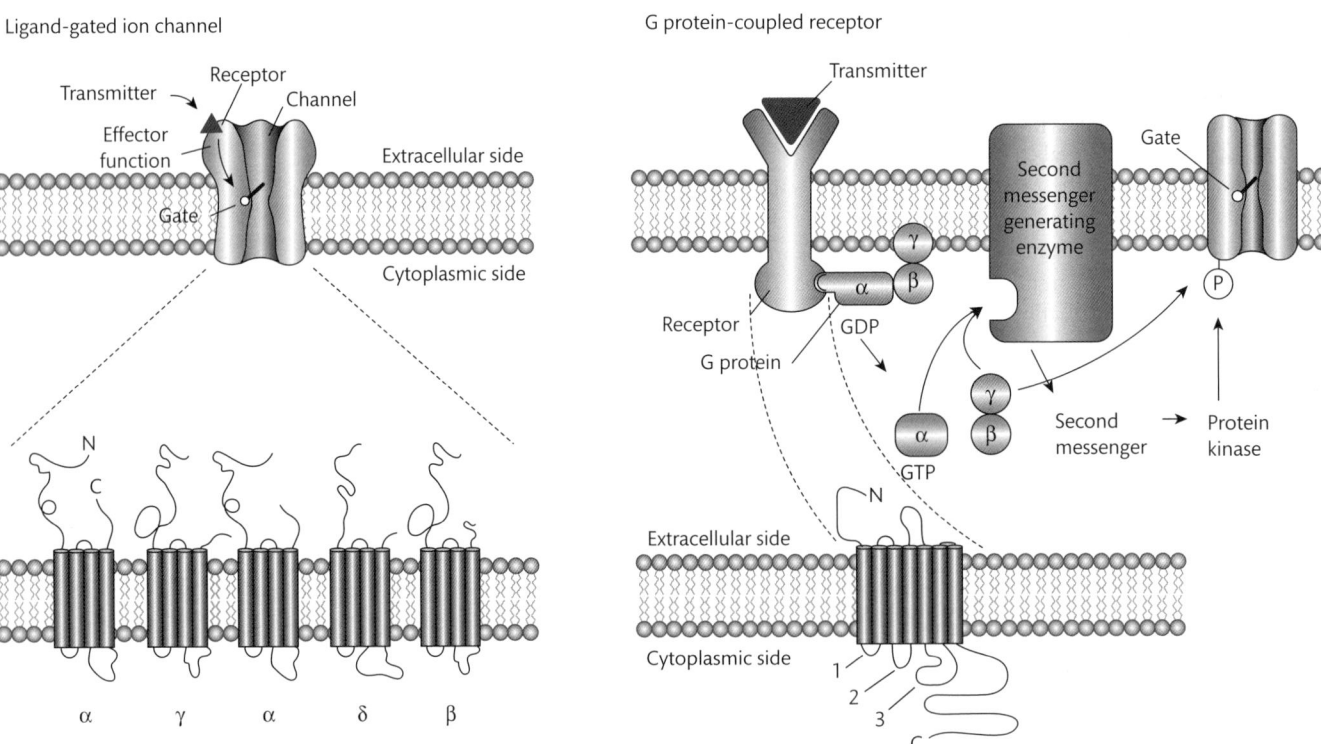

**Fig. 14.2** Diagrammatic representation of ligand-gated ion channel and G protein-coupled receptors. Ligand-gated ion channels comprise multiple protein subunits that form a central pore in the plasma membrane. On binding of the neurotransmitter, this receptor mediates fast excitatory or inhibitory transmission, depending on whether the channel gates cations or chloride ions, respectively. G protein-coupled receptors comprise a single membrane-spanning protein. On binding of the neurotransmitter, this receptor mediates slow transmission by enabling the dissociation of the G protein into an α subunit monomer and a β/γ subunit dimer, both of which may activate an effector enzyme to generate a second messenger. Also, the β/γ subunit dimer may directly interact with ion channels. Second messengers may also indirectly modulate ion channels through phosphorylation by activating protein kinases.

Reproduced from Nestler EJ, Hyman SE, Malenka RC, *Molecular Neuropharmacology*, pp. 64, Copyright (2001), with permission from McGraw-Hill Education.

cAMP formation varies, depending on the form of adenylyl cyclase expressed in neuronal cells.

Both cAMP and cGMP are degraded by phosphodiesterases (PDEs), which are expressed in numerous forms (types 1–11) in brain and peripheral tissues [30]. At high concentrations, caffeine and related methylxanthines inhibit PDE and this action contributes to the pharmacological effects of these drugs. Much effort is being made to develop inhibitors that are selective for brain-specific forms of PDE. Rolipram inhibits all isoforms of PDE4; this drug showed promise as an antidepressant, but its clinical utility was limited by peripheral side effects. However, because PDE4 enzymes comprise a number of isoforms, an inhibitor of one isoform may lead to the development of an effective antidepressant without the side effects of rolipram.

GPCR-induced activation of PLC causes the breakdown of phosphatidylinositol, resulting in the generation and recycling of the second messengers IP$_3$ and DAG, via the phosphoinositide cycle. Both IP$_3$ and DAG produce downstream signalling effects, IP$_3$ through the mobilization of intracellular calcium stores and DAG through activating a protein kinase. There are two major isoforms of PLC in the brain—β and γ, the β isoform being predominantly responsible for mediating the effects of GPCRs linked to G$_q$.

After its formation, IP$_3$ is recycled via a series of dephosphorylations to form inositol, which is used in the regeneration of phosphatidylinositol. Lithium, which is an important drug in the treatment of bipolar disorder, inhibits one of the enzymes involved in the recycling of IP$_3$ [inositol-1-monophosphatase (IMPase)] and causes inositol depletion at therapeutic concentrations. Because inositol does not easily enter the blood–brain barrier, brain inositol levels are thought to fall and the production of the second messengers diminishes. It is a popular hypothesis that inositol depletion is responsible for lithium's clinical effects, but this remains unproven. The recent discovery that the organoselenium antioxidant compound ebselen inhibits IMPase has stimulated interest in the idea that this agent has potential for repurposing, and specifically for use in bipolar depression [42].

In addition to IMPase, lithium interacts (albeit often at high concentrations) with a range of other signalling systems, including various ion channels, adenylyl cyclases, and protein kinases. For example, lithium inhibits glycogen synthase kinase-3β (GSK-3β), which also provides a source of inositol in the brain; certain mood-stabilizing anticonvulsants, such as valproate, also have this effect [43]. This has encouraged the development of GSK-3β inhibitors for bipolar disorder. However, GSK-3β has a range of functions, including a role in trophic mechanisms, and the safety of GSK-3β inhibitors is currently uncertain.

## Downstream signalling cascades

The activation or inhibition of second messenger signalling cascades by GPCRs can profoundly change the intracellular environment of the neuron by regulating the activity of protein kinases and other proteins, including gene transcription factors and even enzymes involved in the regulation of chromatin structure. Consequently, these cascades may regulate gene transcription and protein synthesis and activate multiple downstream effectors, including those that form the cytoskeleton or contribute to mechanisms underlying synaptic

plasticity. Such effects can induce long-lasting changes in neuronal function. Increasing evidence suggests that the neuroadaptive responses to repeated psychotropic drug administration are underpinned by changes in gene expression that result in the remodelling of neural circuit function and structure. This thinking has been applied to explain a multitude of neuropharmacological mechanisms, ranging from compulsive use of recreational drugs to the therapeutic action of antidepressant and antipsychotic drugs.

As an example, recent research has seen the evolution of a fascinating theory to explain the delayed onset of antidepressant effect of drugs like fluoxetine and imipramine that act to inhibit plasma membrane monoamine transporters. It supposes that elevated monoamine levels (through transporter blockade) trigger GPCR signalling cascades that activate gene programmes to enhance neuronal survival and connectivity, the latter having being weakened because of the adverse effects of stress and other environmental factors [18, 44–46]. Some of the key genes involved in this process include trophic factors such as BDNF, which may be a trigger for the production of newly formed neurons and many other forms of neural plasticity that leads to the overall strengthening of synapses and increased information transfer through key neural circuits relevant to mood control. This theory is a driving force for the development of pharmacological strategies for improved antidepressant therapies, even though our knowledge of the key molecules that are changed by antidepressants to bring about the relief of the symptoms of depression is far from complete.

## Non-canonical GPCR signalling

In addition to the classical (canonical) GPCR signalling, it is now recognized that GPCRs signal via a diversity of less well-known (referred to here as non-canonical) pathways, some of which are dependent on 'small G proteins' and others which are G protein-independent. Small G proteins (termed because of their low molecular weight and monomeric composition) comprise a protein superfamily, which also bind GTP and possess intrinsic GTPase activity. These G proteins function as molecular switches that control several cellular processes, ranging from vesicle trafficking and exocytosis (for example, Rab) to assembly of cytoskeletal structures (for example, Rho). Among the best characterized small G proteins are those that comprise the Ras family. Numerous types of cell signals, including those of most neurotrophic factors, converge on Ras and related proteins to regulate mitogen-activated protein (MAP) kinase pathways. Some GPCR signalling is independent of G proteins and often involves the recruitment of members of the arrestin family of proteins, which then trigger downstream pathways such as those involving MAP kinase.

This diversity in GPCR signalling is highly relevant in the context of emerging experimental evidence that different agonists acting at the same receptor can elicit different signals. This phenomenon is sometimes referred to as biased agonism or ligand-dependent signalling. Thus, agonists for a specific receptor may differ not only in terms of potency and efficacy, as given in classical pharmacological accounts, but also in terms of the signal that they elicit. Interestingly, evidence of ligand-dependent signalling through 5-HT$_{2A}$ receptors has relevance to the psychotropic effects of 5-HT$_{2A}$ receptor agonists, some of which are hallucinogenic, but not all, and it may also explain the long-lasting effects of LSD which are difficult to explain on the basis of pharmacokinetics alone [47]. Biased agonism offers intriguing possibilities for therapeutic potential (for example, avoidance of adverse side effects), although this is yet to be explored.

## Concluding remarks

Until recently, studies on the chemistry of synaptic neurotransmission have focused on a relatively small number of neurotransmitters and a narrow group of proteins involved in neurotransmitter function, specifically neurotransmitter receptors, transporters, and enzymes which bring about neurotransmitter synthesis or degradation. Today, powerful molecular and genetic approaches are being used to identify and understand new proteins and mechanisms involved in neurotransmitter function and control. So far, just a few tens of perhaps thousands of neurotransmitter-related proteins have been successfully targeted by pharmacological agents and translated into important treatments of psychiatric disorder, but there is promise of many more such treatments to come. Moreover, this huge diversity of neurotransmitter-related proteins is now emerging as a large resource for studies of genetic risk factors of psychiatric disorder and investigations of biological markers of illness diagnosis and progression and treatment outcome.

### FURTHER INFORMATION

Alexander, S.P., Kelly, E., Marrion, N., et al.; CGTP Collaborators. (2015). The concise guide to pharmacology 2015/16: overview. *British Journal of Pharmacology*, 172, 5729–43.

International Union of Basic and Clinical Pharmacology (IUPHAR) Committee. *Guide to pharmacology* (official database on receptor nomenclature and drug classification). http://www.guidetopharmacology.org

Kandel, E.R., Schwartz, J., Jessell, T., Siegelbaum, S.A., and Hudspeth, A.J. (2013). *Principles of neural science* (5th edn). McGraw-Hill, New York, NY. Further details are available at: http://en.wikipedia.org/wiki/Principles_of_Neural_Science

Nestler, E.J., Hyman, S.E., Holtzman, D.M., and Malenka, R.C. (2015). *Molecular neuropharmacology: a foundation for clinical neuroscience*. McGraw-Hill, New York, NY.

### REFERENCES

1. Maehle, A.H. (2004). 'Receptive substances': John Newport Langley (1852–1925) and his path to a receptor theory of drug action. *Medical History*, 48, 153–74.
2. Langmoen, I.A. and Apuzzo, M.L. (2007). The brain on itself: Nobel laureates and the history of fundamental nervous system function. *Neurosurgery*, 61, 891–907; discussion 907–8.
3. Hokfelt, T., Bartfai, T., and Bloom, F. (2003). Neuropeptides: opportunities for drug discovery. *The Lancet Neurology*, 2, 463–72.
4. Iversen, L. (2006). Neurotransmitter transporters and their impact on the development of psychopharmacology. *British Journal of Pharmacology*, 147(Suppl 1), S82–8.
5. Fremeau, R.T., Jr., Voglmaier, S., Seal, R.P., and Edwards, R.H. (2004). VGLUTs define subsets of excitatory neurons and suggest novel roles for glutamate. *Trends in Neurosciences*, 27, 98–103.
6. Kristensen, A.S., Andersen, J., Jørgensen, T.N., et al. (2011). SLC6 neurotransmitter transporters: structure, function, and regulation. *Pharmacological Reviews*, 63, 585–640.
7. Zhou, Z., Zhen, J., Karpowich, N.K., et al. (2007). LeuT-desipramine structure reveals how antidepressants block neurotransmitter reuptake. *Science*, 317, 1390–3.
8. Coleman, J.A., Green, E.M., and Gouaux, E. (2016). X-ray structures and mechanism of the human serotonin transporter. *Nature*, 532, 334–9.
9. Daws, L.C. (2009). Unfaithful neurotransmitter transporters: focus on serotonin uptake and implications for antidepressant efficacy. *Pharmacology and Therapeutics*, 121, 89–99.
10. Courousse, T. and Gautron, S. (2015). Role of organic cation transporters (OCTs) in the brain. *Pharmacology and Therapeutics*, 146, 94–103.
11. Javitt, D.C. (2012). Glycine transport inhibitors in the treatment of schizophrenia. *Handbook of Experimental Pharmacology*, 213, 367–99.
12. Rothstein, J.D., Patel, S., Regan, M.R., et al. (2005). Beta-lactam antibiotics offer neuroprotection by increasing glutamate transporter expression. *Nature*, 433, 73–7.
13. Sengupta, A., Bocchio, M., Bannerman, D.M., Sharp, T., and Capogna, M. (2017). Control of amygdala circuits by 5-HT neurons via 5-HT and glutamate cotransmission. *Journal of Neuroscience*, 37, 1785–96.
14. Tritsch, N.X., Granger, A.J., and Sabatini, B.L. (2016). Mechanisms and functions of GABA co-release. *Nature Reviews*, 17, 139–45.
15. Scamuffa, N., Calvo, F., Chretien, M., Seidah, N.G., and Khatib, A.M. (2006). Proprotein convertases: lessons from knockouts. *The FASEB Journal*,0 20, 1954–63.
16. Ogren, S.O., Kuteeva, E., Hokfelt, T., and Kehr, J. (2006). Galanin receptor antagonists: a potential novel pharmacological treatment for mood disorders. *CNS Drugs*, 20, 633–54.
17. Chao, M.V. (2003). Neurotrophins and their receptors: a convergence point for many signalling pathways. *Nature Reviews*, 4, 299–309.
18. Castren, E. (2005). Is mood chemistry? *Nature Reviews*, 6, 241–6.
19. Martinowich, K., Manji, H., and Lu, B. (2007). New insights into BDNF function in depression and anxiety. *Nature Neuroscience*, 10, 1089–93.
20. Harmer, C.J., Duman, R.S., and Cowen, P.J. (2017). How do antidepressants work? New perspectives for refining future treatment approaches. *The Lancet Psychiatry*, 4, 409–18.
21. Rostene, W., Kitabgi, P., and Parsadaniantz, S.M. (2007). Chemokines: a new class of neuromodulator? *Nature Reviews*, 8, 895–903.
22. Miller, A.H. and Raison, C.L. (2016). The role of inflammation in depression: from evolutionary imperative to modern treatment target. *Nature Reviews Immunology*, 16, 22–34.
23. Garthwaite, J. and Boulton, C.L. (1995). Nitric oxide signaling in the central nervous system. *Annual Review of Physiology*, 57, 683–706.
24. Calabrese, V., Mancuso, C., Calvani, M., Rizzarelli, E., Butterfield, D.A., and Stella, A.M. (2007). Nitric oxide in the central nervous system: neuroprotection versus neurotoxicity. *Nature Reviews*, 8, 766–75.
25. Lu, H.C. and Mackie, K. (2016). An introduction to the endogenous cannabinoid system. *Biological Psychiatry*, 79, 516–25.
26. Piomelli, D. (2003). The molecular logic of endocannabinoid signalling. *Nature Reviews*, 4, 873–84.

27. Fredholm, B.B., Hokfelt, T., and Milligan, G. (2007). G-protein-coupled receptors: an update. *Acta Physiologica*, 190, 3–7.
28. Rudolph, U. and Mohler, H. (2006). GABA-based therapeutic approaches: GABAA receptor subtype functions. *Current Opinion in Pharmacology*, 6, 18–23.
29. Schuman, E.M. and Seeburg, P.H. (2006). Signalling mechanisms. *Current Opinion in Neurobiology*, 16, 247–50.
30. Alexander, S.P., Mathie, A., and Peters, J.A. (2007). Guide to receptors and channels, 2nd edition (2007 revision). *British Journal of Pharmacology*, 150(Suppl 1), S1.
31. Lynch, G. and Gall, C.M. (2006). Ampakines and the threefold path to cognitive enhancement. *Trends in Neurosciences*, 29, 554–62.
32. Kemp, J.A. and McKernan, R.M. (2002). NMDA receptor pathways as drug targets. *Nature Neuroscience*, 5(Suppl), 1039–42.
33. McKernan, R.M. and Whiting, P.J. (1996). Which GABAA-receptor subtypes really occur in the brain? *Trends in Neurosciences*, 19, 139–43.
34. Farzampour, Z., Reimer, R.J., and Huguenard, J. (2015). Endozepines. *Advances in Pharmacology*, 72, 147–64.
35. Mohler, H. (2012). The GABA system in anxiety and depression and its therapeutic potential. *Neuropharmacology*, 62, 42–53.
36. Skolnick, P. (2012). Anxioselective anxiolytics: on a quest for the Holy Grail. *Trends in Pharmacological Sciences*, 33, 611–20.
37. Barnes, N.M. and Sharp, T. (1999). A review of central 5-HT receptors and their function. *Neuropharmacology*, 38, 1083–152.
38. Lefkowitz, R.J. (2007). Seven transmembrane receptors: something old, something new. *Acta Physiologica*, 190, 9–19.
39. Bockaert, J., Roussignol, G., Becamel, C., *et al.* (2004). GPCR-interacting proteins (GIPs): nature and functions. *Biochemical Society Transactions*, 32(Pt 5), 851–5.
40. Svenningsson, P., Chergui, K., Rachleff, I., *et al.* (2006). Alterations in 5-HT1B receptor function by p11 in depression-like states. *Science*, 311, 77–80.
41. Cooper, D.M. (2003). Regulation and organization of adenylyl cyclases and cAMP. *The Biochemical Journal*, 375(Pt 3), 517–29.
42. Singh, N., Halliday, A.C., Thomas, J.M., *et al.* (2013). A safe lithium mimetic for bipolar disorder. *Nature Communications*, 4, 1332.
43. Gould, T.D. and Manji, H.K. (2005). Glycogen synthase kinase-3: a putative molecular target for lithium mimetic drugs. *Neuropsychopharmacology*, 30, 1223–37.
44. Duman, R.S. (2002). Synaptic plasticity and mood disorders. *Molecular Psychiatry*, 7(Suppl 1), S29–34.
45. Sharp, T. (2013). Molecular and cellular mechanisms of antidepressant action. *Current Topics in Behavioral Neurosciences*, 14, 309–25.
46. Duman, R.S., Aghajanian, G.K., Sanacora, G., and Krystal, J.H. (2016). Synaptic plasticity and depression: new insights from stress and rapid-acting antidepressants. *Nature Medicine*, 22, 238–49.
47. Wacker, D., Wang, S., McCorvy, J.D., *et al.* (2017). Crystal structure of an LSD-bound human serotonin receptor. *Cell*, 168, 377–89 e12.

# 15

# Psychoneuroimmunology

*Juan C. Leza, Javier R. Caso, and Borja García-Bueno*

## Introduction

Psychoneuroimmunology (also known as psychoneuroendocrino-immunology) is a growing scientific discipline that studies the complex bi-directional circuit between the nervous system and the immune system in health and pathological conditions. The study of these interactions requires a multi-disciplinary and convergent approach from psychology, neurosciences, immunology, pharmacology, psychiatry, behavioural medicine, infectious diseases, endocrinology, rheumatology, and other disciplines.

The term was coined around the 1970s by R. Ader and N. Cohen, studying how episodes of stress and anxiety affect a person's immune system and how this activation of the immune system affect mental processes and health in extension.

Along history, a common place for psychoneuroimmunologists is the study of stress exposure and how individuals mount proper responses to cope with it. The mechanism/s implicated in the stress-induced modification of the immune system will be briefly discussed in this chapter, as well as the consequences in the structure and function of the CNS, both at molecular and behavioural/cognitive levels. Some large meta-analytic studies indicate both activation and depression of the immune system after stress exposure, depending on the duration, intensity, and the kind of stressful event (for example, trauma or loss) [1].

## Stress: cross-talk between the brain and the immune system

The term stress has been widely used since a long time ago to define a range of situations and experiences like those in which somebody is suffering from pressure, anxiety, or sadness, for example, being its use correct in all of them. Physiologically, stress is a situation produced subsequent to experiencing an alteration in an organism's homeostasis mainly due to an aversive threat. W. Cannon and H. Selye made some of the initial discoveries in this field and were the first to use the terms stress and 'stress response' [2]. This response, constituted by a three-phase mechanism and defined by Selye as *general adaptation syndrome*, is the result of an adaptation necessary to allow the overcoming of situations in which an organism has to fight or flight to survive. Some of the physiological effects observed in this response are an increase in arousal and concentration capacity, faster cardiac rhythm, higher blood pressure, suppression of the digestive process, redirection of blood to muscles, and a reduction of sexual desire and the immune system activity, among others. All these co-operate to allow the organism to detect the danger and provide it with all the energy available, in order to achieve survival, while depriving the organism from energy necessary for other processes. However, stress is a double-faced phenomenon, since while this fast and reversible response is essential for survival, it may cause adverse effects when secretion of stress hormones is sustained. Indeed, very intense or long-lasting stress results in a new biological equilibrium that can be either beneficial (for example, exercise-induced conditioning of the cardiovascular system) or detrimental, causing damage or disease due to maladaptation. In humans, the treat might be real or not. Although stress is not a disease in itself, continuous exposure to stressful stimuli has been clearly related with the onset, progression, or outcome of many psychopathological processes [3].

Stress response affects many different organs and systems, including the CNS. In the CNS, stress over the course of weeks causes reversible atrophy of hippocampal dendrites and apoptosis, whereas overexposure for months can cause permanent loss of neurons in rodents. Importantly, accumulating evidence of such stress-induced damage in the human brain has been presented [4], particularly in people with PTSD or major depression (that is, decreasing volumes in several brain areas). Studies carried out in animal models or in humans indicate that psychological stress induces a clear inflammatory response in the brain, accompanied by the release of cytokines and oxido-nitrosative mediators and the activation of several intra- and extracellular pathways [5, 6].

## Inflammation: how systemic inflammation reaches the central nervous system

Although stress-induced inflammation occurs in the brain, there is much recent evidence indicating that stress induces a systemic inflammatory response, which suggests possible inflammatory-immune cross-talk between the brain and the periphery. The CNS has long been considered an immune-privileged organ; however, this immune status is far from absolute. There are multiple neuro-immune pathways via which systemic inflammation reaches the CNS (Fig. 15.1).

These could be directly related to behavioural (for example, sickness behaviour, social avoidance, anhedonia) and cognitive alterations (for example, memory disruption), which resemble psychiatric symptomatology. The relative relevance of each one may vary in the function of the type, duration, and severity of the stimuli.

## The humoral pathway: signalling through the blood–brain barrier

The BBB structure is a complex histological, multi-layered structure, formed by a thick, continuous glycocalyx (a complex structure of proteoglycans and sialoproteins in the endothelium), non-fenestrated endothelial cells, linked by tight junctions (TJs), two basement membranes (vascular basement membrane and glia *limitans*), astrocytic end-feet, and two types of perivascular cells (pericytes and perivascular macrophages). All elements of this structure contribute to the functional BBB.

Neuro-immune signalling through the BBB is called the '*humoral pathway*' and occurs via two mechanisms: (1) energy-dependent transportation of immune signals by means of specific/non-specific transporters in the non-fenestrated endothelium of the BBB; and (2) the endothelium and perivascular-associated cells retaining the capacity to detect changes in circulating immune signals (cytokines) and initiating appropriate brain responses by increasing the synthesis and local release of signalling molecules, notably prostaglandins such as prostaglandin $E_2$ (PGE$_2$). Release of cerebrovascular PGE$_2$ activates nearby catecholamine-containing neurons that project to the para-ventricular hypothalamic nucleus (PVN), regulating neuroendocrine responses to stress. Like PGE$_2$, nitric oxide (NO) produced by the endothelium is also considered a second messenger implicated in the *humoral pathway*.

In inflammatory conditions, passage of inflammatory cells (lymphocytes, neutrophils, and monocytes) across the BBB occurs primarily at the post-capillary venules in a process called cellular transmigration through a disrupted endothelium. Once leucocytes reach the perivascular space, a second step requires passage across the glia limitans to enter the brain parenchyma in a process regulated by perivascular cells (macrophages and pericytes).

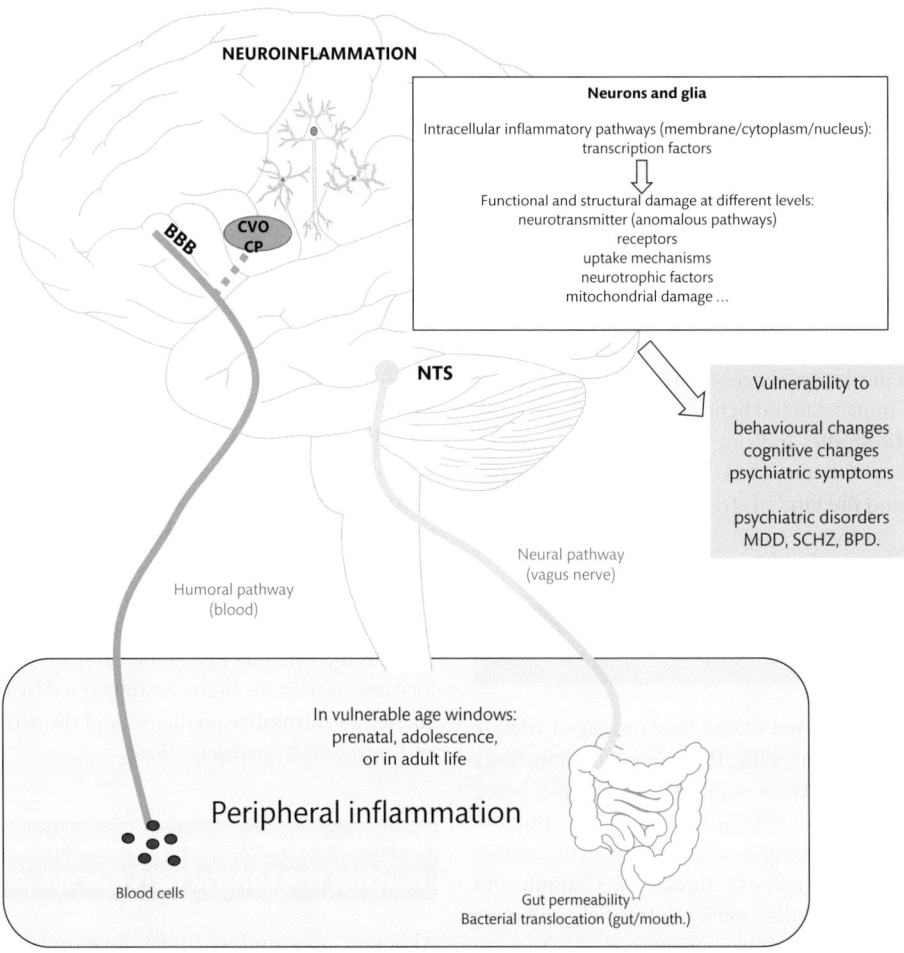

**Fig. 15.1** Multiple neuro-immune pathways by which systemic inflammation can reach the CNS. Possible functional, structural, and clinical consequences. BBB: blood–brain barrier; CVO: circumventricular organs; CP: choroid plexus; NTS: nucleus tractus solitarius; MDD, major depressive disorder; SCHZ, schizophrenia; BPD: bipolar disorder.
Includes images adapted from Motifolio Drawing Toolkits (www.motifolio.com).

## Signalling through structures in the brain that lack a normal blood–brain barrier (circumventricular organs)

The circumventricular organs (CVOs) can be functionally divided in two major types: (1) the sensory organs, including the area postrema (AP), the subfornical organ (SFO), and the vascular organ of the *lamina terminalis*; and (2) the secretory organs, mainly including the subcommissural organ (SCO) and the median eminence. The sensory organs detect and transmit peripheral immune signals to the CNS, and conversely, the secretory organs produce signals (that is, hormones) from the CNS to modulate the activity of peripheral organs and systems. The particular and extensive fenestrated vasculature of these organs allows direct interaction between neurons and glial cells, which also form part of their structure and peripheral blood flow. These organs also possess neuroanatomical connections between them, as well as with other remote brain areas and structures involved in the regulation of the immune system such as the PVN and vagal sensory fibres. The exact contribution of each organ to transduce cytokine-dependent signalling is not known and may vary in function of the intensity of the stimulus. As occurs in the choroid plexus (CP), there are resident macrophage-like cells in the CVOs that respond to circulating stimuli by producing pro-inflammatory cytokines, and also in pathological conditions, there are increased numbers of CD45+ leucocytes in the CVOs, suggesting the recruitment of inflammatory cells into the parenchyma of the CVOs, probably mediated by endothelial adhesion molecules.

## Signalling through the blood–cerebrospinal fluid barrier formed by the choroid plexus and meningeal arachnoid membrane (endothelium and meningeal macrophages)

The CP is located in the brain ventricles and is formed by epithelial cells [with TJs and gap junctions (GJs) between them] that rest upon a basal lamina, and a second stromal structure consisting of central connective tissue and highly fenestrated vascularized tissue populated by diverse cell types (fibroblasts, macrophages, and dendritic cells). Its main function is the production of CSF.

It is accepted that CP response to acute peripheral stimuli is fast and strong but loses magnitude on chronicity. The CP is the preferred site for initial transepithelial leucocyte trafficking from the periphery to the brain, because it contains resident immune cells (the function of CD4+ T cells is especially relevant in this regard) that produce pro-inflammatory cytokines and expresses major histocompatibility complex (MHC) and leucocyte adhesion molecules. The CSF passes into the subarachnoid spaces surrounding the brain and spinal cord. Part of the CSF drains into blood via arachnoid villi in venous sinuses, but the CSF also drains from the cerebral subarachnoid space to cervical lymphatic organs. This pathway also allows traffic of antigen-presenting cells between the brain parenchyma and regional lymph nodes.

## Direct recruitment of immune stimulus-primed peripheral immune cells to brain parenchyma

Peripheral immune cells may act as important modulators of neuroinflammation. Under physiological conditions, several types of immune cells (monocytes, granulocytes, dendritic cells, T cells, and perivascular macrophages) of haematopoietic origin populate specific brain areas (vasculature, CP, and meninges) and exert supportive and immunosurveillance actions. By contrast, in a state of chronic/uncontrolled neuroinflammation (for example, chronic exposure to stress), these cells are potentially detrimental due to their capacity to produce massive levels of pro-inflammatory mediators such as cytokines and chemokines.

In the resolution phase of neuroinflammation after injury, recruitment of blood-derived cells (that is, macrophages) facilitates the resolution of the neuroinflammatory response by displaying an M2-like anti-inflammatory profile. As previously commented, these monocyte-derived macrophages enter the injured brain site through a designated barrier—the CP within the blood–CSF barrier, rather than through the breached BBB.

### Neural pathway

The 'neural pathway' is mainly constituted by the activation of primary sensory afferent nerves such as the *vagus* nerve by macrophages, increased cytokine levels, or direct activation of the innate immune receptors Toll-like receptors (TLRs) by DAMPs (damage-associated molecular patterns) or PAMPs (pathogen-associated molecular patterns). Inflammation signals reach the nucleus tractus solitarius, which interconnects with the dorsal motor nucleus where the majority of efferent vagus nerve fibres originate.

The efferent component of the vagus nerve detects signals from the periphery, and through the release of acetylcholine (ACh) and consequent activation of α7 nicotinic ACh receptors (α7nAChRs) expressed in macrophages and T cells, the production of pro-inflammatory cytokines is markedly inhibited. In addition, stimulation of the vagus nerve induces activation of stress hypothalamus–pituitary–adrenal (HPA) axis, which results in glucocorticoid release by the adrenal cortex, with broad anti-inflammatory actions. This neuro-immune communication is termed '*the* inflammatory reflex'.

In conclusion, the brain and the immune system have mutual dependency. The brain regulates multiple organs, the immune system included, mainly at the level of lymphoid organs. On the other hand, immune cells help to maintain brain homeostasis and plasticity when brain-resident microglia, astroglia, and perivascular macrophages are unable to cope with an exacerbated neuroinflammatory response. Neuro-immune interactions take place through different barriers, each with specific, and often complementary, functions. Elucidation of the multiple interconnections between them will improve the development of new approaches for the treatment of neurodegenerative and psychiatric diseases.

## Inflammation and depression (in animal models and humans)

A biological basis for mood disorders was described as early as the fifth century BC, when Hippocrates referred to *melancholia* as a condition associated with 'aversion to food, despondency, sleeplessness, irritability and restlessness'. Nevertheless, the fundamental pathophysiology of depression still stays elusive. In fact, different studies are indicating that, in some cases, more than 30% of depressed patients fail to achieve remission despite multiple treatment trials [7].

Interestingly, mounting data indicate that inflammation may also play a role in the pathophysiology of major depressive disorder

(MDD). Given the accelerating development of biomarkers and treatments focused on the inflammatory response, there is tremendous promise that these advances, in addition to their relevance to general medicine, may have unique applications in psychiatry.

Different epidemiological studies have demonstrated that MDD is associated with a higher prevalence of elevated markers of inflammation [8], and different meta-analyses have shown that the levels of cytokines and other indicators of an inflammatory scenario are elevated in the periphery of patients with MDD [9–11]. In addition, a recent meta-analysis indicated that elevated peripheral levels of inflammation are contributory to treatment resistance in MDD subjects [12]. Indeed, elevated levels of inflammatory markers predict a poorer response to drugs against depression (antidepressants), and those who do not respond to AD treatments show persistently elevated inflammation.

Thus, inflammation, both in the brain and in the periphery, is being presented as an element worth considering in the aetiology of psychiatric conditions such as MDD. This conception is grounded in the strongly activated inflammatory/immune response detected in these diseases [7, 13–15] and in that patients with MDD who are otherwise medically healthy have been repeatedly observed to have activated inflammatory pathways. In addition to those pathways are worth mentioning increased levels of pro-inflammatory cytokines and acute phase proteins and increased expression of chemokines and adhesion molecules.

Long-term exposure to cytokines also has been shown to lead to marked behavioural alterations in humans. Thus, several studies in humans suggest that immune-targeted therapies may have clinical benefit. For example, medically healthy depressed patients who received the selective cyclo-oxygenase-2 (COX-2) (a key enzyme for the production of prostaglandins and other eicosanoids) inhibitor celecoxib, in combination with reboxetine, showed greater symptomatic improvement vs patients randomized to reboxetine plus placebo [16].

Antidepressant activity of anti-inflammatory therapy has also been observed in patients with autoimmune and inflammatory disorders. For example, in a large double-blind, placebo-controlled trial of the TNFα antagonist etanercept for the treatment of psoriasis, participants who received etanercept exhibited significant improvement in depressive symptoms, compared with placebo-treated subjects, an effect independent of improvement in disease activity [17].

Thus, it seems reasonable to recognize that pro-inflammatory cytokines induce not only symptoms of sickness, but also true MDDs in physically ill patients with no previous history of mental disorders.

Besides, clinical observations and epidemiological data have also demonstrated associations between suicide and inflammatory cytokines in the orbitofrontal cortex, a brain region involved in suicidal vulnerability. Interestingly, the perception of menace that directs suicidal individuals to consider suicide may trigger biological stress responses, including the inflammatory ones [18].

Aside from evidence of increased levels of inflammatory markers in patients with MDD, data from laboratory animals indicate that the administration of innate immune cytokines, including interferon (IFN)-α, or an immunological challenge induced by lipopolysaccharide (LPS) injection (major component of the outer membrane of Gram-negative bacteria which induces the secretion of cytokines) leads to multiple behavioural changes that overlap with MDD, including depressed mood, anhedonia, psychomotor slowing, disrupted sleep, anxiety, etc. This is the so-called *sickness behaviour* [19, 20]. These findings are consistent with a vast literature on laboratory animals, indicating that cytokine antagonists or anti-inflammatory agents can block the development of behavioural changes following immune activation.

On the other hand, it seems fairly recognized nowadays that both genetic and environmental factors (such as stress) contribute to depression. Currently, experimental models of depression are based on exposure to stress, and it has been widely described that experimental stress induces pro-inflammatory actions mediated by glucocorticoids, catecholamines, glutamate, and other mediators released by stress [5]. Thus, experimental data indicate that inflammation is an important component of MDD, and in particular, pro-inflammatory cytokines that are induced by injury and infection, as well as by psychological stress, are implicated in depressive-like behaviour in rodent models.

Some of the mechanisms that might be responsible for inflammation-mediated sickness and depression have now been elucidated. These findings suggest that the brain–cytokine system, which is, in essence, a diffuse system, is the unsuspected conductor of the ensemble of neuronal circuits and neurotransmitters that organize physiological and pathological behaviour. Some of the evidence will be discussed in the next sections.

## Depression, serotonin, and cytokines

Traditionally, the prevailing hypothesis is that depression is caused by some disorganization of brain serotonergic systems, perhaps a deficiency in serotonergic neurotransmission. This hypothesis is based largely on the observation that many effective drugs for depression affect serotonergic transmission. Also, serotonin receptor abnormalities are found in the brain of patients with MDD. While there is no doubt that drugs for depression increase synaptic levels of serotonin, noradrenaline, and (some of the drugs) dopamine, these compounds also suppress pro-inflammatory cytokine production (for example, IL-1β, IL-6, TNFα) and stress hormone release and may additionally stimulate anti-inflammatory cytokine (for example, IL-10) release [21]. These data indicate again that neuro-immune and neuroendocrine system perturbations likely play an important role in the aetiology of depression.

## Depression, immune system activation, and indoleamine 2,3-dioxygenase

As aforementioned, an immunological challenge, such as induced by LPS injection, leads to multiple behavioural changes that overlap with MDD. Thus, a factor which induces an immunological response (such as infection) and subsequent cytokine release could be implicated in the origin of this disease.

An interesting hypothetical mechanism by which infections might induce depression relates to the metabolism of tryptophan and serotonin (5-HT). Infections induce IFN-γ and TNFα, which are potent inducers of indoleamine 2,3-dioxygenase (IDO) in macrophages and certain other cells. This enzyme degrades tryptophan, so IDO enables the conversion of tryptophan to kynurenine. The resulting catabolism of tryptophan decreases its circulating concentrations, and lower plasma concentrations of tryptophan have been associated with depression. It has been postulated that such a decrease may limit the availability of tryptophan to the brain, thus limiting serotonin synthesis and precipitating depression [22].

Furthermore, the induction of IDO through immune system activation could also be playing a role in other theoretical mechanisms implicated in the pathophysiology of MDD such as excitotoxicity and glutamate metabolism. As it has been already mentioned, once activated by pro-inflammatory cytokines, IDO degrades tryptophan. But IDO activation also generates potentially neurotoxic kynurenine metabolites, such as kynurenic acid and quinolinic acid, which could contribute to the pathogenesis of psychiatric diseases through their actions on the glutamate NMDA receptor (that is, kynurenic acid is an endogenous glutamate NMDA receptor antagonist, and quinolinic acid an endogenous glutamate NMDA receptor agonist) [23].

## Depression, bacterial translocation, and innate immunity

Recent studies have postulated that increased gastrointestinal permeability with an increased translocation of LPS from Gram-negative bacteria may play a role in the pathophysiology of MDD. Specifically, it has been suggested that increased LPS translocation may mount an immune response, and thus an inflammatory status, in some patients with MDD and may induce specific sickness behaviour symptoms [24].

Disruptions of the intestinal epithelium allow normally poorly invasive enterobacteria to exploit lipid raft-mediated transcytotic pathways or the enlarged spaces to cross the gut wall. Thus, loss of the epithelial barrier integrity caused by inflammation and/or stress may induce an increased bacterial translocation, provoking increased serum concentrations of LPS. And as it is well known, LPS causes induction of nuclear factor κB (NF-κB), the major upstream intracellular mechanism which regulates inflammatory and oxidative/nitrosative stress mediators, such as COX-2 and inducible NO synthase (iNOS), and also causes cytokine release through its union to the TLR-4 [6].

TLRs are one of main actors of innate immunity, and there are a good number of preclinical studies showing that TLRs are involved in depression-like behaviour induced by experimental models of MDD. Furthermore, there is increasing evidence from the clinical arena suggesting that TLRs are involved in the pathophysiology of MDD. Recently, TLR-4 mRNA expression in peripheral blood has been identified as an independent risk factor related to the severity of MDD. In addition, studies have shown that some elements of the TLR-4 signalling pathway were upregulated at mRNA level in peripheral blood mononuclear cells (PBMCs) of patients with MDD. And importantly, these peripheral alterations of the TLR-4 signalling pathway have been corroborated in post-mortem human brain tissue (dorsolateral prefrontal cortex) from depressed and suicidal patients [25–27].

Based on this, it is plausible to conclude that increased bacterial translocation is another pathway which may explain the inflammatory pathophysiology of MDD. Thus, the TLR-4 pathway may either primarily (increased translocation of LPS inducing inflammation) or secondarily (primary inflammation that may induce bacterial translocation) be involved in the inflammatory pathophysiology of MDD.

Consequently, the study of possible bacterial translocation and the kind of bacteria present in an organism (microbiota) has a crucial importance and represents an area of research in which further investigation is warranted.

The psychoneuroimmunology approach to the study of the pathophysiology of MDD is crucial, as it could expose related biomarkers for the identification and monitoring of potentially responsive patients. From this point of view, there are already compilations of common peripheral biomarkers measured in studies on MDD [28].

Among the inflammatory and immune response peripheral biomarkers, cytokines (for example, TNFα, IL-1β, IL-6, IFN-γ), C-reactive protein, neopterin (released by macrophages and considered a marker of activation of cell-mediated inflammation), and tryptophan catabolites, as well as different elements of the IDO pathway, stand out.

Bearing in mind that inflammation is often followed by oxidative damage, there are other peripheral biomarkers of oxidative and nitrosative stress to consider such as malondialdehyde (a product of lipid peroxidation), superoxide dismutases (SODs) (an important antioxidant defence in nearly all cells exposed to oxidative stress), and glutathione peroxidase and reductase.

## Inflammation and psychosis (in animal models and in humans)

The idea about the existence of alterations of the innate immune system taking part in the aetiology and pathophysiology of psychotic disease is long-standing but has been receiving renewed interest in the last years. Specifically, alterations of the innate immune system could contribute to the pathophysiology of these mental diseases, producing alterations in processes such as dopaminergic and serotonergic metabolism and transmission, neurotrophic factor levels, neurogenesis, and even behaviour and cognition.

There is converging evidence from different fields of knowledge and approaches (genetics, pharmacology, brain imaging, clinical trials), both in experimental animal models and in human biological samples from diverse organic compartments (serum, plasma, PBMCs, and post-mortem human brain tissue samples), as well as from subjects diagnosed with different degrees of psychotic disease.

Most of the evidence supporting peripheral inflammatory changes in schizophrenia involves elevated plasma pro-inflammatory cytokine levels (that is, IL-1β and -6). These effects have been directly associated with certain clinical features such as cognitive impairment and brain volume loss or with negative symptoms. There is less evidence on alterations in the number, activity, and profile of peripheral immune cells in psychotic disease, but some authors have described T cell dysfunction in patients with schizophrenia and an imbalance of immune responses towards a major humoral [T helper 2 (Th2)] response in plasma, correlated with a worse prognosis. In addition, recent studies have reported the existence of anti-NMDA receptor antibodies and surface dopamine-2 receptor antibodies in serum and CSF of subgroups of individuals with psychotic disease.

Inflammatory evidence is also present in the brain. Abnormal CSF cytokine and leucocyte levels have been identified in the brain of schizophrenia patients. Post-mortem evidence for inflammation is growing. Brain microglial activation and abnormal lymphocyte levels have been suggested in post-mortem and PET studies, although novel, highly specific PET ligands for activated microglia are needed. Alterations in other immunity-related systems at the

CNS level have been also reported, such as the case of prostanoids (that is, prostaglandins and related lipid-derived compounds), endocannabinoids, and the tryptophan-degrading enzyme indoleamine 2,3-dioxygenase (IDO) generating potentially neurotoxic kynurenine metabolites such as kynurenic and quinolinic acids. Schizophrenia manifest interrelated peripheral and central symptomatology. Determining the relationship between peripheral and central changes in inflammation-related molecules in subjects with a psychotic disorder could be useful not only for diagnosis and monitoring of the natural course of the disease (trait or state biomarkers, risk/protective factors), but also to reveal possible mechanisms with aetio-pathophysiological relevance.

One relevant question to address is the mechanism/s whereby inflammation leads to brain cell damage in psychotic disease. Some of the putative mechanisms involved include: (1) microglial overactivation or increased microglial cellular density; (2) oxidative/nitrosative stress; (3) uncontrolled activation of the HPA stress axis (hypercortisolism); (4) excitotoxicity and disrupted glutamate metabolism; (5) mitochondrial dysfunction and energy deficits; (6) reduced levels of neurotrophins (that is, BDNF, NGF); (7) impaired neurogenesis; (8) apoptosis; (9) demyelination; (10) impaired glucose transport and metabolism; and (11) functional BBB breakdown and ultrastructural abnormalities affecting a number of brain functions, including excitatory/inhibitory neurotransmission, stress and alarm phase responses, and synaptic plasticity.

Another issue to elucidate is the possible origin of increased inflammation in psychotic disease. There are multiple theories dealing with the origin of increased inflammation in schizophrenia. Five major categories exist:

1. Inflammatory changes before birth (due to prenatal or maternal infections and/or obstetric complications). The common notion is that these factors 'prime' an immature fetal immune system that will remain impaired for a lifetime. This idea is gaining momentum, and schizophrenia is now strongly related to anomalies in neurodevelopment. Currently, the use of maternal immune activation models in rodents is receiving increasing attention in translational psychiatry. These models are relevant because they reproduce in the progeny some functional and structural anomalies in the brain, as well as behavioural alterations and cognitive deficits, characteristic of the pathophysiology of schizophrenia.

2. Inflammatory changes in crucial stages of brain development and maturation (early adulthood) [29]. During early adulthood, the brain undergoes decisive changes, completing the myelination of axon fibres and synaptic pruning in particular areas. These neurodevelopmental changes coincide with the maturation of dopaminergic neurotransmission in cortical structures and may be crucially affected by stimuli triggering potentially detrimental innate immune responses.

3. Inflammatory lifetime changes produced by diverse environmental factors such as episodes of psychosocial stress, infections (viral reactivations, poor hygiene, periodontal problems), dietary deficiencies, alcohol, tobacco, metabolic and autoimmune disorders, medications, etc. In this regard, the family of TLRs have emerged as a possible mechanism involved. TLRs are the first line of defence against invading microorganisms and other immune stimuli. Their expression is modulated in response to pathogens and other environmental stresses. The most studied member of the family TLR-4 orchestrates neuroinflammation in animal models, and its expression is regulated by stress-induced bacterial translocation of gut microflora. Alterations in peripheral TLR activity have been described in schizophrenia and other psychiatric disorders such as depression.

4. Inflammatory changes produced as a consequence of genetic susceptibility due to the existence of hypo-/hyperpolymorphisms in certain immune/inflammatory-related genes as risk factors for this disorder. Genome-wide association studies have identified genes involved in the immune response (MHC, etc.) that correlate with schizophrenia diagnosis.

5. Loss or impairment of protective function in at-risk cell types, such as parvalbumin-expressing cortical interneurons, in relation to oxidative/nitrosative stress.

Several studies have shown that peripheral inflammatory markers may vary with the clinical status of patients and can be used as possible trait/state biomarkers for early diagnosis and also for monitoring disease progression and treatment response. Excellent candidates are pro-/anti-inflammatory cytokines (IL-1β, IL-6, and transforming growth factor-β), oxidative/nitrosative stress mediators [thiobarbituric acid reactive substances (TBARS), SOD], and even some lymphocyte phenotypes (CD4/CD8, CD56). The existence of a 'golden marker' for the disease is highly improbable; rather, studying complete and robust pathways with all elements of intracellular and intercellular pathways, including elements of balancing mechanisms and their relationship with positive/negative symptomatology and cognition deficits, is an interesting approach.

Besides studies for the search of biomarkers, inflammation can be pharmacologically modulated to improve the clinical picture. There are some completed and ongoing double-blind, randomized, placebo-controlled clinical trials with anti-inflammatory augmentation in schizophrenia, but the results are modest and only affecting specific subgroups of patients with schizophrenia. Based on this evidence, future studies should have a change of focus. Current studies propose the control of inflammation via direct inhibition of pro-inflammatory mediators, but pharmacological stimulation of antioxidant/anti-inflammatory pathways to potentiate the endogenous response against disease is emerging as a promising strategy. Complementary pharmacological studies have demonstrated an anti-inflammatory profile of some antipsychotics (that is, paliperidone, clozapine) with reduced expression and release of pro-inflammatory cytokine and stimulated production of anti-inflammatory cytokines such as IL-4, -10, and -17.

We are still far from having a general idea of the role/s of innate immune system/inflammation in the aetiology and pathophysiology of psychotic disease, and consequently from offering an effective and safe treatment for patients based on the modulation of the inflammatory response. There is still a long way to go, with some questions and limitations to resolve:

1. The inflammatory state may vary, depending on the course of the disease. There may be compensatory mechanisms or exhaustion, so it is needed to study different states of psychotic disease, from prodromal stages to first episode to psychosis to full-blown, chronic schizophrenia. Efforts should be made to determine if symptomatic onset of the disease occurs in a vulnerable brain (immunologically/inflammation-primed months/years before

symptoms manifest) or if a genetically prone subject develops symptoms that will increase the deleterious effects of inflammation and/or infection. The search for 'immunophenotypes' is a nascent approach to take into account for the future.

2. The inflammatory response is highly non-specific and is activated in response to multiple endogenous and exogenous factors in the context of psychiatric diseases [30]. Some of the parameters that need to be controlled and considered are: genetic/epigenetic susceptibility, disease state/duration, stress exposure, tobacco/cannabis use, body mass index, type and duration of antipsychotic medication, presence of ongoing infections, etc.

3. The great degree of comorbidity between psychotic disease and inflammation-related diseases, such as depression, obesity, and diabetes, or psychotropic substance abuse, further complicates the scenario.

## The microbiota–gut–brain axis and immunopathogenesis of psychiatric diseases

There is evidence indicating that there is a bi-directional communication between the brain and the enteric nervous system, including the microbiota, which uses neural, hormonal, and immunological routes.

Thus, the microbiota–gut–brain (MGB) axis would be constituted by a complex system of communication between the microbiota, the gut, and the CNS, which would be able to regulate gastrointestinal, immune, and CNS functions. Among those paths of communication between the gut and the CNS are the vagus nerve, the HPA axis, the cytokine network, and tryptophan absorption from the gut into the peripheral bloodstream, as well as the passage of short-chain fatty acids (SCFAs) into the circulatory system [31].

There are multiple pathways guiding the descending and ascending directions of the MGB axis in health and disease. In particular, from the gut to the CNS, studies have revealed that brain activity can be regulated through neural activation of neurons by the gut microbiome, and through endocrine (for example, release of serotonin), metabolic (for example, microbiota synthesis of neuroactive molecules), and immune (for example, systemic inflammation and CNS-infiltrating immune cells) pathways.

The MGB axis is also a key player in neurodevelopment, and consequently it is plausible to consider that the microbiome, and in particular early-life events during initial colonization and microbiota development, can determine general and mental health in later life, which could be playing a crucial role in psychiatric diseases with a neurodevelopmental component such as autism spectrum disorders and schizophrenia.

Furthermore, in inflammatory bowel disease (IBD), comorbidity with mood disorders, such as depression and anxiety, is common, and chronic low-grade inflammation or immune activation that underlies the aetiology of IBD is also a driving risk factor in mood disorders [32]. Importantly, patients with schizophrenia quite often present with gut problems, and irritable bowel syndrome commonly co-occurs with psychiatric disorders. Thus, through diverse mechanisms that can include bacterial translocation, the microbiota from the gut would be able to affect both local and distal locations within the host organism.

Stress, which is a main risk factor for psychiatric diseases, induces intestinal dysfunction and can increase intestinal permeability. But this is not the only factor to consider. Changes in microbiota may lead to brain dysfunction through the production of harmful bacterial products that compromise the integrity of the intestinal tract (permeable intestine or leaky gut syndrome). Here appears a very important concept—the gut microbiota dysbiosis; shifts in microbiota composition and functions from physiological/beneficial states to those pernicious to the host's health are termed dysbiosis, and gut dysbiosis may exert a deleterious impact on brain functioning via the MGB axis. Moreover, it has been recently proposed that dysbiosis might contribute to abnormal brain development, immune regulation, and metabolic function in psychiatric diseases. However, the composition of the gut microbiota has yet to be fully characterized in psychiatric patients, and further research is very much needed.

## Hypersensitivity to food antigens

Among the factors influencing the functioning of the MGB axis, there is one that shows up—hypersensitivity to food antigens. Several studies have found increased immune sensitivity to food-based antigens, namely gluten and milk casein, in psychiatric diseases and, in particular, in patients with schizophrenia [33].

Gluten-dependent disorders have been recently classified into three main groups, based on their pathogenesis [34]: autoimmune reactions, including coeliac disease; allergic reactions, including wheat allergy; and non-autoimmune and non-allergic (innate immunity), which includes non-coeliac gluten sensitivity (NCGS) or intolerance. Schizophrenia has been repeatedly associated with both coeliac disease and NCGS [35]. Indeed, the average prevalence of coeliac disease among patients with schizophrenia is higher than that estimated in the general population [36]. In fact, there are already meta-analyses showing significantly higher levels of some serum biomarkers of gluten hypersensitivity in patients with schizophrenia, although more research is very much needed in this field [37].

On the other hand, elevations in antibodies to milk casein have also been described in subjects with psychiatric diseases, mainly in patients with schizophrenia. The mechanisms mediating the association between heightened antibodies to gluten/casein and the risk of psychiatric disease are not fully understood. For example, in some individuals with a psychotic disorder, comorbidity with coeliac disease/NCGS may disrupt intestinal permeability (that is, 'leaky gut'), thereby allowing these antigens to enter the systemic circulation and generate a humoral immune response, which, in turn, would lead to psychotic symptoms. Indeed, gluten stimulates zonulin release, probably because it is mistaken for a microbial agent and therefore increases gut permeability in humans.

In summary, there is growing evidence supporting that some of the key pathways that are dysfunctional in psychiatric diseases may also be regulated by the MGB axis. Microbiota-targeted therapeutic interventions may include dietary approaches, probiotics, prebiotics, anti-biotherapy, and faecal transplantation. Preclinical studies suggest that strategies manipulating the gut microbiota hold potential preventive applications in psychiatric disorders. Thus, this is a very promising field of research. At this time, human interventions in psychiatry are still scarce and have focused on diet modification, probiotics, and antibiotics. Importantly, all these interventions are currently considered as adjunctive treatments to standard care (for example, drugs for depression, antipsychotics).

## Pharmacology

We are still far from having ideally effective and safe treatments to offer to patients with affective disorders and psychosis. There is therefore a need for a change in the drug discovery strategy, mainly based on a better understanding of the pathophysiology, while, of course, taking into account the overwhelming experimental, epidemiological, and clinical evidence suggesting that prolonged increases in the levels of pro-inflammatory and oxido-nitrosative mediators occur in depression, schizophrenia, and other neuropsychiatric diseases. This fact justifies the ongoing clinical trials on adjunctive therapies with anti-inflammatory and antioxidant drugs in these diseases, including non-steroidal anti-inflammatory drugs and anti-cytokine and antioxidant compounds [38, 39] (that is, aspirin, COX-2 inhibitors, *N*-acetylcysteine, omega-3 fatty acids, and others). Although none of these combinations have demonstrated to be clearly beneficial, much effort has to be made, from basic to clinical research, to address how inflammation and immune dysfunction affect psychopathology. This would contribute to a better understanding of the disease mechanism and to the development of new effective interventions [40].

## REFERENCES

1. Segerstrom, S.C. and Miller, G.E. (2004). Psychological stress and the human immune system: a meta-analytic study of 30 years of inquiry. *Psychological Bulletin*, 130, 601–30.
2. Selye, H. (1936). A syndrome produced by diverse nocuous agents. *Nature*, 32.
3. Madrigal, J.L.M., García-Bueno, B., Cárdenas, A., *et al.* (2004). Oxidative/nitrosative brain damage in stress: possible target for neuropsychopharmacological drugs. *Current Medicinal Chemistry—Central Nervous System Agents*, 4, 235–42
4. Bremner, J.D., Staib, L.H., Kaloupek, D., Southwick, S.M., Soufer, R., and Charney, D.S. (1999). Neural correlates of exposure to traumatic pictures and sound in Vietnam combat veterans with and without posttraumatic stress disorder: a positron emission tomography study. *Biological Psychiatry*, 45, 806–16.
5. García-Bueno, B., Caso, J.R., and Leza, J.C. (2008). Stress as a neuroinflammatory condition in brain: damaging and protective mechanisms. *Neuroscience and Biobehavioral Reviews*, 32, 1136–51.
6. García-Bueno, B., Caso, J.R., Madrigal, J.L., and Leza, J.C. (2016). Innate immune receptor Toll-like receptor 4 signalling in neuropsychiatric diseases. *Neuroscience and Biobehavioral Reviews*, 64, 134–47.
7. Miller, A.H., Maletic, V., and Raison, C.L. (2009). Inflammation and its discontents: the role of cytokines in the pathophysiology of major depression. *Biological Psychiatry*, 65, 732–41.
8. Morris, A.A., Zhao, L., Ahmed, Y., *et al.* (2011). Association between depression and inflammation--differences by race and sex: the META-Health study. *Psychosomatic Medicine*, 73, 462–8.

9. Dowlati, Y., Herrmann, N., Swardfager, W., *et al.* (2010). A meta-analysis of cytokines in major depression. *Biological Psychiatry*, 67, 446–57.
10. Liu, Y., Ho, R.C., and Mak, A. (2012). Interleukin (IL)-6, tumour necrosis factor alpha (TNF-alpha) and soluble interleukin-2 receptors (sIL-2R) are elevated in patients with major depressive disorder: a meta-analysis and meta-regression. *Journal of Affective Disorders*, 139, 230–9.
11. Haapakoski, R., Mathieu, J., Ebmeier, K.P., Alenius, H., and Kivimaki, M. (2015). Cumulative meta-analysis of interleukins 6 and 1beta, tumour necrosis factor alpha and C-reactive protein in patients with major depressive disorder. *Brain Behavior and Immunity*, 49, 206–15.
12. Strawbridge, R., Arnone, D., Danese, A., Papadopoulos, A., Herane Vives, A., and Cleare, A.J. (2015). Inflammation and clinical response to treatment in depression: a meta-analysis. *European Neuropsychopharmacology*, 25, 1532–43.
13. Raison, C.L., Capuron, L., and Miller, A.H. (2006). Cytokines sing the blues: inflammation and the pathogenesis of depression. *Trends in Immunology*, 27, 24–31.
14. Dantzer, R., O'Connor, J.C., Freund, G.G., Johnson, R.W., and Kelley, K.W. (2008). From inflammation to sickness and depression: when the immune system subjugates the brain. *Nature Reviews Neuroscience*, 9, 46–56.
15. Haroon, E., Raison, C.L., and Miller, A.H. (2012). Psychoneuroimmunology meets neuropsychopharmacology: translational implications of the impact of inflammation on behavior. *Neuropsychopharmacology*, 37, 137–62.
16. Muller, N., Schwarz, M.J., Dehning, S., *et al.* (2006). The cyclooxygenase-2 inhibitor celecoxib has therapeutic effects in major depression: results of a double-blind, randomized, placebo controlled, add-on pilot study to reboxetine. *Molecular Psychiatry*, 11, 680–4.
17. Tyring, S., Gottlieb, A., Papp, K., *et al.* (2006) Etanercept and clinical outcomes, fatigue, and depression in psoriasis: double-blind placebo-controlled randomised phase III trial. *The Lancet*, 367, 29–35.
18. Courtet, P., Giner, L., Seneque, M., Guillaume, S., Olie, E., and Ducasse, D. (2015). Neuroinflammation in suicide: toward a comprehensive model. *World Journal of Biological Psychiatry*, 17, 564–86.
19. Kent, S., Bluthe, R.M., Kelley, K.W., and Dantzer, R. (1992). Sickness behavior as a new target for drug development. *Trends in Pharmacological Sciences*, 13, 24–8.
20. Maes, M. (1995). Evidence for an immune response in major depression: a review and hypothesis. *Progress in Neuro-psychopharmacology and Biological Psychiatry*, 19, 11–38.
21. De La Garza, R., 2nd. (2005). Endotoxin- or pro-inflammatory cytokine-induced sickness behavior as an animal model of depression: focus on anhedonia. *Neuroscience and Biobehavioral Reviews*, 29, 761–70.
22. Wichers, M.C. and Maes, M. (2004). The role of indoleamine 2,3-dioxygenase (IDO) in the pathophysiology of interferon-alpha-induced depression. *Journal of Psychiatry and Neuroscience*, 29, 11–17.
23. Schwarcz, R., Bruno, J.P., Muchowski, P.J., and Wu, H.Q. (2012). Kynurenines in the mammalian brain: when physiology meets pathology. *Nature Reviews Neuroscience*, 13, 465–77.
24. Maes, M., Kubera, M., Leunis, J.C., Berk, M., Geffard, M., and Bosmans, E. (2013). In depression, bacterial translocation may drive inflammatory responses, oxidative and nitrosative stress (O&NS), and autoimmune responses directed against

O&NS-damaged neoepitopes. *Acta Psychiatrica Scandinavica*, 127, 344–54.

25. Hajebrahimi, B., Bagheri, M., Hassanshahi, G., *et al.* (2014). The adapter proteins of TLRs, TRIF and MYD88, are upregulated in depressed individuals. *International Journal of Psychiatry in Clinical Practice*, 18, 41–4.

26. Hung, Y.Y., Kang, H.Y., Huang, K.W., and Huang, T.L. (2014). Association between toll-like receptors expression and major depressive disorder. *Psychiatry Research*, 220, 283–6.

27. Pandey, G.N., Rizavi, H.S., Ren, X., Bhaumik, R., and Dwivedi, Y. (2014). Toll-like receptors in the depressed and suicide brain. *Journal of Psychiatric Research*, 53, 62–8.

28. Lopresti, A.L., Maker, G.L., Hood, S.D., and Drummond, P.D. (2014). A review of peripheral biomarkers in major depression: the potential of inflammatory and oxidative stress biomarkers. *Progress in Neuro-psychopharmacology and Biological Psychiatry*, 48, 102–11.

29. Do, K.Q., Cabungcal, J.H., Frank, A., Steullet, P., and Cuenod, M. (2009). Redox dysregulation, neurodevelopment, and schizophrenia. *Current Opinion in Neurobiology*, 19, 220–30.

30. Berk, M., Williams, L.J., Jacka, F.N., *et al.* (2013). So depression is an inflammatory disease, but where does the inflammation come from? *BMC Medicine*, 11, 200.

31. Dinan, T.G. and Cryan, J.F. (2017). Microbes, immunity and behaviour: psychoneuroimmunology meets the microbiome. *Neuropsychopharmacology*, 42, 178–92.

32. O'Malley, D., Quigley, E.M., Dinan, T.G., and Cryan, J.F. (2011). Do interactions between stress and immune responses lead to symptom exacerbations in irritable bowel syndrome? *Brain, Behavior, and Immunity*, 25, 1333–41.

33. Nemani, K., Hosseini Ghomi, R., McCormick, B., and Fan, X. (2015). Schizophrenia and the gut-brain axis. *Progress in Neuro-Psychopharmacology and Biological Psychiatry*, 56, 155–60.

34. Sapone, A., Bai, J.C., Ciacci, C., *et al.* (2012). Spectrum of gluten-related disorders: consensus on new nomenclature and classification. *BMC Medicine*, 10, 13.

35. Severance, E.G., Prandovszky, E., Castiglione, J., and Yolken, R.H. (2015). Gastroenterology issues in schizophrenia: why the gut matters. *Current Psychiatry Reports*, 17, 27.

36. Kalaydjian, A.E., Eaton, W., Cascella, N., and Fasano, A. (2006). The gluten connection: the association between schizophrenia and celiac disease. *Acta Psychiatrica Scandinavica*, 113, 82–90.

37. Lachance, L.R. and McKenzie, K. (2014). Biomarkers of gluten sensitivity in patients with non-affective psychosis: a meta-analysis. *Schizophrenia Research*, 152, 521–7.

38. Leza, J.C. García-Bueno, B., Bioque, M., *et al.* (2015). Inflammation in schizophrenia: a question of balance. *Neuroscience and Biobehavioral Reviews*, 55, 612–26.

39. Rosenblat, J.D., Kakar, R., Berk, M., *et al.* (2016). Anti-inflammatory agents in the treatment of bipolar depression: a systematic review and meta-analysis. *Bipolar Disorders*, 18, 89–101.

40. Khandaker, G.M., Cousins, L., Deakin, J., Lennox, B.R., Yolken, R., and Jones, P.B. (2015). Inflammation and immunity in schizophrenia: implications for pathophysiology and treatment. *The Lancet Psychiatry*, 2, 258–70

# 16

# Functional genomics

*Caleb Webber*

## Introduction

The term functional genomics represents an approach to molecular biology that seeks to generate and exploit a wealth of diverse information about the function of genes in order to understand the relationship between genotype and phenotype. As a genomics approach, the methods employed usually involve efforts to systematically survey every gene or gene product in the genome and thus provide a global view on aspects of gene function. Unlike the static genome, gene function is a dynamic process and thus varies in terms of both space (for example, cell type) and time (for example, development). For example, we may wish to know both which set of genes are switched on in a particular type of neuron and how this set of genes changes with age.

As is often the case in science, our ability to measure is driven largely by technological development. For genomics approaches where scale is important, it is not just the development of technologies that enables us to measure a particular feature, but also further developments that enable us to economically apply this measurement systematically across the genome. Importantly, our ability to measure at the scale of the genome fundamentally changes the nature of the questions we can ask, leading to a step change in discovery. For example, while a quantitative polymerase chain reaction assay allows us to detect changes in the expression of a *pre-specified* gene in diseased tissue, the advent of microarray methodologies enabled us to measure the change in expression across thousands of genes simultaneously. Changing the question from 'is *that* different?' to 'is *anything* different?' enables us to discover disease-associated variation that we might not have thought to look for. This approach has been adopted across psychiatric disorders in recent years and will be covered in detail in the relevant chapters on genetics in this volume. It will form the prelude to understanding the variation in function that is likely to constitute the characteristics of disordered phenotypes.

While functional genomics approaches are often simply scaling up the detection of a known phenomenon, the technologies developed can also extend our knowledge of the basic functional repertoire of the cell. For example, next-generation sequencing approaches enabled the unbiased detection of all expressed RNA molecules in the cell, revealing the existence of tens of thousands of new genes that do not encode proteins and whose roles are currently being elucidated

[1]. Nonetheless, while many genes express RNA molecules that are not templates for translation, the vast majority of our knowledge about the roles of genes comes from studying the functions of proteins, and thus our knowledge is focused towards the subset of genes that encode them. This is an illustration of one bias, and although genomics approaches are innately *less* biased, the biases in each approach to measuring function should be considered when designing and interpreting studies, as discussed in the following sections.

This chapter provides a gene-centric introduction to functional genomics, each section introducing the aspect of gene function being measured and then contextualizing variation in the context of neuropsychiatric disease studies (Fig. 16.1). Each section, namely 'Epigenomics', 'Gene expression', 'Proteomics', and 'Functional annotations', is, in themselves, the subject of dedicated textbooks and dozens of reviews, and thus this chapter provides only a succinct introduction to several large and rapidly growing fields of study.

## Epigenomics

Epigenetic modifications are defined as reversible modifications of DNA or DNA-associated proteins which affect gene expression without altering the DNA sequence. Epigenetics explains why two different cell types possessing exactly the same genetic code execute distinct gene expression programmes and diverge in their roles.

There are two important classes of epigenetics modifications: DNA methylation and histone modification. The transcriptional accessibility of DNA is determined by the condensation state of chromatin, which is formed from structural units called nucleosomes, in which the DNA is wrapped around eight core histone proteins. Post-transcriptional modifications of these histones can alter the regional chromatin state between a transcriptionally active open *euchromatic* state and a transcriptionally silenced closed *heterochromatic* state, thereby impacting gene expression [2, 3]. Active and repressive histone marks delineate coding regions, non-coding regulatory elements including promoter regions near transcriptional initiation sites, and proximal and distal enhancers (Fig. 16.2). In parallel to histone modifications, methylation of the DNA base cytosine within promoter and enhancer regions acts to repress transcription (Fig. 16.2).

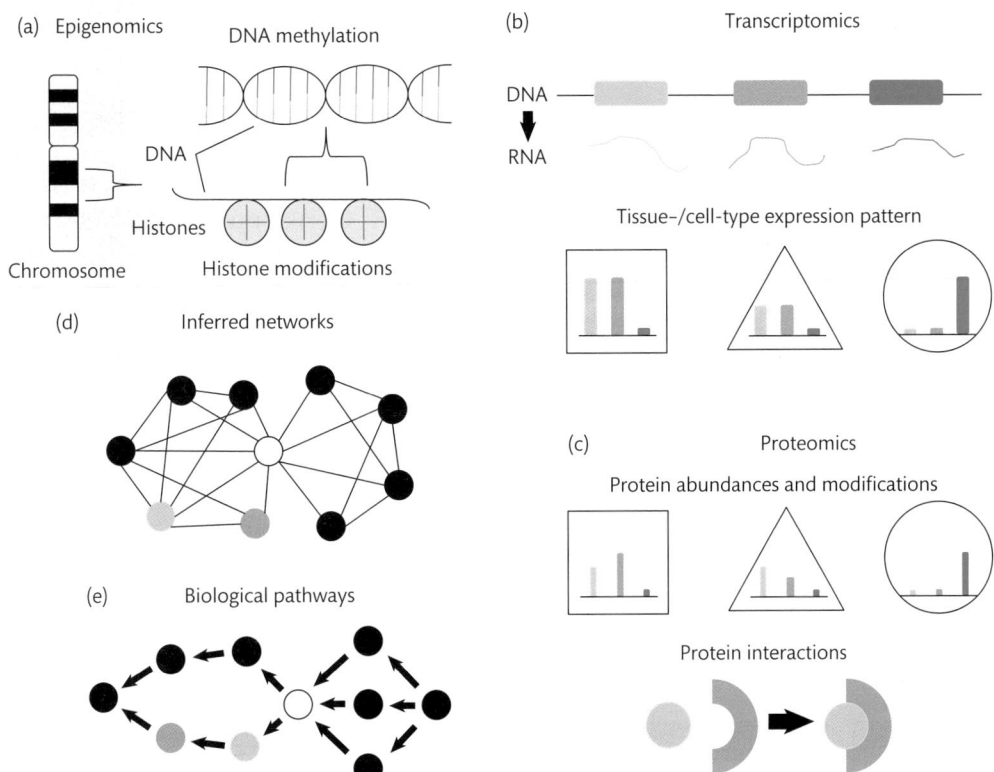

**Fig. 16.1** An overview of functional genomics. (a) Epigenomic analyses can indicate how poised different genes are being transcribed. Different chemical modifications of histones, the proteins that form the scaffold around DNA, and variation in the accessibility of the DNA to proteins that regulate and execute gene expression are associated with active or repressed genes (Fig. 16.2). (b) The variation in gene expression by cell type or with disease state informs on function. Where the expression pattern of genes are similar, it may reflect their co-ordinated regulation as part of the same biological process. (c) While correlated with gene expression level, the abundance of the protein product of a gene can vary due to translational regulation and degradation, while the functioning of a protein can be significantly altered by a range of post-translational chemical modification. A physical interaction detected between two proteins can indicate that they function together in a common role. (d) Functional genomics information, such as the co-ordinated expression of genes, the knowledge that their protein products physically interact, or large-scale information gathered from published literature can be used to infer sets of genes likely to function together in the same biological pathway (e).

Using high-throughput approaches, the Roadmap and ENCODE projects have delivered genome-wide human epigenetic maps that highlight cell-specific regulatory elements, providing a valuable resource for the interpretation of genetic variation [4, 5]. These maps reveal that a large majority of common genetic risk variants identified do not affect the protein-coding sequence but are instead localized in non-coding regions regulating gene expression which these variants are likely to alter. Knowledge of the cell-specific utilization of these regulatory elements enables the identification of the cell type(s) likely affected by variants within them. For example, the 108 genetic risk loci reported so far for schizophrenia (SCZ) are enriched in brain-specific enhancer regions, suggesting these variants affect the expression of genes in the brain, but also within enhancer elements utilized by CD20/CD19 lymphocytes, in turn suggesting a link between SCZ and the immune system [6].

Inter-individual variation in DNA methylation found in fetal brain tissue coincides with SCZ risk loci [7]. However, epigenetic variation is dynamic, varying not just with the cell type, but also over the life of a cell. A study identifying regions of DNA that were differentially methylated in the prefrontal cortex between individuals with and those without SCZ found that these differentially methylated regions were associated with changes in DNA methylation that occurred during the transition from the second fetal trimester to postnatal life, implicating this transition as a key developmental point in the development of the disorder [8].

## Gene expression

The spatiotemporal expression profile of a gene is particularly informative. Knowing when (for example, in development, in disease progression) and where (in which cell types) a gene is switched on, or expressed, is key to understanding both its normal and its aberrant functioning (Fig. 16.1b). Genomic technologies that simultaneously report the expression of thousands of different RNA molecules have advanced rapidly and include microarrays that detect pre-specified RNA molecules and RNA-seq that can sequence the entire population of RNA molecules without pre-selection. However, for neuropsychiatric disorders, access to the relevant living tissue sample or cell population remains challenging. Nonetheless, using post-mortem brains, detailed maps of spatiotemporal gene expression are now available. For example, the BrainSpan atlas of the Developing Human Brain has examined 42 brains to provide the gene expression profiles of up to 16 targeted cortical and subcortical structures across the full course of human brain development [9].

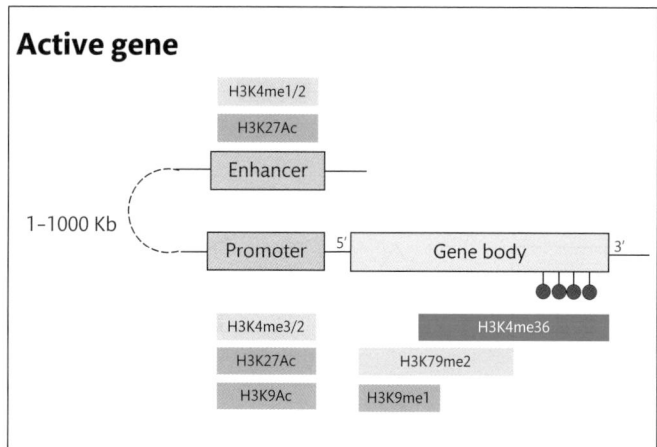

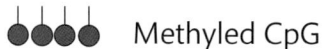

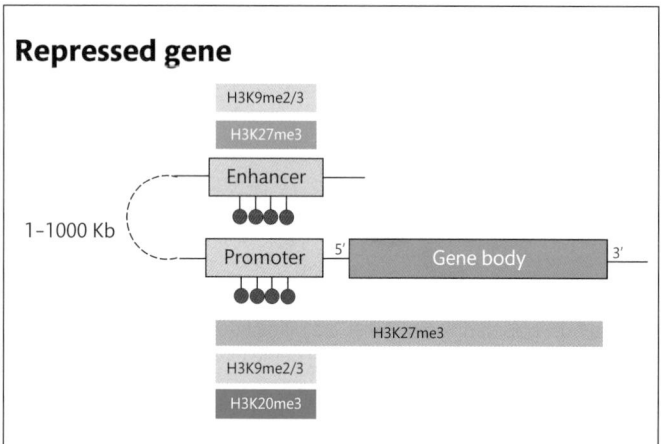

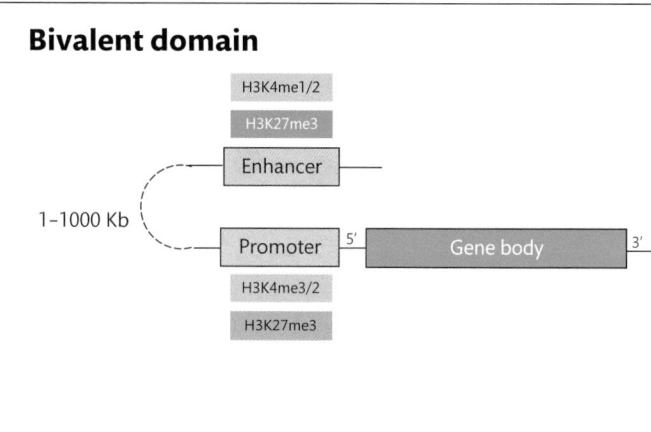

**Fig. 16.2** Epigenetics marks and gene regulation. Different sets of epigenetic modifications, or marks, are associated with three states of gene regulation. The epigenetic marks can map to the full gene body or only the 5′ part or 3′ part to the promoter region or to a (distal or proximal) enhancer [98]. (a) Histone modifications (methylation and acetylations marks) for a transcriptionally active gene. (b) DNA methylation and histone H3 methylation are found in the promoter and enhancer region and surrounding the TSS in transcriptionally repressed genes. (c) Bivalent chromatin domain defined by the simultaneous presence of histone modifications associated with both gene activation and repression [99].

Knowledge of a gene's expression profile helps the causal interpretation of genetic variation observed in patients with neuropsychiatric disorders. In SCZ, for example, newly arising genetic variants that were observed in patients, but not in either parent, and that affected protein-coding sequence tended to affect genes that were expressed prenatally in the dorsolateral prefrontal cortex (DFC) and the hippocampus, with both regions previously implicated in SCZ [10]. Gene expression variation can also be detected directly in the analyses of post-mortem patient brain tissue. Large-scale studies of hippocampal tissue obtained from SCZ, bipolar disorder (BPD), and major depressive disorder (MDD) patients have found evidence for decreased expression of genes involved in antigen processing, GABA signalling, and endocytosis [11]. More specifically for BPD, but also reported in some SCZ studies, an upregulation of metallothionein genes has been observed in the DFC, while reductions in neuropeptide gene expression has been associated with psychosis [12, 13].

Notably, there is little consistency in the observed variation in gene expression for the same disorder across different regions of the brain. Moreover, even within the same region, there is considerable variability among post-mortem gene expression studies, likely due to experimental variation, the relatively small numbers of samples used, and the effects of varying patient medications. For post-mortem studies on neuropsychiatric disorders, and especially so for neurodegenerative disorders, it is also unclear what point in the progression of a disease is being studied, and thus whether any observed variation in gene expression relates to the upstream causes or the downstream consequences. Genetic and epigenetic evidence discussed above points to key prenatal or early postnatal aetiological events for many neuropsychiatric disorders which may be undetectable in adult post-mortem brain tissue. For neurodegenerative disorders, onset precedes the diagnosis by many years, making it hard to discern whether upregulated processes, such as neuroinflammation, are contributing causally to the pathology or are instead protective mechanisms, a vital distinction when targeting therapeutic interventions. Furthermore, the cell type composition can change as a consequence of a disorder, for example with the death of neurons in neurodegeneration, which can then dominate the comparison with healthy tissue [14]. Accordingly, it is reassuring when variation in gene expression in post-mortem tissue can be linked to predisposing genetic variation. For example, genetic variation in *CACNA1C* is associated with an increased risk of BPD, while the expression of this gene has also been found to be downregulated in BPD patients' brains [15, 16]. In other cases, the genetic support can be indirect; *TYROBP* has been found to be upregulated in the brain of late-onset Alzheimer's disease patients and interacts with the Alzheimer's disease-risk gene *TREM2* [17, 18].

## Co-expression networks

The expression of multiple genes can be co-ordinated within the cell, for example in order to deliver all the required subunits necessary to form a functioning protein complex or to put in place all of the enzymes required at each step in a biosynthetic pathway. Thus, the co-expression of genes, that is genes whose variation in expression levels is correlated, is a commonly used approach to divine genes that might function together with a common purpose [19]. The degree of co-expression is measured largely as the correlation coefficient of those gene expressions, as measured at multiple instances, for example their correlated expression across multiple tissues over time during a biological process such as development/ageing or disease progression, or simply from repeated recordings over multiple replicates of the same experiment. Often, co-expression is represented in a network diagram, with genes depicted as nodes and where connections, or edges, between nodes represent the fact that the connected genes are co-expressed (Fig. 16.1d). A group of genes connected together within a network through their correlated expression patterns is often referred to as a co-expression *module* [20]. As compared to variation in a single gene's expression, examining the variation of a group of co-expressed genes that form a module is both more robust to noise affecting the variation of individual genes and also enables the study of variation of the shared functionality captured by the module. Furthermore, following the reasoning that genes that are co-expressed are more likely to function together, genes within a module whose functions are unknown can be inferred from those genes with known functions [21]. This process of inferring function is commonly termed 'guilt by association' and is an often used approach for filling in gaps in knowledge in functional genomics (for example, see the section on protein–protein interactions in this chapter).

Study designs for exploiting gene co-expression methods to understand disease have taken one of two approaches. In the first, gene co-expression modules may be formed from healthy individuals and then changes in expression level of multiple genes within a module within diseased tissue are used to infer up- or downregulation of that pathway. Large-scale gene expression data sets, such as the BrainSpan database, enable the identification of genes whose expression patterns are co-ordinated across regions of the brain and throughout development, enabling the construction of gene-co-expression modules, capturing spatiotemporally co-ordinated gene modules in the healthy developing brain. Mapping mutations observed in SCZ patients onto the genes within these modules identified that these mutations often disrupted module functioning during fetal development within dorsolateral and ventrolateral prefrontal cortex [22]. Within Alzheimer's disease, co-expression analyses of post-mortem tissue have recurrently identified disrupted modules of genes associated with decreasing synaptic plasticity, while those associated with immunity and microglia increased [23, 24]. As noted, care must be taken in the interpretation, as a decrease in the expression of genes across a cell type-specific pathway might be due to the loss of the cell type expressing that pathway, rather than the downregulation of genes within that pathway within the relevant cell type.

In an alternative approach, studies can consider differential co-expression, which looks for changes in the co-ordination of gene expression that suggest that the regulatory relationships between genes that were co-expressed in healthy tissue have been altered in the diseased tissue [25]. For Alzheimer's disease, this approach to identify the rewiring of gene regulation in disease found that many gene modules involved in immunity and microglia function were differentially regulated in patient post-mortem brain tissue [24].

## Proteomics

Proteins are the enactors of the central dogma, and our efforts to measure the expression of genes are largely in order to estimate the abundances of these genes' protein products. The relationship between mRNA abundance and protein abundance is confounded by several factors, including the rates of translation and protein degradation, both of which are highly variable, depending upon the cell state. Nonetheless, in a steady state, studies suggest that gene–gene variation in protein abundances within a cell are primarily determined by those genes' relative mRNA expression. Specifically, upwards of 40% of the variance in protein abundances can be explained by mRNA levels [26–28]. After accounting for the delay between gene expression and protein synthesis, variation in mRNA levels explain around 80% of the change in protein abundance when a cell transitions between states [29, 30]. While this correlation is encouraging, protein activity is not solely determined by abundance. Dynamic post-translational modifications, such as cleavage or reversible covalent additions of chemical side groups or lipids, are key regulators of their activity that are not captured by the transcriptome. For example, as described earlier, acetylation and methylation of histone proteins significantly modify their functional association with DNA. Furthermore, identification of the cellular location(s) of a protein and its molecular partners can reveal much about its role.

Compared to reading the transcriptome, measuring protein abundance is far more challenging due to the diverse physiochemical properties of the constituent amino acids. Nonetheless, over the last 10 years, advances in mass spectrometry-based approaches have enabled the simultaneous estimation of the abundances of over 10,000 proteins. A clear example contributing to the understanding of neuropsychiatric disorders is the proteomic profiling of the neuronal post-synaptic density (PSD) from the human neocortex [31]. While some of the identified PSD proteins were known at the time of the study to have roles in neurological disorders, subsequent genetic studies identifying genes found to be disrupted in individuals with SCZ have found that many of these genes' proteins are found in the PSD, giving a clear indication of the aetiology [32, 33].

As with transcriptomics, the differential abundances of proteins within post-mortem neuronal tissue yield insights into the causes and consequences of neuropsychiatric disease. For the neuropsychiatric disorders SCZ, BPD, and MDD, these studies have revealed hundreds of proteins differentially abundant in patient brain tissue. In common, a meta-study identified a small number of proteins involved in forming and maintaining the myelin sheath, supporting a role for oligodendrocyte dysfunction in these disorders [34–36]. For SCZ more specifically, variation in the abundance of 14-3-3 mediated-signalling proteins was found, for BPD variation in mitochondrial function, and for MDD in oxidative phosphorylation pathways [34]. As with transcriptomics, there is significant variation between individual studies and between the particular brain regions studied, but for proteomics, this is likely amplified by the current variability in multiple reaction monitoring-based proteomic methodologies [28, 37].

### Protein–protein interactions

Knowing which proteins physically interact with each other helps to identify groups of proteins that are functioning together in the same biological process. The set of protein interactions within the cell is commonly referred to as the *interactome*. These interactions can be transient, for example a receptor reversibly binding a ligand, or obligate such as the persistent binding between subunits of a stable protein complex. The causal implication in a disease of multiple genes whose protein products interact provides insight into the perturbed molecular process(es), and the functional concordances between implicated genes give added confidence to their role in the same disease. There are many methods to experimentally determine protein–protein interactions (PPIs) [38–40]. *In vitro* methods often involve the use of a bait or tagged protein that is drawn out of a cell extract, along with any other proteins that are directly or indirectly attached to it [for example, tandem affinity purification and mass spectrometry (TAP-MS), affinity chromatography, co-immunoprecipitation]. *In vivo* methods include the Yeast 2 Hybrid (Y2H) approach. Here, a transcription factor is cleaved into a binding domain and a separated activating domain, and each of a pair of query proteins is fused to one of the two domains. If the two query proteins interact, the two transcription factor domains are brought close to each other and transcription is initiated. However, current methods for detecting PPIs are prone to noise and high rates of false positives, for example due to artefactual interactions detected between proteins that do not reside in the same cellular compartment, and thus corroborative support is often sought to validate PPIs [41, 42].

An early example of the utility of PPIs in providing insights into neuropsychiatric genetics is an interactome study performed for the Disrupted in Schizophrenia 1 (DISC1) protein [43]. Proteins that interacted with DISC1 were identified using Y2H assays, and then a subset of these interactors were selected and their interactors similarly identified. Many of the proteins within the extended DISC1 interactome had roles in synaptic-associated functions such as cytoskeletal stability and organization and intracellular transport, thereby implicating DISC1 in these processes through 'guilt by association' whereby the functionality of a protein is inferred through the known functions of the proteins with which it interacts.

PPIs detected in large- and small-scale studies have been collated within several large, publicly available databases [for example, human protein reference database (HPRD) [44], BioGrid [45]]. Although fewer than 100,000 interactions are currently known, which represents a fraction of the estimated complete interactome [46], these experimentally determined interactions can be supplemented by computationally predicted interactions to provide a key resource for identifying common functions between genes implicated in neurological disease [39]. For example, genome-wide association (GWA) studies have been phenomenally successful in identifying regions of the genome that are associated with the risk of developing SCZ. However, these regions often contain many genes, and so identifying which of these genes is more specifically associated with disease risk remains a current bottleneck in translating these genetic findings into actionable drug targets. By examining the interactions of the proteins expressed by genes within risk loci identified with SCZ GWA studies with the proteins of genes that have been implicated in SCZ in past studies, one study identified interactions between 76 GWA genes and 25 previously implicated SCZ genes [47]. Such studies are able to both propose the causally associated gene within these GWA regions and identify common functions among the sets of interacting proteins, here for example synaptic plasticity, neurotransmission, and inflammation, that may be disrupted in the disease.

The vast majority of human genes express not just one transcript but instead can selectively include or exclude different exons, to generate multiple alternatively spliced transcripts. Alternatively spliced transcripts are expressed in a tissue-specific manner, with many genes expressing a dominant transcript in a particular tissue. Of particular relevance, tissue-specific splicing are most often observed in brain cells with roles in both development and ageing [48–54]. By varying the protein sequence, the set of resulting protein isoforms expressed by a single gene can demonstrate remarkable variation that impacts on function. For example, by varying the inclusion of interaction surface, protein isoforms can interact with alternative sets of proteins, changing the topology of the network [50, 55, 56]. Such tissue-specific, isoform-specific interaction networks are important in understanding cell type-specific gene function, and therefore in understanding the functional impact of genetic variation underlying neuropsychiatric disorders [57].

## Literature annotations

Every day, hundreds of research articles are published, with each article reporting the results of molecular and/or genetic experiments, adding to a body of knowledge about the function of a single gene or a small number of genes. We are unable to read them all and we are unable to remember all that we have read, and what we can remember is highly biased. There is a huge diversity in experimental approaches, reflecting the many questions that might be asked. For example, these articles might report on a study that localizes a protein to a particular cellular structure, identifies a role for a protein within a specific biological function, or details the phenotypic consequences arising from the protein's disruption within a cellular model, a model organism, or a human patient. However, in order to ask questions about groups of genes, such as whether a set of genes found to be disrupted in patients with a particular disease are associated with a particular function, the information about gene function, the language of function, must be consistent between genes.

### Functional annotations

There have been several attempts to organize the wealth of heterogenous information about the function of genes and their expressed proteins. Most commonly, this involves the creation of an ontology, a defined vocabulary that describes a set of entities, or properties, and the interrelationships between them. The most successful and commonly used in molecular biology is Gene Ontology (GO) [58, 59]. Here, the properties of gene products, most commonly proteins, are defined within three ontologies. A protein's action at the molecular level, such as binding or catalysis, is described within *Molecular Function* ontology; where it is located within (or outside) a cell, it is described with *Cellular Component* ontology, while terms within the more abstractly defined *Biological Process* ontology are used to describe the higher-level functioning of a protein such as signal transduction or regulation of gene expression. For example, if we consider the key metabolic enzyme malate dehydrogenase, its Molecular Function terms include *oxidoreductase activity*; its Cellular Component terms include *mitochondrion*, while its *Biological Process* terms include *tricarboxylic acid cycle*. The relationships between terms within the ontology allow proteins to logically acquire additional annotation terms. For example, the GO molecular function ontology defines that the mitochondrion

is a *cytoplasmic part*, which is an *intracellular part*, and thus a gene whose protein is assigned with the GO property of mitochondrion logically inherits both the GO properties of *cytoplasmic part* and *intracellular part*. A fraction of the GO annotation tree for the Biological Process term 'positive regulation of transmission of nerve impulse' is illustrated in Fig. 16.3 where the inherited annotation terms can be seen.

While GO successfully captures a huge amount of information about human gene function, unarguably more than any other single information resource, users exploiting GO functional annotations should be aware of the evidence for a functional annotation. Each GO annotation is associated with an evidence code,

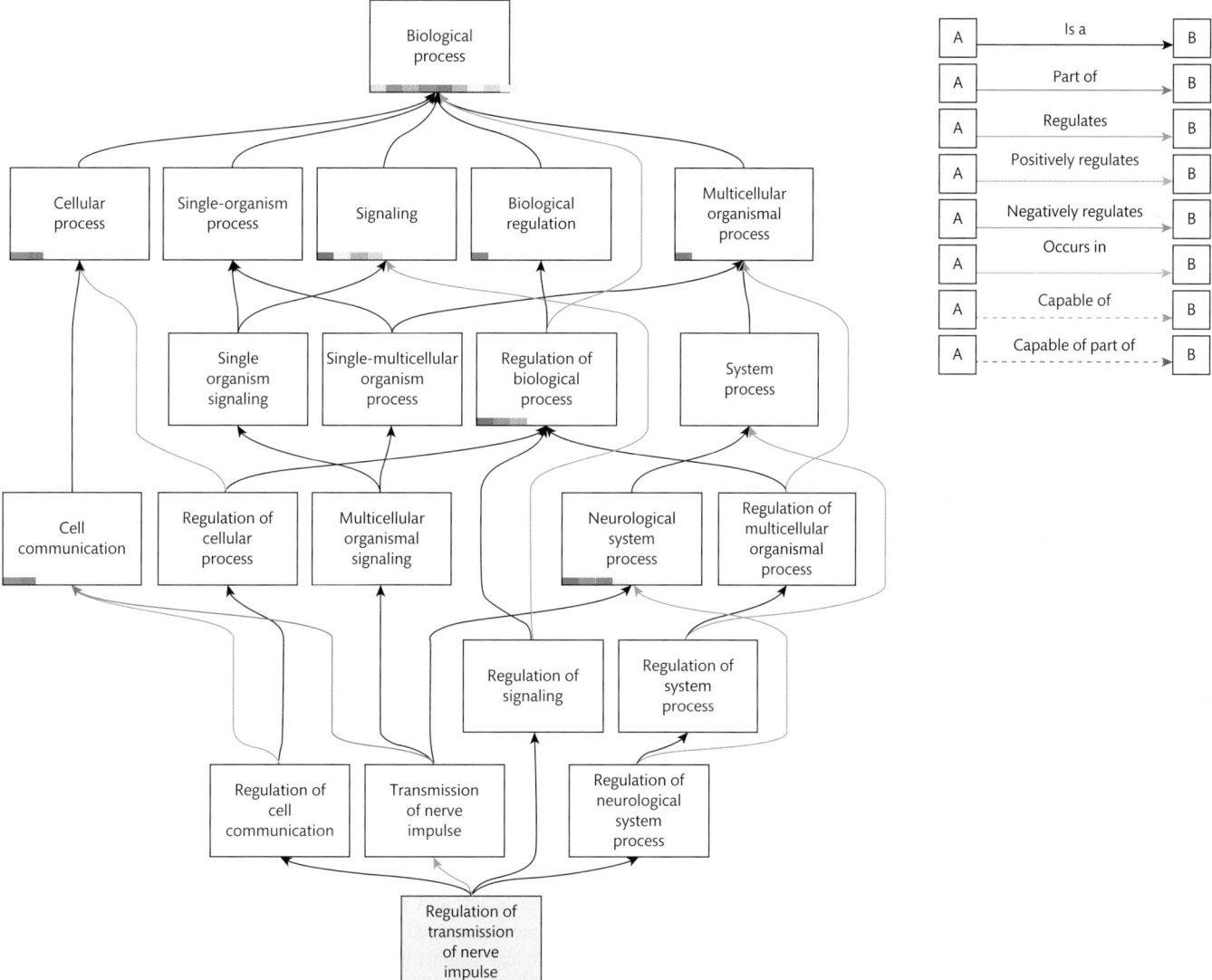

**Fig. 16.3** (see Colour Plate section) An example of hierarchical relationships in the Gene Ontology (GO) [58]. In this example, we show the GO annotation terms that lie above the term 'regulation of transmission of nerve impulse'. Following this GO hierarchy, a gene that was ascribed the function of *regulation of transmission of nerve impulse* would automatically also be assigned all of the functional terms listed. As with other structured ontologies discussed in the main text, an explicit understanding of knowledge relationships between annotation terms makes it possible to identify similarities between gene functions. For example, if we were comparing a gene assigned with the term *regulation of cell communication* to another gene assigned the term *transmission of nerve impulse*, the graph identifies *cell communication* as a common role. Although many of these relationships may seem obvious to a researcher, ontologies are computable, such that we can rapidly compute the similarity between thousands of genes enabling us to statistically identify unusually common functions among sets of genes, for example those found to be dysregulated in a diseased tissue.

Reproduced from *Nature Genetics*, 25(1), Ashburner M, Ball CA, Blake JA, *et al.*, Gene Ontology: tool for the unification of biology, pp. 25–29, Copyright (2000), with permission from Springer Nature.

which can be broadly split into those codes derived from published experiments and those derived by computational predictions. As of writing, almost 16,000 out of a total of 22,000 human protein-coding genes are annotated with at least one GO annotation that has been derived from published experiments. However, for almost 5000 human protein-coding genes, only computationally predicted functional evidence is available, which should be viewed with less confidence. For 1500 genes, GO provides no functional evidence at all, experimental or inferred. Furthermore, while there is thus some functional information ascribed to over 20,000 protein-coding genes, this evidence is likely very incomplete for all but a small fraction of genes, with genes of more interest to the community (for example, those involved in disease) receiving far more experimental attention, and thus acquiring more functional annotations, than those attracting less interest. It is often necessarily assumed in functional genomics that genes that are not annotated with a particular function do not perform that function, but this assumption is flawed: *The absence of evidence is not evidence of absence.* Compounding this, there is a strong bias towards publishing positive, rather than negative, findings, in this case showing what a gene does, rather than what it does not do. Accordingly, more systematically collected functional evidence, such as a genome-wide survey of gene expression, can provide a more robust, albeit significantly less functionally detailed, information source. Despite these concerns, GO remains the current standard for ascribing gene function, and almost all the functional associations of genes with disease described in this chapter, for example sets of genes whose expression or protein abundances are found to be different or dysregulated in diseased tissue, have been identified from the GO annotations of these genes.

## Pathway databases

Although GO aims to capture the function of a gene, it does not embody well the functional relationships between genes. While GO will annotate several genes as belonging to the same biological process, for example the *tricarboxylic acid cycle*, it does not inform on the order in which the enzymes in this fundamental energy cycle act, which is key to understanding the biological process. To address this, pathway databases have been created that map out the constitutive genes, describing a set of interacting genes/products that together perform a particular biological function. Historically, the most well-used of these is the *Kyoto Encyclopaedia of Genes and Genomes* (KEGG), which attempts to map out the literature-reported relationships between genes within a diverse collection of metabolic and cellular processes, including processes associated with specific diseases [60]. More recently initiated databases, for example *Reactome* [61], attempt to more systematically map out the molecular operations of gene products into a hierarchical level of detail, similar to that described previously for GO. However, as discussed for GO annotations, pathway annotations are very incomplete and suffer from significant ascertainment biases. Furthermore, the biological processes that these pathway concepts seek to describe are often active under specific conditions and/or within particular cell types [62], information that is often missing. Nonetheless, from a deterministic perspective, where the aim is to understand the consequences of a genetic variant, understanding the relationship of that gene to the biological process(es) in which it participates will clearly aid in the interpretation.

## Model organism databases

Although far beyond the remit of this chapter to discuss the utility of model organisms for individual neuropsychiatric disorders (for reviews, see [63-70]), the ability to determinedly introduce genetic variation into an organism is a robust approach to understanding the relationship between genotype and phenotype. The evolutionary conservation of the protein-coding sequence of orthologues between two species implies that the function of these genes is similarly conserved between those species, and thus knowledge of the gene in one species can be transferred to the other. This conjecture holds best between unique 1:1 orthologous genes, defined as genes in two species that have been maintained without duplication since those species diverged from a cenancestor [71–73]. While the functional genomics resources described in this chapter thus far are focused on molecular and cellular annotations, from the expression of genes through to the functional roles of their protein products, often it is not immediately obvious how the disruption of a cellular process might manifest a complex behavioural abnormality. Thus, model organisms offer a more direct description of the influence of genetics and environment upon behaviour.

Due to their ready genetic manipulation, easy laboratory management, and study scalability, genotype/phenotype relationships have been extensively explored in the lower model organisms, namely the fruit fly *Drosophila melanogaster*, the nematode *Caenorhabditis elegans*, and the yeast *Saccharomyces cerevisiae*. From a functional genomics perspective, the knowledge amassed about the function of individual genes from studying these model organisms has contributed to a genome-wide body of knowledge that has been collated for each model into community-supported databases (namely FlyBase [74], WormBase [75], Saccharomyces Genome Database [76], and Zfin [77]). Much of this knowledge forms a major contribution to functional and pathway annotation resources.

From a neuropsychiatric perspective, rodent models are pre-eminent in the study of relevant disorders, due both to their more comparable neuroanatomy and to behaviours that are more comparable to neuropsychiatric presentations. From a functional genomics perspective, the systematic collation from published reports by the Mouse Genome Database (MGD) of the phenotypes resulting from determined genetic manipulation of several thousands of mouse genes offers an excellent resource for neurological associations [78]. Currently, the MGD holds phenotypic associations for the unique orthologue of over 9000 human genes and reports this phenotypic information within structured ontology, enabling computational analyses [79]. As with other literature sources of gene functional information, the original studies upon which these data are based were hypothesis-led, and thus only a specific set of phenotypes would have been examined in each study and reported on. Nonetheless, aetiological insights into neuropsychiatric disorders can be robustly obtained, for example an excess of genes whose orthologues' disruption in the mouse yielded synaptic dysfunction has been identified among genes found to be deleted or duplicated in individuals with autism [80, 81]. Of note, for functional genomics approaches, significant efforts are ongoing by the International Mouse Phenotyping Consortium (IMPC) to systematically pass each mutant mouse line through a series of standardized phenotyptic tests of broad relevance to human disease, with results from the first 1750 knockout mouse models recently reported [82–85]. A key criticism of functional annotation resources amassed from individual studies is that where a gene is not annotated with a particular function, researchers might assume that that gene is not associated with that function when, in fact, the association has never been tested. Thus, although the phenotyping of these models is inevitably incomplete, the IMPC's efforts to annotate gene function are hugely powerful, as the systematic testing also provides evidence that a phenotype is not associated with a given gene.

## Future perspectives

Functional genomics is a particularly technology-driven field. New methods are frequently published, enabling new properties of the genome to be assayed or known properties to be examined on an increasing scale. The overwhelming volume of biological data being generated consequently challenges bioinformaticians to develop new analytical techniques able to integrate these diverse data types and make these data coherently available for researchers to query. Thus, while the promises of new technologies are often noisily trumpeted, our organization and standardization of data, for example gene function within GO or organismal phenotype within the Mammalian Phenotype Ontology or the Human Phenotype Ontology, are also important in gaining new biological understanding.

Several current technologies are promising to revolutionize molecular biology and functional genomics and are worth drawing attention to in the context of neuropsychiatric disease. An outstanding problem in the study of the brain is accessibility to brain tissue. As discussed, post-mortem tissue may better reflect the consequences of disease, rather than yield insights into the causes. The development of induced pluripotent stem cells (iPSCs) is enabling researchers to create cultures of patient-derived neurons in the laboratory [86–88]. Here, an accessible non-neuronal tissue is sampled from a patient and then these cells are coerced, through a cocktail of bioagents, into a pluripotent state, able to be subsequently driven down a cell lineage towards a neuronal cell identity. While there are many significant differences between iPSC-derived neurons and native adult neurons, these cell models are promising significant insights into neuropsychiatric disorders, for example, mimicking the differential lithium responsiveness of bipolar patients [89, 90].

While epigenomic, transcriptomic, and proteomic studies have yielded many insights into neuropsychiatric disease, a criticism already discussed when comparing healthy and diseased tissues is that differences in the underlying cell types that form these tissues are obscured when measuring across the whole tissue combined. Recently developed single-cell approaches allow the epigenetic and transcriptomic profiles of individuals cells to be obtained, enabling the cell type to be determined from the cell type-specific marker genes and particular and specific populations of cells to be examined [91–93]. Elsewhere, our ability to manipulate the genetic sequence in disease models to introduce or remove, and thus explore the effects of, disease-predisposing mutations has been revolutionized in terms of ease and scale by the development of the clustered regularly interspaced short palindromic repeat (CRISPR)/Cas system, a prokaryotic antiviral defence mechanism whose constituent proteins are remarkably adept at introducing genome edits [94–96]. By combining these approaches, we might, for example, derive a culture of neuronal cells via iPSCs from a patient. If we have a candidate disease-predisposing genetic variant in that patient, then we could edit the genome of the cells in a parallel culture to remove this variant and then compare the effect of this variant on the individual neuronal cell types (neurons, glial cells). This experiment is certainly not trivial, but remarkably it is now possible.

While these, and many other, developments are exciting, we should resist the urge to generate data simply because we can. These new techniques bring substantial challenges to the bioinformatics interpretation of the data, for example huge variability in cell models and high noise in the single-cell readouts [97], and thus answers may not simply drop out. We must make sure that our applications of functional genomics are both well powered and hypothesis-led and, in particular, that we increase the informatics, mathematic, computational, and statistical expertise required to interpret these fantastical experiments.

## REFERENCES

1. Cech, T.R. and Steitz, J.A. (2014). The noncoding RNA revolution-trashing old rules to forge new ones. *Cell*, 157, 77–94.
2. Jenuwein, T. and Allis, C.D. (2001). Translating the histone code. *Science*, 293, 1074–80.
3. Kouzarides, T. (2007). Chromatin modifications and their function. *Cell*, 128, 693–705.
4. Kundaje, A., *et al.* (2015). Integrative analysis of 111 reference human epigenomes. *Nature*, 518, 317–30.
5. Ecker, J.R., *et al.* (2012). Genomics: ENCODE explained. *Nature*, 489, 52–5.
6. Schizophrenia Working Group of the Psychiatric Genomics Consortium. (2014). Biological insights from 108 schizophrenia-associated genetic loci. *Nature*, 511, 421–7.
7. Hannon, E., *et al.* (2016). Methylation QTLs in the developing brain and their enrichment in schizophrenia risk loci. *Nature Neuroscience*, 19, 48–54.
8. Jaffe, A.E., *et al.* (2016). Mapping DNA methylation across development, genotype and schizophrenia in the human frontal cortex. *Nature Neuroscience*, 19, 40–7.
9. Miller, J.A., *et al.* (2014). Transcriptional landscape of the prenatal human brain. *Nature*, 508, 199–206.
10. Xu, B., *et al.* (2012). *De novo* gene mutations highlight patterns of genetic and neural complexity in schizophrenia. *Nature Genetics*, 44, 1365–9.
11. Darby, M.M., *et al.* (2016). Consistently altered expression of gene sets in postmortem brains of individuals with major psychiatric disorders. *Translational Psychiatry*, 6, e890.
12. Seifuddin, F., *et al.* (2013). Systematic review of genome-wide gene expression studies of bipolar disorder. *BMC Psychiatry*, 13, 213.
13. Choi, K.H., *et al.* (2008). Putative psychosis genes in the prefrontal cortex: combined analysis of gene expression microarrays. *BMC Psychiatry*, 8, 87.
14. Hawrylycz, M.J., *et al.* (2012). An anatomically comprehensive atlas of the adult human brain transcriptome. *Nature*, 489, 391–9.
15. Gershon, E.S., *et al.* (2014). A rare mutation of *CACNA1C* in a patient with bipolar disorder, and decreased gene expression associated with a bipolar-associated common SNP of CACNA1C in brain. *Molecular Psychiatry*, 19, 890–4.
16. Psychiatric GWAS Consortium Bipolar Disorder Working Group. (2011). Large-scale genome-wide association analysis of bipolar disorder identifies a new susceptibility locus near ODZ4. *Nature Genetics*, 43, 977–83.
17. Jiang, T., *et al.* (2013). TREM2 in Alzheimer's disease. *Molecular Neurobiology*, 48, 180–5.

18. Ma, J., *et al.* (2015). TYROBP in Alzheimer's disease. *Molecular Neurobiology*, 51, 820–6.

19. Obayashi, T., *et al.* (2008). COXPRESdb: a database of coexpressed gene networks in mammals. *Nucleic Acids Research*, 36, D77–82.

20. Langfelder, P. and Horvath, S. (2008). WGCNA: an R package for weighted correlation network analysis. *BMC Bioinformatics*, 9, 559.

21. Wolfe, C.J., *et al.* (2005). Systematic survey reveals general applicability of 'guilt-by-association' within gene coexpression networks. *BMC Bioinformatics*, 6, 227.

22. Gulsuner, S., *et al.* (2013). Spatial and temporal mapping of *de novo* mutations in schizophrenia to a fetal prefrontal cortical network. *Cell*, 154, 518–29.

23. Miller, J.A., *et al.* (2008). A systems level analysis of transcriptional changes in Alzheimer's disease and normal aging. *Journal of Neuroscience*, 28, 1410–20.

24. Zhang, B., *et al.* (2013). Integrated systems approach identifies genetic nodes and networks in late-onset Alzheimer's disease. *Cell*, 153, 707–20.

25. de la Fuente, A. (2010). From 'differential expression' to 'differential networking'—identification of dysfunctional regulatory networks in diseases. *Trends in Genetics*, 26, 326–33.

26. Schwanhausser, B., *et al.* (2011). Global quantification of mammalian gene expression control. *Nature*, 473, 337–42.

27. Li, J.J., *et al.* (2014). System wide analyses have underestimated protein abundances and the importance of transcription in mammals. *PeerJ*, 2, e270.

28. Liu, Y., *et al.* (2016). On the dependency of cellular protein Levels on mRNA abundance. *Cell*, 165, 535–50.

29. Lee, M.V., *et al.* (2011). A dynamic model of proteome changes reveals new roles for transcript alteration in yeast. *Molecular Systems Biology*, 7, 514.

30. Lackner, D.H., *et al.* (2012). Regulation of transcriptome, translation, and proteome in response to environmental stress in fission yeast. *Genome Biology*, 13, R25.

31. Bayes, A., *et al.* (2011). Characterization of the proteome, diseases and evolution of the human postsynaptic density. *Nature Neuroscience*, 14, 19–21.

32. Genovese, G., *et al.* (2016). Increased burden of ultra-rare protein-altering variants among 4,877 individuals with schizophrenia. *Nature Neuroscience*, 19, 1433–41.

33. Betancur, C. (2011). Etiological heterogeneity in autism spectrum disorders: more than 100 genetic and genomic disorders and still counting. *Brain Research*, 1380, 42–77.

34. Saia-Cereda, V.M., *et al.* (2017). Psychiatric disorders biochemical pathways unraveled by human brain proteomics. *European Archives of Psychiatry and Clinical Neuroscience*, 267, 3–17.

35. Du, F., *et al.* (2013). Myelin and axon abnormalities in schizophrenia measured with magnetic resonance imaging techniques. *Biological Psychiatry*, 74, 451–7.

36. Lewandowski, K.E., *et al.* (2015). Myelin vs axon abnormalities in white matter in bipolar disorder. *Neuropsychopharmacology*, 40, 1243–9.

37. Davalieva, K., *et al.* (2016). Proteomics research in schizophrenia. *Frontiers in Cellular Neuroscience*, 10, 18.

38. Shoemaker, B.A. and Panchenko, A.R. (2007). Deciphering protein-protein interactions. Part I. Experimental techniques and databases. *PLoS Computational Biology*, 3, e42.

39. Shoemaker, B.A. and Panchenko, A.R. (2007). Deciphering protein–protein interactions. Part II. Computational methods to predict protein and domain interaction partners. *PLoS Computational Biology*, 3, e43.

40. Legrain, P. and Rain, J.C. (2014). Twenty years of protein interaction studies for biological function deciphering. *Journal of Proteomics*, 107, 93–7.

41. Rao, V.S., *et al.* (2014). Protein-protein interaction detection: methods and analysis. *International Journal of Proteomics*, 2014, 147648.

42. Peng, X., *et al.* (2016). Protein–protein interactions: detection, reliability assessment and applications. *Briefings in Bioinformatics*, 18, 798–819.

43. Camargo, L.M., *et al.* (2007). Disrupted in schizophrenia 1 interactome: evidence for the close connectivity of risk genes and a potential synaptic basis for schizophrenia. *Molecular Psychiatry*, 12, 74–86.

44. Peri, S., *et al.* (2004). Human protein reference database as a discovery resource for proteomics. *Nucleic Acids Research*, 32, D497–501.

45. Rual, J.F., *et al.* (2005). Towards a proteome-scale map of the human protein–protein interaction network. *Nature*, 437, 1173–8.

46. Stumpf, M.P., *et al.* (2008) Estimating the size of the human interactome. *Proceedings of the National Academy of Sciences of the United States of America*, 105, 6959–64.

47. Ganapathiraju, M.K., *et al.* (2016). Schizophrenia interactome with 504 novel protein-protein interactions. *npj Schizophrenia*, 2, 16012.

48. Roy, B., *et al.* (2013). Review: alternative splicing (AS) of genes as an approach for generating protein complexity. *Current Genomics*, 14, 182–94.

49. Xu, Q., *et al.* (2002). Genome-wide detection of tissue-specific alternative splicing in the human transcriptome. *Nucleic Acids Research*, 30, 3754–66.

50. Yang, X., *et al.* (2016). Widespread expansion of protein interaction capabilities by alternative splicing. *Cell*, 164, 805–17.

51. Merkin, J., *et al.* (2012). Evolutionary dynamics of gene and isoform regulation in Mammalian tissues. *Science*, 338, 1593–99.

52. Kalsotra, A. and Cooper, T.A. (2011). Functional consequences of developmentally regulated alternative splicing. *Nature Reviews Genetics*, 12, 715–29.

53. Tollervey, J.R., *et al.* (2011). Analysis of alternative splicing associated with aging and neurodegeneration in the human brain. *Genome Research*, 21, 1572–82.

54. Mazin, P., *et al.* (2013). Widespread splicing changes in human brain development and aging. *Molecular Systems Biology*, 9, 633.

55. Buljan, M., *et al.* (2012). Tissue-specific splicing of disordered segments that embed binding motifs rewires protein interaction networks. *Molecular Cell*, 46, 871–83.

56. Ellis, J.D., *et al.* (2012). Tissue-specific alternative splicing remodels protein-protein interaction networks. *Molecular Cell*, 46, 884–92.

57. Corominas, R., *et al.* (2014). Protein interaction network of alternatively spliced isoforms from brain links genetic risk factors for autism. *Nature Communications*, 5, 3650.

58. The Gene Ontology Consortium, *et al.* (2000). Gene ontology: tool for the unification of biology. The Gene Ontology Consortium. *Nature Genetics*, 25, 25–9.

59. The Gene Ontology Consortium, *et al.* (2017). Expansion of the Gene Ontology knowledgebase and resources. *Nucleic Acids Research*, 45, D331–8.

60. Kanehisa, M., *et al.* (2016). KEGG as a reference resource for gene and protein annotation. *Nucleic Acids Research*, 44, D457–62.

61. Fabregat, A., *et al.* (2016). The Reactome pathway Knowledgebase. *Nucleic Acids Research*, 44, D481–7.

62. Khatri, P., *et al.* (2012). Ten years of pathway analysis: current approaches and outstanding challenges. *PLoS Computational Biology*, 8, e1002375.

63. Nestler, E.J. and Hyman, S.E. (2010). Animal models of neuro-psychiatric disorders. *Nature Neuroscience*, 13, 1161–9.

64. Drummond, E. and Wisniewski, T. (2017). Alzheimer's disease: experimental models and reality. *Acta neuropathologica*, 133, 155–75.

65. Ahmari, S.E. (2016). Using mice to model Obsessive Compulsive Disorder: From genes to circuits. *Neuroscience*, 321, 121–37.

66. Kato, T., *et al.* (2016). Animal models of recurrent or bipolar depression. *Neuroscience*, 321, 189–96.

67. Logan, R.W. and McClung, C.A. (2016). Animal models of bipolar mania: the past, present and future. *Neuroscience*, 321, 163–88.

68. Onos, K.D., *et al.* (2016). Toward more predictive genetic mouse models of Alzheimer's disease. *Brain Research Bulletin*, 122, 1–11.

69. Czeh, B., *et al.* (2016). Animal models of major depression and their clinical implications. *Progress in Neuro-psychopharmacology and Biological Psychiatry*, 64, 293–310.

70. Jones, C.A., *et al.* (2011). Animal models of schizophrenia. *British Journal of Pharmacology* 164, 1162–94.

71. Altenhoff, A.M., *et al.* (2012). Resolving the ortholog conjecture: orthologs tend to be weakly, but significantly, more similar in function than paralogs. *PLoS Computational Biology*, 8, e1002514.

72. Chen, X. and Zhang, J. (2012). The ortholog conjecture is untestable by the current gene ontology but is supported by RNA sequencing data. *PLoS Computational Biology*, 8, e1002784.

73. Webber, C. and Ponting, C.P. (2004). Genes and homology. *Current Biology*, 14, R332–3.

74. Gramates, L.S., *et al.* (2017). FlyBase at 25: looking to the future. *Nucleic Acids Research*, 45, D663–71.

75. Howe, K.L., *et al.* (2016). WormBase 2016: expanding to enable helminth genomic research. *Nucleic Acids Research*, 44, D774–80.

76. Cherry, J.M., *et al.* (2012). *Saccharomyces* Genome Database: the genomics resource of budding yeast. *Nucleic Acids Research*, 40, D700–5.

77. Ruzicka, L., *et al.* (2015). ZFIN, The zebrafish model organism database: updates and new directions. *Genesis*, 53, 498–509.

78. Blake, J.A., *et al.* (2017). Mouse Genome Database (MGD)-2017: community knowledge resource for the laboratory mouse. *Nucleic Acids Research*, 45, D723–9.

79. Robinson, P.N. and Webber, C. (2014). Phenotype ontologies and cross-species analysis for translational research. *PLoS Genetics*, 10, e1004268.

80. Gai, X., *et al.* (2012). Rare structural variation of synapse and neurotransmission genes in autism. *Mol Psychiatry*, 17, 402–11.

81. Noh, H.J., *et al.* (2013). Network topologies and convergent aetiologies arising from deletions and duplications observed in individuals with autism. *PLoS Genetics*, 9, e1003523.

82. Brown, S.D. and Moore, M.W. (2012). The International Mouse Phenotyping Consortium: past and future perspectives on mouse phenotyping. *Mammalian Genome*, 23, 632–40.

83. Morgan, H., *et al.* (2012). Accessing and mining data from large-scale mouse phenotyping projects. *International Review of Neurobiology*, 104, 47–70.

84. [No authors listed]. (2014). Still much to learn about mice. *Nature*, 509, 399.

85. Dickinson, M.E., *et al.* (2016). High-throughput discovery of novel developmental phenotypes. *Nature*, 537, 508–14.

86. Brennand, K.J., *et al.* (2012). Modeling psychiatric disorders at the cellular and network levels. *Molecular Psychiatry*, 17, 1239–53.

87. Falk, A., *et al.* (2016). Modeling psychiatric disorders: from genomic findings to cellular phenotypes. *Molecular Psychiatry*, 21, 1167–79.

88. Soliman, M.A., *et al.* (2017). Pluripotent stem cells in neuro-psychiatric disorders. *Molecular Psychiatry*. 22, 1241–9.

89. Mertens, J., *et al.* (2015) Differential responses to lithium in hyperexcitable neurons from patients with bipolar disorder. *Nature*, 527, 95–9.

90. Stern, S., *et al.* (2018) Neurons derived from patients with bipolar disorder divide into intrinsically different sub-populations of neurons, predicting the patients' responsiveness to lithium. *Molecular Psychiatry*. 23, 1453–65.

91. Gawad, C., *et al.* (2016) Single-cell genome sequencing: current state of the science. *Nature Reviews Genetics*, 17, 175–88.

92. Schwartzman, O. and Tanay, A. (2015). Single-cell epigenomics: techniques and emerging applications. *Nature Reviews Genetics*, 16, 716–26.

93. Shapiro, E., *et al.* (2013). Single-cell sequencing-based technologies will revolutionize whole-organism science. *Nature Reviews Genetics*, 14, 618–30.

94. Sander, J.D. and Joung, J.K. (2014). CRISPR-Cas systems for editing, regulating and targeting genomes. *Nature Biotechnology*, 32, 347–55.

95. Dominguez, A.A., *et al.* (2016). Beyond editing: repurposing CRISPR-Cas9 for precision genome regulation and interrogation. *Nature Reviews Molecular Cell Biology*, 17, 5–15.

96. Heidenreich, M. and Zhang, F. (2016). Applications of CRISPR-Cas systems in neuroscience. *Nature Reviews Neuroscience*, 17, 36–44.

97. Stegle, O., *et al.* (2015). Computational and analytical challenges in single-cell transcriptomics. *Nature Reviews Genetics*, 16, 133–45.

98. Barski, A., *et al.* (2007). High-resolution profiling of histone methylations in the human genome. *Cell*, 129, 823–37.

99. Bernstein, B.E., *et al.* (2006). A bivalent chromatin structure marks key developmental genes in embryonic stem cells. *Cell*, 125, 315–26.

# 17

# Cognitive neuroscience
## Principles and methods

*Anna Christina Nobre*

## Introduction

Cognitive neuroscience is the scientific discipline concerned with understanding the neural mechanisms involved in supporting human mental function. The discipline therefore rests on a reductionistic stance, or at least on the assumption that there are principled relationships between the objective, physical brain and the subjective, functional mind. The overarching aim is to build mechanistic bridges connecting the mind to the workings of the organ from which it arises and to the behaviours that arise from it.

Cognitive neuroscience has two primal roots. The first consisted in the observation that damage to the brain can lead to highly selective deficits in high-level human cognitive behaviours such as reasoning and comportment [1], language production and comprehension [2, 3], the recognition of complex objects [4–6], and the comprehension of spatial relations [7, 8]. The second was the development of rigorous quantitative scientific experimental methods to identify and measure elemental processes in human behaviour [9–11]. The two roots came together in the elegant research in neuropsychology and behavioural neurology, which used rigorous psychophysics and cognitive psychology to understand associations and dissociations in elemental cognitive functions in individuals with different patterns of brain damage [12–14].

A third root was being established at around the same time but took longer to mature—the development of methods to measure activity in the human brain. Early attempts were made to measure blood circulation, based on the belief that it was linked to brain activity [15–17]. The coupling between brain activity and local circulatory changes was subsequently scientifically proven [18] and eventually supported the development of effective methods to measure haemodynamic responses using PET [19–21] and fMRI [22]. A complementary set of methods was developed to measure the electrical signals of the brain directly [23, 24]. Once established, modern-day brain imaging and neurophysiological methods provided a significant impetus for the establishment of cognitive neuroscience.

The term 'cognitive neuroscience' was famously coined in a New York taxi in the late 1970s when a renowned neuroscientist (Michael Gazzaniga) and cognitive psychologist (George Miller)

were on the way to a dinner meeting aimed at promoting studies into how the brain enables the mind (https://www.cogneurosociety.org/background/). The name stuck, and the field thrives.

The enormous scope of cognitive neuroscience prevents a comprehensive review. The chapter therefore focuses on highlighting the emerging principles of the brain–mind relationship and the ever improving methods with which to investigate them. The conceptual and methodological breakthroughs provide a foundation for an experimental medicine approach into understanding the neural basis of psychiatric conditions and their treatment.

## Principles

### Levels of organization

The neural mechanisms that contribute to mental function (and dysfunction) can be investigated at various levels of organization. Starting from the most basic unit, it is possible to look for contributing factors linked to molecules, biochemical cascades, cellular structures (for example, synapses), cells, local microcircuits, brain regions, large-scale brain networks, behaviour of individuals, social groups, and culture. There is no leading candidate for the most relevant level of organization. Instead, it is clear that factors at any of these levels can provide important insights into understanding the brain–mind relationship.

As an example, consider the case of human memory. The properties of the NMDA receptor *molecule* are essential for enabling changes in synaptic strength as a function of association between the activities of two interconnected neurons [25, 26]. Donald Hebb [27] had famously proposed such a mechanism to be able to support long-term associative learning in the brain. Similar, though less technically detailed, proposals had also been put forth earlier [28]. *Biochemical cascades*, such as those involving calcium/calmodulin-dependent protein kinase II (CaMKII) are essential for transforming the calcium signal entering via the NMDA receptor channel into stable changes in synaptic transmission and structure [29]. The *synapse* serves as the unit of change, and different algorithms for plasticity may be manifest at different types of synapses, with different consequences for memory. For example, the rules for plasticity differ at the synapse between Schaeffer collaterals between CA3 and CA1 pyramidal neurons vs at the synapse between the mossy fibres from the granule cells of the dentate gyrus and the CA3 pyramidal neurons. What learning properties arise is highly dependent on the way both principle cells and interneurons are interconnected in the *local microcircuitry* of brain regions (for example, entorhinal cortex, dentate gyrus, CA3, and CA1) [30, 31]. For example, in the CA3 region, the sparse pattern of potent connections between mossy fibres and pyramidal cells, together with the dense pattern of recurrent connections among CA3 pyramidal neurons, has been proposed to support sequential learning and auto-associative memory [32, 33]. Different brain *areas* are essential for supporting different types of memory. The hippocampus is essential for forming new long-term episodic memories [12, 34], whereas the cerebellum is required for certain types of sensorimotor forms of conditioning [35]. These brain areas do not operate in isolation, but within large-scale *networks* of brain regions, in which activity injected by other brain areas can modulate the qualities and strength of memories. For example, the prefrontal cortex, which is linked to the hippocampal region, can influence the integrity of source and temporal context of memories [36–38]. None of these neural insights would have come about without the observations of human *behaviour*. The patterns of dissociation among affected vs preserved memory functions in individuals after brain damage were essential to reveal the plurality of memory and to guide its taxonomy. Social, and ultimately cultural, factors strongly influence what individuals end up encoding and storing in memory [39, 40], revealing the fact that memory is biased towards items and events that are relevant to individuals, and therefore proactive and adaptive, rather than passive and impartial.

Given that all levels of organization are informative, research at different levels is equally valid. The ambition is to abstract and formalize the relevant computations at different levels and incorporate their contributions as we move to increasing scales. This is not yet possible with any certainty of capturing the true essence of all biological mechanisms involved, though the use of biophysical and mathematical models is a powerful way to test and refine ideas about computations at different levels. For the empirical scientist conducting research at a given level, the most prudent way forward is to recognize the important constraints and influences brought to bear by the other levels of organization. In the case of human cognitive neuroscience, most of the methods provide access to macroscopic levels of organization, ranging from brain areas to human behaviour. However, these can also be deployed to understand neural changes as a result of molecular manipulations or changes, as in the case of genetic risk factors or pharmacological interventions.

## Structure and function

At all levels of brain organization, structure and function are bound. Thus, in order to understand neural mechanisms of cognition, one must consider the anatomy, physiology, and pharmacology. On a macroscopic scale, the anatomical pathways and connections between areas provide the scaffolding on which neural computations unfold. Furthermore, the anatomical pattern of connections to and from a given brain area is a primary determinant of its functional role [41, 42] for contemporary partitioning of human brain anatomy. The nature, intensity, and timing of physiological signals exchanged within and among brain areas through the anatomical

highways carry the contents of neural information. These determine our behaviours and our mental experience. The carriers of the physiological signals are neurotransmitters and neuromodulators acting through their various receptors. The main excitatory neurotransmitters in the brain—glutamate and GABA—are responsible for the bulk of neuronal communication in the human brain, but neuromodulators such as dopamine, serotonin, noradrenaline, and acetylcholine play essential roles in shaping the specificity, gain, and plasticity of the communications. Thus, when considering the neural basis of psychological functions, it is essential to consider the anatomy, physiology, and pharmacology. As a corollary, when attempting to understand psychological or psychiatric disorders, it is necessary to understand the interplay of these three essential ingredients.

## Networks

The intuitive approach to understanding brain–mind relationships remains stuck in phrenology [43]. We gravitate towards understanding the contributions of individual brain areas to complex cognitive functions, and many scientists continue to focus on individual areas. But it is clear that brain areas are not independent functional modules within the brain. Instead, they are interconnected within large-scale networks. Functional specializations of individual brain areas come together and interact within networks.

Networks can be considered effective functional units in their own right, the integrity of which correlates with complex human psychological functions most directly [3, 44, 45]. Functional brain networks are supported by the patterns of anatomical connectivity in the brain but are also assembled flexibly according to the context of the incoming stimulation and task demands. Some groups of brain areas have a strong and close allegiance with one another, working closely together to support given functions. Examples would be the left hemisphere-dominant language network for speech comprehension and production [46, 47] and the right hemisphere-dominant network for the control of spatial attention [48, 49]. However, new allegiances can be formed flexibly and specific brain areas may be co-opted, depending on the nature of information or computations required for the current task. Indeed, brain areas need not be exclusively dedicated to one network and may contribute to multiple networks that make use of their elemental computational functions. One example is the inferotemporal cortex, noted to contribute to networks involved in visual, working memory, and semantic tasks [50–53].

Large-scale networks have important and distinctive properties. Within networks, the categorical differences between the functions of contributing brain areas can become blurred and difficult to pinpoint. The network architecture can provide resilience to loss of function by providing compensatory mechanisms, unless critical or multiple nodes are damaged. When behavioural deficits occur, these can result from lesions that damage critical brain areas within the network or from lesions that disrupt their connections to other regions. Because of the multiple specialized nodes and their interconnections, behavioural symptoms can be varied and dissociable [49, 54].

The network pattern of organization is recapitulated at lower levels of organization. Individual neurons are embedded within functional ensembles and circuits. In many cases, neuronal ensembles may be assembled flexibly, though constrained by their anatomical connectivity. At an even finer grain, active synapses form dynamic network structures that can support specific patterns of communication and plasticity [55].

## Functional specialization

Although it is no longer sensible to think of brain areas as being fully responsible of delivering specific mental capacities in a phrenological sense, it is clear that brain areas contribute specialized functions to the networks within which they are embedded. The shift from functional localization to functional specialization may appear subtle, but it is fundamental. Functional specialization of brain areas is determined by multiple factors: the pattern of inputs it receives from its various afferent regions, the neuromodulatory influences, the mappings of functional units within the region, the intrinsic microcircuitry that determines how information is transformed locally, and the pattern of outputs to its various efferent regions. Though we have made tremendous progress in sketching the functional contributions of many brain areas, our knowledge of their functional specialization is largely still incomplete.

Functional specialization occurs at different levels of organization. Previously, we considered how brain areas have specialized functions, but the same is true at higher and lower levels of organization. At higher levels of organization, we have functional brain networks that perform different transformations of their characteristic patterns of stimulation. Higher still, in humans, we observe specialization at the level of brain hemispheres. Though the precise origins and determinants of hemispheric specialization remain mysterious, certain brain networks and functions display patterns of hemispheric dominance across the population. Language, for example, tends to be left hemisphere-dominant [2, 15], whereas spatial attention tends to be right hemisphere-dominant [48, 56, 57]. Anatomical differences, such as the torque [58], accompany these functional differences, and disruption during the development of normal hemisphere dominance has been suggested as a possible cause for disorders of mental health [59].

At lower levels of organization, functional specialization occurs within subregions of brain areas, and at cellular and molecular levels. Let us focus on the hippocampal system as an illustration. In the main afferent to the hippocampus proper—the entorhinal cortex—spatial responses of neurons are organized in a grid-like fashion, which has been proposed to provide a scaffolding for constructing maps of spatial relations out of external stimulation [60]. Within individual regions of the hippocampus and closely related structures, neurons display different types of functional specialization, coding for spatial locations within the environment [61, 62], interval durations [63], or head direction [64]. Subcomponents of hippocampal cells are also specialized such as the giant synapses between the dentate mossy fibres and the 'thorny excrescences' on the proximal dendrites of the CA3 neurons and the exuberant pattern of recurrent collaterals within the CA3 region itself. At the molecular level, the NMDA receptor channel, densely packed in some hippocampal subregions, provides a unique molecular logical 'AND' gate, sensing the coincidences of presynaptic and post-synaptic activity, and is thus well suited for gating synaptic plasticity [25, 26, 65]. The computational contributions and implications of these various levels of specialization are not fully understood and remain an area of active research. Interestingly, cognitive neuroscientists are beginning to explore whether some of these specializations, which have been observed within the context of spatial navigation and memory in animal models, may also contribute to the mapping of other types of functional relationships, and therefore underpin cognition more broadly [66–68].

## Concurrent processing

Another hallmark of network organization is the rich, multidirectional, and concurrent flow of information among its various nodes. It is intuitive to think of the brain as operating on simple signals extracted from the external stream of information in an orderly way, reconstructing increasingly more complex and abstracted features and dimensions, and stitching these together into cohesive episodes. But, at best, this is an oversimplification. For example, although there is evidence for increasingly integrated and sophisticated information being coded along sensory hierarchies, it is also well known that information processing does not progress neatly in series through these hierarchies. There are many bifurcations, shortcuts, and re-entrant pathways of information. In vision, the best studied case, multiple paths of visual signal are established already at the first relay. Activity flows from the retina both to the lateral geniculate nucleus of the thalamus and to the superior colliculus. In the cortex, massive interconnections among visual areas are well documented [42, 69]. Bifurcations result in massive concurrent processing. Processing at multiple specialized brain areas proceeds concurrently to extract information about the colour, motion, identity, and spatial relations among items. Analysis in these areas cannot be said to be fully parallel, since many interconnections exist, with the possibility of mutual interaction and cross-talk during concurrent analysis. Re-entrant pathways are also abundant, so that higher-order areas receiving early signals can influence stimulus processing at hierarchically lower-order areas. For example, in vision, prefrontal areas have some of the earliest latencies of stimulation and may influence lower-order areas [70]. One interesting observation, for example, is that there are many times more feedback connections between V1 and the lateral geniculate nucleus than there are feed-forward connections [71]. Information flow in the reverse hierarchical direction may be as important as that in the forward direction [72].

The computational architecture combining functional specialization with distributed, concurrent processing is highly efficient, greatly speeding up perceptual analysis and providing some fault tolerance through compensatory pathways. However, it also poses a major problem, known as the 'binding problem'. How does the brain correctly integrate the various attributes of the individual objects of perception (or thought) to form a cohesive episode? To date, no specific brain repository of fully integrated objects fit for conscious experience has been identified. Most theories posit that the binding problem is solved through the co-ordination of activity across large-scale networks in the brain [73, 74]. These theories are often also invoked to explain the neural basis of perceptual awareness [75, 76]. However, it is fair to say that we still lack an understanding for the exact way in which activity is co-ordinated and integrated throughout brain networks. The questions become particularly thorny when one considers the different timings for information to reach the brain from the different sensory modalities and remembers that we experience the world dynamically as it changes and we move through it.

## Proactive and dynamic modulation

Our conceptualization of the brain is evolving. Instinctively, we have considered the brain as an organ to mirror, or at least construct a good internal model of reality. In this interpretation, the brain is usually a passive organ that reacts to external stimulation, creating a mental percept or construct anew, from scratch, at each moment. Yet, advances in research reveal the brain to be of a very different character. It is a complex dynamical system, ever restless, full of content used proactively and dynamically to interpret incoming signal perturbations to guide adaptive behaviour.

From the very first measurements of electrical signals in the human brain, this organ was found to be full of structured activity [23]. Far from idle, brain activity had rhythms that changed in intensity and frequency with the individuals' state or pursuit. With the advent of modern haemodynamic brain imaging methods, researchers observed that, even at rest, the brain alternates among activated functionally specialized networks [77, 78]. Contemporary electrophysiological methods with good spatial and temporal resolution reveal rapid transitions, with multiple network states per second [79, 80]. At the level of neuronal ensembles, the ebbing and flowing of rhythmic fluctuations in voltage levels is thought to affect neuronal excitability, influencing the timing of neuronal spiking and, ultimately, their communication [81–83].

The earliest psychophysical studies of human behaviour also cast strong doubt on a reactive and bottom–up construction of perception and cognition. For example, when multiple stimuli compete for attention, the resulting percept is strongly dictated by where one wilfully chooses to focus, independently of where one is looking [10]. Over the years, experimental psychology has taught us that, contrary to how it seems, we do not take in the complete and continuous stream of events unfolding around us. Instead, we sample at most a handful of items at any given moment. What ends up being perceived, and subsequently remembered, depends largely on our current task goals, motivations, memories, and emotions [84]. These internal factors influence perception and cognition proactively and dynamically. By combining behavioural studies with measurements of brain activity, cognitive neuroscientists have been charting the brain networks and mechanisms involved in the top–down control of information processing in the brain. Anticipatory signals based on internal states (for example, task goals or memories) carry information about multiple attributes (for example, locations, features, or timings) of expected relevant events. These, in turn, influence multiple stages of sensory and motor processing to determine the objects of perception that occupy the mind or guide action [85].

This continual orchestration of human perception and cognition by internal factors has important repercussions for understanding and treating mental disorders. The delicate regulation and optimization of our mental experience is achieved through fine orchestration of activity in multiple brain areas by large-scale networks involved in attention, memory, motivation, and emotion—often working together. Biased patterns of memories or deficits in motivation can lead to suboptimal or distorted pickup of external information from the environment, for example by prioritizing and selecting items that reinforce negative expectations. In this way, cognitive and emotional biases can compromise the very first exchanges with reality. Furthermore, because these selected items then come to occupy the mind and guide action, they fuel a cognitive vicious cycle that can become difficult to break.

Research into how disruption of proactive top–down control by various types of internal factors contributes to disorders of mental health has great promise. Some researchers are beginning to investigate how mood disorders compromise attention to emotional stimuli [86, 87]. The results are promising and are already leading to some useful cognitive interventions [88, 89]. However, the opportunities remaining to be explored are vast. To make incisive progress, it will help for cognitive neuroscientists to expand their inquiry of attention-related mechanisms to more ecological contexts and to consider the influence of internal factors highlighted by the clinical condition.

## Methods

The last few decades have produced methods for investigating the human brain that would have seemed unimaginable when researchers first started empirical investigations of the brain–mind relationship. Each of the methods has its characteristic strengths and limitations, and so none is superior to others. In order to make advances in understanding how the brain supports cognition, it is always prudent to keep methodological limitations in mind and to employ multiple methods in a complementary fashion, to overcome limitations and guide accurate interpretation. A similar approach should be used to develop biomarkers and treatments for disorders of mental health.

### Psychophysics

Psychophysics is a key term introduced to launch the empirical study of mental functions and to establish psychology as a scientific discipline [90]. Through psychophysics, the researcher investigates how systematic alterations in physical stimulation change an individual's private perceptual experience and behaviour. The use of the term is often confined to studies of perceptual systems, but the methodology applies equally well to investigations of higher-order cognitive functions, such as attention, memory, and emotion, through the systematic manipulation of stimulation.

Careful psychophysical experimentation should be brought to the forefront of understanding the causes of mental health disorders. Their primary and defining symptoms are psychological functions, yet many of the scientific efforts to develop biomarkers and treatments include only coarse psychological assessments or sidestep cognition altogether. Instead, few approaches would make greater inroads to understanding mental disorders than careful psychological testing, enabling reliable, sensitive, and selective quantification of specific cognitive functions.

The establishment of experimental psychology as a scientific field has transformed our understanding of the landscape of mental functions. The constituent elements of cognition are distilled with increasing granularity, and their dissociations, associations, and mutual influences charted. We no longer think of cognitive domains, such as memory, language, executive control, or emotion, as monolithic constructs defined in folk psychological terms. Each of these domains comprises functions with characteristic input streams, functional variables, behavioural consequences, and relationships to other psychological functions.

To dissect the psychological mechanisms of granular cognitive functions, experimental variables are manipulated systematically to measure behavioural consequences. In addition to behavioural responses that explicitly tap into the variables of interest, it is also possible to use indirect behavioural measures, which are altered by the implicit use of the cognitive construct in question. Implicit measures can be very sensitive and circumvent problems related to strategic responding by participants. For example, rather than asking individuals about their reactions to emotional stimuli, it is possible to measure their response times to targets that follow emotional vs neutral stimuli [91] or to name the colour in which emotional vs neutral words are written [92]. The implicit association task [93] is a good example of how implicit measures can reveal instinctive psychological attitudes of prejudice, which would be difficult to assess through explicit judgements. Most behavioural tasks still rely on unitary responses, such as a button response related to detection, discrimination, or choice of a stimulus. In addition to accuracy, response times often add valuable information about the quality of performance. It is possible, however, to obtain much more detailed measures of behavioural performance by using continuous responses in behavioural tasks and by recording the precision and trajectories of responses [94, 95]. For example, rather than indicating whether a particular stimulus held in working memory was on the left or right side of the screen, participants can place the stimulus at its remembered location on the screen. In this way, over trials, it is possible to verify the precision of memory by the dispersion of responses around the correct value, to detect whether participants swap the location of items in mind, or to test whether the response trajectory is influenced by the presence of other stimuli that may have had particular salience or significance [96, 97]. In addition to relying on manual responses, recording eye movements, body movements, facial expressions, and muscle contraction can further add valuable sensitivity to the content and transformation of mental operations. The precise delineation of boundaries among functions, as well as their full characterization, is still a living science and subject to refinement, but current knowledge is sufficiently mature to make significant contributions to the study of mental health.

Our growing insights into psychological functions have not made their way very effectively into the batteries of psychological tasks used for diagnosing mental functions. The challenge is to develop a time-efficient set of tasks that are sensitive, selective, reliable, validated, and easy to administer and quantify. The requirement to use well-validated tasks keeps us tethered to old ways. Some of the most popular neuropsychological tasks combine many psychological functions of different sorts, making interpretation at the granular level problematic. Take, for example, the Wisconsin Card Sorting Task (WCST), used for diagnosing frontal lobe dysfunction. On each trial, participants view three items that can vary along multiple dimensions—colour, shape, and number. They have to learn the rule determining which two items go together. After a series of trials, the categorization rule changes without instruction. Participants must understand that the rule has changed, learn and use the new rule, and inhibit using the previous rule. This simple task therefore requires verbal comprehension, attention to individual features, categorization, learning sensorimotor correspondences, rule switching, inhibition, working memory for the active rule, sustained attention, and more. Most of the favourite neuropsychological tasks, like the WCST, are blunt or, at best, messy tasks from which to interpret the precise functions that may be compromised. But they are also quick and powerful methods for revealing a deficit in the first place, and

over the years, their interpretation has become a science in its own right [98].

Effective behavioural testing is essential. The quality of inference about a given molecular biomarker, brain dysfunction, or experimental treatment for a mental disorder will depend heavily on the quality of behavioural testing. Researchers argue about the best neuropsychological tasks, or combination of tasks, to chart the mental landscape of individuals. The use of a consistent set of tasks is important in order to link research findings from various laboratories around the world. For this reason, efforts are increasingly made to harmonize the use of neuropsychological tasks across research centres, with groups of researchers coming together to thrash out what constitutes the most effective task battery [99]. But even these distilled test batteries still combine old-fashioned and complex tasks that do not isolate and quantify relevant psychological functions with a high level of granularity. Given the state of experimental psychology, much cleaner and more detailed assessments should be possible.

So how do we strike the right level of innovation vs validation? It would be foolish to throw away the old faithful tests, with their many decades of validation. It seems equally foolish not to benefit from the power of precise psychological phenotyping that is currently possible. Multiple components should be considered for striking the right balance. The first step is to acknowledge the importance of cognitive and behavioural phenotyping. Occasionally, major research initiatives or trials of mental disorders use only perfunctory measures of cognition such as administering one of the standard cognitive batteries. What is the logic in downgrading the importance of obtaining high-quality psychological data relative to obtaining other body-based measures? Could this be a lingering prejudice against psychological science? If so, it is high time that we leave this behind. Another contributor could be the lack of access to high-quality cognitive neuroscience, and for this, more cross-fertilization between clinical and basic science training would be highly effective.

Once the importance of sophisticated psychological phenotyping is accepted, it will prove exciting to realize the enormous breakthrough potential that can be achieved through its incorporation into large-scale studies. At this juncture, multiple research approaches should be pursued and interrelated. We should continue to use standardized and well-validated batteries of proven neuropsychological tasks. These are effective at revealing the neuropsychological deficits and tether new studies to the established literature, thus allowing for comparisons. In parallel, we should use contemporary cognitive neuroscience to zoom in on potentially compromised areas in much greater detail. In many cases, it will be worth investing the time to obtain reliable and precise measures through extensive psychological testing that enable the characterization and quantification of cognitive functions at a sufficiently granular level for mapping onto functional brain networks. Granular psychological testing should be ported to digital platforms, which enables testing on massive scales, and therefore greatly accelerates their validation and the development of norms. These tests can be delivered in an engaging, game-lack fashion, in short testing bursts. The opportunity to conduct testing over multiple sessions, such as in a daily fashion, has the added benefit of producing measures of variability, rates of learning, and functions of amelioration or decline. Developing games to measure and track mental health during healthy lifespan development and in the context of disorders is becoming a major enterprise in digital health [100–102]. Finally, we should start using digital technology to measure psychological functions from ongoing natural behaviour in the real world. Patterns and variations in speech, response times, balance, movement, navigation, social contexts, sleep, for example, are likely to provide much more information than constrained psychological tests or games. To understand how the various variables within any one of these behaviours map onto cognitive and brain systems, however, it will be necessary to correlate performance variables during natural behaviour and carefully designed experimental tasks in the first instance.

## Neuropsychology

The first major insights about the relationship between the human mind and brain came from observations of behavioural and cognitive deficits after brain damage. Cases of Phineas Gage [1], Leborgne (Tan) [2, 15], and HM [12 ,34], for example, were pivotal to situating higher-order comportment, language production, and episodic memory in the brain.

Interpreting the functional role of a brain area from a lesion is complicated. The first complication is that naturally occurring lesions, such as after a haemorrhagic stroke, do not follow the boundaries of functional brain areas. Multiple areas may be compromised, and portions of individual areas may be spared. In many cases, therefore, it is impossible to know what exact functional areas have been affected and to what extent. Importantly, lesions also often damage white matter, breaking connections between other, often remote, brain areas.

Lesion location aside, there exist other complications. Psychological functions arise through the co-ordinated activity of large-scale brain networks. In this context, it is important to consider functional inputs and outputs, connections among areas, and possible redundancies or alternative pathways to achieve given functions. It is not possible therefore to conclude that the lesioned area performed the lost function. Instead, one can only infer that the brain cannot support that function in the absence of that area. Rather than the compromised psychological function under observation, a lesioned area could be performing a necessary upstream or downstream function. It is also not possible to conclude that the lesioned brain area does not contribute to a function that remains unaffected, since the given function may also be (or become) supported by an alternative set of brain areas. Lesions to the white matter may disconnect brain areas from their critical inputs and/or outputs. Some have argued that major neurological syndromes result from disconnections caused by lesions to key white matter hubs for inter-areal connections, such as neglect [103], aphasia [44], or amnesia [104].

To complicate matters further, the effects of lesions change over time. Damage to a given area may change the pattern of inputs or outputs to and from other areas, thus changing the levels of effective stimulation at these distant sites. Loss of normal function at these sites can result in neurological damage and atrophy. When studying the effects of chronic lesions, therefore, it is important to consider how other areas and networks have been affected through diaschisis [105, 106]. Complementing the erosion of function in damaged and interconnected areas, there can also be compensatory plasticity in preserved and complementary brain areas.

Despite all its shortcomings and complications, neuropsychology is an essential method for mapping the functional architecture of the human mind and for understanding how brain areas and networks support its various functions. Associations and dissociations among psychological functions affected by different brain lesions are invaluable for identifying the natural kinds of psychological functions, separating those that are strongly interdependent from those that are naturally segregated in the brain. Patterns of dissociation have broken down the previously monolithical constructs into complex systems of constituent functions. Double dissociations are an especially powerful method for identifying neurally independent psychological functions [107]. These have helped us chart the relative independence between syntax and semantics [108], perceptual and motor learning [109–111], and perception for guiding recognition and for guiding action [112]. In addition to carving the psychological landscape at its joints, neuropsychology is also essential to linking psychological function to brain structure. Disruption of a psychological function after damage to a particular area provides confirmation that this area plays a necessary and causal role in supporting the given function. Although it can be problematic to infer the psychological function performed by a given brain area based solely on neuropsychological observation in the first place, for the reasons given, neuropsychological observation is the ultimate testing ground for hypotheses concerning the causal contribution of a brain area to a psychological function.

Most of the neuropsychological literature considers focal brain lesions resulting from haemorrhagic or ischaemic strokes. However, it is also possible to apply neuropsychological methods to understand psychological deficits that result from dysfunctions in brain networks in neurodegenerative and neuropsychiatric conditions. One may argue that network-level neuropsychology is more natural and appropriate, given that psychological functions arise from activity in large-scale networks in the first place. Furthermore, patterns of neurodegeneration and network dysfunction in psychiatric conditions tend to follow the patterns of intrinsic brain connectivity. Patterns of degeneration and dysfunction within networks can be graded along their core nodes and occasionally display focal points. This can reveal interesting focal patterns of relative specialization within large-scale networks. An example is the breakdown of primary progressive aphasia into agrammatic, semantic, and logopenic subtypes, which compromise different aspects of language after pathology weighted to lateral frontal, medial temporal, or lateral temporal regions, respectively [113].

Though, in principle, investigating the cognitive deficits after network-level dysfunction in neuropsychiatric conditions using a neuropsychological approach should be straightforward, in reality, it is very challenging. Some of the reason for the difficulty is that it has taken longer to accept that psychiatric conditions have neural causes. Most efforts in developing neuropsychological methods therefore occurred in the context of neurological disorders. The psychological tests and batteries we have are therefore most sensitive to the psychological consequences of damage in neurological conditions, and especially stroke. Efforts should be increasingly dedicated therefore to develop test batteries that are sensitive to patterns of cognitive and affective breakdown in psychological and psychiatric conditions [114]. The other major difficulty is in identifying the patterns of damage in brain structure, connectivity, and function in psychiatric cases. Without reliable markers of brain dysfunction, the power of the neuropsychological approach is diminished. Identification and quantification of neural markers are likely to improve substantially, as methods for imaging the human brain develop to provide increasing sensitivity to alterations in cortical microstructure, neuromodulation, fine-scale structural connectivity, and integrity and vitality of activity in functional networks.

## Brain stimulation

Transcranial magnetic stimulation (TMS) is a non-invasive method that can simulate the transient effect of a brain lesion [115, 116]. By briefly passing a current through a coil of wires, forming a high-field magnet with a very focal gradient, a strong and rapidly fluctuating magnetic field is formed, which generates electrical currents in the underlying neural tissue and affects the membrane potential of nearby neurons. The result is a brief stimulation of action potentials and interference with the natural pattern of regional neuronal activity. In some cases, TMS elicits positive effects such as the generation of sensations or of motor responses by stimulation of primary sensory or motor areas. Most of the time, however, the result of TMS pulses is to interfere with ongoing neural activity, thus acting as a brief virtual lesion. Virtual TMS lesions have the advantage of being spatially and temporally circumscribed and targeted under experimental control. TMS can be applied in repetitive trains or as single pulses, with varying consequences on the excitability of the targeted region [117]. Because magnetic fields decay rapidly, only superficial cortical brain regions can usually be targeted. The method therefore avoids issues linked to diaschisis and reorganization of function that follow from chronic stroke lesions. However, stimulating one brain area using TMS may also influence activity across the whole network of regions to which the stimulated area is functionally interconnected. By using TMS, it is also possible to get evidence about whether a brain area is causally involved in the psychological function under investigation. By using multiple stimulators, or by combining TMS with brain imaging and recording methods, it also becomes possible to investigate how brain areas causally influence activity in other brain regions and how these modulatory connections, in turn, modify behaviour [118]. Increasingly, other related brain stimulation methods are being developed, which are capable of modifying cortical excitability in subtler and different ways (for example, transcranial direct current stimulation, transcranial alternating current stimulation, and transcranial random noise stimulation) [119]. In addition to their use in testing the causal involvement of brain areas and circuits in particular psychological functions, these methods are being increasingly used to induce plasticity in specific areas and circuits within rehabilitative contexts [120].

## Brain imaging

Methods for imaging structure and function in the human brain *in vivo* and non-invasively have revolutionized the study of psychological function and dysfunction.

The first major technique to be developed was PET [19, 20, 77]. PET measures the concentration of a radioactive substance at different locations within the brain. PET scanners use arrays of detectors to sense the coincidence of gamma rays emitted upon the annihilation of positrons emitted from a radioactive substance. PET can resolve signals at the level of functional brain areas, but its spatial resolution is limited by the dispersion of positrons from their original source. The temporal resolution of PET is dictated by the half-life of the specific radioactive substance being measured.

Some commonly used substances decay very rapidly and thus have a relatively high temporal resolution, while others decay much more slowly and thus have a low temporal resolution.

By using radioactively labelled tracers that mimic or alter the function of neurotransmitters or neuromodulators [for example, 6-$^{18}$F-fluorodopa (FDOPA)], it is possible to investigate neuropharmacological dysfunctions related to psychiatric conditions. PET and the related method of SPECT are the best methods for investigating neuropharmacological alterations associated with psychiatric conditions. The growing availability and specificity of tracers make it possible to study neuropharmacological parameters with ever increasing specificity. In the case of the dopamine system, for example, it is possible to measure synthesis [for example, 6-$^{18}$F-FDOPA and 6-$^{18}$F-fluoro-l-m-tyrosine (FMT)] and transport (for example, $^{11}$C/$^{18}$F-labelled tropane analogues) of dopamine and to isolate multiple dopamine receptor subtypes in the nigrostriatal, mesolimbic, and mesocortical systems (for example, $^{11}$C-SCH 23390 for D1 receptors or $^{11}$C-raclopride for D2/3 receptors).

By using tracers linked to glucose metabolism [for example, 2-deoxyglucose (2-DG] or blood flow (for example, 15-O2), it is possible to investigate patterns of brain activity correlated with psychological states or functions. Neuronal activity is metabolically costly, leading to local increase in glucose metabolism and blood flow. Tracers of glucose metabolism offer the most direct marker of brain activity using brain imaging methods. 2-DG is a glucose analogue that cannot be metabolized. It is taken up by cells with high metabolic demands and remains trapped. The half-life of 2-DG is about 2 hours, and images are typically acquired over 20 minutes. Therefore, although 2-DG imaging provides a good proximal measure of neuronal activity, the time resolution is insufficient for resolving modulations of brain activity within psychological tasks. Measures of blood flow using PET made up some of the first images of brain performing different activities [121]. The most commonly used tracer is 15-O2, which is absorbed into water in blood. It has a short half-life (about 2 minutes), allowing for multiple measurements (usually 8–12) to be taken from one individual during one experimental session, with a temporal resolution of approximately 30 seconds. This method enabled researchers to quantify and compare brain activity within brain regions and to correlate it across task conditions and groups of participants. Haemodynamic-based imaging with 15O2-PET ushered in cognitive neuroscience as we know it today.

PET-based haemodynamic brain imaging was soon to be superseded by fMRI. Most fMRI experiments measure the BOLD signal, which mainly reflects changes in blood flow associated with neuronal activity [22]. The development of the BOLD signal combined many pieces of knowledge about the nature of the MRI signal and its susceptibility to local distortions in the magnetic field. Distortions in the field by the deoxygenated form of haemoglobin [122] lead to signal loss, so that the resulting signal strength is proportional to the ratio of oxygenated-to-deoxygenated haemoglobin [123]. The net increased blood flow into an active brain region leads to an overall increase in the proportion of local oxygenated blood, and therefore of the MRI signal [124]. In addition to being a superb method for investigating brain activity, MRI image sequences can also be used to measure different aspects of brain structure and connectivity (see Chapter 12). This one method—MRI—therefore provides various complementary modalities of brain imaging.

fMRI offers much better spatial and temporal resolution than 15O2-PET, and it allows for many more images to be taken within a given experimental session, thus providing much greater reliability and flexibility. The theoretical spatial resolution of MRI is unlimited, though, in practice, the resolution is limited by coupling between the active neuronal pool and the local source of blood flow, as well as by the requirement to pool over space to increase signal strength. MRI images can be acquired very rapidly, and methodological developments are constantly pushing the time requirements down [125]. However, ultimately, the temporal resolution of fMRI is constrained by the haemodynamic function linking neuronal activity to subsequent changes in the level of oxygenated blood linked to the influx of blood and adjustments to other haemodynamic parameters. Whereas it is possible to obtain a magnetic resonance image within the time frame of local field potentials related to synaptic activity (tens of milliseconds), the haemodynamic response function lags far behind, tracking brain activity with a delay of seconds. Even though the HRF is much slower than its driving impetus by neuronal activity, it is still possible to individuate the responses elicited by different events occurring in rapid succession, if these are appropriately timed and intermixed [126]. Furthermore, the extent to which haemodynamic responses are suppressed by successive stimulation can provide an index of overlap in the neuronal populations activated by these events [127]. MRI-based imaging has been highly successful, and the method is constantly improving, with new hardware advances, imaging sequences, and analysis tools. Arguably, MRI has played a major role in the paradigm shift from a view of the brain as a reactive organ with phrenological units to that of the brain as a proactive dynamical system of complex networks. Initial studies using fMRI in the 1990s focused primarily on brain areas [128, 129]. Soon researchers began investigating the relationships between activity in different brain areas and refining measures of their functional connectivity and interaction [130–132]. Changes in brain activity and functional connectivity by pharmacological manipulations further nuanced our appreciation of modulatory functional interactions in the brain [133]. MRI then enabled the observation that functional brain networks are spontaneously active, even during periods of rest [77, 78]. Resting state networks (RSNs) emphasize the dynamic and active nature of the brain.

Advances in analysis techniques have substantially increased our statistical power and resolution to study the human brain across spatial scales. Going beyond univariate analyses of changes in the magnitude of regional BOLD responses, multivariate analyses can compare patterns of subtle signal variation across voxels [134, 135]. Furthermore, computational approaches are increasingly applied to understand the relationship between patterns of brain activity and their representational content [136], and to arbitrate among competing models about the nature of neural coding supporting psychological functions [137]. At the network level, analyses based on graph theory and network science are increasingly used to estimate parameters related to the patterns and strength of connectivity among various functional nodes on multiple scales [138, 139].

### Electrophysiological recordings

Electrophysiological methods are the most direct way to measure human brain activity. Rather than relying on the relationships between brain activity and metabolic demands and between metabolic demands and blood flow, electrophysiological methods pick up unmediated electrical correlates of neuronal activity. In doing so, these methods have the ability to register changes in brain activity with high temporal fidelity.

Electrical signals generated in the brain were first measured from the exposed animal brain by Richard Caton (1875) [140]. He designed an ingenious voltage-sensitive mechanism to move mirrors—a reflecting galvanometer—and demonstrated systematic changes in the pattern of reflected light upon variation of light stimulation to the eye. Some decades later, Hans Berger (1929) [23] developed the 'electroencephalogram' (EEG), a non-invasive method for recording electrical signals originating from the human brain. The EEG measures fluctuations in voltage over time through electrodes placed on the scalp and a reference electrode. Using his method, Berger described the characteristic frequencies of voltage changes recorded from the human brain in different functional states (for example, sleep, relaxation, intellectual effort, administration of cocaine) and neurological conditions (for example, epilepsy).

Although the EEG records voltage directly, the signals available at the scalp are a macroscopic and distorted summary of activity over large populations of neurons. Voltage signals at the scalp originate mainly from the summation of synaptic potentials of synchronously active neurons that are well aligned spatially [141, 142]. Because voltage decays logarithmically with distance, the measures are heavily biased towards neuronal populations that are close to the active electrode. The orientation of the active neuronal population relative to the electrodes also influences the polarity and amplitude of the signals. The resulting signal therefore reflects the spatial summation of co-active neurons, biased by the degree of co-alignment of contributing neurons, as well as the orientation of the active region within the brain. The skull and scalp further strongly blur the signals before they are recorded [143]. Given these principles, the EEG recordings tend to be biased towards picking up excitatory synaptic potentials from pyramidal neurons in the neocortex [141, 144]. Signals at the scalp have been estimated to reflect the activity in thousands to millions of co-activated neurons [144]. The precise polarity and amplitude of the signals recorded at any given scalp electrode are heavily dependent on the location of the reference electrode.

Magnetoencephalography (MEG) is a more recent electrophysiological method, which uses superconducting quantum interference devices (SQUIDs) to record the magnetic fields that accompany the neuronal voltage signals [145, 146]. Magnetic fields have different properties to voltage potentials, which confer greater spatial resolution to the recordings. The underlying origin of the signal measures with EEG and MEG is the same—summed synaptic potentials over large populations of well-aligned, co-active neurons, but some important details differ in the signals that are measured.

MEG sensors detect local changes in the magnetic field, so the recordings are reference-free. Magnetic fields are unaffected by the conductivity of the skull and scalp, eliminating the problem with blurring and resulting in much sharper gradients of activity measured from the scalp. Magnetic fields decay more sharply than electrical fields with distance, further focusing the activity measured to superficial neocortical sources. Furthermore, the sensors are more sensitive to neuronal activity in sulci, resulting in magnetic fields that are tangentially oriented to the scalp. Altogether, MEG therefore provides more spatially resolved measures of active neuronal populations. The main drawback of MEG, relative to EEG, is its reliance on expensive superconducting technology and on the scarce resource of liquid helium. However, new generations of sensors are being developed to measure MEG with more accessible technologies such as optically pumped magnetometers (OPMs) [147], hybrid quantum interference devices [148], and nitrogen vacancy magnetometers [149].

Compared to haemodynamic imaging methods, EEG and MEG have poorer spatial resolution. Their spatial sensitivity comes from the distribution of voltage or magnetic-field gradients at the scalp, which can be sampled with dense arrays of sensors. It has been known since Helmholtz (1853) [150] that the problem of estimating the sources of signals from within a three-dimensional volume from a pattern on a two-dimensional surface is ill posed. The problem is mathematically underdetermined and impossible to solve uniquely. An infinite number of possible configurations of sources can account for any given surface pattern. Mathematical impossibilities aside, increasingly powerful methods of source reconstruction are being developed, which incorporate knowledge about brain structure and physiology, convergent findings from methods with high spatial resolution, and analytical methods to quantify likelihoods of different possible solutions [151–154].

The direct and time-resolved measures of brain activity from MEG and EEG (M/EEG) can be used to address many important questions relevant to psychiatry [155]. As in Berger's original use of EEG, it is possible to extract useful information just from the raw M/EEG signal. At rest, brains display characteristic patterns of activity within different frequency ranges, thought to reflect the levels of excitability in different neural circuits and on different spatial scales [156]. Disruptions in synaptic function or in the interactions among brain areas within large-scale networks associated with psychiatric conditions can lead to systematic alterations in the characteristic frequencies and power of oscillatory activity. Abnormal patterns of oscillations have been linked to conditions such as schizophrenia [157], autism spectrum disorder [158], and Alzheimer's disease [159]. In addition to characterizing the frequency profile of activity in raw M/EEG, it is also possible to resolve activity in functional networks from the raw MEG signal when individuals are at rest [79]. Investigating the strength in RSNs and connectivity among constituent regions can provide a powerful method to investigate network dysfunctions associated with psychiatric disorders or their risk factors [160, 161]. New analytical methods that identify which functional network is most likely to be active at a given time point enable researchers to quantify the dynamics within functional RSNs [162]. Using such methods, it becomes possible to compare the vitality of networks in psychiatric conditions, for example by determining whether the dwell time of networks indicates excessive rigidity or instability in network states

In addition to general measures of brain activity at rest, M/EEG provide rich information about the brain's response to specific events within tasks. Traditionally, brain activity linked to a perceptual stimulus, a cognitive operation, or a motor response has been studied using event-related potentials (ERPs) or fields (ERFs). These are averages of waveforms triggered by several repetitions of such events, which reinforce the aspects of the signal that are systematically related to the event and average away other artefacts and unrelated brain activity. The resulting waveforms have characteristic patterns of peaks and troughs, known as 'components'. Components are defined by their latency, amplitude, voltage topography over the scalp, and functional modulation by experimental variables

[141, 163]. Their relations to the underlying neural events can be complex. In many cases, there may be no specific single intracranial component, but instead multiple overlapping neural processes that give rise to a macroscopic component at the scalp. These are therefore best understood as sources of controlled observable variability [164] that provide rich, dependent variables to study information processing in the brain during that time period.

Using ERPs and ERFs, it is possible to investigate changes in information processing in the brain on a millisecond-by-millisecond time frame. Such temporal resolution can reveal whether a given psychiatric condition affects early perceptual pickup of information or only later deliberative processes. For example, ERP studies have pointed to early visual deficits in conditions such as schizophrenia [165]. Such conclusions could not be derived from haemodynamic imaging studies showing alterations in the visual cortex, since it would not be clear whether the modulation came from early visual processing or from late feedback modulation of visual areas by re-entrant activity after extensive processing in other areas. Another nice feature of electrophysiological recording methods is that brain responses can be studied without requiring participants to respond. In this way, it is possible to study the extent to which patients with different conditions process irrelevant, distracting stimuli. Such studies can reveal deficits in inhibiting irrelevant information [166] or exaggerated engagement with irrelevant emotional stimuli [167, 168] in different psychiatric and psychological conditions. By focusing on ERPs and ERFs at various stages of processing and by careful experimental design, it is possible to investigate how different psychiatric conditions affect attentional capture, emotional processing, semantic access and integration, memory retrieval, etc, arguably in a more specific and direct way by using brain imaging.

More recently, an increasing number of measures and approaches are being developed to derive and analyse brain signals linked to event processing from raw M/EEG. By relying on trial-by-trial fluctuations in stimulus and behavioural parameters, it is possible to analyse task-related brain signals without having to average brain activity [169], thus providing even greater sensitivity to identify deficits within particular stages of information processing. In addition, task-based analyses are increasingly separating the M/EEG signal into its various frequency components. Changes in the intrinsic oscillatory rhythms induced by stimuli or cognitive operations can suggest alterations in circuit-level activity or connectivity in psychiatric conditions such as schizophrenia and autism spectrum disorders [170, 171].

Because MEG and EEG provide a direct measure of brain activity, unmediated by haemodynamic parameters, they are well suited for investigating pharmacological effects. The powerful combination of pharmacological manipulations with electrophysiology remains under-exploited but is likely to play a major role in investigating pharmacological contributions to psychiatric conditions, as well as developing drug-related treatments [172, 173].

## Biomarkers

By combining neuropsychological batteries and focused cognitive testing with non-invasive measures to image and record brain activity, one dramatically increases the likelihood of identifying relevant biomarkers associated with risk or early stages of psychiatric disorders. It becomes possible to enhance characteristic cognitive profiles with sensitive and selective quantitative measures of speed, accuracy, and variability in specific, relevant cognitive domains. These rich psychological measures can be accompanied by variations in the structure and function of brain areas, their structural and functional connectivity, the strength in activation of large-scale brain networks, the vitality and temporal characteristics of networks, markers of neuronal integration, and communication, the speed and strength of neural responses at various stages of information processing, and altered patterns of information processing at various stages.

Two general approaches can be considered when developing psychiatric biomarkers. The various behavioural and neural measures can be used in a data-driven way to pull out combinations of measures that are predictive of psychiatric risk, condition, or recovery. New multivariate decoding and machine-learning modelling methods are increasingly powerful in identifying combinations of factors associated with particular outcomes. While this chapter strongly endorses the inclusion of factors directly related to cognitive and brain structure and function in biomarker development, it does not exclude the utility of other factors linked to molecular and cellular characteristics. The multivariate decoding approach can easily assimilate all such factors to find the most promising combinations of factors, thus generating high-level composite biomarkers. Much progress can be made in patient stratification, diagnosis, and treatment by using data-driven biomarkers, even without a clear understanding of the mechanisms that link each cognitive or brain factor to the outcome in question. Additionally, these data-driven biomarker candidates can become subjects of enquiry in their own right, yielding new mechanistic hypotheses to be explored.

The other approach is the more traditional, hypothesis-driven experimental-medicine model. In this case, candidate mechanisms of cognitive or brain deficits can be investigated directly. By expanding the methods with which these are investigated, it becomes possible to gain a fuller mechanistic understanding of how a hypothesized deficit is expressed at different levels of analysis, as well as to learn about the breadth of implications of a given deficit and how best to develop treatments.

Good examples of successful hypothesis-driven approaches to psychiatric conditions are found in the context of mood disorders. In the context of depression, Harmer and colleagues [174, 175] have investigated the role of cognitive emotional biases in mediating the effects of drugs for depression (often referred to as antidepressants). By using a sensitive battery of cognitive tests to assess emotional recognition and emotional biases, the researchers have suggested that monoamine reuptake inhibitors influence emotional and social cognition directly, which, in turn, re-dress the mood disorder over time. The proposed mechanism explains why clinical actions of drugs for depression are delayed. By combining cognitive and pharmacological studies with brain imaging methods, the researchers have revealed the neural systems affected by drugs affecting different neuromodulatory systems and have been able to develop effective means to predict individual responses to antidepressant treatment.

A similar experimental medicine approach is being developed in the context of bipolar disorder, which is also benefiting from data-driven discoveries [176]. The guiding hypothesis for this programme of research came as a combination of data-driven and clinical observations. Long-term prospective weekly monitoring of mood levels by patients [177, 178] revealed that individuals with bipolar disorder display high levels of mood instability, rather than the textbook pattern of alternating discrete episodes of mania, depression, and euthymia. Such results from remote monitoring of mood states complement clinical observations and conventional questionnaire findings [179, 180], and also provide rich quantitative data for modelling with machine-learning methods, as well as with novel mathematical techniques [181–183]. These findings raised the intriguing possibility that mood instability may provide a central feature that contributes to bipolar disorder. It occurs in individuals at high risk for bipolar disorder [184], predicts its onset [185], occurs during the prodrome of the disorder [186, 187], and is independently associated with poor prognoses [188–190]. Mood instability may also contribute to other mood disorders, such as borderline personality disorder [191], and may further do so in different ways.

A cognitive neuroscience experimental-medicine programme of work has been launched to characterize the pattern of mood instability associated with the risk for bipolar disorder, to investigate how mood instability is associated with changes in particular cognitive functions and to reveal how altered brain network dynamics may contribute to mood instability and cognitive deficits [176]. If successful, such a programme of research will identify effective biomarkers that will enable the stratification of individuals for trials to investigate the effects of mood-stabilizing drugs, as well as predict and measure their efficacy within individuals. By building on this approach, a double-blind, randomized, placebo-controlled study is investigating changes in mood, cognition, and brain network dynamics after 6 weeks of lithium treatment in participants with bipolar disorder and mood instability [192].

The field can get caught up in debating whether data-driven or hypothesis-driven approaches are the way forward. The answer is simple. They are both useful and can work together effectively, in complementary ways. Ultimately, hypothesis-driven research is essential for developing a deep and nuanced understanding of the mechanism. However, the approach requires building on good initial assumptions and ideas. In any scientific field, there is a danger of building experimental edifices on false starts. The additional challenges in psychiatry related to the lack of simple and tangible phenotypes for grounding the research exacerbate the problem. Data-driven discoveries can help set scientists back on track for better hypothesis-driven research. The process can be iterative, and information can flow in both directions, with data-driven findings informing hypothesis-driven work and results from focused experiments contributing to the pool of data for further mining.

## Acknowledgements

This views in this review were developed during periods of research funding from a Wellcome Trust Senior Investigator Award (104571/Z/14/Z), a European Union FP7 Marie Curie ITN Grant No. 606901 (INDIREA), an MRC UK MEG Partnership Grant, MR/K005464/1a James S. McDonnell Foundation Understanding Human Cognition Collaborative Award 220020448, and the NIHR Oxford Health Biomedical Research Centre. The Wellcome Centre for Integrative Neuroimaging is supported by core funding from the Wellcome Trust (203139/Z/16/Z)

## REFERENCES

1. Harlow JM. *Recovery from the passage of an iron bar through the head.* Massachusetts Medical Society; 1869 (cited 18 September 2017). Available from: https://archive.org/details/66210360R.nlm.nih.gov

2. Broca P. Remarks on the seat of the faculty of articulated language, following an observation of aphemia (loss of speech). *Bull la Société Anat.* 1861;6:330–57. Available from: http://garfield.library.upenn.edu/classics1990/A1990DY08800001.pdf

3. Wernicke C. *Der aphasische Symptomencomplex. Eine psychologische Studie auf anatomischer Basis.* Breslau: M. Cohn und Weigert; 1874 (cited 19 September 2017). Available from: http://www.worldcat.org/title/aphasische-symptomencomplex-eine-psychologische-studie-auf-anatomischer-basis-von-dr-c-wernicke/oclc/458953768

4. Bodamer J. Die Prosop-Agnosie. *Arch für Psychiatr und Nervenkrankheiten Ver mit Zeitschrift für die Gesamte Neurol und Psychiatr.* 1947;179(1–2):6–53. Available from: https://link.springer.com/content/pdf/10.1007%2FBF00352849.pdf

5. Dejerine J. Sur un cas de cecite verbale avec agraphie, suivie d'autopsie. *Mem Soc Biol.* 1891;3:197–201. Available from: http://pubman.mpdl.mpg.de/pubman/item/escidoc:2310098:6/component/escidoc:2453477/Dejerine_1891_Sur_un_cas.pdf

6. Balint R. Seelenlähmung des 'Schauens', optische Ataxie, räumliche störung der Aufmerksamkeit [Soul imbalance of 'seeing', optical ataxia, spatial disturbance of attention]. *Monatsschr Psychiatr Neurol.* 1909;25:51–81.

7. Oppenheim H. Ueber eine durch eine klinisch bisher nicht verwerthete Untersuchungsmethode ermittelte Form der Sensibilitätsstörung bei einseitigen Erkrankungen des Grosshirns. *Neurol Zentralblatt.* 1885;4:529–33.

8. Loeb J. Die elementaren Störungen einfacher Functionen nach oberflächlicher, umschriebener Verletzung des Grosshirns. *Pflügers Arch Eur J Physiol.* 1885;37:51–6.

9. Donders FC. Die Schnelligkeit psychischer Prozesse. *Arch für Anat und Physiol und wissenschaftliche Medizin.* 1868;657–81.

10. von Hemholtz H. *Treatise on Physiological Optics 3.* Leipzig: Voss; 1867.

11. Woodworth RS. Principles of Physiological Psychology. *Science (80-).* London Swan Sonnenschein; 1905 (cited 19 September 2017);22:789–90. Available from: https://ia802604.us.archive.org/11/items/principlesofphys00wundiala/principlesofphys00wundiala.pdf

12. Scoville WB, Milner B. Loss of recent memory after bilateral hippocampal lesions. *J Neurol Neurosurg Psychiatry.* 1957;20:11–21. Available from: https://www.ncbi.nlm.nih.gov/pmc/articles/PMC497229/pdf/jnnpsyc00285-0015.pdf

13. Shallice T, Warrington EK. Independent functioning of verbal memory stores: a neuropsychological study. *Q J Exp Psychol.* 1970;22:261–73. Available from: http://www.tandfonline.com/doi/abs/10.1080/00335557043000203

14. Weiskrantz L, Warrington EK, Sanders MD, Marshall J. Visual capacity in the hemianopic field following a restricted occipital ablation. *Brain.* 1974;97:709–28. Available from: http://www.ncbi.nlm.nih.gov/pubmed/4434190

15. Broca P. Sur la températures morbides locales. *Bull Acad Med.* 1879;2S:1331–47.

16. Mosso A. *Ueber den Kreislauf des Blutes im Menschlichen Gehirn : Untersuchungen.* Leipzig: Veit; 1881 (cited 19 September 2017). Available from: http://www.worldcat.org/title/ueber-den-kreislauf-des-blutes-im-menschlichen-gehirn-untersuchungen/oclc/716184253

17. Berger H. *Zur Lehre von der Blutzirkulation in der Schandelhohle des Menschen.* Jena: von Gustav, Fischer; 1901.

18. Roy CS, Sherrington CS. On the regulation of the blood-supply of the brain. *J Physiol.* 1890;11(1–2):85–108. Available from: https://www.ncbi.nlm.nih.gov/pmc/articles/PMC1514242/pdf/jphysiol02428-0093.pdf

19. Kety, S. S. Measurement of local blood flow by the exchange of an inert, diffusible substance. *Methods Med Res.* 1960;8:228–36. Available from: http://ci.nii.ac.jp/naid/10008368167/

20. Sokoloff L, Reivich M, Kennedy C, et al. The [14c]deoxyglucose method for the measurement of local cerebral glucose utilization: theory, procedure, and normal values in the conscious and anesthetized albino rat. *J Neurochem.* 1977;28:897–916. Available from: http://www.ncbi.nlm.nih.gov/pubmed/864466

21. Fox, P. T., Perlmutter, J. S., and Raichle ME. A stereotactic method of anatomical localization for positron emission tomography. *J Comput Assist Tomogr.* 1985;9:141–53.

22. Ogawa S, Lee TM, Kay AR, Tank DW. Brain magnetic resonance imaging with contrast dependent on blood oxygenation. *Proc Natl Acad Sci U S A.* 1990;87:9868–72. Available from: https://www.ncbi.nlm.nih.gov/pmc/articles/PMC55275/pdf/pnas01049-0370.pdf

23. Berger H. Über das Elektroenzephalogramm des Menschen. *Arch für Psychiatr und Nervenkrankheiten.* 1929;278:527–70. Available from: http://link.springer.com/10.1007/BF01797193

24. Adrian ED, Matthews BHC. The berger rhythm: Potential changes from the occipital lobes in man. *Brain.* 1934;57:355–85. Available from: https://academic.oup.com/brain/article-lookup/doi/10.1093/brain/57.4.355

25. Collingridge GL, Bliss TVP. NMDA receptors—their role in long-term potentiation. *Trends in Neurosciences.* 1987;10:288–93. Available from: http://www.sciencedirect.com/science/article/pii/0166223687901755

26. Collingridge BYGL, Kehl SJ, Mclennan H. Excitatory amino acids in synaptic transmission in the schaffer collateral-commissural pathway of the rat hippocampus. *J Physiol.* 1983;334:33–46. Available from: http://www.ncbi.nlm.nih.gov/pubmed/6306230

27. Attneave F, B, M, Hebb DO. The Organization of Behavior; A Neuropsychological Theory. *Am J Psychol.* 1950;63:633. Available from: http://s-f-walker.org.uk/pubsebooks/pdfs/The_Organization_of_Behavior-Donald_O._Hebb.pdf

28. James W. The Principles of Psychology. *J Hist Philos.* 1890 (cited 19 September 2017). Available from: http://library.manipaldubai.com/DL/the_principles_of_psychology_vol_II.pdf

29. Lisman J, Yasuda R, Raghavachari S. Mechanisms of CaMKII action in long-term potentiation. *Nat Rev Neurosci.* 2012 (cited 19 September 2017). Available from: https://www.ncbi.nlm.nih.gov/pmc/articles/PMC4050655/pdf/nihms585398.pdf

30. Shepherd G, Grillner S. *Handbook of Brain Microcircuits.* 2010 (cited 19 September 2017). Available from: https://brainmaster.com/software/pubs/brain/Handbook of Brain Microcircuts.pdf

31. Treves A, Rolls ET. Computational Analysis of the Role of the Hippocampus in Memory. *Hippocampus.* 1994;4:374–91. Available from: http://www.oxcns.org/papers/186_Treves%2BRolls94.pdf

32. Rolls ET. A theory of hippocampal function in memory. *Hippocampus.* 1996;6:601–20. Available from: http://www.ncbi.nlm.nih.gov/pubmed/9034849

33. Lisman JE. Relating Hippocampal Circuitry to Function. *Neuron.* 1999;22:233–42. Available from: http://www.ncbi.nlm.nih.gov/pubmed/10069330

34. Milner B, Corkin S, Teuber H-L. Further analysis of the hippocampal amnesic syndrome: 14-year follow-up study of

H.M. *Neuropsychologia*. 1968;6:215–34. Available from: http://linkinghub.elsevier.com/retrieve/pii/0028393268900213

35. McCormick D, Thompson R. Cerebellum: essential involvement in the classically conditioned eyelid response. *Science*. 1984;223:296–9. Available from: http://www.ncbi.nlm.nih.gov/pubmed/6701513

36. Milner B, Philip C, Leonard G. Frontal-lobe contribution to regency judgements. *Neuropsychiatr Dis Treat*. 1991;29:601–18. Available from: http://ac.els-cdn.com/002839329190013X/1-s2.0-002839329190013X-main.pdf?_tid=27c5d46a-9d2a-11e7-89f7-00000aacb361&acdnat=1505819184_73e9888f4e07c336386aebaf403c60c2

37. Janowsky JS, Shimamura AP, Squire LR. Source memory impairment in patients with frontal lobe lesions. *Neuropsychologia*. 1989;27:1043–56. Available from: http://www.ncbi.nlm.nih.gov/pubmed/2797412

38. Milner B. Interhemispheric differences in the localization of psychological processes in man. *Br Med Bull*. 1971;27:272–7. Available from: http://www.ncbi.nlm.nih.gov/pubmed/4937273

39. Howard JW, Rothbart M. Social categorization and memory for in-group and out-group behavior. *J Pers Soc Psychol*. 1980;38:301–10. Available from: http://content.apa.org/journals/psp/38/2/301

40. Gutchess AH, Indeck A. Cultural influences on memory. *Prog Brain Res*. 2009;178:137–50.

41. Passingham RE, Stephan KE, Kötter R. The anatomical basis of functional localization in the cortex. *Nat Rev Neurosci*. 2002;3:606–16. Available from: http://www.nature.com/doifinder/10.1038/nrn893

42. Glasser MF, Coalson TS, Robinson EC, *et al*. A multi-modal parcellation of human cerebral cortex. *Nature*. 2016;536:171–8. Available from: http://www.ncbi.nlm.nih.gov/pubmed/27437579

43. Gall FJ, Spurzheim G. *The Anatomy and Physiology of the Nervous System in General, and of the Brain in Particular*. London: Baldwin, Cradock and Joy; 1815.

44. Geschwind N. Disconnexion syndromes in animal and man. *Brain*. 1965;88:237–94. Available from: https://is.muni.cz/el/1423/podzim2011/PSY494_P11/um/28181196/Geschwind__1965_pdf

45. Mesulam M-M. Large-scale neurocognitive networks and distributed processing for attention, language, and memory. *Ann Neurol*. 1990;28:597–613. Available from: http://www.ncbi.nlm.nih.gov/pubmed/2260847

46. Geschwind N. The organization of language and the brain. *Science*. 1970;170:940–4. Available from: http://www.ncbi.nlm.nih.gov/pubmed/5475022

47. Price CJ. Core systems of number. *J Anat*. 2000;197:335–59. Available from: https://www.ncbi.nlm.nih.gov/pmc/articles/PMC1468137/pdf/joa_1973_0335.pdf

48. Mesulam M-Marsel. A cortical network for directed attention and unilateral neglect. *Ann Neurol*. 1981;10:309–25. Available from: http://www.ncbi.nlm.nih.gov/pubmed/7032417

49. Nobre AC, Mesulam M-Marsel. *Large-scale networks for attentional biases*. The Oxford Handbook of Attention; 2014. Available from: http://www.brainandcognition.org/wp-content/uploads/2015/07/Largescale_Networks_for_Attentional_Biases.pdf

50. Gross C. Visual functions of inferotemporal cortex. In: Jung R (ed). *Visual Centers in the Brain. Handbook of Sensory Physiology*; 1973. pp. 451–82. Available from: http://link.springer.com/10.1007/978-3-642-65495-4_11

51. Tanaka K. Inferotemporal cortex and object vision. *Annu Rev Neurosci*. 1996;19:109–39. Available from: http://www.annualreviews.org/doi/10.1146/annurev.ne.19.030196.000545

52. Miller EK, Erickson CA, Desimone R. Neural mechanisms of visual working memory in prefrontal cortex of the macaque. *J Neurosci*. 1996;16:5154–67. Available from: http://www.ncbi.nlm.nih.gov/pubmed/8756444

53. Martin A, Chao LL. Semantic memory and the brain: Structure and processes. *Curr Opin Neurobiol*. 2001;11:194–201. Available from: http://www.ncbi.nlm.nih.gov/pubmed/11301239

54. Mesulam M-Marsel. *Principles of behavioral and cognitive neurology*. Oxford University Press, Oxford; 2000. Available from: https://global.oup.com/academic/product/principles-of-behavioral-and-cognitive-neurology-9780195134759?cc=gb&lang=en&

55. Buonomano D V., Maass W. State-dependent computations: spatiotemporal processing in cortical networks. *Nat Rev Neurosci*. 2009;10:113–25. Available from: http://www.nature.com/doifinder/10.1038/nrn2558

56. Weintraub S, Mesulam MM. Right cerebral dominance in spatial attention. Further evidence based on ipsilateral neglect. *Arch Neurol*. 1987;44:621–5. Available from: http://www.ncbi.nlm.nih.gov/pubmed/3579679

57. Heilman KM, Van Den Abell T. Right hemisphere dominance for attention: the mechanism underlying hemispheric asymmetries of inattention (neglect). *Neurology*. 1980;30:327–30. Available from: http://www.ncbi.nlm.nih.gov/pubmed/7189037

58. Geschwind N, Levitsky W. Human Brain: Left-Right Asymmetries in Temporal Speech Region. *Source Sci New Ser Brain Ser Handb Clin Neurol*. 1968;161:108–293. Available from: http://www.ncbi.nlm.nih.gov/pubmed/5657070

59. Crow TJ, Ball J, Bloom SR, *et al*. Schizophrenia as an anomaly of development of cerebral asymmetry. A postmortem study and a proposal concerning the genetic basis of the disease. *Arch Gen Psychiatry*. 1989;46:1145–50. Available from: http://www.ncbi.nlm.nih.gov/pubmed/2589928

60. Moser EI, Kropff E, Moser M-B. Place Cells, Grid Cells, and the Brain's Spatial Representation System. *Annu Rev Neurosci*. 2008;31:69–89. Available from: http://www.ncbi.nlm.nih.gov/pubmed/18284371

61. O'Keefe J. A review of the hippocampal place cells. *Progr Neurobiol*. 1979;13:419–39. Available from: http://www.ncbi.nlm.nih.gov/pubmed/396576

62. Hartley T, Lever C, Burgess N, O'Keefe J. Space in the brain: how the hippocampal formation supports spatial cognition. *Philos Trans R Soc B Biol Sci*. 2013;369:20120510. Available from: http://dx.doi.org/10.1098/rstb.2012.0510

63. Eichenbaum H. Time cells in the hippocampus: a new dimension for mapping memories. *Nat Rev Neurosci. Nat Res*. 2014;15:732–44. Available from: http://www.nature.com/doifinder/10.1038/nrn3827

64. Taube JS, Muller RU, Ranck JB. Head-direction cells recorded from the postsubiculum in freely moving rats. I. Description and quantitative analysis. *J Neurosci*. 1990;10:420–35. Available from: http://www.ncbi.nlm.nih.gov/pubmed/2303851

65. Kelso SR, Ganong AH, Brown TH. Hebbian synapses in hippocampus. *Proc Natl Acad Sci U S A*. 1986;83:5326–30. Available from: https://www.ncbi.nlm.nih.gov/pmc/articles/PMC323944/pdf/pnas00318-0361.pdf

66. Constantinescu AO, OReilly JX, Behrens TEJ. Organizing conceptual knowledge in humans with a gridlike code. *Science*. 2016;352:1464–8. Available from: http://www.ncbi.nlm.nih.gov/pubmed/27313047

67. Zeidman P, Maguire EA. Anterior hippocampus: the anatomy of perception, imagination and episodic memory. *Nat Rev Neurosci*. 2016;17:173–82. Available from: http://www.ncbi.nlm.nih.gov/pubmed/26865022

68. Kaplan R, Schuck NW, Doeller CF. The Role of Mental Maps in Decision-Making. *Trends in Neurosciences*. 2017;40:256–9. Available from: http://www.ncbi.nlm.nih.gov/pubmed/28365032

69. Felleman DJ, Van Essen DC. Distributed hierachical processing in the primate cerebral cortex. *Cereb Cortex*. 1991;1:1–47. Available from: http://www.cns.nyu.edu/~tony/vns/readings/felleman-vanessen-1991.pdf

70. Bullier J. Integrated model of visual processing. *Brain Res Rev*. 2001;36:96–107. Available from: http://www.ncbi.nlm.nih.gov/pubmed/11690606

71. Sillito AM, Cudeiro J, Jones HE. Always returning: feedback and sensory processing in visual cortex and thalamus. *Trends Neurosci*. 2006;29:307–16. Available from: http://www.ncbi.nlm.nih.gov/pubmed/16713635

72. Hochstein S, Ahissar M. View from the top: Hierarchies and reverse hierarchies in the visual system. *Neuron*. 2002;36:791–804. Available from: http://www.ncbi.nlm.nih.gov/pubmed/12467584

73. Singer W. Neuronal synchronization: A solution to the binding problem. In: *The mind–brain continuum: Sensory processes*. MIT Press, Cambridge, MA; 1996. pp. 101–30. Available from: https://www.tib.eu/de/suchen/id/BLCP%3ACN017542315/Neuronal-Synchronization-A-Solution-to-the-Binding/

74. Von der Malsburg C. The binding problem of neural networks. The mind-brain continuum. *Sens Processes*. 1996;131–46.

75. Dehaene S, Naccache L. Towards a cognitive neuroscience of consciousness:basic evidence. *Cognition* [Internet]. 2001;79:1–37.

76. Baars BJ. In the theatre of consciousness Global Workspace Theory, A Rigorous Scientific Theory of Consciousness. *J Conscious Stud*. 1997;4:292–309. Available from: http://www.wisebrain.org/media/Papers/BaarsTheaterConsciousness.pdf

77. Raichle ME, MacLeod AM, Snyder AZ, Powers WJ, Gusnard DA, Shulman GL. A default mode of brain function. *Proc Natl Acad Sci U S A*. 2001;98:676–82. Available from: http://www.ncbi.nlm.nih.gov/pubmed/11209064

78. Damoiseaux JS, Rombouts SARB, Barkhof F, *et al*. Consistent resting-state networks across healthy subjects. *Proc Natl Acad Sci U S A*. 2006;103:13848–53. Available from: http://www.ncbi.nlm.nih.gov/pubmed/16945915

79. Brookes MJ, Woolrich M, Luckhoo H, *et al*. Investigating the electrophysiological basis of resting state networks using magnetoencephalography. *Proc Natl Acad Sci U S A*. 2011;108:16783–8. Available from: http://www.ncbi.nlm.nih.gov/pubmed/21930901

80. Baker AP, Brookes MJ, Rezek IA, *et al*. Fast transient networks in spontaneous human brain activity. *Elife*. 2014;2014:e01867. Available from: http://www.ncbi.nlm.nih.gov/pubmed/24668169

81. Fries P. Neuronal Gamma-Band Synchronization as a Fundamental Process in Cortical Computation. *Annu Rev Neurosci*. 2009;32:209–24. Available from: http://www.ncbi.nlm.nih.gov/pubmed/19400723

82. Bastos AM, Vezoli J, Fries P. Communication through coherence with inter-areal delays. *Curr Opin Neurobiol*. 2015;31:173–80. Available from: http://dx.doi.org/10.1016/j.conb.2014.11.001

83. Busch NA, Dubois J, VanRullen R. The Phase of Ongoing EEG Oscillations Predicts Visual Perception. *J Neurosci*. 2009;29:7869–76. Available from: http://www.ncbi.nlm.nih.gov/pubmed/19535598

84. Wixted JT. *Stevens' handbook of experimental psychology and cognitive neuroscience*. Available from: http://onlinelibrary.wiley.com/book/10.1002/9781119170174

85. Nobre AC, Kastner S (eds). *The Oxford Handbook of Attention*. Vol. 1. Oxford University Press, Oxford; 2014. Available from: http://oxfordhandbooks.com/view/10.1093/oxfordhb/9780199675111.001.0001/oxfordhb-9780199675111

86. Eysenck MW, Derakshan N, Santos R, Calvo MG. Anxiety and cognitive performance: Attentional control theory. *Emotion*. 2007;7:336–53. Available from: http://www.ncbi.nlm.nih.gov/pubmed/17516812

87. Bar-Haim Y, Lamy D, Pergamin L, Bakermans-Kranenburg MJ, van IJzendoorn MH. Threat-related attentional bias in anxious and nonanxious individuals: A meta-analytic study. *Psychol Bull*. 2007;133:1–24. Available from: http://doi.apa.org/getdoi.cfm?doi=10.1037/0033-2909.133.1.1

88. Linetzky M, Pergamin-Hight L, Pine DS, Bar-Haim Y. Quantitative evaluation of the clinical efficacy of attention bias modification treatment for anxiety disorders. *Depress Anxiety*. 2015;32:383–91. Available from: http://www.ncbi.nlm.nih.gov/pubmed/25708991

89. Blackwell SE, Browning M, Mathews A, *et al*. Positive Imagery-Based Cognitive Bias Modification as a Web-Based Treatment Tool for Depressed Adults. *Clin Psychol Sci*. 2015;3:91–111. Available from: http://www.ncbi.nlm.nih.gov/pubmed/25984421

90. Fechner, G T. Elemente Der Psychophysik. *Br J Stat Psychol*. 1860. Available from: http://doi.wiley.com/10.1111/j.2044-8317.1960.tb00033.x

91. MacLeod C, Mathews A, Tata P. Attentional bias in emotional disorders. *J Abnorm Psychol*. 1986;95:15–20. Available from: http://www.ncbi.nlm.nih.gov/pubmed/3700842

92. Williams JMG, Mathews A, MacLeod C. The emotional Stroop task and psychopathology. *Psychol Bull*. 1996;120:3–24. Available from: http://www.ncbi.nlm.nih.gov/pubmed/8711015

93. Greenwald AG, Greenwald AG, Mcghee DE, Mcghee DE, Schwartz JLK, Schwartz JLK. Measuring Individual Differences in Implicit Cognition: The Implicit Association Test. *J Personal Soclal Psychol*. 1998;74:1464–80. Available from: https://faculty.washington.edu/agg/pdf/Gwald_McGh_Schw_JPSP_1998.OCR.pdf

94. Bays PM, Husain M. Dynamic Shifts of Limited Working Memory Resources in Human Vision. *Science*. 2008;321:851–4. Available from: http://www.ncbi.nlm.nih.gov/pubmed/18687968

95. Theeuwes J, Van der Stigchel S. Saccade trajectory deviations and inhibition-of-return: Measuring the amount of attentional processing. *Vision Res*. 2009;49:1307–15. Available from: http://www.sciencedirect.com/science/article/pii/S0042698908003866

96. Ma WJ, Husain M, Bays PM. Changing concepts of working memory. *Nat Neurosci*. 2014;17:347–56. Available from: http://www.nature.com/doifinder/10.1038/nn.3655

97. Wildegger T, Myers NE, Humphreys G, Nobre AC. Supraliminal But Not Subliminal Distracters Bias Working Memory Recall. *J Exp Psychol Percept Perform*. 2015;41:826–39. Available from: http://www.ncbi.nlm.nih.gov/pubmed/25867502

98. Lezak MD. *Neuropsychological assessment*. Oxford University Press, Oxford; 2012.

99. Weintraub S, Dikmen SS, Heaton RK, *et al*. Cognition assessment using the NIH Toolbox. *Neurology*. 2013;80(Issue 11, Supplement 3):S54–64. Available from: http://www.ncbi.nlm.nih.gov/pubmed/23479546

100. Mishra J, Gazzaley A. Harnessing the neuroplastic potential of the human brain & the future of cognitive rehabilitation. *Front Hum Neurosci*. 2014;8:1–4. Available from: https://www.ncbi.nlm.nih.gov/pmc/articles/PMC3990041/pdf/fnhum-08-00218.pdf

101. Morgan J. Gaming for dementia research: a quest to save the brain. *Lancet Neurol*. 2016;15:1313. Available from: http://linkinghub.elsevier.com/retrieve/pii/S1474442216301235

102. Zokaei N, MacKellar C, Čepukaitytė G, Patai EZ, Nobre AC. Cognitive Training in the Elderly: Bottlenecks and New Avenues. *J Cogn Neurosci*. 2017;29:1473–82. Available from: http://www.mitpressjournals.org/doi/abs/10.1162/jocn_a_01080

103. Bartolomeo P, Thiebaut De Schotten M, Doricchi F. Left unilateral neglect as a disconnection syndrome. *Cerebral Cortex*. 2007;17:2479–90. Available from: http://www.ncbi.nlm.nih.gov/pubmed/17272263

104. Gaffan D, Parker A, Easton A. Dense amnesia in the monkey after transection of fornix, amygdala and anterior temporal stem. *Neuropsychologia*. 2001;39:51–70. Available from: http://www.ncbi.nlm.nih.gov/pubmed/11115655

105. Hillis AE, Wityk RJ, Barker PB, *et al*. Subcortical aphasia and neglect in acute stroke: the role of cortical hypoperfusion. *Brain*. 2002;125(Pt 5):1094–104. Available from: http://www.ncbi.nlm.nih.gov/pubmed/11960898

106. Price CJ, Warburton EA, Moore CJ, Frackowiak RS, Friston KJ. Dynamic diaschisis: anatomically remote and context-sensitive human brain lesions. *J Cogn Neurosci*. 2001;13:419–29. Available from: http://www.ncbi.nlm.nih.gov/pubmed/11388916

107. Teuber H-L. Physiological psychology. *Annu Rev Psychol*. 1955;6:267–96. Available from: http://www.annualreviews.org/doi/10.1146/annurev.ps.06.020155.001411

108. Marslen-Wilson WD, Tyler LK. Dissociating types of mental computation. *Nature*. 1997;387:593. Available from: http://www.ncbi.nlm.nih.gov/pubmed/9177345

109. Knowlton BJ, Mangels JA, Squire LR. A Neostriatal Habit Learning System in Humans. *Science*. 1996;273:1399–402. Available from: http://www.ncbi.nlm.nih.gov/pubmed/8703077

110. Schacter DL. Priming and Multiple Memory Systems: Perceptual Mechanisms of Implicit Memory. *J Cogn Neurosci*. 1992;4:244–56. Available from: https://dash.harvard.edu/bitstream/handle/1/3627272/schacter_primingmultiple.pdf?sequence=2

111. Gabrieli JDE, Fleischman DA, Keane MM, Reminger SL, Morrell F. Double dissociations between memory systems and underlying explicit and implicit memory in the human brain. *Psychol Sci*. 1995;6:76–82. Available from: http://journals.sagepub.com/doi/10.1111/j.1467-9280.1995.tb00310.x

112. Milner AD, Goodale MA. Two visual systems re-viewed. *Neuropsychologia*. 2008;46:774–85. Available from: http://www.ncbi.nlm.nih.gov/pubmed/18037456

113. Gorno-Tempini ML, Hillis AE, Weintraub S, *et al*. Classification of primary progressive aphasia and its variants. *Neurology*. 2011;76:1006–14. Available from: http://www.ncbi.nlm.nih.gov/pubmed/21325651

114. Harmer CJ, Cowen PJ, Goodwin GM. Efficacy markers in depression. *J Psychopharmacol*. 2011;25:1148–58. Available from: http://journals.sagepub.com/doi/10.1177/0269881110367722

115. Walsh V, Cowey A. Transcranial magnetic stimulation and cognitive neuroscience. *Nat Rev Neurosci*. 2000;1:73–80. Available from: http://www.ncbi.nlm.nih.gov/pubmed/11252771

116. Walsh V, Rushworth M. A primer of magnetic stimulation as a tool for neuropsychology. *Neuropsychologia*. 1998;37:125–35. Available from: http://www.ncbi.nlm.nih.gov/pubmed/10080370

117. Sandrini M, Umiltà C, Rusconi E. The use of transcranial magnetic stimulation in cognitive neuroscience: A new synthesis of methodological issues. *Neurosci Biobehav Rev*. 2011;35:516–36. Available from: http://www.ncbi.nlm.nih.gov/pubmed/20599555

118. Bestmann S, Ruff CC, Blankenburg F, Weiskopf N, Driver J, Rothwell JC. Mapping causal interregional influences with concurrent TMS–fMRI. *Exp Brain Res*. 2008;191:383–402. Available from: http://www.ncbi.nlm.nih.gov/pubmed/18936922

119. Inukai Y, Saito K, Sasaki R, *et al*. Comparison of Three Non-Invasive Transcranial Electrical Stimulation Methods for Increasing Cortical Excitability. *Front Hum Neurosci*. 2016;10:668. Available from: http://www.ncbi.nlm.nih.gov/pubmed/28082887

120. Stagg CJ, Jayaram G, Pastor D, Kincses ZT, Matthews PM, Johansen-Berg H. Polarity and timing-dependent effects of transcranial direct current stimulation in explicit motor learning. *Neuropsychologia*. 2011;49:800–4. Available from: http://www.ncbi.nlm.nih.gov/pubmed/21335013

121. Lassen NA, Ingvar DH. Regional cerebral blood flow measurement in man. *Arch Neurol*. 1963;9:615. Available from: http://archneur.jamanetwork.com/article.aspx?doi=10.1001/archneur.1963.00460120065007

122. Pauling L, Coryell CD. The Magnetic Properties and Structure of Hemoglobin, Oxyhemoglobin and Carbonmonoxyhemoglobin. *Proc Natl Acad Sci U S A*. 1936;22:210–16. Available from: https://www.ncbi.nlm.nih.gov/pmc/articles/PMC1076743/pdf/pnas01768-0018.pdf

123. Thulborn KR, Waterton JC, Matthews PM, Radda GK. Oxygenation dependence of the transverse relaxation time of water protons in whole blood at high field. *BBA—Gen Subj*. 1982;714:265–70. Available from: http://www.ncbi.nlm.nih.gov/pubmed/6275909

124. Buxton RB, Wong EC, Frank LR. Dynamics of blood flow and oxygenation changes during brain activation: The balloon model. *Magn Reson Med*. 1998;39:855–64. Available from: http://doi.wiley.com/10.1002/mrm.1910390602

125. Uğurbil K, Xu J, Auerbach EJ, *et al*. Pushing spatial and temporal resolution for functional and diffusion MRI in the Human Connectome Project. *Neuroimage*. 2013;80:80–104. Available from: http://www.ncbi.nlm.nih.gov/pubmed/23702417

126. Dale AM, Buckner RL. Selective averaging of rapidly presented individual trials using fMRI. *Hum Brain Mapp*. 1997;5:329–40. Available from: http://doi.wiley.com/10.1002/%28SICI%291097-0193%281997%295%3A5%3C329%3A%3AAID-HBM1%3E3.0.CO%3B2-5

127. Robson MD, Dorosz JL, Gore JC. Measurements of the temporal fMRI response of the human auditory cortex to trains of tones. *Neuroimage*. 1998;7:185–98. Available from: http://www.ncbi.nlm.nih.gov/pubmed/9597660

128. Morris JS, Ohman A, Dolan RJ. A subcortical pathway to the right amygdala mediating 'unseen' fear. *Proc Natl Acad Sci U S A*. 1999;96:1680–5. Available from: https://www.ncbi.nlm.nih.gov/pmc/articles/PMC15559/pdf/pq001680.pdf

129. Maguire EA, Frackowiak RS, Frith CD. Recalling routes around london: activation of the right hippocampus in taxi drivers. *J Neurosci*. 1997;17:7103–10. Available from: http://citeseerx.ist.psu.edu/viewdoc/download?doi=10.1.1.322.4257&rep=rep1&type=pdf

130. Friston K., Buechel C, Fink G., Morris J, Rolls E, Dolan R. Psychophysiological and Modulatory Interactions in Neuroimaging. *Neuroimage*. 1997;6:218–29. Available from: http://www. ncbi.nlm.nih.gov/pubmed/9344826

131. Büchel C, Coull JT, Friston KJ. The predictive value of changes in effective connectivity for human learning. *Science*. 1999;283:1538–41. Available from: http://www.ncbi.nlm.nih.gov/pubmed/10066177

132. Friston K. Causal modelling and brain connectivity in functional magnetic resonance imaging. *PLoS Biol*. 2009;7:220–5. Available from: http://dx.plos.org/10.1371/journal.pbio.1000033

133. Honey G, Bullmore E. Human pharmacological MRI. *Trends Pharmacol Sci*. 2004;25:366–74. Available from: http://www.ncbi.nlm.nih.gov/pubmed/15219979

134. Norman KA, Polyn SM, Detre GJ, Haxby J V. Beyond mind-reading: multi-voxel pattern analysis of fMRI data. *Trends Cogn Sci*. 2006;10:424–30. Available from: http://www.ncbi.nlm.nih.gov/pubmed/16899397

135. Haynes J-D, Rees G. Decoding mental states from brain activity in humans. *Nat Rev Neurosci*. 2006;7:523–34. Available from: http://www.nature.com/doifinder/10.1038/nrn1931

136. Kriegeskorte N. Representational similarity analysis—connecting the branches of systems neuroscience. *Front Syst Neurosci*. 2008;2:4. Available from: http://www.ncbi.nlm.nih.gov/pubmed/19104670

137. Behrens TEJ, Hunt LT, Rushworth MFS. The Computation of Social Behavior. *Science*. 2009;324:1160–4. Available from: http://www.ncbi.nlm.nih.gov/pubmed/19478175

138. Bullmore E, Sporns O. Complex brain networks: graph theoretical analysis of structural and functional systems. *Nat Rev Neurosci*. 2009;10:186–98. Available from: http://www.ncbi.nlm.nih.gov/pubmed/19190637

139. Stam CJ. Modern network science of neurological disorders. *Nat Rev Neurosci. Nat Res*. 2014;15:683–95. Available from: http://www.nature.com/doifinder/10.1038/nrn3801

140. Caton R. The Electric Currents of the Brain. *Br Med J*. 1875;2:278. Available from: http://echo.mpiwg-berlin.mpg.de/ECHOdocuView?url=/permanent/vlp/lit27690/index.meta

141. Allison T, Wood CC, McCarthy G. The central nervous system. *Psychophysiol Syst Process Appl*. 1986;5–25.

142. Lorente de Nó R. Analysis of the Distribution of the Action Currents of Nerve in Volume Conductors. *Stud from Rockefeller Inst Med Res*. 1947;132:384–477. Available from: https://www.ncbi.nlm.nih.gov/labs/articles/20261890/

143. Srinivasan R, Nunez PL, Tucker DM, Silberstein RB, Peter J. Spatial Sampling and Filtering of EEG with Spline Laplacians to Estimate Cortical Potentials. *Brain Topogr*. 1996;8:355–66. Available from: http://link.springer.com/10.1007/BF01186911

144. Hämäläinen M, Hari R. Magnetoencephalographic (MEG) characterization of dynamic brain activation. *Brain Mapp Methods*. 2002;227–55.

145. Cohen D. Magnetoencephalography: Detection of the Brain's Electrical Activity with a Superconducting Magnetometer. *Science*. 1972;175:664–6. Available from: http://davidcohen.mit.edu/sites/default/files/documents/1972ScienceV175(SquidMEG).pdf

146. Proudfoot M, Woolrich MW, Nobre AC, Turner MR, Turner M. *Magnetoencephalography*. Available from: http://pn.bmj.com/content/practneurol/early/2014/03/19/practneurol-2013-000768.full.pdf

147. Boto E, Meyer SS, Shah V, et al. A new generation of magnetoencephalography: Room temperature measurements using optically-pumped magnetometers. *Neuroimage*. 2017;149:404–14. Available from: http://www.ncbi.nlm.nih.gov/pubmed/28131890

148. Shelly CD, Matrozova EA, Petrashov VT. Resolving thermoelectric "paradox" in superconductors. *Sci Adv*. 2016;2:e1501250–e1501250. Available from: http://advances.sciencemag.org/cgi/doi/10.1126/sciadv.1501250

149. Taylor JM, Cappellaro P, Childress L, et al. High-sensitivity diamond magnetometer with nanoscale resolution. *Nat Phys*. 2008;4:810–16. Available from: http://www.ncbi.nlm.nih.gov/pubmed/16525126

150. Helmholtz H V. Ueber einige Gesetze der Vertheilung elektrischer Ströme in körperlichen Leitern mit Anwendung auf die thierischelektrischen Versuche. *Ann Phys*. 1853;165:211–33.

151. Dale AM, Halgren E. Spatiotemporal mapping of brain activity by integration of multiple imaging modalities. *Curr Opin Neurobiol*. 2001;11:202–8. Available from: http://homes.mpimf-heidelberg.mpg.de/~mhelmsta/pdf/2001 Mapping Rev CurrOpinN.pdf

152. Makeig S, Debener S, Onton J, Delorme A. Mining event-related brain dynamics. *Trends Cogn Sci*. 2004;8:204–10. Available from: http://www.ncbi.nlm.nih.gov/pubmed/15120678

153. Mattout J, Phillips C, Penny WD, Rugg MD, Friston KJ. MEG source localization under multiple constraints: An extended Bayesian framework. *Neuroimage*. 2006;30:753–67. Available from: http://www.ncbi.nlm.nih.gov/pubmed/16368248

154. Woolrich M, Hunt L, Groves A, Barnes G. MEG beamforming using Bayesian PCA for adaptive data covariance matrix regularization. *Neuroimage*. 2011;57:1466–79. Available from: http://www.ncbi.nlm.nih.gov/pubmed/21620977

155. Uhlhaas PJ, Liddle P, Linden DEJ, Nobre AC, Singh KD, Gross J. Magnetoencephalography as a Tool in Psychiatric Research: Current Status and Perspective. *Biol Psychiatry Cogn Neurosci Neuroimaging*. 2017;2:235–44. Available from: http://www.ncbi.nlm.nih.gov/pubmed/28424797

156. Wang X-J. Neurophysiological and Computational Principles of Cortical Rhythms in Cognition. *Physiol Rev*. 2010;90:1195–268. Available from: http://www.ncbi.nlm.nih.gov/pubmed/20664082

157. Uhlhaas PJ, Singer W. Abnormal neural oscillations and synchrony in schizophrenia. *Nat Rev Neurosci*. 2010;11:100–13. Available from: http://www.ncbi.nlm.nih.gov/pubmed/20087360

158. Simon DM, Wallace MT. Dysfunction of sensory oscillations in Autism Spectrum Disorder. *Neurosci Biobehav Rev*. 2016;68:848–61. Available from: http://www.ncbi.nlm.nih.gov/pubmed/27451342

159. de Haan W, Stam CJ, Jones BF, Zuiderwijk IM, van Dijk BW, Scheltens P. Resting-State Oscillatory Brain Dynamics in Alzheimer Disease. *J Clin Neurophysiol*. 2008;25:187–93. Available from: http://www.ncbi.nlm.nih.gov/pubmed/18677182

160. Pineda-Pardo JA, Garcés P, López ME, et al. White matter damage disorganizes brain functional networks in amnestic mild cognitive impairment. *Brain Connect*. 2014;4:312–22. Available from: http://www.ncbi.nlm.nih.gov/pubmed/24617580

161. Cousijn H, Tunbridge EM, Rolinski M, et al. Modulation of hippocampal theta and hippocampal-prefrontal cortex function by a schizophrenia risk gene. *Hum Brain Mapp*. 2015;36:2387–95. Available from: http://www.ncbi.nlm.nih.gov/pubmed/25757652

162. Vidaurre D, Quinn AJ, Baker AP, Dupret D, Tejero-Cantero A, Woolrich MW. Spectrally resolved fast transient brain states in electrophysiological data. *Neuroimage*. 2016;126:81–95. Available from: http://www.sciencedirect.com/science/article/pii/S1053811915010691?via%3Dihub

163. Rugg MD (Michael D., Coles MGH. *Electrophysiology of mind : event-related brain potentials and cognition*. Oxford University Press, Oxford; 1995.

164. Donchin E, Ritter W, McCallum WC. Cognitive Psychophysiology: The endogenous components of the ERP. In: *Event-Related Brain Potentials in Man*. 1978. pp. 349–411. Available from: http://scholarcommons.usf.edu/psy_facpub/224

165. Foxe JJ, Doniger GM, Javitt DC. Early visual processing deficits in schizophrenia: impaired P1 generation revealed by

high-density electrical mapping. *Neuroreport*. 2001;12:3815–20. Available from: http://www.ncbi.nlm.nih.gov/pubmed/11726801

166. Michie PT, Fox AM, Ward PB, Catts S V., McConaghy N. Event-Related Potential Indices of Selective Attention and Cortical Lateralization in Schizophrenia. *Psychophysiology*. 1990;27:209–27. Available from: http://doi.wiley.com/10.1111/j.1469-8986.1990.tb00372.x

167. Fox E, Derakshan N, Shoker L. Trait anxiety modulates the electrophysiological indices of rapid spatial orienting towards angry faces. *Neuroreport*. 2008;19:259–63. Available from: http://content.wkhealth.com/linkback/openurl?sid=WKPTLP:landingpage&an=00001756-200802120-00001

168. Kappenman ES, Farrens JL, Luck SJ, Proudfit GH. Behavioral and ERP measures of attentional bias to threat in the dot-probe task: Poor reliability and lack of correlation with anxiety. *Front Psychol*. 2014;5:1368. Available from: http://www.ncbi.nlm.nih.gov/pubmed/25538644

169. Ratcliff R, Philiastides MG, Sajda P. Quality of evidence for perceptual decision making is indexed by trial-to-trial variability of the EEG. *Proc Natl Acad Sci U S A*. 2009;106(16):6539–44. Available from: http://www.ncbi.nlm.nih.gov/pubmed/19342495

170. Liddle EB, Price D, Palaniyappan L, *et al*. Abnormal salience signaling in schizophrenia: The role of integrative beta oscillations. *Hum Brain Mapp*. 2016;37:1361–74. Available from: http://www.ncbi.nlm.nih.gov/pubmed/26853904

171. Sun L, Gru C, Bo S, *et al*. Impaired Gamma-Band Activity during Perceptual Organization in Adults with Autism Spectrum Disorders: Evidence for Dysfunctional Network Activity in Frontal-Posterior Cortices. *J Neurosci*. 2012;32:9563–73. Available from: http://www.ncbi.nlm.nih.gov/pubmed/22787042

172. Shaw AD, Saxena N, E. Jackson L, Hall JE, Singh KD, Muthukumaraswamy SD. Ketamine amplifies induced gamma frequency oscillations in the human cerebral cortex. *Eur Neuropsychopharmacol*. 2015;25:1136–46. Available from: http://www.ncbi.nlm.nih.gov/pubmed/26123243

173. Schartner MM, Carhart-Harris RL, Barrett AB, Seth AK, Muthukumaraswamy SD. Increased spontaneous MEG signal diversity for psychoactive doses of ketamine, LSD and psilocybin. *Sci Rep*. 2017;7:46421. Available from: http://www.ncbi.nlm.nih.gov/pubmed/28422113

174. Harmer CJ, Duman RS, Cowen PJ. How do antidepressants work? New perspectives for refining future treatment approaches. *Lancet Psychiatry*. 2017;4:409–18. Available from: http://www.ncbi.nlm.nih.gov/pubmed/28153641

175. Warren MB, Pringle A, Harmer CJ. A neurocognitive model for understanding treatment action in depression. *Philos Trans R Soc B Biol Sci*. 2015;370:20140213. Available from: http://www.ncbi.nlm.nih.gov/pubmed/26240428

176. Harrison PJ, Cipriani A, Harmer CJ, *et al*. Innovative approaches to bipolar disorder and its treatment. *Ann N Y Acad Sci*. 2016;1366:76–89. Available from: http://www.ncbi.nlm.nih.gov/pubmed/27111134

177. Geddes JR, Gardiner A, Rendell J, *et al*. Comparative evaluation of quetiapine plus lamotrigine combination versus quetiapine monotherapy (and folic acid versus placebo) in bipolar depression (CEQUEL): A 2 × 2 factorial randomised trial. *Lancet Psychiatry*. 2016;3:31–9. Available from: http://www.ncbi.nlm.nih.gov/pubmed/26687300

178. Bilderbeck AC, Saunders KEA, Glifford GD. Daily and weekly mood ratings: relative contributions to the differentiation of bipolar disorder and borderline personality disorder. *BIPOLAR Disord*. 2015;17:129–30.

179. Henry C, Van den Bulke D, Bellivier F, *et al*. Affective lability and affect intensity as core dimensions of bipolar disorders during euthymic period. *Psychiatry Res*. 2008;159(1–2):1–6. Available from: http://www.ncbi.nlm.nih.gov/pubmed/18295902

180. Ortiz A, Grof P. Electronic monitoring of self-reported mood: the return of the subjective? *Int J Bipolar Disord*. 2016;4:28. Available from: http://www.ncbi.nlm.nih.gov/pubmed/27900735

181. Bonsall MB, Wallace-Hadrill SMA, Geddes JR, Goodwin GM, Holmes EA. Nonlinear time-series approaches in characterizing mood stability and mood instability in bipolar disorder. *Proc R Soc B Biol Sci*. 2012;279:916–24. Available from: http://www.ncbi.nlm.nih.gov/pubmed/21849316

182. Moore PJ, Little MA, McSharry PE, Goodwin GM, Geddes JR. Mood dynamics in bipolar disorder. *Int J Bipolar Disord*. 2014;2:11. Available from: http://www.ncbi.nlm.nih.gov/pubmed/26092397

183. Bonsall MB, Geddes JR, Goodwin GM, Holmes EA. Bipolar disorder dynamics: affective instabilities, relaxation oscillations and noise. *J R Soc Interface*. 2015;12:20150670. Available from: http://www.ncbi.nlm.nih.gov/pubmed/26577592

184. Birmaher, B., B.I. Goldstein DAA. Mood lability among offspring of parents with bipolar disorder and community controls. *BIPOLAR Disord*. 2013;15:253–63.

185. Hafeman DM, Merranko J, Axelson D, *et al*. Toward the definition of a bipolar prodrome: Dimensional predictors of bipolar spectrum disorders in at-risk youths. *Am J Psychiatry*. 2016;173:695–704. Available from: http://www.ncbi.nlm.nih.gov/pubmed/26892940

186. Craddock N, Owen MJ. The Kraepelinian dichotomy—Going, going…but still not gone. *Br J Psychiatry*. 2010;196:92–5. Available from: http://www.ncbi.nlm.nih.gov/pubmed/20118450

187. Howes OD, Lim S, Theologos G, Yung AR, Goodwin GM, McGuire P. A comprehensive review and model of putative prodromal features of bipolar affective disorder. *Psychol Med*. 2011;41:1567–77. Available from: http://www.ncbi.nlm.nih.gov/pubmed/20836910

188. Patel R, Lloyd T, Jackson R, *et al*. Mood instability is a common feature of mental health disorders and is associated with poor clinical outcomes. *BMJ Open*. 2015;5:e007504–e007504. Available from: http://www.ncbi.nlm.nih.gov/pubmed/25998036

189. Strejilevich SA, Martino DJ, Murru A, *et al*. Mood instability and functional recovery in bipolar disorders. *Acta Psychiatr Scand*. 2013;128:194–202. Available from: http://www.ncbi.nlm.nih.gov/pubmed/23331090

190. Gershon A, Eidelman P. Inter-episode affective intensity and instability: Predictors of depression and functional impairment in bipolar disorder. *J Behav Ther Exp Psychiatry*. 2015;46:14–8. Available from: http://www.ncbi.nlm.nih.gov/pubmed/25164093

191. Broome MR, Saunders KEA, Harrison PJ, Marwaha S. Mood instability: significance, definition and measurement. *Br J Psychiatry*. 2015;207:283–5. Available from: http://www.ncbi.nlm.nih.gov/pubmed/26429679

192. Saunders KEA, Cipriani A, Rendell J, *et al*. Oxford Lithium Trial (OxLith) of the early affective, cognitive, neural and biochemical effects of lithium carbonate in bipolar disorder: study protocol for a randomised controlled trial. *Trials*. 2016;17:116. Available from: http://www.ncbi.nlm.nih.gov/pubmed/26936776

# 18

# Ageing and the human brain

*Verena Heise, Enikő Zsoldos, and Klaus P. Ebmeier*

## Introduction

Age is an acknowledged confounder in psychiatric research, most apparent in younger and in older patient groups. There is hardly any study that does not address this variable, usually by matching controls and patients by chronological age, by separating psychiatric disciplines into age groups (viz. child and adolescent or old age psychiatry), or by entering the chronological age as a covariate into regression analyses. Time as a physical category, whether defined as multiples of 9,192,631,770 cycles of radiation (the transition between two energy levels of the caesium-133 atom at rest at a temperature of 0 K (= 1 second [1]) or by the emptying of an hourglass, clearly has no direct mechanistic impact on a person's biological age, nor does our perception of time [2], although chronological time is used as a proxy of ageing. It is understood, moreover, that there is good ageing and bad ageing, depending on genetic and non-genetic factors, which add variability to the association of biological changes with the linear progress of time. This chapter will attempt to identify the time-dependent, that is, cumulative, processes that interfere with the function of the body and, in particular, manifest with changes in behaviour and experience. It will cover genetic and epigenetic mechanisms, the intermediate metabolic changes associated with ageing, as well as changes at a system level that increase the allostatic load and lead to overload. We will pay particular attention to age-related changes in the brain that are likely to be associated with psychiatric disease and that are becoming more and more amenable to examination with *in vivo* imaging techniques. Empirical biology of psychiatric ageing will require a chain of evidence from predisposing variables, longitudinally throughout life to observable brain changes that are associated with changed behaviour and psychiatric illness. We will illustrate this principle with a few examples.

## Mechanisms of ageing

### Cellular ageing

Chronological age is the best predictor of many chronic diseases such as atherosclerosis, type 2 diabetes, most cancers, and neurodegenerative diseases [3]. But how does the passing of time affect the human body? There are many different pathways underlying ageing, but the common denominator is that they affect the accumulation of damage in DNA, proteins, and lipids over time, and thus in organelles, cells, and tissues [4]. This somatic body cell clock determines the fate of individual organisms over weeks, months, and years and is based on mechanisms similar to the germ cell molecular clock that allows us to reconstruct the history of species over hundreds of millennia [5]. It is the balance of two processes that defines how quickly damage occurs—on the one side, external and internal processes that cause cellular damage, and on the other side, systems for maintenance, repair, and turnover.

One example of internal processes associated with age-related damage is the production of reactive oxygen species (ROS). ROS are a normal by-product of cell energy metabolism and are mainly produced in the mitochondria, the power generator of the cell. ROS are chemically very unstable and cause oxidative damage to DNA, proteins, and lipids. This damage, in turn, causes malfunctioning of cells, and ultimately cell death if cells cannot recover [6]. However, there are many systems in the cell to combat oxidative damage, from antioxidants that act as scavengers of ROS to DNA repair mechanisms and degradation pathways for faulty proteins [7]. Accumulation of oxidative damage in cells is the cause of ageing, according to the 'free radical theory' of ageing [8]. However, there is conflicting evidence on the involvement of ROS in shortening or extending the lifespan [9].

Pathways that play a role in the pace of ageing have been extensively studied in the four main model organisms for ageing research: the budding yeast *Saccharomyces cerevisiae*, the nematode worm *Caenorhabditis elegans*, the fruit fly *Drosophila melanogaster*, and the house mouse *Mus musculus musculus/domesticus*. There seem to be converging pathways in these model organisms and humans that not only lead to an extension of the lifespan, but also an improvement of health during ageing—an increased 'health span' [4]. One of the best studied ways of extending life in model organisms is to introduce dietary restriction. This led to the discovery that pathways involved in nutrient sensing are important players in ageing. These pathways are regulated by different proteins: target of rapamycin (TOR), adenosine monophosphate-activated protein (AMP) kinase, sirtuins, and insulin/insulin-like growth factor 1 (IGF-1) [9]. On the one hand, these pathways affect cellular metabolism, which intuitively makes sense; when food is scarce, the organism needs to be able to enter a standby mode of energy-saving to support only those processes that are vital for survival [10]. On the other hand, there is also a link between these pathways and cellular damage because they affect the production of antioxidants and proteins involved in cellular maintenance and repair mechanisms [9]. While it is difficult to establish links between dietary restriction and ageing in humans, studies in rhesus monkeys have shown that it affects ageing in non-human primates as well. Dietary restriction leads to improved insulin sensitivity and inflammatory profiles and protects from age-related diseases such as sarcopenia, cardiovascular disease (CVD), type 2 diabetes, neoplasia, endometriosis, and brain atrophy [11].

## Cellular brain ageing

The brain is particularly susceptible to cellular damage because of its limited capacity for regeneration and its high metabolic demand, which leads to increased ROS production [12]. Many neurodegenerative diseases have in common the fact that postmortem studies show increased oxidative stress and reduced levels of antioxidants in brain regions affected by pathology [6]. Whether this is cause or effect of pathology and the contribution of oxidative stress to brain ageing per se, however, is a matter of intense research [12]. Nevertheless, nutrient-signalling pathways provide a link between cellular damage and the brain. They not only play a role in the periphery, but also mediate signalling in the brain. For example, insulin receptors can be found in the hippocampus and their function depends on insulin transport from the periphery to the brain [13].

One of the direct effects of dietary restriction on the brain is increased production of neurotrophic factors and neurogenesis in the hippocampus [14]. The hippocampus is one of the few areas in the adult human brain that show integration of newly generated neurons into brain circuits. While most studies on neurogenesis have been conducted in rodents, it is reasonable to assume that adult neurogenesis in the human hippocampus serves similar purposes, supporting memory processes and contributing to brain plasticity. Neurogenesis decreases with age, so measures that contribute to increased neurogenesis are thought to be protective [15, 16]. Another mechanism of brain plasticity that decreases with age is synaptic plasticity. It has been extensively studied in non-human primates where age-related cognitive decline is more associated with alterations in synaptic connectivity, particularly highly plastic synapses, than loss of neurons per se [17]. Similar effects have been shown in humans, and research into Alzheimer's disease has shown a high degree of synapse loss, rather than neuron loss at early disease stages, which correlates with cognitive symptoms [18, 19]. Therefore, the loss of synaptic plasticity and connectivity plays a role in the ageing human brain as well. Insights into the mechanisms driving ageing and longevity in humans have focused on two main contributors: genetics and lifestyle and other environmental factors.

## Genetics and epigenetics

The simple concept that some people 'look young' for their age, or vice versa, shows that chronological age, the time that has passed since birth, and biological age, in this case defined by features such as smoothness of the skin, posture, etc., are not necessarily the same. Research into genetic factors that drive the pace of ageing have focused on two extreme ends of the spectrum: those who show accelerated ageing phenotypes due to progeroid syndromes and

centenarians who show exceptional longevity. One example of a progeroid syndrome is Werner syndrome, which is characterized by the development of age-related diseases such as osteoporosis, CVD, and cancer from the age of 20. Research into the genetics of many of these progeroid syndromes has shown the importance of DNA repair and maintenance in ageing [20]. The debate of whether or not familial forms of neurodegenerative diseases, such as Alzheimer's disease, constitute an 'accelerated ageing' phenotype later in life [20] is beyond the scope of this chapter. It is striking, however, that individuals with exceptional longevity seem to escape age-related disorders, including neurodegenerative disorders, altogether and live mostly disease-free until late in life [21]. Longevity clusters in families point towards a link between genetics and lifespan. Additionally, studies have shown that centenarians do not lead a healthier life than the rest of the population, which makes it more likely that it is their genetic makeup that protects them from the development of age-related diseases [21]. However, genome-wide association studies (GWAS) have not yielded very promising results, apart from an association between the apolipoprotein E (APOE) ε2 allele and longevity, which is most likely due to the link between a reduced risk of Alzheimer's disease in carriers of this allele [21]. Some studies have also reported that centenarians are more likely to carry protective alleles for age-related diseases such as cancer, CVD, and type 2 diabetes. However, this appears to depend on the sample source of centenarians because other studies found that centenarians were healthy, even though they carried risk genes for these diseases [21]. More targeted genetic approaches have also shown associations between longevity and genes that are associated with ageing pathways such as forkhead box O3A (FOXO3A) and IGF-1 signalling, genomic stability, in particular telomere protection, and genes that encode antioxidants [21]. The contribution of mitochondria and oxidative stress may implicate mitochondrial DNA. For example, two-thirds of Japanese centenarians were found to carry a mitochondrial gene variant that is possibly associated with decreased mitochondrial leakage of ROS [22]. For an updated list of genes associated with ageing, see The Ageing Gene Database available at: http://genomics.senescence.info/genes/.

One problem with the genetic approaches described is that it is probably too simplistic to assume that all centenarians have the same genetic profile. One could hypothesize that it is again the balance of processes that cause damage vs repair and maintenance pathways that will determine the lifespan in humans. While some centenarians live long and healthy lives because they are resistant to damage in the first place, others profit from systems that efficiently repair damage and allow them to be resilient.

It is not necessarily only the genotype that determines longevity, but also which parts of the DNA are actually transcribed. Epigenetic modifications, such as histone modifications, DNA methylation, and chromatin remodelling, change with age and provide a link between genetics and lifestyle or environmental factors that affect ageing. Members of the sirtuin family of proteins, for example, have been extensively studied as epigenetic factors that influence longevity in model organisms [23]. However, it is unclear whether these proteins also play a role in human longevity [21]. Studies in monozygotic twins have shown that lifestyle or environmental factors contribute to epigenetic differences between twins that increase with age [24]. These factors and the mechanisms underlying their effects on ageing are the subject of extensive research.

## Environmental and lifestyle factors

Studies in model organisms, as mentioned previously, have already provided links between metabolism and ageing. While it is difficult to determine the effects of dietary restriction in randomized controlled trials in humans, several short-term studies have shown beneficial effects, for example a reduction in risk factors for atherosclerosis, that are similar to those observed in animal studies [4]. There are strong links between hypertension, dyslipidaemia, and oxidative stress, with studies showing increased ROS production and decreased antioxidant activity in CVD patients. Indeed, some antihypertensive drugs and cholesterol-lowering statins probably act, at least partly, via decreasing ROS production [25]. As CVD can be seen as a sign of 'unsuccessful' ageing, factors that affect CVD risk, such as diet [26], will also, in turn, affect mechanisms of ageing. Physical activity affects ageing, possibly partly by acting on CVD risk. Even at low levels, physical activity decreases mortality and thus leads to more 'successful' ageing [27]. On a mechanistic level, there is an association between physical activity and leucocyte telomere length, which indicates the effects on pathways that are important for genomic stability [28]. Physical activity also has direct effects on the brain where it leads to increased hippocampal neurogenesis [15]. Another link between the environment and ageing is the immune system. Ageing is associated with upregulated inflammatory markers, possibly because the immune system has to deal with recurrent or chronic systemic infections and imbalances between pro- and anti-inflammatory networks [29]. Following an injury or infection, the immune response to systemic insults is not restricted to the periphery, but also affects the brain. This becomes evident in the associated behavioural symptoms of sickness such as lethargy and poor concentration [30]. Systemic inflammation accompanies many chronic diseases such as rheumatological conditions and CVD. There is also a link between metabolism and the immune system, because increased peripheral insulin levels are associated with increased pro-inflammatory

markers in the cerebrospinal fluid (CSF) [31]. Chronic inflammation leads to an increased state of activation of the brain immune response that accompanies ageing and might, in turn, contribute to neurodegeneration [32]. Not surprisingly, altered immune responses have been described consistently in depressive disorders later in life [33]( see also Chapter 16). Another important lifestyle factor that affects brain ageing is stress, which will be discussed in the next section.

## Stress and ageing (allostatic load)

From first principles, our chance of developing physical and psychological illness increases with time. Any change or challenge within the internal or external environment, no matter how minor it may be, requires temporary adaptations of the internal milieu and a shift in its homeostasis (a process termed allostasis). The repeated demand for allostasis over time can lead to syndromes that are associated with peripheral organ damage, as well as structural and functional brain changes [34], which, in turn, further damage the dysregulated stress response system. These maladaptive responses reflect the 'allostatic load' (AL) and 'overload' [35], physiological dysregulation, and the wear-and-tear of the body, thus representing biological ageing [36, 37] (Fig. 18.1). Common psychological stress, if perceived negatively, rather than as an incentive to strive, is said to accelerate biological ageing and precipitate the onset of age-related diseases [38]. Individual variability in the progressive loss of the ability to deal with stress and the development of age-related distress [39] may also reflect differences in individual potential for brain plasticity and resilience [40].

Chronic stress-related changes accumulate across the lifespan, and challenges faced in later life are associated with intermediate composite markers of AL such as the metabolic syndrome [41]. These, in turn, increase the risk of pathological brain changes and

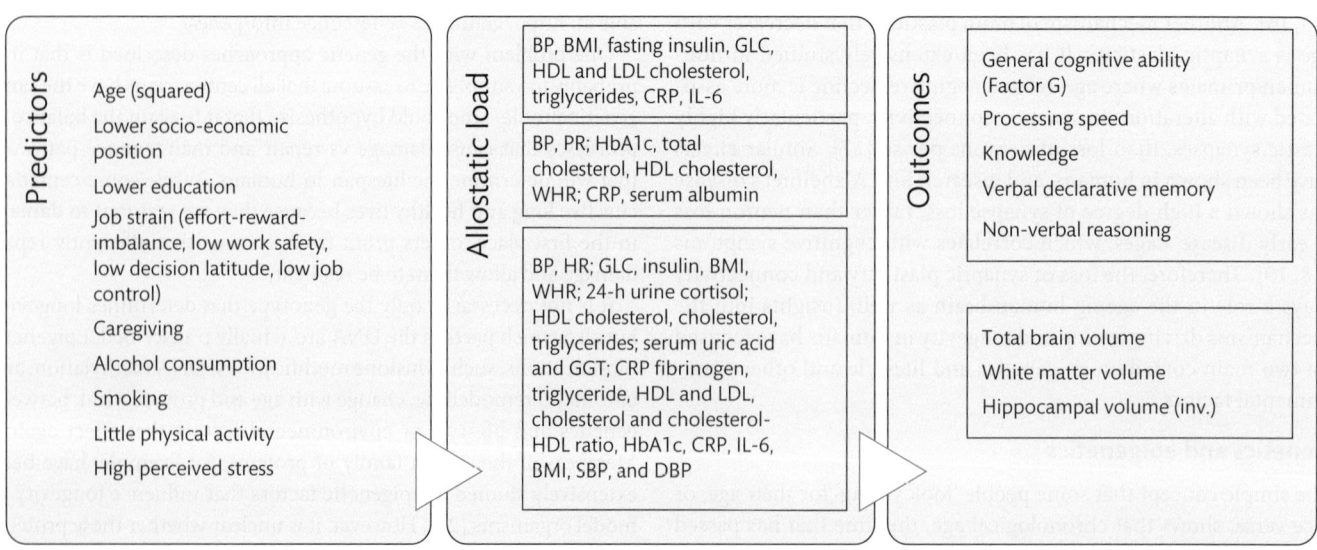

**Fig. 18.1** The secondary stress marker 'allostatic load' with predictors and behavioural and brain outcomes. Three versions of computing the allostatic load from abnormal physiological measures and cited based on the underlying papers [70–75]. BMI, body mass index; BP, blood pressure; CRP, C-reactive protein; DBP, diastolic blood pressure; GGT, gamma-glutamyltranspeptidase; GLC, glucose; HbA1c, glycated haemoglobin; HDL, high-density lipoproteins; HR, heart rate; IL-6, interleukin 6; LDL, low-density lipoproteins; PR, pulse rate; SBP, systolic blood pressure; WHR, waist-to-hip ratio.

age-related diseases such as depression [42], impaired cognitive function [43, 44], and Alzheimer's disease [45].

## Composite measures of biological ageing

The release of stress hormones and their antagonists, along with pro- and anti-inflammatory cytokines, triggers the cardiovascular, metabolic, and inflammatory systems through the HPA axis and the autonomic nervous system to shift their operational ranges in order to sustain allostasis (Table 18.1). While this is adaptive in the short run, prolonged activity results in an increase of AL markers, which predict stress-related illness. Markers include cardiovascular, metabolic, and inflammatory measures, such as summarized in the Framingham risk scores [46] (see also Fig. 18.1), metabolic syndrome [47], or AL index [41], and are better predictors of physical, mental, and cognitive health and mortality risk than individual component measures [48, 49].

**Table 18.1** Composite measures of biological ageing

| | | Allostatic load index [41] | Framingham stroke risk [46] | Metabolic syndrome [47] |
|---|---|---|---|---|
| Cardiovascular | Systolic BP | X | X | X |
| | Diastolic BP | X | | X |
| | CVD | | X | |
| | Atrial fibrillation | | X | |
| | Left ventricular hypertrophy | | X | |
| | BP medication | | X | |
| Metabolic | Diabetes | X | | X |
| | Diabetes medication | | X | |
| | Fasting glucose | | X | |
| | Waist circumference | | X | |
| | Weight | | X | |
| | Fat mass | | X | |
| | % body fat | | X | |
| | Serum triglycerides | X | | X |
| | HDL | | | X |
| | LDL | X | | |
| | Cholesterol | X | | |
| | BMI | X | | |
| | HbA1C | X | | X |
| Immune | C-reactive protein | X | | |
| | Interleukin-6 | X | | |
| Other | Age | | X | |
| | Sex | | X | X |
| | Smoking | | X | |
| | Cortisol | X | | |

BP, blood pressure; BMI, body mass index; CVD, cardiovascular disease; HbA1C, glycated haemoglobin; LDL, low-density lipoprotein.
Allostatic load index below is based on markers available in the Whitehall II study [139, 140].

The effects of psychosocial stress have been most extensively studied in association with cardiovascular health and disease risk in the context of the workplace [50]. Mid-life hypertension is associated with an increased risk of late-onset depression [49] and dementia [51]. It has been linked to atrophy in both occipital and frontal cortical regions [52] and in the hippocampus [53] in cognitively healthy older adults. Consistently high blood pressure across adulthood also predicts structural brain changes in the deep white matter in healthy older adults [54]. Multifactorial cardiovascular and stroke risk scores, such as the Framingham Coronary Heart Disease [55] and stroke risk [46] scores, are associated with cognitive decline [56, 57] and structural brain changes such as grey matter volume reduction [58] and white matter hyperintensities [59]. In turn, patterns of structural brain changes discriminate between those with high vs those with low coronary heart disease risk, as measured by the Framingham Coronary Heart Disease Risk score, even after taking into account the genetic risk for Alzheimer's disease [60].

Metabolic syndrome [47] is a combination of cardiovascular and neuroendocrine factors. It is defined by a number of biomarkers: increased abdominal circumference, increased levels of triglycerides, decreased levels of high-density lipoprotein (HDL) cholesterol, elevated blood pressure (including prehypertension), and fasting glucose levels (prediabetes). A diagnosis of the syndrome is given if at least three of these markers are above their defined thresholds. The effects of workplace psychosocial stress have been shown to manifest as metabolic syndrome [61], besides adverse cardiovascular health, as mentioned in this chapter. In turn, metabolic syndrome is associated with a risk of stroke and CVD mortality [62], telomere shortening [38], and poor mental and cognitive functioning [42, 43, 63]. Our understanding of the association between metabolic syndrome and brain changes, however, is limited [64]. Reduced cortical thickness in distinct areas of both hemispheres, as well as volume reductions in the right nucleus accumbens of middle- to older-aged participants with metabolic syndrome, have been documented [65]. Vascular brain damage in the form of periventricular white matter hyperintensities and subcortical white matter lesions in middle-aged individuals [64], reduced white matter integrity in fronto-temporal regions [66], and silent brain infarction in older individuals [64] have also been reported.

The exact combination of biomarkers that define the AL index is subject to debate [41], as is the way it is computed [67, 68], but it tends to include a combination of stress hormones, inflammatory, cardiovascular, metabolic, dyslipidaemia, and neuroendocrine markers. In combination, they are better predictors of health outcomes and mortality than on their own [69]. Chronological age is a strong predictor of AL increase, and a combination of psychosocial factors, including those at work, predict high levels of the index [70]. A recent systematic review of 16 cross-sectional studies found that occupational stress was positively associated with AL index, in spite of the lack of consensus on its computation and the heterogeneity in study methods and quality [71]. Low socio-economic status is associated with higher AL index across the lifespan [72], which is not surprising, given that the prevalence of stressors is higher in low socio-economic groups. A recent community-based prospective cohort study of middle-aged adults found that material possessions (car and house ownership) and smoking, but not other health behaviours, such as physical activity or alcohol consumption, or psychological factors, mediated the relationship between low socio-economic status and high AL index [73]. Sex differences are present in the association of both socio-economic status and lifestyle with AL index—low occupational position and alcohol abstinence, compared to moderate drinking, is associated with higher AL index levels in women, but the opposite is true for men. Education level, physical activity, and low salt intake seem to be protective against high AL in both sexes [74]. The AL index is a significant predictor of cognitive and physical decline, CVD, and mortality in older adults [48]. In a birth-year cohort, Booth *et al.* [75] reported a negative association of AL index with total brain and white matter volumes, and no association with grey matter volume in participants aged 73 years. In addition, the index was negatively associated with general cognitive ability, processing speed, and knowledge, but not with memory or non-verbal reasoning. Although it is argued that combinations of physiological markers of wear-and-tear are better predictors of brain structure and function than any one of the AL markers [48], the mechanisms in which primary and secondary markers come together to predict cognitive decline are yet to be understood [76].

### Central role of the brain

Several brain structures have a central role in the regulation of the stress response (Fig. 18.2). These regions include the hippocampus, amygdala, and prefrontal cortex. They are important effectors, responding to mediators of allostasis, as well as targets of allostasis, so that chronic dysregulation can result in AL and damage to certain brain structures. Furthermore, they can become central to such dysregulation, stress-related vulnerability, and pathological plasticity [34]. Identifying the precise mechanisms that lead to the wear-and-tear of specific brain structures may lead to effective interventions [37].

The subcortical limbic brain structures, the hippocampus and amygdala, process information arising from less developed brain regions in the diencephalon (such as the hypothalamus) and myelencephalon (parts of the brainstem), along with higher cortical areas, particularly in the prefrontal cortex, to regulate physiological and behavioural responses of allostasis [34]. The formation of synapses and long-term potentiation to facilitate memory can make these responses adaptive. However, neuronal damage caused by chronic elevated glucocorticoid levels can lead to (hippocampal) neuronal death via further dysregulation of glucocorticoid secretion [77]. Although a lack of longitudinal studies makes it challenging to determine the mechanism for this, for example, higher sensitivity to glucocorticoids in PTSD may contribute to hippocampal atrophy [78]. Individuals with smaller hippocampi, on the other hand, may

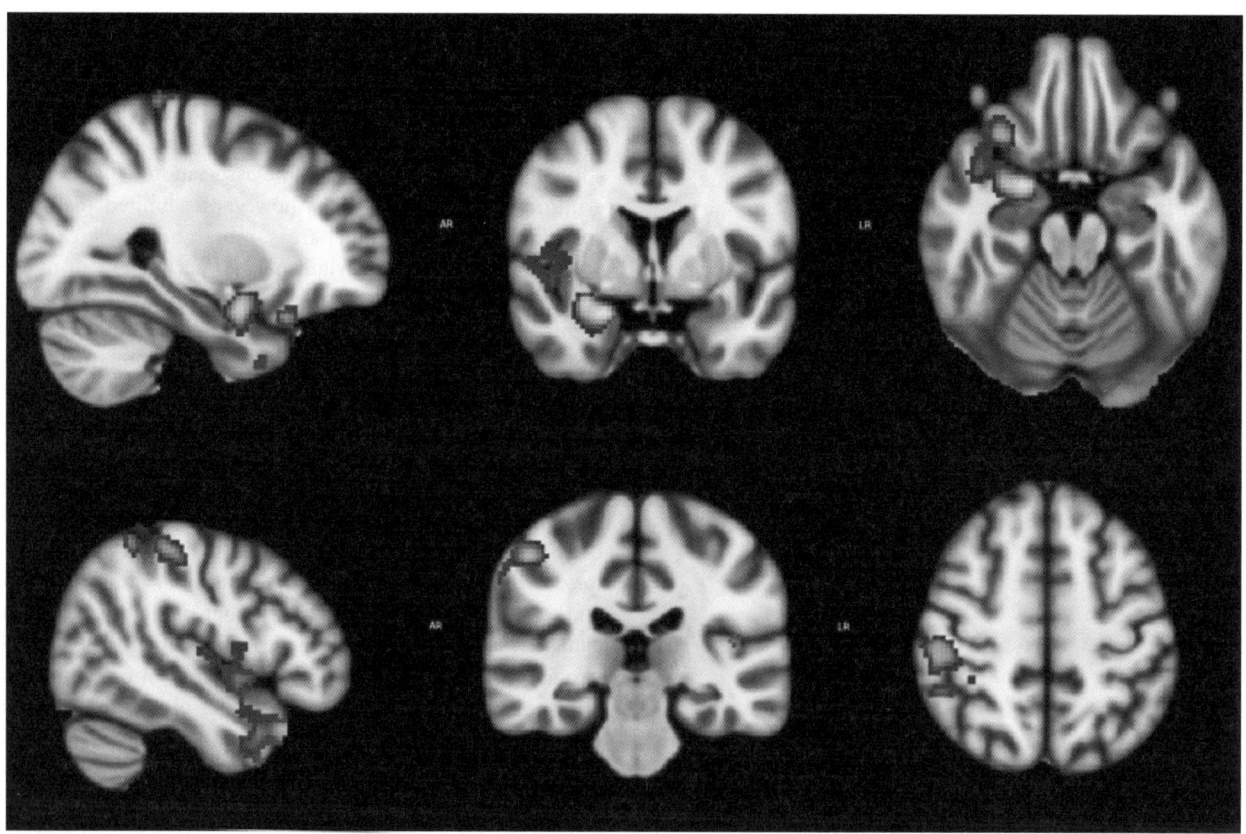

**Fig. 18.2** (see Colour Plate section) Negative association of vascular risk (Framingham Stroke Risk Score) averaged over 20 years from mid- to later life and grey matter density (GMD) in members of the Whitehall II cohort (N = 405). Images were analysed using FSL-VBM, an optimized voxel-based morphometry (VBM) protocol (for more details, see [140]). Using randomized and correcting for multiple comparisons, a voxel-wise general linear model (GLM) was applied between average Framingham Stroke Risk Scores and GMDs, correcting for age and sex. Significance threshold was set at $P$ <0.05, using the threshold-free cluster enhancement (TFCE) method. Significant negative association is present in the right cerebral cortex: in the medial temporal lobe, temporal pole, planum polare (a), and post-central gyrus (b). A = anterior; R = right.
Image courtesy of Dr Enikő Zsoldos.

be more vulnerable to developing PTSD [79]. In older adults, a continuous rise in resting glucocorticoid levels with age seems to be associated with loss of hippocampal volume and memory decline [40]. Changes in white matter microstructure are also present with elevated diurnal and reactive glucocorticoid levels in elderly males [80].

## Psychosocial and severe stress

Common stressful psychosocial and environmental factors, such as socio-economic status and workplace stressors, are predictors of cardiovascular outcomes [81, 82] and mortality [83]. Although attempts to relate specific stressors to specific medical problems have been unsuccessful, stress remains an underlying theme in the development and course of virtually all physical illness [84]. Socio-economic status both in childhood and adulthood is associated with chronic stress [85] and has been linked with negative health outcomes and mortality in later life [86]. Composite measures of AL are often associated with low social status in childhood and adulthood, capturing the long-term effect of chronic stressors, which have a higher prevalence in low socio-economic strata [37]. There is some evidence for the negative association between psychosocial stress in childhood and adulthood [87, 88] and shorter telomere length, which may mediate impaired health in adulthood. Socio-economic status in childhood, however, is not unequivocally associated with telomere length [87]. Negative circumstances in both early and adult life independently predict higher AL index, and so does negative emotional response to stressful life events [89, 90]. There is some evidence that chronic perceived stress and the number of stressful life events is associated with decreased grey matter volumes in the limbic and prefrontal areas in adults without specific psychopathology [91–93]. However, studies like these are scarce and difficult to interpret. In principle, mild or moderately aversive conditions during childhood can shape an individual to be optimally adapted to similar conditions later in life [94] but can also potentiate the effects of further negative events and circumstances—albeit current evidence for this only exists in men [89].

Crises or unexpected traumatic events exerting acute, sudden, or intense stress not only overwhelm coping mechanisms, but may also be associated with psychopathology, such as PTSD [95] or major depression [96]. Extreme life stressors can affect brain structures related to allostasis, such as the hippocampus, amygdala, anterior cingulate cortex, and medial frontal gyrus [93], especially in people with depression [36] and PTSD [78]. In people with major depression or PTSD, childhood neglect or trauma can result in structural and functional brain changes [97]. However, psychopathology itself may already cause these [98, 99].

## Not all stress is bad: potentials for resilience and the slowing of ageing

Mild or moderately aversive conditions during childhood can shape an individual to be optimally adapted to similar conditions later in life [94]. The benefits of mild and limited stressors that result in physiological benefits (so-called 'eustress' or 'hermetic stress') are well documented in laboratory animal studies and can be supportive of successful biological ageing [100, 101]. The relationship between the animal's response to stress and the rate of ageing is extremely complex, and successful translation into human experiments are rare [102]. While the relationship between stressful circumstances (such as daily hassles, workplace stress) and physiological pathways

is plausible, demonstrating and measuring this aspect of biological ageing, independent of disease pathology, is challenged by laboratory and ethical limitations [103]. Healthy eating, including caloric restriction, physical exercise, and gene expression in response to certain stressors, are recommended targets of future biological ageing studies [103]. The advent of longitudinal cohort studies and non-invasive multimodal imaging techniques presents a window of opportunity to bridge the gap between basic and clinical scientific enquiries.

There is some evidence that cumulative adverse circumstances across the lifespan predict physiological dysregulation, measured by the AL index [89]. There is also evidence that this relationship is mediated by the negative emotional response to stressful events [90]. Stress mindset, the extent to which an individual thinks a stressor is debilitating or enhancing is said to be instrumental in the manifestation of the stress response and the acceleration of biological ageing [104]. A key feature of dysfunctional stress adaptation is loss of resilience, which manifests in the form of anxiety and depression. (Mal-)adaptive stress-related brain plasticity, such as dendritic remodelling or shrinkage of dentate gyrus-CA3 pyramidal neurons in the hippocampus or medial prefrontal cortex, dendritic growth in the amygdala, neuronal replacement, and synapse turnover, if reversible, that is, prior to permanent excitotoxic damage [105], can underpin treatment or slowing of age-related changes [106].

# Ageing and the brain

## Structural changes with ageing

That brains change with age has been observed for a long time in the general population. Until recently, this may even have contributed to the clinical neglect of brain imaging in the assessment of pathological changes in higher age groups [107]. Brain size changes with age, declining by 1% every 5 years from the ages of 20 to 80 [108]. Correspondingly, certain domains of cognition, such as memory, reasoning, phonemic and semantic fluency, but not vocabulary, deteriorate from age of 45 at different speeds [109] (see also [110]). Distinct aspects of frontal lobe structure mediate age-related differences in fluid intelligence and multitasking [111]. Structural and functional differences in the medial prefrontal cortex underlie the known distractibility and suppression deficits in ageing [112], known to everybody who has played 'Taboo' with older and younger relatives. This family game requires one player to describe a concept to all other co-players, without using certain given keywords that are commonly linked to the concept, that is, the player has to suppress the 'obvious' responses (the 'performance cut-off' appears to be in the 30s [113]). Objective markers of ageing, such as leucocyte telomere length, have been found to be associated with total and regional brain volumes, in particular the hippocampus, amygdala, and inferior temporal region, in a large population-based cohort [114]. Not only the grey matter, but also the white matter, deteriorates with age [115]. Widespread age-related differences in brain microstructure are demonstrated by quantitative MRI, with an anterior–posterior gradient, for example, more changes in the genu than in the splenium corporis callosi [116]. The aetiology of these changes is not entirely clear, but an important contribution must be from vascular ageing that is also thought to contribute significantly to the development of dementia in Alzheimer's disease [117, 118].

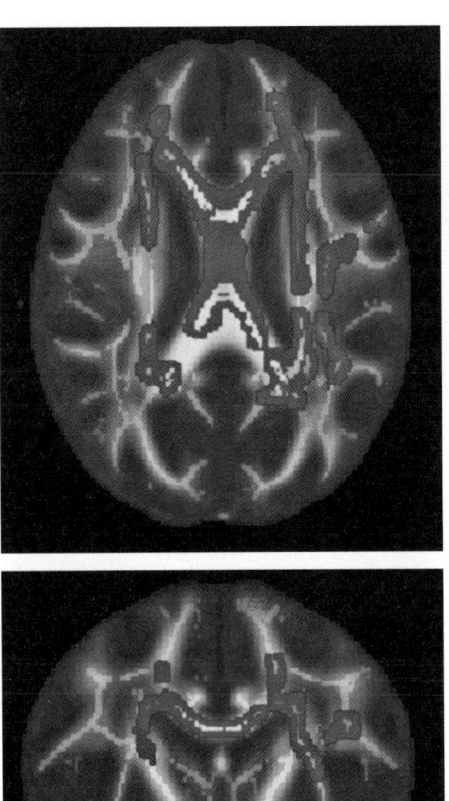
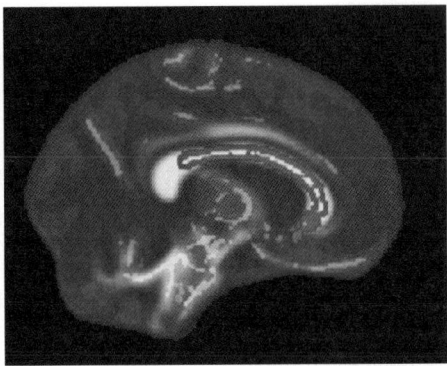
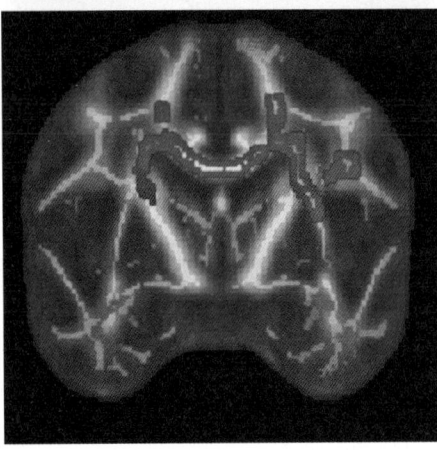

**Fig. 18.3** (see Colour Plate section) Associations of *large vessel elasticity* (from pulse wave velocity data supplied by Eric Brunner, University College London) with mean diffusivity in white matter (a, b, c: negative association) and grey matter density (d: positive association) (*N* = 444). Model: sex, education, mean arterial pressure, alcohol, antihypertensive medication, chronic illness, ethnicity, social class, and FRS (for image acquisition and analysis, see [140]).

Image courtesy of Dr Sana Suri.

Increases in 24-hour systolic blood pressure are associated with arteriolar fragility of the cerebral white matter in people aged over 65. The clinical relevance of such abnormalities in asymptomatic and moderate cardiovascular risk populations is unclear [119].

Figs. 18.2 and 18.3 demonstrate the associations of vascular risk (Framingham stroke risk score) and large vessel elasticity with grey matter density (*N* = 405). Alternative mechanisms underlying age-related white matter changes include excitotoxicity and mitochondrial dysfunction [120]. Also, less decrease over 6 years in C-reactive protein, that is, persistent inflammatory reaction, was significantly associated in octogenarians with poorer white matter integrity in the dorsal and temporal superior longitudinal and uncinate fasciculi (*N* = 276 [121]). Figs. 18.4 and 18.5 summarize the negative associations of grey matter intensity and white matter integrity (fractional isotropy) with age.

### Brain reserve in ageing

Atrophic or regressive brain changes are, however, only half the story [122]—the brain retains plasticity and is able to adapt to damage by reorganization and recruitment of alternative circuits for impaired tasks [123, 124]. A number of mechanisms have been described. Functional activity tends to shift anteriorly with advancing age ('posterior to anterior shift' [125]). This may explain the devastating effect of additionally impaired executive function on patients with primary temporo-parietal lesions in Alzheimer's disease. Particularly within frontal lobes, activation that is lateralized in younger people (as, for example, for verbal and spatial working memory) tends to be distributed more symmetrically with advancing age [126]. This Hemispheric Asymmetry Reduction in Old Adults (HAROLD) model [127] has support in the domains of episodic, semantic, and working memory, perception, and inhibitory control. The large resting brain network that is active when no task is engaged (default mode network) and suppressed during tasks tends to be disrupted with age, in that the link between anterior and posterior sections is weakened [128, 129]. Such changes are associated with poor white matter integrity and cognitive function. While such anterior and posterior uncoupling already occurs in the absence of amyloid [129], it is emphasized in those with amyloid deposits in,

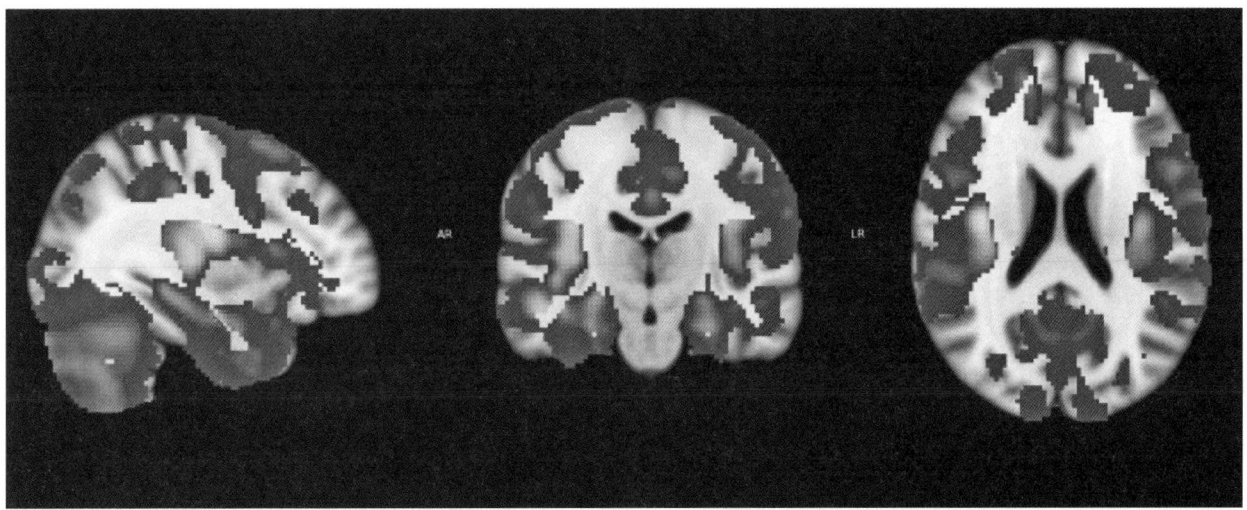

**Fig. 18.4** (see Colour Plate section) Widespread negative association of grey matter density (GMD) with age in members of the Whitehall II cohort (N = 405). Images were analysed using FSL-VBM, an optimized voxel-based morphometry (VBM) protocol. Using randomized and correcting for multiple comparisons, a voxel-wise general linear model (GLM) was applied between age and GMD, correcting for sex and socio-economic status defined by employment grade. Significance threshold was set at P <0.05, using the threshold-free cluster enhancement (TFCE) method [140]. A = anterior; R = right.
Image courtesy of Dr Enikő Zsoldos.

for example, the posterior cingulate gyrus, whether dementing or not [130, 131] (Fig. 18.6).

Cognitive impairment associated with such changes is therefore likely to be due to disruption of brain reserve, rather than damage to networks primarily involved in certain tasks. Apart from functional connectivity documented by PET or resting fMRI, white matter integrity, as recorded by $T_2$-weighted MRI and DTI, is likely to contribute to brain functional reserve [132].

While correlational studies are relatively easy to come by and may reflect a relatively static or pre-existing brain reserve, the mechanisms of brain plasticity supporting cognitive function are more difficult to identify. Valkanova *et al.* [124] cite 36 studies employing a variety of training modalities such as juggling, working memory training, meditation, learning abstract information, and aerobic exercise. There were training-related structural changes, increases or decreases in grey matter volume, a combination of increases and decreases in different brain regions, or no change at all. There was increased white matter integrity (fractional anisotropy) following training, but other patterns of results were also reported. Apart from study-dependent variations in outcome, a number of questions arise in the interpretation of such results. Are changes in the grey or white matter structure simply due to use, or are they associated with learning as such? What are the underlying neural correlates of learning, the temporal dynamics of changes, the relations between structure and function, and the upper limits of improvement? How can gains be maintained [124]? If and how exactly use and training of brain-related skills can contribute to counteract the effect of ageing therefore still awaits clarification.

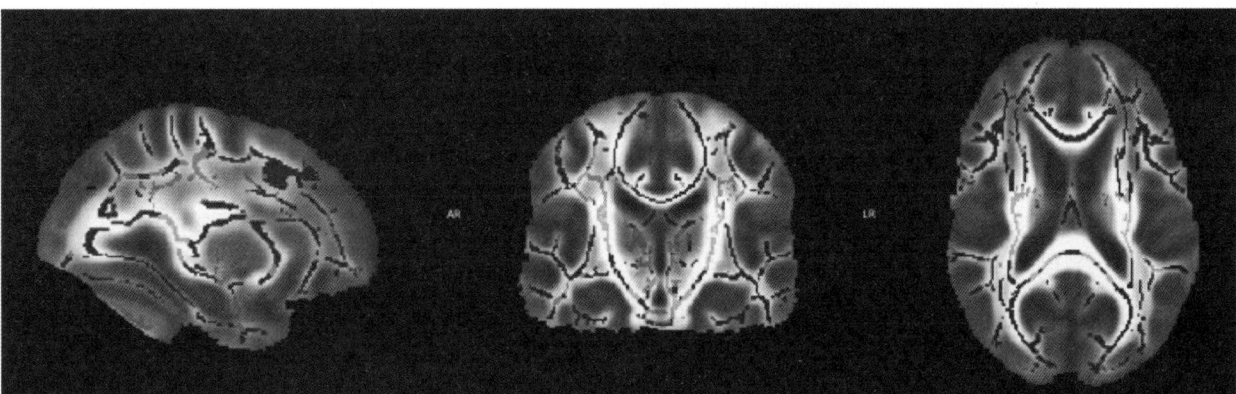

**Fig. 18.5** (see Colour Plate section) Widespread negative association of white matter integrity [fractional anisotropy (FA)] with age (in blue overlaid on green white matter skeleton) in members of the Whitehall II cohort (N = 395). Images were analysed using FSL-TBSS, an optimized tract-based spatial statistics (TBSS) protocol. Using randomized and correcting for multiple comparisons, a voxel-wise general linear model (GLM) was applied between age and FA, correcting for sex and socio-economic status defined by employment grade. Significance threshold was set at P <0.05, using the threshold-free cluster enhancement (TFCE) method [140]. A = anterior; R = right.
Image courtesy of Dr Enikő Zsoldos.

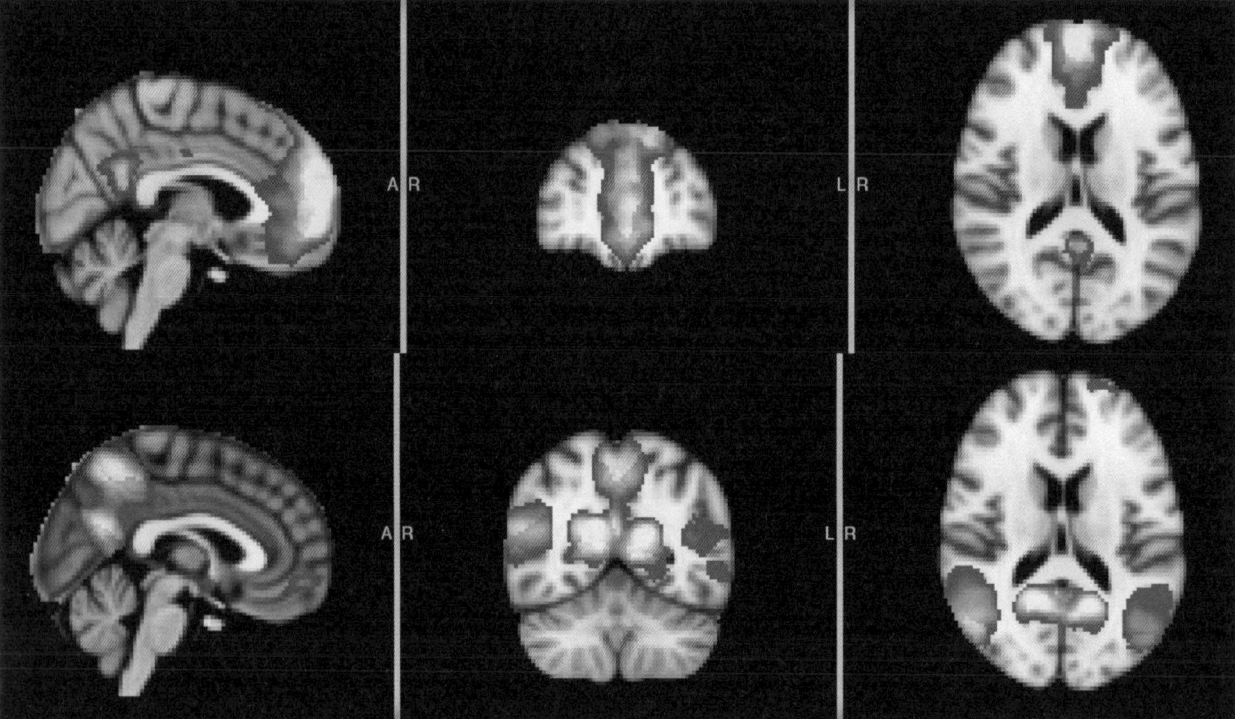

**Fig. 18.6** (see Colour Plate section) Default mode networks generated from 323 Whitehall II participant scans (MoCA >25), showing split between frontal (top) and posterior (bottom) components in older people (mean age 70 years) (for method, see [140]).
Image courtesy of Dr Sana Suri.

## Treatment implications

It is tempting to assume that it might be possible to prevent age-related changes in brain structure and function and cognitive decline by targeting the mechanisms of brain ageing. Indeed, an effect on ageing per se might have knock-on benefits for the host of diseases associated with the ageing process. There are several strategies that are under investigation. Some are aimed at slowing brain ageing with physical exercise, which has been shown in animal models to have beneficial effects on neurogenesis and cerebrovascular health [133]. Cognitive exercise is another preventive strategy that is thought to increase resilience to age-related brain changes [134]. Several pharmacological studies are also under way that target some of the molecular pathways of ageing, such as the TOR or IGF-1 pathways, using repurposed drugs that have already been approved for treatment of other diseases, for example the diabetes drugs metformin and pioglitazone [135,136]. In mouse models, it has been shown that blood transfusions from young mice might lead to rejuvenation of older mouse brains [137], and translation into humans is being tested. However, there is currently not enough evidence to show that any of these strategies can prevent or slow down brain ageing in humans.

## Conclusions

With the advent of sophisticated *in vivo* imaging methods, brain ageing can now be investigated. Naturally, the first available studies are cross-sectional, while large longitudinal studies will be a lifetime in coming. Hypotheses regarding molecular, cellular, and system-level ageing allow for us to start interrogating the available data in a specific fashion. Such multiple testing will always suffer from 'residual confounding'—all samples collected for imaging will be selected in some fashion (willingness to participate, able to enter an MRI scanner), even if they are picked at random from the general population (which most are not). The large number of possible factors contributing to ageing, as well as secular changes in the nature and pattern of causation, will keep researchers busy for decades to come [138].

## REFERENCES

1. Bureau international des poids et mesures. *Le Système international d'unités*. 8 ed. Sèvres: STEDI Media; 2006.
2. Jaspers K. *General Psychopathology*. Baltimore, ML: Johns Hopkins University Press; 1997.
3. Kirkland JL. Translating the Science of Aging into Therapeutic Interventions. Cold Spring Harb Perspect Med. 2016;6:a025908.
4. Gems D, Partridge L. Genetics of longevity in model organisms: debates and paradigm shifts. Annu Rev Physiol. 2013;75:621–44.
5. Benton MJ, Donoghue PC. Paleontological evidence to date the tree of life. Mol Biol Evol. 2007;24:26–53.
6. Andersen JK. Oxidative stress in neurodegeneration: cause or consequence? Nat Med. 2004;10 Suppl:S18–25.
7. Rajawat YS, Hilioti Z, Bossis I. Aging: central role for autophagy and the lysosomal degradative system. Ageing Res Rev. 2009;8:199–213.
8. Harman D. Aging: a theory based on free radical and radiation chemistry. J Gerontology. 1956;11:298–300.

9. Kenyon CJ. The genetics of ageing. Nature. 2010;464:504–12.

10. Fontana L, Partridge L, Longo VD. Extending healthy life span—from yeast to humans. Science. 2010;328:321–6.

11. Kemnitz JW. Calorie restriction and aging in nonhuman primates. ILAR Journal/National Research Council, Institute of Laboratory Animal Resources. 2011;52:66–77.

12. Yeoman M, Scutt G, Faragher R. Insights into CNS ageing from animal models of senescence. Nat Rev Neurosci. 2012;13:435–45.

13. Craft S. Insulin resistance syndrome and Alzheimer's disease: age- and obesity-related effects on memory, amyloid, and inflammation. Neurobiol Aging. 2005;26 Suppl 1:65–9.

14. Maalouf M, Rho JM, Mattson MP. The neuroprotective properties of calorie restriction, the ketogenic diet, and ketone bodies. Brain Res Rev. 2009;59:293–315.

15. Bergmann O, Spalding KL, Frisen J. Adult Neurogenesis in Humans. Cold Spring Harb Perspect Biol. 2015;7:a018994.

16. Winner B, Winkler J. Adult neurogenesis in neurodegenerative diseases. Cold Spring Harb Perspect Biol. 2015;7:a021287.

17. Morrison JH, Baxter MG. The ageing cortical synapse: hallmarks and implications for cognitive decline. Nat Rev Neurosci. 2012;13:240–50.

18. Terry RD, Masliah E, Salmon DP, *et al.* Physical basis of cognitive alterations in Alzheimer's disease: synapse loss is the major correlate of cognitive impairment. Ann Neurol. 1991;30:572–80.

19. Jagust W. Vulnerable neural systems and the borderland of brain aging and neurodegeneration. Neuron. 2013;77:219–34.

20. Martin GM. Genetic modulation of senescent phenotypes in *Homo sapiens*. Cell. 2005;120:523–32.

21. Milman S, Barzilai N. Dissecting the Mechanisms Underlying Unusually Successful Human Health Span and Life Span. Cold Spring Harb Perspect Med. 2016;6:a025098.

22. Tanaka M, Gong J, Zhang J, Yamada Y, Borgeld HJ, Yagi K. Mitochondrial genotype associated with longevity and its inhibitory effect on mutagenesis. Mech Ageing Dev. 2000;116(2–3):65–76.

23. Lopez-Otin C, Blasco MA, Partridge L, Serrano M, Kroemer G. The hallmarks of aging. Cell. 2013;153:1194–217.

24. Talens RP, Christensen K, Putter H, *et al.* Epigenetic variation during the adult lifespan: cross-sectional and longitudinal data on monozygotic twin pairs. *Aging Cell*. 2012;11:694–703.

25. Touyz RM. Reactive oxygen species, vascular oxidative stress, and redox signaling in hypertension: what is the clinical significance? *Hypertension*. 2004;44:248–52.

26. Hu FB, Rimm EB, Stampfer MJ, Ascherio A, Spiegelman D, Willett WC. Prospective study of major dietary patterns and risk of coronary heart disease in men. Am J Clin Nutr. 2000;72:912–21.

27. Woodcock J, Franco OH, Orsini N, Roberts I. Non-vigorous physical activity and all-cause mortality: systematic review and meta-analysis of cohort studies. *Int J Epidemiol*. 2011;40:121–38.

28. Cherkas LF, Hunkin JL, Kato BS, *et al.* The association between physical activity in leisure time and leukocyte telomere length. Arch Intern Med. 2008;168:154–8.

29. Franceschi C, Capri M, Monti D, *et al.* Inflammaging and anti-inflammaging: a systemic perspective on aging and longevity emerged from studies in humans. Mech Ageing Dev. 2007;128:92–105.

30. Holmes C. Review: systemic inflammation and Alzheimer's disease. Neuropathol Appl Neurobiol. 2013;39:51–68.

31. Fishel MA, Watson GS, Montine TJ, *et al.* Hyperinsulinemia provokes synchronous increases in central inflammation and beta-amyloid in normal adults. *Arch Neurol*. 2005;62:1539–44.

32. Perry VH, Newman TA, Cunningham C. The impact of systemic infection on the progression of neurodegenerative disease. Nature Rev Neurosci. 2003;4:103–12.

33. Haapakoski R, Mathieu J, Ebmeier KP, Alenius H, Kivimaki M. Cumulative meta-analysis of interleukins 6 and 1beta, tumour necrosis factor alpha and C-reactive protein in patients with major depressive disorder. Brain Behav Immunity. 2015;49:206–15.

34. McEwen BS, Gianaros PJ. Stress- and allostasis-induced brain plasticity. Annu Rev Med. 2011;62:431–45.

35. McEwen BS, Wingfield JC. The concept of allostasis in biology and biomedicine. Horm Behav. 2003;43:2–15.

36. McEwen BS. Protective and damaging effects of stress mediators. N Engl J Med. 1998;338:171–9.

37. Zsoldos E, Ebmeier KP. Aging and Psychological Stress. In: Fink G, editor. *Stress: Concepts, cognition, emotion and behavior. Handbook of Stress Series.* 1. 1 ed. Burlington: Academic Press; 2016. pp. 311–23.

38. Epel ES. Psychological and metabolic stress: a recipe for accelerated cellular aging? Hormones (Athens). 2009;8:7–22.

39. Zsoldos E, Mahmood A, Ebmeier KP. Occupational stress, bullying and resilience in old age. Maturitas. 2014;78:86–90.

40. Lupien SJ, McEwen BS, Gunnar MR, Heim C. Effects of stress throughout the lifespan on the brain, behaviour and cognition. Nat Rev Neurosci. 2009;10:434–45.

41. Juster RP, McEwen BS, Lupien SJ. Allostatic load biomarkers of chronic stress and impact on health and cognition. Neurosci Biobehav Rev. 2010;35:2–16.

42. Akbaraly TN, Kivimaki M, Brunner EJ, *et al.* Association between metabolic syndrome and depressive symptoms in middle-aged adults: results from the Whitehall II study. Diabetes Care. 2009;32:499–504.

43. Akbaraly TN, Kivimaki M, Shipley MJ, *et al.* Metabolic syndrome over 10 years and cognitive functioning in late midlife: the Whitehall II study. Diabetes Care. 2010;33:84–9.

44. Kim B, Feldman EL. Insulin resistance as a key link for the increased risk of cognitive impairment in the metabolic syndrome. Exp Mol Med. 2015;47:e149.

45. Frisardi V, Solfrizzi V, Seripa D, *et al.* Metabolic-cognitive syndrome: a cross-talk between metabolic syndrome and Alzheimer's disease. Ageing Res Rev. 2010;9:399–417.

46. D'Agostino RB, Wolf PA, Belanger AJ, Kannel WB. Stroke risk profile: adjustment for antihypertensive medication. The Framingham Study. Stroke. 1994;25:40–3.

47. Grundy SM, Brewer HB, Jr., Cleeman JI, *et al.* Definition of metabolic syndrome: report of the National Heart, Lung, and Blood Institute/American Heart Association conference on scientific issues related to definition. Arterioscler Thromb Vasc Biol. 2004;24:e13–18.

48. Seeman TE, McEwen BS, Rowe JW, Singer BH. Allostatic load as a marker of cumulative biological risk: MacArthur studies of successful aging. Proc Natl Acad Sci U S A. 2001;98:4770–5.

49. Valkanova V, Ebmeier KP. Vascular risk factors and depression in later life: a systematic review and meta-analysis. Biol Psychiatry. 2013;73:406–13.

50. Steptoe A, Kivimaki M. Stress and cardiovascular disease. Nat Rev Cardiol. 2012;9:360–70.

51. Gorelick PB, Scuteri A, Black SE, *et al.* Vascular contributions to cognitive impairment and dementia: a statement for healthcare professionals from the American Heart Association/American Stroke Association. Stroke. 2011;42:2672–713.

52. Glodzik L, Mosconi L, Tsui W, et al. Alzheimer's disease markers, hypertension, and gray matter damage in normal elderly. Neurobiol Aging. 2012;33:1215–27.

53. Beauchet O, Celle S, Roche F, et al. Blood pressure levels and brain volume reduction: a systematic review and meta-analysis. J Hypertens. 2013;31:1502–16.

54. Allan CL, Zsoldos E, Filippini N, et al. Lifetime hypertension as a predictor of brain structure in older adults: cohort study with a 28-year follow-up. Br J Psychiatry. 2015;206:308–15.

55. Wilson PW, D'Agostino RB, Levy D, Belanger AM, Silbershatz H, Kannel WB. Prediction of coronary heart disease using risk factor categories. Circulation. 1998;97:1837–47.

56. Dregan A, Stewart R, Gulliford MC. Cardiovascular risk factors and cognitive decline in adults aged 50 and over: a population-based cohort study. Age Ageing. 2013;42:338–45.

57. Kaffashian S, Dugravot A, Elbaz A, et al. Predicting cognitive decline: a dementia risk score vs. the Framingham vascular risk scores. Neurology. 2013;80:1300–6.

58. Debette S, Seshadri S, Beiser A, et al. Midlife vascular risk factor exposure accelerates structural brain aging and cognitive decline. Neurology. 2011;77:461–8.

59. Allan CL, Sexton CE, Kalu UG, et al. Does the Framingham Stroke Risk Profile predict white-matter changes in late-life depression? Int Psychogeriatr. 2012;24:524–31.

60. Rondina JM, Squarzoni P, Souza-Duran FL, et al. Framingham Coronary Heart Disease Risk Score Can be Predicted from Structural Brain Images in Elderly Subjects. Front Aging Neurosci. 2014;6:300.

61. Gimeno D, Tabak AG, Ferrie JE, et al. Justice at work and metabolic syndrome: the Whitehall II study. Occup Environ Med. 2010;67:256–62.

62. Lakka HM, Laaksonen DE, Lakka TA, et al. The metabolic syndrome and total and cardiovascular disease mortality in middle-aged men. JAMA. 2002;288:2709–16.

63. McIntyre RS, Soczynska JK, Konarski JZ, et al. Should Depressive Syndromes Be Reclassified as 'Metabolic Syndrome Type II'? Ann Clin Psychiatry. 2007;19:257–64.

64. Yates KF, Sweat V, Yau PL, Turchiano MM, Convit A. Impact of metabolic syndrome on cognition and brain: a selected review of the literature. Arterioscler Thromb Vasc Biol. 2012;32:2060–7.

65. Song SW, Chung JH, Rho JS, et al. Regional cortical thickness and subcortical volume changes in patients with metabolic syndrome. Brain Imaging Behav. 2015;9:588–96.

66. Segura B, Jurado MA, Freixenet N, Falcon C, Junque C, Arboix A. Microstructural white matter changes in metabolic syndrome: a diffusion tensor imaging study. Neurology. 2009;73:438–44.

67. Wiley JF, Gruenewald TL, Karlamangla AS, Seeman TE. Modeling Multisystem Physiological Dysregulation. Psychosom Med. 2016;78:290–301.

68. Mauss D, Li J, Schmidt B, Angerer P, Jarczok MN. Measuring allostatic load in the workforce: a systematic review. Ind Health. 2015;53:5–20.

69. Karlamangla AS, Singer BH, McEwen BS, Rowe JW, Seeman TE. Allostatic load as a predictor of functional decline. MacArthur studies of successful aging. J Clin Epidemiol. 2002;55:696–710.

70. Dich N, Lange T, Head J, Rod NH. Work stress, caregiving, and allostatic load: prospective results from the Whitehall II cohort study. Psychosom Med. 2015;77:539–47.

71. Mauss D, Li J, Schmidt B, Angerer P, Jarczok MN. [Work-related Stress and the Allostatic Load Index—A Systematic Review]. Gesundheitswesen. 2015.

72. Robertson T, Popham F, Benzeval M. Socioeconomic position across the lifecourse & allostatic load: data from the West of Scotland Twenty-07 cohort study. BMC Public Health. 2014;14:184.

73. Robertson T, Benzeval M, Whitley E, Popham F. The role of material, psychosocial and behavioral factors in mediating the association between socioeconomic position and allostatic load (measured by cardiovascular, metabolic and inflammatory markers). Brain Behav Immun. 2015;45:41–9.

74. Petrovic D, Pivin E, Ponte B, et al. Sociodemographic, behavioral and genetic determinants of allostatic load in a Swiss population-based study. Psychoneuroendocrinology. 2016;67:76–85.

75. Booth T, Royle NA, Corley J, et al. Association of allostatic load with brain structure and cognitive ability in later life. Neurobiol Aging. 2015;36:1390–9.

76. Gruenewald TL, Seeman TE, Ryff CD, Karlamangla AS, Singer BH. Combinations of biomarkers predictive of later life mortality. Proc Natl Acad Sci U S A. 2006;103:14158–63.

77. Sapolsky RM, Romero LM, Munck AU. How do glucocorticoids influence stress responses? Integrating permissive, suppressive, stimulatory, and preparative actions. Endocr Rev. 2000;21:55–89.

78. Deppermann S, Storchak H, Fallgatter AJ, Ehlis AC. Stress-induced neuroplasticity: (mal)adaptation to adverse life events in patients with PTSD—a critical overview. Neuroscience. 2014;283:166–77.

79. Gurvits TV, Shenton ME, Hokama H, et al. Magnetic resonance imaging study of hippocampal volume in chronic, combat-related posttraumatic stress disorder. Biol Psychiatry. 1996;40:1091–9.

80. Cox SR, Bastin ME, Ferguson KJ, et al. Brain white matter integrity and cortisol in older men: the Lothian Birth Cohort 1936. Neurobiol Aging. 2015;36:257–64.

81. Brunner E, Shipley MJ, Blane D, Smith GD, Marmot MG. When does cardiovascular risk start? Past and present socioeconomic circumstances and risk factors in adulthood. J Epidemiol Community Health. 1999;53:757–64.

82. Chandola T, Britton A, Brunner E, Hemingway H, Malik M, Kumari M, et al. Work stress and coronary heart disease: what are the mechanisms? Eur Heart J. 2008;29:640–8.

83. Marmot MG, Smith GD, Stansfeld S, et al. Health inequalities among British civil servants: the Whitehall II study. Lancet. 1991;337:1387–93.

84. Selye J. [The development of the stress theory. Stress and heart diseases]. Orv Hetil. 1969;110:2257–65.

85. McEwen BS, Tucker P. Critical biological pathways for chronic psychosocial stress and research opportunities to advance the consideration of stress in chemical risk assessment. Am J Public Health. 2011;101 Suppl 1:S131–9.

86. Juarez SP, Goodman A, Koupil I. From cradle to grave: tracking socioeconomic inequalities in mortality in a cohort of 11 868 men and women born in Uppsala, Sweden, 1915–1929. J Epidemiol Community Health. 2016;70:569–75.

87. Naess AB, Kirkengen AL. Is childhood stress associated with shorter telomeres? Tidsskr Nor Laegeforen. 2015;135:1356–60.

88. Starkweather AR, Alhaeeri AA, Montpetit A, et al. An integrative review of factors associated with telomere length and implications for biobehavioral research. Nurs Res. 2014;63:36–50.

89. Dich N, Hansen AM, Avlund K, et al. Early life adversity potentiates the effects of later life stress on cumulative physiological dysregulation. Anxiety Stress Coping. 2015;28:372–90.

90. Dich N, Doan SN, Kivimaki M, Kumari M, Rod NH. A non-linear association between self-reported negative emotional response to stress and subsequent allostatic load:

prospective results from the Whitehall II cohort study. Psychoneuroendocrinology. 2014;49:54–61.

91. Cohen RA, Grieve S, Hoth KF, *et al*. Early life stress and morphometry of the adult anterior cingulate cortex and caudate nuclei. Biol Psychiatry. 2006;59:975–82.

92. Gianaros PJ, Jennings JR, Sheu LK, Greer PJ, Kuller LH, Matthews KA. Prospective reports of chronic life stress predict decreased grey matter volume in the hippocampus. Neuroimage. 2007;35:795–803.

93. Papagni SA, Benetti S, Arulanantham S, McCrory E, McGuire P, Mechelli A. Effects of stressful life events on human brain structure: a longitudinal voxel-based morphometry study. Stress. 2011;14:227–32.

94. Nederhof E, Schmidt MV. Mismatch or cumulative stress: toward an integrated hypothesis of programming effects. Physiol Behav. 2012;106:691–700.

95. Cardenas VA, Samuelson K, Lenoci M, *et al*. Changes in brain anatomy during the course of posttraumatic stress disorder. Psychiatry Res. 2011;193:93–100.

96. Koolschijn PC, van Haren NE, Lensvelt-Mulders GJ, Hulshoff Pol HE, Kahn RS. Brain volume abnormalities in major depressive disorder: a meta-analysis of magnetic resonance imaging studies. Hum Brain Mapp. 2009;30:3719–35.

97. Frodl T, Reinhold E, Koutsouleris N, Reiser M, Meisenzahl EM. Interaction of childhood stress with hippocampus and prefrontal cortex volume reduction in major depression. J Psychiatr Res. 2010;44:799–807.

98. Cole J, Chaddock CA, Farmer AE, *et al*. White matter abnormalities and illness severity in major depressive disorder. Br J Psychiatry. 2012;201:33–9.

99. MacQueen G, Frodl T. The hippocampus in major depression: evidence for the convergence of the bench and bedside in psychiatric research? Mol Psychiatry. 2011;16:252–64.

100. Mattson MP. Hormesis defined. Ageing Res Rev. 2008;1:1–7.

101. Selye J. What is stress? Metabolism: clinical and experimental. 1956;5:525–30.

102. Lithgow GJ, Miller RA. Determination of aging rate by co-ordinated resistance to multiple forms of stress. In: Guarente L, Partridge L, Wallace DC (eds). *Molecular Biology of Aging*. New York, NY: Cold Spring Harbour Laboratory Press; 2008. pp. 427–81.

103. Epel ES, Lithgow GJ. Stress biology and aging mechanisms: toward understanding the deep connection between adaptation to stress and longevity. *J Gerontol A Biol Sci Med Sci*. 2014;69 Suppl 1:S10–16.

104. Crum AJ, Salovey P, Achor S. Rethinking stress: the role of mindsets in determining the stress response. J Pers Soc Psychol. 2013;104:716–33.

105. McEwen BS. Stress, sex, and neural adaptation to a changing environment: mechanisms of neuronal remodeling. Ann N Y Acad Sci. 2010;1204 Suppl:E38–59.

106. McEwen BS, Eiland L, Hunter RG, Miller MM. Stress and anxiety: structural plasticity and epigenetic regulation as a consequence of stress. Neuropharmacology. 2012;62:3–12.

107. Dubois B, Feldman HH, Jacova C, Dekosky ST, Barberger-Gateau P, Cummings J, *et al*. Research criteria for the diagnosis of Alzheimer's disease: revising the NINCDS-ADRDA criteria. Lancet Neurol. 2007;6:734–46.

108. Fotenos AF, Mintun MA, Snyder AZ, Morris JC, Buckner RL. Brain volume decline in aging: evidence for a relation between socioeconomic status, preclinical Alzheimer disease, and reserve. Arch Neurol. 2008;65:113–20.

109. Singh-Manoux A, Kivimaki M, Glymour MM, *et al*. Timing of onset of cognitive decline: results from Whitehall II prospective cohort study. BMJ. 2012;344:d7622.

110. Craik FI, Bialystok E. Cognition through the lifespan: mechanisms of change. Trends Cogn Sci. 2006;10:131–8.

111. Kievit RA, Davis SW, Mitchell DJ, Taylor JR, Duncan J, Henson RN. Distinct aspects of frontal lobe structure mediate age-related differences in fluid intelligence and multitasking. Nat Commun. 2014;5:5658.

112. Chadick JZ, Zanto TP, Gazzaley A. Structural and functional differences in medial prefrontal cortex underlie distractibility and suppression deficits in ageing. Nat Commun. 2014;5:4223.

113. Hersch B, Goscinny R, Uderzo A. *Taboo (Party Game)*. Pawtucket, RI: Parker Brothers/Hasbro; 1989.

114. King KS, Kozlitina J, Rosenberg RN, Peshock RM, McColl RW, Garcia CK. Effect of leukocyte telomere length on total and regional brain volumes in a large population-based cohort. JAMA Neurol. 2014;71:1247–54.

115. de Groot M, Cremers LG, Ikram MA, *et al*. White Matter Degeneration with Aging: Longitudinal Diffusion MR Imaging Analysis. Radiology. 2015:150103.

116. Callaghan MF, Freund P, Draganski B, *et al*. Widespread age-related differences in the human brain microstructure revealed by quantitative magnetic resonance imaging. Neurobiol Aging. 2014;35:1862–72.

117. Brun A, Englund E. A white matter disorder in dementia of the Alzheimer type: a pathoanatomical study. Ann Neurol. 1986;19:253–62.

118. Buckner RL. Memory and executive function in aging and AD: multiple factors that cause decline and reserve factors that compensate. Neuron. 2004;44:195–208.

119. Avet J, Pichot V, Barthelemy JC, *et al*. Leukoaraiosis and ambulatory blood pressure load in a healthy elderly cohort study: the PROOF study. Int J Cardiol. 2014;172:59–63.

120. Baltan S. Excitotoxicity and mitochondrial dysfunction underlie age-dependent ischemic white matter injury. Adv Neurobiol. 2014;11:151–70.

121. Bettcher BM, Yaffe K, Boudreau RM, *et al*. Declines in inflammation predict greater white matter microstructure in older adults. Neurobiol Aging. 2015;36:948–54.

122. Greenwood PM. Functional plasticity in cognitive aging: review and hypothesis. Neuropsychology. 2007;21:657–73.

123. Topiwala A, Ebmeier KP. Vascular changes and brain plasticity: a new approach to neurodegenerative diseases. Am J Neurodegener Dis. 2012;1:152–9.

124. Valkanova V, Eguia Rodriguez R, Ebmeier KP. Mind over matter—what do we know about neuroplasticity in adults? Int Psychogeriatr. 2014;26:891–909.

125. Davis SW, Dennis NA, Daselaar SM, Fleck MS, Cabeza R. Que PASA? The posterior-anterior shift in aging. Cereb Cortex. 2008;18:1201–9.

126. Reuter-Lorenz PA, Jonides J, Smith EE, *et al*. Age differences in the frontal lateralization of verbal and spatial working memory revealed by PET. J Cogn Neurosci. 2000;12:174–87.

127. Cabeza R, Anderson ND, Locantore JK, McIntosh AR. Aging gracefully: compensatory brain activity in high-performing older adults. Neuroimage. 2002;17:1394–402.

128. Damoiseaux JS, Beckmann CF, Arigita EJ, et al. Reduced resting-state brain activity in the 'default network' in normal aging. Cereb Cortex. 2008;18:1856–64.

129. Andrews-Hanna JR, Snyder AZ, Vincent JL, et al. Disruption of large-scale brain systems in advanced aging. Neuron. 2007;56:924–35.

130. Sperling RA, Laviolette PS, O'Keefe K, et al. Amyloid deposition is associated with impaired default network function in older persons without dementia. Neuron. 2009;63:178–88.

131. Hedden T, Van Dijk KR, Becker JA, et al. Disruption of functional connectivity in clinically normal older adults harboring amyloid burden. J Neurosci. 2009;29:12686–94.

132. Griebe M, Amann M, Hirsch JG, et al. Reduced functional reserve in patients with age-related white matter changes: a preliminary FMRI study of working memory. PLoS One. 2014;9:e103359.

133. Jagger C, Matthews FE, Wohland P, et al. A comparison of health expectancies over two decades in England: results of the Cognitive Function and Ageing Study I and II. Lancet. 2016;387:779–86.

134. Duzel E, van Praag H, Sendtner M. Can physical exercise in old age improve memory and hippocampal function? Brain. 2016;139:662–73.

135. Lampit A, Hallock H, Valenzuela M. Computerized cognitive training in cognitively healthy older adults: a systematic review and meta-analysis of effect modifiers. PLoS Med. 2014;11:e1001756.

136. Barzilai N, Crandall JP, Kritchevsky SB, Espeland MA. Metformin as a Tool to Target Aging. Cell Metab. 2016;23:1060–5.

137. Femminella GD, Bencivenga L, Petraglia L, et al. Antidiabetic Drugs in Alzheimer's Disease: Mechanisms of Action and Future Perspectives. J Diabetes Res. 2017;2017:7420796.

138. Katsimpardi L, Litterman NK, Schein PA, et al. Vascular and neurogenic rejuvenation of the aging mouse brain by young systemic factors. Science. 2014;344:630–4.

139. Marmot M, Brunner E. Cohort Profile: the Whitehall II study. Int J Epidemiol. 2005;34:251–6.

140. Filippini N, Zsoldos E, Haapakoski R, et al. Study protocol: The Whitehall II imaging sub-study. BMC Psychiatry. 2014;14:159.

# 19

# Development of brain stimulation

*Andrea Crowell, Patricio Riva-Posse, and Helen S. Mayberg*

## History and rationale

The emergence of deep brain stimulation (DBS) as an intervention for treatment-resistant psychiatric disorders is the result of an evolution of understanding of brain function and disease mechanisms across a variety of disciplines within neuroscience and medicine. Refinement of brain imaging strategies has increasingly linked specific symptoms or behaviours with discrete brain regions. Highly sophisticated neuroscience techniques, such as optogenetics, have allowed for an increased understanding of neurocircuitry in awake and behaving animals and the development of more sophisticated translational animal models linking brain and behaviour to human disease. Refinement of neurosurgical techniques led to its expansion into neuropsychiatric disorders, most notably movement disorders. The success of lesioning techniques in Parkinson's disease gave rise to the use of high-frequency DBS at the same target sites, with the initial conception of DBS as a reversible lesion (Fig. 19.1). As these various disciplines evolved in parallel, there is no single rationale for using DBS to treat psychiatric disorders. (See Table 19.1 and Fig. 19.2 [1] for a summary of targets.) For example, use of DBS in the region of the internal capsule for obsessive–compulsive disorder (OCD) and depression largely grew out of the history of performing anterior capsulotomy and other surgical lesions for severe, treatment-resistant cases. Targeting the subcallosal cingulate cortex (SCC) with DBS was the direct extension of neuroimaging findings demonstrating SCC hyperactivity in depression and subsequent normalization of activity following successful treatment, irrespective of treatment modality. Consideration of the nucleus accumbens (NAC) and medial forebrain bundle (MFB) as DBS targets relied heavily on the work in animal models to understand limbic circuitry and reward, implicating the NAC and associated monoaminergic inputs in drive, motivation, and positive reinforcement, all of which are important aspects of nearly any psychiatric syndrome.

Regardless of the target or rationale, all of the data reviewed here represent experimental attempts to treat a subset of patients for whom standard treatments have failed (OCD, depression, eating disorders, addiction) or who suffer from an illness for which there is no treatment that significantly modifies the disease trajectory [Alzheimer's disease (AD)]. Treatment resistance is defined differently for each disorder, although typically it includes non-response or loss of response to multiple medication categories and a validated psychotherapy trial. DBS for OCD does have the CE Mark approval for use in Europe. In the United States, DBS is not US Food and Drug Administration (FDA)-approved for any psychiatric disorder, although the FDA did grant a humanitarian device exemption (HDE) for use in OCD. (For comparison, DBS is FDA-approved for Parkinson's disease and essential tremor, and there is an HDE for dystonia.) The current state of DBS for psychiatric disorders is therefore still very early and largely experimental, driven by the absence of any effective treatment in this subset of patients with severe and treatment-refractory illness. With continued research on brain circuit abnormalities in other conditions, the breadth of potential applications of targeted neuromodulation is likely to increase.

## Disorders and targets

### Obsessive–compulsive disorder

OCD affects approximately 2% of the population. It is a chronic psychiatric disorder, with an estimated 10–20% of affected individuals considered treatment-resistant. Standard treatment includes SSRIs, the tricyclic drug clomipramine, and cognitive behavioural therapy (CBT). Symptoms typically fall into themes such as obsessions, checking, contamination, symmetry, harming, and hoarding. Most patients diagnosed with OCD will also meet criteria for another psychiatric disorder at some point, with major depressive disorder being the most frequent.

The cortico-striato-thalamo-cortical (CSTC) loop has been widely implicated in the pathology of OCD (Fig. 19.3) [2]. This loop includes the lateral orbitofrontal cortex (OFC) projecting, via fibres of the anterior limb of the internal capsule (ALIC), to the head of the caudate, in turn projecting to the globus pallidus and on to the thalamus, which, in turn, projects back to the OFC via fibres of the inferior thalamic peduncle (ITP). In imaging studies of OCD, hyperactivity in the OFC and caudate has been commonly demonstrated and decreases with medication or psychotherapy. Previously, anterior capsulotomy and gamma knife capsulotomy have been used to interrupt fibres reciprocally connecting the mediodorsal thalamus and prefrontal cortex. DBS for treatment of OCD developed from this understanding of the neural circuitry underlying disease pathology, as well as from evidence of effectiveness of other

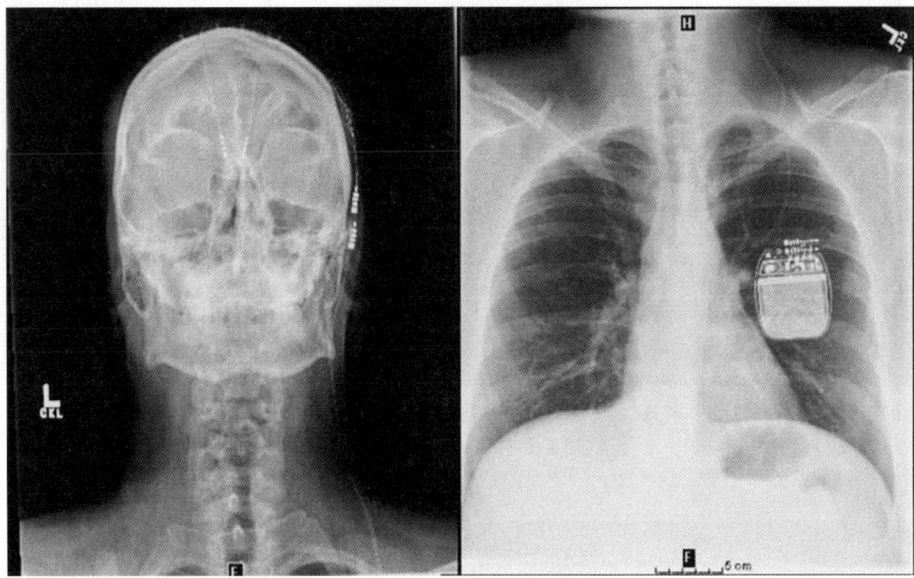

**Fig. 19.1** Radiographs showing DBS leads implanted in the brain (left), with subcutaneous lead extensions connecting the brain leads to the internal pulse generator implanted subcutaneously in the chest wall (right).
Image courtesy of Dr. Helen Mayberg.

neurosurgical procedures that have improved OCD symptoms either intentionally or serendipitously.

### Anterior limb of the internal capsule, ventral striatrum/ventral capsule

The most frequent DBS target for OCD is the ventral portion of the internal capsule, extending into the ventral striatum. The anatomical target of the first DBS for OCD was the ALIC, following the literature on anterior capsulotomy lesions. Initial data came from 15

**Table 19.1** Psychiatric disorders and DBS targets

| | |
|---|---|
| Depression | Subcallosal cingulate |
| | Nucleus accumbens |
| | Ventral capsule/ventral striatum |
| | Medial forebrain bundle |
| | Inferior thalamic peduncle |
| | Lateral habenula |
| Obsessive–compulsive disorder | Ventral capsule/ventral striatum |
| | Nucleus accumbens |
| | Medial forebrain bundle |
| | Subthalamic nucleus |
| | Inferior thalamic peduncle |
| Anorexia | Subcallosal cingulate |
| | Nucleus accumbens |
| Obesity | Lateral hypothalamus |
| Addiction | Nucleus accumbens |
| | Subthalamic nucleus |
| Alzheimer's disease | Fornix/hypothalamus |
| | Nucleus basalis of Meynert |

patients across four studies and case reports [3]; 45% of 11 patients for whom data were tracked showed at least 35% improvement from their baseline Yale-Brown Obsessive Compulsive Scale (Y-BOCS) score, the threshold most commonly used to define treatment response. Collaboration among four work groups at this target demonstrated the effect of a learning curve, such that over time, the target shifted posteriorly to include the ventral internal capsule, caudate nucleus, and NAC [ventral capsule/ventral striatum (VC/VS)]. Results from 34 patients receiving high-frequency stimulation for 36 months showed a 62% response rate. Imaging and animal studies suggest that this more posterior position may more effectively stimulate fibres of the CSTC circuit. In the most recently published cohort of patients, 4 of 6 were responders at 1 year [4]. Full effects of stimulation typically take about 3 months to evolve and plateau. Reports from long-term observational cohorts describe a sustained benefit from VC/VS DBS in OCD.

Stimulation-related side effects are common, at least transiently during stimulation parameter testing. Hypomania affects 35–65% of patients, resolves with changes in parameters, and usually is not severe. Transient sensory effects have also commonly been reported. Other reported effects include: euphoria, giddiness, anxiety, panic attacks, sadness, and stimulation-induced contralateral smile.

DBS at VC/VS appears to be differentially effective on specific symptom subtypes. DBS was 100% effective ($n = 5$) for predominant obsessions and checking, 56% effective ($n = 5/9$) for symmetry and ordering symptoms, and 45% effective ($n = 5/11$) for cleanliness and washing symptoms.

### Nucleus accumbens

The rationale for targeting the NAC directly, rather than as part of the VC/VS approach, stems from evidence of reward system dysfunction in OCD, as well as its role as a relay structure between limbic and cortical areas [5]. Hyperactivity of the NAC specifically, or more generally of limbic activity relative to cortical activity, may lead to fixed thought/action patterns overcoming more flexible and

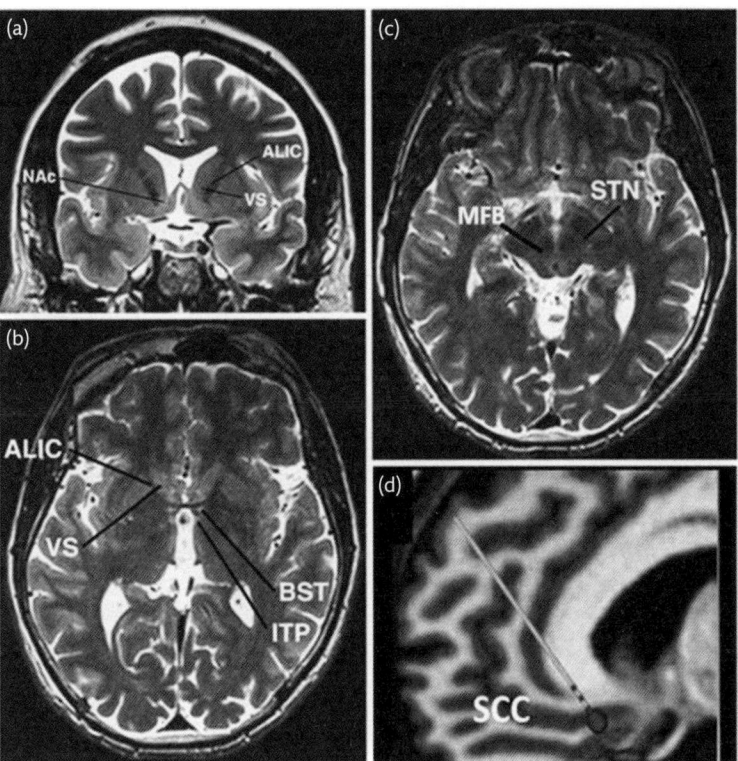

**Fig. 19.2** Deep brain stimulation targets for psychiatric indications. ALIC, anterior limb of the internal capsule; VS, ventral striatum; BST, bed nucleus of the stria terminalis; ITP, inferior thalamic peduncle; NAc, nucleus accumbens; STN, subthalamic nucleus; MFB, medial forebrain bundle; SCC, subcallosal cingulate.

Adapted from *Curr Psychiatry Rep.*, 13(4), de Koning PP, Figee M, van den Munckhof P, *et al.* Current status of deep brain stimulation for obsessive-compulsive disorder: a clinical review of different targets, pp. 274–82, Copyright (2011), with permission from Springer Science Business Media, LLC; *Biol Psychiatry*, 76(12), Riva-Posse P, Choi KS, Holtzheimer PE, *et al.*, Defining critical white matter pathways mediating successful subcallosal cingulate deep brain stimulation for treatment-resistant depression, pp. 963–9, Copyright (2014), with permission from Society of Biological Psychiatry.

appropriate behaviour patterns. Disruption of this aberrant activity with NAC DBS could thus restore behavioural flexibility [5, 6].

Fourteen patients have received right unilateral NAC stimulation; 19 patients have received bilateral NAC DBS. A positive effect of right unilateral NAC stimulation in three of the first four patients reported led investigators to undertake a larger and more rigorous trial, though only one patient in ten met the response criteria of 35% Y-BOCS improvement after 1 year of stimulation. Five additional subjects demonstrated at least 25% improvement [7]. Three case reports of bilateral NAC DBS describe 38–52% improvement after 15–24 months of stimulation. In the largest study of NAC DBS for OCD, 9 of 16 patients (56%) were treatment responders after 8 months of stimulation [8]. Further improvement was seen when CBT was subsequently added, despite the fact that patients had failed CBT prior to DBS [9]. Importantly, four patients with ego-syntonic symptoms of perfectionism, a need for symmetry, reassurance-seeking, and hoarding averaged only a 10% improvement on Y-BOCS, providing additional information about the differential effects of this treatment on different clinical subtypes of OCD.

Similar to VC/VS stimulation, hypomania is the most commonly reported side effect. Transient olfactory phenomena and increased libido were also reported. In the right unilateral cohort, three patients experienced transient agitation due to stimulation. Notably across studies, discontinuation of stimulation was associated with a rapid and poorly tolerated return of negative mood beyond baseline depression ratings, disproportionate to the return of OCD symptoms. This reversed rapidly with resumption of stimulation. The necessity of dose adjustments or evidence of long-term stability of response are not yet reported.

### Medial forebrain bundle

The MFB is a white matter tract that connects the ventral tegmental area and NAC. Based on the rapid antidepressant effects observed with MFB DBS for depression (see next section), two patients with OCD underwent MFB DBS surgery [10]. Both were reported to have acute improvement in affect and compulsions. While one patient met and maintained >35% improvement in Y-BOCS from the first month through the first year of stimulation, the other did not meet response criteria until month 12 of stimulation. In both cases, transient increased heart rate and oculomotor effects typical of stimulation at this target were observed, but hypomania was not.

### Subthalamic nucleus

DBS of the subthalamic nucleus (STN) is an accepted treatment for Parkinson's disease. In a 2002 report on two patients with Parkinson's disease and comorbid OCD who were treated with STN DBS, Parkinson's symptoms improved, as did obsessions and compulsions, with Y-BOCS reductions of 58–64% 2 weeks after surgery and remaining improved over 1 year later. A third, independent case report described similar outcomes.

In a randomized, double-blind trial of STN DBS for patients with severe OCD *without* Parkinson's disease, 12 of 16 patients

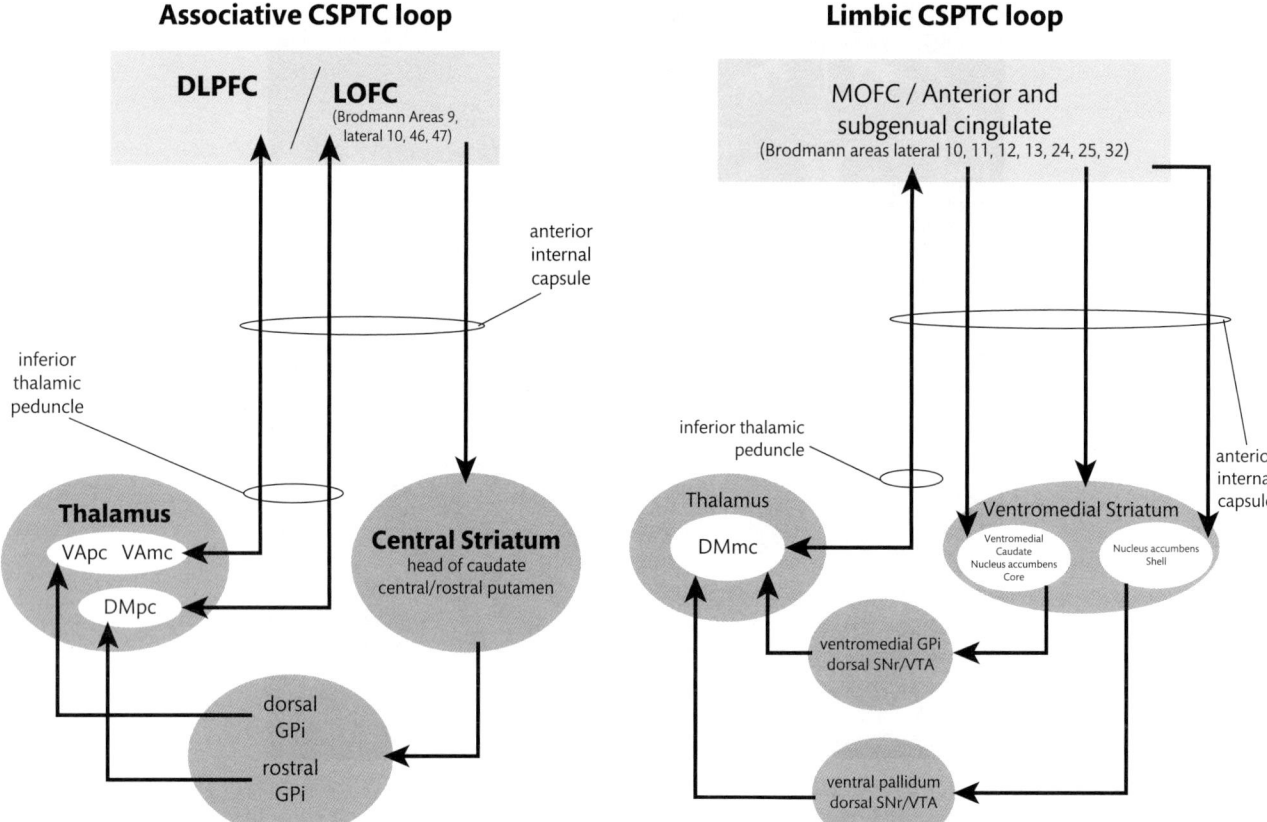

**Fig. 19.3** Cortico-striato-thalamo-cortical loop. DLPFC, dorsolateral prefrontal cortex; LOFC, lateral orbitofrontal cortex; GPi, globus pallidus internus; VAmc, ventral anterior thalamic nucleus magnocellular portion; VApc, ventral antrerior thalmic nucleus parvocellular portion; DMpc, dorsomedial thalamic nucleus parvocellular portion; MOFC, medial orbitofrontal cortex; SNr, substantia nigra pars reticulata; VTA, ventral tegmental area.
Reproduced from *Neuroscience and Biobehavioral Reviews*, 32(3), Kopell BH, Greenberg BD, Anatomy and physiology of the basal ganglia: implications for DBS in psychiatry, pp 408–22, Copyright (2008), with permission from Elsevier Ltd.

randomized to treatment (75%) experienced improvement of at least 25% after 3 months of active stimulation. Three of eight patients in the sham stimulation group responded similarly [11]. Transient mania or hypomania was reported in 6 of 16 (38%). Other side effects were anxiety, dyskinesias/motor effects, and depressed mood and suicidal ideation, which occurred in one patient. Although most adverse events were transient, serious adverse events occurred in 65% of implanted patients. No long-term efficacy data are available. That OCD symptoms improved rapidly in Parkinson's disease, unlike the slower course in OCD patients, across DBS targets likely reflects the pathophysiology of the syndrome in each illness.

### Inferior thalamic peduncle

The ITP was conceived of as a DBS target for OCD because of its location in the CSTC loop, connecting the thalamus to the OFC. A positive experience with ITP DBS in a single patient with MDD who experienced good antidepressant effect for years following DBS surgery, and the fact that many pharmacological and surgical treatments for MDD also treat OCD, also influenced a proof-of-concept study of ITP DBS. Unlike other DBS targets for OCD, the ITP has the advantage of being well defined anatomically and readily identifiable neurosurgically, based on electrophysiological properties. Six patients (100%) with severe, treatment-resistant OCD responded to ITP stimulation, with a 50% average decrease in Y-BOCS scores over 1 year [12]. Improvement

was largely stable after 3 months of stimulation. Three patients were still enrolled in the study 3 years after implantation, all having maintained responder status. No side effects were reported for stimulation on the target contact. However, stimulation above the target, near the fornix, induced confusion in one patient, which resolved when stimulation at that contact was stopped. Additionally, stimulation below the target, at or near the hypothalamus, routinely induced anxiety and dysautonomia. Hypomania was not observed at this target.

Across targets, there is clear evidence that high-frequency stimulation of the orbitofrontal basal ganglia loop system can improve some symptoms of OCD. There has yet to be a systematic study comparing responders to non-responders at a given target or a comparison of the different targets, although OCD symptom subtype appears to be important. PET studies of implanted patients showing increased perfusion in the OFC, subgenual anterior cingulate, striatum, pallidum, and thalamus [13] support CSTC modulation generally as underlying the DBS effect; however, there is not yet a clear understanding of which pathways within the CSTC network mediate either clinical efficacy or side effects.

### Major depressive disorder

MDD is a chronic illness with an episodic course. International surveys have estimated the lifetime prevalence of MDD to be 8–12% typically, although this varies by country, with the lifetime prevalence as high as 17% in the United States. An estimated 27% of individuals will have three or more episodes, while approximately 20% will experience a chronic, unremitting course. An estimated one-third of patients demonstrate some degree of treatment resistance. Definitions of treatment-resistant depression (TRD) include failure to respond to antidepressant medications of adequate dose and duration from multiple pharmacologic classes and/or ECT. The risk of a suicide attempt in patients with MDD is estimated to be 15%, with a 2–12% risk of suicide completion, a risk that increases 7-fold with lack of remission or recurrence of a major depressive episode [14], highlighting the mortality risk in TRD particularly.

The CSTC loop system has also been implicated in the underlying pathology of depression, but involving different cortical components than in OCD. Volumetric and functional abnormalities have been observed in the SCC and ventromedial and dorsolateral prefrontal cortices (DLPFC), as well as the amygdala, hippocampus, and habenula [15]. Studies in non-human primates show white matter connections from medial prefrontal regions to visceromotor output regions, such as the hypothalamus and periaqueductal grey, to limbic areas, including the amygdala and NAC, and to midline thalamic structures. Functional imaging studies have shown overactivity in the SCC and amygdala, and underactivity in the DLPFC, NAC, and ventral striatum—abnormalities reversed with antidepressant treatment. DBS for depression has been guided by these neuroimaging findings, as well as by an understanding of CSTC and reward system anatomy and function from anatomic and animal behaviour studies and from earlier experience with neurosurgical interventions for depression and OCD.

## Subcallosal cingulate cortex

The first brain target for DBS for depression, and the one with the most evidence to date, is the SCC. The rationale for targeting the SCC neurosurgically was functional neuroimaging evidence of pathological hyperactivity of this area in depressed subjects and subsequent normalization of activity with antidepressant treatment. With prevailing theories of the mechanism of DBS being a functional inhibition of the target region, it was hypothesized that inhibition of a hyperactive SCC would enable release from a pathologically negative mood state. Further, connections between the SCC and the insula, hypothalamus, and brainstem would enable changes in neurovegetative symptoms, while connections between the SCC and the medial prefrontal, orbitofrontal, cingulate, and subcortical structures would allow for changes in cognitive, hedonic, and motivational symptoms of depression.

A total of 77 depressed patients (70 MDD, 7 bipolar type 2) from eight clinical sites have been reported to date, most in the context of open-label stimulation experiments, with follow-up of at least 6 months and most for 1 year [16–22]. Clinical response across all studies has been defined as a 50% decrease in the Hamilton Depression Rating Scale (HDRS-17), with a score of <8 defining clinical remission. Combined results of all open-label studies demonstrate a response rate of 53% at 6 months, 47% at 12 months, 69% at 24 months, and 60% at 36 months. Remission rates are 27% at 6 months, 30% at 12 months, 39% at 24 months, and 40% at 36 months. Thus, response/remission is maintained over time and appears to continue to improve over years.

Retrospective analyses of response outcomes, compared to final target placement within the SCC grey matter, were unable to attribute better outcomes to a more specific location within the SCC [23]. More recently, visualization and targeting of specific white matter tracts passing through, and adjacent to, the SCC have been associated with SCC DBS treatment response [24].

Across research groups, it has repeatedly been observed that even sustained antidepressant effects are lost in response to device failure or naturalistic depletion of the battery, evidence that ongoing stimulation is required, even years after implantation. There has been one attempt to study this as a double-blind trial in five SCC DBS patients who were in stable remission over ≥3 months [25]. They were randomized to 3-month blocks of active or sham stimulation in a crossover design. During active stimulation, four patients remained in remission, while one patient lost remission but maintained antidepressant response. During sham stimulation (discontinuation), 2 of 5 patients maintained remission, one patient lost remission but maintained response, and two patients relapsed into a major depressive episode. One subject withdrew from the study during the sham phase due to relapse severity. These results support observations that discontinuation of SCC stimulation typically results in a gradual return of depression symptoms over a period of weeks; a pattern distinct from the rapid change in negative mood described with discontinuation of stimulation at other targets.

Stimulation-related side effects are uncommon, and no mania or hypomania has been reported. On the other hand, there are reports of acute effects of intraoperative stimulation, including an increased sense of calm, increased interest, and 'lightness'. Recent studies suggest that these effects are actually predictable with careful intraoperative testing, and their presence identifies the site for long-term stimulation. Refined analyses of the link between white matter tract location, stimulation-induced acute effects, and long-term efficacy are now emerging [24, 26]. Of the 77 patients described in these reports, there were six suicide attempts (8%) and three completed suicides (4%).

## Ventral capsule/ventral striatum

Stimulation of the VC/VS for treatment of depression extended from earlier studies of VC/VS DBS for OCD and from observations that depressive symptoms decreased in these patients. This region of the internal capsule contains fibre tracts connecting the SCC to the thalamus, and the ventral striatum is linked to motivation and reward. Thus, this target is positioned to affect the neurocircuitry underlying some of the key symptoms of depression.

The initial open-label series described outcomes in 15 depressed patients (14 MDD, 1 bipolar type 1) from three clinical sites [27]. Response rates (decrease in HDRS-24 >50%) were 50% at 3 months and 47% at 6 months; remission rates (HDRS-24 <10) were 20% at 3 and 6 months. Response and remission at the last follow-up (mean 23.5 months) were 53% and 33%, respectively. In five subjects with at least 36 months of follow-up, three had responded and two had remitted, suggesting that, as with the SCC target, response is maintained over time. Subsequently, a double-blind, sham-controlled study randomized 30 patients to either active ($n = 16$) or sham ($n = 14$) stimulation for 16 weeks, followed by an open-label stimulation continuation phase [28]. After the 16-week blinded treatment phase, three subjects in the active stimulation group vs two subjects from the sham stimulation group met response criteria, failing to demonstrate efficacy of VC/VS stimulation. After 8 months of open-label stimulation, 20% of subjects met response criteria and 13% were in remission. This increased to 23.3% response and 20% remission at 24 months. No subject who met responder criteria maintained response for the duration of the follow-up period. In an effort to address study design weaknesses brought to light by the double-blind trial, another group performed a double-blind crossover trial following an open-label optimization phase [29]. Twenty-five subjects at two sites underwent VC/VS DBS. Sixteen subjects participated in a blinded crossover phase. The open-label response rate was 40% (similar to the initial open-label reports), and there was a significant difference in depression rating scores between the active and sham arms of the crossover phase, strengthening the evidence that the antidepressant effect was, in fact, due to stimulation. However, the optimization period was prolonged (52 weeks) and the crossover phase was foreshortened, because 75% of subjects had to be prematurely crossed over due to increased depressive symptoms, often within 1 day of stimulation discontinuation, highlighting the relatively rapid return of depressive symptoms with discontinuation of stimulation at this target.

Intraoperative stimulation in some cases produced improved mood, decreased anxiety, and increased awareness, but also increased anxiety, sweating, speech perseveration, and facial motor effects. Outside of the operating room, two episodes of hypomania were reported in a patient with bipolar disorder, while one unipolar depression patient experienced mania, which resolved with a change in medication and stimulation parameters. During the blinded phase of the later study, irritability, suicidal ideation, hypomania, and mania were described in 1–3 active stimulation subjects but were not observed in any of the sham stimulation subjects. In the 70 subjects described in the VC/VS reports, there were nine suicide attempts (13%) and one completed suicide (1%).

### Nucleus accumbens

The NAC's central role in mediating motivation in reward is key to its appeal as a DBS target for both OCD and depression. If anhedonia is a defining symptom of depression, modulating hedonic centres makes theoretical sense. The NAC is known to be involved in reward processing and reward-seeking behaviours, as well as in drive and motivation. Dysfunctional reward processing has been described in patients with depression, as has abnormal activity of the ventral striatum. Further, the NAC connects with motor, memory, and emotion processing centres, which provides a mechanism by which NAC stimulation may produce antidepressant effects beyond the modulation of anhedonia.

A single study of 11 patients reported a 46% response rate and 30% remission rate at 1 year, with response maintained for up to 4 years [30]. Although patients reported being unable to detect when the stimulation was turned on, initial stimulation induced prompt positive behavioural changes and decreased depression scores. Side effects included erythema, anxiety, sweating, paraesthesiae, hypomania, and, in one case, psychotic symptoms. All such side effects resolved with parameter changes. At times, stimulation parameter changes were associated with acute (2 weeks), but not long term, mood improvement. Discontinuation of stimulation produced a rapid return of depressive symptoms. One suicide attempt and one completed suicide were reported.

### Medial forebrain bundle

From the experience with NAC DBS and the anhedonia/reward modulation rationale, attention turned to the MFB. The superolateral branch of the MFB (slMFB) connects the ventral tegmental area and the NAC. It crosses under the thalamus and joins the ALIC, projecting to the OFC and DLPFC. Animal and imaging studies have supported the MFB as a DBS target. In addition, hypomania that has been seen with STN stimulation for Parkinson's disease has been linked to current spread to the MFB, and electric field modelling has suggested that current spread from the SCC, VC/VS, or NAC may reach the slMFB.

In the first pilot study of seven patients given MFB DBS for TRD, six patients experienced an improvement in depressive symptoms within the first 2 days of stimulation [31]. After 1 week, four patients experienced ≥50% improvement in depression rating scores. After 12 weeks, six patients met this response criteria, four of whom additionally met criteria for remission. In most patients, response was maintained once achieved. The longest follow-up reported for these patients to date is 33 weeks. All patients had acute intraoperative effects suggestive of improved mood and engagement. At higher stimulation amplitudes, all patients experienced blurred vision and strabismus, which limited stimulation parameters. No hypomania was reported in this sample. Notably, the only non-responder in this cohort had suffered an intraoperative haemorrhage, essentially lesioning the slMFB bundle.

An early report on replicability of these findings demonstrated that 3 of 4 subjects implanted with MFB DBS showed acute intraoperative effects, as well as a 50% reduction in depression scores at 1 week [32]. At 6 months, two subjects continued to be responders. Acute intraoperative effects and visual adverse events were as described in the initial study. Long-term follow-up and randomized controlled studies are not yet reported.

### Other targets

In addition to these targets for DBS for depression, two additional regions have been targeted, each with a single case report. As described in the OCD section, one patient was successfully treated with DBS targeting the ITP. The other area targeted is the lateral habenula (LHb). The habenula is a small, midline glutamatergic structure that is well positioned to influence the brain regions implicated in depression symptoms and the neurotransmitter systems modulated by current pharmacotherapies. Convergent lines of evidence support a role for the LHb in negative reward prediction signalling, a possible role in risk-avoidant behaviours, and link LHb hyperactivity with depressed mood states [33]. The single patient implanted at this target had a complicated, but ultimately successful, treatment course.

Across targets, open-label stimulation has been shown to improve symptoms in severe and refractory depression. Failure of large-scale, double-blind trials to replicate these effects warrants consideration of alternate clinical trial designs to better account for the nature and time course of DBS treatment effect. There is clear evidence of target-specific differences in the time course of treatment and discontinuation effects. Suicide is always a concern in the treatment of TRD, but this risk is not exacerbated by DBS.

## Eating disorders

### Anorexia nervosa

Anorexia nervosa (AN) consists of persistent food restriction, an intense fear of gaining weight or behaviour that interferes with weight gain, and a disturbance in self-perceived weight or shape. Lifetime prevalence for women is estimated to be 1–4%, with a ten times greater prevalence in women than in men. It has the highest fatality rate of any psychiatric disorder, with 5.1 deaths per 1000 person-years. One in five AN deaths is from suicide [34]. It also has a high rate of comorbidity with mood and anxiety disorders—68% for MDD and 26% for OCD according to one estimate.

The first reports of DBS for AN were in patients treated for MDD or OCD. One woman treated with SCC DBS for MDD, who had comorbid AN, maintained a relatively stable body mass index (BMI) after DBS surgery, even despite depressive relapses. An increase in disordered eating was successfully treated behaviourally, and no further interventions related to weight in the 3 years of follow-up were needed. A woman with AN who received ALIC DBS for OCD reported feeling differently about food after DBS. She ate more and was less distressed about weight, caloric intake, and sweets. Her BMI after surgery and through 3 years of follow-up was in a healthy range. The authors did not report on OCD symptom improvement.

In the first case series of DBS specifically to treat AN, the SCC DBS target was chosen, based on imaging studies showing similarities in SCC activity in AN and MDD. In addition, treating mood and anxiety comorbidities in patients with AN improves outcomes over treating weight alone. Six adult women with 3–37 years of AN were treated with SCC DBS [35]. All women completed a behavioural treatment programme preoperatively to improve their weight and to be healthy enough for surgery. After 9 months of stimulation, three of six women had maintained their weight at or above their preoperative baseline. In the other half, weight had decreased to near their historical baseline. The three patients who had maintained healthier weights all had comorbid MDD, and all experienced significant improvement in MDD symptoms. These three women also had comorbid OCD, and two were OCD responders as well. Of the four total women who had a depression rating scores in the severe range, all were MDD responders. Five of the six women met criteria for OCD at baseline, of whom three were OCD responders. After 6 months of stimulation, PET imaging demonstrated decreased SCC and medial frontal activity, decreased insula activity, and increased parietal activity, similar to findings in SCC DBS for MDD.

In two Chinese samples, NAC lesions ($n = 6$) and NAC DBS ($n = 2$) were performed in adult women with a BMI of <14.5, and NAC DBS in an additional four women aged 16–17 with a BMI of <13.3. In all cases, BMI improved to 18–22, and comorbid depression, anxiety, and obsessive–compulsive symptoms improved. Weight changes tended to stabilize after 6–12 months of stimulation. No serious adverse events were reported.

### Obesity

While DBS for AN would seem a logical clinical extension of the use of DBS, given the rates of comorbid depression and OCD and the similarities in imaging findings between these illnesses, the rationale for the use of DBS for disorders of overeating comes primarily from animal models of appetite, homeostasis, and self-regulation. Lesions and high-frequency stimulation of the lateral hypothalamus (LHA) decrease food intake in animal models. Given rising obesity rates worldwide, including an estimated 6.6% of persons in the United States having a BMI of >40, it is perhaps no surprise that innovative solutions are being sought to address this epidemic.

The first individual to undergo DBS implantation specifically for obesity was reported by Hamani and colleagues in 2008 [36]. In the course of their intraoperative exploration of the hypothalamic target, they serendipitously elicited remarkable memory effects. Six months of high-frequency stimulation (130 Hz) did not result in any weight change. With low-frequency stimulation (50 Hz) over 5 months, the patient lost 12 kg, without intentional changes to diet or exercise. However, after this weight loss, the patient began to turn the stimulation off in the evenings due to a desire to eat, and he regained the weight. Following this, three patients were implanted with DBS in the LHA, with outcomes reported for up to 39 months [37]. Stimulation raised the resting metabolic rate in two patients. Chronic stimulation on optimized settings for 9–11 months resulted in a modest weight loss of 12.3% and 16.4%. The third patient did not demonstrate an altered resting metabolic rate and experienced negligible weight loss over 16 months. Experientially, patients reported that the best contact settings resulted in a decreased urge to eat, which returned when stimulation was discontinued. Acute stimulation effects included nausea, feeling hot or flushed, anxiety or panic, and increased arousal or activity. Chronic stimulation did not result in any changes in nutritional, hormonal, or neuroendocrine/neuropeptide changes. Psychological testing showed no worsening of binge eating, cognitive restraint, increased hunger, or worsening of body image or quality of life. No significant adverse events were reported over an average follow-up period of 35 months.

### Addiction

Substance use disorders (SUDs) have high prevalence and high relapse rates, despite several proven and effective treatments. In animal models of addiction, behavioural changes have been reported after stimulation of the NAC, LHb, medial prefrontal cortex, and STN. Anecdotally, STN DBS for Parkinson's disease has been described to alleviate impulsivity and behavioural manifestations of dopamine dysregulation syndrome (hypomania, gambling, hypersexuality, punding), as well as drug use [38]. Retrospective observations in patients receiving NAC DBS for Tourette syndrome describe decreased use of nicotine [39].

Despite highly developed animal models to explain the neurobiology of addictive behaviours and behaviour changes in response to stimulation in these animals, the results in human case series are less compelling. Patients selected for DBS, to date, include the most chronic and treatment-resistant patients, all of whom had prior treatment, including multiple admissions to rehabilitation programmes, agonist therapies (such as methadone), and negative reinforcement treatments such as disulfiram. In NAC DBS for opiate dependence in two patients, levomethadone dose and opiate cravings were reduced over a period of 1 year; however, concurrent use of other drugs continued, and one patient relapsed on heroin [40]. In five patients who received NAC DBS for alcohol dependence, all reported decreased craving; however, only two patients remained abstinent [41]. In a single-case report on NAC DBS for cocaine dependence [42], after 2.5 years of chronic stimulation, the patient markedly decreased cocaine use but was not abstinent. As expected, given NAC DBS effects in other disorders, in the cases described, decreased depressive symptoms and possible parameter-dependent hypomania were reported.

Persistent use of substances despite reduced cravings highlights the biggest challenge for trying to treat addiction with neuromodulation of a discrete brain target. While NAC DBS may reduce cravings, SUDs involve more complex behaviours than just reward system dysfunction, with long-standing habits and psychosocial factors that make abstinence difficult and which cannot be captured in animal models.

### Alzheimer's disease

AD is a progressive dementia marked by a gradual, but progressive, decline in memory and cognition, associated with accumulation of beta amyloid plaques and neurofibrillary tangles in the brain. The prevalence of dementia is roughly 24 million cases worldwide and rising, with approximately 70% of cases attributed to AD. The highest rates are in North America and Western Europe. Current treatments do not significantly alter disease progress.

The first series of six patients with mild AD to undergo DBS followed an unexpected intraoperative finding that stimulation near the fornix evoked vivid memories and improvement in verbal recall and spatial associative learning [36]. Based on this incidental finding in an individual without cognitive impairment, the same group performed DBS at the same fornix/hypothalamic target in six individuals with mild AD [43]. The fornix is a large white matter tract connecting the hippocampus and the medial temporal lobe. Lesions here disrupting the Papez circuit are known to produce memory deficits, underscoring its importance in memory function. Of the six patients implanted, only two had the intraoperative stimulation-related recall events demonstrated by the index case. The primary outcome measure was the cognitive subscale of the Alzheimer's Disease Assessment Scale (ADAS-cog). On average, the ADAS-cog score increased by 4.2 points after 1 year of stimulation, an indication of worsened cognition and disease progression. However, as the expected rate of decline may be closer to 6–7 points per year, this outcome may represent a slowing of expected disease progression. The absence of symptoms of hypothalamic dysfunction or serious adverse events prompted the undertaking of a larger double-blind, sham-controlled trial of 42 patients [44]. While there was comparable worsening of cognition after 1 year of active or sham stimulation, subanalysis revealed that AD patients aged <65 years receiving active stimulation had *worse* cognitive scores, compared with those receiving sham stimulation. Patients aged >65 years did appear to have some benefit from active vs sham stimulation.

A second group of six patients with mild to moderate AD underwent DBS targeting the nucleus basalis of Meynert [45]. It should be noted that the specific subregion being targeted—the Ch4 subdivision—was sometimes not able to be stimulated directly due to regional anatomy, thus demonstrating one of the challenges of DBS, that is maximizing benefit while minimizing side effects, a particular challenge in small brain areas where undesirable stimulation in nearby regions is unavoidable. Stimulation settings chosen by this group included low-frequency stimulation (20 Hz), in an effort to exert a potentially excitatory effect on target neurons and stimulate acetylcholine release. No acute stimulation effects were reported. After 11 months of stimulation, the patient group experienced an average increase of 3 points on ADAS-cog. This again indicates worsening of cognition but may represent slowing of expected disease progression. No serious adverse events were reported.

## Summary

There are unique challenges to pursuing DBS within psychiatry. Psychiatric illnesses are complex syndromes with biological and psychological drivers, currently defined categorically, without biologically informed criteria. The complexity of human behaviour cannot be reduced to a single circuit, any more than it can be reduced to a single neurotransmitter. Our current understanding of focal neuromodulation is better suited to treat specific symptoms, rather than broad diagnostic syndromes.

Unlike in DBS for Parkinson's disease, where treatment effect on motor symptoms can be fully realized almost immediately, clinical effects of stimulation on psychiatric symptoms appear to generally take weeks to months, with benefits continuing to accumulate over months to years. This time course does seem to be target-specific, with MFB DBS producing more rapid symptom improvement, but not disease-specific or procedure-specific, with similar response trajectories reported for OCD and MDD following DBS and surgical lesions. Understanding the time course of treatment response has implications for understanding the mechanism of action of DBS, as well as for timing supportive interventions such as psychotherapy.

As reviewed here, much of the experience with DBS for psychiatric disorders to date comes from individual case studies and series. Long-term studies suggest that there is good reason to be optimistic about DBS as a treatment for severe, treatment-refractory psychiatric illness; however, traditional double-blind, sham-controlled clinical trials have been disappointing. Small sample size and suboptimal control for placebo effects are frequent criticisms of DBS trials in psychiatry. Small samples exacerbate the difficulty of designing optimal dose-finding trials, as not only are there many parameters to adjust (pulse width, current, frequency), but the target itself may also have considerable inter-individual variability, precluding the use of standard co-ordinates to guide surgical targeting. One strategy to mitigate concerns about placebo effects is the use of a blinded, staggered-onset of chronic stimulation. The advantage of this approach is the ability to evaluate for a response to sham stimulation without losing statistical power by withholding the intervention entirely from a portion of the subjects. Blinded discontinuation designs similarly preserve statistical power. The other advantage of a blinded discontinuation design is that it allows for optimization of stimulation parameters to occur at the beginning of stimulation. Discontinuing stimulation only after a period of stability has been achieved strengthens the argument that a decline in response is due to the loss of stimulation. The drawbacks to this approach, however, include difficulty in disambiguating whether symptom emergence is truly a return of the illness state vs a stimulation withdrawal syndrome, and also the inability of many subjects to tolerate abrupt discontinuation in some, but not all, of the proposed targets. Reports from multiple targets, most notably the NAC and VC/VS, describe dramatic worsening of symptoms in a short time after discontinuation, including accidental discontinuation. Such symptoms can include suicidal ideation. These challenges highlight the need for thoughtful trial design that takes into account the circumstances particular to DBS as a procedure, as well as the typical patterns of response to stimulation and discontinuation at specific targets. DBS remains a promising intervention for treatment-resistant psychiatric disorders, not only due to its clinical application potential, but also because the discrete modulation of neural circuits sheds light on the underlying neurobiology of these complex illnesses.

## REFERENCES

1. de Koning PP, Figee M, van den Munckhof P, Schuurman PR, Denys D. Current status of deep brain stimulation for obsessive-compulsive disorder: a clinical review of different targets. Curr Psychiatry Rep. 2011;13:274–82.

2. Kopell BH, Greenberg BD. Anatomy and physiology of the basal ganglia: implications for DBS in psychiatry. Neurosci Biobehav Rev. 2008;32:408–22.

3. Greenberg BD, Gabriels LA, Malone DA, Jr., et al. Deep brain stimulation of the ventral internal capsule/ventral striatum for obsessive-compulsive disorder: worldwide experience. Mol Psychiatry. 2010;15:64–79.

4. Goodman WK, Foote KD, Greenberg BD, et al. Deep brain stimulation for intractable obsessive compulsive disorder: pilot study using a blinded, staggered-onset design. Biol Psychiatry. 2010;67:535–42.

5. Sturm V, Lenartz D, Koulousakis A, et al. The nucleus accumbens: a target for deep brain stimulation in obsessive-compulsive- and anxiety-disorders. J Chem Neuroanat. 2003;26:293–9.

6. Franzini A, Messina G, Gambini O, et al. Deep-brain stimulation of the nucleus accumbens in obsessive compulsive disorder: clinical, surgical and electrophysiological considerations in two consecutive patients. Neurol Sci. 2010;31:353–9.

7. Huff W, Lenartz D, Schormann M, et al. Unilateral deep brain stimulation of the nucleus accumbens in patients with treatment-resistant obsessive-compulsive disorder: Outcomes after one year. Clin Neurol Neurosurg. 2010;112:137–43.

8. Denys D, Mantione M, Figee M, et al. Deep brain stimulation of the nucleus accumbens for treatment-refractory obsessive-compulsive disorder. Arch Gen Psychiatry. 2010;67:1061–8.

9. Mantione M, Nieman DH, Figee M, Denys D. Cognitive-behavioural therapy augments the effects of deep brain stimulation in obsessive-compulsive disorder. Psychol Med. 2014;44:3515–22.

10. Coenen VA, Schlaepfer TE, Goll P, et al. The medial forebrain bundle as a target for deep brain stimulation for obsessive-compulsive disorder. CNS Spectr. 2016:1–8.

11. Mallet L, Polosan M, Jaafari N, et al. Subthalamic nucleus stimulation in severe obsessive-compulsive disorder. N Engl J Med. 2008;359:2121–34.

12. Jimenez F, Nicolini H, Lozano AM, Piedimonte F, Salin R, Velasco F. Electrical stimulation of the inferior thalamic peduncle in the treatment of major depression and obsessive compulsive disorders. World Neurosurg. 2013;80(3–4):S30 e17–25.

13. Rauch SL, Dougherty DD, Malone D, et al. A functional neuroimaging investigation of deep brain stimulation in patients with obsessive-compulsive disorder. J Neurosurg. 2006;104:558–65.

14. Oquendo MA, Currier D, Mann JJ. Prospective studies of suicidal behavior in major depressive and bipolar disorders: what is the evidence for predictive risk factors? Acta Psychiatr Scand. 2006;114:151–8.

15. Drevets WC. Neuroimaging and neuropathological studies of depression: implications for the cognitive-emotional features of mood disorders. Curr Opin Neurobiol. 2001;11:240–9.

16. Holtzheimer PE, Kelley ME, Gross RE, et al. Subcallosal cingulate deep brain stimulation for treatment-resistant unipolar and bipolar depression. Arch Gen Psychiatry. 2012;69:150–8.

17. Lozano AM, Giacobbe P, Hamani C, et al. A multicenter pilot study of subcallosal cingulate area deep brain stimulation for treatment-resistant depression. J Neurosurg. 2012;116:315–22.

18. Lozano AM, Mayberg HS, Giacobbe P, Hamani C, Craddock RC, Kennedy SH. Subcallosal cingulate gyrus deep brain stimulation for treatment-resistant depression. Biol Psychiatry. 2008;64:461–7.

19. Mayberg HS, Lozano AM, Voon V, et al. Deep brain stimulation for treatment-resistant depression. Neuron. 2005;45:651–60.

20. Merkl A, Schneider GH, Schonecker T, et al. Antidepressant effects after short-term and chronic stimulation of the subgenual cingulate gyrus in treatment-resistant depression. Exp Neurol. 2013;249:160–8.

21. Puigdemont D, Perez-Egea R, Portella MJ, et al. Deep brain stimulation of the subcallosal cingulate gyrus: further evidence in treatment-resistant major depression. Int J Neuropsychopharmacol. 2012;15:121–33.

22. Ramasubbu R, Anderson S, Haffenden A, Chavda S, Kiss ZH. Double-blind optimization of subcallosal cingulate deep brain stimulation for treatment-resistant depression: a pilot study. J Psychiatry Neurosci. 2013;38:325–32.

23. Hamani C, Mayberg H, Snyder B, Giacobbe P, Kennedy S, Lozano AM. Deep brain stimulation of the subcallosal cingulate gyrus for depression: anatomical location of active contacts in clinical responders and a suggested guideline for targeting. J Neurosurg. 2009;111:1209–15.

24. Riva-Posse P, Choi KS, Holtzheimer PE, et al. Defining critical white matter pathways mediating successful subcallosal cingulate deep brain stimulation for treatment-resistant depression. Biol Psychiatry. 2014;76:963–9.

25. Puigdemont D, Portella M, Perez-Egea R, et al. A randomized double-blind crossover trial of deep brain stimulation of the subcallosal cingulate gyrus in patients with treatment-resistant depression: a pilot study of relapse prevention. J Psychiatry Neurosci. 2015;40:224–31.

26. Choi KS, Riva-Posse P, Gross RE, Mayberg HS. Mapping the 'Depression Switch' During Intraoperative Testing of Subcallosal Cingulate Deep Brain Stimulation. JAMA Neurol. 2015;72:1252–60.

27. Malone DA, Jr., Dougherty DD, Rezai AR, et al. Deep brain stimulation of the ventral capsule/ventral striatum for treatment-resistant depression. Biol Psychiatry. 2009;65:267–75.

28. Dougherty DD, Rezai AR, Carpenter LL, et al. A Randomized Sham-Controlled Trial of Deep Brain Stimulation of the Ventral Capsule/Ventral Striatum for Chronic Treatment-Resistant Depression. Biol Psychiatry. 2015;78:240–8.

29. Bergfeld IO, Mantione M, Hoogendoorn ML, et al. Deep Brain Stimulation of the Ventral Anterior Limb of the Internal Capsule for Treatment-Resistant Depression: A Randomized Clinical Trial. JAMA Psychiatry. 2016;73:456–64.

30. Bewernick BH, Kayser S, Sturm V, Schlaepfer TE. Long-term effects of nucleus accumbens deep brain stimulation in treatment-resistant depression: evidence for sustained efficacy. Neuropsychopharmacology. 2012;37:1975–85.

31. Schlaepfer TE, Bewernick BH, Kayser S, Madler B, Coenen VA. Rapid effects of deep brain stimulation for treatment-resistant major depression. Biol Psychiatry. 2013;73:1204–12.

32. Fenoy AJ, Schulz P, Selvaraj S, *et al*. Deep brain stimulation of the medial forebrain bundle: Distinctive responses in resistant depression. J Affect Disord. 2016;203:143–51.

33. Sartorius A, Henn FA. Deep brain stimulation of the lateral habenula in treatment resistant major depression. Med Hypotheses. 2007;69:1305–8.

34. Arcelus J, Mitchell AJ, Wales J, Nielsen S. Mortality rates in patients with anorexia nervosa and other eating disorders. A meta-analysis of 36 studies. Arch Gen Psychiatry. 2011;68:724–31.

35. Lipsman N, Woodside DB, Giacobbe P, *et al*. Subcallosal cingulate deep brain stimulation for treatment-refractory anorexia nervosa: a phase 1 pilot trial. Lancet. 2013;381:1361–70.

36. Hamani C, McAndrews MP, Cohn M, *et al*. Memory enhancement induced by hypothalamic/fornix deep brain stimulation. Ann Neurol. 2008;63:119–23.

37. Whiting DM, Tomycz ND, Bailes J, *et al*. Lateral hypothalamic area deep brain stimulation for refractory obesity: a pilot study with preliminary data on safety, body weight, and energy metabolism. J Neurosurg. 2013;119:56–63.

38. Witjas T, Baunez C, Henry JM, *et al*. Addiction in Parkinson's disease: impact of subthalamic nucleus deep brain stimulation. Mov Disord. 2005;20:1052–5.

39. Kuhn J, Bauer R, Pohl S, *et al*. Observations on unaided smoking cessation after deep brain stimulation of the nucleus accumbens. Eur Addict Res. 2009;15:196–201.

40. Kuhn J, Moller M, Treppmann JF, *et al*. Deep brain stimulation of the nucleus accumbens and its usefulness in severe opioid addiction. Mol Psychiatry. 2014;19:145–6.

41. Muller UJ, Sturm V, Voges J, *et al*. Nucleus Accumbens Deep Brain Stimulation for Alcohol Addiction—Safety and Clinical Long-term Results of a Pilot Trial. Pharmacopsychiatry. 2016;49:170–3.

42. Goncalves-Ferreira A, do Couto FS, Rainha Campos A, Lucas Neto LP, Goncalves-Ferreira D, Teixeira J. Deep Brain Stimulation for Refractory Cocaine Dependence. Biol Psychiatry. 2016;79:e87–9.

43. Laxton AW, Tang-Wai DF, McAndrews MP, *et al*. A phase I trial of deep brain stimulation of memory circuits in Alzheimer's disease. Ann Neurol. 2010;68:521–34.

44. Lozano AM, Fosdick L, Chakravarty MM, *et al*. A Phase II Study of Fornix Deep Brain Stimulation in Mild Alzheimer's Disease. J Alzheimers Dis. 2016;54:777–87.

45. Kuhn J, Hardenacke K, Lenartz D, *et al*. Deep brain stimulation of the nucleus basalis of Meynert in Alzheimer's dementia. Mol Psychiatry. 2015;20:353–60.

# 20

# Adherence to treatment in psychiatry

*Amy Chan and Rob Horne*

## Adherence: a missing link in psychiatric care?

### The scale of non-adherence

Adherence to treatment is crucial for achieving optimal outcomes [1–3]. Non-adherence to medicines prescribed for mental health conditions is thought to be a common reason for poor treatment outcomes. Reviews of the prevalence of non-adherence in mental health disorders estimate that 25–60% of medicines prescribed for these conditions are not taken as advised [4–6]. Non-adherence is not, of course, unique to psychiatry. It is ubiquitous in medicine, with the WHO estimating that about half of all medicines prescribed for long-term conditions are not taken as prescribed [6]. The consequences of non-adherence are great, both for the individual, society, and the health system [7]. In psychotic disorders, such as schizophrenia, poor adherence is associated with a 3.7 times higher risk of relapse, compared to those who are adherent [8], a greater risk of hospitalization and suicide [7], and an almost three times increase in external service costs [9]. In mood disorders such as depression or bipolar disorder, the statistics are similar. Patients who discontinue their medication early have a higher risk of relapse, hospitalization, and suicide [10]—in a 1-year period, those who were non-adherent to mood stabilizers had an almost four times higher risk of hospitalization than those who were adherent [11], with associated costs being four times or more in non-adherent vs adherent individuals [12, 13].

These figures are, however, reported from published clinical studies, and we should be cautious how we interpret or extrapolate these results, as non-adherence rates and associated consequences vary widely between individuals, across different mental health conditions, and according to how adherence is defined and measured. Nevertheless, non-adherence is an issue which needs to be addressed by those providing, receiving, or funding health care. It not only entails a waste of resources, but also a missed opportunity for health gain [3]. It is the missing link between effective treatment and outcomes in psychiatric care [1, 2]. In a world where resources are limited, it is imperative that we address non-adherence if we are to bridge the gap between treatment efficacy and clinical outcome [3, 6].

Yet despite the vast amount of adherence research published in the last few decades, non-adherence remains a key challenge in clinical practice. Adherence and non-adherence have been defined in various ways, with multiple terms used to describe a similar concept [14], ranging from the traditional paternalistic view of 'compliance' with orders from health care providers to 'adherence' with an agreed plan between the patient and the health care team [6]. Currently, adherence is defined by the WHO as 'the extent to which a person's behaviour (such as taking medication) corresponds with the agreed recommendations from a healthcare provider'. More recently, this overarching concept has been refined by considering three stages of adherence: initiation, implementation, and persistence [14]. Non-adherence can occur at each of these stages. The patient may not initiate treatment (termed primary non-adherence), or they may fail to take the prescribed regimen correctly—where the medication is not taken at the right time, dose, or frequency, or the treatment may be discontinued prematurely (non-persistence). Non-adherence may be used as an umbrella term for each of these specific behaviours [15]. Recent research in schizophrenia seems to suggest that not only is adherence important per se, but the *pattern* of non-adherence may also be significant—different patterns of medication-taking have been associated with different outcomes [2, 16].

Achieving true adherence, where the patient and the provider *agree* to a particular treatment plan, is challenging in psychiatry, as there are unique mitigating factors such as mental health legislation, stigma, discrimination, social isolation, lack of insight, comorbid substance abuse, and cognitive impairment to consider [7, 17].

### Challenges in psychiatry

Although non-adherence is common to all health conditions where long-term adherence is key to outcomes, there are unique challenges in psychiatry. Firstly, patients commonly do not perceive themselves to be ill. The WHO International Pilot Study on Schizophrenia found that lack of insight occurred in 98% of patients and was the most common symptom of schizophrenia [18]. This is similar in patients with bipolar disorder [19]. This lack of illness insight affects not only adherence, but also engagement with health services in general [20, 21]. People who do not perceive themselves to be unwell fail to recognize the need for treatment and care, and as such, poor insight has frequently been associated with non-adherence [8, 20]. Many treatment benefits in psychiatry are silent and long-term, which further reinforces the lack of insight. The 'no symptoms, no problem' view of health is intuitive; thus, adherence is particularly challenging when there is minimal insight and understanding of the illness [20, 21]. Moreover, non-adherence may not lead to an immediate deterioration—relapses may not occur for months, or even years, after stopping medication [21]. Likewise, treatment benefits are often delayed—drugs for depression or psychosis usually take 4–6 weeks before a perceivable benefit is attained. Together, these factors reinforce the perception that medication may not be necessary. As such, early discontinuation of medication is a common manifestation of non-adherence in psychiatry [21], as treatment is stopped when patients judge that the condition has improved.

Secondly, even when patients do gain illness insight, they may not have the capacity to adhere to treatment [2]. This may be due to cognitive impairment that can accompany mental health disorders, the illness itself, or their psychosocial circumstances, which make establishing a regular medication-taking routine or affording long-term medication difficult [2, 22]. Comorbid intellectual disability or substance misuse are other important factors to consider in psychiatry which can influence treatment adherence [20].

Shared decision-making and therapeutic alliance between the clinician and the patient have been shown to be important mediators of adherence—adherence is likely to be higher when there is a positive, trusting clinician–patient relationship [20, 23]. However, this can be difficult to achieve in psychiatry when treatment is started in a compulsory treatment setting and when there is mental health legislation governing this process [24]. In a survey of 104 individuals with schizophrenia, over one-third reported fear of coerced treatment as a barrier to seeking treatment; the use of reminders or warnings about the consequences of non-adherence were perceived negatively as pressures to adhere and were reported as increasing barriers to treatment [25]. Lastly, stigma associated with mental health conditions has consistently been shown to be an adherence barrier [22]. This is common across all mental health conditions, with patient perceptions of stigma influencing treatment behaviours and adherence negatively [26]. These unique challenges need to be considered if we are to promote adherence in psychiatry.

## Interventions to improve adherence in psychiatry: what lessons can be learnt from trials of adherence support?

### What interventions are effective? A review of 20 years of adherence research

Although the problem of non-adherence is well recognized globally, there continues to be no effective solution [27]. A vast amount of research have examined the reasons for non-adherence, and many adherence interventions have been tested in RCTs; yet a sustainable and effective solution remains elusive. In the most recent Cochrane review of adherence interventions, 182 published RCTs were included [27], of which 29 were on psychiatric disorders—primarily in schizophrenia and related psychotic disorders, followed by depression. The quality of these RCTs were low; of these 29 RCTs, only one [28] was considered to have a low risk of bias. Even when all studies are taken into account, the effects of these interventions on adherence are mixed and non-consistent.

There is a general lack of convincing evidence to support one particular intervention over another; where one type of intervention demonstrates positive effects on adherence, the same intervention in a similar population will report negative results. For example, compliance or adherence therapy—a cognitive behavioural intervention using techniques from motivational interviewing to discuss adherence—was reported to improve adherence in patients with psychosis in two studies [29, 30] but failed to demonstrate any effect in two other studies [31, 32]. The wide variability of studies, in terms of study populations, conditions, setting, intervention design, and adherence and outcome measurement, make it difficult to draw comparisons between the different types of interventions. Even when effects are seen on adherence, the benefits are relatively small and effects on clinical outcomes frequently not assessed. Questions on the sustainability and feasibility of implementation into practice also remain. Many of the psychiatric adherence interventions tested are typically very complex—involving multiple resources and intensive follow-up—something that may not be able to be delivered in a real-world clinical setting. Furthermore, details on the actual content and delivery of the interventions are commonly not described in sufficient detail to replicate in practice. These limitations that currently exist with adherence intervention literature make it difficult to design effective interventions in practice; there is a need for more innovative approaches to adherence.

### Lessons learnt from research—there is no 'one size fits all' for adherence interventions

Adherence interventions which have been tested in psychiatry include adherence therapy, education, telemedicine, shared decision-making, family therapy, and pharmacist-led education or medicines management [27]. As the literature highlights, interventions and outcomes are varied and many different approaches have been tried to address non-adherence. There are learnings that can be gained from these 20 years of adherence intervention research. Although there is no evidence to support one particular intervention over another, interventions which have been successful in improving adherence usually consist of: (1) multiple components; (2) ongoing support tailored to address barriers to adherence; and (3) delivery by health care professionals, with additional support from the family or peers [33–36]. Clues can also be provided from adherence studies that investigate relationships between particular patient or illness factors and adherence; although such findings provide little information on how to design effective interventions, they can be useful to help identify groups at risk of non-adherence. For example, patients who lack a support system or have comorbid substance abuse are at a higher risk of non-adherence [20, 21]. This can help target and prioritize adherence interventions to people who need it the most, particularly in limited-resource settings.

However, to design effective interventions on an individual level in practice, one must look beyond population studies and focus on the individual. Study findings may not be easily extrapolated to daily practice. An intervention that may be successful within a particular study population may not be effective for a particular patient. Although some interventions have been able to improve medication adherence, the exact components of the interventions which contributed to its effectiveness are often not known [27]. The lack of detailed, consistent reporting and measurement makes it difficult to draw definitive conclusions to apply in practice. Previous reviews of interventions to improve adherence to psychotropic medicines echo these findings [33–35]. As Kane *et al.* describes—the idea of a 'standardized, universally valid and reliable' approach to promoting adherence is a myth—individualized interventions tailored to the individual are likely needed to improve adherence [21].

## Non-adherence: towards behaviourally intelligent solutions

### Adherence is a behaviour, not a trait

With the vast amount of adherence research, it might seem a wonder why non-adherence still exists. Yet the problem might lie in the approach that has been taken in the past when investigating non-adherence—the limitations of this approach have been discussed previously in Section 2. Prior to the 1970s, much of the research focused on the notion of the 'non-adherent patient'—where attempts to explain non-adherence used 'easily identified and quantifiable dimensions' such as patient, regimen, or illness characteristics [37]. Yet the 'non-adherent patient' is a myth, as most of us are non-adherent some of the time [15]. Associations observed between sociodemographic variables, such as gender and age, and adherence are neither clear nor consistent [15].

Non-adherence is therefore best understood as a variable behaviour, rather than a trait characteristic. For example, studies have reported ethnicity to be a significant predictor of antipsychotic medication non-adherence [38, 39]; yet other literature reports that ethnicity is not a consistent predictor [20]. Likewise, various personality traits have been linked with non-adherence. Extraversion was significantly associated with non-adherence in one study [40], but not another [41]. While understanding some of these factors is important, focusing on sociodemographic factors alone will not fix non-adherence. This is because non-adherence is a feature of the way the individual interacts with their treatment, rather than any particular characteristic of the patient themselves. Non-adherence varies not only between individuals, but even within the same individual over time. Non-adherence does not arise from irrational or misguided behaviour—more often than not, the patient goes through a knowledge process and the way they act come from the attitudes they develop about their condition and medicines, and their personal health experiences [21].

Indeed, patient attitudes, illness perceptions, and health beliefs have been demonstrated to be one of the strongest predictors of adherence [42–44]. Beck *et al.* investigated factors influencing adherence in patients with schizophrenia or schizoaffective disorder and found that patients who viewed antipsychotics as necessary for their treatment had higher adherence; conversely, those who had negative attitudes about medicines in general and were concerned about antipsychotics had poor adherence [43]. The authors called for adherence interventions to focus on treatment attitudes, rather than general education about the illness. These findings make sense when adherence is viewed as a health behaviour—attitudes and beliefs are more likely to be important mediators of behaviour. Adherence interventions should therefore focus on behaviour change principles and techniques. New strategies need to build on this concept of adherence as a health behaviour to allow effective interventions to be developed. Learnings from years of research show that there is no 'adherent personality type' and a 'one size fits all' adherence intervention. There is a need to develop more effective ways of tailoring support to meet the needs of individuals if we are to improve adherence in a sustainable fashion.

### Adherence is a product of motivation and ability

In order to tackle this large-scale problem of non-adherence, it is important to understand why non-adherence occurs from an individual patient perspective. Firstly, non-adherence may be intentional (for example, when we decide not to take the treatment or to take it in a way which differs from the recommendations) and/or unintentional (for example, when we want to follow the recommendations but lack the capability or opportunity to do so). The easiest way to think of this is to consider adherence behaviour as being two-pronged—patients do not adhere to treatment because: either (1) they *do not want to* or (2) they *are not able to*. How non-adherence arises therefore relates to two components which drive the behaviour, respectively—*motivation* and *ability* [15]. This ability, in turn, is affected by the individual's *environment*—both internal factors (for example, knowledge and physical capability to take the medication on time) and external factors (for example, aspects of our environment affecting access to treatment such as not having easy access to a pharmacy) [15, 45].

This forms the basis of the Perceptions and Practicalities Approach (PaPA) to supporting optimal adherence [15], which has been applied to designing interventions in psychiatric disorders [2] and in the National Institute for Health and Care Excellence (NICE) medicines adherence guidelines [46].

### Perceptual or practical barriers to adherence: a Perceptions and Practicalities Approach to designing patient-centred adherence interventions

The PaPA approach to adherence support derives from an analysis of the types of reasons why people do not take their medicines (Fig. 20.1). Recognizing that adherence is a product of motivation and ability, PaPA stipulates that adherence interventions should address both perceptual factors (for example, beliefs about the illness and treatment) as well as practical factors (for example, the ability to remember the medicine, establish a daily routine, and organize or pay for medication supply) [46]. Adherence support should be tailored to the needs of the individual using a menu-based approach where specific intervention components are selected to address specific perceptual and/or practical barriers. The approach also takes account of the social and environmental factors that provide the context around the interaction of the patient with the treatment [15] (Fig. 20.1). The importance of external factors (for example, social and environmental factors) is described in Michie *et al.*'s COM-B conceptual framework for key determinants of behaviour [47]. COM-B describes three components—Capability, Opportunity, and Motivation—which act together to influence behaviour. Capability and opportunity reflect a person's ability; opportunity can also comprise the external factors that make the behaviour possible or prompt it, and thus relates to how environmental and social factors might influence adherence. Together, these relate similarly to the motivation–ability paradigm described previously.

Based on PaPA, adherence support targeted at the level of the individual should be tailored to address the specific perceptions (for

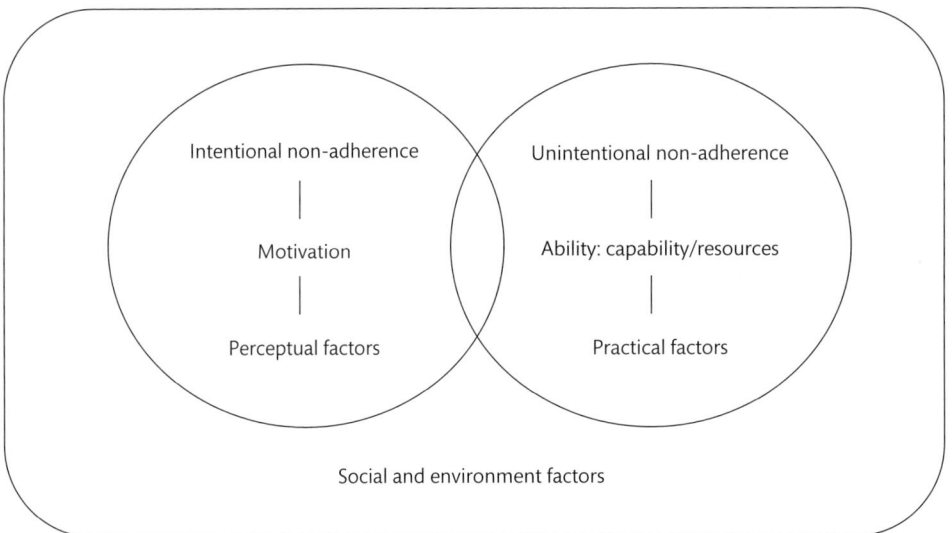

**Fig. 20.1** Figure depicting the interaction between perceptual and practical factors on adherence behaviour.
Reproduced from Horne R, Weinman J, Barber N, *et al., Concordance, adherence and compliance in medicine taking: Report for the National Co-ordinating Centre for NHS Service Delivery and Organisation R & D (NCCSDO),* Copyright (2005), with permission from National Institute of Health Research.

example, beliefs and emotions) and practicalities (for example, capability and resources) influencing a person's motivation and ability to adhere, respectively [15, 46]. As shown in Fig. 20.1, perceptions and practicalities can overlap. For example, motivation may help the individual overcome limitations in capability and opportunity, which might, in turn, influence motivation—hence, the model is depicted as a Venn diagram, rather than two discrete circles (Fig. 20.1).

Adherence is a complex behaviour with multiple determinants—both internal and external (see Fig. 20.2 for a summary). The 'internal' factors influencing motivation and ability may be moderated by 'external' variables, such as the quality of communication between the patient and the health care provider [23], and by the wider societal contexts such as access to treatment and mental health legislation [24].

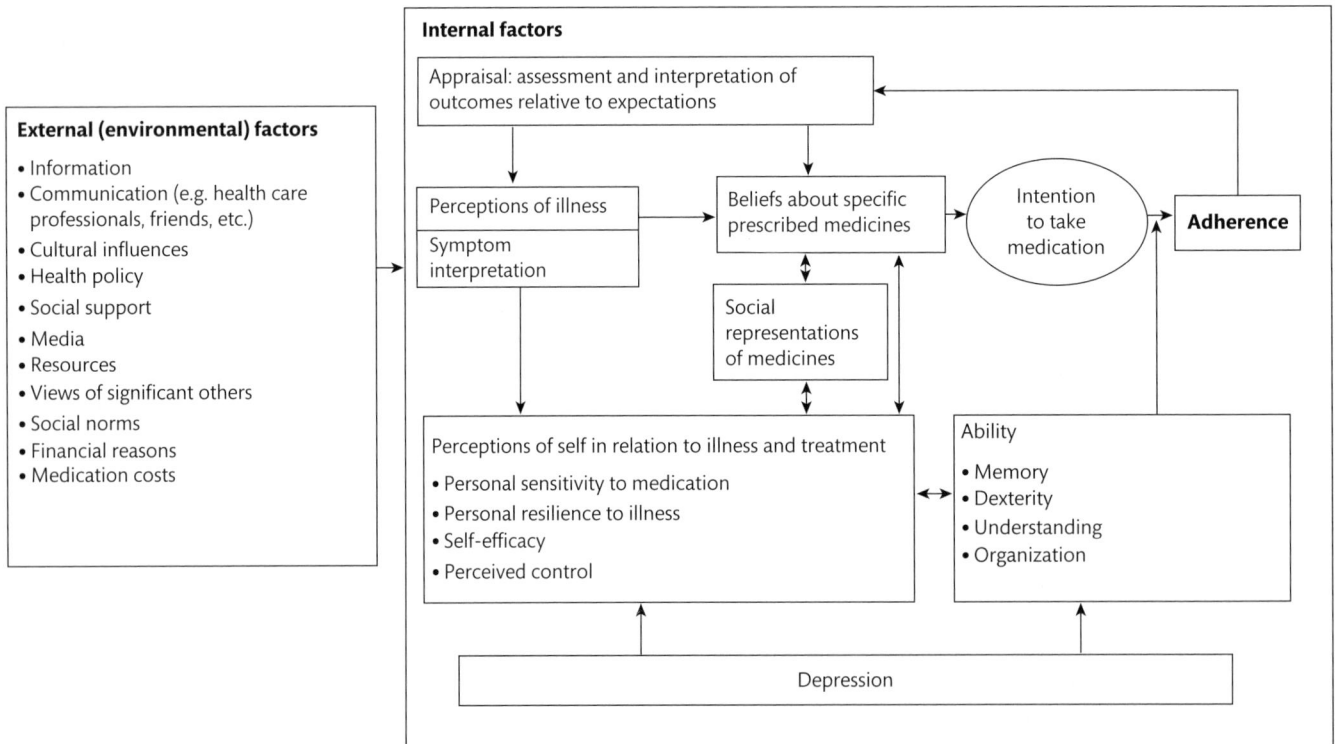

**Fig. 20.2** Conceptual map of determinants of adherence.
Reproduced from Horne R, Weinman J, Barber N, *et al., Concordance, adherence and compliance in medicine taking: Report for the National Co-ordinating Centre for NHS Service Delivery and Organisation R & D (NCCSDO),* Copyright (2005), with permission from National Institute of Health Research.

When considering adherence interventions, various aspects of this adherence behaviour can be targeted. Motivation and ability can be considered separately to help design adherence interventions, based on what factor or factors are driving the behaviour. For example, interventions to improve a patient's *ability* to adhere (such as improving access to treatment) will fail if the patient does not *want* to take the medication (such as when the patient has already decided against the treatment). Understanding what drives a patient's decision to adhere or not to adhere is key to addressing non-adherence.

The following sections explore these two drivers of non-adherence—perceptions and practicalities—in greater detail.

## Perceptions: the role of general and specific beliefs about medication in influencing decisions about treatment

Beliefs about medicines can have a significant impact on adherence—simply providing information is often insufficient to achieve adherence to psychotropic medication [21, 35]. The literature on the effects of education and information provision on adherence shows that giving information about treatment benefits and harms may not impact on decisions to start and continue medication, even though knowledge is increased [48]. One study investigating adherence to tricyclic drugs found that giving treatment leaflets to patients alone, with no counselling, had no effect on adherence [49]; this is supported by a later systematic review which found education interventions demonstrated no clear benefit on adherence and depression outcomes [33]—an association also seen in other psychiatric conditions [43, 50]. Although the quality of the studies do not allow definitive conclusions, together these suggest that information provision and increasing knowledge alone do not overcome non-adherence [15].

Qualitative studies show that many people seem to hold prototypic beliefs about medicines and their capacity to produce harm, as well as benefit, and beliefs about the appropriateness of doctors' prescribing of medicines [51, 52]. These beliefs exist even before a person takes the medication. A review of knowledge and beliefs held by members of the public about psychotropics found that views were generally very negative; this contrasted with positive views about medication for physical disorders [53]. Many were concerned about dependence, lethargy, and brain damage [52, 53], perceiving psychotropics as harmful, addictive substances that should not be taken for long periods of time but tend to be overprescribed by doctors [51].

These beliefs can influence how information is interpreted by patients, what their experiences are, and how they act as a result of this information [15, 53, 54]. Indeed, negative attitudes and beliefs towards medicines used in psychiatry appear to be stronger predictors of non-adherence than demographic or psychosocial factors [20, 42–44]. These attitudes are linked to wider concerns about scientific medicine, a lack of trust in doctors, and an increasing interest in alternative or complementary health care [51, 53]. People also seem to vary in their perceptions of personal sensitivity to medicines [55], with some being more concerned than others about their response to medication.

These *general* beliefs influence the way in which people evaluate a *specific* medication prescribed for a particular condition [51]. These beliefs can affect a person's initial expectations of the outcome of taking a medication, as well as how any subsequent events are interpreted—for example, whether symptoms experienced are attributed to the illness or the medication [56]. These beliefs may even influence the clinical outcome directly via the 'placebo/nocebo' effects of active drugs—terms describing the phenomenon of having beneficial or harmful effects occur when people have positive or negative expectations about the medication, respectively [57]. Beliefs can also be *specific* for a particular medication—for example, concerns around weight gain and extra-pyramidal side effects with dopamine antagonists [21, 58] have been linked with poorer adherence.

## Perceptions: the role of perceived necessity and concerns in influencing decisions about treatment

Once a person has started a new medication, they will begin to form particular beliefs and attitudes towards the treatment, based on their initial and subsequent evaluation of the medication. This evaluation process is captured by the Necessity–Concerns Framework [51]. The framework suggests that the motivation to start and persist with treatment is influenced by the way the individual judges their personal *need* for the treatment, relative to their *concerns* about potential adverse effects. For example, a 2-year prospective study of 254 patients recovering from first-episode psychosis found that the risks of non-adherence was 1.75 times higher in those whose belief in the need for treatment was less, and 2.88 times higher in those who thought medication was of low benefit [59]. Similarly, in a study of 223 individuals prescribed medication for bipolar disorder, the odds of having poor adherence was twice as high in those who had stronger concerns about the negative effects of medication than those who did not—a finding that was independent of mood state, illness, and demographic characteristics [44]. Other studies involving patients from a wide range of other conditions have consistently found similar results—that poor adherence is related to doubts about personal need for medication and concerns about potential adverse effects [60].

Perceived necessity of a treatment is, however, not related to beliefs about treatment efficacy. Although views about medication efficacy are likely to contribute to perceived need, the two are not synonymous. For example, perceived necessity can be influenced by illness beliefs—a patient might believe that a treatment is effective but may not perceive a personal *need* for the treatment. A common situation where this might occur is when the patient lacks illness insight. In this case, the patient may not believe they need any treatment, regardless of its perceived efficacy. Beck *et al.* explored the beliefs about drugs for psychosis in 150 outpatients and found that patients who were aware of their illness were more likely to adhere due to a greater perceived necessity of the treatment [43]. Conversely, a patient might perceive a strong need for a treatment, even though they believe it is only moderately effective—for example, if it is the only treatment that is available or acceptable to the patient. This may be seen with 'natural' remedies such as vitamins or herbs [53] where the patient may express a strong need to take these, instead of the prescribed medicine, despite believing these are only moderately effective.

In terms of perceived concerns, there is much overlap in the type of concerns that patients report about medicines, regardless of the medication type. The experience of symptoms as medication 'side effects' and the disruptive effects of medication on daily living and quality of life are commonly reported concerns [56, 61]. Many patients receiving regular medication who have not experienced adverse effects worry about possible problems in the future—a view that may be related to beliefs that regular medication use can lead to dependence or accumulation within the body and corresponding long-term effects [51, 53]. Concerns also relate to the meaning that being on regular medication has for the individual and their sense of self or identity. Taking a daily treatment may be an unwelcome reminder of their illness, which may have a negative impact on how they view themselves or perceive how they are seen by others. This can be further exacerbated by the stigma associated with taking mental health medication itself [22]. In these circumstances, non-adherence might be seen as an implicit strategy to minimize the impact on their sense of self [62].

These necessity beliefs and concerns can influence adherence separately and in combination, and the effects may be through explicit and implicit processes. For example, in some situations, non-adherence could be part of a deliberate strategy to minimize harm by taking less medication. Alternatively, it might simply reflect the fact that patients who do not perceive their medication to be important are more likely to forget to take it. The impact of perceptions of treatment on adherence may also influenced by beliefs about adherence behaviour itself such as whether or not strict adherence to medication is needed to achieve the desired outcome.

### Practicalities: enhancing capability and opportunity for adherence

Beyond addressing patient perceptions is the need to address factors that determine a patient's *ability* to adhere. Forgetting is the most commonly reported practical reason for medication non-adherence [63]. This may be due to the cognitive effects associated with mental health disorders, as well as a lack of routine and an erratic lifestyle [21]. Reminder systems or medication organizers, such as pill boxes, may be useful, though reported effects are typically modest [64]. Linking medication-taking to specific environmental cues may be more effective than a repeated reminder to help reinforce habits and routine. For example, placing the medication near the toothbrush, so that taking the medication becomes linked to an existing habit, may be useful. However, this is susceptible to changes in the environment or routine such as going on holiday [65].

Linking medication-taking to specific environmental cues may also be useful [66]. This involves planning with the patient how and when they are able to take their medication. Turning a patient's intention to take medication (for example, 'I will take my medicine') into a more specific plan (for example, 'I will take my medicine immediately after I brush my teeth every morning') increases the likelihood of the behaviour being performed [66].

Simplifying the regimen and reducing unnecessary polypharmacy is also important. Complex regimens with a high dosing frequency or complicated instructions for medication-taking can lead to poor adherence [67]. Reducing the dosing frequency to once daily can improve the patient's ability to adhere by making the treatment less intrusive and more convenient. The use of long-acting injections may also promote adherence through this mechanism and reduce the chances of forgetting treatment [68], though patients may have negative perceptions of long-acting injections as these are frequently associated with coercive treatment [69]. Strategies to improve adherence by changing formulation or dosing are therefore likely to be effective only if perceptual barriers to adherence have been addressed [43]. Involving patients in treatment decisions is important to achieve ongoing adherence—patients who were prescribed at least one medication that had been requested by the patient in a psychiatric advance directive had higher adherence at 12 months—with the odds of adhering being 7.8 times higher—than those who did not receive medications as per their advance directive [70]. To achieve adherence, the clinician must therefore aim to elicit the patient's perspective about treatment—including their beliefs and concerns—and ensure that decisions about treatment are informed by fact, rather than misperceptions [17]. Offering a medication choice can be an effective method of involving the patient in prescribing decisions—even as simple as involving the patient in the choice of dosage form can be useful [17, 70]. Medication cost and access to health services and medication may be other factors to consider when addressing practical barriers to adherence [17].

## So . . . you took all your medicines? Methods of assessing adherence

Measuring non-adherence is a complex issue. While self-report is the most practical and convenient method in clinical practice to assess adherence, reports are subjective and often inaccurate. Patients often overestimate adherence [71], yet objective measures have their own shortcomings (Table 20.1). There is a need to remove the negativity surrounding medication non-adherence to encourage honest, non-judgemental communication between the patient and the health care provider. In clinical practice, 'detoxifying' non-adherence and allowing sufficient time in the consultation to discuss barriers to treatment are necessary first steps to improve the assessment of adherence [17, 46]. This may be facilitated by opening up discussions about adherence in a non-judgemental way and explaining the reasons for the discussion. It is helpful to focus the discussions on a specific time period such as 'in the past week' and asking about specific medication-taking behaviours such as skipping or changing the dose or stopping medication [46]. Patients should be encouraged to discuss freely their adherence behaviours and barriers in clinical practice—objective adherence measurement will become less of an issue when this occurs. Until then, however, there remains great interest in measurement, and multiple methods to assess adherence exist (Table 20.1).

## PaPA—a 3-step process towards effective adherence interventions: tailoring support to individual needs

### Informed adherence in practice

Shared decision-marking with the patient and informed choice should be a key facet of clinical practice and adherence. For interventions to be effective, equitable, and efficient, one must facilitate informed choice [15]. A patient can be considered to have made an informed choice if they can demonstrate knowledge of relevant information about the treatment and then act according to their beliefs. This concept of informed choice has been extended to *informed adherence* [72] where evidence-based medicine is used to guide initial treatment recommendations. The recommendations should be presented to patients in a way that takes account of their individual beliefs and preferences, and any incompatibilities between their

**Table 20.1** Summary of adherence measurement methods

**Direct methods**

Direct methods provide evidence that the patient has actually taken the medication and are therefore the most accurate [77].

| Method | Description | Advantages | Disadvantages |
|---|---|---|---|
| Detection of the drug or metabolite in biological fluids | Laboratory testing of drug levels in bodily fluids | Levels are easily quantifiable<br>Can provide data on dose–response | Invasive<br>Low patient acceptability<br>Tests can be costly<br>Time-consuming<br>Difficult to interpret<br>Can only be used if a blood level test exists for the medicine<br>Can exhibit large inter- and intra-patient variability<br>Sampling times need to be accurate<br>Does not provide information on adherence patterns |
| Detection of adjunct biological markers | An additional readily detectable, but inert, stable, and non-toxic, substance is added to the ingested medication, either directly into the drug formulation or taken as an adjunct to therapy | Levels are easily quantifiable<br>Can provide data on dose–response | Not relevant to medicines used in psychiatry, as no biological marker exists<br>Similar disadvantages to detection of drug in biological fluids |
| Direct observation of patient ingestion of treatment | Patient is observed while they take the dose in front of another person, either a health care provider or a family member | Provides direct proof of medication ingestion<br>Allows direct interaction with the patient, which can reveal other aspects of their lifestyle and environment which affect their adherence | Intrusive<br>Resource-intensive as requires repeated health care provider visits<br>Susceptible to patient manipulation (for example, patient can hide medication in the mouth and feign ingestion) |

**Indirect methods**

The majority of adherence measures used are indirect, which measure adherence using patient- or third-party-generated information. These methods are unable to determine whether or not actual medication-taking occurred but are generally more acceptable to patients due to their non-invasive nature.

| Method | Description | Advantages | Disadvantages |
|---|---|---|---|
| Patient self-report | Patient reports on their own adherence behaviour through patient interviews, diary cards, journals, calendars, surveys, or validated adherence questionnaires and rating scales | Simple<br>Cost-effective<br>Convenient<br>Most common method used in the literature and in practice<br>Does not require any extra planning or resources<br>High patient acceptability<br>Easy to use<br>Can provide detailed information on adherence patterns and patient awareness of behaviour if obtained from diaries, journals, or interviews<br>Encourages active patient involvement<br>Facilitates provider–patient discussions | Lack of objectivity—high risk of inaccurate reports of adherence<br>Often overestimates adherence due to patient's desire to be viewed positively by others<br>Risk of recall bias, especially if data reported retrospectively<br>Relies on accuracy of patient records/reports<br>Dependent on patient's ability and willingness to disclose information<br>Patient responses can be affected by how questions are asked and relationship with interviewer |
| Medication counts | Physical count of the number of doses that remain in a patient's medicine bottle, delivery device, or other medication management system, after a pre-determined period of monitoring, and compares this with the expected number of doses that would remain if the patient had taken the medicine exactly as prescribed | Commonly used alternative to self-report<br>Simple, economical<br>Enables medication use to be monitored without the patient<br>Been shown to be more accurate than self-report and prescription refill data, being aware of the parameter being measured<br>Allows some detection of changes in adherence, depending on frequency of counts | Lack of detailed information on the patterns of usage over time<br>Wide variation in accuracy—patients may combine multiple refills in same container, use multiple containers, or share medication with others<br>Difficult to determine the dates of treatment period<br>Need for patients to return medication containers or canisters<br>Patients may suspect adherence is being monitored |
| Prescription refill records | Electronic records of prescription claims made by a pharmacy or a manual process of prescription review | Objective data<br>Easily accessible<br>Readily available in most cases<br>Reduces risk of patients being aware of monitoring<br>Allows large-scale population analyses<br>Enables ease of patient follow-up<br>Can determine trends over prolonged periods | No standard method of data interpretation and analysis<br>Data availability may be delayed<br>Only a proxy measure—dispensed medicines may not be picked up or taken as prescribed<br>Patients may use more than one pharmacy |

(continued)

**Table 20.1**  Continued

| Method | Description | Advantages | Disadvantages |
|---|---|---|---|
| Electronic adherence monitoring | Use of electronic monitoring devices to record medication use through monitoring of the opening of medication bottles, dispensing of drops, or depression of canisters for inhaled medication | Considered as the 'gold standard' of adherence measurement<br>Objective<br>Not reliant on patient self-interpretation<br>Accurate—non-biased data<br>Reliable<br>Less prone to patient deception<br>Provides detailed information about medication taken<br>Allows adherence patterns to be monitored | Inaccurate data recordings or data loss can arise due to device malfunction<br>Devices can be lost or damaged<br>May require patient and practitioner training<br>No confirmation of ingestion<br>Presence of device may change patient behaviour<br>Costly<br>Ethical considerations with monitoring of behaviour<br>Patients may suspect monitoring |

personal beliefs and the prevailing evidence should be resolved by non-judgemental discussion [54].

One approach to achieving informed adherence is to consider the following 'PaPA-based approach to adherence support' in any consultation about treatment:

1. *Facilitate an honest and open discussion.* The discussion should aim to normalize non-adherence and allow patients to report non-adherence and express doubts and concerns. This allows assessment of adherence in a non-judgemental way. Effective communication is important. Factors such as mental state, health literacy, language barriers or visual or hearing impairment may need to be considered to ensure effective communication.

2. *Communicate the **necessity** of treatment.* In psychiatry, many patients do not believe treatment is necessary, as they do not perceive themselves to be ill. Discuss with the patient what their understanding is of the reason for treatment. Explain the condition and how the treatment will influence this, considering the aims of the treatment and what the patient themselves hope to achieve. Focus on how the patient may benefit from the treatment, taking into account the individual motivations the patient may have, which may not be directly related to the illness.

3. *Elicit and address any **concerns** raised about the treatment.* Use open-ended questions to encourage patients to discuss and ask about their condition and treatment. Find out what the patient knows, believes, and understands about their treatment before starting or changing a medicine. Often these concerns centre on dependency and side effects of weight gain and lethargy and how this will affect their daily lives. Discuss and agree a plan of action to manage these concerns with the patient.

4. *Minimize any **practical barriers** to adherence.* It is helpful to discuss how the patient will fit the medication into their daily routine and remember to take the medication. Identify any barriers, and agree a plan of action with the patient.

This approach ensures that both the perceptual barriers (necessity/concern beliefs) and practical barriers are addressed. Previous interventions have had limited effects, partly because either they have not addressed all these factors or the intervention has not been individualized to the patient. Many have focused on single causal factors, whereas adherence is best seen as a complex health behaviour with multiple determinants—both internal and external (see Fig. 20.2 for a summary). By using this approach, interventions can be tailored to the individual while achieving informed adherence.

## Practical considerations in intervention design

When designing and implementing adherence interventions in practice, three dimensions of the intervention need to be optimized for success. This can be remembered as the '3 components to behaviour change' or '3CBC'—content, channel (delivery vehicle), and context.

### Content

This is the basic substance of the intervention and how the specific barriers and enablers of adherence are addressed. Approaches should be tailored to address both the perceptual factors influencing motivation to initiate and persist with treatment, as well as facilitate the ability to adhere, for example by addressing any capacity and resource limitations. The PaPA model described is one method that can be used to ensure all aspects of adherence are addressed.

### Channel

Adherence support should occur, not just at the start of treatment, but also during treatment review, as perceptions, abilities, and adherence can change. For psychiatric disorders, support should extend beyond the prescribing consultation to ongoing medication counselling and review. The increasing use of e-technology (such as smartphone apps) offers the prospect of additional channels to complement practitioner-delivered support [73]. However, despite the plethora of technology and digital solutions available, there is, as yet, little evidence for their efficacy. A recent systematic review found mobile and electronic interventions to be feasible and acceptable in patients with serious mental illness; however, effects on adherence and outcomes are yet to be determined [74]. Applying these principles to develop theory-based content might improve their effectiveness and utility.

### Context

Context considers how appropriate prescribing and adherence support is facilitated by wider contextual factors, such as media representations of treatment and ease of access to treatment. Examples of such strategies include allocating appointments to patients with minimal delay and ensuring medicines are readily accessible and affordable [17]. Organisational and service delivery issues may also impinge on the opportunity to access treatment and support services [75]. The impact of community treatment orders is another contextual factor to consider, particularly as these are widely used in many countries yet the benefits of these on adherence and outcomes remain controversial [76].

## Conclusions

Medication non-adherence is an age-old problem that has existed since the time of Hippocrates; yet it remains a significant problem facing psychiatry today, leading to many lost years of health and livelihood. Despite decades of research, advances made have had limited effect on addressing this issue. The new approach taken in the last few decades where medication adherence is understood as a variable behaviour, rather than a trait characteristic, has shown great potential in paving the way towards an effective intervention. An individualized approach, where each person's unique beliefs, capability, and motivation are taken into account, should be the foundation of every adherence intervention undertaken today. Adherence is everybody's issue—we must endeavour to address this in our everyday practice with every patient we meet. Every small step we take towards targeting this complex behaviour is one step closer to building the missing link between psychiatric treatment and outcome. Only then can we begin to see the gains from the medical advances that our predecessors have achieved many years and decades ago.

## REFERENCES

1. Ascher-Svanum H, Faries DE, Zhu B, Ernst FR, Swartz MS, Swanson JW. Medication adherence and long-term functional outcomes in the treatment of schizophrenia in usual care. Journal of Clinical Psychiatry. 2006;67:453–60.
2. Chapman SCE, Horne R. Medication nonadherence and psychiatry. Current Opinion in Psychiatry. 2013;26:446–52.
3. DiMatteo MR, Giordani PJ, Lepper HS, Croghan TW. Patient adherence and medical treatment outcomes: a meta-analysis. Medical Care. 2002;40:794–811.
4. Nose M, Barbui C, Tansella M. How often do patients with psychosis fail to adhere to treatment programmes? A systematic review. Psychological Medicine. 2003;33:1149–60.
5. Lingam R, Scott J. Treatment non-adherence in affective disorders. Acta Psychiatrica Scandinavica. 2002;105:164–72.
6. Sabaté E. Adherence to long-term therapies: evidence for action. World Health Organization, Geneva; 2003.
7. Higashi K, Medic G, Littlewood KJ, Diez T, Granström O, De Hert M. Medication adherence in schizophrenia: factors influencing adherence and consequences of nonadherence, a systematic literature review. Therapeutic Advances in Psychopharmacology. 2013;3:200–18.
8. Fenton WS, Blyler CR, Heinssen RK. Determinants of medication compliance in schizophrenia: Empirical and clinical findings. Schizophrenia Bulletin. 1997;23:637–51.
9. Knapp M, King D, Pugner K, Lapuerta P. Non-adherence to antipsychotic medication regimens: associations with resource use and costs. British Journal of Psychiatry. 2004;184:509–16.
10. Pompili M, Serafini G, Del Casale A, et al. Improving adherence in mood disorders: the struggle against relapse, recurrence and suicide risk. Expert Review of Neurotherapeutics. 2009;9:985–1004.
11. Scott J, Pope M. Self-reported adherence to treatment with mood stabilizers, plasma levels, and psychiatric hospitalization. American Journal of Psychiatry. 2002;159:1927–9.
12. Svarstad BL, Shireman TI, Sweeney JK. Using drug claims data to assess the relationship of medication adherence with hospitalization and costs. Psychiatric Services (Washington, DC). 2001;52:805–11.
13. Colom F, Vieta E, Tacchi MJ, Sánchez-Moreno J, Scott J. Identifying and improving non-adherence in bipolar disorders. Bipolar Disorders. 2005;7:24–31.
14. Vrijens B, De Geest S, Hughes DA, et al. A new taxonomy for describing and defining adherence to medications. British Journal of Clinical Pharmacology. 2012;73:691–705.
15. Horne R, Weinman J, Barber N, Elliott R, Morgan M, Cribb A. Concordance, adherence and compliance in medicine taking: report for the National Co-ordinating Centre for NHS Service Delivery and Organisation R & D (NCCSDO). NCCSDO, London; 2005.
16. Jaeger S, Pfiffner C, Weiser P, et al. Adherence styles of schizophrenia patients identified by a latent class analysis of the Medication Adherence Rating Scale (MARS): a six-month follow-up study. Psychiatry Res. 2012;200(2–3):83–8.
17. Haddad PM, Brain C, Scott J. Nonadherence with antipsychotic medication in schizophrenia: challenges and management strategies. Patient related outcome measures. 2014;5:43–62.
18. Jablensky A, Sartorius N, Ernberg G, et al. Schizophrenia: manifestations, incidence and course in different cultures. A World Health Organization ten-country study. Psychological Medicine Monograph supplement. 1992;20:1–97.
19. Pini S, Cassano GB, Dell'Osso L, Amador XF. Insight into illness in schizophrenia, schizoaffective disorder, and mood disorders with psychotic features. American Journal of Psychiatry. 2001;158:122–5.
20. Lacro JP, Dunn LB, Dolder CR, Leckband SG, Jeste DV. Prevalence of and risk factors for medication nonadherence in patients with schizophrenia: a comprehensive review of recent literature. Journal of Clinical Psychiatry. 2002;63:892–909.
21. Kane JM, Kishimoto T, Correll CU. Non-adherence to medication in patients with psychotic disorders: epidemiology, contributing factors and management strategies. World Psychiatry. 2013;12:216–26.
22. Hudson TJ, Owen RR, Thrush CR, et al. A pilot study of barriers to medication adherence in schizophrenia. Journal of Clinical Psychiatry. 2004;65:211–16.
23. Thompson L, McCabe R. The effect of clinician-patient alliance and communication on treatment adherence in mental health care: a systematic review. BMC Psychiatry. 2012;12:87.
24. Sheehan KA, Burns T. Perceived Coercion and the Therapeutic Relationship: A Neglected Association? Psychiatric Services. 2011;62:471–6.
25. Swartz MS, Swanson JW, Hannon MJ. Does fear of coercion keep people away from mental health treatment? Evidence from a survey of persons with schizophrenia and mental health professionals. Behavioral Sciences and the Law. 2003;21:459–72.
26. Livingston JD, Boyd JE. Correlates and consequences of internalized stigma for people living with mental illness: A systematic review and meta-analysis. Social Science and Medicine. 2010;71:2150–61.
27. Nieuwlaat R, Wilczynski N, Navarro T, et al. Interventions for enhancing medication adherence. Cochrane Database of Systematic Reviews. 2014;11:CD000011.
28. Farooq S, Nazar Z, Irfan M, et al. Schizophrenia medication adherence in a resource-poor setting: randomised controlled trial of supervised treatment in out-patients for schizophrenia (STOPS). British Journal of Psychiatry. 2011;199:467–72.

29. Kemp R, Hayward P, Applewhaite G, Everitt B, David A. Compliance therapy in psychotic patients: randomised controlled trial. BMJ (Clinical research ed). 1996;312:345–9.

30. Kemp R, Kirov G, Everitt B, Hayward P, David A. Randomised controlled trial of compliance therapy. 18-month follow-up. British Journal of Psychiatry. 1998;172:413–19.

31. Anderson KH, Ford S, Robson D, Cassis J, Rodrigues C, Gray R. An exploratory, randomized controlled trial of adherence therapy for people with schizophrenia. International Journal of Mental Health Nursing. 2010;19:340–9.

32. O'Donnell C, Donohoe G, Sharkey L, et al. Compliance therapy: a randomised controlled trial in schizophrenia. BMJ (Clinical research ed). 2003;327:834.

33. Vergouwen AC, Bakker A, Katon WJ, Verheij TJ, Koerselman F. Improving adherence to antidepressants: a systematic review of interventions. Journal of Clinical Psychiatry. 2003;64:1415–20.

34. Barkhof E, Meijer CJ, de Sonneville LMJ, Linszen DH, de Haan L. Interventions to improve adherence to antipsychotic medication in patients with schizophrenia–A review of the past decade. European Psychiatry. 2012;27:9–18.

35. Chong WW, Aslani P, Chen TF. Effectiveness of interventions to improve antidepressant medication adherence: a systematic review. International Journal of Clinical Practice. 2011;65:954–75.

36. Sajatovic M, Davies M, Hrouda DR. Enhancement of treatment adherence among patients with bipolar disorder. Psychiatric Services. 2004;55:264–9.

37. Becker MH, Maiman LA. Sociobehavioral determinants of compliance with health and medical care recommendations. Medical Care. 1975;13:10–24.

38. Opolka JL, Rascati KL, Brown CM, Gibson PJ. Role of ethnicity in predicting antipsychotic medication adherence. Annals of Pharmacotherapy. 2003;37:625–30.

39. Valenstein M, Blow FC, Copeland LA, et al. Poor Antipsychotic Adherence Among Patients With Schizophrenia: Medication and Patient Factors. Schizophrenia Bulletin. 2004;30:255–64.

40. Cohen NL, Ross EC, Bagby RM, Farvolden P, Kennedy SH. The 5-factor model of personality and antidepressant medication compliance. Canadian Journal of Psychiatry (Revue canadienne de psychiatrie). 2004;49:106–13.

41. Holma IA, Holma KM, Melartin TK, Isometsa ET. Treatment attitudes and adherence of psychiatric patients with major depressive disorder: a five-year prospective study. Journal of Affective Disorders. 2010;127(1–3):102–12.

42. Aikens JE, Nease DE, Nau DP, Klinkman MS, Schwenk TL. Adherence to Maintenance-Phase Antidepressant Medication as a Function of Patient Beliefs About Medication. Annals of Family Medicine. 2005;3:23–30.

43. Beck EM, Cavelti M, Kvrgic S, Kleim B, Vauth R. Are we addressing the 'right stuff' to enhance adherence in schizophrenia? Understanding the role of insight and attitudes towards medication. Schizophrenia Research. 2011;132:42–9.

44. Clatworthy J, Bowskill R, Parham R, Rank T, Scott J, Horne R. Understanding medication non-adherence in bipolar disorders using a Necessity-Concerns Framework. Journal of Affective Disorders. 2009;116:51–5.

45. Piette JD, Heisler M, Horne R, Alexander GC. A conceptually based approach to understanding chronically ill patients' responses to medication cost pressures. Social Science and Medicine. 2006;62:846–57.

46. Nunes V, Neilson J, O'Flynn N, et al. Medicines adherence: involving patients in decisions about prescribed medicines and supporting adherence. National Institute for Health and Clinical Excellence, London; 2009.

47. Michie S, van Stralen MM, West R. The behaviour change wheel: a new method for characterising and designing behaviour change interventions. Implementation science. 2011;6:42.

48. Schwartz A, Crockett RA, Sutton S, et al. Impact on decisions to start or continue medicines of providing information to patients about possible benefits and/or harms: a systematic review and meta-analysis. Medical Decision Making. 2011;31:767–77.

49. Peveler R, George C, Kinmonth AL, Campbell M, Thompson C. Effect of antidepressant drug counselling and information leaflets on adherence to drug treatment in primary care: randomised controlled trial. BMJ (Clinical research ed). 1999;319:612–15.

50. Lincoln TM, Wilhelm K, Nestoriuc Y. Effectiveness of psychoeducation for relapse, symptoms, knowledge, adherence and functioning in psychotic disorders: A meta-analysis. Schizophrenia Research. 2007;96(1–3):232–45.

51. Horne R, Weinman J, Hankins M. The beliefs about medicines questionnaire: the development and evaluation of a new method for assessing the cognitive representation of medication. Psychology and Health. 1999;14:1–24.

52. Britten N, Riley R, Morgan M. Resisting psychotropic medicines: a synthesis of qualitative studies of medicine-taking. Advances in Psychiatric Treatment. 2010;16:207–18.

53. Jorm AF. Mental health literacy. Public knowledge and beliefs about mental disorders. British Journal of Psychiatry. 2000;177:396–401.

54. Horne R, Clatworthy J. Adherence to advice and treatment. Health psychology, 2nd edn. British Psychological Society and Blackwell Publishing: Chichester; 2010. pp. 175–88.

55. Horne R, Faasse K, Cooper V, et al. The perceived sensitivity to medicines (PSM) scale: an evaluation of validity and reliability. British Journal of Health Psychology. 2013;18:18–30.

56. Heller MK, Chapman SC, Horne R. Beliefs about medication predict the misattribution of a common symptom as a medication side effect—Evidence from an analogue online study. Journal of Psychosomatic Research. 2015;79:519–29.

57. Rief W, Bingel U, Schedlowski M, Enck P. Mechanisms involved in placebo and nocebo responses and implications for drug trials. Clinical Pharmacology and Therapeutics. 2011;90:722–6.

58. García S, Martínez-Cengotitabengoa M, López-Zurbano S, et al. Adherence to Antipsychotic Medication in Bipolar Disorder and Schizophrenic Patients: A Systematic Review. Journal of Clinical Psychopharmacology. 2016;36:355–71.

59. Perkins DO, Johnson JL, Hamer RM, et al. Predictors of antipsychotic medication adherence in patients recovering from a first psychotic episode. Schizophrenia Research. 2006;83:53–63.

60. Horne R, Chapman SC, Parham R, Freemantle N, Forbes A, Cooper V. Understanding patients' adherence-related beliefs about medicines prescribed for long-term conditions: a meta-analytic review of the Necessity-Concerns Framework. PLoS One. 2013;8:e80633.

61. Ritsner M, Ponizovsky A, Endicott J, et al. The impact of side-effects of antipsychotic agents on life satisfaction of schizophrenia patients: a naturalistic study. European Neuropsychopharmacology. 2002;12:31–8.

62. Horne R. Treatment perceptions and self-regulation. In: Cameron LD, Leventhal H (eds). The self-regulation of health and illness behaviour. Routledge: New York, NY; 2003. pp. 138–53.

63. Bulloch AG, Adair CE, Patten SB. Forgetfulness: a role in non-compliance with antidepressant treatment. Canadian Journal of Psychiatry. 2006;51:719–22.

64. Boeni F, Spinatsch E, Suter K, Hersberger KE, Arnet I. Effect of drug reminder packaging on medication adherence: a systematic review revealing research gaps. Systematic Reviews. 2014;3:29.

65. Lally P, Gardner B. Promoting habit formation. Health Psychology Review. 2013;7(sup1):S137–58.

66. Gollwitzer PM, Brandstätter V. Implementation intentions and effective goal pursuit. Journal of Personality and social Psychology. 1997;73:186.

67. Pfeiffer PN, Ganoczy D, Valenstein M. Dosing frequency and adherence to antipsychotic medications. Psychiatric Services. 2008;59:1207–10.

68. Kishimoto T, Nitta M, Borenstein M, Kane JM, Correll CU. Long-acting injectable versus oral antipsychotics in schizophrenia: a systematic review and meta-analysis of mirror-image studies. Journal of Clinical Psychiatry. 2013;74:957–65.

69. Jaeger M, Rossler W. Attitudes towards long-acting depot anti-psychotics: a survey of patients, relatives and psychiatrists. Psychiatry Research. 2010;175:58–62.

70. Wilder CM, Elbogen EB, Moser LL, Swanson JW, Swartz MS. Medication preferences and adherence among individuals with severe mental illness and psychiatric advance directives. Psychiatric Services. 2010;61:380–5.

71. Garber MC, Nau DP, Erickson SR, Aikens JE, Lawrence JB. The concordance of self-report with other measures of medication adherence: a summary of the literature. Medical Care. 2004;42:649–52.

72. Horne R, Weinman J. *The theoretical basis of concordance and issues for research. Concordance: a partnership in medicine-taking.* Pharmaceutical Press: London; 2004.

73. Granholm E, Ben-Zeev D, Link PC, Bradshaw KR, Holden JL. Mobile Assessment and Treatment for Schizophrenia (MATS): a pilot trial of an interactive text-messaging intervention for medication adherence, socialization, and auditory hallucinations. Schizophrenia Bulletin. 2012;38:414–25.

74. Naslund JA, Marsch LA, McHugo GJ, Bartels SJ. Emerging mHealth and eHealth interventions for serious mental illness: a review of the literature. Journal of Mental Health. 2015;24:321–32.

75. Horne R, Bell JI, Montgomery JR, Ravn MO, Tooke JE. A new social contract for medical innovation. The Lancet. 2015;385:1153–4.

76. Maughan D, Molodynski A, Rugkåsa J, Burns T. A systematic review of the effect of community treatment orders on service use. Social Psychiatry and Psychiatric Epidemiology. 2014;49:651–63.

77. Farmer KC. Methods for measuring and monitoring medication regimen adherence in clinical trials and clinical practice. Clinical Therapeutics. 1999;21:1074–90.

# SECTION 3
# Intellectual disabilities

# 21

# Core dimensions of intellectual disabilities

*Anthony J. Holland*

## Introduction

This chapter focuses on two main issues: (1) the core dimensions that are part of systems of classification that define what is meant when a person is said to have an intellectual (learning) disability, and how these systems have developed with time; and (2) the behavioural and mental health needs of people with intellectual disabilities (ID) and how such needs might be best conceptualized. The characterization and classification of a group of people as having ID, and including such a classification within the taxonomy of mental disorder, has not been without controversy. The reasons for this relate to the key elements of any classification system—is it valid, and is it reliable? Does it inform and clarify our understanding? To what end is it being used? Does it enhance those it so classifies, or does it demean and contribute to stigma and marginalization? When it comes to illness or disease, accurate diagnosis based on agreed diagnostic criteria is the cornerstone of epidemiological and aetiological research, enabling informed treatment development that can then be generalized to others with similar illnesses. However, an ID is not an illness, and identifying someone as having an ID is not fundamentally a diagnosis because, on its own, the term provides no information about the cause, pathophysiology, or likely prognosis. Rather 'intellectual disability' serves as an umbrella term for a set of 'core dimensions' that describe what is an extremely heterogenous group of people. In addition to the ways we are all different, children and adults with ID also differ extensively in other ways, such as in the cause, nature, and degree of their disabilities and in the presence or absence of secondary sensory, physical, and/or psychiatric comorbidities and/or a pattern of early developmental characteristics of the autistic spectrum disorder. The assessment of children and adults with ID in clinical practice requires that these various strands are integrated into a coherent and comprehensive formulation, which, in turn, informs intervention.

## Background

The initial development of modern systems of classification for 'mental retardation', as it was known then, was reviewed in a special edition of the *American Journal of Psychiatry* in 1972 [1]. The systems referred to used varied terms, and their use and some of the actions that resulted from such labelling would certainly now be seen as unacceptable. However, with time, thinking has developed, and the core dimensions have been reshaped and expanded to better reflect the complexity and interactive nature of the concept of 'intellectual disability', together with a better understanding of the reasons for, and potential pitfalls of, any system of classification. In the 1900s, in the UK, the characterization and classification of people with ID was considered to be necessary to facilitate the segregation of people deemed to be harmful to the population as a whole, or even a major source of criminality, by virtue of their abnormal genetic endowment. The eugenics movement took these ideas to be axiomatic, and they persisted well into the twentieth century. The work of Jack Tizard and others transformed thinking about how people with ID should be supported, leading to the acceptance that people with ID should be, and could be, supported outside of institutions. The 1960s saw the emergence of the concepts of normalization and social role valorization as the principles that should guide the support of people with ID. Within Europe, North America, and other high-resource countries, these changing approaches led to developments in legislation and in policy and practice. With the development of new ways of conceptualizing ID, there was a move away from seeing the nature and extent of the disability as exclusively based in the individual, rather than seeing a person's disability as a consequence of interactions between some innate limitations, the influence of the past and present social and family environments, and importantly educational and life opportunities. Additionally, the nature and extent to which society itself accepted and responded to people with disabilities could ameliorate the disadvantages experienced by those affected.

These social and attitudinal changes occurred during a period in which there were also major advances in areas such as genetics and neurosciences, and in understanding the major environmental causes of ID. The work, for example, of Lionel Penrose and the publication in 1938 of his book the *Biology of Mental Defect* identified the causes of ID [2] (Penrose 1949). The normal human chromosome complement of 23 pairs of chromosomes was identified in the 1950s, and trisomy 21, as the cause of Down's syndrome, was identified shortly afterwards. The sequencing of the human genome was undertaken in the late 1900s and early twenty-first century, and many abnormalities of chromosome number (aneuploidies), chromosomal rearrangements, DNA copy number variations, and single-gene mutations have been described in association with the presence of developmental delay and ID [3].

The recognition of specific environmental causes of ID, as diverse as maternal iodine deficiency, fetal alcohol syndrome, or rubella embryopathy, has all had very clear public health implications in terms of primary prevention. In LMICs, it is recognized that varied environmental and social factors impact on the early cognitive and socio-emotional development of children [4]. These different issues are primarily the province of public health, child health, and maternity services. However, in addition, as findings from studies in the 1970s onwards identified that children and adults with ID have high rates of behavioural problems and mental ill health [5, 6], so the need to address such issues became increasingly apparent. It is primarily for this reason that there is a focus on ID in a textbook of psychiatry. Given research evidence about such comorbidities and with the earlier changes in attitudes and policy, the role of psychiatrists, in particular, has altered beyond recognition from being medical superintendents of large long-stay institutions to being members of community-based interdisciplinary teams undertaking much more focused and nuanced interventions.

## Classification of intellectual disabilities

Given the heterogeneity of people with ID and the potential complexity of the health and support needs of people with ID, what is clear is that no one system of classification is fully adequate and which system is employed, if any, critically depends on the context and the reason for its use. If the question is about the nature and type of support to be offered, this will be better characterized through the lens of a more interactive and dynamic model, in which barriers to that person's full participation and inclusion in society are the focus of enquiry. However, if the question is about the cause of a child's significant developmental delay, then the focus will be more on an accurate description and characterization of his/her unique features—the phenotype, in order to identify the cause. The former approach helps guide educational and service planning and support and is based on what is described as a social model of disability, and the latter is based around a biomedical model. In each of these, the 'core dimensions' will overlap, yet differ in terms of emphasis, as each system of classification has a different purpose.

Historically, there has been a tension between the social and biomedical ways of conceptualizing the needs of people with ID, and in papers advocating these different perspectives, the language and concepts used and the conclusions drawn at times appear irreconcilable. However, such debate has unnecessarily polarized each perspective, and there is a need for a more nuanced understanding [7]. While those from different professional backgrounds may emphasize a different perspective, there is necessarily a coming together of these perspectives, thereby providing the means for structuring our thinking about the needs of people with ID and, in turn, how we might respond to these needs. Diagnostic and classifications systems, such as the *Diagnostic and Statistical Manuals (DSM)* of the APA, first published in 1952, and now as DSM-V [8], and the WHO's *International Classification of Diseases* (soon to be ICD-11), have been developed and modified over time, and newer systems have been developed, which seek to better reflect the nuances required of systems of classification. These aim to both characterize the nature and

extent of a person's impairment and disability on the one hand, and on the other, to be structured enough to be used reliably to compare findings across countries and over time. These include the American Association on Intellectual and Developmental Disabilities' manual *Intellectual Disability: Definition, Classification, and Systems of Support* [9] and the WHO's *Classification of Impairments, Disabilities and Handicaps* [10] and its successor the WHO's *International Classification of Functioning, Disability and Health* [11].

Although, in some areas, the use of systems for classification may be subject to criticism, there are at best very positive benefits to an individual being assessed as having an ID. These include: the prospect of going on to identify the exact cause of a person's ID; awareness of the potential for, and the identification and treatment of, associated health problems; and access to specialized educational support and additional financial support through the benefits system. It is against this background that the defining of what it means to have an ID and the core dimensions that are part of such a definition need to be considered. For the paediatrician, the question may be why this child is developmentally delayed. For the geneticist advising the parents, the questions are: is there a genetic cause, and what is the implication in terms of recurrence risk? For teachers and educational psychologists: what is the nature of the child's intellectual impairment, and how and in what way can education enhance the child's development and acquisition of skills? For public health practitioners: what is the extent and nature of need at a population level, and are there causes that are potentially preventable? For the psychiatrist, clinical psychologists, and community nurses: what is the relationship between the nature and extent of any impairments and disabilities and the emotional and behavioural difficulties that may have brought them in contact with specialist child, adolescent, or adult mental health services? Classification should have a defined purpose, and because the reasons may differ, so then the assessments and classification systems used will vary.

The diagnostic criteria are set out in DSM-V [8], Chapter V of ICD-10 [12], and the American Association of Intellectual Disabilities' *Intellectual Disability; Definition, Classification and Systems of Support* (AAIDD-11) [9]. There are three essential components to all these definitions: (1) evidence of significant intellectual impairment assessed using an established and valid assessment and normally considered to be present when there is a score of less than two standard deviations below the mean; (2) evidence of significant impairment in adaptive functioning, given the age and cultural background of the person concerned; and (3) these features having their origins in childhood, with delays in, or an inability to reach, specific well-recognized developmental milestones and educational attainments, usually with evidence of delay in the first 5 years of life. The exact nature, extent, and severity of the delay will vary across people considered to have an ID but may involve delay in one or more of the following areas: gross motor, sensorimotor, language, and adaptive behaviours. Revisions of the standard classification systems have led to a change in terminology, and 'intellectual developmental disorder' (IDD) is the term now used.

## Intellectual developmental disorder (DSM and ICD systems) (American Psychiatric Association, 2013)

The structure of the classification within DSM-V has been shaped around developmental and lifespan considerations and within a cultural context that recognizes the dimensional nature of psychiatric disorder. It encompasses how factors within an individual's environment in which a person lives influence whether a particular symptom has functional significance or not, thereby moving beyond a simply diagnosis. In DSM-V, IDD is included in a section headed 'Neurodevelopmental disorders', which also includes communication disorders, autism spectrum disorders (without distinguishing between Asperger's syndrome and autism), attention-deficit/hyperactivity disorder (ADHD), specific learning disorders, motor disorders, and other neurodevelopmental disorders. The focus is not primarily one of aetiology, but rather of quantifying the extent of disability by defining the level of intellectual impairment and listing the range of possible adaptive functions that might be impaired. The definition makes it explicit that the onset is within the developmental period and that IDD is the final common pathway of a number of potential aetiologies. Significant sub-average intellectual function is defined as an intelligence quotient (IQ) of 70 or below (using standard IQ tests). IQ is also used to help determine the level of ID (mild, moderate, severe, or profound). Adaptive functioning has to be measured against what would be expected for a person of that age, and the social and cultural experience of the person has to be taken into account. The Wechsler Scales for IQ and the Vineland Adaptive Behaviour Scales or the revised Adaptive Behaviour Scales of the American Association for Mental Retardation for characterizing functioning are established instruments for the measurement of these abilities for which there are normative data for comparison.

Bertelli *et al.* (2016) [13] have reported on development work undertaken to inform ICD-11, specifically whether or not ID should be classified as a health condition. They also proposed the use of the term 'intellectual developmental disorder', defined as 'a group of developmental conditions characterized by a significant impairment of cognitive functions, which are associated with limitations of learning, adaptive behaviour and skills'. They also suggested that the primary category, replacing that of 'Mental retardation', would be 'Neurodevelopmental disorders'. IDD would be a subset of this primary category and encompass 'a broad grouping of heterogeneous developmental conditions which result from significant interference with the growth and maturation of the brain during its early developmental phases including the prenatal and perinatal periods, infancy, childhood, and extending into adolescence'.

These developments in classification systems still use frameworks developed for the classification of illness and are thus unsatisfactory when it comes to ID. However, they do have value in bringing consistency and a degree of rigour to the classification process. Thus, it can be reasonably assumed when the classifications are properly used that there is a degree of reliability to the conclusion that an individual has an ID, and it will not have been based simply on appearance or educational abilities, but rather will have taken into account evidence for a delayed and atypical pattern of development and the continuing presence of intellectual and functional impairments. Depending on circumstances, the next question might well be whether there is a single major cause for such developmental delay (genetic or environmental) or whether that is unlikely and a combination of factors has contributed to a person's atypical developmental history. Given that these approaches have their limitations in terms of characterizing the possible multiple factors that may result in disability, other means of classification with more extensive core dimensions have been proposed.

## Impairments, disabilities, and handicaps (World Health Organization, 1980)

In 1980, the WHO proposed a system of classification that attempted to overcome the limitations of other earlier methods of classification and, most importantly, aimed to guide intervention. Box 21.1 summarizes the terms. In this system, ID can be conceptualized at different levels. At the level of 'impairment', in the case of ID, the organ system involved is the CNS. It is the impairment of this system for genetic, chromosomal, or environmental reasons that primarily affect the acquisition of developmentally related skills and the ability to learn. For the paediatrician or geneticist, a key task is to identify the reasons for any abnormality of brain development, and therefore intellectual impairment. This may have treatment implications, may guide prognosis, and most importantly may help to make sense of the disability for the parents of those affected. It may also have important implications for genetic counselling.

**Box 21.1** World Health Organization's definitions of impairments, disabilities, and handicaps

**Impairment**
- Is any loss or abnormality of psychological, physiological, or anatomical structure or function.
- Represents deviation from some norm in the individual's biomedical status.
- Is characterized by losses or abnormalities that may be temporary or permanent.
- Includes the existence or occurrence of an anomaly, defect, or loss in a limb, organ, tissue, or other structure of the body, or a defect in a functional system or mechanism of the body, including the systems of mental functioning.
- Is not contingent upon aetiology.

**Disability**
- Is any restriction or lack (resulting from impairment) of ability to perform an activity in the manner or within the range considered normal for a human being.
- Is concerned with compound or integrated activities expected of the person or of the body as a whole such as represented by tasks, skills, and behaviours.
- Is the excesses or deficiencies of customarily expected activities and behaviour, which may be temporary or permanent, reversible or irreversible, and progressive or regressive.
- Is the process through which a functional limitation expresses itself as a reality in everyday life.

**Handicap**
- Is a disadvantage for a given individual, resulting from an impairment or a disability that limits or prevents the fulfilment of a role that is normal for that individual.
- Places some value upon this departure from a structural, functional, or performance norm by the individual or his or her peers in the context of their culture.
- Is relative to other people and represents discordance between the individual's performance or status and the expectations of his or her social/cultural group.
- Is a social phenomenon, representing the social and environmental consequences for the individual stemming from his or her impairment and disability.

*Source:* data from World Health Organisation, Definitions of Impairments, Disabilities and Handicaps, Copyright (1980), World Health Organisation.

The associated disability is the effect of the impairment on a person's ability to learn and acquire the new skills that come with development. These, in turn, enable the acquisition of increasingly advanced skills necessary for an independent life. The exact nature and extent of the disability may not only include ID, but also physical and sensory disabilities. The extent to which a given impairment results in a loss of function (disability) may well be influenced by the extent and nature of interventions such as special education or, for example, the correction of hearing loss through treatment and/or the use of a hearing aid.

The final level—that of 'handicap'—is a result of an interaction between the disability and the extent to which support is available or environmental adjustments made at a societal level. It is a measure of disadvantage. The extent of disadvantage can be ameliorated through, for example, the presence of support to enable individuals to go out, or environmental modifications (for example, wheelchair ramps) that diminish the impact of physical disabilities. Such interventions or environmental modifications maximize independence and thereby reduce disadvantage by ensuring that the impact of any given disability on an individual's independence and quality of life is minimized. Shakespeare (2006) [14] has argued that such a structure as this model helps to bring together the biomedical and social models of disability.

## Functioning, disability, and health (ICF) (World Health Organization, 2001)

This new system of classification to replace the 1980 version was published by the WHO in 2001. The focus switched from a system that was seen as just characterizing the negative to a system of classification that also emphasized the positive—what someone is able to do, rather than just what he/she could not do. While the context in this chapter is about people with ID, this system of health classification was developed by the WHO to enable the characterization of 'health domains' across the whole population and therefore should be seen to have universal application. Part 1 is the means whereby body functions, structures, and activities and participation can be characterized. Part 2 relates to 'contextual factors', whether in the environment or the individual. Fig. 21.1 illustrates the relationship between the different components of this classification system. The authors emphasize that it enables a multi-perspective approach and that it can be used by different disciplines as 'building blocks for users who wish to create models and study different aspects of this process'. Part 1 is divided into organ systems. With respect to people with ID, the sections on mental functions and structures of the nervous system may be of particular relevance, but these may be compounded by secondary disabilities, consequent upon abnormalities in structure and function of other organ systems such as those associated with sensory impairments. All of these categories are extensively subdivided. In Part 2, the focus is very much on the specific personal circumstances and the characteristics of the individual environment, including the health system and support available.

This system seeks to do two things. Firstly, it aims to provide a reliable structure for the description of the complex effects of ill health and those factors that might moderate its impact, thereby enabling accurate comparisons across countries, between cultures, and throughout the lifespan. Secondly, it aims to provide a more comprehensive framework to aid intervention, one that moves beyond

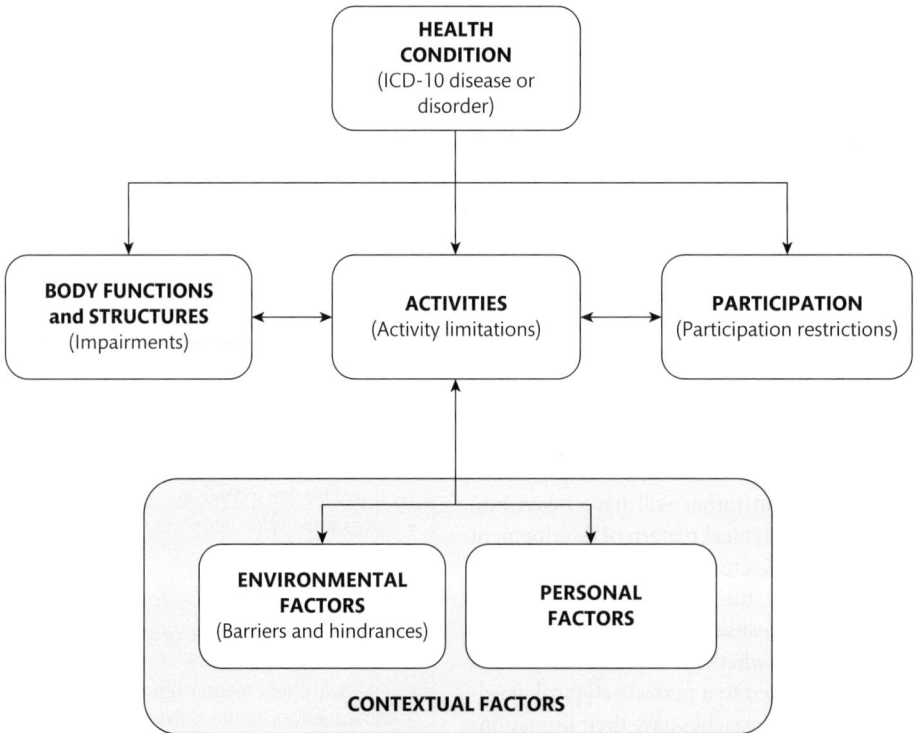

**Fig. 21.1** The World Health Organization's International Classification of Functioning, Disability, and Health model of intellectual disability (WHO ICF model).

Adapted from World Health Organisation, *International Classification of Functioning, Disability and Health,* Copyright (2001), with permission from World Health Organisation.

the single word or brief phrase of classification systems, such as in the ICD and DSM, to a more structured and meaningful description of an individual's strengths and difficulties. In this respect, it seeks to incorporate aspects of the biomedical and social models of disability and an understanding of the person within the context of his or her support network and culture.

This more dynamic and interactive concept of what it means to have an ID and what might contribute to the extent of social inclusions and well-being of that individual is illustrated in the American Association on Intellectual and Developmental Disabilities model of disability (or the AAIDD-11 model). The emphasis is on the moderating effects of individual past and present circumstances and the wider national policy that seeks to ensure that the 'mismatch between competency and environmental demands' is minimized and people with ID are fully included in society. The way in which these formulations influence the approach to treatment is described at greater length in Chapter 35.

## Prevalence and aetiology of intellectual disabilities

As argued, the classification systems described in this chapter are not diagnostic. In addition, these different ways of conceptualizing ID emphasize that the paths to functional impairments are not simply to do with biology; there are interactions with respect to the extent and nature of the statutory provision of education, opportunities in adult life, and societal attitudes, all of which impact on ability and quality of life. Particularly in early life, the biomedical perspective is fundamentally about understanding the reasons for identified problems at birth or in childhood, and in this regard, there have been significant advances. Furthermore, the cause of a person's ID may also inform understanding of behaviour problems and mental ill health, as they affect people with ID and it has become increasingly recognized that this may be an important aspect to psychiatric assessment.

Two broadly distinct groups were identified through population-based studies such as the Aberdeen children's cohort study of the 1950s [15]. Firstly. there are children who have a definite or likely genetic abnormality or specific environmental causes with major effects on subsequent development. Secondly, there are those for whom there is no obvious single major cause for an early developmental delay and subsequent ID. Here, the small effects of many genes combined with social disadvantage may be crucial. The broad difference between these two groups are summarized in Box 21.2. This 'two group' perspective also illustrates the difficulty in arriving at a true prevalence of ID in any given community, given the fact that more than an IQ of below 70 is required when determining if someone should be considered to have an ID. The distribution of IQ in the general population is near normal, with a skew to the left, given the presence of specific neurodevelopmental disorders that are generally associated with a downward shift in IQ. Given this, a figure of 2–2.5% is estimated as the proportion of the population with an IQ of below 70. The problem then is to know how many of this group truly should be considered to have an ID. To address this issue, there have been studies of the administrative prevalence of people with ID, that is the percentage of any given geographic population known to ID services. Figures of between 0.4% to just under 1% are arrived at, depending on a number of factors, including whether

**Box 21.2** Differences between biologically determined and subcultural ID

**Biological**
- Moderate/severe impairment.
- Significant impairment in adaptive functioning.
- Equal distribution across families of different socio-economic status.
- Parents and siblings usually of normal intelligence.
- Dysmorphic characteristics common.
- Other impairments and disabilities common.
- Neglect unusual.

**Subcultural**
- Mild or borderline impairment.
- Minor or no impairment in adaptive functioning.
- More common in families of lower socio-economic status.
- Intellectual ability impaired in family members.
- Dysmorphic characteristics unlikely.
- Other impairments and disabilities unusual.
- Neglect more common.

active screening for people with ID in the population was attempted, whether it was the number of people already known to ID services, whether children and adults were included, and specific geographic factors such as levels of deprivation. Studies indicate that there is a peak in prevalence in childhood and that there may be significant regional variations in any given country. Examples of studies from different countries include that of Sondenaa et al. (2010) [16] in Norway; McConkey et al. (2006) [17] in the island of Ireland; Larson et al. (2001) [18] in the United States; and Wen (1997) [19] in Australia. In an important study in the United States, Fujiura (2003) [20] estimated that there were a further 1.27% of people with mild ID who had very substantial needs and were effectively falling through the net of ID services. A detailed consideration of the epidemiology of ID is presented in Chapter 22.

The striking feature about the ID population is its heterogeneity, both in terms of the nature and severity of disability and also in the presence, or not, of individuals whose ID is due to one of many possible single major causes. Making up this population of people, there are those with specific environmental effects, such as fetal alcohol syndrome, very low birthweight, congenital infections, and maternal iodine deficiency (worldwide, of major significance—see [21]), and those with chromosomal and single-gene disorders which either arise de novo or are inherited. Down's syndrome due to trisomy 21 and fragile X syndrome due to X-linked FMR-1 mutations are two examples that are relatively common. Other neurodevelopmental syndromes due to copy number variations have been identified [22], and advances in genetics using microarray technologies (sometimes referred to as molecular karyotyping) readily enable the identification of copy number variants of various sizes, including chromosomal rearrangements, deletions, and duplications [23]. Some of these are indicative of well-recognized chromosomal deletion neurodevelopmental syndromes (for example, Williams syndrome, cri-du-chat, etc.). Others with previously unrecognized chromosomal abnormalities are still to be properly characterized by phenotypy. Whether such copy number variants should be considered to be pathogenic or a normal polymorphic variation needs to be judged using established databases such as DECIPHER [24].

With improvements in DNA sequencing technology, identification of specific gene mutations is now more readily available, for example, detecting *de novo* or inherited gene mutations such as in the *TSC 1* and *TSC 2* genes that result in the tuberous sclerosis complex. These technologies make possible the characterization and subsequent identification of an increasing number of neurodevelopmental syndromes of genetic origin associated with ID. The specific causes of ID will be considered in more detail in Chapter 23.

The assessment of a child or an adult with ID referred to child and adolescent mental health services or to adult mental health or specialist services because of problem behaviour, and the subsequent formulation, will include any identified major cause of a person's ID such as Down's syndrome. As identification of genetic and environmental causes of ID develops and, with it, our understanding of their specific impact on brain development and functioning, so interventions for mental health and behaviour problems across the lifespan will only become more nuanced and hopefully more effective.

## Core dimensions of disorders of behaviour and mental ill health in children and adults with intellectual disabilities

For health professionals working in mental health or specialist services for children, adolescents, or adults with ID, the primary focus of their work will be on prevention and treatment of secondary disabilities that may arise in the form of challenging behaviours or mental ill health. In people with ID, the development of challenging behaviour may be for a number of reasons, including: being an indication of the development of a comorbid physical or mental disorder, for example, mania presenting with irritability and aggression; changes in the environment and/or in the support provided; or the onset of a physical illness. In contrast, behaviours, such as self-injury or aggression, if long-standing, may be best understood from a developmental or behavioural perspective. In addition, the cause of a person's ID may also inform our understanding of the reasons for particular behavioural or mental health problems that occur. Well-known examples include the excessive eating behaviour and risk of psychopathology associated with Prader–Willi syndrome [25], the high rates of Alzheimer's disease affecting people with Down's syndrome [26], anxiety disorders affecting people with Williams syndrome [27], and severe self-injurious behaviour in people with Lesch–Nyhan and Smith–Magenis syndromes [28]. This observation of an association between specific neurodevelopmental syndromes and a characteristic behaviour was described by Nyhan as 'the behavioural phenotype of organic genetic disease' [29]. Such observations have very significantly altered our understanding of the aetiology and pathophysiology of such behaviours and psychiatric disorders.

Conceptually, comparative studies across different neurodevelopmental syndromes have challenged the orthodoxy of applied behavioural analysis and have required the development of more complex models, which recognize the role of the syndrome-specific developmental profiles and brain mechanisms in the aetiology of syndrome-specific behaviours (see, for example, [30] and [31] on Williams and fragile X syndromes, respectively; and [32]). Oliver and colleagues, for example, have reported very different behavioural and developmental profiles across different

neurodevelopmental syndromes, and they have gone on to propose specific models to account for their occurrence and maintenance [33]. Similarly, studies on Prader–Willi syndrome have proposed specific mechanisms to account for the different components of the behavioural phenotype [25] and the high rates of psychotic illness reported. The latter develops in early adult life but primarily affect those with the chromosome 15 maternal uniparental disomy (UPD) subtype [34]. These observations indicate the importance not only of developmental and bio-psychosocial perspectives, but also of having an understanding of the impact of particular patterns of brain development on behaviour and the risk of comorbid mental disorders. This diverse information informs intervention.

The task of assessment under such circumstances is the bringing together of what is known about the person and his/her behaviour with models of understanding that have been informed by research. This process of assessment and formulation is illustrated in Fig. 21.2 (see also [35] for discussion).

Core dimensions to the understanding of challenging behaviours therefore include establishing how best to conceptualize the problem that has led to the referral (for example, aggressive behaviour, self-injury, apparent loss of skills, etc.). The conceptual models include: (1) that of applied behavioural analysis, with behaviours being identified as having a cause and a function (such as demand avoidant or attention maintained) and being shaped by various contingencies and occurring in the context of certain internal or external setting conditions (for an overview, see [36] O'Reilly et al, 2016); (2) the developmental model, whereby such behaviours (for example, repetitive behaviours) are seen as normally a self-limiting characteristic of typical development and their continuation into later life as a consequence of delayed or an atypical developmental trajectory and/or such behaviours may be syndrome-specific (a

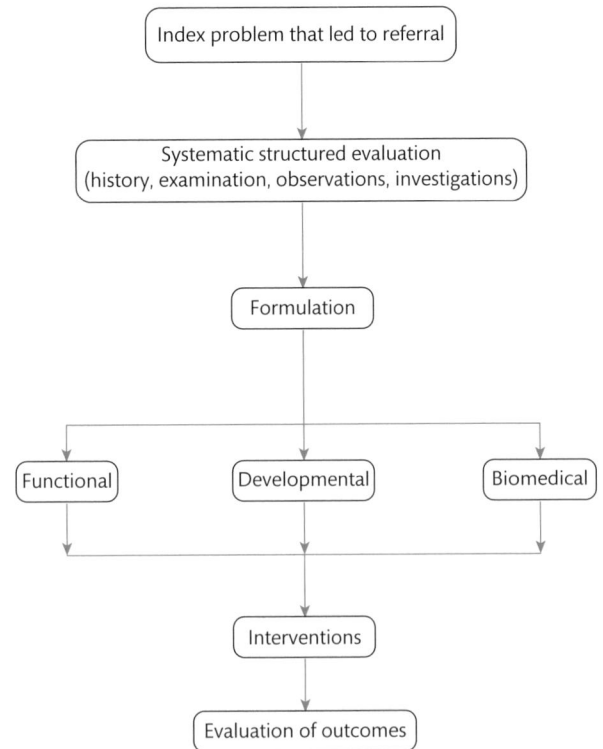

**Fig. 21.2** Developing single or mixed models of understanding that inform intervention.

**Table 21.1** Assessment of behavioural and comorbid psychiatric disorders in people with ID

| Model | Key features | Interventions |
|---|---|---|
| **Applied Behavioural Analysis (ABA)**—also referred to as 'functional analysis', explains the presence of adaptive and challenging behaviours in terms of learning theory and the presence of specific contingencies that increase the probability of such behaviours | Through history and observation, the identification of specific 'functions' for behaviours and the predisposing, precipitating, and maintaining factors and internal and external setting conditions | The development of alternate strategies of support seeking to reinforce positive behaviours and develop adaptive responses to triggering events, and modifying predisposing and maintaining factors and setting conditions |
| **Developmental**—specific patterns of behaviour are explained as a manifestation of atypical and/or delayed development or as a direct consequence of the specific cause of that person's ID (the presence of a 'behavioural phenotype') | Through history-taking and observations, the index behaviours are identified as similar to those that are usually self-limiting and occur as part of normal development or have been shown to occur in excess in those with a specific neurodevelopmental disorder | The development of specific interventions informed by other models that seek to reduce the severity and frequency of such behaviours and/or interventions that are syndrome-specific and informed by knowledge of that syndrome |
| **Biomedical**—a diagnostic approach that seeks to account for challenging behaviour or cognitive abnormalities or abnormalities of mental state on the basis of the co-occurrence of an additional developmental (for example, autism spectrum disorder, ADHD) or acquired comorbidity (for example, affective disorder, dementia, or physical illness) | Through history-taking and additional assessments and investigations, the identification of established signs and symptoms of comorbid psychiatric or physical disorders that the history indicates are likely to account for the development of the index problem that led to referral | The treatment of the specific developmental or acquired comorbid disorder using interventions known to be effective, including, for example, established psychological or pharmacological interventions |

behavioural phenotype); and (3) the possibility that such problems may be integral to, or a consequence of, the development of comorbid physical or psychiatric illness. These different perspectives and their implications are summarized in Table 21.1. They are not necessarily distinct. One example may be a person who has a history of a particular pattern of development characteristic of an autistic spectrum disorder and who finds change difficult to tolerate and anxiety-provoking, who also develops a comorbid illness that additionally impacts on behaviour.

In this context, the assessment of a person with an ID who has exhibited particular problematic behaviours (often referred to as challenging behaviour) is to provide an understanding of such behaviours in order to inform intervention. The core components of any assessment will include history-taking from the patient and/or an informant, a mental state examination and, where appropriate, a physical examination, investigations, and often structured observation over time. The core dimensions will include not only information on the nature, extent, and causation of the person's ID, as described earlier, but also information on the onset and course of the index problem, a diagnostic assessment for the presence, or not, of comorbid mental or physical illness, and observations to indicate whether or not specific factors might precipitate, predispose to, or maintain such behaviours.

The history is crucial—whether some particular behaviour (for example, aggression) is long-standing or new and of recent onset is likely to lead to very different explanations. If long-standing, it may relate more directly to the nature of the person's developmental disability, including emotional dysregulation [37] and environmental triggers. If the behaviour is new and of recent origin, then the possibility that it is a manifestation of the development of a secondary comorbid physical or psychiatric disorder is more likely. The diagnosis of comorbid psychiatric disorders, such as ADHD, severe anxiety, psychotic illness, affective disorder, or dementia, can be problematic where there is limited language development, and information from informants may be crucial. Specific modified diagnostic criteria have been developed, such as the DC-LD [38] and DM-ID [39] (Fletcher et al 2016), to inform the diagnostic process. These modified diagnostic criteria seek to balance

the tension between making them more applicable to the assessment of a population of people with impaired language development on the one hand, and on the other, ensuring that such modified criteria are still valid in terms of the condition they define. While for affective disorders, it may be possible to infer a depressed or manic state on the basis of observation or informant reports (tearfulness, agitation, over-activity, etc.), this is more problematic when it comes to the presence, or not, of thought disorder, hallucinations, or delusions. Illnesses such as schizophrenia are manifestations of disorders of brain mechanisms that underpin thought and perception, and if these have not fully developed, it remains uncertain whether they can be further impaired.

Based on the earlier work of Sovner, Hurley et al. (2016) [35] have summarized the specific problems that may lead to diagnostic uncertainty when assessing a person with an ID. These include: the baseline exaggeration of symptoms (such as self-injury) in times of stress; intellectual distortion in terms of the person's understanding of the questions being asked about his/her mental state and an inability to appreciate the implications of the question; psychosocial masking whereby the symptomatology that occurs may be best understood within a developmental framework but is misconstrued as a manifestation of mental illness; and cognitive disintegration whereby a person with an ID may become grossly disorganized and apparently psychotic due to a lack of cognitive reserve, resulting in a more severe response to the development of a mental illness.

Being aware of these problems and taking a detailed developmental and longitudinal history in order to establish firstly a developmental diagnosis (ID, autistic spectrum disorder, ADHD) and secondly the presence, or not, of a comorbid diagnosis (mood disorder, dementia, etc.) is essential. However, a wider diagnostic approach also draws upon other conceptual models of understanding such as those of applied behavioural analysis.

The purpose of assessment in the context of concerns about a person's behaviour is therefore to arrive at an understanding and to develop a formulation that sets out how the behaviour or problem in question is best understood in terms of these models. This then guides the interventions that follow. These may be as varied as reducing anxiety by improving understanding and reducing the un-predictability of the social environment through the use of visual support, the development of strategies for defusing and best managing challenging behaviour, and the treatment of comorbid physical illness or mental ill health. Formulations should acknowledge the uncertainties that exist and ensure appropriate observations enable a systematic evaluation of the outcomes of a specific approach. Documentation of the assessment and the thinking that led to a particular intervention is essential and of great value, as it allows others now or in the future to better understand how a person's problems at that time were conceptualized.

## Conclusions: the integration of perspectives

The core dimensions that make up the diagnostic criteria that define what is meant by the term 'intellectual disability' have been set out at the beginning of this chapter. The diagnostic criteria do not do justice to the complexity of the issues and have been supplemented by different ways of thinking that have emphasized the multi-dimensional and interactive nature of how we understand the link between impairments in brain development, the impact on function, and, in turn, the effect on quality of life and well-being. It is rarely sufficient simply to state that someone meets the criteria for having an ID. There is the need to consider the barriers that are limiting choice and opportunity. In recent years, there has been a bringing together of social and biomedical models of ID, appreciating that each has its place. Health and social support needs cannot be separated readily, as each depends on the other. With advances in our understanding of the causes of ID, it has also become clear that genetically determined neurodevelopmental syndromes have their own specific atypical developmental trajectories that may also include the emergence of particular patterns of maladaptive behaviours or an increased risk for developing comorbid mental and physical disorders that require treatment in their own right.

While ID falls within the group of disorders known as 'mental disorders', the health and social care needs of the majority of people with ID will not be met through child or adult mental health services, but instead in childhood by paediatric, child development, and family support services, and in adult life, by social services and primary care. However, for those whose mental state or behaviour causes concern and brings them in contact with specialist services for people with ID or with mental health services, there is an additional layer of assessment. The core dimensions of any assessment includes, but is not limited to, only a biomedical diagnostic approach. The application of different theoretical perspectives leading to a wider diagnostic perspective is required that seeks to understand why this problem has affected an individual in a specific way at this time. It is this process of assessment, often requiring expertise from different disciplines and information not only from the person him-/herself, but also his/her family and paid support providers and observations over time, which inform intervention. These interventions are often directly with the family or at the interface with social care and, as has been illustrated, may well take many forms.

## REFERENCES

1. Begab, M.J. and Laveck, G.D. (1972). Mental retardation: development of an international classification scheme. *American Journal of Psychiatry*, 128, 1437–8.
2. Penrose, L. (1949). *The biology of mental defect*. Sidgwick & Jackson Ltd, London.
3. Foster, A., Titheradge, H., and Morton, J. (2015). Genetics of learning disability. *Paediatrics and Child Health*, 25, 450–7.
4. McCoy, D.C., Peet, E.D., Ezzati, M., *et al.* (2016). Early childhood developmental status in low- and middle-income countries: national, regional, and global prevalence estimates using predictive modeling. *PLoS Medicine*, 14, e1002233.
5. Rutter, M., Tizard, J., and Whitmore, K. (1970). *Education, health and behaviour*. Longman Publishing Group, London.
6. Cooper, S.A., Smiley, E., Morrison, J., Williamson, A., and Allan, L. (2007). Mental ill-health in adults with intellectual disabilities: prevalence and associated factors. *British Journal of Psychiatry,* 190, 27–35.
7. Shakespeare, T. and Watson, N. (2001). The social model of disability: an outdated ideology? In: Barnartt, S.N. and Altman, B.M. (eds.) *Exploring theories and expanding methodologies: where we are and where we need to go (Research in Social Science and Disability, Volume 2)*. Emerald Group Publishing Limited, Bingley. pp. 9–28.
8. American Psychiatric Association. (2013). *Diagnostic and statistical manual of mental disorder (DSM-V)*. American Psychiatric Association, Washington, DC.
9. American Association on Intellectual and Developmental Disabilities. (2010). *Intellectual disability: definition, classification, and systems of support*. American Association on Intellectual and Developmental Disabilities, Washington, DC.
10. World Health Organization. (1980). *International Classification of Impairments, Disabilities and Handicaps*. World Health Organization, Geneva.
11. World Health Organization. (2001). *International Classification of Functioning, Disability and Health*. World Health Organization, Geneva.
12. World Health Organization. (1993). *The ICD-10 Classification of Mental and Behavioural Disorders. Clinical descriptions and diagnostic guidelines.* World Health Organization, Geneva.
13. Bertelli, M.O., Munir, K. Harris, J. and Salvador-Carulla, L. (2016). 'Intellectual developmental disorders': reflections on the international consensus document for redefining 'mental retardation-intellectual disability' in ICD-11. *Advances in Mental Health and Intellectual Disabilities*, 10, 36–58.
14. Shakespeare, T. (2006). *Disability rights and wrongs*. Routledge, New York, NY.
15. Birch, H.G., Richardson, S.A., Baird, D., Horobin, G., and Illsley, R. (1970). *Mental subnormality in the community: a clinical and epidemiologic study*. Williams & Wilkins Co., Baltimore, MD.
16. Sondenaa, E., Rasmussen, K., Nottestad, J.A., and Lauvrad, C. (2010). Prevalence of intellectual disabilities in Norway: domestic variation. *Journal of Intellectual Disability Research*, 54, 161–7.
17. McConkey, R., Mulvany, F., and Barron. S. (2006). Adult persons with intellectual disabilities in the island of Ireland. *Journal of Intellectual Disability Research*, 50, 227–36.
18. Larson, S.A., Lakin, C.L., Anderson, L., Kwak, N., Lee, J.H., and Anderson, D. (2001). Prevalence of mental retardation and developmental disabilities: estimates from the 1994/1995 National

Health Interview Survey Disabilities Supplements. *American Journal on Mental Retardation*, 106, 231–54.

19. Wen, X. (1997). *The definition and prevalence of intellectual disabilities in Australia*. Australian Institute of Health and Welfare, Canberra.

20. Fujiura, G.T. and Taylor, S.J. (2003). Continuum of intellectual disability: demographic evidence for the 'forgotten generation'. *Mental Retardation*, 41, 420–9.

21. Zimmerman, M. (2009). Iodine deficiency. *Endocrine Reviews*, 30, 376–408.

22. Kaminsky, E.B., Kaul, V., Paschall, J., *et al.* (2011). An evidence-based approach to establish the functional and clinical significance of copy number variants in intellectual and developmental disabilities. *Genetics in Medicine*, 13, 777–84.

23. Miller, D.T., Adam, M.P., Aradhya, S., *et al.* (2010). Consensus statement: chromosomal microarray is a first-tier clinical diagnostic test for individuals with developmental disabilities or congenital anomalies. *American Journal of Human Genetics*, 86, 749–64.

24. Firth, H.V., Richards, S.M., Bevan, A.P., *et al.* (2009). DECIPHER: Database of Chromosomal Imbalance and Phenotype in Humans using Ensembl Resources. *American Journal of Human Genetics*, 84, 524–33.

25. Holland, A.J., Whittington, J.E. Butler, J., Webb, T., Boer, H., and Clarke, D.J. (2003). Behavioural phenotypes associated with specific genetic disorders: evidence from a population-based study of people with Prader-Willi syndrome. *Psychological Medicine*, 33, 141–53.

26. Holland, A.J., Hon, J., Huppert, F.A., Stevens, F., and Watson, P. (1998). A population-based study of the prevalence and presentation of dementia in adults with Down syndrome. *British Journal of Psychiatry*, 172, 493–8.

27. Woodruff-Borden, J., Kistler, D.J., Henderson, D.R., Crawford, N.A., and Mervis, C.B. (2010). Longitudinal course of anxiety in children and adolescents with Williams syndrome. *American Journal of Medical Genetics Part C: Seminars in Medical Genetics*, 154C, 277–90.

28. Arron, K., Oliver, C., Berg, K., Moss, J., and Burbidge, C. (2011). Prevalence and phenomenology of self-injurious and aggressive behaviour in genetic syndromes. *Journal of Intellectual Disability Research*, 55, 109–20.

29. Nyhan, W. (1972). Behavioral phenotypes in organic genetic disease: presidential address to the Society for Pediatric Research, May 1, 1971. *Pediatric Research*, 6, 1–9.

30. Karmiloff-Smith, A. and Thomas, M. (2003). What can developmental disorders tell us about the neurocomputational constraints that shape development? The case of Williams syndrome. *Development and Psychopathology*, 15, 969–90.

31. Reiss, A.L. and Dant, C.C. (2003). The behavioural neurogenetics of fragile-X syndrome: gene-brain-behaviour relationships in child developmental psychopathologies. *Development and Psychopathology*, 15, 927–68.

32. Harris, J.C. (2003). Social neuroscience, empathy, brain integration, and neurodevelopmental disorders. *Physiology and behavior*, 79, 525–31.

33. Oliver, C., Adams, D., Allen, D., *et al.* (2013). Causal models of clinically significant behaviors in Angelman, Cornelia de Lange, Prader-Willi and Smith-Magenis syndromes. *International Review of Research in Developmental Disabilities*, 44, 167–211.

34. Boer, H., Holland, A.J., Whittington, J., Butler, J., Webb, T., and Clarke, D. (2002). Psychotic illness in people with Prader Willi Syndrome due to chromosome 15 maternal uniparental disomy. *The Lancet*, 359, 135–6.

35. Hurley, A.D., Levitas, A., Luiselli, J.K., Moss, S., Bradley, E.A., and Bailey, N.M. (2016). Assessment and diagnostic procedures. In: Fletcher, R.J., Barnhill, J., and Cooper, S.-A. *Diagnostic manual—intellectual disability: a textbook of diagnosis of mental disorders in persons with intellectual disabilities* (2nd edn). NADD Press, New York, NY.

36. O'Reilly M.F. and Leslie, J.C. (2016). *Behaviour Analysis. Foundations and Applications to Psychology*. Psychology Press, London.

37. Melville, C.A., Johnson, P.C., Smiley, E., Simpson, N., Purves, D., McConnachie, A., and Cooper, S.A. (2016). Problem behaviours and symptom dimensions of psychiatric disorders in adults with intellectual disabilities: an exploratory and confirmatory factor analysis. *Research in Developmental Disabilities*, 55, 1–13.

38. Cooper, S.A., Melville, C.A., and Einfeld, S.L. (2003). Psychiatric diagnosis, intellectual disabilities and Diagnostic Criteria for Psychiatric Disorders for Use with Adults with Learning Disabilities/Mental Retardation (DC-LD) *Journal of Intellectual Disability Research*, 47, 3–15.

39. Fletcher, R.J., Barnhill, J., and Cooper, S.-A. (eds) (2016). *Diagnostic manual—intellectual disability: a textbook of diagnosis of mental disorders in persons with intellectual disability*. NADD Press, New York, NY.

# 22

# Epidemiology and course of intellectual disabilities

*Sally-Ann Cooper*

## Prevalence of intellectual disabilities

Intellectual disabilities are not uncommon. A meta-analysis of 52 studies reported the prevalence of intellectual disabilities to be 10.37/1000 population [1]. Prevalence varied according to age, income group of the country of origin (with higher rates from low-income countries), and study design. In high-income countries, rates for all ages combined were 9.2/1000, with the highest rates in child/young person populations only at 18.3/1000, and the lowest rates in adult-only populations at 4.9/1000. Careful understanding of the nuances is needed though to interpret these findings. Twenty-five of the studies included in the meta-analysis did not provide their age range; a further two did not report their observation period, and some studies were outliers in their findings.

An earlier review of studies between 1960 and 1987 is of lesser relevance to today's population, given cohort effects, almost all were studies in childhood/youth, and some provided very limited methodological information [2].

Studies of prevalence are, of course, challenging to conduct, as they ideally require intelligence to be tested on whole populations and therefore would incur considerable resources and costs. Other approaches can provide useful information, for example:

- Studies of administrative samples, such as people known to local authorities, which account for the majority of studies. These are the people who are making demands upon services, so the information is useful, but there are likely to be some people with intellectual disabilities not included in these samples and some people who do not have intellectual disabilities within the sample. For example, a rate of 4.3/1,000 aged 16+ was reported from Welsh local authorities as being in receipt or in need of intellectual disabilities services [3].
- Studies of people with a record of intellectual disabilities in their general practitioner medical records. In high-income countries, people are likely to have been assessed once their developmental delay was reported, so a record is likely to exist. However, this is complicated by the multiple and changing terminology in use over time. For example, a rate of 5.4/1000 patients aged 18+ was reported from an English database of 451 practices [4].

- Other secondary analysis of data routinely collected for other purposes. These have the attraction that large and whole-country samples can be analysed at relatively little costs, but findings reflect the original definitions used and the ways the data were collected. For example, a rate of 4.9/1000 aged 16+ (self-/proxy report) was reported from an analysis of Scotland's 2011 census [5], and a rate of 23/1000 school-aged children/young persons (teacher report) was reported from Scotland's 2015 pupil census [6].

Population intelligence approximates to a normal distribution, with a mean intelligence quotient of 100 and a standard deviation of 15 points. A statistical definition of intellectual impairments is an intelligence quotient less than two standard deviations from the mean, that is, <70. Simplistically, this would suggest that 2.3% of the population have intellectual impairments. However:

- The greatest deviation from the normal distribution of intelligence is at the extreme ends.
- A test error of 5 points is recognized—and a normal distribution would place 2.5% *within* the range of 70–75, so this can greatly influence identified prevalence.
- There is the Flynn effect (overly high scores due to out-of-date test norms).
- Intellectual disabilities is a social construct, not simply a statistical measure of impairments; the definitions of intellectual disabilities in the standard classificatory manuals ICD-10 [7] and DSM-5 [8] also include the functional requirement of the need for additional support. People learn throughout their lives, and so a child with an intelligence quotient of 69 will need additional educational support at school but, as an adult, may gradually acquire life skills to live independently, maintain relationships, hold employment, raise children, and not identify with intellectual disabilities nor be identified by others as having intellectual disabilities or put demand on services designed for people with intellectual disabilities.
- In countries that provide additional educational support for children with intellectual disabilities, there is a clear advantage to having the label, and flexibility in its use is beneficial for children with abilities that are a little above an intelligence quotient of 70 ('borderline' intellectual disabilities).

- People with intellectual disabilities experience premature death; hence, the proportion of the population with intellectual disabilities progressively falls within older age groups.
- Some children are not identified as having mild intellectual disabilities until they attend school, so rates are lower in pre-schoolers than in school-aged children.
- Cohort effects can influence rates over time, for example, the zika virus epidemic in South America in 2015–2016 causing microcephaly, immunization, iodine, maternal smoking, and alcohol use, changes in termination rates of children with Down syndrome (currently falling, but could possibly increase with the introduction of first-trimester diagnosis) [9], improved antenatal, perinatal, and neonatal health care, increased survival of very low-birthweight infants, identification and treatment of metabolic causes of intellectual disabilities like phenylketonuria, better childhood education, access to cardiac surgery for children with Down syndrome, improved lifestyles, and access to health care.
- Migration and clustering (for example, congregate care and colonies) can influence spatial patterning at local levels and can be influenced by economic factors and local policy.
- Prevalence of mild intellectual disabilities is influenced by many cultural and societal factors that determine whether a mild learning impairment is likely to result in a functional disability, contributing to geographic differences.
- Clearly, there is an intellectual gradient across the population, and the 'cut-off' of 70 is purely arbitrary. Indeed, the accepted 'cut-off' was changed in 1973, substantially affecting rates.

Despite these complexities, there are some reasonably consistent findings across studies:

- In high-income countries, about 5/1000 adults have intellectual disabilities, falling to about 2/1000 over the age of 65 years.
- Prevalence is higher in children and young people than in adults.
- Prevalence is higher in boys/men than girls/women; across the whole of Scotland, 58% of people with intellectual disabilities are male [5].
- Prevalence is higher in low-income countries than in high- and middle-income countries for multiple reasons, including lifestyle and health care, although in areas that are less driven by technology, having mild intellectual impairments may be less disabling.
- The great majority of people with intellectual impairments have mild intellectual impairments (6 mild impairment: 1 moderate to profound impairments), and the majority with intellectual impairments in whom this is disabling have mild, rather than severe, intellectual disabilities.

## Causes of intellectual disabilities

People with intellectual disabilities have some characteristics in common such as needing additional educational support at school, finding it hard to manage money and bills without help as an adult, and having difficulties remembering the temporal sequencing of events. Every person with intellectual disabilities is also unique. Each child inherits a range of genetic information from both their parents which is not shared with other children with intellectual disabilities, and their environment and experiences shape their development, interests, likes, and ambitions. So even people with a clear genetic cause for their intellectual disabilities, such as Down syndrome, are unique from all other persons with Down syndrome, while sharing some characteristics.

Identifying the cause of intellectual disabilities is undertaken by paediatricians and clinical geneticists.

### Genetic factors

Genetic studies indicate intelligence is highly heritable and can itself be conceptualized as a spectrum of syndromes [10]. Additionally, there are many genetic causes of intellectual disabilities, and recent and ongoing studies have found numerous copy number variants associated with developmental disorders, with the challenge of identifying which are clinically relevant. As described in Chapter 23, genetic conditions include:

- Chromosomal anomalies. Examples are trisomies—Down syndrome (trisomy 21), Patau's syndrome (trisomy 13), Edwards' syndrome (trisomy 18); autosomal deletions, for example, cri-du-chat syndrome (terminal deletion of chromosome 15), Williams syndrome (deletion on chromosome 7), and Prader–Willi syndrome and Angelman's syndrome (deletion on chromosome 15 or uniparental disomy); and sex-linked conditions, for example, fragile X syndrome.
- Autosomal and sex-linked recessive conditions (particularly in communities with high rates of consanguinity). Examples are phenylketonuria; homocystinuria; galactosaemia; lipid disorders—Tay–Sachs disease, Gaucher disease, Niemann–Pick disease; and mucopolysaccharidoses—Hunter's disease and Hurler's disease.
- Autosomal and sex-linked dominant conditions. Examples include tuberous sclerosis and neurofibromatosis.

Regarding the prevalence of individual conditions in childhood:

- 1/800 has Down syndrome.
- 1/3600 boys and 1/4000–6000 girls have fragile-X syndrome.
- 1/7500 has Williams syndrome.
- 1/10,000 has Cornelia de Lange.
- 1/10,000–25,000 has Prader–Willi syndrome.
- 1/15,000 has Angelman syndrome.
- 1/20,000 has Smith–Magenis syndrome.
- 1/50,000 has cri-du-chat syndrome.

In addition to causing intellectual disabilities, physical conditions, and influencing trajectories, these genetic conditions can cause a range of other cognitive, behavioural, and mental health problems, for which the term 'behavioural phenotype' is used. Behavioural phenotypes have attracted particular research attention and can inform clinical assessments. Examples include high rates of dementia in middle-aged and older adults with Down syndrome [11, 12]; affective psychosis in Prader–Willi syndrome [13, 14]; self-injurious behaviour in Smith–Magenis syndrome [15]; and depression in phenylketonuria [16]. While these behaviours/mental ill health are genetically driven, it is important to avoid therapeutic nihilism, as interventions may help the individual. Additionally, some genetic syndromes effect physiological differences, which influence treatment choices, for example, the low rates of heart disease and low blood pressure in Down syndrome, differing immunology causing high rates of thyroid disorders and other immunological disorders, and different mechanisms in dementia aetiology (an amyloid model), compared to typical Alzheimer disease. The length of this chapter precludes a detailed consideration of behavioural phenotypes, other than highlighting that clinicians do need to identify if their patient/client has a recognized genetic condition, and its associated physiological patterns.

## Antenatal factors

Antenatal factors include:

- Teratogenic drugs and toxins. Examples include alcohol.
- Infections. Examples include toxoplasmosis, rubella, cytomegalovirus, herpes simplex, syphilis, zika virus, and other infections.
- Fetal growth retardation. Examples include placental dysfunction and hypoxia.
- Endocrine. Examples include iodine deficiency.

## Perinatal factors

Perinatal factors include:

- Birth injury, especially in premature and low-birthweight infants.
- Kernicterus.
- Infections.

## Postnatal factors

Postnatal factors include:

- Infections, encephalitis.
- Toxins.
- Brain tumours.
- Head injury.
- Starvation.

Extreme prematurity has been shown to account for 17% of cases of intellectual disabilities; together, gestational age and birthweight centile have been reported to account for 26.6% of intellectual disabilities [17]. The month of conception (January–March conception, compared with summer conception) has been reported to account for 15% of intellectual disabilities, postulated to be related to vitamin D or infections at the critical first trimester stage of development [18]. Fetal alcohol syndrome is underdiagnosed.

## Mental ill health

Two recent systematic reviews reported that mental ill health is more common in children, young people, and adults with intellectual disabilities than in the general population [19, 20]. Problem behaviours, such as aggressive, self-injurious, and destructive behaviour, are very common in people with intellectual disabilities and do not have an obvious comparator in the general population. Widely reported prevalence rates have been given in view of differences in populations studied (some from mental health services and so their rates are biased and inflated), methods used to identify mental ill health, the types of conditions included within the reported mental ill health (particularly whether or not problem behaviours and/or autism are included), the diagnostic criteria used

(ICD-10 and DSM-5 under-report mental ill health in this population if strictly applied, especially for problem behaviours), and whether studies are reporting point or lifetime prevalences or fail to indicate which [21].

It is not surprising that mental ill health is more common in people with intellectual disabilities, compared with the general population, in view of complex biological factors, psychological and social disadvantages, and additional developmental factors [22].

Population-based studies in children and young people with intellectual disabilities reported the prevalence of mental ill health, including problem behaviours, ranging from 30% [23, 24] to 50% [25]. A robust UK study reported a rate of 36% in 641 children and young people (aged 5–16 years) with intellectual disabilities, compared with 8% of 17,774 children without intellectual disabilities in the same surveys: the children and young people with intellectual disabilities accounted for 14% of all children with mental ill health [26].

Population-based studies in adults with intellectual disabilities reported the prevalence of mental ill health, *excluding* problem behaviours, ranging from 14.5% (when also excluding ADHD, autism, dementia, and personality disorder, people aged 65 and over, and people with severe intellectual disabilities [27]) to 43.8% (adults with moderate to profound intellectual disabilities only [28]). The largest adult population-based prevalence study, in which each person was individually assessed, included 1023 adults with intellectual disabilities [29]. It reported a point prevalence of mental ill health of 40.9%, or 28.3% excluding problem behaviours, and used more robust methods than previous smaller studies [30, 31].

Some types of mental ill health are more common in people with intellectual disabilities, including schizophrenia [32, 33], bipolar disorder [34], dementia (particularly in adults with Down syndrome), but also in adults with intellectual disabilities of other or unknown causes [35, 36], autism [26, 37, 38], ADHD [26], and pica. Prevalence rates of mental ill health in children and young people with intellectual disabilities are reported to be higher than for other children and young people for 27 out of 28 ICD-10 categories [26]. Depression and anxiety are common in people with intellectual disabilities, but probably not more so than in the general population [34, 39].

Problem behaviours are very common in the population with intellectual disabilities. In a large-scale, population-based study of adults aged 16+ years, 22.5% were reported to have problem behaviours [29], and of those, 10% had aggressive behaviour [40] and 5% had self-injurious behaviour [41].

The incidence of mental ill health in adults, excluding problem behaviours, has been reported to be 12.6% over a 2-year period—8.3% for affective disorders, 1.7% for anxiety disorders, and 1.4% for psychotic disorders [42, 33]. The incidence of dementia has also been reported for older adults with intellectual disabilities NOT due to Down syndrome and found to be considerably higher than for the age-matched general population. At the age of 65 years or older, the standardized incidence ratio for dementia was 4.98 [43]. Regarding problem behaviours, the 2-year incidence of aggression was reported as 1.8%, and of self-injury 0.6% [40, 41]. Full remission of psychosis after 2 years was only 14.3% [33], aggression 27.7%, and self-injury 38.2% [40, 41]. These findings suggest that while incidences are higher than those found in the general population, much of the current high prevalence of mental ill health is due to enduring disorders, rather than new episodes, though research on this is limited in quantity.

Studies on common types of mental ill health using general population longitudinal cohorts show high and enduring rates of depression and anxiety in adults with intellectual disabilities, compared with the general population [44–46]. These studies have the attraction of drawing direct comparisons with the general population but included few people with intellectual disabilities, and of those, most had mild learning disabilities and very few severe intellectual disabilities, in view of their design and also with differential loss to follow-up of people with intellectual disabilities, so findings may be biased.

Longitudinal studies have also reported on the mental ill health of children and young people with intellectual disabilities. In an Australian cohort study, children and young people aged 4–19.5 years were followed over four waves of data collection over 14 years. High rates of psychopathology levels were reported, with hyperactivity more prominent at younger ages and persisting for longer in children/young people with more severe degrees of intellectual disabilities. Emotional disorders emerged later in childhood [47–49]. Similar findings have been reported from longitudinal studies in children with intellectual disabilities/borderline intellectual disabilities (excluding those with more severe intellectual disabilities or with additional sensory or physical disabilities) in the Netherlands [50, 51].

### Neurodevelopmental disorders cluster

Gillberg coined the term 'ESSENCE' (Early Symptomatic Syndromes Eliciting Neurodevelopmental Clinical Examination) to describe this [52]. He defined ESSENCE as major problems in: motor skills; general development; speech and language; social interaction and communication; behaviour; hyperactivity or impulsivity; hypoactivity; inattention; and sleep or feeding difficulties. Genetic data also increasingly support clustering of neurodevelopmental (including epilepsy) and mental health problems [53].

## Physical ill health, disabilities, and multi-morbidity

Additional physical ill health and disabilities are common in people with intellectual disabilities. Indeed multi-morbidity is typical for people with intellectual disabilities [4, 54], and hence too is polypharmacy. This has implications, as it adds complexity to mental and physical health assessments (for example, distinguishing between complex partial seizures, depression, and anti-epileptic drug side effects), in assessments that are also challenging due to communication needs, impairment of understanding, and visual and hearing impairments, all of which are common in people with intellectual disabilities. This probably contributes to the under-recognition of mental ill health that occurs in this population. It also means that there are more disease–disease, drug–disease, and drug–drug interactions to take account of when managing conditions. For example, postural problems and deformities (common in people with cerebral palsy and people with profound intellectual disabilities) impact upon gastro-oesophageal reflux disease (GORD), which is extremely common in people with intellectual disabilities, more so the more severe their intellectual disabilities, and can cause anxiety. GORD

occurs in about 50% of adults with intellectual disabilities; a consequence is that drugs to manage osteoporosis cannot be tolerated, and osteoporosis is common in this population. Many psychotropic drugs, commonly prescribed for people with intellectual disabilities, lower the seizure threshold, and epilepsy is common. People with intellectual disabilities may not be able to self-report drug side effects and are reliant on others observing these; hence, pharmacovigilance is essential. Anticholinergic burden due to polypharmacy of drugs with these side effects is an issue for people with intellectual disabilities, with potential negative side effects such as further impairment of cognition [55].

Long-term conditions are more common for adults with intellectual disabilities, compared to the general population. Children, young people, and adults with intellectual disabilities have higher rates of epilepsy (25% [56]), visual impairment (50%), hearing impairment (40%), impacted cerumen, GORD (50% [57]), dysphagia [58], constipation, diabetes, thyroid dysfunction, osteoporosis, contractures, mobility and balance impairments, injuries, eczema, xerosis, obesity, and heart failure, compared with the general population [4, 54, 59, 60]. Asthma is also reported to be more common in people with intellectual disabilities and may be due to obesity, but it is possible that some of this is a misdiagnosis of reflux pneumonitis or aspiration pneumonia. In some cases, the excess physical ill health burden relates to the person's underlying cause of intellectual disabilities (for example, thyroid dysfunction and Down syndrome), but lifestyle and environmental factors and suboptimal support and health care are also important contributors. Some problems predispose to others. For example, psychotropic drugs (prescribed to about 20% of the adult population with intellectual disabilities) [61] can increase diabetes risk, as can obesity which is common [62], and sedentary lifestyles, also common [63]).

In view of the shorter life expectancy of people with more severe intellectual disabilities and those with syndromal causes for their intellectual disabilities, older adults with intellectual disabilities have different characteristics, compared with younger adults. Older adults as a group have milder levels of intellectual disabilities and lesser quantities of additional physical ill health. The profile of their health needs changes, as they have lower rates of the physical ill health and disabilities associated with severe intellectual disabilities but start to acquire physical ill health associated with ageing. In extreme old age, the health characteristics of people with intellectual disabilities becomes more like those of the general population.

## Lifespan

People with intellectual disabilities do not live as long as other people; and life expectancy is shorter, the more severe the person's intellectual disabilities. A recent systematic review included 27 studies and found that although life expectancy has improved in recent decades, it is lower, compared with the general population, by about 20 years, with no evidence of any closure of the inequality gap [64]. More severe intellectual disabilities and/or additional comorbidities were associated with the shortest life expectancy. Standardized mortality rates showed a greater inequality for women than for men, for reasons that are unknown. The main causes of death differed from the general population, with respiratory disease the most common, then circulatory diseases (with greater congenital, and lesser ischaemic, disease compared with the general population). Cancer was less common, compared with the general population, and the cancer profile differed from that in the general population.

Specific syndromes can also shorten life expectancy, including death *in utero* and in infancy and childhood. Life expectancy for people with Down syndrome has improved markedly over the last 50 years, with access to treatments for congenital heart disorders and improved surgical techniques and post-operative care accounting for much of this [65], but is still reported to be 30 years less than in the general population. Down syndrome has been reported to occur in 1.2/1000 pregnancies, of which 78.1% are live births. Survival at 1 year for live births in 1995–1999 was 91.6% [66], and 85% are estimated to survive to 10 years [67]. The proportion of people with Down syndrome reduces in older cohorts; 75% survive to 50 years, 50% to 58.6 years, and 25% to 62.9 years [68].

The shorter life expectancy of people with intellectual disabilities does not just relate to syndromal causes of death and multimorbidity. Some deaths are potentially avoidable, being amenable to good-quality care. A confidential inquiry reviewed 247 deaths of people with intellectual disabilities, finding that 22% were aged less than 50 years [69]. Avoidable deaths from causes that could have been amenable to good-quality health care occurred in 37%, compared with only 13% of the general population [69]. A further large-scale study (16,666 people with intellectual disabilities—656 deaths, compared with age-, gender-, and practice-matched controls, $n = 113,562$—1358 deaths) also found high rates of deaths amenable to good-quality health care at 37.0%, compared with 22.5% in the general population [70]. The authors also pointed out the standard definition of amenable deaths they used did not include some types of death that could be considered amenable to health care and which they found occurred more commonly in people with intellectual disabilities, including deaths from urinary tract infections and aspiration pneumonitis [70]. Hence, these disturbing figures are actually an undercount of the deaths amenable to good care that people with intellectual disabilities experience.

Improving health care for people with intellectual disabilities needs to become a priority for clinicians, service commissioners, and policymakers.

## REFERENCES

1. Maulik PK, Mascarenhas MN, Mathers CD, Dua T, Saxena S. Prevalence of intellectual disability: A meta-analysis of population-based studies. *Research in Developmental Disabilities*, 2011;32:419–36.
2. Roeleveld N, Zielhuis GA, Gabreels F. The prevalence of mental retardation: A critical review of recent literature. *Developmental Medicine and Child Neurology*, 1997;39:125–32.
3. Felce D. *Interpretation of intellectual disability in Wales for policy and strategic purposes*. Welsh Centre for Intellectual Disabilities, Cardiff. 12; 2004.
4. Carey, IM, Shah SM, Hosking FJ, *et al*. Health characteristics and consultation patterns of people with intellectual disability: a cross-sectional database study in English general practice. *British Journal of General Practice*, 2016;66:e264–70.
5. Scottish Learning Disabilities Observatory. *Scotland: population characteristics*. https://www.sldo.ac.uk/census-2011-information/learning-disabilities/topics/population/
6. Scottish Learning Disabilities Observatory. *Children and young people with disabilities and autism spectrum disorders identified through the Scottish Pupil Census*. https://www.sldo.ac.uk/projects/children-and-young-people-health/pupil-census/
7. World Health Organization. *The ICD-10 Classification of Mental and Behavioural Disorders*. Geneva: World Health Organization; 1990.
8. American Psychiatric Association. *Diagnostic and Statistical Manual of Mental Disorders*, fifth edition. Arlington, VA: American Psychiatric Association; 2013.
9. Jacobs M, Cooper S-A, McGowan R, Nelson S, Pell J. Pregnancy outcome following prenatal diagnosis of chromosomal anomaly: a record linkage study of 26,261 pregnancies. *PLoS One*. 2016;11:e0166909.
10. Davies G, Tenesa, A, Payton A, *et al*. Genome-wide association studies establish that human intelligence is highly heritable and polygenic. *Molecular Psychiatry*, 2011;16:996–1005.
11. Oliver C, Holland AJ. Down's syndrome and Alzheimer's disease: a review. *Psychological Medicine*, 1986;16:307–22.
12. Prasher VP. Age-specific prevalence, thyroid dysfunction and depressive symptomatology in adults with down syndrome and dementia. International *Journal of Geriatric Psychiatry*, 1995;10:25–31.
13. Beardsmore A, Dorman T, Cooper S-A, Webb T. Affective psychosis and Prader-Willi syndrome. *Journal of Intellectual Disabilities Research*, 1998;42:463–71.
14. Soni S, Whittington J, Holland AJ, *et al*. The course and outcome of psychiatric illness in people with Prader-Willi syndrome: implications for management and treatment. *Journal of Intellectual Disability Research*, 2007;51:32–42.
15. Taylor L, Oliver C. The behavioural phenotype of Smith-Magenis syndrome. Evidence for a gene-environment interaction. *Journal of Intellectual Disabilities Research*, 2008;52:830–41.
16. Pietz J, Fätkenheuer B, Burgard P, Armbruster M, Esser G, Schmidt H. Psychiatric Disorders in Adult Patients With Early-treated Phenylketonuria. *Pediatrics*, 1997;99:345–50.
17. Mackay DF, Smith GCS, Dobbie R, Cooper S-A, Pell JP. Obstetrics factors and different causes of special educational need: Retrospective cohort study of 407,503 schoolchildren. *British Journal of Obstetrics and Gynaecology*, 2013;120:297–308.
18. Mackay DF, Smith GCS, Cooper S-A, *et al*. Month of conception and developmental disorders: A record-linkage study of 801,603 children. *American Journal of Epidemiology*, 2016;184:485–93.
19. Buckles J, Luckasson R, Keefe, E. A Systematic Review of the Prevalence of Psychiatric Disorders in Adults With Intellectual Disability, 2003–2010. *Journal of Mental Health Research in Intellectual Disabilities*, 2013;6:181–207.
20. Einfeld SL, Ellis LA, Emerson E. Comorbidity of intellectual disability and mental disorder in children and adolescents: a systematic review. *Journal of Intellectual and Developmental Disabilities*, 2011;36:137–43.
21. Smiley E. Epidemiology of mental health problems in adults with learning disability: an update. *Advances in Psychiatric Treatment*, 2005;11:214–22.
22. Simpson N, Mizen L, Cooper S-A. Intellectual disabilities. *Medicine*, 2016;44:679–82.
23. Rutter M, Tizard J, Whitmore K. *Education, Health and Behaviour*. London: Longman; 1970.
24. Birch HG, Richardson SA, Baird D, Horobin G, Illsley R. *Mental Subnormality in the Community: A Clinical and Epidemiological Study*. Baltimore, MD: Williams and Wilkins; 1970.

25. Dekker MC, Koot HM, van der Ende J, Verhulst FC. Emotional and behavioural problems in chidren and adolescents with and without intellectual disabilities. *Journal of Child Psychology and Psychiatry*, 2002;43:1087–98.

26. Emerson E, Hatton C. Mental health of children and adolescents with intellectual disabilities in Britain. *British Journal of Psychiatry*, 2007;191:493–9.

27. Deb S, Thomas M, Bright, C. Mental disorder in adults with intellectual disability. 1: Prevalence of functional psychiatric illness among a community-based population aged between 16 and 64 years. *Journal of Intellectual Disability Research*, 2001;45:495–505.

28. Bailey N. Prevalence of psychiatric disorders in adults with moderate to profound learning disabilities, *Advances in Mental Health and Learning Disabilities*, 2007;1:36–44.

29. Cooper S-A, Smiley E, Morrison J, Allan L, Williamson, A. Prevalence of and associations with mental ill-health in adults with intellectual disabilities. *British Journal of Psychiatry*, 2007;190:27–35.

30. Cooper S- A, Bailey NM. Psychiatric disorders amongst adults with learning disabilities: prevalence and relationship to ability level. *Irish Journal of Psychological Medicine*, 2001;18:45–53.

31. Corbett JA. Psychiatric morbidity and mental retardation. In: James FE, Snaith RP (eds). *Psychiatric Illness and Mental Handicap*, pp. 11–25. London: Gaskell Press; 1979.

32. Turner TH. Schizophrenia and mental handicap: an historical review, with implications for further research. *Psychological Medicine*, 1989;19:301–14.

33. Cooper S-A, Smiley E, Morrison J, *et al*. Psychosis and adults with intellectual disabilities. Prevalence, incidence, and related factors. *Social Psychiatry and Psychiatric Epidemiology*, 2007;42:530–6.

34. Cooper S-A, Smiley E, Allan L, Morrison J. The incidence of unipolar and bipolar depression and mania in adults with intellectual disabilities. Prospective cohort study. *British Journal of Psychiatry*, 2018;212:295–300.

35. Cooper S-A. High prevalence of dementia amongst people with learning disabilities not attributed to Down's syndrome. *Psychological Medicine*, 1997;27:609–16.

36. Strydom A, Livingston G, King M, Hassiotis A. Prevalence of dementia in intellectual disability using different diagnostic criteria. *British Journal of Psychiatry*, 2007;191:150–7.

37. Baird G, Simonoff E, Pickles A, et al. Prevalence of disorders of the autism spectrum in a population cohort of children in South Thames: the Special Needs and Autism Project (SNAP). *The Lancet*, 2006;368:210–15.

38. Brugha TS, Spiers N, Bankart J, *et al*. Epidemiology of autism in adults across age groups and ability levels. *British Journal of Psychiatry*, 2016;209:498–503.

39. Reid K, Smiley E, Cooper S-A. Prevalence and associations with anxiety disorders in adults with intellectual disabilities. *Journal of Intellectual Disability Research*, 2011;55:172–81.

40. Cooper S-A, Smiley E, Jackson A, *et al*. Adults with intellectual disabilities. Prevalence, incidence, and remission of aggressive behaviour, and related factors. *Journal of Intellectual Disability Research*, 2009;53:217–32.

41. Cooper S-A, Smiley E, Allan L, *et al*. Adults with intellectual disabilities. Prevalence, incidence and remission of self-injurious behaviour, and related factors. *Journal of Intellectual Disability Research*, 2009;53:200–16.

42. Smiley E, Cooper S-A, Finlayson J, *et al*. The incidence, and predictors of mental ill-health in adults with intellectual disabilities. Prospective study. *British Journal of Psychiatry*, 2007;191:313–19.

43. Strydom A, Chan T, King M, Hassiotis A, Livingston G. Incidence of dementia in older adults with intellectual disabilities. *Research in Developmental Disabilities*, 2013;34:1881–5.

44. Maughan B, Collishaw S, Pickles A. Mild mental retardation: psychosocial functioning in adulthood. *Psychological Medicine*, 1999;29:351–66.

45. Collishaw S, Maughan B, Pickles A. Affective problems in adults with mild learning disability: the roles of social disadvantage and ill health. *British Journal of Psychiatry*, 2004;185:350–1.

46. Richards M, Maughan B, Hardy R, Hall I, Strydom A, Wadsworth M. Long-term affective disorder in people with learning disability. *British Journal of Psychiatry*, 2001;170:523–7.

47. Einfeld SL, Tonge, BJ. Population prevalence of psychopathology in children and adolescents with intellectual disability: II epidemiological findings. *Journal of Intellectual Disability Research*, 1996;40:99–109.

48. Tonge BJ, Einfeld SL. Psychopathology and Intellectual Disability: The Australian Child to Adult Longitudinal Study. *International Review of Research in Mental Retardation*, 2003;26:61–91.

49. Einfeld SL, Piccinin AM, Mackinnon A, *et al*. Psychopathology in Young People With Intellectual Disability. *Journal of the American Medical Association*, 2006;296:1981–9.

50. Wallander JL, Dekker MC, Koot HM. Risk factors for psychopathology in children with intellectual disability: a prospective longitudinal population-based study. *Journal of Intellectual Disability Research*, 2006;50:259–68.

51. De Ruiter KP, Dekker MC, Frank C. Verhulst FC, Koot HM. Developmental course of psychopathology in youths with and without intellectual disabilities. *Journal of Child Psychology and Psychiatry*, 2007;48:498–507.

52. Gillberg C. The ESSENCE in child psychiatry: Early Symptomatic Syndromes Eliciting Neurodevelopmental Clinical Examinations. *Research in Developmental Disabilities*, 2010;31:1543–51.

53. Moreno-De-Luca A, Myers SM, Challman TD, Moreno-De-Luca D, Evans DW, Ledbetter DH. Developmental Brain Dysfunction: Revival and Expansion of Old Concepts Based on New Genetic Evidence. *The Lancet Neurology*, 2013;12:406–14.

54. Cooper S-A, McLean G, Guthrie B, *et al*. Multiple physical and mental health comorbidity in adults with intellectual disabilities: population-based cross-sectional analysis. *BMC Family Practice*, 2015;16:110.

55. O'Dwyer M, Peklar J, McCallion P, McCarron M, Henman MC. Factors associated with polypharmacy and excessive polypharmacy in older people with Intellectual Disability differ from the general population; a cross-sectional observational nationwide study. *BMJ Open*, 2016;6:e010505.

56. Bowley C, Kerr M. Epilepsy and intellectual disability: invited review. *Journal of Intellectual Disability Research*, 2000;44:529–43.

57. Böhmer CJ, Niezen-de Boer MC, Klinkenberg-Knol EC, Deville WL, Nadorp JH, Meuwissen SG. The prevalence of gastroesophageal reflux disease in institutionalized intellectually disabled individuals. *American Journal of Gastroenterology*, 1999;94:804–10.

58. Robertson J, Chadwick D, Baines S, Emerson E, Hatton C. People with intellectual disabilities and dysphagia. *Disability Rehabilitation*. 2017;12:1–16.

59. McCarron M, Swinburne J, Burke E, McGlinchey E, Carroll R, McCallion P. Patterns of multimorbidity in an older population

of persons with an intellectual disability: results from the intellectual disability supplement to the Irish longitudinal study on aging (IDS-TILDA). *Research in Developmental Disabilities*, 2013;34:521–7.

60. Hermans H, Evenhuis HM. Multimorbidity in older adults with intellectual disabilities. *Research in Developmental Disabilities*, 2014;35:776–83.

61. Sheehan R, Hassiotis A, Walters K, Osborn D, Strydom A, Horsfall L. Mental illness, challenging behaviour, and psychotropic drug prescribing in people with intellectual disability: UK population based cohort study. *BMJ*, 2015;351:h4326.

62. Melville CA, Cooper S-A, Morrison J, Allan L, Smiley E, Williamson A. The prevalence and determinants of obesity in adults with intellectual disabilities. *Journal of Applied Research in Intellectual Disabilities*, 2008;21:425–37.

63. Finlayson J, Jackson A, Cooper S-A, *et al.* Understanding predictors of low physical activity in adults with intellectual disabilities. *Journal of Applied Research in Intellectual Disabilities*, 2009;22:236–47.

64. O'Leary L, Hughes-McCormack L, Cooper S-A. Life expectancy and causes of death of people with intellectual disabilities: a systematic review. *Journal of Applied Research in Intellectual Disabilities*, 2018;31:325–42.

65. Hijii T, Fukushige J, Igarashi H, *et al.* Life expectancy and social adaptation in individuals with Down syndrome with and without surgery for congenital heart disease. *Clinical Pediatrics*, 1997;37:327–32.

66. Bell R, Rankin J., Donaldson LJ. Northern congenital Abnormality Survey Steering Group. Down's syndrome: occurrence and outcome in the North of England 1985-99. *Paediatric and Perinatal Epidemiology*, 2003;17:33–39.

67. Leonard S, Bower C, Petterson B, Leonard H. Survival of infants born with Down's syndrome: 1980–96. *Paediatric and Perinatal Epidemiology*, 2000;14:163–71.

68. Glasson EJ, Sullivan SG, Hussain R, *et al.* The changing survival profile of people with Down syndrome: implications for genetic counseling. *Clinical Genetics*, 2002;62:390–3.

69. Heslop P, Blair PS, Fleming P, Hoghton M, Marriott A, Russ L. The Confidential Inquiry into premature deaths of people with intellectual disabilities in the UK: a population-based study. *The Lancet*, 2014;383:889–95.

70. Hosking FJ, Carey IM, Shah SM, *et al.* Mortality Among Adults With Intellectual Disability in England: Comparisons With the General Population. *American Journal of Public Health*, 2016;106:1483–90.

# 23

# Aetiology of intellectual disability and its clinical features

*Judith L. Rapoport, Dale Zhou, and Kwangmi Ahn*

## Causation

### The complexity of causes

Intellectual disability (ID) can follow many biological, environmental, and psychological events. Most do not directly, or inevitably, lead to ID. Genetic causes may be hereditary or non-hereditary and may or may not produce specific syndromes. It is no longer easy to separate genetic from non-genetic causes; for example, some environmental causes, such as lead, contribute to ID and can produce heritable epigenetic changes. In other disorders, environmental factors are more prominent or perhaps more easily measured. This is a rapidly changing area, as advances in genetic methodology and thr ability to share large samples have greatly increased the identification of genetic determinants of severe ID [1].

It is presumed that abnormality in prenatal brain development accounts for many, if not most, cases of ID. Neurological symptoms during the neonatal period are strongly associated with prenatal developmental disturbances. Placental insufficiency may lead to malnutrition, intrauterine growth retardation, and prematurity. One of the most important examples of impaired prenatal brain development is that of fetal alcohol spectrum disorders (FASD). Research on this very common cause of ID has focused on several neurotransmitters, insulin resistance, alterations of the hypothalamic–pituitary–adrenal (HPA) axis, oxidative stress, and epigenetic factors [2]. Other toxic substances, such as lead, not only contribute to intellectual impairment, but may also produce heritable epigenetic changes [3–5].

As discussed elsewhere, ID frequently coexists with other medical, neurological, and psychiatric disorders, which may further restrict interactions with the environment and further delay the development of the individual.

### Classifying causes

It is difficult to establish the prevalence of ID, as perhaps 70% of those so classified have relatively mild disturbance. Rates are higher among very low-birthweight infants, with substantial variations in rates of mild ID by socio-economic status, but similar rates for severe ID [6]. There are many possible bases for classifying causes. Here too, the issue is complex with respect to underlying brain abnormalities. Both genetic and non-genetic forms of ID share cellular and cortical neurophysiological pathogenetic signatures that result in anomalous function of pyramidal neurons [7].

Classification by timing may be more successful, although here too pre-existing risk factors, such as low iodine in certain geographic regions, complicate recommendations for screening for thyroid dysfunction [8, 9]. Thus, screening of environmental, maternal prenatal, and neonatal measures may all be indicated (for example, folic acid deficiency). Separating a group with known genetic syndromes has been useful to date, but because these syndromes are proliferating and often overlap substantially, it may be unclear in the future how helpful these will be as primary classifiers as the number of syndromes continue to *increase*.

This chapter is divided into four sections:

1. ID in which there are well-documented external prenatal environmental factors.
2. ID with salient genetic causes.
3. ID treatment and prevention.
4. ID-associated syndromes in which multiple clinical manifestations are apparent, in addition to ID (see Chapter 22).

The section on treatment and prevention focus on the nature and timing of treatment and preventive efforts.

## Prominent environmental causes

### External prenatal factors

*Fetal alcohol exposure*

Fetal alcohol spectrum disorder (as it is commonly called in the literature) is one of the main causes of ID worldwide and the leading non-hereditary cause of ID in Western geographic regions, with 1% of children in the United States affected. It is now identified in DSM-V through a specifier and is no longer a separate entity in ICD-11. Part of the reason for this diagnostic change is the variability in, and non-specificity of, neurological and physiognomic features. Research has focused on a broad array of physiological abnormalities, as well as epigenetic pathways [2]. Current treatment involves support to the families with symptom-focused cognitive and psychiatric remediation [10]. Future efforts must prepare for better strategies for the prevention of this major societal problem.

## Congenital hypothyroidism

The essential role of thyroid hormone in CNS maturation has been clearly demonstrated, and the critical period for this CNS dependency extends from fetal life to 24–36 months of age [9]. The benefit of early treatment was apparent, and with the availability of congenital hypothyroidism (CH) screening through assays for thyroxine and thyroid-stimulating hormone and an adaptation of these methods to the filter paper blood spots used for phenylketonuria (PKU) screening, CH screening is now a standard of care. The majority of children who were treated early experience normal growth and normal-range IQ values [11]. Widespread micronutrient deficiencies exist with pregnant women and their children under 5 years at highest risk. Iron, iodine, foliate, and zinc deficiencies are the most widespread and all contribute to poor growth and intellectual impairments [12].

## External postnatal factors

### Brain injury

Traffic accidents are a major source of brain trauma. Here too, multiple factors are involved in recovery [13, 14].

### Meningitis

Meningitis after the neonatal period can result in ID, particularly in severe cases. Lead is a potent neurotoxicant, with demonstrated effects on the brain of children and adults. There is a documented association between early life exposure to lead and impaired cognitive function in children. These impairments are influenced by the degree of exposure, indicated by childhood blood lead levels and sociodemographic factors, with impairment generally falling in the milder range [15, 16]. Early treatment is of great importance, alongside environmental monitoring.

## Salient genetic causes

Twin and family studies in various populations and patient cohorts revealed a strong genetic basis, with 30–90% heritability, depending on the diagnostic category and study design [17, 18]. Similar to IQ, mild ID (50 < IQ < 70) is heritable and caused by many genes of small effect [17, 19–22]. However, a major cause of severe ID could be rare, non-inheritable *de novo* point mutations [23–25], along with environmental factors [26, 27].

Genetic causes of ID are thought to account for 25–50% of ID cases and are more frequently observed in the group of severe ID, accounting for up to 65% [28–33]. Genetic causes of severe ID include chromosome aneusomies (aneuploidy and translocation), chromosome structural abnormalities, and monogenic disease. Unfortunately, ID displays extreme genetic locus heterogeneity, and about 50% of ID still remain without any molecular diagnosis [34]. ID shares some genetic mechanisms with the broader group of

neurodevelopmental disorders [30]. The combination of novel technology, such as next-generation sequencing (NGS), and increased biological understanding is rapidly increasing the diagnostic yield of genetic tests in ID and improving the usefulness of genetic test results for patients and families involved [35–37]. In addition, it is providing possibilities for carrier testing and prenatal screening, as well as new targets for treatment [25].

## Chromosome aneusomies

As chromosome aneusomies are the most common known causes of ID, several new methods, based on high-density microarray techniques or NGS followed by karyotype analysis, have been developed and widely used over recent years to increase detection rate of subtle aneusomies [21, 38–40]. These causes explain up to 15% of severe cases [41, 42]. Trisomy 21, or Down's syndrome, is the most common chromosomal aneuploidy associated with ID, with an estimated frequency of 1.5 in 1000 pregnancies and accounting for 6–8% of all ID. Other common chromosomal abnormalities include X chromosome aneusomies and a variety of cytogenetically balanced and unbalanced translocations. The most frequent X chromosomal aneusomies are XXY (Klinefelter's syndrome), XO (Turner's syndrome), and XYY syndrome, accounting for 1% of severe ID. There is also a wide range of recurrent sub-chromosomal deletions or duplications such as Prader–Willi and Angelman syndromes (15q11.2–q13 deletion), Williams–Beuren syndrome (7q11.23 deletion), Smith–Magenis syndrome (17p11.2 deletion), and di George syndrome (22q11.2 deletion). The wide application of high-density microarrays increases the identification of copy number variants (CNVs) associated with ID. Approximately 15–20% of patients with ID had microdeletions and duplications revealed by array-based CNV analyses [39, 43–45]. These CNVs include both rare *de novo*, as well as rare inherited, mutations. It is anticipated that clinical overlap will make their syndromal phenotypic distances less useful, as more genetic events are identified.

## Single-gene causes

It has been estimated that mutations in more than 700 different genes may cause ID [25]. These mutations include X-linked, autosomal dominant, and autosomal recessive ID and can be inherited or arise through *de novo* events. Until NGS methods came into use, only a handful of autosomal ID-associated recessive genes were discovered, possibly due to limitations of cytogenetic and sequencing technology and the absence of large families with autosomal forms of ID [25]. Most metabolic disorders belong to autosomal recessive forms of ID (ARID), caused by single mutated genes that disturb metabolism by deficient enzyme activity. These diseases include PKU and homocystinuria. For the last decade, over 300 genes have been identified for ARID, mostly by homozygosity mapping using single-nucleotide polymorphism (SNP) microarrays in large consanguineous families and subsequent follow-up of candidate genes by Sanger sequencing [46, 47]. In outbred populations, ARID may account for about 10–20% of the cases, while autosomal recessive disorders were found to be up to 3-fold more frequent among inbred, compared to non-inbred, cases [48, 49].

Autosomal dominant genes cause tuberous sclerosis, myotonic dystrophy, Gorlin syndrome, neurofibromatosis type 1, Apert syndrome, Menes syndrome, and Huntington's disease. The trio-based exome sequencing design allowed the identification of dominant *de novo* mutations (heterozygous) or small indels associated with severe, sporadic non-syndromic ID, accounting for 13–55% of patients with high locus heterogeneity [17, 35, 50]. Exome sequencing also rapidly identified autosomal dominant sporadic syndromes associated with ID such as Schinzel–Giedion syndrome [51], Kabuki syndrome [52], and Bohring–Opitz syndrome [53].

For many years, research into the molecular causes of ID has focused on the X chromosome because males are affected more often than females [54–56]. Mutations in more than 100 X-linked genes are now known to cause ID, accounting for 10–12% of males with ID, with none of these genes individually explaining more than 0.1% of ID [57–59]. The most well-known example is fragile X syndrome, which is caused by expansion of a CGG repeat in the *FMR1* gene (fragile X mental retardation 1) and is the second most common genetic cause of intellectual disability, accounting for about 0.5% of ID, after Down syndrome [60].

The genetic causes of ID are rapidly being uncovered and will be essential for genetic counselling, diagnostics, and treatment in the future. Microarrays for mutation screening of known disease genes, as well as exome and whole-genome sequencing, will likely become essential tools, both for clinical diagnostic purposes and research.

## Treatment and prevention

### Screening/prevention/preatment

Newborn screening—tests that can be done within the first hours or days of life and have a potential for preventing severe health problems— has evolved from simple blood or urine tests to a comprehensive and complex system, detecting over 50 different conditions, including those relevant to ID such as CH and several amino acid deficiencies. The newborn blood spot taken from a heel stick is mandated in most of North America and Europe [61].

Table 23.1 shows the timing and nature of screening for genetic disorders and those with prominent environmental factors. Box 23.1 lists the diagnostic examinations for presumed or established intellectual disabilities.

### Environmental/social assessment

FASD—prenatal counselling of the mother and family, family counselling, and prenatal care.

**Table 23.1** Aetiology of intellectual disability based on time and mechanism of the injury to the central nervous system and history for timing of diagnosis and treatment

| Aetiology | History |
|---|---|
| Genetic causes: chromosomal, CNV, single gene, single base pair Mitochondrial disorders | Family history: recurrent miscarriages, consanguinity |
| External prenatal factors: infections, maternal illness, for example, hypothyroidism, micronutrient deficiency | Gestational history: maternal infection, trauma, drugs, alcohol, exposure |
| Postnatally acquired disorders Infection Brain trauma Psychosocial, for example, environmental stimuli | Social history History of meningitis, rubella Trauma, toxicity, for example, lead |

**Box 23.1** Diagnostic examination of presumed or established intellectual disability

- General examination for dysmorphic features.
- Neurological, ophthalmological, audiological, cardiological, and neuropsychological assessments.
- Full blood count, thyroid function.
- Genetic screening (Table 23.1).
- Blood/urine.
- Neuroimaging.
- Neurophysiological EEG.

### Prenatal screening/maternal assessment

There have been potentially revolutionary changes to prenatal diagnosis and screening and include both imaging and tissue diagnoses. The discovery of cell-free fetal DNA in maternal plasma opened up a new frontier in the quest for a non-invasive prenatal screening strategy [62], since validated in several studies [63, 64]. Future population studies will be essential to evaluate these data, as the overall cumulative prevalence of many genetic risk markers is not established.

### Newborn/infant tests and treatments (for example, thyroid)

Newborn screening for CH—awareness of an iodine-poor environment and CH screening at birth now permit levothyroxine therapy by 4–6 weeks of life, which represents the standard of care.

## Syndromes causing intellectual disability

Classic syndromes are usually associated with chromosomal abnormalities and large structural variations, since this type of alteration is more likely to lead to additional phenotypic presentations other than ID alone. This section deals with some of the syndromes that increase to have ID. In syndromic ID, patients present with one or multiple clinical features or comorbidities, in addition to ID. However, symptoms of some syndromes may be so subtle that they are extremely difficult to diagnose, unless the features are looked for specifically in the context of a known genetic defect previously associated with these features. Thus, the distinction between syndromic ID and non-syndromic ID is often blurred [30].

Table 23.2 describes the most well-known syndromes causing ID.

*Tuberous sclerosis* occurs in 1 in 7000 people, with a majority arising from spontaneous mutations to 9q34 and 16p13. This syndrome is characterized by a triad of epilepsy, intellectual deficiency, and a characteristic facial skin lesion.

*Turner's syndrome* occurs in 1 in 10,000 female births and is caused by a loss or an abnormality of one X chromosome in women. Ninety-nine per cent of affected fetuses miscarry. Affected women exhibit normal intelligence and verbal abilities, with significant variation. They show deficits in spatial perception, visual motor integration, affect recognition, visual memory, and attention. Furthermore, they tend to display hyperactivity and distractibility during childhood, poor social skills, immature social relationships, and low self-esteem in adolescence. Dysmorphic features include: a webbed neck, a low hairline at the rear of the head, widely spaced nipples, and multiple pigmented naevi. Some have cardiovascular abnormalities.

**Table 23.2** Most prevalent syndromes associated with intellectual disability

| Classification | Prevalence | Genetic abnormality | Behavioural and cognitive features | Physical features |
|---|---|---|---|---|
| Klinefelter's syndrome | 1 in 660 live births (possibly increasing) | Additional X chromosome(s) in phenotypic males | IQ score ranges from 60 to 130, with greater impairment to verbal IQ. High rate of learning disability, speech and motor delays, and impairment in language processing. Adults may have increased impulsiveness and rate of antisocial behaviour | Small testes; hypergonadotropic hypogonadism; azoospermia; infertility; increased luteinizing hormone and follicle-stimulating hormone; hypogonadism; gynaecomastia<br><br>Below-average height, weight, and head circumference at birth; accelerated growth and increased height from 3 years onwards<br><br>Increased risk of diabetes and metabolic syndrome, abdominal obesity, autoimmune diseases, osteopenia, cryptorchidism, decreased penile size (children), congenital malformations (for example, clinodactyly), cardiovascular abnormalities, breast cancer, osteoporosis, mediastinal cancers |
| XXX syndrome | 1 in 1000 female births | 47,XXX resulting from primary non-disjunction of a maternal or paternal X chromosome during meiosis. Only 40 cases of 48,XXXX reported<br><br>Risk increases with advanced maternal age | Affected women have IQs of between 80 and 90, with increasing severity of IQ deficits corresponding to additional X aneuploidies. Women with XXXX syndrome have IQs of 55–75<br><br>Developmental delay; motor and speech delays; higher risk of cognitive deficits and learning disabilities in school-age years. Some experience relatively poor short-term auditory memory<br><br>Under-activity and withdrawal have been reported; slowed emotional development | Hypotonia, low birthweight, and small head circumference in newborns. Increased height in adulthood, with a low body mass index, epicanthal folds, hypotonia, and clinodactyly<br><br>Unimpaired fertility, but possible premature ovarian failure and recurrent spontaneous abortions<br><br>Seizures, renal, and genitourinary abnormalities |
| XYY syndrome | 1 in 1000 live male births | Primary non-disjunction of the Y chromosome; 10% have mosaic 46,XY/47,XYY chromosome complement. Offspring with two Y chromosomes are rare | Affected men have lower mean intelligence scores, but with large overlap with the normal distribution<br><br>Poor social adaptation, distractibility, hyperactivity, temper tantrums, and speech and language problems are relatively common in childhood<br><br>Increased frequency of XYY men among inmates in special prisons<br><br>Balance and co-ordination minimally compromised | Increase in body and leg length between years 4 and 9. As adults, most are over 10 cm taller than their fathers<br><br>Sexual development and fertility are unaffected |
| Down's syndrome | 1 in 2000 at maternal age of 30<br>1 in 100 at maternal age of 40 | Additional chromosome 21. Rarer cases caused by chromosomal translocation or mosaicism | Adults have moderate ID<br><br>Affected children have some degree of specific speech and language delay<br><br>Stubbornness and obsessional features over-represented | Muscular hypotonia that typically improves with development, short stature in adulthood, with characteristic facial appearance, eyes sloping upwards and outwards, wide nose bridge and unusually shaped head, transverse crease on the arm, large cleft between first and second toes, relatively short upper arms<br><br>Thyroid abnormalities, heart abnormality, gastrointestinal abnormality, changes in blood cells |
| Velo-cardio-facial syndrome | 1 in 2000 people | Microdeletions at 22q11 (90% of cases arise *de novo*; 10% inherited) | Learning disability, as well as speech and language problems are common<br><br>Difficulties with social interaction. Anxiety, social withdrawal, and other disorders have also been reported | Physical features include cardiac abnormalities, including ventriculoseptal deficits, pulmonary stenosis, and cardiac outlet abnormalities<br><br>Prominent nose with broad bridge and squared tip, small head, or small lower jaw; ocular abnormalities; cleft palate; short stature and long, thin, hyperextensible fingers |

**Table 23.2**   Continued

| Classification | Prevalence | Genetic abnormality | Behavioural and cognitive features | Physical features |
|---|---|---|---|---|
| Neurofibromatosis type 1 | 1 in 3000 births | Associated with 17q11.2, which produces neurofibromin and is involved in regulating cell division and tumour suppression; 50% of all new cases arise in unaffected families due to high spontaneous mutation | Speech or language abnormalities, learning disability, specific developmental disorders involving reading writing, or numeracy Distractibility, impulsiveness; visuospatial abnormalities, lack of co-ordination | Diagnosis usually requires two or more of the following symptoms: six or more light brown skin lesions of >5 mm in diameter before puberty or 15 mm after puberty; two or more neurofibromas or one plexiform neurofibroma; freckling of the inguinal or axillary regions; two or more Lisch nodules; optic nerve glioma; bony lesions; a first-degree relative with the disorder Non-enhancing hyperintensities on MRI located at the cerebellum, basal ganglia, brainstem, and thalamus Tumours from connective tissue of nerve sheaths |
| Fetal alcohol syndrome* | 0.33 per 1000 births | Exposure to alcohol at any stage of fetal development inhibits $N$-methyl-$D$-aspartate receptors, which mediate post-synaptic excitatory effects of glutamate, and affects cell proliferation and causes cognitive impairment | Usually mild to moderate ID, but may be severe Reduction in attention span, over-activity, irritability in infancy, and co-ordination problems | Facial dysmorphology: thin upper lip and smooth philtrum, small jaw, low-set abnormal ears, and palate abnormalities. Growth retardation, skeletal abnormalities, for example, deformed ribs and sternum, spinal curvature, dislocated hips, fused or webbed or missing fingers or toes, limited joint movement, small head Heart abnormalities and urinary tract anomalies Small brain with abnormally arranged cells |
| Fragile X syndrome | 0.3 in 1000 | X-linked trinucleotide repeats eventually halt function of the *FMR1* gene Healthy individuals have around 50 repeats; carriers with 50–100 repeats are considered to have the pre-mutation, and carriers with over 230 repeats are considered to have the full mutation | Mild to moderate ID. Severity of ID in women depends on the random proportion of cells with X inactivation. Pre-mutation carriers are intellectually unimpaired Problems with attention and concentration may be disproportionate to the severity of ID Speech and language delay; disorganized speech Some degree of social impairment. Men with fragile X syndrome are usually affectionate, without the aloof quality typical of autism Self-injury; stereotyped behaviour, for example, hand flapping | Large testes apparent after puberty; long face; high-arched palate; large forehead, ears, and lower jaw; hyper-extensible joints, flat feet; cardiovascular abnormalities; ear infections; cataracts |
| Congenital hypothyroidism | 1 in 4000. Occurs more commonly in females | Majority of cases caused by deficiency of iodine in mother or infant. Some cases due to mutations in genes involved in thyroid development and hormonogenesis such as *PAX8, TSHR, TSHB, DUOX2, TG, TPO,* and *SLCA5* | If untreated, even mild cases may lead to failure of cognitive development, resulting in ID Sleep disorder | Severely affected children have a characteristic appearance, with a puffy face, large and protruding tongue, dry and brittle hair, low hairline, and low muscle tone Constipation and jaundice |
| Duchenne muscular dystrophy | 1 in 4000 male births | X-linked recessive, with 30% of cases due to new mutations Deletions, duplications, and mutations at Xp21 result in failure to produce dystrophin, a protein component of muscle tissue | Some affected people have IQs within normal range Specific reading disorder and learning disability Low mood, anxiety, and social abnormalities | Typical onset is from 2 to 6 years. Progressive muscle weakness, affecting the pelvis, upper leg, and upper arm first Respiratory muscles and cardiovascular muscle abnormalities may occur later Severity is initially greater in the legs and torso, eventually moving up to the arms and respiratory muscles |

* No longer separate in DSM-V.

*Angelman syndrome* occurs in 1 in 10,000 births and is associated with deletions at the 15q11–q13 region of maternal origin (see Prader–Willi syndrome). Affected patients exhibit severe ID, markedly delayed motor milestones, little speech development, and over-activity associated with short attention span. Physical features include hypopigmentation, a small head, characteristic face with wide mouth, 'hooked' nose, prominent lower jaw, widely spaced teeth, and tongue protrusion. Voluntary movements are jerky, and gait is ataxic with stiff legs. Affected patients tend to enjoy social and physical contact, mouthing objects, and display a fascination with water.

*PKU* occurs in 1 in 10,000 live births and is caused by a mutation at 12q22–24.1, which results in deficiency of the enzyme phenylalanine hydroxylase. Affected patients exhibit moderate to severe learning disability, displaying deficits in mathematical, visuospatial, and language skills. Physical features include a small head, blond hair, blue eyes, and eczema. Behavioural features include over-activity, self-injury, irritability, and marked social impairments. They are often affected by tremor and movement disorders.

*Rett's syndrome* occurs in 1 in 10,000 women and is associated with a mutation at Xq28, which is usually lethal in males but may persist in a small number of surviving males. Affected patients exhibit severe learning disability. Physical features include cessation of development, lack of muscle tone, scoliosis, spasticity, reduction in brain size with reduced cortical thickness, reduced neuronal branching, and depigmentation of the basal ganglia. Behavioural features include immobility at infancy, loss of skills from around 18 months onwards, stereotyped movements, over-breathing or cessation of breathing, sleep disturbances, and withdrawal.

*Williams syndrome* occurs in 1 in 15,000 infants and is associated with a deletion at 7q11.3. Affected children have moderate or severe learning disability. Behavioural features include difficulty feeding, irritability, constipation, and failure to thrive at infancy. Affected children display social disinhibition, over-activity, poor concentration, eating and sleeping abnormalities, abnormal anxiety, poor peer relationships, and abnormal hearing sensitivity. Physical features include prominent cheeks, wide mouth, flat nasal bridge, growth retardation, high serum calcium concentrations, and kidney and heart lesions.

*Smith–Lemli–Opitz syndrome* mostly affects males, occuring in 1 in 30,000 live births, and is due to abnormalities at 11q12–13. Affected patients have moderate to severe learning disability. Physical features include growth retardation of the fetus during pregnancy, small head, drooping eyelids, squint, forward-facing nostrils, small lower jaw, abnormalities of external genitalia, hypospadias, undescended testes, cleft palate, finger abnormalities, and abnormalities of almost all major organ systems. Behavioural features include aggressive and self-injurious behaviour.

*Cri-du-chat syndrome* occurs in 1 in 35,000 births and is associated with deletions at the 5p terminal. Affected patients have mild to severe intellectual deficiency, with markedly delayed language development. Behavioural features include hyperactivity, feeding difficulties, and an abnormally high-pitched cry at infancy. Physical features include ear abnormalities, round face with widely spaced slanting eyes, small head, flat broad nose, small lower jaw, and premature greying of hair. They sometimes have an asymmetrical face, cleft lip or palate, curved fingers, hernias, and orthopaedic abnormalities.

*Prader–Willi syndrome* occurs in 1 in 40,000 live births and is associated with a deletion at 15q11-q13 of paternal origin. Physical features include hypotonia, short stature, small hands and feet, a characteristic pattern of facial appearance, and lack of sexual development at adulthood. Behavioural features include feeding problems in infancy, overeating in early childhood, insatiety, sleep abnormalities, lower threshold for loss of temper, scratching or picking at skin, insistence on routines, and compulsive behaviours. Obesity may result due to overeating.

*Smith–Magenis syndrome*, occurring 1 in 50,000 births, is associated with deletions at 17p11.2 and commonly results in moderate ID. Behavioural and cognitive features include placid newborns, difficulty with feeding, hyperactivity, self-injury, self-hugging, midline handclapping, sleep disorder, absence of rapid eye movement

(REM) sleep, and insensitivity to pain. Physical features include flattened mid face, abnormally shaped upper lip, short hands and feet, single transverse palmar crease, abnormally shaped or placed ears, and sometimes a high-arched palate or protruding tongue. Otitis media and squint are common.

*De Lange syndrome* occurs in 1 in 60,000 live births and is associated with mutations in chromosome 5 at the *NIPBL* gene. It results in severe learning disability, with very limited speech. Physical features include hearing impairments, gut malformations, congenital heart defects, gastrointestinal pain, growth retardation, well-defined arched eyebrows meeting in the middle, long and curled eyelashes, small nose with forward-facing nostrils, down-turned mouth with thin lips, and small or shortened limbs. Behavioural features include self-injury, autistic features, and pleasurable responses to vestibular stimulation.

*Mucopolysaccharidoses* are autosomal recessive (except for Hunter's syndrome, which is X-linked) that occur in around 1 in 100,000 to 1 in 500,000 births. ID ranges from absent to severe. Physical features include gargoylism, hepatosplenomagaly, joint stiffness, eye abnormalities, and short statures. Behavioural and cognitive features include sleep problems, aggression, over-activity, restlessness, and anxiety.

*Rubinstein–Taybi syndrome* occurs in 1 in 125,000 live births and is associated with microdeletions at 16p13.3. Patients have moderate learning disability. Physical features include congenital heart defects, urinary tract abnormalities, decreased height, inadequate weight at infancy, small head, beaked or straight nose, downward-slanting eyes, stiff gait, and thumbs or first toes with broad terminal phalanges, sometimes with an angulation deformity. Behavioural cognitive features include constipation, friendly disposition, propensity to self-stimulatory activities, and reduced attention span.

*Lesch–Nyhan syndrome* occurs in 1 in 380,000 births and is an X-linked recessive trait which results in hyperuricaemia. It can also be caused by complete and partial deletions, insertions, and duplications of Xp26q27. Patients with this syndrome have mild to severe ID. Physical features include hypotonia, hyperreflexia, and clonus during the first year, growth retardation, and gout. Behavioural features include compulsive behaviours, self-injury, spasticity and choreo-athetoid movements at 9 months, dystonic movements, dysarthria, and athetoid and movement abnormalities.

## REFERENCES

1. Girirajan S, Rosenfeld JA, Coe BP, *et al.* Phenotypic Heterogeneity of Genomic Disorders and Rare Copy-Number Variants. N Engl J Med. 2012;367(14):1321–31.
2. Bakoyiannis I, Gkioka E, Pergialiotis V, *et al.* Fetal alcohol spectrum disorders and cognitive functions of young children. Rev Neurosci. 2014;25(5):631–9.
3. Faulk C, Barks A, Liu K, Goodrich JM, Dolinoy DC. Early-life lead exposure results in dose- and sex-specific effects on weight and epigenetic gene regulation in weanling mice. Epigenomics. 2013;5(5):487–500.
4. Bihaqi SW, Huang H, Wu J, Zawia NH. Infant exposure to lead (Pb) and epigenetic modifications in the aging primate brain: implications for Alzheimer's disease. J Alzheimers Dis. 2011;27(4):819–33.

5. Li Y, Xie C, Murphy SK, *et al*. Lead Exposure during Early Human Development and DNA Methylation of Imprinted Gene Regulatory Elements in Adulthood. Environ Health Perspect. 2016;124(5):666–73.

6. Kliegman RM SB, Geme JS, Schor NF, Behrman RE. *Nelson Textbook of Pediatrics*. Elsevier Health Sciences, Philadelphia, PA; 2011.

7. Granato A, De Giorgio A. Alterations of neocortical pyramidal neurons: turning points in the genesis of mental retardation. Front Pediatr. 2014;2:86.

8. Rayman MP, Bath SC. The new emergence of iodine deficiency in the UK: consequences for child neurodevelopment. Ann Clin Biochem. 2015;52:705–8.

9. Bath SC, Combet E, Scully P, Zimmermann MB, Hampshire-Jones KH, Rayman MP. A multi-centre pilot study of iodine status in UK schoolchildren, aged 8–10 years. Eur J Nutr. 2016;55:2001–9.

10. Petrenko CL. Positive Behavioral Interventions and Family Support for Fetal Alcohol Spectrum Disorders. Curr Dev Disord Rep. 2015;2(3):199–209.

11. Fisher DA. The importance of early management in optimizing IQ in infants with congenital hypothyroidism. J Pediatr. 2000;136(3):273–4.

12. Bailey R, West K, Black R. The epidemiology of global micronutrient deficiencies. Ann Nutr Metab. 2015;66(Suppl 2):22–33.

13. Bigler ED, Jantz PB, Farrer TJ, *et al*. Day of injury CT and late MRI findings: Cognitive outcome in a paediatric sample with complicated mild traumatic brain injury. Brain Inj. 2015;29(9):1062–70.

14. Bigler ED, Stern Y. Traumatic brain injury and reserve. Handb Clin Neurol. 2015;128:691–710.

15. Williams NM, Franke B, Mick E, *et al*. Genome-wide analysis of copy number variants in attention deficit hyperactivity disorder: the role of rare variants and duplications at 15q13.3. Am J Psychiatry. 2012;169(2):195–204.

16. Mazumdar M, Bellinger DC, Gregas M, Abanilla K, Bacic J, Needleman HL. Low-level environmental lead exposure in childhood and adult intellectual function: a follow-up study. Environ Health. 2011;10:24.

17. Haworth CM, Wright MJ, Martin NW, *et al*. A twin study of the genetics of high cognitive ability selected from 11,000 twin pairs in six studies from four countries. Behav Genet. 2009;39(4):359–70.

18. Pettersson E, Anckarsater H, Gillberg C, Lichtenstein P. Different neurodevelopmental symptoms have a common genetic etiology. J Child Psychol Psychiatry. 2013;54(12):1356–65.

19. Cherny SS, Cardon LR, Fulker DW, DeFries JC. Differential heritability across levels of cognitive ability. Behav Genet. 1992;22(2):153–62.

20. Thompson LA, Detterman DK, Plomin R. Differences in heritability across groups differing in ability, revisited. Behav Genet. 1993;23(4):331–6.

21. Mefford HC, Batshaw ML, Hoffman EP. Genomics, intellectual disability, and autism. N Engl J Med. 2012;366:733–43.

22. Plomin R, Deary IJ. Genetics and intelligence differences: five special findings. Mol Psychiatry. 2015;20(1):98–108.

23. Deary IJ, Spinath FM, Bates TC. Genetics of intelligence. Eur J Hum Genet. 2006;14(6):690–700.

24. Bouchard TJ, Jr., McGue M. Familial studies of intelligence: a review. Science. 1981;212(4498):1055–9.

25. Vissers LELM, Gilissen C, Veltman JA. Genetic studies in intellectual disability and related disorders. Nat Rev Genet. 2016;17(1):9–18.

26. Kiser DP, Rivero O, Lesch KP. Annual research review: The (epi)genetics of neurodevelopmental disorders in the era of whole-genome sequencing—unveiling the dark matter. J Child Psychol Psychiatry. 2015;56(3):278–95.

27. Reichenberg A, Cederlof M, McMillan A, *et al*. Discontinuity in the genetic and environmental causes of the intellectual disability spectrum. Proc Natl Acad Sci U S A. 2016;113(4):1098–103.

28. McLaren J, Bryson SE. Review of recent epidemiological studies of mental retardation: prevalence, associated disorders, and etiology. Am J Ment Retard. 1987;92(3):243–54.

29. Moeschler JB, Shevell M; American Academy of Pediatrics Committee on Genetics. Clinical genetic evaluation of the child with mental retardation or developmental delays. Pediatrics. 2006;117(6):2304–16.

30. Kaufman L, Ayub M, Vincent JB. The genetic basis of non-syndromic intellectual disability: a review. J Neurodev Disord. 2010;2(4):182–209.

31. Lundvall M, Rajaei S, Erlandson A, Kyllerman M. Aetiology of severe mental retardation and further genetic analysis by high-resolution microarray in a population-based series of 6- to 17-year-old children. Acta Paediatr. 2012;101(1):85–91.

32. Karam SM, Riegel M, Segal SL, *et al*. Genetic causes of intellectual disability in a birth cohort: A population-based study. American Journal of Medical Genetics Part A. 2015;167(6):1204–14.

33. Grozeva D, Carss K, Spasic-Boskovic O, *et al*. Targeted Next-Generation Sequencing Analysis of 1,000 Individuals with Intellectual Disability. Hum Mutat. 2015;36(12):1197–204.

34. Gilissen C, Hehir-Kwa JY, Thung DT, *et al*. Genome sequencing identifies major causes of severe intellectual disability. Nature. 2014;511(7509):344–7.

35. de Ligt J, Willemsen MH, van Bon BW, *et al*. Diagnostic exome sequencing in persons with severe intellectual disability. N Engl J Med. 2012;367(20):1921–9.

36. Gilissen C, Hoischen A, Brunner HG, Veltman JA. Disease gene identification strategies for exome sequencing. Eur J Hum Genet. 2012;20(5):490–7.

37. Rabbani B, Tekin M, Mahdieh N. The promise of whole-exome sequencing in medical genetics. J Hum Genet. 2014;59(1):5–15.

38. Flint J, Knight S. The use of telomere probes to investigate submicroscopic rearrangements associated with mental retardation. Curr Opin Genet Dev. 2003;13(3):310–16.

39. Cooper GM. A copy number variation morbidity map of developmental delay. Nat Genet. 2011;43:838–46.

40. Newman S, Hermetz KE, Weckselblatt B, Rudd MK. Next-generation sequencing of duplication CNVs reveals that most are tandem and some create fusion genes at breakpoints. Am J Hum Genet. 2015;96(2):208–20.

41. Michelson DJ. Evidence report: genetic and metabolic testing on children with global developmental delay: report of the Quality Standards Subcommittee of the American Academy of Neurology and the Practice Committee of the Child Neurology Society. Neurology. 2011;77:1629–35.

42. van Karnebeek CD, Jansweijer MC, Leenders AG, Offringa M, Hennekam RC. Diagnostic investigations in individuals with mental retardation: a systematic literature review of their usefulness. Eur J Hum Genet. 2005;13:6–25.

43. Wagenstaller J. Copy-number variations measured by single-nucleotide-polymorphism oligonucleotide arrays in patients with mental retardation. Am J Hum Genet. 2007;81:768–79.
44. Hochstenbach R, van Binsbergen E, Engelen J, *et al*. Array analysis and karyotyping: workflow consequences based on a retrospective study of 36,325 patients with idiopathic developmental delay in the Netherlands. Eur J Med Genet. 2009;52(4):161–9.
45. Miller DT. Consensus statement: chromosomal microarray is a first-tier clinical diagnostic test for individuals with developmental disabilities or congenital anomalies. Am J Hum Genet. 2010;86:749–64.
46. Ropers HH. Genetics of early onset cognitive impairment. Annu Rev Genomics Hum Genet. 2010;11:161–87.
47. Musante L, Ropers HH. Genetics of recessive cognitive disorders. Trends Genet. 2014;30:32–9.
48. Hoodfar E, Teebi AS. Genetic referrals of Middle Eastern origin in a western city: inbreeding and disease profile. J Med Genet. 1996;33(3):212–15.
49. Hamamy HA, Masri AT, Al-Hadidy AM, Ajlouni KM. Consanguinity and genetic disorders. Profile from Jordan. Saudi Med J. 2007;28(7):1015–17.
50. Rauch A. Range of genetic mutations associated with severe non-syndromic sporadic intellectual disability: an exome sequencing study. Lancet. 2012;380:1674–82.
51. Hoischen A. *De novo* mutations of SETBP1 cause Schinzel-Giedion syndrome. Nat Genet. 2010;42:483–5.
52. Ng SB. Exome sequencing identifies *MLL2* mutations as a cause of Kabuki syndrome. Nat Genet. 2010;42:790–3.
53. Hoischen A. *De novo* nonsense mutations in ASXL1 cause Bohring-Opitz syndrome. Nat Genet. 2011;43:729–31.
54. Lehrke R. A theory of X-linkage of major intellectual traits. Response to Dr. Anastasi and to the Drs. Nance and Engel. Am J Ment Defic. 1972;76(6):626–31.
55. Lehrke R. Theory of X-linkage of major intellectual traits. Am J Ment Defic. 1972;76(6):611–19.
56. Leonard H, Wen X. The epidemiology of mental retardation: challenges and opportunities in the new millennium. Ment Retard Dev Disabil Res Rev. 2002;8:117–34.
57. Lubs HA, Stevenson RE, Schwartz CE. Fragile X and X-linked intellectual disability: four decades of discovery. Am J Hum Genet. 2012;90:579–90.
58. Tarpey PS, Smith R, Pleasance E, *et al*. A systematic, large-scale resequencing screen of X-chromosome coding exons in mental retardation. Nat Genet. 2009;41(5):535–43.
59. Hu H, Haas SA, Chelly J, *et al*. X-exome sequencing of 405 unresolved families identifies seven novel intellectual disability genes. Mol Psychiatry. 2016;21(1):133–48.
60. Coffee B. Incidence of fragile X syndrome by newborn screening for methylated FMR1 DNA. Am J Hum Genet. 2009;85:503–14.
61. Therrell BL, Padilla CD, Loeber JG, *et al*. Current status of newborn screening worldwide: 2015. Semin Perinatol. 2015;39(3):171–87.
62. Lo YM, Corbetta N, Chamberlain PF, *et al*. Presence of fetal DNA in maternal plasma and serum. Lancet. 1997;350(9076):485–7.
63. Porreco RP, Garite TJ, Maurel K, *et al*. Noninvasive prenatal screening for fetal trisomies 21, 18, 13 and the common sex chromosome aneuploidies from maternal blood using massively parallel genomic sequencing of DNA. Am J Obstet Gynecol. 2014;211(4):365 e1–12.
64. Evans MI, Andriole S, Evans SM. Genetics: update on prenatal screening and diagnosis. Obstet Gynecol Clin North Am. 2015;42(2):193–208.

# 24

# Management and treatment of intellectual disability

*José L. Ayuso-Mateos and Cary S. Kogan*

## Introduction

The advent of a model of disorders of intellectual development/intellectual disability that emphasizes inclusiveness and participation in society for affected individuals brought with it a greater emphasis on considerations of the influence of contextual factors that facilitate or impede functioning within society (see also Chapter 21). The WHO revision of the International Classification of Diseases (ICD), the most widely used health classification worldwide, was approved by the World Health Assembly in May 2019. The focus of the revision of the ICD Mental and Behavioural Disorders chapter led by the WHO Department of Mental Health and Substance Abuse is the incorporation of current scientific evidence in a set of diagnostic guidelines that will maximize clinical utility and global applicability [1, 2]. Consistent with the overarching goal of the classification revision to enhance clinical utility, the ICD guidelines for disorders of intellectual development were written to facilitate more pervasive, efficient, and accurate identification of affected individuals, with the ultimate goal of enhancing access to appropriate services in varied settings globally [3].

Disorders of intellectual development is a term proposed for the first time in ICD to replace the label of mental retardation that appeared in ICD-10. Although intellectual disability is frequently used and indeed appears in DSM-5 [4], inclusion of the word 'disability' in the label would be at odds with the approach promoted by the WHO Family of International Classifications that distinguishes between health conditions classified in the ICD from the consequences of those conditions (that is, disabilities) classified in the ICF. The 'Disorders of intellectual development' title also reflects that the onset of the condition is during the developmental period and focuses on the broad construct of 'intellect' that is well understood in policy circles, as well as among researchers and clinicians [3]. Disorders of intellectual development is classified among other neurodevelopmental disorders, and its guidelines are used in concert with the guidelines for autism spectrum disorder to characterize the degree of impairments in intellectual functioning in individuals affected by that disorder.

Disorders of intellectual development are defined by three essential features in ICD: (1) significant limitations in intellectual functioning generalized to various domains (for example, perceptual reasoning, working memory, etc.); (2) significant limitations in adaptive behaviour, which is the set of conceptual, social, and practical skills; and (3) onset of both of these limitations during the developmental period. ICD-11 preserves the existing four levels of severity that appear in ICD-10 (that is, mild, moderate, severe, and profound), largely due to evidence that increasing severity is associated with a number of important support needs, including choice of living arrangements [5]. ICD-11 will propose an approach that requires consideration of both intellectual and adaptive behaviour functioning to determine the level of severity. Each level of severity is defined by the expected range of performance on measures of intellectual and adaptive behaviour functioning, with a caveat stipulating that differentiation between severe and profound levels on the basis of intellectual functioning is unreliable and therefore should be guided by findings on measures of adaptive behaviour skills. There is also a qualifier to indicate a provisional diagnosis that is used when a comprehensive assessment has not been, or cannot be, performed (for example, sensory limitations) or if a child is 4 years or younger. Poor reliability of the assessment of intellectual and adaptive behaviour functioning in young children preclude a definitive assignment of severity.

In recognition of the fact that, in many settings worldwide, particularly in low- and middle-income countries, patients are unlikely to be assessed by mental health or developmental specialists, the ICD-11 guidelines also include a set of tables that outline concrete behavioural indicators of intellectual and adaptive behaviour functioning at each severity level expected of individuals falling into one of three age ranges (early childhood, childhood/adolescence, and adulthood) [6]. These tables were developed primarily to assist non-specialists to determine the level of severity of a disorder of intellectual development. Although the use of standardized, normed measures of intellectual and adaptive behaviour functioning is preferable for determining the level of severity, the WHO recognizes that availability of such measures in local languages in many global settings is limited. Thus, the behavioural indicator tables provide an alternative means of establishing severity on the basis of observed or informant-reported behaviours. This system represents a considerable improvement over the idiosyncratic determination of severity or overreliance on the use of a provisional diagnosis, practices that limit patients' access to appropriate services. Clinicians are instructed to assign the level of severity on the basis of the level at which the majority of the individual's intellectual ability and adaptive behaviour across all three domains fall, using various sources of data and clinical judgement.

### Co-occurring disorders in ICD-11

Chapter 24 has outlined the common comorbidities seen between intellectual disability and other psychiatric disorders. The ICD-11 proposals for the disorders of intellectual development guidelines provide users with comprehensive guidance on the detection of commonly co-occurring disorders in affected individuals. Identification of these co-occurring conditions is of vital importance in understanding the needs for, and developing, an appropriate treatment plan for affected individuals. Therefore, ICD-11 proposals outline guidance on the more commonly comorbid conditions, including autism spectrum disorder (ASD), attention-deficit/hyperactivity disorder (ADHD), and various other mental and behavioural disorders.

ASD frequently presents with limitations in intellectual and adaptive behaviour functioning, and when both are found to be two or more standard deviations below the mean, a diagnosis of ASD with intellectual impairment is assigned co-concurrently with a disorder of intellectual development qualified according to the determined level of severity. However, in these circumstances, the ICD-11 guidance indicates that determination of the level of severity of the intellectual disability should be more reliant on the conceptual and practical domains of adaptive behaviour functioning, giving less weight to social skill abilities, because social communication deficits are a hallmark feature of ASD and better accounted for by that diagnosis.

Rates of co-occurring ADHD in individuals with a disorder of intellectual development diagnosis are significantly higher than in the general population (for example, [7]). When inattention and/or hyperactivity–impulsivity are significantly affected in an individual with a disorder of intellectual development beyond what is expected, based on age and the level of intellectual functioning, a co-occurring diagnosis of ADHD can be assigned.

A variety of other mental and behavioural disorders are known to occur at the same, or perhaps higher, rates among individuals affected by disorders of intellectual development, as compared to the general population (for example, mood disorder, anxiety and fear-related disorders, impulse-control disorders, and psychotic disorders) [8]. ICD-11 guidelines caution clinicians to ensure that assessments are conducted with methods that are appropriate to individuals' level of intellectual functioning and to be aware that self-report is less reliable among affected individuals and may lead to underreporting of co-occurring psychopathology. Therefore, observable signs or reports by caregivers or individuals close to the person being assessed may provide a more accurate understanding of the presence of co-occurring ICD-11 mental and behavioural disorders.

## Management

The general approach to management of persons with an intellectual disability is educational and psychosocial, with use of specific appropriate management interventions for mental health and behavioural problems when needed. Psychiatric comorbidities in persons with an intellectual disability are often under-detected. Comorbidities are typically suspected when patients exhibit changes in behaviour, particularly disruptive behaviour. The Royal College of Psychiatrists (2016) [9] has recently summarized three broad situations in which people with an intellectual disability and mental health or behavioural problems might come into contact with primary or secondary care: (1) the presence of challenging behaviour that is not associated with a mental disorder; (2) the presence of challenging behaviour that is associated with symptoms that meet the diagnostic criteria for a mental disorder; and (3) the presence of challenging behaviour that is associated with some psychiatric symptoms that do not quite fulfil the diagnostic criteria for a mental disorder. In many circumstances, changes in behaviour can be attributed to physical illness, difficulties in communication, or environmental changes, or can be a reaction to stressful circumstances or frustration. The clinical assessment should consider all the aforementioned factors, and the diagnostic formulation that serves as the basis for a management plan should reflect not only the severity and known aetiology of the intellectual disability, but also any co-occurring mental and physical disorders, as well as information gathered about psychosocial stressors and behavioural problems. If the clinician considers the presence of a physical health problem as the main factor explaining the behavioural symptoms, appropriate intervention for the physical conditions should follow promptly.

Proper identification of co-occurring disorders is essential in addressing the needs of affected individuals. When assessing for co-occurrence, clinicians should be familiar with the concept of diagnostic 'overshadowing', whereby emotional and behavioural symptoms or frank psychopathology are misattributed to the features of the disorder of intellectual development, rather than a separable disorder. Overlooking co-occurring disorders deprives affected individuals of potentially helpful interventions. A mitigating strategy is to use modified diagnostic criteria sets to differentiate symptoms of disorders of intellectual development from those better attributable to co-occurring conditions [for example, Diagnostic Manual-Intellectual Disabilities (DM-ID) [10]]. A general guiding principle in the assessment of mental and behavioural disorders in individuals with a disorder of intellectual development is that clinicians employ methods that are appropriate to the individual's level of development and intellectual functioning, which may require a greater reliance on signs in combination with collateral reports. Reporting of internal states is more difficult for affected individuals, particularly those with more severe forms of disorders of intellectual development.

### Psychosocial interventions

Psychosocial interventions that target behavioural and emotional difficulties, as well as diagnosable co-occurring mental and behavioural disorders, can be effective tools in the overall management plan for individuals with intellectual disability. Formulation and implementation of a treatment plan, even when it is meant to reduce or eliminate disruptive behaviours (for example, self-injurious or aggressive behaviours) should be undertaken, with the goal of improving affected individuals' quality of life and, in doing so, respect the principles of equality, non-discrimination, and self-determination. Intervention selection that promotes the acquisition of academic skills, beneficial habits, and general development should be based on the results of a functional behaviour analysis and often include psychoeducation, skills training, positive behavioural support (for example, differential and non-contingent reinforcement, altering triggers for undesirable behaviour, minimal use of aversive strategies, and reactive strategies such as the use of distraction [11]), carer involvement and training, and, in children, token economies [12]. Furthermore, when appropriate, cognitive behavioural therapy may be indicated. Many of the same psychosocial interventions that apply to redressing adaptive skill deficits among affected individuals are relevant to the management and modification of challenging behaviours and co-occurring mental and behavioural disorders. This approach views all systems of supports as ultimately serving to improve human functioning outcomes such as socio-economic status, health status, and subjective well-being of the individual [13, 14].

Challenging behaviours refer to those that interfere with the affected individual's quality of life, including their ability to function in social, academic, and employment contexts. They typically refer to self- and other oriented aggression, destruction of property, and behavioural stereotypies [15]. In a large population-based study conducted in Sweden, behaviour problems, which are considered to be less severe forms of challenging behaviours not necessarily requiring intervention, were observed in 62% of affected individuals [16]. Typically, co-occurring challenging behaviours vary according to the level of severity of the disorder of intellectual development and with age [17–19]. Although prevention strategies that anticipate the need for establishing effective communication strategies, modifications to environmental stimuli, and awareness of consequences that might reinforce challenging behaviour are preferable [20], usually consultation requests focus on existing behaviours that significantly interfere with the patient's functioning or are affecting the ability of the individual to function within specific contexts.

Optimal management strategies often require the co-ordination of services across multiple disciplines that include, but are not limited to, psychiatry, psychology, occupational therapy, speech and language therapy, genetic counselling, and nursing. In addition to these professionals, parents, teachers, supervisors, and other caregivers should be consulted to provide their perspectives on the individual's functioning within the various contexts that they frequent. Although some challenging behaviours may generalize across contexts, some may not. Furthermore, modification of contextual factors (for example, specific stimuli in the environment) independent of other management strategies may reduce or eliminate challenging behaviours.

A comprehensive diagnostic assessment typically involves integration of data from genetic testing, physical assessment, interviews of the patient and his or her caregivers, and consultation with multidisciplinary team members. Furthermore, challenging behaviours are most effectively addressed after a functional behaviour assessment has been conducted. The rationale for functional behaviour assessments emerges from research demonstrating that challenging behaviours serve a functional role for the individual and become established through operant principles of contingent reinforcement. Therefore, an explanation of the relationship between antecedent factors, challenging behaviours, and consequences provides a rational basis for intervention. Indeed, meta-analyses consistently support the effectiveness of functional behaviour assessments in improving treatment outcomes across all severity levels over those that do not

include such evaluations (for example, [21]). Challenging behaviours may be found to function as social positive reinforcers (for example, to obtain attention), social negative reinforcers (for example, to avoid having to complete a task), or sensory reinforcers (for example, repetitive self-stimulatory behaviours) [22]. Thus, interventions to reduce the frequency of challenging behaviours can centre on removing antecedent factors, altering identified reinforcers, or modifying reinforcement schedules. Early intervention to address challenging behaviours is beneficial in preventing these from becoming entrenched in the individual's repertoire.

### Addressing comorbid psychopathology

Behavioural management strategies predicated on the results of a thorough functional behaviour assessments are also helpful in addressing co-occurring externalizing disorders (for example, oppositional defiant disorder). Supplementing clinician-administered behavioural management with parent/caregiver skills training is often more effective than direct intervention with the affected individual (for example, Stepping Stones Triple-P, [23, 24]). With respect to emotional disorders, there is emerging evidence that psychological treatments, in particular cognitive behavioural therapy, may be as efficacious in addressing mood, anxiety, stress-related disorders (that is, PTSD) in people with disorders of intellectual development as in the general population [25, 26]. The ability to engage in cognitive behavioural interventions depends, in part, on the capacity of the individual to understand the relationship between internal states, behaviours, and cognitions, a task that is more likely achievable for those with mild to moderate forms of disorders of intellectual development.

### Pharmacological interventions

In general, the indications for the use of psychotropic drugs in this population are the same as in populations with normal intellectual functioning. In clinical practice, the administration of psychotropic agents in patients with intellectual disability is very common. A recent population-based cohort study of adults with intellectual disabilities in the UK showed that almost half were taking some form of psychotropic drug and that the proportion of participants with intellectual disability being prescribed psychotropic drugs exceeded the proportion with recorded mental illness [27]. Rather, many were prescribed these drugs to address challenging behaviours.

Psychiatric drug treatments are generally effective at the same doses and for the same indications than in the general population without this condition. Once a medication is selected on the basis of being properly indicated, the prescriber is confronted with a series of additional challenges. The most salient of these are: the coexistence of medical comorbidities, the concomitant use of other therapeutic substances, issues related to adherence to the medications, and the need to carefully monitor the impact of the pharmacological interventions in terms of efficacy and side effects in patients who may have communications problems.

There is no clear evidence that those with intellectual disability have more side effects when prescribed psychiatric treatments [28]. However, affected individuals have higher rates of physical health comorbidities and premature mortality [29]. Major health risk factors, such as obesity, metabolic syndrome, and diabetes, are highly prevalent in this population [30]. The monitoring of patients with intellectual disability receiving psychotropic drugs should consider not only the elevated risk of specific drugs, such as dopamine serotonin antagonists that increase the risk of metabolic syndrome and extra-pyramidal symptoms, but also assess medical status, dietary regimen, changes in the environment, and polypharmacy. Furthermore, with greater severity of intellectual impairment, sensory deficits and neurological comorbidities (for example, epilepsy) are very frequent, increasing the risk of severe side effects at lower doses, as well as special sensitivities to the neurological side effects of these drugs.

Involvement of the caregiver should be incorporated in any management plan, because adherence, as well as reporting of response to treatment and side effects, often relies on their co-operation. Their prejudices against medication may be a contributing factor in cases of non-adherence to the prescription. The likely effects of the intervention on the patient's and carer's quality of life should also be considered. During the required monitoring period after the prescription of psychotropic drugs, efforts should be made to solicit and incorporate objective information from the carers, as well as the patients. As a general rule, the lowest possible dose should be prescribed, with the physician assessing the need for treatment continuation once the target symptoms have improved or when there is non-response and/or side effects that have an impact on the patient's functioning and quality of life.

### Use of dopamine antagonists/partial agonists

Dopamine antagonists/partial agonists (meaning the so-called typical and atypical antipsychotics) are used frequently in the management of a variety of presenting symptoms, even when the evidence for efficacy is not available. Concerns about inadequate prescribing of these agents have been raised, in particular, in relation to the management of challenging behaviours [31]. While there is limited evidence that suggests that dopamine antagonists may be effective in treating behavioural disturbances in adults with intellectual disability with comorbid autism [32], evidence supporting the use of such medication outside this clinical situation is lacking [33]. The NICE guidelines (2015) [34] recommend that clinicians consider dopamine antagonists to manage challenging behaviour only if 'psychological or other interventions alone do not produce change within an agreed time; or treatment for any coexisting mental or physical health problem has not led to a reduction in the behaviour or the risk to the person or others is very severe (for example, because of violence, aggression or self-injury)' (National Institute for Health and Care Excellence, 2015).

Use of dopamine antagonists for the pharmacological treatment of aggression specifically is controversial. Once properly indicated, the follow-up of the patient should take anticipate that adverse effects may be more likely due to the higher incidence of comorbid conditions (for example, neurological disorders) and should consider that some patients may have an elevated baseline cardio-metabolic risk profile. Dopamine/serotonin antagonists have less risk of side effects like dyskinesia, but they have been associated with weight gain, metabolic syndrome, and increases in prolactin level. In practice, use in the intellectual disability population may be at lower doses than for other groups of psychiatric patients and is not necessarily associated with worse metabolic profiles. However, prolactin elevation (most marked with amisulpride and risperidone) is common and often associated with secondary hypogonadism in women [28]. Hypogonadism may, in turn, lead to bone loss in a population already at risk for osteoporosis and fractures. Management of hypogonadism is indicated, although there is currently too little awareness of this risk, which should be screened for more regularly. In cases with treatment-resistant psychosis, clozapine could be considered, but only when blood test monitoring can be ensured.

### Use of drugs for depression

Selective serotonin reuptake inhibitors (SSRIs) are the most commonly used medication in patients with intellectual disability, both for depressive disorders and anxiety disorders. They are also frequently prescribed for the management of obsessive–compulsive symptomatology. During the first few weeks of treatment, some patients report nervousness and agitation. Changes in behaviour (for example, increased aggression, self-injury, repetitive behaviour) may indicate adverse effects or a switch to a manic phase [35]. The prescription of these drugs should start with a low dose, and increases should be slower than in the population without intellectual disability. Treatment guidelines based on evidence collected in clinical populations without intellectual disability also stress the need for monitoring emerging suicidality and suicide attempts during treatment with antidepressants in children and adolescents with depression [36, 37]. Because the potential for drug interactions with SSRIs, the clinician should be vigilant when using these agents simultaneously with other drugs that are metabolized by cytochrome P450 enzymes.

### Benzodiazepines

These agents should only be used for a limited period of time, and long-term treatment with these agents should be avoided. Paradoxical reactions to benzodiazepines (disinhibition) can manifest in this clinical population in the form of impulsivity, aggression, or rage.

### Mood-stabilizing drugs

In addition to their use in bipolar disorder and acute mania, lithium and anti-epileptic drugs have been shown to be effective in the management of affective instability, which can manifest in the form of irritability, rage, and outburst of aggression [38]. Many patients with intellectual disability also have seizures that may increase the behavioural problems. As in the general population, therapy must be guided by regular serum monitoring, as lithium and anti-epileptic drugs are correlated with therapeutic and toxic effects.

There are ongoing concerns among users, carers, health care providers, and researchers that psychotropic drugs are too often used inappropriately in people with intellectual disability. It is not unusual to observe overuse of psychotropic drugs to treat challenging behaviour, excessive dosages, and polypharmacy. The off-label use of psychotropics is common practice in this area of medicine, as is the fact that once psychotropic drugs are prescribed for a particular challenging behaviour, they are incorporated in the long-term management of the case, without proper consideration as to whether long-term treatment is indicated. Current evidence suggests that comprehensive and personalized functional assessment of behaviours in their context with an overarching goal of optimizing integration and normal functioning leads to better outcomes. With these assessment data, it is easier to develop a treatment plan that is amenable to psychological and environmental management of mental illness and challenging behaviour, which, in turn, is likely to reduce or, in some cases, obviate the need for presciption of psychotropic drugs.

## Conclusions

Revised diagnostic guidelines, such as those in the forthcoming ICD-11, have focused on enhancing clinical utility and international applicability. These characteristics of the classification are expected to improve early and accurate diagnosis of disorders of intellectual development, thereby permitting a greater number of persons to be eligible for treatment. Although effective psychosocial and pharmacological interventions are available for the management of challenging behaviours and comorbid psychopathology in affected individuals, these often depend on specialized behavioural interdisciplinary teams, a luxury in most settings across the world. Future research should focus on improving universal accessibility of biopsychosocial services across the lifespan through training of non-specialist staff, as well as carers, in evidence-based approaches such as positive behavioural support.

## REFERENCES

1. First, M.B., Reed, G.M., Hyman, S.E., and Saxena, S. (2015). The development of the ICD-11 Clinical Descriptions and Diagnostic Guidelines for Mental and Behavioural Disorders. *World Psychiatry*, 14, 82–90.
2. International Advisory Group for the Revision of ICD-10 Mental and Behavioural Disorders. (2011). A conceptual framework for the revision of the ICD-10 classification of mental and behavioural disorders. *World Psychiatry*, 10, 86–92.
3. Salvador-Carulla, L., Reed, G.M., Vaez-Azizi, L.M., *et al.* (2011). Intellectual developmental disorders: towards a new name, definition and framework for 'mental retardation/intellectual disability' in ICD-11. *World Psychiatry*, 10, 175–80.
4. American Psychiatric Association. (2013). *Diagnostic and statistical manual of mental disorders* (5th edn). American Psychiatric Association, Washington, DC.
5. Stancliffe, R.J., Lakin, K.C., Larson, S., Engler, J., Taub, S., and Fortune, J. (2011). Choice of living arrangements. *Journal of Intellectual Disability Research*, 55, 746–62.
6. Tassé, M.J., Balboni, G., Navas, P., *et al.* (2019). Developing behavioural indicators for intellectual functioning and adaptive behaviour for ICD-11 disorders of intellectual development. *Journal of Intellectual Disability Research*, 63, 386–407.
7. Oxelgren, U.W., Myrelid, A., Anneren, G., *et al.* (2017). Prevalence of autism and attention-deficit-hyperactivity disorder in Down syndrome: a population-based study. *Developmental Medicine and Child Neurology*, 59, 276–83.
8. Munir, K.M. (2016). The co-occurrence of mental disorders in children and adolescents with intellectual disability/intellectual developmental disorder. *Current Opinion in Psychiatry*, 29, 95–102.
9. Royal College of Psychiatrists. (2016). *Psychotropic drug prescribing for people with intellectual disability, mental health problems and/or behaviours that challenge: practice guidelines*. Royal College of Psychiatrists, London.
10. Fletcher, R., Loschen, E., Stavrakaki, C., and First, M.B. (2007). *Diagnostic manual-ID: a textbook of diagnosis of mental disorders in persons with intellectual disability*. NADD Press, New York, NY.
11. Allen, D., James, W., Evans, J., Hawkins, S., and Jenkins, R. (2005). Positive behavioural support: definition, current status, and future directions. *Tizard Learning Disability Review*, 10, 4–11.
12. Matson, J.L. and Boisjoli, J.A. (2009). The token economy for children with intellectual disability and/or autism: a review. *Research in Developmental Disabilities*, 30, 240–8.
13. Luckasson, R. and Schalock, R.L. (2013). Defining and applying a functionality approach to intellectual disability. *Journal of Intellectual Disability Research*, 57, 657–68.
14. Schalock, R.L., Borthwick-Duffy, S.A., Bradley, V.J., *et al.* (2010). *Intellectual Disability: Definition, Classification, and Systems of Supports* (11th edn). American Association on Intellectual and Developmental Disabilities, Silver Spring, MD.
15. Luiselli, J.K. (2012). *The handbook of high-risk challenging behaviors in people with intellectual and developmental disabilities*. Paul H. Brookes Publishing, Baltimore, MD.
16. Lundqvist, L.O. (2013). Prevalence and risk markers of behavior problems among adults with intellectual disabilities: a total population study in Orebro County, Sweden. *Research in Developmental Disabilities*, 34, 1346–56.
17. Lloyd, B.P. and Kennedy, C.H. (2014). Assessment and treatment of challenging behaviour for individuals with intellectual disability: a research review. *Journal of Applied Research in Intellectual Disabilities*, 27, 187–99.
18. Lowe, K., Allen, D., Jones, E., Brophy, S., Moore, K., and James, W. (2007). Challenging behaviours: prevalence and topographies. *Journal of Intellectual Disability Research*, 51, 625–36.
19. Poppes, P., Van der Putten, A.J., and Vlaskamp, C. (2010). Frequency and severity of challenging behaviour in people with profound intellectual and multiple disabilities. *Research in Developmental Disabilities*, 31, 1269–75.
20. Carr, E.G., Horner, R.H., Turnbull, A.P., *et al.* (1999). *Positive behavior support for people with developmental disabilities: a research synthesis*. American Association on Mental Retardation, Washington, DC.
21. Didden, R., Korzilius, H., Van Oorsouw, W., Sturmey, P., and Bodfish, J. (2006). Behavioral treatment of challenging behaviors in individuals with mild mental retardation: meta-analysis of single-subject research. *American Journal on Mental Retardation*, 111, 290–8.
22. Carr, E.G. (1977). The motivation of self-injurious behavior: a review of some hypotheses. *Psychological Bulletin*, 84, 800.
23. Sanders, M.R., Mazzucchelli, T.G., and Studman, L.J. (2004). Stepping Stones Triple P: the theoretical basis and development of an evidence-based positive parenting program for families with a child who has a disability. *Journal of Intellectual and Developmental Disability*, 29, 265–83.
24. Tellegen, C.L. and Sanders, M.R. (2013). Stepping Stones Triple P-Positive Parenting Program for children with disability: a systematic review and meta-analysis. *Research in Developmental Disabilities*, 34, 1556–71.
25. Brown, M., Duff, H., Karatzias, T., and Horsburgh, D. (2011). A review of the literature relating to psychological interventions and people with intellectual disabilities: issues for research, policy, education and clinical practice. *Journal of Intellectual Disability*, 15, 31–45.
26. Vereenooghe, L. and Langdon, P.E. (2013). Psychological therapies for people with intellectual disabilities: a systematic review and meta-analysis. *Research in Developmental Disabilities*, 34, 4085–102.
27. Sheehan, R., Hassiotis, A., Walters, K., Osborn, D., Strydom, A., and Horsfall, L. (2015). Mental illness, challenging behaviour,

and psychotropic drug prescribing in people with intellectual disability: UK population based cohort study. *BMJ*, 351, h4326.

28. Frighi, V., Stephenson, M.T., Morovat, A., *et al.* (2011). Safety of antipsychotics in people with intellectual disability. *British Journal of Psychiatry*, 199, 289–95.

29. Heslop, P., Blair, P.S., Fleming, P., *et al.* (2014). The Confidential Inquiry into premature deaths of people with intellectual disabilities in the UK: a population-based study. *The Lancet*, 383, 889–95.

30. Haveman, M., Heller, T., Lee, L., Maaskant, M., Shooshtari, S., and Strydom, A. (2010). Major health risks in aging persons with intellectual disabilities: an overview of recent studies. *Journal of Policy and Practice in Intellect Disabilities*, 7, 59–69.

31. Tyrer, P., Cooper, S.A., and Hassiotis, A. (2014). Drug treatments in people with intellectual disability and challenging behaviour. *BMJ*, 349, g4323.

32. Sawyer, A., Lake, J.K., Lunsky, Y., Liu, S.-K., and Desarkar, P. (2014). Psychopharmacological treatment of challenging behaviours in adults with autism and intellectual disabilities: a systematic review. *Research in Autism Spectrum Disorders*, 8, 803–13.

33. Tyrer, P., Oliver-Africano, P.C., Ahmed, Z., *et al.* (2008). Risperidone, haloperidol, and placebo in the treatment of aggressive challenging behaviour in patients with intellectual disability: a randomised controlled trial. *The Lancet*, 371, 57–63.

34. National Institute for Health and Care Excellence (NICE). (2015). *Challenging behaviour and learning disabilities: prevention and interventions for people with learning disabilities whose behaviour challenges.* NICE guideline [NG11]. NICE, London.

35. Trollor, J.N., Salomon, C., and Franklin, C. (2016). Prescribing psychotropic drugs to adults with an intellectual disability. *Australian Prescriber*, 39, 126–30.

36. Birmaher, B., Brent, D., AACAP Work Group on Quality Issues, *et al.* (2007). Practice parameter for the assessment and treatment of children and adolescents with depressive disorders. *Journal of the American Academy of Child and Adolescent Psychiatry*, 46, 1503–26.

37. National Institute for Health and Care Excellence (NICE). (2009). *The treatment and management of depression in adults.* Clinical guideline [CG90]. NICE, London.

38. Campbell, M. and Cueva, J.E. (1995). Psychopharmacology in child and adolescent psychiatry: a review of the past seven years. Part II. *Journal of the American Academy of Child and Adolescent Psychiatry*, 34, 1262–72.

SECTION 4

Autism spectrum disorders

# 25

# Core dimensions of autism spectrum disorders

*Fred R. Volkmar and Scott L.J. Jackson*

## Introduction

Autism spectrum disorder (ASD) is a neurodevelopmental disorder that manifests during the early developmental period of childhood. This disorder is behaviourally defined by impairments in social interaction and communication, in combination with restricted and stereotyped patterns of behaviour and/or interest. There is, however, a diverse range of symptom presentation and severity among diagnosed individuals, including a range of cognitive ability that spans IQ scores representative of profound intellectual disability through to average and well above-average levels of intelligence. As a result, in less severe cases, symptoms may not become fully apparent until later stages of life when social demands surpass the individual's limited abilities. ASD is a new diagnostic label, chosen by the American Psychiatric Association for the 2013 release of the fifth edition of their *Diagnostic and Statistic Manual* (DSM-5) [1]. This label was designed to provide a singular diagnosis to individuals who would have previously been categorized by one of the pervasive developmental disorders (PDDs), as defined in the fourth edition of the DSM [2, 3] and the WHO's counterpart to DSM-IV—the tenth edition of the International Classification of Diseases (ICD-10) [4]. Resultantly, the previously unique PDD diagnoses of autistic disorder (childhood autism in ICD-10), Asperger's syndrome, childhood disintegrative disorder, and PDD-not otherwise specified (PDD-NOS) (PDD-unspecified in ICD-10), are no longer present as diagnostic options for new cases based on DSM-5 criteria but can be 'grandfathered' in by those who were already holding one of these diagnoses prior to this categorical shift.

The ASD section of this textbook will examine and discuss this disorder from a variety of perspectives. This will include chapters addressing current understandings of treatment planning, prevention and epidemiology, genetics, imaging, and management of ASD. Chapter 25, however, will provide an overview of ASD, covering topics of disorder history, prevalence estimates, demographic patterns, clinical features, diagnostic criteria, and differential diagnosis, and close with a discussion on the criticisms and concerns surrounding the DSM-5 classification of ASD and expectations for how this disorder will be defined in the forthcoming eleventh edition of the ICD (ICD-11).

## History of autism spectrum disorders

Leo Kanner, an Austrian-born child psychiatrist, working at Johns Hopkins University, is credited with the first clinical portrayal of ASD in his 1943 paper entitled *Autistic disturbances of affective contact* [5]. In this paper, Kanner details the behaviour of 11 children displaying a pattern of symptoms which included intense resistance to change, insistence on 'aloneness', and impairments in both communication skills and social interaction. Meanwhile, in 1944, independent of the work being conducted by Kanner, Hans Asperger (a psychiatrist working in Austria) produced his own clinical accounts of four cases of what he referred to as autistic personality disorder in his paper *Die Autistischen Psychopathe im Kindesalter* [6]. Similar to what was being described by Kanner, Asperger notes impairments in social and emotional relationships, abnormalities in speech and non-verbal communication, and restricted, but intense, focus on special interests. The primary difference between their accounts is that Asperger additionally discusses the presence of extraordinary skills in particular cognitive domains (for example, mathematics) in the children he was observing. Unfortunately, due to the fact that his work was published in German, Asperger's clinical findings did not become widely disseminated in English-speaking regions until nearly 40 years later.

The first widely utilized label for this disorder ('early infantile autism') was provided in a 1956 paper co-authored by Kanner and Leon Eisenberg [7]. In this paper, the authors proposed that two core features define early infantile autism: 'obsessive insistence on sameness' and 'extreme self-isolation'. Kanner had observed that parents of the patients visiting his clinic presented with similar social disinterest and emotionally distant characteristics to those expressed by their children. Based on these observations, Eisenberg and Kanner proposed that emotional deprivation, as a result of this distant and 'cold' parenting, could play a role in the development of early infantile autism. However, they also went on to express that emotional deprivation could not solely account for the development of early infantile autism, as it was their belief that this disorder was a state that was present at birth and, as such, was likely to be the result of a combination of biological, psychological, and social factors. Unfortunately, it was their declaration regarding the potential role of socially detached, 'cold' parenting that got the most attention initially, and eventually resulted in what becomes known as the 'refrigerator mother' theory of autism. In the 1960s, this theory was furthered in publications by Bruno Bettelheim [8, 9], who, for many years, was considered as one of the leading experts in the field of autism, resulting in the 'refrigerator mother' theory becoming widely disseminated and accepted by many in the lay population, as well as in medical fields.

Beginning in the late 1960s, and more significantly in the 1970s, research in the field of autism moved away from the clinical descriptions and/or theory presentations that previously dominated the landscape of autism literature, and began applying more scientifically stringent methodologies to the study of this disorder. Works produced during this period presented serious challenges to the psychogenic theories of autism (for example, the 'refrigerator mother' theory), by providing empirically supported evidence for a biological and neurological basis of the disorder [10, 11]. In addition, evidence was produced against the then-held position that autism was a form of childhood schizophrenia, with comparative studies clearly distinguishing the two disorders by their associated symptoms, phenomenology, age of onset, and family history [12, 13]. Following these scientific advances, 'infantile autism' was introduced as a formal diagnostic category by the American Psychiatric Association in the 1980 release of DSM-III [14]. Infantile autism was classified as a PDD, a term developed specifically for DSM-III, and defined as being characterized by pervasive and severe impairment in multiple basic functions, including socialization and communication.

In 1981 [15], Lorna Wing introduces the findings of Hans Asperger to the English-speaking world and describes 'Asperger's syndrome', a milder manifestation of the clinical symptoms of infantile autism, often paired with strong cognitive abilities in fields such as mathematics, and excluding the significant language development delays associated with autism. In DSM-IV [2] and DSM-IV-TR [3], the association between this Asperger's syndrome and autism (then labelled as 'autistic disorder') was officially recognized by the American Psychiatric Association, with the decision to expand the diagnostic category of PDDs to include five disorders that were thought to be related to, or share, many of the same features of one another: autistic disorder, Asperger's syndrome, Rett's syndrome, childhood disintegrative disorder, and PDD-NOS. Following this expansion, this group of disorders (with the exception of Rett's syndrome) began to be discussed under the umbrella term of 'autism spectrum disorders' in much of the autism literature.

In 2013, the fifth, and most recent, edition of the DSM (DSM-5) [1] was released and was met with a great deal of controversy regarding its alterations to the diagnostic categorizations of autism and its related disorders. In DSM-5, the previously distinct categories of autistic disorder—childhood disintegrative disorder, Asperger's syndrome, and PDD-NOS—have been reconceptualized as a singular 'autism spectrum disorder' and are defined by more rigid diagnostic criteria. This change was made in an effort to provide a more unified and rigorous definition of what autism is; however, it was met with a number of concerns and criticisms from medical professionals, as well as autism advocacy groups (see Concerns and criticisms of DSM-5 classification of autism spectrum disorder, p. 242, which contains further discussion on this topic), including negative impacts on the sense of community and identity that had been gained through specific diagnostic labels and potential issues with impaired

children not meeting the more stringent diagnostic criteria and losing access to critical services as a result. To address the former of these concerns, while Asperger's syndrome and PDD-NOS are no longer diagnostic options for clinicians within the framework of DSM-5, it was decided that a 'grandfather' clause would be introduced, allowing these labels to remain in individuals who received their diagnosis prior to this change. Meanwhile, to address the concerns over diagnostic sensitivity, DSM-5 introduced a new condition called social communication disorder, intended to provide a label for children without the repetitive and stereotyped behaviour components of ASD but who do express significant social/communicative impairments.

## Prevalence estimates

The first study to present data regarding an estimated prevalence rate for autism was performed by Victor Lotter in 1966 [16]. To provide this estimate, Lotter screened the entire population of 8- to 10-year-old children from a county in the south east of England (78,000 children in total) for behavioural markers of early infantile autism, as then defined by Eisenberg and Kanner [6]. The findings of this screening resulted in an estimate that autism was present in 4.5 of every 10,000 children. From this point until as late as the 1990s, autism was considered to be a rare condition, with subsequent published prevalence reports suggesting rates of 2–5 per 10,000 children [17, 18]. Following the inclusion of 'Infantile autism' in DSM-III in 1980 [14], and the subsequent expansion of diagnostic criteria in the 1987 release of the revised DSM-III-R [19], reported epidemiological studies began documenting dramatic increases in the estimated rates of prevalence for this disorder [20-24, 29].

Beginning in the early 2000s, the Center for Disease Control and Prevention (CDC) began collecting large data samples of 8-year old children from across the United States and producing highly detailed prevalence reports for autism based on their findings every 2–4 years. The most recent of these reports was released in 2014 and documented findings from a sample of 363,749 children (roughly 9% of the total population of 8-year olds in the United States) that was collected across 11 different sites in 2010 [20]. Based on the findings of this report, the overall prevalence of ASD (based on DSM IV-TR diagnostic criteria for autistic disorder, Asperger's syndrome, or PDD-NOS) for children aged 8 years in the United States is 147 per 10,000 (or 1 in 68). That figure was 29% higher than their previous estimate based on data from 2008 [22], 64% higher than their estimate based on data from 2006 [23], and a staggering 123% higher than their estimate based on data from 2002 [24]. In combination with earlier prevalence studies, the findings produced by the CDC suggest a continuous and exponential growth pattern in ASD prevalence over the past 4–5 decades (Fig. 25.1).

This trend of dramatic increases in the reported prevalence of ASD has led some to the conclusion that these findings are evidence of an 'autism epidemic' and, as a result, has encouraged increases in research focused on identifying potential environmental factors to help explain this phenomenon. However, a majority of practitioners and researchers within the ASD field have issued caution against interpreting these findings in this manner and instead suggested that the majority of these increases can be explained by a combination of alternative factors, including: broadening of diagnostic

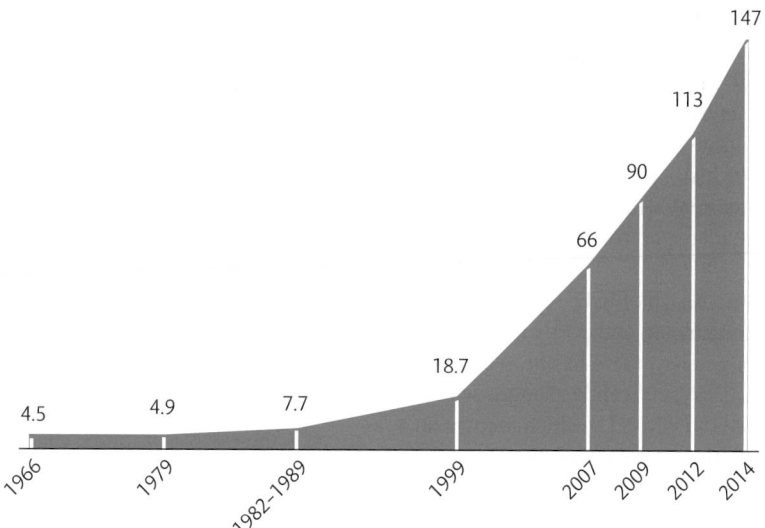

**Fig. 25.1** Time trend of estimated autism prevalence rates (number of children per 10,000). Prevalence estimates for the reported years are from the following studies: 1966 [16], 1979 [18], 1982-1989 [21], 1999 [29], 2007 [24], 2009 [23], 2012 [22], 2014 [20].

criteria, increased availability of diagnostic services, increased disorder awareness, and diagnostic transference/substitution of children who may have previously received an alternative diagnosis (for example, intellectual disability). Though the combination of these factors may be able to account for a large portion of these increases over the years, there may yet be true increases in ASD incidence as well. As such, continued work in this area, and in the identification of potential environmental factors associated with an increased ASD liability, is warranted.

Of note, there is frequently a discrepancy between the current high prevalence rates of ASD among samples of children and the generally lower observed prevalence rates in adults. For some, this discrepancy has been viewed as support to the idea that there has been, in fact, an increase in ASD incidence in recent decades. In contrast to this position, however, it is becoming more apparent that these discrepancies are likely the result of less accurate diagnostic and identification practices in the past [25, 26]. Providing support to these beliefs, and perhaps one of the more compelling findings in opposition to the 'autism epidemic' theory, a recent large community survey estimated that prevalence rates of ASD for adults in the UK should be roughly 1.1% (essentially the same as those found in samples of children), but many of these adults are currently misdiagnosed or completely unidentified [27]. Regardless of whether there has been a true increase in incidence of ASD or not, recent reports suggest that, of all mental disorders, ASD is now the leading cause of disability in children below 5 years of age, affecting somewhere between 1% and 2%, or 52 million children [28], and a roughly equivalent proportion of adults [27] across the globe.

## Demographics

One thing which has remained consistent since the earliest epidemiological studies of ASD is a disproportionate gender ratio. From Kanner's first cohort in 1943 [4] to the first reported prevalence study in 1966 [17], and all the way through to the most recent CDC report released in 2014 [20], autism has been notably more prevalent among males than females, with estimated ratios of 2.5–5:1 [20, 30].

A number of different hypotheses have been proposed to account for the presence of this gender difference. This includes ascertainment bias or altered phenotypical expression in females, resulting in issues with underdiagnosis [31, 32], increased susceptibility of males due to elevated prenatal and early postnatal testosterone levels [33], or the existence of a female protective effect requiring a greater aetiologic load in girls before ASD behavioural symptoms will manifest [34]. At the moment, however, no definitive explanation for why ASD is more prevalent in males than females has emerged. Based on current estimates [20], the male:female gender ratio for ASD is 4.5:1, with a slight increase in this discrepancy when specifically examining individuals without co-occurring intellectual disability (4.9:1).

Unlike gender ratios, one aspect of the demographics of individuals with ASD that has changed over the years is intellectual ability. In particular, over the last decade or so, there have been notable increases in individuals identified with ASD with average or above-average intellectual ability. Likely a result of improved awareness and detection of the often subtler behavioural manifestations of ASD in this more intellectually able cohort, recent findings suggested that 46% of children with an ASD diagnosis have IQ scores in the average to above-average range (>85), 23% in the borderline range (IQ = 71–85), and 31% considered to be in the range of intellectual disability (IQ ≤70). Finally, estimated prevalence rates of ASD tend to be higher among white/Caucasian children, compared to other ethnic/racial groups [20]. However, much of this variation can be accounted for by the significantly higher rates among white children of ASD diagnoses without co-occurring intellectual disability (a diagnosis that can be more difficult to recognize) and thus is likely more suggestive of the influence of socio-economic variables on the quality and quantity of diagnostic and treatment services available to families than of a true discrepancy of ASD prevalence between ethnic/racial groups [35].

## Clinical features and diagnostic criteria

Although there is a general consensus that there is a strong genetic and biological basis to ASD, currently no definitive biological, neurological, or genetic markers for this disorder have been identified. As a result, clinical definitions of ASD remain fundamentally behavioural and historical, reliant on observations (by the clinician or caregiver) of characteristic problems of social interaction, communication, and unusual behaviours which are of early onset (hence the importance of history). Complicating the task of diagnosis (and probably consistent with emerging genetic research [36]), it is clear that a broader spectrum of condition(s) are involved [37].

For the past two decades, the approach of ICD-10 [4] and DSM-IV [2, 3] have been generally concurrent, and partly as a result of this international diagnostic consistency, there has been an explosion of knowledge and research. This has recently changed with the rather different approach adopted in DSM-5 [1] which focuses on a rather narrower view of autism, in the more classic sense of Kanner's autism, resulting in many more cognitively able or less 'prototypical' cases being excluded from an ASD diagnosis [38]. Further complicating the matter are the 'grandfather' clauses (adopted, in part, as a result of criticism of the increased diagnostic stringency) that allow older cases with 'well-established' DSM-IV diagnoses to retain their diagnosis.

Current diagnostic criteria for ASD, as defined by DSM-5, necessitate the presentation of impairments in the following two areas [1]:

1. Persistent deficits in social interaction and social communication (including impaired social–emotional reciprocity, deficits in non-verbal social communicative behaviours, and impaired ability to develop, maintain, and understand age-appropriate social relationships).

2. Restricted and repetitive patterns of activities, behaviours, or interests (including repetitive or stereotyped motor movements, speech, or use of objects; inflexibility with regard to routine adherence, insistence on consistency, or ritualized patterns of behaviour; highly restricted interests that are atypical in focus or intensity; and hypo- or hyper-reactivity to sensory input or atypical interest in sensory features of their environment).

For a diagnosis to be received, the presence of these symptoms must be present during a child's 'early developmental period' and result in clinically significant impairment in some critical area of functioning (for example, occupational, social, academic). The first of these requirements, however, includes the caveat that explicit symptoms of impairment may not become fully apparent until in later stages of life when social demands surpass an individual's limited abilities [1].

The DSM-5 approach has been extensively critiqued [38], and a recent meta-analysis has confirmed the consensus that it represents a move to a more stringent diagnostic concept [39], somewhat undercutting the significance of the name change from the previous category of 'Pervasive developmental disorder' to 'Autism spectrum disorder'. Although perhaps intended to provide a diagnostic option to those individuals not captured by this more stringent diagnostic approach, the inclusion of a new communication disorder—social communication disorder—was introduced in DSM-5. However, the introduction of social communication disorder presents with its own issues, given the very small amount of work supporting such a concept and the complexities involved in its application [40, 41].

## Differential diagnosis

ASD must be differentiated from other developmental disorders—most frequently from intellectual disability (which co-occurs in roughly 30% of cases of ASD [20]) and language/communication disorders. In intellectual disability without ASD, developmental skills (including social ones) are generally relatively evenly developed (or impaired), as compared to the more typical pattern of marked areas of strength (non-verbal abilities) and weakness (verbal and social abilities) seen in ASD. The tasks of differential diagnosis can be most complicated in individuals with severe or profound intellectual disabilities, as differences in relative areas of strength and weakness can be less discernible at these levels of cognitive impairment. Conversely, for more cognitively able individuals, such as those with a DSM-IV diagnosis of Asperger's syndrome, receiving a new diagnosis of ASD may become an unnecessarily complicated task due to the grandfather clause component of DSM-5 [1]. In communication disorders, social vulnerabilities are usually not particularly prominent and the desire to communicate often is clearly present. The new diagnosis of social communication disorder allows for a diagnosis when social and communication problems (but not restrictive behaviours) are present, but not as severe as in the more classic ASD [41].

Some individuals who go on, in later adolescence or young adulthood, to develop schizophrenia may exhibit social oddities earlier in life, similar to, but not typically as severe as, those seen in ASD. Occasionally, severe social anxiety problems may initially be confused with ASD; however, these cases will generally not present with the restricted and repetitive behaviours and interests found in ASD. Conversely, the unusual (often due to intensity or repetitive nature) behaviours or interests of individuals with obsessive–compulsive disorder may be taken to suggest ASD; however, in these cases, the social and language communication skills will be preserved. Sometimes, in cases of severe neglect, a range of symptoms suggestive of ASD may be present; however, in these cases, a history of neglect will often be observed and the social vulnerabilities will begin to abate once appropriate care is provided [42].

## Concerns and criticisms of DSM-5 classification of autism spectrum disorders

Both Kanner's original description of early infantile autism [5, 7] and Asperger's description of autistic personality disorder [6] have been somewhat modified over time. For Kanner's autism, Rutter's 1978 synthesis of subsequent work [43] focused on both social and language/communication deficits of a specific kind (not just explained by overall developmental delay) associated with problems in dealing with change and 'insistence on sameness'. Similarly, Wing's 1981 paper [15] introduced, in large part, Asperger's clinical reports to the English-speaking world, but also modified and broadened it in important ways in her definition of Asperger's syndrome [44]. Kanner's autism was officially recognized in DSM-III [14] and, up until the release of DSM-5 [1], maintained this traditional grouping of diagnostic features/criteria. Of note was the inclusion of other disorders with autism in the PDD category in DSM-IV [2, 3], including Asperger's syndrome, and the convergence of ICD-10 [4] and DSM-IV definitions of these categories. For autism (or autistic disorder/childhood autism, as were then the labels), the DSM-IV/ICD-10 definition proved quite flexible, with many possible combinations of criteria resulting in a diagnosis.

A number of overall changes impacted the DSM-5 review process. Several decisions were made at a programmatic level (for example, to avoid having an entire child section, to change approaches to multi-axial classifications and 'not otherwise specified' conditions) that impacted the process. A further consideration was the decision to primarily rely on data from commonly utilized ASD diagnostic instruments, rather than on field trial data, to provide the new definitions for disorder criteria. Early on, the decision was made to move to a new diagnostic label—autism spectrum disorder (although note the singular term)—and avoid finer-grained classifications like Asperger's syndrome, etc. The use of modified codes and measures of severity were incorporated and were meant to provide the important detailed information otherwise lost with the unification of the previously distinct disorders under a singular label. The decision to eliminate Asperger's syndrome was most controversial, given that despite continued disagreements about the best diagnostic approach to use, research on that condition had increased significantly and meta-analyses were just beginning to appear that showed important differences from more classic Kanner's autism, which can have critical impacts on effective treatment options and strategies [45, 46].

Factor analysis of an extensive data set using measures of both current functioning and past history was utilized to come to the decision to adopt a 'two-factor' approach for the ASD diagnostic criteria in DSM-5. The two factors, determined by this analysis, included one set of monothetic criteria (that is, all four features must be present) focused on social communication problems, and a second set of polythetic criteria (that is, two of four features must be present) focused on restricted, repetitive, or atypical interests and behaviours. Post hoc analyses of the data suggested this to be a well-functioning criteria set. However, some problems have quickly become evident. In the first place, the combinations of criteria that resulted in a diagnosis of ASD were drastically reduced. Secondly, the inclusion of a new diagnostic feature associated with hypo- and hypersensitivity to sensory input did not appear well justified, as a similar feature had produced little predictive value in DSM-IV field trials [47]. In the latter, a factor analysis had shown that two-, three-, or five-factor solutions worked reasonably well (the two-factor solution paralleling the DSM-5 approach, and the five-factor solution providing additional sub-factors based on the repetitive behaviour category) [47]. It should be noted, however, that interpretations of factor analyses can be particularly susceptible to some significant issues, particularly if important data are not included and thus are unable to influence the factors being produced (see [48] for a discussion of the uses and misuses of factor analysis). Some recent studies have now questioned aspects of the factor solution proposed for DSM-5 [49, 50].

As a practical matter, it was quickly apparent that the approach adopted would disqualify many individuals from a diagnosis—particularly those who were younger or more cognitively able (see [51] for a recent meta-analysis). As a result, a decision was made to 'grandfather' in those cases with well-established previous diagnoses, thus resulting in both DSM-IV and DSM-5 diagnostic categories being in effect simultaneously. Some aspects of the approach adopted by DSM-5 are welcome. In fact, the current diagnostic definition is, in many ways, more consistent with Kanner's classic

definition of autism than the broader autism spectrum adopted in DSM-IV, which has a considerable body of support from both genetic and psychological research [38]. As noted previously, the inclusion of a new communication disorder—'social communication disorder'—was not well justified and, as a practical matter, may not succeed in its purpose of capturing those individuals who will fall outside the more stringent DSM-5 diagnostic criteria for ASD, as it was not developed to be convergent with previous diagnoses of Asperger's syndrome or PDD-NOS.

## Expectations for ICD-11

The eleventh edition of the WHO's International Classification of Diseases (ICD-11) is currently being developed and likely will be approved in 2018. A major focus of this effort has been the desire to make the manual (or at least the clinical version) more user-friendly. There has been some attempt to encourage the use of a standard template for clinical decisions and diagnostic guidelines [52]. On balance, it likely will have areas of convergence with DSM-5, with some potential differences as well. A draft version is available, and efforts to evaluate it are now under way [53]. It seems likely that the ICD-11 diagnosis will certainly include individuals with ASD in DSM-5; at this point, the questions centre more around the approach to grouping certain conditions, for example, cases with regression or the more prototypical Asperger's phenotype, and whether the 'grandfathering' rule of DSM-5 will also be adopted.

It should be noted that, in addition to official systems like ICD and DSM, adoption of the Research Domain Criteria (RDoC) approach, proposed by the National Institute of Mental Health, attempts to cut across traditional definitions and focuses on domains of neurobiology and behaviour [54]. The RDoC approaches are organized around several domains of functioning and various approaches of units of study [55]. The latter can range from genes to behaviour to self-report. This approach has been extensively critiqued [56, 57] but has stimulated new lines of enquiry in fields such as co-occurring conditions in traditional approaches. As such, it may have some utility for clinical and treatment studies in which the focus or target behaviour(s) cut across transitional diagnostic categories [54, 58, 59].

## REFERENCES

1. American Psychiatric Association. (2013). *Diagnostic and statistical manual for mental disorders*, fifth edition. American Psychiatric Press, Washington, DC.
2. American Psychiatric Association. (1994). *Diagnostic and statistical manual for mental disorders*, fourth edition. American Psychiatric Press, Washington, DC.
3. American Psychiatric Association. (2000). *Diagnostic and statistical manual for mental disorders*, fourth edition (text revision). American Psychiatric Press, Washington, DC.
4. World Health Organization. (1992). *The ICD-10 classification of mental and behavioural disorders: clinical descriptions and diagnostic guidelines*. World Health Organization, Geneva.
5. Kanner, L. (1943). Autistic disturbances of affective contact. *Nervous Child*, 2, 217–50.
6. Asperger, H. (1944). Die 'Autistischen Psychopathe' im Kindesalter. *European Archives of Psychiatry and Clinical Neuroscience*, 117, 76–136.

7. Eisenberg, L. and Kanner, L. (1956). Childhood schizo-phrenia: symposium, 1955: 6. early infantile autism, 1943–55. *American Journal of Orthopsychiatry*, 26, 556.

8. Bettelheim, B. (1959). Feral children and autistic children. *American Journal of Sociology*, 455–67.

9. Bettelheim, B. (1967). *Empty fortress: infantile autism and the birth of the self.* Simon and Schuster, New York, NY.

10. Rimland, B. (1964). *Infantile autism: the syndrome and its implications for a neural theory of behavior.* Appleton-Century-Crofts, New York, NY.

11. Wing, J.K. (ed.). (1966). *Early childhood autism: clinical, educational and social aspects.* Pergamon, Oxford.

12. Kolvin, I. (1971). Studies in the childhood psychoses. I. Diagnostic criteria and classification. *British Journal of Psychiatry*, 118, 381.

13. Kolvin, I., Ounsted, C., Humphrey, M., and McNay, A. (1971). The phenomenology of childhood psychoses. *British Journal of Psychiatry*, 118, 385–95.

14. American Psychiatric Association. (1980). *Diagnostic and statistical manual for mental disorders*, third edition. American Psychiatric Press, Washington, DC.

15. Wing, L. (1981). Asperger's syndrome: a clinical account. *Psychological Medicine*, 11, 115–29.

16. Lotter, V. (1966). Epidemiology of autistic conditions in young children. *Social Psychiatry*, 1, 124–35.

17. Wing, L. and Potter, D. (2002). The epidemiology of autistic spectrum disorders: is the prevalence rising? *Mental Retardation and Developmental Disabilities Research Reviews*, 8, 151–61.

18. Wing, L. and Gould, J. (1979). Severe impairments of social interaction and associated abnormalities in children: epidemiology and classification. *Journal of Autism and Developmental Disorders*, 9, 11–29.

19. American Psychiatric Association. (1987). *Diagnostic and statistical manual for mental disorders*, third edition (revised). American Psychiatric Press, Washington, DC.

20. Centers for Disease Control and Prevention. (2014). Prevalence of autism spectrum disorder among children aged 8 years—autism and developmental disabilities monitoring network, 11 sites, United States, 2010. *Morbidity and Mortality Weekly Report Surveillance Summaries*, 63, 1–21.

21. Gillberg, C. and Wing, L. (1999). Autism: not an extremely rare disorder. *Acta Psychiatrica Scandinavica*, 99, 399–406.

22. Baio, J. and Centers for Disease Control and Prevention. (2012). Prevalence of autism spectrum disorders: Autism and Developmental Disabilities Monitoring Network, 14 Sites, United States, 2008. *Morbidity and Mortality Weekly Report Surveillance Summaries*, 61(3).

23. Rice, C. and Centers for Disease Control and Prevention. (2009). Prevalence of autism spectrum disorders: Autism and Developmental Disabilities Monitoring Network, United States, 2006. *Morbidity and Mortality Weekly Report Surveillance Summaries*, 58, Number SS–10.

24. Centers for Disease Control and Prevention. (2007). Prevalence of autism spectrum disorders—autism and developmental disabilities monitoring network, 14 sites, United States, 2002. *Morbidity and Mortality Weekly Report Surveillance Summaries*, 56, 2–28.

25. Happé, F. and Charlton, R.A. (2012). Aging in autism spectrum disorders: a mini-review. *Gerontology*, 58, 70–8.

26. Klaiman, C., Fernandez-Carriba, S., Hall, C., and Saulnier, C. (2015). Assessment of autism across the lifespan: a way forward. *Current Developmental Disorders Reports*, 2, 84–92.

27. Brugha, T.S., McManus, S., Bankart, J., *et al.* (2011). Epidemiology of autism spectrum disorders in adults in the community in England. *Archives of General Psychiatry*, 68, 459–65.

28. Hahler, E.M. and Elsabbagh, M. (2015). Autism: a global perspective. *Current Developmental Disorders Reports*, 2, 58–64.

29. Fombonne, E. (1999). The epidemiology of autism: a review. *Psychological Medicine*, 29(4), 769–786.

30. Idring, S., Lundberg, M., Sturm, H., *et al.* (2015). Changes in prevalence of autism spectrum disorders in 2001–2011: findings from the Stockholm youth cohort. *Journal of Autism and Developmental Disorders*, 45, 1766–73.

31. Zwaigenbaum, L., Bryson, S.E., Szatmari, P., *et al.* (2012). Sex differences in children with autism spectrum disorder identified within a high-risk infant cohort. *Journal of Autism and Developmental Disorders*, 42, 2585–96.

32. Lai, M.C., Lombardo, M.V., Auyeung, B., Chakrabarti, B., and Baron-Cohen, S. (2015). Sex/gender differences and autism: setting the scene for future research. *Journal of the American Academy of Child and Adolescent Psychiatry*, 54, 11–24.

33. Auyeung, B., Taylor, K., Hackett, G., and Baron-Cohen, S. (2010). Foetal testosterone and autistic traits in 18 to 24-month-old children. *Molecular Autism*, 1, 1–8.

34. Robinson, E.B., Lichtenstein, P., Anckarsäter, H., Happé, F., and Ronald, A. (2013). Examining and interpreting the female protective effect against autistic behavior. *Proceedings of the National Academy of Sciences of the United States of America*, 110, 5258–62.

35. Dickerson, A.S., Rahbar, M.H., Pearson, D.A., *et al.* (2016). Autism spectrum disorder reporting in lower socioeconomic neighborhoods. *Autism*, 21, 470–80.

36. Rutter, M. and Thapar, A. (2014*). Genetics of autism spectrum disorders.* In: Volkmar, F., Rogers, S., Paul, R., and Pelphrey, K. (eds). *Handbook of autism and pervasive developmental disorders* (4th edn), Vol. II. Wiley Press, Hoboken NJ. pp. 411–23.

37. Ingersoll, B. and Wainer, A. (2014). *The broader autism phenotype.* In: Volkmar, F., Rogers, S., Paul, R., and Pelphrey, K. (eds). *Handbook of autism and pervasive developmental disorders* (4th edn), Vol. I. Wiley Press, Hoboken NJ. pp. 28–56.

38. McPartland, J.C., Reichow, B., and Volkmar, F.R. (2012). Sensitivity and specificity of proposed DSM-5 diagnostic criteria for autism spectrum disorder. *Journal of the American Academy of Child and Adolescent Psychiatry*, 51, 368–83.

39. Smith, I.C., Reichow, B., and Volkmar, F.R. (2015). The effects of DSM-5 criteria on number of individuals diagnosed with autism spectrum disorder: a systematic review. *Journal of Autism and Developmental Disorders*, 45, 2541–52.

40. Tufan, E. (2014). The relationship between social communication disorder (SCD) and broad autism phenotype (BAP). *Journal of the American Academy of Child and Adolescent Psychiatry*, 53, 1130.

41. Ozonoff, S. and Miller, M. (2014). The relationship between social communication disorder (SCD) and broad autism phenotype (BAP): reply. *Journal of the American Academy of Child and Adolescent Psychiatry*, 53,1130–1.

42. Rutter, M., Kumsta, R., Schlotz, W., and Sonuga-Barke, E. (2012). Longitudinal studies using a 'natural experiment' design: the case of adoptees from Romanian institutions. *Journal of the American Academy of Child and Adolescent Psychiatry*, 51, 762–70.

43. Rutter, M. (1978). Diagnosis and definition of childhood autism. *Journal of Autism and Childhood Schizophrenia*, 8, 139–61.

44. Volkmar, F.R., Klin, A., and McPartland, J.C. (2014). *Asperger syndrome: an overview.* In: McPartland, J.C, Klin, A., and

Volkmar, F.R. (eds). *Asperger syndrome: assessing and treating high-functioning autism spectrum disorders*. Guilford Press, New York, NY. pp. 1–42.

45. Chiang, H.M., Tsai, L.Y., Cheung, Y.K., Brown, A., and Li, H. (2014). A meta-analysis of differences in IQ profiles between individuals with Asperger's disorder and high-functioning autism. *Journal of Autism and Developmental Disorders*, 44, 1577–96.

46. Volkmar, F.R., Klin, A., and McPartland, J.C.(2014). *Treatment and intervention guidelines for Asperger syndrome*. In: McPartland, J.C, Klin, A., and Volkmar, F.R. (eds). *Asperger syndrome: assessing and treating high-functioning autism spectrum disorders*. Guilford Press, New York, NY. pp. 143–78.

47. Volkmar, F.R., Klin, A., Siegel, B., *et al.* (1994). Field trial for autistic disorder in DSM-IV. *American Journal of Psychiatry*, 151, 1361–7.

48. Gould, S.J. (1996). *The mismeasure of man*. Norton, New York, NY.

49. Bölte, S. and Poustka, F. (2001). [Factor structure of the Autism Diagnostic Interview-Revised (ADI-R): a study of dimensional versus categorical classification of autistic disorders]. *Zeitschrift fur Kinder-und Jugendpsychiatrie und Psychotherapie*, 29, 221–9.

50. Wade, J. and Reeves, R. Examination of the factor structure of the Autism Diagnostic Interview-Revised (ADI-R) within a simplex population. *Journal of Autism and Developmental Disorders* (in press).

51. Smith, I.C., Reichow, B., and Volkmar, F.R. (2015). The effects of DSM-5 criteria on number of individuals diagnosed with autism spectrum disorder: a systematic review. *Journal of Autism and Developmental Disorders*, 45, 2541–52.

52. First, M.B., Reed, G.M., Hyman, S.E., and Saxena, S. (2015). The development of the ICD-11 clinical descriptions and diagnostic guidelines for mental and behavioural disorders. *World Psychiatry*, 14, 82–90.

53. Reed, G.M., First, M.B., Elena Medina-Mora, M., Gureje, O., Pike, K.M., and Saxena, S. (2016). Draft diagnostic guidelines for ICD-11 mental and behavioural disorders available for review and comment. *World Psychiatry*, 15, 112–13.

54. Lilienfeld, S.O. (2014). The Research Domain Criteria (RDoC): an analysis of methodological and conceptual challenges. *Behaviour Research and Therapy*, 62, 129–39.

55. Insel, T., Cuthbert, B., Garvey, M., *et al.* (2010). Research Domain Criteria (RDoC): toward a new classification framework for research on mental disorders. *American Journal of Psychiatry*, 167, 748–51.

56. Cuthbert, B.N. (2014). The RDoC framework: facilitating transition from ICD/DSM to dimensional approaches that integrate neuroscience and psychopathology. *World Psychiatry*, 13, 28–35.

57. Cuthbert, B.N. (2015). Research Domain Criteria: toward future psychiatric nosologies. *Dialogues in Clinical Neuroscience*, 17, 89–97.

58. Sukhodolsky, D.G., Scahill, L., Gadow, K.D., *et al.* (2008). Parent-rated anxiety symptoms in children with pervasive developmental disorders: frequency and association with demographic and clinical characteristics. *Journal of Abnormal Child Psychology*, 36, 117–28.

59. Sukhodolsky, D.G., Vander Wyk, B., Eilbott, J., *et al.* (2016). Neural mechanisms of cognitive-behavioral therapy for aggression in children: design of a randomized controlled trail within the RDoC construct of frustrative non-reward. *Journal of Child and Adolescent Psychopharmacology*, 26, 38–48.

# 26

# Basic mechanisms and treatment targets for autism spectrum disorders

*Emily J.H. Jones*

## Introduction to autism spectrum disorder

Autism spectrum disorder (ASD) is a neurodevelopmental disorder characterized by difficulties with social communication, and the presence of restrictive interests, repetitive behaviours, and sensory symptoms [1]. Symptoms must be apparent from early childhood for a diagnosis to be made. ASD is 3–4 times more common in boys than girls, which likely represents a combination of biological differences and under-identification of girls in community settings. The name 'autism *spectrum* disorder' reflects the huge variability in the degree and nature of the symptoms that people with ASD experience and the likely heterogeneity in their underlying causal mechanisms. While some individuals with ASD have highly successful professional and personal lives, others may never live independently, have a job, or form strong peer relationships. Developing new treatment options for individuals with ASD requires determining the mechanisms that underlie the emergence, consolidation, and maintenance of core symptoms throughout the lifespan. This chapter will describe the approaches used to study the basic mechanisms underlying ASD, review our current understanding of the processes that contribute to symptoms, and indicate the value of this work for identifying new treatment targets.

## Approaches to identifying the mechanisms that underlie symptoms of ASD

When searching for treatment targets, we need to identify the biological or neurodevelopmental pathways that cause the emergence or maintenance of clinical symptoms of ASD. Such causal mechanisms need to be distinguished from secondary or compensatory processes and be separated from differences related to co-occurring symptoms (like anxiety or ADHD), in order to target core domains of ASD symptomatology. We must understand how mechanisms relate to both strengths and weaknesses in ASD, in order to avoid unwanted effects of targeted treatments. To address these pressing goals, researchers have taken a range of approaches that I shall summarize now.

## Case-control studies

The vast majority of efforts to delineate the mechanisms underlying ASD symptoms rely on comparing neurocognitive function in people with and without ASD. Any difference in the ASD group is usually interpreted as atypicality and considered to be a candidate causal mechanism. Such 'case-control' designs can provide a rapid assessment of whether a particular measure is likely to have value for further investigation. However, they have many limitations. Firstly, the interpretation of group differences always relies on the selection of an appropriate control group, but finding the 'perfect' control group is very difficult (and perhaps impossible). Groups may differ on both core and associated symptoms (for example, anxiety and depression); examining whether variables associated with case/control differences are dimensionally related to autism symptomatology can mitigate this concern but require large group sizes. Dealing with IQ is similarly problematic; uneven cognitive profiles in individuals with ASD can make matching difficult, and the considerable neurobiological heterogeneity in children with general developmental delays can limit our understanding of the differences we see in the ASD group. There is also a degree of genetic overlap between developmental disability and ASD [2], so we could be 'controlling' for variation in which we are interested. An alternative option is to contrast how performance on a neurocognitive task relates to variables, such as chronological age, mental age, or social communication skill, in both the ASD and comparison groups. This 'developmental trajectories' approach has been used to show that face-processing skills co-vary with broader social communication skills in the same way in children with and without ASD, such that children with ASD were showing patterns resembling those in younger typically developing children [3]. This approach is very promising but is yet to be widely adopted. In light of such limitations, research has moved away from traditional case-control designs and towards other approaches.

## Trait-based approaches

Trait-based approaches, like the Research Domain Criteria (RDoC) framework, address some of the limitations of case-control designs [4]. Moving beyond the clinical diagnosis, the RDoc specifies a number of domains that can be described at multiple levels of analysis (from genetics to behaviour). Focusing on particular key domains within heterogenous participant groups may be fruitful in identifying the neural mechanisms that are associated with variation in a particular symptom cluster. Since most genetic risk for ASD lies with common variation [5] and genes carrying risk for ASD co-vary with typical variation in social communication skills in childhood [6], studying the neurocognitive underpinnings of ASD-related traits in the general population could be very fruitful. Given the developmental nature of ASD, studies in infancy are particularly important. Indeed, we recently showed that infant measures of social attention that predict later ASD also co-vary with parental ASD-related traits in a large group of typically developing infants [7] (Fig. 26.1). Such studies provide great potential for understanding the neurodevelopmental processes that mediate between genetic risk and phenotypic expression of ASD-related traits.

The RDoc framework is not without limitations. The developmental aspects of the framework need elaborating [8], which is critical to increasing its applicability to neurodevelopmental disorders like ASD. This can be challenging, because neural functions may be less specialized or differentiated in early infancy and the mapping between brain function and cognitive process may be different [9]. A further challenge to fully implementing trait-based approaches is the relative fragility of our current neurocognitive batteries. Many lack acceptable basic psychometric properties like test–retest reliability, or context insensitivity, which may be a critical limitation to their use in indexing individual differences in a clinical context. One way to mitigate these concerns is to select tasks for investigation that produce robust replicable responses in individuals. However, will these be sensitive to ASD-related differences? A number of recent studies have linked ASD to increased intra-individual variability in responses [10, 11] or greater idiosyncrasy in functional activation patterns [12, 13]. If ASD is characterized not by stably different (trait-like) neurocognitive function, but by greater 'state' variation in activation patterns, simple tasks that achieve high test–retest reliability in individuals with ASD may actually be those that are least likely to identify deficits. In general, the field may need to

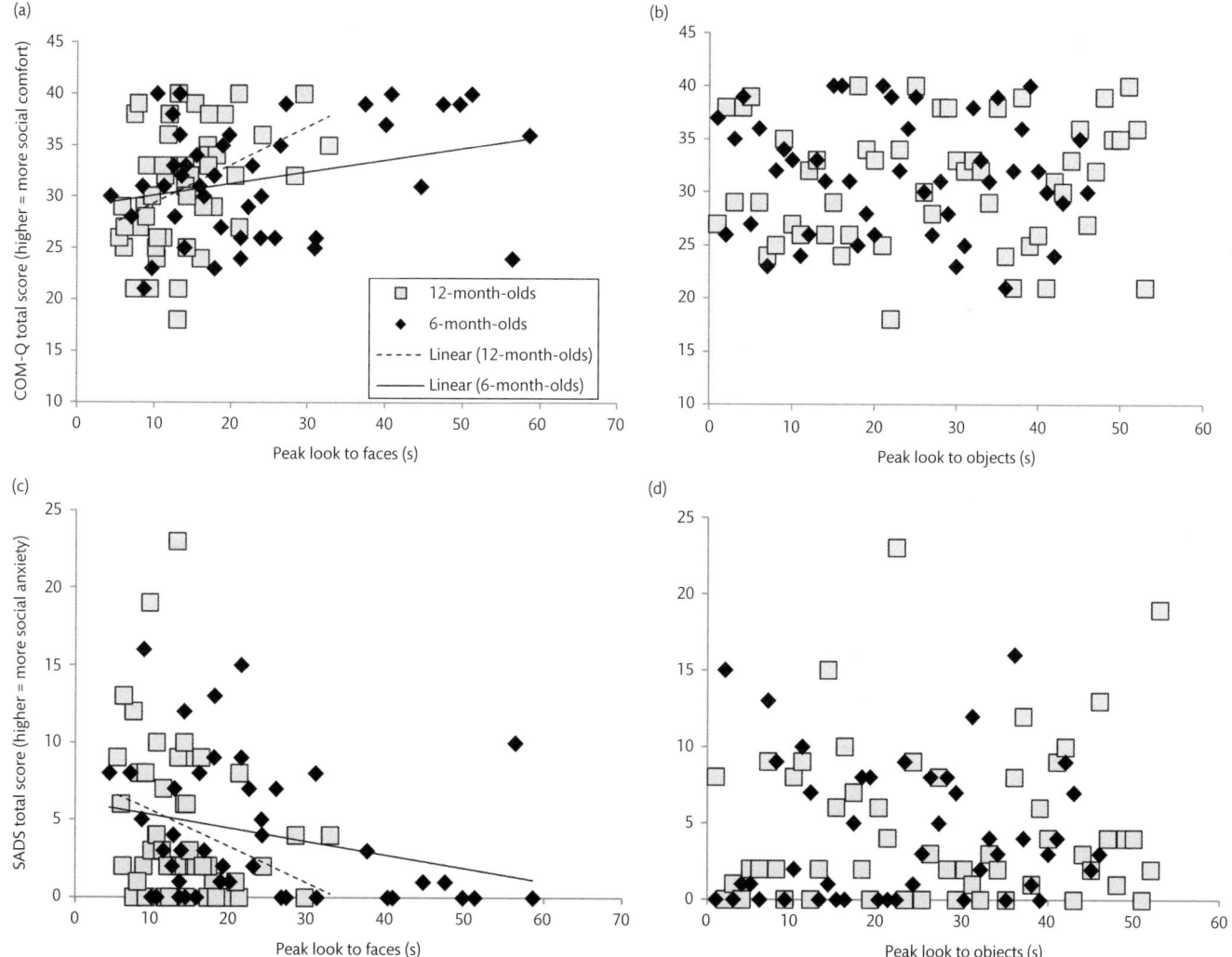

**Fig. 26.1** Higher parent social anxiety (SADS, social anxiety, and distress) and lower social comfort (COMQ, Social Competence Questionnaire) relate to shorter peak look to faces (a, c), but not objects (b, d) in 6- and 12-month-old infants. Shorter peak looks to faces have been previously associated with later ASD.

Reproduced from *J. Child Psychol. Psychiatry*, 58(3), Jones EJH, Venema K, Earl RK., *et al.*, Infant social attention: an endophenotype of ASD-related traits? pp. 270–281, Copyright (2017), with permission from John Wiley and Sons.

develop more sophisticated neurocognitive methodologies rooted in neurobiology to find metrics that circumvent these issues. This may include a shift of approach from static cognitive traits towards identifying markers of state-related changes in brain responses.

## Longitudinal prospective studies

Longitudinal studies of children with ASD allow the identification of neural mechanisms that predict later symptom variation. In a recent example, Neuhaus and colleagues showed that more normative neural responses to faces at the age of 3 years predicted greater improvement in core ASD symptoms between the age of 3 and adolescence [14] (Fig. 26.2). Although these associations do not prove causality, they provide a more powerful way of identifying good candidate mechanisms to subject to more rigorous testing. Prospective studies of infants at familial risk for ASD go one step further by allowing investigators to identify mechanisms that may underpin symptom *emergence*. Such studies follow groups of infants with older siblings with ASD, who have a 20% chance of developing ASD themselves [15]. Researchers use a battery of measures to assess early neural, cognitive, and behavioural development in these infants, which can then be examined in light of their ASD outcome status from toddlerhood (Fig. 26.3). Recent reviews of this literature highlight the accumulation of behavioural autism symptoms in the second year of life, preceded by more subtle, but apparently more

domain-general, atypicalities [16, 17]; early reports from parent-mediated interventions for high-risk infants suggest that some of these domains can be successfully targeted [18–20] (Fig. 26.4).

## Genetics

Given the high heritability of ASD, genetic information is critical to building causal models of symptom emergence. Advances in technology have rapidly expanded our ability to extract and interpret information about genetic variation associated with ASD, although there is still much to discover [21]. However, turning genetic information into meaningful hypotheses about causal mechanisms remains challenging. Many genetic studies still use coarse phenotypes like the presence or absence of a clinically determined ASD diagnosis, which shares many of the limitations of case-control studies of neurocognitive measures described (including the common failure to consider co-occurring syndromes like depression, ADHD, or anxiety). Further, the path between genotype and phenotype is not static but emerges through a developmental interaction between the gene and the environment on the substrate of the developing brain (Fig. 26.5). Substantial compensatory and adaptive mechanisms exist to buffer early disruptions, and these likely include epigenetic modifications that produce significant changes in gene expression over development [22]. In order to understand how genetic variation underpins ASD symptom emergence, prospective studies are required that measure genetic variation, epigenetic

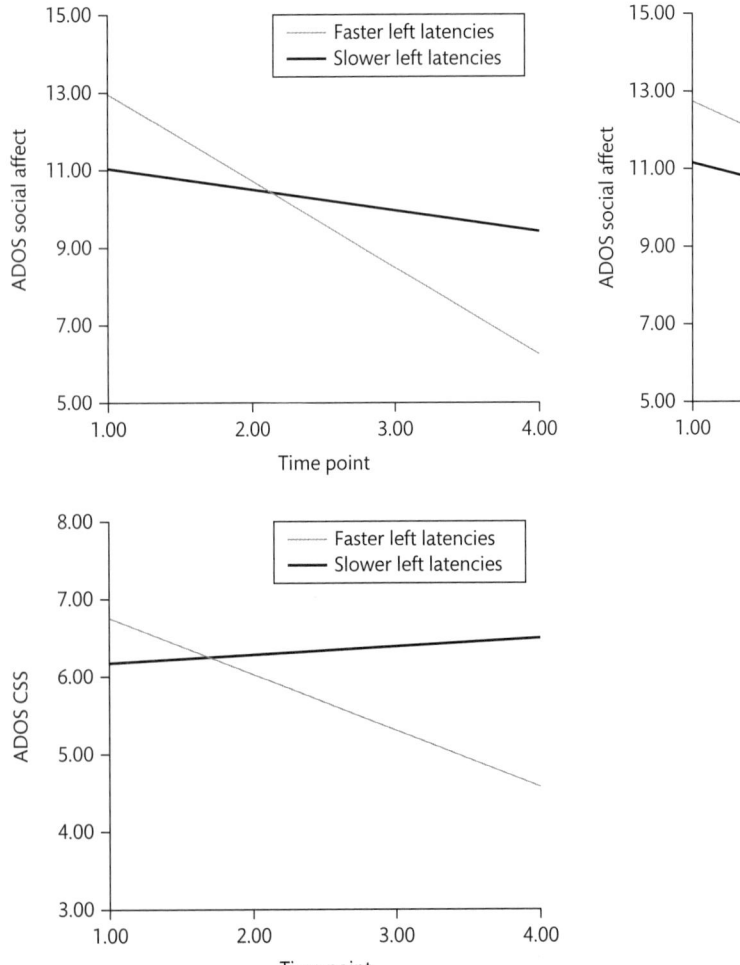
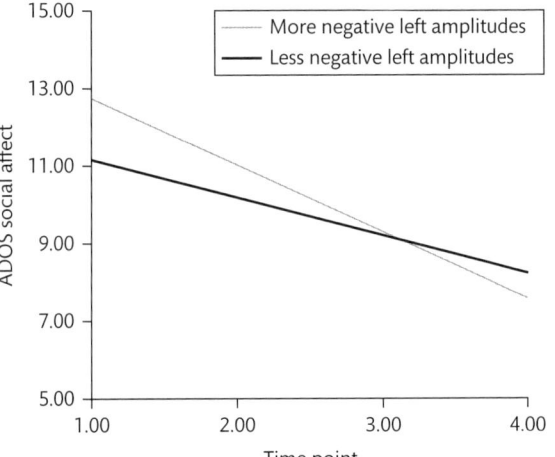

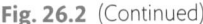

**Fig. 26.2** (Continued)

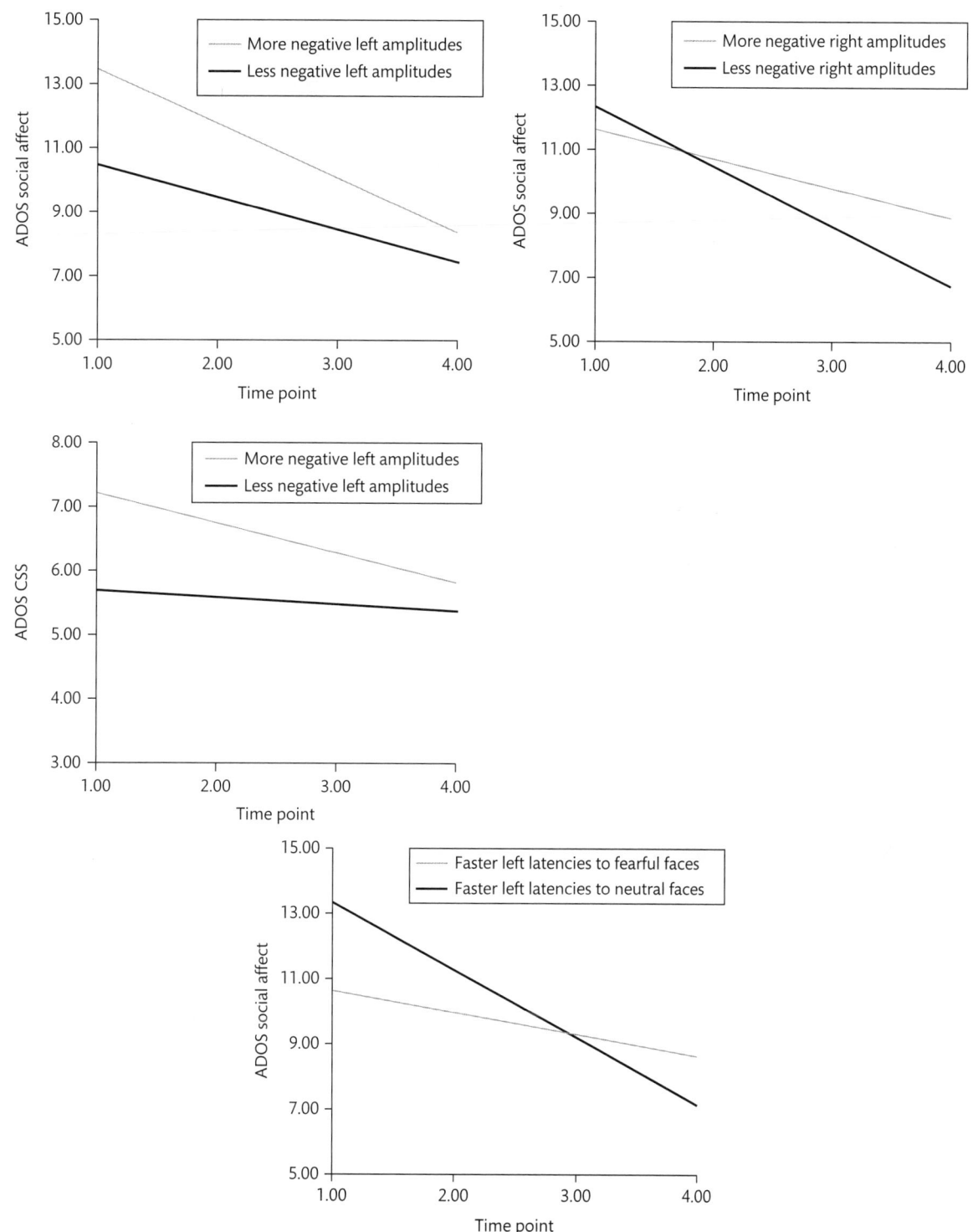

**Fig. 26.2** ADOS social affect symptom trajectories over time by N290 response (median split) to neutral faces. Time point 1 = 3 years, 2 = 6 years, 3 = 9 years, 4 = 14 years.

Reproduced from *J. Autism Dev. Disord.*, 46(7), Neuhaus E, Jones EJ, Barnes K, *et al.*, The Relationship Between Early Neural Responses to Emotional Faces at Age 3 and Later Autism and Anxiety Symptoms in Adolescents with Autism, pp. 2450–2463, Copyright (2016), with permission from Springer Science Business Media New York.

regulation, the developing brain, and emerging behavioural symptoms over time.

A complementary approach to incorporating information about genetics into models of ASD emergence is to study children with genetic syndromes associated with high rates of ASD like fragile X, tuberous sclerosis, or Cohen's syndrome [23]. Animal models of some of these conditions are available, allowing clearer links to be drawn between human research and basic neurobiology and allowing identification of putative treatment targets. However, medications targeted at mechanisms in conditions like fragile X produce

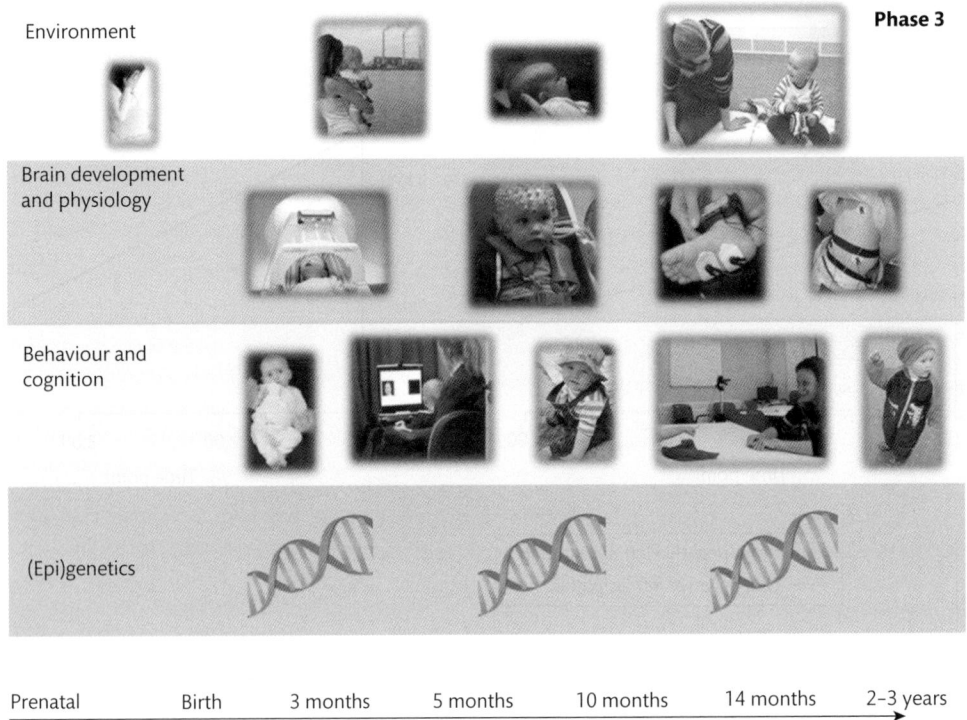

**Fig. 26.3** Prospective infant sibling studies using broad batteries of measures to assess the emergence of ASD over developmental time. Note: N290 responses were modelled as continuous predictors. For ease of visualization, lines shown represent symptom trajectories for participants divided on median value of N290 responses.

Image courtesy of Emily Gold.

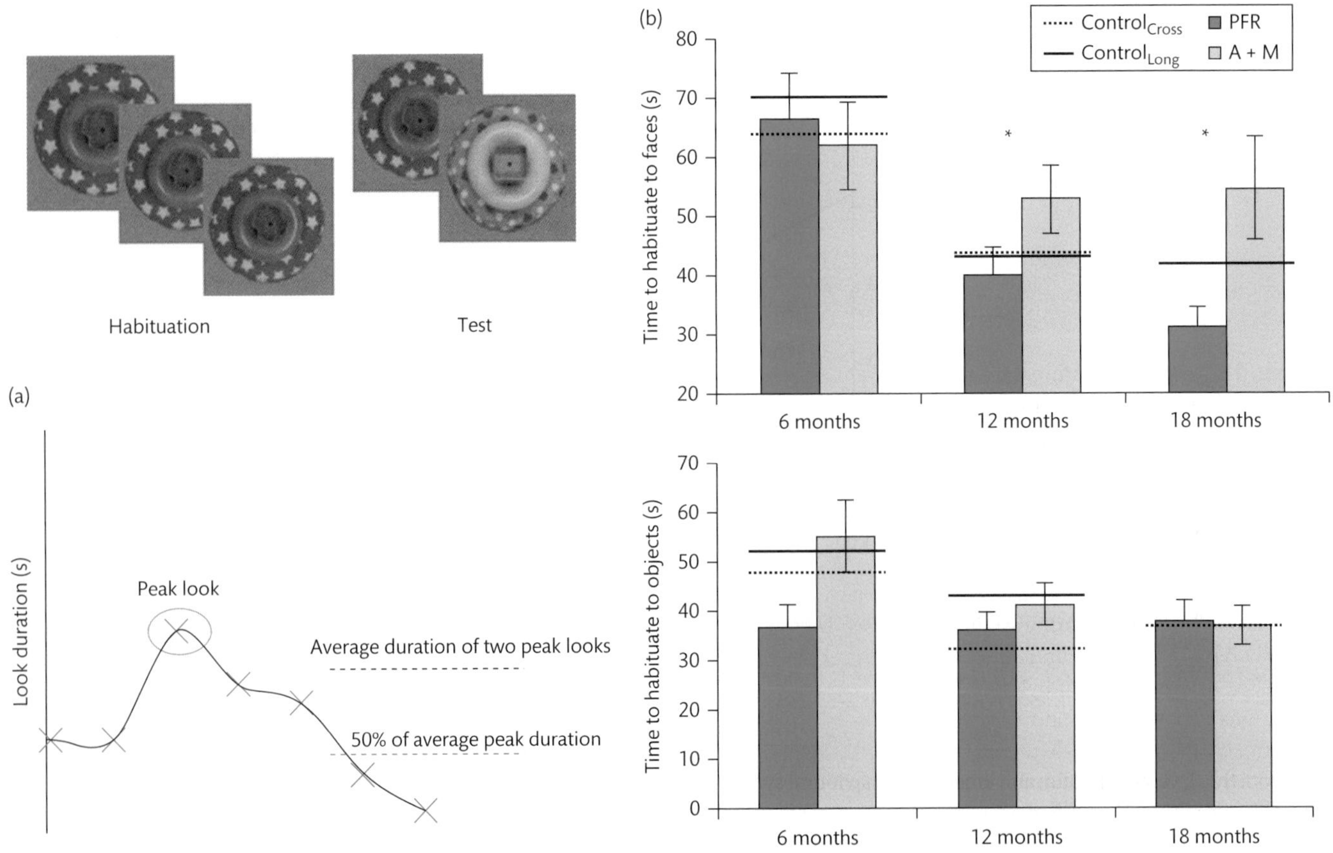

**Fig. 26.4** Effects of parent-mediated intervention on time to habituate to faces (a) in infants at high familial risk for ASD. Infants who received the Promoting First Relationships (PFR) intervention showed greater developmental improvements in habituation time than infants who only received assessment and monitoring. Data from low-risk control infants are shown as solid (longitudinal) and dotted (cross-sectional) lines.

Adapted from *Autism Res.*, 10(5), Jones EJH, Dawson G, Estes A, *et al.*, Parent-delivered early intervention in infants at risk for ASD: Effects on electrophysiological and habituation measures of social attention, pp.961–972, Copyright (2017), with permission from John Wiley and Sons.

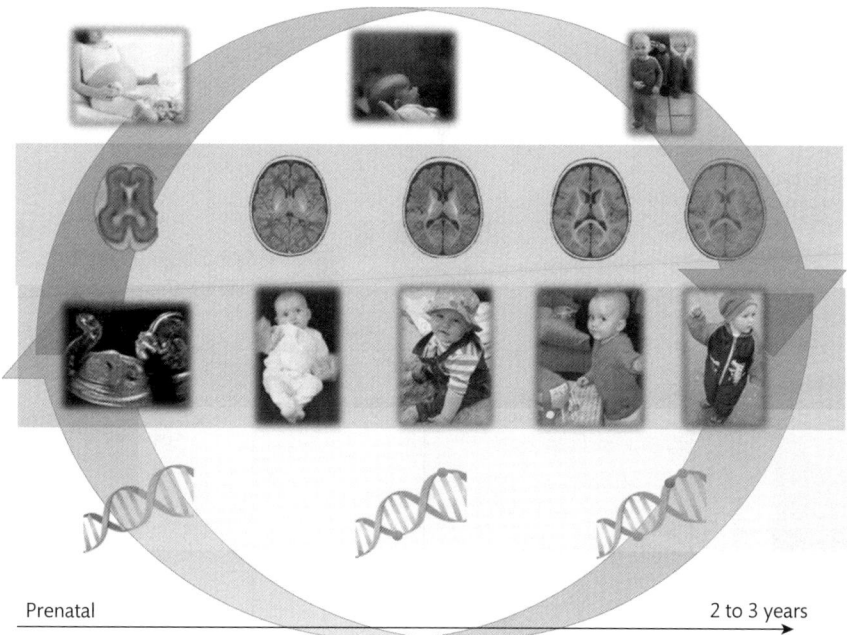

**Fig. 26.5** Symptoms of ASD emerge through a complex interaction between genes and environment, which interact in the context of the child's developing body and brain.
Image courtesy of Emily Gold.

impressive effects in rodents but have yet to show promise in human trials [24]. The significant limitations of mouse and rat models in modelling social and communication domains may play a role. Further, little is known about which of the neurodevelopmental paths underlying symptoms of ASD in genetic disorders are shared with children with idiopathic ASD. Fortunately, a number of investigators have recently begun longitudinal prospective studies of infants with conditions like tuberous sclerosis or neurofibromatosis type 1, which will go some way to addressing these questions.

## Current understanding of the mechanisms underlying ASD symptoms

The rapidly expanding literature on ASD constantly produces new hypotheses about its underpinning mechanisms. I have selected three explanations in the following sections that illustrate the necessity of both theories derived from 'top–down' clinical studies of individuals with ASD and those with a strong emphasis on genetics and neurobiology. I will point to areas of interface between these levels of explanation, which hold promise for the eventual reconciliation of these frameworks. However, it is important to note that there may or may not be one 'final causal path' to autism symptoms—it is probable that autism represents the combination of several risk pathways that happen to co-occur in some individuals, and the number of possible combinations may be many and varied (the 'autisms' [25]). There is very unlikely to be one single explanation for autism, and indeed the following accounts contain many different specific routes to differences in a very broadly defined area of neurocognitive function.

### Social attention, motivation, and affiliation

Social communication impairment is one of the most distinctive features of ASD. 'Social first' theories propose that children with ASD find social stimuli less engaging than they should (for a variety of

possible reasons), which may compromise learning about the social world and the ongoing development of the social brain [26–28]. Routes to diminished engagement may include a failure to assign reward value to social stimuli, altered responsivity to complex and unpredictable stimuli, or difficulties with specific aspects of social cognition. Children may experience one or more of these specific difficulties, but the common end result posited is a gradual withdrawal from the social world. Given that self-directed experience is likely very important in social communication development, children's initial difficulties are compounded by this social withdrawal.

### Evidence for the role of social attention

A range of evidence exists for the early emergence of differences in social attention. While 'innate' social subcortical orienting may be intact [29], putatively 'cortical' aspects of social attention are altered early in infants with later ASD. By 6 months, infants with later ASD show altered temporal profiles of attention engagement with faces [30] (Fig. 26.6), reduced interest in speaking faces [31], reduced interest in social scenes [32], and declining interest in the eyes [33]. Differences in social behaviours like joint attention accumulate through the second year, resulting in a profile of a gradually decreasing interest in other people that matches that hypothesized in developmental accounts [34]. Taken together, data from prospective studies indicate that differences in social attention are observed from early development of infants with later ASD. One critical next step is to establish whether such differences are simply a signature of ASD unfolding [35] or whether they additionally contribute to later emerging social communication problems.

Studies of newly diagnosed toddlers confirm differences in social attention. For example, when viewing naturalistic social scenes, toddlers with ASD pay less attention to other people's activities [36] and show reduced interest in faces and people when speech and eye contact are introduced [37]. Further, toddlers with ASD show reduced attention to stimuli depicting biological motion [38, 39], a

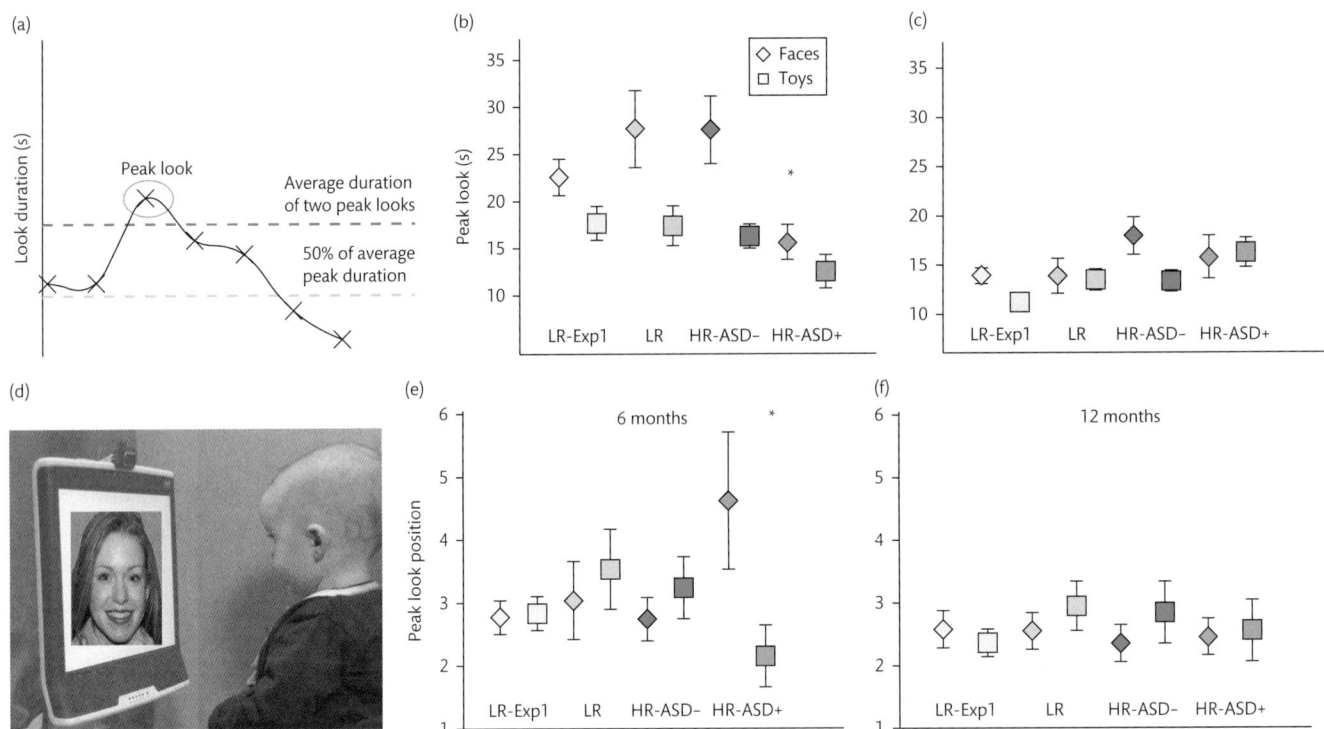

**Fig. 26.6** Shorter (b) and delayed (e) peak looks to faces relate to later autism at 6 months in high-risk infants. Data taken from a habituation paradigm illustrated in (a) and (d).
Adapted from *J. Neurodev. Disord.*, 8(7), Jones EJH, *et al.*, Reduced engagement with social stimuli in 6-month-old infants with later autism spectrum disorder: a longitudinal prospective study of infants at high familial risk, Copyright (2016), Jones *et al.* Reproduced under the Creative Commons Attribution License CC BY 4.0.
Image courtesy of Emily Gold.

highly conserved ability typically present from birth [40]. By the time of diagnosis, differences in social attention are accompanied by alterations in face processing. Expert face processing relies on experience with faces in early development [41], and thus, early alterations in face processing could represent downstream consequences of diminished social attention. For example, pre-schoolers with ASD show altered neural responses to familiar faces [42] and faces displaying emotional expressions [43] that predicted symptom trajectories into adolescence [14], indicating broad disruption to social brain systems. Toddlers with ASD also take longer to learn about faces [44] and show delays in neural responses to face familiarity that are in line with their broader social delays [3] (Fig. 26.7). Of note, basic face-processing components like the N290 appear typical in earlier development [30, 45]. Taken together, disruptions in social attention may be associated with downstream effects on aspects of social cognition by the time of diagnosis.

Moving forward, the potential role of social attention in the emergence of ASD makes it a suitable target for developing proxy markers of treatment outcome. This may be particularly important in developmental populations in which symptoms may not have fully emerged. However, the likelihood that there is heterogeneity in the processes that underlie alterations in social attention means that we will likely need a range of 'biomarkers' if we wish to target the underlying neural systems. Measures like eye-tracking responses to complex social scenes may be closer to the symptoms used to diagnose ASD and may thus show shared alterations across a broader range of individuals. In contrast, EEG or fMRI studies may target

systems that are only altered in a subset of individuals and may thus be more suited to identifying meaningful subgroups of participants. Whether or not these subgroups require different treatment approaches remains an open question and relates to whether or not alterations in particular neurocognitive systems can be linked to particular aspects of molecular pathophysiology. It may be EEG- or fMRI-derived subgroups can be used to define measures that are used to test the effects of treatments on the systems that appear altered in that individual, but the underpinning pathophysiological alterations may not fall into the same categories. For example, one might determine that social reward networks are underpinning social difficulties in one subgroup, while differences in social cognition are most problematic for another. The same treatment might be tested, but its effects on social reward used as the primary outcome in one group and its effects on social cognition as the primary outcome in another. Alternatively, a treatment may specifically target social cognition, in which case participants may be screened on the basis of neurocognitive measures for trial entry. New efforts to use EEG to identify participants for clinical trials are an important step in testing such ideas.

### Treatment targets

Although neurodevelopmental studies with humans do not examine the primary distal causes of autism (genetic and environmental), they can identify developmental processes that serve to canalize or consolidate development down an atypical path. Targeting such processes may provide valuable ways of ameliorating later symptom

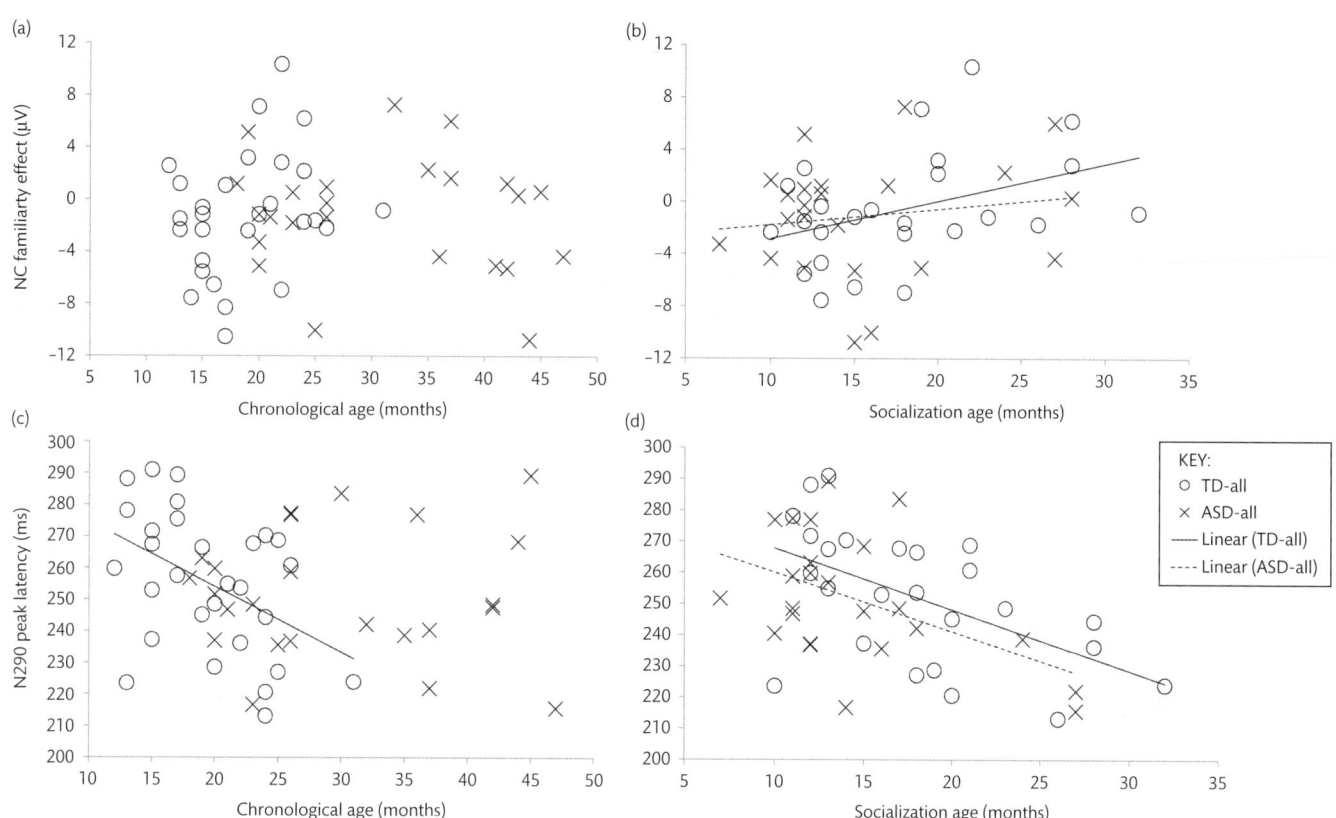

**Fig. 26.7** Relationship between the Nc event-related potential familiarity effect (response to familiar minus unfamiliar face) and (a) chronological age and (b) socialization age, taken from the Vineland Adaptive Behavior Scales. Relationship between the N290 event-related potential peak latency and (c) chronological age and (d) socialization age. Findings show that in toddlers with autism, responses to faces develop in line with social, but not chronological, age.

Adapted from *Child Dev.* 82(6), Webb SJ, Jones EJ, Merkle K, *et al.* Developmental Change in the ERP Responses to Familiar Faces in Toddlers with Autism Spectrum Disorders Versus Typical Development, pp. 1868–1886, Copyright (2011), with permission from John Wiley and Sons.

trajectories. Joint attention is a construct that illustrates the potential for developing causal models of ASD emergence that can be used to develop new treatments. Joint attention refers to the ability to 'co-ordinate attention between interactive social partners with respect to objects or events in order to share an awareness of the objects or events' [46]. Most typically developing infants are able to share attention, follow another's direction of attention, and direct another's attention by pointing themselves by around 12 months. Early joint attention skills predict individual differences in later language development [47], consistent with the idea that shared attention scaffolds early language development. Toddlers with ASD show marked impairments in aspects of joint attention [46, 48] that relate both to concurrent and future language skills [49]. Building on this research, Connie Kasari and colleagues have developed programmes targeted at joint attention, in addition to other symbolic play and engagement skills [Joint Attention, Symbolic Play, Engagement and Regulation (JASPER)], and shown significant effects on social communication, emotion regulation, and language in pre-schoolers [50, 51]. Indeed, JASPER is one of two interventions recommended by NICE in the UK as evidence-based. The progress in this research field highlights the power of a developmental approach.

Social engagement (broadly defined) has been the target of other successful behavioural intervention approaches for children with ASD. For example, Dawson and Rogers have developed comprehensive and intensive programmes (the Early Start Denver Model)

that also feature inter-personal exchange and shared engagement as a core target; these have improved both communication skills [52] and neural responses to social stimuli [53] in young children with ASD. Green and colleagues have developed the less intensive Preschool Autism Communication Trial (PACT) model, which focused on increasing the engagement and reciprocity of interactions between children and their parents [54]. This intervention can produce long-term improvements in symptoms in children with ASD [55]; improvements are likely mediated through changes in parental synchrony and child initiations [56]. Plasticity in early development has the potential to be even greater, and so researchers have also developed parent-mediated programmes for infants at high familial risk for ASD. These typically focus on boosting sensitivity to early communicative cues, encouraging the child's efforts to enter the social world. Though replication is needed, early results are promising and suggest there may be effects on emerging autism symptoms [18, 20] and the neurocognitive correlates of social attention [19]. One key limitation of psychosocial trials is that parents and caregivers are aware of treatment status, making the use of caregiver questionnaire measures (the most common outcome measures used in pharmaceutical trials) very problematic. Blinded behavioural or neurocognitive outcome assessments are thus critically important in this field. However, the relevance of many of these measures to everyday functioning for individuals has not been demonstrated. Ongoing efforts to develop new objective biomarkers for social cognition [57] and analysis approaches for common diagnostic assessments that are more sensitive to treatment change [58] will facilitate progress in this area. Further, testing whether changes in social attention/social cognition predict longer-lasting change in social functioning will be an important test of causal frameworks and will indicate whether such measures could form proxy outcome measures for future trials.

Pharmacological treatment targets in the domain of social cognition have also been identified. One promising line of investigation is the neuropeptides oxytocin and vasopressin. These are highly conserved mediators of complex social cognition and behaviour and, with appropriate caution, could thus prove valuable translational targets [59, 60]. Several trials of the effects of oxytocin have been reported in people with autism, with some predicted effects on social cognition and behaviour [61–63]. One challenge to be addressed is the mode of oxytocin administration, since effects on the brain of intranasal administration (the most common method) may be limited to high doses and within certain time windows after administration [64]. The developmental window during which oxytocin is administered may also be critical. For example, mice with a mutation in *Cntnap2* display deficits in social behaviour and reduced oxytocin; daily application of oxytocin improved later social engagement, but this was most pronounced when treatment occurred earlier in development [65]. These results are promising, but in wildtype mice, chronic application of oxytocin developmentally can produce compensatory mechanisms that *reduce* sociability in adulthood [66]. Such results illustrate the importance of considering compensatory systems and the need for individualized treatment approaches. Vasopressin (which differs in only two amino acids from oxytocin) has been less well investigated, but in addition to core functions in regulating blood pressure, it also has an important function in mediating social behaviours [4]. Vasopressin enters the CNS after intranasal administration and can modulate brain networks involved in processing emotional information [67]. Thus, a number of clinical trials targeting vasopressin in ASD are under way (https://clinicaltrials.gov). Interestingly, while some investigators are testing the effects of increasing levels of vasopressin (http://med.stanford.edu/clinicaltrials/trials/NCT01962870), others have reasoned that suppressing vasopressin activity may be more appropriate [68]. Taken together, neuropeptides show some promise as translational targets for further work.

### Inhibition/excitation balance

#### Evidence

Network and clustering-based approaches to genetic data have identified common functions that appear to be compromised by a range of risk variants for ASD, which include neural signalling and development, synaptic transmission, chromatin remodelling, neural–glial signalling, and transcriptional regulation [69]. Examination of expression patterns of risk genes by brain region and developmental stage has identified transcriptional regulation and synaptic development during pre- and early postnatal development as loci of alteration, with concentrations in superficial cortical layers and glutamatergic synapses [70]. Taken together, such work indicates (perhaps unsurprisingly) that ASD is related to differences in the formation and specialization of brain networks. One specific line of investigation has focused on disruptions in either glutamate or

GABA-ergic systems, which could lead to alterations in the co-ordination of inhibition/excitation in the brain [71]. The high co-occurrence of epilepsy in individuals with ASD forms one line of evidence for this hypothesis [72], in addition to the high rates of ASD in disorders that disturb glutamatergic or GABA-ergic functioning like 15q11–13, fragile X, or neurofibromatosis type 1 [73]. Alterations in GABA and glutamate levels have been identified in individuals with ASD using magnetic resonance spectroscopy, though findings are somewhat inconsistent and limited by lack of spatial precision [74, 75]. Emerging evidence from stem cell models implicate an over-production of GABA-ergic neurons [76]. Theoretical models indicate the important role of GABA in maintaining brain networks [77], and evidence from animal models suggests that GABA or glutamatergic dysfunction could contribute to maintenance of concurrent ASD symptoms [78]. Thus, a range of evidence indicates that GABA/glutamate systems may be appropriate treatment targets for targeting current symptomatology.

Developmental actions of GABA and glutamate are also critical to consider. GABA has well-defined roles in controlling processes, including cell proliferation, neuroblast migration, dendritic maturation, and synapse elimination [79, 80]. Activity-dependent GABA signalling is thought to be critical in optiziming the balance between excitation and inhibition in the developing cortex [79] and has a critical role in shaping cortical-sensitive periods [81]. Such sensitive periods are important in tuning brain responses to the faces and voices infants encounter in their environment, a process called perceptual narrowing [82]. Disruptions to GABA-ergic signalling processes could thus impact early experience-dependent specialization of the social brain, potentially resulting in ASD symptoms. Further, a wide body of research indicates that GABA initially has a depolarizing function, with a switch to a hyperpolarizing function somewhere around the end of the first postnatal week in rodents, though there has been some debate [83, 84]. Other neurotransmitter systems with significant developmental roles include serotonin, which has also been implicated in autism and is particularly involved in early development of sensory systems [85]. Understanding how key neurotransmitter systems contribute to the emergence of autism symptoms will be assisted by longitudinal prospective studies of populations of human infants with genetic syndromes associated with alterations in key neurotransmitter systems.

#### Treatment targets

A number of therapeutic targets have been identified that may modulate GABA or glutamatergic functioning. For example, acamprosate is a GABAa agonist and a glutamate antagonist, which has shown some benefit in open-label trials [86]. The GABAb agonist arbaclofen has successfully reversed symptoms in animal models of fragile X syndrome, but human trials have been disappointing [24]. Vigabatrin inhibits the breakdown of GABA and increases GABA concentration; its use for seizures in infants with tuberous sclerosis has been associated with some improvement in ASD symptoms in later development [87]. Gabapentin increases GABA concentration and is sometimes used to manage disruptive behaviours in adults with ASD [88]. Other anti-epileptic drugs like topiramate, levetiracetam, and lamotrigine have been trialled, with limited effects on core symptoms [89]. D-cycloserine is a partial glutamatergic agonist, which has had limited efficacy for core symptoms [90] but may support long-term effects of targeted social skills training in children with ASD [91]. Bumetanide enhances GABA-ergic inhibition and again has shown some promise [92]. Targeting the serotonin system, SSRIs like fluoxetine and citalopram have been trialled in older populations, with mixed results [93]. Clearly, further work on turning promising genetic findings into drug targets is required. One key step is to develop better neurocognitive markers of targeted neurotransmitter systems that can be used as outcome measures in clinical trials.

## Oxidative stress and immune activation

### Evidence

Emerging evidence suggests a role for maternal immune activation/inflammation and oxidative stress in causing ASD [94–96]. Prenatal risk factors for ASD include infection, maternal gestational diabetes and medication use, exposure to significant pollution, neonatal anaemia, meconium aspiration or exposure, and respiratory distress [97–99], many of which cause some degree of hypoxia and/or a strong maternal immune response in pre- or early postnatal development. Mutations or alterations in mitochondrial functioning have also been linked to ASD [100], which may compromise energy available to neurons. With regard to inflammation, epidemiological studies indicate correlations between autism and familial history of atopic diseases like asthma, eczema, allergies, and food intolerance, all associated with inflammatory responses [96]. Prenatal immune activation may produce changes in methylation (particularly in the prefrontal cortex) that could contribute to later ASD symptoms [101]. Effects of oxidative stress or inflammation may also depend on the presence of particular risk genes in influencing outcome [102, 103]. Interestingly, gene expression studies show that individuals with ASD exhibit upregulated expression of genes associated with inflammatory responses that are correlated with downregulation of synaptic transmission genes [104]. Developmental analyses suggest that these inflammatory responses may be secondary consequences of early dysregulation associated with changes in synaptic function or brain activity across the first decades of life [22]. However, such changes may still contribute to maintenance of core and associated symptoms of autism and thus represent appropriate targets for intervention.

### Treatment targets

There have been some promising signals of the antioxidant *N*-acetyl cysteine (also involved in regulation of extracellular glutamate) during adolescence in animal models of schizophrenia [105]. Early trials in ASD are not promising [106] but may have selected insufficiently sensitive outcome measures (questionnaire-based, rather than mechanistic, as in the animal model); application at a prodromal stage of the disorder may be more effective but, of course, would be associated with significant ethical hurdles. Other investigators have shown promising effects of sulforaphane (in combination with other compounds), a component of broccoli that also has significant antioxidant properties; effects were apparently reversed when the participants stopped taking the treatments [107]. Concerns have been raised about the unusually small 'placebo' response in the control group, although one of the key measures is not commonly used in ASD trials (the Social Responsiveness Scale). There have also been some supportive findings in animal models [108], suggesting that this kind of approach may be worthy of further investigation.

## Linking top-down and bottom-up models

To date, attempts to link the literature derived from top–down dissections of the clinical difficulties experienced by children with ASD and emerging 'bottom–up' findings from genetic studies and animal models have been relatively exploratory. There are domain-general explanations of ASD within the cognitive literature that may map more readily onto the emerging neurobiological literature; these include ideas about neural variability [11], reduced influence of prior information on current processing [109], or alterations in weighting of errors within predictive coding frameworks [110]. However, while these explanations map relatively clearly onto some of the perceptual experiences of individuals with ASD, they generally provide relatively underspecified accounts of both core social communication symptoms of ASD. Moving forward requires rigorous experimental and theoretical and computational approaches to understanding the interfaces between these literatures. Nonetheless, there are some potential points of convergence. Firstly, effects of early widespread neuronal disruption on sensitive periods in early brain specialization may be one possibility for why the difficulties in ASD are so pronounced in the social domain. Experience-dependent learning is clearly very important in the development of social communication, since infants are not born knowing what language they will speak or what faces they will see; many ASD-associated genes converge on processes like neural signalling and development, synaptic transmission, activity-dependent chromatin remodelling, neural–glial signalling, and transcriptional regulation that would be expected to affect experience-dependent specialization. Higher-order association 'nexus' regions that are critical in social processing may be particularly vulnerable to altered inhibition/excitation balance, because they integrate signals from several regions [111]. Gene expression studies are also beginning to reveal degrees of anatomical specificity in observed changes that may help guide human neuroimaging studies; for example, disordered cortical patterning of gene expression has been observed in frontal and temporal cortices, critical to the social brain network. Greater refinement of genetic, neurobiological, and human phenotyping studies may converge on meaningful explanations of how apparently domain-general alterations produce the relatively specific symptoms experienced by individuals with ASD.

An alternative possibility is that the disruptions associated with highly penetrant genes or environmental risk factors may not directly cause the social symptoms associated with ASD. Some of the more penetrant genetic variants may simply cause the brain to work less effectively, which only produces symptoms of ASD when on a genetic background that predisposes children towards poorer social skills [112]. Similar hypotheses have been advanced for environmental factors like maternal immune activation [113]. Indeed, most copy number variations associated with ASD have also been associated with a wide range of other conditions. Genetic evidence suggests that copy number variations and common variation associated with ASD may affect different biological processes [114]. Larger mutations may alter the degree to which neurodevelopmental trajectories are buffered against environmental or other genetic perturbation [115, 116], with specificity then linked to those perturbations. If this is the case, trying to figure out how mutations that apparently have widespread effects lead to relatively specific symptoms may be a fruitless endeavour. Indeed, robust 'autistic-like' phenotypes in mice with fragile X syndrome mutations are only seen on a limited range of genetic backgrounds [117], potentially critical to understanding the failure of recent trials inspired by mechanisms affected by the fragile X syndrome mutation. However, such accounts need to explain why some genetic syndromes like Williams syndrome are not associated with high rates of ASD.

Thirdly, it is critical to understand the role of adaptation in shaping the ASD phenotype. The brain is an organ of adaptation at multiple spatial and temporal scales [111]. These adaptive processes could be relevant to ASD in a number of ways. Firstly, deficits in adaptation could directly contribute to ASD. For example, homeostatic processes act to regulate inhibition/excitation ratios, and disorders/insufficiency of homeostasis [118] or autoregulation in general [71] have been posited as unifying frameworks in ASD. Neurotransmitter systems like GABA or neuropeptides like vasopressin may thus need to be balanced within an optimal range, rather than generally up- or downregulated by treatment. Secondly, alterations that occur during particular time windows could cause long-term effects but be rapidly masked by subsequent compensatory processes [119]. In this case, adaptive processes would make it impossible to identify the original causes of ASD in the mature brain. Thirdly, adaptive processes may produce symptoms of ASD that represent optimal functioning for that individual brain, given its early processing constraints [111]. If this is the case, boosting adaptation may actually result in more symptoms of ASD. Finally, adaptive or compensatory processes may not be specific to ASD but may produce co-occurring symptoms. For example, recent gene expression studies indicate that immune-related markers emerge over the first two decades of life [22]. Increased cytokine and other inflammatory responses have been linked to depression [120], and so these responses may relate (as cause or consequence) to the common co-occurrence of conditions like depression in individuals with ASD. The likely critical role of adaptation indicates that pharmaceutical development will require us to disentangle adaptive or compensatory responses from primary causal pathways.

## Summary

Although the number of clinical trials of novel therapies for ASD is increasing, there has been much discussion of how to accelerate the pace of translation to the clinic [121, 122]. We need better measures with which to stratify participants for inclusion in trials and to measure the effects of those trials on the processes we think are impaired. This involves moving from group-level neuroimaging measures that are inconsistent across studies and have low reliability to identifying robust proxy biomarkers of treatment success. Such biomarkers should be developed not only from theoretical models of what we think underpins autism symptoms, but also from bottom-up measures of the pathophysiological processes implicated by genetic work and animal models. We also need translatable biomarkers that are sensitive to the same systems across species and can move with a drug from preclinical to clinical work; public–private partnerships can be valuable in this endeavour [123]. Further, we need a deeper understanding of how genetic and pathophysiological variation maps onto brain circuits and then onto emergent cognitive functions during development, and how this shapes final common pathways to symptom development. This will require emphasis on longitudinal studies that measure brain and behavioural development in genetically characterized populations, coupled with computational models and use of large normative data sets on gene expression and circuit function. Finally, we need to understand the complex interactions between different neurotransmitter and neuropeptide systems over developmental time, including the role of compensatory changes, and an appropriate target may be to achieve balance, rather than to uniformly boost or suppress activity in particular systems. Despite these challenges, new insights mean that treatment development for ASD is poised to enter a new frontier of translational opportunity.

## REFERENCES

1. American Psychiatric Association. *Diagnostic and statistical manual of mental disorders.* (2013). American Psychiatric Association, Arlington, VA.
2. Vissers, L. E., Gilissen, C. & Veltman, J. A. Genetic studies in intellectual disability and related disorders. *Nat. Rev. Genet.* **17**, 9–18 (2016).
3. Webb, S. J. *et al.* Developmental Change in the ERP Responses to Familiar Faces in Toddlers With Autism Spectrum Disorders Versus Typical Development. *Child Dev.* **82**, 1868–86 (2011).
4. Insel, T. *et al.* Research Domain Criteria (RDoC): Toward a New Classification Framework for Research on Mental Disorders. *Am. J. Psychiatry* **167**, 748–51 (2010).
5. Gaugler, T. *et al.* Most genetic risk for autism resides with common variation. *Nat. Genet.* **46**, 881–5 (2014).
6. St Pourcain, B. *et al.* ASD and schizophrenia show distinct developmental profiles in common genetic overlap with population-based social communication difficulties. *Mol. Psychiatry* **23**, 263–70 (2018).
7. Jones, E. J. H., Venema, K., Earl, R. K., Lowy, R. & Webb, S. J. Infant social attention: an endophenotype of ASD-related traits? *J. Child Psychol. Psychiatry* **58**, 270–81 (2017).
8. Casey, B. J., Oliveri, M. E. & Insel, T. A Neurodevelopmental Perspective on the Research Domain Criteria (RDoC) Framework. *Biol. Psychiatry* **76**, 350–3 (2014).
9. Johnson, M. H. Interactive specialization: a domain-general framework for human functional brain development? *Dev. Cogn. Neurosci.* **1**, 7–21 (2011).
10. Butler, J. S., Molholm, S., Andrade, G. N. & Foxe, J. J. An Examination of the Neural Unreliability Thesis of Autism. *Cereb. Cortex* **27**, 185–200 (2017).
11. Milne, E. Increased intra-participant variability in children with autistic spectrum disorders: evidence from single-trial analysis of evoked EEG. *Front. Percept. Sci.* **2**, 51 (2011).
12. Byrge, L., Dubois, J., Tyszka, J. M., Adolphs, R. & Kennedy, D. P. Idiosyncratic Brain Activation Patterns Are Associated with Poor Social Comprehension in Autism. *J. Neurosci.* **35**, 5837 (2015).
13. Hahamy, A., Behrmann, M. & Malach, R. The idiosyncratic brain: distortion of spontaneous connectivity patterns in autism spectrum disorder. *Nat. Neurosci.* **18**, 302–9 (2015).
14. Neuhaus, E. *et al.* The Relationship Between Early Neural Responses to Emotional Faces at Age 3 and Later Autism and Anxiety Symptoms in Adolescents with Autism. *J. Autism Dev. Disord.* **46**, 2450–63 (2016).
15. Ozonoff, S. *et al.* Recurrence Risk for Autism Spectrum Disorders: A Baby Siblings Research Consortium Study. *Pediatrics* **128**, e488–95 (2011).

16. Jones, E. J. H., Gliga, T., Bedford, R., Charman, T. & Johnson, M. H. Developmental pathways to autism: a review of prospective studies of infants at risk. *Neurosci. Biobehav. Rev.* **39**, 1–33 (2014).

17. Varcin, K. J. & Nelson, C. A. A developmental neuroscience approach to the search for biomarkers in autism spectrum disorder. *Curr. Opin. Neurol.* **29**, 123–9 (2016).

18. Green, J. *et al.* Parent-mediated intervention versus no intervention for infants at high risk of autism: a parallel, single-blind, randomised trial. *Lancet Psychiatry* **2**, 133–40 (2015).

19. Jones, E. J. H., Dawson, G., Estes, A., Kelly, J. & Webb, S. J. Parent-delivered early intervention in infants at risk for ASD: Effects on electrophysiological and habituation measures of social attention. *Autism Res.* **10**, 961–72 (2017).

20. Rogers, S. J. *et al.* Autism treatment in the first year of life: a pilot study of infant start, a parent-implemented intervention for symptomatic infants. *J. Autism Dev. Disord.* **44**, 2981–95 (2014).

21. de la Torre-Ubieta, L., Won, H., Stein, J. L. & Geschwind, D. H. Advancing the understanding of autism disease mechanisms through genetics. *Nat. Med.* **22**, 345–61 (2016).

22. Parikshak, N. N. *et al.* Genome-wide changes in lncRNA, splicing, and regional gene expression patterns in autism. *Nature* **540**, 423–7 (2016).

23. Sztainberg, Y. & Zoghbi, H. Y. Lessons learned from studying syndromic autism spectrum disorders. *Nat. Neurosci.* **19**, 1408–17 (2016).

24. Berry-Kravis, E. *et al.* Mavoglurant in fragile X syndrome: Results of two randomized, double-blind, placebo-controlled trials. *Sci. Transl. Med.* **8**, 321ra5 (2016).

25. Geschwind, D. H. & Levitt, P. Autism spectrum disorders: developmental disconnection syndromes. *Curr. Opin. Neurobiol.* **17**, 103–11 (2007).

26. Chevallier, C., Kohls, G., Troiani, V., Brodkin, E. S. & Schultz, R. T. The social motivation theory of autism. *Trends Cogn. Sci.* **16**, 231–9 (2012).

27. Dawson, G., Meltzoff, A. N., Osterling, J., Rinaldi, J. & Brown, E. Children with Autism Fail to Orient to Naturally Occurring Social Stimuli. *J. Autism Dev. Disord.* **28**, 479–85 (1998).

28. Pelphrey, K. A., Shultz, S., Hudac, C. M. & Vander Wyk, B. C. Research Review: Constraining heterogeneity: the social brain and its development in autism spectrum disorder. *J. Child Psychol. Psychiatry* **52**, 631–44 (2011).

29. Johnson, M. H. Autism: demise of the innate social orienting hypothesis. *Curr. Biol.* **24**, R30–1 (2014).

30. Jones, E. J. H. *et al.* Reduced engagement with social stimuli in 6-month-old infants with later autism spectrum disorder: a longitudinal prospective study of infants at high familial risk. *J. Neurodev. Disord.* **8**, 7 (2016).

31. Shic, F., Macari, S. & Chawarska, K. Speech Disturbs Face Scanning in 6-Month-Old Infants Who Develop Autism Spectrum Disorder. *Biol. Psychiatry* **75**, 231–7 (2014).

32. Chawarska, K., Macari, S. & Shic, F. Decreased Spontaneous Attention to Social Scenes in 6-Month-Old Infants Later Diagnosed with Autism Spectrum Disorders. *Biol. Psychiatry* **74**, 195–203 (2013).

33. Jones, W. & Klin, A. Attention to eyes is present but in decline in 2-6-month-old infants later diagnosed with autism. *Nature* **504**, 427–31 (2013).

34. Ozonoff, S. *et al.* A Prospective Study of the Emergence of Early Behavioral Signs of Autism. *J. Am. Acad. Child Adolesc. Psychiatry* **49**, 256–66.e2 (2010).

35. Klin, A., Shultz, S. & Jones, W. Social visual engagement in infants and toddlers with autism: Early developmental transitions and a model of pathogenesis. *Neurosci. Biobehav. Rev.* **50**, 189–203 (2015).

36. Shic, F., Bradshaw, J., Klin, A., Scassellati, B. & Chawarska, K. Limited activity monitoring in toddlers with autism spectrum disorder. *Brain Res.* **1380**, 246–54 (2011).

37. Chawarska, K., Macari, S. & Shic, F. Context modulates attention to social scenes in toddlers with autism. *J. Child Psychol. Psychiatry* **53**, 903–13 (2012).

38. Falck-Ytter, T., Rehnberg, E. & Bölte, S. Lack of Visual Orienting to Biological Motion and Audiovisual Synchrony in 3-Year-Olds with Autism. *PLoS One* **8**, e68816 (2013).

39. Klin, A., Lin, D. J., Gorrindo, P., Ramsay, G. & Jones, W. Two-year-olds with autism orient to non-social contingencies rather than biological motion. *Nature* **459**, 257–61 (2009).

40. Simion, F., Regolin, L. & Bulf, H. A predisposition for biological motion in the newborn baby. *Proc. Natl. Acad. Sci. U. S. A.* **105**, 809–13 (2008).

41. Le Grand, R., Mondloch, C. J., Maurer, D. & Brent, H. P. Neuroperception: Early visual experience and face processing. *Nature* **410**, 890–90 (2001).

42. Dawson, G. *et al.* Neural Correlates of Face and Object Recognition in Young Children with Autism Spectrum Disorder, Developmental Delay, and Typical Development. *Child Dev.* **73**, 700–17 (2002).

43. Dawson, G., Webb, S. J., Carver, L., Panagiotides, H. & McPartland, J. Young children with autism show atypical brain responses to fearful versus neutral facial expressions of emotion. *Dev. Sci.* **7**, 340–59 (2004).

44. Webb, S. J. *et al.* Toddlers with elevated autism symptoms show slowed habituation to faces. *Child Neuropsychol. J. Norm. Abnorm. Dev. Child. Adolesc.* **16**, 255–78 (2010).

45. Elsabbagh, M. *et al.* Infant Neural Sensitivity to Dynamic Eye Gaze Is Associated with Later Emerging Autism. *Curr. Biol.* **22**, 338–42 (2012).

46. Mundy, P., Sigman, M., Ungerer, J. & Sherman, T. Defining the Social Deficits of Autism: The Contribution of Non-Verbal Communication Measures. *J. Child Psychol. Psychiatry* **27**, 657–69 (1986).

47. Morales, M. *et al.* Responding to Joint Attention Across the 6- Through 24-Month Age Period and Early Language Acquisition. *J. Appl. Dev. Psychol.* **21**, 283–98 (2000).

48. Dawson, G. *et al.* Early social attention impairments in autism: social orienting, joint attention, and attention to distress. *Dev. Psychol.* **40**, 271–83 (2004).

49. Sigman, M. *et al.* Continuity and change in the social competence of children with autism, Down syndrome, and developmental delays. *Monogr. Soc. Res. Child Dev.* **64**, 1–114 (1999).

50. Kasari, C., Gulsrud, A., Paparella, T., Hellemann, G. & Berry, K. Randomized comparative efficacy study of parent-mediated interventions for toddlers with autism. *J. Consult. Clin. Psychol.* **83**, 554–63 (2015).

51. Kasari, C., Paparella, T., Freeman, S. & Jahromi, L. B. Language outcome in autism: Randomized comparison of joint attention and play interventions. *J. Consult. Clin. Psychol.* **76**, 125–37 (2008).

52. Dawson, G. *et al.* Randomized, Controlled Trial of an Intervention for Toddlers With Autism: The Early Start Denver Model. *Pediatrics* **125**, e17–23 (2010).

53. Dawson, G. *et al.* Early behavioral intervention is associated with normalized brain activity in young children with autism. *J. Am. Acad. Child Adolesc. Psychiatry* **51**, 1150–9 (2012).

54. Green, J. *et al.* Parent-mediated communication-focused treatment in children with autism (PACT): a randomised controlled trial. *Lancet* **375**, 2152–60 (2010).

55. Pickles, A. *et al.* Parent-mediated social communication therapy for young children with autism (PACT): long-term follow-up of a randomised controlled trial. *Lancet* **388**, 2501–9 (2016).

56. Pickles, A. *et al.* Treatment mechanism in the MRC preschool autism communication trial: implications for study design and parent-focussed therapy for children. *J. Child Psychol. Psychiatry* **56**, 162–70 (2015).

57. RFA-MH-15-800: *Consortium on Biomarker and Outcome Measures of Social Impairment for Use in Clinical Trials in Autism Spectrum Disorder (U19).* Available at: https://grants.nih.gov/grants/guide/rfa-files/RFA-MH-15-800.html (accessed 8 February 2017).

58. Kitzerow, J., Teufel, K., Wilker, C. & Freitag, C. M. Using the brief observation of social communication change (BOSCC) to measure autism-specific development. *Autism Res. Off. J. Int. Soc. Autism Res.* **9**, 940–50 (2016).

59. Chang, S. W. C. & Platt, M. L. Oxytocin and social cognition in rhesus macaques: Implications for understanding and treating human psychopathology. *Brain Res.* **0**, 57 (2014).

60. Meyer-Lindenberg, A., Domes, G., Kirsch, P. & Heinrichs, M. Oxytocin and vasopressin in the human brain: social neuropeptides for translational medicine. *Nat. Rev. Neurosci.* **12**, 524–38 (2011).

61. Domes, G. *et al.* Effects of intranasal oxytocin on the neural basis of face processing in autism spectrum disorder. *Biol. Psychiatry* **74**, 164–71 (2013).

62. Gordon, I. *et al.* Oxytocin enhances brain function in children with autism. *Proc. Natl. Acad. Sci. U. S. A.* **110**, 20953–8 (2013).

63. Guastella, A. J. *et al.* Intranasal Oxytocin Improves Emotion Recognition for Youth with Autism Spectrum Disorders. *Biol. Psychiatry* **67**, 692–4 (2010).

64. Freeman, S. M. *et al.* Plasma and CSF oxytocin levels after intranasal and intravenous oxytocin in awake macaques. *Psychoneuroendocrinology* **66**, 185–94 (2016).

65. Peñagarikano, O. *et al.* Exogenous and evoked oxytocin restores social behavior in the Cntnap2 mouse model of autism. *Sci. Transl. Med.* **7**, 271ra8 (2015).

66. Huang, H. *et al.* Chronic and acute intranasal oxytocin produce divergent social effects in mice. *Neuropsychopharmacology.* **39**, 1102–14 (2014).

67. Zink, C. F., Stein, J. L., Kempf, L., Hakimi, S. & Meyer-Lindenberg, A. Vasopressin modulates medial prefrontal cortex-amygdala circuitry during emotion processing in humans. *J. Neurosci.* **30**, 7017–22 (2010).

68. Umbricht, D. *et al.* A Single Dose, Randomized, Controlled Proof-Of-Mechanism Study of a Novel Vasopressin 1a Receptor Antagonist (RG7713) in High-Functioning Adults with Autism Spectrum Disorder. *Neuropsychopharmacology* **42**, 1924 (2017).

69. De Rubeis, S. *et al.* Synaptic, transcriptional and chromatin genes disrupted in autism. *Nature* **515**, 209–15 (2014).

70. Parikshak, N. N. *et al.* Integrative functional genomic analyses implicate specific molecular pathways and circuits in autism. *Cell* **155**, 1008–21 (2013).

71. Mullins, C., Fishell, G. & Tsien, R. W. Unifying Views of Autism Spectrum Disorders: A Consideration of Autoregulatory Feedback Loops. *Neuron* **89**, 1131–56 (2016).

72. Bolton, P. F. *et al.* Epilepsy in autism: features and correlates. *Br. J. Psychiatry* **198**, 289–94 (2011).

73. Coghlan, S. *et al.* GABA system dysfunction in autism and related disorders: From synapse to symptoms. *Neurosci. Biobehav. Rev.* **36**, 2044–55 (2012).

74. Gaetz, W. *et al.* GABA estimation in the brains of children on the autism spectrum: Measurement precision and regional cortical variation. *NeuroImage* **86**, 1–9 (2014).

75. Horder, J. *et al.* Reduced subcortical glutamate/glutamine in adults with autism spectrum disorders: a [1H]MRS study. *Transl. Psychiatry* **3**, e279 (2013).

76. Mariani, J. *et al.* FOXG1-Dependent Dysregulation of GABA/Glutamate Neuron Differentiation in Autism Spectrum Disorders. *Cell* **162**, 375–90 (2015).

77. Turkheimer, F. E., Leech, R., Expert, P., Lord, L.-D. & Vernon, A. C. The brain's code and its canonical computational motifs. From sensory cortex to the default mode network: A multi-scale model of brain function in health and disease. *Neurosci. Biobehav. Rev.* **55**, 211–22 (2015).

78. Yizhar, O. *et al.* Neocortical excitation/inhibition balance in information processing and social dysfunction. *Nature* **477**, 171–8 (2011).

79. Le Magueresse, C. & Monyer, H. GABAergic Interneurons Shape the Functional Maturation of the Cortex. *Neuron* **77**, 388–405 (2013).

80. Represa, A. & Ben-Ari, Y. Trophic actions of GABA on neuronal development. *Trends Neurosci.* **28**, 278–83 (2005).

81. Hensch, T. K. Critical period plasticity in local cortical circuits. *Nat. Rev. Neurosci.* **6**, 877–88 (2005).

82. Maurer, D. & Werker, J. F. Perceptual narrowing during infancy: A comparison of language and faces. *Dev. Psychobiol.* **56**, 154–78 (2014).

83. Ben-Ari, Y. *et al.* Refuting the challenges of the developmental shift of polarity of GABA actions: GABA more exciting than ever! *Front. Cell. Neurosci.* **6**, 35 (2012).

84. Bregestovski, P. & Bernard, C. Excitatory GABA: How a Correct Observation May Turn Out to be an Experimental Artifact. *Front. Pharmacol.* **3**, 65 (2012).

85. Muller, C. L., Anacker, A. M. J. & Veenstra-VanderWeele, J. The serotonin system in autism spectrum disorder: From biomarker to animal models. *Neuroscience* **321**, 24–41 (2016).

86. Erickson, C. A. *et al.* Impact of acamprosate on behavior and brain-derived neurotrophic factor: an open-label study in youth with fragile X syndrome. *Psychopharmacology (Berl.)* **228**, 75–84 (2013).

87. Jambaqué, I., Chiron, C., Dumas, C., Mumford, J. & Dulac, O. Mental and behavioural outcome of infantile epilepsy treated by vigabatrin in tuberous sclerosis patients. *Epilepsy Res.* **38**, 151–60 (2000).

88. Guglielmo, R., Ioime, L., Grandinetti, P. & Janiri, L. Managing disruptive and compulsive behaviors in adult with autistic disorder with gabapentin. *J. Clin. Psychopharmacol.* **33**, 273–4 (2013).

89. Hirota, T., Veenstra-Vanderweele, J., Hollander, E. & Kishi, T. Antiepileptic medications in autism spectrum disorder: a systematic review and meta-analysis. *J. Autism Dev. Disord.* **44**, 948–57 (2014).

90. Minshawi, N. F. *et al.* A randomized, placebo-controlled trial of d-cycloserine for the enhancement of social skills training in autism spectrum disorders. *Mol. Autism* **7**, 2 (2016).

91. Wink, L. K. *et al.* d-Cycloserine enhances durability of social skills training in autism spectrum disorder. *Mol. Autism* **8**, 2 (2017).

92. Lemonnier, E. *et al.* A randomised controlled trial of bumetanide in the treatment of autism in children. *Transl. Psychiatry* **2**, e202 (2012).

93. Williams, K., Brignell, A., Randall, M., Silove, N. & Hazell, P. Selective serotonin reuptake inhibitors (SSRIs) for autism spectrum disorders (ASD). *Cochrane Database Syst. Rev.* **8**, CD004677 (2013).

94. Johnson, A. W. *et al.* Cognitive and motivational deficits together with prefrontal oxidative stress in a mouse model for neuropsychiatric illness. *Proc. Natl. Acad. Sci. U. S. A.* **110**, 12462–7 (2013).

95. Smaga, I. *et al.* Oxidative stress as an etiological factor and a potential treatment target of psychiatric disorders. Part 2. Depression, anxiety, schizophrenia and autism. *Pharmacol. Rep.* **67**, 569–80 (2015).

96. Theoharides, T. C., Tsilioni, I., Patel, A. B. & Doyle, R. Atopic diseases and inflammation of the brain in the pathogenesis of autism spectrum disorders. *Transl. Psychiatry* **6**, e844 (2016).

97. Froehlich-Santino, W. *et al.* Prenatal and perinatal risk factors in a twin study of autism spectrum disorders. *J. Psychiatr. Res.* **54**, 100–8 (2014).

98. Lyall, K., Schmidt, R. J. & Hertz-Picciotto, I. Maternal lifestyle and environmental risk factors for autism spectrum disorders. *Int. J. Epidemiol.* **43**, 443–64 (2014).

99. Willfors, C. et al. Medical history of discordant twins and environmental etiologies of autism. *Transl. Psychiatry* **7**, e1014 (2017).

100. Rossignol, D. A. & Frye, R. E. Evidence linking oxidative stress, mitochondrial dysfunction, and inflammation in the brain of individuals with autism. *Front. Physiol.* **5**, 150 (2014).

101. Richetto, J. *et al.* Genome-wide DNA Methylation Changes in a Mouse Model of Infection-Mediated Neurodevelopmental Disorders. *Biol. Psychiatry* **81**, 265–76 (2017).

102. Ehninger, D. *et al.* Gestational immune activation and Tsc2 haploinsufficiency cooperate to disrupt fetal survival and may perturb social behavior in adult mice. *Mol. Psychiatry* **17**, 62–70 (2012).

103. Tyzio, R. *et al.* Oxytocin-Mediated GABA Inhibition During Delivery Attenuates Autism Pathogenesis in Rodent Offspring. *Science* **343**, 675–9 (2014).

104. Gupta, S. *et al.* Transcriptome analysis reveals dysregulation of innate immune response genes and neuronal activity-dependent genes in autism. *Nat. Commun.* **5**, 5748 (2014).

105. Cabungcal, J.-H. *et al.* Juvenile antioxidant treatment prevents adult deficits in a developmental model of schizophrenia. *Neuron* **83**, 1073–84 (2014).

106. Wink, L. K. *et al.* A randomized placebo-controlled pilot study of N-acetylcysteine in youth with autism spectrum disorder. *Mol. Autism* **7**, 26 (2016).

107. Singh, K. *et al.* Sulforaphane treatment of autism spectrum disorder (ASD). *Proc. Natl. Acad. Sci. U. S. A.* **111**, 15550–5 (2014).

108. Shirai, Y. *et al.* Dietary Intake of Sulforaphane-Rich Broccoli Sprout Extracts during Juvenile and Adolescence Can Prevent Phencyclidine-Induced Cognitive Deficits at Adulthood. *PLoS One* **10**, e0127244 (2015).

109. Pellicano, E. & Burr, D. When the world becomes 'too real': a Bayesian explanation of autistic perception. *Trends Cogn. Sci.* **16**, 504–10 (2012).

110. Lawson, R. P., Rees, G. & Friston, K. J. An aberrant precision account of autism. *Front. Hum. Neurosci.* **8**, 302 (2014).

111. Johnson, M. H., Jones, E. J. H. & Gliga, T. Brain adaptation and alternative developmental trajectories. *Dev. Psychopathol.* **27**, 425–42 (2015).

112. Moreno-De-Luca, A. *et al.* Developmental brain dysfunction: revival and expansion of old concepts based on new genetic evidence. *Lancet Neurol.* **12**, 406–14 (2013).

113. Careaga, M., Murai, T. & Bauman, M. D. Maternal Immune Activation and Autism Spectrum Disorder: From Rodents to Nonhuman and Human Primates. *Biol. Psychiatry* **81**, 391–401 (2017).

114. Iossifov, I. *et al.* The contribution of *de novo* coding mutations to autism spectrum disorder. *Nature* **515**, 216–21 (2014).

115. Félix, M.-A. & Barkoulas, M. Pervasive robustness in biological systems. *Nat. Rev. Genet.* **16**, 483–96 (2015).

116. Gandal, M. J., Leppa, V., Won, H., Parikshak, N. N. & Geschwind, D. H. The road to precision psychiatry: translating genetics into disease mechanisms. *Nat. Neurosci.* **19**, 1397–407 (2016).

117. Spencer, C. M. *et al.* Modifying behavioral phenotypes in Fmr1KO mice: genetic background differences reveal autistic-like responses. *Autism Res.* **4**, 40–56 (2011).

118. Nelson, S. B. & Valakh, V. Excitatory/Inhibitory Balance and Circuit Homeostasis in Autism Spectrum Disorders. *Neuron* **87**, 684–98 (2015).

119. Meredith, R. M., Dawitz, J. & Kramvis, I. Sensitive time-windows for susceptibility in neurodevelopmental disorders. *Trends Neurosci.* **35**, 335–44 (2012).

120. Setiawan, E. *et al.* Role of translocator protein density, a marker of neuroinflammation, in the brain during major depressive episodes. *JAMA Psychiatry* **72**, 268–75 (2015).

121. Krystal, J. H. & State, M. W. Psychiatric Disorders: Diagnosis to Therapy. *Cell* **157**, 201–14 (2014).

122. Szatmari, P., Charman, T. & Constantino, J. N. Into, and Out of, the 'Valley of Death': Research in Autism Spectrum Disorders. *J. Am. Acad. Child Adolesc. Psychiatry* **51**, 1108–12 (2012).

123. Loth, E., Spooren, W. & Murphy, D. G. New treatment targets for autism spectrum disorders: EU-AIMS. *Lancet Psychiatry* **1**, 413–15 (2014).

# 27

# Epidemiology of autism

*Charles R. Newton*

## Introduction

The epidemiology of autism has generated much interest recently, mainly because of the reported dramatic increases in the prevalence of autism in the last few decades and the controversy surrounding vaccines and autism. These reports have led to speculation of the causes and intensive study of the changing epidemiology of autism in some countries. This chapter provides a background to the epidemiology, particularly the global burden of disease and changes in the prevalence of autism in the last few decades and the risk factors that may contribute to these changes in epidemiology. In addition, financial burden and premature mortality are discussed.

## Epidemiological concepts of autism

The epidemiology of autism is complicated by the difficulty in determining its onset and the changes in the criteria used for the diagnosis over time. Autism is widely considered as a lifelong condition that occurs in genetically susceptible individuals, who may be exposed to other influences either *in utero* or after birth. The diagnosis of autism is rarely made before 18 months of age, although parents will often have concerns before that age. The age of diagnosis varies considerably, being influenced by the presence of symptom severity (particularly earlier in those with greater intellectual disability), socio-economic status (later in those with lower socio-economic status), parental concerns, and geographical region since this is determined by public awareness, expertise, and facilities for diagnosis [1]. Thus, determination of the onset is difficult, which makes calculating the incidence (new cases per population per unit time) problematic. The incidence is a more robust epidemiological measurement than prevalence (number of cases per population at point in time), particularly when examining the secular trends and identifying risk factors. However, incidence measurements may underestimate the burden of a condition if there is premature mortality (see Premature mortality, p. 267) or if there is spontaneous remission (this is rare in autism, since the diagnosis is stable throughout life, although the severity of symptoms may change). Most of the epidemiological studies have reported prevalence, since they are conducted on referral databases (which are susceptible to

bias, particularly ascertainment and assessment bias) or cross-sectional surveys with differing methodologies (postal surveys, community door-to-door surveys). Comparison between cross-sectional surveys are problematic, since the results are influenced by different methodologies, including identifying all the people within the denominator, tools used to screen for autism, age of the subjects, expertise of the final diagnosis, and diagnostic criteria. Comparison of the subjects identified with autism from surveys and established databases of autism may show significant discrepancies [2]. Birth cohorts may be more informative but are expensive and difficult to conduct.

## Prevalence of autism

The initial studies measuring the prevalence of autism in the 1960s and 1970s reported low frequencies, with prevalences from 0.7 to 4.6 per 10,000, mainly using Kanner's description of the diagnosis [3] (Table 27.1). The DSM-III criteria published in 1980 [4] was used in most studies of that decade, with prevalences reported from 2.0 to 13.8 per 10,000 (Fig. 27.1). In this era, the comparison between the studies was complicated by use of varying methods for case ascertainment, different age groups studied, and some studies using the Kanner's criteria, Lorna Wing's triad [5], or Rutter's definition [6]. In the 1990s, the prevalences reported were considerably higher, with a prevalence of 60/10,000 reported from Sweden [7]. The analysis of the secular trends was complicated by the use of ICD-10 [8] and the introduction of DSM-IV published in 1994 (Table 27.1). From the year 2000, the reported prevalence of autism was consistently and considerably higher, ranging from 11.0 to 157 per 10,000. Most of these studies used either DSM-IV or ICD-10 criteria for autism. Since 2010, the prevalence of autism in some countries has been reported as even higher, with a prevalence of 140/10,000 in the United States across all age groups [9] and 260/10,1000 in South Korean children [10].

## Causes of reported increased prevalence of autism

Since the original delineation of autism by Kanner in 1943 [3], the conceptualization of autism has undergone significant changes

**Table 27.1** Studies measuring the prevalence of autism in the 1960s and 1970s

| | Kanner (1943)[1] | Rutter and Schopler (1978)[2] | Wing and Gould (1978)[3] | DSM-III[4] | DSM-IIIR[5] | DSM-IV[6] |
|---|---|---|---|---|---|---|
| Social communication | 1. Profound lack of affective contact | 1. Impaired social development which is out-of-keeping with the child's intellectual level | 1. Impairment in social communication | 1. Lack of responsiveness to others | 1. Impairment in reciprocal social interaction (at least two from a list of five items, comprising specified clinical examples) | (A) Qualitative impairment in social interaction, as manifested by at least two of the following: 1. Marked impairments in the use of multiple non-verbal behaviours such as eye-to-eye gaze, facial expression, body posture, and gestures to regulate social interaction 2. Failure to develop peer relationships appropriate to the developmental level 3. Lack of spontaneous seeking to share enjoyment, interests, or achievements with other people, (for example, by lack of showing, bringing, or pointing out objects of interest to other people) 4. Lack of social or emotional reciprocity (note: in the description, it gives the following as examples: not actively participating in simple social play or games, preferring solitary activities or involving others in activities only as tools or 'mechanical' aids) |
| Language | | 2. Delayed and deviant language development that also has certain defined features and is out of keeping with the child's intellectual level | 2. Impairment in verbal and non-verbal communication | 2. Language absence or abnormalities | 2. Impairment in verbal and non-verbal communication (at least one from a list of six items) | (B) Qualitative impairments in communication, as manifested by at least one of the following: 1. Delay in, or total lack of, the development of spoken language (not accompanied by an attempt to compensate through alternative modes of communication such as gesture or mime) 2. In individuals with adequate speech, marked impairment in the ability to initiate or sustain a conversation with others 3. Stereotyped and repetitive use of language or idiosyncratic language 4. Lack of varied, spontaneous make-believe play or social imitative play appropriate to the developmental level |
| Behaviour | 2. Repetitive, ritualistic behaviour, which must be of an elaborate kind | 3. 'Insistence on sameness', as shown by stereotyped play patterns, preoccupations, or resistance to change | 3. Repetitive, ritualistic behaviour | 3. Resistance to change or attachment to objects | 3. Markedly restricted repertoire of activities and interests (at least one from a list of five items) | (C) Restricted, repetitive, and stereotyped patterns of behaviour, interests, and activities, as manifested by at least two of the following: 1. Encompassing preoccupation with one or more stereotyped and restricted patterns of interest that is abnormal either in intensity or focus 2. Apparently inflexible adherence to specific, non-functional routines or rituals 3. Stereotyped and repetitive motor mannerisms (for example, hand or finger flapping or twisting, or complex whole body movements) 4. Persistent preoccupation with parts of objects |

*(continued)*

**Table 27.1**    Continued

|  | Kanner (1943)[1] | Rutter and Schopler (1978)[2] | Wing and Gould (1978)[3] | DSM-III[4] | DSM-IIIR[5] | DSM-IV[6] |
|---|---|---|---|---|---|---|
| Other features | Other features include:<br>3. An anxiously obsessive desire for the preservation of sameness in the child's routines and environment<br>4. A fascination for objects, which are handled with skill in fine motor movements<br>5. Mutism or a kind of language that does not seem intended for inter-personal communication<br>6. Good cognitive potential shown in feats of memory or skills on performance tests, especially the Séguin form board |  |  | 4. Absence of schizophrenic features | 4. In a total of at least eight from among the 16 items listed | A total of six (or more) items from (A), (B), and (C), with at least two from (A) and one each from (B) and (C)<br>(III) The disturbance is not better accounted for by Rett's disorder or childhood disintegrative disorder |
| Onset | Kanner also emphasized the onset from birth or before 30 months | 4. Onset before 30 months |  | 5. Onset before 30 months |  | (II) Delays or abnormal functioning in at least one of the following areas, with onset prior to age of 3 years:<br>(A) Social interaction<br>(B) Language as used in social communication<br>(C) Symbolic or imaginative play |

Source: data from *Nervous Child*, 2, Kanner L, Autistic disturbances of affective contact, pp. 217–250, Copyright (1943); Rutter M, Diagnosis and definition. In: Rutter M, Schopler E, [eds], *Autism: A Reappraisal of Concepts and Treatment*, pp. 1–25, Copyright (1978), Plenum Press; *J Autism Child Schizophr.*, 8(1), Wing L, Gould J, Systematic recording of behaviors and skills of retarded and psychotic children, pp. 79–97, Copyright (1978); Spitzer RL, Gibbon M, Skodol AE, *et al.*, *DSM-III. Diagnostic and Statistical Manual of Mental Disorders* (Third Edition), Copyright (1989), American Psychiatric Press; Perry S, Allen F, Clarkin JC, *DSM-III-R Casebook of Treatment Selection*, Copyright (1996), Routledge; *DSM-IV-TR: Diagnostic and Statistical Manual of Mental Disorders (Diagnostic & Statistical Manual of Mental Disorders)*, 4th Revised edition, Copyright (1994), American Psychiatric Association.

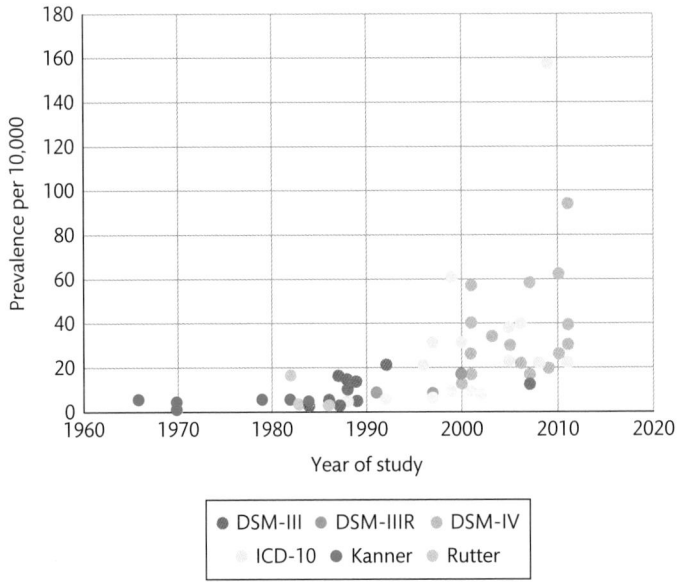

**Fig. 27.1** (see Colour Plate section) Prevalence of autism since the 1960s to 2015 according to the diagnostic criteria.

[11]. The definition has changed from a discrete disorder, based upon Kanner's description, to the concept that autism is part of a spectrum of disorders characterized by impaired social communication with differing degrees of severity. More recently, autism has been considered as a continuum, in which the diagnosis depends upon the number and severity of autistic traits. These differences in the concepts of autism have largely brought about the changes in the diagnostic criteria but have been influenced by changing conceptualization of mental health disorders and the complexity of the genetic basis.

The changes in the diagnostic criteria have had a major impact on the epidemiology of autism, from subjects with intellectual disability defined in Kanner's original description to DSM-IV and ICD-10 which are much more inclusive, encompassing higher-functioning individuals such as those with Asperger's syndrome. Thus, the prevalence of autism in London in the UK was three times higher with the reclassification of cases by ICD-10 criteria, compared to those defined by Kanner's criteria in the original study [12]. Many of these additional cases are a result of diagnostic substitution, in which cases of autism were previously diagnosed as other conditions. In the 1960s and 1970s, many cases of autism would have been classified as intellectual disability. In an analysis of special education requirements across the United States, Shattuck showed that many children initially diagnosed with intellectual disability were subsequently diagnosed with autism, and the increase in prevalence of autism was associated with a reduction in intellectual disability during this period [13]. In the UK, analysis of the General Practitioner Research Database demonstrated that the incidence of autism from the 1988 birth cohort rose from 4/10,000/year to 25/10,000/year in the 1997 birth cohort, and again this increase was attributed to changes in the diagnostic criteria [14].

Increased public and medical awareness of autism is likely to have increased the prevalence of autism over time. Parents of children with communication difficulties are more likely to take their children for assessment and ask about the diagnosis of autism. The formation of advocacy groups, for example Autism Speaks in the United States and the National Autism Society in the UK, has certainly increased public awareness and possibly led to an increase in referrals for assessment. Furthermore, parents are more likely to have their children assessed for autism nowadays, since in many Western countries, there is an increase in financial, psychological, and therapeutic support for families with autism than previously. Health care workers are more likely to entertain the diagnosis, and autism is now an established component of undergraduate teaching for health and educational professionals. Autism diagnostic services has increased, which, although they may be self-servicing, have arisen for perceived needs in communities. There has been an increase in national (Denmark [15]), medical [16], and educational [13, 17] registries in the 1990s. However, interpretation of the secular trends in these registries is problematic, since the reports often do not account for the many confounding factors such as increasing population, decreasing age of diagnosis, or changes in referral patterns and availability of services.

## Changes in biological risk factors and in the prevalence of autism

The changes in a number of biological risk factors may have influenced the secular changes in the prevalence of autism. Increasing paternal age is associated with an increased risk of developing autism [18], and the paternal age has increased. Some drugs, for example sodium valproate, or alcohol use during pregnancy are associated with autism, and these may have contributed to the increase in the 1980s and 1990s. The influence of these factors in the last decade is likely to have decreased, given the increased awareness of the effects on the fetus [19]. The incidence of perinatal factors, for example prematurity, associated with autism has increased, and survival of affected neonates has improved [20]. Migration is associated with autism in some countries, for example Sweden, and this has increased in the last few decades [21]. In contrast, the incidence of other risk factors associated with autism, for example rubella and thalidomide exposure, has decreased.

## Prevalence of autism across the world

The global burden of autism has not yet been defined accurately. Although there are many epidemiological studies from North America, Europe, and Japan, there are few studies from the remainder of the world. Thus, in a recent review of mental disorders of children, there were no data on any disorders in 124 of the 187 countries [22]. In particular, there were no studies on the prevalence of autism in Africa, South and Central Asia, Central and Latin America, and Eastern and Central Europe. In another review, the median prevalence from the available studies was 17 (range 3–94) per 10,000 in 36 studies conducted since 2000, with the median prevalence of all pervasive disorders as 62 (range 1–189) per 10,000 from 32 studies during the same time period [23]. There was no significant difference between these estimates between the studies conducted in Europe, North America, and Western Pacific.

## Global burden of autism

The Global Burden of Disease (GBD) was set up in the 1990s to compare the burden between countries and monitor secular trends. The GBD is usually presented in disability-adjusted life years (DALYs), which is the sum of years lost to life (YLLs) + years lived with disability (YLDs). The latter, in turn, is derived from incidence × disability weight. The disability weight in the 1990s was determined by expert opinion, but in the most recent estimations, the disability weight has been derived from interviews conducted across the world [24]. However, these interviews did not assess the disability weights associated with autism.

The global burden of autism, as measured with DALYs, was 337.8 million in 1990 and had increased by 38% to 467.6 million in 2010; however, this increase could be attributed to the population growth, with no increase in DALYs per capita [25]. Standardized by age and sex, this equated to 111 DALYs per 100,000 population [95%

uncertainty interval (UI) 77–154], but with 170 DALYs per 100,000 males (95% UI 119–237) and 50 DALYs per 100,000 females (95% UI 35–68).

## Sex ratio

The male predominance of autism was recognized by Kanner, and subsequently confirmed by later studies. Overall the ratio of males to females is 4.2:1 [26], but it depends upon the phenotype, in particular the degree of intellectual disability. As the intelligence quotient decreases, the ratio between males to females also decreases.

## Risk factors

Autism has high heritability, with twin studies suggesting that heritability ranges from 64% to 91% [27], with the estimate partially explained by the phenotype being studied. However, the genetic basis of autism is complex, with multiple genes involved by a variety of abnormalities such as copy number variants, common genetic variants, etc. It is likely that a multitude of genetic factors influence the susceptibility of an individual to develop autism, but there may be environmental factors that influence the genetic propensity [28]. The complex genetic basis of autism is outside the scope of this chapter, and the reader is referred to some excellent reviews [29–31].

There are a number of risk factors associated with autism, including parental acquired risk factors, and intrauterine, perinatal, and postnatal risk factors. Increasing paternal age (>50 years) is associated with a small, but significant, risk (relative risks of 1.5) of autism [18, 32, 33]. Advanced maternal age (>40 years) is also associated with an increased risk, but the relative risk is smaller than that with older fathers. In addition, young mothers (<20 years) have an increased risk [18]. However, given the relatively low relative risks and the inconsistency between studies, the importance of these factors is not well established.

Exposure to intrauterine infections, drugs, and other insults is also associated with autism. Rubella infection during pregnancy was the first infection to be associated with the development of autism. Initial studies suggested that 4–7% of affected fetuses develop autism [34], and the risk is increased in those children who had other features of congenital rubella syndrome. Further studies report the prevalence may be as high as 12% [35]. Other infections, such as cytomegalovirus [36], influenza, and parvovirus, have been documented with autism, but the epidemiological data are weaker than those with rubella. Likewise, some parasitic infections, such as toxoplasmosis and tick-borne infections, have weak and inconsistent associations with autism [37].

In a meta-analysis of papers published by 2007, maternal infection during pregnancy (OR 1.18; 95% CI 0.76–1.83), vaginal infections (OR 0.49; 95% CI 0.22–1.09), and maternal fever (OR 1.24; 95% CI 0.76–2.04) were not associated with autism [38]. However, when the analysis was limited to the four studies that controlled for multiple covariates or used sibling controls; exposure to intrauterine infections was significantly associated with autism (OR 1.82; 95% CI 1.01–3.30). Two recent population-based studies from Denmark and Taiwan have similar results. In the Danish study, admission to hospital due to maternal viral infection in the first trimester [adjusted

hazard ratio (aHR) 2.98; 95% CI 1.29–7.15] and maternal bacterial infection in the second trimester (aHR 1.42; 95% CI 1.08–1.87) was associated with autism in the children, but no association was found between any maternal infection and autism (aHR 1.14; 95% CI 0.96–1.34) [39]. In the Taiwanese study of 4184 children with autism, two or more outpatient visits for genital infection [adjusted odds ratio (aOR) 1.34; 95% CI 1.12, 1.60] and bacterial infection (aOR 1.24; 95% CI 1.06, 1.43) were associated with autism [40].

More recently, considerable interest has been generated by immunological activation during pregnancy. Maternal autoantibodies to fetal brain proteins are associated with the development of autism [41]. Immunoglobulin G (IgG) reactivity against fetal brain proteins was found in the plasma of 7 of 61 American mothers (11.5%) of children with autism, but not in 62 mothers of typically developing children ($p = 0.006$) or 40 mothers of children with non-ASD developmental delay ($p = 0.04$) [41]. Further studies have identified that the antibodies are against fetal brain tissue, and not adult brains. In addition, in a systematic review, maternal autoimmune diseases were associated with autism (pooled OR 1.34; 95% CI 1.23–1.46), including maternal thyroid disease [42].

The association between vaccines and the development of autism has been controversial, with a highly publicized study discredited [43]. Vaccination of children occurs at the ages when children are most likely to first show the features of autism. Thus, it is not surprising that many people think that there is an association between vaccination and autism. Since the original, but discredited, publication suggesting a link between mumps, measles, and rubella vaccination and the development of autism, there has been considerable work to assess the association with this vaccine. The most robust studies have not found an association, in particular the analysis of the Danish national database [15] and a case-control study based upon the British General Practice Register [44].

In addition, a meta-analysis of a number of vaccines have not found an association between any of these vaccines and autism [45]. The cohort data revealed no relationship between vaccination and autism (OR 0.99; 95% CI 0.92–1.06), and there was no relationship between autism and the measles, mumps, and rubella vaccine (OR 0.84; 95% CI 0.70–1.01) or the adjuvants used such as thimerosal (OR 1.00; 95% CI 0.77–1.31) or mercury (OR 1.00; 95% CI 0.93–1.07). The case-control data found similar results. Although the immunological activation induced by vaccination may lead to CNS manifestations, currently there is no evidence to support vaccination is associated with autism.

Other maternal factors thought to be associated with autism include gestational diabetes, nausea/vomiting, and bleeding during pregnancy. Gestational diabetes is associated with autism in a number of studies, and a recent retrospective longitudinal cohort study in California in the United States found that the risk of autism was associated with maternal type 2 diabetes (birth year aHR 1.33; 95% CI 1.07–1.66) and gestational diabetes diagnosed at 26 weeks or earlier (1.42; 95% CI 1.16–1.75) adjusted for maternal age, parity, education, household income, race/ethnicity, history of comorbidity, and sex of the offspring [46]. In a meta-analysis using a random effects model to calculate the summary effects, nausea/vomiting (1.48; 95% CI 1.03–2.14) and bleeding during pregnancy (1.81; 95% CI 1.14–2.86) were associated with autism [38].

Prematurity (gestational age <37 weeks) and low birthweight (<2.5 kg) often occur together, and without accurate estimates

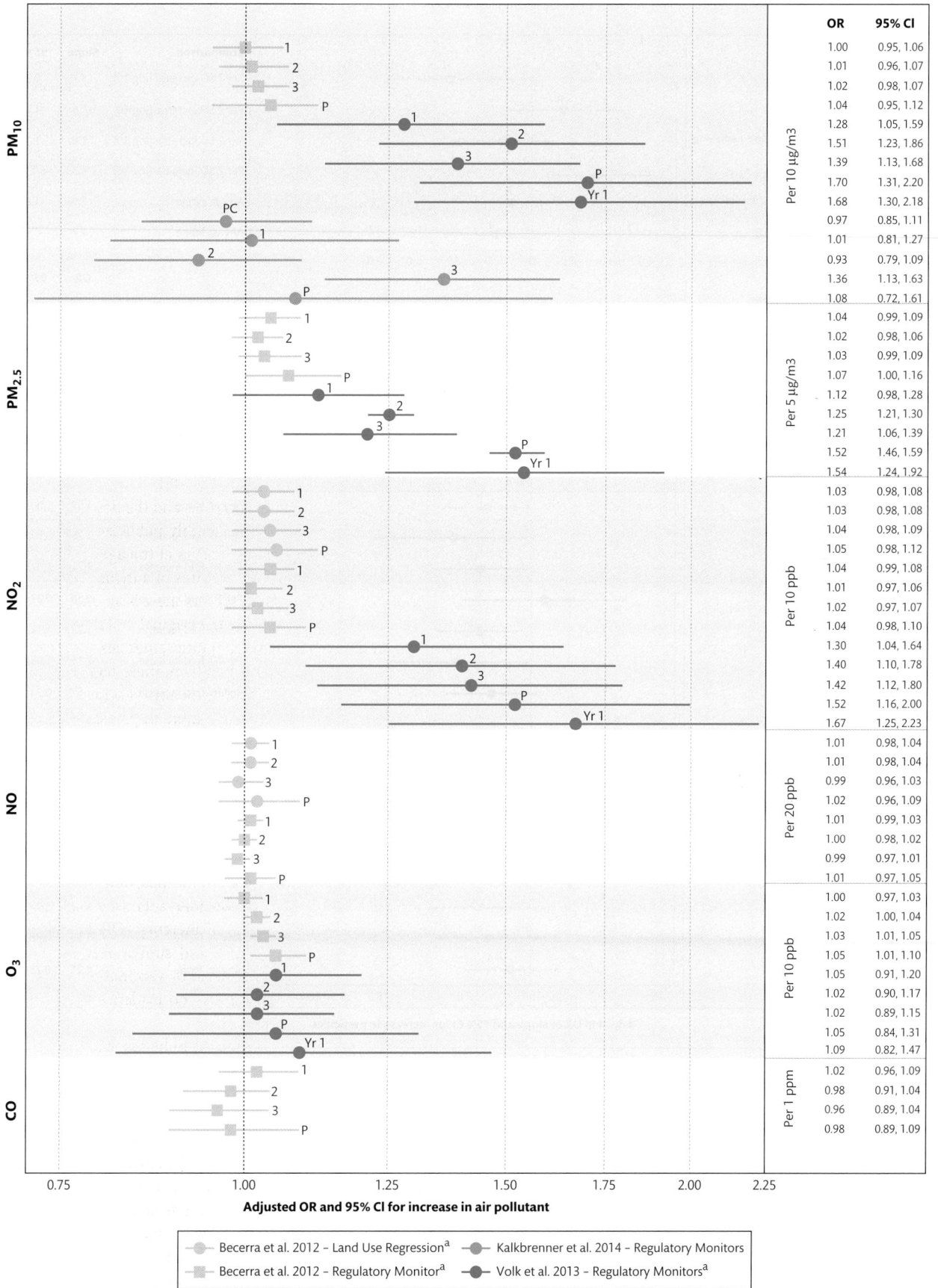

**Fig. 27.2** (see Colour Plate section) Associations between autism and estimates of exposure to individual traffic-related and criteria air pollutants. PM$_{10}$, particulate matter <10 μm in diameter; PM$_{2.5}$, particulate matter <2.5 μm in diameter; NO$_2$, nitrogen dioxide; NO, nitrogen oxide; O$_3$, ozone; CO, carbon monoxide. Exposure measured during developmental windows: PC, peri-conceptual; 1, trimester 1; 2, trimester 2; 3, trimester 3; P, pregnancy; Yr 1, first postnatal year. We recalculated parameters to reflect a change in the exposure comparison, to be consistent with other comparisons in the figure, involving calculations assuming that parameters were normally distributed.

Reproduced from *Curr Probl Pediatr Adolesc Health Care*, 44(10), Kalkbrenner AE, Schmidt RJ, Penlesky AC, Environmental chemical exposures and autism spectrum disorders: a review of the epidemiological evidence, pp. 277–318, Copyright (2014), with permission from Mosby, Inc.

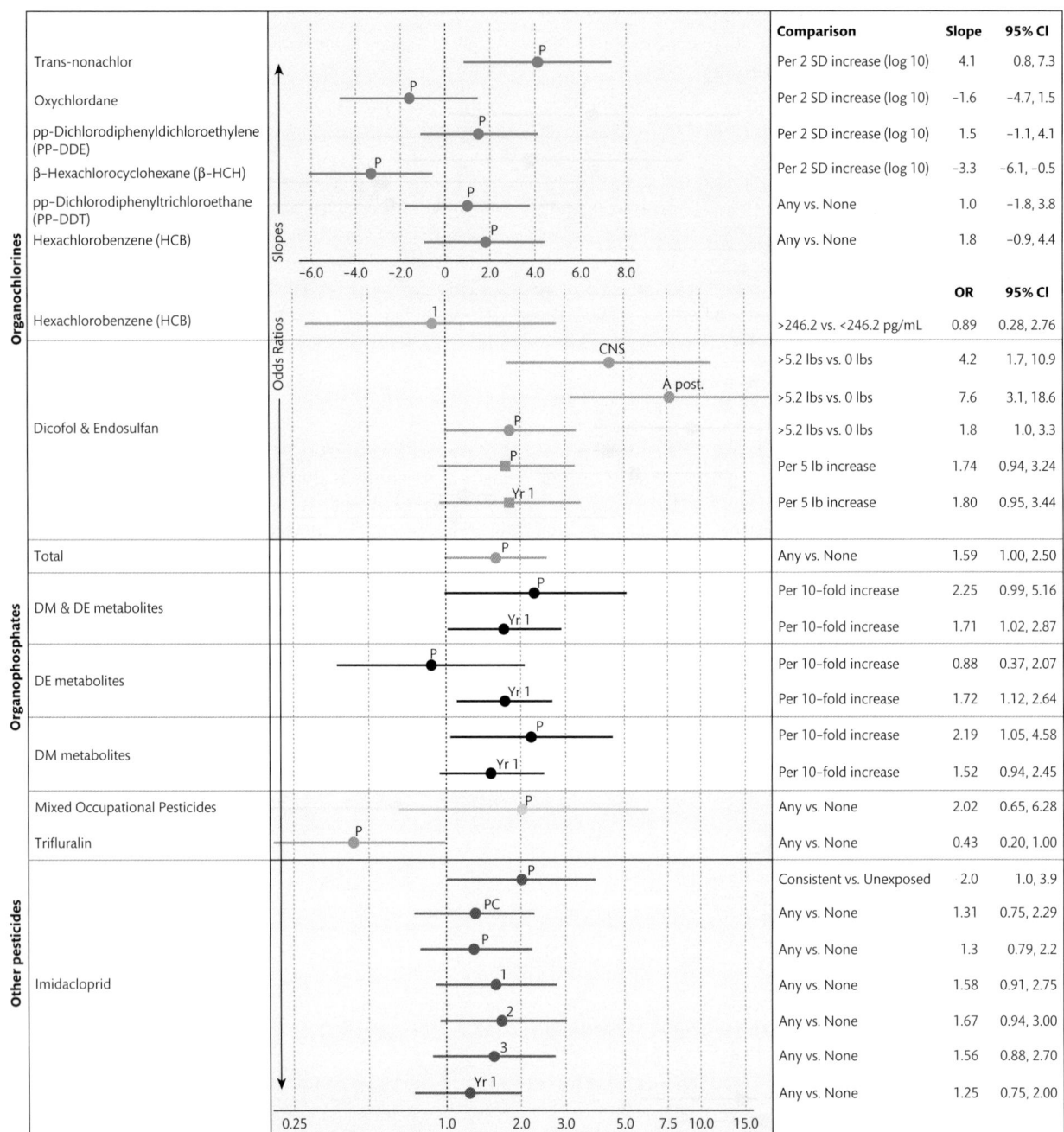

**Fig. 27.3** (see Colour Plate section) Associations between autism and estimates of exposure to pesticides.
DE metabolites, diethyl phosphate metabolites of organophosphate pesticides; DM metabolites, dimethyl phosphate metabolites of organophosphate pesticides. Exposure measured during developmental windows: CNS, a priori period of central nervous system development (7 days pre-fertilization to 49 days post-fertilization); a period of development (26–81 days post-fertilization); 1, trimester 1; 2, trimester 2; 3, trimester 3; P, pregnancy; Yr 1, first postnatal year. Other results not reported as measures of association with confidence intervals included pesticides that were determined not to be associated with increased autism risk and were not included in subsequent analyses from Roberts *et al.* 138: pesticide classes (cholinesterase inhibitors, copper-containing compounds, fumigants, avermectins, halogenated organics, N-methyl carbamates, pyrethroids, and thiocarbamates) and individual pesticide compounds (1,3-dichloropropene, chloropicrin, cypermethrin, fenarimol, methyl bromide, norflurazon, bromacil acid, chlorpyrifos, dazomet, glyphosate, molinate, oxadiazon, bifenthrin, diuron, metam-sodium, myclobutanil, and paraquat).

Reproduced from *Curr Probl Pediatr Adolesc Health Care*, 44(10), Kalkbrenner AE, Schmidt RJ, Penlesky AC, Environmental chemical exposures and autism spectrum disorders: a review of the epidemiological evidence, pp. 277–318, Copyright (2014), with permission from Mosby, Inc.

of gestational age and monitoring growth during the intrauterine period, it is difficult to differentiate between the risks associated with these factors. Although prematurity has been shown to be associated with autism in some studies, it was not significantly associated with autism in a meta-analysis [47]. A meta-analysis of studies has shown that intrauterine growth retardation is also associated with autism, with risk ratios from 1 to 2 [47, 48]. Other perinatal factors associated with autism identified in the meta-analysis include multiple births [summary effect size 1.77 (1.23–2.55)], being born in summer [1.14 (1.02–1.26)], breech presentation [1.81 (1.21–2.71)], cord complications [1.50 (1.00–2.24)], fetal distress [1.32 (1.09–2.12)], birth injury [4.90 (1.41–16.94)], maternal haemorrhage [2.39 (1.35–4.21)], low Apgar score at 5 minutes [1.67 (1.24–2.26)] [47].

There is considerable interest in the relationship between toxins and autism. In a rigorously conducted review on autism and toxins, the authors selected papers on the following criteria: population-based human (epidemiological) research, robust statistical tools, individual-level data on autism diagnoses, environmental–chemical measurements with exposures around conception or during pregnancy or the first postnatal year, and with valid comparison, including appropriate sample selection and accounting for confounders and adequate sample sizes to generate precise measures of association [49]. In this study, there was an association between autism and measures of mixed air pollutant exposures and diesel particulate matter (Fig. 27.2) and different-size air pollutants and nitrogen dioxide, but not with ozone or carbon monoxide. Associations were stronger for exposures in the third trimester of pregnancy and the first year of life, compared to earlier in pregnancy. In this review, there was a suggestion that volatile organic compounds, for example benzene and heavy metals (lead, mercury, manganese), may be associated with autism, but the ORs were not high or consistent across studies. The evidence for an association between a number of pesticides and autism was more convincing (Fig. 27.3). There was little evidence of the association between polychlorinated biphenyls, flame retardants, non-stick chemicals, or biphenol-A; evidence for some phthalates are more suggestive [49].

## Premature mortality

There has been little research on the premature mortality associated with autism. Standard mortality ratio (SMR) is used to compare mortality of a condition with the background population adjusted for age and sex. In early studies, the SMR of autism ranged from 1.9 in Denmark to 2.6 in the United States.

In a recent update of the Danish study, the SMR was 1.93 (CI 1.26–2.82), with the SMR higher for females (SMR 4.01; CI 1.73–7.90) than for males (SMR 1.57; CI 0.93–2.48) [50]. During the 45 years of follow-up, the SMR varied between 1.42 and 1.98, while the SMR for females varied between 3.17 and 5.22. The most common causes of the 26 deaths in this cohort were unnatural causes (suicide = 2, suffocation = 2), epilepsy (8 had epilepsy, with 4 stating that epilepsy contributed to their death), and infections.

In an analysis of a population database in Sweden, the authors compared 27,122 ASD probands, diagnosed between 1987 and 2009, with sex-, age-, and county of residence-matched controls ($n$ = 2,672,185) [51]. They found that 706 (2.60%) of people with autism died, compared to 24,358 controls (OR 2.56; 95% CI

2.38–2.76). Mortality occurred in most diagnostic categories, with the patterns of mortality influenced by sex and intellectual disability.

## Financial costs

Autism, as a life-long disorder, is associated with significant costs to the family and society. It was estimated that the annual total costs in 2011 associated with autism was about £3.1 billion in the UK and 250 billion USD in the United States, assuming 40% have intellectual disability [52]. The presence of intellectual disability increases the costs up to five times, compared to those without intellectual disability, depending upon age. The discounted lifetime costs of autism without intellectual disability were £0.92 million in the UK and 1.43 million USD in the United States, while those of autism with intellectual disability were £1.5 million in the UK and 2.44 million USD in the United States [52]. These costs are likely to be underestimates, since autism is often not diagnosed in older people. Thus, one forecast suggests that the total ASD-attributable costs in the United States will rise to over 450 billion USD by 2025 [53].

## Conclusions

The burden of autism is well established in North America and Europe, but data from other continents, particularly Africa and Asia, are limited. The apparent increase in the prevalence of autism in North America and Europe is likely to be caused mainly by an increase in awareness and a change in diagnostic criteria. The interaction between genetic susceptibility to autism and environmental factors needs further examination. There is no evidence that autism is associated with vaccines, but its relationship with immunological responses needs further examination. Autism is associated with premature mortality and engenders considerable costs.

## REFERENCES

1. Daniels AM, Mandell DS. Explaining differences in age at autism spectrum disorder diagnosis: a critical review. Autism. 2014;18(5):583–97.
2. Harrison MJ, O'Hare AE, Campbell H, Adamson A, McNeillage J. Prevalence of autistic spectrum disorders in Lothian, Scotland: an estimate using the 'capture-recapture' technique. Arch Dis Child. 2006;91(1):16–19.
3. Kanner L. Autistic disturbances of affective contact. Nervous Child. 1943;2:217–50.
4. American Psychiatric Association. *Diagnostic and statistical manual of mental disorders*, 3rd edition. Washington, DC: American Psychiatric Association; 1984.
5. Wing L, Gould J. Systematic recording of behaviors and skills of retarded and psychotic children. Journal of Autism and Childhood Schizophrenia. 1978;8(1):79–97.
6. Rutter M. Diagnosis and definition. In: Rutter M, Schopler E, editors. *Autism: A Reappraisal of Concepts and Treatment*. New York, NY: Plenum Press; 1978. pp. 1–25.
7. Kadesjo B, Gillberg C, Hagberg B. Brief report: autism and Asperger syndrome in seven-year-old children: a total population study. J Autism Dev Disord. 1999;29(4):327–31.

8. World Health Organization. *International Classification of Diseases*, 10th edition. Geneva: World Health Organization; 1990.

9. Baio J, Wiggins L, Christensen DL, *et al*. Prevalence and Characteristics of Autism Spectrum Disorder Among Children Aged 8 Years—Autism and Developmental Disabilities Monitoring Network, 11 Sites, United States, 2012. MMWR Surveill Summ. 2016;65(3):1–23.

10. Kim YS, Leventhal BL, Koh YJ, *et al*. Prevalence of autism spectrum disorders in a total population sample. Am J Psychiatry. 2011;168(9):904–12.

11. Volkmar FR, McPartland JC. From Kanner to DSM-5: autism as an evolving diagnostic concept. Ann Rev Clin Psychol. 2014;10:193–212.

12. Gillberg C, Wing L. Autism: not an extremely rare disorder. Acta Psychiatr Scand. 1999;99(6):399–406.

13. Shattuck PT, Durkin M, Maenner M, *et al*. Timing of identification among children with an autism spectrum disorder: findings from a population-based surveillance study. J Am Acad Child Adolesc Psychiatry. 2009;48(5):474–83.

14. Hagberg K, Jick H. Autism in the UK for birth cohorts 1988–2001. Epidemiology. 2010;21(3):426–7.

15. Madsen KM, Hviid A, Vestergaard M, *et al*. A population-based study of measles, mumps, and rubella vaccination and autism. N Engl J Med. 2002;347(19):1477–82.

16. Howe YJ, Yatchmink Y, Viscidi EW, Morrow EM. Ascertainment and gender in autism spectrum disorders. J Am Acad Child Adolesc Psychiatry. 2014;53(6):698–700.

17. Gal G, Abiri L, Reichenberg A, Gabis L, Gross R. Time trends in reported autism spectrum disorders in Israel, 1986–2005. J Autism Dev Disord. 2012;42(3):428–31.

18. Sandin S, Schendel D, Magnusson P, *et al*. Autism risk associated with parental age and with increasing difference in age between the parents. Mol Psychiatry. 2016;21:693–700.

19. Gentile S. Risks of neurobehavioral teratogenicity associated with prenatal exposure to valproate monotherapy: a systematic review with regulatory repercussions. CNS Spectr. 2014;19(4):305–15.

20. Mahoney AD, Minter B, Burch K, Stapel-Wax J. Autism spectrum disorders and prematurity: a review across gestational age subgroups. Adv Neonatal Care. 2013;13(4):247–51.

21. Crafa D, Warfa N. Maternal migration and autism risk: systematic analysis. Int Rev Psychiatry. 2015;27(1):64–71.

22. Erskine HE, Baxter AJ, Patton G, *et al*. The global coverage of prevalence data for mental disorders in children and adolescents. Epidemiol Psychiatr Sci. 2016:1–8.

23. Elsabbagh M, Divan G, Koh YJ, *et al*. Global prevalence of autism and other pervasive developmental disorders. Autism Res. 2012;5(3):160–79.

24. Salomon JA, Haagsma JA, Davis A, *et al*. Disability weights for the Global Burden of Disease 2013 study. Lancet Global health. 2015;3(11):e712–23.

25. Baxter AJ, Brugha TS, Erskine HE, Scheurer RW, Vos T, Scott JG. The epidemiology and global burden of autism spectrum disorders. Psychol Med. 2015;45(3):601–13.

26. Fombonne E. Epidemiological trends in autism. Mol Psychiatry. 2002;7:S4–46.

27. Tick B, Bolton P, Happe F, Rutter M, Rijsdijk F. Heritability of autism spectrum disorders: a meta-analysis of twin studies. J Child Psychol Psychiatry. 2016;57(5):585–95.

28. Tordjman S, Somogyi E, Coulon N, *et al*. Gene x Environment interactions in autism spectrum disorders: role of epigenetic mechanisms. Front Psychiatry. 2014;5:53.

29. Ziats MN, Rennert OM. The Evolving Diagnostic and Genetic Landscapes of Autism Spectrum Disorder. Front Genetics. 2016;7:65.

30. Robinson EB, Neale BM, Hyman SE. Genetic research in autism spectrum disorders. Curr Opin Pediatr. 2015;27(6):685–91.

31. AlSagob M, Colak D, Kaya N. Genetics of autism spectrum disorder: an update on copy number variations leading to autism in the next generation sequencing era. Discovery Med. 2015;19(106):367–79.

32. Idring S, Magnusson C, Lundberg M, *et al*. Parental age and the risk of autism spectrum disorders: findings from a Swedish population-based cohort. Int J Epidemiol. 2014;43:107–15.

33. Sandin S, Hultman CM, Kolevzon A, Gross R, MacCabe JH, Reichenberg A. Advancing maternal age is associated with increasing risk for autism: a review and meta-analysis. J Am Acad Child Adolesc Psychiatry. 2012;51(5):477–86 e1.

34. Chess S. Follow-up report on autism in congenital rubella. J Autism Child Schizophr. 1977;7(1):69–81.

35. Hutton J. Does Rubella Cause Autism: A 2015 Reappraisal? Front Hum Neurosci. 2016;10:25.

36. Yamashita Y, Fujimoto C, Nakajima E, Isagai T, Matsuishi T. Possible association between congenital cytomegalovirus infection and autistic disorder. J Autism Dev Disord. 2003;33(4):455–9.

37. Ornoy A, Weinstein-Fudim L, Ergaz Z. Prenatal factors associated with autism spectrum disorder (ASD). Reprod Toxicol. 2015;56:155–69.

38. Gardener H, Spiegelman D, Buka SL. Prenatal risk factors for autism: comprehensive meta-analysis. Br J Psychiatry. 2009;195:7–14.

39. Atladottir HO, Thorsen P, Ostergaard L, *et al*. Maternal infection requiring hospitalization during pregnancy and autism spectrum disorders. J Autism Dev Disord. 2010;40(12):1423–30.

40. Fang SY, Wang S, Huang N, Yeh HH, Chen CY. Prenatal Infection and Autism Spectrum Disorders in Childhood: A Population-Based Case-Control Study in Taiwan. Paediatr Perinat Epidemiol. 2015;29(4):307–16.

41. Braunschweig D, Van de Water J. Maternal autoantibodies in autism. Arch Neurol. 2012;69(6):693–9.

42. Chen SW, Zhong XS, Jiang LN, *et al*. Maternal autoimmune diseases and the risk of autism spectrum disorders in offspring: A systematic review and meta-analysis. Behav Brain Res. 2016;296:61–9.

43. [No authors listed]. Retraction—Ileal-lymphoid-nodular hyperplasia, non-specific colitis, and pervasive developmental disorder in children. Lancet. 2010;375(9713):445.

44. Smeeth L, Cook C, Fombonne E, *et al*. MMR vaccination and pervasive developmental disorders: a case-control study. Lancet. 2004;364(9438):963–9.

45. Taylor LE, Swerdfeger AL, Eslick GD. Vaccines are not associated with autism: an evidence-based meta-analysis of case-control and cohort studies. Vaccine. 2014;32(29):3623–9.

46. Xiang AH, Wang X, Martinez MP, *et al*. Association of maternal diabetes with autism in offspring. JAMA. 2015;313(14): 1425–34.

47. Gardener H, Spiegelman D, Buka SL. Perinatal and neonatal risk factors for autism: a comprehensive meta-analysis. Pediatrics. 2011;128(2):344–55.

48. Kolevzon A, Gross R, Reichenberg A. Prenatal and perinatal risk factors for autism: a review and integration of findings. Arch Pediatr Adolesc Med. 2007;161(4):326–33.

49. Kalkbrenner AE, Schmidt RJ, Penlesky AC. Environmental chemical exposures and autism spectrum disorders: a review of the epidemiological evidence. Curr Probl Pediatr Adolesc Health Care. 2014;44(10):277–318.

50. Mouridsen SE, Bronnum-Hansen H, Rich B, Isager T. Mortality and causes of death in autism spectrum disorders: an update. Autism. 2008;12(4):403–14.

51. Hirvikoski T, Mittendorfer-Rutz E, Boman M, Larsson H, Lichtenstein P, Bolte S. Premature mortality in autism spectrum disorder. Br J Psychiatry. 2016;208(3):232–8.

52. Buescher AV, Cidav Z, Knapp M, Mandell DS. Costs of Autism Spectrum Disorders in the United Kingdom and the United States. JAMA Pediatrics. 2014;168(8):721–8.

53. Leigh JP, Du J. Brief Report: Forecasting the Economic Burden of Autism in 2015 and 2025 in the United States. J Autism Dev Disord. 2015;45(12):4135–9.

# 28

# Genetics of autism spectrum disorders

*Abha R. Gupta, Thomas V. Fernandez, and Ellen J. Hoffman*

## ASD heritability and early genetic investigations

Autism spectrum disorder (ASD) has long been recognized as a heritable disorder, based on family and twin studies. Monozygotic twin concordance rates have been reported to be approximately 60% for the full syndrome and 90% for the broad spectrum. In contrast, dizygotic twin concordance has been reported to be relatively low, approximately 3–15%, depending on the diagnostic criteria used. These data support the conclusion that the observed familial clustering is largely the result of genetic factors and translate into an estimate of heritability that places ASD among the most strongly genetic of all neuropsychiatric conditions [1–7].

Establishing high heritability has encouraged the search for genetic variants that are enriched in ASD. Early insights into ASD risk genes came from recognition that children with rare syndromes of known genetic causes (for example, fragile X syndrome, tuberous sclerosis complex, Angelman syndrome) have high rates of ASD diagnosis, ranging from approximately 10% (Duchenne muscular dystrophy) to 80% (Phelan–McDermid syndrome) [8–10]. Initially, there was great hope that genetic linkage and candidate gene association studies would complement these syndromic observations and rapidly yield a wealth of new insights about ASD genetic susceptibility loci.

Linkage analysis assesses the probability that a given phenotype and particular genetic markers are transmitted together from one generation to the next. Association studies typically investigate one or a number of known, common genetic polymorphisms that lie within or near pre-determined candidate genes of interest, comparing allele frequencies in cases vs controls. Such association studies have been popular over the last few decades, owing, in part, to the practicalities of subject recruitment and greater theoretical power to detect common susceptibility variants of relatively small effect, compared to linkage studies [11–14]. However, linkage and candidate gene association studies in ASD, and in nearly all complex neuropsychiatric disorders, have yielded very few reproducible findings. This is likely due to previously underappreciated factors such as locus and allelic heterogeneity, clinical heterogeneity, and differing inclusion criteria, inadequate control for population stratification, and insufficiently powered study cohorts, especially when studying common alleles with small effect sizes [15–17].

Due to these limitations, and coinciding with microarray technological advancements that delivered affordable high-density genotyping platforms, about 10 years ago, there was a shift in methodology from candidate gene association to genome-wide association studies (GWAS), simultaneously testing hundreds of thousands to millions of common single-nucleotide polymorphisms (SNPs) for association with disease. Querying SNPs throughout the genome eliminates the need to previously select candidate variants, allowing for hypothesis-neutral investigations. This method also yields data that allow rigorous matching for ancestry between cases and controls, an aforementioned confounder in earlier association studies. The primary challenge in GWAS is the large number of independent comparisons performed, requiring a widely accepted genome-wide significance threshold of $p \leq 5 \times 10^{-8}$. Given the heterogeneity of complex disease, large sample sizes are required to achieve this level of significance. Nevertheless, this technique led to renewed excitement in the field around the potential for variant and risk gene discovery. However, in ASD, none of the candidate genes emerging from earlier association or linkage studies have reached the statistical threshold for genome-wide significance using GWAS [18, 19], suggesting either that these candidate genes had initial false-positive associations or that the current GWAS cohorts lack sufficient statistical power to detect common variant association. Nevertheless, efforts on this front continue; recent data suggest that one promising way to reduce genetic heterogeneity in ASD, and thereby improve statistical power, under the GWAS framework may be to focus analysis on intermediate core phenotypes that accompany the disorder [20].

## A windfall of success in ASD risk gene discovery

To date, the most fruitful studies for identifying risk genes in ASD have been those focusing on rare, large-effect variants in the protein-coding regions (exome) of the genome. In addition to the genes implicated in rare syndromic forms of ASD, rare point mutations in the *NLGN3X* and *NLGN4X* genes (*Neuroligin 3X* and *4X*) were the first replicated findings in non-syndromic (idiopathic) ASD [21, 22]. Soon after, driven by technological advances that allowed for the detection of genome-wide rare *de novo* mutations (detected in the probands, but not the parents), several studies reported an increased rate of *de novo* copy number variants (CNVs) in ASD and confirmed risk loci identified by the clustering of such variants in certain genomic regions among unrelated individuals with ASD [23–39].

Similarly, *de novo* coding single nucleotide variants (SNVs) and insertion–deletions (indels) have been found by whole-exome sequencing studies to contribute to ASD risk. In particular, likely gene disrupting (LGD) *de novo* variants (for example, nonsense, splice site, frameshift) are enriched in ASD and have proven to be a powerful avenue for identifying individual risk genes by the finding of multiple such variants in the same gene in unrelated individuals [40–45].

Owing mainly to *de novo* genotyping and sequencing studies, dozens of high-confidence ASD risk genes have been discovered, out of an estimated target of 500–1000 genes underlying ASD risk [46]. A recent analysis of all available *de novo* whole-exome sequencing and CNV data from >5000 families in the Autism Genome Project and the Simons Simplex Collection identified 65 ASD risk genes and six CNV regions [32]. Several online databases are updated regularly with the latest findings regarding ASD risk genes and loci, supported by evidence from ongoing sequencing and genotyping studies [47–50].

Based on currently available data, there is an important contribution to ASD risk from rare *de novo* and rare inherited variation. Rare genetic variants are believed to cause approximately 10–30% of ASD [32, 46, 51], and each individual variant can confer significant risk on its own, for example, making an individual 30–50 times more likely to develop ASD. Despite the fact that all of the ASD risk genes and loci to date have emerged from rare variant studies, the largest component of genetic risk in ASD is believed to derive from common genetic variants of additive effect. When considered as a whole, the contribution of common genetic variation is estimated between 15% and 50% [52–54]. Yet, the increase in ASD risk by an individual common variant is very small, on the order of 5–10%, and no common risk loci have yet been definitively identified. To find common variants of small effect, future efforts will need to study even larger cohorts than those included in studies to date.

## Stepping towards an understanding of ASD biology

Now that there are clear, successful avenues for risk gene discovery in ASD, it is possible to begin asking whether identified genes are involved in common biological processes, whether they are expressed in particular brain regions, during certain developmental time periods, and whether their gene products are enriched in certain cell types. Already, we are seeing that ASD risk genes are more likely to be expressed in cortical pyramidal neurons during mid-fetal development [55, 56]. Furthermore, gene set enrichment analyses are showing that ASD risk genes and loci are converging onto a smaller number of biological processes, including chromatin remodelling, transcriptional regulation, synaptic functioning, Wnt and MAPK signalling, and interactions with the *FMR1* (*fragile X mental retardation 1*) gene [24, 27, 30, 41, 42, 57]. In this way, variant discovery provides an important foothold for identifying risk genes and for beginning to understand ASD neurobiology. However, it is critically important to study the downstream consequences of the identified variants to refine our understanding of disease pathophysiology and pave the way for earlier diagnosis, therapeutic interventions, and novel treatments.

## Importance of modelling ASD variants

Once candidate genes have been identified, the most important and challenging next step is gaining an understanding of how disruption of these risk genes affects basic processes of nervous system development, resulting in behavioural dysfunction. That is, identification of ASD-associated genes has the potential to provide a critical window into neurobiological mechanisms underlying ASD. For example, some of the earliest insights into the neurobiology of ASD came from animal models of monogenic syndromes that are associated with an increased risk of ASD, including fragile X syndrome (FXS) and tuberous sclerosis complex (TSC). Here, 'knockout' mouse models lacking the function of the genes that are causative for these syndromes provided the first evidence for pathophysiological mechanisms underlying ASD and revealed possible pathways for therapeutic targeting. However, recent large-scale whole-exome sequencing efforts of affected individuals have led to a rapidly expanding list of 'high-confidence' ASD risk genes, which has made modelling ASD-associated variants increasingly challenging. While these risk genes represent seemingly disparate functions, ranging from ion channels and cell adhesion molecules to chromatin remodellers and transcription factors, there is emerging evidence that they converge on common mechanistic pathways such as synapse function, chromatin modification, transcriptional regulation, Wnt signalling, and targets of the fragile X mental retardation protein (FMRP) [42, 57–60]. In this way, these studies have revealed pathways that are likely to play a key role in ASD. Moreover, to keep pace with the increased rate of gene discovery, scientists are now employing new cellular, molecular, and computational strategies, which allow for the simultaneous analysis of multiple risk genes and are beginning to shed light on fundamental questions in ASD neurobiology. For example, these studies aim to elucidate the specific developmental stages and neuronal cell types, that is, when and where ASD risk gene function is most critical for brain development. Another objective of functional studies is to leverage the growing number of risk genes to uncover neurobiological pathways that can serve as targets for novel pharmacotherapies. Therefore, recent studies modelling ASD-associated variants are playing a pivotal role in advancing the field from risk gene discovery to the elucidation of neurodevelopmental mechanisms and targeted pharmacological treatments.

## Insights from models of monogenic ASD-associated syndromes

Early insights into the neurobiology of ASD came from animal models of monogenic syndromes that are associated with increased autism risk, as mentioned. FXS is the most common inherited cause of ASD and is a notable example of how modelling the loss of function of a single gene can result in the identification of novel biological pathways and potential therapeutic targets [61]. Studies of mice lacking the function of the *FMR1* gene, which is disrupted in FXS, led to the metabotropic glutamatergic receptor (mGluR) theory of FXS. Specifically, mouse knockouts of *FMR1* were found to exhibit an increase in a form of synaptic plasticity—long-term depression (LTD), which is dependent on protein synthesis and mGluR activation [62]. Therefore, excessive mGluR signalling and LTD were proposed as a potential mechanism underlying abnormal structural and behavioural phenotypes in mice lacking *FMR1* function [62], including altered dendritic spine structure in adult cortical neurons, hyperactivity, and learning deficits [63, 64]. Indeed, multiple studies have shown that inhibition of mGluR signalling is able to reverse physiological, structural, and behavioural abnormalities in animal models of FXS, ranging from the mouse to the fly [65–70] (reviewed in [71]), leading to clinical trials of mGluR antagonists [72]. While the efficacy of these agents has yet to be demonstrated in human patients with FXS, modifications in clinical trial design, such as administering the medication to younger patients for a longer duration and developing more precise efficacy measurements, may improve outcomes [73].

TSC, which is caused by heterozygous mutations in the *TSC1* or *TSC2* genes, is another example of a syndrome associated with an increased risk of ASD that led to the identification of an important signalling pathway with relevance to ASD. Specifically, these genes encode proteins that function as negative regulators of the mammalian target of rapamycin (mTOR) pathway, which is involved in protein synthesis and cell proliferation [74]. This discovery led to the hypothesis that inhibitors of mTOR, such as rapamycin, might serve as potential therapeutic agents. Interestingly, rapamycin was found to reverse learning and social deficits in mouse models of TSC [75, 76], paving the way for clinical trials of this class of medications. In addition, mutations in the *PTEN* gene (*Phosphatase and Tensin Homolog*), which also negatively regulates mTOR, are associated with an increased risk of ASD and macrocephaly [77–80], providing further evidence for this pathway in the neurobiology of ASD. Rapamycin was also found to reverse macrocephaly and behavioural abnormalities, including anxiety and social deficits, in a conditional mouse knockout in which *PTEN* function was disrupted in post-mitotic neurons [81]. Clinical trials are currently under way to investigate the effect of mTOR inhibitors on cognition in children and adolescents with *PTEN* mutations (http://www.clinicaltrials.gov).

Other examples of monogenic syndromes associated with ASD that have shed light on relevant molecular mechanisms include Rett syndrome, caused by mutations in the *MECP2* gene (*Methyl-CpG binding domain-2*), and neurofibromatosis type 1, caused by disruption of the *NF1* gene (*Neurofibromin 1*) [61]. In addition, with the increased rate of gene discovery in idiopathic ASD from whole-exome sequencing, together with more detailed clinical characterization of individuals carrying variants in specific risk genes, there is growing evidence that each of these ASD-associated genes may represent a subtype of ASD with shared clinical features [57]. For example, recent studies have suggested that the high-confidence ASD genes *CHD8* (*Chromodomain Helicase DNA Binding Protein 8*), *DYRK1A* (*Dual Specificity Tyrosine Phosphorylation Regulated Kinase 1A*), *POGZ* (*Pogo Transposable Element Derived with ZNF Domain*), and *GRIN2B* (*Glutamate Ionotropic Receptor NMDA Type Subunit 2B*) may represent distinct ASD syndromes [82–85]. Therefore, animal models of each of these genes have the potential to reveal biological pathways that are uniquely disrupted due to gene loss and to identify specific pharmacological targets, providing a 'personalized medicine' approach to developing new treatments. For example, point mutations in the *SHANK3* gene (*SH3 and multiple ankyrin repeat domains 3*), which encodes a post-synaptic scaffolding protein at excitatory synapses, as well as deletions of the chromosome region 22q13.3, which includes this gene, are associated with Phelan–McDermid

syndrome, which is characterized by ASD, intellectual disability, seizures, and dysmorphic features [86]. Physiological and motor deficits in mice in which *SHANK3* function was disrupted were rescued by treatment with insulin-like growth factor 1 (IGF-1) [87], which promotes synaptogenesis [88]. IGF-1 was also found to reverse deficits in excitatory signalling in an induced pluripotent stem cell (iPSC) model of Phelan–McDermid syndrome [89] and rescued abnormal phenotypes in mouse and iPSC models of Rett syndrome [90, 91]. These preclinical studies led to a pilot clinical trial of nine individuals with Phelan–McDermid syndrome, in which IGF-1 showed some benefit in treating social deficits and repetitive behaviours, though larger studies are needed [92].

## Modelling ASD risk genes in animal systems

Animal models offer distinct advantages for the functional analysis of ASD risk genes. Firstly, animal models allow for the investigation of the role of risk genes in neural circuits in a live, behaving organism, which is not possible using *in vitro* approaches [93]. Secondly, risk gene function can be studied along a developmental trajectory, including embryonic stages in animal models [94], which is critical for understanding the role of ASD risk genes, given that many of these genes are expressed embryonically. Thirdly, animal knockouts provide a platform for identifying novel pharmacological pathways and studying the *in vivo* effects of drugs targeting these pathways [93]. Moreover, emerging cellular and molecular technologies are expanding the range of scientific questions that can be addressed using animal models. For example, a recently developed method CLARITY allows for high-resolution, three-dimensional imaging of intact mouse brains [95]. Other new techniques, such as optogenetics and genetically encoded calcium indicators, allow scientists to assess the circuit-level and behavioural effects of activating a subset of neurons (engineered to express a light-activated channel) [96–98] and to visualize neural activity in an awake, behaving animal [99, 100]. Further, CRISPR (clustered regularly interspaced short palindromic repeats)/Cas9 technology, a highly efficient and flexible method for generating targeted mutations [101], has revolutionized the ability to model ASD-associated mutations in both *in vivo* and *in vitro* systems. In addition, there is increasing interest in using smaller, less complex organisms, such as the zebrafish and *Drosophila*, to model ASD risk genes, given their experimental tractability for conducting large-scale phenotyping analyses and high-throughput pharmacological screens [70, 93, 102]. While these systems are less conserved than mice, in comparison to humans, at the genetic and structural levels, it is anticipated that future studies will capitalize on the advantages of multiple animal models for the functional analysis of ASD genes.

At the same time, there are clear limitations to modelling ASD-associated genes in animal systems. Firstly, it is impossible to fully recapitulate human behaviours in animals, given the limits of face validity [93, 94, 103]. Secondly, pharmacological candidates identified in animal models may not translate to effective treatments in humans. The example of mGluR antagonists in FXS highlights these challenges, including identifying the optimal age, duration of medication administration, and outcome measurements in human studies, which are not easily translated from preclinical studies [73]. Thirdly, animal systems cannot fully recapitulate the genetic diversity of an individual, which may shape clinical presentation. Despite these drawbacks, animal models provide an important *in vivo* approach for elucidating the role of ASD risk genes in basic mechanisms of neurodevelopment and circuit-level function.

## Human induced pluripotent stem cell modelling of ASD risk genes

Another approach to modelling ASD-associated mutations is the use of human iPSCs. The scientific basis for iPSC generation was reported in a landmark study which demonstrated that adult human dermal fibroblasts could be reprogrammed into a pluripotent state by four transcription factors: Oct3/4, Sox2, Klf4, and c-Myc [104]. These cells could, in turn, be differentiated into any cell type, including neural cells. Protocols have been developed to differentiate iPSCs into specific neural populations, including electrically active GABAergic, glutamatergic, and dopaminergic neurons; astrocytes; and oligodendrocytes [105, 106]. This approach also enables the analysis of patient-derived cells during the course of neural differentiation, from iPSCs to neural progenitor cells (NPCs) to mature neurons. In addition, a series of assays can be performed on these cells, including transcriptional profiling studies; analyses of neuronal morphology; synapse formation and function; and neuronal migration, differentiation, and proliferation—providing a rich database for assessing the effect of patient mutations on cellular and physiological phenotypes. Further, neural cells can be grown as three-dimensional organoids, which, to some extent, can recapitulate features of early human brain development and allow for the analysis of simple network activity [105, 107]. To model ASD-associated mutations using iPSCs, scientists have adopted two main experimental strategies: (1) generating iPSCs from cells obtained from individuals with ASD carrying a mutation in a particular risk gene; and (2) genetically engineering iPSCs generated from the cells of an unaffected individual using the CRISPR/Cas9 system to introduce a mutation identified in an individual with ASD. The former approach captures the genetic background of the patient, which is highly relevant to ASD, where clinical presentation may be influenced by a combination of rare *de novo* and transmitted variants, along with common variants, while the latter method allows scientists to compare ASD-associated mutations in an isogenic background, providing a readout of the effects of the variants alone on cellular phenotypes. Another approach utilizes morphological analysis and transcriptional profiling of iPSCs generated from individuals with idiopathic ASD (unknown aetiology), which has also provided insights into neurobiological mechanisms in ASD [108].

There are several notable advantages of using iPSCs for the functional analysis of ASD risk genes. Firstly, unlike animal models, iPSCs allow for the analysis of cellular phenotypes in the genetic background of a patient, which can play a critical role in shaping the clinical presentation [109]. Secondly, multiple sequence variants or large CNVs found in an individual with ASD are difficult to model in animals but are present in patient-derived iPSCs [110]. Thirdly, the use of iPSCs offers key advantages over studies of post-mortem tissue [110, 111], which can be confounded by environmental or treatment effects over the lifetime of an individual and cannot provide electrophysiological or other functional information. Fourthly, iPSCs are amenable to high-throughput pharmacological screens

to identify compounds that reverse cellular or electrophysiological phenotypes associated with a particular variant, which can complement drug screens in animal models where the same risk gene has been disrupted. Consistent with the goals of personalized medicine, patient-derived iPSCs provide an individualized platform for the discovery of potential new treatments. Nonetheless, limitations of iPSC modelling include the inability to assess the effect of mutations on circuit-level or behavioural phenotypes in an intact nervous system. In addition, generating iPSCs, NPCs, and mature neurons is a time-intensive process, such that it may take 2 months to reprogramme source cells into iPSCs and differentiate iPSCs into NPCs, and 3–4 months to generate neural cells. Further, because reprogramming cells involves inducing genome-wide epigenetic changes [112], it is important to analyse epigenetic patterns before and after iPSC generation, though iPSCs from individuals with Angelman and Prader–Willi syndromes were found to retain the appropriate patterns of DNA methylation [113]. Taken together, iPSC modelling of ASD-associated variants has enabled scientists to, at least partially, overcome the challenge of obtaining living human brain tissue for study, revolutionizing the functional analysis of ASD risk genes at the cellular and molecular levels.

## ASD risk gene network analysis

While ASD risk genes may be associated with distinct clinical features that define subtypes of the disorder [57], there is evidence that many of these genes converge on common neurodevelopmental pathways that provide critical insights into ASD biology, as mentioned [42, 57–60]. Despite the important mechanistic insights gained by modelling individual risk genes, one at a time, in animal or iPSC models, given the rapid rate of ASD gene discovery, this single-gene approach is becoming increasingly challenging. Here, advances in computational tools, which allow for the simultaneous analysis of hundreds of ASD-associated genes using a systems or network-based approach, are beginning to illuminate common neurodevelopmental mechanisms across these genes [60]. Specifically, studies have harnessed the BrainSpan transcriptome data set, which includes human gene expression data from the brains of 57 typically developing individuals and encompasses multiple anatomical regions and a range of developmental stages, from early fetal stage to late adulthood [114, 115], to elucidate when and where ASD risk genes might play critical roles in the developing brain [60]. In one study, researchers constructed gene co-expression networks around high-confidence ASD genes utilizing the BrainSpan data set and assessed these networks for enrichment of an additional set of probable ASD-associated genes, identifying mid-fetal glutamatergic projection neurons in cortical layers V–VI as a point of convergence [56]. Another study used weighted gene co-expression network analysis to construct co-expression networks using the BrainSpan data set and mapped ASD-associated genes onto these networks [116]. This study found enrichment of ASD risk genes in glutamatergic projection neurons in superficial cortical layers II–IV, though a weaker enrichment signal was also detected in deep layers [116]. Therefore, these types of analyses provide a spatiotemporal readout of when and where ASD genes are likely to function in brain development, which is expected to inform future functional studies of these genes in model systems [60]. Taken together, network-based approaches,

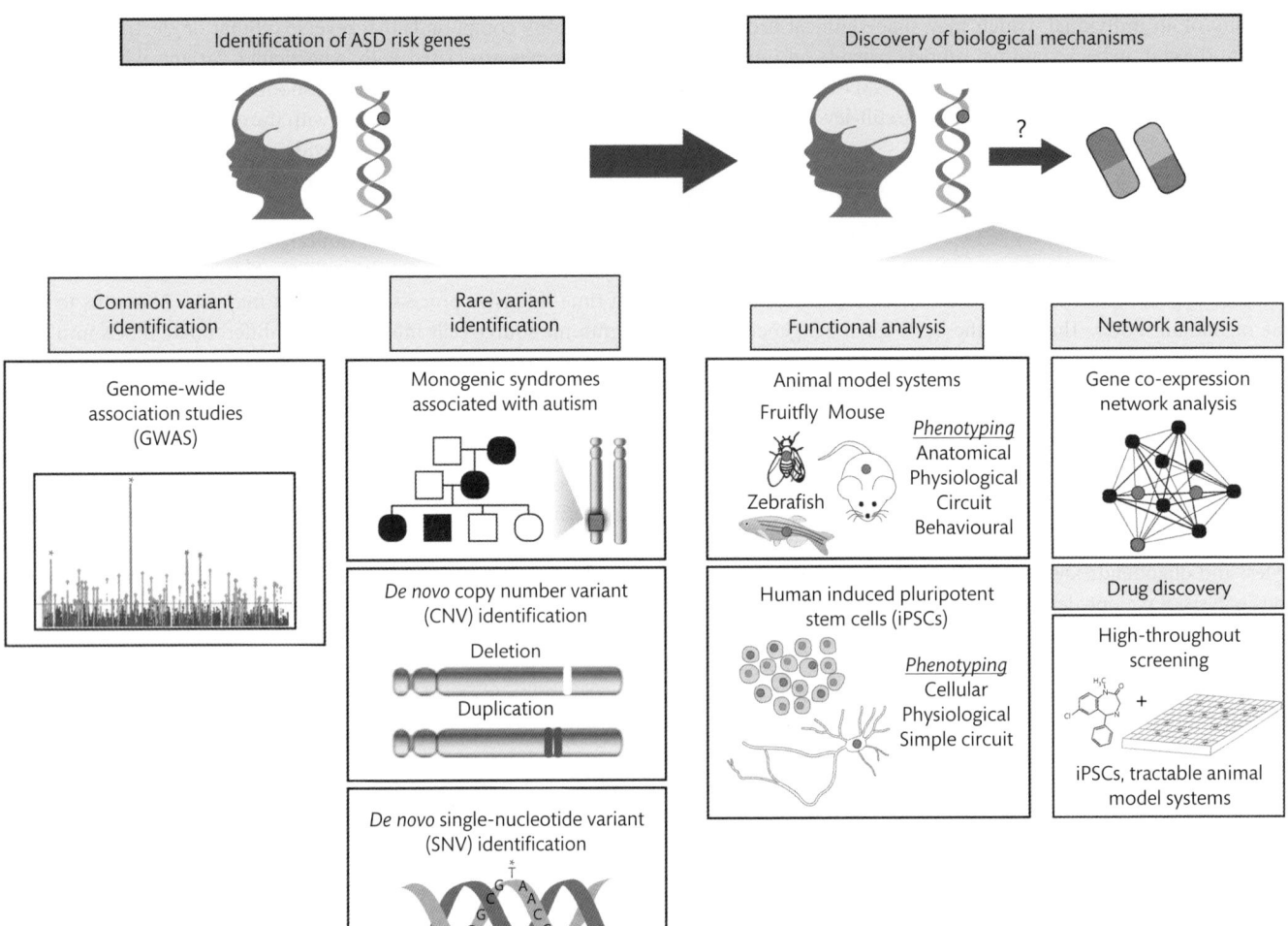

**Fig. 28.1** Schematic representation of the pathway from the identification of risk genes to the discovery of biological mechanisms in ASD. Risk genes associated with ASD are identified by a variety of techniques: genome-wide association studies, linkage analysis, chromosomal microarray (to identify CNVs), and whole-exome/genome sequencing (to identify sequence variants). Functional analysis aims to bridge genetics and neurobiology by determining the impact of variants on biological systems through *in vivo* and *in vitro* approaches such as animal model systems and induced pluripotent stem cells. Network analysis aims to accomplish this through computational approaches such as gene co-expression studies. The discovery of biological mechanisms is expected to identify novel targets for pharmacological intervention in ASD, the ultimate goal of this research.

along with *in vivo* and *in vitro* models of ASD-associated genes, are anticipated to advance our understanding of the basic neurobiology of ASD and provide a path towards the development of mechanism-based treatments. Fig. 28.1 summarizes the pathway from the identification of risk genes to the discovery of biological mechanisms in ASD.

## Clinical genetics testing in ASD

Although the genetic contribution to ASD is well established, there has been much debate over the years as to the most appropriate laboratory tests to pursue in individuals with ASD. Clinical genetics testing is an important component of the medical evaluation of all patients with a diagnosis on the spectrum, from severely to mildly impaired, for a number of reasons. As has been described, there is substantial overlap between ASD and some genetic syndromes such as FXS and TSC. The identification of a known genetic syndrome allows the clinician to provide anticipatory guidance regarding

medical and developmental trajectories to caregivers. This is especially critical if there is additional organ involvement. For example, FXS can also cause vision problems, such as strabismus and amblyopia, and hypotonia. The benign tumours which characterize TSC can disrupt the function of not only the brain, but also multiple other vital organs such as the heart, lungs, liver, and kidneys. Establishing a genetic aetiology can help in obtaining needed care and services and avoid the pursuit of further, unnecessary diagnostic tests. Another important reason for clinical genetic testing is that the identification of variants and whether they are *de novo* or inherited through the testing of family members can have implications for genetic counselling. The parents of an affected child may want to know their chances of having subsequent affected children, and aunts and uncles may want to know if a variant is being passed through a family.

The American College of Medical Genetics and Genomics (ACMG) has provided the most detailed guidelines for clinical genetics testing in ASD [117]. These guidelines are structured as two tiers of tests, with the first tier expected to have higher diagnostic yield. If first-tier tests are negative, second-tier tests may be pursued.

After completion of a three-generation family history to identify a potential mode of inheritance for the disorder, clinical geneticists should determine if a known genetic syndrome is present, guided by a thorough history and physical examination which includes a detailed dysmorphology exam. If a specific syndrome or metabolic disorder is suspected, targeted testing should be performed. If a syndrome that is firmly associated with ASD is diagnosed, the ACMG does not consider further testing necessary. These syndromes include 22q11.2 deletion, Angelman, CHARGE, FXS, Prader–Willi, Rett, and TSC, among others [117]. In the absence of a known syndrome, chromosomal microarray analysis (CMA) should be obtained. Either through array-comparative genomic hybridization (aCGH) or an SNP array, CMA will detect chromosomal deletions and duplications. This test has replaced karyotypes since the International Standard Cytogenomic Array Consortium has concluded that CMA has a higher yield than karyotyping [118]. DNA testing for FXS is recommended for all male patients and for those female patients with clinical features of FXS or a positive family history. If all first-tier tests are negative, clinical geneticists can consider specific gene tests, such as looking for variants in *MECP2* and *PTEN*, and brain magnetic resonance imaging (MRI) if indicators are present.

The ACMG estimates that, for idiopathic ASD, a minimal clinical genetics evaluation consisting of CMA and FXS testing will have a combined diagnostic yield of approximately 10–15%. A comprehensive evaluation, guided by the two-tiered approach, is estimated to identify an aetiology in 30–40% of individuals with ASD [117]. Although the ACMG does not currently recommend specific gene testing in idiopathic ASD other than for FXS, *MECP2*, and *PTEN*, it is expected that ASD gene panels will become increasingly valid as researchers continue to dissect the genetic aetiology of ASD, as discussed in this chapter.

## REFERENCES

1. Folstein S, Rutter M. Infantile autism: a genetic study of 21 twin pairs. J Child Psychol Psychiatry. 1977;18(4):297–321.
2. Hallmayer J, Cleveland S, Torres A, *et al.* Genetic heritability and shared environmental factors among twin pairs with autism. Arch Gen Psychiatry. 2011;68(11):1095–102.
3. Sandin S, Lichtenstein P, Kuja-Halkola R, Larsson H, Hultman CM, Reichenberg A. The familial risk of autism. JAMA. 2014;311(17):1770–7.
4. Bailey A, Le Couteur A, Gottesman I, *et al.* Autism as a strongly genetic disorder: evidence from a British twin study. Psychol Med. 1995;25(1):63–77.
5. Lichtenstein P, Carlstrom E, Rastam M, Gillberg C, Anckarsater H. The genetics of autism spectrum disorders and related neuropsychiatric disorders in childhood. Am J Psychiatry. 2010;167(11):1357–63.
6. Ronald A, Hoekstra RA. Autism spectrum disorders and autistic traits: a decade of new twin studies. Am J Med Genet B Neuropsychiatr Genet. 2011;156(3):255–74.
7. Robinson EB, Neale BM, Hyman SE. Genetic research in autism spectrum disorders. Curr Opin Pediatr. 2015;27(6):685–91.
8. Vorstman JAS, Parr JR, Moreno-De-Luca D, Anney RJL, Nurnberger JI, Jr., Hallmayer JF. Autism genetics: opportunities and challenges for clinical translation. Nat Rev Genet. 2017;18(6):362–76.
9. Zafeiriou DI, Ververi A, Dafoulis V, Kalyva E, Vargiami E. Autism spectrum disorders: the quest for genetic syndromes. Am J Med Genet B Neuropsychiatr Genet. 2013;162b(4):327–66.
10. Betancur C. Etiological heterogeneity in autism spectrum disorders: more than 100 genetic and genomic disorders and still counting. Brain Res. 2011;1380:42–77.
11. Rutter M, Silberg J, O'Connor T, Simonoff E. Genetics and child psychiatry: I Advances in quantitative and molecular genetics. J Child Psychol Psychiatry. 1999;40(1):3–18.
12. Sanders AR, Duan J, Gejman PV. Complexities in psychiatric genetics. Int Rev Psychiatry. 2004;16(4):284–93.
13. Risch N, Merikangas K. The future of genetic studies of complex human diseases. Science. 1996;273(5281):1516–17.
14. Risch NJ. Searching for genetic determinants in the new millennium. Nature. 2000;405(6788):847–56.
15. Altshuler D, Daly MJ, Lander ES. Genetic mapping in human disease. Science. 2008;322(5903):881–8.
16. Manolio TA, Collins FS, Cox NJ, *et al.* Finding the missing heritability of complex diseases. Nature. 2009;461(7265):747–53.
17. Hirschhorn JN, Lohmueller K, Byrne E, Hirschhorn K. A comprehensive review of genetic association studies. Genet Med. 2002;4(2):45–61.
18. Anney R, Klei L, Pinto D, *et al.* Individual common variants exert weak effects on the risk for autism spectrum disorderspi. Hum Mol Genet. 2012;21(21):4781–92.
19. Chaste P, Klei L, Sanders SJ, *et al.* A genome-wide association study of autism using the Simons Simplex Collection: Does reducing phenotypic heterogeneity in autism increase genetic homogeneity? Biol Psychiatry. 2015;77(9):775–84.
20. Cantor RM, Navarro L, Won H, Walker RL, Lowe JK, Geschwind DH. ASD restricted and repetitive behaviors associated at 17q21.33: genes prioritized by expression in fetal brains. Mol Psychiatry. 2018;23:993–1000.
21. Jamain S, Quach H, Betancur C, *et al.* Mutations of the X-linked genes encoding neuroligins NLGN3 and NLGN4 are associated with autism. Nat Genet. 2003;34(1):27–9.
22. Laumonnier F, Bonnet-Brilhault F, Gomot M, *et al.* X-linked mental retardation and autism are associated with a mutation in the *NLGN4* gene, a member of the neuroligin family. Am J Hum Genet. 2004;74(3):552–7.
23. Marshall C, Noor A, Vincent J, *et al.* Structural variation of chromosomes in autism spectrum disorder. Am J Hum Genet. 2008;82(2):477–88.
24. Pinto D, Pagnamenta AT, Klei L, *et al.* Functional impact of global rare copy number variation in autism spectrum disorders. Nature. 2010;466(7304):368–72.
25. Sanders SJ, Ercan-Sencicek AG, Hus V, *et al.* Multiple recurrent *de novo* CNVs, including duplications of the 7q11.23 Williams syndrome region, are strongly associated with autism. Neuron. 2011;70(5):863–85.
26. Levy D, Ronemus M, Yamrom B, *et al.* Rare *De Novo* and Transmitted Copy-Number Variation in Autistic Spectrum Disorders. Neuron. 2011;70(5):886–97.
27. Pinto D, Delaby E, Merico D, *et al.* Convergence of genes and cellular pathways dysregulated in autism spectrum disorders. Am J Hum Genet. 2014;94(5):677–94.
28. Weiss L, Shen Y, Korn J, *et al.* Association between microdeletion and microduplication at 16p11.2 and autism. N Engl J Med. 2008;358(7):667–75.
29. Kumar R, KaraMohamed S, Sudi J, *et al.* Recurrent 16p11.2 microdeletions in autism. Human molecular genetics. 2008;17(4):628–38.
30. Szatmari P, Paterson A, Zwaigenbaum L, *et al.* Mapping autism risk loci using genetic linkage and chromosomal rearrangements. Nat Genet. 2007;39(3):319–28.

31. Moreno-De-Luca D, Sanders SJ, Willsey AJ, *et al.* Using large clinical data sets to infer pathogenicity for rare copy number variants in autism cohorts. Mol Psychiatry. 2013;18(10):1090–5.

32. Sanders SJ, He X, Willsey AJ, *et al.* Insights into Autism Spectrum Disorder Genomic Architecture and Biology from 71 Risk Loci. Neuron. 2015;87:1215–33.

33. Sebat J, Lakshmi B, Malhotra D, *et al.* Strong association of *de novo* copy number mutations with autism. Science. 2007;316(5823):445–9.

34. Bucan M, Abrahams BS, Wang K, *et al.* Genome-wide analyses of exonic copy number variants in a family-based study point to novel autism susceptibility genes. PLoS Genet. 2009;5(6):e1000536.

35. Glessner J, Wang K, Cai G, *et al.* Autism genome-wide copy number variation reveals ubiquitin and neuronal genes. Nature. 2009;459(7246):569–73.

36. Itsara A, Wu H, Smith JD, *et al. De novo* rates and selection of large copy number variation. Genome Res. 2010;20:1469–81.

37. Griswold AJ, Ma D, Cukier HN, *et al.* Evaluation of copy number variations reveals novel candidate genes in autism spectrum disorder-associated pathways. Hum Mol Genet. 2012;21(15):3513–23.

38. O'Roak BJ, Deriziotis P, Lee C, *et al.* Exome sequencing in sporadic autism spectrum disorders identifies severe *de novo* mutations. Nat Genet. 2011;43(6):585–9.

39. Dong S, Walker MF, Carriero NJ, *et al. De novo* insertions and deletions of predominantly paternal origin are associated with autism spectrum disorder. Cell Rep. 2014;9(1):16–23.

40. Neale BM, Kou Y, Liu L, *et al.* Patterns and rates of exonic *de novo* mutations in autism spectrum disorders. Nature. 2012;485(7397):242–5.

41. De Rubeis S, He X, Goldberg AP, *et al.* Synaptic, transcriptional and chromatin genes disrupted in autism. Nature. 2014;515(7526):209–15.

42. Iossifov I, O'Roak BJ, Sanders SJ, *et al.* The contribution of *de novo* coding mutations to autism spectrum disorder. Nature. 2014;515(7526):216–21.

43. Sanders SJ, Murtha MT, Gupta AR, Murdoch JD, Raubeson MJ, Willsey AJ, et al. *De novo* mutations revealed by whole-exome sequencing are strongly associated with autism. Nature. 2012;485(7397):237–41.

44. O'Roak BJ, Vives L, Girirajan S, *et al.* Sporadic autism exomes reveal a highly interconnected protein network of *de novo* mutations. Nature. 2012;485(7397):246–50.

45. Gilman SR, Iossifov I, Levy D, Ronemus M, Wigler M, Vitkup D. Rare *de novo* variants associated with autism implicate a large functional network of genes involved in formation and function of synapses. Neuron. 2011;70(5):898–907.

46. Ronemus M, Iossifov I, Levy D, Wigler M. The role of *de novo* mutations in the genetics of autism spectrum disorders. Nat Rev Genet. 2014;15(2):133–41.

47. Abrahams BS, Arking DE, Campbell DB, *et al.* SFARI Gene 2.0: a community-driven knowledgebase for the autism spectrum disorders (ASDs). Mol Autism. 2013;4(1):36.

48. Basu SN, Kollu R, Banerjee-Basu S. AutDB: a gene reference resource for autism research. Nucleic Acids Res. 2009;37(Database issue):D832–6.

49. Turner TN, Yi Q, Krumm N, *et al.* denovo-db: a compendium of human *de novo* variants. Nucleic Acids Res. 2017;45(D1):D804–11.

50. Li J, Cai T, Jiang Y, *et al.* Genes with *de novo* mutations are shared by four neuropsychiatric disorders discovered from NPdenovo database. Mol Psychiatry. 2016;21(2):290–7.

51. Buxbaum JD. Multiple rare variants in the etiology of autism spectrum disorders. Dialogues Clin Neurosci. 2009;11(1):35–43.

52. Lee SH, Ripke S, Neale BM, *et al.* Genetic relationship between five psychiatric disorders estimated from genome-wide SNPs. Nat Genet. 2013;45(9):984–94.

53. Gaugler T, Klei L, Sanders SJ, *et al.* Most genetic risk for autism resides with common variation. Nat Genet. 2014;46(8):881–5.

54. Klei L, Sanders SJ, Murtha MT, *et al.* Common genetic variants, acting additively, are a major source of risk for autism. Mol Autism. 2012;3(1):9.

55. Parikshak NN, Swarup V, Belgard TG, *et al.* Genome-wide changes in lncRNA, splicing, and regional gene expression patterns in autism. Nature. 2016;540(7633):423–7.

56. Willsey AJ, Sanders SJ, Li M, *et al.* Coexpression networks implicate human midfetal deep cortical projection neurons in the pathogenesis of autism. Cell. 2013;155(5):997–1007.

57. Krumm N, O'Roak BJ, Shendure J, Eichler EE. A *de novo* convergence of autism genetics and molecular neuroscience. Trends Neurosci. 2014;37(2):95–105.

58. De Rubeis S, He X, Goldberg AP, *et al.* Synaptic, transcriptional and chromatin genes disrupted in autism. Nature. 2014;515(7526):209–15.

59. Sanders SJ, He X, Willsey AJ, *et al.* Insights into Autism Spectrum Disorder Genomic Architecture and Biology from 71 Risk Loci. Neuron. 2015;87(6):1215–33.

60. Willsey AJ, State MW. Autism spectrum disorders: from genes to neurobiology. Curr Opin Neurobiol. 2015;30:92–9.

61. Krueger DD, Bear MF. Toward fulfilling the promise of molecular medicine in fragile X syndrome. Annu Rev Med. 2011;62:411–29.

62. Huber KM, Gallagher SM, Warren ST, Bear MF. Altered synaptic plasticity in a mouse model of fragile X mental retardation. Proc Natl Acad Sci U S A. 2002;99(11):7746–50.

63. Comery TA, Harris JB, Willems PJ, *et al.* Abnormal dendritic spines in fragile X knockout mice: maturation and pruning deficits. Proc Natl Acad Sci U S A. 1997;94(10):5401–4.

64. Fmr1 knockout mice: a model to study fragile X mental retardation. The Dutch-Belgian Fragile X Consortium. Cell. 1994;78(1):23–33.

65. Dolen G, Osterweil E, Rao BS, *et al.* Correction of fragile X syndrome in mice. Neuron. 2007;56(6):955–62.

66. Vinueza Veloz MF, Buijsen RA, Willemsen R, Cupido A, Bosman LW, Koekkoek SK, et al. The effect of an mGluR5 inhibitor on procedural memory and avoidance discrimination impairments in Fmr1 KO mice. Genes Brain Behav. 2012;11(3):325–31.

67. Min WW, Yuskaitis CJ, Yan Q, *et al.* Elevated glycogen synthase kinase-3 activity in Fragile X mice: key metabolic regulator with evidence for treatment potential. Neuropharmacology. 2009;56(2):463–72.

68. Yan QJ, Rammal M, Tranfaglia M, Bauchwitz RP. Suppression of two major Fragile X Syndrome mouse model phenotypes by the mGluR5 antagonist MPEP. Neuropharmacology. 2005;49(7):1053–66.

69. Thomas AM, Bui N, Perkins JR, Yuva-Paylor LA, Paylor R. Group I metabotropic glutamate receptor antagonists alter select behaviors in a mouse model for fragile X syndrome. Psychopharmacology. 2012;219(1):47–58.

70. McBride SM, Choi CH, Wang Y, *et al.* Pharmacological rescue of synaptic plasticity, courtship behavior, and mushroom body defects in a Drosophila model of fragile X syndrome. Neuron. 2005;45(5):753–64.

71. Bhakar AL, Dolen G, Bear MF. The pathophysiology of fragile X (and what it teaches us about synapses). Annu Rev Neurosci. 2012;35:417–43.

72. Berry-Kravis E. Mechanism-based treatments in neurodevelopmental disorders: fragile X syndrome. Pediatr Neurol. 2014;50(4):297–302.

73. Berry-Kravis E, Des Portes V, Hagerman R, et al. Mavoglurant in fragile X syndrome: Results of two randomized, double-blind, placebo-controlled trials. Sci Transl Med. 2016;8(321):321ra5.

74. Tee AR, Fingar DC, Manning BD, Kwiatkowski DJ, Cantley LC, Blenis J. Tuberous sclerosis complex-1 and -2 gene products function together to inhibit mammalian target of rapamycin (mTOR)-mediated downstream signaling. Proc Natl Acad Sci U S A. 2002;99(21):13571–6.

75. Ehninger D, Han S, Shilyansky C, et al. Reversal of learning deficits in a Tsc2+/− mouse model of tuberous sclerosis. Nat Med. 2008;14(8):843–8.

76. Sato A, Kasai S, Kobayashi T, et al. Rapamycin reverses impaired social interaction in mouse models of tuberous sclerosis complex. Nat Comm. 2012;3:1292.

77. Goffin A, Hoefsloot LH, Bosgoed E, Swillen A, Fryns JP. PTEN mutation in a family with Cowden syndrome and autism. Am J Med Genet. 2001;105(6):521–4.

78. Butler MG, Dasouki MJ, Zhou XP, et al. Subset of individuals with autism spectrum disorders and extreme macrocephaly associated with germline PTEN tumour suppressor gene mutations. J Med Genet. 2005;42(4):318–21.

79. Varga EA, Pastore M, Prior T, Herman GE, McBride KL. The prevalence of PTEN mutations in a clinical pediatric cohort with autism spectrum disorders, developmental delay, and macrocephaly. Genet Med. 2009;11(2):111–17.

80. McBride KL, Varga EA, Pastore MT, et al. Confirmation study of PTEN mutations among individuals with autism or developmental delays/mental retardation and macrocephaly. Autism Res. 2010;3(3):137–41.

81. Zhou J, Blundell J, Ogawa S, et al. Pharmacological inhibition of mTORC1 suppresses anatomical, cellular, and behavioral abnormalities in neural-specific Pten knock-out mice. J Neurosci. 2009;29(6):1773–83.

82. Bernier R, Golzio C, Xiong B, et al. Disruptive CHD8 Mutations Define a Subtype of Autism Early in Development. Cell. 2014;158(2):263–76.

83. van Bon BW, Coe BP, Bernier R, et al. Disruptive de novo mutations of DYRK1A lead to a syndromic form of autism and ID. Mol Psychiatry. 2016;21(1):126–32.

84. Dentici ML, Niceta M, Pantaleoni F, et al. Expanding the phenotypic spectrum of truncating POGZ mutations: Association with CNS malformations, skeletal abnormalities, and distinctive facial dysmorphism. Am J Med Genet A. 2017;173:1965–9.

85. Platzer K, Yuan H, Schutz H, et al. GRIN2B encephalopathy: novel findings on phenotype, variant clustering, functional consequences and treatment aspects. J Med Genet. 2017;54:460–70.

86. Harony-Nicolas H, De Rubeis S, Kolevzon A, Buxbaum JD. Phelan McDermid Syndrome: From Genetic Discoveries to Animal Models and Treatment. J Child Neurol. 2015;30(14):1861–70.

87. Bozdagi O, Tavassoli T, Buxbaum JD. Insulin-like growth factor-1 rescues synaptic and motor deficits in a mouse model of autism and developmental delay. Mol Autism. 2013;4(1):9.

88. O'Kusky JR, Ye P, D'Ercole AJ. Insulin-like growth factor-I promotes neurogenesis and synaptogenesis in the hippocampal dentate gyrus during postnatal development. J Neurosci. 2000;20(22):8435–42.

89. Shcheglovitov A, Shcheglovitova O, Yazawa M, et al. SHANK3 and IGF1 restore synaptic deficits in neurons from 22q13 deletion syndrome patients. Nature. 2013;503(7475):267–71.

90. Tropea D, Giacometti E, Wilson NR, et al. Partial reversal of Rett Syndrome-like symptoms in MeCP2 mutant mice. Proc Natl Acad Sci U S A. 2009;106(6):2029–34.

91. Marchetto MC, Carromeu C, Acab A, et al. A model for neural development and treatment of Rett syndrome using human induced pluripotent stem cells. Cell. 2010;143(4):527–39.

92. Kolevzon A, Bush L, Wang AT, et al. A pilot controlled trial of insulin-like growth factor-1 in children with Phelan-McDermid syndrome. Mol Autism. 2014;5(1):54.

93. McCammon JM, Sive H. Challenges in understanding psychiatric disorders and developing therapeutics: a role for zebrafish. Dis Models Mech. 2015;8(7):647–56.

94. Stevens HE, Vaccarino FM. How animal models inform child and adolescent psychiatry. J Am Acad Child Adolesc Psychiatry. 2015;54(5):352–9.

95. Chung K, Wallace J, Kim SY, et al. Structural and molecular interrogation of intact biological systems. Nature. 2013;497(7449):332–7.

96. Cardin JA, Carlen M, Meletis K, et al. Targeted optogenetic stimulation and recording of neurons in vivo using cell-type-specific expression of Channelrhodopsin-2. Nature Protoc. 2010;5(2):247–54.

97. Ferenczi EA, Zalocusky KA, Liston C, et al. Prefrontal cortical regulation of brainwide circuit dynamics and reward-related behavior. Science. 2016;351(6268):aac9698.

98. Sohal VS, Zhang F, Yizhar O, Deisseroth K. Parvalbumin neurons and gamma rhythms enhance cortical circuit performance. Nature. 2009;459(7247):698–702.

99. Akerboom J, Chen TW, Wardill TJ, et al. Optimization of a GCaMP calcium indicator for neural activity imaging. J Neurosci. 2012;32(40):13819–40.

100. Dunn TW, Gebhardt C, Naumann EA, et al. Neural Circuits Underlying Visually Evoked Escapes in Larval Zebrafish. Neuron. 2016;89(3):613–28.

101. Jinek M, Chylinski K, Fonfara I, Hauer M, Doudna JA, Charpentier E. A programmable dual-RNA-guided DNA endonuclease in adaptive bacterial immunity. Science. 2012;337(6096):816–21.

102. Hoffman EJ, Turner KJ, Fernandez JM, et al. Estrogens Suppress a Behavioral Phenotype in Zebrafish Mutants of the Autism Risk Gene, CNTNAP2. Neuron. 2016;89(4):725–33.

103. Robertson HR, Feng G. Annual Research Review: Transgenic mouse models of childhood-onset psychiatric disorders. Journal Child Psychol Psychiatry. 2011;52(4):442–75.

104. Takahashi K, Tanabe K, Ohnuki M, et al. Induction of pluripotent stem cells from adult human fibroblasts by defined factors. Cell. 2007;131(5):861–72.

105. Nestor MW, Phillips AW, Artimovich E, Nestor JE, Hussman JP, Blatt GJ. Human Inducible Pluripotent Stem Cells and Autism Spectrum Disorder: Emerging Technologies. Autism Res. 2016;9(5):513–35.

106. Wen Z, Christian KM, Song H, Ming GL. Modeling psychiatric disorders with patient-derived iPSCs. Curr Opin Neurobiol. 2016;36:118–27.

107. Ben-Reuven L, Reiner O. Modeling the autistic cell: iPSCs recapitulate developmental principles of syndromic and nonsyndromic ASD. Dev Growth Differ. 2016;58(5):481–91.

108. Mariani J, Coppola G, Zhang P, et al. FOXG1-Dependent Dysregulation of GABA/Glutamate Neuron Differentiation in Autism Spectrum Disorders. Cell. 2015;162(2):375–90.

109. Kim DS, Ross PJ, Zaslavsky K, Ellis J. Optimizing neuronal differentiation from induced pluripotent stem cells to model ASD. Front Cell Neurosci. 2014;8:109.

110. Habela CW, Song H, Ming GL. Modeling synaptogenesis in schizophrenia and autism using human iPSC derived neurons. Mol Cell Neurosci. 2016;73:52–62.

111. Acab A, Muotri AR. The Use of Induced Pluripotent Stem Cell Technology to Advance Autism Research and Treatment. Neurotherapeutics. 2015;12(3):534–45.

112. Brix J, Zhou Y, Luo Y. The Epigenetic Reprogramming Roadmap in Generation of iPSCs from Somatic Cells. J Genet Genomics. 2015;42(12):661–70.

113. Chamberlain SJ, Chen PF, Ng KY, et al. Induced pluripotent stem cell models of the genomic imprinting disorders Angelman and Prader-Willi syndromes. Proc Natl Acad Sci U S A. 2010;107(41):17668–73.

114. Kang HJ, Kawasawa YI, Cheng F, et al. Spatio-temporal transcriptome of the human brain. Nature. 2011;478(7370):483–9.

115. Miller JA, Ding SL, Sunkin SM, et al. Transcriptional landscape of the prenatal human brain. Nature. 2014;508(7495):199–206.

116. Parikshak NN, Luo R, Zhang A, et al. Integrative functional genomic analyses implicate specific molecular pathways and circuits in autism. Cell. 2013;155(5):1008–21.

117. Schaefer GB, Mendelsohn NJ, Professional P, Guidelines C. Clinical genetics evaluation in identifying the etiology of autism spectrum disorders: 2013 guideline revisions. Genet Med. 2013;15:399–407.

118. Miller DT, Adam MP, Aradhya S, et al. Consensus statement: chromosomal microarray is a first-tier clinical diagnostic test for individuals with developmental disabilities or congenital anomalies. Am J Hum Genet. 2010; 86(5):749–64.

# 29

# Imaging of autism spectrum disorders

*Christine Ecker and Declan Murphy*

## Introduction

Autism spectrum disorders (ASD) encompass a group of life-long neurodevelopmental conditions that are characterized by deficits in social communication, social reciprocity, and repetitive and stereotyped behaviours and interests [1]. ASD are typically diagnosed during early childhood using behavioural observations and/or clinical interviews, with clinical symptoms persisting across the human lifespan in roughly 90% of all cases [2]. Over the last decade, prevalence estimates for ASD have consistently been rising—from about 2–4 individuals per 10,000 children in the 1960s and 1970s to about 1 in 68 children in 2014 (that is, roughly 1.4% of the general population) [3]. While this increase in prevalence may partially be due to modifications to diagnostic criteria, improved assessment tools, and/or increased awareness, the rise in prevalence also highlights the growing need for developing novel pharmacotherapies and behavioural interventions designed to effectively target the core symptoms of ASD. Yet, developing treatment and interventions for ASD remains a challenge. ASD is accompanied by a large degree of inter-individual variability, both phenotypic and causative, which has so far hampered large-scale clinical trials. For example, genetic studies implicate more than 100 different genetic and genomic loci in ASD [4], which, in turn, interact with environmental factors to give rise to complex behavioural phenotypes. Consequently, there is a large degree of heterogeneity in the time course, severity, and profile of symptoms expressed by ASD individuals. Current research efforts are thus directed towards disentangling the large degree of complexity associated with ASD, and to establish homogenous subgroups or 'strata' of individuals with a common genetic and (neuro)biological make-up. Here, neuroimaging studies employing magnetic resonance imaging (MRI) are absolutely crucial, as they offer unique insights into the anatomy and functioning of the brain *in vivo*.

In this chapter, we review and critically discuss 'state-of-the-art' *in vivo* neuroimaging findings examining ASD, with a particular focus on studies investigating brain structure and connectivity. Firstly, we will review the findings of neuroimaging studies examining early brain development in ASD. These studies predominantly focus on the neurodevelopmental trajectory of global brain measures that may underpin regional differences in brain anatomy typically observed during late childhood and adolescence in ASD. We will then examine how the atypical developmental trajectory during early brain development may lead to differences in brain connectivity in ASD, which are accompanied by atypical patterns of cortical gyrification. Last, we will present the findings of a growing number of neuroimaging studies examining differences in the neurobiology of ASD between men and women.

## Atypical brain development during early childhood in ASD

It is well established that ASD is accompanied by an atypical development of the brain and developmental perturbations to the formation of the brain's micro- and macro-circuitry. Early cross-sectional studies show that the brain of toddlers with ASD is—on average—larger in total volume than the brain of typically developing (TD) children between the ages of 2–4 years [5]. This increase in total brain volume is paralleled by an increase in head circumference, which has been reported in several cross-sectional and longitudinal studies (for example, [6]). The early enlargement of the brain seems to disappear between 5 and 6 years of age, when developmental trajectories of ASD individuals and TD controls intersect [7]. After this age, no significant increase in total brain volume is typically reported in ASD. Taken together, these early findings led to the suggestion that the brain in ASD may undergo an atypical trajectory of maturation, which is characterized by a period of increased growth during toddlerhood, followed by a period of reduced or arrested growth during childhood, and possibly a period of accelerated decline in total brain volume over the remaining lifespan [8] (Fig. 29.1). These early cross-sectional studies have been confirmed by more recent longitudinal studies of brain development in ASD. For example, a recent investigation by Lange *et al.* (2015) examined atypical brain development in ASD from early childhood into adolescence and found: (1) significantly increased brain volumes in young children with ASD; (2) intersecting growth curves between 10 and 15 years of age; and (3) significantly decreased brain volume during adolescence [9]. While there is some variability with regard to the reported age range, when growth curves intersect, these findings suggest that the size of the brain in ASD lies within the 'normal' range during early adolescence, when between-group differences in total brain volume are minimal. However, how this relates to the

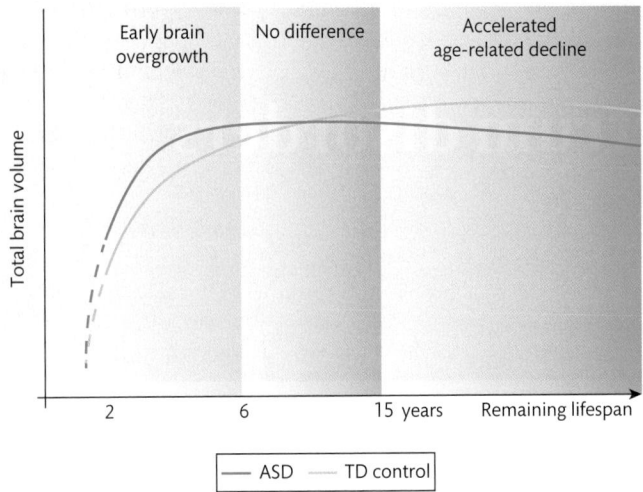

**Fig. 29.1** Differences in the neurodevelopmental trajectory of brain maturation in ASD individuals and TD controls across the human lifespan.

remains unclear whether the early brain overgrowth in toddlers with ASD reflects an ongoing neurodevelopmental process, which is accompanied by an accelerated rate of growth during early childhood, or—alternatively—constitutes the end result of an early developmental perturbation prior to the age of 2 years.

## Early brain overgrowth in ASD—a biomarker or simply 'the tip of the iceberg'?

Despite the large body of evidence supporting the original reports of an early overgrowth of the brain in ASD, it remains contentious how relevant macrocephaly is for ASD and whether an early increase in total brain volume may potentially be used as an early biomarker for the condition. For instance, while the brain in ASD may—on average—be larger than the brain in TD individuals, macrocephaly (that is, an increase in head circumference of >2 standard deviations above the average for that age, or larger than the 98th percentile) is only observed in about 20% of all individuals with ASD across studies [14]. This implies that in about 80% of ASD individuals, significant clinical enlargement of the head or brain is absent. Thus, early markers of total brain volume or head circumference may not reflect a neurobiological mechanism that is common to all individuals on the ASD spectrum. As pointed out by Lainhart *et al.* (2006), it may therefore be that the early brain overgrowth occurs in a specific neurobiological subtype (or 'stratum') of ASD individuals only and may hence be used for stratification, rather than for diagnostic purposes. Alternatively, macrocephaly may represent the 'tip of the iceberg', that is a general tendency towards an increased head and brain size in ASD individuals [17]. In this case, an increase in head size may be indicative of the risk for ASD, rather than of the condition itself. A number of recent studies also call for a revision of population norms, which are used to define what is clinically 'abnormal'. For example, a study by Raznahan *et al.* (2013) suggested that the increased head circumference in ASD might reflect a bias in population norm, rather than a replicable pattern of dysregulated brain growth [18], particularly when examining patient populations in the mental health setting. In future investigations, it will thus be of importance to account for variations in population norms, which may affect the size of expected effects when comparing psychiatric populations with normative populations.

Head circumference is also correlated with various epidemiological measures such as biological sex, age, weight and height, and genetic ancestry. Such non-ASD measures may therefore also impact on population norms, and hence significant between-group differences, and so need to be accounted for in the statistical model [19]. Based on these findings, there is also some evidence to suggest that the early brain overgrowth in ASD may reflect an early pattern of general physical (that is, somatic) overgrowth, rather than being specific to the brain, and particularly in boys with the condition [20]. Taken together, these studies highlight the importance of considering wider contextual issues when interpreting the findings of traditional studies reporting early brain overgrowth in ASD. Overall, therefore, it seems that measures of total brain volume and/or head size may offer neither sufficient sensitivity (that is, ability to detect an effect or disease if it is present) nor specificity (that is, ability to detect the absence of an effect or disease if it is not present) to be employed as a biomarker for ASD.

severity of autistic symptoms is currently unknown. Furthermore, despite the absence of significant between-group differences in total volume around adolescence, it is likely that the atypical developmental trajectory of brain maturation prior to this time interferes with the development of large-scale neural systems, which reflects regional, rather than global, differences in ASD.

Typical brain development occurs in a highly 'orchestrated' fashion where the development of phylogenetically younger cortical areas (for example, higher-order association areas in frontal and temporal lobes) builds on the development of phylogenetically older brain regions (for example, occipital and parietal regions) [10]. However, evidence suggests that frontal–temporal regions mature earlier and faster in ASD individuals than in TD controls [11]. These early deviations from the typically synchronized developmental trajectory would therefore also be expected to impact on the development of brain connectivity. For example, a study by Wolff *et al.* (2012) examined structural brain connectivity in 6-month-old infants at high genetic (that is, familial) risk of ASD (for example, siblings of individuals with a confirmed diagnosis of ASD). In high-risk infants who receive a diagnosis of ASD at the age of 2 years, perturbations in the development of white matter fibre tracts are already visible at 6 months, relative to low-risk infants without ASD [12]. Moreover, a more recent study by the same research group also reported a significant increase in area and thickness of the corpus callosum, which structurally connects the two hemispheres of the brain, in infants with ASD scanned at 6 months of age [13]. Taken together, these studies suggest that the early atypical development of the cortical grey matter in ASD is accompanied by differences in white matter fibre tracts that can be observed as early as 6 months of age—that is, before the first symptoms typically manifest (around 1–2 years of age). Yet, there remains some debate on the particular time point during early development when grey matter differences first arise in ASD. For example, no significant increase in head circumference has been reported in ASD during the first year of life [14]. There are two studies reporting an enlargement of the brain in 2-year olds [15, 16], but direct evidence of a significant enlargement of the brain during the first year of life remains missing. It thus

## Brain structure and functioning across later childhood and adolescence in ASD

While the neurodevelopmental trajectory of brain maturation during early development is well characterized in ASD, less is known about the trajectory of brain development during late childhood and adolescence. In contrast to the differences in total brain volume observed during early life, brain development during later childhood and adolescence in ASD seems to be dominated by an accelerated age-related decline in volume. Typically, the pre-pubertal increase in grey matter volume is followed by a post-pubertal loss, resulting in an inverted U-shaped trajectory across the human lifespan [21]. There is evidence to suggest that the typical attrition of grey matter volume after reaching its peak during early adolescence is accelerated in ASD individuals during adolescence and adulthood. For example, the longitudinal study by Lange *et al.* (2015) noted previously found an accelerated decrease in total grey matter in ASD individuals after the age of approximately 15 years, which was accompanied by a reduced growth rate of total white matter [9]. These findings are in agreement with a previous longitudinal study by Hardan *et al.* (2009) in a smaller sample, who also reported a significantly greater decrease in total grey matter volume during late childhood and early adolescence in ASD 8- to 12-year olds over a period of 30 months [22]. Notably, the study by Hardan *et al.* (2009) also reported that the accelerated decrease in total grey matter volume is accompanied by significant reductions in cortical thickness. This is of importance, as total grey matter volume is, by definition, a product of two separate neuroanatomical features, namely cortical thickness and surface area, both of which: (1) are mediated by different sets of genes; (2) have a different phylogeny; and (3) represent distinct aspects of the cortical architecture (for example, [23]). Accelerated age-related cortical thinning has also been reported by cross-sectional studies investigating regional, rather than global, differences (for example, in temporal and parietal brain regions) [24, 25]. The age-related decrease in cortical thickness also seems to be accompanied by a

decrease in surface area. For instance, a more rapid decline in surface area in ASD with increasing age has been reported on the global [26], as well as regional, level [27]. Taken together, these findings suggest that the trajectory of brain maturation in ASD differs across distinct stages of development, which are dominated by an accelerated increase in volume, followed by an accelerated age-related decline in adulthood (Fig. 29.1).

Moreover, while neuroimaging studies investigating early brain development in ASD have predominantly focused on age-related differences in total brain volume, studies examining the neurobiological underpinnings of ASD during late childhood and/or adolescence mostly focus on regional differences in brain anatomy and functioning. Using more 'fine-grained' techniques such as voxel-based morphometry (VBM) or functional magnetic resonance imaging (fMRI), it is also possible to link specific autistic symptoms and traits to neuroanatomical or functional abnormalities in individual brain regions. Overall, the core components of wider neurocognitive systems that mediate the cluster of behavioural symptoms typically observed in ASD are well established. By large, these include: (1) fronto-temporal and fronto-parietal regions; (2) the amygdala–hippocampal complex; (3) the cerebellum and basal ganglia; and (4) the anterior and posterior cingulate cortices (for a review, see [28]) (Fig. 29.2). As might be expected, many of these brain regions include the set of brain regions that mediate functions related to social cognition and emotional processing, which are also commonly termed the 'social' and 'emotional' brain [29]. The core components of the 'emotional brain' include: (1) subcortical regions such as the amygdala, nucleus accumbens, and hypothalamus; and (2) cortical regions such as the orbitofrontal cortex (OFC), the anterior cingulate cortex (ACC), and the medial prefrontal cortex (mPFC) (reviewed in [30]). Furthermore, the extended neural systems mediating social–emotional processing include the superior and anterior temporal lobes (STL and ATL), the posterior cingulate cortex (PCC), the temporo-parietal junction (TPJ), the somatosensory cortex, and the intraparietal sulcus (see also [29]). Many of these regions have also been found to be atypical

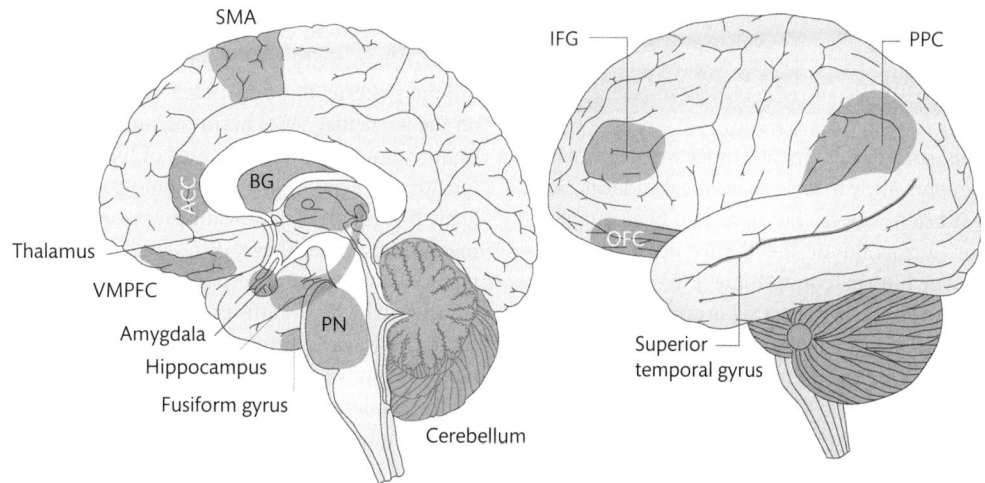

**Fig. 29.2** The neurocognitive systems underlying ASD. Core ASD regions (orange areas) include the ventromedial prefrontal cortex (VMPFC), the orbitofrontal cortex (OFC), the superior temporal gyrus (STS), the amygdala, and the anterior cingulate cortex (ACC). Extended ASD regions (green areas) include the inferior frontal gyrus (IFG), the posterior parietal cortex (PPC), the cerebellum, the hippocampus, the fusiform gyrus, the pons (PN), the basal ganglia (BG), the thalamus, and the supplementary motor area (SMA).
Adapted from *Trends Neurosci.*, 31(3), Amaral DG, Schumann CM, Nordahl CW, Neuroanatomy of autism, pp. 137–45, Copyright (2008), with permission from Elsevier Ltd.

in ASD not only structurally (as described previously), but also functionally. For example, fMRI studies examining deficits in theory of mind [31], face processing [32], perception of biological motion [33], self-referential cognition, and empathy [34] in ASD have reported functional abnormalities in many of the regions that mediate social and emotional processing.

In addition, there is large degree of overlap between the neural systems implicated in ASD and the neural circuitry mediating obsessive–compulsive disorder (OCD), which highlights the close symptomatic link between ASD and OCD. For example, a study by Russell *et al.* (2005) showed that individuals with ASD and OCD had similar frequencies of obsessive–compulsive symptoms, despite at a lower level of symptom severity, with only somatic obsessions and repeating rituals being more common in the OCD group [35]. In OCD, obsessive–compulsive symptoms have been linked to the so-called cortico-striato-thalamo-cortical (CSTC) circuitry (also known as the frontostriatal or corticostriatal model), which comprises the thalamus, the OFC, ACC, and striatum [36]. Neuroanatomical differences in these regions have also been reported in ASD. For instance, individuals with ASD show an increase in the rate of growth of the caudate nucleus, one of the two integral parts of the striatum, which was observed between 10 and 12 years of age [37]. Moreover, the increased rate of growth in the caudate nucleus was significantly correlated with the severity of repetitive behaviours in ASD, thus suggesting that the neurodevelopmental trajectory of the caudate nucleus may offer a neurobiological marker for stereotypic and repetitive behaviours in ASD [37]. Comparison between the neurobiological underpinnings of OCD and ASD shows that the cortical abnormalities observed in ASD may not be unique to, nor causal for, the condition. Rather, similarities and/or differences in neurobiological phenotypes may be associated with similarities/differences in clinical symptom profiles. New research frameworks, such as the Research Domain Criteria (RDoC) initiative (http://www.nimh.nih.gov/research-priorities/rdoc/index.shtml) that considers mental disorders along dimensions of symptoms and neurobiological measures, rather than distinct categories, will thus be crucial for future investigations aimed at establishing distinct and common genetic or molecular pathways across disorders.

## Atypical brain connectivity in ASD

The early perturbations to the developmental trajectory of brain maturation in ASD are not only likely to yield anatomical and functional differences in isolated brain regions, but have also been suggested to interfere with the formation of the brains neurocircuitry—commonly known as the human 'connectome' [38]. However, the notion of atypical brain connectivity in ASD is complex, involving abnormalities with the grey and white matter (for example, [39]), and different levels of integration [40]. Consequently, there is significant heterogeneity in analytical frameworks used to examine brain connectivity in ASD, and in reported results. Overall, however, connectivity analysis methods may be subdivided into: (1) approaches aimed at investigating structural brain connectivity; and (2) approaches aimed at examining functional brain connectivity (Fig. 29.3).

Structural connectivity (that is, the existence and degree of structural white matter connection in the brain) has so far mostly been examined using voxel-wise analysis of the white matter and diffusion tensor imaging (DTI). For instance, VBM studies showed that individuals with ASD have spatially distributed reductions in regional white matter volume during childhood [41], adolescence [42], and adulthood [43]. The results of such voxel-wise analyses are, however, inherently difficult to interpret due to methodological limitations (for example, issues related to image registration and/or segmentation) and cannot also unequivocally be linked to particular fibre tracks. For localization purposes, techniques such as DTI are better suited, as they allow the three-dimensional reconstruction of particular fibre tracks in order to examine tract-specific measures of structural white matter connectivity. In ASD, DTI studies have reported neuroanatomical differences in a number of white matter tracts that include the corpus callosum [44], the arcuate fasciculus [45], the limbic pathways [46], and the amygdala–hippocampal complex [47]. A number of DTI studies have also reported differences in the basal ganglia [48], the cerebellum [49], and the corticospinal tract [50]. In many of these tracts, reports point towards a reduced degree of structural white matter connectivity in ASD, and this contributed to the notion of ASD being a 'neurodevelopmental disconnection' syndrome [51] that is characterized by deficits in global (that is, large-scale) brain connectivity. Such deficits in connectivity have also been observed on the functional level.

Functional connectivity is generally defined as the degree of 'temporal coherence' between two neurophysiological signals and can be quantified, based on correlations between fMRI or EEG time series acquired in the presence of a stimulation paradigm or while the brain is 'at rest'. Early fMRI studies examining functional connectivity during task performance suggested that the brain of individuals with ASD may exhibit a reduced degree of long-distance functional connectivity, and this has been reported during executive functioning [52], sentence comprehension [53], and working memory tasks [54]. However, more recent studies show that patterns of both hypo- and hyperconnectivity can be observed when combining findings across studies [55]. Taken together, this indicates: (1) either that findings are inconsistent across studies; or (2) that the concept of atypical brain connectivity is more complex than originally assumed. A similar picture of mixed results comes from studies examining resting-state fMRI connectivity in ASD—with researchers arguing in favour of under-connectivity [56], over-connectivity (for example, [57]), or unique patterns of both under- and over-connectivity, depending on the particular set of brain regions examined [58]. It is important to note, however, that measures of functional connectivity are very sensitive to even minor methodological differences, and this most likely underpins a significant proportion of the variability in findings. For example, Thai *et al.* (2009) highlighted the influence of differences in activation response between ASD individuals and TD controls, which may affect the degree of functional connectivity observed within and across groups, in addition to the selection of particular regions of interests and general constraints in temporal and spatial resolution [59]. Choices in some aspects of image processing can also affect the results [55]. Finally, there is evidence to suggest that the size (and sign) of the effects of connectivity analyses are age-dependent and may therefore vary as a function of the particular developmental stage under investigation [60]. Such methodological factors thus need to be accounted for in future studies examining functional connectivity in ASD. So far, however, the large variability in findings across studies has hampered the interpretability of the

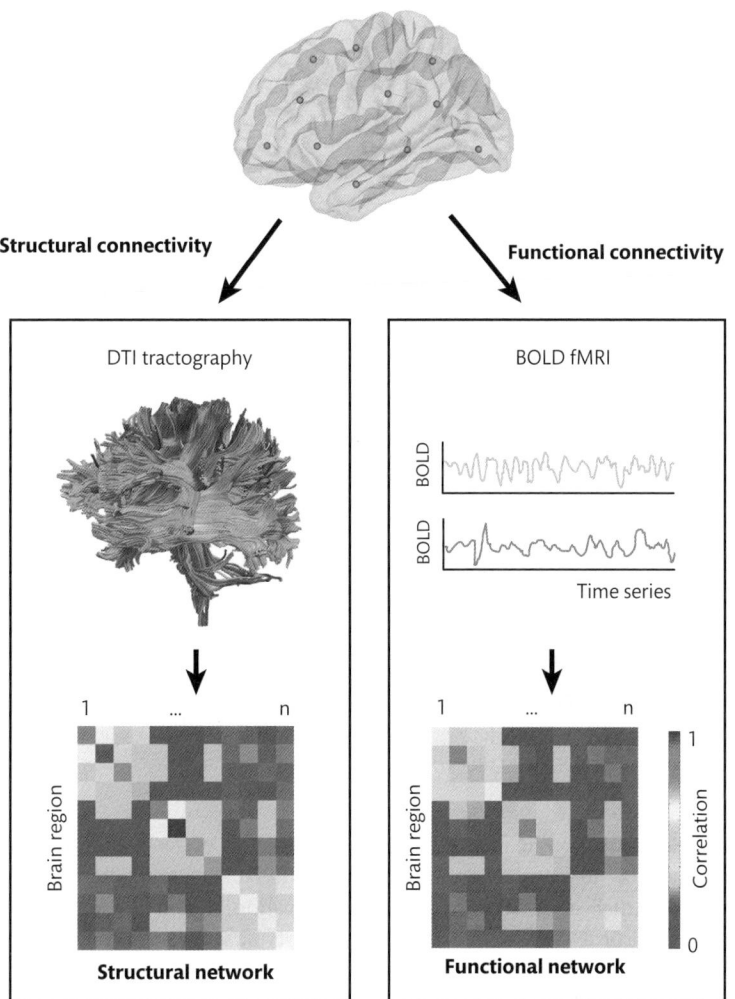

Structural connectivity

Functional connectivity

DTI tractography

BOLD fMRI

Structural network

Functional network

**Fig. 29.3** (see Colour Plate section) Schematic illustration of the underlying concepts behind atypical structural and functional brain connectivity in ASD.

results, and a consistent overarching concept that can explain atypical functional brain connectivity in ASD has yet to emerge.

## Atypical cortical gyrification in ASD—a retrospective window into early cortical expansion

The notion of atypical brain connectivity has also been discussed in light of recent studies examining cortical gyrification in ASD. As the cortex expands during development, it eventually needs to fold to fit an increasing surface area into the restricted space of the skull. Based on the evidence of early brain overgrowth in ASD (see previous section), which seems to be driven by an accelerated expansion of the cortex [61], it is therefore likely that the brain in ASD not only differs in structure and connectivity, but also in shape (that is, geometry). More specifically, an accelerated and more pronounced expansion of the cortex is expected to be associated with a higher degree of cortical folding, as well as atypical patterns of cortical gyrification. Yet, studies investigating measures of cortical geometry, rather than volume, are rare, and the few existing studies have led to variable findings. Most of these studies are based on the so-called gyrification index (or GI) [62]. This measures the degree

of cortical folding (Fig. 29.4). Using the GI, Hardan *et al.* (2004) examined gyrification in a coronal slice of the prefrontal cortex in ASD. They reported that children and adolescents with ASD showed greater prefrontal cortical folding than TD controls, while no significant between-group differences were observed in adults [63]. This early report thus agrees with the notion that early expansion of the cortical surface in ASD might result in increased cortical folding.

The findings of more recent investigations examining cortical gyrification in ASD are, however, variable. Most of these recent studies utilized high-resolution surface reconstructions of the left and right hemispheres of the brain that can subsequently be used to estimate the degree of gyrification at each location on the cortical surface. For example, the so-called local gyrification index (*l*GI) measures gyrification at more than 300,000 different locations (that is, vertices) where the *l*GI at a given vertex is computed as the ratio between the surface of a circular patch on the outer smooth surface of the brain and the surface of the corresponding patch on the inner pial surface (Fig. 29.4). Hence, similar to the original GI, the *l*GI at a point reflects the amount of cortex buried within the sulcal folds in the surrounding area [64]. Studies utilizing the *l*GI have so far reported: (1) significant increases in gyrification in bilateral posterior brain regions in males with ASD, compared to TD controls

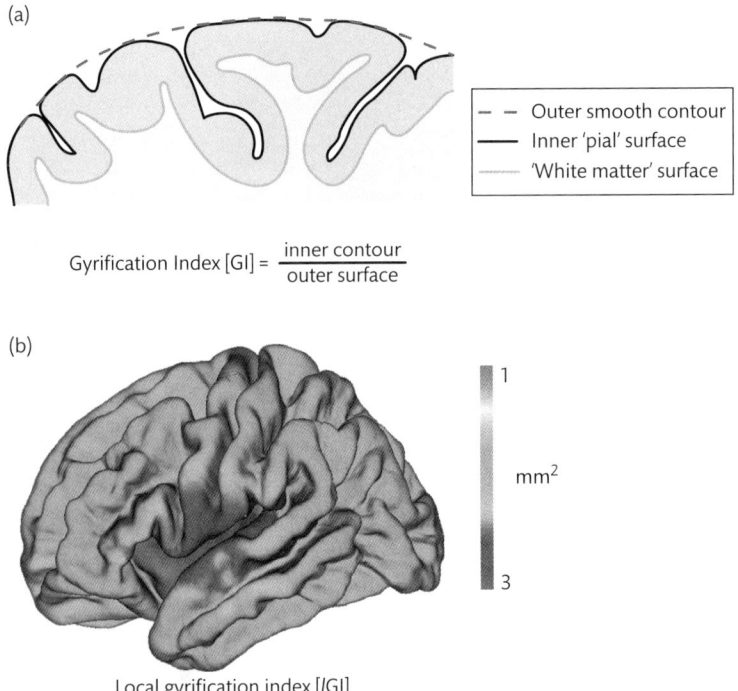

$$\text{Gyrification Index [GI]} = \frac{\text{inner contour}}{\text{outer surface}}$$

Local gyrification index [*l*GI]

**Fig. 29.4**  (see Colour Plate section) Computation of the gyrification index (GI) as the ratio between the inner (i.e. pial) surface of the brain and the outer smooth contour. The GI can be calculated within brain slices in 2D (a) and at each location on the cortical surface in 3D (b).

(12–23 years of age) [65], and significant reductions in the *l*GI (2) in the left supramarginal gyrus in males aged 8–40 years [66] and (3) in the right inferior frontal and medial parieto-occipital cortices in children with ASD [67]. Last, atypical cortical gyrification in ASD has been demonstrated, using a variety of alternative metrics of cortical folding, including measures of sulcal morphometry [68], sulcal depth [69], and gyral complexity [70]. Thus, there is considerable variability in findings reported by existing neuroimaging studies, with regard to both the degree of atypical gyrification and the particular regional pattern of gyrification in ASD.

While these divergent findings can be partially explained by differences in sample size, participant demographics, and analytical techniques, evidence also suggests that patterns of cortical gyrification are highly variable across individuals, even in normative populations, and that both genetic and non-genetic factors contribute to the formation of cortical gyri [71]. For example, Kates *et al.* (2009) examined the amount of GI concordance in monozygotic twin pairs, in which only one had a diagnosis of ASD, and in typically developing unrelated controls. It was found that cortical folding patterns across most brain regions are highly discordant within monozygotic twin pairs, although children with ASD and their co-twins both exhibited increased cortical folding in the right parietal lobe [72]. This finding is in contrast to conventional measures of brain anatomy (for example, total or regional brain volumes), which are highly concordant between twins and might thus be largely genetically determined [73]. Moreover, cortical folding is not significantly correlated with total brain weight or volume, or with body weight and length, which are under strict genetic control [62]. Measures of gyrification thus seem to be particularly sensitive to environmental (that is, non-genetic) factors and reflect a degree of plasticity that is independent of overall brain size [74]. Thus, to elucidate the

contribution of genetic and non-genetic factors to brain development in ASD, various cortical features, including those of cortical gyrification, should be examined to account for the large amount of phenotypic inter-individual variability typically noted between individuals with ASD.

## Neuroimaging studies examining sex differences in ASD

As mentioned in the introduction, ASD is accompanied by a large degree of inter-individual heterogeneity. Recent research efforts are thus directed towards establishing genetically and/or biologically homogenous subgroups of individuals that might, in turn, benefit from the same—or a similar—approach to treatment. One way of reducing the phenotypic heterogeneity associated with ASD is to stratify individuals by demographic characteristics such as age, intellectual ability, and also biological sex. An increasing number of studies are therefore now directed at establishing whether the neurobiology of ASD significantly differs between men and women. However, studies examining females with ASD are relatively rare.

So far, most of our understanding of the neurobiological underpinnings of ASD comes from studies examining male participants exclusively. For instance, it is estimated that there are about eight structural, and 15 functional, neuroimaging studies in males for every one neuroimaging study examining females [75]. The overrepresentation of studies examining males is primarily due to the increased prevalence of ASD in males, with an average male-to-female prevalence ratio of approximately 4:1 [76]. Thus, females with ASD are relatively rare and hence more difficult to recruit than males. The reasons for the male-preponderant prevalence of ASD is largely unknown. However, it has been suggested that there are sex differences in the clinical phenotype of ASD, which may impede the diagnosis in females. For example, males with ASD have been reported to show more 'externalizing' behavioural problems (that is, actions directed towards the external environment) than females. Such externalizing behaviours include aggressive behaviour, hyperactivity, reduced pro-social behaviours, and repetitive/restricted behaviours and interests [77]. Females with ASD, on the other hand, have been suggested to show more 'internalizing' behaviours such as anxiety and depression and/or other affective symptoms [78]. Also, females with ASD may have a greater ability to camouflage difficulties, particularly in the social domain [79]. Taken together, such differences in terms of the clinical phenotype of ASD may impact on our ability to diagnose the condition in females, which will, in turn, affect prevalence estimates. Consequently, little is currently known about the neurobiology of ASD in females.

In terms of brain anatomy, some of the early neuroimaging studies suggest that the degree of cortical abnormality observed in girls with ASD may be significantly greater, as compared to boys. For instance, Bloss and Courchesne (2007) reported a larger deviation from same-sex TD controls among girls vs boys with ASD, in temporal grey and white matter volumes and in grey matter volume of the cerebellum [80]. Girls with ASD have also been reported to differ more robustly in amygdala volume from TD girls between the ages of 1 and 5 years, in comparison to the differences between boys with ASD and TD boy controls [81]. While there are also reports of a similar degree of cerebral enlargement for both boys and girls (for example, [82]), findings across studies suggest that girls may need to deviate more from their respective normative population than boys in order to demonstrate a clinical ASD phenotype. This observation also supports aetiological models proposing that while females are likely to carry a higher genetic load for ASD than males, females may also have a higher 'threshold' (that is, minimum liability sufficient to cause ASD) for reaching affection status than males (reviewed in [83]). Alternatively, female-specific protective factors that may include environmental, biological, and/or epigenetic mechanisms may counteract the genetic liability for ASD in females overall, so that a comparable threshold would affect a smaller proportion of females in comparison to males (see also [84]). In this case, one would expect the cortical pathology of ASD to be significantly modulated by biological sex.

There are few imaging studies to date that have examined the degree to which biological sex modulates the regional anatomy of the brain, and of those that are available, most are based on assessing sex-by-diagnosis interactions within a general linear model (GLM). For instance, Lai et al. (2013) performed a VBM analysis and found significant sex-by-diagnosis interactions in several white matter clusters that also showed a significant difference in white matter volume between males and females [85]. Notably, no significant sex-by-diagnosis interactions were reported when examining regional grey matter volume. Similarly, Beacher et al. (2012) reported significant sex-by-diagnosis interaction in: (1) total white matter volume; (2) regional grey matter volume of the right inferior parietal lobe; and (3) diffusion measures in the corpus callosum, cingulum, and corona radiata [86]. Last, a recent study examined local gyrification in males and females with ASD and TD controls—reporting that the degree of gyrification in the ventromedial/orbitofrontal cortices was significantly modulated by biological sex [64]. Overall, these studies suggest that the neuroanatomy of ASD differs significantly between males and females and that biological sex attenuates the cortical pathology of ASD. Treating biological males and females as distinct genetic and/or biological subgroups may thus reduce the large degree of phenotypic heterogeneity that is characteristic for ASD and also help us better examine the neurobiological underpinnings that undermine risk and resilience for neurodevelopmental conditions.

## Conclusions

Over the last two decades, human neuroimaging studies have played a crucial role in establishing the cortical mechanisms that underlie the cluster of behavioural deficits typically observed in ASD. Most importantly, it is known from neuroimaging studies that ASD is accompanied by an atypical developmental trajectory of brain maturation, which leads to differences in brain anatomy and connectivity. In turn, insights arising from the examination of the brain in vivo can inform genetic and/or molecular investigations, to help elucidate the underlying genetic and/or molecular mechanisms of ASD. This also demonstrates that the role of neuroimaging in mental health research is transitioning into being an integral part of 'translational research', which integrates findings across multiple disciplines and translates them into the real-world clinical settings (that is, 'from bench to bedside'). For instance, in the future, neuroimaging approaches may be used to assist (for example, in combination with clinical interview) the diagnosis/stratification of ASD into more biologically homogenous subtypes and/or to predict response to treatment. Here, it will be crucial to shift the analytical focus from the group-level statistical inference to the individual (that is, case) level—for example, using multivariate pattern classification (MVPC) techniques (for example, [87]). Moreover, such techniques make it possible to take into account complex and multivariate biological features and are hence particularly well suited to characterize conditions with a complex genetic and neurobiological architecture such as ASD. However, the application of these approaches in the clinical setting remains a vision for the future, and there is currently a lack of studies validating models established in the research (that is, investigative) setting on independent clinical validation samples. If successful, however, these new approaches may one day prove invaluable in helping to diagnose, treat, and characterize ASD.

### REFERENCES

1. Wing L. The autistic spectrum. Lancet. 1997;350(9093):1761–6.
2. Lord C, Risi S, Lambrecht L, et al. The autism diagnostic observation schedule-generic: a standard measure of social and communication deficits associated with the spectrum of autism. J Autism Dev Disord. 2000;30(3):205–23.
3. Baio J; Centers for Disease Control and Prevention. Prevalence of autism spectrum disorder among children aged 8 years—Autism and Developmental Disabilities Monitoring Network, 11 Sites, United States, 2010. MMWR Surveill. Summ. 2014;63(2):1–21.
4. Betancur C. Etiological heterogeneity in autism spectrum disorders: more than 100 genetic and genomic disorders and still counting. Brain Res. 2011;22;1380:42–77.
5. Courchesne E. Abnormal early brain development in autism. Mol Psychiatry. 2002;7 Suppl 2:S21–3.

6. Lainhart JE, Piven J, Wzorek M, *et al.* Macrocephaly in children and adults with autism. J Am Acad Child Adolesc Psychiatry. 1997;36:282–90.

7. Courchesne E, Karns CM, Davis HR, *et al.* Unusual brain growth patterns in early life in patients with autistic disorder: an MRI study. Neurology. 2001 24;57:245–54.

8. Courchesne E, Campbell K, Solso S. Brain growth across the life span in autism: age-specific changes in anatomical pathology. Brain Res. 2011;1380:138–45.

9. Lange N, Travers BG, Bigler ED, *et al.* Longitudinal volumetric brain changes in autism spectrum disorder ages 6–35 years. Autism Res. 2015;8(1):82–93.

10. Gogtay N, Giedd JN, Lusk L, *et al.* Dynamic mapping of human cortical development during childhood through early adulthood. Proc Natl Acad Sci U S A. 2004;101(21):8174–9.

11. Carper RA, Courchesne E. Localized enlargement of the frontal cortex in early autism. Biol Psychiatry. 2005;57(2):126–33.

12. Wolff JJ, Gu H, Gerig G, *et al.* Differences in white matter fiber tract development present from 6 to 24 months in infants with autism. Am J Psychiatry. 2012;169(6):589–600.

13. Wolff JJ, Gerig G, Lewis JD, *et al.* Altered corpus callosum morphology associated with autism over the first 2 years of life. Brain. 2015;138(Pt 7):2046–58.

14. Zwaigenbaum L, Young GS, Stone WL, *et al.* Early head growth in infants at risk of autism: a baby siblings research consortium study. J Am Acad Child Adolesc Psychiatry. 2014;53(10):1053–62.

15. Hazlett HC, Poe MD, Gerig G, *et al.* Early brain overgrowth in autism associated with an increase in cortical surface area before age 2 years. Arch Gen Psychiatry. 2011;68(5):467–76.

16. Schumann CM, Bloss CS, Barnes CC, *et al.* Longitudinal magnetic resonance imaging study of cortical development through early childhood in autism. J Neurosci. 2010;30(12):4419–27.

17. Lainhart JE, Bigler ED, Bocian M, *et al.* Head circumference and height in autism: a study by the Collaborative Program of Excellence in Autism. Am J Med Genet A. 2006;140(21):2257–74.

18. Raznahan A, Wallace GL, Antezana L, *et al.* Compared to what? Early brain overgrowth in autism and the perils of population norms. Biol Psychiatry. 2013;74(8):563–75.

19. Chaste P, Klei L, Sanders SJ, *et al.* Adjusting head circumference for covariates in autism: clinical correlates of a highly heritable continuous trait. Biol Psychiatry. 2013;74(8):576–84.

20. Campbell DJ, Chang J, Chawarska K. Early generalized overgrowth in autism spectrum disorder: prevalence rates, gender effects, and clinical outcomes. J Am Acad Child Adolesc Psychiatry. 2014;53(10):1063–5.

21. Giedd JN, Blumenthal J, Jeffries NO, *et al.* Brain development during childhood and adolescence: a longitudinal MRI study. Nat Neurosci. 1999;2(10):861–3.

22. Hardan AY, Libove RA, Keshavan MS, Melhem NM, Minshew NJ. A preliminary longitudinal magnetic resonance imaging study of brain volume and cortical thickness in autism. Biol Psychiatry. 2009;66(4):320–6.

23. Rakic P. Evolution of the neocortex: a perspective from developmental biology. Nat Rev Neurosci. 2009;10(10):724–35.

24. Wallace GL, Dankner N, Kenworthy L, Giedd JN, Martin A. Age-related temporal and parietal cortical thinning in autism spectrum disorders. Brain. 2010;133(Pt 12):3745–54.

25. Wallace GL, Eisenberg IW, Robustelli B, *et al.* Longitudinal cortical development during adolescence and young adulthood in autism spectrum disorder: increased cortical thinning but comparable surface area changes. J Am Acad Child Adolesc Psychiatry. 2015;54(6):464–9.

26. Mak-Fan KM, Taylor MJ, Roberts W, Lerch JP. Measures of Cortical Grey Matter Structure and Development in Children with Autism Spectrum Disorder. J Autism Dev Disord. 2011;42(3):419–27.

27. Ecker C, Shahidiani A, Feng Y, *et al.* The effect of age, diagnosis, and their interaction on vertex-based measures of cortical thickness and surface area in autism spectrum disorder. J Neural Transm. 2014;121(9):1157–70.

28. Amaral DG, Schumann CM, Nordahl CW. Neuroanatomy of autism. Trends Neurosci. 2008;31(3):137–45.

29. Blakemore S-J. The social brain in adolescence. Nat Rev Neurosci. 2008;9(4):267–77.

30. Pessoa L. On the relationship between emotion and cognition. Nat Rev Neurosci. 2008;9(2):148–58.

31. Castelli F, Frith C, Happé F, Frith U. Autism, Asperger syndrome and brain mechanisms for the attribution of mental states to animated shapes. Brain. 2002;125(Pt 8):1839–49.

32. Scherf KS, Elbich D, Minshew N, Behrmann M. Individual differences in symptom severity and behavior predict neural activation during face processing in adolescents with autism. Neuroimage Clin. 2015;7:53–67.

33. Pelphrey KA, Mitchell TV, McKeown MJ, Goldstein J, Allison T, McCarthy G. Brain activity evoked by the perception of human walking: controlling for meaningful coherent motion. J Neurosci. 2003;23(17):6819–25.

34. Lombardo MV, Chakrabarti B, Lai M-C, MRC AIMS Consortium, Baron-Cohen S. Self-referential and social cognition in a case of autism and agenesis of the corpus callosum. Mol Autism. 2012;3(1):14.

35. Russell AJ, Mataix-Cols D, Anson M, Murphy DGM. Obsessions and compulsions in Asperger syndrome and high-functioning autism. Br J Psychiatry. 2005;186(6):525–8.

36. Pauls DL, Abramovitch A, Rauch SL, Geller DA. Obsessive-compulsive disorder: an integrative genetic and neurobiological perspective. Nat Rev Neurosci. 2014;15(6):410–24.

37. Langen M, Bos D, Noordermeer SDS, Nederveen H, van Engeland H, Durston S. Changes in the Development of Striatum Are Involved in Repetitive Behavior in Autism. Biol Psychiatry. 2013;76(5):405–11.

38. Courchesne E, Pierce K. Why the frontal cortex in autism might be talking only to itself: local over-connectivity but long-distance disconnection. Curr Opin Neurobiol. 2005;15(2):225–30.

39. Ecker C, Andrews D, Dell'Acqua F, *et al.* Relationship Between Cortical Gyrification, White Matter Connectivity, and Autism Spectrum Disorder. Cereb Cortex. 2016;26(7):3297–309.

40. Belmonte MK, Allen G, Beckel-Mitchener A, Boulanger LM, Carper RA, Webb SJ. Autism and abnormal development of brain connectivity. J Neurosci. 2004;24(42):9228–31.

41. McAlonan GM, Cheung V, Cheung C, *et al.* Mapping the brain in autism. A voxel-based MRI study of volumetric differences and intercorrelations in autism. Brain. 2005;128(Pt 2):268–76.

42. Waiter GD, Williams JHG, Murray AD, Gilchrist A, Perrett DI, Whiten A. Structural white matter deficits in high-functioning individuals with autistic spectrum disorder: a voxel-based investigation. Neuroimage. 2005;24(2):455–61.

43. Ecker C, Suckling J, Deoni SC, *et al.* Brain anatomy and its relationship to behavior in adults with autism spectrum disorder: a multicenter magnetic resonance imaging study. Arch Gen Psychiatry. 2012;69(2):195–209.

44. Freitag CM, Luders E, Hulst HE, *et al*. Total brain volume and corpus callosum size in medication-naïve adolescents and young adults with autism spectrum disorder. Biol Psychiatry. 2009;66(4):316–19.

45. Sahyoun CP, Belliveau JW, Mody M. White matter integrity and pictorial reasoning in high-functioning children with autism. Brain Cogn. 2010;73(3):180–8.

46. Pugliese L, Catani M, Ameis S, *et al*. The anatomy of extended limbic pathways in Asperger syndrome: a preliminary diffusion tensor imaging tractography study. Neuroimage. 2009 15;47(2):427–34.

47. Conturo TE, Williams DL, Smith CD, Gultepe E, Akbudak E, Minshew NJ. Neuronal fiber pathway abnormalities in autism: an initial MRI diffusion tensor tracking study of hippocampo-fusiform and amygdalo-fusiform pathways. J Int Neuropsychol Soc. 2008;14(6):933–46.

48. Langen M, Leemans A, Johnston P, *et al*. Fronto-striatal circuitry and inhibitory control in autism: Findings from diffusion tensor imaging tractography. Cortex. 2011;48(2):183–93.

49. Catani M, Jones DK, Daly E, *et al*. Altered cerebellar feedback projections in Asperger syndrome. Neuroimage. 2008;41(4):1184–91.

50. Brito AR, Vasconcelos MM, Domingues RC, *et al*. Diffusion tensor imaging findings in school-aged autistic children. J Neuroimaging. 2009;19(4):337–43.

51. Geschwind DH, Levitt P. Autism spectrum disorders: developmental disconnection syndromes. Curr Opin Neurobiol. 2007;17(1):103–11.

52. Just MA, Cherkassky VL, Keller TA, Kana RK, Minshew NJ. Functional and anatomical cortical underconnectivity in autism: evidence from an FMRI study of an executive function task and corpus callosum morphometry. Cereb Cortex. 2007;17(4):951–61.

53. Just MA, Cherkassky VL, Keller TA, Minshew NJ. Cortical activation and synchronization during sentence comprehension in high-functioning autism: evidence of underconnectivity. Brain. 2004;127(Pt 8):1811–21.

54. Koshino H, Kana RK, Keller TA, Cherkassky VL, Minshew NJ, Just MA. fMRI investigation of working memory for faces in autism: visual coding and underconnectivity with frontal areas. Cereb Cortex. 2008;18(2):289–300.

55. Müller R-A, Shih P, Keehn B, Deyoe JR, Leyden KM, Shukla DK. Underconnected, but how? A survey of functional connectivity MRI studies in autism spectrum disorders. Cereb Cortex. 2011;21(10):2233–43.

56. Abrams DA, Lynch CJ, Cheng KM, *et al*. Underconnectivity between voice-selective cortex and reward circuitry in children with autism. Proc Natl Acad Sci U S A. 2013;110(29):12060–5.

57. Di Martino A, Kelly C, Grzadzinski R, *et al*. Aberrant striatal functional connectivity in children with autism. Biol Psychiatry. 2011;69(9):847–56.

58. Noonan SK, Haist F, Müller R-A. Aberrant functional connectivity in autism: evidence from low-frequency BOLD signal fluctuations. Brain Res. 2009;1262:48–63.

59. Thai NJ, Longe O, Rippon G. Disconnected brains: what is the role of fMRI in connectivity research? Int J Psychophysiol. 2009;73(1):27–32.

60. Uddin LQ, Supekar K, Menon V. Reconceptualizing functional brain connectivity in autism from a developmental perspective. Front Hum Neurosci. 2013;7:458.

61. Hazlett HC, Poe MD, Gerig G, *et al*. Early brain overgrowth in autism associated with an increase in cortical surface area before age 2 years. Arch Gen Psychiatry. 2011;68(5):467–76.

62. Zilles K, Armstrong E, Schleicher A, Kretschmann HJ. The human pattern of gyrification in the cerebral cortex. Anat Embryol. 1988;179(2):173–9.

63. Hardan AY, Jou RJ, Keshavan MS, Varma R, Minshew NJ. Increased frontal cortical folding in autism: a preliminary MRI study. Psychiatry Res. 2004;131(3):263–8.

64. Schaer M, Cuadra MB, Tamarit L, Lazeyras F, Eliez S, Thiran J-P. A surface-based approach to quantify local cortical gyrification. IEEE Trans Med Imaging. 2008;27(2):161–70.

65. Wallace GL, Robustelli B, Dankner N, Kenworthy L, Giedd JN, Martin A. Increased gyrification, but comparable surface area in adolescents with autism spectrum disorders. Brain. 2013;136(Pt 6):1956–67.

66. Libero LE, DeRamus TP, Deshpande HD, Kana RK. Surface-based morphometry of the cortical architecture of autism spectrum disorders: volume, thickness, area, and gyrification. Neuropsychologia. 2014;62C:1–10.

67. Schaer M, Ottet M-C, Scariati E, *et al*. Decreased frontal gyrification correlates with altered connectivity in children with autism. Front Hum Neurosci. 2013;7:750.

68. Levitt JG, Blanton RE, Smalley S, *et al*. Cortical sulcal maps in autism. Cereb Cortex. 2003;13(7):728–35.

69. Nordahl CW, Dierker D, Mostafavi I, *et al*. Cortical folding abnormalities in autism revealed by surface-based morphometry. J Neurosci. 2007;27(43):11725–35.

70. Williams EL, El-Baz A, Nitzken M, Switala AE, Casanova MF. Spherical harmonic analysis of cortical complexity in autism and dyslexia. Transl Neurosci. 2012;3(1):36–40.

71. Bartley AJ, Jones DW, Weinberger DR. Genetic variability of human brain size and cortical gyral patterns. Brain. 1997;120 (Pt 2):257–69.

72. Kates WR, Ikuta I, Burnette CP. Gyrification patterns in monozygotic twin pairs varying in discordance for autism. Autism Res. 2009;2(5):267–78.

73. White T, Andreasen NC, Nopoulos P. Brain volumes and surface morphology in monozygotic twins. Cereb Cortex. 2002;12(5):486–93.

74. Zilles K, Palomero-Gallagher N, Amunts K. Development of cortical folding during evolution and ontogeny. Trends Neurosci. 2013;36(5):275–84.

75. Philip RCM, Dauvermann MR, Whalley HC, Baynham K, Lawrie SM, Stanfield AC. A systematic review and meta-analysis of the fMRI investigation of autism spectrum disorders. Neurosci Biobehav Rev. 2012;36(2):901–42.

76. Fombonne E. Epidemiology of autistic disorder and other pervasive developmental disorders. J Clin Psychiatry. 2005;66 Suppl 10:3–8.

77. Bölte S, Duketis E, Poustka F, Holtmann M. Sex differences in cognitive domains and their clinical correlates in higher-functioning autism spectrum disorders. Autism. 2011;15(4):497–511.

78. Mandy W, Chilvers R, Chowdhury U, Salter G, Seigal A, Skuse D. Sex differences in autism spectrum disorder: evidence from a large sample of children and adolescents. J Autism Dev Disord. 2012;42(7):1304–13.

79. Dworzynski K, Ronald A, Bolton P, Happé F. How different are girls and boys above and below the diagnostic threshold for

autism spectrum disorders? J Am Acad Child Adolesc Psychiatry. 2012;51(8):788–97.

80. Bloss CS, Courchesne E. MRI neuroanatomy in young girls with autism: a preliminary study. J Am Acad Child Adolesc Psychiatry. 2007;46(4):515–23.

81. Schumann CM, Barnes CC, Lord C, Courchesne E. Amygdala enlargement in toddlers with autism related to severity of social and communication impairments. Biol Psychiatry. 2009;66(10):942–9.

82. Sparks BF, Friedman SD, Shaw DW, et al. Brain structural abnormalities in young children with autism spectrum disorder. Neurology. 2002;59(2):184–92.

83. Werling DM, Geschwind DH. Sex differences in autism spectrum disorders. Curr Opin Neurol. 2013;26(2):146–53.

84. Reich R, Cloninger CR, Guze SB. The multifactorial model of disease transmission: I. Description of the model and its use in psychiatry. Br J Psychiatry. 1975;127:1–10.

85. Lai M-C, Lombardo MV, Suckling J, et al. Biological sex affects the neurobiology of autism. Brain. 2013;136(Pt 9):2799–815.

86. Beacher FD, Minati L, Baron-Cohen S, et al. Autism attenuates sex differences in brain structure: a combined voxel-based morphometry and diffusion tensor imaging study. AJNR Am J Neuroradiol. 2012;33(1):83–9.

87. Ecker C, Marquand A, Mourão-Miranda J, et al. Describing the brain in autism in five dimensions--magnetic resonance imaging-assisted diagnosis of autism spectrum disorder using a multiparameter classification approach. J Neurosci. 2010;30(32):10612–23.

# 30

# Management and treatment of autism spectrum disorders

*Emily Simonoff*

## Introduction

Autism spectrum disorder (ASD) is characterized by pervasive impairments in reciprocal social communication and restricted and repetitive behaviours and interests (RRBIs). These characteristics are typically evident early in life, and while the course is variable, impairments persist across the life course. Diagnostic terminology has recently changed in the US DSM-5 [1], in which childhood autism, Asperger's syndrome, atypical autism, and pervasive developmental disorders are all subsumed under the umbrella category of ASD. This change occurred because of inconsistency in the use of different diagnostic subtypes within ASD [2] and also in recognition of the broad spectrum of severity, both across and within individuals over their life course. Life course variability in the manifestations of ASD may reflect changes emanating from within the individual, such as acquisition of language, or the implementation of environmental accommodations such as an ASD-oriented education or employment.

While the diagnostic criteria for ASD are based on the core symptoms of social communication and RRBIs, co-occurring disorders of development and mental health are the rule. In relation to cognition, approximately half of those with ASD also have an intellectual disability (ID), as defined by an intelligence quotient (IQ) of below 70 [3], and over half of those with normal non-verbal intelligence have a specific language impairment [4]. Motor co-ordination problems are more loosely defined, but population studies indicate that three-quarters of children with ASD score in the impaired range on structured assessments [5]. Psychiatric disorders are also highly prevalent, with aggregate rates in the region of 70% [6–9]. A heterogenous range of medical conditions are also common in ASD, with about 15% of people having a causal medical/genetic disorder [10, 11] and a further proportion having coexisting, but not causal, conditions such as epilepsy. Finally, people with ASD have impairments in adaptive function, the competence to undertake a range of everyday activities, including personal care, communication with others, and organization, and these impairments exceed that expected on the basis of their IQ. This impacts significantly on the degree of independence achieved by people with ASD across the full IQ range. Hence, the comprehensive management and treatment of

people with ASD requires a wide-ranging approach to a diverse set of conditions.

Because ASD is a developmental disorder starting in early life but continuing throughout life, the manifestations often vary considerably and the goals of parents/carers and people with ASD often change over time in relation to treatment goals (Fig. 30.1). In early childhood, following diagnosis, there is often a focus on interventions that will minimize or eradicate core ASD symptoms, including the development of effective communication strategies and optimization of learning. In later childhood, co-occurring mental health problems are more obvious. The importance of peers and the challenges experienced in initiating and maintaining these relationships are more evident. During later adolescence and adulthood, concern may focus on improving adaptive function and increasing independence (both typically lagging behind learning), and widening participation in education, employment, or community life. Although some behaviour problems may ameliorate, often anxiety depression become more prominent. In early childhood, ASD is often viewed by parents as a condition to 'eradicate'; however, many adults living with ASD embrace their autistic identity but want help with specific concerns, such as employment and other aspects of the 'neurotypical' environment, and with managing their mental health [12]. This changing perspective means that clinicians and services need to be patient-centred and flexible in their approach, as well as help to shape realistic goals and targets.

Many individuals with ASD, including those with average to above average intellectual ability, need support throughout their lives. The ethos in adult mental health services is to enable patient independence and ensure confidentiality. However, people with ASD are frequently anxious about health appointments and find it difficult to tolerate busy waiting rooms. Their difficulties with communication, emotional literacy, and perspective-taking can interfere with their ability to give a full and accurate account of their symptoms and experiences. Their need for support in health care appointments is recognized in the National Institute for Health and Care Excellence (NICE) guidelines for adults with ASD [13]. Throughout this chapter, we refer to 'patients and their families,' recognizing that

| Mid childhood/early adolescence | Mid childhood/early adolescence | Adulthood |
|---|---|---|
| • Manage mental health problems<br>• Optimize education, including extra<br>• help/special school placement<br>• Facilitate friendships<br>• Maintain harmonious family life | • Manage mental health problems<br>• Optimize education, including extra<br>• help/special school placement<br>• Facilitate friendships<br>• Maintain harmonious family life | • Manage mental & physical health<br>• Identify employment opportunities<br>• Develop independence<br>• Identify social and support outside family<br>• Find ways to improve quality of life |

**Fig. 30.1** Management and treatment priorities change across development.

in childhood, this is typically parents and in adulthood, it may involve other family members or carers.

## General approach to treatment and management of ASD

The focus of this chapter is on the management of both core symptoms of ASD and co-occurring psychiatric conditions. These can be extremely variable, and a personalized approach is required.

### The autism team

Because of the range of core and co-occurring symptoms, clinical input is needed from multiple disciplines within health, as well as from education, employment, social care, and the voluntary sector. Furthermore, as ASD is a chronic condition, services should recognize that the needs of people with ASD are long term and that models of care developed for episodic conditions may not meet their needs. In England, therefore, the NICE has recommended that every local authority should have an 'ASD team', which may be virtual, but where the relevant professionals can be brought together to consider and manage the needs of individual patients [14].

The diversity of needs mandates that health services are multidisciplinary in their composition. When younger children are involved, paediatric input is essential to consider underlying and associated medical/genetic disorders. Neurological expertise should be available across the lifespan. From mid childhood onwards, psychiatrists and psychologists are core members of the autism team, in relation to the diagnosis and management of ASD and additional mental health problems. Speech and language therapists are also essential to work with ASD patients with varying levels of verbal communication. Occupational therapists play an important role in the management of motor impairments and the sensory atypicalities that are often distressing and impairing. Occupational therapists may also provide useful input in relation to employment. Usually outwith the clinical team, but essential to meeting the needs of patients, are close links with education, including special education, and social care.

### Principles of intervention

#### Building on strengths

The cognitive profiles and learning styles of people with ASD, while diverse, are often different from those of non-autistic, typically developing people of the same age and ability level. Often these differences are viewed as impairments that will interfere with effective treatment, but a neurodiversity perspective would instead highlight the strengths to be enhanced and drawn upon. These may include good visuo-spatial memory, attention to detail, and willingness to

follow rules and instructions carefully. In developing an intervention plan, individual strengths should be systematically elicited through interviews, questionnaires, and cognitive assessment of the patient.

#### Identifying and prioritizing intervention targets and goals

ASD is a severe and pervasive disorder that affects every aspect of life. As discussed in the following sections, while there is emerging evidence that some interventions may improve core symptoms, these are far from curative, and the overwhelming majority of people with ASD continue to experience significant impairment. Treatment of co-occurring mental health problems typically results in less amelioration than might be expected in other patient groups. The reasons for this reduction in effectiveness remain uncertain. One possibility is that co-occurring conditions have a different aetiology in ASD, and hence the target(s) or underpinning mechanisms for intervention are different. Another possibility, particularly for non-pharmacological treatments, is that people with ASD are not able to use the intervention in the way intended because of ASD-related differences such as cognitive strategies. Alternatively, it is possible that the true effect of such interventions is similar in people with ASD, but the effects are difficult to detect and measure in the context of their ASD. Regardless of the reason, a general observation is that people with ASD often remain significantly impaired in their functioning, following a course of evidence-based intervention. Therefore, clinicians should work with patients to set realistic goals.

An additional challenge is the typical presentation of co-occurring conditions may mean that patients and their families have multiple treatment targets. The establishment of a sequence of priorities should consider which symptoms are most impairing, most likely to respond to interventions, and likely to have a knock-on impact on other symptoms.

#### Monitoring of treatment benefits and adverse effects

The co-occurrence of core ASD symptoms and additional mental health problems may hinder the ability of patients and family informants to identify improvement in target symptoms. A first step is psychoeducation about which of the patient's symptoms are related to core ASD symptoms and which to co-occurring disorders. Treatment planning should include a discussion of which symptoms are targeted by specific interventions. In monitoring treatment benefits, structured scales, whether standardized or bespoke, are helpful for both patients and clinicians. Autistic patients frequently find it useful to rate their symptoms on a Likert scale, which provides the clinician with quantitative information about improvement. A baseline measure should be obtained before initiating treatment.

Similarly, structured and systematic monitoring for possible adverse effects is essential. The impairments experienced by ASD patients in communication, emotional literacy, and verbalizing physical sensations may mean that they do not recognize these and volunteer this information at clinical reviews. At the same time, patients with ASD may have more day-to-day variability, which can affect the assessment of benefit and also lead to misattribution of variability as adverse effects. The use of routine monitoring measures can help to disentangle variability from treatment-related benefits and adverse effects.

### Specific considerations for pharmacological interventions

Over and above the principles outlined, patients with ASD may be more sensitive to psychoactive medications. This means that they should be commenced on low doses, titrated more gradually to a therapeutic dose (which is sometimes lower than for other patient populations), and monitored more frequently. It is good practice in all patients to use as few medications as possible to manage symptoms. This is even more the case in ASD where drug interactions could be more likely to precipitate adverse effects. Hence, every attempt should be made to optimize the dose of individual medications. Notwithstanding this, many patients require multiple medications and a distinction should be made between the use of multiple drugs for a single symptom complex (polypharmacy) and the need to use drugs targeting different, co-occurring symptoms, which may be essential to a comprehensive approach to management.

Particularly in younger patients and those with ID, it can be difficult to undertake routine medical investigations, such as blood tests, that are normally expected for the initiation and monitoring of medication. In discussion with parents or legal guardians, the clinician should make a judgement and recommendation about the relative risks and benefits of an intervention when routine monitoring is difficult or impossible. It is also often possible to be opportunistic in obtaining investigations when the patient is undergoing other medical procedures.

### General considerations for psychological interventions

As with other groups, patients with ASD and their families are keen to have access to psychological interventions. Clinicians are sometimes concerned about the appropriateness of talking treatments with patients whose communication skills are impaired. However, strategies for adaptation, for example modified cognitive behavioural therapy (CBT), are now available and have been evaluated in clinical trials, with positive effects, as described in the following sections. Before commencing psychological work, it is helpful to undertake a cognitive assessment to gain a better understanding of the patient's cognitive level. Clinicians may be misled by patients' 'chattiness' into assuming they have good receptive language when, in fact, their abilities are significantly compromised. The principles of adapted CBT for people with ASD include establishing emotional literacy, using visual materials to support the work, both in sessions and as part of the intervention, and additional practice in multiple settings to aid generalization. Autistic patients may continue to benefit into adult life from family members as co-therapists, as often used with younger children.

### Other non-pharmacological interventions

Clinicians should be aware of the importance of other modalities of support or intervention. While there is increasing interest in neuromodulation, there is at present no evidence for its use in ASD. However, education for youth and appropriate supported (where necessary) employment for adults are among the most important ways of optimizing life chances and improving quality of life. The acquisition of educational levels and adaptive skills is often slower in people with ASD but continues into adult life. In recognition of this, many countries have legislated that people with ASD have the right to state-supported education past the age mandated for typically developing people. Clinicians often have a key role in highlighting elements of the educational or employment environment that will foster development and well-being.

## Specific treatments and interventions

The following sections on treatment are organized by symptom domain, and within each section, interventions are considered according to type. Where evidence is stratified or limited by age, this is indicated.

### Treatment of core symptoms of ASD

Although the diagnosis of an ASD requires the presence of both social communication impairments and restricted RRBIs, there is evidence that these domains are underpinned by separate, correlated genetic architecture [15]. Furthermore, the current evidence suggests that the effects of interventions are relatively specific. Psychological interventions have focused on social communication and learning, with little evidence of transfer of effects to RRBIs. Conversely, the limited evidence for pharmacological interventions suggests that may be principally useful in managing RRBIs.

### Social communication

At present, there is no good evidence that pharmacological interventions improve social communication, although a number are being investigated. While there is evidence suggesting secondary improvement in social communication when co-occurring disorders, for example attention-deficit/hyperactivity disorder (ADHD) [16] or irritability [17, 18], are treated, this is likely to be mediated by improvement in the original target symptoms, rather than having a direct effect. They should not be used in the absence of the primary symptoms.

There is emerging evidence for psychological interventions aimed at improving social communication in young children, from toddlers through the early school years. In evaluating the evidence in relation to psychological interventions, it is important to focus on studies with objective and/or blinded outcome measures, as unblinded parent reports are subject to bias and placebo effects [19]. In relation to parent-mediated interventions, a randomized controlled trial (RCT) in the UK that aimed to improve parental sensitivity to their children's behaviour failed to find a significant effect on child social communication at the end of the trial but did find an effect on parental sensitivity [20]. Interestingly, a follow-up 5–6 years later demonstrated significant benefit for the treatment group on a blinded outcome measure of social communication (but not language level) [21]. Several RCTs in the United States have reported similar findings [22–24].

There is also emerging evidence for the benefits of structured social skills programmes, whether parent-mediated [25–27] or school-based [28]. This evidence applies from early to mid childhood, for example age 5–6 years, through to adolescence.

Applied behavioural analysis (ABA) is a popular approach with a focus on intensive behavioural work to help autistic children acquire specific skills. Early evaluation suggested that while specific skills might be learnt, the intervention did not generalize to meaningful improvements in ASD [29]. In line with the early findings, a structured variation—the Early Start Denver Model (ESDM)—has been more carefully evaluated recently, with follow-up findings at 1 and 2 years. This revealed improvements in the treated group in IQ and adaptive function, but not in ASD symptoms [30], with these gain no longer being significant at the 4-year follow-up [31]. Studies combining classical ABA and joint attention training approaches have reported benefits for proximal target symptoms, but it is unclear whether these effects generalize to outcomes more closely linked to real-life functioning [32, 33].

In adults, observational studies suggest that behavioural or social learning approaches may be helpful, but the evidence from RCTs is very weak, with only one study which failed to find significant benefit of a social learning programme [34]. There are a range of other interventions to consider for adults with ASD which may benefit their adaptive function and quality of life, without specifically improving social communication skills. These include structured life skills programmes for those who have difficulty with organization or social isolation and CBT-based programmes to reduce the risk of victimization [35]. However, the evidence base is weak.

Research shows that the following treatments are *not* of benefit, exclusion diets have no benefit, and the once-touted treatments of secretin, hyperbaric oxygen, and chelation therapy may be harmful [36].

### Restricted and repetitive behaviours and interests

Despite early findings suggestive of benefit, selective serotonin reuptake inhibitors (SSRIs) should not be used to treat RRBIs. Early, but small, studies of fluoxetine in children [37] and adults [38] and fluvoxamine in adults [39] were superseded by a large trial of citalopram in youth, which failed to identify beneficial effects and demonstrated adverse effects in the treated group [40]. These aggregate findings, along with a few other studies, were combined in a Cochrane review that did not support the use of SSRIs for RRBIs in ASD [41]. As for social symptoms, both risperidone [42] and aripiprazole [43, 44] significantly reduced stereotypic behaviour in secondary analyses where autistic children were selected, based on high levels of irritability. The interpretation of these findings should be that where high levels of irritability are present, such drugs may have wide-ranging benefits. There are no trials suggesting psychological interventions directed at RRBIs are useful.

### Sensory symptoms

The recent revision of DSM-5 included for the first time sensory atypicalities as part of the diagnostic criteria [1]. They are subsumed under the domain of RRBIs. Sensory atypicalities include both hyper- and hyposensitivity, as well as unusual interests to one or more domains of sensation. The study of sensory atypicalities has been held back by a lack of good measures of sensory experiences and behaviours. Recommendations from occupational therapists include the use of stimuli that provide alternative sensations such as squeezy balls, weighted blankets and vests, eye protectors, and massage. There is weak (because of small sample size and non-blinded outcomes) RCT evidence for the benefit of occupational therapy

in one structured intervention of 30 sessions [45] and similarly for massage [46]. Although they have been popular, the evidence on weighted vests does not support their use [47].

### Treatment of common co-occurring mental disorders

As highlighted previously, co-occurring psychiatric disorders are the rule in people with ASD. The reasons for this are only partly understood. Twin studies indicate that co-occurrence with other neurodevelopmental disorders, such as ADHD, tics/Tourette's syndrome, and ID is predominantly due to shared genetic risk factors [48]. This does not apply to co-occurring emotional symptoms where shared genetic factors are very small [49]. For the latter group of symptoms, it is more likely that features of ASD, impairments in cognitive processing, including social cognition, and executive function are mediators for emotional disorders [50]. Differences in behavioural style may render people with ASD more likely to experience adverse environmental and life events, including bullying [51], and they may have greater difficulty in adaptive responses when they have occurred. Others have argued that the high level of co-occurring psychopathology merely reflects inaccuracies in diagnostic boundaries and that these should be broader and more inclusive to reflect the patterns of observed symptoms. A benefit of conceptualizing these symptom domains as co-occurring disorders is that it encourages clinicians to identify and treat them, drawing upon the wider intervention evidence base in the absence of ASD-specific studies.

### Attention-deficit/hyperactivity disorder

Population studies suggest 30–50% of children with ASD meet criteria for ADHD [8, 9]. Diagnostic classification systems prior to DSM-5 precluded the diagnosis of ADHD (hyperkinetic disorder in the International Classification of Disease) in the context of ASD; hence, much of the relevant research refers to people with high levels of ADHD or hyperactivity symptoms. For all practical purposes, the patients included in pharmacological trials would meet formal diagnostic criteria for ADHD or hyperkinetic disorder and they are referred to in the following sections as having ADHD for ease of discussion.

There are RCTs supporting the benefits of methylphenidate, atomoxetine, and guanfacine in youth with ASD and ADHD. Methylphenidate has been evaluated in four RCTs, with a meta-analytic effect size of 0.66 [52] and about half being classified as responders [53]. This contrasts with effect sizes in the region of 0.8–1.0 in typically developing youth with ADHD [54] and 80–90% of responders [55]. Furthermore, rates of adverse effects are higher, with 18% in the largest study being withdrawn due to adverse effects in one study [53].

Atomoxetine has been evaluated in a small [56] and medium-sized [57] trial. Both reported significant improvements with active treatment over placebo, but effect sizes were not reported. In the larger study, only 21% were responders under the usual criteria (vs 9% in the placebo group) [57], compared to 57% and 25%, respectively, in the smaller study [56]. However, rates of adverse effects were low, with only two withdrawals across both studies. A two-by-two RCT (atomoxetine vs placebo, parent training vs no psychological intervention) showed benefits for all three active arms (atomoxetine plus parent training, atomoxetine alone, and parent training alone), with effect sizes of between 0.57 and 0.98, compared to no treatment. The active arms could not be distinguished statistically [58].

Most recently, guanfacine has been evaluated in ASD and ADHD in a medium-sized study showing a large effect size (>1), with 50% of the active group classed as responders vs 9% of the placebo group [59]. Adverse effects leading to withdrawal were present in 13%, and lethargy early in treatment was prominent.

The only RCT evidence for psychological intervention comes from the atomoxetine/parent training study described, in which the effect size against no active treatment was 0.6 [58]. In contrast to the pharmacological trials, this was not a blinded outcome, as parents were the recipients of the intervention, as well as the informants on ADHD, so the magnitude should be viewed with caution [60].

In summary, there is good evidence for pharmacological interventions in ADHD among youth with ASD. However, the effects are mostly smaller than in typically developing youth and the rate of adverse effects is higher. Therefore, careful monitoring is required when prescribing. Different classes of medication should be tried sequentially if benefits are inadequate or the drug is poorly tolerated. There are no adult studies to draw upon; therefore, extrapolation from the experience in children and adolescents is necessary. The findings of parent training highlight the importance of including psychological approaches to intervention and is consistent with the NICE update on ADHD, in which it is recommended that parent training is offered to all parents of children with ADHD [61].

### Anxiety and obsessive–compulsive disorders

Rates of anxiety disorders vary widely across studies, from about 30% to 80%, depending on populations and measurement [62]. With regard to pharmacological interventions, there have been no RCTs targeting anxiety disorders among patients with ASD. Trials of both fluoxetine and citalopram failed to show an impact on obsessional symptoms [37, 40], and these trials were likely measuring RRBIs, rather than obsessive–compulsive disorder (OCD).

A meta-analysis of eight RCTs of adapted cognitive behavioural therapy (CBT) for anxiety in children and adolescents indicates benefits, with an aggregate effect size of 1.2 [63]. Child-reported outcomes from five studies revealed a lower meta-analytic effect size of 0.68. As above, these large effects should be viewed with caution, as the informants were not blind to treatment allocation and four of the trials used waitlist controls. In addition, the samples are selected to include youth of higher intellectual ability. In adults, the evidence for CBT is more anecdotal. One medium-sized trial of CBT for OCD in adolescents and adults with ASD failed to find a treatment effect against generic anxiety management [64]. The sample sizes was probably not large enough for a comparison against an active intervention, and both the rate of response (45% vs 20%) and effect sizes (0.33 vs 0.05) were suggestive of superiority for CBT that warrants further investigation.

When possible, CBT should be the first-line treatment. Pharmacologically, in the absence of ASD-specific data, treatment should follow that used in typically developing individuals, with the provisos described in relation to low doses and gradual titration. Medication should be considered when CBT is ineffective or unsuitable because of patient characteristics, including anxiety that is too severe for such an approach.

### Depression

Rates of depression appear to be low in children with ASD [9] but affects up to 50% of adults [7]. There is even less evidence base for ASD-specific treatment of depression. One extremely small study of fluoxetine in adults failed to find an effect but was underpowered to reach any conclusions [65]. There is a similar lack of evidence in relation to psychological interventions for depression. Treating depression should follow recommendations for people without ASD, but when psychological interventions are used, they should be adapted to be ASD-specific.

### Tics

Tics are common in ASD [8, 9] but importantly need to be differentiated from mannerisms, stereotypies, repetitive behaviours, and complex rituals. This usually requires direct observation. As in typically developing people, tics should only be treated when they are impairing and then the aim of treatment should be to manage impairment, rather than eradicate the tics. Psychoeducation is important, as families and teachers often do not appreciate the involuntary nature of tics. In individuals without ASD, a recent meta-analysis of RCTs reported good to moderate quality evidence for the benefits of the alpha-2 adrenergic receptor agonists clonidine and guanfacine and dopamine antagonists/partial agonists [66]. This review also judged the trials for habit reversal to be of good quality and demonstrating efficacy. These findings should guide intervention in ASD.

### Behaviours that challenge

One of the most common and impairing presentations among people with ASD is that of 'behaviours that challenge others' or 'challenging behaviour'. Over the years, a number of terms have been used to reflect these behaviours, which comprise aggressions directed at the self or others and severe non-compliant behaviour, frequently with high levels of irritability. These behaviours may vary in their intensity and frequency but are of concern when they impact on an individual's ability to participate in everyday activities such as family life, school attendance, employment, or leisure activities. Such behaviours are common in people with ASD and more frequent than in other conditions causing similar impact on intellectual functioning [67, 68]. Behaviours that challenge have been conceptualized in different theoretical perspectives, which are not mutually exclusive. In the comprehensive approach to their management, all need to be considered.

Social learning models of behaviours that challenge view these as maladaptive learnt responses. Applied behaviour analysis (ABA) aims to identify the causes and responses that are driving its reinforcement. There is an extensive ABA literature of individual patients and case series demonstrating how learning principles can be used to break the cycle of these behaviours. Although there is a lack of group-based RCTs, the literature includes examples demonstrating the causal role of contingent response, in which the response to a challenging behaviour is modified, leading to a reduction in the behaviour, followed by a return to the original contingencies, which leads to a return of the unwanted behaviour. All clinicians working with these patients demonstrating challenging behaviour should have a good understanding of functional behavioural analysis in order to take a history that elicits antecedents, behaviours, and consequences. ABA in its classical form is undertaken by psychologists and behaviour modification therapists who make use of a range of operant conditioning principles; it can be time-consuming but is an important treatment modality for behaviour that challenges.

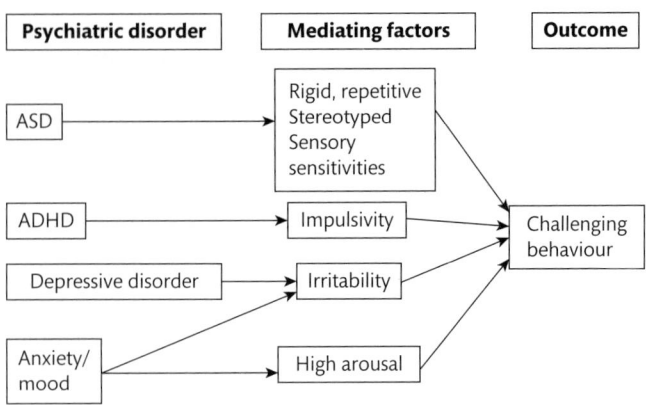

**Fig. 30.2** Conceptual framework linking psychiatric disorders to behaviour that challenges.

Behaviours that challenge may also arise as a consequence of conditions causing pain or discomfort. Painful conditions are more common in ASD, either due to the high rates of causal or associated medical conditions. Even higher-functioning autistic individuals often have difficulty identifying bodily sensations and linking them to their emotional state and behaviour. Hence, these should always be considered, especially when there is a sudden increase in challenging behaviour.

Behaviour that challenges may also be an external manifestation of an underlying psychiatric disorder (Fig. 30.2). The presentation of psychiatric disorders may be atypical and more difficult to identify because of poor communication skills and emotional literacy. For example, in autistic individuals, anxiety may present as irritability [69]. The link between different psychiatric disorders and behaviours that challenge has been demonstrated in adults with ID [70]. Clinicians should assess for psychiatric disorders that may underpin behaviours that challenge.

In the absence of identifying another psychiatric disorder, there is evidence for treating behaviour that challenge described as 'irritability' with dopamine antagonists/partial agonists, most notably risperidone and aripiprazole. Both drugs have robust acute and medium-term benefits [71, 72]. However, they may also have significant adverse effects, which include weight gain and somnolence, and for risperidone, raised prolactin levels [73, 74]. Clinical impressions that aripiprazole may have fewer adverse effects are not at present confirmed by research; a small head-to-head comparison, which was likely underpowered, failed to detect differences in rates of short-term adverse effects [75].

A trial comparing risperidone alone vs risperidone and parent training in children revealed significantly greater improvement in adaptive function in those receiving the combination intervention, and medication doses were marginally (not significantly) lower than in the medication only arm [76]. Based on all these findings, in conjunction with clinical consensus, NICE recommends that behavioural treatment should be the first-line intervention for behaviour that challenges. Medication should only be first line when circumstances do not permit a behavioural intervention, and where this is the case, a behavioural intervention should be added as soon as possible. Conversely, if a behavioural intervention is inadequate, medication augmentation should be considered. Although medication retains its effectiveness in the medium term, there are real concerns about long-term safety. Ideally, the use of antipsychotic medication should be seen as an opportunity to develop other strategies for behavioural management, with the aim of reducing or eliminating medication, wherever possible.

### Sleep problems

Although sleep problems are very common in people with ASD, particularly those with associated ID [77], research on their management is very limited. Sleep onset and maintenance are the most common problems. The causes are likely multifactorial; there is emerging evidence for biological differences in melatonin production and circadian patterns. Co-occurring medical disorders may play a role, and sleep apnoea should be considered. Psychiatric disorders, such as anxiety, depression, and ADHD, are all linked to sleep problems in people without ASD, and these are of higher prevalence in ASD. People with ASD often have maladaptive bedtime routines that cause or exacerbate sleep problems.

One trial of melatonin in children with developmental disabilities included a large proportion with ASD [78]. The protocol required that eligible families first receive a manual on behavioural management of sleep. Following this, over one-third of children no longer met inclusion criteria, highlighting the benefits of psychosocial intervention. Among those completing the trial, parent diaries indicated a benefit of melatonin for sleep latency and total sleep time, while actigraphy on a subsample confirmed the effect on sleep latency only. Recommendations from NICE place priority on behavioural management strategies, particularly the implementation of a sleep hygiene programme. Where this is insufficient, melatonin can be considered but should only be extended when there is clear benefit and then for a limited time period [36].

## Conclusions and research directions

ASD is a severe, pervasive, and lifelong disorder. Although there is an increasing understanding of its aetiology, this has only begun to translate into theoretically derived approaches to intervention. In relation to core symptoms of ASD, most promising at present are psychosocial interventions aimed at improving social communication. A better understanding of their long-term impact is required. Pharmacological approaches to core symptoms have recently focused on molecules implicated in biological pathways that appear to be different in people with ASD, but there is insufficient evidence to recommend their use in clinical practice. A programme of clinical trials is needed to escalate the rate of progress.

Co-occurring psychiatric disorders are exceedingly common in ASD and form an important consideration in the comprehensive management of ASD. There is a good evidence base for the treatment of ADHD and 'irritability' or behaviour that challenges, and some evidence to guide practice for anxiety disorders. However, for many other psychiatric disorders, there is a lack of therapeutic research in ASD, leaving clinicians reliant on the evidence base for patients without ASD. Because of the differences in biology and cognitive make-up, such extrapolation may be inappropriate. There is an urgent need for treatment trials in affective and sleep disorders. Different intervention modalities should be considered, both on their own and in combination.

The development of new, reliable, sensitive, and unbiased objective outcome measures should aid the progress and interpretation of clinical trials. Finally, environmental interventions, including those based in education and employment, have the potential to produce large gains in well-being and quality of life.

## REFERENCES

1. American Psychiatric Association. *Diagnostic and Statistical Manual of Mental Disorders* (DSM-5`). American Psychiatric Association, Washington, DC; 2013.
2. Lord C, Petkova E, Hus V, *et al.* A multisite study of the clinical diagnosis of different autism spectrum disorders. Archives of General Psychiatry. 2012;69(3):306–13.
3. Charman T, Pickles A, Simonoff E, Chandler S, Loucas T, Baird G. IQ in children with autism spectrum disorders: Data from the SNAP project. Psychological Medicine 2011;41(3):619–27.
4. Loucas T, Charman T, Pickles A, *et al.* Autistic symptomatology and language ability in autism spectrum disorder and specific language impairment. Journal of Child Psychology and Psychiatry. 2008;49(11):1184–92.
5. Green D, Charman T, Pickles A, *et al.* Impairment in movement skills of children with autistic spectrum disorders. Developmental Medicine and Child Neurology. 2009;51(4):311–16.
6. Gjevik E, Eldevik S, Fjaeran-Granum T, Sponheim E. Kiddie-SADS reveals high rates of DSM-IV disorders in children and adolescents with autism spectrum disorders. Journal of Autism and Developmental Disorders. 2011;41(6):761–9.
7. Hofvander B, Delorme R, Chaste P, *et al.* Psychiatric and psychosocial problems in adults with normal-intelligence autism spectrum disorders. BMC Psychiatry. 2009;35:1–9.
8. Salazar F, Baird G, Chandler S, *et al.* Co-occurring psychiatric disorders in preschool and elementary school-aged children with autism spectrum disorder. Journal of Autism and Developmental Disorders. 2015;45(8):2283–94.
9. Simonoff E, Pickles A, Charman T, Chandler S, Loucas T, Baird G. Psychiatric disorders in children with autism spectrum disorders: prevalence, comorbidity and associated factors. Journal of the American Academy of Child and Adolescent Psychiatry. 2008;47(8):921–9.
10. Fombonne E. Epidemiology of pervasive developmental disorders. Pediatric Research. 2009;65(6):591–8.
11. Oron O, Elliott E. Delineating the common biological pathways perturbed by ASD's genetic etiology: Lessons from network-based studies. International Journal of Molecular Sciences. 2017;18(4):882.
12. Wallace S, Parr J, Hardy A. *One in a hundred: Putting families at the heart of autism research.* Autistica, London; 2014.
13. National Institute of Health and Care Excellence. *Autism spectrum disorder in adults: diagnosis and management.* National Institute of Health and Care Excellence, London; 2012.
14. National Institute for Health and Care Excellence. *Autism: recognition, referral, diagnosis and management of adults on the autism spectrum.* National Institute of Health and Care Excellence, London; 2012.
15. Ronald A, Happe F, Bolton P, *et al.* Genetic heterogeneity between the three components of the autism spectrum: a twin study. Journal of the American Academy of Child and Adolescent Psychiatry. 2006;45(6):691–9.
16. Jahromi LB, Kasari CL, McCracken JT, *et al.* Positive effects of methylphenidate on social communication and self-regulation in children with pervasive developmental disorders and hyperactivity. Journal of Autism and Developmental Disorders. 2009;39(3):395–404.
17. Aman MG, Hollway JA, Leone S, *et al.* Effects of risperidone on cognitive-motor performance and motor movements in chronically medicated children. Research in Developmental Disabilities. 2009;30(2):386–96.
18. McCracken JT, McGough J, Shah B, *et al.* Risperidone in children with autism and serious behavioral problems. New England Journal of Medicine. 2002;347(5):314–21.
19. Grzadzinski R, Carr T, Colombi C, *et al.* Measuring changes in social communication behaviors: Preliminary development of the Brief Observation of Social Communication Change (BOSCC). Journal of Autism and Developmental Disorders. 2016;46(7):464–79.
20. Green J, Charman T, Pickles A, *et al.* Parent-mediated intervention versus no intervention for infants at high risk of autism: a parallel, single-blind, randomised trial. The Lancet Psychiatry. 2015;2(2):133–40.
21. Pickles A, Le Couteur A, Leadbitter K, *et al.* Parent-mediated social communication therapy for young children with autism (PACT): long-term follow-up of a randomised controlled trial. The Lancet. 2016;388(10059):2501–9.
22. Carter AS, Messinger DS, Stone WL, Celimli S, Nahmias AS, Yoder P. A randomized controlled trial of Hanen's 'More Than Words' in toddlers with early autism symptoms. Journal of Child Psychology and Psychiatry. 2011;52(7):741–52.
23. Kasari C, Gulsrud AC, Wong C, Kwon S, Locke J. Randomized controlled caregiver mediated joint engagement intervention for toddlers with autism. Journal of Autism and Developmental Disorders. 2010;40(9):1045–6.
24. Wetherby AM, Guthrie W, Woods J, *et al.* Parent-implemented social intervention for toddlers with autism: an RCT. Pediatrics. 2014;134(6):1084–93.
25. Frankel F, Myatt R, Sugar C, Whitham C, Gorospe CM, Laugeson E. A randomized controlled study of parent-assisted children's friendship training with children having autism spectrum disorders. Journal of Autism and Developmental Disorders. 2010;40(7):827–42.
26. Laugeson EA, Frankel F, Mogil C, Dillon AR. Parent-assisted social skills training to improve friendships in teens with autism spectrum disorders. Journal of Autism and Developmental Disorders. 2009;39(4):596–606.
27. Laugeson EA, Frankel F, Gantman A, Dillon AR, Mogil C. Evidence-based social skills training for adolescents with autism spectrum disorders: the UCLA PEERS program. Journal of Autism and Developmental Disorders. 2012;42(6):1025–36.
28. Kasari C, Dean M, Kretzmann M, *et al.* Children with autism spectrum disorder and social skills groups at school: a randomized trial comparing intervention approach and peer composition. Journal of Child Psychology and Psychiatry and Allied Disciplines. 2016;57:171–9.
29. Howlin P, Magiati I, Charman T, MacLean JWE. SystematicrReview of early intensive behavioral interventions for children With autism. American Journal on Intellectual and Developmental Disabilities. 2009;114(1):23–41.
30. Dawson G, Rogers S, Munson J, *et al.* Randomized, controlled trial of an intervention for toddlers with autism: the Early Start Denver Model. Pediatrics. 2010;125(1):e17–23.

31. Estes A, Munson J, Rogers SJ, Greenson J, Winter J, Dawson G. Long-term outcomes of early intervention in 6-year-old children with autism spectrum disorder. Journal of the American Academy of Child and Adolescent Psychiatry. 2015;54(7):580–7.

32. Kasari C, Freeman S, Paparella T. Joint attention and symbolic play in young children with autism: a randomized controlled intervention study. Journal of Child Psychology and Psychiatry. 2006;47(6):611–20.

33. Landa RJ, Holman KC, O'Neill AH, Stuart EA. Intervention targeting development of socially synchronous engagement in toddlers with autism spectrum disorder: a randomized controlled trial. Journal of Child Psychology and Psychiatry. 2011;52(1):13–21.

34. Golan O, Baron-Cohen S. Systemizing empathy: Teaching adults with Asperger syndrome or high-functioning autism to recognize complex emotions using interactive multimedia. Development and Psychopathology. 2006;18(02):591–617.

35. Khemka I. Increasing independent decision-making skills of women with mental retardation in simulated interpersonal situations of abuse. American Journal on Mental Retardation. 2000;105(5):387–401.

36. National Collaborating Centre for Mental Health. *The management and support of children and young people on the autism spectrum*. 2013. https://www.nice.org.uk/guidance/cg170/documents/autism-management-of-autism-in-children-and-young-people-nice-version2

37. Hollander E, Phillips A, Chaplin W, et al. A placebo-controlled crossover trial of liquid fluoxetine on repetitive behaviors in childhood and adolescent autism. Neuropsychopharmacology. 2005;30(3):582–9.

38. Hollander E, Soorya L, Chaplin W, et al. A double-blind placebo-controlled trial of fluoxetine for repetitive behaviors and global severity in adult autism spectrum disorders. American Journal of Psychiatry. 2012;169(3):292–9.

39. McDougle CJ, Naylor ST, Cohen DJ, Volkmar FR, Heninger GR, Price LH. A double-blind, placebo-controlled study of fluvoxamine in adults with autistic disorder. Archives of General Psychiatry. 1996;53(11):1001–8.

40. King BH, Hollander E, Sikich L, et al. Lack of efficacy of citalopram in children with autism spectrum disorders and high levels of repetitive behavior. Archives of General Psychiatry. 2009;66(6):583–90.

41. Williams K, Brignell A, Randall M, Silove N, Hazell P. Selective serotonin reuptake inhibitors (SSRIs) for autism spectrum disorders (ASD). Cochrane Database of Systematic Reviews. 2013;8:CD004677.

42. McDougle CJ, Scahill L, Aman MG, et al. Risperidone for the core symptom domains of autism: results from the study by the autism network of the research units on pediatric psychopharmacology. American Journal of Psychiatry. 2005;162(6):1142–8.

43. Aman MG, Kasper W, Manos G, et al. Line-item analysis of the Aberrant Behavior Checklist: results from two studies of aripiprazole in the treatment of irritability associated with autistic disorder. Journal of Child and Adolescent Psychopharmacology. 2010;20(5):415–22.

44. Marcus RN, Owen R, Kamen L, et al. A placebo-controlled, fixed-dose study of aripiprazole in children and adolescents with irritability associated with autistic disorder. Journal of the American Academy of Child and Adolescent Psychiatry. 2009;48(11):1110–19.

45. Schaaf RC, Benevides T, Mailloux Z, et al. An intervention for sensory difficulties in children with autism: a randomized trial. Journal of Autism and Developmental Disorders. 2014;44(7):1493–506.

46. Silva LM, Cignolini A, Warren R, Budden S, Skowron-Gooch A. Improvement in sensory impairment and social interaction in young children with autism following treatment with an original Qigong massage methodology. American Journal of Chinese Medicine. 2007;35(3):393–406.

47. Stephenson J, Carter M. The use of weighted vests with children with autism spectrum disorders and other disabilities. Journal of Autism and Developmental Disorders. 2009;39(1):105–14.

48. Lichtenstein P, Carlstrom E, Rastam M, Gillberg C, Anckarsater H. The genetics of autism spectrum disorders and related neuropsychiatric disorders in childhood. American Journal of Psychiatry. 2010;167(11):1357–63.

49. Hallett V, Ronald A, Rijsdijk F, Happe F. Association of autistic-like and internalizing traits during childhood: A longitudinal twin study. American Journal of Psychiatry. 2009;167:809–17.

50. Hollocks, Jones CR, Pickles A, et al. The association between social cognition and executive functioning and symptoms of anxiety and depression in adolescents with autism spectrum disorders. Autism Research. 2014;7(2):216–28.

51. van Roekel E, Scholte RH, Didden R, van Roekel E, Scholte RHJ, Didden R. Bullying among adolescents with autism spectrum disorders: prevalence and perception. Journal of Autism and Developmental Disorders. 2010;40(1):63–73.

52. Reichow B, Volkmar FR, Bloch MH. Systematic review and meta-analysis of pharmacological treatment of the symptoms of attention-deficit/hyperactivity disorder in children with pervasive developmental disorders. Journal of Autism and Developmental Disorders. 2013;43(10):2435–41.

53. Research Units on Pediatric Psychopharmacology Autism Network. Randomized, controlled, crossover trial of methylphenidate in pervasive developmental disorders with hyperactivity. Archives of General Psychiatry. 2005;62(11):1266–74.

54. Faraone SV. Using meta-analysis to compare the efficacy of medications for Attention-Deficit/Hyperactivity Disorder in youths. Pharmacy and Therapeutics. 2009;34(12):678–94.

55. Jensen PS. A 14-month randomized clinical trial of treatment strategies for attention-deficit/hyperactivity disorder. Archives of General Psychiatry. 1999;56(12):1073–86.

56. Arnold LE, Aman MG, Cook AM, et al. Atomoxetine for hyperactivity in autism spectrum disorders: placebo-controlled crossover pilot trial. Journal of the American Academy of Child and Adolescent Psychiatry. 2006;45(10):1196–205.

57. Harfterkamp M, van de Loo-Neus G, Minderaa RB, et al. A randomized double-blind study of atomoxetine versus placebo for attention-deficit/hyperactivity disorder symptoms in children with autism spectrum disorder. Journal of the American Academy of Child and Adolescent Psychiatry. 2012;51(7):733–41.

58. Handen BL, Aman MG, Arnold LE, et al. Atomoxetine, parent training, and their combination in children With autism spectrum disorder and attention-deficit/hyperactivity disorder. Journal of the American Academy of Child and Adolescent Psychiatry. 2015;54(11):905–15.

59. Scahill L, McCracken JT, King BH, et al. Extended-release guanfacine for hyperactivity in children with autism spectrum disorder. American Journal of Psychiatry. 2015;172(12):1197–206.

60. Sonuga-Barke E, Brandeis D, Cortese S, et al. Non-pharmacological interventions for attention-deficit/hyperactivity disorder: systematic review and meta-analyses of randomised

controlled trials of dietary and psychological treatments. American Journal of Psychiatry. 2013;170(3):275–89.

61. National Institute for Health and Care Excellence. *Attention deficit hyperactivity disorder: diagnosis and management: update.* National Institute for Health and Care Excellence, London; 2018.

62. White SW, Oswald D, Ollendick T, Scahill L. Anxiety in children and adolescents with autism spectrum disorders. Clinical Psychology Review. 2009;29:216–29.

63. Sukhodolsky DG, Bloch MH, Panza KE, Reichow B. Cognitive-behavioral therapy for anxiety in children with high-functioning autism: A meta-analysis. Pediatrics. 2013;132(5):e1341–50.

64. Russell AJ, Jassi A, Fullana MA, *et al.* Cognitive behavior therapy for comorbid obsessive-compulsive disorder in high-functioning autism spectrum disorders: a randomized controlled trial. Depress Anxiety. 2013;30(8):697–708.

65. Buchsbaum MS, Hollander E, Haznedar MM, *et al.* Effect of fluoxetine on regional cerebral metabolism in autistic spectrum disorders: a pilot study. International Journal of Neuropsychopharmacology. 2001;4(2):119–25.

66. Whittington C, Pennant M, Kendall T, *et al.* Practitioner Review: Treatments for Tourette syndrome in children and young people–a systematic review. Journal of Child Psychology and Psychiatry. 2016;57(9):988–1004.

67. Brereton AV, Tonge BJ, Einfeld SL. Psychopathology in children and adolescents with autism compared to young people with intellectual disability. Journal of Autism and Developmental Disorders. 2006;36(7):863–70.

68. Richards C, Oliver C, Nelson L, Moss J. Self-injurious behaviour in individuals with autism spectrum disorder and intellectual disability. Journal of Intellectual Disability Research. 2012;56(5):476–89.

69. Mikita N, Hollocks MJ, Papadopoulos AS, *et al.* Irritability in boys with autism spectrum disorders: an investigation of physiological reactivity. Journal of Child Psychology and Psychiatry. 2015;56(10):1118–26.

70. Moss S, Emerson E, Kiernan C, Turner S, Hatton C, Alborz A. Psychiatric symptoms in adults with learning disability

and challenging behaviour. British Journal of Psychiatry. 2000;177:451–6.

71. Findling RL, Aman MG, Eerdekens M, Derivan A, Lyons B, Risperidone Disruptive Behavior Study G. Long-term, open-label study of risperidone in children with severe disruptive behaviors and below-average IQ. American Journal of Psychiatry. 2004;161(4):677–84.

72. Marcus RN, Owen R, Manos G, *et al.* Aripiprazole in the treatment of irritability in pediatric patients (aged 6–17 years) with autistic disorder: results from a 52-week, open-label study. Journal of Child and Adolescent Psychopharmacology. 2011;21(3):229–36.

73. Aman MG, Arnold LE, McDougle CJ, *et al.* Acute and long-term safety and tolerability of risperidone in children with autism. Journal of Child and Adolescent Psychopharmacology. 2005;15(6):869–84.

74. Anderson GM, Scahill L, McCracken JT, McDougle CJ, Aman MG, Tierney E. Effects of short- and long-term risperidone treatment on prolactin levels in children with autism. Biological Psychiatry. 2007;61(4):545–50.

75. Ghanizadeh A, Sahraeizadeh A, Berk M. A head-to-head comparison of aripiprazole and risperidone for safety and treating autistic disorders, a randomized double blind clinical trial. Child Psychiatry and Human Development. 2014;45(2): 185–92.

76. Scahill L, McDougle CJ, Aman MG, *et al.* Effects of risperidone and parent training on adaptive functioning in children with pervasive developmental disorders and serious behavioral problems. Journal of the American Academy of Child and Adolescent Psychiatry. 2012;51(2):136–46.

77. Richdale AL, Schreck KA. Sleep problems in autism spectrum disorders: prevalence, nature, and possible biopsychosocial aetiologies. Sleep Medicine Reviews. 2009;13(6):403–11.

78. Gringras P, Gamble C, Jones AP, *et al.* Melatonin for sleep problems in children with neurodevelopmental disorders: randomised double masked placebo controlled trial. British Medical Journal. 2012;345:e6664.

# SECTION 5

# Attention-deficit/hyperactivity disorder

SECTION 5

Attention-deficit hyperactivity
disorder

# 31

# Core dimensions of attention-deficit/hyperactivity disorder

*Eric Taylor*

## Introduction

The concept of attention-deficit/hyperactivity disorder (ADHD) arose from neurological formulations but does not entail them, and the modern definition describes a set of behavioural traits. A condition consisting of pervasive and persistent inattention and/or impulsiveness is validated by its predictive power. It is associated with the presence of brain changes and genetic inheritance, as well as treatment response and prognosis [1]. The historical evolution of the concept is described by Taylor [2]; it began with the idea that some behavioural problems in children arose, not from social and familial adversity, but from subtle changes in brain development. Nowadays, however, the definition comes from specific and observable behaviour traits without assumption of cause. 'Attention Deficit/Hyperactivity Disorder' (ADHD) in DSM-5 [3] and 'Hyperkinetic Disorder' in ICD-10 [4] describe a constellation of *overactivity, impulsivity*, and *inattentiveness*.

These core problems often coexist with other difficulties of learning, behaviour, or mental life, and the coexisting problems may dominate the presentation. This coexistence, to the psychopathologist, emphasizes the multi-faceted nature of the disorder; to the sociologist, a doubt about whether it should be seen as a disorder at all; to the developmentalist, the shifting and context-dependent nature of childhood traits. For clinicians, ADHD symptoms usually need to be disentangled from a complex web of problems. It is worthwhile to do so because of the strong developmental impact of ADHD and the existence of effective treatments. Public controversy continues, but professional practice in most countries makes ADHD one of the most commonly diagnosed problems of child mental health.

## Clinical features

### Hyperactivity

The idea of hyperactivity is an excess of undirected movement. It is not totally dependent on context and cannot be reduced to non-compliance; physical measures of activity level have indicated that it is higher in children with ADHD than in controls, even during

sleep [5]. It is, however, partly dependent upon context—it is often inhibited by a novel environment, creating a pitfall for the inexperienced diagnostician who may exclude it incorrectly because it is not manifest during observation at a first clinic visit. It may not be shown in situations where high activity is expected such as the games field or energetic play. The key situations where it is evident are familiar to the child and where calm is expected, such as visiting family friends, attending church, at mealtimes, during homework, and—often the most troublesome—at school, during class.

### Impulsiveness

Impulsiveness means action without reflection—often described as a failure to 'stop and think'. The term covers premature, unprepared, and poorly timed behaviours—such as interrupting others and giving too little time to appreciate what is involved in a school task or a social situation.

It can also refer to several neuropsychological changes such as failure to inhibit inappropriate responses, aversion to delay, and speed/accuracy tradeoffs. These are indeed more common in children with ADHD and may well underlie some of the observed behaviour changes, but they are not constant and are not part of the diagnosis.

DSM-5 sets out a list of observable behaviours that together define a dimension of hyperactivity–impulsiveness. They can be summarized as:

- Often fidgeting.
- Often leaving seat.
- Often running or climbing inappropriately.
- Often unable to play quietly.
- Often unable to be still when required.
- Often talking excessively.
- Often blurting out answers prematurely.
- Often having difficulty in waiting.
- Often interrupting or intruding on others.

Six of these nine problems need to be present—or five of them for people aged over 17—as a criterion for the diagnosis. Experienced clinicians will sometimes find it infeasible, or even misleading, to make a pedantic count and may be guided by the overall impression of an unmistakeable deviation from what is expected for an individual of given chronological and developmental age.

## Inattentiveness

Inattentiveness means disorganized and forgetful behaviour—short-sequence activities, changing before they are completed, with lack of attention to detail and failure to correct mistakes. These are behavioural observations, not psychological constructs. On a cognitive level, 'attention deficit' is not always an accurate description; the performance of affected children does not always fade with time on a task any more than that of ordinary people, and the presence of irrelevant information ('distractors') does not necessarily worsen their performance disproportionately to that of other people [6]. Cognitive changes of several kinds are indeed seen more frequently than in typically developing people. These changes go beyond attention and executive function [7]; the recognition of inattentiveness depends on descriptions and observations of behaviour, rather than on tests of performance.

DSM-5 provides a list of nine possible features that are often present to excess. They can be summarized briefly as:

- Lack of close attention to details; careless mistakes.
- Difficulty in sustaining attention on tasks or play.
- Not listening when spoken to.
- Not following instructions or finishing tasks.
- Difficulty organizing tasks and activities.
- Avoiding tasks that require effort.
- Losing things that are needed for activities.
- Distractible by outside stimuli.
- Forgetfulness in daily activities.

Six of the problems should be present for the full diagnosis (or five in adult life). Care is needed to avoid confusion with oppositional behaviour. For example, 'not following instructions' is intended to imply that instructions are forgotten or not attended to, but the behaviour can also be shown for reasons of wilfulness and defiance. Careful description, or witnessing the behaviours complained of, is necessary to identify the quality of disorganization. The recognition of the disability therefore needs an experienced professional. The diagnostician also needs to recognize that the behaviours can be modified by the context. Tasks with a strong incentive, or that are inherently rewarding and engaging, may well elicit a much improved performance. Good focus on a shoot-em-up computer game, or good self-control at the first visit to the office, should not be taken to exclude the diagnosis.

## Further requirements for diagnosis

### Developmental inappropriateness

Inattention and impulsive over-activity both need to be judged in terms of what is clearly excessive for the individual's developmental level. Either is sufficient for a diagnosis; when both are present, then the combination should be noted. In the previous version of DSM-IV, there was an expectation that predominantly inattentive, predominantly impulsive, and mixed subtypes should be distinguished. A longitudinal study, however, has found that they do not behave as subtypes over time—one tends to turn into another. They are,

accordingly, now referred to only as 'presentations'. Nevertheless, clinical experience suggests that there are important differences in children who are not just 'predominantly', but *exclusively*, inattentive. Dreamy children, who are sluggish, rather than excitable, in temperament can still have enough problems in their attention that their education is seriously compromised. They will need much more focus on educational progress, and less on risk for antisocial development, than their disruptive contemporaries—and indeed much more psychological research than has yet been forthcoming.

### Pervasiveness and persistence

Pervasiveness across situations and over time is another important part of the clinical picture. One is trying to identify a trait in the person, not simply a quality of the environment that elicits restlessness. The extent of pervasiveness is the main distinction between the DSM-5 definition of ADHD and the ICD-10 definition (currently under revision) of hyperkinetic disorder (HKD). The latter specifies that all three of the cardinal features—impulsiveness, over-activity, and inattentiveness—should be present, pervasively and persistently, across home, school, or work, and in other situations. HKD is therefore, in effect, a subtype of ADHD [8].

### Disability

Impairment in social, academic, or occupational functioning is also a necessary condition for the full diagnosis. The necessity for this is somewhat controversial. The extent to which the features of ADHD impose a disability is very variable. Careful parents and responsive teachers can help a child to achieve their potential, in spite of the struggle to focus and self-organize. Conversely, a highly academic school may impose demands for achievement that entail a real disability for children who have only minor difficulties in concentrating. Furthermore, in comorbid cases, it can be hard to tell whether the impairment is due to the ADHD itself or to the coexisting difficulties (see Associated features, p. 302).

The level of impairment of function that is required for the diagnosis accounts for a good deal of the great variation in prevalence between different studies and different places [9] (see Chapter 33). A full assessment will separate caseness and impairment, and accept both as important in making the formulation and clinical plan.

## Associated features

Many other behavioural changes characterize some children with ADHD. They are, for instance, often irritable and their emotions can flash very rapidly when provoked. They may sleep badly (and this, in turn, can contribute to poor concentration). They can be aggressive to other people and non-compliant to authority. They can also be charming, humorous, inquisitive, and intuitive. None of these, however, are either constant in ADHD or confined to those with ADHD. They are worth noting, but they do not make the diagnosis.

## Modifying features

Inattention and impulsive over-activity both need to be assessed in light of the effects of age, gender, and developmental level.

## The first 3 years

A 'difficult temperament' in early childhood includes over-activity and poor self-regulation and can have a harmful effect on parent–child relationships. Some children do indeed present a whirlwind of activity, but the normal range is very great and the concept of inattentiveness is hard to apply at this age. The exploration of the world by toddlers is typically short-lived, but intense. A diagnosis of ADHD would be insecure.

## Age 3–6 years

ADHD behaviours are clearly recognizable by this age, and there is a strong likelihood of persistence into the school years [10]. It can still be difficult to distinguish between behaviour problems at home resulting from impulsiveness and those from headstrongness and anger. The presence or absence of inattentiveness is therefore important for diagnosis, but the issue is often not pressing because parent training is an effective intervention for behaviour problems at home and should be available for parents with children at risk, without waiting for a formal diagnosis.

## Age 7–11 years

Attention span increases during the early school years, and most children with ADHD will be able to sustain interest for some 3 minutes—more, if the activity is unusually attractive. Hyperactivity is reflected in running and climbing in situations that expect calm. School and peer demands make ADHD behaviours impairing; the tolerance of families and culture at large help to determine whether ADHD is seen as a problem, and this is a very common age for referral and diagnosis. Hyperactivity (as opposed to inattentiveness alone) becomes important in generating aggressive and antisocial behaviour and delinquency. The extent to which there is a poor social outcome depends upon both genetic and environmental influences [11], including gene–environment interactions such as that found in a study in which a catechol-O-methyltransferase (COMT) gene polymorphism, together with low birthweight, predicted the development of antisocial symptoms in those with ADHD [12].

## Age 12–18 years

During adolescence, there is maturing in the abilities of self-control. Attention span may well have risen to 10 minutes at a time, but the demands of classrooms will typically expect much more. Academic failure becomes increasingly salient in the young people's lives. Hyperactivity may now be reflected only in fidgeting and a strong feeling of a need to be 'up and away'. Emotions can become unregulated in most teenagers, but especially so in those with ADHD. Some children with ADHD will become more reflective, but the demands for self-control rise as well, and so the young people still tend to be more impulsive and inattentive than their peers. Indeed, even those who had never been clinically diagnosed or referred for help were still four times as likely to merit a psychiatric diagnosis by the time they were 17 years old in a longitudinal population study [13]. Those who continue to show hyperactivity are at increased risk for other problems, notably aggressive and antisocial behaviour, delinquency, and motor traffic accidents. Substance misuse may be appearing, largely attributable to coexisting problems of conduct and social dysfunction.

## Adult life

By adult life, most will no longer meet full diagnostic criteria for ADHD, but most will retain some functional impairment related to hyperactivity and the impairment is present at lower levels of the number of criteria than is the case in chidhood [14]. DSM-5 therefore adjusted the number of symptoms expected for diagnosis, from six to five. Inattention may now be reflected in incomplete assignments, procrastination, and mind-wandering. Over-activity may be confined to an inner feeling of restlessness. Impulsiveness may now be a matter of recklessness and poor decision-making. Emotional lability is often a major part of the presentation and is closely linked to the level of the ADHD problems themselves [15].

There is also an expectation that the symptoms should have started in childhood, that is, before the age of 12 years. They may well not have been diagnosed at the time, and indeed they may not even have been impairing. Bright children may have been able to achieve satisfactory academic progress, and those without significant oppositional problems may well have fitted harmoniously into family life. ADHD features may only have become impairing when adult life presented greater demands for responsibility and scheduling. Recent research from a longitudinally studied cohort has identified adults who presented ADHD features but did not show them when they were studied in their childhood [16]. These 'adult-onset' people were different from those whose ADHD had been continuous throughout development, in ways that cast doubt on whether they could be considered as showing a neurodevelopmental disorder—they were less likely to have affected family members and cognitive deficits, and more likely to have used cannabis and other drugs.

A key difficulty in current knowledge is that of making an accurate diagnosis when adults present for the first time [17]. Adults may be mistaken in their recall of their childhoods, and the subjective aspects of their condition may be rather different from those that other people observe. The account of somebody who knows the patient well—perhaps a spouse or a work partner—is very desirable but does, of course, need interpreting in light of their own interests in a diagnosis. People who knew the individual as a child can be very helpful informants, for example through a telephone interview, and there may be school records available. Simply the giving of a diagnosis comes as a relief to some who have puzzled over the reasons for their failures and can liberate problem-solving approaches

## Gender

Females are less likely than males to be rated as over-active, impulsive, or inattentive during childhood. The ratio is usually about 2–3:1 in population surveys, and those girls who are affected are no less likely than affected males to become impaired in social and academic functioning [18]. Diagnostic rates in series of children referred to clinics usually yield much wider ratios, and it may well be that boys are preferentially identified in the community as needing help. Affected girls are often more troubled by inattention than over-activity and may often suffer more than boys from impairment of peer relationships. In current knowledge, the same criteria should be applied to both genders. Clinicians, however, should guard against dismissing girls who are not disruptive as being unaffected by ADHD.

## Developmental level

The diagnosis should only be made when the problems are out of keeping with the developmental level. Intellectual disability is very likely to include problems of concentration. Psychometric assessment is therefore advised before assuming that attentiveness is disproportionately affected in such cases or that this deficit is responsible for poor achievement. Over-activity/impulsiveness is usually assessed with reference to what would be expected in a typically developing child whose chronological age would correspond to the developmental age of the child being assessed. The validity of this approach deserves the attention of researchers.

## Diagnostic problems

Description of the symptoms makes them sound easy to recognize, and indeed the problems are usually very salient, disruptive to other people, and common causes of referral to health and special education services. Nevertheless, there are pitfalls in the diagnosis, making it necessary for a specialist assessment to be undertaken before the diagnosis is given.

### Differentiation from normality

The behaviours of ADHD are continuously distributed in the population (see Chapter 33). The level that is considered normal or acceptable will vary from one culture to another and from one rater to another. To be diagnosed, it should be excessive not only for the child's age but also for the developmental level, present across situations and time, and giving rise to significant distress or dysfunction.

### Confusion of cardinal and associated features

Many behavioural problems—such as temper tantrums, sleeplessness, aggression, and disobedience to adult authority—are common in children with ADHD and may be the key reasons for presentation. It is easy to make the mistake of diagnosing ADHD when only disruptive behaviour is present. Some of the confusion comes from the ambiguity of 'impulsiveness'. Behaviours, such as calling out in class and interrupting others, can indeed come from a difficulty in holding oneself back, but they can also represent deliberate flouting of the rules. Direct observation can usually make the distinction—watching either the children tackling tasks requiring them to stop and think in the clinic or their natural behaviour in the classroom. Inattentive behaviour also helps to make the diagnosis of ADHD and is less confounded by oppositionality.

### Reliance on non-expert judgements

Judgements about whether behaviours occur 'often' and are atypical demand considerable familiarity with the usual range of variation. The diagnostician will acquire this in the course of training and experience; experienced teachers will be excellent judges, but inexperienced or overstressed parents may identify the problems at a low level of hyperactive behaviour or suppose that an abnormal level is only to be expected in childhood. It is usually helpful to obtain a detailed behavioural account, rather than rely on an overall judgment of 'over-activity' or 'failure to concentrate'.

Contradiction between sources may occur and lead to arguments between parents and teachers. This may be due to different expectations, the emotional relationship of raters with the child, or children behaving very differently in contexts that vary in the demands placed on the children. The clinician needs to understand the full context of the way involved adults describe the child.

### Difficulties in recognition in the presence of coexisting problems

It is commonplace for children whose problems meet the criteria for ADHD to show other patterns of disturbance as well. This is often, confusingly, called 'comorbidity'—confusing because it implies that the other pattern is a distinct disorder, which is only one of the explanations for coexisting problems. Clinicians need to understand the relationships for two reasons, so that they do not make or miss the diagnosis of ADHD and so that they can make good strategies for treating ADHD in the presence of other disorders and other disorders in the presence of ADHD.

#### Conduct and oppositional disorders

The most common association, and the best researched, is with conduct and oppositional disorders. Nearly half the children with hyperactive behaviour in a community survey showed high levels of defiant and aggressive conduct as well, but the associations of the two problems were different, with hyperactivity (but not conduct problems) being associated with delays in motor and language development [19]. When both ADHD and conduct problems were present, the combined condition ('hyperkinetic conduct disorder' in ICD-10) showed the associations of both disorders. ADHD is therefore not to be diagnosed by the absence of conduct disorder features, but by the clear presence of the core problems of inattentiveness and disorganization.

#### Tourette's disorder and multiple tics

A different kind of differential is presented by children with Tourette's disorder. Their motor restlessness may indeed represent the coexistence of ADHD but can result directly from tics. If a child's tics are very frequent and numerous, then their repetitive and stereotyped nature may not be apparent and they may be seen simply as restless fidgetiness. Again, direct observation of the pattern of over-activity is the key. When there is doubt, filming the child and subsequent slow-motion review may make repetitive patterns evident.

#### Autism spectrum disorders

Children with autism have clear and characteristic impairments of language, communication, and social development. Spectrum disorders, however, can raise diagnostic challenges. Children with ADHD alone often show language delays (usually of an expressive nature with oversimple utterances, by contrast with the receptive difficulties and idiosyncratic patterns of autism). Their attention difficulties may make them unresponsive to the overtures of others in a way that can simulate the social obliviousness of people in the spectrum of autism, and they are often friendless—not because of lack of interest in others, but because of the capacity of hyperactive behaviour to irritate other people. Indeed, attention problems can extend to perseveration on certain activities, such as video games, which may be mistaken for the restricted interests of autism. All these factors can lead to ADHD being mistaken for autism, but the reverse can happen too. There are other reasons for over-active behaviour in autism. Firstly, stereotyped patterns of driven over-activity can be seen; they are not disorganized or impulsiveness and are often made worse by change and novelty (which usually reduce the over-activity of ADHD). Secondly, episodic bursts of extreme activity can be seen and may be best regarded and treated as catatonic. Thirdly, akathisia may result from neuroleptic medication, or irritable restlessness from anticonvulsants, and it will be necessary to establish a clear history that ADHD has been a persistent trait.

### Attachment disorders

Reactive attachment disorder (RAD) may share with ADHD a disinhibited style of relating to other people (an unreserved, but shallow, making of social contact). Children with RAD, however, tend to be controlling rather than disorganized, and vigilant rather than inattentive, and inattention and impulsiveness are not cardinal features of RAD—so it is not difficult to recognize both patterns when present in an individual child. The confusion in practice often comes from theoretical misconceptions. Those caring for neglected or abandoned children may consider that the diagnosis of ADHD cannot be accurate because the cause of the children's problems is clearly to be found in their early deprivation. The causal pathway may indeed be that of neglect (though genetic inheritance and fetal damage also need considering); but ADHD is a descriptive category, not an explanatory one. If the pattern of ADHD is present, it still needs recognizing—not least because the cause of the ADHD behaviour does not seem to determine the response to stimulant medication and children who have encountered neglect or abnormal early attachment may still have their ADHD problems reduced by medication.

### Bipolar disorders

Both ADHD and manic conditions are characterized by over-activity, overtalkativeness, a sensation of whirling thoughts, and often irritable mood. The distinction is made by the presence in bipolar disorder of episodicity, euphoria, and grandiosity.

In all these differential diagnoses, the principle is to establish that the individual shows not only over-active or inattentive behaviour, but also the specific pattern of ADHD. Experienced judgement may be required, and the practice of diagnosing on the basis of questionnaire scores alone carries risks of both overidentification and missing cases.

In adult life, there are still more possibilities for misdiagnosis. The most common reasons for uncertainty are in distinguishing from atypical bipolar disorder and the effects of substance misuse. 'Personality disorder' is sometimes applied, and indeed ADHD shares with personality disorders a long-standing trait quality but can also be a more precise way of describing the difficulties presented. Differentiation from the normal range of variation can be difficult in the absence of clear standards. The task of the diagnostician is harder when adults are presenting for the first time if only self-report is available; the self-description of hyperactivity may be a form of self-depreciation.

## Methods of recognition

### Rating scales

Questionnaire ratings by parents or teachers are very useful for screening purposes and monitoring interventions. Many are available; the most famous are those from Conners which yield several different scoring systems [20], derivatives such as the Iowa Conners, and the Strengths and Weaknesses of ADHD-symptoms and Normal-behavior (SWAN) and Swanson, Nolan, and Pelham (SNAP) scales [21]. Other scales were developed directly from the DSM criteria such as the ADHD Rating Scale [22] and the Vanderbilt ADHD Rating Scale [23]. Furthermore, several general-purpose scales include subscales comprising problems of over-activity and inattention such as the widely used Child Behavior Problems Checklist (CBCL) [24] and the Strengths and Difficulties Questionnaire (SDQ) [25]. They are particularly suitable for initial screening and triage. Free access from the Internet is available for SNAP-IV and SWAN (http://www.myadhd.com/snap-iv-6160-18sampl.html) and SDQ (http://www.sdqinfo.org).

Many of these rating scales have similar strengths and weaknesses [26]. In group studies, they give a reasonably good discrimination between people with a clinical diagnosis of ADHD and controls from the ordinary population, with an effect size of about two standard deviations, implying a substantial overlap. This discrimination is probably somewhat better for the special-purpose ADHD scales than for the general-purpose scales. Test–retest reliability is typically around 0.7; all are sensitive to the effects of medication. Agreement between teachers and parents is typically rather low. The SWAN scale was developed with a wider range of scores for each item (including both 'far above average' and 'far below average')—so it will yield a more Gaussian distribution in a population survey than most other instruments. All scales, used as a population screen, leave a fair number of individuals misclassified and are liable to many false positives. The questionnaires are best seen as a first stage of screening, not as defining casehood.

For adults, a variety of self-report measures have been developed and are reviewed by Davidson [27]. The Wender Utah scales were particularly important in the early conceptualization of adult ADHD [28], but—like other rating scales—they tend to overidentify. An Adult ADHD Self-Report Scale (ASRS-v1.1) [29] is a symptom checklist developed for the WHO. It can be downloaded from: http://www.caddra.ca/pdfs/Guidelines_ENG_ChangesJuly2012.pdf

### Informant interview

A detailed interview with parents (or other main caregivers) is the most informative single method for assessing children and adolescents. The aim is to go beyond their overall ratings of problems to an understanding of what actual behaviours are the basis for ratings. It is helpful to obtain a description of key situations such as getting ready for school, playing with toys, drawing, mealtimes, homework, and family excursions. Parents will usually have very good recall of attention and activity control, even if their knowledge about the normal range is limited. Professional judgement can then be applied to whether those descriptions indicate abnormality of development.

Standardized interview schedules are also available. Some are highly structured and can be delivered by non-clinicians such as the Diagnostic Interview Schedule for Children (DISC) [30]. Others are more interactive, can be delivered flexibly, and expect the interviewer, rather than the respondent, to be the specifier of what is rated (as described previously). Examples of these 'semi-structured' instruments would be the Child and Adolescent Psychiatric Assessment (CAPA) [31] and the Schedule for Affective Disorders and Schizophrenia for School Age Children (K-SADS) [32]. They are time-consuming, sometimes too much so for routine clinical practice, but can ensure a full cover of salient features.

Interviewing should, of course, go beyond the making of a single diagnosis. It should include other problems, social and intellectual development, emotional life, and any physical problems. It can also be helpful—when possible—to interview teachers, not only to gain a full impression of the child in the classroom, but also to be seen to do so lest teachers form the impression of a less-than-comprehensive evaluation.

### Psychiatric interview

Interview with the child is valuable for the observation of attention and social interaction that it yields, and for understanding a child's view of their predicament. Children, however, are not good witnesses about their own concentration and impulse control, and even affected adults are not good at describing themselves in these terms. The experience of ADHD is usually one of suffering the reactions evoked from other people, or one of repeated failure. Adults often describe an experience of whirling and interrupted thoughts (in the absence of manic features), and some children will say the same, especially if treatment has enabled them to make a comparison with another way of being.

### Observation

Direct observation of the child in the clinic, or during psychometric testing, can give a vivid idea of the nature of their problems in attending. Do they take time to appreciate what they are being asked to do? Is the tempo of their activity increased? Can they slow down when asked? Are they distracted by the setting? Do they complete tasks or play activities? Similarly, observation of play and task performance in natural settings can be valuable in confirming or qualifying the accounts of informants. The effect of the presence of the observer needs to be taken into account in making judgements.

### Investigations

Assessment needs not only to distinguish ADHD from related disorders, but also to consider whether the ADHD pattern may result from remediable causes. The anamnestic history is by far the most productive investigation. It should include whether hearing problems have been excluded by previous testing (and if not, an expert assessment should be arranged), and any injuries or diseases potentially damaging to the brain. The strengths and weaknesses of the family environment need to be assessed; they may dictate the choices of treatment. Physical examination should be sufficient to detect congenital anomalies, skin lesions, and motor abnormalities that can be the pointers to a neurological cause. Psychometric assessment is desirable whenever there are problems at school, both to generate an idea of developmental level against which the 'developmental inappropriateness' of behavioural symptoms can be judged and to detect barriers to learning that may be the reason for inattentiveness. Special physical investigations are not routinely necessary. EEG often yields evidence of immaturity, but this does not advance assessment much and is not routinely indicated. It is valuable in the investigation of epilepsy and in the rare cases when deterioration of function suggests the possibility of a degenerative disorder. Blood tests should be planned only on the basis of history and examination but may include tests of thyroid function, lead (in high-lead areas), chromosomal integrity (including fragile-X probe) when there is

other evidence of developmental delay, and specific DNA tests when there is clinical suspicion of a phenotype such as that of Williams syndrome.

## Communicating the diagnosis

Unlike most psychiatric conditions, a diagnosis of ADHD is often sought by parents and welcomed by them. Its image of being a physically caused neurological disease is often perceived as a relief from the stigma of mental disorder. On the other hand, the media controversy over whether it is a 'real' disorder and over the use of controlled drugs leaves some parents confused and fearful.

Assessment on the principles described will have led to an individual formulation of the nature and causes of the impairment. Extended explanation is worthwhile in the longer term. An oversimple description in terms of a chemical deficiency in the brain may seem a useful starting point but can lead to unrealistic expectations for treatment and frustration with the doctor or, worse, with the child. A model of chronic disability is in keeping with the evidence from longitudinal studies but needs to be modulated by the good outcome for some children, the improvement for most, and the ability of warm and encouraging parenting to reduce the risks for antisocial behaviour in later childhood and adolescence.

Children's understanding of their problems is also worth a good deal of effort. Little research has so far addressed the issue, but it is important to their ability to cope. They need to know that their problem is understood, that treatments are available, that they can influence their outcome by their own actions, and that the people around them understand all this and can be encouraging. Positive role models are useful—some successful sports stars, performers, politicians, and business people have outed themselves as having, and sometimes using, ADHD. Explanations need to be repeated, as the young people mature and expect a fuller and more interactive discussion.

Explanation is often needed by teachers as well. They may need to revise their expectations of the level of challenge with which the child can cope, and for some, frustration can lead to antagonism towards the child's family. If they already see ADHD as a neurological disease, then the frequent observations of changeability in the children and of the ability to cope sometimes with difficult tasks may make them reject a neurological cause—and, with it, the diagnosis and validity of drug treatment. They may need to know that physical and psychological factors can both enter into the child's presentation and that the effect of medication does not depend on the aetiology.

Explanation often leads on to basic advice about helping the children's development. The first steps with parents are to establish whether there is already a framework of frequent warm interactions and effective ways of giving instructions and following up children's actions with consistent patterns of reward or loss of reward. If this does not already exist, then a parent training group is often helpful. Both a supportive atmosphere and the teaching of skills in behaviour modification seem to be necessary. The target behaviours for modification are often the ones most troublesome to parents—disobedience and aggression—rather than restlessness or inattentiveness specifically.

Liaison with schools should include advice on the severity of the problem and the intensity and nature of extra help that will be required. Teachers will often be able to share good practice in classroom management. One of the principles is to maintain good stimulus control, for instance by having the affected child at the front of the class under the teacher's eye. Another is to find opportunities for the children to let off physical energy (they can sometimes be used as messengers between classrooms) and to learn in short chunks. Variety and interest in the material to be learnt or understood are useful. Transitions between activities in the classroom are often the time for children to become disorganized, and the child with ADHD should be the first to change activity, with the teacher's supervision. Individual attention is probably the most effective resource in the classroom, but it is also very demanding—a classroom assistant may help to achieve it. Star charts for younger children and token economy systems for older ones are often recommended but usually depend upon the system used for the rest of the class.

In summary, this section has presented a picture of ADHD and a severe form—HKD—as disabilities that change with development and are often accompanied by other problems that can mask it or themselves be masked by it. They are rewarding challenges for diagnosis and treatment in adulthood, as well as during childhood and adolescence.

## REFERENCES

1. National Institute for Health and Care Excellence. *Attention Deficit Hyperactivity Disorder: diagnosis and management.* https://www.nice.org.uk/guidance/CG72; 2008.
2. Taylor E. Antecedents of ADHD: a historical account of diagnostic concepts. ADHD Attention Deficit and Hyperactivity Disorders. 2011;3(2):69–75.
3. American Psychiatric Association. *Diagnostic and statistical manual of mental disorders (DSM-5®).* Washington DC: American Psychiatric Association; 2013.
4. World Health Organization. *The ICD-10 classification of mental and behavioural disorders: clinical descriptions and diagnostic guidelines.* Geneva: World Health Organization; 1992.
5. Porrino LJ, Rapoport JL, Behar D, Sceery W, Ismond DR, Bunney Jr WE. A naturalistic assessment of the motor activity of hyperactive boys: I. Comparison with normal controls. Archives of General Psychiatry. 1983;40(6):681.
6. Sonuga-Barke EJ, Halperin JM. Developmental phenotypes and causal pathways in attention deficit/hyperactivity disorder: potential targets for early intervention? Journal of Child Psychology and Psychiatry. 2010;51(4):368–89.
7. Castellanos FX, Sonuga-Barke EJ, Milham MP, Tannock R. Characterizing cognition in ADHD: beyond executive dysfunction. Trends in cognitive sciences. 2006;10(3):117–23.
8. Santosh PJ, Taylor E, Swanson J, et al. Refining the diagnoses of inattention and overactivity syndromes: A reanalysis of the Multimodal Treatment study of attention deficit hyperactivity disorder (ADHD) based on ICD-10 criteria for hyperkinetic disorder. Clinical Neuroscience Research. 2005;5(5):307–14.
9. Willcutt EG. The prevalence of DSM-IV attention-deficit/hyperactivity disorder: a meta-analytic review. Neurotherapeutics. 2012;9(3):490–9.
10. Lahey BB, Pelham WE, Loney J, et al. Three-year predictive validity of DSM-IV attention deficit hyperactivity disorder in children diagnosed at 4–6 years of age. American Journal of Psychiatry. 2004;161:2014–20.
11. Greven CU, Asherson P, Rijsdijk FV, Plomin R. A longitudinal twin study on the association between inattentive and hyperactive-impulsive ADHD symptoms. Journal of Abnormal Child Psychology. 2011;39(5):623–32.
12. Thapar A, Langley K, Fowler T, et al. Catechol O-methyltransferase gene variant and birth weight predict early-onset antisocial behavior in children with attention-deficit/hyperactivity disorder. Archives of General Psychiatry. 2005;62(11):1275–8.
13. Taylor E, Chadwick O, Heptinstall E, Danckaerts M. Hyperactivity and conduct problems as risk factors for adolescent development. Journal of the American Academy of Child and Adolescent Psychiatry. 1996;35(9):1213–26.
14. McGough JJ, Barkley RA. Diagnostic controversies in adult attention deficit hyperactivity disorder. American Journal of Psychiatry. 2004;161(11):1948–56.
15. Skirrow C, Asherson P. Emotional lability, comorbidity and impairment in adults with attention-deficit hyperactivity disorder. Journal of Affective Disorders. 2013;147(1):80–6.
16. Moffitt TE, Houts R, Asherson P, et al. Is adult ADHD a childhood-onset neurodevelopmental disorder? Evidence from a four-decade longitudinal cohort study. American Journal of Psychiatry. 2015: 172(10): 967–77.
17. Asherson P. Clinical assessment and treatment of attention deficit hyperactivity disorder in adults. Expert review of neurotherapeutics. 2005;5(4):525–39.
18. Young S, Heptinstall E, Sonuga-Barke EJ, Chadwick O, Taylor E. The adolescent outcome of hyperactive girls: self-report of psychosocial status. Journal of Child Psychology and Psychiatry. 2005;46(3):255–62.
19. Taylor E, Sandberg S, Thorley G. *The epidemiology of childhood hyperactivity.* New York, NY: Oxford University Press; 1991.
20. Conners, CK. *Conners' Rating Scales*, 3rd edition. Toronto: Multi Health Systems; 2008.
21. Swanson JM, Schuck S, Porter MM, et al. Categorical and Dimensional Definitions and Evaluations of Symptoms of ADHD: History of the SNAP and the SWAN Rating Scales. International Journal of Educational and Psychological Assessment. 2012;10(1):51.
22. DuPaul GJ. Parent and teacher ratings of ADHD symptoms: Psychometric properties in a community-based sample. Journal of Clinical Child and Adolescent Psychology. 1991;20(3):245–53.
23. Bard DE, Wolraich ML, Neas B, Doffing M, Beck L. The psychometric properties of the Vanderbilt attention-deficit hyperactivity disorder diagnostic parent rating scale in a community population. Journal of Developmental and Behavioral Pediatrics. 2013;34(2):72–82.
24. Achenbach TM, Ruffle TM. The Child Behavior Checklist and related forms for assessing behavioral/emotional problems and competencies. Pediatrics in Review. 2000;21(8):265–71.
25. Goodman R. The Strengths and Difficulties Questionnaire: a research note. Journal of Child Psychology and Psychiatry. 1997;38(5):581–6.
26. Burns GL, Walsh JA, Servera M, Lorenzo-Seva U, Cardo E, Rodríguez-Fornells A. Construct validity of ADHD/ODD rating scales: recommendations for the evaluation of forthcoming DSM-V ADHD/ODD scales. Journal of Abnormal Child Psychology. 2013;41(1):15–26.
27. Davidson MA. ADHD in adults: a review of the literature. Journal of Attention Disorders. 2008;11(6):628–41.

28. McCann BS, Scheele L, Ward N, Roy-Byrne P. Discriminant validity of the Wender Utah Rating Scale for attention-deficit/hyperactivity disorder in adults. Journal of Neuropsychiatry and Clinical Neurosciences. 2000;12:240–5.

29. Adler LA, Kessler RC, Spencer T. *Adult ADHD Self-Report Scale-v1.1 (ASRS-v1.1) Symptom Checklist*. Geneva: World Health Organization; 2003.

30. Shaffer D, Fisher P, Lucas CP, Dulcan MK, Schwab-Stone ME. NIMH Diagnostic Interview Schedule for Children Version IV (NIMH DISC-IV): description, differences from previous versions, and reliability of some common diagnoses. Journal of the American Academy of Child and Adolescent Psychiatry. 2000;39(1):28–38.

31. Angold A, Costello EJ. The child and adolescent psychiatric assessment (CAPA). Journal of the American Academy of Child and Adolescent Psychiatry. 2000;39(1):39–48.

32. Ambrosini PJ. Historical development and present status of the schedule for affective disorders and schizophrenia for school-age children (K-SADS). Journal of the American Academy of Child and Adolescent Psychiatry. 2000;39(1):49–58.

# 32

# Basic mechanisms and treatment planning/targets for attention-deficit/hyperactivity disorder

*Barbara Franke and Jan K. Buitelaar*

## Introduction to ADHD biology

Although the first description of an ADHD-like disorder dates back nearly 250 years to 1775 [1], the aetiology of ADHD and the basic mechanisms underlying the disorder are still relatively poorly understood. Hypotheses about mechanisms have been defined at different levels, including cognitive, neurophysiologic, and molecular theories and models.

### Cognitive functioning in ADHD

As explained in Chapter 31, ADHD is a behaviourally defined disorder. However, cognitive deficits have been studied as an integral part of it. Individuals with ADHD have, on average, a 7- to 12-point lower IQ than non-ADHD matched controls [2]. This association seems to be partly explained by shared genetic risk factors between ADHD and IQ [2]. Initial theories claimed ADHD to be due to a single core cognitive deficit, for example in sustained attention [3], non-optimal regulation of the energetic state, and selected problems in activation [4], weak inhibitory control, that is, the capacity to voluntarily inhibit or regulate prepotent attentional or behavioural responses [5] or delay aversion and/or altered sensitivity to reward [6]. However, from more recent work in both children and adults, it is clear that ADHD is characterized by deficits in relatively independent cognitive domains, and that there is a large heterogeneity in the cognitive deficits across individual patients (for example, [7, 8]). Executive functioning deficits are seen in visuo-spatial and verbal working memory, inhibitory control, vigilance, and planning. Reward dysregulation in patients with ADHD is reflected in suboptimal and more risky decisions and preference for immediate, compared with delayed, rewards. Other domains impaired in ADHD are temporal information processing and timing, speech and language, memory span, speed processing, response time variability, arousal/activation, and motor control [1]. Although most ADHD patients show deficits in one or two domains, some have no deficits, and very few show deficits in all domains. Attempts to identify subgroups with homogenous cognitive profiles have revealed four cognitive subtypes in a community sample of control children and among subjects with ADHD [9]. This was replicated in a sample of adults with ADHD and adult controls [10]. It supports the view that at least part of ADHD's cognitive heterogeneity is nested within normal variation. It is, however, unclear whether these subtypes predict treatment response or course. It is also unclear whether cognitive deficits cause ADHD symptoms, though cognitive deficits appear to moderate the development of the clinical phenotype [11, 12].

### Neuroimaging findings in ADHD

Chapter 35 summarizes our current understanding of the brain structural and functional correlates of ADHD (see also [1, 13]). Briefly, alterations have been observed in virtually all neuroimaging modalities applied to the study of the ADHD brain, including structural and fMRI, EEG, and MEG. Grey matter structure, both cortical (thickness and surface area) and subcortical (volume), seems to be less affected in adults than in children with ADHD [14, 14a]. In functional activation studies in children with ADHD, hypoactivation relative to comparison subjects was observed mostly in systems involved in executive function (fronto-parietal network) and attention (ventral attentional network). Significant hyperactivation in ADHD relative to comparison subjects was observed predominantly in the default, ventral attention, and somatomotor networks. In adults, ADHD-related hypoactivation was predominant in the fronto-parietal system, while ADHD-related hyperactivation was present in the visual, dorsal attention, and default networks [15]. Most central to the mechanistic models of ADHD are MRI findings showing structural differences between patients with ADHD and normally developing individuals in the basal ganglia, especially the different components of the striatum (for example, [14]) and a potential structural and/or functional dysregulation of fronto-subcortical-cerebellar connections, which are of importance in controlling attention and salience thresholds, motor behaviour, inhibitory control, and response to reward [1, 13].

Atypical brain activity underlying multiple cognitive processes and resting state activity has further been reported in EEG and ERP studies. Abnormal ERP activity has been found in both children and adults with ADHD, in association with attentional allocation, inhibition, response preparation, and error processing [16]. Preparation–vigilance measures were also predictive of remission of ADHD over adolescence into adulthood [16]. Similarly, atypical patterns of quantitative EEG frequency have been observed, mostly as increased power of low-frequency theta activity and/or decreased power of fast beta activity [17]. Excessive theta/beta ratio cannot be considered a reliable diagnostic measure of ADHD but may be useful as a prognostic measure [18].

Importantly, the brain alterations seen in ADHD are heterogenous, with individual patients showing different patterns of alterations and individual neuroimaging findings having very limited effect sizes. As a result, neuroimaging has not found its way into diagnostic protocols for ADHD, nor has it been predictive for treatment planning [19, 20].

## Molecular neurobiology of ADHD

Knowledge about the molecular neurobiology of ADHD has so far largely relied on serendipity and coincidental findings, for example from medication studies and work on animal models. Additional evidence for the involvement of particular pathways comes from genetics as well as first metabolite biomarker studies. For example, a comprehensive meta-analysis of potential biomarkers found several measures, specifically noradrenaline, monoamine oxidase, 3-methoxy-4-hydroxyphenylethylene glycol, and cortisol, to be significantly altered in blood and urine of drug-naïve/drug-free patients with ADHD, compared to healthy individuals [21]. Some of the metabolites were also associated with symptom severity of ADHD and/or the response to ADHD medication.

### Monoaminergic neurotransmission pathways in ADHD

The serendipitous finding that methylphenidate (MPH) treats ADHD symptoms originally directed research into the role of dopaminergic neurotransmission in the aetiology of the disorder. This effort was soon extended to include noradrenaline pathways, given the realization that MPH is not selective to the dopamine synapse, but also blocks noradrenaline transporter function. Later, serotonergic neurotransmission has also been found to be involved.

### Dopamine

The neurotransmitter dopamine is involved in regulation of motor activity and limbic functions, but also in attention and cognition, especially executive functioning [22] and reward processing [23–25]. It is a key contributor to behavioural adaptation and to anticipatory processes necessary for preparing voluntary action following intention [26]. Thus, the function of dopamine maps well onto those domains implicated by the signs and symptoms observed in people with ADHD. Further, dopamine circuit dysfunction has been implicated in ADHD by different experimental evidence [27].

Dopamine-producing cells are localized in the midbrain substantia nigra pars compacta and the ventral tegmental area. From there, three projection pathways can be distinguished: the nigrostriatal pathway, which originates from the substantia nigra and projects to the dorsal striatum (caudate nucleus and putamen); the mesolimbic pathway, which projects from the ventral tegmentum to limbic system structures, in particular the ventral striatum (nucleus accumbens), hippocampus, and amygdala; and the mesocortical pathway also originating in the ventral tegmental area, which projects to the cerebral cortex (the medial prefrontal areas, in particular) [28].

As indicated previously, the dopamine transporter—which is the most important molecule in the regulation of dopamine signalling in most areas of the brain—is the main target of stimulants like MPH and also dexamphetamine, the most frequently used prescription drugs for the treatment of ADHD symptoms. Blockade of the dopamine transporter leads to an increase in dopamine concentration, particularly in parts of the basal ganglia that have the highest expression of the transporter, that is, the striatum [29, 30]. This effect is due to the blockade of the transporter molecule in the case of MPH [31] and due to both transporter blockade and stimulation of dopamine release/block of breakdown through monoamine oxidase in the case of dexamphetamine [32]. The dopamine transporter protein (DAT) and its gene *DAT1* (official name *SLC6A3*) have thus received the most attention in research of mechanisms underlying ADHD. In animal models, knockout of the *DAT1* gene produces elevated dopaminergic tone and hyperactivity in the mouse [33]; the latter is also observed upon knock-down of the dopamine transporter in the fruit fly *Drosophila melanogaster* [34]. The neonatal 6-hydroxy-dopamine lesioned rat model also implicates the dopaminergic system in ADHD-like behaviour [35]. Neuroimaging studies of the dopamine transporter in humans with PET suggest increased dopamine transporter activity in ADHD, compared with healthy individuals [36, 37], and evidence for depressed dopamine signalling has been inferred from alterations in dopamine receptors seen in PET [38]. Disturbed dopamine signalling has also been suggested by findings of genetic studies. Genetic polymorphism in the 3′-regulatory region of the *DAT1* gene has been the subject of most studies. Meta-analyses have supported significant associations of this genetic variation in the gene, albeit different versions of the gene in children and adults with ADHD [39–41]. Furthermore, an analysis of genetic variants in a larger group of genes involved in ADHD suggested an association of this set of genes with the severity of symptoms in children with the disorder [42].

### Noradrenaline

Noradrenaline signalling is intimately linked to the dopamine system because noradrenaline is a downstream product of the metabolism of dopamine. Noradrenaline neurotransmission regulates important higher cognitive functions, such as working memory and inhibitory control, primarily through its projections originating in the locus coeruleus and innervating multiple areas of the cortex, the thalamus, and cerebellum [27]. Innervation of the prefrontal cortex (PFC) by noradrenaline pathways is thought to be particularly important for understanding ADHD. Noradrenaline and dopamine signalling are intimately linked in the PFC, that is, they influence each other in optimizing PFC performance in cognitive tasks [43–45]. A role of noradrenaline in ADHD is implied by the inhibition of the noradrenaline transporter (NET) by MPH and dexamphetamine (in addition to DAT) [27, 44]. Moreover, atomoxetine, a selective NET inhibitor, is effective in the treatment of the cardinal symptoms of ADHD and some of its comorbidities [46, 47], as are several other prescription drugs with noradrenergic, but not dopaminergic, properties, like guanfacine and clonidine [27]. While this is potent evidence that altering noradrenaline signalling can ameliorate the symptoms of ADHD, less evidence is available to link it to ADHD aetiology per se. This may primarily be due to the concentration of research effort on the dopaminergic pathways and the large overlap between dopamine and noradrenaline synthesis and function. No animal models for ADHD based on altering genes involved directly in noradrenaline signalling have yet been described, but many models actually implicate both dopamine and noradrenaline neurotransmission circuits [48]. PET of the NET has been inconclusive, thus far [49]. Genetic studies of a number of noradrenaline receptors and the NET have not produced convincing evidence for the involvement of these genes either [40, 50].

## Serotonin

Serotonin is involved in regulating mood and emotion, and also plays an important role in inhibition, one of the executive cognitive deficits observed in ADHD [51]. The neurons of the raphe nuclei in the midline of the brainstem are the main source of serotonin in the brain. Axons of neurons in the higher raphe nuclei spread out to the entire brain, with strong projections, for example, into the PFC, while axons originating in the lower raphe nuclei project to the cerebellum and spinal cord (see also Chapters 11 and 14). Serotonin signalling is known to affect the regulation of other neurotransmitters, including that of dopamine, which may occur through several mechanisms [52]. Neurotransmission through serotonin was first implicated in ADHD based on paradoxical calming effects of MPH observed in a mouse model lacking DAT [53]; the drug was shown to act by blocking the serotonin transporter in the absence of DAT [54]. Also other animal models with altered serotonin signalling show ADHD-like symptoms and inattention, as well as hyperactivity [51]. In humans, studies have reported reduced levels of peripheral serotonin in patients with ADHD (for example, [55]), but other studies did not find such effects [51]. The exact role of serotonin in ADHD still has to be defined in humans. Serotonin neurotransmission may modulate the severity of ADHD symptoms, rather than being related to ADHD onset [42]. Other theories suggest that it may be the comorbidity, especially with antisocial behaviours (conduct disorder, obsessive–compulsive disorder, aggression) and mood disorders (major depression and/or anxiety), rather than the core symptoms of ADHD, which is influenced by serotonin [51]. Genetic studies of the contribution of the serotonergic system to ADHD have not been fully convincing. However, in a meta-analysis, the serotonin receptor gene HTR1B and the gene encoding the serotonin transporter (SLC6A4, 5-HTT, SERT) have been implicated in the disorder [40].

Gene–environment interactions may explain some of the observed inconsistency across studies, as the effect of stress on ADHD symptoms seems to be influenced by genetic variation in the serotonin transporter gene [56]. A recent analysis of a gene set related to serotonergic neurotransmission suggests that variation in serotonergic genes may be associated with disease severity [42]. Tryptophan depletion, which causes reduction in brain 5-HT synthesis, was associated with increases of aggression, inattention, and impulsivity [51]. A retrospective pilot study on the administration of precursors of serotonin and dopamine led to promising results in 85 children and adolescents with ADHD [57]. However, in spite of this supportive evidence for serotonergic involvement in

ADHD, findings from clinical trials with SNRIs, such as venlafaxine and duloxetine, in adults with ADHD are rather mixed (for review, see [51]).

## Other neurotransmission pathways in ADHD aetiology

### Glutamate

Glutamate is the most abundant excitatory neurotransmitter in the human CNS and is involved in many neuronal functions, including synaptic transmission, neuronal migration, excitability, plasticity, and long-term potentiation [58] (see Chapter 14). The fronto-striatal circuits implicated in impulsivity and compulsivity are notable for their relatively rich glutamatergic receptor density. Glutamatergic projections from the various frontal subregions (orbitofrontal, infralimbic cortex, and prelimbic cortex) to the striatum (and vice versa) play a key role in the regulation of various compulsive behaviours. Glutamate receptor proteins are expressed on the surface of neurons in such a way that they can only be activated from the outside, so glutamate exerts its neurotransmitter function from the extracellular fluid. Glutamate levels are regulated by releasing glutamate to the extracellular fluid and then removing glutamate from it. There are no enzymes located extracellularly that can degrade glutamate, so low extracellular concentrations require active reuptake. Several families of glutamate receptor proteins have been identified and classified as NMDA, AMPA, kainate, and metabotropic receptors [59]. Most, if not all, cells in the nervous system express at least one type of glutamate receptor.

Several candidate genes within the glutamatergic system have been associated with ADHD. For instance, associations have been found for variation in the GRIN2B gene with both inattention and hyperactivity symptoms in ADHD [60]. A genome-wide study investigating rare variants found overrepresentation of variants belonging to the metabotropic glutamate receptor genes in several ADHD cohorts [61]. An analysis of a glutamate gene set showed significant association with the severity of hyperactivity/impulsivity of patients with ADHD [62]. Proton magnetic resonance spectroscopy (MRS) studies suggest a possible increase in Glx (a combination of glutamate, glutamine, and GABA) in the striatum across ADHD, OCD, and ASD, and further, an increased Glx signal in the anterior cingulate cortex in children with ADHD and ASD, but a lower Glx signal in adults with ADHD and ASD. This suggests neurodevelopmental changes in fronto-striatal glutamatergic circuits across the lifespan [63]. Glutamatergic agents, such as memantine, an antagonist of the NMDA receptor, are of potential value in the treatment of impulsivity in children and adolescents, including ADHD [64, 65], but large-scale positive trials have not yet been published.

### Histamine

Histamine is one of the key neurotransmitters regulating arousal and attention. The cell bodies of histamine neurons are found in the posterior hypothalamus, in the tuberomammillary nuclei. From here, these neurons project throughout the brain, including to the cortex, through the medial forebrain bundle. Histamine neurons increase wakefulness and prevent sleep [66]. In addition, histamine is an important agent in (neuro)immune reactions. Interest in the role of histamine in ADHD has resulted from observations that allergies have an increased incidence in people with ADHD. Indeed, a recent meta-analysis showed that children with ADHD are more likely to develop asthma, allergic rhinitis, atopic dermatitis, and allergic conjunctivitis than healthy individuals [67]. Similarly, children with allergies appear to have higher ADHD symptom ratings than non-affected children [68]. The histamine H3 receptor subtype is mainly distributed in the CNS and functions as a presynaptic autoreceptor (that reduces histamine release) and a heteroreceptor (that regulates the release of other neurotransmitters). Histamine H3 receptor antagonists and inverse agonists increase the release of brain histamine and other neurotransmitters. The H3 receptor antagonists have been shown to promote arousal in various species, without the psychomotor activation seen with stimulants [69]. Potent histamine H3 receptor antagonists are currently being developed and tested for the treatment of ADHD [70].

### Nicotinic acetylcholinergic system

Nicotinic acetylcholine receptors are receptor proteins that respond to the neurotransmitter acetylcholine. Nicotinic receptors also respond to drugs, including the nicotinic receptor agonist nicotine. Nicotine use has been associated with improvement in cognition, attention in particular, in different animal species, healthy human volunteers, and patients with ADHD [71–75]. In addition, the nicotinic acetylcholine neurotransmission system is also implicated in ADHD through genetic findings; a large study of copy number variants found duplications of the gene encoding the α7-nicotinic acetylcholine receptor (*CHRNA7*), located in the mutation-prone region on chromosome 15q13.3, to contribute to the risk for the disorder [76]. The nicotinic acetylcholine system may be one of the new targets for the development of alternative drugs for ADHD. Nicotine appears to exert its beneficial effect selectively on behavioural inhibition and delay aversion tasks, which are known to have good discriminant validity in distinguishing subjects with ADHD from controls [75, 77]. Stimulation of neuronal nicotinic acetylcholine receptors by nicotine may be mediated directly via changes of cholinergic neurotransmission and/or by modulating the activity of other neurotransmitters, including dopamine (see Dopamine, p. 310). Trials of nicotinic drugs demonstrated beneficial effects in adults with ADHD, with evidence for positive effects on cognitive and emotional domains [78]. There are no approved medications yet for ADHD that target nicotinic acetylcholine receptor function.

### The genetic architecture of ADHD

ADHD is a highly heritable disorder, both in children and in adults, with heritability estimates of around 60–80%, based on twin studies [79, 80]. As discussed in Chapter 34, the genetic architecture of ADHD is complex and multifactorial, such that most patients probably carry many genetic risk factors, which are individually of small effect size. Importantly, twin studies as well as molecular genetic studies suggest that there is incomplete overlap between the genetic factors that are involved in ADHD onset and those that are relevant for the persistence of ADHD across adolescence into adulthood [39, 81–83]. Genetic studies can be an ideal starting point to understand the molecular and cellular processes involved in a disease. As for other disorders, genetic approaches include hypothesis-based candidate gene approaches and hypothesis-free genome-wide studies [84]. The first candidate gene-based studies for ADHD, dating back to the 1980s, mainly concentrated on genes related to monoaminergic neurotransmission, based on information on the drugs effective in treating ADHD symptoms described in previous paragraphs [1, 79].

Genome-wide association studies [50] and genome sequencing are now becoming available in increasingly large samples and will eventually allow new hypotheses regarding the basic biological mechanisms of the disorder [1, 84, 85].

### The role of the environment

The behaviour of any individual develops from an interplay of nature and nurture; neither genetic nor environmental factors are likely to act in isolation [86]. Different forms of gene–environment interplay (see review in [87]) and gene–environment correlation [88–91] are relevant to ADHD and are also described in Chapter 34. Environmental factors known to increase ADHD risk and/or disease severity and persistence include pre-/perinatal as well as postnatal factors (for example, [1]). Exposures occurring *in utero* and in the early years of life, which are major windows of developmental vulnerability, have the strongest effects on ADHD. The brain is then growing at maximal speed, and the blood–brain barrier provides only partial protection against the entry of substances into the CNS [92]. Prenatal exposures to neurotoxicants, such as organic solvents, pesticides, and flame retardants [93–95], as well as the heavy metals zinc and lead [21], are linked to ADHD. Additional risk from maternal smoking and alcohol use during pregnancy may be partly mediated by genetic factors [96] (see Chapter 34). Postnatally, stressful events like early deprivation [97], harsh parenting practices [88], and composites of early adversity (low social class, marital discord, large family size, paternal criminality, maternal mental disorder, and foster care) [98] are of importance. Particularly informative is a follow-up study of Romanian adoptees, who had experienced severe early deprivation in orphanages during early life prior to adoption. This showed a dose-dependent relationship of the length of deprivation with the risk for development of ADHD-like symptoms [97]. Exposure to increased stress due to negative life events or daily hassles has been shown to exacerbate ADHD core symptoms [56] and may contribute to ADHD persistence. Like genetic risk factors, the effects of any one environmental risk factor are small and, rather than being specific to ADHD, these environmental risks are associated with several psychiatric disorders.

The environmental contribution to ADHD is viewed as an increasingly important target of research, because environmental factors may, in principle, be modifiable, though not always easily in practice. Identification of protective factors is as important as scrutinizing the risk factors, and this may contribute to therapy and prevention in ADHD.

## Mechanistic theories underlying ADHD

Hypotheses about the mechanisms underlying ADHD have been defined at molecular, brain neurophysiologic, and cognitive levels. A number of models have been put forward, based on this work, which aim at vertical integration of the information across these domains of function. We mention the more prominent ones here, although there is insufficient evidence yet as to what the most accurate model is to describe the processes underlying ADHD and how the different models relate to each other. In all of them, dopamine and noradrenaline, in some cases in their relation to glutamate, play a central role. Taking into account the important regulatory activities of the monoaminergic neurotransmitters in glutamate signalling (as

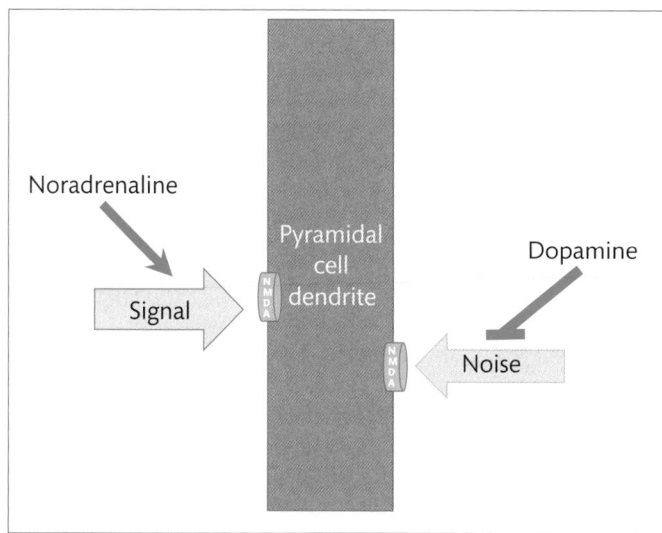

**Fig. 32.1** Dopamine and noradrenaline are important in regulating glutamatergic neurotransmission in cortical neurons. Noradrenaline amplifies signals coming in from other neurons via NMDA-type glutamatergic receptors, while dopamine reduces background noise. In this way, specificity of signalling of the pyramidal neurons is ensured.
Adapted from *J Am Acad Child Adolesc Psychiatry*, 51(4), Arnsten AF, Rubia K, Neurobiological circuits regulating attention, cognitive control, motivation, and emotion: disruptions in neurodevelopmental psychiatric disorders, pp. 356–367, Copyright (2012), with permission from American Academy of Child and Adolescent Psychiatry.

depicted in the schematic in Fig. 32.1 and described in [99]), this is not surprising.

The dynamic developmental model of ADHD was largely based on research on an animal model for ADHD—the spontaneous hypertensive rat. Published by Sagvolden and coworkers in 2005, it supposes low tonic and low phasic dopamine in cortico-striatal loops, resulting in an ineffectiveness to regulate signalling of other neurotransmitter systems. Through the mesolimbic dopaminergic pathway, this is thought to produce altered reinforcement of behaviour and deficient extinction of previously reinforced behaviour, resulting in the rise to delay aversion, development of hyperactivity in novel situations, impulsiveness, deficient sustained attention, increased behavioural variability, and failure to 'inhibit' responses ('disinhibition'). Hypofunction of the mesocortical dopamine pathway is thought to cause attention problems and poor executive functions. Altered nigrostriatal dopamine is linked to impaired modulation of motor functions and deficient non-declarative habit learning and memory [100].

A model for cognitive deficits in ADHD, in which the dopamine and noradrenaline systems and the basal ganglia are central, was proposed by Frank and coworkers, based on computational modelling [101]. They suggested that tonic and phasic dopamine in the striatum is low in people with ADHD and that tonic noradrenaline is high, causing a lowered phasic noradrenaline. According to the model, the lowered dopamine levels should lead to deficits in learning from positive reinforcement. The altered noradrenaline levels may underlie the intra-individual variability observed in people with ADHD. Alterations in the levels dopamine and noradrenaline are viewed as occurring independently [28].

The moderate brain arousal model poses the combination of low tonic with increased phasic dopamine to cause the symptoms of ADHD [102, 103]. This is in contrast to the dynamic developmental model and the basal ganglia model, which suppose both tonic and phasic dopamine to be low in ADHD. The low tonic dopamine results in hypo-arousal when few stimuli are provided to the brain, but also in increased stimulus responsivity of cells in terms of phasic dopamine, resulting in exaggerated responses to environmental stimuli. Since dopamine shows an inverted-U dose–response relationship with performance, both too little and too much dopamine will result in underperformance of the brain, as seen in ADHD [28].

The dopamine transfer theory—a purely theoretical model to explain some of the symptoms of ADHD—supposes that the dopamine response to a reward at the cellular level is normal in people with ADHD, but that it cannot be transferred to a reward-predictive cue due to an insufficient (low) phasic dopamine level [104]. This was hypothesized to result in a delay in the dopamine signal at the level of the cell and the observed reduction of the anticipatory striatal brain activity in people with ADHD [105].

The neuroenergetics model is defined at the cellular level and postulates that neurons function suboptimally in people with ADHD because they cannot adequately recruit lactate from astrocytes [106]. The putative cause is altered noradrenaline and glutamate neurotransmission, which is needed to stimulate astrocytes to release the necessary lactate. Lactate is produced in astrocytes by glycolysis and, after uptake by neurons, is converted into pyruvate and glucose. The astrocyte–neuron lactate transfer shuttle system ensures a supply of substrates for brain metabolism. There is increasing evidence for lactate acting as a signalling molecule in the brain, to link metabolism, substrate availability, blood flow, and neuronal activity [107]. The suboptimal use of the shuttle system is proposed to result in lack of energy, which causes attention drifts, mental fatigue, and response variability, as observed in ADHD.

## Future prospects for novel targets in ADHD

In the coming years, the hypothesis-generating data coming from genome-wide analyses can be expected to identify the mechanisms underlying the disorder; they may also contribute to developing treatment that goes beyond the current approach, which can only dampen the symptoms of the disorder. The first papers implicating novel biological processes and mechanisms in ADHD have now been published. This work has implicated the neurodevelopmental process of neurite outgrowth in the aetiology of the disorder [85]. More recently, integration of genome-wide association studies of common and rare genetic variants found several additional biological processes to be involved, including ligand-gated ion channel activity and oxidative stress-related pathways [108, 109]. Such processes are known to be druggable and thus may represent the first candidates for the development of novel therapeutic approaches. Since the field of genetics research is currently upscaling strongly, more interesting findings can be expected in the coming years. Ultimately, we will need interdisciplinary approaches integrating research across different levels of organismal complexity, including genetics, genomics, and cell- and/or animal-based model systems, as recently discussed in [50], to really understand the biology of ADHD and increase the chances of developing curative treatment options.

## REFERENCES

1. Faraone, S.V., Asherson, P., Banaschewski, T., *et al.* (2015). Attention-deficit/hyperactivity disorder. *Nature Reviews Disease Primers*, 1, 15020.

2. Mill, J., Caspi, A., Williams, B.S., *et al.* (2006). Prediction of heterogeneity in intelligence and adult prognosis by genetic polymorphisms in the dopamine system among children with attention-deficit/hyperactivity disorder: evidence from 2 birth cohorts. *Archives of General Psychiatry*, 63, 462–9.

3. Sykes, D.H., Douglas, V.I., and Morgenstern, G. (1973). Sustained attention in hyperactive children. *Journal of Child Psychology and Psychiatry and Allied Disciplines*, 14, 213–20.

4. Sergeant, J. (2000). The cognitive-energetic model: an empirical approach to attention-deficit hyperactivity disorder. *Neuroscience and Biobehavioral Reviews*, 24, 7–12.

5. Barkley, R.A. (1997). Behavioral inhibition, sustained attention, and executive functions: constructing a unifying theory of ADHD. *Psychological Bulletin*, 121, 65–94.

6. Sonuga-Barke, E.J., Houlberg, K., and Hall, M. (1994). When is 'impulsiveness' not impulsive? The case of hyperactive children's cognitive style. *Journal of Child Psychology and Psychiatry and Allied Disciplines*, 35, 1247–53.

7. Sjowall, D., Roth, L., Lindqvist, S., and Thorell, L.B. (2013). Multiple deficits in ADHD: executive dysfunction, delay aversion, reaction time variability, and emotional deficits. *Journal of Child Psychology and Psychiatry and Allied Disciplines*, 54, 619–27.

8. Sonuga-Barke, E., Bitsakou, P., and Thompson, M. (2010). Beyond the dual pathway model: evidence for the dissociation of timing, inhibitory, and delay-related impairments in attention-deficit/hyperactivity disorder. *Journal of the American Academy of Child and Adolescent Psychiatry*, 49, 345–55.

9. Fair, D.A., Bathula, D., Nikolas, M.A., and Nigg, J.T. (2012). Distinct neuropsychological subgroups in typically developing youth inform heterogeneity in children with ADHD. *Proceedings of the National Academy of Sciences of the United States of America*, 109, 6769–74.

10. Mostert, J.C., Hoogman, M., Onnink, A.M., *et al.* (2018). Similar subgroups based on cognitive performance parse heterogeneity in adults with ADHD and healthy controls. *Journal of Attention Disorders*, 22, 281–92.

11. van Lieshout, M., Luman, M., Buitelaar, J., Rommelse, N.N., and Oosterlaan, J. (2013). Does neurocognitive functioning predict future or persistence of ADHD? A systematic review. *Clinical Psychology Review*, 33, 539–60.

12. van Lieshout, M., Luman, M., Twisk, J.W., *et al.* (2017). Neurocognitive predictors of ADHD outcome: a 6-year follow-up study. *Journal of Abnormal Child Psychology*, 45, 261–72.

13. Franke, B., Michelini, G., Asherson, P., *et al.* (2018). Live fast, die young? A review on the developmental trajectories of ADHD across the lifespan. *European Neuropsychopharmacology*, 28, 1058–88.

14. Hoogman, M., Bralten, J., Hibar, D.P., *et al.* (2017). Subcortical brain volume differences in participants with attention deficit hyperactivity disorder in children and adults: a cross-sectional mega-analysis. *The Lancet Psychiatry*, 4, 310–19.

14a. Hoogman, M., Muetzel, R., Guimaraes, J.P., *et al.* (2019). Brain imaging of the cortex in ADHD: a coordinated analysis of large-scale clinical and population-based samples. *American Journal of Psychiatry*, 176(7), 531–42.

15. Cortese, S., Kelly, C., Chabernaud, C., *et al.* (2012). Toward systems neuroscience of ADHD: a meta-analysis of 55 fMRI studies. *American Journal of Psychiatry*, 169, 1038–55.

16. Cheung, C.H., Rijsdijk, F., McLoughlin, G., *et al.* (2016). Cognitive and neurophysiological markers of ADHD persistence and remission. *British Journal of Psychiatry*, 208, 548–55.

17. Tye, C., Rijsdijk, F., Greven, C.U., Kuntsi, J., Asherson, P., and McLoughlin, G. (2012). Shared genetic influences on ADHD symptoms and very low-frequency EEG activity: a twin study. *Journal of Child Psychology and Psychiatry, and Allied Disciplines*, 53, 706–15.

18. Arns, M., Conners, C.K., and Kraemer, H.C. (2013). A decade of EEG theta/beta ratio research in ADHD: a meta-analysis. *Journal of Attention Disorders*, 17, 374–83.

19. Marquand, A.F., Wolfers, T., Mennes, M., Buitelaar, J., and Beckmann, C.F. (2016). Beyond lumping and splitting: a review of computational approaches for stratifying psychiatric disorders. *Biological Psychiatry Cognitive Neuroscience and Neuroimaging*, 1, 433–47.

20. Wolfers, T., Buitelaar, J.K., Beckmann, C.F., Franke, B., and Marquand, A.F. (2015). From estimating activation locality to predicting disorder: a review of pattern recognition for neuroimaging-based psychiatric diagnostics. *Neuroscience and Biobehavioral Reviews*, 57, 328–49.

21. Scassellati, C., Bonvicini, C., Faraone, S.V., and Gennarelli, M. (2012). Biomarkers and attention-deficit/hyperactivity disorder: a systematic review and meta-analyses. *Journal of the American Academy of Child and Adolescent Psychiatry*, 51, 1003–19 e1020.

22. Nieoullon, A. (2002). Dopamine and the regulation of cognition and attention. *Progress in Neurobiology*, 67, 53–83.

23. Arnsten, A.F. (2006). Fundamentals of attention-deficit/hyperactivity disorder: circuits and pathways. *Journal of Clinical Psychiatry*, 67(Suppl 8), 7–12.

24. Prince, J. (2008). Catecholamine dysfunction in attention-deficit/hyperactivity disorder: an update. *Journal of Clinical Psychopharmacology*, 28, S39–45.

25. Volkow, N.D., Wang, G.J., Kollins, S.H., *et al.* (2009). Evaluating dopamine reward pathway in ADHD: clinical implications. *JAMA*, 302, 1084–91.

26. Nieoullon, A. and Coquerel, A. (2003). Dopamine: a key regulator to adapt action, emotion, motivation and cognition. *Current Opinion in Neurology*, 16(Suppl 2), S3–9.

27. Del Campo, N., Chamberlain, S.R., Sahakian, B.J., and Robbins, T.W. (2011). The roles of dopamine and noradrenaline in the pathophysiology and treatment of attention-deficit/hyperactivity disorder. *Biological Psychiatry*, 69, e145–57.

28. Ziegler, S., Pedersen, M.L., Mowinckel, A.M., and Biele, G. (2016). Modelling ADHD: a review of ADHD theories through their predictions for computational models of decision-making and reinforcement learning. *Neuroscience and Biobehavioral Reviews*, 71, 633–56.

29. Kuczenski, R. and Segal, D.S. (2002). Exposure of adolescent rats to oral methylphenidate: preferential effects on extracellular norepinephrine and absence of sensitization and cross-sensitization to methamphetamine. *Journal of Neuroscience*, 22, 7264–271.

30. Kuczenski, R. and Segal, D.S. (2005). Stimulant actions in rodents: implications for attention-deficit/hyperactivity disorder treatment and potential substance abuse. *Biological Psychiatry*, 57, 1391–6.

31. Zetterstrom, T., Sharp, T., Collin, A.K., and Ungerstedt, U. (1988). *In vivo* measurement of extracellular dopamine and DOPAC in rat striatum after various dopamine-releasing drugs: implications for the origin of extracellular DOPAC. *European Journal of Pharmacology*, 148, 327–34.

32. Kuczenski, R. and Segal, D.S. (1975). Differential effects of D- and L-amphetamine and methylphenidate on rat striatal dopamine biosynthesis. *European Journal of Pharmacology*, 30, 244–51.

33. Giros, B., Jaber, M., Jones, S.R., Wightman, R.M., and Caron, M.G. (1996). Hyperlocomotion and indifference to cocaine and amphetamine in mice lacking the dopamine transporter. *Nature*, 379, 606–12.

34. van der Voet, M., Harich, B., Franke, B., and Schenck, A. (2016). ADHD-associated dopamine transporter, latrophilin and neurofibromin share a dopamine-related locomotor signature in *Drosophila*. *Molecular Psychiatry*, 21, 565–73.

35. van der Kooij, M.A. and Glennon, J.C. (2007). Animal models concerning the role of dopamine in attention-deficit hyperactivity disorder. *Neuroscience and Biobehavioral Reviews*, 31, 597–618.

36. Faraone, S.V., Spencer, T.J., Madras, B.K., Zhang-James, Y., and Biederman, J. (2014). Functional effects of dopamine transporter gene genotypes on in vivo dopamine transporter functioning: a meta-analysis. *Molecular Psychiatry*, 19, 880–9.

37. Fusar-Poli, P., Rubia, K., Rossi, G., Sartori, G., and Balottin, U. (2012). Striatal dopamine transporter alterations in ADHD: pathophysiology or adaptation to psychostimulants? A meta-analysis. *American Journal of Psychiatry*, 169, 264–72.

38. Volkow, N.D., Wang, G.J., Newcorn, J., et al. (2007). Depressed dopamine activity in caudate and preliminary evidence of limbic involvement in adults with attention-deficit/hyperactivity disorder. *Archives of General Psychiatry*, 64, 932–40.

39. Franke, B., Vasquez, A.A., Johansson, S., et al. (2010). Multicenter analysis of the SLC6A3/DAT1 VNTR haplotype in persistent ADHD suggests differential involvement of the gene in childhood and persistent ADHD. *Neuropsychopharmacology*, 35, 656–64.

40. Gizer, I.R., Ficks, C., and Waldman, I.D. (2009). Candidate gene studies of ADHD: a meta-analytic review. *Human Genetics*, 126, 51–90.

41. Li, D., Sham, P.C., Owen, M.J., and He, L. (2006). Meta-analysis shows significant association between dopamine system genes and attention deficit hyperactivity disorder (ADHD). *Human Molecular Genetics*, 15, 2276–84.

42. Bralten, J., Franke, B., Waldman, I., et al. (2013). Candidate genetic pathways for attention-deficit/hyperactivity disorder (ADHD) show association to hyperactive/impulsive symptoms in children with ADHD. *Journal of the American Academy of Child and Adolescent Psychiatry*, 52, 1204–12 e1201.

43. Arnsten, A.F. (2011). Catecholamine influences on dorsolateral prefrontal cortical networks. *Biological Psychiatry*, 69, e89–99.

44. Arnsten, A.F. and Pliszka, S.R. (2011). Catecholamine influences on prefrontal cortical function: relevance to treatment of attention deficit/hyperactivity disorder and related disorders. *Pharmacology, Biochemistry, and Behavior*, 99, 211–16.

45. Xing, B., Li, Y.C., and Gao, W.J. (2016). Norepinephrine versus dopamine and their interaction in modulating synaptic function in the prefrontal cortex. *Brain Research*, 1641, 217–33.

46. Fredriksen, M., Halmoy, A., Faraone, S.V., and Haavik, J. (2013). Long-term efficacy and safety of treatment with stimulants and atomoxetine in adult ADHD: a review of controlled and naturalistic studies. *European Neuropsychopharmacology*, 23, 508–27.

47. Hutchison, S.L., Ghuman, J.K., Ghuman, H.S., Karpov, I., and Schuster, J.M. (2016). Efficacy of atomoxetine in the treatment of attention-deficit hyperactivity disorder in patients with common comorbidities in children, adolescents and adults: a review. *Therapeutic Advances in Psychopharmacology*, 6, 317–34.

48. de la Peña, J.B., Dela Peña, I.J., Custodio, R.J., Botanas, C.J., Kim, H.J., and Cheong, J.H. (2018). Exploring the validity of proposed transgenic animal models of attention-deficit hyperactivity disorder (ADHD). *Molecular Neurobiology*, 55, 3739–54.

49. Vanicek, T., Spies, M., Rami-Mark, C., et al. (2014). The norepinephrine transporter in attention-deficit/hyperactivity disorder investigated with positron emission tomography. *JAMA Psychiatry*, 71, 1340–9.

50. Klein, M., Onnink, M., van Donkelaar, M., et al. (2017). Brain imaging genetics in ADHD and beyond: mapping pathways from gene to disorder at different levels of complexity. *Neuroscience and Biobehavioral Reviews*, 80, 115–55.

51. Banerjee, E. and Nandagopal, K. (2015). Does serotonin deficit mediate susceptibility to ADHD? *Neurochemistry International*, 82, 52–68.

52. Oades, R.D. (2008). Dopamine-serotonin interactions in attention-deficit hyperactivity disorder (ADHD). *Progress in Brain Research*, 172, 543–65.

53. Kuntsi, J., McLoughlin, G., and Asherson, P. (2006). Attention deficit hyperactivity disorder. *Neuromolecular Medicine*, 8, 461–84.

54. Gainetdinov, R.R., Wetsel, W.C., Jones, S.R., Levin, E.D., Jaber, M., and Caron, M.G. (1999). Role of serotonin in the paradoxical calming effect of psychostimulants on hyperactivity. *Science*, 283, 397–401.

55. Spivak, B., Vered, Y., Yoran-Hegesh, R., et al. (1999). Circulatory levels of catecholamines, serotonin and lipids in attention deficit hyperactivity disorder. *Acta Psychiatrica Scandinavica*, 99, 300–4.

56. van der Meer, D., Hartman, C.A., Richards, J., et al. (2014). The serotonin transporter gene polymorphism 5-HTTLPR moderates the effects of stress on attention-deficit/hyperactivity disorder. *Journal of Child Psychology and Psychiatry, and Allied Disciplines*, 55, 1363–71.

57. Hinz, M., Stein, A., Neff, R., Weinberg, R., and Uncini, T. (2011). Treatment of attention deficit hyperactivity disorder with monoamine amino acid precursors and organic cation transporter assay interpretation. *Neuropsychiatric Disease and Treatment*, 7, 31–8.

58. Zhou, Y., and Danbolt, N.C. (2014). Glutamate as a neurotransmitter in the healthy brain. *Journal of Neural Transmission*, 121, 799–817.

59. Gregory, K.J., Noetzel, M.J., and Niswender, C.M. (2013). Pharmacology of metabotropic glutamate receptor allosteric modulators: structural basis and therapeutic potential for CNS disorders. *Progress in Molecular Biology and Translational Science*, 115, 61–121.

60. Dorval, K.M., Wigg, K.G., Crosbie, J., et al. (2007). Association of the glutamate receptor subunit gene GRIN2B with attention-deficit/hyperactivity disorder. *Genes, Brain, and Behavior*, 6, 444–52.

61. Elia, J., Glessner, J.T., Wang, K., et al. (2012). Genome-wide copy number variation study associates metabotropic glutamate receptor gene networks with attention deficit hyperactivity disorder. *Nature Genetics*, 44, 78–84.

62. Naaijen, J., Bralten, J., Poelmans, G., et al. (2017). Glutamatergic and GABAergic gene sets in attention-deficit/hyperactivity disorder: association to overlapping traits in ADHD and autism. *Translational Psychiatry*, 7, e999.

63. Naaijen, J., Lythgoe, D.J., Amiri, H., Buitelaar, J.K., and Glennon, J.C. (2015). Fronto-striatal glutamatergic compounds in compulsive and impulsive syndromes: a review of magnetic resonance spectroscopy studies. *Neuroscience and Biobehavioral Reviews*, 52, 74–88.

64. Findling, R.L., McNamara, N.K., Stansbrey, R.J., *et al.* (2007). A pilot evaluation of the safety, tolerability, pharmacokinetics, and effectiveness of memantine in pediatric patients with attention-deficit/hyperactivity disorder combined type. *Journal of Child and Adolescent Psychopharmacology*, 17, 19–33.

65. Mechler, K., Hage, A., Schweinfurth, N., *et al.* (2017). Glutamatergic agents in the treatment of compulsivity and impulsivity in child and adolescent psychiatry: a systematic review of the literature. *Zeitschrift für Kinder- und Jugendpsychiatrie und Psychotherapie*, 1–18.

66. Brown, R.E., Stevens, D.R., and Haas, H.L. (2001). The physiology of brain histamine. *Progress in Neurobiology*, 63, 637–72.

67. Miyazaki, C., Koyama, M., Ota, E., *et al.* (2017). Allergic diseases in children with attention deficit hyperactivity disorder: a systematic review and meta-analysis. *BMC Psychiatry*, 17, 120.

68. Yang, M.T., Lee, W.T., Liang, J.S., *et al.* (2014). Hyperactivity and impulsivity in children with untreated allergic rhinitis: corroborated by rating scale and continuous performance test. *Pediatrics and Neonatology*, 55, 168–74.

69. Sadek, B., Saad, A., Sadeq, A., Jalal, F., and Stark, H. (2016). Histamine H3 receptor as a potential target for cognitive symptoms in neuropsychiatric diseases. *Behavioural Brain Research*, 312, 415–30.

70. Moorthy, G., Sallee, F., Gabbita, P., Zemlan, F., Sallans, L., and Desai, P.B. (2015). Safety, tolerability and pharmacokinetics of 2-pyridylacetic acid, a major metabolite of betahistine, in a phase 1 dose escalation study in subjects with ADHD. *Biopharmaceutics and Drug Disposition*, 36, 429–39.

71. Conners, C.K., Levin, E.D., Sparrow, E., *et al.* (1996). Nicotine and attention in adult attention deficit hyperactivity disorder (ADHD). *Psychopharmacology Bulletin*, 32, 67–73.

72. Levin, E.D. (2002). Nicotinic receptor subtypes and cognitive function. *Journal of Neurobiology*, 53, 633–40.

73. Levin, E.D., Conners, C.K., Sparrow, E., *et al.* (1996). Nicotine effects on adults with attention-deficit/hyperactivity disorder. *Psychopharmacology (Berlin)*, 123, 55–63.

74. Potter, A.S. and Newhouse, P.A. (2008). Acute nicotine improves cognitive deficits in young adults with attention-deficit/hyperactivity disorder. *Pharmacology, Biochemistry, and Behavior*, 88, 407–17.

75. Potter, A.S., Newhouse, P.A., and Bucci, D.J. (2006). Central nicotinic cholinergic systems: a role in the cognitive dysfunction in attention-deficit/hyperactivity disorder? *Behavioural Brain Research*, 175, 201–11.

76. Williams, N.M., Franke, B., Mick, E., *et al.* (2012). Genome-wide analysis of copy number variants in attention deficit hyperactivity disorder: the role of rare variants and duplications at 15q13.3. *American Journal of Psychiatry*, 169, 195–204.

77. Potter, A.S., Bucci, D.J., and Newhouse, P.A. (2012). Manipulation of nicotinic acetylcholine receptors differentially affects behavioral inhibition in human subjects with and without disordered baseline impulsivity. *Psychopharmacology (Berlin)*, 220, 331–40.

78. Potter, A.S., Schaubhut, G., and Shipman, M. (2014). Targeting the nicotinic cholinergic system to treat attention-deficit/hyperactivity disorder: rationale and progress to date. *CNS Drugs*, 28, 1103–13.

79. Faraone, S.V., Perlis, R.H., Doyle, A.E., *et al.* (2005). Molecular genetics of attention-deficit/hyperactivity disorder. *Biological Psychiatry*, 57, 1313–23.

80. Larsson, H., Chang, Z., D'Onofrio, B.M., and Lichtenstein, P. (2014). The heritability of clinically diagnosed attention deficit hyperactivity disorder across the lifespan. *Psychological Medicine*, 44, 2223–9.

81. Chang, Z., Lichtenstein, P., Asherson, P.J., and Larsson, H. (2013). Developmental twin study of attention problems: high heritabilities throughout development. *JAMA Psychiatry*, 70, 311–18.

82. Greven, C.U., Rijsdijk, F.V., and Plomin, R. (2011). A twin study of ADHD symptoms in early adolescence: hyperactivity-impulsivity and inattentiveness show substantial genetic overlap but also genetic specificity. *Journal of Abnormal Child Psychology*, 39, 265–75.

83. Pingault, J.B., Viding, E., Galera, C., *et al.* (2015). Genetic and environmental influences on the developmental course of attention-deficit/hyperactivity disorder symptoms from childhood to adolescence. *JAMA Psychiatry*, 72, 651–8.

84. Franke, B., Neale, B.M., and Faraone, S.V. (2009). Genome-wide association studies in ADHD. *Human Genetics*, 126, 13–50.

85. Poelmans, G., Pauls, D.L., Buitelaar, J.K., and Franke, B. (2011). Integrated genome-wide association study findings: identification of a neurodevelopmental network for attention deficit hyperactivity disorder. *American Journal of Psychiatry*, 168, 365–77.

86. Rutter, M., Dunn, J., Plomin, R., *et al.* (1997). Integrating nature and nurture: implications of person-environment correlations and interactions for developmental psychopathology. *Development and Psychopathology*, 9, 335–64.

87. Franke, B. and Buitelaar, J.K. (2018). Gene–environment interactions. In: Banaschewski, T., Coghill, D., and Zuddas, A. (eds). *Oxford Textbook of Attention Deficit Hyperactivity Disorder*. Oxford University Press, Oxford. pp. 35–56.

88. Harold, G.T., Leve, L.D., Barrett, D., *et al.* (2013). Biological and rearing mother influences on child ADHD symptoms: revisiting the developmental interface between nature and nurture. *Journal of Child Psychology and Psychiatry, and Allied Disciplines*, 54, 1038–46.

89. Knafo, A. and Jaffee, S.R. (2013). Gene-environment correlation in developmental psychopathology. *Development and Psychopathology*, 25, 1–6.

90. Plomin, R., DeFries, J.C., and Loehlin, J.C. (1977). Genotype-environment interaction and correlation in the analysis of human behavior. *Psychological Bulletin*, 84, 309–22.

91. Scarr, S. and McCartney, K. (1983). How people make their own environments: a theory of genotype greater than environment effects. *Child Development*, 54, 424–35.

92. Zheng, W., Aschner, M., and Ghersi-Egea, J.F. (2003). Brain barrier systems: a new frontier in metal neurotoxicological research. *Toxicology and Applied Pharmacology*, 192, 1–11.

93. Grandjean, P. and Landrigan, P.J. (2014). Neurobehavioural effects of developmental toxicity. *The Lancet Neurology*, 13, 330–8.

94. Pele, F., Muckle, G., Costet, N., *et al.* (2013). Occupational solvent exposure during pregnancy and child behaviour at age 2. *Occupational and Environmental Medicine*, 70, 114–19.

95. Rauh, V.A. and Margolis, A.E. (2016). Environmental exposures, neurodevelopment, and child mental health—new paradigms for the study of brain and behavioral effects. *Journal of Child Psychology and Psychiatry, and Allied Disciplines*, 57, 775–93.

96. Thapar, A., Cooper, M., Eyre, O., and Langley, K. (2013). What have we learnt about the causes of ADHD? *Journal of Child Psychology and Psychiatry, and Allied Disciplines*, 54, 3–16.

97. Stevens, S.E., Sonuga-Barke, E.J., Kreppner, J.M., *et al.* (2008). Inattention/overactivity following early severe institutional deprivation: presentation and associations in early adolescence. *Journal of Abnormal Child Psychology*, 36, 385–98.

98. Ostergaard, S.D., Larsen, J.T., Dalsgaard, S., *et al.* (2016). Predicting ADHD by assessment of Rutter's indicators of adversity in infancy. *PLoS One*, 11, e0157352.

99. Arnsten, A.F. and Rubia, K. (2012). Neurobiological circuits regulating attention, cognitive control, motivation, and emotion: disruptions in neurodevelopmental psychiatric disorders. *Journal of the American Academy of Child and Adolescent Psychiatry*, 51, 356–67.

100. Sagvolden, T., Johansen, E.B., Aase, H., and Russell, V.A. (2005). A dynamic developmental theory of attention-deficit/hyperactivity disorder (ADHD) predominantly hyperactive/impulsive and combined subtypes. *Behavioral and Brain Sciences*, 28, 397–419.

101. Frank, M.J., Santamaria, A., O'Reilly, R.C., and Willcutt, E. (2007). Testing computational models of dopamine and noradrenaline dysfunction in attention deficit/hyperactivity disorder. *Neuropsychopharmacology*, 32, 1583–99.

102. Grace, A.A. (1991). Phasic versus tonic dopamine release and the modulation of dopamine system responsivity: a hypothesis for the etiology of schizophrenia. *Neuroscience*, 41, 1–24.

103. Sikstrom, S. and Soderlund, G. (2007). Stimulus-dependent dopamine release in attention-deficit/hyperactivity disorder. *Psychological Review*, 114, 1047–75.

104. Tripp, G. and Wickens, J.R. (2009). Neurobiology of ADHD. *Neuropharmacology*, 57, 579–89.

105. Plichta, M.M. and Scheres, A. (2014). Ventral-striatal responsiveness during reward anticipation in ADHD and its relation to trait impulsivity in the healthy population: a meta-analytic review of the fMRI literature. *Neuroscience and Biobehavioral Reviews*, 38, 125–34.

106. Killeen, P.R., Russell, V.A., and Sergeant, J.A. (2013). A behavioral neuroenergetics theory of ADHD. *Neuroscience and Biobehavioral Reviews*, 37, 625–57.

107. Riske, L., Thomas, R.K., Baker, G.B., and Dursun, S.M. (2017). Lactate in the brain: an update on its relevance to brain energy, neurons, glia and panic disorder. *Therapeutic Advances in Psychopharmacology*, 7, 85–9.

108. Mooney, M.A., McWeeney, S.K., Faraone, S.V., *et al.* (2016). Pathway analysis in attention deficit hyperactivity disorder: an ensemble approach. *American Journal of Medical Genetics Part B*, 171, 815–26.

109. Thapar, A., Martin, J., Mick, E., *et al.* (2016). Psychiatric gene discoveries shape evidence on ADHD's biology. *Molecular Psychiatry*, 21, 1202–7.

# 33

# Epidemiology of attention-deficit/hyperactivity disorder and the implications for its prevention

*Guilherme V. Polanczyk*

## Introduction

Since the publication of the third edition of the *Diagnostic and Statistical Manual of Mental Disorders*, third edition (DSM-III) in 1980, when the first reliable operational diagnostic criteria for attention-deficit/hyperactivity disorder (ADHD) appeared, the scientific literature on the various aspects of the disorder has been expanding significantly. Rigorous and informative epidemiological studies have been conducted to describe the distribution and natural course of the disorder. The familial nature of ADHD and the importance of genetic risk have also been recognized, as described in Chapter 34. Nevertheless, as for any complex disorder for which no single risk factor is either necessary or sufficient to cause the disorder, longitudinal—mainly retrospective—and case-control studies have suggested that certain environmental factors increase the risk for ADHD. As is usual in medicine, epidemiological findings have contributed to shed light on aetiological mechanisms and temporal and cultural effects, to plan services, and to monitor delivery of treatment, among other clinical and research advances. It has the potential to contribute to the next challenge of the field—to prevent the development of the disorder.

## Prevalence

Studies investigating the prevalence of ADHD emerged soon after DSM-III was published in 1980. As the studies accumulated, the overall result was of a significant variability on reported rates, ranging from as low as 1% to as high as nearly 20% among school-age children. This variability raised debates of whether broad cultural and societal modifications, mediated by changes in family structure and habits and also by increasing academic expectations and failing educational models, were producing the disorder. As described in Chapter 31, these debates fuelled concerns about the validity of ADHD. However, it was important, and initially underestimated, that surveys adopted a variety of methods (in regard of sampling

strategy and study design), case definitions (for example, diagnostic criteria), and strategies to collect information (for example, instrument, informant), and several studies were of low or very low quality. The conclusion that prevalence rates varied across settings was, in fact, premature, because methodologies influence the findings and direct comparisons between individual results were not possible. Therefore, the appreciation of study methods and the empirical assessment of their effect are key to interpret prevalence rates of ADHD.

### Study methods

Sampling is the process of selecting study participants. This is a fundamental process in an epidemiological study, because the sample must accurately represent the target population. If, for any reason, selected participants do not represent the specific population of interest, results cannot be generalized to that population and are valid only for the specific sample studied. A probabilistic sampling strategy, in which, by the principle of randomization, each eligible member of the population has a defined chance to be identified and included, is essential. Nevertheless, it is necessary to have an objective list of all of the units in the target population, that is, a sampling frame. Examples of sampling frames are telephone directories, census data, and schools. For studies investigating the prevalence of childhood mental disorders, including ADHD, schools are frequently used as the sampling frame. However, if virtually all children from the population of interest are not enrolled in ordinary schools, or if individuals are enrolled in schools but are not attending classes (which may be closely linked to the presence of mental disorders), this strategy is likely to produce biased results. Different probabilistic sampling strategies can be adopted to select the units within the frame such as simple random, stratified random, and systematic random. As the sampling frame and eligible participants are identified, it is possible to identify and study the individuals who refuse to participate. Among eligible individuals, the proportion who give consent to participate and are actually assessed (that is, the response rate of a study) is an important indicator of the success of the sampling procedure. If a substantial proportion of eligible participants do not take part in a survey, or if refusal to participate is non-random (that is, associated with specific characteristics of participants), results may be biased and inferences about the whole population of interest may not be possible.

In one-stage design studies, diagnostic interviews are used to assess the whole sample. In two-stage design studies, a screening instrument is answered by the whole sample and individuals are selected for further assessment by diagnostic interviews based on its results. It is fundamental that not only individuals who are considered to have screened positive, but also a proportion of individuals who screen negative, are assessed with the diagnostic interview, so that rates of false and true positives (and negatives) at the screening phase can be determined and prevalence rates for the whole sample estimated.

In terms of case definition, the inconsistencies between diagnostic criteria presented by DSM and the International Classification of Diseases (ICD) may also have reduced the homogeneity of prevalence rates. The background to the overall approach to the diagnosis of ADHD has been described in detail in Chapter 31. Research diagnosis of hyperkinetic disorder requires symptoms of both inattention and hyperactivity–impulsivity, whereas DSM-III-R, DSM-IV, and DSM-5 require symptoms of only one of the symptom dimensions. Therefore, prevalence rates according to ICD are consistently lower than those according to DSM. Differences between DSM-III-R and DSM-IV were subtle. DSM-5 introduced three important modifications to DSM-IV criteria: extended the upper limit of the age of onset of symptoms from 7 to 12 years of age; decreased the symptom threshold for adults (18 years of age and older) from six to five symptoms; and indicated that ADHD could be diagnosed in comorbidity with autism spectrum disorder. The impact of the modification of the age of onset of symptoms on prevalence rates was investigated in a representative sample of the population prospectively followed during childhood. Results showed that extending the age of onset criterion to age 12 resulted in an increase in ADHD prevalence by age 12 of only 0.1% [1]. As for adult ADHD, uncertainties regarding the most valid definition of the disorder (for example, reflected by modifications of symptom threshold, developmental manifestations of symptoms such as hyperactivity) and the most appropriate strategy to assess the disorder (for example, reflected by the requirement, or not, of collateral informants) are very important for case definition in epidemiological studies. Reduction of the symptom threshold for diagnosing adults is expected to increase the expected prevalence rates by 27% [2].

Also in terms of case definition, diagnostic assessment, informant, and requirement for functional impairment for the diagnosis are all important. As for mental disorders generally, standardized assessment by using a diagnostic interview is a key component to guaranteeing consistency within and between studies (see Chapter 7). Interviews vary in the way questions are constructed, on the presence of gate/skip questions, and on the emphasis on the respondent's understanding and interpretation of the questions (structured interviews, usually administered by lay interviewers) or on the interviewers' interpretation of the responses (semi-structured interviews, usually administered by trained mental health professionals). Informants more frequently reporting ADHD symptoms are parents, children (usually older than 11 years), and teachers. The correlation between different informants is low to moderate, which suggests that symptoms are modulated by settings and/or different informants emphasize different aspects of behaviour. Thus, it is indicated to use multiple informants and integrate

information using different strategies such as the 'best estimate procedure', 'and rule', and 'or rule'. The best estimate procedure implies that data from different sources and instruments are integrated by clinicians, who define the presence of a diagnosis, based on their best judgement of available information. The 'and rule' implies that a symptom should be considered positive if both informants endorse the symptom. The 'or rule' implies that a symptom should be considered positive if one out of two informants endorses the symptom.

Requirement of functional impairment for the diagnosis is an important parameter for case definition, as individuals frequently meet symptomatic criteria but have minimal or no impairment criteria but have optimal functioning. This may be dependent upon the structure of the environment they are part of, the support they receive, the demands they are faced to, the expectations placed on their performance, and the very specific definition of impairment. Different definitions of functional impairment may be adopted such as measures of impairment specifically related to ADHD or global measures of impairment [such as the Child Global Assessment Scale [CGAS]]. The former has the advantage to be related specifically to the identified disorder, and the latter, although not specifying the source of impairment, is a good predictor of adaptative functioning and need of service.

## Prevalence rates in childhood and adolescence

The first comprehensive literature review and meta-analysis on the prevalence rates of ADHD [3] was based on an extensive search strategy, and studies were included based on the following inclusion criteria: (1) original surveys on ADHD/hyperkinetic disorder prevalence (point prevalence); (2) diagnoses based on any DSM (III, III-R, or IV) or ICD (9 or 10) versions; (3) probabilistic sample from the general population or from schools; and (4) participants up to the age of 18 years. One hundred and two studies were included, which represented populations from North America ($k$ = 32), Europe ($k$ = 32), Asia ($k$ = 15), South America ($k$ = 9), Oceania ($k$ = 6), Middle East ($k$ = 4), and Africa ($k$ = 4). Most studies had their samples ascertained from schools ($k$ = 60), with a one-stage assessment ($k$ = 61), adopting DSM-IV criteria ($k$ = 44), with no impairment criterion ($k$ = 68), and with parents as the most frequent source of information ($k$ = 33). A meta-regression analysis was performed to empirically investigate the methodological approaches that impacted the detected rates. Multivariate meta-regression identified diagnostic criteria, source of information, and requirement of functional impairment for the diagnosis as methodological procedures significantly associated with variability of estimates. The analysis identified that study location was associated with heterogeneity only when estimates from Africa and the Middle East were compared to estimates from North America. Estimates from Europe, Oceania, South America, and Asia did not differ from estimates from North America. It is noteworthy that Africa and the Middle East were the continents with the fewest number of studies ($k$ = 4 in each continent). A meta-analysis resulted in a pooled prevalence rate of 5.29% [95% confidence interval (CI) 5.01–5.56] (Fig. 33.1).

A second comprehensive review of the literature on the prevalence of ADHD and a meta-analysis including only studies that adopted DSM-IV diagnostic criteria were published in 2012 [4]. Eighty-six studies were included, and pooled estimates ranged from 5.9% to 7.1%, depending on the source of information for the diagnosis. Further results detected significant heterogeneity between estimates, but once again, the country or region where the study was

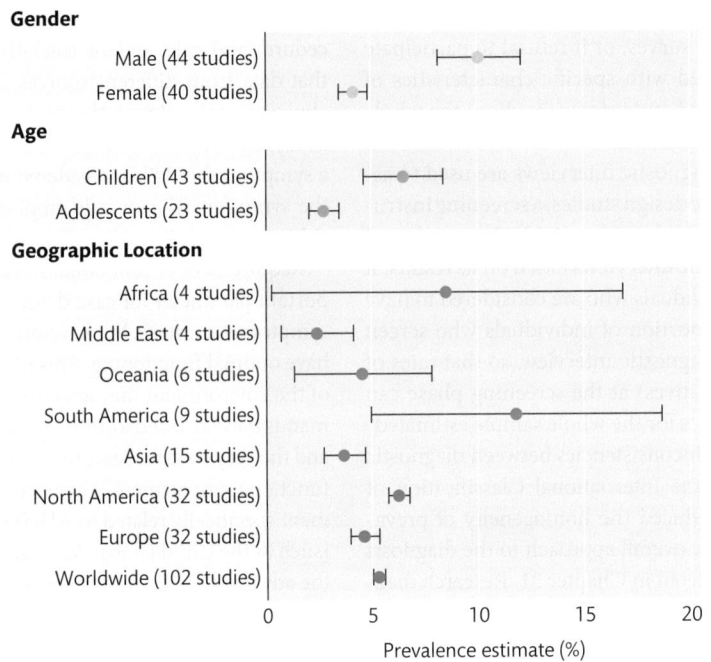

**Fig. 33.1** ADHD/HD pooled prevalence according to demographic characteristics and geographic location.
Reproduced from *American Journal of Psychiatry*, 164(6), Polanczyk G, Silva de Lima M, Horta BL, *et al.*, The Worldwide Prevalence of ADHD: A Systematic Review and Metaregression Analysis, pp. 942–948, Copyright (2007), with permission from American Psychiatric Association.

conducted did not explain the variability, supporting the previous findings.

A third comprehensive review of the literature aggregated studies included in the first two meta-analyses [3, 4] and updated the search aiming to follow up the previous finding that estimates from Africa and the Middle East were different from those from North America [5]. As the influence of time on prevalence of ADHD was still a matter of controversy, this study also aimed to investigate time-effects on prevalence rates. The third review detected 154 studies, and 135 were included in the multivariate statistical models. The 25th, 50th, and 75th percentiles of distribution of studies, based on year of publication, corresponded, respectively, to years 1997, 2001, and 2005. The studies represented populations from North America ($k = 48$), Europe ($k = 42$), Asia ($k = 12$), South America ($k = 10$), Oceania ($k = 7$), the Middle East ($k = 11$), and Africa ($k = 5$). Univariate analysis revealed that diagnostic criteria, impairment criterion, source of information, and geographical location of studies (but not year of study publication) were significantly associated with heterogeneity of prevalence estimates. Multivariate analysis indicated that source of information, impairment criterion, and diagnostic criteria remained significantly associated with heterogeneity of results. Rates based on teacher reports were an estimated 5.47% higher than those based on best estimate procedure, and those rates with no requirement for impairment were an estimated 2.32% higher than when impairment was required. Regarding diagnostic criteria, rates based on DSM-III-R and ICD-10 were an estimated 2.42% and 4.09%, respectively, lower than rates based on DSM-IV. Study location was no longer significant when methodological variables were accounted for. Year of publication was not associated with heterogeneity, indicating the absence of time-effect on prevalence of ADHD (Fig. 33.2). No significant interaction was detected between year of publication and diagnostic criteria (Fig. 33.3), other methodological variables,

and geographic location (Fig. 33.4), ruling out a possible increase in prevalence estimates over time in specific geographic locations or for specific study methods [5].

The lack of time-effect on prevalence rates detected is in accordance with studies that have investigated rates of inattentive and/or hyperactive symptoms, using equivalent rating scales and parents or teachers as informants across time. They found no evidence for a systematic variation in prevalence of ADHD symptoms, with symptom levels and the proportion of children with clinical scores remaining stable or presenting small reductions over recent decades [6].

One important limitations of the existing epidemiological literature is the scarcity of studies outside Europe and North America. In this regard, the Global Burden of Disease Study 2010 (GBD 2010) and 2013 (GBD 2013) systematically reviewed the literature and employed an imputation method to derive prevalence estimates by age and sex in three time periods (1990, 2005, and 2010) for 21 world regions, including those with little or no data. For each of the time period, ADHD prevalence for boys was estimated in 2.2% (95% CI 2.0–2.3) and for girls in 0.7% (95% CI 0.6–0.7), indicating that prevalence remained stable over time [7]. Nevertheless, a very concerning scenario is the small proportion of the global population of children and adolescents represented in prevalence studies for any mental disorder. From the GBD data, it is estimated that only 5.47% of children and adolescents around the world are covered by ADHD surveys. This proportion is hugely discrepant between high-income and low-/middle-income regions—36.47% and 2%, respectively [8].

Other meta-analyses conducted on the prevalence of ADHD detected discrepant findings such as higher [9] or variable [10] rates across regions. Nevertheless, these analyses had different inclusion criteria that explained the contrasting findings, such as the inclusion of studies that relied on questionnaires for diagnosis and the

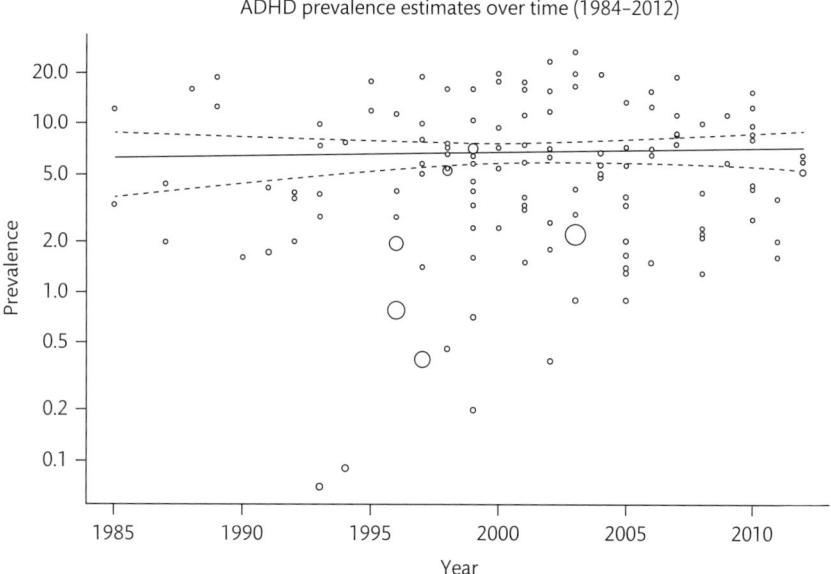

**Fig. 33.2** ADHD prevalence rates as a function of the year of study publication. The point sizes are drawn proportional to the inverse of the standard errors. The predicted average prevalence estimate rate based on a mixed-effects model is added to the plot (with corresponding 95% confidence interval bounds).

Reproduced from *International Journal of Epidemiology*, 43(2), Polanczyk G, Guilherme V, Willcutt, EG, ADHD prevalence estimates across three decades: an updated systematic review and meta-regression analysis, pp. 434–442, Copyright (2014) with permission from Oxford University Press.

exclusion of studies using ICD criteria [9] and the inclusion of studies using regional diagnostic criteria for mental disorders [10].

More recently, a systematic review of surveys estimating the prevalence of any mental disorder in the community across the world, including ADHD, was published [11]. The systematic search identified 23,191 abstracts; 198 studies were selected for review, 48 studies met inclusion criteria, and 41 studies were included. The studies were published from 1985 to 2012 and represented populations from North America ($k = 14$), Europe ($k = 14$), Asia ($k = 8$), South America

($k = 5$), Oceania ($k = 3$), the Middle East ($k = 2$), and Africa ($k = 2$). A pooled rate of prevalence of any mental disorder was estimated in 13.4% (95% CI 11.3–15.9). The final multivariate meta-regression model identified sample representativeness, sample frame, and diagnostic interview as significant moderators of prevalence estimates. Study geographic location and sample age range were not significant moderators. Secondary meta-analysis focusing on ADHD included 33 studies, representing a sample of 77,297 individuals, and resulted in a pooled prevalence of 3.4% (95% CI 2.6–4.5) [11].

## Prevalence rates in adulthood

Prevalence studies of ADHD in adulthood emerged approximately a decade after studies in childhood, and significant fewer surveys have been conducted so far. A systematic review published in 2009 identified seven samples eligible for a meta-analysis, which yielded a prevalence rate of 2.5% (95% CI 2.1–3.1). Mean age of participants ranged from 19 to 45 years, but mostly up to 28 years, with only one sample with a mean age of 45 years [12]. Prevalence rates were detected to have a significant negative association with age, and this association was moderated by the gender composition of the sample. In a study investigating individuals from 60 to 94 years, the estimated prevalence rates of ADHD weighted back to the general population was 2.8% (95% CI 0.86–4.64) using a cut-off point of six symptoms, and 4.2% (95% CI 2.05–6.39) using a cut-off point of four symptoms [13].

Recently, the WHO's World Mental Health (WMH) Survey Initiative reported estimated prevalence rates for adults 18 to 44 years of age in 20 WMH surveys. These surveys were conducted in 11 high-income, 5 upper middle-income, and 4 low- and lower middle-income countries. Estimated rates were based on retrospective self-report of childhood ADHD, the presence of current symptoms and related impairment, and a multiple imputation method to assign clinical diagnoses of adult ADHD. Prevalence of

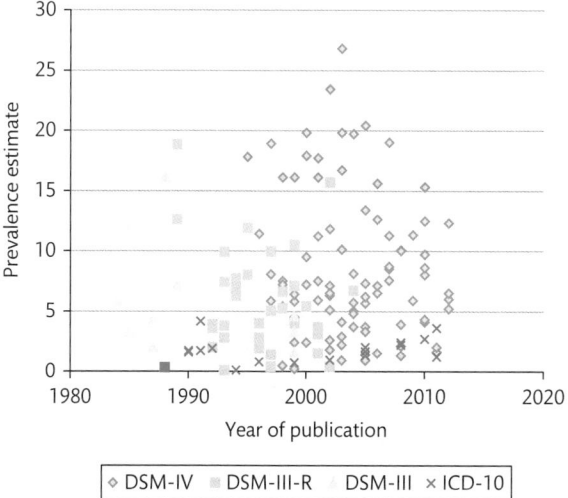

**Fig. 33.3** ADHD prevalence estimates over time as a function of diagnostic criteria.

Reproduced from *International Journal of Epidemiology*, 43(2), Polanczyk G, Guilherme V, Willcutt, EG, ADHD prevalence estimates across three decades: an updated systematic review and meta-regression analysis, pp. 434–442, Copyright (2014) with permission from Oxford University Press.

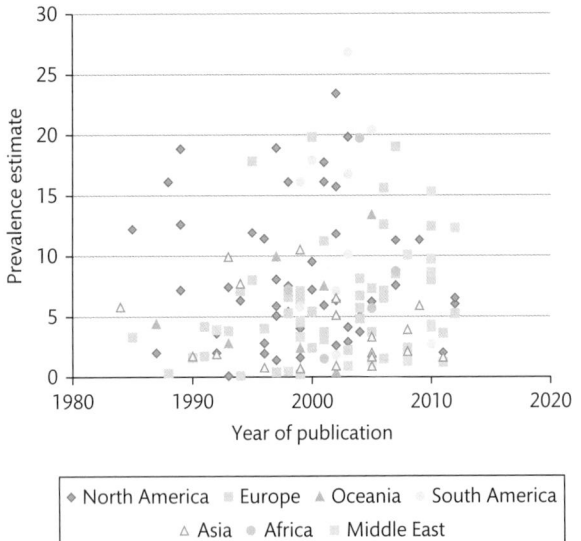

**Fig. 33.4** (see Colour Plate section) ADHD prevalence estimates over time as a function of geographic location of the studies.

Reproduced from *International Journal of Epidemiology*, 43(2), Polanczyk G, Guilherme V, Willcutt, EG, ADHD prevalence estimates across three decades: an updated systematic review and meta-regression analysis, pp. 434–442, Copyright (2014) with permission from Oxford University Press.

DSM-IV ADHD in childhood averaged 2.2% across surveys (range 0.1–8.1%). Estimates had a positive correlation with country income. Current prevalence of adult ADHD averaged 2.8% across surveys (range 0.6–7.3%), a higher rate than childhood ADHD. Higher estimates in adulthood were also detected in high-income (3.6%) than in low- and lower middle-income (1.4%) countries [14].

## Developmental changes

The first prospective longitudinal studies that investigated the natural course of ADHD across development included clinically referred children and clearly documented that symptoms declined over time. An early systematic review initially estimated an exponential decline during development, suggesting that virtually all children with ADHD would improve over time [15]. Subsequent studies have confirmed that remission of full diagnostic status was indeed common but that a substantial number of children remained symptomatic and most of them remained impaired as early adults [16]. Longitudinal studies documented that decline is more pronounced for hyperactive and impulsive symptoms, and less pronounced for inattention [16]. Indeed, cross-sectional studies assessing adults with ADHD indicated that inattention and executive dysfunction are the most common symptoms [17].

A meta-analysis of longitudinal studies confirmed that rates of ADHD persistence across development depended on its conceptual definition. The pooled rate for persistence at a mean age of 25 years according to full criteria (syndromatic persistence) for DSM-III, DSM-III-R, or DSM-IV adult ADHD was approximately 15%, and according to partial remission (symptomatic persistence) approximately 65% [18]. The study with the longest prospective follow-up conducted until now evaluated adults at a mean age of 41 years who were clinically referred and diagnosed with ADHD as children, at a mean age of 8 years [19]. Among them, 22% met adult ADHD criteria (vs 5% in the comparison group). Individuals with childhood ADHD had worse educational, occupational, economic, and social outcomes as adults, as well as increased rates of antisocial personality disorder and substance use disorders [19].

More recently, prospective longitudinal studies following representative community samples of children to adolescence and adulthood challenged the notion that ADHD always begins early in life. Moffitt *et al.* [20], studying the Dunedin Multidisciplinary Health and Development Study in New Zealand, documented ADHD cases prospectively from childhood to 38 years of age. The authors reported a follow-forward analysis of ADHD cases diagnosed in childhood and a follow-back analysis of ADHD cases diagnosed in adulthood. Follow-forward analysis revealed that only 5% of children with ADHD still met diagnostic criteria at the age of 38 but continued to experience difficulties in life adjustment. Follow-back analysis showed that only 10% of adults with ADHD had the diagnosis as children [20]. Surprisingly, these results were replicated in two other prospective longitudinal studies of community samples from the UK [21] and Brazil [22]. Analysis of the E-Risk Study (UK) demonstrated that 21.9% of children with ADHD met diagnostic criteria at the age of 18 years. At the age of 18 years, only 32.5% of those with ADHD met criteria for ADHD during childhood [21]. Analysis of the Pelotas Study (Brazil) demonstrated that 17.2% of children with ADHD met diagnostic criteria at the age of 18–19 years. At the age of 18 years, only 12.6% of those with ADHD met criteria for ADHD during childhood [22]. Adult ADHD cases without a history of childhood ADHD were not fully explained by comorbidities, subthreshold symptoms, and information bias. A possible explanation is that subthreshold cases in childhood emerge as cases in adulthood when demands exceed capacities [23]. Alternatively, child-onset and adult-onset ADHD may be distinct disorders, with possible distinct aetiologies. In this direction, polygenic risk score for ADHD (see Chapter 34) predicts childhood-, but not adult-, onset forms of ADHD [20]. Also, the likelihood of adult-onset ADHD arising in a monozygotic twin is not increased when the co-twin has childhood-onset ADHD [21]. The questions of whether adult-onset ADHD represents the late expression of early-onset neurogenetic risk factors or if it constitutes a distinct syndrome are yet to be answered [24].

## Risk factors

### Sociodemographic risk

ADHD affects predominantly males, with a male:female ratio of 3–4:1 in clinical samples [25] and 2.4:1 in community samples [26], suggesting a significant referral bias. Among adults, this sex difference is attenuated, probably also due to referral biases (in the opposite direction) or sex-specific developmental trajectories of ADHD. Cross-sectional studies and administrative data detected associations with ethnicity, which are not detected by community-based studies. Low socio-economic status in early childhood is associated with increased likelihood of ADHD, but it is not clear if it is a marker or risk, since there is a strong genetic risk and the disorder leads to low educational and occupational achievement, or if there is a causal relationship [27], possibly interacting with other risk factors [28].

## Genetics

Evidence from different approaches support the strong genetic influences on ADHD, which are mostly of small individual effect. Genetic variants underlie multiple molecular, neural, and cognitive trajectories, partially shared with other neurodevelopmental disorders, that lead to behavioural phenotypes currently defined as ADHD [29, 30]. A detailed description is given in Chapter 34.

## Environmental risk

Twin studies indicate that shared environmental risks are not relevant to the aetiology of ADHD. Environmental risk factors seem to exert their effect in the non-shared familial environment, that is, parental influences that are specific to a child, peer, and school influences and exposure to individual risks. Exposure to environmental stressors may result in biological changes, such as brain structure and function, and also in modifications of gene expression. Environmental risk can also interact with genetic variants and, depending on them, can have different effects, that is, gene–environment interaction. Also, environmental risks can arise due to behaviours that are genetically influenced and may have partial or no effect on the outcome once the genetic effects are taken into account, that is, gene–environment correlation. Environmental risks have been investigated by different epidemiological methods, some of them suited to infer causality, but most of them not. Exposures to risk factors can be influenced by confounders, some of which are not identified and controlled for (for example, genetic effects), and also by the very presence of ADHD that can lead to the risk exposure (reverse causation). Selection bias is also an important methodological caveat that may lead to false positive associations.

## Prenatal and perinatal factors

Low birthweight, prematurity, obstetric complications, *in utero* exposure to maternal stress, tobacco, and alcohol and substances (medications and illicit drugs) are risk factors associated with ADHD. There are no studies to date demonstrating their causal effect. Associations between maternal stress and smoking during pregnancy and ADHD have been demonstrated by genetically sensitive studies to be explained mainly by genetic or other shared risk factors [31].

## Toxins

The association with prenatal exposure to toxins, such as organophosphate pesticides, polychlorinated biphenyls, and lead, has been studied in longitudinal studies, and also in cross-sectional studies which demonstrated higher levels in children affected by ADHD. Their causal association is biologically plausible, and animal studies have supported their negative effect over several domains of cognitive function. Nevertheless, their causal effect in humans has yet to be demonstrated.

## Diet

Extreme nutritional deficits impair neurodevelopmental processes globally, but the effects of specific nutrients and how mild deficits at specific moments of development affect cognitive functions are not yet clear [32]. The associations between zinc, magnesium, and polyunsaturated fatty acids and ADHD have been studied in cross-sectional studies, and there is no convincing evidence indicating that they are risk factors, and not correlates. Sugar and artificial food colourings have also been identified so far as correlates.

## Other factors

Obesity [33], sleep disorders [34, 35], and television exposure [36] have been associated with attentional problems and ADHD by cross-sectional, prospective, and retrospective longitudinal studies, with insufficient data to characterize the temporal ordering; at the moment, they are also understood as correlates.

## Family adversity

Family adversity and harsh or hostile parent–child interactions have been consistently associated with ADHD but may arise as consequences of the disorder, rather than increase the risk of it [37]. The English and Romanian Adoptees study has followed children exposed to early severe institutional deprivation in Romania who were subsequently adopted by English families and studied their long-term emotional and cognitive developmental. Deprivation had strong effects immediately after adoption, followed by substantial catch-up for some children at the age of 6 [38]. At the age of 15 years, children exposed to more than 6 months of deprivation were four times more likely to present with ADHD than those with less than 6 months of deprivation, and those children exposed to more than 6 months of deprivation had persistently higher rates of inattention and hyperactivity through to the ages of 23 to 25 [39]. These results point to a causal role of very severe early deprivation in the development of ADHD with particular characteristics. Deprivation-related ADHD was not as likely as non-deprivation-related ADHD to affect boys and to present with comorbid conduct problems; it presented with high levels of comorbid social disinhibition and autistic features and severe neuropsychological impairment [40].

# Prevention

## Conceptual and methodological issues

Preventive actions target causal risk factors to reduce incidence, that is, new cases of disorders. Therefore, by definition, preventive interventions are those implemented before the onset of the disorder. Those implemented after the onset are referred to as treatment or rehabilitation. There are three levels of preventive interventions: universal, selective, and indicated. Universal interventions target the general public or a whole population group that has not been identified on the basis of increased risk. Selective interventions target individuals or subgroups of the population whose risk of developing a disorder is significantly higher than average, as evidenced by biological, psychological, or social risk factors. Indicated interventions target high-risk people who are identified as having minimal, but detectable, signs or symptoms or biological markers, indicating a predisposition for a disorder, but who do not meet diagnostic criteria at that time. Also preceding the disease onset, measures to enhance well-being (by increasing protective factors such as supportive family, school, and community environments) may also function as preventive measures [41].

In the past decades, significant investment has been directed to the prevention science of mental, emotional, and behavioural disorders affecting youth. Researchers have successfully developed and tested interventions targeting depression, suicide, schizophrenia, and conduct disorder. These studies have begun to define the methodological challenges and strategies for the success of preventative interventions for mental disorders. Firstly, the causal mechanisms or origins of the disorder should be clear enough to be manipulated by strategies that are effective in reducing their occurrence or buffering their effects. Secondly, the disorder itself must be well characterized, together with the boundaries between the disorder and normalcy and its trajectory. Thirdly, methods to screen and identify individuals who are not affected by the disorder but are likely to develop it within a specific period of time should be available. Fourthly, the risks and costs related to the screening and intervention processes should be well balanced and not be higher than their potential benefits. Once all these challenges have been overcome, randomized controlled studies with adequate statistical power must demonstrate the benefits of the intervention. Statistical power reflects the necessary sample size to demonstrate reductions in incidence of the disorder, which may vary from hundreds to tens of thousands. It will depend on the base rate of new cases for the particular population studied and the magnitude of the effect of the intervention [42]. Preventive interventions are not necessarily ready to be used once their effectiveness has been demonstrated, but they must be implemented, sustained, and scaled up within clinical and community systems and offered to the target populations. At this stage, elements such as programme contents, delivery strategy, intensity and duration, personnel training and supervision, compliance, fidelity, and funding need to be addressed, so that they can be translated into real-world programmes [43–45].

### Challenges of preventive interventions for ADHD

The development of preventive strategies for ADHD, such as for any neurodevelopmental disorder, is a challenging endeavour. ADHD arises as a consequence of multiple mechanistic causal processes, for which no component has been identified so far as sufficient or necessary. More importantly, as reviewed before, only a few environmental exposures—components that can be manipulated—have been identified so far as likely causal. Early severe institutional deprivation is likely to be causal but is mercifully uncommon in developed societies. Pre- and perinatal conditions and environmental toxins have been demonstrated to be risk factors with an unclear causal role. No other manipulable causal risk factor has been identified so far. In addition, genetic influences seem to be substantial, explaining a large proportion of heritability. The effects of genetic variants possibly interact with environmental exposures occurring early in life (some of them in the prenatal period) and lead to early emerging psychopathological processes. In addition, there are no current technologies to identify molecular and neural psychopathological processes at their early stages, before the manifestation of behavioural symptoms. Therefore, with obscure causal mechanisms and early arising psychopathological processes, at the present moment, ADHD becomes identifiable at a stage when strategies can no longer prevent its development. Early diagnosis and interventions have an important potential to prevent cumulative impairments and comorbidities over development but are not conceptually defined as preventive interventions.

Therefore, preventive interventions that might reduce the incidence of ADHD and that are readily available are universal or selective programmes to act on the initial stages of common multi-disease mechanisms. In fact, compartmentalized programmes that focus on specific aspects of behavioural, educational, or social problems are unlikely to be adopted as public policies, which is an argument in favour of universal and selective prevention programmes [46]. These interventions potentially produce multiple benefits, which increase their cost–benefit and consequently their implementation and scale. Several intervention programmes in early childhood have been developed and tested worldwide [47, 48]. Some of the most studied interventions focus on programmes for the development of parental competences [49], on the stimulation of infants during the first 3 years of life [50], or on school curricula for the development of social and emotional competencies of children from 4 years of age [51]. Important features of a successful early childhood intervention programme include integrated models that combine elements geared to physical health, cognitive, emotional, and social development, sufficient duration and intensity, modelling learning, structured curriculum, adequate material support for learning, systematic supervision, and clear incorporation of theories of change [52].

A number of issues arise from the experience to date [52, 53]. Firstly, is there a distinction between promotion and prevention strategies, and can the incidence of mental disorders be reduced with promotion strategies? It is hypothesized that the promotion of skills is one of the possible mechanisms through which mental disorders can be prevented [54]. Thus, as social–emotional skills are developed generally, there would be a secondary reduction in the occurrence of mental disorders. This is an example of the Rose prevention paradox and refers to the hypothesis that an intervention benefiting a large number of people at moderate risk may be of more value than an intervention benefiting only a small number of people at high risk [46]. However, it is a consensus that positive mental health and mental disorders are not just opposing poles of the same dimension, but two overlapping and interrelated components of the concept of mental health. Other important issues to be addressed are implementation characteristics, even for those programmes that have evidence of their effectiveness [43]. Among the main barriers are the limited description of the interventions, the overlap between elements of prevention and promotion in the same programmes. the limited theoretical conceptualization of the desired changes and how they can lead to the desired outcomes, and the external validity of the evidence. In addition, poor understanding of the mechanisms involved in the effect of interventions and the lack of evidence of sustained effects beyond their initial implementation constitute significant barriers to the success of prevention science.

## Conclusions

ADHD is an impairing neurodevelopmental disorder that affects approximately 5% of children and adolescents worldwide, irrespective of their country of origin. In childhood, it affects predominantly males, although there is significant referral bias in their favour. In adulthood, sex differences are attenuated. ADHD is a long-lasting disorder, with symptoms or diagnosis persisting in approximately

70% of children as early adults. Cross-sectional studies estimate the adult ADHD prevalence in 2.5%.

Emerging evidence suggests that ADHD may arise in adulthood, challenging the notion that the disorder has always a neurodevelopmental origin. Currently, there are no definitive explanations for the so-called 'ADHD adult-onset cases', and hypotheses suggest that clinical cases in adulthood are preceded by childhood subclinical cases that emerge because of increasing demands or decreasing support or that child-onset and adult-onset ADHD are distinct disorders. In any case, no sufficient or necessary causal components (in terms of genetic risk, but also environmental influences and their interaction) have yet been implicated. Indeed, there are no environmental risks for ADHD identified so far of important magnitude and population-attributable fraction. In addition, molecular, neural, and cognitive psychopathological processes underlying the emergence of ADHD cannot yet be precisely identified, although, as explained in Chapters 32 and 34, the field is evolving rapidly.

Prevention is especially appealing for childhood mental disorders, which emerge temporally close to putative risk exposures. However, aetiological mechanisms probably operate during the perinatal period, are dominated by genetic risk, and have very few established environmental causal risk factors. Future elucidation of specific causal mechanisms will be required to inform the development of effective preventive interventions. Until then, the science of prevention of childhood mental disorders can be best further developed by accommodation with the growing interdisciplinary field of early childhood development.

## REFERENCES

1. Polanczyk, G., Caspi, A., Houts, R., Kollins, S.H., Rohde, L.A., and Moffitt, T.E. (2010). Implications of extending the ADHD age-of-onset criterion to age 12: results from a prospectively studied birth cohort. *Journal of the American Academy of Child and Adolescent Psychiatry*, 49, 210–16.

2. Matte, B., Anselmi, L., Salum, G.A., *et al.* (2014). ADHD in DSM-5: a field trial in a large, representative sample of 18- to 19-year-old adults. *Psychological Medicine*, 45, 361–73.

3. Polanczyk, G., de Lima, M.S., Horta, B.L., Biederman, J., and Rohde, L.A. (2007). The worldwide prevalence of ADHD: a systematic review and metaregression analysis. *American Journal of Psychiatry*, 164, 942–8.

4. Willcutt, E.G. (2012). The prevalence of DSM-IV attention-deficit/hyperactivity disorder: a meta-analytic review. *Neurotherapeutics*, 9, 490–9.

5. Polanczyk, G.V., Willcutt, E.G., Salum, G.A., Kieling, C., and Rohde, L.A. (2014). ADHD prevalence estimates across three decades: an updated systematic review and meta-regression analysis. *International Journal of Epidemiology*, 43, 434–42.

6. Collishaw, S. (2014). Annual Research Review: Secular trends in child and adolescent mental health. *Journal of Child Psychology and Psychiatry*, 56, 370–93.

7. Erskine, H.E., Ferrari, A.J., Nelson, P., *et al.* (2013). Epidemiological modelling of attention-deficit/hyperactivity disorder and conduct disorder for the Global Burden of Disease Study 2010. *Journal of Child Psychology and Psychiatry*, 54, 1263–74.

8. Erskine, H.E., Baxter, A.J., Patton, G., *et al.* (2017). The global coverage of prevalence data for mental disorders in children and adolescents. *Epidemiology and Psychiatric Sciences*, 26, 395–402.

9. Thomas, R., Sanders, S., Doust, J., Beller, E., and Glasziou, P. (2015). Prevalence of attention-deficit/hyperactivity disorder: a systematic review and meta-analysis. *Pediatrics*, 135, e994–1001.

10. Wang, T., Liu, K., Li, Z., *et al.* (2017). Prevalence of attention deficit/hyperactivity disorder among children and adolescents in China: a systematic review and meta- analysis. *BMC Psychiatry*, 17, 32.

11. Polanczyk, G.V., Salum, G.A., Sugaya, L.S., Caye, A., and Rohde, L.A. (2015). A meta-analysis of the worldwide prevalence of mental disorders in children and adolescents. *Journal of Child Psychology and Psychiatry*, 56, 345–65.

12. Simon, V., Czobor, P., Balint, S., Meszaros, A., and Bitter, I. (2009). Prevalence and correlates of adult attention-deficit hyperactivity disorder: meta-analysis. *British Journal of Psychiatry*, 194, 204–11.

13. Michielsen, M., Semeijn, E., Comijs HC, *et al.* (2012). Prevalence of attention-deficit hyperactivity disorder in older adults in The Netherlands. *British Journal of Psychiatry*, 201, 298–305.

14. Fayyad, J., Sampson, N.A., Hwang, I., *et al.* (2017). The descriptive epidemiology of DSM-IV Adult ADHD in the World Health Organization World Mental Health Surveys. *ADHD Attention Deficit and Hyperactivity Disorders*, 9, 47–65.

15. Hill, J.C. and Schoener, E.P. (1996). Age-dependent decline of attention deficit hyperactivity disorder. *American Journal of Psychiatry*, 153, 1143–6.

16. Biederman, J., Mick, E., and Faraone, S.V. (2000). Age-dependent decline of symptoms of attention deficit hyperactivity disorder: impact of remission definition and symptom type. *American Journal of Psychiatry*, 157, 816–18.

17. Kessler, R.C., Green, J.G., Adler, L.A., *et al.* (2010). Structure and diagnosis of adult attention-deficit/hyperactivity disorder: analysis of expanded symptom criteria from the Adult ADHD Clinical Diagnostic Scale. *Archives of General Psychiatry*, 67, 1168–78.

18. Faraone, S.V., Biederman, J., and Mick, E. (2006). The age-dependent decline of attention deficit hyperactivity disorder: a meta-analysis of follow-up studies. *Psychological Medicine*, 159–65.

19. Klein, R.G., Mannuzza, S., Olazagasti, M.A.R., *et al.* (2012). Clinical and functional outcome of childhood attention-deficit/hyperactivity disorder 33 years later. *Archives of General Psychiatry*, 69, 1295–303.

20. Moffitt, T.E., Houts, R., Asherson, P., *et al.* (2015). Is adult ADHD a childhood-onset neurodevelopmental disorder? Evidence from a four-decade longitudinal cohort study. *American Journal of Psychiatry*, 172, 967–77.

21. Agnew-Blais, J.C., Polanczyk, G.V., Danese, A., Wertz, J., Moffitt, T.E., and Arseneault, L. (2016). Evaluation of the persistence, remission, and emergence of attention-deficit/hyperactivity disorder in young adulthood. *JAMA Psychiatry*, 73, 713–20.

22. Caye, A., Rocha, T.B.-M., Anselmi, L., *et al.* (2016). Attention-deficit/hyperactivity disorder trajectories from childhood to young adulthood: evidence from a birth cohort supporting a late-onset syndrome. *JAMA Psychiatry*, 73, 705–12.

23. Faraone, S.V. and Biederman, J. (2016). Can attention-deficit/hyperactivity disorder onset occur in adulthood? *JAMA Psychiatry*, 73, 655–6.

24. Shaw, P. and Polanczyk, G.V. (2017). Combining epidemiological and neurobiological perspectives to characterize the lifetime trajectories of ADHD. *European Child and Adolescent Psychiatry*, 20, 1–3.

25. Faraone, S.V. (2009). Using meta-analysis to compare the efficacy of medications for attention-deficit/hyperactivity disorder in youths. *Physical Therapy*, 34, 678–94.

26. Polanczyk, G., de Lima, M.S., Horta, B.L., Biederman, J., and Rohde, L.A. (2007). The worldwide prevalence of ADHD: a systematic review and metaregression analysis. *American Journal of Psychiatry*, 164, 942–8.

27. Larsson, H., Sariaslan, A., Långström, N., D'Onofrio, B., and Lichtenstein, P. (2013). Family income in early childhood and subsequent attention deficit/hyperactivity disorder: a quasi-experimental study. *Journal of Child Psychology and Psychiatry*, 55, 428–35.

28. Rowland, A.S., Skipper, B.J., Rabiner, D.L., *et al.* (2017). Attention-deficit/hyperactivity disorder (ADHD): interaction between socioeconomic status and parental history of ADHD determines prevalence. *Journal of Child Psychology and Psychiatry*, 36, 1204.

29. Faraone, S.V., Asherson, P., Banaschewski, T., *et al.* (2015). Attention-deficit/hyperactivity disorder. *Nature Reviews Disease Primers*, 1, 15020.

30. Thapar, A. and Cooper, M. (2015). Attention deficit hyperactivity disorder. *The Lancet*, 387, 1240–50.

31. Thapar, A., Cooper, M., Eyre, O., and Langley, K. (2013). What have we learnt about the causes of ADHD? *Journal of Child Psychology and Psychiatry*, 54, 3–16.

32. Gómez-Pinilla, F. (2008). Brain foods: the effects of nutrients on brain function. *Nature Reviews Neuroscience*, 9, 568–78.

33. Rankin, J., Matthews, L., Cobley, S., *et al.* (2016). Psychological consequences of childhood obesity: psychiatric comorbidity and prevention. *Adolescent Health, Medicine, and Therapeutics*, 7, 125–46.

34. Bonuck, K., Freeman, K., Chervin, R.D., and Xu, L. (2012). Sleep-disordered breathing in a population-based cohort: behavioral outcomes at 4 and 7 years. *Pediatrics*, 129, e857–65.

35. Fischman, S., Kuffler, D.P., and Bloch, C. (2015). Disordered sleep as a cause of attention deficit/hyperactivity disorder: recognition and management. *Clinical Pediatrics (Phila)*, 54, 713–22.

36. Christakis, D.A., Zimmerman, F.J., DiGiuseppe, D.L., and McCarty, C.A. (2004). Early television exposure and subsequent attentional problems in children. *Pediatrics*, 113, 708–13.

37. Lifford, K.J., Harold, G.T., and Thapar, A. (2009). Parent–child hostility and child ADHD symptoms: a genetically sensitive and longitudinal analysis. *Journal of Child Psychology and Psychiatry*, 50, 1468–76.

38. O'Connor, T.G., Rutter, M., Beckett, C., Keaveney, L., and Kreppner, J.M. (2000). The effects of global severe privation on cognitive competence: extension and longitudinal follow-up. English and Romanian Adoptees Study Team. *Child Development*, 71, 376–90.

39. Sonuga-Barke, E.J.S., Kennedy, M., Kumsta, R., *et al.* (2017). Child-to-adult neurodevelopmental and mental health trajectories after early life deprivation: the young adult follow-up of the longitudinal English and Romanian Adoptees study. *The Lancet*, 389, 1539–48.

40. Kennedy, M., Kreppner, J., Knights, N., *et al.* (2016). Early severe institutional deprivation is associated with a persistent variant of adult attention-deficit/hyperactivity disorder: clinical presentation, developmental continuities and life circumstances in the English and Romanian Adoptees study. *Journal of Child Psychology and Psychiatry*, 57, 1113–25.

41. National Research Council and Institute of Medicine. (2009). *Preventing mental, emotional, and behavioral disorders among young people: progress and possibilities*. The National Academies Press, Washington, DC.

42. Muñoz, R.F., Cuijpers, P., Smit, F., Barrera, A.Z., and Leykin, Y. (2010). Prevention of major depression. *Annual Review of Clinical Psychology*, 6, 181–212.

43. Yousafzai, A.K. and Aboud, F. (2013). Review of implementation processes for integrated nutrition and psychosocial stimulation interventions. *Annals of the New York Academy of Sciences*, 1308, 33–45.

44. Betancourt, T.S. and Chambers, D.A. (2016). Optimizing an era of global mental health implementation science. *JAMA Psychiatry*, 73, 99.

45. Gold, R., Bunce, A.E., Cohen, D.J., *et al.* Reporting on the strategies needed to implement proven interventions: an example from a 'real-world' cross-setting implementation study. *Mayo Clinic Proceedings*, 91, 1074–83.

46. Chiolero, A., Paradis, G., and Paccaud, F. (2015). The pseudo-high-risk prevention strategy. *International Journal of Epidemiology*, 44, 1469–73.

47. Daelmans, B., Black, M.M., Lombardi, J., *et al.* Effective interventions and strategies for improving early child development. *BMJ*, 351, h4029.

48. Britto, P.R., Lye, S.J., Proulx, K., *et al.* (2017). Nurturing care: promoting early childhood development. *The Lancet*, 389, 91–102.

49. Olds, D., Henderson, C.R., Cole, R., *et al.* (1998). Long-term effects of nurse home visitation on children's criminal and antisocial behavior: 15-year follow-up of a randomized controlled trial. *JAMA*, 280, 1238–44.

50. Walker, S.P., Chang, S.M., Powell, C.A., and Grantham-McGregor, S.M. (2005). Effects of early childhood psychosocial stimulation and nutritional supplementation on cognition and education in growth-stunted Jamaican children: prospective cohort study. *The Lancet*, 366, 1804–7.

51. Campbell, F., Conti, G., Heckman, J.J., *et al.* (2014). Early childhood investments substantially boost adult health. *Science*, 343, 1478–85.

52. Aboud, F.E. and Yousafzai, A.K. (2015). Global health and development in early childhood. *Annual Review of Psychology*, 66, 433–57.

53. Black, M.M., Walker, S.P., Fernald, L.C.H., *et al.* (2017). Early childhood development coming of age: science through the life course. *The Lancet*, 389, 77–90.

54. World Health Organization (2004). *Prevention of mental disorders: effective interventions and policy options*. World Health Organization, Geneva.

# 34

# Genetics of attention-deficit/hyperactivity disorder

*Kate Langley and Anita Thapar*

## Overview

Attention-deficit/hyperactivity disorder (ADHD) is a phenotypically heterogenous disorder and, like other psychiatric disorders, is multifactorial in origin; multiple genetic, as well as environmental, influences contribute risk. The multifactorial liability model is one useful approach to conceptualizing complex disorders such as ADHD. This considers disorders, including ADHD, as manifestations of an underlying continuously distributed liability, with the diagnosis lying above a certain threshold on this liability curve (Fig. 34.1). Multiple risk factors contribute to this liability, and the additive effects of genetic and environmental risk and protective factors shift individuals along this population liability. This chapter will look at the role of genetic factors in the aetiology of ADHD and those factors that have already been identified as being relevant, highlighting our current understanding regarding its genetic architecture. It will also discuss the methodological and phenotypic challenges that have influenced our current understanding. The heterogeneity of the ADHD phenotype has been discussed in more detail in Chapter 31.

## Familial risk and heritability estimates from twin and family studies

Traditional genetic studies that infer, rather than directly assess, genetic contribution have overwhelmingly found ADHD to be a highly familial and heritable disorder. Family studies have shown that the risk of ADHD is increased in first-degree relatives of those with the disorder, with modest relative risks of between 4.0% and 5.4% [1]. Similarly, adoption studies of ADHD have suggested that adopted children have ADHD behaviour scores that are more similar to their biological than adoptive parents [2–5].

Numerous twin studies have also indicated the importance of genetic factors in the aetiology of ADHD, with meta-analyses reporting heritability estimates of between 70% and 80% [6]. The remainder of the variance is generally found to be due to unique environmental effects, with only a very small proportion attributable to shared environmental factors [6]. These studies suggest ADHD is one of the more heritable of psychiatric disorders, on a par with autism spectrum disorder (ASD), bipolar disorder, and schizophrenia [7, 8].

These estimates are similar for the ADHD symptom dimensions of inattention and hyperactivity/impulsivity, with both common and separate genetic factors relevant to each dimension [6, 9–11]. There is also evidence from twin studies that genetic factors influencing ADHD act on a continuum, whereby heritability estimates are similar between those with a clinical diagnosis of the disorder and the traits seen within the general population (for example, [12, 13–15]). The informant utilized to ascertain ADHD symptoms appears to be important here and is an important consideration for genetic studies of ADHD. Twin studies using self-reported ADHD symptoms in adulthood have reported significantly lower heritability estimates of between 30% and 40% [16] than studies of children or adolescents that have generally utilized parent or teacher reports. The low self-report heritability estimates may reflect findings that affected individuals are less accurate than others at describing their own ADHD behaviours [17]. However, investigations have suggested that the drop-off in heritability estimates is likely due to the fact that (unlike with parent and, frequently, teacher reports) self-reported measures involve different individuals rating each twin. Studies where different parents or teachers reported on twins in childhood (for example, [18, 19]) have seen this same drop-off in heritability rates, while studies utilizing composite measures of parent and teacher reports and self-report in adulthood have observed high heritability rates of 60–70% [17]. While the initial findings of adult ADHD twin studies are no longer considered a challenge to the view that ADHD is highly heritable throughout the lifespan, they do highlight that methodological issues, such as the choice of informant, can impact upon our conclusions and understanding regarding the genetics of ADHD.

## Rare genetic variants and copy number variants

While traditional twin and family studies are unable to identify which specific genetic factors might be involved in the disorder, they do indicate that molecular genetic studies should aid our

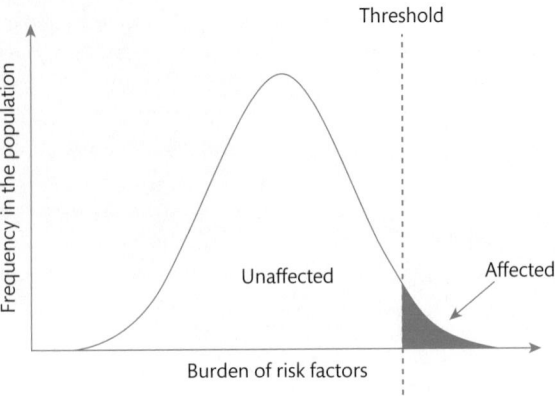

**Fig. 34.1** Threshold liability model. Multiple risk factors, both genetic and environmental, are continuously distributed across the population. Individuals with a burden of risk factors above a certain threshold are considered to have a clinical diagnosis of the disorder.

understanding of the aetiology and pathogenesis of ADHD. To date, such studies have involved investigation of different classes of gene variants, both rare and common, across the whole genome and at specific candidate locations. It has been known for some time that some types of rare genetic syndromes are associated with ADHD phenotypes. For example, 22q11.2 deletion syndrome, as well as being a known risk factor for schizophrenia, is commonly associated with ADHD in childhood [20]. Other rare genetic syndromes associated with ADHD include fragile X syndrome [21] and tuberous sclerosis [22]. It is not inevitable that affected individuals show intellectual disability, but these syndromes are commonly characterized by additional phenotypic characteristics (for example, congenital heart defect, dysmorphic features, epilepsy). A number of studies have investigated the contribution of rare chromosomal deletions and duplications known as CNVs to ADHD risk. As observed for schizophrenia, ASD, and intellectual disability, a higher burden of large, rare CNVs has been identified in individuals with ADHD, compared to control individuals [23–26] (see Chapters 23, 28, and 59).

The burden of large, rare CNVs is especially elevated in those who have intellectual disability, as well as ADHD, but findings are not restricted to this IQ group [25]. Not all studies have individually observed an excess of CNVs in those with ADHD (for example, [27–29]). However, a pooled analysis of multiple data sets suggests overall there is an increased burden of CNVs in children with ADHD and a significant excess of duplications at chromosomes 15q13.3 and 16p13.11 [24, 25]. ADHD-associated CNVs show significant overlap with those implicated in ASD and schizophrenia [25, 27]. These findings highlight that even though these disorders are clinically very different, there are shared genetic risk factors. Genetic findings provide a window into biology that is otherwise difficult to directly access for psychiatric disorders, including ADHD. CNVs associated with ADHD have started to provide some clues on pathogenesis. These chromosomal duplications and deletions span genes that encode proteins involved in multiple biological pathways that also partially overlap with those implicated in autism and schizophrenia. Results to date from ADHD CNV studies [27, 30–32] suggest significant evidence of enrichment for genes involved in the brain (for example, neurite outgrowth, ion channel pathways). However, the

genes and biological mechanisms implicated in ADHD are not identical to those in other disorders. That is perhaps unsurprising, given their phenotypic manifestations are dissimilar and also medications that are effective in reducing ADHD symptoms do not benefit core symptoms of schizophrenia and autism.

Rare genetic mutations, including CNVs, can either be inherited from a parent with the same mutation (transmitted) or arise as the result of a spontaneous mutation in the individual (*de novo*). There have been some suggestions that spontaneous *de novo* CNVs may provide especially useful clues on genetic risk loci for disorders [33] and are associated with a larger effect size than transmitted CNVs [34]. While not all studies of ADHD have parental DNA to identify the origin of CNVs (for example, [32]), it seems that both transmitted and *de novo* CNVs have been identified in those with ADHD [25, 27–29]. Interestingly, some inherited CNVs seem to originate from parents who are also affected by ADHD [27–29] and involve regions previously implicated as risk loci for ADHD and other neurodevelopmental disorders [27, 28]. While further work is needed to replicate these findings and further elucidate their potential role in the aetiology of ADHD, they highlight the relevance of looking beyond the individual at the wider family to further understand the genetic aetiology of ADHD.

As one would expect for a multifactorial disorder, these rare genetic syndromes and CNVs are not observed in all affected individuals and CNV carriers do not necessarily show ADHD alone. CNVs are one class of rare genetic variant involving chromosomal alterations. To date, rare variations in DNA *sequence* have not been examined in ADHD. However, common gene variants have been investigated, and this will be discussed next.

## Candidate gene studies

Initial molecular genetic studies were restricted to genotyping genetic variants at specific locations, rather than across the whole genome. In psychiatry, such candidate gene-based approaches are now regarded with scepticism, given the high likelihood of false positives. Also, the pathogenesis of psychiatric disorders is unknown, meaning that the selection of candidate genes is not based on a firm hypothesis. Nevertheless, for ADHD, some candidate gene variant findings were replicated and withstood meta-analysis. Meta-analyses have shown associations for variants within *DRD4, DAT1, DRD5, 5HTT*, and *SNAP25* [35]. As the candidate gene methods have been replaced by newer hypothesis-free genome-wide association studies (GWAS), the relevance of these putative risk variants needs to be reconfirmed. While none of these findings have been upheld by GWAS to date, this might be observed in the future as sample sizes for such studies increase. This has been seen for schizophrenia; variants within the *DRD2* gene that had been associated with schizophrenia in candidate gene studies were not replicated in smaller GWAS, but *DRD2* has now been implicated by the largest schizophrenia GWAS to date [36].

## Findings from ADHD GWAS

GWAS use case-control or similar types of design to investigate the association between a disorder and a large number of single-nucleotide polymorphisms (SNPs), a type of common genetic variant, across the genome simultaneously. This method is advantageous, as it looks at multiple variants in a hypothesis-free (and therefore unbiased) manner, but requires stringent corrections for multiple testing as so many variants are tested for association [37]. This means that such studies require extremely large samples for associations to reach genome-wide significance [38].

GWAS of ADHD have generally been undertaken on small, underpowered samples. In the first nine reported studies [23, 39–45], sample sizes for ADHD cases ranged from 343 to 1013, with a meta-analysis of four separate studies [46], including just over 3000 individuals with ADHD. None of these studies reported any genome-wide significant findings, and there was little overlap in the top hits across studies. Although the small sample sizes were acknowledged to be an issue (for example, [47, 48]), as for similarly sized samples investigating schizophrenia or bipolar disorder [46], the lack of findings initially led some to question the relevance of common gene variants in the aetiology of ADHD [49].

However, recently, the ADHD sample size assembled by the Psychiatric Genetics Consortium (PGC) ADHD subgroup has risen to over 20,000 ADHD cases and 35,000 controls. Initial reports suggest twelve genome-wide significant loci (PGC-ADHD subgroup report, International Society of Psychiatric Genetics meeting, Toronto, October 2015) [49a]. This is an exciting development and, given the increased sample size in comparison to previous studies of ADHD, demonstrates the frequently cited need for large samples to find genome-wide significant risk loci [38, 50]. It is too early to understand the implications of these findings. Each of these variants will need to be looked at in more detail to identify the specific causal variant, as has been undertaken in other complex disorders (for example, [51]). It will also be important to ascertain whether the genes implicated by the associated SNPs highlight specific biological functions or pathways [36]. Furthermore, it is clear that these putative risk loci are only the 'tip of the iceberg' in understanding the aetiology of ADHD, as a multifactorial disorder influenced by multiple genetic *and* non-genetic risk factors. Also, a much larger number of common and rare genetic loci remain to be identified. Although the latest ADHD GWAS includes a much larger sample size, it is still small in comparison to those utilized for studies of other medical and some psychiatric disorders. Indeed, in the study of schizophrenia, where the largest GWAS study has identified 128 genome-wide significant hits [36], it is recognized that this is not the full extent of the common genetic variance accountable for the disorder [50].

However, because these studies were sufficiently powered to identify genetic loci with an effect size of 1.3 [37], we can conclude that there are no ADHD common genetic risk variants with a large effect size. This suggests that, as with other disorders such as schizophrenia (for example, [36]), the genetic architecture of ADHD is explained by a large number of common gene variants, each of small effect size, as well as rare mutations that have larger effect size. Environmental risks may also make an important contribution.

## Composite measures of common genetic risk

While the recent GWAS findings are promising, any single SNP has a small effect size on its own. This has led to methods that involve generating composite measures of multiple common genetic risk variants [37, 52]. One such method is genomic relationship–matrix restricted maximum likelihood (GRML), which is often referred to by the software programme used to implement it—GCTA. Using genome-wide SNP data, this method estimates the genetic similarity between unrelated individuals. This makes it possible to identify SNP heritability, which ranges between 17% and 45% [45, 53–55] (although not all are in agreement [56]). Schizophrenia polygenic risk scores derived from much larger studies account for only 7% of the variance [36]. Common gene variants appear to account for only a proportion of the heritability identified by twin studies, and this will, in part, be due to the role of additional risks, including rare variants such as CNVs.

A further method used to obtain a composite measure of common genetic risk is polygenic risk score analysis, which involves summing multiple risk alleles (SNPs) identified by a 'discovery' GWAS, including those at a very nominal level of significance. Putative risk alleles in individuals in an independent sample are then combined to give an individual polygenic risk score. ADHD polygenic risk scores have been shown to predict ADHD caseness [57], which highlighted, prior to the PGC genome-wide significant findings, that common gene variants contribute to risk.

ADHD is a multifactorial liability disorder whereby genetic and other risks are on a continuum throughout the population, with clinical diagnosis as one extreme (for example, [12–15]). Polygenic risk scores derived from the general population's ADHD trait scores predict ADHD diagnosis in a case-control sample [58], while the opposite is also observed; ADHD polygenic risk scores derived from patients with the diagnosis (case-control samples) predict ADHD trait levels in the general population [30, 59].

Polygenic risk scores (across all disorders) currently account for a very small proportion of the phenotype variance—0.1–2.0% in the current studies of ADHD (for example, [49a, 57, 59]). Therefore, while polygenic risk score analyses can give some insight into the genetic architecture of ADHD, they only provide one indicator of genetic risk and alone cannot be used as diagnostic prediction tools. As sample sizes increase and our ability to identify loci more accurately from GWAS increases, measurement of genetic risk should improve, and when coupled with other measures of genetic risk (for example, family history), predictive ability should also improve [60].

## Gene–environment interplay

Environmental exposures often believed to be risk factors for ADHD are described in Chapter 34. It will be explained in more detail here why the epidemiological findings may be a further expression of genetic, rather than simply environmental, risk. Environmental exposure in ADHD is not independent of an individual's genes—a phenomenon known as gene–environment correlation. Gene–environment correlation arises for environmental exposures (for example, quality of relationships) that are shaped by individuals' behaviours or dispositions (active and evocative gene–environment correlation) or through their parents' attributes (passive gene–environmental correlation). Further explanations and examples of gene–environment correlation can be seen in Table 34.1. Even if an environmental risk has genetic origins, the impact on ADHD could still be environmental, although designs that go beyond observation

**Table 34.1** Types of gene–environment correlations: descriptions and examples

| Type of gene–environment correlation | Description | Example |
| --- | --- | --- |
| Passive | An individual inherits genotypes from their parents who also provide the rearing environment | A disorganized parent may provide a more chaotic home environment, which reinforces the child's own disorganized tendencies |
| Active (niche picking) | Individuals seek environments that are compatible with, and reinforce, their genetic propensities | An impulsive child may seek out more risky situations or choose friends who engage in risky behaviour |
| Evocative | An individual's genetic tendencies elicit reactions from others which reinforce these tendencies | An irritable child will elicit more negative interactions from those around them |

(for example, genetically informative twin studies) are required to test this. For example, cigarette smoking is an environmental risk that is strongly genetically influenced (that is, has genetic origins), but it is an exposure that still has environmentally 'mediated' causal risk effects on lung cancer.

There is evidence to suggest that some of the environmental risks thought to contribute to ADHD (for example, maternal lifestyle during pregnancy) do have partly genetic origins. The next question is whether the genetic factors that impact on ADHD environmental exposures (for example, maternal lifestyle) overlap with the ones that contribute to offspring ADHD. If that is the case, it would mean these environmental exposures, rather than being true causal risk factors for ADHD, represent expressions of the same genetic liability. Maternal smoking in pregnancy is a risk factor that is robustly associated with ADHD [61] but that is also under strong genetic influence. Multiple genetically informative studies, including discordant sibling pair designs (where the mother smokes in one pregnancy, and not in the other) [62], children of twins [63], and a design based on children born by assisted production [64], suggest that while the links between maternal smoking in pregnancy and offspring low birthweight are 'environmentally mediated', as one would expect, for ADHD, the association appears to be entirely, or mainly, explained by shared genetic liability in mother and child (manifest as smoking in pregnancy and offspring ADHD) [64a]. Clearly, smoking cessation is advisable for offspring and maternal health, but these findings suggest that this policy is unlikely to reduce the numbers affected by ADHD.

Mother–child hostility is another apparent environmental risk factor for ADHD. However, a number of genetically informative [65, 66] and treatment designs [67] suggest that it again is a consequence of ADHD symptoms and child genetic liability. Nevertheless, parent–child hostility has environmentally mediated links with conduct disorder [68] so might be important in terms of modifying ADHD outcomes. In contrast to these findings, very extreme early privation, as experienced by a group of children initially reared in Romanian orphanages and then adopted away, is an exposure that impacts on ADHD-like symptoms [69]. The links cannot be explained by shared genetic liabilities because the environmental exposure was imposed, rather than selected or evoked.

Gene–environment interaction provides another example of how genes and the environment work together. This has been demonstrated most clearly in animal models where the observable manifestation (phenotype) of a gene depends on the environmental context (for example, diet, exposure to a pathogen). Interaction extends to the molecular level; DNA codes for proteins, and there are multiple complex molecular mechanisms, including epigenetic ones, that modify the biological function of the same DNA sequence. Gene–environment interaction in humans is much more challenging to assess robustly at a molecular level. Traditional behavioural genetic designs that involve separation of G and E and capture all genetic liability via design (for example, children adopted away at birth) have shown repeatedly that the clinical manifestations of genetic liability (for example, for criminal behaviour, schizophrenia) are modified by the rearing environment and/or adoptive context (for example, [70, 71]). However, ADHD has not been studied in this way. Although there are published reports of interaction between specific candidate gene variants and environmental exposures (for example, [72, 73]), convincing findings on ADHD have yet to emerge. Similar methodological issues apply to the concept of 'differential susceptibility' whereby some individuals are more susceptible to the benefits of positive enriched environments, as well as more vulnerable to environmental risks.

Another example of gene–environment interaction comes from pharmacogenetics when the effects of medication (the environmental exposure) vary according to genotype, for example, slow and ultra-rapid metabolizers of drugs metabolized by the enzyme CYP2D6 [74]. So far, there have been no consistent and robust pharmacogenenetic findings in relation to ADHD medications that would have clinical practice implications. Despite the research challenges, it remains important at a conceptual level to appreciate the interplay of genes and the environment in understanding the aetiology of ADHD.

## Phenotype heterogeneity and ADHD

As described in detail in Chapter 31, ADHD is a highly heterogenous clinical disorder, with individuals frequently presenting with comorbid ASD, conduct disorder, anxiety, or depression.

Heterogeneity is very likely to be influenced by the underlying genetic architecture of the disorder. For example, the degree of genetic risk loading appears to vary for different subgroups of individuals with ADHD. Family and twin studies of ADHD suggest that individuals with comorbid conduct disorder have an increased genetic load, in comparison to those with ADHD alone [75, 76]. The relative risk (RR) of ADHD in biological relatives of those with ADHD plus conduct disorder is almost twice as high (RR 9.5) as that among first-degree relatives of individuals with ADHD alone (RR 5.4) [75]. At a molecular level, ADHD polygenic risk scores have also been observed to be higher in those individuals who have ADHD with comorbid conduct disorder, when compared to those with ADHD alone [57].

Previous candidate gene studies have suggested that there may be additional genetic variants which are specifically related to the subgroup of individuals with ADHD and conduct disorder, rather than all individuals with ADHD (for example, associations with the COMT val158met variant which have been identified in numerous replicated studies and a pooled analysis) (for example, [77, 78–80]). Time will tell whether or not this pattern of different genetic risks contributing to ADHD subtypes (and these specific associations) is confirmed, but such studies highlight the potential association of clinical heterogeneity to the genetic architecture of ADHD and the need to take this into account in the future.

While initially considered to be a childhood disorder, it is now recognized that ADHD persists into later adolescence and adulthood in a substantial number of individuals [81, 82]. Twin studies suggest that heritability estimates for ADHD are relatively stable throughout the lifespan (for example, [17–19]). Indeed, longitudinal studies following individuals throughout childhood to early adulthood suggest that heritability rates for ADHD remain stable, although the influence of specific genetic factors may change over time [83]. This change in the specific genetic factors potentially relevant at different ages may introduce a further element of heterogeneity in studies attempting to identify specific ADHD loci and may need to be considered. This is especially because, as larger samples are sought for GWAS, samples of children and adults with ADHD may be pooled. However, family and twin studies suggest that persistence of ADHD into adult life is more strongly familial [84] and highly heritable than childhood ADHD alone. To date, genome-wide gene discovery studies of adult ADHD have not yielded unique findings. Recent reports have suggested a further source of heterogeneity in adult ADHD; three population cohorts have shown that new cases of ADHD can present for the first time in late adolescence or adulthood [85–87]; future studies may consider the extent to which genetic factors are relevant to this group and how this may be the same or different to those for childhood-onset ADHD. The first of these studies [86] found that ADHD polygenic risk score did not significantly predict this later-onset group, although the sample size was small and an older discovery GWAS was used to generate risk alleles. Replication will be required.

## Shared genetic risks across disorders

Given that ADHD is known frequently to co-occur with other disorders, there has been interest in whether or not there is an overlap between the genetic risk for different psychiatric disorders. Twin studies suggest that there is considerable overlap of ADHD genetic risk factors with those that contribute to ASD [9], conduct disorder [76], and other neurodevelopmental disorders [88], although the extent of this overlap may vary somewhat, depending upon whether age or hyperactive/impulsive or inattentive symptoms are considered [9]. Although there are some shared genetic effects, twin studies also demonstrate genetic risks that are unique to each disorder. ADHD polygenic risk score studies have shown some overlap with other disorders (schizophrenia, bipolar disorder, and depression [54, 57]) and with other neurodevelopmental traits, including cognitive and language ability in the general population [89].

The large PGC Cross Disorder Group investigates the overlap between eight psychiatric disorders: ADHD, ASD, schizophrenia, bipolar disorder, major depressive disorder, anorexia nervosa, obsessional compulsive disorder, and Tourette syndrome. Using GWAS data, this group has found four genome-wide significant genetic loci appearing to be in common across disorders [54]. Interestingly, ADHD genetic overlap was strongest between ADHD and major depressive disorder [90, 90a].

## Summary and clinical implications

While it has been known for some time that ADHD is highly heritable, progress to date in identifying specific gene variants has been slow until recently. However, now is an exciting time. The findings of the first twelve genome-wide significant loci from the largest GWAS study to date give a glimpse of the specific common genetic risk variants that might be involved in the disorder and provide future insights into biology. Genetic findings confirm what clinicians have long supposed—that ADHD lies at the end of a population continuum. However, individual genetic loci have very small effect sizes, and at present, even composite measures cannot be used to predict who has or will get ADHD [90b].

CNV studies have demonstrated the relevance of rare variants to ADHD that have much greater effect size than individual common variants. These CNV findings have further highlighted the neurodevelopmental origins of ADHD and overlap between different neurodevelopmental traits as well as disorders. Overall genetics research findings are strongly supportive of the DSM-5 approach whereby ADHD is classified under the group of neurodevelopmental disorders, along with autism. Major efforts will be required to move research on ADHD genetic discoveries into clinically meaningful findings. This includes investigating the biological impacts of gene mutations, especially rare, highly penetrant ones. This can be achieved using a variety of approaches, including animal studies and cellular models (see Chapter 32). Other research will involve assessing the impact of gene variants (composite measures of common gene variants or rare, highly penetrant mutations) on brain/cognitive function (for example, [91]) and population health (for example, [92]).

Finally, genetic testing will become an issue. At present, although rare mutations are associated with ADHD, routine genetic testing for CNVs in those with ADHD alone is not indicated in any country, unless the affected individual also has intellectual disability. While genetic understanding cannot currently influence clinical practice, it is likely that as rare genetic subforms of ADHD are identified, policies for genetic investigation in practice might alter. Increased understanding will enable researchers to investigate the pathogenesis of ADHD in more detail, with positive benefits for the treatment of ADHD.

## REFERENCES

1. Thapar A, Langley K, Owen MJ, O'Donovan MC. Advances in genetic findings on attention deficit hyperactivity disorder. Psychological Medicine. 2007;37(12):1681–92.
2. Cantwell DP. Genetics of hyperactivity. Journal of Child Psychology and Psychiatry and Allied dDisciplines. 1975;16(3):261–4.
3. Cunningham L, Cadoret RJ, Loftus R, Edwards JE. Studies of adoptees from psychiatrically disturbed biological parents:

psychiatric conditions in childhood and adolescence. British Journal of Psychiatry. 1975;126:534–49.

4. Alberts-Corush J, Firestone P, Goodman JT. Attention and impulsivity characteristics of the biological and adoptive parents of hyperactive and normal control children. American Journal of Orthopsychiatry. 1986;56(3):413–23.

5. Sprich S, Biederman J, Crawford MH, Mundy E, Faraone SV. Adoptive and biological families of children and adolescents with ADHD. Journal of the American Academy of Child and Adolescent Psychiatry. 2000;39(11):1432–7.

6. Nikolas MA, Burt SA. Genetic and environmental influences on ADHD symptom dimensions of inattention and hyperactivity: a meta-analysis. Journal of Abnormal Psychology. 2010;119(1):1–17.

7. Uher R. The role of genetic variation in the causation of mental illness: an evolution-informed framework. Molecular Psychiatry. 2009;14(12):1072–82.

8. Sullivan PF, Daly MJ, O'Donovan M. Genetic architectures of psychiatric disorders: the emerging picture and its implications. Nature Reviews Genetics. 2012;13(8):537–51.

9. Rommelse NN, Hartman CA. Review: changing (shared) heritability of ASD and ADHD across the lifespan. European Child and Adolescent Psychiatry. 2016;25(3):213–15.

10. Greven CU, Rijsdijk FV, Plomin R. A twin study of ADHD symptoms in early adolescence: hyperactivity-impulsivity and inattentiveness show substantial genetic overlap but also genetic specificity. Journal of Abnormal Child Psychology. 2011;39(2):265–75.

11. McLoughlin G, Ronald A, Kuntsi J, Asherson P, Plomin R. Genetic support for the dual nature of attention deficit hyperactivity disorder: substantial genetic overlap between the inattentive and hyperactive-impulsive components. Journal of Abnormal Child Psychology. 2007;35(6):999–1008.

12. Thapar A. Attention deficit hyperactivity disorder: new genetic findings, new directions. In: Plomin RDJ, Craig I, McGuffin P (eds). *Behavioural Genetics in the Postgenomic Era*. Washington, DC: American Psychological Association; 2002. pp. 445–62.

13. Levy F, Hay DA, McStephen M, Wood C, Waldman I. Attention-deficit hyperactivity disorder: a category or a continuum? Genetic analysis of a large-scale twin study. Journal of the American Academy of Child and Adolescent Psychiatry. 1997;36(6):737–44.

14. Larsson H, Anckarsater H, Råstam M, Chang Z, Lichtenstein P. Childhood attention-deficit hyperactivity disorder as an extreme of a continuous trait: a quantitative genetic study of 8,500 twin pairs. Journal of Child Psychology and Psychiatry. 2011;53(1):73–80.

15. Greven CU, Merwood A, van der Meer JM, Haworth CM, Rommelse N, Buitelaar JK. The opposite end of the attention deficit hyperactivity disorder continuum: genetic and environmental aetiologies of extremely low ADHD traits. Journal of Child Psychology and Psychiatry, and Allied Disciplines. 2016;57(4):523–31.

16. Franke B, Faraone SV, Asherson P, et al. The genetics of attention deficit/hyperactivity disorder in adults, a review. Molecular Psychiatry. 2012;17(10):960–87.

17. Chang Z, Lichtenstein P, Asherson PJ, Larsson H. Developmental twin study of attention problems: high heritabilities throughout development. JAMA Psychiatry. 2013;70(3):311–18.

18. Merwood A, Greven CU, Price TS, et al. Different heritabilities but shared etiological influences for parent, teacher and self-ratings of ADHD symptoms: an adolescent twin study. Psychological Medicine. 2013;43(9):1973–84.

19. Pettersson E, Anckarsater H, Gillberg C, Lichtenstein P. Different neurodevelopmental symptoms have a common genetic etiology. Journal of Child Psychology and Psychiatry, and Allied Disciplines. 2013;54(12):1356–65.

20. Niarchou M, Martin J, Thapar A, Owen MJ, van den Bree MB. The clinical presentation of attention deficit-hyperactivity disorder (ADHD) in children with 22q11.2 deletion syndrome. American Journal of Medical Genetics Part B, Neuropsychiatric Genetics, 2015;168(8):730–8.

21. Farzin F, Perry H, Hessl D, et al. Autism spectrum disorders and attention-deficit/hyperactivity disorder in boys with the fragile X premutation. Journal of Developmental and Behavioral Pediatrics. 2006;27(2 Suppl):S137–44.

22. Curatolo P, Bombardieri R, Jozwiak S. Tuberous sclerosis. The Lancet. 2008;372(9639):657–68.

23. Stergiakouli E, Hamshere M, Holmans P, et al. Investigating the contribution of common genetic variants to the risk and pathogenesis of ADHD. American Journal of Psychiatry. 2012;169(2):186–94.

24. Williams NM, Franke B, Mick E, et al. Genome-wide analysis of copy number variants in attention deficit hyperactivity disorder: the role of rare variants and duplications at 15q13. 3. American Journal of Psychiatry. 2012;169(2):195–204.

25. Williams NM, Zaharieva I, Martin A, et al. Rare chromosomal deletions and duplications in attention-deficit hyperactivity disorder: a genome-wide analysis. The Lancet. 2010;376(9750):1401–8.

26. Yang L, Neale BM, Liu L, et al. Polygenic transmission and complex neuro developmental network for attention deficit hyperactivity disorder: genome-wide association study of both common and rare variants. American Journal of Medical Genetics Part B, Neuropsychiatric Genetics, 2013;162B(5):419–30.

27. Lionel AC, Crosbie J, Barbosa N, et al. Rare Copy Number Variation Discovery and Cross-Disorder Comparisons Identify Risk Genes for ADHD. Science Translational Medicine. 2011;3(95):95–75.

28. Elia J, Gai X, Xie HM, et al. Rare structural variants found in attention-deficit hyperactivity disorder are preferentially associated with neurodevelopmental genes. Molecular Psychiatry. 2010;15(6):637–46.

29. Lesch KP, Selch S, Renner TJ, et al. Genome-wide copy number variation analysis in attention-deficit/hyperactivity disorder: association with neuropeptide Y gene dosage in an extended pedigree. Molecular Psychiatry. 2011;16(5):491–503.

30. Martin J, Hamshere ML, Stergiakouli E, O'Donovan MC, Thapar A. Genetic risk for attention-deficit/hyperactivity disorder contributes to neurodevelopmental traits in the general population. Biological Psychiatry. 2014;76(8):664–71.

31. Thapar A, Martin J, Mick E, et al. Psychiatric gene discoveries shape evidence on ADHD's biology. Molecular Psychiatry. 2016;21:1202–7.

32. Jarick I, Volckmar AL, Pütter C, et al. Genome-wide analysis of rare copy number variations reveals *PARK2* as a candidate gene for attention-deficit/hyperactivity disorder. Molecular Psychiatry. 2014;19:115–21.

33. State M, Thapar A. Genetics. In: Thapar A, Pine DS, Leckman JF, Scott S, Snowling M, Taylor E (eds). *Rutter's Child and Adolescent Psychiatry*, 6th edn. Chichester: Wiley Blackwell; 2015. pp. 303–16.

34. Malhotra D, Sebat J. CNVs: harbingers of a rare variant revolution in psychiatric genetics. Cell. 2012;148(6):1223–41.

35. Gizer IR, Ficks C, Waldman ID. Candidate gene studies of ADHD: a meta-analytic review. Human Genetics. 2009;126(1):51–90.

36. Schizophrenia Working Group of the Psychiatric Genomics Consortium. Biological insights from 108 schizophrenia-associated genetic loci. Nature. 2014;511(7510):421–7.

37. Wray NR, Lee SH, Mehta D, Vinkhuyzen AA, Dudbridge F, Middeldorp CM. Research review: Polygenic methods and their application to psychiatric traits. Journal of Child Psychology and Psychiatry, and Allied Disciplines. 2014;55(10):1068–87.

38. Manolio TA, Collins FS, Cox NJ, et al. Finding the missing heritability of complex diseases. Nature. 2009;461(7265):747–53.

39. Hinney A, Scherag A, Jarick I, et al. Genome-wide association study in German patients with attention deficit/hyperactivity disorder. American Journal of Medical Genetics Part B, Neuropsychiatric Genetics, 2011;156B(8):888–97.

40. Neale BM, Lasky-Su J, Anney R, et al. Genome-wide association scan of attention deficit hyperactivity disorder. American Journal of Medical Genetics, Neuropsychiatric Genetics. 2008;147B(8):1337–44.

41. Neale BM, Medland S, Ripke S, et al. Case-control genome-wide association study of attention-deficit/hyperactivity disorder. Journal of the American Academy of Child and Adolescent Psychiatry. 2010;49(9):906–20.

42. Lesch KP, Timmesfeld N, Renner TJ, et al. Molecular genetics of adult ADHD: converging evidence from genome-wide association and extended pedigree linkage studies. Journal of Neural Transmission (Vienna). 2008;115(11):1573–85.

43. Mick E, Todorov A, Smalley S, et al. Family-based genome-wide association scan of attention-deficit/hyperactivity disorder. Journal of the American Academy of Child and Adolescent Psychiatry. 2010;49:898–905.

44. Elia J, Glessner JT, Wang K, et al. Genome-wide copy number variation study associates metabotropic glutamate receptor gene networks with attention deficit hyperactivity disorder. Nature Genetics. 2011;44:78–84.

45. Zayats T, Athanasiu L, Sonderby I, et al. Genome-wide analysis of attention deficit hyperactivity disorder in Norway. PLoS One. 2015;10(4):e0122501.

46. Neale BM, Medland SE, Ripke S, Asherson P, Franke B, Lesch KP, et al. Meta-analysis of genome-wide association studies of attention-deficit/hyperactivity disorder. Journal of the American Academy of Child and Adolescent Psychiatry. 2010;49(9):884–97.

47. Franke B, Neale BM, Faraone SV. Genome-wide association studies in ADHD. Human Genetics. 2009;126(1):13–50.

48. Neale BM, Kou Y, Liu L, et al. Patterns and rates of exonic de novo mutations in autism spectrum disorders. Nature. 2012;485(7397):242–5.

49. James O. Not in your genes. The Psychologist. 2015;28:950–7.

49a. Demontis et al. Discovery of the first genome-wide significant risk loci for attention deficit/hyperactivity disorder. Nature Genetics. 2019;51:63–75.

50. Flint J, Munafo M. Schizophrenia: genesis of a complex disease. Nature. 2014;511(7510):412–13.

51. Stranger BE, Stahl EA, Raj T. Progress and promise of genome-wide association studies for human complex trait genetics. Genetics. 2011;187(2):367–83.

52. Thapar A, Harold G. Editorial perspective: Why is there such a mismatch between traditional heritability estimates and molecular genetic findings for behavioural traits? Journal of Child Psychology and Psychiatry, and Allied Disciplines. 2014;55(10):1088–91.

53. Yang L, Neale BM, Liu L, et al. Polygenic transmission and complex neurodevelopmental network for attention deficit hyperactivity disorder: Genome-wide association study of both common and rare variants. American Journal of Medical Genetics Part B: Neuropsychiatric Genetics. 2013;162B:419–30.

54. Cross-Disorder Group of the Psychiatric Genomics Consortium. Identification of risk loci with shared effects on five major psychiatric disorders: a genome-wide analysis. The Lancet. 2013;381(9875):1371–9.

55. Pappa I, Fedko IO, Mileva-Seitz VR, et al. Single Nucleotide Polymorphism Heritability of Behavior Problems in Childhood: Genome-Wide Complex Trait Analysis. Journal of the American Academy of Child and Adolescent Psychiatry. 2015;54(9):737–44.

56. Trzaskowski M, Yang J, Visscher PM, Plomin R. DNA evidence for strong genetic stability and increasing heritability of intelligence from age 7 to 12. Molecular Psychiatry. 2014;19(3):380–4.

57. Hamshere ML, Langley K, Martin J, et al. High loading of polygenic risk for ADHD in children with comorbid aggression. American Journal of Psychiatry. 2013;170(8):909–16.

58. Stergiakouli E, Martin J, Hamshere ML, et al. Shared genetic influences between attention-deficit/hyperactivity disorder (ADHD) traits in children and clinical ADHD. Journal of the American Academy of Child and Adolescent Psychiatry. 2015;54(4):322–7.

59. Groen-Blokhuis MM, Middeldorp CM, Kan KJ, et al. Attention-deficit/hyperactivity disorder polygenic risk scores predict attention problems in a population-based sample of children. Journal of the American Academy of Child and Adolescent Psychiatry. 2014;53(10):1123–9 e6.

60. Chatterjee N, Wheeler B, Sampson J, Hartge P, Chanock SJ, Park JH. Projecting the performance of risk prediction based on polygenic analyses of genome-wide association studies. Nature Genetics. 2013;45(4):400–5, 5e1–3.

61. Langley K, Rice F, van den Bree MB, Thapar A. Maternal smoking during pregnancy as an environmental risk factor for attention deficit hyperactivity disorder behaviour. A review. Minerva Pediatrica. 2005;57(6):359–71.

62. Obel C, Zhu JL, Olsen J, et al. The risk of attention deficit hyperactivity disorder in children exposed to maternal smoking during pregnancy—a re-examination using a sibling design. Journal of Child Psychology and Psychiatry, and Allied Disciplines. 2016;57(4):532–7.

63. Knopik VS, Heath AC, Jacob T, et al. Maternal alcohol use disorder and offspring ADHD: disentangling genetic and environmental effects using a children-of-twins design. Psychological Medicine. 2006;36(10):1461–71.

64. Thapar A, Rice F, Hay D, et al. Prenatal smoking might not cause Attention-Deficit/Hyperactivity Disorder: Evidence from a novel design. Biological Psychiatry. 2009;66(8):722–7.

64a. Rice et al. Identifying the contribution of prenatal risk factors to offspring development and psychopathology: What designs to use and a critique of literature on maternal smoking and stress in pregnancy. Developmental Psychopathology. 2018;30(3);1104–28.

65. Harold GT, Leve LD, Barrett D, et al. Biological and rearing mother influences on child ADHD symptoms: revisiting the developmental interface between nature and nurture. Journal of Child Psychology and Psychiatry, and Allied Disciplines. 2013;54(10):1038–46.

66. Lifford KJ, Harold GT, Thapar A. Parent-child relationships and ADHD symptoms: a longitudinal analysis. Journal of Abnormal Child Psychology. 2008;36(2):285–96.

67. Schachar R, Taylor E, Weiselberg M, Thorley G, Rutter M. Changes in family function and relationships in children who respond to methylphenidate. Journal of the American Academy of Child and Adolescent Psychiatry. 1987;26(5):728–32.

68. Jaffee SR, Caspi A, Moffitt TE, Taylor A. Physical maltreatment victim to antisocial child: evidence of an environmentally mediated process. Journal of Abnormal Psychology. 2004;113(1):44–55.

69. Stevens SE, Sonuga-Barke EJ, Kreppner JM, et al. Inattention/overactivity following early severe institutional deprivation: presentation and associations in early adolescence. Journal of Abnormal Child Psychology. 2008;36(3):385–98.

70. Kendler KS, Larsson Lonn S, Morris NA, Sundquist J, Langstrom N, Sundquist K. A Swedish national adoption study of criminality. Psychological Medicine. 2014;44(9):1913–25.

71. Wynne LC, Tienari P, Nieminen P, et al. I. Genotype-environment interaction in the schizophrenia spectrum: genetic liability and global family ratings in the Finnish Adoption Study. Family process. 2006;45(4):419–34.

72. Langley K, Turic D, Rice F, et al. Testing for Gene-environment interaction effects in Attention deficit hyperactivity disorder and associated antisocial behavior. American Journal of Medical Genetics Part B: Neuropsychiatric Genetics. 2008;147B(1):49–53.

73. Neuman RJ, Lobos E, Reich W, Henderson CA, Sun LW, Todd RD. Prenatal Smoking Exposure and Dopaminergic Genotypes Interact to Cause a Severe ADHD Subtype. Biological Psychiatry. 2007;61(12):1320–8.

74. Phillips KA, Veenstra DL, Oren E, Lee JK, Sadee W. Potential role of pharmacogenomics in reducing adverse drug reactions: a systematic review. JAMA. 2001;286(18):2270–9.

75. Faraone SV, Biederman J, Monuteaux MC. Toward guidelines for pedigree selection in genetic studies of attention deficit hyperactivity disorder. Genetic Epidemiology. 2000;18(1):1–16.

76. Thapar A, Harrington R, McGuffin P. Examining the comorbidity of ADHD-related behaviours and conduct problems using a twin study design. British Journal of Psychiatry. 2001;179:224–9.

77. Caspi A, Langley K, Milne B, et al. A replicated molecular genetic basis for subtyping antisocial behavior in children with attention-deficit/hyperactivity disorder. Archives of General Psychiatry. 2008;65(2):203–10.

78. Langley K, Heron J, O'Donovan MC, Owen MJ, Thapar A. Genotype Link With Extreme Antisocial Behavior: The Contribution of Cognitive Pathways. Archives of General Psychiatry. 2010;67(12):1317.

79. Thapar A, Langley K, Fowler T, et al. Catechol O-methyltransferase gene variant and birth weight predict early-onset antisocial behavior in children with attention-deficit/hyperactivity disorder. Archives of General Psychiatry. 2005;62(11):1275–8.

80. Salatino-Oliveira A, Genro JP, Guimaraes AP, et al. Catechol-O-methyltransferase Val(158)Met polymorphism is associated with disruptive behavior disorders among children and adolescents with ADHD. Journal of Neural Transmission. 2012;119(6):729–33.

81. Kessler RC, Green JG, Adler LA, et al. Structure and diagnosis of adult attention-deficit/hyperactivity disorder: analysis of expanded symptom criteria from the Adult ADHD Clinical Diagnostic Scale. Archives of General Psychiatry. 2010;67(11):1168–78.

82. Klein RG, Mannuzza S, Olazagasti MA, et al. Clinical and functional outcome of childhood attention-deficit/hyperactivity disorder 33 years later. Archives of General Psychiatry. 2012;69(12):1295–303.

83. Posthuma D, Polderman TJ. What have we learned from recent twin studies about the etiology of neurodevelopmental disorders? Current Opinion in Neurology. 2013;26(2):111–21.

84. Faraone SV, Biederman J, Spencer T, et al. Attention-deficit/hyperactivity disorder in adults: an overview. Biological Psychiatry. 2000;48(1):9–20.

85. Agnew-Blais JC, Polanczyk GV, Danese A, Wertz J, Moffitt TE, Arseneault L. Evaluation of the Persistence, Remission, and Emergence of Attention-Deficit/Hyperactivity Disorder in Young Adulthood. JAMA Psychiatry. 2016;73:713–20.

86. Moffitt TE, Houts R, Asherson P, et al. Is Adult ADHD a Childhood-Onset Neurodevelopmental Disorder? Evidence From a Four-Decade Longitudinal Cohort Study. American Journal of Psychiatry. 2015;172(10):967–77.

87. Caye A, Rocha TB, Anselmi L, et al. Attention-Deficit/Hyperactivity Disorder Trajectories From Childhood to Young Adulthood: Evidence From a Birth Cohort Supporting a Late-onset Syndrome. JAMA Psychiatry. 2016;73:705–12.

88. Lichtenstein P, Carlström E, Råstam M, Gillberg C, Anckarsäter H. The genetics of autism spectrum disorders and related neuropsychiatric disorders in childhood. American Journal of Psychiatry. 2010;167(11):1357–63.

89. Martin J, Cooper M, Hamshere ML, et al. Biological overlap of attention-deficit/hyperactivity disorder and autism spectrum disorder: evidence from copy number variants. Journal of the American Academy of Child and Adolescent Psychiatry. 2014;53(7):761–70 e26.

90. Cross-Disorder Group of the Psychiatric Genomics Consortium; Lee SH, Ripke S, Neale BM, et al. Genetic relationship between five psychiatric disorders estimated from genome-wide SNPs. Nature Genetics. 2013;45(9):984–94.

90a. Cross-Disorder Group of the Psychiatric Genetics Consortium. Gemone wide meta-analysis identifies genomic relationships, novel loci and pleiotropic mechanisms across eight psychiatric disorders. bioRxiv: https://www.biorxiv.org/content/10.1101/528117v1 [in press].

90b. Thapar A. Discoveries on the Genetics of ADHD in the 21st Century: New Findings and Their Implications. American Journal of Psychiatry. 2018;175(10):943–50.

91. van Goozen SH, Langley K, Northover C, et al. Identifying mechanisms that underlie links between COMT genotype and aggression in male adolescents with ADHD. Journal of Child Psychology and Psychiatry, and Allied Disciplines. 2016;57(4):472–80.

92. Martin J, Hamshere ML, Stergiakouli E, O'Donovan MC, Thapar A. Neurocognitive abilities in the general population and composite genetic risk scores for attention-deficit hyperactivity disorder. Journal of Child Psychology and Psychiatry, and Allied Disciplines. 2015;56(6):648–56.

# 35

# Insights from neuroanatomical imaging into attention-deficit/hyperactivity disorder throughout the lifespan[1]

*Philip Shaw and Eszter Szekely*

## Introduction

Early models of attention-deficit/hyperactivity disorder (ADHD) sometimes viewed the disorder as a result of 'minimal' damage to brain structure and function [1]. This was partly based on a comparison with the effects of lesions of certain brain structures. For example, damage to the prefrontal cortex (PFC) is linked to deficits in motor and impulse control [2, 3]. The advent of magnetic resonance imaging (MRI), a non- invasive imaging tool that is free of ionizing radiation, accelerated the study of brain–behaviour relationships. It provided direct access into the developing brain. Here we review the literature, exploring the insights into ADHD throughout the lifespan provided by neuroanatomical imaging.

To outline this chapter, firstly, models of ADHD are briefly reviewed to aid in the interpretation of the neuroanatomical findings. Secondly, the literature on structural brain differences found in ADHD is summarized, adopting a developmental perspective, as childhood, adolescent, and adult ADHD are considered. Finally, looking to the future, we consider possible clinical applications of this work and likely research directions.

## Neurocognitive models of ADHD

There is a near consensus that there are multiple neuropsychological pathways to ADHD [4–7]. These are discussed in greater depth elsewhere (see Chapters 32 and 33). Here, we sketch these models to aid with the interpretation of the major neuroanatomical findings. The models are illustrated in Fig. 35.1. Firstly, ADHD has long been associated with anomalies in the *fronto-striato-thalamic*

circuitry, that is, the rich, sometimes bidirectional, interconnections between the prefrontal/parietal cortices, basal ganglia, and thalamic nuclei [8]. These circuits mediate a host of cognitive functions that are disrupted in ADHD such as working memory, response inhibition, and sustained attention. Secondly, children with ADHD also often show deficits in processing information about the temporal structure of the environment, making errors in time estimation, perception, and temporal foresight [9, 10]. In turn, this implicates the *corticocerebellar circuitry* spanning the cerebellum and its projections to the PFC, cingulate, and some parietal regions.

Thirdly, an aversion to delayed reinforcement, expressed as atypical processing of rewards, has been found in ADHD [6, 11]. This feature, along with anomalies in brain activation during anticipation of rewards, has spurred interest in connections between the *ventral striatum* and the *ventromedial cortex/orbitofrontal cortex (OFC)* in ADHD [12]. Fourthly, emotion dysregulation is increasingly recognized as a common, if not core, problem in ADHD [13]. It implicates the paralimbic circuitry, particularly interactions between the *amygdala, medial PFC, and OFC*. Finally, it has been argued that children with ADHD are not so much consistently worse at certain cognitive functions as they are more variable in performance, perhaps due to anomalies in vigilance or motivation [14–16]. This model has been linked most closely with atypical neurophysiology, specifically anomalies in the patterns of synchronized brain activity that arise during periods free from task demands [17]. However, there are also some possible neuroanatomical correlates, with increased within-subject variability associated with decreased white matter and prefrontal grey matter anomalies.

Most cognitive models of ADHD derive from research in children. However, it is increasingly clear that we need to consider the neural and cognitive anomalies that underpin ADHD throughout the lifespan. This is because, while some children 'grow out' of ADHD, many do not. Recent prospective studies find that 20–45% of children with ADHD will have the full syndrome into adulthood

---

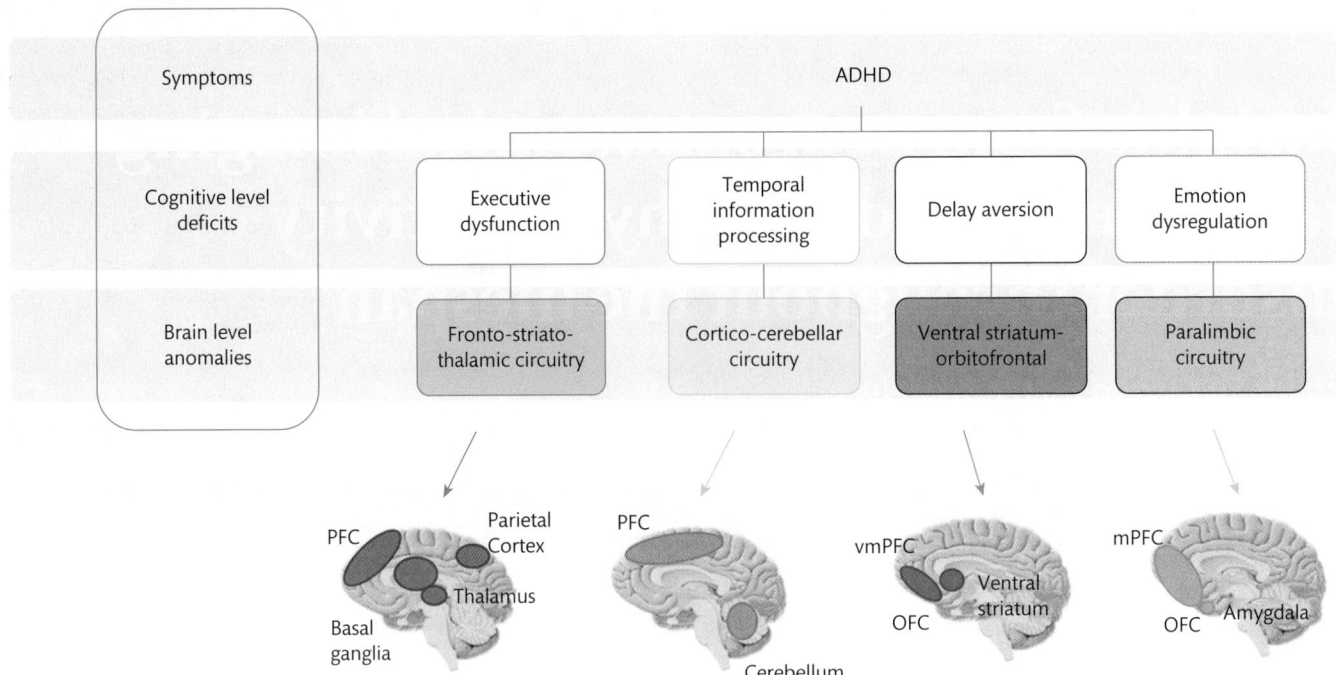

**Fig. 35.1** A sketch of some current neurocognitive models of ADHD. m, medial; OFC, orbitofrontal cortex; PFC, prefrontal cortex; vm, ventromedial.

and a further 25–48% have impairing symptoms [18, 19] (see also Chapter 34).

## A review of the neuroanatomy of ADHD throughout the lifespan

This is a selective, but comprehensive, review of the structural neuroimaging literature of ADHD, highlighting some landmark studies and key concepts. Systematic reviews and meta-analyses are referenced throughout, where appropriate. We first review childhood ADHD, summarizing findings for the three main compartments of the brain: deep brain structures, the cerebral cortex, and the cerebellum. We then review the literature on adolescent and adult ADHD.

### Childhood ADHD: the basal ganglia and other deep structures

The basal ganglia are perhaps the most widely studied brain structures in ADHD. This reflects their status as pivotal components in nearly all of the circuitry implicated in the disorder. Neuroimaging studies in the 1990s focused mainly on the caudate, often using manual tracing to chart volumetric alterations. The findings were mixed, with reports of increase [20], decrease [21, 22], and no difference [23]. The next wave of imaging studies has employed methods unconstrained by a priori regions of interest. These include voxel- based morphometry, which allows change in grey matter volume and density to be measured at thousands of points (or voxels) throughout the entire brain. In a landmark quantitative meta-analysis, Nakao and colleagues found that 14 such studies converged to find reduction in the dimensions of the right putamen and globus pallidus extending to the head of the caudate [24]. This effect was more pronounced in childhood and could not be attributed

to psychostimulant medication (which attenuated diagnostic group differences). The findings lend support to the 'classic' models of ADHD as stemming from anomalies in the fronto-striatal circuitry which mediates many executive functions.

Conventional MRI, at the currently used field strength of 1.5 and 3 T, has great difficulty in resolving the individual subnuclei of deep brain structures such as the striatum and thalamus. Thus, localized compromise of subnuclei could be missed. One strategy to circumvent this limitation is to examine the surface morphology of these deep structures. This is defined by the degree to which an individual's basal ganglia (or thalamic) surface contours have to be 'deformed' (stretched or shrunk) to fit a template [25, 26]. Surface expansions are generally interpreted as reflecting volume increase in underlying nuclei, and surface contractions as indicative of volume loss. The identity of the underlying nuclei is inferred through reference to surface maps of the structures, created by expert neuroanatomists.

One of the first studies to use this approach found that smaller basal ganglia volumes in boys with ADHD were driven by compression bilaterally in the head of the caudate and the anterior putamen, with relative sparing of more posterior regions [27]. A somewhat similar pattern was reported by a separate group [28].

The basal ganglia are richly interconnected with the thalamus, and here too localized surface anomalies have been delineated using this surface mapping technique [29]. Specifically, marked surface contraction in the region of the pulvinar nuclei bilaterally was noted in a group of 105 children with ADHD and controls. The pulvinar nuclei link action and vision, and the pulvinar's lateral portions, where the morphological anomalies were most prominent, support circuitry that detects salient somatosensory stimuli. Such morphological disruption of the pulvinar could contribute to the inefficient allocation of attentional resources seen in ADHD [30]. Notably, these complex surface changes and associated underlying volumetric perturbations did not lead to a change in the overall volume of the thalamus in youths with ADHD, relative to typically developing youths. Thus, a traditional region-of-interest study examining the volume of the thalamus would have missed these subtle, but important, diagnostic signals.

Others have looked beyond striatothalamic regions and delineated similarly localized changes that can inform cognitive models of ADHD. One study of 114 children delineated components of the limbic system, specifically the amygdala and the interconnected OFC [31]. It detected anomalies in amygdala shape— but not volume—and a disruption of the typical correlation between the amygdala and orbitofrontal volumes, suggesting a breakdown in the connectivity between components of the limbic system. The limbic system underlies affective processes such as emotion perception and emotion regulation. Thus, these findings lend support to the emotion regulation difficulties often seen in the disorder.

The basal ganglia develop throughout childhood [32]. This raises the question of whether the growth trajectories of the basal ganglia are altered in childhood ADHD. While cross-sectional data can be used to define trajectories, longitudinal data are better suited for capturing dynamic processes. In part, this is because longitudinal data focus on within-subject variation over time (which is of central interest) and remove much between-subject variance (which can confound). Indeed, theoretically, the only situation in which individual trajectories can be correctly inferred from cross-sectionally derived curves of mean values is when all entrances or exits from the study are random and the trajectories of the ADHD and control groups are parallel [33]. Neither requirement is likely to be met in ADHD.

One study used a mix of longitudinal and cross-sectional data to chart the development of the basal ganglia, comparing 270 children with ADHD against 270 well-matched typically developing controls [34]. Age-related change was mapped using surface-based morphological methods. The study confirmed prior findings of a general increase in surface area of the basal ganglia throughout childhood into mid adolescence. Children with ADHD similarly showed an increase in surface area but started from a 'lower' point, as they had a decreased surface area at study entry in the head of the caudate and the body of the putamen. Only one region showed a diagnostic difference in trajectories—the ventral striatum. Here, the typically developing group showed surface area expansion with age, whereas the ADHD group showed progressive contraction. In cognitive terms, the atypical development of the ventral striatum supports cognitive models implicating anomalous reward processing as a key contributor to childhood ADHD.

## Childhood ADHD and the cerebral cortex

Different areas of the cerebral cortex have also been implicated in most neurocognitive models of ADHD, partly through their rich interactions with striatal, thalamic, and cerebellar regions. An early landmark study of 152 children with ADHD and 139 well-matched typically developing controls established that there was a 4–6% reduction in the volume of the cerebral cortex, affecting all the major lobes [35]. Advances in analytical techniques provide more precise localization of change, allowing a closer alignment of neuroanatomical findings with cognitive models. Many studies have used methods that extract the cortical mantle and then measure the thickness, surface area, and curvature at thousands of points across the cerebrum [36, 37]. In childhood ADHD, ten studies have converged

to find a predominantly thinner cortex with reduced surface area, albeit with less agreement on the precise location of change [38–47]. Thus, widespread reduction of cortical dimensions in children with ADHD have been reported in the PFC, superior parietal cortex, and medial and anterior temporal regions. One study has reported increased dimensions confined to the primary somatosensory cortex [48]. Direct links between this compromised cortical substrate and cognitive deficits have been found. Thus, one study reported that at a group (but not individual) level, deficits in inhibitory control found in ADHD were accompanied by a thinner inferior frontal cortex [44]. A separate study using voxel-based morphometry found that age-related deficits in response inhibition in children with ADHD improved in tandem with increasing volumes in a network comprising the anterior cingulate cortex, striatum, and medial temporal lobes [49].

The cerebral cortex also develops during childhood, again prompting us to ask if trajectories differ in ADHD. Using data from over 500 children, many with repeated observations, the velocity of cortical development of both cortical thickness and surface area was defined [42, 50]. The key finding was a slower rate of cortical change in childhood ADHD. This altered velocity entailed a 'delay' in some prefrontal regions, as defined by the age at which each cortical vertex attained its peak dimensions. More recent work suggests that these differential trajectories may be moderated by intelligence, with slower rates of cortical development being more prominent in ADHD children with lower intelligence [51].

## Childhood ADHD and the cerebellum

Although the cerebellum has traditionally been considered a site of motor control, lesion studies and functional imaging studies in healthy subjects have demonstrated a wide range of cognitive and affective functions in cerebellar structures, particularly temporal information processing (but also attention shifting, verbal working memory, and emotional regulation [52, 53]). Dysfunction in each of these cognitive domains has, in turn, been implicated in the aetiology of ADHD. Anatomically, there are reciprocal loops that interconnect cerebral cortical areas, including the PFC, with the cerebellum by way of the pons, dentate nucleus, and thalamus. Structural anomalies of the cerebellum are among the most consistently reported features of ADHD [54–57]. A recent meta-analysis found that the regions most reduced in ADHD—lobule IX and VIIIB, Crus 1—were entirely distinct from those compromised among children with autism or developmental dyslexia [58]. These ADHD-related cerebellar regions interact richly with prefrontal and striatal regions to form networks involved not only in temporal information processing, but also in the effortful allocation of attention.

Dividing a literature overview into sections on different brain regions should not be taken to diminish the importance of discerning the coherent patterns of change that occur across the entire brain [5]. Large-scale brain networks in ADHD have largely (and appropriately) been mainly delineated using imaging modalities that more directly measure structural (for example, diffusion tensor imaging) and functional connections (for example, resting state fMRI) [59]. Nonetheless, the ways in which different brain structures co-vary in their dimensions can provide a more indirect index of anatomical networks [60]. One study adopting this approach found anomalous anatomical network structures in children with ADHD, centred on the OFC and insula [61]. Future work will usefully integrate such approaches with other modalities of imaging.

## Adolescent and adult ADHD

Most studies have focused on childhood or adult ADHD, with a relative neglect of adolescence. This gap has been filled by a recent large study of 307 adolescents with ADHD, 169 of their unaffected siblings, and 196 typically developing controls [62]. Two major neuroanatomical findings have emerged. Firstly, during adolescence, there is a fixed, non-progressive reduction in total brain volume in ADHD, echoing earlier childhood studies [63]. By contrast, there was progressive volume loss in adolescence in the right caudate and putamen (unlike childhood studies). Many of these changes were present in an attenuated form in the unaffected siblings, suggesting that they represent shared familial, perhaps genetic, risk factors. Cortical dimensions were also examined, and the ADHD group showed global thinning, compared to controls, with the medial temporal cortex being particularly compromised [45]. This effect was found throughout the adolescent to the adult age range and held even when psychostimulant medication was considered. This finding might suggest a developmental shift from the fronto-parietal anomalies that are prominent in early childhood ADHD towards more medial temporal/limbic anomalies in adolescents and adults.

In addition, the medial temporal anomalies are consonant with the prominent emotional dysregulation seen in young adults with ADHD (although direct evidence of a link was not found).

Studies into adults with ADHD have addressed two central issues. Firstly, are the neuroanatomical changes seen in childhood ADHD fixed and thus carried forward into adulthood, or do novel neuroanatomical changes emerge in adult ADHD? Secondly, is the variable clinical course of ADHD reflected in neuroanatomical change?

Most adult studies have focused on cortical structure and reported decreased volumes of predominantly prefrontal regions (dorsolateral, anterior cingulate, and OFC) [64, 65]. Cortical thinning in adult ADHD has also been found in the right inferior prefrontal, cingulate, and medial frontal cortices, in keeping with childhood findings [66, 67]. This would suggest that many of the anomalies of childhood are carried forward to adulthood. However, a more complex picture emerges, particularly when we consider the highly variable clinical course of ADHD.

One study clinically followed a large group of males with childhood ADHD into late adulthood (mean age 41 years) [68]. By this stage, 17 individuals had ADHD persisting into adulthood and 26 had remitted ADHD; contrasts were drawn against 57 never-affected controls. Neuroimaging was added at the adult assessment to allow an examination of the cerebral cortical structure and grey matter density. The study found a globally thinner cortex in both the persistent and remitted ADHD groups, compared to controls, particularly in the parietal, temporal, and frontopolar regions and the precuneus. The ADHD outcome groups mostly did not differ significantly from one another, compatible with fixed 'trait' deficits possibly carried forward from childhood. However, some changes did reflect outcome. The right middle frontal and limbic cortices were thinner, and the right cerebellum and thalamus had lower grey matter density in the persistent, compared to the remitted and never-affected, groups.

A separate study of clinical course used a fully longitudinal design and acquired neuroanatomical data in tandem with clinical assessments, both in childhood (mean age 10 years) and in early adulthood (mean age 24 years) [69]. Such longitudinal data provided the ideal tool for delineating the neuroanatomical trajectories that are tied to the variable clinical course. By adulthood, 55 of the 92 members of the ADHD group had remitted and the remainder still met diagnostic criteria. Contrasts were made against 184 never-affected controls. Regions were identified where change in cortical structure—specifically cortical thickness—was tied to this variable outcome. A link emerged in the cingulate cortex bilaterally, the right inferior parietal cortex and dorsolateral PFC, and the left sensorimotor region. Here, increasing severity of adult inattention, but not hyperactivity–impulsivity, was linked with higher rates of cortical thinning. The net effect of these differences was that those whose ADHD symptoms improved showed a significant convergence during adolescence towards typical cortical dimensions, rectifying early anomalies. By contrast, those with persisting symptoms had childhood cortical anomalies that persisted into adulthood. Importantly, these outcome-related differences in trajectories held when psychostimulant treatment history was entered as a covariate. These regions where the trajectory was tied to outcome span several of the brain networks most closely linked with ADHD. For example, outcome was linked with trajectories of the fronto-parietal cortical regions that guide much goal-directed behaviour through cortico-striato-thalamic circuits.

Do the trajectories of other brain regions also mirror the clinical course? Such a link was found for the developmental trajectories of some, but not all, cerebellar regions [70]. Studying 72 participants from the study just discussed, the trajectories of cerebellar development were defined from at least three scans. Outcome was assessed in adolescence. Some cerebellar trajectories were sensitive to outcome. There was atypical progressive volume loss in the inferior–posterior cerebellar lobes in those with worse clinical outcome, and a convergence to typical dimensions in the anterior hemisphere in those who improved. Not all cerebellar change reflected outcome—a reduced volume of the superior vermis persisted, regardless of outcome.

In summary, there is regional heterogeneity in the neuroanatomical trajectories of variable adult outcome. While different prefrontal cortical and cerebellar hemispheric development may be tied to different clinical outcome, more posterior cortical regions and the cerebellar vermis may show more fixed, trait-like deficits.

To summarize this section, meta-analyses and some of the larger individual studies converge to find anomalies in the basal ganglia in ADHD, some of which appear developmentally fixed while others may be progressive. Compromise of the cerebral cortex is commonly found, albeit with less consensus on the exact regions affected. Again, some of these anomalies may vary with age in ADHD and may be tied to the clinical course of the disorder. Finally, while the morphology of the cerebellum is relatively understudied, it may also show a mix of fixed and dynamic anomalies, some of which show diagnostic specificity.

## Towards future clinical application

Clinicians are often interested in two questions. Firstly, can neuroimaging aid with the diagnosis or prognosis of ADHD? Secondly, what are the effects, if any, of psychostimulants given as treatment for ADHD on brain structure?

At present, neuroimaging remains a research tool and the diagnosis of ADHD remains a clinical skill. Neuroimaging can define robust differences at the group level and provides rich insights into neurobiological mechanisms. However, to realize clinical utility, the next wave of studies will need to be able to detect changes at the individual level with high sensitivity and specificity. It seems unlikely that 'one-shot', one-modality imaging will suffice for this purpose, and multimodal imaging may be required. Biomarkers are not only needed to inform diagnosis, but also prognosis. We currently cannot accurately predict an individual child's likely outcome using clinical, sociodemographic, and neuropsychological data. For example, while baseline symptom severity and multiple comorbidities are significantly associated with long-term course, one study found these factors combined account for only 15–20% of the variance in outcome [71–73]. There are mixed findings on whether or not socioeconomic status, general intelligence, family environment, and cognitive skills are associated with adult outcome [71, 73–79]. In this context, future studies will increasingly turn to objective measures of the brain and the genome to inform diagnosis and prognosis.

Psychostimulants appear to normalize brain activity in ADHD during the performance of tasks and while the subject is at rest [80, 81]. What about neuroanatomy? Nearly all studies found that either there is no clear association between anatomy and psychostimulant treatment or treatment is associated with more normative dimensions (reviewed in [82]). One report found psychostimulant treatment to be associated with a smaller hippocampus, although this was not found in a larger study [63, 83]. However, it is critical to remember that all of the neuroanatomical studies discussed here are observational and causality cannot be inferred. For example, other factors, such as socio-economic status, access to care, or comorbidities, could influence the likelihood of receiving psychostimulant medication and brain structure. Statements about causality await imaging within the context of randomized medical trials.

## Future research directions

What does the future hold for neuroanatomical imaging in ADHD? Four major shifts are already discernible: (1) a shift from diagnostic categories towards considering underlying dimensions; (2) a move to 'big data' partly attained through collaborative efforts; (3) the rise of novel imaging modalities and their integration; and (4) the use of brain structure as a phenotype in genetic studies into ADHD and related disorders.

### The shift from categorical approaches to dimensionality

The National Institute of Mental Health has recently proposed a shift in research focus away from the use of DSM-5 diagnostic categories towards objectively defined constructs that are continuously distributed throughout the population [84]. In line with this concept, epidemiological and neuropsychological evidence suggests that ADHD can be considered dimensionally, lying at the extreme end of a continuous distribution of symptoms and underlying cognitive processes [85, 86]. Thus, it becomes pressing to ask if such dimensionality is also present in the brain changes associated with the categorical disorders.

To date, studies have only asked if the symptom dimensions of ADHD are tied to neuroanatomical change. Three studies have found such links. The first built on the earlier finding of a slower rate of cortical change in those with a diagnosis of ADHD. It found that this slower rate of cortical thinning during late childhood and adolescence was also associated with the severity of symptoms of hyperactivity and impulsivity in typically developing children [87]. As symptoms of hyperactivity–impulsivity increased in 193 typical children (with 389 neuroanatomical scans), the rate of cortical thinning decreased, approaching that seen in a group of 197 children with the clinical syndrome. Thus, similar, but attenuated, disruptions to trajectories are found in children who exhibit behavioural problems characteristic of ADHD, even when these do not pass the threshold for making a diagnosis. This finding was replicated in a separate cohort of 357 typically developing children among whom higher-attention problems were associated with a thinner cortex at baseline and slower cortical thinning with ageing in multiple areas involved in attention processes [88]. Finally, a population-based imaging study of 444 children found that greater problems with hyperactivity and impulsivity were associated with a thinner postcentral cortex bilaterally [89]. The next stage is to define how cognitive domains pertinent to ADHD and related diagnostic entities might also impact on the brain and its development.

### Big data

Several meta-analytic studies have already demonstrated the power of quantitative summaries of several smaller studies. Such meta-analyses are being facilitated by international collaborative efforts such as the Enhancing Neuroimaging in Genetics through Meta-Analyses initiative (http://enigma.ini.usc.edu). This collaboration has already provided initial reports on subcortical compromise in ADHD in over 3200 participants [90]. Such meta-analyses are not without their limitations. Foremost is the integration of data acquired using different scanners, with different sequences, and with often slight, but important, variations in image processing. This includes consensus protocols on how to assess the quality of images for motion and other imaging artefacts. The requisite methods are being developed to allow the integration of diverse data collected on different platforms.

### Novel imaging modalities and their integration

We are already seeing a shift towards imaging at field strengths (7 T and above) that can distinguish, for the first time, the layers of the cortex, the subfields of the hippocampus, and the subnuclei of deep structures. These data will quickly surpass existing data, extending and refining our current conclusions. Integration of these multimodal images is under way, often using multivariate methods that detect patterns or 'motifs' across multiple data sets that characterize ADHD [91].

### Brain structure and genomics

While ADHD is highly heritable ($h_2$ >0.7), there has been limited progress in understanding the mode of action of susceptibility genes [92, 93] (see Chapter 35). It has been argued that the phenotype for genetic studies should not always be the diagnostic category of ADHD per se but should also include quantitative brain-based traits that are pertinent to the disorder [94, 95]. Such quantitative traits have the advantage of containing more information about inter-individual trait variability than a dichotomous diagnostic category. The brain also lies closer to gene action and may be genetically less complex than the more distal clinical phenotypes of outcome.

Finally, progress in genetics might also be aided by parsing ADHD according to its highly variable clinical outcome. Developmental phenotypes that capture the dynamic nature of ADHD might better reflect its biology and provide better targets for genetic understanding. This developmental perspective is particularly important, given that a longitudinal study of 8395 twin pairs found that over half of the genetic contributors to variance in clinical course were distinct to those genetic factors driving the onset of ADHD [96].

What is the evidence that the brain alterations associated with ADHD are genetically determined? Comparing monozygotic and dizygotic twins is the ideal design for parsing the relative contribution to aetiology of genetics and unique and shared environmental factors. While no study has yet adopted this design in ADHD per se, one group used a variant of this design [97]. It found that volumes of the PFC were likely under genetic control (through a contrast of concordantly affected against concordantly unaffected monozygotic twins), whereas striatal volumes were more likely under environmental control (differing within discordant twin pairs). Several studies have also reported that some of the brain changes seen in children with ADHD, such as decreased prefrontal grey volume, are also found in their unaffected siblings in an attenuated form [63, 98]. Similarly, a study of 169 unaffected siblings found they had reduced volumes of total and cerebral grey, but not white, matter that lay between their siblings with ADHD and unaffected controls [63]. Interestingly, the finding of compromise in unaffected siblings does not extend to the cerebellum, one of the least heritable brain structures [99]. These unaffected sibling studies point to familial factors—either genetic or shared environment—as pivotal in determining some, but not all, brain dimensions pertinent to ADHD.

The next step is to identify the specific genes driving this heritability. To date, candidate genes implicated by a priori knowledge have been studied. Among structural studies, most have focused on common polymorphisms of the dopaminergic system. Risk-conferring variants of the dopamine transporter gene and the dopamine D4 receptor were associated, respectively, with decreased volume of the caudate nucleus and volumes and thickness of the prefrontal and parietal regions [100–102], with some studies finding this effect was confined to those with ADHD [102]. However, several studies do not report associations. A notable negative finding came from a population-based study of 1871 children, of whom 344 had neuroimaging [103]. It tested for additive effects of genetic variation in dopamine, serotonin, and neurite outgrowth pathways on both the severity of ADHD-related problems and the volume of the basal ganglia. While a modest association between ADHD symptom severity and putamen volume was found, none of the genetic pathways were related to clinical or brain features.

The future lies in studying the impact of common and rare genetic variants across the entire genome on the brain in ADHD. Given the large numbers that are needed for such studies (usually tens of thousands), it is likely that the primary phenotypes used for gene discovery will have to be relatively cheap and quick to ascertain, and entail minimal inconvenience—such as online questionnaires and testing. The deep phenotyping provided by multimodal imaging may prove prohibitively expensive when focused on just one disorder. Thus, the neural phenotyping of ADHD might be most usefully employed to characterize the most promising signals to emerge from larger studies using more readily available clinical and behavioural phenotypes.

Understanding the impact of DNA sequence variation on the brain in ADHD is only the first step. Interactions between the environment and genes are critical to consider, not least as the high heritability estimates include not only the main effect of genes, but also gene–environment interactions. There are a handful of pertinent studies. One of the most studied and controversial gene–environment interactions is between variants of the serotonin transporter gene (a variable number tandem repeat polymorphism in the promoter region) and early life adversity in producing vulnerability to depression [104, 105]. A study of 701 youths found that this interaction between the serotonin transporter gene variants and chronic life stressors was also associated with the severity of ADHD symptoms [106]. Using mediation analyses, the study further found that decreased volume of the OFC and anterior cingulate cortex could be the mechanism underlying this interaction.

The environment can also alter gene expression through epigenetic modifications such as methylation of DNA sequences. A recent study found that high levels of methylation of the serotonin transporter gene in 102 children with ADHD were associated with more severe symptoms and decreased thickness of the right occipitotemporal cortex [107]. Clearly, such preliminary findings require replication, but the studies illustrate how we can take well-characterized gene–environment interactions into the brain in an effort to map out the pathways to ADHD.

## Conclusions

Structural neuroimaging in ADHD is surprisingly young; large-scale research applications of MRI only started in the 1990s. Imaging has already moved beyond delineating morphometric change in entire lobes or deep structures, to consider how the disorder might be characterized by highly localized alterations in volume, shape, and surface complexity. The future holds challenges. Group-level differences can richly inform our models of ADHD, which could, in turn, impact on treatment approaches. However, direct clinical application of imaging to diagnosis or prognosis awaits the delineation of specific and sensitive alterations among individuals with ADHD. Chances of attaining this goal may be boosted by integrating neuroanatomical imaging with other imaging modalities and neuropsychological, clinical, and environmental data. Multimodal imaging will also prove vital if we are to define the neural mechanisms through which genetic variants confer risk for ADHD. While many challenges lie ahead, given the advances already made, it appears that the future of neuroanatomical imaging in ADHD is shaping up well.

## REFERENCES

1. Eisenberg, L. Commentary with a historical perspective by a child psychiatrist: when 'ADHD' was the 'brain- damaged child'. *Journal of Child and Adolescent Psychopharmacology*. 2007;17:279–83.
2. Aron, A.R., Robbins, T.W., and Poldrack, R.A. Inhibition and the right inferior frontal cortex. *Trends in Cognitive Sciences*. 2004;8:170–7.
3. Bechara, A. and Van Der Linden, M. Decision- making and impulse control after frontal lobe injuries. *Current Opinion in Neurology*. 2005;18:734–9.

4. Durston, S., van Belle, J., and de Zeeuw, P. Differentiating frontostriatal and fronto- cerebellar circuits in attention-deficit/hyperactivity disorder. *Biological Psychiatry*. 2011;69:1178–84.

5. Castellanos FX, Proal E. Large- scale brain systems in ADHD: beyond the prefrontal- striatal model. *Trends in Cognitive Sciences*. 2012;16(1):17–26.

6. Sonuga- Barke EJ. Causal models of attention- deficit/ hyperactivity disorder: from common simple deficits to multiple developmental pathways. *Biological Psychiatry*. 2005;57(11):1231–8.

7. Nigg JT, Casey BJ. An integrative theory of attention- deficit/hyperactivity disorder based on the cognitive and affective neurosciences. *Development Psychopathology*. 2005;17(3):785–806.

8. Alexander GE, DeLong MR, Strick PL. Parallel organization of functionally segregated circuits linking basal ganglia and cortex. *Annual Reviews of Neuroscience*. 1986;9:357–81.

9. Castellanos FX, Sonuga- Barke EJS, Milham MP, Tannock R. Characterizing cognition in ADHD: beyond executive dysfunction. *Trends in Cognitive Sciences*. 2006;10(3):117–23.

10. Noreika V, Falter CM, Rubia K. Timing deficits in attention-deficit/hyperactivity disorder (ADHD): evidence from neurocognitive and neuroimaging studies. *Neuropsychologia*. 2013;51(2):235–66.

11. Sagvolden T, Johansen EB, Aase H, Russell VA. A dynamic developmental theory of attention- deficit/ hyperactivity disorder (ADHD) predominantly hyperactive/ impulsive and combined subtypes. *Behavioral and Brain Sciences*. 2005;28(3):397–418.

12. Plichta MM, Scheres A. Ventral—striatal responsiveness during reward anticipation in ADHD and its relation to trait impulsivity in the healthy population: a meta- analytic review of the fMRI literature. *Neuroscience and Biobehavioral Reviews*. 2014;38:125–34.

13. Shaw P, Stringaris A, Nigg J, Leibenluft E. Emotion dysregulation in attention deficit hyperactivity disorder. *American Journal of Psychiatry*. 2014;171:276–93.

14. Klein C, Wendling K, Huettner P, Ruder H, Peper M. Intra-subject variability in attention- deficit hyperactivity disorder. *Biological Psychiatry*. 2006;60(10):1088–97.

15. Tamm L, Narad ME, Antonini TN, O'Brien KM, Hawk LW Jr, Epstein JN. Reaction time variability in ADHD: a review. *Neurotherapeutics*. 2012;9(3):500–8.

16. Kofler MJ, Rapport MD, Sarver DE, *et al.* Reaction time variability in ADHD: a meta- analytic review of 319 studies. *Clinical Psychology Review*. 2013;33(6):795–811.

17. Castellanos FX, Sonuga- Barke EJ, Scheres A, Di Martino A, Hyde C, Walters JR. Varieties of attention- deficit/ hyperactivity disorder- related intra- individual variability. *Biological Psychiatry*. 2005;57(11):1416–23.

18. Klein RG, Mannuzza S, Olazagasti MaAR, *et al.* Clinical and functional outcome of childhood attention- deficit/ hyperactivity disorder 33 years later. *Archives of General Psychiatry*. 2012;69(12):1295–303.

19. Faraone SV, Biederman J, Mick E. The age- dependent decline of attention deficit hyperactivity disorder: a meta- analysis of follow- up studies. *Psychological Medicine*. 2006;36(2):159–65.

20. Mataro M, Garcia- Sanchez C, Junque C, Estevez- Gonzalez A, Pujol J. Magnetic resonance imaging measurement of the caudate nucleus in adolescents with attention- deficit hyperactivity disorder and its relationship with neuropsychological and behavioral measures. *Archives of Neurology*. 1997;54(8):963–8.

21. Castellanos FX, Lee PP, Sharp W, *et al.* Developmental trajectories of brain volume abnormalities in children and adolescents with attention- deficit/ hyperactivity disorder. *JAMA*. 2002;288(14):1740–8.

22. Filipek PA, Semrud- Clikeman M, Steingard RJ, Renshaw PF, Kennedy DN, Biederman J. Volumetric MRI analysis comparing subjects having attention- deficit hyperactivity disorder with normal controls. *Neurology*. 1997;48(3):589–601.

23. Greven CU, Bralten J, Mennes M, *et al.* Developmentally stable whole- brain volume reductions and developmentally sensitive caudate and putamen volume alterations in those with attention-deficit/ hyperactivity disorder and their unaffected siblings. *JAMA Psychiatry*. 2015;72(5):490–9.

24. Nakao T, Radua J, Rubia K, Mataix- Cols D. Gray matter volume abnormalities in ADHD: voxel- based meta- analysis exploring the effects of age and stimulant medication. *American Journal of Psychiatry*. 2011;2011:24.

25. Chakravarty MM, Steadman P, van Eede MC, *et al.* Performing label- fusion- based segmentation using multiple automatically generated templates. *Human Brain Mapping*. 2013;34(10):2635–54.

26. Van Essen DC. Windows on the brain: the emerging role of atlases and databases in neuroscience. *Current Opinion in Neurobiology*. 2002;12(5):574–9.

27. Qiu A, Crocetti D, Adler M, *et al.* Basal ganglia volume and shape in children with attention deficit hyperactivity disorder. *American Journal of Psychiatry*. 2009;166(1):74–82.

28. Sobel LJ, Bansal R, Maia TV, *et al.* Basal ganglia surface morphology and the effects of stimulant medications in youth with attention deficit hyperactivity disorder. *American Journal of Psychiatry*. 2010;167(8):977–86.

29. Ivanov I. Morphological abnormalities of the thalamus in youths with attention deficit hyperactivity disorder. *American Journal of Psychiatry*. 2010;167(4):397.

30. Grieve KL. The primate pulvinar nuclei: vision and action. *Trends in Neurosciences*. 2000;23(1):35.

31. Plessen KJ, Bansal R, Zhu H, *et al.* Hippocampus and amygdala morphology in attention- deficit/ hyperactivity disorder. *Archives of General Psychiatry*. 2006;63(7):795–807.

32. Lenroot RK, Giedd JN. Brain development in children and adolescents: insights from anatomical magnetic resonance imaging. *Neuroscience and Biobehavioral Reviews*. 2006;30(6):718–29.

33. Kraemer HC, Yesavage JA, Taylor JL, Kupfer D. How can we learn about developmental processes from cross- sectional studies, or can we? *American Journal of Psychiatry*. 2000;157(2):163–71.

34. Shaw P, De Rossi P, Watson B, *et al.* Mapping the development of the basal ganglia in children with attention- deficit/ hyperactivity disorder. *Journal of the American Academy of Child and Adolescent Psychiatry*. 2014;53(7):780–9.

35. Castellanos F, Lee P, Sharp W, *et al.* Developmental trajectories of brain volume abnormalities in children and adolescents with attention- deficit/ hyperactivity disorder. *JAMA*. 2002;288:1740–8.

36. Lerch JP, Evans AC. Cortical thickness analysis examined through power analysis and a population simulation. *Neuroimage*. 2005;24(1):163–73.

37. Thompson PM, Lee AD, Dutton RA, *et al.* Abnormal cortical complexity and thickness profiles mapped in Williams syndrome. *Journal of Neuroscience*. 2005;25(16):4146–58.

38. Narr KL, Woods RP, Lin J, *et al.* Widespread cortical thinning is a robust anatomical marker for attention- deficit/ hyperactivity disorder. *Journal of the American Academy of Child and Adolescent Psychiatry*. 2009;48(10):1014–22.

39. Almeida LG, Ricardo-Garcell J, Prado H, *et al.* Reduced right frontal cortical thickness in children, adolescents and adults with ADHD and its correlation to clinical variables: a cross- sectional study. *Journal of Psychiatric Research*. 2011;44(16):1214–23.

40. Yang X- R, Carrey N, Bernier D, MacMaster FP. Cortical thickness in young treatment- naive children with ADHD. *Journal of Attention Disorders*. 2015;19(11):925–30.

41. Hoekzema E, Carmona S, Ramos-Quiroga JA, et al. Laminar thickness alterations in the fronto- parietal cortical mantle of patients with attention- deficit/hyperactivity disorder. *PLoS One*. 2012;12:e48286.

42. Shaw P, Malek M, Watson B, Sharp W, Evans A, Greenstein D. Development of cortical surface area and gyrification in attention-deficit/ hyperactivity disorder. *Biological Psychiatry*. 2012;72(3):191–7.

43. Shaw P, Lerch J, Greenstein D, et al. Longitudinal mapping of cortical thickness and clinical outcome in children and adolescents with attention deficit/hyperactivity disorder. *Archives of General Psychiatry*. 2006;63(5):540–9.

44. Batty MJ, Liddle EB, Pitiot A, et al. Cortical gray matter in attention- deficit/hyperactivity disorder: a structural magnetic resonance imaging study. *Journal of the American Academy of Child and Adolescent Psychiatry*. 2010;49(3):229–38.

45. Schweren LJ, Hartman CA, Heslenfeld DJ, et al. Thinner medial temporal cortex in adolescents with attention- deficit/hyperactivity disorder and the effects of stimulants. *Journal of the American Academy of Child and Adolescent Psychiatry*. 2015;54(8):660–7.

46. Sowell ER, Thompson PM, Welcome SE, Henkenius AL, Toga AW, Peterson BS. Cortical abnormalities in children and adolescents with attention-deficit hyperactivity disorder. *The Lancet*. 2003;362(9397):1699–707.

47. Wolosin SM, Richardson ME, Hennessey JG, Denckla MB, Mostofsky SH. Abnormal cerebral cortex structure in children with ADHD. *Human Brain Mapping*. 2009;30(1):175–84.

48. Duerden EG, Tannock R, Dockstader C. Altered cortical morphology in sensorimotor processing regions in adolescents and adults with attention- deficit/hyperactivity disorder. *Brain Research*. 2012;1445:82–91.

49. McAlonan GM, Cheung V, Chua SE, et al. Age- related grey matter volume correlates of response inhibition and shifting in attention-deficit hyperactivity disorder. *British Journal of Psychiatry*. 2009;194(2):123–9.

50. Shaw P, Eckstrand K, Sharp W, et al. Attention- deficit/hyperactivity disorder is characterized by a delay in cortical maturation. *Proceedings of the National Academy of Sciences of the United States of America*. 2007;104(49):19649–54.

51. de Zeeuw P, Schnack HG, van Belle J, et al. Differential brain development with low and high IQ in attention-deficit/hyperactivity disorder. *PLoS One*. 2012;7(4):e35770.

52. Schmahmann JD. Disorders of the cerebellum: ataxia, dysmetria of thought, and the cerebellar cognitive affective syndrome. *Journal Neuropsychiatry Clinical Neuroscience*. 2004;16(3):367–78.

53. Stoodley CJ. The cerebellum and cognition: evidence from functional imaging studies. *The Cerebellum*. 2012;11(2):352–65.

54. Hill D, Yeo R, Campbell R, Hart B, Vigil J, Brooks W. Magnetic resonance imaging correlates of attention- deficit/ hyperactivity disorder in children. *Neuropsychology*. 2003;17:496–506.

55. Berquin PC, Giedd JN, Jacobsen LK, et al. Cerebellum in attention-deficit hyperactivity disorder: a morphometric MRI study. *Neurology*. 1998;50(4):1087–93.

56. Bussing R, Grudnik J, Mason D, Wasiak M, Leonard C. ADHD and conduct disorder: an MRI study in a community sample. *World Journal of Biological Psychiatry*. 2002;3(4):216–20.

57. Mostofsky SH, Reiss AL, Lockhart P, Denckla MB. Evaluation of cerebellar size in attention- deficit/hyperactivity disorder. *Journal of Child Neurology*. 1998;13(9):434–9.

58. Stoodley CJ. Distinct regions of the cerebellum show gray matter decreases in autism, ADHD, and developmental dyslexia. *Frontiers in Systems Neuroscience*. 2014;8:92.

59. Konrad K, Eickhoff SB. Is the ADHD brain wired differently? A review on structural and functional connectivity in attention deficit hyperactivity disorder. *Human Brain Mapping*. 2010;31(6):904–16.

60. Mechelli A, Friston KJ, Frackowiak RS, Price CJ. Structural covariance in the human cortex. *Journal of Neuroscience*. 2005;25(36):8303–10.

61. Li X, Cao Q, Pu F, et al. Abnormalities of structural covariance networks in drug- naïve boys with attention deficit hyperactivity disorder. *Psychiatry Research: Neuroimaging*. 2015;231(3):273–8.

62. von Rhein D, Mennes M, van Ewijk H, et al. The NeuroIMAGE study: a prospective phenotypic, cognitive, genetic and MRI study in children with attention-deficit/hyperactivity disorder. Design and descriptives. *European Child and Adolescent Psychiatry*. 2014;24(3):265–81.

63. Greven CU, Bralten J, Mennes M, et al. Developmentally stable whole- brain volume reductions and developmentally sensitive caudate and putamen volume alterations in those with attention-deficit/ hyperactivity disorder and their unaffected siblings. *JAMA Psychiatry*. 2015;72(5):490–9.

64. Hesslinger B, Tebartz van Elst L, Thiel T, Haegele K, Hennig J, Ebert D. Frontoorbital volume reductions in adult patients with attention deficit hyperactivity disorder. *Neuroscience Letters*. 2002;328(3):319–21.

65. Seidman LJ, Valera EM, Makris N. Structural brain imaging of attention- deficit/ hyperactivity disorder. *Biological Psychiatry*. 2005;57(11):1263–72.

66. Makris N, Biederman J, Valera EM, et al. Cortical thinning of the attention and executive function networks in adults with attention- deficit/ hyperactivity disorder. *Cerebral Cortex*. 2007;17(6):1364–75.

67. Almeida LG, Ricardo- Garcell J, Prado H, et al. Reduced right frontal cortical thickness in children, adolescents and adults with ADHD and its correlation to clinical variables: a cross- sectional study. *Journal of Psychiatric Research*. 2010;44(16):1214–23.

68. Proal E, Reiss PT, Klein RG, et al. Brain gray matter deficits at 33- year follow-up in adults with attention-deficit/hyperactivity disorder established in childhood. *Archives of General Psychiatry*. 2011;68(11):1122–34.

69. Shaw P, Malek M, Watson B, Greenstein D, de Rossi P, Sharp W. Trajectories of cerebral cortical development in childhood and adolescence and adult attention-deficit/hyperactivity disorder. *Biological Psychiatry*. 2013;74(8):599–606.

70. Mackie S, Shaw P, Lenroot R, et al. Cerebellar development and clinical outcome in attention deficit hyperactivity disorder. [see comment]. *American Journal of Psychiatry*. 2007;164(4):647–55.

71. Cheung CH, Rijdijk F, McLoughlin G, Faraone SV, Asherson P, Kuntsi J. Childhood predictors of adolescent and young adult outcome in ADHD. *Journal of Psychiatric Research*. 2015;62:92–100.

72. Taylor E, Chadwick O, Heptinstall E, Danckaerts M. Hyperactivity and conduct problems as risk factors for adolescent development. *Journal of the American Academy of Child and Adolescent Psychiatry*. 1996;35(9):1213–26.

73. Biederman J, Petty CR, Clarke A, Lomedico A, Faraone SV. Predictors of persistent ADHD: an 11-year follow-up study. *Journal of Psychiatric Research*. 2011;45(2):150–5.

74. Molina BS, Hinshaw SP, Swanson JM, et al. The MTA at 8 years: prospective follow-up of children treated for combined-type ADHD in a multisite study. *Journal of the American Academy of Child and Adolescent Psychiatry*. 2009;48(5):484–500.

75. Hart EL, Lahey BB, Loeber R, Applegate B, Frick PJ. Developmental change in attention-deficit hyperactivity disorder in boys: a four-year longitudinal study. *Journal of Abnormal Child Psychology*. 1995;23(6):729–49.

76. Langley K, Fowler T, Ford T, *et al*. Adolescent clinical outcomes for young people with attention-deficit hyperactivity disorder. *British Journal of Psychiatry*. 2010;196(3):235–40.

77. Biederman J, Petty CR, Ball SW, *et al*. Are cognitive deficits in attention deficit/hyperactivity disorder related to the course of the disorder? A prospective controlled follow-up study of grown up boys with persistent and remitting course. *Psychiatry Research*. 2009;170(2):177–82.

78. Brocki KC, Nyberg L, Thorell LB, Bohlin G. Early concurrent and longitudinal symptoms of ADHD and ODD: relations to different types of inhibitory control and working memory. *Journal of Child Psychology and Psychiatry*. 2007;48(10):1033–41.

79. Weiss G, Hechtman LT. *Hyperactive children grown up: ADHD in children, adolescents, and adults*. London: Guilford Press; 1993.

80. Rubia K, Alegria AA, Cubillo AI, Smith AB, Brammer MJ, Radua J. Effects of stimulants on brain function in attention-deficit/hyperactivity disorder: a systematic review and meta-analysis. *Biological Psychiatry*. 2014;76(8):616–28.

81. Spencer TJ, Brown A, Seidman LJ, *et al*. Effect of psychostimulants on brain structure and function in ADHD: a qualitative literature review of magnetic resonance imaging-based neuroimaging studies. *Journal of Clinical Psychiatry*. 2013;74(9):902–17.

82. Friedman LA, Rapoport JL. Brain development in ADHD. *Current Opinion in Neurobiology*. 2015;30:106–11.

83. Frodl T, Stauber J, Schaaff N, *et al*. Amygdala reduction in patients with ADHD compared with major depression and healthy volunteers. *Acta Psychiatrica Scandinavica*. 2010;121(2):111–18.

84. Insel T, Cuthbert B, Garvey M, *et al*. Research domain criteria (RDoC): toward a new classification framework for research on mental disorders. *American Journal of Psychiatry*. 2010;167(7):748–51.

85. Lubke GH, Hudziak JJ, Derks EM, van Bijsterveldt TCEM, Boomsma DI. Maternal ratings of attention problems in ADHD: evidence for the existence of a continuum. *Journal of the American Academy of Child and Adolescent Psychiatry*. 2009;48(11):1085–93.

86. Polderman TJC, Derks EM, Hudziak JJ, Verhulst FC, Posthuma D, Boomsma DI. Across the continuum of attention skills: a twin study of the SWAN ADHD rating scale. *Journal of Child Psychology & Psychiatry and Allied Disciplines*. 2007;48(11):1080–7.

87. Shaw P, Gilliam M, Liverpool M, *et al*. Cortical development in typically developing children with symptoms of hyperactivity and impulsivity: support for a dimensional view of attention deficit hyperactivity disorder. *American Journal of Psychiatry*. 2011;168(2):143–51.

88. Ducharme S, Hudziak JJ, Botteron KN, *et al*. Decreased regional cortical thickness and thinning rate are associated with inattention symptoms in healthy children. *Journal of the American Academy of Child and Adolescent Psychiatry*. 2012;51(1):18–27. e2.

89. Mous S, Muetzel R, El Marroun H, *et al*. Cortical thickness and inattention/hyperactivity symptoms in young children: a population-based study. *Psychological Medicine*. 2014;44(15):3203–13.

90. Hoogman M, Bralten J, Zwiers M, Van Hulzen K, Schweren L; The ENIGMA-ADHD Working Group. Subcortical volumes across the lifespan in ADHD: an ENIGMA collaboration. *European Neuropsychopharmacology*. 2015;25 (Supplement 2):S189. doi: http://dx.doi.org/10.1016/S0924-977X(15)30184-X.

91. Zhao Y, Castellanos FX. Annual research review: discovery science strategies in studies of the pathophysiology of child and adolescent psychiatric disorders: promises and limitations. *Journal of Child Psychology and Psychiatry*. 2016:57(3):421–39.

92. Schachar R. Genetics of attention deficit hyperactivity disorder: recent updates and future prospects. *Current Developmental Disorders Reports*. 2014;1(1):41–9.

93. Hawi Z, Cummins T, Tong J, *et al*. The molecular genetic architecture of attention deficit hyperactivity disorder. *Molecular Psychiatry*. 2015;20(3):289–97.

94. Gottesman II, Gould TD. The endophenotype concept in psychiatry: etymology and strategic intentions. *American Journal of Psychiatry*. 2003;160(4):636–45.

95. Meyer-Lindenberg A, Weinberger DR. Intermediate phenotypes and genetic mechanisms of psychiatric disorders. *Nature Reviews Neuroscience*. 2006;7(10):818–27.

96. Pingault JB, Viding E, Galera C, *et al*. Genetic and environmental influences on the developmental course of attention-deficit/hyperactivity disorder symptoms from childhood to adolescence. *JAMA Psychiatry*. 2015;72(7):651–8.

97. van't Ent D, Lehn H, Derks EM, *et al*. A structural MRI study in monozygotic twins concordant or discordant for attention/hyperactivity problems: evidence for genetic and environmental heterogeneity in the developing brain. *Neuroimage*. 2007;35(3):1004–20.

98. Durston S. Imaging genetics in ADHD. *Neuroimage*. 2010;53(3):832–8.

99. Wallace GL, Eric Schmitt J, Lenroot R, *et al*. A pediatric twin study of brain morphometry. *Journal of Child Psychology and Psychiatry*. 2006;47(10):987–93.

100. Durston S, Fossella J, Casey B, *et al*. Differential effects of DRD4 and DAT1 genotype on fronto-striatal gray matter volumes in a sample of subjects with attention deficit hyperactivity disorder, their unaffected siblings, and controls. *Molecular Psychiatry*. 2005;10(7):678–85.

101. Shaw P, Gornick M, Lerch J, *et al*. Polymorphisms of the dopamine D4 receptor, clinical outcome, and cortical structure in attention-deficit/hyperactivity disorder. *Archives of General Psychiatry*. 2007;64(8):921–31.

102. Monuteaux MC, Seidman LJ, Faraone SV, *et al*. A preliminary study of dopamine D4 receptor genotype and structural brain alterations in adults with ADHD. *American Journal of Medical Genetics Part B: Neuropsychiatric Genetics*. 2008;147(8):1436–41.

103. Mous SE, Hammerschlag AR, Polderman TJC, *et al*. A population-based imaging genetics study of inattention/hyperactivity: basal ganglia and genetic pathways. *Journal of the American Academy of Child and Adolescent Psychiatry*. 54(9):745–52.

104. Risch N, Herrell R, Lehner T, *et al*. Interaction between the serotonin transporter gene (5-HTTLPR), stressful life events, and risk of depression: a meta-analysis. *JAMA*. 2009;301(23):2462–71.

105. Karg K, Burmeister M, Shedden K, Sen S. The serotonin transporter promoter variant (5-HTTLPR), stress, and depression meta-analysis revisited: evidence of genetic moderation. *Archives of General Psychiatry*. 2011;68(5):444–54.

106. van der Meer D, Hoekstra PJ, Zwiers M, *et al*. Brain correlates of the interaction between 5-HTTLPR and psychosocial stress mediating attention deficit hyperactivity disorder severity. *American Journal of Psychiatry*. 2015;172(8):768–75.

107. Park S, Lee J-M, Kim J-W, *et al*. Associations between serotonin transporter gene (SLC6A4) methylation and clinical characteristics and cortical thickness in children with ADHD. *Psychological Medicine*. 2015;45(14):3009–17.

# 36

# Management and treatment of attention-deficit/hyperactivity disorder

*Alessandro Zuddas and Sara Carucci*

## Assessment

As explained at length in Chapter 32, attention-deficit/hyperactivity disorder (ADHD) assessment involves the integration of information from different sources and an appropriate clinical decision-making process able to resolve conflicting observations and information. The full assessment includes information collected by validated instruments documenting present problems, health and developmental history, comorbid psychiatric conditions, and global functioning; intruments and procedures include questionnaires, interviews, and, when apropriate, direct observation and neuropsychological testing. Assessment of cardiac risk factors needs to be recorded at assessment before prescribing medications and routinely thereafter. At the end of the assessment process, the clinician will determine a principal and differential diagnosis and the presence of any comorbidity, and will develop a formulation that places these diagnoses in context.

ADHD treatment guidelines and algorithms have been developed in Europe [1–4] and North America [5–7], proposing evidence-based approaches for ADHD assessment and management. Model templates for planning services for ADHD assessment and intervention, such as the Dundee ADHD Clinical Care Pathway (DACCP) [8], have also been tested and are currently used in many countries; it includes specific stages for: (1) referral and pre-assessment; (2) assessment, diagnosis, and treatment planning; (3) initiating treatment; and (4) monitoring and continuing care.

## Clinical management

Treatment for ADHD is based on a multimodal approach combining behavioural and pharmacological treatment [2, 9]. European guidelines highly recommend a stepwise approach, with psychobehavioural interventions as first-line treatments, especially for pre-school children and subjects affected by a mild form of the disorder. American guidelines do not preclude pharmacotherapy as a first therapeutic approach, even in the youngest and mildest cases.

If pharmacological treatment is prescribed first line, it should be combined with behavioural interventions in any case. However, it is largely accepted that pharmacological treatment for ADHD is highly effective, either alone or in combination with behavioural interventions, that it has greater benefits than behavioural intervention alone, and that outcomes are much improved when a structured approach to medication management is adopted [10]. There is not a unique strategy for management; individual circumstances, comorbidities, and medical history have to be considered as an integral part of the treatment plan [11]; after appropriate information, parents' and patients' preference should always be taken into account.

When concomitant medical or psychiatric conditions such as conduct disorders, specific learning disorder, and social difficulties are present, psychosocial, psychoeducational, and environmental interventions centred on the family and school are often required.

The main objectives of any comprehensive treatment are:

- To improve *core* ADHD symptoms.
- To improve interpersonal relationships with parents, siblings, teachers, and peers.
- To decrease disruptive behaviours.
- To improve school learning abilities.
- To increase personal autonomy and self-esteem.
- To improve social acceptability of the disorders and the quality of life of children/adolescents suffering from the disorder.

## Non-pharmacological interventions

The most common non-pharmacological treatments are behavioural interventions both for children and carers [that is, parent training (PT), educator/teacher training, cognitive behavioural therapy (CBT), support groups, and social skills training], cognitive training, neurofeedback, and nutraceutics. The objective is to improve global functioning and reduce ADHD symptoms.

### Parent training

PT programmes are psychoeducational interventions providing parents with information about ADHD and adequate strategies to target and monitor problematic behaviours, in order to better manage their children. The intervention is typically delivered to groups of parents and covers positive reinforcement skills, reward systems, the use of 'time out', liaison with teachers, and planning ahead to anticipate problems.

According to recent studies, PT has positive effects on the behaviour of ADHD children by increasing parents' behaviour management skills, as well as reducing stress and improving parents' sense of efficacy [12].

## Cognitive behavioural therapy

CBT is a structured psychotherapeutic approach to help subjects in recognizing their dysfunctional patterns of thought and behaviour. It aims to help subjects to learn new skills and strategies to achieve their objectives, improve self-esteem, and deal with their emotions and social difficulties.

Objective evidence for the efficacy of psychosocial interventions is problematic. A recent meta-analysis by the European ADHD Guideline Group (EAGG) showed good effect sizes when outcome measures were based on ADHD assessments by raters closest to the therapeutic setting. There was an overall standardized mean difference (SMD) of 0.40 (95% CI 0.20, 0.60). However, when only ratings by assessors blind to treatment allocation were considered, treatment effects almost disappeared (SMD 0.02, 95% CI −0.30, 0.34) [13].

In contrast with the lack of sufficient evidence on ADHD core symptoms, a more recent meta-analysis showed a significant positive effect of behavioural interventions on parenting skills and conduct problems in ADHD children [14, 15].

## Cognitive training

In recent years, also cognitive training aimed at targeting specific deficits (for example, attention, working memory, inhibitory control) has been investigated as potential ADHD treatment [16]. The effects of cognitive training on ADHD, as addressed in a recent meta-analysis performed by the same EAGG, were significant when calculated using unblinded ratings (SMD 0.64, 95% CI 0.33–0.95) but, as reported for psychoeducational interventions, became statistically non-significant (SMD 0.24, 95% CI 0.24–0.72) when measures generated by probably blinded observers were used [17].

A more recent meta-analysis, including a larger number of trials, showed a more reliable estimate of the effects of cognitive training on specific functions (working memory, sustained attention, and inhibition); when measured by blinded raters, cognitive training mainly improved working memory, with limited effects on ADHD core symptoms [17].

## Neurofeedback

Neurofeedback is based on the training of self-regulation of brain activity; it has been considered a promising ADHD treatment by targeting aberrant patterns of brain activity putatively underpinning the disorder. The results of a recent meta-analysis on 13 controlled trials did not show neurofeedback to be an effective treatment for ADHD when evaluated by probably blinded raters [18]. A recent study in adults confirmed these results [19], although some more promising preliminary results have been reported with innovative techniques [20, 21].

Behavioural interventions have also been provided as useful treatments for managing comorbid disorders in ADHD subjects. Recently, a multi-centre RCT conducted in 159 adolescents, investigating two new individual, short-term cognitive behavioural

therapies (one including skills teaching, while the other was solution-focused), showed significant improvements in comorbid depression, anxiety, and disruptive disorder symptoms with both approaches [22]. Weaker evidence is available for the efficacy of behavioural sleep interventions in children with ADHD, although about 70% of ADHD subjects display mild to severe sleep problems. Behavioural treatments for insomnia are clearly effective in children in general [23], and ADHD should be considered not only a day-time disorder, but also better as a 24-hour ongoing process including sleep difficulties. Given the well-known consequences of poor sleep on memory and cognition, behavioural approaches to improve sleep may represent an important resource needing more specific research [24]. Some clinicians already recommend initiating behavioural treatment for poor sleep early in management, since it is a non-contentious symptom, carrying none of the stigma of a psychiatric diagnosis.

## Nutraceutics

There has been growing interest in the roles of the n-3 polyunsaturated fatty acids (PUFAs) docosahexaenoic acid (DHA) and the precursor eicosapentaenoic acid (EPA) as potential treatments for ADHD symptoms. The longest-chain n-3 PUFA DHA is the most abundant PUFA in brain membrane phospholipids; it has an important role in membrane fluidity and associated metabolic and neural activities. DHA appears to be particularly concentrated at synapses, influencing dopaminergic, serotonergic, noradrenergic, and gabaergic neurotransmission [25]. Recent meta-analyses [26–28] suggest that omega supplementation may improve ADHD symptoms to a modest degree, with an effect size of about a quarter as large as that seen for pharmacological treatment; whether subnormal blood concentrations should be an indication for treatment is still not clearly established.

In summary, evidence from meta-analyses investigating RCTs of non-pharmacological interventions indicate that non-pharmacological treatments should not be recommended as the only interventions for core ADHD symptoms. The wider adoption of such approaches requires better evidence reported using blinded assessments [17]. This does not mean that pharmacological therapy necessarily represents the first choice for all subjects; in some children, psychosocial interventions alone are associated with recovery [29]. However, consistent evidence across studies confirms the utility of adding appropriate pharmacological therapy to existing psychosocial therapy, while only small benefits emerge from the addition of current psychosocial therapy to an ongoing drug treatment.

## Pharmacological treatments

Drug treatment for ADHD represents an intervention of specific value and relevance to patients within multimodal treatment. Methylphenidate (MPH), dexamfetamine, or amphetamine (AMP), derivatives, and 'noradrenergic' medications atomoxetine (ATX) and guanfacine are the most effective psychopharmacological treatments for ADHD. As a class the first three are usually referred to as stimulants. As explained in Chapter 11, terms based on mechanism of action are much preferable. This is especially true in this case because the objective of treatment in ADHD is almost the opposite of stimulation.

## Drugs for ADHD

AMP and MPH have been proved to be the most effective drugs for ADHD; their use is well established and consistently recommended in evidence-based clinical guidelines across the world [1–9], with a response rate of around 70%, rising to 95% when non-responders are treated with a second drug [30]. It is a significant problem that amphetamine is a controlled substance as a result of the United Nations decree in 1971. In a number of countries, it is classed along with drugs like heroin, which has inevitably retarded its adoption for the treatment of children.

### Molecular mechanism of action of drugs for ADHD

AMP and MPH enhance the efflux and function of noradrenaline (NA) and dopamine (DA) in the CNS, with a rapid onset of action; they act by blocking (or even reversing) reuptake in their respective monoamine transporters [31]. AMP also increases catecholamine release from synaptic vesicles [32]. The therapeutic effects on behaviour and attention are presumed to be related to the enhanced neurotransmission of these catecholamines, especially in the prefrontal cortex [33].

Racemic AMP (α-methylphenetylamine) contains equal amounts of d-(dextroamphetamine) and l-amphetamine isomers. In vitro, the affinity of AMP is higher for noradrenaline transporters (NETs) in the prefrontal cortex than for DA (in the striatum) [34].

MPH is significantly less potent than AMP at inhibiting vesicular accumulation of DA or NA, but a similarly potent inhibitor of synaptic reuptake of DA and a slightly less potent inhibitor of NA reuptake.

At therapeutic doses, DA and NA have a complementary effect on the firing rate of catecholamine neurons, which results in improved signalling, especially in the prefrontal cortex [35]. During cognitive tasks, MPH has been shown to increase cerebral blood flow in dorsolateral prefrontal and posterior parietal cortices in healthy controls [36] and in the prefrontal cortex in adults with ADHD [37], with a significant decrease in other regions. This suggests decreased metabolic activation in task-irrelevant brain regions, with, in turn, more focused activation in task-relevant areas and improved performance [38].

More recently, drugs for ADHD have been shown to modulate functional connectivity; MPH normalizes activation and functional connectivity deficits in the brain networks supporting attention and motivation. This has been shown in medication-naïve children with ADHD during a rewarded continuous performance task, together with normalization of fronto-cingulate under-activation during error processing [39]. In adolescents with ADHD, the drugs demonstrated effects on the functional connectivity of fronto-parietal networks, with beneficial effects on working memory performance [40]. During inhibitory tasks, children with ADHD exhibit a raised motivational threshold at which task-relevant stimuli become sufficiently salient to deactivate the default mode network (DMN); treatment with MPH normalizes this threshold [41].

### Pharmacokinetics

Absorption of AMP is rapid, with peak plasma levels about 3 hours after oral administration. AMP is metabolized through the liver by various P450 enzymes. Food does not affect total absorption but can delay it.

Consistently with its pharmacokinetic profile, the onset of action of AMP is rapid, within 1 hour after administration. For immediate-release preparations, the duration of action is slightly longer than for MPH (around 405 hours), but still requiring at least twice-daily administration to ensure adequate coverage. Mixtures of different d-AMP and dl-AMP salt formulations (that is, Adderal*) are available in the United States, but not in Europe.

Lisdexamfetamine (LDX) is dextroamphetamine (DEX) covalently attached to the essential amino acid L-lysine. LDX itself is not pharmacodynamically active nor does it result in high DEX levels when injected or snorted, thus having a lower abuse potential. Following oral administration, the amide linkage between the two molecules is enzymatically hydrolysed, releasing active DEX. Most of this hydrolysis takes place within red blood cells. Pharmacokinetics of d-AMP after single-dose oral administration is linear; in adults, there is no accumulation of DEX at steady state nor accumulation of LDX dimesylate after once-daily dosing for 7 consecutive days. The mean plasma half-life of d-AMP is about 11 hours.

Oral MPH is rapidly absorbed from the gastrointestinal tract, with peak plasma concentrations occurring about 1.5–3 hours after administration. The elimination plasma steady half-life of d-threo-MPH is about 3–3.5 hours. Because of this short-half life, steady state for MPH is not achieved during regular treatment, although there is a theoretical possibility of steady state developing with high doses of extended-release preparations or in poor metabolizers. Classroom studies suggest a close relationship between the pharmacokinetic profile and pharmacodynamic properties [42]. Optimal clinical effect appears to be associated with rapidly increasing levels in the morning, followed by a steadily increasing plasma level across the rest of the day.

Concerta XL*, Matoride XL*, Equasym XL*, Medikinet Retard*, and Ritalin LA* all provide a mixture of immediate- and extended-release MPH; they differ in the mechanics of the delayed-release system and in the proportion of immediate-release to delayed-release MPH. Concerta XL* and Matoride XL* effects last 10–12 hours, while Equasym XL*, Ritalin LA*, and Medikinet Retard* can be considered mid-release formulations lasting between 6 and 8 hours.

Transdermal patches (Daytrana*) allow about 12 hours of effect if worn for 9 hours and are available in the United States. This formulation exhibits minimal first-pass metabolism, resulting in high bioavailability of MPH. Quillivant XR* (5 mg/mL) is a recent long-lasting liquid preparation of MPH. Peak plasma levels occur approximately 5 hours after dosing, with effects marketed to last for up to 12 hours.

These differing delivery profiles provide the clinician with increased options when choosing which preparation to use. They allow a more flexible and sensitive individualized adjustment, while retaining the benefits of an extended-release preparation. Pharmacokinetic profiles may, however, show considerable inter-individual variation, and caution should be observed when generalizing from aggregated profiles to individual cases.

### Interaction with other drugs

Drugs for ADHD show little interference with the metabolism and pharmacokinetics of other medications. There is, however, a potential to inhibit the metabolism of anticonvulsant drugs, such as phenobarbital, phenytoin, and primidone, and of tricyclics. Drugs for ADHD may potentiate stimulating effects of other drugs on the cardiovascular or central nervous system and can increase pressor response to vasopressor agents. There are potentially dangerous interactions with substances of abuse like cocaine and other sympathomimetic agents, including ATX.

## Clinical efficacy

Strong evidence supports the efficacy of drugs for ADHD in reducing ADHD core symptoms over treatment periods of up to a year, and numerous placebo-controlled randomized trials confirm their effectiveness in the short term, with effect sizes of between 0.8 and 1.1 on hyperactivity symptoms [2].

Drugs for ADHD reduce restlessness, inattentiveness, and impulsiveness markedly and rapidly, but they also have an important role in improving the quality of social interactions and decreasing aggression. Beneficial effects also extend to a broad range of associated functional impairments and comorbidities, including increased academic achievement [43], reduced risk of emergency admission to hospital for trauma [44], lower risk of depression [45] and suicidal events [46], and decreased rates of substance abuse [47] and criminality [48], although effect sizes are generally somewhat smaller than for symptom reduction per se.

Knowledge about the effectiveness of medication in ADHD children and adolescents has also been expanded in specific spopulations.

Within the Preschoolers with ADHD Treatment Study (PATS) trial, 160 children younger than 6 years were randomized to placebo or immediate-release MPH. The magnitude of MPH effect (dose range 2.5–7.5 mg) was lower than typically observed in school-aged children, with an increased frequency and severity of adverse events (that is, greater mood lability or reduced growth rate and treatment discontinuation in about 11% of cases) [49].

Positive results, but with more frequent and severe adverse effects have also been observed in ADHD children with comorbid autism spectrum disorder (ASD). A meta-analysis showed MPH to be effective (effect size 0.67) for treating ADHD symptoms in children with pervasive developmental disorders, but its relatively lower tolerability must be taken into account [50].

Although early studies suggested that children with comorbid anxiety or internalizing symptoms displayed lower response rates on ADHD symptoms, more recent studies, including the MTA study, do not support this. Drugs for ADHD at a group level show a beneficial effect on anxiety [51], and several recent studies showed that they are quite effective in controlling ADHD in the context of Tourette's disorder.

A recent meta-analysis also shows that MPH is clearly an important potential therapeutic option for comorbid disruptive behavioural problems and aggression in patients with ADHD and conduct disorder. Studies of MPH efficacy on aggression in conduct disorder without ADHD are still lacking [52].

LDX has been shown to be more effective than placebo on ADHD symptoms (effect size 1.8). LDX was also effective in treating day-to-day problems associated with ADHD, significantly improving quality of life [53]. The randomized withdrawal of treatment after 24 weeks of open-label treatment indicated the continued benefit of LDX treatment, with treatment-emerging adverse events generally consistent with those associated with the MPH preparation, used as the active comparator [54].

## Long-term efficacy of drugs for ADHD

Although the short-term benefit of drugs for ADHD has been repeatedly confirmed within several studies, its long-term effects have been less well investigated. The MTA study still represents the most valid source of information on the long-term effects of MPH. Within this large-scale, random-allocation, non-blind trial, a comparison was made between careful medication management, intensive behaviourally oriented psychosocial therapy, a combination of the two, and a simple referral back to community (usually medication) [10]. The main conclusions after 14 months were that careful medication was more effective than behavioural treatment. The combination of behavioural therapy and medication did have some benefits: better control of aggressive behaviour at home, improved overall sense of satisfaction of parents, and possibly reduced medication dosage.

The follow-up at 36 months, by which time parents and children were free to choose the actual treatment, showed that all four original groups had a similar outcome; similar results were observed at up to 16 years' follow-up [55]. Various explanations are possible—the effects of more intensive therapy disappear when intensive treatment is stopped; self-selection of patients to treatments at the end of the randomization phase may lead to similar outcome (many children assigned to behavioural intervention started medication, and a significant percentage of those on intensive medication management actually withdrew medication). The most favourable overall development was found in children initially randomized to the MTA medication regime, whether or not they were taking medication at 36 months, thus suggesting some lasting benefit for some children with ADHD.

## Non-dopaminergic medications

Currently, two classes of non-dopaminergic agents are approved for ADHD treatment: the selective NA reuptake inhibitor ATX and the α2 agonists guanfacine and clonidine. The main clinical differences between these agents and dopaminergic drugs are their more favourable legal status, their potential for a long (up to 24 hours) duration of clinical efficacy, and a generally slower onset of action (at least several weeks).

### Mechanism of action and pharmacokinetics

*ATX* is a selective inhibitor of NA synaptic reuptake. *In vitro*, it shows high affinity with NETs, and *in vivo*, it induces an increase in NA extracellular concentrations in the prefrontal cortex. In this region, despite its low affinity for its transporters, it also results in a strong increase in the extraneuronal concentration of DA, which remains stable in the nucleus accumbens and striatum [56], making abuse or triggering of tics by ATX unlikely.

ATX is metabolized mainly through the hepatic cytochrome P450 2D6 enzymatic system (CYP2D6), resulting in metabolites with clinically significant activity. Once-daily ATX is associated with a decrease in 3,4-dihydroxyphenylethylene glycol (DHPG), which is the main brain metabolite of NA and a biomarker of central NET inhibition, persisting for at least 24 hours. Interestingly, there also appears to be a dissociation between the pharmacokinetic and pharmacodynamic profiles for ATX, with evidence that, despite the relatively short half-life, even once-daily dosing can result in clinical effects lasting throughout the day.

*Guanfacine* is a selective α2 noradrenergic agonist, with 15–20 times higher affinity for α2A adrenergic receptors than for α2B or α2C receptors. Extended-release guanfacine (matrix-s tablets, GXR) is well absorbed; after oral administration, the time to peak plasma concentration is approximately 5 hours. GXR half-life is 16–17 hours, allowing once-daily administration. The pharmacokinetic profile of guanfacine is linear (first-order) and dose-proportional. The profile of GXR differs from that of immediate-release (IR) guanfacine, with GXR resulting in 60% lower $C_{max}$ and up to 43% lower area under the curve (AUC), compared to IR tablets [57].

*Clonidine* is an α2 receptor agonist, which modulates adrenergic transmission. Reducing sympathetic activity can give rise to hypotension, sedation, and irritability. Clonidine appears to be less efficacious than conventional drugs in the treatment of ADHD. The effectiveness in reducing tics in children with ADHD is comparable to dopaminergic drugs. In addition to the effects of sedation and symptomatic hypotension, clonidine can cause bradycardia and dry mouth.

### Clinical efficacy of non-dopaminergic medications

The clinical efficacy of ATX has been well documented in short- and long-term studies, with an effect size of approximately 0.7 across studies [58, 59]. The onset of clinical effectiveness of ATX is slower than that of dopaminergic drugs, varying between 2 and 4 weeks. Full therapeutic effect can take up to 6–8 (or even 12) weeks, but responders typically show some degree of improvement by 4 weeks [60]. Some patients may continue to improve for 36 weeks [61].

Guanfacine showed significant improvement of clinician- and teacher-rated symptoms, functional impairment, and positive continuous performance outcome measures in a series of controlled trials [62]. A recent randomized withdrawal trial showed long-term maintenance of efficacy [63]. In adults, guanfacine modulates the influence of emotion control on cortical activation for cognitive control [64].

### Other drugs

*Bupropion* acts as a weak inhibitor of presynaptic reuptake of NA, DA, and 5-HT; it has been licensed for depression and smoking cessation. It showed better efficacy than placebo in reducing ADHD symptoms in children, although lower than dopaminergic drugs. Bupropion can cause nausea, insomnia, and palpitations; it can also trigger tics and cause dermatological reactions, at times severe enough to lead to discontinuation of the drug. Three head-to-head trials found bupropion had efficacy comparable to that of MPH, although a large double-blind, placebo-controlled multi-centre study found smaller effect sizes for bupropion, compared to MPH. In terms of tolerability, a head-to-head trial found that headache was more frequent in the MPH group than in the bupropion-treated group, with no difference in other adverse events [65].

*Tricyclic antidepressants*: the mechanism of action of tricyclics involve inhibition of presynpatic NA reuptake, with poor selectivity. None of them is approved by the FDA or European Medicines Agency (EMA) for the treatment of ADHD; they were prescribed off-label for children with ADHD, but after the introduction of ATX, they are rarely used because of concerns about their potential cardiovascular toxicity.

*Modafinil* is a '*wakefulness-promoting agent*' marketed for the treatment of narcolepsy; it has been occasionally used for the management of inattention in adults. Its mechanism is poorly defined as a non-dopaminergic activating action on the frontal cortex. A recent meta-analysis on five RCTs showed an effect size of 0.7 on ADHD symptoms and a significantly higher incidence of decreased appetite and insomnia, but non-significant cardiovascular adverse events, compared to placebo [66].

## Medication safety and management of adverse effects

Medications for ADHD are generally safe and well tolerated; adverse effects are mild, transitory, reversible, and easily manageable by the ADHD specialist [3, 4]. The most common side effects of dopaminergic agents include sleep difficulties, irritability, appetite and weight loss, headache, tachycardia, and increased blood pressure (BP) and heart frequency. Side effects of non-dopaminergic drugs mainly include nausea, sedation, and appetite loss, dry mouth, insomnia, constipation, and mood swings. Additionally, urinary retention and sexual dysfunction have been observed in adult patients. Most of these adverse effects diminish over the first months of treatment, with no significant differences between normal and poor metabolizers [2].

More severe adverse reactions, like psychotic symptoms or allergic reactions, have rarely been observed in association with dopaminergic or non-dopaminergic medications [3, 4]. Despite this, the tolerability and safety of medications used to treat ADHD have recently been raised as a concern to some regulatory authorities. In January 2009, the European Union (EU) Committee for Medicinal Products for Human Use (CHMP) concluded that the benefit of MPH outweighs the risk when prescribed to ADHD children over 6 years and recommended to standardize prescribing and to provide safety information across all EU members. They further concluded that research was needed on the long-term effects of MPH [67]. As a result of these recommendations, the Attention Deficit Hyperactivity Disorder Drugs Use Chronic Effects (ADDUCE) consortium was established to confirm MPH safety; it included experts in the fields of ADHD, drug safety, neuropsychopharmacology, and cardiovascular research (http://www.adhd-adduce.org).

### Cardiovascular effects

MPH, AMP, and ATX are sympathomimetic agents that increase noradrenergic and dopaminergic transmission; an effect on heart rate (HR) and BP is therefore an intrinsic feature of their pharmacological activity [68, 69]. MPH and ATX may be associated with generally small elevations of BP (≤5 mmHg) and HR [≤10 beats/minute (bpm)] at a group level; a subset of children and adolescents (around 5–15%) may experience greater treatment-related increases in HR or BP, over the 95th centile, or may report a cardiovascular-type complaint during drug treatment [69].

The 10-year follow-up of the MTA study [70] found no effect of treatment on either systolic or diastolic BP; however, use of dopaminergic drugs was associated with a higher HR at years 3 and 8. A recent meta-analysis conducted in ADHD children and adolescents treated with MPH, AMP, or ATX, including 18 trials with data from 5837 participants (80.7% boys) and an average treatment duration of 28.7 weeks, revealed that all three medications were associated with a small, but statistically significant, pre–post-increase of systolic BP (SBP). Compared to AMP and ATX, MPH did not show a pre–post-effect on diastolic BP (DBP) and HR. Only 2% of patients discontinued their medication due to any cardiovascular effect. In the majority of patients, the cardiovascular effects resolved spontaneously or with medication dose changes [71]. A meta-analysis in adult patients with ADHD reported that treatment is associated with small, but significant, increases in SBP (+2.0 mmHg) and HR (+5.7 bpm), but no effect on DBP [72]. No changes in ECG parameters, including PR, QRS, and QT intervals, have been associated with the use of MPH and ATX [69]. However, it is a concern that even small, but persistent, BP and/or HR increases may increase the risk for serious cardiovascular events, including sudden cardiac death, acute myocardial infarction, and stroke, in the long term. The magnitude of this risk remains to be established.

The available epidemiological studies, summarized by Hammerness *et al.* [65], do not show a significant association between ADHD drugs and serious cardiovascular events. A recent large study of 1,200,438 children and young adults between 2 and 24 years found no evidence that ADHD drugs increased the risk of serious cardiovascular events [73]. Similarly, several large registry studies of adults [74] and children (3–17 years) [75] suggest that ADHD medication, when medically supervised, was not associated with an increased risk of severe cardiovascular events.

Current guidelines [3] recommend that patients being considered for ADHD medication should have a clinical assessment, including identification of any known heart disease, any history of syncope with exercise, and any family history of sudden unexpected death under the age of 40 years. HR and BP should be taken at baseline and repeated every 3–6 months. It is important to make a referral for further assessment when indicated, and for patients with pre-existing cardiac conditions, dopamine or NA-releasing drugs should be used cautiously and only after consultation with a cardiologist.

### Growth and developmental effects

One of the most common side effects of drugs for ADHD is appetite loss, with consequent reduced weight gain and possible growth reduction with prolonged use. The mechanism by which growth is affected has not yet been fully clarified. The decrease in appetite and the consequent reduction in caloric intake represent the obvious probable cause of the growth slowdown [76]. Other possible mechanisms include medication effects on hepatic and/or CNS growth factors and direct effects on cartilage.

Studies providing longitudinal data suggest the height deficit is approximately 1 cm/year during the first 3 years of treatment, while some other data suggest that these effects tend to attenuate over time and ultimate adult growth parameters are generally not affected [72, 77].

In the recently published MTA follow-up into adulthood [55], prolonged use of MPH in the ADHD group resulted in an average height of 1.29 ± 0.55 cm shorter than the control group ($p < 0.01$, $d = 0.21$). Within the treated sample, adherence to drug treatment was classed as consistent, inconsistent, or negligible: participants with the consistent or inconsistent pattern were 2.55 ± 0.73 cm shorter than the subgroup with the negligible pattern ($p < 0.0005$, $d = 0.42$).

Preliminary analysis of the large 2-year naturalistic pharmacovigilance ADDUCE study [67] shows a lower height velocity standard deviation score (SDS) in medicated ADHD subjects than in unmedicated ones, roughly equivalent to a reduction in height velocity of about 0.35 cm/year for a 9.6-year-old boy (mean age of subjects in the study). In post hoc analyses, the impact on a child's height velocity SDS was apparently associated with the severity of illness, suggesting a possible dose-dependent effect of MPH.

With regard to ATX, a meta-analysis of seven double-blind/placebo-controlled and six open-label studies found that the mean actual weight and height at 24 months were, respectively, 2.5 kg and 2.7 cm lower than the expected values [78]. The difference occurred mostly during the first 18 months of treatment.

In order to prevent growth suppression and ensure an adequate growth pattern to subjects in the age of development, current guidelines [3] recommend:

* Monitoring appetite, weight, height, and BMI every 6 months.
* Differentiating between pretreatment eating problems and medication-induced eating problems.
* Giving medication after meals, rather than before.
* Encouraging the use of high-calorific snacks and late evening meals.
* Reducing the dose or switching to an alternative class or formulation.
* Discontinuing medication on weekends to prevent weight loss or longer drug holidays to allow for catch-up growth.
* Referring to a paediatric endocrinologist/growth specialist if height and weight values are below critical thresholds.

### Neurological effects

#### Tics

Drugs for ADHD might, from a theoretical point of view, exacerbate tic severity as they can increase DA activity in the basal ganglia [79]. A meta-analysis, including nine DBRPC trials, examining the efficacy of medications for ADHD in children with comorbid tic (a total of 477 subjects) concluded that MPH does not worsen tic severity in the short term, although it is possible that MPH may worsen tics in individual cases and that ATX can, on the other hand, significantly improve comorbid tics [80]. The recent Cochrane group systematic review [81] concluded the same. With regard to ATX, although it can have a positive effect on tic frequency, some case reports have described exacerbation of tics during ATX treatment [4]. Thus, tics are no longer a contraindication for the use of ADHD drugs in the EU, but caution is still recommended [82] (EMA, 2010).

The management of tics should include: (1) observation of the intensity of tics over a 3-month period before any decision regarding ADHD treatment; (2) dose reduction; (3) substitution; and (4) if the previous measures are not effective, an antipsychotic can be added to control tics.

#### Sleep problems

Sleep problems are common in individuals with ADHD, and it is also important to rule out primary sleep disorders that may mimic or exacerbate ADHD. Both AMP and MPH may increase the latency to sleep onset, shorten sleep duration, and decrease sleep efficiency [83]. It is necessary to assess sleep at baseline and to continually monitor throughout treatment, as all ADHD medications can affect sleep. Dose timing adjustments, switching drug formulations, or adding an evening dose of melatonin are often helpful strategies for drug-exacerbated insomnia in children displaying a good medication response [84].

### Seizures and epilepsy

Although longer-term effects of MPH and its effects in children with frequent seizures need further study, current evidence supports the use of MPH for the treatment of ADHD in patients with well-controlled epilepsy and even in those with infrequent seizures [85]. When epilepsy is poorly controlled, the frequency of seizures should be carefully monitored; if their frequency increases, or seizures develop *de novo*, then ADHD medication should be stopped.

## Psychiatric effects

### Psychotic, mood, and other psychiatric symptoms

Drugs for ADHD have been associated rarely with possible severe psychiatric effects, including psychotic symptoms (hallucinations). A review of the literature does not strongly indicate an association between MPH treatment for ADHD and psychosis. However, some open-label trial extension studies reported discontinuations due to psychotic symptoms. In contrast, some positive clinical experience (drugs for ADHD being helpful) have been reported for managing ADHD symptoms in the context of a psychotic disorder. A single study also found that medication with MPH in childhood could show a protective effect by reducing schizotypic features in adults.

Suicide-related events have also been investigated during treatment with drugs for ADHD, with symptoms sometimes anecdotally improving following discontinuation of medication. A recent population-based electronic medical records study showed that, in fact, the incidence of suicide attempts was higher in the period immediately *before* the start of MPH treatment. The risk remained elevated immediately after the start of MPH treatment but returned to baseline levels during continuation of the treatment. The observed higher risk of suicide attempts *before* treatment may reflect emerging psychiatric symptoms that trigger medical consultations, resulting in MPH treatment [86].

Population-based studies indicate that medication for ADHD is associated with a reduced long-term risk (that is, 3 years later) for depression [45] and a potential protective effect on suicidal behaviour [87]. However, individual patients being treated with medications for ADHD should be observed for the emergence of psychotic symptoms, depression, irritability, and suicidal ideation, as part of routine monitoring.

Mood lability, dysphoria, anxiety, hostility, and explosive outbursts may be observed in 5–10% of children taking drugs for ADHD. Among children whose aggressive behaviour develops in the context of ADHD and oppositional defiant disorder or conduct disorder, systematic, well-monitored titration of monotherapy often reduces aggression considerably, thus averting the need for additional medications [88].

### Substance misuse

DA-releasing drugs have the potential for misuse and can be diverted by patients or families to this end [89]. The extended-release formulations of drugs for ADHD are less prone to diversion, because they do rapidly increase blood drug levels and are also less easily crushed into powder for injection or snorting. Once-a-day administration also makes parental supervision easier to enforce. Non-dopaminergic medications (that is, ATX) are another option with low abuse potential.

Concern has been raised that therapeutic use of drugs for ADHD may result in 'sensitization' and possibly increase the risk for substance use disorder (SUD) later in life. However, ADHD is associated with impulsivity and conduct disturbances, and represents itself a risk factor for SUD. Naturalistic follow-up studies do not support the contention that drugs for ADHD increase the risk for SUD (for example, Swedish registry studies found drug treatment associated with decreased rates in patients with ADHD) [48].

## Management and treatment of ADHD in adulthood

ADHD is a chronic condition with symptoms frequently persisting into adulthood. About 60% of affected children have, as adults, significant ADHD-related impairments, including social dysfunction, educational and occupational underachievement, substance abuse, increased risk for accidents, and legal difficulties [90]. Although awareness, recognition, and diagnostic criteria of ADHD in adults have improved in recent years, there is still the need to increase physician support and specialized services for the clinical management of this disorder, as patients make the transition to the adult health care system [91, 92].

The NICE guidelines in the UK provide strong support for the provision of adult ADHD services, recommending that young people with ADHD and receiving treatment from child and adolescent mental health services (CAMHS) or paediatric services should be reassessed at school-leaving age to establish whether treatment should continue into adulthood.

Adult ADHD symptomatology differs from the typical childhood presentations; hyperactivity/impulsivity may diminish over time, while inattention tends more often to persist, with a greater impact in adults. Optimal strategies for ADHD in adulthood are, as in childhood, multimodal, with the main goals of improving symptoms and optimizing functional performance [93]. Adults respond well to the same classes of medication used in children, and MPH and AMP are confirmed as first-line pharmacologic interventions [94]. Adults with ADHD have, in fact, reported improved social relationships, academic/work functionality, and driving, together with reduced criminal behaviour, as a consequence of ADHD medications [95]. Additionally, adults with ADHD treated with drugs prior to 18 years have been shown to have better outcomes across broad quality of life measurements, as compared with subjects not previously so treated [96].

Just as for children and adolescents, drug treatment of adult ADHD consistently yields positive short-term effects, but few trials have evaluated their long-term efficacy and safety. Poor compliance and comorbid psychiatric disorders may further complicate the determination of treatment benefits in adults with ADHD [97]. ADHD medications can cause side effects also during adulthood. The most worrying include increases in both BP and HR. However, as confirmed by a recent large population cohort study [70], there is no increased risk for acute myocardial infarction, sudden cardiac death, or stroke for current ADHD medication users, compared to non-users. While the risks of serious side effects are thought to be low for healthy adults, physicians should, however, be cautious when prescribing for patients with cardiovascular disease, seizure disorders, and psychosis [98].

Even though pharmacologic interventions are considered first-line treatments for ADHD, some adults with ADHD continue to experience significant residual and impairing symptoms. CBT has been shown helpful in the treatment of adult ADHD, alone and in combination with psychopharmacology [99].

Another psycoeducational approach that has gained increasing popularity in the last year is coaching. It is a highly individualized intervention, in which a personally assigned coach guides the patient in accomplishing tasks and goals. Coaching differs from traditional CBT, because it is more focused on solving specific problems or reaching specific goals and is more accessible to the patient on an as-needed basis [100].

## Conclusions

ADHD is a chronic, heterogenous condition, with a high prevalence and persistence into adult life and the potential for serious functional impairment extending beyond the affected individual. Established efficient assessment methods and good treatment evidence help clinicians in monitoring and managing this disorder in childhood and adulthood. ADHD drugs, available in different formulations, are, especially in the short term, currently among the more effective drugs in psychiatry and perhaps in general medicine [101], with a good safety profile. Long-term treatment efficacy and tolerability and safety data are still insufficient and need more research. On the basis of the current evidence, however, there does not seem to be any necessity to change current clinical guidelines for the monitoring of the main possible adverse events.

## REFERENCES

1. Taylor E, Dopfner M, Sergeant J, et al. European clinical guidelines for hyperkinetic disorder—first upgrade. Eur Child Adolesc Psychiatry. 2004;13(Suppl 1):i7–30.
2. Banaschewski T, Coghill D, Santosh P, et al. Long-acting medications for the hyperkinetic disorders. A systematic review and European treatment guideline. Eur Child Adolesc Psychiatry. 2006;15:476–95.
3. Cortese S, Holtmann M, Banaschewski T, et al. Practitioner review: current best practice in the management of adverse events during treatment with ADHD medications in children and adolescents. J Child Psychol Psychiatry. 2013;54:227–46.
4. Graham J, Banaschewski T, Buitelaar J, et al. European guidelines on managing adverse effects of medication for ADHD. Eur Child Adolesc Psychiatry. 2011;20:17–37.
5. McClellan J, Kowatch R, Findling RL. Practice parameter for the assessment and treatment of children and adolescents with bipolar disorder. J Am Acad Child Adolesc Psychiatry. 2007;46:107–25.
6. Wolraich M, Brown L, Brown RT, et al. ADHD: clinical practice guideline for the diagnosis, evaluation, and treatment of attention-deficit/hyperactivity disorder in children and adolescents. Pediatrics. 2011;128:1007–22.
7. Pliszka SR, Crismon ML, Hughes CW, et al. The Texas Children's Medication Algorithm Project: revision of the algorithm for pharmacotherapy of attention-deficit/hyperactivity disorder. J Am Acad Child Adolesc Psychiatry. 2006;45:642–57.
8. Coghill D, Seth S. Effective management of attention-deficit/hyperactivity disorder (ADHD) through structured re-assessment: the Dundee ADHD Clinical Care Pathway. Child Adolesc Psychiatry Ment Health. 2015;9–52.
9. Pliszka S, and the AACAP Work Group on Quality Issues. Practice parameter for the assessment and treatment of children and adolescents with attention-deficit/hyperactivity disorder. J Am Acad Child Adolesc Psychiatry. 2007;46:894–921.
10. MTA Cooperative Group. A 14-month randomized clinical trial of treatment strategies for attention-deficit/hyperactivity disorder. The MTA cooperative group multimodal treatment study of children with ADHD. Arch Gen Psychiatry. 1999;56(12):1073–86.
11. Thapar A, Cooper M. Attention deficit hyperactivity disorder. Lancet. 2016; 19;387(10024):1240–50.
12. Zwi M, Jones H, Thorgaard C, York A, Dennis JA. Parent training interventions for Attention Deficit Hyperactivity Disorder (ADHD) in children aged 5 to 18 years. Cochrane Database Syst Rev. 2011;12:CD003018.
13. Sonuga-Barke EJ, Brandeis D, Cortese S, et al. Nonpharmacological interventions for ADHD: systematic review and meta-analyses of randomized controlled trials of dietary and psychological treatments. Am J Psychiatry. 2013;170:275–89.
14. Daley D, van der Oord S, Ferrin M, et al. EAGG. Behavioral interventions in attention-deficit/hyperactivity disorder: a meta-analysis of randomized controlled trials across multiple outcome domains. J Am Acad Child Adolesc Psychiatry. 2014;53(8):835–47.
15. Daley D, Van Der Oord S, Ferrin M, et al. Practitioner Review: Current best practice in the use of parent training and other behavioural interventions in the treatment of children and adolescents with attention deficit hyperactivity disorder (ADHD). J Child Psychology Psychiatry. 2017;59:932–47.
16. Rapport MD, Orban SA, Kofler MJ, Friedman LM. Do programs designed to train working memory, other executive functions, and attention benefit children with ADHD? A meta-analytic review of cognitive, academic, and behavioral outcomes. Clin Psychol Rev. 2013;33:1237–52.
17. Cortese S., Ferrin M., Brandeis D., et al. Cognitive Training for Attention Deficit/Hyperactivity Disorder: Meta-Analysis of Clinical and Neuropsychological Outcomes From Randomized Controlled Trials. J Am Acad Child Adolesc Psychiatry. 2015;54(3):164–74.
18. Cortese S, Ferrin M, Brandeis D, et al. Neurofeedback for Attention-Deficit/Hyperactivity Disorder: Meta-Analysis of Clinical and Neuropsychological Outcomes From Randomized Controlled Trial. J Am Acad Child Adolesc Psychiatry. 2016;55(6):444–55.
19. Schönenberg M, Wiedemann E, Schneidt A, et al. Neurofeedback, sham neurofeedback, and cognitive-behavioural group therapy in adults with attention-deficit hyperactivity disorder: a triple-blind, randomised, controlled trial. Lancet Psychiatry. 2017;4:673–84.
20. Alegria AA, Wulff M, Brinson H, et al. Real-time fMRI neurofeedback in adolescents with attention deficit hyperactivity disorder. Hum Brain Mapp. 2017;38(6):3190–209.
21. Zilverstand A, Sorger B, Slaats-Willemse D, Kan CC, Goebel R, Buitelaar JK. fMRI Neurofeedback Training for Increasing Anterior Cingulate Cortex Activation in Adult Attention Deficit Hyperactivity Disorder. An Exploratory Randomized, Single-Blinded Study. PLoS One. 2017;12(1):e0170795.

22. Boyer BE, Geurts HM, Prins PJ, Van der Oord S. Two novel CBTs for adolescents with ADHD: the value of planning skills. European Child and Adolescent Psychiatry. 2015;24(9):1075–90.

23. Min dell JA, Kuhn B, Lewin DS, Meltzer LJ, Sadeh A. Behavioral treatment of bedtime problems and night wakings in infants and young children. Sleep. 2006;29:1263–76.

24. Cortese S, Brown TE, Corkum P, et al. Assessment and management of sleep problems in youths with attention-deficit/hyperactivity disorder. J Am Acad Child Adolesc Psychiatry. 2013;52(8):784–96.

25. Sinn N. Nutritional and dietary influences on attention deficit hyperactivity disorder. Nutr Rev. 2008;66(10):558–68.

26. Hawkey E, Nigg JT. Omega-3 fatty acid and ADHD: blood level analysis and meta-analytic extension of supplementation trials. Clin Psychol Rev. 2014;34:496–505.

27. Chang JC, Su KP, Mondelli V and Pariante CM. Omega-3 Polyunsaturated Fatty Acids in Youths with Attention Deficit Hyperactivity Disorder: a Systematic Review and Meta-Analysis of Clinical Trials and Biological Studies. Neuropsychopharmacology. 2018;43:534–45.

28. Bloch MH, Qawasmi A. Omega-3 Fatty Acid Supplementation for the Treatment of Children WithAttention-Deficit/Hyperactivity Disorder Symptomatology: Systematic Review and Meta-Analysis. J Am Acad Child Adolesc Psychiatry. 2011;50(10):991–1000.

29. Swanson JM, Kraemer HC, Hinshaw SP, Arnold LE, Conners CK. Clinical relevance of the primary findings of the MTA: success rates based on severity of ADHD and ODD symptoms at the end of treatment. J Am Acad Child Adolesc Psychiatry. 2001;40(2):168–79.

30. Hodgkins P, Shaw M, Coghill D, Hechtman L. Amfetamine and methylphenidate medications for attention-deficit/hyperactivity disorder: complementary treatment options. Eur Child Adolesc Psychiatry. 2012;21(9):477–92.

31. Arnsten AF, Pliszka SR. Catecholamine influences on prefrontal cortical function: relevance to treatment of attention deficit/hyperactivity disorder and related disorders. Pharmacol Biochem Behav. 2011;99(2):211–16.

32. Robertson SD, Matthies HJ, Galli A. A closer look at amphetamine-induced reverse transport and trafficking of the dopamine and norepinephrine transporters. Mol Neurobiol. 2009;39(2):73–80.

33. Arnsten AF. Catecholamine influences on dorsolateral prefrontal cortical networks. Biological Psychiatry. 2011;69(12):e89–99.

34. Easton N, Steward C, Marshall F, Fone K, Marsden C. Effects of amphetamine isomers, methylphenidate and atomoxetine on synaptosomal and synaptic vesicle accumulation and release of dopamine and noradrenaline in vitro in the rat brain. Neuropharmacology. 2007;52(2):405–14.

35. Arnsten AF. The Emerging Neurobiology of Attention Deficit Hyperactivity Disorder: The Key Role of the Prefrontal Association Cortex. J Pediatr. 2009;154(5):I-S43.

36. Mehta MA, Owen AM, Sahakian BJ, Mavaddat N, Pickard JD, Robbins TW. Methylphenidate enhances working memory by modulating discrete frontal and parietal lobe regions in the human brain. J Neurosci. 2000;20(6):RC65.

37. Schweitzer JB, Lee DO, Hanford RB, et al. Effect of methylphenidate on executive functioning in adults with attention-deficit/hyperactivity disorder: normalization of behavior but not related brain activity. Biol Psychiatry. 2004;56(8):597–606.

38. Volkow ND, Fowler JS, Wang GJ, et al. Methylphenidate decreased the amount of glucose needed by the brain to perform a cognitive task. PLoS One. 2008;3(4):e2017.

39. Rubia K, Halari R, Mohammad AM, Taylor E, Brammer M. Methylphenidate normalizes frontocingulate underactivation during error processing in attention-deficit/hyperactivity disorder. Biol Psychiatry. 2011;70(3):255–62.

40. Wong CG, Stevens MC. The effects of stimulant medication on working memory functional connectivity in attention-deficit/hyperactivity disorder. Biol Psychiatry. 2012;71(5):458–66.

41. Liddle EB, Hollis C, Batty MJ, et al. Task-related default mode network modulation and inhibitory control in ADHD: effects of motivation and methylphenidate. J Child Psychol Psychiatry. 2011;52(7):761–71.

42. Swanson JM, Wigal SB, Wigal T, et al. A comparison of once-daily extended-release methylphenidate formulations in children with attention-deficit/hyperactivity disorder in the laboratory school (the Comacs Study). Pediatrics. 2004;113(3 Pt 1):e206–16.

43. Barbaresi WJ, Katusic SK, Colligan RC, Weaver AL, Jacobsen SJ. Modifiers of long-term school outcomes for children with attention-deficit/hyperactivity disorder: does treatment with stimulant medication make a difference? Results from a population-based study. J Dev Behav Pediatr. 2007;28(4):274–87.

44. Man KK, Chan EW, Coghill D, et al. Methylphenidate and the risk of trauma. Pediatrics. 2015;135(1):40–8.

45. Chang Z, D'Onofrio BM, Quinn PD, Lichtenstein P, Larsson H. Medication for Attention-Deficit/Hyperactivity Disorder and Risk for Depression: A Nationwide Longitudinal Cohort Study. Biol Psychiatry. 2016;80:916–22.

46. Chen Q, Sjolander A, Runeson B, D'Onofrio BM, Lichtenstein P, Larsson H. Drug treatment for attention-deficit/hyperactivity disorder and suicidal behaviour: register based study. BMJ. 2014;348:g3769.

47. Chang Z, Lichtenstein P, Halldner L, et al. Stimulant ADHD medication and risk for substance abuse. J Child Psychol Psychiatry. 2014;55(8):878–85.

48. Lichtenstein P, Halldner L, Zetterqvist J, et al. Medication for attention deficit-hyperactivity disorder and criminality. N Engl J Med. 2012;367(21):2006–14.

49. Greenhill L, Kollins S, Abikoff H, et al. Efficacy and safety of immediate-release methylphenidate treatment for preschoolers with ADHD. J Am Acad Child Adolesc Psychiatry. 2006;45(11):1284–93.

50. Reichow B, Volkmar FR, Bloch MH. Systematic review and meta-analysis of pharmacological treatment of the symptoms of attention-deficit/hyperactivity disorder in children with pervasive developmental disorders. J Autism Dev Disord. 2013;43(10):2435–41.

51. Coughlin CG, Cohen SC, Mulqueen JM, Ferracioli-Oda E, Stuckelman ZD, Bloch MH. Meta-Analysis: Reduced Risk of Anxiety with Psychostimulant Treatment in Children with Attention-Deficit/Hyperactivity Disorder. J Child Adolesc Psychopharmacol. 2015;25(8):611–17.

52. Balia C, Carucci S, Coghill D, Zuddas A. The pharmacological treatment of aggression in children and adolescents with conduct disorder. Do callous-unemotional traits modulate the efficacy of medication? Neurosci Biobehav Rev. 2018;91:218–38.

53. Banaschewski T, Soutullo C, Lecendreux M, et al. Health-related quality of life and functional outcomes from a randomized, controlled study of lisdexamfetamine dimesylate in children and adolescents with attention deficit hyperactivity disorder. CNS Drugs. 2013;27(10):829–40.

54. Coghill DR, Banaschewski T, Lecendreux M, *et al.* Maintenance of efficacy of lisdexamfetamine dimesylate in children and adolescents with attention-deficit/hyperactivity disorder: randomized-withdrawal study design. J Am Acad Child Adolesc Psychiatry. 2014;53(6):647–57 e1.

55. Swanson JM, Arnold LE, Molina BSG. Young adult outcomes in the follow-up of the multimodal treatment study of attention-deficit/hyperactivity disorder: symptom persistence, source discrepancy, and height suppression. J Child Psychol Psychiatry. 2017;58(6):663–78.

56. Garnock-Jones K P and Keating G. Atomoxetine A Review of its Use in Attention-Deficit Hyperactivity Disorder in Children and Adolescents. Pediatr Drugs. 2009;11(3):203–26.

57. Elbe D, Reddy D. Focus on Guanfacine Extended-release: A Review of its Use in Child and Adolescent Psychiatry. Journal of the Canadian Academy of Child and Adolescent Psychiatry. 2014;23(1):48–60.

58. Faraone SV. Using meta-analysis to compare the efficacy of medications for attention-deficit/hyperactivity disorder in youths. Pharmacy and Therapeutics. 2009;34(12):678.

59. Schwartz S, Correll CU. Efficacy and safety of atomoxetine in children and adolescents with attention-deficit/hyperactivity disorder: results from a comprehensive meta-analysis and metaregression. J Am Acad Child Adolesc Psychiatry. 2014;53(2):174–87.

60. Dickson RA, Maki E, Gibbins C, Gutkin SW, Turgay A, Weiss MD. Time courses of improvement and symptom remission in children treated with atomoxetine for attention-deficit/hyperactivity disorder: analysis of Canadian open-label studies. Child Adolesc Psychiatry Ment health. 2011;5:14.

61. Marchant BK, Reimherr FW, Halls C, *et al.* Long-term open-label response to atomoxetine in adult ADHD: influence of sex, emotional dysregulation, and double-blind response to atomoxetine. Atten Defic Hyperact Disord. 2011;3:237–44.

62. Hervas A, Huss M, Johnson M, *et al.* Efficacy and safety of extended-release guanfacine hydrochloride in children and adolescents with attention-deficit/hyperactivity disorder: a randomized, controlled, phase III trial. Eur Neuropsychopharmacol. 2014;24(12):1861–72.

63. Newcorn JH, Harpin V, Huss M, *et al.* Extended-release guanfacine hydrochloride in 6-17-year olds with ADHD: a randomised-withdrawal maintenance of efficacy study. J Child Psychol Psychiatry. 2016;57(6):717–28.

64. Schulz KP, Clerkin SM, Fan J, *et al.* Guanfacine modulates the influence of emotional cues on prefrontal cortex activation for cognitive control. Psychopharmacology. 2013;226:261–71.

65. Ng QX. A Systematic Review of the Use of Bupropion for Attention-Deficit/Hyperactivity Disorder in Children and Adolescents. J Child Adolesc Psychopharmacol. 2017;27(2):112–16.

66. Wang SM, Han C, Lee SJ, *et al.* Modafinil for the treatment of attention-deficit/hyperactivity disorder: A meta-analysis. J Psychiatr Res. 2017;84:292–300.

67. Inglis SK, Carucci S, Garas P, *et al.* Prospective observational study protocol to investigate long-term adverse effects of methylphenidate in children and adolescents with ADHD: the Attention Deficit Hyperactivity Disorder Drugs Use Chronic Effects (ADDUCE) study. BMJ Open. 2016;6:e010433.

68. Volkow ND, Wang GJ, Fowler JS, *et al.* Cardiovascular effects of methylphenidate in humans are associated with increases of dopamine in brain and of epinephrine in plasma. Psychopharmacology. 2003;166(3):264–70.

69. Hammerness PG, Perrin JM, Shelley-Abrahamson R, Wilens TE. Cardiovascular risk of stimulant treatment in pediatric attention-deficit/hyperactivity disorder: update and clinical recommendations. J Am Acad Child Adolesc Psychiatry. 2011;50(10):978–90.

70. Vitiello, B., Elliott, G.R., Swanson, J.M., *et al.* Blood pressure and heart rate over 10 years in the multimodal treatment study of children with ADHD. American Journal of Psychiatry. 2012;169:167–77.

71. Hennissen L, Bakker MJ, Banaschewski T, *et al.* Cardiovascular Effects of Stimulant and Non-Stimulant Medication for Children and Adolescents with ADHD: A Systematic Review and Meta-Analysis of Trialsof Methylphenidate, Amphetamines and Atomoxetine. CNS Drugs. 2017;31:199–215.

72. Mick E, McManus DD, Goldberg RJ. Meta-analysis of increased heart rate and blood pressure associated with CNS stimulant treatment of ADHD in adults. Eur Neuropsychopharmacol. 2013;23(6):534–41.

73. Cooper WO, Habel LA, Sox CM, *et al.* ADHD drugs and serious cardiovascular events in children and young adults. N Engl J Med. 2011;365(20):1896–904.

74. Habel LA, Cooper WO, Sox CM, *et al.* ADHD medications and risk of serious cardiovascular events in young and middle-aged adults. JAMA. 2011;306(24):2673–83.

75. Schelleman H, Bilker WB, Strom BL, *et al.* Cardiovascular events and death in children exposed and unexposed to ADHD agents. Pediatrics. 2011;127(6):1102–10.

76. Vitiello B. Understanding the risk of using medications for attention deficit hyperactivity disorder with respect to physical growth and cardiovascular function. Child Adolesc Psychiatr Clin N Am. 2008;17(2):459–74.

77. Peyre H., Hoertel N., Cortese S., *et al.* Long-term effects of ADHD medication on adult height: results from the NESARC. J Clin Psychiatry. 2013;74:1123–4.

78. Kratochvil CJ, Wilens TE, Greenhill LL, Gao H, Baker KD, Feldman PD, Gelowitz DL. Effects of long-term atomoxetine treatment for young children with attention-deficit/hyperactivity disorder. J Am Acad Child Adolesc Psychiatry. 2006;45(8):919–27.

79. Albin, R.L. Neurobiology of basal ganglia and Tourette syndrome: Striatal and dopamine function. Advances in Neurology. 2006;99:99–106.

80. Bloch MH, Panza KE, Landeros-Weisenberger A, Leckman JF. Meta-analysis: Treatment of attention-deficit/hyperactivity disorder in children with comorbid tic disorders. J Am Acad Child Adolesc Psychiatry. 2009;48:884–93.

81. Pringsheim T, Steeves T. Pharmacological treatment for Attention Deficit Hyperactivity Disorder (ADHD) in children with comorbid tic disorders. Cochrane Database Syst Rev. 2011;4:CD007990.

82. European Medicines Agency. (2010). *Overview of comments received on 'Guideline on the clinical investigation of medicinal products for the treatment of attention deficit hyperactivity disorder (ADHD)' (EMEA/CHMP/EWP/431734/2008).* Available from: http://www.ema.europa.eu/docs/en_GB/document_library/Other/2010/08/WC500095687.pdf

83. Kidwell KM, Van Dyk TR, Lundahl A, Nelson TD. Stimulant Medications and Sleep for Youth With ADHD: A Meta-analysis. Pediatrics. 2015;136(6):1144–53.

84. Cortese S, Brown TE, Corkum P, *et al.* Assessment and management of sleep problems in youths with attention-deficit/hyperactivity disorder. J Am Acad Child Adolesc Psychiatry. 2013;52(8):784–96.

85. Torres AR, Whitney J, Gonzalez-Heydrich J. Attention-deficit/hyperactivity disorder in pediatric patients with epilepsy: review of pharmacological treatment. Epilepsy Behav. 2008;12(2):217–33.

86. Man KKC, Coghill D, Chan EW, et al. Association of Risk of Suicide Attempts With Methylphenidate Treatment. JAMA Psychiatry. 2017;74:1048–55.

87. Chen Q, Sjolander A, Runeson B, D'Onofrio BM, Lichtenstein P, Larsson H. Drug treatment for attention-deficit/hyperactivity disorder and suicidal behaviour: register based study. BMJ. 2014;348:g3769.

88. Blader JC, Pliszka SR, Jensen PS, Schooler NR, Kafantaris V. Stimulant-responsive and stimulant-refractory aggressive behavior among children with ADHD. Pediatrics. 2010;126(4):e796–806.

89. Wilens TE, Adler LA, Adams J, et al. Misuse and diversion of stimulants prescribed for ADHD: a systematic review of the literature. J Am Acad Child Adolesc Psychiatry. 2008;47(1):21–31.

90. Biederman J, Faraone SV, Spencer TJ, et al. Functional impairments in adults with self-reports of diagnosed ADHD: a controlled study of 1001 adults in the community. J Clin Psychiatry. 2006;67(4):524–40.

91. Hall CL, Newell K, Taylor J, Sayal K, Swift KD, Hollis C. 'Mind the gap'—mapping services for young people with ADHD transitioning from child to adult mental health services. BMC Psychiatry. 2013;13:186.

92. Young JL, Goodman DW. Adult Attention-Deficit/Hyperactivity Disorder Diagnosis, Management, and Treatment in the DSM-5 Era. Prim Care Companion CNS Disord. 2016;18(6).

93. Felt BT, Biermann B, Christner JG, et al. Diagnosis and management of ADHD in children. Am Fam Physician. 2014;90(7):456–64.

94. Wigal SB. Efficacy and safety limitations of attention-deficit hyperactivity disorder pharmacotherapy in children and adults. CNS Drugs. 2009;23(suppl 1):21–31.

95. McCarthy S. Pharmacological interventions for ADHD: how do adolescent and adult patient beliefs and attitudes impact treatment adherence? Patient Prefer Adherence. 2014;8:1317–27.

96. Rasmussen K, Palmstierna T, Levander S. Differences in psychiatric problems and criminality between individuals treated with central stimulants before and after adulthood. J Atten Disord. 2019;23:173–80.

97. Newcorn JH, Weiss M, Stein MA. The complexity of ADHD: diagnosis and treatment of the adult patient with comorbidities. CNS Spectr. 2007;12(suppl 12):1–14, quiz 15–6.

98. Volkow ND, Swanson JM. Clinical practice: adult attention deficit-hyperactivity disorder. N Engl J Med. 2013;369(20):1935–44.

99. Knouse LE, Safren SA. Current status of cognitive behavioral therapy for adult attention-deficit hyperactivity disorder. Psychiatr Clin North Am. 2010;33(3):497–509.

100. Knouse LE, Cooper-Vince C, Sprich S, et al. Recent developments in the psychosocial treatment of adult ADHD. Expert Rev Neurother. 2008; 8(10):1537–48.

101. Leucht S, Hierl S, Kissling W, Dold M, Davis JM. Putting the efficacy of psychiatric and general medicine medication into perspective: review of meta-analyses. Br J Psychiatry. 2012;200(2):97–106.

# SECTION 6
# Motor disorders

SECTION C
MOTOR DISORDERS

# 37

# Neurodevelopmental motor disorders

*Davide Martino and Antonella Macerollo*

## Introduction

Neurodevelopmental motor disorders are a group of conditions characterized by developmental deficits in learning, control, and execution of motor skills. These deficits may manifest as difficulties in programming and executing fine and gross motor tasks that are crucial for routine activities of daily living and social and academic abilities, as well as an inability to control excessively repetitive or unwanted motor behaviours. The appropriate realization of a motor programme or a sequence of movements requires the convergence of numerous pathways [sensory (somatosensory, proprioceptive, visual, vestibular) pathways, motor pathways, and regulatory pathways, for example cortico-basal ganglia, cerebello-thalamo-cortical and intracortical networks]. This neuroanatomical substrate involves cortical and subcortical structures regulating the correct integration of sensory inputs and motor outputs, which allows the successful execution and learning of advantageous goal-directed movements. The correct functional development of motricity is strongly supported by experience, with appropriate synaptic circuits being reinforced and established as a result of recurrent practice of efficient movement patterns.

The most common neurodevelopmental motor disorders are tic disorders, stereotypic motor disorder, and developmental coordination disorder (DCD), which will be the object of this chapter.

## Tic disorders

### Phenomenology

Tic disorders are characterized by the recurrent presence of tics, which can be defined as unwanted, discrete, non-goal-directed, non-rhythmic movements (*motor* tics) or vocalizations (*vocal* tics). The basic features of tics which help distinguish them from other abnormal behaviours include: repetitive and patterned character; variability of the type of movement/vocalization and severity; association with premonitory urges; and partial or complete suppressibility on demand. Three tic disorders are included in DSM-5: Tourette's disorder [also called Tourette's syndrome (TS)], persistent (also called chronic) motor or vocal tic disorder; and provisional tic disorder [1]. The core diagnostic criteria of tic disorders are listed in Box 37.1.

The repetitive and patterned character of tics is an important feature to differentiate them from other unwanted movements such as chorea or myoclonus. Regardless of their repetitive quality, tics are highly variable within and across subjects, as regards to muscle groups involved (and thus body location), complexity, and interference with normal voluntary behaviour. The overall severity of tics fluctuates over time, and each tic may wax and wane over the course of time. Their changing pattern is one of the main differences with stereotypies, discussed later in this chapter.

Although virtually any striatal muscle group in the body can be involved in a tic, a cranio-caudal gradient of frequency is typically observed, with the face, head, and proximal upper limbs being the most commonly affected. At the same time, the ability to suppress tics voluntarily is maximal where tics are least frequent (trunk and lower limbs), and minimal in the most cranial body areas [2].

Tics are also classified as simple and complex, depending on whether they involve a single muscle group or consist of coordinated sequences or combinations of movements/vocalizations involving several muscle groups. Motor tics may therefore range from very rapid, simple motor twitches (for example, blinking, facial grimacing, head flicks, shoulder shrugs, etc.) to orchestrated sequences of movements, sometimes resembling purposeful behaviour. Likewise, vocal tics may range from monosyllabic, meaningless vocal utterances to longer fragments of verbal language with a semantic content. Complex tic-like repetitive behaviours include also: echophenomena (echopraxia, echolalia) and paliphenomena, that is, non-voluntary repetition of movements or vocalizations made by another person or his/her own; and socially inappropriate words or gestures, which can also have obscene content, as in coprophenomena (coprolalia, copropraxia). When severe enough, tics may cause impairment in social, academic, and professional functioning. Some tics may have a violent and potentially (although not deliberately) self-harming quality, for example, head banging, hitting, etc.

Premonitory urges (PUs) are uncomfortable sensations that build up in intensity immediately before tics and are markedly alleviated immediately after tic release. Often the linked PUs and tics occur in the same body region. In some patients, PUs are described more as a poorly defined feeling of pressure, tension, or restlessness around the body part associated with a certain tic. Only about 25% of pre-pubertal children are able to describe PUs, whereas this

**Box 37.1** DSM-5 criteria for tic disorders

Tourette's syndrome (TS)

For a person to be diagnosed with TS, he or she must:

- Have two or more motor tics (for example, blinking or shrugging the shoulders) and at least one vocal tic (for example, humming, clearing the throat, or yelling out a word or phrase), although they might not always happen at the same time.
- Have had tics for at least a year; the tics can occur many times a day (usually in bouts) nearly every day, or off and on.
- Have tics that begin before he or she is 18 years of age.
- Have symptoms that are not due to taking medicine or other drugs or due to having another medical condition (for example, seizures, Huntington disease, or post-viral encephalitis).

Persistent (chronic) motor or vocal tic disorder

For a person to be diagnosed with a persistent tic disorder, he or she must fulfil the same criteria of TS, apart from the first criterion, which is as follows:

- The person must have one or more motor tics (for example, blinking or shrugging the shoulders) or vocal tics (for example, humming, clearing the throat, or yelling out a word or phrase), *but not both.*

Provisional tic disorder

For a person to be diagnosed with this disorder, he or she must fulfil the same criteria of persistent (chronic) tic disorder, with the only difference that tics have been present for no longer than 12 months in a row.

*Source:* data from the *Diagnostic and Statistical Manual of Mental Disorders,* Fifth Edition, DSM-5, Copyright (2013), American Psychiatric Association.

self-awareness increases dramatically to about 60% during late teen years [3]. Fig. 37.1 summarizes the differences in the main antecedents between tics, compulsions, and impulsive actions.

Patients with tics may also report 'just-right' phenomena, in which they reiterate actions that may or may not involve sensory experiences (for example, repeatedly touching an object or a body part) until these feel 'just right'. 'Just-right' phenomena are more common in patients with comorbid obsessive–compulsive disorder [3].

Another relevant sensory feature associated with tics is the unusual focus of attention on external stimuli which are repetitive, faint, and poorly salient. This phenomenon has been named somatic hypersensitivity or site sensitization and is not related to abnormalities in the ability to discriminate between sensory stimuli of different intensities [4]. Some patients may become easily and disproportionately irritated by excessive irritation by environmental noise (misophonia). The origin of somatic hypersensitivity in tic disorders is still not very well understood but may be related to abnormalities of sensorimotor gating.

The ability to suppress tics is higher in adults than in children and varies across patients. Although suppressing tics leads to a rise in PU intensity, the quality or severity of PUs is not associated with the ability to hold tics in [2]. Although a proportion of patients may experience a rebound worsening of tics, following prolonged tic suppression, this is not a constant feature. More rapid tics, for example eye movements or blinking, are often too quick to be suppressed. Active tic suppression demands attention and may distract from complex cognitive activities, including school-based learning activities. Voluntary suppression of tics is facilitated by reward, for example in social situations where inhibiting tics may lead to greater social acceptance. Relaxation, physical exercise, engagement in attention-demanding tasks, and reduced sympathetic tone may also reduce tic severity. At the same time, psychosocial stress is the most effective contextual factor that modulates tic severity. Raised

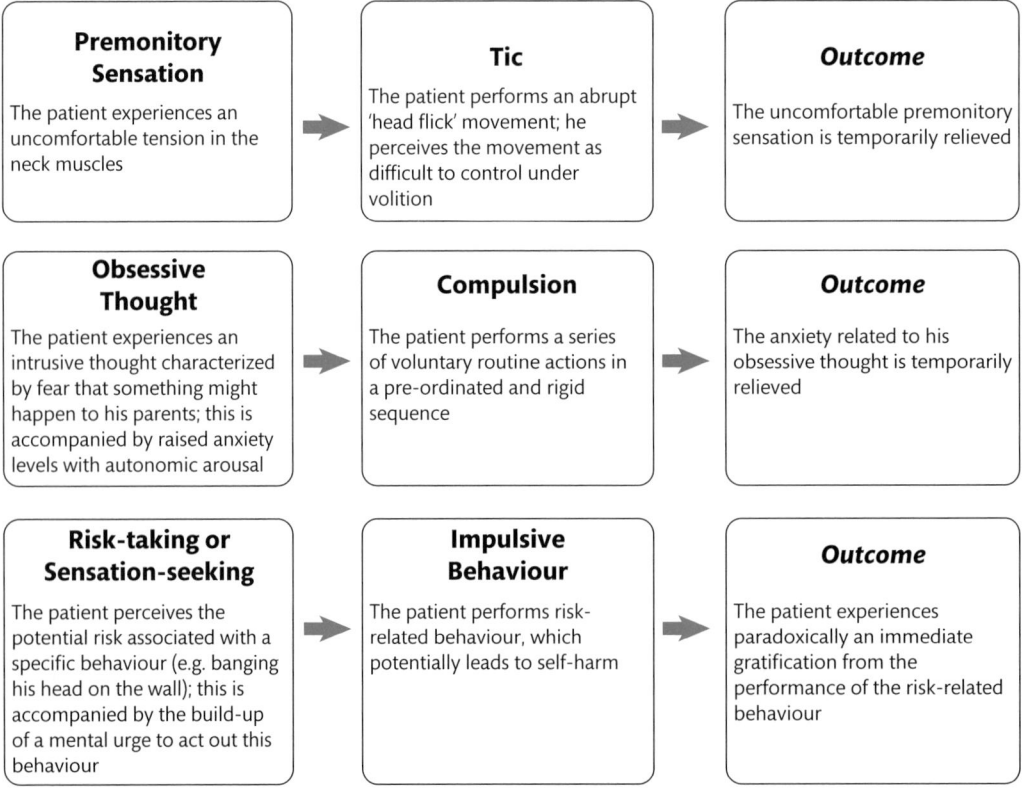

**Fig. 37.1** Basic phenomenologic differences between tics, compulsions, and impulsive behaviours.

anxiety levels and fatigue are also important precipitants of tics. Moreover, in some cases, tics and PUs may be precipitated by talking or thinking about them (metacognitive inducibility) [5].

Tic-like rapid movements presenting in adulthood may be labelled as tics, but at least a proportion of them are considered to have a *functional* origin. Apart from age at onset, these abnormal movements differ from typical 'organic' tics for their female predominance, sudden onset often precipitated by minor trauma or panic attacks, uncommon association with PUs or suppressibility, common suggestibility, lack of association with a family history of tic disorders or a personal history of ADHD or OCD, and no response to anti-tic medications such as dopamine antagonists [6].

Tics typically begin between 5 and 8 years of age, and in up to 95% between ages 4 and 13. The first tics are more frequently simple and involve cranial muscles, usually facial (blinking, sniffing, etc.). Severity peaks around puberty (age 10–12) when complex tics usually appear, and tics may spread beyond the cranio-cervical region. Tics usually decrease in the second decade. Persistence of clinically relevant tics in adulthood was found to be associated with higher tic severity in childhood, lower caudate volumes, and poorer performance on tasks involving visuomotor skills during childhood [7].

Most prevalence studies on tic disorders have focused on paediatric populations. A meta-analysis of prevalence data from 1985 to 2011 found that studies applying a school-based assessment yielded a combined prevalence of 0.77% for TS, 1.61% for chronic tic disorders, 2.99% for transient tic disorders, and 2.82% for the 'all tic disorders' category in the population of up to 16 years of age [8]. There is, however, large variability of estimates across studies, due to differences in design and conduct. A male predominance was detectable only in TS, but not in other chronic and transient (provisional) tic disorders. Cohort studies of youth with TS report that half to two-thirds of these patients experience a significant decline of tic symptoms that roughly coincides with late adolescence. In contrast with this, a study in which adults previously diagnosed with TS in childhood were evaluated again after age 20 found that 90% still had tics, suggesting that tic disorders are not rare in adulthood [9].

The lifetime prevalence of any psychiatric comorbidity among TS patients was estimated at 85–90%, with almost 60% suffering from two or more psychiatric disorders, and more than 70% meeting criteria for OCD or ADHD [2, 3]. Overall, other symptoms/behaviours are often a greater cause of distress than tics and have a negative impact on TS patients' quality of life.

ADHD is the most common comorbidity, affecting up to 60% of TS patients, particularly male children. ADHD typically begins before the onset of tics, and its presence is associated with earlier tic onset (5.8 vs 6.2 years in TS patients without ADHD). ADHD is associated with a higher likelihood of reduced social functioning, anxiety disorder, anger control and sleep problems, mood disorders, and conduct or oppositional defiant disorder.

Obsessive–compulsive symptomatology in TS is most often associated with symmetry behaviours, 'just-right' experiences, and repetitive touching, although other types of obsessive–compulsive behaviours may also be observed. In a large sample of more than 5000 children and adolescents with TS, comorbid OCD was associated with ADHD, mood and anxiety disorders, conduct disorder/oppositional defiant disorder, and autism spectrum disorder (ASD) [10].

Self-injurious behaviour is encountered in up to 60% of TS patients. TS patients are 1.4 times more likely to suffer from anxiety than the general population, independent of comorbid OCD and ADHD. Up to 30% of patients may develop mood disorders in their lifetime, although this seems mostly accounted for by comorbid OCD. About 10% of youth with chronic tic disorders experience suicidal thoughts and/or behaviours [11]. Prevalence estimates of ASD in TS may be as high as 13%. Of note, ASD were found to be associated with a higher risk of rage attacks/explosive outbursts. Finally, 64% of adult TS patients were found to have at least one comorbid personality disorder, with borderline, depressive, obsessive–compulsive, paranoid, passive aggressive, and avoidant being the most common [10].

### Pathogenesis

Structural and functional abnormalities were detected in TS patients at numerous levels of the cortico-striato-thalamo-cortical (CSTC) network, which is fundamental for the programming and execution of motor actions and habit formation [12]. On a microscopic level, one transcriptomics and two neuropathological studies of previously medicated TS adults showed reduced numbers and gene expression within inhibitory GABAergic and cholinergic interneurons in sensorimotor parts of the striatum and internal segment of the globus pallidus. A functional imbalance between inhibition/excitation in these structures was hypothesized. Animal model work on rodents and monkeys have shown that injection of the $GABA_A$ antagonist bicuculline in sensorimotor parts of the striatum leads to disinhibition of the CSTC loops and to generation of tic-like rapid movements, whereas injection in the nucleus accumbens (ventral or limbic part of the striatum) leads to vocal utterances resembling vocal tics. Tic-like generation in one of these models followed the somatotopical distribution of respective disinhibited striatal motor areas [13, 14].

Structural neuroimaging studies in TS patients have provided further evidence of abnormalities in CSTC circuits (in particular, in sensorimotor and limbic loops). Voxel-based morphometry studies reported volumetric changes of the caudate, putamen, midbrain, and hippocampus, whereas diffusion tensor imaging tractography showed reduced connectivity between the supplementary motor area and the basal ganglia, as well as in frontal cortico-cortical circuits [15]. Event-related fMRI revealed activation of the sensorimotor area and posterior parietal cortex at tic onset, whereas premotor areas, the anterior cingulate cortex, and the insula were activated in the 2 seconds prior to tic (hence, possibly corresponding to the urge to tic). It has thus been speculated that urge activity in the insula could influence the primary motor cortex to produce tics, bypassing the premotor cortex [16].

There is evidence for defective inhibitory mechanisms in TS brains, at the level of both intracortical inhibitory microcircuits and sensorimotor gating. The latter is classically explored, assessing prepulse inhibition, where an initial small sensory stimulus inhibits a reflex response to a second stronger stimulus. Prepulse inhibition defects have been reported in a proportion of patients with tic disorders and could be associated with the somatic hypersensitivity exhibited by these patients [17].

Another important theory at the basis of tic generation supports the involvement of overactive dopaminergic systems. This is suggested by the observation of excessive phasic dopamine release following stimulation with amphetamine in nuclear imaging studies. It also gives support to the idea that tics represent a form of habit, arising from a dopaminergically mediated reward associated with the relief of the uncomfortable urge induced by the tic movement [12].

A long list of conditions and psychotropic substances may give rise to secondary tics. A later age at onset (late adolescence or adulthood), abrupt onset, and association with other neurological manifestations should prompt to exclude these secondary causes. Box 37.2 provides a comprehensive list of these causes.

## Management

A comprehensive history, collected from patients and reliable informants, and assessment using validated rating instruments for tics and associated behavioural symptoms are crucial in guiding the management of tic disorders (Fig. 37.2). Appropriate education of patients and families is a necessary phase of management, which aims at optimizing the understanding and acceptance of symptoms and identifying the best coping strategies with the disorder. Both thorough assessment and education help the clinician in selecting patients who require more active interventions for their tics, when these are needed, and whether and which comorbidities should be treated with priority.

Tics typically require active interventions when they are stigmatizing, socially or academically impairing, influencing mood and self-esteem, and generating situational anxiety. Also, a smaller proportion of cases experience violent tics that are potentially harmful or physically exhausting, leading to pain, headaches, or fatigue. Fig. 37.3 presents a therapeutic algorithm adapted from recently published guidelines [18, 19].

The first line of interventions for tics encompasses pharmacological and behavioural approaches. The choice of a specific intervention is not only guided by evidence, but relies also on the predicted compliance of each individual to a given treatment, as well as on the need to obtain a rapid effect and the direct availability of certain interventions (for example, behavioural).

Dopamine antagonist drugs have been in the therapeutic arsenal for tics for more than 40 years. Pimozide (0.5–6 mg) and haloperidol (0.5–10 mg) were shown to be superior to placebo by six and three RCTs of fair quality, respectively, although haloperidol showed a worse tolerability profile. The use of fluphenazine (0.5–20 mg) is supported by open-label studies, retrospective case series, and one single-blind, placebo-controlled crossover study. Benzamides like tiapride and sulpiride (50–200 mg) are also used, especially in some European countries. However, there is limited evidence of their efficacy; moreover, sedation is frequently reported by patients on sulpiride (Table 37.1) [20].

Among second-generation antipsychotics, the use of risperidone is supported by five RCTs that confirmed its superiority to placebo in treating tics. A meta-analysis showed that risperidone (daily dose range 1–6 mg) does not differ in efficacy from haloperidol, pimozide, and ziprasidone. Initial evidence shows that risperidone could be helpful as an augmentation strategy for associated obsessive–compulsive symptoms and impulse-control disorder. The efficacy of aripiprazole (5–30 mg) is supported by one fair-quality RCT, five prospective open-label studies on relatively large clinical samples, and one meta-analysis. About two-thirds of treated patients across different ages show clinically significant improvement of their tics with this medication, with effects lasting over 1 year in up to 50% of responders. Cardiac safety may also be larger for aripiprazole,

**Box 37.2** Secondary causes of tics

- **Neurodevelopmental disorders**
  - Mental retardation
  - Autistic spectrum disorders (including Asperger's syndrome)
  - Rett's syndrome
  - Genetic and chromosomal abnormalities
  - X-linked mental retardation (*MRX23*)
  - Albright hereditary osteodystrophy
  - Duchenne muscular dystrophy
  - Factor VIII haemophilia
  - Fragile X syndrome
  - Lesch–Nyhan syndrome
  - Triple X and 9p mosaicism
  - 47,XXY karyotype
  - Partial trisomy 16
  - 9p monosomy
  - Beckwith–Wiedemann syndrome
  - Tuberous sclerosis
  - Congenital adrenal hyperplasia due to 21-hydroxylase deficiency
  - Phenylketonuria
  - Corpus callosum dysgenesis
  - Craniosynostosis
  - Klinefelter's syndrome
  - Neurofibromatosis
  - Developmental stuttering
- **Acute brain lesions**
  - Post-traumatic
  - Vascular
  - Infectious
  - Varicella-zoster virus
  - Herpes simplex encephalitis
  - *Mycoplasma pneumoniae*
  - Lyme disease
- **Post-infectious**
  - Sydenham's chorea
  - Paediatric autoimmune neuropsychiatric disorder associated with streptococcal infections (PANDAS)
  - Neurodegenerative diseases
  - Huntington's disease
  - Neuroacanthocytosis syndromes
  - Neurodegeneration with brain iron accumulation
- **Other systemic diseases**
  - Behçet's syndrome
  - Antiphospholipid syndrome
- **Peripheral trauma**
- **Amphetamines**
- **Cocaine**
- **Heroin**
- **Methylphenidate**
- **Pemoline**
- **Antipsychotics (D2 blockers)**
  - Fluphenazine
  - Perphenazine
  - Thiothixene
- **Antidepressants**
- **Antiepileptics**
  - Carbamazepine
  - Phenytoin
  - Phenobarbital
  - Lamotrigine
- **L-dopa**

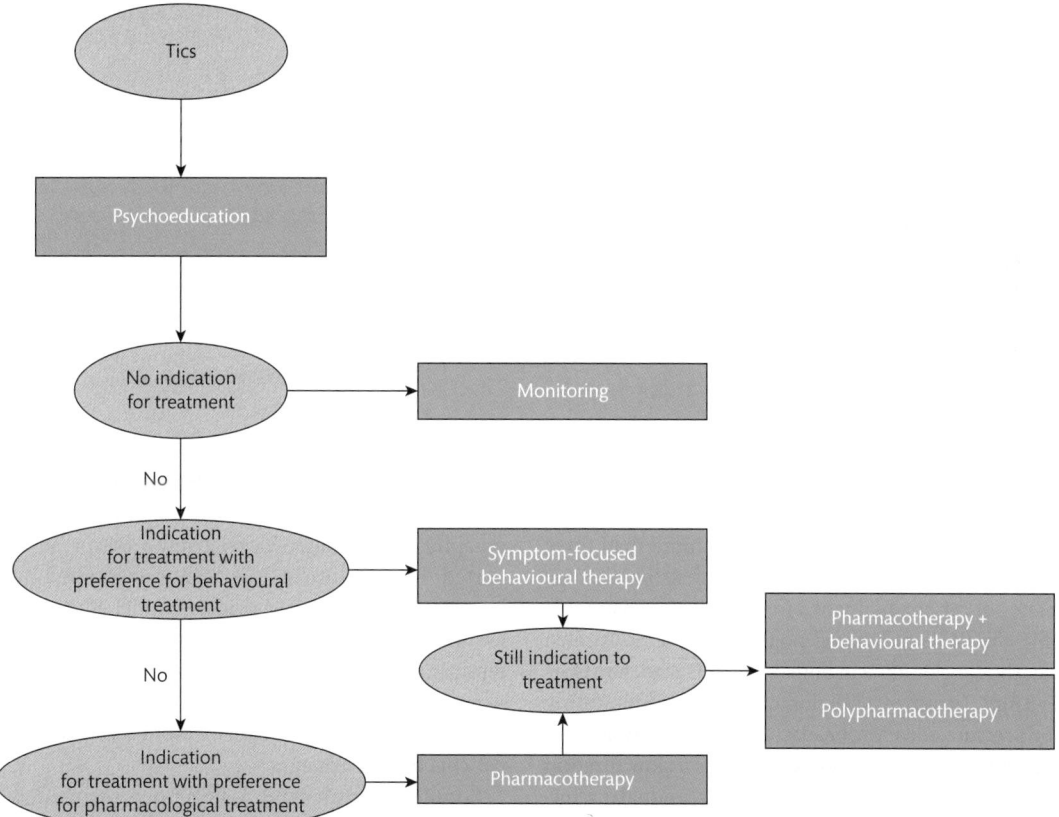

**1. DEMOGRAPHICS**
(age, gender, ethnicity, education level, SES, marital status [parental or pts])

**2. TIC EVALUATION**
- **YALE GLOBAL TIC SEVERITY SCALE** (checklist + severity + overall impairment) – **PUTS**
- **Engage and listen to parents/partners**
- **CONTEXTUAL FACTORS** (*no standardized instrument available*)

**3. COMORBIDITIES**
- **OCD**: [C]Y- BOCS
- **ADHD**: SNAP
- **Anxiety/depression**: SCARED – BDI/BAI
- **Disruptive behaviours**: DBRS
- **Autism**: ASSQ

**4. AREA OF FUNCTIONING**
**Engage and listen to parents/partners** (academic and professional proficiency; hobbies and recreational interests; aspirations)
**GTS-QoL**
**Sleep diary** (if required)

**Fig. 37.2** Assessment plan in Tourette's syndrome. PUTS, Premonitory Urge for Tics Scale (Woods *et al.*, 2005); OCD, obsessive–compulsive disorder; [C]Y-BOCS: [Children]Yale–Brown Obsessive–Compulsive Scale (Scahill *et al.*, 1997); SNAP, Swanson, Nolan and Pelham questionnaire (Bussing *et al.*, 2008); SCARED, Screen for Child Anxiety and Related Emotional Disorders (Birmaher *et al.*, 1997); BDI, Beck Depression Inventory (Joe *et al.*, 2008); BAI, Beck Anxiety Inventory (Steer *et al.*, 1986); DBRS, Disruptive Behavior Rating Scale (Silva *et al.*, 2005); ASSQ, Autism Spectrum Screening Questionnaire (Ehlers *et al.*, 1999).§

**Fig. 37.3** Decision tree for the treatment of tics (specifically focused on Tourette's syndrome and other primary tic disorders).

Adapted from *Eur Child Adolesc Psychiatry*, 20(4), Roessner V, Plessen KJ, Rothenberger A, *et al.*, European clinical guidelines for Tourette syndrome and other tic disorders. Part II: pharmacological treatment, pp. 173–196, Copyright (2011), The Author(s).

**Table 37.1** Medications for the treatment of tics

| Medication | Daily dose (mg) | Adverse effects | Level of evidence |
|---|---|---|---|
| Clonidine | 0.05–3 | Sedation, dry mouth, headache, irritability, mid-sleep awakenings, rebound hypertension, tics and anxiety following abrupt discontinuation | CG: moderate quality, strong recommendation<br>ESSTS: level A evidence |
| Guanfacine | 0.5–4 | Orthostatic hypotension, bradycardia, sedation, headache | CG: moderate quality, strong recommendation<br>ESSTS: level A evidence |
| Haloperidol | 0.5–10 | Rigidity, parkinsonism, tardive involuntary movements and akathisia; appetite changes; weight gain; salivary changes; constipation; depression, anxiety; fatigue, sedation; hyperprolactinaemia (galactorrhoea, gynaecomastia, irregular menses, sexual dysfunction) | CG: high quality, weak recommendation<br>ESSTS: level A evidence |
| Pimozide | 0.5–6 | Similar to haloperidol, but with less movement disorders; QTc interval prolongation | CG: high quality, weak recommendation<br>ESSTS: level A evidence |
| Risperidone | 0.5–16 | Sedation, fatigue, depression and acute phobic reactions, weight gain | CG: high quality, weak recommendation<br>ESSTS: level A evidence |
| Aripiprazole | 5–30 | Weight gain, increase in BMI and waist circumference, nausea, fatigue, sedation, akathisia, movement disorders, sleep problems; probably lower risk of QT prolongation than with other antipsychotics | CG: moderate quality, weak recommendation<br>ESSTS: level B evidence |
| Ziprasidone | 5–40 | Sedation, anxiety, akathisia, movement disorders | CG: low quality, weak recommendation<br>ESSTS: level B evidence |
| Olanzapine | 2.5–20 | Sedation, weight gain and increased appetite, dry mouth, transient hypoglycaemia | CG: low quality, weak recommendation<br>ESSTS: level B evidence |
| Fluphenazine | 0.5–20 | Similar to haloperidol, but less frequent | CG: low quality, weak recommendation<br>ESSTS: not evaluated |
| Sulpiride Tiapride | 50–200 | Sedation; less commonly, paradoxical depression, restlessness, sleep problems, weight gain, hyperprolactinaemia | CG: not evaluated<br>ESSTS: level B evidence |
| Topiramate | 50–150 | Weight loss, paraesthesiae | CG: low quality, weak recommendation<br>ESSTS: not evaluated |
| Botulinum toxin |  | Focal weakness, hypophonia | CG: low quality, weak recommendation |
| Delta-9-THC | 10 | Anxiety, dizziness, fatigue, dry mouth, mood changes, memory loss, psychosis, blurred vision | CG: low quality, weak recommendation |
| Quetiapine | 50–250 | Sedation | CG: very low quality, weak recommendation<br>ESSTS: level C evidence |
| Tetrabenazine | 25–150 | Sedation, fatigue, nausea, insomnia, akathisia, parkinsonism, depression | CG: very low quality, weak recommendation |

Adapted from Martino, D. and Mink, J.W. (2013). Tic disorders. *Continuum (Minneap Minn)*, 19(5 Movement Disorders), 1287–311.
CG: Canadian guidelines (Pringsheim I., 2012).
ESSTS: European Society for the Study of Tourette Syndrome guidelines (Roessner *et al.*, 2011).

compared to other dopamine antagonist drugs, in patients with tics [20].

Alpha-2 agonists have been used to treat tics for more than three decades. Clonidine and guanfacine are considered first-line therapy in the United States and Canada, thanks for their more favourable tolerability profile. Six RCTs of heterogenous quality demonstrated superiority to placebo for clonidine in both oral and transdermal formulations (0.05–3 mg). Treatment with clonidine requires monitoring for reduced blood pressure, sedation, headache, irritability, dysphoria, and interrupted night sleep. It is also advisable to use a slow titration of clonidine in order to improve tolerability, as well as gradual discontinuation to prevent rebound hypertension. Guanfacine has a longer half-life than clonidine and can be administered only once daily (0.5–4 mg); it has a similar side effect profile to clonidine. Two RCTs and two open-label studies confirmed the efficacy of guanfacine, especially in children with tic disorders. Importantly, one meta-analysis confirmed superiority to placebo for both alpha-2-agonists only for youngsters with comorbid ADHD [21].

Tetrabenazine is a presynaptic dopamine depletor that acts by blocking the vesicular VMAT2 protein and displays minor postsynaptic D2 blockage. Its relatively widespread use in tics is supported by its greater tolerability, compared to antipsychotics; however, there is limited evidence of its efficacy, mainly supported by a single small open-label trial and by retrospective cohort studies reporting improvement of tic severity sustained for up to 2 years. Among GABA agonists, baclofen and topiramate were found to be moderately effective in two medium-sized double-blind RCTs on patients of different ages.

Botulinum toxin type A injections represent a very useful resource in older adolescents and adults for the treatment of persistent, simple motor tics located to the upper face or neck, as well as for a number of vocal tics, including coprolalic utterances. However, as with tetrabenazine, its large use is not supported by a strong evidence of efficacy, which consists only of case reports or small series, three retrospective cohort studies, and one RCT. Hypophonia is a very common side effect of botulinum toxin injections for vocal tics.

Delta-9-tetrahydrocannabinol, the main active compound of cannabis, has been tested in two small RCTs on adults with TS, showing a modest, but promising, benefit on some outcome measures and acceptable tolerability. Nicotine has been investigated as an add-on treatment to haloperidol in a number of studies, but its mild efficacy is outweighed by intolerable gastrointestinal side effects [20].

Complementary and alternative medicine approaches in TS have recently attracted growing interest. Among the most promising interventions, there is interesting evidence of safety and moderate efficacy on tics or tic-related impairment for omega-3 fatty acids and chinese traditional medicine approaches that include Ningdong and 5-Ling granules. The efficacy on tic severity of 5-Ling granules has recently been reported by a large double-blind RCT [22].

Investigation and application of behavioural therapies specifically targeting tics have remarkably increased in the last decade. The most effective treatment approaches of this kind are habit reversal training (HRT), a related and expanded version of the HRT package called Comprehensive Behavioral Intervention for Tics (CBIT), and exposure and response prevention (ERP) for tics [23, 24]. HRT for tics is built on *awareness training*, during which patients learn to recognize in real time their urges and tics; *competing response training*, whereby non-pervasive motor behaviours physically incompatible with tics are selected and implemented to diminish tic production; and *social support*, based on the engagement of a support person in promoting the deployment of competing motor responses outside of therapy. Six RCTs and other smaller observational studies demonstrated the efficacy of HRT in diminishing tic severity. This was confirmed by meta-analyses, which detected a large treatment effect size, similar to that observed in other widely used behavioural interventions for conditions like OCD or anxiety disorders. A combination of HRT and acceptance and commitment therapy (ACT) has also been proposed but is still not supported by sufficient evidence of efficacy. ACT consists of exercises helping patients to gain distance from distressing cognitions, emotions, and urges.

CBIT is the most popular and, to date, effective extension of HRT. CBIT complements HRT with: (1) *function-based assessment*, which targets contextual factors predictably worsening tics and facilitates support persons and patients to identify strategies to counteract tic-prone situations; (2) *relaxation training*, primarily acting on stress management; and (4) and *psychoeducational interventions*. CBIT consists of 11 1-hour long sessions, six of which weekly, two scheduled every 2 weeks, followed by three booster monthly sessions, with a fixed protocol of homework assignments. This treatment protocol was three times superior to supportive therapy plus psychoeducation in two large multi-site RCTs, one with children and one with adults with TS, demonstrating very good tolerability and low attrition, sustained improvements for more than 6 months, and amelioration of familial distress, obsessive–compulsive symptoms, and anxiety [23]. Preliminary evidence demonstrated the non-inferiority of HRT administration via a tele-health approach, compared to face-to-face administration.

ERP is largely used in OCD. Its adaptation for tic treatment relies on prolonged exposure to urges associated with sustained suppression of tics, thus generating habituation to the urge and a progressive decrease in the motivation of the patient to tic. Only one RCT has shown non-inferiority of ERP to HRT [24].

A cognitive psychophysiological model, aiming to change the background activity against which tics occurs and treat associated metacognitive and perfectionist beliefs, has recently been tested in an open trial [25]. Other therapeutic approaches focusing on stress modulation that have recently been tested in open-label studies include mindfulness-based stress reduction programmes in small group classes, which yielded a promising percentage of responders, or aerobic exercise sessions such as kickboxing routines. Neurofeedback modulation of EEG oscillatory activity of cortical areas involved in cognitive control has also been tested in preliminary open-label studies and found to attenuate ADHD and tic symptoms. Controlled trials for these approaches are lacking. More research is also needed to increase knowledge of predictors of good response to CBT and patient selection criteria.

Within the realm of neuromodulation strategies for more severe cases of TS, deep brain stimulation (DBS) remains the only active intervention that is extensively being investigated for adult TS patients who are deemed refractory to pharmacological and behavioural interventions. The main patient selection criteria for DBS in TS proposed by recommendation documents [26] are listed in Box 37.3.

Consensus on the ideal anatomical target has not yet been reached to date, mostly due to the lack of adequately powered active comparator trials. The most frequently used targets, supported by crossover RCTs, are the centromedian/parafascicular-substantia periventricularis-nucleus ventralis oralis internus crosspoint of the thalamus and the globus pallidus pars interna (more frequently the anteromedial, or limbic, portion) [27, 28]. Although DBS of TS has not raised major safety concerns to date, its efficacy appears to be still quite variable across patients, and long-term observation is warranted. The application of adaptive approaches using looped paradigms that adapt stimulation parameters to real-time brain oscillatory activities associated with tic generation is currently being investigated.

---

**Box 37.3** Recommendation on patient selection for deep brain stimulation in Tourette's syndrome

- Diagnosis of TS or other chronic tic disorder.
- Age 18 or above (according to some authors, 25 or above).
- Tics as prominent feature of the clinical presentation.
- High tic severity (proposed as ≥35 on the Yale Global Tic Severity Subscore for a stable period of time, suggested by some authors of at least 12 months) and/or presence of potentially highly disabling or harmful tics (for example, tics associated with a clear self-injurious component).
- Tics are considered refractory to pharmacological and behavioural interventions. Failure of pharmacological treatment implies having tried a course with medications from at least three different pharmacological classes (for example, antipsychotics, α2-agonists, benzodiazepines), lasting at least 12 weeks (according to other authors, 6 months) for each drug, at adequate dosage and with proven compliance. Failure of behavioural therapy implies having tried at least ten sessions of behavioural treatment (either HRT-based or ERP-based).
- Stable and optimized treatment of medical, cognitive, and behavioural comorbidities.
- Expected compliance during monitoring (stable psychosocial environment).

## Stereotypic motor disorder

### Phenomenology

Stereotypies are repetitive, non-goal-directed actions predominantly seen in childhood. Unlike tics, they can be highly consistent over time (≥4 weeks), are generally not preceded by sensory or mental experiences, and may be distracted by surrounding stimuli (for example, by calling the child's name) [29]. *Common stereotypies* are the most frequent, occurring in 20–50% of children. These comprise non-disabling habits which change pattern during development, including (in order of the most frequent time of appearance) thumb sucking, body rocking, nail biting, foot tapping, head banging, chewing, or hair twisting. Common stereotypies only seldom require medical intervention, and this is usually related to medical sequelae caused by their persistance and intensity such as dental malocclusion, digital deformities, paronychia, skin abrasions, or temporomandibular disorders. *Complex motor stereotypies* consist of different limb movements (flapping, waving, fisting, finger or wrist movements). These are subdivided into *primary* (stable or remitting, occurring in developmentally normal children) and *secondary* (occurring in conjunction with a neurologic or behavioural disorder), which, in some cases, may develop into self-injurious behaviours (for example, eye poking, biting, head banging, complex hand movements) [30, 31]. Other secondary stereotypies include atypical gazing, pacing, running, and jumping, all typically associated with autism. *Head nodding* begins earlier, is a quasi-rhythmic stereotypy which may also involve the shoulders, and often regresses in later childhood. In general, intense emotional states (particularly excitement), being engrossed in demanding activities, fatigue, or boredom may trigger stereotypies. Movements related to intense imagery have also recently been identified as a subtype of primary complex motor stereotypies.

The DSM-5 defines repetitive habit behaviours that cause impairment to the child as a stereotypic movement disorder (Box 37.4) [1]. Complex motor stereotypies and head nodding fulfil the DSM-5 criteria for stereotypic movement disorder.

Birth and developmental history, including defective communication and social skills, may be very helpful to identify disorders underlying secondary complex stereotypies. Family history of complex motor stereotypies may be present in as many as 40% of cases. Drug history is also relevant; for example, toxic effects of amphetamines include severe head banging and hand biting stereotypies [29].

Complex motor stereotypies have been estimated to occur in up to 3–4% of the general population of pre-school children, but in more than 60% of autistic pre-schoolers and 25% of non-autistic pre-schoolers with similar intellectual abilities [32]. The prevalence of complex motor stereotypies may be as high as 40–60% in institutionalized children with severe learning disabilities, with self-harming forms estimated to be 5–6 times less common. More than 80% of complex motor stereotypies begin before age 2; one-third of cases improve or resolve, in most cases during the first year, and 60% stabilize, although often persisting at least through the teenage years. If the behaviour persists through childhood, it is more likely that it will become a substantial problem with age. Overall, there is a male predominance in complex motor stereotypies, in part confounded by the different prevalence of underlying diagnoses between the two genders.

---

**Box 37.4** DSM-5 criteria for stereotypic motor disorder

- Repetitive, seemingly driven, and apparently purposeless motor behaviour (for example, handshaking or waving, body rocking, head banging, self-biting, or hitting one's own body).
- The repetitive motor behaviour interferes with social, academic, or other activities and may result in self-injury.
- Onset in the early developmental period.
- The repetitive motor behaviour is not attributable to the physiologic effects of a substance or neurologic condition and cannot be better explained by another neurodevelopmental or mental disorder (for example, trichotillomania or OCD).

The following *specifiers* are used:

- With self-injurious behaviour (or behaviour that would be self-injurious if not prevented).
- Without self-injurious behaviour.

Whether the stereotypy is associated with a known medical or genetic condition, developmental disorder, or environmental factor is also specified, and an additional code is used to identify the associated element. *Severity* is specified as follows:

- Mild—symptoms are easily suppressed by sensory stimulus or distraction.
- Moderate—symptoms necessitate explicit protective measures and behavioural modification.
- Severe—continuous monitoring and protective measures are required to prevent serious injury.

*Source*: data from the *Diagnostic and Statistical Manual of Mental Disorders*, Fifth Edition, DSM-5, Copyright (2013), American Psychiatric Association.

---

The main causes of secondary stereotypies are neurodevelopmental disorders including severe learning disabilities and autistic spectrum disorders (Fig. 37.4). Therefore, identification of intellectual disability or developmental delay is crucial in the differential diagnosis of stereotypies. Some forms are associated with chromosomal aberrations (for example, Down's syndrome, Williams syndrome, fragile X syndrome, cri-du-chat syndrome) or with Smith–Magenis syndrome. Deprivation stereotypies are permanent and observed in patients with congenital sensory deprivation.

Another important genetic cause of stereotypies is Rett's syndrome, an X-linked, neurodegenerative illness that typically presents with stereotypies in the developmental period [33]. Rett's syndrome is caused by mutations in the *MECP2* gene, which codes for a protein that acts as a transcriptional repressor binding to methylated DNA. Whereas stereotypies in ASD are more intermittent, randomly distributed with preference for distal extremities, and associated frequently with visual inspection and flickering of the fingers, the stereotypies in Rett's syndrome are more continuous, predominantly located in the hands, mouth, and axial districts, and commonly involve objects.

Genetically inherited neurometabolic causes of stereotypies include, among others, phenylketonuria and adenylosuccinate lyase deficiency. Among acquired causes of stereotypies, autoimmune encephalopathies such as anti-NMDA receptor antibody-mediated encephalitis have been reported and may be triggered by emotional stimuli. These stereotypies are typically located to the upper limbs and bucco-linguo-facial regions, and sometimes may be difficult to differentiate from chorea. When rarer forms of repetitive actions are present, epileptic automatisms should be considered.

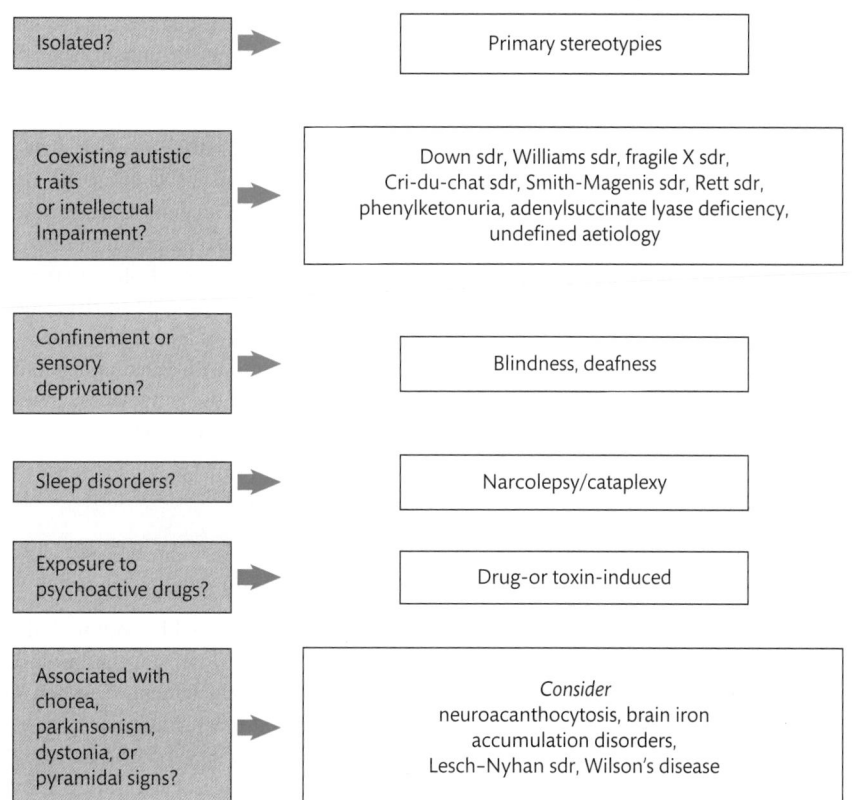

**Fig. 37.4** Aetiology of motor stereotypies.

Adapted from Martino D, Espay AJ, Fasano A, *et al.*, Unvoluntary Motor Behaviours. In: Chapter 3: Disorders of Movement, pp. 97–153, Copyright (2016), with permission from Springer-Verlag.

## Pathogenesis

Abnormalities of dopaminergic transmission in the basal ganglia are involved in the generation of stereotypies. Systemic or intrastriatal infusion of amphetamines and dopamine agonists in rats may cause highly repetitive behaviours (sniffing, gnawing, licking, biting), which resemble stereotypies in humans, and can be antagonized by dopamine D1 receptor blockers. Amphetamines and other psychostimulants, particularly cocaine, potentiate dopaminergic release and transmission and are known to be able to cause stereotypies in the developmental period. Tardive stereotypies are very rare in the developmental period. In general, specific movements involving the arms (rhythmical extensions of the elbow), trunk, and pelvis, such as 'copulatory dyskinesias', may be considered stereotypies [34].

## Management

Overall, a functional behavioural assessment by a psychologist may be helpful to determine the impact of stereotypies on the youngster's routine daily life and can aid in identifying the types of activities that may occur jointly with, or exacerbate, stereotypies. Family members and significant others will urge to seek specialist attention when they recognize typical stereotyped behaviours. The aetiologic diagnosis relies primarily on a complete medical history and physical examination, complemented by a series of instrumental tests, primarily biochemical or genetic.

Isolated primary stereotypies can be regarded as developmental variants of physiological habits that often do not require specific treatment, apart from appropriate psychoeducation. The main aim of psychoeducational interventions in motor stereotypies is to diminish parental anxiety and correct inaccurate beliefs and perceptions in order to avoid unnecessary distress or stigmatization related to these motor behaviours. The management of stereotypies, as for other developmental motor disorders, should be tailored to the characteristics of the patient, in particular his/her age, behavioural comorbidities, and the aetiology of the stereotypies. Similar to standard practice in tic disorders, motor stereotypies require an active intervention when, after accurate psychopathological screening, these cause social isolation or stigma, predispose to physical injury directly associated with the self-injurious character of the movements, and when these generate substantial familial distress. In these cases, referral to a child psychologist or psychiatrist or to a developmental–behavioural paediatrician is advisable.

The mainstay of active treatment of common or primary complex motor stereotypies (Fig. 37.5) is behavioural therapy [35]. This includes two components: intervention on the context of environmental surroundings, and direct intervention on the patient. The principle of intervening on the environmental context is to adjust the surroundings in order to minimize the risks of injury and the vulnerability associated with more violent or erratic movements. Environmental interventions may target antecedents and consequences. Antecedent-based strategies have originally included providing visual or verbal cues to forewarn the patient of a change in the activity, engaging in calming (for example, taking a nap) or highly preferred activities prior to a difficult or less preferred activity. Physical exercise has also been used. Other examples of

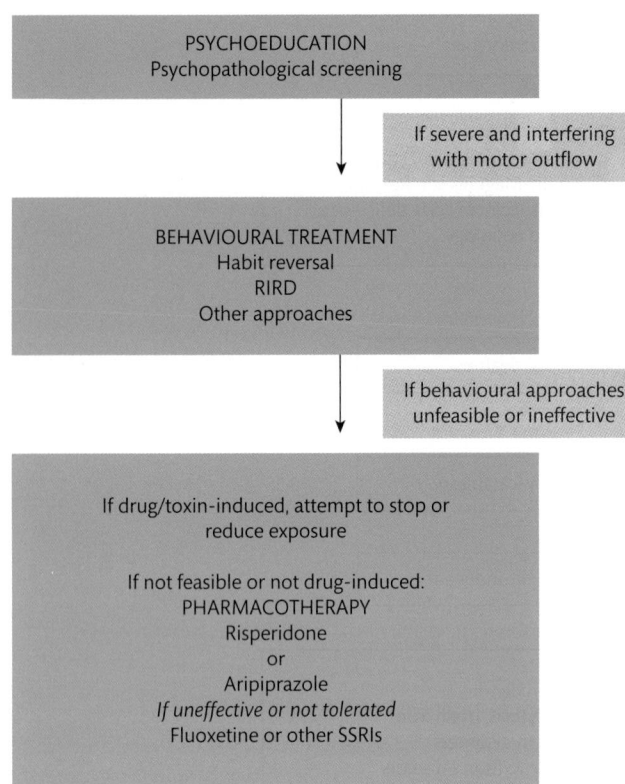

**Fig. 37.5** Decision tree for the treatment of stereotypies.
Adapted from Martino D, Espay AJ, Fasano A, *et al.*, Unvoluntary Motor Behaviours. In: Chapter 3: Disorders of Movement, pp. 97–153, Copyright (2016), with permission from Springer-Verlag.

antecedent-based strategies include: the removal of stimuli triggering stereotypies, as, for example, using gloves or adhesive plasters to prevent thumb sucking; contingency manipulation, for example using bitter- or aversive-tasting substances to prevent nail biting or thumb sucking; and non-contingent stimulation or environmental enrichment, consisting of providing the patient access to appropriate, competing sources of reinforcement such as preferred objects. The safety of the environment can be increased also by protecting from physical consequences such as using a helmet in cases of severe head banging or dental occlusion splints for tooth clenching.

Several behavioural approaches have been applied to primary complex motor stereotypies, whereas these usually show lower efficacy and feasibility in secondary stereotypies. More recently, it was shown that behavioural treatments may retain their efficacy also when provided in a home-based, parent-administered fashion through an instructional DVD [36]. Habit reversal therapy using differential reinforcement has demonstrated efficacy lasting more than 12 months. Evidence is less strong for other approaches, including response interruption and redirection in secondary stereotypies associated with ASD, relaxation training, or response blocking [35].

Pharmacological interventions are taken into account only when behavioural strategies are either unfeasible or ineffective (Fig. 37.5) [34, 37]. Most of the data concerning drug therapies refer to secondary stereotypies associated with learning disabilities and/or autism. Evidence of efficacy is overall limited. Drugs for depression, in particular fluoxetine and clomipramine, are the family of psychotropic agents probably the most investigated. A meta-analysis has

documented a small, but significant, effect of SSRIs in decreasing stereotyped behaviours in autism. The effect of naltrexone, an opioid receptor competitive antagonist, in ASD was systematically reviewed, showing that this drug may improve hyperactivity and irritability, whereas its actual effect on stereotyped behaviours remains uncertain. Drugs for psychosis have also been explored. A meta-analysis of three RCTs demonstrated that risperidone may decrease stereotypies subscale scores in autism [38]. Aripiprazole showed effect in the treatment of stereotypies in autistic children, with better tolerability, compared to risperidone or haloperidol. Finally, a Cochrane review of five double-blind RCTs on self-injurious behaviours in adults with learning disabilities concluded for a weak evidence for any of the active drugs investigated, clomipramine and naltrexone among others [34].

## Developmental co-ordination disorders

### Phenomenology

DCDs are characterized by motor skills deficits, with onset in the early developmental period, that are not explained by intellectual disability, visual impairment, or other neurologic motor problems such as cerebral palsy, muscular dystrophies, or degenerative disorders. The specific DSM-5 criteria for DCDs are listed in Box 37.5 [1]. DCDs constitute a broad clinical spectrum, in which the severity of motor impairment and the burden of comorbidities vary considerably. Their prevalence also varies widely across different studies, falling within a conservative estimate range of 1.5–5% of children below age 10, with an additional 10% of children possibly affected by minor forms of DCDs. A 1.7:1 male-to-female ratio has been reported in a study on more than 7000 British children, but no well-documented interracial or inter-ethnic differences [39].

In line with the introductory considerations at the beginning of this chapter, the pathogenesis of DCDs can be related to abnormal maturation and/or integration of the different building blocks of motor functioning, for example muscular tone and strength, gross

> **Box 37.5** DSM-5 criteria for developmental co-ordination disorder
>
> - Acquisition and execution of co-ordinated motor skills are below what would be expected at a given chronologic age and opportunity for skill learning and use; difficulties are manifested as clumsiness (for example, dropping or bumping into objects) and as slowness and inaccuracy of performance of motor skills (for example, catching an object, using scissors, handwriting, riding a bike, or participating in sports).
> - The motor skills deficit significantly or persistently interferes with activities of daily living appropriate to the chronologic age (for example, self-care and self-maintenance) and impacts academic/school productivity, prevocational and vocational activities, leisure, and play.
> - Onset in the early developmental period.
> - The motor skills deficits cannot be better explained by intellectual disability or visual impairment and are not attributable to a neurologic condition affecting movement (for example, cerebral palsy, muscular dystrophy, or a degenerative disorder).
>
> *Source*: data from the *Diagnostic and Statistical Manual of Mental Disorders*, Fifth Edition, DSM-5, Copyright (2013), American Psychiatric Association.

and fine motor skills, planning and kinematic monitoring of movement, and sensory–motor integration. These functional blocks depend on the normal maturation and connectivity of integrated pathways, involving the motor cortex, cerebellum, and sensory systems (proprioceptive, visual, vestibular). Different forms of DCDs may differ, according to which of the core processes of motor development is primarily dysfunctional, although subtyping of DCDs is still under investigation. Some disorders referring to specific core neuromotor developmental processes, such as 'sensory integration disorder', might, in fact, represent subtypes of DCDs, rather than different conditions.

## Pathogenesis

Like other developmental motor disorders, DCDs are also believed to result from alterations in the global organization of brain networks, which is demonstrated by structural and functional differences in sensory–motor tract connectivity between DCDs and typically developing children [40]. DCDs have a multifactorial aetiology, involving genetic, pre-/perinatal, and environmental factors. The heritability of DCDs has been estimated to be between 0.47 and 0.69, with a likely polygenic architecture of the genetic contribution to their pathogenesis. Intrauterine exposure to alcohol, and possibly to stimulants like cocaine or methamphetamine, is an important risk factor for the development of DCDs, as the overlap between DCDs and fetal alcohol spectrum disorder suggests [41]. Likewise, extremely pre-term infants (particularly those born at <37 weeks of gestational age) have a substantially higher risk for developing DCDs, compared to infants born at term [39]. Postnatal exposure, including exposure to lead, manganese, and iron deficiency, may also be contributing factors.

Several comorbidities may be associated with DCDs. Common problems that aggravate motor co-ordination difficulties in children include problems with attention and concentration such as those in ADHD [39]. Children with ASD have also been reported to exhibit frequently 'motor clumsiness', although there is little overlap in connectivity abnormalities between these two groups of disorders [42, 43]. Many children with motor difficulties have language difficulties, including stuttering and orofacial dyspraxia, and may have problems in written expression and other learning disabilities.

## Assessment

The diagnosis of DCDs is based on an accurate history and physical examination of the fine and gross motricity of the child. Presentation varies with age, and therefore, information on specific motor co-ordination problems should be sought across the different stages of the neurodevelopmental period. Table 37.2 summarizes the main manifestations of motor co-ordination abnormalities.

The physical examination of the child in the context of DCDs can be divided into two main parts: (1) the observation of motor co-ordination within daily activities, including playing; and (2) dedicated manoeuvres aiming at the assessment of specific motor tasks and abilities. The first part includes assessment of routines associated with academic activities or activities of daily living, for example cutting with scissors, tying shoes, drawing or colouring, throwing or kicking a ball, putting on or taking off a coat or a pair of trousers. The second part of the assessment may involve different manoeuvres that have not, to date, been operationalized in a universally accepted assessment protocol. Examples of these manoeuvres are performing sequential finger tapping in search of sequential errors and adventitious or mirror movements; finger-to-nose or finger-chase tasks; testing energy investment in a given sequential motor task (for example, drawing, writing, etc.) when sustained for 2–3 minutes; searching for 'motor clumsiness', indicating visuospatial deficits; testing the accuracy of fine motor tasks, for example activities involving small or miniature toys (miniature domestic utensils, small blocks for building activities, etc.); and testing co-ordination in gross motricity typically associated with sports or physical play activities.

Overall, children with DCDs typically underperform in many activities of daily living, when compared to typically developing children of the same age. Interestingly, limited physical activity levels resulting from DCDs may increase the risk for cardiovascular disease and predispose to obesity [44], as well as predispose to reduced self-esteem and problems with peer relation and depression, in addition to the learning difficulties that may occur in comorbidity with DCDs [45–47]. In addition, children with DCDs may exhibit a range of gait abnormalities and an increased risk of falls, associated with altered control of the centre of mass and a diminished limit of stability in the backward direction [48, 49].

**Table 37.2** Main motor manifestations associated with developmental co-ordination disorders throughout the developmental period

| Stage of development | Manifestations potentially associated with DCDs |
| --- | --- |
| First year of life | • Hypertonic reactions to auditory or visual stimuli<br>• Persistence of primitive (Moro, plantar, rooting) reflexes<br>• Delayed ability to roll over or sit without head-lag; tendency to slip through the examiner's grasp<br>• Ability to self-correct posture and sit unassisted by 9 months of age<br>• Persisting Babinski sign at the end of the first year of life<br>• Persisting crossed-adductor reflexes and ankle clonus |
| Second and third years of life | • Difficulty in making a pincer grasp (that is, picking up a small object with the index and thumb)<br>• Inability to furniture-walk by 18 months of age<br>• Refusal of foods requiring greater chewing ability by the end of the third year of life |
| Pre-school and school years | • Obvious delay in ability to jump and hop<br>• Complete lack of, or premature, hand dominance (although true ambidexterity is possible)<br>• Difficulty in pencil grasp<br>• Inco-ordination in playing with a ball<br>• Inco-ordination in other fine motor tasks such as tying shoes, drawing, colouring, etc. |

A normative functional skills assessment may be used to evaluate the breadth and severity of the DCD. This relies on commonly used tests of motor impairment, which include: the Bruininks–Oseretsky Test of Motor Proficiency (BOTMP), suitable for youth aged 4–21years and frequently administered by therapists to monitor the efficacy of a treatment course; the Movement Assessment Battery for Children (MABC), which evaluates comprehensively manual dexterity, static and dynamic balance, and the functional inter-actions between the child and the surrounding environment; and the Test for Gross Motor Development, second edition (TGMD-2), used in children aged 3–10 years and focused on locomotor and object control abilities. Additional commonly used instruments for a broader neurodevelopmental evaluation are, among others, the Touwen Test for children with minor neurologic dysfunction and the Physical and Neurological Examination for Soft Signs (PANESS).

The diagnostic workup of DCDs should also include investiga-tions aiming to rule out alternative causes for motor skills deficits. Among these, laboratory and neurophysiological tests to rule out muscle and peripheral nerve disorders and screening for metal toxicity and iron deficiency and metabolic abnormalities, such as thyroid dysfunction, may be warranted. Brain imaging and gen-etic screening for ataxias, myopathies, peripheral neuropathies, and metabolic syndromes could be necessary in specific cases, and neurological consultation is advised.

## Management

The large inter-individual variability of adaptive functioning prob-lems generated by DCDs requires a treatment approach that is highly personalized. A recent meta-analysis has identified strong effects in improving motor performance for task-oriented interven-tions and physical or occupational therapy, compared to process-oriented therapies, with insufficient evidence in support of chemical supplementation [50].

Physiotherapists and occupational therapists administer task-oriented interventions, often in collaboration with supporting figures like teachers and the direct engagement of parents. Task-oriented interventions exploit a top–down approach, employing specific techniques that target difficulties with specific motor challenges, for example catching a ball, performing fine digital tasks, handwriting, etc. Cognitive motor intervention is an ex-ample of these task-oriented treatments. It is based on designing a set of exercises that children should practise, with the assistance and supervision of parents, until the motor skills are mastered. The possibility of measuring objectively the treatment goal repre-sents an important advantage of this approach. Cognitive motor intervention builds substantially also on motivational and cog-nitive reinforcers as crucial drivers of motor learning and aims at generating a schema that could be reused later also in other situations [51].

An alternative (bottom–up) approach that has been used by physiotherapists and occupational therapists is based on the as-sumption that general mechanisms like dysfunctional sensory in-tegration or abnormal kinaesthetic perception subdue the motor co-ordination difficulties. This approach modulates the exposure to external stimuli (visual, auditory, tactile, proprioceptive) that influ-ence motor performance in children with DCDs, who may be either hypersensitive or hyposensitive to endogenous and exogenous stimulation. It also exploits techniques that foster self-regulatory mechanisms of sensory–motor integration. The efficacy of sensory integration therapies could be higher in combination with occupa-tional therapy, although a recent meta-analysis has demonstrated a weak effect in improving motor performance, and doubts have been casted on their overall value [50, 52].

More recently, specific programmes aiming at improving balance strategies in DCDs have been tested in RCTs. Task-specific balance training approaches, such as functional movement training and a specific adaptation of the latter—functional movement-power training, showed efficacy in enhancing balance strategies and neuromuscular performance in children with DCDs [53]. The effi-cacy of other treatment approaches, including kinaesthetic or visual training and neurodevelopmental treatment, has a weak or insuffi-cient evidence base.

Finally, there are no pharmacologic approaches that showed consistent efficacy in improving motor performance in DCDs. Methylphenidate showed a moderate effect size in three studies and represents the most explored medication in this context [50]. Other pharmacologic strategies may help specific comorbidities that affect motor co-ordination; for example, propranolol or other beta-blockers may ameliorate severe hand tremor when this is ag-gravating co-ordination problems.

## REFERENCES

1. American Psychiatric Association. (2013). *Diagnostic and statis-tical manual of mental disorders* (5th ed.). American Psychiatric Association, Washington, DC.
2. Ganos C, Martino D. Tics and Tourette syndrome. Neurol Clin 2015;33:115–36.
3. Martino D, Madhusudan N, Zis P, Cavanna AE. An introduction to the clinical phenomenology of Tourette syndrome. Int Rev Neurobiol 2013;112:1–33.
4. Belluscio BA, Jin L, Watters V, Lee TH, Hallett M. Sensory sen-sitivity to external stimuli in Tourette syndrome patients. Mov Disord 2011;26:2538–43.
5. Conelea CA, Woods DW. The influence of contextual factors on tic expression in Tourette's syndrome: a review. J Psychosom Res 2008;65:487–96.
6. Demartini B, Ricciardi L, Parees I, Ganos C, Bhatia KP, Edwards MJ. A positive diagnosis of functional (psychogenic) tics. Eur J Neurol 2015;22:527–36.
7. Cohen SC, Leckman JF, Bloch MH. Clinical assessment of Tourette syndrome and tic disorders. Neurosci Biobehav Rev 2013;37:997–1007.
8. Knight T, Steeves T, Day L, Lowerison M, Jetté N, Pringsheim T. Prevalence of tic disorders: a systematic review and meta-analysis. Pediatr Neurol 2012;47:77–90.
9. Pappert EJ, Goetz CG, Louis ED, Blasucci L, Leurgans S. Objective assessments of longitudinal outcome in Gilles de la Tourette's syndrome. Neurology 2003;61:936–40.
10. Cavanna AE, Rickards H. The psychopathological spectrum of Gilles de la Tourette syndrome. Neurosci Biobehav Rev 2013;37:1008–15.
11. Johnco C, McGuire JF, McBride NM, Murphy TK, Lewin AB, Storch EA. Suicidal ideation in youth with tic disorders. J Affect Disord 2016;200:204–11.

12. Ganos C, Roessner V, Munchau A. The functional anatomy of Gilles de la Tourette syndrome. Neurosci Biobehav Rev 2013;37:1050–62.

13. Israelashvili M, Bar-Gad I. Corticostriatal divergent function in determining the temporal and spatial properties of motor tics. J Neurosci 2015;35:16340–51.

14. McCairn KW, Nagai Y, Hori Y, et al. A primary role for nucleus accumbens and related limbic network in vocal tics. Neuron 2016;89:300–7.

15. Worbe Y, Lehericy S, Hartmann A. Neuroimaging of tic genesis: present status and future perspectives. Mov Disord 2015;30:1179–83.

16. Hallett M. Tourette syndrome: update. Brain Dev 2015;37:651–5.

17. Zebardast N, Crowley MJ, Bloch MH, et al. Brain mechanisms for prepulse inhibition in adults with Tourette syndrome: initial findings. Psychiatry Res 2013;214:33–41.

18. Roessner V, Plessen KJ, Rothenberger A, et al. European clinical guidelines for Tourette syndrome and other tic disorders. Part II: pharmacological treatment. Eur Child Adolesc Psychiatry 2011;20:173–96.

19. Pringsheim T, Doja A, Gorman D, et al. Canadian guidelines for the evidence–based treatment of tic disorders: pharmacotherapy. Can J Psychiatry 2012;57:133–43.

20. Mogwitz S, Buse J, Ehrlich S, Roessner V. Clinical pharmacology of dopamine-modulating agents in Tourette's syndrome. Int Rev Neurobiol 2013;112:281–349.

21. Weisman H, Qureshi IA, Leckman JF, Scahill L, Bloch MH. Systematic review: pharmacological treatment of tic disorders—efficacy of antipsychotic and alpha-2 adrenergic agonist agents. Neurosci Biobehav Rev 2013;37:1162–71.

22. Zheng Y, Zhang ZJ, Han XM, et al. A proprietary herbal medicine (5-Ling granule) for Tourette syndrome: a randomized controlled trial. J Child Psychol Psychiatry 2016;57:74–83.

23. Piacentini J, Woods DW, Scahill L, et al. Behavior therapy for children with Tourette disorder: a randomized controlled trial. JAMA 2010;303:1929–37.

24. van de Griendt JM, Verdellen CW, van Dijk MK, Verbraak MJ. Behavioural treatment of tics: habit reversal and exposure with response prevention. Neurosci Biobehav Rev 2013;37:1172–7.

25. O'Connor K, Lavoie M, Blanchet P, St-Pierre-Delorme ME. Evaluation of a cognitive psychophysiological model for management of tic disorders: an open trial. Br J Psychiatry 2016;209:76–83.

26. Schrock LE, Mink JW, Woods DW, et al. Tourette syndrome deep brain stimulation: a review and updated recommendations. Mov Disord 2015;30:448–71.

27. Kefalopoulou Z, Zrinzo L, Jahanshahi M, et al. Bilateral globus pallidus stimulation for severe Tourette's syndrome: a double-blind, randomised crossover trial. Lancet Neurol 2015;14:595–605.

28. Ackermans L, Duits A, van der Linden C, et al. Double-blind clinical trial of thalamic stimulation in patients with Tourette syndrome. Brain 2011;134:832–44.

29. Singer HS. Motor stereotypies. Semin Pediatr Neurol 2009;16:77–81.

30. Ghosh D, Rajan PV, Erenberg G. A comparative study of primary and secondary stereotypies. J Child Neurol 2013;28:1562–8.

31. Oakley C, Mahone EM, Morris-Berry C, Kline T, Singer HS. Primary complex motor stereotypies in older children and adolescents: clinical features and longitudinal follow-up. Pediatr Neurol 2015;52:398–403.

32. Maski KP, Jeste SS, Spence SJ. Common neurological co-morbidities in autism spectrum disorders. Curr Opin Pediatr 2011;23:609–15.

33. Goldman S, Temudo T. Hand stereotypies distinguish Rett syndrome from autism disorder. Mov Disord 2012;27:1060–2.

34. Martino D, Espay AJ, Fasano A, Morgante. Unvoluntary motor behaviours. In: Martino D, Espay AJ, Fasano A, Morgante (eds). *Disorders of Movement—a guide to diagnosis and treatment.* Springer-Verlag, Berlin Heidelberg; 2016. pp. 97–206.

35. Miller JM, Singer HS, Bridges DD, Waranch HR. Behavioral therapy for treatment of stereotypic movements in nonautistic children. J Child Neurol 2006;21:119–25.

36. Specht MW, Mahone EM, Kline T, et al. Efficacy of parent-delivered behavioral therapy for primary complex motor stereotypies. Dev Med Child Neurol 2016 Jun 4. doi: 10.1111/dmcn.13164. [Epub ahead of print].

37. Carrasco M, Volkmar FR, Bloch MH. Pharmacologic treatment of repetitive behaviors in autism spectrum disorders: evidence of publication bias. Pediatrics 2012;129:e1301–10.

38. Lemmon ME, Gregas M, Jeste SS. Risperidone use in autism spectrum disorders: a retrospective review of a clinic-referred patient population. J Child Neurol 2011;26:428–32.

39. Lingam R, Hunt L, Golding J, Jongmans M, Emond A. Prevalence of developmental coordination disorder using the DSM-IV at 7 years of age: a UK population-based study. Pediatrics 2009;123:e693–700.

40. Peters LH, Maathuis CG, Hadders-Algra M. Neural correlates of developmental coordination disorder. Dev Med Child Neurol 2013;55 Suppl 4:59–64.

41. Doney R, Lucas BR, Jones T, Howat P, Sauer K, Elliott EJ. Fine motor skills in children with prenatal alcohol exposure or fetal alcohol spectrum disorder. J Dev Behav Pediatr 2014;35:598–609.

42. Kopp S, Beckung E, Gillberg C. Developmental coordination disorder and other motor control problems in girls with autism spectrum disorder and/or attention-deficit/hyperactivity disorder. Res Dev Disabil 2010;31:350–61.

43. Caeyenberghs K, Taymans T, Wilson PH, Vanderstraeten G, Hosseini H, van Waelvelde H. Neural signature of developmental coordination disorder in the structural connectome independent of comorbid autism. Dev Sci 2016;19:599–612.

44. Hendrix CG, Prins MR, Dekkers H. Developmental coordination disorder and overweight and obesity in children: a systematic review. Obes Rev 2014;15:408–23.

45. Lingam R, Jongmans MJ, Ellis M, Hunt LP, Golding J, Emond A. Mental health difficulties in children with developmental coordination disorder. Pediatrics 2012;129:e882–91.

46. Farmer M, Echenne B, Bentourkia M. Study of clinical characteristics in young subjects with developmental coordination disorder. Brain Dev 2016;38:538–47.

47. Van den Heuvel M, Jansen DE, Reijneveld SA, Flapper BC, Smits-Engelsman BC. Identification of emotional and behavioral problems by teachers in children with developmental coordination disorder in the school community. Res Dev Disabil 2016;51–2:40–8.

48. Wilmut K, Du W, Barnett AL. Gait patterns in children with developmental coordinatio disorder. Exp Brain Res 2016;234:1747–55.

49. Fong SS, Ng SS, Chung LM, Ki WY, Chow LP, Macfarlane DJ. Direction-specific impairment of stability limits and falls in

children with developmental coordination disorder: implications for rehabilitation. Gait Posture 2016;43:60–4.

50. Smits-Engelsman BC, Blank R, van der Kaay AC, *et al*. Efficacy of interventions to improve motor performance in children with developmental coordination disorder: a combined systematic review and meta-analysis. Dev Med Child Neurol 2013;55:229–37.

51. Blank R, Smits-Engelsman B, Polatajko H, Wilson P. European Academy for Childhood Disability (EACD): recommendations on the definition, diagnosis and intervention of developmental coordination disorder (long version). Dev Med Child Neurol 2012;54:54–93.

52. Zimmer M, Desch L. Sensory integration therapies for children with developmental and behavioral disorders. Pediatrics 2012;129:1186–9.

53. Fong SS, Guo X, Cheng YT, *et al*. A novel balance training program for children with developmental coordination disorder: a randomized controlled trial. Medicine (Baltimore) 2016;95:e3492.

# SECTION 7
# Delirium, dementia, and other cognitive disorders

# 38

# Pathways of neurodegeneration underlying dementia

*Noel J. Buckley and George K. Tofaris*

## Shared mechanisms of neurodegeneration

Dementia has become the most prevalent disease burden of our time. In the UK alone, there are currently over 850,000 sufferers, a figure that is predicted to rise to 1 million by 2025 and 2 million by 2050. This presents an enormous societal and economic burden (currently £26 billion per annum). Globally, the figures are even more staggering with around 47 million sufferers and an associated economic cost of close to $1 trillion (https://www.alzheimers.org.uk/download/downloads/id/2323/dementia_uk_update.pdf; https://www.alz.co.uk/research/WorldAlzheimerReport2015.pdf). Neurodegenerative diseases are progressive, age-related multifactorial diseases with increasing prevalence and no cure or lasting symptomatic therapy. The need to understand the cellular and molecular mechanisms that underpin dementia has never been more urgent.

There are many causes of dementia, but most are due to neurodegenerative diseases (NDDs), principally Alzheimer's disease (AD), Parkinson's disease (PD), Huntington's disease (HD), and fronto-temporal dementia (FTD). Historically, these diseases have been studied in isolation as separate entities, but recently a consensus has arisen that, despite arising from distinct aetiologies, NDDs share many common underlying mechanisms that can be exploited to identify novel therapeutic targets. In broad strokes, these common cellular mechanisms include misfolded protein aggregation, endoplasmic reticulum (ER) stress, mitochondrial dysfunction, synaptic dysfunction, cellular transport, and inflammation. These cellular functions share overlapping molecular aetiologies, so, for example, cellular stressors, such as α-synuclein or β-amyloid (Aβ), may give rise to misfolded proteins that, in turn, generate ER stress and disrupt cellular transport, resulting in disruption to cellular trafficking and mitochondrial and synaptic function. Accordingly, discovering the underlying molecular players, their mechanisms, and how their interactions disrupt cellular function, leading to neuronal dysfunction and subsequent loss, has become a major goal in understanding the molecular and cellular aetiology of NDDs. One caveat to bear in mind is that even if the ultimate symptoms of NDDs primarily reflect loss of synaptic function, neuronal connectivity, and neuronal death, nevertheless disease pathogenesis takes place in a complex cellular milieu and requires interactions among astrocytes, microglia, and the cerebral vasculature. Indeed the 'neurovascular unit' has been proposed as a term to encompass this complexity. Although this parsimony of common mechanism is an attractive concept, it is equally important to recognize that each NDD does have its own distinct signature, so we need to be cognizant of both disease-specific and disease-common mechanisms. Here, we focus on mechanisms common among NDDs, but the following chapters in this book complement this approach and adopt a disease-specific focus.

### Pathology and genetics

At first sight, the pathologies of NDDs such as AD and PD appear distinct. On the one hand, AD is associated with progressive deficits in memory, cognition, and behaviour, while, on the other hand, PD is primarily considered a dysfunction of motor control. However, 30% of AD sufferers develop PD, and a similar proportion of PD patients develop dementia. This overlap extends to the primary molecular pathology of both diseases; AD is characterized by extracellular deposits of Aβ plaques and intracellular accumulations of tau neurofibrillary tangles distributed throughout the forebrain, whereas PD is characterized by accumulation of α-synuclein in Lewy bodies (LBs) within the dopaminergic neurons of the midbrain. However, LBs are not restricted to PD and are also found in the amygdala of over half of patients diagnosed with familial or sporadic AD, as well as those suffering from dementia with Lewy bodies (DLB) [1]. Similarly, neuronal inclusions of TDP43 (TAR-DNA binding protein 43) are common to AD, FTD, and amyotrophic lateral sclerosis (ALS) [2–4], while tau (encoded by the *MAPT* gene) neurofibrillary tangles are present in the brains of AD, DLB, and FTD [5]. Further evidence of common aetiology among NDDs is provided by the overlap of the underlying genetics of NDDs. An example is provided by the microtubule-associated protein (MAPT) H1 haplotype that is associated with both AD and PD, with the suggestion that these *MAPT* variants increase the risk of PD by a crossover of the mechanisms governing aggregations in LBs and neurofibrillary tangles [6]. More recently, several loss-of-function variants in the

ATP-binding cassette transporter A7 (*ABCA7*) (required for protein aggregate clearance) have been associated with both AD and PD [7]. Common genetic association goes beyond AD and PD; a notable example is *C9orf72* (chromosome 9 open reading frame 72) bearing hexanucleotide GGGGCC repeat expansions as a causative gene in both FTD and ALS [8, 9] and even more prevalently in FTD-ALS [10]. Further common genetic causality of multiple NDDs is evidenced by mutations in Fused in Sarcoma (*FUS*), an RNA-binding protein, valosin-containing protein (*VCP*), and Ubiquitin 2 (UBQLN2), all of which are associated with a minority of ALS and FTD cases [11–14]. The commonality of function of many risk genes associated with AD and other NDDs can be seen in Fig. 38.1.

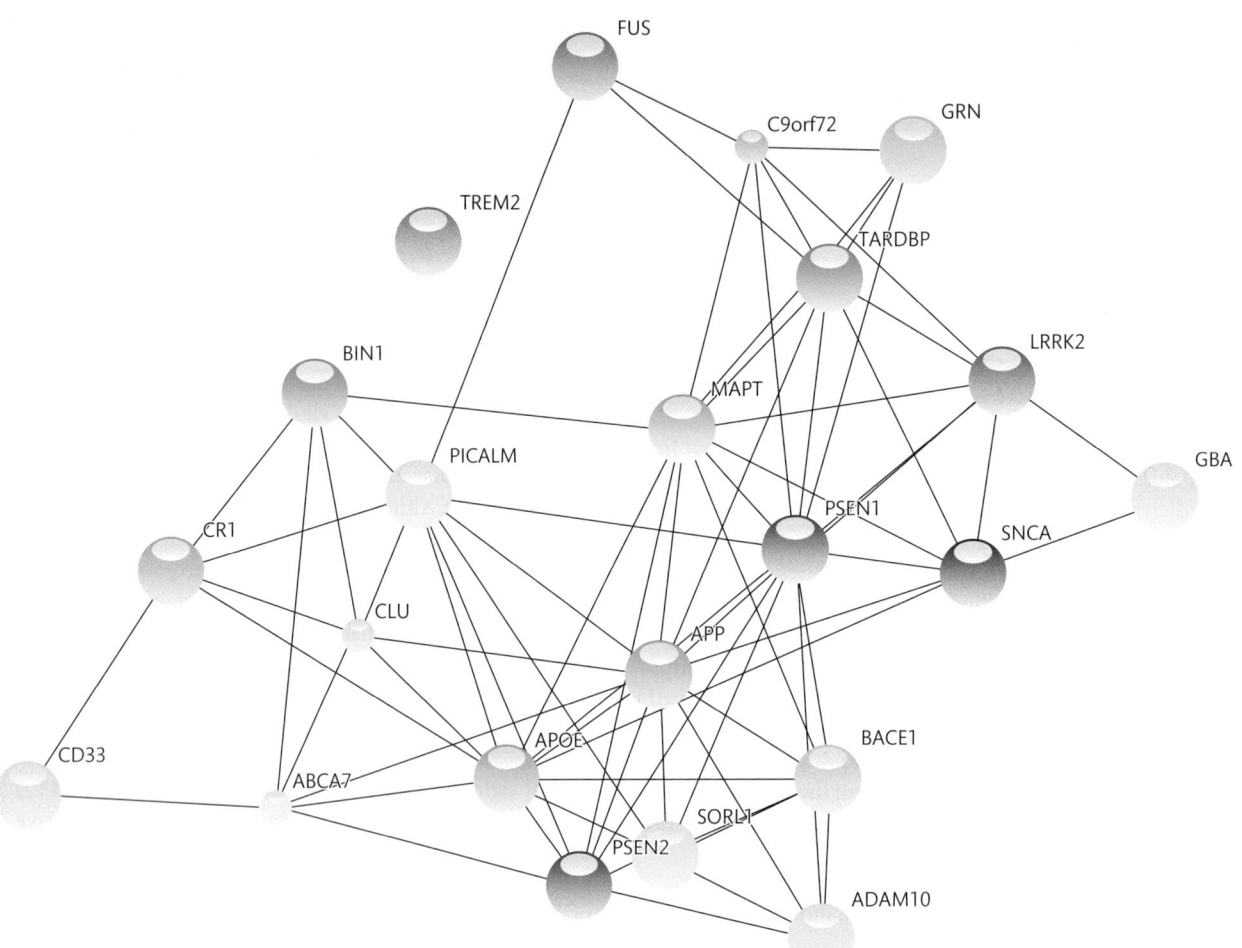

**Fig. 38.1** Associations among genes linked to AD, PD, FTD, PDD, DLB, using the functional protein association network tool STRING (https://string-db.org). APP represents a clear hub in this network. The primary known function of genes are shown below (information extracted from STRING and AlzPedia (http://www.alzforum.org/alzpedia)), but in many cases, links between pathogenic mechanisms and associated genes are unknown or poorly characterized.

**ABCA7**—ATP-binding cassette, sub-family A (ABC1), member 7; expressed in macrophages and microglia. Plays a role in phagocytosis by macrophages of apoptotic cells. Binds APOA1 and may function in apolipoprotein-mediated phospholipid efflux from cells.

**ADAM10**—ADAM metallopeptidase domain 10. A sheddase thought to be the physiological α-secretase for APP.

**APOE**—apolipoprotein E; a secreted lipoprotein that mediates binding, internalization, and catabolism of lipoprotein particles. Involved in clearance of Aβ from the brain and cerebral vasculature.

**APP**—amyloid beta (A4) precursor protein; a type I transmembrane protein whose proteolysis gives rise to β-amyloid peptides.

**BACE1**—beta-site APP-cleaving enzyme 1; a transmembrane aspartyl protease responsible for β-secretase processing of APP.

**BIN1**—bridging integrator 1; functions in clathrin-mediated synaptic vesicle endocytosis and endocytic recycling.

**CD33**—mediates sialic acid-dependent binding to cells. Slows phagocytosis and Aβ clearance.

**PSEN1**—presenilin 1; probable catalytic subunit of the gamma-secretase complex, an endoprotease complex that catalyses the intramembrane cleavage of integral membrane proteins, including APP, in a processive fashion that releases Aβ peptides of different lengths.

**PSEN2**—presenilin 2; probable catalytic subunit of the gamma-secretase complex, an endoprotease complex that catalyses the intramembrane cleavage of integral membrane proteins, including APP.

**CLU**—clusterin; isoform 1 functions as an extracellular chaperone that prevents aggregation of non-native proteins. Inhibits the formation of amyloid fibrils by APP, APOC2, B2M, CALCA, CSN3, SNCA, and aggregation-prone LYZ variants. Functions primarily as an extracellular chaperone but also mediates neurotoxicity of β-amyloid.

**CR1**—complement component (3b/4b) receptor 1. Mediates cellular binding of particles and immune complexes that have activated complement. Effects inflammation and amyloid accumulation.

## Proteostasis

The realization that a neurodegenerative phenotype, very similar to the corresponding sporadic disease, can result from single genotypes has led to the identification of the key effector proteins in these diseases and a common theme that may explain their role in the progression of diverse pathologies, that is, the idea that specific proteins accumulate within or outside neurons and misfold into toxic conformers, which may also spread to distant brain regions within interconnected neuronal networks. Several genes that cause monogenic AD, such as amyloid beta precursor protein (*APP*), presenilin1 (*PSEN1*), and presenilin2 (*PSEN2*), as well as variants in the genome, such as phosphatidylinositol binding clathrin assembly protein (*PICALM*), have mapped out the pathway of Aβ clearance and suggested that increased production and deposition of Aβ$_{1-42}$ in the brain of patients with sporadic AD may be the initiating pathogenic event [15]. Similarly, tau mutations were identified in familial cases of FTD, and tau fibrils in neurofibrillary tangles is a cardinal feature of sporadic AD. α-synuclein mutations or multiplications are rare causes of PD that share the same pathology with sporadic PD, namely the misfolding of α-synuclein into LBs.

These pathological changes are thought to predate the clinical presentation by several years. For example, studies of a familial AD cohort (the Dominantly Inherited Alzheimer Network [DIAN]) suggest that Aβ$_{1-42}$ levels in the CSF begin to decline as early as 25 years before the onset of symptoms [16]. This is followed by the appearance of fibrillar amyloid deposits in the brain detected by Pittsburgh compound B (PiB)-PET, increased levels of tau in the CSF, and progressive brain atrophy roughly 15 years before clinical presentation [16]. Cerebral hypometabolism and subtle episodic verbal memory impairment seem to begin about 10 years before overt dementia [16]. This time course may be generally similar to that of sporadic AD, based on cross-sectional studies [17], suggesting that detectable biochemical and histopathological abnormalities occur at least two decades before clinical symptoms.

Fibrillar assemblies of Aβ$_{1-42}$, tau, and α-synuclein also exert non-cell autonomous effects, which are reminiscent of 'prion-like' phenomena. The strongest evidence that this may occur in the human brain comes from the identification of LB pathology in embryonic neural grafts 12–16 years after transplantation into the brain of people with PD [18, 19]. Direct inoculation of human brain extracts or human brain-extracted fibrils from patients with LB pathology or multi-system atrophy led to progressive α-synuclein aggregation and neurodegeneration in connected areas of the brain in animal models, including non-human primates [20–22]. The propagation of α-synuclein in mouse brain has also been demonstrated with recombinant fibrils, but cell loss in this model was not always seen [20, 23, 24]. Similarly, tau pathology without neurodegeneration was observed in wild-type or transgenic mice expressing human tau, after seeding with fibrils extracted from human brain or mouse brain expressing the pathogenic P301S tau mutation [25, 26]. Intracerebral infusion of dilute Aβ-rich brain extracts from AD patients or from aged APP-transgenic mice also stimulated the premature formation of plaques and amyloid angiopathy in these models [27]. Spreading of α-synuclein and tau aggregates from the periphery to the brain has also been demonstrated [25, 26, 28].

Progress in identifying pathogenic proteins and their mode of propagation opened up the possibility for targeted therapies aimed at preventing their spread or promoting the clearance of their misfolded conformers. However, the most widely tested therapeutic approach to date—the use of active or passive immunotherapy—has not shown adequate clinical efficacy, even though there was evidence in some trials that such approaches promote the clearance of Aβ$_{1-42}$ [15]. A similarly poor response was detected in a larger trial that examined the effect of Aβ$_{1-42}$ immunotherapy in a group of patients with mild cognitive impairment. Whether such therapies need to be given at the pre-symptomatic phase of the disease to be effective is currently being investigated in around 300 pre-symptomatic members of a large Colombian pedigree with the *PSEN1* E280 → A280 missense mutation and a smaller number of pre-symptomatic American participants from the DIAN cohort who carry other presenilin mutations. In contrast to the disappointing results in humans, immunotherapies in preclinical models effectively reduced

---

**C9orf72**—chromosome 9 open reading frame 72; may play a role in endosomal trafficking and autophagy. Sequesters critical RNA-binding proteins in RNA foci.

**FUS**—fused in sarcoma; binds both single-stranded and double-stranded DNA and participates in transcription, processing, and nucleus-to-cytoplasm transport of mRNA.

**GBA**—glucosidase-beta acid; a lysosomal hydrolase that digests glycolipids. Impairment leads to lipid build-up in lysosomes, leading to cellular damage and inflammation.

**LRRK2**—leucine-rich repeat kinase 2; regulates autophagy and protein trafficking via phosphorylation of Rab proteins. Common PD-linked mutations in *LRRK2* activate its kinase activity.

**PICALM**—phosphatidyl inositol-binding clathrin assembly protein; accessory protein in the endocytic pathway—assembles clathrin and adapter protein complex 2 (AP2) to cell membranes at sites of coated pit formation and clathrin vesicle assembly. Also affects internalization of APP, and thus production of Aβ.

**GRN**—granulin; a secreted growth factor with cytokine-like activity involved in inflammation, wound healing, and cancer. Has neurotrophic properties.

**SNCA**—synuclein alpha. Fibrillar assemblies of alpha-synuclein are the main component of Lewy bodies and Lewy neurites. Its normal function is unclear, but it is implicated in synaptic vesicle recycling, SNARE assembly, and neurotransmitter release.

**SORL1**—sortilin-related receptor, L. A multi-functional endocytic receptor that may be implicated in the uptake of lipoproteins and proteases. Binds to APP and traffics APP between the secretory pathway, cell surface, and endosome.

**MAPT**—microtubule-associated protein tau; promotes microtubule assembly and stability, and might be involved in the establishment and maintenance of neuronal polarity.

**TARDBP**—TAR DNA-binding protein; DNA- and RNA-binding protein which regulates transcription and many aspects of RNA processing such as splicing, trafficking, stabilization, and miRNA production.

**TREM2**—triggering receptor expressed on myeloid cells 2; may have a role in chronic inflammation and may play a role in amyloid-related neuroinflammation via phagocytosis of amyloid and neuronal debris.

the burden of pathological aggregates. The reason for this discrepancy is currently unclear but suggests that the complex cellular states of the human diseased brain beyond the culprit protein need to be considered.

One limitation of targeted therapies against misfolded proteins, as exemplified by immunotherapies, is the assumption that during 'degenerative' cellular states in the sporadic forms of these diseases, the neuronal mechanisms that normally handle misfolded proteins will rapidly recover and respond adequately to further protein aggregation, which *in vivo* may actually occur over a period of hours [29]. Age-related deficiencies in protein homeostasis (proteostasis) could contribute to the accumulation of aggregating proteins [30]. For example in AD or PD brains, there is upregulation of chaperones and accumulation of proteasomal and autophagic components [31].

Accumulation of misfolded proteins typically triggers the activation of chaperones, which either attempt to refold proteins or help redirect non-native conformers towards degradation by proteasomes or lysosomes. Proteasomes are large multi-subunit complexes that consist of a 19S regulatory cap and a 20S proteolytic core. The 19S regulatory particle recognizes ubiquitinated substrates, removes ubiquitin chains, and unfolds the substrate to allow entry into the 20S core where it is rapidly degraded into peptides [32]. Although the proteasome is the primary source of protein degradation in the cell, restricted entry into the proteolytic chamber of the 20S component does not permit the degradation of misfolded or large protein complexes. One way to bypass this limitation is to employ chaperone complexes, such as the BAG1-HSP70 or cytosolic VCP/p97, that retrieve misfolded proteins from aggregates and then direct them to the proteasome. Alternatively, larger aggregates can be directed en masse to the lysosome via autophagy. Autophagy complements the proteasome in three forms: macroautophagy, chaperone-mediated autophagy (CMA), and microautophagy. Macroautophagy is the best-understood form and entails the sequestration of organelles or aggregates into a double-membrane structure known as the autophagosome. The resulting autophagosome is then transported to, and fuses with, the lysosome, thereby delivering its cargo for degradation. In contrast, microautophagy occurs by direct engulfment of the cytosol at the lysosome membrane, and CMA occurs through HSC70-mediated delivery of proteins across the lysosomal membrane via the LAMP2A receptor [33].

Selective targeting of misfolded proteins to the proteasome or lysosome is initiated by the addition of polyubiquitin chains in a three-step enzymatic process involving E1 ubiquitin-activating enzymes, E2 ubiquitin-conjugating enzymes (E2s), and E3 ubiquitin ligases (E3s). There are more than 650 E3s and 30 E2s that regulate the degradation of protein substrates, making this system highly specialized. Ubiquitin chains are formed through conjugation of ubiquitin monomers to protein substrates via distinct lysine residues; K48- and K11-linked ubiquitin chains are the main linkages that direct substrates to the proteasome, whereas K63-linked chains mediate trafficking to the lysosome. This is achieved by the action of adaptor complexes, which recognize the ubiquitin chain and direct the ubiquitinated proteins to the relevant pathway. Deubiquitinating enzymes (DUBs) remove ubiquitin chains and may determine commitment to degradation or trim ubiquitin chains to fine-tune the degradation process. The relevance of ubiquitin-dependent quality control is well established in PD, especially in a subgroup of *familial* cases that are caused by mutations in the E3 ligases Parkin or FBXO7.

Ubiquitin signalling also regulates α-synuclein degradation and counteracts its proteotoxicity. For example, the E3 ligase CHIP that normally eliminates cytosolic misfolded proteins was implicated in the clearance of oligomeric α-synuclein [34]. The E3 ligase NEDD4 exerts a protective effect in diverse models of α-synuclein toxicity, at least in part, by directly promoting the ubiquitination and lysosomal degradation of α-synuclein [35, 36]. Interestingly, a small molecule activator of NEDD4 protects induced pluripotent stem cell (iPSC)-derived dopaminergic neurons expressing the pathogenic A53T mutation [37]. Ubiquitination in LBs is significantly reduced in the pigmented neurons of the substantia nigra, compared to other brain regions, and this pattern inversely correlates with the upregulation of the deubiquitinase USP8 [38]. USP8 deubiquitinates α-synuclein and opposes its lysosomal degradation *in vitro*, whereas USP8 knockdown in fly models prevents α-synuclein accumulation and toxicity [38]. The role of Parkin in mitophagy is discussed in Mitochondrial dysfunction, p. 377.

### Endoplasmic reticulum stress

Defects in protein trafficking between organelles, especially the ER to Golgi and endosomes to lysosomes, are also critical in neurodegeneration. For example, mutations in VPS35, a component of the retromer complex which functions in endosomal protein sorting cause late-onset forms of familial PD and AD [39]. Heterozygous mutations in the lysosomal enzyme glucocerebrosidase (GBA), which, when biallelic, cause Gaucher's disease, are the most common risk factors for PD; and mutations in the kinase LRRK2, which is the most common form of autosomal dominant PD with LB pathology impair endosomal trafficking and autophagy [39]. The significance of these pathways for the viability of vulnerable neuronal subpopulations in PD and AD is reinforced by genome-wide analysis of variants in common sporadic forms of these diseases (for example, GAK and RAB7L in PD and PICALM in AD) that function in these pathways. Misfolded proteins accumulating in the ER lumen are normally recognized by ER membrane-associated complexes and retrotranslocated to the cytoplasm by the AAA ATPase VCP/p97–NPL4–UFD-1 complex. The retrotranslocated protein is then ubiquitinated and delivered to the proteasome for degradation, thereby eliminating terminally misfolded proteins from the ER. In neurodegenerative diseases, ER stress due to accumulation of misfolded proteins in the ER lumen activates the unfolded protein response (UPR), a protective cellular response that aims to reduce unfolded protein load and restore protein-folding homeostasis. The UPR has three arms, which initiate signalling cascades through protein kinase RNA (PKR)-like ER kinase (PERK), inositol-requiring enzyme 1 (IRE1), and activating transcription factor 6 (ATF6). Paradoxically, persistent activation of the PERK-eIF2α branch of the UPR is detrimental, as it causes uncompensated decline in global translation rates, leading to synaptic failure and neuronal death [40]. Restoring translation by targeting PERK or more selectively eIF2α, using repurposed drugs such as trazodone, was neuroprotective and enhanced memory in animal models of prion disease and tauopathy despite the accumulation of misfolded proteins [41]. In this respect, specialized enzyme complexes that function in protein folding, trafficking, or degradation are emerging at the frontier of experimental therapeutics in neurodegenerative diseases.

## Mitochondrial dysfunction

Mitochondria are responsible for ATP generation, intracellular calcium ($Ca^{2+}$) homeostasis, reactive oxygen species (ROS) formation, and apoptosis. Neurons are exquisitely sensitive to mitochondrial dysfunction because of their high energy demands, and it is not surprising that many NDDs are linked to mitochondrial dysfunction. Numerous studies have shown mitochondrial structural changes that precede pathology in AD brain [42] and expression of β-amyloid leads to loss of activity of several key mitochondrial enzymes involved in the tricarboxylic acid (TCA) cycle or the electron transport chain, including the α-ketoglutarate dehydrogenase complex, the pyruvate dehydrogenase complex, and cytochrome oxidase [43].

Early evidence for the role of mitochondrial dysfunction in dopaminergic neurons came from observations in methyl-4-phenyl-1,2,3,6-tetrahydropyridine (MPTP) users who developed parkinsonism. Subsequent studies showed that MPTP is rapidly taken up by astrocytes, metabolized to 1-methyl-4-phenylpyridinium (MPP+), which is taken by dopaminergic neurons and inhibits complex I in the electron transport chain, thereby inhibiting ATP production, decreasing intracellular $Ca^{2+}$-buffering capacity, and increasing ROS production, all of which lead to neurotoxicity. Complex I activity is also lowered in PD brain, and several genes linked to PD are all linked to mitochondrial function, including *SNCA* (*PARK1/4*), *Parkin* (*PARK2*), *PINK1* (*PARK6*), *PARK7*, *LRRK2* (*PARK8*), and *HTRA2* (*PARK13*) [44]. Dissipation of the mitochondrial membrane potential induces translocation of the kinase pink1 to mitochondria and activation of Parkin through phosphorylation of ubiquitin and the ubiquitin-like domain of Parkin. This cascade initiates the degradation of mitochondrial proteins by the proteasome in a p97-dependent fashion or mitophagy, a process opposed by the mitochondrial deubiquitinase USP30 [45].

In HD brain, the activities of Complex I, II, and II are all inhibited. HD is a monogenic disorder, so the primacy of mutant huntingtin (HTT) in disease aetiology is beyond dispute, but still the mechanism of action remains unclear. There is evidence of direct interaction of mutant HTT with mitochondria, resulting in depolarization [46]; again these mitochondrial changes preceded overt disease symptomology. In addition, it is likely that some of the mutant HTT interaction with mitochondria is mediated indirectly via dysregulation of key transcription factors such as p53 and CREB-binding protein [47]. These examples serve to illustrate the mitochondria as the recipient of cellular stressors, but mitochondrial dysfunction and mitophagy can ultimately amplify inflammatory responses by releasing ROS into the cytoplasm and extracellular space—once again muddying the relationship of cause and effect of NDD pathology.

## Common molecular pathways in NDD: REST

In the preceding sections, we have illuminated common pathologies, genetics, and cellular processes that accompany all NDDs. Here, we explore the idea that common molecular mechanisms may also be at play in driving or protecting against neurodegeneration. Our exemplar is the transcriptional repressor RE1-silencing transcription factor (REST), a key regulatory factor that has been implicated in the pathogenesis of several NDDs, including HD, PD, and AD [48–51]. REST was discovered over 20 years ago [52], and its role was initially seen as that of a transcriptional silencer of differentiated neuronal genes in neural progenitors and non-neural tissue. Initially, it was thought that REST was silenced during neuronal differentiation, thereby allowing the expression of differentiated neuronal genes. However, REST's role is now seen as much more multi-faceted, and we now know that REST is not silenced during neuronal differentiation but continues to be expressed at low levels in several areas of the adult brain, notably the cerebral cortex where it represses the expression of many neuronal genes [53–57]. However, the role of REST during neurodegeneration is controversial, since it has been shown to be both pro-apoptotic and neuroprotective, depending on circumstances. In HD, in the presence of mutant HTT, levels of nuclear REST are increased, leading to repression of numerous REST target genes, including *BDNF*, an essential neurotrophic factor required for survival of medium spiny GABAergic neurons in the striatum [50, 51]. REST has also been shown to be pro-apoptotic in hippocampal CA1 neurons subjected to ischaemic insults, resulting in increased levels of nuclear REST and enrichment at the miR-132 promoter, leading to silencing of miR-132 expression and subsequent neuronal death [58]. The role of REST in PD is less clear. Administration of the dopaminergic neurotoxin MPTP to REST-null mice led to enhanced loss of dopaminergic neurons, indicating that REST was normally neuroprotective [48], whereas earlier studies showed that MPTP increased migration of REST from the nucleus to the cytosol, accompanied by subsequent increase in REST target gene expression and increased cell death [59]. This apparent contradiction can be resolved by considering that, in both cases, REST levels at their target genes are decreased either due to ablation of the REST gene or migration of the REST protein from the nucleus, and both result in increased susceptibility to MPTP toxicity. Stated otherwise normal (nuclear) levels of REST are neuroprotective. This neuroprotective action of REST has been more directly interrogated in a recent study that indicates a neuroprotective role for REST in the ageing brain that is lost in the brain of patients with mild cognitive impairment and AD, FTD, and DLB [49]. Further, using SHSY5Y neuroblastoma cells, they showed that REST bound the promoters of many cell death genes, including p38 MAP kinase, FAS, FADD, and TRADD, as well as the presenilin 2 promoter. Moreover, REST was induced in both cultured mouse and human cortical neurons in response to challenges with $A\beta_{1-42}$ or $H_2O_2$, and ablation of REST in mouse cortical neurons led to an increase in the expression of pro-apoptotic genes and increased neurodegeneration in response to Aβ challenge. So how can these studies be reconciled?

WNT signalling has long been associated with AD pathogenesis, and numerous studies have shown that canonical wnt signalling protects against β-amyloid toxicity [60–62]. Acute exposure of rat cortical neurons to Aβ activates non-canonical wnt signalling via the JNK/PCP pathway and subsequent activation of several transcription factors, including EGR1 and KLF10, as part of a pro-apoptotic pathway [63]. Furthermore, this pathway is also detectable in the brain of people and in animal models with amyloidopathy, but not tauopathy, adding weight to the evidence that this non-canonical pathway is activated by Aβ in AD. Since REST is known to be directly regulated by canonical wnt signalling [64, 65], then when taken together, these observations suggest a model whereby exposure to Aβ controls a bipartite signalling cascade, with canonical wnt signalling controlling an anti-apoptotic arm, in which REST represses pro-apoptotic genes, and non-canonical wnt signalling controlling an antagonistic pro-apoptotic arm in which JNK/PCP activates pro-apoptotic genes.

This model supports the suggestion that high levels of REST in the ageing brain play a neuroprotective role and may be sufficient to protect against dementia, even when the brain shows significant structural pathology, including Aβ deposits [49]. This conditionality of Aβ-induced neurodegeneration is also reflected in the levels of Aβ *in vivo*, which fluctuate as a function of neuronal activity [66], diurnal cycle [67, 68], and ageing [67]. Importantly, diurnal variation of Aβ occurs in the brain of APPswe/PS1ΔE9 mice before the appearance of Aβ plaques. Furthermore, in the human brain, increases in Aβ also precede the appearance of Aβ plaques or any symptoms of AD. In other words, neurons are constantly exposed to fluctuating levels of Aβ, yet this does not immediately result in an increase in Aβ plaque formation or neuronal death. REST could thus act as a gatekeeper in this bipartite response to Aβ and could act as an essential component of a homeostatic response to neurodegenerative stressors such as Aβ, perhaps as an inhibitory node of a feed-forward inhibition loop, a widespread regulatory motif that homeostatically regulates many molecular pathways [69] by modulating the dynamic response of network output to a varying input, that is, they buffer a gene network against fluctuations in input, whether as signal or noise. This would allow a neuron to tolerate low Aβ exposure without committing to an irreversible apoptotic response, yet still permit apoptosis in the presence of persistent Aβ exposure. Taken together, these observations indicate that REST occupies a unique position as a key regulator of neuroprotective pathways induced in the ageing brain, offering protection against β-amyloid-induced neurodegeneration. Since REST is induced in response to several stressors, including $Fe^{2+}$, $H_2O_2$, and the glutathione synthesis inhibitor buthione sulfoxide [49], then this may provide a model whereby REST provides neuroprotection against a wide range of neurodegenerative stressors. More generally, this multifaceted role of REST may reflect the perspective that although the molecular function of a gene may be largely fixed, the biological process that this function subserves is highly context-dependent. This system's perspective is reflected in the different gene modules and networks in which a gene may be embedded, which will, in turn, depend on the cell type and cell state, that is, it is the network interactions and output that determine the 'function' of the gene.

## Novel cellular models of neurodegeneration

The underlying cause of most NDDs is a complex cocktail of genetic and environmental risk factors, and this is nowhere clearer than in AD [70]. The predominant hypothesis to date has been that of the 'amyloid cascade', the initial evidence for which came from the observations that autosomal dominant AD arises from mutations in either the amyloid β precursor protein (*APP*) gene or in genes encoding APP secretases. In brief, the amyloid cascade hypothesis posits that faulty processing of APP generates neurotoxic Aβ fragments and consequent neurodegeneration and other hallmarks of AD pathology, including aggregation of phosphorylated tau and synaptic loss [71]. However, as stated earlier, clinical trials of immunotherapies targeting $Aβ_{1-42}$ have failed. Although these failures may be most related to clinical trials being conducted too late or on participants without amyloid pathology, they nonetheless serve to emphasize that late-onset AD is likely to be complex and that a fuller understanding of the molecular mechanisms of the canonical amyloid cascade, as well as associated processes, including inflammation, for example,

is an essential prerequisite to developing therapeutic interventions. This amyloid cascade hypothesis has led to the development of numerous animal models as investigative tools to interrogate disease mechanism and as screens to identify therapeutic targets. The majority of these are murine and based on the introduction of cocktails of mutations targeting *APP*, *PSEN1*, *PSEN2*, and *MAPT* [72]. However, rodent models have several severe limitations, especially in relation to AD. Firstly, there are numerous important intrinsic differences between human and rodent neurons, including marked differences in the transcriptome of the ageing brain [73, 74], human-specific transcriptional modules in AD brain [75], neuronal size and complexity of the dendritic tree [76], protein composition of the post-synaptic density [77], and speed of synaptic information transfer [78]. Secondly, overexpression of mouse APP does not aggregate in amyloid plaques, a striking difference between mice and humans. Subsequent generation of mouse transgenic lines, such as PDAPP and Tg2576, which bear mutant human *APP* genes, still fail to exhibit cardinal hallmarks of AD, including neurofibrillary tangle formation and neuronal death [79, 80]. Thirdly, more recent mouse models based on the 3×Tg triple mutation (APP Swedish; *MAPT P301L; PSEN1 M146V*) offer some improvement, including synaptic dysfunction preceding the deposition of plaques and tangles [79], but only by forcing the overexpression of a set of mutations that do not have any pathophysiological counterpart in humans. Fourthly, animal amyloid modes show cognitive deficits in the absence of discernible neuronal pathology; yet in humans, cognitive impairment is accompanied by neuronal pathology and death. This profound incongruity undermines the usefulness of animal models in a myriad of AD drug development programmes. Fifthly, there is a tacit assumption that the underlying regulatory molecular machinery is conserved between mouse and human. Whereas this is true on a coarse-grained analysis, it is demonstrably untrue at a detailed level; comparison of the cistromes of numerous transcription factors shows only a small conservation of transcription factor binding sites (TFBS) between mouse and human [80], and furthermore, genes associated with hominid-specific TFBS are specifically enriched in neurological pathways [81]. This latter issue is brought into sharp focus by a recent study on the transcriptional repressor REST, elevated levels of which are found in the normal ageing brain, but not in AD brain (see earlier), and which confer neuroprotection by repressing pro-apoptotic genes in the normal ageing brain [49]. However, close inspection of human and mouse REST cistromes [82] shows that many of the genes conferring protection in the human brain are REST targets only in humans, but not in mice. These differences in the underlying topology of mouse and human gene networks may result in potentially critical species-specific gene–gene interactions that undermine the relevance of mouse systems as tools to investigate molecular mechanisms and the discovery of therapeutic targets in human cells. This has led to searches for human cellular neuronal models that obviate these limitations and reduce our reliance on rodent models. Until recently, human cellular models were dominated by non-neuronal cell lines, such as HEK293, or neuroblastoma lines, such as SH-SY5Y, all of which suffer from many limitations, including their non-neuronal origin, aberrant cell signalling, and chromosomal abnormalities, serious concerns that curb any enthusiasm for their usage. However, the twin developments of cellular reprogramming and gene editing have completely changed the experimental landscape of modelling disease using human cells.

## Induced pluripotent stem cells

Yamanaka's groundbreaking discovery of reprogramming somatic cells [83] to become iPSCs has revolutionized much of biology. iPSCs have the cardinal properties of an embryonic stem cell: (1) they can self-renew and maintain their pluripotent state; and (2) they can differentiate to (almost) any lineage. Equally importantly, iPSCs obviate many ethical concerns over the use of primary human embryonic stem cells, since they do not require the destruction of human embryos. Unlike immortalized human cell lines, iPSCs are 'normal', can be derived from any personal genetic background, and can be produced by reprogramming a wide range of somatic cells, including readily available skin fibroblasts and hair follicle cells, making it possible to readily make patient-specific iPSCs. These, in turn, can be differentiated towards multiple neuronal (and glial) types relevant to individual NDDs, associated with loss of specific neuronal populations such as cortical neurons in AD, medium spiny GABAergic neurons of the basal ganglia in HD, and dopaminergic neurons of the substantia nigra in PD. iPSC neurons have many features that lend themselves to modelling neurodegeneration *in vitro* [84–86], including: (1) acquisition of electrical excitability, as evidenced by the expression of voltage-sensitive sodium ($Na^+$) and potassium ($K^+$) channels; (2) firing of action potentials; and (3) physical evidence of synapses on the basis of juxtaposition of pre- and post-synaptic markers [3]. Not only do these iPSC-derived neurons offer potential to generate cells for replacement of damaged tissue, but they also offer unparalleled human cellular models of disease and discovery tools for therapeutic target identification and drug screening [84, 87].

## Gene editing

The advent of gene editing, particularly by use of CRISPR/CAS9 [88, 89] offers the possibility of introducing, or reversing, disease-associated mutations. As with iPSCs, this development opens up possibilities for repair and replacement and for generating new cellular models. The most widely used CRISPR/CAS9 system can be thought of as comprising a dual module made up of a unique genomic address delivery system [provided by single-guide RNAs (sgRNAs) and a cargo (CRISPR-associated protein 9 (CAS9)]. The sgRNA binds to its unique genomic address and then takes delivery of the CAS9 cargo. CAS9, in its native form, then introduces double-stranded DNA breaks, which are subsequently repaired by endogenous DNA repair mechanisms and, as a consequence, introduces discrete mutations into the targeted locus. More recently, numerous engineered forms of CAS9 have been introduced that use CAS9 simply as a delivery vehicle to introduce novel genome-modifying activities to greatly expand the repertoire of genomic and epigenomic changes, including: (1) reversion of specific disease-associated SNPs; (2) exerting local control of transcriptional activation or silencing; and (3) manipulation of specific epigenetic marks [90, 91]. The combined power of iPSCs and gene editing now lets us derive neurons from any patient-specific background, study their behaviour before and after making highly discrete changes to the genome or epigenome, and attribute any changes in behaviour to a specific genetic locus. An example of this power can be seen in studies of iPSCs derived from a familial AD background. iPSC neurons derived from patients carrying a duplication of the *APP* gene have higher levels of $A\beta_{1-40}$, increased tau phosphorylation, and raised levels of GSKβ, relative to normal iPSCs, all of which are seen in AD brain [92]. Use of CRISPR/CAS9 to introduce AD disease causing mutations in the *APP* gene (*APP^swe*)

and the *PSEN1* gene (*PSEN1^{M146V}*) of iPSC neurons also gave rise to elevations in Aβ, and in this latter case, use of gene editing allowed unambiguous attribution of the change in cellular phenotype to specific disease mutations [93].

## Outlook

The primacy of any of the biological processes discussed here in the aetiology and pathogenesis of NDDs is an ongoing source of contention, and undoubtedly it varies within and among diseases. More likely is that pathogenesis is not a linear cascade, but any of these processes can act as a driver and recruit other processes into tipping neurons into a neurodegenerative state. Although the brain has only a limited capacity to replenish lost neurons, it does exhibit remarkable plasticity, which ensures that the myriad of its neuronal connections continues to function until a critical threshold is eventually reached. It is now considered likely that a prolonged period of neuronal compensated dysfunction may precede cell loss. Identifying stages on this neurodegenerative trajectory that are reversible and irreversible will be key to developing future therapeutic targeting strategies. Similar to the approaches that have been so successful in cancer, a deeper understanding of the fundamental biology that drives neuronal degeneration, rather than a focus on a singular cellular process, is likely to lead to successful targeted therapies.

## REFERENCES

1. Hamilton RL. Lewy Bodies in Alzheimer's Disease: A Neuropathological Review of 145 Cases Using -Synuclein Immunohistochemistry. Brain Pathology. 2000;(10):378–84.
2. Cook C, Zhang Y-J, Xu Y-F, Dickson DW, Petrucelli L. TDP-43 in neurodegenerative disorders. Expert Opinion on Biological Therapy. 2008;8(7):969–78.
3. Shi Y, Kirwan P, Livesey FJ. Directed differentiation of human pluripotent stem cells to cerebral cortex neurons and neural networks. Nat Protoc. 2012;7(10):1836–46.
4. Neumann M, Sampathu DM, Kwong LK, et al. Ubiquitinated TDP-43 in frontotemporal lobar degeneration and amyotrophic lateral sclerosis. Science. 2006;314(5796):130–3.
5. Hall B, Mak E, Cervenka S, Aigbirhio FI, Rowe JB, O'Brien JT. In vivo tau PET imaging in dementia: Pathophysiology, radiotracer quantification, and a systematic review of clinical findings. Ageing Research Reviews. 2017;36:50–63.
6. Shulman JM, De Jager PL. Evidence for a common pathway linking neurodegenerative diseases. Nat Genet. 2009;41(12):1261–2.
7. Nuytemans K, Maldonado L, Ali A, et al. Overlap between Parkinson disease and Alzheimer disease in ABCA7 functional variants. Neurol Genet. 2016;2(1):e44.
8. A Hexanucleotide Repeat Expansion in C9ORF72 Is the Cause of Chromosome 9p21-Linked ALS-FTD. 2011;72(2):257–68.
9. DeJesus-Hernandez M, Mackenzie IR, Boeve BF, et al. Expanded GGGGCC hexanucleotide repeat in noncoding region of C9ORF72 causes chromosome 9p-linked FTD and ALS. Neuron. 2011;72(2):245–56.
10. Po K, Leslie FVC, Gracia N, et al. Heritability in frontotemporal dementia: more missing pieces? J Neurol. 2014;261(11):2170–7.
11. Johnson JO, Mandrioli J, Benatar M, et al. Exome sequencing reveals VCP mutations as a cause of familial ALS. Neuron. 2010;68(5):857–64.

12. Blair IP, Williams KL, Warraich ST, *et al.* FUS mutations in amyotrophic lateral sclerosis: clinical, pathological, neurophysiological and genetic analysis. J Neurol Neurosurg Psychiatr. 2010;81(6):639–45.

13. Kwiatkowski TJ, Bosco DA, Leclerc AL, *et al.* Mutations in the FUS/TLS gene on chromosome 16 cause familial amyotrophic lateral sclerosis. Science. 2009;323(5918):1205–8.

14. Deng H-X, Chen W, Hong S-T, *et al.* Mutations in UBQLN2 cause dominant X-linked juvenile and adult-onset ALS and ALS/dementia. Nature. 2011;477(7363):211–15.

15. Selkoe DJ. Preventing Alzheimer's disease. Science. 2012;337(6101):1488–92.

16. Bateman RJ, Xiong C, Benzinger TLS, Fagan AM, Goate A, Fox NC, *et al.* Clinical and biomarker changes in dominantly inherited Alzheimer's disease. N Engl J Med, 2012;367(9):795–804.

17. Jack CR, Knopman DS, Jagust WJ, *et al.* Hypothetical model of dynamic biomarkers of the Alzheimer's pathological cascade. Lancet Neurology, 2010;9(1):119–28.

18. Li J-Y, Englund E, Holton JL, *et al.* Lewy bodies in grafted neurons in subjects with Parkinson's disease suggest host-to-graft disease propagation. Nat Med. 2008;14(5):501–3.

19. Kordower JH, Chu Y, Hauser RA, Freeman TB, Olanow CW. Lewy body-like pathology in long-term embryonic nigral transplants in Parkinson's disease. Nat Med. 2008;14(5):504–6.

20. Masuda-Suzukake M, Nonaka T, Hosokawa M, *et al.* Prion-like spreading of pathological α-synuclein in brain. Brain. 2013;136(Pt 4):1128–38.

21. Recasens A, Dehay B, Bové J, *et al.* Lewy body extracts from Parkinson disease brains trigger α-synuclein pathology and neurodegeneration in mice and monkeys. Ann Neurol. 2014;75(3):351–62.

22. Prusiner SB, Woerman AL, Mordes DA, *et al.* Evidence for α-synuclein prions causing multiple system atrophy in humans with parkinsonism. Proc Natl Acad Sci U S A. 2015;112(38):E5308–17.

23. Luk KC, Kehm V, Carroll J, *et al.* Pathological α-synuclein transmission initiates Parkinson-like neurodegeneration in nontransgenic mice. Science. 2012;338(6109):949–53.

24. Osterberg VR, Spinelli KJ, Weston LJ, Luk KC, Woltjer RL, Unni VK. Progressive aggregation of alpha-synuclein and selective degeneration of lewy inclusion-bearing neurons in a mouse model of parkinsonism. Cell Rep. 2015;10(8):1252–60.

25. Clavaguera F, Akatsu H, Fraser G, *et al.* Brain homogenates from human tauopathies induce tau inclusions in mouse brain. Proc Natl Acad Sci U S A, 2013;110(23):9535–40.

26. Clavaguera F, Bolmont T, Crowther RA, *et al.* Transmission and spreading of tauopathy in transgenic mouse brain. Nat Cell Biol. 2009;11(7):909–13.

27. Meyer-Luehmann M, Coomaraswamy J, Bolmont T, *et al.* Exogenous induction of cerebral beta-amyloidogenesis is governed by agent and host. Science. 2006;313(5794):1781–4.

28. Peelaerts W, Bousset L, Van der Perren A, *et al.* α-Synuclein strains cause distinct synucleinopathies after local and systemic administration. Nature. 2015;522(7556):340–4.

29. de Calignon A, Polydoro M, Suárez-Calvet M, *et al.* Propagation of tau pathology in a model of early Alzheimer's disease. Neuron. 2012;73(4):685–97.

30. Labbadia J, Morimoto RI. The biology of proteostasis in aging and disease. Annu Rev Biochem. 2015;84(1):435–64.

31. Nixon RA. The role of autophagy in neurodegenerative disease. Nat Med. 2013;19(8):983–97.

32. Goldberg AL. Protein degradation and protection against misfolded or damaged proteins. Nature. 2003;426(6968):895–9.

33. Rubinsztein DC. The roles of intracellular protein-degradation pathways in neurodegeneration. Nature. 2006;443(7113):780–6.

34. Tetzlaff JE, Putcha P, Outeiro TF, *et al.* CHIP targets toxic alpha-Synuclein oligomers for degradation. J Biol Chem. 2008;283(26):17962–8.

35. Tofaris GK, Kim HT, Hourez R, Jung J-W, Kim KP, Goldberg AL. Ubiquitin ligase Nedd4 promotes alpha-synuclein degradation by the endosomal-lysosomal pathway. Proc Natl Acad Sci U S A. 2011;108(41):17004–9.

36. Davies SE, Hallett PJ, Moens T, *et al.* Enhanced ubiquitin-dependent degradation by Nedd4 protects against α-synuclein accumulation and toxicity in animal models of Parkinson's disease. Neurobiol Dis. 2014;64:79–87.

37. Chung CY, Khurana V, Auluck PK, *et al.* Identification and rescue of α-synuclein toxicity in Parkinson patient-derived neurons. Science. 2013;342(6161):983–7.

38. Alexopoulou Z, Lang J, Perrett RM, *et al.* Deubiquitinase Usp8 regulates α-synuclein clearance and modifies its toxicity in Lewy body disease. Proc Natl Acad Sci U S A. 2016;113(32):E4688–97.

39. Perrett RM, Alexopoulou Z, Tofaris GK. The endosomal pathway in Parkinson's disease. Mol Cell Neurosci. 2015;66(Pt A):21–8.

40. Moreno JA, Radford H, Peretti D, *et al.* Sustained translational repression by eIF2α-P mediates prion neurodegeneration. Nature. 2012;485(7399):507–11.

41. Halliday M, Radford H, Zents KAM, *et al.* Repurposed drugs targeting eIF2α-P-mediated translational repression prevent neurodegeneration in mice. Brain. 2017;140(6):1768–83.

42. la Monte de SM, Luong T, Neely TR, Robinson D, Wands JR. Mitochondrial DNA damage as a mechanism of cell loss in Alzheimer's disease. Lab Invest. 2000;80(8):1323–35.

43. Swerdlow RH, Burns JM, Khan SM. The Alzheimer's disease mitochondrial cascade hypothesis. J Alzheimers Dis. 2010;20 Suppl 2(S2):S265–79.

44. Lezi E, Swerdlow RH. Mitochondria in neurodegeneration. Adv Exp Med Biol. 2012;942:269–86.

45. Pickrell AM, Youle RJ. The roles of PINK1, parkin, and mitochondrial fidelity in Parkinson's disease. Neuron. 2015;85(2):257–73.

46. Panov AV, Gutekunst C-A, Leavitt BR, *et al.* Early mitochondrial calcium defects in Huntington's disease are a direct effect of polyglutamines. Nat Neurosci. 2002;5(8):731–6.

47. Sugars KL, Rubinsztein DC. Transcriptional abnormalities in Huntington disease. Trends Genet. 2003;19(5):233–8.

48. Yu M, Suo H, Liu M, *et al.* NRSF/REST neuronal deficient mice are more vulnerable to the neurotoxin MPTP. Neurobiol Aging. 2013;34(3):916–27.

49. Lu T, Aron L, Zullo J, *et al.* REST and stress resistance in ageing and Alzheimer's disease. Nature. 2014;507(7493):448–54.

50. Zuccato C, Tartari M, Crotti A, *et al.* Huntingtin interacts with REST/NRSF to modulate the transcription of NRSE-controlled neuronal genes. Nat Genet. 2003;35(1):76–83.

51. Zuccato C, Zuccato C, Belyaev N, *et al.* Widespread disruption of repressor element-1 silencing transcription factor/neuron-restrictive silencer factor occupancy at its target genes in Huntington's disease. J Neurosci. 2007;27(26):6972–83.

52. Chen ZF, Paquette AJ, Anderson DJ. NRSF/REST is required in vivo for repression of multiple neuronal target genes during embryogenesis. Nat Genet. 1998;20(2):136–42.

53. Ballas N, Grunseich C, Lu DD, Speh JC, Mandel G. REST and Its Corepressors Mediate Plasticity of Neuronal Gene Chromatin throughout Neurogenesis. Cell. 2005;121(4):645–57.

54. Johnson R, Teh CH-L, Kunarso G, et al. REST Regulates Distinct Transcriptional Networks in Embryonic and Neural Stem Cells. PLoS Biol. 2008;6(10):e256.

55. Gao Z, Ure K, Ding P, et al. The master negative regulator REST/NRSF controls adult neurogenesis by restraining the neurogenic program in quiescent stem cells. J Neurosci. 2011;31(26):9772–86.

56. Aoki H, Hara A, Era T, Kunisada T, Yamada Y. Genetic ablation of Rest leads to in vitro-specific derepression of neuronal genes during neurogenesis. Development. 2012;139(4):667–77.

57. Covey MV, Streb JW, Spektor R, Ballas N. REST regulates the pool size of the different neural lineages by restricting the generation of neurons and oligodendrocytes from neural stem/progenitor cells. Development. 2012;139(16):2878–90.

58. Hwang J-Y, Kaneko N, Noh K-M, Pontarelli F, Zukin RS. The gene silencing transcription factor REST represses miR-132 expression in hippocampal neurons destined to die. J Mol Biol. 2014;426(20):3454–66.

59. Yu M, Cai L, Liang M, Huang Y, Gao H, Lu S, et al. Alteration of NRSF expression exacerbating 1-methyl-4-phenyl-pyridinium ion-induced cell death of SH-SY5Y cells. Neurosci Res. 2009;65(3):236–44.

60. Purro SA, Dickins EM, Salinas PC. The secreted Wnt antagonist Dickkopf-1 is required for amyloid β-mediated synaptic loss. J Neurosci. 2012;32(10):3492–8.

61. De Ferrari GV, Chacón MA, Barría MI, et al. Activation of Wnt signaling rescues neurodegeneration and behavioral impairments induced by beta-amyloid fibrils. Mol Psychiatry. 2003;8(2):195–208.

62. De Ferrari GV, Inestrosa NC. Wnt signaling function in Alzheimer's disease. Brain Res Brain Res Rev. 2000;33(1):1–12.

63. Killick R, Ribe EM, Al-Shawi R, et al. Clusterin regulates β-amyloid toxicity via Dickkopf-1-driven induction of the wnt-PCP-JNK pathway. Mol Psychiatry, 2014;19(1):88–98.

64. Nishihara S, Tsuda L, Ogura T. The canonical Wnt pathway directly regulates NRSF/REST expression in chick spinal cord. Biochem Biophys Res Comm. 2003;311(1):55–63.

65. Lee M, Ji H, Furuta Y, Park J-I, McCrea PD. p120-catenin regulates REST and CoREST, and modulates mouse embryonic stem cell differentiation. J Cell Sci. 2014;127(Pt 18):4037–51.

66. Cirrito JR, Yamada KA, Finn MB, et al. Synaptic activity regulates interstitial fluid amyloid-beta levels in vivo. Neuron. 2005;48(6):913–22.

67. Lesné SE, Sherman MA, Grant M, et al. Brain amyloid-β oligomers in ageing and Alzheimer's disease. Brain. 2013;136(Pt 5):1383–98.

68. Kang J-E, Lim MM, Bateman RJ, et al. Amyloid-beta dynamics are regulated by orexin and the sleep-wake cycle. Science. 2009;326(5955):1005–7.

69. Savageau MA, Jacknow G. Feedfoward inhibition in biosynthetic pathways: inhibition of the aminoacyl-tRNA synthetase by intermediates of the pathway. J Theor Biol. 1979;77(4):405–25.

70. De Strooper B, Karran E. The Cellular Phase of Alzheimer's Disease. Cell. 2016;164(4):603–15.

71. Hardy J, Selkoe DJ. The amyloid hypothesis of Alzheimer's disease: progress and problems on the road to therapeutics. Science. 2002;297(5580):353–6.

72. Webster SJ, Bachstetter AD, Nelson PT, Schmitt FA, Van Eldik LJ. Using mice to model Alzheimer's dementia: an overview of the clinical disease and the preclinical behavioral changes in 10 mouse models. Front Genet. 2014;5:88.

73. Loerch PM, Lu T, Dakin KA, et al. Evolution of the aging brain transcriptome and synaptic regulation. PLoS ONE. 2008;3(10):e3329.

74. Bishop NA, Lu T, Yankner BA. Neural mechanisms of ageing and cognitive decline. Nature. 2010;464(7288):529–35.

75. Wang P, Zhao D, Rockowitz S, Zheng D. Divergence and rewiring of regulatory networks for neural development between human and other species. Neurogenesis. 2016;3(1):e1231495.

76. Mohan H, Verhoog MB, Doreswamy KK, et al. Dendritic and Axonal Architecture of Individual Pyramidal Neurons across Layers of Adult Human Neocortex. Cereb Cortex. 2015;25(12):4839–53.

77. Bayés A, Collins MO, Croning MDR, van de Lagemaat LN, Choudhary JS, Grant SGN. Comparative study of human and mouse postsynaptic proteomes finds high compositional conservation and abundance differences for key synaptic proteins. PLoS One. 2012;7(10):e46683.

78. Testa-Silva G, Verhoog MB, Linaro D, et al. High bandwidth synaptic communication and frequency tracking in human neocortex. PLoS Biol. 2014;12(11):e1002007.

79. Chin J. Selecting a mouse model of Alzheimer's disease. Methods Mol Biol. 2011;670:169–89.

80. Villar D, Flicek P, Odom DT. Evolution of transcription factor binding in metazoans—mechanisms and functional implications. Nat Rev Genet. 2014;15(4):221–33.

81. Yokoyama KD, Zhang Y, Ma J. Tracing the evolution of lineage-specific transcription factor binding sites in a birth-death framework. PLoS Comput Biol. 2014;10(8):e1003771.

82. Rockowitz S, Zheng D. Significant expansion of the REST/NRSF cistrome in human versus mouse embryonic stem cells: potential implications for neural development. Nucleic Acids Res. 2015;43(12):5730–43.

83. Takahashi K, Yamanaka S. Induction of Pluripotent Stem Cells from Mouse Embryonic and Adult Fibroblast Cultures by Defined Factors. Cell. 2006;126(4):663–76.

84. Haston KM, Finkbeiner S. Clinical Trials in a Dish: The Potential of Pluripotent Stem Cells to Develop Therapies for Neurodegenerative Diseases. Annu Rev Pharmacol Toxicol. 2015;56(1):489–510.

85. Hung SSC, Khan S, Lo CY, Hewitt AW, Wong RCB. Drug discovery using induced pluripotent stem cell models of neurodegenerative and ocular diseases. Pharmacol Ther. 2017;177:32–43.

86. Payne NL, Sylvain A, O'Brien C, Herszfeld D, Sun G, Bernard CCA. Application of human induced pluripotent stem cells for modeling and treating neurodegenerative diseases. New BIOTECHNOLOGY. 2015;32(1):212–28.

87. Sandoe J, Eggan K. Opportunities and challenges of pluripotent stem cell neurodegenerative disease models. Nature. 2013;16(7):780–9.

88. Doudna JA, Charpentier E. The new frontier of genome engineering with CRISPR-Cas9. Science. 2014;346(6213):1258096–6.

89. Jinek M, Chylinski K, Fonfara I, Hauer M, Doudna JA, Charpentier E. A programmable dual-RNA-guided DNA endonuclease in adaptive bacterial immunity. Science. 2012;337(6096):816–21.

90. Yang MG, West AE. Editing the Neuronal Genome: a CRISPR View of Chromatin Regulation in Neuronal Development, Function, and Plasticity. Yale J Biol Med. 2016;89(4):457–70.

91. Thakore PI, Black JB, Hilton IB, Gersbach CA. Editing the epigenome: technologies for programmable transcription and epigenetic modulation. Nature. 2016;13(2):127–37.

92. Israel MA, Yuan SH, Bardy C, et al. Probing sporadic and familial Alzheimer's disease using induced pluripotent stem cells. Nature. 2012;482(7384):216–20.

93. Paquet D, Kwart D, Chen A, et al. Efficient introduction of specific homozygous and heterozygous mutations using CRISPR/Cas9. Nature. 2016;533(7601):125–9.

# 39

# Delirium

*Ravi S. Bhat and Kenneth Rockwood*

## Introduction

Delirium is a common term; it has been used to name creations as varied as a waltz, a book series, and an alcoholic beverage. Delirium is also a common condition; while no age is unaffected, elderly people are most often affected, especially those in long-term care (LTC) or admitted to hospitals. In such people, it is associated with very poor outcomes. While about half do not remember, those who do live with the anxiety evoked by their experience [1]. Delirium is associated with more in-hospital complications, longer stays in hospital, a greater likelihood of transfer to nursing homes, and higher mortality. Hospitals incur greater costs in managing delirium. Despite its common usage, frequency of occurrence, and impact on people and health care systems, delirium remains poorly diagnosed.

Delirium has been recognized and described for two millennia [2]. The stability of description is remarkable. Delirium was thought to be an acute and transient mental disorder, associated mostly with febrile illnesses and alcohol. It is still considered to be a disorder of acute onset, but now it is recognized that its course is not always transient [3].

Research on delirium has progressed in the past couple of decades [4]. There is greater confidence in our ability to prevent delirium than in our ability to treat it [5]. The problem in translation of current research is held back by the consistent and widespread reports of persistently high rates of diagnostic error [6]. To this end, delirium needs to be better understood, so that we can provide better care to the most vulnerable older people [7], especially in the context of a rapidly ageing society and our increasingly refined understanding of frailty and dementia subtypes.

## The delirium concept—evolution and classificatory systems

The key conceptual change of delirium reflects how populations are ageing. Something that was likely observed in adults with acute illnesses, intoxications, or withdrawals is now seen mainly in older people in hospitals and nursing homes or in adults with very severe or terminal illnesses; this age and specialty distribution is reflected in a recent delirium prevalence study in a university hospital in Ireland [8].

In the first available descriptions, delirium was distinguished from insanity [2]. Transiency was an important contrasting feature between delirium and insanity, with the latter seen to be a permanent condition [9]. Since the beginning of the nineteenth century, delirium began to be conceptualized as a disorder of consciousness, with 'clouding' coming to represent both an alteration in the level and fragmentation of consciousness [2]. The literature from this era is rich in clinically descriptive detail, but problematic in its application. Delirium has been seen either as not being a problem of consciousness or as a problem of content of consciousness [10]. The clinical features of delirium are such that it does not allow for it to be operationalized either on a binary measure, as in present or not present, or to be thought of as being along a continuum. The modern approach to the problem has been to work by trial and error (Table 39.1), with the word 'consciousness' being finally removed in DSM 5. The European Delirium Association and the American Delirium Association have jointly critiqued this change, asserting that '*conceptualisation of delirium must extend beyond what can be assessed through cognitive testing (attention) and accept that altered arousal is fundamental*' [11] (2014). It might be that the essence of consciousness is not readily captured and is in need still of both a better description and, with it, quantification.

Attention is easier to define than consciousness, though seemingly hard to standardize for routine clinical examination. Impairments in attention have been as a reduced ability to direct, focus, shift, and sustain attention, which incorporates most aspects of what is currently known about it [12]. However, there are problems in both addressing it in research and translating this into clinical practice, not the least because of overlap between the constructs of attention, working memory, and executive control [13]. DSM-5 certainly achieves high inter-rater reliability [14], but when interpreted strictly, it may miss many cases [15], as might be expected when a key component is missed. In contrast, the ICD-10 rigid criteria achieve high specificity at the cost of low sensitivity, because of the requirement of a number of mandatory features [14].

Regardless, it is important not to limit our understanding of a phenomenon because of artificially imposed constraints by definitions and rating scales derived thereof. Recognizing this limitation, Paula Trzepacz, David Meagher, and José Franco have proposed their Trzepacz, Meagher, and Franco (TMF) research criteria for delirium, based on an analysis of data from the Delirium Rating

**Table 39.1** Comparison of diagnostic systems

| | ICD-10 | DSM-III | DSM-III-R | DSM-IV | DSM-5 |
|---|---|---|---|---|---|
| **Clouding of consciousness** | Reduced clarity of awareness of the environment | Reduced clarity of awareness of the environment | Not stated | Not stated | Not stated |
| **Consciousness** | As above | As above | Reduced level of consciousness | Reduced clarity of awareness of environment | Not required |
| **Attention** | Reduced ability to focus, sustain, or shift attention | Reduced ability to focus, sustain, or shift attention to environmental stimuli | Reduced ability to maintain attention *and* to shift attention to *new* external stimuli | Reduced ability to focus, sustain, or shift attention | Reduced ability to focus, sustain, or shift attention |
| **Awareness** | As above | As above | Not stated | As above | Reduced orientation to the environment |
| **Disturbances in cognition** | Both immediate recall and recent memory and disorientation in time, place, or person required | Disorientation and memory impairment. Required feature if testable | Disorientation to time, place, or person and memory impairment | *Change* in cognition (memory deficit, disorientation, language disturbance) or … | Change in cognition (memory deficit, disorientation, language, *and* visuospatial ability) or … |
| **Disturbances in perception** | Not required | Defined as misinterpretations, illusions, or hallucinations | Defined as misinterpretations, illusions, or hallucinations | … development of perceptual disturbance not accounted for by dementia | … perception (included in 'change in cognition' above) |
| **Disturbances in speech/thinking** | Not required | Defined as 'at times incoherent' | Disorganized thinking: rambling, irrelevant or incoherent speech | Not required | Not required |
| **Sleep–wake cycle disturbances** | One of three features: insomnia, nocturnal worsening of symptoms, and disturbing dreams | Defined as insomnia or daytime drowsiness | Defined as insomnia or daytime sleepiness | Not required | Not required |
| **Psychomotor disturbances** | One of following: shifts from hypo- to hyperactivity; ↑ reaction time; ↑ or ↓ flow of speech; enhanced startle reaction | Defined as ↑ or ↓ psychomotor activity | Defined as ↑ or ↓ psychomotor activity | Not required | Not required |
| **Onset** | Developing rapidly; time course not defined | Developing over a short period of time—hours to days | Developing over a short period of time—hours to days | Developing over a short period of time—hours to days | Disturbance in attention and awareness defined developing over a short period of time—hours to days |
| **Presence of fluctuation** | Diurnal pattern | Diurnal pattern | Diurnal pattern | Diurnal pattern | Diurnal pattern of fluctuating severity of inattention and ↓ awareness |
| **Requirement of cause** | Cerebral or systemic disease | Evidence or presumption of organic factor judged to be aetiologically related allowed | And presumption of aetiology if symptoms not accounted for by a 'non-organic mental disorder' | Direct physiological consequences of a general medical condition | Broader categories |
| **Exclusion** | Not stated | Not stated | Not stated | Dementias | Other major neurocognitive disorders and coma |

☐ Essential    ☐ Either/or (use ambiguous)    ▨ Additional    ▨ Not stated/not required

Source: data from World Health Organization, *The ICD-10 Classification of Mental and Behavioural Disorders*, Copyright (1996), World Health Organization; *Diagnostic and Statistical Manual of Mental Disorders*, (Third Edition, DSM-III, Copyright (1980); Third Edition-Revised, DSM-III-R, Copyright (1987); *Fourth Edition, DSM-IV*, Copyright (1994); Fifth Edition, DSM-5, Copyright (2013)), American Psychiatric Association.

Scale-Revised-98 (DRS-R-98) [7]. These criteria have three domains of impairment: attentional/cognitive, circadian, and higher-level thinking [7]. The TMF criteria had high sensitivity and specificity (87.4% and 89.2%, respectively) and were better balanced than DSM-III-R (100% and 31.6%, respectively), DSM-IV (97.7% and 74.1%, respectively), DSM-5 (97.7% and 72.6%, respectively), and ICD-10 (66.2% and 100%, respectively).

## Epidemiology of delirium

Elderly people will make up approximately 16% of the world population by 2050 [16]. While, at any given time, about 4–6% of older adults are in nursing homes, around 30–50% of them will use a nursing home before their deaths [17]. Older people are high users of hospitals; around 40% of acute hospital stays were for people aged 65 years and older. A recent study suggested that hospitalization appears to be related to the proximity to death and nursing home use to ageing, which, if true, implies that nursing home use is likely to grow more rapidly than hospital use as populations age [18]. Another study found that multi-morbidity and neuropsychiatric diagnoses were the highest risks for LTC dependency [19]. If correct, these findings imply two things. Firstly, that people in hospitals and nursing homes are more likely to be the oldest old, to have higher rates of cognitive impairment, and to be frail and closer to death—all factors associated with high rates of delirium. Secondly, an understanding of delirium, the problems of its diagnosis, and management must broaden to include delirium in nursing homes and other settings.

In the general population, delirium is more common with advancing age and in the presence of dementia. In people ≥65 years, the point prevalence of delirium is estimated to be around 2% [20]. A population-based study examining the 30-day prevalence in the oldest old diagnosed delirium in 17% among the 85-year olds, 21% among the 90-year olds, and 39% among participants aged 95 years and older [21]. Overall, delirium was present in 52% of those with dementia, compared to only 5% of those without dementia. LTC is variably defined in studies [20]; when defined narrowly to include nursing homes, the prevalence estimates are still quite varied, ranging from just over 1% to 70% [20].

Eleven to 25% of hospitalized elder patients have delirium on admission, and a further 30% will develop it during the course of hospitalization [22]. The former is inaccurately termed 'prevalent' delirium, missing points in patient flow in and out of the hospital through emergency departments (EDs). Delirium occurs in 8–10% of older patients presenting to EDs, and 15% still have delirium at ED discharge [22]. Two-thirds of people with ' excited delirium', a poorly recognized state, die at the scene or during transport by paramedics or police [23]. Excited delirium is a term used most often in the forensic literature to refer to patients who, in other contexts, might have been referred to having hyperactive delirium. A key difference seems to be the context, with ingestion of drugs or toxins by community-dwelling people, many of whom are not elderly and whose initial encounter is frequently with the police, being the characteristic case. The mortality rate is non-trivial, and the term is meant also to suggest extreme adrenergic activation, for a variety of reasons. Given our limited experience with, and understanding of, this special case, we will not be referring to it further (see [23]).

Of the 11% of patients who had delirium in the ED on day 1, in nearly three-quarters, it persisted into day 2 and for about half of them for all 3 days [24]. Thus, the timing of delirium assessments can miss cases.

Once admitted, one study found a point prevalence of delirium of approximately 20% of adults evaluated [8]. The highest rate (>50%) was unsurprisingly found in the geriatrics ward and the lowest in surgical wards, with intermediate rates in both medical and orthopaedic wards (around 25%). When only older adults were examined in a nationwide study in Italy, the point prevalence of delirium was estimated to be approximately 23% [25]. The highest rates were detected in neurology and geriatrics wards. There are three caveats to consider from these studies. Firstly, a number of patients may be excluded because of untestability and lack of consent. Secondly, the relatively lower rate of delirium in surgical wards may be an artefact of the point prevalence estimation, especially if done on a weekend [8]. Surgery is a risk for delirium—the type of surgery, whether it was elective or emergency, and the duration of surgery appear to be important determinants of post-operative delirium [22]. Finally, both these studies excluded intensive care units (ICUs) [8, 25] and one excluded palliative care units [25]. The prevalence of delirium in ICU cohort studies can range from a low of 20–30% to as high as 70–80% [26], and in palliative care units, the delirium prevalence increases closer to death: 13.3–42.3% on admission, 26–62% during admission, and 58.8–88% in the weeks or hours preceding death [27]. This dramatic rise in delirium closer to death raises a pragmatic question—how do we distinguish between delirium as a part of dying and delirium as a sign of preventable death [28]? Prevalence estimates may rise further by 8–13% if subsyndromal delirium, a prognostically important milder state that does not meet the full diagnostic criteria, is included [29].

## Clinical features and diagnosis

History taking and learning to interview and observe a patient who might not be very co-operative is critical to both the diagnosis of delirium and its differential diagnosis. Every effort must be made to obtain collateral information from the patient's family members, caregivers, general practitioner, and past clinical records.

Delirium is an acute-onset condition. About half of older patients with delirium in hospitals already have it at admission, so this is an important part of the history to ascertain. The key questions are whether the current presentation of the older person *represents a change for them* and, if so, *the time course of that change*. Responses from family members such as ' ... this isn't my mum', or ' ... my father is off with the fairies' should be taken seriously. It is also useful to find out if the patient had had a cognitive assessment in the past year, since most high-income countries now require periodic cognitive assessments for older people. In hospital, baseline cognitive assessment and change indicate delirium [30].

Once onset, delirium characteristically fluctuates, often in a diurnal pattern, within as little as 3 hours [31]. This can be missed if examinations are less frequent (for example, every 3 days) [32]. Experts rely on fluctuation of motor symptoms wherein changes to physical activity of the patient appear important [33]. This may be particularly helpful in diagnosing delirium superimposed on dementia, both in the hospital [34] and in nursing homes [35].

Delirium presents as a mental disorder; it typically shows gross disturbance of mental functions and consciousness. Schiff and Plum noted that the primary neuropsychological components of consciousness are arousal, attention, intention, memory, awareness, and mood/emotion [10]. Research on clinical features of delirium demonstrates impairments in all of these components of consciousness. In addition, there are often profound disturbances in both the form and content of thought and perception. Overall there is considerable fragmentation of the conscious experience, which was one of the meanings held by the phrase 'clouding of consciousness'.

Generalized arousal is considered to be the most powerful and essential activity in any vertebrate nervous system [36]. Arousal is essential for the organism to be both aware and attentive [37]. In delirium, arousal is both diminished and heightened, as manifest when patients are hypoactive and hyperactive. Hypoactive and mixed subtypes are usually more common than the hyperactive subtype and more likely to be missed. Two-thirds of subtypes appear to maintain stability over time [38]. There is some evidence that arousal may predict both delirium and inattention [39]. Testing attention and other cognitive functions is difficult when arousal is reduced, so it is useful to become clinically adept at observing changes to arousal. Rating scales such as the modified Richmond Agitation and Sedation Scale (mRASS) [33] and the Observational Scale of Level of Arousal [39] may assist.

Attention is commonly impaired during clinical examination; global attention, when measured as the patient's ability to participate in a conversation over a short period of time, is the most common impairment [40, 41]. Of the available tests of attention, months backwards, defined as the ability to name months backwards from December to July without error, appears to perform the best, both in hospitals [41] and in nursing homes [42]. These measures are easy to use by the bedside, but practice is essential in learning both to administer and to observe patients as they perform. An app is also available to assist in this process [43], although how it will be employed in routine practice is unclear [44]. To a certain extent, the ability to direct attention is an act of intention; however, intention has, as such, not been studied in delirium. The ability to direct the mind towards an object and the capacity to act on the object are typically impaired.

Awareness of both self and the environment is grossly impaired. While the diagnostic systems do not guide us in how this is to be either understood or measured, research into the subjective experience in delirium demonstrates this impairment to a startling degree. Patients talked of experiencing themselves as being in a vacuum or a torpor and/or slumbering and that the surroundings were experienced through a mist [1]. Time-orderedness of this awareness too was impaired; patients encountered a mix of events from past and present, and visualization interpreted as imagination or fantasizing in a borderline state. These experiences were typically frightening when experienced and, when remembered, evoked a variety of emotions, from feelings of suspiciousness to shame, and between 19% and 22% develop post-traumatic stress disorder [45]. Examining these experiences relies on developing nuanced interview and analytic skills.

Delirious people feel turbulent emotions, from anxiety and sadness to irritability and anger. Sadness and anxiety, along with diminished activity of the hypoactive subtype of delirium, prompt a diagnosis of depression in such patients and lead to inappropriate treatment [46]. Psychotic symptoms are fragmented; judgements about, or perceptual misinterpretations of, the immediate external world are common, and when hallucinations occur, they are short-lasting and frightening. Thus, delusions, unlike those seen in schizophrenia, are liable to change and rarely systematized. Delusions and psychomotor agitation appear to predict the severity of distress after delirium [45]. The persistence of memories and distress may remind the clinician of delusions, but its certainty relates to the experience at the time and, unlike those seen in schizophrenia, is not an ongoing experience of the world. Hallucinations are typically visual and may occur in up to 50% of patients; rates are higher (nearly three-fourths) in patients referred to consultation–liaison psychiatry services [47]. It is clinical lore that delirium must be considered in an elderly person with first-onset visual hallucinations; however, one must be cautious in passively accepting it because it is not informed by research, and visual hallucinations are common in Lewy body dementias (LBDs).

Standard electroencephalography (EEG) is neither recommended for, nor feasible in, routine clinical practice. A recent study has shown that it may be possible to derive useful information from just two electrodes [48]. How this will influence routine practice has yet to be established.

## Differential diagnosis

The differential diagnosis of delirium is influenced by the settings in which the patient is examined; in hospitals, dementias, depression, and alcohol use disorders (AUDs) are important to consider, whereas in nursing homes, dementias, behavioural and psychological symptoms of dementia (BPSD), and depression are likely more important. The task is made challenging because of the frequent co-occurrence of these disorders.

Dementia and cognitive impairment are consistently identified as risk factors for delirium. In approximately 50% of patients, delirium is superimposed on dementia [34]. The problem then is not just to differentiate delirium from dementias, but also to diagnose it when dementia is present; there appears to be no consensus among experts as to how to do this [49] (Table 39.2). Three issues must be considered. Firstly, there is considerable overlap of symptoms between delirium and those of dementias such as LBD and some rare forms of dementias such as those caused by infections and prions. Two-thirds of experts found it challenging to diagnose delirium superimposed on dementia with Lewy bodies (DLB) [49]. While estimates of prior probability in a setting is a useful guide to differential diagnosis, the risk of missed diagnoses and potential harm from treatment makes it important to ensure accuracy of diagnosis. Secondly, BPSD are not included in the diagnostic criteria for the most common dementias [AD and vascular dementia (VaD)], but these are common and add to the challenge of a delirium diagnosis. Finally, in a fifth of cases, delirium persists at 6 months after diagnosis [50]; where does delirium end and dementia begin?

Dementias can onset acutely [51], though the proportion of those that onset over hours to days might be small. Cerebrovascular disease, including VaD, is an important differential diagnosis because of possible acuity of onset and common co-occurrence. Around 11% of dementia patients in acute hospitals may have VaD [52]; while the frequency of strategic infarct VaD in this population is not known, it

**Table 39.2** Prevalence and comparison between delirium and dementias

| | Delirium | | Dementias | | BPSD | | AD/mixed | VaD | DLB |
|---|---|---|---|---|---|---|---|---|---|
| Setting | Hospitals | LTC | Hospitals | LTC | Hospitals | LTC | Hospitals | Hospitals | Hospitals |
| Prevalence | 17–30% | 1.4–70% | 3–63% | 58% | 62% | 78% | 80% | ?11% | ?3% |
| Onset | Acute (hours to days) | | Typically insidious | | Acute to subacute onset | | Insidious | Acute to insidious | Insidious |
| Arousal | Impaired | | Typically unimpaired | | May be impaired | | Typically unimpaired | May be impaired | Impaired |
| Attention | 97% | | Impaired | | Impaired | | Impaired | Impaired | Grossly impaired |
| Orientation | 75% | | Impaired | | Impaired | | Impaired | Impaired | Impaired |
| Memory | 88% | | Impaired | | Impaired | | Impaired | May not be in early stages | Impaired |
| Sleep–wake cycle | 97% | | May be impaired | | 6–11% | | May be impaired | May be impaired | Impaired |
| Hallucinations | 50% | | May be present | | 0–18% | | May be present | May be present | Present |
| Delusions | 31% | | May be present | | 9–40% | | Present (later stages) | Present (earlier stages) | Present |
| Fluctuation | Present | | May be present | | May be present | | May be present (20%) | May be present (35–50%) | Present (90%) |
| Course | Persistent in 20% at end of 6 months | | Progressive | | Persistent | | Progressive | Stable to progressive | Progressive |

may account for 10% of all VaD diagnoses at autopsy [53]. Delirium can also be present in 10-30% of patients with stroke [54]. The presence of focal neurological signs should trigger requests for brain imaging. When absent, repeat assessment focusing on arousal levels, attention, and focal higher cognitive signs can be helpful. Other dementias, typically those of infective causes or due to prions, can be acute in onset, but the prevalence is unknown. A high index of suspicion generated by experience of a curious mind is possibly vital.

LBD in general, but DLB in particular, has a clinical presentation that is most similar to delirium. Global cognitive impairment (in this case, dementia), fluctuation in cognition, with pronounced variations in attention and alertness, and visual hallucinations are core criteria for DLB [55]. The prevalence of DLB in hospital settings and in nursing homes is not known; it may be present in approximately 3% of inpatients [56], and 2% of patients with delirium during hospitalization were diagnosed with DLB at 3 months' follow-up [57]. Parkinson's disease, which is associated with both hallucinations and delirium, is perhaps more common in hospitals and nursing homes [58]. The time course over which symptoms evolve and the presence of Parkinsonian signs help differentiate. Treatment of hyperactive delirium may involve the use of dopamine antagonist drugs, such as haloperidol, which may be fatal in patients with DLB.

BPSD are common in dementias and especially so in nursing homes and perhaps also in hospitals; a recent study estimated that around 70% of hospitalized patients with dementia will show at least one BPSD [59]. The phenomenon of sundowning can mimic delirium, and delirium worsens BPSD [60]. BPSD tend to be persistent, so once again attempts to obtain a history from family members or staff at the nursing home are important in distinguishing delirium from BPSD.

Depression is common in hospitalized elderly patients [46], and delirium, depression, and dementia commonly co-occur in nursing homes [61]. Patients with hypoactive delirium and those with significant disturbance in mood and emotion can appear depressed on cross-sectional examination, leading to misdiagnosis. Efforts to obtain a history and, in the fast-paced environment of an acute ward, avoid conflating a symptom with a syndrome are important to

an accurate diagnosis. Depression onsets over days to weeks, rather than hours to days; severe melancholic depression can show fluctuation, but it is typically predictable, with characteristic worsening of symptoms in the morning; while sleep-offset insomnia is characteristic of severe depression, insomnia in depression can also be of sleep-onset and sleep-maintenance. However, it is rarely fragmented or reversed, as seen in delirium; when psychotic symptoms occur in depression, they tend to be delusions, which are typically delusions of poverty, guilt, and nihilism.

The number of people with substance use disorders aged 50+ years are likely to double by 2020 [62]. Almost 50% of older adults (≥65 years) and almost 25% of subjects over 85 years drink alcohol; AUDs afflict 1–3% of elderly subjects [62]. In addition, up to 30% of older patients hospitalized in general medicine wards and up to 50% of those hospitalized in psychiatric wards have AUDs. Standardized rating scales are recommended for the identification and prediction of withdrawal symptoms [62].

Late-onset schizophrenia and late-onset schizophrenia like psychosis are relatively rare. People with these disorders are less likely than young-onset schizophrenia to demonstrate cognitive symptoms [63]; indeed cognitive impairment is felt sometimes to exclude a diagnosis [64]. Where it does not, impairments in attention and memory are common [65]. Base rates of diagnoses are a useful guide to diagnostic reasoning.

In summary, careful history taking and interview, along with collateral information focused on premorbid cognition and behaviour and examination, are key, but no guarantee, to an accurate diagnosis.

## Instruments

Given the rate of misdiagnosis of delirium, bedside use is as important a feature of a tool as it is for research. Two systematic reviews have examined the role of delirium assessment instruments [66, 67]. Wong et al. [66] reported that positive findings on the Global Attentiveness Rating (GAR), Memorial Delirium Assessment Scale (MDAS), Confusion Assessment Method (CAM), Delirium Rating

Scale Revised-98 (DRS-R-98), Clinical Assessment of Confusion (CAC), and Delirium Observation Screening Scale (DOSS) each had a likelihood ratio of >5 for diagnosing delirium. They determined that the Mini-Mental State Examination (MMSE) was the least useful for identifying patients with delirium [66]. The other brief cognitive screening instruments likely perform similarly. However, it is clinically relevant and important to conduct routine cognitive assessments, where possible, on all older patients admitted to hospital and those in post-acute care and nursing homes. Such instruments [for example, the Abbreviated Mental Test Score (AMTS)] might be helpful in the following ways in identifying delirium: (1) to detect dementia, possibly the most important risk factors for delirium, in hospitalized older patients [68]; (2) given its sensitivity, the MMSE may be useful in ruling out delirium [69]; (3) a change from baseline cognition may help predict delirium [30]; or (4) specific items such as disorientation to time and place on the MMSE on admission could predict delirium. Impairment in these two items classified nearly 90% of patients, and these two measures, along with visuoconstructional impairment, were each associated with either hypoactive or mixed subtype [70].

A problem when instruments are used in isolation is that they have to fit into hospital clinicians' available time. Even the CAM, which takes only 5 minutes to complete, may be too long for the busy clinician [66]. Besides, almost all instruments require training; in untrained clinicians, CAM has a low sensitivity [71–73]. Instruments may have to be suitably matched to clinicians using them. For example, the DRS-R-98 might be more suitable for use by suitably trained clinicians such as old age psychiatrists and geriatricians. On the other hand, the Nursing Delirium Screening Scale (Nu-DESC), which has shown good psychometric properties in two systematic reviews, might be a good observational tool for routine use by nurses [66, 67]. Two new instruments have taken on the challenge of being both brief and capable of wider use: 4AT [74] and RADAR (*Repérage Actif du Delirium Adapté à la Routine* or Recognizing Acute Delirium As Part of Your Routine) [35]. The 4AT has four items: (1) alertness; (2) four questions from the AMTS on age, date of birth, place (name of the hospital or building), and current year; (3) attention as tested by months of the year backwards; and (4) acute change or fluctuating course (http://www.the4at.com/). The RADAR has just three questions: 'When you gave the patient his/her medication: 1) Was the patient drowsy?; 2) Did the patient have trouble following your instructions?; 3) Were the patient's movements slowed down?' [35]. Of the two, the 4AT has so far shown a good balance between sensitivity and specificity when used by geriatricians [74] (Bellelli et al., 2014) and nurses without training in its use [75]. The RADAR had lower levels of both sensitivity and specificity, but participating nursing staff took only 7 seconds, on average, to complete the tool and almost all received it very well [35]. Additionally, it is important to note that the RADAR was tested across five nursing homes where the misdiagnosis of delirium is typically higher than in hospitals [76].

## Natural history of delirium

Delirium is associated with an increased risk of post-discharge mortality, institutionalization, and dementia [77]. Hypoactive delirium, increased severity, and persistent delirium, pre-existing dementias, and depression may all be predictive of these negative outcomes [78].

Delirium has been for long thought of as a transient disorder; most modern studies demonstrated that this is not the case. One review found the combined proportions with persistent delirium at discharge, 1, 3, and 6 months to be approximately 45%, 30%, 25%, and 20%, respectively [50]. Persistence was associated with dementia, increasing numbers of medical conditions, increasing severity of delirium, hypoactive symptoms, and hypoxic illnesses [3]. It is unclear what proportion of these outcomes are attributable to factors other than delirium. Mortality in delirium may be mediated by the severity of illness and frailty in the short term [79] and through cognitive impairment in the long term [80]. Other negative outcomes may be mediated through persistence, which, in turn, is likely due to pre-existing dementia [78] and the presence of other geriatric syndromes [81]. Delirium, especially hypoactive delirium, is likely to predispose to deconditioning, falls, dehydration, pressure ulcers, and urinary retention, which, in turn, send the patient into a vicious spiral [81].

The outcomes of delirium from ICU settings are no less grim. Patients with delirium had significantly higher mortality during admission, longer durations of mechanical ventilation, and longer lengths of stay in the ICU and in hospital [82].

In nursing homes, symptoms of delirium predict incident delirium [83]. Baseline delirium and subsyndromal symptoms of delirium, depression, and dementia interact to lead to increased mortality and functional and cognitive decline [61].

Examination of outcomes of delirium requires further work. Adamis *et al.* [84] noted that recovery is not well defined for delirium; they proposed sustained improvement in cognitive function to define therapeutic outcomes in delirium. Following generally accepted nomenclature in psychiatry, they defined 'response' as when baseline cognitive function is re-established for at least one full day of assessment and 'recovery' when this baseline cognitive function is sustained for at least a week [84].

## Aetiopathogenesis of delirium

Causality in medicine is commonly conceptualized, such that they can be reduced to biology, with preference for bottom–up explanations that focus on generative physiological mechanisms [85]. Outside of geriatrics and psychiatry, causality is commonly required to be parsimonious; multiple causes are eschewed. For the researcher, the attraction is the idea that a single cause can lead to a single treatment, and for the busy clinician, a clear direction for action. These ideas can be problematic when applied to the common and complex presentations of later life, including delirium.

Considering the pathogenesis of delirium, many causal hypotheses/models have been articulated [86]. A closer look reveals two broad categories: (1) those that reduce the cause of delirium to a single final common pathway operating in and through the brain; and (2) those that address complexity by other means. Complexity is usually addressed by attempting to either integrate two or more 'final common pathways' together or use a framework such as the vulnerability–stress model to either empirically derive or theorize a model. There is a varying degree of strength of assumption in these models as to whether the brain is the organ of dysfunction. A metaphorical understanding of delirium and related geriatric giants would consider the human organism as a complex system, however.

When complex systems fail, their highest-order functions fail first. In humans, consciousness, one of the higher-order functions, and its failure are signalled by delirium. In this metaphor, the brain is simply a bystander to a set of processes occurring throughout the body [37].

To be valid, the single common pathway theories should be able to describe the mechanisms that lead to the delirium in particular, and not something else, either dementia or one of the other complex presentations in older adults. These should also explain the occurrence of delirium subtypes, especially the occurrence of the mixed subtype of delirium. The more complex theories should not be setting-specific; they should be able to account for delirium in an older adult, regardless of the setting. They should also be able to describe the occurrence of delirium in older adults of varying levels of fitness within the same setting. Finally, they should serve utility.

## Single final common pathway hypotheses

### Oxidative stress

Engel and Romano [9], in their now classic paper, hypothesized that delirium could result from two processes: failure of function or failure of structure. In this schema, the former is reversible and the latter permanent, drawing to the distinction between transient delirium and permanent dementia. Presciently, they noted it was too early to 'regard these states as any more than different degrees or stages of similar processes'. Their hypothesis was that delirium resulted from low cerebral oxygen consumption. In its modern iteration, delirium is thought to result from brain damage resulting from oxidative stress [87]. Neopterin produced by microglia in the brain is a marker for both cell-mediated immunity and oxidative stress and was found to be higher in both the preoperative samples of CSF and the serum of delirious patients than in those with no delirium. Those with both delirium and chronic cognitive impairment had the highest levels of neopterin, and those with neither had the lowest [87]. In those without cognitive impairment, there was a correlation between delirium severity and neopterin levels. The association between obstructive sleep apnoea and delirium is seen as further evidence of the role of oxidative stress [88]. The fact that neopterin also has a role in cell-mediated immunity (though, in their study, the correlations persisted, even when those with infection and malignancies were removed from analysis) suggests more complex pathways. Importantly, elevated levels have been found in other neuropsychiatric disorders.

### Neuroendocrine hypothesis

Kral hypothesized that delirium was the result of age-linked decline of stress resistance mediated through the hypothalamo–pituitary–adrenal (HPA) axis [89]. Some recent support for this hypothesis has come from a positive association between raised perioperative plasma cortisol concentrations post-coronary artery bypass graft surgery [90]. However, unlike other recent studies examining anticholinergic activity, this study did not adjust for confounders [91]. Moreover, intraoperative dexamethasone failed to reduce the incidence of post-operative delirium [92]. The important issue here is that impaired HPA activity has not only profound systemic effects, but also effects on the brain, and it is through their pro-inflammatory effects that they can be usefully integrated into a more complex hypothesis [93].

### Cholinergic hypothesis

Tune *et al.* proposed the cholinergic hypothesis, based on the finding of an association between the use of anticholinergic drugs and post-operative delirium [94]. The hypothesis is attractive because of both the basal forebrain degenerative changes in dementias and the role that acetylcholine plays in arousal and attention. Much work has been done since the 1980s to prove the hypothesis by attempting to demonstrate associations between anticholinergic drug burden and serum anticholinergic activity and delirium. However, both an early [95] and recent studies cast doubt on this hypothesis [5, 91, 96, 97]. In one cohort study, anticholinergic drugs were not associated with an increased risk of delirium [96], while in another cohort study, the associations disappeared after adjusting for confounders [91]; in the first study examining CSF (and serum) anticholinergic activity, there was no association between either of these measures and delirium [97], and finally cholinesterase inhibitors have not demonstrated a role in preventing delirium [5]. Acetylcholine is but one important component in the modulation of attention and arousal [12]; disturbances in other neurotransmitters, such as dopamine, noradrenaline, GABA, and glutamate, are posited as well [86]. It is not that cholinergic systems have no role in delirium; instead they are likely to be part of more complex dysfunction that leads to delirium [98].

### Melatonin hypothesis

Rooij and van Munster [99], noting the prominent disturbance of the circadian rhythm in the sundowning phenomenon seen in dementia and delirium, posited that melatonin deficiency triggers delirium and thus could be used to prevent it from occurring. The potential efficacy of melatonin in reducing symptoms of sundowning to this idea [100]; unfortunately, a large randomized clinical trial by the same group found no evidence for melatonin in reducing post-operative delirium [101]. Melatonin is implicated in the modulation of inflammation in the brain, and there are associations between sleep dysregulation and decreased proportions of natural killer cells, reduced lymphokine-activated killer activity, and reduced IL-2 production [86]. As with other pathways considered here, the picture points to complex interactions between inflammation, neurotransmitters, and neuroendocrine activity [86], which leads us to consider complex models that have attempted to integrate these findings in a systematic manner. Although additional investigations have been proposed, there is little evidence to recommend the use of melatonin at this time [102].

## Complex models

### Neuroinflammatory hypothesis

The most common hypotheses attempt to integrate theory and available data in different ways [98, 103, 104].

Pro-inflammatory cytokines generated in the periphery, such as interleukin 1β (IL-1β), tumour necrosis factor α (TNFα), and interleukin 6 (IL-6), communicate with the brain through several routes, including autonomic afferents, across the blood–brain barrier (BBB), and via the circumventricular region [103]. Increased TNFα is thought to activate microglia, which, in turn, release cytokines and prostaglandins. One postulate is that, with ageing and dementia, microglia are 'primed' due to loss of cholinergic inhibition resulting in their heightened response [98]. There is evidence that increasing severity of dementia may be associated with higher likelihood of delirium [105]. This microglial priming and resulting uncontrolled inflammation causes further neurodegeneration leading to a vicious cycle of brain change [98]. Even though cytokines are known to be increased in delirium [106], this hypothesis, while explaining why neuroinflammation could be associated with dementia, does not quite explain the occurrence of delirium [98]. Cerejeira et al. [103] and Cunningham and Maclullich [104] go further, using an explicitly stated vulnerability–stress framework to provide mechanistically plausible accounts for the occurrence of delirium. In their comprehensive review, Cerejeira et al. [103] concluded delirium symptoms may be accounted for by the widespread dysregulation of brain homeostasis, neurotransmission, and neurophysiological functions, resulting 'in a reduced capacity to interact with the environment and to integrate stimuli within the cognitive experience'. In a more nuanced analysis, Cunningham and Maclullich [104] stated that their model accounts for the characteristic symptoms of hypoactive delirium, but not for the presence of psychotic symptoms. Intriguingly, in a longitudinal study of community-dwelling older adults with AD, raised IL-6 was associated with hallucinations, but not with delirium [107].

### Network disconnection hypothesis

The network disconnection hypothesis, also using the vulnerability–stress framework, proposes that acute breakdown of network connectivity within the brain results in delirium [86]. Two recent studies have attempted to characterize this hypothesized disconnection through fMRI and a within-patients design [108] and EEG using a between-patients design [109]. They both demonstrated disconnection, but one showed an increase in functional connectivity between the prefrontal cortex and the posterior cingulate cortex [108], while the other found reduced corticocortical connectivity [109]. Manshour and Avidan urge caution in interpreting these findings as evidence of disconnection given the assumptions made [110]. Post-operative delirium may be predicted by increased white matter hyperintensities (WMHs), offering a structural basis for this apparent functional disconnection [111], though in another study, WMHs did not predict post-operative delirium in those without dementia [112]. This latter group of researchers did find an association between diffusion tensor imaging abnormalities observed in the corpus callosum, cingulum, and temporal lobe and delirium [113], suggesting that disconnection may yet play an important role in delirium.

### Multifactorial model

At the level of the human organism, Inouye's multifactorial model is widely regarded. It too employs the vulnerability–stress framework, furnishing empirically derived factors to populate vulnerabilities and stressors [114]. It has clinical and pedagogic utility. The lack of temporal separation between, and lack of clarity of, vulnerabilities and stressors poses a problem, as does a failure to provide an explanation as to why delirium is caused. A recent study found preoperative risk factors, such as impaired cognition, thus more clearly temporally separated vulnerabilities, clearly modify the response to post-operative factors, such as post-operative pain and opioid use, to result in delirium [115]. This model may not work well in nursing homes [116]. In addition, there is some evidence that deficit accumulation, and thus systems failure, may account for delirium [79], but this has not been tested more widely.

In summary, current models integrate available evidence and may explain at least one of the subtypes of delirium and provide a mechanism for accounting for the influence of age and pre-existing dementia in being a vulnerability to delirium. Most do not explain why the complex impairments lead to the characteristic symptoms of delirium, and not dementia, however. The multifactorial model and clinical and pedagogic utility may not be applicable outside hospital settings.

## Treatment and management of delirium

The treatment and management of delirium are as much about prevention as it is about treating the condition once it has occurred. Management strategies that use single and multiple components, reflecting the multifactorial causation of delirium, have been trialled.

Multicomponent interventions typically include some combination of the following: staff education, orientation protocols, avoidance of sensory deprivation, multi-disciplinary team approach to care, sleep protocols, early mobilization, hydration, nutrition, medication reviews, oxygen delivery, and pain control [117]. The quality of evidence from the four randomised clinical trials reviewed in a recent systematic overview was considered to be very low [117]. There appears to be no evidence for efficacy of multicomponent interventions in the treatment of delirium. No new trials of multicomponent interventions in acute care appear to have been published after 2006 [118]; a pragmatic trial in post-acute care too failed to show an effect [119]. Does this mean that we should give up on treating delirium? What one of us wrote more than a decade ago is still relevant: '...the care provided to the intervention group is how most of us would like our loved ones to be cared for, with enough attention paid to them that health care professionals would at least recognize alterations in their mental state. The unattractive but real alternative is that these patients are consigned to a poor quality of care for 'confusion' that demoralizes families and health care professionals alike. Let me press the point further: to fail to recognize delirium is to practise with an unsatisfying disengagement with one's patients' lives' [120].

Dopamine antagonists and other psychotropics are commonly used to treat delirium and agitation in acute hospitals. The (at least) four systematic reviews/meta-analysis published in 2015–2016 vary in their recommendations in using dopamine antagonist medications to treat delirium [121–124]. What is clear is that routine use of such medications cannot be recommended for the treatment of delirium. In routine use, the harms from this class of drugs outweigh any potential benefit. However, there will be times in a busy hospital ward when behavioural control of agitation is required for the safety of the patient and others. In each single case, a risk–benefit analysis must be done before using a dopamine antagonist. On the positive side, a majority of the studies show some benefit, in contrast to use of pro-cholinergic drugs or benzodiazepines [125]. Most treatment guidelines recommend haloperidol, and some include olanzapine [125]. The problem with haloperidol is that it is reputed to cause extra-pyramidal side effects (EPSEs), and it is not quite known how it helps. EPSEs may well be caused by higher doses; for example, in one recent clinical trial, the haloperidol dose, which is roughly equivalent to risperidone, was four times higher than the risperidone dose [126]. When used in equivalent doses (chlorpromazine equivalent dose of approximately 60 mg/day), haloperidol (approximately 1 mg/day) was equally efficacious as newer dopamine antagonists without EPSEs [127]. The problem discovered in this trial was that the efficacy of all the dopamine antagonists tested was poor in those aged 75 years and over [127]. Benzodiazepines are not recommended in the treatment of typical delirium in an older person. However, they will need to be considered in cases where alcohol withdrawal is the cause of the delirium. In such cases, in order to avoid risks of oversedation, short-acting benzodiazepines should be considered. Lorazepam (1–2 mg orally or intramuscularly or intravenously every 4 hours) or oxazepam (30–60 mg orally every 4 hours for the first day, and then tapering the dose by 50% on days 2 and 3) are recommended [128].

If a dopamine antagonist is deemed necessary to use, then it is best to first trial haloperidol. The typical dosing should be 0.25 mg 3–4 times a day, resulting in stable drug levels from the outset. The important act is to review the use of the medication daily and to taper and cease it as soon as possible. Ideally, this would be part of a hospital routine to match the use of dopamine antagonist medications to an indication for their use.

In summary, multicomponent interventions continue to be important in ensuring older adults receive good quality of care during their hospitalization. Routine use of dopamine antagonist medications is not recommended for the treatment of delirium; they should be used when necessary to provide safe care in a hospital setting.

There is better evidence of effect for multicomponent interventions in the prevention of delirium. A recent Cochrane review found moderate-quality evidence that multicomponent interventions reduce the incidence of delirium, compared to usual care, with similar effect sizes across medical and surgical settings. However, the evidence was less for efficacy in patients with pre-existing dementia [5]. It is not clear which combination of components works best for patients and for patients in a given setting [117], but based on the very limited evidence from trials that used single components, it is possible that staff education, reorientation protocols, and geriatric consultations may be important components to include [117]. A pragmatic clinical trial in 283 older patients admitted for hip fracture repair found good adherence to pre-printed post-operative orders, but more importantly, significantly less delirium in the intervention group (33% vs 51% in controls) and a stronger effect in people with pre-existing dementia [129].

Multicomponent interventions are not without problems; it is unclear if they actually work in reducing delirium in the most frail [130], and implementation of *all elements* in a hospital setting *over time* may be problematic. This requires change in the thinking of what hospitals do, from the coal-face to the board [131]; a frail older adult-friendly hospital is likely to be friendly for all patients.

There is no evidence for the use of cholinesterase inhibitors, melatonin agonists, or dopamine antagonist medications in the prevention of delirium [5]. In the ICU setting, dexmedetomidine appears to reduce the incidence of delirium, agitation, and confusion in critically ill patients [132]. Placement of earplugs in patients admitted to the ICU, either in isolation or as part of a bundle of sleep hygiene improvement, appears to reduce the risk of delirium [133]. However, these short-term gains have to be considered against the finding that interventions do not reduce short-term mortality [134].

There is little evidence of systematic interventions in nursing homes [135]. In their review, Clegg *et al.* [135] found one large cluster randomized trial of a computerized system to identify medications that may contribute to delirium risk and trigger a pharmacist-led medication review. This study showed a large reduction in delirium incidence, but not in other measures such as reduction in hospital admissions, mortality, or falls risk. Despite this, it is heartening to see the reduction in delirium incidence alone. While the system may not be either available or affordable in all countries, consideration for deprescribing is important. Canada has now established a deprescribing network, and information available on its website http://deprescribing.org/ would be a useful resource to consider.

## Closing remarks and future

Interest in delirium, both in research and policy, has dramatically increased in the past decade. This bodes well. However, despite this heightened interest, diagnostic error rate for delirium remains high and outcomes poor. Josef Strauss wrote his waltz *Delirien* for a medical ball; as beautiful as it is, after the first minute and 40 seconds, it contains little in its music to suggest the turbulence of delirium. Perhaps it is time for us to dance to a different tune for, and with, our patients.

## Acknowledgements

Our thanks to A. Ryan Bhat for his musical analysis of *Delirien*, Opus 212, Josef Strauss.

## REFERENCES

1. Andersson, E. M., Hallberg, I. R., Norberg, A., and Edberg, A. K. 2002. The meaning of acute confusional state from the perspective of elderly patients. *Int J Geriatr Psychiatry*, 17, 652–63.
2. Lipowski, Z. J. *Delirium: Acute Confusional States*. Oxford University Press, New York, NY; 1990.
3. Dasgupta, M. and Hillier, L. M. 2010. Factors associated with prolonged delirium: a systematic review. *Int Psychogeriatr*, 22, 373–94.
4. Maclullich, A. M., Anand, A, Davis, D. H., *et al.* 2013. New horizons in the pathogenesis, assessment and management of delirium. *Age Ageing*, 42, 667–74.
5. Siddiqi, N., Harrison, J. K., Clegg, A., *et al.* 2016. Interventions for preventing delirium in hospitalised non-ICU patients. *Cochrane Database Syst Rev*, 3, CD005563.
6. Bhat, R. S. and Rockwood, K. 2016. The role of diagnosis in delirium. *Int Psychogeriatr*, 28, 1579–86.
7. Trzepacz, P. T., Meagher, D. J., and Franco, J. G. 2016. Comparison of diagnostic classification systems for delirium with new research criteria that incorporate the three core domains. *J Psychosom Res*, 84, 60–8.
8. Ryan, D. J., O'regan, N. A., Caoimh, R. O., *et al.* 2013. Delirium in an adult acute hospital population: predictors, prevalence and detection. *BMJ Open*, 3, pii: e001772.
9. Engel, G. L. and Romano, J. 1959. Delirium, a syndrome of cerebral insufficiency. *J Chronic Dis*, 9, 260–77.
10. Schiff, N. D. and Plum, F. 2000. The role of arousal and "gating" systems in the neurology of impaired consciousness. *J Clin Neurophysiol*, 17, 438–52.
11. European Delirium Association; American Delirium Society. 2014. The DSM-5 criteria, level of arousal and delirium diagnosis: inclusiveness is safer. *BMC Med*, 12, 141.

12. Petersen, S. E. and Posner, M. I. 2012. The attention system of the human brain: 20 years after. *Annu Rev Neurosci*, 35, 73–89.

13. Tieges, Z., Brown, L. J., and Maclullich, A. M. 2014. Objective assessment of attention in delirium: a narrative review. *Int J Geriatr Psychiatry*, 29, 1185–97.

14. Sepulveda, E., Franco, J. G., Trzepacz, P. T., *et al.* 2016. Delirium diagnosis defined by cluster analysis of symptoms versus diagnosis by DSM and ICD criteria: diagnostic accuracy study. *BMC Psychiatry*, 16, 167.

15. Meagher, D. J., Morandi, A., Inouye, S. K., *et al.* 2014. Concordance between DSM-IV and DSM-5 criteria for delirium diagnosis in a pooled database of 768 prospectively evaluated patients using the delirium rating scale-revised-98. *BMC Med*, 12, 164.

16. World Health Organization, 2011. *World report on ageing and health*. World Health Organization, Geneva.

17. Broad, J. B., Ashton, T., Gott, M., McLeod, H., Davis, P. B., and Connolly, M. J. 2015. Likelihood of residential aged care use in later life: a simple approach to estimation with international comparison. *Aust N Z J Public Health*, 39, 374–9.

18. Murphy, M. and Martikainen, P. 2013. Use of hospital and long-term institutional care services in relation to proximity to death among older people in Finland. *Soc Sci Med*, 88, 39–47.

19. Koller, D., Schön G, Schäfer I, Glaeske G, van den Bussche H, and Hansen H. 2014. Multimorbidity and long-term care dependency--a five-year follow-up. *BMC Geriatr*, 14, 70.

20. De Lange, E., Verhaak, P. F., and Van der Meer, K. 2013. Prevalence, presentation and prognosis of delirium in older people in the population, at home and in long term care: a review. *Int J Geriatr Psychiatry*, 28, 127–34.

21. Mathillas, J., Olofsson B, Lövheim H, and Gustafson Y. 2013. Thirty-day prevalence of delirium among very old people: a population-based study of very old people living at home and in institutions. *Arch Gerontol Geriatr*, 57, 298–304.

22. Vasilevskis, E. E., Han, J. H., Hughes, C. G., and Ely, E. W. 2012. Epidemiology and risk factors for delirium across hospital settings. *Best Pract Res Clin Anaesthesiol*, 26, 277–87.

23. Takeuchi, A., Ahern, T. L., and Henderson, S. O. 2011. Excited delirium. *West J Emerg Med*, 12, 77–83.

24. Hsieh, S. J., Madahar, P., Hope, A. A., Zapata, J., and Gong, M. N. 2015. Clinical deterioration in older adults with delirium during early hospitalisation: a prospective cohort study. *BMJ Open*, 5, e007496.

25. Bellelli, G., Morandi, A., Di Santo, S. G., *et al.* 2016. 'Delirium Day': a nationwide point prevalence study of delirium in older hospitalized patients using an easy standardized diagnostic tool. *BMC Med*, 14, 106.

26. Salluh, J. I., Soares, M., Teles, J. M., *et al.* 2010. Delirium epidemiology in critical care (DECCA): an international study. *Crit Care*, 14, R210.

27. Hosie, A., Davidson, P. M., Agar, M., Sanderson, C. R., and Phillips, J. 2013. Delirium prevalence, incidence, and implications for screening in specialist palliative care inpatient settings: a systematic review. *Palliat Med*, 27, 486–98.

28. Rockwood, K. and Lindesay, J. 2002. Delirium and dying. *Int Psychogeriatr*, 14, 235–8.

29. Meagher D, O'Regan N, Ryan D, *et al.* 2014. Frequency of delirium and subsyndromal delirium in an adult acute hospital population. *Br J Psychiatry*, 205, 478–85.

30. O'Keefe, S. T., Mulkerrin, E. C., Nayeem, K., Varughese, M., and Pillay, I. 2005. Use of serial Mini-Mental State Examinations to diagnose and monitor delirium in elderly hospital patients. *J Am Geriatr Soc*, 53, 867–70.

31. Andersson, E. M., Gustafson, L., and Hallberg, I. R. 2001. Acute confusional state in elderly orthopaedic patients: factors of importance for detection in nursing care. *Int J Geriatr Psychiatry*, 16, 7–17.

32. Meagher, D., Adamis, D., Trzepacz, P., and Leonard, M. 2012. Features of subsyndromal and persistent delirium. *Br J Psychiatry*, 200, 37–44.

33. Morandi, A., McCurley, J., Vasilevskis, E. E., *et al.* 2012. Tools to detect delirium superimposed on dementia: a systematic review. *J Am Geriatr Soc*, 60, 2005–13.

34. Morandi, A., Davis, D., Bellelli, G., *et al.* 2017. The Diagnosis of Delirium Superimposed on Dementia: An Emerging Challenge. *J Am Med Dir Assoc*, 18, 12–18.

35. Voyer, P., Champoux, N., Desrosiers, J., *et al.* 2015. Recognizing acute delirium as part of your routine [RADAR]: a validation study. *BMC Nurs*, 14, 19.

36. Quinkert, A. W., Vimal, V., Weil, Z. M., *et al.* 2011. Quantitative descriptions of generalized arousal, an elementary function of the vertebrate brain. *Proc Natl Acad Sci U S A*, 108 Suppl 3, 15617–23.

37. Bhat, R. and Rockwood, K. 2007. Delirium as a disorder of consciousness. *J Neurol Neurosurg Psychiatry*, 78, 1167–70.

38. Meagher, D. J., Leonard, M., Donnelly, S., Conroy, M., Adamis, D., and Trzepacz, P. T. 2012. A longitudinal study of motor subtypes in delirium: frequency and stability during episodes. *J Psychosom Res*, 72, 236–41.

39. Tieges, Z., McGrath, A., Hall, R. J., and Maclullich, A. M. 2013. Abnormal level of arousal as a predictor of delirium and inattention: an exploratory study. *Am J Geriatr Psychiatry*, 21, 1244–53.

40. O'Keeffe, S. T. and Gosney, M. A. 1997. Assessing attentiveness in older hospital patients: global assessment versus tests of attention. *J Am Geriatr Soc*, 45, 470–3.

41. Adamis, D., Meagher, D., Murrah, O., *et al.* 2016. Evaluating attention in delirium: A comparison of bedside tests of attention. *Geriatr Gerontol Int*, 16, 1028–35.

42. Voyer, P., Champoux, N., Desrosiers, J., *et al.* 2016. Assessment of inattention in the context of delirium screening: one size does not fit all! *Int Psychogeriatr*, 28, 1293–301.

43. Tieges, Z., Stíobhairt, A., Scott, K., *et al.* 2015. Development of a smartphone application for the objective detection of attentional deficits in delirium. *Int Psychogeriatr*, 27, 1251–62.

44. Rockwood, K. 2015. Bringing delirium into the 21st century: will physicians get the app out? *Int Psychogeriatr*, 27, 1247–9.

45. Partridge, J. S., Martin, F. C., Harari, D., and Dhesi, J. K. 2013. The delirium experience: what is the effect on patients, relatives and staff and what can be done to modify this? *Int J Geriatr Psychiatry*, 28, 804–12.

46. O'Sullivan, R., Inouye, S. K., and Meagher, D. 2014. Delirium and depression: inter-relationship and clinical overlap in elderly people. *Lancet Psychiatry*, 1, 303–11.

47. Grover, S., Agarwal, M., Sharma, A., *et al.* 2013. Symptoms and aetiology of delirium: a comparison of elderly and adult patients. *East Asian Arch Psychiatry*, 23, 56–64.

48. Van der Kooi, A. W., Zaal, I. J., Klijn, F. A., *et al.* 2015. Delirium detection using EEG: what and how to measure. *Chest*, 147, 94–101.

49. Richardson, S., Teodorczuk, A., Bellelli, G., *et al.* 2016. Delirium superimposed on dementia: a survey of delirium specialists shows a lack of consensus in clinical practice and research studies. *Int Psychogeriatr*, 28, 853–61.

50. Cole, M. G., Ciampi, A., Belzile, E., and Zhong, L. 2009. Persistent delirium in older hospital patients: a systematic review of frequency and prognosis. *Age Ageing*, 38, 19–26.

51. King, P., Devichand, P., and Rockwood, K. 2006. Dementia of acute onset in the Canadian Study of Health and Aging. *Int Psychogeriatr*, 17, 451–9.

52. Mukadam, N. and Sampson, E. L. 2011. A systematic review of the prevalence, associations and outcomes of dementia in older general hospital inpatients. *Int Psychogeriatr*, 23, 344–55.

53. Jellinger, K. A. and Attems, J. 2010. Prevalence of dementia disorders in the oldest-old: an autopsy study. *Acta Neuropathol*, 119, 421–33.

54. Shi, Q., Presutti, R., Selchen, D., and Saposnik, G. 2012. Delirium in acute stroke: a systematic review and meta-analysis. *Stroke*, 43, 645–9.

55. McKeith, I. G., Dickson, D. W., Lowe, J., et al. 2005. Diagnosis and management of dementia with Lewy bodies: third report of the DLB Consortium. *Neurology*, 65, 1863–72.

56. Vann Jones, S. A. and O'Brien, J. T. 2014. The prevalence and incidence of dementia with Lewy bodies: a systematic review of population and clinical studies. *Psychol Med*, 44, 673–83.

57. Jackson, T. A., Maclullich, A. M., Gladmad, J. R., Lord, J. M., and Sheehan, B. 2016. Undiagnosed long-term cognitive impairment in acutely hospitalised older medical patients with delirium: a prospective cohort study. *Age Ageing*, 45, 493–9.

58. Vardy, E. R., Teodorczuk, A., and Yarnall, A. J. 2015. Review of delirium in patients with Parkinson's disease. *J Neurol*, 262, 2401–10.

59. Sampson, E. L., White, N., Leurent, B., et al. 2014. Behavioural and psychiatric symptoms in people with dementia admitted to the acute hospital: prospective cohort study. *Br J Psychiatry*, 205, 189–96.

60. Landreville, P., Voyer, P., and Carmichael, P. H. 2013. Relationship between delirium and behavioral symptoms of dementia. *Int Psychogeriatr*, 25, 635–43.

61. McCusker, J., Cole, M. G., Voyer, P., et al. 2014. Six-month outcomes of co-occurring delirium, depression, and dementia in long-term care. *J Am Geriatr Soc*, 62, 2296–302.

62. Wu, L. T. and Blazer, D. G. 2014. Substance use disorders and psychiatric comorbidity in mid and later life: a review. *Int J Epidemiol*, 43, 304–17.

63. Rajji, T. K., Ismail, Z., Mulsant, B. H. 2009. Age at onset and cognition in schizophrenia: meta-analysis. *Br J Psychiatry*, 195, 286–93.

64. Sin Fai Lam, C. C., Reeves, S. J., Stewart, R., and Howard, R. 2016. Service and treatment engagement of people with very late-onset schizophrenia-like psychosis. *BJPsych Bull*. 40, 185–6.

65. Ting, C., Rajji, T. K., Ismail, Z., et al. 2010. Differentiating the cognitive profile of schizophrenia from that of Alzheimer disease and depression in late life. *PLoS One*, 5, e10151.

66. Wong, C. L., Holroyd-Leduc, J., Simel, D. L., and Straus, S. E. 2010. Does this patient have delirium?: value of bedside instruments. *JAMA*, 304, 779–86.

67. Van Velthuijsen, E. L., Zwakhalen, S. M., Warnier, R. M., Mulder, W. J., Verhey, F. R., and Kempen, G. I. 2016. Psychometric properties and feasibility of instruments for the detection of delirium in older hospitalized patients: a systematic review. *Int J Geriatr Psychiatry*, 31, 974–89.

68. Jackson, T. A., Gladman, J. R., Harwood, R. H., et al. 2017. Challenges and opportunities in understanding dementia and delirium in the acute hospital. *PLoS Med*, 14, e1002247.

69. Mitchell, A. J., Shukla, D., Ajumal, H. A., Stubbs, B., and Tahir, T. A. 2014. The Mini-Mental State Examination as a diagnostic and screening test for delirium: systematic review and meta-analysis. *Gen Hosp Psychiatry*, 36, 627–33.

70. Gabriel Franco, J., Santesteban, O., Trzepacz, P., et al. 2014. MMSE items that predict incident delirium and hypoactive subtype in older medical inpatients. *Psychiatry Res*, 220, 975–81.

71. Rolfson, D. B., McElhaney, J. E., Jhangri, G. S., and Rockwood, K. 1999. Validity of the confusion assessment method in detecting postoperative delirium in the elderly. *Int Psychogeriatr*, 11, 431–8.

72. Inouye, S. K., Foreman, M. D., Mion, L. C., Katz, K. H., and Cooney, L. M. Jr. 2001. Nurses' recognition of delirium and its symptoms: comparison of nurse and researcher ratings. *Arch Intern Med*, 161, 2467–73.

73. Ryan, D. J., O'Regan, N. A., Caoimh, R. Ó., et al. 2009. Delirium in an adult acute hospital population: predictors, prevalence and detection. *BMJ Open*, 3, pii: e001772.

74. Bellelli, G., Morandi, A., Davis, D. H., et al. 2014. Validation of the 4AT, a new instrument for rapid delirium screening: a study in 234 hospitalised older people. *Age Ageing*, 43, 496–502.

75. De, J., Wand, A. P. F., Smerdely, P. I., and Hunt, G. E. 2016. Validating the 4A's test in screening for delirium in a culturally diverse geriatric inpatient population. *Int J Geriatr Psychiatry*, 32, 1322–9.

76. Voyer, P., Richard, S., McCusker, J., et al. 2012. Detection of delirium and its symptoms by nurses working in a long term care facility. *J Am Med Dir Assoc*, 13, 264–71.

77. Witlox, J., Eurelings, L. S., De Jonghe, J. F., Kalisvaart, K. J., Eikelenboom, P., and Van Gool, W. A. 2010. Delirium in elderly patients and the risk of postdischarge mortality, institutionalization, and dementia: a meta-analysis. *JAMA*, 304, 443–51.

78. Jackson, T. A., Wilson, D., Richardson, S., and Lord, J. M. 2016. Predicting outcome in older hospital patients with delirium: a systematic literature review. *Int J Geriatr Psychiatry*, 31, 392–9.

79. Lin, H. S., Peel, N. M., and Hubbard, R. E. 2016. Baseline Vulnerability and Inpatient Frailty Status in Relation to Adverse Outcomes in a Surgical Cohort. *J Frailty Aging*, 5, 180–2.

80. Muresan, M. L., Adamis, D., Murray, O., O'Mahony, E., and McCarthy, G. 2016. Delirium, how does it end? Mortality as an outcome in older medical inpatients. *Int J Geriatr Psychiatry*, 31, 349–54.

81. Marcantonio, E. R., Kiely, D. K., Simon, S. E., et al. 2005. Outcomes of older people admitted to postacute facilities with delirium. *J Am Geriatr Soc*, 53, 963–9.

82. Salluh, J. I., Wang, H., Schneider, E. B., et al. 2015. Outcome of delirium in critically ill patients: systematic review and meta-analysis. *BMJ*, 350, h2538.

83. Cole, M. G., McCusker, J., Voyer, P., et al. 2013. Symptoms of delirium predict incident delirium in older long-term care residents. *Int Psychogeriatr*, 25, 887–94.

84. Adamis, D., Devaney, A., Shanahan, E., McCarthy, G., and Meagher, D. 2015. Defining 'recovery' for delirium research: a systematic review. *Age Ageing*, 44, 318–21.

85. Reiss, J. and Ankeny, R. A. 2016. Philosophy of medicine. In: Zalta, E. N. (ed.) *The Stanford Encyclopedia of Philosophy*. 06/06/2016 ed.

86. Maldonado, J. R. 2013. Neuropathogenesis of delirium: review of current etiologic theories and common pathways. *Am J Geriatr Psychiatry*, 21, 1190–222.

87. Hall, R. J. and Watne, L. O. 2016. Cerebrospinal fluid levels of neopterin are elevated in delirium after hip fracture. *J Neuroinflammation*, 13, 170.

88. Flink, B. J., Rivelli, S. K., Cox, E. A., *et al.* 2012. Obstructive sleep apnea and incidence of postoperative delirium after elective knee replacement in the nondemented elderly. *Anesthesiology*, 116, 788–96.

89. Kral, V. A. 1973. Psychiatric problems in the aged: a reconsideration. *Can Med Assoc J*, 108, 584 passim.

90. Kazmierski, J., Banys, A., Latek, J., Bourke, J., and Jaszewski, R. 2013. Cortisol levels and neuropsychiatric diagnosis as markers of postoperative delirium: a prospective cohort study. *Crit Care*, 17, R38.

91. Van Munster, B. C., Thomas, C., Kreisel, S. H., *et al.* 2012. Longitudinal assessment of serum anticholinergic activity in delirium of the elderly. *J Psychiatr Res*, 46, 1339–45.

92. Sauër, A. M., Slooter, A. J., Veldhuijzen, D. S., van Eijk, M. M., Devlin, J. W., and van Dijk, D. 2014. Intraoperative dexamethasone and delirium after cardiac surgery: a randomized clinical trial. *Anesth Analg*, 119, 1046–52.

93. Maclullich, A. M., Ferguson, K. J., Miller, T., de Rooij, S. E., and Cunningham, C. 2008. Unravelling the pathophysiology of delirium: a focus on the role of aberrant stress responses. *J Psychosom Res*, 65, 229–38.

94. Tune, L. E., Damlouji, N. F., Holland, A., Gardner, T. J., Folstein, M. F., and Coyle, J. T. 1981. Association of postoperative delirium with raised serum levels of anticholinergic drugs. *Lancet*, 2, 651–3.

95. Schor, J. D., Levkoff, S. E., Lipsitz, L. A., *et al.* 1992. Risk factors for delirium in hospitalized elderly. *JAMA*, 267:827–31.

96. Campbell, N., Perkins, A., Hui, S., Khan, B., and Boustani, M. 2011. Association between prescribing of anticholinergic medications and incident delirium: a cohort study. *J Am Geriatr Soc*, 59 Suppl 2, S277–81.

97. Watne, L. O., Hall, R. J., Molden, E., *et al.* 2014. Anticholinergic activity in cerebrospinal fluid and serum in individuals with hip fracture with and without delirium. *J Am Geriatr Soc*, 62, 94–102.

98. Van Gool, W. A., Van de Beek, D., and Eikelenboom, P. 2010. Systemic infection and delirium: when cytokines and acetylcholine collide. *Lancet*, 375, 773–5.

99. de Rooij, S. E. and van Munster, B. C. 2013. Melatonin deficiency hypothesis in delirium: a synthesis of current evidence. *Rejuvenation Res*, 16, 273–8.

100. De Jonghe, A., Korevaar, J. C., Van Munster, B. C., and De Rooij, S. E. 2010. Effectiveness of melatonin treatment on circadian rhythm disturbances in dementia. Are there implications for delirium? A systematic review. *Int J Geriatr Psychiatry*, 25, 1201–8.

101. de Jonghe, A., van Munster, B. C., Goslings, J. C., *et al.* 2014. Effect of melatonin on incidence of delirium among patients with hip fracture: a multicentre, double-blind randomized controlled trial. *CMAJ*, 186, E547–56.

102. Walker, C. K. and Gales, M. A. 2017. Melatonin Receptor Agonists for Delirium Prevention. *Ann Pharmacother*, 51, 72–8.

103. Cerejeira, J., Firmino, H., Vaz-Serra, A., and Mukaetova-Ladinska, E. B. 2010. The neuroinflammatory hypothesis of delirium. *Acta Neuropathologica*, 119, 737–54.

104. Cunningham, C. and Maclullich, A. M. 2013. At the extreme end of the psychoneuroimmunological spectrum: delirium as a maladaptive sickness behaviour response. *Brain Behav Immun*, 28, 1–13.

105. Davis, D. H., Skelly, D. T., Murray, C., *et al.* 2015. Worsening cognitive impairment and neurodegenerative pathology progressively increase risk for delirium. *Am J Geriatr Psychiatry*, 23, 403–15.

106. Khan, B. A., Zawahiri, M., Campbell, N. L., and Boustani, M. A. 2011. Biomarkers for delirium--a review. *J Am Geriatr Soc*, 59 Suppl 2, S256–61.

107. Holmes, C., Cunningham, C., Zotova, E., Culliford, D., and Perry, V. H. 2011. Proinflammatory cytokines, sickness behavior, and Alzheimer disease. *Neurology*, 77, 212–18.

108. Choi, S. H., Lee, H., Chung, T. S., *et al.* 2012. Neural network functional connectivity during and after an episode of delirium. *Am J Psychiatry*, 169, 498–507.

109. Van Dellen, E., Van der Kooi, A. W., Numan, T., *et al.* 2014. Decreased functional connectivity and disturbed directionality of information flow in the electroencephalography of intensive care unit patients with delirium after cardiac surgery. *Anesthesiology*, 121, 328–35.

110. Mashour, G. A. and Avidan, M. S. 2014. Postoperative delirium: disconnecting the network? *Anesthesiology*, 121, 214–16.

111. Hatano, Y., Narumoto, J., Shibata, K., *et al.* 2013. White-matter hyperintensities predict delirium after cardiac surgery. *Am J Geriatr Psychiatry*, 21, 938–45.

112. Cavallari, M., Hshieh, T. T., Guttmann, C. R., *et al.* 2015. Brain atrophy and white-matter hyperintensities are not significantly associated with incidence and severity of postoperative delirium in older persons without dementia. *Neurobiol Aging*, 36, 2122–9.

113. Cavallari, M., Dai, W., Guttmann, C. R., *et al.* 2016. Neural substrates of vulnerability to postsurgical delirium as revealed by presurgical diffusion MRI. *Brain*, 139, 1282–94.

114. Inouye, S. K. 1999. Predisposing and precipitating factors for delirium in hospitalized older patients. *Dement Geriatr Cogn Disord*, 10, 393–400.

115. Leung, J. M., Sands, L. P., Lim, E., Tsai, T. L., and Kinjo, S. 2013. Does preoperative risk for delirium moderate the effects of postoperative pain and opiate use on postoperative delirium? *Am J Geriatr Psychiatry*, 21, 946–56.

116. Voyer, P., Richard, S., Doucet, L., Cyr, N., and Carmichael, P. H. 2010. Examination of the multifactorial model of delirium among long-term care residents with dementia. *Geriatr Nurs*, 31, 105–14.

117. Abraha, I., Trotta, F., Rimland, J. M., *et al.* 2015. Efficacy of non-pharmacological interventions to prevent and treat delirium in older patients: a systematic overview. The SENATOR project ONTOP Series. *PLoS One*, 10, e0123090.

118. Pitkälä, K. H., Laurila, J. V., Strandberg, T. E., and Tilvis, R. S. 2006. Multicomponent geriatric intervention for elderly inpatients with delirium: a randomized, controlled trial. *J Gerontol A Biol Sci Med Sci*, 61, 176–81.

119. Marcantonio, E. R., Bergmann, M. A., Kiely, D. K., Orav, E. J., and Jones, R. N. 2010. Randomized trial of a delirium abatement program for postacute skilled nursing facilities. *J Am Geriatr Soc*, 58, 1019–26.

120. Rockwood, K. J. 2002. Out of the furrow and into the fire: where do we go with delirium? *CMAJ*, 167, 763–4.

121. Fok, M. C., Sepehry, A. A., Frisch, L., *et al.* 2015. Do antipsychotics prevent postoperative delirium? A systematic review and meta-analysis. *Int J Geriatr Psychiatry*, 30, 333–44.

122. Schrijver, E. J., De Graaf, K., De Vries, O. J., Maier, A. B., and Nanayakkara, P. W. 2016. Efficacy and safety of haloperidol for in-hospital delirium prevention and treatment: a systematic review of current evidence. *Eur J Intern Med*, 27, 14–23.

123. Kishi, T., Hirota, T., Matsunaga, S., and Iwata, N. 2016. Antipsychotic medications for the treatment of delirium: a systematic review and meta-analysis of randomised controlled trials. *J Neurol Neurosurg Psychiatry*, 87, 767–74.

124. Neufeld, K. J., Yue, J., Robinson, T. N., Inouye, S. K., and Needham, D. M. 2016. Antipsychotic medication for prevention

and treatment of delirium in hospitalized adults: a systematic review and meta-analysis. *J Am Geriatr Soc*, 64, 705–14.

125. Meagher, D. J., McLoughlin, L., Leonard, M., Hannon, N., Dunne, C., and O'Regan, N. 2013. What do we really know about the treatment of delirium with antipsychotics? Ten key issues for delirium pharmacotherapy. *Am J Geriatr Psychiatry*, 21, 1223–38.

126. Boettger, S., Jenewein, J., and Breitbart, W. 2015. Haloperidol, risperidone, olanzapine and aripiprazole in the management of delirium: a comparison of efficacy, safety, and side effects. *Palliat Support Care*, 13, 1079–85.

127. Yoon, H. J., Park, K. M., Choi, W. J., *et al.* 2013. Efficacy and safety of haloperidol versus atypical antipsychotic medications in the treatment of delirium. *BMC Psychiatry*, 13, 240.

128. Caputo, F., Vignoli, T., Leggio, L., Addolorato, G., Zoli, G., and Bernardi, M. 2012. Alcohol use disorders in the elderly: a brief overview from epidemiology to treatment options. *Exp Gerontol*, 47, 411–16.

129. Freter, S., Koller, K., Dunbar, M., Macknight, C., and Rockwood, K. 2017. Translating delirium prevention strategies for elderly adults with hip fracture into routine clinical care: a pragmatic clinical trial. *J Am Geriatr Soc*, 65, 567–73.

130. Teale, E. and Young, J. 2015. Multicomponent delirium prevention: not as effective as NICE suggest? *Age Ageing*, 44, 915–17.

131. O'Hanlon, S., O'Regan, N., Maclullich, A. M., *et al.* 2014. Improving delirium care through early intervention: from bench to bedside to boardroom. *J Neurol Neurosurg Psychiatry*, 85, 207–13.

132. Pasin, L., Landoni, G., Nardelli, P. *et al.* 2014. Dexmedetomidine reduces the risk of delirium, agitation and confusion in critically Ill patients: a meta-analysis of randomized controlled trials. *J Cardiothorac Vasc Anesth*, 28, 1459–66.

133. Litton, E., Carnegie, V., Elliott, R., and Webb, S.A. 2016. The Efficacy of Earplugs as a Sleep Hygiene Strategy for Reducing Delirium in the ICU: A Systematic Review and Meta-Analysis. *Crit Care Med*, 44, 992–9.

134. Al-Qadheeb, N. S., Balk, E. M., Fraser, G. L., *et al.* 2014. Randomized ICU trials do not demonstrate an association between interventions that reduce delirium duration and short-term mortality: a systematic review and meta-analysis. *Crit Care Med*, 42, 1442–54.

135. Clegg, A., Siddiqi, N., Heaven, A., Young, J., and Holt, R. 2014. Interventions for preventing delirium in older people in institutional long-term care. *Cochrane Database Syst Rev*, 1, CD009537.

# 40

# Alzheimer's disease

*Ivan Koychev and John Gallacher*

## Introduction

Worldwide, 47.5 million people have dementia. The total number of people with dementia is expected to reach 75.5 million by 2030 and 135.5 million by 2050 [1, 2]. In the UK, dementia has become the leading cause of death in women and is second to heart disease for men [3]. The most common cause of dementia is Alzheimer's disease (AD), being implicated in up to 70% of dementia cases [4]. The tragic combination of symptoms present in AD has a profound emotional and resource-intensive impact on patients, family, friends, and carers.

## Clinical features

Typical early symptoms include absent-mindedness, difficulty re-calling names and words, difficulty learning new information, disorientation in unfamiliar surroundings, and reduced social en-gagement. Atypical, non-amnestic forms also exist where the ini-tial presentation is dominated by visual agnosia (posterior cortical atrophy), word-finding difficulties (logopenic—primary progressive aphasia), or dysexecutive syndrome (presents as fronto-temporal dementia phenocopy). As the disease progresses, there is marked memory loss and loss of other cognitive skills, including a reduced vocabulary and less complex speech patterns. This may be accom-panied by mood swings, apathy, a decline in social skills, and the emergence of psychotic phenomena. Advanced AD is character-ized by monosyllabic speech, psychotic symptoms, behavioural dis-turbance, loss of bladder and bowel control, and reduced mobility. Nevertheless, due to the mixed nature of dementia pathologies, the differential diagnosis of AD is inexact. For example, AD frequently occurs in the presence of vascular changes, indicating a coexisting vascular dementia. Without imaging and neurocognitive test evi-dence, the early stages in atypical AD may not be distinguishable from other neuropathologies. The lack of certainty is reflected in the NINDS-ADRDRA diagnostic category of 'probable AD' [5]. Post-mortem examination reveals that AD brains are characterized by the aggregation and accumulations of inter-neuronal amyloid (de-scribed as amyloid plaques) and intra-neuronal tau (described as neurofibrillary tangles) proteins.

There are two separate AD expressions, based on their age of onset and underlying genetics. In early-onset AD, also known as dominantly inherited or familial AD (fAD) due to its high inherit-ability, symptoms can begin in a person's late 20s through to their 50s. Late-onset AD, also known as sporadic AD (sAD), has more varied genetic determinants, but they individually and collectively have less impact. In sAD, there is a greater influence of environmental risk factors such as exercise, alcohol consumption, and obesity. In sAD, symptoms rarely occur before the age of 65. Although the range and complexity of causal factors may be greater in sAD, the disease pro-cesses are sufficiently similar for both to result in comparable symp-tomatology and neuropathology. This has allowed fAD to be used as a model for sAD [6].

Current convention set by the National Institute on Aging–Alzheimer's Association Workgroup differentiates core clinical and research diagnostic criteria [7]. In clinical practice, the diagnosis of probable AD requires the presence of dementia (either amnestic or non-amnestic in terms of affected cognitive domain) that is of in-sidious onset, represents a deterioration from the individual's base-line, and is not more likely to be accounted for by another cause (for example, other types of dementia or other neurological or med-ical comorbidities). The term mild cognitive impairment (MCI) has additionally been introduced to recognize states of pre-dementia where cognitive impairment does not interfere to a significant extent in the patient's function. The research AD criteria see the addition of two sets of biomarkers: pathophysiology and neuronal injury. The former is defined by the presence of AD pathology (low CSF Aβ-42 levels or positive PET amyloid imaging). The major neuronal injury biomarkers are elevated levels of CSF tau, reduced temporo-parietal glucose uptake, as measured by [18]fluorodeoxyglucose PET, and disproportionate atrophy in the temporal and parietal lobes using structural neuroimaging. The current recommendation is that the biomarker-enhanced AD diagnosis is not used in routine clinical practice, as the core clinical criteria have good diagnostic accuracy for the majority of patients, while the biomarker criteria require fur-ther validation and standardization across laboratories.

## Epidemiology

fAD accounts for less than 5% of AD cases, and due to its herit-ability, most cases are easily identified [8]. Characterizing the preva-lence, incidence, and risk factor profile of sAD, however, is more challenging due to the subtle and insidious onset of symptoms, the stigma associated with a dementia diagnosis, and the limited availability of diagnostic tools. Accurate diagnosis, particularly in the early disease stages, is difficult and requires (preferably serial) structural and molecular brain imaging, as well as CSF analysis. These highly specialized data are rarely available in population studies, being confined to clinical studies.

In a systematic review of 45 studies of sAD, with 20 studies eligible for meta-analysis of participants aged 60+ years, the overall prevalence was 4%, ranging from 1.5% in India to 20% in Israel. In community settings, the prevalence was 3%, while in institutional settings, the prevalence ranged between 10% and 23%. Age-specific prevalence of sAD increases from around 1% at age 60 years to 2% at age 65, 5% at age 70, 10% at age 75, and 20% at age 80 to rates of around 30% at age 90 [9, 10].

In a systematic review of 30 studies, with 11 studies eligible for meta-analysis of participants aged 60+ years, the pooled annual incidence of sAD was 1.6%. All studies in this meta-analysis were in community settings, with estimates ranging between 0.7% in an Italian study to 3% in an American study. Age-specific incidence rates go from around 0.2% at 65 years to 6% at 90 years [9]. A more sophisticated analysis, adjusting for competing morbidities and attrition, but using non-specified dementia as an outcome, confirms these systematic review estimates [11].

Until the age of 85, AD incidence rates for men and women are comparable [12]. Beyond the age of 85, incident AD is lower in men, although vascular dementia risk in men rises. The resulting balance of risk is for an overall increased risk of incident dementia in women at older age. The extent to which this is due to greater female survival is unknown.

A comparison of dementia across 20 years (1989–2008) in the UK shows a recent and modest decline in annual incidence from 2% to 1.7% [13]. This is more pronounced in men and is attributed to an improvement in lifestyle over this period. Although these numbers refer to dementia, given the mixed pathology of many dementias, similar changes are unlikely not to be reflected in sAD. This drop in incidence, although encouraging, will do little to ameliorate the population impact of sAD. Due to the increasing numbers of older people, the overall numbers of sAD cases will continue to rise. Similar trends are found elsewhere [14]. These findings are consistent with the fall in AD after the age of 98 found in post-mortem studies [15].

## Neuropathology

AD is a protein abnormality resulting in relentlessly progressive neurodegeneration. The molecular biology underlying AD is complex and incompletely understood. Interest has focused on the two main brain protein accumulations that are characteristic of AD: amyloid and tau. The β-amyloid protein (Aβ) is prone to aggregation when it fails to fold into the three-dimensional structure that is essential to its function. The misfolded Aβ monomers progressively aggregate, forming oligomers, then fibrils, and then into relatively disordered clumps of fibrils known as plaque. Tau protein stabilizes extracellular clumps, which are essential to a number of cellular processes. It has a number of phosphorylation sites. Hyperphosphorylation at these sites inhibits microtubule assembly

and sequesters normally phosphorylated tau, causing microtubule disassembly. Hyperphosphorylated tau self-assembles into paired helices and straight filaments, which aggregate as tangles.

These accumulations of misfolded proteins are intracellular tangles of protein processing abnormalities. Although these endpoints are unlikely to represent the initial neuropathological triggers, with time (and increasing age), accumulation of misfolded proteins may result in further cellular changes to oxidative and inflammatory pathways, leading to energy failure, axonal transportation failure, synaptic dysfunction, and neuronal death.

## Genetics

The genetic variants causing fAD are found in the β-amyloid precursor protein (*APP*), presenilin-1 (*PSEN1*), and presenilin-2 (*PSEN2*) genes [16]. These genes are located on chromosomes 21, 14, and 1, respectively. Of the 30 known coding mutations in the *APP* gene, 25 result in over-production of Aβ, resulting in AD. Most of these variants are highly penetrant, that is, almost all individuals carrying the variant will develop AD. One variant (A673T) reduces Aβ production and is protective against AD [17]. PSEN1 and PSEN2 contribute to the γ-secretase complex, which processes APP. The *PSEN1* and *PSEN2* genes each contains ten coding exons, several variants of which increase the production of the longer forms of Aβ, that is, those which are more likely to misfold.

The genetics of sAD are more complex, involving a greater variety of genes, each with lower penetrance. The apolipoprotein E (*APOE*) gene is the strongest genetic risk factor for sAD [18]. Of the three common alleles, ε4 is associated with a higher risk of AD relative to ε3, while ε2 is associated with a lower risk relative to ε3 [19]. The three alleles are expressed unevenly in the general population, with 60–90% being ε3 carriers, 10–20% carrying ε4, and 0–20% ε2 [20]. A single ε4 allele confers a 3-fold greater risk, while two ε4 alleles confer a 12-fold greater risk. APOE binds to Aβ and is involved on the clearance of Aβ from the brain. Genome-wide association studies (GWAS) have identified other genetic variants related to AD risk [21–23]. These genes affect a wide range of mechanisms. Although these risk variants can be relatively common in the general population (3–50%), their individual contribution to AD risk is small. Although the specific AD-related functionality of the risk variants is largely unknown, likely areas of action can be identified. Reduced expression of the clusterin gene (*CLU*) is associated with a higher risk of AD, clusterin being involved in Aβ clearance [16]. Variants in the ATP-binding cassette transporter A7 (*ABCA7*) gene that reduce gene expression are associated with an increased AD risk. *ABCA7* deletion facilitated the processing of APP to Aβ by increasing the levels of the β-site APP cleaving enzyme 1 (BACE1) [16]. Several genes have been associated with the immune response (*CR1*, *CD33*, *MS4A*, *TREM2*). The relationship between the immune response and AD is complex, but in general, upregulation of the immune response is associated with a raised AD risk. A further constellation of AD risk genes is associated with endocytosis (*BIN1*, *PICAML*, *CD2AP*, *SORL1*). Endocytosis is critical to many aspects of neuronal health, including APP processing (*BIN1*), Aβ clearance (*PICALM*), synapse formation (*CD2AP*), and APP cleavage and APOE uptake (*SORL1*). Although each of these GWAS-identified genes contributes only a small degree of AD risk, in combination,

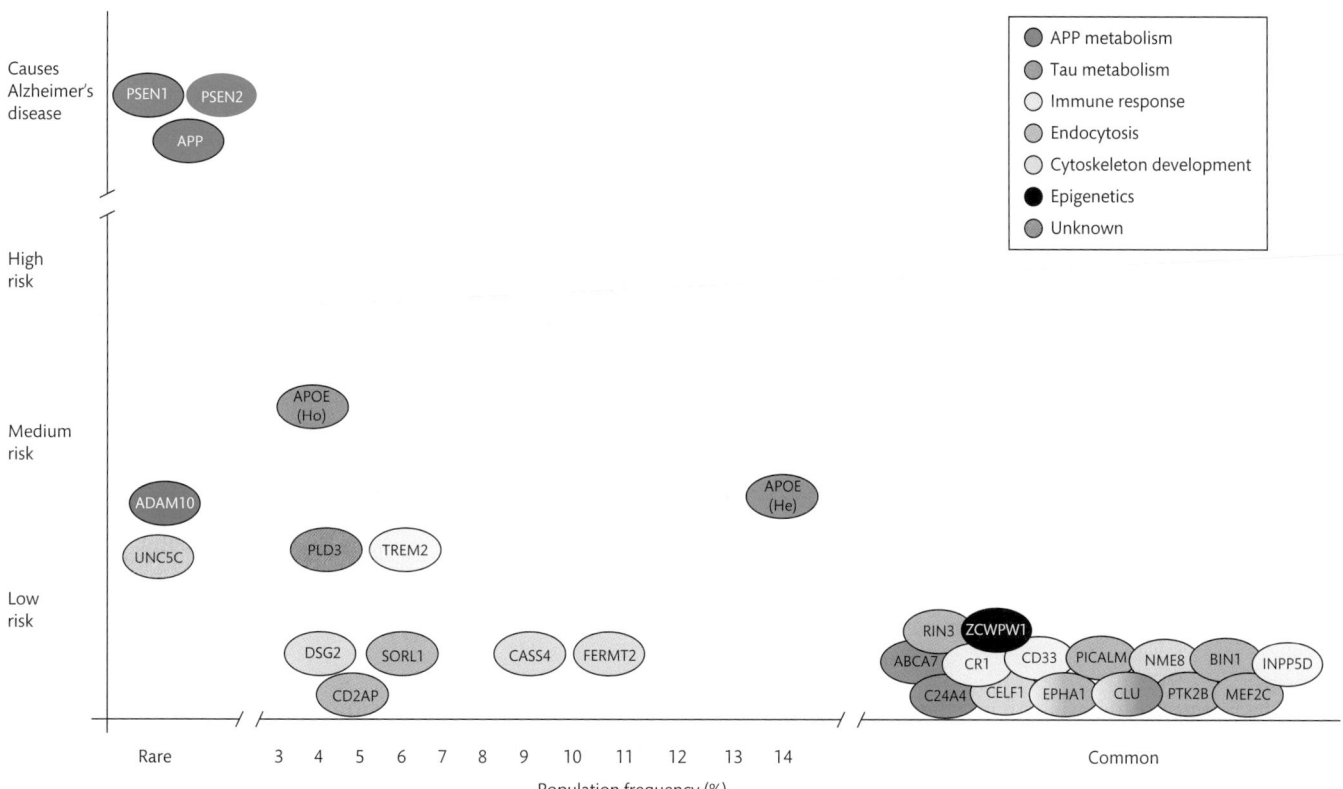

**Fig. 40.1** (see Colour Plate section) Risk genes for Alzheimer's disease identifying the primary mechanism, risk conferred, and population allele frequency.

Adapted from *Biol Psychiatry*, 77(1), Karch CM, Goate AM, Alzheimer's disease risk genes and mechanisms of disease pathogenesis, pp. 43–51, Copyright (2015), with permission from Society of Biological Psychiatry.

the risk increases. Although the patterns of association are complex, put simply, if APOE is included in the polygenic risk estimate, comparison of the extremely high and extremely low polygenic risk score groups can predict AD with >80% accuracy [24–26]. The range of risk genes is summarized in Fig. 40.1 (adapted from Karch and Goate [16]), giving the primary mechanism, risk conferred, and population allele frequency.

## Mechanisms

That sAD is genetically heterogenous suggests it is unlikely that a single mechanism will fully explain the variety of protein–protein interactions underlying the disease. AD may best be considered as a multifactorial disorder—a common outcome from multiple neuropathologic pathways. A parsimonious and necessarily simplistic working model would be the expression of amyloid and tau protein folding abnormalities which not only exert direct neurotoxic effects, but also promote an innate immune response, leading to synaptic failure, neurodegeneration, and apoptosis. Tau and amyloid may have a synergistic impact on the immune response, serving to accelerate neurodegeneration. Injury to the neurovascular unit may increase susceptibility to AD through large-vessel atheroma and disruption to the blood–brain barrier. Finally, the systematic spread of amyloid and tau suggests that extracellular misfolded amyloid and tau protein may 'seed' protein misfolding in surrounding cells.

### Beta amyloid

AD-specific initiating events include Aβ processing [27]. Aβ is an albumoid (albumin-like) peptide synthesized from APP. Aβ peptides are natural products of metabolism. Aβ is formed by the processing of APP by sequential enzymatic cleavage involving α, β, and γ-secretase. There are six known isoforms of Aβ, which vary in length from 36 to 43 peptides [4]. The amyloid hypothesis is that the longer isoforms, that is, Aβ ≥42 peptides, which are more self-aggregating, are over-produced intracellularly throughout life in fAD and gradually rise extracellularly with age due to faulty clearance mechanisms in sAD. From this perspective, both fAD and sAD point to APP processing as being the trigger for AD.

### Transmembrane APP processing

APP produced within the cell is cleaved, as it passes through the cell membrane (Fig. 40.2). Non-amyloidogenic cleavage of APP begins with α-secretase cleavage of APP, leading to the release of the fragment sAPPα into the intercellular space; sAPPα contributes to synapse formation and repair. sAPPα includes part of the Aβ sequence and so precludes the formation of Aβ. The remaining APP (in the form of the C83 fragment), still tethered to the cell membrane, is cleaved by γ-secretase, releasing P3 fragment into the intercellular space and the APP intracellular domain (AICD) back into the cell.

Amyloidogenic cleavage begins with β-secretase activity, leading to the release of a shortened fragment (sAPPβ) into the extracellular space, leaving the Aβ peptide intact. The remaining APP (in the form of the C99 fragment), still tethered to the cell membrane, is

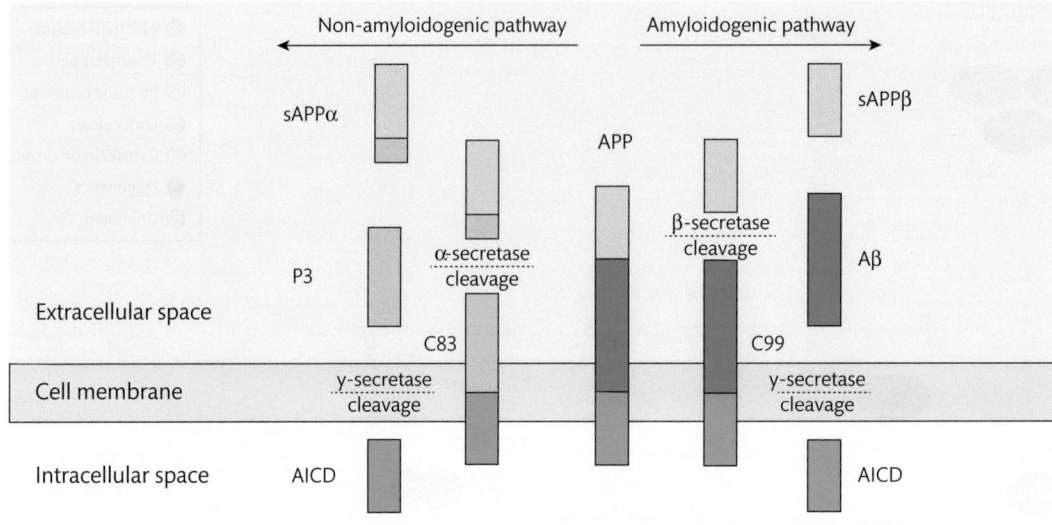

**Fig. 40.2** (see Colour Plate section) Schematic of amyloidogenic and non-amyloidogenic APP processing pathways.

cleaved by γ-secretase, releasing Aβ into the intercellular space and AICD back into the cell. γ Mitochondrial mass changes occur in the AD brain -secretase cleavage proceeds in a number of steps, beginning with ε-cleavage releasing either Aβ48 or Aβ49, which are then processed, leading to the release of extracellular Aβ [28].

Newly cleaved monomeric Aβ aggregates into oligomers, which, in turn, become fibrils and then plaques. Plaque formation is a dynamic process, with individual oligomers aggregating and disaggregating. Relatively diffuse plaques occur in normal ageing. In AD, plaques are Aβ42 rich, more frequent, and more compact, consisting of a central core of amyloid fibrils. Apart from stimulating an inflammatory response, it is difficult to see how plaques affect cell function, and plaque formation may be thought of as a compensatory mechanism to isolate harmful species. That plaques are surrounded by dystrophic neurites and astrocytes suggests they are not entirely inert, and the dynamic nature of Aβ aggregation suggests that it is the presence of aggregating oligomers that is neurotoxic and stimulates an immune response. Extracellular oligomeric Aβ has been shown to interfere with synaptic function, adversely affecting long-term potentiation (LTP). This, in turn, downregulates the translation of neurotransmitters at the synapse, leading to the withdrawal of dendritic spines. In the case of the hippocampus, this effectively inhibits new memories from forming and established memories being retained.

For fAD, genetic variants that are related to AD risk increase the level of either Aβ42 or the Aβ42/Aβ40 ratio. For sAD, the key genetic risk factor is APOE. In the brain, most APOE is expressed by astrocytes. Although its function and activity are not fully understood, APOE has an affinity for Aβ, binding to form a protein complex. APOE alleles vary in their Aβ binding ability, with E2 > E3 > E4. The production of Aβ does not appear to vary according to APOE genotype. The lack of variation in production, combined with variation in binding, suggests that for sAD, it is the amyloid clearance mechanism that is not operating efficiently [18]. This is consistent with evidence that in AD, CNS Aβ is lower, suggesting that Aβ is being retained in the brain.

## Intracellular APP processing

APP in the cytosol is also processed within the cell, although this process is less well understood. Several studies have demonstrated that α- and β-secretases are present in the ER, enabling APP cleavage [29, 30]. As in the plasma membrane, α- and β-secretases compete with each other for intracellular APP cleavage; this competition modulates the production of Aβ. It has also been shown that γ-secretase activity is located predominantly in a specialized subcompartment of the ER—the mitochondria-associated membrane (MAM). MAM is an intracellular lipid, raft-like structure intimately involved in cholesterol and phospholipid metabolism and is physically and biochemically connected to mitochondria. The area of close apposition between mitochondria and MAM is substantially enlarged in AD. Release of Aβ from the ER into the cytosol and exposure of Aβ to mitochondria suggest intracellular neurotoxic mechanisms.

Mitochondrial mass changes occur in the AD brain. Although the total amount of mitochondria may increase, in hippocampal neurons, there is a decline in the number of intact mitochondria and an increase in the number of degraded mitochondria. A case can be made that the brain of AD subjects show perturbed mitochondrial function and a subsequent compensatory response. The bioenergetics evidence has led to the mitochondrial cascade hypothesis, where mitochondrial dysfunction initiates the preferential production of intracellular Aβ42. However, the balance of evidence is in favour of APP processing as an initiating event and that an effect of mitochondrial function on intracellular Aβ is subsequent to the initial production of Aβ oligomers.

## Tau

Tau is more closely associated with cognitive performance than Aβ [31–33], and porcine evidence suggests tau is required for Aβ-mediated toxicity [34]. Furthermore, extracellular and intracellular Aβ do not immediately explain the development of the tau-based neurofibrillary tangles that are characteristic of AD [35].

Tau is a soluble protein found abundantly in neurons and is one of three microtubule-associated proteins (MAPs) which promote the assembly and stability of microtubules in the neuron, microtubules being essential to axoplasmic flow which is critical for neuronal activity. The ability of tau to support microtubule structure is dependent on the level of phosphorylation [36]. Optimal phosphorylation occurs with the phosphorylation of around 30 of the 85 potential sites. Hyperphosphorylated tau has several cytotoxic effects. As the number of phosphorylated sites increase beyond 30, tau loses the ability to bind with microtubules. Hyperphosphorylated tau also sequesters normal tau and other MAPs from the microtubule lattice into the cytosol. This destabilizes the microtubule, leading to disassembly. Microtubule network dysfunction leads to loss of axonal transportation and neurodegeneration. Apart from affecting normal microtubule function, hyperphosphorylated tau is associated with conformational changes, leading to misfolding and increased aggregation. As with mature Aβ plaques, mature neurofibrillary tangles are relatively inert, suggesting that it is monomeric and oligomeric hyperphosphorylated tau that is cytotoxic, that is, it is the soluble species, rather than the neurofibrillary tangle itself [37].

A link between tau phosphorylation and APP processing in the cell membrane has been shown, although the full pathway is not clear [36]. In stem cell models, changes in tau production and tau phosphorylation are associated with APP processing through β- and γ-secretase activity. Inhibition of β-secretase reduced tau levels and phosphorylation, while inhibition of γ-secretase was associated with increased tau and tau phosphorylation [29]. Modulation (enhancement) of γ-secretase was associated with reduced tau production. Limiting β-secretase function reduces the release of APP-C99, while limiting γ-secretase function reduces the release of both APP-C99 and APP-C83 (Fig. 40.2). Enhancing γ-secretase function increases the release of APP-99 and APP-83, which accumulate in the cell. These findings suggest that tau production and tau phosphorylation occur as part of an APP processing pathway, which is independent of extracellular Aβ levels. How phosphorylated tau affects cell function is largely unknown. One possible mechanism is a gradual loss of axonal function through the disassembly of microtubules, leading to an immune response and apoptosis. APOE4 is associated with increased tau phosphorylation [38]. Although the mechanisms are unclear, that APOE4 acts independently on both tau and Aβ opens the possibility that tau and Aβ may act synergistically to accelerate neurodegeneration.

## Immune response

Several strands of evidence suggest a general upregulation of the immune response, associated with a raised AD risk. Genetic evidence for an immune response to plaque comes from the overexpression of genes (*Trem2, CR1, CD33*) that are associated with plaque phagocytosis [39–42]. The co-location of plaque with astrocytes and other glial elements and the presence of inflammatory and complement cascade components implicate an innate and adaptive immune response to the presence of plaque. This response is likely to be subsequent to the triggering events surrounding APP processing but serves to accelerate AD pathology. Although the immune response may be targeted at plaque removal, by microglial phagocytosis, for example, it is unlikely not to affect the surrounding neurons. The associated increasing concentrations of reactive oxygen species and inflammatory cytokines, for example, will affect the function and

integrity of the plasma membrane. As described, the increased susceptibility to AD, associated with an upregulated immune response, may be largely a response to abnormal APP processing. However, it may be that upregulation provides a cellular environment that also facilitates abnormal APP processing.

## Synaptic failure

Although proteinopathy may initiate neurodegeneration, AD is functionally a reflection of synaptic failure leading to neuronal loss [43]. Synaptic loss is more prevalent in the vicinity of Aβ plaques, suggesting plaques are a source of synaptotoxic molecules [44]. Hippocampal synapses begin to decline in patients with mild cognitive impairment in whom the remaining synaptic profiles show compensatory increases in size. In mild AD, there is a reduction of about 25% in the presynaptic vesicle protein synaptophysin. With advancing disease, synapses are disproportionately lost, relative to neurons, and this loss is the best correlate with clinical symptoms of dementia. Experimental application and expression of Aβ, especially oligomers, impair synaptic plasticity by altering the balance between LTP and long-term depression (LTD) in favour of LTD. LTP refers to the increase in dendritic spine development, while LTD causes spine shrinkage and collapse, thus reducing the number of dendritic spines [45]. At high concentrations, oligomers may suppress basal synaptic transmission. From *in vitro* studies, Aβ is associated with disruption of the release of presynaptic neurotransmitters and postsynaptic glutamate receptor ion currents [46, 47]. For example, Aβ binds to α-7 nicotinic acetylcholine receptors, impairing the release of acetylcholine and the maintenance of LTP. Although a reduction in LTP is found in normal ageing, it may be that Aβ triggers synaptic deficits earlier.

## Circulatory and metabolic factors

Vascular injury and the resulting parenchymal inflammation perpetuate the cycle of protein misfolding. Although cases of 'pure' AD are recognized, most AD cases are mixed, combining features of both AD and vascular disease [4]. This has led to an increased interest in the neurovascular unit—the close anatomical and functional relationship between the cellular components of the brain [48]. Aβ is toxic to endothelial and smooth muscles cells and compromises the Aβ influx and efflux mechanisms of the blood–brain barrier [49]. A further factor is the reduced cerebral blood flow typically found in AD [50]. The extent to which this reflects reduced demand or inadequate supply is moot.

Metabolic factors focus on the insulin signalling pathway. Glucose intolerance and type 2 diabetes are risk factors for AD. Several models have been proposed to explain the increased insulin resistance underlying these associations [51]. These focus on deregulated insulin signalling affecting the energy available to the cell, increased inflammatory response, increased Aβ production, and compromised synaptic transmission. However, the direction of causality involved in these associations is unclear.

## Propagation

Mechanisms underlying the spread of AD pathology, typically beginning in the entorhinal cortex have focused on the prion hypothesis, which is that the process is dependent on the nucleating properties of misfolded protein and the transmission of misfolded protein between cells [52, 53]. In this model, misfolded protein acts as a template for further misfolding, accelerating the misfolding process. If the misfolded protein is released into the extracellular space and endocytosed into a neighbouring cell, the misfolding process is transmitted independently of the receiving cell's intrinsic ability to misfold the protein [54, 55]. In AD, there is evidence that both Aβ and tau can be transmitted between cells. This 'prion' model does not replace the basic trigger mechanism of APP processing. It is likely that populations of cells, subject to proteolytic 'stresses' (genetic or otherwise), independently produce misfolded protein and that the seeding of these proteins further distributes pathology.

## Treatment

Significant advances in the understanding of AD pathophysiology and corresponding investment in the development of potential disease-modifying treatment have so far not led to effective aetiological therapy, with several notable failed agents. The only licensed treatment of AD is therefore symptomatic, with two drug classes available: acetylcholinesterase inhibitors (donepezil, rivastigmine, and galantamine) and the NMDA receptor antagonist galantamine. The former are licensed for mild to moderate AD, while memantine can be used in moderate to severe AD. The most recent guidelines recommend a combination between the two classes in moderate and severe AD cases [56]. The expected benefit is stabilization of cognitive decline for a period of 6–12 months, with, on average, nine patients needed to be treated for one of them to experience significant benefit (that is, number needed to treat of 9). Despite the modest immediate benefits associated with these drugs, they appear to have some additional effects in those treated long term. In the Donepezil and Memantine in Moderate to Severe Alzheimer's Disease (DOMINO) study, Howard and co-authors examined the effects of continuing symptomatic treatment beyond the stage of moderate to severe dementia; a sample of patients on stable donepezil dose were randomized to: (1) continue the drug; (2) discontinue the drug; or (3) switch to, or add, memantine. In this study, the group that discontinued symptomatic treatment had faster cognitive decline and worse functional outcomes [57] and were admitted to care more quickly [58]. These results led to the current consensus guideline that 'cholinesterase inhibitors should not be stopped just because the point of severe dementia has been reached' [59].

The transition of prodromal and subclinical AD is accompanied by the emergence of a variety of behavioural and psychological symptoms of dementia (BPSD). These include depression (comorbidity of AD and depression in up to 50%), psychosis, agitation, aggression, sleep disturbance, wandering, apathy, and a variety of socially inappropriate behaviours. Some of these symptoms affect practically all patients with dementia at some point of the illness and are a major cause of loss of independence, carer burden, and early placement into nursing care [60]. Current guidelines advocate the use of non-pharmacological strategies to prevent and address problem behaviours in dementia [61]. Pharmacological treatment of aggression through sedation is limited to acute settings to prevent injury with long-term use of dopamine antagonists, which is being actively discouraged due to a 3-fold elevation in risk for cerebrovascular events. Drugs for psychosis, such as risperidone, offer some efficacy in terms of improving recurrent agitation and psychosis symptoms, which warrants careful consideration of risk/benefits.

SSRIs may be a better alternative, with evidence of citalopram and sertraline, in particular, for beneficial effects on agitation and psychosis. Also, long-term treatment with a drug for depression should be a consideration where there is comorbid depression, although the evidence for efficacy is weak [60]. Careful risk/benefit consideration is also applicable here, given the higher likelihood of SSRIs causing hyponatraemia and gastrointestinal bleeding in the elderly.

## Care

The care for individuals with dementia is a major societal challenge, with an estimation of care costs in the United States alone standing at $203 billion in 2013 and expected to rise to $1.2 trillion in 2050 [63]. This is due to individuals with dementia requiring significantly higher levels of care than other chronic conditions. This level of need, as a rule, leads to care in nursing homes, with four-fifths of all residents suffering from dementia. Still, the majority of dementia patients are being looked after by their families in their homes. Such informal care is associated with significant carer strain, with higher levels of stress, less time for social interaction, and high prevalence of dropping out of work or otherwise missing job opportunities, relative to carers of other chronic conditions [63]. Carers are also at significantly higher risk for psychological problems (for example, depression risk is 3–39 times higher than age-matched controls [64]) and physical deterioration (carers experiencing stress have a 60% higher risk of mortality over 4 years, relative to those who do not report stress [65]). Informal care, however, is and will remain critical to the sustainability of looking after dementia. Long-term strategies therefore focus on reducing carer burden through complex interventions, focusing on education, training, practical support, and respite. A typical intervention lasts 8–12 weeks and includes individual or family counselling, case management, education on strategies for managing behaviours, and environmental modifications. Such interventions result in improvement of carer mental health and increase the time to institutionalization by up to a year [66].

## Prevention

Prevention of sAD has been identified by the WHO and G8 as a key element in the strategy to counter the dementia epidemic. Economic analyses have shown that delaying the onset of the disease by even 1 year would reduce its prevalence by up to 11%, while a delay of 5 years would halve it [67].

### Risk factors

A number of risk factors for sAD have been identified. Non-modifiable risk factors can be used for targeting therapies in appropriate groups. The best established non-modifiable risk factors for sAD are age, genetics, and female sex. These are discussed in the relevant Epidemiology and Genetics sections of this chapter. Modifiable risk factors are the logical focus of prevention strategies. Attributing population risk estimates, that is, the proportion of the population for whom a risk factor has caused a disease, is particularly challenging for sAD. Apart from most risk factor studies focusing on non-specific dementia as an outcome, rather than sAD, the major modifiable risk factors for sAD (lifestyle, comorbidities, education) are unlikely to impact sAD independently of each other. Nevertheless, an overall estimate is that between a third and a half of all sAD cases are attributable to modifiable risk factors [68].

Lifestyle risk factors, such as exercise, diet, smoking, excessive alcohol use, and associated cardiovascular risk, are the main focus of prevention programmes in sAD. This focus predicates a life course approach to dementia prevention, as these risk factors frequently represent chronic exposures and exposure at some life stages may be more harmful than at others.

## Cardiovascular factors

The major modifiable cardiovascular risk factors (hypertension, diabetes, obesity) increase the likelihood of not only the vascular subtype of dementia, but also sAD. This is due to the two conditions frequently sharing neurodegenerative pathologies—it is likely that cardiovascular disease potentiates sAD pathology through disruption of the blood–brain barrier and atherosclerotic, inflammatory, and/or thrombotic mechanisms. Hypertension was identified as a major risk factor through cohorts such as the Goteborg Longitudinal Study [69] and the Honolulu Asia Aging Study [70]. They demonstrated a strong relationship between mid-life hypertension and dementia in later life, but also that a decline in blood pressure levels frequently precedes the development of sAD. This had previously led to the distorted view that low blood pressure predisposes to sAD. Direct evidence of sAD-protective effects of long-term blood pressure control is currently lacking, despite significant evidence of the benefit of blood pressure therapies on overall mortality and morbidity [71]. Late-life diabetes has been consistently linked to both sAD and vascular dementia. Trials exploring the protective effect of strict diabetic control on cognition had conflicting results; this may have been due to tighter control being associated with cognitive benefits, but also increasing the risk of hypoglycaemic episodes, a known risk factor for dementia onset [72]. The evidence for up to 50% increase in sporadic dementia risk by mid-life diabetes comes from health record studies, for example an American study of 8845 patient records [73]. While obesity and associated hypercholesterolaemia in middle age have not been shown to directly increase the risk for sAD [72], it is nonetheless a rational target for prevention, given their established role as cardiovascular risk factors. In later life, perhaps counterintuitively, body mass index reduction precedes the development of sAD by 5–15 years [74]. Current research therefore demonstrates the importance of addressing cardiovascular risk factors from a life course perspective, with emphasis on mid-life risk factor control.

## Alcohol and smoking

Smoking is a major risk factor for sAD and the only one with a good level of evidence for the protective effect of intervention. Specifically, current smokers have a 50% increase in their sAD risk, relative to never-smokers. The effect appears to be mediated by a direct effect on amyloid metabolism (reduction in microglia-mediated amyloid clearance), as well as the well-described effect of increasing cardiovascular risk. It is plausible that the true risk for sAD is underestimated due to the greatly reduced life expectancy associated with smoking—analyses aiming to account for the missing smokers support this. In addition, heavy smokers who survive to old age are likely to be biologically unusual individuals who have a variety of protective factors against cardiovascular risks that may also confer

protection against sAD. Importantly, smoking cessation leads to a reduction of sAD risk to the level of never-smokers [72], which is hugely encouraging for prevention programmes.

The association with alcohol consumption is less clear. A recent meta-analysis demonstrated a modest protective effect for moderate drinkers vs abstainers, while heavy drinkers had comparable risk with abstainers [72]. This 'J'-shaped curve, reminiscent of that found between alcohol and cardiovasular disease, likely reflects several competing mechanisms. These include the 'sick-quitter' effect where higher-risk individuals stop drinking prior to the onset of symptoms, the underreporting of alcohol consumption at high levels of intake, and under-representation of high-risk individuals with high alcohol of intake. Although plausible protective mechanisms for a protective effect of moderate alcohol on the cerebrovascular system exist, population-based 30-year follow-up imaging evidence showed no benefits of light drinking, with hippocampal atrophy rising dose-dependently [75].

## Physical exercise and cognitive stimulation

Regular exercise is recommended as a means of reducing cardiovascular, as well as broader health, risk and therefore has the potential for indirectly reducing sAD risk. In addition, exercise improves cerebral perfusion, has anti-inflammatory properties, improves synaptic function, and stimulates neurogenesis [76]. It also has a social and cognitive element, which is protective in terms of mental health more broadly. A systematic review of the effects of physical effects on sAD risk in older adults showed a 50% sAD risk reduction in those exercising regularly [77]. Interpretation of these data, however, is limited by the possibility that lower physical activity may be part of the dementia prodrome, either through apathy or through broader functional impairment (reverse causality).

Similarly, cognitively stimulating activities are of great interest as potential protective strategies. The available studies point to a consistent reduction of sAD risk in older adults who engage in intellectually challenging activities vs passive activities such as watching TV. These effects suffer from the same limitation as physical exercise where a gradual reduction in engagement with intellectual activities may be the first sign of incipient dementia. Some evidence, however, exists linking intellectual activity in early and mid life and a reduced risk for sporadic dementia (Rush Memory and Aging study Project [78]). Whether the benefits of cognitive stimulation are due to a slowing of pathology or an improved efficiency of remaining function due to training is unclear.

## Psychological factors

Psychiatric disorders are of particular interest in relation to prevention of sAD, given their high prevalence across the lifespan and the availability of effective psychological and pharmacological treatments. There is a robust link between depression in late life and the incidence of sporadic dementia, whereby having depression increases nearly 2-fold the risk of developing dementia [72, 79]. Having depression also increases the risk of transitioning from MCI to dementia [80]. The interpretation that late-life depression is a risk factor for depression was discounted recently by the 28-year-long follow-up Whitehall II cohort study [81]. It is instead more likely that low mood forms part of the dementia prodrome or that the two conditions share a common cause. The same study discounted a role for mid-life depression as a risk factor for sAD, even where it was of a recurrent/chronic nature. Personality factors, schizophrenia, and other psychiatric factors have been investigated, but the evidence for a link with sAD is so far lacking [72]. While this shows that treating depression is unlikely to delay the onset of sAD, the well-established deleterious effects of depression on memory, sleep, and social functioning makes treating depression in the stage of established cognitive impairment an important clinical consideration.

### Education and occupational attainment

Higher educational and occupational attainments have consistently been implicated as protective for developing dementia in later life. For education, a recent meta-analysis reported an approximately 40% risk reduction for high vs low education attainers [72]. Similarly, there was an 80% increased risk for dementia in low-paid workers, although a significant part of the variance appeared to be accounted for by their level of education [72]. The protective effects of education may be due to prolonged period of learning, stimulating the development, or being the result, of larger brain volume or neural networks of greater complexity. These potential physical and functional factors could be related to a greater capacity to compensate the underlying sAD pathology and thus delay the onset of clinical symptoms (the 'cognitive reserve' theory). Equally, an inborn characteristic of the nervous system that is protective of sAD may also increase the capacity to learn at a young age and thus predispose to longer education.

## Future trends

The importance of conducting effective primary and secondary prevention of sAD has led to the development of population-based programmes specifically designed to translate sAD risk factor research into public health benefit. The clustering of lifestyle risk factors in sAD lends itself to complex interventions where several risk factors are addressed simultaneously. The Finnish Geriatric Intervention Study to Prevent Cognitive Impairment and Disability (FINGER) is one of the first such initiatives aimed at secondary prevention [82]. FINGER recruited non-demented individuals in the 60–77 years range who had an elevated dementia risk score (based on age, sex, education, blood pressure, BMI, cholesterol levels, and physical activity), as well as a minor degree of cognitive impairment. This therefore selected an ultra-high-risk population for dementia and allowed the trial of a multi-domain intervention involving changes to nutrition, physical activity, education, and cognitive training. The intervention group's cognitive outcomes improved at 25–150%, compared to the control group (health advice only). Future studies would need to demonstrate the benefit of such interventions on the key public health outcome—time to dementia onset. A further key question to be addressed is the extent to which addressing risk factors in mid life results in effective primary prevention of sAD. However, indirect evidence of this effect is already available through the observed decline in the projected dementia incidence rate—a trend attributed to improved cardiovascular risk control [11].

Despite the huge societal gains that are likely to accrue from risk factor control, it is likely that disease-modifying treatments will be required to affect the global burden of dementia. The realization that the disease process starts decades before the first symptoms has led to a number of initiatives aimed at identifying the condition either

at its preclinical (that is, a state with evidence of sAD pathology) or prodromal (that is, a state of minimal symptoms and sAD pathology) stages.

Development in these disease stages rests on the increased knowledge of mechanisms for the development of new compounds, access to biomarkers for risk stratification for targeting treatments to those who will benefit the most, the development of more sensitive outcome measures allowing benefits to be more efficiently detected, and a trials-ready infrastructure enabling new compounds to be tested more rapidly. These challenges are increasingly being met through large-scale collaborative platform science projects. In relation to mechanisms, these include the UK Dementia Research Institute (https://ukdri.ac.uk/). For biomarker development, there is the Deep and Frequent Phenotyping Study [83], while for risk stratification and trials, there are the Dementias Platform UK (https://www.dementiasplatform.uk/), the European Prevention of Alzheimer's Dementia Consortium (EPAD) (http://ep-ad.org/), and the American-based Global Alzheimer's Platform Foundation (http://globalalzplatform.org/). Powerful digital technologies are also being harnessed for sAD research, including the Dementias Platform UK (https://www.dementiasplatform.uk/), the European Medical Informatics Framework (http://www.emif.eu/), and the Real world Outcomes across the Alzheimer's Disease spectrum for better care: Multi-modal data Access Platform (ROADMAP) project for the assessment of real-world evidence in sAD (http://roadmap-alzheimer.org/).

Arguably, a culture shift in the public perception of AD and dementia in general will be required before full benefit of preventative and treatment strategies will be realized. Moving from dementia to a framework of brain health would help de-stigmatize cognitive decline, empower the public to take greater responsibility for prevention, and encourage society at large to generate inclusive solutions for maintaining functional independence. To reimagine dementia care in terms of brain health centres, rather than memory clinics, would not be an idle reverie.

## REFERENCES

1. World Health Organization. *Dementia fact sheet. Secondary WHO Dementia fact sheet 2017*. http://www.who.int/mediacentre/factsheets/fs362/en/
2. Prince M, Bryce R, Albanese E, et al. The global prevalence of dementia: a systematic review and metaanalysis. Alzheimers Dement 2013;**9**(1):63–75 e2.
3. Office for National Statistics. *Deaths registered in England and Wales: 2015*. 2016.
4. Querfurth HW, LaFerla FM. Alzheimer's disease. N Engl J Med 2010;**362**(4):329–44.
5. McKhann G, Drachman D, Folstein M, et al. Clinical diagnosis of Alzheimer's disease: report of the NINCDS-ADRDA Work Group under the auspices of Department of Health and Human Services Task Force on Alzheimer's Disease. Neurology 1984;**34**(7):939–44.
6. Scheuner D, Eckman C, Jensen M, et al. Secreted amyloid beta-protein similar to that in the senile plaques of Alzheimer's disease is increased in vivo by the presenilin 1 and 2 and APP mutations linked to familial Alzheimer's disease. Nat Med 1996;**2**(8):864–70.
7. McKhann GM, Knopman DS, Chertkow H, et al. The diagnosis of dementia due to Alzheimer's disease: recommendations

from the National Institute on Aging-Alzheimer's Association workgroups on diagnostic guidelines for Alzheimer's disease. Alzheimers Dement 2011;7(3):263–9.

8. Lambert MA, Bickel H, Prince M, et al. Estimating the burden of early onset dementia; systematic review of disease prevalence. Eur J Neurol 2014;21(4):563–9.

9. Fiest KM, Roberts JI, Maxwell CJ, et al. The Prevalence and Incidence of Dementia Due to Alzheimer's Disease: a Systematic Review and Meta-Analysis. Can J Neurol Sci 2016;43 Suppl 1:S51–82.

10. Masters CL, Bateman R, Blennow K, et al. Alzheimer's disease. Nat Rev Dis Primers 2015;1:15056.

11. Ahmadi-Abhari S, Guzman-Castillo M, Bandosz P, et al. Temporal trend in dementia incidence since 2002 and projections for prevalence in England and Wales to 2040: modelling study. BMJ 2017;358:j2856.

12. Ruitenberg A, Ott A, van Swieten JC, et al. Incidence of dementia: does gender make a difference? Neurobiol Aging 2001;22(4):575–80.

13. Matthews FE, Stephan BC, Robinson L, et al. A two decade dementia incidence comparison from the Cognitive Function and Ageing Studies I and II. Nat Commun 2016;7:11398.

14. Schrijvers EM, Verhaaren BF, Koudstaal PJ, et al. Is dementia incidence declining?: trends in dementia incidence since 1990 in the Rotterdam Study. Neurology 2012;78(19):1456–63.

15. Nelson PT, Schmitt FA, Lin Y, et al. Hippocampal sclerosis in advanced age: clinical and pathological features. Brain 2011;134(Pt 5):1506–18.

16. Karch CM, Goate AM. Alzheimer's disease risk genes and mechanisms of disease pathogenesis. Biol Psychiatry 2015;77(1):43–51.

17. Jonsson T, Atwal JK, Steinberg S, et al. A mutation in APP protects against Alzheimer's disease and age-related cognitive decline. Nature 2012;488(7409):96–9.

18. Kim J, Basak JM, Holtzman DM. The role of apolipoprotein E in Alzheimer's disease. Neuron 2009;63(3):287–303.

19. Corder EH, Saunders AM, Risch NJ, et al. Protective effect of apolipoprotein E type 2 allele for late onset Alzheimer disease. Nat Genet 1994;7(2):180–4.

20. Corbo RM, Scacchi R. Apolipoprotein E (APOE) allele distribution in the world. Is APOE*4 a 'thrifty' allele? Ann Hum Genet 1999;63(Pt 4):301–10.

21. Harold D, Abraham R, Hollingworth P, et al. Genome-wide association study identifies variants at CLU and PICALM associated with Alzheimer's disease. Nat Genet 2009;41(10):1088–93.

22. Hollingworth P, Harold D, Sims R, et al. Common variants at ABCA7, MS4A6A/MS4A4E, EPHA1, CD33 and CD2AP are associated with Alzheimer's disease. Nat Genet 2011;43(5):429–35.

23. Lambert JC, Ibrahim-Verbaas CA, Harold D, et al. Meta-analysis of 74,046 individuals identifies 11 new susceptibility loci for Alzheimer's disease. Nat Genet 2013;45(12):1452–8.

24. Escott-Price V, Shoai M, Pither R, et al. Polygenic score prediction captures nearly all common genetic risk for Alzheimer's disease. Neurobiol Aging 2017;49:214 e7–14 e11.

25. Escott-Price V, Sims R, Bannister C, et al. Common polygenic variation enhances risk prediction for Alzheimer's disease. Brain 2015;138(Pt 12):3673–84.

26. Morgan AR, Touchard S, O'Hagan C, et al. The Correlation between Inflammatory Biomarkers and Polygenic Risk Score in Alzheimer's Disease. J Alzheimers Dis 2017;56(1):25–36.

27. Selkoe DJ, Hardy J. The amyloid hypothesis of Alzheimer's disease at 25 years. EMBO Mol Med 2016;8(6):595–608.

28. Weidemann A, Eggert S, Reinhard FB, et al. A novel epsilon-cleavage within the transmembrane domain of the Alzheimer amyloid precursor protein demonstrates homology with Notch processing. Biochemistry 2002;41(8):2825–35.

29. Moore S, Evans LD, Andersson T, et al. APP metabolism regulates tau proteostasis in human cerebral cortex neurons. Cell Rep 2015;11(5):689–96.

30. Placido AI, Pereira CM, Duarte AI, et al. The role of endoplasmic reticulum in amyloid precursor protein processing and trafficking: implications for Alzheimer's disease. Biochim Biophys Acta 2014;1842(9):1444–53.

31. Maccioni RB, Lavados M, Guillon M, et al. Anomalously phosphorylated tau and Abeta fragments in the CSF correlates with cognitive impairment in MCI subjects. Neurobiol Aging 2006;27(2):237–44.

32. Maccioni RB, Lavados M, Maccioni CB, et al. Biological markers of Alzheimer's disease and mild cognitive impairment. Curr Alzheimer Res 2004;1(4):307–14.

33. Mudher A, Lovestone S. Alzheimer's disease-do tauists and baptists finally shake hands? Trends Neurosci 2002;25(1):22–6.

34. Ittner LM, Ke YD, Delerue F, et al. Dendritic function of tau mediates amyloid-beta toxicity in Alzheimer's disease mouse models. Cell 2010;142(3):387–97.

35. Maccioni RB, Farias G, Morales I, et al. The revitalized tau hypothesis on Alzheimer's disease. Arch Med Res 2010;41(3):226–31.

36. Noble W, Hanger DP, Miller CC, et al. The importance of tau phosphorylation for neurodegenerative diseases. Front Neurol 2013;4:83.

37. Sheng M, Sabatini BL, Sudhof TC. Synapses and Alzheimer's disease. Cold Spring Harbor Perspectives in Biology 2012;4:pii:a005777.

38. Small SA, Duff K. Linking Abeta and tau in late-onset Alzheimer's disease: a dual pathway hypothesis. Neuron 2008;60(4):534–42.

39. International Genomics of Alzheimer's Disease Consortium. Convergent genetic and expression data implicate immunity in Alzheimer's disease. Alzheimers Dement 2015;11(6):658–71.

40. Hakobyan S, Harding K, Aiyaz M, et al. Complement Biomarkers as Predictors of Disease Progression in Alzheimer's Disease. J Alzheimers Dis 2016;54(2):707–16.

41. Jones L, Holmans PA, Hamshere ML, et al. Genetic evidence implicates the immune system and cholesterol metabolism in the aetiology of Alzheimer's disease. PLoS One 2010;5(11):e13950.

42. Sims R, van der Lee SJ, Naj AC, et al. Rare coding variants in PLCG2, ABI3, and TREM2 implicate microglial-mediated innate immunity in Alzheimer's disease. Nat Genet 2017;49:1373–84.

43. Coleman PD, Yao PJ. Synaptic slaughter in Alzheimer's disease. Neurobiol Aging 2003;24(8):1023–7.

44. Koffie RM, Hyman BT, Spires-Jones TL. Alzheimer's disease: synapses gone cold. Mol Neurodegener 2011;6(1):63.

45. Bastrikova N, Gardner GA, Reece JM, et al. Synapse elimination accompanies functional plasticity in hippocampal neurons. Proc Natl Acad Sci U S A 2008;105(8):3123–7.

46. Marcello E, Epis R, Di Luca M. Amyloid flirting with synaptic failure: towards a comprehensive view of Alzheimer's disease pathogenesis. Eur J Pharmacol 2008;585(1):109–18.

47. Marcello E, Epis R, Saraceno C, et al. Synaptic dysfunction in Alzheimer's disease. Adv Exp Med Biol 2012;970:573–601.

48. De Strooper B, Karran E. The Cellular Phase of Alzheimer's Disease. Cell 2016;164(4):603–15.

49. Deane R, Zlokovic BV. Role of the blood-brain barrier in the pathogenesis of Alzheimer's disease. Curr Alzheimer Res 2007;**4**(2):191–7.
50. Ruitenberg A, den Heijer T, Bakker SL, *et al.* Cerebral hypoperfusion and clinical onset of dementia: the Rotterdam Study. Ann Neurol 2005;**57**(6):789–94.
51. De Felice FG, Lourenco MV, Ferreira ST. How does brain insulin resistance develop in Alzheimer's disease? Alzheimers Dement 2014;**10**(1 Suppl):S26–32.
52. Brettschneider J, Del Tredici K, Lee VM, *et al.* Spreading of pathology in neurodegenerative diseases: a focus on human studies. Nat Rev Neurosci 2015;**16**(2):109–20.
53. Walker LC, Jucker M. Neurodegenerative diseases: expanding the prion concept. Annu Rev Neurosci 2015;**38**:87–103.
54. Takahashi M, Miyata H, Kametani F, *et al.* Extracellular association of APP and tau fibrils induces intracellular aggregate formation of tau. Acta Neuropathol 2015;**129**(6):895–907.
55. Hasegawa M. Molecular Mechanisms in the Pathogenesis of Alzheimer's disease and Tauopathies-Prion-Like Seeded Aggregation and Phosphorylation. Biomolecules 2016;**6**(2).
56. Schmidt R, Hofer E, Bouwman FH, *et al.* EFNS-ENS/EAN Guideline on concomitant use of cholinesterase inhibitors and memantine in moderate to severe Alzheimer's disease. Eur J Neurol 2015;**22**(6):889–98.
57. Howard R, McShane R, Lindesay J, *et al.* Donepezil and memantine for moderate-to-severe Alzheimer's disease. N Engl J Med 2012;**366**(10):893–903.
58. Howard R, McShane R, Lindesay J, *et al.* Nursing home placement in the Donepezil and Memantine in Moderate to Severe Alzheimer's Disease (DOMINO-AD) trial: secondary and post-hoc analyses. Lancet Neurol 2015;**14**(12):1171–81.
59. O'Brien JT, Holmes C, Jones M, *et al.* Clinical practice with anti-dementia drugs: A revised (third) consensus statement from the British Association for Psychopharmacology. J Psychopharmacol 2017;**31**(2):147–68.
60. Kales HC, Gitlin LN, Lyketsos CG. Assessment and management of behavioral and psychological symptoms of dementia. BMJ 2015;**350**:h369.
61. National Institute for Health and Care Excellence. *Dementia: supporting people with dementia and their carers in health and social care.* 2016. https://www.nice.org.uk/guidance/cg42
62. Schneider LS, Dagerman K, Insel PS. Efficacy and adverse effects of atypical antipsychotics for dementia: meta-analysis of randomized, placebo-controlled trials. Am J Geriatr Psychiatry 2006;**14**(3):191–210.
63. Prince M, Prina M, Guerchet M. *World Alzheimer Report 2013. Secondary World Alzheimer Report 2013.* 2013. https://www.alz.co.uk/research/WorldAlzheimerReport2013.pdf
64. Cuijpers P. Depressive disorders in caregivers of dementia patients: a systematic review. Aging Ment Health 2005;**9**(4):325–30.
65. Schulz R, Beach SR. Caregiving as a risk factor for mortality: the Caregiver Health Effects Study. JAMA 1999;**282**(23):2215–19.
66. Pinquart M, Sorensen S. Helping caregivers of persons with dementia: which interventions work and how large are their effects? Int Psychogeriatr 2006;**18**(4):577–95.
67. Brookmeyer R, Johnson E, Ziegler-Graham K, *et al.* Forecasting the global burden of Alzheimer's disease. Alzheimers Dement 2007;**3**(3):186–91.
68. Norton S, Matthews FE, Barnes DE, *et al.* Potential for primary prevention of Alzheimer's disease: an analysis of population-based data. Lancet Neurol 2014;**13**(8):788–94.
69. Skoog I, Lernfelt B, Landahl S, *et al.* 15-year longitudinal study of blood pressure and dementia. Lancet 1996;**347**(9009):1141–5.
70. Stewart R, Xue QL, Masaki K, *et al.* Change in blood pressure and incident dementia: a 32-year prospective study. Hypertension 2009;**54**(2):233–40.
71. Musini VM, Tejani AM, Bassett K, *et al.* Pharmacotherapy for hypertension in the elderly. Cochrane Database Syst Rev 2009;**4**:CD000028.
72. Prince M, Albanese E, Guerchet M, *et al. World Alzheimer Report 2014. Secondary World Alzheimer Report 2014.* 2014.
73. Whitmer RA, Sidney S, Selby J, *et al.* Midlife cardiovascular risk factors and risk of dementia in late life. Neurology 2005;**64**(2):277–81.
74. Tolppanen AM, Ngandu T, Kareholt I, *et al.* Midlife and late-life body mass index and late-life dementia: results from a prospective population-based cohort. J Alzheimers Dis 2014;**38**(1):201–9.
75. Topiwala A, Allan CL, Valkanova V, *et al.* Moderate alcohol consumption as risk factor for adverse brain outcomes and cognitive decline: longitudinal cohort study. BMJ 2017;**357**:j2353.
76. Rolland Y, Abellan van Kan G, Vellas B. Physical activity and Alzheimer's disease: from prevention to therapeutic perspectives. J Am Med Dir Assoc 2008;**9**(6):390–405.
77. Hamer M, Chida Y. Physical activity and risk of neurodegenerative disease: a systematic review of prospective evidence. Psychol Med 2009;**39**(1):3–11.
78. Wilson RS, Begeny CT, Boyle PA, *et al.* Vulnerability to stress, anxiety, and development of dementia in old age. Am J Geriatr Psychiatry 2011;**19**(4):327–34.
79. Diniz BS, Butters MA, Albert SM, *et al.* Late-life depression and risk of vascular dementia and Alzheimer's disease: systematic review and meta-analysis of community-based cohort studies. Br J Psychiatry 2013;**202**(5):329–35.
80. Ismail Z, Elbayoumi H, Fischer CE, *et al.* Prevalence of Depression in Patients With Mild Cognitive Impairment: A Systematic Review and Meta-analysis. JAMA Psychiatry 2017;**74**(1):58–67.
81. Singh-Manoux A, Dugravot A, Fournier A, *et al.* Trajectories of Depressive Symptoms Before Diagnosis of Dementia: A 28-Year Follow-up Study. JAMA Psychiatry 2017;**74**(7):712–18.
82. Ngandu T, Lehtisalo J, Solomon A, *et al.* A 2 year multidomain intervention of diet, exercise, cognitive training, and vascular risk monitoring versus control to prevent cognitive decline in at-risk elderly people (FINGER): a randomised controlled trial. Lancet 2015;**385**(9984):2255–63.
83. Koychev I, Gunn RN, Firouzian A, *et al.* PET Tau and Amyloid-beta Burden in Mild Alzheimer's Disease: Divergent Relationship with Age, Cognition, and Cerebrospinal Fluid Biomarkers. J Alzheimers Dis 2017;**60**:283–93.

# 41

# Frontotemporal dementias

*Akitoshi Takeda and Bruce Miller*

## Introduction

Arnold Pick first reported in 1892 a case of dementia with symptoms of aphasia and atrophy of the frontal and temporal lobes [1]. By the 1920s, the clinicopathological entity named Pick's disease had been established [2]. It was soon realized that many patients with progressive degeneration of the frontotemporal regions did not have classical Pick bodies. In 1994, the Lund–Manchester groups developed a consensus to delineate the clinical and neuropathological criteria for what they called frontotemporal lobar degeneration (FTLD) [3]. The criteria encompassed each of the major clinical syndromes of FTLD: frontotemporal dementia (FTD) [currently called behavioural-variant FTD (bvFTD)], progressive non-fluent aphasia, and semantic dementia. These criteria have been replaced by the international criteria for FTD [4-14] and primary progressive aphasia (PPA) [5-27].

## Epidemiology

FTD is recognized as one of the leading causes of early-onset dementia and typically presents in people in their late fifties. The onset of symptoms is usually between the fourth and eighth decades, but cases that begin in the third and ninth decades are seen. About 10% of FTD cases present in patients aged less than 45 years, and about 60% of FTD cases present in those aged between 45 and 64 years [6]. Approximately 30–50% of cases are familial, and 10–15% of FTD cases appear to be associated with an autosomal dominant pattern of inheritance. The prevalence of FTD in individuals between 45 and 64 years of age is estimated to be 2–22 per 100,000 but varies widely, ranging from 4–31 per 100,000 in Europe [4] and 15–22 per 100,000 in the United States [6] to 2–9.5 per 100,000 in Japan [5, 7]. The estimated incidence of FTD is between 2.7 and 4.1 per 100,000 person-years, based on population studies from the United States and Europe [4]. Regarding the gender distribution of FTD, some studies have reported a significantly higher prevalence among men, whereas other studies have reported almost the same prevalence in men and women [4]. The median survival after onset is 6.0–11.8 years [8–10]. In FTD subtypes, semantic dementia has longer median survival (12 years) [9], while FTD and motor neuron disease (FTD-MND) has the shortest median survival (3 years) [8, 11].

## Classification

FTD is a neurodegenerative disorder that primarily affects the frontal and temporal lobes and leads to distinct clinical syndromes. FTD is classified into three clinical variants, according to the FTD consensus criteria: (1) bvFTD, which is characterized by early and significant changes in behaviour, emotion, personality, and executive control; (2) non-fluent-variant PPA (nfvPPA), which is characterized by progressive deficits in speech, grammar, and word output; and (3) semantic-variant PPA (svPPA), which is a progressive disorder of semantic knowledge and naming. Some patients present with features of both FTD and amyotrophic lateral sclerosis (ALS)/MND (ALS/MND). In addition, behavioural and cognitive symptoms of progressive supranuclear palsy (PSP) and cortico-basal syndrome (CBS) often overlap with FTD. These clinical syndromes are closely linked to specific molecular pathologies that affect the frontal and temporal lobes [12] (Fig. 41.1).

A new classification for cognitive disorders (including dementia) was established in the *Diagnostic and Statistical Manual of Mental Disorders*, fifth edition (DSM-5). FTD is referred to as a frontotemporal neurocognitive disorder (NCD) in DSM-5. Frontotemporal NCDs are subdivided into mild or major frontotemporal NCD, according to the severity of cognitive impairment. Frontotemporal NCD is characterized by the progressive development of behavioural and personality changes and/or language impairments. According to the DSM-5 criteria, the prerequisite for a diagnosis of behavioural-variant frontotemporal NCD is a progressive decline in social cognition and/or executive abilities. In addition, three or more of the following behavioural features must be present: behavioural disinhibition, apathy/inertia, loss of empathy, perseverative/ritualistic behaviour, and hyperorality/dietary changes. The diagnosis is categorized as 'possible' or 'probable' frontotemporal NCD, according to the severity of cognitive and functional impairment. If there is supporting evidence from genetic mutations or neuroimaging, the diagnosis is described as probable; otherwise, it is designated as possible [13]. The behavioural variant and three language variants (agrammatic/non-fluent, semantic, and logopenic) exhibit distinct patterns of brain atrophy and some distinctive forms of neuropathology. The necessary criteria must be met to make a diagnosis of either the behavioural or the language variant, but many individuals present with features of both.

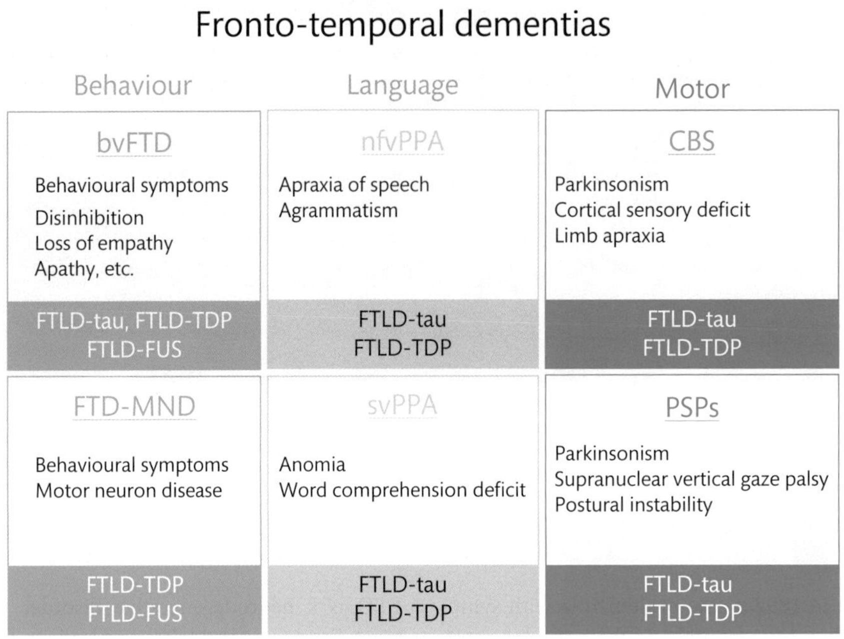

# Fronto-temporal dementias

| Behaviour | Language | Motor |
|---|---|---|
| **bvFTD** | **nfvPPA** | **CBS** |
| Behavioural symptoms | Apraxia of speech | Parkinsonism |
| Disinhibition | Agrammatism | Cortical sensory deficit |
| Loss of empathy | | Limb apraxia |
| Apathy, etc. | | |
| FTLD-tau, FTLD-TDP FTLD-FUS | FTLD-tau FTLD-TDP | FTLD-tau FTLD-TDP |
| **FTD-MND** | **svPPA** | **PSPs** |
| Behavioural symptoms | Anomia | Parkinsonism |
| Motor neuron disease | Word comprehension deficit | Supranuclear vertical gaze palsy |
| | | Postural instability |
| FTLD-TDP FTLD-FUS | FTLD-tau FTLD-TDP | FTLD-tau FTLD-TDP |

**Fig. 41.1** Clinical and pathological spectrum of frontotemporal dementias. Frontotemporal dementia encompasses three canonical syndromes: behaviour syndrome, language syndrome, and motor syndrome. These clinical syndromes can overlap in the disease course.

Despite recent advances in the characterization of bvFTD, the diagnosis of the syndrome remains challenging. Some patients with bvFTD are misdiagnosed as having psychiatric disorders or Alzheimer's disease (AD). In the absence of definitive biomarkers, clinical diagnostic criteria are more important in the diagnosis of bvFTD. The International Behavior-variant FTD Criteria Consortium (FTDC) developed revised guidelines for the diagnosis of bvFTD in 2011. A diagnosis of bvFTD is categorized as 'possible', 'probable', or 'definite' bvFTD, based on this hierarchical classification system, with support from radiological findings, genetic studies, and neuropathological data. The FTDC criteria have been changed by prescribing specific criteria for diagnosis, while excluding patients with biomarkers for AD or other neurodegenerative disease [14].

## Behavioural-variant frontotemporal dementia

The most pronounced behavioural symptoms of bvFTD are loss of empathy, apathy, and disinhibition, which typically precede any obvious cognitive impairment. Therefore, bvFTD can be mistaken for depression or other psychiatric disorders in the early stages. In bvFTD, behavioural changes can lead to job loss and financial problems. The families of patients with bvFTD report high levels of distress from the very early stages, compared with families of patients who have AD [15]. Most behavioural symptoms are caused by disruptions to the brain networks involved in emotions and social function. Patients with bvFTD show loss of empathy towards family and other people. They cannot interpret the emotional state of other people and show decreased responsiveness to emotions (emotional blunting). Family members of patients with bvFTD often describe their loss of empathy as selfish or self-centred. Loss of empathy is associated with human brain networks that include the medial orbitofrontal cortex (OFC), anterior temporal lobe, and anterior insula, and these regions match those affected by the pattern of

atrophy characteristic of bvFTD [16, 17]. The loss of empathy seems to be lateralized to the right anterior temporal lobe, OFC, and anterior insula [16, 18].

Apathy is defined as loss of interest or emotion and loss of motivation [19], and in patients with bvFTD, this presents as reduced interest in work, hobbies, and hygiene that leads to a decline in personal hygiene. Apathy is associated with atrophy of the anterior cingulate cortex (ACC) and ventromedial superior frontal cortex [20]. The ACC (especially the dorsal ACC) also plays an important role in both the motor and cognitive domains. The dorsal ACC is involved with the supplemental motor area in the planning of complex movements. ACC lesions can cause dramatic reductions in spontaneous speech and movement (akinetic mutism) in extreme cases [21]. In terms of the cognitive domain, the dorsal ACC and dorsolateral prefrontal cortex are associated with executive functions such as set maintenance.

Disinhibition is a distinctive feature of bvFTD, and the OFC plays an important role in modifying behaviour, depending on the principle of receiving rewards and avoiding punishment [22]. Avoiding inappropriate behaviour is a key component of successful social functioning. The OFC is one of the earliest regions affected in bvFTD, and its atrophy leads to disinhibition [22]. Dysfunction of the right OFC in bvFTD manifests as marked behavioural disinhibition [20], which is associated with inappropriate behaviours such as hugging or kissing strangers, urinating in public, or telling sexual jokes. Behavioural disinhibition may also manifest as impulsivity such as reckless driving, excessive purchasing of unnecessary items, or criminal behaviour such as shoplifting. Loss of insight is defined as a lack of awareness of mental symptoms due to frank denial or unconcern for the consequences [23]. Patients with bvFTD show even more severely diminished insight into their symptoms and overestimate their performance. Loss of insight is associated with ventromedial and frontopolar prefrontal atrophy [23].

Alterations in eating behaviour occur in patients with bvFTD, including changes in appetite and food preferences. Patients with bvFTD tend to display sugar cravings and binge eating, often associated with significant weight gain. Changes in food preferences are due to dysfunction in neural networks that include the hypothalamus, right insula, bilateral nucleus accumbens, and OFC [24]. Binge eating is associated with loss of function in the right ventral insula, striatum, OFC, thalamus, and anterior cingulate [24, 25]. In terms of neuropsychological testing, patients with bvFTD tend to show deficits in executive function, although visuo-spatial function, and often episodic memory, is relatively spared, compared with AD [26].

### Language-variant frontotemporal dementia

PPA is a progressive language disorder that is often associated with disproportionate atrophy of the left frontal and temporal lobes, and is classified as language-variant frontotemporal NCD in DSM-5 [13]. Language dysfunction is the main symptom for the first 2 years of the illness. Deficits in language production, object naming, syntax, or word comprehension are apparent during conversation or in speech and language assessments [27]. Patients with language-variant frontotemporal NCD present with PPA with gradual onset, with three subtypes being commonly described—semantic-variant, agrammatic/non-fluent-variant, and logopenic-variant—and each variant has distinctive features and corresponding neuropathology [27]. nfvPPA and svPPA are associated with FTD, and logopenic-variant PPA is associated with AD. 'Probable' is distinguished from 'possible' frontotemporal NCD by the presence of causative genetic factors (such as mutations in the gene coding for microtubule-associated protein tau) or by the presence of a distinctive pattern of atrophy or reduced activity in frontotemporal regions on structural or functional imaging [13].

### Non-fluent-variant primary progressive aphasia

nfvPPA is characterized by non-fluent and effortful speech production, and agrammatism (omission or misuse of grammar) is usually, but not always, present. Agrammatism and effortful speech are core symptoms of nfvPPA [27]. Apraxia of speech (AOS) is also common in nfvPPA. AOS causes inconsistent speech sound errors such as distortions, insertions, deletions, substitutions, and transpositions of speech sounds. Word-finding difficulties are relatively mild, compared with svPPA. Single-word and object comprehension are relatively spared, although patients can have mild anomia that may be more pronounced for verbs than for nouns. Deficits in syntax comprehension are evidenced by impairments in sentence comprehension, initially only for the most difficult syntactic constructions [27]. nfvPPA is associated with atrophy predominantly in the left inferior frontal and insular regions, which is necessary for making a diagnosis of the imaging-supported non-fluent variant. Clinically, nfvPPA patients exhibit few behavioural changes.

### Semantic-variant primary progressive aphasia

Patients with svPPA present with deficits in comprehension and word-finding abilities (anomia) due to impairments in semantic knowledge; however, these patients retain a fluent expressive speech pattern, with correct use of grammar. Anomia and single-word comprehension deficits are the core features [27]. These deficits reflect a gradual loss of semantic knowledge, which is observed irrespective of modality. Anomia tends to be more pronounced for nouns than for verbs or pronouns. Semantic deficits are usually present for most categories (that is, tools, animals, and people), although rare cases have been described with greater, or even selective, deficits for people and animals. A common feature among svPPA patients is surface dyslexia and dysgraphia, impairments in which words with atypical spelling or pronunciation are regularized. Anatomically, svPPA is associated with atrophy in the ventral and lateral portions of the bilateral anterior temporal lobes, although damage is usually greater on the left side. The clinical presentation of predominantly right-sided semantic dementia cases is heterogenous and includes inappropriate behaviour, loss of knowledge about familiar faces, loss of empathy, and/or semantic deficits [28].

### Motor symptoms

In patients with FTD syndromes that overlap with MND, behavioural and cognitive symptoms can develop before, after, or simultaneously with motor symptoms. Patients with FTD often present with parkinsonism, including bradykinesia, rigidity, tremor, and/or postural instability. The prevalence of parkinsonism in FTD varies from 12.5% to 30% [29]. Early parkinsonism is observed in 16% of FTD patients [30], with bradykinesia being the most common manifestation in 84% of patients, followed by a parkinsonian gait (71%), rigidity and postural instability (35.5%), and resting tremor (6.5%) [31]. PSP and CBS are two atypical parkinsonian syndromes demonstrating cognitive and behavioural features that overlap with FTD. Patients with FTD often have concomitant ALS/MND. In some instances, FTD precedes ALS by many years; in other instances, ALS occurs before FTD. The incidence of FTD in patients with bulbar-onset ALS is reported to be as high as 48% [32]. Although 10–15% of patients with FTD develop MND [32, 33], there is an even higher prevalence of 'subclinical' MND, with evidence from electromyography (EMG) of MND or mild motor signs such as fasciculations in 30–60% of patients with FTD [32, 33]. Among the FTD variants, MND arises frequently in patients with bvFTD, and less often in patients with svPPA or nfvPPA.

## Genetics

Approximately 40% of FTD cases have a family history, and 10–15% of FTD cases show an autosomal dominant pattern. Mutations have currently been associated with bvFTD in genes encoding the following proteins: chromosome 9 open reading frame 72 (C9ORF72), microtubule-associated protein tau (MAPT), granulin (GRN), transactive response DNA-binding protein 43 (TARDBP, otherwise known as TDP-43), fused in sarcoma (FUS), valosin-containing protein (VCP), and charged multivesicular body protein 2b (CHMP2B) [34] (Table 41.1). Mutations in C9ORF72, MAPT, and GRN account for the majority of familial FTD cases [35].

### C9ORF72

The C9ORF72 mutation results in a recently identified hexanucleotide repeat expansion on chromosome 9 [36]. The largest proportion of familial FTD (about 25%) is caused by

**Table 41.1** Clinical and neuroimaging features of hereditary frontotemporal dementia

| | Prevalence | Mean age of onset | Clinical presentation | Atrophy pattern |
|---|---|---|---|---|
| C9ORF72 | 25% of familial FTD | 45 years | bvFTD<br>ALS<br>FTD-MND<br>Parkinsonism | Symmetrical frontal atrophy with temporal and parietal involvement<br>Thalamus and cerebellar atrophy |
| MAPT | 2–11% of familial FTD | 49 years | bvFTD<br>PPA<br>CBS<br>PSP | Symmetric anteromedial temporal lobe atrophy |
| GRN | 20% of familial FTD | 58 years | bvFTD<br>PPA<br>CBS<br>PSP | Asymmetric frontal, temporal, and parietal lobe atrophy |
| FUS | 3% of familial FTD-MND | 46 years | FTD-MND<br>ALS | Frontal and temporal atrophy |
| VCP | 1–2% of familial FTD-MND | 57 years | bvFTD<br>FTD-MND<br>Inclusion body myopathy<br>Paget's disease of the bone | Frontal, temporal, and parietal lobes, especially prefrontal and superior temporal cortices |
| TARDP | 1.3% of familial FTD-MND | 63 years | FTD-MND<br>ALS | Frontal and temporal atrophy |
| CHMP2B | 1% of familial FTD-MND | 58 years | bvFTD<br>FTD-MND | Frontal and temporal atrophy |
| TBK1 | 0.5–4% of ALS | 67 years | FTD-MND<br>ALS<br>nfvPPA<br>svPPA<br>CBS | Asymmetric anterior temporal atrophy and frontal involvement |

pathogenic expansions of *C9ORF72* [35]. Cases with *C9ORF72* mutations are characterized by underlying TDP-43 pathology [36]. The most common clinical phenotypes associated with *C9ORF72* mutations are bvFTD, ALS, or both. *C9ORF72* mutations are the most common genetic cause of familial FTD and ALS [37]. Thirty to 50% of patients with *C9ORF72* expansions present with hallucinations and delusions [36].

## MAPT

The microtubule-associated protein tau is encoded by *MAPT* and plays an important role in microtubule assembly and stabilization in neurons. *MAPT* mutations account for between 2% and 11% of familial FTD cases [34]. An *MAPT* mutation was identified as the first causative genetic mutation in several families with FTD and associated parkinsonism in 1998 [38]. *MAPT* mutations are associated with an underlying tauopathy. Clinically, cases with *MAPT* mutations usually present with bvFTD and may include parkinsonism. PPA syndromes, including nfvPPA and svPPA, can also be seen in patients with *MAPT* mutations [39]. Variability in the normal haplotypes of *MAPT* has also been associated with an increased risk for the development of the syndromes PSP and CBS that overlap with FTD [40].

## GRN

*GRN* encodes granulin, a secreted protein that may function in inflammation, wound repair, and cell cycling [41]. The neuropathology of patients with *GRN* mutations is characterized by tau-negative, TDP-43-positive inclusions. *GRN* mutations account for up to 20% of familial FTD cases and are occasionally seen in sporadic cases

[42]. *GRN* mutations are found in 24.7% of FTLD-TDP cases [41] and are associated with an earlier age of symptom onset and an earlier age of death, compared with FTLD-TDP patients without *GRN* mutations [41]. The clinical presentation of patients with *GRN* mutations is bvFTD, with nfvPPA or CBS seen less frequently [34]. Episodic memory deficits occur in 10–30% of those with *GRN* mutations and may lead to the clinical diagnosis of an amnestic variant of MCI, with parietal deficits similar to AD [42]. *GRN* mutations are seldom seen in association with MND [41].

## Others

Mutations in the genes encoding five other proteins, including VCP, CHMP2B, TARDP, FUS, and TBK-1, have been identified in a minority of cases [34]. *VCP* mutations result in a rare syndromic combination of bvFTD with inclusion body myopathy and Paget's disease of bone (known as IBMPFD). Pathologically, *VCP* mutations have TDP-43 type D pathology [43]. *CHMP2B* mutations are a genetic cause of FTD linked to chromosome 3 (FTD-3), which was originally identified in a large Danish family. The phenotype of *CHMP2B* mutations is usually a behavioural syndrome similar to bvFTD, although several cases with FTD-MND have been described [44]. *TARDBP* mutations on chromosome 1 have been reported in FTD and FTD-MND cases [45], and are found in 5% of those with familial ALS [42]. *FUS* mutations were originally described in familial ALS, accounting for 3% of cases [46]; however, most FTD cases with FUS pathology are sporadic and do not have *FUS* mutations [47]. Finally, recent studies suggest that loss-of-function mutations in *TBK1* (encoding TANK-binding kinase 1) can cause FTD-MND. In addition, svPPA and nfvPPA can be manifestations of *TBK1* mutations and should be considered in patients with PPA associated with ALS.

Semantic and non-fluent aphasic variants, secondarily associated with ALS, are predominant FTLD phenotypes in TBK1 carriers [48, 49].

## Pathology

To distinguish the neuropathology from the clinical diagnosis, the term FTD is used for the clinical syndrome, whereas the term FTLD is used when referring to the neuropathological classification [50]. AD pathology can be responsible for bvFTD syndrome, although if the international research criteria for this disorder are applied carefully, this is rare [51]. One pathological finding of FTLD is regional atrophy of the frontal and temporal cortices, with neuronal loss and microvacuolation predominantly involving the superficial cortical layers II and III [52]. FTLD is a neuropathologically heterogenous disorder, which can be divided into two major subtypes, according to the characteristic pattern of abnormal protein deposition: FTLD with tau-positive inclusions (FTLD-tau) subtype and FTLD with ubiquitin-positive and TDP-43-positive subtype. FTLD-FUS is seen in a small minority of tau-negative, ubiquitin-positive cases [12] (Table 41.2).

### FTLD-tau

FTLD-tau accounts for 36–50% of all cases of FTLD, according to different pathological series, and varies widely across the different FTD syndromes [35]. The defining characteristic of FTLD-tau is the accumulation of filamentous aggregates of pathological tau in neurons, astrocytes, and oligodendrocytes, which are collectively known as tauopathies (Fig. 41.2a–c). Primary tauopathies include Pick's disease, FTD with *MAPT* mutations (FTDP-17), PSP, CBD, argyrophilic grain disease (AGD), and neurofibrillary tangle dementia (NTD). The most common primary tauopathy is CBD, accounting for 35% of cases, followed by PSP with 31%, Pick's disease with 30%, and AGD accounting for the remaining 4% of all cases of FTLD-tau [12]. Pick's disease is characterized by the presence of Pick bodies, cytoplasmic inclusions composed primarily of three-repeat isoforms of abnormal tau protein (Fig. 2a). PSP, CBD, and AGD are tauopathies with predominantly four-repeat tau isoforms. There are very good clinicopathological associations between FTLD-tau as a group, particularly for PSP. nfvPPA is usually a primary tauopathy, with CBD accounting for approximately 50% of cases with PSP and Pick's disease also seen [12, 53]. At our institution, University of California, San Francisco, approximately one-third of all bvFTD cases are due to tau.

### FTLD-TDP

TDP-43 is a ubiquitously expressed nuclear protein that functions as a repressor of transcription. It also regulates gene expression and splicing. FTLD-TDP is represented in about 50% of all cases of FTD [35]. TDP-43 pathology is seen in sporadic and familial cases of FTLD involving mutations in the genes for GRN and VCP, and in FTD with or without MND and the C9ORF72 hexanucleotide repeat, as well as familial and sporadic cases of ALS [52]. Four major subtypes of FTLD-TDP are recognized (types A, B, C, and D), based on the pattern of cytoplasmic or intranuclear pathology [54] (Fig. 2d) (Table 41.2).

### FTLD-FUS

FTLD-FUS accounts for about 10% of all bvFTD cases [35, 55]. The majority of tau-negative/TDP-43-negative, ubiquitin-positive FTLD cases have positive immunohistochemical staining for the FUS protein, thus distinguishing a third category of FTLD neuropathology that includes the categories formerly called atypical FTLD with ubiquitinated inclusions (aFTLD-U), basophilic inclusion body disease (BIBD), and neuronal intermediate filament inclusion disease (NIFID) [55]. This last entity is characterized by sporadic, early-onset (<40 years) bvFTD or FTD-MND [35].

### Others

The FTLD-other category is reserved for diseases in which the major protein associated with the disease entity remains unknown [12]. FTLD without inclusions (FTLD-ni) is diagnosed when there is histological evidence of frontotemporal neuronal loss and gliosis, but no presence of any inclusions by immunostaining. FTLD with immunohistochemistry against proteins of the ubiquitin proteosomal system (FTLD-UPS) is diagnosed when there are ubiquitin or p62 immunoreactive inclusions that are negative for tau, alpha-synuclein, alpha-internexin, TDP-43, and FUS [12]. The majority of FTLD-UPS cases are associated with *CHMP2B* mutations [12, 44].

## Investigations

### Neuroimaging

Structural MRI shows distinct patterns of atrophy in FTD. Brain atrophy in FTD predominantly affects the frontal or temporal lobes, and atrophy of the ACC and frontal insular cortex are particularly characteristic of FTD, while medial and posterior temporo-parietal and occipital lobe atrophy is indicative of AD, rather than FTD [56]. The genetic forms of FTD have their own typical patterns of atrophy. *GRN* mutations are more likely to show strongly asymmetrical atrophy, predominantly affecting one hemisphere and involving the inferior frontal, temporal, and inferior parietal lobes [34]. *MAPT* mutations are associated with a more symmetrical pattern of atrophy, localized predominantly in the anterior temporal lobes and also involving the OFC [34]. With *C9ORF72* mutations, thalamic, and sometimes cerebellar, atrophy is a distinguishing feature, and a slightly more generalized pattern of atrophy is evident than with the other genetic forms of FTD.

**Table 41.2** Correlations between clinical presentation, pathology, and genetics in frontotemporal dementia

|  |  | Common clinical presentation | Associated gene mutation |
|---|---|---|---|
| FTLD-tau |  | bvFTD, nfvPPA, svPPA, CBS, PSP | *MAPT* |
| FTLD-TDP | Type A | bvFTD, nfvPPA | PGRN |
|  | Type B | bvFTD, FTD-MND | C9ORF72 |
|  | Type C | svPPA, bvFTD |  |
|  | Type D | IBMPFD | VCP |
| FTLD-FUS |  | bvFTD, FTD-MND | FUS |
| FTLD-UPS |  | bvFTD, FTD-MND | CHMP2B |

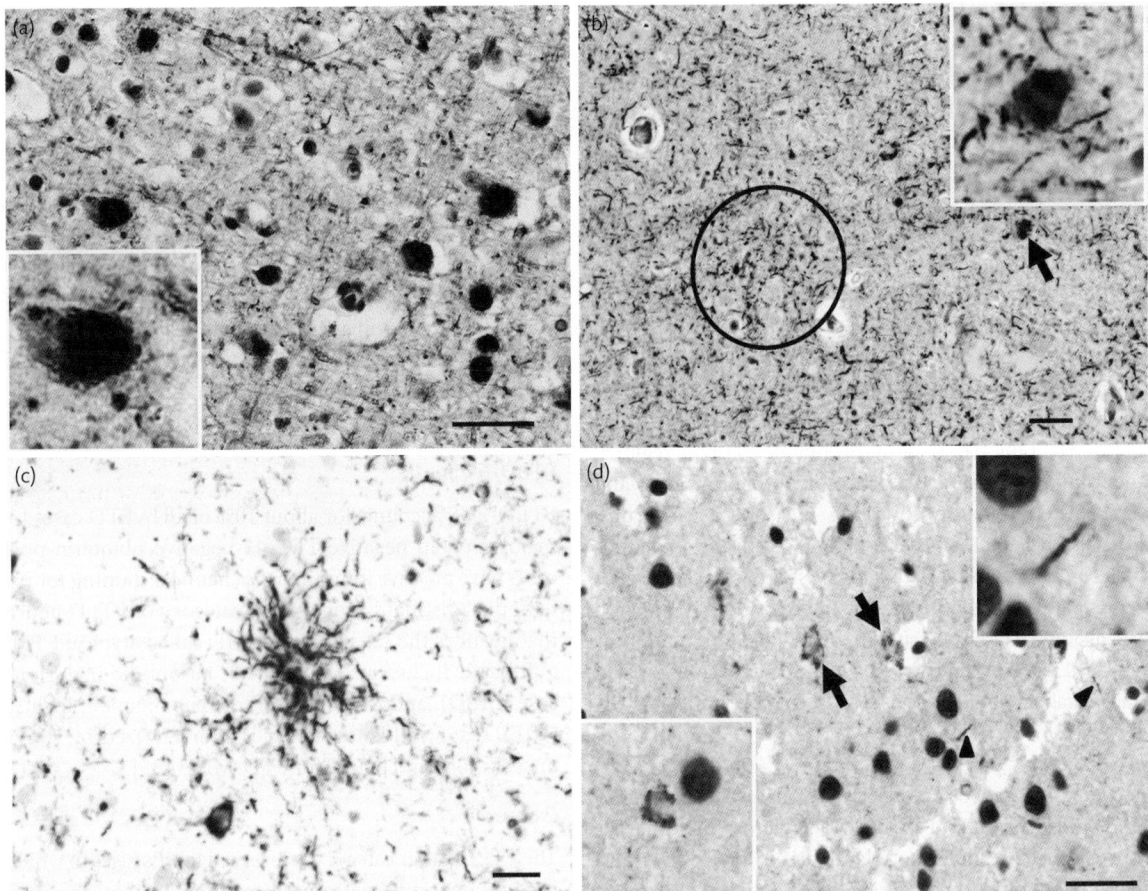

**Fig. 41.2** (see Colour Plate section) Histological features of FTLD-tau and FTLD-TDP. (a) Pick's disease. Pick bodies (lower inset) in the inferior temporal gyrus. (b) Cortico-basal degeneration. Astrocytic plaque (circle) and neuronal cytoplasmic inclusions (arrow and upper inset) in the precentral gyrus. (c) Progressive supranuclear palsy. Tufted astrocyte in the sensorimotor cortex. (d) FTLD-TDP type B. Neuronal cytoplasmic inclusions (arrow and lower inset) and neuropil threads (arrowheads and upper inset) in the middle frontal gyrus. Immunostains are phospho-tau (a–c) and TDP-43 (d). All scale bar represents 10 μm.

PET imaging is also useful for distinguishing AD and FTD. In FDG-PET studies, a pattern of hypometabolism in the frontal, anterior temporal, and anterior cingulate cortices characterizes FTD, while hypometabolism in the temporoparietal and posterior cingulate cortices characterizes AD [57]. Amyloid imaging may also be useful to distinguish FTD from AD. The novel PET tracer [11]C-PiB selectively binds to amyloid plaques and identifies cortical lesions affected by AD pathology [58]. A variety of tau tracers are being tested in patients with AD [59]. Tau imaging could potentially differentiate between AD, FTLD-tau, and FTLD with ubiquitinated inclusions, although at least with the svPPA form of FTD where TDP-43 is usually the underlying pathology, tau imaging markers have proven disappointing.

Functional connectivity network mapping using resting state fMRI is a novel technique for identifying specific brain networks. In patients with bvFTD, intrinsic connectivity within the salience network is decreased, while increased activity is seen in the default mode network. By contrast, the opposite pattern of intrinsic connectivity is seen in AD [60].

### *In vivo* biomarkers

To date, no serum or CSF biomarkers have been identified that distinguish patients with FTD from normal controls. Similarly, there

is no biomarker that enables the differentiation of FTD subtypes. By contrast, biomarkers that help to differentiate AD from FTD are well accepted. tau, phosphorylated tau (pTau181), and Aβ42 in combination help to differentiate FTD from AD [61]. Aβ42 in the CSF is reduced, and tau and pTau181 are increased in AD, compared with FTD. Combined CSF analysis of the ratios of Aβ42/Aβ40 [62], total tau/Ab42, or phosphorylated tau/Aβ42 [63] can be used to improve the diagnostic accuracy and enable AD to be differentiated from FTD.

### Differential diagnosis

A careful history, which includes the progression of behavioural changes and family and social history, is one of the most effective ways to distinguish FTD from other dementias. Performance on neuropsychological testing, laboratory studies, and neuroimaging also help to differentiate FTD from other causes of dementia such as inflammation or infectious disease. Among the subtypes of FTD, the differential diagnosis of early bvFTD is the most challenging. The possibility of AD needs to be considered, especially the behavioural/dysexecutive variant that also affects the frontal lobes. Some 10–40%

of patients clinically diagnosed with bvFTD have subsequently been found to have AD pathology on amyloid PET or post-mortem evaluations [64], although our recent studies suggest that bvFTD diagnosed in an expert centre is almost never due to AD pathology. Patients with behavioural variant AD showed worse memory deficits than those with bvFTD but did not differ from patients with typical AD, while their executive function was more impaired, compared to patients with bvFTD and typical AD [64].

Another important differential diagnosis is late-onset psychiatric disease. In the early stage of bvFTD, behavioural changes, including disinhibition, apathy, and compulsive behaviour, can occur in the absence of neurological signs or cognitive impairment. These behavioural changes in bvFTD can overlap with specific psychiatric disorders. The initial diagnosis in 6% of patients with bvFTD is schizophrenia, schizoaffective disorder, bipolar disorder, depression, or an unspecified psychotic state [65]. A few forms of genetic bvFTD have been associated with psychotic symptoms. Patients with bvFTD and *C9ORF72* mutations often exhibit psychosis as a dominant presenting problem, resulting in initial diagnoses of obsessive–compulsive disorder, schizophrenia, or bipolar disorder [36]. Patients with bvFTD and *GRN* mutations also present with psychiatric manifestations, including bulimia, personality changes, sexual disinhibition, ritualistic behaviours, and paranoia [66].

There is a subset of bvFTD patients in whom disease progression following clinical diagnosis does not appear to occur despite a clear history from caregivers of initial personality and behavioural changes. These patients are said to suffer from bvFTD phenocopy syndrome [67]. Patients with phenocopy syndrome should be distinguishable because they do not show a functional decline or imaging changes [14]. As the long-term prognosis is good, it seems less likely that phenocopy syndrome is caused by a neurodegenerative disorder [14]. Recent work suggests that some phenocopy subjects carry a genetic form of bvFTD [68].

## Treatment and care

Currently, no disease-modifying treatments can alter the course of FTD. Therefore, pharmacological treatments have focused on the modulation of behavioural and cognitive symptoms of FTD [35, 69]. Recent randomized controlled trials have shown that cholinesterase inhibitors, galantamine, and memantine, which are effective for treating cognitive or behavioural symptoms in AD patients, have no efficacy in patients with FTD [69, 70]. Some drugs for depression, including SSRIs and trazodone, have shown efficacy in improving the behavioural symptoms of bvFTD such as disinhibition, depression, compulsive behaviour, and carbohydrate cravings [35, 70]. A few studies have shown that olanzapine is effective for aggression, agitation, and psychosis, although the adverse events associated with dopamine antagonists include parkinsonism [69, 70].

To manage the behavioural symptoms of bvFTD, environmental modification and education for caregivers are also necessary. Educating caregivers about the best non-pharmacological behavioural strategies, identification of triggers for problematic behaviours, and increasing their coping skills have shown success in reducing caregiver stress and improving caregiver tools for managing behavioural symptoms [70, 71]. Resources, such as The Association for Frontotemporal Degeneration, and the development of strategies to maintain emotional and physical safety have been shown to minimize caregiver burden [70].

## REFERENCES

1. Pick A. Über die Beziehungen der senilen Hirnatrophie zur Aphasie. Prager Medizinische Wochenschrift. 1892;17:165–7.
2. Schneider C. Über Picksche Krankheit. Monatschrift für Psychiatrie und Neurologie. 1927;65:230–75.
3. Neary D, Snowden JS, Gustafson L, et al. Frontotemporal lobar degeneration: a consensus on clinical diagnostic criteria. Neurology. 1998;51(6):1546–54.
4. Onyike CU, Diehl-Schmid J. The epidemiology of frontotemporal dementia. Int Rev Psychiatry. 2013;25(2):130–7.
5. Ikejima C, Yasuno F, Mizukami K, Sasaki M, Tanimukai S, Asada T. Prevalence and causes of early-onset dementia in Japan: a population-based study. Stroke. 2009;40(8):2709–14.
6. Knopman DS, Roberts RO. Estimating the number of persons with frontotemporal lobar degeneration in the US population. J Mol Neurosci. 2011;45(3):330–5.
7. Wada-Isoe K, Ito S, Adachi T, et al. Epidemiological survey of frontotemporal lobar degeneration in tottori prefecture, Japan. Dement Geriatr Cogn Dis Extra. 2012;2(1):381–6.
8. Hodges JR, Davies R, Xuereb J, Kril J, Halliday G. Survival in frontotemporal dementia. Neurology. 2003;61(3):349–54.
9. Roberson ED, Hesse JH, Rose KD, et al. Frontotemporal dementia progresses to death faster than Alzheimer disease. Neurology. 2005;65(5):719–25.
10. Nunnemann S, Last D, Schuster T, Forstl H, Kurz A, Diehl-Schmid J. Survival in a German population with frontotemporal lobar degeneration. Neuroepidemiology. 2011;37(3–4):160–5.
11. Hu WT, Seelaar H, Josephs KA, et al. Survival profiles of patients with frontotemporal dementia and motor neuron disease. Arch Neurol. 2009;66(11):1359–64.
12. Josephs KA, Hodges JR, Snowden JS, et al. Neuropathological background of phenotypical variability in frontotemporal dementia. Acta Neuropathol. 2011;122(2):137–53.
13. American Psychiatric Association. *Diagnostic and statistical manual of mental disorders*, fifth edition. American Psychiatric Association, Washington, DC; 2013.
14. Rascovsky K, Hodges JR, Knopman D, et al. Sensitivity of revised diagnostic criteria for the behavioural variant of frontotemporal dementia. Brain. 2011;134(Pt 9):2456–77.
15. Ranasinghe KG, Rankin KP, Lobach IV, et al. Cognition and neuropsychiatry in behavioral variant frontotemporal dementia by disease stage. Neurology. 2016;86(7):600–10.
16. Rankin KP, Gorno-Tempini ML, Allison SC, et al. Structural anatomy of empathy in neurodegenerative disease. Brain. 2006;129(Pt 11):2945–56.
17. Seeley WW, Zhou J, Kim EJ. Frontotemporal dementia: what can the behavioral variant teach us about human brain organization? Neuroscientist. 2012;18(4):373–85.
18. Perry RJ, Rosen HR, Kramer JH, Beer JS, Levenson RL, Miller BL. Hemispheric dominance for emotions, empathy and social behaviour: evidence from right and left handers with frontotemporal dementia. Neurocase. 2001;7(2):145–60.
19. Marin RS. Apathy: a neuropsychiatric syndrome. J Neuropsychiatry Clin Neurosci. 1991;3(3):243–54.
20. Rosen HJ, Allison SC, Schauer GF, Gorno-Tempini ML, Weiner MW, Miller BL. Neuroanatomical correlates of behavioural disorders in dementia. Brain. 2005;128(Pt 11):2612–25.

21. Cummings JL. Frontal-subcortical circuits and human behavior. Arch Neurol. 1993;50(8):873–80.

22. Viskontas IV, Possin KL, Miller BL. Symptoms of frontotemporal dementia provide insights into orbitofrontal cortex function and social behavior. Ann N Y Acad Sci. 2007;1121:528–45.

23. Hornberger M, Yew B, Gilardoni S, et al. Ventromedial-frontopolar prefrontal cortex atrophy correlates with insight loss in frontotemporal dementia and Alzheimer's disease. Hum Brain Mapp. 2014;35(2):616–26.

24. Ahmed RM, Irish M, Henning E, et al. Assessment of Eating Behavior Disturbance and Associated Neural Networks in Frontotemporal Dementia. JAMA Neurol. 2016;73(3):282–90.

25. Woolley JD, Gorno-Tempini ML, Seeley WW, et al. Binge eating is associated with right orbitofrontal-insular-striatal atrophy in frontotemporal dementia. Neurology. 2007;69(14):1424–33.

26. Perry RJ, Hodges JR. Differentiating frontal and temporal variant frontotemporal dementia from Alzheimer's disease. Neurology. 2000;54(12):2277–84.

27. Gorno-Tempini ML, Hillis AE, Weintraub S, et al. Classification of primary progressive aphasia and its variants. Neurology. 2011;76(11):1006–14.

28. Chan D, Anderson V, Pijnenburg Y, et al. The clinical profile of right temporal lobe atrophy. Brain. 2009;132(Pt 5):1287–98.

29. Park HK, Chung SJ. New perspective on parkinsonism in frontotemporal lobar degeneration. J Mov Disord. [Review]. 2013;6(1):1–8.

30. Seelaar H, Kamphorst W, Rosso SM, et al. Distinct genetic forms of frontotemporal dementia. Neurology. 2008 14;71(16):1220–6.

31. Baizabal-Carvallo JF, Jankovic J. Parkinsonism, movement disorders and genetics in frontotemporal dementia. Nat Rev Neurol. 2016;12(3):175–85.

32. Lomen-Hoerth C, Anderson T, Miller B. The overlap of amyotrophic lateral sclerosis and frontotemporal dementia. Neurology. 2002;59(7):1077–9.

33. Burrell JR, Kiernan MC, Vucic S, Hodges JR. Motor neuron dysfunction in frontotemporal dementia. Brain. 2011;134(Pt 9):2582–94.

34. Rohrer JD, Warren JD. Phenotypic signatures of genetic frontotemporal dementia. Curr Opin Neurol. 2011;24(6):542–9.

35. Bang J, Spina S, Miller BL. Frontotemporal dementia. Lancet. 2015;386(10004):1672–82.

36. Rohrer JD, Isaacs AM, Mizielinska S, et al. C9orf72 expansions in frontotemporal dementia and amyotrophic lateral sclerosis. Lancet Neurol. 2015;14(3):291–301.

37. De Jesus-Hernandez M, Mackenzie IR, Boeve BF, et al. Expanded GGGGCC hexanucleotide repeat in noncoding region of C9ORF72 causes chromosome 9p-linked FTD and ALS. Neuron. 2011;72(2):245–56.

38. Hutton M, Lendon CL, Rizzu P, et al. Association of missense and 5'-splice-site mutations in tau with the inherited dementia FTDP-17. Nature. 1998;393(6686):702–5.

39. Ghetti B, Oblak AL, Boeve BF, Johnson KA, Dickerson BC, Goedert M. Invited review: Frontotemporal dementia caused by microtubule-associated protein tau gene (MAPT) mutations: a chameleon for neuropathology and neuroimaging. Neuropathol Appl Neurobiol. 2015;41(1):24–46.

40. Houlden H, Baker M, Morris HR, et al. Corticobasal degeneration and progressive supranuclear palsy share a common tau haplotype. Neurology. 2001;56(12):1702–6.

41. Chen-Plotkin AS, Martinez-Lage M, Sleiman PM, et al. Genetic and clinical features of progranulin-associated frontotemporal lobar degeneration. Arch Neurol. 2011;68(4):488–97.

42. Seelaar H, Rohrer JD, Pijnenburg YA, Fox NC, van Swieten JC. Clinical, genetic and pathological heterogeneity of frontotemporal dementia: a review. J Neurol Neurosurg Psychiatry. 2011;82(5):476–86.

43. Kimonis VE, Fulchiero E, Vesa J, Watts G. VCP disease associated with myopathy, Paget disease of bone and frontotemporal dementia: review of a unique disorder. Biochim Biophys Acta. 2008;1782(12):744–8.

44. Isaacs AM, Johannsen P, Holm I, Nielsen JE. Frontotemporal dementia caused by CHMP2B mutations. Curr Alzheimer Res. 2011;8(3):246–51.

45. Benajiba L, Le Ber I, Camuzat A, et al. TARDBP mutations in motoneuron disease with frontotemporal lobar degeneration. Ann Neurol. 2009;65(4):470–3.

46. Blair IP, Williams KL, Warraich ST, et al. FUS mutations in amyotrophic lateral sclerosis: clinical, pathological, neurophysiological and genetic analysis. J Neurol Neurosurg Psychiatry. 2010;81(6):639–45.

47. Neumann M, Rademakers R, Roeber S, Baker M, Kretzschmar HA, Mackenzie IR. A new subtype of frontotemporal lobar degeneration with FUS pathology. Brain. 2009;132(Pt 11):2922–31.

48. Caroppo P, Camuzat A, De Septenville A, et al. Semantic and nonfluent aphasic variants, secondarily associated with amyotrophic lateral sclerosis, are predominant frontotemporal lobar degeneration phenotypes in TBK1 carriers. Alzheimers Dement. 2015;1(4):481–6.

49. Freischmidt A, Wieland T, Richter B, et al. Haploinsufficiency of TBK1 causes familial ALS and fronto-temporal dementia. Nat Neurosci. 2015 May;18:631–6.

50. McKhann GM, Albert MS, Grossman M, Miller B, Dickson D, Trojanowski JQ. Clinical and pathological diagnosis of frontotemporal dementia: report of the Work Group on Frontotemporal Dementia and Pick's Disease. Arch Neurol. 2001;58(11):1803–9.

51. Alladi S, Xuereb J, Bak T, et al. Focal cortical presentations of Alzheimer's disease. Brain. 2007;130(Pt 10):2636–45.

52. Cairns NJ, Bigio EH, Mackenzie IR, et al. Neuropathologic diagnostic and nosologic criteria for frontotemporal lobar degeneration: consensus of the Consortium for Frontotemporal Lobar Degeneration. Acta Neuropathol. 2007;114(1):5–22.

53. Deramecourt V, Lebert F, Debachy B, et al. Prediction of pathology in primary progressive language and speech disorders. Neurology. 2010;74(1):42–9.

54. Mackenzie IR, Neumann M, Baborie A, et al. A harmonized classification system for FTLD-TDP pathology. Acta Neuropathol. 2011;122(1):111–13.

55. Mackenzie IR, Munoz DG, Kusaka H, et al. Distinct pathological subtypes of FTLD-FUS. Acta Neuropathol. 2011;121:207–18.

56. Rabinovici GD, Seeley WW, Kim EJ, et al. Distinct MRI atrophy patterns in autopsy-proven Alzheimer's disease and frontotemporal lobar degeneration. Am J Alzheimers Dis Other Demen. 2007 Dec–2008 Jan;22(6):474–88.

57. Foster NL, Heidebrink JL, Clark CM, et al. FDG-PET improves accuracy in distinguishing frontotemporal dementia and Alzheimer's disease. Brain. 2007;130(Pt 10):2616–35.

58. Klunk WE, Engler H, Nordberg A, et al. Imaging brain amyloid in Alzheimer's disease with Pittsburgh Compound-B. Ann Neurol. 2004;55(3):306–19.

59. Maruyama M, Shimada H, Suhara T, et al. Imaging of tau pathology in a tauopathy mouse model and in Alzheimer patients compared to normal controls. Neuron. 2013;79(6):1094–108.

60. Zhou J, Greicius MD, Gennatas ED, et al. Divergent network connectivity changes in behavioural variant frontotemporal dementia and Alzheimer's disease. Brain. 2010;133(Pt 5):1352–67.

61. Oeckl P, Steinacker P, Feneberg E, Otto M. Cerebrospinal fluid proteomics and protein biomarkers in frontotemporal lobar degeneration: Current status and future perspectives. Biochim Biophys Acta. 2015;1854(7):757–68.

62. Spies PE, Slats D, Sjogren JM, et al. The cerebrospinal fluid amyloid beta42/40 ratio in the differentiation of Alzheimer's disease from non-Alzheimer's dementia. Curr Alzheimer Res. 2010;7(5):470–6.

63. de Souza LC, Lamari F, Belliard S, et al. Cerebrospinal fluid biomarkers in the differential diagnosis of Alzheimer's disease from other cortical dementias. J Neurol Neurosurg Psychiatry. 2011;82(3):240–6.

64. Ossenkoppele R, Pijnenburg YA, Perry DC, et al. The behavioural/dysexecutive variant of Alzheimer's disease: clinical, neuroimaging and pathological features. Brain. 2015;138(Pt 9):2732–49.

65. Lanata SC, Miller BL. The behavioural variant frontotemporal dementia (bvFTD) syndrome in psychiatry. J Neurol Neurosurg Psychiatry. 2016;87(5):501–11.

66. Le Ber I, Camuzat A, Hannequin D, et al. Phenotype variability in progranulin mutation carriers: a clinical, neuropsychological, imaging and genetic study. Brain. 2008;131(Pt 3):732–46.

67. Kipps CM, Hodges JR, Hornberger M. Nonprogressive behavioural frontotemporal dementia: recent developments and clinical implications of the 'bvFTD phenocopy syndrome'. Curr Opin Neurol. 2010;23(6):628–32.

68. Khan BK, Yokoyama JS, Takada LT, et al. Atypical, slowly progressive behavioural variant frontotemporal dementia associated with C9ORF72 hexanucleotide expansion. J Neurol Neurosurg Psychiatry. 2012;83(4):358–64.

69. Seltman RE, Matthews BR. Frontotemporal lobar degeneration: epidemiology, pathology, diagnosis and management. CNS Drugs. 2012;26(10):841–70.

70. Bott NT, Radke A, Stephens ML, Kramer JH. Frontotemporal dementia: diagnosis, deficits and management. Neurodegener Dis Manag. 2014;4(6):439–54.

71. Merrilees J. A model for management of behavioral symptoms in frontotemporal lobar degeneration. Alzheimer Dis Assoc Disord. 2007;21(4):S64–9.

# 42

# Prion disease

*Akin Nihat, TzeHow Mok, and John Collinge*

## Introduction

Human prion diseases, also known as subacute spongiform encephalopathies, have been traditionally classified into Creutzfeldt–
Jakob disease (CJD), Gerstmann–Sträussler syndrome (GSS) (also
known as Gerstmann–Sträussler–Scheinker disease), and kuru,
although this has largely been superseded by aetiological categorization. Although rare, with an annual incidence of 1–2 per million
worldwide (accounting for 1 in 5000 deaths in the UK), remarkable attention has been focused on these diseases. This is because
of the unique biology of the transmissible agent, or prion, and also
because bovine spongiform encephalopathy (BSE), an epidemic
bovine prion disease, was transmitted to humans as variant CJD
(vCJD), leading to fears of a significant public health threat through
dietary exposure.

The transmissibility of the human diseases was first demonstrated
with the transmission of kuru and then CJD in 1966 and 1968, respectively, [1, 2] by intracerebral inoculation of brain homogenates
into chimpanzees. Transmission of GSS followed in 1981. The prototypic prion disease is scrapie, a common naturally occurring disease
of sheep and goats, recognized in Europe for over 200 years and present in sheep flocks of many countries. Scrapie was demonstrated
to be transmissible by inoculation in 1936 [3], and the recognition
that kuru, and then CJD, resembled scrapie in its histopathological
appearances led to the suggestion that these diseases may also be
transmissible [4]. Kuru reached epidemic proportions among the
Fore linguistic group in the Eastern Highlands of Papua New Guinea
and was transmitted by consumption of human tissues at mortuary
feasts. Since the cessation of cannibalism in the 1950s, the disease
has declined, but a few cases were still occurring into the 2010s as
a result of long incubation periods, which may exceed 50 years [5].

The term Creutzfeldt–Jakob disease was introduced by Spielmeyer
in 1922, bringing together the case reports published by Creutzfeldt
and Jakob. Several of these cases would not meet modern diagnostic
criteria for CJD; indeed, it was not until the demonstration of transmissibility allowing diagnostic criteria to be refined that a clear diagnostic entity developed. Prion diseases of both humans and animals
are associated with the accumulation in the brain of disease-related
isoforms of a host-encoded protein known as prion protein (PrP),
and all share common histopathological features: the classical triad
of spongiform vacuolation (affecting any part of the cerebral grey

matter), astrocytic proliferation, and neuronal loss, accompanied by
PrP deposits which may form amyloid plaques.

## Aetiology

According to the widely accepted 'protein-only' hypothesis, prions are
devoid of significant nucleic acid and consist of multichain assemblies
of misfolded, host-encoded PrP, a cell surface glycoprotein expressed
in most tissues, but at its highest levels in the CNS. Cellular PrP (PrP$^C$)
is present in all vertebrates and highly conserved in mammals. Prions
are thought to propagate by acting as a template to recruit PrP monomers in an autocatalytic process of seeded protein polymerization and
fission, mimicking propagation of a biological pathogen. Biophysical
experiments established that PrP$^C$, rich in α-helical structure, needs to
largely unfold in order to adopt the β-sheet-rich structure of the infectious amyloid form, arguing that prions propagate by recruitment of
at least partially unfolded PrP. Disease-related PrP isoforms have been
classically referred to as PrP$^{Sc}$ (for the scrapie form of PrP), which was
originally defined by its partial resistance to proteolytic digestion.
However, it is now established that there are multiple disease-related
forms of PrP, some of which are protease-sensitive, and the term PrP$^{Sc}$
should not be used synonymously with prion infectivity.

Human prion diseases have three distinct aetiologies: (1) autosomal dominant inheritance, whereby coding mutations in the PrP
gene (*PRNP*) result in PrP$^C$ predisposed to form seeds; (2) sporadic CJD, following the spontaneous production of seeds as a rare
stochastic event and representing the large majority of CJD cases;
and (3) acquired by environmental exposure to prions. While this
aetiological triumvirate was thought unique, it is now being widely
considered whether this is relevant to much more common diseases.
Notably, the principal neurodegenerative diseases are all associated
with accumulation of misfolded proteins; they also occur primarily as
sporadic conditions, but with rare inherited forms generally associated with mutations in the genes encoding or processing the relevant
accumulating proteins or peptides. Recent data are challenging the
assumption that these conditions do not have acquired forms, with
a developing interest in understanding whether the so-called 'prion-
like' mechanisms are involved, notably in Alzheimer's disease [6].

The human PrP gene (*PRNP*) is a single-copy gene located on the
short arm of chromosome 20. A turning point in understanding

human prion diseases was the identification of mutations in *PRNP* in familial CJD and GSS in 1989. The first mutation to be identified in *PRNP* was in a family with CJD and constituted a 144-bp insertion into the coding sequence [7]. A second mutation was reported in two families with GSS, and genetic linkage was confirmed between this missense variant at codon 102 and GSS, confirming that GSS was an autosomal dominant Mendelian disorder [8]. Current evidence suggests that around 15% of prion diseases are inherited and over 40 coding mutations in *PRNP* are now recognized.

A common PrP polymorphism at residue 129, where either methionine or valine can be encoded, is a key determinant of genetic susceptibility to acquired and sporadic prion diseases—the large majority of which occur in homozygous individuals [9, 10]. This protective effect of *PRNP* codon 129 heterozygosity is also seen in some of the inherited prion diseases.

### Prion strains and transmission characteristics

Although devoid of a nucleic acid genome, prions exist as multiple strains which can be serially propagated in laboratory animals and produce distinct patterns of disease. Strains are associated with specific types of PrP$^{Sc}$, and it is thought they represent structurally distinct seeds that are able to recruit host PrP$^{C}$ into their discrete polymeric forms. Understanding how a protein-only infectious agent could encode such phenotypic information has been of considerable biological interest and represents a non-Mendelian form of transmission.

Prion strain diversity appears to be encoded by differences in PrP conformation and pattern of glycosylation [11]. Molecular strain typing approaches, based on these characteristics, have allowed the identification of multiple types among CJD cases. Two classifications are in use; no internationally agreed classification has yet emerged, and it is likely that additional PrP$^{Sc}$ types or strains will be identified [12, 13]. According to the London classification, four main types of PrP$^{Sc}$ are recognized—sporadic and iatrogenic CJD being of PrP$^{Sc}$ types 1–3, while all variant CJD cases are associated with a distinctive type 4 PrP$^{Sc}$ [11, 12].

Transmission of prion diseases between different mammalian species is limited by a so-called 'species barrier'. Early studies of the molecular basis of the species barrier argued that it principally resided in differences in PrP primary structure between the inoculating species and the host. Transgenic mice expressing hamster PrP were, unlike wild-type mice, highly susceptible to infection with hamster prions [14]. That most sporadic and acquired CJD occurred in individuals homozygous at *PRNP* polymorphic codon 129 supported the view that prion propagation proceeded most efficiently when interacting PrP$^{Sc}$ and PrP$^{C}$ were of identical primary structure [12]. However, it has been long recognized that prion strain type affects ease of transmission to another species. Interestingly, with BSE prions, the strain component to the barrier seems to predominate, with BSE not only transmitting efficiently to a range of species, but maintaining its transmission characteristics, even when passaged through an intermediate species with a distinct PrP gene [15]. The term 'transmission barrier' is therefore preferable [15]. Both the PrP amino acid sequence and strain type affect the three-dimensional structure of glycosylated PrP, which will presumably, in turn, affect the efficiency of the protein–protein interactions thought to determine prion propagation.

Mammalian PrP genes are highly conserved. Presumably only a restricted number of different PrP$^{Sc}$ conformations (that are highly stable and can therefore be serially propagated) will be permissible thermodynamically and will constitute the range of prion strains seen in mammals. While a significant number of different PrP$^{Sc}$ conformations may be possible among the range of mammalian PrPs, only a subset of these would be allowable for a given single mammalian PrP. Substantial overlap between the favoured conformations for PrP$^{Sc}$ derived from species A and species B might therefore result in relatively easy transmission of prion diseases between these two species, while two species with no preferred PrP$^{Sc}$ conformations in common would have a large barrier to transmission (and indeed transmission would necessitate a change of strain type). According to such a *conformational selection model* [16] of a prion transmission barrier, BSE may represent a thermodynamically highly favoured PrP$^{Sc}$ conformation that is permissive for PrP expressed in a wide range of different species, accounting for the remarkable promiscuity of this strain in mammals. Contribution of other components to the transmission barrier is possible and may involve interacting co-factors which mediate the efficiency of prion propagation, although no such factors have yet been identified.

Additional data have further challenged our understanding of transmission barriers [17], the assessment of which has relied on the development of a clinical disease in inoculated animals. However, it is now clear that *subclinical prion infections* are sometimes established on prion inoculation of a second species [18]. Such animals harbour high levels of prion infectivity but do not develop clinical disease during a normal lifespan. The existence of such subclinical carrier states of prion infection has important potential animal and public health implications and argues against direct neurotoxicity of prions. Indeed, recent studies have demonstrated uncoupling of prion propagation and neurotoxicity [19].

The transmission barrier between cattle BSE and humans cannot be directly measured but can be modelled in transgenic mice expressing human PrP$^{C}$, which produce human PrP$^{Sc}$ when challenged with human prions. While these transgenic mouse models have been able to faithfully propagate human prion strains [11, 20, 21] and recapitulate the characteristic neuropathology of vCJD [22], there are important caveats in extrapolating from such animal models to human susceptibility. However, these studies have found a much higher infection rate in transgenic mice expressing human PrP M129 than mice expressing human PrP V129 when challenged with either BSE or vCJD prions, and demonstrated that BSE prion infection can produce disease phenotypes resembling sporadic CJD and also novel prion strain phenotypes. Most recently, these studies have argued that the vCJD phenotype may only be expressed in the presence of the M form of human PrP [23]. While implying that only those humans expressing PrP M129 may develop the vCJD phenotype, this does not mean that VV individuals are completely resistant to BSE prion infection—but rather that if infected, they would show a different phenotype [23]. Modelling of susceptibility of the MV genotype suggests that several different phenotypes may be possible when infected with BSE or vCJD prions [24].

### Clinical features and diagnosis

Human prion diseases can be divided aetiologically into inherited, sporadic, and acquired forms, which largely share one or more core clinical features: progressive cognitive deterioration, ataxia, myoclonus, and pyramidal or extra-pyramidal motor signs. Focal cognitive deficits (for example, executive or memory impairment) may present in isolation for weeks or months, as can isolated ataxia. There is inevitably progression to global cognitive dysfunction, and the common pre-terminal clinical state is akinetic mutism.

Nevertheless, there is wide phenotypic variability both between and within aetiological groups. Indeed, kindreds with inherited prion disease that segregate the same mutation can manifest remarkably diverse clinical presentations. Approximately 85–90% of human prion disease cases in the UK are sporadic, and psychiatric symptoms in the form of agitation, anxiety, hallucinations, or depression are present in the majority early in disease course. A subset of patients develop a more discrete psychiatric syndrome, such as florid psychosis, and may first present to psychiatric services without common motor features.

Broadly, prion disease should be considered in all cases of early-onset or rapidly progressive dementia or ataxia. Significant clinical overlap exists with other neurodegenerative syndromes, including Alzheimer's disease, dementia with Lewy bodies, and fronto-temporal dementia. A definite diagnosis can only be made via neuropathological examination, commonly post-mortem (or with a confirmed *PRNP* mutation in inherited prion disease). However, the rapid advancement in diagnostic markers, in particular diffusion-weighted MRI and CSF prion seeding assays for sporadic prion disease, coupled with the availability of *PRNP* genotyping, now permits accurate ante mortem diagnosis in the large majority of cases. Brain biopsy is now rarely required and is usually reserved for cases with highly atypical features or a strong suspicion of a treatable mimic. The key clinical features and investigations for the diagnosis of prion disease are given in Box 42.1.

## Sporadic CJD

The onset is usually in the 45- to 90-years age group, peaking around 65 years. Sporadic CJD (sCJD) classically presents with rapidly progressive multifocal dementia, myoclonus, and gait ataxia. The condition typically progresses over weeks to akinetic mutism and death, often in 2–3 months; around 70% of cases die in under 6 months and 90% by 1 year. Prodromal features such as headache, fatigue, or weight loss are reported in about a third of cases; the other key features of sCJD include pyramidal and extra-pyramidal signs and visual signs. For case classification for epidemiological purposes, the appropriate clinical picture, in combination with at least one typical investigation finding (MRI, EEG, or CSF), would allow ante mortem classification as *probable* sCJD, without histological confirmation (Box 42.1). Probable CJD is almost always (>95%) confirmed as definite if autopsy is performed.

Routine blood investigations are usually within the normal range and, even when abnormal, possess no particular value diagnostically. MRI brain with diffusion-weighted sequences has emerged as the most sensitive non-invasive diagnostic tool for sCJD [25]; sCJD patients typically demonstrate restricted diffusion in the basal ganglia and thalami and cortical ribboning, but the regional combinations vary from case to case (Fig. 42.1). Signal hyperintensity on T2-weighted and FLAIR sequences in the corresponding regions may also be present, but this is less striking. CSF examination is essential to exclude other causes of rapid cognitive decline, and both cell count and routine biochemistry remain normal in sCJD cases.

---

**Box 42.1** Diagnosis of prion disease

**Sporadic CJD (MRI-CJD diagnostic criteria [25])**

I. *Clinical signs (rapidly progressive dementia\* with additional features)*
  − Myoclonus.
  − Cerebellar or visual signs.
  − Pyramidal or extra-pyramidal signs.
  − Akinetic mutism.

II. *Tests*
  − Periodic sharp waves complexes on EEG.
  − 14-3-3 protein detected in CSF.
  − High signal abnormalities in caudate nucleus/striatum, or at least two cortical regions (temporal/parietal/occipital), either in diffusion-weighted imaging (DWI) or fluid attenuation inversion recovery (FLAIR) MRI sequences.
  − Positive RT-QuIC in CSF or other tissues

*Probable sCJD*
- Rapidly progressive dementia and two of I and at least one of II. Progressive neurological syndrome and positive RT-QuIC in CSF or other tissues

*Possible sCJD*
- Rapidly progressive dementia and two of I and duration of less than 2 years.

**Iatrogenic CJD**
- Progressive predominantly cerebellar syndrome and behavioural disturbance in a recipient of human pituitary hormones (growth hormone or gonadotrophin). Limb dysaesthesiae is also a frequent feature.
- Probable CJD with exposure to a recognized iatrogenic CJD risk factor: human pituitary hormones; human dura mater graft; corneal graft from a recipient with definite/probable human prion disease; exposure to neurosurgical instruments used in a case with definite/probable human prion disease.
- Incubation periods may be over 40 years from exposure.
- MRI findings are similar to those seen in sporadic CJD; EEG periodic sharp waves are rarely seen.
- CSF 14-3-3 protein can be detected in approximately half of cases; RTQuIC can also be positive, but sensitivity is much reduced, compared with sporadic CJD.

**Variant CJD**
- Progressive neuropsychiatric syndrome: depression, anxiety, withdrawal, delusions.
- Peripheral sensory symptoms (pain or dysaesthesiae), cerebella ataxia, and myoclonus/chorea/dystonia often precede dementia.
- Mostly young adults, with a longer disease course (>6 months).
- EEG: non-specific slow waves, CSF 14-3-3 may be elevated or normal.
- MRI: pulvinar sign present in approximately 90% (particularly FLAIR sequence) but may be a late feature and not pathognomonic.
- Tonsil biopsy: characteristic PrP immunostaining and PrP$^{Sc}$ on western blot.

**Inherited prion disease**
- Varied clinical syndromes between and within kindreds: consider in all pre-senile dementias and ataxias, irrespective of family history.
- *PRNP* analysis: diagnostic, codon 129 genotype may predict age at onset in pre-symptomatic testing.

\* This is typically 6 months or less, but there is high variability; approximately 10% have a duration of >2 years. No other cause identified, including no pathogenic *PRNP* mutations.

Incorporates data from Lloyd, S., Mead, S., & Collinge, J. (2011). Genetics of prion disease. In *Prion Proteins* (pp. 1–22). Springer Berlin Heidelberg.

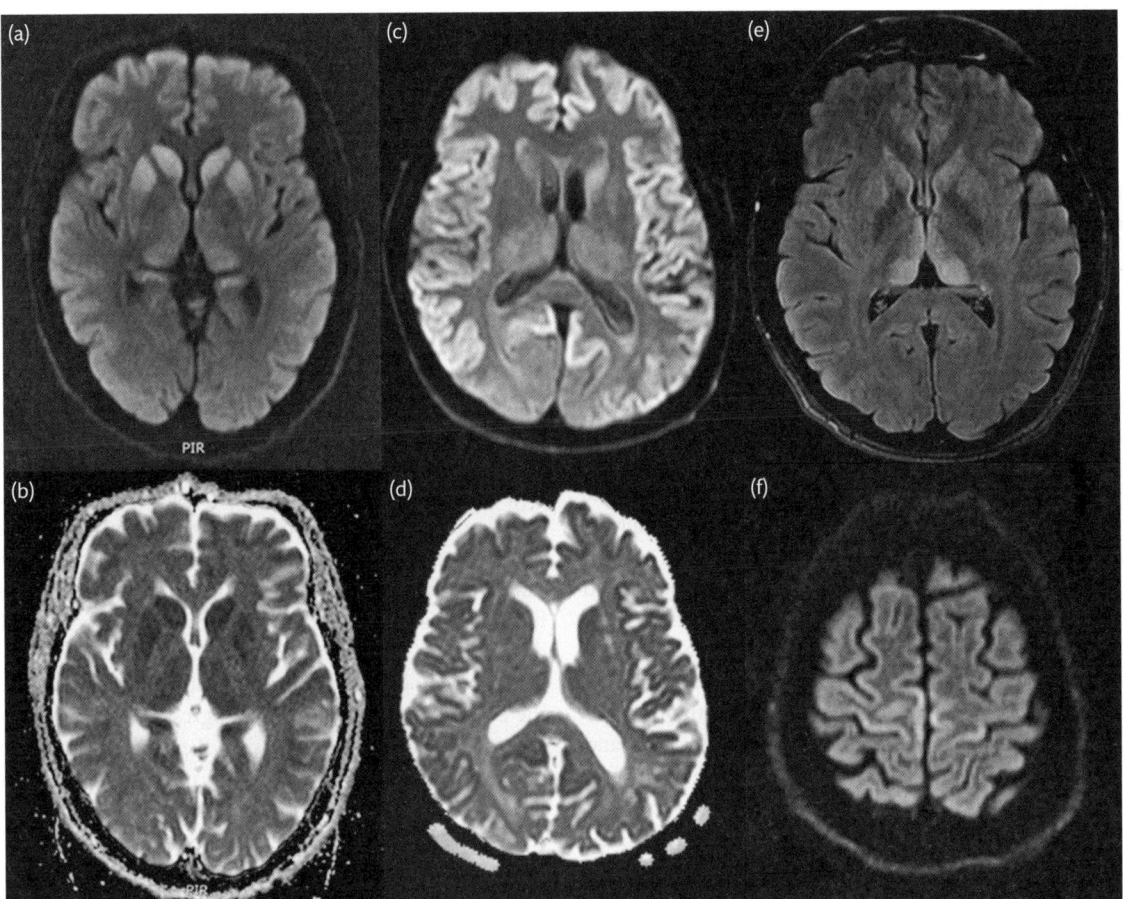

**Fig. 42.1** Typical MRI features of sporadic CJD (sCJD), variant CJD (vCJD), and iatrogenic CJD. (a) Diffusion-weighted (DW) imaging showing the basal ganglia, thalamic, and hippocampal tail increased signal in sCJD, with corresponding restriction (b) in apparent diffusion coefficient (ADC) sequence. (c) and (d) DW and ADC images in sCJD, showing cortical ribboning and restricted diffusion. (e) FLAIR image in vCJD showing the pulvinar sign (thalamic high signal more prominent than in the basal ganglia). (f) DW image in iatrogenic CJD, showing high signal in the motor strip.

The presence of protein 14-3-3, raised S100B levels, and highly elevated total tau levels in the CSF are useful adjunctive tests for sCJD. However, they have been superseded by the development of the real-time quaking-induced conversion (RT-QuIC) assay in recent years. RT-QuIC is an amyloid-seeding assay that uses repeated mechanical sample shaking and incubation to amplify prion seeds in patient CSF, using recombinant PrP as a substrate and a fluorescent thioflavin T readout. A positive CSF RT-QuIC possesses a comparable sensitivity to a positive protein 14-3-3 in the CSF, but more importantly it has a specificity for sCJD approaching 100% [26]. The RT-QuIC assays seeded by nasal brushings and, more recently, skin from sCJD patients also yield high sensitivities and specificities approaching (and reaching) 100%, although neither of these have yet been incorporated into routine clinical practice [27, 28]. EEG in sCJD may show characteristic pseudoperiodic sharp wave activity, but this is demonstrated in less than 50% of patients [25], the large majority of whom are *PRNP* codon 129 MM. To some extent, demonstration of a typical EEG is dependent on the number of serial EEGs performed.

Neuropathological confirmation of sCJD is by demonstration of the classical spongiform change, neuronal loss, astrocytosis, and positive PrP immunohistochemistry. PrP amyloid plaques are usually not present in sCJD, although protease-resistant PrP$^{Sc}$ types 1–3 can be demonstrated by immunoblotting of brain homogenates

(molecular strain typing; see Aetiology, p. 414). *PRNP* analysis is important to exclude pathogenic mutations. By definition, there is no family history in these cases, although rarely mutations are seen due to late-onset disease or non-paternity. It is possible some cases might arise from somatic mutation of *PRNP* or unidentified environmental exposure to human or animal prions.

## Atypical forms of sCJD

Atypical forms of sCJD with distinct clinical syndromes and durations of survival are well recognized. Those with the so-called ataxic variant of sCJD present with slowly evolving gait ataxia in the initial months before the onset of cognitive impairment. These individuals are typically *PRNP* codon 129 MV and have a longer duration of illness, with a good proportion living beyond 2 years from the time of symptom onset. In the Heidenhain variant of sCJD, which affects individuals who are *PRNP* codon 129 MM, cortical visual symptoms and signs predominate in the early course of the illness, while memory remains intact; patients can progress rapidly to cortical blindness and death in as short as 4 weeks from symptom onset, often accompanied by severe agitation.

Other clinical syndromes at presentation encountered in sCJD patients include pure cognitive syndromes, neuropsychiatric syndromes, cortico-basal syndrome, and stroke-like syndromes;

the former two can progress slowly with late emergence of typical sCJD signs and are frequently mistaken for Alzheimer's disease and behavioural-variant fronto-temporal lobar degeneration, respectively.

## Acquired prion diseases

While human prion diseases can be transmitted to experimental animals by inoculation, they are not contagious in humans. Documented case-to-case spread has only occurred during endo-cannibalistic practices (kuru) or following accidental inoculation with prions during medical or surgical procedures (iatrogenic CJD).

### Kuru

Kuru reached epidemic proportions among the Fore linguistic group and their neighbours in the Eastern Highlands of Papua New Guinea [29]. It predominantly affected women and children, as they were the principal participants in the practice of consuming dead relatives at mortuary feasts, as a mark of respect and mourning.

The clinical course typically lasts between 1 and 2 years and begins with a constitutional prodrome of headaches and limb and joint pain, followed by progressive cerebellar ataxia, often with other features such as tremor, diplopia, dysarthria, social withdrawal, and depression. Patients subsequently develop global dementia and frequently pyramidal and extra-pyramidal motor signs.

Kuru incidence has been in decline since its peak in the 1950s, following the cessation of endocannabalism in the late 1950s, and the last recorded case was 2012. However, the study of kuru continues to reveal valuable insights, the most recent being the identification of the protective G127V polymorphism in kindreds at the epicentre of the kuru epidemic. This polymorphism appeared to provide complete protection against kuru [30], and this was supported by transgenic mouse modelling and inoculation experiments which showed that mice expressing human PrP 127V were completely resistant to all known human prion strains [31].

### Iatrogenic CJD

Iatrogenic transmission of CJD has occurred by accidental inoculation with human prions as a result of medical procedures. Such iatrogenic routes include the use of inadequately sterilized neurosurgical instruments, dura mater and corneal grafting, and use of human cadaveric pituitary-derived growth hormone or gonadotrophin. It is of considerable interest that cases arising from intracerebral or optic inoculation manifest clinically as classical CJD, with rapidly progressive dementia, while those resulting from peripheral inoculation, most notably following pituitary-derived growth hormone exposure, typically present with a progressive cerebellar syndrome and are, in that respect, somewhat reminiscent of kuru. Unsurprisingly, the incubation period in intracerebral cases is short (less than 2 years for depth electrodes and neurosurgery), as compared to peripheral cases (typically 15 years or more). There is evidence for genetic susceptibility to iatrogenic CJD with an excess of codon 129 homozygotes [9] (see Aetiology, p. 414).

### Variant CJD

The appearance of an unusual form of CJD in the UK was heralded by a spate of cases in teenagers and young adults in 1995–1996, with a surprisingly consistent, but unique, histological pattern [32]. There was considerable concern over the possibility that they might suggest a link with BSE. These cases were named 'new variant' CJD, and eventually 'variant' CJD (vCJD), although it was clear that they were also rather atypical in their clinical presentation; in fact, most cases did not meet the accepted clinical diagnostic criteria for probable CJD.

Direct experimental evidence that vCJD is caused by BSE was provided by molecular analysis of human prion strains and transmission studies in transgenic and wild-type mice (see Aetiology, p. 414), with the most likely explanation being exposure to specified bovine offal (notably CNS tissues) prior to the ban on its inclusion in human foodstuffs in 1989. While it is now clear that vCJD is caused by infection with BSE prions, it is unclear why this particular age group should be predominantly affected.

vCJD has an insidious clinical onset, and its early features are highly non-specific. The clinical presentation is often with behavioural and psychiatric disturbance, commonly depression, but also anxiety, social withdrawal, and behavioural change, complex unsustained delusions, and visual and auditory hallucinations. Initial referral is consequently often to a psychiatrist. Persistent limb or face dysaesthesiae and pain are also prominent early features. In most cases, neurological features are not apparent until some months into the clinical course, whereby a progressive cerebellar syndrome develops with gait and limb ataxia. Overt dementia then occurs, with inevitable progression to akinetic mutism. Myoclonus is seen in most patients, and chorea is often present, which may be severe in some patients. The age at onset ranges from 12 to 74 years, with a mean of around 28 years. Clinical course is usually prolonged, compared to sCJD (9–35 months, median 14 months).

The EEG is abnormal, most frequently showing generalized slow wave activity, but without the pseudoperiodic pattern seen in sCJD cases. CSF 14-3-3 protein may be elevated or normal. Neuroimaging by CT is either normal or shows only mild atrophy. The most useful non-invasive investigation in advanced cases is magnetic resonance neuroimaging, in which FLAIR hyperintensity has been demonstrated in the pulvinar nuclei of the thalamus, designated the 'pulvinar sign', in 91% of vCJD cases [33]. The pulvinar sign is not exclusive to vCJD but can also be seen in sCJD, paraneoplastic limbic encephalitis, idiopathic intracranial hypertension, status epilepticus associated with cat-scratch disease, Alper's disease, and post-infectious encephalitis. The absence of the pulvinar sign does not exclude a diagnosis of vCJD, and in fact, the MRI in older patients with histologically confirmed vCJD seems less likely to possess the pulvinar sign [34]. Remarkably, up until early 2016, all definite cases of vCJD have been of the *PRNP* codon 129 MM genotype; a case of vCJD in an individual who is *PRNP* codon 129 MV was previously described, but the first case of pathologically confirmed vCJD in whom the *PRNP* codon 129 genotype was MV was reported in 2017 [35]. MRI features in this case were reminiscent of sCJD; the pulvinar sign was absent. Crucially, this patient did not fulfil diagnostic criteria for probable or possible vCJD in life.

Tonsillar biopsy is a sensitive and specific diagnostic procedure for vCJD and obviates the need for brain biopsy, based on the presence of prion replication in lymphoreticular tissue prior to neurological onset [36–39]. Tonsillar PrP$^{Sc}$ is uniformly present in clinically affected cases of vCJD, but not in other forms of prion disease. Prior to tonsil biopsy, *PRNP* analysis is essential to rule out pathogenic mutations, which may clinically mimic vCJD.

Several biofluid-based techniques have been in development for diagnostic use in vCJD. The blood-based direct detection assay (DDA) exploits the steel binding affinity of prions with a capture matrix, coupled with immunodetection; this had a sensitivity of 71% and a specificity of 100% and is available at the UK National Prion Clinic [40]. More recently, the protein misfolding cyclic amplification (PMCA) assay, which is analogous to the RT-QuIC technique but uses repetitive cycles of sonication, instead of shaking and western blot as a readout, has been adapted with success for historical vCJD blood and urine samples. The sensitivities and specificities achieved were between 90% and 100%, but neither has yet been applied in routine clinical practice or for screening purposes [41–43].

The neuropathological appearances of vCJD are striking and relatively consistent. While there is widespread spongiform change and gliosis and neuronal loss, most severe in the basal ganglia and thalamus, the most remarkable feature is abundant 'florid' PrP amyloid plaques (in which the plaques are surrounded by vacuoles) in the cerebral and cerebellar cortices. Western blot analysis of brain tissue demonstrates PrP$^{Sc}$ type 4, which is pathognomonic of vCJD.

Important lessons predicting the evolution of vCJD epidemiology can be drawn from kuru research and large-scale studies of archived appendix tissue in the UK. Firstly, kuru studies highlighted the profound effect of *PRNP* codon 129 genotype on incubation period with individuals who are 129 MV, having incubation periods which can exceed 50 years [5]; a similar effect of codon 129 genotype on incubation period is also seen in iatrogenic CJD cases secondary to human cadaveric growth hormone [44]. Secondly, screening of archived appendix studies led to estimates that approximately 1 in 2000 of the UK population carry subclinical vCJD infection [45]. While numbers of vCJD cases have steadily fallen since their peak in 2000, it is possible that a second wave of cases may occur in 129 MV individuals. Furthermore, given the atypical clinical features of the MV vCJD case and results from animal modelling studies (see Aetiology, p. 414), assiduous autopsy surveillance may be required to establish the true extent of BSE-related human prion disease, some of which might present as sCJD.

### Secondary (iatrogenic) vCJD

The prominent lymphoreticular involvement raised early concerns that vCJD may be transmissible by blood transfusion. Indeed the tissue distribution is similar to that of ovine scrapie where prionaemia has been demonstrated experimentally. In 2004, two transfusion-associated cases of vCJD prion infection were reported among a small cohort of patients identified as having received blood from a donor who subsequently developed vCJD. One patient had a typical clinical course of vCJD, although the diagnosis was not made until autopsy, and had the *PRNP* codon 129 MM genotype. The second, who died of an unrelated condition, was found to have prion infection at autopsy. This patient had the *PRNP* codon 129 MV genotype, which is associated with relative resistance to prion disease. Subsequently, two further patients have been diagnosed with vCJD during life from this group of 23 known surviving recipients of implicated blood. That four of 23 patients have been infected, three dying of vCJD, in each case following transfusion with a single unit of implicated red cells, suggests the risk to recipients of blood from a silently infected donor is substantial. The incubation period in the clinical cases was 6–7 years. Since 2003, all known recipients of implicated blood have been notified of their status. Over 6000 individuals in the UK have been exposed to blood products prepared from large donor pools containing blood from a donor who went on to develop vCJD. None of these individuals, predominantly haemophiliacs, have yet developed vCJD.

## Inherited prion diseases

Approximately 10–15% of human prion disease cases are inherited in an autosomal dominant fashion. Over 40 pathogenic mutations are reported in the human PrP gene (Fig. 42.2) and consist of: (1) point mutations within the coding sequence, resulting in amino acid substitutions in PrP or the production of a stop codon resulting in the expression of a truncated PrP; (2) insertions encoding additional integral copies of an octapeptide repeat present in a tandem array of five copies in the normal protein [octapeptide repeat insertion (OPRI)]; and (3) insertions or deletions resulting in a frameshift mutation. Some reportedly pathogenic mutations may, in fact, represent benign or risk-conferring polymorphisms [46].

Phenotypes can be widely variable, even within kindreds; hence, *PRNP* analysis should be considered in all early-onset dementing or ataxic disorders and is available from the UK National Prion Clinic (see Further information, p. 421). Brief details of the more commonly seen types are given in the following sections. For a more comprehensive review, see reference [47].

### P102L (commonly presenting as Gerstmann–Sträussler–Scheinker syndrome)

This is the most common mutation seen in the UK, usually presenting as GSS, as originally described in 1936 in a family, prior to the discovery of *PRNP* mutations [48]. Progressive ataxia is the dominant clinical feature, with dementia, pyramidal features, and lower limb dysaesthesiae occurring later. The mean age of onset is 49 years (range 25–70), and the mean clinical duration 4 years. Rarely, the clinical course is shorter and can closely mimic sCJD.

### Octapeptide repeat insertion mutations

The first PrP mutation reported was a 6-OPRI mutation, found in a small UK family with familial CJD [7], now known to form part of the largest known kindred with an inherited prion disease caused by an OPRI mutation. Kindreds segregating for pathogenic mutations encompassing 4–9 and 12-OPRI mutations are described (see, for example, [49–52]). Insertions of 1–3 OPRI repeats have been rarely reported, often with clinical and neuropathological features indistinguishable from sCJD [53]; it remains to be seen whether these reflect true pathogenic mutations or benign polymorphisms in the context of sporadic disease.

The 6-OPRI mutation is the most commonly seen in the UK; the initial presentation is usually of cortical cognitive deficits such as apraxia, acalculia, language impairment, frontal dysexecutive features, and episodic memory loss. Physically, there is a varying combination of cerebellar ataxia and dysarthria, pyramidal signs, myoclonus, and occasionally extra-pyramidal signs, chorea, and seizures. A well-described behavioural prodrome can include personality disorder, aggression, hypersexuality, and impulsivity, often manifesting in childhood or long before any overt neurodegenerative syndrome; patients are frequently in contact with the criminal justice system prior to diagnosis [54]. The mean age of onset is 34 years

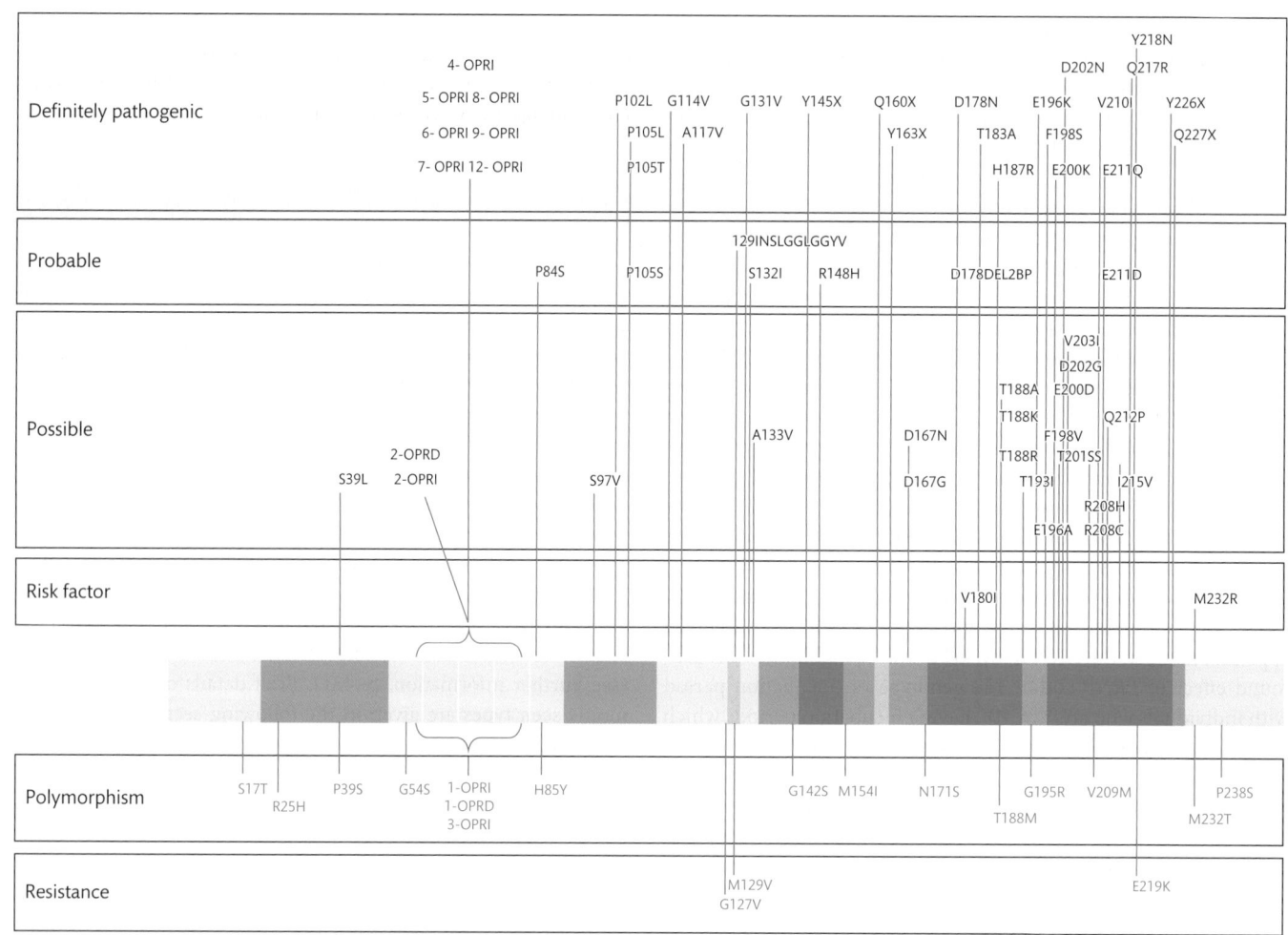

**Fig. 42.2** Pathogenic mutations (above) and polymorphic variants of the human prion protein gene.

(range 20–53), with a mean clinical duration of 8–10 years. Codon 129 heterozygotes have an age of onset of approximately 10 years later than homozygotes [51].

### A117V

This mutation has been described in families from France, the United States, and the UK [55]. The clinical features are of progressive cortical dementia that can often present as expressive language dysfunction. There is associated Parkinsonism, which may predominate in the early stages and mimic Parkinson's disease. Pyramidal signs, pseudobulbar features, and cerebellar ataxia are also seen. The mean age of onset is 39 years, and the mean clinical duration of around 4 years.

### D178N (fatal familial insomnia)

The D178N mutation has been documented widely in kindreds throughout Europe [56, 57], and the clinical phenotype is modified by the codon 129 status of the mutant allele. When the mutation is encoded on a methionine 129 allele, the clinical picture is usually of fatal familial insomnia (FFI); the cardinal feature is insomnia, often with a preceding period of inattentiveness. There may be initially compensatory daytime somnolence that masks early symptoms. Autonomic features invariably develop, including hypertension, excessive salivation, hyperhidrosis, diurnal pyrexia. and impotence.

Hallucinations are a frequent feature, and with progression, there is ataxia, dementia, and myoclonus. The mean age of onset is 50 years (range 20–72). When the codon 178 mutation occurs on a valine 129 allele, the clinical picture closely mimics sCJD [58], as do MRI diffusion-weighted imaging sequence appearances, albeit with a more prolonged course of about 15 months.

### E200K

This mutation is the most common cause of inherited prion disease worldwide, particularly in closely segregated communities, for example in Chile and Slovakia, and among Sephardic Jews in Libya and Israel [59, 60]. The clinical picture and imaging findings are indistinguishable from sCJD, although there is often peripheral neuropathy, and seizures are more frequently seen. The mean age at onset is a little earlier than in sCJD, at around 61 years, but there is a wide range of 31–78 years in the UK. The clinical duration is, on average, 5 months.

### Y163X (PrP systemic amyloidosis)

First described in 2013 in a large family from the south of England, this truncation mutation usually manifests in the fourth decade with insidious diarrhoea, nausea, autonomic disturbance, neurogenic bladder, and recurrent urinary infections, followed much later by length-dependent axonal neuropathy and cognitive decline. The clinical course is progressive over approximately 20 years, and pathology is remarkable for the extent of peripheral prion amyloid deposition, primarily in the gut, in addition to the CNS [61].

## Pre-symptomatic and antenatal testing

Direct gene testing allows unequivocal diagnosis in patients with inherited forms of the disease and pre-symptomatic testing of unaffected, but at-risk, family members, as well as antenatal testing after appropriate genetic counselling. Pre-implantation genetic diagnosis and transfer of unaffected embryos via *in vitro* fertilization (IVF) were successfully used to remove the risk of inherited prion disease in the offspring of a parent carrying the F198S mutation in the United States [62].

Because age of clinical onset in some mutations is affected by *PRNP* codon 129 genotype, it is often possible to determine within a family whether a carrier of a mutation will have an early or late onset of disease. However, biomarkers indicating a more specific age of onset are sorely needed and are the focus of determined investigation.

Most of the common mutations appear to be fully penetrant; however, experience with some is extremely limited. In some families, for example with E200K or D178N (FFI), there are examples of elderly unaffected gene carriers who appear to have escaped the disease; the wide age of onset may indicate complete penetrance at a very advanced age, which may not be practically relevant for many patients. Recent work comparing the expected incidence of clinical disease with the frequency of reportedly pathogenic mutations in large control populations suggests the penetrance of several to be 10% or lower; at this level, they may be better classified as risk-conferring variants [46], with important implications for genetic counselling discussions.

Genetic counselling is essential prior to pre-symptomatic testing. A positive PrP gene analysis has important consequences for other family members, and it is preferable to have discussed these issues with others in the immediate family before testing. Following the identification of a mutation, the wider family should be referred for genetic counselling. It is vital to counsel both those testing positive for mutations and those untested but at-risk that they should not be blood or organ donors and should inform surgeons, including dentists, of their risk status prior to significant procedures, as precautions may be necessary to minimize the risk of iatrogenic transmission.

## Treatment

All recognized prion diseases are invariably fatal, following a progressive course. There have been few robust therapeutic trials in human prion disease. These are challenging due to the combination of difficulty recruiting adequate patient numbers, a paucity of validated outcome measures beyond mortality, and widely variable disease patterns in the absence of longitudinal natural history data. Many of these barriers to meaningful controlled clinical trials have now been largely overcome [63, 64].

A double-blind RCT of flupertine, a non-opioid analgesic, suggested some benefit in cognitive scores, but not mortality, albeit in a small sample size and with borderline statistical significance [65]. A patient preference trial (PRION-1) of quinacrine, an anti-malarial agent, in 107 patients with prion disease did not significantly alter the disease course [66]. A more recent randomized, double-blind, placebo-controlled trial of doxycycline, an antibiotic with positive reports in previous observational studies, similarly did not show any effect on disease progression or mortality [67]. The effects of a variety of other agents have been reported anecdotally or in small case series, including pentosan polysulfate, a glycosaminoglycan administered to a handful of patients with vCJD, with anecdotal reports of some longer disease courses [68].

More recently, many groups have turned their attention to targeting the PrP itself; interference with PrP$^C$ expression in the adult brain is without serious effect and blocks the onset of neurological disease in animal models [69]. Anti-PrP monoclonal antibodies, or small molecules that interfere with the conversion of PrP$^C$ to PrP$^{Sc}$, appear to slow or arrest the disease course in mouse models of CJD if given prophylactically, during the incubation period [70]. They represent a promising therapeutic avenue in humanized form. New methods for early diagnosis—and their timely use—will therefore be vital, as arresting prion propagation will not reverse neuronal cell loss, which may be considerable by the time a clinical diagnosis is typically reached.

Symptom management is crucial and, for specific indications, can be highly effective. Myoclonus is generally of cortical origin and responds well to levetiracetam, or a benzodiazepine (commonly clonazepam), or sodium valproate at normal therapeutic doses. Visual hallucinations can be managed with a centrally acting anticholinesterase such as donepezil, and aggression or agitation with a dopamine antagonist, such as risperidone or quetiapine, or benzodiazepines; extra-pyramidal symptoms are common in prion disease, and the risk of these should be taken into account when prescribing (see Chapter 64 for details).

Patients and their families require early and consistent support, given the likely rapid pace of clinical change and the variety of functional deficits in cognition, mobility, toileting, and behaviour. Good community or residential nursing care is essential, and the involvement of a palliative care team is often of great benefit. Supportive medical therapies, such as parenteral nutrition, may prolong survival, with no appreciable improvement in quality of life.

## FURTHER INFORMATION

CJD Support Network. http://www.cjdsupport.net/
Medical Research Council Prion Unit at University College London, Institute of Prion Diseases. http://www.prion.ucl.ac.uk/
The National CJD Research and Surveillance Unit, Western General Hospital, Edinburgh. http://www.cjd.ed.ac.uk/
Public Health England. *Creuztfeldt–Jakob disease (CJD): guidance, data and analysis*. 2008. https://www.gov.uk/government/collections/creutzfeldt-jakob-disease-cjd-guidance-data-and-analysis
UK National Prion Clinic at the National Hospital for Neurology and Neurosurgery, London. http://www.nationalprionclinic.org

## REFERENCES

1. Gajdusek, D.C., Gibbs, C.J. Jr, and Alpers, M.P. (1966). Experimental transmission of a kuru-like syndrome to chimpanzees. *Nature*, **209**, 794–6.
2. Gibbs, C.J. Jr, Gajdusek, D.C., Asher, D.M., *et al.* (1968). Creutzfeldt-Jakob disease (spongiform

encephalopathy): transmission to the chimpanzee. *Science*, **161**, 388–9.

3. Cuillé, J. and Chelle, P.L. (1936). La maladie dite tremblante du mouton est-elle inocuable? *C R Acad Sci*, **203**, 1552–4.

4. Hadlow, W.J. (1959). Scrapie and kuru. *Lancet*, **2**, 289–90.

5. Collinge, J., Whitfield, J., McKintosh, E., *et al.* (2006). Kuru in the 21st century—an acquired human prion disease with very long incubation periods. *Lancet*, **367**, 2068–74.

6. Collinge, J. (2016). Mammalian prions and their wider relevance in neurodegenerative diseases. *Nature*, **539**, 217–26.

7. Owen, F., Poulter, M., Lofthouse, R., *et al.* (1989). Insertion in prion protein gene in familial Creutzfeldt-Jakob disease. *Lancet*, **1**, 51–2.

8. Hsiao, K., Baker, H.F., Crow, T.J., *et al.* (1989). Linkage of a prion protein missense variant to Gerstmann–Straussler syndrome. *Nature*, **338**, 342–5.

9. Collinge, J., Palmer, M.S., and Dryden, A.J. (1991). Genetic predisposition to iatrogenic Creutzfeldt-Jakob disease. *Lancet*, **337**, 1441–2.

10. Palmer, M.S., Dryden, A.J., Hughes, J.T., *et al.* (1991). Homozygous prion protein genotype predisposes to sporadic Creutzfeldt-Jakob disease. *Nature*, **352**, 340–2.

11. Collinge, J., Sidle, K.C.L., Meads, J., *et al.* (1996). Molecular analysis of prion strain variation and the aetiology of 'new variant' CJD. *Nature*, **383**, 685–90.

12. Hill, A.F., Joiner, S., Wadsworth, J.D., *et al.* (2003). Molecular classification of sporadic Creutzfeldt-Jakob disease. *Brain*, **126**(Pt 6), 1333–46.

13. Parchi, P., Giese, A., Capellari, S., *et al.* (1999). Classification of sporadic Creutzfeldt-Jakob disease based on molecular and phenotypic analysis of 300 subjects. *Annals of Neurology*, **46**, 224–33.

14. Prusiner, S.B., Scott, M., Foster, D., *et al.* (1990). Transgenetic studies implicate interactions between homologous PrP isoforms in scrapie prion replication. *Cell*, **63**, 673–86.

15. Bruce, M., Chree, A., McConnell, I., *et al.* (1994). Transmission of bovine spongiform encephalopathy and scrapie to mice: strain variation and the species barrier. *Philosophical Transactions of the Royal Society of London. Series B, Biological Sciences*, **343**, 405–11.

16. Collinge, J. (1999). Variant Creutzfeldt-Jakob disease. *Lancet*, **354**, 317–23.

17. Hill, A.F., Joiner, S., Linehan, J., *et al.* (2000). Species barrier independent prion replication in apparently resistant species. *Proceedings of the National Academy of Sciences of the United States of America*, **97**, 10248–53.

18. Hill, A.F. and Collinge, J. (2003). Subclinical prion infection. *Trends in Microbiology*, **11**, 578–84.

19. Sandberg, M. K., Al-Doujaily, H., Sharps, B., Clarke, A. R., and Collinge, J. (2011). Prion propagation and toxicity in vivo occur in two distinct mechanistic phases. *Nature*, **470**, 540–2.

20. Hill, A.F., Desbruslais, M., Joiner, S., *et al.* (1997). The same prion strain causes vCJD and BSE. *Nature*, **389**, 448–50.

21. Collinge, J., Palmer, M.S., Sidle, K.C.L., *et al.* (1995). Unaltered susceptibility to BSE in transgenic mice expressing human prion protein. *Nature*, **378**, 779–83.

22. Asante, E.A., Linehan, J.M., Desbruslais, M., *et al.* (2002). BSE prions propagate as either variant CJD-like or sporadic CJD-like prion strains in transgenic mice expressing human prion protein. *EMBO Journal*, **21**, 6358–66.

23. Wadsworth, J.D., Asante, E.A., Desbruslais, M., *et al.* (2004). Human prion protein with valine 129 prevents expression of variant CJD phenotype. *Science*, **306**, 1793–6.

24. Asante, E.A., Linehan, J.M., Gowland, I., *et al.* (2006). Dissociation of pathological and molecular phenotype of variant Creutzfeldt-Jakob disease in transgenic human prion protein 129 heterozygous mice. *Proceedings of the National Academy of Sciences of the United States of America*, **103**, 10759–64.

25. Zerr, I., Kallenberg, K., Summers, D. M., *et al.* (2009). Updated clinical diagnostic criteria for sporadic Creutzfeldt-Jakob disease. *Brain*, **132**, 2659–68.

26. Zanusso, G., Monaco, S., Pocchiari, M., *et al.* (2016). Advanced tests for early and accurate diagnosis of Creutzfeldt-Jakob disease. *Nature Reviews Neurology*, **12**, 325–33.

27. Orrú, C. D., Bongianni, M., Tonoli, G., *at al.* (2014). A test for Creutzfeldt–Jakob disease using nasal brushings. *New England Journal of Medicine*, **371**, 519–29.

28. Orrú, C. D., Yuan, J., Appleby, B. S., *et al.* (2017). Prion seeding activity and infectivity in skin samples from patients with sporadic Creutzfeldt-Jakob disease. *Science Translational Medicine*, **9**, eaam7785.

29. Alpers, M.P. (1987). Epidemiology and clinical aspects of kuru. In: S.B. Prusiner and M.P. McKinley (eds). *Prions: novel infectious pathogens causing scrapie and Creutzfeldt-Jakob disease*, pp. 451–65. Academic Press, San Diego, CA.

30. Mead, S., Whitfield, J., Poulter, M., *et al.* (2009). A novel protective prion protein variant that colocalizes with kuru exposure. *New England Journal of Medicine*, **361**, 2056–65.

31. Asante, E. A., Smidak, M., Grimshaw, A., *et al.* (2015). A naturally occurring variant of the human prion protein completely prevents prion disease. *Nature*, **522**, 478–81.

32. Britton, T.C., Al-Sarraj, S., Shaw, C., *et al.* (1995). Sporadic Creutzfeldt-Jakob disease in a 16-year-old in the UK. *Lancet*, **346**, 1155.

33. Heath, C. A., Cooper, S. A., Murray, K., *at al.* (2010). Validation of diagnostic criteria for variant Creutzfeldt–Jakob disease. *Annals of neurology*, **67**, 761–70.

34. El Tawil, S., Mackay, G., Davidson, *et al.* (2015). Variant Creutzfeldt-Jakob disease in older patients. *J Neurol Neurosurg Psychiatry*, **86**, 1279–80.

35. Mok, T., Jaunmuktane, Z., Joiner, S., *et al.* (2017). Variant Creutzfeldt–Jakob disease in a patient with heterozygosity at PRNP codon 129. *New England Journal of Medicine*, **376**, 292–4.

36. Siddique, D., Kennedy, A., Thomas, D., *et al.* (2005). Tonsil biopsy in the investigation of suspected variant Creutzfeldt-Jakob disease—a cohort study of 50 pts. *Journal of the Neurological Sciences*, **238**(Suppl. 1), S1–570.

37. Hill, A.F., Zeidler, M., Ironside, J., *et al.* (1997). Diagnosis of new variant Creutzfeldt-Jakob disease by tonsil biopsy. *Lancet*, **349**, 99–100.

38. Wadsworth, J.D.F., Joiner, S., Hill, A.F., *et al.* (2001). Tissue distribution of protease resistant prion protein in variant CJD using a highly sensitive immuno-blotting assay. *Lancet*, **358**, 171–80.

39. Hilton, D.A., Sutak, J., Smith, M.E., *et al.* (2004). Specificity of lymphoreticular accumulation of prion protein for variant Creutzfeldt-Jakob disease. *Journal of Clinical Pathology*, **57**, 300–2.

40. Edgeworth, J. A., Farmer, M., Sicilia, A., *et al.* (2011). Detection of prion infection in variant Creutzfeldt-Jakob disease: a blood-based assay. *The Lancet*, **377**, 487–93.

41. Moda, F., Gambetti, P., Notari, S., *et al.* (2014). Prions in the urine of patients with variant Creutzfeldt–Jakob disease. *New England Journal of Medicine*, **371**, 530–9.

42. Concha-Marambio, L., Pritzkow, S., Moda, F., *et al.* (2016). Detection of prions in blood from patients with variant Creutzfeldt-Jakob disease. *Science Translational Medicine*, **8**, 370ra183.

43. Bougard, D., Brandel, J. P., Bélondrade, M., *et al.* (2016). Detection of prions in the plasma of presymptomatic and symptomatic patients with variant Creutzfeldt-Jakob disease. *Science Translational Medicine*, **8**, 370ra182.

44. Rudge, P., Jaunmuktane, Z., Adlard, P., *et al.* (2015). Iatrogenic CJD due to pituitary-derived growth hormone with genetically determined incubation times of up to 40 years. *Brain*, **138**, 3386–99.

45. Gill, O.N., Spencer, Y., Richard-Loendt, A., *et al.* Prevalent abnormal prion protein in human appendixes after bovine spongiform encephalopathy epizootic: large scale survey. *BMJ*, **347**, f5675.

46. Minikel, E. V., Vallabh, S. M., Lek, M., *et al.* (2016). Quantifying prion disease penetrance using large population control cohorts. *Science Translational Medicine*, **8**, 322ra9.

47. Lloyd, S., Mead, S., and Collinge, J. (2011). Genetics of prion disease. In: Tatzelt, J. (ed). *Prion Proteins*, pp. 1–22. Springer, Berlin Heidelberg.

48. Webb, T. E. F., Poulter, M., Beck, J., *et al.* (2008). Phenotypic heterogeneity and genetic modification of P102L inherited prion disease in an international series. *Brain*, **131**, 2632–46.

49. Kaski, D. N., Pennington, C., Beck, J., *et al.* (2011). Inherited prion disease with 4-octapeptide repeat insertion: disease requires the interaction of multiple genetic risk factors. *Brain*, **134**, 1829–38.

50. Mead, S., Webb, T. E. F., Campbell, T. *et al.* (2007). Inherited prion disease with 5-OPRI Phenotype modification by repeat length and codon 129. *Neurology*, **69**, 730–8.

51. Mead, S., Poulter, M., Beck, J., *et al.* (2006). Inherited prion disease with six octapeptide repeat insertional mutation—molecular analysis of phenotypic heterogeneity. *Brain*, **129**, 2297–317.

52. Paucar, M., Xiang, F., Moore, R., *et al.* (2013). Genotype-phenotype analysis in inherited prion disease with eight octapeptide repeat insertional mutation. *Prion*, **7**, 501–10.

53. Nishida, Y., Sodeyama, N., Toru, Y., *et al.* (2004). Creutzfeldt–Jakob disease with a novel insertion and codon 219 Lys/Lys polymorphism in PRNP. *Neurology*, **63**, 1978–9.

54. Collinge, J., Brown, J., Hardy, J., *et al.* (1992). Inherited prion disease with 144 base pair gene insertion. II. Clinical and pathological features. *Brain*, **115**, 687–710.

55. Mallucci, G. R., Campbell, T. A., Dickinson, A., *et al.* (1999). Inherited prion disease with an alanine to valine mutation at codon 117 in the prion protein gene. *Brain*, **122**, 1823–37.

56. Zarranz, J. J., Digon, A., Atares, B., *et al.* (2005). Phenotypic variability in familial prion diseases due to the D178N mutation. *Journal of Neurology, Neurosurgery and Psychiatry*, **76**, 1491–6.

57. Gallassi, R., Morreale, A., Montagna, P., *et al.* (1996). Fatal familial insomnia Behavioral and cognitive features. *Neurology*, **46**, 935–9.

58. Goldfarb, L.G., Petersen, R.B., Tabaton, M., *et al.* (1992). Fatal familial insomnia and familial Creutzfeldt-Jakob disease: disease phenotype determined by a DNA polymorphism. *Science*, **258**, 806–8.

59. Goldfarb, L.G., Korczyn, A.D., Brown, P., *et al.* (1990). Mutation in codon 200 of scrapie amyloid precursor gene linked to Creutzfeldt-Jakob disease in Sephardic Jews of Libyan and non-Libyan origin. *Lancet*, **336**, 637–8.

60. Brown, P., Galvez, S., Goldfarb, L.G., *et al.* (1992). Familial Creutzfeldt-Jakob disease in Chile is associated with the codon 200 mutation of the PRNP amyloid precursor gene on chromosome 20. *Journal of Neurological Sciences*, **112**, 65–7.

61. Mead, S., Gandhi, S., Beck, J., *et al.* (2013). A novel prion disease associated with diarrhea and autonomic neuropathy. *New England Journal of Medicine*, **369**, 1904–14.

62. Uflacker, A., Doraiswamy, P. M., Rechitsky, S., *et al.* (2014). Preimplantation genetic diagnosis (PGD) for genetic prion disorder due to F198S mutation in the PRNP gene. *JAMA Neurology*, **71**, 484–6.

63. Thompson, A. G., Lowe, J., Fox, Z., *et al.* (2013). The Medical Research Council Prion Disease Rating Scale: a new outcome measure for prion disease therapeutic trials developed and validated using systematic observational studies. *Brain*, **136**, 1116–27.

64. Mead, S., Burnell, M., Lowe, J., *et al.* (2016). Clinical trial simulations based on genetic stratification and the natural history of a functional outcome measure in Creutzfeldt-Jakob disease. *JAMA Neurology*, **73**, 447–55.

65. Otto, M., Cepek, L., Ratzka, P., *et al.* (2004). Efficacy of flupirtine on cognitive function in patients with CJD A double-blind study. *Neurology*, **62**, 714–18.

66. Collinge, J., Gorham, M., Hudson, F., *et al.* (2009). Safety and efficacy of quinacrine in human prion disease (PRION-1 study): a patient-preference trial. *The Lancet Neurology*, **8**, 334–44.

67. Haïk, S., Marcon, G., Mallet, A., *et al.* (2014). Doxycycline in Creutzfeldt-Jakob disease: a phase 2, randomised, double-blind, placebo-controlled trial. *The Lancet Neurology*, **13**, 150–8.

68. Rainov, N. G., Tsuboi, Y., Krolak-Salmon, P., *et al.* (2007). Experimental treatments for human transmissible spongiform encephalopathies: is there a role for pentosan polysulfate? *Expert Opinion on Biological Therapy*, **7**, 713–26.

69. Aguzzi, A., and Collinge, J. (1997). Post-exposure prophylaxis after accidental prion inoculation. *Lancet*, **350**, 1519–20.

70. White, A. R., Enever, P., Tayebi, M., *et al.* (2003). Monoclonal antibodies inhibit prion replication and delay the development of prion disease. *Nature*, **422**, 80–3.

# 43

# Dementia with Lewy bodies

*Anto P. Rajkumar and Dag Aarsland*

## Introduction

Dementia with Lewy bodies (DLB) is the second most common neurodegenerative dementia [1]. Lewy bodies are abnormal aggregates of several proteins that form eosinophilic spherical neuronal intracytoplasmic inclusions. Lewy bodies are found in the cerebral cortex, brainstem, various subcortical structures, and peripheral nervous system. Clinical manifestations of DLB include cognitive impairment, extra-pyramidal symptoms, neuropsychiatric symptoms, and autonomic dysfunction.

DLB has been known by other names, which include diffuse Lewy body disease, Lewy body dementia, dementia associated with cortical Lewy bodies, senile dementia of Lewy body type, and the Lewy body variant of Alzheimer's disease [2]. The current consensus is that 'Lewy body dementia' term includes DLB and Parkinson's disease dementia (PDD) [3]. DLB and PDD are clinically differentiated only by the timing of onset of dementia and Parkinson's disease (PD), using an arbitrary 1-year rule. PDD starts at least 1 year after well-established PD, but people with DLB develop dementia before, concurrently, or within 1 year of onset of Parkinsonism. Some people with DLB never develop Parkinsonism. Once both dementia and Parkinsonism are well established, DLB and PDD seldom differ clinically. As increasing evidence suggests common pathophysiological processes underlying the two disorders [3], DLB and PDD can also be viewed together as a single nosological continuum [4]. However, this chapter focuses only on DLB, and Chapter 44 presents PDD in detail.

## Brief history

Fritz Heinrich Lewy, later known as Frederic Henry Lewey, first reported eosinophilic intracytoplasmic inclusions in 1912, while he was studying the neuropathology of PD in the team of Alois Alzheimer at Munich University. He observed the inclusions in the dorsal vagal nuclei and substantia innominata of people with PD, but he concluded that the inclusion bodies are not pathognomonic of PD [5]. Konstantin Tretiakoff, a Russian neuropathologist, coined the term 'Corps de Lewy' (Lewy bodies) and presented it as one of the major hallmarks of PD pathology in 1919. Lewy also observed swellings of axon cylinders of the neurons with the inclusions, and

they were called 'Lewy neurites' later. The interest in Lewy bodies was renewed in 1960 when Bethlem and Den Haltog Jager diligently documented the distribution of Lewy bodies in the central and autonomic nervous systems. Later, Haruo Okazaki reported in 1961 autopsies of two people with progressive dementia and rigidity, who had widely disseminated Lewy bodies in their cerebral cortex.

Over the next two decades, Kenji Kosaka and other researchers from Japan reported autopsies of more than 20 people, who clinically presented with varying degrees of extra-pyramidal symptoms, cognitive impairment, and neuropsychiatric symptoms and had variable distribution of Lewy bodies in their brainstem and cerebral cortex. They proposed the term 'Lewy body disease' in 1980 and classified it into brainstem, transitional, and diffuse types. Yoshimura reported more autopsies of people with the diffuse type and proposed the term 'diffuse Lewy body disease' in 1983 [6]. Hansen and Perry reported more autopsies from North America and Europe, respectively, in 1990. Their studies have confirmed that diffuse Lewy body disease is not rare and that at least 15–20% of older people with dementia have Lewy bodies. Later, more autopsies that found Lewy bodies almost exclusively in the cerebral cortex were reported. The first international workshop on DLB was held in Newcastle in the UK in 1995, and the consensus guidelines for the clinical and pathological diagnosis of DLB were published in 1996. Maria Spillantini identified the major component of Lewy bodies as α-synuclein in 1997. The Third International Workshop on DLB was held in 2003, and the revised consensus diagnostic guidelines for DLB were published in 2005. The fourth consensus report of the DLB Consortium and the revised criteria for the clinical diagnosis of DLB was published in 2017. Studies investigating the epidemiology, pathophysiology, clinical diagnosis, and management of DLB have been exponentially increasing over the past two decades, and this chapter attempts to provide a brief overview of this expanding knowledge base.

## Epidemiology

Robust data on the prevalence and incidence of DLB remain sparse. However, DLB is no longer considered to be a rare disorder, and its prevalence is second only to Alzheimer's dementia (AD) among older adults with neurodegenerative dementia. A recent systematic review, including 22 studies that investigated the prevalence and/or incidence of DLB, has reported that the incidence rates ranged from 0.5 to 1.6 per 1000 person-years among the community-dwelling older adults aged 65 years and above [7]. 3.2–7.1% of all incident dementias are due to DLB. The incidence of DLB is nearly twice more common in men than in women. The prevalence of DLB has been reported from 0.02 to 0.06 per 1000 adults younger than 65 years of age, and from 0.3 to 6.5 per 1000 older adults aged 65 and above. Studies that included only people older than 70 years have reported the prevalence of DLB as from 8.6 to 33.3 per 1000 people, and one study that included only people older than 81 years has reported the prevalence as 63.5 per 1000 people. The mean prevalence of DLB is 4.2% in community studies, and it is 7.5% in clinical samples.

DLB remains underdiagnosed in many clinical settings, so the prevalence of DLB could be higher than the reported estimates [8, 9]. Studies including detailed neurological examinations, neuroimaging, and screening for rapid eye movement (REM) sleep behaviour disorder (RBD) have reported the prevalence of DLB as high as 24%. Advancing age, hypertension, dyslipidaemia, and a past history of depression and anxiety have been reported to increase the risk of DLB. People with DLB reportedly have poorer quality of life than those with AD. Quality of life in DLB has been directly associated with the independency in instrumental activities of daily living and inversely associated with neuropsychiatric symptoms, especially apathy and delusions [10]. People with DLB may utilize more health resources, and their costs of care are reportedly higher than those of people with AD [11].

## Pathology

### Neuropathology

Subcortical and cortical Lewy bodies differ in their appearance and immunohistochemical staining. Subcortical Lewy bodies have the characteristic appearance of dense eosinophilic cores, surrounded by concentric lamellar bands and pallid halos. They can be visualized by immunohistochemical staining for α-synuclein and ubiquitin. Cortical Lewy bodies do not have the surrounding halo. They can be visualized by immunohistochemical staining for ubiquitin, but less than one-third of cortical Lewy bodies can be detected by α-synuclein immunostaining [12]. Lewy neurites are abnormal neuronal projections, including aggregates of α-synuclein and other proteins. They are more extensively distributed in various cortical and subcortical regions than the Lewy bodies, and they can be visualized by immunohistochemical staining for α-synuclein and ubiquitin. They are believed to represent earlier stages of neurodegeneration and to lead to synaptic dysfunction when they are present in the presynaptic terminals.

It remains uncertain whether Lewy bodies play a neurotoxic or neuroprotective role [3]. Moreover, the relationship between cortical Lewy body burden and the clinical severity of DLB is not linear. However, a pathological classification system including three subtypes of DLB has been proposed on the basis of a semi-quantitative scoring system assessing the pattern of distribution of Lewy bodies and Lewy neurites. Brainstem-predominant DLB has Lewy pathology principally within the substantia nigra, dorsal nucleus of the vagus, and the locus caeruleus. Limbic or transitional DLB includes Lewy pathology in the anterior cingulate and transtentorhinal cortices. The third subtype—neocortical or diffuse DLB—has disseminated Lewy pathology in the cerebral cortex, with or without involvement of the brainstem. Braak has introduced a pathological staging system for PD, and he has suggested caudorostral progression of Lewy pathology that starts from the brainstem and then spreads to the neocortex. Some people with DLB may follow the caudorostral progression of Lewy pathology, but many do not follow this kind of spread. Hence, the importance of Braak staging is limited to DLB, and an additional 'cerebral' subtype of DLB has been proposed.

Eighty to 90% of older adults with DLB have varying degrees of coexisting Alzheimer's-like pathology. They often have diffuse β-amyloid plaques, but neocortical neurofibrillary tangles are less common in DLB. The neocortical type of DLB is more likely to have substantial coexisting Alzheimer's-like pathology. Increasing evidence support that β-amyloid deposition also contributes to the pathology of DLB. Loss of cholinergic neurons in the basal nucleus of Meynert and decreased cortical choline acetyltransferase indicate that the deficits in cholinergic neurotransmission are common in DLB. Such deficits occur earlier and are more severe in DLB than in AD. Minor cerebrovascular lesions are found in around 30% of older adults with DLB, but their contribution to DLB pathology is uncertain. Depletion of dopaminergic neurons and deficits in GABA and serotonergic neurotransmission have been reported in older adults with DLB [1].

### Neuroimaging

Neuroimaging of people with DLB not only helps to enhance our understanding of the underlying pathology, but also has direct clinical implications [13]. Structural neuroimaging in DLB with MRI often reveals diffuse, but relatively mild global, grey matter atrophy with relatively preserved medial temporal lobes, when compared to people with AD. However, if there is substantial coexisting Alzheimer's-like pathology, medial temporal lobes may not be spared. The volume of the substantia innominata and putamen may be less in DLB than in AD. Atrophy in the temporal, occipital, and parietal lobes is often more pronounced in DLB than in PDD. Diffusion tensor imaging (DTI) studies have documented the loss of parieto-occipital white matter tracts in DLB, when compared with people without cognitive impairment [14]. Several studies have investigated DLB using magnetic resonance spectroscopy (MRS) [15]. They have documented reduced $N$-acetyl aspartate/creatine ratio in the centrum semiovale, occipital grey matter, and temporal lobes in DLB, when compared to healthy controls. Findings on choline/creatine ratios in DLB have been inconsistent. A recent study has reported that people with mild cognitive impairment (MCI) and lower $N$-acetyl aspartate/creatine ratio in their posterior cingulate cortex were significantly more likely to develop AD, but not DLB [16].

$^{123}$I-2β-carbomethoxy-3β-4-iodophenyl-$N$-3-fluoropropyl nortropane single-photon emission computed tomography ($^{123}$FP-CIT SPECT) can demonstrate low dopamine transporter uptake in the basal ganglia in people with DLB. This can distinguish DLB from AD, before one develops clinically observable extra-pyramidal symptoms. This has been evaluated in a multi-centre phase III trial, and it has been incorporated in the DLB Consortium revised criteria for the clinical diagnosis of DLB [17]. SPECT studies investigating regional cerebral blood flow by using radionucleotides, such as $^{99m}$Tc hexamethylpropyleneamineoxime, have reported global cortical hypoperfusion in DLB, when compared to healthy controls, and occipital hypoperfusion in DLB, when compared to people with AD. PET studies using $^{18}$F-fluorodeoxyglucose (FDG) have confirmed occipital hypometabolism in DLB, when compared to AD. An association between the frequency of visual hallucinations and occipital hypometabolism in DLB has been reported. Besides, metabolism in the posterior cingulate cortex is relatively preserved in DLB, when compared to AD, and this 'posterior cingulate island sign' can distinguish DLB from AD. Amyloid PET studies have documented variable degrees of cortical β-amyloid ligand binding in DLB. β-amyloid deposition is usually more in DLB, when compared to healthy controls and people with PDD, but it is relatively less than that in AD [18]. A recent tau PET study that employed $^{18}$F-labelled AV-1451 ligand has demonstrated variable tau pathology, especially in the inferior temporal gyrus and precuneus, in people with DLB [19]. Cholinergic PET studies have reported reduced cortical and thalamic acetylcholinesterase activity in DLB. $^{123}$I-metaiodobenzylguanidine (MIBG) scintigraphy can demonstrate the involvement of the autonomic nervous system in DLB. Reduced myocardial MIBG uptake due to the involvement of post-ganglionic cardiac sympathetic nerves can distinguish DLB from AD very accurately, and it has been recently included in the diagnostic criteria for DLB [20]. Fig. 43.1 presents representative coronal MRI, FDG PET, and $^{123}$FP-CIT SPECT images in DLB and AD.

## Molecular biology

Lewy bodies are complex structures, and they are made of at least 90 distinct molecules [21]. They comprise α-synuclein, α-synuclein binding proteins, such as tau, agrin, synphilin-1, 14-3-3, and microtubule-associated proteins, and synphilin-1 binding proteins such as parkin, dorfin, and glycogen synthase kinase-3β. They include proteins from the ubiquitin proteasome system, such as ubiquitin, ubiquitin-activating enzyme, ubiquitin-conjugating enzyme, ubiquitin C-terminal hydrolase, ubiquitin ligase, proteasome, and proteasome activators, and from the autophagosome lysosome system such as glucocerebrosidase, LC3, GATE-16, and NBR1. Many aggresome-related proteins, such as γ-tubulin, HDAC6, and pericentrin, several cellular stress response proteins including heat-shock proteins, clusterin, glutathione peroxidase, heme oxygenase-1, αB-crystallin, and superoxide dismutase 1 and 2, and various protein phosphorylation and signal transduction proteins including calcium/calmodulin-dependent protein kinase II, cyclin-dependent kinase 5, G-protein coupled receptor kinase 5, leucine-rich repeat kinase 2 (LRRK2), and phospholipase C-δ, are found in Lewy bodies. Lewy bodies include mitochondria-related proteins, such as cox IV, cytochrome C, and PTEN-induced putative kinase 1 (PINK1), cell cycle proteins, such as cyclin B and retinoblastoma protein, and cytoskeletal proteins, such as neurofilament, and tubulin. Several cytosolic proteins, including amyloid precursor protein, calbindin, choline acetyltransferase, chromogranin A, synaptophysin, synaptotagmin, tyrosine hydroxylase, and vesicular monoamine transporter 2, immunoglobulins, and lipids are present in Lewy bodies [21].

It is widely accepted that aggregation of α-synuclein is the key initial step in the formation of Lewy bodies [12]. DLB, along with PD and multiple system atrophy, is recognized as a primary α-synucleinopathy. Made of 140 amino acids, α-synuclein normally exists as an unfolded protein without a typical secondary structure or as a stable folded tetramer. It is principally localized in the presynaptic terminals of neurons. Molecular functions of α-synuclein remain uncertain, but they may include trafficking of synaptic vesicles, formation of SNARE complexes that mediate the fusion of vesicles with their target membranes, regulation of synaptic vesicle recycling, and regulation of presynaptic release of several neurotransmitters, including dopamine [22]. Presynaptic α-synuclein aggregation leads to synaptic dysfunction that may explain the neurodegeneration in DLB. Conformational changes and aggregatory properties of α-synuclein have been extensively investigated over the last decade. α-synuclein is susceptible to undergo various post-translational modifications, such as phosphorylation, ubiquitination, nitration, oxidation, and sumoylation [23]. Such post-translational modifications, binding with polyamines, and cross-linking by tissue transglutaminase promote oligomerization of α-synuclein; this leads to the formation of protofibrils and mature aggregates [24]. α-synuclein oligomers and protofibrils are neurotoxic. However, the formation of Lewy bodies with other proteins may protect the involved neurons and prolong their survival [12]. There are at least two more alternatively spliced isoforms of α-synuclein. α-synuclein that has 126 amino acids (α-synuclein 126) is less prone for aggregation, but α-synuclein that has 112 amino acids (α-synuclein 112) has increased propensity for aggregation [25].

α-synuclein oligomers can be released into the extracellular space either by exocytosis or by the formation of exosomes, which are 30–100 nm-sized extracellular vesicles [26]. Exosomes carry a complex cargo of proteins, lipids, and nucleic acids from the brain to the peripheral systems, and they lead to cell-to-cell transport of several biologically active molecules, including α-synuclein. An increasing number of cell culture, animal, and post-mortem studies have shown that exogenous α-synuclein can instigate Lewy pathology in the recipient cells, and the possibility of prion-like propagation of α-synuclein in DLB has been hypothesized [27]. Extracellular α-synuclein can activate neighbouring microglia and astrocytes. Possible mechanisms of microglial activation by α-synuclein, and consequent chronic neuroinflammation in DLB, have been studied over the past decade [28]. Activated microglia release pro-inflammatory cytokines, such as interleukin-1β, interleukin-2, interleukin-6, and tumour necrosis factor-α, nitric oxide, and reactive oxygen molecules and trigger an apoptotic process of affected neurons [29]. Besides, the ubiquitin proteasome system and the autophagy lysosome pathway are the two most essential pathways that repair or degrade several abnormal neuronal proteins, including α-synuclein. Accumulating evidence suggests that these two pathways are dysfunctional in DLB and that such deficits lead to an increased release of extracellular α-synuclein and an uncontrolled propagation of associated pathology. β-glucocerebrosidase 1 (GCase), a lysosomal hydrolase, has received special attention recently [30]. Lysosomal dysfunction, secondary to GCase deficiency, may lead to misprocessing and aggregation of α-synuclein [31]. GCase deficiency also contributes to mitochondrial dysfunction [32], and other mitochondria-related proteins, such as parkin and PINK1, are involved in the pathology of DLB. Mitochondrial energy metabolism dysfunction increases the vulnerability of neurons to oxidative damage [33], and α-synuclein pathology can directly damage mitochondria [34].

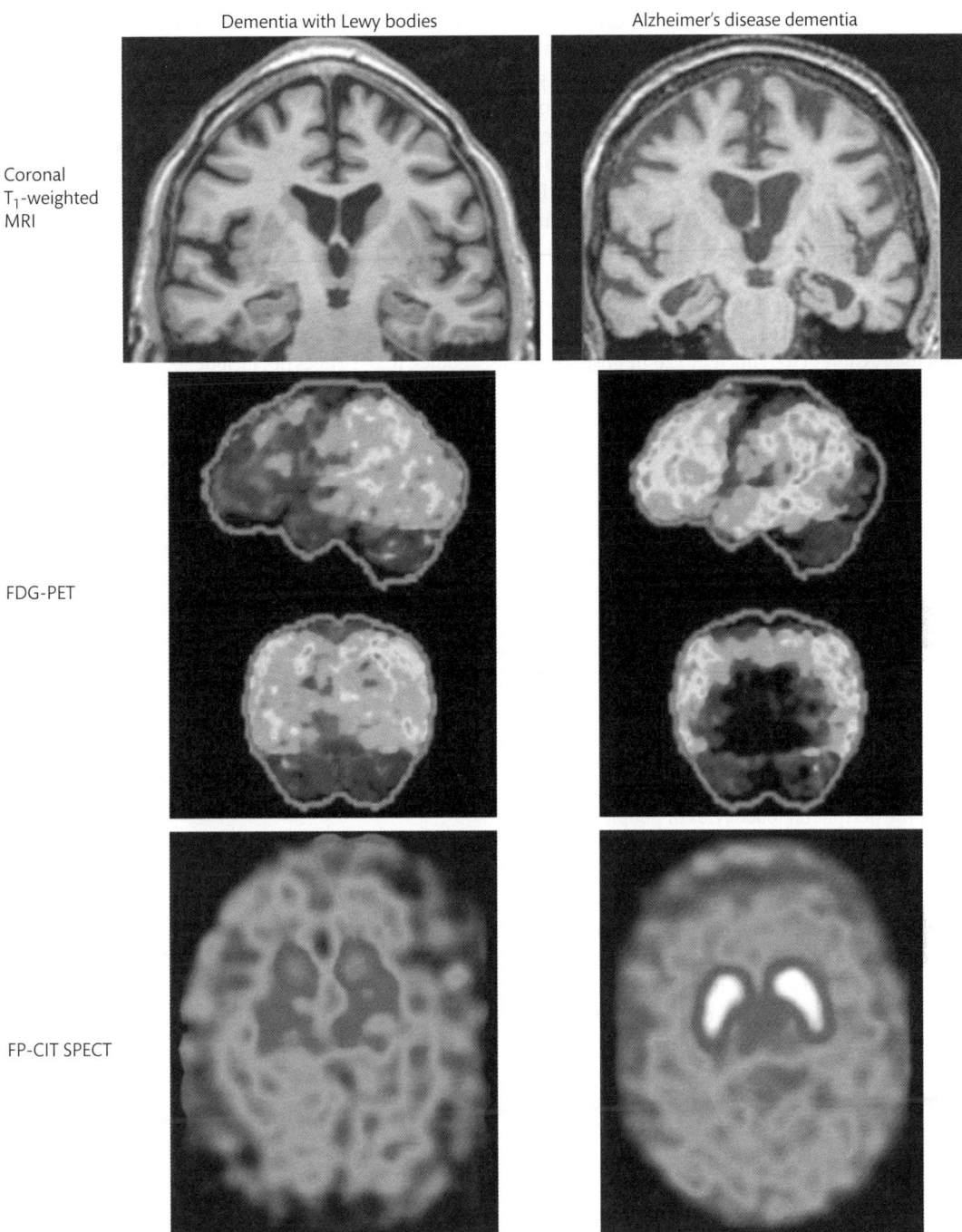

Dementia with Lewy bodies        Alzheimer's disease dementia

Coronal T₁-weighted MRI

FDG-PET

FP-CIT SPECT

**Fig. 43.1** (see Colour Plate section) Representative coronal MRI, FDG-PET, and FP-CIT SPECT images in DLB and AD.
Reprinted from *The Lancet* 386(10004), Walker Z, Possin KL, Boeve BF, Aarsland D., Lewy body dementias, Pages 1683–97. Copyright 2015 with permission from Elsevier.

## Genetics

Although DLB is mostly sporadic, there is evidence for familial aggregation of DLB [35]. A genome-wide linkage study in an autosomal dominant family with autopsy confirmed DLB has mapped the chromosomal locus for DLB at 2q35–q36 [36]. *SNCA* codes for α-synuclein, and *SNCA* triplications and missense mutations have been associated with DLB [37]. *GBA* (glucosylceramidase beta) encodes GCase, and the genetic associations between DLB and polymorphisms in *GBA* have been replicated by several studies [38–40]. A large multi-centre study has reported that pathogenic

*GBA* mutations increase the risk of DLB by more than eight times and that they are associated with an earlier age of onset of DLB and disease severity [39]. A recent study has found that the pathogenic *GBA* mutation carriers have significantly less GCase activity in their brain [41]. Another large study that investigated 788 people with DLB and 2624 controls has reported false-discovery adjusted statistically significant genetic associations of DLB with *APOE, SNCA,* and *SCARB2* (scavenger receptor class B member 2) [42]. Along with *GBA* and *SCARB2* mutations that lead to lysosomal dysfunction, two more lysosome-related genes *SMPD1* and *MCOLN1* have been associated with Lewy pathology [41]. Available evidence suggests that *APOE* ε4 allele increases the risk of DLB and that *APOE* ε2 allele reduces the risk and delays the onset of DLB by 4 years [43]. Evidence supporting the associations between DLB and other AD-related genes, such as *APP* and *PSEN1*, are weak [37]. The first genome-wide association study (GWAS) investigating DLB was published in January 2018. It estimated 36% heritability of DLB, and it confirmed the associations between DLB and variants in *APOE*, *SNCA*, and *GBA* [43a].

Gene expression studies in DLB have confirmed the importance of alternative splicing of α-synuclein and the differential expression of the isoforms. Increased expression of α-synuclein 112 and decreased expression of α-synuclein 126 in post-mortem frontal cortical samples from people with DLB have been reported [25]. A study investigating the expression of all small ribonucleic acids (RNAs) in post-mortem temporal cortical samples of people with DLB did not find any differentially expressed small RNA. However, another study that investigated post-mortem anterior cingulate cortical samples from people with DLB using next-generation RNA sequencing technology has documented 490 differentially expressed genes, including many downregulated genes, which are implicated in neurogenesis, myelination, and regulation of nervous system development [44]. Another study that investigated the primary visual cortex post-mortem, using gene expression microarrays, has reported that several genes, associated with GABAergic neurotransmission, were differentially expressed in people with DLB who experienced recurrent complex visual hallucinations. Lower levels of DNA methylation in the *SCNA* intron 1 has been found in the peripheral leucocytes of people with DLB, but studies evaluating the epigenetics of DLB remain sparse [45].

### Other biological correlates

Theta and delta wave activity and frequency variation in EEG, especially in the posterior leads, are more frequent in DLB than in AD and PDD [46]. Quantitative EEG may predict conversion of MCI to DLB accurately. RBD is a core clinical feature of DLB. Video polysomnographic investigation of people with DLB has revealed increased sleep latency, reduced sleep efficiency, and altered non-REM sleep architecture. Several studies have investigated potential biomarkers of DLB in the CSF for helping an early and accurate clinical diagnosis, as well as for monitoring prognosis and treatment effectiveness [47]. A meta-analysis including 13 studies and 2728 people has established that α-synuclein concentration in the CSF is significantly lower in DLB than in AD [48]. Akin to AD, CSF β-amyloid 1-42 concentration is often reduced in DLB and has been shown to predict a more rapid cognitive decline in DLB [49]. However, CSF tau and phosphorylated tau concentrations are less in DLB than in AD. The oxidized form of β-amyloid 1-40 in the CSF is higher in DLB than in PDD and healthy controls. CSF levels of homovanillic acid, 5-hydroxyindoleacetic acid, 3-methoxy-4-hydroxy phenylethyleneglycol levels, and neurosin, as well as cocaine and amphetamine-regulated transcript, have been reported to be less in DLB than in AD. Other CSF studies have reported elevated levels of neurofilaments, calcium, and magnesium, as well as reduced levels of soluble neuron glia 2 in DLB [47]. Studies evaluating potential biomarkers of DLB in other biological fluids remain sparse. Unlike AD, serum fatty acid-binding protein levels are elevated in DLB. Preliminary evidence suggests elevated serum

magnesium levels in DLB. Although Lewy pathology often involves minor salivary glands, reliable salivary biomarkers for DLB have not been found so far.

## Diagnosis

Although a definite diagnosis of DLB can be confirmed only by neuropathological verification, a probable or possible diagnosis of DLB can be made clinically. DLB is currently diagnosed by using either the DLB Consortium revised criteria for the clinical diagnosis of DLB [50] or the DSM-5 diagnostic criteria for major neurocognitive disorder with Lewy bodies. ICD-10 does not include specific diagnostic criteria for DLB.

### The DLB consortium criteria

DLB diagnoses are missed more often than not in clinical settings when standard diagnostic criteria are not used routinely. A large study that evaluated the accuracy of clinical diagnoses of DLB, in comparison with autopsy findings, has reported 95% specificity, but only 32% sensitivity [51]. The third DLB Consortium revised criteria for the clinical diagnosis of DLB have been reported to increase the clinical diagnoses of probable DLB by nearly 24%. Table 43.1 presents the current revised criteria for the clinical diagnosis of probable and possible DLB [50]. Meeting the general criteria for dementia is essential for the diagnosis of possible or probable DLB. Two of the four core clinical features (fluctuating cognition, recurrent visual hallucinations, RBD and spontaneous Parkinsonism) are sufficient for a diagnosis of probable DLB, and only one of them is sufficient for a diagnosis of possible DLB. If one or more of the indicative biomarkers is present in the presence of one or more core clinical features, probable DLB can be diagnosed. A diagnosis of probable DLB cannot be made on the basis of indicative biomarkers alone. In the absence of any core clinical features, one or more indicative biomarkers are sufficient for a diagnosis of possible DLB. Possible DLB is an unstable diagnosis, and some develop probable DLB, whereas others develop AD or other diseases. The revised criteria list supportive clinical features and supportive biomarkers that are commonly present in DLB, but their diagnostic specificity are uncertain. Hence, these supportive features do not have any diagnostic weighting. There are ongoing endeavours to improve the sensitivity of the criteria without compromising their specificity.

### DSM-5 diagnostic criteria

As the term 'dementia' is replaced by the term 'major neurocognitive disorder' in DSM-5, DLB is called 'major neurocognitive disorder with Lewy bodies' (NCDLB). The DSM-5 diagnostic criteria for probable and possible major NCDLB mirrors the 2005 version of third DLB Consortium revised criteria for the clinical diagnosis of DLB, but there are a few differences between the two. Three core features (fluctuating cognition, recurrent visual hallucinations, and spontaneous Parkinsonism) are included, and RBD and severe neuroleptic sensitivity are mentioned as two suggestive features in DSM-5. The neuroimaging biomarker demonstrating low dopamine transporter uptake in the basal ganglia is not included in DSM-5, and this may compromise the sensitivity of the criteria further. At least two core features or one core feature with one or two suggestive features

**Table 43.1** The DLB Consortium revised criteria for the clinical diagnosis of probable and possible DLB

| Feature of DLB | Criteria |
|---|---|
| Essential feature | Dementia that is defined by progressive cognitive decline of sufficient magnitude to interfere with normal social or occupational function. Prominent or persistent memory impairment may not occur in the early stages but is usually evident with progression. Deficits on tests of attention, executive function, and visuo-spatial ability may be especially prominent |
| Core clinical features | 1. Fluctuating cognition with pronounced variations in attention and alertness<br>2. Recurrent visual hallucinations that are typically well formed and detailed<br>3. Spontaneous features of Parkinsonism<br>4. REM sleep behaviour disorder that may precede cognitive decline |
| Supportive clinical features | Severe sensitivity to antipsychotic agents, postural instability, repeated falls, syncope or other transient episodes of unresponsiveness, severe autonomic dysfunction, hypersomnia, hyposmia, hallucinations in other modalities, systematized delusions, apathy, anxiety, and depression |
| Indicative biomarkers | 1. Reduced dopamine transporter uptake in basal ganglia demonstrated by SPECT or PET<br>2. Abnormal (low uptake) [123]iodine-MIBG myocardial scintigraphy<br>3. Polysomnographic confirmation of REM sleep without atonia |
| Supportive biomarkers | 1. Relative preservation of medial temporal lobe structures on CT/MRI<br>2. Generalized low uptake on SPECT/PET perfusion/metabolism scan with reduced occipital activity with or without the cingulate island sign on FDG-PET imaging<br>3. Prominent posterior slow-wave activity on EEG with periodic fluctuations in the pre-alpha/theta range |
| A diagnosis of DLB is less likely | 1. In the presence of a physical illness or brain disorder including cerebrovascular disease sufficient to account in part or in total for the clinical picture<br>2. If Parkinsonism only appears for the first time at a stage of severe dementia |
| Temporal sequence of symptoms | DLB should be diagnosed when dementia occurs before or concurrently with Parkinsonism. The term PDD should be used to describe dementia that occurs in the context of well-established Parkinson's disease. In clinical settings, the term that is most appropriate to the clinical situation should be used, and generic terms such as Lewy body disease are often helpful. In research studies in which distinction needs to be made between DLB and PDD, the existing 1-year rule between the onset of dementia and Parkinsonism for DLB continues to be recommended |

Adapted from Neurology, 89(1), McKeith IG, Bradley F, Boeve BF, et al., Diagnosis and management of dementia with Lewy bodies: fourth consensus report of the DLB Consortium, pp. 88-100. Copyright (2017), with permission from American Academy of Neurology

are needed to diagnose probable major NCDLB. Only one core feature or one or two suggestive features are needed to diagnose possible major NCDLB. Besides, there is no consensus on the definition of prodromal or pre-dementia phase of DLB, but DSM-5 has introduced probable and possible mild neurocognitive disorder with Lewy bodies. Nosological validity of these two diagnostic categories remains uncertain. DSM-5 has also provided further coding for major NCDLB with or without behavioural disturbance. However, DSM-5 does not include a list of supportive features of NCDLB but mentions many supportive features as 'diagnostic markers' with uncertain diagnostic weighting.

## Clinical presentation

As the initial clinical presentation of DLB varies widely, people with DLB may first present to primary care, psychiatric, neurology, internal medicine, or emergency services. DLB may initially present with memory impairment, impairment of other cognitive functions, visual hallucinations, psychosis, depression, fall, syncope, loss of consciousness, acute confusion, sleep disorders, autonomic dysfunction, or extra-pyramidal symptoms. Such heterogenous clinical presentation contributes to the underdiagnosis of DLB in clinical settings. DLB is not clinically diagnosed, until people develop cognitive impairments that are severe enough to interfere with their functions. People with DLB have varying degrees of cortical and subcortical neuropsychological deficits. People with DLB often have greater impairment of their attention, visuo-spatial skills, and executive functions than people with AD [52]. DLB usually presents with recurrent episodes of confusional states on

a background of progressive cognitive deterioration. Fluctuating cognition with pronounced variations in attention and alertness is a core feature of DLB. Fluctuating cognition is present in 50–75% of people with DLB but is difficult to elicit reliably in the clinical setting. Scales, such as clinician assessment of fluctuation, the one-day fluctuation assessment scale, the Mayo fluctuations composite scale, and the dementia cognitive fluctuation scale, may help, but they need further validation and they are seldom used routinely. Visuo-spatial impairment occurs more frequently and earlier in DLB than in AD. Executive function deficits in DLB include impairments in cognitive flexibility, planning, abstraction, conceptualization, judgement, self-monitoring, and reinforcement learning. Episodic memory and verbal memory impairments are often less severe in DLB than in AD. Recognition of information is better preserved than recall in DLB, and this indicates impaired retrieval mechanisms in DLB.

Spontaneous Parkinsonism may occur in 60–92% of people with DLB [53], and 25–50% of people with DLB may have them at the time of their diagnoses. Missing the clinical diagnosis of DLB is more likely in those lacking clinically observable extra-pyramidal symptoms. Detailed neurological examination and scales, such as the unified PD rating scale, facilitate the detection of extra-pyramidal symptoms in DLB. Extra-pyramidal symptoms in DLB often include bilaterally symmetrical limb rigidity, symmetrical postural tremor, bradykinesia, facial impassivity, axial rigidity, and shuffling gait. Prominent tremors, asymmetrical resting tremors, and asymmetrical limb rigidity are less common in DLB [2]. [123]FP-CIT SPECT and PET neuroimaging can demonstrate reduced dopamine transporter uptake in the basal ganglia, before the occurrence of clinically observable extra-pyramidal symptoms. A meta-analysis including four studies and 419 people has reported that [123]FP-CIT SPECT has 86.5% sensitivity and 93.6% specificity to diagnose DLB [54]. [123]FP-CIT SPECT is not necessary once Parkinsonism is well established clinically. Missing a clinical diagnosis of DLB and the presence of associated psychotic symptoms often set the stage for revealing severe sensitivity to dopamine antagonist drugs in DLB. Challenge with a dopamine antagonist must not be used for the diagnosis of DLB, because of the associated risks.

Almost 85% of people with DLB experience recurrent complex visual hallucinations that usually feature people, children, and animals [53]. The images are often vivid, colourful, well formed, three-dimensional, and mute. Visuoperceptual deficits predispose people with DLB to experience visual hallucinations [55]. A combination of faulty perception of environmental stimuli, impaired recollection of prior experience, and intact generation of images may lead to visual hallucinations. Studies that evaluated the neurocognitive processes underlying visual hallucinations in DLB have proposed a disconnection between the prefrontal cortex and the visual cortex, as well as improper activation of the inferior temporal cortex [56]. Hallucinations involving other modalities are less common. People with DLB may have other neuropsychiatric symptoms, including apathy, paranoid delusions, depression, anxiety, and aggression [57]. Besides, RBD is a parasomnia that presents with a lack of motor inhibition during REM sleep, leading to potentially harmful simple or complex dream-enacting vocalizations and motor behaviours. Although a formal diagnosis of RBD can be confirmed only by polysomnography, diligent history taking and standardized questionnaires, such as the Mayo sleep questionnaire, can elicit RBD reliably in clinical settings. The prevalence of RBD among people with DLB has been suggested to be as high as 77%, and RBD often precedes the onset of DLB by several years. Additionally, autonomic dysfunction, including orthostatic hypotension, and carotid sinus hypersensitivity are common in DLB, and they may lead to constipation, urinary incontinence, syncope, and falls.

## Differential diagnosis

Differentiating DLB from other conditions with overlapping clinical presentations is essential for accurate diagnosis and appropriate management, and for minimizing the use of dopamine antagonists. Differential diagnosis of DLB include AD, PDD, vascular dementia, fronto-temporal dementia, other dementias, delirium, PD, adverse effects of anti-parkinsonian medications, progressive supranuclear palsy, multiple system atrophy, cortico-basal degeneration, other neurodegenerative diseases, prion diseases, complex partial seizures, late-onset psychosis, and psychotic depression. Diligent history taking, neurological examination, neuropsychological assessments, neuroimaging, EEG, and CSF biomarkers aid to clarify diagnostic dilemmas [53]. Fluctuating cognition and RBD are likely to be missed, unless specifically asked for, and eliciting them is vital for an accurate clinical diagnosis of DLB. If fluctuating cognition is the principal clinical presentation, a detailed systemic examination and investigations for potential causes for delirium should be carried out. Polypharmacy and associated adverse effects in older adults can mimic many clinical features of DLB. Hence, a comprehensive medication review is essential.

AD is the most common clinical misdiagnosis of people with DLB. The neuropsychological profiles of AD and DLB differ, and people with DLB may perform relatively worse on tests of attention, working memory, figure copying, spatial judgement, and set-shifting. SPECT and PET can help differentiating DLB from other dementias by revealing low dopamine transporter uptake in the basal ganglia and occipital hypoperfusion, as well as hypometabolism. [123]FP-CIT SPECT may be positive in fronto-temporal dementia, but associated occipital hypometabolism favours the diagnosis of DLB. A meta-analysis including eight studies and 346 people has reported that MIBG scintigraphy can differentiate DLB from other dementias, with 98% sensitivity and 94% specificity [20]. CSF biomarkers may not help the differential diagnosis of DLB, but they may predict a more severe clinical course. Besides, DLB may initially present only with neuropsychiatric symptoms, so it should be considered as one of the differential diagnoses for all older adults presenting with late-onset psychosis, especially if they have associated cognitive deficits or extra-pyramidal symptoms.

## Clinical course

Pathological processes underlying DLB may begin several years earlier than their clinical manifestations. A heterogenous, potentially long prodromal phase of DLB is widely recognized but has been poorly defined so far. RBD is likely to be the most common feature of prodromal DLB. Many longitudinal studies have confirmed the association between idiopathic RBD and later DLB diagnosis [58]. Features of prodromal DLB may include MCI, subtle neuropsychological deficits, olfactory dysfunction, dysautonomia, constipation, hypersalivation, mild extra-pyramidal symptoms, and neuropsychiatric symptoms. Among people presenting with MCI, non-amnestic deficits, fluctuating cognition, visual hallucinations, extra-pyramidal symptoms, EEG changes, low dopamine transporter uptake in the basal ganglia, reduced myocardial MIBG uptake, occipital hypoperfusion, and occipital hypometabolism have been associated with progression to DLB. The clinical onset of DLB is often insidious. Typical clinical course is gradually progressive, and the rate of cognitive decline is similar to that of AD. Initial studies have suggested that DLB and AD do not differ in their prognosis, but recent evidence indicates a worse prognosis for DLB. Longitudinal studies evaluating the courses of DLB and AD have associated DLB with an increased risk of mortality [59], shorter median survival time, and earlier admission to nursing homes by nearly 2 years [60]. DLB also places a high burden on the caregivers, even compared to AD [61]. *APOE* ε4 allele has been associated with a rapid decline in DLB, and increased CSF tau levels have been associated with shorter survival in DLB.

## Management

Good clinical management of DLB begins with an early accurate diagnosis. As treatments that can alter the progression of DLB pathology are not currently available, contemporary management focuses on symptomatic treatment, treatment of comorbidity, and providing holistic supportive care. Patients, their families, and carers need to be educated about the nature of the illness and should be involved in

**Table 43.2** Summary of available pharmacological options for DLB

| Symptoms | Medications |
|---|---|
| Cognitive symptoms | Donepezil*<br>Rivastigmine<br>Galantamine<br>Memantine |
| Hallucinations and delusions | Donepezil<br>Rivastigmine<br>Memantine<br>Clozapine<br>Quetiapine<br>Pimavanserin<br>Olanzapine (poorly tolerated) |
| Depression | Antidepressant medications |
| Anxiety | Antidepressant medications |
| REM sleep behaviour disorder | Rivastigmine<br>Memantine<br>Melatonin<br>Clonazepam |
| Restless legs syndrome | Gabapentin |
| Excessive daytime sedation | Modafinil/armodafinil |
| Postural hypotension | Fludrocortisone |
| Urinary incontinence | Trospium |

* Level I evidence is available.

all clinical decisions. Individualized care plans should be formulated after comprehensive assessments of the needs, risks, disability, and wishes of people with DLB. Well-co-ordinated multi-disciplinary management involving general practitioners, psychiatrists, neurologists, psychologists, nurses, physiotherapists, occupational therapists, and social workers is preferred. Good-quality RCTs specifically recruiting people with DLB are few, and people with DLB are very sensitive to drug-related adverse effects. Hence, treating psychiatrists should adhere diligently to the general principles of geriatric psychopharmacology such as very low-dose initiation, slow titration, periodic monitoring, dose reduction at the earliest possible opportunity, and minimizing polypharmacy. Therapeutic decision-making is not easy when distressing psychotic symptoms and neuroleptic sensitivity coexist in DLB. It is tough for patients and their carers to make a choice between mobility and psychosis. Risks and benefits of all available treatment options should be discussed in such scenarios. Table 43.2 presents a summary of available pharmacological management options for DLB.

## Cognitive symptoms

Available evidence supports the use of acetylcholinesterase inhibitors in standard doses to treat cognitive symptoms in DLB. There have been two RCTs evaluating donepezil, and one RCT investigating the effects of rivastigmine in DLB [62]. Donepezil was significantly more effective in both RCTs, with a pooled mean difference of nearly 2 Mini-Mental State Examination (MMSE) points, and cognitive improvements were maintained for 52 weeks in both RCTs. Both RCTs have reported that people receiving donepezil were significantly more likely to have absence of deterioration on clinical global impression. People taking rivastigmine showed nearly 1-point improvement of their MMSE scores during the study period, but this effect was not statistically significant. An uncontrolled trial

investigating the efficacy of galantamine in DLB has reported improvements in cognitive fluctuations. There have been two RCTs investigating the effects of memantine in mixed DLB and PDD samples [63]. Subgroup analyses revealed small, but statistically significant, improvements among the participants with DLB. Moreover, meta-analyses have supported the use of anti-dementia drugs in DLB [64].

## Neuropsychiatric symptoms

Evidence supporting the use of donepezil, rivastigmine, and memantine to treat neuropsychiatric symptoms in DLB is not robust. Some people with DLB may be on anti-parkinsonian medications. If they develop distressing visual hallucinations or other neuropsychiatric symptoms, the possibility of reducing anti-parkinsonian medications should be considered first. One RCT has provided evidence for the efficacy of donepezil to treat delusions, hallucinations, apathy, and depression in DLB, but a subsequent larger RCT has not confirmed this effect [62]. Another RCT has showed that rivastigmine could mitigate delusions, hallucinations, apathy, and depression in DLB, but the effects were not statistically significant. There have been two RCTs providing debatable evidence for and against the efficacy of memantine to treat neuropsychiatric symptoms in DLB. After considering a trial of an acetylcholinesterase inhibitor, the option of a low-dose dopamine antagonist may be considered. As already noted, dopamine antagonists are poorly tolerated by people with DLB, and there is insufficient evidence justifying their use. A small RCT has shown that risperidone was poorly tolerated, and it worsened cognition and neuropsychiatric symptoms in DLB [65]. People with DLB tolerate olanzapine poorly, but a small RCT has reported that olanzapine 5 mg/day could significantly reduce the severity of delusions and hallucinations [66]. A case series supported the use of quetiapine, but the only RCT investigating the effects of quetiapine in DLB was negative. There have not been any studies investigating the efficacy of clozapine to treat psychotic symptoms in DLB. However, extrapolating the evidence for its efficacy to treat psychotic symptoms in PDD suggests that low-dose clozapine (6.25–50 mg/day) may be the drug of choice in DLB also [57]. Similarly, pimavanserin, a selective serotonin 5-HT$_{2A}$ inverse agonist, has not been evaluated in DLB, but level I evidence exists for its efficacy to reduce psychosis in PD. Future studies investigating its efficacy and safety in people with DLB are awaited with interest.

Drugs may be used to treat depression or anxiety symptoms in DLB, but the evidence supporting their use is weak. Citalopram is the only drug for depression that has been investigated by an RCT for its efficacy in DLB. The RCT did not show any benefit, and it showed that citalopram was poorly tolerated [65]. Drugs with anticholinergic adverse effects should be avoided. Other drugs for depression may be used in DLB after careful consideration of their adverse effect profiles and potential drug interactions. Besides, a case series each for zonisamide and ramelteon, as well as a very small RCT for the herbal medicine yokukansan, has provided weak evidence for their efficacy to lessen neuropsychiatric symptoms in DLB.

## Other symptoms

Anti-parkinsonian medications are used in DLB to manage the extra-pyramidal symptoms, but they may worsen visual hallucinations and other neuropsychiatric symptoms. Moreover, levodopa response is variable in DLB. Assessing and managing the risk of falls is essential for all people with DLB and mobility problems. Rivastigmine and memantine may reduce the frequency of RBD in DLB. Melatonin and low-dose clonazepam can be used to manage RBD. Gabapentin may be helpful in people with DLB presenting with restless legs syndrome. There is weak evidence to support the use of modafinil and armodafinil for managing excessive daytime sedation in DLB. Obstructive sleep apnoea is not uncommon in DLB, and its treatment may improve excessive daytime sedation in DLB. Fludrocortisone can be used to manage postural hypotension in DLB. Review of antihypertensive medications, salt supplementation, and compression stockings should be considered. Trospium may help with urinary incontinence. Constipation in people with DLB can be managed by dietary changes, exercise, stool softeners, psyllium, or polyethylene glycol.

### Non-pharmacological interventions

There have not been many systematic trials evaluating the efficacy of non-pharmacological interventions for managing various symptoms in DLB. Electroconvulsive therapy may be considered for people with DLB presenting with severe depression and psychosis, and a few case reports, as well as a small case series, support its efficacy and safety in DLB [67]. Repetitive transcranial magnetic stimulation may be helpful in DLB. A case study employing a novel structured intervention model—'skill building through task-oriented motor practice'—has reported functional gains in a woman with DLB [68]. Physical exercise, social interactions, person-centred care, cognitive training, and cognitive behavioural therapy may help people with DLB, but further research is needed to investigate their efficacy.

## Future research

A consensus should be reached on the definition of prodromal DLB. It will help future research for identifying novel biomarkers to help with early diagnosis and for developing potential neuroprotective therapies [69]. Large, robust RCTs are needed for addressing many unanswered questions regarding the efficacy of available pharmacological and non-pharmacological options for the symptomatic treatment of DLB. Genetics, transcriptomics, and epigenetics of DLB should be investigated further. Further research on extracellular α-synuclein and circulating exosomes may enhance our understanding of neurobiology of DLB and may reveal novel therapeutic avenues. Research on extracellular α-synuclein has already provided the impetus for developing immunotherapeutic approaches for DLB [70].

## REFERENCES

1. Mayo MC, Bordelon Y. Dementia with Lewy bodies. Semin Neurol. 2014;34(2):182–8.
2. McKeith I, Mintzer J, Aarsland D, *et al.* Dementia with Lewy bodies. Lancet Neurol. 2004;3(1):19–28.
3. Walker Z, Possin KL, Boeve BF, Aarsland D. Lewy body dementias. Lancet. 2015;386(10004):1683–97.
4. McKeith I. Dementia with Lewy bodies and Parkinson's disease with dementia: where two worlds collide. Pract Neurol. 2007;7(6):374–82.
5. Holdorff B, Rodrigues e Silva AM, Dodel R. Centenary of Lewy bodies (1912-2012). J Neural Transm (Vienna). 2013;120(4):509–16.
6. Kosaka K. Latest concept of Lewy body disease. Psychiatry Clin Neurosci. 2014;68(6):391–4.
7. Hogan DB, Fiest KM, Roberts JI, *et al.* The Prevalence and Incidence of Dementia with Lewy Bodies: a Systematic Review. Can J Neurol Sci. 2016;43 Suppl 1:S83–95.
8. Zaccai J, McCracken C, Brayne C. A systematic review of prevalence and incidence studies of dementia with Lewy bodies. Age Ageing. 2005;34(6):561–6.
9. Vann Jones SA, O'Brien JT. The prevalence and incidence of dementia with Lewy bodies: a systematic review of population and clinical studies. Psychol Med. 2014;44(4):673–83.
10. Bostrom F, Jonsson L, Minthon L, Londos E. Patients with dementia with lewy bodies have more impaired quality of life than patients with Alzheimer disease. Alzheimer Dis Assoc Disord. 2007;21(2):150–4.
11. Vossius C, Rongve A, Testad I, Wimo A, Aarsland D. The use and costs of formal care in newly diagnosed dementia: a three-year prospective follow-up study. Am J Geriatr Psychiatry. 2014;22(4):381–8.
12. Beyer K, Domingo-Sabat M, Ariza A. Molecular pathology of Lewy body diseases. Int J Mol Sci. 2009;10(3):724–45.
13. Mak E, Su L, Williams GB, O'Brien JT. Neuroimaging characteristics of dementia with Lewy bodies. Alzheimers Res Ther. 2014;6(2):18.
14. Taylor JP, O'Brien J. Neuroimaging of dementia with Lewy bodies. Neuroimaging Clin N Am. 2012;22(1):67–81, viii.
15. Magierski R, Sobow T. Magnetic resonance spectroscopy in the diagnosis of dementia with Lewy bodies. Biomed Res Int. 2014;2014:809503.
16. Zhang B, Ferman TJ, Boeve BF, *et al.* MRS in mild cognitive impairment: early differentiation of dementia with Lewy bodies and Alzheimer's disease. J Neuroimaging. 2015;25(2):269–74.
17. Brigo F, Turri G, Tinazzi M. 123I-FP-CIT SPECT in the differential diagnosis between dementia with Lewy bodies and other dementias. J Neurol Sci. 2015;359(1–2):161–71.
18. Donaghy P, Thomas AJ, O'Brien JT. Amyloid PET Imaging in Lewy body disorders. Am J Geriatr Psychiatry. 2015;23(1):23–37.
19. Gomperts SN, Locascio JJ, Makaretz SJ, *et al.* Tau Positron Emission Tomographic Imaging in the Lewy Body Diseases. JAMA Neurol. 2016;73(11):1334–41.
20. Treglia G, Cason E. Diagnostic performance of myocardial innervation imaging using MIBG scintigraphy in differential diagnosis between dementia with lewy bodies and other dementias: a systematic review and a meta-analysis. J Neuroimaging. 2012;22(2):111–17.
21. Wakabayashi K, Tanji K, Odagiri S, Miki Y, Mori F, Takahashi H. The Lewy body in Parkinson's disease and related neurodegenerative disorders. Mol Neurobiol. 2013;47(2):495–508.
22. Kim WS, Kagedal K, Halliday GM. Alpha-synuclein biology in Lewy body diseases. Alzheimers Res Ther. 2014;6(5):73.
23. Beyer K, Ariza A. Alpha-aynuclein posttranslational modification and alternative splicing as a trigger for neurodegeneration. Mol Neurobiol. 2013;47(2):509–24.
24. Beyer K. Alpha-synuclein structure, posttranslational modification and alternative splicing as aggregation enhancers. Acta Neuropathol. 2006;112(3):237–51.

25. Beyer K, Humbert J, Ferrer A, *et al*. Low alpha-synuclein 126 mRNA levels in dementia with Lewy bodies and Alzheimer disease. Neuroreport. 2006;17(12):1327–30.

26. Marques O, Outeiro TF. Alpha-synuclein: from secretion to dysfunction and death. Cell Death Dis. 2012;3:e350.

27. Lee HJ, Bae EJ, Lee SJ. Extracellular alpha—synuclein-a novel and crucial factor in Lewy body diseases. Nat Rev Neurol. 2014;10(2):92–8.

28. Surendranathan A, Rowe JB, O'Brien JT. Neuroinflammation in Lewy body dementia. Parkinsonism Relat Disord. 2015;21(12):1398–406.

29. Fellner L, Stefanova N. The role of glia in alpha-synucleinopathies. Mol Neurobiol. 2013;47(2):575–86.

30. Kurzawa-Akanbi M, Hanson PS, Blain PG, *et al*. Glucocerebrosidase mutations alter the endoplasmic reticulum and lysosomes in Lewy body disease. J Neurochem. 2012;123(2):298–309.

31. Cullen V, Sardi SP, Ng J, *et al*. Acid beta-glucosidase mutants linked to Gaucher disease, Parkinson disease, and Lewy body dementia alter alpha-synuclein processing. Ann Neurol. 2011;69(6):940–53.

32. Cleeter MW, Chau KY, Gluck C, *et al*. Glucocerebrosidase inhibition causes mitochondrial dysfunction and free radical damage. Neurochem Int. 2013;62(1):1–7.

33. Nunomura A, Moreira PI, Castellani RJ, Lee HG, Zhu X, Smith MA, et al. Oxidative damage to RNA in aging and neurodegenerative disorders. Neurotox Res. 2012;22(3):231–48.

34. Spano M, Signorelli M, Vitaliani R, Aguglia E, Giometto B. The possible involvement of mitochondrial dysfunctions in Lewy body dementia: a systematic review. Funct Neurol. 2015;30(3):151–8.

35. Nervi A, Reitz C, Tang MX, Santana V, Piriz A, Reyes D, et al. Familial aggregation of dementia with Lewy bodies. Arch Neurol. 2011;68(1):90–3.

36. Bogaerts V, Engelborghs S, Kumar-Singh S, *et al*. A novel locus for dementia with Lewy bodies: a clinically and genetically heterogeneous disorder. Brain. 2007;130(Pt 9):2277–91.

37. Meeus B, Theuns J, Van Broeckhoven C. The genetics of dementia with Lewy bodies: what are we missing? Arch Neurol. 2012;69(9):1113–18.

38. Clark LN, Kartsaklis LA, Wolf Gilbert R, *et al*. Association of glucocerebrosidase mutations with dementia with lewy bodies. Arch Neurol. 2009;66(5):578–83.

39. Nalls MA, Duran R, Lopez G, *et al*. A multicenter study of glucocerebrosidase mutations in dementia with Lewy bodies. JAMA Neurol. 2013;70(6):727–35.

40. Tsuang D, Leverenz JB, Lopez OL, *et al*. GBA mutations increase risk for Lewy body disease with and without Alzheimer disease pathology. Neurology. 2012;79(19):1944–50.

41. Clark LN, Chan R, Cheng R, *et al*. Gene-wise association of variants in four lysosomal storage disorder genes in neuropathologically confirmed Lewy body disease. PLoS One. 2015;10(5):e0125204.

42. Bras J, Guerreiro R, Darwent L, *et al*. Genetic analysis implicates APOE, SNCA and suggests lysosomal dysfunction in the etiology of dementia with Lewy bodies. Hum Mol Genet. 2014;23(23):6139–46.

43. Berge G, Sando SB, Rongve A, Aarsland D, White LR. Apolipoprotein E epsilon2 genotype delays onset of dementia with Lewy bodies in a Norwegian cohort. J Neurol Neurosurg Psychiatry. 2014;85(11):1227–31.

43a. Guerreiro R, Ross OA, Kun-Rodrigues C, *et al*. Investigating the genetic architecture of dementia with lewy bodies: A two-stage genome-wide association study. Lancet Neurol. 2018;17(1):64–74.

44. Pietrzak M, Papp A, Curtis A, *et al*. Gene expression profiling of brain samples from patients with Lewy body dementia. Biochem Biophys Res Commun. 2016;479(4):875–80.

45. Funahashi Y, Yoshino Y, Yamazaki K, *et al*. DNA methylation changes at SNCA intron 1 in patients with dementia with Lewy bodies. Psychiatry Clin Neurosci. 2017;71:28–35.

46. Bonanni L, Franciotti R, Nobili F, *et al*. EEG Markers of Dementia with Lewy Bodies: A Multicenter Cohort Study. J Alzheimers Dis. 2016;54(4):1649–57.

47. Schade S, Mollenhauer B. Biomarkers in biological fluids for dementia with Lewy bodies. Alzheimers Res Ther. 2014;6(5–8):72.

48. Lim X, Yeo JM, Green A, Pal S. The diagnostic utility of cerebrospinal fluid alpha-synuclein analysis in dementia with Lewy bodies—a systematic review and meta-analysis. Parkinsonism Relat Disord. 2013;19(10):851–8.

49. Abdelnour C, van Steenoven I, Londos E, *et al*. Alzheimer's disease cerebrospinal fluid biomarkers predict cognitive decline in lewy body dementia. Mov Disord. 2016;31(8):1203–8.

50. McKeith IG, Boeve BF, Dickson DW, *et al*. Diagnosis and management of dementia with Lewy bodies: Fourth consensus report of the DLB Consortium. Neurology. 2017; 89(1): 88–100.

51. Nelson PT, Jicha GA, Kryscio RJ, *et al*. Low sensitivity in clinical diagnoses of dementia with Lewy bodies. J Neurol. 2010;257(3):359–66.

52. Bronnick K, Breitve MH, Rongve A, Aarsland D. Neurocognitive Deficits Distinguishing Mild Dementia with Lewy Bodies from Mild Alzheimer's Disease are Associated with Parkinsonism. J Alzheimers Dis. 2016;53(4):1277–85.

53. Morra LF, Donovick PJ. Clinical presentation and differential diagnosis of dementia with Lewy bodies: a review. Int J Geriatr Psychiatry. 2014;29(6):569–76.

54. Papathanasiou ND, Boutsiadis A, Dickson J, Bomanji JB. Diagnostic accuracy of (1)(2)(3)I-FP-CIT (DaTSCAN) in dementia with Lewy bodies: a meta-analysis of published studies. Parkinsonism Relat Disord. 2012;18(3):225–9.

55. Carter R, Ffytche DH. On visual hallucinations and cortical networks: a trans-diagnostic review. J Neurol. 2015;262(7):1780–90.

56. Tsukada H, Fujii H, Aihara K, Tsuda I. Computational model of visual hallucination in dementia with Lewy bodies. Neural Netw. 2015;62:73–82.

57. Ballard C, Aarsland D, Francis P, Corbett A. Neuropsychiatric symptoms in patients with dementias associated with cortical Lewy bodies: pathophysiology, clinical features, and pharmacological management. Drugs Aging. 2013;30(8):603–11.

58. Fujishiro H, Nakamura S, Sato K, Iseki E. Prodromal dementia with Lewy bodies. Geriatr Gerontol Int. 2015;15(7):817–26.

59. Oesterhus R, Soennesyn H, Rongve A, Ballard C, Aarsland D, Vossius C. Long-term mortality in a cohort of home-dwelling elderly with mild Alzheimer's disease and Lewy body dementia. Dement Geriatr Cogn Disord. 2014;38(3–4):161–9.

60. Rongve A, Vossius C, Nore S, Testad I, Aarsland D. Time until nursing home admission in people with mild dementia: comparison of dementia with Lewy bodies and Alzheimer's dementia. Int J Geriatr Psychiatry. 2014;29(4):392–8.

61. Svendsboe E, Terum T, Testad I, *et al*. Caregiver burden in family carers of people with dementia with Lewy bodies and Alzheimer's disease. Int J Geriatr Psychiatry. 2016;31(9):1075–83.

62. Stinton C, McKeith I, Taylor JP, *et al*. Pharmacological Management of Lewy Body Dementia: A Systematic Review and Meta-Analysis. Am J Psychiatry. 2015;172(8):731–42.

63. Matsunaga S, Kishi T, Iwata N. Memantine for Lewy body disorders: systematic review and meta-analysis. Am J Geriatr Psychiatry. 2015;23(4):373–83.

64. Wang HF, Yu JT, Tang SW, *et al*. Efficacy and safety of cholinesterase inhibitors and memantine in cognitive impairment in Parkinson's disease, Parkinson's disease dementia, and dementia with Lewy bodies: systematic review with meta-analysis and trial sequential analysis. J Neurol Neurosurg Psychiatry. 2015;86(2):135–43.

65. Culo S, Mulsant BH, Rosen J, *et al*. Treating neuropsychiatric symptoms in dementia with Lewy bodies: a randomized controlled-trial. Alzheimer Dis Assoc Disord. 2010;24(4):360–4.

66. Cummings JL, Street J, Masterman D, Clark WS. Efficacy of olanzapine in the treatment of psychosis in dementia with lewy bodies. Dement Geriatr Cogn Disord. 2002;13(2):67–73.

67. Burgut FT, Kellner CH. Electroconvulsive therapy (ECT) for dementia with Lewy bodies. Med Hypotheses. 2010;75(2):139–40.

68. Inskip M, Mavros Y, Sachdev PS, Fiatarone Singh MA. Exercise for Individuals with Lewy Body Dementia: A Systematic Review. PLoS One. 2016;11(6):e0156520.

69. Zhang Q, Kim YC, Narayanan NS. Disease-modifying therapeutic directions for Lewy-Body dementias. Front Neurosci. 2015;9:293.

70. Valera E, Masliah E. Immunotherapy for neurodegenerative diseases: focus on alpha-synucleinopathies. Pharmacol Ther. 2013;138(3):311–22.

# 44

# Dementia in Parkinson's disease

*Michele Hu and Fahd Baig*

## Pathogenesis and pathophysiology

### Neuropathology

The neurobiological basis for Parkinson's disease (PD) is the degeneration of nigrostriatal dopamine neurons and the pathological depositon of the protein, α-synuclein in intra-neuronal Lewy inclusions within vulnerable populations of neurons in the brain. Lewy bodies (LBs) (aggregations of proteins, including α-synuclein) and neurites (degenerating neurites with α-synuclein) have been considered to be pathological hallmarks of PD (see Chapter 43). Braak and colleagues have proposed a staging schema by which the distribution of Lewy pathology spreads through the brainstem in a prion-like fashion into the midbrain and subsequently throughout the cortex [1] (Table 44.1; Fig. 44.1). These pathological changes occur gradually and progressively over many years, with a significant period of clinically silent cell dysfunction and cell death or autonomic/sleep/mood symptoms before the onset of Parkinson's motor symptoms.

In the elderly, pathologies often occur on a background of age-related pathologies, which are extremely common in the over-75 age group. The pathologic substrate for Parkinson's disease dementia (PDD) and Parkinson's disease with mild cognitive impairment (PD-MCI) appears to be heterogenous and includes LBs, Alzheimer's disease (AD) pathology, cerebrovascular disease, and other findings, including cerebral amyloid angiopathy (Fig. 44.2) [2].

The most compelling evidence to date suggests that Lewy-related pathology is the most important factor in the development of cognitive impairment in PD. The distribution of synuclein pathology has been shown, to some extent, to map the clinical symptoms [3–5]. However, neuronal loss can be present in the absence of Lewy pathology [6], leading to the investigation of smaller α-synuclein aggregates [7]. Further uncertainty about the role of synuclein pathology is caused by the presence of LBs in the absence of Parkinsonian symptoms, termed incidental Lewy body disease. There also appears to be a synergistic relationship between α-synuclein, amyloid peptide, and tau proteins [8]. The additional presence of Alzheimer's pathology is associated with a shorter time to dementia and a higher burden of Lewy pathology in the cortex. There are also some data suggesting that chronological ageing may be an important driving factor in the onset of dementia in PD

patients [9], a factor also related to the prevalence of AD pathology in patients with dementia.

Neuropathologic studies have also linked tau deposition to Lewy body diseases, with the following observations. In both patients with DLB and those with PDD, the presence of tau pathologic changes, in combination with Aβ and α-synuclein, has been shown to potentiate dementia [10]. Furthermore, as in patients with AD [11], tau aggregates in those with PD have been found to correlate with the severity of cognitive impairment [12], and tau aggregates measured at autopsy late in the course of the disease are commonly observed in both patients with PDD and those with DLB. However, greater tau burden has been noted in the tissue of patients with DLB than in those with PDD [13], raising the possibility of a difference during life. The contribution of brain tau aggregates during life to the clinical manifestations and course of these diseases has only recently been delineated due to new imaging tracers (see Imaging under Biomarkers for PDD, p. 443, for imaging correlates).

In summary, it is very likely that there is a synergistic effect between α-synuclein pathology, age, and other pathologies, including AD and tau pathology, that is the main driver of cognitive decline in PD.

### Neurotransmitter systems

Multiple neurotransmitter deficits have long been emphasized as of major importance in PD, and particularly in underlying the cognitive deficits. An understanding of these deficits has led to current management options for PDD, namely cholinesterase inhibitors and changes to dopamine medication use.

### Dopamine and PDD

Dopaminergic neurons in the brain are found in three main midbrain dopamine regions, projecting to the *basal ganglia* (nigrostriatal system), *limbic regions* (mesolimbic system), and *cortical regions* (mesocortical system; Fig. 44.3).

The largest group of dopaminergic neurons are found in the substantia nigra (SN), which project upwards to the striatum (largely the putamen) in an important feedback loop controlling actions and thoughts. The ventrolateral portion (red-VLa SN) of this loop degenerates early in PD before LB formation and dementia, leading to progressive motor deficits of bradykinesia, rigidity, and tremor helped by dopamine replacement. In PDD, there is greater

**Table 44.1** Stages in the evolution of PD-related pathology

| Area of pathology | Possible clinical correlate | Subregions affected |
|---|---|---|
| Stage I: medulla oblongata | Constipation, hyposmia | Lesions in dorsal IX/X motor nucleus |
| Stage 2: medulla oblongata and pons | Sleep, depression, anxiety | Pathology of stage 1 plus lesions in raphe, reticular, and caeruleus–subcaeruleus nuclei |
| Stage 3: midbrain | Motor PD | Pathology of stage 2 plus midbrain lesions, especially substantia nigra |
| Stage 4: basal prosencephalon and mesocortex | PD-MCI | Pathology of stage 3 plus prosencephalic lesions, temporal mesocortex |
| Stage 5: neocortex | PD-MCI/PDD | Pathology of stage 4 plus higher-order sensory neocortical lesions |
| Stage 6: neocortex | PDD | Pathology of stage 5 plus first-order sensory association areas of neocortex |

Source: data from *Neurology*, 64(8), Braak H, Rüb U, Jansen Steur ENH, *et al.*, Cognitive status correlates with neuropathologic stage in Parkinson disease, pp.1404–10, Copyright (2005), American Academy of Neurology.

degeneration of the medial SN dopamine neurons [orange—medial SN and ventral tegmental area (VTA)], which project through the mesolimbic pathway and are involved in behavioural selection and impulsivity. Dopamine agonist use may enhance this pathway, contributing to impulse control disorders (ICDs) in PD. Degeneration of dopaminergic neurons in the VTA (yellow) may lead to a reduction in cortical dopamine through the mesocortical system, affecting cognitive function.

### Other monoamine systems and PDD

Marked degeneration of noradrenergic neurons in the locus caeruleus projecting to the forebrain are well described in PDD. Degeneration of serotonergic neurons in the median raphe nucleus as the disease progresses, with reduced serotonin innervation, is described.

### Acetylcholine and PDD

An approximate 40% loss of cholinergic pedunculopontine neurons, which project to the thalamus, is observed. However, degeneration is most marked in the nucleus basalis, leading to severe, widespread cortical reductions in choline acetyltransferase, which correlate with the extent of cognitive impairment and can be demonstrated with functional imaging studies. Anticholinergic medications accelerate

PD cognitive impairment, while cholinesterase inhibitors, such as donepezil and rivastigmine, benefit PDD.

### Summary of neurotransmitter systems

In summary, the emergence of PDD occurs on a background of severe dopamine deficits and correlates with a marked loss of limbic and cortically projecting dopaminergic, noradrenergic, serotonergic, and acetylcholinergic neurons.

## Epidemiology and risk factors

The heterogeneity of cognitive deficits found in PDD, coupled with a variability in cognitive tests and diagnostic criteria, cause significant problems when comparing published studies. Recent attempts to address this have included the publication of diagnostic standards, which have included the introduction of the concept of PD-MCI. This classification system is drawn from the study of AD as a means of classifying cognitive problems which do not meet the criteria for dementia.

Dementia is common in PD; while the point prevalence of PDD is estimated to be 31.3% (95% CI 29.2–33.6%) [14], the risk of developing dementia increases with time. While not all suffering

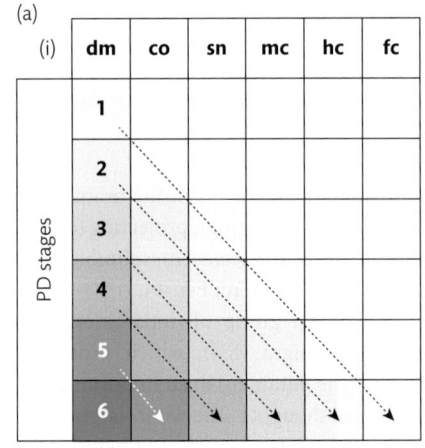
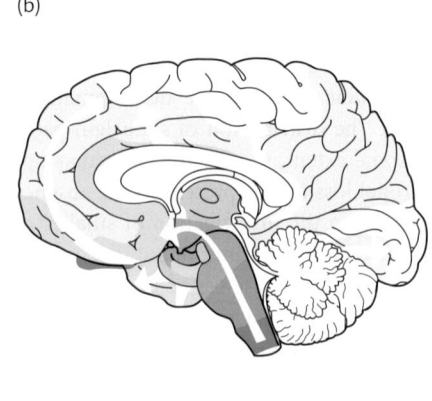

**Fig. 44.1** How PD pathology spreads upwards in PD.
Reproduced from *Neurology*, 64(8), Braak H, Rüb U, Jansen Steur ENH, *et al.*, Cognitive status correlates with neuropathologic stage in Parkinson disease, pp. 1404–10, Copyright (2005), with permission from American Academy of Neurology.

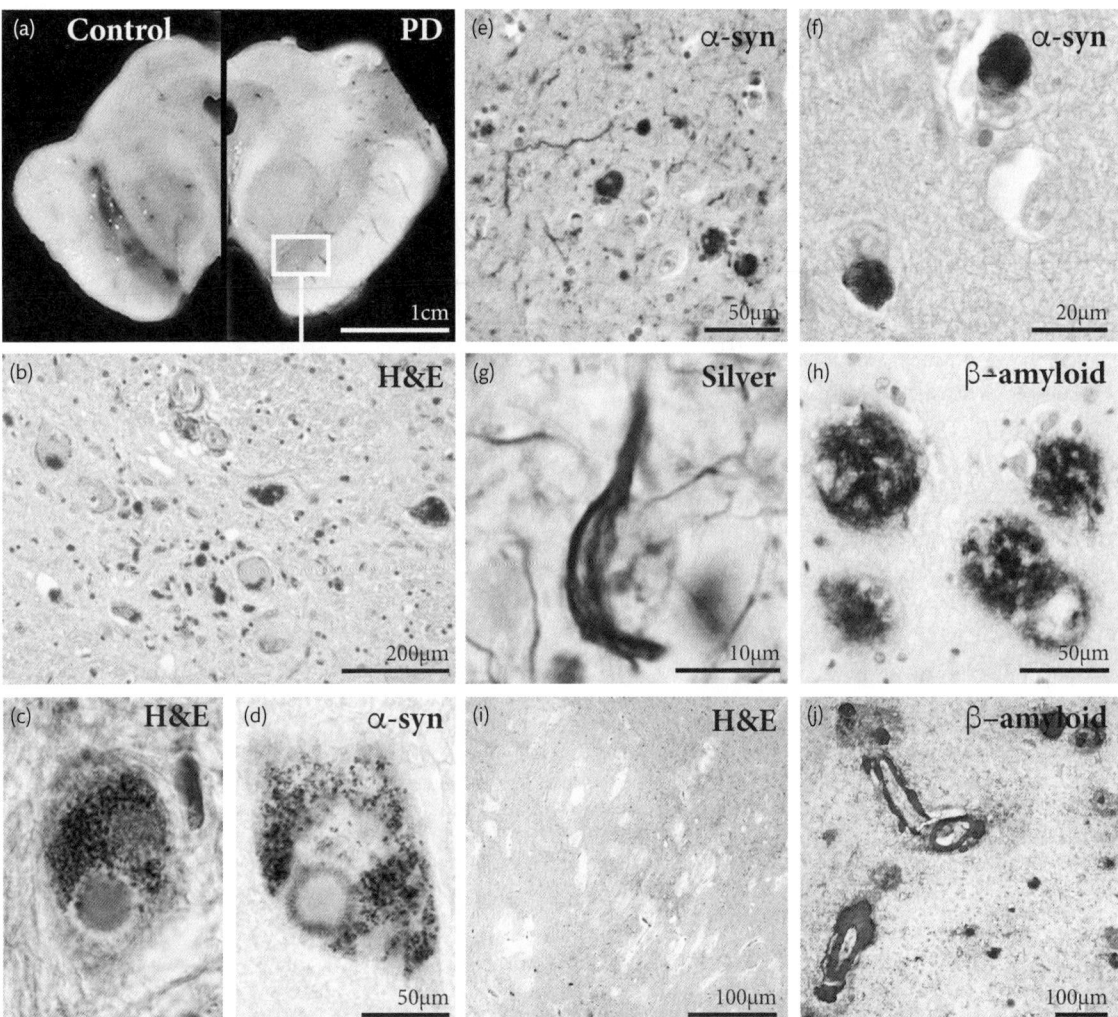

**Fig. 44.2** (see Colour Plate section) Tissue histopathology of PD and PDD. (a) Transverse section through the midbrain of a control (at left) showing the darkly pigmented SN in the ventral aspect of the midbrain, whereas the pigmented neurons in this structure are lost in patients with PD (at right). (b) Higher magnification (box in (a)) of a haematoxylin and eosin-stained section through the SN, showing only a few pigmented neurons remaining with many smaller phagocytic microglia. (c) and (d) Higher magnification of a haematoxylin and eosin-stained (c) and an a-Syn-immunoreactive (d) pigmented neuron in the SN of a PD patient containing an LB. (e) and (f) a-Syn-immunoreactive LBs and Lewy neurites in the amygdala (e) and anterior cingulate cortex (f) of a patient with PDD. (g) Silver-stained neurofibrillary tangle in the cortex of a patient with PDD. (h) Beta-amyloid-immunoreactive plaques in the cortex of a patient with PDD. (i) Vascular ischaemic tissue damage identified in a haematoxylin and eosin-stained section of the globus pallidus in a patient with PDD. (j) Beta-amyloid-immunoreactive congophilic angiopathy in the cortex of a patient with PDD.
Reproduced from *Mov Disord.*, 29(5), Halliday GM, Leverenz JB, Schneider JS, *et al.*, The neurobiological basis of cognitive impairment in Parkinson's disease, pp. 634–50, Copyright (2014), with permission from John Wiley and Sons.

dementia, even in the earliest stages of the disease, up to half will have a degree of cognitive impairment. The onset of dementia itself is highly variable, with a mean onset of 6 years and up to half of patients developing dementia within 10 years from diagnosis in a community study followed up from diagnosis [15]. By 20 years, most (the long-term cumulative prevalence is up to 80%) will have developed dementia, although not all [16, 17].

While the cognitive decline is progressive, it is non-linear and heterogenous. The pattern of cognitive deficits (including visuo-spatial, executive, and memory domains early on) varies considerably between individuals, as does the rate of the evolution of the symptoms. Overall, however, allowing for this inter-individual variability, the rate of global decline (as measured by global cognitive tasks) is slower initially and increases with disease duration and the onset of dementia [18]. This may be because the global cognition scores are not sensitive enough to pick up the subtle changes earlier in the disease course but has been a consistent finding. The decline is overall faster than reported in age-matched control groups.

Studies consistently agree that older age increases the risk of more rapid cognitive impairment [15, 19]. Other features, such as vascular risk factors [20], the presence of REM sleep behaviour disorder [21], motor impairment, poor fluency, and visuo-spatial dysfunction [15] may also predict an earlier dementia. The impact of PDD is substantial, with major consequences for functioning, institutionalization, psychiatric comorbidity, caregiver burden, and mortality [22]. Once dementia has developed, progression of physical and cognitive decline to death is similar across all groups, lasting on average 3 years (range 1–9).

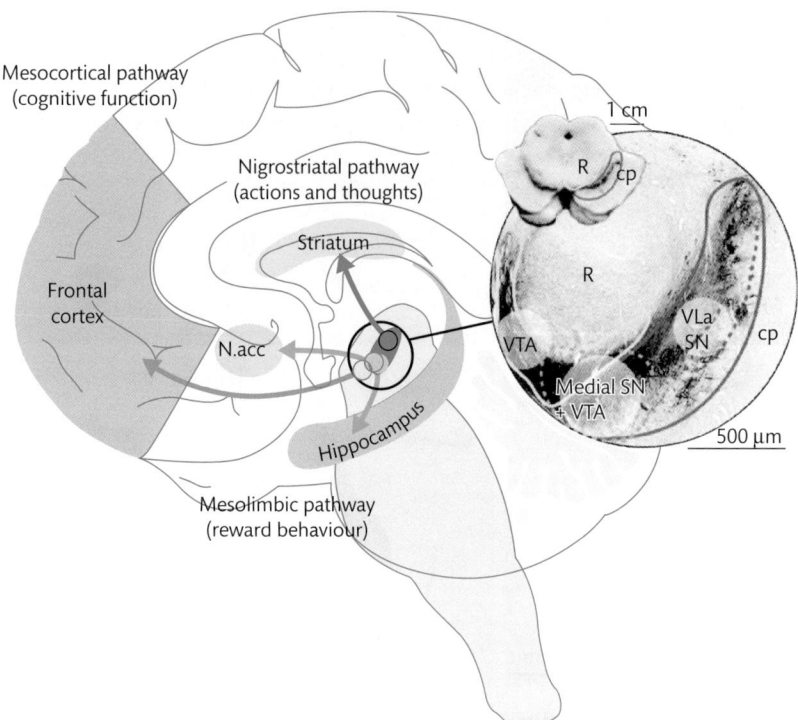

**Fig. 44.3** (see Colour Plate section) Dopamine pathways affected in PD and PDD. Red outline: SN, which contains both dopamine neurons in the pars compacta that give rise to the nigrostriatal projections, and GABA neurons in the pars reticulate, which innervate the thalamus. Dotted red line: ventrolateral (VLa) SN, which is selectively damaged in patients with PD. Yellow outline: ventral tegmental area (VTA), which contains both dopamine and non-dopamine neurons that project to limbic and cortical regions. Dotted orange outline: medial SN and VTA, which give rise to mesolimbic projections affected in patients with PDD. cp, cerebral peduncle; N. acc, nucleus accumbens; R, red nucleus.

Reproduced from *Mov Disord.*, 29(5), Halliday GM, Leverenz JB, Schneider JS, *et al.*, The neurobiological basis of cognitive impairment in Parkinson's disease, pp. 634–50, Copyright (2014), with permission from John Wiley and Sons.

## Genetic risk factors and PDD

### Familial PD

Several mutations have been found to be associated with PD, and it is generally accepted that interplay of genetic and environmental factors in an ageing brain are influencing disease development and progression. However, despite clear evidence for monogenetic and susceptibility genes in PD, the role of genetic factors in the development of dementia in PD is less clear [23]. Dementia is more common in patients with PD with a strong family association of PD probably reflecting the influence of genetic factors in the development of dementia in PD [24]. Mutations in the α-synuclein gene (*SNCA*) can be found even in sporadic PD. Functional studies on brain tissue revealed that *SNCA* genomic copy number and gene expression are related, as an increasing number of *SNCA* copies leads to an increase in α-synuclein expression, as well as LB formation. Consistent with these findings, a relationship between *SNCA* dosage and clinical phenotype, including age at onset, progression, and development of dementia, has been reported.

Mutations in the leucine-rich repeat kinase 2 gene (*LRRK2*) and *parkin* are the two most common genetic causes of Parkinsonism. Patients displaying various mutations in *LRRK2* have a low rate of cognitive dysfunction and dementia. In *parkin* mutations, progression of the disease tends to be rather slow, and dementia is not a common feature. Much less is known regarding the association with dementia of two other mutations associated with PD—*Pink1* and

*DJ-1*. It should be noted, however, that these monogenic forms of PD are generally rare and will occur with an overall frequency of <5% in community-ascertained, unselected Caucasian PD cohorts.

### Cognition and risk genes

Mutations in the genes transcribing microtubule-associated protein tau (MAPT), apolipoprotein E (APOE), glucocerebrosidase (GBA), and SNCA have all been associated with increased dementia risk in PD. MAPT helps assemble and stabilize microtubules throughout the central nervous system, predominantly found in the axons of neurons. The gene encoding MAPT is located on chromosome 17q21, part of a 900-kb fragment which is commonly inverted, causing two common haplotypes H1 and H2. Despite the fact that tau pathology is not a neuropathological feature of PD, the *MAPT* gene (H1/H1 MAPT haplotype) has been consistently identified as a risk gene for both PD and PDD [15, 25, 26] Interestingly, a gene–gene interaction between *MAPT* and *SNCA* was also reported [27].

Mutations in the *GBA* gene have been found to increase both PD risk and the risk of PDD, with affected patients presenting at a younger age and developing dementia earlier. Visuo-spatial deficits specifically have been associated with this haplotype, even prior to the onset of dementia, with regionally specific changes in cortical activation [28–30] The link between dementia risk and the APOE ε4 genotype is strongly established, with the ε4 allele associated with a higher risk and an earlier onset of AD. In PD, however, there is no association between the APOE ε4 genotype and PD risk. However, this genotype is an independent predictor of PDD, even when controlling for AD pathology severity [31]. The enzyme catechol-*O*-methyltransferase (COMT) is an important regulator of synaptic dopamine, particularly in the frontal and prefrontal cortices. A common functional polymorphism causing lower enzymatic activity is linked to poor attention and executive performance in early PD subjects; however, this genotype is not predictive of future dementia [32]. Lastly, a recent study characterized the *SNCA* gene locus in PDD and DLB, and found a PDD risk haplotype that was distinct from DLB, with association profiles in single-nucleotide polymorphisms across the *SNCA* gene for Parkinsonism and dementia [33].

## Classification, clinical criteria, and controversies

Cognitive impairment in PD is heterogenous both in severity and pattern and is subject to influences both integral and external to the disease. Diagnostic criteria have been developed by the Movement Disorders Society that help to guide clinicians and researchers to an accurate diagnosis of PD-MCI [34] or PDD [35]. These criteria largely meet the *Diagnostic and Statistical Manual of Mental Disorders*, fourth edition criteria for dementia. In both PD-MCI and PDD, gradual cognitive decline within the context of established PD and objectively demonstrated cognitive deficits are core features (Table 44.2).

In PDD, cognitive deficits in more than one domain are required, whereas in PD-MCI, a single domain may be affected. In PDD, the deficits must be severe enough to impair activities of daily living, whereas in PD-MCI, they must not be sufficiently severe to interfere with functional independence (although minor difficulties may be present). To operationalize these criteria and to assess the pattern and severity of cognitive dysfunction, we need: (1) valid measures of cognitive abilities covering the major domains of cognition; (2) a method to determine whether or not the performance represents a decline from a person's previous level of functioning; and (3) an assessment of how the individual's cognitive abilities enable (or disable) function in day-to-day activities. These will be further discussed in Diagnosis and differential diagnosis, p. 441 later in this chapter.

Although cognitive impairment in PD exists on a continuum of severity, it is often divided into two categories—mild cognitive impairment and PDD, based on the extent to which the impairment interferes with activities of daily living (Table 44.2). This classification system risks oversimplifying a very complex entity but has been fundamental to clinical trials of therapies for cognitive dysfunction in PD, which have been largely devoted to the treatment of PDD. Currently, therefore, evidence-based treatment of cognitive impairment in PD is restricted to PDD and depends on making a diagnosis of this entity. Identifying mild cognitive impairment is also useful, however, because it has prognostic significance. Several longitudinal studies have demonstrated that PD-MCI is a risk factor for developing PDD. There is also evidence that the pattern of cognitive deficit is prognostically important(see [36] for review).

### Controversies: the 1-year rule

With advances in knowledge, disease boundaries may change and require redefinition of the disease. In the case of PD, as diagnostic criteria currently stand, dementia developing before the second year of Parkinsonism is an exclusion criterion for PD; the diagnosis is DLB.

If dementia starts after 1 year, the diagnosis is PDD. Beyond the arbitrary nature of the 1-year rule, there is increasing controversy about whether the distinction itself is valid. PDD and DLB share many similarities in dementia presentation, neuropsychological findings, non-motor profile (olfactory loss, depression, sleep disorders, and autonomic dysfunction in both), imaging, genetics, and pathology (Fig. 44.4). However, broad differences do exist and are summarized in Fig. 44.3. Fig. 44.5 illustrates how the type of cortical pathology and clinical presentation of PDD and DLB might interact. A recent MDS task force proposed that the 1-year rule separating PDD and DLB be omitted [37]. The authors argued that rather, when a patient presents with motor signs and meets full clinical criteria for PD, the diagnosis of PD is applied, regardless of the presence or timing of dementia. In other words, dementia is no longer an exclusion criterion for PD. For those patients who already carry a DLB diagnosis (according to consensus criteria [38]), the authors argued that the diagnosis can optionally be qualified as 'PD (DLB subtype)'. Note that this proposal would not invalidate the diagnostic category

**Table 44.2** Criteria for PDD

| | Core features | Associated features | Exclusions |
|---|---|---|---|
| Probable PDD | 1. PD diagnosis | 1. Typical cognitive deficits in two of four domains (attention, executive function, visuo-spatial function, and free recall) | 1. Vascular disease on imaging or other abnormality that may cause cognitive impairment, but not dementia<br>2. Unknown time interval between motor and cognitive symptoms |
| | 2. Slowly progressive dementia syndrome | 2. At least one behavioural symptom (apathy, depression/anxious mood, hallucinations, delusions, or excessive daytime sleepiness) | 3. Acute confusion resulting from systemic diseases or abnormalities or drug intoxication<br>4. Features compatible with probable vascular dementia |
| Possible PDD | 1. PD diagnosis | 1. Atypical cognitive deficits in one or more domain (fluent aphasia or storage-failure amnesia) with preserved attention | 1. Acute confusion resulting from systemic diseases or abnormalities or drug intoxication |
| | 2. Slowly progressive dementia syndrome | Vascular disease on imaging or other abnormality that may cause cognitive impairment, but not dementia, and/or unknown time interval between motor and cognitive symptoms | 2. Features compatible with probable vascular dementia |

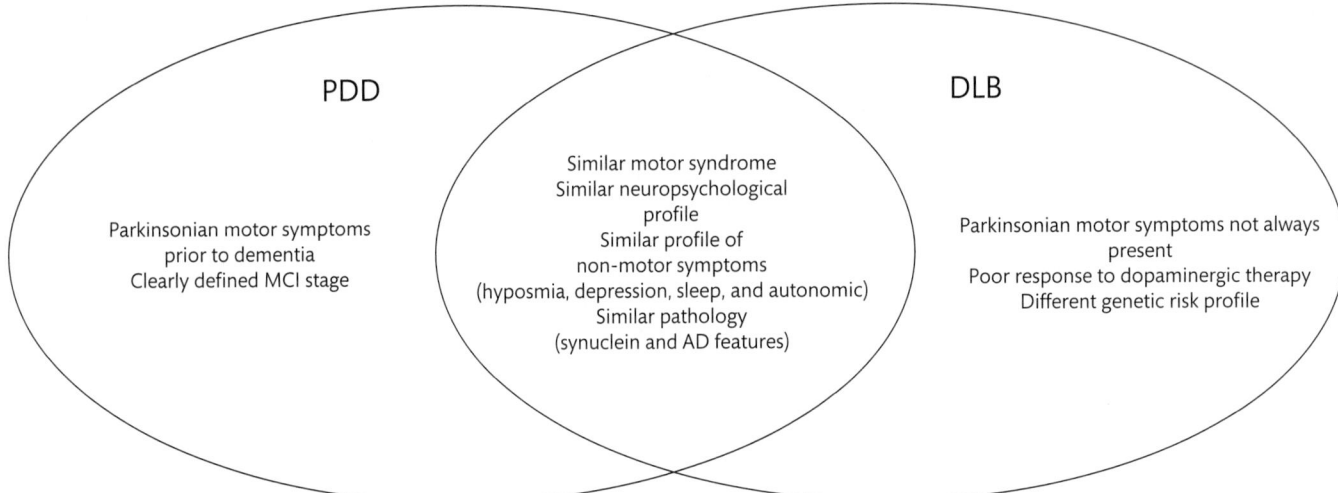

**Fig. 44.4** Similarities and differences between PDD and DLB.

of DLB. In clinical communication with patients with the DLB subtype, the diagnostic term DLB could continue to be used [37].

Contrary to this, others have argued that the 1-year rule distinguishing PDD from DLB is worth maintaining because it serves an important purpose in clinical practice, clinical and basic science research and when helping the lay community understand the complexity of these different clinical phenotypes. Furthermore, opponents believed that adding an additional diagnostic label 'PD (dementia with Lewy bodies subtype)' will confuse, rather than clarify, the distinction between DLB and PD or PDD and will not improve management or expedite therapeutic development [39].

## Clinical features

### Cognitive syndrome

#### PD-MCI

The spectrum of impairment ranges broadly in phenotype, as well as in timing in the disease course. Cognitive deficits can occur in one or more domains, vary in severity, and present differently at various

stages of the disease. Studies of incident PD indicate that cognitive impairment is not just a late-stage problem but occurs in up to 50% of early cases, including untreated individuals, who manifest PD-MCI [40–43]. Executive function represents the most common cognitive domain affected in PD early on, as well as later, in the disease. Deficits can be detected on tests that are sensitive to frontal dysfunction (for example, tests of planning, spatial working memory, and attentional set shifting). However, impairments in attention, explicit memory, and visuo-spatial function also are demonstrable in early PD. Executive dysfunction may occur individually as a single-domain impairment or in combination with other cognitive deficits as multiple-domain impairments. Some, but not all, studies investigating clinical features and frequencies of cognitive impairment in PD patients without dementia revealed that non-memory (non-amnestic) single-domain deficits are the most frequent cognitive subtype.

#### PDD

The cognitive profile of PDD remains variable, although it often affects cognitive domains similar to those affected in PD-MCI, but with more severe deficits and with the disruption of multiple areas. The onset of PDD is insidious. In one prospective study, the mean

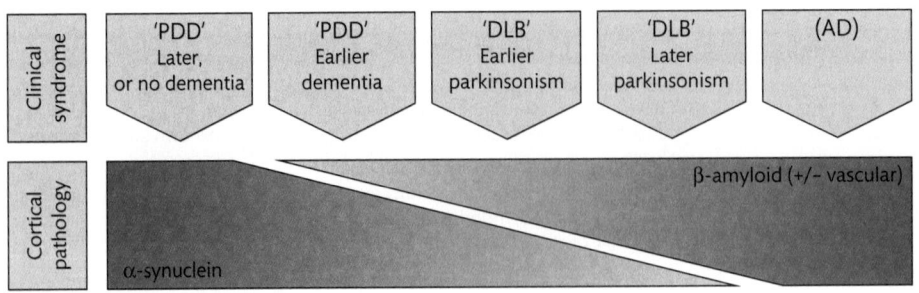

**Fig. 44.5** Cortical pathology and clinical presentation of PDD and DLB. Dementia in DLB/PD is associated with two major pathologies: synucleinopathy (a-Syn, i.e. Parkinson pathology) and neuritic amyloidopathy (i.e. Alzheimer pathology). In PD patients who develop dementia very late in their illness, or not at all (far left), neuritic amyloid deposition is minimal (or absent), and cortical pathology is mainly that of a-Syn deposition. At the other extreme, DLB patients with predominant neuritic amyloid deposition and very minimal a-Syn deposition would usually be diagnosed as AD during life, developing clinical DLB hallmarks late (if at all). Between these two extremes of the spectrum lie the most patients with PD and DLB.

annual decline on the MMSE during 4 years was 1 point in the non-demented and 2.3 points in the PDD group, the latter figure being similar to the decline observed in patients with AD. A similar rate of decline was reported in another longitudinal study; the mean decline in MMSE over 2 years was 4.5 and was comparable to that seen in patients with DLB, with a mean decline of 3.9 points [35].

By definition, PDD includes impairment in at least two cognitive domains but, as per MDS criteria, does not require memory deficits. The predominant cognitive deficits in late PDD are similar to those in DLB, with marked visuo-spatial dysfunction and fluctuating attention. Impairments in executive function, working memory, and episodic memory are also common in PDD, although language, particularly as measured by object naming, tends to be relatively preserved (see [44] for review).

### Longitudinal relationship between PD-MCI and PDD

The CamPaIGN study, a longitudinal population-based cohort of incident PD, recently reported 10-year follow-up data [15]. Analyses at multiple time points in this cohort (n = 142) indicated that, aside from age, the most significant baseline predictors of later dementia were impaired semantic fluency and pentagon copying (hazard ratios of 3.1 and 2.6, respectively, for dementia at 10 years from diagnosis). There was no association between 'fronto-striatal-based' executive dysfunction and later dementia and, in fact, there was no decline in executive function performance over this time.

### Neurological findings

By definition, the PDD patient will have features of established motoric Parkinsonism, of which *bradykinesia* is key—characterized by a progressive *decrement* in the amplitude or velocity of movement (or both), rather than the generalized slowness seen with cerebellar or pyramidal disorders. Rigidity and tremor are common, and in general, motor Parkinsonism will be more severe than that seen in DLB or the mild extra-pyramidal features associated with AD. Parkinsonism is typically levodopa-responsive, with levodopa-induced dyskinesias common at this advanced stage and other features such as wearing-off periods. As the disease progresses, severe Parkinsonian symptoms with gait freezing are common, so that the patient frequently falls and becomes wheelchair-bound. The quality of the dementia resembles a subcortical pattern, with pronounced psychomotor slowing, not usually accompanied by severe aphasia, agnosia, or apraxia. Patients perform disproportionately poorly on timed tests and visuo-spatial tasks.

### Psychiatric issues

A variety of neuropsychiatric symptoms, including depression, anxiety, hallucinations, apathy, psychosis, and ICDs, occur commonly in up to 90% of PDD patients [45]. Psychotic symptoms affect 60% of PD patients long term and include hallucinations and delusion. The occurrence of these symptoms are predictors of nursing home placement and mortality. Complex visual hallucinations, often of animals or people, are the most typical manifestation, occurring in 40–90% of PDD patients, but other visuoperceptual disturbances can occur, including illusionary experiences, sensations of movement in the periphery (passage hallucination), and a feeling of presence (extracampine hallucination). Auditory, tactile, and olfactory hallucinations are less common. Delusions manifest when insight is compromised, so they are associated with a degree of cognitive impairment. Delusions in PD tend to be paranoid in nature, and other phenomena, including delusional misidentification (for example, Capgras and Fregoli syndromes), can occur in a minority.

Depression is one of the most common non-motor symptoms in PD, with clinically relevant symptoms occurring in 35% of PD patients. Rates are higher in PD-MCI, and there is a known association between depression and cognitive impairment. Generalized anxiety disorder (GAD) is the most commonly diagnosed anxiety condition in PD, followed by panic attacks and phobias. Anxiety is also strongly linked to depressive symptoms but appears to be less common in PDD than PD, and is also related to motor symptoms, particularly occurring in the off condition in patients with motor fluctuations. Apathy, defined as a decrease in goal-directed behaviour, verbalization, and mood, is common in a range of neurodegenerative diseases, including PD. It is usually accompanied by reduced self-awareness, so changes are noticed and brought to the attention of clinicians by caregivers. A common assumption is that the patient is depressed, although a lack of endorsement of sad mood suggests apathy instead. Apathy can occur independently of cognitive impairment in PD, but overlap is common. Some studies estimate the prevalence of apathy in PDD to be up to 50%.

ICDs (for example, compulsive gambling, buying, sexual behaviour, and eating) are increasingly recognized as common and clinically significant disorders in PD. Given that research suggests that the strongest risk factors for ICD development in PD are dopamine agonist treatment and younger age, and given that cognitively impaired patients are more likely to be older and less likely to be prescribed a dopamine agonist, it is not surprising that ICDs are not commonly reported in PDD patients. In one single-centre study of 805 PD patients, ICD symptoms were less common in PD patients with dementia (3.8%), compared with non-demented patients (9.6%) [46].

## Diagnosis and differential diagnosis

As mentioned in Classification, clinical criteria, and controversies, p. 439, the clinical diagnosis of PDD requires: (1) valid measures of cognitive abilities covering the major domains of cognition; (2) a method to determine whether or not the performance represents a decline from a person's previous level of functioning; and (3) an assessment of how the individual's cognitive abilities enable (or disable) function in day-to-day activities. Core features are established PD (clinical diagnosis usually made by a physician) and objectively demonstrated cognitive deficit.

### Clinical evaluation

The cornerstone in the evaluation of a patient with suspected PDD is detailed clinical and neurological history and examination, including interview with a close informant. Assessment of social functions and activities of daily living, as well as psychiatric and behavioural symptoms, is part of the basic evaluation.

### Measuring cognitive function

Cognitive function in PD is generally measured in one of three settings: (1) in the course of an evaluation by a physician or an occupational or speech therapist; (2) by a neuropsychologist performing a dedicated clinical cognitive evaluation; or (3) in a research study. These assessments require different tools; a physician or an occupational therapist usually requires a relatively short global cognitive scale with adequate sensitivity to screen for the presence of cognitive impairment or to follow changes over time (Table 44.3). A neuropsychologist uses multiple tests, each emphasizing a specific cognitive domain, to provide a detailed assessment of the pattern of cognitive dysfunction. Research studies require variable detail, depending on the goals of the study, but generally necessitate an instrument with good specificity for an accurate diagnosis and often responsiveness to change over time. Thus, methods for assessing cognitive function in PD need to be selected with careful thought to the goals of the assessment [36]. A useful summary of cognitive screening measures and their approximate administration time is given later in this chapter.

In terms of selecting a brief bedside screening tool, the author would generally favour the MoCA over the MMSE for assessing PD cognition, as it has greater sensitivity across a range of cognitive subdomains, shows less ceiling effects, and is more sensitive than the MMSE in detecting longitudinal change over time [41].

### Establishing cognitive decline

As described previously, to establish a diagnosis, it is critical to understand whether or not any impairment represents a decline from a premorbid level of cognitive functioning. Subjective reports of decline are often spontaneously reported during clinical and research contacts and can be elicited with general questions about concerns related to memory or thinking. A more formal method is to use a cognitive complaint interview. However, patients are not very insightful into their own difficulties, questioning the reliability of this approach. Work in AD has suggested that patients with earlier dementia, but not MCI, underreport cognitive difficulties, compared with caregivers, suggesting that incorporating caregiver report of cognitive complaints is important.

To the author's knowledge, this issue has not been evaluated in PD; however, the use of a caregiver-reported questionnaire—the short form of the Informant Questionnaire on Cognitive Decline in the Elderly (SHORT IQ-CODE) [47]—is currently being evaluated, to assess for cognitive decline in the Oxford Discovery PD cohort. Lastly, cognitive decline can be established on the basis of serial performance on cognitive testing by a clinician or on the basis of results from neuropsychological test performance that is poorer than expected based on an estimate of a person's premorbid cognitive abilities. Estimating premorbid verbal IQ can be accomplished using a reading test such as the Wechsler Test of Adult Reading or the National Adult Reading Test, which are relatively resistant to change in the face of common neurodegenerative conditions.

### Assessing function in relation to cognition

Impairment on the patient's ability to carry out instrumental activities of daily living (IADLs) is an essential feature for establishing the severity of cognitive impairment. This is especially relevant for non-demented PD subjects in whom some aspects of altered functioning in IADLs may appear unnoticeable before the diagnosis of dementia without a formal examination.

As described, the presence of significant functional deficiency due to cognitive impairment is embedded in the current criteria to support the diagnosis of PDD. Moreover, the major formal differentiation of PD-MCI from PDD has typically required cognitive deficits not to interfere significantly with the patient's ability to implement IADLs. Presently, judgement as to the PD patient's ability to adapt to the demands of the environment and execute IADLs is mostly derived from indirect methods (for example, cognitive testing), unstructured interviews with relatives or other caregivers, or the use of functional scales intended for other dementias.

Scales not specific for PD do not take into account the motor impact of the disease and can overestimate the extent to which cognitive dysfunction is contributing to problems carrying out IADLs. The lack of a recommendable instrument, capable of measuring the specific impact of cognitive decline in PD, minimizing the motor symptoms of the disease, has made it challenging to set a standard for what is meant by 'significantly' (that is, dementia) or 'subtly reduced' (that is, MCI) functional performance. Two new PD-specific instruments—the PD-Cognitive Function Rating Scale (PD-CFRS) [48] and the brief Penn Daily Activities Questionnaire (PDAQ) [49]—may help fill the need for assessments of IADLs that are sensitive to cognitive impairment in PD, while minimizing the motor aspects of the disease.

**Table 44.3** Generic and non-Parkinson's disease specific cognitive screening measures

| Scale name | Assessed cognitive domains | Approximate administration time |
|---|---|---|
| Mini-Mental State Examination (MMSE) | Orientation, verbal registration and recall, attention, naming and repetition, verbal comprehension, praxis, visuo-spatial | 10 min |
| Montreal Cognitive Assessment (MoCA) | Orientation, attention, memory, naming, fluency, verbal repetition, visuo-spatial/executive | 10 min |
| Addenbrooke Cognitive Examination (Revised)—ACE(R) | Attention/orientation, memory, fluency, language, visuo-spatial | 20 min |
| Cambridge Cognitive Assessment (Revised)—CAMCOG(R) | Orientation, language, memory, attention, praxis, calculations, abstract reasoning, perception | 25 min |
| Dementia Rating Scale (2nd edition)/Mattis Dementia Rating Scale—DRS (2) | Attention, initiation/perseveration, construction, conceptualization, memory | 30 min |
| Repeatable Battery for the Assessment of Neuropsychological Status (RBANS) | Attention, language, visuo-spatial/construction, immediate memory, delayed memory | 30 min |
| Alzheimer's Disease Assessment Scale—Cognition (ADAS-Cog) | Memory, language, praxis | 30 min |

## Differential diagnosis

The differential diagnosis of PD is extensive; of particular note, those that are also degenerative are associated with dementia/MCI, including progressive supranuclear palsy (PSP), multiple system atrophy (MSA), DLB, and cortico-basal degeneration (CBD). Occsaionally, frontal lobe disorders nay be mistaken for Parkinsonian disorders, such as Pick's disease, and non-degenerative aetiologies such as frontal lobe meningiomas or drug-induced Parkinsonism. Other progressive, non-degenerative diseases that have some Parkinsonian features include multi-infarct dementia and normal pressure hydrocephalus, usually excluded on an MRI brain scan. Occasionally, Parkinsonian features occur in patients with AD.

## Biomarkers for PDD

The point prevalence of dementia in patients with PD is 25%, and it riscs to 80% in patients who live for >20 years with the disorder. Cognitive decline in PD worsens the patient's prognosis more than any other non-motor symptoms. A prognostic marker delineating the probability for those patients at risk for cognitive decline would be of utmost importance. While PD-MCI is a risk factor for PDD, it is a heterogenous entity, and it is not known which types of PD-MCI confer a higher risk of progression to dementia. In this sense, useful biomarkers are needed that can predict future outcome or that are useful to longitudinally track the underlying disease pathology in an objective way. In this section, we summarize the current knowledge on cerebrospinal fluid (CSF) and blood proteins, imaging, and the impairment of gait/postural instability as risk markers for cognitive decline in PD. Genetic predictors of PDD have been discussed elsewhere.

### Cerebrospinal fluid

The presence of LBs, amyloid plaques, and neurofibrillary tangles in the neocortex and limbic system is associated with dementia and MCI in PD. Hence, the levels of amyloid-β (Aβ), tau protein, and α-synuclein have been studied in the CSF of PD patients (see [50, 51] for review). In most studies, there was less Aβ in PDD than in healthy controls, and lower levels of Aβ were associated with progression to dementia in PD and cognitive measures. By contrast, data for total (t-tau) and phosphorylated tau (p-tau) are less consistent, with increased or unchanged levels in PDD patients. Although total α-synuclein was similar in PDD and controls in initial studies, technically more advanced analyses showed that PDD patients have more oligomeric forms of α-synuclein, and a higher total α-synuclein concentration was associated with a faster decline in cognitive performance in de novo patients. However, most studies have failed to find any association between total or oligomeric α-synuclein and cognition in PD patients.

Proteins involved in inflammatory processes, oxidative stress, and neuronal viability have also been investigated in the CSF, with elevated C-reactive protein, IL-6, and IL-1b in PD-MCI compared to PD normal-cognition patients or controls. Uric acid (UA), a scavenger of free radicals, and cystatin C, which has anti-amyloidogenic properties, were also reduced in PDD and DLB patients. Despite some variability, reduced Aβ in PDD patients and those who progress to PDD is consistent, and this suggests that the Aβ protein

might represent a useful biomarker to identify specific types of PD-MCI that might be at higher risk of suffering dementia.

### Plasma/serum and urine

Plasma or serum levels of proteins involved in inflammation (C-reactive protein), oxidative stress (UA), or neuroprotection (vitamin D, transthyretin) were not different in PDD and cognitively normal PD patients [50, 51]. However, in PD patients with normal cognition, low UA concentrations were associated with a worse outcome in global cognition, attention, and memory; high vitamin D levels with better semantic fluency and memory; and high concentrations of IL-6, tumour necrosis factor-α, and interferon-γ-induced protein 10, with lower cognitive scores. Importantly, low levels of epidermal growth factor (EGF) and insulin-like growth factor (IGF) have certain predictive values for the development of dementia and cognitive decline, and IGF positively correlates with global cognition and executive function.

There is no consistent relationship between plasma homocysteine and dementia or worse cognitive outcome. Lipids have also been evaluated because abnormal lipid peroxidation may play a role in the pathogenesis of PD and other neurodegenerative diseases. Whereas plasma levels of phospholipids were higher in PD-MCI than in normal cognition PD subjects, prostaglandin isomers derived from free radical peroxidation of polyunsaturated fatty did not differ. In keeping with findings in plasma, low UA levels are associated with poor neuropsychological performance. These findings are consistent with recent data linking neurodegeneration and ageing with disturbances in lipid metabolism and neuroinflammation.

### Imaging

(See [50] for a review of this topic.)

#### MRI grey matter changes

Although there are many studies in this field, the most valuable are those with larger cohorts and more advanced analytic approaches, especially the longitudinal studies. Accordingly, reduced cortical volume or thickness in several areas, and especially in the hippocampus, appears to be associated with progression to dementia and MCI. This is a promising avenue to be followed, in which well-designed prospective studies using modern analytical models might help to validate these findings or identify new patterns that could serve as potential biomarkers.

#### White matter microstructure

##### Diffusion tensor imaging

Reduced fractional anisotropy (FA) or increased mean diffusivity (MD) in diffusion tensor imaging studies can indicate alterations in the microstructure of white matter (WM) tracts. Both approaches show that dementia and MCI in PD are associated with extensive areas of modified WM microstructure, with reduced FA being widespread in PDD along the main tracts.

#### Functional MRI

##### Cerebral blood flow

Functional MRI (fMRI) in resting state or during the execution of tasks indirectly measures neural activity and is used to study regional activation of the brain and the association or dependency between two or more anatomic locations, termed functional connectivity. One interesting approach is to study the default network that reflects the predominant activity at rest, which is dampened when switching to a cognitive task. In PDD patients, this network has weaker connectivity in the right inferior frontal gyrus and is less intensely deactivated than in controls when confronted with a complex visual task. Considering the data available, it can be speculated that there are two main functional networks in the resting state: one more anterior that seems to be related to executive dysfunction, and another more posterior one that might herald the evolution to dementia. This would also be consistent with observations derived from the longitudinal CamPAIGN cohort (see Longitudinal relationship between PD-MCI and PDD, p. 441).

### PET and single-photon emission computed tomography (SPECT) imaging

#### Cholinergic ligands

Pathological studies and pharmacological trials with acetylcholinesterase inhibitors indicate that cholinergic dysfunction is relevant in dementia in PD. Studies using different radiotracers show that the cholinergic activity in PDD patients was weaker in the whole cortex and in the occipital, precentral, parietal, temporal, and posterior cingulate cortices than in healthy controls. PET studies indicate that assessing the cholinergic state might be useful as a biomarker of dementia in PD, but current accessibility limits their clinical and research use.

#### Aβ ligands

Fibrils of Aβ can be assessed *in vivo* by Pittsburgh compound B (PiB) PET imaging [52]. Studies showed that cortical Aβ deposition is common in individuals with PD and PDD, that high levels of Aβ are observed in most cases of DLB [53], and that greater deposition of Aβ is a risk factor for cognitive impairment in patients with PD, accelerating cognitive decline once established [54]. These findings were consistent with prior neuropathologic reports. In AD, disease progression occurs in the context of high Aβ levels and is associated with the spread of tau deposits from the medial temporal lobe to the basal temporal neocortex and then to other neocortical regions [55], in association with regional neuronal loss. From the few such studies undertaken in PD patients, the *in vivo* results of PiB-PET studies are rather variable, with low sensitivity and specificity in the diagnosis of dementia and MCI in PD patients.

#### Regional blood flow/glucose uptake ligands

Reduced regional cerebral blood flow and FDG-PET uptake in the posterior cortical areas seem to be useful biomarkers of dementia in PD, in line with fMRI data.

#### Tau ligands

In the last year, the radioligand fluorine 18-labelled AV-1451, also known as [18F]T807, has been used to image tau in patients with LB diseases because of its high affinity, selectivity, and favourable kinetics for imaging tau. Two recent studies have shown: (1) AD patients can be distinguished from DLB patients on the basis of significantly higher AV-1451 uptake, representing cortical tau, particularly in the medial temporal lobes [56]; and (2) patients with DLB and

PDD manifest a spectrum of tau pathology, with cortical tau aggregates associated with cognitive impairment [52].

### Gait and cognition in PD

Gait disturbance in PD shares neurochemical, pathological, structural, and genetic relationships with cognitive risk factors [51, 57]. It is believed that gait disturbance associated with the postural instability gait disorder (PIGD) motor PD phenotype and dementia is underpinned by a common neurochemical deficit in cholinergic function. Brain imaging highlights shared structural correlates of gait and cognitive impairment. Combined with evidence in older adults that gait changes may precede cognitive decline, these findings add validity to the role of gait as a surrogate marker of cognitive impairment. Longitudinal follow-up is required to explore the temporal relationship between these risk factors and their sensitivity and specificity.

## Treatment

In recent years, there have been important advances regarding clinical characterizations, definitions, associated biomarkers, and risk factors for both MCI in PD and PDD. However, there is a paucity of effective therapies for cognitive impairment in PD, whether for mild symptoms or for moderate to severe dementia [58]. At present, only rivastigmine is U.S. Food and Drug Administration-approved for PDD, an indication received nearly a decade ago. Given the frequency of PD cognitive impairment and its substantial impact on both patients and families, the lack of available and effective treatments represents a striking gap in the field, especially when compared to the large number of available therapies. Improved symptomatic therapies, as well as potential disease-modifying agents, for PD cognitive impairment are needed.

Treatments can be broadly divided into pharmacological and non-pharmacological and are summarized here. However, special considerations apply to the management of PDD. Firstly, dopaminergic therapy is more likely to cause hallucinations and delusions in Parkinsonian patients with dementia than in those with uncomplicated PD. Secondly, neuroleptic therapy is more likely to cause an exacerbation of Parkinsonian symptoms, hence should be avoided unless absolutely clinically necessary. Third, on–off motor fluctuations may commonly be accompanied by mild fluctuations in cognitive state as well.

### Pharmacological treatments

Modest symptomatic effect of the cholinesterase inhibitor rivastigmine for PDD has been shown, in particular for patients with accompanying visual hallucinations [59]. Other cholinesterase inhibitors, such as donepezil, have been shown to produce similar modest improvements in cognition and behaviour in PDD and DLB [60]. A naturalistic study indicated that amantadine may increase the time from onset of PD to dementia [61]. Several studies have used memantine to show benefit in patients with both PDD and DLB combined [62]. PD psychosis can be difficult to treat; practically, however, removal of anti-parkinsonian medications may help ameliorate psychotic symptoms, particularly in the earlier stages of the disease, and a specific order of withdrawal has been suggested, beginning with anticholinergic agents through to dopamine agonists/COMT inhibitors, and then finally, if required, levodopa [45]. However, reductions in dopamine therapies can be challenging, given the need to adequately treat motor symptoms.

Specific pharmacological interventions include the use of drugs for psychosis; however, as mentioned, these are more likely to cause an exacerbation in motor symptoms in PD patients. Dopamine antagonists, such as haloperidol, can provoke severe neuroleptic sensitivity reactions and therefore are contraindicated in this population. Similar reactions or worsening of parkinsonism can also be observed with most of the newer drugs such as risperidone, olanzapine, and aripiprazole [63], which should be avoided because of the risk. While there have been numerous RCTs of antipsychotics for PD psychosis, there is a paucity of data looking at the benefits of these agents in PD patients with cognitive impairment specifically. The exception is clozapine where one major study with a positive outcome included some PD patients with possible dementia (mean baseline MMSE: placebo group, 21.7; clozapine group, 23.8) [64]. However, subgroup data for PDD patients were not provided, and widespread use of clozapine is limited due to its potential to induce agranulocytosis and the necessity for regular blood monitoring. Quetiapine is used most frequently for PD psychosis, but there is no evidence from controlled studies for its efficacy in PDD [65] Additionally, prolonged use of dopamine antagonists may have deleterious effects on cognition, and they significantly increase cerebrovascular events and mortality in older people with dementia in general (see [45] for review), so these agents should be used cautiously in PD patients with cognitive impairment until demonstrated not to increase morbidity and mortality in this population.

A promising new drug for PD psychosis is pimavanserin (selective 5-HT2A inverse agonist). A recent controlled trial found a significant benefit of pimavanserin on all endpoints, including the Scale for Assessment of Positive Symptoms in Parkinson's Disease (SAPS-PD) score, with additional improvement in night-time sleep and daytime somnolence [66]. Overall pimavanserin was well tolerated and did not worsen motor symptoms.

Cholinesterase inhibitors, in particular rivastigmine, may be an alternative first-line treatment option, as these agents can improve cognition, function, and neuropsychiatric symptoms. Other drugs, such as memantine (NMDA antagonist) and ondansetron (5-HT3 antagonist), have also been considered for the treatment of PD psychosis. Overall the therapeutic benefit of memantine remains inconclusive, and from a psychosis perspective, improvements in the neuropsychiatric inventory (NPI) in patients with PDD have not been observed, although there may be some benefit in DLB patients.

### Non-pharmacological treatments

There are no systematic studies evaluating non-pharmacological interventions for PD psychosis, although a small study suggested benefit for ECT in patients refractory to dopamine antagonists [67]. As mentioned, removal of anti-parkinsonian medications can help ameliorate psychotic symptoms, but often at the cost of motor control. Phased reduction, followed by withdrawal, if necessary, of dopamine agonist medication, in particular, is critical to the management of ICDs. Abrupt withdrawal of dopamine agonist medication should be avoided, due to the risk of causing dopamine agonist withdrawal syndrome (DAWS), an unpleasant syndrome characterized by agitation, motor restlessness, worsening of symptoms,

dysphoria, and anxiety. Similarly, abrupt withdrawal of levodopa or any dopaminergic medication can cause neuroleptic malignant syndrome and should always be contemplated with the full support and involvement of a PD physician.

Non-pharmacological interventions for PDD include several ongoing studies of deep brain stimulation (DBS) surgery in PD, targeting the bilateral nucleus basalis of Meynert, a cholinergic-innervated basal forebrain site involved in attention, learning, and memory processes, which is impaired in dementia. Non-pharmacological strategies for treating PD cognitive impairment represent an area of growing interest and include cognitive training, physical exercise and physical therapy, music and art therapy, and non-invasive brain stimulation techniques (see [58] for review). To date, many studies are open-label pilot studies; though there are several small RCTs, 'double blinding' of study personnel and patients in these types of interventions can be challenging. There is great heterogeneity in study methodologies [for example, different types of cognitive tasks and means of assessments (computerized interventions, neuropsychological tests, and word games, along with the duration of study and practice), physical exercises and methods (aerobic, dance, strength, and so on), and cognitive targets (attention, executive function, memory, and so on)].

Studies in PD have generally focused on cognitively intact or non-demented, but mildly cognitively impaired, PD patients, rather than those with PDD. Cognitive therapies include cognitive training exercises, computerized brain training, and non-physical leisure activities which have the potential to improve cognitive outcomes and IADLs (see [58] for review). Physical exercise and activity have reported benefits on motor PD symptoms, while studies investigating their effects on cognition are growing. Beneficial effects of combined physical activity and cognitive training therapies may be potentially additive [68, 58 ].

### Prognosis and future perspectives

The cumulative incidence of PDD from longitudinal studies of incident PD cohorts is remarkably consistent, suggesting that around half will develop dementia within 10 years from diagnosis. The onset of PDD is insidious, with a similar reported mean annual decline on the MMSE to that seen in AD and DLB [35]. However, disease progression varies considerably, with some patients declining rapidly, while others have a more benign course. The determinants underpinning this variability are poorly understood. Post-mortem studies showed that concurrent AD neuropathology is associated with a more rapid cognitive decline in LBD patients, shorter time between parkinsonism and dementia onset, and a worse prognosis. There also appears to be a synergistic relationship between tau, α-synuclein, and amyloid pathology (see earlier). However, it is still unclear whether *in vivo* surrogate biomarkers (amyloid/tau imaging, CSF protein quantification) can predict LBD endophenotype in terms of disease progression. Response to current symptomatic treatments is also variable in PD, and a better understanding of the mechanisms of response and non-response to these agents will be key in informing who to target with a new range of emerging symptomatic drugs.

There is major pharma investment into disease-modifying treatments in early AD targeting amyloid and tau, with recent data, excitingly, suggesting benefit. Aggregation of these brain proteins also occur in LBD and may have deleterious effects, as well as synergistically promote α-synuclein aggregation (the core aggregate in LB disease). Developing relevant stratification of biomarkers could therefore mean that any effective near-future anti-amyloid/tau treatments could also be offered to selected PDD and DLB patients. Furthermore, anti-α-synuclein therapies, protein degradation enhancers, and mitochondrial stabilizers are all in development, and stratification in PDD would be highly apposite to de-risking trials of these agents.

Lastly, the earlier any intervention, the more effective it is likely to be. Therefore, intervention at the PD-MCI stage, to prevent the inexorable progression to PDD, must be a key focus of future treatments in PD if they are to be effective. Biomarkers, in particular, the emerging imaging biomarkers outlined, could be especially useful to identify those PD-MCI patients at high risk of developing dementia in the short to mid term.

## REFERENCES

1. Braak H, Rub U, Jansen Steur EN, Del Tredici K, de Vos RA. Cognitive status correlates with neuropathologic stage in Parkinson disease. *Neurology*. 2005;64:1404–10.
2. Halliday GM, Leverenz JB, Schneider JS, Adler CH. The neurobiological basis of cognitive impairment in Parkinson's disease. *Mov Disord*. 2014;29:634–50.
3. Doty RL. Olfactory dysfunction in Parkinson disease. *Nat Rev Neurol*. 2012;8:329–39.
4. Kempster PA, O'Sullivan SS, Holton JL, Revesz T, Lees AJ. Relationships between age and late progression of Parkinson's disease: a clinico-pathological study. *Brain*. 2010;133:1755–62.
5. Kalia LV, Lang AE, Hazrati L, et al. CLinical correlations with lewy body pathology in lrrk2-related parkinson disease. *JAMA Neurol*. 2015;72:100–5.
6. Dijkstra AA, Voorn P, Berendse HW, Groenewegen HJ, Rozemuller AJ, van de Berg WD. Stage-dependent nigral neuronal loss in incidental Lewy body and Parkinson's disease. *Mov Disord*. 2014;29:1244–51.
7. Kalia LV, Lang AE. Parkinson disease in 2015: evolving basic, pathological and clinical concepts in PD. *Nat Rev Neurol*. 2016;12:65–6.
8. Irwin DJ, Lee VMY, Trojanowski JQ. Parkinson's disease dementia: convergence of [alpha]-synuclein, tau and amyloid-[beta] pathologies. *Nat Rev Neurosci*. 2013;14:626–36.
9. Reid WG, Hely MA, Morris JG, Loy C, Halliday GM. Dementia in Parkinson's disease: a 20-year neuropsychological study (Sydney Multicentre Study). *J Neurol Neurosurg Psychiatry*. 2011;82:1033–7.
10. Howlett DR, Whitfield D, Johnson M, et al. Regional multiple pathology scores are associated with cognitive decline in Lewy body dementias. *Brain Pathol*. 2015;25:401–8.
11. Arriagada PV, Growdon JH, Hedley-Whyte ET, Hyman BT. Neurofibrillary tangles but not senile plaques parallel duration and severity of Alzheimer's disease. *Neurology*. 1992;42(3 Pt 1):631–9.
12. Horvath J, Herrmann FR, Burkhard PR, Bouras C, Kovari E. Neuropathology of dementia in a large cohort of patients with Parkinson's disease. *Parkinsonism Relat Disord*. 2013;19:864–8; discussion 864.
13. Walker L, McAleese KE, Thomas AJ, et al. Neuropathologically mixed Alzheimer's and Lewy body disease: burden of pathological protein aggregates differs between clinical phenotypes. *Acta Neuropathol*. 2015;129:729–48.
14. Aarsland D, Zaccai J, Brayne C. A systematic review of prevalence studies of dementia in Parkinson's disease. *Mov Disord*. 2005;20:1255–63.
15. Williams-Gray CH, Mason SL, Evans JR, et al. The CamPaIGN study of Parkinson's disease: 10-year outlook in an incident population-based cohort. *J Neurol Neurosurg Psychiatry*. 2013;84:1258–64.
16. Aarsland D, Kurz MW. The epidemiology of dementia associated with Parkinson disease. *J Neurol Sci*. 2010;289:18–22.
17. Hely MA, Reid WG, Adena MA, Halliday GM, Morris JG. The Sydney multicenter study of Parkinson's disease: the inevitability of dementia at 20 years. *Mov Disord*. 2008;23:837–44.
18. Maetzler W, Liepelt I, Berg D. Progression of Parkinson's disease in the clinical phase: potential markers. *Lancet Neurol*. 2009;8:1158–71.
19. Muslimovic D, Post B, Speelman JD, De Haan RJ, Schmand B. Cognitive decline in Parkinson's disease: a prospective longitudinal study. *J Int Neuropsychol Soc*. 2009;15:426–37.
20. Malek N, Lawton MA, Swallow DM, et al. Vascular disease and vascular risk factors in relation to motor features and cognition in early Parkinson's disease. *Mov Disord*. 2016;31:1518–26.
21. Rolinski M, Szewczyk-Krolikowski K, Tomlinson PR, et al. REM sleep behaviour disorder is associated with worse quality of life and other non-motor features in early Parkinson's disease. *J Neurol Neurosurg Psychiatry*. 2014;85:560–6.
22. Hu MT, Szewczyk-Krolikowski K, Tomlinson P, et al. Predictors of cognitive impairment in an early stage Parkinson's disease cohort. *Mov Disord*. 2014;29:351–9
23. Aarsland D, Beyer MK, Kurz MW. Dementia in Parkinson's disease. *Curr Opin Neurol*. 2008;21:676–82.
24. Kurz MW, Larsen JP, Kvaloy JT, Aarsland D. Associations between family history of Parkinson's disease and dementia and risk of dementia in Parkinson's disease: a community-based, longitudinal study. *Mov Disord*. 2006;21:2170–4.
25. Lill CM, Roehr JT, McQueen MB, et al. Comprehensive research synopsis and systematic meta-analyses in Parkinson's disease genetics: The PDGene database. *PLoS Genetics*. 2012;8:e1002548.
26. Seto-Salvia N, Clarimon J, Pagonabarraga J, et al. Dementia risk in Parkinson disease: disentangling the role of MAPT haplotypes. *Arch Neurol*. 2011;68:359–64.
27. Goris A, Williams-Gray CH, Clark GR, et al. Tau and alpha-synuclein in susceptibility to, and dementia in, Parkinson's disease. *Ann Neurol*. 2007;62:145–53.
28. Neumann J, Bras J, Deas E, et al. Glucocerebrosidase mutations in clinical and pathologically proven Parkinson's disease. *Brain*. 2009;132:1783.
29. Winder-Rhodes SE, Evans JR, Ban M, et al. Glucocerebrosidase mutations influence the natural history of Parkinson's disease in a community-based incident cohort. *Brain*. 2013;136:392–9.
30. Zokaei N, McNeill A, Proukakis C, et al. Visual short-term memory deficits associated with GBA mutation and Parkinson's disease. *Brain*. 2014;137:2303–11.
31. Irwin DJ, White MT, Toledo JB, et al. Neuropathologic substrates of Parkinson disease dementia. *Ann Neurol*. 2012;72:587–98.
32. Williams-Gray CH, Hampshire A, Barker RA, Owen AM. Attentional control in Parkinson's disease is dependent on COMT val 158 met genotype. *Brain*. 2008;131(Pt 2):397–408.
33. Guella I, Evans DM, Szu-Tu C, et al. alpha-synuclein genetic variability: a biomarker for dementia in Parkinson disease. *Ann Neurol*. 2016;79:991–9.
34. Litvan I, Goldman JG, Troster AI, et al. Diagnostic criteria for mild cognitive impairment in Parkinson's disease: Movement Disorder Society Task Force guidelines. *Mov Disord*. 2012;27:349–56.

35. Emre M, Aarsland D, Brown R, *et al*. Clinical diagnostic criteria for dementia associated with Parkinson's disease. *Mov Disord*. 2007;22:1689–707; quiz 837.

36. Marras C, Troster AI, Kulisevsky J, Stebbins GT. The tools of the trade: a state of the art 'How to Assess Cognition' in the patient with Parkinson's disease. *Mov Disord*. 2014;29:584–96.

37. Berg D, Postuma RB, *et al*. Time to redefine PD? Introductory statement of the MDS Task Force on the definition of Parkinson's disease. *Mov Disord*. 2014;29:454–62.

38. McKeith IG, Dickson DW, Lowe J, Emre M, O'Brien JT, Feldman H, *et al*. Diagnosis and management of dementia with Lewy bodies: third report of the DLB Consortium. *Neurology*. 2005;65:1863–72.

39. Boeve BF, Dickson DW, Duda JE, *et al*. Arguing against the proposed definition changes of PD. *Mov Disord*. 2016;31:1619–22.

40. Aarsland D, Bronnick K, Larsen JP, Tysnes OB, Alves G; Norwegian ParkWest Study Group. Cognitive impairment in incident, untreated Parkinson disease: the Norwegian ParkWest study. *Neurology*. 2009;72:1121–6.

41. Hu MT, Szewczyk-Krolikowski K, Tomlinson P, *et al*. Predictors of cognitive impairment in an early stage Parkinson's disease cohort. *Mov Disord*. 2014;29:351–9.

42. Williams-Gray CH, Foltynie T, Brayne CE, Robbins TW, Barker RA. Evolution of cognitive dysfunction in an incident Parkinson's disease cohort. *Brain*. 2007;130(Pt 7):1787–98.

43. Yarnall AJ, Breen DP, Duncan GW, *et al*. Characterizing mild cognitive impairment in incident Parkinson disease: the ICICLE-PD study. *Neurology*. 2014;82:308–16.

44. Goldman JG, Williams-Gray C, Barker RA, Duda JE, Galvin JE. The spectrum of cognitive impairment in Lewy body diseases. *Mov Disord*. 2014;29:608–21.

45. Aarsland D, Taylor JP, Weintraub D. Psychiatric issues in cognitive impairment. *Mov Disord*. 2014;29:651–62.

46. Poletti M, Logi C, Lucetti C, *et al*. A single-center, cross-sectional prevalence study of impulse control disorders in Parkinson disease: association with vdopaminergic drugs. *J Clin Psychopharmacol*. 2013;33:691–4.

47. Jorm AF. A short form of the Informant Questionnaire on Cognitive Decline in the Elderly (IQCODE): development and cross-validation. *Psychol Med*. 1994;24:145–53.

48. Kulisevsky J, Fernandez de Bobadilla R, Pagonabarraga J, *et al*. Measuring functional impact of cognitive impairment: validation of the Parkinson's disease cognitive functional rating scale. *Parkinsonism Relat Disord*. 2013;19:812–17.

49. Brennan L, Siderowf A, Rubright JD, *et al*. The Penn Parkinson's Daily Activities Questionnaire-15: Psychometric properties of a brief assessment of cognitive instrumental activities of daily living in Parkinson's disease. *Parkinsonism Relat Disord*. 2016;25:21–6.

50. Delgado-Alvarado M, Gago B, Navalpotro-Gomez I, Jimenez-Urbieta H, Rodriguez-Oroz MC. Biomarkers for dementia and mild cognitive impairment in Parkinson's disease. *Mov Disord*. 2016;31:861–81.

51. Mollenhauer B, Rochester L, Chen-Plotkin A, Brooks D. What can biomarkers tell us about cognition in Parkinson's disease? *Mov Disord*. 2014;29:622–33.

52. Gomperts SN, Locascio JJ, Makaretz SJ, *et al*. Tau positron emission tomographic imaging in the Lewy body diseases. *JAMA Neurol*. 2016;73:1334–41.

53. Gomperts SN, Rentz DM, Moran E, *et al*. Imaging amyloid deposition in Lewy body diseases. *Neurology*. 2008;71:903–10.

54. Gomperts SN, Locascio JJ, Rentz D, *et al*. Amyloid is linked to cognitive decline in patients with Parkinson disease without dementia. *Neurology*. 2013;80:85–91.

55. Spillantini MG, Goedert M. Tau pathology and neurodegeneration. *Lancet Neurol*. 2013;12:609–22.

56. Kantarci K, Lowe VJ, Boeve BF, *et al*. AV-1451 tau and beta-amyloid positron emission tomography imaging in dementia with Lewy bodies. *Ann Neurol*. 2017;81:58–67.

57. Rochester L, Yarnall AJ, Baker MR, *et al*. Cholinergic dysfunction contributes to gait disturbance in early Parkinson's disease. *Brain*. 2012;135(Pt 9):2779–88.

58. Goldman JG, Weintraub D. Advances in the treatment of cognitive impairment in Parkinson's disease. *Mov Disord*. 2015;30:1471–89.

59. Burn D, Emre M, McKeith I, *et al*. Effects of rivastigmine in patients with and without visual hallucinations in dementia associated with Parkinson's disease. *Mov Disord*. 2006;21:1899–907.

60. Thomas AJ, Burn DJ, Rowan EN, *et al*. A comparison of the efficacy of donepezil in Parkinson's disease with dementia and dementia with Lewy bodies. *Int J Geriatr Psychiatry*. 2005;20:938–44.

61. Inzelberg R, Bonuccelli U, Schechtman E, *et al*. Association between amantadine and the onset of dementia in Parkinson's disease. *Mov Disord*. 2006;21:1375–9.

62. Aarsland D, Ballard C, Walker Z, *et al*. Memantine in patients with Parkinson's disease dementia or dementia with Lewy bodies: a double-blind, placebo-controlled, multicentre trial. *Lancet Neurol*. 2009;8:613–18.

63. Emre M, Ford PJ, Bilgic B, Uc EY. Cognitive impairment and dementia in Parkinson's disease: practical issues and management. *Mov Disord*. 2014;29:663–72.

64. Low-dose clozapine for the treatment of drug-induced psychosis in Parkinson's disease. The Parkinson Study Group. *N Engl J Med*. 1999;340:757–63.

65. Seppi K, Weintraub D, Coelho M, *et al*. The Movement Disorder Society Evidence-based medicine review update: treatments for the non-motor symptoms of Parkinson's disease. *Mov Disord*. 2011;26 Suppl 3:S42–80.

66. Cummings J, Isaacson S, Mills R, *et al*. Pimavanserin for patients with Parkinson's disease psychosis: a randomised, placebo-controlled phase 3 trial. *Lancet*. 2014;383:533–40.

67. Ueda S, Koyama K, Okubo Y. Marked improvement of psychotic symptoms after electroconvulsive therapy in Parkinson disease. *J ECT*. 2010;26:111–15.

68. Thom JM, Clare L. Rationale for combined exercise and cognition-focused interventions to improve functional independence in people with dementia. *Gerontology*. 2011;57:265–75.

# 45

# Dementia due to Huntington's disease

*Russell L. Margolis*

## Introduction

Huntington's disease (HD) was first described in 1872 by George Huntington, an American physician living on Long Island, New York. His father and grandfather practised medicine in the same community, so that he had access to case notes from several generations of families who lived there. This long period of record-keeping allowed him to document a hereditary form of chorea, similar to 'common (Sydenham's) chorea', but progressing over many years to death. Its sufferers had a tendency to insanity and suicide. Huntington's brief essay, which also included a clear description of autosomal dominant inheritance, remains one of the classic descriptions of a medical disorder [1].

## Clinical features and course of illness

HD is an inherited neuropsychiatric disorder prominently affecting the striatum and its direct connections. It is characterized by a triad of clinical features that are common to diseases of this region: a non-aphasic *dementia, depression* and other disorders of affect, and a variety of *dyskinesias*, most typically chorea [2, 3]. Chorea, from the Greek word for 'dance', describes involuntary, non-stereotyped jerky movements. The illness, insidious in onset, may begin with all or any one of these three features. Patients who present initially to psychiatrists usually have dementia, personality changes (such as apathy, irritability, or loss of temper), or depression, often with suicidal thoughts or attempts. Symptoms may appear at any time from early childhood to old age, most frequently between 35 and 45 years of age. Once the illness begins, sufferers gradually deteriorate over many years in their cognitive and motor functioning and end in a persistent vegetative state, with almost complete loss of voluntary motor function. Death occurs after about 15–20 years and is usually caused by inanition or aspiration pneumonia. Some patients die earlier from suicide or from injuries such as subdural haematomas caused by a fall. Patients with early onset seem to progress more rapidly than those whose symptoms begin later in life.

## Pathology and genetics

The earliest visible neuropathology is in the striosomes of the caudate/putamen [4], followed by a dorsal-to-ventral progressive loss of almost all striatal output neurons. The deep layers of multiple cortical regions are also prominently affected, and there can also be milder neuronal loss in some brainstem nuclei. Protein aggregates, most easily detectable in neuronal nuclei, are prominent. Neuroimaging studies have shown that neuropathological changes typically begin before the onset of clinically detectable disease. In particular, the extent of striatal loss in pre-symptomatic individuals, as measured by MRI, correlates with the predicted time until disease onset [5]. Cortical thinning [6] and white matter loss and disorganization [7, 8] have also been detected in pre-symptomatic gene carriers. Subtle changes possibly related to abnormal brain development have also been reported.

The prevalence of HD ranges from about 6 to 14 cases per 100,000 population in North America, Western Europe, and Australia, with much lower prevalence in Asia [9]. HD is caused by the expansion of an unstable triplet repeat sequence (CAG) in the first exon of a gene near the telomere of chromosome 4p [10]. It is transmitted as an autosomal dominant trait; if one parent carries the mutation, each offspring (regardless of sex) has an independent 50% chance of inheriting the abnormal gene. Normal repeat lengths range from about 7 to 28 triplets. Individuals with 29–35 triplets will not develop HD (with possible rare exceptions) but may pass an expanded allele to an offspring, while individuals with 40 or more triplets will develop HD. Repeat lengths of 36–39 triplets may or may not cause disease. The rate of mutation from a normal-length allele to an expanded one is low, so that most patients have an affected parent. Family history, however, can be obscured by multiple factors, including misdiagnosis of the parent, death of the parent before disease onset, adoption, and incorrect assignment of paternity. The repeat length does not remain stable at meiosis. In HD, the number of CAG triplets is more likely to increase when the gene is transmitted by fathers. As the number of repeats increases, the age at onset is earlier. Thus, paternal transmission is often associated with 'anticipation', earlier onset in the subsequent generation; most individuals with childhood onset have affected fathers [11].

The pathogenesis of HD is not well understood but appears to be multi-faceted [12]. The gene *huntingtin*, with the expanded repeat, is expressed as the protein huntingtin. The CAG repeat expansion is translated as an expanded polyglutamine tract, which appears to have neurotoxic properties. The region of the huntingtin protein with the polyglutamine tract may be cleaved from the rest of the protein and adopt an abnormal configuration, or it may be abnormally modified by post-translational processes such as phosphorylation. These changes, in turn, are thought to lead to disruption of cellular functions, including transcriptional machinery, protein degradation processes, metabolism, and cellular transport. Other proposed pathogenic mechanisms include toxicity derived from huntingtin RNA transcripts containing the expanded CAG repeat, atypical translation of the *huntingtin* gene leading to proteins with long stretches of other amino acids, and loss of the normal function of the huntingtin protein.

## Diagnosis

The clinical diagnosis of HD remains dependent on a thorough psychiatric history, including a detailed family history and history of changes in social adjustment, mental state examination, cognitive examination, and neurological examination. The features vary, depending on how long the patient has been ill [13]. Once the disease is suspected on clinical grounds, genetic testing, available through many commercial laboratories, provides the definitive diagnosis. A number of large completed and ongoing longitudinal studies of HD, including PREDICT, PHAROS, COHORT, REGISTRY, and Enroll-HD, have greatly enhanced knowledge of the signs, symptoms, and course of HD.

## Diagnosis of patients with early symptoms

Patients with HD who initially consult psychiatrists may present with a variety of psychiatric syndromes, including depression, bipolar disorder, obsessive–compulsive disorder, schizophrenia, or excessive anxiety. Irritability or apathy may be a manifestation of one of these syndromes or may appear separately. The psychiatric syndromes seen in HD are clinically indistinguishable from idiopathic disorders, and in perhaps 20% of cases, neurological signs may not be present. Suicide is a risk in this prodromal phase, even if the patient is unaware of their risk for HD [14]. Presenting symptoms and problems with functioning at work or at home must often be elicited from an informant; the patient may minimize them through embarrassment or fear, or even be unaware of them. Common changes include decline in work speed or accuracy, which may result in demotion or warnings from superiors, a tendency to become irritated or physically aggressive in response to annoying stimuli that would not have elicited such a response in the past, and a decreased interest in activities. Most of these symptoms and behaviours are common in psychiatric disorders, but cognitive inefficiency and irritability may seem disproportionately extreme relative to the patient's other symptoms. On cognitive examination, the patient may have difficulty recalling dates of important life events and more difficulty than expected with 'serial sevens'. Cognitive changes are often easier to notice after the psychiatric disorder is treated, which can usually be accomplished using standard medications. However, unlike the typical response to treatment of idiopathic disorders, cognitive inefficiency and difficulties at work, apathy (if present), and sometimes irritability remain, even after the HD patient's mood, energy, and sleep patterns have improved.

On neurological examination, motor restlessness is usually present but is easily misinterpreted as a manifestation of anxiety. Motor signs may be subtle: slightly slow saccadic eye movements [15],

writhing movements of the protruded tongue or of the fingertips when the arms are held at 90°, or mild dysdiadochokinesia.

Diagnosis can be further complicated by the apparent lack of a family history of HD. The family may not have been informed about the affected parent's diagnosis or may know only that a parent died in a psychiatric institution or committed suicide. In other cases, the paternity is uncertain. If the family history is actually negative (this is quite uncommon) or unobtainable (often the case for adopted individuals who frequently present in childhood), the diagnosis may be confirmed by testing for the HD gene expansion.

HD with onset in childhood or early adolescence [16] most often presents with cognitive and behavioural features, including speech and language problems, a decline in school performance, deterioration of handwriting, and loss of interest in school and social activities [17]. These non-motoric disturbances may be the only clinical features for several years before motor impairment begins. The motor impairment in a majority of juvenile-onset patients will include prominent parkinsonism, bradykinesia, very slow saccades, lead pipe or cogwheel rigidity, and dystonia, with chorea less prominent or even absent. However, many affected juveniles have motor signs similar to typical HD. Myoclonus and epilepsy are observed in as many as 50% of early-onset HD, and some children develop a coarse tremor.

Even though it can be difficult, it is important to make the diagnosis of HD as early as possible, particularly in employed persons. Poor function at work (or in schoolwork or household duties) occurs early, and patients can lose their jobs or support of their family, often on suspicion of drug or alcohol abuse or of indifference to the work or home environment. This is usually avoided if the diagnosis is made known to the family and employer, allowing modification of the work environment or retirement on the basis of disability and family education about the illness. Prompt diagnosis does not always mean that the patient needs to be immediately informed of the diagnosis. Occasionally, patients are too depressed to do this safely; others indicate that they do not wish to be told. Treatment can usually proceed despite the patient's reluctance to label the disorder.

## Diagnosis of patients with well-established signs and symptoms

After a few years of illness, diagnosis is easier. The signs and symptoms will have worsened, and usually the motor disorder is obvious. A typical patient who has been ill for about 5–7 years is unable to work or manage finances but lives at home and is able to manage personal needs. Some patients remain active and energetic, continuing to participate as fully in life as their cognitive and motor disabilities allow; others are apathetic most of the time, but irritable when disturbed; still others may have a depressive syndrome, at times complicated by delusions, obsessions, or compulsions. Many patients are anxious and easily upset by changes of routine. An uncommon, but very troublesome, feature of HD is sexual abnormality. While most patients become impotent or uninterested in sex, a few are hypersexual and may develop paraphilias [18]. It is important to inquire about these specifically because neither the patient nor his or her spouse will likely mention problems.

Cognitively, patients complain of forgetfulness and distractibility. Thinking is slow; patients have difficulty following a conversation and cannot complete a multistaged task. On cognitive examination,

Mini-Mental State Examination scores [19] may still be above the cut-off score of 23 for dementia, but serial sevens will be very poor, and one or two items will be missed on recalling words after a distraction. On neuropsychological testing, the IQ will be lower than expected for education, and there will be difficulty learning word lists and performing tests that require changing sets.

Most patients will have obvious involuntary choreic movements, as well as difficulty with control of voluntary motor movements, as seen by clumsiness, slowness, dysarthria, and an unsteady gait. The involuntary movements will wax and wane with the level of arousal; it can be worsened by performing serial sevens or by fine motor tasks. Speech will have an irregular staccato, often laboured, quality. Saccadic eye movements will be slow or irregular, and the patient will be obviously clumsy on tests of dysdiadochokinesia and rapid movements such as finger–thumb tapping, although finger-to-nose testing is normal. Gait will be wide-based and irregular, with difficulty with tandem walking. Reflexes are usually brisk, and a history of falls can be elicited.

## Diagnosis of patients with advanced disease

After 10 years of illness, dementia is more severe, with poor performance on all aspects of the cognitive examination, except naming. Speech is dysfluent, with long lapses between the examiner's question and the patient's reply, rather like Broca's (expressive) aphasia. Some patients will be almost unable to speak, although language comprehension is relatively preserved. Patients (if they are co-operative) can carry out simple commands and will recognize relatives and nursing staff. Patients may be irritable, particularly when their verbal requests cannot be understood or routines altered. Psychiatric syndromes are more difficult to discern, but most can be diagnosed by observing behaviour such as hoarding, sleeplessness, or diurnal variation in mood. Physical disabilities are much worse. Patients often need to be fed, toileted, and helped with most daily needs. They have difficulty walking and may fall, causing further disability through broken limbs or subdural haematomas. Chorea often stabilizes or subsides [13], but the ability to carry out voluntary movements becomes seriously disabling. If they survive long enough, patients become unable to initiate speech or to walk, swallow only with great difficulty, and have such severely rigid muscle tone that they may be nearly unable to move their bodies. Clonus and positive Babinski signs are present. Patients in this sort of 'persistent vegetative state' [20] are difficult to distinguish from individuals in the late stages of other movement disorders or dementias; as in early disease, diagnosis will depend on eliciting a family history or genetic testing.

## Differential diagnosis

The differential diagnosis of HD is extensive [3], but only a few of the disorders for which it can be mistaken are common [2]. These include other dementias, other movement disorders, and other psychiatric disorders. The most common subcortical dementia is *Parkinson's disease* (PD), in which motor slowness resembles that of HD, but the characteristic pill-rolling tremor and festinating gait of PD are rare in HD. The dementia associated with *late-life depression* can look very similar to HD, including motor slowness. *Alzheimer's disease*

is easily distinguished by the lack of motor signs during the first several years of illness and more prominent difficulty with memory and language, as opposed to attention and calculation. Perhaps most difficult to distinguish clinically are the *fronto-temporal dementias*, which present with prominent behavioural disturbances and a positive family history. The clinical presentation may be insufficient to distinguish these various dementias in patients with advanced disease, since they may all progress to a persistent vegetative state. The family history and duration of illness (which is longer for HD than for Alzheimer's disease or fronto-temporal dementia) can be helpful. The C9ORF72 expansion mutation, a common cause of amyotrophic lateral sclerosis and fronto-temporal dementia, can also lead to a HD-like phenotype.

Several *less common diseases classified as movement disorders* may closely resemble HD. They often have an autosomal dominant inheritance pattern, and some, like HD, are caused by expansion of unstable triplet repeat sequences. Examples include Fahr's syndrome (calcification of the striatum), some forms of spinocerebellar degeneration and benign familial chorea, neuroacanthocytosis, HD-like 2 (HDL2), and dentatorubropallidoluysian atrophy (*DRPLA*). These disorders, while much rarer than HD (except for DRPLA in Japan), can so closely resemble HD that they can only be distinguished by genetic testing.

The most common movement disorder that resembles HD is *tardive dyskinesia*. Patients with HD occasionally have several years of a schizophrenia syndrome before the movement disorder begins. If they have been treated with dopamine antagonist medicines, the subsequent onset of involuntary movements can be mistaken for tardive dyskinesia. On the other hand, the choreoathetotic involuntary movements of severe tardive dyskinesia, which may involve the trunk and extremities, as well as the face, may be mistaken for HD. Usually, it is possible to distinguish patients with tardive dyskinesia by their normal saccadic eye movements, normal tandem gait, and fluid and fluent speech [21]. However, genetic testing may be necessary in some cases. Wilson's disease also presents with the subcortical triad and should be considered when neither parent is affected. It is recessively inherited, so that the only affected relatives are siblings. Very late-onset HD may be diagnosed as 'senile chorea' because the family history appears to be negative. Family members will also present with symptoms only late in life and may have died before their manifestation.

The differential diagnosis of nearly all psychiatric disorders includes HD, as described.

## Treatment and management

Currently, there is no treatment that influences the fundamental course of illness of HD, though much work is now directed in that direction (see Future of HD research and treatment, p. 452). However, it is possible to alleviate some of the symptoms of HD through judicious use of pharmacological interventions [22]. Chorea can be diminished with tetrabenazine, low doses of dopamine antagonist medicines (though probably with less effect in advanced disease), and occasionally benzodiazepines, though risks and benefits with all of these treatments must be carefully weighed. The recently available modified versions of tetrabenazine, deutetrabenazine, and valbenazine may prove more convenient to administer or less of a risk for depression than tetrabenazine itself [23]. Given the potential side effects of haloperidol, particularly at doses of more than 5 mg, newer dopamine antagonist medicines are now increasingly recommended for chorea suppression if tetrabenazine or its derivatives are contraindicated or ineffective. Dystonia may be treated with botulinum toxin injections or benzodiazepines, and there is evidence that deep brain stimulation may prove helpful in some cases [24]. Muscle rigidity and consequent contractions occur in late HD, causing pain and difficulty in positioning the patient to avoid pressure sores. Amantadine (which also has a positive effect on mood) can somewhat decrease the rigidity; chairs and beds must be padded and tailored to each patient's specific needs. In the setting of falls or unexpected worsening of movement or cognition, clinicians need to consider the possibility of a subdural haematoma.

Psychiatric manifestations are present to some extent in a vast majority of HD patients and may become severe in more than one-third. Appropriate pharmacological and non-pharmacological treatment has the potential to significantly improve the quality of life for HD patients and their families, and may help decrease the high rate of suicide observed in HD. Clinical experience suggests that depression, anxiety, and obsessive–compulsive disorder associated with HD usually respond to pharmacological treatments used for the similar idiopathic disorders, though there have been few systematic treatment trials of psychiatric syndromes in HD [25]. Because some patients are unaware of their depressed mood (just as they can be unaware of their involuntary movements), an informant is often needed to elicit the symptoms and monitor response to treatment. It is also important to distinguish depression (from which the patient is miserable and sleepless) and apathy, which does not cause distress. Occasionally, mood and anxiety disorders are chronic and unresponsive to treatment. Severe, unresponsive depression can be treated successfully with electroconvulsive therapy [26]. Bipolar disorder in patients with HD may not respond to lithium but may improve with carbamazepine or valproic acid. In addition, lithium is difficult to administer because of the risk of lithium toxicity related to insufficient fluid intake. Valproic acid, serotonin-specific reuptake inhibitors, and low-dose dopamine antagonist agents may also be helpful in the treatment of irritability. In one case report, high doses of sertraline were effective for intractable aggression [27]. Schizophrenic-like syndromes, while not particularly common, can be difficult to treat but may respond to a standard dopamine antagonist medicine, with a preference towards newer agents with less $D_2$ receptor affinity. Clozapine remains an option in patients not responding to other drugs. Apathy, when not part of a depression syndrome, does not respond well to pharmacological interventions.

As with most dementias, psychopathology influences, and is influenced by, the patient's environment. Patients do best in a calm, highly predictable environment where cognitive expectations are not too complicated. When the environment is too taxing, patients become irritable, especially towards their family. HD seriously damages family relationships, which, in turn, affects the patient. The well spouse becomes responsible for supporting the family, caring for the children and the patient, and making family and financial decisions. Spouses' lives are further complicated by patients' unwillingness to relinquish financial and family decision-making; patients usually make poor decisions that can damage family relationships and finances. Some patients neglect their children or treat them badly. If the other parent cannot prevent this, it is wisest to remove the patient from the home. There is no research on the treatment of sexual aggression, which occasionally occurs in males, but a few men have been successfully treated with depot anti-androgen agents. Supportive psychotherapy for the patient should focus on minimizing demoralization at lost abilities. Spouses can be helped with reorganizing family life to maximize predictability of the patient's environment, diplomatically decreasing the patient's domestic responsibilities, and assuring that the spouse has time away from the patient.

## Helping persons at risk for HD

People at risk for HD vary in their abilities to deal with the burden of uncertainty, depending on their personal attributes and their experience with the illness in a relative. A few consult physicians for reassurance, but most avoid doctors until they become ill, and even then many resist medical attention, claiming against all evidence that they are perfectly well. Currently, a minority of asymptomatic persons at risk for HD decide to have genetic testing, but these individuals, skewed towards those whose anxiety is lessened by planning for the future, have usually handled the test results well, regardless of whether positive or negative [28]. As more clinical trials are launched for individuals with the HD mutation who are without detectable symptoms, the incentive for pre-symptomatic testing will likely increase, with a concomitant change in the nature of individuals seeking testing. Fetal and pre-implantation genetic testing is now available in some centres, each with its own set of potentially complicated ethical and practical issues that must be sorted out prior to testing.

Pre-symptomatic genetic testing [29] of any sort should always be preceded by genetic counselling, provided either by a genetic counsellor or by a clinician familiar with HD genetics and the potential practical and psychological consequences of both positive and negative test results. Counselling should include a discussion of the motivations for seeking testing, which may include decisions about childbearing, education, employment, finances, participation in clinical trials, or the potential at-risk status of offspring. Many individuals who come for testing have not seriously considered the possibility that they will test positive for the mutation, so that role-playing about various outcome scenarios is important. Occasionally, persons request testing who have learnt only recently that they are at risk for HD. Others apply who are depressed or under unusual stress for other reasons. Such persons should be encouraged to delay testing until their situation becomes more settled. Finally, some people who request testing already have symptoms of HD, yet do not wish to have a diagnosis. Considerable care is required to decide how best to support such individuals, and family members or close friends of the person should be consulted.

## Future of HD research and treatment

While efforts to explore the course of HD and to improve symptomatic HD treatment continue, the focus of HD research is moving towards finding treatments that can stop, slow, or prevent the development and progression of the neuronal dysfunction and neurodegeneration that underlie the disease. New tools for modelling HD, including a variety of animal models and induced pluripotent stem cells, should facilitate preclinical work [30]. HD investigators are also attempting to develop increasingly sensitive biomarkers, measurable correlates of disease progression that can facilitate the detection of efficacious therapies in individuals who do not have clinically manifest HD and that can lead to clinical study designs that require fewer subjects and a shorter duration of treatment [31, 32]. Recent studies have demonstrated that some agents thought to be of general neuroprotective value, such as co-enzyme Q10, likely lack significant clinical efficacy in HD [33], while other protective agents still under investigation, such as PBT2, may have benefit [34]. Attention and funding have increasingly emphasized the development of methods for suppressing the expression of the mutant HD allele [35], with antisense oligonucleotide strategies just reaching the stage of clinical trials. The potential power of such therapeutic approaches, or even more sophisticated methods such as gene editing to remove the mutation from the genome, has generated considerable optimism among HD investigators and HD families.

## REFERENCES

1. Huntington, G. (1872). On chorea. Reprinted in *Advances in Neurology*, **1**, 33–5 (1973).
2. Walker, R.H. (ed) (2011). *The differential Diagnosis of Chorea*. Oxford University Press, Oxford.
3. Bates, G., Harper, P.S., Jones, L. (2002). *Huntington's disease*. Oxford University Press, Oxford.
4. Hedreen, J.C., Folstein, S.E. (1995). Early loss of neostriatal striosome neurons in Huntington's disease. *Journal of Neuropathology and Experimental Neurology*, **54**, 105–20.
5. Aylward E.H., Codori, A.M., Rosenblatt, A., *et al.* (2000). Rate of caudate atrophy in presymptomatic and symptomatic stages of Huntington's disease. *Movement Disorders*, **15**, 552–60.
6. Nopoulos, P.C., Aylward, E.H., Ross, C.A., *et al.*; PREDICT-HD Investigators and Coordinators of the Huntington Study Group (HSG) (2010). Cerebral cortex structure in prodromal Huntington disease. *Neurobiology of Disease*. **40**, 544–54.
7. Paulsen, J.S., Magnotta, V.A., Mikos, A.E., *et al.* (2006). Brain structure in preclinical Huntington's disease. *Biological Psychiatry*, **59**, 57–63.
8. Matsui J.T., Vaidya, J.G., Wassermann, D., *et al.*; PREDICT-HD Investigators and Coordinators of the Huntington Study Group. (2015). Prefrontal cortex white matter tracts in prodromal Huntington disease. *Human Brain Mapping*, **36**, 3717–32.
9. Baig, S.S., Strong, M., Quarrell, O.W. (2016). The global prevalence of Huntington's disease: a systematic review and discussion. *Neurodegenerative Disease Management*, **6**, 331–43.
10. Huntington's Disease Collaborative Research Group. (1993). A novel gene containing a trinucleotide repeat that is expanded and unstable on Huntington's disease chromosomes. *Cell*, **72**, 971–83.
11. Ranen, N.G., Stine, O.C., Abbott, M.H., *et al.* (1995). Anticipation and instability of (CAG)*n* repeats in IT-15 in parent–offspring pairs with Huntington's disease. *American Journal of Human Genetics*, **57**, 593–602.
12. Bates, G.P., Dorsey, R., Gusella, J.F., *et al.* (2015). Huntington disease. *Nature Reviews Disease Primers*, **1**,15005
13. Dorsey, E.R., Beck, C.A., Darwin, K., *et al.*; Huntington Study Group COHORT Investigators. (2013). Natural history of Huntington disease. JAMA Neurology. **70**,1520–30.
14. Folstein, S.E., Abbott, M.H., Franz, M.L., Huang, S., Chase, G.A., Folstein, M.F. (1983). The association of affective disorder with

15. Lasker A., Zee D.S. (1994). Ocular Motor Abnormalities in Huntington's Disease. *Vision Research*, **34**, 3639–45.
16. Quarrell, O.W., Nance, M.A., Nopoulos, P., *et al.* (2013). Managing juvenile Huntington's disease. *Neurodegenerative Disease Management*. 2013;**3**(3).
17. Nance, M. (1997). Genetic testing of children at risk for Huntington's disease. *Neurology*, **49**, 1048–53.
18. Federoff, J.O., Peyser, C.E., Franz, M.L., Folstein, S.E. (1994). Sexual disorders in Huntington's disease. *Journal of Neuropsychiatry and Clinical Neuroscience*, **6**, 147–53.
19. Folstein, M.F., Folstein, S.E., McHugh, P.R. (1975). 'Mini-Mental State': a practical method for grading the cognitive state of patients for the clinician. *Journal of Psychiatric Research*, **2**, 189–98.
20. Walshe, T.M., Leonard, C. (1985). Persistent vegetative state: extension of the syndrome to include chronic disorders. *Archives of Neurology*, **42**, 1045–7.
21. David, A.S., Jeste, D.V., Folstein, M.F., Folstein, S.E. (1987). Voluntary movement dysfunction in Huntington's disease and tardive dyskinesia. *Acta Neurologica Scandinavica*, **75**, 130–9.
22. Venuto, C.S., McGarry, A., Ma, Q., Kieburtz, K. (2012). Pharmacologic approaches to the treatment of Huntington's disease. *Movement Disorders*, **27**, 31–41.
23. Huntington Study Group. (2016). Effect of Deutetrabenazine on Chorea Among Patients With Huntington Disease: A Randomized Clinical Trial. *JAMA*, **316**, 40–50.
24. Sharma, M, Deogaonkar, M. (2015). Deep brain stimulation in Huntington's disease: assessment of potential targets. *Journal of Clinical Neuroscience*, **22**, 812–17.
25. Anderson, K.E., Marder, K.S. (2001). An overview of psychiatric symptoms in Huntington's disease. *Current Psychiatry Reports*. **3**, 379–88.
26. Cusin, C., Franco, F.B., Fernandez-Robles, C., DuBois, C.M., Welch, C.A. (2013). Rapid improvement of depression and psychotic symptoms in Huntington's disease: a retrospective chart review of seven patients treated with electroconvulsive therapy. *Journal of General Hospital Psychiatry*, **35**, 678e3-5.
27. Ranen, N.G., Lipsey, J.R., Treisman, G., Ross, C.A. (1996). Sertraline in the treatment of severe aggressiveness in Huntington's disease. *Journal of Neuropsychiatry and Clinical Neuroscience*, **8**, 338–40.
28. Baig, S.S., Strong, M., Rosser, E., *et al.*; UK Huntington's Disease Prediction Consortium, Quarrell, O.W. (2016). 22 Years of predictive testing for Huntington's disease: the experience of the UK Huntington's Prediction Consortium. *European Journal of Human Genetics*, **24**, 1396–402.
29. Nance, M.A. (2017). Genetic counseling and testing for Huntington's disease: A historical review. *American Journal of Medical Genetics Part B: Neuropsychiatric Genetics*, **174**, 75–92.
30. HD iPSC Consortium. (2012). Induced pluripotent stem cells from patients with Huntington's disease show CAG-repeat-expansion-associated phenotypes. *Cell Stem Cell*, **11**, 264–78.
31. Paulsen, J.S., Long, J.D, Johnson, H.J., *et al.*; PREDICT-HD Investigators and Coordinators of the Huntington Study Group. (2014). Clinical and Biomarker Changes in Premanifest Huntington Disease Show Trial Feasibility: A Decade of the PREDICT-HD Study. *Frontiers in Aging Neuroscience*, **6**, 78.
32. Ross, C.A., Aylward, E.H., Wild, E.J., *et al.* (2014). Huntington disease: natural history, biomarkers and prospects for therapeutics. *Nature Reviews Neurology*, **10**, 204–16.

33. McGarry, A., McDermot, M., Kieburtz, K., *et al.* (2017). A Randomized, Double-Blind, Placebo-Controlled Trial of Coenzyme Q10 in Huntington's Disease. *Neurology*, **88**, 152–9.

34. Huntington Study Group Reach2HD Investigators, (2015). Safety, tolerability, and efficacy of PBT2 in Huntington's disease: a phase 2, randomised, double-blind, placebo-controlled trial. *The Lancet Neurology*. **14**, 39–47.

35. Aronin, N., DiFiglia, M. (2014). Huntingtin-lowering strategies in Huntington's disease: antisense oligonucleotides, small RNAs, and gene editing. *Movement Disorders*, **29**, 1455–61.

# 46

# Vascular cognitive impairment

*Joanne A. Byars and Ricardo E. Jorge*

## Introduction

Vascular cognitive impairment (VCI), known as vascular dementia (VasD) in its more severe form, is cognitive impairment due to pathology of blood vessels in the brain. This pathology encompasses both ischaemic and haemorrhagic disease; however, most literature focuses on ischaemic disease, as this is the far more prevalent form.

Various sets of diagnostic criteria for VCI and VasD exist, but all share some factors in common—the patient must have evidence of cognitive impairment, evidence of cerebrovascular disease, and evidence of an association between the two [1]. The *Diagnostic and Statistical Manual of Mental Disorders*, fifth edition (DSM-5) outlines criteria for major and mild vascular neurocognitive disorder, the term DSM-5 uses for VCI [2] (Box 46.1).

Aggressive modification of vascular risk factors has a greater potential to modify the course of VCI than the progression of neurodegenerative disorders such as Alzheimer's disease (AD). This makes an early and accurate diagnosis of VCI critically important.

## Epidemiology

VasD is the second leading cause of dementia in the United States, affecting 1.2–4.2% of people over the age of 65 years and representing 15–20% of dementia cases. The prevalence of VasD increases with age [1]. It is unclear whether the prevalence of VasD differs by sex [1]. Currently, there are no reliable statistics on the prevalence of VCI not rising to the level of dementia.

Encouragingly, the rate of VasD appears to be falling. Recent data from the Framingham Heart Study found that the overall incidence of dementia has declined over the past 40 years, falling by 20% every 10 years [3]. The rate of VasD has fallen faster than that of AD [3]. The risk of developing dementia after a stroke has also decreased, from nine times higher to less than twice higher than that in individuals without a stroke [3]. While some evidence suggests that improved control of vascular risk factors may have contributed to the decline in dementia, this does not account for all the reduction seen [3].

Individuals with stroke are at higher risk for VCI than the general population. Following a stroke, 6–32% of patients develop dementia of some type [4]. Even small strokes substantially increase the risk of cognitive impairment. One study of patients with lacunar ischaemic CVA, without large-vessel strokes, found that 47% had mild cognitive impairment (MCI), making MCI more common than physical disability [5].

## Subtypes of VCI

Most classifications divide VCI into three subtypes: multi-infarct VCI, strategic infarct VCI, and small-vessel VCI [4]. Some authors refer to small-vessel VCI as subcortical VCI or Binswanger disease [4].

Patients with multi-infarct VCI may show the classic 'stepwise decline' pattern, in which each stroke adds a new cognitive burden, with periods of relative cognitive stability in between strokes. However, the other forms of VCI typically follow a different course.

In strategic infarct VCI, a single stroke affects a region critical for cognitive functioning and produces VCI after the single event. Classic strategic infarct locations include the thalamus, mesial frontal lobe, caudate, mesial temporal lobe, left angular gyrus, and genu of the left internal capsule [1]. However, strokes in other locations can also produce strategic infarct VCI, and due to individual variations in brain anatomy and connectivity, clinical findings may not always correlate with classic syndromes.

Notably, patients can show progressive cognitive decline following a single stroke; this may be due to disruption of brain networks resulting in ongoing worsening, though this hypothesis still lacks definitive proof [4]. In any case, this finding indicates a complex relationship between stroke and cognitive decline, which goes beyond the impact of neuronal demise resulting from stroke. However, reducing rates of stroke likely constitutes a very effective way to reduce rates of VasD.

In small-vessel VCI, patients typically show gradually progressive cognitive decline. They may never experience a 'clinical' stroke that produces an obvious and immediate change in neurologic function. However, physical examination may reveal abnormal neurologic findings such as hyperreflexia, Parkinsonism, and gait disturbance [6]. Small-vessel VCI can occur due to lacunar strokes or ischaemic demyelination [7].

As individuals with cerebrovascular disease commonly have involvement of both small and large vessels, patients can have

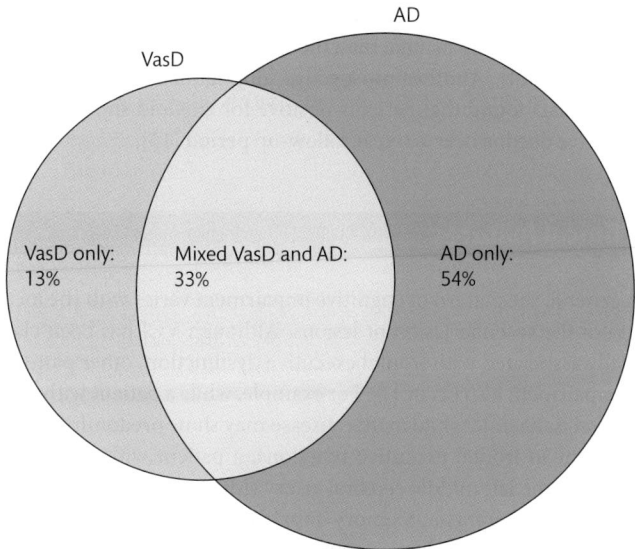

**Fig. 46.1** Overlap between VasD and AD.

combinations of multi-infarct, strategic infarct, and small-vessel VCI. One study found that lacunar infarcts represent the most common type of stroke seen in VasD [8].

Some studies have found that 70% of individuals with VasD also have comorbid AD-type pathology, a condition referred to as mixed dementia [9]. Most VCI is sporadic, but familial forms, such as VCI due to cerebral autosomal dominant arteriopathy with subcortical infarcts and leukoencephalopathy (CADASIL), also exist [4].

## Overlap between VCI and Alzheimer's disease

Although VCI can occur in isolation, cerebrovascular disease and AD can co-occur and synergistically worsen each other.

One large community-based study found that, among individuals with either VasD, AD, or both, 13% had only VasD, 54% had only AD, and 33% had both [9] (Fig. 46.1). Notably, 83% of these patients with VasD and/or mixed VasD-AD had no clinical history of stroke and likely would have received an incorrect diagnosis if MRI had not been performed, underscoring the critical importance of neuroimaging for the correct determination of the dementia type [9].

In post-mortem studies, many individuals with dementia show a mix of cerebrovascular and AD neuropathology. Amyloid plaques, neurofibrillary tangles, cerebral amyloid angiopathy (CAA), and white matter lesions are found in both disorders [8]. About 10% of individuals with pure VasD show evidence of CAA, and CAA could contribute to further damage of blood vessels and progression of cerebrovascular disease, large intracerebral hemorrhages, and microbleeds [1, 8]. In AD, amyloid-β builds up around blood vessels in the brain, causing impairment of vascular functioning [1].

Almost 30% of individuals with VasD have hippocampal sclerosis, possibly related to hippocampal neurons being especially vulnerable to ischaemia [8]. Both vascular disease and AD-type pathology are associated with hippocampal atrophy [1].

Recent imaging advances—namely, the development of Pittsburgh compound B (PIB), a radiotracer used with PET—allow for the non-invasive assessment of amyloid-β burden. This technique permits a more accurate classification of pure VasD (VasD without evidence of amyloid-β burden) vs mixed VasD-AD (VasD with excessive amyloid-β burden) and has led to new insights into how these two subcategories of VasD resemble and diverge from each other.

Some studies have observed different patterns of MRI findings in individuals with VasD with and without concomitant amyloid-β burden. For instance, among patients with small-vessel VasD, those who are amyloid-positive may have smaller hippocampal volumes and those who are amyloid-negative may have more lacunar infarcts [10, 11]. One study found that individuals with small-vessel VasD, without evidence of amyloid burden, showed damage to the white matter throughout the entire cerebrum, as opposed to the regional pattern seen in AD without vascular disease [12].

Vascular risk factors not only increase the risk of VasD, but also the risk of AD. Hypertension, diabetes mellitus (DM), metabolic syndrome, coronary artery disease (CAD), smoking, atrial fibrillation, atherosclerosis, and obesity are all associated with an increased risk for AD, and having a stroke may double the risk for AD [4].

Vascular disease also worsens the severity of neurodegenerative dementia. One neuropathologic study found that, among individuals with AD or Parkinsonian neurodegenerative diseases, those who also had cerebrovascular disease required less primary neurodegenerative pathology (neurofibrillary tangles or Lewy bodies) to reach the same severity of clinical dementia as individuals with neurodegeneration only [13]. As cerebrovascular disease is common in individuals with neurodegenerative dementia, these findings suggest that tight control of vascular risk factors could potentially help in these conditions as well [13].

Conversely, neurodegenerative pathology can worsen VCI. One cross-sectional study of MCI due to subcortical vascular disease found that individuals with excessive amyloid-β burden showed more cognitive impairment than those with only ischaemic vascular pathology [14]. Another prospective longitudinal study of small-vessel VasD found that patients positive for amyloid showed faster cognitive decline over a 3-year follow-up period [15].

## Clinical features

In general, the pattern of cognitive impairment varies with the location of the vascular lesion or lesions. Although VCI has been classically associated with frontal executive dysfunction, other patterns of impairment also occur [1]. For example, while a patient with subcortical ischaemic white matter disease may show predominant impairment in frontal executive functions, a patient with a strategic infarct in the left middle cerebral artery (MCA) territory may show aphasia and/or apraxia. Memory impairment in VCI may occur due to stroke affecting the hippocampus or to the concomitant presence of AD-type pathology. Although lacunar strokes are often associated with impairments in frontal executive functions, one study found that episodic memory impairment was just as common in this stroke type [5].

Depending on the location of their strokes, individuals with VCI can also show deficits in elementary neurologic function such as hemiparesis, visual field cuts, urinary incontinence, and gait disturbance. They may also show other neurologic signs such as hyperreflexia and Parkinsonism.

Individuals with VCI also frequently experience neuropsychiatric symptoms. Up to 95% of patients with VCI may have at least one psychiatric or behaviour symptom [16]. Depression and apathy represent the most common symptoms, with depression present in 50–75% and apathy in one-third to two-thirds of individuals with VCI [16–18]. Apathy becomes more common with increasing severity of cognitive impairment [16, 17, 19]. Irritability, anxiety, and agitation each occur in about half of patients, disinhibition in about 10–30%, and psychotic symptoms in 20–30% [16, 17].

Individuals with VasD show poorer sleep than those with AD, and one cross-sectional study of subcortical VasD found that patients with more white matter hyperintensities (WMHs) experienced worse sleep [20].

## Diagnosis

The diagnosis of VCI is based on history, neurological examination, cognitive testing, and neuroimaging. Neuroimaging can reveal evidence of cerebrovascular disease and 'asymptomatic' ischaemic or haemorrhagic damage, even in the absence of a clinical history of stroke.

Clinicians should be aware that patients who have never had a clinical stroke can still have VCI, as some forms of VCI (such as small-vessel VCI) do not necessarily cause any obvious abrupt neurologic changes.

### Neuroimaging

In recognition of the variety of international practice settings, most criteria sets require *either* clinical (clinical history of stroke and/or findings of focal neurological deficits consistent with stroke on neurological examination) *or* radiologic evidence of cerebrovascular disease.

However, in a country with ready availability of neuroimaging, clinicians should certainly obtain it to confirm evidence of cerebrovascular disease. Even if the history and examination are compatible with stroke, other aetiologies such as a tumour could, in some circumstances, produce a similar clinical picture but need drastically different treatment. Additionally, imaging distinguishes between ischaemic and haemorrhagic stroke—an important determination to make, as their secondary prevention strategies may differ significantly.

To diagnose VCI, MRI is preferable to CT, unless there is a contraindication, given its greater sensitivity. Specialized MRI sequences, such as susceptibility-weighted imaging (SWI) and gradient echo (GRE) sequences, detect the presence of blood with high sensitivity and specificity, including microbleeds related to amyloid angiopathy [21]. By evaluating the integrity of white matter tracts, diffusion tensor imaging (DTI) can identify white matter damage not seen on conventional MRI sequences such as T2 and fluid-attenuated inversion recovery (FLAIR) [12].

Common imaging findings in VCI include evidence of large-vessel ischaemic stroke(s), lacunar ischaemic stroke(s), extensive WMHs, white matter atrophy, and/or large or small haemorrhages. Microhaemorrhages are very common in ischaemic VasD—occurring in two-thirds to four-fifths of patients, a higher percentage than in other dementias such as AD [21]. Of note, individuals without VCI, cognitive impairment, cerebrovascular disease, or other structural brain disease can also show WMHs, for instance, patients with migraine or some individuals with healthy ageing [7]. When long tract signs, such as weakness or hyperreflexia, accompany WMHs, the WMHs more likely reflect genuine pathology [7]. However, there is no clear cut-off for the size or amount of vascular lesions required to cause VCI, as substantial inter-individual variability exists.

Dementia or cognitive impairment—of any type—cannot be diagnosed solely on an imaging basis. Some individuals have more cognitive reserve than others, so two people with the same imaging findings could have very different levels of cognitive functioning.

### Cognitive evaluation

Cognitive evaluation should encompass both a thorough clinical history of cognitive and functional changes, and cognitive testing [20]. To diagnose VCI, there should be evidence that the patient has experienced a cognitive decline relative to his or her baseline functioning.

The clinical history provides key information about the patient's prior functional level, the time course and nature of the cognitive changes, associated symptoms, and performance of activities of daily living and instrumental activities of daily living [22]. The clinical history does have limitations, however. The patient and/or other informants may dismiss worrisome events—such as getting lost while driving in a familiar area—as normal ageing, even though they are not. Sometimes, a similarly aged family member, such as a spouse, may also have cognitive impairment and thus not accurately perceive or remember the patient's recent functioning.

In addition to a thorough history, appropriate cognitive testing—taking into account the patient's age and educational, occupational, and cultural background—is essential for diagnosing VCI. However, the test results must be interpreted in light of the overall clinical context, as no test is 100% sensitive or specific for cognitive impairment.

No cognitive test is entirely free of cultural and socio-economic bias. Typical cognitive batteries fail to capture important domains of cognition—such as social cognition, artistic creativity, and mechanical ability—and the clinical history may be more useful in uncovering decline in these areas. Patients functioning at a high occupational level may experience a decline in job performance as an early symptom of VCI; while this decline may have significant real-world importance, insufficiently challenging or occupationally specific cognitive tests may not detect any problems. For example, if a theoretical physicist comes to clinic complaining of recent difficulty solving problems in her field, very few physicians or neuropsychologists could determine if this was objectively true through office-based testing! Consultation with a professional colleague of the patient—with the patient's consent—may help establish whether there is an actual decline in functioning, even when cognitive test scores are in the normal range.

Some patients' premorbid functioning may have been higher or lower than predicted by standard test norms or by estimates of premorbid intellectual functioning, and thus isolated test results may mislead as to whether a decline from baseline has occurred. For instance, a patient may have limited formal education due to socio-economic circumstances but be self-taught, well read, and functioning at a high intellectual level prior to his or her current problems. Conversely, due to variation in educational quality, some individuals may have graduated from high school without achieving functional literacy. Additionally, no tests to estimate premorbid intellectual functioning have complete immunity to decline from the effects of an acquired cognitive disorder; the data do not support the idea that some areas of cognitive functioning are 'crystallized' and do not decline in dementia.

However, in most cases, the results of appropriately interpreted norm-based cognitive testing significantly help in clarifying the presence, severity, and nature of cognitive impairment.

Given the heterogeneity of cognitive deficits in VCI, testing should assess both overall cognitive function—using a test of general cognitive function such as the Folstein Mini-Mental Status Exam (MMSE) or the Montreal Cognitive Assessment (MoCA)—as well as multiple specific cognitive domains, including tests of frontal executive function, memory, attention and concentration, orientation, visuo-spatial function, and language, and assessment for neglect.

All tests have strengths and weaknesses. The MMSE depends heavily on the assessment of orientation, memory, and language and show less sensitivity for detecting impairment in patients whose primary problems may involve other domains; clinicians should supplement these tests with other instruments which better assess other cognitive functions. The MoCA may assess a broader variety of domains than the MMSE but may misclassify cognitively normal individuals with low educational attainment as having dementia.

One useful approach is to assess overall cognitive functioning with a general test such as the MMSE or the MoCA, and then use tests of specific domains to interrogate further into areas of possible impairment. Box 46.2 lists several brief domain-specific assessments useful for administration at the bedside or in the clinic

---

**Box 46.2** Tests of cognition for bedside and clinic

ATTENTION/CONCENTRATION
- Digit span forward and backward
- Months backward

FRONTAL EXECUTIVE FUNCTIONS
- Frontal assessment battery
- Antisaccades

LANGUAGE
- Bedside Western Aphasia Battery-Revised
- Boston Naming Test

MEMORY
- Hopkins Verbal Learning Test

NEGLECT
- Line bisection
- Target cancellation

VISUO-SPATIAL FUNCTION
- Clock-drawing test
- Navon figures

---

## Differential diagnosis

The differential diagnosis for VCI includes neurodegenerative dementias such as AD and fronto-temporal dementia; multiple sclerosis and other autoimmune neurologic conditions; chronic infections such as HIV or neurosyphilis; vitamin deficiencies; endocrinopathies; leukodystrophies; and toxic exposures such as medications which impair cognition, alcohol, opioids, heavy metals, and volatile substances. Of note, some of these disorders can cause white matter changes which may be difficult to distinguish from those of VCI without further investigation such as cerebrospinal fluid (CSF) analysis or enzyme testing.

When evaluating a patient for a cognitive disorder—whether suspected VCI or another condition—the most important task is to rule out potentially reversible or modifiable causes. If a patient with AD receives a misdiagnosis of VCI, that patient will not miss out on a disease-modifying treatment, as none currently exists for AD. However, if a patient with multiple sclerosis, severe B12 deficiency, or neurosyphilis is misdiagnosed with VCI, this could result in a lost opportunity to halt or reverse the progression of these treatable diseases.

Serum laboratory testing for reversible causes of cognitive impairment should include assessment of B12, thyroid function tests, complete blood count (CBC), comprehensive metabolic panel (CMP), ammonia, vitamin D, folate, thiamine, HIV, treponemal syphilis testing, erythrocyte sedimentation rate (ESR), and antinuclear antibody (ANA) [22, 23]. Depending on clinical circumstances (for example, a history of gastric bypass or other condition affecting nutrient absorption, or an occupational history of heavy metal exposure), additional testing may be needed to fully evaluate for potentially reversible causes.

Unfortunately, many older individuals use medications known to impair cognition and increase risk for dementia, such as anticholinergic medications (for example, allergy medications, over-the-counter sleeping aids, antispasmodic bladder medications, and certain drugs for depression, anxiety, and psychosis) and benzodiazepines. Alcohol and recreational drugs can also cause cognitive impairment. Fortunately, the cognitive harm done by these exogenous factors is at least potentially reversible. Before diagnosing a cognitive disorder, clinicians should make all efforts to eliminate the use of these agents and then reassess cognition and functioning. Even if the patient does have VCI, these substances will likely worsen impairment and should be eliminated in any case.

Individuals with a history of stroke or ischaemic white matter disease show increased rates of depression, which can contribute to functional impairment and may resemble a neurocognitive disorder but which is reversible with appropriate treatment [1]. Clinicians assessing a patient for cognitive impairment should always evaluate for depression and treat it whenever present, regardless of whether or not it caused the cognitive problems—comorbid untreated depression can substantially worsen cognitive function. In addition to causing emotional suffering, post-stroke depression is associated with increased mortality, more disability, slower neurologic recovery, an increased risk of suicide, and worse quality of life [24]. The cognitive deficits most consistently associated with depression are impairment of attention/concentration, frontal executive function, working memory, and processing speed; depression would be very unlikely to cause other deficits such as aphasia or neglect [25].

Sometimes, it may not be possible to determine whether cerebrovascular disease or another condition such as AD is the primary determinant of cognitive impairment. However, in either case, uncontrolled vascular risk factors can cause worsening of functioning and cognition, so vascular risk factor modification should be undertaken regardless. Any patient with cerebrovascular disease needs vascular risk factor modification, regardless of cognitive status or type of cognitive disorder.

## Mechanisms of VCI

Although strokes can produce cognitive impairment by direct damage to brain regions involved in cognition, additional mechanisms likely can also give rise to VCI.

Small-vessel VCI may disrupt the neurovascular unit, that is, the vascular endothelium, perivascular cells, glia, and neurons, which work together and influence each other to maintain cerebral homeostasis—via inflammation and damage to the blood–brain barrier, as shown in Fig. 46.2 [1, 7]. Injury to the neurovascular unit may play key role in the progression of white matter injury in small-vessel VCI and occurs more frequently in VCI than when white matter changes occur in the context of AD [6]. Neuropathologic findings in small-vessel VCI include abnormalities in and around small vessels, including endothelial dysfunction, vessel fibrosis, and inflammation [6]. These changes may cause cerebrovascular resistance and decreased cerebral blood flow, thereby potentially contributing to hypoperfusion and further vascular damage [4].The CSF of individuals with small-vessel VCI shows elevations in albumin and matrix metalloproteinases, consistent with inflammation and blood–brain barrier disruption; specialized MRI also reveals evidence of damage to the blood–brain barrier [6, 26]. Damage to the neurovascular unit may impair perfusion during cognitive activities and thus further exacerbate neuronal dysfunction in vascular cognitive impairment [4].

In addition to the classic findings of ischaemia or haemorrhage, VCI may cause other brain changes which could adversely affect cognition. VCI may cause changes in the corpus callosum, such as decreased white matter integrity and perhaps decreased size, potentially affecting interhemispheric transmission of information [27]. One study also found decreased white matter integrity in the corpus callosum in VasD [27]. One study found that strategic-infarct VCI from isolated left thalamic stroke was associated with decreased cerebral blood flow in both hemispheres, suggesting that even a single small stroke can have far-reaching consequences, perhaps by disrupting broader networks involved in cognition [28].

A cross-sectional study found that individuals with 'asymptomatic' subcortical lacunar infarcts showed more cortical and subcortical atrophy and more cognitive impairment than healthy controls [29].

Though classically associated with AD, cholinergic deficits may occur in VCI as well [1]. Neuropathologic case-control studies found impairment of cholinergic pathways in small-vessel VasD and CADASIL [30]. However, another neuropathologic case-control study found that individuals with 'pure' VasD, without any evidence of AD-type pathology, did not show evidence of temporal lobe cholinergic deficits, as compared to healthy controls; on the other hand, individuals with mixed VasD-AD did show cholinergic deficits comparable to those seen in 'pure' AD [31].

## Outcomes and consequences of VCI

There is contradictory evidence on whether VasD progresses faster or more slowly than AD. Some studies have found that individuals with VasD survive for a mean of 5–6 years following diagnosis, a slightly shorter survival than in AD; however, these studies are over 20 years old and may not reflect changes in diagnosis (that is, increased detection sensitivity with more widespread use of MRI) and advances in vascular risk factor control, which could potentially improve survival in the current era [32]. One large cohort study of memory clinic patients seen found that individuals with VasD show slower progression of functional decline than those with AD [33]. However, only 2% of study participants had VasD, a far lower number than their proportion among dementia cases in the general population, raising questions about the generalizability of this finding.

VasD increases the risk of subsequent stroke and adversely affects stroke recovery. Individuals with VasD, but no prior history of clinical stroke or transient ischaemic attack (TIA), show a 2-fold higher risk for subsequent ischaemic stroke and TIA and a 4-fold higher risk for subsequent haemorrhagic stroke [34]. One study of patients hospitalized for acute stroke found that those with VasD have less functional recovery at 1 year follow-up than those with normal cognition; however, VCI not rising to the level of dementia did not worsen functional outcomes [35].

Individuals with VasD also show higher rates of other vascular diseases—namely, atherosclerosis, heart failure, and atrial fibrillation—as well as higher rates of non-vascular comorbidities such as sepsis, injuries, lung diseases including chronic obstructive pulmonary disease, and urinary diseases [36].

VasD increases the risk for delirium, which can worsen dementia outcomes [37]. One study of memory clinic outpatients found that one-third of patients with VasD had superimposed

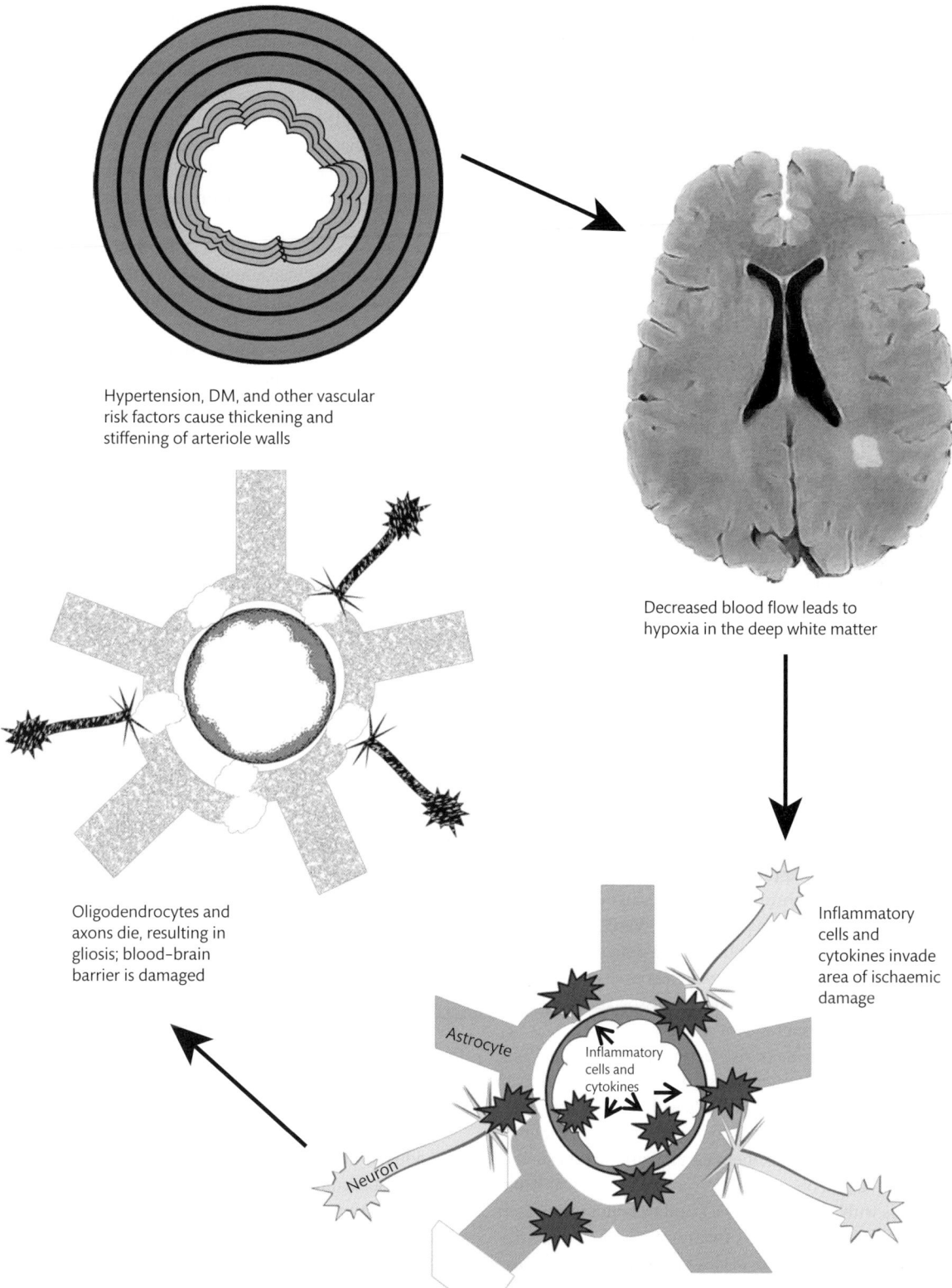

Hypertension, DM, and other vascular risk factors cause thickening and stiffening of arteriole walls

Decreased blood flow leads to hypoxia in the deep white matter

Oligodendrocytes and axons die, resulting in gliosis; blood–brain barrier is damaged

Inflammatory cells and cytokines invade area of ischaemic damage

Astrocyte

Inflammatory cells and cytokines

Neuron

**Fig. 46.2** Schematic diagram of the pathophysiology of small-vessel VCI.

delirium at the time of their clinic visit [37]. Among individuals with neurodegenerative dementias such as AD, those with imaging evidence of comorbid cerebrovascular disease had higher rates of delirium than those without cerebrovascular disease [37]. Clinicians

treating patients with VasD should carefully monitor for delirium and educate family members and other caregivers about the symptoms and significance of delirium, so that they can seek treatment promptly if it occurs.

## Risk factors

### Stroke

Stroke, whether clinically apparent or silent, whether haemorrhagic or ischaemic, is a major risk factor for VCI. Having a clinical stroke doubles the risk for dementia [1]. Among people with stroke, 7% develop new-onset dementia within the first year after the stroke and nearly 50% develop dementia over the next 2 years [1]. Forty per cent of patients with first ever ischaemic or haemorrhagic stroke, who do not have severe aphasia, have VCI at 3-months' follow-up [38].

Individuals with silent ischaemic strokes, WMHs, and/or 'asymptomatic' cerebral microbleeds also show an increased risk for subsequently developing cognitive impairment [1, 8]. Among patients with MCI, those with more WMHs are more likely to convert to VasD [39].

All else being equal, patients with more brain territory affected by infarcts are more likely to have cognitive impairment than those with less affected territory. However, since other factors, such as stroke location, vary significantly between patients, overall there is no clear relationship between the number/volume of strokes and cognitive impairment [1]. For instance, even a small lacunar infarct in the thalamus could produce major cognitive consequences, while a larger infarct in the deep white matter could go largely unnoticed.

### Other vascular risk factors

In addition to stroke itself, vascular risk factors associated with stroke also increase the risk for VCI. Even in the absence of stroke or dementia, individuals with more vascular risk factors show worse cognitive performance [4].

One large population-based prospective study of factors important for good vascular health—not smoking, maintaining a healthy body weight, engaging in regular physical activity, eating a healthy diet, and having blood pressure, cholesterol, and fasting glucose at goal—found that the more of these factors an individual had, the lower his or her risk for subsequent stroke, VasD, or cognitive decline [40]. Importantly, all of these factors are potentially modifiable, suggesting a strategy for preventing dementia.

Multiple longitudinal studies support an association between mid-life hypertension and subsequent development of VasD [1]. Hypertension appears to be a major risk factor for small-vessel VasD, found in a significant majority of patients [6]. However, one study in South Korea found that 25% of individuals with small-vessel VasD did not have any current or previous hypertension [41]. These individuals also had lower rates of other vascular risk factors such as DM, hyperlipidaemia, and obesity and lower rates of clinical stroke than other patients with subcortical VasD, and were not more likely to smoke [41]. Potentially, they have other novel risk factors predisposing them to small-vessel VasD [41]. One cross-sectional case-control study found that individuals with a history of hypertension had decreased cortical blood flow in the temporal and occipital lobes; this finding suggests an additional pathway by which hypertension could contribute to VCI, but the study did not actually measure cognition, making it impossible to draw a firm conclusion [42].

Most, but not all, studies have found that atrial fibrillation increases the risk for VasD; in the studies that did not find an increase risk, it is possible that participants were more effectively anticoagulated, thus attenuating their risk [1].

Diseases of other blood vessels—including CAD, peripheral arterial disease, carotid atherosclerosis, and carotid thickening or stiffening—are associated with an increased risk for VasD [1]. Some studies have found that increased carotid artery thickening and stiffness are associated with worse cognitive performance; although one study found that carotid artery stiffness predicted subsequent cognitive worsening, it is not known whether carotid artery changes cause or contribute to cognitive impairment or whether they are both related to some other factors [1].

Smoking is associated with a 1.4-times greater risk for subsequently developing VasD; however, former smokers who have quit do not have an elevated risk [43]. Similar relationships with smoking are seen for AD and all-cause dementia as well [43]. This pattern suggests that smoking increases the risk for developing VasD—as well as dementia in general—but that quitting smoking can eliminate this excess risk [43].

Type 2 DM (T2DM) increases the risk for subsequently developing VasD by 2.5 times; T2DM also increases the risk for AD, but not by as much [42]. Insulin resistance also increases the risk for VasD [8].

The role of hyperlipidaemia in VCI remains unclear [1].

### Genetic risk factors

CADASIL is a Mendelian genetic disorder caused by mutations in the *NOTCH3* gene and markedly increases the risk for VCI [43]. CADASIL is the most common hereditary stroke syndrome, with a prevalence of up to 1 in 20,000 adults [43]. One epidemiologic study found that 48% of individuals with CADASIL had cognitive impairment [43].

Apolipoprotein E (APOE) is a protein involved in lipid metabolism, including CNS cholesterol transport, among other functions; it is well known that APOE 4 polymorphism increases the risk for AD [8]. The role of APOE polymorphisms in VasD risk is still unclear; a majority of studies have found that the APOE 4 allele does increase the risk for VasD, though the magnitude of increased risk is less than that for AD [8]. However, a significant minority of studies have found no relationship [8]. As the negative studies were conducted in areas where people may be more likely to eat a Mediterranean diet or a diet high in fish, diet could potentially moderate the relationship between APOE genotype and VasD, such that individuals with APOE 4 alleles who consume a heart-healthy diet do not face an increased risk, while those with APOE 4 alleles who eat more saturated fat and cholesterol do; however, no study has yet investigated this question [8].

### Other risk factors

Individuals with depression late in life have a 2.5 times greater likelihood of subsequently developing VasD [46].

Inflammation and oxidative stress may also increase the risk for VCI. Increased blood levels of inflammatory proteins, such as α-1-chymotrypsin, C-reactive protein, and interleukin-6, are associated with an increased risk for subsequently developing VasD [1]. Chronic kidney disease—typically accompanied by inflammation, in addition to other adverse physiologic changes—is also associated with an increased risk for VasD [1]. One cross-sectional case-control study found that individuals with VasD showed a biomarker pattern consistent with increased oxidative stress, as compared to healthy controls, even after adjusting for other vascular risk factors [47]. Individuals with VasD may also show hyperhomocysteinaemia and hyperuricaemia [47].

One cross-sectional case-control study found lower serum levels of brain-derived neurotrophic factor (BDNF) in individuals with VasD than in healthy controls [46]. BDNF plays an important role in synaptic plasticity and neuronal survival, so loss of BDNF could plausibly contribute to dementia [46]. However, a prior study found that BDNF levels were not decreased in VasD; this may possibly reflect the different levels of VasD severity in the two studies [46].

## Prevention and disease-modifying treatment

As VCI is caused by damage to the brain from vascular causes, that is, strokes and ischaemic demyelination—interventions to reduce the risk of stroke and improve vascular health can help prevent VCI and help arrest disease progression once VCI is present. Rates of VasD are falling, a hopeful finding which appears due, in part, to improvements in vascular risk factor modification [3].

Hypertension is the single most common modifiable stroke risk factor, and hypertension should be treated to reduce the risk for VasD [1]. One RCT in patients with a history of stroke found that reducing blood pressure with antihypertensives reduced the risk for developing dementia, and a prospective cohort study found an inverse relationship between VasD and antihypertensive drug use [1, 8]. White matter lesions increase when hypertension is not controlled, while treatment of hypertension reduces their progression [6].

Numerous observational studies of the Mediterranean diet, as well as one RCT of a Mediterranean diet supplemented with olive oil or nuts, have found that this diet reduces the risk of cognitive decline [49]. Although these studies did not specifically target individuals with VCI, other studies have found that a Mediterranean diet and olive oil can both reduce the risk of clinical stroke, WMHs, and silent stroke, making it very plausible that this diet could reduce the risk of VCI and even potentially slow disease progression in those who have it [49]. Theories for why a Mediterranean diet could benefit cognition and reduce vascular disease include its high levels of antioxidant and anti-inflammatory substances, including polyphenols and omega-3 fatty acids [49].

A meta-analysis of prospective longitudinal studies found that people who regularly exercise are less likely to get VasD [50]; however, these non-RCT studies do not permit a determination of causality. One cohort study of patients with white matter lesions found that increased physical activity was associated with lower rates of cognitive impairment [6].

RCTs of antioxidant and B vitamin supplementation—albeit not focusing on individuals with VCI—have, in general, found no effects on cognitive function, though some subgroup analyses suggest that some particular individuals (for example, those with poor dietary intake of vitamin B) may potentially experience some benefit [1].

Patients with VCI, a history of stroke or TIA, or imaging evidence of cerebrovascular disease should be worked up for modifiable risk factors—most importantly, hypertension, DM, and atrial fibrillation. Patients without these classic vascular risk factors—particularly young individuals—should undergo work-up for hypercoaguable states and other causes of cryptogenic stroke. All clinicians should encourage smoking cessation, as quitting smoking reduces the risk for subsequent VCI to the level of that seen in never-smokers [43]. Aggressive secondary stroke prevention measures—such

those delineated in the American Heart Association/American Stroke Association guidelines—should be undertaken to prevent worsening of cognitive impairment and disability and to lessen the risk for future stroke.

## Symptomatic treatment

Although there are no FDA-approved treatments for VCI, there is reasonably good evidence to support the off-label use of medications approved for other conditions to ameliorate the symptoms of VCI.

Cognitive-enhancing drugs approved for AD—cholinesterase inhibitors and memantine—appear to show benefit in VCI as well. Donepezil has the best evidence base for use in VasD without concomitant AD [1]. Multiple double-blind, placebo-controlled RCTs have shown that donepezil improves cognition in VasD; however, different studies have differed on whether donepezil also improves functional outcomes [1]. In one study of donepezil, the 10 mg/day dose showed superiority to the 5 mg/day dose on the measure of dementia severity, but the doses did not differ on other measures [51].

Galantamine also has evidence supporting its use in VasD, with RCTs showing it improves cognition; however, the evidence is more robust for mixed AD-VasD than for pure VasD [1].

One large placebo-controlled trial found that oral rivastigmine improved cognitive outcomes, though not overall functional status, in individuals with VasD; however, a subgroup analysis found that the cognitive benefit was driven by participants aged 75 years old or above, who may have been more likely to have concomitant AD pathology [52]. Two small studies of rivastigmine in VCI did not find any benefits; however, it is possible they were underpowered, and in addition, one study used a smaller dose (6 mg/day) than the study which did find cognitive benefit (mean dose 9.4 mg/day) [53].

Overall, cholinesterase inhibitors appear to be safe and well tolerated in VasD, with rates and severity of adverse effects similar to those observed in AD [1].

Two double-blind, placebo-controlled RCTs examined the uncompetitive NDMA inhibitor memantine in VasD. Both found that memantine improved cognitive outcomes but did not affect functional status [54, 55]. Memantine was safe and well tolerated in these studies [54, 55].

In addition to their benefits in VasD, donepezil, galantamine, and memantine have RCT evidence that they are effective for post-stroke aphasia, again suggesting these agents can improve cognitive deficits due to cerebrovascular disease [56].

Some preliminary data suggest that SSRIs may improve cognition in VCI. A small randomized, open-label trial of fluoxetine in non-depressed patients with VasD found that participants in the fluoxetine group showed a small, but statistically significant, increase in cognitive function following 12 weeks of treatment [57]. Serum BDNF levels in the fluoxetine group also increased more and positively correlated with the degree of cognitive improvement, suggesting an SSRI-induced BDNF increase as one potential mechanism for the cognitive benefit [57]. A double-blind study of escitalopram in patients with stroke, but not necessarily VasD, and a retrospective open-label case series examining sertraline in VCI found similar cognitive improvement [57, 58]. Further studies are needed to help elucidate whether SSRIs may play a role in the treatment of cognitive impairment due to cerebrovascular disease, but these results suggest

SSRIs may represent one additional potential avenue of therapy. Fluoxetine has randomized, double-blind, placebo-controlled trial evidence that it can improve motor function following stroke, which suggests another way in which SSRIs could benefit individuals with VCI, many of whom also have motoric deficits [59].

One small double-blind, randomized, placebo-controlled trial for the treatment of aphasia in acute stroke found that dextroamphetamine improved language function in the subacute period [60]. It is unknown if stimulants could improve other post-stroke cognitive deficits.

Some individuals with dementia may develop severe behaviour problems and often receive dopamine antagonist drugs as treatment, though given their potential for adverse side effects, they should be reserved for situations in which non-pharmacologic means have failed. While dopamine antagonist drugs appear to improve behavioural disturbance in the short term in AD, there are no high-quality data on whether they are effective in VasD [61]. However, a retrospective cohort study of individuals with VasD, followed up for a mean of 2 years, found that patients who were prescribed risperidone, quetiapine, or olanzapine did not show an increased mortality risk; of note, the study did not examine the use of other dopamine antagonist drugs and did not evaluate adverse outcomes other than death [61].

Standard rehabilitation therapies for post-stroke cognitive deficits, for example speech therapy for aphasia, prism glasses for neglect, etc., may also be useful in patients with VCI who have these deficits, though they have not been specifically studied in the VCI population. Nonetheless, given the favourable benefit/risk ratio, if a patient with VCI has a cognitive deficit with a known post-stroke rehabilitation strategy, the patient should be offered the intervention.

Thus far, psychosocial interventions for VCI have received little study. One uncontrolled trial of recreation therapy—playing games, dancing, and playing music—improved cognitive function in patients with VasD, and the benefit increased with increasing number of sessions [62]. Given the potential for benefit and the very low risk of harm, it is reasonable to try psychosocial strategies with evidence for efficacy in dementia in general such as environmental enrichment, animal therapy, baby doll therapy, physical activity, social engagement, and provision of enjoyable activities [63].

## Conclusions

VCI represents a leading cause of cognitive impairment, but vascular risk factor modification may reduce VCI risk and decrease disease progression. Individuals without a history of clinical stroke may still have VCI, so clinicians should consider this diagnosis in any patient with acquired cognitive impairment. Cholinesterase inhibitors and possibly memantine may improve cognitive functioning in individuals with VCI.

## REFERENCES

1. Gorelick, P.B., et al. Vascular contributions to cognitive impairment and dementia: a statement for healthcare professionals from the american heart association/american stroke association. Stroke, 2011. 42(9): 2672–713.

2. American Psychiatric Association. Diagnostic and statistical manual of mental disorders: DSM-5, fifth edition. Washington, DC: American Psychiatric Association; 2013.

3. Satizabal, C.L., et al. Incidence of Dementia over Three Decades in the Framingham Heart Study. N Engl J Med, 2016. 374(6): 523–32.

4. Wiesmann, M., A.J. Kiliaan, and J.A. Claassen. Vascular aspects of cognitive impairment and dementia. J Cereb Blood Flow Metab, 2013. 33(11): 1696–706.

5. Jacova, C., et al. Cognitive impairment in lacunar strokes: the SPS3 trial. Ann Neurol, 2012. 72(3): 351–62.

6. Huisa, B.N. and G.A. Rosenberg. Binswanger's disease: toward a diagnosis agreement and therapeutic approach. Expert Rev Neurother, 2014. 14(10): 1203–13.

7. Rosenberg, G.A., M. Bjerke, and A. Wallin. Multimodal markers of inflammation in the subcortical ischemic vascular disease type of vascular cognitive impairment. Stroke, 2014. 45(5): 1531–8.

8. Rohn, T.T. Is apolipoprotein E4 an important risk factor for vascular dementia? Int J Clin Exp Pathol, 2014. 7(7): 3504–11.

9. Kuller, L.H., et al. Determinants of vascular dementia in the Cardiovascular Health Cognition Study. Neurology, 2005. 64(9): 1548–52.

10. Lee, J.H., et al. Identification of pure subcortical vascular dementia using 11C-Pittsburgh compound B. Neurology, 2011. 77(1): 18–25.

11. Kim, G.H., et al. Seoul criteria for PiB(-) subcortical vascular dementia based on clinical and MRI variables. Neurology, 2014. 82(17): 1529–35.

12. Kim, Y.J., et al. White matter microstructural changes in pure Alzheimer's disease and subcortical vascular dementia. Eur J Neurol, 2015. 22(4): 709–16.

13. Toledo, J.B., et al. Contribution of cerebrovascular disease in autopsy confirmed neurodegenerative disease cases in the National Alzheimer's Coordinating Centre. Brain, 2013. 136(Pt 9): 2697–706.

14. Lee, M.J., et al. Synergistic effects of ischemia and beta-amyloid burden on cognitive decline in patients with subcortical vascular mild cognitive impairment. JAMA Psychiatry, 2014. 71(4): 412–22.

15. Ye, B.S., et al. Effects of amyloid and vascular markers on cognitive decline in subcortical vascular dementia. Neurology, 2015. 85(19): 1687–93.

16. Gupta, M., et al. Behavioural and psychological symptoms in poststroke vascular cognitive impairment. Behav Neurol, 2014. 2014: 430128.

17. Johnson, D.K., et al. Neuropsychiatric profiles in dementia. Alzheimer Dis Assoc Disord, 2011. 25(4): 326–32.

18. Robinson, R.G. and R.E. Jorge. Post-Stroke Depression: A Review. Am J Psychiatry, 2016. 173(3): 221–31.

19. Jorge, R.E., S.E. Starkstein, and R.G. Robinson. Apathy following stroke. Can J Psychiatry, 2010. 55(6): 350–4.

20. Cheng, C.Y., et al. Sleep disturbance correlates with white matter hyperintensity in patients with subcortical ischemic vascular dementia. J Geriatr Psychiatry Neurol, 2013. 26(3): 158–64.

21. Haller, S., et al. Neuroimaging of dementia in 2013: what radiologists need to know. Eur Radiol, 2013. 23(12): 3393–404.

22. Galasko, D. The diagnostic evaluation of a patient with dementia. Continuum (Minneap Minn), 2013. 19(2 Dementia): 397–410.

23. Annweiler, C., et al. 'Vitamin D and cognition in older adults': updated international recommendations. J Intern Med, 2015. 277(1): 45–57.

24. Ayerbe, L., *et al*. The long-term outcomes of depression up to 10 years after stroke; the South London Stroke Register. J Neurol Neurosurg Psychiatry, 2014. 85(5): 514–21.

25. McIntyre, R.S., *et al*. Cognitive deficits and functional outcomes in major depressive disorder: determinants, substrates, and treatment interventions. Depress Anxiety, 2013. 30(6): 515–27.

26. Hermann, P., *et al*. CSF biomarkers and neuropsychological profiles in patients with cerebral small-vessel disease. PLoS One, 2014. 9(8): e105000.

27. Wu, X.P., *et al*. Quantitative measurement to evaluate morphological changes of the corpus callosum in patients with subcortical ischemic vascular dementia. Acta Radiol, 2015. 56(2): 214–18.

28. Meguro, K., *et al*. Vascular dementia with left thalamic infarction: neuropsychological and behavioral implications suggested by involvement of the thalamic nucleus and the remote effect on cerebral cortex. The Osaki-Tajiri project. Psychiatry Res, 2013. 213(1): 56–62.

29. Thong, J.Y., *et al*. Association of silent lacunar infarct with brain atrophy and cognitive impairment. J Neurol Neurosurg Psychiatry, 2013. 84(11): 1219–25.

30. Tomimoto, H., *et al*. Loss of cholinergic pathways in vascular dementia of the Binswanger type. Dement Geriatr Cogn Disord, 2005. 19(5–6): 282–8.

31. Perry, E., *et al*. Absence of cholinergic deficits in 'pure' vascular dementia. Neurology, 2005. 64(1): 132–3.

32. Kua, E.H., *et al*. The natural history of dementia. Psychogeriatrics, 2014. 14(3): 196–201.

33. Gill, D.P., *et al*. Differences in rate of functional decline across three dementia types. Alzheimers Dement, 2013. 9(5 Suppl): S63–71.

34. Imfeld, P., *et al*. Risk of incident stroke in patients with Alzheimer disease or vascular dementia. Neurology, 2013. 81(10): 910–19.

35. Park, Y.H., *et al*. Executive function as a strong predictor of recovery from disability in patients with acute stroke: a preliminary study. J Stroke Cerebrovasc Dis, 2015. 24(3): 554–61.

36. Habeych, M.E. and R. Castilla-Puentes. Comorbid Medical Conditions in Vascular Dementia: A Matched Case-Control Study. J Nerv Ment Dis, 2015. 203(8): 604–8.

37. Hasegawa, N., *et al*. Prevalence of delirium among outpatients with dementia. Int Psychogeriatr, 2013. 25(11): 1877–83.

38. Arauz, A., *et al*. Vascular cognitive disorders and depression after first-ever stroke: the Fogarty-Mexico Stroke Cohort. Cerebrovasc Dis, 2014. 38(4): 284–9.

39. Bombois, S., *et al*. Vascular subcortical hyperintensities predict conversion to vascular and mixed dementia in MCI patients. Stroke, 2008. 39(7): 2046–51.

40. Pase, M.P., *et al*. Association of Ideal Cardiovascular Health With Vascular Brain Injury and Incident Dementia. Stroke, 2016. 47(5): 1201–6.

41. Chung, S.J., *et al*. Subcortical vascular dementia (SVaD) without hypertension (HTN) may be a unique subtype of vascular dementia (VaD). Arch Gerontol Geriatr, 2014. 58(2): 231–5.

42. Alosco, M.L., *et al*. The impact of hypertension on cerebral perfusion and cortical thickness in older adults. J Am Soc Hypertens, 2014. 8(8): 561–70.

43. Zhong, G., *et al*. Smoking is associated with an increased risk of dementia: a meta-analysis of prospective cohort studies with investigation of potential effect modifiers. PLoS One, 2015. 10(3): e0118333.

44. Cheng, G., *et al*. Diabetes as a risk factor for dementia and mild cognitive impairment: a meta-analysis of longitudinal studies. Intern Med J, 2012. 42(5): 484–91.

45. Moreton, F.C., *et al*. Changing clinical patterns and increasing prevalence in CADASIL. Acta Neurol Scand, 2014. 130(3): 197–203.

46. Diniz, B.S., *et al*. Late-life depression and risk of vascular dementia and Alzheimer's disease: systematic review and meta-analysis of community-based cohort studies. Br J Psychiatry, 2013. 202(5): 329–35.

47. Cervellati, C., *et al*. Oxidative balance, homocysteine, and uric acid levels in older patients with Late Onset Alzheimer's Disease or Vascular Dementia. J Neurol Sci, 2014. 337(1–2): 156–61.

48. Ventriglia, M., *et al*. Serum brain-derived neurotrophic factor levels in different neurological diseases. Biomed Res Int, 2013. 2013: 901082.

49. Valls-Pedret, C., *et al*. Mediterranean Diet and Age-Related Cognitive Decline: A Randomized Clinical Trial. JAMA Intern Med, 2015. 175(7): 1094–103.

50. Aarsland, D., *et al*. Is physical activity a potential preventive factor for vascular dementia? A systematic review. Aging Ment Health, 2010. 14(4): 386–95.

51. Wilkinson, D., *et al*. Donepezil in vascular dementia: a randomized, placebo-controlled study. Neurology, 2003. 61(4): 479–86.

52. Ballard, C., *et al*. Efficacy, safety and tolerability of rivastigmine capsules in patients with probable vascular dementia: the VantagE study. Curr Med Res Opin, 2008. 24(9): 2561–74.

53. Birks, J., B. McGuinness, and D. Craig. Rivastigmine for vascular cognitive impairment. Cochrane Database Syst Rev, 2013. 5: CD004744.

54. Orgogozo, J.M., *et al*. Efficacy and safety of memantine in patients with mild to moderate vascular dementia: a randomized, placebo-controlled trial (MMM 300). Stroke, 2002. 33(7): 1834–9.

55. Wilcock, G., *et al*. A double-blind, placebo-controlled multicentre study of memantine in mild to moderate vascular dementia (MMM500). Int Clin Psychopharmacol, 2002. 17(6): 297–305.

56. Allen, L., *et al*. Therapeutic interventions for aphasia initiated more than six months post stroke: a review of the evidence. Top Stroke Rehabil, 2012. 19(6): 523–35.

57. Liu, X., *et al*. Effects of fluoxetine on brain-derived neurotrophic factor serum concentration and cognition in patients with vascular dementia. Clin Interv Aging, 2014. 9: 411–18.

58. Jorge, R.E., *et al*. Escitalopram and enhancement of cognitive recovery following stroke. Arch Gen Psychiatry. 67(2): 187–96.

59. Chollet, F., *et al*. Fluoxetine for motor recovery after acute ischaemic stroke (FLAME): a randomised placebo-controlled trial. Lancet Neurol, 2011. 10(2): 123–30.

60. Walker-Batson, D., *et al*. A double-blind, placebo-controlled study of the use of amphetamine in the treatment of aphasia. Stroke, 2001. 32(9): 2093–8.

61. Sultana, J., *et al*. Associations between risk of mortality and atypical antipsychotic use in vascular dementia: a clinical cohort study. Int J Geriatr Psychiatry, 2014. 29(12): 1249–54.

62. Nagaya, M., *et al*. Recreational rehabilitation improved cognitive function in vascular dementia. J Am Geriatr Soc, 2005. 53(5): 911–12.

63. Cohen-Mansfield, J. Nonpharmacologic treatment of behavioral disorders in dementia. Curr Treat Options Neurol, 2013. 15(6): 765–85.

# 47

# Traumatic brain injury

*Christian Lepage, Inga K. Koerte, Vivian Schultz, Michael J. Coleman, and Martha E. Shenton*

## Introduction

Traumatic brain injury (TBI) is the result of blunt trauma, acceleration–deceleration forces, rotational forces, or blast exposure to the head. The injury involves a heterogenous pattern of focal and/or diffuse damage to the brain. The severity of the injury covers the spectrum from mild to moderate to severe, with severe injury leading to possible coma and even death. In addition, the range of symptoms, the variability in treatment options, and the prognosis of TBI, as well as the psychosocial implications, make it a complex injury that often calls upon the services of neurosurgeons, neurologists, psychiatrists, psychologists, and rehabilitation specialists to help patients achieve the best outcome possible.

The aim of this chapter is to provide an overview of TBI that includes the classification, epidemiology, aetiology, and pathophysiology of TBI. This is followed by an overview of clinical symptoms and long-term outcome. We then review diagnostic implications and treatment options. This is followed by a review of other neuropsychiatric disorders that evince overlapping symptoms such as post-traumatic stress disorder (PTSD) and depression. We end with a summary that emphasizes evidence-based diagnosis and the need for more research focused on recovery over time.

## Classification of mild, moderate, and severe TBI

TBIs are commonly classified into mild, moderate, and severe, using the Glasgow Coma Scale (GCS) score [1]. The GCS measures patient responsiveness along three dimensions: eye opening, verbal performance, and motor response. GCS scores range from 3 to 15, with higher scores reflecting greater functioning. GCS scores indicate TBI severity as follows: GCS scores of 13–15 are considered mild, 9–12 moderate, and 8 and below severe (Table 47.1). Further, duration of loss of consciousness, along with time span of post-traumatic amnesia (PTA), is also used to classify the degree of severity. The term 'concussion' is often used as a synonym for mild TBI (mTBI), both in general and in the field of sports-related brain injury. For a review of TBI classification approaches, see [2].

## Epidemiology

TBI is a leading cause of disability and mortality [3] throughout the world. In the United States, an estimated 2% of the population lives with disability resulting from TBI. The annual incidence of TBI is approximately 1.7 million [4]. Fortunately, approximately 80% of these injuries are considered to be 'mild'. The prevalence of mTBI is, however, likely greatly underestimated, as the extant statistics frequently exclude cases of TBI treated in non-hospital and military settings. Additionally, it is not known how many individuals do not seek medical care or whose diagnoses are missed altogether. Thus, the true prevalence is likely much higher for those with mTBI.

The annual direct costs associated with TBI are estimated to be $13 billion, while the indirect costs, which include missing days of work, are estimated to be $65 billion, making TBI one of the most costly health problems needing rehabilitation services [5]. Of further note, longterm disability is estimated to affect 43% of post-acute hospitalization cases [5]. Further, within 1 year of TBI, nearly a third of patients report difficulties with two or more activities of daily living, while about 40% require the assistance of another person due to cognitive and/or physical disability (mainly those with moderate or severe TBI). For example, a prospective study by Ponsford *et al.* [6] showed that, of patients employed prior to moderate or severe TBI, only 40% returned to work in some capacity (either to pre-injury or modified duties) when assessed at 2, 5, and 10 years post-injury. Thus, the outcome for those with more moderate and severe TBI is worse than for the majority of patients who are diagnosed with mTBI.

## Aetiology

### Sources of injury and mortality

The leading causes of TBI based on emergency department visits in the United States are falls (41%), a head strike by or against an object (19%), motor vehicle traffic accidents (15%), and assaults (11%) [7]. Falls associated with TBI are most common in children under 4 years of age and in adults 75 years and older, while TBI resulting

**Table 47.1** Traumatic brain injury severity classification

| Severity | GCS score | Alteration in consciousness | Loss of consciousness | Post-traumatic amnesia |
|---|---|---|---|---|
| Mild | 13–15 | ≤24 hours | 0–30 minutes | ≤24 hours |
| Moderate | 9–12 | >24 hours | >30 minutes, <24 hours | >24 hours, <7 days |
| Severe | 3–8 | >24 hours | ≥24 hours | ≥7 days |

GCS. Glasgow Coma Scale.

from motor vehicle accidents is most common between the ages of 15 and 34 years, and TBI resulting from assault is most common between the ages of 20 and 34 years [4]. Additionally, head impacts by or against an object are most common from childbirth to 19 years and peak again between the ages of 25 and 34 [4]. Finally, TBI-related mortality is most commonly caused by firearms (35%), motor vehicle accidents (31%), and falls (17%) [8].

### Risk factors for TBI

The incidence of TBI is affected by a number of variables, including sex, age, socio-economic status, race and ethnicity, alcohol and other substance use, and experiencing a previous TBI. More specifically, across the sexes and over the lifespan, TBI is most common in children age 0 to 4, adolescents age 15 to 19, and adults over the age of 75 years [4]. Males have a higher incidence of TBI than females across all age groups [4, 9], with the exception of those who are aged 75 years or older where females have a higher incidence. The greater number of TBIs in males has been attributed to increased risk-taking behaviours and activities.

The incidence of TBI also varies by socio-economic status, with a higher incidence of TBI in families with lower income. The incidence of TBI is also increased in non-white ethnic groups in the United States [4, 8]. Moreover, African Americans, Native Americans, and Alaska Natives are reported to have the highest incidence of assault TBI [10]. The use of alcohol and other substances is also often associated with an increased risk for TBI [11]. It has also long been recognized that an initial TBI carries a greater risk than the general population for subsequent TBI(s) [12]. In fact, individuals who incur a first TBI are three times more likely to incur a second TBI, and those who incur a second TBI are 7.8 (males) to 9.3 (females) times at greater risk for a third TBI [13].

### Pathophysiology

TBI may lead to shear deformation of the brain with stretching of axons and the surrounding myelin sheath. This stretching may result in changes in cell membrane permeability, which may, in turn, result in ionic shifts, including an influx of calcium. Calcium may then accumulate in the mitochondria where it leads to impaired oxidative metabolism, with subsequent energy failure of the cell, and eventually to the breakdown of microtubules. In addition, there may be other factors that contribute to brain injury such as sudden changes in cerebral blood flow and decreases in inhibitory neurotransmitters such as GABA and/or activation of NMDA receptors. [14, 15].

Brain injury following TBI is characterized by focal and/or diffuse neuropathologies that, depending upon their localization and severity, can lead to dysfunction at physiologic, cellular, and subcellular

levels. The initial effects of a head injury include scalp and skull lesions, cerebral contusions, haemorrhages, intracranial haematomas, and diffuse traumatic axonal injuries [16]. The primary injury may also initiate processes that lead to secondary damage, which can evolve over the course of recovery and may result in later effects of injury. Such secondary damage is more likely in moderate and severe TBI and may include ischaemia, elevated intracranial pressure, neuroinflammation, cell death, infection, and gliosis [16]. In mTBI, there are generally no visible brain alterations observed on CT scans or conventional MRI scans, although there is evidence of brain injury in post-mortem studies of those diagnosed with mTBI who died from other causes [17].

### Clinical presentation

#### Moderate and severe TBI

TBI is associated with a range of neurologic, neuropsychiatric, cognitive, and behavioural disturbances where the degree of impairment typically reflects the severity of the injury. In the acute phase following injury, the symptoms observed often reflect the location and severity of damage to brain tissue and blood vessels, as well as the presence of concomitant injuries, e.g., skull fracture. Acute symptoms may include headache, nausea, dizziness, disorientation, and disturbances of consciousness or even coma [18]. In the subacute phase following injury, seizures are common and carry the added risk of a secondary injury to the brain [19]. In the chronic phase, moderate to severe TBI may result in alterations in consciousness, paresis, neuropathies, speech impairments, seizure disorders, attention, memory, and concentration problems, sleep disturbances, changes in personality, depression, irritability, impulsivity, fatigue, and other emotional and behavioural problems [20].

#### Mild TBI

Acute symptoms following mTBI may include nausea, headache, neck pain, blurred vision, insomnia, dizziness, postural instability, fatigue, memory, attention, concentration problems, and slowed processing speed, among other symptoms such as light and sound sensitivity [18]. These symptoms are typically most prominent in the acute stage of post-injury and, in most cases, resolve over days and weeks (Fig. 47.1). It is important to note, however, that not all symptoms are present in all patients who suffer from mTBI, and in the absence of radiological evidence from CT or MRI, the diagnosis is generally made based on the occurrence of a head trauma and self-reported symptoms.

In the event that there are radiological findings in mTBI, for example cerebral contusion or haematoma, such an injury is often referred to as 'complicated mTBI' [21]. Of note here, there appear to

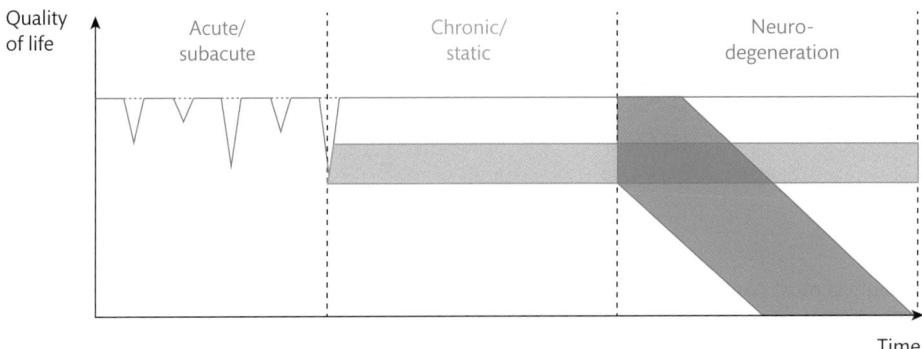

**Fig. 47.1** This is a schematic multistage disease model of possible short- and long-term sequelae, following single and repetitive brain trauma. There are three possible trajectories: an acute/subacute phase, a chronic/static phase, and a neurodegeneration phase. Subconcussive head impacts usually do not result in acute symptoms indicated by the horizontal dotted line in the acute/subacute stage. Some patients may experience chronic post-concussive symptoms that resolve over time (black line) or continue (light grey band). A small subgroup will develop a neurodegenerative disease (darker grey band).

Adapted from *Brain Pathol.*, 25(3), Koerte IK, Lin AP, Willems A, *et al.*, A review of neuroimaging findings in repetitive brain trauma, pp. 318–49, Copyright (2015), with permission from John Wiley and Sons.

be no differences in reported symptoms, neurocognitive measures, or long-term prognosis in those diagnosed with complicated mTBI vs mTBI. Notably however, as a group, those with complicated mTBI tend to take longer to return to work than those with mTBI without radiological findings [21]. Moreover, a recent study by Panenka and colleagues [22] reported that while there were no differences between mTBI and complicated mTBI with respect to reported symptoms, neurocognitive functioning, or clinical outcome, there were differences in DTI findings 6–8 weeks following injury. Thus, diffusion imaging measures may be a more sensitive measure of diffuse axonal injury, which is one of the most characteristic findings in mTBI.

## Long-term outcome

### Post-concussive syndrome

While most individuals recover completely from mTBI, there are up to 15–30% who continue to experience cognitive and behavioural symptoms that may persist for months or even years [23] (Fig. 47.1). These individuals have been referred to as the 'miserable minority' [24]. The term 'post-concussion syndrome' (PCS), or persistent post-concussive symptoms, has been used to describe these patients where there is often a combination of non-specific symptoms that persist beyond 3 months post-injury. Symptoms may include headache, fatigue, dizziness, blurred vision, nausea, irritability, sleep disturbances, hypersensitivity to light and noise, depression, and anxiety, in addition to deficits in attention, memory, concentration, executive function, and speed of processing (for example, [25]). PCS is presumed to result from a dysfunctional cognitive feedback loop [26] where acute TBI-related symptoms disrupt cognition and cause anxiety, which, in turn, results in further cognitive disruption. The literature suggests that there may also be premorbid risk factors that contribute to the development of PCS. These risk factors may include neurologic findings, psychological and personality factors, psychosocial issues, and/or being a participant in litigation (for a review, see [27]). Cognitive biases and misattribution of symptoms, as well as excessive cognitive and physical rest, may also contribute to prolonged recovery from mTBI. The problem is further compounded by the fact that the symptoms in mTBI in general, and in PCS in particular, also overlap with other disorders such as depression and PTSD. Nonetheless, taken together, the possible explanations for PCS are many. It is also clear that radiological evidence that goes beyond conventional MRI and CT is needed because these more conventional measures lack sufficient sensitivity to detect diffuse axonal injuries, which, as noted previously, are the most common brain injury in mTBI [28].

### Psychosocial issues

TBI-related alterations in cognition, behaviour, and emotion can also adversely affect psychosocial adjustment across multiple domains, including life satisfaction, social functioning, employment and school, independent living, and leisure activities (for reviews, see [29, 30]). For example, moderate to severe TBI is often associated with lower overall life satisfaction, both in the acute and long term post-injury phases. Changes in life roles (for example, work, hobbies, relationships) and depression are common following such TBI, and they are strong predictors of life satisfaction across the first 5 years post-injury [31], making these important targets for early intervention.

Several pre-injury variables are also noted to increase the risk for poor psychosocial outcome following TBI. Pre-injury psychiatric burden and a history of substance abuse are, for example, both associated with decreased employment and independent living status following moderate to severe TBI. Furthermore, both pre-injury functioning (including education and employment) and pre-injury condition (including psychiatric disorder, substance abuse, sensory dysfunction, and learning difficulties) are associated with less post-injury life satisfaction and function [32].

Families and caregivers are also an integral part of rehabilitation following TBI. Unfortunately rates of distress, including anxiety, depression, and poor social adjustment, are common in adult caregivers of individuals with TBI (for a review, see [33]). Such interpersonal challenges, initiated by TBI, may change family roles, and relationships may become strained. In mild to moderate TBI, better family functioning, including reduced caregiver distress, is associated with greater home and social integration [34]. In severe TBI, increased social support of the caregiver is associated with improved productivity and social integration in the patient [34]. Thus, support for TBI patients, as well as for their families and caregivers, is a critical part of any rehabilitation programme.

## Neurodegenerative disorders

Neurodegenerative disorders have been associated with a *history* of TBI (Fig. 47.1). There is evidence to suggest that a history of TBI is associated with a greater risk for Parkinson's disease [35], amyotrophic lateral sclerosis [36], and Alzheimer's disease [37]. In general, a history of TBI is believed to increase the risk for later-life proteinopathies, which are the underlying pathophysiology of these three neurodegenerative disorders [36]. Another proteinopathy with a strong link to a history of repetitive TBI is chronic traumatic encephalopathy (CTE).

In post-mortem studies, CTE is characterized by a pathognomonic pattern of perivascular deposition of hyperphosphorylated tau (p-tau) in neurons and astrocytes. In early stages of the disease, more focal perivascular accumulations can be detected at the depths of the cortical sulci. As the disease progresses, widespread distribution is detected throughout the brain [38]. In later stages of the disease, brain atrophy may be extant [38]. At present, CTE is diagnosed post-mortem. Moreover, a history of exposure to repetitive head impacts is assumed to be a necessary, but not sufficient, cause for the development of CTE (for a review, see [39]).

CTE has most often been reported in athletes participating in contact sports involving repetitive head impacts (for example,

boxing, ice hockey, American football, and soccer) and in military service members who are exposed to blast and/or direct head impacts [38, 40]. The clinical presentation of CTE, however, is not well understood [38, 41, 42]. Via next-of-kin interviews and medical record review of neuropathologically confirmed CTE, a constellation of prodromal symptoms appears to herald the disease. These symptoms include disturbances in behaviour (e.g., increased impulsivity and aggression), mood (e.g., depression), and cognition (e.g., difficulties with memory and executive function, as well as eventual dementia) [42]. In addition, symptoms associated with CTE may begin years following exposure to repetitive head impacts. At this point, it is not known why some individuals experience symptoms earlier and in closer proximity to the repetitive head impacts. At present, knowledge regarding the course of neurodegenerative brain alterations that result from repetitive blows to the head is sparse.

## Repetitive subconcussive head impacts

Subconcussive head impacts generally do not result in acute symptoms but may lead to structural and functional brain changes similar to those caused by mTBI [43]. Using diffusion MRI, a study by Koerte and colleagues detected microstructural brain alterations in active soccer players without a history of concussion or mTBI. However, professional soccer players experience a large number of repetitive head impacts while heading the ball [44] (Fig. 47.2).

Another study reports impaired brain function using task-based functional MRI in contact sports athletes without a history of concussion. Further studies also demonstrate cognitive, functional, and biochemical changes in athletes participating in contact sports, despite the absence of clinical symptoms associated with mTBI (for a review, see [45]). These findings may be due to cumulative effects of repetitive head impacts or they may reflect the beginning stages of a neurodegenerative disease, including CTE [46]. It is also not known if these observed brain changes are reversible, although one

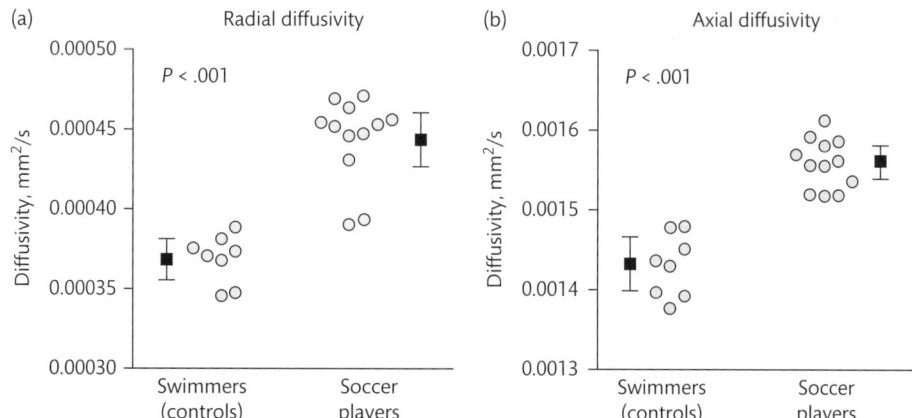

**Fig. 47.2** Diffusion tensor imaging was used to compare professionally trained young adult soccer players with age- and gender-matched controls engaged in a non-contact sport (swimming). Increased radial diffusivity was observed in the white matter in soccer players, compared to swimmers, suggesting structural changes similar to those changes observed after mTBI.

recent study of college football players suggests that following a rest period of 6 months, subtle microstructural changes reverted to baseline [47].

## Diagnostic implications

### Neuroimaging

In the acute setting, neuroimaging modalities such as CT and non-contrast MRI are often used to rule out complications in TBI, including fracture of the skull, haemorrhage in the intracranial compartments, and oedema. However, only 10% of CT scans and 30% of magnetic resonance scans reveal abnormalities in mTBI [28]. Moreover, CT and conventional MRI are not sensitive enough to detect subtle brain alterations, including traumatic axonal injury, which is commonly observed following mTBI [28]. Most importantly, information based on conventional CT and MRI is not associated with long-term prognosis following mTBI. There is thus a critical need to follow these individuals over time in future studies.

Indeed, radiological evidence for mTBI is needed using highly sensitive and objective measures to ensure early diagnosis and provide accurate prognosis. Currently there are advanced neuroimaging modalities being developed to understand better brain abnormalities following TBI, and especially mTBI and repetitive brain trauma (for a review, see [28, 45]). These imaging modalities include techniques to investigate brain structure

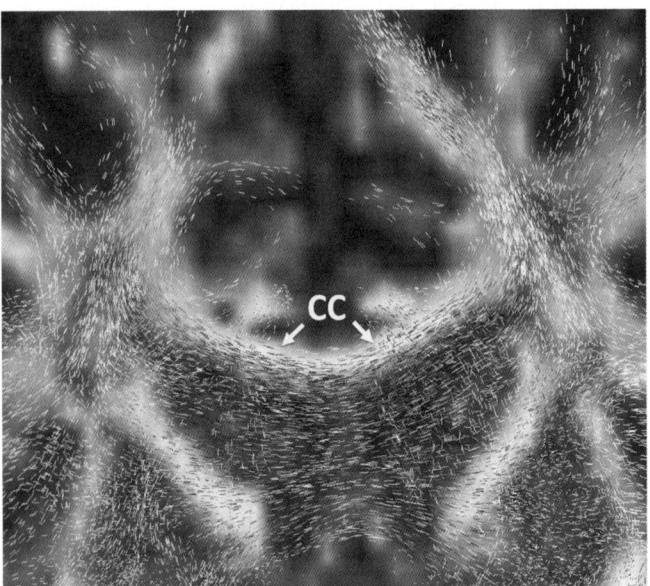

**Fig. 47.3** (see Colour Plate section) Diffusion tensor imaging measures the preferred direction of diffusion of water molecules. High directionality of diffusion can be observed in well-organized regions of the brain such as in the corpus callosum, as depicted here (see arrows). Diffusion tensor imaging provides information about the microstructure of brain tissue and thus may provide useful information in patients with TBI where diffuse axonal injury that involves the white matter is common.
Reproduced from Koerte IK, Hufschmidt J, Muehlmann M, *et al.*, Advanced Neuroimaging of Mild Traumatic Brain Injury. In: Laskowitz D, Grant G [Eds.], *Translational Research in Traumatic Brain Injury*, pp. 277–299, Copyright (2016), with permission from Taylor & Francis Group LLC.

(structural MRI) and tissue microstructure (DTI) (Fig. 47.3), as well as blood flow (arterial spin-labelling, single-photon emission tomography) and to detect micro-haemorrhages (susceptibility-weighted imaging). There are also techniques to measure indirectly brain function (fMRI) and brain metabolism (PET, MRS) (for reviews, see [28, 45]).

### Neuropsychological evaluation

A neuropsychological assessment may also contribute to understanding cognitive functioning in TBI, including psychiatric and neurobehavioural sequelae. Such an evaluation typically includes the assessment of cognitive, emotional, and psychosocial domains. In the acute stage of recovery from TBI, comprehensive assessments are not typically carried out because in cases of moderate to severe TBI, patients often exhibit various symptoms, such as variable or absent responsiveness, disorientation and/or delirium, and disrupted comprehension, each of which can interfere with accurate neuropsychological assessment [48]. Instead, a brief evaluation at the bedside may help to determine the patient's level of consciousness, the magnitude of PTA and confusion, general cognitive functioning, language functioning, and the emotional state. Several such bedside evaluations may reveal changes in the patient's status and also inform early clinical care. These assessments may also help to provide feedback to the patient, family, and caregivers, as well to monitor treatment interventions (for example, medication) and decision-making capacity (for an in-depth review, see [49]).

The cognitive sequelae of TBI are also variable and are influenced by pre-, peri-, and post-injury factors [50, 51]. Thus, when indicated, comprehensive neuropsychological assessments may play an important role in characterizing specific cognitive deficits and strengths, as well as aid in educating both patients and families, establishing treatment goals, developing rehabilitation plans, and informing prognosis [52]. In moderate to severe TBI, such assessments are recommended once patients have recovered from states of confusion and/or at 3- and 6-month intervals [53]. In mTBI, cognitive disruption, if any, is generally resolved within days of post-injury [54, 55], which has led some to recommend that comprehensive neuropsychological assessments are indicated only after this time period [56]. In sports-related concussion, on the other hand, baseline neuropsychological data are increasingly collected, albeit from briefer assessment batteries such as the Immediate Post-Concussion Assessment and Cognitive Testing (ImPACT) [57]. Here, repeat testing informs concussion management, including return-to-play decisions. Concussed athletes are usually removed from both play and practice until they are asymptomatic and neuropsychological testing demonstrates baseline performances [52].

### Electroencephalography

EEG is an important assessment tool for the clinical management of moderate and severe TBI in the acute phase of injury. More specifically, EEG is used to determine the depth of coma and to diagnose cerebral death [58]. Continuous EEG monitoring is recommended, particularly in the acute period following moderate to severe injury, in order to detect (subclinical) seizures which are common and carry the risk for secondary injuries to the brain [59]. Alterations in EEG in these patients also provide prognostic information regarding outcome. In subacute to chronic phases following moderate to severe

TBI, EEG is important for the diagnosis of post-traumatic epilepsy. The severity of TBI is, in fact, a strong risk factor for post-traumatic epilepsy [60]. Although the risk is highest within 6 months after injury, it is important to note that post-traumatic epilepsy can manifest even years after trauma [60, 61]. Finally, in subacute and chronic phases following moderate to severe injury, EEG biofeedback is sometimes used in the rehabilitation process [62].

In contrast to moderate and severe TBI, the application of EEG in mTBI has not been established for clinical use. Recent research suggests, however, that EEG may provide information on brain abnormalities associated with mTBI [63]. Alterations in EEG are more likely seen with a history of longer periods of loss of consciousness (LOC) or PTA and usually manifest as focal or generalized slowing, accompanied by a decrease in frequency of the posterior alpha [64]. In the subacute phase after mTBI, weeks to months after injury, a frequency increase of 1–2 Hz in the posterior alpha can be observed [64, 65]. This may reflect a return to baseline after the aforementioned slowing in frequency. Notably, most EEG abnormalities resolve within weeks to months post-injury [63]. In chronic phases of mTBI, 6 months or more following injury, EEG abnormalities can still be observed in a subgroup of patients. Of note, left temporal slowing may be associated with PCS [66]. It is, however, important to note that such EEG abnormalities may also occur in other psychiatric disorders such as PTSD, depression, and anxiety disorders and are therefore not specific to mTBI [67–69]. These abnormalities may also reflect comorbid illnesses with mTBI. Furthermore, and as noted previously, standardization for the use of EEG for mTBI in the clinic has not been established.

## Treatment

### Psychopharmacotherapy

TBI at all levels of severity can initiate a cascade of neurobiological processes responsible for neurotransmitter dysregulation that contributes to cognitive impairment and neuropsychiatric sequelae (for a review, see [70]). Accordingly, pharmacotherapy has long been part of the treatment and rehabilitation of TBI-related cognitive and neuropsychiatric dysfunction (for example, see [71]). Moreover, by alleviating neurocognitive symptoms, pharmacotherapy can increase the benefits from other non-pharmacological treatments (for example, cognitive rehabilitation). However, to date, there is a lack of RCTs that could form the basis for evidence-based clinical practice [72, 73]. Thus, although pharmacological interventions are common after TBI, there exists considerable variability among the specific agents administered between and within cognitive and neuropsychiatric domains [74, 75].

Despite a shortage of guidelines, comprehensive reviews of the literature offer the following recommendations [70, 72, 74, 76]. Specifically, methylphenidate and, to a lesser extent, cholinesterase inhibitors have shown efficacy in treating deficits in attention and information processing speed. Similarly, cholinesterase inhibitors and neurostimulants have demonstrated limited recovery of memory and executive function. With respect to neurobehavioural and psychiatric symptoms, β-blockers can improve agitation and aggression, while limited evidence suggests that sertraline can alleviate depression, particularly in the later phases of recovery. Beyond

these, clinicians may prescribe medications based on common practice for similar dysfunctions. However, this is based on limited evidence and mainly on subjective clinical impressions and expert opinion (see [75]). As a result, some authors have offered clinical practice directives for the delivery of pharmacotherapy—initial dosing should be lower than in non-brain-injured populations, and increased doses should occur at a more conservative pace (that is, start low, go slow). Also, reassessment of both direct and side effects should be frequent. Further, a partial response can be met by the introduction of a second agent with a separate mechanism of action, and if targeted symptoms worsen upon the introduction of the pharmacological agent, doses should be lowered, or ceased, if the symptoms intensify [76, 77].

### Cognitive rehabilitation

As noted previously, TBI-related disturbances in neurocognitive and psychiatric functioning can interfere with psychosocial functioning, independent living, and vocational and educational pursuits. Cognitive rehabilitation (CR) includes interventions aimed at assisting patients, as well as their families, to cope with cognitive and behavioural deficits following TBI. The evidence of CR has burgeoned over the last 30 years, leading to many options for clinicians seeking to improve the cognitive and psychosocial functioning of TBI patients (for reviews, see [78–81]).

Clinician-directed CR interventions may also improve cognitive functioning across many domains, including memory, attention, and executive function [82]. Deficits in memory are best addressed using external memory aids, such as journals, notebooks, and planners, as well as electronic aids like smartphones and electronic calendars [83, 84]. Although generally thought of as distinct cognitive abilities, within the context of CR, attention and executive function have been thought of as a unitary construct [78]. Accordingly, cognitive abilities within the purview of attention and executive functions include goal setting, planning, organization, initiation, and maintenance of activities, as well as executive control of attention (that is, selective attention, alternating attention, and working memory) [78]. Attention and executive function interventions demonstrate efficacy when they include direct attention (that is, repetition, hierarchical strategy development) and metacognitive training [85, 86]. Thus, these components are recommended practice standards for the rehabilitation of attention and executive function [82].

### Interventions for mild TBI

Although, as previously mentioned, mTBI is associated with a constellation of cognitive, affective, and neurologic symptoms, for most individuals, injury-related impairments tend to resolve within days to weeks, with a smaller number resolving in 3 months. Historically, rest has been considered the gold standard for clinical management. However, there is little consensus on the definition and duration of rest following mTBI, and the benefits of rest are not based on empirical evidence. Prolonged rest may, in fact, even increase the risk for post-concussion-like symptoms [87]. Silverberg and Iverson, for example, noted the possible deleterious effects of too much bed rest in their guidelines for the clinical management of mTBI. Their guidelines include: (1) bed rest for more than 3 days is not recommended; (2) pre-injury activities should resume gradually; (3) for the first 2 weeks following post-acute injury, there should be a reduction in physical and cognitive demands; and (4) for patients symptomatic after 1 month, supervised exercise should be considered. Marshall and colleagues [88] provide similar guidelines for athletes who have suffered a sports-related concussion. These include: (1) players should be medically evaluated on site by a licensed health provider who will determine the appropriate disposition of the player; (2) in the absence of a health provider, the player should be removed from practice or play and a referral to a physician should be arranged; (3) after first aid, an objective assessment of concussion should be administered; (4) the player should be accompanied and monitored over the first few hours post-injury; and (5) diagnosed or suspected concussions should prohibit return to play or practice [88]. It is important to note, however, that while elite athletes may experience significant cognitive and psychological sequelae from concussions, they are more likely to minimize the short- and long-term consequences of head impacts. A clear example is an anonymous NFL nation survey conducted by ESPN. In this survey, 320 NFL players were asked if they would play in the Super Bowl 2014 with a concussion; 85% responded 'yes' [89].

Beyond rest in the acute stage (for example, 3 days post-injury), there is accumulating evidence to suggest that education and support, provided shortly after mTBI, can be helpful, especially for somatic and psychological complaints (for reviews, see [27, 90–92]). Education should be both verbal and in print, and should include information about the symptoms common to mTBI and the time course of convalescence. Moreover, the impact of educational interventions are optimal when delivered to patients and their families, friends, employers, insurers, and/or significant others [90]. Support may take the form of validation of the patient's complaints, normalization of the symptoms, and reassurance about expected positive recovery, along with techniques to manage stress [88].

For patients with significant and prolonged complaints (that is, PCS), education and reassurance have been efficacious in shortening the duration of post-concussive symptoms (for a review, see [27]). Marshall and colleagues [88] further recommended that, for patients with chronic post-concussive symptoms, primary care providers must consider the multi-factorial nature of these complaints and management strategies should be developed with all contributing factors in mind. Notably, there is little evidence that cognitive rehabilitation and cognitive behavioural therapy are effective interventions for patients with persistent post-concussive symptoms [92, 93]. Importantly, highly sensitive neuroimaging techniques have recently become available that might shed light on the nature of post-concussive symptoms.

## Differential diagnoses

It is important to note that there is an overlap among the symptoms of mTBI and other disorders, including depression, anxiety, and PTSD. This overlap in symptoms creates diagnostic and treatment challenges for the clinician. Thus, an important first step towards differential diagnosis is to understand both the intersection and delineation of symptoms following TBI and common comorbidities. As mentioned previously, common causes of TBI include motor vehicle accidents, assaults, and combat. In addition to the increased risk for extracranial injury, such traumatic events can initiate pathological

anxiety and stress reactions, some of which may develop into PTSD, independent of TBI [94–96]. In addition, there is the issue of a differential diagnosis of depression and anxiety vs depression and anxiety being a consequence of TBI [97]. Here, we highlight important features of anxiety and depression, to aid in the differential diagnosis of mTBI (readers are referred to Chapters 74 to 92 for in-depth reviews of these topics).

## Summary and future directions

The diagnosis of moderate and severe TBI is typically clear, as are the acute treatment interventions, e.g., neurosurgical intervention. Nonetheless, the prognosis is less clear, although there are guidelines regarding what to expect at different stages of progression or recovery. With mTBI, however, the picture becomes more complex, as even the diagnosis is not always clear. More studies are thus needed to understand better the neurobiological underpinnings of mTBI and to develop more sensitive methods to detect brain alterations associated with brain dysfunction. The previously mentioned advances in neuroimaging, including diffusion MRI and MRS, are among the most promising imaging modalities for providing sensitive measures of brain alterations following mTBI, which may become biomarkers for diagnosis and prognosis and for predicting treatment efficacy as new pharmacological treatments become available. Further, it is critical to characterize subject-specific injury profiles to move towards a more personalized medicine approach tailored to each patient. Moreover, it is important to identify risk factors for poor long-term outcome and to develop individualized interventions and potential preventative strategies. The development of reliable biomarkers for the diagnosis, prognosis, and monitoring of treatment efficacy is an important area for future research that will transform what we know about the underlying pathomechanisms, as well as what we know about the short- and long-term sequelae of TBI, and these developments will lead to more informed personalized medicine approaches to treatment by health care providers.

## Acknowledgements

The authors of this study were supported by the NIH (U01 NS 093334 (IKK, MES (R01 NS100952)(IKK)))), the Veterans Affairs (VA Merit Award I01 RX00928 (MES), the Department of Defense Congressionally Directed Medical Research Programs (W81XWH-08-2-0159 (MES)), German Academic Exchange Service PROMOS award (VS), and the Canadian Institutes of Health Research Frederick Banting and Charles Best Doctoral Award (CL).

## REFERENCES

1. Teasdale G, Jennett B. Assessment of coma and impaired consciousness. A practical scale. Lancet. 1974;2(7872):81–4.
2. Saatman KE, Duhaime AC, Bullock R, et al. Classification of traumatic brain injury for targeted therapies. J Neurotrauma. 2008;25(7):719–38.
3. Roozenbeek B, Maas AI, Menon DK. Changing patterns in the epidemiology of traumatic brain injury. Nat Rev Neurol. 2013;9(4):231–6.

4. Faul M, Likang X. Wald MM, Coronado VG. *Traumatic Brain Injury in the United States: Emergency Department Visits, Hospitalizations and Deaths 2002–2006*. Atlanta, GA: Centers for Disease Control and Prevention, National Center for Injury Prevention and Control; 2010.

5. Ma VY, Chan L, Carruthers KJ. Incidence, prevalence, costs, and impact on disability of common conditions requiring rehabilitation in the United States: stroke, spinal cord injury, traumatic brain injury, multiple sclerosis, osteoarthritis, rheumatoid arthritis, limb loss, and back pain. Arch Phys Med Rehabil. 2014;95(5):986–95 e1.

6. Ponsford JL, Downing MG, Olver J, et al. Longitudinal follow-up of patients with traumatic brain injury: outcome at two, five, and ten years post-injury. J Neurotrauma. 2014;31(1):64–77.

7. Centers for Disease Control and Prevention. *Report to Congress on Traumatic Brain Injury in the United States: Epidemiology and Rehabilitation*. Atlanta, GA: National Center for Injury Prevention and Control; 2015.

8. Coronado VG, Xu L, Basavaraju SV, et al. Surveillance for traumatic brain injury-related deaths—United States, 1997–2007. MMWR Surveill Summ. 2011;60(5):1–32.

9. Tagliaferri F, Compagnone C, Korsic M, Servadei F, Kraus J. A systematic review of brain injury epidemiology in Europe. Acta Neurochir (Wien). 2006;148(3):255–68; discussion 68.

10. Langlois JA, Kegler SR, Butler JA, et al. Traumatic brain injury-related hospital discharges. Results from a 14-state surveillance system, 1997. MMWR Surveill Summ. 2003;52(4):1–20.

11. Bjork JM, Grant SJ. Does traumatic brain injury increase risk for substance abuse? J Neurotrauma. 2009;26(7):1077–82.

12. Salcido R, Costich JF. Recurrent traumatic brain injury. Brain Inj. 1992;6(3):293–8.

13. Annegers JF, Grabow JD, Kurland LT, Laws ER, Jr. The incidence, causes, and secular trends of head trauma in Olmsted County, Minnesota, 1935–1974. Neurology. 1980;30(9):912–19.

14. Giza CC, Hovda DA. The Neurometabolic Cascade of Concussion. J Athl Train. 2001;36(3):228–35.

15. Serbest G, Burkhardt MF, Siman R, Raghupathi R, Saatman KE. Temporal profiles of cytoskeletal protein loss following traumatic axonal injury in mice. Neurochem Res. 2007;32(12):2006–14.

16. Smith C. Neuropathology. In: Silver JM, McAllister TW, Yudofsky SC (eds). *Textbook of Traumatic Brain Injury*, second edition. Arlington, VA: American Psychiatric Publishing; 2011. pp. 23–36

17. Bigler ED. Neuropsychological results and neuropathological findings at autopsy in a case of mild traumatic brain injury. J Int Neuropsychol Soc. 2004;10(5):794–806.

18. Zasler ND, Katz DI, Zafonte RD (eds). *Brain Injury Medicine, 2nd Edition: Principles and Practice*. New York, NY: Demos Medical Publishing; 2012.

19. Vespa PM, Nuwer MR, Nenov V, et al. Increased incidence and impact of nonconvulsive and convulsive seizures after traumatic brain injury as detected by continuous electroencephalographic monitoring. J Neurosurg. 1999;91(5):750–60.

20. Nampiaparampil DE. Prevalence of chronic pain after traumatic brain injury: a systematic review. JAMA. 2008;300(6):711–19.

21. Iverson GL, Lange RT, Waljas M, et al. Outcome from Complicated versus Uncomplicated Mild Traumatic Brain Injury. Rehabilitation research and practice. 2012;2012:415740.

22. Panenka WJ, Lange RT, Bouix S, et al. Neuropsychological outcome and diffusion tensor imaging in complicated versus uncomplicated mild traumatic brain injury. PLoS One. 2015;10(4):e0122746.

23. Konrad C, Geburek AJ, Rist F, et al. Long-term cognitive and emotional consequences of mild traumatic brain injury. Psychol Med. 2011;41(6):1197–211.

24. Ruff RM, Camenzuli L, Mueller J. Miserable minority: emotional risk factors that influence the outcome of a mild traumatic brain injury. Brain Inj. 1996;10(8):551–65.

25. Bigler ED. Neuropsychology and clinical neuroscience of persistent post-concussive syndrome. J Int Neuropsychol Soc. 2008;14:1–22.

26. Silver JM. Neuropsychiatry of persistent symptoms after concussion. Psychiatr Clin North Am. 2014;37(1):91–102.

27. Broshek DK, De Marco AP, Freeman JR. A review of post-concussion syndrome and psychological factors associated with concussion. Brain Inj. 2015;29(2):228–37.

28. Shenton ME, Hamoda HM, Schneiderman JS, et al. A review of magnetic resonance imaging and diffusion tensor imaging findings in mild traumatic brain injury. Brain Imaging Behav. 2012;6(2):137–92.

29. Blais MC, Boisvert JM. Psychological and marital adjustment in couples following a traumatic brain injury (TBI): a critical review. Brain Inj. 2005;19(14):1223–35.

30. Cassidy JD, Cancelliere C, Carroll LJ, et al. Systematic review of self-reported prognosis in adults after mild traumatic brain injury: results of the International Collaboration on Mild Traumatic Brain Injury Prognosis. Arch Phys Med Rehabil. 2014;95(3 Suppl):S132–51.

31. Juengst SB, Adams LM, Bogner JA, et al. Trajectories of life satisfaction after traumatic brain injury: Influence of life roles, age, cognitive disability, and depressive symptoms. Rehabil Psychol. 2015;60(4):353–64.

32. Davis LC, Sherer M, Sander AM, et al. Preinjury predictors of life satisfaction at 1 year after traumatic brain injury. Arch Phys Med Rehabil. 2012;93(8):1324–30.

33. Sander AM, Maestas KL, Clark AN, Havins WN. Predictors of Emotional Distress in Family Caregivers of Persons with Traumatic Brain Injury: A Systematic Review. Brain Impairment. 2013;14(1):113–29.

34. Sady MD, Sander AM, Clark AN, Sherer M, Nakase-Richardson R, Malec JF. Relationship of preinjury caregiver and family functioning to community integration in adults with traumatic brain injury. Arch Phys Med Rehabil. 2010;91(10):1542–50.

35. Jafari S, Etminan M, Aminzadeh F, Samii A. Head injury and risk of Parkinson disease: a systematic review and meta-analysis. Mov Disord. 2013;28(9):1222–9.

36. Gupta R, Sen N. Traumatic brain injury: a risk factor for neurodegenerative diseases. Rev Neurosci. 2016;27(1):93–100.

37. Washington PM, Villapol S, Burns MP. Polypathology and dementia after brain trauma: Does brain injury trigger distinct neurodegenerative diseases, or should they be classified together as traumatic encephalopathy? Exp Neurol. 2016; 275 Pt 3:381–8.

38. McKee AC, Stern RA, Nowinski CJ, et al. The spectrum of disease in chronic traumatic encephalopathy. Brain: a journal of neurology. 2013;136(Pt 1):43–64.

39. Baugh CM, Stamm JM, Riley DO, et al. Chronic traumatic encephalopathy: neurodegeneration following repetitive concussive and subconcussive brain trauma. Brain Imaging Behav. 2012;6(2):244–54.

40. Goldstein LE, Fisher AM, Tagge CA, et al. Chronic traumatic encephalopathy in blast-exposed military veterans and a blast neurotrauma mouse model. Science Transl Med. 2012;4(134):134ra60.

41. Montenigro PH, Baugh CM, Daneshvar DH, *et al*. Clinical sub-types of chronic traumatic encephalopathy: literature review and proposed research diagnostic criteria for traumatic encephalopathy syndrome. Alzheimers Res Ther. 2014;6(5):68.

42. Stern RA, Daneshvar DH, Baugh CM, *et al*. Clinical presentation of chronic traumatic encephalopathy. Neurology. 2013;81(13):1122–9.

43. Bailes JE, Petraglia AL, Omalu BI, Nauman E, Talavage T. Role of subconcussion in repetitive mild traumatic brain injury. J Neurosurg. 2013;119(5):1235–45.

44. Koerte IK, Ertl-Wagner B, Reiser M, Zafonte R, Shenton ME. White matter integrity in the brains of professional soccer players without a symptomatic concussion. JAMA. 2012;308(18):1859–61.

45. Koerte IK, Lin AP, Willems A, *et al*. A review of neuroimaging findings in repetitive brain trauma. Brain Pathol. 2015;25(3):318–49.

46. Stern RA, Riley DO, Daneshvar DH, Nowinski CJ, Cantu RC, McKee AC. Long-term consequences of repetitive brain trauma: chronic traumatic encephalopathy. PM R. 2011;3(10 Suppl 2):S460–7.

47. Mayinger MC, Merchant-Borna K, Hufschmidt J, *et al*. White matter alterations in college football players: a longitudinal diffusion tensor imaging study. Brain Imaging Behav. 2018;12:44–53.

48. Lezak MD, Howieson DB, Bigler ED, Tranel D. Neuropathology for neuropsychologists. In: Lezak MD, Howieson DB, Bigler ED, Tranel D. *Neuropsychological Assessment*, fifth edition. New York, NY: Oxford University Press; 2012. .

49. Sherer M, Giacino JT, Doiron M, LaRussa A, Taylor S. Bedside evaluations. In: Barr B (ed). *Handbook on the Neuropsychology of Traumatic Brain Injury*. New York, NY: Springer; 2014. pp. 49–76.

50. Belanger HG, Curtiss G, Demery JA, Lebowitz BK, Vanderploeg RD. Factors moderating neuropsychological outcomes following mild traumatic brain injury: a meta-analysis. J Int Neuropsychol Soc. 2005;11(3):215–27.

51. Dikmen SS, Corrigan JD, Levin HS, Machamer J, Stiers W, Weisskopf MG. Cognitive outcome following traumatic brain injury. J Head Trauma Rehabil. 2009;24(6):430–8.

52. Vanderploeg RD. Neuropsychological assessment. In: Arciniegas DB, Zasler ND, Vanderploeg RD, Jaffee MS, Garcia TA (eds). *Management of Adults With Traumatic Brain Injury*. Arlington, VA: American Psychiatric Association; 2013.

53. Sherer M, Novack TA. Neuropsychological assessment after traumatic brain injury in adults. In: Prigatano GP, Pliskin NH (eds). *Clinical Neuropsychology and Cost Outcome Research: A Beginning*. New York, NY: Psychology Press; 2003.

54. Belanger HG, Vanderploeg RD. The neuropsychological impact of sports-related concussion: a meta-analysis. J Int Neuropsychol Soc. 2005;11(4):345–57.

55. Schretlen DJ, Shapiro AM. A quantitative review of the effects of traumatic brain injury on cognitive functioning. Int Rev Psychiatry. 2003;15(4):341–9.

56. Management of Concussion/mTBI Working Group. VA/DoD Clinical Practice Guideline for Management of Concussion/Mild Traumatic Brain Injury (mTBI). J Rehabil Res Dev. 2009;46:CP1–68.

57. Schatz P, Pardini JE, Lovell MR, Collins MW, Podell K. Sensitivity and specificity of the ImPACT Test Battery for concussion in athletes. Arch Clin Neuropsychol. 2006;21(1):91–9.

58. Schmitt S, Dichter MA. Electrophysiologic recordings in traumatic brain injury. Handb Clin Neurol. 2015;127:319–39.

59. Zimmermann LL, Diaz-Arrastia R, Vespa PM. Seizures and the role of anticonvulsants after traumatic brain injury. In: Vespa PM, Hirt D, Manley GT (eds). *Traumatic Brain Injury, An Issue of Neurosurgery Clinics of North America*. Philadelphia, Pennsylvania: Elsevier; 2016.

60. Christensen J. The Epidemiology of Posttraumatic Epilepsy. Semin Neurol. 2015;35(3):218–22.

61. Mahler B, Carlsson S, Andersson T, Adelow C, Ahlbom A, Tomson T. Unprovoked seizures after traumatic brain injury: A population-based case-control study. Epilepsia. 2015;56(9):1438–44.

62. Thornton KE, Carmody DP. Traumatic brain injury rehabilitation: QEEG biofeedback treatment protocols. Appl Psychophysiol Biofeedback. 2009;34(1):59–68.

63. Haneef Z, Levin HS, Frost JD, Jr, Mizrahi EM. Electroencephalography and quantitative electroencephalography in mild traumatic brain injury. J Neurotrauma. 2013;30(8):653–6.

64. Nuwer MR, Hovda DA, Schrader LM, Vespa PM. Routine and quantitative EEG in mild traumatic brain injury. Clin Neurophysiol. 2005;116(9):2001–25.

65. Koufen H, Dichgans J. [Frequency and course of posttraumatic EEG-abnormalities and their correlations with clinical symptoms: a systematic follow up study in 344 adults (author's transl)]. Fortschr Neurol Psychiatr Grenzgeb. 1978;46(4):165–77.

66. McClelland RJ, Fenton GW, Rutherford W. The postconcussional syndrome revisited. J R Soc Med. 1994;87(9):508–10.

67. Franke LM, Walker WC, Hoke KW, Wares JR. Distinction in EEG slow oscillations between chronic mild traumatic brain injury and PTSD. Int J Psychophysiol. 2016;106:21–9.

68. Canali P, Casarotto S, Rosanova M, *et al*. Abnormal brain oscillations persist after recovery from bipolar depression. Eur Psychiatry. 2016;41:10–15.

69. Bandelow B, Baldwin D, Abelli M, *et al*. Biological markers for anxiety disorders, OCD and PTSD: A consensus statement. Part II: Neurochemistry, neurophysiology and neurocognition. World J Biol Psychiatry. 2016:1–53.

70. Arciniegas DB, Silver JM. Pharmacotherapy of posttraumatic cognitive impairments. Behav Neurol. 2006;17(1):25–42.

71. Gualtieri CT. Pharmacotherapy and the neurobehavioural sequelae of traumatic brain injury. Brain Inj. 1988;2(2):101–29.

72. Neurobehavioral Guidelines Working Group, Warden DL, Gordon B, McAllister TW, *et al*. Guidelines for the pharmacologic treatment of neurobehavioral sequelae of traumatic brain injury. J Neurotrauma. 2006;23(10):1468–501.

73. Waldron-Perrine B, Hanks RA, Perrine SA. Pharmacotherapy for postacute traumatic brain injury: a literature review for guidance in psychological practice. Rehabil Psychol. 2008;53(4):426–44.

74. Chew E, Zafonte RD. Pharmacological management of neurobehavioral disorders following traumatic brain injury—a state-of-the-art review. J Rehabil Res Dev. 2009;46(6):851–79.

75. Hammond FM, Barrett RS, Shea T, *et al*. Psychotropic Medication Use During Inpatient Rehabilitation for Traumatic Brain Injury. Arch Phys Med Rehabil. 2015;96(8 Suppl):S256–3 e14.

76. Arciniegas DB, Silver JM. Psychopharmacology. In: Silver JM, McAllister TW, Yudofsky SC (eds). *Textbook of Traumatic Brain Injury, second edition*. Washington, DC: American Psychiatric Publishing, Inc.; 2011.

77. Arciniegas DB, Frey KL, Newman J, Wortzel HS. Evaluation and Management of Posttraumatic Cognitive Impairments. Psychiatr Ann. 2010;40(11):540–52.

78. Cicerone KD, Maestas, K. . Rehabilitation of attention and executive function impairments. In: Sherer M, Sander AM (eds). *Handbook on the Neuropsychology of Traumatic Brain Injury*. New York, NY: Springer; 2014.

79. O'Neil-Pirozzi TM, Kennedy MR, Sohlberg MM. Evidence-Based Practice for the Use of Internal Strategies as a Memory Compensation Technique After Brain Injury: A Systematic Review. J Head Trauma Rehabil. 2016;31(4):E1–11.

80. Rohling ML, Faust ME, Beverly B, Demakis G. Effectiveness of cognitive rehabilitation following acquired brain injury: a meta-analytic re-examination of Cicerone et al.'s (2000, 2005) systematic reviews. Neuropsychology. 2009;23(1):20–39.

81. Tsaousides T, Gordon WA. Cognitive rehabilitation following traumatic brain injury: assessment to treatment. Mt Sinai J Med. 2009;76(2):173–81.

82. Cicerone KD, Langenbahn DM, Braden C, *et al*. Evidence-based cognitive rehabilitation: updated review of the literature from 2003 through 2008. Arch Phys Med Rehabil. 2011;92(4):519–30.

83. Dowds MM, Lee PH, Sheer JB, *et al*. Electronic reminding technology following traumatic brain injury: effects on timely task completion. J Head Trauma Rehabil. 2011;26(5):339–47.

84. Evald L. Prospective memory rehabilitation using smartphones in patients with TBI: What do participants report? Neuropsychol Rehabil. 2015;25(2):283–97.

85. Cantor J, Ashman T, Dams-O'Connor K, *et al*. Evaluation of the short-term executive plus intervention for executive dysfunction after traumatic brain injury: a randomized controlled trial with minimization. Arch Phys Med Rehabil. 2014;95(1):1–9 e3.

86. Tornas S, Lovstad M, Solbakk AK, *et al*. Rehabilitation of Executive Functions in Patients with Chronic Acquired Brain Injury with Goal Management Training, External Cuing, and Emotional Regulation: A Randomized Controlled Trial. J Int Neuropsychol Soc. 2016;22(4):436–52.

87. Silverberg ND, Iverson GL. Is rest after concussion 'the best medicine?': recommendations for activity resumption following concussion in athletes, civilians, and military service members. J Head Trauma Rehabil. 2013;28(4):250–9.

88. Marshall S, Bayley M, McCullagh S, *et al*. Updated clinical practice guidelines for concussion/mild traumatic brain injury and persistent symptoms. Brain Inj. 2015;29(6):688–700.

89. Keim J. *Most would play Super Bowl with concussion*. 2014. http://www.espn.com/nfl/story/_/id/10358874/majority-nfl-players-play-super-bowl-concussion-espn-survey

90. Arciniegas DB, Anderson CA, Topkoff J, McAllister TW. Mild traumatic brain injury: a neuropsychiatric approach to diagnosis, evaluation, and treatment. Neuropsychiatr Dis Treat. 2005;1(4):311–27.

91. Comper P, Bisschop SM, Carnide N, Tricco A. A systematic review of treatments for mild traumatic brain injury. Brain Inj. 2005;19(11):863–80.

92. Snell DL, Surgenor LJ, Hay-Smith EJ, Siegert RJ. A systematic review of psychological treatments for mild traumatic brain injury: an update on the evidence. J Clin Exp Neuropsychol. 2009;31(1):20–38.

93. Potter S, Brown RG. Cognitive behavioural therapy and persistent post-concussional symptoms: integrating conceptual issues and practical aspects in treatment. Neuropsychol Rehabil. 2012;22(1):1–25.

94. Bryant RA, Marosszeky JE, Crooks J, Gurka JA. Posttraumatic stress disorder after severe traumatic brain injury. Am J Psychiatry. 2000;157(4):629–31.

95. Levin HS, Brown SA, Song JX, *et al*. Depression and post-traumatic stress disorder at three months after mild to moderate traumatic brain injury. J Clin Exp Neuropsychol. 2001;23(6):754–69.

96. Vasterling JJ, Brailey K, Proctor SP, Kane R, Heeren T, Franz M. Neuropsychological outcomes of mild traumatic brain injury, post-traumatic stress disorder and depression in Iraq-deployed US Army soldiers. Br J Psychiatry. 2012;201(3):186–92.

97. Bombardier CH, Fann JR, Temkin NR, Esselman PC, Barber J, Dikmen SS. Rates of major depressive disorder and clinical outcomes following traumatic brain injury. JAMA. 2010;303(19):1938–45.

# SECTION 8
# Substance use disorders

# 48

# Substance use disorders and the mechanisms of drug addiction

*Trevor W. Robbins and Barry J. Everitt*

## Introduction

Substance use disorders and the underlying problem of drug addiction have been affected by two major developments: firstly, the revolution in understanding provided by neuroscientific research, aided by arguably the most successful animal model of psychiatric disorder; and secondly, a recent significant change in the diagnostic criteria for 'substance use disorder' provided by DSM-5 (Box 48.1). Relevant to the present chapter, under DSM-IV, *substance dependence* was preferred to the term 'addiction', emphasizing the psychological and physiological concomitants of withdrawal phenomena. For opioid dependence, caused, for example, by abstinence in humans or by treatment with an opioid receptor antagonist, such as naloxone, in animal experimental studies, these withdrawal symptoms are classically manifest as a group of severe autonomic responses such as palpitations, sweating, and cramps, and in rats, by 'wet dog shakes' and piloerection, as well as by psychological dysphoria in humans and elevations of the reward threshold in rats [1]. This constellation of aversive symptoms can theoretically be considered as constituting *negative reinforcement*, an event increasing the probability of behaviour reducing its future occurrence (see Glossary of key terms, p. 488)—hence the drive to obtain more drug to avoid or escape from these withdrawal symptoms. This view of drug addiction thus accounts for the *maintenance* of drug-seeking and drug-taking behaviour, complementing the common sense view that the *initiation* of drug-taking is supported by positive subjective effects, before drug addiction sets in. These latter effects are thus described as positive reinforcement increasing the probability of behaviour producing them (see Glossary of key terms, p. 488). Such positive and negative effects are characteristic of all drugs of abuse, including stimulants such as cocaine and amphetamine, alcohol, nicotine, cannabis, ketamine, and benzodiazepines. However, the precise pattern of withdrawal effects varies considerably across compounds; the physical signs of withdrawal following cocaine are much less significant than the accompanying psychological dysphoria, for example. At this point, it is important to distinguish objective measures of behavioural and autonomic responses, from which much may be deduced about the underlying subjective motivational states, and the subjective symptoms themselves, which are more difficult to measure (Box 48.2).

These positive and negative effects of drugs can be linked by opponent motivational theories, such as that by Solomon [2], as applied by Koob and Le Moal [3], to explain addiction (Fig. 48.1). These authors postulate that positive effects of drugs are counteracted by negative effects as the drugs wear off, and moreover that, with repetition, the positive effects become progressively smaller, perhaps, in part, caused by tolerance (that is, reduced efficacy of repeated drug treatments), whereas the negative effects become progressively greater, so that negative reinforcing events predominate. According to Koob and Le Moal [4], this process ultimately progresses to a state of 'allostasis', by which the drug abuser is unable to attain normal bodily and subjective 'homeostasis' by moderate drug-taking—leading to a vicious circle of drug bingeing and dependence, which is further exacerbated by its stressful sequelae.

This theory appears to be a compelling account of addiction and yet does not apparently explain why DSM-5 criteria of addiction have so radically moved away from substance dependence as its defining element. This is partly because it is evident from the study of other drug effects, such as those of caffeine, that a withdrawal syndrome per se is not necessary for the serious sequelae of drug addiction. Additionally, although withdrawal and tolerance are important potential symptoms of substance use disorder, they constitute only two of about 11 symptoms by which addiction is now defined (Box 48.1). From Box 48.1, it can be noted that the other symptoms are mainly those associated with 'top–down' cognitive control, especially exemplified by the compulsive drug-seeking and drug-taking that occurs, for example, during relapse. These responses apparently occur almost reflexively to cues that have become associated with the drugs, including even people and places, and are exceedingly difficult to bring under conscious restraint [5]. The other quality of compulsive responses is the tendency for such behaviour to be performed despite evident aversive consequences. This pattern of behaviour has thus been associated with a rather different theory that emphasizes positive reinforcement and a progressive loss of top–down control from higher brain centres in addiction [6, 7].

## The positive reinforcement or reward-based theory of addiction

The idea that the positive subjective effects of drugs play a greater part in addiction gained much from the discovery of an apparent reward system in the brain. This was initially supported by the observation that rats would perform responses such as lever-pressing, leading to intracranial stimulation ('self-stimulation' behaviour), an obvious manifestation of positive reinforcement which was, however, limited to certain brain regions [8]. Eventually, it was realized that the regions coincided to a considerable degree, though not exclusively, with the location of dopamine (DA)-containing neurons in such areas as the ventral tegmental area (VTA) of the midbrain which innervate structures, including the nucleus accumbens (part of the ventral striatum), amygdala, and medial prefrontal cortex (Fig. 48.2). Focusing on stimulant drugs, such as d-amphetamine and cocaine, which were already known to be indirect agonists of the catecholamine neurotransmitter systems DA and noradrenaline (NA), Wise and others showed from pharmacological studies using DA and NA receptor antagonists that rodents appeared to regulate the amount of drug that could be self-administered intravenously via implanted jugular vein catheters to some sort of optimal level [9]. This regulation was selectively affected by DA receptor antagonists (such as haloperidol) [10]. Thus, a small dose of haloperidol would actually increase the rates of self-administration, presumably as the animal strives to overcome the effects of DA receptor blockade. This self-administration paradigm has subsequently become the gold standard for research studies of the reinforcing effects of drugs. Evidence of its validity comes from the fact that virtually all drugs of abuse in humans are self-administered by experimental

**Box 48.2**  Subjective feelings contributing to drug addiction

What is the underlying nature of positive and negative reinforcement? Positive reinforcers are defined according to Thorndike's Law of Effect which posits that they are events that increase the probability of responses that produced them. Early textbook theories of motivation, suggested that reinforcers have several functions including: (1) a reduction in drive or need reduction in relation to homeostatic regulation; (2) consolidation of learning or memory of associative or contingent relationships between environmental stimuli and responses or actions (leading, for example, to relatively automatic stimulus-response habits); (3) incentive-motivational effects leading to appropriate preparatory (appetitive) responses, such as approach behavior, or physiological adjustments in expectation of outcome or goal (such as eating food). Negative reinforcers are more difficult to characterize as they are defined as aversive events that increase the likelihood of their postponement or omission. Clearly both positive and negative reinforcement may play a role in drug abuse and addiction. But how do these aspects of reinforcement theory relate to the subjective effects of drugs that presumably play some part in addiction?

Incentive-motivational theories emphasize the hedonic properties of the reinforcer, especially when there is no obvious deficit or need state: for example, reinforcers such as intracranial electrical self-stimulation of the brain, cocaine, sex, sweet foods or novel objects. Thus reinforcers may have yet another function, to generate a subjective appraisal of their effects in terms of pleasure or aversion. This conceptualization has encouraged the use of terms such as 'reward' and 'liking' that connote hedonic subjective responses associated with positive reinforcers. Hedonic reactions are certainly important in early responses to drugs—for example, the subjective euphoria or 'high' initially associated with early experiences with the drug, which however may show a gradual reduction with repeated experience ('tolerance'). Moreover, it can be argued that behaviour governed by reinforcement is not always necessarily accompanied by conscious pleasure, as in the case, for example, of habits. Negative reinforcement may also be associated with subjective responses such as 'relief' (e.g. on avoiding an electric shock or escaping the pangs of withdrawal). Withdrawal itself is often accompanied by subjective craving for drug; however the precise causal, as distinct from correlative, role of such craving (also often called 'wanting') in motivating drug seeking behaviour remains unclear.

These issues are difficult to address because experimental animals, of course, do not have verbal responses to express any subjective feelings they may experience, whereas we can infer much about reinforcement processes from their overt behaviour. A causal analysis of the neural basis of subjective responses in humans is also only in a relatively early stage. Presumably, this must involve an attributional system which connects thoughts to actions and also may involve interactions with language based processing.

Indiscriminate substitution of the term 'reward' for 'reinforcement' therefore may therefore sometimes lead to mistaken assumptions about the neural nature of the human 'reward system'. This system undoubtedly includes those regions such as the nucleus accumbens, and its dopaminergic innervation, as determined from animal studies, but may well extend to other interactive cortical areas within a greater neural network. The orbitofrontal cortex is linked to sensory and value-based representations of reinforcers and the relative utility of different courses of action producing them, as well visual, auditory or olfactory cues which predict them through conditioning processes. Feelings of pleasure presumably arise from the visceral feedback provided from the autonomic nervous system which are integrated into emotional reactions by such structures as the insular cortex, and labelled as pleasant (or otherwise) according to the social and cognitive context in which they are experienced. This is in accordance with many studies of how environmental context may affect attributions of pleasure or aversion to what may be physiologically similar responses to drugs. Consequently, although it is important to take subjective responses into account, it is also a viable strategy to measure objectively how animal and human subjects actually behave in relation to repeated drug exposure.

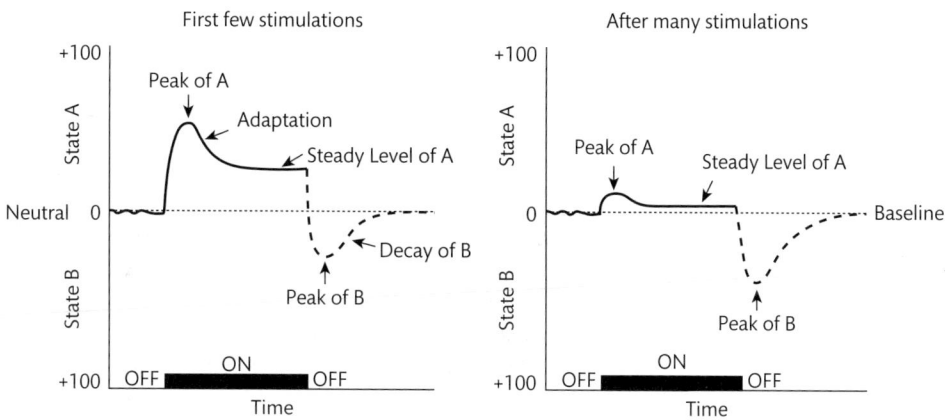

**Fig. 48.1** Opponent motivational processing. A theory of affective dynamics which suggests that the positive emotional State A arising from a stimulating (standard square wave) rewarding event undergoes several transitions, both after a few presentations and after many. The peak emotional impact of the event is experienced soon after its presentation and then exhibits sensory adaptation, declining over time while the stimulation is still ON. The hypothetical opponent negative or aversive experience (State B) comes after the event has been completed (that is, is OFF). This might relate to the effects of any reward (or, inversely speaking, of any punisher); in the case of a drug of abuse, it most obviously relates to the euphoric 'high', experienced soon after the drug takes effect (for example, almost immediately after intravenous self-administration), and the 'low' after the drug has worn off. Note that State B is always less marked than State A during the first few stimulations, so that the initial emotional state is positive. After many rewarding 'stimulations', the positive effects of State A have hypothetically markedly diminished, compared with their peak during the first few stimulations. In the case of drugs of abuse, this relates to the well-known *tolerance* (progressive diminution) of pharmacological effects with repeated experience. However, the aversive after-effects in State B have increased, and so the net impact is negative. For drugs of abuse, this stage hypothetically corresponds to the state of 'withdrawal' (see text) and motivates avoidance behaviour controlled by negative reinforcement.
Reproduced from *Psychol Rev.*, 81(2), Solomon RL, Corbit JD, An Opponent- Process Theory of Motivation: I. Temporal Dynamics of Affect, pp. 119–145, Copyright (1974) with permission from American Psychological Association.

animals [11]. (A notable exception is that of LSD; however, there are good grounds for believing that the psychomimetic use of this drug by humans is not typical of drug abuse.) More recently, drug self-administration has been incorporated into behavioural models of addiction that have some measure of face validity [1, 12, 13].

Further significant observations supporting a central dopaminergic mediation of the effects of stimulant drugs included findings that the depletion of DA in the so-called mesolimbic projections from the VTA to the nucleus accumbens reduced self-administration rates for cocaine [14]. Perhaps more dramatically, it was also shown that d-amphetamine was self-administered directly into the nucleus accumbens by rats through an implanted cannula [15], but not significantly into other brain regions (Fig. 48.2). Moreover, these effects were demonstrated to be DA-dependent, in that concurrent treatment with DA receptor antagonists again produced an upregulation of self-administration [16].

The implication of mesolimbic DA in the positive reinforcing effects of drugs was consistent with evidence that natural rewards, such as food and sex, also exerted their reinforcing effects via this pathway [11]. However, even more significant was that the positive reinforcing effects of other drugs of abuse whose primary mechanisms of actions were not dopaminergic could also potentially be indirectly mediated by this system because of their modulatory effects on other receptors present in the VTA or nucleus accumbens—for example, nicotine, opioids (Fig. 48.2), cannabinoids, and, via GABA and glutamate receptors, alcohol and benzodiazepines [11]. This hypothesis was supported by evidence obtained using *in vivo* microdialysis which showed that many of these drugs upregulated DA levels in the nucleus accumbens. The hypothesis that the DA system was a 'final common pathway' in mediating the positive reinforcing effects of drugs of abuse has been an attractive hypothesis, not least because

it provided a potential basis for understanding polydrug abuse, by which human drug abusers will readily switch between different combinations of drugs when the supply of one of them is cut off.

The implication of a positive reinforcement system focused on the VTA that mediated effects of opioidergic agents, such as morphine and heroin, was exploited by Bozarth and Wise to test the opponent motivational process account of opioid addiction described here. They showed that intracranial self-administration of morphine could be maintained into the VTA region, supporting the positive reinforcement hypothesis, but that the self-administering rats did not exhibit the symptoms of physical withdrawal when challenged with naloxone [17]. Therefore, the maintenance of self-administration could not be attributed simply to overcoming negative reinforcement. By contrast, administration of morphine to the periaqueductal grey in the hindbrain did lead to physical symptoms on challenge with naloxone [17]. Therefore, it appears that the positive reinforcing effects of morphine and heroin and their actions on autonomic centres can be dissociated; the fact that opioid receptors are involved in these different responses is coincidental and not inextricably related. Nevertheless, some form of the opponent theory can be supported, as a subsequent study showed that the antagonism of opioid receptors within the nucleus accumbens could produce conditioned aversion to the place where heroin was experienced, suggesting that the drug was producing aversive after-effects in this mesolimbic reward system [18]. The additional assumption that the positive effects were mediated by the DA reinforcement system was also contradicted by the fact that the self-administration of heroin was incompletely blocked by DA depletion from the nucleus accumbens, suggesting that at least some of its positive reinforcing action was DA-independent [19]. This picture is probably true for other drugs of abuse such as alcohol and nicotine; DA mechanisms

(a)                                                          (b)

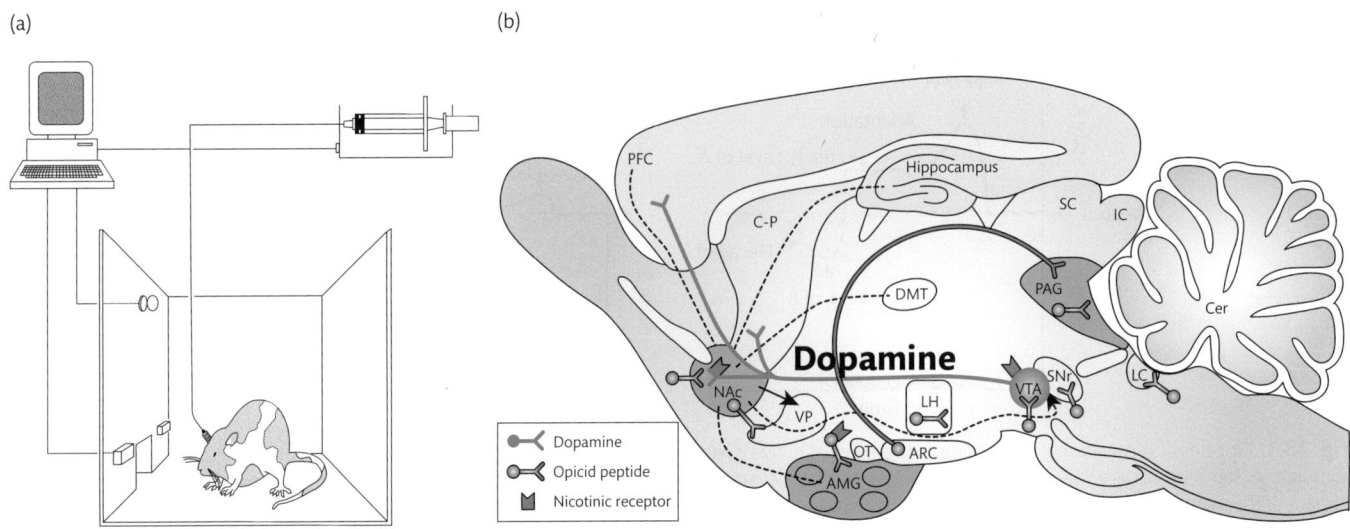

**Fig. 48.2** (see Colour Plate section) (a) Intracerebral drug self-administration. By pressing a lever in an operant chamber, rats can deliver microlitre and microgram quantities of drugs, such as amphetamine, directly into the brain. A major neural locus that supports such drug self-administration is the nucleus accumbens. (b) A schematic sagittal section of the rat brain showing the mesolimbic dopamine system, comprising cell bodies in the ventral tegmental area (VTA), axons that run in the medial forebrain bundle in the lateral hypothalamus, and terminals in the nucleus accumbens (NAc), medial prefrontal cortex (PFC), and amygdala (AMG), among other forebrain structures. Nicotinic and opioid receptors are shown on both dopamine neuron cell bodies and terminals in the nucleus accumbens. Some major cortical afferents to the nucleus accumbens are also shown and include the amygdala, hippocampal formation, and prefrontal cortex. Opioidergic (beta-endorphin-containing) projections are shown originating in the hypothalamic arcuate nucleus (ARC) and innervating the midbrain periaqueductal grey matter (PAG). Small enkephalin-containing interneurons are represented in green. There is widespread agreement that all drugs of abuse, in addition to actions on their specific molecular targets, can increase activity in the mesolimbic dopamine system and dopamine release in the nucleus accumbens and is often therefore referred to as the common reward pathway. (See [90].)

Reproduced from *Trends Pharmacol Sci.*, 13(5), Koob G, Drugs of abuse: anatomy, pharmacology and function of reward pathways, pp. 177–84, Copyright (1992) with permission from Elsevier Ltd.

may indeed play a role and be a part of a 'final common pathway' leading to rewarding effects, but these are not the only source of the positive reinforcing actions of these compounds.

## The importance of conditioning and associative learning

One of the properties of reinforcers is that they support new learning, and there are many indications that drug addiction may represent aberrant associative learning. An implication of this hypothesis is that cues and contexts (places) associated with drugs may gain salience via association with drugs through Pavlovian conditioning and thus exert important control over behaviour. Such cues may be the sight of needles or drug-taking paraphernalia, which have been reported to produce euphoric 'highs' in their own right in some addicted individuals. Drugs, such as amphetamine and cocaine, can enhance the salience of stimuli paired with other rewards, such as food, water, and brain stimulation, and such stimuli can even act as reinforcers themselves after conditioning, when they are termed conditioned reinforcers [20]. The potentiation of rewarding properties of environmental stimuli has been shown to depend on an interaction between two major factors: the integrity of the basolateral amygdala (BLA), which enables the association between the conditioned stimulus (CS) (for example, a predictive noise or light) and the unconditioned stimulus (US) (for example, food, sex, or addictive drug) and the dopaminergic innervation of the nucleus accumbens (which is responsible for the behavioural activation produced by such stimuli in responding under the influence

of the stimulant drug) [21, 22]. These factors have been shown to influence drug-seeking behaviour to a considerable extent. Thus, in a schedule in which rats work to obtain intravenous infusions of drugs by their instrumental lever-pressing, drug-seeking behaviour can be maintained for long periods, even before drug delivery by the presentation of brief stimuli (for example, lights or noises) associated with the ultimate delivery of the drug [23–25]. The same phenomenon has been demonstrated in humans [26]. The use of the conditioned reinforcers to maintain behaviour in this way can be termed a second-order schedule of reinforcement, its special utility being that it is then feasible to measure the motivational effects of the drug in terms of the responding made during the drug-seeking period prior to drug self-infusion [23]. Subsequent to that first infusion, the motivational salience of the drug-paired cues presumably becomes even greater as a consequence of the actions of the drug itself. This schedule has been used in several ways: (1) to define the neural pathways responsible for drug-seeking behaviour; and (2) as a method for screening possible remediative drug therapies that reduce drug-seeking and may therefore be employed potentially to combat craving and relapse in human drug abusers [27].

## Neural basis of drug-seeking behaviour

(See Fig. 48.3.)

Based on the previous findings implicating the BLA in CS–US association, it was perhaps not surprising to find that excitotoxic lesions of this structure significantly impaired the acquisition of cocaine-seeking dependent on drug CS to mediate delays to

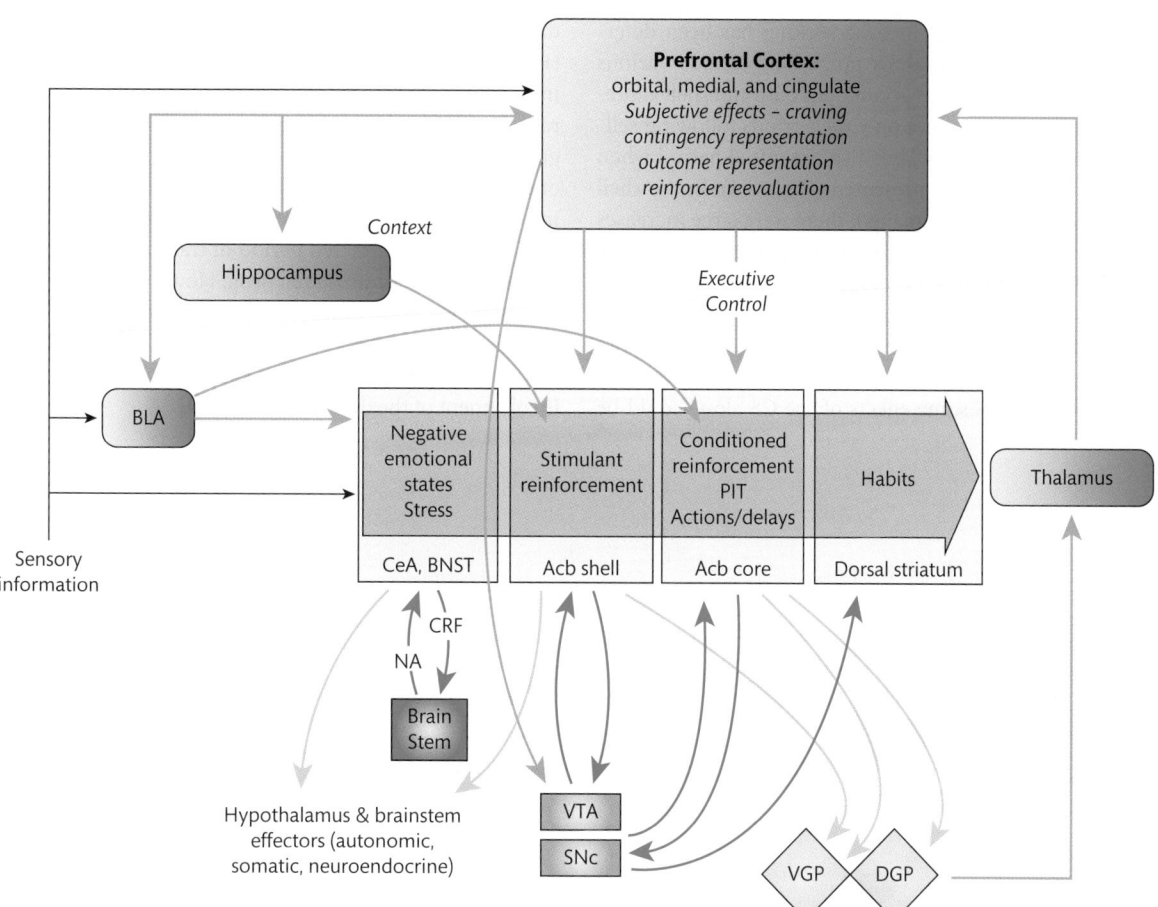

**Fig. 48.3** (see Colour Plate section) Representation of key components of limbic cortico-striatal circuitry in which psychological and physiological processes important in drug addiction are indicated. These include: (1) the processing of conditioned reinforcement (and Pavlovian associations between environmental stimuli and drugs in general) by the basolateral amygdala and of contextual information by the hippocampus; (2) goal-directed actions involve interactions between prefrontal cortical areas (orbitofrontal, ventromedial) and the dorsomedial striatum; (3) habits (stimulus–response associations) depend on interactions between the prefrontal cortex (sensorimotor) and dorsolateral striatum; (4) 'executive control' depends on the prefrontal cortex and includes representation of contingencies and outcomes and their value and subjective states (craving and feelings) associated with drugs; (5) in functional imaging studies, drug craving involves activation of the orbital, anterior cingulate, and insular cortices and temporal lobe structures, including the amygdala; (6) connections between dopaminergic neurons and the striatum, linking the ventral with the dorsal striatum via interactions organized in a striato-midbrain-striatal spiralling cascade of neuronal interconnections; (7) reinforcing effects of drugs may engage stimulant Pavlovian influences on behaviour such as Pavlovian-instrumental transfer, or conditioned motivation, and conditioned reinforcement processes in the nucleus accumbens shell and core and then engage stimulus–response habits that depend on the dorsal striatum; (8) the extended amygdala is composed of several basal forebrain structures, including the bed nucleus of the stria terminalis, the centromedial amygdala, and, more controversially, the medial portion (or shell) of the nucleus accumbens. A major transmitter in the extended amygdala is the corticotropin-releasing factor, which projects to the brainstem where noradrenergic neurons provide a major projection reciprocally to the extended amygdala. Activation of this system is closely associated with the negative affective state that occurs during withdrawal. Green/blue arrows, glutamatergic projections; orange arrows, dopaminergic projections; pink arrows, GABAergic projections. Acb, nucleus accumbens; BLA, basolateral amygdala; VTA, ventral tegmental area; SNc, substantia nigra pars compacta. VGP, ventral globus pallidus; DGP, dorsal globus pallidus; BNST, bed nucleus of the stria terminalis; CeA, central nucleus of the amygdala; NA, noradrenaline; CRF, corticotropin-releasing factor; PIT, Pavlovian-instrumental transfer. (See [91].)
Reproduced from Koob GE, Everitt BJ, Robbins TW, Chapter 43: Reward, Motivation, and Addiction. In: Squire L, Berg D, Bloom F, et al. [Eds]., *Fundamental Neuroscience*, Third Edition, pp. 987–1016, Copyright (2008), with permission from Elsevier Inc.

self-administration [28] (Fig. 48.2). Also thematic was the finding that similar lesions of the so-called core subregion of the nucleus accumbens produced similar effects, reflecting, in part, the innervation by the BLA of this structure [29], as later confirmed by disconnection of these two structures [30]. Intriguingly, lesions of the other major subregion of the nucleus accumbens—the shell—also affected performance, but mainly to reduce the rate of responding produced by the response-contingent conditioned reinforcers [29]. On the basis of these findings, it could be concluded that the acquisition of cocaine-seeking was controlled by an amygdala–accumbens

pathway. Whether this is also true for other drugs of abuse is not quite clear, as second-order schedule performance maintained by heroin was shown to be less susceptible to BLA lesions [31]. There are several other afferent pathways to the nucleus accumbens, including from the hippocampus, insula, anterior cingulate, and prefrontal cortex, so it is possible that other pathways also contribute to the effects of conditioned stimuli in various contexts, including stress. There is indeed evidence from a specific model of relapse, termed reinstatement following extinction of drug-seeking, that these other structures participate in different forms of relapse [32].

The possible role of DA itself in drug-seeking has been determined by using *in vivo* microdialysis probes directed to various striatal sites, including the nucleus accumbens core and shell subregions. Of particular interest are not only the periods following self-administered infusions of cocaine, but also the initial period when only conditioned reinforcers are presented (Fig. 48.4). In the shell region (as well as other striatal domains), there were large increases following cocaine infusions, but no significant increases during the initial period. Presumably, this is one of the initial sites of the unconditioned reinforcing effects of stimulant drugs, consistent with the earlier evidence of effects of lesions described previously. In the core region, there was a similar picture, although the levels of DA were lower than in the shell, and some effects of the CS alone could be discerned, but only if such stimuli were presented in a novel context (Fig. 48.4). Of greatest significance, however, was the finding that in the dorsal striatum (that is, the caudate–putamen of the rat), the release of DA in the periods producing the CS was approximately as great as for the drug itself (Fig. 48.4). This was one of the first pieces of evidence to suggest that the dorsal striatum also has a role to play in cocaine-seeking under the control of conditioned reinforcers, especially after a protracted period of training and increasing experience of the self-administered drug. However, other observations are consistent with this view. For example, autoradiographic evidence of changes in DA receptors in the striatum in rhesus monkeys chronically self-administrating cocaine showed a gradual, all-encompassing involvement of the dorsal striatum [33].

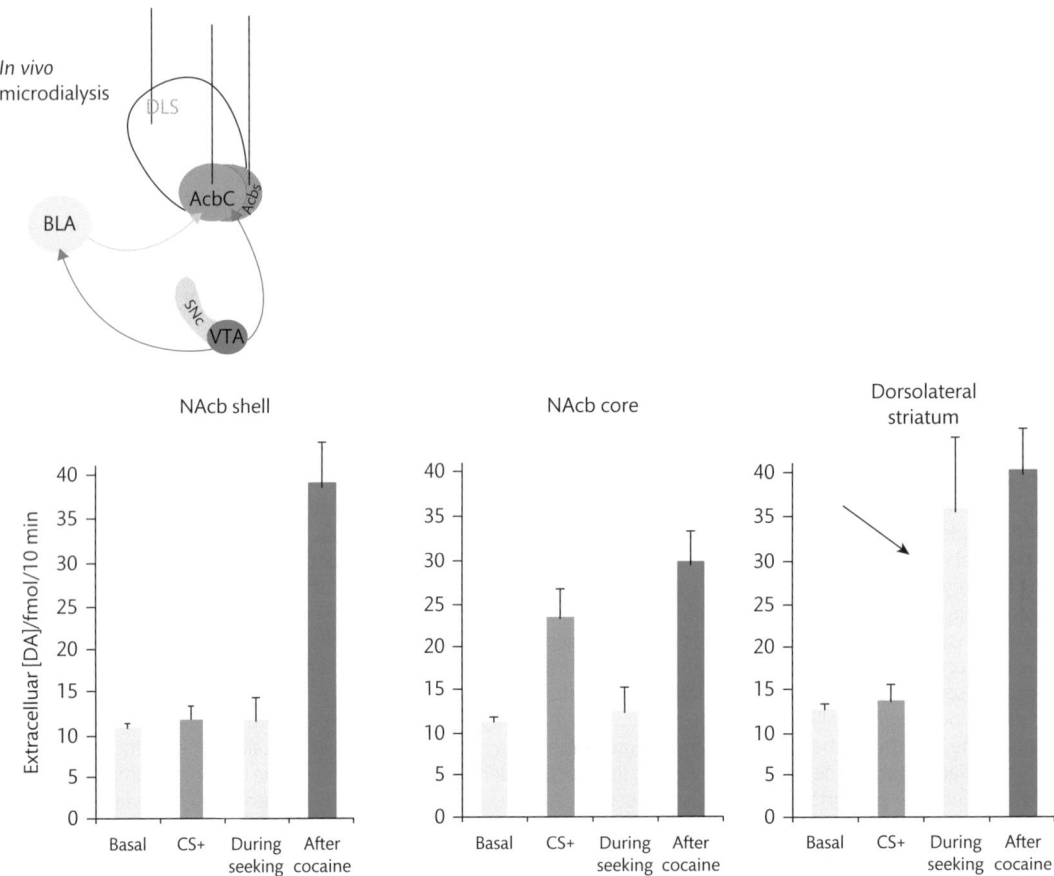

**Fig. 48.4** In this study, rats were trained to respond for intravenous cocaine under a so-called second-order schedule of reinforcement, in which their drug-seeking behaviour depended on the response-contingent presentation of cocaine-associated conditioned stimuli (acting as conditioned reinforcers) during delays to reward. After a prolonged period of training, dopamine extracellular levels in three areas of the striatum were measured (at the end of 1-hour seeking sessions): the nucleus accumbens core, the shell, and the dorsolateral striatum. Following the infusion of cocaine, dopamine release was increased in all areas, indicating the effects of the drug on these richly dopamine-innervated striatal areas. However, there were no increases in dopamine in the nucleus accumbens core and shell following the prolonged bout of drug-seeking responding, but instead marked increases in the dorsolateral striatum. This area is strongly implicated in stimulus–response or habit behaviour, and this dopaminergic correlate of cocaine-seeking is a key part of the evidence in favour of the development of the habitual nature of drug-seeking after prolonged experience. Also of note is the increase in dopamine in the nucleus accumbens core when the cocaine-associated conditioned stimulus was presented surprisingly (that is, in a different context to previously), indicating that this component of the dopamine system is responsive to cues associated with drug reward but is less engaged by habitual drug-seeking behaviour. (See [92, 93].)

Source: data from *J Neurosci.*, 20(19), Ito R, Dalley JW, Howes SR, *et al.*, Dissociation in Conditioned Dopamine Release in the Nucleus Accumbens Core and Shell in Response to Cocaine cues and during Cocaine-Seeking Behavior in rats, pp. 7489–95, Copyright (2000), Society for Neuroscience; *J Neurosci.*, 22(14), Ito R, Dalley JW, Robbins TW, *et al.*, Dopamine release in the dorsal striatum during cocaine-seeking behavior under the control of a drug-associated cue, pp. 6247–53, Copyright (2002), Society for Neuroscience.

## Neuropsychological theories of drug addiction

(See Fig. 48.5.)

The evidence of dorsal striatal involvement can be interpreted to suggest a devolution of control over behaviour, from the ventral to the dorsal striatum, with chronic drug exposure. In psychological terms, this might be construed as a shift in balance between two learning systems—a goal-directed system in which behaviour is controlled by its consequences (that is, rewarding drug effects), and a relatively unconscious stimulus–response habit-based learning system, which is more automatic and depends on stimuli that simply elicit responses without reference to the goal. Therefore, the hypothesis has been advanced [6, 7, 34] that drug-seeking behaviour eventually becomes less goal-directed and more habitual with drug experience—in other words, that habitual drug-seeking is at the basis

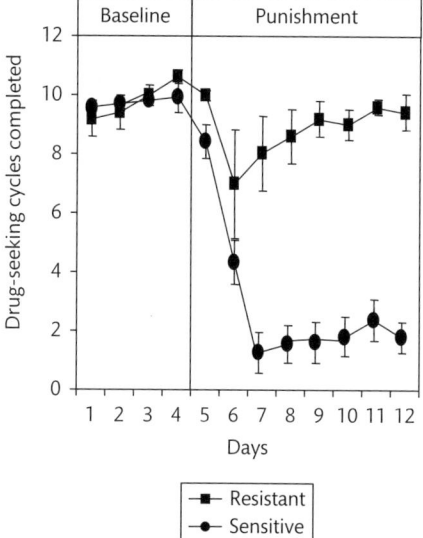

**Fig. 48.5** Compulsive drug-seeking in an animal model of addictive behaviour. In this study, rats were trained on a task in which responding on one lever in an operant chamber gives access to a second lever, responding on which delivers an intravenous infusion of cocaine. These levers are therefore designated 'seeking lever' (on which responding is never reinforced) and 'taking lever' (on which responding is always reinforced), and the rats perform 'cycles' of seeking and taking. Then, either after a short or long drug-seeking-taking history, a cycle of seeking responses was unpredictably punished, rather than giving access to the taking lever and hence intravenous cocaine. Thus, in this procedure, rats must run the 'risk' of punishment in order to gain the opportunity to take cocaine; the analogy with humans foraging for cocaine is obvious. After a brief history of taking cocaine, all rats suppressed their seeking behaviour when punishment was introduced (they abstained). However, after a long history, the figure shows that although the majority of rats abstained, a subpopulation of about 20% of rats continued to seek cocaine in the face of punishment, that is, were compulsive (therefore meeting key DSM-5 criteria for 'addiction'). Rats with a behavioural trait of high impulsivity expressed before any cocaine experience are much more likely to become compulsive, that is, they are vulnerable to develop compulsive cocaine-seeking. (See [94].)

Source: data from *Psychopharmacology*, 194(1), Pelloux Y, Everitt BJ, Dickinson A, Compulsive drug seeking by rats under punishment: effects of drug taking history, pp. 127–37, Copyright (2007), Springer-Verlag; *Psychopharmacology*, 232(1), Pelloux Y, Murray JE, Everitt BJ, Differential vulnerability to the punishment of cocaine related behaviours: effects of locus of punishment, cocaine taking history and alternative reinforcer availability, pp. 125–34, Copyright (2015), Springer-Verlag.

of compulsive drug-seeking symptoms, according to DSM-5 criteria (Box 48.1). However, such a theory requires some understanding of how habitual behaviour can become compulsive, despite adverse consequences, and this may require additional factors. One of these is the concept of loss of top–down control, especially by so-called executive mechanisms of the prefrontal cortex. There is considerable evidence that chronic drug-taking compromises prefrontal functioning in experimental animals and, as will be seen from evidence to be considered later, also in humans, and therefore, a mechanistic basis for habits to become compulsive [35–38]. A parallel, competing hypothesis is that compulsive behaviour arises from a gradual sensitization of the mesolimbic reward system by repeated drug exposure, leading to excessive motivation for drugs [39]. Although there is no doubt that effects of drugs can gradually augment over time and can be manifest in responses, such as enhanced locomotor activity, it is less clear how such augmentation can occur to enhance compulsive instrumental drug-seeking, leading to drug-taking. A further suggestion has been that stress can exacerbate the transition from goal-directed responding to habits [40] and may cross-sensitize with the effects of stimulant drugs. It should be noted that both drug-induced sensitization and stress have been shown directly to influence dorsal striatal mechanisms of habitual responding [40, 41].

How does one begin to distinguish among these various accounts of addiction to stimulant drugs? And to what extent does it apply to other drugs of abuse? These two issues, as well as the opponent motivational theory, are at the forefront of current research attempts to understand the theoretical basis of drug addiction. A possible reconciliation of habit with the opponent motivational theory would suggest that negatively reinforced behaviour is especially subject to habitual control [7].

Learning theory has advanced several methods for diagnosing the contribution of habits and goal-directed actions to behavioural output, with both playing a part (Fig. 48.5). Habits tend to emerge with extended training, and the nature of the reinforcement schedule is also important [42]. Habitual behaviour persists if: (1) goals are devalued, for example by satiety or counterconditioning with toxins, in the case of food reward; or (2) the contingent (that is, predictive) relationship between actions and goals is degraded in any way. Some of these tests have been used to probe the habitual nature of chronic drug self-administration for cocaine, alcohol, and nicotine in experimental animals, with, in every case, habitual control predominating (see [7, 43] for reviews). For example, it has been shown that overtraining of cocaine-seeking under a second-order schedule of reinforcement makes performance more vulnerable to suppression by DA receptor blockade of the dorsal striatum, compared with infusions into the ventral striatum [44]. This pattern contrasts markedly with that observed following the acquisition of drug-seeking behaviour, which, as we have seen, implicates especially the nucleus accumbens core (which mediates Pavlovian influences on instrumental behaviour [45]) and the dorsomedial striatum (which mediates action–outcome learning [46]). The nucleus accumbens core circuitry likely continues to play a part in the control of this behaviour, which can be assumed to be at least partly habitual in nature. A study that disconnected the nucleus accumbens core and the dorsolateral striatum by combining unilateral manipulations of each structure on opposite sides of the brain showed that a circuit functionally linking these two structures was implicated [47]. An obvious candidate for their interaction is the cascading circuitry that links the ventral striatum to the dorsal striatum in a unidirectional manner, via backward and forward projections to and from successive sectors of the striatum, beginning in the accumbens shell and terminating in the putamen, a possible site of stimulus–response habit-based learning [48]. This circuitry provides the basis for the BLA, via its direct projections to the nucleus accumbens core, to influence the dorsolateral striatum, and hence stimulus–response habits—circuitry that has been demonstrated electrophysiologically [49].

Another way of measuring compulsive behaviour is to make it 'risky' by unpredictably punishing drug-seeking behaviour on one lever which, on other occasions, gives access to a second taking lever, responding on which results in drug self-administration. After a short cocaine history, all rats suppressed their drug-seeking. However, after a long history of cocaine exposure, a proportion of rats continued to respond (the majority suppressed their drug-seeking), despite these adverse consequences, and this therefore fulfils an operational definition of compulsive drug-seeking [12] (Fig. 48.5). Intriguingly, the proportion of rats showing such compulsive cocaine-seeking (about 15–20%) is rather similar to the proportion of human drug abusers thought to make the transition to cocaine addiction. Drug-seeking under punishment is associated with reduced forebrain levels of serotonin [(37] and depends on the dorsolateral striatum [50], consistent with the view that compulsive drug-seeking reflects loss of control over habitual behaviour. Moreover, optogenetic stimulation of the medial prefrontal cortex (which is hypoactive in compulsive rats) restores sensitivity to punishment and reduces compulsive cocaine-seeking [38].

## Impulsivity vs compulsivity

The issue of individual differences in the propensity for addiction has led to the search for biobehavioural markers of possible vulnerability. An early suggestion for stimulant drug susceptibility was that those rats exhibiting behavioural hyperactivity in a novel test environment would subsequently respond for lower doses of d-amphetamine, perhaps as a consequence of their risky 'sensation-seeking' which hypothetically promoted drug-seeking [51]. Another finding has been that rats consistently responding prematurely in an attentional task (in other words, responding prior to the presentation of visual targets needing detection for food rewards) also had an increased tendency to self-administer cocaine, when allowed binge access to the drug, although there were no obvious differences in acquisition of this behaviour [52].They also exhibited compulsive drug-seeking in a procedure that measures addiction-like behavioural criteria (compulsivity, increased motivation, and persistent seeking in the signalled absence of the drug) [53]. Moreover, when behavioural hyperactivity was used to stratify the same population, there was no obvious effect in parallel with what had been shown earlier to affect the acquisition of drug-seeking; indeed 'high responder' rats were actually resistant to developing addiction-like behavioural criteria [53, 54]. Thus, it is possible that different phenotypes contribute to different aspects of drug addiction, for example to the tendencies to sample drug effects and for drug-seeking to become compulsive [7, 55]. Further analyses have been made of other predisposing factors that contribute to drug abuse in experimental animals, and other influences have been suggested to include the temporal discounting of reward (that is, choosing small, immediate rewards in preference to larger, delayed ones), risky decision-making, individual differences in Pavlovian conditioning, novelty seeking, and anxiety [55]. Different predisposing influences may exist for different drugs or for different components of abusing the same drug. For example, the propensity for stimulant self-administration in male rhesus monkeys has been shown to depend on factors such as social dominance (submissive monkeys being more susceptible) [56]. Moreover, although high impulsivity has been shown to predict nicotine [57], as well as cocaine susceptibility, it does not predict vulnerability to self-administer heroin [58]. This is an area in which it is clearly important to explore possible parallels with humans, and one feature of research into addiction using experimental animals has been how well the principles so gained from appropriate behavioural models sometimes appear to apply also to human drug addiction.

## Translation of experimental research on addiction in animals to humans

Striking parallels of research in experimental animals and humans addicted to drugs exist in both the behavioural and neural domains. Although much human research has revolved around relapse and its subjective correlates, which include the 'craving' or urge to take drugs, this has not handicapped application of the basic research findings to any great degree, as long as operational principles have been applied. An important example of how behavioural analysis is at least as important in humans as in experimental animals has been the observation of consistent drug preferences in drug-experienced humans for low doses of heroin that appear to occur without detecting any subjective drug effect [59]. It would appear that preference for certain drug effects may be occurring below the threshold for conscious detection of those effects, strongly implicating implicit factors at work, perhaps also involving brain regions not directly involved in conscious experience itself. Another intriguing connection is between the pharmacological studies described earlier, suggesting that drug-taking may begin as a form of self-medication by which rodents strive to attain an optimal level of functioning of the DA systems, and studies of the status of the central striatal DA function in healthy volunteers in relation to drug preference. Thus, volunteers without a history of drug abuse, but exhibiting low striatal D2/3 receptor binding, tended to find the effects of the psychomotor stimulant methylphenidate pleasurable, whereas those with high D2/3 striatal binding found them aversive [60, 61].

Research using experimental animals that has highlighted the role of the mesolimbic DA system and limbic–striatal mechanisms has stimulated parallel investigations in the human drug abuse literature. One of the main examples has been the work on DA receptors in human drug addicts by Volkow and colleagues. The authors were able to find, using a radioligand for DA D2/3 receptors with positron emission tomography (PET), that stimulant and heroin abusers, as well as alcoholics, all exhibited reductions in D2/3 DA receptor availability in the dorsal striatum [62], a striking endorsement of earlier animal work supporting a common role for DA in mediating the effects of a number of drugs of abuse. Important as these observations are, they entail a number of interpretative difficulties. These include whether the prime change is in D2 or D3 receptors (the radioligand in question being non-selective), whether it is pre- or post-synaptic (while acknowledging the much higher concentration of post-synaptic D2 receptors in the human striatum), and consequently the precise status of DA function, given the opposite effects that inhibitory presynaptic receptors and post-synaptic receptors have on DA function. These issues can all be addressed, and a current consensus is that the reduced D2/3 receptor function may be correlated with reduced DA activity (at least in chronic drug abusers) [63]. An additional finding of interest is that the reductions in D2/3 DA receptors are correlated with hypometabolism in the orbitofrontal cortex [64], a prefrontal region of great importance for reward function and decision-making cognition in humans. Therefore, it is evident that the changes in striatal DA status are associated with impaired cortical function—and may represent one of the deficits leading to impaired top–down control of behaviour, in this case impaired goal-directed behaviour, and suggestive of an alteration in the balance between goal-directed and habitual behaviour, favouring the latter, in drug addiction [7, 43].

However, a yet more difficult consideration to resolve is whether the changes in D2/3 DA receptors are effects of excessive drug exposure or actually predisposing causes of drug abuse, a question evidently difficult to address in humans without the aid of a prospective longitudinal study. A behavioural issue posing an analogous cause-and-effect quandary is whether impulsive decision-making and compulsive drug use arise from possible 'neurotoxic' effects of excessive drug-taking or again whether it is a predisposing factor. The presence of such predisposing factors in experimental animals described here suggests the latter [53]. Equally, studies of D2/3 DA receptors using microPET in high-impulsive rats showed that they exhibit reduced D2/3 receptors in the ventral striatum, suggesting that this change may, in part, reflect a pre-existing state in the rats, perhaps caused by some combination of genetic or environmental

factors [52]. It is possible, of course, that both predisposing and drug-induced factors combine to drive down D2/3 receptor availability.

The study of human drug abusers using other state-of-the-art neuroimaging methods, including structural magnetic resonance imaging (MRI), functional MRI, and diffusion tensor imaging, combined with sensitive behavioural indicators, is beginning to unravel the causes and effects of drug abuse. For example, it has been shown that measures of response inhibitory control (in which subjects have to cancel or restrain an already initiated response) are impaired in individuals with DSM-IV-defined stimulant drug dependence. However, of even greater significance was the fact that their siblings who did not abuse drugs were similarly impaired, as compared to age- and IQ-matched controls and to recreational drug abusers not attaining DSM-IV criteria of drug dependence [65]. This strongly implies an intermediate phenotype or endophenotype of impulsivity predicting vulnerability to stimulant drug addiction, in parallel with the animal model described previously. The hypothesis of an impulsivity endophenotype has been further supported using questionnaires to measure impulsivity and sensation-seeking; whereas the former scores were elevated in both the stimulant-dependent individuals and their siblings, elevated sensation-seeking was confined to the stimulant-dependent and recreational groups only [66].

What factors then protect the siblings from becoming drug-addicted and thus confer resilience? A functional MRI study may provide some insight, as this shows reduced activity in a region of the prefrontal cortex implicated in inhibitory response control (in the region of the right inferior frontal cortex) in stimulant-dependent individuals, contrasting with enhanced activity in the same region in their siblings (Fig. 48.6) [67]. Hypothetically, the siblings may be attempting to exert enhanced restraint over predispositions to

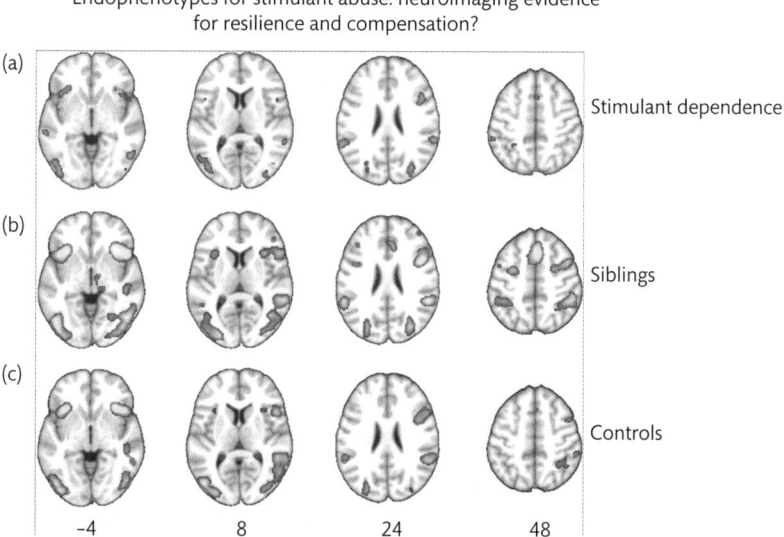

Endophenotypes for stimulant abuse: neuroimaging evidence for resilience and compensation?

**Fig. 48.6** (see Colour Plate section) Evidence of hypothetical resilience factors operating in siblings of stimulant-dependent individuals (bottom row scans) in terms of BOLD response overactivation of the right inferior frontal gyrus during functional magnetic resonance imaging study of the stop-signal reaction time task, as compared with healthy control volunteers (middle row scans) and stimulant-dependent individuals (top row)—the latter showing significant reductions, compared with controls. Significant brain activation maps were associated with stopping in each group ($P < 0.05$, family-wise error). Axial brain slices demonstrate main activation clusters per group at family-wise error, $P < 0.05$. The z-co-ordinate slices are: –4, 8, 24, and 48. The right side of each slice corresponds to the right side of the brain.

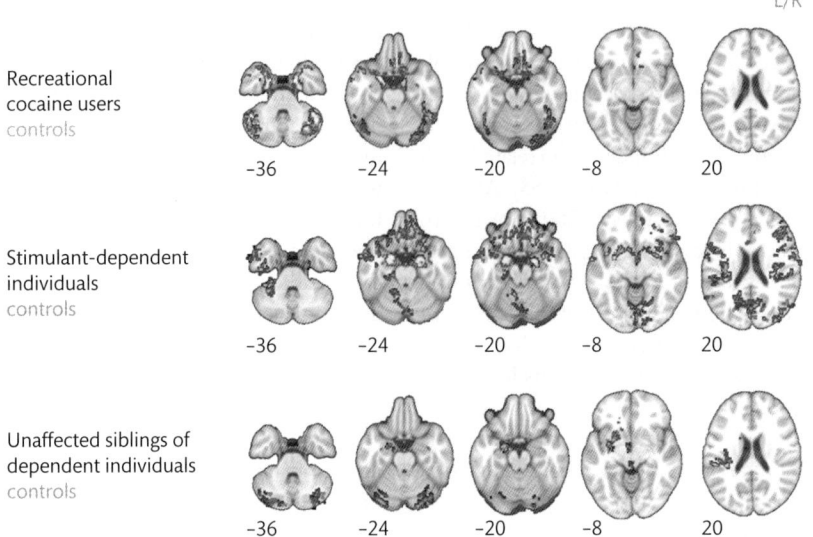

**Fig. 48.7** (see Colour Plate section) Structural brain abnormalities associated with stimulant exposure and familial risk. Blue voxels indicate a decrease, and red voxels indicate an increase, in grey matter volume, compared with control volunteers. Both recreational and dependent stimulant users showed significant increases in the parahippocampal gyrus, compared with healthy control volunteers, but differed with regard to abnormalities in the orbitofrontal cortex. Recreational users did not show any of the changes in brain regions associated with familial risk such as increased volume of the amygdala and putamen and decreased volume in the posterior insula. Siblings of stimulant-dependent stimulant abusers showed larger grey matter volumes in the basal ganglia, particularly the putamen. Sections and horizontal numbers below each section of the image refer to its plane position (mm) relative to the origin in MNI stereotactic space. L, left; R, right.

impulsive responding (although this may not always be successful). These attempts occur in the context of both the stimulant-dependent group as well as the siblings exhibiting reduced white matter innervation of the inferior frontal cortex via the arcuate fasciculus that correlates significantly with their performance on the inhibitory control task. There is, in fact, a burgeoning literature of failures in inhibitory control in drug abusers associated with cortical impairment (reviewed in [68]). Such factors could contribute to compulsive behaviour, in tandem with the hypothesized deficits in learning and conditioned drug responses observed in experimental animals.

There has been, by now, extensive confirmation that Pavlovian conditioned cues elicit disruptive craving responses and concomitant neural changes in activity in drug abusers in brain regions, consistent with what has been found in experimental animals. Thus, for example, Grant and Childress were among the first to demonstrate excessive activation of limbic regions, including the amygdala, in response to drug-related cues in drug abusers, compared with healthy volunteers [69, 70]. Consistent with stimulus–response habit-based dorsal striatal mediation of such effects, Volkow and colleagues found in functional MRI studies that drug cues associated with cocaine activated the dorsal, rather than the ventral, striatum [71]. Another study revealed similar findings for alcoholics, although, revealingly, recreational drinkers showed activation of the ventral striatum [72], clearly consistent in this cross-sectional study with a transition to dorsal striatal mechanisms in the drug-dependent individual.

Structural MRI has also shown that the amygdala and striatum tend to be larger in both stimulant-dependent individuals and their non-drug-abusing siblings, whereas the stimulant-dependent individuals (though not recreational users) have reduced cortical grey matter in regions such as the orbitofrontal and temporal cortices [65] (Fig. 48.7). The extent of reductions in grey matter in the ventromedial prefrontal cortex has been shown to be related to the duration of stimulant drug use, suggesting that the drug has exerted a cumulative toxic effect, as well as to measures of compulsive drug use obtained using the Obsessive Compulsive Drug Use Scale (OCDUS). Indeed, a significant correlation between grey matter volume in the inferior frontal and rectal gyri and measures of compulsive cocaine-taking (OCDUS) has been demonstrated in a group of chronic cocaine users [73] (Fig. 48.8). These findings suggest that stimulant drug abuse does impair cortical functioning, although it is not known to what extent these changes are permanent and irreversible, for example, following abstinence. Other evidence can be cited in support of the shift in balance between systems of goal-directed control vs habit learning in stimulant drug abusers [74]. Comparable analyses exist of the sequelae of chronic alcoholism, as well as other drugs of abuse [72].

Behavioural studies of human stimulant drug addiction using the devaluation method and other computational paradigms are compatible with the hypothesis of habit-based learning in stimulant-dependent individuals. Thus, for example, stimulant abusers were slower to learn goal-directed responses that earned points leading to monetary reward but exhibited more robust appetitive habits than controls. They were also impaired in learning to avoid electric shocks, although their aversive habitual responding was normal [74]. These results suggest that there might be specific behavioural approaches to treatment.

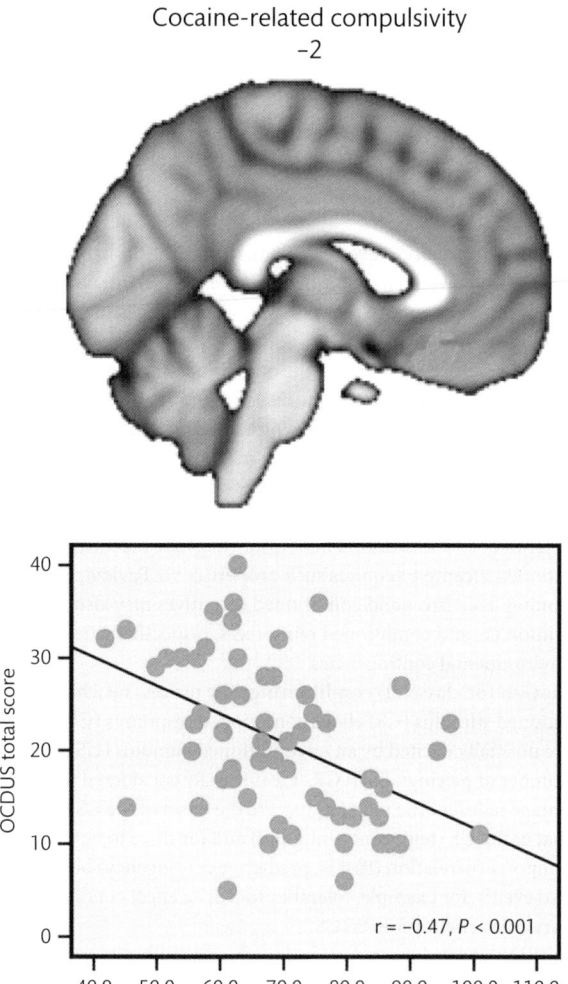

**Fig. 48.8** Significant association between grey matter volume and measures of compulsivity in a group of chronic cocaine users. Regions that correlated significantly with compulsive cocaine-taking (as assessed by OCDUS) are coloured in green. The scatter plot below the brain image shows the correlation between this measure and grey matter volume for each drug user in those regions. The probability threshold for significance was P ~0.002 for each analysis. The statistical results are overlaid on the FSL MNI152 standard T1 image, and the numbers above each section of the image refer to its plane position (mm) relative to the origin in MNI stereotactic space. L, left; R, right.

Reproduced from *Brain*, 134(Pt 7), Ersche KD, Barnes A, Jones PS, *et al.*, Abnormal structure of frontostriatal brain systems is associated with aspects of impulsivity and compulsivity in cocaine dependence, pp. 2013–24, Copyright (2011), with permission from Oxford University Press.

## Treatment of drug addiction via translational studies

Despite the evident progress in understanding the behavioural and neural mechanisms underlying drug addiction, we are still some way from finding effective treatments for this heterogenous and difficult patient group. This may arise, in part, from the habitual nature of addiction and its relapsing nature, which are antithetical to mainline cognitive behavioural therapy techniques, although motivational enhancement programmes may prove useful. Substitution

pharmacotherapy with the long-acting opioid methadone has long been a staple procedure for heroin abuse, although this can have several deleterious side effects, and there is certainly scope for promising alternative opioid treatments such as buprenorphine. For nicotine addiction, there is a variety of substitution therapies based on the nicotine patch, gum, and lozenges, and now nicotine vaping devices, as well the partial nicotinic receptor agonist varenicline [75]. Nalmephene, an opioid receptor antagonist, has recently been introduced for the treatment of alcoholism through its ability to reduce volumes of alcohol drunk in a binge [76]. No such effective substitution treatments exist for stimulant drugs, although the atypical stimulant modafinil may offer some promise.

These are important and effective harm reduction strategies that might, though not necessarily, open the door to abstinence and the prevention of relapse, which are major goals in the treatment of addiction. However, it should be possible to develop such treatments and there are different targets in this regard, for example to reduce the impact of stress and anxiety associated with relapse to alcohol use or to medicate dysphoric and anhedonic states that can persist long into withdrawal from stimulants, nicotine, and opiates [77], or treatments that reduce the impact of drug-associated stimuli on craving and relapse [78]. Many treatment leads have been identified in a wide range of animal studies in the context of drug discovery programmes, well reviewed in the recent surveys by Koob and Mason [75] and Everitt [27]. Some have been licensed by the FDA, such as the opiate receptor antagonist naltrexone and acamprosate (a partial agonist at glutamate NMDA receptors/glutamate metabotropic receptor antagonist), for alcohol abuse. Experimental agents based on combating the effects of stress (corticotrophin-releasing factor receptor antagonist or dynorphin-kappa opioid receptor antagonists) or impulsivity (atomoxetine) or related anti-relapse actions by putative actions on top–down circuitry (gabapentin, *N*-acetylcysteine) have so far been shown to have limited effects in human trials but remain under experimental investigation. Despite a range of pharmacological agents having the ability to reduce drug cue-elicited cocaine-seeking and relapse in animal models, including a D3 dopamine receptor antagonist, a μ-opioid receptor antagonist, and drugs interfering with glutamate transmission, none has yet successfully made it to the clinic [27].

The evident overlap of neural circuitry controlling responses to emotional cues and memories with those implicated in addiction has led to the revisiting of extinction [79], as well as the application of memory reconsolidation methodologies [80] (Fig. 48.9), by which the associative links between drugs and associated cues that help to maintain drug-seeking behaviour can be disrupted in experimental animals by a combination of behavioural procedure and pharmacological intervention. While it has been shown that drug cue extinction can be achieved in a clinical setting, with consequent reductions in cue-elicited craving, it is clear that this provides, at best, a mildly effective relapse prevention treatment because of the context dependence of extinction (therapy in the clinic does not extend to real-life environments), such that spontaneous recovery, renewal, and reinstatement of the extinguished response are common [81, 82]. However, the recent demonstration of 'super-extinction' [83], achieved by combining a brief drug cue memory retrieval with a conventional CS extinction protocol followed after a brief delay (30 minutes), has re-awoken interest in extinction therapies, since, in this case, a more complete and long-term extinction of the CS is

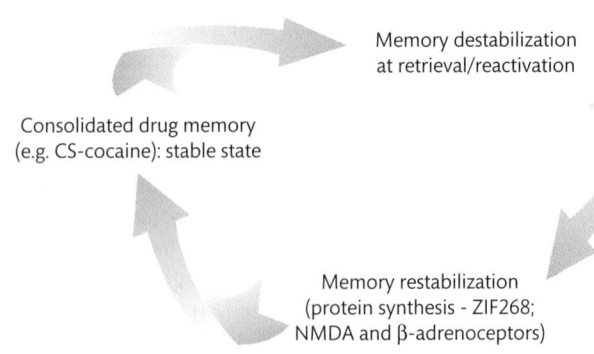

**Fig. 48.9** Illustration of the concept of memory reconsolidation. The consolidated drug memory, established by repeated Pavlovian association with an environmental stimulus (CS) and self-administered drug effect, is stored in a stable state. Brief presentations of the drug CS (called 'reactivation') can result in destabilization of the memory in the brain (in the case of a CS–drug memory, in the basolateral amygdala). The memory can persist in the brain if it is restabilized through *de novo* protein synthesis. The expression of the protein ZIF268 is a requirement of cued drug memory reconsolidation in the basolateral amygdala and is regulated by activation of NMDA receptors. Memory reconsolidation can be prevented by inhibiting protein synthesis in the amygdala or knocking down ZIF268 by infusing *zif268* antisense oligonucleotides or by blocking NMDA or β-adrenoceptors. Systemic NMDA or β-adrenoceptor blockade also prevents drug memory reconsolidation. The result is drug memory 'erasure', with the consequence that the drug-associated CS can no longer support drug-seeking, and this thereby reduces the propensity to relapse [27].

Reproduced from *Eur J Neurosci.*, 40(1), Everitt BJ, Neural and psychological mechanisms underlying compulsive drug seeking habits and drug memories--indications for novel treatments of addiction, pp. 2163–82, Copyright (2014), with permission from John Wiley and Sons. Reproduced under the Creative Commons Attribution License (CC BY).

achieved. Although most often shown in conditioned fear studies, an impressive demonstration of the super-extinction of a CS–drug memory in animals self-administering cocaine or heroin, as well as, most remarkably, in a heroin-addicted inpatient population, with evidence of a decrement in craving and physiological responses to heroin cues 6 months later [84], suggests further detailed investigation is warranted. The neural basis of these effects remains unknown.

Targeting memory reconsolidation (Fig. 48.9) also holds translational promise [80, 85]. It is now widely accepted that under specific circumstances, memory retrieval (or, more appropriately, 'reactivation') that is too brief to engage extinction learning causes the memory trace to become labile in the brain, from which it must undergo protein synthesis-dependent restablization if it is to persist [86]. Reconsolidation can be prevented by treatment with an amnestic agent, such as an NMDA receptor antagonist or a β-adrenergic receptor antagonist, given just once in conjunction with the brief memory reactivation [27, 87]. This results in amnesia and apparent erasure of the memory trace, or a great diminution of the strength of the memory, such that presenting the CS subsequently no longer elicits conditioned fear (in the case of aversive conditioning) or instrumental drug-seeking (in the case of animals seeking cocaine or alcohol) [27, 87, 88]. While the effects to reduce conditioned fear in animals has been successfully translated to the clinic in the successful treatment of phobias [89], to date, attempts to do so in the treatment of addiction have met with only limited, or sometimes no, success. It seems that a major obstacle to deploying reconsolidation strategies in the treatment of addiction is defining precisely the conditions under which retrieval results in the destabilization of the memory. If the behavioural parameters can be defined precisely—a challenge when the conditioning history is so variable and of such long duration—then this approach to relapse prevention holds great promise.

## GLOSSARY OF KEY TERMS

**Positive reinforcer.** An event which increases the probability of a response upon which it is contingent, for example, intravenous drug infusions maintaining lever pressing, alcohol ingestion maintaining licking or drinking.

**Negative reinforcer.** An event, the omission or termination of which increases the probability of the response upon which it is contingent, for example, withdrawal symptoms precipitated by scheduled administration of naloxone in morphine-dependent animals avoided by lever pressing which postpones the naloxone.

**Incentive.** A stimulus that elicits an approach behaviour (positive incentive) or a withdrawal behaviour (negative incentive). A conditioned incentive acquires such properties via Pavlovian conditioning. Incentives and conditioned incentives may also function as reinforcers and conditioned reinforcers, respectively, depending on environmental contingencies.

**Pavlovian (or classical) conditioning.** The process by which a conditioned stimulus (CS) elicits conditioned responses (CRs) that are normally elicited by an unconditioned stimulus (US) after a number of pairings. Such CRs are normally considered to be involuntary reflexes. The pairings require the onset of the CS to precede that of the US (temporal contiguity) and for there to be a positive temporal correlation (that is, predictive contingency) between the two events, for example, tolerance to a drug effect conditioned to a particular environmental CS.

**Conditioned reinforcer.** A stimulus which acquires its reinforcing properties (positive or negative) by pairings with other, generally primary, reinforcers such as food, drugs, sex, or electric shock. A stimulus can function as a conditioned reinforcer or as a discriminative stimulus in the same situation.

**Contingency.** A consistent temporal relationship between two (or more) events that reduces the uncertainty of the subsequent event, for example, between particular stimuli and particular responses.

**Action–outcome learning.** When instrumental actions are goal-directed, the actions (for example, lever-pressing) are made with the intention of obtaining the goal. The actions are sensitive to the devaluation of the goal; for example, an animal that has learnt to lever-press for food will respond much less or not at all for that food if it is devalued either by making it ill after ingesting the food or by pre-feeding to satiety with the same food. This is called **reinforcer devaluation**. It is very easy to devalue ingestive reinforcers, but not intravenously self-administered drugs such as cocaine.

**Stimulus–response or 'habit' learning.** In habit learning, instrumental performance is acquired through the association of responses with stimuli present during training. It therefore reflects the formation of stimulus–response associations, and reinforcers primarily serve the function of strengthening the stimulus–response association, but they do not become encoded as a goal. Therefore, devaluing the reinforcer does not affect instrumental responding.

**Drug-taking.** A term used to describe drug self-administration when the drug is readily available, for example, following each instrumental response on a lever or the simple drinking of alcohol (so-called continuous reinforcement). The subject does not need to forage or to work for the drug nor mediate delays in acquiring, that is, does not actively need to 'seek' the drug.

**Drug-seeking.** This is instrumental or foraging behaviour performed to give access to the opportunity to take a drug, as measured under second-order schedules of reinforcement, in seeking-taking, and extinction–reinstatement tasks in animal models.

**Compulsive drug-seeking.** This is instrumental behaviour that persists in the face of adverse consequences such as punishment or the risk of punishment.

## REFERENCES

1. Koob GF, Le Moal M. *Neurobiology of Addiction*. San Diego, CA: Academic Press; 2005.
2. Solomon RL, Corbit JD. An opponent-process theory of motivation. I. Temporal dynamics of affect. *Psychol Rev*. 1974;81:119–45.
3. Koob GF, Le Moal M. Drug abuse: hedonic homeostatic dysregulation. *Science*. 1997;278:52–8.
4. Koob G, Le Moal M. Drug addiction, dysregulation of reward, and allostasis. *Neuropsychopharmacology*. 2001;24:97–129.
5. O'Brien CP, Childress AR, Mclellan A, Ehrman R. A learning model of addiction. *Res Publ Assoc Res Nerv Ment Dis*. 1992;70:157–77.
6. Everitt BJ, Robbins TW. Neural systems of reinforcement for drug addiction: from actions to habits to compulsion. *Nat Neurosci*. 2005;8:1481–9.
7. Everitt BJ, Robbins TW. Drug addiction: updating actions to habits to compulsions ten years on. *Annu Rev Psychol*. 2016;67:23–50.
8. Olds J, Milner P. Positive reinforcement produced by electrical stimulation of septal area and other regions of rat brain. *J Comp Physiol Psychol*. 1954;47:419–27.
9. Gerber GJ, Wise RA. Pharmacological regulation of intravenous cocaine and heroin self-administration in rats: a variable dose paradigm. *Pharmacol Biochem Behav*. 1989;32:527–31.
10. De Wit H, Wise RA. Blockade of cocaine reinforcement in rats with the dopamine receptor blocker pimozide, but not with the noradrenergic blockers phentolamine or phenoxybenzamine. *Can J Psychol*. 1977;31:195–203.
11. Wise RA, Rompre PP. Brain dopamine and reward. *Annu Rev Psychol*. 1989;40:191–225.
12. Pelloux Y, Everitt BJ, Dickinson A. Compulsive drug seeking by rats under punishment: effects of drug taking history. *Psychopharmacology*. 2007;194:127–37.
13. Deroche-Gamonet V, Belin D, Piazza PV. Evidence for addiction-like behavior in the rat. *Science*. 2004;305:1014–17.
14. Roberts DC, Corcoran ME, Fibiger HC. On the role of ascending catecholaminergic systems in intravenous self-administration of cocaine. *Pharmacol Biochem Behav*. 1977;6:615–20.
15. Hoebel BG, Monaco AP, Hernandez L, Aulisi EF, Stanley BG, Lenard L. Self-injection of amphetamine directly into the brain. *Psychopharmacology*. 1983;81:158–63.
16. Phillips GD, Robbins TW, Everitt BJ. Bilateral intra-accumbens self-administration of d-amphetamine: antagonism with intra-accumbens SCH-23390 and sulpiride. *Psychopharmacology*. 1994;114:477–85.
17. Bozarth MA, Wise RA. Anatomically distinct opiate receptor fields mediate reward and physical dependence. *Science*. 1984;224:516–17.
18. Koob G, Maldonado R, Stinus L. Neural substrates of opiate withdrawal. *Trends Neurosci*. 1992;15:186–91.
19. Ettenberg A, Pettit HO, Bloom FE, Koob GF. Heroin and cocaine intravenous self-administration in rats: Mediation by separate neural systems. *Psychopharmacology*. 1982;78:204–9.
20. Mackintosh N. *The Psychology of Animal Learning*. Oxford: Academic Press; 1974.
21. Cador M, Robbins TW, Everitt BJ. Involvement of the amygdala in stimulus-reward associations: interaction with the ventral striatum. *Neuroscience*. 1989;30:77–86.
22. Taylor JR, Robbins T. 6-Hydroxydopamine lesions of the nucleus accumbens, but not of the caudate nucleus, attenuate enhanced responding with reward-related stimuli produced by intra-accumbens d-amphetamine. *Psychopharmacology (Berl)*. 1986;90:390–7.
23. Everitt B, Robbins T. Second-order schedules of drug reinforcement in rats and monkeys: measurement of reinforcing efficacy and drug-seeking behaviour. *Psychopharmacology*. 2000;153:17–30.
24. Goldberg SR, Morse WH, Goldberg DM. Behavior maintained under a second-order schedule by intramuscular injection of morphine or cocaine in rhesus monkeys. *J Pharmacol Exp Ther*. 1976;199:278–86.
25. Schindler C, Panlilio L, Goldberg S. Second-order schedules of drug self-administration in animals. *Psychopharmacology (Berl)*. 2002;163(3–4):327–44.
26. Panlilio L, Yasar S, Nemeth-Coslett R, *et al.* Human cocaine-seeking behavior and its control by drug-associated stimuli in the laboratory. *Neuropsychopharmacology*. 2005;30:433–43.
27. Everitt BJ. Neural and psychological mechanisms underlying compulsive drug seeking habits and drug memories—indications for novel treatments of addiction. *Eur J Neurosci*. 2014;40:2163–82.
28. Whitelaw RB, Markou A, Robbins TW, Everitt BJ. Excitotoxic lesions of the basolateral amygdala impair the acquisition of cocaine-seeking behaviour under a second-order schedule of reinforcement. *Psychopharmacology (Berl)*. 1996;127: 213–24.
29. Ito R, Robbins T, Everitt B. Differential control over cocaine-seeking behavior by nucleus accumbens core and shell. *Nat Neurosci*. 2004;7:389–97.
30. Di Ciano P, Everitt BJ. Direct interactions between the basolateral amygdala and nucleus accumbens core underlie cocaine-seeking behavior by rats. *J Neurosci*. 2004;24:7167–73.
31. Alderson HL, Robbins TW, Everitt BJ. The effects of excitotoxic lesions of the basolateral amygdala on the acquisition of heroin-seeking behaviour in rats. *Psychopharmacology*. 2000;153:111–19.
32. Kalivas PW, McFarland K. Brain circuitry and the reinstatement of cocaine-seeking behavior. *Psychopharmacology*. 2003;168(1–2):44–56.
33. Moore RJ, Vinsant SL, Nader MA, Porrino L, Friedman DP. Effect of cocaine self-administration on dopamine D2 receptors in rhesus monkeys. *Synapse* 1998;30:88–96
34. Robbins TW, Everitt BJ. Drug addiction: bad habits add up. *Nature*. 1999;398:567–70.
35. Jentsch J, Taylor J. Impulsivity resulting from frontostriatal dysfunction in drug abuse: implications for the control of

behavior by reward-related stimuli. *Psychopharmacology (Berl)*. 1999;146:373–90.

36. Schoenbaum G, Shaham Y. The role of orbitofrontal cortex in drug addiction: s review of preclinical studies. *Biol Psychiatry*. 2008;63:256–62.

37. Pelloux Y, Dilleen R, Economidou D, Theobald D, Everitt B. Reduced forebrain serotonin transmission is causally involved in the development of compulsive cocaine seeking in rats. *Neuropsychopharmacology*. 2012;37:2505–14.

38. Chen B, Yau H, Hatch C, et al. Rescuing cocaine-induced prefrontal cortex hypoactivity prevents compulsive cocaine seeking. *Nature*. 2013;496:359–62.

39. Robinson TE, Berridge KC. The neural basis of drug craving: an incentive-sensitization theory of addiction. *Brain Res Brain Res Rev*. 1993;18:247–91.

40. Dias-Ferreira E, Sousa J, Melo I, et al. Chronic stress causes frontostriatal reorganization and affects decision-making. *Science*. 2009;325:621–5.

41. Nelson A, Killcross S. Amphetamine exposure enhances habit formation. *J Neurosci*. 2006;26:3805–12.

42. Dickinson A. Actions and habits: the development of behavioural autonomy. *Philosophical Transactions of the Royal Society of London B Biological Sciences*. 1985;308:67–78.

43. Hogarth L, Balleine B, Corbit L, Killcross S. Associative learning mechanisms underpinning the transition from recreational drug use to addiction. *Ann N Y Acad Sci*. 2013;1282:12–24.

44. Vanderschuren L, Di Ciano P, Everitt B. Involvement of the dorsal striatum in cue-controlled cocaine seeking. *J Neurosci*. 2005;25:8665–70.

45. Cardinal R, Parkinson JA, Hall J, Everitt B. Emotion and motivation: the role of the amygdala, ventral striatum, and prefrontal cortex. *Neurosci Biobehav Rev*. 2002;26:321–52.

46. Murray JE, Belin D, Everitt BJ. Double dissociation of the dorsomedial and dorsolateral striatal control over the acquisition and performance of cocaine seeking. *Neuropsychopharmacology*. 2012;37:2456–66.

47. Belin D, Everitt BJ. Cocaine seeking habits depend upon dopamine-dependent serial connectivity linking the ventral with the dorsal striatum. *Neuron*. 2008;57:432–41.

48. Haber S, Fudge J, McFarland N. Striatonigrostriatal pathways in primates form an ascending spiral from the shell to the dorsolateral striatum. *J Neurosci*. 2000;20:2369–82.

49. Murray JE, Belin-Rauscent A, Simon M, et al. Basolateral and central amygdala differentially recruit and maintain dorsolateral striatum-dependent cocaine-seeking habits. *Nat Commun*. 2015;6:10088.

50. Jonkman S, Pelloux Y, Everitt B. Differential roles of the dorsolateral and midlateral striatum in punished cocaine seeking. *J Neurosci*. 2012;32:4645–50.

51. Piazza P, Deminiere J, Le Moal M, Simon H. Factors that predict individual vulnerability to amphetamine self-administration. *Science*. 1989;245:1511–13.

52. Dalley JW, Fryer TD, Brichard L, et al. Nucleus accumbens D2/3 receptors predict trait impulsivity and cocaine reinforcement. *Science*. 2007;315:1267–70.

53. Belin D, Mar AC, Dalley JW, Robbins TW, Everitt BJ. High impulsivity predicts the switch to compulsive cocaine-taking. *Science*. 2008;320:1352–5.

54. Vanhille N, Belin-Rauscent A, Mar AC, Ducret E, Belin D. High locomotor reactivity to novelty is associated with an increased propensity to choose saccharin over cocaine: new insights

into the vulnerability to addiction. *Neuropsychopharmacology*. 2015;40:577–89.

55. Belin D, Belin-Rauscent A, Everitt BJ, Dalley JW. In search of predictive endophenotypes in addiction: insights from preclinical research. *Genes Brain Behav*. 2016;15:74–88.

56. Morgan D, Grant KA, Gage HD, et al. Social dominance in monkeys: dopamine D2 receptors and cocaine self-administration. *Nat Neurosci*. 2002;5:169–74.

57. Diergaarde L, Pattij T, Poortvliet I, et al. Impulsive Choice and impulsive action predict vulnerability to distinct stages of nicotine seeking in rats. *Biol Psychiatry*. 2008;63:301–8.

58. McNamara R, Dalley J, Robbins T, Everitt B, Belin D. Trait-like impulsivity does not predict escalation of heroin self-administration in the rat. *Psychopharmacology (Berl)*. 2010;212:453–64.

59. Lamb RJ, Preston KL, Schindler CW, et al. The reinforcing and subjective effects of morphine in post-addicts: a dose-response study. *J Pharmacol Exp Ther*. 1991;259:1165–73.

60. Volkow ND, Wang GJ, Fowler JS, et al. Prediction of reinforcing responses to psychostimulants in humans by brain dopamine D2 receptor levels. *Am J Psychiatry*. 1999;156:1440–3.

61. Volkow N. The addicted human brain viewed in the light of imaging studies: brain circuits and treatment strategies. *Neuropharmacology*. 2004;47:3–13.

62. Volkow N, Fowler J, Wang G, Swanson J, Telang F. Dopamine in drug abuse and addiction: results of imaging studies and treatment implications. *Arch Neurol*. 2007;64:1575–9.

63. Martinez D, Kim J-H, Krystal J, Abi-Dargham A. Imaging the neurochemistry of alcohol and substance abuse. *Neuroimag Clin N Am*. 2007;17:539–55.

64. Volkow N, Fowler J, Wang G, Hitzemann R. Decreased dopamine D2 receptor availability is associated with reduced frontal metabolism in cocaine abusers. *Synapse*. 1993;14:169–77.

65. Ersche K, Jones P, Williams G, Turton A, Robbins T, Bullmore E. Abnormal brain structure implicated in stimulant drug addiction. *Science*. 2012;335:601–4.

66. Ersche K, Jones P, Williams G, Smith D, Bullmore E, Robbins T. Distinctive personality traits and neural correlates associated with stimulant drug use versus familial risk of stimulant dependence. *Biol Psychiatry*. 2013;74:137–44.

67. Morein-Zamir S, Simon Jones P, Bullmore ET, Robbins TW, Ersche KD. Prefrontal hypoactivity associated with impaired inhibition in stimulant-dependent individuals but evidence for hyperactivation in their unaffected siblings. *Neuropsychopharmacology*. 2013;38:1945–53.

68. Morein-Zamir S, Robbins TW. Fronto-striatal circuits in response-inhibition: relevance to addiction. *Brain Research*. 2014;21:488–97.

69. Grant S, London ED, Newlin DB, et al. Activation of memory circuits during cue-elicited cocaine craving. *Proc Natl Acad Sci U S A*. 1996;93:12040–5.

70. Childress A, Mozley P, McElgin W, Fitzgerald J, Reivich M, O'Brien C. Limbic activation during cue-induced cocaine craving. *Am J Psychiatry*. 1999;156:11–18.

71. Volkow N, Wang GJ, Telang F, et al. Cocaine cues and dopamine in dorsal striatum: mechanism of craving in cocaine addiction. *J Neurosci*. 2006;26:6583–8.

72. Vollstadt-Klein S, Wichert S, Rabinstein J, et al. Initial, habitual and compulsive alcohol use is characterized by a shift of cue processing from ventral to dorsal striatum. *Addiction*. 2010;105:1741–9.

73. Ersche K, Barnes A, Simon Jones P, Morein-Zamir S, Robbins T, Bullmore E. Abnormal structure of frontostriatal brain systems is associated with aspects of impulsivity and compulsivity in cocaine dependence. *Brain.* 2011;134(Pt 7):2013–24.

74. Ersche KD, Gillan CM, Jones PS, *et al.* Carrots and sticks fail to change behavior in cocaine addiction. *Science.* 2016;352:1468–71.

75. Koob GF, Mason BJ. Existing and future drugs for the treatment of the dark side of addiction. *Annu Rev Pharmacol Toxicol.* 2016;56:299–322.

76. Soyka M. Nalmephene for the treastment of alcohol depdendence: a current update. *J Neuropsychopharmacol.* 2014;17:675–84.

77. Koob G, Le Moal M. Addiction and the brain antireward system. *Annu Rev Psychol.* 2008;59:29–53.

78. O'Brien CP. Anticraving medications for relapse prevention: a possible new class of psychoactive medications. *Am J Psychiatry.* 2005;162:1423–31.

79. Myers KM, Carlezon WA, Jr. Extinction of drug- and withdrawal-paired cues in animal models: relevance to the treatment of addiction. *Neurosci Biobehav Rev.* 2010;35:285–302.

80. Milton A, Everitt B. The psychological and neurochemical mechanisms of drug memory reconsolidation: implications for the treatment of addiction. *Eur J Neurosci.* 2010;31:2308–19.

81. Carter BL, Tiffany ST. Meta-analysis of cue-reactivity in addiction research. *Addiction.* 1999;94:327–40.

82. Conklin CA, Tiffany ST. Applying extinction research and theory to cue-exposure in addiction treatments. *Addiction.* 2002;97:155–67.

83. Monfils MH, Cowansage KK, Klann E, LeDoux JE. Extinction-reconsolidation boundaries: key to persistent attenuation of fear memories. *Science.* 2009;324:951–5.

84. Xue Y, Luo Y, Wu P, *et al.* A memory retrieval-extinction procedure to prevent drug craving and relapse. *Science.* 2012;336:241–5.

85. Taylor J, Olausson P, Quinn J, Torregrossa M. Targeting extinction and reconsolidation mechanisms to combat the impact of drug cues on addiction. *Neuropharmacology.* 2009;56(Suppl 1):186–95.

86. Nader K, Schafe G, Le Doux J. Fear memories require protein synthesis in the amygdala for reconsolidation after retrieval. *Nature.* 2000;406:722–6.

87. Nader K, Hardt O. A single standard for memory: the case for reconsolidation. *Nature Rev Neurosci.* 2009;10:224–34.

88. Schramm MJW, Everitt BJ, Milton AL. Bidirectional modulation of alcohol-associated memory reconsolidation through manipulation of adrenergic signaling. *Neuropsychopharmacology.* 2016;41:1103–11.

89. Soeter M, Kindt M. An abrupt transformation of phobic behavior after a post-retrieval amnesic agent. *Biol Psychiatry.* 2015;78:880–6.

90. Koob G. Drugs of abuse: anatomy, pharmacology and function of reward pathways. *Trends Pharmacol Sci.* 1992;13:177–84.

91. Koob GF, Everitt BJ, Robbins TW. Reward, motivation and addiction. In: Squire LR, Bloom FE, du Lac S, Ghosh A, Spitzer NC (eds). *Fundamental Neuroscience.* San Diego, CA: Elsevier; 2008. pp. 987–1016.

92. Ito R, Dalley J, Howes SR, Robbins T, Everitt B. Dissociation in conditioned dopaminer release in the nucleus accumbens core and shell in response to cocaine cues and during cocaine-seeking behavior in rats. *J Neurosci.* 2000;20:7489–95.

93. Ito R, Dalley J, Robbins T, Everitt B. Dopamine release in the dorsal striatum during cocaine-seeking behavior under the control of a drug-associated cue. *J Neurosci.* 2002;22:6247–53.

94. Pelloux Y, Murray JE, Everitt BJ. Differential vulnerability to the punishment of cocaine related behaviours: effects of locus of punishment, cocaine taking history and alternative reinforcer availability. *Psychopharmacology (Berl).* 2015;232:125–34.

# 49

# Genetics of substance use disorders

*Yann Le Strat, Nicolas Ramoz, and Philip Gorwood*

## Genetics of substance use disorders: a historical perspective

The currently accepted claim that 'addiction is a brain disease with a genetic component' would sound familiar to a nineteenth-century alienist. While Esquirol had already mentioned the importance of heredity in the physiopathology of mental disorders, it was in 1860 that Morel gave heredity a central place within nosography by coining the term 'degeneration theory'. Morel separated psychiatric disorders into two categories, depending on whether they are hereditary or not. Magnan and other French psychiatrists retained this nomenclature. If the scientific rationale is sometimes surprising, or even fanciful, some questions remain relevant in the twenty-first century. Thus, Bouchereau discusses the impact of placental transfer of alcohol as a possible confounding factor in the heritability of alcohol use disorder (AUD), and Morel evokes the possible inheritance of a diathesis, that is, a predisposition to the disease close to the modern concept of endophenotype. Finally, the 'law of double fertilization' of the same author attributes an identical importance to the 'moral elements and organic conditions' in the development of a mental disorder such as AUD, which could be compared to the gene × environment interactions at the forefront of our current thinking.

## Heritability of substance use disorders

It has been over 50 years since Kaij *et al.*'s first twin study on AUD, which suggested substance use disorders to be, at least in part, due to genetic variance. Subsequent twin and family studies have continued to support a genetic component to substance use disorders (SUD). Having a first-degree relative with SUD confers a greater risk than any individual environmental factor.

Heritability is defined as the proportion of the phenotypic variance attributed to additive genetic factors. Several methods have been used to calculate heritability. The data from twin studies are most often presented as pair and proband concordance in monozygotic (MZ) and dizygotic (DZ) twins. Pair concordance represents the percentage of all twin pairs within the sample who are concordant for disease.

Twin studies remain key to estimates of heritability in SUD, and their basis can be simply stated. Falconer's equation of heritability states that $h^2 = 2(rMZ - rDZ)$, with $h^2$ = heritability, rMZ = intraclass correlation of MZ twins, and rDZ = intraclass correlation of DZ twins.

This equation assumes that:

1. The presence or absence of the disease is determined by genetic and normally distributed environmental factors.
2. All genetic influences are additive.
3. MZ twins share 100% of segregating genes.
4. DZ twins share, on average, 50% of segregating genes.
5. MZ and DZ twin pairs have a similar shared environment.
6. Genetic and environmental variations act independently of each other.

These assumptions are likely to be an oversimplification of the real genetic and environmental actions, and the estimations of heritability using this model are generally considered to be too narrowed, given that they include neither gene × gene nor gene × environment interactions.

Twin studies also assume random mating. However, a predisposition for SUD may be more frequently observed than expected in the parents of twins, and therefore, the genetic correlation between DZ twins is increased as a function of such assortive mating, biasing the estimation of heritability.

The estimations of heritability for alcohol, nicotine, cannabis, and illicit SUD across selected samples of twins are reported in Table 49.1 [1–3].

The recent twin literature suggests that this heritability of the completed stage of addiction (that is, the genetic influence on the diagnosis of SUD) lumps together genetic factors involved at different stages of an addiction. Firstly, some genetic factors increase the risk that individuals are exposed to a substance and experiment with it. Secondly, other genetic factors are involved in the reinforcing effect of the substance. Thirdly, genetic variants might also modify the risk for developing an SUD after regular use. Fourthly, individual variation in the metabolism or pharmacological action of the substance may modulate the risk for addiction. Heritability will be a complex composite of the genetic factors operating early and late in the exposure to the substance of interest.

Heritability of addictions is specific to the population and varies by gender, is influenced by the cultural environment, and will also

**Table 49.1** Heritability of alcohol use disorder, nicotine dependence, cannabis use disorder, and illicit substance use disorder among twin cohorts

| Sample | Alcohol use disorder | Nicotine dependence | Cannabis use disorder | Illicit substance use disorder |
|---|---|---|---|---|
| VATSPUD | 52% | 52% | | 60–80% |
| Vietnam era twins | 0–65% | 60% | 33% | 34% |
| National Swedish register | 22–57% | 48–62% | 70% | |
| Meta-analysis of twin studies | 43–53% [1] | 37% [2] | 51–59% [3] | |

be modified by exposure to the substance. If a trait or behaviour has no variability, even if it is strongly supported by genetic factors, its heritability cannot be estimated. For example, in the western adult population, it is not meaningful to examine the heritability of lifetime alcohol use, since most adults are likely to report at least one drink in their lifetime. Similarly, the heritability of nicotine dependence has 'increased' in women from zero in those born at the beginning of the twentieth century to levels comparable to those seen in men for those born after 1940, because of the greater opportunity for tobacco use in women in the second part of the twentieth century. The expression of the involved susceptibility genes could not be estimated when women had very limited access to tobacco [4].

## Endophenotypes

SUD constitute a broad category of heterogenous phenotypes, with patients exhibiting a large range of biomarkers and symptom severity, which has further complicated efforts to identify genetic variants. Employing more specific definitions of phenotypes may be more important than using larger sample sizes for detecting true genetic associations. The use of endophenotypes or objective measures of specific neurobiological functions may be particularly helpful in reducing clinical heterogeneity.

Neurobehavioural phenotypes associated with SUD include impulsivity and novelty seeking, stress reactivity, behavioural disinhibition, trait anxiety, and attention allocation, among many others. The expression of these traits varies through the lifespan and during the addiction's stages. For example, impulsivity is higher during adolescence, a period associated with enhanced experimentation with psychoactive substances. Moreover, drug use increases impulsivity, which may, in turn, promote continuous use of the substance. Delay discounting (DD), a decline in the subjective value of reward with increasing delay until its receipt, is an established model to determine one's location on the continuum from impulsive decision-making to self-control, and constitutes a promising endophenotype in the study of SUD [5]. Patients with SUD exhibit a greater DD (a tendency to choose lower, but quicker, rewards rather than higher, but delayed, ones) than controls. A positive relationship between DD and subsequent initiation or increased use of tobacco has been described. DD is also improved in substance users in response to therapeutic interventions. Given that the heritability of DD varies between 46% and 56% [6], it provides an avenue of future research as a candidate behavioural marker of SUD.

Subjective responses to initial substance use have also been considered as a plausible endophenotype. Individuals vary widely in their subjective experience of a psychoactive substance, and this

may play a role in the development of an SUD. Such subjective response represents a heritable endophenotype. Among the most important findings, the literature consistently shows that individuals who demonstrated low response to alcohol in an alcohol challenge test are more likely to develop an AUD at 8-year follow-up [7]. Low sensitivity might be unique to this drug, because it leads to higher consumption. Other studies have confirmed that positive experiences in early use of other substances are important risk factors for later SUD [8, 9].

## Candidate genes

The candidate gene approach was the first strategy to investigate the genetic factors involved in SUD. This approach means searching for mutations, or screening for polymorphic markers, in one or more genes selected for their potential role in SUD. Such strategy requires recruiting patients with and without SUD, as: (1) a case-control study (to see if the studied allele is more frequent in the affected population, compared to the healthy control group); or (2) a trio approach (including affected patients and their fathers and mothers, in order to check if the vulnerability allele is more transmitted from the heterogenous parent(s) to the affected proband); or (3) siblings (where affected sibs should have the vulnerability allele more frequently in common than expected by chances only); or (4) multiplex families (calculating if the vulnerability allele is more frequently transmitted to affected cases, and not transmitted to healthy relatives). Several national and international cohorts have been implemented, following at least one of these strategies. Some examples are the Collaborative Studies on Genetics of Alcoholism (COGA) from the National Institute on Alcohol Abuse and Alcoholism (NIAAA), the Family Study of Cocaine Dependence (FSCD), and the Collaborative Genetic Study of Nicotine Dependence (COGEND).

Current research suggests that a major gene effect on SUD vulnerability is unlikely [9], but some plausible positive findings have been obtained. The candidate genes involved in the reward pathway, especially dopamine receptors, have been widely investigated in SUD. Several studies reported that the Taq1A variant (corresponding to rs1800497) of the gene encoding the dopamine D2 receptor (the *DRD2* gene) is associated with alcohol dependence. Interestingly, this genetic variant changes an amino acid in a novel gene *ANKK1*, which encodes an X-kinase that regulates the presence of the dopamine D2 receptor at the cellular membrane [10]. Some genetic variants of the enzymes involved in the metabolism of ethanol, namely the alcohol dehydrogenase (*ADH*) and acetaldehyde dehydrogenase (*ALDH*) genes, have also been associated with a lower risk for developing AUD, mainly in South Eastern Asian populations [11].

## Genome-wide association studies

The first genome-wide association studies (GWAS) were published in 2006. SNPs are used as markers of a genomic region, with the majority of them having minimal or no impact on the biological system. A minority can have functional consequences, by causing amino acid changes, altering mRNA transcript stability, or improving transcription factor binding affinity. SNPs are the most frequent form of genetic variation in the genome. The paradigm underlying GWAS is that complex disorders, including SUD, are polygenic, driven by multiple common genetic polymorphisms, and follow a non-Mendelian pattern of inheritance (Fig. 49.1).

In the GWAS approach, it is assumed that common disorders are likely to be influenced by genetic variation that is also common in the general population. The discovery of several susceptibility variants for common diseases with high minor allele frequency (including the *APOE* gene for Alzheimer's disease [12, 13] or the *PPARg* gene for type 2 diabetes) led to the development of what is now called the 'common disease/common variant hypothesis' [14].

Contrasting with the candidate gene approach, GWAS do not require any assumption on the genomic location of the causal variants and use the strengths of association studies, even in the absence of convincing literature on the location of involved genes. The first GWAS strategy was published in 2014 [15].

The first GWAS of AUD was initially published in 2006 [16] in a sample of 1024 cases and 996 controls, using more than 500,000 SNPs (Fig. 49.2). Complete analysis reported that no associations were genome-wide significant [17]. The largest independent GWAS published to date involved more than 16,000 participants, providing information on about a million autosomal SNPs [18]. This study added to the evidence for the association of variants in the *ADH* gene coding for an alcohol-metabolizing enzyme and provided insight on the role of new loci mapping to the *ADH* gene cluster [18].

As for other similar analyses in psychiatry, a recent review of 12 published AUD GWAS [19] concluded that larger samples will be required to detect loci, in addition to those encoding the genes already mentioned.

A first GWAS on heroin published in 2019 and performed on 325 methadone stabilized, former severe heroin addicts and 250 controls showed an association with the the cytosolic dual-specificity phosphatase 27 encoded by the *DUSP27* gene [20]. Three GWAS reported genome-wide significant SNP association with opioid use disorder. These results included SNPs that mapped to *KCNG2*, which encodes a potassium voltage-gated ion channel [21], and *CNIH3*, which encodes a glutamate receptor-associated regulatory protein [21]. A recent genome-wide study on cannabis dependence has been performed on three large independent cohorts including 15,000 subjects and detected interesting associations in novel genes, including a novel antisense transcript RP11-206M11.7, the solute carrier family 35 member G1, the *SLC35G1* gene, and the CUB and Sushi multiple domains 1 gene *CSMD1* [21]. The first GWAS on cocaine use disorder detected a significant role of the *FAM53B* gene, the product of which is involved in the regulation of cell proliferation, but with an unclear biological role in the development of cocaine dependence [21].

The most compelling evidence has come from GWAS and GWAS meta-analyses on nicotine use disorder, showing an association between the nicotinic acetylcholine receptor gene cluster CHRNA5-A3-B4 on chromosome 15 (15q25) and both nicotine dependence and smoking cumulative quantity [22]. This is highly relevant, given that while there are thousands of compounds in cigarette smoke, nicotine is the principal component responsible for nicotine dependence and exerts its action in the brain through neuronal nicotinic acetylcholine receptors, which are widely distributed in both the central and the peripheral nervous systems [22]. Two associations between nicotine dependence and genetic variants was published in 2007, one in a candidate gene study [23] and one GWAS

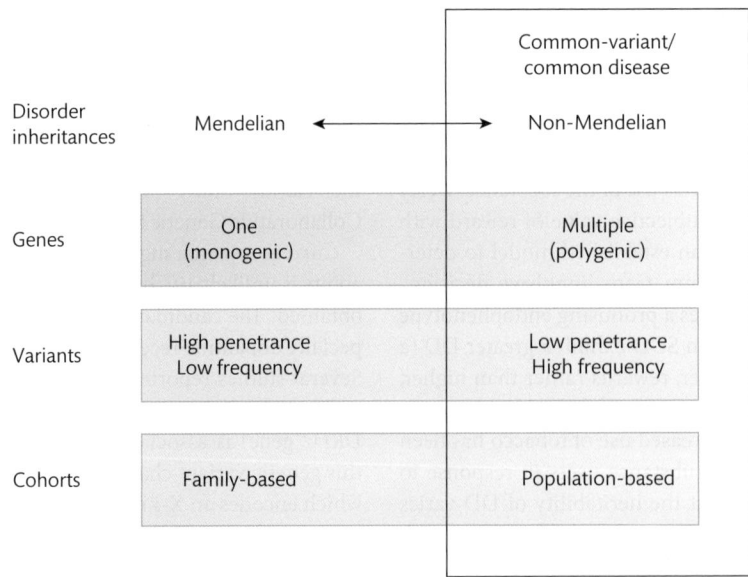

**Fig. 49.1** Schematic representation of the hypotheses of genes and variants involved in disorder inheritance according to their Mendelian and non-Mendelian status. The paradigm is that Mendelian-inherited disorders should involve genetic variants with a high penetrance and a low frequency in one gene, while non-Mendelian-inherited disorders should involve variants with a low penetrance but a high frequency in different genes. Thus, Mendelian disorders could be studied with family-based cohorts, while non-Mendelian disorders could be studied with population-based cohorts.

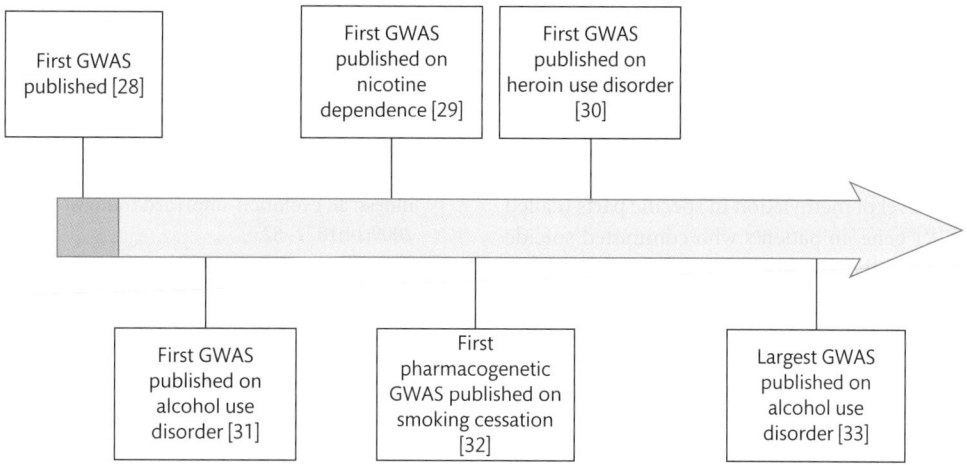

**Fig. 49.2** Historical GWAS discoveries on substance use disorders.

on nicotine [24]. In this preliminary study, examining 3713 SNPs in more than 300 candidate genes and involving 879 light smokers and 1050 heavy smokers, multiple SNPs within the CHRNA5-A3-B4 were associated with nicotine dependence [23]. In the GWAS study, 1050 dependent smokers and 879 non-dependent smokers as controls allowed to associated *CHRNB3* gene [24]. In 2008, two GWAS, considering smoking quantity, but also smoking-related disease (lung cancer and peripheral arterial disease), confirmed the association of variants within this locus and smoking-related phenotypes [25]. Further studies demonstrated the impact of a non-synonymous SNP in the α5-nicotinic acetylcholine receptor gene (*CHRNA5*) on behaviours associated with the risk of developing tobacco dependence, including a decrease in the aversive effect of nicotine [26]. This genetic assessment for nicotine abstinence could be helpful to use as a biomarker of pharmacogenetics in smoking cessation [27].

## Pharmacogenetics of substance use disorders

Recent interventions emphasize the importance of early and intensive treatment for SUD. These studies also demonstrate additional factors that influence outcome such as psychiatric comorbidity (including post-traumatic stress disorder or schizophrenia, among many others) or medical conditions associated with substance use. This has called for treatment elements, such as the choice of psychotherapy and medication, and the goal (abstinence vs controlled use, among many others) to be individualized, so that optimal patient outcomes can be met. It is also tempting to hope that recent genetic findings can help to develop an individualized approach in the clinical management of patients with SUD.

Pharmacogenetic studies may provide the first examples for innovation. In AUD, there appears to be important moderating effects of variation in *OPRM1* on the response to the opioid antagonist naltrexone [28]. The Asp40 allele of Asn40Asp, encoded by the A118G SNP, predicts a significantly lower rate of relapse in four RCTs, while the others were not significant. A meta-analysis confirmed that naltrexone-treated patients carrying the ASP40 allele of the A118G SNP had lower rates of relapse [29]. Human laboratory studies also suggested that the A118G SNP moderates the effects of alcohol, including a differential reduction of the alcohol euphoric effect or craving. Other dopaminergic, serotonergic, GABAergic, and

glutamatergic genes have been studied, but no other specific candidate polymorphism has to date yielded replicable findings [28].

A number of studies have examined the association of genetic variants on features of opioid use disorder and treatment outcome. Methadone and buprenorphine are two common and effective maintenance medications for opioid use disorder. The *DRD2* gene, coding for the D2 dopaminergic receptor and located on chromosome 11 (region 11q23), displays a polymorphism known as Taq1A and has been the subject of over 300 studies [30, 31]. Meta-analyses confirmed a modest, but significant, higher prevalence of the A1 allele in patients with opiate use disorder [30]. Taq1A has also been associated with greater heroin craving. In predicting the outcome of an opioid maintenance treatment, the results have been less conclusive so far. Indeed, in four studies including 404 participants with a maintenance medication, three failed to find an association of this variant with a significant difference in outcome. Similarly, several variants within the *OPRM1* gene (including the A118G SNP) and the *OPRD1* gene have provided inconclusive results so far in pharmacogenetic trials.

## Conclusions and perspectives

National and international consortia, recruiting large samples of controls and affected patients, have been successfully used in the genetics of SUD. GWAS have demonstrated the role of variants of nicotinic receptor genes in tobacco dependence and confirmed the involvement of genes encoding enzymes in charge of the metabolism of ethanol in AUD. Furthermore, genes involved in the dopamine pathway have been found associated with several SUDs, although how they increase the vulnerability to SUDs is not entirely deciphered.

The development of new tools to investigate the genome, such as next-generation sequencing (NGS), now make it possible to sequence all exons of the 25,000 genes of the human genome. This technique will identify genetic variations within exons, including rare *de novo* mutations (detected in patients while absent in their parents), which was almost impossible with previous approaches. Analysis of the exome, or genome-wide exome sequencing (GWES), has indeed been a diagnostic tool in common pathologies, but not yet in SUDs. However, GWES is only sequencing about 1.5% of the entire human genome, and other variants, for example those located in the regulatory regions of genes, may impact the risk of the disorder. Furthermore, genetic studies can now be combined with other analyses to investigate the epigenetics of SUD. Epigenetics relate to the modification of DNA chemistry (but not the DNA sequence), which leads to modifications of gene expression in response to different environmental factors. Early life trauma has been found, for example to increase the level of methylation in specific parts (called CpG islands) of the *GR1* gene, in patients who committed suicide and were abused during childhood [32].

Epigenetics could be the missing link between high heritability and the important role of purely environmental factors, that is, explaining, in part, the 'missing heritability', a concept focusing on the gap between high heritability and the weak role of any individual associated gene.

Future directions should therefore combine the study of developmental and environmental factors with genetic and epigenetic factors. Since the substratum of methylation sites (epigenetic regulation) is purely genetic, the impact of different trauma may vary according to individual genetic polymorphisms. This approach also places clinical evidence at the forefront when studying the genetic vulnerability of SUD.

## REFERENCES

1. Walters GD. The heritability of alcohol abuse and dependence: a meta-analysis of behavior genetic research. *Am J Drug Alcohol Abuse*. 2002;28:557–84.
2. Li MD, Cheng R, Ma JZ, Swan GE. A meta-analysis of estimated genetic and environmental effects on smoking behavior in male and female adult twins. *Addiction*. 2003;98:23–31.
3. Verweij KJ, Zietsch BP, Lynskey MT, *et al*. Genetic and environmental influences on cannabis use initiation and problematic use: a meta-analysis of twin studies. *Addiction*. 2010;105:417–30.
4. Kendler KS, Thornton LM, Pedersen NL. Tobacco consumption in Swedish twins reared apart and reared together. *Arch Gen Psychiatry*. 2000;57:886–92.
5. Bickel WK. Discounting of delayed rewards as an endophenotype. *Biol Psychiatry*. 2015;77:846–7.
6. Anokhin AP, Golosheykin S, Grant JD, Heath AC. Heritability of delay discounting in adolescence: a longitudinal twin study. *Behav Genet*. 2011;41:175–83.
7. Schuckit MA. A brief history of research on the genetics of alcohol and other drug use disorders. *J Stud Alcohol Drugs*. 2014;75(Suppl 17):59–67.
8. Le Strat Y, Ramoz N, Horwood J, *et al*. First positive reactions to cannabis constitute a priority risk factor for cannabis dependence. *Addiction*. 2009;104:1710–17.
9. Baggio S, Studer J, Deline S, Mohler-Kuo M, Daeppen JB, Gmel G. The relationship between subjective experiences during first use of tobacco and cannabis and the effect of the substance experienced first. *Nicotine Tob Res*. 2014;16:84–92.
10. Gorwood P, Le Strat Y, Ramoz N, Dubertret C, Moalic JM, Simonneau M. Genetics of dopamine receptors and drug addiction. *Hum Genet*. 2012;131:803–22.
11. Wall TL, Luczak SE, Hiller-Sturmhofel S. Biology, genetics, and environment: underlying factors influencing alcohol metabolism. *Alcohol Res*. 2016;38:59–68.
12. Chouraki V, Seshadri S. Genetics of Alzheimer's disease. *Adv Genet*. 2014;87:245–94.
13. Cuyvers E, Sleegers K. Genetic variations underlying Alzheimer's disease: evidence from genome-wide association studies and beyond. *Lancet Neurol*. 2016;15:857–68.
14. Uher R. The role of genetic variation in the causation of mental illness: an evolution-informed framework. *Mol Psychiatry*. 2009;14:1072–82.
15. Klein RJ, Zeiss C, Chew EY, *et al*. Complement factor H polymorphism in age-related macular degeneration. *Science*. 2005;308:385–9.
16. Johnson C, Drgon T, Liu QR, *et al*. Pooled association genome scanning for alcohol dependence using 104,268 SNPs: Validation and use to identify alcoholism vulnerability loci in unrelated individuals from the collaborative study on the genetics of alcoholism. *Am J Med Genet B Neuropsychiatr Genet*. 2006;141B:844–53.
17. Treutlein J, Cichon S, Ridinger M, *et al*. Genome-wide association study of alcohol dependence. *Arch Gen Psychiatry*. 2009;66:773–84.
18. Gelernter J, Kranzler HR, Sherva R, *et al*. Genome-wide association study of alcohol dependence:significant findings in African- and European-Americans including novel risk loci. *Mol Psychiatry*. 2014;19:41–9.
19. Hart AB, Kranzler HR. Alcohol dependence genetics: lessons learned from genome-wide association studies (GWAS) and post-GWAS analyses. *Alcohol Clin Exp Res*. 2015;39:1312–27.
20. Nielsen DA, Ji F, Yuferov V, *et al*. Genome-wide association study identifies genes that may contribute to risk for developing heroin addiction. *Psychiatr Genet*. 2010;20:207–14.
21. Jensen KP. A review of genome-wide association studies of stimulant and opioid use disorders. *Mol Neuropsychiatry*. 2016;2:37–45.
22. Berrettini WH, Doyle GA. The CHRNA5-A3-B4 gene cluster in nicotine addiction. *Mol Psychiatry*. 2012;17:856–66.
23. Saccone SF, Hinrichs AL, Saccone NL, *et al*. Cholinergic nicotinic receptor genes implicated in a nicotine dependence association study targeting 348 candidate genes with 3713 SNPs. *Hum Mol Genet*. 2007;16:36–49.
24. Bierut LJ, Madden PA, Breslau N, *et al*. Novel genes identified in a high-density genome wide association study for nicotine dependence. *Hum Mol Genet*. 2007;16:24–35.
25. Wen L, Jiang K, Yuan W, Cui W, Li MD. Contribution of variants in CHRNA5/A3/B4 gene cluster on chromosome 15 to tobacco smoking: from genetic association to mechanism. *Mol Neurobiol*. 2016;53:472–84.
26. Fowler CD, Kenny PJ. Nicotine aversion: neurobiological mechanisms and relevance to tobacco dependence vulnerability. *Neuropharmacology*. 2014;76 Pt B:533–44.
27. Uhl GR, Drgon T, Johnson C, Rose JE. Nicotine abstinence genotyping: Assessing the impact on smoking cessation clinical trials. *Pharmacogenomics J*. 2009;9:111–15.
28. Heilig M, Goldman D, Berrettini W, O'Brien CP. Pharmacogenetic approaches to the treatment of alcohol addiction. *Nat Rev Neurosci*. 2011;12:670–84.
29. Chamorro AJ, Marcos M, Miron-Canelo JA, Pastor I, Gonzalez-Sarmiento R, Laso FJ. Association of micro-opioid receptor (*OPRM1*) gene polymorphism with response to naltrexone in alcohol dependence: a systematic review and meta-analysis. *Addict Biol*. 2012;17:505–12.

30. Le Foll B, Gallo A, Le Strat Y, Lu L, Gorwood P. Genetics of dopamine receptors and drug addiction: a comprehensive review. *Behav Pharmacol*. 2009;20:1–17.

31. Patriquin MA, Bauer IE, Soares JC, Graham DP, Nielsen DA. Addiction pharmacogenetics: a systematic review of the genetic variation of the dopaminergic system. *Psychiatr Genet*. 2015;25:181–93.

32. McGowan PO, Sasaki A, D'Alessio AC, *et al*. Epigenetic regulation of the glucocorticoid receptor in human brain associates with childhood abuse. *Nat Neurosci*. 2009;12:342–8.

# 50

# Alcohol use disorder

*Wim van den Brink and Falk Kiefer*

## Introduction

Alcohol is the most frequently used addictive substance in the world, with large regional variations in the amount of alcohol that is consumed and related variations in damage due to excessive use and alcohol use disorders. About half of the global adult population (48%) has never consumed alcohol, whereas 14% was drinking in the past but has ceased alcohol consumption and 'only' 38% is currently drinking [1]. There are, however, large regional differences, with 80–90% of lifetime abstainers in Islamic countries and only 20% of lifetime abstainers and 60–70% of current drinkers in North America and Europe. Worldwide, mean alcohol consumption among people aged 15 years and older is about 6.2 L of pure alcohol per person per year, which translates into about 13.5 g of pure alcohol per person per day, which is clearly within the WHO range for low-risk alcohol drinking (1–20 g/day for women and 1–40 g/day for men). However, there are large inter-personal and regional differences in the level of alcohol consumption. People in the Eastern Mediterranean region (for example, Jordan: mean 0.7 L) and the South East Asian region (for example, Pakistan: mean 0.1 L) generally drink much less, whereas people in North America (mean 9.5 L) and Europe (mean 10.9 L) drink much more than the worldwide average, with the highest drinking levels in Central and Eastern European countries (for example, Russian Federation: mean 16.1 L).[1]

There is no officially defined safe drinking level, and the amount and type of damage due to alcohol are mainly dependent on the volume of alcohol consumed, the drinking pattern, and the quality of the alcohol that is used. For example, alcohol consumption has been identified as a component cause for more than 200 diseases, injuries, and other health conditions, and for most of these diseases and injuries, there is a clear dose–response relationship [2]. Also the pattern of drinking affects the risks [3]; for example, drinking while eating is associated with less harm from chronic diseases than the same pattern of drinking at other times [4], whereas heavy episodic or binge drinking is linked to unintentional injuries (accidents), intentional injuries (suicides) [5], and ischaemic heart disease and ischaemic stroke [6]. Finally, the quality of alcoholic beverages may impact on health and mortality; for example, home-made or illegally produced alcoholic beverages can be contaminated with methanol or other toxic substances. However, there is no evidence that consumption of illegally produced alcohol is markedly linked at a population level to morbidity or mortality over and above the effects of the level of ethanol use [7].

Worldwide, there are 3.3 million deaths every year resulting from the harmful use of alcohol representing 5.9% of all deaths, including 33% of cardiovascular diseases and diabetes, 17% of unintentional injuries, 16% of gastrointestinal diseases, 13% of cancers, and 21% of other diseases. These deaths occur early in life, and in the age group of 20–39 years, approximately 25% of total deaths are alcohol-attributable. Therefore, it comes as no surprise that 5.1% of the global burden of disease and injury in terms of disability-adjusted life years (DALYs) is attributable to alcohol [1]. Finally, the harmful use of alcohol brings significant social and economic losses to individuals and society at large.

It is important to realize that about two-thirds of all alcohol-related deaths are caused by 4–7% of drinkers, that is, drinkers with an alcohol use disorder and often with chronic, excessive alcohol consumption [8]. Like the level of alcohol consumption in the population, the 12-month prevalence of alcohol use disorders (harmful use/abuse and dependence) shows considerable regional variation, with low rates in the Eastern Mediterranean region (0.3%) and the South East Asian region (2.2%) and much higher rates in the Americas (6.0%) and Europe (7.5%) [1]. In this chapter, we focus on these people with an alcohol use disorder.

## Classification and diagnosis of alcohol use disorders

The concept of addiction, later called dependence and now substance use disorder, is long, complex, and full of controversies. Alcohol use and alcohol use problems are already known from ancient biblical, Egyptian, and Babylonian sources. In the seventeenth and early eighteenth centuries, regular alcohol use was very common in Europe since alcohol represented a cheap and useful combination of clean water and calories. With the change from a mainly agricultural society to an industrial society in the middle of the eighteenth century, regular intoxication became problematic and 'habitual drunkards' were seen as morally weak and in need of re-education in a correctional centre that generally took the shape of a prison (*moral model*). This view changed in the beginning of the nineteenth century with the start of the temperance movement. Habitual drunkards were no longer seen as morally weak, but as victims of the highly addictive substance alcohol, and regulation, or even prohibition, of the production, trade, and consumption of alcohol was seen as the best solution for the problem of excessive alcohol use (*pharmacological model*). The term 'alcoholism' was first used in 1849 by the Swedish physician Magnus Huss to describe the detrimental effects of alcohol. In the early twentieth century, psychoanalytic theorists proposed that alcoholism was not a separate problem, but just a symptom of a character neurosis/personality disorder (*symptomatic model*). Successful treatment of the underlying personality disorder (in a therapeutic community) would also resolve the alcohol problem. Between 1946 and 1960, E. Morton Jellinek performed a series of studies among AA members, and based on the results of these studies, he coined the term 'disease of alcoholism' with five different subtypes (*biological or disease model*). It was only in the 1970s that psychologists and sociologists developed theoretical and treatment models for problematic alcohol use, with psychologists proposing that alcoholism was a form of maladapted learnt behaviour that could be redressed during psychological interventions (*psychological or learning model*) and sociologists stating that alcoholism is a normal response to abnormal circumstances and that normalization of these circumstances would solve the problem (*social model*). In 1975, a WHO steering group discussed the latest developments, and based on this discussion, Edwards and Gross proposed a new model integrating biological, psychological, and social aspects [9]—the alcohol dependence syndrome with the following symptoms: narrowing of drinking repertoire; salience of drink-seeking behaviour; increased tolerance; repeated withdrawal; repeated relief/avoidance of withdrawal by drinking; subjective awareness of compulsion to drink (craving); and reinstatement of the syndrome after abstinence (*biopsychosocial model*). In 1997, Alan Leshner, then the director of the National Institute of Drug Abuse (NIDA), made a final contribution to the history of the concept of addiction when he wrote a paper with the challenging title 'Addiction is a brain disease, and it matters' (*brain disease model*) [10]. The brain disease model states that addiction is a chronic, relapsing disease that results from biological vulnerabilities and the prolonged effects of drugs on the brain. However, as with many other brain diseases, addiction has embedded behavioural and social context aspects that are important parts of the disorder itself. Therefore, effective treatments should include biological, behavioural, and social context components.

The history of the classification of alcohol use problems runs partly parallel with the history of the concept of alcoholism. In the first two editions of the *Diagnostic and Statistical Manual of Mental Disorders* of the American Psychiatric Association (DSM-I, 1952; DSM-II, 1968), alcoholism was classified as a subcategory of the sociopathic personality disorder, and thus reminiscent of the moral or symptomatic model [11, 12]. In DSM-III (1980), the term 'alcoholism' was dropped in favour of two distinct, but loosely defined, categories labelled 'alcohol abuse' and 'alcohol dependence' and these new disorders were placed in a separate category 'Substance use disorders', rather than as subsets of personality disorders [13]. DSM was revised again in 1987 (DSM-III-R) [14]. This time, the alcohol dependence syndrome [9] was used as a starting point and explicit diagnostic criteria were provided. As a consequence, the category of dependence (≥3 out of nine criteria) was expanded to include some criteria that, in DSM-III, were considered symptoms

of abuse, and the category 'Abuse' (≥1 out of 2 criteria) became a residual category for diagnosing those who never met criteria for dependence but who drank despite alcohol-related physical, social, psychological, or occupational problems or who repeatedly drank in dangerous situations such as in conjunction with driving. In 1994, the fourth edition of DSM (DSM-IV) was published, with some minor changes in the criteria sets for dependence (≥3 out of seven criteria) and abuse (≥2 out of four criteria) [15]. The latest revision of DSM (DSM-5) was introduced in 2013 and contained important changes with regard to the classification of alcohol-related problems [16]. In DSM-5, the dependence criterion 'legal problems' was eliminated and replaced by 'craving' as a new criterion. In addition, alcohol abuse and alcohol dependence were integrated into a single disorder called 'alcohol use disorder' (AUD) with 11 criteria (ten old criteria and one new criterion—craving) and three levels of disorder severity, based on the number of criteria present in the last 12 months: mild AUD (2–3 out of 11 criteria), moderate AUD (4–5 out of 11 criteria), and severe AUD (≥6 out of 11 criteria). Table 50.1 presents a summary of the criteria for the DSM-5 classification of an AUD [16] (also discussed in relation to mechanisms of addiction in Chapter 48).

Similar to DSM, there were also substantial and largely parallel changes in the definition of alcohol use problems in the International Classification of Diseases (ICD) of the WHO. Early definitions of alcoholism in ICD-7 (1958) and ICD-8 (1968) stressed the sociological, rather than the physical, aspects of dependence [17, 18]. However, in ICD-9 (1978), the term alcoholism was dropped in favour of alcohol dependence syndrome [19]. Similar to DSM-IV (1994), ICD-10 (1992) defined two mutually exclusive alcohol diagnoses: harmful use and dependence [20]. However, in contrast to DSM-IV where abuse was defined by alcohol-induced social impairments, inter-personal problems, legal problems, and/or hazardous use, in ICD-10, harmful use was determined by alcohol-induced psychological or physical harm. ICD-10 dependence (≥3 out of six criteria) was very similar to DSM-IV dependence but ICD-10 already included craving as one of the criteria. In the draft version of the latest version of ICD (ICD-11), the two mutually exclusive categories of harmful use and dependence are retained, but harmful use will now include the criterion 'family harmed by substance use', whereas the six dependence criteria of ICD-10 will be reduced to only three criteria: physical dependence (tolerance or withdrawal), priority of use (much time or reduced activities, or psychological/physical harm), and impaired control (quit/cut or larger/longer or craving) [21]. Symptoms from at least two of the three proposed ICD-11 dependence criteria are needed for a diagnosis of alcohol dependence (Table 50.1).

There are some early findings comparing DSM-IV to DSM-5 and ICD-11 (draft) to DSM-5. These findings show that the prevalence of AUD in the general population according to DSM-5 is somewhat higher than according to DSM-IV (abuse and dependence), but that very similar prevalence rates are obtained in clinical settings [22]. Furthermore, the threshold for DSM-IV alcohol dependence (≥3 out of seven criteria) seems to be very similar to the threshold for DSM-5 moderate alcohol use disorder (≥4 out of 11 criteria) [23]. In a general population study from Australia, the prevalence of alcohol dependence according to ICD-10, ICD-11, and DSM-IV was very similar, but the prevalence of DSM-5 moderate/severe AUD was substantially higher [24]. Finally, a study among American

**Table 50.1** Classification of alcohol use disorders in DSM-IV, DSM-5, ICD-10, and ICD-11

| | DSM-IV<br>Alcohol dependence (≥3/7) | DSM-5<br>Alcohol use disorder (≥2/11)<br>(mild 2–3/11; moderate 4–5/11;<br>severe ≥6/11) | ICD-10<br>Alcohol dependence (≥3/6) | ICD-11<br>Alcohol dependence (≥2/3) |
|---|---|---|---|---|
| 1 | | Craving | Craving | 1. Impaired control over substance use often accompanied by craving |
| 2 | Persistent desire or unsuccessful attempts to reduce or stop alcohol use | Persistent desire or unsuccessful attempts to reduce or stop | | |
| 3 | Alcohol use more or longer than intended | Alcohol use more or longer than intended | Alcohol use more or longer than intended | |
| 4 | Reduced social, occupational, and recreational activities due to alcohol use | Failure to fulfil role obligations due to alcohol use | Neglect of other pleasures and responsibilities due to time needed to obtain and recover from alcohol use | 2. Substance becomes increasing priority in life and relegates other areas of life to periphery; continued alcohol use despite problems |
| 5 | Lots of time spent to obtain, use, or recover from the effects of alcohol | Lots of time spent to obtain, use, or recover from the effects of alcohol | (Subsumed in above criterion) | |
| 6 | Continued alcohol use despite recurrent or persistent physical or psychological problems due to alcohol use | Continued alcohol use despite recurrent or persistent physical or psychological problems due to alcohol use | Continued alcohol use despite harmful consequences | |
| 7a | Tolerance indicated by increased use to obtain same effect or reduced effect with the same amount | Tolerance indicated by increased use to obtain same effect or reduced effect with the same amount | Tolerance indicated by increased use to obtain same effect | 3. Physiological features, including tolerance, withdrawal, and/or alcohol use to prevent or alleviate withdrawal symptoms (not just hangover) |
| 7b | Withdrawal manifested by specific withdrawal syndrome or alcohol use to relieve or avoid withdrawal symptoms | Withdrawal manifested by specific withdrawal syndrome or alcohol use to relieve or avoid withdrawal symptoms | Withdrawal manifested by specific withdrawal syndrome or alcohol use to relieve or avoid withdrawal symptoms | |
| | **Alcohol abuse (≥1/4)** | | **Harmful alcohol use (≥1/2)** | |
| 8 | Continued alcohol use despite recurrent or persistent social or inter-personal problems due to alcohol use | Continued alcohol use despite recurrent or persistent social or inter-personal problems due to alcohol use | Continued alcohol use despite recurrent or persistent social or inter-personal problems due to alcohol use | (Partly in criterion 2) |
| 9 | Hazardous drinking (for example, while driving) | Hazardous drinking (for example, while driving) | | |
| 10 | Failure to fulfil major role obligations due to drinking | Failure to fulfil major role obligations due to drinking | | (Partly in criterion 2) |
| 11 | Recurrent alcohol-related legal problems | | | |
| 12 | | | Continued alcohol use despite recurrent or persistent physical or psychological problems due to alcohol use (see also criterion 6) | |

Source: data from: *Diagnostic and Statistical Manual of Mental Disorders*, (Fourth Edition, DSM-IV, Copyright (1994); Fifth Edition, DSM-5, Copyright (2013)), American Psychiatric Association; World Health Organization, *The ICD-10 Classification of Mental and Behavioural Disorders*, Copyright (1996), World Health Organization; Poznyak V, *An Update on ICD-11 Taxonomy of Disorders Due to Psychoactive Substance Use and Related Health Conditions*, International Society of Research on Alcoholism (ISBRA), Copyright (2016), World Health Organization.

adolescents admitted for intensive outpatient addiction treatment showed that ICD-11 produced a lower prevalence of AUD, but a much higher prevalence of alcohol dependence than DSM-IV alcohol dependence and DSM-5 moderate/severe AUD, with very low levels of intersystem diagnostic agreement [25]. These findings show that the final word about the classification of alcohol use-related problems is still not spoken and that further studies are needed.

## Mechanism of action of alcohol and neurobiology of alcohol use disorders

Alcohol modulates neural activity directly via ethanol-binding sites on several membrane receptors, including the N-methyl-D-aspartate (NMDA) receptor, the gamma-aminobutyric acid A (GABA-A) receptor, the 5-hydroxytryptamine-3 (5-HT$_3$) receptor, and ion channels [26]. In addition to these primary targets, indirect effects on neurochemical and neuroendocrine systems trigger reinforcing and stress-related effects. The main indirect targets are the dopamine system, the opioid system, and the hypothalamus–pituitary–adrenocortical (HPA) axis [27–30].

Following chronic administration of alcohol, several neurobiological adaptations (for example, changes in gene expression, molecular alterations, synaptic and cellular changes) take place that may result eventually in long-lasting alterations in neuronal network activity [31]. These alterations persist during abstinence. Corresponding behavioural effects become evident when the recently abstinent subject is exposed to alcohol-related stimuli or stress. Thus, even after successful detoxification and abstinence treatment, somebody with an AUD remains at risk for relapse. Animal models have assisted in identifying the molecular mechanisms that are primarily involved in alcohol reward and compulsive alcohol intake behaviour [32]. For example, a sensitization process within the dopaminergic reward system, especially in response to alcohol-related cues, drives relapse behaviour, even after protracted abstinence [33]. It is suggested that in the non-addicted, but vulnerable, brain, a phasic dopamine signal within the ventral striatum/nucleus accumbens (VS/NcAcc) leads to incentive salience and acts as a form of stimulus–reward learning, in which incentive salience is assigned to alcohol-related reward cues [34]. In the transition to addictive behaviour, VS/NcAcc-driven incentive salience to reward transforms into repetitive, automatized stimulus–reaction schemata that are mainly mediated by the recruitment of the dopaminergic dorsal striatum (DS), a change that is here referred to as the 'ventral–dorsal striatal shift' [10–37]. In addition, preclinical studies suggest a critical involvement of prefrontal cortical–striatal connectivity with glutamate–dopamine interactions in the transition from recreational to compulsive alcohol-seeking behaviour [38, 39]. The loss of type 2 metabotropic glutamate receptors (mGluR2) in the cortico-accumbal neurocircuitry due to chronic alcohol use is important for the increased propensity to relapse [40]. Loss of these auto-receptors is accompanied by a loss of neuronal plasticity, that is, the mGluR2-mediated long-term depression (LTD) is abolished in the addicted brain, resulting in reduced prefrontal cognitive control over the hyperactive reward system [41]. Due to this reduced prefrontal control and the progressive recruitment of a striatal dopaminergic mechanism ('VS-DS shift'), automatized behaviour and repetitive and compulsive uncontrolled alcohol use are facilitated [36, 42]. Human neuroimaging studies are supporting the importance of prefrontal regions in the alcohol-addicted brain [43, 44]. Further detail on animal models and human experimental studies underlying this formulation is given in Chapter 48.

At the psychological level, relapse can be understood using the negative reinforcement theory. Thus, avoidance of an aversive state during withdrawal—which is characterized by depressed mood and elevated anxiety—triggers a relapse to alcohol use [45]. In most patients, these symptoms abate over 3–6 weeks of abstinence, while relapse risk persists long beyond this period. However, more subtle changes, such as increased behavioural sensitivity to stress, support the clinical relevance of negative emotionality for protracted abstinence and relapse [46]. Modelling this process of alcohol-induced negative emotionality in laboratory animals has led to the discovery of augmented corticotropin-releasing hormone (CRH) signalling in the amygdala as a pathological mechanism that drives negative emotionality, and thereby relief drinking. It has been postulated that CRH signalling via its CRH1 receptor is a key element of the neuroadaptive changes driving relapse behaviour [47]. Pathological engagement of CRH signalling in the amygdala leads to negative emotionality during protracted abstinence and subsequently to relief drinking. Another mechanism that leads to relief drinking is an upregulation of the dynorphin/kappa opioid receptor (KOR) system in the brain [48–50]. It is important to note that activation of the dynorphin/KOR system, especially in the NcAcc [51], induces a dysphoric state [52], which may also drive relief drinking.

These findings are important to better understand the nature of substance use disorders and the problems that patients with these disorders experience and to guide the development of new treatments.

Psychological treatments can be directed at increased motivation to reduce or stop the use of alcohol (for example, motivational interviewing), while pharmacological treatments can be directed at reducing the rewarding effects of alcohol (for example, opioid receptor antagonists). Psychological and pharmacological treatments can also be used to reduce negative emotions related to substance use (CBT, α-adrenergic antagonists), to reduce craving (for example, cue-exposure treatment, glutamate antagonists), to improve cognitive control (for example, CBT, stimulants), and finally to replace alcohol with less toxic substitutes (for example, high-dose baclofen). In the following paragraphs, these approaches will be discussed in greater detail.

## Psychological treatments for patients with an alcohol use disorder

A crucial step in the treatment of patients with an alcohol use disorder is motivation for treatment. Many people with an alcohol use disorder are not aware of the fact that their alcohol use is causing problems (*precontemplation stage*), or they do recognize that alcohol is causing problems but they feel that there is still a reasonable balance between the short-term gains and the long-term problems (*contemplation stage*). In both cases, there is no perceived need to change one's behaviour. At a certain time or after appropriate motivational stimulation, people with an alcohol problem may realize that the balance between pros and cons begins to tip in the direction of change (*preparation stage*), which may actually result in concrete changes in behaviour and in changes of the environment (*action stage*). However, even after a period of reduced drinking or abstinence, relapse is still very likely to occur if no measures are taken to prevent this (*maintenance stage*).

Until the 1980s, the common way to deal with 'unmotivated' patients was a harsh and confrontational strategy to overcome 'pathological denial'. Since then, a more effective approach has been developed—motivational interviewing. It combines a supportive and empathic counselling style with a directive method for resolving the perceived ambivalence in the direction of change, that is, reduced drinking or total abstinence [53]. In the latest version of motivational enhancement therapy (MET), the intervention mainly tries to evoke 'change talk' and to prevent 'counterchange talk' [54]. In a recent fMRI study, it was shown that in patients with an alcohol use disorder, listening to their own change talk significantly reduced activation of the cingulate cortex and the insula during a priming dose of alcohol and that this reduction in brain activation was associated with a reduction in subjective craving [55]. MET is currently accepted as an evidence-based treatment for patients with an alcohol use disorder, with similar effects in patients in different stages of motivation.

In addition to MET, there are several other evidence-based psychological treatments for patients with an alcohol use disorder, including cognitive behavioural therapy (CBT), often with a strong emphasis on social skills training, although without clear support that improved coping skills mediate the benefit [56]; cue-exposure treatment (CET; often as part of CBT); 12-step facilitation (TSF), a professional intervention intended to make patients join a self-help group, for example Alcohol Anonymous (AA) meetings; contingency management (CM) with rewards for negative alcohol breath tests or attendance of therapy sessions (often as part of a community reinforcement approach); community reinforcement approach (CRA), generally including an amalgam of different techniques, for example social skills training, medication compliance support, medication, vocational training, marital therapy, and/or CM; and behavioural couple therapy [57]. It should be noted, however, that behavioural couple therapy is probably not more effective than individual CBT [58].

There are also several interventions with no proven effectiveness or with proven non-effectiveness, including psychodynamic psychotherapy, experientially oriented therapies, and system-theoretically based approaches [57].

Finally, there are some new treatments with some empirical support, but without conclusive evidence of their effectiveness. The most promising of these are: mindfulness-based relapse prevention [59]; acceptance and commitment therapy [60]; approach bias retraining [61]; and counterconditioning [62].

According to most authors, MET and CBT should be available to all patients with an alcohol use disorder as the standard treatment, with other treatments being available for special patients or as an additional treatment for those who do not or insufficiently respond to MET or CBT. However, other authors claim that CRA, as a more comprehensive treatment, should be the standard with a different set of treatment modules for different patients. Unfortunately, there are very few studies directly comparing these different approaches.

With regard to MET/CBT, it is important to notice that group and individual CBT are equally effective [64] and that MET/CBT offered as an online self-help intervention is also effective, although an online self-help intervention blended with chat sessions with a professional is more effective and more cost-effective than online self-help-only intervention [65]. These findings show that MET and CBT can be effectively and cost-effectively offered in different treatment settings and even to people who are not (yet) ready to seek contact with an official addiction treatment service.

An unresolved question is the effectiveness and cost-effectiveness of treatment according to the time-honoured Minnesota model, that is, a comprehensive inpatient 12-step treatment followed by long-term AA attendance. In a review for the Netherlands' National Health Care Institute, it was concluded that the evidence for the efficacy of inpatient and day care treatments according to this model was weak at best (only two RCTs), that these treatments are probably not (much) more effective than standard outpatient treatments (for example, MET, CBT), and that these treatments are almost certainly less cost-effective than standard outpatient treatments [63].

## Pharmacological treatments for patients with an alcohol use disorder

The first medication for the treatment of alcohol use disorder was disulfiram. Disulfiram and similar compounds were originally used for the industrial vulcanization of rubber. Some workers noticed that exposure to disulfiram, in combination with alcohol, made them feel sick. In 1948, Danish researchers made the connection and proposed disulfiram for the treatment of patients with an alcohol use disorder. Normally, alcohol is broken down in the liver by the enzyme alcohol dehydrogenase (ADH) to acetaldehyde, which is then converted by the enzyme acetaldehyde dehydrogenase (ALDH) to

harmless acetate. Disulfiram (125–250 mg/day) blocks ALDH, and after alcohol intake, the concentration of acetaldehyde in the blood may become 5–10 times higher than during metabolism of the same amount of alcohol alone. As a consequence, patients using alcohol while under the influence of disulfiram will experience a set of very unpleasant symptoms, including flushing of the skin, accelerated heart rate, shortness of breath, nausea, vomiting, throbbing headache, and sometimes even visual disturbances, mental confusion, postural syncope, and circulatory collapse.

In a recent meta-analysis, disulfiram was more effective than placebo in open-label, non-blinded studies (effect size g = 0.70), but not in blinded studies (g = 0.01), suggesting that the effect of disulfiram depends directly on the patient's anxious anticipation of its adverse effects [66]. Therefore, disulfiram seems to be a form of assisted psychotherapy, rather than pharmacotherapy per se. In the same meta-analysis, supervised disulfiram was more effective than acamprosate and naltrexone in establishing abstinence and to prevent relapse. However, it does not reduce alcohol craving, and (thus) there is poor compliance and the medication seems to be effective only when taken under supervision [67]. Moreover, disulfiram has many contraindications, including brain damage, heart failure, liver cirrhosis, and psychosis—conditions that are relatively frequent in patients with an alcohol use disorder.

From the introduction of disulfiram, it took about 40 years before new medications for the treatment of alcohol dependence entered the market in the early 1990s: acamprosate first in Europe and—much later—in America, and naltrexone first in America and—somewhat later—in Europe. Acamprosate changes the balance between the GABA and glutamate systems probably by its action on the NMDA receptor. It reduces withdrawal and craving, and it promotes long-term abstinence in compliant patients. It has to be taken at 333 mg three times a day, and the main contraindication is severe kidney impairment. Naltrexone is a non-selective opioid receptor antagonist that reduces alcohol reward and craving and results in reduced drinking with less heavy drinking days, and in some patients, it also promotes abstinence. Naltrexone is taken once a day (50 mg), and the main contraindications are the use of (prescribed or illicit) opioids, acute hepatitis, and liver failure. However, with the dose that is used, interference with liver function is rare, and if alcohol intake is reduced, liver function may actually improve. In a recent meta-analysis [67], acamprosate and naltrexone were equally effective, with no significant differences in drinking outcomes in studies where the two medications were directly compared. In placebo-controlled trials, acamprosate was mainly effective in the prevention of any drinking [number needed to treat (NNT) = 12], whereas naltrexone was mainly effective in the prevention of heavy drinking (NNT = 12) and much less so for the prevention of any drinking (NNT = 20).

Recently, a fourth medication—nalmefene—was registered in Europe for the treatment of alcohol dependence. Nalmefene is a mu (MOR) and delta opioid receptor (DOR) antagonist and a kappa opioid receptor (KOR) partial agonist. Since in alcohol-dependent patients, the KOR is already overstimulated, nalmefene is functionally a KOR antagonist. Nalmefene reduces alcohol reward (MOR antagonist), and it may reduce dysphoria (KOR partial agonist) in chronic alcohol-dependent patients [68]. In the recommended dose, nalmefene is quickly absorbed, with a maximum plasma concentration reached within 1 hour, occupation of almost all MORs within less than 3 hours, and full receptor occupancy remaining for at least 26 hours [69]. In contrast to the other registered medications, nalmefene is used 'as needed' (that is, only when the patient exprience the risk of relapse); the goal is reduction of (heavy) alcohol use, rather than total abstinence, and the medication should only be prescribed to heavy-drinking patients. The strategy to take the medication 'as needed' puts the responsibility for the treatment clearly on the patient. As such, it synergizes with strategies that try to empower patients. Moreover, the goal of reduced drinking allows patients who are not ready or not willing to stop drinking completely to enter treatment. In a meta-analysis [68], nalmefene was shown to be effective in the reduction of the number of heavy drinking days, with a small effect in alcohol-dependent patients (g = 0.20) and a somewhat larger effect in alcohol-dependent patients with (very) heavy drinking risk levels (g = 0.33).

There are also other medications, often with different molecular targets, that have been tested for the treatment of alcohol dependence. Since none of these compounds have relevant marketing authorization, their prescription for alcohol dependence is off-label. The most promising so far is topiramate (150–300 mg/day), an atypical anti-epileptic drug that probably blocks voltage-gated sodium channels and high-voltage-activated calcium channels, strongly stimulates specific GABA-A receptor isoforms, and somewhat inhibits glutamatergic AMPA/kainate receptors. In a meta-analysis of seven RCTs [70], topiramate was effective in both the prevention of any drinking (g = 0.47) and the reduction of the number of heavy drinking days (g = 0.41). Topiramate has many frequently occurring side effects (for example, weight loss, paraesthesia, fatigue, dizziness, sleepiness, depression), and titration can take up to 8 weeks, making it less suitable for weakly motivated and/or impulsive patients.

Other promising medications include [71, 72] gabapentin (GABAergic medication registered for epilepsy, neuropathic pain, and restless legs), sodium oxybate (GABAergic medication registered for narcolepsy), varenicline [nicotinic acetylcholine receptor (partial) agonist registered for nicotine dependence], doxasozine (α1-adrenergic antagonist registered for hypertension and urinary retention due to benign prostate hyperplasia), modafinil (a wakefulness-promoting dopamine reuptake inhibitor registered for narcolepsy), and baclofen (a GABA-B agonist registered for spasticity). In France, more than 200,000 patients with an alcohol use disorder have already been treated with baclofen at low (up to 60 mg/day) or (very) high doses (up to 330 mg/day), despite a paucity of evidence for efficacy at low doses and for efficacy and safety at (very) high doses. This is a very promising medication, but further studies are needed to learn more about the most adequate dose, the most suited patient profile, and the long-term safety [73].

## Improving treatment outcomes

In the previous paragraphs, it has been shown that there many proven effective treatments available for patients with an alcohol use disorder. However, effect sizes are small to moderate (g = 0.20–0.50; NNT 10–20), and many patients do not respond to these treatments.

One of the main determinants of outcome is the stage of the illness when patients enter treatment. Most patients are in a relatively late stage, and thus a rather advanced state of the disease with more

complex neural consequences of their chronic and excessive alcohol use (for example, VS-DS shift) and with serious physical, psychological, and social consequences, including liver impairment, depression, homelessness, etc. Their response to treatment is generally less good than in patients with a short illness history. This situation can only be improved by interventions directed at destigmatization [74] and increased availability of (anonymous) online self-help and online blended interventions [75].

Other strategies to improve the effect of treatments for alcohol use disorders are: improving treatment compliance, combining psychotherapy and pharmacotherapy, combining medications with a different mechanism of action (polypharmacy), and personalized medicine, that is, matching specific patients to specific treatments [71].

For improved compliance, attempts have been made to produce long-acting medications, including subcutaneous disulfiram implants and intramuscular naltrexone injections. However, so far no positive results have been reported.

In the combination of psychotherapy and pharmacotherapy, it is clear that pharmacotherapy adds to the effect of psychotherapy (all pharmacotherapy registration trials used the medication/placebo as an add-on to some form of psychotherapy or psychosocial support), whereas psychotherapy does not seem to add substantially to the effect of pharmacotherapy, neither in terms of compliance nor in terms of alcohol use outcomes [76, 77].

Combined use of medications may hold more promise. Acamprosate plus naltrexone has been shown to be more effective than either medication alone [78, 79], and the same was true for acamprosate plus disulfiram, compared to acamprosate alone [80]. The main question that remains here is when combined use of different medications should be considered: (1) right at the start of treatment to prevent treatment dropout due to non-response, but with the risk of more side effects; or (2) only after treatment with a single medication failed, but with the risk of further damage during the unsuccessful single medication treatment.

In our view, the most promising way to improve the (cost-)effectiveness of alcohol use disorder treatments is the use of personalized medicine, that is, tailoring treatments to specific patients based on direct observable clinical characteristics (phenotype), indirectly observable brain functions (endophenotype), and/or genetic indicators (genotype). With regard to the intensity of treatment, it is well known that inpatient treatment is generally more expensive, but not more effective than (intensive) outpatient treatment [81], probably with the exception of some very severely alcohol-dependent patients and those with serious social problems, especially those with unstable housing or being homeless [82].

With regard to psychotherapy, there have been some (very) large studies looking at patient–treatment matching, but none of these studies have found that patients with certain patient and/or environment characteristics (level of alcohol involvement, cognitive impairment, conceptual level, gender, meaning seeking, motivational stage, psychiatric comorbidity, sociopathy, social support for drinking, alcoholism typology) do clearly better with specific types of psychotherapy [83, 84]. However, in a re-analysis of the study MATCH, there were some indications that MET was performing better than CBT in patients with lower baseline motivation for change [85].

With regard to the pharmacotherapy of alcohol dependence, there are some very promising matching findings (Table 50.2).

**Table 50.2** Personalized pharmacotherapy model for alcohol dependence

| Treatment goal | First choice | Second choice | Third choice |
|---|---|---|---|
| Abstinence | **Acamprosate** *(anxiety, withdrawal, GATA4)* <br>**Naltrexone**[*] *(FH +, ASPD, SL, OPRM1)* | **Disulfiram** *(partner)* | Baclofen HD *(anxiety, withdrawal)* <br>Gabapentin *(sleep problems)* <br>GHB[#] |
| Reduced drinking | Naltrexone *(FH +, ASPD, SL, OPRM1)* <br>**Nalmefene** *(dysphoria?)* | Topiramate *(GRIK1)* | Modafinil *(high impulsivity)* <br>Varenicline *(smoking)* <br>Doxazosin *(FH +)* |

Personal characteristics for treatment choice within brackets in italics; bold medications are registered for the treatment of alcohol dependence.
GATA4, gene encoding a member of the GATA family of zinc finger transcription factors; FH +, positive family history of alcohol use disorder; ASPD, antisocial personality disorder; SL, sweet-liking; OPRM1, mu opioid receptor gene; GRIK1, gene encoding the glutamate ionotropic receptor kainate type subunit 1; GHB, gamma-hydroxybutyric acid/sodium oxybate.
[*] Naltrexone is registered for indication 'abstinence', but seems to work better for indication 'reduced drinking'.
[#] Only used for treatment of alcohol dependence in Austria and Italy.

For example, in a review of studies on the use of naltrexone in the treatment of alcohol dependence, it was shown that patients with one or more of the following characteristics tended to do better with naltrexone: positive family history of alcohol problems, Asn40Asp polymorphism of the MOR (*OPRM1*) gene, pretreatment abstinence, and sweet-liking [86]. Genetic variations in the *GATA4* gene seem to have an effect on the treatment response to acamprosate in alcohol-dependent patients via modulation of atrial natriuretic peptide (ANP) plasma levels [87]. Probably the most robust pharmacogenetic finding so far is the moderating effect of the glutamatergic *GRIK1* gene on the effect of topiramate in treating patients with alcohol dependence [88]; in a prospective placebo-controlled RCT, topiramate was only effective in rs2832407 C allele homozygotic patients (42%), and not in A allele carriers (58%). Finally, modafinil has been shown in one study to have a favourable effect in alcohol-dependent patients with high motor impulsivity, whereas it had a detrimental effect in alcohol-dependent patients with low motor impulsivity, indicating that individual patient characteristics cannot only be predictive of benefits, but also of potential harms [89].

These and similar findings may explain why trials find no or only very small treatment effects in unstratified, heterogenous patient populations. On the other hand, such findings often arise in secondary analysis of trial data and thus require replication. For example, a prospective RCT failed to confirm the matching effect of the Asn40Asp polymorphism of the *OPRM1* gene [90]. All future studies must clearly be informed by our growing understanding of individual or subgroup differences in complex disorders.

## Conclusions

Alcohol use disorders are frequently occurring problems that involve severe personal suffering and create substantial societal costs. The definition of these disorders is still under debate, but the existing working definitions have made it possible to investigate their neurobiology and to study the effectiveness and cost-effectiveness of psychotherapeutic and pharmacological interventions. These studies have shown that there are many proven effective interventions, albeit with limited effect sizes. Research has also shown that early detection and treatment (for example, with online interventions), combinations of treatments (polypharmacy), and a better system of patient–treatment matching can lead to a better outcome and a better future for patients with an alcohol use disorder.

## REFERENCES

1. World Health Organization. *Global status report on alcohol and health 2014*. Geneva: World Health Organization; 2014.
2. Rehm J, Mathers C, Popova S, Thavorncharoensap M, Teerawattananon Y, Patra J. Global burden of disease and injury and economic cost attributable to alcohol use and alcohol use disorders. Lancet. 2009; 373:2223–33.
3. Rehm J, Room R, Graham K, Monteiro M, Gmel G, Sempos CT. The relationship of average volume of alcohol consumption and patterns of drinking to burden of disease: An overview. Addiction. 2003; 98:1209–28.
4. Stranges S, Wu T, Dorn JM, et al. Relationship of alcohol drinking pattern to risk of hypertension: a population-based study. Hypertension. 2004; 44:813–19.
5. Macdonald S, Greer A, Brubacher J, Cherpitel C, Stockwell T, Zeisser C. Alcohol consumption and injury. In: Boyle P, Boffetta P, Lowenfels AB, et al. (eds). *Alcohol: Science, policy and public health*. Oxford: Oxford University Press; 2013. pp. 171–8.
6. Roerecke M, Rehm J. Irregular heavy drinking occasions and risk of ischemic heart disease: A systematic review and meta-analysis. Am J Epidemiol. 2010;171:633–44.
7. Rehm J, Kailasapillai S, Larsen E, et al. A systematic review of the epidemiology of unrecorded alcohol consumption and the chemical composition of unrecorded alcohol. Addiction. 2014; 109:880–93.
8. Rehm J, Shield KD, Gmel G, Rehm MX, Frick U. Modeling the impact of alcohol dependence on mortality burden and the effect of available treatment interventions in the European Union. Eur Neuropsychopharmacol. 2013; 23:89–97.
9. Edwards G, Gross MM. Alcohol dependence: provisional description of a clinical syndrome. Br Med J. 1976; 1:1058–61.
10. Leshner AI. Addiction is a brain disease, and it matters. Science. 1997; 278:45–7.
11. American Psychiatric Association. *Diagnostic and Statistical manual of Mental Disorders*, first edition (DSM-I). Washington DC, American Psychiatric Press; 1952.
12. American Psychiatric Association. *Diagnostic and Statistical Manual of Mental Disorders*, second edition (DSM-II). Washington DC, American Psychiatric Press; 1968.
13. American Psychiatric Association. *Diagnostic and Statistical Manual of Mental Disorders*, third edition (DSM-III). Washington DC, American Psychiatric Press; 1980.
14. American Psychiatric Association. *Diagnostic and Statistical Manual of Mental Disorders*, third edition—Revised (DSM-II-R). Washington DC, American Psychiatric Press; 1987.

15. American Psychiatric Association. *Diagnostic and Statistical Manual of Mental Disorders*, fourth edition (DSM-IV). Washington DC, American Psychiatric Press; 1994.

16. American Psychiatric Association. *Diagnostic and Statistical Manual of Mental Disorders*, fifth edition (DSM-5). Washington DC, American Psychiatric Press; 2013.

17. World Health Organization. *Manual of the International Classification of Diseases, Injuries, and Causes of Death*, seventh edition (ICD-7). Geneva, World Health Organization; 1958

18. World Health Organization. *Manual of the International Classification of Diseases, Injuries, and Causes of Death*, eight edition (ICD-8). Geneva, World Health Organization; 1968.

19. World Health Organization. *Manual of the International Classification of Diseases, Injuries, and Causes of Death*, ninth edition (ICD-9). Geneva, World Health Organization; 1979.

20. World Health Organization. *Manual of the International Classification of Diseases, Injuries, and Causes of Death*, tenth edition (ICD-10). Geneva, World Health Organization; 1999.

21. Poznyak V. *An Update on ICD-11 Taxonomy of Disorders Due to Psychoactive Substance Use and Related Health Conditions.* International Society of Research on Alcoholism (ISBRA), Berlin; 2016.

22. Bartoli F, Carra G, Crocamo C, Clerici M. From DSM-IV to DSM-5 alcohol use disorder: an overview of epidemiological data. Addict Behav. 2015; 41:46–50.

23. Compton WM, Dawson DA, Goldstein RB, Grant BF. Crosswalk between DSM-IV dependence and DSM-5 substance use disorders for opioids, cannabis, cocaine and alcohol. Drug Alcohol Depend. 2013; 132:387–90.

24. Lago L, Bruno R, Degenhardt L. Concordance of ICD-11 and DSM-5 definitions of alcohol and cannabis use disorders: a population survey. Lancet Psychiatry. 2016; 3:673–84.

25. Chung T, Cornelius J, Clark D, Martin C. Greater Prevalence of Proposed ICD-11 Alcohol and cannabis dependence compared to ICD-10, DSM-IV, and DSM-5 in treated adolescents. Alcohol Clin Exp Res. 2017; 41:1584–92.

26. Olsen RW, Li GD, Wallner M, Trudell JR, et al. Structural models of ligand-gated ion channels: sites of action for anesthetics and ethanol. Alcohol Clin Exp Res. 2014; 38: 595–603.

27. Spanagel R. Alcoholism: a systems approach from molecular physiology to behaviour. Physiol Rev. 2009; 89:649–705.

28. Le Merrer J, Becker JA, Befort K, Kieffer BL. Reward processing by the opioid system in the brain. Physiol Rev. 2009; 89:1379–412.

29. Benyamina A, Kebir O, Blecha L, Reynaud M, Krebs MO. CNR1 gene polymorphisms in addictive disorders: a systematic review and a meta-analysis. Addict Biol. 2011; 16:1–6.

30. Eisenhardt M, Hansson AC, Spanagel R, Bilbao A. Chronic intermittent ethanol exposure in mice leads to an up-regulation of CRH/CRHR1 signaling. Alcohol Clin Exp Res. 2015; 39:752–62.

31. Jangra A, Sriram CS, Pandey S, et al. Epigenetic Modifications, Alcoholic Brain and Potential Drug Targets. Ann Neurosci. 2016; 23:246–60.

32. Sanchis-Segura C, Spanagel R. Behavioural assessment of drug reinforcement and addictive features in rodents: an overview. Addict Biol. 2006; 11:2–38.

33. Robinson TE, Berridge KC. Addiction. Annu Rev Psychol. 2003; 54:25–53.

34. Flagel SB, Clark JJ, Robinson TE, et al. A selective role for dopamine in stimulus-reward learning. Nature. 2011; 469:53–7.

35. Vollstädt-Klein S, Wichert S, Rabinstein J, et al. Initial, habitual and compulsive alcohol use is characterized by a shift of cue

36. Everitt BJ, Robbins TW. Neural systems of reinforcement for drug addiction: from actions to habits to compulsion. Nat Neurosci. 2005; 8:1481–9.

37. Belin-Rauscent A, Everitt BJ, Belin D. Intrastriatal shifts mediate the transition from drug-seeking actions to habits. Biol Psychiatry. 2012; 72:343–5.

38. Russo SJ, Dietz DM, Dumitriu D, Morrison JH, Malenka RC, Nestler EJ. The addicted synapse: mechanisms of synaptic and structural plasticity in nucleus accumbens. Trends Neurosci. 2010; 33:267–76.

39. van Huijstee AN, Mansvelder HD. Glutamatergic synaptic plasticity in the mesocorticolimbic system in addiction. Front Cell Neurosci. 2015; 20; 8:466.

40. Meinhardt M, Hansson AC, Perreau-Lenz S, et al. Rescue of infralimbic mGluR2 deficit restores control over drug-seeking behavior in alcohol dependence. J Neurosci. 2013; 13; 33:2794–806.

41. Kasanetz F, Lafourcade M, Deroche-Gamonet V, et al. Prefrontal synaptic markers of cocaine addiction-like behavior in rats. Mol Psychiatry. 2013; 18:729–37.

42. Willuhn I, Burgeno LM, Everitt BJ, Phillips PE. Hierarchical recruitment of phasic dopamine signaling in the striatum during the progression of cocaine use. Proc Natl Acad Sci U S A. 2012; 109:20703–8.

43. Goldstein RZ, Volkow ND. Dysfunction of the prefrontal cortex in addiction: neuroimaging findings and clinical implications. Nat Rev Neurosci. 2011; 12:652–69.

44. Reiter AM, Deserno L, Kallert T, Heinze HJ, Heinz A, Schlagenhauf F. Behavioral and Neural Signatures of Reduced Updating of Alternative Options in Alcohol-Dependent Patients during Flexible Decision-Making. J Neurosci. 2016; 26;36(43):10935–48.

45. Koob GF. Theoretical frameworks and mechanistic aspects of alcohol addiction: alcohol addiction as a reward deficit disorder. Curr Top Behav Neurosci. 2013; 13:3–30.

46. Heilig M, Egli M, Crabbe JC, Becker HC. Acute withdrawal, protracted abstinence and negative affect in alcoholism: are they linked? Addict Biol. 2010; 5:169–84.

47. Heilig M, Koob GF. A key role for corticotropin-releasing factor in alcohol dependence. Trends Neurosci. 2007; 30:399–406.

48. Shippenberg TS, Zapata A, Chefer VI. Dynorphin and the pathophysiology of drug addiction. Pharmacol Ther. 2007; 116:306–21.

49. D'Addario C, Caputi FF, Rimondini R, et al. Different alcohol exposures induce selective alterations on the expression of dynorphin and nociceptin systems related genes in rat brain. Addict Biol. 2013; 18:425–33.

50. Bazov I, Kononenko O, Watanabe H, et al. The endogenous opioid system in human alcoholics: molecular adaptations in brain areas involved in cognitive control of addiction. Addict Biol. 2013; 18:161–9.

51. Spanagel R, Herz A, Shippenberg TS. Opposing tonically active endogenous opioid systems modulate the mesolimbic dopaminergic pathway. Proc Natl Acad Sci U S A. 1992; 89:2046–50.

52. Pfeiffer A, Brantl V, Herz A, Emrich HM. Psychotomimesis mediated by kappa opiate receptors. Science. 1986; 233:774–6.

53. Miller, W. Motivational Interviewing with problem drinkers. Behav Psychother. 1983; 11:147–72.

54. Miller WR, Rollnick S. *Motivational Interviewing. Helping people change*, third edition. New York, NY, Guilford Press; 2013.

55. Feldstein Ewing SW, Filbey FM, Hendershot CS, McEachern AD, Hutchison KE. Proposed model of the neurobiological

mechanisms underlying psychosocial alcohol interventions: the example of motivational interviewing. J Stud Alcohol Drugs.2011; 72:903–16.

56. Morgenstern J, Longabaugh R. Cognitive-behavioral treatment for alcohol dependence: a review of evidence for its hypothesized mechanisms of action. Addiction. 2000; 95:1475–90.

57. Emmelkamp PMG, Vedel E. *Evidence-based treatment for alcohol and drug abuse. A practitioner's guide to theory, methods, and practice*. New York, NY, Routledge; 2006.

58. Vedel E, Emmelkamp PM, Schippers GM. Individual cognitive-behavioral therapy and behavioral couples therapy in alcohol use disorder: a comparative evaluation in community-based addiction treatment centers. Psychother Psychosom. 2008; 77:280–8.

59. Bowen S, Witkiewitz K, Clifasefi SL, et al. Relative efficacy of mindfulness-based relapse prevention, standard relapse prevention, and treatment as usual for substance use disorders: a randomized clinical trial. JAMA Psychiatry. 2014; 71:547–56.

60. Lee EB, An W, Levin ME, Twohig MP. An initial meta-analysis of Acceptance and Commitment Therapy for treating substance use disorders. Drug Alcohol Depend. 2015; 155:1–7.

61. Wiers RW, Eberl C, Rinck M, Becker ES, Lindenmeyer J. Retraining automatic action tendencies changes alcoholic patients' approach bias for alcohol and improves treatment outcome. Psychol Sci. 2011; 22:490–7.

62. Das RK, Lawn W, Kamboj SK. Rewriting the valuation and salience of alcohol-related stimuli via memory reconsolidation. Transl Psychiatry. 2015; 5:e645.

63. Latta JM, Welten D. *Standpunt Minnesota Model. Diemen, College voor zorgverzekeringen*, 2013. https://www.zorginstituutnederland.nl/publicaties/standpunten/2013/06/10/standpunt-minnesota-model

64. Sobell LC, Sobell MB, Agrawal S. Randomized controlled trial of a cognitive-behavioral motivational intervention in a group versus individual format for substance use disorders. Psychol Addict Behav. 2009; 23:672–83.

65. Blankers M, Koeter MW, Schippers GM. Internet therapy versus internet self-help versus no treatment for problematic alcohol use: A randomized controlled trial. J Consult Clin Psychol. 2011; 79:330–41.

66. Skinner MD, Lahmek P, Pham H, Aubin HJ. Disulfiram efficacy in the treatment of alcohol dependence: a meta-analysis. PLoS One. 2014; 9:e87366.

67. Jonas DE, Amick HR, Feltner C, et al. Pharmacotherapy for adults with alcohol use disorders in outpatient settings: a systematic review and meta-analysis. JAMA. 2014; 311:1889–900.

68. Mann K, Torup L, Sørensen P, Gual A, Swift R, Walker B, van den Brink W. Nalmefene for the management of alcohol dependence: review on its pharmacology, mechanism of action and meta-analysis on its clinical efficacy. Eur Neuropsychopharmacol. 2016; 26:1941–9.

69. Ingman K, Hagelberg N, Aalto S, et al. Prolonged central mu-opioid receptor occupancy after single and repeated nalmefene dosing. Neuropsychopharmacology. 2005; 30:2245–53.

70. Blodgett JC, Del Re AC, Maisel NC, Finney JW. A meta-analysis of topiramate's effects for individuals with alcohol use disorders. Alcohol Clin Exp Res. 2014; 38:1481–8.

71. van den Brink W. Evidence-based pharmacological treatment of substance use disorders and pathological gambling. Curr Drug Abuse Rev. 2012; 5:3–31.

72. Soyka M, Müller CA. Pharmacotherapy of alcoholism—an update on approved and off-label medications. Expert Opin Pharmacother. 2017; 18:1187–99.

73. Beraha EM, Salemink E, Goudriaan AE, et al. Efficacy and safety of high-dose baclofen for the treatment of alcohol dependence: A multicentre, randomised, double-blind controlled trial. Eur Neuropsychopharmacol. 2016; 26:1950–9.

74. Stuart H. Reducing the stigma of mental illness. Glob Ment Health (Camb). 2016; 10:e17.

75. Sundström C, Blankers M, Khadjesari Z. Computer-Based Interventions for Problematic Alcohol Use: a Review of Systematic Reviews. Int J Behav Med. 2016 [Epub ahead of print].

76. De Wildt WA, Schippers GM, Van Den Brink W, Potgieter AS, Deckers F, Bets D. Does psychosocial treatment enhance the efficacy of acamprosate in patients with alcohol problems? Alcohol Alcohol. 2002; 37:375–82.

77. Agosti V, Nunes EV, O'Shea D. Do manualized psychosocial interventions help reduce relapse among alcohol-dependent adults treated with naltrexone or placebo? A meta-analysis. Am J Addict. 2012; 21:501–7.

78. Kiefer F, Jahn H, Tarnaske T, et al. Comparing and combining naltrexone and acamprosate in relapse prevention of alcoholism: a double-blind, placebo-controlled study. Arch Gen Psychiatry. 2003; 60:92–9.

79. Feeney GF, Connor JP, Young RM, Tucker J, McPherson A. Combined acamprosate and naltrexone, with cognitive behavioural therapy is superior to either medication alone for alcohol abstinence: a single centres' experience with pharmacotherapy. Alcohol Alcohol. 2006; 41:321–7.

80. Besson J, Aeby F, Kasas A, Lehert P, Potgieter A. Combined efficacy of acamprosate and disulfiram in the treatment of alcoholism: a controlled study. Alcohol Clin Exp Res. 1998; 22: 73–9.

81. McCarty D, Braude L, Lyman DR, et al. Substance abuse intensive outpatient programs: assessing the evidence. Psychiatr Serv. 2014; 65:718–26.

82. Tiet QQ, Ilgen MA, Byrnes HF, Harris AH, Finney JW. Treatment setting and baseline substance use severity interact to predict patients' outcomes. Addiction. 2007; 102:432–40.

83. Matching Alcoholism Treatments to Client Heterogeneity: Project MATCH posttreatment drinking outcomes. J Stud Alcohol. 1997; 58:7–29.

84. UKATT Research Team. UK Alcohol Treatment Trial: client-treatment matching effects. Addiction. 2008; 103:228–38.

85. Witkiewitz K, Hartzler B, Donovan D. Matching motivation enhancement treatment to client motivation: re-examining the Project MATCH motivation matching hypothesis. Addiction. 2010; 105:1403–13.

86. Garbutt JC, Greenblatt AM, West SL, et al. Clinical and biological moderators of response to naltrexone in alcohol dependence: a systematic review of the evidence. Addiction. 2014; 109: 1274–84.

87. Kiefer F, Witt SH, Frank J, et al. Involvement of the atrial natriuretic peptide transcription factor GATA4 in alcohol dependence, relapse risk and treatment response to acamprosate. Pharmacogenomics J. 2011; 11:368–74.

88. Kranzler HR, Covault J, Feinn R, et al. Topiramate treatment for heavy drinkers: moderation by a GRIK1 polymorphism. Am J Psychiatry. 2014; 171:445–52.

89. Joos L, Goudriaan AE, Schmaal L, et al. Effect of modafinil on impulsivity and relapse in alcohol dependent patients: a randomized, placebo-controlled trial. Eur Neuropsychopharmacol. 2013; 23:948–55.

90. Oslin DW, Leong SH, Lynch KG, et al. Naltrexone vs placebo for the treatment of alcohol dependence: A randomized clinical trial. JAMA Psychiatry. 2015; 72:430–7.

# 51

# Opioids
## Heroin, methadone, and buprenorphine

*Michael Farrell, Briony Larance, and Courtney Breen*

## What are opioids?

The term *opioid* is a general term applied to drugs derived from the opium poppy (*Papaver somniferum*) and the range of naturally occurring, synthetic, and semi-synthetic compounds derived from them [1]. These drugs relieve pain (*analgesic* effect) and create a sense of euphoria (*narcotic* effect). Opioids produce most of their effects by binding to three main opioid receptor subtypes in the brain: mu (μ), delta (δ), and kappa (κ) [1]. There are also endogenous opioids, such as endorphins, that help the body regulate the sensation of pain, although mostly, the term *opioid* is used to describe a class of exogenous drugs (such as heroin and morphine). Examples of different opioids and their mode of action (that is, *agonists, partial agonists, antagonists*, and *agonist–antagonists*) [1] are provided in Table 51.1. Opioid *agonists* include heroin, morphine, and methadone; a *partial agonist* is buprenorphine, and opioid *antagonists* include naltrexone and naloxone.

### The role of opioid medications

Pharmaceutical opioids have an important, legitimate role in medical practice and contribute to the health and well-being of many patients. There are two broad clinical indications for their use: (1) the management of pain that is either acute or chronic; and (2) the management of opioid dependence through opioid substitution therapy (OST). The World Health Organization (WHO) states that opioid medications are '*absolutely necessary*' for the management of severe cancer pain [2, p. 7] and '*essential medicines*' for the treatment of opioid dependence [3]. Although the optimal use of opioids in the management of chronic non-cancer pain is increasingly debated and a subject of significant controversy in North America [4], there are clear statements from pain organizations supporting their continuing use [5, 6].

### Common opioids

Opium is extracted from the opium poppy, and heroin (diacetylmorphine) is synthesized from the extraction; both are short-acting opioid agonists [1, 7]. Heroin has medical applications in some countries, with a long tradition of medical use for analgesia in England (for example, [8, 9]). In other countries, including Australia, both heroin and opium are illegal and their use is heavily stigmatized because of the health and social harms associated with illicit use [10]. A large number of pharmaceutical opioids have been developed for medical purposes.

Many of the opioid medications used most commonly in the management of pain (both acute and chronic) are longer acting than heroin and include morphine, oxycodone, hydromorphone, propoxyphene, fentanyl, pethidine, codeine, and less commonly methadone and buprenorphine (Table 51.1) [11]. Methadone and buprenorphine are the most commonly used opioids for the management of opioid dependence.

### The effects of opioids—desirable and adverse

The desirable effects of opioid agonists and partial agonists include euphoria, analgesia, and sedation [10]. The more common adverse effects associated with opioid use include nausea, vomiting, respiratory depression, constipation, drowsiness, and confusion [14, 15]. These side effects often limit the dosing and effectiveness of opioids, leading to early discontinuation, under-dosing, and adequate analgesia [14]. Prolonged use of opioids may result in additional adverse consequences such as tolerance hyperalgesia, decreases in testosterone, oestrogen, and other hormones, and immunosuppression [14]. Higher doses, particularly deliberate overdoses, can produce severe respiratory depression, circulatory failure, coma, and death [10, 16, 17].

When opioid medications are used outside the guidelines for safe and effective use, adverse effects are more likely, particularly those associated with higher doses and injection. Additional risks are associated with concurrent use of sedative drugs (for example, [18, 19–21]) and the presence of pre-existing conditions like impairment of liver function in which medicinal opioid use may be contraindicated [1, 17]. The injection of opioids also carries risks such as the potential transmission of blood-borne virus (BBV) infection if injecting equipment is shared, as well as harms related to injection of a non-sterile medication that is intended for administration by another route. The risk of developing opioid dependence may also be greater if used outside of, or without, medical supervision.

**Table 51.1** Common pharmaceutical opioids

| Type of opioid | Common drug names | Main medical indication | Half-life* |
|---|---|---|---|
| **Agonist** | Codeine | Pain | 3 hours |
| | Fentanyl | Pain | 3 hours[1] |
| | Hydromorphone | Pain | 2.5 hours |
| | Methadone | Pain/opioid dependence | 15–60 hours |
| | Morphine | Pain | 3 hours |
| | Oxycodone | Pain | 2.5 hours |
| | Pethidine | Pain | 3 hours |
| | Dextropropoxyphene | Pain | 6–12 hours |
| **Partial agonist** | Buprenorphine | Pain/opioid dependence | 35 hours[2] |
| **Antagonist** | Naltrexone | Opioid dependence | 4–13 hours |
| | Naloxone | Emergency treatment of opioid overdose | 1–1.5 hours |

* Half-life for immediate-release formulation.
[1] Following an intravenous dose.
[2] Following a sublingual dose.
Source: data from Brunton L, Chabner B, Knollman B, *Goodman & Gilman's The Pharmacological Basis of Therapeutics*, 11th ed., Copyright (2006), McGraw-Hill; *Pain Physician*, 11(2 Suppl), Trescot AM, Datta S, Lee M, *et al.*, Opioid pharmacology, S133–53, Copyright (2008), American Society of Interventional Pain Physicians.

**Table 51.2** Criteria for past year ICD-10/DSM-IV opioid dependence

| *Both classifications require three or more of the following criteria to have been present together during the previous 12 months:* | ICD-10 | DSM-IV |
|---|---|---|
| Compulsive use | ✓ | |
| Loss of control (onset, termination, or levels of use) | ✓ | |
| Escalation in dose or length of use | | ✓ |
| Unsuccessful attempts to cease or control use | | ✓ |
| Withdrawal | ✓ | ✓ |
| Tolerance | ✓ | ✓ |
| Progressive neglect of usual interests/responsibilities | ✓ | ✓ |
| Continued use despite harm | ✓ | ✓ |
| Increased time spent obtaining, using, or recovering from use | | ✓ |

*Source:* data from: World Health Organization, *The ICD-10 Classification of Mental and Behavioural Disorders*, Copyright (1996), World Health Organization; *Diagnostic and Statistical Manual of Mental Disorders*, Fourth Edition, DSM-IV, Copyright (1994), American Psychiatric Association.

Regardless of whether opioids are used with or without medical supervision, tolerance will develop following a period of regular use [22]. Opioid tolerance is a predictable pharmacological adaptation, and patients may require increasing amounts of the drug to maintain the same pharmacological effects [22, 23]. Tolerance develops to the analgesic, euphoric, sedative, respiratory depressant, and nauseating effects of opioids, but not to their peripheral effects on miosis (constriction of the pupils) and constipation [22].

If use ceases after tolerance has developed, withdrawal symptoms usually occur. Common withdrawal symptoms include body aches, diarrhoea, gooseflesh, loss of appetite, nervousness, restlessness, runny nose, sneezing, tremors or shivering, stomach cramps, nausea, insomnia, increased sweating, lethargy, tachycardia, and fever [16, 22]. With appropriate medical supervision and gradual withdrawal, these symptoms are usually mild. When opioids are stopped abruptly, however, these symptoms are more severe.

## Opioid dependence

### The clinical features of opioid dependence

The repeated, ongoing use of heroin, opium, or pharmaceutical opioids can result in people developing the chronic, often relapsing, condition known as *opioid dependence*. Opioid dependence causes significant burden to the user, their family, and the broader community [10]. It can result in significant costs to society through unemployment, homelessness, family disruption, loss of economic productivity, social instability, criminal activity, and/or ill health [24, 25]. It is typically characterized by the symptoms of tolerance, withdrawal upon cessation, compulsive use, loss of control over use, escalation in dose or length of use, unsuccessful quit attempts, progressive neglect of usual interests and responsibilities, continued use despite harm, and/or increased time spent obtaining, using, or recovering from use (Table 51.2) [26, 27].

The major health consequences of illicit opioid dependence include an increased risk of blood-borne infections such as HIV, HCV, and HBV through injection [24], overdose, and highly elevated risks of premature mortality [28–30]. In the 2000 WHO Global Burden of Disease estimates, it was thought that illicit drug use caused around 200,000 deaths worldwide, of which opioid overdose was estimated to account for around 70,000 (around 35%), and AIDS around 105,000 (around 53%) [28].

People affected by opioid dependence frequently fluctuate between the physical states of intoxication and withdrawal [31]. This pharmacological instability can disrupt the neurobiological systems that regulate, among other things, emotion, mood, and sleep, and the individual can experience dysphoria and persistent drug cravings [32, 33]. Comorbid psychiatric disorders are common, including elevated levels of depression, anxiety, suicidality, personality disorders, and post-traumatic stress disorder [34, 35]. Among people who are opioid-dependent, the daily challenge of obtaining opioids tends to dominate their experience and activities. The chaotic lifestyle of opioid dependence has profound social effects on the person and the people around them—managing dependence and the associated harms is often a long-term issue [10].

Currently, there are two main systems of classification for the diagnosis of opioid use disorders internationally: (1) the International Classification of Diseases, tenth revision (ICD-10) produced by the WHO and typically preferred in health epidemiology; and (2) the *Diagnostic and Statistical Manual of Mental Disorders* (DSM-IV-TR, DSM-5) preferred by the mental health sector and the United States in particular [26, 27]. Both ICD-10 and DSM-IV-TR historically used the term *opioid dependence* to describe a pattern of 'maladaptive behaviours', such as loss of control over use, craving, preoccupation with use, and continued use despite causing harm [26, 27], but both classification systems have recently undergone revisions, with ICD-11 still in draft form.

The newest edition of the *Diagnostic and Statistical Manual of Mental Disorders* (DSM-5) made substantial changes to the way in which opioid use disorders were conceptualized. DSM-5 no longer uses the terms 'abuse' and 'dependence', in favour of a single continuum of opioid use disorders classified as mild, moderate, or severe, depending on the number of diagnostic criteria met [36]. In addition, tolerance and withdrawal were previously included as features of the drug use disorder *opioid dependence* but, on their own, were not sufficient for the opioid dependence diagnosis. In DSM-5, tolerance and withdrawal are excluded as features of an opioid use disorder where an individual is prescribed an opioid and taking it as directed [36].

## Epidemiology and natural history of problematic opioid use

Illicit opioid use, typically involving heroin, but increasingly involving the extra-medical use of other pharmaceutical opioids, is a significant health problem internationally. In many developed countries, dependent heroin users are typically daily, or near daily, injectors of heroin, and other opioid and sedative drugs in combination with, or as an alternative to, heroin. They continue to use heroin despite the significant social and health problems arising from use, such as being arrested for drug or property crimes, with subsequent imprisonment, exposure to BBVs and increased potential for contracting infectious diseases, and fatal or non-fatal opioid overdose. Increasingly, in countries such as the United States, there are new populations of people who developed opioid dependence through the extra-medical use of pharmaceutical opioids [37] and there is evidence of people transitioning from problematic use of pharmaceutical opioids to heroin injection [38].

Research with prospective cohort studies of dependent opioid users in the United Kingdom, Australia, and the United States indicates that many dependent heroin users who seek treatment or come to attention through the legal system continue to use heroin for decades [39–42]. In this population, daily heroin use is punctuated by periods of abstinence, drug treatment, and imprisonment [10]. When periods of voluntary and involuntary abstinence during treatment or imprisonment are included, it has been estimated that dependent heroin users use heroin daily for 40–60% of their 20-year use careers [43, 44]. 'Remission' rates for heroin dependence are half those for other illicit drugs [45]. It is this long-term pattern of problematic opioid use that presents challenges to clinicians and researchers in determining the best management approaches and in ensuring that the extent of the adverse social and health consequences are minimized.

The illegality of opioids, such as heroin, makes the accurate assessment of how many people use these drugs difficult; however, recent estimates suggest there are 15.5 million problem opioid users worldwide [46, 47], and although the prevalence of opioid dependence is low (0.7–0.9% of the global population [48]), it is the largest direct contributor to the burden of illicit drug use [46, 48]. The harms to the individual and the community are significant, with large burden associated with infectious diseases (for example, HIV, HBV, and HBC) and overdose deaths [30, 46].

### Risk factors for opioid use and dependence

Very few studies have examined the risk factors and life pathways that lead young people to use, and become dependent on, heroin. This makes strong statements about the precursors of illicit opioid use difficult. There is, however, a large literature on risk factors for early use of alcohol and cannabis which indicates that young people who are the earliest initiators and heaviest users of alcohol and cannabis are those who are most likely to use heroin [49–51].

Two aspects of the family environment are associated with increased rates of licit and illicit drug use among children and adolescents. The first is the extent to which the child is exposed to a disadvantaged home environment, with parental conflict and poor discipline and supervision [52]. The second is the extent to which the child's parents and siblings use alcohol and other drugs [52]. These family environment factors can give rise to chronic childhood adversity but specifically predispose to drug use.

Children who perform poorly in school, those with impulsive or problem behaviour or conduct disorder in childhood, and those who are early users of alcohol and other drugs are more likely to use drugs like heroin [52, 53]. The nature of the relationship between peer affiliations and adolescent substance use remains controversial, but affiliation with drug-using peers is an important risk factor for drug use, which operates independently of individual and family risk factors [49].

Exposures to these family and social risk factors are highly correlated. Young people who initiate substance use at an early age have often been exposed to multiple social and family disadvantages. They also tend to be impulsive, to have performed poorly at school, to come from families with problems and a history of parental substance use, and to affiliate with delinquent peers [49, 51, 52]. These psychosocial factors are confounded by genetic factors predisposing to substance use. The genetics of addiction are described in more detail in Chapter 49.

North America is currently experiencing escalating pharmaceutical opioid use and harm [37], recently labelled a 'public health emergency' by the Trump administration, with substantial increases in opioid-related deaths [54] and strain upon the health and drug treatment system [55]. The problems observed across North America appear to have been driven by widespread prescribing of controlled-release and 'strong opioids' such as oxycodone and fentanyl [56]. In this context, non-medical use of pharmaceutical opioids in childhood and early adolescence is a strong predictor of heroin use onset among adolescents and young adults [57]. Other countries, such as Australia, have also documented increasing opioid exposure across the general population, paralleled by increasing harms, including opioid-related hospital admissions, overdose, and opioid dependence and treatment-seeking [58].

## Treatment of opioid dependence

Worldwide, of all the illicit drugs, the demand for treatment is highest for opioids. The chronic, relapsing nature of opioid dependence often results in repeated treatment episodes and prolonged treatment need. The aims of any opioid treatment programme should be guided by the principles of reducing or ceasing opioid use, preventing future harms associated with opioid use, minimizing mortality risk, and improving quality of life and well-being [59].

### Treatment ideologies

Like alcohol, the dependence or addiction to illicit opioids has sometimes been viewed as a moral fault; however, increasingly, heroin dependence is being managed as a medical disorder. While early attempts to achieve abstinence were prominent, the recognition that opioid dependence is a chronic, relapsing disorder led to a focus on methods that would address the issue of relapse. Pharmacological treatments using methadone were viewed as a means of achieving neurobiological stability, thus maintaining the person in treatment, minimizing their relapse to illicit opioid use, and reducing the risk of fatal opioid overdose.

Other than methadone maintenance clinics, the treatment approaches for opioid dependence in many countries (for example, the United States) were largely non-medically orientated, predominantly focusing on psychosocial approaches to achieving and maintaining abstinence. There is a long tradition of using residential rehabilitation through a range of models and philosophies including Concept House and 12-Step models derived from Alcoholics Anonymous (usually referred to as Narcotics Anonymous). More recently, the introduction of buprenorphine for use in general practice was viewed in many countries (including the United States and France) as an opportunity to move away from more specialist clinics into primary care and to broaden access to opioid maintenance treatment [60]. Pharmacotherapies, such as methadone and buprenorphine, have been and remain the mainstays of effective management of opioid dependence.

### Opioid agonist (maintenance) treatments

Opioid agonist (maintenance) treatments, typically oral methadone or sublingual buprenorphine (± naloxone), used at the optimal dose range, are effective in treating opioid dependence. Maintenance treatment is designed to be an ongoing treatment. Maintenance use of pharmaceutical-grade opioids with a long duration of action, in known doses and purity, provides an opportunity to stabilize the person by eliminating withdrawal, craving, participation in obtaining illegal opioids, and the need for frequent (and risky) drug injection. When provided in the context of high-quality treatment services, these medications interrupt the cycle of intoxication and withdrawal, greatly reducing heroin and other illicit opioid use, crime, and the risk of death through overdose [59].

#### Methadone

The real breakthrough in the treatment of opioid dependence was the development of opioid agonists for maintenance treatment. Methadone was the first of these agonist drugs, introduced by Dole and Nyswander in New York in the early 1960s. They defined opioid dependence as a 'physiological disease characterised by a permanent metabolic deficiency', which was best managed by administering the opioid-dependent person 'a sufficient amount of drug to stabilise the metabolic deficiency' [61]. They introduced orally administered high or 'blockade' oral methadone doses at stabilization levels of between 50 mg to 150 mg/day as maintenance treatment [62]. Methadone treatment was administered as a component of a long-term supporting programme with maintenance, rather than opioid abstinence, as the original treatment goal [63].

This original maintenance model has sometimes been altered by lowering methadone doses, time-limiting treatment programmes, and responding to 'treatment failure' (for example, ongoing illicit opioid use) in a punitive fashion such as expelling the individual from treatment [63]. A systematic review found methadone doses of 60–100 mg/day are more effective than lower dosages in retaining patients and in reducing the use of heroin and cocaine during treatment. The optimal dose will vary for individuals and requires clinical judgement, but clinical guidelines should reflect the evidence [64].

The most effective methadone programmes are those that follow the original Dole and Nyswander dose range [63]. There have been a small number of RCTs on the efficacy of methadone treatment in comparison to control conditions, and they have shown that methadone maintenance was more effective than detoxification, no treatment, or placebo at retaining subjects in treatment and in reducing opioid use [65, 66]. To confirm these findings, similar efficacy has been noted in observational studies, with the additional finding that methadone-maintained individuals report reduced participation in criminal activity and reduced mortality [30, 67, 68].

With the spread of HIV/AIDS in the 1980s, methadone treatment received additional support and funding in countries around the world in the effort to slow the spread of the virus among the population of injecting drug users. There is reasonable evidence that methadone treatment was effective in this goal, if given at adequate dose levels and if patients remained in treatment [69, 70]. Its efficacy in helping reduce the prevalence of other established blood-borne epidemics such as HCV and HBV was and remains less clear, although there is evidence that good coverage of opioid maintenance treatment, combined with needle-syringe programmes, results in lower HCV incidence [71, 72]. Partly in recognition of its role in reducing the spread of HIV, methadone was included in the WHO's *Model List of Essential Medicines* in 2005 [73].

### Buprenorphine

The partial opioid agonist buprenorphine was developed in the 1970s as an analgesic and was soon after investigated for the treatment of opioid dependence. Early work using buprenorphine administered by the subcutaneous route characterized it as an opioid with low physical dependence liability, with minimal withdrawal syndrome [74]. Subsequently, evidence has suggested that buprenorphine does produce mild to moderate withdrawal syndrome [75]. Substantial international research effort has established the efficacy of buprenorphine maintenance therapy in RCTs [76].

France went from having no opioid maintenance treatments to registering both methadone and buprenorphine in 1995. By the next year, all registered doctors in France were able to prescribe buprenorphine without any additional training or licensing (the number of places in methadone treatment remained limited) [77]. This has resulted in approximately 65,000 patients per year being treated with buprenorphine, ten times the number treated there with methadone [78]. While other countries have not adopted France's more liberal buprenorphine-prescribing policies, it has been registered for use in the maintenance treatment of opioid dependence in Australia since 2001 and the United States since 2002, and many European countries. In Australia, medical practitioners have to be registered as buprenorphine prescribers in a similar accreditation process to methadone prescribing. In the United States, buprenorphine is less strictly regulated than methadone [79].

Buprenorphine is poorly absorbed when taken orally, so the usual route of administration is sublingual. Because the opioid effects plateau at increasing doses, buprenorphine carries a lower overdose risk than methadone, even if taken with other opioids [80]. It may still cause respiratory depression, however [81], particularly if taken with other sedative drugs such as alcohol or benzodiazepines [20, 21]. Buprenorphine dissociates from opioid receptor binding sites very slowly, possibly explaining the limited withdrawal syndrome observed with its use [82, 83]. Like methadone, buprenorphine has applications in both the management of pain and the treatment of opioid dependence. High-dose formulations have been used increasingly as maintenance treatment, and buprenorphine joined methadone in 2005 on the WHO's *Model List of Medicines* [84] as maintenance treatment for opioid dependence.

## Buprenorphine–naloxone

A newer formulation, also developed as a sublingual tablet and, more recently, as a sublingual film, contains both buprenorphine and naloxone (a μ , κ, and δ-receptor antagonist with no agonist effects) in a 4:1 ratio [85]. Buprenorphine–naloxone was specifically designed to minimize the risk of intravenous misuse among people who are opioid-dependent [85].

Buprenorphine–naloxone has clinical actions that are similar to those of buprenorphine. Addition of naloxone reduces the abuse liability of buprenorphine by attenuating the effects of its opioid agonist action and impacting withdrawal in certain circumstances [85]. When *injected* by opioid-tolerant individuals (an unintended route of administration), the formulation can precipitate unpleasant withdrawal symptoms [86]. This is because a sublingual dose of naloxone has a potent antagonist effect if injected, consistent with its use in emergency reversal of acute adverse opioid effects [1].

## Long-acting (depot and implant) formulations of buprenorphine

There is considerable interest in the development of long-acting (depot and implant) preparations of buprenorphine that would potentially improve adherence and pharmacological stability and allow the patient to undertake activities without having to attend their local pharmacy/clinic on a daily basis. Studies are under way to evaluate a number of different long-acting formulations. This is likely to become a significant treatment option in many countries over the next few years.

## Other opioid agonist treatments

The use of diacetylmorphine (heroin) as maintenance treatment was investigated decades ago, and again more recently [87]. Unfortunately, the stigma associated with heroin use means reasoned debate about its utility as a maintenance agent has been limited. Its use as a therapeutic agent is limited by its illicit status in many countries, but some countries have adopted the use of heroin as a maintenance agent for heroin dependence [88, 89].

Other opioid agonist treatments include dihydrocodeine and long-acting morphine [90]. Some countries have opted for introducing injectable opioid treatment for those people who do not respond well in first-line treatment with oral methadone or sublingual buprenorphine, for example the UK [87], Switzerland [91], and the Netherlands [88].

## Benefits and risks of agonist maintenance treatments

Opioid agonist treatments result in significant reductions in the negative health consequences and adverse effects of heroin dependence on public order [92]. There is strong evidence that methadone and buprenorphine are effective in reducing drug use [65, 93] and the spread of HIV [94]. Opioid agonist treatments have been demonstrated to improve physical and mental health and social functioning [65, 93] and to substantially reduce criminality [65, 95].

Demand for treatment, however, typically far exceeds the number of treatment places that are needed [96].

Despite its advantages, methadone is a full opioid agonist, and there is no ceiling to the level of respiratory depression or sedation which methadone can induce; thus, an overdose can be fatal [97]. In some countries and settings, the inconvenience of daily dosing and clinic visits may be unattractive to clients, and restrictions imposed by the daily dosing schedule on clients' general lifestyle and on opportunities to sustain employment may also limit its acceptance by people who are opioid-dependent.

The provision of unsupervised doses of methadone or buprenorphine results in diversion of the drug for illicit use by those not in treatment. The extent of this problem varies within and between countries, reflecting different policy and regulatory approaches. Under supervised dosing conditions, buprenorphine may be easier to divert than methadone, given its tablet formulation. It may also be easier to prepare for injection (an unintended route of administration), hence the development of buprenorphine–naloxone. Since buprenorphine is a partial agonist, it is safer in overdose [98]. Other benefits of buprenorphine may include an easier withdrawal phase and, because of a longer duration of action, the option of alternate-day dosing.

## Management of opioid withdrawal

In opioid-dependent patients, management of opioid withdrawal alone does not represent a treatment in and of itself, since relapse to opioid use is common following medication cessation [99]. Symptomatic treatment of the physical effects of opioid withdrawal with clonidine or lofexidine is sometimes used in settings where it is not possible to prescribe effective opioid substitution. However, buprenorphine is more effective than clonidine or lofexidine for the management of opioid withdrawal and may offer some advantages over methadone in terms of quicker resolution of withdrawal symptoms and possibly slightly higher rates of completion of withdrawal [100].

## Naltrexone for relapse prevention

Naltrexone is an opioid receptor antagonist and so can prevent an individual who was formerly using opioids from experiencing the desired effects. Oral naltrexone is not widely used; its effects are not attractive to the target population, achieves limited adherence, and does not provide any additional benefits to other standards of care in terms of relapse prevention [101]. Individuals can only commence naltrexone following a withdrawal programme; otherwise, it can result in severe and prolonged withdrawal symptoms. It appears to be suited only to a small and highly motivated formerly opioid-dependent people seeking to maintain abstinence [102]. Depot and implant formulations of naltrexone may have greater utility, but current data are only preliminary.

## Psychosocial interventions

In the absence of evidence for the effectiveness of psychosocial treatments alone, they are usually adjunctive to opioid maintenance treatment [95, 103–104].

### Psychological interventions

Psychological interventions can range from unstructured supportive counselling and motivational interviewing to highly structured techniques. The choice will depend on the available resources, appropriateness to the individual's situation, patient acceptability, staff training, and cultural appropriateness.

The two main evidence-based therapy approaches include cognitive behavioural therapy (CBT) [105] and contingency management [106]. Applied to opioid dependence, CBT is based on the principle that addictions are learnt behaviours that can be modified most effectively by changing the faulty cognitions that maintain behaviour and by promoting positive cognitions and behaviour change. Variants of this approach include 'cognitive therapy' and 'motivational enhancement therapy'. CBT is typically delivered by trained clinicians [107].

Somewhat differently, contingency management assumes that behaviours are underpinned by conditioned learning, specifically classical and operant conditioning [106]. This approach aims to extinguish the classically conditioned responses using techniques like cue exposure, and to reinforce positive behaviour using instrumental conditioning where behaviours, such as abstinence, are rewarded using strategies such as contingency management. Typically, contingency management programmes clearly define the desired behaviour (for example, opioid-free days), conduct regular monitoring (for example, urine drug screening), specify rewards such as money or vouchers, and provide personalized, positive feedback from the treating staff.

### Social interventions

Social interventions provide practical assistance in addressing basic needs, such as food or housing, as well as education and employment support, and access to broader community resources (such as government benefits, recreational/leisure opportunities, etc.) [107, 108]. Typically, the patient's needs are assessed and met using a key worker or a case management system outside the treatment service) [107, 108].

### Self-help groups

Typically, these groups are abstinence-based and provide emotional support. Many also promote a particular ideology or values through which members may develop a strong sense of identity. The most common framework for self-help groups is the 12-Step programme (for example, Narcotics Anonymous). Little research has been conducted on this approach, but observational studies indicate positive treatment effects. Self-help groups are inexpensive and are a valued source of psychosocial support among participants. An important component is voluntary participation.

## Clinical management and considerations

### Assessment and diagnosis of opioid dependence
#### Substance use

A detailed substance use history takes into account the use of all psychoactive substances, including illicit and pharmaceutical opioids, alcohol, cannabis, stimulants, and benzodiazepines. The assessment should establish past and current substance use, duration of use, quantity and frequency of recent use, route of administration, and time of last use [107–109]. In addition to current substance use, it is important to assess the patient's experiences of previous treatment episodes, including their perspectives on what worked previously, the factors leading to relapse, and the types of treatment they are prepared to consider [107].

#### Physical examination

Physical examination should include assessment of intoxication and withdrawal (as observable indicators of neuroadaptation), relative to the patient's report of last drug use. Withdrawal severity can assist in indicating the severity of dependence, as well as the timing and amount of the first dose of methadone or buprenorphine [109]. Recent use of opioids increases the likelihood of withdrawal being precipitated by buprenorphine or naloxone. Intoxication with central nervous system depressants, such as alcohol or benzodiazepines, in combination with methadone or buprenorphine, increases the risk of overdose [109]; this is a critical consideration during induction and needs ongoing assessment and review.

Among people who inject opioids, physical examination of injection sites can also provide useful information on the timing and duration of injecting drug use, as well as any related complications such as site infections [107–109]. A combination of recent and old injection sites will normally be seen in an opioid-dependent patient with current neuroadaptation [107].

#### Urine drug screening

Urine drug screening is useful to corroborate patient history and establish recent opioid and other substance use [107–109]. Negative urine drug screening, combined with the absence of withdrawal symptoms, indicates caution is needed in the initiation of opioid maintenance therapy or other sedative medication [109] due to increased risk of overdose. Urine testing, in combination with patient history, is also useful in identifying other substances that have recently been consumed. International guidelines recommend against using a naloxone challenge to confirm current neuroadaptation, as this can induce significant withdrawal effects unnecessarily [107]. Delays in obtaining urine drug screening results should not delay treatment initiation where the diagnosis can be clearly established [107–109]. Urine drug screening can be perceived as punitive by patients, so it is important to explain the purpose clearly [109].

#### Other investigations

Investigations for other conditions, either related to the presenting condition or related to the patient's drug use (for example, BBVs, liver disease) should also be undertaken to inform future care planning. A high proportion of people who inject drugs may also be infected with HBV or HCV. This is unlikely to pose problems for induction of methadone or buprenorphine, unless advanced liver disease is detectable at clinical examination [109], but it is an important clinical consideration. Voluntary testing for HIV, hepatitis C, and common infectious diseases should be offered as part of an individual assessment, accompanied by counselling before and after the test [107]. Serology testing and vaccination for hepatitis B are also recommended [107]. Other infectious diseases that should be taken into consideration include tuberculosis and sexually transmitted infections.

Pregnancy testing should be offered to all women, particularly those contemplating opioid withdrawal, because it may influence the choice of treatment [107].

## Diagnosis of opioid dependence

Typically, opioid dependence is established according to standard definitions in the ICD or DSM [107–109]. It can be more challenging to assess dependence in a patient using pharmaceutical opioids for chronic pain. Tolerance and withdrawal can arise due to neuroadaptation associated with regular use of opioids for pain, and on their own, these features are not sufficient to diagnose dependence in this context. Features consistent with diminished control over opioid use (for example, multiple dose escalations, unsanctioned routes of administration, use for reasons other than pain, etc.) should also be examined. The diagnosis of opioid dependence is typically based on the patient history, corroborated by physical examination and/or other investigations [107].

## Other biopsychosocial considerations

### General health

Beyond establishing substance use and opioid dependence, it is good practice to assess the general health of patients being considered for methadone or buprenorphine maintenance treatment. The aim is to identify unmet health care needs and any health problems that could interact with methadone or buprenorphine [108]. Such assessments might include: past medical issues, operations, injuries, and periods in hospital; current prescription medications; psychiatric history; drug-related complications such as injection-related injuries or diseases; family planning and contraception; sexual health; dental health; and allergies or sensitivities [108]. Additional investigations may include liver, thyroid, and renal function and haematological indices [108].

Patients with prolongation of the QTc interval (that is, >500 ms between the onset of ventricular depolarization and completion of ventricular repolarization) who are treated with methadone and, less commonly, buprenorphine are at increased risk of adverse cardiac-related events [109].

### Psychiatric comorbidity

Depression, anxiety, and post-traumatic stress disorder are common among people who are opioid-dependent [110], and psychiatric assessment and referral should be incorporated into care planning.

### Social issues

Social exclusion and issues, such as housing, financial, and relationship problems, are also important clinical considerations and may impact on the choice of treatment and setting.

### Risk assessment

Assessing risks that may impact on the safety or efficacy of treatment is essential, including risk behaviours such as overdose, polydrug use, problematic alcohol use, unsafe injecting practices, and unsafe sex. Wider risk may include self-harm or risk of harm to others. Risks to dependent children should also be assessed and responded to, according to local child protection requirements [108]. Risk assessments should be ongoing throughout treatment and involve the relevant health and welfare providers.

### Care planning

The challenge in the management of opioid dependence does not simply come from the need for knowledge and expertise around diagnosing and managing opioid dependence. A structured and compassionate approach to some of the more complex aspects of drug dependence and related lifestyle complications is required to assess and plan sensible care. In the first instance, current injectors will need advice about harm reduction, safer injection practices, and overdose prevention and management. Discussion about the choice of agonist maintenance treatment should take into account patient preferences, but local policies and guidelines will also be important factors.

Current evidence suggests that key treatment outcomes for methadone and buprenorphine are comparable under optimal treatment conditions. Other factors that may impact upon treatment choice include patient or clinician preferences and previous responses to treatment. There may be considerable individual variation in absorption, metabolism, and clearance of methadone or buprenorphine. Patients who continue to use opioids, while receiving high doses of buprenorphine, may be better suited to higher doses of a full agonist like methadone. On the other hand, the less sedating effects of buprenorphine may be preferred by some patients.

## Specific groups and issues

There are some patient groups with additional or complex needs, and specific treatment settings that may raise important considerations in planning treatment of opioids dependence.

### Adolescents

Some adolescents are brought to the clinic by families concerned about their drug use. Others come from socially disadvantaged backgrounds, may be homeless, and may have more severe presentations. Assessment of adolescents should include medical, psychological, education, family, and other aspects of the adolescent's life.

Treatment approaches should take into account the higher levels of risk-taking, novelty-seeking, and peer pressure among adolescents, compared to older people. Treatment needs to be individualized and comprehensive, taking into consideration an adolescent's strengths, psychosocial supports, education, legal status, health, and pattern of illicit drug use. Agonist maintenance treatments in adolescent populations need further study, but early findings are promising [111, 112]. The clinical profile of opioid-dependent adolescents can be complex, with a high prevalence of comorbid depression, post-traumatic stress disorder, conduct disorder, and attention-deficit/hyperactivity disorder. Where there is supportive family or carers, family counselling may be helpful.

### Women

Women may be more vulnerable to the adverse medical and social consequences of opioid dependence. Compared to men, women with opioid dependence tend to have lower levels of education, fewer financial resources, and elevated histories of childhood trauma and physical and sexual abuse [113, 114].

Women typically use less quantity of opioids than men but transition more rapidly to dependence and treatment-seeking, with more benzodiazepine use [109]. They are more likely to have childcare responsibilities that could impede their access to treatments, and they may be reluctant to participate in group support activities with men [113]. Some evidence indicates that women are less likely to drop out of women-only programmes, which is likely to lead to better outcomes [113]. However, data are lacking on the relative efficacy of gender-specific services for women. To be responsive to the needs of women, it has been suggested services need to provide individual or female-only group counselling and childcare facilities and take measures to prevent sexual harassment of female patients by male staff [109].

### Pregnancy and breastfeeding

Maintaining or initiating opioid agonist maintenance treatment is the preferred approach to the management of opioid dependence in women who are pregnant or breastfeeding [108, 115]. Methadone is frequently preferred to buprenorphine because it has been in use longer in this context [107, 109]. Among opioid-dependent women who are pregnant, methadone is associated with improved maternal and neonatal outcomes, compared to the pregnancies of women not receiving opioid agonist treatment. Although both methadone and buprenorphine are associated with neonatal abstinence syndrome, this can be resolved by administering morphine with supportive care [108].

Detoxification during pregnancy is not recommended. In the first trimester, detoxification carries significant risk of miscarriage. In the third trimester, it can cause significant fetal distress and premature labour [109]. Typically, pregnant women are encouraged to remain on agonist maintenance therapy during pregnancy and the postnatal period [107]. Agonist maintenance treatment is thought to have minimal long-term developmental impacts on children, when compared to the risk of maternal heroin use and resulting harms [109].

Both methadone and buprenorphine are detectable in breast milk at low levels, which are not thought to affect infant outcomes [107]. Thus, opioid-dependent mothers are normally encouraged to breastfeed; however, where there is polydrug dependence, caution may be necessary.

### Blood-borne virus infections and tuberculosis

Early in the HIV epidemic of the 1980s, it was established that provision of sterile injecting equipment and increased coverage of opioid dependence treatment could reduce the spread of BBVs. This approach combines a public health strategy with a high standard of individual treatment.

England and Australia, for example, have achieved major success, with <2% of people who inject drugs contracting HIV over the past few decades [116]. Unfortunately there are many countries, particularly in the Asia Pacific region, Eastern Europe, and Russia, that still report major rates of HIV infection among injecting drug users [116].

For those who are infected, combined treatment of both HIV with available antiretroviral medications and agonist maintenance treatment to manage the opioid dependence can achieve reasonable levels of adherence [116].

The new treatments for hepatitis C are also acceptable to patients and are associated with very high levels of clearance [117]. The challenge for treatment systems is to develop integrated approaches that enable all current and former injectors to benefit.

Tuberculosis is a new and increasing concern because of multi-resistant cases in vulnerable populations of prisoners [118], the homeless, and migrant populations.

### Forensic and prison populations

Between a third and a half of most prison populations have a history of opioid dependence.

This poses risks for individuals both at the point of entry and at the point of departure from prison. On entry, there is a need for a proper assessment of both physical and mental health status and plans for appropriate care and management of their drug dependence. Ideally, the provision of ongoing maintenance should be made available [119, 120]. This will reduce the risk of both suicide and unnatural death during the period of imprisonment [119]. It will also reduce very significantly the risk of overdose death in the first month after release [121]. In addition, provision of this treatment should help to engage individuals in help and support and care for other aspects of their mental and physical well-being, including possible treatment for hepatitis C [122].

Most individuals are in prison for short periods of time. A system works best when it aims to create continuity between treatment in the prison and treatment in the community that works to promote health and well-being and to assist in the reintegration into the community after prison release.

### Psychiatric comorbidity and polysubstance use

There are well-recognized overlaps between substance dependence and psychiatric comorbidity, so all assessments need to take into consideration the risks for self-harm and suicide and manage appropriately. However, polysubstance use poses a significant challenge for treatment planning and ensuring appropriate prescribing. Such individuals require careful assessment, ideally by a specialist practitioner who has both inpatient facilities and community arrangements where daily supervision of prescribed medication can be undertaken. Careful and cautious approaches can stabilize such individuals and reduce the immediate risk of overdose death.

## Conclusions

Over the past few decades, the treatment of opioid dependence has been well developed and the benefits and outcomes of treatment have been well documented. It has, however, remained a controversial treatment. The advent of prescription opioid dependence has further highlighted some of the complexities for doctors prescribing opioids in the longer term. The lifesaving benefits of good management of opioid dependence are beyond question. The opportunity to use such treatment to engage individuals in a broader range of medical and social interventions that will assist them to get their lives back on track is substantial. The issues of addiction in modern medicine are such that they require all competent and trained clinicians to have a full knowledge of basic assessment and management of drug dependence as core clinical skills. We look forward to the day when all doctors grasp this opportunity and extend it to their most vulnerable patients.

### REFERENCES

1. Trescot AM, Datta S, Lee M, Hansen H. Opioid pharmacology. *Pain Physician*. 2008;11:S133–53.
2. World Health Organization. *Achieving balance in national opioid drugs control policy: a guideline for assessment*. Geneva: World Health Organization; 2000.
3. World Health Organization. *WHO Model List of Essential Medicines*, 15th edition. 2007. http://www.who.int/medicines/publications/essentialmedicines/en/index.html

4. Ballantyne JC. Regulation of opioid prescribing. *BMJ*. 2007;334:811–12.

5. American Academy of Pain Medicine and American Pain Society. *The use of opioids for the treatment of chronic pain: a consensus statement from the American Academy of Pain Medicine and the American Pain Society*. 2007. http://www.painmed.org/productpub/statements/pdfs/opioids.pdf

6. Beubler E, Jaksch W, Devulder J, *et al.* The European white paper on the use of opioids in chronic pain management. *Journal of Pain and Palliative Care Pharmacotherapy*. 2006;20:79–87.

7. United Nations Office on Drugs and Crime. *World Drug Illicit Report 2009*. Vienna: United Nations; 2009.

8. Ferri M, Davoli M, Perucci CA. Heroin maintenance for chronic heroin dependents (review). *Cochrane Database of Systematic Reviews*. 2005;2:CD003410.

9. Ferri M, Davoli M, Perucci CA. Heroin maintenance treatment for chronic heroin-dependent individuals: a Cochrane systematic review of effectiveness. *Journal of Substance Abuse Treatment*. 2006;30:63–72.

10. Darke S. *The Life of the Heroin User: Typical Beginnings, Trajectories and Outcomes*. Cambridge: Cambridge University Press; 2011.

11. Degenhardt L, Larance B, Mathers B, *et al. Benefits and risks of pharmaceutical opioids: essential treatment and diverted medication. A global review of availability, extra-medical use, injection and the association with HIV*. Thematic paper undertaken on behalf of the Reference Group to the United Nations on HIV and injecting drug use. Sydney: National Drug and Alcohol Research Centre, University of New South Wales; 2008.

12. Brunton L, Chabner B, Knollman B. *Goodman & Gilman's The Pharmacological Basis of Therapeutics*, 11th edition. New York, NY: McGraw-Hill; 2006.

13. Trescot AM, Datta S, Lee M, Hansen H. Opioid pharmacology. *Pain Physician*. 2008;11(2 Suppl):S133–53.

14. Benyamin R, Trescot AM, Datta S, *et al.* Opioid complications and side effects. *Pain Physician*. 2008;11:S105–20.

15. McNicol E, Horowicz-Mehler N, Fisk RA, *et al.* Management of opioid side effects in cancer-related and chronic noncancer pain: a systematic review. *Journal of Pain*. 2008;5:231–56.

16. MIMS Online. 2007. https://www.mimsonline.com.au/Search/QuickSearch.aspx?ModuleName=Product%20Info&searchKeyword=2007

17. Darke S, Degenhardt L, Mattick RP. *Mortality amongst Illicit Drug Users*. Cambridge: Cambridge University Press; 2007.

18. Caplehorn JRM, Drummer OH. Fatal methadone toxicity: signs and circumstances, and the role of benzodiazepines. *Australian and New Zealand Journal of Public Health*. 2002;26:358–62.

19. Mueller MR, Shah NG, Landen MG. Unintentional prescription drug overdose deaths in New Mexico, 1994–2003. *American Journal of Preventive Medicine*. 2006;30:423–9.

20. Nielsen S, Dietze P, Lee N, Dunlop A, Taylor D. Concurrent buprenorphine and benzodiazepines use and self-reported opioid toxicity in opioid substitution treatment. *Addiction*. 2007;102:616–22.

21. Reynaud M, Petit G, Potard D, Courty P. Six deaths linked to concomitant use of buprenorphine and benzodiazepines. *Addiction*. 1998;93:1385–92.

22. Mitra S, Sinatra RS. Perioperative management of acute pain in the opioid-dependent patient. *Anesthesiology*. 2004;101:212–27.

23. Savage SR. Opioid therapy of chronic pain: assessment of consequences. *Acta Anaesthesiologica Scandinavica*. 1999;43:909–17.

24. World Health Organization/United Nations Office of Drugs and Crime/Joint United Nations Programme on HIV/AIDs. *WHO/UNODC/UNAIDS position paper: substitution maintenance therapy in the management of opioid dependence and HIV/AIDs prevention*. Geneva: World Health Organisation; 2004.

25. Wall R, Rehm J, Fischer B, *et al.* Social costs of untreated opioid dependence. *Journal of Urban Health*. 2000;77:688–722.

26. American Psychiatric Association. *Diagnostic and Statistical Manual for Mental Disorders (DSM-IV-TR)*. Washington, D.C.: American Psychiatric Association; 2000.

27. World Health Organization. *The International Classification of Diseases, Version 10*. Geneva: World Health Organization; 1993.

28. Degenhardt L, Hall W, Lynskey M, Warner-Smith M. Illicit drug use. In: Ezzati M, Lopez AD, Rodgers A, Murray R (eds). *Comparative Quantification of Health Risks: Global and Regional Burden of Disease Attributable to Selected Major Risk Factors*, 2nd edition. Geneva: World Health Organization; 2004. pp. 1109–76.

29. Degenhardt L, Hall W, Warner-Smith M. Using cohort studies to estimate mortality among injecting drug users that is not attributable to AIDS. *Sexually Transmitted Infections*. 2006;82:56–63.

30. Degenhardt L, Bucello C, Mathers B, *et al.* Mortality among regular or dependent users of heroin and other opioids: a systematic review and meta-analysis of cohort studies. *Addiction*. 2011;106:32–51.

31. Royal Australian College of Physicians (Adult Medicine Division). *Australasian Chapter of Addiction Medicine. Clinical Guidelines: Assessing suitability for unsupervised medication doses in the treatment of opioid dependency*. Sydney: Adult Medicine Division, The Royal Australian College of Physicians; 2006.

32. Kosten TR. Neurobiology of abused drugs: opioids and stimulants. *Journal of Nervous and Mental Disease*. 1990;178:217–27.

33. Stimmel B. Maintenance for opioid addiction with buprenorphine and methadone: 'The only thing new in the world is the history you don't know'. *Journal of Addictive Diseases*. 2005;24:1–6.

34. Mills KL, Lynskey M, Teesson M, Ross J, Darke S. Post-traumatic stress disorder among people with heroin dependence in the Australian treatment outcome study (ATOS): prevalence and correlates. *Drug and Alcohol Dependence*. 2005;77:243–9.

35. Darke S, Ross J, Williamson A, Mills KL, Havard A, Teesson M. Borderline personality disorder and persistently elevated levels of risk in 36-month outcomes for the treatment of heroin dependence. *Addiction*. 2007;102:1140–6.

36. American Psychiatric Association. *Diagnostic and Statistical Manual of Mental Disorders (DSM-5). DSM-5 Development: Proposed Draft Revisions to DSM Disorders and Criteria: Substance-Related Disorders*. 2010. http://www.dsm5.org/ProposedRevisions/Pages/Substance-RelatedDisorders.aspx

37. Fischer B, Rehm J. Revisiting the 'paradigm shift' in opioid use: Developments and implications 10 years later. *Drug and Alcohol Review*. 2017;37(Suppl 1):S199–202.

38. Carlson RG, Nahhas RW, Martins SS, Daniulaityte R. Predictors of transition to heroin use among initially non-opioid dependent illicit pharmaceutical opioid users: a natural history study. *Drug and Alcohol Dependence*. 2016;160:127–34.

39. Hser YI, Hoffman V, Grella CE, Anglin MD. A 33-year follow-up of narcotics addicts. *Arch Gen Psychiatry*. 2001;58:503–8.

40. Goldstein A, Herrera J. Heroin addicts and methadone treatment in Alburquerque: a 22 year follow-up. *Drug and Alcohol Dependence*. 1995;40:139–50.

41. Hser YI, Hunag D, Chou C, Anglin MD. Trajectories of heroin addiction. Growth mixture modelling results based on a 33-year follow-up study. *Evaluation Review*. 2007;6:548–63.

42. Teesson M, Marel C, Darke S, *et al*. Long-term mortality, remission, criminality and psychiatric comorbidity of heroin dependence: 11-year findings from the Australian Treatment Outcome Study. *Addiction*. 2015;110:986–93.

43. Maddux J, Desmond D. Methadone maintenance and recovery from opioid dependence. *American Journal of Drug and Alcohol Abuse*. 1992;18:63–74.

44. Ball J, Shaffer J, Nurco D. The day-to-day criminality of heroin addicts in Baltimore—a study in the continuity of offence rates. *Drug and Alcohol Dependence*. 1983;12:119–42.

45. Calabria B, Degenhardt L, Briegleb C, *et al*. Systematic review of prospective studies investigating 'remission' from amphetamine, cannabis, cocaine or opioid dependence. *Addictive Behaviors*. 2010;35:741–9.

46. Degenhardt L, Charlson F, Mathers B, *et al*. The global epidemiology and burden of opioid dependence: results from the global burden of disease 2010 study. *Addiction*. 2014;109:1320–33.

47. Degenhardt L, Hall W. Extent of illicit drug use and dependence, and their contribution to the global burden of disease. *The Lancet*. 2012;379:55–70.

48. United Nations Office on Drugs and Crime. *World Drug Report 2017*. 2017. https://www.unodc.org/wdr2017/

49. Fergusson DM, Horwood LJ. Early onset cannabis use and psychosocial adjustment in young adults. *Addiction*. 1997;92:279–96.

50. Chen K, Kandel DB. The natural history of drug use from adolescence to the mid-thirties in a general population sample [see comments]. *American Journal of Public Health*. 1995;85:41–7.

51. Fergusson DM, Horwood LJ. Does cannabis use encourage other forms of illicit drug use? *Addiction*. 2000;95:505–20.

52. Hawkins J, Catalano R, Miller J. Risk and protective factors for alcohol and other drug problems in adolescence and early adulthood: implications for substance abuse prevention. *Psychological Bulletin*. 1992;112:64–105.

53. Hawkins J, Graham J, Maguin E, Abbott R, Hill K, Catalano R. Exploring the effects of age of alcohol use initiation and psychosocial risk factors on subsequent alcohol misuse. *Journal of Studies on Alcohol*. 1997;58:280–90.

54. Kassebaum NJ, Arora M, Barber RM, *et al*. Global, regional, and national disability-adjusted life-years (DALYs) for 315 diseases and injuries and healthy life expectancy (HALE), 1990–2015: a systematic analysis for the Global Burden of Disease Study 2015. *The Lancet*. 2016;388:1603–58.

55. Hsu DJ, McCarthy EP, Stevens JP, Mukamal KJ. Hospitalizations, costs and outcomes associated with heroin and prescription opioid overdoses in the United States 2001–12. *Addiction*. 2017;112:1558–64.

56. Rudd RA, Seth P, David F, Scholl L. Increases in drug and opioid-involved overdose deaths—United States, 2010–2015. *Morbidity and Mortality Weekly Report*. 2016;65:1445–52.

57. Cerdá M, Santaella J, Marshall BDL, Kim JH, Martins SS. Nonmedical prescription opioid use in childhood and early adolescence predicts transitions to heroin use in young adulthood: a national study. *Journal of Pediatrics*. 2015;167:605–12.e2.

58. Larance B, Degenhardt L, Peacock A, *et al*. Pharmaceutical opioid use and harm in Australia: the need for proactive and preventative responses. *Drug and Alcohol Review*. 2018;37(Suppl 1): S203–5.

59. World Health Organization. *Guidelines for the Psychosocially Assisted Pharmacological Treatmentof Opioid Dependence*. Geneva: World Health Organization; 2009.

60. Coffey C, Carlin JB, Degenhardt L, Lynskey M, Sanci L, Patton GC. Cannabis dependence in young adults: an Australian population study. *Addiction*. 2002;97:187–94.

61. Dole VP, Nyswander M. A medical treatment for diacetylmorphine (heroin) addiction: a clinical trial with methadone hydrochloride. *JAMA*. 1965;193:80–4.

62. Dole V, Nyswander M. A medical treatment for diacetylmorphine (heroin) addiction. *JAMA*. 1965;193:80–4.

63. Hall W, Ward J, Mattick RP. The effectiveness of methadone maintenance treatment 1: heroin use and crime. In: Ward J, Mattick RP, Hall W (eds). *Methadone Maintenance Treatment and Other Opioid Replacement Therapies*. Amsterdam: Harwood Academic Publishers; 1998. pp. 17–57.

64. Faggiano F, Vigna-Taglianti F, Versino E, Lemma P. Methadone maintenance at different dosages for opioid dependence. *Cochrane Database of Systematic Reviews*. 2003;3:CD002208.

65. Mattick RP, Breen C, Kimber J, Davoli M. Methadone maintenance therapy versus no opioid replacement therapy for opioid dependence. *Cochrane Database of Systematic Reviews*. 2009;2:CD002209.

66. Amato L, Davoli M, A.Perucci C, Ferri M, Faggiano F, P. Mattick R. An overview of systematic reviews of the effectiveness of opiate maintenance therapies: available evidence to inform clinical practice and research. *Journal of Substance Abuse Treatment*. 28:321–9.

67. Clausen T, Anchersen K, Waal H. Mortality prior to, during and after opioid maintenance treatment (OMT): A national prospective cross-registry study. *Drug and Alcohol Dependence*. 2008;94:151–7.

68. Lind B, Chen S, Weatherburn D, Mattick R. The effectiveness of methadone maintenance treatment in controlling crime. An Australian aggregate-level analysis. *Journal of Criminology*. 2005;45:201–11.

69. Gowing L, Farrell MF, Bornemann R, Sullivan LE, Ali R. Oral substitution treatment of injecting opioid users for prevention of HIV infection. *Cochrane Database of Systematic Reviews*. 2011;8:CD004145.

70. MacArthur GJ, Minozzi S, Martin N, *et al*. Opiate substitution treatment and HIV transmission in people who inject drugs: systematic review and meta-analysis. *BMJ*. 2012;345:e5945.

71. Ward J, Mattick RP, Hall W. The effectiveness of methadone maintenance treatment 2: HIV and infectious hepatitis. In: Ward J, Mattick RP, Hall W, editors. *Methadone maintenance treatment and other opioid replacement therapies*. Amsterdam: Harwood Academic Publishers; 1998. pp. 59–74.

72. Turner KME, Hutchinson S, Vickerman P, *et al*. The impact of needle and syringe provision and opiate substitution therapy on the incidence of hepatitis C virus in injecting drug users: pooling of UK evidence. *Addiction*. 2011;106:1978–88.

73. World Health Organization. *WHO Model List of Essential Medicines*, 20th edition. 2017. https://www.who.int/medicines/publications/essentialmedicines/en/

74. Jasinski D, Pevnick J, Griffith J. Human pharmacology and abuse potential of the analgesic buprenorphine. *Arch Gen Psychiatry*. 1978;35:501–6.

75. Fudala PJ, Jaffe, J.H., Dax, E.M., Johnson, R.E. Use of buprenorphine in the treatment of opioid addiction. II. Physiologic and behavioral effects of daily and alternateday

administration and abrupt withdrawal. *Clinical Pharmacology and Therapeutics*. 1990;47:525–34.

76. Mattick RP, Breen C, Kimber J, Davoli M. Buprenorphine maintenance versus placebo or methadone maintenance for opioid dependence. *Cochrane Database of Systematic Reviews*. 2014;2:CD002207.

77. Thirion X, Lapierre V, Micallef J, et al. Buprenorphine prescription by general practitioners in a French region. *Drug and Alcohol Dependence*. 2002;65:197–204.

78. Auriacombe M, Fatseas M, Dubernet J, Daulouede JP, Tignol J. French field experience with buprenorphine. *American Journal on Addictions*. 2004;13:S17-28.

79. Vastag B. In-office opiate treatment 'not a panacea': physicians slow to embrace therapeutic option. *JAMA*. 2003;290:731–5.

80. Elkader AS, B. Buprenorphine: clinical pharmacokinetics in the treatment of opioid dependence. *Clinical Pharmacokinetics*. 2005;44:661–80.

81. Geib A-J, Babu K, Ewald MB, Boyer EW. Buprenorphine/naloxone. CNS depression and respiratory insufficiency after inadvertant administration in infants: 5 case reports. *Pediatrics*. 2006;118:1746–51.

82. Dum J, Blasig J, Herz A. Buprenorphine: demonstration of physical dependence liability. *European Journal of Pharmacology*. 1981;70:293–300.

83. Quinn DI, Wodak A, Day RO. Pharmacokinetic and pharmacodynamic principles of illit drug use and treatment of illicit drug users. *Clinical Pharmacokinetics*. 1997;33:344–400.

84. World Health Organization. *WHO Model List of Essential Medicines*, 20th edition. 2017. https://www.who.int/medicines/publications/essentialmedicines/en/

85. Mammen K, Bell J. The clinical efficacy and abuse potential of combination buprenorphine-naloxone in the treatment of opioid dependence. *Expert Opinion on Pharmacotherapy*. 2009;10:2537–44.

86. Chiang CN, Hawks RL. Pharmacokinetics of the combination tablet of buprenorphine and naloxone. *Drug and Alcohol Dependence*. 2003;70(2, Supplement 1):S39–47.

87. Strang J, Metrebian N, Lintzeris N, et al. Supervised injactable heroin or injectable methadone versus optimised oral methadone as treatment for chronic heroin addicts in England after persistent failure of orthodox treatment (RIOTT): a randomised trial. *The Lancet*. 2010;375:1885–95.

88. Blanken P, Hendriks VM, Van Ree JM, Van Den Brink W. Outcome of long-term heroin-assisted treatment offered to chronic, treatment-resistant heroin addicts in the Netherlands. *Addiction*. 2010;105:300–8.

89. Farrell M, Hall W. Heroin-assisted treatment: has a controversial treatment come of age? *British Journal of Psychiatry*. 2015;207:3–4.

90. White JM, Lopatko OV. Opioid maintenance: a comparative review of pharmacological strategies. *Expert Opinion on Pharmacotherapy*. 2007;8:1–11.

91. Rehm J, Gschwend P, Steffen T, Gutzwiller F, Dobler-Mikola A, Uchtenhagen A. Feasibility, safety, and efficacy of injectable heroin prescription for refractory opioid addicts: a follow-up study. *The Lancet*. 2001;358:1417–20.

92. Hall W, Lynskey M, Degenhardt L. *Heroin use in Australia: its impact on public health and public order*. NDARC Monograph Number 42. Sydney: National Drug and Alcohol Research Centre, University of New South Wales; 1999.

93. Mattick RP, Kimber J, Breen C, Davoli M. Buprenorphine maintenance versus placebo or methadone maintenance for

94. Gowing L, Farrell M, Bornemann R, Sullivan LE, Ali R. Oral substitution treatment of injecting drug users for prevention of HIV infection. *Cochrane Database of Systematic Reviews*. 2011;10:CD004145.

95. Amato L, Davoli M, Perucci CA, Ferri M, Faggiano F, Mattick RP. An overview of systematic reviews of the effectiveness of opiate maintenance therapies: available evidence to inform clinical practice and research. *Journal of Substance Abuse Treatment*. 2005;28:321–9.

96. Mathers B, Degenhardt L, Ali H, et al. HIV prevention, treatment and care services for people who inject drugs: a systematic review of global, regional and national coverage. *The Lancet*. 2010;375:1–15.

97. Drummer OH, Opeskin K, Syrjanen M, Cordner SM. Methadone toxicity causing death in ten subjects starting on a methadone maintenance program. *American Journal of Forensic Medicine and Pathology*. 1992;13:346–50.

98. Kimber J, Larney S, Hickman M, Randall D, Degenhardt L. Mortality risk of opioid substitution therapy with methadone versus buprenorphine: a retrospective cohort study. *The Lancet Psychiatry*. 2015;2:901–8.

99. Ling W, Smith D. Buprenorphine: blending practice and research. *Journal of Substance Abuse Treatment*. 2002;23:87–92.

100. Gowing L, Ali R, White JM. Buprenorphine for the management of opioid withdrawal. *Cochrane Database of Systematic Reviews*. 2009;3:CD002025.

101. Minozzi S, Amato L, Vecchi S, Davoli M, Kirchmayer U, Verster A. Oral naltrexone maintenance treatment for opioid dependence. *Cochrane Database of Systematic Reviews*. 2011;4:CD001333.

102. Mattick RP, Oliphant D, Ward J, Hall W. The effectiveness of other opioid replacement therapies: LAAM, heroin, buprenorphine, naltrexone and injectable maintenance. In: Ward J, Mattick RP, Hall W (eds). *Methadone Maintenance Treatment and Other Opioid Replacement Therapies*. Amsterdam: Harwood Academic Publishers; 1998. pp. 123–60.

103. Amato L, Minozzi S, Davoli M, Vecchi S. Psychosocial and pharmacological treatments versus pharmacological treatments for opioid detoxification. *Cochrane Database of Systematic Reviews*. 2011;9:CD005031.

104. Amato L, Minozzi S, Davoli M, Vecchi S. Psychosocial combined with agonist maintenance treatments versus agonist maintenance treatments alone for treatment of opioid dependence. *Cochrane Database of Systematic Reviews*. 2011;10:CD004147.

105. Moore BA, Fiellin DA, Cutter CJ, et al. Cognitive behavioral therapy improves treatment outcomes for prescription opioid users in primary care buprenorphine treatment. *Journal of Substance Abuse Treatment*. 2016;71:54–7.

106. Weinstock J, Alessi SM, Petry NM. Regardless of psychiatric severity the addition of contingency management to standard treatment improves retention and drug use outcomes. *Drug and Alcohol Dependence*. 2007;87:288–96.

107. World Health Organization. *Guidelines for the psychosocially assisted pharmacological treatment of opioid dependence*. Geneva: World Health Organization; 2009.

108. Department of Health (England) and the devolved administrations. *Drug misuse and dependence: UK guidelines on clinical management*. London: Department of Health (England), the Scottish Government, Welsh Assembly Government and Northern Ireland Executive; 2007.

109. Gowing L, Ali R, Dunlop A, Farrell M, Lintzeris N. National guidelines for medication-assisted treatment of opioid dependence. Canberra: Department of Health, Commonwealth of Australia; 2014.

110. Mills KL, Teesson M, Ross J, Peters L. Trauma, PTSD, and substance use disorders: findings from the Australian National Survey of Mental Health and Well-Being. *Am J Psychiatry*. 2006;163:652–8.

111. Minozzi S, Amato L, Bellisario C, Davoli M. Maintenance treatments for opiate-dependent adolescents. *Cochrane Database of Systematic Reviews*. 2014;6:CD007210.

112. Committee on Substance Use and Prevention. Medication-assisted treatment of adolescents with opioid use disorders. *Pediatrics*. 2016;138:pii:e20161893.

113. Prendergast ML, Messina NP, Hall EA, Warda US. The relative effectiveness of women-only and mixed-gender treatment for substance-abusing women. *Journal of Substance Abuse Treatment*. 2011;40:336–48.

114. Shand FL, Degenhardt L, Slade T, Nelson EC. Sex differences amongst dependent heroin users: Histories, clinical characteristics and predictors of other substance dependence. *Addictive Behaviors*. 2011;36:27–36.

115. Department of Health and Ageing. *National pharmacotherapy policy for people dependent on opioids*. Canberra: Commonwealth of Australia; 2007.

116. Mathers BM, Degenhardt L, Ali H, *et al*. HIV prevention, treatment, and care services for people who inject drugs: a systematic review of global, regional, and national coverage. *The Lancet*. 2010;375:1014–28.

117. Nelson PK, Mathers BM, Cowie B, *et al*. Global epidemiology of hepatitis B and hepatitis C in people who inject drugs: results of systematic reviews. *The Lancet*. 2011;378:571–83.

118. Dolan K, Wirtz AL, Moazen B, *et al*. Global burden of HIV, viral hepatitis, and tuberculosis in prisoners and detainees. *The Lancet*. 2016;388:1089–102.

119. Larney S, Gisev N, Farrell M, *et al*. Opioid substitution therapy as a strategy to reduce deaths in prison: retrospective cohort study. *BMJ Open*. 2014;4:e004666.

120. Hedrich D, Alves P, Farrell M, Stöver H, Møller L, Mayet S. The effectiveness of opioid maintenance treatment in prison settings: a systematic review. *Addiction*. 2012;107:501–17.

121. Degenhardt L, Larney S, Kimber J, *et al*. The impact of opioid substitution therapy on mortality post-release from prison: retrospective data linkage study. *Addiction*. 2014;109:1306–17.

122. Larney S. Does opioid substitution treatment in prisons reduce injecting-related HIV risk behaviours? A systematic review. *Addiction*. 2010;105:216–23.

# 52

# Cannabis and mental illness

*David J. Castle*

## Introduction

*Cannabis sativa* has long been of interest to psychiatrists, mostly, it is reasonable to say, for its perceived negative effects on mental health in certain key domains, including mood, psychosis, and cognition. The last decade, in particular, has seen a flurry of activities aimed at trying to understand the associations between psychotic disorders, such as schizophrenia, and exposure to cannabis. There has also been increasing concern about negative effects on cognitive functioning in people who use large quantities of high-potency cannabis.

This occurs in the context of major changes to the potency of the plant product, as new strains and hydroponically grown cannabis have increasingly higher concentrations of the main psychotomimetic constituent delta-9-tetrahydrocannabinol (THC) and less of the putatively antipsychotic constituent cannabidiol (CBD). Also, the evolution of numerous synthetic cannabinoids makes tracking and policing of THC-like chemicals very difficult.

On the other side is a broader global debate about decriminalization, and even legalization, of cannabis. In part, this is driven by the clear failure of the 'war on drugs' to curb cannabis consumption and the understanding that criminal legislation and policing approaches to curtailing use are too simplistic and take up massive policing and legal resources. Also, many people believe that for most people, modest consumption of cannabis is not particularly harmful; one could argue that alcohol is a far more destructive drug at a population level and is associated with a myriad of physical and mental health problems.

Also, there is a resurgence of interest in cannabis as medicine. There is a long history of cannabis being used for various medical indications, including certain severe epilepsies, chronic pain syndromes, nausea associated with chemotherapy, painful spasm associated with multiple sclerosis, and appetite stimulation in people with cancer and HIV-AIDS. Thus, numerous jurisdictions around the globe are making cannabis available as a medication, and some are going further than this and essentially legalizing it. All these aspects are important in appreciating the place of cannabis in society and in informing debate about its availability. For a thoughtful discussion of these matters, including policy implications, the reader is referred to Hall and Degenhardt [1].

Henceforth, this chapter focuses on the psychiatric aspects of cannabis. A brief overview is provided of the cannabis plant and its constituents, followed by a discussion about the human cannabinoid system. The impact of cannabis on anxiety and mood symptoms is then covered, followed by a consideration of cannabis as a psychotomimetic agent and its impact on psychotic disorders, including whether it can be considered a cumulative causal factor for schizophrenia. Finally, the impact of cannabis on cognitive functioning, both short- and long-term, is discussed.

## The cannabis plant

*Cannabis sativa* has been used for centuries by humans for its effects on the mind. Mostly it is smoked, sometimes mixed with tobacco. As it burns very hot, the smoke is often bubbled through water to cool it for ease of inhalation. It can also be eaten, usually cooked in a cookie or cake. It can also be made into an oily formulation that can be imbibed as an oil or in capsule form. Inhaled cannabis enters the brain within seconds and has a very abrupt onset of CNS effects, while eating the product results in a much slower onset of action.

The plant is constituted of numerous chemicals, the most important of which, for psychiatry at least, is THC, the major psychotomimetic agent in the plant. There is also growing psychiatric interest in another cannabinoid, namely CBD, which appears to have some antipsychotic properties [2], as well as anti-inflammatory and neuroprotective effects [3]. Thus, the ratio of CBD to THC in the plant can be construed as an indicator of its potency in terms of its ability to induce psychotic symptoms.

There is a wide variation in the THC content of *Cannabis sativa*, dependent upon the precise strain, the manner in which it is grown, the part of the plant imbibed, and the manner in which it is prepared. Generally speaking, the leaves are less potent than the flowering parts [4]. The age of the plant is also of relevance, as the chemical constituents change with age; for example, THC is degraded to CBD. There is some confusion about the terms used to describe various preparations of cannabis. Here we follow the suggestion of Slade *et al.* [5]—thus, marijuana (also known as 'herbal') is a combination of buds and leaves of pollinated female plants, usually cultivated outdoors; sinsemilla (also known as 'skunk') comprises unfertilized buds of the female plant, usually cultivated indoors; and cannabis oil (also known as 'hash oil') is an oily product produced by solvent extraction or distillation of the plant product.

There are good longitudinal data to suggest that street cannabis is becoming more potent in terms of THC content, expressly over the last two decades. Slade and colleagues [5] provide a comprehensive overview of longitudinal drug seizure data from the United States covering the period 1975–2009. Two main trends emerge, namely that an increasingly higher proportion of products is sinsemilla, rather than herbal marijuana and that the THC content of cannabis of all forms (that is, marijuana, sinsemilla, and hash oil) has increased, from under 1% in 1975 to around 10% in 2009. In terms of the CBD:THC ratio, for sinsemilla, this was around 9.5% over the period 1981–1996, dropping to 5.6% in 1997–2009 [5]. Thus, in terms of both THC content and DBD:THC ratio, street cannabis is becoming more potent. Data from jurisdictions other than the United States point in the same direction. This has important implication for psychiatry, as described in the next section.

## The cannabinoid system

The human cannabinoid system is increasingly better understood. This has been spurred inter alia by the synthesis of THC and the discovery of the cannabinoid CB1 and CB2 receptors and the naturally occurring substrate of the CB1 receptor, anadamide. The CB2 receptor is expressed mainly in the spleen and testis and seems to be associated with immune function and, to a lesser extent, in the CNS where it has a role in inflammatory and degenerative processes [6]. We shall not address the CB2 system further here.

The CB1 receptor is expressed diffusely throughout the CNS, including the frontal cortex, basal ganglia, caudate, anterior cingulate cortex, cerebellum, hippocampus, and hypothalamus. The receptor is predominantly presynaptic and plays a role in the mediation of release of a number of neurotransmitters, including dopamine, noradrenaline, acetylcholine, glutamate, serotonin, and GABA. It is the receptor subtype relevant to the drug's psychotropic effects.

The advent of antagonists at the CB1 receptor allows a dissection of cause and effect in terms of what is mediated by the CB1 system. In particular, the CB1 receptor antagonist rimonabant (also referred to as SR141716) was employed in a number of such studies and showed great promise in its effects on weight reduction and reduction in hypercholesterolaemia and diabetes in animal and human experiments. Unfortunately, it carried a risk of depression and suicidality, so it was withdrawn from the market [7].

The cannabinoid system has a wide range of functions, including the modulation of pain (there are close interactions with the opiate system), memory, psychomotor control, and sleep and appetitive functions. Iversen [6] has summarized these main effects and outlined the major neural networks involved; this is summarized here, and the reader is referred to Iversen [6] for a full list of references. THC has acute effects on *motor control*, with a tendency to impaired fine motor movements and a wide-based gait, suggestive of cerebellar pathology. Impaired *short-term memory* is well described in the setting of cannabis intoxication, with particular impairment of attention, presumably mediated by hippocampal pathways. There has been a suggestion that this might indicate a role for THC in the extinction of aversive memories in post-traumatic stress disorder. There is a well-established association of THC exposure with a *craving for high-fat, high-sugar foods* (the so-called 'munchies'), operating via hypothalamic mechanisms. This has led to the use

of THC and synthetic cannabinoids in the stimulation of appetite in people with HIV-AIDS and some cancers. The appetitive effect and weight gain are blocked by rimonabant, which had therapeutic use in weight reduction, interestingly initially through a reduction in craving such foodstuffs, but after a number of weeks via direct metabolic effects. THC also has established *anti-nausea* properties and has been used in amelioration of nausea associated with chemotherapy.

Cascio and Pertwee [7] provided an overview of the effects of THC on *acute and chronic pain syndromes*, pointing out the distribution of CB1 (and CB2) receptors on pain pathways in the brain and spinal cord, as well as peripheral sensory nerves. There is an intricate interaction between the cannabinoid and opioid systems which might explain some of the analgesic effects. The synthetic cannabinoid receptor agonist nabilone has been shown to ameliorate chronic neuropathic pain, headache, and fibromyalgic pain, while Sativex˚ (which contains both THC and CBD) has been employed in the management of pain associated with multiple sclerosis and advanced malignancies (for references, see [7]).

A matter which is still debated is whether THC is an addictive substance. Certainly, animal models show that tolerance develops to many of the behavioural and other effects of THC, and there is a withdrawal syndrome [8]. A dependence syndrome has also been shown in humans, albeit tolerance does not necessarily occur for all its effects and many users do not increase their use once they have reached some sort of plateau. Withdrawal is not as rapid and dramatic as with substances such as nicotine or alcohol—the highly lipophilic nature of THC means that it remains for weeks in the brain and is excreted only slowly upon cessation in regular heavy users. This said, withdrawal effects which have been reliably documented include sleep difficulties, loss of appetite and weight loss, and, in some individuals, restlessness, irritability, and anger [9]. This syndrome can be precipitated by rimonabant in animal models [10].

## Effects on anxiety and mood

Many users of cannabis report that it reduces anxiety, enhances mood, and results in a relaxed sense of well-being. Its sedative properties are also reportedly helpful in individuals with chronic sleep disorders, albeit this has not been an area of rigorous scientific study.

In terms of anxiety, animal work has found that CB1 receptor knockout mice show increased anxiety-related behaviours, while CB1 receptor antagonists can reduce such behaviours in animal models of anxiety [7]. Also, rimonabant caused substantial anxiety symptoms in some individuals. This suggests that the cannabinoid system might have a potential therapeutic role in anxiety disorders; however, this has not been a major focus of scientific endeavour to date. Also, paradoxically, some individuals suffer extreme anxiety, and even panic attacks, upon exposure to THC; presumably this is mediated, in part at least, by tachycardia induced by THC, which could precipitate panic in vulnerable individuals.

The mood effects of cannabis are complex. It is very well known that acute intoxication is associated with a child-like mirthful laughter which is very intoxicating, but short-lived. Some early reports of cannabis having more enduring mood effects, and even being effective for some people with treatment-resistant depression, have not been supported by rigorous studies. Indeed, most work on mood effects of cannabis has reported an association with depression. However, albeit there is an established increased risk of depressive disorders in habitual cannabis users, the association is confounded by numerous psychosocial factors, including socio-economic status, as well as by the use of other substances such as alcohol. The most informative studies in this area are cohort studies, which follow large groups of people prospectively and attempt to control for confounders, as well as establish the temporal sequence between exposure (that is, cannabis) and the putative outcome (depression). Degenhardt *et al.* [11] reviewed such studies and concluded that there is a lack of consistent evidence supporting a causal relationship between cannabis exposure and depression or suicide. They point out the inconsistency in the data and variable methodology. Most such studies have been performed in young people, and cannabis/depression associations that do appear to survive controlling for confounding factors are strongest for young females.

There has been surprisingly little scientific scrutiny of cannabis in relation to bipolar disorder, despite its widespread use by people with this malady, and reports of benefits in both mood and sleep modulation. Again, large prospective studies are required to inform our understanding of cannabis use in the context of a bipolar diathesis. Silberberg *et al.* [12] selectively reviewed some such studies and found fairly mixed results, albeit the larger and more methodologically robust studies suggested worse outcomes for people with bipolar disorder who use cannabis. For example, van Rossum *et al.* [13] studied 3459 bipolar patients and found that those who were cannabis users had more manic relapses and worse psychosocial outcomes, but they were also less likely to adhere to medications, and one cannot exclude the possibility that people with more severe illness are inherently more likely to use cannabis.

There is more debate about whether cannabis use can independently increase the risk of bipolar disorder and/or bring forward the onset. In a general population study of 4815 people, Henquet *et al.* [14] reported an association between cannabis consumption and later manic symptoms, which was robust after controlling for a number of sociodemographic confounders, as well as for the evolution of psychotic symptoms. Similarly, van Laar *et al.* [15] reported a 5-fold increased risk of bipolar disorder associated with cannabis use in a sample of 3881 individuals from the general population. Some evidence suggests that cannabis use is associated with an earlier onset of bipolar disorder. Overall, it seems sage to suggest that cannabis might increase the risk of bipolar disorder in vulnerable individuals and also result in an earlier first manifestation. Also, cannabis use in people with an established illness should be strongly discouraged. That said, attention to other substances of abuse, as well as broader psychosocial and illness-related parameters and adherence to medication, is very important.

## Cannabis and psychosis

Arguably, consumption of cannabis can produce psychotic phenomena in anybody, but individual predisposition depends upon experience with the drug, the context in which it is consumed, the THC content (and the CBD:THC ratio), and crucially the individual's psychosis proneness. The latter is a measure of how vulnerable the individual is to the manifestation of psychotic symptoms. It is well known that anything up to 15% of the population have experienced psychotic phenomena at

some time, and elegant work from Verdoux and colleagues [16] has shown that increased psychosis proneness is associated with a higher likelihood of psychotic symptoms on exposure to cannabis.

People with established psychotic illnesses, such as schizophrenia, have a very high psychotic predisposition and thus are likely to manifest psychotic symptoms when imbibing cannabis. This has been confirmed in people with schizophrenia given intravenous TCH [17]. This is certainly seen clinically, and the negative impact of cannabis on the longitudinal course of schizophrenia is well recognized in longitudinal studies, albeit there is still some debate about the direction of causality and the contribution of confounding factors such as other illicit substances [18].

What is also of interest is that people with psychotic disorders still remain liable to psychotic relapse upon using cannabis, even if they are taking medications which effectively block dopamine D2 receptors. Indeed, D'Souza and colleagues [17] found that people with schizophrenia were more likely than healthy controls to experience psychotic symptoms when exposed to intravenous THC, even when they were on dopamine antagonist drugs. Thus, the induction of psychotic symptoms by THC is more complex than simply a release of dopamine. What is clear is that the effects are mediated by the CB1 receptor. Thus, Huestis and colleagues [19] administered rimonabant to volunteers, then gave them a cannabis cigarette to smoke, and found that rimonabant effectively blocked the psychotomimetic effects of cannabis.

An important area of investigation is to understand why people with established psychotic disorders smoke cannabis to the extent that they do. A number of studies have explored this and have generally concluded that the motivation lies largely in the area of alleviation of negative affect (for example, boredom, insomnia, anxiety, depression) [14, 20]. Importantly, very little support has been found for the notion that people with schizophrenia 'self-medicate' positive symptoms or try to alleviate medication side effects with cannabis; if there is a 'self-medication' component, it is the negative, rather than the positive, symptoms of psychosis that are targeted by users. This has clinical applicability in that understanding the reasons for use can help engage individuals in effective programmes to assist them in reducing their cannabis use [21].

There are also fairly consistent data to support the notion that cannabis use in youth can 'bring forward' the onset of schizophrenia. For example, using a large Australian data set, Stefanis and colleagues [22] estimated this effect to be of the order of 7–8 years, which obviously has a major impact on the individual, as they stand to lose a substantial period of early adulthood to the illness. Not all studies [23] have reported this effect, and controlling for all potential confounders is difficult.

A rather more contentious aspect of the cannabis/schizophrenia debate is whether cannabis consumption can actually contribute causally to schizophrenia—that is, do some people who have used cannabis and who later develop schizophrenia only manifest the disorder because they used cannabis? Clearly the vast majority of people who do use cannabis do not go on to develop schizophrenia, and the rate of schizophrenia across the globe does not vary in alignment with the rates of use of cannabis. Any studies in this area face the fact that some of the genes involved in the predisposition to schizophrenia also predispose to cannabis consumption [24]; there are many potential confounding factors, including socio-economic factors and the use of other illicit drugs—and even the licit drugs alcohol and tobacco—and it is hard to establish the true temporal sequence of exposure (that is, cannabis) and outcome (that is, schizophrenia). Many people with schizophrenia have very protracted prodromes (which may last for years) and are characterized largely by negative affect, which could (as outlined previously) directly lead to the consumption of cannabis and spurious assumptions about the direction of causality [25, 26]

Nevertheless, high-quality longitudinal cohort studies are now available that have fairly consistently reported an association between the use of cannabis in youth and later psychotic symptoms, and so support a causal connection [27]. There are fewer such studies with a specific schizophrenia outcome, but Zammit and colleagues [27] have provided a thorough overview of this area and suggest there is sufficient evidence to support public health campaigns regarding the potential risk of cannabis use and later schizophrenia, albeit conceding that the 'number needed to prevent' (NNP) one case of schizophrenia is very high; Hickman et al. [28] suggested that for every prevented case, some 2800 males (95% confidence limits 2018, 4530) aged 20–24 would need to become entirely abstinent (the estimates are even higher for older people and females). These estimates do not account for the fact that higher-potency cannabis (that is, sinsemilla) appears to carry a particularly strong association with schizophrenia [29], and this might be a specific focus of public health education and regulation where cannabis is effectively legalized.

Health campaigns could also target those individuals who seem particularly liable to develop schizophrenia upon exposure to cannabis. It seems obvious to warn people with psychosis proneness, those who have experienced a particularly strong psychotic reaction to acute exposure to cannabis, and those with a family history of schizophrenia. Certain genetic profiles may also signal vulnerability. For example, Caspi et al. [30] reported that, in the Dunedin cohort study, individuals homozygous for the valine allele at Val-158-Met within the catechol-$O$-methyltransferase (COMT) gene were more vulnerable than those with other variants to develop a psychotic disorder upon exposure to cannabis before the age of 18 years. This finding has not been convincingly replicated, but more recent interest in the AKT1 gene does seem to be bearing fruit in terms of our understanding of interaction effects between certain genotypes and the use of cannabis [31].

## Cannabis and cognition

As outlined in previous sections, acute intoxication with cannabis carries with it associated impairment in cognitive functions, notably registration and short-term memory. What is more contentious and more worrying from a general and public health perspective is whether cannabis can cause lasting cognitive dysfunction.

Solowij and Pesa [32] reviewed animal and human investigations of the effects of cannabis on cognition in both short- and long-term studies. They confirm that in the short term, there are effects on attention, memory, executive, and inhibitory processes. They also cite evidence of some longer-lasting effects in heavy users where early use (that is, adolescence) of high-potency cannabis seems most concerning. This reflects increasing concern about high-THC cannabis use at sensitive stages of brain development [33].

There is a well-described 'amotivational' syndrome associated with chronic heavy use of cannabis. Characteristics include elements

of dependence, such as craving, salience, and prioritization of drug acquisition above other pursuits, as well as some cognitive impairment in the domains outlined previously [34]. A debated issue is whether these cognitive problems revert if the individual stops using cannabis. The weight of evidence is that most of the effects do not endure, as long as the cannabis is given sufficient time to wash out of the brain (and this might take up to a month) [35, 36]. However, some research suggests not all cognitive functioning returns to baseline.

Neuroimaging studies have been highly inconsistent regarding structural brain abnormalities in association with prolonged heavy cannabis consumption. It is very difficult to control for the amount of exposure to cannabis, as well as to all potential confounding factors, not least the use of other drugs, such as alcohol, which are known brain toxins. Yucel et al. [37] have reported a unique group of individuals who were heavy long-term cannabis users but who apparently had no history of the use of other drugs; there were subtle volume reduction in the hippocampus and amygdala. Other studies have failed to replicate these findings, and particularly when alcohol exposure has been controlled for [33]. What is rather more consistent has been the finding of abnormalities in the white matter and impaired neuronal connectivity, including hippocampal connections and axons in the corpus callosum [38].

## Conclusions

*Cannabis sativa* remains the most widely used illicit drug worldwide. Its relevance to psychiatry lies in balancing its potentially harmful effects vs its potentially therapeutic benefits. Certainly, it is a drug of potential dependence but is less habit-forming than, for example, tobacco, and the withdrawal syndrome less dangerous than for, say, alcohol. It has effects on anxiety (these effects are somewhat dose-dependent), and it may have a therapeutic place in the treatment of some aspects of post-traumatic stress disorder. The association with depression has probably been overstated, and cohort studies suggest the association is more reverse causality than direct causality, and the population-attributable fraction (PAF) is very modest at around 2%. Effects on people with bipolar disorder have been under-researched, but the weight of evidence is that it is associated with an increased risk of manic relapse. THC, acting via CB1 receptors, can produce psychotic phenomena, notably in individuals with psychosis proneness and particularly in people with schizophrenia. It may also 'bring forward' the onset of schizophrenia by some years and be a cumulative causal factor for schizophrenia, albeit again the PAF is low (the highest estimates are 15%, but many researchers would put it around the 8% mark). Acute cognitive effects of cannabis are well described, as is an amotivational syndrome which appears largely reversible with cessation of the drug. Some evidence suggests enduring neurocognitive effects in heavy users, but the extent of the effect is much lower than, for example, sustained heavy alcohol use.

All this needs to be balanced by a consideration of the established and potential medical benefits of the cannabinoids. The role of CBD in the management of psychotic disorders is particularly alluring, as is the potential role of other non-THC cannabinoids in various disease states. It is hoped that moves to reignite the role of cannabis as medicine will have therapeutic benefits for many, and that the ongoing exploration of the cannabinoid systems will enhance our understanding and treatment of a number of psychiatric disorders.

# REFERENCES

1. Hall W, Degenhardt L. (2012). What are the policy implications of the evidence on cannabis and psychosis? In: Castle DJ, Murray RM, D'Souza C (eds). *Marijuana and Madness*, 2nd edition. Cambridge: Cambridge University Press, pp. 55–65.

2. Leweke FM, Piomelli D, Pahlisch F, *et al.* (2012). Cannabidiol enhances anandamide signaling and alleviates psychotic symptoms of schizophrenia. *Translational Psychiatry*, 2, e94.

3. Mechoulam R, Hanus L. (2012). Other cannabinoids. In: Castle DJ, Murray RM, D'Souza C (eds). *Marijuana and Madness*, 2nd edition. Cambridge: Cambridge University Press, pp. 17–22.

4. McLaren J, Swift W, Dillon P, Allsop S. (2008). Cannabis potency and contamination: a review of the literature. *Addiction*, 103, 1100–9.

5. Slade D, Mehmedic Z, Chandra S, ElSohly M. (2012). Is cannabis becoming more potent? In Castle DJ, Murray RM, D'Souza C (eds). *Marijuana and Madness*, 2nd edition. Cambridge: Cambridge University Press, pp. 35–54.

6. Iversen L. (2012). How cannabis works in the brain. In: Castle DJ, Murray RM, D'Souza C (eds). *Marijuana and Madness*, 2nd edition. Cambridge: Cambridge University Press, pp. 1–16.

7. Cascio MG, Pertwee R. (2012). The function of the endocannabinoid system. In: Castle DJ, Murray RM, D'Souza C (eds). *Marijuana and Madness*, 2nd edition. Cambridge: Cambridge University Press, pp. 23–34.

8. Pertwee RG. (1991). Tolerance to and dependence on psychotropic cannabinoids. In: Pratt J (ed). *The Biological Basis of Drug Tolerance*. London: Academic Press, pp. 232–65.

9. Budney AJ, Hughes JR, Moore BA, Vandrey R. (2004). Review of the validity and significance of the cannabis withdrawal syndrome. *American Journal of Psychiatry*, 161, 1967–77.

10. Cooper ZD, Haney M. (2009). Actions of delta-9-tetrahydrocannbinol in cannabis. *International Review of Psychiatry*, 21, 104–21.

11. Degenhardt L. Hall W, Lynskey M, Coffey C, Patton G. (2012). The association between cannabis use and depression: a review of the evidence. In: Castle DJ, Murray RM, D'Souza C (eds). *Marijuana and Madness*, 2nd edition. Cambridge: Cambridge University Press, pp. 114–28.

12. Silberberg C, Castle D, Koethe D. (2012). Cannabis, cannabinoids and bipolar disorder. In: Castle DJ, Murray RM, D'Souza C (eds). *Marijuana and Madness*, 2nd edition. Cambridge: Cambridge University Press, pp. 129–36.

13. Van Rossum I, Boomsma M, Tenback D, Reed C, van Os J. (2009). Does cannabis use affect treatment outcomes in bipolar disorder? A longitudinal analysis. *Journal of Nervous and Mental Disease*, 197, 35–40.

14. Henquet C, Krabbendam L, de Graaf R, ten Have M, van Os J (2006) Cannabis use and expression of mania in the general population. *Journal of Affective Disorders*, 95. 103–10.

15. Van Laar M, van Dorsselaer S, Monshouwer K, de Graaf R. (2007). Does cannabis use predict the first incidence of mood and anxiety disorders in the adult population? *Addiction*, 102, 1251–60.

16. Verdoux H, Sorbara F, Gindre C, Swendsen JD, van Os J. (2003). Cannabis use and dimensions of psychosis in a nonclinical population of female subjects. *Schizophrenia Research*, 59, 77–84.

17. D'Souza DC, Abi-Saab WM, Madonick S, *et al.* (2005). Delta-9-tetrahydrocannabinol effects in schizophrenia: implications for cognition, psychosis and addiction. *Biological Psychiatry*, 57, 594–608.

18. Linzen D, van Amelsvoort T. (2012). Cannabis abuse and the course of schizophrenia. In: Castle DJ, Murray RM, D'Souza C (eds). *Marijuana and Madness*, 2nd edition. Cambridge: Cambridge University Press, pp. 210–17.

19. Huestis MA, Gorelick DA, Heishman SJ, *et al.* (2001). Blockade of effects of smoked marijuana by the CB1-selective cannabinoid receptor antagonist SR141716. *Archives of General Psychiatry*, 58, 322–8.

20. Spencer C, Castle DJ, Mitchie P. (2002). An examination of the validity of a motivational model for understanding substance use among individuals with psychotic disorders. *Schizophrenia Bulletin*, 28, 233–47.

21. James W, Preston N, Koh G, *et al.* (2004). A group intervention which assists patients with dual diagnosis reduce their drug use: a randomized controlled trial. *Psychological Medicine*, 34, 983–90.

22. Stefanis N, Dragovic M, Power BD, Jablensky V, Castle D, Morgan V. (2013). Age at initiation of cannabis use predicts age at onset of psychosis: the 7–8 year trend. *Schizophrenia Bulletin*, 39, 251–4.

23. Cantor-Graae E, Nordström LG, McNeil TF. (2001). Substance abuse in schizophrenia: a review of the literature and a study of correlates in Sweden. *Schizophrenia Research*, 48, 69–82.

24. Power RA, Verweij KZ, Zuhair M, *et al.* (2014). Genetic predisoposition to schizophrenia associated with increased used of cannabis. *Molecular Psychiatry*, 19, 1201–4.

25. Castle D. (2013). Cannabis and psychosis: what causes what? *F1000 Medicine Reports*, 5, 1.

26. Moore TH, Zammit S, Lingford-Hughes A, *et al.* (2007). Cannabis use and risk of psychotic or affective mental health outcomes. *The Lancet*, 370, 319–28.

27. Zammit S, Areneault L, Cannon M, Murray RM. (2012). Does cannabis cause schizophrenia? The epidemiological evidence. In: Castle DJ, Murray RM, D'Souza C (eds). *Marijuana and Madness*, 2nd edition. Cambridge: Cambridge University Press, pp. 169–83.

28. Hickman M, Vickerman P, Macleod J, Kirkbride J, Jones PB. (2007). Cannabis and schizophrenia: model projections of the impact of the rise in cannabis use on historical and future trends in schizophrenia in England and Wales. *Addiction*, 102, 597–606.

29. Di Forti M, Morgan C, Dazzan P, *et al.* (2009). High-potency cannabis and the risk of psychosis. *British Journal of Psychiatry*, 195, 488–91.

30. Caspi A, Moffitt TE, Cannon M, *et al.* (2005). Moderation of the effect of adolescent-onset cannabis use on adult psychosis by a functional polymorphism in the catechol-*O*-methyltransferase gene: longitudinal evidence of a gene X environment interaction. *Biological Psychiatry*, 57, 1117–27.

31. Di Forti M, Henquet C, Verdoux H, Murray RM, van Os J. (2012). Which cannabis users develop psychosis? In: Castle DJ, Murray RM, D'Souza C (eds). *Marijuana and Madness*, 2nd edition. Cambridge: Cambridge University Press, pp. 137–43.

32. Solowij N, Pesa N. (2012). Cannabis and cognition:short and long term effects. In: Castle DJ, Murray RM, D'Souza C (eds). *Marijuana and Madness*, 2nd edition. Cambridge: Cambridge University Press, pp. 91–102.

33. Lubman DI, Cheetham A, Yucel M. (2015). Cannabis and adolescent brain development. *Pharmacological Therapies*, 148, 1–16.

34. Volkow ND, Wang GJ, Telang F, *et al.* (2014). Decreased dopamine brain activity in marijuana abusers is associated with negative emotionality and addiction severity. *Proceedings of the*

*National Academy of Sciences of the United States of America,* 111, E3149–56.

35. Pope HG, Gruber AJ, Hudson JI, Huestis MA, Yurgelun-Todd D. (2001). Neuropsychological performance in long-term cannabis users. *Archives of General Psychiatry*, 58, 909–15.

36. Weiland BJ, Thayer RE, Depue BE, Sabbineni A, Bryan AD, Hutchinson KE. (2015). Daily marijuana use is not associated with brain morphometric measures in adiloscents or adults. c*Journal of Neuroscience*, 35, 1505–12.

37. Yucel M, Solowij N, Respondek C, *et al.* (2008). Regional brain abnormalities associated with long-term heavy cannabis use. *Archives of General Psychiatry*, 65, 694–701.

38. Zalesky A, Solowji N, Yucel M, *et al.* (2012). Effect of long-term cannabis use on axonal fibre connectivity. *Brain*, 135(pt7), 2245–55.

# 53

# Stimulants, ecstasy, and other 'party drugs'

*Adam R. Winstock and Remy Flechais*

## Introduction

Stimulant drugs, such as cocaine, amphetamine, and 3,4-methylenedioxymethamphetamine (MDMA), remain the most commonly used group of illicit psychoactive drugs after cannabis. Their use crosses cultures, age groups, functions, and socio-economic profiles. For most users, the risks related to acute intoxication will be the most commonly experienced harm, with dependence being relatively rare. While variations in precise neuropharmacological action, potency, preparations, route of synthesis, and administration lead to discrete populations of users adopting diverse patterns of use with associated risks and harms, stimulant drugs share a common neurobiology, with similar effect profile and treatment options. Dose-related intoxication with these drugs can result in acute psychopathology that may require assessment, treatment, and follow-up by the general psychiatrist. It is important to note that few people will use these drugs in isolation and that polydrug use contributes significantly to the harm profiles associated with these drugs. In recent years, the appearance of a wide range of novel psychoactive substances (NPS) that mimic the effects of more traditional drugs has posed a challenge to policy-makers and added a level of unpredictability for both users and treatment providers [1]. The appearance of a more robust 'chem-sex' (this refers to the use of drugs to chemically enhance sexual experience) scene in the UK has led to drugs such as crystal methamphetamine, gamma hydroxybutyrate (GHB), and mephedrone being added to the list of those drugs psychiatrists need to be able to assess and treat most effectively within a multidisciplinary team [2].

## ICD/DSM classifications

The ICD-10 definition for a dependence syndrome to any substance revolves around having at least three of the following symptoms present together for at least 1 month, or if lasting less than 1 month have been present together repeatedly in the last 12 months: a strong desire to take the drug, difficulties in controlling its use, persisting in its use despite harmful consequences, a higher priority given to drug use than to other activities and obligations, increased tolerance, and sometimes a physical withdrawal state. The ICD codes then vary according to substances, and relevant to this chapter are: F14—mental and behavioural disorder due to the use of cocaine; and F15—mental and behavioural disorder due to the use of other stimulants, including caffeine. There are further specifiers such as .0 acute intoxication, .1 harmful use, .2 dependence syndrome, .3 withdrawal state, .4 withdrawal state with delirium, .5 psychotic disorder (and many more; see ICD 10 for further details).

DSM-5 classifies substance use disorders according to symptoms of dependence similar in nature to ICD, but there are 11 of them. DSM-5 describes a continuum of substance use disorders and divides this into mild (2–3), moderate (4–5), and severe (>6) categories, based on how many symptoms are present at the same time. The codes relevant to this chapter are: mild 305.70 (amphetamine-type substance) 305.60 (cocaine); moderate 304.40 (amphetamine-type substance) 304.20 (cocaine); and severe 304.40 (amphetamine-type substance) 304.20 (cocaine). There are other specifiers in DSM-5 such as acute intoxication, withdrawal, and other substance-induced disorders (for example, psychotic disorder, anxiety disorder, etc.) (see DSM-5 for further details).

## Assessment and investigations

Assessing a person who reports the use of stimulant or other party drugs follows the same principles as for other drug use assessments. A focus on the type of drug/s, pattern, and frequency of use, including the amount used on the day of use (usually in grams or fractions thereof, or monetary spend), the preparation used, polydrug use, including route of use, is mandatory. Asking about key psychosocial and life event determinants that accompanied the progress from initial use to current use patterns, combined with assessment of perceived function (for example, work, managing stress/anxiety, enhanced sexual function, partying) and the level of control over use, are useful. Any history of overdose, treatment-seeking, and involvement in associated high-risk behaviours, such as sex, crimes, and violence, should be noted. Specific assessment to determine the presence of dependence and withdrawal can usually be done by enquiring about a typical day of use, from waking to sleep, with assessment of risk behaviours, drug use prioritization, and craving. Asking what happens if the person goes without the drug for more than a day or two can help you identify the levels of control over use and the presence of withdrawal. Withdrawal needs to be differentiated from a shorter-lived comedown that many users of stimulants experience in the days following use more akin to a hangover. Blood-borne virus (BBV) screening should be offered routinely to injectors and those involved in high-risk sexual activities. Urinary drug screens (UDS) may be useful to corroborate which substances were used or confirm abstinence, though drugs such as GHB and many NPS may not be detected on routine UDS. Most stimulant drugs will be detectable in the urine for 2–3 days following use.

## Amphetamine (speed) and methamphetamine—'crystalline methamphetamine hydrochloride' (ice, crystal, shabu, yaba, meth, tina)

### Background

Amphetamine-type stimulants are the most commonly used synthetic stimulant drugs in the world. Originally developed as medicines (initially as nasal decongestants, appetite suppressants/weight loss agents, and mood enhancers), their abuse potential and ability to induce a range of psychopathologies, most notably transient psychotic episodes, are well recognized. Still used in the treatment of narcolepsy and ADHD, dexamphetamine differs from methamphetamine only by the addition of a methyl group, which lowers its melting point (allowing it to be smoked) and increases its potency and ability to cross the blood–brain barrier. Despite observed differences in the way the drugs are used, the problems they cause, and their clinical presentations, in laboratory double-blind conditions, the subjective experience of the two drugs is remarkably similar [3].

Until recently, the dominant form of amphetamine seen in the UK was low-purity amphetamine sulfate (typically 4–10% purity, comprising both D- and L-isomers). While methamphetamine use has historically been problematic in the United States, Australia, and South East Asian countries, such as Thailand, Japan, and Korea, for many years, its appearance in the UK is actually a recent phenomenon. Its arrival coincides with the rise of the gay 'chem-sex' scene in major cities in the UK, and methamphetamine is now starting to make its presence felt within both emergency departments and sexual health and addiction services. In the UK, methamphetamine was reclassified as a Class A drug in 2007, and amphetamine is a Class B drug. In the UK, a gram of amphetamine sulfate costs about £10, and a gram of methamphetamine sulfate between £100 and £150.

### Preparation, purity, and routes of use

Amphetamine sulfate (speed) is usually sold as a white/off white/beige crystalline powder and is most commonly snorted or taken orally, dissolved in a drink, or wrapped in cigarette paper and swallowed (known as bombing or parachuting). Amphetamine sulfate is water-soluble and can be injected, though because of its high melting point, it cannot be effectively smoked. Purities are typically very low in the UK, with common bulking agents being caffeine and lactose. Purities of over 30% are not uncommon across the European Union. Diversion of prescribed dexamphetamine tablets (and the closely related methylphenidate) occurs and is a major problem in countries such as the United States where rates of prescription for conditions such as ADHD are much higher than in the UK.

Unlike illicit amphetamine sulfate powder, methamphetamine is often of very high purity. Its physical form varies, depending on its route of synthesis and purity. Crystalline methamphetamine hydrochloride (known as ice because it can resemble shards of glass) can be up to 80% pure. Base amphetamine (sometimes known as paste), is an oily, waxy intermediate product on the way to the manufacture of the crystalline hydrochloride salt of methamphetamine and has a lower purity of about 40–50%. Methamphetamine is a versatile drug and can be smoked, snorted, injected, and taken orally.

### Mechanism of action and metabolism

Methamphetamine closely resembles amphetamine sulfate (commonly referred to as speed) in structure and mechanism of action but is more potent in its sympathomimetic effects and has a longer duration of action (half-life of about 12 hours, compared to 2–4 hours for amphetamine sulfate). Amphetamine has both direct sympathomimetic effects secondary to disruption of vesicular storage of monoamines and inhibition of their breakdown by MAOIs and indirect actions through inhibition of central presynaptic reuptake of catecholamines.

### Prevalence and patterns of use

The use of amphetamine in the UK is less common than that of either cocaine or MDMA. A total of 0.6% of 16- to 59-year olds report using amphetamine in the last year, and 1.3% of 16- to 24-year olds—0.1% and 0.2%, respectively, of those age groups for methamphetamine. Lifetime ever use in 16- to 59-year olds is 10.1% for amphetamine and 0.9% for methamphetamine [4]. As noted in Background, p. 526, in the UK, methamphetamine is becoming more prevalent among certain segments of the population, particularly in association with the gay and dance music scene, but compared to the use of MDMA and cocaine in all its forms, the prevalence of methamphetamine use at present is still low [5].

### Doses and typical patterns of use

Most consumers will use infrequently, with daily use, even among dependent users, being uncommon. Typical consumption amounts vary widely, but doses of somewhere between 0.25 g and 1 g in a session would not be uncommon. Heavier users develop tolerance and can consume considerably higher doses. Because these drugs energize people and reduce the need for sleep, use sessions can extend over several days, with prolonged insomnia being associated with the development of paranoia and hostility.

### Physical and psychological effects and complications

The effects of all amphetamines are dose-related. They induce euphoria, elevation of mood and alertness, increased speed of thought and speech, and heightened perceptual awareness and lead to reduction in appetite and need for sleep. The physical manifestations of amphetamine and methamphetamine are broadly similar, characterized by sympathetic arousal with tachycardia, hypertension, hyperthermia, and increased respiration, accompanied by sweating, pupillary dilatation, increased motor activity, dry mouth, tremor, and blurred vision. Occasionally, serious medical complications arise, including malignant hyperthermia, coronary artery syndrome, seizures, and cerebral bleeds (Table 53.1). Route-related harms, such as local trauma, septal ulceration, abscesses, and BBVs from snorting and injecting, can combine with more chronic physiological tolls, including malnutrition from prolonged anorexia and hyperactivity, poor dentition, skin picking, and gastrointestinal tract ulceration, leaving users in very poor physical health.

**Table 53.1** Clinical signs of intoxication with amphetamine

| Physical | Psychological | Behavioural |
|---|---|---|
| Elevated pulse, blood pressure, temperature | Euphoria/energized | Motor hyperactivity |
| Increased respiratory rate | Anxious/irritable | Restless/twitching |
| Sweating/dehydrated | Rapid thoughts | Talkative, pressured speech |
| Dilated pupils | Paranoia | Aggressive |
| Tremor/shakiness/bruxism | Perceptual disturbance | Stereotyped movements |

The acute sought-after effects of increased energy and euphoria, enhanced stamina, confidence, disinhibition, and heightened awareness can easily give way to a range of dose-related unwanted psychological effects. These include anxiety, panic, extreme agitation, paranoia, hostility, aggression, hallucinations, confusion, disorientation, and psychosis.

## Other consequences of use

### Dependence and withdrawal

Dependence may occur and is more common among heavy users who are male and in those who smoke or inject the drug. Methamphetamine is considered to have a higher abuse liability and potential for harm than amphetamine. Although dependent users may use every day to avoid withdrawal, more typically users tend to consume a large amount of the drug (often several grams) over several days, going without sleep (a binge) before ceasing use through physical exhaustion or an exhaustion of funds. 'Crashing' refers to the period following a binge, which is characterized by fatigue, hypersomnia, hyperphagia, and low mood due to acute monoamine depletion. The crash and subsequent comedown period may last 2–7 days. If abstinence persists, a longer-term withdrawal period may be seen, characterized by craving, low mood, anergia, irritability, sleep, and appetite disturbance. Similar neurobiological mechanisms involving alterations in the function and activity of monoamine neurotransmitters are responsible for the overlap between the symptoms of depression and those of stimulant withdrawal [6, 7]. Typically, the withdrawal gradually diminishes over 2–4 weeks, though dysphoric symptoms may persist for up to 10 weeks.

### Withdrawal management and relapse prevention

Management of withdrawal is largely supportive and preferably within a safe, well-supported home environment. Inpatient admission is rarely required, other than in those with polyuse dependence and where use is accompanied by severe mental or physical illness. Despite decades of research, there are currently no widely accepted evidence-based pharmacotherapy regimes for the treatment of psychostimulant withdrawal [8]. The patient should be placed in quiet surroundings for several days and allowed to sleep and eat as much as is needed. Because a significant component of the withdrawal syndrome is probably related to neurotransmitter depletion, recovery may be delayed because of anorexia associated with amphetamine use. It may be useful in some to provide nutritional supplements or a well-balanced diet rich in monoamine precursors—phenylalanine, tyrosine, L-tryptophan, which are found in, for example, pumpkin seeds, chocolate, Marmite®, and

bananas. Benzodiazepines may be prescribed on a short-term basis for agitation, though these may delay the return to normal sleep architecture. Some patients may become markedly despondent during withdrawal, and a suicide assessment may be necessary. Relapse prevention, based on cognitive behavioural therapeutic (CBT) principles and mutual aid groups, has shown to be effective in reducing relapse and should be part of any treatment intervention. Given the high rates of ADHD comorbidity among stimulant users, it is of note that there is growing interest and evidence to support the use of substitute prescribing in those with concurrent stimulant dependence and ADHD. Some of the most promising results have come from correctional facilities where methylphenidate has been used successfully to reduce both ADHD symptoms and relapse to stimulant drug use [9] (see Cocaine/crack cocaine (charlie, coke, chang, snow, white, crack), p. 528).

### Low mood and depression: assessment and management

The mainstay of treatment for those with dependence on amphetamines is psychological, with medication-based treatment having a limited role in the management of withdrawal and relapse prevention, other than in addressing underlying comorbidities such as depression and ADHD. While amphetamine use can exacerbate depression in those with a primary underlying disorder, antidepressants have no specific anti-craving effects, and the efficacy of antidepressants in reducing depression is confined to those stimulant users who are depressed. Clinicians should avoid diagnosing and initiating medication-based treatment for a primary depressive disorder in those presenting during active periods of use or withdrawal. Patients should have the difficulties of making an accurate diagnosis explained to them and should be supported to achieve a period of 2–4 weeks' abstinence and have their mood reassessed before a decision is made to commence antidepressants. The advantages of waiting before deciding whether or not to prescribe antidepressants are improved diagnostic accuracy, avoidance of potentially unnecessary medication and the inaccurate attribution of low mood to drug use and not to an intrinsic disorder, and almost certainly an improvement in compliance and efficacy. Persistence of depressive symptoms beyond 2–4 weeks after stopping amphetamine use may suggest that there is an underlying depressive illness, and this should be treated [10]; left unmanaged, its presence represents a high risk for relapse. Psychosocial treatments, including CBT and motivational enhancement therapy (MET), for stimulant abuse and dependence have been found to be effective in reducing levels of use [11], with their efficacy enhanced through combining them with contingency management approaches offering non-drug reinforcers for engagement and abstinence.

### Stimulant-induced psychosis

The use of high doses of methamphetamine may lead to the induction of a temporary psychotic state that may be clinically indistinguishable from paranoid schizophrenia. First recognized in 1938 in association with Benzedrine® nasal inhalers, it was not until Connell's classic 1958 study that the syndrome was well described. Acute transient psychotic episodes (typically characterized by suspiciousness, hostility, unusual thought content, and hallucinations) occur in about 10–15% of users. Psychotic episodes are more common in dependent users, users of methamphetamine, men, injectors, polydrug users, those with a past history of psychosis, and following a binge in association with prolonged insomnia [12].

Amphetamine-induced psychosis is characterized by persecutory delusions and hallucinations which are typically auditory but may be visual or tactile (typically formication, or the sensation of insects crawling under the skin; this can rarely lead to secondary delusions such as Ekbom's syndrome of delusional parasitosis). Little has changed in the way of management since Connell's time—he recommended 'removal of the drug and appropriate sedation'. Often, patients present with high levels of hostility and violence secondary to persecutory delusions or hallucinations, and safe containment and management of the disturbed individual can require enormous levels of both physical and chemical restraint. Benzodiazepines (often required in very high doses) should be the first-line medication, with antipsychotics used only where additional tranquillization is required. A diagnosis of a possible underlying or persistent psychotic disorder must be deferred until a reassessment can be made in a drug-free state. These often florid psychoses usually remit within a few days, and the user returns to normal functioning, although some retain a vulnerability to such episodes [13]. Only a minority (1–15%) persist beyond 1 month, and many of these patients will have underlying psychiatric disorders [14].

The prognosis is variable, with those who have experienced stimulant-induced psychotic episodes being more vulnerable to future episodes (possibly through behavioural sensitization) on re-exposure to the drug, often at lower levels. Recent PET imaging studies in chronic methamphetamine users have demonstrated a reduction in dopamine transporter concentration, and this reduction was significantly associated with the duration of methamphetamine use and closely related to the severity of persistent psychiatric symptoms. Moreover, the severity of psychiatric symptoms was significantly correlated with the duration of methamphetamine use. Cessation is still potentially important since there does appear to be some recovery of dopamine transporter function with abstinence.

From a neurotoxicity perspective, preclinical studies have shown amphetamines to be toxic to dopaminergic axon terminals in the striatum, in particular the nigrostriatal pathway. Other neurotransmitter systems (GABA, glutamate, serotonin, and ACh) may also be affected, and the underlying mechanisms causing such damage are thought to be multiple, including oxidative stress, excitotoxicity, neuroinflammation, and others [15]. Amphetamine use in humans (in particular, methamphetamine) has been associated with abnormal morphology of the substantia nigra and possible vulnerability to Parkinson's disease (PD) [16]. Epidemiological studies have suggested an increased rate (2- to 3-fold) of PD in amphetamine users [17–19]. Similarities in methamphetamine-associated dopaminergic neural damage to that seen in PD have resulted in some animal models used in PD research being based on methamphetamine exposure [20].

### Stimulant overdose

Dose-related toxicity results from excessive levels of extracellular dopamine, noradrenaline, and serotonin. Acute sympathomimetic toxicity is primarily manifested through neurological and cardiovascular effects, though pathology can extend to the gastrointestinal, renal, musculoskeletal, and pulmonary systems. Clinically, stimulant overdose is recognized by a constellation of psychological (anxiety, panic, paranoia, hallucinations, confusion, and hostility), behavioural (aggression, agitation, and hyperactivity), and physiological (mydriasis, hyperthermia, dehydration, sweating, tremor, hyperreflexia, hypertension,

tachycardia, movement disorders, and seizures) symptoms. The management of sympathomimetic overdose is largely supportive, with cessation of stimulant consumption typically leading to resolution over a few hours or days. Where there is risk to self or others, either as a result of physiological overstimulation or aggressive behaviours, benzodiazepines (often in high doses) and, in some cases, medications to stabilize cardiovascular overstimulation are required. In cases where agitation, delirium, and movement disorders are unresponsive to benzodiazepines, second-line therapies, such as antipsychotics, intravenous sedation, and muscle relaxants, can be considered. Rapid cooling may be required in cases of malignant hyperthermia.

## Harm reduction for stimulant users

The risks of acute harm from stimulant-type drugs are related to the dose, length of current use episode, route of use, and polydrug use and are greater among heavy frequent users. As a result, the key safer use strategies include avoiding injecting and smoking, not mixing with other drugs or alcohol, limiting the amount used during a session, avoiding the development of tolerance through taking regular breaks from use (giving both the body and brain time to recover), trying to limit periods of use to 1–2 days, avoiding prolonged insomnia which markedly increases the risks of developing psychosis, and eating and sleeping well between episodes of use.

## Cocaine/crack cocaine (charlie, coke, chang, snow, white, crack)

### Background

Cocaine is a major alkaloid constituent of the Andean bush *Erythroxylum coca*. Originally used for millennia to increase stamina, suppress appetite, and manage altitude sickness by indigenous groups in South America, cocaine hydrochloride (powder) production and distribution is a multi-billion dollar industry, thought to underpin much of the violence and corruption that ravages countries such as Mexico. Used recreationally to induce euphoria, energy, and confidence, cocaine is frequently combined with depressants such as alcohol and opioids. It is sold either as a water-soluble crystalline hydrochloride powder or as a smokable free alkaloid base form (no longer the salt—therefore, no longer water-soluble) known as crack. In both forms, the mechanisms of action and potential for cocaine to cause harm are remarkably similar. In fact, it is the differences in routes of use (smoking/injecting vs snorting), socio-economic status (rich vs poor), and ethnicity (white vs black) and involvement in criminality and heroin use that are mostly responsible for the observed differences in the presentation and harms seen among users of these two different preparations. In the UK, cocaine in all its forms is a Class A drug.

### Mechanism of action

Cocaine is an indirect sympathomimetic agent that causes an acute, but transient, blockade of the dopamine transporter (DAT), causing an acute elevation of dopamine levels, resulting in the experienced pleasure burst. Chronic cocaine administration leads to a compensatory increase in DAT levels, such as that with abstinence, and these increased transporter levels lead to a relative reduction in levels of dopamine outside nerve cells. Neuroimaging studies suggest that there is persistent reorganization of reward pathways, which may underlie the persistence of craving, even after many months of abstinence. Its half-life is about 50 minutes.

## Route of administration

Intranasal use of cocaine powder is the major route of administration in the general population. Purity in the UK has increased in recent years, with street deals varying between 10 and 70%, giving rise to a two-tier market, with 'economy' cocaine selling for £50–60/gram and 'premium' cocaine for over £100 in some places. Intranasally, cocaine lasts about 1–3 hours and is re-dosed every 1–2 hours in small amounts (known as lines) over the course of a session. Typical amounts used on the day of use would be 0.5–1 g/day; much larger amounts can be seen in those dependent upon the drug. Intravenous use is associated with a shorter duration of action, more intense effects, and greater morbidity. Cocaine injectors sometimes administer 20 times or more in a day. In combination with heroin (known as speedballing), it has high associated mortality rates. Smoked as crack cocaine, the high lasts a matter of minutes. Intense, short-lived euphoria, followed by a rapid return to baseline or an overshoot to feeling lousy, is a recipe for enormous reinforcement and is often a gateway into heroin use, which is marketed by dealers as a way of managing the comedown from crack cocaine. Crack cocaine users can often consume many grams of the drug over a session, with the rate-limiting factor being money.

Many people may use powdered cocaine in a recreational fashion for many years and without significant problems. Others may insidiously develop problematic use, characterized by increasingly regular dosing, development of tolerance, craving, and loss of control. Concurrent consumption of alcohol is common and can lead to increased rates of acute harm and dependence. At population level in England and Wales, in 18- to 59-year olds, the reported lifetime ever use is 9.7% for cocaine powder and 1.2% for crack. Last year use in 16- to 24-year olds was 4.8% for powder and 0.1% for crack, and in the 18- to 59-year olds, 2.3% for powder and 0.1% for crack [4]. Frequently seen as a way of enhancing confidence and performance, attempts at reducing use are often accompanied by a rebound fall in self-esteem and energy and the development of depression. It is of note that crack is sold in small unit cost deals (£5–10), compared to the costlier dealing unit of cocaine. Within UK drug treatment services, coexisting crack cocaine and heroin use are common, with typical users reporting smoking 3–4 'bags' per day, equating to approximately half a gram. Although dealers usually provide the user with the preparation of their choice, some users will 'wash' their own cocaine powder with a base (ammonia or bicarbonate of soda) to make their own crack, while cocaine injectors are sometimes left with having to inject crack if powder cocaine is unavailable. It may be that there are groups of 'functional' occasional users of crack, but in those with substance use disorders, the pattern of use is often uncontrolled and leads to significant harm.

## Dependence and withdrawal

Dependence to cocaine can occur with both powder and crack but is potentially more likely if smoked as crack. This is due to the more rapid onset of action, intense highs, and early withdrawals, which are very reinforcing. Features of escalating use over time, loss of control, tolerance, withdrawal symptoms, cravings, salience, and continued use despite knowledge of harm can all manifest. Dependent users may not necessarily have to use every day—typically crack users tend to use in binges over a few days, then rest—but there are rarely many consecutive days off, and even then, dependent users often use other substances to combat the withdrawal symptoms.

The withdrawal syndrome is similar to that seen in amphetamine withdrawal, with common symptoms including dysphoric mood, fatigue, irritability, increased appetite, hypersomnia/insomnia (reflecting a homeostatic resetting response to acute intoxication-related insomnia and anorexia), irritability, craving, lethargy, or agitation. Secondary to a hypo-dopaminergic state, the predominant psychological symptoms peak on days 2–7, reducing gradually over the following 3–6 weeks.

## Effects and toxicity

These are similar to those seen with amphetamines and include signs of sympathetic arousal (tachycardia, hypertension, severe agitation, hyperthermia, seizures) and severe cardiac problems such as coronary artery spasm, congestive cardiac failure, arrhythmias, ischaemia, and myocarditis. Cocaine, when consumed with alcohol, results in the formation of the less anxiogenic, but more cardiotoxic, reinforcing, and longer-lasting, cocaethylene. Concurrent consumption of alcohol, and then cocaine, leads to a 30% increase in peak plasma cocaine levels, which may increase the risk of sudden death in a vulnerable minority. Chronic use has more recently been associated with accelerated cerebrovascular ischaemia and strokes in young users.

Psychiatric comorbidity with cocaine dependence is high. About 25% have coexisting ADHD; 50% experience alcohol use disorders, and rates of depression are much higher than that of the general population. Depression predicts poorer outcome in cocaine dependence and, untreated, can lead to an increased risk of relapse. Although adverse psychological experiences are less common than among users of methamphetamine, because of cocaine's shorter half-life, transient episodes related to sympathomimetic hyperarousal, such as anxiety, panic, agitation, paranoia, and aggression (especially when consumed with alcohol), are not uncommon. Acute adverse effects are seen with crack, because of its greater intensity of effect and the dose of drug consumed.

## Route-related harms

Persistent intranasal use can result in nosebleeds, with the risk of viral BBV transmission. Smoking the free alkaloid base as 'crack' is associated with a shorter, more intense high and can lead to acute lung injury in the form of 'crack lung', a progressive fibrotic condition of the lung. Users present with haemoptysis, hypoxaemia, fever, and cough, with pulmonary interstitial inflammation and peripheral eosinophilia. Injecting cocaine is associated with higher rates of sharing of intravenous equipment and HIV transmission and can also cause significant local trauma secondary to local anaesthesia that precludes pain-associated restriction in damaging injecting behaviour. Cocaine use, especially via the smoking route, is associated with marked increase in risk of stroke (once controlled for tobacco and alcohol use, odds ratio of >5) in the 24 hours following use among young adults [21].

## Treatment

Hospital admission for withdrawal may be necessary in some clients, such as those with unstable living conditions, comorbid mental health or severe physical illness, or polydrug dependence, or those in whom severe withdrawal has been experienced and attempts at outpatient detoxification have proved ineffective. Optimized nutrition, rest, and symptomatic relief with short-term, low-dose benzodiazepines [for example, diazepam 5 mg three times daily (tds)] may be helpful.

However, as with other stimulant drugs, there is little evidence to support the routine use of any specific pharmacotherapy either in the management of cocaine withdrawal or in maintaining abstinence from it, apart from situations where a comorbid psychiatric condition has been identified (see Medication-based treatments for stimulant use disorders/dependence, p. 530). The evidence suggests the most effective interventions are based on CBT (see below).

## Medication-based treatments for stimulant use disorders/dependence

Despite decades of research on a wide variety of different therapeutic agents, there is still no evidence-based pharmacotherapy available for the general treatment of cocaine dependence. In the absence of primary depressive disorders, antidepressants are not useful as a treatment for cocaine dependence. In those with a primary depressive disorder, the efficacy of antidepressant medication will be very limited if the person continues to use cocaine. Untreated depression, however, is a risk factor for relapse to cocaine use, and careful assessment is required, even after several weeks of abstinence, to ensure it does not emerge late and be left untreated. There is also no evidence for the use of antipsychotics, anti-epileptics, or opioid antagonists in the treatment of cocaine dependence. There is no widely utilized or evidence-based substitute medication, as is the case for opioid dependence. However, there is growing interest in the possible role of stimulant replacement therapy in the treatment of carefully selected groups, combined with psychosocial interventions. Promising results for such approaches have been seen among those with comorbid ADHD where the provision of an oral alternative stimulant (for example, dexamphetamine or methylphenidate) has been initiated as a harm reduction approach in persistent high-risk injectors. In such groups, with appropriate assessment and monitoring (for unwanted cardiovascular and psychological effects), stimulant medications can be safe and effective. Concerns over prescribing a drug with abuse liability, risk of diversion, and difficulty with ensuring compliance mean the use of substitute prescribing is not straightforward. It is likely, however, that in combination with psychological support, including contingency management, such approaches may be currently among the most effective available [22]. Extended-release preparations may be the most effective, being less reinforcing and requiring lower levels of supervision.

Although rates of stimulant dependence are high among those with adult ADHD, there is no evidence to suggest they are significantly higher than in those with other substance use disorders, with rates among those with substance use dependence being between 20% and 25% [23]. There is growing interest in the role of substitute prescribing in those with concurrent stimulant dependence and ADHD [24]. Some of the most promising results have come from correctional facilities where methylphenidate has been used successfully to reduce both ADHD symptoms and relapse to stimulant drug use [25]. It may therefore be the case that selective treatment of adults with coexisting stimulant dependence and ADHD may have specific therapeutic benefits. Screening for ADHD in those

with stimulant disorders is therefore clinically useful. Some adults may give clues to their primary diagnosis by reporting a paradoxical response to stimulant drugs as adults (for example, feeling calm and 'normal'), as opposed to hyper and aroused which would be the normal subjective response to drugs like cocaine in those without ADHD. There is also interest in the use of non-stimulant medications in the treatment of stimulant use disorders, including modafinil, a wakefulness-promoting agent approved for the treatment of narcolepsy and shift-work sleep disorders. With both dopaminergic and glutamatergic activity, early work suggests it might be useful in the treatment of cocaine dependence, with studies showing a reduction in subjective effects, use, and craving [26].

A more recent development in the treatment of those with drug dependence has been the provision of non-drug rewards (for example, a voucher or monetary incentive) for engagement in treatment and confirmed abstinence from drugs. Such approaches are referred to as contingency management (CM). In trials where CM has been used in the treatment of stimulant use disorders, combined with other psychological approaches, such as CBT or MET, CM has been shown to increase retention in treatment, increase abstinence, and possibly enhance the efficacy of pharmacological interventions [27]. Although still uncommon in routine practice, the evidence suggests that CM should be offered as part of routine clinical interventions, in conjunction with other therapies.

Interest and clinical trial research into a vaccine for cocaine dependence continue, with the development of antibodies to bind to cocaine and prevent it from reaching receptor sites. To date, clinical trials suggest such interventions are some way off and, once developed, will no doubt face a series of ethical and biological hurdles before immunization of vulnerable groups, such as the young or those with addiction histories, becomes part of treatment anytime soon.

## Ecstasy (3,4-methylenedioxymethamphetamine) (MDMA, E, X, XTC, pills, beans, Molly, Mandy)

### Background

MDMA is a synthetic stimulant drug characterized by pro-social effects, euphoria, energy, and empathy. First synthesized in 1912 by Merck Pharmaceuticals, MDMA remained largely ignored until the 1950s when the United States army explored its potential as a military agent (though, unlike methamphetamine, it lacked an aggressive edge and was more likely to make someone hug their enemies than kill them!). In the late 1960s and early 1970s, recreational drug users on the west coast of America began to recognize the desirable effect profile of MDMA and the closely related drug MDA (methylenedioxyamphetamine). In the mid to late 1970s, some clinicians—influenced by the biochemist and psychopharmacologist Alexander Shulgin who had resynthesized MDMA in his laboratory in 1976—started exploring its therapeutic potential to facilitate marriage counselling and individual therapy. Such usage was dismissed by the United States government, and what followed were three decades of research focusing on MDMA-related harms, with MDMA being branded a potent neurotoxin with no place in medicine. The last 10 years, however, have seen a gradual resetting and revision of both its acute harms and longer-term neurotoxicity, as well as its therapeutic potential.

Although MDMA may claim its place as the pre-eminent dance drug and possessor of the best branding in terms of name ('Ecstasy'), MDMA is only one of a large number of synthetic amphetamine-type drugs possessing varying degrees of stimulant, hallucinogenic, and empathogenic effects that are used within the dance scene. As with most stimulant drugs, desirable effects and the risk of harm are dose-related. As seen in other illicit drugs, inconsistent preparations and variations in quality (for example, the amount of MDMA in a pill) and the presence of more dangerous contaminants [such as paramethoxymethamphetamine (PMMA)] mean that informed dosing and safer use strategies have their limitations. Overall, MDMA can be considered a relatively safe drug; acutely, it has a low risk of death, and although tolerance and loss of control are reported by users [28], few, if any, users will ever seek help for problems associated with its use in isolation from other drugs. Understanding its effects and risk profile is most useful to the clinician in ensuring an accurate assessment of mood and other psychological symptoms that can occur in the presence of MDMA use or that can be worsened by its use. In the UK, MDMA is classified as a Class A drug.

## Preparations, purity, and routes of use

MDMA is most commonly sold as tablets (pills) or powder (crystals) and taken orally, though it may be snorted, taken rectally, or injected. MDMA tablets vary in size, shape, and colour and are typically branded with an imprinted logo (for example, of a cartoon character, a car manufacturer, or a luxury brand). The size and shape of the tablet give no clue to its content, though, since 2015, in the UK and across much of Europe, tablets sold as ecstasy do contain MDMA, though the dose and precise composition vary. In recent years, it appears that the average dose of MDMA found in a pill has increased, with the average ecstasy pill containing 80–150 mg, though pills containing over 300 mg have been identified. These higher-dose pills have almost certainly contributed to both an escalation in the number of users seeking emergency medical treatment following the use of MDMA and an escalation in MDMA-related fatalities (from eight in 2010 to 63 in 2016, and over 56 in 2017 [29]). It is of note that while MDMA deaths are not clearly dose-related (the relationship between consumed dose and the risk of death is inconsistent and unpredictable on an individual level), higher doses of MDMA make you more vulnerable to environmental factors such as high temperature and overcrowding. The average dose of MDMA to give the user an optimal balance of positive vs negative effects is about 80–150 mg in divided doses (1.5 mg/kg). Higher-dose tablets can make it easy to take too much and expose people to dose-related unwanted effects, including agitation, panic, chest pain, overheating, hallucinations, and confusion. MDMA crystals are white, beige, or brownish in colour and can look very similar to other white crystalline drugs such as crystal meth. Typically swallowed either by wrapping in cigarette paper (known as parachuting or bombing) or taken by licking a finger and dipping it in MDMA powder (known as dabbing), MDMA powder can also be snorted or, rarely, injected. In the UK, an ecstasy tablet costs £5–10, with a gram of MDMA crystals costing around £40.

## Pill testing

Because of the variations in quality, some users utilize drug testing methods (such as the Marquis test which gives colorimetric results by mixing the substance with a reagent) and websites (http://

www.EcstasyData.org) which provide the contents of different pills following more elaborate analytical methods. Although these approaches have some role, not least in getting users to consider the risks and engage in conversations about harm reduction practices, these approaches are limited by accuracy of data, especially regarding the amount of each active drug present. More sophisticated analytical techniques can help in identification of more psychoactive contents such as paramethoxyamphetamine (PMA) [30]. There is a good case for an early warning system to ensure that information about high-dose MDMA pills or pills found to contain dangerous contaminants is made available to the drug-using community, though exactly what approach is the best, given resource limitations, is uncertain. However, in recent years, across many countries in Europe, the availability of on-site sophisticated analytical processes [for example, gas chromatography–mass spectrometry (GCMS), high-performance liquid chromatography (HPLC)] are offering the possibility of integrated harm reduction and chemical composition analysis, including the amount of active drug which can help people change their drug using behaviour. However, the majority of drug-related deaths remain unpredictable, and individual behaviour the biggest modifiable risk behaviour. Knowing the content of your tablet never guarantees the user a positive experience and can never reduce the risk associated with use to zero [31].

## Prevalence and patterns of MDMA use as ecstasy

British population studies show that 54% of 20- to 22-year olds have been offered ecstasy at some time and 15% have tried it at least once [32]. The current prevalence in 16- to 24-year olds has increased to 5.4% in terms of last year use [4]. Use appears higher in those associated with the dance music drug scene, with over 90% reporting lifetime ever use. Similar findings have been reported from Europe [33], Australia [34], and the United States.

The typical pattern of use in the UK and Europe is 1–2 tablets a night (equivalent to 100–250 mg of MDMA powder). Most people use less than ten times per year. Tolerance develops with regular use and is associated with higher-dose consumption and higher levels of polydrug use. Ecstasy, especially within the context of dance clubs, is rarely taken in isolation, and polydrug use is the norm, with different adjunctive substances taken at different times over the course of a night [35]. For example, alcohol is taken with ecstasy at the beginning of the night to get a stronger/better high [36]. Cocaine, amphetamines, and/or additional ecstasy tablets are taken to maintain arousal and a state of alertness (the MDMA entactogenic effects fade away in 2–4 hours). Finally, depressants such as cannabis, alcohol, benzodiazepines, and more rarely opiates may be taken in the last part of the night to calm down before going home, since the untoward after-effects of ecstasy (namely irritability, insomnia, and restlessness) may persist well beyond its 'pleasurable' effects. With chronic high dosage, ecstasy users develop tolerance and experience a decrease in the desired effects over time, which could lead to use of other stimulants and hallucinogens [35].

## Physical effects and complications

Physiologically sympathomimetic properties similar to amphetamine predominate, including tachycardia, anorexia, increased respiratory rate and blood pressure, increased motor activity, tremor, mydriasis, increased temperature, and sweating. Jaw tightening (bruxism), xerostomia, and teeth grinding with molar erosion may also be seen (Table 53.2). Sleep architecture modification [37] and sexual activity alteration [38, 39] have also been described.

After MDMA intake, a number of untoward effects (often part of the 'coming up' phase when the effects of MDMA first manifest) may commonly occur, including nausea, vomiting, diarrhoea, tachycardia, and palpitations. Pathologies less commonly seen include arrhythmias, hypertension, potentially life-threatening metabolic acidosis, cerebral haemorrhage, convulsions, coma, rhabdomyolysis, thrombocytopenia, disseminated intravascular coagulation, syndrome of inappropriate antidiuretic hormone (SIADH), acute kidney failure, acute liver failure, dehydration, and malignant hyperthermia [40–44].

Hyperthermia, although enhanced by exertional activity and poorly ventilated environments, may occur somewhat independently from the setting in which the drug is taken, because MDMA has thermal dysregulation effects in its own right. However, in clubs, dehydration is common and thirst naturally prompts individuals to replace body fluids lost during sweating sensibly with fruit juices, other isotonic fluids, or water, or less sensibly, but quite commonly, with alcohol. Very rarely, excessive intake of hypotonic fluids, coupled with an increase in vasopressin levels, has led to the occurrence of lethal hyponatraemia [45]. Deaths as a result of SIADH are very rare but may be most associated with excessive hypotonic fluid consumption, with MDMA potentially leading to urinary retention and impairing awareness of the need to micturate. In normal subjects who take MDMA and do not develop SIADH, there does appear to be an increase in both antidiuretic hormone (ADH) (greater in females than males) and oxytocin levels [46], the latter perhaps responsible for the drug's pro-social effects. Ninety per cent of cases of SIADH are seen in women.

MDMA is a potentially damaging cardiac stimulant [47], with reports suggesting long-term MDMA use may possibly lead to a fenfluramine-like valvular heart disease condition. Between 0.5% and 1% of last year users of MDMA report seeking emergency medical treatment in the previous 12 months, with the rate among young women being 2–3 times greater than among men. Presentations are more common in heavy regular users and those combining MDMA with alcohol and/or other drugs.

## MDMA's psychological effects and problems

(See Table 53.2 [48].) Being structurally related to both amphetamine and mescaline, 'empathogens' or 'entactogens' [49] like MDMA possess both stimulant and hallucinogenic properties, which allow them to be discriminated from other related substances. After MDMA ingestion, enhanced mood, increased energy, openness, heightened sensory perception, and mild perceptual alterations are reported [40, 42, 48].

MDMA is described as evoking 'an easily controlled altered state of consciousness with emotional and sensual overtones' [50], with the substance's appeal resting in its 'dramatic and consistent ability to induce in the user a profound feeling of attachment and connection'. With this in mind, it is perhaps not surprising that the Los Angeles dealer who coined the street name 'ecstasy' for MDMA would have preferred the name 'empathy', but he did not feel that his typical customer would know what it meant. These qualities were also what has led to recent research into its use within a clinical psychotherapeutic setting in the treatment of PTSD [51–54].

**Table 53.2** Psychological and physical effects of MDMA

| Physical | Psychological |
|---|---|
| Increase in physical and emotional energy | Relaxation/euphoria |
| Dilated pupils, dry mouth | Feelings of well-being |
| Tachycardia, hypertension, increased respiratory rate | Enhanced closeness and sociability |
| Increased sweating, dehydration | Heightened perceptual awareness |
| Increased motor activity, tremor | Disinhibition |
| Blurred/double vision | Increased response to touch/empathy |
| Anorexia, nausea, weight loss | Anxiety/panic/paranoia |
| Teeth grinding, jaw clenching (bruxism) | Agitation and restlessness |

Adapted from *J Nerv Ment Dis.*, 180(6), Liester MB, Grob CS, Bravo GL, *et al.*, Phenomenology and sequelae of 3,4-methylenedioxymethamphetamine use, pp. 345–54, Copyright (1992), with permission from Wolters Kluwer Health, Inc.

## Acute psychological problems associated with MDMA use

There have been reports of acute episodes of anxiety, panic, paranoia, excessive agitation, confusion, hallucinations, and rarely brief psychotic episodes following the consumption of MDMA. Many users of MDMA report 'mid-week blues', with some individuals reporting clinically borderline levels of depression in the days following MDMA [55], which could reflect the depletion of serotonin following the acute elevation that follows ingestion of MDMA. This could be seen as a parallel to the 'crash' reported after abstinence of cocaine use or as a hangover effect from all-night dancing, excessive alcohol, and minimal sleep. Although depression, anxiety, and mood fluctuations attributed to ecstasy are reported to be strongly related to the number of occasions of MDMA use [56, 57], Morgan *et al.* [58] found that higher depression scores among current heavy ecstasy users, in comparison to drug-naïve and polydrug controls, were no longer significant after treating cannabis use as a covariate.

## Other consequences of use

### Neurotoxicity, neuropsychological impairments, and psychiatric presentations

Significant research into MDMA has been ongoing for around 30 years. Much of the evidence for MDMA causing 5-HT neurotoxicity comes from preclinical studies in rodents and non-human primates where findings of depleted 5-HT brain tissue levels, reduced 5-hydroxyindoleacetic acid (5-HIAA) levels, reduced tyrosine hydroxylase activity, and reduction in serotonin transporter (SERT) binding have been consistently reported [59].

With regard to MDMA having 5-HT neurotoxic effects in humans, there is ongoing debate. Given the preclinical data, it is likely that similar effects would occur in humans; however, there are issues around inter-species scaling and dosing regimes (animal studies often dose multiple times per day on consecutive days, which is quite different from human recreational MDMA use patterns, and also often in higher milligrams per kilogram than humans would typically consume), which mean extrapolation from animal studies is complicated [60].

In a recent meta-analysis of both preclinical and human molecular imaging studies on MDMA, the main finding was a reduction in

SERT binding across the cerebral cortex and parts of the forebrain, especially in heavy users, but there is evidence of some recovery after cessation of MDMA use [61]. This reduction in SERT binding is thought to be indicative of serotonergic neurotoxicity; however, downregulation of SERT cannot be excluded. In a systematic review of imaging studies in moderate users (<100 tablets lifetime, or <50 lifetime episodes of MDMA use), there was no convincing evidence that moderate MDMA use was associated with structural or functional brain alterations in neuroimaging measures [62].

From a functional perspective, MDMA use in humans has been associated with a number of neuropsychological deficits which are thought to be underpinned by 5-HT system dysfunction; however, the evidence for specific MDMA-attributable deficits remains a little controversial due to inherent confounds such as purity of tablets taken, use mainly of cross-sectional studies, and comorbid polydrug use often seen in MDMA users. The latter issue has benefited from use of non-MDMA-using polydrug control groups, rather than drug-naïve controls, in more recent studies. A recent meta-analysis has shown that MDMA users show impaired executive function, relative to non-users, in particular in its sub-domains: accessing long-term/semantic memory, 'switching', and 'updating' [63]. Other functional deficits associated with MDMA use have been described in prospective memory, higher cognitive processing, such as logical reasoning, problem-solving, organizational control, and social intelligence. Other psychobiological domains affected by MDMA are sleep apnoea, visual information processing, immunocompetence, pain perception, psychomotor skill, and damage to emergent children of pregnant women [64].

MDMA intake may put users at significant risk for developing psychiatric problems [65], although some have suggested that this may occur only in vulnerable individuals [66]. Studies suggest that ecstasy users may report both childhood emotional/physical abuse [67] and a history of familial depression, anxiety, and panic attacks [68] more frequently than ecstasy-naïve controls. Many studies also report increases in psychopathology in MDMA users, relative to non-MDMA-using polydrug controls, in self-reported measures of anxiety, depression, memory, and impulsivity [69].

### Depression and its management in MDMA users

In a patient presenting with psychological problems who has a history of MDMA use, the crucial assessment issues are the identification of any premorbid disorders, their position in the cycle of use/post-use, and the persistence of any symptoms beyond a 2- to 4-week period following cessation of use. As with amphetamine use, in the days after taking MDMA, there may be symptoms attributable to monoamine depletion and subsequent repletion. A period of acute 5-HT depletion due to vesicular monoamine depletion (mid-week blues) is likely to be the most potent cause for the relative reduction in monoamine neurotransmitters. Repeated use of MDMA over several days will be associated with markedly diminished effects. Recovery is delayed further by inhibition of the rate-limiting enzyme (tyrosine hydroxylase in the case of MDMA) and the relative absence, especially in chronic users, of a good source of monoamine precursors following stimulant-induced anorexia and malnutrition. It is likely that, as with other stimulant drugs, including cocaine, a period of extended, but less intense, withdrawal symptoms (mood, sleep) may be seen with persistent abstinence, which may take weeks or months to recede and are associated with the more gradual

reversal of neuroadaptive changes in dopaminergic receptor sensitivity/expression [70].

As with amphetamine and cocaine users, antidepressant treatments should usually not be commenced until 2–4 weeks after cessation of MDMA use, in order to allow for reassessment and confirmation of any disorder. There are also at least theoretical causes for concern over potentially fatal interactions between MDMA and SSRIs that have been reported very rarely, possibly because some SSRIs (that is, citalopram) can inhibit the CYP2D6 enzyme [71]. The precise effects of combining SSRIs and MDMA appear to be related to whether use of the SSRI was before or after MDMA and whether SSRI dosing is acute or chronic. For example, SSRIs given acutely after MDMA (taken by users to intensify the ecstasy effects) may theoretically increase the risk of precipitating a serotonergic syndrome. It is probable that SSRIs and other classes of antidepressants can be used effectively in this group if a diagnosis of responsive affective/anxiety disorder is confirmed and abstinence is maintained. CBT may be useful in this group, both to address their underlying drug use as well as to address any coexisting anxiety/depressive disorders.

Dependence with the development of heavy regular use patterns is possible, though there are unlikely to be any specific signs or symptoms that differentiate diagnosis or management significantly from other forms of stimulant dependence.

## Assisted psychotherapy and the potential therapeutic role of MDMA

While this chapter has concentrated on the recreational use and dangers of MDMA, interest in MDMA as an empathogen predates its incarnation as a party drug. There is now serious interest in the medical use of MDMA to treat PTSD. The initiative has evolved over many years as the Multidisciplinary Association for Psychedelic Studies (MAPS) project (http://www.maps.org/research/mdma). Agreement has been reached with the FDA to designate MDMA as a 'breakthrough medicine'. A definitive RCT is planned, supported by philanthropic donations, and the objective is an approval by 2021.

## Novel psychoactive drugs

Since the mid 2000s, a dizzying array of diverse novel psychoactive drugs have appeared in the UK and across the world. Unhelpfully labelled 'legal high' by the media, until recently, many were openly sold on the UK high streets as smokable herbal preparations, pills, and powders. They were carefully branded and labelled with 'not for human consumption' to ensure they did not contravene the law. Often attempting to mimic the effects of traditional drugs—most commonly, cannabis, stimulants, and hallucinogens—they vary widely in their desirability, potency, effect, and risk profile. These new compounds are often undetected by UDS, and statutory services are often unaware of their presence in the community until they cause clinical problems in emergency departments or are found in police seizures. Such triangulation of data sources is required to keep abreast of this rapidly developing area.

The Psychoactive Substances Bill passed in the UK in May 2016 is an attempt to reduce their widespread availability and has led to closure of over 300 'headshops' across the UK. While reducing easy access on high streets will lead to a reduction in use, it is probable that distribution and supply will continue either through illicit street dealing networks or dark-net drugs markets. Where the effect profile, demand, and profit are attractive enough, it is likely that some classes of these drugs will remain in circulation. For the psychiatrist, the important issues are that these drugs are not picked up on routine drug screening; hence, clinicians should remain alert to the possibility that young people who present with disturbed behaviour or psychopathology may have used them. Offering a relatively cheap, but generally less desirable, high, many people who use these drugs could be considered vulnerable in other ways, through their young age, coexisting mental illness, or homelessness. At the time of writing, synthetic cannabinoid products, which are a particular problem within prisons, pose some of the greatest risks. These potent CB1 receptor agonists not only carry the risk of dependence and withdrawal, but their acute use is also at least 30 times more likely to lead to emergency medical treatment than high-potency herbal cannabis [72]. Symptoms include extreme agitation and a transient psychotic state, which will often resolve after cessation of use but may persist in some cases for weeks and may require antipsychotics. Acute psychotic mental states need appropriate monitoring and follow-up. Although deaths are still relatively rare, some of these NPS can cause significant physical harms such as seizures and arrhythmias. Collaborative management with general medical colleagues and good clinical documentation, combined with appropriate investigations such as ECGs and biochemical screens, should be undertaken.

## Mephedrone (meow meow, M-CAT, 4MMC)

### Background

Mephedrone (4-methylmethcathinone) is one of a number of cathinone compounds (methylone, methcathinone, MDPV, and others), which derive from the natural herbal stimulant khat (*Catha edulis*) and are β-keto analogues of amphetamine. Mephedrone came to prominence in the UK in 2009 as a cheap and easily accessible alternative to MDMA and cocaine (it was legally sold and marketed in the UK until April 2010) [73], both of which had been of poor quality in years prior to its appearance. After it was made illegal, its use among the general population diminished significantly, though access through street dealers and online markets has continued. It is most commonly associated with the gay music and 'chem-sex' scenes where it is often taken in conjunction with other drugs, including GHB and crystal methamphetamine.

### Preparation and routes of use

Mephedrone hydrochloride is typically sold as a white crystalline powder. It is water-soluble and is most commonly snorted intranasally, with single doses being between 50 and 150 mg. Taken intranasally, effects come on swiftly (within 10–20 minutes) and last approximately 1–2 hours, with users re-dosing every 30–120 minutes over the course of a session; some heavy users are capable of consuming over 5 g. It can also be taken orally, often wrapped in cigarette paper, a practice known as bombing, for a slower onset of action and less intense onset of effect. It can also be used rectally and by intravenous injection—the latter being associated with

significant tissue damage. Injection among naïve injecting groups can be a particular risk factor for HIV where the sexualized injection of drugs such as mephedrone and crystal methamphetamine (known as 'slamming') can be seen in association with other risky sexual practices.

### Mechanism of action and effect profile

Mephedrone consumption results in typical stimulant-related effects—euphoria, increased concentration, talkativeness, urge to move, empathy, jaw clenching, reduced appetite, and insomnia are most commonly reported. At higher doses, mephedrone has the potential to cause a toxic sympathetic syndrome, with agitation, panic, dehydration, overheating, seizures, cardiovascular dysregulation, and paranoid episodes, leading to emergency medical presentations [74]. Its mechanism of action is similar to other stimulant drugs: extracellular release of monoamine neurotransmitters (dopamine and serotonin) and inhibition of their reuptake (dopamine, serotonin, and noradrenaline). Overall, mephedrone has an effect profile similar to MDMA, but with a duration of action and abuse liability similar to that of cocaine. Animal models confirm its potential to cause dependence with mephedrone (high levels of self-administration in rat models [75]). With a short duration of action and rapid development of tolerance, dependence will be seen among a proportion of regular users. The comedown after mephedrone appears to be worse than with either cocaine or MDMA. Lowering of mood following use (presumably due to acute monoamine depletion) may be marked and can be associated with elevated suicide risk, especially in those with underlying psychiatric conditions [76].

### Treatment

Treatment interventions are broadly similar to those for other stimulant drugs, with emphasis on harm reduction, self-regulation, management of acute toxicity, differentiation between drug intoxication/withdrawal, and primary underlying psychiatric condition and relapse prevention [77].

## Gamma hydroxylbutyrate (GHB, GBH, G, fantasy, liquid ecstasy, and GBL)

### Background

GHB is an endogenous short-chain fatty acid found in the central nervous system and elsewhere in the body. It is a putative neurotransmitter, and specific binding sites have been identified in the hippocampus (linked to dopamine neurons), but its precise role is yet to be identified. Trace amounts may also be found in certain fruits such as guava. In the UK, GHB is a Class C drug. Along with its precursors, including the psychoactive pro-compounds GBL (gamma butyrolactone) and 1,4-butanediol, GHB is a colourless, odourless, slightly acidic-tasting liquid that, when consumed orally, is used for pro-social, sexual, and sedating effects.

GHB was originally developed as an anaesthetic in the 1960s. In the 1980s, it had found clinical utility as a sedative, as a treatment for narcolepsy, and as a detoxification agent (it is effective in the management of alcohol withdrawal). It is also used (with little evidence of effect) to promote muscle growth in bodybuilders (through its effect on increasing slow-wave sleep). Since the 1990s, however, it has become best known for its place among the smorgasbord of drugs commonly used by those involved in the dance/rave scene, especially those from the LGBT community where its pro-social and aphrodisiac qualities have made it popular, particularly in conjunction with crystal methamphetamine and mephedrone. Almost unique among liquid drugs of abuse, GHB is typically consumed in doses of only 1–2 mL; combined with its narrow therapeutic index, this implies a high risk of overdose, which is increased in combination with alcohol [78].

## Preparation (pro-drugs), purity, and routes of use

Until the late 1990s, GHB and its precursors were widely available in shops and the Internet as a clear liquid. As an industrial solvent and a cleaning product, it was also easy to come across these drugs in other guises. For example, GBL was sold in high-street chemists as nail polish remover and websites offered litre bottles as alloy cleaners. Because of its relative ease of manufacture, attempts at home production also occur but can result in preparations of widely varying concentrations; high concentrations can be quite caustic, resulting in gastrointestinal discomfort and nausea, with a risk of vomiting and aspiration.

## Doses and typical patterns of use

Most users of GHB are not daily dependent users and will use for 1–2 days in association with other drugs, most commonly alcohol, methamphetamine, poppers, and sexual enhancers such as sildenafil. Typical doses are 1–2 mL dispensed via an eye dropper or a syringe, often mixed with juice or alcohol to disguise the taste, and taken every 2–3 hours. Heavy users may dose 3–4 mL every hour, with bigger doses at night to aid sleep. While most users will limit their use to situations which exploit its pro-social, disinhibitory, and aphrodisiac qualities, a minority of users (less than 5%) will extend their use over periods of weeks or months. Daily use for more than 1–2 weeks can lead users to developing tolerance and withdrawal symptoms upon cessation, which drives further use.

## Mechanism of action

GHB readily crosses the blood–brain barrier and acutely leads to a transient decrease, followed by an increase, in dopamine levels (and an increase in endogenous opioid release). Increases in other neurotransmitters, such as GABA, ACh, and 5-HT, are also seen. At higher doses, it exhibits some partial action at GABA-B receptors (epileptogenic). GHB is usually taken orally, often mixed in fruit juice or an alcoholic beverage. It has a very rapid onset of action, with noticeable effects occurring within 15 minutes of administration; it has a relatively short duration of action (half-life 27 minutes), with effects peaking at 30–60 minutes and being over within 2–4 hours, being eliminated through its breakdown to carbon dioxide and water.

## Physical effects and complications

GHB exhibits a very narrow therapeutic index, and as a result of wide inter-personal variation in tolerance and significantly enhanced toxicity (depressant effects) when combined with alcohol, overdose with GHB has been reported more frequently than for any other dance drug [79, 80]. Overdose should be suspected in someone who presents with nystagmus, ataxia, nausea, vomiting, sedation, weakness, bradycardia, hypotension, and rapid onset of unconsciousness (quite similar to severe alcohol intoxication, but without alcohol on the breath). Management should include placing the person in the recovery position, airway management, and pulse oximetry. GCS scores may be very low (<6). If oxygen saturation drops or the patient is so unconscious that they can tolerate a Guedel airway, then ventilation should be considered. Overdoses are short-lived, and most awake somewhat aroused and disorientated after a few hours. Other clinical presentations include agitation, anxiety, coma, amnesia, seizures, and collapse. These patients, when in a coma, may require ventilation and typically suddenly emerge from their coma with high levels of agitation, arousal, and violence.

## Longer-term use, behavioural risks, and dependence

GHB can cause marked disinhibition and amnesia. This can result in people engaging in high-risk sexual practices or falling victim to sexual assault. Shame and uncertainty over what may or may not have happened can cause significant emotional distress to individuals. Until recently, dependence on GHB was considered rare among users, but with the apparent escalation in use across many countries, increasing numbers of people are coming forward, seeking treatment for dependence and the management of withdrawal. Tolerance and withdrawal can be seen among users who persist with daily use for more than a few weeks. Continued use outside party environments may be motivated by GHB's amelioration of the comedown from other drugs, facilitation of sleep, or improved anxiety and confidence in social situations. Dependence is characterized by the development of tolerance (bigger doses taken at shorter intervals), intense craving, continued use despite evident harms, and a well-defined withdrawal syndrome. Withdrawal from GHB, like alcohol, sits on a spectrum and is dominated by autonomic and psychological arousal. Among severely dependent users, withdrawal commences within 2–4 hours and can escalate rapidly, from early symptoms of craving, anxiety, sweating, and tremor to confusion, disorientation, hallucinations, and seizures. Untreated/unplanned withdrawal can be life-threatening, and unplanned withdrawal can require huge doses of benzodiazepines to manage the high levels of autonomic instability, delirium, and seizure risk. Planned withdrawal can be safely done on an outpatient basis by experienced clinical teams. The basic principles of treatment are an initial planning and assessment phase, with encouragement to stop any concurrent stimulant use (as it tends to lead to larger GHB usage). A tapered reduction in dose over the following week is sometimes supported by preloading with baclofen, which seems to reduce craving for GHB and subsequently reduce the need for high-dose benzodiazepines during the active detoxification phase. The aim is to lower total daily doses to below 25 mL/day before cessation. At cessation of GHB use, the acute withdrawal syndrome is managed by diazepam (typically in the region of 30–60 mg/day), given in 3–4 divided doses, tapering down over 7–10 days. Baclofen may be continued throughout the detoxification period and can be useful to continue for 2–3 weeks following detoxification completion, to aid sleep and manage residual craving and withdrawal.

## Harm reduction strategies for GHB users

Given the small difference between a dose that induces euphoria and stimulation and a toxic dose, measuring doses with a syringe (1.0–1.5 mL would be a typical dose) or using pre-filled capsules can reduce the risk of accidental overdose. Variations in preparation purity suggest test dosing from new batches is advisable. Avoiding mixing with alcohol, which increases the risk of overdose through synergistic respiratory depressant effects, is advisable, as is additional stimulant use, which is often associated with increased GHB consumption. Finally, avoiding use on more than 2–3 consecutive days can avoid the development of tolerance and of dependence and withdrawal in the first place.

## Conclusions

MDMA, cocaine, methamphetamine, and GHB are all capable of producing acute adverse psychological experiences in normal users and exacerbating symptoms in those with underlying psychological disorders. They vary widely in their ability to induce dependence and in their long-term neuropsychiatric consequences. For the psychiatrist, the most common problems will be assisting in managing acute time-limited adverse psychological reactions, including withdrawal, and ensuring adequate follow-up assessment is provided. This is required to review the need for longer-term medication and to ensure that the differentiation between an underlying primary/precipitated disorder or a *de novo* condition that is time-limited and resolved with maintained abstinence is made. Because of the significant potential of the drug to cause physical harm, attention should also be paid to clinical examination, biochemical investigation, BBV screening, and liaison with medical specialists. The provision of harm reduction advice and strategies to support self-regulation, combined with the treatment of underlying conditions that may be driving continued use, will also form important aspects of clinical practice. In those who present with acute drug-related psychological symptoms, there should be an emphasis on follow-up since, in some cases, the symptoms will represent the onset of a persistent independent disorder which requires treatment. Users who have experienced acute psychological problems should be encouraged to make the attribution that there may be something inherent in them that makes them susceptible to experiencing unpleasant reactions with a drug; they are likely to remain vulnerable to those adverse experiences. This may be difficult to accept for potentially vulnerable young people who may prefer to think that the experience was not enjoyable because the drugs were not good—'it was a bad pill'.

### FURTHER INFORMATION

Erowid. http://www.erowid.org
European Monitoring Centre for Drugs and Drug Addition. http://www.emcdda.europa.eu
Global Drug Survey. http://www.globaldrugsurvey.com
NEPTUNE. http://www.neptune-clinical-guidance.co.uk

### REFERENCES

1. Winstock A.R., Ramsey J.D. (2010). Legal highs and the challenges for policy makers. *Addiction*, **105**, 1685–7.
2. Winstock A.R., Mitcheson L. (2012). New recreational drugs and the primary care approach to patients who use them. *BMJ*, **344**, e288.
3. Kirkpatrick M.G., Gunderson E.W., Johanson C.E., *et al.* (2012). Comparison of intranasal methamphetamine and d-amphetamine self-administration by humans. *Addiction*, **107**, 783–91.
4. Home Office National Statistics. (2015). *Drug misuse: Findings from the 2014/15 Crime Survey for England and Wales*, second edition. Home Office National Statistics.
5. Bolding, G., Hart, G., Sherr, L., *et al.* (2006). Use of crystal methamphetamine among gay men in London. *Addiction*, **101**, 1622–30.
6. Kosten, T.R., Markou, A., Koob, G.F. (1998). Depression and stimulant dependence: neurobiology and pharmacotherapy. *Journal of Nervous and Mental Disease*, **186**, 737–45.
7. Lambert, G., Johansson, M., Agren, H., *et al.* (2000). Reduced brain norepinephrine and dopamine release in treatment-refractory depressive illness: evidence in support of the catecholamine hypothesis of mood disorders. *Archives of General Psychiatry*, **57**, 787–93.
8. Shearer, J., Gowing, L.R. (2004). Pharmacotherapies for problematic psychostimulant use: a review of current research. *Drug and Alcohol Review*, **23**, 203–11.
9. Konstenius, M., Jayaram-Lindström, N., Guterstam, J., *et al.* (2014). Methylphenidate for attention deficit hyperactivity disorder and drug relapse in criminal offenders with substance dependence: a 24-week randomized placebo-controlled trial. *Addiction*, **109**, 440–9.
10. Kosten, T.R., Markou, A., Koob, G.F. (1998). Depression and stimulant dependence: neurobiology and pharmacotherapy. *Journal of Nervous and Mental Disease*, **186**, 737–45.
11. Baker, A., Lee, N.K., Jenner, L. (eds.) (2004). *Models of intervention and care for psychostimulant users*, second edition. Canberra: Department of Health and Ageing.
12. McKetin, R., McLaren, J., Lubman, D.I., *et al.* (2006). The prevalence of psychotic symptoms among methamphetamine users. *Addiction*, **101**, 1473–8.
13. Harris, D., Batki, S.L. (2000). Stimulant psychosis: symptom profile and acute clinical course. *American Journal on Addictions*, **9**, 28–37.
14. McKetin, R., McLaren, J., Lubman, D.I., *et al.* (2006). The prevalence of psychotic symptoms among methamphetamine users. *Addiction*, **101**, 1473–8.
15. Moratalla, R., Khairnar, A., Simola, N., *et al.* (2015). Amphetamine-related drugs neurotoxicity in humans and in experimental animals: main mechanisms. *Progress in Neurobiology*, **pii**, S0301–82.
16. Todd, G., Pearson-Dennett, V., Wilcox, R.A., *et al.* (2016). Adults with a history of illicit amphetamine use exhibit abnormal substantia nigra morphology and parkinsonism. *Parkinsonism and Related Disorders*. **25**, 27–32.
17. Callaghan, R.C., Cunningham, J.K., Sajeev, G., *et al.* (2010). Incidence of Parkinson's disease among hospital patients with methamphetamine-use disorders. *Movement Disorders*, **25**, 2333–9.
18. Callaghan, R.C., Cunningham, J.K., Sykes, J., *et al.* (2012). Increased risk of Parkinson's disease in individuals hospitalized with conditions related to the use of methamphetamine or other amphetamine-type drugs. *Drug and Alcohol Dependence*, **120**, 35–40.
19. Curtin, K., Fleckenstein, A.E., Robison. R.J., *et al.* (2015). Methamphetamine/amphetamine abuse and risk of Parkinson's disease in Utah: a population-based assessment. *Drug and Alcohol Dependence*, **146**, 30–8.
20. Thrash, B., Thiruchelvan, K., Ahuja, M., *et al.* (2009). Methamphetamine-induced neurotoxicity: the road to Parkinson's disease. *Pharmacological Reports*, **61**, 966–77.
21. Sordo L., Indave B.I., Barrio G., *et al.* (2014). Cocaine use and risk of stroke: a systematic review. *Drug and Alcohol Dependence*, **142**, 1–13.

22. van Emmerik-van Oortmerssen, K., van de Glind, G., van den Brink, W., et al. (2012). Prevalence of attention-deficit hyperactivity disorder in substance use disorder patients: a meta-analysis and meta-regression analysis. Drug and Alcohol Dependence, 122, 11–19.

23. Mariani, J.J., Levin, F.R. (2012). Psychostimulant treatment of cocaine dependence. Psychiatric Clinics in North America, 35, 425–39.

24. Levin, F.R., Mariani, J.J., Specker, S., et al. (2015). Extended-Release Mixed Amphetamine Salts vs Placebo for Comorbid Adult Attention-Deficit/Hyperactivity Disorder and Cocaine Use Disorder: A Randomized Clinical Trial. JAMA Psychiatry, 72, 593–602.

25. Konstenius, M., Jayaram-Lindström, N., Guterstam, J., et al. (2014). Methylphenidate for attention deficit hyperactivity disorder and drug relapse in criminal offenders with substance dependence: a 24-week randomized placebo-controlled trial. Addiction, 109, 440–9.

26. Kampman, K.M., Lynch, K.G., Pettinati, H.M., et al. (2015). A double blind, placebo controlled trial of modafinil for the treatment of cocaine dependence without co-morbid alcohol dependence. Drug and Alcohol Dependence, 155, 105–10.

27. Schierenberg, A., van Amsterdam, J., van den Brink, W., et al. (2012). Efficacy of contingency management for cocaine dependence treatment: a review of the evidence. Current Drug Abuse Reviews. 5, 320–31.

28. Uosukainen, H., Tacke, U., Winstock, A.R. (2015). Self-reported prevalence of dependence of MDMA compared to cocaine, mephedrone and ketamine among a sample of recreational poly-drug users. International Journal of Drug Policy, 26, 78–83.

29. Office of National Statistics (2016). Deaths related to drug poisoning in England and Wales: 2015 registrations. London: Office of National Statistics.

30. Byard, R.W., Gilbert, J., James, R., et al. (1998). Amphetamine derivative fatalities in South Australia: is 'ecstasy' the culprit? American Journal of Forensic Medicine and Pathology, 19, 261–5.

31. Winstock, A.R., Wolff, K., Ramsey, J. (2001). Ecstasy pill testing: harm minimization gone too far? Addiction, 96, 1139–48.

32. Webb, E., Ashton, C.H., Kelly, P., et al. (1996). Alcohol and drug use in UK university students. The Lancet, 348, 922–5.

33. Condon, J., Smith, N. (2003). Prevalence of drug use: key findings from the 2002/2003 British Crime Survey. 229. London: Home Office.

34. Copeland, J., Dillon, P., Gascoigne, M. (2006). Ecstasy and the concomitant use of pharmaceuticals. Addictive Behaviors, 31, 367–70.

35. Winstock, A.R., Griffiths, P., Stewart, D. (2001). Drugs and the dance music scene: a survey of current drug use patterns among a sample of dance music enthusiasts in the UK. Drug and Alcohol Dependence, 64, 9–17.

36. Schifano, F. (2004). A bitter pill. Overview of ecstasy (MDMA, MDA) related fatalities. Psychopharmacology, 173, 242–8.

37. McCann, U.D., Eligulashvili, V., Ricaurte, G.A. (2000). (±)3,4 Methylenedioxymethamphetamine ('Ecstasy')-induced serotonin neurotoxicity in clinical studies. Neuropsychobiology, 42, 11–16.

38. Topp, L., Hando, J., Dillon, P., et al. (1999). Ecstasy use in Australia: patterns of use and associated harm. Drug and Alcohol Dependence, 55, 105–15.

39. Parrott, A.C. (2001). Human psychopharmacology of ecstasy (MDMA): a review of 15 years of empirical research. Human Psychopharmacology, 16, 557–77.

40. Schifano, F., Oyefeso, A., Corkery, J., et al. (2003). Death rates from ecstasy (MDMA, MDA) and polydrug use in England and Wales 1996–2002. Human Psychopharmacology Clinical Experimental, 18, 519–24.

41. Tancer, M., Johanson, C.E. (2003). Reinforcing, subjective, and physiological effects of MDMA in humans: a comparison with d-amphetamine and mCPP. Drug and Alcohol Dependence, 72, 33–44.

42. de la Torre, R., Farré, M., Ortuño, J., et al. (2000). Non-linear pharmacokinetics of MDMA ("ecstasy") in humans. British Journal of Clinical Pharmacology, 49, 104–9.

43. Harris, D.S., Baggott, M., Mendelson, J.H., et al. (2002). Subjective and hormonal effects of 3,4-methylenedioxymethamphetamine (MDMA) in humans. Psychopharmacology, 162, 396–405.

44. Hernandez-Lopez, C., Farre, M., Roset, P.N., et al. (2002). 3,4-Methylenedioxymethamphetamine (ecstasy) and alcohol interactions in humans: psychomotor performance, subjective effects, and pharmacokinetics. Journal of Pharmacology and Experimental Therapeutics, 300, 236–44.

45. Budisavljevic, M.N., Stewart, L., Sahn, S.A., et al. (2003). Hyponatremia associated with 3,4-methylenedioxymethylamphetamine ('ecstasy') abuse. American Journal of the Medical Sciences, 326, 89–93.

46. Wolff, K., Tsapakis, E.M., Winstock, A.R., et al. (2006). Vasopressin and oxytocin secretion in response to the consumption of ecstasy in a clubbing population. Journal of Psychopharmacology, 20, 400–10.

47. Parrott, A.C. (2007). Ecstasy versus alcohol: Tolstoy and the variations of unhappiness. Journal of Psychopharmacology, 21, 3–6.

48. Liester, M.B., Grob, C.S., Bravo, G.L., et al. (1992). Phenomenology and sequelae of 3,4-methylenedioxymethamphetamine use. Journal of Nervous and Mental Disease, 180, 345–54.

49. Nichols, D.E. (1986). Differences between the mechanism of action of MDMA, MBDB, and the classic hallucinogens. Identificationof a new therapeutic class: entactogens. Journal of Psychoactive Drugs, 18, 305–13.

50. Shulgin, A.T. (1978). Characterization of three new psychotomimetics. In: Stillman, N.C., Willete, N.E. (eds.) The Pharmacology of Hallucinogens. Oxford: Pergamon Press. pp. 74–83.

51. Mithoefer, M.C., Wagner, T.M., Mithoefer, A.T., et al. (2011). The safety and efficacy of ±3,4-methylenedioxymethamphetamine-assisted psychotherapy in subjects with chronic, treatment-resistant posttraumatic stress disorder: the first randomized controlled pilot study. Journal of Psychopharmacology, 25, 439–52.

52. Mithoefer, M.C., Wagner, M.T., Mithoefer, A.T., et al. (2013). Durability of improvement in post-traumatic stress disorder symptoms and absence of harmful effects or drug dependency after 3 4-methylenedioxymethamphetamine-assisted psychotherapy: a prospective long-term follow-up study. Journal of Psychopharmacology, 27, 28–39.

53. Oehen, P., Traber, R., Widmer, V., et al. (2013). A randomized, controlled pilot study of MDMA (±3,4-Methylenedioxymethamphetamine)-assisted psychotherapy for treatment of resistant, chronic Post-Traumatic Stress Disorder (PTSD). Journal of Psychopharmacology, 27, 40–52.

54. Sessa B. (2017). MDMA and PTSD treatment: "PTSD: from novel pathophysiology to innovative therapeutics". Neuroscience Letters, 649, 176–80.

55. Curran, H.V., Travill, R.A. (1997). Mood and cognitive effects of ±3,4-methylenedioxymethamphetamine (MDMA, 'ecstasy'): weekend 'high' followed by mid-week low. *Addiction*, **92**, 821–31.

56. Guillot, C., Greenway, D. (2006). Recreational ecstasy use and depression. *Journal of Psychopharmacology*, **20**, 411–16.

57. Schifano, F., Di Furia, L., Forza, C., *et al.* (1998). MDMA ('ecstasy') consumption in the context of polydrug abuse: a report on 150 patients. *Drug and Alcohol Dependence*, **52**, 85–90.

58. Morgan, M.J., McFie, L., Fleetwood, H., *et al.* (2002). Ecstasy (MDMA): are the psychological problems associated with its use reversed by prolonged abstinence? *Psychopharmacology*, **159**, 294–303.

59. Lyles, J., Cadet, J.L. (2003). Methylenedioxymethamphetamine (MDMA, Ecstasy) neurotoxicity: cellular and molecular mechanisms. *Brain Research. Brain Research Reviews*, **42**, 155–68.

60. Baumann, M.H., Wang, X., Rothman, R.B. (2006). 3,4-Methylenedioxymethamphetamine (MDMA) neurotoxicity in rats: a reappraisal of past and present findings. *Psychopharmacology (Berlin)*, **189**, 407–24.

61. Vegting, Y., Reneman, L., Booij, J. (2016). The effects of ecstasy on neurotransmitter systems: a review on the findings of molecular imaging studies. *Psychopharmacology (Berlin)*, **233**, 19–20.

62. Mueller, F., Lenz, C., Steiner, M., *et al.* (2016). Neuroimaging in moderate MDMA use: a systematic review. *Neuroscience and Biobehavioural Reviews*, **62**, 21–34.

63. Roberts, C.A., Jones, A., Montgomery, C. (2016). Meta-analysis of executive functioning in ecstasy/polydrug users. *Psychological Medicine*, 46,1581–96.

64. Parrott, A.C. (2013). Human psychobiology of MDMA or 'Ecstasy': an overview of 25 years of empirical research. *Human Psychopharmacology*, **28**, 289–307.

65. Verheyden, S.L., Henry, J.A., Curran, H.V. (2003). Acute, sub-acute and long-term subjective consequences of 'ecstasy' (MDMA) consumption in 430 regular users. *Human Psychopharmacology Clinical Experimental*, **18**, 507–17.

66. Gerra, G., Zaimovic, A., Giucastro, G., *et al.* (1998). Serotonergic function after (+/−)3,4-methylene-dioxymethamphetamine ('Ecstasy') in humans. *International Clinical Psychopharmacology*, **13**, 1–9.

67. Singer, L.T., Linares, T.J., Ntiri, S., *et al.* (2004). Psychosocial profiles of older adolescent MDMA users. *Drug and Alcohol Dependence*, **74**, 245–52.

68. Guillot, C.R., Berman, M.E. (2007). MDMA (Ecstasy) use and psychiatric problems. *Psychopharmacology*, **189**, 575–6.

69. Rogers, G., Elston, J., Garside, R., *et al.* (2009). The harmful health effects of recreational ecstasy: a systematic review of observational evidence. *Health Technology Assessment*, **13**, 1–315.

70. Kosten, T.R., Markou, A., Koob, G.F. (1998). Depression and stimulant dependence: neurobiology and pharmacotherapy. *Journal of Nervous and Mental Disease*, **186**, 737–45.

71. Liechti, M.E. and Vollenweider, F.X. (2000). The serotonin uptake inhibitor citalopram reduces acute cardiovascular and vegetative effects of 3,4 methylenedioxymethamphetamine ('ecstasy') in healthy volunteers. *Journal of Psychopharmacology*, **14**, 269–74.

72. Winstock A., Lynskey M., Borschmann R., *et al.* (2015). Risk of emergency medical treatment following consumption of cannabis or synthetic cannabinoids in a large global sample. *Journal of Psychopharmacology*, **29**, 698–703.

73. Winstock, A., Mitcheson, L., Ramsey, J., *et al.* (2011). Mephedrone: use, subjective effects and health risks. *Addiction*, **106**, 1991–6.

74. Wood, D. M., Davies, S., Puchnarewicz, M., *et al.* (2010). Recreational use of mephedrone (4-methylmethcathinone, 4-MMC) with associated sympathomimetic toxicity. *Journal of Medical Toxicology*, **6**, 327–30.

75. Motbey C.P., Clemens K., Apetz N., *et al.* (2013). High levels of intravenous mephedrone (4-methylmethcathinone) self-administration in rats: neural consequences and comparison with methamphetamine. *Journal of Psychopharmacology*, **27**, 823–36.

76. Schifano, F., Corkery J., Ghodse A.H. (2012). Suspected and confirmed fatalities associated with mephedrone (4-methylmethcathinone, 'meow meow') in the United Kingdom. *Journal of Clinical Psychopharmacology*, **32**, 710–14.

77. Winstock, A. R., Mitcheson, L. (2012). New recreational drugs and the primary care approach to patients who use them. *BMJ*, **344**, e288.

78. Rodgers, J., Ashton, C.H., Gilvarry, E., *et al.* (2004). Liquid ecstasy: a new kid on the dance floor. *British Journal of Psychiatry*, **184**, 104–6.

79. Degenhardt, L., Darke, S., Dillon, P. (2003). The prevalence and correlates of gamma-hydroxybutyrate (GHB) overdose among Australian users. *Addiction*, **98**, 199–204.

80. Deveaux, M., Renet, S., Renet, V., *et al.* (2002). Utilisation de l'acide gamma-hydroxybutyrique (GHB) dans les rave-parties et pour la soumission chimique en France: mythe ou realité? *Acta Clinica Belgica—Supplementum*, **1**, 37–40.

# 54

# Psychedelics and dissociative substances

*Adam R. Winstock and James Rucker*

## Psychedelics

The psychedelics are a distinct group of drugs, the primary effects of which are alterations in perception, mood, and thought processing in clear consciousness and usually with retained insight. They do not cause dependence, are physiologically non-toxic, and harms to the end user and society are notably low in comparison to other illicit drugs [1].

The term 'psychedelic' literally translates from the Greek as 'mind-manifesting', a term chosen by the psychiatrist Humphrey Osmond in 1957 to denote a curious and putatively therapeutic tendency to 'unmask' repressed elements of the psyche. The two most commonly used psychedelics in the UK are LSD (d-lysergic acid diethylamide), a semi-synthetic compound discovered in 1938 by Albert Hofman, and psilocybin (N,N-dimethyl-4-phosphoryloxytryptamine), which is found in, among others, the psilocybe group of 'magic' mushrooms that grow throughout the UK and worldwide. Less commonly encountered are mescaline (3,4,5-trimethoxyphenethylamine), found in the North American peyote cactus, and DMT (N,N-dimethyltryptamine), the principal component of the South American ceremonial sacrament ayahuasca. Other examples include the '2C' group of psychedelics (for example, 2C-B, 2C-B-FLY, 2C-I, and 2C-E) and a wide range of recently developed synthetic psychedelics, including the NBOMes.

Classical psychedelics are divided into members of three chemical classes (Fig. 54.1): (1) tryptamines (for example, psilocybin); (2) ergolines (for example, LSD); and (3) phenethylamines (for example, mescaline and 2C-B). There are scores, if not hundreds, of compounds subsumed within these classes that have psychedelic effects. All classical psychedelics are active at the 2a subtype of the serotonin receptor (5-HT2a), with effects being strongly dose-related. Users of psychedelics typically report changes under five distinct phenomenological categories:

1. Perceptual distortions, most commonly visual, including synaesthesia (crossing of sensory modalities, for example, hearing colours).
2. Changes in somatic experience—visceral, tactile, and interoceptive.
3. Changes in affect and mood, including, but not limited to, elation, euphoria, anxiety, and paranoia.
4. Distortions in thought processing, from changes in semantic attribution and belief structures to blurring and dissolution of conceptual boundaries (for example, between 'self' and 'other', also known as 'ego dissolution'). Increasing confusion occurs at higher doses or in cognitively destabilizing environments.
5. Entheogenic experiences: spiritual, transcendent, often ineffable experiences.

### History

Psychedelics have a long relationship with the human species, which contextualizes current and evolving attitudes towards them. Evidence for the use of psychedelics (particularly psilocybin and mescaline) dates back further than for any other psychoactive substance, particularly in ceremonial, healing, and spiritual rituals. Depictions of mushrooms and temples built to mushroom 'deities' and use of the word *teonanácatl*, or 'flesh of God', to denote psilocybin-containing mushrooms in indigenous cultures in Mexico and Guatemala date back to around 7000 BC. Records of the Greek 'Eleusian Mysteries' suggest that the ceremony surrounding them was based on a psychedelic compound. The modern history of psychedelic use began when Arthur Heffter, a German chemist, isolated mescaline from the peyote cactus in 1897. However, it was not until the development of LSD that the medical use of psychedelics began to be investigated in earnest.

LSD was first synthesized by the Swiss chemist Albert Hofman in 1938, as part of a systematic investigation of compounds related to the 5-HT1 receptor agonist ergotamine [2]. Ergotamine, one of the ergot alkaloids, is produced by the parasitic rye fungus *Claviceps purpurea* and was responsible for the outbreaks of mass poisoning from consumption of spoilt stocks of rye in the Middle Ages, a condition known as *St. Anthony's fire*. LSD was found to be unremarkable in animal testing; however, Hofman resynthesized it on a hunch in 1943. After accidentally contaminating himself with a small amount, he experienced what was probably the world's first 'acid trip'. Further investigation of LSD found it to be extremely potent (the threshold dose for subjective effects is approximately 50 μg), but notably physiologically safe, with animals surviving overdoses that were relatively much larger than other psychoactive drugs.

Reassured by its physiological safety and recognizing that it might be of much interest to psychiatrists, LSD was marketed under the tradename Delysid". Between 1947 and 1967, LSD and, to a lesser

| Classical psychedelic chemical classes | | | |
| --- | --- | --- | --- |
| Class | Ergolines | Phenethylamines | Tryptamines |
| Basic structure | 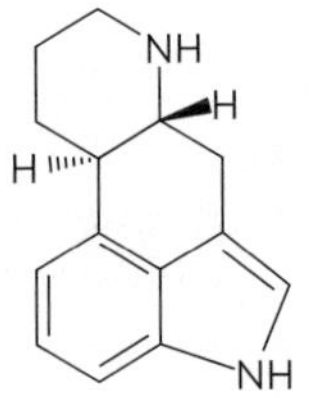 | 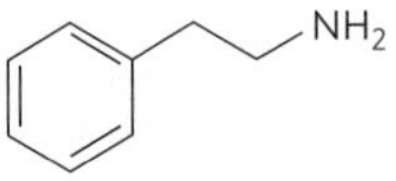 | 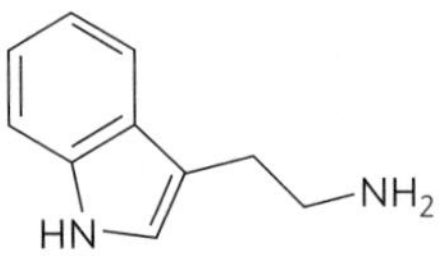 |
| Common example | LSD (d-lysergic acid diethylamide) | Mescaline (3,4,5-trimethoxy-phenethylamine) | Psilocybin (N,N-dimethyl-4-phosphoryloxytryptamine) |

**Fig. 54.1** Three chemically distinct classes of classical psychedelic compounds.

extent, mescaline and psilocybin were widely used as therapeutic agents, particularly as 'catalysts' in psychotherapy [3]. LSD also came to the attention of the American secret service where it was investigated as an agent of 'mind control' under the notorious *MK Ultra* programme, which was finally shut down in 1973 [4]. LSD was found to be ineffective for such purposes, instead rendering civilians and troops liable to disorganized behaviour and indifference to authority. The proselytization of LSD by the disgraced Harvard professor Timothy Leary led to its increasing recreational use, and it became a counter-cultural symbol against the status quo. Medical concern was raised for psychological toxicity in certain vulnerable groups [5].

Partly because of medical concern, and partly because of the counter-cultural opposition to the Vietnam War and conservative values in general, the Nixon administration of the time heavily criminalized psychedelics, along with many other psychoactive drugs. This dramatic escalation of the so-called 'war on drugs' stopped all medical use and scientific research, while pushing recreational use underground. A systematic media-led campaign of demonization in the 1960s and 1970s led psychedelics, particularly LSD, to be among the most heavily stigmatized of all psychoactive drugs, a stigma that is still present today.

### Legal status in the UK

Almost all classical psychedelics fall under the remit of the UK Misuse of Drugs Act, 1971, where they are generally Schedule 1, Class A compounds. As such, they are legally defined as having the maximum potential for harm and dependence and no identified medical use, a definition that does not survive objective scientific scrutiny [1, 6]. Until the passing of the Psychoactive Substances Act, 2016, a number of chemical analogue compounds (for example, 2C-B-FLY and 1P-LSD) with similar effect profiles were legally available for purchase online and from so-called 'head shops'. While head shops have now closed, the simple act of possession of these substances for personal use, unlike those classified under the 1971 Act, is not considered an offence under the 2016 Act.

### Preparation, purity, and routes of use

Psilocybin occurs in a wide variety of mushrooms, including (but not limited to) the genus *Psilocybe*, which grow throughout the UK.

They are most profligate in wet periods during early autumn. Liberty cap mushrooms are the species most commonly encountered in the UK, with doses of 10–20 mushrooms being a typical starting dose. The greatest risk of harm comes from picking the wrong type of mushroom, as some are poisonous. Psilocybin-containing mushrooms can be eaten raw, cooked, or dried and are often infused in hot water or added to other foodstuffs. Psilocybin is heat-sensitive, and prolonged cooking or boiling results in its degradation. Possession of psilocybin-containing mushrooms is an offence under the Misuse of Drugs Act, 1971.

LSD can be chemically derived from the ergot alkaloids that occur in the parasitic grain fungus *Claviceps purpurea*. However, cultivation of the fungus is unusually difficult, and the sequelae of accidental ingestion potentially fatal. It is usually chemically synthesized from lysergic acid or 3-indolepropionic acid. LSD is extremely potent, with 1 g making 10,000 moderate (100 µg) oral doses. It is soluble in either water or alcohol and is colourless and tasteless; it is therefore difficult to detect without sophisticated testing apparatus and is easily concealed and transported. Drops of liquid LSD can be sold for immediate consumption from dropper bottles or, more commonly, drops are absorbed onto squares ('tabs') of blotting paper, gelatin, sugar cubes, or small volumes of a binding material to form what is known as a 'microdot'. In recent years, novel potent psychedelics with a riskier effect profile have been sold as LSD tabs, such as 2-(4-iodo-2,5-dimethoxyphenyl)-*N*-[(2-methoxyphenyl)methyl] ethanamine (25I-NBOMe).

### Mechanism of action and metabolism

Classical psychedelics are broad serotonergic agonists. However, the subjective effect appears to be derived from partial agonism at 5-HT2a receptors that are predominantly expressed on pyramidal neurons within layer V of the human neocortex [7]. Thus, cross-tolerance occurs between different psychedelics, the degree of subjective potency is robustly associated with affinity at the 5-HT2a receptor, and antagonists at the 5-HT2a receptor (for example, risperidone) abolish the subjective effects of psychedelics. However, some 5-HT2a agonists (for example, lisuride) fail to produce psychedelic effects, suggesting that 5-HT2a agonism, while necessary, is not sufficient [8]. The psychedelic effect may also be dependent on the type 2 metabotropic glutamate receptor, as mice deficient in the corresponding gene are unresponsive to psychedelics [9]. A summation of the current evidence suggests that psychedelics may act via a heteroreceptor complex of these two receptor types, modulating the balance of downstream second messenger systems and changing the phase of firing of layer V pyramidal neurons. Within cortical neural networks, there is widening of the measured local field potentials and human EEG recordings shows characteristic suppression of alpha waves; how this leads to the observed neuroimaging changes, subjective effects, and putative therapeutic effects is far from clear. While other subtypes of the 5-HT receptor are also stimulated by psychedelics, their contribution to the subjective effect is likely to be only minor.

Approximately 50% of ingested psilocybin is absorbed through the digestive tract. Psilocybin is biologically inactive but is rapidly dephosphorylated to the active molecule psilocin. Psilocin is hepatically metabolized by monoamine oxidase; however, some undergoes glucuronidation and is excreted renally. The elimination half life of psilocybin is 50 minutes and for psilocin is 1.25 - 2.5 hours, depending on whether psilocybin is administered intravenously or orally, respectively [10].

LSD is completely absorbed in the digestive tract, with a maximal plasma concentration achieved after about 90 minutes. LSD has a half-life of approximately 3.5 hours in both men and women and shows first-order kinetics. It is hepatically metabolized to a variety of different compounds, and only about 1% of the original drug is excreted in its original form in the urine. The principal metabolite is probably 2-oxo-3-hydroxy-LSD [11].

### Recent brain scanning findings

Modern neuroimaging research suggests that psychedelics are neither stimulants nor depressants of brain activity. Instead, fMRI measures of 'functional connectivity' have suggested that brain network integrity is decreased under psychedelics and cross-talk between normally well-differentiated brain regions and networks is increased. There is some evidence that these effects correlate with the subjective effects of psychedelics; decreased default-mode network integrity and increased global connectivity have been found to correlate with ratings of ego dissolution under LSD, and increased communication between the primary visual cortex and the rest of the brain correlated with ratings of eyes-closed visual imagery [12].

### Prevalence

Of the classical psychedelics, the lifetime prevalence of LSD and psilocybin ingestion is largely similar, while more users report past year usage of psilocybin than LSD. Use is more common among those in the dance music and rave scenes. The most recent British Crime Survey (2017/2018) suggested that, while lifetime use has remained static over the last 20 years at about 9% among 16- to 59-year olds, past year reported use of psychedelics by this group has fallen from 1.3% in 1996 to 0.7% in 2017/2018 (average 0.7%). The fall in use appears most marked in younger groups, with 6.6% of 16- to 24-year olds reporting lifetime use of psychedelics in 2017/2018, compared to 16.1% reporting lifetime usage in 1996. Past year use among younger age groups has also fallen from 5.3% in 1996 to 2.3% in 2017/2018. In the UK, psychedelic use is notably rare among Asian, Black, and Chinese ethnic groups. Psychedelic usage does not tend to cluster in particular social classes. The most common pattern of use is one of episodic experimentation fading into abstinence. Chronic use is very uncommon, but of those who have used

psychedelics for decades, it is usual that they claim no lasting harms and claim considerable benefits.

### Harms

#### LSD, psilocybin, and mescaline

Despite politically led and media-driven rhetoric and the general lay perception that the classical psychedelics are dangerous, they are objectively one of the safest known classes of CNS drugs, and death due to direct toxicity of LSD, psilocybin, or mescaline is almost unknown in the literature despite well over 50 years of recreational use [7, 13]. This is likely attributable to their lack of activity on neurotransmitter systems that control basic physiological functions and their partial agonist property at serotonin receptors [14]. Overdose generally requires cardiac monitoring and supportive management in a comfortable, low-stimulus, reassuring environment. Benzodiazepines, such as lorazepam or diazepam, are the first-line treatment for symptomatic relief from emotional distress or behavioural disturbance. Significant behavioural disturbance after benzodiazepine treatment should raise the suspicion that other drugs have been taken.

### Other psychedelics

#### The classical '2C' phenethylamine compounds

There are a large number of synthetically derived psychedelics. The classical '2C' phenethylamine compounds, such as 2C-B, 2C-I, and 2C-E, as well as various tryptamine-derived psychedelics, were synthesized and self-administered by the chemist Alexander Shulgin in the 1960s and 1970s. His experiences and the chemical synthesis were described in the books *TiHKAL* and *PiHKAL* and in many online reports of use. Of these, 2C-B is the most popular and is generally well tolerated. Treatment of overdose is as per the other classical psychedelics.

#### 25I-NBOMe

A number of substituted 2C compounds have been developed since the turn of the century, and concern for physical toxicity exists for 25I-NBOMe (N-Bomb), which is the N-benzyl derivative of 2C-I. It is exceptionally potent, to the extent that it can be used as a substitute for LSD on blotter papers [15]. Unlike classical psychedelics, it is a full agonist at the 5-HT2a receptor. It appears to promote both vascular constriction and platelet aggregation in overdose, placing the user at risk of acute cardiac, CNS, and limb ischaemia, as well as serotonin syndrome. Reports of deaths directly attributable to 25I-NBOMe have accumulated since its emergence as a recreationally used substance in around 2010, and it remains a concern at the time of writing. LSD is tasteless, and therefore users should be advised to be suspicious of LSD blotters tasting of anything other than the blotter paper itself.

#### Dimethyltryptamine

Dimethyltryptamine (DMT), the active component of ayahuasca, has recently become increasingly popular with the rise of smoked DMT and the commercialization of the ceremonial aspects of the drugs [16]. When smoked, it leads to a short-lived (less than 2 hours), but intense, psychedelic experience. Ayahuasca is an oral preparation usually derived from the *Banisteriopsis caapi* vine. DMT when taken orally needs to be consumed with harmine or another compound with monoamine oxidase-inhibiting (MAOI) activity.

## Psychological effects and complications

The psychological effects of psychedelics are dependent on the psychological mind 'set' of the user and the environmental 'setting' of the experience. Experienced recreational drug users rank psilocybin and LSD as having low harm and high benefit potential in comparison to other drugs [17]. However, recreational use is not without its risks, particularly in psychologically sensitive individuals and in psychologically destabilizing environments. Those with a personal or family history of severe and enduring psychotic disorders should be particularly discouraged from experimentation with psychedelics.

In a recent web-based survey of difficult or negative experiences during psilocybin use, 62% of 1993 respondents rated the experience as being within the top ten most challenging experiences of their lives; yet 84% reported that they benefited in some way from this, and 76% reported increases in current well-being or life satisfaction. Thirty-four per cent and 31% reported the experience to be in the top five most personally meaningful and spiritually significant experiences in their lives, respectively. In contrast, 8% reported a decrease in well-being or life satisfaction as a result of the difficult experience, and three respondents reported that they had attempted suicide or suffered prolonged psychotic experiences [18]. This result is consistent with the observation that psychedelics unmask repressed (and hence somewhat unpredictable) elements of the psyche, but that the successful integration of such elements within conscious experience can be beneficial to the overall psychological well-being. This underlines the importance of set and setting and speaks to the possible therapeutic potential of psychedelics in medically controlled settings where both set and setting can be optimized and the risks minimized.

### Hallucinogen persisting perceptual disorder

Hallucinogen persisting perceptual disorder (HPPD) was included in DSM-IV as an attempt to capture a syndrome whereby users of psychedelics report distressing residual effects long after the drug has cleared from the body. A summation of the evidence for HPPD in 2002 concluded that while the disorder probably existed, it was poorly defined, rare, and aetiologically opaque [19]. A variety of theories have been put forward, ranging from a direct neurotoxic effect of the drug to a negative psychological reaction to the effect of the drug. Direct neurotoxicity appears unlikely, particularly since experience with recreational use is extensive and massive overdoses of psychedelics have been survived without apparent clinical sequelae. An idiosyncratic premorbid biological sensitivity in some individuals cannot be ruled out, but it appears more likely that some users are psychologically sensitive to the effects of the psychedelic experience, perhaps becoming more 'aware' of the fluctuating functioning of various aspects of experiential processing. Consequently, the symptomatology reported within the scope of HPPD is widely variable and no particular medical treatment has become prominent. In most cases, HPPD appears to resolve over time with psychological support.

## Other consequences of use

### Dependence and withdrawal

There is no evidence that psychedelics cause physiological or psychological dependence. Indeed they may be a treatment for physical dependence, with the evidence most strong for alcoholism [20]. Complete tolerance to the classical psychedelics develops, usually within 72 hours, and full resensitization takes 1 week or longer. No defined withdrawal syndrome has been identified, although tension headaches responsive to simple analgesia are common in the 24 hours after use.

### Psychedelic-induced psychosis

Brief, self-limiting psychotic episodes can occur while intoxicated with psychedelics and are more common in naïve users, those with a past history of psychiatric illness, and users of longer-acting, more potent substances such as LSD. Such episodes, subsumed along with anxiety and panic reactions under the term 'bad trip', can be more likely if the drug is consumed in unfavourable environments or at a time when the person feels uncertain or unsafe.

Many people report negative or difficult-to-deal-with experiences when taking psychedelics. For many, working through the experience with the support of a caring, empathic other can itself be a useful and enriching experience. Medical management is supportive, with cessation of drug consumption, psychological support, and sedation with benzodiazepines, if necessary.

In the pre-prohibition era, psychedelic drugs were used on a wide variety of psychiatric patients and disorders. While some observed that they appeared to 'unmask' psychotic disorders in high-risk individuals, this was tempered by evidence from observational studies suggesting that the rate of psychedelic-induced schizophrenia was probably no higher than chance. Even so, the current clinical consensus is that psychedelic drugs should be avoided by those at high risk of developing psychotic disorders.

### Use in therapy

Prior to prohibition in the late 1960s, thousands of patients, reported in many hundreds of academic papers, were treated with psychedelics (usually LSD) in Europe and the United States, with six international conferences on psychedelic-catalysed psychotherapy organized during this period [21]. Their use was much wider than is usually appreciated today [13]. This use swiftly declined after the 1967 United Nations declaration on drugs, which legally defined them, paradoxically, as having no medical use and placing stringent restrictions on their manufacture, supply, and prescription. While pre-prohibition studies of the therapeutic efficacy of psychedelics, in common with many clinical studies at the time, were of suboptimal standard, good-quality evidence for efficacy was found in alcoholism. A modern meta-analysis of six controlled trials found a substantial therapeutic effect of LSD over placebo in objective measures of alcohol use [20]. A recent systematic review of pre-prohibition evidence in unipolar mood disorders was also broadly encouraging [22]. Since 2006, small pilot studies have shown promising results in anxiety associated with advanced cancer [23], obsessive–compulsive disorder [24], tobacco [25] and alcohol [26] addiction, cluster headaches [27], and treatment-resistant unipolar depression (TRD) [28]. Two RCTs of psilocybin in existential distress associated with life threatening cancer were published in 2016 [29, 30]. RCTs with psilocybin for TRD are now under way [13].

## Ketamine

### Introduction

Ketamine is a dissociative anaesthetic that exerts its action primarily through non-competitive antagonism at the NMDA receptor. It is almost unique as an anaesthetic in its ability to produce a 'dissociative' state, which results in higher brain structures being prevented from perceiving auditory, visual, or painful stimuli, leading to 'a lack of responsive awareness' [31]. Over the last 20 years, its use as a recreational drug has spread, and although there are concerns that longer-term use may be associated with serious physical (urinary tract) and psychological (cognitive impairment) harms, ketamine does benefit from having a wide margin of safety in overdose, with the greatest risk for most users being that of trauma or accidental harm while intoxicated.

## Background and legal status

Ketamine is a versatile medication and is in widespread use in both general, paediatric, and emergency medicine (in anaesthesia and pain management). It is also a remarkably safe drug in clinical practice where the pronounced analgesia and amnesia occur without any significant depression of cardiac or respiratory function and maintenance of the gag reflex. The WHO has listed it as an essential medicine. Emergence phenomena (experienced as people recover from anaesthetic doses of the drug) encompass a range of unusual psychological experiences, including hallucinations, near-death and out-of-body experiences, delirium, and confusion; these have limited its use in wider clinical settings [32]. Ketamine has been part of the illicit drug scene in the UK since the 1990s. Currently, it is most commonly seen among those involved in the clubbing scene, especially trance music events. In June 2014, ketamine changed from a class C to a class B controlled drug in the UK.

## Preparation, purity, and routes of use

Ketamine is typically sold as a crystalline powder for intranasal use (usual doses 50–250 mg), though it can also be found in liquid, tablet, or capsular form for ingestion. When obtained from diverted licit sources, the formulation of the drug is a solution prepared for intravenous use, which is then dried and taken intranasally. Ketamine may be adequately absorbed via the intranasal, intravenous, subcutaneous, intramuscular, rectal, and intrathecal routes, with snorting and injecting being the most common recreational routes of use.

## Mechanism of action and metabolism

The most significant pharmacological action of ketamine is non-competitive antagonist binding at the cation channel of the NMDA receptor. Ketamine has a range of other actions; it is a weak μ receptor agonist, induces the release of dopamine, blocks muscarinic acetylcholine receptors, and may potentiate the effects of GABA synaptic inhibition. Ketamine undergoes marked first-pass metabolism with the production of its less potent metabolite norketamine. Orally ketamine results in a more sedative and less psychedelic experience. Most of the parent drug will be eliminated from the body within 24 hours.

## Prevalence

Findings from the 2017/2018 Crime Survey of England and Wales suggest that the lifetime use of ketamine among 16- to 59-year olds (2.8%). Past year rates of use are on par with these more traditional hallucinogenic drugs, with 0.8% of those aged 16–59 years reporting use in the last 12 months. Rates are higher among younger users and those involved in the clubbing scene where last year rates of over 25% have been reported [33].

## Patterns of use

Compared to commonly used stimulant drugs, the abuse liability of ketamine is low, but compared to LSD and psilocybin, ketamine is far more likely to be associated with compulsive patterns of use, the development of tolerance, and acute problems [34]. Ketamine may also lend itself to binge use due to its shorter duration of action, compared to LSD and psilocybin. Typically, users will consume less than 0.5 g/day, though because tolerance can develop quickly, chronic regular users may use in excess of 5 g/day. Ketamine is taken in combination with other club drugs, with polyuse typically increasing the risk of acute harm.

## Psychological effects and complications

Effects are highly sensitive to age, dose, route, set, and setting. While low doses can be stimulating with elevation in mood, distortion of time and space, and enhanced sensory perception, feelings of 'melting into one's surroundings' are common. At higher doses, ketamine induces the full range of psychedelic effects with emotional, cognitive, and perceptual distortion, including out-of-body experiences and visual hallucinations [35] (Table 54.1). The Harvard academic Timothy Leary described it as 'the ultimate psychedelic journey'. Users describe entering the 'K hole' where they experience visits to god, aliens, their birth, past lives, and the 'experiences of evolution'. Some users report taking issues of set and setting into careful consideration prior to using ketamine. Such preparation cannot be performed if the drug is consumed unwittingly when it has been marketed under the guise of another drug such as ecstasy. Being an amnestic, it may become difficult to remember the total doses consumed.

The relationship between long-term ketamine use and elevated depression scores has been investigated among both current and ex-users. Although heavier users were more likely to score more highly, these were not at clinically significant levels and there was no relationship with changes in ketamine use [36].

Ketamine can also produce a psychotic picture that superficially mimics schizophrenia [37]. Both positive and negative symptoms of schizophrenia can be transiently seen in normal users, and its use can exacerbate symptoms in those with pre-existing psychotic disorders. Other adverse effects can include frightening hallucinations/out-of-body experiences, thought disorder, confusion, and dissociation. Such episodes tend to be short-lived, resolving in a few hours or at the most a few days. In many respects, these are like those adverse effects seen with LSD, though with ketamine, they come on after a shorter period following use and recede more quickly. (Table 54.1).

## Acute complications and harms

Ketamine has a wide margin of safety within medical settings, and although relatively safe in overdose, in combination with ethanol or other CNS depressants, the use of ketamine can result in death. In recreational settings, the greatest risk of harm is from accidental injury, for example trauma, drowning and hypothermia secondary to immobility, and vulnerability to assault [38]. Rarely, more severe complications are reported, including severe agitation and rhabdomyolysis. Within accident and emergency departments, the most common presentations are impaired consciousness, abdominal pain (known as K cramps), lower urinary tract symptoms, and dizziness. Ketamine's cardiovascular risks are enhanced when it is taken

**Table 54.1**  Ketamine: psychological and physical effects

| Psychological | Physical |
|---|---|
| Rapid onset, short duration of action (1 hour), wide safety margin | |
| Dissociative anaesthesia, 'somatosensory blockade' analgesia | Dilated pupils |
| Perceptual distortion/hallucinations/near death | Tachycardia |
| Out-of-body experience | Hypertension |
| Thought disorder/synaesthesia | Ataxia |
| Emergence phenomena | Paralysis |
| Cognitive impairment | Sweating |
| Amnesia | Hypersalivation |
| Derealization/depersonalization | Little effect on cough reflex |

with stimulant drugs. Because of its fast urinary excretion (within 2 hours), the ability to identify ketamine in urine screens is almost impossible, and thus a level of clinical suspicion is required, especially if a history of its use is not forthcoming. Detection by clinical examination relies on identifying elevated blood pressure, moderate tachycardia, abdominal tenderness, and white powder rings on the nose [39].

### Ketamine bladder

Heavy regular use of ketamine can result in progressive inflammation, ulceration, and scarring of the bladder. Known as ketamine-induced cystitis or ketamine bladder, ketamine, or one of its metabolites, is thought to induce apoptosis (cell death). Early detection and harm reduction should be part of any clinical consultation with ketamine users. Any clinical assessment of ketamine users must include enquiry as to the presence of symptoms suggestive of bladder damage, including frequency, dysuria, lower abdominal pain, and haematuria [33]. Early referral to urologists and addiction specialists for co-ordinated interventions is recommended. Complete cessation of use in cases of ketamine bladder must be encouraged, since in the worst cases, the bladder may be lost, which is an exceedingly unpleasant outcome.

### Harm reduction

Like other harms, 'ketamine bladder' appears to be dose-related and is more likely to occur in heavy, dependent users. It may be more likely to be seen in those who drink alcohol when they use ketamine, and it is wise to remain well hydrated when using the drug. Purity between batches can vary, and given the marked dose–response effect of the drug, careful measurement of doses using milligram scales and test dosing new batches are advisable [40]. Intravenous use is to be avoided, being a risk for overdose and prolonged immobility, with associated vulnerability to environmental harms. Rapid referral to specialist services for those reporting bladder symptoms is advised.

### Dependence and withdrawal

Animals models suggest that ketamine has the potential to cause dependence, with rats showing re-administration, conditioned place preference, and locomotor sensitization following repeated administration. However, in man, dependence on ketamine is rare, with

most of the literature coming from small case reports [41]. Regular users of ketamine report the rapid development of tolerance and compulsive patterns of use with loss of control and continued use despite harms. Evidence for a specific withdrawal syndrome is lacking, though upon cessation use, some dependent users report craving and sympathomimetic lability with shaking, sweaty, irritability, and insomnia [42]. Among those with pain associated with bladder damage, persistent use may be driven by a desire for analgesia. While cessation can be associated with mood and behavioural disturbances, a well-defined physical withdrawal syndrome is not seen. Symptomatic relief of agitation and insomnia, along with analgesia, if required, combined with good psychological support, remains the mainstay of managing withdrawal. There are no specific psychological therapies, but relapse prevention can be supported by the adaptation of CBT and MET, while addressing comorbid conditions and any other individual psychological needs.

### Cognitive impairment

There has been considerable research into the neurocognitive consequences of ketamine. Among infrequent users, ketamine does not appear to be associated with any significant impairment. However, frequent, heavy use is associated with marked deficits in both short- and long-term memory [43], most notably deficits in visual recognition and spatial working memory. Cognitive impairments may not only interfere with a person's ability to perform in their normal working or social roles but can also interfere with their treatment.

### Ketamine in treatment-resistant depression and alcohol dependence

Recent work has highlighted the potential of ketamine as a therapeutic agent in those with TRD, typically using intravenous infusions 2–3 times per week, usually over several weeks. Initial results have been promising [44] and suggest the drug is well tolerated and effective (see Chapter 72). An intranasal formulation of an isomer of ketamine (esketamine) has recently been licensed for the treatment of depression in the United States. Ketamine is also being explored as a treatment for those with dependence, in particular alcohol [42].

### FURTHER READING

Hofmann A. (2013). *LSD: My Problem Child*. Oxford University Press, Oxford.

Nichols DE. (2016). Psychedelics. *Pharmacol Rev*, 68, 264–355. http://doi.org/10.1124/pr.115.011478

Rucker JJH, Iliff J, Nutt DJ. (2018). Psychiatry & the psychedelic drugs. Past, present & future. *Neuropharmacology*, 142, 200–18.

Shulgin A, Shulgin A. (1995). *Pihkal (Phenethylamines I Have Known and Loved): A Chemical Love Story*. Transform Press, Berkeley, CA.

Shulgin A, Shulgin A. (1997). *TiHKAL (Tryptamines I Have Known and Loved): The Continuation*. Transform Press, Berkeley, CA.

### REFERENCES

1. Nutt DJ, King LA, Phillips LD. (2010). Drug harms in the UK: a multicriteria decision analysis. *Lancet*, 376, 1558–65.
2. Hofmann A. (2013). *LSD: My Problem Child*. Oxford University Press, Oxford.
3. Grof S. (1980). *LSD Psychotherapy*. Hunter House, Pomona, CA.

4. Lee M, Shlain B. (2007). *Acid Dreams*. Grove Press/Atlantic, New York, NY.

5. Cohen S. (1960). Lysergic acid diethylamide: side effects and complications. *J Nerv Ment Dis*, 130, 30–40.

6. Rucker JJH. (2015). Psychedelic drugs should be legally reclassified so that researchers can investigate their therapeutic potential. *BMJ*, 350, h2902–2.

7. Nichols DE. (2016). Psychedelics. *Pharmacol Rev*, 68, 264–355.

8. González-Maeso J, Weisstaub NV, Zhou M, *et al.* (2007). Hallucinogens recruit specific cortical 5-HT2A receptor-mediated signaling pathways to affect behavior. *Neuron*, 53, 439–52.

9. Moreno JL, Holloway T, Albizu L, Sealfon SC, González-Maeso J. (2011). Metabotropic glutamate mGlu2 receptor is necessary for the pharmacological and behavioral effects induced by hallucinogenic 5-HT2A receptor agonists. *Neurosci Lett*, 493, 76–9.

10. Tylš F, Páleníček T, Horáček J. (2014). Psilocybin—summary of knowledge and new perspectives. *Eur Neuropsychopharmacol*, 24, 342–56.

11. Dolder PC, Schmid Y, Haschke M, Rentsch KM, Liechti ME. (2016). Pharmacokinetics and concentration-effect relationship of oral LSD in humans. *Int J Neuropsychopharmacol*, 19, pyv072.

12. Carhart-Harris RL, Muthukumaraswamy S, Roseman L, *et al.* (2016). Neural correlates of the LSD experience revealed by multimodal neuroimaging. *PNAS*, 113, 4853–8.

13. Rucker JJH, Iliff J, Nutt DJ. (2018). Psychiatry & the psychedelic drugs. Past, present & future. *Neuropharmacology*, 142, 200–18.

14. Ray TS. (2010). Psychedelics and the human receptorome. *PLoS One*, 5, e9019.

15. Lawn W, Barratt M, Williams M, Horne A, Winstock A. (2014). The NBOMe hallucinogenic drug series: patterns of use, characteristics of users and self-reported effects in a large international sample. *Psychopharmacol*, 28, 780–8.

16. Winstock AR, Kaar S, Borschmann R. (2014). Dimethyltryptamine (DMT): prevalence, user characteristics and abuse liability in a large global sample. *J Psychopharmacol*, 28, 49–54.

17. Carhart-Harris RL, Nutt DJ. (2013). Experienced drug users assess the relative harms and benefits of drugs: a web-based survey. *J Psychoactive Drugs*, 45, 322–8.

18. Carbonaro TM, Bradstreet MP, Barrett FS, *et al.* (2016). Survey study of challenging experiences after ingesting psilocybin mushrooms: acute and enduring positive and negative consequences. *J Psychopharmacol*, 30, 1268–78.

19. Halpern JH, Pope HG. (2003). Hallucinogen persisting perception disorder: what do we know after 50 years? *Drug Alcohol Depend*, 69, 109–19.

20. Krebs TS, Johansen PO. (2012). Lysergic acid diethylamide (LSD) for alcoholism: meta-analysis of randomized controlled trials. *J Psychopharmacol*, 26, 994–1002.

21. Grinspoon L, Bakalar J. (1997). *Psychedelic Drugs Reconsidered* (first edition). The Lindesmith Center, New York, NY.

22. Rucker JJH, Jelen LA, Flynn S, Frowde KD, Young AH. (2016). Psychedelics in the treatment of unipolar mood disorders: a systematic review. *J Psychopharmacol*, 30, 1220–9.

23. Grob CS, Danforth AL, Chopra GS, *et al.* (2011). Pilot study of psilocybin treatment for anxiety in patients with advanced-stage cancer. *Arch Gen Psychiatry*, 68, 71–8.

24. Moreno FA, Wiegand CB, Taitano EK, Delgado PL. (2006). Safety, tolerability, and efficacy of psilocybin in 9 patients with obsessive-compulsive disorder. *J Clin Psychiatry*, 67, 1735–40.

25. Johnson MW, Garcia-Romeu A, Cosimano MP, Griffiths RR. (2014). Pilot study of the 5-HT2AR agonist psilocybin in the treatment of tobacco addiction. *J Psychopharmacol*, 28, 983–92.

26. Bogenschutz MP, Forcehimes AA, Pommy JA, Wilcox CE, Barbosa PCR, Strassman RJ. (2015). Psilocybin-assisted treatment for alcohol dependence: a proof-of-concept study. *J Psychopharmacol*, 29, 289–99.

27. Sewell RA, Halpern JH, Pope HG. (2006). Response of cluster headache to psilocybin and LSD. *Neurology*, 66, 1920–2.

28. Carhart-Harris RL, Bolstridge M, Rucker J, Day C. (2016). Psilocybin with psychological support for treatment-resistant depression: an open-label feasibility study. *Lancet*, 3, 619–27.

29. Griffiths RR, Johnson MW, Carducci MA, *et al.* (2016). Psilocybin produces substantial and sustained decreases in depression and anxiety in patients with life-threatening cancer: a randomized double-blind trial. *J Psychopharmacol*, 30, 1181–97.

30. Ross S, Bossis A, Guss J, *et al.* (2016). Rapid and sustained symptom reduction following psilocybin treatment for anxiety and depression in patients with life-threatening cancer: a randomized controlled trial. *J Psychopharmacol*, 30, 1165–80.

31. Wolff K, Winstock AR. (2006). Ketamine: from medicine to misuse. *CNS Drugs*, 20, 199–218.

32. Morgan CJ, Curran HV. (2012). Independent Scientific Committee on Drugs. *Addiction*, 107, 27–38.

33. Winstock AR, Mitcheson L, Gillatt DA, Cottrell AM. (2012). The prevalence and natural history of urinary symptoms among recreational ketamine users. *BJU Int*, 110, 1762–6.

34. Uosukainen H, Tacke U, Winstock AR. (2015). Self-reported prevalence of dependence of MDMA compared to cocaine, mephedrone and ketamine among a sample of recreational polydrug users. *Int J Drug Policy*, 26, 78–83.

35. Stewart CE. (2001). Ketamine as a street drug. *Emerg Med Serv*, 30: 30, 32, 44 passim.

36. Morgan CJ., Muetzelfeldt L, Curran HV. (2010). Consequences of chronic ketamine self-administration upon neurocognitive function and psychological wellbeing: a 1-year longitudinal study. *Addiction*, 105, 121–33.

37. Fletcher PC, Honey GD. (2006). Schizophrenia, ketamine and cannabis: evidence of overlapping memory deficits. *Trends Cogn Sci*, 10, 167–74.

38. Jansen KL. (2000). A review of the nonmedical use of ketamine: use, users and consequences. *J Psychoact Drugs*, 32, 419–33.

39. Ng SH, Tse ML, Ng HW, Lau FL. (2010). Emergency department presentation of ketamine abusers in Hong Kong: a review of 233 cases. *Hong Kong Med J*, 16, 6–11.

40. Taylor CF, Winstock AR, Olsburgh J. (2014). Where next in ketamine uropathy? Dedicated management centres? *BJU Int*, 114, 637–8.

41. Pal HR, Berry N, Kumar R, Ray R. (2002). Ketamine dependence. *Anaesth Intensive Care*, 30, 382–4.

42. Critchlow DG. (2006). A case of ketamine dependence with discontinuation symptoms. *Addiction*, 101, 1212–13.

43. Morgan CJ, Curran HV. (2006). Acute and chronic effects of ketamine upon human memory: a review. *Psychopharmacology (Berl)*, 188, 408–24.

44. Singh JB, Fedgchin M, Daly EJ, *et al.* (2016). A double-blind, randomized, placebo-controlled, dose-frequency study of intravenous ketamine in patients with treatment-resistant depression. *Am J Psychiatry*, 173, 816–26.

# 55

# Tobacco addiction

*Marcus Munafò and Meryem Grabski*

## Epidemiology

### The tobacco epidemic

Tobacco use is the main preventable cause of premature death worldwide. Currently, about 5 million people die from smoking-related disease each year, and this number continues to grow. In most high-income countries, smoking rates have declined dramatically in the last 20 years, but they are increasing in many low- and middle-income countries [1]. The tobacco epidemic within high-income countries has been described in four stages [2] (Fig. 55.1). The first is marked by the widespread uptake of smoking in a population, especially by men, and almost no smoking-related deaths. In the second, uptake from men continues to increase and women start taking up smoking too, while smoking-related deaths begin to occur. In the third, smoking rates in men start declining, as do rates in women towards the end of this phase, and smoking-related deaths rise to about 25–30% of all deaths in men. In the fourth, smoking-related deaths in men peak early in this period, and a couple of decades later the same happens in women. Smoking rates keep declining in a similar fashion in men and women, although the rate of the decline begins to slow down. This model was developed based on observations in high-income countries, but it has been suggested that it is still largely applicable to low- and middle-income countries, although it may not be as applicable to women; the gender gap seems to remain large in many of these countries.

### Smoking prevalence

The UK, along with most high-income countries, is in the fourth stage of the tobacco epidemic. Smoking rates in the UK have declined considerably—from the early 1970s when 45% of all adults were smokers to below 20% today. In particular, the UK has seen a marked narrowing of the gap between the prevalence of male and female smoking. The prevalence of smoking is highest in young adults (25- to 34-year olds), and lowest in adults over 60 years (although this is, in part, due to differential mortality between smokers and non-smokers as they age). The uptake of smoking usually occurs in mid adolescence, with two-thirds of smokers starting before the age of 18. Whereas smoking is nearly absent in 11-year olds, regular smoking (that is, at least once per week) begins to be seen among 15-years olds. Smoking prevalence is strongly patterned by socio-economic position, with the highest proportion of smokers being from less affluent socio-economic backgrounds. Smoking is therefore a strong driver of health inequalities between the rich and the poor today [3]. Smoking rates in the UK are comparable to most other high-income countries, but there are examples of high-income countries where smoking rates are higher (for example, Russia and Greece). Many low- and middle-income countries are at the second stage of the tobacco epidemic model and have some of the highest smoking rates in males today (for example, Indonesia, China, and Jordan), whereas smoking rates in females are much lower in these countries [1].

### Tobacco constituents

Tobacco is made from the cured leaves of the tobacco plant. It is predominantly consumed in the form of manufactured cigarettes (making up the vast majority of worldwide sales), but it can also be chewed, inhaled, or smoked in other forms (for example, pipes or cigars). Burning tobacco produces further chemicals as a result of the combustion process; over 7000 different chemicals and compounds have been identified in tobacco smoke from cigarettes. Many are toxic, and over 70 are carcinogenic [4]. The primary psychoactive addictive substance in tobacco is nicotine, a nicotinic acetylcholine receptor (nAChR) agonist. There is some evidence that other components of tobacco, or their metabolites, such as acetaldehyde, nornicotine, myosmine, cotinine, anabasine, and anatabine, have synergistic effects with nicotine or have reinforcing effects on their own. The investigation of the effects of these substances presents several methodological challenges such as disentangling the direct effect of the substances from the effects of nicotine and their interactions with nicotine and one another. Moreover, these substances usually occur in tobacco smoke in very low doses and are therefore difficult to model experimentally.

### Morbidity and mortality related to tobacco smoking

Diseases caused by tobacco smoking include various cancers, cardiovascular disease, and pulmonary disease, and it also has marked effects on prenatal development. Smoking is believed to be responsible for the majority of lung cancers and has also been linked to cancer of the mouth, bladder, kidney, cervix, stomach, and other organs. Smoking is responsible for much ischaemic heart disease and is a risk factor for heart attack and stroke. Two types of lung

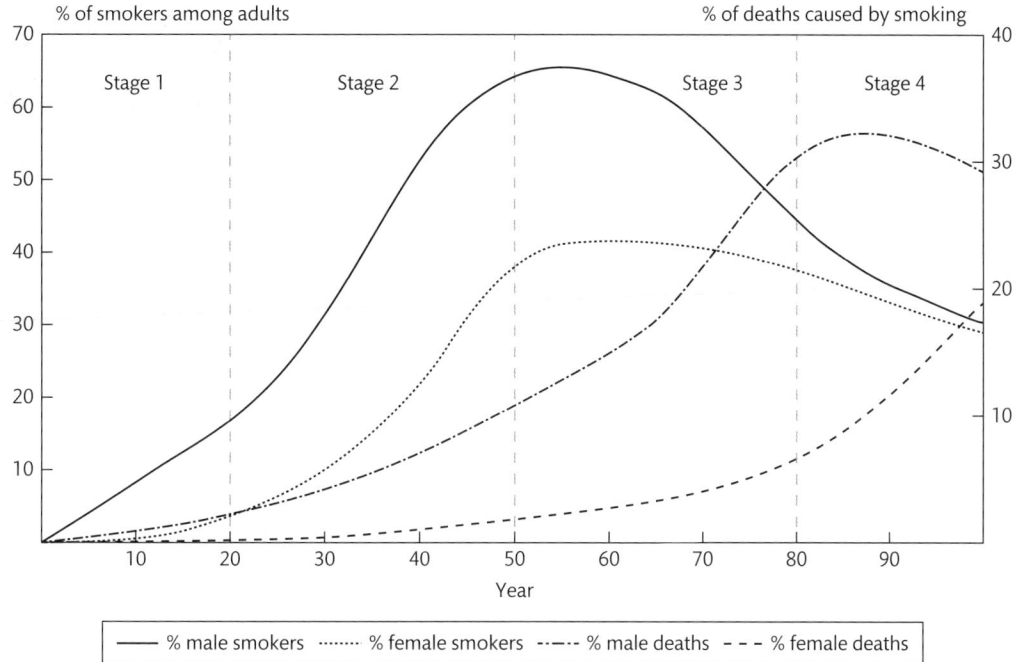

**Fig. 55.1** The different stages of the tobacco epidemic in men and women.
Reproduced from *Tobacco Control*, 3(3), Lopez AD, Collishaw NE, Piha T, A descriptive model of the cigarette epidemic in developed countries, pp. 242–247, Copyright (1994), with permission from *British Medical Journal*.

disease—chronic bronchitis and emphysema—are also caused mainly by smoking. Inhalation of tobacco smoke damages the airway and lung tissue, which also leaves the lungs more vulnerable to environmental pollutants and infections. Smoking during pregnancy doubles the risk of pre-term delivery and stillbirth, and is linked to low birthweight, increased birth defects, and birth complications, as well as negative long-term health outcomes of the infant such as asthma, breathing problems, and learning difficulties. It is still unclear whether tobacco exposure in the prenatal environment is a direct cause of these long-term outcomes. For example, exposure to smoking during pregnancy increases the risk of the offspring becoming a smoker, but genetic predisposition or the postnatal environment, such as sharing a household with smoking parents, could be responsible for these associations. Conclusive evidence on whether the effect of prenatal tobacco exposure on offspring smoking outcomes is causal or associative, or a mixture of both, requires genetically informed investigation.

## Neurobiology and pharmacokinetics

### Routes of administration

Tobacco can be consumed in different ways, and the route of administration affects its addictiveness, as well as its health risk profile. Most tobacco is smoked in the form of cigarettes, but it can also be smoked in the form of water pipes, traditional pipes, and cigars, or consumed as smokeless tobacco by chewing or inhaling it through the nose or mouth. Cigarettes are manufactured from flue-cured tobacco; this lowers the pH of the saliva in the mouth, and therefore, nicotine cannot be absorbed through the oral mucosa, in contrast to tobacco used in pipes and cigars or chewing tobacco. It necessitates

the inhalation of cigarette smoke into the lungs, in order to absorb nicotine at these pH levels. Nicotine levels then rise sharply in blood returning to the heart and quickly reach the brain. The delivery of nicotine via cigarette smoking has the most immediate, strong, and addictive effect of all tobacco delivery systems. It is also related to the most negative health outcomes, due to the production of carcinogens through the burning of tobacco and the release of carbon monoxide, as well the wide distribution of these substances into the body via the lungs. Other forms of administration of nicotine, via the oral mucosa or nasal cavities (in the case of dry snuff), do not result in such sharp increases in nicotine blood levels (Fig. 55.2). However, forms of tobacco use other than cigarette smoking also carry health risks. Pipe and cigar smoking and smokeless tobacco are related to oral and pancreatic cancers, as well as lung and heart disease.

Nicotine-containing products can be considered to lie on a continuum of harm to the user where combustible cigarettes are the most harmful and pharmaceutical nicotine replacement products the least harmful. Other products such as smokeless tobacco products and unregulated nicotine products such as nicotine lollipops occupy intermediate positions. Although the subject of some controversy, e-cigarettes are generally considered to be much less harmful than cigarettes, and closer in levels of harm to nicotine replacement products [5].

### Tobacco in the brain

Nicotine binds to nAChRs, which are expressed throughout the brain. They are ligand-gated ion channels consisting of α and β subunits, which have differential profiles in their response to nicotine. Their stimulation indirectly releases a variety of neurotransmitters [6]. The primary reinforcing effect of nicotine is ascribed to the activation of nAChRs in the mesolimbic pathway, specifically those

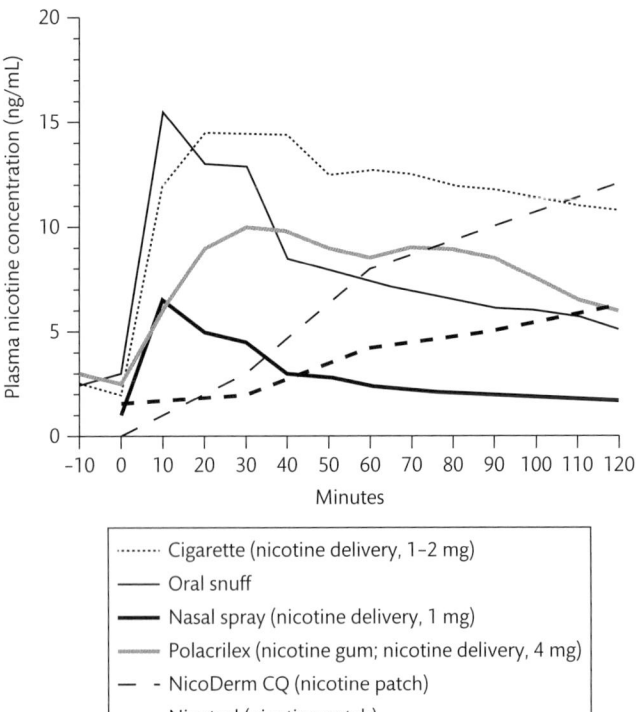

**Fig. 55.2** Venous blood concentrations of nicotine over time for various nicotine delivery systems.

Reproduced from *Clinics in Office Practice*, 26(3), Fant RV, Owen LL, Henningfield JE, Nicotine Replacement Therapy, pp. 633–652, Copyright (1999), with permission from W. B. Saunders Company.

projecting from the ventral tegmental area (VTA) into the nucleus accumbens (NAcc) where they release dopamine (DA). nAChR subtypes thought to be involved in this process include α4, α6, and β2. The release of DA into the NAcc plays an important role in the processing of natural rewards and reinforcers, such as food and sex, and is a locus for the action of drugs of abuse like cocaine. Several studies using animal models have shown that nAChRs located within the VTA are involved in reinforcement behaviour to nicotine. Increases in DA after nicotine exposure have also been shown in brain imaging studies using human participants, although results are equivocal regarding the magnitude of the DA release [7]. Nicotine also promotes the release of serotonin linked to mood regulation and appetite, noradrenaline linked to arousal and appetite, and vasopressin linked to memory enhancement [8]. Other constituents of tobacco smoke also appear to play an important role in tobacco addiction. Much research has been conducted on the chronic effect of cigarette smoking on the inhibition of monoamine oxidase (MAO) A and B, which seems to enhance the direct effect of nicotine by leading to an increase of DA, noradrenaline, and serotonin in the brain [9, 10].

### Tobacco reward and reinforcement

Many smokers report that smoking is pleasurable and reduces negative affect and stress, although there is conflicting evidence against such effects [11, 12]. Once tobacco dependence is established, the discontinuation of smoking causes withdrawal symptoms. Smoking is therefore associated with both positive reinforcement (that is, obtaining pleasurable consequences) and negative reinforcement (that is, avoiding aversive consequences). The primary reinforcing

constituent of tobacco is nicotine; animals will preferentially self-administer nicotine intravenously relative to placebo [13], as will humans [14, 15]. However, other factors contribute to the reinforcing effects of tobacco use. In classic nicotine self-administration studies in animals, the delivery of nicotine is often paired with a neutral stimulus such as light or noise. These studies show that after repeated pairing, this neutral stimulus becomes as important as nicotine in the maintenance, extinction, and reacquisition of self-administration of nicotine. Similarly, in humans, smokers tend to associate specific cues, such as certain moods, situations, and environmental factors, with the positive effect of smoking (see Environmental drivers of relapse, p. 549). Through conditioning, these smoking-related cues acquire motivational properties and therefore increase craving for nicotine and trigger relapse. In cue reactivity studies, nicotine-dependent individuals exhibit increases in affect, heart rate, skin conductivity, and subjective craving, following the presentation of smoking-related stimuli [16]. Other substances present in tobacco smoke may also contribute to its reinforcing actions. Much research has focused on monoamine oxidase A inhibitors, present in tobacco and tobacco smoke, which may enhance the rewarding effect of nicotine [9, 10]. Acetaldehydes, present in tobacco, also have reinforcing properties and may enhance the reinforcing properties of nicotine [17].

### Genetics of nicotine addiction

Like other addictive habits, smoking behaviours are under a substantial degree of genetic influence (see Chapter 49). Twin studies suggest most smoking-related traits, such as smoking initiation [18], the development of tobacco dependence [19], and cessation [20], are genetically influenced. However, the identification of specific genetic variants that influence smoking behaviour has been challenging. Candidate gene studies have met with limited success, despite genes encoding nicotine receptor subtypes, DA receptors, and GABA receptors being plausible candidates [21]. Genome-wide association studies have identified several promising genetic variants associated with smoking behaviour, most prominently the *CHRNA5-CHRNA3-CHRNB4* gene cluster on chromosome 15 [22, 23]. These genetic variants influence consumption and titration (adjustment of nicotine intake according to the strength of the cigarette). Thus, α5 knockout mice (a model for humans who carry the rs16969968 risk allele) with delivery of self-administered nicotine were less able than normal mice to titrate the delivery of nicotine to a consistent, desired level [24]. Similarly, humans carrying the rs16969968 risk allele show a reduced aversive response to high doses of nicotine [25]. Therefore, deficient α5 signalling may attenuate the negative effects of nicotine, leading to heavier use. Nevertheless, the proportion of variance explained by such variants is much lower than the estimates of heritability indicated by twin studies. Larger sample sizes and refinement of the methodology of genotyping may enable the identification of proper pathways in the future.

## Dependence and withdrawal

### Tobacco withdrawal syndrome

After several hours of smoking abstinence, dependent smokers will experience tobacco withdrawal. The primary tobacco withdrawal symptoms reported by the fifth edition of *Diagnostic and Statistical*

*Manual of Mental Disorders* (DSM-5) are irritability/anger/frustration, anxiety, depressed mood, difficulty concentrating, increased appetite, insomnia, and restlessness [26]. Other symptoms can include constipation, dizziness, nausea, and disrupted cognitive function such as impairment of working memory [27]. Tobacco craving is also usually observed after smoking abstinence. As with most drugs of abuse, withdrawal symptoms are one of the main drivers for relapse and reinstatement of smoking behaviour following abstinence. They can persist for several months after smoking cessation, but the time course of withdrawal symptoms varies considerably between individuals. Increases in craving and negative affect are the most common symptoms after smoking cessation, and the intensity of these symptoms is predictive of relapse. Furthermore, smokers who experience more *variable* symptoms have been found to be more likely to relapse.

### Environmental drivers of relapse

Environmental stimuli associated with smoking can promote smoking behaviour in several ways. Firstly, a stimulus that has repeatedly been paired with smoking (for example, the look, feel, and taste of a cigarette, a lighter, an ashtray, the effects of alcohol or coffee, etc.) can elicit a conditioned response and tobacco craving. The effect of smoking-related stimuli has been investigated experimentally with cue–exposure paradigms. Here smoking stimuli, or photographs or videos of these, are presented to the participant. Differences in outcomes, while the participant is subjected to a smoking stimulus (as compared to a neutral stimulus), can indicate which domains are influenced by smoking cues. The most reliable responses to smoking cues are increases in craving levels and heart rate [16]. Secondly, environmental stimuli related to smoking can become primary reinforcers in their own right. In animals, a formerly extinguished nicotine self-administration behaviour can be reinstated when the animal is presented with a nicotine-related cue (in this case, a neutral light or sound that was paired with nicotine administration) [28]. In humans, denicotinized cigarettes lead to a greater reduction in the consumption of nicotine-containing cigarettes than nicotine gum [29], supporting the conclusion that nicotine withdrawal is driven not only by the absence of nicotine, but also by the absence of smoking-related stimuli.

These findings have important implications for the development of smoking cessation treatments—dissociating smoking cues from the reinforcing effect of nicotine might extinguish the learnt connection between nicotine administration and the smoking cue, reducing the risk of relapse. One approach is to substitute regular cigarettes with denicotinized cigarettes; once smoking does not provide any more nicotine reinforcement, the sensorimotor cues of smoking should lose their hedonic value. The reduction of withdrawal symptoms has been found to be even more pronounced when the administration of denicotinized cigarettes is combined with nicotine replacement therapy (NRT). Similarly, varenicline, a nicotinic partial agonist, exerts its effect partly by blocking receptors that facilitate the rewarding experience of smoking. It is prescribed to be taken by smokers for a short period *before* a quit attempt, which may help to extinguish these associations. The number of cigarettes smoked per day decreases during the pre-cessation period, and cessation rates are higher than for other smoking cessation pharmacotherapies [30]. Smoking cues seem to vary in their impact on different groups of smokers; for example, females respond more strongly to smoking cues than males.

### Psychological drivers of relapse

Psychological factors, such as stress and negative affect, are often cited by smokers as reasons for smoking and for relapse during a cessation attempt. Smokers often attribute the stress- and anxiety-reducing properties of cigarettes as one of the main drivers for smoking and often attribute relapse to acute stress and negative affect. An alternative explanation is that this perceived relief of stress and negative affect through smoking is actually a misattribution of withdrawal relief [31]. In recent years, ecological momentary assessment (EMA) studies have advanced our understanding of the role of negative affect and stress on acute smoking behaviour. Participants are provided with a device (for example, a smartphone-app) that allows them to provide information about craving, mood, or stress levels in real time in their everyday environment. These studies have not found a systematic relationship between negative states and acute 'regular' smoking behaviour. In smokers attempting to quit, on the other hand, acute negative affect, as well as stress, has been found to play an important role in smoking lapses [32]. Rapid increases in negative affect precede lapse episodes, and lapses that are triggered by stress progress more quickly to another lapse. However, studies investigating stress levels and negative affect among successful quitters have found that, even though stress initially increases after quitting, in the long run, stress levels decrease even below pre-cessation levels [33]. This could mean that smoking, in fact, *increases* stress-levels, which are then reduced back to normal after quitting, although a recent Mendelian randomization meta-analysis did not find any evidence that smoking heaviness causally influenced anxiety or depression [33]. The results may be driven by other factors, for example the adaptation of a healthier lifestyle in successful quitters. The presence of clinically significant negative affect has also been related to poor cessation success [34], and several studies found that a history of depression increases the risk for relapse [35]. Smokers diagnosed with multiple episodes of depression (rather than one) may be at higher risk for relapse [36]. The causal relationship between smoking and depression (and other mental health issues) remains unclear (see Smoking in psychiatric populations, pp.550–1).

### Cognition and relapse

Many smokers report perceived cognitive benefits from smoking, and cognitive impairment during abstinence. However, it is unclear whether smoking results in genuine cognitive benefits, rather than simply relieving withdrawal symptoms that include impaired cognition. Laboratory research on tobacco addiction and cognition has focused on two issues: (1) the potentially positive effect of tobacco smoking (and specifically nicotine) on cognitive performance; and (2) the negative effect of tobacco withdrawal on cognitive performance. A meta-analysis on the effect of cigarette smoking and/or nicotine administration in non-smokers and non-deprived smokers on cognitive performance found an improvement on fine motor abilities and certain measures of attention and working memory [37]. Much of the interest in the cognition-enhancing effect of nicotine has been fuelled by its potential as a treatment for cognitive dysfunction; early research suggested benefits from nAChR agonist treatment for Alzheimer's disease, schizophrenia, and attention-deficit/hyperactivity disorder (ADHD) but have not translated into clinical practice. The effect of withdrawal on cognitive performance is usually investigated using an acute abstinence paradigm, in which cognitive task performance is compared between smokers who are subjected to a period of acute abstinence (of 8 hours or more) and smokers who smoke as per usual. A recent meta-analysis of these tasks found that abstinent smokers showed higher delay discounting of monetary rewards, lower response inhibition, and impaired arithmetic and recognition memory performance, compared with non-abstinent smokers [38]. Cognitive performance tasks that are sensitive to withdrawal in smokers might be useful in assessing the efficacy of novel treatments to ameliorate withdrawal symptoms. The advantage of objective cognitive performance task outcomes, such as reaction times or error rates, over self-report is that they are less biased. Nevertheless, the results of cognitive performance task studies, both investigating cognitive-enhancing effects of nicotine, as well as the effect of nicotine abstinence on task performance, should be interpreted with caution. The tasks used to assess cognitive performance are usually quite heterogenous, even if indicated for the same cognitive domain. This is even true for the same tasks, as standardized guidelines on presentation times, stimuli, selection of participants, etc., are currently lacking.

## Smoking in psychiatric populations

### Schizophrenia

Even though smoking rates in the general population are declining, they remain high in people with mental illness. In particular, among people with schizophrenia, the prevalence of smoking is substantially higher than in the general population [39]. Smokers with schizophrenia are also more dependent, smoke more heavily, and have greater difficulties quitting than smokers from the general population [40, 41]. There are several hypotheses for why smoking is so common in patients with schizophrenia. The self-medication hypothesis suggests that smoking might ameliorate some of the negative symptoms of schizophrenia [42] and cognitive deficits common in schizophrenia such as reduced visuo-spatial working memory. Smoking could also counteract the effects of dopamine antagonist medications; for example, smoking rates increase after smokers with schizophrenia begin treatment with haloperidol. However, there is also emerging evidence that smoking could be an aetiological risk factor for schizophrenia [43]. Smoking usually predates the onset of psychotic symptoms, and cohort studies have found that there is a dose–response relationship between smoking and the onset of schizophrenia, so that people who smoke more heavily have a higher risk of developing schizophrenia [44, 45]. A recent genome-wide association study identified a variant in the nAChR gene cluster CHRNA5-A3-B4 (associated with smoking intensity) to be also associated with schizophrenia [46]. This association could be interpreted in two ways—smoking and schizophrenia might be influenced by this genetic variant independently, or this genetic variant may reflect a causal link between smoking and schizophrenia.

### Depression and anxiety

Depression and anxiety are both associated with higher levels of smoking, and smokers are also more likely to receive a diagnosis of clinical depression or anxiety. Smoking rates among adults diagnosed with major depressive disorder (MDD) are higher than in the general population, while greater nicotine dependence is associated

with higher rates of a diagnosis of MDD [47]. Furthermore, attempts to quit smoking are more likely to fail in smokers with MDD than without [36]. In anxiety disorders, comorbidity estimates vary strongly with regard to the specific disorder investigated, the sample under investigation, and the definition of smoking behaviour. One study found a high prevalence of smoking in people with social phobia and panic disorders, whereas it was markedly lower than in the general population among people with obsessive–compulsive disorder [48]. Several hypotheses have been proposed regarding the nature of the relationship between smoking and depression/anxiety. The self-medication hypothesis suggests that depressed or anxious people smoke in order to manage their symptoms, so that symptoms lead to smoking, including smoking initiation and subsequent heaviness of use [49]. However, the misattribution hypothesis suggests that the relief of stress and negative affect attributed to smoking is actually due to relief of withdrawal symptoms, rather than the relief of the underlying emotional psychopathology [31].

Smoking could be a risk factor for the onset of depression, for example by influencing a person's response to environmental stressors via its effect on the pituitary system, as has been suggested in animal models. Evidence against this hypothesis was cited previously [33]. It is also possible that a bi-directional relationship between smoking and anxiety or depression may exist, whereby smoking initiation might be motivated by the desire to manage symptoms, but chronic smoking might negatively influence outcomes. This is supported by two meta-analyses, one of which found that mental health symptoms generally improve after smoking cessation [50], and one that concluded that compelling evidence for either hypothesis is currently lacking [51]. Finally, shared genetic influences on both smoking levels and anxiety and depression could also be responsible for the high comorbidity of smoking and depression [52].

### Other mental health problems

Higher rates of smoking than in the general population have been recorded in people with several other mental health problems such as ADHD, conduct disorder, bipolar disorder (BP), and eating disorders [53]. In ADHD, the self-medication hypothesis has been suggested as a potential reason for smoking uptake. As dopaminergic function is altered in ADHD, this might be related to higher initial rewarding effects of nicotine, which could lead to higher rates of smoking uptake. Nicotine has also been shown to improve some of the typical deficits in executive function seen in ADHD [54]. Epidemiological research has focused on the consistent association between maternal smoking during pregnancy and ADHD, as well as conduct disorder (which shows comorbidity with ADHD). Whether smoking during pregnancy is a risk factor for later development of these disorders in offspring or whether a common environment or common genetic variants drive this relationship is unclear [55]. A high rate of maternal smoking in people diagnosed with ADHD and conduct disorder could explain the high rates of smoking in later life in these populations. High rates of smoking have been found in people diagnosed with BP. It has been proposed that the mechanisms are similar to those underlying depression, such as mood dysregulation and heavy dependence, which lead to difficulties in quitting, but comparatively little research has been done in BP patients yet [56]. The relationship between smoking and eating disorders has typically been investigated in the context of smoking as an appetite and weight control method. Smoking rates are higher in people with eating disorders [57] and concerns about weight gain following cessation are cited by many smokers as a major reason for continued smoking.

## Smoking in mental health service settings

As smoking is the greatest single contributor to the 10 to 20 year reduced life expectancy among people with severe mental illness, special attention should be given to smoking cessation in patients in mental health settings [58]. In the UK, mental health units have been required by law to ban smoking in all enclosed spaces since July 2008. A survey in 2014 in medium- and low-secure mental health facilities showed that 83% prohibited smoking within buildings but allowed it within gardens and outside of the secure perimeter such as hospital grounds. A complete ban on smoking in all hospital buildings and grounds has been recommended but is currently enforced by only 9% of facilities [59]. However, implementing smoking bans in mental health service settings brings specific challenges. There is often a long-standing culture of smoking among both patients and staff; cigarettes may be used as rewards for patients for meeting therapeutic goals, and smoking together may help staff and patients to create therapeutic relationships. Other potential barriers to the introduction of smoking bans may include increased aggression and stress in patients, weight gain in patients, unpredictable interactions of smoking cessation with psychotic medication, security issues (for example, due to patients smoking in their bedroom), and increased costs for implementation of smoking-free facilities. Several of these concerns have been reviewed in recent years and could either be alleviated or are unfounded. For example, disruptive behaviour and verbal aggression decrease after the implementation of smoking bans in many cases, while stress and anxiety levels have been found to decrease after smoking cessation in many studies and may only be a concern in the short term (see Dependence and withdrawal, pp. 548–9). Smoking cessation often leads to improved efficacy of psychotropic medication, as smoking increases the metabolism of many drugs [60]. The dose should be carefully monitored during a smoking cessation attempt, but a reduction of antipsychotic medication is typically seen as a positive outcome, as it may lead to a reduction of negative side effects.

## Interventions: treatment and prevention

### Pharmacological treatments

Several pharmacological treatments to support smoking cessation are available today. The most widely used are NRT, varenicline, and bupropion, which are available as first-line treatments in many countries, including the UK. In the UK, NRT is available over the counter and in several formulations. The most commonly used method is the transdermal patch, which is available in several doses and strengths and allows nicotine to be absorbed slowly through the skin. Other forms of NRT include chewing gum, lozenges, sublingual tablets, sprays, and inhalers. With these, nicotine is absorbed via the nasal or oral mucosa; the rate of nicotine absorption is more rapid than with transdermal patches, but not as rapid as when smoking a cigarette. The aim of NRT is to provide nicotine during smoking cessation attempts in order to ameliorate physiological and psychological withdrawal symptoms and the motivation to smoke. The combination of different methods of NRT, such as patch and nasal spray

or patch and gum, may be more effective than using any of these methods alone [61]. Varenicline is a selective nicotinic receptor partial agonist, licensed as a prescription-only treatment. It binds to the α4β2-nAChR, which is responsible for mediating the reinforcing properties of nicotine. This alleviates craving and withdrawal during smoking cessation. During nicotine exposure, the receptor occupancy of varenicline blocks reinforcing effects of smoking [62]. Since varenicline is prescribed to be taken for 2 weeks prior to a quit attempt, during which the smoker continues to smoke as usual, this may lead to extinction of the conditioned cues associated with smoking and may contribute, in part, to its superior efficacy relative to NRT. Bupropion was originally developed as a drug for depression and is now licensed in sustained-release formulation for use in smoking cessation. Its antidepressant properties may make bupropion helpful for smoking cessation if nicotine withdrawal produces depressive symptoms. Nicotine itself may also have antidepressant properties, which are substituted for by bupropion [63]. The efficacy of varenicline for smoking cessation is somewhat greater than that of NRT or bupropion, while NRT and bupropion have similar efficacy [61]. However, the absolute quit rates achieved remain low—only about 20% of smokers using any of these methods are able to quit successfully and remain abstinent [64]. There are many reasons for this such as the importance of smoking cues and the sensorimotor stimulation in maintaining smoking behaviour (see Environmental drivers of relapse, p. 549), which are both lacking in pharmacological treatment.

### E-cigarettes

Electronic cigarettes, or 'e-cigarettes', are handheld electronic devices that heat a liquid ('e-liquid') to create an aerosol, which the user inhales ('vaping'). The e-liquid usually comprises propylene glycol and flavourings, with or without nicotine; there is wide variation in the exact composition of the fluid and in the different models of e-cigarettes available. The common features include a cartridge, which holds the e-liquid, a heating device, and a power source. Some e-cigarettes are manufactured for one time-use only, while others are refillable.

Currently, there are considerable differences between countries in the regulation of the sale of e-cigarettes; their sale is completely banned in some countries. In Europe, new regulations concerning e-cigarettes have been introduced into the European Tobacco Products Directive (TPD). These new regulations came into force in May 2016, and all products now have to be fully compliant with the TPD since May 2017. The major changes in the regulation of e-cigarette products were as follows: (1) new products and changes to existing products must be notified to the Medicines and Healthcare products Regulatory Agency (MHRA); (2) information on the content and safety of the products must be provided to the MHRA; (3) products will have to be child-safe, so that they do not leak or break easily; (4) newspapers, radio, and TV advertisement for e-cigarette products are now banned (but not billboard and poster advertisement); and (5) e-liquids containing more than 20 mg of nicotine per millilitre need a medical licence authorized by the MHRA.

Since their widespread introduction in 2006, the use of e-cigarettes has grown rapidly and many smokers report successfully using e-cigarettes as an alternative form of nicotine delivery. There are some reasons to believe that they will be superior to other smoking cessation methods, as they give the smoker a sensory and behavioural experience, with rapid delivery of nicotine to the brain, which resembles that achieved from a conventional cigarette. Experienced users of second- and third-generation e-cigarettes have been found to achieve nicotine levels very similar to those achieved through regular cigarette use. A recent Cochrane review concluded that e-cigarettes containing nicotine are effective for smoking cessation [65], and a recent randomized controlled trial found that e-cigarettes were more effective for smoking cessation than nicotine-replacement therapy, when both products were accompanied by behavioural support [65a].

At the same time, there has been controversy surrounding e-cigarettes. One concern has been the potential uptake of e-cigarettes by non-smokers, particularly children, and their potential as a gateway to smoking conventional cigarettes. Current evidence suggests that while children and young people are experimenting with e-cigarettes, this is rare in never-smokers. Thus, there is little evidence that vaping will readily progress to smoking. The long-term health consequences of using e-cigarettes are also unknown, so definitive statements about the toxicity of e-cigarettes are currently impossible. The range of products and liquids available and the length of time most tobacco-related diseases take to become apparent are problematic. However, the models of e-cigarettes tested to date have been found to provide the users with substantially lower levels of potentially harmful chemicals than conventional cigarettes [5, 66]. A recent report of the Royal College of Physicians concluded that the using risk of e-cigarettes 'is unlikely to exceed 5% of the harm from smoking tobacco' [67]. The risk of second-hand exposure is likely to be correspondingly low as well.

### Behavioural treatments

Behavioural treatments also play a role in smoking cessation; the combination of pharmacological and behavioural treatments is more effective than any one treatment method alone [68, 69]. There is evidence for the efficacy of low-level interventions such as providing smokers with print-based self-help materials about cessation [70] and telephone support [71]. However, more intensive counselling and behavioural therapies are generally superior to these low-level interventions [72–74]. Motivational interviewing (MI) is a client-centred counselling style, with the aim of eliciting behaviour change by exploring and resolving ambivalence. The MI approach was originally developed for use in substance abuse and has since been applied specifically to smoking cessation. A recent review on the current evidence found that MI is superior to brief advice and usual care when provided by a general practitioner. Interestingly, shorter sessions were found to be more effective than longer ones [75]. Other methods, such as mindfulness training and meditation, have claimed positive results, but the evidence is currently preliminary. A positive effect of exercise interventions on smoking cessation has also been reported in several studies, but more substantial evidence of positive long-term effects is still needed [76]. Determining the ideal intervention in terms of content and intensity for each smoking population is challenging due to the difficulty of identifying the specific aspects that make an intervention effective and the specific needs of different smoking populations.

### Prevention and policy

Tobacco control policies have contributed to the fall in smoking prevalence since the post-war period in many high-income countries. Within Europe, the strength of tobacco control policies varies across countries and is considered strongest in the UK. Specific policies that have been found to be effective in decreasing smoking rates include taxation, bans on smoking in public places, bans on the advertising of tobacco products, health warnings on tobacco products, and plain (or standardized) packaging. The retail price of tobacco products can be increased by governments by raising taxes on them. The amount to which consumers will continue or cease to buy a product depending on its price is referred to as 'price elasticity'. Compared to many other consumer products, the demand for tobacco products is only moderately elastic. A meta-analysis estimated the average price elasticity of demand for tobacco products at about −0.48, which is consistent with other findings [77, 78]. This means that a 10% increase in price will be followed by a decrease in consumption of about 4.8%. Nevertheless, as increases in tobacco taxes result in higher prices of tobacco for a whole population, even small reductions have a big impact. Increasing tobacco taxes has, in fact, been found to be the most effective way to decrease consumption in a population [79, 80]. Currently, 77% of the price of a packet of cigarettes account for taxes in the UK, and taxes have increased by 30% over the last 10 years.

Banning smoking in public enclosed places has several obvious benefits. Apart from the fact that non-smokers are not subjected to second-hand smoke, it also decreases opportunities for smokers to smoke, thus supporting smoking cessation. It also makes smoking less socially acceptable, which, in turn, reduces smoking and exposure to tobacco smoke. The banning of advertisement of tobacco products is another important step in order to decrease smoking rates, specifically in teenagers and young people. In order to be effective, an advertisement ban has to be comprehensive and include all types of media and outdoor advertisement. In the UK, all forms of tobacco advertising and promotion are banned since the Tobacco Advertising and Promotion Act 2002. This now includes the display of tobacco products at the point of sale since 2015 and the implementation of standardized plain packaging for all tobacco products since May 2017, which requires the removal of all branding on any tobacco product. Finally, health warnings on tobacco packaging, as well as in media campaigns, have been found to increase health awareness in the population and to change the image of smoking. The last point is crucial in order to prevent young people from taking up smoking. In the UK, picture warnings on tobacco products have been implemented in 2008.

### FURTHER READING

Caponnetto P, Polosa R, Russo C, Leotta C, Campagna D. Successful smoking cessation with electronic cigarettes in smokers with a documented history of recurring relapses: a case series. *Journal of Medical Case Reports.* 2011;5:585.

Fant RV, Owen LL, Jack E. Henningfield JE. Nicotine replacement therapy. *Clinics in Office Practice.* 1999;26:633–52.

### REFERENCES

1. World Health Organization. *WHO global report on trends in prevalence of tobacco smoking 2018*: World Health Organization, Geneva; 2018.
2. Lopez AD, Collishaw NE, Piha T. A descriptive model of the cigarette epidemic in developed countries. *Tobacco Control.* 1994;3:242.

3. Office for National Statistics. *General lifestyle survey*. The Stationary Office, London; 2013.

4. US Food and Drug Administration. Harmful and potentially harmful constituents in tobacco products and tobacco smoke; established list. *Federal Register*. 2012;77:20034–7.

5. McNeill A, Brose L, Calder R, Hitchman S, Hajek P, McRobbie H. *E-cigarettes: an evidence update: a report commissioned by Public Health England*. Public Health England, London; 2015.

6. Court JA, Martin-Ruiz C, Graham A, Perry E. Nicotinic receptors in human brain: topography and pathology. *Journal of Chemical Neuroanatomy*. 2000;20:281–98.

7. Brody AL. Functional brain imaging of tobacco use and dependence. *Journal of Psychiatric Research*. 2006;40:404–18.

8. Benowitz NL. Nicotine addiction. *New England Journal of Medicine*. 2010;362:2295–303.

9. Berlin I, Anthenelli RM. Monoamine oxidases and tobacco smoking. *International Journal of Neuropsychopharmacology*. 2001;4:33–42.

10. Fowler JS, Logan J, Wang GJ, Volkow ND. Monoamine oxidase and cigarette smoking. *Neurotoxicology*. 2003;24:75–82.

11. Shiffman S, Paty JA, Gwaltney CJ, Dang Q. Immediate antecedents of cigarette smoking: an analysis of unrestricted smoking patterns. *Journal of Abnormal Psychology*. 2004;113:166–71.

12. Shiffman S, Gwaltney CJ, Balabanis MH, *et al.* Immediate antecedents of cigarette smoking: an analysis from ecological momentary assessment. *Journal of Abnormal Psychology*. 2002;111:531.

13. Donny EC, Caggiula AR, Knopf S, Brown C. Nicotine self-administration in rats. *Psychopharmacology*. 1995;122:390–4.

14. Harvey DM, Yasar S, Heishman SJ, Panlilio LV, Henningfield JE, Goldberg SR. Nicotine serves as an effective reinforcer of intravenous drug-taking behavior in human cigarette smokers. *Psychopharmacology*. 2004;175:134–42.

15. Henningfield JE, Goldberg SR. Nicotine as a reinforcer in human subjects and laboratory animals. *Pharmacology Biochemistry and Behavior*. 1983;19:989–92.

16. Carter BL, Tiffany ST. Meta-analysis of cue-reactivity in addiction research. *Addiction*. 1999;94:327–40.

17. Talhout R, Opperhuizen A, van Amsterdam JG. Role of acetaldehyde in tobacco smoke addiction. *European Neuropsychopharmacology*. 2007;17:627–36.

18. Heath AC, Cates R, Martin NG, *et al.* Genetic contribution to risk of smoking initiation: comparisons across birth cohorts and across cultures. *Journal of Substance Abuse*. 1993;5:221–46.

19. Maes HH, Sullivan PF, Bulik CM, *et al.* A twin study of genetic and environmental influences on tobacco initiation, regular tobacco use and nicotine dependence. *Psychological Medicine*. 2004;34:1251–61.

20. Carmelli D, Swan GE, Robinette D, Fabsitz R. Genetic influence on smoking—a study of male twins. *New England Journal of Medicine*. 1992;327:829–33.

21. Ho MK, Tyndale RF. Overview of the pharmacogenomics of cigarette smoking. *Pharmacogenomics Journal*. 2007;7:81–98.

22. Saccone SF, Hinrichs AL, Saccone NL, *et al.* Cholinergic nicotinic receptor genes implicated in a nicotine dependence association study targeting 348 candidate genes with 3713 SNPs. *Human Molecular Genetics*. 2007;16:36–49.

23. Thorgeirsson TE, Geller F, Sulem P, *et al.* A variant associated with nicotine dependence, lung cancer and peripheral arterial disease. *Nature*. 2008;452:638–42.

24. Fowler CD, Lu Q, Johnson PM, Marks MJ, Kenny PJ. Habenular [agr] 5 nicotinic receptor subunit signalling controls nicotine intake. *Nature*. 2011;471:597–601.

25. Jensen KP, Devito EE, Herman AI, Valentine GW, Gelernter J, Sofuoglu M. A CHRNA5 smoking risk variant decreases the aversive effects of nicotine in humans. *Neuropsychopharmacology*. 2015;40:2813–21.

26. American Psychiatric Association. *Diagnostic and Statistical Manual of Mental Disorders*, fifth edition. American Psychiatric Association, Washington, DC; 2013.

27. Heishman SJ, Kleykamp BA, Singleton EG. Meta-analysis of the acute effects of nicotine and smoking on human performance. *Psychopharmacology*. 2010;210:453–69.

28. Le Foll B, Goldberg SR. Control of the reinforcing effects of nicotine by associated environmental stimuli in animals and humans. *Trends in Pharmacological Sciences*. 2005;26:287–93.

29. Johnson MW, Bickel WK, Kirshenbaum AP. Substitutes for tobacco smoking: a behavioral economic analysis of nicotine gum, denicotinized cigarettes, and nicotine-containing cigarettes. *Drug and Alcohol Dependence*. 2004;74:253–64.

30. Hajek P, McRobbie HJ, Myers KE, Stapleton J, Dhanji A-R. Use of varenicline for 4 weeks before quitting smoking: decrease in ad lib smoking and increase in smoking cessation rates. *Archives of Internal Medicine*. 2011;171:770–7.

31. DiFranza JR, Wellman RJ. A sensitization-homeostasis model of nicotine craving, withdrawal, and tolerance: integrating the clinical and basic science literature. *Nicotine and Tobacco Research*. 2005;7:9–26.

32. Shiffman S, Paty JA, Gnys M, Kassel JA, Hickcox M. First lapses to smoking: within-subjects analysis of real-time reports. *Journal of Consulting and Clinical Psychology*. 1996;64:366–79.

33. Taylor AE, Fluharty ME, Bjørngaard JH, *et al.* Investigating the possible causal association of smoking with depression and anxiety using Mendelian randomisation meta-analysis: the CARTA consortium. *BMJ Open*. 2014;4:e006141.

34. Glassman AH, Helzer JE, Covey LS, *et al.* Smoking, smoking cessation, and major depression. *JAMA*. 1990;264:1546–9.

35. Hitsman B, Papandonatos GD, McChargue DE, *et al.* Past major depression and smoking cessation outcome: a systematic review and meta-analysis update. *Addiction*. 2013;108:294–306.

36. Hitsman B, Borrelli B, McChargue D, Spring B, Niaura R. History of depression and smoking cessation outcome: a meta-analysis. *Journal of Consulting and Clinical Psychology*. 2003;71:657.

37. Heishman SJ, Kleykamp BA, Singleton EG. Meta-analysis of the acute effects of nicotine and smoking on human performance. *Psychopharmacology*. 2010;210:453–69.

38. Grabski M, Curran HV, Nutt DJ, et al. Behavioral tasks sensitive to acute abstinence and predictive of smoking cessation success: a systematic review and meta-analysis. *Addiction*. 2016;111:2134–44.

39. de Leon J, Diaz FJ. A meta-analysis of worldwide studies demonstrates an association between schizophrenia and tobacco smoking behaviors. *Schizophrenia Research*. 2005;76:135–57.

40. Olincy A, Young DA, Freedman R. Increased levels of the nicotine metabolite cotinine in schizophrenic smokers compared to other smokers. *Biological Psychiatry*. 1997;42:1–5.

41. Salokangas RK, Honkonen T, Stengård E, Koivisto A-M, Hietala J. Cigarette smoking in long-term schizophrenia. *European Psychiatry*. 2006;21:219–23.

42. Kumari V, Postma P. Nicotine use in schizophrenia: the self medication hypotheses. *Neuroscience and Biobehavioral Reviews*. 2005;29:1021–34.

43. Gage SH, Munafò MR. Rethinking the association between smoking and schizophrenia. *The Lancet Psychiatry*. 2015;2:118.

44. Weiser M, Reichenberg A, Grotto I, *et al*. Higher rates of cigarette smoking in male adolescents before the onset of schizophrenia: a historical-prospective cohort study. *American Journal of Psychiatry*. 2003;161:1219–23.

45. Kendler KS, Lönn SL, Sundquist J, Sundquist K. Smoking and schizophrenia in population cohorts of Swedish women and men: a prospective co-relative control study. *American Journal of Psychiatry*. 2015;172:1092–100.

46. Ripke S, Neale BM, Corvin A, *et al*. Biological insights from 108 schizophrenia-associated genetic loci. *Nature*. 2014;511:421.

47. Dierker LC, Avenevoli S, Merikangas KR, Flaherty BP, Stolar M. Association between psychiatric disorders and the progression of tobacco use behaviors. *Journal of the American Academy of Child and Adolescent Psychiatry*. 2001;40:1159–67.

48. Himle J, Thyer BA, Fischer DJ. Prevalence of smoking among anxious outpatients. *Phobia Practice and Research Journal*. 1988;1:25–31.

49. Chaiton MO, Cohen JE, O'Loughlin J, Rehm J. A systematic review of longitudinal studies on the association between depression and smoking in adolescents. *BMC Public Health*. 2009;9:1.

50. Taylor G, McNeill A, Girling A, Farley A, Lindson-Hawley N, Aveyard P. Change in mental health after smoking cessation: systematic review and meta-analysis. *BMJ*. 2014;348:g1151.

51. Fluharty M, Taylor AE, Grabski M, Munafò MR. The association of cigarette smoking with depression and anxiety: a systematic review. *Nicotine and Tobacco Research*. 2016:ntw140.

52. Kendler KS, Neale MC, MacLean CJ, Heath AC, Eaves LJ, Kessler RC. Smoking and major depression: a causal analysis. *Archives of General Psychiatry*. 1993;50:36–43.

53. Lasser K, Boyd JW, Woolhandler S, Himmelstein DU, McCormick D, Bor DH. Smoking and mental illness: a population-based prevalence study. JAMA. 2000;284:2606–10.

54. McClernon FJ, Kollins SH. ADHD and smoking: from genes to brain to behavior. *Annals of the New York Academy of Sciences*. 2008;1141:131–47.

55. Thapar A, Fowler T, Rice F, *et al*. Maternal smoking during pregnancy and attention deficit hyperactivity disorder symptoms in offspring. *American Journal of Psychiatry*. 2003;160:1985–9.

56. Heffner JL, Strawn JR, DelBello MP, Strakowski SM, Anthenelli RM. The co-occurrence of cigarette smoking and bipolar disorder: phenomenology and treatment considerations. *Bipolar Disorders*. 2011;13:439–53.

57. Anzengruber D, Klump KL, Thornton L, *et al*. Smoking in eating disorders. *Eating Behaviors*. 2006;7:291–9.

58. Brown S, Kim M, Mitchell C, Inskip H. Twenty-five year mortality of a community cohort with schizophrenia. *British Journal of Psychiatry*. 2010;196:116–21.

59. Public Health England. *Smoking cessation in secure mental health settings: guidance for commissioners*. Public Health England, London; 2015.

60. Schein JR. Cigarette smoking and clinically significant drug interactions. *Annals of Pharmacotherapy*. 1995;29:1139–48.

61. Cahill K, Stevens S, Perera R, Lancaster T. Pharmacological interventions for smoking cessation: an overview and network meta-analysis. *Cochrane Database of Systematic Reviews*. 2013;CD009329.

62. Jorenby DE, Hays JT, Rigotti NA, *et al*. Efficacy of varenicline, an α4β2 nicotinic acetylcholine receptor partial agonist, vs placebo or sustained-release bupropion for smoking cessation: a randomized controlled trial. *JAMA*. 2006;296:56–63.

63. Hurt RD, Sachs DP, Glover ED, *et al*. A comparison of sustained-release bupropion and placebo for smoking cessation. *New England Journal of Medicine*. 1997;337:1195–202.

64. Schnoll RA, Lerman C. Current and emerging pharmacotherapies for treating tobacco dependence. *Expert Opinion on Emerging Drugs*. 2006;11:429–44.

65. Hartmann-Boyce J, McRobbie H, Bullen C, Begh R, Stead LF, Hajek P. Electronic cigarettes for smoking cessation. *Cochrane Database of Systematic Reviews*. 2016;CD010216.

65a. Hajek P, Phillips-Waller A, Przulj D, et al. A randomized trial of e-cigarettes versus nicotine-replacement therapy. *N Engl J Med*. 2019;380(7):629–37.

66. Hajek P, Etter JF, Benowitz N, Eissenberg T, McRobbie H. Electronic cigarettes: review of use, content, safety, effects on smokers and potential for harm and benefit. *Addiction*. 2014;109:1801–10.

67. Royal College of Physicians Tobacco Advisory Group. *Nicotine without smoke-tobacco harm reduction*. Royal College of Physicians, London; 2016.

68. Stead LF, Koilpillai P, Fanshawe TR, Lancaster T. Combined pharmacotherapy and behavioural interventions for smoking cessation. *Cochrane Database of Systematic Reviews*. 2016;3:CD008286.

69. Stead LF, Koilpillai P, Lancaster T. Additional behavioural support as an adjunct to pharmacotherapy for smoking cessation. *Cochrane Database of Systematic Reviews*. 2015;10:CD009670.

70. Hartmann-Boyce J, Lancaster T, Stead LF. Print-based self-help interventions for smoking cessation. *Cochrane Database of Systematic Reviews*. 2014;6:CD001118.

71. Whittaker R, McRobbie H, Bullen C, Borland R, Rodgers A, Gu Y. Mobile phone-based interventions for smoking cessation. *Cochrane Database of Systematic Reviews*. 2016;4:CD006611.

72. Fiore M, Jaen CR, Baker T, *et al. Treating tobacco use and dependence: 2008 update*. US Department of Health and Human Services, Rockville, MD; 2008.

73. Fiore MC, Bailey WC, Cohen SJ, *et al. Treating tobacco use and dependence: clinical practice guideline*. US Department of Health and Human Services, Rockville, MD; 2000.

74. Lancaster T, Stead LF. Individual behavioural counselling for smoking cessation. *Cochrane Database of Systematic Reviews*. 2005;2:CD001292.

75. Lindson-Hawley N, Thompson TP, Begh R. Motivational interviewing for smoking cessation. *Cochrane Database of Systematic Reviews*. 2015;3:CD006936.

76. Ussher MH, Taylor AH, Faulkner GEJ. Exercise interventions for smoking cessation. *Cochrane Database of Systematic Reviews*. 2014;8:CD002295.

77. Forster M, Jones AM. The role of tobacco taxes in starting and quitting smoking: duration analysis of British data. *Journal of the Royal Statistical Society: Series A (Statistics in Society)*. 2001;164:517–47.

78. Gallet CA, List JA. Cigarette demand: a meta-analysis of elasticities. *Health Economics*. 2003;12:821–35.

79. Jha P, Peto R. Global effects of smoking, of quitting, and of taxing tobacco. *New England Journal of Medicine*. 2014;370:60–8.

80. Chaloupka FJ, Hu T-W, Warner KE, Jacobs R, Yurekli A. The taxation of tobacco products. In: Jha P, Chaloupka F (eds). *Tobacco Control in Developing Countries*. Oxford University Press, Oxford; 2000. pp. 237–72.

# 56

# Comorbidity of substance use and psychiatric disorders

*Julia M.A. Sinclair and Anne Lingford-Hughes*

## Introduction

For any individual, it is likely that a number of factors contribute to the comorbidity of psychiatric and substance use disorder (SUD). These may include genetics, family history, environmental factors (for example, stress, childhood experiences, current life events), and personality traits (for example, impulsivity). Such vulnerability factors may be common to both the psychiatric disorder and the SUD, rather than one being a consequence of the other (Fig. 56.1). For instance, higher levels of impulsivity are seen in alcohol use disorder (AUD) and bipolar disorder and likely contribute to their high comorbidity [1]. The same symptom may also be either a cause or a consequence; for instance, depression or anxiety may increase the likelihood of substance use, which then is likely to exacerbate the mental state, resulting in greater anxiety and depression symptoms and fuelling further alcohol or other substance use which patients may regard as treating their anxiety or depression. Epidemiological studies in major depressive disorder (as opposed to depressive symptoms) and AUD have shown that either may predate the other. It appears that such independent mood disorder may be common in those with SUD who present for treatment [2]. Consequently, it should be determined how any substance use may be contributing to a patient's psychiatric symptoms and discussed with them in order to optimize a treatment approach. It may be unhelpful to refer to either the psychiatric disorder or SUD as primary or secondary, since this may imply that treating one will improve the other; this is not borne out in many studies and so has limited clinical utility. Both disorders will need to be treated concurrently for any improvement to be robust.

## Assessment principles

The assessment of patients who have AUD or SUD comorbid with one or more other psychiatric disorder follows the same principles as those highlighted in other sections, including the importance of a collateral history from family members or carers. The priority is to ensure that a full history is taken to identify the range of comorbidities, and an accurate assessment of the frequency and levels of use of any substances. The evidence is that this is, in general, poorly done [3], and patient outcomes are likely to be substantially worse where an AUD or SUD is not identified accurately [4].

Screening for nicotine, alcohol, and drug use should be a routine part of any psychiatric assessment and integrated into the history of the presenting complaint, given the impact these substances have on the mental state. For patients not presenting primarily with an SUD, it is especially important that these questions are asked in an objective, non-judgemental way, explaining to the patient that it is important that you fully understand the factors that may be contributing to their current distress in order to most effectively help them. Patients may (understandably) be hesitant to disclose their alcohol or substance use if they believe that it may result in sanctions or being denied treatment.

Clinicians need to be competent in understanding how to calculate units of alcohol in order to accurately assess levels of use, understand the likely contribution that alcohol is making to the presenting complaint (both acutely and chronically), and make a competent risk assessment of the likelihood of symptoms on alcohol withdrawal [3, 5]. Full assessment of the need for alcohol detoxification is covered elsewhere (see Chapter 52) and is no different for patients with comorbid conditions.

## Quantifying substance use

This is potentially more challenging given both the range and routes of consumption of other drugs. The terminology for substances may be unfamiliar to clinicians and frequently changes. Illicitly obtained drugs also vary in strength and purity, frequently containing fillers or adulterants, which may themselves have psychotropic properties. Patients can be reluctant to disclose their level of use or over-report it through fear of withdrawal and being undertreated, or as a form of active drug-seeking behaviour. There is no practical and reliable way to reconcile these issues. Record what is reported, ask for a collateral history, and regularly reassess the patient if they are presenting in an acutely disturbed state. Urine drug screens (where available) may be helpful to detect opioids, some stimulants, and cannabis, but the availability of novel psychoactive substances (NPS) means that

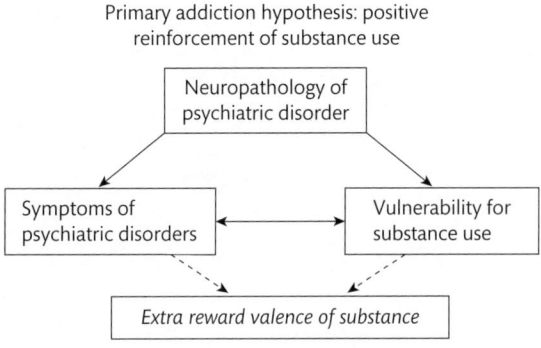

Primary addiction hypothesis: positive
reinforcement of substance use

**Fig. 56.1** Comorbid addiction vulnerability.

increasingly clinicians will need to rely on the history and empirical observation of the effect of the psychopharmacological properties of any substance use on the patient's presentation. These can be divided broadly into three main categories: sedatives, stimulants, and hallucinogens—the properties and management of which are covered elsewhere (see Chapters 53, 54, 55, and 56).

## Diagnosis and goals of treatment

One major challenge in the management of patients with comorbidity is that they may present requesting treatment for one condition (for example, depression) and not be aware, or willing to consider, the impact that comorbid alcohol or other substance use has on their presentation or outcome.

A patient-centred approach to treatment needs to begin where the patient is, in terms of their own explanation for their illness, and to agree on some preliminary, achievable goals that build trust in the therapeutic relationship and increase the patient's self-efficacy.

For patients who are not physically dependent on alcohol or other substances, psychosocial approaches may be sufficient; brief interventions, based on motivational interviewing principles for behaviour change, are as appropriate for patients with a comorbid psychiatric disorder and can be delivered within general psychiatric settings as part of a holistic management plan. Essentially, what works in other settings should be tried but may be less effective [6].

Patients presenting with comorbid substance dependence (particularly with alcohol) require a clear management plan, integrating a combination of psychosocial and pharmacological treatments targeted at BOTH conditions, which is likely to be more effective for patients who have often tried and failed with a less co-ordinated approach.

Establishing patients who are dependent on nicotine or opioids on some form of substitution therapy is beneficial, but there is no evidence for any pharmacological approaches in the management of comorbid cannabis use, stimulant use, or any of the NPS. For these, psychosocial approaches are the mainstay of treatment.

## The individual substances

### Nicotine dependence

Individuals with severe mental illness (SMI) have among the highest prevalence rates of current nicotine smoking, at 50–85% [7]. Tobacco smoking is a substantial contributor to the reduction in

life expectancy for such individuals. The introduction of a smoking ban in hospitals presented some challenges to inpatient psychiatric units, particularly where individuals may be residing involuntarily for some time. Individuals with schizophrenia are three times more likely to initiate smoking, and although they are equally as interested in quitting smoking, including taking nicotine replacement therapy (NRT), they are five times less likely to be successful at so doing than the general population [7]. It is therefore important that support to stop or change smoking behaviour should be offered. The role of e-cigarettes in helping such individuals change is not currently clear.

In a meta-analysis of efficacy and tolerability of adjunctive pharmacotherapy for smoking cessation in adults with SMI, trials included schizophrenia, schizoaffective disorder, and bipolar disorder, and both bupropion and varenicline were superior to placebo, with no differences in tolerability [8]. However, the quality of the trials was noted as low. Systematic reviews of varenicline concluded that it is superior to placebo in smoking cessation in individuals with SMI [8, 9]. Varenicline increased the chances of successful long-term smoking cessation by between 2–3 times, compared with pharmacologically unassisted quit attempts [9]. The most common side effect reported was nausea. However, it is the risk of neuropsychiatric side effects from varenicline that has been debated. One systematic review and meta-analysis did not find a significant difference in risk of suicide, attempted suicide or suicidal ideation, depression, or death between varenicline and placebo, and no evidence that the presence of psychiatric illness impacted on depression or suicidal ideation [10]. The Evaluating Adverse Events in a Global Smoking Cessation Study (EAGLES) investigated neuropsychiatric complications from varenicline in over 8000 motivated-to-quit individuals with and without a psychiatric disorder [11]. There was no significant increase in neuropsychiatric adverse events attributable to varenicline or bupropion relative to nicotine patch or placebo. Varenicline was more effective than placebo, nicotine patch, and bupropion in helping smokers with a psychiatric disorder (including psychosis and mood and anxiety disorders) achieve abstinence, and bupropion and nicotine patch were more effective than placebo. It is therefore suggested that all patients quitting smoking should be told about the small chance they may experience severe mood changes and all clinicians should be alert for these changes. It is notable that the majority of trials only included those who were motivated to quit and whose psychiatric disorder was stable and so may not be generalizable to all individuals or psychiatric patients.

### Alcohol dependence

Usual medication regimens for alcohol detoxification can be used in patients with comorbid psychiatric illness, with due consideration for doses required to avoid complications, for example seizures, and any liver or renal impairment altering pharmacokinetics. Mentally ill patients are more likely to require inpatient admission for detoxification, and so relapse prevention plans should be established and implemented at this time.

There are three main relapse prevention medications to be considered for patients with AUD: acamprosate, naltrexone, and disulfiram [12]. The limited evidence for their use in different comorbid conditions will be considered later, but the principle of active treatment of alcohol dependence as part of overall patient management and treatment plan is key [13]. Where there is no specific evidence for use in an individual comorbid condition, data on the drug's pharmacokinetics and other safety data can be used to extrapolate from the treatment of AUD alone to help determine a risk–benefit profile of treatment with a specific medication in individual patients.

## Opioid dependence

The most robust evidence for the pharmacological treatment of opioid dependence in patients with a range of psychiatric condtions is to engage in opiate substitution therapy (OST) programmes such as methadone or buprenorphine [13].

## Psychiatric disorders

### Schizophrenia

Managing patients with schizophrenia who also use substances is a common and substantial challenge. While the focus is often on cannabinoids, comorbidity with nicotine and alcohol is more common and, as such, has a significant impact on life expectancy. Stimulant use disorder, which can be associated with psychotic phenomena, has been reported to be higher in the schizophrenia spectrum than in the general population at 10.4% but varies considerably, depending on the setting, geographical location, etc.; notably, cannabis use disorder was strongly linked with stimulant use disorder [14]. While there is some evidence that residential 'dual diagnosis' treatment programmes may lead to improvements, their availability is likely to be very limited, at least in the UK. Most individuals will be treated in the community, with occasional admissions to a general psychiatric ward and varying input from specialist addiction services.

There are a range of clinical guidelines providing approaches to treating individuals with SUD and schizophrenia [15, 16]. Negative symptoms and cognitive impairment can make it particularly challenging to engage an individual with schizophrenia in psychological approaches to reduce their drug use or prevent relapse, as well as contributing to poor adherence to medication. The UK NICE guidelines for such comorbidity recommend that the severity of both disorders, the individual's social and treatment context, and their readiness to change should be considered [16]. In addition, clear advice about reducing the risk of their substance abuse (for example, by not injecting, avoiding to use multiple drugs concurrently, etc.) and reminders of adverse consequences of their substance abuse, as well as not taking their drugs for psychosis, should not be forgotten [15].

#### Psychosocial approaches

Cochrane reviews have concluded that there was no good evidence for effectiveness of any one particular psychosocial treatment in psychotic spectrum disorders comorbid with substance abuse or for those with serious mental illness, of which the majority had schizophrenia or psychotic illness [17]. However, this should be seen in the context of a very limited evidence base. Motivational interviewing is the most common approach studied, often in addition to CBT, and other models investigated include contingency management and skills training.

In the UK, a trial in schizophrenia, schizophreniform disorder, or schizoaffective disorder and substance (drug and/or alcohol) use disorder did not find that integrated motivational interviewing and CBT plus standard care were superior to standard care alone in improving outcomes, for example hospitalization, symptom outcomes, and functioning [18]. Alcohol was the most commonly

misused substance, followed by cannabis. Integrated therapy resulted in a reduction in the amount of substance used for at least 1 year after completion of therapy. It is interesting to note that this reduction in substance use was not associated with improvements in outcomes for their psychotic illness and is in keeping with other studies. To test the theory that more prolonged treatment was needed, a further trial compared treatment as usual with shorter-term intervention (12 sessions over 4.5 months) and with a longer-term delivery (24 sessions over 9 months) [19]. This again showed no differences between groups in any of the outcomes regarding psychosis or cannabis use. Though no association was found between sessions attended and outcome, the median number of sessions attended was 12 of the 24 available, despite good therapeutic relationships and meeting in the patient's home. The authors note that this result is in keeping with trials treating cannabis use disorder alone; focus on associated problems, rather than cannabis use itself, may be more helpful.

#### Pharmacological approaches to treating schizophrenia

There are few randomized trials comparing different medications to guide clinical practice. Published studies mostly describe uncontrolled designs with small numbers of participants, comparison of the impact of switching the type of medicines, or case series. Dopamine-blocking activity in the dopaminergic mesolimbic pathway was originally seen as an appropriate therapeutic strategy for substance misuse, since it would reduce their rewarding effects; it is now recognized that dopaminergic activity may be blunted in patients with SUD. Thus, further blockade is likely to be counterproductive, with the potential to increase substance use as a way to boost the hypodopaminergic mesolimbic system. It was hypothesized that newer drugs with weaker DRD2 antagonism (and less impact on the dopaminergic system) would result in less substance misuse when used to treat patients with schizophrenia. The Clinical Antipsychotic Trial of Intervention Effectiveness (CATIE) compared olanzapine, risperidone, ziprasidone, quetiapine, and perphenazine; the CATIE study participants included 37% with a current SUD, and of these, 87% drank alcohol, 44% used cannabis, and 36% used cocaine. While the CATIE study showed that olanzapine was superior to other drugs on the primary outcome of 'time to all-cause discontinuation' over 18 months, illicit drug use attenuated this superiority [20]. There was little between the different drugs for psychosis on measures of smoking, alcohol, and drug use in multiple subgroups with reductions evident across all groups. Nevertheless, there is no large randomized trial a priori comparing different dopamine antagonists on substance use outcomes.

The role of clozapine in treating schizophrenia comorbid with SUD is of considerable interest, given its efficacy in treatment-resistant populations. In routine clinical practice, these patients would include those with comorbidity and there are case reports and case series describing beneficial effects of clozapine [13]. However, there has been no randomized prospective trial of clozapine in this clinical population. In summary, clinical guidance is that the choice of drugs for psychosis can be based on the side effect profile and tolerability for each patient without regard to their SUD.

#### Treating SUD in the context of schizophrenia

##### Alcohol dependence

There are a number of alcohol relapse prevention medications that should be considered to improve drinking behaviour, but there is limited evidence to guide practice [13]. For both acamprosate and naltrexone, no adverse effects are apparent of additional particular relevance, compared with a non-comorbid population. A placebo-controlled RCT reported that the opiate antagonist naltrexone was associated with fewer drinking days, fewer heavy drinking days, and less craving, though psychosis did not concurrently improve [21].

Use of disulfiram in patients with psychosis is relatively contra-indicated because its use in high doses will result in higher dopamine levels and potentially acutely increase psychosis [22]. However, more recent studies in patients with psychosis—not all with schizophrenia [13, 21]—have reported disulfiram reduced alcohol consumption, with limited adverse events.

### Cannabis use disorders

A systematic review and meta-analysis reported that motivational interviewing, with or without CBT, reduced the quantity of cannabis use (but not the frequency) and positive symptoms of schizophrenia; however, there was limited impact on negative symptoms [23]. Delivery of MI + CBT to a group, rather than an individual, did not improve cannabis or psychotic outcomes, though the quality of life did improve [24]. One trial compared 'treatment as usual' with combined MI and CBT in patients with schizophrenia spectrum psychosis and cannabis use disorder [25]. The combined intervention showed a possible reduction in the number of monthly joints, but not days of cannabis use, and did not reduce psychotic symptoms. However, further analysis revealed that those who received the combined intervention had more visits to a psychiatric emergency department and hospitalizations but spent less time in hospital.

If focusing on the patient alone may not be particularly beneficial, does involving the family improve outcomes? A recent trial in recent-onset schizophrenia with cannabis use found that family-based MI and interaction skills were superior to routine family support for some outcomes. Thus, training parents helped reduce cannabis use but did not reduce the parent's stress and sense of burden or their general level of functioning. Notably, this benefit in reducing cannabis use was maintained at 15-month follow-up. While statistically there was no difference between groups or during trial of follow-up in other substance use, it is interesting to note that alcohol use did increase in the intervention group where a reduction in cannabis use was seen [26].

No single medicine has superiority over another; for example, olanzapine and risperidone are similar in impact on substance use and psychosis [13]. A pilot study comparing clozapine (mean: 225 mg/day) with ziprasidone (mean: 200 mg/day) in patients with schizophrenia and cannabis use disorder found that cannabis use similarly decreased in both groups over 12 months [27]. While clozapine was associated with fewer positive symptoms, it also incurred more side effects and poorer compliance. Thus, the available data support clinical guidance that the choice of drugs for psychosis can be based on the side effect profile and tolerability for each patient without consideration of their SUD.

### Stimulant use disorder

Psychological approaches are the mainstay of treatments for stimulant use disorders, with contingency management showing effectiveness [13]. An RCT compared 3 months of contingency management for stimulant abstinence plus treatment as usual, and treatment as usual with reinforcement for study participation only in patient with serious mental illness [28]. Of the participants, about 33% had

schizoaffective spectrum disorder, 34% had bipolar disorder, and 27% had major depression. Though they were less likely to remain in the 3-month trial, those who received contingency management were 2.4 times more likely to have a stimulant-negative urine. In addition, they had less use of stimulants in the following 3 months and significantly lower levels of alcohol use, injection drug use, and psychiatric symptoms, and were less likely to be admitted for psychiatric hospitalization.

### Bipolar disorder

Substance misuse in bipolar disorder provides clinical, diagnostic, and management challenges [15, 16]. AUDs are particularly highly prevalent in bipolar disorder and may complicate both manic and depressive presentations. There is no evidence that a particular mood stabilizer is superior to another in improving either substance misuse or bipolar disorder [13]. The combination of sodium valproate and lithium may be better than lithium alone in improving alcohol outcomes, though not necessarily manic and depressive symptoms. Due to the scant evidence base, clinical guidance generally recommends following usual practice in managing their bipolar disorder.

### Treatment of substance use disorder

Again, there is limited evidence and it mainly applies to alcohol dependence. There is evidence to suggest that naltrexone or disulfiram are superior to placebo in improving drinking behaviours in those with alcohol dependence and a psychotic disorder, of whom the majority (73%) had bipolar disorder [21]. However, they did complain more about side effects. Acamprosate has been used safely in patients with bipolar disorder and alcohol dependence, in addition to their mood-stabilizing medication, but without benefit in a preliminary report [29]. Despite such limited evidence, medication should be considered for management of comorbid alcohol dependence. In addition and also for other substances, psychosocial approaches should be used. As with other psychiatric disorders, the key is assessing and diagnosing any substance misuse and how it may contribute to their bipolar disorder in order to manage it optimally.

### Depression

The co-occurrence of mood and SUD is common, yet studies specifically investigating effective management of both conditions are limited. There have been three systematic reviews [30–32], all examining slightly different, but related, questions. These used the same 11 RCTs (published between 1990 and 2010), evaluating the efficacy of different medicines in depression with comorbid alcohol dependence, as the basis of their analysis. Nunes and Levin (2004) [30] analysed 14 studies, eight with depression and comorbid alcohol dependence, two with depression and cocaine use, and four with depression and comorbid opioid dependence (on methadone maintenance treatment). They concluded that overall, drugs for depression had a modest beneficial effect, but that 'concurrent therapy directly targeting the addiciton was also required'. The meta-analysis by Torrens et al (2005) [31] investigated whether sertraline, tricyclic reuptake inhibitors, and nefazadone were an effective treatment for patients with SUD in a wider range of studies (nine with depression and comorbid alcohol dependence, five with cocaine, and seven with opioid dependence comorbid with depression), combined with another 40 studies examining the efficacy of drugs for depression in nicotine, cocaine, and alcohol dependence alone. They concluded there was no significant effect for sertraline on depressive symptoms in the comorbid alcohol group. There was some benefit for medicines with broader pharmacology (imipramine, desipramine, and nefazodone) on depressive symtoms in the comorbid group, although safety concerns in overdose limit their usefulness. In terms of reducing alcohol consumption, neither SSRIs nor the other drugs for depressiom on their own had any significant impact. The most recent meta-analysis [32] compared 11 RCTs of drug efficacy in alcohol and comorbid depression (involving 891 patients), with the clinical trial data of over 46,000 patients with depression alone. Response rates to the active treatment was 50–60% in both the depression-only group and the depression comorbid with alcohol use group. However, placebo response differed significantly across the groups, with 37.7–39.3% in the non-comorbid depression group and 47.1–53.1% in the comorbid alcohol group. A limitation with all three meta-analyses is that they do not include any data on SSRIs (other than sertraline and fluoxetine), mirtazapine, or venlafaxine. A recent small ($N = 14$) double-blind, placebo-controlled pilot trial of mirtazapine in depressed patients and comorbid AUD suggests that it is safe and tolerated, and may have an effect on depressive symptoms, but not alcohol consumption, although it was extremely underpowered for confidence in its conclusions [33].

### Treatment of substance use disorder

While drugs for depression have a modest effect on levels of depression in the comorbid group, they have not been shown to cause a direct or consequent reduction in alcohol consumption [30], and similarly use of relapse prevention medication alone (without treating the underlying psychiatric disorder) had minimal effect on outcomes [21]. Improved outcomes have been shown by combined treatment for depression (with sertraline 200 mg daily) and alcohol dependence (naltrexone 100 mg daily) in a placebo-controlled four-arm study. Only the active combination of both drugs was significantly better in improving drinking behaviour and also had a marginally better effect on depression, relative to placebo [34]. Overall the safety profile for use of acamprosate and naltrexone in patients with comorbid depression is good; a thorough risk assessment needs to be undertaken prior to the use of disulfiram, due to potential dangers of interaction with alcohol in suicidal patients [35], but active treatment of both conditions is recommended [13].

It is less common for patients dependent on opioids to present with depression, and beyond establishing them on OST, there is limited benefit of treating patients with a drug for depression [31, 36]. For patients with depression and use of dopamine-releasing drugs ('stimulants') or cannabis, there is no evidence for the benefit of pharmacological treatment for their substance use, and management is primarily psychosocial.

### PTSD and other anxiety disorders

Anxiety symptoms are common in patients with SUD and may be present as part of intoxication, withdrawal, or early abstinence from substances, depending on the substance used, and a thorough history is required to ascertain the role that they play in the presenting mental state. For example, patients with severe alcohol dependence frequently develop panic symptoms, which resolve on detoxification and abstinence. Patients with anxiety disorders also frequently have SUD, and the temporal relationship between the two conditions are frequently difficult to untangle, as PTSD has often been present for many years before patients present.

In PTSD, SUD is 2–3 times more likely than in the general population, and outcomes in the comorbid population are worse that outcomes for either disorder alone. A recent review of the evidence base for PTSD co-occurring with AUD [37] showed that pharmacological interventions for AUD (naltrexone, disulfiram, and topiramate) or PTSD (sertraline, desipramine, prazosin) were mainly effective in reducing drinking outcomes (including one study with adjuvant psychotherapy), but only one study with sertaline demonstrated an effect over placebo in the reduction of PTSD symptoms. The review concludes that the safety profile for topiramate is likely to limit its usefulness in clinicial practice, but that naltrexone and disulfiram are relatively safe to use, although further studies are required to test the efficacy of pharmacological and psychotherapeutic interventions in combination for both disorders [13, 37].

Patients with social anxiety disorder (SAD) have often had symptoms from childhood and start using substances (especially alcohol) as a form of self-management during adolescence, with SAD being the primary condition in 80% of cases. Despite the significant comorbidity between the two conditions, the only studies conducted have been with paroxetine, and a recent Cochrane review found the quality of studies to be low [38]. The same review found a single RCT for the treatment of generalized anxiety disorder comorbid with AUD using buspirone but reported the quality of study design and reporting to be low, such that limited conclusions can be drawn.

Overall, anxiety disorders, despite substantial comorbidity with SUD, especially alcohol, have a very limited evidence base for treatment, and extrapolation from what works in the non-comorbid condition is needed in clinical settings, in the absence of clear research evidence.

There is some evidence that the GABA agonist baclofen may have a role to play in relapse prevention from alcohol in patients with anxiety symptoms, and at time of writing, it has a 'temporary recommendation for use' in France for the maintenance of alcohol abstinence or for the reduction of consumption to low levels in patients with alcohol dependence who have not responded to other treatments. However, evidence for its effectivenss has yet to be fully demonstrated, and there are concerns about its safety profile in overdose [35].

### Attention-deficit/hyperactivity disorder

Substance use is six times more common in adolescents with ADHD than the general population. Atomoxetine is recommended as a first-line treatment in adults with ADHD comorbid with SUD due to the lack of abuse potential, although evidence of efficacy is limited. A single study of ADHD adults with comorbid AUD found significant effects on ADHD symptoms, but inconsistent effects on drinking behaviour; more research is required to investigate effective treatments [39].

## Training needs

While professionals working in psychiatric services are highly likely to have had sufficient training and experience in managing mood and psychotic disorders, as well as other less common psychiatric disorders, the same is not the case for substance use and addiction.

For example, in the UK, the reduced psychiatric expertise in specialist addiction services also means that general psychiatric services are more likely to have to be involved in managing individuals with comorbidity.

While there is a small evidence base for the effectiveness of treatments targeting comorbid SUD and psychiatric disorder, the frequency of their occurrence and the negative impact on outcomes mean that psychiatrists need to develop a degree of clinical expertise in managing these complex conditions. Being aware of the evidence available, extrapolating from what is known to be effective in the single condtion, and making a balanced risk assessment prior to a trial of treatment will be necessary to optimize treatments.

## REFERENCES

1. Strakowski SM, DelBello MP. The co-occurrence of bipolar and substance use disorders. *Clin Psychol Rev*. 2000;20:191–206.
2. Tolliver BK, Anton RF. Assessment and treatment of mood disorders in the context of substance abuse. *Dialogues Clin Neurosci*. 2015;17:181–90.
3. Paton C, Chee S, Drummond C, et al. Medically assisted withdrawal from alcohol: an audit of practice in acute adult psychiatric wards in the UK conducted by the Prescribing Observatory for Mental Health (POMH-UK). *J Psychopharmacol*. 2015;29:A109.
4. King E, Baldwin DS, Sinclair JMA, et al. The Wessex Recent Inpatient Suicide Study, 1: case-control study of 234 recently discharged psychiatric patient suicides. *Br J Psychiatry*. 2001;178:531–6.
5. Royal College of Psychiatrists. *Alcohol and other drugs: core medical competencies. Final report of the working group of the medical Royal Colleges*. Royal College of Psychiatrists; 2012. http://www.aomrc.org.uk/wp-content/uploads/2016/05/Alcohol_Drugs_Competencies_0612.pdf
6. Tiet QQ, Mausbach B. Treatment for patients with dual diagnosis: a review. *Alcohol Clin Exp Res*. 2007;31:513–36.
7. de Leon J, Diaz FJ. A meta-analysis of worldwide studies demonstrates an association between schizophrenia and tobacco smoking behaviors. *Schizophr Res*. 2005;76:135–57.
8. Roberts E, Eden Evins A, McNeill A, Robson D. Efficacy and tolerability of pharmacotherapy for smoking cessation in adults with serious mental illness: a systematic review and network meta-analysis. *Addiction*. 2016;111:599–612.
9. Cahill K, Lindson-Hawley N, Thomas KH, Fanshawe TR, Lancaster T. Nicotine receptor partial agonists for smoking cessation. *Cochrane Database Syst Rev*. 2016;5:CD006103.
10. Thomas KH, Martin RM, Knipe DW, Higgins JP, Gunnell D. Risk of neuropsychiatric adverse events associated with varenicline: systematic review and meta-analysis. *BMJ*. 2015;350:h1109.
11. Anthenelli RM, Benowitz NL, West R, et al. Neuropsychiatric safety and efficacy of varenicline, bupropion, and nicotine patch in smokers with and without psychiatric disorders (EAGLES): a double-blind, randomised, placebo-controlled clinical trial. *Lancet*. 2016;387:2507–20.
12. National Institute for Health and Care Excellence. *Alcohol dependence and harmful alcohol use*. NICE clinical guideline [CG115]. National Institute for Health and Care Excellence, London; 2011.
13. Lingford-Hughes AR, Welch S, Peters L, Nutt DJ; British Association for Psychopharmacology, Expert Reviewers Group. BAP updated guidelines: evidence-based guidelines for the pharmacological management of substance abuse, harmful use, addiction and comorbidity: recommendations from BAP. *J Psychopharmacology*. 2012;26:899–952.
14. Sara GE, Large MM, Matheson SL, et al. Stimulant use disorders in people with psychosis: a meta-analysis of rate and factors affecting variation. *Aust N Z J Psychiatry*. 2015;49:106–17.
15. Marel C, Mills KL, Kingston R, et al. *Guidelines on the management of co-occurring alcohol and other drug and mental health conditions in alcohol and other drug treatment settings* (2nd edition). Centre of Research Excellence in Mental Health and Substance Use, National Drug and Alcohol Research Centre, University of New South Wales, Sydney; 2016.
16. National Institute for Health and Care Excellence. *Psychosis with coexisting substance misuse*. NICE clinical guideline [CG120]. National Institute for Health and Care Excellence, London; 2011.
17. Hunt, G, Siegfried, N, Morley, K, Sitharthan, T, and Cleary, M. Psychosocial interventions for people with both severe mental illness and substance misuse *Cochrane Database Syst Rev*. 2013;10:CD001088.
18. Barrowclough C, Haddock G, Wykes T, et al. Integrated motivational interviewing and cognitive behavioural therapy for people with psychosis and comorbid substance misuse: randomised controlled trial. *BMJ*. 2010;341:c6325.
19. Barrowclough C, Marshall M, Gregg L, et al. A phase-specific psychological therapy for people with problematic cannabis use following a first episode of psychosis: a randomized controlled trial. *Psychol Med*. 2014;44:2749–61.
20. Swartz MS, Wagner HR, Swanson JW, et al.; CATIE Investigators. The effectiveness of antipsychotic medications in patients who use or avoid illicit substances: results from the CATIE study. *Schizophr Res*. 2008;100:39–52.
21. Petrakis IL, Nich C, Ralevski E. Psychotic spectrum disorders and alcohol abuse: a review of pharmacotherapeutic strategies and a report on the effectiveness of naltrexone and disulfiram. *Schizophr Bull*. 2006;32:644–54.
23. Hjorthoj CR, Baker A, Fohlmann A, Nordentoft M. Intervention efficacy in trials targeting cannabis use disorders in patients with comorbid psychosis systematic review and meta-analysis. *Curr Pharm Des*. 2014;20:2205–11.
24. Madigan K, Brennan D, Lawlor E, et al. A multi-center, randomized controlled trial of a group psychological intervention for psychosis with comorbid cannabis dependence over the early course of illness. *Schizophr Res*. 2013;143:138–42.
25. Hjorthøj CR, Orlovska S, Fohlmann A, Nordentoft M. Psychiatric treatment following participation in the CapOpus randomized trial for patients with comorbid cannabis use disorder and psychosis. *Schizophr Res*. 2013;151:191–6.
26. Smeerdijk M, Keet R, Dekker N, et al. Motivational interviewing and interactional skills training for parents to change cannabis use in young adults with recent-onset schizophrenia: a randomized controlled trial. *Psychol Med*. 2012;42:1627–36.
27. Schnell T, Koethe D, Krasnianski A, et al. Ziprasidone versus clozapine in the treatment of dually diagnosed (DD) patients with schizophrenia and cannabis use disorders: a randomized study. *Am J Addict*. 2014;23:308–12.
28. McDonell MG, Srebnik D, Angelo F, et al. Randomized controlled trial of contingency management for stimulant use in community mental health patients with serious mental illness. *Am J Psychiatry*. 2013;170:94–101.

29. Tolliver BK, Desantis SM, Brown DG, Prisciandaro JJ, Brady KT. A randomized, double-blind, placebo-controlled clinical trial of acamprosate in alcohol-dependent individuals with bipolar disorder: a preliminary report. *Bipolar Disord*. 2012;14:54–63.

30. Nunes EV, Levin FR. Treatment of depression in patients with alcohol or other drug dependence: a meta-analysis. *JAMA*. 2004;291:1887–96.

31. Torrens M, Fonseca F, Mateu G, Farré M. Efficacy of antidepressants in substance use disorders with and without comorbid depression. A systematic review and meta-analysis. *Drug Alcohol Depend*. 2005;78:1–22.

32. Iovieno N, Tedeschini E, Bentley KH, Evins AE, Papakostas GI. Antidepressants for major depressive disorder and dysthymic disorder in patients with comorbid alcohol use disorders: a meta-analysis of placebo-controlled randomized trials. *J Clin Psychiatry*. 2011;72:1144–51.

33. Cornelius JR, Chung T, Douaihy AB, *et al.* Mirtazapine in comorbid major depression and an alcohol use disorder: a double-blind placebo-controlled pilot trial. *Psychiatry Res*. 2016;242;326–30.

34. Pettinati HM, Oslin DW, Kampman KM, *et al.* A double blind, placebo controlled trial combining sertraline with naltrexone for treating co-occuring depression with alcohol dependence. *Am J Psychiatry*. 2010;167:668–75.

35. Sinclair JMA, Chambers SE, Shiles CJ, Baldwin DS. Safety and tolerability of pharmacological treatment of alcohol dependence: comprehensive review of evidence. *Drug Saf*. 2016;39:267–245.

36. Stein MD, Herman D, Kettavong B, *et al.* Antidepressant treatment does not improve buprenorphine retention among opioid-dependent persons. *J Subst Abuse Treat*. 2010;39:157–66.

37. Taylor M, Petrakis I, Ralevski E. Treatment of alcohol use disorder and co-occuring PTSD. *Am J Drug Alcohol Abuse*. 2017;43:391–401.

38. Ipser JC, Wilson D, Taiwo, Akindipe TO, Sager C, Stein DJ. Pharmacotherapy for anxiety and comorbid alcohol use disorders. *Cochrane Database Syst Rev*. 2015;1:CD007575.

39. Bolea-Alamañac B, Nutt DJ, Adamou M, *et al.* Evidence-based guidelines for the pharmacological management of attention deficit hyperactivity disorder: update on recommendations from the British Association for Psychopharmacology. *J Psychopharmacol*. 2014;28:179–203.

# 57

# The core dimensions of schizophrenia

*Nancy C. Andreasen*

## Introduction

Schizophrenia is probably the most devastating illness that psychiatrists treat. An estimated 1% of the population has schizophrenia, which claims its victims at a youthful age and often prevents their full participation in society. Schizophrenia also creates an enormous economic burden, calculated at $65 billion annually in direct and indirect costs [1]. Despite its emotional and economic costs, schizophrenia has yet to receive sufficient recognition as a major public health concern or adequate research support to investigate its causes, treatments, and prevention.

## History

Schizophrenia and other psychotic disorders have been recognized in almost all cultures and described and/or portrayed throughout much of recorded time.

Although schizophrenia was only demarcated as a specific diagnostic entity at the end of the nineteenth century, earlier accounts appear in the literature. Many characters 'become mad' in classical tragedy, although the patterns of illness do not map precisely on the modern conceptions of schizophrenia—a fact probably due to both literary licence and to the fact that the nosology of mental illness was not highly refined at that time. By the era of Elizabethan drama, however, we have portrayals of schizophrenia that closely resemble the modern concept. The madness of Ophelia in Hamlet is quite similar to modern schizophrenia, and the portrayal of 'Poor Tom', son of Gloucester pretending to be a 'Bedlam beggar' escaped from the large Bethlehem Hospital where mental patients were housed, is a near-perfect portrayal of both hallucinations and disorganized speech:

> Who gives anything to Poor Tom? Whom the foul fiend
> hath led through fire and through flame ... ? Tom's
> a-cold,— O, do de, do de, do de ... Do poor Tom some
> charity, whom the foul fiend vexes. There I could have
> him now,—and there, and there again, and there.
>
> King Lear III.iv.51

Its modern history dates to Emil Kraepelin, who is credited with identifying schizophrenia [2]. His original term for schizophrenia

*dementia praecox* was based on his observations that these patients developed their illness at a relatively early age (praecox) and were likely to have a chronic and deteriorating course (dementia). Kraepelin was also instrumental in separating dementia praecox from manic–depressive illness, which had its onset distributed throughout life and a more episodic course.

Dementia praecox was eventually renamed *schizophrenia*, a term coined by Eugen Bleuler to emphasize the cognitive impairment that occurs, which he conceptualized as a splitting of the psychic processes [3]. Bleuler believed that certain symptoms were fundamental to the illness, including affective blunting, disturbances of association (that is, fragmented thinking), autism, and ambivalence (for example, fragmented emotional responses). These eventually enjoyed widespread acceptance as 'Bleuler's four As'. Other symptoms, such as delusions and hallucinations, were considered by him to be 'accessory symptoms', which occurred in other disorders such as manic–depressive illness.

Bleuler's ideas enjoyed widespread acceptance, and generations of psychiatrists were taught the importance of his fundamental symptoms (the four As). Unlike hallucinations and delusions, these symptoms are on a continuum with normality and can be present in relatively mild forms, even in psychiatrically healthy persons. Consequently, the conceptualization of schizophrenia in the United States became increasingly broad. Later, the ideas of the German psychiatrist Kurt Schneider, who emphasized first-rank or specific psychotic symptoms, were introduced, helping to reshape the concept of schizophrenia into one of a relatively severe psychotic disorder, bringing it back to the original ideas of Kraepelin [4]. DSM-5 represents a convergence of various points of view, with its Kraepelinian emphasis on course, specific delusions, and hallucinations thought important by Kurt Schneider, and acknowledgement of the importance of Bleuler's fundamental symptoms.

## Definition

In DSM-5, schizophrenia is defined by a group of characteristic positive or negative symptoms; deterioration in social, work, or interpersonal relationships; and continuous signs of the disturbance for at least 6 months [5]. In addition, schizoaffective disorder and mood disorder with psychotic features have been ruled out, and the disturbance is not due to the direct physiological effects of a substance or a general medical condition. When an illness otherwise meets the criteria but has a duration of less than 6 months, it is called *schizophreniform disorder*. When the duration is less than 4 weeks, it may be classified as either a *brief psychotic disorder* or a *psychotic disorder not otherwise specified*, which is a residual category for psychotic disturbances that cannot be better classified.

## Differential diagnosis

Schizophrenia should be thought of as a diagnosis of exclusion because the consequences of the diagnosis are severe and limit therapeutic options. There are no definitive tests for schizophrenia, so the diagnosis rests on historical and clinical information.

A thorough physical examination and history are required to rule out other medical causes for schizophrenic symptoms. Psychotic symptoms are found in many other illnesses, including substance abuse (for example, hallucinogens, phencyclidine, amphetamines, cocaine, alcohol), intoxication due to commonly prescribed medications (for example, corticosteroids, anticholinergics, levodopa), infections, metabolic and endocrine disorders, tumours and mass lesions, and temporal lobe epilepsy. Laboratory tests may be helpful in ruling out these aetiologies, and magnetic resonance imaging may be useful in selected patients to rule out alternative diagnoses or during the initial workup for new-onset cases.

The major differential diagnosis involves separating schizophrenia from mood disorder, delusional disorder, or personality disorder. The chief distinction from mood disorders is that with schizophrenia, a full depressive or manic syndrome is either absent or develops after the psychotic symptoms, or is brief in duration relative to the duration of psychotic symptoms. Unlike delusional disorder, schizophrenia is characterized by bizarre delusions and hallucinations are common. Patients with personality disorders, particularly those disorders within the eccentric cluster (for example, schizoid, schizotypal, or paranoid), may be characterized by indifference to social relationships and have a restricted affect, bizarre ideation, or odd speech but are not psychotic.

Other psychiatric disorders also must be ruled out, including schizophreniform disorder, brief psychotic disorder, factitious disorder with psychological symptoms, and malingering. When symptoms persist for more than 6 months, schizophreniform disorder can be ruled out. The history of how the illness presents will help to rule out a brief psychotic disorder, because schizophrenia generally has an insidious onset and there are usually no precipitating stressors. Factitious disorder may be difficult to distinguish from schizophrenia, especially when the patient is knowledgeable about mental illness or is medically trained, but careful observation should enable the clinician to make the distinction between real or feigned psychosis. Likewise, a malingerer could attempt to simulate schizophrenia, but careful observation and history-taking will help to distinguish the disorders. With the malingerer, there will be evidence of obvious secondary gain, such as avoiding incarceration or severe punishment, and the history may suggest antisocial personality disorder.

## Dimensional approaches

A variety of methods have been developed to describe and classify the symptoms in schizophrenia. Traditionally, schizophrenia is considered to be a type of 'psychosis', yet the definition of psychosis has been elusive. Older definitions stressed the subjective and internal psychological experience and defined psychosis as an 'impairment in reality testing'. Moreover, psychosis has been defined objectively and operationally as the occurrence of hallucinations and delusions. Because schizophrenia is characterized by so many different types of symptoms, clinicians and scientists have tried to simplify the description of the clinical presentation by categorizing symptoms along dimensions, rather than discrete categories of psychopathology.

Recent research suggests there are three symptom dimensions. The first—psychoticism—involves hallucinations and delusions, the classic symptoms of psychosis. The second—disorganization—involves bizarre speech and behaviour and incongruous affect. The third—negative symptoms—involves alogia, affective blunting, anhedonia, and avolition. The author has developed the Scale for the Assessment of Positive Symptoms (SAPS) and the Scale for the Assessment of Negative Symptoms (SANS) to evaluate these symptoms [6, 7]. (See Table 57.1 for a description of the frequencies of positive and negative symptoms.)

### The psychotic dimension

This symptom dimension refers to two classic 'psychotic' symptoms that reflect a patient's confusion about the loss of boundaries between himself or herself and the external world: hallucinations and delusions. Both symptoms reflect a 'loss of ego boundaries'—the patient is unable to distinguish between his or her own thoughts and perceptions and those that he or she obtains by observing the external world.

*Hallucinations* have sometimes been considered to be the hallmark of schizophrenia, although they may occur in other disorders, including mood disorders and disorders induced by medical illness or various substances. Hallucinations are perceptions experienced without an external stimulus to the sense organs and with a quality similar to a true perception. Schizophrenic patients commonly report auditory, visual, tactile, gustatory, or olfactory hallucinations, or a combination of these. Auditory hallucinations are the most frequent; they are commonly experienced as voices but may also be noises or music. The voices come from outside the person's head, and they usually speak words, phrases, or sentences. Visual hallucinations may be simple or complex and include flashes of light, persons, animals, or objects. Olfactory and gustatory hallucinations are often experienced together, especially as unpleasant tastes or odours. Tactile hallucinations may be experienced as sensations of being touched or pricked, electrical sensations, or sensations of insects crawling under the skin, which is called *formication*.

*Delusions* involve disturbance in thought, rather than perception; they are firmly held beliefs that are untrue, as well as contrary to a person's educational and cultural background. Delusions occurring in schizophrenic patients may have somatic, grandiose, religious, nihilistic, or persecutory themes. The type and frequency of delusions tend to differ according to culture. For example, in the United States,

**Table 57.1** Frequency of symptoms in schizophrenia patients

| Symptoms | % | Symptoms | % |
|---|---|---|---|
| NEGATIVE SYMPTOMS | | POSITIVE SYMPTOMS | |
| Affective flattening | | Hallucinations | |
| Unchanging facial expression | 96 | Auditory | 75 |
| Decreased spontaneous movements | 66 | Voices commenting | 58 |
| Few expressive gestures | 81 | Voices conversing | 57 |
| Poor eye contact | 71 | Somatic–tactile | 20 |
| Affective non-responsivity | 64 | Olfactory | 6 |
| Inappropriate affect | 63 | Visual | 49 |
| Lack of vocal inflections | 73 | | |
| | | Delusions | |
| Alogia | | Persecutory | 81 |
| Poverty of speech | 53 | Jealous | 4 |
| Poverty of content of speech | 51 | Guilt, sin | 26 |
| Blocking | 23 | Grandiose | 39 |
| Increased response latency | 31 | Religious | 31 |
| | | Somatic | 28 |
| Avolition–apathy | | Delusions of reference | 49 |
| Impaired grooming and hygiene | 87 | Delusions of being controlled | 46 |
| Lack of persistence at work or school | 95 | Delusions of mind reading | 48 |
| Physical anergia | 82 | Thought broadcasting | 23 |
| | | Thought insertion | 31 |
| Anhedonia–asociality | | Thought withdrawal | 27 |
| Few recreational interests/ activities | 95 | | |
| Little sexual interest/activity | 69 | Bizarre behaviour | |
| Impaired intimacy/closeness | 84 | Clothing, appearance | 20 |
| Few relationships with friends | 96 | Social, sexual behaviour | 33 |
| Peers | | Aggressive–agitated | 27 |
| | | Repetitive–stereotyped | 28 |
| Attention | | | |
| Social inattentiveness | 78 | Positive formal thought disorder | |
| Inattentiveness during testing | 64 | Derailment | 45 |
| | | Pressure of speech | 24 |
| | | Tangentiality | 5 |
| | | Distractible speech | 23 |
| | | Clanging | 3 |
| | | Incoherence | 23 |
| | | Illogicality | 23 |
| | | Circumstantiality | 35 |

Adapted from *Schizophr Bull*, 13(1), Andreasen NC, The diagnosis of schizophrenia, pp. 9–22, Copyright (1987), with permission from Oxford University Press.

a patient might worry about being spied on by the FBI or CIA; in sub-Saharan Africa, a Bantu or Zulu patient is more likely to worry about persecution by demons or spirits. (See Table 57.2 for a detailed description of the various types of delusions.)

**Table 57.2** Varied content in delusions

| Delusions | Foci of preoccupation |
|---|---|
| Grandiose | Possessing wealth or great beauty, or having a special ability (for example, extrasensory perception); having influential friends; being an important figure (for example, Napoleon, Hitler) |
| Nihilistic | Believing that one is dead or dying; believing that one does not exist or that the world does not exist |
| Persecutory | Being persecuted by friends, neighbours, or spouses; being followed, monitored, or spied upon by the government |
| Somatic | Believing that one's organs have stopped functioning (for example, that the heart is no longer beating) or are rotting away; believing that the nose or other body part is terribly misshapen or disfigured |
| Sexual | Belief that one's sexual behaviour is commonly known; that one is a prostitute, paedophile, or rapist; that masturbation has led to illness or insanity; that one's sexual abilities are legendary |
| Religious | Belief that one has sinned against God; that one has a special relationship to God or some other deity; that one has a special religious mission; that one is the Devil or is condemned to burn in Hell |

Certain types of hallucinations and delusions were considered 'first rank' by Kurt Schneider [4]. These hallucinations include clearly audible voices commenting on a person's actions, or arguing with each other about a patient, or repeating aloud the patient's thoughts. The delusions include thought broadcasting, thought withdrawal, thought insertion, or being controlled. These symptoms commonly occur in schizophrenic patients but are also found in patients with psychoses due to mood disorders, medical illness, or the effect of substances. (See Table 57.3 for a description of Schneider's 'first-rank' symptoms.)

## The disorganization dimension

The disorganization dimension includes disorganized speech, disorganized or bizarre behaviour, and incongruous affect.

Disorganized speech, or *thought disorder*, was regarded as the most important symptom of schizophrenia by Bleuler. Historically, the types of thought disorder have included associative loosening, illogical thinking, over-inclusive thinking, and loss of the ability to engage in abstract thinking. Standard definitions for various types of thought disorders have been developed that stress objective aspects of language and communication (which are empirical indicators of 'thought'), such as derailment, poverty of speech, poverty of content of speech, or tangential replies, and all have been found to occur in both schizophrenia and mood disorders. Manic patients often have a thought disorder characterized by tangentiality, derailment (loose associations), and illogicality. Depressed patients manifest thought disorder less frequently than manic patients but may display poverty of speech, tangentiality, or circumstantiality. Other types of formal thought disorder include perseveration, distractibility, clanging, neologisms, echolalia, and blocking; with the possible exception of clanging in mania, none appears to be disorder-specific.

An example of speech from a schizophrenia patient with a prominent thought disorder, especially derailment, follows:

Let's see, there was one I would have liked if it wasn't for the instructor, well I go along with his, he was always wanted me to do the worse in the class, it seemed, like, and I'd always get bad, the grade,

**Table 57.3** Schneider's first-rank symptoms

| Thought echo | Hearing one's thoughts being spoken aloud |
| --- | --- |
| Voices commenting | Hearing a voice making a running commentary about oneself |
| Voices conversing | Hearing several voices talking or arguing about oneself |
| Somatic hallucination | A hallucination involving the perception of a physical experience within the body |
| Thought withdrawal or insertion | Belief that thoughts are being withdrawn or inserted into the patient's mind by an outside force |
| Thought broadcasting | Belief that the person's thoughts are being broadcast so that his/her private thoughts are known to others |
| Delusional perceptions | A true perception, to which the person attributes a false meaning |
| Delusions of passivity | Being influenced or forced to do things or want things the patient does not wish to do and does not want |
| Delusions of control | Being made to feel emotions or sensations that are not the patient's own |

in my grading, and he tried to make other people like they were good enough to be in Hollywood or something, you know I's be the last one down the ladder. That, that's the way they wanted the grading to be in the first place according to whose, theirs, they, they have all different reasons than I, I, I think that they use that they want one, won't come out.[1]

Many schizophrenic patients display various types of disorganized motor and social behaviour, another aspect of this dimension. Abnormal motor behaviours range from catatonic stupor to excitement. In a *catatonic stupor*, the patient may be immobile, mute, and unresponsive, yet fully conscious. With catatonic excitement, the patient may exhibit uncontrolled and aimless motor activity. Patients sometimes assume bizarre or uncomfortable postures, such as squatting, and maintain them for long periods. Patients may exhibit a *stereotypy*, which is repeated, but non-goal-directed, movement such as back and forth rocking. They may also display *mannerisms*, which are normal goal-directed activities, but are either odd in appearance or out of context such as grimacing. Other common symptoms are *echopraxia*, or imitating the movements and gestures of another person; *automatic obedience*, or carrying out simple commands in a robot-like fashion; and *negativism*, or refusing to cooperate with simple requests for no apparent reason.

*Deterioration of social behaviour* often occurs along with social withdrawal. Patients may neglect themselves, become messy or unkempt, and wear dirty or inappropriate clothing. Patients may ignore their surroundings, so that they become cluttered and untidy. Patients may develop other odd behaviours that break social conventions such as masturbating in public, foraging through garbage bins, or shouting obscenities. Many of today's street people suffer from schizophrenia.

*Incongruity of affect* is another component of the disorganized dimension. Patients may smile inappropriately when speaking of neutral or sad topics, or giggle for no apparent reason. This symptom

---

1. Reproduced from Andreasen NC, *The Broken Brain: The biological revolution in psychiatry*, pp. 61, Copyright (1984), with permission from HarperCollins Publishers.

should not be confused with the nervous smiling or giggling that sometimes occurs in anxious patients.

**The negative dimension**

DSM-5 lists two negative symptoms as characteristic of schizophrenia: affective blunting (diminished emotional expression) and avolition. Other negative symptoms that are common in schizophrenia include alogia (poverty of speech), anhedonia, and attentional impairment. Taken together, they may be considered to represent a new 'five As'. Negative symptoms reflect a deficiency of mental functioning that is normally present.

*Affective flattening or blunting* is a reduced intensity of emotional expression and response. It is manifested by unchanging facial expression, decreased spontaneous movements, poverty of expressive gestures, poor eye contact, lack of voice inflections, and slowed speech.

*Avolition* is a loss of the ability to initiate goal-directed behaviour and carry it through to completion. Patients seem to have lost their will or drive. They may initiate a project and then abandon it for a few days or weeks, and then fail to appear or wander aimlessly away while at work. This symptom is sometimes interpreted as laziness but, in fact, represents the loss or diminution of basic drives and the capacity to formulate and pursue long-range plans.

*Alogia* is characterized by a diminution in the amount of spontaneous speech, as well as a tendency to produce speech that is empty or impoverished in content when the amount is adequate. It is the external expression in language of the impoverishment of thought that occurs in many patients with schizophrenia. Patients may have great difficulty in producing fluent responses to questions.

*Anhedonia*, or the inability to experience pleasure, is also very common. Many patients describe themselves as feeling emotionally empty. They are no longer able to enjoy activities that previously gave them pleasure such as playing sports or seeing family or friends. Their awareness that they have lost the capacity to enjoy themselves may be a source of great psychological pain.

*Attentional impairment* is reflected in an inability to concentrate or by stimuli that they cannot process or filter; this, in turn, causes them to feel confused or to experience fragmented thoughts.

Another aspect of this dimension is a *reduced intensity of emotional response* that leaves schizophrenic patients indifferent and apathetic.

Depressive symptoms occur in up to 60% of schizophrenic patients. Depression is often difficult to diagnose because symptoms of schizophrenia and depression frequently overlap. Dopamine antagonists may also cause what may appear to be depression but is actually drug-induced akinesia.

**Other symptoms**

*Lack of insight* is common in schizophrenia. A patient may not believe that he or she is ill or abnormal in any way. To the patient, the hallucinations and delusions are real, not imagined. Poor insight is one of the most difficult symptoms to treat, and it may persist even when other symptoms, such as hallucinations or delusions, respond to treatment. Orientation and memory are usually normal, unless they are impaired by the patient's psychotic symptoms, inattention, or distractibility.

Non-localizing neurological soft signs occur in a substantial proportion of patients and include abnormalities in stereognosis, graphesthesia, balance, and proprioception [11]. A disorder of the visual tracking of smoothly moving targets (that is, smooth pursuit eye movement) has been observed in both schizophrenia patients and their relatives. Other ocular abnormalities commonly include the absence and avoidance of eye contact and staring for long periods. Decreased or rapid blink rates and bouts of rapid blinking may occur. Some patients display disturbances of sleep, sexual interest, and other bodily functions. A variety of disrupted sleep measures have been reported, but decreased delta sleep with diminished stage 4 is the most consistent finding. Many schizophrenia patients have inactive sex drives and derive little or no pleasure from sexual activity.

### Premorbid personality

Several early writers, including Kraepelin and Bleuler, observed that patients with schizophrenia often had abnormal premorbid personalities. A review of early studies of personality and schizophrenia showed that premorbid schizoid traits were present in one-fourth of schizophrenic patients, but one-sixth had a range of other personality disturbances [12]. Poor premorbid adjustment has been shown to correlate with early disease onset, poor overall prognosis, negative symptoms, cognitive deficits, and poor social functioning.

### Alcohol and drug abuse

Alcohol and drug abuse is especially common in patients with schizophrenia. Drug-using patients tend to be young, male, and poorly compliant with treatment; they also tend to have frequent hospitalizations. It is believed that many abuse drugs in an attempt to treat their depression or their medication side effects (for example, akinesia) or to ameliorate their lack of motivation and pleasure.

### Other problems

People who suffer from schizophrenia are at high risk of committing suicidal acts [13]. About one-third will attempt suicide, and 1 in 10 will eventually complete suicide. Risk factors for suicide include male gender, age under 30 years, unemployment, chronic course, prior depression, past treatment for depression, history of substance abuse, and recent hospital discharge.

Recent research shows that patients with schizophrenia and other severe mental disorders exhibit relatively high rates of violent behaviour and criminality. In the Epidemiologic Catchment Area study [14], schizophrenic patients had rates of violent behaviour five times higher than persons without mental illness, although the rate was about half that seen in persons with alcohol abuse or dependence. Schizophrenic patients with coexisting alcoholism are even more likely to commit violent acts.

## Course of illness

Schizophrenia is typically viewed as a chronic disorder that begins early in life and has a poor long-term outcome. Its onset generally begins with a *prodromal phase* characterized by social withdrawal and other subtle changes in behaviour and emotional responsiveness, peculiar behaviour, deterioration in personal hygiene and grooming, and strange ideation. The prodrome varies in length but typically lasts from months to years.

The prodrome is followed by an *active phase*, in which psychotic symptoms first appear. At this point, the clinical disorder becomes evident, and a diagnosis of schizophrenia can be made. This phase is characterized by hallucinations and delusions, alarming both friends and family members, and often leading to medical intervention. A *residual phase* follows the resolution of the active phase and is similar to the prodrome. Psychotic symptoms may persist during this phase, but at a lower level of intensity, and they may not be as troublesome to the patient. Active phase symptoms may occur episodically ('acute exacerbations'), with variable levels of remission seen between episodes. The frequency and timing of these episodes are unpredictable, although stressful situations may precede these relapses or, in some instances, drug abuse. The stages of schizophrenia are described in Table 57.4.

Relapses are often preceded by changes in thought, feeling, or behaviour noticed by the patient and family members. Symptoms preceding relapse may include dysphoria, seclusiveness, sleep disturbance, anxiety, and ideas of reference. Patients gradually accrue increased levels of morbidity in the form of residual or persistent symptoms and decrements in function from their premorbid status. Relatively severe psychosis is continuous and unrelenting in some patients. Schizophrenia may reach a plateau of severity at about 5 years without further deterioration.

Several long-term follow-up studies have been published using contemporary definitions of schizophrenia [15, 16]. One of the best known is the 'Iowa 500', in which 186 schizophrenic patients admitted to the University of Iowa Psychiatric Hospital between 1934 and 1944 were followed up [15]. Twenty per cent were reported to be psychiatrically well at follow-up, but 54% had incapacitating psychiatric symptoms; 21% were married or widowed, but 67% had never married; 34% lived in their own home or with a relative, but 18% were in mental institutions (including transitional institutions such as halfway houses); 35% were economically productive, but 58% had never worked. The group experienced excessive mortality from both natural and unnatural causes, and more than 10% committed suicide.

In summary, modern outcome studies show that schizophrenia can be a devastating illness that may affect multiple aspects of a patient's life. However, some patients with schizophrenia will have a relatively good outcome and do not experience the severe deterioration sometimes considered to be a hallmark of the disorder.

### Outcome predictors

It is difficult to predict outcome in individual patients based on these studies. However, factors associated with a good outcome include

Table 57.4 Typical stages of schizophrenia

| Stages | Typical features |
| --- | --- |
| Prodromal | Insidious onset over months or years; subtle behaviour changes, including social withdrawal, work impairment, inappropriate affect, avolition, and strange ideation |
| Active phase | Psychotic symptoms develop, including hallucinations, delusions, or disorganized speech and behaviour. These florid symptoms are alarming and lead to medical intervention. Acute phase symptoms may re-emerge during the residual phase ('acute exacerbation') |
| Residual phase | Active phase symptoms are absent or no longer prominent. There is role impairment, negative symptoms, or attenuated positive symptoms |

**Table 57.5** Features associated with good and poor outcome

| Feature | Good outcome | Poor outcome |
| --- | --- | --- |
| Onset | Acute | Insidious |
| Duration | Short | Chronic |
| Mood symptoms | Present | Absent |
| Sensorium | Clouded | Clear |
| Premorbid function | Good | Poor |
| Marital functioning | Married | Never married |
| Psychosexual functioning | Good | Poor |
| Neurological functioning | Normal | Soft signs present |
| Structural brain abnormalities | None | Present |
| Parental education | High | Low |
| Family history/schizophrenia | Negative | Positive |

acute onset, short duration of illness, lack of prior psychiatric history, presence of affective symptoms or confusion, good premorbid adjustment, steady work history, marriage, and older age at onset. Poor prognostic features include insidious onset, long duration of symptoms, affective blunting, obsessive–compulsive symptoms, assaultiveness, premorbid personality disorder, poor work history, celibacy, and young age at onset. Prognostic features in schizophrenia are summarized in Table 57.5.

Schizophrenic patients are more likely to experience a good outcome now than 100 years ago. There are several possible explanations for this finding: (1) the illness has changed; (2) neuroleptic medication and other treatments have altered the natural history of the illness; or (3) our definitions of good outcome have changed. For example, good outcome now may include patients living in care facilities who have minimal symptoms but are clearly not well. For reasons that are not well understood, cross-cultural studies have shown that patients in less developed countries tend to have better outcomes than those in more developed countries [17]. It may be that a person suffering from schizophrenia is better accepted in less developed societies, has fewer external demands, and is more likely to be taken care of by family members. Women, in general, tend to have a better outcome than men in their response to medication and in long-term course.

## Mechanisms of schizophrenia

Many thinkers have considered schizophrenia to be a neurocognitive disorder, with the various signs and symptoms reflecting the downstream effects of a fundamental cognitive deficit. Schizophrenia poses special challenges to the development of cognitive models because of its breadth and diversity of symptoms. The symptoms include nearly all domains of cognitive function: perception (hallucinations), inferential thinking (delusions), fluency of thought and speech (alogia), clarity and organization of thought and speech (formal thought disorder), motor activity (catatonia), emotional expression (affective blunting), ability to initiate and complete goal-directed behaviour (avolition), and ability to seek out and experience emotional gratification (anhedonia).

An initial survey of the diversity of symptoms might suggest that multiple brain regions are involved in schizophrenia, in a spotty

pattern much as once occurred in neurosyphilis. In the absence of visible lesions and known pathogens, investigators have turned to the exploration of models that could explain the diversity of symptoms through a single cognitive mechanism. The convergent conclusions of these different models are striking.

An approach some investigators have taken is to divide the symptoms into three broad groups: (1) disorders of willed action (which lead to symptoms such as alogia and avolition); (2) disorders of self-monitoring (which lead to symptoms such as auditory hallucinations of alien control); and (3) disorders in monitoring the intentions of others ('mentalizing') (which lead to symptoms such as formal thought disorder and delusions of persecution). These could represent a more general underlying mechanism—a disorder of consciousness or self-awareness that impairs the ability to think with 'meta-representations' (higher-order abstract concepts that are representations of mental states) [18–24].

One popular model suggests that the fundamental impairment in schizophrenia is an inability to guide behaviour by representations, often referred to as a defect in working memory [19]. *Working memory* involves the ability to hold a representation 'online' and perform cognitive operations in a flexible manner, to formulate and modify plans, and to base behaviour on internally held ideas and thoughts, rather than being driven by external stimuli. A defect in this ability can explain a variety of symptoms in schizophrenia. For example, the inability to hold a discourse plan in mind and monitor speech output may lead to disorganized speech and thought disorder; the inability to maintain a plan for behavioural activities could lead to negative symptoms such as avolition or alogia; the inability to reference a specific external or internal experience against associative memories (mediated by cortical and subcortical circuitry involving frontal/parietal/temporal regions and the thalamus) could lead to an altered consciousness of sensory experience that would be expressed as delusions or hallucinations. The model also explains the perseverative behaviour observed in studies using the Wisconsin Card Sorting Test and is consistent with the compromised blood flow to the prefrontal cortex in these patients. Overall, this model suggests a major role for prefrontal regions and their multiple distributed cortical, thalamic, and striatal connections in a fundamental cognitive function—representationally guided behaviour—that permits organisms to adapt flexibly to a changing environment and to achieve temporal and spatial continuity between past experiences and present and future actions.

Alternatively (or complementarily), the chapter author has used the clinical presentation of schizophrenia as a point of departure, postulating that the symptoms arise from 'cognitive dysmetria' [25, 26]. This refers to impaired connectivity between frontal, cerebellar, and thalamic regions as a consequence of a neurodevelopmental defect or perhaps a series of them. Motor dysmetria has been observed in schizophrenia since its original description by Kraepelin, and soft signs of poor co-ordination are reported in more contemporary studies [11].

More injurious, however, is the related 'cognitive dysmetria', which produces 'poor co-ordination' of mental activities. The word *metron* literally means 'measure'—a person with schizophrenia has a fundamental deficit in taking measure of time and space and in making inferences about interrelationships between him- or herself and others, or between the past, present, and future. He or she cannot accurately time input and output, and therefore cannot co-ordinate the perception, prioritization, retrieval, and expression of experiences and ideas. This model has received extensive support from work with magnetic resonance imaging and positron emission tomography. (See Chapter 60 for more detail.)

The common thread in these observations is that schizophrenia reflects a disruption in a fundamental cognitive process that affects a specific circuitry in the brain [23, 24]. Various research teams may use different terminology and somewhat different concepts—meta-representations, representationally guided behaviour, information processing/attention, cognitive dysmetria—but they convey a common theme. Cognitive dysfunction in schizophrenia is an inefficient temporal and spatial referencing of information and experience as the person attempts to determine boundaries between self and non-self and to formulate effective decisions or plans that will guide him or her through the small-scale (speaking a sentence) or large-scale (finding a job) manoeuvres of daily living. This capacity is sometimes referred to as *consciousness*.

Investigators also converge on similar conclusions about the neuroanatomic substrates of the cognitive dysfunction. All agree that it must involve distributed circuits, rather than a single specific 'localization', and all suggest a key role for interrelationships among the prefrontal cortex, other interconnected cortical regions, and subcortical regions, particularly the thalamus and striatum (see Chapter 60).

## Pathophysiology and aetiology

A consensus now exists among many clinicians and research investigators that schizophrenia is best conceptualized as a 'multiple-hit' illness similar to cancer. Individuals may carry a genetic predisposition, but this vulnerability is not 'released' unless other factors also intervene. Although the majority of these factors are considered environmental, in the sense that they are not encoded in DNA and could potentially produce mutations or influence gene expression, the majority are also biological, rather than psychological, and include factors such as birth injuries or nutrition [27]. Current studies of the neurobiology of schizophrenia examine a multiplicity of factors, including genetics, anatomy (primarily through structural neuroimaging)), functional circuitry (through functional neuroimaging), neuropathology, electrophysiology, neurochemistry and neuropharmacology, and neurodevelopment.

### Genetics

Evidence for a genetic contribution to schizophrenia is based on family studies, twin studies, studies of adoptees, and molecular genetic techniques. Summaries of individual family studies have shown siblings of schizophrenic patients to have about a 10% chance of developing schizophrenia, whereas children who have one parent with schizophrenia have a 5–6% chance. The risk of family members developing schizophrenia increases markedly when two or more family members have the illness. The risk of developing schizophrenia is 17% for persons with one sibling and one parent with schizophrenia, and 46% for children of two schizophrenic parents. Twin studies have been remarkably consistent in demonstrating high concordance rates for identical twins averaging 46%, compared to 14% concordance in non-identical twins. Adoption studies show that the risk for schizophrenia is greater in the biological relatives of

index adoptees who had schizophrenia than in the biological relatives of mentally healthy control adoptees.

Studies are now under way to illuminate the genetic underpinnings of schizophrenia at the molecular level (see Chapter 61 for more details). Researchers have implicated several different gene regions, but none has emerged as conclusive as yet. Because of implications for solving multiple key problems (diagnostic, prognostic, treatment choices), this is one of the central topics for schizophrenia research and it is likely to remain so for some time [28].

### Neuropathology

A better understanding of neurodevelopment has helped shape contemporary post-mortem studies. During the second trimester, neurons in the fetal brain must migrate to the appropriate layers of the cortex, then connect with other groups of neurons to form functional networks. Other developmental processes include excessive proliferation of cells and dendrites, subsequently followed by pruning and programmed cell death (apoptosis) of subplate neurons; surviving cells remain as interstitial neurons (or 'interneurons') of the white matter. The resulting network of neurons and cytoplasmic processes is called the *neuropil*. Research suggests that schizophrenia could be related to disturbances in any of these phases of brain maturation, ranging from migration to apoptosis. Failure of the cells to migrate to their proper position may show up as ectopic grey matter or neuronal disarray in specific regions of the hippocampus.

Displacement of neurons and a paucity of neurons in the superficial layers in the rostral and intermediate portions of the entorhinal cortex of the parahippocampal gyrus have also been reported and have been attributed to faulty neuronal migration. More recently, researchers have observed displacement of interneurons in the frontal lobe cortex, including decreased cell density in the superficial white matter and increased cell density in the deeper white matter, findings also thought consistent with an alteration in the migration of subplate neurons or in the pattern of programmed cell death [29].

Neuropathology has also been used to explore whether abnormalities can be found in key candidate regions such as the thalamus or prefrontal cortex. Decreased cell density in the medial dorsal nucleus of the thalamus, a crucial nucleus that projects to the prefrontal cortex, thalamic abnormalities, and increased cell packing density in the prefrontal cortex have all been described. The latter finding is consistent with a loss of the surrounding neuropil and consequent shrinkage of the interneuronal space. A convergence of findings is beginning to emerge from the variable perspectives of structural and functional neuroimaging and neuropathology. These perspectives are all consistent with neurodevelopmental mechanisms and with abnormalities in frontal, temporal, and thalamic regions.

### Neurodevelopmental influences

Several lines of evidence have supported speculation that schizophrenia is a neurodevelopmental disorder resulting from brain injury occurring early in life. For example, schizophrenic patients are more likely than non-schizophrenic control subjects to have a history of birth injury and perinatal complications, which could result in subtle brain injury, setting the stage for the development of schizophrenia [27]. Seasonality of birth in schizophrenic patients has also suggested to some a neurodevelopmental aetiology. Throughout the temperate northern latitudes, more people with schizophrenia are born in winter months than at any other time. This suggests that some schizophrenic persons could have sustained central nervous system damage in the womb from a viral illness.

## Evolutionary aspects

That schizophrenia persists in the human population despite the fact that the majority of people who develop it do not marry or procreate is fascinating. This observation should perhaps be coupled with another that has been less frequently noted and has not yet been systematically investigated—a substantial number of highly creative individuals have family members who are in the schizophrenia spectrum. The association between manic–depressive illness and creativity is well established, but most of this work has focused on literary or artistic creativity [30].

In the case of schizophrenia, there may be a link with scientific creativity, although the evidence at present is only anecdotal. However, an impressive number of Nobel laureates have an association with schizophrenia. Bertrand Russell had a son and a granddaughter who suffered from schizophrenia, as well as an aunt and an uncle who probably also suffered from this illness when it was simply called 'insanity'. Albert Einstein had a son by his first wife who developed schizophrenia. John Nash, a recent Nobel laureate in economics, developed schizophrenia himself in his early 30s and also had a son who suffers from schizophrenia. James Joyce was emotionally aloof and cold and became increasingly disorganized artistically; his daughter Lucia suffered from hebephrenic schizophrenia. Isaac Newton was a solitary, chronically suspicious, and socially aloof man who had a variety of unusual interests and beliefs; he would probably be called schizotypal using modern nomenclature; however, he also had a psychotic break at age 40.

Coupled with the persistence of schizophrenia throughout history despite decreased fertility and procreation, this modest association between schizophrenia and 'genius' suggests that, perhaps like sickle-cell anemia, a predisposition to schizophrenia may convey a biological advantage in some situations.

## REFERENCES

1. Murray, C.J., Lopez, A.D. (1996). *The global burden of disease: a comprehensive assessment of mortality and disability from diseases, injuries, and risk factors in 1990 and projected to 2020*. World Health Organization, Geneva.
2. Kraepelin, E. (1919). *Dementia Praecox and Paraphrenia* (Barclay, R.M. Robertson, G.M., trans.). E and S Livingstone, Edinburgh.
3. Bleuler, E. (1950). *Dementia Praecox of the Group of Schizophrenias* (Zinkin, J., trans.). International Universities Press, New York, NY.
4. Schneider, K. (1974). Primary and secondary symptoms in schizophrenia. In: Hirsch, S.R., Shepherds, M. (eds). *Themes and Variations in European Psychiatry*. John Wright, Bristol; pp. 40–6.
5. American Psychiatric Association. (2013). *Diagnostic and Statistical Manual of Mental Disorders*, fifth edition. American Psychiatric Association, Arlington, VA; pp. 99–108.
6. Andreasen, N.C. (1984). *The Scale for Assessment of Negative Symptoms (SANS)*. University of Iowa, Iowa City, IA.
7. Andreasen, N.C. (1984). *The Scale for the Assessment of Positive Symptoms (SAPS)*. University of Iowa, Iowa City, IA.
8. Andreasen, N.C., Arndt, S., Miller, D., Flaum, M., Nopoulos, P. (1995). Correlational studies of the scale for the assessment of negative symptoms and the scale for the assessment of positive symptoms: an overview and update. *Psychopathology*, 28, 7–17.
9. O'Leary, D.S., Flaum, M., Kesler, M.L., Flashman, L.A., Arndt, S., Andreasen, N.C. (2000). Cognitive correlates of the negative, disorganized, and psychotic symptom dimensions of schizophrenia. *Journal of Neuropsychiatry and Clinical Neurosciences*, 12, 4–15.
10. Andreasen, N.C. (1984). *The Broken Brain: The biological revolution in psychiatry* (first edition). Harper & Row, New York, NY; p. 61.
11. Flashman, L.A., Flaum, M., Gupta, S., Andreasen, N.C. (1996). Soft signs and neuropsychological performance in schizophrenia. *American Journal of Psychiatry*, 153, 526–32.
12. Nicholson, R., Lenane, M., Singaracharlu, S., et al. (2000). Premorbid speech and language impairment in childhood-onset schizophrenia—associated with risk factors. *American Journal of Psychiatry*, 157, 794–800.
13. Breier, A., Astrachan, B.M. (1984). Characterization of schizophrenic patients who commit suicide. *American Journal of Psychiatry*, 141, 206–9.
14. Regier, D.A., Farmer, M.E., Rae, D.S., et al. (1990). Comorbidity of mental disorders with alcohol and other drug abuse. Results from the Epidemiologic Catchment Area (ECA) Study. *JAMA*, 264, 2511–18.
15. Winokur, G., Tsuang, M.T. (1996). *The Natural History of Mania, Depression, and Schizophrenia*. American Psychiatric Press, Washington, DC.
16. McGlashan, T.H. (1984). The Chestnut Lodge follow-up study, II: long-term outcome in schizophrenia and the affective disorders. *Archives of General Psychiatry*, 41, 586–601.
17. Jablensky, A., Sartorius, N., Ernberg, G., et al. (1992). Schizophrenia: manifestations, incidence and course in different cultures. A World Health Organization Ten-Country Study. *Psychological Medicine Monograph Supplement*, 20, 1–97.
18. McGuire, P.K., Frith, C.D. (1996). Disordered functional connectivity in schizophrenia. *Psychological Medicine*, 26, 663–7.
19. Goldman-Rakic, P.S. (1994). Working memory dysfunction in schizophrenia. *Journal of Neuropsychiatry and Clinical Neurosciences*, 64, 348–57.
20. Frith, C.D. (2004). Schizophrenia and theory of mind. *Psychological Medicine*, 34, 385–9.
21. Frith, C.D. (1992). *The Cognitive Neuropsychology of Schizophrenia*. Lawrence Erlbaum, Hove.
22. Frith, C.D., Friston, K.J., Herold, S., et al. (1995). Regional brain activity in chronic schizophrenic patients during performance of a verbal fluency task. *British Journal of Psychiatry*, 167, 343–9.
23. Goldman-Rakic, P.S. (1988). Changing concepts of cortical connectivity: parallel distributed cortical networks. In: Rakic, P., Singer, W. (eds). *Neurobiology of Neocortex*. Wiley, New York, NY; pp. 177–202.
24. Goldman-Rakic, P.S. (1988). Topography of cognition: parallel distributed networks in primate association cortex. *Annual Review of Neuroscience*, 11, 137–56.
25. Andreasen, N.C., Paradiso, S., O'Leary, D.S. (1998). 'Cognitive dysmetria' as an integrative theory of schizophrenia: a dysfunction in cortical-subcortical-cerebellar circuitry? *Schizophrenia Bulletin*, 24, 203–18.
26. Andreasen, N.C., Nopoulos, P., O'Leary, D.S., Miller, D.D., Wassink, T., Flaum, M. (1999). Defining the phenotype of schizophrenia: cognitive dysmetria and its neural mechanisms. *Biological Psychiatry*, 46, 909–20.

27. McNeil, T.F., Cantor-Graae, E., Weinberger, D.R. (2000). Relationship of obstetric complications and differences in size of brain structure in monozygotic twin pairs discordant for schizophrenia. *American Journal of Psychiatry*, 157, 203–12.

28. Riley, B., Kendler, K.S. (2006). Molecular genetic studies of schizophrenia. *European Journal of Human Genetics*, 14, 669–80.

29. Selemon, L.D., Rajkowska, G., Goldman-Rakic, S. (1995). Abnormally high neuronal density in the schizophrenic cortex. *Archives in General Psychiatry*, 52, 805–18.

30. Andreasen, N.C. (2014). *Secrets of the Creative Brain*. The Atlantic. https://www.theatlantic.com/magazine/archive/2014/07/secrets-of-the-creative-brain/372299/

# 58

# Epidemiology and course of schizophrenia

*Assen Jablensky*

## Introduction

Epidemiological research into schizophrenia aims to answer four essential questions:

- What is the 'true' frequency of the disorder in various populations, and how is it distributed across the various groups within populations?
- Do the incidence, manifestations, and course of schizophrenia vary in relation to factors of the physical and social environment?
- Who is at risk, and what forces determine or influence the risk of developing schizophrenia?
- Can the answers to these questions help explain what causes the disorder and how to prevent it?

Schizophrenia has been studied extensively from an epidemiological perspective since Kraepelin [1] introduced the concept of *dementia praecox* in 1896 [1–6]. In the first half of the twentieth century, epidemiological research into schizophrenia took two divergent paths. While European studies tended to focus on population distributions and genetic risks, North American researchers investigated the social ecology of the disorder. A variety of methods were explored and successfully applied by the pioneers of psychiatric epidemiology, and the contours of the epidemiological map of schizophrenia in Europe and North America were effectively laid down between the two World Wars. The early studies were carried out by dedicated researchers who often spent months or years collecting data 'door-to-door' in small communities. Close knowledge of the respondents, access to multigenerational records from local parish registers, and the co-operation of the community resulted in studies that remain landmarks of psychiatric epidemiology (Table 58.1).

During the last several decades, the scope of epidemiological studies of schizophrenia has expanded to include populations in Asia, Africa, and South America, about which little had been known previously. The World Health Organization (WHO) International Pilot Study of Schizophrenia [7] and its successor—the WHO 10-country epidemiological study [8]—were the first systematic investigations of the comparative incidence, clinical manifestations, and course of schizophrenia in both developing and developed countries. The WHO programme was an impetus for similar studies in India, China, the Caribbean, and Australia. Two major studies of psychiatric morbidity in the United States—the Epidemiological Catchment Area project [9] and the National Comorbidity Survey [10]—generated data on the prevalence of DSM-III/IIIR schizophrenia and related disorders in representative population samples. In the 1980s and 1990s, epidemiological studies increasingly utilized existing large databases, such as cumulative case registers or birth cohorts, to test hypotheses about risk factors and began to include methods of genetic epidemiology. There is a current tendency towards integrating epidemiological approaches with other types of aetiological research in schizophrenia. This predicts an important role for epidemiology in the era of genetics and molecular biology of mental disorders.

## Epidemiological methods in the study of schizophrenia

Measurement of the prevalence, incidence, and disease expectancy of schizophrenia depends critically on the sensitivity of the case-finding method (that is, its capacity to identify all affected persons in a given population) and the availability of a diagnostic instrument or procedure that selects 'true' cases (that is, those corresponding to an established clinical concept).

### Case-finding

Case-finding designs fall into three broad groups: case detection in clinical populations, door-to-door surveys of population samples or whole communities, and birth cohort studies. Each method has its advantages and limitations.

While case-finding through the mental health services provides relatively easy access to a substantial proportion of all persons with schizophrenia, the cases in treatment may not be fully representative of all individuals with the disorder. Bias related to gender, marital status, socio-economic factors, culture, or ethnicity is known to affect the probability of being in treatment at a given time in a given setting, and generalizations about schizophrenia from hospital or clinic samples are liable to error. Some of the deficiencies of case-finding through service contacts are avoided in cumulative national or regional psychiatric case registers, which cover large, well-defined populations and can be linked to other population databases (for example, birth records). This makes registers efficient research instruments in low-incidence disorders such as schizophrenia.

**Table 58.1** Historical landmarks in the epidemiology of psychoses

| Author | Method | Target population | Case finding | Assessment |
|---|---|---|---|---|
| Koller (1895) [2] | The first case-control study of psychoses | Cases of psychosis and normal controls | Hospital and clinic records | Genealogical inquiry |
| Luxenburger (1928) [3] | Twin concordance analysis | Monozygotic and dizygotic twin pairs | Search of birth registers | Diagnosis: 'definite' and 'probable' |
| Brugger (1931) [4] | Census (door-to-door survey) | Area in Thuringia (population 37,561) | Hospital records and key informants | Personal examination of 'suspected' cases and controls |
| Klemperer (1933) [5] | Birth cohort study | Random sample (n = 1000) of all births in Munich, 1881–1890 | Tracing of cohort members (44% successfully traced) | Personal examination or key informant interview (271 examined) |
| Essen-Möller et al. (1956) [6] | Census and follow-up surveys | Rural community (n = 2550 + 1013 new residents during follow-up) | Complete census; tracing of persons who had migrated out | Personal examination and re-examination of all residents |

Surveys involve accounting for every person at risk within a defined community or a population sample in terms of either being or not being a case. Face-to-face interviews (and follow-up) of all residents in defined communities has been a feature of some high-quality research, especially in Scandinavian countries [6]. However, since the size of the populations surveyed in this way is limited, the number of detected cases of schizophrenia is usually too small to generate stable estimates of epidemiological parameters. Surveys of large populations involve two basic designs: a single-phase survey of a probability sample drawn from the general population; and a two-phase survey where a validated screening test is first applied to the entire population and only those scoring as screen-positive proceed to a full assessment. In the instance of schizophrenia, logistics dictates a choice between assessing large numbers less rigorously and investigating a smaller sample in greater depth. In the absence of a simple and valid screening procedure for schizophrenia, such as a biological or psychological test, the advantages of the two-phase survey may be offset by poor sensitivity or specificity of the screening device, which is usually a questionnaire or checklist.

The study of birth cohorts at ages when their members have passed through the greater part of the period of risk for onset of schizophrenia is usually done by face-to-face interviewing or by analysing available case register data. Well-characterized birth cohorts are among the best tools for the study of the incidence of schizophrenia and associated risk factors [11]. However, even in settings where the population is stable and mortality and morbidity are adequately monitored, the size of birth cohorts with prospectively collected data may not be sufficient for conclusive epidemiological inferences.

All this suggests that there is no single 'gold standard' of case-finding for schizophrenia that could be applied across all possible settings, and the assets and liabilities of particular case-finding procedures need to be evaluated in the context of each study. This makes the detailed reporting of case-finding methods a mandatory prerequisite for an 'evidence-based' epidemiology of schizophrenia.

## Diagnosis

Variation in diagnostic concepts and practices always explains a proportion of the variation in the results of schizophrenia studies, especially if they involve different populations or different periods. In the late 1960s, the WHO International Pilot Study of Schizophrenia [7] examined diagnostic variation in schizophrenia across nine countries by comparing the diagnoses made by psychiatrists using a clinical interview and diagnostic classification by a computer algorithm [12] utilizing the same interview data. The results demonstrated that in the majority of settings, psychiatrists were using comparable diagnostic concepts. The introduction of explicit diagnostic criteria and rules with the consecutive editions of DSM and the WHO's ICD-10 improved further the reliability of diagnosis but did not resolve all diagnostic issues, with implications for epidemiology. While ICD-10 and DSM-IV tended to agree well on the core cases of schizophrenia, they agree less well on the classification of atypical or milder cases. Such differences may be less important in clinical practice, but they present a problem for epidemiological and genetic studies. By providing more restrictive criteria for schizophrenia, both classifications aim to identify clinically similar cases and to minimize false-positive diagnoses. This is not an unequivocal advantage, since applying such criteria at case-finding may result in the rejection of potential cases which fail to meet the full set of criteria at initial assessment. Therefore, it is desirable to develop less restrictive screening versions of the DSM and ICD criteria for epidemiological research.

## Instruments

The diagnostic instruments used in surveys which involve interviewing fall into two categories: fully structured interviews such as the Diagnostic Interview Schedule (DIS) [9] and the Composite International Diagnostic Interview (CIDI) [13], both written to match exactly the diagnostic criteria of DSM-IIIR/IV and ICD-10; and semi-structured interview schedules, such as the Present State Examination (PSE) [12] and the Schedules for Clinical Assessment in Neuropsychiatry (SCAN) [14], which cover a broad range of psychopathology.

The DIS/CIDI type of instrument is reliable and capable of generating standard diagnoses of common mental disorders in a single-phase survey design. Its clinical validity in schizophrenia is less certain because symptoms may not be reported accurately or impairment may be underestimated by the respondent. In contrast, the PSE/SCAN allows a greater amount of psychopathological data to be elicited in a flexible clinical interview format, but its use in epidemiological studies presupposes the availability of clinically trained interviewers. While SCAN and other similar interviews are suitable as second-stage diagnostic instruments, there is still a need for a relatively simple and effective screening procedure for case-finding of schizophrenia in field surveys.

The epidemiological description of schizophrenia draws on extensive evidence available today on its frequency, age, and sex distribution in relatively large populations or geographical areas. Less than complete information is available on variations in its epidemiological characteristics that may be found in unusual or isolated populations.

## Prevalence

Prevalence provides an estimate of the proportion of cases per 1000 persons at risk present in a population at a given time or over a defined period. Point prevalence refers to the 'active' (that is, symptomatic) cases on a given date or within a brief census period. Since asymptomatic cases (for example, persons in remission) will be missed in a point prevalence survey, it is useful to supplement the assessment of the present mental state with an enquiry about past episodes of the disorder to obtain a lifetime prevalence index. In schizophrenia, which tends to be a chronic course, estimates of point and lifetime prevalence will be closer to each other than in remitting illnesses.

An overview of selected prevalence studies of schizophrenia spanning over seven decades is presented in Table 58.2 and in two systematic reviews of the literature [15, 16]. The studies differ in many aspects of methodology, but in the majority, they feature a high intensity of case-finding. Several studies are repeat surveys in which the original population was reassessed following an interval of 10 or more years (the resulting consecutive prevalence figures are indicated by arrows).

Most studies have produced point prevalence estimates in the range of 2.1–7.0 per 1000 population at risk and a lifetime prevalence of schizophrenia in the range of 15.0–19.0 per 1000. These figures should be considered with caution because of demographic differences between populations related to factors such as age-specific mortality and migration. A systematic review of 188 studies in 46 countries, published between 1965 and 2002 [15], estimated the median value for point prevalence at 4.6 per 1000 persons and for a lifetime prevalence at 7.2 per 1000.

Certain populations and groups deviate markedly from the central tendency. A strikingly high prevalence of schizophrenia (2–3 times the national or regional average) has been found in geographically and genetically isolated populations, including small communities in northern Sweden and Finland [19, 25], while at the other extreme, virtual absence of schizophrenia and a high rate of depression have been claimed for the Hutterites of South Dakota, a Protestant sect whose members live in close-knit endogamous communities sheltered from the outside world [27]. Negative social selection for schizoid individuals who fail to adjust to the lifestyle of the majority and eventually migrate without leaving progeny has been suggested (but not definitively proven) as an explanation. Results of two surveys in Taiwan [28], separated by 15 years, pointed to a falling prevalence of schizophrenia (from 2.1 to 1.4 per 1000) in the context of major socio-economic change and an overall increase in total mental morbidity in the population.

The question about the extent of true variation in the prevalence of schizophrenia across populations has no simple answer. Methodological differences among studies, related to sampling, case-finding, and diagnostic assessment, are likely to account for a good deal of the observed variation [29].

Notwithstanding such caveats in the interpretation of survey findings, the prevalence rates are fairly similar in the majority of studies, though certain specific populations clearly deviate from the modal value. Even in those instances, however, the magnitude of the deviation is modest, compared with the 10- to 30-fold differences in prevalence observed in other multifactorial diseases (for example, diabetes, ischaemic heart disease, multiple sclerosis) across populations.

**Table 58.2** Selected prevalence studies of schizophrenia

| Author | Country | Population | Method | Prevalence per 1000 population at risk |
|---|---|---|---|---|
| Bøjholm and Strömgren (1983) [17] | Denmark | Island of Bornholm (n = 50,000) | Census interviews, repeat census | 3.9 → 3.3 |
| Böök (1953) [18] Böök et al. (1978) [19] | Sweden | Genetic isolate (n = 9000); age 15–50 | Census interviews, repeat census | 9.5 → 17.0 |
| Crocetti et al. (1971) [20] | Croatia | Sample of 9201 households | Census of hospital records and interviews | 5.9 |
| Dube and Kumar (1972) [21] | India | Four areas in Agra (n = 29,468) | Census based on hospital and clinic records | 2.6 |
| Keith et al. (1991) [22] | United States | Aggregated population across five ECA sites | Sample survey; interviews | 7.0 (point); 15.0 (lifetime) |
| Jeffreys et al. (1997) [23] | UK | London health district (n = 112,127) | Census; interview of sample (n = 172) | 5.1 |
| Jablensky et al. (2000) [24] | Australia | Four urban areas (n = 1,084,978) | Census, screen for psychosis; patient interviews | 4.7 (point); 5.8[a] (12 months) |
| Perälä et al. (2007) [25] | Finland | National sample (n = 8028) | Screen for psychosis, interviews, register and casenote data | 10.0 (lifetime) |
| Morgan et al. (2014) [26] | Australia | Catchment areas with total population (n = 1,464,921; | Sample (n = 1642) of patients with psychoses in contact with mental health services | 3.1 (point) 3.45[b] (lifetime) |

[a] Schizophrenia and spectrum disorders.
[b] All psychoses.

## Incidence

While prevalence is a proportion, incidence is a rate (an estimate of the annual number of new cases in a defined population per 1000 persons at risk). Incidence is of greater interest for the study of risk factors than prevalence, since it represents the so-called force of morbidity (the probability of disease occurrence) in a given population and is closer in time to the action of antecedent or precipitating factors. The estimation of incidence depends critically on the ability to determine reliably the point of onset of the disorder. In the case of schizophrenia, the long prodromal period and the fuzzy boundary between the premorbid state and the onset of psychosis make this particularly difficult. In the absence of an objective biomarker of the disease, onset is usually defined as the point in time when clinical manifestations become recognizable and diagnosable according to specified criteria. The first hospital admission, which has been used as a proxy for disease onset in many studies, is not a robust indicator because of the variable time lag between the earliest appearance of symptoms and the first admission across treatment facilities and settings. A better approximation is provided by the first contact, that is, the point at which any psychiatric, general medical, or alternative 'helping' agency is accessed by symptomatic individuals for the first time. A limitation common to both first-admission and first-contact studies is that they produce rates of 'treated' incidence and miss symptomatic cases that do not present for assessment or treatment. This limitation can be overcome by periodically repeated door-to-door surveys of the same population or by longitudinal cohort studies.

Table 58.3 presents the essential features and findings of seven historical incidence studies of schizophrenia. Although these studies vary in details of their methodology, the variation of the reported rates in settings as different as Barbados and Dublin is relatively modest, in the range of 0.32 [38] to 0.57 [33] per 1000 population at risk. Studies using more stringent criteria, such as DSM-IIIR, DSM-IV, ICD-10, or *Catego* S+ [12], have reported incidence rates 2–3 times lower than those based on 'broad' criteria. A systematic review of data from some 160 studies from 33 countries, published between 1965 and 2001 [30] yielded a median value of 0.15 and mean value of 0.24 per 1000, with a 5-fold range of the rates and a tendency for more recent studies to report lower rates. Similar results have been reported in a systematic review and meta-analyses of schizophrenia incidence studies in England [31].

Considering the methodological differences among studies, generalizing about the incidence of schizophrenia from pooled data may be problematic [29]. To date, the only investigation that had applied a uniform design and common research tools to generate directly comparable incidence data for different populations was the WHO 10-country study [8]. Incidence counts in the WHO study were based on first-in-lifetime contacts with any 'helping agency' within defined areas (including traditional healers in the developing countries) which were monitored for new cases over a 2-year period. Potential cases and key informants were interviewed by clinicians using standardized instruments, and the timing of onset was ascertained for the majority of the patients. In 86% of the 1022 patients, the onset of diagnostic symptoms of schizophrenia was within the year preceding the first contact, and therefore, the first-contact incidence rate was adopted as a reasonable approximation to the 'true' onset rate. Two definitions of 'caseness' were used to determine incidence: a 'broad' clinical definition comprising ICD-9 schizophrenia and paranoid psychoses; and a more restrictive definition of PSE/*Catego* S + 'nuclear' schizophrenia manifesting with Schneiderian first-rank symptoms. The rates for eight of the catchment areas are shown in Table 58.4.

While the differences between the rates for 'broadly' defined schizophrenia (0.16–0.42 per 1000) were significant ($P$ <0.001), those for 'nuclear' schizophrenia were not, suggesting that the frequency of this diagnostic subgroup varies less across different populations. Replications of the design of the WHO 10-country study, including its research procedures and instruments, have been carried out, with similar results in India [36] and the Caribbean [38].

### Disease expectancy (morbid risk)

This is the probability that an individual born into a defined population will develop the disease if he or she survives the period of risk for that disease. In the instance of schizophrenia, the period of risk is usually defined as 15–54 years. If age- and sex-specific incidence rates are known, disease expectancy can be estimated directly by a summation of the age-specific rates within the period of risk. Alternatively, disease expectancy can be estimated indirectly from prevalence data (Table 58.5).

**Table 58.3** Selected incidence studies of schizophrenia

| Author | Country | Population | Method | Rate per 1000 population at risk |
|---|---|---|---|---|
| Ödegaard (1946) [32] | Cumulative national case register | Total population of Norway | All first admissions 1926–1935 ($n$ = 14,231); statistical analysis | 0.24 (hospital diagnoses) |
| Walsh (1969) [33] | Ireland | City of Dublin ($n$ = 720,000) | First admissions | 0.57 (males), 0.46 (females) |
| Murphy and Raman (1971) [34] | Mauritius | Total population ($n$ = 257,000) | First admissions | 0.24 (Africans); 0.14 Indian Hindus); 0.09 (Indian Moslems) |
| Helgason (1977) [35] | Iceland | Total population ($n$ = 221,799) | First admissions (case register) | 0.27 |
| Rajkumar *et al.* (1993) [36] | India | Area in Chennai (Madras) ($n$ = 43,097) | Key informants; door-to-door survey | 0.41 |
| Brewin *et al.* (1997) [37] | UK | City of Nottingham | Two cohorts of first contacts (1978–1980 and 1992–1994) | 0.25 → 0.29 0.14 → 0.09 |
| Mahy *et al.* (1999) [38] | Barbados | Total population ($n$ = 262,000) | First contacts, interviews | 0.32 (ICD-9) |

**Table 58.4** WHO ten-country study of schizophrenia

| Country | Area | 'Broad' definition (ICD-9) | | | 'Narrow' definition (CATEGO S+) | | |
|---|---|---|---|---|---|---|---|
| | | Male | Female | All | Male | Female | All |
| Denmark | Aarhus | 0.18 | 0.13 | 0.16 | 0.09 | 0.05 | 0.07 |
| India | Chandigarh (rural area) | 0.37 | 0.48 | 0.42 | 0.13 | 0.09 | 0.11 |
| India | Chandigarh (urban area) | 0.34 | 0.35 | 0.35 | 0.08 | 0.11 | 0.09 |
| Ireland | Dublin | 0.23 | 0.21 | 0.22 | 0.10 | 0.08 | 0.09 |
| Japan | Nagasaki | 0.23 | 0.18 | 0.20 | 0.11 | 0.09 | 0.10 |
| Russia | Moscow | 0.25 | 0.31 | 0.28 | 0.03 | 0.03 | 0.02 |
| UK | Nottingham | 0.28 | 0.15 | 0.22 | 0.17 | 0.12 | 0.14 |
| United States | Honolulu | 0.18 | 0.14 | 0.16 | 0.10 | 0.08 | 0.09 |

Reproduced from *Psychol Med Monogr* Suppl., 20, Jablensky A, Sartorius N, Ernberg G, *et al.*, Schizophrenia: manifestations and course in different cultures. A World Health Organization ten-country study, pp. 1–97, Copy-right (1992), with permission from Cambridge University Press.

The estimates of disease expectancy produced by a number of studies are fairly consistent across populations and over time. Excluding outliers, such as the northern Swedish isolate [18, 19], they vary about 5-fold; in the WHO study [8], they range from 0.59% (Aarhus) to 1.8% (Chandigarh, rural area) for ICD-9 schizophrenia and from 0.26% (Honolulu) to 0.54% (Nottingham) for *Catego S +* 'nuclear' schizophrenia. The frequently cited modal estimate of lifetime disease expectancy for broadly defined schizophrenia at around 1% seems to be consistent with the evidence.

### Associations with age and sex

Schizophrenia may have its onset at any age—in childhood as well as past middle age—although the vast majority of onsets fall within the 15–54 years of age interval. Onsets in men peak steeply in the age group of 20–24 years; thereafter, the rate of inception remains more or less constant at a lower level. In women, a less prominent peak in the age group of 20–24 years is followed by another increase in incidence in age groups older than 35. While the age-specific incidence up to the mid-thirties is significantly higher in men, the male-to-female ratio becomes inverted with age, reaching 1:1.9 for onsets after the age of 40 and 1:4, or even 1:6, for onsets after the age of 60. There seems to be no real 'point of rarity' between the symptomatology of late-onset schizophrenia and schizophrenia of early onset.

The sex differences in mean age at onset are unlikely to be an invariant biological characteristic of schizophrenia. For example, within families carrying high genetic risk (two or more affected members), no significant differences in age at onset have been found between male and female siblings with schizophrenia. In some populations (for example, India and China), the male predominance in the frequency of onsets in the younger age groups is attenuated or even inverted [39, 40].

The question of whether the total lifetime risks for men and women are about the same, or different, has not been answered definitively. In the WHO 10-country study, the cumulated risks for males and females up to the age of 54 were found to be approximately equal [8]. Scandinavian studies which followed up population cohorts into very old age (over 80) reported a higher cumulated lifetime risk in women than in men [41].

Male–female differences have been described in relation to the premorbid history (better premorbid functioning in women), the occurrence of brain abnormalities (more frequent in men), course (a higher percentage of remitting illness episodes and shorter hospital stay in women), and outcome (higher survival rate in the community, less disability in women). However, there is no unequivocal evidence of consistent sex differences in the symptom profiles of schizophrenia, including the frequency of positive and negative symptoms. Generally, the sex differences described in schizophrenia are more likely to result from normal sexual dimorphism in brain development, as well as from gender-related social roles, rather than from sex-specific aetiological factors.

**Table 58.5** Selected course and outcome studies of schizophrenia

| Author | Country | Sample size | Follow-up years | Proportion of good outcome |
|---|---|---|---|---|
| Bleuler M (1978) [107] | Switzerland | 208 | 23 | 20% complete remission; 33% 'mild defect' |
| Tsuang *et al.* (1979) [108] | United States | 186 | 35 | 46% recovered or improved significantly |
| Ciompi (1980) [109] | Switzerland | 289 | 37 | 20% recovered, 43% 'definitely improved' |
| Huber *et al.* (1980) [110] | Germany | 502 | 22 | 26% recovered, 31% remission, 'mild defect' |
| Johnstone *et al.* (1990) [73] | UK | 530 | 13 | 14% 'excellent'; 18.5% 'very good social adjustment' |
| WHO (2007) [74] | Developing countries | 467 | 15–26 | 62.7% complete remissions; 55.5% never hospitalized during follow-up; 42.9% unimpaired social functioning during 75% of follow-up |
| WHO (2007) [74] | Developed countries | 603 | 15–26 | 36.8% complete remissions; 8.1% never hospitalized during follow-up; 31.6% unimpaired social functioning during follow-up |

## Fertility, mortality, and comorbidity

Earlier studies reported low fertility in both men and women diagnosed with schizophrenia. The mean number of children fathered by men with schizophrenia in Sweden was 0.9, and the average number of live births over the entire reproductive period of women treated for schizophrenia in Norway between 1936 and 1975 was 1.8, compared with 2.2 for the general female population [42]. Yet this phenomenon is neither universal nor consistent over time. In the WHO 10-country study [8], the fertility of women with schizophrenia in India did not differ from that of women in the general population within the same age groups and geographic areas. Although men with schizophrenia continue to be reproductively disadvantaged, the fertility of women with schizophrenia has increased over the last decades, and this trend is likely to be sustained as a result of deinstitutionalization and the greater number of people with mental disorders being able to live in the community.

Excess mortality associated with schizophrenia has been well documented by studies on large cohorts. National case register data for Norway, 1926–1941 and 1950–1974, indicated that while the total mortality of psychiatric patients was decreasing, the relative mortality of patients with schizophrenia remained unchanged at a level higher than twice that of the general population [32]. A meta-analysis of 18 studies [43] estimated a crude mortality rate of 189 deaths per 10,000 population per year and a 10-year survival rate of 81%. Mortality among males was significantly higher than among females, and the difference was primarily due to an excess in suicides and accidents. Unnatural causes apart, the leading causes of death among schizophrenia patients are similar to those in the general population, with the exception of significantly lower-than-expected cancer morbidity and mortality, especially for tobacco-related malignancies in males with schizophrenia [44]. This puzzling phenomenon has been replicated by several case register and record linkage studies [45, 46] and does not appear to be an artefact. Its causes remain unknown, though protective effects of both genes and antipsychotic pharmacological agents have been proposed.

The single most common cause of death among schizophrenia patients at present is suicide (aggregated standardized mortality ratios of 9.6 for males and 6.8 for females), which accounts for 28% of the excess mortality in schizophrenia [47]. The suicide rate in schizophrenia patients is at least equal to, or may indeed be higher than, the suicide rate in major depression. Several risk factors, relatively specific to schizophrenia, have been suggested: being young and male; experiencing multiple relapses and remissions; comorbid substance use; awareness of the deteriorating course of the condition; and loss of faith in treatment. Data from successive patient cohorts in Denmark [48], Scotland [49], and Western Australia [50] suggested an alarming trend of increasing mortality in first-admission patients with schizophrenia. Particularly striking was the standardized mortality ratio of 16.4 for males with schizophrenia in the first year after diagnosis. In the Australian study, suicide risk was highest in the first 7 days after discharge from inpatient care. These trends seem to parallel the significant reductions in the number of psychiatric beds and the concomitant pressure for early patient discharge. Whether the increases in suicide mortality are associated with the shift in the management of schizophrenia from hospital to community care remains to be established.

## Comorbidity

There is significant comorbidity in schizophrenia, comprising: (1) common medical problems and diseases that affect schizophrenia patients more frequently than attributable to chance; and (2) certain rare conditions or abnormalities which tend to co-occur with the disorder.

Physical disease is common but tends to remain often undetected and underdiagnosed. Between 46% and 80% of inpatients with schizophrenia, and between 20% and 43% of outpatients, have been found in different surveys to have concurrent medical illnesses [51]. Persons with schizophrenia, and especially those who are homeless or injection drug users, are at increased risk for potentially life-threatening communicable disease, such as HIV/AIDS, hepatitis C, and tuberculosis [52]. Among the chronic non-communicable diseases, patients with schizophrenia have significantly higher-than-expected rates of diabetes, arteriosclerosis, and ischaemic heart disease, which are increasingly contributing to their high mortality rate [54–56]. Obesity and concomitant metabolic syndrome involving insulin resistance are at present common problems in schizophrenia patients. Although a high incidence of diabetes in schizophrenia patients had been described long before the introduction of neuroleptic treatment, a contributing role for some of the drugs with antagonist properties at histamine and serotonin receptors has not been ruled out.

Some rare genetic or idiopathic disorders, such as metachromatic leukodystrophy, acute intermittent porphyria, and coeliac disease, as well as dysmorphic features such as high-steepled palate, malformed ears, and other minor physical anomalies, have also been reported to co-occur with schizophrenia [57, 58]. On the other hand, several studies have found a lower-than-expected rate of rheumatoid arthritis in schizophrenia patients [59]. A recent joint study by the Psychiatric Genomic Consortium and the Rheumatoid Arthritis Consortium analysed a large sample of cases and controls for the two disorders and concluded that the negative relationship between them reflects, 'at least in part', genetic factors [60].

## Substance abuse

Substance abuse is at present by far the most common associated health problem among patients with schizophrenia [61] and may involve any drug of abuse or a polydrug combination. It seems, however, that the addictive use of cannabis, stimulants, and nicotine is disproportionately high among schizophrenia patients and may be linked to the underlying neurobiology of the disorder. In a nationwide sample of patients with psychotic disorders in Australia [24], a lifetime diagnosis of comorbid drug abuse or dependence was made in 36.3% of males and 15.7% of females with schizophrenia (compared to 3.1% and 1.3%, respectively, in the general population). In addition to poor prognosis of schizophrenia in patients with heavy cannabis use, a systematic review of published data on cannabis exposure and the onset of schizophrenia [62] concluded that early use increased the risk of psychosis in a dose-related manner, especially in persons at high genetic risk of schizophrenia [63]. Similarly, stimulants tend to exacerbate acute psychotic symptoms in over 50% of schizophrenia patients [64]. The prevalence of cigarette smoking among schizophrenia patients is, on average, 2–3 times higher than in the general population [24], but the evidence regarding any effects of nicotine use specifically on the onset and course of schizophrenia is equivocal.

## Geographical and cultural variation

To date, no population or culture has been identified in which schizophrenic illnesses do not occur. There is also no strong evidence that the incidence of schizophrenia either is uniform or varies widely across populations, provided that the populations being compared are large enough to minimize the effects of small-area variation. The evidence that specific psychosocial or cultural factors play an aetiological role in schizophrenia is also inconsistent [65–67]. However, there are well-replicated findings of variations in the course and outcome of schizophrenia across populations and cultures that involve, above all, a higher rate of symptomatic recovery and a lower rate of social deterioration in traditional rural communities. Data supporting this conclusion were provided by the WHO studies [7, 8], which found a higher proportion of recovering or improving patients in developing countries such as India and Nigeria than in developed countries. Sampling bias (for example, a higher percentage of acute-onset schizophreniform illnesses of good prognosis among Third World patients) was not a likely explanation. A better outcome in developing countries was found in patients with various modes of onset, and the initial symptoms of the disorder did not distinguish good-outcome from poor-outcome cases. What causes such differences in the prognosis of schizophrenia remains largely unknown. The follow-up in the WHO studies demonstrated that the outcome of paranoid psychoses and affective disorders was also better in developing countries. Such a general effect on the outcome of psychiatric disorders may result from psychosocial factors such as availability of social support networks, non-stigmatizing beliefs about mental illness, and positive expectations during the early stages of psychotic illness, as well as from unknown genetic or ecological (including nutritional) factors influencing brain development.

# Variations in the course and outcome of schizophrenia

The course of schizophrenia is as variable as its symptoms. Since the great majority of schizophrenic patients are today receiving pharmacological treatment, current and recent studies may not reflect the 'natural' course and outcome of the disorder.

## The 'natural history' of schizophrenia before the neuroleptic era

Studies in urban communities in Scotland [68] and India [69] and a study in a rural community in China [70] estimated the proportions of never-hospitalized schizophrenic patients at 6.7%, 28.7%, and 30.6%, respectively. About half of the Scottish patients had been prescribed neuroleptics by their general practitioners, while the Indian and Chinese patients had been virtually untreated. In all three settings, the outcomes of these samples were heterogenous, but they did not differ much from the outcomes in treated patients. In a historical study of 70 Swedish patients with first admissions in 1925, lifetime records were retrieved and re-diagnosed in accordance with DSM-III criteria [71]. The outcome was rated as 'good' in 33% (but no patient was considered as completely recovered), as 'profoundly deteriorated' in 43%, and as intermediate in 24%.

A long-term perspective on the course of schizophrenia over successive generations is provided by a meta-analysis of 320 outcome studies on schizophrenia or *dementia praecox* published between 1895 and 1992, including a total of 51,800 subjects [72]. Overall, about 40% of the patients were reported as improved after an average length of follow-up of 5.6 years. There was a significant increase in improvement during the period 1956–1985, compared to 1895–1955, clearly related to the introduction of neuroleptic treatment, but a secular trend towards better outcomes with every successive decade had been present for much longer. Coupled with the virtual disappearance of the most 'catastrophic' forms of schizophrenia (for example, 'lethal catatonia'), these observations suggest that a transition to a less deteriorating course of the disorder had occurred prior to modern pharmacological treatment. Among the factors explaining this shift, one should consider improvements in general care and progressive changes in attitudes and hospital regime which occurred in a number of institutions on both sides of the Atlantic in the 1930s and 1940s, as well as heightened expectations that psychosocial measures, such as psychotherapy or rehabilitation, could result in a cure in some cases.

## Patterns and stages in the course of schizophrenia

The marked heterogeneity in the course of schizophrenia can be reduced to a limited number of patterns into which cases tend to cluster over time. In earlier long-term follow-up studies, 8–12 different categories of course had been described. These classifications were derived from empirical observation, rather than statistical modelling. They conflated into single categories: the mode of onset, longitudinal aspects such as frequency and duration of psychotic episodes, remissions, and end states. Treating these various aspects of the longitudinal profile of the illness as independent dimensions is today recommended [73]. However, the complexity of statistical modelling of the course of schizophrenia is such that the development of a classification of course that would be both useful in clinical practice and rigorous in a statistical sense may not be easy to achieve. Therefore, a heuristic compromise between these two requirements should, as a minimum, define operationally and assess separately: (1) the number and duration of discrete episodes of illness; (2) the predominant clinical features of each episode (for example, psychotic or affective); and (3) the number and length of remissions and their quality (presence/absence of residual negative or deficit symptoms and signs). By combining these variables, several patterns of course have been derived that have found good empirical support in international follow-up studies: (1) single psychotic episode followed by complete remission; (2) single psychotic episode followed by incomplete remission; (3) two or more psychotic episodes, with complete remissions between episodes; (4) two or more psychotic episodes, with incomplete remissions between episodes; and (5) continuous (unremitting) psychotic illness. With some modifications, these longitudinal patterns have been incorporated into research tools such as the SCAN [14].

## WHO studies on course and outcome of schizophrenia

A transcultural investigation co-ordinated by the WHO [74]—the International Study of Schizophrenia (ISoS)—which involved 18 research centres in 14 countries, achieved the tracing of 75% of cases that had been assessed in the earlier WHO studies and also included additional patient cohorts from mainland China, Hong Kong, and

India. Follow-up data were collected on a total of 1633 cases, and 890 patients were re-interviewed at either 15- or 25-year follow-up since their first assessment. The main results were as follows. Firstly, there was striking heterogeneity in the course of schizophrenia. Patients with similar baseline clinical characteristics developed a spectrum of outcomes, ranging from clinical and social recovery after a single psychotic episode to chronic unremitting psychosis and severe impairment. However, the overall rate of recovery was 48% at the 15-year follow-up and as high as 54% at the 25-year follow-up. Secondly, the frequency of both relapses and remissions increased over time. Regardless of this, the cumulative proportion of time during which patients had psychotic symptoms tended to remain stable or decrease. At 15- and 25-year follow-up, 42% and 41%, respectively, had been free of psychotic symptoms for the past 2 years. Thirdly, while the percentage of patients with continuous deteriorating illness was similar across the sites of the WHO studies, the outcome was generally better in the developing countries. This could not be attributed to any particular clinical subtype of the disorder, for example to cases of acute onset, since it applied equally to cases of slow, insidious onset. The main outcome difference across the study areas was in the average length of symptom-free remissions. No single factor accounting for this difference could be identified, but better integration of the mentally ill person in the domestic economy of traditional rural communities could be part of the explanation. It should be noted, however, that increasing social and economic stresses experienced by both urban and rural communities in many developing countries may have eroded the traditional support systems, resulting in worse outcomes, as suggested by several recent studies. Fourthly, whether the better outcome of schizophrenia in developing countries is 'transportable' following migration to other settings remains unclear. Data on immigrants treated for first episodes of schizophrenia in the UK suggest that while Asian patients have lower relapse and readmission rates than British-born whites, Afro-Caribbean immigrants show a higher rate. Marked social and family structure differences between the Asian and Afro-Caribbean immigrant communities suggest that the likelihood of a more benign course may depend on the degree to which the immigrant group has retained its traditional values and intra-group cohesion [75].

## Factors maintaining the incidence of schizophrenia in populations

Coupled with the evidence that the lifetime risk of the disorder (about 1%) is similar across populations, the question about factors that sustain the incidence of schizophrenia despite reduced reproductive fitness remains open. Schizophrenia is a complex polygenic disorder, with incomplete or variable penetrance of the genotype and widespread locus and allelic heterogeneity. The polygenic model implies that loss of risk alleles resulting from the lower reproductive fitness of affected individuals would have a negligible effect on the overall gene pool in the population. Previous conjectures that *de novo* germ-line mutations inherited from an ageing father may be responsible for a substantial proportion of incident cases of schizophrenia [76] is difficult to reconcile with current knowledge that mutation rates for most human genes are within the range of $10^{-6}$–$10^{-5}$ per generation, that is, their contribution to the maintenance of schizophrenia in the population would be insignificant. Considering that both multiple genes and multiple exogenous factors are likely to be involved in the causation of schizophrenia, neither increased fertility in asymptomatic carriers of the risk genes nor paternal inheritance of germ-line mutations appear to be either necessary or sufficient for the persistence of the disorder.

### Genetic risk: necessary and sufficient?

Family aggregation of schizophrenia is at present the only epidemiologically well-established risk factor for the disorder, with a relative risk for first-degree relatives of persons with schizophrenia in the range of 6–17% [78]. Allowing for diagnostic variation, the risk estimates generated by different studies are similar and suggest a general pattern of descending risk as the proportions of shared genes between any two individuals decrease. Although heritability of schizophrenia (commonly estimated at about 80%) provides the basis for the search of specific genes, gene networks, and regulatory polymorphisms involved in schizophrenia causation, the extent to which genetic vulnerability alone is necessary and sufficient to produce the disorder remains unclear. While an environmental contribution to the aetiology of schizophrenia is highly plausible, the evidence in support of it is inferential, typically proceeding from the early observation that the concordance for schizophrenia in monozygotic twins (sharing 100% of their genes) is only about 50%. The majority of investigators now agree that genes and environments should be studied jointly, and three models of conjunction have been proposed [79]: (1) the effects of predisposing genes and environmental factors are additive and increase the risk of disease in a linear fashion; (2) genes modulate the sensitivity of the brain to environmental insults; and (3) by fostering certain personality traits and associated behaviour, genes influence the likelihood of an individual's exposure to stressful environments.

### Environmental insults during gestation and fetal development

A winter–spring excess of schizophrenic births was first described in 1929 [80] and since then reported by numerous studies, mostly in the northern hemisphere (southern hemisphere data are less consistent). Though some of these studies did not definitively prove or rule out a seasonal effect, winter–spring births were associated with a mild, but significant, increase in the relative risk (RR) for schizophrenia (RR = 1.11; CI 1.06–1.18) in a large population cohort from Denmark [81]. Thus, birth seasonality appears to be a robust finding, though few biologically testable hypotheses have been advanced to explain it. One of them is the seasonally increased risk of intrauterine exposure to viral infection *in utero*. Exposure to influenza has been implicated as a risk factor since a report that a significant proportion of adult schizophrenia in Helsinki was associated with presumed second-trimester *in utero* exposure to the 1957 A2 influenza epidemic [82]. Numerous studies, attempting to replicate the link between maternal influenza and schizophrenia, have since reached conflicting results, with negative findings reported from an increasing number of studies based on large population samples [83], as well as studies including data on schizophrenia risk in the offspring of women with prospectively recorded influenza infection during pregnancy [84]. However, positive associations between schizophrenia in the offspring and maternal infection during pregnancy has been reported for rubella [85] and toxoplasmosis [86], and the issue of prenatal infection contributing to schizophrenia risk merits further study. Maternal obstetric complications, ranging from placental abnormalities in the first trimester of pregnancy to diabetes, pre-eclampsia, perinatal hypoxia, and low birthweight, are widely regarded to be risk factors in schizophrenia. Population-based studies [87] using prospectively recorded obstetric data tend to report conflicting or inconclusive results, with generally small effect sizes (odds ratio of <2) for any positive findings [88]. However, several birth cohort studies with long-term follow-up have found significantly increased risk of adult schizophrenia in individuals who had survived severe, mainly hypoxic perinatal brain damage [88]. Birthweight (adjusted for gestation) is another factor that may have a complex relationship with schizophrenia risk. A large cohort study in Sweden [89] found significant hazard ratios of 7.03 for males of low birthweight (<2500 g) and 3.37 for those of high birthweight (>4000 g). It remains unclear, however, if severe obstetric complications, such as perinatal hypoxia or low birthweight, are capable of raising substantially the risk of schizophrenia in an adult in the absence of increased genetic risk. Maternal schizophrenia is associated with a higher rate of pregnancy complications, including low birthweight [90], but it is not known if the effects of genetic liability and obstetric complications on schizophrenia risk in the offspring are additive or interactive. It is also possible that genetic predisposition sensitizes the developing brain to lesions resulting from randomly occurring, less severe obstetric complications. Such gaps in knowledge or inconsistencies among research findings point to the clarification of these issues as a priority for epidemiological research.

### Early developmental antecedents of schizophrenia

Children at high genetic risk for schizophrenia (that is, having parents or other first-degree relatives with the disorder) tend to show early signs of aberrant neurodevelopment, including ventricular enlargement on computerized tomography [91] and decreased activation in the prefrontal and parietal regions of the heteromodal association cortex on functional magnetic resonance imaging [92]. The results of such imaging studies are limited by small sample size and may not be generalizable. However, population-based or cohort studies, such as the National Child Development Study in the UK, have demonstrated a higher incidence of abnormal motor and speech development before 2 years of age and of soft neurological signs (poor motor control, co-ordination, and balance), non-right-handedness, and speech defects between the ages of 2–15 [93]. Cognitive deficits involving verbal memory, sustained attention, and executive functions, as well as abnormalities in event-related brain potentials and oculomotor control [94–96], are common in patients with schizophrenia and antedate the onset of clinical symptoms. They also occur in a proportion of their clinically normal biological relatives but are rare in control subjects drawn from the general population. Their specificity to schizophrenia needs to be investigated in larger population samples. Should such *endophenotypes* be validated as biological markers of schizophrenia, the power of risk prediction at the level of the individual is likely to increase substantially. In a Swedish cohort study [97] involving a 15-year follow-up of 109,643 men conscripted into the army at the age of 18–20, the individuals who subsequently developed schizophrenia were compared with the rest of the cohort on the performance of IQ-related tests and tasks at the time of conscription. Controlling for potential confounders, the risk of schizophrenia was found to increase linearly with the decrement of IQ. The effect was mainly attributable to poor performance on verbal tasks and tests of reasoning.

### Premorbid social impairment

Individuals who develop schizophrenia as adults are more likely to manifest difficulties in social interaction during childhood and adolescence than individuals who do not develop schizophrenia. Population-based evidence of early socialization difficulties (school problems, social anxiety, and preference for solitary play) in children who develop schizophrenia as adults is provided by the prospective study of a national birth cohort in the UK [93]. It should be noted, however, that the early behavioural traits that tend to be associated with schizophrenia in adult life have low specificity and their predictive value is limited.

### Early rearing environment

Support for an effect of the early rearing family environment on the risk of developing schizophrenia is provided by a study of a Finnish sample of adopted children born to mothers with schizophrenia (a high-risk group) and a control sample of adoptees at no increased genetic risk [98]. Though the rates of adult psychosis or severe personality disorder were significantly higher in the high-risk group, compared with the control group, the difference was entirely attributable to a subset of the high-risk children who grew up in dysfunctional or otherwise disturbed adoptive families—a result consistent with the gene–environment model of genetic influence on a person's sensitivity to psychosocial adversity.

### The urban environment

Earlier hypotheses that urban environments increase the risk of psychosis, either by contributing to causation (the breeder effect) or by attracting vulnerable individuals (the drift effect), have been more recently revived in the light of epidemiological findings suggesting that urban birth is associated with a moderate, but statistically significant, increase in the incidence of schizophrenia, affective psychoses, and other non-affective psychoses [99]. It remains unclear whether the effect is linked to a factor operating pre- or perinatally, or a factor influencing postnatal development.

### Socio-economic disadvantage

Since the 1930s, numerous studies in North America and Europe have consistently found that the economically disadvantaged social groups contribute disproportionately to the first-admission rate for schizophrenia. Two explanatory hypotheses of social causation ('breeder') and of social selection ('drift') were originally proposed [100]. According to the social causation theory, greater socio-economic adversity, characteristic of lower-class living conditions, could precipitate psychosis in genetically vulnerable individuals who have a restricted capacity to cope with complex or stressful situations. However, another study [101] found that the social class distribution of fathers of schizophrenic patients did not deviate from that of the general population, and that the excess of low socio-economic status among schizophrenic patients was mainly attributable to individuals who had drifted down the occupational and social scale prior to the onset of psychosis. As a result, aetiological research in schizophrenia in recent decades has tended to ignore such 'macrosocial' variables. However, the possibility remains that social stratification, socio-economic status, and acculturation stress are contributing factors in the causation of schizophrenia.

## Migrants and ethnic minorities

An exceptionally high incidence rate of schizophrenia (about 6.0 per 1000) has been reported to be found in the African–Caribbean population in the UK [102, 103]. The excess morbidity is not restricted to recent immigrants and is higher in the British-born second generation of migrants. Similar findings of nearly 4-fold excess over the general population rate have been reported for the Dutch Antillean and Surinamese immigrants in Holland [104]. The causes of this phenomenon remain obscure. Incidence studies in the Caribbean do not indicate any excess morbidity in the indigenous populations from which migrants are recruited. Explanations in terms of biological risk factors have found little support. A finding in need of replication is the significant increase of schizophrenia among the siblings of second-generation African–Caribbean schizophrenia patients, compared with the incidence of schizophrenia in the siblings of white patients [105]. Such 'horizontal' increase in the morbid risk suggests that an environmental factor may be modifying the penetrance of the genetic predisposition to schizophrenia carried by a proportion of the African–Caribbean population. Psychosocial hypotheses involving acculturation stress, demoralization due to racial discrimination, and blocked opportunities for upward social mobility have been suggested but not yet definitively tested.

## Can schizophrenia be prevented?

Increasing investment in early diagnosis and treatment of schizophrenia raises important questions of whether people likely to develop schizophrenia can be reliably recognized at the prodromal stage, prior to the onset of symptoms, or even earlier, with a view to pharmacological, cognitive, or social interventions aiming to primary prevention of the disorder [111]. Early diagnosis and treatment of symptomatic cases can have an effect on the short- or medium-term outcome, but the population-wide detection of people at risk is problematic. Screening young age groups in the population for predictors, such as family history of psychosis, obstetric complications, or abnormal eye tracking, is likely to end up in multiple false-positive and false-negative results and a generally low positive predictive value. Problems of reliability of measurement apart, population-based screening will pose huge practical and ethical problems of having to treat a large number of individuals who do not have the disorder and missing many others who eventually will develop the disorder. While pre-symptomatic detection and preventative intervention in schizophrenia do not, at present, appear to be feasible, secondary prevention, aiming at optimizing the treatment of early symptomatic cases and supporting their social, educational, or occupational functioning, has the potential for improving the prognosis and outcome of the disorder.

## Summary and conclusions

After many decades of epidemiological research, essential questions about the nature and causes of schizophrenia still await answers [106]. However, two major conclusions stand out.

- Schizophrenia is characterized by phenotypic variability and likely genetic heterogeneity. While the clinical concept of schizophrenia as a broad syndrome with some internal cohesion and characteristic patterns of course over time is well supported by epidemiological evidence, its dissection into modular subtypes with specific neurocognitive and neurophysiological underpinnings is beginning to be perceived as a promising approach in schizophrenia genetics. The study of endophenotypes cutting across the conventional diagnostic boundaries may reveal unexpected patterns of associations with symptoms, personality traits, or behaviours, as well as genetic polymorphisms, providing epidemiology with rich material for future hypothesis testing at the population level.

- No single environmental risk factor of major effect on the incidence of schizophrenia has yet been established. Further studies using large samples are required to evaluate potential risk factors, antecedents, and predictors for which the present evidence is inconclusive. Assuming that multiple environmental risk factors of small to moderate effect will eventually be identified, the results will complement those of genetic research.

## REFERENCES

1. Kraepelin, E. (1896). *Psychiatrie. Ein Lehrbuch für Studirende und Aerzte*. Barth, Leipzig (reprint edition 1976 by Arno Press Inc., New York, NY).
2. Koller, J. (1895). Beitrag zur Erblichkeitsstatisyik der Geisteskrankheiten in Canton Zürich. *Archiv für Psychiatrie*, 27, 269–94.
3. Luxenburger, H. (1928). Vorläufiger Bericht über psychiatrische Serienuntersuchungen an Zwillingen. *Zeitschrift für die gesamte Neurologie und Psychiatrie*, 116, 297–326.
4. Brugger, C. (1931). Versuch einer Geisteskrankenzählung in Thüringen. *Zeitschrift für die gesamte Neurologie und Psychiatrie*, 133, 252–390.
5. Klemperer, J. (1933). Zur Belastungsstatistik der Durchschnittbevölkerung. Psychosenhäufigkeit unter 1000 stichprobenmässig ausgelesenen Probanden. *Zeitschrift für die gesamte Neurologie und Psychiatrie*, 146, 277–316.
6. Essen-Möller, E., Larsson, H., Uddenberg, C.E. *et al.* (1956). Individual traits and morbidity in a Swedish rural population. *Acta Psychiatrica et Neurologica Scandinavica*, 100 (Suppl), 1–136.
7. World Health Organization. (1973). *The International Pilot Study of Schizophrenia*, Vol. 1. World Health Organization, Geneva.
8. Jablensky, A., Sartorius, N., Ernberg, G. *et al.* (1992). Schizophrenia: manifestations and course in different cultures. A World Health Organization ten-country study. *Psychological Medicine*, Monograph Supplement, 20, 1–97.
9. Robins, L.N. and Regier, D.A. (eds.) (1991). *Psychiatric Disorders in America. The Epidemiologic Catchment Area Study*. Free Press, New York, NY.
10. Kessler, R.C., McGonagle, K.A., Zhao, S. *et al.* (1994). Lifetime and 12-month prevalence of DSM-IIIR psychiatric disorders in the United States. Results from the National Comorbidity Survey. *Archives of General Psychiatry*, 51, 8–19.
11. Morgan, V.A., Valuri, G.M., Croft, M.L. *et al.* (2011). Cohort profile: pathways of risk from conception to disease: the Western Australian schizophrenia high-risk e-cohort. *International Journal of Epidemiology*, 40, 1477–85.

12. Wing, J.K., Cooper, J.E., and Sartorius, N. (1974). *The Measurement and Classification of Psychiatric Symptoms.* Cambridge University Press, Cambridge.

13. Robins, L.N., Wing, J., Wittchen, H.U. *et al.* (1988). The Composite International Diagnostic Interview: an epidemiological instrument suitable for use in conjunction with different diagnostic systems and in different cultures. *Archives of General Psychiatry*, 45, 1069–77.

14. Wing, J.K., Babor, T., Brigha, T. *et al.* (1990). SCAN. Schedules for clinical assessment in neuropsychiatry. *Archives of General Psychiatry*, 47, 589–93.

15. Saha, S., Chant, D., Welham, J., and McGrath, J. (2005). A systematic review of the prevalence of schizophrenia. *PLoS Medicine*, 2, e141.

16. Simeone, J.C., Ward, A.J., Rotella, P. *et al.* (2015). An evaluation of published estimates of schizophrenia prevalence from 1990–2013: a systematic literature review. *BMC Psychiatry*, 15, 193.

17. Bøjholm, S. and Strömgren, E. (1989). Prevalence of schizophrenia on the island of Bornholm in 1935 and in 1983. *Acta Psychiatrica Scandinavica*, 79 (Suppl. 348), 157–66.

18. Böök, J.A. (1953). A genetic and neuropsychiatric investigation of a North Swedish population (with special regard to schizophrenia and mental deficiency). *Acta Genetica*, 4, 1–100.

19. Böök, J.A., Wettenberg, L., and Modrzewska, K. (1978). Schizophrenia in a North Swedish geographical isolate, 1900–1977: epidemiology, genetics and biochemistry. *Clinical Genetics*, 14, 373–94.

20. Crocetti, G.J., Lemkau, P.V., Kulcar, Z. *et al.* (1971). Selected aspects of the epidemiology of psychoses in Croatia, Yugoslavia, II. The cluster sample and the results of the pilot survey. *American Journal of Epidemiology*, 94, 126–34.

21. Dube, K.V. and Kumar, N. (1972). An epidemiological study of schizophrenia. *Journal of Biosocial Science*, 4, 187–95.

22. Keith, S.J., Regier, D.A., and Rae, D.S. (1991). Schizophrenic disorders. In: *Psychiatric Disorders in America. The Epidemiologic Catchment Area Study* (eds. L.N. Robins and D.A. Regier), pp. 33–52. Free Press, New York, NY.

23. Jeffreys, S.E., Harvey, C.A., NcNaught, A.S. *et al.* (1997). The Hampstead schizophrenia survey 1991. I. Prevalence and service use comparisons in an inner London health authority, 1986–1991. *British Journal of Psychiatry*, 170, 301–6.

24. Jablensky, A., McGrath, J., Herrman, H. *et al.* (2000). Psychotic disorders in urban areas: an overview of the Study on Low Prevalence Disorders. *Australian and New Zealand Journal of Psychiatry*, 34, 221–36.

25. Perälä, J., Suvisaari, J. Saarni, S.I. *et al.* (2007). Lifetime prevalence of psychotic and bipolar I disorders in a general population. *Archives of General Psychiatry*, 64, 19–28.

26. Morgan, V.A., McGrath, J.J., Jablensky, A. *et al.* (2014). Psychosis prevalence and physical, metabolic and cognitive co-morbidity: data from the second Australian national survey of psychosis. *Psychological Medicine*, 44, 2163–76.

27. Eaton, W. and Weil, R.J. (1955). *Culture and Mental Disorder. A Comparative Study of the Hutterites and Other Populations.* Free Press, Glencoe, IL.

28. Lin, T.Y., Chu, H.M., Rin, H. *et al.* (1989). Effects of social change on mental disorders in Taiwan: observations based on a 15-year follow-up survey of general population in three communities. *Acta Psychiatrica Scandinavica*, 79 (Suppl. 348), 11–34.

29. Messias E.L., Chen, C.Y., and Eaton, W.W. (2007). Epidemiology of schizophrenia: review of findings and myths. *Psychiatric Clinics of North America*, 30, 323–38.

30. McGrath, J., Saha, S. Welham, J. *et al.* (2004). A systematic review of the incidence of schizophrenia: the distribution of rates and the influence of sex, urbanicity, migrant status and methodology. *BMC Medicine*, 2, 13.

31. Kirkbride, J.B., Errazuriz, A., Croudace, T.J. *et al.* (2012). Incidence of schizophrenia and other psychoses in England, 1950–2009: a systematic review and meta-analyses. *PLoS One*, 7, 3.

32. Ödegaard, Ö. (1946). A statistical investigation into the incidence of mental disorders in Norway. *Psychiatric Quarterly*, 20, 381–401.

33. Walsh, D. (1969). Mental illness in Dublin—first admissions. *British Journal of Psychiatry*, 115, 449–56.

34. Murphy, H.B.M. and Raman, A.C. (1971). The chronicity of schizophrenia in indigenous tropical people. Results of a twelve-year follow-up survey in Mauritius. *British Journal of Psychiatry*, 118, 489–97.

35. Helgason, I., (1977). Psychiatric services and mental illness in Iceland. *Acta Psychiatrica Scandinavica*, 53 (Suppl. 268), 1–140.

36. Rajkumar, S. Padmavati, R., Thara, R. *et al.* (1993). Incidence of schizophrenia in an urban community in Madras. *Indian Journal of Psychiatry*, 35, 11–17.

37. Brewin, J., Cantwell, R. Dalkin, T. *et al.* (1997). Incidence of schizophrenia in Nottingham. *British Journal of Psychiatry*, 171, 140–4.

38. Mahy, G.E., Mallett, R., Leff, J. *et al.* (1999). First-contact incidence rate of schizophrenia on Barbados. *British Journal of Psychiatry*, 175, 28–33.

39. Murthy, G.V.S., Janakiramaiah, N., Gangadhar, B.N. *et al.* (1998) Sex difference in age at onset of schizophrenia: discrepant findings from India. *Acta Psychiatrica Scandinavica*, 97, 321–5.

40. Phillips, M.R., Yang, G., Li, S. *et al.* (2004) Suicide and the unique prevalence pattern of schizophrenia in mainland China: a retrospective observational study. *The Lancet*, 364, 1062–8.

41. Helgason T. and Magnusson, H. (1989). The first 80 years of life. A psychiatric epidemiological study. *Acta Psychiatrica Scandinavica*, 79 (Suppl. 348), 85–94.

42. Ödegaard, Ö. (1980). Fertility of psychiatric first admissions in Norway, 1936–1975. *Acta Psychiatrica Scandinavica*, 62, 212–20.

43. Brown, S. (1997). Excess mortality in schizophrenia. A meta-analysis. *British Journal of Psychiatry*, 171, 502–8.

44. Dupont, A., Jensen, O.M., Strömgren, E. *et al.* (1986). Incidence of cancer in patients diagnosed as schizophrenia in Denmark. In: *Psychiatric Case Registers in Public Health* (eds. S.H. Ten Horn, R. Giel, and W. Gulbinat), pp. 229–39, Elsevier, Amsterdam.

45. Dalton, S.O., Mellemkjaer L., Thomassen, L. *et al.* (2005). Risk for cancer in a cohort of patients hospitalized for schizophrenia in Denmark, 1969–1993. *Schizophrenia Research*, 75, 315–24.

46. Grinspoon, A., Barchana, M., Ponizovsky, A. *et al.* (2005). Cancer in schizophrenia: is the risk higher or lower? *Schizophrenia Research*, 73, 333–41.

47. Heilä, H. and Lönqvist, J. (2003). The clinical epidemiology of suicide in schizophrenia. In: *The Epidemiology of Schizophrenia* (eds. R.M. Murray, P. Jones, E. Susser, J. van Os, and M. Cannon), pp. 288–314. Cambridge University Press, Cambridge.

48. Mortensen, P.B. and Juel, K. (1993). Mortality and causes of death in first admitted schizophrenia patients. *British Journal of Psychiatry*, 163, 183–9.

49. Geddes, J.R. and Juszczak, E. (1995). Period trends in rate of suicide in first 28 days after discharge from psychiatric hospital in Scotland, 1968–92. *BMJ*, 311, 357–60.

50. Lawrence, D., Holman, C.D.J., Jablensky A. *et al.* (2001). Increasing rates of suicide in Western Australian psychiatric

patients: a record linkage study. *Acta Psychiatrica Scandinavica*, 104, 443–51.

51. Jeste D.V., Gladsjo, J.A., Lindamer, L.A. *et al.* (1966). Medical comorbidity in schizophrenia. *Schizophrenia Bulletin*, 22, 413–30.

52. Susser E., Valencia, E., and Conover, S. (1993). Prevalence of HIV infection among psychiatric patients in a New Yorl City men's shelter. *American Journal of Public Health*, 83, 568–70.

53. Mortensen, P.B. (2003). Mortality and physical illness in schizophrenia. In: *The Epidemiology of Schizophrenia* (eds. R.M. Murray, P. Jones, E. Susser, J. van Os, and M. Cannon), pp. 275–87. Cambridge University Press, Cambridge.

54. Lawrence, D.M., Holman, C.D.J., Jablensky, A.V. *et al.* (2003). Death rate from ischaemic heart disease in Western Australian psychiatric patients 1980–1998. *British Journal of Psychiatry*, 182, 32–6.

55. Goff, D.C., Sullivan, L.M., McEvoy, J.P. *et al.* (2005). A comparison of ten-year cardiac risk estimates in schizophrenia patients from the CATIE study and matched controls. *Schizophrenia Research*, 80, 45–53.

56. Saari, K.M., Lindeman, S.M., Viilo, K.M. *et al.* (2005). A 4-fold risk of metabolic syndrome in patients with schizophrenia: the Northern Finland 1966 birth cohort study. *Journal of Clinical Psychiatry*, 66, 559–63.

57. Hyde, T.M., Ziegler, J.C., and Weinberger, D. (1992). Psychiatric disturbances in metachromatic leucodystrophy. *Archives of Neurology*, 49, 401–6.

58. Murphy, K.C. and Owen, M.J. (1996). Minor physical anomalies and their relationship to the aetiology of schizophrenia. *British Journal of Psychiatry*, 168, 139–42.

59. Eaton, W.M., Hayward, C., and Ram, R. (1992). Schizophrenia and rheumatoid arthritis: a review. *Schizophrenia Research*, 6, 181–92.

60. Lee, S.H., Byrne, E.M., Hultman, C.M. *et al.* (2015). New data and an old puzzle: the negative association between schizophrenia and rheumatoid arthritis. *International Journal of Epidemiology*, 44, 1706–21.

61. Murray, R.M., Grech, A., Phillips, P. *et al.* (2003). What is the relationship between substance abuse and schizophrenia? In: *The Epidemiology of Schizophrenia* (eds. R.M. Murray, P. Jones, E. Susser, J. van Os, and M. Cannon), pp. 317–42. Cambridge University Press, Cambridge.

62. Semple, D.M., McIntosh, A.M., and Lawrie, S.M. (2005). Cannabis as a risk factor for psychosis: systematic review. *Journal of Psychopharmacology*, 19, 187–94.

63. Stefanis, N.C., Dragovic, M., Power, B.D. *et al.* (2013). Age at initiation of cannabis use predicts age at onset of psychosis: the 7- to 8-year trend. *Schizophrenia Bulletin*, 39, 251–4.

64. Curran, C., Byrappa, N., and McBride, A. (2004). Stimulant psychosis: systematic review. *British Journal of Psychiatry*, 185, 196–204.

65. Jablensky, A. (2000). Epidemiology of schizophrenia: the global burden of disease and disability. *European Archives of Psychiatry and Clinical Neuroscience*, 250, 274–85.

66. Boydell, J. and Murray, R. (2003). Urbanization, migration and risk of schizophrenia. In: *The Epidemiology of Schizophrenia* (eds. R.M. Murray, P. Jones, E. Susser, J. van Os, and M. Cannon), pp. 49–67. Cambridge University Press, Cambridge.

67. Murray, C.J.L. and Lopez, A.D. (eds.) *The Global Burden of Disease. A Comprehensive Assessment of Mortality and Disability from Diseases, Injuries, and Risk Factors in 1990 and Projected to 2020.* Harvard School of Public Health, Cambridge, MA.

68. Geddes, J.R. and Kendell, R.E. (1995). Schizophrenic subjects with no history of admission to hospital. *Psychological Medicine*, 25, 859–68.

69. Padmavathi, R., Rajkumar, S., and Srinivasan, T.N. (1998). Schizophrenic patients who were never treated—a study in an Indian urban community. *Psychological Medicine*, 28, 1113–17.

70. Ran, M., Xiang, M., Huang, M. *et al.* (2001). Natural course of schizophrenia: 2-year follow-up study in a rural Chinese community. *British Journal of Psychiatry*, 178, 154–8.

71. Jonsson, S.A.T. and Jonsson, H. (1992). Outcome of untreated schizophrenia: a search for symptoms and traits with prognostic meaning in patients admitted to a mental hospital in the preneuroleptic era. *Acta Psychiatrica Scandinavica*, 85, 313–20.

72. Hegarty, J.D., Baldessarini, R.J., Tohen, M. *et al.* (1994). One hundred years of schizophrenia: a meta-analysis of the outcome literature. *American Journal of Psychiatry*, 151, 1409–16.

73. Johnstone, E.C., Macmillan, J.E., Frith, C.D. *et al.* (1990). Further investigation of the predictors of outcome following first schizophrenic episodes. *British Journal of Psychiatry*, 157, 182–9.

74. Hopper, K, Harrison, G., and Wanderling, J.A. (2007). An overview of course and outcome in ISoS. In: *Recovery from Schizophrenia. An International Perspective. A report from the WHO Collaborative Project, the International Study of Schizophrenia* (eds. K. Hopper, G. Harrison, A. Janca, and N. Sartorius), pp. 23–38. World Health Organization, Geneva.

75. Borque, F., van der Ven, E., and Malla, A. (2011). A meta-analysis of the risk for psychotic disorders among first- and second-generation immigrants. *Psychological Medicine*, 5, 897–910.

76. Sipos, A., Rasmussen, F., Harrison, G. *et al.* (2004). Paternal age and schizophrenia: a population based cohort study. *BMJ*, 330, 147–8.

78. Gottersman II, Laursen, T.M., Bertelsen, A., and Mortensen, P.B. (2010). Severe mental disorders in offspring with 2 psychiatrically ill parents. *Archives of General Psychiatry*, 67, 252–7.

79. Kendler, K.S. and Eaves, L.J. (1986). Models for the joint effect of genotype and environment on liability to psychiatric illness. *American Journal of Psychiatry*, 143, 279–89.

80. Tramer, M. (1929). Über die biologische Bedeutung des Geburtsmonates, insbesondere für die Psychoseerkrankung. *Schweizerischer Archiv für Neurologie und Psychiatrie*, 24, 17–24.

81. Mortensen, P.B., Pedersen, C.B., Westergaard, T. *et al.* (1999). Effects of family history and place and season of birth on the risk of schizophrenia. *New England Journal of Medicine*, 340, 603–8.

82. Mednick, S.A., Machon, R.A., Huttunen, M.O. *et al.* (1988). Adult schizophrenia following prenatal exposure to an influenza epidemic. *Archives of General Psychiatry*, 45, 189–92.

83. Morgan, V., Castle, D., Page, A. *et al.* (1997). Influenza epidemic and incidence of schizophrenia, affective disorders and mental retardation in Western Australia: no evidence of a major effect. *Schizophrenia Research*, 26, 25–39.

84. Cannon, M., Cotter, D., Coffey, V.P. *et al.* (1996). Prenatal exposure to the 1957 influenza epidemic and adult schizophrenia: a follow-up study. *British Journal of Psychiatry*, 168, 368–71.

85. Brown, A.S., Cohen, P., Harkavy-Friedman, J. *et al.* (2001). Prenatal rubella, premorbid abnormalities, an adult schizophrenia. *Biological Psychiatry*, 49, 473–86.

86. Brown, A.S., Schaefer, C.A., Quesenberry, C.P. *et al.* (2005). Maternal exposure to toxoplasmosis and risk of schizophrenia in the offspring. *American Journal of Psychiatry*, 162, 767–73.

87. Buka, S.L., Tsuang, M.T., and Lipsitt, L.P. (1993). Pregnancy/delivery complications and psychiatric diagnosis: a prospective study. *Archives of General Psychiatry*, 50, 151–6.

88. Zornberg, G.L., Buka, S.L., and Tsuang, M.T. (2000). Hypoxic-ischemia-related fetal/neonatal complications and risk of schizophrenia and other nonaffective psychoses: a 19-year longitudinal study. *American Journal of Psychiatry*, 157, 96–202.

89. Bennedsen, B.E., Mortensen, P.B., Olesen, A.V. *et al.* (2001). Obstetric complications in women with schizophrenia. *Schizophrenia Research*, 47, 167–75.

90. Jablensky, A.V., Morgan, V., Zubrick, S.R. *et al.* (2005). Pregnancy, delivery, and neonatal complications in a population cohort of women with schizophrenia and major affective disorders. *American Journal of Psychiatry*, 50, 551–64.

91. Cannon, T.D., Mednick, S.A., Parnas, J. *et al.* (1993). Developmental brain abnormalities in the offspring of schizophrenic mothers. *Archives of General Psychiatry*, 50, 551–64.

92. Keshavan, M.S., Diwadkar, V.A., Spencer, S.M. *et al.* (2002). A preliminary functional magnetic resonance imaging study in offspring of schizophrenia patients. *Progress in Neuro-Psychopharmacology and Biological Psychiatry*, 26, 1143–9.

93. Leask, S.J., Done, D.J., and Crow, T.J. (2002). Adult psychosis, common childhood infections and neurological soft signs in a national birth cohort. *British Journal of Psychiatry*, 181, 387–92.

94. Thaden, E., Rhinewine, J.P., Lencz, T. *et al.* (2006). Early-onset schizophrenia is associated with impaired adolescent development of attentional capacity using the identical pairs continuous performance test. *Schizophrenia Research*, 81, 157–66.

95. Winterer, G., Egan, M.F., Raedler, T. *et al.* (2003). P300 and genetic risk for schizophrenia. *Archives of General Psychiatry*, 60, 1158–67.

96. Calkins, M.E., Curtis, C.E., Iacono, W.G. *et al.* (2004). Antisaccade performance is impaired in medically and psychiatrically healthy biological relatives of schizophrenia patients. *Schizophrenia Research*, 71, 167–78.

97. Zammitt, S., Allebeck, P., David, A.S. *et al.* (2004). A longitudinal study of premorbid IQ score and risk developing schizophrenia, bipolar disorder, severe depression, and other nonaffective psychoses. *Archives of General Psychiatry*, 61, 354–60.

98. Wahlberg, K.E., Wynne, L.C., Oja, H. *et al.* (1997). Gene-environment interaction in vulnerability to schizophrenia: findings from the Finnish adoptive family study of schizophrenia. *American Journal of Psychiatry*, 154, 355–62.

99. van Os, J., Hanssen, M., Bak, M. *et al.* (2003). Do urbanicity and familial liability coparticipate in causing psychosis? *American Journal of Psychiatry*, 160, 477–82.

100. Goldberg, E.M. and Morrison, S.L. (1963). Schizophrenia and social class. *British Journal of Psychiatry*, 109, 785–802.

101. Mischler, E.G. and Scotch, N.A. (1983). Sociocultural factors in the epidemiology of schizophrenia: a review. *Psychiatry*, 26, 315–51.

102. Bhugra, D., Leff, J., Mallett, R. *et al.* (1997). Incidence and outcomes of schizophrenia in Whites, African-Caribbeans, and Asians in London. *Psychological Medicine*, 27, 791–8.

103. Harrison, G., Glazebrook, C., Brewin, J. *et al.* (1997). Increased incidence of psychotic disorders in migrants from the Caribbean to the United Kingdom. *Psychological Medicine*, 27, 799–806.

104. Selten, J.P., Slaets, J.P.I., and Kahn, R.S. (1997). Schizophrenia in the Surinamese and Dutch Antillean immigrants to the Netherlands; evidence of an increased incidence. *Psychological Medicine*, 27, 807–11.

105. Hutchinson, G., Takei, N., Fahy, T.A. *et al.* (1998). Morbid risk of schizophrenia in first-degree relatives of White and African-Caribbean patients with psychosis. *British Journal of Psychiatry*, 169, 776–80.

106. Heilbronner, U., Samara, M., Leucht, S. *et al.* (2016). The longitudinal course of schizophrenia across the lifespan: clinical, cognitive, and neurobiological aspects. *Harvard Review of Psychiatry*, 24, 118–28.

107. Bleuler, M. (1978). *The Schizophrenic Disorders. Long-term Patient and Family Studies.* Yale University Press, New Haven, CA.

108. Tsuang, M, Woolson, R., and Fleming, J. (1979). Long-term outcome of major psychoses. I. Schizophrenia and affective disorders compared with psychiatrically symptom-free surgical conditions. *Archives of General Psychiatry*, 36, 1295–301.

109. Ciompi, I. (1980). Catamnestic long-term study on the course of life and aging of schizophrenics. *Schizophrenia Bulletin*, 6, 606–18.

110. Huber, G., Gross, G., Schüttler, R. *et al.* (1980). Longitudinal studies of schizophrenic patients. *Schizophrenia Bulletin*, 6, 592–605.

111. Brown, A.S. and McGrath, J.J. (2010). The prevention of schizophrenia. *Schizophrenia Bulletin*, 37, 257–61.

# 59

# Genetics of schizophrenia

*Kimberley M. Kendall, James T.R. Walters, and Michael C. O'Donovan*

## Genetic epidemiology

The main focus of this chapter is the progress that has occurred over the past 10 years in identifying molecular genetic risk factors for schizophrenia. The recent successes have required persistence in the face of considerable adversity. Some of the barriers to progress reflect difficulties inherent in genetic studies of almost any complex disorder, medical or psychiatric. Others reflect the particular challenges of studying heterogenous psychiatric disorders where the diagnostic categories are, at best, of uncertain validity (see Chapters 7 and 8). That molecular genetic research in schizophrenia has been allowed to continue, and ultimately flourish, owes much to the work of genetic epidemiologists who, over many decades, have consistently documented a substantial heritable component to variation in liability to schizophrenia. This section provides a brief consideration of that essential underpinning work; readers with a particular interest in this work, much of it historical, are directed to authoritative reviews elsewhere [1–3].

### Family studies

Family studies spanning much of the 1900s demonstrated that first-degree relatives of index cases with schizophrenia (probands) had a higher risk, about 10-fold, of developing the disorder than the population at large [1]. The validity of these early studies was often questioned, given methodological shortcomings, for example lack of control groups, biased ascertainment, diagnoses that were not blind to family relationships, and diagnoses which were unreliable in the absence of operational diagnostic criteria. However, from the 1980s onwards, a wave of more sophisticated studies addressed these deficiencies; overall, they consistently supported the earlier work [1, 3]. For example, the risk for siblings of probands with schizophrenia is around 8–10% (Fig. 59.1). At first inspection, the lifetime risk of schizophrenia among parents of an affected individual (6%) seems low, compared with other first-degree relatives (siblings and offspring). However, due to low fecundity associated with schizophrenia [4], parents as a general class have a low risk of the disorder, and when risk is expressed relative to population baseline rates, the relative risk is similar (around 9–10) for parents, siblings, and children of an affected individual [5].

Compared with earlier plots of morbid risk [1], the inclusion of newer data in Fig. 59.1 results in two major differences. One concerns the risk in twins (see Twin studies, p. 587). The other concerns the risk to offspring of two affected parents, which was previously estimated to be around 48%, based on a small number of observations, but a more recent (large) study puts this at around 28%, increasing to 39% when schizophrenia-related disorders are included [6].

### Twin studies

The principles underlying the many twin studies conducted in psychiatric disorders are the same. Monozygotic (MZ) twins are perfectly correlated for all genetic loci that show variation in the population, whereas dizygotic (DZ) twins are, on average, 50% correlated. Assuming that the extent to which MZ and DZ twins share their environment is roughly equal, higher concordance in MZ twins suggests the disorder is, at least partly, genetic. Concordance of less than 100% in MZ twins suggests environmental factors or chance (including *de novo* mutation) also play a role. Early twin studies showed higher concordance in MZ twins, compared to DZ twins, but as with family studies, methodological concerns left these open to criticism. However, the most recent wave of studies have addressed earlier methodological limitations.

In a pooled sample analysis of four modern-era twin studies, proband-wise concordance rates for (strict and probable) DSM-III-R schizophrenia were 50% in MZ twins and 4.1% in DZ twins [7]. Modelling suggested that variance in population risk was best attributed to additive genetic factors acting together with specific (in the sense of exposures affecting only one twin) environmental factors. Heritability, the component attributable to genes, was 88%, although a more recent meta-analysis of a larger number of twins provided a lower estimate of around 81% [8]. Surprisingly, the lifetime risk for schizophrenia among DZ co-twins of affected probands seems considerably lower than that for non-twin siblings for reasons that are not fully established. The substantial difference in concordance between MZ and DZ twins is suggestive of influences from gene–environment correlation and/or non-additive genetic inheritance [9].

### Adoption studies

As both the genetic and environmental backgrounds of family member twins are, at least in part, correlated, it is difficult to separate definitively the contributions of genetic and environmental factors through family and twin study designs alone. Moreover, the

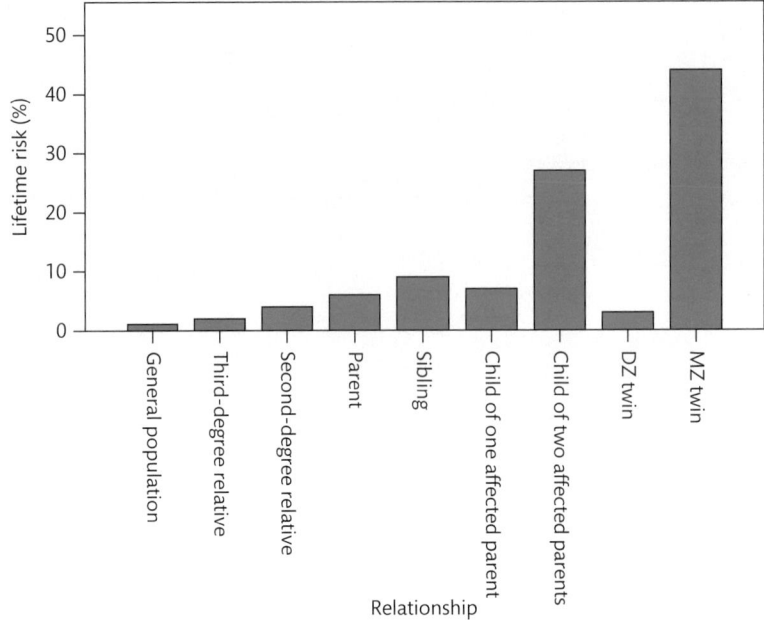

**Fig. 59.1** Lifetime risk of schizophrenia according to the relationship to an affected individual.

Source: data from Gottesman II, *Schizophrenia Genesis: The Origins of Madness*, Copyright (1991), WH Freeman; *Am J Med Genet*, 97(1), Cardno AG, Gottesman II, Twin studies of schizophrenia: from bow-and-arrow concordances to star wars Mx and functional genomics, pp. 12–17, Copyright (2000), John Wiley and Sons; *Arch Gen Psychiatry*, 67(3), Gottesman II, Laursen TM, Bertelsen A, *et al.*, Severe mental disorders in offspring with 2 psychiatrically ill parents, pp. 252–7, Copyright (2010), American Medical Association.

validity of twin studies has repeatedly been criticized, based on the possibility of greater correlations between the prenatal and postnatal environments of MZ than DZ twins. Thus, a third design based on adoption studies has formed an important foundation for the hypothesis of an important role for genes in the aetiology of schizophrenia. The premise underpinning the adoption design is that if genes play a role in a phenotype, adoptees should show evidence for phenotypic correlation with their biological relatives, despite being removed from a correlated environment.

Detailed discussion of the early adoption literature is given elsewhere [1, 10]. Briefly, adoptee studies have shown that the adopted-away children of people with schizophrenia have higher rates of schizophrenia and schizophrenia spectrum disorder than adoptees of controls. Adoptive family studies have shown that the biological relatives of affected adoptees have higher rates of the disorder than either their adoptive relatives or the relatives of unaffected adoptees. And one cross-fostering study showed that adoptees of control parents raised by a parent with schizophrenia had a lower risk of the disorder than the biological offspring of a person with schizophrenia raised by adoptive parents without the disorder.

Most adoption studies were conducted prior to the use of modern operational diagnostic criteria, so particularly notable is a study based on the Finnish national register, which used such criteria from the outset. Narrowly defined schizophrenia only showed a trend level difference in the adopted-away children of mothers with the disorder, compared with those of controls (5.3% vs 1.7%, respectively). However, the risk for schizophrenia spectrum disorders (22.46%) among adoptees whose mothers had schizophrenia spectrum disorder was much higher than the adoptees of controls (4.36%), supporting the hypothesis of a genetic contribution to a broader schizophrenia-related phenotype [11]. In the most recent study incorporating adoption data, adoptees with an affected

biological parent had an elevated relative risk (13.7) of developing schizophrenia [12] in the range expected for first-degree relatives of an affected proband.

Overall, the findings from adoption studies of multiple designs are consistent with those from other genetic epidemiological approaches; while the validity of the assumptions underpinning each study design can be debated, this consistency provides a strong and coherent body of evidence for an important contribution of genetic inheritance to the aetiology of schizophrenia.

## Genetic epidemiology and risk across disorders

The challenges of psychiatric diagnosis, and the evidence for the validity or otherwise of the boundaries that separate diagnostic categories or that delineate subtypes, are discussed in Chapters 7 and 8. However, to appreciate the context of recent genomic findings, this topic requires brief consideration. Genetic research has generally treated schizophrenia as a fully distinct entity from major mood disorders, based on both Kraepelinian tradition and also evidence from family studies that suggested the disorders breed true (that is, they segregate in different families). The status of schizoaffective disorder has historically been unclear. Some have considered it to be a categorical error, others a form of bipolar disorder, of schizophrenia, a distinct entity, or a state of comorbidity [13]. Moreover, although schizophrenia is now widely considered to be a neurodevelopmental disorder, it has been regarded as completely distinct from other neurodevelopmental categories such as intellectual disability (ID), autism spectrum disorder (ASD), and attention-deficit/hyperactivity disorder (ADHD). However, the idea that the disorders, in particular schizophrenia and mood disorders, breed true is not fully supported by historical family studies [3] and recent genetic epidemiology now offers substantial challenges to this view.

One study that has been particularly influential was based on over 2 million families from Sweden [12]. As expected, first-degree relatives of probands with schizophrenia had around a 9- to 10-fold increase in the risk for the disorder. However, they also had a substantially increased risk (3- to 6-fold, depending on the class of relative) of bipolar disorder, as did the adopted-away biological children of parents with schizophrenia. Modelling suggested around half of the heritability of schizophrenia comes from genetic effects that also contribute to bipolar disorder. Strong evidence for overlaps in the genetics of schizophrenia, schizoaffective disorder, and bipolar disorder were also found in an innovative twin study [14] in which individuals were allowed to have multiple diagnoses (that is, symptoms of one disorder were not used to exclude another disorder), and similar conclusions can be drawn from a study showing that the heritability of narrowly defined schizophrenia is essentially unchanged when other psychotic disorders are included [9].

Regarding possible overlaps among neurodevelopmental disorders, a study of three different data sets supported an earlier Danish study in finding that first-degree relatives of people with schizophrenia had more than twice the expected risk for ASD [15]. The parents and sibs of probands with bipolar disorder also had an increased risk for ASD, albeit to a lesser degree. Extending the findings to ID, an Australian study found the children of mothers with schizophrenia, bipolar affective disorder, and unipolar depression to be at an increased risk of ID [odds ratio (OR) 2.9–3.1] [16]. As we have discussed, familial clustering does not imply shared genes, but the findings are consistent with the hypothesis of genetic overlap, a theme we consider later when discussing the molecular genetics data.

## Paternal age and fecundity

People with schizophrenia have fewer children than the general population, an effect that is quite substantial, with men and women with the disorder reproducing at rates of 75% and 50%, respectively, lower than expected [4]. Low fecundity associated with schizophrenia has led to speculation about how risk alleles, and therefore the disorder, remain apparently impervious to removal from the population by natural selection [4]. It has also been established that children of older fathers are at increased risk of developing schizophrenia, a recent study estimating the risk to be 1.5-fold higher than expected in children of fathers over the age of 45 [17]. A hypothesis that has tried to link these two observations and has become a topic of sufficient interest to deserve special mention is that the answer to the persistence of the disorder lies in *de novo* or new mutation. The hypothesis is largely founded upon the fact that, like the risk of schizophrenia, the rate of *de novo* point mutation also increases with paternal age [18]. It is clear that *de novo* mutation does indeed contribute to schizophrenia (discussed later), but this contribution is minor and is unlikely to explain either the persistence of the disorder in the population or the effect of paternal age. The true explanations for the paternal age effect are not fully resolved, but a credible alternative may be that unaffected men who have a higher genetic loading (and therefore whose children are at higher genetic risk) may also tend to have children later, perhaps as a result of subclinical behavioural or personality traits [19]. This is of more than theoretical interest, given the potential to give incorrect advice about the risks that might accompany delayed fatherhood,

based upon a model where the directions of cause and effect are incorrectly specified.

## Molecular genetics

### Linkage, association, and genetic architecture

Linkage performs best when applied to genetic disorders with simple (dominant, recessive, sex-linked) patterns of inheritance but rapidly loses power in the face of marked locus heterogeneity (that is, there are large numbers of distinct genomic regions with pathogenic variants). This is particularly true if the heterogeneity cannot be constrained by selecting families with particular phenotypic features. It is also not suited to disorders where the risk alleles are numerous and common and have small effects because even in a single family, the risk is likely to be due to multiple alleles, none of which is required to be co-transmitted with the phenotype. Under that scenario, association studies offer a more powerful approach.

Linkage allows researchers to survey the whole genome for disease-causing variants, using only a few hundreds of genetic markers, whereas hundreds of thousands of markers are required to screen the whole genome by association. In the late twentieth century, technological limitations in the speed and cost of genome analysis meant that linkage was perceived to have a huge advantage since researchers trying to apply association methodologies were forced to select specific candidate genes. Candidates were selected on the basis of being located within a region of putative linkage (positional candidates) or because they were postulated to be involved on the basis of their role in biological processes (functional candidates).

### Linkage

While linkage studies routinely delivered hundreds of pathogenic genes for single-gene disorders, they did not deliver replicable findings in schizophrenia, or indeed many other common medical disorders. Even a meta-analysis of over 3200 separate pedigrees [20] failed to identify high-confidence linked loci. With the benefit of hindsight, it is now clear that the genetic and phenotypic architectures of schizophrenia are probably as unfavourable for linkage as it is possible to be.

It is true that large numbers of statistically significant linkages were observed in individual pedigrees or groups of pedigrees (for an example, see [21]) and that genuine linkages are difficult to replicate in the face of extensive locus heterogeneity. These two factors mean we cannot be certain whether the failures to replicate initial linkages reflect the greater-than-expected locus heterogeneity of the disorder or whether they were simply false positives. For now, what we can say with certainty is that no Mendelian forms of schizophrenia have yet been identified. Interest in applying (modified) principles of linkage is likely to be rekindled by the new genome-wide sequencing methods which, at single base, rather than mega-base, resolution, may deal better with heterogeneity.

### Candidate gene association

In the 1990s and early 2000s, large numbers of candidate genes and variants were tested in schizophrenia. In Table 59.1, we present the findings for some of the most widely discussed genes from the candidate gene literature [22], based upon results from the largest

**Table 59.1** Associations to the most widely discussed genes from the candidate literature (*p* values represent the best association within, or close to, the gene)

| Gene | Minimum *p* value |
| --- | --- |
| DRD2 | $2.7 \times 10^{-11}$ |
| NRG1 | $6.2 \times 10^{-4}$ |
| RGS4 | $2.4 \times 10^{-2}$ |
| COMT | $6.5 \times 10^{-3}$ |
| DTNBP1 | $2.5 \times 10^{-4}$ |
| HTR2A | $5.3 \times 10^{-4}$ |
| DAOA | 0.015 |
| DISC1 | $4.5 \times 10^{-4}$ |
| DRD3 | $3.3 \times 10^{-3}$ |

*Source*: data from *Mol Psychiatry*, 20(5), Farrell M, Werge T, Sklar P, *et al.*, Evaluating historical candidate genes for schizophrenia, pp. 555–62, Copyright (2015), Springer Nature; *Nature*, 511, Schizophrenia Working Group of the Psychiatric Genomics Consortium (PGC), Biological insights from 108 schizophrenia-associated genetic loci, pp. 421–27, Copyright (2014), Springer Nature.

published genome-wide association study (GWAS) [23] of schizophrenia, which included most of the data sets that were considered supportive of the earlier associations, and the findings can therefore be considered to largely supersede the earlier evidence. In the vast majority of cases, the candidate genes are not supported at what is now considered an appropriately stringent threshold (*p* $<5 \times 10^{-8}$). However, there are caveats to this conclusion. In some cases (*DTNBP1, NRG1, RGS4*), the strongest findings depended on marker combinations (haplotypes), which are not specifically evaluated in GWAS data. Whether this is an important caveat is unclear, since the high-density coverage of markers in the GWAS is likely to have covered the markers presumed to drive the haplotype associations. Secondly, for one locus—*DRD2* encoding the dopamine D2 receptor, there is now strong evidence for an association in the vicinity of this gene, although not to an allele that was identified in the candidate gene literature. For those particularly interested in candidate genes, and the differences in approach that systematic coverage of candidate genes has enabled, we recommend two papers: one pre-GWAS [22] and one post-GWAS [24]. As the latter concludes, the current evidence suggests that the historical candidate gene literature did not yield clear insights into the genetic basis of schizophrenia.

With hindsight, there are several reasons why this phase of genetic study did not deliver. Major limitations in our understanding of schizophrenia meant the choice of candidates did not constrain the enormous variation of the genome to a substantially smaller number of genes with a high prior probability of being associated. Moreover, how small the association effect sizes were likely to be, and therefore what constitutes adequate sample sizes, was not widely appreciated until the landmark work of the Wellcome Trust Case Control Consortium [25]. Together, small effect sizes and the low prior probability for any candidate variant meant the studies were substantially underpowered to detect true associations at the stringent levels of significance necessary to control for type I errors. For example, a candidate gene study of 2000 subjects (a large study for most of the candidate gene era) has power of only 0.001 to detect an effect size at the upper end of the range (OR 1.2) that has subsequently been shown to operate for schizophrenia, at genome-wide significance. Moreover, even if some of the candidate associations were true, subsequent replication studies would have been underpowered to confirm them.

## Genome-wide association studies

Human variant mapping studies, such as The HapMap Project, have documented the nature and genomic location of a high fraction of all common DNA sequence variation that is present in the human population. This knowledge, coupled with novel genomic technology and statistical methodology, made it possible around 15 years ago to undertake the so-called GWAS, in which millions of SNPs are comprehensively assayed in an individual in a single experiment. In contrast to earlier association approaches, the GWAS design does not rely on prior knowledge of the most likely candidate genes or candidate genes, making GWAS seem an ideal tool for disorders of unknown pathophysiology such as schizophrenia.

The first GWAS studies of schizophrenia, based on small samples, failed to identify associations, leading some to suggest that the class of genetic variant accessible to this study design, that is, common alleles, plays no role in the disorder. However, an alternative view, informed by similar developments in complex genetics as a whole, was that the early studies were underpowered; other than suggesting that no common risk alleles operate in the disorder with large effect sizes (ORs >2; equivalent to *APOE* in Alzheimer's disease), the main message was that success would require extremely large samples that could realistically only be obtained by collaboration. How large GWAS studies might have to be was shown by the study of O'Donovan and colleagues (2008) [26]. Like those that preceded it, this study was based on what would now be considered a very small-discovery GWAS sample, but the top findings were pursued sequentially in large replication cohorts into a final meta-analysis, which included 7308 schizophrenia cases and 12,834 controls. This led to highly suggestive evidence for association to a locus containing the gene *ZNF804A*, but genome-wide significant evidence was only obtained when the affected phenotype was broadened to include bipolar disorder, allowing an analysis of 9173 cases and 12,834 controls. Association to schizophrenia on its own at genome-wide significance was not obtained for a further 3 years, by which time the analysis was based on almost 60,000 subjects [27].

In terms of gene discovery, the early work was disappointing, but it did point to some of the key features that have emerged from much larger GWAS. Firstly, the effect size of the associated common variant at *ZNF804A* was small, with an OR of 1.1, an effect size typical of the findings that have followed. Secondly, while it was difficult to obtain genome-wide significance, the study demonstrated an excess of nominally significant replications when the top GWAS associations were tested in large independent samples. This suggested that large numbers of true associations lay among the markers showing moderate evidence of association in GWAS that even large meta-analyses were underpowered to unequivocally implicate. And thirdly, the enhanced evidence for association between a variant at the gene *ZNF804A* and a combined schizophrenia–bipolar phenotype tends to support the findings from epidemiology for genetic overlaps between these two disorders.

A major insight into the role of common variants in schizophrenia came not from specific associations, but from patterns of data from large groups of markers. Seminal here was the work of the International Schizophrenia Consortium [28] that proposed large numbers of common risk alleles exist for schizophrenia, but in the GWAS sample they had available (about 3000 cases and 4000 controls), these could not be identified at the required levels of significance due to small effect sizes. To test this, the ISC considered all alleles in their study to be possible risk alleles if they were associated with schizophrenia at a very loose threshold of significance (for example, $p$ <0.5). The ISC postulated that under a highly polygenic model, although most such associated alleles will be false, there would also be large numbers of true risk alleles captured at this threshold. They further postulated that if the disorder were polygenic enough, in independent data sets, individuals with the disorder would, on average, carry a larger burden of the presumed risk alleles than those without the disorder. In their landmark study, not only did the ISC confirm this to be true, they also showed by testing a range of models of genetic architecture that it was likely that the component of risk conferred by common risk alleles was distributed across at least 1000 alleles, and quite possibly many more than this. Modelling also suggested that the common polygenic SNP component to the disorder contributed around a third of the genetic risk to the disorder. The approach developed by the ISC, variously known as polygenic risk scoring (PRS), risk profile scoring (RPS), and genetic risk scoring (GRS), has, as we shall discuss later, become an important tool in psychiatric research extending beyond discovery genetics.

Since these early studies, approximately 20 risk alleles were identified from studies conducted by informal groupings of investigators and structured consortia (see [29]). However, the main breakthrough in detecting common alleles for the disorder required the international community to pool their resources into a super-consortium, which is now known as the Schizophrenia Working Group of the Psychiatric Genomics Consortium. The effect of this has been dramatic; in its first paper in 2011, the PGC reported ten associations using a sample of 9394 cases, but only 3 years later, based on a discovery GWAS sample of approximately 35,500 cases and 45,000 controls and with additional follow-up in another sample of 1513 cases and 66,236 controls, 128 independent genetic associations spanning 108 physically distinct genomic loci were identified [23].

Associations were particularly enriched for genes expressed in the brain, confirming schizophrenia is primarily a CNS disorder, rather than a manifestation of peripheral dysfunction, although the findings do not exclude a role for the latter. Some of the associations appear to give support to classical neurotransmission hypotheses of schizophrenia, including associations to loci containing *DRD2* (encoding the dopamine receptor D2) and genes involved in glutamatergic neurotransmission (for example, *GRM3* encoding metabotropic glutamate receptor type 3, *GRIN2A* encoding subunit 2A of the ionotropic NMDA receptor, and *GRIA1* encoding subunit 1 of the ionotropic AMPA receptor). The finding of associations to the locus encoding DRD2, the only known effective therapeutic target in schizophrenia, also holds out the possibility that other associations highlight drug treatment targets. However, the vast majority of the findings are not so plausibly interpreted and likely hold clues to novel aspects of pathophysiology. In particular, multiple associations to genes (*CACNA1C*, *CACNB2*, and *CACNA1I*) encoding calcium channels point to the likely importance of this family of proteins in the disorder.

As is characteristic of GWAS, the vast majority of the associations (including those to the loci containing the candidate genes discussed) could not be credibly ascribed to DNA variants that are predicted to change the amino acid sequences of proteins, and it seems most likely that the majority of susceptibility alleles exert their effects by altering gene expression. This makes interpreting the functional significance of the associations a challenging task and researchers are still mining the findings, aiming to develop a deeper understanding of their implications for pathophysiology.

A recent example of the sort of work required was recently reported by Sekar and colleagues (2016) [30], who dissected the source of an association at the extended MHC region of chromosome 6. This region spans about 8 million bases, contains hundreds of genes, and represents the most robustly associated locus in the PGC study and the locus with the largest (though still modest) effect size (OR = 1.2) [23]. The authors showed that much of the association at this locus was driven by a complex chromosomal structural rearrangement, which affects expression of the gene complement component C4A. How this finding potentially fits with emerging insights into the biological basis of schizophrenia is discussed later.

Despite the undoubted successes of the PGC study, only a small fraction of all common variation has been identified, representing 3–4% of the variance for the disorder. However, the PGC and GWAS that preceded it do provide a clear strategy for success; notwithstanding the enhanced heterogeneity that most investigators assume comes from pooling samples from a diverse range of ancestries (the PGC study was based on individuals of European and Asian ancestry from over 30 countries), diagnostic methods, and ascertainment strategies, large samples clearly deliver. It is a certainty that in the next few years, the number of associated loci will increase considerably. Developing methods and resources that accelerate the rate by which those findings can be converted to biological insights into the aetiology will be critical if the wealth of findings are to be translated into benefits for patients.

### Genomic copy number variants

CNVs are deletions and duplications of chromosomal segments of at least 1000 bases (1 kb); they are highly relevant to autism and other forms of ID, as discussed in Chapter 28. Prior to the GWAS era, a deletion CNV at chromosome 22q11.2 (22q11.2del) was the only DNA variant, common or rare, that was indisputably pathogenic for schizophrenia [22]. This deletion is also known to cause a congenital syndrome variously called velo-cardio-facial syndrome (VCFS), di George syndrome, or Shprintzen syndrome. The fact that carriers of this CNV usually have recognizable clinical and dysmorphic features was critical to the early discovery of its involvement in schizophrenia, since it was possible to demonstrate an elevated rate of psychosis in those with the clinical features of VCFS.

Although few doubted that the rate of psychosis was elevated in those with VCFS, it was not uncommon for it to be argued that the associated psychiatric phenotype represented a symptomatic form of psychosis secondary to ID, rather than a disorder that should be considered true schizophrenia. However, it has now become more widely accepted that those with VCFS have schizophrenia for reasons that we touch on here, as they are relevant more generally to any discussion of rare variants in schizophrenia. Firstly, studies using research diagnoses showed that the psychosis that occurs in VCFS meets operational diagnostic criteria for schizophrenia, the only criterion for schizophrenia that we currently have. Secondly, studies of 'routine' clinical cases of schizophrenia have demonstrated that those with operationally diagnosed schizophrenia also have a greatly elevated rate (about 40- to 60-fold) of 22q11.2del [31]. Thirdly, the elevated risk of schizophrenia in VCFS is not restricted to those with obvious ID. Fourthly, cognitive impairment is increasingly accepted as a core feature of schizophrenia, rather than a primary cause of the disorder (see Chapter 57). Finally, as the number of CNVs associated with both cognitive impairment and schizophrenia has increased, so the idea that the psychosis in 22q11.2del is distinct from the rest of schizophrenia seems less tenable, and more so since it has been recently shown that people with CNVs and schizophrenia also have elevated burdens of the sorts of common schizophrenia risk alleles derived from GWAS in general (that is, non-CNV carrier) patient populations [32].

Beyond 22q11.2del, the recognition of a wider role for CNVs in schizophrenia had to await the development of genome-wide technologies that allow a genotype-, rather than a phenotype-led, approach. Evidence for a role of CNVs in schizophrenia comes from three main sources.

Firstly, as we already discussed, risk alleles such as CNVs that confer large effects on risk of the disorder are likely to be under strong negative (natural) selection, leading some to the hypothesis that risk alleles of large effect might be maintained by new or *de novo* mutations. Consistent with this prediction, CNVs have been observed to occur as new or *de novo* mutations more frequently in cases (about 5% at the current resolution for detecting CNVs) relative to controls (about 1–2%) [33]. Secondly, at a genome-wide level, large studies have consistently shown that the total burden of large (>100 kb) and rare (frequency <1%) CNVs (both deletions and duplications) is increased around 1.15-fold in patients with schizophrenia in comparison with controls [34]. Finally, and most conclusively, there is now strong evidence implicating multiple specific loci in the disorder.

The earliest genotype-led study to suggest the role of a CNV in schizophrenia was a small study of parent–proband trios in which the aim was to discover *de novo* mutations [35]. Two candidate CNVs were identified—one a *de novo* duplication spanning a number of genes, including *APBA2*, and the other was a transmitted deletion at *NRXN1*. Both CNVs had been previously implicated in neurodevelopmental phenotypes, suggesting they may be pathogenic. Moreover, APBA2 and neurexin 1 are members of a complex, which mediates interactions between pre- and post-synaptic structures in the brain. Promising though these findings were, they were no more than suggestive, and it took a larger case-control study to convincingly implicate deletions at the neurexin 1 locus in the disorder, with a substantial OR of around 9 [36].

The most robust early evidence implicating specific CNVs, however, came from simultaneous publications from two consortia—the SGENE+ consortium [37] and the International Schizophrenia Consortium [34]. Hitherto unprecedented in psychiatric genetics, the two studies had almost identical results. Both implicated deletions at 15q13.3 and 1q21.1, while the SGENE+ study additionally reported evidence supporting deletions at 15q11.2 that the ISC study had excluded for technical reasons. Since this early work, a number of additional, strongly supported schizophrenia-associated CNVs have been identified (Fig. 59.2). All the CNV loci implicated

so far are rare (population frequency usually <0.1%), each occurring in fewer than 1% of cases, and those that have been discovered have considerably larger effect sizes than SNPs, with ORs ranging between about 2 and 60 [38]. It should be noted that power considerations imply that rare variants can only be convincingly associated if they have large effect sizes, and therefore, the profile of effect sizes documented to date may be more a feature of the current sample sizes than an intrinsic property of CNVs as a mutation class.

One of the most notable features of schizophrenia risk CNVs is that they are also risk factors for other neurodevelopmental disorders, including ID, ASD, epilepsy, and ADHD, and a range of congenital malformations, that is, they are often pleiotropic. Indeed, every CNV known to increase the risk of schizophrenia also does so for ID [39]. The theme of shared risk factors across disorders is taken up further under Sequencing studies, p. 592 and Applications of polygenic methodology, p. 594.

### Sequencing studies

For the present purposes, although CNVs and other chromosomal arrangements are detectable by sequencing, the primary aim of sequencing studies is to identify variants similar in structure to those detected by GWAS (that is, single nucleotide and small insertion/deletion variants), but which are too rare to be captured by GWAS. Cost implications have led researchers to focus on the coding exome, so we will refer to these as rare coding variants (RCVs) that change the DNA sequence at single or a few nucleotides. As for studies of CNVs, exome sequencing studies have been prosecuted along two main designs: family-based seeking a contribution from *de novo* RCVs and case-control. Even though the largest of the first wave of studies were grossly underpowered to detect individual pathogenic single nucleotide variants (SNVs), they did show that groups of genes that had prevously been identified as likely related to the disorder were enriched for very rare, non-synonymous RCVs in cases, compared with controls, and among mutations occuring as *de novo* mutations [40, 41]. Just as elevated burdens of rare CNVs [34] and common risk alleles [28] heralded the identification of specific risk alleles of those classes, this burden of RCVs provided for optimism that the same would be true for this class of alleles when sample sizes are adequate.

Sample sizes are still too small to expect large-scale discovery, but nevertheless, this optimism has already been shown to be well founded. A meta-analysis of 4264 cases, 9343 controls, and 1077 parent–proband trios obtained strong evidence for a single gene enriched for very damaging (so-called loss of function, or LoF) mutations in schizophrenia [42]. The gene *SETD1A* encodes a protein that methylates histone proteins, a process believed to be important in regulating gene expression. Identifying which genes are regulated by *SETD1A* is the next step in understanding how loss of activity of this protein leads to disease.

Sequencing studies have also recapitulated the findings from CNVs of overlaps between neurodevelopmental disorders. As a group, genes impacted by LoF *de novo* mutations in schizophrenia are enriched for those affected by this same class of mutation in people with ASD and ID [40], while at an even finer level of resolution, the same LoF mutation in *SETD1A* that contributes high risk to schizophrenia also does so for severe ID and developmental delay [42].

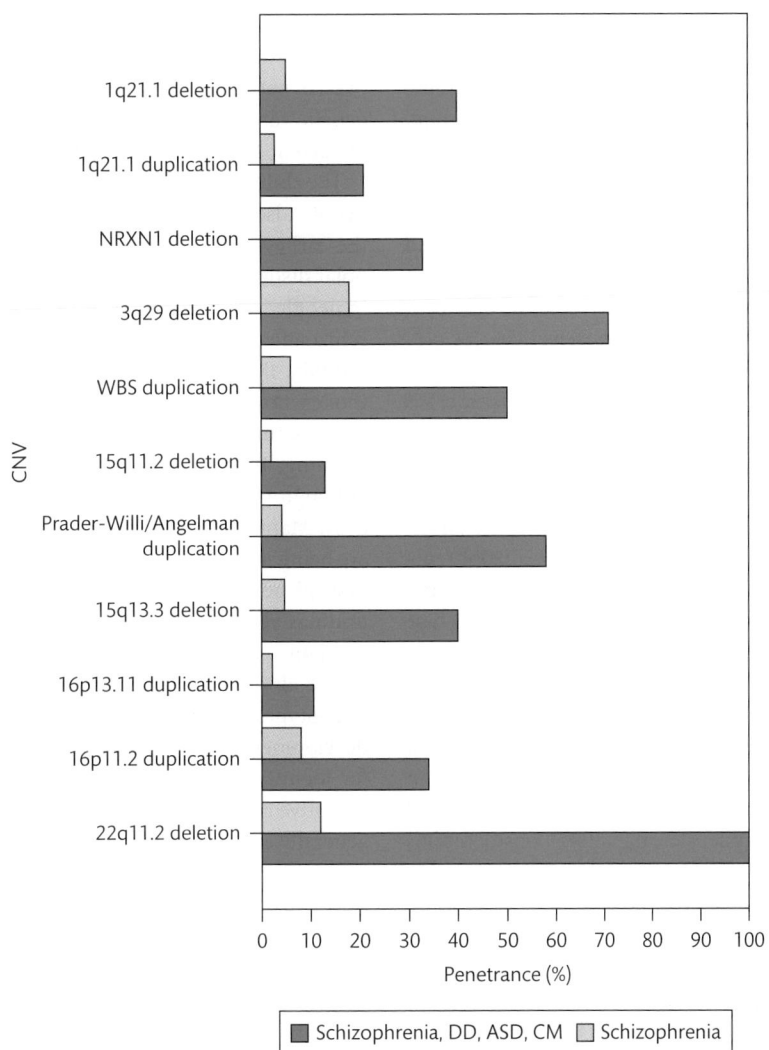

**Fig. 59.2** Penetrance of schizophrenia-associated CNVs for schizophrenia and other developmental disorders [38]. DD, developmental delay; ASD, autism spectrum disorders; CM, congenital malformation.

## Glimpses of the biological basis of schizophrenia

Most of the genetic risk for schizophrenia is not yet linked to specific DNA variants, and even the majority of robust associations do not implicate individual genes at high levels of certainty. This is because GWAS implicates chromosomal regions, rather than definitively pointing to only a single gene, and CNVs usually span multiple genes. Nevertheless, there is already strong evidence that many of the findings converge onto plausible pathophysiological processes. System genomics studies (analyses that determine if certain types of mutations are overrepresented in groups of genes that have related functions) show that in people with schizophrenia, rare mutations of all classes (CNVs and RCVs, transmitted and *de novo*) tend to cluster in genes encoding post-synaptic components of excitatory synapses. In particular, an excess of mutations have been found repeatedly in genes encoding proteins affiliated with the *N*-methyl-*D*-aspartate receptor (NMDAR) and those affiliated with the neuronal activity-regulated cytoskeleton-associated (ARC) protein which regulates post-synaptic strength at glutamatergic synapses [40, 41, 43, 44]. Studies have also documented that rare mutations and, to a lesser extent, common variant associations are enriched among genes encoding proteins whose synthesis is inhibited by fragile X mental retardation protein (FMRP) [23, 40, 41]. Genes encoding voltage-gated calcium channels are similarly implicated both by GWAS and by one study of rare genetic variation [23, 41, 45], and more recently, evidence has emerged for enrichment of case CNVs in genes encoding GABA$_A$ receptor affiliated proteins [44], which has strong functional links with the glutamatergic system. All these sets of genes are important components or regulators of synaptic plasticity, a set of processes that are known to be critical for a range of cognitive processes, including learning, memory, and, it now seems highly likely, schizophrenia [44, 46].

These convergent findings point to some general biological hypotheses, but they do not capture the totality of the association signal. There is evidence from the association between schizophrenia and rare variants at *SETD1A*, as well as from common GWAS signals [47] that chromatin modification is also implicated, while the identification of complement C4A as a susceptibility factor highlights the involvement of immune mechanisms. It is unclear if the findings discussed here also converge on the general area of synaptic plasticity, but it is notable that in the brain, much of C4 protein co-localizes with glutamatergic markers. There is also evidence that mice lacking C4 show abnormalities of plasticity in visual pathways, perhaps through synaptic pruning. It is therefore possible that these apparently disparate biological pathways converge onto a coherent, and yet broad, set of pathogenic processes.

### Genetic prediction and testing

Here we briefly consider the implications of the findings discussed previously. In people with schizophrenia entering genetic studies (which are biased towards chronicity and severity), the rate of known pathogenic CNVs is around 2.5%, implying low sensitivity for prediction. In the general population, the penetrance for schizophrenia in carriers (the proportion of carriers developing the disorder) is between 2% and 18% (Fig. 59.2) [38], implying low specificity for prediction. While the screening value of CNVs for prediction is therefore low for the proportion of cases who are carriers, that knowledge may have value for patients who often are desperate for an explanation for their illness. Moreover, as we have seen, schizophrenia is not the only possible outcome in CNV carriers; considering developmental delay, ASD, and congenital malformations, the average penetrance for any of these disorders is around 40% (Fig. 59.2). So for the 50% of the offspring of CNV carriers who themselves are carriers, the risk for a range of neurodevelopmental outcomes is high. CNVs may also lead to comorbidity for medical phenotypes, which may be overlooked in people with psychosis who often do not gain good access to physical health care but that are treatable if detected (for example, cardiac defects, epilepsy, cataracts). Considerations such as these have led to calls for CNV testing to be offered to people with schizophrenia [48], although at the time of writing, as far as we are aware, this is not routine practice in any part of the world.

The principles of PRS are discussed previously. This method provides researchers with a tool that allows an unaffected individual's liability to the disorder to be estimated. While this has many research applications, currently, the degree of liability captured by PRS is not of clinical value; its sensitivity and specificity for predicting affected status are inadequate, and the predictive power as depicted by area under the curve (AUC) analysis is only 0.62 [23].

### Applications of polygenic methodology

As perhaps the first valid biomarker for liability to the disorder, PRS is opening up interesting areas for research [49]. In the first paper to exploit this, the ISC (2009) [28] showed the burden of common schizophrenia-associated alleles, as measured by PRS, was not just increased in people with schizophrenia, but it was also increased in people with bipolar disorder. This finding points to a shared genetic contribution between the two disorders and is consistent with some of the newer genetic epidemiology discussed earlier in the chapter [12]. Subsequently, RPS and other polygenic approaches [49] have documented substantial sharing of risk alleles between schizophrenia and major depression, as well as significant, and perhaps more unexpected, overlaps with autism, ADHD, anorexia nervosa, obsessive–compulsive disorder, and neuroticism. More controversially, polygenic risk for schizophrenia (in unaffected people) has been linked to poor cognitive performance yet, simultaneously, to higher educational performance and creativity [50]. Given the large number of risk alleles involved in schizophrenia, and the likelihood that these, in turn, influence multiple domains of brain function, it is perhaps not surprising that overlaps exist for common alleles across multiple psychiatric, behavioural, and cognitive phenotypes. Nevertheless, considered alongside results of studies showing overlap between neurodevelopmental disorders with respect to rare genetic variation [51], these findings pose challenges to the validity of current classification systems.

The ability to measure, imperfectly, genetic liability in unaffected people also offers new opportunities for patient stratification. In the earliest such application, it was shown that in people with bipolar disorder, loading for schizophrenia polygenic risk was higher in people with psychotic features and in those who met criteria for schizoaffective disorder [52]. Conversely, in people with schizophrenia, the polygenic burden of bipolar risk alleles is higher in those who have co-occurrence of manic symptoms [53]. Findings such as these suggest a biological structure of psychosis corresponding, in part, to symptom domains, rather than categories, although much more work is required to establish this unequivocally. Many other approaches to stratification based on risk alleles are being investigated, including treatment response, outcome after first episode, and predicting functional impairment, but none of the findings yet have the robustness of those documenting phenotype overlaps.

PRS also offers the potential for looking in unaffected people for phenotypes that correspond to increased liability, for studying the developmental trajectory of individuals at elevated risk, and perhaps for identifying modifiable environmental factors or psychological cognitive traits that alter trajectories to illness. Again, these findings generally are not yet entirely robust, but it has been shown that elevated PRS relates to negative, rather than positive, symptom dimensions, suggesting the former may be better markers for detecting those at risk of the disorder [54].

Finally, PRS also offers the possibility of evaluating putative intermediate phenotypes that might mediate the link between genes and disorder. In schizophrenia, clear positive findings have yet to emerge, and for now, perhaps the most interesting of this type of study concerns negative studies. A particularly notable example of this, given the size and power of the study, was one that found no overlap between genes that influence the size of subcortical brain structures and those that influence schizophrenia [55], implying that the volume of those brain structures (for example, striatum, hippocampus) is not an important mediating factor of genetic risk for schizophrenia.

## Conclusions

After a lengthy period of apparent advances and retreats, molecular genetic studies of schizophrenia have recently delivered robust findings in large number. These, in turn, are beginning to provide insights into general areas of pathophysiology, challenge the validity of psychiatric nosology, and provide novel tools for research more widely. Thus far, there has been limited clinical translation of these results, though some of the findings implicating rare genetic variants may be of direct relevance in the clinic. On a cautionary note, the current findings represent only a fraction of the total genetic contribution to schizophrenia. While there are grounds to believe that much more will be uncovered and that the process of doing so will accelerate, there remains much to be done to convert the genetic findings to a deep mechanistic understanding that will be required if genetics is to fulfil its promise of driving the development of novel treatments.

## REFERENCES

1. Gottesman, II. (1991). *Schizophrenia Genesis: The Origins of Madness*. WH Freeman, New York, NY.

2. Gottesman, II, McGuffin, P, Farmer, AE. (1987). Clinical genetics as clues to the 'real' genetics of schizophrenia (a decade of modest gains while playing for time). *Schizophr Bull* 13: 23.

3. Kendler, KS, Diehl SR. (1993). The genetics of schizophrenia: a current, genetic-epidemiologic perspective. *Schizophr Bull* 19: 261.

4. Power, RA, Kyaga, S, Uher, R, *et al.* (2013). Fecundity of patients with schizophrenia, autism, bipolar affective disorder, depression, anorexia nervosa, or substance abuse vs their unaffected siblings. *JAMA Psychiatry* 70: 22.

5. Lichtenstein, P, Björk, C, Hultman, CM, Scolnick, E, Sklar, P, Sullivan, PF. (2006). Recurrence risks for schizophrenia in a Swedish national cohort. *Psychol Med* 36: 1417.

6. Gottesman, II, Laursen, TM, Bertelsen, A, Mortensen, PB. (2010). Severe mental disorders in offspring with 2 psychiatrically ill parents. *Arch Gen Psychiatry* 67: 252.

7. Cardno, AG, Gottesman, II. (2000). Twin studies of schizophrenia: from bow-and-arrow concordances to star wars Mx and functional genomics. *Am J Med Genet* 97: 12.

8. Sullivan, PF, Kendler, KS, Neale, MC. (2003). Schizophrenia as a complex trait: evidence from a meta-analysis of twin studies. *Arch Gen Psychiatry* 60: 1187.

9. Kläning, U, Trumbetta, SL, Gottesman, II, Skytthe, A, Kyvik, KO, Bertelsen, A. (2015). A Danish twin study of schizophrenia liability: investigation from interviewed twins for genetic links to affective psychoses and for cross-cohort comparisons. *Behav Genet* 46: 193.

10. Gottesman, II, Shields, J. (1976). A critical review of recent adoption, twin and family studies of schizophrenia: behavioral genetics perspectives. *Schizophr Bull* 2: 360.

11. Tienari, P, Wynne, LC, Läksy, K, *et al.* (2003). Genetic boundaries of the schizophrenia spectrum: evidence from the Finnish adoptive family study of schizophrenia. *Am J Psychiatry* 160: 1587.

12. Lichtenstein, P, Yip, BH, Björk, C, *et al.* (2009). Common genetic influences for schizophrenia and bipolar disorder: a population-based study of 2 million nuclear families. *Lancet* 373: 234.

13. Malaspina, D, Owen, MJ, Heckers, S, *et al.* (2013). Schizoaffective disorder in the DSM-5. *Schizophr Res* 150: 21.

14. Cardno, AG, Rijsdijk, FV, Sham, PC, *et al.* (2002). A twin study of genetic relationships between psychotic symptoms. *Am J Psychiatry* 159: 539.

15. Sullivan, PF, Magnusson, C, Reichenberg, A et al, 2012a. Family history of schizophrenia and bipolar disorder as risk factors for autism. *Arch Gen Psychiatry* 69(11): 1099.

16. Morgan, VA, Croft, ML, Giuletta, M, *et al.* (2012). Intellectual disability and other neuropsychiatric outcomes in high-risk children of mothers with schizophrenia, bipolar disorder and unipolar major depression. *Br J Psychiatry* 200: 282.

17. McGrath, JJ, Petersen, L, Agerbo, E, *et al.* (2014). A comprehensive assessment of parental age and psychiatric disorders. *JAMA Psychiatry* 71: 301.

18. Malaspina, D, Corcoran, C, Fahim, C, *et al.* (2002). Paternal age and sporadic schizophrenia: evidence for *de novo* mutations. *Am J Med Genet* 114: 299.

19. Gratten, J, Wray, NR, Peyrot, WJ, *et al.* (2016). Risk of psychiatric illness from advanced paternal age is not predominantly from *de novo* mutations. *Nat Genet* 48, 718–24.

20. Ng, MY, Levinson, DF, Faraone, SV, *et al.* (2009). Meta-analysis of 32 genome-wide linkage studies of schizophrenia. *Mol Psychiatry* 14: 774.

21. Sherrington, R, Brynjolfsson, J, Petursson, H, *et al.* (1988). Localization of a susceptibility locus for schizophrenia on chromosome 5. *Nature* 336: 164.

22. Owen, MJ, Williams, NM, O'Donovan, MC. (2004). The molecular genetics of schizophrenia: new findings promise new insights. *Mol Psychiatry* 9: 14.

23. Schizophrenia Working Group of the Psychiatric Genomics Consortium (PGC). (2014). Biological insights from 108 schizophrenia-associated genetic loci. *Nature* 511; 421.

24. Farrell, M, Werge, T, Sklar, P, *et al.* (2015). Evaluating historical candidate genes for schizophrenia. *Mol Psychiatry* 20: 555.

25. Wellcome Trust Case Control Consortium. (2007). Genome-wide association study of 14,000 cases of seven common diseases and 3,000 shared controls. *Nature* 447: 661.

26. O'Donovan, MC, Craddock, N, Norton, N, *et al.* (2008). Identification of loci associated with schizophrenia by genome-wide association and follow-up. *Nat Genet* 40: 1053.

27. Williams, HJ, Norton, N, Dwyer, S, *et al.* (2011). Fine mapping of *ZNF804A* and genome-wide significant evidence for its involvement in schizophrenia and bipolar disorder. *Mol Psychiatry* 16: 429–41.

28. International Schizophrenia Consortium (ISC). (2009). Common polygenic variation contributes to risk of schizophrenia and bipolar disorder. *Nature* 460: 748.

29. Sullivan, PF, Daly, MJ, O'Donovan, MC. (2012). Genetic architectures of psychiatric disorders: the emerging picture and its implications. *Nat Rev Genet* 13: 537.

30. Sekar, A, Bialas, AR, de Rivera, H, *et al.* (2016). Schizophrenia risk from complex variation of complement component 4. *Nature* 530: 177.

31. Rees, E, Walters, JT, Georgieva, L, *et al.* (2014). Analysis of copy number variations at 15 schizophrenia-associated loci. *Br J Psychiatry* 204: 108.

32. Tansey, KE, Rees, E, Linden, DE, *et al.* (2016). Common alleles contribute to schizophrenia in CNV carriers. *Mol Psychiatry* 21: 1085–9.

33. Rees, E, Kirov, G, O'Donovan, MC, Owen, MJ. (2012). *De novo* mutation in schizophrenia. *Schizophr Bull* 38: 377.

34. International Schizophrenia Consortium (ISC). (2008). Rare chromosomal deletions and duplications increase risk of schizophrenia. *Nature* 455: 237.

35. Kirov, G, Gumus, D, Chen, W, *et al.* (2008). Comparative genome hybridization suggests a role for *NRXN1* and *APBA2* in schizophrenia. *Hum Mol Genet* 17: 458.

36. Rujescu, D, Ingason, A, Cichon, S, *et al.* (2009). Disruption of the neurexin 1 gene is associated with schizophrenia. *Hum Mol Genet* 18: 988.

37. Stefansson, H, Rujescu, D, Cichon, S, *et al.* (2008). Large recurrent microdeletions associated with schizophrenia. *Nature* 455: 232.

38. Kirov, G, Rees, E, Walters, JT, *et al.* (2014). The penetrance of copy number variations for schizophrenia and developmental delay. *Biol Psychiatry* 75: 378.

39. Rees, E, Kendall, K, Pardiñas, AF, *et al.* (2016). Analysis of intellectual disability copy number variants for association with schizophrenia. *JAMA Psychiatry* 73: 963–9.

40. Fromer, M, Pocklington, AJ, Kavanagh, DH, *et al.* (2014). *De novo* mutations in schizophrenia implicate synaptic networks. *Nature* 506: 179.

41. Purcell, SM, Moran, JL, Fromer, M, *et al.* (2014). A polygenic burden of rare disruptive mutations in schizophrenia. *Nature* 506: 185.

42. Singh, T, Kurki, MI, Curtis, D, *et al.* (2016). Rare loss-of-function variants in *SETD1A* are associated with schizophrenia and developmental disorders. *Nat Neurosci* 19: 571.

43. Kirov, G, Pocklinglington, AJ, Holmans, P, *et al.* (2012). *De novo* CNV analysis implicates specific abnormalities of postsynaptic signalling complexes in the pathogenesis of schizophrenia. *Mol Psychiatry* 17: 142.

44. Pocklington, AJ, Rees, E, Walters, JT, *et al.* (2015). Novel findings from CNVs implicate inhibitory and excitatory signalling complexes in schizophrenia. *Neuron* 86: 1203.

45. Ripke, S, O'Dushlaine, C, Chambert, K, *et al.* (2013). Genome-wide association analysis identifies 13 new risk loci for schizophrenia. *Nat Genet* 45: 1150.

46. Hall, J, Trent, S, Thomas, KL, O'Donovan, MC, Owen, MJ. (2015). Genetic risk for schizophrenia: convergence on synaptic pathways involved in plasticity. *Biol Psychiatry* 77: 52.

47. The Network and Pathway Analysis Subgroup of the Psychiatric Genomics Consortium. (2015). Psychiatric genome-wide association study analyses implicate neuronal, immune and histone pathways. *Nat Neurosci* 18: 199.

48. Costain, G, Lionel, AC, Merico, D, *et al.* (2013). Pathogenic rare copy number variants in community-based schizophrenia suggest a potential role for clinical microarrays. *Hum Mol Genet* 22: 4485.

49. Wray, NR, Lee, SH, Mehta, D, Vinkhuyzen, AA, Dudbridge, F, Middeldorp, CM. (2014). Research review: polygenic methods and their applications to psychiatric traits. *J Child Psychol Psychiatry* 55: 1068.

50. Power, RA, Steinberg, S, Bjornsdottir, G, *et al.* (2015). Polygenic risk scores for schizophrenia and bipolar disorder predict creativity. *Nat Neurosci* 18: 953.

51. Owen, MJ. (2014). New approaches to psychiatric diagnostic classification. *Neuron* 84: 564.

52. Hamshere, ML, O'Donovan, MC, Jones, IR, *et al.* (2011). Polygenic dissection of the bipolar phenotype. *Br J Psychiatry* 198: 284.

53. Ruderfer, DM, Fanous, AH, Ripke, S, McQuillin, A, Amdur, RL; Schizophrenia Working Group of the Psychiatric Genomics Consortium, *et al.* (2014). Polygenic dissection of diagnosis and clinical dimensions of bipolar disorder and schizophrenia. *Mol Psychiatry* 19: 1017.

54. Jones, HJ, Stergiakouli, E, Tansey, KE, *et al.* (2016). Phenotypic manifestation of genetic risk for schizophrenia during adolescence in the general population. *JAMA Psychiatry* 73: 221.

55. Franke, B, Stein, JL, Ripke, S, *et al.* (2016). Genetic influences on schizophrenia and subcortical brain volumes: large-scale proof of concept. *Nat Neurosci* 19: 420.

# 60

# Structural and functional neuroimaging of schizophrenia

*Andreea O. Diaconescu, Sandra Iglesias, and Klaas E. Stephan*

## Historical origins of neuroimaging in schizophrenia

Neuroimaging has played a pivotal role in the scientific investigation of schizophrenia. In particular, imaging provided empirical evidence that the brain of patients with schizophrenia exhibits structural and functional differences, compared to both controls and patients with other diseases. This evidence was crucial for the long-standing debate of whether schizophrenia has biological roots or is purely social and psychological in origin (for example, as hypothesized by theories of 'double-bind' [1] or the concept of the 'schizophrenogenic mother' [2]). This introductory section provides a brief overview of seminal neuroimaging studies of schizophrenia across different modalities.

Historically, an early and extremely influential *in vivo* demonstration of structural brain changes in schizophrenia was provided by a computed tomography (CT) study by Johnstone and colleagues (1976). This study demonstrated significant enlargement of ventricles in patients with schizophrenia, compared to matched healthy controls; furthermore, ventricular size correlated significantly with cognitive impairment [3]. One concern was that these structural changes might have arisen from the long-term institutionalization of these particular patients and the often invasive treatments they had received (including insulin coma therapy). However, the finding of enlarged ventricles was subsequently replicated in multiple CT and magnetic resonance imaging (MRI) studies (Fig. 60.1) [4–6] and confirmed by meta-analyses [7].

Early functional neuroimaging studies of schizophrenia examined basic physiology, using radioactive measurements of cerebral perfusion and metabolism, respectively, as provided by single-photon emission computed tomography (SPECT) and positron emission tomography (PET). A seminal SPECT study found that older (but not younger) patients with chronic schizophrenia had decreased perfusion in their frontal lobes, compared to a control group of alcoholic patients [8]. This 'hypofrontality' was also detected using PET and was related to poor performance in cognitive tests [5]. Together with increased metabolic activity in the basal ganglia, hypofrontality

offered an explanation for the '[ … ] simultaneous generation of positive and negative symptoms [ . . . ]' [9]. However, subsequent PET studies failed to find hypofrontality [10, 11]; this discrepancy may have arisen from several factors, including performance differences between patients and controls in particular, but also differences in whether studies examined 'resting' conditions or cognitive tasks and differences in statistical analysis techniques (for discussions of hypofrontality, see [12, 13]).

Electroencephalography (EEG) played an important role in early brain activity investigations of schizophrenia, providing high temporal resolution of normal and pathological brain processes. Early studies reported multiple abnormalities in the electrical brain activity of patients with schizophrenia, for example epileptic-like potentials, reduced alpha activity, and/or enhanced fast-wave activity [14]. The investigation of evoked EEG responses to sensory events [event-related potentials (ERPs)] received particular interest. Notable findings in schizophrenia patients included reductions in N100 [15, 16] and P300 amplitudes [17], irrespective of the sensory modality. Since the early 1990s, the auditory mismatch negativity (MMN) has been widely investigated in schizophrenia. The MMN is the difference potential between responses to unpredictable stimuli ('deviants') and predictable stimuli ('standards'). In the first study of MMN in schizophrenia, Shelley *et al.* (1991) found an attenuation of the auditory MMN amplitude in schizophrenia patients, as compared to controls [18]. This finding has since been replicated by a large number of studies (for a meta-analysis, see [19]) and continues to play a major role in contemporary schizophrenia research.

Prior to the advent of functional MRI (fMRI), PET played a critical role in assessing regional activation changes in schizophrenia during cognitive tasks *in vivo* [20–24]. Given the long-standing notions of schizophrenia as resulting from abnormal connectivity [25] (see The dysconnection theory of schizophrenia, p. 602), particular attempts were made to link aberrant activity in neural networks to symptoms of schizophrenia [23, 26–28]. For instance, the concept of 'cognitive dysmetria'—'the difficulty in prioritizing, processing, coordinating, and responding to information' [29]—was linked to alterations of a prefrontal–thalamic–cerebellar circuit measured with PET in schizophrenia patients [30].

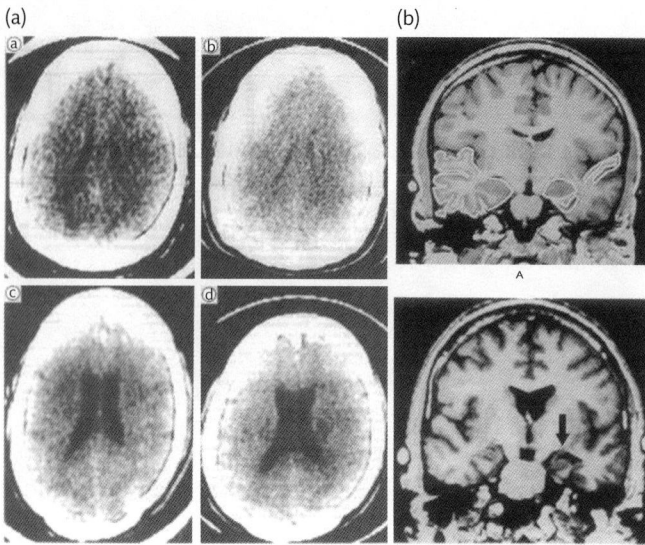

**Fig. 60.1** Structural brain differences in schizophrenia.
(a) An 8-year follow-up CT scan in two patients (panels a and b, and panels c and d are the same patients) showing ventricular size and configuration.
Reproduced from *J Neurol Neurosurg Psychiatry*, 51(2), Illowsky BP, Juliano DM, Bigelow LB, *et al.*, Stability of CT scan findings in schizophrenia: results of an 8 year follow-up study, pp. 209–13, Copyright (1988), with permission from *British Medical Journal*.
(b) Upper panel: control subject and outlined regions of interest in the temporal lobe. Lower panel: schizophrenia patient; increased ventricle size, increased tissue loss in the parahippocampal gyrus imaged with MRI.
Reproduced from *New Engl J Med*, 327(9), Shenton ME, Kikinis R, Jolesz FA, *et al.*, Abnormalities of the Left Temporal Lobe and Thought Disorder in Schizophrenia, pp. 604–612, Copyright (1992), with permission from Massachusetts Medical Society.

Finally, the development of fMRI in the 1990s led to a breakthrough in neurophysiological research on schizophrenia *in vivo*. While the non-quantitative nature of the blood–oxygen level-dependent (BOLD) signal and the complexities of data analysis induced an initial delay in the uptake of fMRI, its considerably higher temporal and spatial resolution, compared to PET, as well as its radioactive-free nature, radically increased the utility and availability of functional neuroimaging for schizophrenia research. The earliest fMRI applications to schizophrenia included neurological soft signs, as probed by simple motor tasks [31], auditory hallucinations [32], and working memory [33]. Since then, the vast majority of functional imaging studies on schizophrenia have used fMRI, as reflected by the literature covered in the following sections.

Following the early milestone neuroimaging studies described previously, the neuroimaging research in schizophrenia has virtually exploded, resulting in a vast body of literature that is impossible to cover in a single chapter. In the following, we partition the neuroimaging literature on schizophrenia into two broad classes: discovery-oriented and theory-driven approaches. With regard to the latter, we use four major contemporary pathophysiological theories in order to structure the imaging literature on schizophrenia and focus on studies with a direct connection to proposed disease mechanisms. We conclude with an outlook on computational neuroimaging approaches that strive for mechanistic interpretability, as opposed to descriptive accounts of neuroimaging data [34].

## Discovery-oriented neuroimaging approaches

The introduction of non-invasive neuroimaging with MRI enabled the systematic search for structural and functional differences in the brain of patients with schizophrenia. Most of the initial work, beginning in the early 1980s [35, 36], used structural MRI to identify neuroanatomical abnormalities. Two main approaches have been used: region of interest (ROI) analyses, which are based on a priori chosen regions delineated by atlases or manual tracing, and whole-brain approaches such as voxel-based morphometry (VBM) [37].

Some of the most notable replicated findings include: ventricular enlargement [38], cerebral atrophy [39], grey matter reductions in the amygdala, hippocampus, parahippocampal gyrus, and anterior cingulate gyrus [40, 41], and frontal lobe abnormalities, particularly in prefrontal and orbitofrontal subregions [42]. Whole-brain approaches, such as VBM, that are not biased to one particular region, have pointed to grey matter decreases in patients with schizophrenia, compared to healthy controls, in several regions, including the thalamus, insula, superior temporal gyrus (in particular, in the left hemisphere, which is associated with auditory information processing and language), anterior and posterior cingulate, and medial frontal gyrus [43, 44].

Longitudinal studies addressed the question of whether these volumetric abnormalities were present before the onset of the illness or materialized only after its onset. A particular focus has been on individuals at risk for schizophrenia; here, longitudinal studies found volumetric reductions of the temporal, cingulate, insular, prefrontal, and parahippocampal cortices in those individuals who later developed first-episode psychosis symptoms [45]. In a large multi-site early prevention study of at-risk mental state (ARMS) individuals, larger reductions in grey matter volume of the parahippocampal gyrus were detected in ARMS individuals who transitioned to psychosis, compared to those who maintained a subclinical symptom level [46]. Grey matter abnormalities also progressed after the onset of schizophrenia. Longitudinal studies in chronically ill patients suggest that progressive brain changes continue for up to 20 years after the first symptoms [7, 47]. These changes include lateral ventricle volume increases and grey matter density decreases in specific brain regions, including the superior frontal gyrus, superior temporal gyrus (particularly in the left hemisphere), right caudate nucleus, and right thalamus [7, 47].

The development of diffusion-weighted imaging (DWI) has made it possible to investigate white matter *in vivo* and derive estimates of connectivity by tractography. Meta-analyses of DWI studies in schizophrenia suggested that white matter abnormalities are apparent in two main regions—the left frontal deep white matter tract linking the frontal lobe, thalamus, and cingulate gyrus, and the left temporal deep white matter tract linking the frontal lobe, hippocampus, amygdala, and temporal and occipital lobes [48, 49]. DWI-derived connectivity matrices have fuelled the emerging field of connectomics, which uses graph-theoretical methods to examine the topology of networks. Applications of the graph theory to DWI data from patients with schizophrenia suggested reduced network capacity for integration, as reflected by longer path lengths [50], reduced network efficiency [51], and reduced 'rich club' organization [52].

A parallel line of research has assessed these putative functional integration abnormalities in schizophrenia by corresponding analyses of functional connectivity. While reduced functional connectivity—in particular fronto-temporal connectivity [27]—has featured prominently in the literature [52, 53], enhanced functional connectivity has also been reported [54, 55], even in the presence of reduced structural connectivity in patients [56]. However, this diversity may, at least in part, also result from methodological differences across studies. For example, Yang *et al.* (2014) showed that global signal regression strongly affected coupling estimates (see [56] for discussion).

Graph-theoretical investigations of functional connectivity matrices have provided important insights into network alterations in schizophrenia [56]. Notable findings include reductions in clustering, small worldness, and the probability of high-degree hubs [53]. Interestingly, meta-analyses of fMRI activity in schizophrenia have shown that abnormal activations are concentrated in hubs of a 'normative connectome' such as the thalamus, middle cingulate gyrus, and the dorsolateral prefrontal cortex (PFC) [57].

An alternative approach to examining large-scale functional connectivity without a priori parcellation is independent component analysis (ICA). This method identifies networks as spatially distinct maps of voxels which share a common time course. This approach has shown across both 'resting state' conditions and cognitive paradigms that schizophrenia is characterized by altered global connectivity patterns [58, 59].

## Theory-driven neuroimaging approaches

The short summary of discovery-oriented analyses of structural and functional neuroimaging data in the previous section outlined alterations of global brain organization that are largely descriptive and do not specify a specific disease mechanism. We now turn to imaging studies that were motivated by a particular pathophysiological theory. These include: (1) the neurodevelopmental theory; (2) the dopamine theory; (3) GABAergic and glutamatergic theories; and (4) the dysconnection theory of schizophrenia.

### The neurodevelopmental theory of schizophrenia

The *neurodevelopmental theory of schizophrenia* postulates an aberrant development of the central nervous system as the cause of the disorder [60, 61]. In brief, this theory assumes that a disruption occurs during early (pre-/perinatal) or late (puberty and adolescence) neurodevelopmental processes that impacts on the biochemistry, function, and structure (including connectivity) of the brain. Possible environmental factors include (social) stressors that result in endocrine and metabolic changes and/or infections, presumably interacting with specific genetic predispositions [62].

One starting point for the neurodevelopmental theory was the finding, from the early neuroimaging studies described previously, of structural brain differences in schizophrenia, especially increased lateral ventricles (Fig. 60.1). For example, intrigued by the finding that enlarged ventricles were already present at the earliest stage of schizophrenia, Murray and Lewis (1987) speculated that these changes represented possible consequences of earlier developmental disturbances [60]. Furthermore, this structural abnormality was initially thought not to be associated with the duration of the disease or type of therapy [63]. (Later studies showed, however, that the enlargement of ventricles continues during the course of schizophrenia;

for a meta-analysis and review, see [7, 64], respectively). These structural findings were hypothesized to result from the interaction between genetic predisposition and environmental insults. One model suggested that disruptions in normal neurodevelopment may take place in the pre- or perinatal period, through infections or obstetric complications which impact globally on the normal development of the nervous system, including proliferation and migration of neurons, and the growth and pruning of axonal connections [60, 62, 63]. This was supported by studies showing that individuals who developed schizophrenia were more likely to have experienced pre- or perinatal adverse events, compared to healthy subjects (for review, see [65]); mixed evidence (reviewed in [66]) exists for a similar risk role of perinatal infections.

An alternative to a more 'global lesion' is that the early damage of circumscribed brain regions may affect the development of other regions such as the PFC [61]. One particular candidate for such an initial lesion is the hippocampus, which contributes to regulating the activity of midbrain dopamine neurons; indeed, animal models with prenatal hippocampal lesions found increased activity of dopaminergic neurons in the midbrain [67]. The ensuing change in neuromodulatory projections might impact on the development of prefrontal (and other) regions.

A non-trivial challenge for the neurodevelopmental account of schizophrenia is to explain why morphological changes are not confined to the time of the hypothetical insult but continue to unfold in time. As noted by Kempton *et al.* (2010), the finding of continuously accelerated enlargements of the lateral ventricles '[ … ] challenges an exclusively neurodevelopmental model of schizophrenia' [64]. Beyond simple volumetric changes, several longitudinal structural MRI studies have demonstrated that schizophrenia has a progressive nature, with pronounced grey matter changes occurring over at least 20 years after disease onset; comprehensive reviews and meta-analyses can be found in [7, 68–70]. For example, an early study by Thompson and colleagues (2001) observed accelerated grey matter loss over 5 years in very early-onset schizophrenia, compared to healthy controls, starting in parietal brain regions and motor and supplementary motor cortices, and progressing later to the superior frontal gyri, dorsolateral PFC, and temporal cortices, including the superior temporal gyrus (Fig. 60.2) [71]. This progressive grey matter loss was correlated with an overall decrease in global functioning in the patient group. In particular, faster loss rates of grey matter in temporal regions were associated with more severe positive symptoms, and faster loss rates of frontal grey matter loss with negative symptoms.

Consistent with these results, a more rapid grey matter reduction relative to age-related loss in healthy controls was found in subsequent longitudinal MRI studies across different clinical stages and medication status. This included first-episode schizophrenia patients [72], medicated patients [73], and, to a lesser extent, drug-naïve patients [74] (Fig. 60.2). Generally, medication appears to modulate, but not explain, accelerated grey matter loss in patients with schizophrenia [68, 75].

### The dopamine theory of schizophrenia

The *dopamine (DA) theory of schizophrenia* was initially based upon the thesis that the efficacy of neuroleptic drugs to attenuate psychosis symptoms depended on striatal D2 antagonism [76]. Since then, a substantial number of PET and SPECT studies have provided

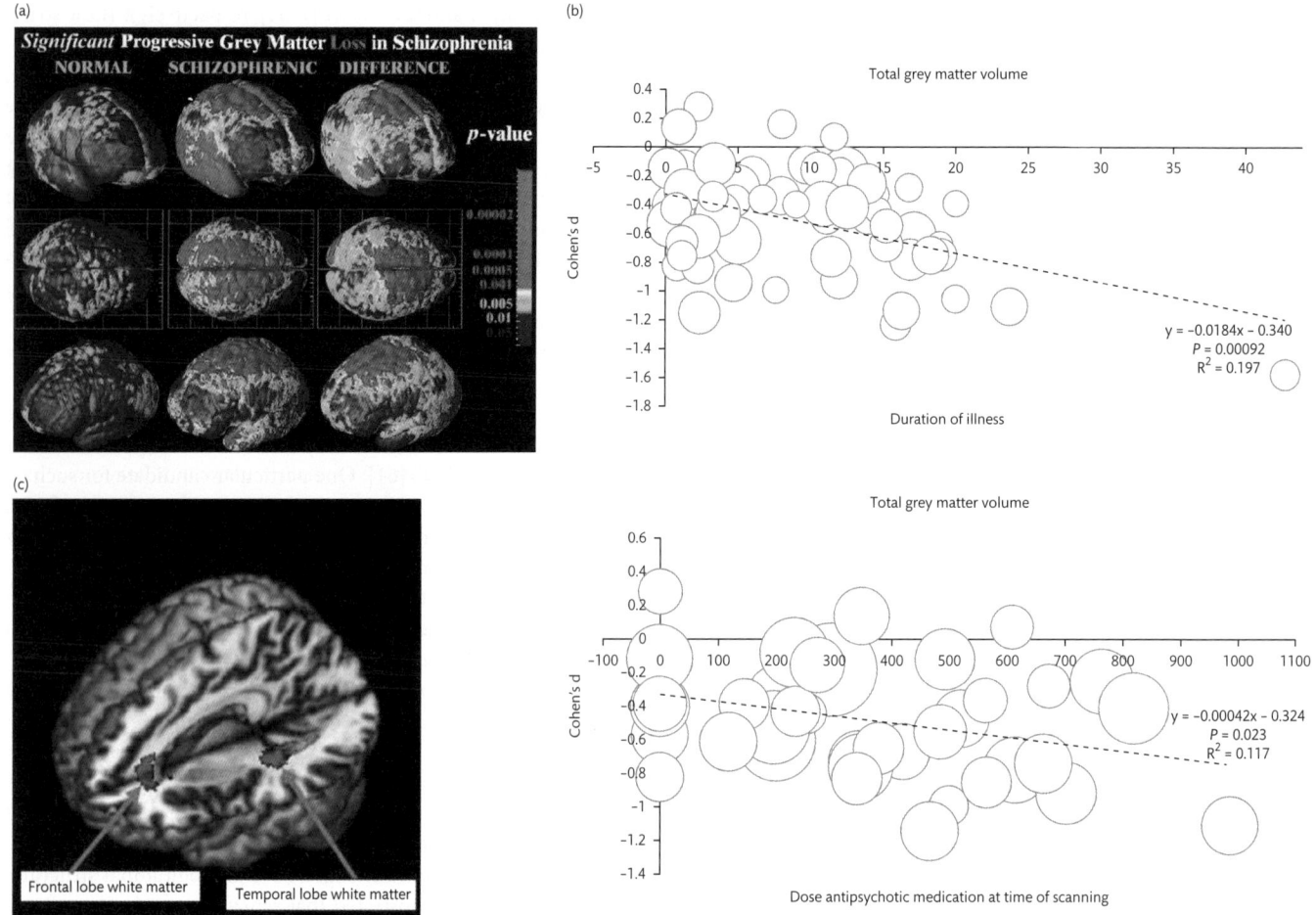

**Fig. 60.2** Progressive grey and white matter loss in schizophrenia.

(a) Significant grey matter loss in normal adolescents and schizophrenia (see Colour Plate section).

Reproduced from *Proc Natl Acad Sci U S A*, 98(20), Thompson PM, Vidal C, Giedd JN, *et al.*, Mapping adolescent brain change reveals dynamic wave of accelerated gray matter loss in very early-onset schizophrenia, pp. 11650–5, Copyright (2001), with permission from National Academy of Sciences.

(b) Upper panel: total grey matter volume reduction depends on duration of illness; lower panel: total grey matter volume reduction was more pronounced in patients using a higher dose of atypical antipsychotics.

Reproduced from *Schizophr Bull.*, 39(5), Haijma SV, Haren NV, Cahn W, *et al.*, Brain Volumes in Schizophrenia: A Meta-Analysis in Over 18 000 Subjects, pp. 1129–38, Copyright (2013), with permission from Oxford University Press.

(c) Regional fractional anisotropy reductions in the deep white matter of the left frontal and left temporal lobes in schizophrenia (see Colour Plate section).

Reproduced from *Schizophr Res*, 108(1–3), Ellison-Wright I, Bullmore E, Meta-analysis of diffusion tensor imaging studies in schizophrenia, pp. 3–10, Copyright (2009), with permission from Elsevier B.V.

compelling evidence of elevated presynaptic DA levels in the striatum (for example, [77]). Presynaptic DA can be investigated using tracers like $^{18}$F-dihydroxyphenyl-$L$-alanine ($^{18}$F-DOPA), which are taken up by dopaminergic terminals and probe DA synthesis capacity. Beyond individual studies, evidence of elevated DA synthesis capacity in the striatum was provided by meta-analyses of patients with schizophrenia [78, 79]. This elevation was also found in individuals at risk for psychosis [80, 81], including medication-naïve prodromal individuals [82]. When followed longitudinally, a subset of the ultra-high-risk subjects who transitioned from the prodromal stage to frank psychosis showed a progressive increase in DA synthesis [83]. In addition to the striatum, corresponding findings were also recently made for the midbrain [84].

Another argument in favour of a central role of DA relates to the role of the DA system in learning and plasticity. DA modulates glutamatergic plasticity in several ways; for example, activation of D1 receptors enhances, and of D2 receptors diminishes, NMDA receptor-mediated long-term potentiation [85]. Referring to the importance of DA in learning and plasticity, one theory of psychosis holds that individuals with schizophrenia attribute aberrant salience to irrelevant information due to inappropriate, 'chaotic' phasic firing of DA neurons [86–89]. This theory posits a key role of the DA system in mediating the misattribution of salience [90] and is supported by a host of fMRI studies in patients with schizophrenia. Firstly, empirical support for this theory comes from Pavlovian conditioning experiments where neutral cues were associated with appetitive or aversive events [91–93]. Behaviourally and autonomically, schizophrenia patients exhibited reduced differences in responding to paired cues (that is, cues that predict reinforcement) relative to unpaired ones. These behavioural effects were related to increased activity in the dopaminergic midbrain and dopaminoceptive regions, including the ventral striatum, across both aversive and appetitive contexts [91, 92]. Secondly, in the context of instrumental learning, BOLD activation in the ventral striatum in response to reward-predicting cues was shown to be blunted in medicated patients [94], medication-free patients [95–97], unaffected patient siblings [98], and healthy controls with subclinical psychosis-like symptoms [99]. In some studies (for example, [94]), attenuated responses to reward prediction error, but increased responses to prediction error, on neutral trials were also found in the dopaminergic midbrain.

Blunted striatal activations in response to task-relevant stimuli may be specifically linked to negative symptoms [100], even in unmedicated patients [95], whereas enhanced midbrain and striatal response to task-irrelevant stimuli appear to be related to positive symptoms in both unmedicated [94, 101] and medicated patients [93]. fMRI studies that specifically tested salience attributions [102] provide further support for aberrant signals in the midbrain and ventral striatum, as accounting for positive symptoms in schizophrenia [103].

## The GABAergic and glutamatergic theories of schizophrenia

The *NMDA* (*N*-methyl-*D*-aspartate) *and GABA* (gamma aminobutyric acid) *receptor hypofunction theory of schizophrenia* was based on the finding that dissociative anaesthetics, including ketamine, an NMDA receptor (NMDAR) antagonist [104], can induce a transient psychosis-like state in healthy volunteers that is characterized by perceptual alterations, delusion-like ideas, thought disorder, and blunted affect [105]. Ketamine can also aggravate psychosis in patients with schizophrenia [106].

A single dose of ketamine leads to a significant reduction in the auditory MMN, an electrophysiological response to rule violations. This was first shown using invasive recordings in monkeys [107], followed by multiple demonstrations in humans, based on EEG (for example, [108–110]). Importantly, the auditory MMN is also significantly reduced in patients with schizophrenia, in a comparable manner as under ketamine application [111], and represents one of the most robust group-level physiological indices of the clinical diagnosis of schizophrenia. Reduced auditory MMN amplitude in schizophrenia was first described by Shelley *et al.* (1991), a finding that has since been replicated by dozens of studies (for a meta-analysis, see [19]).

The auditory MMN is reduced not only in schizophrenia patients, but also among ARMS individuals with subclinical symptoms, and substantially more reduced in those who transition to psychosis [112]. A recent fMRI study also demonstrated auditory mismatch impairments in schizophrenia patients, as reflected by reduced BOLD responses to mismatch blocks in auditory regions (primary auditory cortex and superior temporal gyrus), anterior cingulate, and medial prefrontal gyri [113] (Fig. 60.3).

In addition to NMDARs, GABAergic receptors have been implicated in the pathophysiology of schizophrenia [114–116]. Both processes may be closely connected—given that NMDARs provide a major source of excitatory input to inhibitory interneurons [117, 118], NMDAR antagonism may lead to disinhibition of their post-synaptic target neurons, with less coherent pyramidal cell firing as a possible consequence (for review, see [119]). Indirect empirical evidence for this process in schizophrenia is provided by studies examining neuronal oscillations with EEG/MEG recordings [120]. For example, gamma-band oscillations in the dorsolateral PFC,

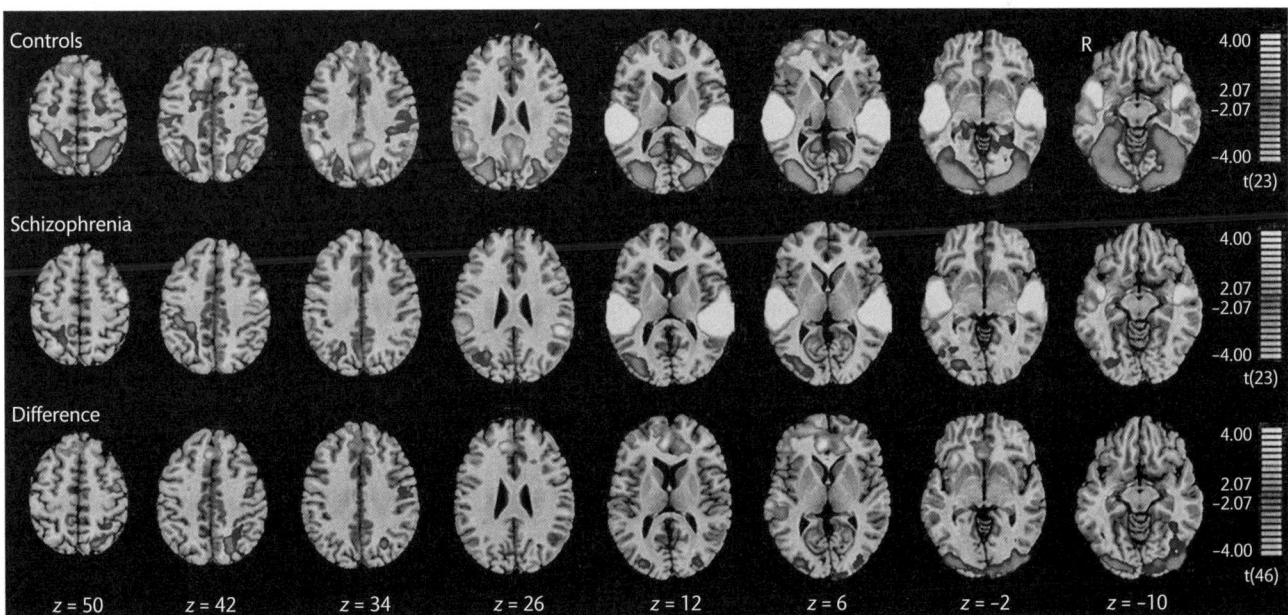

**Fig. 60.3** (see Colour Plate section) Haemodynamic response to mismatch blocks (*P* <0.05). A corrected cluster size threshold was based on a Monte Carlo simulation. First row: healthy controls; second row: schizophrenia patients; third row: difference between healthy controls and schizophrenia patients for the contrast mismatch > standard (baseline) condition. Schizophrenia patients exhibited less activity in the auditory cortex and prefrontal and salience network (bilateral ACC, medial frontal gyrus, and right insula). Enhanced activity was found in schizophrenia patients in the pre- and postcentral gyri, compared to the control group. *z*-co-ordinates refer to the Talairach system.

which are in the 30- to 80-Hz range and scale with working memory load [121], are significantly reduced in schizophrenia patients, compared to controls [122].

A more direct, but static, readout of GABA levels can be obtained by magnetic resonance spectroscopy (MRS) (for review, see [123]). MRS can be implemented in different ways; most commonly, it focuses on hydrogen nuclear spins ($^1$H MRS). These hydrogen nuclear spins are reflected by specific radiofrequency signals that are determined by the chemical environment of the hydrogen spins. This allows, in principle, for the detection of certain endogenous metabolites, including GABA and glutamate.

MRS is increasingly being applied to schizophrenia. For example, Yoon *et al.* (2010) found reduced GABA levels in the visual cortex of patients with schizophrenia [124]. This reduction correlated with orientation-specific surround suppression, a psychophysical measure that is believed to reflect cortical inhibition. Kegeles *et al.* (2012) employed MRS to measure GABA and glutamate levels in the dorsolateral and medial PFC, respectively, contrasting both medicated and non-medicated patients with schizophrenia to healthy controls. They found a significant increase of both GABA and glutamate levels in the medial prefrontal region in unmedicated, but not medicated, patients. By contrast, there were no group differences in the dorsolateral PFC for either transmitter [125].

The practical application of MRS to schizophrenia, however, is aggravated by various methodological challenges [126]. One of the most obvious practical limitations is that most presently used MRS techniques are limited spatially to a small ROI (although alternatives are emerging such as chemical exchange saturation transfer (CEST) techniques; see, for example, [127]). Variations in the ROIs across reports may provide one partial explanation for why the MRS literature on alterations of GABA levels in schizophrenia is diverse and difficult to reconcile. Put differently, 'MRS assays of GABA concentration have yielded equivocal evidence of large-scale alteration in GABA concentration' in schizophrenia [126]. The most comprehensive review to date that we are aware of (that is, [128]) failed to find significant alterations in GABA levels in schizophrenia, as assessed by MRS.

## The dysconnection theory of schizophrenia

The proposition that schizophrenia represents a mental condition characterized by cognitive disintegration dates back to Wernicke, who proposed that the disorder arises due to a disruption of association fibre tracts, and later to Bleuler (1911) who described the 'splitting' of mental functions [129]. The dysconnection theory of schizophrenia follows this tradition. It arose from the initial thesis that positive symptoms in schizophrenia might be explained as a consequence of disrupted temporo-prefrontal functional connectivity, as had been observed in early PET studies [130]. This led to conceptualizing schizophrenia initially as a disconnection syndrome [27, 131].

However, although most structural and functional connectivity analyses in schizophrenia tend to report a decrease in connectivity, especially with the frontal cortex [132], enhanced connectivity is also a frequent finding, as discussed previously. This motivated a replacement of the Latin prefix 'dis' (apart) by the Greek prefix 'dys' (bad or ill) [133] and led to a more concrete specification of the pathophysiology that underlies aberrant functional coupling of schizophrenia. Specifically, the dysconnection hypothesis postulates that the central disease mechanism in schizophrenia is an aberrant neuromodulatory regulation (dopaminergic and/or cholinergic) of NMDAR-dependent synaptic plasticity [131]. This explains both functional and structural connectivity in schizophrenia as the consequences of disturbances in 'NMDAR-neuromodulator interactions' (NNI) [133, 134].

Abnormal NNI is consistent with the other pathophysiological theories described previously and may offer a unifying theme for their integration (for details, see [134]). For example, NMDAR hypofunction due to aberrant neuromodulatory regulation can explain progressive grey matter loss (as NMDARs provide a potent neurotrophic signal); it naturally incorporates the NMDAR hypofunction and DA theories and it relates to GABAergic dysfunction, given the role of the latter in post-synaptic gain control, and thus the encoding of precision. Equally importantly, NNI is affected by both genetic [135] and environmental (hormonal, immunological, and metabolic) risk factors for schizophrenia. This makes NNI a key target of gene–environmental interactions and could help explain the clinical heterogeneity across patients [134].

What distinguishes the dysconnection theory from other theories of schizophrenia, however, is that it proposes a specific computational patho-mechanism—an abnormal hierarchical Bayesian inference in the cortex, as a result of aberrant NNI [133, 136]. In hierarchical Bayesian theories of brain function, such as predictive coding [137, 138], the brain is assumed to construct a hierarchical model of the world in order to infer the environmental causes of its sensory inputs. In this predictive coding framework, hierarchically related levels of cortical processing streams exchange predictions and prediction errors in order to estimate states of the world given sensory input (perceptual inference) and adjust the model's predictions (learning). Critically, prediction errors are weighted by how uncertain or precise both predictions and sensory inputs are. This ensures that perception and learning are influenced by the relative reliability of sensory information and prior beliefs.

Importantly, in addition to physiological studies in animals (for example, [139]), human pharmacological neuroimaging studies have disclosed likely relations between the computational quantities in predictive coding and physiological processes (for reviews, see [34, 136, 140]). In brief, prediction errors are thought to be conveyed by ascending connections via both AMPA (α-amino-3-hydroxyl-5-methyl-4-isoxazole propionate) and NMDA receptors, while predictions are signalled via NMDARs by descending connections. Finally, precision weighting is likely implemented by neuromodulatory, as well as GABAergic, influences, both of which regulate the gain of glutamatergic post-synaptic responses.

The physiological–computational links suggested by the dysconnection theory are important for at least two reasons. Firstly, they suggest that the heterogenous spectrum nature of schizophrenia could be resolved by tools that infer subject-specific abnormalities of NNI from measured brain activity and behaviour [133]. Secondly, they highlight the connections of the dysconnection hypothesis to the other theories of schizophrenia discussed previously. In particular, precision provides an important bridge to the theory of DA-induced 'aberrant salience' in schizophrenia [87]. Put differently, precision offers a formal definition of salience that can help explain prominent symptoms such as hallucinations and delusions [136, 141, 142].

Neuroimaging studies have provided several lines of empirical evidence for the physiological (NNI) and computational (hierarchical Bayesian inference) aspects of the dysconnection theory. Reviews can be found elsewhere [134, 136, 143]; here, for lack of space, we focus on three particular aspects from the recent literature.

Firstly, according to the dysconnection hypothesis, the empirically observed reduction in the auditory MMN should be understood as resulting from abnormal NNI and reflecting impaired hierarchical Bayesian inference [133]. This has been corroborated by recent studies. For example, computational modelling of empirical EEG data demonstrated that a Bayesian inference process [144] provides a better explanation of trial-by-trial changes in the auditory MMN than conventional theories such as change detection or adaptation. Physiologically, reduced MMN in schizophrenia patients is reflected by abnormal connectivity in auditory hierarchies, as shown by a dynamic causal model (DCM) of EEG data that revealed both abnormal ascending and descending connection strengths at the time when surprising stimuli (deviants) were presented [145].

Secondly, from the perspective of the dysconnection hypotheses, hallucinations would arise naturally when prior expectations (about the occurrence of human voices) in higher areas of the auditory hierarchy become abnormally tight (for example, due to a cholinergic abnormality; cf. [137]). One consequence of such overly precise priors would be a down-weighting of prediction errors computed in lower areas. This is precisely what was found in a recent fMRI study on schizophrenia patients with auditory hallucinations that showed a reduced prediction error signal in the auditory cortex [146]. Interestingly, the putative hyper-precision of auditory priors could reflect a compensatory response to initially abnormally high sensory precision.

Thirdly, an imbalance in the precision weighting of bottom–up signals and top–down predictions—in this case, reduced precision of predictions relative to sensory precision—would also explain the empirically observed reduced sensitivity of patients with schizophrenia to visual illusions [147]. This has been studied in patients with schizophrenia, using an identical 'hollow mask' illusion paradigm for both fMRI and EEG. In both modalities, DCM demonstrated that, consistent with reduced precision of predictions (in this case about facial stimuli), the patients' pronounced lack of susceptibility to the 'hollow mask' illusion could be explained by increased strengths of bottom–up connections, combined with reduced strengths of top–down connections, compared to healthy controls [148, 149].

## Outlook

Neuroimaging studies have provided invaluable insights into the structural and functional changes associated with schizophrenia. In spite of their scientific success, neuroimaging and electrophysiological techniques have not provided concrete diagnostic tools for psychiatry so far [150]. One explanation for this lack of translation is that conventional analysis methods have remained mostly descriptive—they describe patterns of activations, connections, or changes in brain structure, but they do not allow for quantifying the probability that a particular disease mechanism is present. This, however, is the basis for differential diagnosis and targeted treatment.

In the following, we briefly outline two complementary strategies for addressing this problem. A first possibility is to invest in the development of neuroimaging techniques that provide more direct physiological interpretability than the available structural or functional contrasts in MRI. A prime candidate for this purpose is MRS. Despite its potential, it has, somewhat surprisingly, not made decisive contributions to schizophrenia research so far. Reasons include variability in ROIs across studies, as discussed previously, but also technical limitations since at lower field strengths, the separation of different peaks in the spectrum is difficult. Advances in high-field MRI and the development of CEST techniques—which make MRI sensitive to concentrations of a host of endogenous metabolites [151, 152] and provide whole-brain coverage of neurotransmitter systems—are beginning to change the clinical utility of MRS, as illustrated by recent applications to epilepsy [127].

A second option is to pursue a neuromodelling strategy. This usually takes one of two forms: biophysical network models (BNMs) and generative models (for review, see [34]). The former consist of regional circuit models that are connected by long-range connections, typically informed by DWI data (for review, see [153]). While BNMs have found application for schizophrenia (for example, [54]), their complexity makes parameter estimation from fMRI or EEG data difficult; often, only a single global scaling parameter of connection strengths is estimated. This has restricted the potential of BNMs to provide clinical tests. 'Generative models' (Fig. 60.4) [163] represent an alternative. These describe potential neural mechanisms that could have generated the measured neuroimaging data (EEG or fMRI), including noise. Put differently, generative models embody a probabilistic mapping from the (hidden) neural states to the measured data; this mapping can, in principle, be inverted to uncover disease mechanisms in individual patients [154]. One example of such an approach is DCM, which describes the dynamics of neuronal populations using differential equations [155]. DCMs explain measured brain activity as arising circuit dynamics that is a function of: (1) intrinsic connectivity; (2) experimentally induced perturbations; and (3) modulatory inputs that invoke contextual changes in synaptic strengths (that is, short-term plasticity during learning or neuromodulatory influences). In conjunction with suitably defined observation models, DCMs can be applied to either fMRI or electrophysiological data. Importantly, such models require a prior distribution, indicating the possible range of parameter values. Techniques such as DWI or MRS can be used to provide anatomical or physiological constraints on the variance of these prior distributions in individual patients (for proof of concept, see [156]). As has been demonstrated in various validation studies in humans and animals (for example, [109, 157–159]), DCM can potentially detect alterations in glutamatergic, GABAergic, and neuromodulatory (for example, dopaminergic and cholinergic) synaptic transmission and thus provide a considerably more detailed assessment of pathophysiology than a phenomenological account of changes in function coupling.

A complementary approach within a computational approach to neuroimaging-based differential diagnosis is provided by generative models of behaviour. These can be fitted to individual behavioural responses in order to infer on trajectories of computational quantities such as prediction errors. While this approach has featured prominently in the investigation of dopaminergic abnormalities in schizophrenia, as discussed previously, recent results based on hierarchical Bayesian models have suggested the possibility of assessing trial-wise activity in both dopaminergic and cholinergic regions

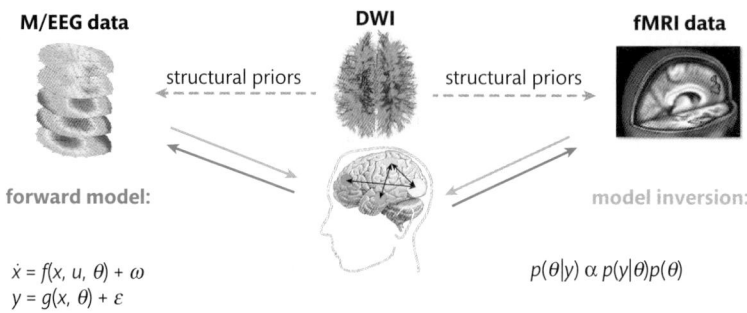

**Fig. 60.4** (see Colour Plate section) Generative models for neuroimaging data.
Generative models applied to neuroimaging data propose that we can infer on neural activity (for example, firing rate) from the measured signal. Constrained by priors that define neuroanatomical connectivity obtained by DWI techniques, generative models comprise neural state equations, which describe the hidden dynamics in terms of differential equations that are parameterized, and a forward model that describes a mapping from the neural state to the measured signal. To estimate how neural states translate into the measured signal, the model is inverted, that is, fitted to the neuroimaging data and the connectivity parameters that generated the observed data are estimated. DWI, diffusion-weighted imaging; M/EEG, magneto-/electroencephalography.

Reproduced from *NeuroImage*, 45(2), Chen CC, Henson RN, Stephan KE, *et al.*, Forward and backward connections in the brain: A DCM study of functional asymmetries, pp. 453–62, Copyright (2009), with permission from Elsevier Inc.; *Neuron*, 87(4), Stephan KE, Iglesias S, Heinzle J, *et al.*, Translational Perspectives for Computational Neuroimaging, pp. 716–32, Copyright (2015), with permission from Elsevier Inc.

under the same paradigm [160, 161]. This may provide a powerful approach for classifying patients with schizophrenia into different NNI subgroups.

The utility of generative models for detecting physiologically defined subgroups within schizophrenia has been demonstrated previously. For example, Brodersen and colleagues (2014) applied a simple DCM of interactions between visual, parietal, and prefrontal regions to fMRI data from 41 patients with schizophrenia who performed a working memory task [162]. Using a variational Gaussian mixture model, they found that three clusters provided an optimal explanation of variability in connectivity estimates across patients. Remarkably, these subgroups, defined in an entirely unsupervised way, exhibited significant differences in negative symptoms, thus establishing a link between physiology and clinical symptoms. While this finding did not constitute a clinically relevant solution, as it only predicted symptoms that were already known to the clinician, it illustrates the potential of a 'generative embedding' approach. The hope is that more sophisticated models, such as DCMs capable of inferring transmitter-specific synaptic properties from electrophysiological data [157], could convey real clinical utility such as predictions about treatment responses [34].

While generative modelling approaches open up exciting opportunities for neuroimaging research on schizophrenia, validation studies are needed to determine their clinical utility. In other words, regardless of how well a model may capture a putative pathophysiology, it needs to support differential diagnosis or predict treatment response with sufficient accuracy and in individual patients. This can only be tested in prospective studies where patients are followed up after a clinical intervention and which target clinically relevant questions such as predicting the response to specific drugs for psychosis.

## REFERENCES

1. Bateson G, Jackson DD, Haley J, Weakland J. Toward a theory of schizophrenia. Behav Sci. 1956;1:251–64.
2. Harrington A. The fall of the schizophrenogenic mother. Lancet. 2012;379:1292–3.
3. Johnstone EC, Crow TJ, Frith CD, Husband J, Kreel L. Cerebral ventricular size and cognitive impairment in chronic schizophrenia. Lancet. 1976;2:924–6.
4. Illowsky BP, Juliano DM, Bigelow LB, Weinberger DR. Stability of CT scan findings in schizophrenia: results of an 8 year follow-up study. J Neurol Neurosurg Psychiatry. 1988;51:209–13.
5. Kotrla KJ, Weinberger DR. Brain imaging in schizophrenia. Annu Rev Med. 1995;46:113–22.
6. Shenton ME, Kikinis R, Jolesz FA, *et al.* Abnormalities of the left temporal lobe and thought disorder in schizophrenia. N Engl J Med. 1992;327:604–12.
7. Pol HEH, Kahn RS. What happens after the first episode? A review of progressive brain changes in chronically ill patients with schizophrenia. Schizophr Bull. 2008;34:354–66.
8. Ingvar DH, Franzén G. Abnormalities of cerebral blood flow distribution in patients with chronic schizophrenia. Acta Psychiatr Scand. 1974;50:425–62.
9. Andreasen NC. Brain imaging: applications in psychiatry. Science. 1988;239:1381–8.
10. Ebmeier KP, Lawrie SM, Blackwood DH, Johnstone EC, Goodwin GM. Hypofrontality revisited: a high resolution single photon emission computed tomography study in schizophrenia. J Neurol Neurosurg Psychiatry. 1995;58:452–6.
11. Gur R, Gur R. Hypofrontality in schizophrenia: RIP. Lancet. 1995;345:1383–4.
12. Andreasen NC, O'Leary DS, Flaum M, *et al.* Hypofrontality in schizophrenia: distributed dysfunctional circuits in neuroleptic-naïve patients. Lancet. 1997;349:1730–4.
13. Weinberger DR, Berman KF, Frith C. Prefrontal function in schizophrenia: confounds and controversies [and discussion]. Philos Trans R Soc Lond B Biol Sci. 1996;351:1495–503.
14. Itil TM. Qualitative and quantitative EEG findings in schizophrenia. Schizophr Bull. 1977;3:61–79.
15. Saletu B, Itil TM, Saletu M. Auditory evoked response, EEG, and thought process in schizophrenics. Am J Psychiatry. 1971;128:336–44.
16. Shagass C, Straumanis JJ, Roemer RA, Amadeo M. Evoked potentials of schizophrenics in several sensory modalities. Biol Psychiatry. 1977;12:221–35.

17. Roth WT, Cannon EH. Some features of the auditory evoked response in schizophrenics. Arch Gen Psychiatry. 1972;27:466–71.
18. Shelley AM, Ward PB, Catts SV, Michie PT, Andrews S, McConaghy N. Mismatch negativity: an index of a preattentive processing deficit in schizophrenia. Biol Psychiatry. 1991;30:1059–62.
19. Umbricht D, Krljes S. Mismatch negativity in schizophrenia: a meta-analysis. Schizophr Res. 2005;76:1–23.
20. Berman KF, Ostrem JL, Randolph C, et al. Physiological activation of a cortical network during performance of the Wisconsin Card Sorting Test: A positron emission tomography study. Neuropsychologia. 1995;33:1027–46.
21. Carter CS, Mintun M, Nichols T, Cohen JD. Anterior Cingulate Gyrus Dysfunction and Selective Attention Deficits in Schizophrenia: [15O]H2O PET Study During Single-Trial Stroop Task Performance. Am J Psychiatry. 1997;154:1670–5.
22. Dolan RJ, Fletcher P, Frith CD, Friston KJ, Frackowiak RS, Grasby PM. Dopaminergic modulation of impaired cognitive activation in the anterior cingulate cortex in schizophrenia. Nature. 1995;378:180–2.
23. Frith CD, Friston KJ, Herold S, et al. Regional brain activity in chronic schizophrenic patients during the performance of a verbal fluency task. Br J Psychiatry. 1995;167:343–9.
24. Liddle PF, Friston KJ, Frith CD, Hirsch SR, Jones T, Frackowiak RS. Patterns of cerebral blood flow in schizophrenia. Br J Psychiatry. 1992;160:179–86.
25. Wernicke C. Grundriss der psychiatrie in klinischen vorlesungen. Leipzig: G. Thieme; 1894. Available from: https//catalog.hathitrust.org/Record/008857220
26. Fletcher P, McKenna PJ, Friston KJ, Frith CD, Dolan RJ. Abnormal cingulate modulation of fronto-temporal connectivity in schizophrenia. NeuroImage. 1999;9:337–42.
27. Friston KJ, Frith CD. Schizophrenia—a Disconnection Syndrome. Clin Neurosci. 1995;3:89–97.
28. Frith CD, Friston KJ, Liddle PF, Frackowiak RSJ. Pet Imaging and Cognition in Schizophrenia. J R Soc Med. 1992;85:222–4.
29. Andreasen NC, Paradiso S, O'Leary DS. "Cognitive Dysmetria" as an Integrative Theory of Schizophrenia: A Dysfunction in Cortical-Subcortical-Cerebellar Circuitry? Schizophr Bull. 1998;24:203–18.
30. Andreasen NC, O'Leary DS, Cizadlo T, et al. Schizophrenia and cognitive dysmetria: a positron-emission tomography study of dysfunctional prefrontal-thalamic-cerebellar circuitry. Proc Natl Acad Sci U S A. 1996;93:9985–90.
31. Schröder J, Wenz F, Schad LR, Baudendistel K, Knopp MV. Sensorimotor cortex and supplementary motor area changes in schizophrenia. A study with functional magnetic resonance imaging. Br J Psychiatry. 1995;167:197–201.
32. David AS, Woodruff PW, Howard R, et al. Auditory hallucinations inhibit exogenous activation of auditory association cortex. Neuroreport. 1996;7:932–6.
33. Callicott JH, Ramsey NF, Tallent K, et al. Functional Magnetic Resonance Imaging Brain Mapping in Psychiatry: Methodological Issues Illustrated in a Study of Working Memory in Schizophrenia. Neuropsychopharmacology. 1998;18:186–96.
34. Stephan KE, Iglesias S, Heinzle J, Diaconescu AO. Translational Perspectives for Computational Neuroimaging. Neuron. 2015;87:716–32.
35. Andreasen N, Nasrallah HA, Dunn V, et al. Structural Abnormalities in the Frontal System in Schizophrenia: A Magnetic Resonance Imaging Study. Arch Gen Psychiatry. 1986;43:136–44.
36. Smith RC, Calderon M, Ravichandran GK, et al. Nuclear magnetic resonance in schizophrenia: A preliminary study. Psychiatry Res. 1984;12:137–47.
37. Ashburner J, Friston KJ. Voxel-Based Morphometry—The Methods. NeuroImage. 2000;11:805–21.
38. Andreasen NC, Ehrhardt JC, Swayze VW, et al. Magnetic Resonance Imaging of the Brain in Schizophrenia: The Pathophysiologic Significance of Structural Abnormalities. Arch Gen Psychiatry. 1990;47:35–44.
39. Andreone N, Tansella M, Cerini R, et al. Cerebral atrophy and white matter disruption in chronic schizophrenia. Eur Arch Psychiatry Clin Neurosci. 2007;257:3–11.
40. Fornito A, Yücel M, Dean B, Wood SJ, Pantelis C. Anatomical Abnormalities of the Anterior Cingulate Cortex in Schizophrenia: Bridging the Gap Between Neuroimaging and Neuropathology. Schizophr Bull. 2009;35:973–93.
41. Lawrie SM, Abukmeil SS. Brain abnormality in schizophrenia. A systematic and quantitative review of volumetric magnetic resonance imaging studies. Br J Psychiatry. 1998;172:110–20.
42. Shenton ME, Dickey CC, Frumin M, McCarley RW. A review of MRI findings in schizophrenia. Schizophr Res. 2001;49:1–52.
43. Ellison-Wright I, Glahn DC, Laird AR, Thelen SM, Bullmore E. The Anatomy of First-Episode and Chronic Schizophrenia: An Anatomical Likelihood Estimation Meta-Analysis. Am J Psychiatry. 2008;165:1015–23.
44. Honea R, Crow TJ, Passingham D, Mackay CE. Regional Deficits in Brain Volume in Schizophrenia: A Meta-Analysis of Voxel-Based Morphometry Studies. Am J Psychiatry. 2005;162:2233–45.
45. Borgwardt SJ, McGuire PK, Aston J, et al. Reductions in frontal, temporal and parietal volume associated with the onset of psychosis. Schizophr Res. 2008;106:108–14.
46. Fusar-Poli P, Borgwardt S, Bechdolf A, et al. The Psychosis High-Risk State. JAMA Psychiatry. 2013;70:107–20.
47. van Haren NEM, Hulshoff Pol HE, Schnack HG, et al. Focal Gray Matter Changes in Schizophrenia across the Course of the Illness: A 5-Year Follow-Up Study. Neuropsychopharmacology. 2007;32:2057–66.
48. Bora E, Fornito A, Radua J, et al. Neuroanatomical abnormalities in schizophrenia: A multimodal voxelwise meta-analysis and meta-regression analysis. Schizophr Res. 2011;127:46–57.
49. Ellison-Wright I, Bullmore E. Meta-analysis of diffusion tensor imaging studies in schizophrenia. Schizophr Res. 2009;108:3–10.
50. Heuvel MP van den, Mandl RCW, Stam CJ, Kahn RS, Pol HEH. Aberrant Frontal and Temporal Complex Network Structure in Schizophrenia: A Graph Theoretical Analysis. J Neurosci. 2010;30:15915–26.
51. Zalesky A, Fornito A, Seal ML, et al. Disrupted axonal fiber connectivity in schizophrenia. Biol Psychiatry. 2011;69:80–9.
52. van den Heuvel MP, Sporns O, Collin G, et al. Abnormal Rich Club Organization and Functional Brain Dynamics in Schizophrenia. JAMA Psychiatry. 2013;70:783–92.
53. Lynall ME, Bassett DS, Kerwin R, et al. Functional connectivity and brain networks in schizophrenia. J Neurosci Off J Soc Neurosci. 2010;30:9477–87.
54. Anticevic A, Hu X, Xiao Y, et al. Early-Course Unmedicated Schizophrenia Patients Exhibit Elevated Prefrontal Connectivity Associated with Longitudinal Change. J Neurosci. 2015;35:267–86.
55. Yang GJ, Murray JD, Repovs G, et al. Altered global brain signal in schizophrenia. Proc Natl Acad Sci U S A. 2014;111:7438–43.

56. Fornito A, Bullmore ET. Reconciling abnormalities of brain network structure and function in schizophrenia. Curr Opin Neurobiol. 2015;30:44–50.

57. Crossley NA, Mechelli A, Ginestet C, Rubinov M, Bullmore ET, McGuire P. Altered Hub Functioning and Compensatory Activations in the Connectome: A Meta-Analysis of Functional Neuroimaging Studies in Schizophrenia. Schizophr Bull. 2016;42:434–42.

58. Calhoun VD, Eichele T, Pearlson G. Functional brain networks in schizophrenia: a review. Front Hum Neurosci. 2009;3:17.

59. Jafri MJ, Pearlson GD, Stevens M, Calhoun VD. A method for functional network connectivity among spatially independent resting-state components in schizophrenia. NeuroImage. 2008;39:1666–81.

60. Murray RM, Lewis SW. Is Schizophrenia a Neurodevelopmental Disorder. BMJ. 1987;295:681–2.

61. Weinberger DR. Implications of normal brain development for the pathogenesis of schizophrenia. Arch Gen Psychiatry. 1987;44:660–9.

62. Fatemi SH, Folsom TD. The Neurodevelopmental Hypothesis of Schizophrenia, Revisited. Schizophr Bull. 2009;35:528–48.

63. Frangou S, Murray RM. Imaging as a tool in exploring the neurodevelopment and genetics of schizophrenia. Br Med Bull. 1996;52:587–96.

64. Kempton MJ, Stahl D, Williams SCR, DeLisi LE. Progressive lateral ventricular enlargement in schizophrenia: A meta-analysis of longitudinal MRI studies. Schizophr Res. 2010;120:54–62.

65. Rapoport JL, Addington AM, Frangou S, Psych MRC. The neurodevelopmental model of schizophrenia: update 2005. Mol Psychiatry. 2005;10:434–49.

66. Khandaker GM, Zimbron J, Lewis G, Jones PB. Prenatal maternal infection, neurodevelopment and adult schizophrenia: a systematic review of population-based studies. Psychol Med. 2013;43:239–57.

67. Lodge DJ, Grace AA. Aberrant Hippocampal Activity Underlies the Dopamine Dysregulation in an Animal Model of Schizophrenia. J Neurosci. 2007;27:11424–30.

68. Fusar-Poli P, Smieskova R, Kempton MJ, Ho BC, Andreasen NC, Borgwardt S. Progressive brain changes in schizophrenia related to antipsychotic treatment? A meta-analysis of longitudinal MRI studies. Neurosci Biobehav Rev. 2013;37:1680–91.

69. Olabi B, Ellison-Wright I, McIntosh AM, Wood SJ, Bullmore E, Lawrie SM. Are There Progressive Brain Changes in Schizophrenia? A Meta-Analysis of Structural Magnetic Resonance Imaging Studies. Biol Psychiatry. 2011;70:88–96.

70. Vita A, De Peri L, Deste G, Sacchetti E. Progressive loss of cortical gray matter in schizophrenia: a meta-analysis and meta-regression of longitudinal MRI studies. Transl Psychiatry. 2012;2:e190.

71. Thompson PM, Vidal C, Giedd JN, et al. Mapping adolescent brain change reveals dynamic wave of accelerated gray matter loss in very early-onset schizophrenia. Proc Natl Acad Sci U S A. 2001;98:11650–5.

72. Cahn W, Pol HEH, Lems EBTE, et al. Brain Volume Changes in First-Episode Schizophrenia: A 1-Year Follow-up Study. Arch Gen Psychiatry. 2002;59:1002–10.

73. van Haren NEM, Pol HEH, Schnack HG, et al. Progressive Brain Volume Loss in Schizophrenia Over the Course of the Illness: Evidence of Maturational Abnormalities in Early Adulthood. Biol Psychiatry. 2008;63:106–13.

74. Haijma SV, Haren NV, Cahn W, Koolschijn PCMP, Pol HEH, Kahn RS. Brain Volumes in Schizophrenia: A Meta-Analysis in Over 18 000 Subjects. Schizophr Bull. 2013;39:1129–38.

75. Vita A, De Peri L, Deste G, Barlati S, Sacchetti E. The Effect of Antipsychotic Treatment on Cortical Gray Matter Changes in Schizophrenia: Does the Class Matter? A Meta-analysis and Meta-regression of Longitudinal Magnetic Resonance Imaging Studies. Biol Psychiatry. 2015;78:403–12.

76. Carlsson A. Does dopamine play a role in schizophrenia? Psychol Med. 1977;7:583–97.

77. Abi-Dargham A, Gil R, Krystal J, et al. Increased Striatal Dopamine Transmission in Schizophrenia: Confirmation in a Second Cohort. Am J Psychiatry. 1998;155:761–7.

78. Fusar-Poli P, Meyer-Lindenberg A. Striatal Presynaptic Dopamine in Schizophrenia, Part II: Meta-Analysis of [18F/11C]-DOPA PET Studies. Schizophr Bull. 2013;39:33–42.

79. Howes OD, Kambeitz J, Kim E, et al. The Nature of Dopamine Dysfunction in Schizophrenia and What This Means for Treatment: Meta-analysis of Imaging Studies. Arch Gen Psychiatry. 2012;69:776–86.

80. Egerton A, Chaddock CA, Winton-Brown TT, et al. Presynaptic Striatal Dopamine Dysfunction in People at Ultra-high Risk for Psychosis: Findings in a Second Cohort. Biol Psychiatry. 2013;74:106–12.

81. Howes OD, Montgomery AJ, Asselin M, et al. Elevated striatal dopamine function linked to prodromal signs of schizophrenia. Arch Gen Psychiatry. 2009;66:13–20.

82. Hietala J, Syvälahti E, Vuorio K, et al. Presynaptic dopamine function in striatum of neuroleptic-naive schizophrenic patients. Lancet. 1995;346:1130–1.

83. Howes O, Bose S, Turkheimer F, et al. Progressive increase in striatal dopamine synthesis capacity as patients develop psychosis: a PET study. Mol Psychiatry. 2011;16:885–6.

84. Howes OD, Williams M, Ibrahim K, et al. Midbrain dopamine function in schizophrenia and depression: a post-mortem and positron emission tomographic imaging study. Brain. 2013;136:3242–51.

85. Tseng KY, O'Donnell P. Dopamine–Glutamate Interactions Controlling Prefrontal Cortical Pyramidal Cell Excitability Involve Multiple Signaling Mechanisms. J Neurosci. 2004;24:5131–9.

86. Heinz A. Dopaminergic dysfunction in alcoholism and schizophrenia—psychopathological and behavioral correlates. Eur Psychiatry. 2002;17:9–16.

87. Kapur S. Psychosis as a state of aberrant salience: a framework linking biology, phenomenology, and pharmacology in schizophrenia. Am J Psychiatry. 2003;160:13–23.

88. King R, Barchas JD, Huberman BA. Chaotic behavior in dopamine neurodynamics. Proc Natl Acad Sci U S A. 1984;81:1244–7.

89. Shaner A. Delusions, superstitious conditioning and chaotic dopamine neurodynamics. Med Hypotheses. 1999;52:119–23.

90. Winton-Brown TT, Fusar-Poli P, Ungless MA, Howes OD. Dopaminergic basis of salience dysregulation in psychosis. Trends Neurosci. 2014;37:85–94.

91. Diaconescu AO, Jensen J, Wang H, et al. Aberrant Effective Connectivity in Schizophrenia Patients during Appetitive Conditioning. Front Hum Neurosci. 2011;4:239.

92. Jensen J, Willeit M, Zipursky RB, et al. The Formation of Abnormal Associations in Schizophrenia: Neural and Behavioral Evidence. Neuropsychopharmacology. 2007;33:473–9.

93. Romaniuk L, Honey GD, King JR, *et al.* Midbrain activation during Pavlovian conditioning and delusional symptoms in schizophrenia. Arch Gen Psychiatry. 2010;67:1246–54.

94. Murray GK, Corlett PR, Clark L, *et al.* Substantia nigra/ventral tegmental reward prediction error disruption in psychosis. Mol Psychiatry. 2008;13:239, 267–76.

95. Juckel G, Schlagenhauf F, Koslowski M, *et al.* Dysfunction of ventral striatal reward prediction in schizophrenia. NeuroImage. 2006;29:409–16.

96. Nielsen MØ, Rostrup E, Wulff S, *et al.* Alterations of the Brain Reward System in Antipsychotic Naïve Schizophrenia Patients. Biol Psychiatry. 2012;71:898–905.

97. Schlagenhauf F, Sterzer P, Schmack K, *et al.* Reward Feedback Alterations in Unmedicated Schizophrenia Patients: Relevance for Delusions. Biol Psychiatry. 2009;65:1032–9.

98. Leeuw M de, Kahn RS, Vink M. Fronto-striatal Dysfunction During Reward Processing in Unaffected Siblings of Schizophrenia Patients. Schizophr Bull. 2015;41:94–103.

99. Simon JJ, Cordeiro SA, Weber M-A, *et al.* Reward System Dysfunction as a Neural Substrate of Symptom Expression Across the General Population and Patients With Schizophrenia. Schizophr Bull. 2015;41:1370–8.

100. Waltz JA, Schweitzer JB, Ross TJ, *et al.* Abnormal Responses to Monetary Outcomes in Cortex, but not in the Basal Ganglia, in Schizophrenia. Neuropsychopharmacology. 2010;35:2427–39.

101. Esslinger C, Englisch S, Inta D, *et al.* Ventral striatal activation during attribution of stimulus saliency and reward anticipation is correlated in unmedicated first episode schizophrenia patients. Schizophr Res. 2012;140:114–21.

102. Roiser JP, Stephan KE, den Ouden HE, Friston KJ, Joyce EM. Adaptive and aberrant reward prediction signals in the human brain. NeuroImage. 2010;50:657–64.

103. Roiser JP, Howes OD, Chaddock CA, Joyce EM, McGuire P. Neural and Behavioral Correlates of Aberrant Salience in Individuals at Risk for Psychosis. Schizophr Bull. 2013;39:1328–36.

104. Coyle JT. NMDA Receptor and Schizophrenia: A Brief History. Schizophr Bull. 2012;38:920–6.

105. Krystal JH, Karper LP, Seibyl JP, *et al.* Subanesthetic Effects of the Noncompetitive NMDA Antagonist, Ketamine, in Humans: Psychotomimetic, Perceptual, Cognitive, and Neuroendocrine Responses. Arch Gen Psychiatry. 1994;51:199–214.

106. Lahti AC, Koffel B, LaPorte D, Tamminga CA. Subanesthetic Doses of Ketamine Stimulate Psychosis in Schizophrenia. Neuropsychopharmacology. 1995;13:9–19.

107. Javitt DC, Steinschneider M, Schroeder CE, Arezzo JC. Role of cortical N-methyl-D-aspartate receptors in auditory sensory memory and mismatch negativity generation: implications for schizophrenia. Proc Natl Acad Sci U S A. 1996;93:11962–7.

108. Gunduz-Bruce H, Reinhart RMG, Roach BJ, *et al.* Glutamatergic Modulation of Auditory Information Processing in the Human Brain. Biol Psychiatry. 2012;71:969–77.

109. Schmidt A, Diaconescu AO, Kometer M, Friston KJ, Stephan KE, Vollenweider FX. Modeling Ketamine Effects on Synaptic Plasticity During the Mismatch Negativity. Cereb Cortex. 2013;23:2394–406.

110. Umbricht D, Schmid L, Koller R, Vollenweider FX, Hell D, Javitt DC. Ketamine-induced deficits in auditory and visual context-dependent processing in healthy volunteers: implications for models of cognitive deficits in schizophrenia. Arch Gen Psychiatry. 2000;57:1139–47.

111. Umbricht D, Koller R, Schmid L, *et al.* How specific are deficits in mismatch negativity generation to schizophrenia? Biol Psychiatry. 2003;53:1120–31.

112. Shaikh M, Valmaggia L, Broome MR, *et al.* Reduced mismatch negativity predates the onset of psychosis. Schizophr Res. 2012;134:42–8.

113. Gaebler AJ, Mathiak K, Koten JW, *et al.* Auditory mismatch impairments are characterized by core neural dysfunctions in schizophrenia. Brain. 2015;138:1410–23.

114. Benes FM, Vincent SL, Alsterberg G, Bird ED, SanGiovanni JP. Increased GABAA receptor binding in superficial layers of cingulate cortex in schizophrenics. J Neurosci. 1992;12:924–9.

115. Benes FM, Vincent SL, Marie A, Khan Y. Up-regulation of GABA(A) receptor binding on neurons of the prefrontal cortex in schizophrenic subjects. Neuroscience. 1996;75:1021–31.

116. Lewis DA, Gonzalez-Burgos G. Pathophysiologically based treatment interventions in schizophrenia. Nat Med. 2006;12:1016–22.

117. Buhl EH, Szilágyi T, Halasy K, Somogyi P. Physiological properties of anatomically identified basket and bistratified cells in the CA1 area of the rat hippocampus in vitro. Hippocampus. 1996;6:294–305.

118. Homayoun H, Moghaddam B. NMDA Receptor Hypofunction Produces Opposite Effects on Prefrontal Cortex Interneurons and Pyramidal Neurons. J Neurosci. 2007;27:11496–500.

119. Rotaru DC, Lewis DA, Gonzalez-Burgos G. The role of glutamatergic inputs onto parvalbumin-positive interneurons: relevance for schizophrenia. Rev Neurosci. 2012;23:97–109.

120. Uhlhaas PJ, Haenschel C, Nikolic D, Singer W. The role of oscillations and synchrony in cortical networks and their putative relevance for the pathophysiology of schizophrenia. Schizophr Bull. 2008;34:927–43.

121. Howard MW, Rizzuto DS, Caplan JB, *et al.* Gamma Oscillations Correlate with Working Memory Load in Humans. Cereb Cortex. 2003;13:1369–74.

122. Uhlhaas PJ, Singer W. Abnormal neural oscillations and synchrony in schizophrenia. Nat Rev Neurosci. 2010;11:100–13.

123. Puts NAJ, Edden RAE. *In vivo* magnetic resonance spectroscopy of GABA: A methodological review. Prog Nucl Magn Reson Spectrosc. 2012;60:29–41.

124. Yoon JH, Maddock RJ, Rokem A, *et al.* GABA Concentration Is Reduced in Visual Cortex in Schizophrenia and Correlates with Orientation-Specific Surround Suppression. J Neurosci. 2010;30:3777–81.

125. Kegeles LS, Mao X, Stanford AD, *et al.* Elevated Prefrontal Cortex γ-Aminobutyric Acid and Glutamate-Glutamine Levels in Schizophrenia Measured *In Vivo* With Proton Magnetic Resonance Spectroscopy. Arch Gen Psychiatry. 2012;69:449–59.

126. Taylor SF, Tso IF. GABA abnormalities in schizophrenia: A methodological review of in vivo studies. Schizophr Res. 2015;167:84–90.

127. Davis KA, Nanga RPR, Das S, *et al.* Glutamate imaging (GluCEST) lateralizes epileptic foci in nonlesional temporal lobe epilepsy. Sci Transl Med. 2015;7:309ra161.

128. Schür RR, Draisma LWR, Wijnen JP, *et al.* Brain GABA levels across psychiatric disorders: A systematic literature review and meta-analysis of 1H-MRS studies. Hum Brain Mapp. 2016;37:3337–52.

129. Bleuler E. *Dementia Praecox or the Group of Schizophrenias.* New York, NY: International Universities Press; 1911.

130. Friston KJ, Liddle PF, Frith CD, Hirsch SR, Frackowiak RSJ. The Left Medial Temporal Region and Schizophrenia—a Pet Study. Brain J Neurol. 1992;115:367–82.

131. Friston KJ. The disconnection hypothesis. Schizophr Res. 1998;30:115–25.

132. Pettersson-Yeo W, Allen P, Benetti S, McGuire P, Mechelli A. Dysconnectivity in schizophrenia: where are we now? Neurosci Biobehav Rev. 2011;35:1110–24.

133. Stephan KE, Baldeweg T, Friston KJ. Synaptic plasticity and dysconnection in schizophrenia. Biol Psychiatry. 2006;59:929–39.

134. Stephan KE, Friston KJ, Frith CD. Dysconnection in schizophrenia: from abnormal synaptic plasticity to failures of self-monitoring. Schizophr Bull. 2009;35:509–27.

135. Schizophrenia Working Group of the Psychiatric Genomics Consortium. Biological insights from 108 schizophrenia-associated genetic loci. Nature. 2014;511:421–7.

136. Adams RA, Stephan KE, Brown HR, Frith CD, Friston KJ. The Computational Anatomy of Psychosis. Front Psychiatry. 2013;4:47.

137. Friston K. A theory of cortical responses. Philos Trans R Soc Lond B Biol Sci. 2005;360:815–36.

138. Rao RPN, Ballard DH. Predictive coding in the visual cortex: a functional interpretation of some extra-classical receptive-field effects. Nat Neurosci. 1999;2:79–87.

139. Self MW, Kooijmans RN, Supèr H, Lamme VA, Roelfsema PR. Different glutamate receptors convey feedforward and recurrent processing in macaque V1. Proc Natl Acad Sci U S A. 2012;109:11031–6.

140. Corlett PR, Taylor JR, Wang X-J, Fletcher PC, Krystal JH. Toward a neurobiology of delusions. Prog Neurobiol. 2010;92:345–69.

141. Corlett PR, Honey GD, Krystal JH, Fletcher PC. Glutamatergic model psychoses: prediction error, learning, and inference. Neuropsychopharmacology. 2011;36:294–315.

142. Fletcher PC, Frith CD. Perceiving is believing: a Bayesian approach to explaining the positive symptoms of schizophrenia. Nat Rev Neurosci. 2009;10:48–58.

143. Friston K, Brown HR, Siemerkus J, Stephan KE. The dysconnection hypothesis (2016). Schizophr Res. 2016;176:83–94.

144. Lieder F, Stephan KE, Garrido MI, Daunizeau J, Friston KJ. A neurocomputational model of the mismatch negativity. PLoS Comput Biol. 2013;9:e1003288.

145. Dima D, Frangou S, Burge L, Braeutigam S, James AC. Abnormal intrinsic and extrinsic connectivity within the magnetic mismatch negativity brain network in schizophrenia: A preliminary study. Schizophr Res. 2012;135:23–7.

146. Horga G, Schatz KC, Abi-Dargham A, Peterson BS. Deficits in Predictive Coding Underlie Hallucinations in Schizophrenia. J Neurosci. 2014;34:8072–82.

147. Notredame C-E, Pins D, Deneve S, Jardri R. What visual illusions teach us about schizophrenia. Front Integr Neurosci. 2014;8:63.

148. Dima D, Roiser JP, Dietrich DE, et al. Understanding why patients with schizophrenia do not perceive the hollow-mask illusion using dynamic causal modelling. NeuroImage. 2009;46:1180–6.

149. Dima D, Dietrich DE, Dillo W, Emrich HM. Impaired top-down processes in schizophrenia: A DCM study of ERPs. NeuroImage. 2010;52:824–32.

150. Kapur S, Phillips AG, Insel TR. Why has it taken so long for biological psychiatry to develop clinical tests and what to do about it? Mol Psychiatry. 2012;17:1174–9.

151. Ward KM, Aletras AH, Balaban RS. A New Class of Contrast Agents for MRI Based on Proton Chemical Exchange Dependent Saturation Transfer (CEST). J Magn Reson. 2000;143:79–87.

152. Zhou J, Zijl PCM van. Chemical exchange saturation transfer imaging and spectroscopy. Prog Nucl Magn Reson Spectrosc. 2006;48:109–36.

153. Deco G, Ponce-Alvarez A, Mantini D, Romani GL, Hagmann P, Corbetta M. Resting-State Functional Connectivity Emerges from Structurally and Dynamically Shaped Slow Linear Fluctuations. J Neurosci. 2013;33:11239–52.

154. Stephan KE, Schlagenhauf F, Huys QJM, et al. Computational neuroimaging strategies for single patient predictions. NeuroImage. 2017;145, Part B:180–99.

155. Friston KJ, Harrison L, Penny W. Dynamic causal modelling. NeuroImage. 2003;19:1273–302.

156. Stephan KE, Tittgemeyer M, Knösche TR, Moran RJ, Friston KJ. Tractography-based priors for dynamic causal models. Neuroimage. 2009;47:1628.

157. Moran RJ, Symmonds M, Stephan KE, Friston KJ, Dolan RJ. An in vivo assay of synaptic function mediating human cognition. Curr Biol. 2011;21:1320–5.

158. Moran RJ, Jung F, Kumagai T, et al. Dynamic Causal Models and Physiological Inference: A Validation Study Using Isoflurane Anaesthesia in Rodents. PLoS One. 2011;6:e22790.

159. Moran RJ, Campo P, Symmonds M, Stephan KE, Dolan RJ, Friston KJ. Free Energy, Precision and Learning: The Role of Cholinergic Neuromodulation. J Neurosci. 2013;33:8227–36.

160. Diaconescu AO, Mathys CD, Weber LAE, Kasper L, Mauer J, Stephan KE. Hierarchical prediction errors in midbrain and septum during social learning. Soc Cogn Affect Neurosci. 2017;12:618–34.

161. Iglesias S, Mathys C, Brodersen KH, et al. Hierarchical Prediction Errors in Midbrain and Basal Forebrain during Sensory Learning. Neuron. 2013;80:519–30.

162. Brodersen KH, Deserno L, Schlagenhauf F, et al. Dissecting psychiatric spectrum disorders by generative embedding. NeuroImage Clin. 2014;4:98–111.

163. Chen CC, Henson RN, Stephan KE, Kilner JM, Friston KJ. Forward and backward connections in the brain: A DCM study of functional asymmetries. NeuroImage. 2009;45:453–62.

# 61

# Schizoaffective and schizotypal disorders/ acute and transient psychotic disorders

*William S. Stone, Stephen V. Faraone, and Ming T. Tsuang*

## Introduction

This chapter focuses on several disorders that show similarities to schizophrenia, including schizoaffective disorder, schizotypal personality disorder, and brief psychotic states. Areas of emphasis include the clinical features, classification, diagnosis, epidemiology, course, and prognosis for each disorder. Some aspects will be underscored to reflect critical issues such as levels of heterogeneity, reliability, and validity. These issues are related to the accurate classification of the disorders, which are important for at least three related reasons. Firstly, it is essential to develop reliable and valid diagnostic criteria in order to study the aetiology of the disorders and then utilize that knowledge to develop rational and testable intervention strategies. Heterogeneity adds variance to the process that reduces both the reliability of diagnosis and also the statistical power of experimental designs to detect intervention/treatment effects.

Secondly, the development of newer generations of psychopharmacological treatments holds the promise of matching more appropriate and efficacious medications with specific syndromes or types of symptoms. This trend underscores the importance of differential diagnosis in determining what treatment a patient will receive. Heterogeneity within a diagnostic category complicates the achievement of this goal. Thirdly, as psychiatry inches closer to the inclusion of dimensional and trans-diagnostic models in the conceptualization, assessment, and treatment of psychopathology, diagnostic reliability and validity are increasingly critical components of translational efforts to integrate clinical, behavioural, cognitive, biological, and genetic markers/phenotypes across psychiatric disorders [1, 2]. Each disorder will be considered separately, starting with a review of schizoaffective disorder, the most severe of the three conditions.

## Schizoaffective disorder

### Clinical features

Each edition of the *Diagnostic and Statistical Manual of Mental Disorders* (DSM) described a version of a disorder that afflicts patients with both schizophrenic and affective symptoms. The term 'schizoaffective disorder' first appeared in DSM, third edition (DSM-III) in 1980 [3], but without operational diagnostic criteria. DSM-III-Revised (DSM-III-R) introduced four diagnostic criteria and depressive and bipolar subtypes [4]. DSM-IV retained the diagnostic criteria and added a mixed subtype [5] that did not change in the DSM-IV 'Text Revision' (DSM-IV-TR). Criterion A in DSM-IV required an uninterrupted mood episode that could be major depressive (and must include depressed mood), manic, or mixed in nature. During the same period, Criterion B required a period of at least 2 weeks with hallucinations or delusions that were not associated with prominent mood disturbances. Criterion C specified that the symptoms comprising the mood disturbance persisted for significant portions of the active and residual stages of the disorder. Criterion D required that symptoms of the disorder were not attributable to substance use/abuse or to general medical conditions.

Schizoaffective disorder in DSM-5 does not differ radically from its conception in DSM-IV [6, 7] but is defined more stringently. Criterion C, in particular, now requires that symptoms of a major mood episode must be present for over half of the total duration of the active and residual phases of the illness (that is, the entire course of illness). This change is also significant because DSM-IV did not define the required duration of the mood disturbance. Moreover, DSM-5 requires the mood disturbance to meet diagnostic criteria for a major mood episode for a majority of the illness. Affective disorders that do not meet full criteria for a major mood episode do not meet the criterion. One effect of the change in Criterion C may be to reduce an apparent bias in clinical diagnosis towards less severe diagnoses, as shown, for example, by a study that compared clinical diagnoses with research diagnoses of hospitalized psychiatric inpatients [8]. In that study, treating clinicians diagnosed 36% of the sample (*n* = 134) with schizophrenia, 37% with schizoaffective disorder, and 27% with psychotic bipolar disorder. By contrast, diagnoses made by trained research personnel using the Structured Clinical Interview of DSM-IV-TR included 48% with schizophrenia, 28% with schizoaffective disorder, and 24% with psychotic bipolar disorder.

Like schizophrenia, Criterion A in DSM-5 schizophrenia must be met at some point in schizoaffective disorder. Unlike schizophrenia,

Criterion B, which involves functional declines in social, interpersonal relations, or work, and Criterion F, which involves the exclusion of autistic spectrum disorder or communication disorder in childhood, are not required in DSM-5 schizoaffective disorder. At any point in time, affective and non-affective symptoms may or may not occur simultaneously, which underscores the importance of considering the course of the illness longitudinally, in addition to its cross-sectional presentation. Symptom clusters that are primarily affective, schizophrenic, or mixed predominate at different times.

Compared to patients with schizophrenia, patients with schizoaffective disorder often (though not always) demonstrate relatively high levels of premorbid function [9, 10]. This trend partly reflects the absence of a required functional decline in schizoaffective disorder. Nevertheless, premorbid vulnerabilities in multiple cognitive and clinical functions are common [11]. Patients with schizoaffective disorder also tend to show more identifiable precipitating events. The nature of the precipitating stressor may vary widely; for example, it may be physical (for example, recently giving birth or experiencing a head injury) or interpersonal (for example, a change in an important relationship). The clinical course of the disorder is often characterized by a periodic, rapid onset of symptoms that shows a relatively high degree of remission after several weeks or months. As Vaillant pointed out in the 1960s, many of these patients 'recover' completely after an episode and resume their lives at premorbid levels of function [12]. As will be further noted later in this chapter, the clinical features of some cases of schizoaffective disorder mainly resemble those of schizophrenia, while the features of other cases are more similar to those of bipolar disorder. Regardless of the subtype or variant of the disorder, however, the mortality rate is of special concern. Rates of death due mainly to suicide or accident show elevations in this disorder that are similar to those observed in schizophrenia and major affective disorders [13]. A recent study showed, however, that even when schizophrenia and schizoaffective disorder subjects were matched for age, gender, and race, schizoaffective subjects showed higher rates of suicide attempts, were hospitalized for suicidality more frequently, and showed higher rates of anxiety disorders, compared to schizophrenia subjects [14].

Schizoaffective disorder is more common in females than in males [6, 9]. The age of onset varies but tends to be younger than that of unipolar or bipolar disorder. Tsuang *et al.* found the median age of onset for schizoaffective disorder was 29 years, which was significantly lower than groups with bipolar or unipolar affective disorder, but similar to a group with schizophrenia. Marneros *et al.* [10] also reported that a median age of onset of 29 years for schizoaffective disorder was lower than the median age for groups with affective disorders (35 years), but reported that it was higher than a group with schizophrenia (24 years). In contrast, Reichenberg *et al.* [11] reported no differences in the age of first hospitalization between patients with schizophrenia, schizoaffective disorder, or non-psychotic bipolar disorder. These differences between studies reflect differences in both the diagnostic criteria employed and the heterogeneity of the disorder.

## Classification

The classification of schizoaffective disorder has always been controversial. Kraepelin reported in 1919 that patients with both affective and schizophrenic symptoms complicated the differential diagnosis

due to the 'mingling of morbid symptoms of both psychoses'. Kasanin first employed the term 'acute schizophrenic psychoses' in 1933 to describe a group of patients who experienced a rapid onset of emotional turmoil and psychotic symptoms but who recovered after several weeks or months [9, 15]. These symptoms appeared similar to schizophrenia during periods of exacerbation, but unlike schizophrenia, they showed a greater tendency to remit between episodes. Kasinin's view of schizoaffective disorder as a (chronic) schizophrenia-like condition with a better outcome was not adopted by DSM-5 or earlier editions [7], though it is more consistent generally with the notion of acute and transient psychotic disorders described later in this chapter. Nevertheless, ongoing debates about the nature of schizoaffective disorder have persisted since Kraepelin's division of psychoses into affective and schizophrenia types, with most conceptualizations focusing on the following possibilities: (1) it is a type of schizophrenia; (2) it is a type of affective disorder; (3) it is a unique disorder that is separate from both schizophrenia and bipolar disorder; (4) it reflects an arbitrary categorization of clinical symptoms that masks a continuum of pathology between schizophrenia and affective illness; and (5) it contained a heterogenous collection of 'interforms' between schizophrenia and affective disorder (that is, symptoms of both disorders).

The last possibility is not mutually exclusive of the first four; for example, one or more variants of schizoaffective disorder may be related closely to schizophrenia, while another may be related more closely to an affective disorder. The issue has yet to be resolved. Classification problems reflect conceptual difficulties about the nature of schizoaffective disorder, its diagnosis, and its reliability and validity. Compared to schizophrenia, bipolar disorder, and unipolar depression, both test–retest reliability and inter-rater reliability are low [16, 17]. It is too soon to know whether DSM-5 attempts to tighten diagnostic criteria will improve inter-rater reliability, especially in clinical settings [8]. Different conceptual assumptions and research strategies also lead to different conclusions about the nature of the disorder. Several meta-analyses by Baethge and colleagues showed, for example, that subjects with schizoaffective disorder showed clinical and demographic characteristics that fell between schizophrenia and bipolar disorder [18] and between schizophrenia and unipolar depression [19]. Levels of heterogeneity were also intermediate between schizophrenia and both bipolar disorder and unipolar depression [19, 20]. These findings were interpreted as consistent with the Kraepelinian dichotomy.

Family and outcome studies provide useful ways of assessing the relative merits of each of the possibilities outlined previously. These approaches are informative and will be reviewed later in this chapter, although interpretations of such studies are complicated at times by the use of different diagnostic criteria across investigations.

### Family studies

Family studies employ a behavioural genetic method that assumes that related disorders co-aggregate more frequently in biologically related individuals than they do in the general population. Thus, a disorder more likely belongs in the schizophrenia spectrum if it occurs more frequently in biological relatives of schizophrenia patients, compared with appropriate controls. Similarly, a disorder more likely belongs in the affective spectrum if it occurs more frequently among the relatives of patients with affective disorders. Consideration of evidence directly pertinent to the question of where schizoaffective disorder belongs in the schizophrenia spectrum, which includes a growing number of genetic studies, is beyond the scope of the current discussion. Instead, only representative findings pertinent to the present discussion about the clinical classification of schizoaffective disorder will be summarized here.

Bertelsen and Gottesman [21] summarized a series of seven family studies published between 1979 and 1993, using structured diagnostic criteria. Analyses of risk to the development of schizophrenia, schizoaffective disorder, and affective disorder in the first-degree relatives of patients with schizoaffective disorder were included. In all seven studies, the relatives showed a higher risk of developing an affective disorder than of developing schizoaffective disorder. In five of the seven studies, the risks of developing schizophrenia was equal to, or greater than, the risk of developing schizoaffective disorder. Thus, the relatives of schizoaffective patients showed generally higher risks of developing disorders other than the one with which their ill relatives were diagnosed. These findings were consistent with a heterogenous view of schizoaffective disorder, in which individual cases represented subtypes of either schizophrenia or affective disorder. The findings were also consistent with the possibility that schizoaffective disorder represents a chance collection of 'interforms' between schizophrenia and affective disorder.

This latter view also found a measure of support in a more recent report that utilized the Danish National Register [22] where the relative risk of schizoaffective disorder was elevated significantly (relative risk = 2.76) if a first-degree relative had any history of mental illness. The relative risk increased further if the disorder demonstrated by the first-degree relative included schizophrenia (2.57), bipolar disorder (3.23), or schizoaffective disorder itself (1.92). Notably, the relative risk for schizophrenia was highest when a first-degree relative had schizophrenia (3.22), and the relative risk for bipolar disorder was highest when a first-degree relative had bipolar disorder (5.19). These findings show further that schizoaffective disorder may be related genetically to both schizophrenia and bipolar disorder, either as a subtype or as an interform.

These findings were not consistent with the view that schizoaffective disorder represented a continuum between the other two disorders, because in that case, the rate of schizoaffective disorder in first-degree relatives would have been higher, compared with the rates at which these relatives developed schizophrenia or affective disorder. The findings were also inconsistent with the possibility that schizoaffective disorder represented a unique disorder that was independent of either schizophrenia or an affective disorder. In that case, the first-degree relatives of patients with schizoaffective disorder should show relatively high rates of schizoaffective disorder itself, but relatively low rates of the other disorders. In a series of studies reviewed by Bertelsen and Gottesman [21], the morbid risk for schizoaffective disorder itself ranged from 1.8% to 6.1% in first-degree relatives of patients with schizoaffective disorder, which was still higher than the rate observed in the general population (see Epidemiology, p. 612). These results, taken together with the higher risks for both schizophrenia and affective disorder, suggest that schizoaffective disorder is a heterogenous condition. Recent reviews of family studies, including those that considered depressed (that is, unipolar) and bipolar subtypes, have also underscored both the heterogeneity of schizoaffective disorder and the controversial nature of its classification [23, 24].

## Outcome studies

A majority of outcome studies show that schizoaffective disorder has a better course than schizophrenia, but a poorer course than affective disorder [25–27]. Other researchers reported similar findings. Kendler et al., for example, showed intermediate levels of clinical impairment for schizoaffective disorder in an epidemiological family study. Marneros et al. reported on outcomes as part of the Cologne Longitudinal Study, using modified DSM-III-R diagnoses [28]. The outcomes were measured by symptoms in five dimensions (psychotic symptoms, reduction of energetic potential, qualitative and quantitative disturbances of affect, and other disturbances of behaviour) that persisted for at least 3 years. Consistent with the pattern described thus far, poor outcomes in the schizoaffective group occurred at a rate (49.5% of the sample) that was intermediate between those observed in the schizophrenic (93.2%) and affective groups (35.8%), and differed significantly from both of them. In a more recent study, Jäger et al. studied 241 patients at the time of their first hospitalization, and then again 15 years later [29, 30]. Again, schizoaffective subjects presented a less impaired clinical picture than the one shown by schizophrenic subjects, but more impaired than the one shown by affective subjects.

While these studies show schizoaffective disorder to have intermediate outcomes generally, there are categories in which it resembles schizophrenia or affective disorder more closely. For example, Samson et al. [25] and Reinares et al. [27] noted that outcomes for schizoaffective disorder were equivalent to those for affective disorder in several dimensions. Marneros et al. showed that 70% of a schizoaffective group were rated as good or excellent on a measure of social adjustment, which did not differ significantly from 84% of an affective group who received the same rating (reviewed in [27]). Both groups differed significantly from a schizophrenic group, however, in which only 44% of the group demonstrated good or excellent outcomes. Moreover, the schizoaffective and affective disorder groups did not differ on a rating scale of psychological impairments (for example, body language, affect display, conversation skills, and co-operation), although both were rated as significantly less impaired than the schizophrenic group.

Other studies, however, such as Kendler et al. [28], reported similarities between some types of psychotic symptoms in schizoaffective disorder and schizophrenia, including the severity of delusions and positive thought disorder and the frequency of hallucinations. Each of these groups showed higher levels of these symptoms than an affective disorder group. Hizdon et al. reported recently that individuals with schizoaffective disorder did not differ from individuals with schizophrenia on basic cognitive measures of executive function, memory, and processing speed, although the schizoaffective group did perform better on measures of social cognition [31]. Reichenberg et al. showed that individuals with schizophrenia and schizoaffective disorder who were assessed premorbidly performed similar to each other, but lower than individuals who later developed non-psychotic bipolar disorder, on selected tests of intellectual and academic functions [11].

These overall differences in outcome serve to validate the classification of schizoaffective disorder as a separate syndrome further. Its heterogeneity, however, raises the issue of whether such intermediate outcomes might reflect the mean of a combination of mainly good and mainly poor outcomes. This, in turn, leads to the question of whether schizoaffective disorder can be subtyped in a useful and valid manner. If so, are better and worse outcomes associated with different variants of the syndrome?

Vaillant suggested in the 1960s that prognostic indicators, including a good premorbid level of adjustment, the presence of precipitating factors, an acute onset, confusion, the presence of affective symptoms, and a family history of affective disorder (or the absence of a schizophrenic history), could predict remission in approximately 80% of cases of 'remitting schizophrenia' [31]. The inclusion of affective symptoms and a positive family history for affective illness on the list contributed (later) to hypotheses that variants of schizoaffective disorder were related to affective illness and to better outcomes. In contrast, variants associated more with schizophrenic symptoms or family histories were associated more with schizophrenia and relatively poor outcomes. [32].

There have been a variety of attempts to subtype schizoaffective disorders, based on whether affective or schizophrenic symptoms predominate. The validity of many of these attempts, however, is inconclusive [21, 28]. Conversely, a latent class analysis of psychotic patients from the Roscommon Study showed that most cases of DSM-III-R schizoaffective disorder were categorized in either a bipolar schizomania class ($n = 19$) or a schizodepression class ($n = 13$), rather than in schizophrenia ($n = 1$), major depression ($n = 0$), schizophreniform ($n = 3$), or hebephrenia ($n = 3$) classes [33]. Moreover, Reinares *et al.* reviewed evidence showing that bipolar and depressive subtypes differed from each other in ways consistent with differences between bipolar and unipolar affective disorders [27]. For example, the bipolar schizoaffective subtype was associated with more total episodes, more episodes with shorter periods and cycles, and higher frequency of cycles. Higher numbers of cycles were associated with poorer long-term outcomes. Taken together, these studies show at least some recent support for the subtyping of schizoaffective disorder into mainly affective and mainly schizophrenic variants.

Other factors associated with poor outcomes include poor interepisode recoveries [28], persistent psychotic symptoms in the absence of affective features, poor premorbid social adjustment, chronicity, a higher number of schizophrenia-like symptoms [34], and the presence of schizoaffective mixed states [27].

### Differential diagnosis

The major feature of DSM-5 schizoaffective disorder [6] involves a mood disorder occurring concurrently with Criterion A of schizophrenia for a continuous period of time. Many other disorders that present with psychotic or mood symptoms should be considered in the differential diagnosis of schizoaffective disorder, including, for example, other psychiatric or neurological disorders involving psychotic symptoms, acquired substance or toxin-induced psychotic conditions, cognitive disorders, prodromal syndromes, personality disorders, anxiety disorders, neurodevelopmental disorders, and states of delirium. Particular concern involves the differential diagnosis between schizoaffective disorder and schizophrenia, and between schizoaffective disorder and either bipolar disorder or a depressive disorder with psychotic symptoms. In DSM-5, Criterion C distinguishes schizoaffective disorder from schizophrenia by requiring that the prominent mood disorder in schizoaffective disorder characterizes over half the period spanning the active and residual phases of the disorder. Criterion B distinguishes schizoaffective

disorder from other mood disorders involving psychosis by requiring the presence of delusions or hallucinations for at least 2 weeks in the absence of prominent depressive or manic symptoms. Notably, these diagnostic criteria may be met during some phases of the disorder, but not others. Thus, the presence of a prominent mood disturbance occurring over half the time could shift, for example, to occur less than half the time during the course of the disorder, which might necessitate a valid change in diagnosis from schizoaffective disorder to schizophrenia.

### Epidemiology

#### Incidence

Earlier studies showed that new cases of 'schizomanic' patients (that is, manic patients who also demonstrated schizophrenic or paranoid symptoms) numbered approximately 1.7 per 100,000 per year [35]. This was less than the 4 per 100,000 per year shown by 'schizodepressive' patients. The number of schizoaffective cases in this study exceeded the number of manic patients and made up half of the number of schizophrenia cases. Since then, Tien and Eaton analysed data from the Epidemiologic Catchment Area Study for three non-overlapping groups with psychotic symptoms [36]. One of these groups comprised individuals with 'psychotic affective syndrome', which was similar to schizoaffective disorder, except that most members of the group (59%) demonstrated psychotic symptoms only in conjunction with a mood disturbance (essentially DSM-III-R mood disturbance with psychotic symptoms). The incidence of this disorder was 1.7 per 1000 per year, which was approximately equal to the rate for schizophrenia (2.0 per 1000 per year). Even if the 59% of the group who met the criteria for a mood disorder with psychotic features were excluded, the remaining 41% would still comprise a higher incidence rate than that detected by earlier studies. Differences in sampling procedures (treated vs non-treated samples) may have contributed to the differences observed in the rates. More importantly, however, these studies showed that schizoaffective disorder occurred at 50–85% of the rate of schizophrenia, thus confirming that patients with this disorder comprise a clinically significant population. One current, but long-standing, issue involves questions about the temporal stability of incidence rates in schizophrenia-related disorders, as reflected by reports of both increases and decreases.

#### Prevalence

Until recently, prevalence estimates for schizoaffective disorder relied mainly on samples that were treated in clinics or other psychiatric settings. Because a variety of factors influence the decision to enter and remain in treatment, the estimates varied substantially. For example, Okasha reviewed studies that reported rates varying between 2% and 29% [23]. A recent epidemiological study in Finland using 8028 people who were at least 30 years old showed a lifetime prevalence rate of 0.32% for schizoaffective disorder (compared to 0.87% for schizophrenia), which accounted for 10.5% of all psychotic disorders [37]. This is a lower estimate than many earlier studies reported and likely results from a combination of factors (including a narrowing of diagnostic criteria and increased utilization of multiple sources of information such as case notes and registers, in addition to interview data) that together have improved diagnostic accuracy.

## Review of evidence

Treatments for schizoaffective disorder are the same as those for schizophrenia and affective disorders alone. As the nature and efficacy of those treatments are discussed elsewhere, they will not be considered here. Rather, this section will focus on management issues related to the need to treat symptoms of both disorders simultaneously or sequentially.

## Management

Psychopharmacological treatments may be viewed in terms of DSM-5 schizoaffective disorder subtypes, including the bipolar type and the depressive type. Treatment of the bipolar type will include dopamine antagonist medication (for example, clozapine, risperidone, quetiapine, ziprasidone, or olanzapine), particularly if psychotic symptoms are present. In addition, drugs for unipolar depression, mood stabilizers (for example, lithium), or anticonvulsants (for example, valproate or carbamazepine) may be useful with this group. It will be necessary in such cases to weigh the potential risks of such medications, such as elevated toxicity and metabolic abnormalities, against the potential benefits.

In the depressive subtype, combination treatments may also be more effective than a single treatment. Dopamine antagonist treatments alone may be more efficient, however, if affective symptoms (that is, depression) are largely secondary to the experience of having a psychotic condition and its attendant interpersonal, social, and financial difficulties. In these cases, remediation of the psychotic symptoms may also ameliorate the affective problems. For other cases, which include more of a treatment-refractory depression, drugs for psychosis may be augmented with a mood stabilizer or antidepressant medication. Moreover, electroconvulsive therapy may reduce mortality rates in schizoaffective patients.

As was true in earlier versions of DSM, the bipolar subtype (including a manic episode and possibly major depressive episodes) may be difficult to distinguish from the depressive subtype (including major depressive episodes in the absence of manic episodes), especially in the presence of psychotic symptoms. In these cases, treatment decisions may rest on the presenting symptoms of the patient. At any point, treatment is partly dependent on the presence or absence of psychotic symptoms. As noted previously, psychotic episodes in this period are associated with relatively poorer outcomes and are likely to require chronic drug therapy.

## Schizotypal personality disorder

### Clinical features

Like schizoaffective disorder, schizotypal personality disorder (PD) is a complex and chronic condition that includes some, but not all, of the features of schizoaffective disorder and schizophrenia. Changes from DSM-IV to DSM-5 reflect a growing recognition that, while this disorder should still be viewed as a personality disorder, it should also be classified as a schizophrenia spectrum condition [6, 38]. Most notably, persistent psychosis is not part of the syndrome in individuals with schizotypal PD, although milder forms of thought disorder may occur such as magical thinking or ideas

of reference (as opposed to delusions of reference, which indicate psychosis). Moreover, brief episodes of psychosis may occur in times of stress but will not persist.

Schizotypal patients show pervasive deficits in social and interpersonal traits. They often demonstrate aloofness, poor eye contact, affective constriction, and suspiciousness. Consequently, close interpersonal relationships either are avoided or cause discomfort and anxiety. This social anxiety persists despite familiarity and is often related to suspiciousness or attenuated psychotic paranoia, rather than to fears of negative evaluations by others. Individuals with schizotypal PD usually have few friends and demonstrate deficiencies in social cognition such as problems in sensing social cues or affective signals accurately from others. These problems in social cognition exacerbate suspiciousness or paranoia and contribute to the persistence of anxiety over time.

Schizotypal patients may show magical thinking, ideas of reference, unusual perceptions (for example, sensing the presence of another person or that people are talking about them), and/or perceptual illusions (for example, often perceiving a dimly lit lamp post as a person). Both their social deficits and these cognitive–perceptual problems contribute to an overall impression of oddness. However, this feature may occur independently of other clinical symptoms [39] and manifest itself in odd speech or unusual appearance. The oddness or eccentricities evident in these patients are often ego-syntonic (that is, they are not experienced as problems). Moreover, schizotypal patients show deficits in attention, long-term verbal memory, and executive functions. These cognitive deficits are qualitatively similar to those seen in schizophrenia (and schizoaffective disorder), but like many other clinical manifestations of this disorder, they are quantitatively milder [40, 41].

Like schizophrenia, schizotypal PD is often evident by early adulthood, but schizotypal traits may be evident in late childhood or adolescence. Once it appears, the disorder tends to show a chronic course, but one that includes periodic exacerbations and attenuations of symptoms. A study that followed individuals with schizotypal PD for 2 years showed that paranoid thoughts and unusual perceptual experiences were among the most stable and least malleable DSM-IV symptoms, while the most changeable were odd behaviours and restricted affect [40]. The former symptoms were thus more trait-like, and the latter were more intermittent. The same group also showed that in the course of 2 years (with treatment), 61% of schizotypal patients no longer met DSM-IV diagnostic criteria for the disorder [42]. With a more stringent definition of improvement (12 months with two or fewer symptoms meeting criteria), the rate of remission dropped to 23%. These studies show that both the severity and the expression of the disorder vary over time and probably as a function of treatment. A recent study that assessed twins with either schizotypal or paranoid PD over a 10-year period showed much of the observed stability of the disorders (about 67%) was attributable to shared genetic factors between early and middle adulthood, while the effects of environmental risk factors were more transient [43]. Consistent with previous studies, subjects with schizotypal PD also showed moderate declines in symptom levels over time [44, 45].

### Classification

In contrast to the controversy surrounding the classification of schizoaffective disorder, family, twin, and adoption studies clearly support the view that schizotypal PD is best classified in the schizophrenia spectrum [38, 46, 47]. Nevertheless, it is a complex and chronic disorder that, in all likelihood, is also heterogenous. Kendler pointed out that this heterogeneity was at least partly related to the two primary methods used to study the disorder [48]. One of these involves the 'clinical method', which identifies patients with mild forms of schizophrenic or psychotic-like symptoms. This type of patient, for example, is often characterized by relatively high levels of positive psychiatric symptoms (for example, magical thinking and perceptual distortions). Patients identified in this manner often comprise a heterogenous group themselves, however, involving patients with schizotypal symptoms, together with patients with other types of severe personality problems such as borderline personality disorder [47].

In contrast, the 'family research method' identifies relatives of patients with schizophrenia who have subtle schizophrenia-like symptoms. Features associated more with familial than with clinical schizotypal PD include a predominance of negative symptoms (for example, social withdrawal and impairment, and higher levels of anxiety and poor rapport), cognitive or electrophysiological impairments (for example, impaired language comprehension, eye-tracking, and attentional dysfunctions, though all of these also occur in clinical PD), and elevated rates of schizophrenia and related disorders in family members [46]. Thaker et al. reported that familial and clinical schizotypal PDs were similar on measures of physical or social anhedonia [49].

The concept of familial schizotypal disorder is particularly important because it may share a common genetic basis with schizophrenia. Paul Meehl first proposed the term 'schizotaxia' to describe the genetic vulnerability to schizophrenia and suggested that individuals with schizotaxia would eventually develop either schizotypal PD or schizophrenia, depending on the protection or liability afforded by environmental circumstances [50]. As the concept evolved, Meehl reformulated it to allow for the possibility that some people with schizotaxia would develop neither schizophrenia nor schizotypal PD. In fact, evidence now shows that the clinical symptoms observed in many non-psychotic first-degree relatives of people with schizophrenia are similar to those observed in familial schizotypal PD [46, 51]. Psychiatric features in such relatives frequently include an aggregation of negative symptoms that are qualitatively similar to, but milder than, those often cited in schizophrenia. Positive symptoms, however, are usually less evident in these relatives than they are in schizophrenia or schizotypal PD. Neuropsychological impairments in biological relatives of people with schizophrenia are also qualitatively similar to, but milder than, those seen in people with schizophrenia [41].

Faraone et al. suggested a reformulation of Meehl's concept of schizotaxia that focuses on these features of negative symptoms and neuropsychological deficits [46]. Unlike schizotypal PD, which occurs in less than 10% of adult relatives of patients diagnosed with schizophrenia, the basic symptoms of schizotaxia occur in 20–50% of adult relatives, suggesting further that the genetic liability to schizophrenia does not lead inevitably to schizophrenia, schizotypal PD, or schizoid PD. More recent studies showed that operational definitions of schizotaxia in non-psychotic adult relatives, based on neuropsychological deficits and negative symptoms, were supported by cluster analyses and were partially amenable to pharmacological intervention [41].

## Diagnosis and differential diagnosis

The DSM-5 diagnostic criteria for schizotypal PD do not differ substantially from the criteria used in DSM-IV. While an alternative, more dimensional model of PDs is included in the DSM-5 manual that structures these symptoms somewhat differently, the categorical system of previous versions remains in place [6]. In this context, DSM-5 Criterion A includes deficits in personality that involves ideas (but not delusions) of reference (A1), unusual ideas or types of thought such as magical thinking (unrelated to cultural norms) or beliefs in special powers such as clairvoyance (A2), unusual perceptual experiences such as illusions or transitory hallucinations (A3), unusual forms of thinking or speech (such as frequent use of vague, tangential, metaphorical, or stereotyped language) (A4), frequent suspiciousness or paranoid thoughts (A5), constricted or inappropriate affect (A6), odd or unusual behaviours, manners of dress or other aspects of appearance (A7), constricted interpersonal relationships that often include few, if any, close friends or other non-familial relationships (A8), and acute anxiety in social situations that does not decline with familiarity and is related primarily to suspiciousness of others, rather than to self-consciousness or fear of negative evaluations by others (as is typical in social anxiety) (A9).

As in DSM-IV, five out of the nine symptoms are required to meet Criterion A. These symptoms emerge by early adulthood and occur in a variety of contexts. Criterion B requires that symptoms in Criterion A do not occur only during the periods of disorders involving sustained psychosis, such as schizophrenia, bipolar disorder, or depression with psychotic features, or autism spectrum disorder (ASD).

The differential diagnosis includes a variety of other disorders. A key difference between schizotypal PD and schizophrenia, psychotic mood disorders, or presentations of psychosis in ASD involves the transient nature of psychotic symptoms in schizotypal PD. It may be distinguished from ASD (though sometimes with difficulty) by the relatively greater deficits in social awareness, lack of emotional reciprocity, or frequent presence of stereotyped behaviours or interests in ASD. Schizotypal PD may be distinguished from neurodevelopmental disorders involving language or other forms of communication by the presence of relatively more specific problems in language reception or production that are usually identified by specialized testing. Such problems are not typically present in schizotypal PD. It also differs from communication disorders by its oddness of its content, rather than by the deficiencies of its form.

Schizotypal PD may be confused with several other PDs but can be distinguished from them. It differs from schizoid and from paranoid PD, for example, by its pattern of cognitive and perceptual distortions and by the eccentricities in appearance, language, or behaviour shown frequently by schizotypal patients. Schizotypal individuals who show transient psychotic symptoms may resemble individuals with borderline PD, but the pattern differs in that psychotic-like symptoms and social isolation in schizotypal PD are more likely to persist in the absence of affective turmoil, and schizotypal individuals are less likely to display the impulsive and manipulative traits that are often associated with borderline PD. Some individuals with narcissistic PD may demonstrate suspiciousness or social alienation, but, unlike in schizotypal PD, these symptoms/traits are related to underlying fears of exposing imperfections or flaws. Individuals with avoidant PD may be aversive to, or anxious in, social interactions, but it reflects a fear of rejection in the context of a desire for such relationships in avoidant PD, whereas it reflects suspicion and a lack of desire for such relationships in schizotypal PD.

## Epidemiology

### Incidence

A literature search did not identify incidence studies for schizotypal PD.

### Prevalence

A review by Tsuang *et al.* showed prevalence rates in non-clinical samples ranged from 0.7% to 5.1%, with a median nearing 3.0% [52]. Higher rates occurred in clinical samples—2.0–64.0%, with a median of 17.5%. More recently, Torgersen *et al.* reported a rate of 0.6% for DSM-III-R in a community sample, which is lower than the rates in studies reviewed by Tsuang *et al.* [53]. In contrast to non-clinical samples, the prevalence of schizotypal PD among the relatives of schizophrenic individuals is as high as 10%. More recently, the lifetime prevalence of schizotypal PD in the United States was reported to be near 4.0%, with modestly higher rates for men (4.2%) than women (3.7%) [54].

## Treatment

There is unfortunately a continuing dearth of outcome studies involving psychotherapy, psychosocial, or psychopharmacological treatments for schizotypal PD [47]. Older published studies often show methodological limitations (for example, small samples, subjects with mixed diagnoses, inadequate controls, and problems with internal validity) or provide outcome data on only limited aspects of the disorder. Despite these caveats, it is clear that few treatment gains are evident in earlier studies [55]. Recent evidence for the efficacy of psychotherapy for PDs is more promising but is limited mainly to other PDs [56].

Several earlier studies investigated the usefulness of medications in treating schizotypal PD, although they typically employed small numbers of subjects, combined samples of schizotypal and borderline PDs, and showed little clinical improvement. Dopamine antagonist drugs were proposed to reduce positive symptoms or depressed mood in times of acute stress, but the high incidence of adverse side effects discouraged their widespread use at other times, including the more chronic stable (that is, non-crisis) phases of the disorder. Other types of medication, including fluoxetine, have shown generally non-specific effects of treatment.

Hymowitz *et al.* administered a low dose of haloperidol to 17 outpatients with DSM-III diagnoses of schizotypal PD for 6 weeks [57]. The initial dose of 2.0 mg was intended to rise to 12.0 mg, but side effects prevented increases beyond a mean dose of 3.6 mg. Even with lower doses, 50% of the sample withdrew from the study because of side effects. The 17 subjects who completed 2 weeks of the protocol improved somewhat in ratings of ideas of reference, odd communications, social isolation, and overall functioning.

More recently, Koenigisberg *et al.* employed a double-blind protocol to administer low doses of risperidone (0.25–2.0 mg/day), a medication with serotonin antagonist properties, to 25 patients with DSM-IV schizotypal PD, for 9 weeks [58]. Compared to a placebo control group, patients who received risperidone demonstrated significant reductions in positive and negative symptoms, with

no difference in dropout rates between groups. These findings are encouraging and consistent with evidence described previously that schizotypal symptoms are amenable to change [40, 42]. Hopefully, findings like these will stimulate additional research into pharmacological treatments for this disorder.

## Management

Though trust and rapport with a therapist are often difficult to establish in schizotypal PD, the therapeutic relationship may be used to mitigate the marked deficits in interpersonal relationships that characterize this syndrome [58]. The frequent occurrence of paranoia and suspiciousness, together with social aloofness and constricted affect, may make exploratory psychotherapeutic approaches less effective than supportive cognitive behavioural therapies. In fact, these patients may only seek treatment to alleviate circumscribed problems like anxiety or somatic complaints. Approaches that emphasize concrete interim goals and stipulate explicit means of attaining them thus have the best chances of success. Because individuals with this disorder are vulnerable to decompensation during times of stress and may experience transient episodes of psychosis, they may also benefit from techniques to facilitate stress reduction (for example, relaxation techniques, exercise, yoga, and meditation). Fortunately, some people with schizotypal features are likely to seek treatment in times of stress [59, 60]. In the short term, brief courses of dopamine antagonist treatment may be useful if symptoms of psychosis appear. It is important to note, however, that individuals with schizotypal PD may receive unwarranted diagnoses of schizophrenia and receive longer-term treatment [47].

Cognitive problems are also frequently amenable to concrete goal-oriented approaches to treatment. Patients benefit from understanding their cognitive strengths and weaknesses because it helps them confront and cope with long-standing difficulties in their lives. For example, problems in attention, verbal memory, or organizational skills contribute to failures in educational, occupational, and social endeavours, while reinforcing negative self-images and increasing performance anxiety. Knowledge of circumscribed cognitive problems allows patients to reframe their difficulties in a more positive manner and facilitate the selection of realistic personal, educational, and occupational goals. While cognitive deficits in schizotypal PD are well established [47], there have been few trials of medications to improve cognition, though the administration of guanfacine and dopamine agonists may show promise.

## Brief psychotic disorder

### Clinical features

Brief psychotic episodes have long been a source of interest [61] but have defied simple classifications. Consequently, different versions of this condition have been proposed and utilized. Brief psychotic disorder in DSM-5 involves at least one symptom from a group that includes delusions, hallucinations, disorganized speech, and/or grossly disorganized or catatonic behaviour [6]. The onset of these symptoms is rapid, with the transition from a non-psychotic state to a psychotic one occurring within 2 weeks. Typically, a prodromal period is not present. The duration of symptoms lasts from 1 day to 1 month. This diagnosis does not require associated social or occupational dysfunction. Symptoms may not be attributable to substance abuse or therapeutic medications or to other medical conditions, nor can they be explained better by other psychiatric disorders that involve psychotic symptoms such as schizophrenia or bipolar disorder. Specifiers may be added that note that the episode followed a stressful incident (that is, with marked stressors) or did not (that is, without marked stressors). The episode may also be specified as post-partum, meaning it occurred during pregnancy or within a month of giving birth, and it may be specified as involving catatonia. The severity of the episode may be recorded on a 5-point scale that ranges from 0 (absent) to 4 for the previous 7 days. At the conclusion of the episode, individuals return to premorbid levels of function.

The International Classification of Diseases, tenth edition (ICD-10) defines a similar diagnostic category—the acute and transient psychotic disorders (ATPDs), with six subtypes [62]. One difference involves a longer period, compared to the DSM-5 version (3 months, compared to 1 month). ATPDs should also show a fully developed episode within 2 weeks.

In addition to classifications as psychotic disorders, brief psychotic episodes are also classified as clinical high-risk states. The Structured Interview for Prodromal Syndromes (SIPS) operationalizes a syndrome [Brief Intermittent Psychotic Symptoms (BIPS)] which may last up to 3 months and include at least one symptom of psychosis (at least one of the scales P1–P5 is rated a 6) in that period. The symptom(s) must last at least several minutes per day at least once per month, but less than 1 hour per day for at least 4 days per week for the last month [63, 64]. No decline in social or occupational functioning is required to meet the diagnostic criteria for this syndrome. The Comprehensive Assessment of At-Risk Mental State (CAARMS) defines a similar clinical high-risk syndrome [Brief Limited Intermittent Psychotic Symptoms (BLIPS)] that also requires at least one symptom of psychosis (at least one of the scales P1, P2, or P4 is rated 6 or P3 is rated ≥5) [65–67]. CAARMS BLIPS symptoms differ from those in the SIPS BIPS syndrome in that symptoms should have been evident in the previous 12 months, though not for more than 5 years. They occur 3–4 times per week when they persist for at least an hour, or they occur daily when they persist for less than an hour. Unlike BIPS, CAARMS symptoms are associated with at least a 30% drop in functioning on the Social and Occupational Functioning Assessment Scale (SOFAS), lasting at least 1 month in the previous year, or show a low score for over a year.

The risk of recurrent psychotic features in individuals who meet criteria for either the disorders described previously or the clinical high-risk syndromes is significant, though not as high as individuals who demonstrate first-episode schizophrenia [61, 68]. Differences between rates of recurrence in these different brief conditions are small.

### Differential diagnosis

Brief psychotic disorders may be differentiated from chronic disorders with psychotic features, such as schizophrenia, bipolar disorder, and depression with psychotic features, both by the persistence of the symptoms and the loss of function in multiple domains and by the failure to resolve fully, even with treatment. It is important to note, however, that some individuals, despite the generally favourable outcomes associated with brief psychotic symptoms, may develop a chronic psychotic disorder subsequently (especially those with longer symptom durations such as BLIPS cases). Problems involving substance abuse, traumatic brain injury, delirium, and other medical conditions should be considered and assessed. If forensic circumstances exist, the possibility of malingering or other forms of symptom magnification should be considered. Some PDs may also present with brief psychotic symptoms that may be distinguished (for example, borderline PD) by their chronicity and symptom history.

### Management

In line with the brief course of these symptoms/disorders, crisis management is a first line of response and may include short-term hospitalization and treatments with dopamine antagonist medications. Behavioural treatments, such as cognitive behavioural therapy, may be useful to reduce or minimize stress and emotional dysregulation and thereby reduce the likelihood of future episodes. Nevertheless, it will be important to monitor individuals who have demonstrated brief psychotic disorders or episodes to assess their stability of clinical functions and the possible emergence of additional brief or chronic psychotic disorders.

### Possibilities for prevention

Current early intervention programmes involve secondary prevention, which includes early identification and treatment of clinical (usually psychotic or psychotic-like) symptoms. While intervention is necessary to alleviate clinical symptoms at any point during the disorder, it is particularly important early on because it might alter the trajectory of illness. Patients treated with drugs for psychosis during their first or second hospital admission, for example, show better outcomes than those who are not treated until later.

Primary prevention, which involves treatment before the disorder manifests itself clinically, is not yet available for schizophrenia, schizoaffective disorder, schizotypal PD, brief psychotic disorder, or other disorders in the schizophrenia spectrum. To develop such treatments, it will be necessary to predict first who is most likely to develop a disorder and who is not. There are a few encouraging approaches, including ongoing genetic 'high-risk' studies that follow the offspring of schizophrenic parents longitudinally. Such studies help to identify traits early in life that predict which individuals are most likely to experience emergent clinical symptoms in adulthood. This type of study is particularly important because it can facilitate the formation of homogenous high-risk groups, which, in turn, can facilitate the development of focused prevention strategies. Similarly, longitudinal studies of clinical high-risk patients also provide critical information about the nature of 'conversion' to psychosis.

With our current knowledge, however, it is difficult to justify preventive treatments—especially medication—for people without symptoms. The authors have argued elsewhere, however, that if people in high-risk groups (like first-degree biological relatives of patients with schizophrenia, or clinical high-risk patients) show clinically meaningful symptoms that can be organized into valid liability syndromes, then intervention attempts may become appropriate [46, 51]. The authors proposed this course of action for people with 'schizotaxia' and suggested preliminary research guidelines [69].

# REFERENCES

1. Keshavan MS. Nosology of psychoses in DSM-5: inches ahead but miles to go. *Schizophrenia Research*. 2013;150:40–1.
2. Cuthbert BN, Insel TR. Toward new approaches to psychotic disorders: the NIMH Research Domain Criteria project. *Schizophrenia Bulletin*. 2010;36:1061–2.
3. American Psychiatric Association. *Diagnostic and Statistical Manual of Mental Disorders (DSM-III)*, third edition. Washington, DC: American Psychiatric Association; 1980.
4. American Psychiatric Association. *Diagnostic and Statistical Manual of Mental Disorders (DSM-IIIR)*, third edition. Washington, DC: American Psychiatric Association; 1987.
5. American Psychiatric Association. *Diagnostic and Statistical Manual of Mental Disorders (DSM-IV)*, fourth edition. Washington, DC: American Psychiatric Association; 1994.
6. American Psychiatric Association. *Diagnostic and Statistical Manual of Mental Disorders (DSM-5)*. Washington, DC: American Psychiatric Association; 2013.
7. Malaspina D, Owen MJ, Heckers S, et al. Schizoaffective disorder in DSM-5. *Schizophrenia Research*. 2013;150:21–5.
8. Wilson JE, Nian H, Heckers S. the schizoaffective disorder diagnosis: a conundrum in the clinical setting. *European Archives of Psychiatry and Clinical Neuroscience*. 2014;264:29–34.
9. Tsuang MT, Simpson SJC, Fleming JA. Diagnostic criteria for subtyping schizoaffective disorder. In: Marneros A, Tsuang MT (eds). *Schizoaffective Psychoses*. Berlin: Springer-Verlag; 1986. pp. 50–62.
10. Marneros A, Deister A, Rohde A. Sociodemographic and premorbid features of schizophrenic, schizoaffective and affective psychoses. In: Marneros A, Tsuang MT (eds). *Affective and Schizoaffective Disorders*. Berlin: Springer-Verlag; 1990. pp. 130–45.
11. Reichenberg A, Weiser M, Rabinowitz J, et al. A population-based cohort study of premorbid intellectual, language and behavioral functioning in patients with schizophrenia, schizoaffective disorder, and nonpsychotic bipolar disorder. *American Journal of Psychiatry*. 2002;159:2027–35.
12. Vaillant G. The prediction of recovery in schizophrenia. *Journal of Nervous and Mental Disease*. 1962;135:534–43.
13. Simpson J. Mortality studies in schizophrenia. In: Tsuang MT, Simpson JC (eds). *Nosology, Epidemiology and Genetics of Schizophrenia*. Amsterdam, New York, Oxford: Elsevier Science Publishers BV; 1988. pp. 245–73.
14. Seldin K, Armstrong K, Schiff ML, Heckers S. Reducing the diagnostic heterogeneity of schizoaffective disorder. *Frontiers in Psychiatry*. 2017;8:18.
15. Kasanin J. The acute schizoaffective psychoses. *American Journal of Psychiatry*. 1933;90:97–126.
16. Santelmann H, Franklin J, Busshoff J, Baethge C. Test-retest reliability of schizoaffective disorder compared with schizophrenia, bipolar disorder, and unipolar depression—a systematic review and meta-analysis. *Bipolar Disorders*. 2015;17:753–68.
17. Santelmann H, Franklin J, Busshoff J, Baethge C. Interrater reliability of schizoaffective disorder compared with schizophrenia, bipolar disorder, and unipolar depression—a systematic review and meta-analysis. *Schizophrenia Research*. 2016;176:357–63.
18. Pagel T, Baldessarini RJ, Franklin J, Baethge C. Characteristics of patients diagnosed with schizoaffective disorder compared with schizophrenia and bipolar disorder. *Bipolar Disorders*. 2013;15:229–39.
19. Rink L, Pagel T, Franklin J, Baethge C. Characteristics and heterogeneity of schizoaffective disorder compared with inipolar depression and schizophrenia—a systematic literature review and meta-analysis. *Journal of Affective Disorders*. 2016;191:8–14.
20. Pagel T, Baldessarini RJ, Franklin J, Baethge C. Heterogenity of schizoaffective disorder compared with schizophrenia and bipolar disorder. *Acta Psychiatrica Scandinavica*. 2013;128:238–50.
21. Bertelsen A, Gottesman, II. Schizoaffective psychoses: genetical clues to classification. *American Journal of Medical Genetics (Neuropsychiatric Genetics)*. 1995;60:7–11.
22. Laursen TM, Labouriau R, Licht RW, et al. Family history of psychiatric illness as a risk factor for schizoaffective disorder: a Danish register-based cohort study. *Archives of General Psychiatry*. 2005;62:841–8.
23. Okasha A. The concept of schizoaffective disorder: utility versus validity and reliability—a transcultural perspective. In: Marneros A, Akiskal AH (eds). *The Overlap of Affective and Schizophrenic Spectra*. Cambridge: Cambridge University Press; 2007. pp. 104–32.
24. Coryell W. Phenomenological approaches to the schizoaffective spectrum. In: Marneros A, Akiskal AH (eds). *The Overlap of Affective and Schizophrenic Spectra*. Cambridge: Cambridge University Press; 2007. pp. 133–44.
25. Samson JA, Simpson JC, Tsuang MT. Outcome of schizoaffective disorders. *Schizophrenia Bulletin*. 1988;14:543–54.
26. Angst J. The course of schizoaffective disorders. In: Marneros A, Tsuang MT (eds). *Schizoaffective Psychoses*. Berlin: Springer-Verlag; 1986. pp. 63–93.
27. Reinares M, Vieta E, Benabarre A, Marneros A. Clinical course of schizoaffective disorders. In: Marneros A, Akiskal AH (eds). *The Overlap of Affective and Schizophrenic Spectra*. Cambridge: Cambridge University Press; 2007. pp. 145–55.
28. Kendler KS, McGuire M, Gruenberg AM, Walsh D. Examining the validity of DSM-III-R schizoaffective disorder and its putative subtypes in the Roscommon Family Study. *American Journal of Psychiatry*. 1995;152:755–64.
29. Marneros A, Rohde A, Deister A. Frequency and phenomenology of persisting alterations in affective, schizoaffective and schizophrenia disorders: a comparison. *Psychopathology*. 1998;31:23–8.
30. Jager M, Bottlender R, Strauss A, Moller J. Fifteen-year follow-up of ICD-schizoaffective disorders compared to schizophrenia and affective disorders. *Acta Psychiatrica Scandinavica*. 2004;109:30–7.
31. Fiszdon JM, Richardson R, Greig T, Bell MD. A comparison of basic and social cognition between schizophrenia and schizoaffective disorder. *Schizophrenia Research*. 2007;91:117–21.
32. Vaillant G. Prospective prediciton of schizophrenic remission. *Archives of General Psychiatry*. 1964;11:509–18.
33. Levitt JJ, Tsuang MT. The heterogeneity of schizoaffective disorder: implications for treatment. *American Journal of Psychiatry*. 1988;145:926–36.
34. Kendler KS, Karkowski LM, Walsh D. The structure of psychosis: latent class analysis of probands from the Roscommon Family Study. *Archives of General Psychiatry*. 1998;55:492–9.
35. Tsuang MT, Levitt JJ, Simpson JC. Schizoaffective disorder. In: Hirsch SR, Weinberger DR (eds). *Schizophrenia*. Oxford: Blackwell Scientific; 1995. pp. 46–58.
36. Tien AY, Eaton WW. Psychopathologic precursors and sociodemographic risk factors for the schizophrenia syndrome. *Archives of General Psychiatry*. 1992;49:37–46.

37. Perala J, Suvisaari J, Saarni SI, *et al*. Lifetime prevalence of psychotic and bipolar I disorders in a general population. *Archives of General Psychiatry*. 2007;64:19–28.

38. Chemerinski E, Triebwasser J, Roussos P, Siever LJ. Schizotypal personality disorder. *Journal of Personality Disorders*. 2013;27:652–79.

39. Battaglia M, Cavallini MC, Macciardi F, Bellodi L. The structure of DSM-III-R schizotypal personality disorder diagnosed by direct interviews. *Schizophrenia Bulletin*. 1997;23:83–92.

40. McGlashan TH, Grilo CM, Sanislow CA, *et al*. Two-year prevalence and stability of individual DSM-IV criteria for schizotypal, borderline, avoidant, and obsessive-compulsive personality disorders: toward a hybrid model of axis II disorders. *American Journal of Psychiatry*. 2005;162:883–9.

41. Stone WS, Seidman LJ. Neuropsychological and structural imaging endophenotypes in schizophrenia. In: Cicchetti D (ed). *Developmental Psychopathology*, third edition. Hoboken, NJ: John Wiley and Sons; 2016. pp. 931–65.

42. Grilo CM, Sanislow CA, Gunderson JG, *et al*. Two-year stability and change of schizotypal, borderline, avoidant and obsessive-compulsive personality disorders. *Journal of Clinical and Consulting Psychology*. 2004;72:767–75.

43. Kendler KS, Aggen SH, Neale MC, *et al*. A longitudinal twin study of cluster A personality disorders. *Psychological Medicine*. 2015;45:1531–8.

44. Sanislow CA, Little TD, Ansell EB, *et al*. Ten-year stability and latent structure of the DSM-IV schizotypal, borderline, avoidant, and obsessive-compulsive personality disorders. *Journal of Abnormal Psychology*. 2009;118:507–19.

45. Johnson JG, Cohen P, Kasen S, Skodol AE, Hamagami F, Brook JS. Age-related change in personality disorder trait levels between early adolescence and adulthood: a community-based longitudinal investigation. *Acta Psychiatrica Scandinavica*. 2000;102:265–75.

46. Faraone SV, Green AI, Seidman LJ, Tsuang MT. 'Schizotaxia': clinical implications and new directions for research. *Schizophrenia Bulletin*. 2001;27:1–18.

47. Rosell DR, Futterman SE, McMaster A, Siever LJ. Schizotypal personality disorder: a current review. *Current Psychiatry Reports*. 2014;16:452.

48. Kendler KS. Diagnostic approaches to schizotypal personality disorder: a historical perspective. *Schizophrenia Bulletin*. 1985;11:538–53.

49. Thaker G, Moran M, Adami H, Cassady S. Psychosis proneness scales in schizophrenia spectrum personality disorders: familial vs. nonfamilial samples. *Psychiatry Research*. 1993;46:47–57.

50. Meehl PE. Schizotaxia revisited. *Archives of General Psychiatry*. 1989;46:935–44.

51. Stone WS, Giuliano AJ. Development of liability syndromes for schizophrenia: where did they come from and where are they going? *American Journal of Medical Genetics Part B: Neuropsychiatric Genetics*. 2013;162B:687–97.

52. Tsuang MT, Gilbertson MW, Faraone SV. Genetic transmission of negative and positive symptoms in the biological relatives of schizophrenics. In: Marneros A, Tsuang MT, Andreasen N (eds). *Positive vs Negative Schizophrenia*. New York, NY: Springer-Verlag; 1991. pp. 265–91.

53. Torgersen S, Kringlen E, Cramer V. The prevalence of personality disorders in a community sample. *Archives of General Psychiatry*. 2001;58:590–6.

54. Pulay AJ, Stinson FS, Dawson DA, *et al*. Prevalence, correlates, disability, and co-morbidity of DSM-IV schizotypal personality disorder: results from the wave 2 national epidemiologic survey on alcohol and related conditions. *Primary Care Companion to the Journal of Clinical Psychiatry*. 2009;11:53–7.

55. Battaglia M, Torgersen S. Schizotypal disorder: at the crossroads of genetics and nosology. *Acta Psychiatrica Scandinavica*. 1996;94:303–10.

56. Tsuang MT, Stone WS, Faraone SV. Overview for treatment for schizotypal and schizoid personality disorders: present and future. *NOOS Aggiornamenti in Psichiatria*. 1998;4:201–15.

57. Hymowitz P, Frances A, Jacobsberg LB, Sickles M, Hoyt R. Neuroleptic treatment of schizotypal personality disorders. *Comprehensive Psychiatry*. 1986;27:267–71.

58. Koenigsberg HW, Reynolds D, Goodman M, *et al*. Risperidone in the treatment of schizotypal personality disorder. *Journal of Clinical Psychiatry*. 2003;64:628–34.

59. Bender S. The therapeutic alliance in the treatment of personality disorders. *Journal of Psychiatric Practice*. 2005;11:73–87.

60. Poreh A, Whitman D. MMPI-2 schizophrenia spectrum profiles among schizotypal college students and college students who seek psychological treatment. *Psychological Reports*. 1993;73:987–94.

61. Fusar-Poli P, Cappucciati M, Bonoldi I, *et al*. Prognosis of brief psychotic episodes: a meta-analysis. *JAMA Psychiatry*. 2016;73:211–20.

62. World Health Organization. *The ICD-10 classification of mental and behavioural health disorders*. Geneva: World Health Organization; 1993.

63. Miller TJ, McGlashan TH, Rosen JL, *et al*. Prodromal assessment with the Structured Interview for Prodromal Syndromes and the Scale of Prodromal Symptoms: predictive validity, interrater reliability and training to reliability. *Schizophrenia Bulletin*. 2003;29:703–15.

64. McGlashan TH, Walsh B, Wood SJ. *The Psychosis-Risk Syndrome: Handbook for Diagnosis and Follow-up*. New York, NY: Oxford University Press; 2010.

65. Yung AR, Nelson B, Stanford C, *et al*. Validation of 'prodromal' criteria to detect individuals at ultra high risk of psychosis: 2 year follow-up. *Schizophrenia Research*. 2008;105:10–17.

66. Yung AR, Phillips LJ, Yuen HP, *et al*. Psychosis prediction: a 12-month follow-up of a high risk ('prodromal') group. *Schizophrenia Research*. 2003;60:21–32.

67. Yung AR, Yuen HP, McGorry PD, *et al*. Mapping the onset of psychosis: the Comprehensive Assessment of At-Risk Mental States. *New Zealand Journal of Psychiatry*. 2005;39:964–71.

68. Fusar-Poli P, Cappucciati M, De Micheli A, *et al*. Diagnostic and prognostic significance of brief limited psychotic symptoms (BLIPS) in individuals at ultra high risk. *Schizophrenia Bulletin*. 2017;43:48–56.

69. Tsuang MT, Stone WS, Seidman LJ, *et al*. Treatment of nonpsychotic relatives of patients with schizophrenia: four case studies. *Biological Psychiatry*. 1999;41:1412–18.

# 62

# Delusional disorders

*Andreas Marneros*

## Definition

*Delusional disorder is a psychotic disorder, characterized by well-systematized and long-lasting delusions, whereas other mental and personality domains usually remain intact.*

Although modern diagnostic systems (DSM-5 297.1, ICD-10 F22, and presumably also ICD-11) [1–3] categorize it in a spectrum with schizophrenia and other psychotic disorders, it is autochthonous and autonomous, that is, a disorder by its own and independent with its specific clinical features and rules. A shift to schizophrenia in the course of the disease is rare [4, 5].

## A very short history

There is a plethora of literature dealing with delusional disorders and paranoia, most of which is historical or in the form of case reports. It is beyond the scope of this chapter to deal with it in its entirety, so the basic conclusions drawn from it are included. Many of these original papers are quoted within references provided in this chapter [4–6]. The concept we nowadays call delusional disorder has a long history, as long as psychiatry itself. The term delusional disorder presents a new name for the old concept of paranoia and was 'officially' introduced with DSM-III-R in 1987, but it was created by George Winokur as early as in 1977 [7]. Delusional disorder, in fact, is nothing else than the latest successor, or the new name, of paranoia as defined in their final version by Emil Kraepelin in 1915, which was the successor of concepts like 'monomania' in French psychiatry and 'primary insanity' in German psychiatry [4]. The concept of paranoia has a long history which is closely connected with the development of psychiatry itself. Nevertheless, the debate on, and the interest in, paranoia lost its vim and vigour after the first decades of the twentieth century and came to a near standstill in the middle of that century. A wave of overdiagnosing schizophrenia was one of the main reasons of its marginalization, as well as the beginning of operationalized diagnostics and the introduction of new treatments, which are mostly refused by patients with paranoia. As mentioned previously, George Winokur introduced the term delusional disorder in 1977, aiming to bring clarity to the equivocal and diffuse use of the term paranoia, especially in the anglophone literature.

Winokur's term covers, in fact, the same as Emil Kraepelin's concept of paranoia.

## Diagnosis

The ICD-10 category 'persistent delusional disorder' is likely to change into 'delusional disorder' in ICD-11 [3]. However, the major diagnostic criteria, according to ICD-11 Beta Draft, will probably remain unchanged, with the addition of a specifier for the present state of the condition (symptomatic—partial remission—full remission) (see Box 62.1).

The diagnostic criteria of DSM-5 are very similar to that of ICD. The most important difference regards the duration of delusions (ICD at least 3 months; DSM-5 at least 1 month).

## Prevalence and demography

Prevalence and demography of delusional disorder within the general population are not exactly known. The base rate of delusional disorder is unclear. The most important reasons why this psychotic condition is difficult to uncover and little is known so far about treatment, prognosis, etc. are patients with delusional disorder do not feel ill or disabled and many other psychosocial abilities usually remain intact, so they do not seek medical or psychological help. In addition, the disorder is usually monosymptomatic and monothematic, so distinction between delusions, overvalued ideas, and reality is difficult, sometimes even impossible. The impairments in psychosocial functioning can be more circumscribed, as seen in other psychotic disorders; behaviour is not obviously bizzare or odd, and patients often show sufficient integration in relevant domains of social life, so there is no necessity for their families or authorities to initiate contact with mental services. However, boundaries between delusional disorder, other psychotic disorders, and paranoid personality are often elusive. The fact that delusions are common in a number of different mental disorders makes it difficult to estimate the prevalence of pure delusional disorder. Epidemiological investigations reporting on 'paranoid' symptoms in the general population refer to a great spectrum of phenomena, which are rarely symptoms of delusional disorder [4].

**Box 62.1** Persistent delusional disorder in ICD-10 (F22) (presumably delusional disorder in ICD-11)

A. A delusion or a set of related delusions, other than those listed as typically schizophrenic in criterion G1(1)b or d for F20.0–F20.3 (that is, other than completely impossible or culturally inappropriate), must be present. The most common examples are persecutory, grandiose, hypochondriacal, jealous (zelotypic), or erotic delusions.

B. The delusion(s) in criterion A must be present for at least 3 months.

C. The general criteria for schizophrenia (F20.0–F20.3) are not fulfilled.

D. There must be no persistent hallucinations in any modality (but there may be transitory or occasional auditory hallucinations that are not in the third person or giving a running commentary).

E. Depressive symptoms (or even a depressive episode (F32) may be present intermittently, provided that the delusions persist at times when there is no disturbance of mood.

F. *Most commonly used exclusion clause.* There must be no evidence of primary or secondary organic mental disorder, as listed under F00–F09, or of a psychotic disorder due to psychoactive substance use (F1x.5).

Reproduced from World Health Organization, *The ICD-10 Classification of Mental and Behavioural Disorders*, Copyright (1996), with permission from World Health Organization.

Nevertheless, based on available findings, the *lifetime prevalence* of delusional disorder in the general population may be estimated to be somewhat between 0.03% and 0.2%, while their prevalence in a clinical population is approximately 0.5–1% of all admissions (older investigations reported up to 4%) and approximately 2–3% of all psychotic disorders. Reported *gender* differences are not significant. *Age at onset* is usually middle to late adult life, with a peak between ages 35 and 50. Concerning *sociodemographic characteristics*, the majority of patients are married or in a stable partnership and they represent all social classes and levels of education, though lower socio-educational levels and, among these patients, immigrants, are more frequently represented. Similar to other psychotic disorders, many patients come from a broken home [4, 8–11].

## Aetiopathogenesis

Various efforts are made to explain how delusional disorder arises, yet all are mainly speculative. The main approaches include the following:

1. The *phenomenological approach* describes preconditions and pre-delusional states, as well as formation, consolidation, and recovery or chronicity of delusional states [4, 12].

2. The *psychodynamic approach* tries to explain delusional disorders (paranoia) as a defence against awareness of vulnerability, having projection as the main mechanism. Libidinous allocations being connected to homosexuality, anality, etc. play an important role [4].

3. The *neuropsychological approach* uses cognitive deficit theories, involving cognitions, attributions, and emotions as an explanatory model [4].

4. Other *psychological approaches* assume that interactions of special personality features, stressful life events, and the social environment are essential for the development of delusional disorder. The many findings regarding *personality features* in patients with delusional disorder are inconsistent. According to psychological approaches, patients with delusional disorder often show strong introversion and anancastic features, little openness to experience, lack of concern for others, and lability of self-esteem and of self-concepts [4].

5. The *genetic approach* contributes only marginally, mainly because of very small samples [13].

6. The same applies to other *biological approaches*. Some investigations provide evidence of brain abnormality in the medial frontal/anterior cingulate cortex and insula [14]. But it is not certain whether such findings are specific for delusional disorder. Some delusional types can be present in brain damages, but that is an exclusion criterion for the autochthonous disorder [4].

## Symptoms and differential diagnosis

The disorder, as already pointed out, is usually *monosymptomatic*, having as main symptom autochthonous, *monothematic delusions* of long duration. This means that: (1) the delusions are not associated, derivable, or embedded into a net of other psychopathological symptoms; some other symptoms, like hallucinations, can occur, although very rarely, but they are transient, not intensive, and derivable from the delusions—actually they are delusional misinterpretations, and not real hallucinations; (2) the delusions usually deal exclusively or predominantly with only one theme, that is, they are monothematic; only seldom—in a mixed type—more than one topic is evident with equal presence and intensity, none of which predominating over the others; the most common theme is persecution and related ideas; (3) their duration is long—months, years, or even decades, sometimes lifelong; (4) the consciousness is always clear and signs of dementia or of any other central nervous system disease are not present; and (5) they are not due to medical conditions or substances.

The first and second of these aspects differentiate delusional disorder from *schizophrenia, schizoaffective disorder, psychotic bipolar or depressive disorders* and (together with the third aspect) *the polymorphous type of brief psychotic disorder* [4, 6]. If occasionally mood episodes occur, the delusions are of longer duration and not derivable from the mood symptoms. In cases of *obsessive–compulsive disorder* with lack of insight respectively with delusional beliefs, the obsessive–compulsive behaviour is the differentiating feature. But one has to be aware that some types of delusional disorder, especially the querulous–litigious form, can be associated with obsessive behaviour. In *paranoid personality disorder*—in contrast to delusional disorder—paranoid thinking is usually diffuse and affects many areas of life; it does not have a priori evidence and is accompanied by a general suspiciousness during the lifespan [4]. The fourth and fifth aspects differentiate delusional disorder from organic psychosis.

## Subtypes

The DSM-5 identifies seven *subtypes* of delusional disorder—erotomanic, grandiose, jealous, persecutory, somatic, mixed, and unspecified type, while ICD-10 also names a litigious and a self-referential type. But according to other views, the litigious form belongs to the persecutory type, whereas the self-referential aspect is associated with all types [4, 5]. However, all subtypes basically focus on the following three 'arche-themes', that is, existential, essential, and universal groups of concerns, fears, and desires of human beings:

• Sexuality and mating: focusing on Eros.
• Fears or desires regarding one's own body as carrier of health, image, performance, and reproduction: focusing on Soma.
• Survival and safety: focusing on Security.

Delusional disorder can be therefore divided, according to their 'arche-theme', into three groups [4]:

• Erotocentric (erotomania, jealousy),
• Securocentric (persecutory and related delusions, Capgras syndrome, etc.), and
• Somatocentric (delusions of health threat, parasitosis, dysmorphia, own odour, pregnancy, Cotard's syndrome, etc.).

### Erotocentric group

#### Erotomanic type

*Patients with delusions of erotomanic type are imperturbably convinced of being loved by someone*, mostly by a celebrity or someone of higher social standing. That person usually is completely unaware and out of reach for the erotomanic, which may cause intense stalking behaviour from the patient [4, 5].

Although this syndrome has been known since the ancient Greek period, it found its first scientific reference as an autonomous syndrome by the German psychiatrist Ernst Kretschmer in 1918 [4]. The detailed descriptions of the French psychiatrist de Clérambault, however, contributed to connecting erotomania to his name ('de Clérambault syndrome'), although he mainly described patients with delusions of being loved as a symptom of schizophrenia [15]. Erotomanic and jealous types can occur together, creating a common erotocentric group [4].

The *epidemiology* of the erotomanic type is unknown but seems to be rare. Delusions of being loved, however, can be found as symptoms in other psychotic conditions. The 'Halle study on Delusional Disorders' [4, 10, 11] found that out of 9969 inpatients at the Halle Psychiatric University Clinic in Germany between 1994 and 2007, and among 4753 non-organic psychotic disorders, only two patients had an erotomanic subtype of delusional disorder, both of whom were men. Although an earlier study [16] identified 15 patients with erotomanic delusions in a catchment area of approximately 400,000 people within a year, only three of these patients had an erotomanic delusional disorder.

Summarizing the data available, it can be concluded that the erotomanic type of delusional disorder is rare, more frequently—but not exclusively—occurring in unmarried females, with the first manifestation usually after the age of 30. But young men, even when married, may also be affected. The object of love usually is heterosexual, sometimes also homosexual. Stalking behaviour is not

unusual. The delusion may occur suddenly or develop gradually, and although the course and outcome are uncertain, they are usually long-lasting; sometimes the disorder may last several decades [4, 5, 17].

#### Jealous type

*The jealous type is characterized by the delusion that the patient's own sexual partner is being unfaithful.* Delusional jealousy can also be a symptom of other psychotic disorders. As already mentioned, it can co-occur with the erotomanic type, building a common erotocentric group [4].

A synonym of the disorder is *Othello syndrome*, after the character in Shakespeare's drama Othello who murdered his wife, based on his false belief that she had been disloyal. However, it is wrong to name delusional jealousy Othello syndrome. Othello's belief that his wife was not faithful to him was not delusional, but based on false facts deliberately arranged by others, especially by Jago [4]. Othello never had delusions of jealousy.

Patients' beliefs are sometimes bizarre or obscure; for example, even a high age of 80 or even higher is not an obstacle. Patients change their usual behaviour, become irritable, and show rough, aggressive, or even violent behaviour towards the partner. Their conviction cannot be disproven by any counter-argument or counter-evidence.

The prevalence of the jealous type is hard to be estimated for the same reasons as for other delusional disorders. Presumably it is approximately less than 10% within the group of delusional disorder. It remains unclear if there is a gender imbalance; some studies found more females, others more males. Previous assumptions that delusional jealousy is exclusively or predominantly an alcoholic syndrome could not be confirmed by modern authors [4, 5]. It is important to keep in mind that the disorder tends to be chronic and may be dangerous for the partner or the delusional rival.

### Securocentric group

#### Persecutory and related types

*The persecutory type is characterized by the delusion of being persecuted or harmed.* The theme of persecution and the kind of persecutors are very broad. In the eyes of the deluded individual, everything can be perceived as an indication of persecution and everybody as a persecutor, even persons trying to help. Patients tend to relate mutual activities of everyday life to themselves (as self-reverential delusions). Patients experience problems in interpersonal relationships and sometimes with the law. In some rare cases, the subject of persecution is not the patient himself, but a related person, hence 'persecutory delusional disorder by proxy'.

The phenomenology of persecutory delusional disorder can be classified into three types, according to the patient's behaviour and reactions [4]:

1. The flight type.
2. The fight type.
3. The height type.

The '*flight type*' is the most common and is characterized by 'fleeing from the danger', that is avoidance, isolation, and anxiety.

The '*fight type*' is characterized by sthenic reactions, aggression, and sometimes also violence. It can be divided into two subtypes:

1. The '*assaultive*' subtype is characterized by violent accusations against the assumed persecutors.
2. The '*querulous-litigious*' subtype is characterized by convictions of being treated unjustly and incorrectly and of being discriminated against, insofar patients feel persecuted by institutions or persons, or even by the legal system.

The '*height type*' is characterized by compensation of delusional persecutions by delusions of grandiosity.

Regarding prevalence and demography, the majority of cases of delusional disorder (approximately 60%) are included among the persecutory type, affecting more frequently men. Psychosocial adversity, like perceived ethnicity discrimination, may play a role in the development of persecutory symptomatology [18]. Though the diagnosis in many cases is stable over years, the persecutory type may change more often into schizophrenia than other types [4].

## Querulous-litigious subtype

Although ICD-10 names a querulous-litigious subtype, this can be seen as a form of the persecutory subtype, as mentioned previously. *The affected individual fights against delusional injustice, seeking help of the courts or authorities or, in some cases, by debating.* This behaviour can sometimes be dangerous, showing the 'Nemesis syndrome'—which means a subjective justified penalty, named according to Nemesis, the Greek goddess of high and divine vengeance. Patients with querulous-litigious delusions have sthenic and combative personalities, not seldom also showing obsessive features, and are willing to fight for their own satisfaction and compensation. But they are also isolated, because they usually do not win favours from their environments.

In a clinical setting, this subtype is rare. The 'Halle study on Delusional Disorders' found a querulous-litigious subtype in only three patients (0.03%) out of all 9969 admissions between 1994 and 2008—that is 7.0% out of all patients diagnosed with having a delusional disorder, which is in accordance with the findings of other authors [4]. A decrease in treated cases has been reported after the first half of the twentieth century [19]. At the University Clinic of Bern (Switzerland), the prevalence of patients with litigious symptomatology was 0.275% between 1922 and 1951, but only 0.09% between 1964 and 1993. Regarding psychotic querulous-litigious behaviour, the decrease in diagnoses was calculated as 74% between those two time periods [20]. One reason has to be taken into account—that patients with querulous-litigious delusions mostly contact the police or legal authorities, not the medical system. Another reason is probably that psychiatrists, on the other hand, do not have great interest in dealing with querulous-litigious patients because the psychiatrists themselves experience a number of difficulties with these patients—they fight doctors and their institutions through letters, emails, telephone calls, legal complaints, and even stalking behaviour. Another reason might be the difficulty in precisely distinguishing between querulous-litigious delusions, paranoid personality, and reality.

## Grandiose type

*Patients with this type show delusions of inflated worth, power, knowledge, identity, or special relationship to a deity or famous person.* Although the official diagnostic systems define a grandiose type, experienced clinicians and researchers question its independent existence [4, 5]. Munro, for example, an expert in the topic, only remembers two cases in his long period of clinical experience. Also the author of the present chapter encountered, over 40 years, primary delusions of grandiosity only in patients with mania, schizomania, schizophrenia, ecstatic forms of brief psychotic disorders, and organic psychosis, but never a primary grandiose type of delusional disorder. Nor did the 'Halle study on Delusional Disorders' find any case [4, 11, 12]. Possibly, the phenomenon could be explained by the following:

1. An independent 'grandiose delusional disorder' is so extremely rare that it practically does not exist.
2. Patients with grandiose type feel healthy, glorious, and superior and are self-confident. Hence, they do not seek help and usually do not harm anybody, and their social functioning is not impaired. So there is no reason to contact medical authorities.
3. There is a change in today's delusional themes, in comparison to earlier times, and grandiosity has become rare or presents only in psychotic disorders with manic or hyperthymic mood.
4. Modern operational diagnostic systems allocate states previously diagnosed as 'grandiose delusional disorder' to other categories like mania, schizomania, schizophrenia, etc.
5. A thorough analysis of the background of delusion of grandiosity could reveal them as the 'height' reaction type or the persecutory type.

Grandiosity and persecution can be the opposite sides of the same coin, as illustrated by related and generally inseparable beliefs: 'I am important enough to be singled out for persecution' and 'I am singled out for persecution because I am so important'; 'they persecuted me, because I am such an important person' or 'they persecuted me, because I am such an intelligent person' or 'such a powerful person', etc.; and 'as I am so superior, they are not able to harm me. There is no danger for me. I don't need to be afraid'. A flight into grandiosity may be one of the possibilities to compensate not only feelings of worthlessness and other negative thoughts and feelings, but also fear of persecution.

Thus, there is strong evidence that the very rare cases of the 'grandiose type' are simply a variation of the persecutory type, as it was presented previously [4, 5].

## Delusional misidentification

Delusional misidentification is characterized by misidentification of persons, but sometimes also of animals or inanimate things.

It is a non-specific phenomenon, symptom of various psychotic disorders, but obviously very rare as an independent delusional disorder. The content of the delusion is almost always threatening to the existence of the individual, related persons, or even the whole human race. Hence it could be mostly allocated to the securogenic type. The group of delusional misidentification syndromes do not include states in which the patient misjudges his environment due to clouded consciousness.

Delusional misidentification has varying phenomenology, giving rise to the following subtypes.

*Capgras syndrome* (named according to the French psychiatrist Joseph Capgras, one of its descriptors in the twentieth century—although it was already repeatedly described in the nineteenth century [4]) is the core of the group of misidentification syndromes. The main belief of a patient with Capgras syndrome is that someone in their environment, usually a close relative or a significant other, has been replaced by an identical-looking double. Only subtle details reveal the double; some hair behind the ear, some small movements, some minor details of the smile, etc. may be hints that the person is not the real one, but a replacement. The real person who has been replaced is thought to be absent. Patients usually indicate 'dark powers', 'the evil', 'secret services', 'the Mafia', or 'enemies' as having initiated the replacement. The 'double' is usually believed to be a spy or to be instructed to persecute and harm the patient, the city, the country, or even the whole world. The patient is occupied by uncertainties, is increasingly suspicious, feels great internal tensions, and is anxious, agitated, perplexed, and hostile against the 'double'.

Other phenomenological variations of the misidentification syndromes are extremely rare, or even exotic, like the following:

*Frégoli syndrome*: the patient believes that imposters frequently alter their facial appearance to resemble familiar people in his environment. It is named after Léopoldo Frégolian, an Italian actor famous for his ability to transform himself on stage into various characters. The patient thus identifies the imposter (usually as the persecutor) in several persons, for example the doctor, next time the nurses or fellow inpatients, then perhaps in neighbours, the postman, and so on. However, the persecutor is always one and the same.

*Intermetamorphosis*: a delusion that people around the patient have transformed physically and psychologically into one another. The transformation may concern also animals, as well as objects. It also implies the transformation of one's own person into someone else.

*Subjective doubles*: the patient believes in the existence of exact doubles of themselves. Although the syndrome of doubles of the self has superficial similarities to *heautoscopy*, the two phenomena are far from being identical. In cases of subjective doubles, the patients are convinced of the existence of another person associated with the delusional belief of being his or her double, while heautoscopy is a sort of hallucination, seeing oneself outside one's own body.

*Clonal doubles* or *clonal pluralization*: it is characterized by the delusion that there are several persons looking very much alike, that is, as clones of one and the same person.

*Zoocentric misidentification*: the patient is convinced that pets have been replaced by others.

*Inanimate misidentification*: the patient is convinced that things have been replaced by other things or by their doubles.

*Misidentification of time*: it is characterized by the patient's conviction that the present time has been substituted or that the usual passage of time has been changed in the sense of permanently repeating itself.

## Somatocentric group

The somatocentric delusional disorders, somewhat broader than the somatic type of DSM-5 or ICD-10 (-11), focus on one's own body and its functions. *The delusional theme concerns negative alterations of one's own body image, bodily functions, and bodily health*, as in the following syndromes:

- Delusional parasitosis.
- Cotard's syndrome.

- Delusional syndrome of one's own odour (olfactory reference syndrome).
- Delusional pregnancy.
- Health threat and dysmorphia delusional syndrome.
- Lycanthropy and zooanthropy.

### Delusional parasitosis

*Delusional parasitosis is the delusion of being infested with parasites.* The infested organ is usually the skin, but sometimes also the intestines, vagina, mouth, nose, etc.

The syndrome is known under various names: delusions of infestation, Ekbom's syndrome, *präseniler Dermatazoenwahn* (this is the original name given to the syndrome by Ekbom and means pre-senile delusional parasitosis), chronic tactile hallucinosis, delusional infestation, monosymptomatic hypochondriasis, monosymptomatic hypochondriacal psychosis, acarophobia, and *névrodermie parasitophobique*.

The Swedish psychiatrist Karl Ekbom introduced the German term *Dermatozoenwahn* in 1938, describing seven cases, mainly women, aged between 50 and 60, who were complaining of itching and paraesthesiae and were stubbornly and fixedly convinced that the discomfort was caused by small animals (for example, insects, parasites). However, the phenomenon had already been described many decades before Ekbom [4]. But it is his main contribution—that he described it as a delusional syndrome.

The *phenomenology* of delusional parasitosis is very homogenous and extremely alike in all affected patients. Almost all patients describe very intense itching as the key symptom. They complain about little creatures or microorganisms crawling, biting, stinging, hopping, or running on or under their skin. They show a high level of suffering, but only few report actual pain. The skin sensations usually persist the whole day and may also disturb the patient's sleep. More than one-third of the patients additionally describe sensations inside body openings or in the interior of their body: in their mouth, nose, inner ear, anus, intestines, lungs, or genitals. More than two-thirds of the patients present illusionary misidentifications or visual hallucinations related with the skin or parasites. Some patients even approach local health authorities or their general practitioners, carrying small containers with the 'parasites' with them, attempting to provide evidence of the cause of their torment. Thorough investigations of those objects usually reveal that they are small fragments of skin, hair, dried blood, scabs, dried nasal mucus, lint, textile fibres, dust, or excrement particles, etc., but in spite of such explanations, the patients are utterly convinced that these are parasites or their excretions.

The visual phenomena usually do not fulfil the definition of real hallucinations, because they are not perceptions without a stimulus; there is a stimulus—the small signs mentioned previously, which are misidentified by the patients as parasites. This can be defined as *illusionary misidentifications secondary to the tactile sensations or to the delusion of parasitosis*.

Other delusions secondary to the primary delusion (for example, delusions of reference) are possible, but based on, and derivable from, the primary delusional conviction. Other associated hallucinatory phenomena or misinterpreted perceptions (for example, visual, auditory, olfactory, or gustatory) are rare and without diagnostic relevance.

The prevalence of delusional parasitosis is not exactly known. Psychiatrists are likely to be the last specialists contacted by patients with delusional parasitosis. Most patients first seek help from dermatologists, general practitioners, or local health authorities. Only when distress and suffering seem to become unbearable do they seek a psychiatrist's advice. Nevertheless, delusional parasitosis, with approximately 0.5% of psychiatric inpatients, is not common. Females seem to be more frequently affected than males.

Although delusional parasitosis can manifest itself in every period of adult life, it is more frequent after the fifth decade, but not exclusively 'pre-senile', as Ekbom supposed.

Perhaps delusional parasitosis is the most common delusion that can be 'infectious'. Although the so-called *shared psychosis*, mostly in the form of '*folie à deux*', is rare, the ratio of shared psychosis in delusional parasitosis seems to be higher than in other psychotic disorders [4, 5].

There has been long discussions, mostly in the anglophone literature, of whether delusional parasitosis is a type of hypochondriasis or whether it is more correct to define it as *hypochondriacal delusion of parasitosis*. However, only a minority of patients with delusional parasitosis fulfil the essential criterion of hypochondriasis, that is, excessive preoccupation with anxious self-observation and worries about having a serious disease. In contrast to such concerns regarding one's own health, many patients with delusional parasitosis deny every kind of disease; they empathetically underline that they do not have any physical or mental disorder; they are 'just attacked by parasites'. This is why many patients do not seek the help of a doctor, but of an exterminator, a parasitologist, or even of local health and hygiene authorities.

But it is also true that some patients, although not the majority, have a hypochondriacal background. Also, during the long-term course of their illness, some patients may move towards the hypochondriacal pole. From a theoretical point of view, it seems important to differentiate between delusions and tactile hallucinations. Some authors believe that delusions are secondary, whereas tactile hallucinations are primary. But as mentioned, in contrast to other types of hallucinations, it is extremely difficult to define a patient's bodily sensation as being hallucinatory or not.

Summarizing the literature on the topic, it can be concluded that both mechanisms—hallucinatory and delusional—may occur in the sense of *organic hallucinosis* or *delusional disorder*.

Delusions of parasitosis may manifest as symptoms of schizophrenia, of organic psychotic disorders such as delirium and cocaine abuse, or of other psychotic disorders. The distinction between autonomous delusional disorder of parasitosis and symptomatic delusional parasitosis due to other conditions usually is easy, assuming the other defining criteria of the previously mentioned disorders are fulfilled, that is, the criteria of schizophrenia, psychotic affective disorders, organic psychotic disorders, etc.

*Treatment* is that of the underlying condition (somatic or psychotic). Clinical evidence has shown the effectiveness of dopamine antagonists, occasionally in combination with antidepressants, in some cases of autochthonous and autonomous delusional disorder of parasitosis.

In regard to *prognosis*, it can be concluded, that although in some cases the syndrome can become chronic, in many cases the prognosis seems to be benign following adequate treatment.

## Cotard's syndrome

Cotard's syndrome is a rare clinical condition, the most prominent symptom of which is the nihilistic delusion of denial of one's own body or parts of the body or even the delusion of being dead.

The syndrome was called after Jules Cotard, a French psychiatrist, to whom we owe the first systematic description in 1880, although the syndrome had been known before [4].

Patients hold the distinct delusion of being dead, not existing, putrefying, or having lost body parts, blood, internal organs, or very rarely their own soul. Symptoms of negation sometimes extend to the environment and even to the whole cosmos. Initially, the symptomatology is quite similar to that of derealization and/or depersonalization. The delusional beliefs determine the patient's behaviour. Patients being convinced that they do not have a stomach or any intestinal organs will refuse to eat or drink. Patients with the delusional conviction that their legs are dead or 'lifeless' will refuse to walk and will stay in bed for a long period of time, sometimes extending to several months. In severe cases, the patients no longer communicate with their surroundings. They present total negativism with mutism, in more severe cases even stupor. Thus, it is recommendable in patients with severe delusional depression, who develop stupor in the form of catatonic depression, to find out whether this is a consequence or a result of the patients' delusional conviction of negation. Analgesia, or even anaesthesia, has been observed in some patients.

Cotard's symptomatology is rare and can accompany severe psychotic depression but can also be observed in schizophrenia and organic brain damage; as an autonomous delusional disorder, it is apparently extremely rare. Insofar *treatment* of the syndrome depends on the underlying illnesses, it is symptomatic. Dopamine antagonists, alone or in combination with antidepressants and ECT treatment, could be effective.

## Delusions of one's own odour (olfactory reference syndrome)

Delusions of one's own odour can be defined as the unfounded and uncorrectable conviction of a patient to emit a bad or foul odour.

There are several synonyms, which only partially are correct and identical with the delusional disorder of one's own odour: olfactory reference syndrome, delusions of bromosis or of smell, delusional halitosis, hallucinatory halitosis, imaginary halitosis, etc.

If the delusions of one's own odour are the only prominent symptom and there's no indication for another type of psychosis like schizophrenia, schizoaffective or depressive disorder, and if they are not caused by organic factors, they fulfil the criteria of an autonomous delusional disorder. Delusions of one's own odour must also be distinguished from social anxiety spectrum disorders in which the respective believes are not delusional.

Olfactory delusional disorder is not only very rare, but also very difficult to be identified as such. If the patients report on smells from other people or things of the environment, it usually indicates olfactory hallucinations. But when the patient reports on own body odours, distinction between delusion and hallucination is needed. If the patient reports *perceptions* of smell originating from their own body or body fluids and the smell cannot be perceived by other people, the patient may have hallucinations. In contrast, patients with symptoms of delusions of their own odour normally phrase it like: "No, I do not perceive any strange or other extraordinary odour coming from my body, but I am sure that I give off such smells.

I notice it from other people's reactions when I enter a room or when I am close to people. They look at me very strangely; their facial expressions change; they move away, they talk to each other meaningfully. It can only be related to my own odour, which I personally do not perceive. This is logical because people usually do not perceive their own odours."

The patients also give a reason for their strange and bad odours perceived by others: they have done or thought something wrong or immoral. For instance, a 28-year-old male patient believed that people knew he masturbated because the next day his body smelled strange and extraordinary. He never perceived that smell, but could conclude it from the reactions of his colleagues in the office. So even if a patient reports on own odours it needs to be differentiated whether it is an olfactory hallucinosis, which—other than delusions—often is related to temporal lobe epilepsy or other temporal lobe damages [4].

There are no statistical surveys on the prevalence of the autonomous delusional disorder, but only case reports, and even those are very rare.

Psychogenic factors, especially sensitive and anxious personality features, are reported to have pathogenetic or pathoplastic relevance.

*Treatment* with drugs for psychosis and psychotherapy may be effective, but findings are inconsistent. As a result of their condition patients suffer from severe impairment in work and social relationships [21].

## Delusional pregnancy and Couvade syndrome

Delusional pregnancy (or delusional pseudocyesis) is characterized by the delusion to be pregnant (even in women with no sexual relations or in non-reproductive phases of life).

Although delusional pregnancy is not an extremely rare syndrome within major psychotic disorders, especially in schizophrenia, schizoaffective disorder, or psychotic mood disorders, it is extremely rare as autonomous delusional disorder. Delusions of pregnancy may last over a course of many years—in some reports over 25 years—and also in women over the age of 60.

Couvade syndrome is defined as the phenomenon in which husbands, boyfriends, or other exceptionally related persons of pregnant women develop symptoms of pregnancy too.

Couvade syndrome has apparently been well known since ancient times; it was even mentioned in the Greek myth of the 'Argonauts', and 2000 years ago, the Greek geographer Strabon reported on that phenomenon too [4].

The name *Couvade syndrome* was derived from the early French verb *couver*, which means *to brood* or *to hatch*. Couvade syndrome is a very rare syndrome in clinical reality, although some publications state the opposite. A reason for this discrepancy might be the fact that in some studies, certain symptoms having none or only little association with pregnancy (like toothache) are assumed to be an indicator for Couvade syndrome. There is no evidence that such symptoms are delusional. In contrast to Couvade syndrome, which is usually non-delusional, there are only few reports on *real delusions of pregnancy in men*, but as a symptom of psychotic or organic disorders, among other symptoms, especially in epilepsy, and post-ictal psychosis.

There is a plethora of theories trying to explain the phenomenon, for instance psychodynamic ones, but none of which has been proven.

## Lycanthropy or zooanthropy

*Lycanthropy or zooanthropy is a mainly delusional conviction that one has been transformed into a wolf or another animal (lýkos is the Greek word for wolf).*

Lycanthropy or zooanthropy is extremely rare. In international literature, over the last two centuries, only a few cases reported lycanthropic delusions. They are usually of short duration, lasting a few days or weeks, sometimes only hours, and seldom over a longer time. Mostly it is considered a symptom of major psychiatric disorders, especially of mood disorders, schizophrenia, or organic brain disorders, also involving alcohol and drug abuse, or psychogenic (dissociative or hysterical). Therefore, there is only little support to define lycanthropy as an autonomous delusional disorder [4].

## Delusional disorders of health threat and dysmorphia (somatic type)

*Patients with delusional disorder of health threat have unsubstantiated and uncorrectable convictions of having a severe illness or any other threat to their health.*

Hypochondriac delusions is a usual synonym for the disorder, but the term is not only discriminating and inexact, but it also does not cover the broad spectrum of health threat delusions [4].

Diagnosis, especially differential diagnosis, of delusional disorder of health threat is really difficult, mainly because the boundaries to non-delusional (hypochondriacal) fears are diffuse, uncertain, and difficult to draw.

The spectrum of themes of delusions of health threat are as broad and variable as there are organic diseases. Delusional ideas may focus on all parts and organs of the human body. They may occur as an autonomous delusional disorder, but more often they develop as symptoms of a major psychotic disorder (schizophrenia, schizoaffective disorder, delusional depression, or organic psychosis). Delusional disorders of health threat may be based on the patient's own or the family's experiences. A successfully treated 'real' medical condition in the past can be the source of the theme of a later delusional disorder.

*Delusional dysmorphia is characterized by the unsubstantiated and uncorrectable conviction that the body schema is unattractive or disproportioned.*

Delusional forms of the conviction of being misshapen have to be distinguished from phobic fears with that content. Nevertheless, patients with delusions of dysmorphia—usually younger than in other types of delusional disorder—are very unhappy people. The adverse influence of the disorder on their social interactions is massive; patients isolate themselves and are irritable, envious, and insecure, with low self-esteem.

Unlike other somatocentric delusions, delusions of dysmorphia usually begin early in life, mostly in adolescence, sometimes even in childhood. Adolescence is a fruitful soil for ideas of dysmorphia or dysmorphophobia, which may, in some cases, develop into delusions of dysmorphia.

In summary, it can be concluded that presumably there might never be reliable statistics on the prevalence of delusional disorder of health threat or of dysmorphia. Most patients from the first category will seek help from various physicians, but not from psychiatrists or psychologists. And patients not only with delusions of dysmorphia, but also any kind of dysmorphophobia, will most likely seek advice from an aesthetic surgeon, rather than from a psychiatrist.

Delineation of delusional disorders of health threat or of dysmorphia from non-delusional health threat syndromes (hypochondria or hypochondriacal disorder) and body dysmorphic disorder remains difficult—this is one of the reasons why we do not have—and do not get—reliable epidemiological data.

Delusions of health threat and of dysmorphia are rare as autonomous and autochthonous disorders but are usually associated with depression, schizophrenia, schizoaffective disorder, or disorders of the brain.

Prognosis is largely related to response to treatment, which mostly consists of a multimodal therapy setting of drugs for psychosis and/or depression and psychotherapy. Some authors report better response to treatment in somatocentric delusional disorders than in other types [5].

It is no surprise that in somatocentric syndromes, the relevance of culturally accepted fears and beliefs has to be taken into account. Some *culture-related somatocentric syndromes* are phobic, rather than delusional—for example, koro syndrome (acute fear or conviction of patients of having a genital retraction, which leads to death), in South East Asia; Kaza basolo (fear of women that their clitoris has been stolen, in Central Africa; *Dhat syndrome* with anxiety and somatocentric contents, like weakness and exhaustion, associated with convictions that their cause is loss of semen, in India; or *taijin kyofusho* (fear concerning mainly dysmorphia), in Japan.

## Prognosis

The prognosis of delusional disorder is discussed controversially, moving between pessimistic and optimistic views [4, 5]. According to evidence collected to date, the following can be concluded.

Delusional disorders are *highly stable* over many years, that is, in the great majority of patients, there is no syndrome shift in the course of the illness.

Symptoms usually *persist* over years or decades, and in some patients lifelong. Nevertheless, cases of some specific types of somatocentric delusional disorder, like delusional parasitosis, can have a benign prognosis after treatment with neuroleptics.

Although a number of patients suffer interactional problems with the social environment, which leads to early retirement, *autarky* remains intact in the great majority. This means patients are not impaired or disabled, live independently, and do not need any kind of support.

There exists *comorbidity* with depressive episodes, but reports vary considerably—approximately 30% to more than 70% of patients develop temporarily during course also depressive episodes; comorbidity with alcoholism seems to be lower, approximately 10%.

Controversially discussed in recent literature is an association of delusional disorder and dementia. Some studies found patients with delusional disorder at higher risk than the general population [22, 23], but others not [4, 11, 12].

## Treatment

There is a lack of systematic, double-blind, randomized controlled trials on this topic, using methods similar to those in other psychotic

disorders. What we know about the efficacy of treatment is mainly from anecdotic reports or very small heterogenous samples.

Whereas some authors expressed therapeutic optimism mainly regarding dopamine antagonists [5], other investigations, as well as clinical experience, do not share such over-optimistic views [4]. Comparative trials did not find a better outcome in the group admitted after the introduction of dopamine antagonists in modern psychiatry, in comparison to the time before their introduction [24]. Nevertheless, some somatocentric delusional disorders, like delusional parasitosis, respond positively to treatment with dopamine antagonists [4, 5].

All reports on *electroconvulsive therapy* are anecdotal [4], just like reviews on the efficacy of *psychotherapy* in delusional disorder. One of the rare comparative psychotherapeutic trials [25] included only a small number of patients ($n$ = 11 allocated to a cognitive behavioural therapy group; $n$ = 6 to an attention placebo control group) for a relatively short treatment period of 24 weeks. Completers in both groups showed clinical improvement, but those in the cognitive behavioural group improved in more aspects.

Notwithstanding, long-term investigations proved that in spite of occasional or even continuous treatment in the majority of patients (up to 80%), the delusions remained for a long time unremitted [4, 11, 12].

The enormous difficulties associated with the treatment of patients with delusional disorder have to be taken into consideration, mainly because patients do not feel ill or disturbed and so refuse any kind of therapeutic help. Usually, such patients become dissatisfied, noncompliant, and suspicious, discontinue therapy, regard hospitalization as a hostile act, and often set off a long-lasting war of nerves against the treating staff, even after their discharge from hospital.

Any patient with delusional disorder might be difficult, but querulous-litigious patients are perhaps the most difficult and unpleasant ones—not only for their social environment and the legal system, but also for therapists. Their psychotherapists or psychiatrists are frequently persecuted by querulous-litigious patients and reported to university authorities, hospital administrations, ministries, or even legal representatives.

Nevertheless, some authors recommend an integrated method for treating 'paranoia', using a multimodal therapeutic approach of combination of psychodynamic (uncovering), interpersonal, cognitive behavioural, and pharmacological therapeutic techniques [26].

## REFERENCES

1. American Psychiatric Association (2013). *Diagnostic and Statistical Manual of Mental Disorders* (5th edn). American Psychiatric Association, Washington, DC.
2. World Health Organization (1991). *ICD-10 Classification of Mental and Behavioural Disorders: Clinical Descriptions and Diagnostic Guidelines*. World Health Organization, Geneva.
3. Gaebel W, Zielasek J, Cleveland H-R (2012). Classifying psychosis: challenges and opportunities. *Int Rev Psychiatry.* 24:538–48.
4. Marneros A (2012). *Persistent Delusional Disorders: Myths and Realities.* Nova Science, New York, NY.
5. Munro A (1999). *Delusional Disorder: Paranoia and Related Illnesses.* Cambridge University Press, Cambridge.
6. Marneros A, Pillmann F (2004). *Acute and Transient Psychoses.* Cambridge University Press, Cambridge.

7. Winokur G (1977). Delusional disorder (paranoia). *Compr Psychiatry*. 18:511–21.

8. Perälä J, Suvisaari J, Saarni SI, *et al.* (2007). Lifetime prevalence of psychotic and bipolar I disorders in a general population. *Arch Gen Psychiatry*. 64:19–28.

9. Grover S, Biswas P, Avasthi A (2007). Delusional disorder: study from North India. *Psychiatry Clin Neurosci*. 61:462–70.

10. Wustmann T, Pillmann F, Marneros A (2011). Gender-related features of persistent delusional disorder. *Eur Arch Psychiatry Clin Neurosci*. 261:29–36.

11. Wustmann T, Pillmann F, Friedemann J, Piro J, Schmeil A, Marneros A (2012). The clinical and sociodemographic profile of persistent delusional disorders. *Psychopathology*. 45:200–2.

12. Fuentenebro F, Berrios GE (1995). The predelusional state: a conceptual history. *Compr Psychiatry*. 36:251–9.

13. Cardno AG, McGuffin P (2006). Genetics and delusional disorder. *Behav Sci Law*. 24:257–76.

14. Vicens V, Radua J, Salvador R, *et al.* (2016). Structural and functional brain changes in delusional disorder. *Br J Psychiatry*. 208:153–9.

15. Berrios GE, Kennedy N (2002). Erotomania: a conceptual history. *Hist Psychiatry*. 13:381–400.

16. Kennedy N, McDonough M, Kelly B, Berrios GE (2002). Erotomania revisited: clinical course and treatment. *Compr Psychiatry*. 43:1–6.

17. Jordan HW, Lockert EW, Johnson-Warren M, *et al.* (2006). Erotomania revisited: thirty-four years later. *J Natl Med Assoc*. 98:787–93.

18. Shaikh M, Ellett L, Dutt A, *et al.* (2016). Perceived ethnic discrimination and persecutory paranoia in individuals at ultra-high risk for psychosis. *Psychiatry Res*. 12:309–14.

19. Mullen PE, Lester G (2006). Vexatious litigants and unusually persistent complainants and petitioners: from querulous paranoia to querulous behaviour. *Behav Sci Law*. 24:333–49.

20. Caduff F (1995). Querulanz—ein verschwindendes psychopathologisches Verhaltensmuster? *Fortschr Neurol Psychiatr*. 63:504–10.

21. Greenberg JL, Shaw AM, Reuman L, Schwartz R, Wilhelm S (2016). Clinical features of olfactory reference syndrome: an Internet-based study. *J Psychosom Res*. 80:11–16.

22. Korner A, Lopez AG, Lauritzen L, Andersen PK, Kessing LV (2008). Delusional disorder in old age and the risk of developing dementia—a nationwide register-based study. *Aging Ment Health*. 12:625–9.

23. Leinonen E, Santala M, Hyotyla T, Santala H, Eskola N, Salokangas RKR (2004). Elderly patients with major depressive disorder and delusional disorder are at increased risk of subsequent dementia. *Nord J Psychiatry*. 58:161–4.

24. Opjordsmoen S, Retterstøl N (1993). Outcome in delusional disorder in different periods of time—possible implications for treatment with neuroleptics. *Psychopathology*. 26:90–4.

25. O'Connor K, Stip E, Pelissier MC, *et al.* (2007). Treating delusional disorder: a comparison of cognitive-behavioural therapy and attention placebo control. *Can J Psychiatry*. 52:182–90.

26. Kantor M (2004). *Understanding Paranoia: A Guide for Professionals, Families, and Sufferers*. Praeger Publishers, Westport, CT.

# 63

# Prevention and early intervention in psychotic disorders

*Emre Bora, Mahesh Jayaram, and Christos Pantelis*

## Introduction

### What is early psychosis?

Psychosis is a severe mental illness that most often begins in late adolescence or early adulthood, though it can affect people across the lifespan. Early psychosis refers to the onset of symptoms or prodromal features that begin during early neurodevelopment. The term first-episode psychosis (FEP) is often used to refer to the first time psychosis is manifest, though this may be later in life (beyond adolescence). Psychosis is associated with a distinct break from reality and characterized by disorganized thinking and sometimes speech, delusions, hallucinations, and disturbances in behaviour and affect. It can also be associated with prominent motor/volitional disturbances, cognitive disturbances, and impaired insight (for discussion about the types of psychosis, see [1]). Early psychosis may be preceded by prodromal stages before full-blown psychosis is apparent. This may include changes to thought and perception, which are often vague, yet can be distressing. It is, however, important to consider these phenomena carefully across the stages, from prodrome (and even earlier) to psychosis, so that effective strategies for illness prevention and intervention can be put in place. In this chapter, we discuss the importance of early identification and treatment of early psychosis and its prodrome.

### What are the prodromal symptoms of psychosis?

The 'prodrome' of psychosis (which includes, but is not limited to, schizophrenia) constitutes a period of change from baseline premorbid levels of functioning and may progress to a stage where patients are experiencing perceptual, mood, and behavioural changes prior to the onset of frank psychotic symptoms. Thus often, these are only recognized in hindsight, rather than ahead of time. Patients who develop schizophrenia, with the benefit of hindsight, are able to recall that they experienced prodromal symptoms about 80–90% of the time. Ten to 20% of patients with schizophrenia can develop the illness 'out of the blue', that is, without prodromal symptoms [2, 3].

In order to better understand and accurately identify prodromal symptoms, various groups have defined sets of phenomena that characterize the prodrome and earlier stages. Some of these approaches were based on identifying individuals showing higher conversion rate, based on genetic risk, together with other vulnerabilities, including familial risk and functional decline, multiple affected family members, and familial risk together with cognitive deficits or negative symptoms [4, 5]. Other approaches aim to recognize individuals who are help-seeking due to emerging psychotic symptoms, who have not met psychotic disorder criteria as yet but are potentially in the prodromal phase [clinical high-risk (CHR) or ultra-high-risk (UHR) for psychosis]. An approach that seems to encompass all of these varied symptoms can be found in a key paper [6], which describes the contemporary thinking around CHR psychosis states. Broadly, there are two key concepts—the UHR criteria and basic symptoms (BS), both of which have similar criteria, with a goal of identifying those who would be more likely to transition to psychosis within a short time period (12–24 months). Preceding the CHR phase is the period relating to other factors leading to increased vulnerability. This is outlined further in Fig. 63.1.

The notion of very early signs of psychosis has been evident in the literature for over 40 years. Gerd Huber introduced the concept of BS of psychosis, a relatively well-known concept in Germany, but less widely used elsewhere, which describes the early prodromal phases of psychosis [7, 8]. BS are subtle and sometimes vague (ill-defined) features experienced by the individual and may include elusive disturbances in thought, speech, mood, or bodily perceptions, and can also include cognitive–perceptive and/or cognitive disturbances [9]. The individual may use personalized coping strategies, such as avoidance of certain situations and social isolation, and may overcome them for at least a period of time. The development of psychosis and cognitive deficits are often associated with partial or complete loss of insight [10]. Together with more recent conceptualizations of prodromal symptoms, the approach of identifying the earliest prodromal stages of schizophrenia has provided the tantalizing possibility for early identification and treatment, with the hope of delaying, or even preventing, the illness. This approach also allows for the identification of brain changes and potential mechanisms in early psychosis and schizophrenia [11].

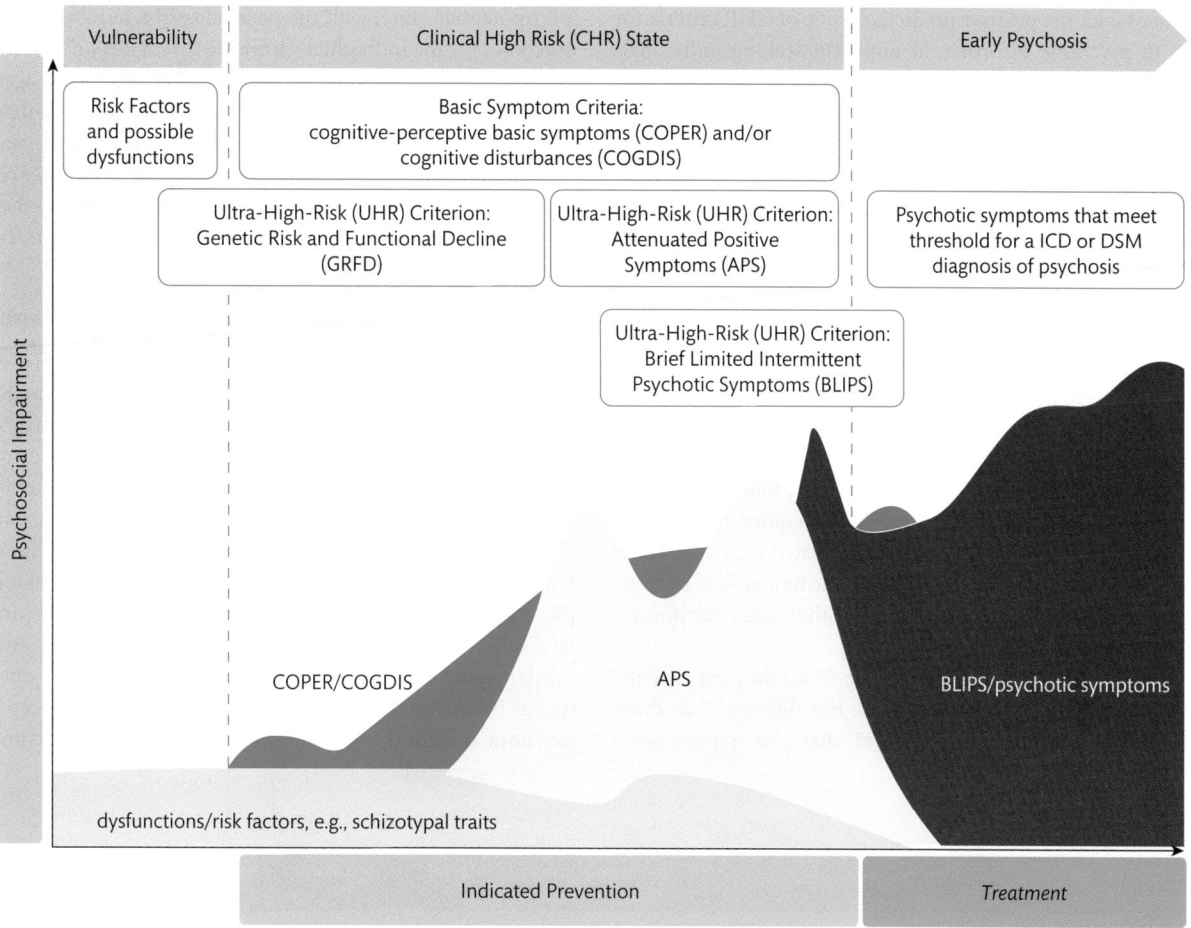

**Fig. 63.1** Model of transition from CHR states to psychosis [6].
Reproduced from *Eur Psychiatry*, 30(3), Schultze-Lutter F, Michel C, Schmidt SJ, *et al.*, EPA guidance on the early detection of clinical high risk states of psychoses, pp. 405–16, Copyright (2015), with permission from Elsevier Masson SAS.

The original concept of UHR for psychosis was defined according to the presence of state [psychotic-like experiences (PLEs), brief psychotic symptoms] and trait risk factors (schizotypy, family history), associated with a clinically significant drop in function, assessed using the Global Assessment of Functioning (GAF) scale [12]. Early studies indicated that 37% converted to psychosis within 12 months [13] A meta analysis of more recent studies using such criteria has identified the transition rate to be 22% [14]. The importance of this notion was the possibility of early/pre-onset identification and intervention to prevent or ameliorate psychosis and the possibility to examine neurobiological changes around the transition to active illness [11, 15, 16]. Important criticisms of this approach, however, are the focus on psychotic-like experiences (PLEs) and the lack of a clear boundary for transition to psychosis. Thus, to date, it is unclear that there is a discontinuity between the UHR state and psychosis, which requires longitudinal mapping of trajectories from pre-psychosis onset [17]. More recent conceptualizations suggest that a dimensional approach may be more appropriate [18].

The UHR criteria over the last two decades encompass other related concepts such as Brief Limited Intermittent Psychotic Symptoms (BLIPS), Attenuated Psychotic Symptoms (APS), Genetic Risk and Deterioration Syndrome (GRDS) Subgroup, and the Unspecified Prodromal Symptoms (UPS) group. Other groups have defined genetic high-risk individuals, which potentially allows for an even earlier identification of pre-psychotic individuals at high risk for psychosis [19]. There is no consensus as to whether these are distinct entities or fall under the umbrella of UHR, as outlined in this detailed review [20].

### Detection of individuals at ultra-high risk and conversion rates for psychosis

In recent years, there has been increasing effort to develop a greater focus on specific risk paradigms to identify individuals who have a higher risk and transition rate, in comparison to psychometric schizotypy, PLEs, and familial high-risk approaches. A number of structured interview methods, including Comprehensive Assessment of At-Risk Mental States (CAARM) and Structured Interview for Psychosis-Risk Syndromes (SIPS), have been developed to detect CHR groups [21]. In practice, the predominant presentation of the majority of individuals meeting CHR criteria is APS (85%) in a recent meta-analysis [22]. The same study also found that the conversion rate for developing psychosis was considerably higher across these risk paradigms, compared with psychometric schizotypy, PLEs, and family history (for example, the transition risk within 36 months was 20% for APS and 26% for APS + GRDS) Transition rate of BLIPS was much higher (39% within 24 months).

On the other hand, the positive predictive value of CHR criteria for transition to psychotic disorders in non-help-seeking individuals was only 5.7%. Similarly, the annual risk of PLEs for psychotic outcome was relatively low (0.56% per year) [23].

### Staging model for psychosis

Following on from the work in defining UHR and psychosis transition, McGorry and colleagues [24] have proposed a staging model of psychosis (Table 63.1), which incorporates the earliest stages of psychosis and considers the onset and progression of the illness to chronicity. This model borrows from notions developed for cancer staging and treatment, and is appealing as it suggests that each stage may require different interventions/treatment strategies. The central concept for the psychoses is that earlier stages are characterized by differences neurobiologically and better functional abilities, and require different interventions. Thus, earlier stages may warrant less extreme measures, while later stages will likely require more radical interventions. Further, each stage may be associated with differences neurobiologically and there may be identifiable biomarkers by stage [25], though it is yet to be demonstrated that there are clear boundaries between the proposed stages.

McGorry and colleagues [26] have gone on to propose that the earliest stages, namely UHR or earlier, are less differentiated diagnostically, prompting them to consider that this represents a 'pluripotential' state, with the possibility of a number of diagnostic outcomes for the individual. However, it remains unclear if the condition at this stage is truly 'pluripotential' or whether progression to one or other psychotic condition has already been pre-determined by factors yet to be identified (for example, genetic). Current initiatives are attempting to use machine-learning and other analytical approaches to examine if features of the illness at its earliest stages may predict the onset of psychosis, diagnosis, long-term course, or functional outcomes [27].

### Why is early intervention for psychosis important?

In general medicine, early intervention (EI) targeting prevention or disease modification has been a topic of interest for some time for a number of conditions such as diabetes, cancer, and cardiovascular diseases. EI aims to target pathophysiological processes causing a disorder, with the aim to cease or slow its progression before symptoms emerge or become chronic and untreatable. While the ideal goal of EI is prevention, in most cases, modification of the illness course is a more realistic outcome. The proposed staging model for schizophrenia and other psychotic disorders, as discussed, appears to have face validity as an appealing notion, to intervene early and reduce the damaging impacts of the illness, in terms of clinical outcome, as well as brain structure and function. However, the concept of EI in psychotic disorders is perhaps not as straightforward, compared to

**Table 63.1** Staging model

| Stage | Definition | Target populations and referral sources | Potential interventions |
|---|---|---|---|
| 0 | Increased risk of psychotic or severe mood disorder and no symptoms currently | First-degree teenage relatives of probands | 1. Improved mental health literacy<br>2. Family education, drug education<br>3. Brief cognitive skills training |
| 1a | Mild/non-specific symptoms (including neurocognitive deficits) of psychosis or severe mood disorder. Mild functional change or decline | Screening of teenage populations. Referral by: primary care physicians; school counsellors | 1. Formal mental health literacy<br>2. Family psychoeducation, formal CBT<br>3. Active substance misuse reduction |
| 1b | Ultra-high risk: moderate but subthreshold symptoms, with moderate neurocognitive changes and functional decline to caseness (GAF, <70) | Referral by: educational agencies; primary care physicians; emergency departments; welfare agencies | 1. Family psychoeducation, formal CBT<br>2. Active substance misuse reduction<br>3. Omega-3 fatty acids<br>4. Dopamine antagonists/partial agonists<br>5. Antidepressant agents or mood stabilizers |
| 2 | First episode of psychotic or severe mood disorder Full-threshold disorder with moderate to severe symptoms, neurocognitive deficits, and functional decline (GAF 30–50) | Referral by: primary care physicians; emergency departments; welfare agencies; specialist care agencies; drug and alcohol services | 1. Family psychoeducation, formal CBT<br>2. Active substance misuse reduction<br>3. Dopamine antagonists/partial agonists<br>4. Antidepressant agents or mood stabilizers<br>5. Vocational rehabilitation |
| 3a | Incomplete remission from first episode of care; patient's management could be linked or fast-tracked to Stage 4 | Primary and specialist care services | 1. As for Stage 2, but with additional emphasis on medical and psychosocial strategies to achieve full remission |
| 3b | Recurrence or relapse of psychotic or mood disorder, which stabilizes with treatment at a GAF level, or with residual symptoms or neurocognition below the best level achieved after remission from the first episode | Primary and specialist care services | 1. As for Stage 3a, but with additional emphasis on relapse prevention and strategies to detect 'early warning signs' |
| 3c | Multiple relapses, provided worsening in clinical extent and impact of illness is objectively present | Specialist care services | 1. As for Stage 3b, but with emphasis on long-term stabilization |
| 4 | Severe, persistent, or unremitting illness (based on symptoms, neurocognition, and disability criteria). Patient's management could be fast-tracked to this stage at first presentation, based on specific clinical and functional criteria (from Stage 2) or because of failure to respond to treatment (from Stage 3a) | Specialized care services | 1. As for Stage 3c, but with emphasis on clozapine, other tertiary treatments, and social participation despite ongoing disability |

Adapted from *Aust N Z J Psychiatry*, 40(8), McGorry, PD, Hickie IB, Yung AR, *et al.*, Clinical staging of psychiatric disorders: a heuristic framework for choosing earlier, safer and more effective interventions, pp. 616–622, Copyright (2006), with permission from SAGE Publications.

other medical conditions, due to the complexity of factors involved, the diagnostic difficulties given the reliance on psychopathology, which may be ill-defined at illness onset, the variable trajectory, and the importance of other comorbid prognostic factors (for example, stress, substance use, and other environmental insults). Further, EI programmes require substantial resources. Therefore, it is important to review the available evidence of efficacy and effectiveness of available EI models for psychosis, which should complement resources needed for those with established schizophrenia.

### Interventions in the prenatal period and infancy

The greatest single risk factor for schizophrenia is genetic load [28], and recent studies attempt to delineate the genes relevant to the disorder [29], which provide clues for a number of potential treatment targets. Genetic susceptibility factors are likely to cause schizophrenia, with their negative influence on brain development from the prenatal period to later phases of brain development [11, 30]. Other critical events during early brain development, such as prenatal infection and starvation, and perinatal hypoxia are well-established risk factors for schizophrenia, while a range of other insults during early neurodevelopment, such as vitamin D deficiency, are also implicated [31], suggesting that public health measures at the population level may be important. Recent studies focus on the importance of gene–environment interactions [32], which should be examined across neurodevelopment. However, there is a lack of preclinical/animal research that examines gene–environment interactions across development and the impact on brain maturation. Such strategies would inform the development of novel pharmacological strategies relevant to the emergence of the disorder.

### Public health measures to reduce the burden of psychotic illness

General non-specific public health measures, including nutritional health and better prenatal and perinatal care, can have a potential effect on reducing the risk for schizophrenia and co-occurring neurodevelopmental cognitive deficits. Another approach can be prenatal dietary supplementation to prevent schizophrenia, similar to the use of folate to reduce the risk of spina bifida and other disorders related to failure of closing of midline structures. Some authors have argued that prenatal choline supplementation, based on α-7 nicotinic receptor-related effects on neuronal inhibition deficits in schizophrenia, can reduce the incidence of schizophrenia. Low levels of vitamin D, folate, and retinol and increased homocysteine levels in early life have been proposed as risk factors for schizophrenia and neurodevelopmental disorders [33–35]. However, methodological difficulties, particularly the low population prevalence and the late onset around the beginning of the third decade of life, provide a significant challenge in testing the role of dietary supplementation during early development in reducing the risk of schizophrenia. Strategies to examine this question include long-term population-based studies where data are available at, or prior to, birth and/or targeting high-risk groups of individuals (for example, those with a positive family history).

A few RCTs have investigated the effect of prenatal choline supplementation on biological markers that have been associated with future schizophrenia risk (cognitive abilities and inhibition of P50 potential) in infants and children. In a placebo controlled trial of choline supplementation in pregnant women, babies in the choline group had better P50 inhibition than controls at 1 month, but no difference was found at 3 months [36]. Another study found no evidence of cognitive differences at age of 1 year between choline and placebo groups [37]; however, maternal choline intake above 400 mg/day had significant effects on cognition at 7-year follow-up [38]. In a Finnish birth cohort study, vitamin D supplementation during the first year of life was associated with a reduced risk of schizophrenia in males [39]. Another Danish population-based case-controlled study found that both increased and reduced levels of vitamin D in neonates were associated with a higher risk of developing schizophrenia, suggesting a non-linear relationship [40]. Correcting abnormal levels of vitamin D and other deficiencies during early life may potentially reduce the incidence of schizophrenia. However, there is a need for longitudinal studies investigating the role of dietary supplements as an EI strategy, which could target high-risk subjects (for example, those with a positive family history).

It is also important to consider the possibility that the interaction of familial risk and environmental risks factors (nutritional, obstetric problems, stress) can increase the risk for infants, as women with psychosis are less likely to receive adequate prenatal care than healthy women. Multi-disciplinary teams (for example, obstetricians, neonatologists, nutritionists, psychiatrists, adult- and infant–parent-trained psychologists, and social workers) could address problematic prenatal issues, including nutritional deficiencies, lifestyle concerns such as the use of tobacco, alcohol, or other drug use, or life stresses including housing or violence in the home [41]. Enhancing parenting skills, supporting parents, and effective treatment of symptoms and cognitive rehabilitation in parents can potentially improve the resilience of a child at genetic risk for developing psychotic disorders [41]. Other than children of a parent with schizophrenia, strategies to identify high-risk children (for example, those with 22q11.2 deletion and other schizophrenia-related CNVs) might be appropriate for such interventions.

### Intervention for specific and non-specific at-risk groups in childhood/early adolescence

An alternative approach involves interventions targeting non-specific risk factors such as trauma and stress, bullying, drug abuse, and migration in childhood and teenage years, which are associated with an increased risk of mental disorders, including schizophrenia. For example, evidence suggests that interventions for teens and their parents, which improve family communication and rule setting, can reduce the rate of subsequent drug abuse and associated problem behaviours [42]. Reducing peer rejection and bullying with social (anti-bullying programs) and individual (social skills training) interventions might be another potential strategy [43, 44].

The use of treatments as early as possible in the premorbid phase of the illness may also improve outcomes. Such intervention strategies are currently being investigated in those individuals identified as at CHR for psychosis; however, such studies are relatively few. Very few studies and case reports have provided evidence of short-term CBT and a web-based self-help programme in reducing PLEs [45]. However, there are some efforts to develop psychosocial intervention programmes targeting children with familial high and low risk presenting with developmental delays, PLEs, and emotional problems [46]. Cognitive remediation in children with neuropsychological difficulties can also potentially improve resilience of children at risk. Studies investigating trajectories of PLEs, social withdrawal, cognitive development, and other potential antecedents of psychosis can help to identify target populations. For example, emerging evidence suggests that, while PLEs in children might be mostly benign and temporary, persistence of such symptoms are more likely to precede psychotic disorders and might be indicators of a need for interventions.

The strategy and focus in the last two decades on CHR for psychosis have provided the possibility to explore EI strategies in adolescence; however, there is currently only a limited focus on early (pre-emptive) intervention in childhood. This presents an important area of endeavour for future studies. Importantly, most of the proposed interventions have low risk and can benefit in enhancing resilience in a relatively large population, as childhood antecedents of psychosis have low specificity and can be associated with other psychopathologies.

## Early intervention in adolescence and young adults

### Goals and challenges for early intervention in individuals at clinical high risk for psychosis

Improving long-term outcome is the main goal for EI in individuals at high risk for psychosis. It is also hoped that EI in individuals at high risk can prevent or delay a first psychotic episode, which is often a very stressful experience for the individual and their family. Supporting individuals with mental illness and their families during late adolescence and early adulthood is also critical for helping individuals in pursuing academic or vocational goals, developing social and sexual relationships and developing skills necessary for independent living. EI programmes also emphasize the concept of phase-specific treatment, suggesting that treatments that have limited benefits in chronic patients can be helpful in at-risk individuals (for example, CBT, fish oil).

There are a number of conceptual and practical challenges in developing and implementing EI programmes in individuals at high risk for psychosis. The main challenge is the low positive predictive value of the current construct of high risk for psychosis. The majority of individuals who meet CHR criteria never develop psychotic disorders. Even though some of these help-seeking individuals might have subclinical psychotic conditions with a good prognosis, most (false-positives) would have non-psychotic conditions, including affective disorders, dissociative symptoms, trauma cluster B personality traits, and substance use. The heterogeneity of individuals meeting current CHR criteria has important implications for research and treatment of early psychosis. The problem of high false-positive rates leads to ethical problems, including use of drugs for psychosis and stigmatization in individuals who have no underlying psychotic disorder. For true positives, the current CHR criteria, including the condition of being a help-seeking individual, together with the demands of EI programmes, would lead to recruitment of individuals with milder psychotic disorders, rather than individuals with poor insight, non-adherence, and poor prognosis. Also, current criteria for detecting CHR omit negative and disorganized symptoms and cognitive deficits, which might be beneficial for identifying those individuals with the highest need for help. The heterogeneity of CHR is also a challenge for assessing the efficacy of treatment methods, as the individuals with different underlying psychopathological conditions can respond to different components of EI programmes. That it is called 'phase-specific' treatment for CHR

might be simply a reflection of the relationship between the heterogeneity of individuals with CHR and treatment response. Thus, some individuals might respond to treatments that do not work in chronic psychotic patients, as they have no underlying psychosis. On the other hand, dopamine antagonist drugs would remain as the main treatment of choice for true positives, if we were able to detect these individuals with sufficiently high accuracy. Stigma associated with psychotic disorder is another challenge in managing individuals with CHR.

### Current evidence for efficacy of early intervention programmes

CHR has been by far the most commonly used high-risk paradigm in EI studies. Only a few studies have investigated the role of intervention in other high-risk paradigms. Several studies with small sample sizes have investigated the role of low-dose risperidone on first-degree relatives of individuals with schizophrenia presenting with negative symptoms and/or neurocognitive deficits (schizotaxia). These studies have provided evidence for a reduction of negative symptoms and cognitive deficits in these individuals [5, 47, 48]. Another study of standard vs integrated treatment (assertive community treatment, social skills training, and psychoeducation groups to patients and families) in schizotypal personality disorder individuals found lower transition rates to FEP in the integrated treatment group at 2-year follow-up (25% vs 48%) [49].

In accordance with the popularity of the CHR concept, a number of studies have investigated the effects of interventions with psychosocial and medication/dietary supplements in help-seeking individuals meeting CHR criteria. Many of these studies included control groups (that is, standard treatment and placebo). Some studies have reported reductions in symptom severity in both EI and control groups; however, most used conversion to psychosis as their primary outcome. Importantly, several meta-analyses of RCTs suggested that EI has generally produced significantly reduced conversion rates at 6- to 48-month follow-up [50, 51].

The use of dopamine antagonists in CHR individuals has been trialled early but has led to controversy about the ethics of this approach at such an early 'pre-psychosis' stage. Various drugs have been examined, including risperidone, aripiprazole, perospirone, and amisulpride, as a standalone or in combination with psychological treatment [50, 51], with few of these studies being RCTs [52–55]. These studies provided some evidence for efficacy of drugs in reducing the transition rate at follow-up. The ethical issues in prescribing dopamine antagonists in CHR include exposure of false-positive individuals to these medications and their side effects.

Alternative, less invasive pharmacological interventions showed initial promise and did not suffer from such ethical issues. These include the use of dietary supplementation with long-chain omega-3 polyunsaturated fatty acids (PUFAs/fish oil), which do not have any clinically relevant adverse effects. Initial findings suggested that PUFAs can be beneficial in improving outcomes, as suggested by the Vienna Omega-3 Study. This was the first RCT of omega-3 PUFAs in CHR, demonstrating that a 12-week intervention was associated with a significantly reduced risk of experiencing an FEP during a 12-month follow-up (5% for omega-3 PUFAs vs 28% for placebo) and with significant symptomatic and functional improvements [56]. Recently, findings from a longer follow-up (median = 6.7 years) of the same individuals suggested that benefits of this intervention might be sustained. The cumulative conversion rate to psychosis at the longer-term follow-up was 9.8% (4/41) of subjects in the omega-3 PUFA group, and 40% (16/40) of subjects in the placebo group. This study was followed by two larger replication studies that investigated the effect of omega-3 PUFAs as an EI strategy. NEURAPRO-E is a multi-centre RCT (involving 304 participants), which compared outcome in one group treated with omega-3 PUFAs plus cognitive behavioural case management (CBCM) with a placebo plus CBCM group. Unfortunately, the outcome of NEURAPRO-E has not replicated the findings of the Vienna trial. In this study, there was no advantage of PUFAs, in comparison to placebo, for change in symptoms and functioning and 12-month transition rates (11.2% vs 11.5%) [57]. Similarly, the rate of psychotic conversion did not differ in the omega-3 fatty acid (13%) vs placebo (8%) samples in the recent NAPLS Omega-3 Fatty Acid Versus Placebo Study [58].

As a summary, studies in CHR suggest that psychological treatments and dopamine antagonists might reduce the incidence of developing a full-blown psychotic episode at 6- to 48-month follow-up. The findings regarding the effect of PUFAs are controversial; however, the larger multi-centre studies would suggest there is limited benefit. Importantly, the long-term effects of these psychosocial and pharmacological interventions on transition rates, functioning, and symptoms have not been clarified. Given the ethical issues of using potentially invasive treatments to groups of individuals with relatively low transition rates, psychosocial approaches are the mainstay of EI in CHR.

## Early intervention in first-episode psychosis

### Treatment of early psychosis

#### Pharmacological

Dopamine antagonists are the mainstay of treatment of psychosis and have an important role in treating acute episodes and reducing relapse rates in schizophrenia. Large multi-centre trials provide support for their use in early psychosis, as demonstrated by the European First Episode Schizophrenia Trial (EUFEST) [59]. In this study ($N = 498$), second-generation antipsychotics (SGAs) (also referred to as atypical antipsychotics) were tolerated better and were associated with lower discontinuation rates. The term 'second-generation antipsychotic' was the terminology used at the time to distinguish a heterogenous group of new drugs from classical or 'first-generation' drugs for psychosis. This terminology will be used to describe the results of the trial, but it is not otherwise to be encouraged for reasons given in Chapter 10. While an initial analysis did not find significant differences between SGAs and low-dose haloperidol [a first-generation antipsychotic (FGA), classical or typical antipsychotic], subsequent analysis demonstrated a higher response and remission rate for most SGAs, compared to low-dose haloperidol [60], while there was a similar level of improvement in cognition [61]. A meta-analysis of drugs for psychosis in FEP indicated that olanzapine and amisulpride were relatively more effective than older drugs [62]. In considering the evidence in FEP, however, it is important to consider issues such as compliance and engagement with treatment strategies. Further, there are important decisions about duration of use of medication in young people, given the issue of diagnostic uncertainty at this stage of illness and the impact of adverse events caused by these medications. Thus, milder forms of the illness will be apparent at this early stage; symptom remission will be more likely, and affective psychoses or substance-related psychotic disorders may have differing outcomes. Therefore, smaller doses might be sufficient in many patients with FEP, compared to chronic patients, and early dose reduction, in comparison to maintenance, might be associated with better functional outcome [63] and reduced side effect burden. In the short term, younger people might be susceptible to developing extra-pyramidal side effects, especially with older dopamine antagonist drugs, while the newer dopamine antagonists have histamine and serotonin-blocking properties associated with weight gain and metabolic syndrome. Weight gain is a particularly important issue in young people (that is, negative effect on self-esteem and peer relations) that can lead to non-adherence. Further, weight gain and metabolic syndrome can be associated with increased cognitive deficits, morbidity, and mortality in the long term. Most drugs for psychosis, with some exceptions (for example, ziprasidone), are associated with weight gain in FEP [64].

Like in chronic schizophrenia, psychological treatments might benefit individuals with FEP. Evidence suggests that CBT and family interventions are effective in FEP [65]. Recently, a number of studies have investigated the role of cognitive remediation in FEP, summarized in a meta-analysis [66], which confirmed significant, but modest, gains for verbal memory and social cognition, although the domain being examined may be important to consider [67]. Social skills training, psychoeducation, and vocational training have also been used in early psychosis [68, 69].

#### Psychosocial interventions

Most of the available early interventions in CHR studies used psychological interventions, with CBT being most commonly employed. Others [70] examined family-focused therapy (FFT), including a study investigating the effects of psychoeducational multifamily group treatment [71]. A number of these studies combined elements of various CBT, social skills training, psychoeducation, and family intervention and support (integrated treatments) [72–74]. A few studies investigating the effect of cognitive remediation in CHR [75, 76] have found that psychological interventions and cognitive remediation are associated with improved outcomes during the intervention period. Such studies are consistent with the notion that less invasive interventions would be appropriate at earlier illness stages, as proposed in the staging model. However, it should be noted that such interventions may also be useful at later illness stages.

## Early intervention services

### Specialized early intervention programmes for FEP

Programmes providing interventions for FEP are becoming commonplace in a number of developed countries. These services provide specialized assertive EI to improve outcomes in psychotic disorders. While implementing these programmes is costly and resource-intensive, it has been hypothesized that they can improve long-term outcomes (and decrease overall costs) as the first 3–5 years after FEP have been suggested to be a critical period for making a meaningful change to the future course of the illness. Another important concept for EI in FEP is the duration of untreated psychosis (DUP). Patients with psychotic symptoms typically seek help for their symptoms after a considerable delay. Evidence suggests that longer DUP might be associated with poor prognosis [77]. Therefore, it is hoped that reducing DUP can improve long-term outcomes in FEP. EI in early psychosis can also reduce complications of onset of illness, including substance abuse, suicide, and inter-personal problems and family burden. EI programmes include intensive case management with low caseloads, assertive outreach, psychiatric treatment, and easy access to staff, providing psychoeducation, family interventions, and other psychosocial supports, which might include psychological treatments, social skills training, and vocational training. In most of these models, a specialist/standalone multi-disciplinary team provides EIs. Several alternative approaches, including the 'Hub and Spoke' model and enhanced community mental health care, also exist [78]. 'Hub and Spoke' models aim to overcome the challenges of providing EI in remote and rural areas, in which specialist staff within community systems are supported by a central 'hub'. In the enhanced community mental health care ('specialist within a generalist') model, staff in the community team have an EI role for some clients, in addition to their usual role.

It is also important to note that integrative treatment for psychotic disorders was initially developed in chronic patients. The original integrative treatment approach is based on a 'chronic disease' model, in which individuals need to be supported by intensive case management and specialist services, in order to function in the society or residential units. Studies on chronic schizophrenia have shown benefits of integrative treatment, in comparison to treatment as usual [79]. In the chronic disease model, it is not expected that long-term functioning of individuals would significantly improve a few years following discharge from such services. However, the promise of integrative treatment in EI services is changing the illness course and improving long-term functioning by intervening in the 'critical period' and by reducing the need of individuals for such services in the coming years. Therefore, it is important to test the long-term functioning of individuals and their capacity to maintain gains once the EI programme is ceased.

### Evidence for short-term efficacy of EI in FEP

Currently, there are many EI services in Australia, North America, Europe, and Asia. A number of RCTs have investigated the efficacy of such programmes in comparison to treatment as usual (TAU). The Danish OPUS trial, which randomized 547 patients with FEP to either a 2-year specialized assertive EI programme or standard treatment, is the most comprehensive study to date that has examined short- and long-term outcomes [80]. Results of the OPUS trial showed positive effects on psychotic and negative symptoms, treatment non-adherence, level of functioning, secondary substance abuse, level of user, and family satisfaction in the EI group, in comparison to the TAU group. There was a reduction in the number of days patients used beds in the EI group, compared to the TAU group. A more recent EI trial—the Recovery After an Initial Schizophrenia Episode Early Treatment Program [NIMH RAISE-ETP (NAVIGATE)]—included 404 individuals with FEP. This study reported greater improvement in quality of life and symptoms, in comparison to usual community care. A number of smaller trials, including the smaller Lambeth Early Onset (LEO) study [82], the International Optimal Treatment (IOT) study subset [83], the

Croydon Outreach and Assertive Support Team (COAST) [84], the Specialized Treatment Early in Psychosis (STEP) [85], the Psychosis early Intervention and Assessment of Needs and Outcome (PIANO) [86], and the Early Psychosis Intervention Center (EPICENTER) [87] studies, had already reported similar benefits during the intervention period. Several studies recruited individuals who already completed an EI service [OPUS, Early Assessment Service for Young People with Psychosis (EASY) and Canadian Prevention and Early Intervention Program for Psychoses (PEPP)] and randomized them to prolonged EI (additional 1–3 years) and regular care groups [88, 89]. These studies found that prolonged EI was associated with sustained benefits, in comparison to the regular care group within the intervention period. It has been suggested that EI services might be cost-effective, as increased costs of integrated treatment are balanced by reduced days of inpatient admissions [85, 90]. In summary, the current evidence suggests that EI services are better than TAU in ordinary community mental health teams during the intervention period. This finding is similar to the outcome of integrative treatment studies in chronic schizophrenia [91].

### Evidence for long-term efficacy of EI in FEP after ceasing intervention

Evidence suggests that EI can significantly reduce the DUP, however, the clinical significance of this finding is unclear. The Treatment and Intervention in Psychosis Study (TIPS) attempted to answer this question using a quasi-experimental design (92). The TIPS study compared the outcome of individuals living in areas where public information campaigns and low-threshold early detection teams were established, compared to individuals living in other areas. In early detection areas, DUP was significantly reduced (from 16 to 4 weeks), but the clinical significance of this finding was dubious. At 10 years, half of the individuals in both areas were not remitted [93]. In the same study, the recovery rate was better in individuals in the early detection area, as they were more likely to be in full-time employment (27% vs 11%). However, it is likely that baseline differences between groups can explain the observed findings, as patients from the early detection area had fewer positive and negative symptoms at presentation. Thus, low-threshold early detection approaches are likely to recruit a higher percentage of individuals with milder psychotic illness and shorter DUP. Clearly, better controlled studies are required to address this important question.

RCT studies comparing the long-term outcome of EI services and TAU can be more informative. A critical question for EI outcome research is whether time-limited intervention during a 'critical period', unlike similar interventions in chronic patients, dramatically improves long-term outcomes, in comparison to TAU, after individuals are discharged to regular services. To date, several groups have reported their findings regarding long-term outcomes. In contrast to findings suggesting short-term benefits of EI, a number of 5- to 12-year follow-up findings reported in the OPUS [80, 94], IOT [95], and LEO [96] RCTs have not found evidence for sustained benefits in EI groupa, in comparison to TAU groups. Current evidence does not support the long-term sustaining benefits of EI after ceasing treatment. It was suggested that the duration of treatment in the EI service can be important for maintaining outcomes in the long term and that 2–3 years of intervention might be insufficient. As discussed, several recent ongoing studies investigated the effect of prolonged EI and recently completed prolonged intervention periods

[89, 97]. The Jockey Club Early Psychosis (JCEP) project is another ongoing study comparing effectiveness of 4 years and 2 years of EI and standard care [98]. When completed, 5- and 10-year post-intervention outcome findings of these studies may show whether prolonged EI, unlike the 2-year intervention, has sustained bene-fits after intervention is ceased. The findings to date therefore raise important questions about the benefits of EI services, unless such intervention can be sustained in the long term, perhaps even beyond an extended EI programme. Evidence is needed to inform decisions about the configuration of services and the balance between EI vs post-EI services.

## Conclusions

Current evidence suggests that integrative treatment in early psych-osis is more successful than 'treatment as usual' care in reducing symptoms and relapse rates and improving engagement. Offering high-quality, integrative, intensive, needs-based services that in-corporate age-specific/relevant goals at all stages of psychotic dis-orders, including early, medium, or late stages, is the best service we can offer at this point in time. Emphasizing the importance of optimism and instilling hope for symptomatic and functional re-covery should be implemented across all stages of psychosis. Early detection and intervention services and public awareness cam-paigns are important to increase the possibility for individuals with psychotic disorders to access help in the early stages of the illness. For individuals having potential prodromal symptoms, given the significant issue of false-positives identified by CHR cri-teria, together with the clinical heterogeneity of this population, a generic psychological treatment approach remains the main inter-vention for the foreseeable future. Studies investigating the tra-jectory of developmental antecedents of psychotic disorders and the effectiveness of pre-emptive interventions are clearly needed. Continuing research efforts to develop better and highly accurate markers of psychotic disorders and other mental disorders at pre-morbid and prodromal stages are critical for true EI, which could reduce the incidence and/or improve long-term outcomes for psychotic disorders.

## Acknowledgements

Prof C. Pantelis was supported by a NHMRC Senior Principal Research Fellowship (ID: 1105825). The authors contributed equally in the preparation of this chapter.

## REFERENCES

1. Thomas N, Pantelis C. Psychotic disorders. In: Cautin R, Lilienfeld S (eds). *The Encyclopedia of Clinical Psychology*. John Wiley & Sons, New York, NY; 2015. p. 16.
2. Yung AR, McGorry PD. The initial prodrome in psych-osis: descriptive and qualitative aspects. Aust N Z J Psychiatry. 1996;30:587–99.
3. Yung AR, Phillips LJ, McGorry PD, *et al*. Prediction of psych-osis. A step towards indicated prevention of schizophrenia. Br J Psychiatry Suppl. 1998;172:14–20.
4. Johnstone EC, Lawrie SM, Cosway R. What does the Edinburgh high-risk study tell us about schizophrenia? Am J Med Genet. 2002;114:906–12.
5. Tsuang MT, Stone WS, Tarbox SI, Faraone SV. Treatment of nonpsychotic relatives of patients with schizophrenia: six case studies. Am J Med Genet. 2002;114:943–8.
6. Schultze-Lutter F, Michel C, Schmidt SJ, *et al*. EPA guidance on the early detection of clinical high risk states of psychoses. Eur Psychiatry. 2015;30:405–16.
7. Huber G, Gross G. The concept of basic symptoms in schizo-phrenic and schizoaffective psychoses. Recenti Prog Med. 1989;80:646–52.
8. Schultze-Lutter F. Subjective symptoms of schizophrenia in re-search and the clinic: the basic symptom concept. Schizophr Bull. 2009;35:5–8.
9. Klosterkotter J, Schultze-Lutter F, Ruhrmann S. Kraepelin and psychotic prodromal conditions. Eur Arch Psychiatry Clin Neurosci. 2008;258 Suppl 2:74–84.
10. Quee PJ, van der Meer L, Bruggeman R, *et al*. Insight in psych-osis: relationship with neurocognition, social cognition and clinical symptoms depends on phase of illness. Schizophr Bull. 2011;37:29–37.
11. Pantelis C, Yücel M, Wood SJ, *et al*. Structural brain imaging evidence for multiple pathological processes at different stages of brain development in schizophrenia. Schizophr Bull. 2005;31:672–96.
12. American Psychiatric Association. *Diagnostic and statistical manual of mental disorders: DSM-IV-TR*, fourth edition, text revi-sion. American Psychiatric Association, Washington, DC; 2000.
13. Yung AR, McGorry PD. The prodromal phase of first-episode psychosis: past and current conceptualizations. Schizophr Bull. 1996;22:353–70.
14. Fusar-Poli P, Bonoldi I, Yung AR, *et al*. Predicting psych-osis: meta-analysis of transition outcomes in individuals at high clinical risk. Arch Gen Psychiatry. 2012;69:220–9.
15. Fusar-Poli P, Radua J, McGuire P, Borgwardt S. Neuroanatomical maps of psychosis onset: voxel-wise meta-analysis of antipsychotic-naive VBM studies. Schizophr Bull. 2012;38:1297–307.
16. Pantelis C, Velakoulis D, McGorry PD, *et al*. Neuroanatomical abnormalities before and after onset of psychosis: a cross-sectional and longitudinal MRI comparison. Lancet. 2003;361:281–8.
17. Cropley VL, Pantelis C. Using longitudinal imaging to map the 'relapse signature' of schizophrenia and other psychoses. Epidemiol Psychiatr Sci. 2014;23:219–25.
18. van Os J, Guloksuz S. A critique of the "ultra-high risk" and "transition" paradigm. World Psychiatry. 2017;16:200–6.
19. Johnstone EC, Ebmeier KP, Miller P, Owens DG, Lawrie SM. Predicting schizophrenia: findings from the Edinburgh High-Risk Study. Br J Psychiatry. 2005;186:18–25.
20. Fusar-Poli P, Borgwardt S, Bechdolf A, *et al*. The psychosis high-risk state: a comprehensive state-of-the-art review. JAMA Psychiatry. 2013;70:107–20.
21. Yung AR, Yuen HP, McGorry PD, *et al*. Mapping the onset of psychosis: the Comprehensive Assessment of At-Risk Mental States. Aust N Z J Psychiatry. 2005;39:964–71.
22. Fusar-Poli P, Cappucciati M, Borgwardt S, *et al*. Heterogeneity of Psychosis Risk Within Individuals at Clinical High Risk: A Meta-analytical Stratification. JAMA Psychiatry. 2016; 73:113–20.

23. Kaymaz N, Drukker M, Lieb R, *et al*. Do subthreshold psychotic experiences predict clinical outcomes in unselected non-help-seeking population-based samples? A systematic review and meta-analysis, enriched with new results. Psychol Med. 2012;42:2239–53.

24. McGorry PD, Hickie IB, Yung AR, Pantelis C, Jackson HJ. Clinical staging of psychiatric disorders: a heuristic framework for choosing earlier, safer and more effective interventions. Aust N Z J Psychiatry. 2006;40:616–22.

25. Wood SJ, Yung AR, McGorry PD, Pantelis C. Neuroimaging and treatment evidence for clinical staging in psychotic disorders: from the at-risk mental state to chronic schizophrenia. Biol Psychiatry. 2011;70:619–25.

26. McGorry PD. Risk syndromes, clinical staging and DSM V: new diagnostic infrastructure for early intervention in psychiatry. Schizophr Res. 2010;120:49–53.

27. Koutsouleris N, Gaser C, Bottlender R, *et al*. Use of neuroanatomical pattern regression to predict the structural brain dynamics of vulnerability and transition to psychosis. Schizophr Res. 2010;123:175–87.

28. Gottesman, II, Shields J. A polygenic theory of schizophrenia. Proc Natl Acad Sci U S A. 1967;58:199–205.

29. Schizophrenia Working Group of the Psychiatric Genomics Consortium. Biological insights from 108 schizophrenia-associated genetic loci. Nature. 2014;511:421–7.

30. Bora E. Neurodevelopmental origin of cognitive impairment in schizophrenia. Psychol Med. 2015;45:1–9.

31. McGrath JJ, Murray RM. Risk factors for schizophrenia: from conception to birth. In: Hirsch SR, Weinberger DR, editors. *Schizophrenia*, second edition. Blackwell Science, Oxford; 2003. pp. 232–50.

32. Van Os J, Rutten BP, Myin-Germeys I, *et al*. Identifying gene-environment interactions in schizophrenia: Contemporary challenges for integrated, large-scale investigations. Schizophr Bull. 2014;40:729–36.

33. Bao Y, Ibram G, Blaner WS, *et al*. Low maternal retinol as a risk factor for schizophrenia in adult offspring. Schizophr Res. 2012;137:159–65.

34. Brown AS, Bottiglieri T, Schaefer CA, *et al*. Elevated prenatal homocysteine levels as a risk factor for schizophrenia. Arch Gen Psychiatry. 2007;64:31–9.

35. Picker JD, Coyle JT. Do maternal folate and homocysteine levels play a role in neurodevelopmental processes that increase risk for schizophrenia? Harv Rev Psychiatry. 2005;13:197–205.

36. Ross RG, Hunter SK, McCarthy L, *et al*. Perinatal choline effects on neonatal pathophysiology related to later schizophrenia risk. Am J Psychiatry. 2013;170:290–8.

37. Cheatham CL, Goldman BD, Fischer LM, da Costa KA, Reznick JS, Zeisel SH. Phosphatidylcholine supplementation in pregnant women consuming moderate-choline diets does not enhance infant cognitive function: a randomized, double-blind, placebo-controlled trial. Am J Clin Nutr. 2012;96:1465–72.

38. Boeke CE, Gillman MW, Hughes MD, Rifas-Shiman SL, Villamor E, Oken E. Choline intake during pregnancy and child cognition at age 7 years. Am J Epidemiol. 2013;177:1338–47.

39. McGrath J, Saari K, Hakko H, *et al*. Vitamin D supplementation during the first year of life and risk of schizophrenia: a Finnish birth cohort study. Schizophr Res. 2004;67:237–45.

40. McGrath JJ, Eyles DW, Pedersen CB, *et al*. Neonatal vitamin D status and risk of schizophrenia: a population-based case-control study. Arch Gen Psychiatry. 2010;67:889–94.

41. Newman L, Judd F, Olsson CA, *et al*. Early origins of mental disorder—risk factors in the perinatal and infant period. BMC Psychiatry. 2016;16:270.

42. Patnode CD, O'Connor E, Rowland M, Burda BU, Perdue LA, Whitlock EP. Primary care behavioral interventions to prevent or reduce illicit drug use and nonmedical pharmaceutical use in children and adolescents: a systematic evidence review for the U.S. Preventive Services Task Force. Ann Intern Med. 2014;160:612–20.

43. Stoltz S, van Londen M, Dekovic M, de Castro BO, Prinzie P, Lochman JE. Effectiveness of an individual school-based intervention for children with aggressive behaviour: a randomized controlled trial. Behav Cogn Psychother. 2013;41:525–48.

44. Waasdorp TE, Bradshaw CP, Leaf PJ. The impact of schoolwide positive behavioral interventions and supports on bullying and peer rejection: a randomized controlled effectiveness trial. Arch Pediatr Adolesc Med. 2012;166:149–56.

45. Stafford E, Hides L, Kavanagh DJ. The acceptability, usability and short-term outcomes of Get Real: a web-based program for psychotic-like experiences (PLEs). Internet Interventions. 2015;2:266–71.

46. Uher R, Cumby J, MacKenzie LE, *et al*. A familial risk enriched cohort as a platform for testing early interventions to prevent severe mental illness. BMC Psychiatry. 2014;14:344.

47. Rybakowski JK, Drozdz W, Borkowska A. Long-term administration of the low-dose risperidone in schizotaxia subjects. Hum Psychopharmacol. 2007;22:407–12.

48. Stone WS, Hsi X, Giuliano AJ, *et al*. Are neurocognitive, clinical and social dysfunctions in schizotaxia reversible pharmacologically?: Results from the Changsha study. Asian J Psychiatr. 2012;5:73–82.

49. Nordentoft M, Thorup A, Petersen L, *et al*. Transition rates from schizotypal disorder to psychotic disorder for first-contact patients included in the OPUS trial. A randomized clinical trial of integrated treatment and standard treatment. Schizophr Res. 2006;83:29–40.

50. Schmidt SJ, Schultze-Lutter F, Schimmelmann BG, *et al*. EPA guidance on the early intervention in clinical high risk states of psychoses. Eur Psychiatry. 2015;30:388–404.

51. van der Gaag M, Smit F, Bechdolf A, *et al*. Preventing a first episode of psychosis: meta-analysis of randomized controlled prevention trials of 12 month and longer-term follow-ups. Schizophr Res. 2013;14956–62.

52. Ruhrmann S, Bechdolf A, Kuhn KU, *et al*. Acute effects of treatment for prodromal symptoms for people putatively in a late initial prodromal state of psychosis. Br J Psychiatry Suppl. 2007;51:s88–95.

53. McGorry PD, Nelson B, Phillips LJ, *et al*. Randomized controlled trial of interventions for young people at ultra-high risk of psychosis: twelve-month outcome. J Clin Psychiatry. 2013;74:349–56.

54. McGorry PD, Yung AR, Phillips LJ, *et al*. Randomized controlled trial of interventions designed to reduce the risk of progression to first-episode psychosis in a clinical sample with subthreshold symptoms. Arch Gen Psychiatry. 2002;59:921–8.

55. McGlashan TH, Zipursky RB, Perkins D, *et al*. Randomized, double-blind trial of olanzapine versus placebo in patients prodromally symptomatic for psychosis. Am J Psychiatry. 2006;163:790–9.

56. Amminger GP, Schafer MR, Papageorgiou K, *et al*. Long-chain omega-3 fatty acids for indicated prevention of psychotic disorders: a randomized, placebo-controlled trial. Arch Gen Psychiatry. 2010;67:146–54.

57. McGorry PD, Markulev C, Nelson B, *et al.* The NEURAPRO-E study: a multicentre RCT of omega 3 fatty acids and cognitive behavioural case management for patients at ultra high risk of schizophrenia and other psychotic disorders. Schizophr Bull. 2015;41(Suppl 1):S322–3.

58. Cadenhead K, Addington J, Cannon T, *et al.* Omega-3 Fatty Acid Versus Placebo in a Clinical High-Risk Sample From the North American Prodrome Longitudinal Studies (NAPLS) Consortium. Schizophr Bull. 2017;43(suppl 1):S16.

59. Kahn RS, Fleischhacker WW, Boter H, *et al.*; EUFEST study group. Effectiveness of antipsychotic drugs in first-episode schizophrenia and schizophreniform disorder an open randomised clinical trial. Lancet. 2008;371:1085–97.

60. Boter H, Peuskens J, Libiger J, *et al.* Effectiveness of antipsychotics in first-episode schizophrenia and schizophreniform disorder on response and remission: an open randomized clinical trial (EUFEST). Schizophr Res. 2009;115:97–103.

61. Davidson M, Galderisi S, Weiser M, *et al.* Cognitive effects of antipsychotic drugs in first-episode schizophrenia and schizophreniform disorder: a randomized, open-label clinical trial (EUFEST). Am J Psychiatry. 2009;166:675–82.

62. Zhang JP, Gallego JA, Robinson DG, Malhotra AK, Kane JM, Correll CU. Efficacy and safety of individual second-generation vs. first-generation antipsychotics in first-episode psychosis: a systematic review and meta-analysis. Int J Neuropsychopharmacol. 2013;16:1205–18.

63. Wunderink L, Nieboer RM, Wiersma D, Sytema S, Nienhuis FJ. Recovery in remitted first-episode psychosis at 7 years of follow-up of an early dose reduction/discontinuation or maintenance treatment strategy: long-term follow-up of a 2-year randomized clinical trial. JAMA Psychiatry. 2013;70:913–20.

64. Tek C, Kucukgoncu S, Guloksuz S, Woods SW, Srihari VH, Annamalai A. Antipsychotic-induced weight gain in first-episode psychosis patients: a meta-analysis of differential effects of antipsychotic medications. Early Interv Psychiatry. 2016;10:193–202.

65. Bird V, Premkumar P, Kendall T, Whittington C, Mitchell J, Kuipers E. Early intervention services, cognitive-behavioural therapy and family intervention in early psychosis: systematic review. Br J Psychiatry. 2010;197:350–6.

66. Revell ER, Neill JC, Harte M, Khan Z, Drake RJ. A systematic review and meta-analysis of cognitive remediation in early schizophrenia. Schizophr Res. 2015;168:213–22.

67. Pantelis C, Wannan C, Bartholomeusz CF, Allott K, McGorry PD. Cognitive Intervention in Early Psychosis—Preserving abilities versus remediating deficits. Curr Opin Behav Sci. 2015;4:63–72.

68. Rinaldi M, Perkins R, McNeil K, Hickman N, Singh SP. The Individual Placement and Support approach to vocational rehabilitation for young people with first episode psychosis in the UK. J Ment Health. 2010;19:483–91.

69. Liu P, Parker AG, Hetrick SE, Callahan P, de Silva S, Purcell R. An evidence map of interventions across premorbid, ultra-high risk and first episode phases of psychosis. Schizophr Res. 2010;123:37–44.

70. Miklowitz DJ, O'Brien MP, Schlosser DA, *et al.* Family-focused treatment for adolescents and young adults at high risk for psychosis: results of a randomized trial. J Am Acad Child Adolesc Psychiatry. 2014;53:848–58.

71. McFarlane WR, Levin B, Travis L, *et al.* Clinical and functional outcomes after 2 years in the early detection and intervention for the prevention of psychosis multisite effectiveness trial. Schizophr Bull. 2015;41:30–43.

72. Addington J, Epstein I, Liu L, French P, Boydell KM, Zipursky RB. A randomized controlled trial of cognitive behavioral therapy for individuals at clinical high risk of psychosis. Schizophr Res. 2011;125:54–61.

73. Bechdolf A, Wagner M, Veith V, *et al.* Randomized controlled multicentre trial of cognitive behaviour therapy in the early initial prodromal state: effects on social adjustment post treatment. Early Interv Psychiatry. 2007;1:71–8.

74. Thompson E, Millman ZB, Okuzawa N, *et al.* Evidence-based early interventions for individuals at clinical high risk for psychosis: a review of treatment components. J Nerv Ment Dis. 2015;203:342–51.

75. Loewy R, Fisher M, Schlosser DA, *et al.* Intensive Auditory Cognitive Training Improves Verbal Memory in Adolescents and Young Adults at Clinical High Risk for Psychosis. Schizophr Bull. 2016;42 Suppl 1:S118–26.

76. Piskulic D, Barbato M, Liu L, Addington J. Pilot study of cognitive remediation therapy on cognition in young people at clinical high risk of psychosis. Psychiatry Res. 2015;225:93–8.

77. Addington J, Van Mastrigt S, Addington D. Duration of untreated psychosis: impact on 2-year outcome. Psychol Med. 2004;34:277–84.

78. Behan C, Masterson S, Clarke M. Systematic review of the evidence for service models delivering early intervention in psychosis outside the stand-alone centre. Early Intervention in Psychiatry. 2017;11:3–13.

79. Lenroot R, Bustillo JR, Lauriello J, Keith SJ. Integrated treatment of schizophrenia. Psychiatr Serv. 2003;54:1499–507.

80. Kane JM, Robinson DG, Schooler NR, *et al.* Comprehensive versus usual community care for first-episode psychosis: 2-year outcomes from the NIMH RAISE Early Treatment Program. Am J Psychiatry. 2016;173:362–72.

81. Bertelsen M, Jeppesen P, Petersen L, *et al.* Five-year follow-up of a randomized multicenter trial of intensive early intervention vs standard treatment for patients with a first episode of psychotic illness: the OPUS trial. Arch Gen Psychiatry. 2008;65:762–71.

82. Craig TK, Garety P, Power P, *et al.* The Lambeth Early Onset (LEO) Team: randomised controlled trial of the effectiveness of specialised care for early psychosis. BMJ. 2004;329:1067.

83. Grawe RW, Falloon IR, Widen JH, Skogvoll E. Two years of continued early treatment for recent-onset schizophrenia: a randomised controlled study. Acta Psychiatr Scand. 2006;114:328–36.

84. Kuipers E, Holloway F, Rabe-Hesketh S, Tennakoon L; Croydon Outreach and Assertive Support Team (COAST). An RCT of early intervention in psychosis: Croydon Outreach and Assertive Support Team (COAST). Soc Psychiatry Psychiatr Epidemiol. 2004;39:358–63.

85. Srihari VH, Tek C, Kucukgoncu S, *et al.* First-Episode Services for Psychotic Disorders in the U.S. Public Sector: A Pragmatic Randomized Controlled Trial. Psychiatr Serv. 2015;66:705–12.

86. Ruggeri M, Bonetto C, Lasalvia A, *et al.* Feasibility and Effectiveness of a Multi-Element Psychosocial Intervention for First-Episode Psychosis: Results From the Cluster-Randomized Controlled GET UP PIANO Trial in a Catchment Area of 10 Million Inhabitants. Schizophr Bull. 2015;41:1192–203.

87. Breitborde NJ, Bell EK, Dawley D, *et al.* The Early Psychosis Intervention Center (EPICENTER): development and six-month outcomes of an American first-episode psychosis clinical service. BMC Psychiatry. 2015;15:266.

88. Albert N, Melau M, Jensen H, *et al.* Five years of specialised early intervention versus two years of specialised early intervention followed by three years of standard treatment for patients with a

first episode psychosis: randomised, superiority, parallel group trial in Denmark (OPUS II). BMJ. 2017;356:i6681.

89. Chang WC, Chan GH, Jim OT, et al. Optimal duration of an early intervention programme for first-episode psychosis: randomised controlled trial. Br J Psychiatry. 2015;206:492–500.

90. Hastrup LH, Kronborg C, Bertelsen M, et al. Cost-effectiveness of early intervention in first-episode psychosis: economic evaluation of a randomised controlled trial (the OPUS study). Br J Psychiatry. 2013;202:35–41.

91. Reilly S, Planner C, Gask L, et al. Collaborative care approaches for people with severe mental illness. Cochrane Database Syst Rev. 2013;11:CD009531.

92. Friis S, Vaglum P, Haahr U, et al. Effect of an early detection programme on duration of untreated psychosis: part of the Scandinavian TIPS study. Br J Psychiatry Suppl. 2005;48:s29–32.

93. Hegelstad WT, Larsen TK, Auestad B, et al. Long-term follow-up of the TIPS early detection in psychosis study: effects on 10-year outcome. Am J Psychiatry. 2012;169:374–80.

94. Secher RG, Hjorthoj CR, Austin SF, et al. Ten-year follow-up of the OPUS specialized early intervention trial for patients with a first episode of psychosis. Schizophr Bull. 2015;41:617–26.

95. Sigrunarson V, Grawe RW, Morken G. Integrated treatment vs. treatment-as-usual for recent onset schizophrenia; 12 year follow-up on a randomized controlled trial. BMC Psychiatry. 2013;13:200.

96. Gafoor R, Nitsch D, McCrone P, et al. Effect of early intervention on 5-year outcome in non-affective psychosis. Br J Psychiatry. 2010;196:372–6.

97. Albert N, Melau M, Jensen H, et al. Five years of specialised early intervention versus two years of specialised early intervention followed by three years of standard treatment for patients with a first episode psychosis: randomised, superiority, parallel group trial in Denmark (OPUS II). BMJ. 2017;356:i6681.

98. Hui CL, Chang WC, Chan SK, et al. Early intervention and evaluation for adult-onset psychosis: the JCEP study rationale and design. Early Interv Psychiatry. 2014;8:261–8.

# 64

# Antipsychotic and anticholinergic drugs

*Herbert Y. Meltzer and William V. Bobo*

## Introduction

The discovery by Delay and Denicker in 1953 that chlorpromazine was highly effective in alleviating delusions, hallucinations, and disorganized thinking was the seminal breakthrough in the treatment of schizophrenia, the first agent to produce sufficient relief of core psychotic symptoms to permit life outside of institutions for many patients with schizophrenia, and even a return to a semblance of normal function for those individuals with relatively little cognitive impairment. Chlorpromazine and the other typical (first generation) antipsychotic drugs introduced over the next 30 years were of immense benefit to people who experience psychotic symptoms as a component of a diverse group of neuropsychiatric and medical disorders, as well as drug-induced psychoses. Clinical and basic studies of these and the subsequent classes of drugs for psychosis have contributed to understanding the pathophysiology of schizophrenia and other forms of mental illness with psychotic features. The first generation of drugs for psychosis led to identifying the role of dopamine in psychosis, motor function, and some endocrine functions. This group of drugs led to the development of drugs with minimal motor side effects. These were marketed as 'atypical antipsychotics', as opposed to the older 'typical' drugs; they are also sometimes referred to as second- and third-generation antipsychotic drugs, and clozapine is the prototype. Their pharmacology is much more complex and involves, beyond interactions with dopamine receptors, direct and indirect effects on a variety or neurotransmitters, especially serotonin, glutamate, GABA, acetylcholine, histamine, and neuromodulators, such as brain-derived neurotrophic factor (BDNF), affecting synaptic structure and function. This chapter will describe the various classes of antipsychotic agents, with emphasis on the drugs with minimal motor side effects, their benefits and adverse effects, recommendations for use in clinical practice, and their mechanism of action (MOA). The drugs used to treat the extrapyramidal side effects (EPS) produced mainly by the typical dopamine antagonist drugs are also considered.

## Classes of antipsychotic drugs

As explained in Chapter 10, the broad classification of psychotropic drugs has usually been on the basis of indication. It has been argued there that we should move away from such classification to one based on the MOA. However, the present chapter explains how thinking around the MOA developed. The indication (antipsychotic) preceded the understanding of the MOA. Therefore, the conventional terminology is used here to illustrate how the field has developed. In most other chapters, which describe the many uses of these drugs, the older terminology is avoided where possible.

Antipsychotic drugs have been classified into two broad categories: typical and atypical [1]. Typical antipsychotic drugs are those which 'typically' produce EPS at clinically effective doses, including parkinsonism (muscle rigidity, tremor, bradykinesia), acute dystonic reactions, akathisia (restlessness), and tardive dyskinesia. The efficacy of typical antipsychotics is mediated by blockade of dopamine D2 receptors in the dorsal striatum and limbic system, which includes the nucleus accumbens, stria terminalis, and amygdala [2, 3]. However, their blockade of D2 receptors in the dorsal striatum leads to the motor side effects described previously [3].

The typical antipsychotic drugs are members of a variety of chemical families (Table 64.1). They vary in their affinity for the D2 receptor, with low-affinity drugs such as chlorpromazine, which require high doses for clinical efficacy, to high-affinity drugs, such as haloperidol, which are effective at lower doses (Table 64.1). Whereas typical antipsychotics are associated with EPS at therapeutic doses, atypical antipsychotic drugs are associated with a lower (but not absent) risk of EPS at clinically effective doses. As such, 'atypicality' of antipsychotic drugs is based on clinical effects on motor system functioning. Kapur and Seeman [4] proposed that the rate of dissociation of all antipsychotic drugs from the D2 receptor provides the basis for the distinction between typical and atypical antipsychotic drugs, with atypical antipsychotic drugs dissociating more rapidly. While this is true for clozapine and quetiapine, the atypical drugs risperidone, sertindole, olanzapine, and asenapine dissociate no more rapidly or even slower than haloperidol. As such, 'fast dissociation' cannot provide the pharmacological basis for atypicality for most of the drugs that are considered atypical. The pharmacologic basis for atypicality will be discussed subsequently. Sertindole is a phenylindole compound with a receptor profile which places it in the class of 5-HT2A/D2 antagonist atypical antipsychotic drugs [5]. Concerns about it causing QTc prolongation have limited its use [6].

Low-potency typical agents are those in which the usual dose range in schizophrenia is ≥200 mg/day, whereas mid- to high-potency agents are those in which the usual dose range is between

**Table 64.1** Selected antipsychotic drugs and classification

| Drug name | Trade name (examples from pharmaceutical companies in the United States) | Chemical class | General class | D2 potency* |
|---|---|---|---|---|
| Aripiprazole | Abilify® | Dihydrocarbostyril | Atypical | |
| Asenapine | Saphris® | Dibenzo-oxepino pyrrole | Atypical | |
| Blonaserin | Lonasen® | 4-phenyl-2-(1-piperazinyl) pyridine | Atypical | |
| Brexpiprazole | Rexulti® | 4-piperazin-1-yl-4-benzo[B]thiophene | Atypical | |
| Cariprazine | Vraylar® | Dichloro-phenyl-piperazine | Atypical | |
| Chlorpromazine | Thorazine® | Phenothiazine | Typical | Low |
| Clozapine | Clozaril® | Dibenzazepine | Atypical | |
| Droperidol | Inapsine® | Butyrophenone | Typical | Mid |
| Fluphenazine | Prolixin® | Phenothiazine | Typical | High |
| Haloperidol | Haldol® | Butyrophenone | Typical | High |
| Iloperidone | Fanapt® | Piperidinyl-benzisoxazole derivative | Atypical | |
| Loxapine | Loxitane® | Dibenzazepine | Typical | Mid |
| Lurasidone | Latuda® | Piperidinyl-benzisoxazole derivative | Atypical | |
| Mesoridazine | Serentil® | Phenothiazine | Typical | Low |
| Molindone | Moban® | Dihydroindolone | Typical | Mid |
| Olanzapine | Zyprexa® | Thiobenzodiazepine | Atypical | |
| Paliperidone | Invega® | 9-hydroxy metabolite of risperidone | Atypical | |
| Perphenazine | Trilafon® | Phenothiazine | Typical | Mid |
| Pimozide | Orap® | Butyrophenone | Typical | Mid |
| Promazine | | Phenothiazine | Typical | Mid |
| Quetiapine | Seroquel® | Dibenzothiazepine | Atypical | |
| Risperidone | Risperdal®, Risperdal CONSTA® | Benzisoxazole | Atypical | |
| Sertindole | Serdolect® | Phenylindole | Atypical | |
| Thioridazine | Mellaril® | Phenothiazine | Typical | Low |
| Tiotixene | Navane® | Thioxanthene | Typical | High |
| Trifluoperazine | Stelazine® | Phenothiazine | Typical | Mid |
| Ziprasidone | Geodon® | Benzisothiazole | Atypical | |

* Classification on the basis of potency of D2 receptor binding for typical antipsychotic drugs only.

2 mg/day and 175 mg/day. In general, the low-potency drugs are associated with more sedative, orthostatic hypotensive, and anticholinergic adverse effects than the high-potency agents, but also have less of a tendency to produce EPS. All typical antipsychotics are equally effective to reduce psychosis, but because of secondary pharmacologic features, they differ from one another with regard to their adverse effect profiles, for example EPS, weight gain, sedation, hypotension, etc. [7].

Atypical antipsychotics are characterized by a more diverse and complex pattern of pharmacological activity. Most are serotonin [5-hydroxytryptamine (5-HT)] 2A and dopamine D2 antagonists or D2 partial agonists, and many have a variety of activities at other receptors whose contribution to their mode of action is still being elucidated [2]. Substituted benzamides, for example amisulpride, also produce low EPS at clinically effective doses and may constitute another class of atypical agents. The prototypical atypical antipsychotic drug is clozapine, a dibenzodiazepine (Table 64.1) [8]. Other atypical antipsychotic drugs are shown in Table 64.1 [8–11]. These drugs are all more potent 5-HT2A than D2 receptor antagonists, as well

as multi-receptor antagonists [12, 13], except for aripiprazole and brexpiprazole, which act as dopamine D2 receptor partial agonists [14, 15]. Amisulpride is a unique atypical antipsychotic drug that acts as an antagonist at dopamine D2 and D3 receptors and at the serotonin 5-HT7 receptor. Cariprazine is a dopamine D2 and D3 receptor partial agonist, with high selectivity towards the D3 receptor [16]. As will be discussed, the atypical antipsychotic drugs differ not only with regard to pharmacological activity and adverse effects, but also with regard to efficacy [17, 18]. Atypical antipsychotic agents have been shown to have advantages, albeit modest, in treating negative and mood symptoms [19–21] and to improve some domains of cognitive dysfunction in patients with schizophrenia, related primary psychotic disorders, and perhaps other psychiatric disorders [22–24].

## Pharmacology

There is abundant evidence that dopamine plays a key role in the aetiology of psychosis and the action of antipsychotic drugs [25].

The doses of typical antipsychotic drugs is highly correlated with their affinities for D2 receptors. Amphetamine and methamphetamine, which increase synaptic concentrations of dopamine, exacerbate delusions and hallucinations in some patients with schizophrenia, due to stimulation of a subgroup of D2 receptors in mesolimbic nuclei [26, 27] and the dorsal striatum. The cell bodies of mesolimbic and dorsal striatal dopamine neurons reside in the ventral tegmentum and substantia nigra, respectively [28]. The outflow of these regions to the thalamus and the cortex has been postulated to mediate psychotic symptoms. As such, blockade of mesolimbic and striatal dopamine D2 receptors is thought to be the basis for drugs to ameliorate psychotic symptoms, although the firing rate of the mesolimbic dopaminergic neurons is subject to multiple influences, including stimulatory serotonergic input from the median raphe nucleus [29].

A group of ventral tegmental dopamine neurons project to various regions of the cortex and comprise the mesocortical dopamine system. There is extensive evidence that these neurons are important for cognition, especially working memory [30], as well as negative symptoms [31]. Typical drugs occupy 80–95% of striatal D2 receptors in patients with schizophrenia at clinically effective doses,

though much lower occupancy can lead to control of psychosis [32]. EPS occurs at above 80% occupancy of these receptors. Blockade of D2 receptors in the anterior pituitary gland is the basis for their ability to stimulate prolactin secretion [33].

The prefrontal cortex has relatively low concentrations of D2 receptors and has a higher density of D1, D3, and D4 dopamine receptors [27]. The activation of D1 receptors in the prefrontal cortex may be especially critical for normal working memory and other executive-type functions subserved by this brain region. However, no D1 agonists are currently approved. D1-positive allosteric modulators have shown promise in preclinical studies as cognitive enhancers. Drugs which selectively block D4 receptors have not been found to have an antipsychotic effect [34]. There is extensive evidence that selective D3 receptor partial agonists and antagonists show promise to treat cognitive impairment and negative symptoms [35, 36]. The typical antipsychotic drugs vary in their *in vitro* and *in vivo* affinities for receptors such as the dopamine D1, histamine H1, muscarinic, α1- and α2-adrenergic, and serotonergic receptors (Table 64.2), which mediate effects on arousal, extra-pyramidal, cognitive, cardiovascular, gastrointestinal, and genitourinary function (Table 64.3) [15, 16, 37–42].

**Table 64.2** Affinities of selected antipsychotic drugs at various neuroreceptors

| Drug name | D2 | 5-HT1A | 5-HT2A | 5-HT2C | α-1 | α-2 | H-1 | M-1 |
|---|---|---|---|---|---|---|---|---|
| Aripiprazole | 0.95 | 5.6 | 4.6 | 181.0 | 25.0 | 74.0 | 29.0 | ≥6K |
| Asenapine | 2.0 | 15.0 | 0.8 | 0.3 | 1.1 | 16.1 | 9.3 | 24.3 |
| Blonanserin | 0.7 | 804.0 | 0.8 | 26.0 | 27 | 530.0 | 765.0 | 100.0 |
| Brexpiprazole | 0.3 | 0.1 | 0.5 | | 0.2 | 0.6 | 19.0 | Negligible |
| Cariprazine | 9.2 | 8.6 | 7.7 | 6.9 | 6.7 | <6.0 | 7.6 | Negligible |
| Chlorpromazine | 2.0 | ≥3K | 3.2 | 26.0 | 0.28 | 184.0 | 0.18 | 47.0 |
| Clozapine | 431.0 | 105.0 | 13.0 | 29.0 | 1.6 | 142.0 | 2.0 | 14.0 |
| Fluphenazine | 0.54 | 145.0 | 7.4 | 418.0 | 6.4 | 314.0 | 7.3 | ≥1K |
| Haloperidol | 2.0 | ≥1K | 73.0 | ≥10K | 12.0 | ≥1K | ≥3K | ≥10K |
| Iloperidone | 3.3 | 33.0 | 0.2 | 14.0 | 0.3 | 3.0 | 12.3 | >1K |
| Lurasidone | 1.7 | 6.8 | 2.0 | | 47.9 | 40.7 | >1K | >1K |
| Loxapine | 10.0 | ≥2K | 3.9 | 21.0 | 31.0 | 151.0 | 2.8 | 175.0 |
| Molindone | 63.0 | ≥3K | 320.0 | ≥10K | ≥2K | ≥1K | ≥2K | NA |
| Olanzapine | 72.0 | ≥2K | 3.0 | 24.0 | 109.0 | 314.0 | 4.9 | 24.0 |
| 9-OH risperidone* | 9.4 | 637.8 | 1.9 | 100.3 | 2.5 | 4.7 | 5.6 | ≥10K |
| Perphenazine | 1.4 | 421.0 | 5.6 | 132.0 | 10.0 | 810.5 | 8.0 | NA |
| Pimozide | 0.65 | 650.0 | 19.0 | ≥3K | 197.7 | ≥1K | 692.0 | 800.0 |
| Quetiapine | 567.0 | 431.0 | 366.0 | ≥1K | 22.0 | ≥3K | 7.5 | 858.0 |
| Risperidone | 4.9 | 427.0 | 0.19 | 94.9 | 5.0 | 151.0 | 5.2 | ≥10K |
| Sertindole | 6.6 | >1K | 0.6 | 6.0 | 3.9 | 190.0 | 320.0 | >1K |
| Thioridazine | 10.0 | 108.0 | 11.0 | 69.0 | 1.3 | 134.0 | 14.0 | 33.0 |
| Tiothixene | 1.4 | 410.0 | 111.0 | ≥1K | 12.0 | 80.0 | 12.0 | ≥10K |
| Trifluoperazine | 1.3 | 950.0 | 13.0 | 378.0 | 24. | 653.7 | 63.0 | NA |
| Ziprasidone | 4.0 | 76.0 | 2.8 | 68.0 | 18.0 | 160.0 | 130.0 | ≥10K |

All receptor-binding affinities are reported as Ki (nM) using National Institutes of Mental Health (NIMH) Psychoactive Drug Screening Program (PDSP) certified data, available online at http://pdsp.cwru.edu/pdsp.php, unless otherwise specified. In general, the lower the Ki (nM) value, the higher the binding affinity for the drug at a given receptor site.
NA, human cloned receptor data not available.
* 9-hydroxy (9-OH) risperidone is marketed as paliperidone.

**Table 64.3** Hypothesized therapeutic and adverse effects of receptor occupancy by antipsychotic drugs

| Target receptor | Pharmacological activity | Therapeutic effect(s) | Adverse effect(s) |
|---|---|---|---|
| Dopamine D2 | Antagonism or partial agonist effects | Reduction of positive symptoms | Extrapyramidal effects (EPS) Hyperprolactinemia |
| Serotonin (5-HT) 1A | Full or partial agonist effects | Cognitive enhancement Reduction of mood and anxiety symptoms | |
| 5-HT2A | Antagonism | Reduction of negative symptoms Reduction of EPS Reduction of mood and anxiety symptoms Increased deep sleep | |
| 5-HT2C | Antagonism | Reduced anxiety symptoms | Weight gain |
| Adrenergic α-1 | Antagonism | | Orthostatic hypotension Dizziness |
| Adrenergic α-2 | Antagonism | | Reflex tachycardia |
| Histamine H-1 | Sedation | Sedation Drowsiness Weight gain | |
| Muscarinic (cholinergic) M-1 | Antagonism | Reduction of EPS | Blurry vision Exacerbation of acute angle closure glaucoma Sinus tachycardia Constipation Urinary retention Memory dysfunction |

Source: data from *Psychopharmacol Bull.*, 35(4), Kelly DL, Love RC, Ziprasidone and the QTC interval: phar-macokinetic and pharmacodynamic considerations, pp. 66–79, Copyright (2001), MedWorks Media Global, LLC.

Thioridazine is a relatively potent antimuscarinic agent. Most of the low-potency drugs for psychosis are potent α-1 and H1 antagonists, which contribute to orthostatic hypotension and weight gain, respectively.

The receptor-binding affinities of the atypical antipsychotic drugs have been related to their efficacy and side effect profiles. As noted previously, the most important determinant of atypicality for most of the currently available agents of this type is that they are more potent 5-HT2A than D2 receptor antagonists. An exception is aripiprazole, which combines potent 5-HT2A antagonism and 5-HT1A agonism, with partial D2 receptor agonism. Another exception is amisulpride, which is a selective D2/3 antagonist, with little pharmacological activity at 5-HT2A receptors. Combined 5-HT2A and less potent D2 antagonism is the most consistent principle yet discovered to produce a separation between antipsychotic action and interference with motor function [43]. The low potential for EPS with clozapine, and subsequently olanzapine, quetiapine, risperidone, iloperidone, ziprasidone, paliperidone, and asenapine is, in part, due to their relatively stronger 5-HT2 antagonist and weaker D2 antagonist properties. Direct and indirect 5-HT1A partial and full agonist effects of the atypical antipsychotic drugs have also been shown to contribute to their low EPS profile. The atypical antipsychotic agents have the ability to increase prefrontal cortical dopaminergic activity, compared with subcortical dopaminergic activity [44]. The ability to increase the release of dopamine in the prefrontal cortex may be to improve cognition and negative symptoms. It may also contribute to decreasing the release of dopamine in the mesolimbic region, because prefrontal dopamine neurons modulate the activity of corticolimbic glutamatergic neurons that regulate the activity of ventral and dorsal striatal DA neurons [30]. Clozapine and some of the other atypical antipsychotic drugs that are also potent 5-HT2A antagonists also produce marked increases in prefrontal cortical and hippocampal acetylcholine efflux [45]. These atypical agents also produce marked increases in noradrenaline efflux in the prefrontal cortex, which is correlated in time and magnitude with the increase in extracellular dopamine [46]. It is of interest that in rodents, combining ritanserin (a mixed 5-HT2A/2B/2C antagonist) or M-100907 (a selective 5-HT2A antagonist) with a selective D2/3 antagonist resulted in increased prefrontal dopamine release [47, 48]. The importance of serotonin receptors other than 5-HT2A for antipsychotic action has received considerable attention. Activation of 5-HT1A receptors are believed to have a dopamine-modulating effect similar to that of 5-HT2A antagonism [49]. Under experimental conditions, 5-HT1A agonists have been shown to stimulate cortical dopamine release [50, 51], and in schizophrenic patients who were stabilized on haloperidol, the addition of tandospirone, a 5-HT1A partial agonist, resulted in improved neurocognitive performance [52]. This effect has also been demonstrated for buspirone, another 5-HT1A partial agonist [53]. Antagonism of 5-HT2C receptors also appears to result in cortical dopamine and noradrenaline release, as well as in the nucleus accumbens [54]. As is the case with 5-HT1A activity, not all atypical antipsychotic drugs are active at 5-HT2C receptors (Table 64.2). Like antagonism at histamine H1 receptors [55], 5-HT2C antagonist activity may be related to weight gain [56].

Clozapine, olanzapine, risperidone, and quetiapine are able to block the interference in prepulse inhibition produced by d-amphetamine, apomorphine, or phencyclidine at doses that do not interfere with locomotor function [57]. Clozapine and M100907 are able to block the effects of phencyclidine, an N-methyl-D-aspartate (NMDA) receptor antagonist, on locomotor activity in rodents [58].

The extent of involvement of other atypical relative to typical drugs at NMDA receptors and other glutamatergic targets is an area of active interest. Other receptor targets that are of special interest in terms of improving cognitive functioning and selected psychotic symptoms include M1 muscarinic, α-7 nicotinic, and α-1 and α-2 adrenergic receptors [59].

## Administration, pharmacokinetics, and dosage

### Administration

#### Typical antipsychotic drugs

The major use is for the treatment of schizophrenia. Other major uses that will be touched on briefly in this chapter include treatment of mood disorders such as major depression (as an adjunct to antidepressants) and bipolar disorder. Indications discussed in other chapters of this textbook include Tourette's syndrome and aggression. The major advantage of the typical drugs is their ability to improve positive symptoms in patients with schizophrenia, that is, delusions and hallucinations, and to rapidly reduce psychotic symptoms, as well as the core non-psychotic signs and symptoms of manic episodes (including agitation, hostility, aggressive behaviour, psychomotor agitation, and severe insomnia). Administration of typical drugs leads to the complete or nearly complete elimination of positive symptoms and disorganization of thought and affect in about 60–70% of patients with schizophrenia and an even higher proportion of those with psychotic mania and psychotic depression [60]. The antipsychotic response in schizophrenia and mania is sometimes apparent within a few days in many patients, but maximum benefit usually takes up to several weeks or months to unfold. A reasonable duration for a therapeutic trial with one of these agents is 4–6 weeks. It is not appropriate to switch medications after 1 or 2 weeks, even if a response is not apparent, unless side effects pose a serious problem. Positive symptoms (delusions and hallucinations) do not respond to typical drugs in about 10% of schizophrenic patients, even during the first episode [61]. Another 20% of patients with schizophrenia develop resistance to these agents during the subsequent course of their illnesses [62]. Development of resistance to typical drugs may occur at any time during the course of treatment, even after many years of control of positive symptoms. Such patients may respond to clozapine [63] or one of the other atypical drugs [61, 62]. The average doses of the typical neuroleptic drugs are given in Table 64.4. The best results with these drugs in terms of efficacy and side effects may be expected with the lowest dose needed to produce control of positive symptoms with the fewest EPS [7, 64].

Controlled studies have failed to find benefits from high-dose strategies or combining two or more typical antipsychotics. Increasing the dose of these agents when patients fail to respond rapidly, for example within days, should be avoided. Augmentation with a benzodiazepine may be useful to decrease anxiety until the lower doses of drugs produce adequate control of positive symptoms [7, 64]. Patients who receive high doses of these drugs adequately are at greater risk of hyperprolactinaemic effects, EPS, and tardive dyskinesia and are generally better treated with an atypical antipsychotic drug.

However, improvement in positive symptoms is only one element in the treatment of schizophrenia. Additional efficacy factors of major importance are summarized in Table 64.5.

Tolerability and safety factors, such as compliance, tardive dyskinesia, weight gain, and medical morbidity, are also major elements in outcome and influence the choice of a typical or atypical drug. Typical drugs are not as effective as atypical drugs for improving primary negative symptoms [65]. Abnormalities in specific domains of cognition (Table 64.5) are present in first-episode schizophrenic patients at a moderate to severe level and show additional deterioration during the course of illness [66]. Approximately 85% of patients with schizophrenia are clinically impaired in one or more domains of cognition [67, 68]. Cognition has been shown to be the most critical determinant of functional capacity among patients with schizophrenia, even more so than positive symptoms [67]. Typical antipsychotic drugs usually do not improve cognitive function [70]. Development of tardive dyskinesia may diminish the possibility of obtaining benefit from atypical antipsychotic to improve cognition [71].

All of the typical drugs are likely to be equally effective in treating either the initial presentation or recurrent psychosis due to breakthrough of symptoms, despite compliance, or because of having stopped medication [7, 62, 64]. First-episode patients with schizophrenia usually require much lower doses than patients with two or more episodes, suggesting some progression of the disease process or the development of tolerance to the mechanism of action of these drugs [72]. Doses for more chronic patients should be in the range of 5–10 mg of haloperidol equivalents per day (Table 64.4) for up to 4–6 weeks, unless there is a major need for chemical means to prevent harm to self or others, to decrease excitement, or to induce sleep [73]. Auxiliary medications for anxiety and sleeplessness, for example benzodiazepines, may supplement these low doses [74].

Parenteral injections of haloperidol, chlorpromazine, or other dopamine antagonists/partial agonists may be needed for patients who refuse oral medication or where very rapid onset of action is needed to control acutely dangerous behaviours if less restrictive means either fail or cannot be utilized safely. Commonly, haloperidol (2–10 mg) with or without lorazepam (2–4 mg) is delivered intramuscularly every 30–60 minutes, as required, up to three doses. Doses of haloperidol given intramuscularly in such situations generally should not exceed 18 mg per day. Oral medication should be substituted as soon as feasible. If positive symptoms fail to respond to a single trial of a typical drug at adequate doses in patients with schizophrenia, there is evidence that switching to another typical antipsychotic, even of a different chemical class, is unlikely to produce greater control [7, 60, 62]. This is likely to be true for other indications for the use of antipsychotic agents as well.

In cases of repeated illness relapse due to poor compliance or when patients prefer it, the use of long-acting (for example, depot) injectable medications, typically administered once every 2–4 weeks, should be used. The use of injectable antipsychotic medication has been associated with lower rates of relapse and rehospitalization and greater global improvement, compared with oral typical antipsychotics [75], possibly as a result of ensured drug delivery. Long-acting injectable drugs should not be given to ameliorate acute behavioural disturbances.

In summary, typical antipsychotic drugs may be less desirable than typical antipsychotic drugs for some patients because of their greater risk for EPS, tardive dyskinesia, and prolactin elevations and lower adherence. On the other hand, typical antipsychotics are less expensive, on average, than atypical antipsychotic drugs.

**Table 64.4** Oral dosing of antipsychotic drugs

| Typical antipsychotic drugs | | | | |
| --- | --- | --- | --- | --- |
| | Equivalent doses (mg/day) | Starting dose | Titration schedule | Dose range (mg/day) |
| Chlorpromazine[a] | 100 | 15–50 mg 2–4 times daily | As clinically indicated | 300–1000 (divided once daily to four times daily) |
| Fluphenazine[b] | 2 | 0.5–10 mg/day (divided every 6–8 hours) | As clinically indicated | 5–20 |
| Haloperidol[c] | 2 | 0.5–5 mg twice daily | As clinically indicated | 5–20 |
| Loxapine | 10 | 10 mg twice daily | As clinically indicated | 30–100 |
| Mesoridazine | 50 | | | 150–400 |
| Molindone | 10 | 50–75 mg/day divided 3–4 times daily | As clinically indicated | 30–100 |
| Perphenazine[d] | 10 | 4–8 mg three times daily (8–16 mg 2–4 times daily if hospitalized) | As clinically indicated | 16–64 |
| Thioridazine | 100 | 50–100 mg three times daily | As clinically indicated | 300–800 |
| Tiotixene | 5 | 2 mg three times daily | As clinically indicated | 15–50 |
| Trifluoperazine | 5 | 2–5 mg twice daily | As clinically indicated | 15–50 |

For elderly patients or those with renal or hepatic problems, the doses of drug may need to be reduced by one-half or more.

[a] Short-acting IM formulation may be given 25–50 mg (may repeat after 1–4 hours, as required); may gradually increase the dose up to 400 mg IM every 4–6 hours (maximum of 2000 mg/day)—may be needed for severe cases.

[b] Short-acting IM formulation may be given 2.5–10 mg/day at every 6- to 8-hour intervals; depot IM formulation may be given 12.5–25 mg every 3 weeks.

[c] Short-acting IM formulation may be given 2–5 mg every 1–4 hours; depot IM formulation may be given at approximately 10–20 times the stable oral dose every 4 weeks.

[d] Short-acting IM formulation may be given 5–10 mg every 6 hours (maximum of 30 mg/day).

| Atypical antipsychotic drugs | | | |
| --- | --- | --- | --- |
| | Starting dose | Titration schedule | Dose range (mg/day) |
| Asenapine | 5 mg twice daily | As clinically indicated, to usual effective dose range of 5–10 mg twice daily | 5–10 mg twice daily |
| Aripiprazole[a,b] | 10–15 mg daily | As clinically indicated, every 2 weeks | 10–30 |
| Blonanserin | 4 mg twice daily | As clinically indicated, to usual effective dose range of 4–12 mg twice daily | 4–12 mg twice daily |
| Brexpiprazole | 1 mg daily | Increase to 2 mg/day on days 5–7, 2 mg/day or 4 mg/day on days 8+ | 2–4 |
| Cariprazine | 1.5 mg daily | As clinically indicated, to usual effective dose range of 1.5–6.0 mg/day | 1.5–6.0 |
| Clozapine | 12.5 mg once daily to twice daily | Increase by 25–50 mg/day until usual effective dose of 300–450 mg/day after 2–4 weeks | 150–600 |
| Iloperidone | 1 mg twice daily | Increase to 2, 4, 6, 8, and 12 mg twice daily on treatment days 2, 3, 4, 5, 6, and 7 (respectively) | 6–12 mg twice daily |
| Lurasidone | 40 mg daily (with food) | As clinically indicated, to usual effective dose range of 40–160 mg/day (all doses with food) | 40–160 |
| Olanzapine[c,d] | 5–10 mg daily | As clinically indicated, by 5 mg/day every 7 days | 10–30 |
| Paliperidone[e] | 6 mg/day | As clinically indicated, by 3 mg/day every 2–4 week increments, up to 12 mg daily | 6–12 |
| Quetiapine | 25 mg twice daily | Increase by 25–50 mg 2–3 times daily on days 2 and 3, to target dose of 300–400 mg daily (QD –TID) by day 4. Further increases as clinically indicated by 25–50 mg twice daily every 2 days | 300– 800 |
| Risperidone[f] | 0.5–1 mg twice daily | Increase by 0.5–1 mg twice daily on days 2 and 3, with further dose increases thereafter by 0.5–1 mg increments every 7 days as required | 2–8 |
| Ziprasidone[g] | 20 mg twice daily with food | Increase by 20–40 mg twice daily every 2 days to target dose of 80 mg (all doses with food) | 120–200 |

For elderly patients or those with renal or hepatic problems, doses of drug may need to be reduced by one-half or more and titration may be slower.

[a] Short-acting IM formulation may be given at 9.75 mg, though the lower 5.25 mg dose may be indicated in some situations.

[b] There are two long-acting IM formulations. Aripiprazole monohydrate may be initiated at 400 mg as a gluteal or deltoid injection (continue oral aripiprazole for 2 weeks), with once-monthly dosing at 400 mg (160–300 mg once monthly if there are adverse reactions, in pharmacogenetic CYP2D6 poor metabolizers, or if taken with drugs that inhibit CYP2D6 or 3A4). Aripiprazole lauroxil may be initiated at 441–882 mg (continue oral aripiprazole for 3 weeks), followed by repeated administration every 4 weeks [441 mg (deltoid or gluteal injection), 662 mg (gluteal injection only), or 882 mg doses (gluteal injection only)] or every 6 weeks (882 mg dose only).

[c] Short-acting IM formulation may be given 10 mg as required (may be repeated after 2 hours, up to 30 mg/day).

[d] Long-acting IM formulation may be initiated at 210 mg or 300 mg every 2 weeks for a total of 8 weeks, followed by maintenance dosing (150–405 mg every 2–4 weeks).

[e] There are two long-acting IM formulations of paliperidone. The once-monthly long-acting injectable form is may be initiated at 234 mg (deltoid injection), followed by a 156 mg deltoid injection on day 8. Maintenance doses are given by deltoid or gluteal injection once monthly in the 39–234 mg dose range. The once-quarterly (every 3 months) long-acting injectable form can be considered after successful treatment with the once-monthly form for at least 4 months and may be initiated at 273–819 mg.

[f] Long-acting IM formulation may be initiated at 25 mg Q 2 weeks (continue oral risperidone dose for 3 weeks), with increases as clinically indicated every 4 weeks up to a dose of 50 mg Q 2 weeks.

[g] Short-acting IM formulation may be given 10–20 mg as required (may be repeated Q 2–4 hours as needed, up to 40 mg/day).

**Table 64.5** Target signs and symptoms for the pharmacological management of schizophrenia

| Target | Description | |
|---|---|---|
| Positive syndrome | Hallucinations | Typically the most amenable to treatment with all antipsychotic drugs |
| | Delusions | |
| Negative syndrome | Avolition | Robustly correlated with functional impairment in schizophrenia |
| | Apathy | More difficult to treat pharmacologically and may require longer to respond than positive signs and symptoms |
| | Anhedonia | |
| | Lack of responsiveness | Pharmacological adjuncts may be needed, though understudied |
| | Poor rapport with others | Atypical antipsychotic drugs are believed to be more efficacious than typical antipsychotics |
| | Passive social withdrawal | |
| | Poverty of speech | |
| | Affective flattening | |
| Hostility/excitement | Verbal or physical aggression | Typically amenable to treatment with all antipsychotic drugs |
| | | Use of parenteral formulation may be required |
| Mood and anxiety symptoms | Depressed mood | Believed to be more responsive to treatment with atypical antipsychotic drugs |
| | Anxious mood | Clozapine has demonstrated superiority for treating chronic suicidality in schizophrenia |
| | Nervousness | |
| | Panic symptoms | |
| | Suicidal ideation | |
| Cognitive impairment (psychopathological definition) | Disorientation | Some domains respond favourably to antipsychotic drug treatment, though response is often incomplete |
| | Problems with abstraction | |
| | Attentional problems | |
| | Preoccupations | |
| | Disorganized thought processes | |
| Cognitive impairment (neuropsychological testing definition) | Working memory | Neuropsychological deficits, like negative signs and symptoms, are robustly correlated with functional outcome in schizophrenia |
| | Attention/vigilance | Very difficult to treat with medication alone |
| | Verbal learning/memory | Atypical antipsychotic drugs are believed to be superior to typical antipsychotics, though effect sizes are only mild to moderate for the former |
| | Visual learning/memory | |
| | Problem-solving | |
| | Processing speed | |

## Atypical antipsychotic drugs

There are major advantages for the atypical drugs, and these agents are recommended as first-line treatment [76, 77]. They are the most widely prescribed drug treatment for schizophrenia, mania, and psychotic depression in clinical practice in many parts of the world. There are many such drugs which share some pharmacology but also have unique features. New ones are still being added, some with markedly different core features. With one exception—pimavanserin, recently approved for treatment of the psychosis of Parkinson's disease [78], all the atypical antipsychotic drugs directly affect dopamine D2 receptors, usually as antagonists, but also as partial agonists, for example aripiprazole and brexpiprazole. However, D2 receptor actions are part of a multi-receptor profile, which includes actions on multiple dopamine, serotonin, and other receptors. Some atypical antipsychotic drugs (for example, clozapine, olanzapine, quetiapine in its immediate-release form, risperidone, and ziprasidone) are no longer patent-protected and are available in less expensive generic brands. Most of the atypical drugs will be off patent by 2020. Although the conversion from branded to generic (and vice versa) forms of antipsychotic drugs is relatively easy in most patients, not requiring cross-titration, close monitoring is required during the switch, particularly with clozapine [79].

The relative effectiveness of atypical, compared with typical, antipsychotics for the treatment of schizophrenia has been the subject of some controversy, particularly after the publication of the initial phase results of three large studies—the Clinical Antipsychotic Trial of Intervention Effectiveness (CATIE) conducted in the United States [80], the Cost Utility of the Latest Antipsychotic drugs in Schizophrenia Study (CUtLASS) conducted in the UK [81] and the European First Episode Schizophrenia Trial (EUFEST) conducted at numerous clinical sites across Europe and in Israel [82]. Broadly, these trials had less stringent inclusion criteria than those typically encountered in experimental randomized trials and focused on outcome measures other than symptom change such as time to study drug discontinuation for any reason and quality of life. In general, these studies failed to demonstrate the superiority of atypical over typical antipsychotics across these effectiveness outcomes, although the second phases of two of these trials showed superior effectiveness of clozapine over comparator antipsychotics for patients considered to have treatment-resistant schizophrenia [83, 84], and olanzapine was shown to have superior effectiveness to comparator drugs in CATIE phase 1 (CATIE-1). Although the pragmatic and comparative effectiveness aspects of these trials were innovative, their methodologies and results have been subject to criticism, based on dosing imbalances between individual antipsychotics in CATIE-1, the inclusion of sulpiride (which has atypical properties) and long-acting injectable antipsychotics in the 'first-generation' antipsychotic drug treatment arm (no long-acting injectable agents in the 'second-generation' antipsychotic arm) in CUtLASS phase 1 (CUtLASS-1), questionable sensitivity of the chosen effectiveness endpoints to between-drug differences in outcome, the channelling of patients with tardive dyskinesia away from treatment with typical antipsychotics, and high rates of cross-contamination between treatment arms owing to antipsychotic drug switching (CUtLASS-1) [85–88].

### Clozapine

Clozapine was synthesized in 1959 as part of a project to discover antipsychotic drugs with low potential for EPS. It proved to be one of the most interesting and clinically important compounds ever discovered. It was labelled as being 'atypical' because of its ability to block amphetamine-induced locomotor activity, one of the most widely accepted models for antipsychotic effects, without producing catalepsy in rodents, the leading model for causation of EPS in humans. Subsequent clinical studies showed it to have the lowest EPS liability of any antipsychotic drug [89]. Clinical trials in the 1960s and 1970s demonstrated efficacy for positive symptoms [90]. In 1975, 6 years after its introduction in Europe, clozapine was reported to produce a high rate of agranulocytosis. Six deaths occurred in clozapine-treated patients in a geographically restricted area of Finland over a short period of time. Clozapine was withdrawn from general use, although it remained available for humanitarian use [91].

Clozapine was reintroduced in 1989 after it was demonstrated to be superior to chlorpromazine to improve positive and negative symptoms in 300 patients who were resistant to the action of at least three typical antipsychotics [92]. Thirty per cent of the patients treated with clozapine responded after 6 weeks of treatment, compared to 4% of the chlorpromazine-treated patients. Subsequent studies have shown that 40–60% of patients will respond within 6 months of initiating clozapine treatment. Other predictors of response include weight gain and absence of atrophy in the prefrontal cortex [61]. Clozapine has been shown to uniquely reduce the risk of suicide in schizophrenia [63, 93]. It has also been shown to improve some aspects of cognitive function, especially verbal fluency, immediate and delayed verbal learning and memory, and attention [22–24]. N-desmethylclozapine is the major metabolite of clozapine. It is an M1 muscarinic receptor agonist and has been shown to have beneficial effects on working memory [94].

Because of the side effect profile of clozapine and because it has not been shown to be superior to other drugs for treatment-responsive schizophrenia [95], it is not generally used as a first-line drug. On the other hand, monitoring neutrophil counts for the development of agranulocytosis or granulocytopenia and improved methods of treating agranulocytosis have made it much safer to use. Clozapine is under-utilized in many parts of the world. All schizophrenia patients with persistent psychotic symptoms after two adequate trials of other drugs should be considered for a trial of clozapine, which should be 6 months in duration, before concluding it is ineffective.

Clozapine is usually given twice daily, but sometimes more than half of the dose or the entire dose is given at bedtime to minimize daytime sedation. The daily dosage is gradually titrated to the target range described in Table 64.4. Patients who are treatment-resistant usually require doses of 400 mg/day or higher, or a minimum blood concentration of 350 µg/L [96]. Typical or non-clozapine atypical antipsychotic drugs should be discontinued either before beginning clozapine or by eliminating them over a 1- to 2-week period as the

dose of clozapine is increased. Typical antipsychotic drugs would be predicted to interfere with some of the benefits of clozapine and should not ordinarily be prescribed with clozapine.

Determination of clozapine plasma levels is useful whenever patients are not responding adequately. It may be useful to augment clozapine treatment with valproic acid or other mood stabilizers (such as lithium, carbamazepine, lamotrigine, or topiramate), anxiolytic drugs, or an antidepressant [63]. The choice of augmenting agent is largely driven by symptomatic considerations, or pharmacokinetic interactions in the case of fluvoxamine. However, none of these strategies have strong empiric support. One exception may be the addition of sulpiride, which may result in a significant reduction in symptom burden when added to clozapine [97]. Electroconvulsive therapy (ECT) also resulted in a modest further reduction in symptoms when used in conjunction with clozapine and appears to be well tolerated [98]. It is difficult to postulate a rationale for adding another atypical drug, with the exception of amisulpride, because of their similarity in pharmacology to clozapine, although a modest number of short-term studies have shown modest benefit with adjunctive aripiprazole for attenuating psychotic symptoms when combined with clozapine [99]. It should be discontinued if side effects are intolerable or if there is no apparent response after a 6-month trial of clozapine alone and subsequent trials with augmentation therapy. Clearly, further studies involving clozapine partial- or non-responders are urgently needed. It should be noted that discontinuation of clozapine can precipitate a severe relapse, even when clozapine is slowly tapered [100].

### Risperidone

Risperidone is a first-line drug for the treatment of schizophrenia [101]. Definitive data are lacking for its efficacy in patients who have treatment-resistant schizophrenia, although preliminary evidence suggests that the use of higher doses of long-acting injectable risperidone [up to 100 mg intramuscularly (IM) every 2 weeks] may be effective [102]. Risperidone may be useful in patients who fail to tolerate other antipsychotic agents because of side effects not shared by risperidone such as anticholinergic effects. Risperidone is well tolerated in low doses by the elderly and has been widely used in the United States for the treatment of a variety of senile psychoses [103, 104]. Its efficacy against haloperidol was established in a series of multi-centre trials which demonstrated advantages for risperidone in overall psychopathology in mainly chronic schizophrenic patients in an acute exacerbation at doses in the 6–8 mg/day range. However, these doses have proven to be higher than is needed for most patients in clinical practice, possibly reflecting some of the problems in generalizing from controlled clinical trials. The doses for schizophrenia most often used in non-elderly adults are now 4–6 mg/day. First-episode patients may not tolerate higher doses (for example, above 5 mg/day), and some may respond to as little as 1–2 mg/day. Treatment-resistant patients have been shown to respond to long-acting risperidone at doses of 50 or 100 mg every 2 weeks [105].

Beyond treatment of acute symptoms, risperidone is also effective for long-term maintenance phase and relapse prevention. For instance, relative to haloperidol, risperidone has also been associated with a lower risk of relapse (34% vs 60%) over a minimum of 12 months of treatment [106]. In another study that retrospectively compared rates of rehospitalization for patients who received treatment with risperidone, olanzapine, or typical antipsychotics, rehospitalization rates for risperidone and olanzapine were similar and both were significantly less than those of patients treated with typical antipsychotics [107].

Risperidone is usually initiated at low doses (for example, 1–2 mg daily) and is titrated into the dosage range provided in Table 64.4. The medication is often initiated in twice-daily dosing; however, because its primary active metabolite 9-OH risperidone is pharmacologically equivalent to its parent drug and because it has a longer elimination half-life, once-daily dosing is also possible. Risperidone is available in soluble water and liquid forms, which may be advantageous for patients who have swallowing difficulties or require taking their medication in a non-pill form for other reasons, including their own preference.

For patients who have a history of poor compliance leading to frequently relapsing illness, or for those who prefer it, a long-acting injectable form of risperidone is available (Table 64.1) for administration every 2 weeks. Response may be expected to occur in the 25–50 mg (per every 2-week dose) range [108]; however, oral risperidone must be continued through at least the first 3 weeks of treatment with the long-acting injectable form before being slowly tapered. Supplementation with oral medication may be required when the dose of the long-acting drug is upwardly adjusted due to breakthrough psychotic symptoms.

Risperidone has more of a tendency to produce EPS than other atypical antipsychotics, but this can be minimized by using the lowest dose which controls positive symptoms and adding an anticholinergic drug, if necessary [109]. Among atypical drugs, risperidone and paliperidone produce the greatest increases in serum prolactin, particularly in women [110]. Elevations in prolactin levels as a result of treatment with risperidone do not always translate into clinical symptoms such as sexual dysfunction or gynaecomastia in men and menstrual changes and breast discharge in women [110].

A meta-analysis of six studies comparing risperidone to typical antipsychotic treatment indicated risperidone was superior for treating negative symptoms [111]. Risperidone has also been shown to improve cognition in schizophrenia, more so than typical antipsychotic drugs [23]. Improvement in working memory was greater than that of other domains.

In summary, risperidone is a first-line pharmacological treatment of schizophrenia. It may have advantages over typical drugs with regard to negative symptoms, cognition, and EPS, but it does produce dose-dependent increases in EPS risk and large increases in serum prolactin levels, even compared to typical antipsychotic drugs. The long-acting injectable form of risperidone is preferred in patients with problems with oral drug compliance. Risperidone in its long-acting injectable form has also been shown to be effective for the prevention of relapse or hospitalization during bipolar maintenance treatment, although it may be more effective for preventing manic or mixed episodes than depressive episodes [112].

### Olanzapine

Olanzapine is also a first-line treatment for schizophrenia [77]. Some treatment-resistant patients respond to olanzapine at doses in the 20–40 mg/day range, but the side effect burden may be treatment-limiting for some patients, especially weight gain and related metabolic effects [113].

The efficacy of olanzapine in treating psychosis and negative symptoms in patients with an acute exacerbation of schizophrenia has been established in multiple large-scale, multi-centre trials [114]. In these trials, olanzapine at doses of 10–20 mg/day has been superior to placebo and equivalent or superior to haloperidol in some measures of total psychopathology and positive or negative symptoms. For example, in one North American multi-centre trial, olanzapine (15 ± 5 mg/day) was superior to haloperidol (15 ± 5 mg/day) in the treatment of negative symptoms [115]. Olanzapine improves primary negative symptoms, rather than secondary negative symptoms [116].

Olanzapine has also been found to be effective as a maintenance treatment of schizophrenia [117]. The estimated relapse rates, defined as the need for hospitalization, during a 1-year period in three studies of patients receiving olanzapine for maintenance treatment were 19.6–28.6% [117].

Olanzapine has been reported to improve cognitive dysfunction [23, 24] in patients with schizophrenia or schizoaffective disorder. Pharmacoeconomic studies and investigations of medication effects on quality of life measures indicate that olanzapine has a beneficial cost–outcome profile. For instance, in one investigation, the higher cost of olanzapine, relative to haloperidol, was offset by olanzapine treatment-associated reductions in rehospitalization and overall treatment costs [118].

The average clinical dose of olanzapine is 12.5–20 mg/day, but many patients respond to lower doses (for example, 10 mg daily) [119]. A principle advantage of olanzapine is its once-daily dosing and the feasibility of starting the medication at a dose that is clinically effective for most patients. For acute situations where rapid control of agitation, hostility, or other dangerous behaviours is required, olanzapine is available as a short-acting injectable medication (Table 64.1) [120]. For patients with frequent relapses owing to poor adherence to oral medication, a long-acting injectable form of olanzapine is available. A small number of patients experienced excessive sedation, fatigue, dizziness, or delirium owing to inadvertent *intravascular* injection of long-acting injectable olanzapine [120]. Olanzapine long-acting injectable must therefore be administered by trained individuals, along with close observation and additional safety measures (such as avoidance of driving) that address the risk of developing post-injection syndrome symptoms.

In summary, olanzapine is an effective atypical drug with specific advantages in terms of its once-a-day administration, low risk for EPS, and efficacy for cognitive dysfunction and negative symptoms. Clinically significant weight gain and related dysmetabolic adverse effects may be a problem for some patients, as will be discussed. Olanzapine has been shown to effectively reduce manic symptoms in adults with bipolar I disorder [21] and to effectively reduce depressive symptoms when used as a pharmacological adjunct for the treatment of refractory unipolar major depression and acute depressive episodes in patients with bipolar I disorder [121, 122].

### Quetiapine

Quetiapine has been shown to be as effective as typical antipsychotics in the acute treatment of schizophrenia, with low EPS risk and no effect on serum prolactin levels [123, 124]. Quetiapine and clozapine both appear to bind more loosely to striatal D2 receptors than other antipsychotic drugs, and both drugs show antipsychotic activity at D2 receptor occupancies that are well below the 60% threshold identified for most other antipsychotic drugs [125]. In spite of this similarity with clozapine, quetiapine does not appear to have efficacy comparable to clozapine for treatment-resistant patients.

The efficacy of quetiapine for acute-phase schizophrenia is supported by results from several RCTs that documented superiority of quetiapine, relative to placebo, across several doses, with some patients responding to 150 mg/day and others requiring 750 mg/day [123]. For instance, in one high- (750 mg/day) vs low-dosage (250 mg/day) study, both dosage groups evidenced greater reduction in positive symptoms, relative to placebo; however, the differences were significant only for the high-dose group [124]. In another study that assessed multiple fixed doses of quetiapine (75–750 mg/day), compared with haloperidol and placebo, significant differences in improvement over placebo for quetiapine were observed in the dosage range of 150–750 mg/day [123].

Quetiapine's effect on negative symptoms continue to be investigated. One placebo-controlled comparison documented improvements in negative symptoms with quetiapine treatment across a wide range of doses, with the greatest improvement reported at 300 mg daily [123]. In the high- vs low-dose study reviewed previously, the high-dose group also experienced greater improvement in negative symptoms, relative to placebo [124]. Like risperidone and olanzapine, quetiapine appears to improve depressive symptoms and certain cognitive deficits [23, 24] associated with schizophrenia or schizoaffective disorder. The improvements in cognition with quetiapine appear to be superior to those of haloperidol [126].

These results suggest that overall the greatest improvement in positive and negative symptoms may occur when quetiapine is used at the higher end of its dosage range. The average clinical dose appears to be between 300 and 500 mg/day, usually given twice daily, though some benefit from the medication when given only once daily. The effects of using higher doses for patients who do not respond adequately to these doses are uncertain. A titration of the dosage is required after initiating the medication. From the viewpoint of EPS and hyperprolactinaemic effects, quetiapine appears to confer only low risk. As such, like clozapine, it appears to be well tolerated, even among patients with idiopathic Parkinson's disease [127]. Sedation may be a limiting side effect for some, especially during dosage titration. Weight-related, metabolic, and other adverse effects will be discussed in greater detail.

Quetiapine is one of the best studied pharmacotherapies for bipolar disorders. In addition to its effectiveness for reducing the acute symptoms of mania [128], quetiapine is effective for the acute treatment of depressive episodes in patients with bipolar I and II disorders [129, 130]. Quetiapine has also been shown to be effective as a bipolar maintenance treatment [131].

In summary, quetiapine also appears to be effective for a wide range of schizophrenia-associated symptoms and confers a lower level of risk in terms of antidopaminergic adverse effects. The dosage range of this medication may be quite wide, though patients may have a greater chance of benefiting from the medication at the higher end of this range. Quetiapine is a first-line option for treating acute manic episodes in patients with bipolar I disorder, and depressive episodes in patients with bipolar I or II disorder. Quetiapine has also been shown to reduce depressive symptoms in adults with inadequate response to some antidepressants such as selective serotonin reuptake inhibitors (for example, fluoxetine,

etc.) and serotonin–noradrenaline reuptake inhibitors (for example, venlafaxine, etc.) [132].

### Ziprasidone

Ziprasidone has a varied receptor occupancy profile. Like most atypical antipsychotic drugs, it displays high-affinity 5-HT2A binding, coupled with relatively lower-affinity D2 receptor binding. Ziprasidone is also a 5-HT1A agonist, as well as both a serotonin and a noradrenaline reuptake pump inhibitor [133]. This profile predicts a wide range of pharmacological activity against core psychotic symptoms and negative and affective symptoms, as well as neurocognition.

Ziprasidone, like quetiapine, has been shown to be superior to placebo for the reduction of total psychopathology and positive and negative symptoms in patients with schizophrenia [134, 135]. There is limited evidence to suggest superiority over typical antipsychotics with regard to improvement in positive and negative symptoms [134, 136]. Studies of multiple fixed doses of ziprasidone vs haloperidol at conventional doses indicate that ziprasidone yields similar efficacy to haloperidol for reducing positive symptoms and global psychopathology at a dose of 160 mg/day [136].

Ziprasidone significantly improved negative symptoms and reduced the risk of relapse, compared to placebo, in a 1-year maintenance study in stable hospitalized chronic schizophrenic patients [137]. These maintenance-phase effects were not dependent on the daily dose of ziprasidone. In a 28-week comparison with haloperidol, the two groups evidenced similar overall effects for positive symptoms; however, between-group differences were documented, favouring ziprasidone for negative symptoms and EPS [138]. Ziprasidone was effective against depressive symptoms associated with schizophrenia in one study at a dose of 160 mg/day [139]. Significant improvements in multiple cognitive domains have been reported among ziprasidone-treated patients in a variety of treatment contexts [140]. Such changes appear to be unrelated to improvements in other symptoms of schizophrenia. Ziprasidone treatment has been associated with significant improvement in quality of life measures in one post hoc data analysis [141]. Further investigation of the effect of ziprasidone on health-related quality of life and similar outcomes are warranted. Ziprasidone treatment of schizophrenia appears to be cost-effective, relative to no treatment [142]. Further cost–benefit studies are needed.

The dose range of ziprasidone for acute treatment appears to be between 80 mg/day and 160 mg/day, and higher doses within this range may be more effective (Table 64.4). Doses greater than 120 mg/day appear to be required to achieve approx. 60% dopamine D2 receptor blockade [143], the D2 receptor occupancy threshold that appears to coincide with efficacy against positive symptoms, as presented earlier. The medication is usually given twice daily, although some may take the medication once daily at night-time. Titration of the total daily dose into the recommended range is required after initiating the medication. One critical aspect of medication administration for ziprasidone is the requirement that the medication be taken with food. There appear to be profound differences in bioavailability at equivalent doses between the fed and unfed state [144]. A full meal, as opposed to a light snack, appears to be required. Therefore, patients are encouraged to take their medication with meals.

A short-acting intramuscular formulation of ziprasidone has been developed, which should be useful in situations where more rapid action is needed. This formulation is available in two doses (10 mg and 20 mg), the preferred dosage being 20 mg due to a significantly greater reduction in agitation, relative to the lower dose [145]. Use of the short-acting injectable form can facilitate a transition to oral medication and may reduce the time required to titrate the daily dose of ziprasidone to one that is likely to be effective.

Ziprasidone appears to be well tolerated. Treatment-emergent EPS burden is low [135, 136]. Initial problems with somnolence or behavioural activation are usually self-limited, although temporary use of clonazepam or other benzodiazepine at low doses may improve tolerability, especially during the titration phase, should the latter occur. Importantly, data from both short- and long-term studies indicated that ziprasidone is not associated with clinically significant changes in weight, glycaemic measures, or markers of lipid homeostasis [146].

Ziprasidone can result in partial blockade of the slow potassium rectifier current in the cardiac conduction system, which may result in prolongation of the QTc interval [147]. On the other hand, ziprasidone was not shown to be associated with an elevated risk of non-suicidal mortality, relative to olanzapine, in a large simple trial of over 18,000 patients with schizophrenia [148]. Under routine circumstances, screening electrocardiograms are not required. Nevertheless, caution may be warranted for individuals who are at risk for significant prolongation of the QTc interval, including patients who take medications other than ziprasidone that prolong the QTc interval. Concomitant use of CYP450 3A4 inhibitors does not appear to pose a significant risk [149].

In summary, ziprasidone appears to be a useful additional atypical antipsychotic agent because of its favourable side effect profile, including no weight gain—a major problem with olanzapine and clozapine—and no prolactin elevation, which is a less serious side effect of risperidone. Patients should be instructed to take the medication with food. Ziprasidone treatment may result in an increase in the QTc interval; however, in a great majority of cases, this is not clinically significant. Although it is effective for treating acute manic episodes in patients with bipolar I disorder [128], it has not been shown to be clearly effective for bipolar depression when used as an adjunct to mood stabilizers [150].

### Aripiprazole

Aripiprazole is pharmacologically distinct from the drugs reviewed previously in that it combines partial D2 receptor agonism with high-potency 5-HT2A antagonism. As a partial D2 receptor agonist with low intrinsic activity, it will generally reduce dopamine D2 receptor stimulation [151]. Conversely, it should act primarily as an agonist when endogenous dopamine is limited, as may be the case in the prefrontal cortex in patients with schizophrenia [30]. For this reason, aripiprazole is sometimes referred to as a 'dopamine stabilizer'. Aripiprazole also functions as a potent 5-HT1A partial agonist [152].

The efficacy of aripiprazole in the treatment of acute schizophrenia at doses ranging between 10 mg and 30 mg (taken once daily) was established on the basis of four short-term randomized controlled studies [153]. Relative to placebo, efficacy against negative symptoms was also demonstrated [154]. Long-term superiority of aripiprazole (vs placebo) for relapse over 26 weeks [155] and medication compliance and symptom response (vs haloperidol) for up to 52 weeks has also been established [156]. One study reported on the effectiveness of flexibly dosed aripiprazole (15–30 mg daily) among patients with schizophrenia with a history of resistance to treatment with olanzapine or risperidone [157]. Aripiprazole is an effective maintenance treatment with a favourable side effect profile, particularly for weight gain [158, 159]. However, it does cause akathisia and some nausea, particularly early in its usage. Aripiprazole has been reported to have beneficial effects on neurocognitive performance, but the data are rather limited [160].

Treatment with aripiprazole is usually initiated with 10–15 mg daily, although some patients may not be able to tolerate these doses due to agitation, nausea, or vomiting. Doses as high as 30 mg are sometimes indicated. An oral solution form is also available. Aripiprazole is also available in a water-soluble, as well as an acute intramuscular, form. The acute injectable form appears to be effective in the dosage range of 5.25–15 mg [161]. The recommended dose is 9.75 mg.

Several long-acting injectable forms of aripiprazole are available for patients who prefer or require long-acting injectable medications [162]. The first is aripiprazole monohydrate, a once-monthly injectable form of aripiprazole. The recommended starting and monthly maintenance dose of once-monthly long-acting injectable aripiprazole is 400 mg in the absence of interacting medications [163]. Oral aripiprazole (10–20 mg daily) must be taken for at least the first 14 days of long-acting aripiprazole initiation. More recently, aripiprazole lauroxil, a prodrug of aripiprazole, has also become available as a once-monthly injectable medication [164]. The recommended starting and monthly maintenance doses are 441 mg, 662 mg, or 882 mg, which correspond roughly to oral aripiprazole daily doses of 10 mg, 15 mg, and 20 mg or more. The highest dose (882 mg) can be administered once every 6 weeks via gluteal injection. Oral aripiprazole must be taken for at least the first 21 days of aripiprazole lauroxil.

For mood disorders, aripiprazole has been shown to be effective as an adjunctive treatment in adults with major depressive disorder who responded poorly to antidepressants [165]. Aripiprazole has been shown to effectively reduce manic symptoms in adults with bipolar I disorder—both alone and as an adjunct to mood stabilizers [166]. However, aripiprazole has not demonstrated clear benefit for treating bipolar depression [167].

Aripiprazole is generally well tolerated, with an adverse effect profile similar to placebo in short-term studies involving patients with acute schizophrenia and in longer-term studies of chronic, stable patients [153]. As is the case with all atypical antipsychotic drugs, the EPS burden is lower than that of typical antipsychotics. In summary, aripiprazole appears to be effective as an acute and long-term maintenance treatment for schizophrenia and related psychotic disorders at recommended doses, though some patients may require higher doses. Aripiprazole was initiated in most studies at doses of 10–15 mg once daily; however, some patients may require a slower titration following a lower starting dose. This medication is available in many forms, all of which appear to be very well tolerated. Aripiprazole is effective as an adjunctive treatment for patients with major depression who respond suboptimally to antidepressants and as monotherapy or adjunctive treatment for acute manic episodes in patients with bipolar I disorder. Important benefits from a tolerability viewpoint include very low rates of prolactin elevation and a low risk of weight gain and metabolic adverse effects.

*Paliperidone*

Paliperidone is the 9-OH metabolite of risperidone, which has a longer elimination half-life than the parent compound, as reviewed previously. Paliperidone, which is pharmacologically similar with regard to receptor occupancy profile to risperidone, is available commercially in an extended-release oral form and in two long-acting injectable forms.

The short-term efficacy of oral paliperidone has been established on the basis of multiple randomized, placebo-controlled studies [168]. In these studies, all doses of paliperidone were superior to placebo for reducing global psychopathology and positive symptoms, as well as negative symptoms, anxious/depressive symptoms associated with schizophrenia, and hostility/excitement. The recommended starting dose of oral paliperidone is 6 mg, given once daily. Doses may be upwardly adjusted at 3 mg/day increments, up to 12 mg daily. Elevations in prolactin levels are like those observed with risperidone treatment.

Paliperidone is available in once-monthly and 3-monthly long-acting injectable formulations. Long-acting injectable paliperidone has been shown to be effective for maintenance treatment in patients with schizophrenia [169, 170]. The paliperidone once-monthly long-acting injectable formulation is initiated at 234 mg (paliperidone palmitate salt) IM (deltoid muscle) on day 1, followed by 156 mg IM (deltoid muscle) 7 days later. The typical maintenance dose is 117 mg IM (deltoid or gluteal muscle) once monthly, with a range of 39–234 mg IM 1-monthly, depending on effectiveness and tolerability.

In summary, paliperidone appears to be safe and effective for both short- and long-term treatment of schizophrenia. The EPS and prolactinaemic adverse effect burden may resemble that of risperidone, but this notion requires prospective investigation. Oral paliperidone can be started at a clinically effective dose. Long-acting injectable forms are also currently available.

*Amisulpride*

The efficacy of amisulpride for the treatment of positive symptoms has been established over a wide dosage range (200–1200 mg daily) in treatment studies of up to 12 months' duration [171]. In general, it appears that higher doses (above 400 mg/day) are effective for treating patients with predominantly positive symptoms, although efficacy against negative symptoms has also been demonstrated [172, 173]. Low-dose amisulpride (approx. 300 mg/day) has been reported to be effective in treating negative symptoms in schizophrenics with predominantly negative symptoms [174, 175]. Amisulpride may improve primary negative symptoms [174, 175]. Amisulpride produces minimal EPS but may result in increased prolactin levels [176]. There are some data which suggest it can improve depressive symptoms in schizophrenia [177]. There are no data on its efficacy in treatment-resistant patients. Because its pharmacology is quite distinct from that of the 5-HT2A-based receptor antagonists previously discussed, amisulpride may be useful in patients who fail to tolerate that class of drugs. Amisulpride has also been demonstrated as being superior to haloperidol on quality of life measures and global functioning [178] and to significantly improve quality of life over 12 months of treatment [179] in patients with schizophrenia. Sulpiride is closely related to amisulpride and is widely used in the UK and some other regions of the world, but it is not licensed in the United States. Information about its typical and atypical properties are not as clear as for amisulpride and will not be discussed here.

*Lurasidone*

Lurasidone, like most other atypical antipsychotic drugs, exhibits potent 5-HT2A blockade, coupled with D2 receptor blockade [39]. In addition, lurasidone is a potent 5-HT7 receptor antagonist and a 5-HT1A partial agonist, with moderate affinity for α1-adrenergic receptors and negligible binding activity at other monoamine receptors and at dopamine and serotonin transporters [10, 39]. Lurasidone is metabolized almost entirely by CYP3A4 and has a mean elimination half-life of 18 hours. Similar to ziprasidone, lurasidone must be taken with food in order to ensure adequate exposure to the medication [10].

The short-term efficacy of lurasidone for treating schizophrenia is established on the basis of multiple acute-phase randomized, placebo-controlled studies [180–183]. In these studies, lurasidone was superior to placebo for reducing global psychopathology, positive symptoms, and negative symptoms in the 40–160 mg dose range. The efficacy of lurasidone (40–80 mg/day) for the maintenance treatment of schizophrenia was recently demonstrated in a randomized, placebo-controlled withdrawal study [184]. During the double-blind maintenance phase of the study, lurasidone significantly delayed time to relapse, as compared with placebo. Lurasidone is associated with mild dose-dependent akathisia, but a low risk of weight gain and associated dysmetabolic effects [185].

The recommended starting dose of lurasidone is 40 mg, given once daily. The typical effective dose range is 40–80 mg daily. The maximum recommended dose is 160 mg daily with meals.

Lurasidone is also indicated for treatment of depressive episodes in patients with bipolar I disorder. The short-term efficacy of lurasidone monotherapy for bipolar I depression was demonstrated in a 6-week randomized, placebo-controlled trial [186]. Lurasidone at both 20–60 mg/day and 80–120 mg/day showed significantly greater improvement in depressive symptoms than placebo. In a second 6-week randomized trial, lurasidone was superior to placebo as adjuncts to lithium or valproate in adults with bipolar I depression [187]. Lurasidone was also shown to improve depressive symptoms and overall illness severity in adults with major depressive disorder and subthreshold hypomanic symptoms in short-term (6 week) randomized, placebo-controlled trials [188, 189].

In summary, lurasidone appears to be efficacious and safe for the short- and long-term treatment of schizophrenia. All doses must be taken with food to ensure adequate exposure to the medication. Its side effect profile appears to be favourable, compared with many other atypical antipsychotic drugs. Lurasidone is effective for treating acute depressive episodes in patients with bipolar I disorder, both as monotherapy and as an adjunct to lithium or valproate.

*Asenapine*

Asenapine is also a potent antagonist at dopamine D2 and serotonin 5-HT2A receptors [10]. Asenapine also binds with relatively high potency to serotonin 5-HT2C, 5-HT6, 5-HT7, histamine H1, and α1-noradrenergic receptors where it acts as an antagonist, but has negligible affinity for muscarinic M1 receptors [10, 12, 190]. Asenapine also binds with high affinity to 5-HT1A receptors where it acts as a partial agonist [191].

The efficacy of asenapine for acute-phase treatment of schizophrenia was demonstrated in two randomized, double-blind, placebo-controlled trials [192, 193]. In these studies, asenapine at doses of 5–10 mg twice daily demonstrated superiority over placebo for reducing psychotic and negative symptoms. The longer-term efficacy of asenapine in adults with schizophrenia was investigated in two published randomized studies [194, 195], including one relapse prevention study [196]. In the relapse prevention study, patients who were clinically stable at the end of an open-label pre-randomization phase were randomized to double-blind continuation treatment with sublingual asenapine 10 mg twice daily or placebo for an additional 26 weeks. During double-blind treatment, relapse rates were significantly lower and mean time to relapse was significantly longer with asenapine than placebo.

Asenapine has also been shown to be an effective treatment for manic and mixed episodes in adults with bipolar I disorder on the basis of four randomized trials [196]. Efficacy for this indication has been demonstrated at both the 5 mg and 10 mg twice-daily doses in adults [197].

Asenapine is available as a rapidly dissolving tablet formulated for absorption via the buccal mucosa [10]. Swallowing asenapine tablets renders the drug ineffective. For adults, asenapine is initiated at a dose of 5 mg sublingually twice daily. The recommended dose range across indications in adults is 5–10 mg twice daily.

### Iloperidone

Iloperidone exhibits high affinity for dopamine D2 and D3 and serotonin 5-HT2A receptors where it acts as an antagonist [8, 10]. Iloperidone binds with moderate affinity to dopamine D4, serotonin 5-HT6 and 5-HT7, and α1-noradrenergic receptors, and with low affinity to dopamine D1, serotonin 5-HT1A, and histamine H1 receptors [10]. Iloperidone has no significant affinity for muscarinic cholinergic M1 receptors, but its antagonism of α1-noradrenergic receptors leads to orthostatic hypotension [10]. Thus, even though the clinically effective dose range of iloperidone for treating adults with schizophrenia is 6–12 mg twice daily, the recommended starting dose is low (1 mg twice daily). Dose titration is required in order to lower the risk of treatment-emergent orthostatic hypotension [10].

The 6–12 mg twice-daily dose range of iloperidone has been shown to be effective for treating acute symptoms of schizophrenia [198–200]. The long-term safety and efficacy of iloperidone were established in three 52-week, randomized, double-blind, multi-centre trials, and pooled data from these studies have been published [201]. Iloperidone is available as solid oral tablets. As indicated earlier, iloperidone must be started at a low dose (1 mg twice daily) and slowly increased to a target dose of 6–12 mg twice daily over several days in order to reduce the risk of treatment-emergent orthostatic hypotension.

### Brexpiprazole

Brexpiprazole is a partial agonist at 5-HT1A and D2 receptors and an antagonist at 5-HT2A and α1B/2C-adrenergic receptors [202]. It acts as a moderate antagonist at serotonin 5HT7 and 5HT2C receptors and histamine H1 receptors, and has only negligible binding activity at muscarinic M1 receptors [15]. Brexpiprazole thus shares with aripiprazole high-affinity partial agonist effects at D2 and 5-HT1A receptors, although brexpiprazole has higher intrinsic activity at 5-HT1A receptors.

The efficacy of brexpiprazole for acute treatment of schizophrenia in adults is supported by two 6-week randomized trials [203, 204]. In one study, only the 4 mg brexpiprazole dose group (not the 1 or 2 mg dose groups) was significantly more effective than placebo [204]. Brexpiprazole was associated with significantly lower relapse rates than placebo (14% vs 39%) during a 12-month maintenance period in one study [205].

The most common and dose-dependent side effects of brexpiprazole include nausea, akathisia, headache, and modest weight gain. Brexpiprazole was associated with modest and dose-dependent increases in prolactin levels. No significant differences with placebo in the risk of adverse changes in glucose or lipid profiles were observed in short-term trials.

The results of randomized short-term trials also support the efficacy of brexpiprazole as an adjunct to antidepressants for major depressive disorder [206–208]. These studies enrolled patients with major depression and inadequate response to antidepressants who then failed to respond to a prospective trial of conventional antidepressant plus placebo, before being randomized to adjunctive brexpiprazole or placebo for 6 more weeks. In each of these studies, adjunctive brexpiprazole (1.5–3 mg) resulted in significantly greater reduction in depressive symptoms than placebo.

The recommended starting dose for schizophrenia is 1 mg/day. After 7 days, the dose should be increased to 2 mg/day, with further adjustment based on clinical response and tolerability, up to a maximum daily dose of 4 mg/day. For major depression, the recommended starting dose is 0.5 mg/day, followed by weekly dose titration up to 1.0 mg/day, and then to an initial target dose of 2 mg/day. The maximum recommended dose for adjunctive treatment of major depressive disorder is 3 mg/day.

### Cariprazine

Cariprazine is a partial agonist at dopamine D3 receptors and a weaker partial agonist at D2 and serotonin 5-HT1A receptors. Its mechanism of action is therefore distinct from that of most other atypical antipsychotics, so it may be a reasonable alternative treatment when other drugs fail and the patient is not clearly treatment-refractory. Cariprazine is a weak antagonist at 5-HT2A, α1-noradrenergic, and histamine H1 receptors [16, 209]. Efficacy for acute treatment of schizophrenia in adults has been demonstrated in multiple randomized trials across a wide range of doses (1.5–9.0 mg/day) [210–212]. Cariprazine has been shown to significantly reduce relapse rates in longer-term studies of patients with schizophrenia [213].

The efficacy of cariprazine has also been demonstrated for acute manic or mixed episodes in patients with bipolar I disorder. In these studies, cariprazine demonstrated significantly greater reduction in manic symptoms than placebo across a variety of doses, ranging from 3 mg/day to 12 mg/day [214–216] after 3 weeks of treatment. One 8-week randomized trial also demonstrated significantly greater improvement in depressive symptoms at a daily dose of 1.5 mg than placebo in adults with bipolar I depression [217].

In conclusion, cariprazine has demonstrated efficacy in multiple randomized trials for treating acutely exacerbated schizophrenia and acute manic or mixed episodes in patients with bipolar I disorder. For acute schizophrenia, higher cariprazine doses may be more effective than lower doses. Cariprazine has shown promise as a treatment for acute bipolar I depression and as an adjunct to conventional antidepressants for patients with major depressive disorder who are responding poorly to treatment with antidepressants alone. Additional studies of cariprazine for bipolar depression and poorly responding major depression are needed to reach definitive conclusions about its role in treating each of these conditions.

## Pharmacokinetics, metabolism, and drug interactions

### Typical antipsychotic drugs

Typical antipsychotics are well absorbed when administered orally or parenterally. IM injection leads to more rapid and higher plasma levels. Peak plasma levels are reached in 30 minutes after IM injection and 1–4 hours after oral injection. Steady state is achieved in 3–5 days. The half-life for elimination is in the range of 10–30 hours. Metabolism of typical and atypical drugs occurs mainly in the liver, via the hepatic cytochrome (CYP)450 enzymes, particularly the 2D6 and 3A4 sub-families for most drugs. Dosing of typical medications are determined by clinical effects, and less by pharmacokinetic factors.

Pharmacokinetic drug–drug interactions at the level of protein binding are expected to be minimal, even though most typical antipsychotics are tightly bound to plasma proteins. Even so, appropriate therapeutic monitoring of drugs that are also tightly bound to plasma proteins but have a narrow therapeutic index (for example, warfarin, digoxin, phenytoin) when used in conjunction with typical antipsychotics is warranted. Interactions at the level of the CYP450 system are also thought to be minimal for most agents. Because smoking is so common among patients with schizophrenia and because smoking can be associated with potent induction of CYP450 1A2 isoenzymatic activity, dosage adjustments may be needed for selected antipsychotic drugs during any changes in smoking status. Other combinations with typical antipsychotics may be worth avoiding for other reasons such as increased central nervous system effects (for example, anxiolytics, other central nervous system depressants, anticholinergics, certain antihypertensive drugs), increased EPS (for example, metoclopramide, D2-blocking anti-nausea drugs, caffeine), impaired cardiac conduction (certain drugs combined with typical antipsychotics known to prolong the QTc interval), and neurotoxicity (lithium), especially among individuals who are more advanced in age.

### Atypical antipsychotic drugs

#### Clozapine

There are wide variations in the pharmacokinetics of clozapine in patients. The average half-life is 6–12 hours. Plasma concentrations are higher in Chinese patients than in Caucasian patients, in non-smokers than smokers, and in females than males. The metabolism of clozapine occurs mainly in the liver. Clozapine's chief metabolite is N-desmethylclozapine, which has some biological activity. Clozapine is metabolized by CYP1A2, and several potential drug–drug interactions are thus possible. When agents that induce CYP1A2 are prescribed or ingested, close monitoring of patients for a worsening of symptoms is warranted. Plasma levels of clozapine of approximately 350 ng/mL are more often associated with good response than lower levels [218] and should be checked in such cases. Upward adjustment of the clozapine daily dosage will typically correct the problem. On the other hand, if a CYP1A2 inducer is discontinued (for example, sudden abstinence

from cigarette smoking, etc.) or a potent inhibitor is added, this may result in a rise in clozapine concentration and an increase in adverse effect risk [219]. Caution may also be warranted for drugs that are potent inhibitors of CYP2C19 and CYP3A4 [220]. In addition, caution is warranted when considering concomitant use of drugs which can also cause bone marrow suppression (for example, carbamazepine) or precipitously drop the seizure threshold.

#### Risperidone

Risperidone is well absorbed from the gut and is extensively metabolized in the liver by CYP2D6 to 9-hydroxyrisperidone in approximately 92–94% of Caucasians [221]. Thus, 9-OH risperidone is an active species in the majority of patients. About 6–8% of Caucasians and a small proportion of Asians have a polymorphism of the CYP2D6 gene, which leads to poor metabolism of risperidone. For poor metabolizers of risperidone, the active moiety is mainly the parent compound. The half-life of the 9-OH metabolite is about 21 hours, whereas the half-life of risperidone is about 3 hours. Thus, risperidone can be used on a once-a-day schedule for normal metabolizers, whereas multiple doses are needed for those who are poor metabolizers. Risperidone should be titrated from 2 to 5 mg/day over at least a 3-day period to minimize hypotensive and neuromuscular side effects. Drugs known to induce or inhibit CYP2D6 and 3A4 may alter plasma levels of risperidone; thus, close monitoring is advised when such agents are added to ongoing risperidone treatment.

#### Olanzapine

Oral olanzapine has a half-life of 24–30 hours, which indicates that single daily administration is adequate [222]. The metabolic pathways of olanzapine involves CYP2D6, CYP1A2, and flavin-containing mono-oxygenases, as well as N-glucuronidation. It has a low potential for drug–drug interactions and requires extremely high concentrations, not likely to be achieved under clinical conditions, to inhibit CYP450 systems. Plasma levels of approximately 9.3 mg/mL have been reported to predict better clinical response to olanzapine in inpatients with an acute exacerbation [223]. Olanzapine is detectable in plasma immediately following the first injection of its long-acting injectable formulation; therefore, oral olanzapine is not required during the initiation of olanzapine long-acting injection therapy. Drugs that are known inducers or inhibitors of CYP1A2 may significantly affect plasma levels of olanzapine and alter its clinical effects at a given dosage; thus, active monitoring of symptoms and adverse effects is indicated if such agents are added. As is the case with clozapine, gender and smoking status may influence olanzapine levels, leading to adjustment in dosage [224].

#### Quetiapine

Quetiapine is well absorbed and is approximately 83% protein-bound [223]. Quetiapine is better absorbed after eating [225]. It has a half-life of 6 hours and is metabolized in the liver by CYP3A4 to inactive metabolites. Quetiapine has significant interactions with inducers and inhibitors of CYP3A4. Co-administration with these agents may require dosage adjustment. Once-daily dosing, a common dosing strategy for quetiapine, is also supported in the literature [226].

## Ziprasidone

Ziprasidone has a half-life of 4–10 hours. Twice-daily administration is possible despite this relatively short half-life. Ziprasidone should always be taken after eating in order to facilitate absorption. About two-thirds of ziprasidone is metabolized by aldehyde oxidase into inactive metabolites. The remainder is metabolized by CYP3A4 and CYP1A2 into inactive metabolites. At the current time, there are no known drug interactions with ziprasidone at the level of aldehyde oxidase, since enzymatic activity does not appear to be altered by co-administered drugs. Although CYP3A4 appears to play only a minor role in the metabolism of ziprasidone, potent inhibitors or inducers of CYP3A4 may significantly alter plasma concentrations of ziprasidone [227] and may thus necessitate an adjustment in dosage. The use of concomitant medications that may prolong the QTc interval should be avoided. Ziprasidone is contraindicated for patients with a history of known QT prolongation, recent myocardial infarction, or uncompensated heart failure.

## Aripiprazole

Oral aripiprazole is well absorbed from the gut and has an elimination half-life of 75 hours. It is metabolized primarily by CYP3A4 and 2D6 isoenzymes into an active metabolite dehydro-aripiprazole, which has a half-life of 94 hours. This pharmacokinetic pattern supports once-daily dosing. Aripiprazole is also available in a long-acting injectable form. The absorption of long-acting injectable aripiprazole following IM injection is slow; therefore, oral aripiprazole must be co-administered during the first 2 weeks of long-acting injectable aripiprazole therapy. The mean elimination half-life of aripiprazole is dose-proportional (approximately 30 days following 300-mg injections provided every 4 weeks; approximately 47 days following 400-mg injections given every 4 weeks). Because aripiprazole is metabolized by CYP3A4 and 2D6, known inhibitors or inducers of these isoenzymes may result in increased or decreased clearance of aripiprazole and dehydro-aripiprazole [228].

## Paliperidone

Oral paliperidone is marketed in an osmotically controlled extended-release formulation, which results in steady release of active drug over a 24-hour period. Long-acting injectable paliperidone is available as a palmitate ester. Because the active moiety paliperidone is detectable in plasma after the first injection, co-administration of oral paliperidone is not required. The elimination half-life of paliperidone palmitate is variable, ranging from 25 to 49 days. Regardless of how it is formulated, hepatic metabolism is not considered a major route of clearance for paliperidone. Paliperidone is converted into metabolites that are not believed to contribute significantly to its overall pharmacological activity. Few significant drug–drug interactions at the level of the CYP450 system are therefore anticipated. Even so, the plasma concentration of paliperidone may be altered by drug interactions at CYP3A4 [229].

## Amisulpride

Amisulpride has a half-life of 10–15 hours. It is well tolerated. As yet, there are no known drug interactions.

## Lurasidone

Lurasidone is available as a solid oral tablet. The absorption of lurasidone is significantly increased when administered with food; the area under the curve and Cmax are increased 2- to 3-fold, respectively, in the fed vs the fasting state [10]. Lurasidone is extensively metabolized in the liver via the CYP3A4 isoenzyme. The mean elimination half-life of lurasidone is 18 hours.

## Asenapine

Asenapine is available as a rapidly dissolving tablet for sublingual or buccal administration. Asenapine is absorbed by the oral mucosa, which results in a bioavailability of approximately 35%. Swallowing the tablet reduces bioavailability to <2% [10]. The consumption of liquids within 10 minutes of administration of asenapine can also significantly reduce its bioavailability, so it is recommended that eating or drinking be avoided within 10 minutes of asenapine administration. Asenapine undergoes direct glucuronidation by UGT1A4 and is metabolized in the liver by the CYP1A2 isoenzyme (and, to a lesser degree, by CYP3A4 and CYP2D6).

## Iloperidone

Iloperidone has a half-life of 12–15 hours. Its absorption is not affected by food. Iloperidone is approximately 95% protein-bound and is extensively metabolized in the liver via CYP2D6 and CYP3A4 [230]. The mean elimination half-life of iloperidone is 18 hours for CYP2D6 extensive metabolizers, and 33 hours for slow metabolizers [10].

## Brexpiprazole

Brexpiprazole is rapidly absorbed after oral administration and is eliminated primarily by hepatic metabolism (CYP3A4 and 2D6). The mean half-life of brexpiprazole at steady-state is approximately 91 hours.

## Cariprazine

Cariprazine is rapidly absorbed after oral administration, and it is eliminated primarily by hepatic metabolism via CYP3A4 and, to a lesser degree, via CYP2D6. The mean elimination half-life of cariprazine is 2–5 days in the dose range of 1.5–12.5 mg/day.

## Side effects

(See Table 64.6.)

### Typical antipsychotics

The adverse effects that are most routinely concerning for typical antipsychotic drug treatment are EPS. High-potency dopamine antagonist drugs, such as haloperidol and fluphenazine, are more likely to produce EPS than low-potency agents such as chlorpromazine and thioridazine. There are a wide range of EPS produced by typical antipsychotics, including dystonic reactions when first administered, akathisia during the first 2–3 weeks, parkinsonism during the first several weeks with variable persistence, neuroleptic malignant syndrome at any time point but usually in the initial weeks, and tardive dyskinesia.

*Dystonic reactions* due to dopamine antagonist drugs can be treated with parenteral anticholinergic agents or diphenhydramine, an antihistamine with some anticholinergic properties. The use of anticholinergic and other agents to manage parkinsonism due to typical dopamine antagonist drugs will be discussed subsequently.

**Table 64.6** Adverse effects of selected antipsychotic drugs

| Typical antipsychotic drugs | | | | | | | | |
|---|---|---|---|---|---|---|---|---|
| | EPS | Tardive dyskinesia | Prolactin elevation | Sedation | Weight gain | Orthostasis | Anticholinergic | Diabetes exacerbation and dyslipidaemia |
| Chlorpromazine<br>Fluphenazine<br>Haloperidol<br>Loxapine<br>Mesoridazine<br>Molindone<br>Perphenazine<br>Thioridazine<br>Tiotixene<br>Trifluoperazine | Mild to moderate (for low-potency* drugs) to high (for high-potency* drugs) | Moderate to high | Moderate to high (risk higher for high-potency drugs) | Mild to moderate (for high-potency drugs) to high (for low-potency drugs); lowest risk for molindone | Mild to moderate (for high-potency drugs) to high (for low-potency drugs); least for molindone | Mild to moderate (for high-potency drugs) to high (for low-potency drugs) | Mild to moderate (for high-potency drugs) to high (for low-potency drugs) | Low to moderate |

* See Table 64.1 for list of low-, mid-, and high-potency (with respect to dopamine D2 receptor blockade) antipsychotic drugs.
Estimates were derived by the chapter authors.
Source: data from the *International Psychopharmacology Algorithm Project (IPAP)*, *Algorithm for the treatment of schizophrenia*, Copyright (2008), International Psychopharmacology Algorithm Project (IPAP).

| Atypical antipsychotic drugs | | | | | | | | |
|---|---|---|---|---|---|---|---|---|
| | EPS | Tardive dyskinesia | Prolactin elevation | Sedation | Weight gain | Orthostasis | Anticholinergic | Glucose dysregulation and dyslipidaemia |
| Amisulpride | Low | Rare | High | Low | Low | Low | Rarely | Rarely |
| Aripiprazole | Low (moderate at higher doses) | Rarely to low | Rarely | Rarely to low | Low | Low to moderate | Rarely | Rarely |
| Asenapine | Low (moderate at higher doses) | ? | Low to moderate | Low to moderate | Low to moderate | Rarely | Rarely | Low |
| Brexpiprazole | Low (moderate at higher doses) | ? | Low (risk may increase at higher doses) | Low | Moderate | Rarely | Rarely | Low |
| Cariprazine | Low (moderate at higher doses) | ? | Rarely to low | Low to moderate | Low | Rarely | Rarely | Low |
| Clozapine | Rarely | Rarely | Transient | High | High | High | High | High |
| Iloperidone | Low | ? | Rarely to low | Low | Moderate | High | Rarely | Low |
| Lurasidone | Low (moderate at higher doses) | ? | Rarely to low | Low to moderate | Low | Rarely | Rarely | Low |
| Olanzapine | Moderate (low if ≤10 mg/day) | Rare | Low (if <20 mg/day) | Moderate to high | High | Low | Low | High |
| Paliperidone | Moderate | ? | High | Low | Low to moderate | Moderate | Rarely | Low |
| Quetiapine | Rarely | Rarely | Rarely | Moderate | Moderate | Moderate | Rarely to low | Moderate |
| Risperidone | Moderate (less if <4 mg/day) | Rarely | High | Low | Moderate | Moderate | Rarely | Low |
| Ziprasidone | Rarely to low | Rarely | Rarely to low | Rarely to moderate | Low | Low to moderate | Rarely | Rarely |

Estimates were derived by the chapter authors. In many cases, only limited data were available, particularly for newer agents.
Additional information based on references [10, 168, 185, 203, 253, and 254], and US drug label information (available online at https://dailymed.nlm.nih.gov/dailymed/index.cfm) for asenapine, brexpiprazole, cariprazine, iloperidone, lurasidone, and paliperidone.
There are insufficient data regarding the risk of tardive dyskinesia for asenapine, brexpiprazole, cariprazine, iloperidone, lurasidone, or paliperidone.
Source: data from the *International Psychopharmacology Algorithm Project (IPAP)*, *Algorithm for the treatment of schizophrenia*, Copyright (2008), International Psychopharmacology Algorithm Project (IPAP).

*Akathisia* may be the most common EPS, occurring in up to 70% of patients treated long term with haloperidol [231]. The term refers to a subjective uncomfortable experience of motor restlessness which is relieved by movement. As such, patients will complain of discomfort and manifest increases in psychomotor behaviour. These symptoms can be distressing enough to cause agitation or suicidal behaviours [232]. Patient age does not seem to influence the risk of developing akathisia, but women are believed to be at higher risk. Diagnosis of this condition is necessary to prevent inadvertent increases in doses due to mistaken conclusion that discomfort from akathisia is due to worsening psychosis. This effect may be managed by reduction in dosage and switching to an atypical antipsychotic drug or a drug that is less likely to cause akathisia. Akathisia may respond to anticholinergic medications, usually within 3–7 days. Other options include low doses of benzodiazepines or β-adrenergic blockers, assuming no contraindications to either.

*Parkinsonism* caused by dopamine antagonist drugs resembles idiopathic parkinsonism. Diagnostically, severe dopamine antagonist-induced parkinsonism may resemble depression or negative symptoms of schizophrenia; however, the associated motor signs and time course of symptoms in relation to starting antipsychotic treatment distinguish the former. Like akathisia, the onset and severity of drug-induced parkinsonism is related to dosage; thus, a lowering of the dose or switching to a medication that is less likely to cause this effect may provide significant relief or ameliorate the parkinsonian signs and symptoms altogether. When this is not feasible, anticholinergic medications may provide relief, typically within 3–7 days. The response to anticholinergic medication is quite variable, however.

*Tardive dyskinesia* emerges at various rates, depending upon age, sex, and diagnosis [233, 234]. The rate in younger patients is between 3% and 5% per year. It is higher in bipolar than schizophrenic patients and much higher in people above the age of 60. It is related to the dose and will be less likely with lower doses of typical antipsychotics. Tardive dyskinesia is ordinarily reversible, although irreversible and/or extremely severe and rarely life-threatening forms can occur. The best way to minimize its occurrence is to use an atypical antipsychotic drug in lieu of a typical agent, since these drugs as a class are associated with a much lower risk of tardive dyskinesia [234]. Patients with mood disorders should generally not receive maintenance treatment with typical antipsychotic drugs, unless clinically necessary. There are no definitive treatments for tardive dyskinesia, though some controlled evidence supports the use of adjunctive gingko biloba extracts, amantadine, tetrabenazine, and valbenazine [235–240]. Generally, the best strategy is prevention through the use of atypical drugs and periodic screening with a structured assessment tool such as the Abnormal Involuntary Movement Scale (AIMS). There is some suggestion in the literature that continuation of antipsychotic treatment does not worsen tardive dyskinesia and may eventually result in stabilization and improvement of tardive symptoms. Switching to clozapine is useful to control tardive symptoms when they are very severe.

*Neuroleptic malignant syndrome (NMS)* is a rare, life-threatening side effect related to an apparent compromise of the neuromuscular and sympathetic nervous systems [241]. It usually occurs at the initiation of treatment with a high-potency dopamine antagonist but may occur with any of the typical (or atypical) agents at any point.

NMS is characterized by muscle rigidity, breakdown of muscle fibres leading to large increases in plasma creatine kinase concentration, fever, autonomic instability, changing levels of consciousness, and sometimes death. It is treated by immediately discontinuing all dopamine antagonist drugs, applying external hypothermia, and supporting blood pressure. Administering a direct-acting dopamine agonist, such as bromocriptine or pergolide, and dantrolene sodium, which blocks the release of intracellular stored calcium ions, may be useful adjuncts. After successful treatment of NMS, an atypical antipsychotic should be used, even though these agents, including clozapine, may also induce NMS.

The typical dopamine antagonist drugs produce a wide variety of other side effects, including weight gain, seizures (especially pimozide), sedation, hypotension, elevated liver enzymes, retinitis pigmentosa (thioridazine), orthostatic hypotension, prolongation of the QTc interval (low-potency phenothiazines, pimozide), and anticholinergic effects (mesoridazine, chlorpromazine, thioridazine). All of the typical dopamine antagonist drugs produce marked increases in serum prolactin levels, with increases being greater in females than males [33]. Prolactin elevations may affect sexual function in both males and females, with difficulty achieving erection or orgasm being among the most common side effects [33].

## Atypical antipsychotic drugs

### Clozapine

#### Agranulocytosis

It has now been reliably established that clozapine produces agranulocytosis in slightly <1 per 100 patients [242, 243]. The peak of agranulocytosis with clozapine occurs between 4 and 18 weeks and then falls off sharply. Weekly monitoring of the white cell or absolute neutrophil count is required for 26 weeks in most countries, with the frequency decreasing to biweekly or monthly thereafter, sometimes on a voluntary basis. In the United States, monthly monitoring is required, assuming no haematological abnormalities after 1 year of treatment. With monitoring, agranulocytosis can usually be detected before infection sets in or becomes overwhelming. Discontinuation of clozapine, beginning treatment with colony cell-stimulating factors, and the usual procedures for treating an infection are usually effective in restoring the white cell line.

#### Other side effects

Clozapine produces a wide range of side effects [243]. These can generally be managed by dose adjustment and concomitant medications. Clozapine produces hypotension because of its potent α1-adrenoceptor antagonism and must be slowly titrated in most patients. Low-dose glucocorticoid treatment may be helpful in some patients with severe hypotension. Clozapine rarely, if ever, produces significant EPS, although some cases of akathisia and NMS have been reported.

Major motor seizures are another important side effect of clozapine. They are dose-related, with the incidence being about 2% in patients at low doses and 6% at doses >600 mg/day. They are sometimes preceded by myoclonic jerks. Valproic acid and dose reductions are usually effective in preventing the progression of myoclonic jerks or treating major motor seizures. Other anticonvulsants can be combined with clozapine, if needed, though caution would be clearly warranted with the use of carbamazepine due to its potential for bone marrow suppression.

Hypersalivation is a common side effect that usually responds to anticholinergic therapy or clonidine. Exacerbation of obsessive–compulsive symptoms has been reported with clozapine. Augmentation with an SSRI or lithium carbonate is usually effective.

Weight gain is a frequent side effect of clozapine, with about 30% of patients gaining >7% of body weight [243]. Dietary changes and exercise are useful in minimizing this effect. A related problem is the emergence of insulin resistance or type 2 diabetes or exacerbation of existing diabetes, with or without atherogenic changes in the serum lipid profile. There have also been reports of diabetic ketoacidosis that emerged in the context of clozapine treatment. Of the atypical drugs, clozapine and olanzapine are associated with the highest risk for clinically significant weight gain, as well as abnormalities in glycaemic control and lipid homeostasis [146].

Somnolence, tachycardia, hypertension, constipation, and stuttering are also side effects of clozapine. Tachycardia is treated only when the pulse is >100 beats/minute. β-blockers are effective to reduce the heart rate but may also result in synergism of hypotensive effects [243].

There have been reports of clozapine-associated myocarditis and cardiomyopathy [244]. The presence of eosinophilia accompanied by cardiotoxic signs, such as tachycardia, fatigue, orthostasis, or respiratory problems (many of which are adverse effects of clozapine), should alert the clinician to the possibility of myocarditis and the need for medical evaluation.

Finally, treatment with clozapine may not uncommonly result in an asymptomatic mild elevation in hepatic transaminase levels; however, there have also been reports of hepatotoxicity in the setting of clozapine treatment. Polypharmacy appears to be a risk factor. Cases of fulminant hepatotoxicity leading to liver failure are rare.

## Risperidone

Risperidone is associated with moderate weight gain, comparable to that of typical dopamine antagonist drugs in most cases and less than that of clozapine and olanzapine [146]. Risperidone also produces some postural hypotension because of its α1-adrenoceptor-blocking properties. Risperidone produces greater increases in serum prolactin secretion than any of the other atypical antipsychotic drugs [33]. The increases appear to be at least comparable to those of typical antipsychotics [245]. At higher doses, particularly above 6 mg daily in most adults, the incidence of EPS also increases [246], though typically not to the degree observed when using typical dopamine antagonist drugs in clinical practice. Risperidone, like clozapine and other agents of this type, can sometimes exacerbate or induce symptoms of obsessive–compulsive disorder and tics, probably due to its antiserotonergic properties. This can be counteracted in some patients by the addition of an SSRI. Risperidone is not associated with agranulocytosis or increased risk of seizures. Because of its low affinity for muscarinic receptors, risperidone treatment is not associated with significant anticholinergic effects.

## Olanzapine

Olanzapine also produces dose-dependent EPS, including some dystonic reactions in patients with schizophrenia, but these are less frequent and severe than those produced by typical dopamine antagonist drugs or risperidone [245]. Olanzapine is less well tolerated than clozapine in patients with Parkinson's disease. Olanzapine, like other atypical drugs, is associated with a lower risk of tardive dyskinesia than typical antipsychotics.

The major side effect of olanzapine is weight gain [245]. Large weight gains due to increased appetite occur in 10–15% of olanzapine-treated patients during the first 6 months of treatment. Another 20–35% gain between 7% and 10% of baseline body weight. These gains tend to persist for as long as patients continue the medication. Like clozapine, olanzapine is also associated with higher risk of insulin resistance, glycaemic changes, and the development of atherogenic dyslipidaemias [146]. Cases of diabetic ketoacidosis associated with olanzapine treatment have been reported.

Olanzapine is also associated with an increase in liver enzymes, orthostatic hypotension, anticholinergic side effects, and sedation. Many of these adverse effects are time-limited and reduce in intensity or resolve over the first few weeks of treatment with continuous use. Olanzapine produces transient increases in serum prolactin levels, which are smaller in magnitude than those produced by typical dopamine antagonist drugs or risperidone [33, 245].

Olanzapine, like other agents of this type, can occasionally exacerbate or induce symptoms of obsessive–compulsive disorder and tics, probably due to its antiserotonergic properties. This can be counteracted in some patients by the addition of an SSRI. Olanzapine is not associated with agranulocytosis or increased risk of seizures.

## Quetiapine

Quetiapine appears to have fewer EPS than either risperidone or olanzapine [225, 245]. Quetiapine is tolerated in patients with Parkinson's disease to a much greater extent than risperidone or olanzapine. The incidence of EPS with quetiapine in schizophrenic patients appears to be comparable to placebo. The major side effects with quetiapine are headache, agitation, dry mouth, dizziness, weight gain, and postural hypotension [245].

With regard to weight gain and other metabolic effects, quetiapine treatment appears to confer moderate risk—similar to that of risperidone, but less than that associated with clozapine or olanzapine treatment [146]. Far less is known about the long-term effects of quetiapine on markers of glycaemic and lipid homeostasis. Nevertheless, clinically significant changes in serum lipids have been reported.

Decreased serum thyroid hormone levels, increased hepatic transaminases, and elevated serum lipids have been reported. Decreases in total and free thyroxine, when they occur, are mild and non-progressive and are not believed to be clinically significant. The effect may be dose-dependent. Similar to clozapine, asymptomatic elevations in hepatic transaminases may be encountered early in the course of treatment, followed by a return to baseline values. Animal studies suggest an increased risk of cataracts [245]. Periodic ophthalmological screening for lenticular opacities is recommended by the manufacturer, though no causal relationship between the use of quetiapine and the development of cataracts has been demonstrated to date.

## Ziprasidone

Ziprasidone does not appear to significantly increase serum prolactin concentration and has a very low risk of EPS, weight gain, and changes in markers of glucose handling and lipid metabolism. Its major side effects are nasal congestion and somnolence [245], the latter of which is usually transient. There has been some concern of cardiac arrhythmias related to increased QTc interval; however, perusal of the available data does not reveal a significant problem in this regard. However, caution is warranted when considering the co-administration of ziprasidone with other drugs that are known to prolong the QTc interval, since ziprasidone has been associated with a significant increase in the QTc interval of 16.6 ms, which was greater than that with other atypical antipsychotics and haloperidol, but less than that with thioridazine [247]. Screening for electrolyte abnormalities and cardiac disease (including recent myocardial infarction, congestive heart failure symptoms, and arrythmias, with or without syncope) may be indicated prior to starting ziprasidone.

## Aripiprazole

Aripiprazole is well tolerated and does not appear to routinely cause hyperprolactinaemic changes at recommended dosages, although EPS has been reported to occur with aripiprazole, particularly for patients with affective disorders (major depression, bipolar disorders) [248]. Aripiprazole is also not associated with lower risk of clinically significant increases in weight or changes in markers of glucose handling or lipid homeostasis, relative to several other atypical drugs such as clozapine, olanzapine, quetiapine, and risperidone [146]. Aripiprazole, ziprasidone, and lurasidone are believed to have the most advantageous metabolic risk profiles [146, 185].

## Paliperidone

Paliperidone was also well tolerated, with the most common side effect being tachycardia. Rates of discontinuation due to adverse effects are very low. The risk of hyperprolactinaemia with paliperidone appears to resemble that of risperidone, although no head-to-head comparisons have been carried out. The changes in prolactin levels may be dose-related [168]. The EPS burden associated with paliperidone during short-term studies was low for the 6-mg dose; however, at higher doses, the incidence of EPS appears to be higher [168]. Short-term weight gain in a meta-analysis of 15 randomized trials was shown to be +1.2 kg; however, measures of metabolic effects with paliperidone showed no significant changes from baseline [185]. Similar results were found for paliperidone during medium-term treatment [249].

## Lurasidone

The most common adverse effects of lurasidone are somnolence, akathisia, nausea, and parkinsonism. The occurrence of akathisia appears to increase in a dose-dependent manner, up to 120 mg/day [10], and appears to be higher with lurasidone than with aripiprazole or asenapine, based on indirect comparisons vs placebo [250]. Minimal changes in body weight were observed among lurasidone-treated subjects in short-term studies [185]. In a pooled analysis of longer-term studies, there were only minimal changes from baseline in body weight, and the incidence rates of clinically significant weight gain (an increase of ≥7% above baseline) and weight loss (a decrease from baseline by the same amount) were 16% and 19%, respectively [251].

## Asenapine

The most common adverse effects of asenapine are insomnia, somnolence, and EPS, including dose-dependent risk of akathisia [10]. Transient oral hypoesthesias (usually resolved within 1 hour) have also been reported. Preliminary data suggest that asenapine may be associated with a similar degree of short-term body weight gain as paliperidone (+1.2 kg), but with low risk of clinically significant short-term changes in metabolic measures [185]. The relative risk of clinically significant weight gain (defined as a ≥7% weight increase from baseline) vs placebo was 4.1 (95% CI 2.3–7.4) [185].

## Iloperidone

The most common side effects from short-term studies of iloperidone were dizziness, dry mouth, somnolence, and dyspepsia. Iloperidone was not shown to increase the risk of EPS during short-term follow-up [10]. Iloperidone was associated with numerically higher rates of orthostatic hypotension (20%) than haloperidol (15%) and risperidone (12%), although orthostatic hypotension with iloperidone generally did not persist past the first 7 days of treatment. Statistically significant increases in the QTc interval were observed with iloperidone treatment at all tested dose ranges [252]. Iloperidone has been associated with a statistically significant increase in body weight and changes in lipid profiles, relative to placebo, but these results were based on analysis of only one clinical trial [185]. Additional studies of iloperidone's anthropometric and metabolic effects are needed.

## Brexpiprazole

Dose-dependent adverse effects of brexpiprazole include nausea, akathisia, and headache [253]. Brexpiprazole has also been associated with modest weight gain, but as yet no significant differences from placebo with respect to adverse changes in glycaemic or lipid profiles have been observed in short-term randomized trials [253]. There is no consistent evidence yet of clinically relevant short-term changes in prolactin concentration with brexpiprazole therapy. Brexpiprazole 2 mg has been associated with decreases in prolactin levels, while the 4-mg dose has been associated with increased prolactin concentrations [203]. Additional studies are needed to clarify brexpiprazole's anthropometric, prolactinaemic, and metabolic risk profile.

## Cariprazine

Common adverse effects of cariprazine include insomnia, extrapyramidal symptoms, akathisia, sedation, dizziness, anxiety, and gastrointestinal distress [254]. Cariprazine appears to be associated with greater risk of clinically significant weight gain than placebo [254]; however, no statistically significant differences in adverse metabolic parameters or cardiovascular-related events have been observed. Additional studies are needed to better define the adverse effect profile of cariprazine, particularly over longer-term treatment.

## Indications and contraindications

The main indication for antipsychotic drugs is the treatment of all phases of schizophrenia, including acute, florid symptoms of psychosis, and the prevention of relapse. Important other uses include the acute treatment and prophylaxis of mania, the acute treatment of depressive episodes in patients with bipolar disorders (for some agents such as quetiapine, olanzapine, lurasidone, and cariprazine) and major depression with psychotic features, the psychosis, agitation, and aggression of various dementias, the treatment of psychoses due to L-dopa or other dopamine agonists in Parkinson's disease, Tourette's syndrome, treatment-resistant obsessive–compulsive disorder, self-injurious behaviour, porphyria, anti-emesis, intractable hiccoughs, and in some cases as antipruritics. Some current research has suggested that antipsychotic drugs may be of use to prevent the onset of schizophrenia by administering them to individuals who are in the prodromal phase of the illness. Several atypical antipsychotic drugs are being trialled on an experimental basis for various character disorders such as borderline, schizoid, and schizotypal personality disorders. Clozapine, which has the lowest incidence of EPS of any of the antipsychotic drugs, has some special applications in neurological conditions such as essential tremor and the treatment of water intoxication syndrome in schizophrenic patients. Uses in other psychiatric and neurological conditions may be expected to emerge, as the safety profile of these agents is better described.

## Anti-parkinsonian agents

### Anticholinergic drugs

Anticholinergic, antihistaminic, benzodiazepines, dopamine agonists, and β-blockers are of importance in the management of EPS. They are usually needed with typical dopamine antagonist drugs, but some patients will require such treatment when taking atypical antipsychotic drugs. Anticholinergics and antihistaminics (for example, diphenhydramine) are used to treat acute dyskinesias and dystonias, parkinsonian side effects, and akathisia [255]. These agents block the effects of increased acetylcholine release due to D2 receptor blockade in the basal ganglia. The most widely used anticholinergic drugs are benztropine (1–6 mg/day, usually in divided doses), biperiden (2–16 mg/day in two or three doses), procyclidine (5–30 mg/day), and trihexyphenidyl (1–15 mg/day in a single or divided doses).

These anticholinergic agents are competitive antagonists of the five subtypes of muscarinic receptors (M1 through to M5). They have minimal antagonist effects at nicotinic cholinergic receptors. Blockade of cholinergic receptors on intrastriatal neurons by these agents restores the cholinergic balance, which is disrupted by blockade of D2 dopamine receptors. Other central effects include impairment of various forms of memory. Elderly patients, in particular, may develop anticholinergic-induced agitation, irritability, disorientation, hallucinations, and delirium because of the natural loss of cholinergic neurons with ageing.

### Side effects

These agents have some preference for the central nervous system, but peripheral anticholinergic effects are to be expected. Blockade of vagal tone in the heart produces tachycardia. Other adverse effects include decreased bladder function, urinary retention, and decreased bowel motility leading to constipation and impaction. Decreased saliva and bronchial secretions contribute to dry mouth and increased dental caries, while decreased sweating increases the risk of heat stroke. Blockade of muscarinic receptors in the eye cause pupillary dilatation and inhibition of accommodation, leading to photophobia and blurred vision. The muscarinic receptors in the basal ganglia are predominantly M2, whereas those in the periphery are M1. The rank order of anticholinergic drugs for relative selectivity for the M2 receptor is biperiden, procyclidine, trihexyphenidyl, and benztropine. All these agents can cause dry mouth, blurred vision, urinary retention, constipation, and increased intraocular pressure. They may cause anticholinergic delirium in elderly patients or after taking high doses. Biperiden is less likely to cause peripheral anticholinergic effects. Benztropine, biperiden, and trihexyphenidyl may cause euphoria because of their ability to inhibit dopamine reuptake and they may be subject to abuse.

### Indications

Anticholinergic drugs or the antihistamine diphenhydramine are given IM for the treatment of acute dystonic reactions. They are usually effective within minutes and may have to be repeated. It is usually not necessary to prescribe an oral anticholinergic following a dystonic reaction, though some may require their brief use, depending on which antipsychotic is prescribed. These agents should not be given prophylactically, unless the patient is at established risk for EPS at the dose of antipsychotic which is being started. If akathisia or parkinsonism develops following treatment with a typical dopamine antagonist drug, the first consideration should be whether to continue to use the offending agent, drop the dosage, or substitute with an atypical antipsychotic drug. If decreasing the dose of antipsychotic drugs is not clinically feasible, substituting with an atypical agent is clearly the recommended choice since it avoids all the unpleasant side effects of anticholinergic agents.

### Other drugs

Amantadine, which also has antiviral actions, is able to increase the release of dopamine in the basal ganglia, which diminishes the release of acetylcholine. It may improve drug-induced EPS [255, 256]. It has also been reported to improve sexual function and decrease weight gain due to dopamine antagonist drugs. But it may also cause worsening psychosis, increased arousal, agitation, and indigestion. As such, caution is warranted when using amantadine to treat EPS. The usual oral dose is 100–400 mg/day.

β-blockers, such as propranolol, atenolol, and pindolol, are useful for treating akathisia and tremor [255]. They may cause bradycardia, and particularly immediate-release forms should not be stopped abruptly due to rebound tachycardia.

Benzodiazepines, such as clonazepam, lorazepam, and diazepam, are useful for treating akathisia, acute dystonias, and acute dyskinesias. They can cause drowsiness and lethargy, and have abuse potential.

## Conclusions

Dopamine antagonist/partial agonist drugs are the principle treatment for schizophrenia, and selected agents are widely used in other psychotic and non-psychotic disorders such as bipolar disorder and major depression. Their main benefits are to treat psychotic symptoms across various illnesses. The atypical drugs have largely displaced the typical ones because of lower EPS and tardive dyskinesia risk profiles. However, several atypical drugs are associated with higher risk of weight gain and dysmetabolic effects. Atypical, but not typical, drugs appear to improve negative symptoms and cognition. New atypical drugs for psychosis continue to be developed, including those with partial agonist activity on presynaptic dopamine receptors and more extensive interactions with serotonergic receptors [257]. Several atypical drugs have established effectiveness—or have shown promise—for treating bipolar depression and major depression (as adjunctive therapy). Long-term treatment of affective disorders with typical antipsychotics is generally avoided, owing to heightened risk of tardive dyskinesia in such patients.

Dopamine antagonist/partial agonist drugs are useful as both acute and maintenance treatment to prevent the recurrence of psychotic symptoms in patients with schizophrenia and related psychotic disorders. The greater EPS and tardive dyskinesia risk of the typical antipsychotics, coupled with their lesser efficacy to improve negative symptoms and cognition, suggest that atypical agents are preferred, whenever possible, for long-term treatment. These advantages must be balanced against the greater long-term risk of weight gain and adverse metabolic effects associated with some atypical antipsychotic drugs. Clozapine, despite its risk of agranulocytosis and adverse metabolic effects, is the treatment of choice for patients with treatment-resistant schizophrenia. Although they have been considered together here as a single group, atypical antipsychotics have somewhat different pharmacologic profiles. Outside of clozapine for refractory schizophrenia, it is not yet clear which of these agents should be trialled in a given patient, but ongoing research may clarify this. These compounds, as well as others expected to be approved for use in the near future, will need to be compared with each other to determine if differential indications exist. Side effect differences among these drugs, as well as the availability of long-acting preparations, may help clinicians choose among them. As long as the typical drugs remain in use and for some patients who receive atypical agents, anticholinergic and other anti-parkinsonian drugs will continue to be necessary to treat EPS.

Because of the high rates of poor adherence to drugs in patients with schizophrenia and other disorders, it is important to develop more long-acting injectable atypical antipsychotics. Fortunately, several typical and atypical antipsychotic drugs have long-acting injectable formulations that are currently available for clinical use.

While the current group of atypical antipsychotic drugs is predominantly characterized by relatively more potent 5-HT2A than D2 receptor antagonism, or by partial D2 agonist effects, new pharmacological strategies will emerge for drugs with lower EPS liability than the typical antipsychotics. Because newer antipsychotic drugs are so effective in treating core psychotic symptoms, while limiting the risk for EPS, the remaining challenge rests in the development of agents that effectively treat other important features of schizophrenia, such as cognitive impairment and negative symptoms, without the metabolic and other side effects associated with these agents. Finally, the development of biomarkers, particularly genetic measures, to enable personalized medicine and reduce the number of therapeutic trials required to find optimal treatments for patients requiring drug treatment for psychosis remains a long-sought goal in the field that may be achievable in the near term [258–260].

## FURTHER INFORMATION

Haddad, P, Lambert, T., Lauriello, J. (2010). *Antipsychotic Long-Acting Injections*. Oxford: Oxford University Press.

Schatzberg, A.F. and Nemeroff, C.B. (eds.) (2017). *American Psychiatric Association Publishing Textbook of Psychopharmacology*, fifth edition. Washington, DC: American Psychiatric Association.

Weinberger, D.R. and Harrison, P.J. (2011). *Schizophrenia*, third edition. Chichester: Wiley-Blackwell.

## REFERENCES

1. Meltzer, H. (1995). The concept of atypical antipsychotics. In: *Advances in the Neurobiology of Schizophrenia* (eds. J.A. den Boer, H.G.M. Westenberg, H.M. van Praag), pp. 265–73. Chichester: Wiley.

2. Xiberas, X., Martinot, J.L., Mallet, L., *et al.* (2001). Extrastriatal and striatal D(2) dopamine receptor blockade with haloperidol or new antipsychotic drugs in patients with schizophrenia. *British Journal of Psychiatry*, **179**, 503–8.

3. Kapur, S., Zipursky, R., Jones, C., Remington, G., Houle, S. (2000). Relationship between dopamine D(2) occupancy, clinical response, and side effects: a double-blind PET study of first-episode schizophrenia. *American Journal of Psychiatry*, **157**, 514–20.

4. Kapur, S. and Seeman, P. (2001). Does fast dissociation from the dopamine D(2) receptor explain the action of atypical antipsychotics? A new hypothesis. *American Journal of Psychiatry*, **158**, 360–9.

5. Muscatello, M.R., Bruno, A., Pandolfo, G., *et al.* (2010). Emerging treatments in the management of schizophrenia—focus on sertindole. *Drug Design, Development and Therapy*, **4**, 187–201.

6. Thomas, S.H., Drici, M.D., Hall, G.C., *et al.* (2010). Safety of sertindole versus risperidone in schizophrenia: principal results of the sertindole cohort prospective study (SCoP). *Acta Psychiatrica Scandinavica*, **122**, 345–55.

7. Dixon, L., Lehman, A., Levine, J. (1995). Conventional antipsychotic medications for schizophrenia. *Schizophrenia Bulletin*, **21**, 567–78.

8. Fitton, A. and Heel, R. (1990). Clozapine: a review of its pharmacological properties, and therapeutic use in schizophrenia. *Drugs*, **40**, 722–47.

9. Kusumi, I., Boku, S., Takahashi, Y. (2015). Psychopharmacology of atypical antipsychotic drugs: from the receptor binding profile to neuroprotection and neurogenesis. *Psychiatry and Clinical Neurosciences*, **69**, 243–58.

10. Bobo, W.V. (2013). Asenapine, iloperidone and lurasidone: critical appraisal of the most recently approved pharmacotherpies for schizophrenia in adults. *Expert Review of Clinical Pharmacology*, **6**, 61–91.

11. Citrome, L. (2013). A review of the pharmacology, efficacy and tolerability of recently approved and upcoming oral antipsychotics: an evidence-based medicine approach. *CNS Drugs*, **27**, 879–911.

12. Richelson, E. and Souder, T. (2000). Binding of antipsychotic drugs to human brain receptors; focus on newer generation compounds. *Life Science*, **68**, 29–39

13. Meltzer, H.Y., Li, Z., Kaneda, Y., Ichikawa, J. (2003). Serotonin receptors: their key role in drugs to treat schizophrenia. *Progress in Neuropsychopharmacology and Biological Psychiatry*, **27**, 1159–72.

14. Burris, K.D., Molski, T.F., Xu, C., *et al.* (2002) Aripiprazole, a novel antipsychotic, is a high-affinity partial agonist at human dopamine D2 receptors. *Journal of Pharmacology and Experimental Therapeutics*, **302**, 381–9.

15. Maeda, K., Sugino, H., Naoki, A., *et al.* (2014). Brexpiprazole I: *in vitro* and *in vivo* characterization of a novel serotonin-dopamine activity modulator. *Journal of Pharmacology and Experimental Therapeutics*, **350**, 589–604.

16. Kiss, B., Horvath, A., Nemethy, Z., *et al.* (2010). Cariprazine (RGH-188), a dopamine D3 receptor-preferring, D3/D2 dopamine receptor antagonist–partial agonist antipsychotic candidate: *in vitro* and neurochemical profile. *Journal of Pharmacology and Experimental Therapeutics*, **333**, 328–40.

17. Anonymous (1998). Adverse effects of the atypical anti-psychotics. Collaborative Working Group on Clinical Trial Evaluations. *Journal of Clinical Psychiatry*, **59**, 17–22.

18. Luft, B. and Taylor, D. (2006). A review of atypical antipsychotic drugs versus conventional medication in schizophrenia. *Expert Opinion on Pharmacotherapy*. **7**, 1739–48.

19. The Collaborative Working Group (1998). Atypical anti-psychotics for treatment of depression in schizophrenia and affective disorders. *Journal of Clinical Psychiatry*, **12**, 41–6.

20. Cruz, N., Sanchez-Moreno, J., Torres, F., *et al.* (2010). Efficacy of modern antipsychotics in placebo-controlled trials in bioplar depression: a meta-analysis. *International Journal of Neuropsychopharmacology*, **13**, 5–14.

21. Perlis, R.H., Welge, J.A., Vornik, L.A., *et al.* (2006). Atypical antipsychotics in the treatment of mania: a meta-analysis of ranodmized, placebo-controlled trials. *Journal of Clinical Psychiatry*, **67**, 509–16.

22. Keefe, R.S., Silva, S.G., Perkins, D.O., *et al.* (1999). The effects of atypical antipsychotic drugs on neurocognitive impairment in schizophrenia: a review and meta-analysis. *Schizohrenia Bulletin*, **25**, 201–22.

23. Woodward, N.D., Purdon, S.E., Meltzer, H.Y., *et al.* (2005). Meta-analysis of neuropsychological change to clozapine, olanzapine, quetiapine, and risperidone in schizophrenia. *International Journal of Neuropsychopharmacology*, **8**, 457–72.

24. Keefe, R., Silva, S., Perkins, D., *et al.* (1999). The effects of atypical antipsychotic drugs on neurocognitive impairment in schizohprenia. *Schizophrenia Bulletin*, **25**, 201–32.

25. Toda, M., Abi-Dargham, Al. (2007). Dopamine hypothesis of schizophrenia: making sense of it all. *Current Psychiatry Reports*, **2**, 329–36.

26. Meltzer, H.Y. and Stahl, S.M. (1976). The dopamine hypothesis of schizophrenia: a review. *Schizophrenia Bulletin*, **2**, 19–76.

27. Davis, K., Kahn, R., Ko, G., *et al.* (1992). Dopamine in schizo-phrenia: a review and reconceptualization. *American Journal of Psychiatry*, **148**, 1474–86.

28. Kegeles, L.S., Abi-Darghan, A., Frankle, W.G., *et al.* (2010). Increased synaptic dopamine function in associative regions of the striatum in schizophrenia. *Archives of General Psychiatry*, **67**, 231–9.

29. Meltzer, H. (1999). The role of serotonin in antipsychotic drug action. *Neuropsychopharmacology*, **21**, 106–15.

30. Goldman–Rakic, P. and Selemon, L. (1997). Functional and anatomical aspects of prefrontal pathology in schizophrenia. *Schizophrenia Bulletin*, **23**, 437–58.

31. Abi-Dargham, A. and Moore, H. (2003). Prefrontal DA trans-mission at D1 receptors and the pathology of schizophrenia. *Neuroscientist*, **9**, 404–16.

32. Farde, L., Nordstrom, A., Wiesel, F., *et al.* (1992). Positron emis-sion tomographic analysis of central D1 and D2 dopamine re-ceptor occupancy in patients treated with classical antipsychotics and clozapine. Relation to extrapyramidal side effects. *Archives of General Psychiatry*, **49**, 538–44.

33. Haddad, P.M., Wieck, A. (2004). Antipsychotic-induced hyperprolactinemia: mechanisms, clinical features and manage-ment. *Drugs*, **64**, 2291–314.

34. Kramer, M., Last, B., *et al.*; the D4 Dopamine Antagonist Group (1997). The effects of a selective D4 dopamine receptor antag-onism. (L-745, 870) in acutely psychotic inpatients with schizo-phrenia. *Archives of General Psychiatry*, **54**, 567–72.

35. Gross, G., Wicke, K., Drescher, K.U. (2013). Dopamine D3 re-ceptor antagonism—still a therapeutic option for the treatment of schizophrenia. *Naunyn-Schmiedeberg's Archives of Pharmacology*, **386**, 155–66.

36. Neill, J.C., Grayson, B., Kiss, B., *et al.* (2016). Effects of cariprazine, a novel antipsychotic, on cognitive deficit and nega-tive symptoms in a rodent model of schizophrenia symptom-atology. *European Neuropsychpharmacology*, **26**, 3–14.

37. Richelson, E. (1988). Neuroleptic binding to human brain recep-tors: relation to clinical effects. *Annals of the New York Academy of Sciences*, **537**, 435–42.

38. Une, T., Kurumiya, S. (2007). Pharmacological profile of blonanserin. *Japanese Journal of Clinical Psychopharmacology*, **10**, 1263–72.

39. Ishibashi, T., Horisawa, T., Tokuda, K., *et al.* (2010). Pharmacological profile of lurasidone, a novel antipsychotic agent with potent 5-hydroxytryptamine 7 (5-HT7) and 5-HT1A receptor activity. *Journal of Pharmacology and Experimental Therapeutics*, **334**, 171–81.

40. Kroeze, W.K., Hufeisen, S.J., Popadak, B.A., *et al.* (2003). H1-histamine receptor affinity predicts short-term weight gain for typical and atypical antipsychotic drugs. *Neuropsychopharmacology*, **28**, 519–26.

41. Collaborative Working Group. (1998). Adverse effects of the atypical antipsychotics. *Journal of Clinical Psychiatry*, **12**, 17–22.

42. Kelly, D.L. and Love, R.C. (2001). Ziprasidone and the QTc interval: pharmacokinetic and pharmacodynamic considerations. *Psychopharmacology Bulletin*, **35**, 66–79.

43. Meltzer, H.Y., Matsubara, S., Lee, M. (1989). Classification of typical and atypical antipsychotic drugs on the basis of dopamine D-1, D-2 and serotonin 2 pKi values. *Journal of Pharmacology and Experimental Therapeutics*, **251**, 238–46.

44. Kuroki, T., Meltzer, H., Ichikawa, J. (1998). Effects of anti-psychotic drugs on extracellular dopamine levels in rat medial prefrontal cortex and nucleus accumbens. *Journal of Pharmacology and Experimental Therapeutics*, **288**, 774–81.

45. Parada, M., Hernande, L., Puig de Parada, M., *et al.* (1997). Selection action of acute systemic clozapine on acetylcholine release in the rat prefrontal cortex by reference to the nu-cleus accumbens and striatum. *Journal of Pharmacology and Experimental Therapeutics*, **281**, 582–8.

46. Li, X., Perry, K., Wong, D., *et al.* (1998). Olanzapine increases *in vivo* dopamine and norepinephrine release in rat prefrontal cortex, nucleus accumbens and striatum. *Psychopharmacology*, **136**, 153–61.

47. Andersson, J.L., Nomikos, G.G., Marcus, M., *et al.* (1995). Ritanserin potentiates the stimulatory effects of raclopride on neuronal activity and dopamine release selectivity in the mesolimbic dopaminergic system. *Naunyn- Schmiedeberg's Archives of Pharmacology*, **352**, 374–85.

48. Westerink, B.H., Kawahara, Y., De Boer, P., *et al.* (2001). Antipsychotic drugs classified by their effects on the release of dopamine and noradrenaline in the prefrontal cortex and stri-atum. *European Journal of Pharmacology*, **412**, 127–38.

49. Araneda, R. and Andrade, R. (1991). 5-Hydroxytryptamine 2 and 5-hydroxytryptamine1A receptors mediate opposing responses on membrane excitability in rat association cortex. *Neuroscience*, **40**, 399–412.

50. Ichikawa, J. and Meltzer, H.Y. (1999). R(+)-8-OH-DPAT, a serotonin1A receptor agonist, potentiated S(−) sulpiride-induced dopamine release in rat medial prefrontal cortex and nucleus accumbens but not striatum. *Journal of Pharmacology and Experimental Therapeutics*, **291**, 1227–32.

51. Sakaue, M., Somboonthum, P., Nishihara, B., *et al.* (2000). Postsynaptic 5-hydroxytryptamine(1A) receptor activation increases *in vivo* dopamine release in rat prefrontal cortex. *British Journal of Pharmacology*, **129**, 1028–34.

52. Sumiyoshi, T., Matsui, M., Yamashita, I., *et al.* (2001). Enhancement of cognitive performance in schizophrenia by addition of tandospirone to neuroleptic treatment. *American Journal of Psychiatry*, **158**, 1722–5.

53. Sumiyoshi, T., Park, S., Jayathilake, K., *et al.* (2007). Effect of buspirone, a serotonin(1A) partial agonist, on cognitive function in schizophrenia: a randomized, double-blind, placebo-controlled study. *Schizophrenia Research*, **95**, 158–68.

54. Bonaccorso, S., Meltzer, H.Y., Li, Z., *et al.* (2002). SR46349-B, a 5-HT(2A/2C) receptor antagonist, potentiates haloperidol-induced dopamine release in rat medial prefrontal cortex and nucleus accumbens. *Neuropsychopharmacology*, **27**, 430–41.

55. Kroeze, W.K., Hufeisen, S.J., Popadak, B.A., *et al.* (2003). H1-histamine receptor affinity predicts short-term weight gain for typical and atypical antipsychotic drugs. *Neuropsychopharmacology*, **28**, 519–26.

56. Reynolds, G.P., Templeman, L.A., Zhang, Z.J. (2005). The role of 5-HT2C receptor polymorphisms in the pharmacogenetics of antipsychotic drug treatment. *Progress in Neuropsychopharmacology and Biological Psychiatry*, **29**, 1021–8.

57. Geyer, M.A. and Ellenbroek, B. (2003). Animal behavior models of the mechanisms undelrying antipsychotic atypicality. *Progress in Neuro-Psychopharmacology and Biological Psychiatry*, **27**, 1071–9.

58. Maurel-Remy, S., Bervoets, K., Millan, M.J. (1995). Blockade of phencyclidine-induced hyperlocomotion by clozapine and MDL 100,907 in rats reflects antagonism of 5-HT2A receptors. *European Journal of Pharmacology*, **280**, R9–11.

59. Ahmed, A.O. and Bhat, I.A. (2014). Psychopharmacological treatment of neurocognitive deficits in people with schizophrenia: a review of old and new targets. *CNS Drugs*, **28**, 301–18.

60. Kane, J. and Marder, S. (1993). Psychopharmacologic treatment of schizophrenia. *Schizophrenia Bulletin*, **19**, 287–302.

61. Lieberman, J., Jody, D., Geisler, S., *et al.* (1993). Time course and biologic correlates of treatment response in fi rst–episode schizophrenia. *Archives of General Psychiatry*, **50**, 369–76.

62. Meltzer, H., Lee, M., Cola, P. (1998). The evolution of treatment resistance. Biological implications. *Journal of Clinical Psychopharmacology*, **18**, 5–11.

63. Meltzer, H. (1997). Treatment-resistant schizophrenia: the role of clozapine. *Current Medical Research Opinion*, **14**, 1–20.

64. Kane, J. and Marder, S. (1992). Psychopharmacologic treatment of schizophrenia. *Schizophrenia Bulletin*, **19**, 287–302.

65. Fusar-Poli, P., Papanastasiou, E., Stahl, D., *et al.* (2015). Treatments of negative symptoms in schizophrenia: meta-analysis of 168 randomized placebo-controlled trials. *Schizophrenia Bulletin*, **41**, 892–9.

66. Rajji, T.K., Miranda, D., Mulsant, B.H. (2014). Cognition, function, and disability in patients with schizophrenia: a review of longitudinal studies. *Canadian Journal of Psychiatry*, **59**, 13–17.

67. Saykin, A., Shtasel, D., Gur, R., *et al.* (1994). Neuropsychological deficits in neuroleptic naïve patients with first-episode schizophrenia. *Archives of General Psychiatry*, **51**, 124–31.

68. Palmer, B., Heaton, R., Paulsen, J., *et al.* (1997). Is it possible to be schizophrenic yet neuropsychologically normal? *Neuropsychology*, **11**, 437–46.

69. Green, M. (1996). What are the functional consequences of neurocognitive deficits in schizophrenia? *American Journal of Psychiatry*, **153**, 321–30.

70. Meltzer, H.Y. and McGurk, S. (1999). The effect of clozapine, risperidone and olanzapine on cognitive function in schizophrenia. *Schizophrenia Bulletin*, **25**, 233–56.

71. Caroff, S.N., Davis, V.G., Miller, D.D., *et al.* (2011). Treatment outcomes of patients with tardive dyskinesia and chronic schizophrenia. *Journal of Clinical Psychiatry*, **72**, 295–303.

72. Sheitman, B., Lee, H., Strauss, R., *et al.* (1997). The evaluation and treatment of first–episode psychosis. *Schizophrenia Bulletin*, **23**, 653–61.

73. McEvoy, J., Hogarty, G., Steingard, S. (1991). Optimal dose of neuroleptic in acute schizophrenia. A controlled study of the neuroleptic threshold and higher haloperidol dose. *Archives of General Psychiatry*, **48**, 739–45.

74. Carpenter, W., Buchanan, R., Kirkpatrick, B., *et al.* (1999). Diazepam treatment of early signs of exacerbation in schizophrenia. *American Journal of Psychiatry*, **156**, 299–303.

75. Schooler, N.R. (2003). Relapse and rehospitalization: comparing oral and depot antipsychotics. *Journal of Clinical Psychiatry*, **64** (suppl 16), 14–17.

76. Lehman, A.F., Kreyenbuhl, J., Buchanan, R.W., *et al.* (2004). The Schizophrenia Patient Outcomes Research Team (PORT): updated treatment recommendations 2003. *Schizophrenia Bulletin*, **30**, 193–217.

77. Lehman, A.F., *et al.* American Psychiatric Association; Steering Committee on Practice Guidelines. (2004). Practice guideline for the treatment of patients with schizophrenia, second edition. *American Journal of Psychiatry*, **161** (2 suppl), 1–56.

78. Cummings, J., Isaacson, S., Mills, R., *et al.* (2014). Pimavanserin for patients with Parkinson's disease psychosis: a randomised, placebo-controlled phase 3 trial. *Lancet*, **383**, 533–40.

79. Bobo, W.V., Stovall, J.A., Knostman, M., *et al.* (2010). Converting from brand-name to generic clozapine: a review of effec-tiveness and tolerability data. *American Journal of Health Systems Pharmacy*, **67**, 27–37.

80. Lieberman, J.A., Stroup, T.S., McEvoy, J.P., *et al.* (2005). Effectiveness of antipsychotic drugs in patients with chronic schizophrenia. *New England Journal of Medicine*, **353**, 1209–23.

81. Jones, P.B., Barnes, T.R., Davies, L., *et al.* (2006). Randomized controlled trial of the effect on quality of life of second- vs first-generation antipsychotic drugs in schizophrenia: Cost Utility of the Latest Antipsychotic Drugs in Schizophrenia Study (CUtLASS 1). *Archives of General Psychiatry*, **63**, 1079–87.

82. Kahn, R.S., Fleischhacker, W.W., Boter, H., *et al.* (2008). Effectiveness of antipsychotic drugs in first-episode schizophrenia and schizophreniform disorder: an open randomised clinical trial. *Lancet*, **371**, 1085–97.

83. McEvoy, J.P., Lieberman, J.A., Stroup, T.S., *et al.* (2006). Effectiveness of clozapine versus olanzapine, quetiapine, and risperidone in patients with chronic schizophrenia who did not respond to prior atypical antipsychotic treatment. *American Journal of Psychiatry*, **163**, 600–10.

84. Davies, L.M., Barnes, T.R., Jones, P.B., *et al.* (2008). A randomized controlled trial of the cost-utility of second-generation antipsychotics in people with psychosis and eligible for clozapine. *Value in Health*, **11**, 549–62.

85. Meltzer, H.Y. and Bobo, W.V. (2006). Interpreting the efficacy findings in the CATIE study: what clinicians should know. *CNS Spectrums*, **11** (7 suppl. 7), 14–24.

86. Kraemer, H.C., Glick, I.D., Klein, D.F. (2009). Clinical trials design lessons from the CATIE study. *American Journal of Psychiatry*, **166**, 1222–8.

87. Naber, D. and Lambert, M. (2009). The CATIE and CUtLASS studies in schizophrenia: results and implications for clinicians. *CNS Drugs*, **23**, 649–59.

88. Agius, M., Davis, A., Gilhooley, M., *et al.* (2010). What do large scale studies of medication in schizophrenia add to our management strategies? *Psychiatria Danubina*, **22**, 323–8.

89. Tarsy, D., Baldessarini, R.J., Tarazi, F.I. (2002). Effects of newer antipsychtoics on extrapyramidal function. *CNS Drugs*, **16**, 23–45.

90. Baldessarini, R. and Frankenberg, F. (1991). Clozapine: a novel antipsychotic agent. *New England Journal of Medicine*, **324**, 746–54.

91. Meltzer, H. (1979). The clozapine story. In: *The Handbook of Psychopharmacology Trials* (eds. M. Hertzman and D. Feltner), pp. 137–56. New York, NY: New York University Press.

92. Kane, J., Honigfeld, G., *et al.*; Clozaril Collaborative Study Group (1988). Clozapine for the treatment resistant schizophrenic: a double-blind comparison with chlorpromazine. *Archives of General Psychiatry*, **45**, 789–96.

93. Meltzer, H.Y., Alphs, L., *et al.*; International Suicide Prevention Trial Study Group. (2003). Clozapine treatment for suicidality in schizophrenia: International Suicide Prevention Trial (InterSePT). *Archives of General Psychiatry*, **60**, 82–91.

94. Weiner, D.M., Meltzer, H.Y., Veinbergs, I., *et al.* (2004). The role of M1 muscarinic receptor agonism of N-desmethylclozapine in the unique clinical effects of clozapine. *Psychopharmacology (Berlin)*, **177**, 207–16.

95. Meltzer, H.Y., Bobo, W.V., Lee, M.A., *et al.* (2010). A randomized trial comparing clozapine and typical neuroleptic drugs in non-treatment-resistant schizophrenia. *Psychiatry Research*, **177**, 286–93.

96. Schulte, P. (2003). What is an adequate trial with clozapine?: therapeutic drug monitoring and time to response in treatment-refractory schizophrenia. *Clinical Pharmacokinetics*, **42**, 607–18.

97. Shiloh, R., Zemishlany, Z., Aizenberg, D., *et al.* (1997). Sulpiride augmentation in people with schizophrenia partially responsive to clozapine. A double-blind, placebo-controlled study. *British Journal of Psychiatry*, **171**, 569–73.

98. Lally, J., Tully, J., Robertson, D., *et al.* (2016). Augmentation of clozapine with electroconvulsive therapy in treatment resistant schizophrenia: a systematic review and meta-analysis. *Schizophrenia Research*, **171**, 215–24.

99. Srisurapanont, M., Suttajit, S., Maneeton, H., Maneeton, B. (2015). Efficacy and safety of aripiprazole augmentation of clozapine in schizophrenia: a systematic review and meta-analysis of randomized-controlled trials. *Journal of Psychiatric Research*, **62**, 38–47.

100. Meltzer, H., Lee, M., Ranjan, R., *et al.* (1996). Relapse following clozapine withdrawal: effect of cyproheptadine plus neuroleptic. *Psychopharmacology*, **124**, 176–87.

101. Glick, I.D., Lemmens, P., Vester-Blokland, E. (2001). Treatment of the symptoms of schizophrenia: a combined analysis of double-blind studies comparing risperidone with haloperidol and other antipsychotic agents. *International Clinical Psychopharmacology*, **16**, 165–74.

102. Meltzer, H.Y., Lindenmayer, J.P., Kwentus, J., *et al.* (2014). A six month randomized controlled trial of long acting injectable risperidone 50 and 100mg in treatment resistant schizophrenia. *Schizophrenia Research*, **154**, 14–22.

103. Kumar, V. and Brecher, M. (1999). Psychopharmacology of atypical antipsychotics and clinical outcomes in elderly patients. *Journal of Clinical Psychiatry*, **60**, 10–16.

104. Simpson, G. and Lindenmayer, J. (1997). Extrapyramidal symptoms in patients treated with risperidone. *Journal of Clinical Psychopharmacology*, **17**, 194–201.

105. Meltzer, H.Y., Lindenmayer, J.P., Kwenhus, J., *et al.* (2014). A six month randomized controlled trial of long acting injectable risperidone 50 and 100 mg in treatment resistant schizophrenia. *Schizophrenia Research*, **154**, 14–22.

106. Csernansky, J.G., Mahmoud, R., Brenner, R. (2002). A comparison of risperidone and haloperidol for the prevention of relapse in patients with schizophrenia. *New England Journal of Medicine*, **346**, 16–22.

107. Rabinowitz, J., Lichtenberg, P., Kaplan, Z., *et al.* (2001). Rehospitalization rates of chronically ill schizohprenic patients discharged on a regimen of risperidone, olanzapine, or conventional antipsychotics. *American Journal of Psychiatry*, **158**, 266–9.

108. Moller, H.J. Long-acting injectable risperidone for the treatment of schizophrenia: clinical perspectives. *Drugs*, **67**, 1541–66.

109. Rummel-Kluge, C., Komossa, K., Schwarz, S., *et al.* Second-generation antipsychotic drugs and extrapyramidal side effects: a systematic review and meta-analysis of head-to-head comparisons. *Schizophrenia Bulletin*, **38**, 167–77.

110. Peuskens, J., Pani, L., Detraux, J., De Hert, M. (2014). The effects of novel and newly approved antipsychotics on serum prolactin levels: a comprehensive review. *CNS Drugs*, **28**, 421–53.

111. Carman, J., Peuskens, J., Vangeneugden, A. (1995). Risperidone in the treatment of negative symptoms of schizophrenia: a meta-analysis. *International Clinical Psychopharmacology*, **10**, 207–13.

112. Bobo, W.V. and Shelton, R.C. (2010). Risperidone long-acting injectable (Risperdal Consta®) for maintenance treatment in patients with bipolardisorder. *Expert Review of Neurotherapeutics*, **10**, 1637–58.

113. Meltzer, H.Y., Bobo, W.V., Roy, A., *et al.* (2008). A randomized, double-blind comparison of clozapine and high-dose olanzapine in treatment-resistant patients with schizophrenia. *Journal of Clinical Psychiatry*, **69**, 274–85.

114. Komossa, K., Rummel-Kluge, C., Hunger, H., *et al.* (2010). Olanzapine versus other atyipcal antipsychotics for schizophrenia. *Cochrane Database of Systematic Reviews*, **3**, CD006654.

115. Beasley, C., Tollefson, G., Tran, P., *et al.* (1996). Olanzapine versus placebo and haloperidol acute phase results of the North American double-blind olanzapine trial. *Neuropsychopharmacology*, **14**, 111–23.

116. Tollefson, G. and Sanger, T. (1997). Negative symptoms, a path analytic approach to a double-blind, placebo- and haloperidol-controlled clinical trial with olanzapine. *American Journal of Psychiatry*, **54**, 466–74.

117. Tran, P., Dellva, M., Tollefson, G., *et al.* (1998). Oral olanzapine versus oral haloperidol in the maintenance treatment of schizophrenia and related psychoses. *British Journal of Psychiatry*, **172**, 499–505.

118. Almond, S. and O'Donnell, O. (1998). Cost analysis of the treatment of schizophrenia in the UK: a comparison of olanzapine and haloperidol. *Pharmacogenomics*, **13**, 575–88.

119. Kinon, B.J., Ahl, J., Stauffer, V.L., *et al.* (2004). Dose response and atypical antipsychotics in schizophrenia. *CNS Drugs*, **18**, 597–616.

120. Wagstaff, A.J., Easton, J., Scott, L.J. (2005). Intramuscular olanzapine: a review of its use in the management of acute agitation. *CNS Drugs*, **19**, 147–64.

121. Bobo, W.V., Shelton, R.C. (2009). Fluoxetine and olanzapine combination therapy in treatment-resistant major depression: review of efficacy and safety data. *Expert Opinion on Pharmacotherapy*, **10**, 2145–59.

122. Silva, M.T., Zimmermann, I.R., Galvao, T.F., Pereira, M.G. (2013). Olanzapine plus fluoxetine for bipolar disorder: a systematic review and meta-analysis. *Journal of Affective Disorders*, **146**, 310–18.

123. Arvanitis, L. and Miller, B. (1997). Multiple fixed dose of 'Seroquel' (quetiapine) in patients with acute exacerbation of schizophrenia: a comparison with haloperidol and placebo. The Seroquel Trial 13 Study Group. *Biological Psychiatry*, **42**, 233–46.

124. Small, J., Hirsch, S., et al.; the Seroquel Study Group (1997). Quetiapine in patients with schizophrenia: a high- and low-dose double-blind comparison with placebo. *Archives of General Psychiatry*, **54**, 549–57.

125. Gefvert, O., Lundberg, T., Wieselgren, I.M., et al. (2001). D(2) and 5HT(2A) receptor occupancy of different doses of quetiapine in schizophrenia: a PET study. *European Neuropsychopharmacology*, **11**, 105–10.

126. Velligan, D.I., Newcomer, J., Pultz, J., et al. (2002). Does cognitive function improve with quetiapine in comparison to haloperidol? *Schizophrenia Research*, **53**, 239–48.

127. Fernandez, H.H., Trieschmann, M.E., Friedman, J.H. (2003). Treatment of psychosis in Parkinson's disease: safety considerations. *Drug Safety*, **26**, 643–59.

128. Yildiz, A., Nikodem, M., Vieta, E., et al. (2015). A network meta-analysis on comparative efficacy and all-cause discontinuation of antimanic treatments in acute bipolar mania. *Psychological Medicine*, **45**, 299–317.

129. Chiesa, A., Chierzi, F., De Ronchi, D., Serretti, A. (2012). Quetiapine for bipolar depression: a systematic review and meta-analysis. *International Clinical Psychopharmacology*, **27**, 76–90.

130. Suppes, T., Hirschfeld, R.M., Vieta, E., et al. (2008). Quetiapine for the treatment of bipolar II depression: analysis of data from two randomized, double-blind, placebo-controlled studies. *World Journal of Biological Psychiatry*, **9**, 198–211.

131. Ketter, T.A., Miller, S., Dell'Osso, B., Wang, P.W. (2016). Treatment of bipolar disorder: Review of evidence regarding quetiapine and lithium *Journal of Affective Disorders*, **191**, 256–73.

132. Bauer, M., Demyttenaere, K., El-Khalili, N., et al. (2014). Pooled analysis of adjunct extended-release quetiapine fumarate in patients with major depressive disorder according to ongoing SSRI or SNRI treatment. *International Clinical Psychopharmacology*, **29**, 16–25.

133. Stahl, S.M. and Shayegan, D.K. (2003). The psychopharmacology of ziprasidone: receptor-binding properties and real-world psychiatric practice. *Journal of Clinical Psychiatry*, **64** (Suppl 19), 6–12.

134. Davis, R. and Markham, A. (1997). Ziprasidone. *CNS Drugs*, **8**, 153–9.

135. Tandon, R., Harrigan, E., Zorn, S. (1997). Ziprasidone: a novel antipsychotic with unique pharmacology and therapeutic potential. *Journal of Serotonin Research*, **4**, 159–77.

136. Swainston, H.T. and Scott, L.J. (2006). Ziprasidone: a review of its use in schizophrenia and schizoaffective disorder. *CNS Drugs*, **20**, 1027–52.

137. Arato, M., O'Connor, R., Meltzer, H.Y. (2002). A 1-year, double-blind, placebo-controlled trial of ziprasidone 40, 80 and 160 mg/day in chronic schizophrenia: the Ziprasidone Extended Use in Schizophrenia (ZEUS) study. *International Clinical Psychopharmacology*, **17**, 207–15.

138. Hirsch, S.R., Kissling, W., Bauml, J., et al. (2002). A 28-week comparison of ziprasidone and haloperidol in outpatients with stable schizophrenia. *Journal of Clinical Psychiatry*, **63**, 516–23.

139. Daniel, D.G., Zimbroff, D.L., Potkin, S.G., et al. (1999). Ziprasidone 80 mg/day and 160 mg/day in the acute exacerbation of schizophrenia and schizoaffective disorder: a 6-week placebo-controlled trial. Ziprasidone Study Group. *Neuropsychopharmacology*, **20**, 491–505.

140. Harvey, P.D. (2003). Ziprasidone and cognition: the evolving story. *Journal of Clinical Psychiatry*, **64** (suppl 19), 33–9.

141. Phillips, G.A., Van Brunt, D.L., Roychowdhury, S.M., et al. (2006). The relationship between quality of life and clinical efficacy from a randomized trial comparing olanzapine and ziprasidone. *Journal of Clinical Psychiatry*, **67**, 1397–403.

142. Bernardo, M., Ramon Azanza, J., Rubio-Terres, C., et al. (2006). Cost-effectiveness analysis of schizophrenia relapse prevention: an economic evaluation of the ZEUS (Ziprasidone-Extended-Use-In- Schizophrenia) study in Spain. *Clinical Drug Investigation*, **26**, 447–57.

143. Mamo, D., Kapur, S., Shammi, C.M., et al. (2004). A PET study of dopamine D2 and serotonin 5-HT1 receptor occupancy in patients with schizophrenia treated with therapeutic doses of ziprasidone. *American Journal of Psychiatry*, **161**, 818–25.

144. Hamelin, B.A., Allard, S., Laplante, L., et al. The effect of timing of a standard meal on the pharmacokinetics and pharmacodynamics of the novel atypical antipsychotic agent ziprasidone. *Pharmacotherapy*, **18**, 9–15.

145. Daniel, D.G., Potkin, S.G., Reeves, K.R., et al. (2001). Intramuscular (IM) ziprasidone 20 mg is effective in reducing acute agitation associated with psychosis: a double-bline, randomized trial. *Psychopharmacology*, **155**, 128–34.

146. Newcomer, J.W. and Haupt, D.W. (2006). The metabolic effects of antipsychotic medications. *Canadian Journal of Psychiatry*, **51**, 480–91.

147. Haddad, P.M. and Anderson, I.M. (2002). Antipsychotic-related QTc prolongation, torsade de pointes and sudden death. *Drugs*, **62**, 1649–71.

148. Strom, B.L., Eng, S.M., Faich, G., et al. Comparative mortality associated with ziprasidone and olanzapine in real-world use among 18,154 patients with schizophrenia: The Ziprasidone Observational Study of Cardiac Outcomes (ZODIAC). *American Journal of Psychiatry*, **168**, 193–201.

149. Harrigan, E.P., Miceli, J.J., Anziano, R., et al. (2004). A randomized evaluation of the effects of six antipsychotic agents on QTc, in the absence and presence of metabolic inhibition. *Journal of Clinical Psychopharmacology*, **24**, 62–9.

150. Sachs, G.S., Ice, K.S., Chappell, P.B., et al. Efficacy and safety of adjunctive oral ziprasidone for acute treatment of depression in patients with bipolar I disorder: a randomized, double-blind, placebo-controlled trial. *Journal of Clinical Psychiatry*, **72**, 1413–22.

151. Burris, K.D., Molski, T.F., Xu, C., et al. (2002). Aripiprazole, a novel antipsychotic, is a high-affinity partial agonist at human dopamine D2 receptors. *Journal of Pharmacology and Experimental Therapeutics*, **302**, 381–9.

152. Jordan, S., Koprivica, V., Chen, R., et al. (2002). The antipsychotic aripiprazole is a potent, partial agonist at the human

5-HT1A receptor. *European Journal of Pharmacology*, **441**, 137–40.

153. El-Sayeh, H.G., Morganti, C., Adams, C.E. (2006). Aripiprazole for schizophrenia. Systematic review. *British Journal of Psychiatry*, **189**, 102–8.

154. Potkin, S.G., Saha, A.R., Kujawa, M.J., *et al.* (2003). Aripiprazole, an antipsychotic with a novel mechanism of action, and risperidone vs placebo in patients with schizophrenia and schizoaffective disorder. *Archives of General Psychiatry*, **60**, 681–90.

155. Piggott, T.A., Carson, W.H., *et al.*; Aripiprazole Study Group. (2003). Aripiprazole for the prevention of relapse in stabilized patients with chronic schizophrenia: a placebo-controlled 26-week study. *Journal of Clinical Psychiatry*, **64**, 1048–56.

156. Kasper, S., Lerman, M.N., McQuade, R.D., *et al.* (2003). Efficacy and safety of aripiprazole vs. haloperidol for long-term maintenance treatment following acute relapse of schizophrenia. *International Journal of Neuropsychopharmacology*, **6**, 325–37.

157. Kane, J.M., Meltzer, H.Y., *et al.*; Aripiprazole Study Group. (2007). Aripiprazole for treatment-resistant schizophrenia: results of a multicenter, randomized, double-blind, comparison study versus perphenazine. *Journal of Clinical Psychiatry*, **68**, 213–23.

158. Tandon, R., Marcus, R.N., Stock, E.G., *et al.* (2006). A prospective, multicenter, randomized, parallel-group, openlabel study of aripiprazole in the management of patients with schizophrenia or schizoaffective disorder in general psychiatric practice: Broad Effectiveness Trial With Aripiprazole (BETA). *Schizophrenia Research*, **84**, 77–89.

159. Chrzanowski, W.K., Marcus, R.N., Torbeyns, A., *et al.* (2006). Effectiveness of long-term aripiprazole therapy in patients with acutely relapsing or chronic, stable schizophrenia: a 52-week, open-label comparison with olanzapine. *Psychopharmacology*, **189**, 259–66.

160. Kern, R.S., Green, M.F., Cornblatt, B.A., *et al.* (2006). The neurocognitive effects of aripiprazole: an open-label comparison with olanzapine. *Psychopharmacology*, **187**, 312–20.

161. Tran-Johnson, T.K., Stack, D.A., Marcus, R.N., *et al.* (2007). Efficacy and safety of intramuscular aripiprazole in patients with acute agitation: a randomized, double-blind, placebo-controlled trial. *Journal of Clinical Psychiatry*, **68**, 111–19.

162. Fleischhacker, W.W., Sanchez, R., Perry, P.P., *et al.* (2014). Aripiprazole once-monthly for treatment of schizophrenia: double-blind, randomised, non-inferiority study. *British Journal of Psychiatry*, **205**, 135–44.

163. Citrome, L. (2016). Aripiprazole long-acting injectable formulations for schizophrenia: aripirazole monohydrate and aripiprazole lauroxil. *Expert Reviews of Clinical Pharmacology*, **9**, 169–86.

164. Meltzer, H.Y., Risinger, R., Nasrallah, H.A., *et al.* (2015). A randomized, double-blind, placebo-controlled trial of aripiprazole lauroxil in acute exacerbation of schizophrenia. *Journal of Clinical Psychiatry*, **76**, 1085–90.

165. Nelson, J.C., Thase, M.E., Bellocchio, E.E., *et al.* (2012). Efficacy of adjunctive aripiprazole in patients with major depressive disorder who showed minimal response to initial antidepressant therapy. *International Clinical Psychopharmacology*, **27**, 125–33.

166. Brown, R., Taylor, M.J., Geddes, J. (2013). Aripiprazole alone or in combination for acute mania. *Cochrane Database of Systematic Reviews*, **12**, CD005000.

167. Thase, M.E., Jonas, A., Khan, A., *et al.* (2008). Aripiprazole monotherapy in nonpsychotic bipolar I depression: results of 2 randomized, placebo-controlled studies. *Journal of Clinical Psychopharmacology*, **28**, 13–20.

168. Meltzer, H.Y., Bobo, W.V., Nuamah, I.F., *et al.* Efficacy and tolerability of oral paliperidone extended-release tablets in the treatment of acute schizophrenia: pooled data from three 6-week, placebo-controlled studies. *Journal of Clinical Psychiatry*, **69**, 817–29.

169. Nussbaum, A.M. and Stroup, T.S. (2012). Paliperidone palmitate for schizophrenia. *Cochrane Database of Systematic Reviews*, **6**, CD008296.

170. Carpiniello, B. and Pinna, F. (2016). Critical appraisal of 3-monthly paliperidone depot injections in the treatment of schizophrenia. *Drug Design, Development and Therapy*, **10**, 1731–42.

171. McKeage, K. and Plosker, G.L. (2004). Amisulpride: a review of its use in the management of schizophrenia. *CNS Drugs*, **18**, 933–56.

172. Möller, J., Boyer, P., *et al.*; the PROD–ASLP Study Group. (1997). Improvement of acute exacerbations of schizophrenia with amisulpride: a comparison with haloperidol. *Psychopharmacology*, **132**, 396–401.

173. Freeman, H. (1997). Amisulpride compared with standard antipsychotics in acute exacerbations of schizophrenia: three efficacy studies. *International Clinical Psychopharmacology*, **12**, 11–17.

174. Paillere–Martinot, M., Lecrubier, Y., Martinot, J., *et al.* (1995). Improvement of some schizophrenic deficit symptoms with low doses of amisulpride. *American Journal of Psychiatry*, **152**, 130–4.

175. Boyer, P., Lecrubier, Y., Pucch, A., *et al.* (1995). Treatment of negative symptoms in schizophrenia with amisulpride. *British Journal of Psychiatry*, **166**, 68–72.

176. Kopecek M., Bears M., Svarc J., Dockery C., Horacek J. (2004). Hyperprolactinemia after low dose of amisulpride. *Neuroendocrinology Letters*, **25**, 419–22.

177. Peuskens, J., Moller H.J., Puech, A. (2002). Amisulpride improves depressive symptoms in acute exacerbations of schizophrenia: comparison with haloperidol and risperidone. *European Neuropsychopharmacology*, **12**, 305–10.

178. Colonna, L., Saleem, P., Dondey-Nouvel, L., *et al.* (2000). Long-term safety and efficacy of amisulpride in subchronic or chronic schizophrenia. Amisulpride Study Group. *International Clinical Psychopharmacology*, **15**, 13–22.

179. Surguladze, S., Patel, A., Kerwin, R.W., *et al.* (2005). Cost analysis of treating schizophrenia with amisulpride: naturalistic mirror image study. *Progress in Neuropsychopharmacology and Biological Psychiatry*, **29**, 517–22.

180. Nakamura, M., Ogasa, M., Guarino, J., *et al.* (2009). Lurasidone in the treatment of acute schizophrenia: a double-blind, placebocontrolled trial. *Journal of Clinical Psychiatry*, **70**, 829–36.

181. Meltzer, H.Y., Cucchiaro, J., Silva, R., *et al.* (2011). Lurasidone in the treatment of schizophrenia: a randomized, double-blind, placebo- and olanzapine-controlled study. *American Journal of Psychiatry*, **168**, 957–67.

182. Kane, J.M. (2011). Lurasidone: a clinical overview. *Journal of Clinical Psychiatry*, **72**(Suppl. 1), 24–8.

183. Yasui-Furukori, N. (2012). Update on the development of lurasidone as a treatment for patients with acute schizophrenia. *Drug Design, Development and Therapy*, **6**, 107–15.

184. Tandon, R., Cucchiaro, J., Phillips, D., *et al.* (2016). A double-blind, placebo-controlled, randomized withdrawal study of

lurasidone for the maintenance of efficacy in patients with schizophrenia. *Journal of Psychopharmacology*, **30**, 69–77.

185. De Hert, M., Yu, W., Detraux, J., *et al.* (2012). Body weight and metabolic adverse effects of asenapine, iloperidone, lurasidone and paliperidone in the treatment of schizophrenia and bipolar disorder: a systematic review and exploratory meta-analysis. *CNS Drugs*, **26**, 733–59.

186. Loebel, A., Cucchiaro, J., Silva, R., *et al.* (2014). Lurasidone monotherapy in the treatment of bipolar I depression: a randomized, double-blind, placebo-controlled study. *American Journal of Psychiatry*, **171**, 160–8.

187. Loebel, A., Cucchiaro, J., Silve, R., *et al.* (2014). Lurasidone as adjunctive therapy with lithium or valproate for the treatment of bipolar I depression: a randomized, double-blind, placebo-controlled study. *American Journal of Psychiatry*, **171**, 169–77.

188. Suppes, T., Silva, R., Cucchiaro, J. *et al.* (2016). Lurasidone for the treatment of major depressive disorder with mixed features: a randomized, double-blind, placebo-controlled study. *American Journal of Psychiatry*, **173**, 400–7.

189. McIntyre, R.S., Cucchiaro, J., Pikalov, A., *et al.* (2015). Lurasidone in the treatment of bipolar depression with mixed (subsyndromal hypomanic) features: post hoc analysis of a randomized placebo-controlled trial. *Journal of Clinical Psychiatry*, **76**, 398–405.

190. Schotte, A., Janssen, P.F., Gommeren, W., *et al.* (1996). Risperidone compared with new and reference antipsychotic drugs: *in vitro* and *in vivo* receptor binding. *Psychopharmacology (Berlin)*, **124**, 57–73.

191. Ghanbari, R., El Mansari, M., Shahid, M., Blier, P. (2009). Electrophysiological characterization of the effects of asenapine at 5-HT(1A), 5-HT(2A), alpha(2)-adrenergic and D(2) receptors in the rat brain. *European Neuropsychopharmacology*, **19**, 177–87.

192. Potkin, S.G., Cohen, M., Panagides, J. (2007). Efficacy and tolerability of asenapine in acute schizophrenia: a placebo- and risperidonecontrolled trial. *Journal of Clinical Psychiatry*, **68**, 1492–500.

193. Kane, J.M., Cohen, M., Zhao, J., *et al.* (2010). Efficacy and safety of asenapine in a placebo- and haloperidolcontrolled trial in patients with acute exacerbation of schizophrenia. *Journal of Clinical Psychopharmacology*, **30**, 106–15.

194. Kane, J.M., Mackle, M., Snow-Adami, L., *et al.* (2011). A randomized placebo-controlled trial of asenapine for the prevention of relapse of schizophrenia after long-term treatment. *Journal of Clinical Psychiatry*, **72**, 349–55.

195. Schoemaker, J., Naber, D., Vrijland, P., *et al.* (2010). Long-term assessment of asenapine vs. olanzapine in patients with schizophrenia or schizoaffective disorder. *Pharmacopsychiatry*, **43**, 138–46.

196. Vita, A., De Peri, L., Siracusano, A., *et al.* (2013). Efficacy and tolerability of asenapine for acute mania in bipolar I disorder: meta-analyses of randomized-controlled trials. *International Clinical Psychopharmacology*, **28**, 219–27.

197. Landbloom, R.L., Mackle, M., Wu, X., *et al.* Asenapine: Efficacy and safety of 5 and 10mg bid in a 3-week, randomized, double-blind, placebo-controlled trial in adults with a manic or mixed episode associated with bipolar I disorder. *Journal of Affective Disorders*, **190**, 103–10.

198. Potkin, S.G., Litman, R.E., Torres, R., Wolfgang, C.D. (2008). Efficacy of iloperidone in the treatment of schizophrenia: initial phase 3 studies. *Journal of Clinical Psychopharmacology*, **28**(2 Suppl. 1), S4–11.

199. Cutler, A.J., Kalali, A.H., Weiden, P.J., *et al.* (2008). Four-week, double-blind, placebo- and ziprasidonecontrolled trial of iloperidone in patients with acute exacerbations of schizophrenia. *Journal of Clinical Psychopharmacology*, **28**(2 Suppl. 1), S20–8.

200. Potkin, S.G., Litman, R.E., Torres, R., Wolfgang, C.D. (2008). Efficacy of iloperidone in the treatment of schizophrenia: initial phase 3 studies. *Journal of Clinical Psychopharmacology*, **28**(2 Suppl. 1), S4–11.

201. Kane, J.M., Lauriello, J., Laska, E., *et al.* (2008). Long-term efficacy and safety of iloperidone: results from 3 clinical trials for the treatment of schizophrenia. *Journal of Clinical Psychopharmacology*, **28**(2 Suppl. 1), S29–35.

202. Citrome, L., Stensbol, T.B., Maeda, K. (2015). The preclinical profile of brexpiprazole: what is its clinical relevance for the treatment of psychiatric disorders? *Expert Review of Neurotherapeutics*, **15**,1219–29.

203. Correll, C.U., Skuban, A., Ouyang, J., *et al.* (2015). Efficacy and safety of brexpiprazole for the treatment of acute schizophrenia: a 6-week randomized, double-blind, placebo-controlled trial. *American Journal of Psychiatry*, **172**, 870–80.

204. Kane, J.M., Skuban, A., Ouyang, J., *et al.* (2015). A multi-center, randomized, double-blind, controlled phase 3 trial of fixed-dose brexpiprazole for the treatment of adults with acute schizophrenia. *Schizophrrenia Research*, **164**, 127–35.

205. Fleischhacker, W.W., Hobart, M., Ouyang, J., *et al.* (2016). Efficacy and safety of brexpiprazole (OPC-34712) as maintenance treatment in adults with schizophrenia: a randomized, double-blind, placebo-controlled study. *International Journal of Neuropsychopharmacology*, **20**, 11–21.

206. Thase, M.E., Fava, M., Hobart, M., *et al.* (2011). Efficacy of adjunctive OPC-34712 across multiple outcome measures in major depressive disorder: a phase II randomized, placebo-controlled study. *Neuropsychopharmacology*, **36**, S302–4.

207. Thase M.E., Youakim, J.M., Skuban, A., *et al.* Efficacy and safety of adjunctive brexpiprazole 2 mg in major depressive disorder: a phase 3, randomized, double-blind study in patients with inadequate response to antidepressants. *Journal of Clinical Psychiatry*, **76**, 1224–31.

208. Thase, M.E., Youakim, J.M., Skuban, A., *et al.* Adjunctive brexpiprazole 1 and 3 mg for patients with major depressive disorder following inadequate response to antidepressants: a phase 3, randomized, double-blind study. *Journal of Clinical Psychiatry*, **76**, 1232–40.

209. Newman-Tancredi, A. and Kleven, M.S. (2011). Comparative pharmacology of antipsychotics possessing combined dopamine D2 and serotonin 5-HT1A receptor properties. *Psychopharmacology (Berlin)*, **216**, 451–73.

210. Durgam, S., Starace, A., Migliore, R., *et al.* (2014). An evaluation of the safety and efficacy of cariprazine in patients with acute exacerbation of schizophrenia: a phase II, randomized clinical trial. *Schizophrenia Research*, **152**, 450–7.

211. Kane, J.M., Zukin, S., Wang, Y., *et al.* (2015). Efficacy and safety of cariprazine in acute exacerbation of schizophrenia: results from an international, phase III clinical trial. *Journal of Clinical Psychopharmacology*, **35**, 367–73.

212. Durgam, S., Cutler, A.J., Lu, K., *et al.* Cariprazine in acute exacerbation of schizophrenia: a fixed-dose, phase 3, randomized, double-blind, placebo- and active-controlled trial. *Journal of Clinical Psychiatry*, **76**, e1574–82.

213. Durgam, S., Earley, W., Li, R., *et al.* (2016). Long-term cariprazine treatment for the prevention of relapse in patients

with schizophrenia: a randomized, double-blind, placebo-controlled trial. *Schizophrenia Research*, **176**, 264–71.

214. Calabrese, J.R., Keck, P.E., Jr., Starace, A., *et al.* (2015). Efficacy and safety of low- and high-dose cariprazine in acute and mixed mania associated with bipolar I disorder: a double-blind, placebo-controlled study. *Journal of Clinical Psychiatry*, **76**, 284–92.

215. Sachs, G.S., Greenberg, W.M., Starace, A., *et al.* (2015). Cariprazine in the treatment of acute mania in bipolar I disorder: a double-blind, placebo-controlled, phase III trial. *Journal of Affective Disorders*, **174**, 296–302.

216. Durgam, S., Starace, A., Li, D., *et al.* (2015). The efficacy and tolerability of cariprazine in acute mania associated with bipolar I disorder: a phase II trial. *Bipolar Disorders*, **17**, 63–75.

217. Durgam, S., Earley, W., Lipschitz, A., *et al.* (2016). An 8-week randomized, double-blind, placebo-controlled evaluation of the safety and efficacy of cariprazine in patients with bipolar I depression. *American Journal of Psychiatry*, **173**, 271–81.

218. Bell, R., McLaren, A., Glanos, J., *et al.* (1998). The clinical use of plasma clozapine levels. *Australian and New Zealand Journal of Psychiatry*, **32**, 567–74.

219. Prior, T.I., Chue, P.S., Tibbo, P., *et al.* (1999). Drug metabolism and atypical antipsychotics. *European Neuropsychopharmacology*, **9**, 301–9.

220. Olesen, O.V. and Linnet, K. (2001). Contributions of five human cytochrome P450 isoforms to the *N*-demethylation of clozapine *in vitro* at low and high concentrations. *Journal of Clinical Pharmacology*, **41**, 823–32.

221. He, H. and Richardson, J. (1995). A pharmacological, pharmacokinetic and clinical overview of risperidone, a new antipsychotic that blocks serotonin 5-HT2 and dopamine D2 receptors. *International Clinical Psychopharmacology*, **10**, 19–30.

222. Tollefson, G. and Kuntz, A. (1999). Review of recent clinical studies with olanzapine. *British Journal of Psychiatry*, **37**, 30–5.

223. Aravagiri, M., Ames, D., Wirshing, W., *et al.* (1997). Plasma level monitoring of olanzapine in patients with schizophrenia: determination by high-performance liquid chromatography with electrochemical detection. *Therapeutic Drug Monitoring*, **19**, 307–13.

224. Tsuda, Y., Saruwatari, J., Yasui-Furukori, N. (2014). Meta-analysis: the effects of smoking on the disposition of two commonly used antipsychotic agents, olanzapine and clozapine. *BMJ Open*, **4**, e004216.

225. Casey, D. (1996). 'Seroquel'(quetiapine): preclinical and clinical findings of a new atypical antipsychotic. *Experimentation, Opinion and Investigation of Drugs*, **5**, 939–57.

226. Chengappa, K.N., Parepally, H., Brar, J.S., *et al.* (2003). A random-assigment, double-blind, clinical trial of once- vs twice-daily administration of quetiapine fumarate in patients with schizophrenia or schizoaffective disorder: a pilot study. *Canadian Journal of Psychiatry*, **48**, 187–94.

227. Beedham, C., Miceli, J.J., Obach, R.S. (2003). Ziprasidone metabolism, aldehyde oxidase, and clinical implications. *Journal of Clinical Psychopharmacology*, **23**, 229–32.

228. Swainston, H.T. and Perry, C.M. (2004). Aripiprazole: a review of its use in schizophrenia and schizoaffective disorder. *Drugs*, **64**, 1715–36.

229. Jung, S.M., Kim, K.A., Cho, H.K., *et al.* (2005). Cytochrome P450 3A inhibitor itraconazole affects plasma concentrations of risperidone and 9-hydroxyrisperidone in schizophrenic patients. *Clinical Pharmacology and Therapeutics*, **78**, 520–8.

230. Sheehan, J.J., Sliwa, J.K., Amatniek, J.C., *et al.* (2010). Atypical antipsychotic metabolism and excretion. *Current Drug Metabolism*, **11**, 516–25.

231. Sachdev, P. (1995). The epidemiology of drug-induced akathisia: Part I. Acute akathisia. *Schizophrenia Bulletin*, **21**, 431–49.

232. Atbasoglu, E.C., Schultz, S.K., Andreasen, N.C. (2001). The relationship of akathisia with suicidality and depersonalization among patients with schizophrenia. *Journal of Neuropsychiatry and Clinical Neuroscience*, **13**, 336–41.

233. Cavallaro, R. and Smeraldi, E. (1995). Antipsychotic-induced tardive dyskinesia. *CNS Drugs*, **4**, 278–93.

234. Kane, J.M. (2004). Tardive dyskinesia rates with atypical antipsychotics in adults: prevalence and incidence. *Journal of Clinical Psychiatry*, **65** (suppl 9), 16–20.

235. Zhang, W.F., Tan, Y.L., Zhang, X.Y., *et al.* (2011). Extract of Ginkgo biloba treatment for tardive dyskinesia in schizophrenia: a randomized, double-blind, placebo-controlled trial. *Journal of Clinical Psychiatry*, **72**, 615–21.

236. Pappa, S., Tsouli, S., Apostolou, G., *et al.* (2010). Effects of amantadine on tardive dyskinesia: a randomized, double-blind, placebo-controlled study. *Clinical Neuropharmacology*, **33**, 271–5.

237. Angus, S., Sugars, J., Koskewich, S., Schneider, N.M. (1997). A controlled trial of amantadine hydrochloride and neuroleptics in the treatment of tardive dyskinesia. *Journal of Clinical Psychopharmacology*, **17**, 88–91.

238. Muller, T. (2015). Valbenazine granted breakthrough drug status for treating tardive dyskinesia. *Expert Opinion on Investigational Drugs*, **24**, 737–42.

239. Kaur, N., Kumar, P., Jamwal, S., *et al.* Tetrabenazine: spotlight on drug review. *Annals of Neurosciences*, **23**, 176–85.

240. O'Brien, C.F., Jiminez, R., Hauser, R.A., *et al.* NBI-98854, a selective monoamine transport inhibitor for the treatment of tardive dyskinesia: a randomized, double-blind, placebo-controlled study. *Movement Disorders*, **30**, 1681–7.

241. Velamoor, V. (1998). Neuroleptic malignant syndrome. Recognition, prevention and management. *Drug Safety*, **19**, 73–81.

242. Alvir, J., Lieberman, J., Safferman, A., *et al.* (1993). Clozapine-induced agranulocytosis: incidence and risk factors in the United States. *New England Journal of Medicine*, **329**, 162–7.

243. Lieberman, J. and Safferman, A. (1992). Clinical profile of clozapine: adverse reactions and agranulocytosis. *Psychiatric Quarterly*, **63**, 51–70.

244. Merrill, D.B., Dec, G.W., Goff, D.C. (2005). Adverse cardiac effects associated with clozapine. *Journal of Clinical Psychopharmacology*, **25**, 32–41.

245. Collaborative Working Group. (1998). Adverse effects of the atypical antipsychotics. *Journal of Clinical Psychiatry*, **12**, 17–22.

246. Marder, S., Meibach, R. (1994). Risperidone in the treatment of schizophrenia. *American Journal of Psychiatry*, **151**, 825–35.

247. Kelly, D.L. and Love, R.C. (2001). Ziprasidone and the QTc interval: pharmacokinetic and pharmacodynamic considerations. *Psychopharmacology Bulletin*, **35**, 66–79.

248. Pae, C.U. (2009). A review of the safety and tolerability of aripiprazole. *Expert Opinion on Drug Safety*, **8**, 373–86.

249. Kramer, M., Simpson, G., Maciulis, V., *et al.* (2007). Paliperidone extended-release tablets for prevention of symptom recurrence in patients with schizophrenia: a randomized, double-blind, placebo-controlled study. *Journal of Clinical Psychopharmacology*, **27**, 6–14.

250. Thomas, J.E., Caballero, J., Harrington, C.A. (2015). The incidence of akathisia in the treatment of schizophrenia with aripirazole, asenapine, and lurasidone: a meta-analysis. *Current Neuropharmacology*, **13**, 681–91.

251. Meyer, J.M., Mao, Y., Pikalov, A., *et al.* (2015). Weight change during long-term treatment with lurasidone: pooled analysis of studies in patients with schizophrenia. *International Clinical Psychopharmacology*, **30**, 342–50.

252. Weiden, P.J., Cutler, A.J., Polymeropoulos, M.H., Wolfgang, C.D. (2008). Safety profile of iloperidone: a pooled analysis of 6-week acute-phase pivotal trials. *Journal of Clinical Psychopharmacology*, **28**(2 Suppl. 1), S12–19.

253. Citrome, L. (2015). Brexpiprazole for schizophrenia and as adjunct for major depressive disorder: a systematic review of the efficacy and safety profile for this newly approved antipsychotic—what is the number needed to treat, number needed to harm and likelihood to be helped or harmed? *International Journal of Clinical Practice*, **69**, 978–97.

254. Lao, K.S., He, Y., Wong, I.C., *et al.* (2016). Tolerability and safety profile of cariprazine in treating psychotic disorders, bipolar disorder and major depressive disorder: a systematic review with meta-analysis of randomized controlled trials. *CNS Drugs*, **30**, 1043–54.

255. Holloman, L.C. and Marder, S.R. (1997). Management of acute extrapyramidal effects induced by antipsychotic drugs. *American Journal of Health System Pharmacy*, **54**, 2461–77.

256. Konig, P., Chwatal, K., Havelec, L., *et al.* (1996). Amantadine versus biperiden: a double-blind study of treatment efficacy in neuroleptic extrapyramidal movement disorders. *Neuropsychobiology*, **33**, 80–4.

257. Lieberman, J.A., Davis, R.E., Correll, C.U., *et al.* (2016). ITI-007 for the treatment of schizophrenia: a 4-week randomized, double-blind, controlled trial. *Biological Psychiatry*, **79**, 952–61.

258. Light, G.A. and Swerdlow, N.R. (2015). Future clinical uses of neurophysiologicla biomarkers to predict and monitor treatment response for schizophrenia. *Annals of the New York Academy of Sciences*, **1344**, 105–19.

259. Sethi, S. and Brietzke, E. (2015). Omics-based biomarkers: application of metabomics in neuropsychiatric disorders. *International Journal of Neuropsychopharmacology*, **19**, pyv096.

260. Souza, R.P., Meltzer, H.Y., Lieberman, J.A., *et al.* (2010). Influence of neurexin 1 (NRXN1) polymorphisms in clozapine response. *Human Psychopharmacology*, **25**, 582–5.

# 65

# Treatment and management of patients with schizophrenia

*Joseph P. McEvoy, Kammarauche Asuzu, Daniel W. Bradford, Oliver Freudenreich, and Katherine H. Moyer*

## Overview

In this chapter, *treatment* will be defined as 'medical care given to a patient for an illness or injury' [1]. The treatment section will focus on biological aspects of schizophrenia and comorbid medical illnesses for which efficacious somatic treatments are available, including:

1. Positive psychopathology (delusional beliefs, hallucinatory perceptions, and disorganization of thinking and behaviour) associated with excessive dopamine release, which responds adequately to first-line antipsychotic medication (FL-APM.)
2. Positive psychopathology which does not respond adequately to FL-APM, for which a trial of clozapine is indicated.
3. Comorbid medical illnesses that shorten the lifespan of patients with schizophrenia, including those caused or worsened by treatment with FL-APM or clozapine.

In this chapter, *management* will be defined as 'the manner in which someone behaves toward or deals with someone or something' [1]. The management section will focus on:

1. Dealing with enduring deficits in cognition, motivation/expression, and sensorimotor function resulting from biological processes for which no somatic treatments are currently available, that are prominent in a subset of patients.
2. Dealing with enduring deficits in self-control, manifest in comorbid substance use disorder (SUD), impulsive character traits, and high-risk and disruptive behaviours, that are prominent in a subset of patients.
3. Dealing with enduring distress from adverse childhood experiences, ongoing life stress, and external and internalized stigma.

*Treatment* (medical care) can only be delivered effectively if clinical care systems modify their expectations of patients' functional capacities and accommodate clinical interactions and environments to *manage* (deal with) the enduring attributes of patients with schizophrenia.

Team-based care, for example, comprehensive first-episode psychosis (FEP) treatment programmes, integrated mental health care/primary care treatment programmes, and assertive community treatment (ACT) programmes, may offer the greatest benefit for the majority of patients with schizophrenia.

The enduring attributes of patients with schizophrenia interfere with chronic illness self-management. Family and important others (for example, partners, friends, and certified peer specialists) can assist where patients' functional capacities are limited; they should be welcome as members of care teams.

## Treatment

### Medical care for dopamine-related positive psychopathology (FL-APM)

Dopamine release in the terminal fields of ventral tegmental area (VTA) neurons is increased in the majority of unmedicated patients experiencing FEP or recurrent psychosis and is correlated with the severity of positive psychopathology [2]. Dopamine release in these regions is involved in the assignment of salience to items of sensory experience and intrapsychic life [3].

Patients entering FEP report experiences compatible with inappropriate assignment of salience to random observations and thoughts—'There is a brightness and clarity of outline of things around me. Last week I was with a girl and suddenly she seemed to get bigger and bigger', 'The sun seemed too big for me and it was coming closer', 'Big, magnified thoughts come into my head when I am speaking and put away the words I want to say, and make me stray away from what was in my mind' [4].

FL-APM act by binding, as antagonists or partial agonists, to dopamine D2 receptors in the terminal fields of VTA dopamine neurons, shielding them from excessive dopamine. These dopamine neurons subsequently reduce their activity, shifting into depolarization block [5].

The efficacy of FL-APM is greatest early in the illness. Therapeutic benefit occurs at lower doses of FL-APM in FEP, and a higher percentage of patients achieve remission of positive psychopathology (all items rated 'mild' or less, that is, they are uncommon and non-intrusive and do not drive behaviour), in comparison to chronic, multi-episode patients [6].

The goal of treatment with FL-APM is the achievement and maintenance of sustained remission, which is associated with better quality of life. For most patients, uninterrupted treatment with FL-APM is necessary for sustained remission.

Treatment with FL-APM should be initiated early. Longer duration of unmedicated psychosis (DUP) prior to FL-APM for FEP is associated with reduced likelihood of remission, more prominent negative psychopathology, and poorer functioning [7]. Longer cumulative duration of unmedicated relapses during the years following FEP is associated with loss of brain volume, more prominent cognitive impairment, and more FL-APM-resistant positive psychopathology [8].

The benefits of sustained remission with uninterrupted FL-APM are large. The risks of relapse are grievous, including derailment from trajectories of development (school, work, independent living, and relationships), violence, self-injury, hospitalization, or incarceration.

It appears that a minority of patients in sustained remission can be withdrawn from FL-APM after FEP and maintain good function and quality of life [9]. However, clinicians cannot identify these patients prospectively.

If a remitted patient insists on FL-APM discontinuation, gradual tapering over several months, with close observation by others (for example, family) and regular clinical contact, may permit early detection of relapse and re-initiation of FL-APM before grievous consequences occur.

Non-remitted patients are highly likely to rapidly relapse after FL-APM discontinuation, and FL-APM discontinuation should be discouraged [10].

Interruptions in treatment with FL-APM following FEP are common (50% in the first year), delay the achievement of remission, and increase the likelihood of relapse 5-fold [11]. Factors associated with relapse include comorbid SUD, lack of insight, and lack of engaged family [12], all acting through the final common pathway of interrupted FL-APM.

Impaired insight, an enduring deficit, is associated with higher levels of psychopathology and cognitive impairment, and reduced brain volumes, in patients with FEP [13].

Long-acting injected (LAI) FL-APM provide real-time, accurate information regarding treatment interruption. If patients fail to present for, or refuse, scheduled injections, clinicians and engaged family/others can express concern. Shared decision-making is undertaken with shared facts.

## Tolerability

There is little difference in efficacy, but substantial differences in side effects (and the ease with which side effects can be mitigated) among the FL-APM. Many FL-APM and many strategies to mitigate their side effects are available. It is reasonable to propose to patients the goal of minimal or no subjective distress or objective toxicity with FL-APM.

Clinicians may select 2–3 FL-APM to prescribe regularly, so as to become experienced and skilled in their use. Characteristics to consider include:

1. Side effects that can be mitigated by sensible dosing or well-tolerated concomitant medications.
2. Once-daily dosing of oral preparations.
3. Availability of LAI preparations.
4. Affordability.

Clinicians should describe common potential side effects of any FL-APM prescribed and strategies to monitor for, and mitigate, them. Patients should have contact information for clinicians, so that relief of side effects is quickly achieved and FL-APM discontinuation avoided.

### Early-onset extra-pyramidal side effects (EPSEs)

*Dystonic reactions* are spasmodic contractions of the face, neck, trunk, and/or extremities that can be frightening and uncomfortable, occurring most commonly in young male patients receiving high doses of FL-APM with preponderant dopamine D2 antagonism (for example, haloperidol). Dystonic reactions can be rapidly relieved by intramuscular anticholinergic or benzodiazepine medications. Clinicians may then consider switching the FL-APM or lowering the dose.

*Restlessness (akathisia)* occurs most commonly during treatment with haloperidol-like FL-APM or dopamine D2 partial agonists (for example, aripiprazole). Unrelenting restlessness has been associated with suicide and violence. Clinicians should inquire about, and observe for, (pacing, foot-tapping) restlessness. Clinicians may consider switching the FL-APM. Otherwise, extended treatment with β-blocking agents or benzodiazepines may be necessary to mitigate restlessness.

*Bradykinesia–rigidity* indicates excessive dopamine D2 receptor antagonism (calling for reduced FL-APM dose) or intrinsic susceptibility (suggesting consideration of clozapine). Tailoring individualized doses of haloperidol-like FL-APM to the 'neuroleptic threshold', at which point minimal bradykinesia–rigidity can be detected on examination, but no coarse EPSE is present, offers the therapeutic benefit of these agents with good tolerability [14].

Anticholinergic medications prescribed to treat early EPSE of FL-APM have dose-related side effects, including dry mouth, blurred vision, constipation, and cognitive impairment [15]. Reduction in coarse EPSE produced by anticholinergic medication is not accompanied by a reduced risk for tardive dyskinesia (TD). Dose reduction of FL-APM is the preferred approach to coarse EPSE.

### Late-onset EPSE

*Tardive dyskinesia* (TD) is manifest as involuntary, purposeless, repetitive movements commonly involving the lips (for example, pursing or smacking), jaw, and/or tongue, but also the upper regions of the face (blinking), distal extremities, and trunk. Patients with TD have difficulty not moving.

The movements can be disfiguring and stigmatizing. 'Mild' movements in a patient whose job requires social interaction may have 'severe' repercussions.

TD is believed to result from enhanced sensitivity of striatal dopamine D2 receptors (after years of deprivation of dopamine), which respond excessively to ambient synaptic dopamine.

Patients with FL-APM-resistant schizophrenia, especially those who are violent, may receive high doses of FL-APM, leading to TD.

Clozapine may relieve FL-APM-resistant positive psychopathology and TD in such patients [16].

Inhibitors of vesicular monoamine transporter-2 (VMAT2) block the uptake of dopamine into presynaptic vesicles of nigrostriatal dopamine neurons; these agents significantly reduce the severity of TD [17].

*Neuroleptic malignant syndrome* (NMS) is characterized by muscle rigidity that may be intense, creating heat and dissipating moisture. Immobility prevents fluid intake and increases the risk for infection and thromboembolism. Muscle fibre breakdown releases myoglobin that can precipitate in renal tubules in the setting of dehydration. FL-APM should be discontinued until NMS is resolved.

Supportive care focusing on hydration, identification and treatment of infection, prevention of thromboembolism, and treatment with dopamine agonists (for example, amantadine) and benzodiazepines reduces morbidity and mortality [18].

In severe cases that do not respond to supportive care, dantrolene (reduces excitation–contraction coupling in skeletal muscle) or electroconvulsive therapy should be considered. Extended muscle rigidity may result in persistent contractures.

### Prolactin-related side effects

Elevated prolactin levels result from antagonism at tubero-infundibular dopamine D2 receptors, located outside the blood–brain barrier (BBB), by FL-APM that penetrate the BBB poorly (for example, risperidone). Breast enlargement/lactation and sexual dysfunction may result in men and women, and menstrual cycling may be suppressed in women. Bone demineralization may result from reductions in oestrogen levels [19].

Clinicians may consider preferentially prescribing FL-APM that do not elevate prolactin.

Weight gain and metabolic side effects are discussed in Antipsychotic medications may cause or worsen modifiable risk factors , p. 671.

### Medical care for positive psychopathology that responds inadequately to FL-APM

Approximately 80% of FEP patients achieve remission of positive psychopathology over months of uninterrupted treatment with FL-APM; in most, substantial improvement is apparent within days. Approximately 20% are *treatment-resistant* at FEP and remain so thereafter [20]. *Earlier onset of FEP and longer DUP* prior to initiation of FL-APM reduce the likelihood of remission.

During the years following FEP, the *duration of unmedicated psychotic relapses* is associated with accrued FL-APM-resistant positive psychopathology and reduced brain volume [8]. Approximately 33% of patients become FL-APM-resistant, no longer demonstrating correlations between dopamine release and positive psychopathology [21].

Clozapine reduces positive psychopathology and mortality [22] in at least 40% of FL-APM-resistant patients, reduces aggression in patients selected for aggressiveness [23], and reduces self-injury in patients selected for self-injury [24]. Community tenure (avoidance of hospitalization or incarceration) is increased with clozapine.

Clozapine is under-utilized. Clinicians unfamiliar with the use of clozapine may consider referring FL-APM-resistant patients to clinicians who are experienced in its use.

Clozapine should be considered after two FL-APM trials have failed to produce adequate therapeutic benefit. Olanzapine may offer the greatest therapeutic benefit among FL-APM and should be considered for the second trial [25]. For early-onset psychosis or if aggression or self-injury is prominent, clozapine should be considered after one failed FL-APM trial. Patients who prove to be exquisitely susceptible to EPSE or who have experienced NMS may do best with clozapine.

Augmentation of clozapine with *electroconvulsive therapy* may reduce positive psychopathology, aggression, or self-injury in incomplete responders to clozapine alone [26].

### Clozapine side effects

*Agranulocytosis* occurs in approximately 1% of clozapine-treated patients, most commonly during the first 3 months of treatment [27]. Risk evaluation and mitigation strategies (REMS) guide monitoring.

*Myocarditis* occurs in approximately 0.2%, most commonly during weeks 3–4 of treatment. Monitoring eosinophil count, inflammation (for example, C-reactive protein), and muscle damage (for example, troponin) at baseline and at weeks 1–4 permits early detection and discontinuation of clozapine prior to extensive heart damage [28]. Slower titration of clozapine dose may reduce risk.

*Seizures* occur in 2–6%; risk is greater with prior seizures (for example, febrile seizures in childhood), head injury, and higher clozapine dose [28]. Therapeutic drug monitoring may avoid excessive clozapine blood levels. Myoclonus during dose titration foreshadows seizures [29].

*Salivary pooling*, related to increased salivation and decreased swallowing, may increase the risk for aspiration, especially during sleep. Quaternary anticholinergic agents (for example, glycopyrrolate) reduce salivation and do not penetrate the BBB [30].

*Constipation* is common and can lead to adynamic ileus and death. Daily stool softeners (for example, docusate) and a weekly osmotic laxative can be started when clozapine is initiated [31]. A stimulant laxative can be prescribed as needed.

*Venous thromboembolism* risk is increased 30-fold with clozapine [32]. Daily aspirin should be considered when starting clozapine.

There is *no therapeutic alternative* to clozapine in patients whose positive psychopathology, aggression, or self-injurious behaviour are resistant to FL-APM. Clinicians must strive to mitigate clozapine side effects for patients who benefit from its use, because few, if any, other therapeutic options exist.

### Accelerated mortality

Patients with schizophrenia die more than 20 years earlier than general population controls, primarily from medical causes of death that are similar to those of the general population (heart attacks, strokes, cancer, and complications of diabetes mellitus) [33]. *Modifiable risk factors* (MRFs) (for example, insulin resistance, dyslipidaemia, hypertension, cigarette smoking) for these causes of death are more prevalent and more severe, at any age, among patients with schizophrenia than among general population controls [34].

Children later diagnosed with schizophrenia are less physically active than general population children. Medication-naïve FEP patients have higher rates of obesity, insulin resistance, and smoking than general population controls [35].

Patients with schizophrenia and comorbid SUD (*vide infra*) engage in more high-risk behaviours, resulting in higher rates of infection with bloodborne viruses [HIV, hepatitis B virus (HBV), and hepatitis C virus (HCV)] than general population controls.

Rates of suicide, homicide, and accidental death are also increased.

## Antipsychotic medications may cause or worsen modifiable risk factors

FL-APM have varying propensities to cause or worsen weight gain, insulin resistance, or dyslipidaemia, or to reduce physical activity through sedation or EPSEs [35]. Clinicians may consider preferentially prescribing FL-APM with minimal propensities to cause or worsen MRFs.

Olanzapine and clozapine have high propensities and should not be prescribed for patients who achieve adequate therapeutic benefit from more benign FL-APM. If olanzapine or clozapine are necessary to achieve adequate therapeutic benefit, pre-emptive mitigation strategies (see Interventions to mitigate modifiable risk factors, p. 671) should be considered when these agents are started.

## Patients with schizophrenia commonly receive poor medical care

Rates of adherence to practice guidelines in general medical care settings are 'considerably lower' for patients with schizophrenia than for non-schizophrenic patients [33, 34]. Patients with schizophrenia and diabetes mellitus or hypertension [36] are less likely to receive guideline-concordant screenings, testing, and treatments. Following myocardial infarction, patients with schizophrenia are less likely to receive indicated reperfusion procedures [37].

Patients with schizophrenia and cancer die sooner than those with cancer alone. Including a psychiatrist in the cancer care team, ongoing prescription of antipsychotic medications, and prevention of relapse after cancer diagnosis significantly reduce the likelihood of disruption in cancer care [38].

The 'chronic care model' for optimal treatment and management of chronic biological illnesses envisions 'informed, activated patients' interacting productively with 'prepared, proactive practice teams' [39]. Patients with schizophrenia have difficulties being informed and activated because of distracting positive psychopathology and enduring deficits in cognition, motivation, and expression. Few medical care systems accommodate to make interactions with patients with schizophrenia more productive.

## Interventions to mitigate modifiable risk factors

Providing uninterrupted antipsychotic medications is associated with decreased all-cause mortality in schizophrenia [40].

Co-localization of primary care in mental health care facilities simplifies the cognitive/motivational challenges that patients with schizophrenia must overcome (for example, appointments at multiple locations and different times), facilitates communication among treating clinicians, and improves primary care outcomes [41].

Embedding nurses in mental health care facilities to assist patients with schizophrenia in overcoming obstacles to care (for example, making primary care appointments and arranging transportation), instruct patients and their families in chronic illness self-management, and co-ordinate prescribing across mental health and primary care providers reduces MRFs and mortality risk [42]. Certified peer specialists may also assist patients with chronic illness self-management, in particular through increased physical activity and medication compliance [43].

Efforts at smoking cessation should include both individual or group psychosocial support and adjunctive pharmacotherapy.

Efforts without pharmacotherapy are rarely successful in patients with schizophrenia. In 12-week trials, varenicline is superior to bupropion/nicotine replacement therapy (B/NRT), and B/NRT is superior to placebo in achieving smoking cessation in patients with schizophrenia [44], but post-trial relapse rates are high. Maintenance treatment with varenicline is significantly superior to placebo in sustaining smoking cessation [45]. Neither varenicline nor B/NRT has been associated with worsening of psychopathology or suicide, relative to placebo. Clinicians treating patients with schizophrenia may consider becoming skilled in the use of varenicline and B/NRT.

Metformin [46] and liraglutide [47] are associated with weight loss and reduced insulin resistance in patients receiving dopamine antagonist medications with high propensities to cause or worsen MRFs. Clinicians may consider becoming skilled in their use. Topiramate reduces weight gain associated with antipsychotic medications [48].

Patients with schizophrenia are more sedentary than the general population. Diet and exercise programmes targeting weight and fitness may reduce MRFs in patients with schizophrenia, but they are not commonly available.

### Women's issues

Women with schizophrenia report more lifetime sexual partners and higher rates of being raped or engaging in prostitution, but are less likely to have been tested for HIV, than general population women. They report fewer planned pregnancies, more unwanted pregnancies, and more abortions [49].

Sexual violence is associated with more severe positive psychopathology, comorbid SUD, and homelessness. Among homeless women with schizophrenia, sexual violence (97% lifetime incidence) 'amounts to normative experience' [50].

The benefits of continuing antipsychotic medications through pregnancy to prevent relapse outweigh the low risks of teratogenicity. However, antipsychotic medications throughout pregnancy is associated with greater weight gain and risks for gestational diabetes. Women with schizophrenia have higher rates of preterm birth.

Clozapine treatment during pregnancy is associated with over 2-fold increase in gestational diabetes. Infants born to mothers taking clozapine are more likely to be 'floppy' and to experience seizures, and they must be checked for agranulocytosis [51].

## Management

### Enduring deficits in cognition, motivation/expression, and sensorimotor function

A subset of the offspring of patients with schizophrenia, including many who will later become psychotic, display deficits in cognition, motivation/expression, and /or sensorimotor function in infancy and childhood, long before the onset of psychosis [52].

In large population cohorts, characterized in childhood and followed through adulthood, a subset of those children who will later become psychotic display deficits in cognition, motivation/expression, and/or sensorimotor function [53].

At adult-onset FEP, prominent impairments in cognition, motivation/expression, and/or sensorimotor function are present in a subset of patients and are associated with poor subsequent social and occupational function [54]. In early-onset FEP, prominent impairments are present in >80% of patients, in association with brain volume loss and FL-APM-resistant positive psychopathology [55].

During the years following FEP, increasing deficits in cognition and motivation/expression occur in a subset of patients, accompanied by brain volume loss and increasing FL-APM-resistant positive psychopathology [8].

Many, but not all, studies suggest that prominent impairments in cognition, motivation/expression, and sensorimotor function tend to occur in the same patients. Parsimony suggests the unproven possibility that the deficits share a common pathophysiology with variable distribution throughout the central nervous system. The deficits are enduring. They do not go away.

## Cognitive deficits

At FEP, patients perform at a level 1.5 standard deviations below the general population, with particular deficits in learning and memory [56]. Patients with chronic schizophrenia perform at a level 1.5–2.5 standard deviations below the general population (in the range of the lowest 5–10% of the general population), substantially limiting their abilities to engage successfully in real-world tasks [57], for example, self-management of chronic mental and physical illnesses.

Patients with schizophrenia show pronounced hypoactivation of circuitry in the 'multiple demand network' of the left lateral prefrontal cortex, including portions servicing initial, rudimentary processes (for example, updating, set shifting, and inhibition), compatible with a broad disruption of neuropsychological performance encompassing multiple cognitive domains [58]. Structural imaging studies also demonstrate disruption of white matter tracts 'facilitating information processing in the cortico-basal ganglia network' in patients with chronic schizophrenia [59].

The effects of APM on cognition in schizophrenia appear to be minimal. Adjunctive pharmacotherapies targeting cholinergic, glutamatergic, or serotonergic neurotransmissions have, so far, failed to improve cognition. Cognitive remediation has shown benefit in improving function in some, but not all, trials and may be of greatest value in supported employment settings [60]. Long-term durability of effects is not established.

Cognitive function is associated with cardio-respiratory function in patients with schizophrenia. Twelve-week programmes that engage patients with schizophrenia in vigorous physical exercise appear to improve cognitive function [61] and brain volume. These gains do not persist after the exercise programmes end, as patients resume their pre-programme activity levels.

Modifications/accommodations to deal with cognitive deficits are discussed in Modifications and accommodations, p. 672.

## Motivation/expression deficits

The assessment of 'primary' deficits in motivation/expression should be preceded by detection and correction of superficially similar phenomena, for example, akinesia or somnolence due to prescribed medications or SUD, catatonia, social withdrawal due to positive psychopathology (for example, paranoia), depression and anxiety, or behavioural regression due to isolation or social deprivation [62].

Deficits in motivation most powerfully predict social and occupational function [63]. Patients with schizophrenia appear able to experience pleasure when exposed to pleasant experiences but

have 'difficulty using mental representation of affective value to guide decision-making and goal-directed behavior' [63]. Areas of 'dysconnectivity associated with reward responsivity' have been identified in functional imaging studies [64].

At present, there is no convincing evidence regarding efficacy for any treatment for enduring deficits in motivation/expression [65].

## Neurological soft signs

Neurological soft signs (NSS) are 'non-localizing neurological abnormalities that cannot be related to impairment of a specific brain region' [66]. Typical NSS include impairments in motor coordination, the sequencing of complex movements, and sensory integration (for example, right–left discrimination).

NSS are observed in dopamine antagonist medication-naïve FEP patients and in the majority of patients with chronic schizophrenia. NSS are strongly associated with cognitive and motivation/expression deficits and with FL-APM-resistant positive psychopathology [67].

## Modifications and accommodations

Modifications are reductions in expectations as to what patients with schizophrenia can do, relative to general population controls. For example, patients with schizophrenia recall, on average, half as many words as general population controls after a single presentation of a word list [56]. They may do best with educational processes (for example, illness self-management information) that provide them with half as much information as the general population would be expected to remember. The information must be thoughtfully selected and include the critical facts to be transmitted.

Accommodations are adaptions in clinical interactions (for example, offering multiple brief sessions over time to transmit illness self-management information gradually) and in clinical environments (for example, co-localization of mental health and primary care) to achieve desired outcomes despite enduring deficits.

Modifications and accommodations are recommended for the informed consent process [68] in patients with schizophrenia, including adequate time for repeated presentations in minimally distracting settings, involving family members, consideration of multiple media (written, spoken, figures), and feedback testing: 'Professionals … and patients cannot be assured that they have understood one another—especially in the case of persons already known to suffer problems of comprehension—without some form of checking' [69]. Clinicians may consider more widespread use of such procedures.

Clinical staff and family/important others may also provide functions that patients cannot offer (for example, activity therapists initiating outings that patients with motivation deficits do not initiate but may enjoy).

Patients with schizophrenia display a wide range of severity of enduring deficits. In an optimal system, safe and comfortable housing options, offering a range of independence (matched to patients' cognitive function and initiative), would be available. However, the type of housing provided appears to be mostly driven by regional approaches to health planning [70]. Discussions about independence should include the risks of loneliness and of relapse [71].

In an optimal system, a range of opportunities for productive activities would be available, from sheltered workshops through accommodated work placements without pay (disability benefits are preserved) and supported employment programmes. Only approximately 10% of patients with schizophrenia can support themselves through competitive employment, but approximately 70% can participate in productive activities with accommodations [72]. Patients who successfully manage their illness can serve as Certified Peer Specialists, trained to share their experiences and coping strategies with other patients, providing support with illness management, communication with clinicians, and overall health—maintaining hope and reducing internalized stigma [73].

## Self-control

Across the general population, there is a gradient of self-control—'an effortful regulation of the self by the self' [74]. Self-control, assessed in early childhood, predicts multiple health, relationship, and achievement outcomes in adult life [75, 76].

Those in the lowest quintile of self-control display more SUD and criminality and poorer mental and physical health than the remainder of the general population, and they utilize disproportionate amounts of society's health care and criminal justice resources [75].

Those in the highest quintile are characterized by conscientiousness—'a large class of personality traits that include responsibility, industriousness, and orderliness' [74]—which is associated with higher incomes and occupational prestige, more stable and satisfying relationships, better health, and greater longevity [75].

A subset of patients with schizophrenia display enduring deficits in self-control, manifest in comorbid SUD, disruptive behaviours leading to hospitalization or incarceration, poor engagement with treatment, poor illness self-management, poor physical health, and accelerated mortality.

Patients with schizophrenia appear more likely to mate [77, 78] and to cohabitate with [79] deviant individuals, including those with deficits in self-control. These pairings may result in offspring with schizophrenia and deficits in self-control and in environments in which high rates of adverse childhood experiences (ACEs) and adult trauma occur.

## Comorbid substance use disorder

At FEP, at least 40% of patients use substances, predominantly marijuana or alcohol. Approximately half of those using substances cease without specific interventions. Patients who cease substance use are more likely to have engaged families, and their outcomes are as good as those of FEP patients without substance use [80].

Patients who continue substance use despite FEP, now diagnosed with comorbid SUD, have higher rates of first-degree relatives with SUD than other FEP patients [81]. They are predominantly male and demonstrate impulsiveness, sensation-seeking, and behavioural disinhibition [82], similar to general population individuals with SUD, features that are antithetical to conscientiousness. They are more likely to display features of conduct disorder in childhood and antisocial personality disorder (ASPD) as adults [83]. Risk for violence is modestly increased in schizophrenia, but substantially increased with comorbid SUD and ASPD [84].

Patients with schizophrenia and SUD have more frequent interruptions in antipsychotic medication, more severe positive psychopathology at cross-sectional assessments, higher rates of relapse and service utilization, lower rates of remission, and higher rates of completed suicide than patients with schizophrenia alone. Their all-cause mortality rate is substantially higher (SMR 8.46 versus 3.61) than that of patients with schizophrenia alone [85].

## Management and treatment of comorbid substance use disorder

Patients with schizophrenia and deficits in self-control are not help-seeking. Engagement may be initiated during hospitalization or incarceration, or through assertive outreach in the community.

Sustained engagement is simplified if patients reside with the family (who should also be engaged and supported) or have a residence (which may need to be provided as an initial priority).

Non-compliance with prescribed oral medication is to be expected. Some trials report reduced hospitalization or incarceration with LAI antipsychotic medication [86]. If compliance with oral medication and REMS procedures can be assured, clozapine may reduce substance use and positive psychopathology [87]. Trials with agents such as LAI naltrexone are needed.

A small percentage of patients with schizophrenia and SUD will engage in intensive, team-based approaches, for example Behavioural Treatment for Substance Abuse in Severe and Persistent Mental Illness (BTSAS) offering small groups twice a week for 6 months, motivational interviewing, monetary rewards for negative urine screens, and social skills training, that have been associated with a higher percentage of negative urine screens and fewer hospitalizations than standard care [88].

ACT teams bring treatment to patients with schizophrenia and deficits in self-control who are not help-seeking. Multi-disciplinary, well-staffed teams go out and find (assertive outreach) patients who do not come to clinic appointments, are available around the clock for crisis support, and directly provide (as opposed to making referrals for which patients will not show up) a broad range of services—'helping with illness management, medication management, housing, finances, and anything else critical to the individual's community adjustment' [89]. In clinical trials, patients assigned to ACT teams have fewer hospital days and better patient and family satisfaction (and connection) than patients in standard care.

Incorporation of Certified Peer Specialists in ACT teams may improve the functioning of patients receiving ACT services and leads to fewer days of homelessness or hospitalization [90].

## Adverse childhood experiences

In the general population, ACEs (for example, physical or sexual abuse, observed domestic violence, parental mental illness, death or separation/divorce, or placement in foster care) are associated with SUD, depression, and poorer health and quality of life in adulthood [91]. Environments in which one ACE occurs may also offer others, and 'accumulating levels of adversity often produce graded decrements in development and functioning' [92].

Patients with schizophrenia report more ACEs than the general population, and more ACEs are associated with more SUD, homelessness, incarceration, suicidal thoughts, and health problems (for example, HIV infection) [93].

## Interventions to mitigate adverse childhood experiences

Early nutritional [94] and psychosocial enrichment [95, 96] programmes supporting mothers and children at genetic and/or environmental risk may improve outcomes.

Resilience, 'defined as a dynamic process encompassing positive adaptions (not merely the absence of pathology or dysfunction) within the context of significant adversity' [97], may explain variance in outcomes after ACEs. Early conceptualizations of resilience focused on traits within individuals presumed to impart hardiness. Later conceptualizations also highlight 'affectional ties within the family and with extra-familial informal support systems' [98] that can be protective and potentially restorative. Resilience is not a fixed set of attributes, but a dynamic process that can change in response to new challenges, opportunities, and emerging competencies. Resilience-enhancing interventions are discussed in Individual resilience training, p. 675.

## Internalized stigma

'Stigma', directly translated, refers to a visible mark usually made by a pointed instrument. Current usage derives from the mark tattooed or branded into the skin of slaves or prisoners, denoting their undesirable status.

Internalized stigma, the degree to which patients accept that they are marked as less desirable, with less value or power, because of the presence of schizophrenia, is associated with greater feelings of depression, alienation, and perceived discrimination, and greater endorsement of unflattering mental illness stereotypes [99]. Clinicians may directly challenge internalized stigma through cognitive behavioural therapy [100].

## Stigma resistance

Stigma resistance, the degree to which patients reject derogatory self-assessments, is associated with higher self-esteem and reported empowerment, higher levels of hope and quality of life, and less depression [101]. Having social contacts (family and friends) and being in outpatient treatment—perceiving that one 'matters' to others—are associated with greater stigma resistance [102, 103]. Better cognitive functioning and higher levels of the personality trait of self-directedness are associated with greater stigma resistance.

Stigma resistance and resilience overlap. Sustaining connectedness with family and important others and providing the experience of productive activities may be important strategies for strengthening stigma resistance.

## Internalized stigma in caregivers

Caregivers of patients with schizophrenia report more internalized stigma than caregivers of patients with bipolar disorder or depression. Earlier age of onset of psychosis and longer duration of illness (markers of the degree of enduring impairment) are associated with higher levels of internalized stigma in caregivers [104]. Higher levels of internalized stigma are associated with higher levels of psychological morbidity in caregivers [105] and should be a target of family psychoeducation and support.

## Assignment of stigma by the public

The public assigns stigma based upon diagnosis (the most severe, for example, schizophrenia, assigned the most stigma), judgements of the intensity of treatment needed (for example, hospitalization vs outpatient care), and judgements of the level of associated psychosocial disabilities [106]. Efforts to improve the public's opinions of patients with schizophrenia have shown little effectiveness [107].

Non-psychiatric physicians responding to vignettes depicting various clinical populations expressed their least positive attitudes towards patients with schizophrenia and personality disorder and those classified as criminals. Mental health clinicians may preferentially refer patients with schizophrenia for non-psychiatric care to clinicians who have demonstrated more positive views of patients with schizophrenia.

## The right beginning: comprehensive FEP treatment programmes

Comprehensive FEP treatment programmes are team-based and offer evidence-based pharmacological treatment, involvement of family, support for patients' education/employment goals, and individual psychosocial treatments, usually for a period of 2 years. Patients assigned to comprehensive FEP treatment programmes are more likely to remain in treatment, have less psychopathology and fewer hospitalizations, and have improved functioning, while receiving lower doses of antipsychotic medications, relative to patients assigned to TAU (treatment as usual). They report better quality of life and satisfaction with treatment and are more likely to be in school or working. Their families report less burden than the families of patients assigned to TAU [10].

## Evidence-based pharmacological treatment

Sustained remission of positive psychopathology is the goal of pharmacological treatment. LAI FL-APM may be considered in patients with comorbid SUD, lack of insight, and/or no engaged family [108]. Use of the fewest medications, at the lowest effective doses, may offer treatment, with minimal or no side effects.

Interruptions in antipsychotic medication that lead to relapse can be detected quickly by team members (including family), and antipsychotic medication restarted. The duration of unmedicated relapse, not the occurrence, is associated with decline [8].

Monitoring of physical health and interventions to mitigate MRFs begins immediately in FEP treatment programmes [109]. Aerobic exercise may assist in managing weight and metabolic side effects and may benefit cognition and functioning [110].

## Engagement of families

Family members fear relapse [111] and struggle with their relative's enduring deficits. They should be included in shared decision-making about medications. They should be encouraged to provide cognitive and motivational functioning that patients lack, for example, assisting with illness management and including patients in enjoyable activities.

Family members are a resource that clinicians strengthen through knowledge and support through appreciation and encouragement. Real-world successes—the prevention of relapse, the achievement of productive activity by their relatives—may reduce their internalized stigma.

## Education/employment support

Assistance with education/employment may be the most attractive aspect of FEP treatment programmes for patients. Returning to productive activity (school or work) provides purpose and supports self-esteem, and offers opportunities for social engagement. Work may bring patients and their families additional income.

Current approaches place patients into productive activity rapidly as psychosis is controlled, in the hope of forestalling dependency and demoralization [112]. With team support, many patients successfully manage the challenges of school and work.

### Individual resilience training

Patients in individual resilience training (IRT) 'matter'—IRT focuses on their strengths and the achievement of their individual goals in recovery. Education about the psychotic episode and assistance in processing that experience are provided, and patients are taught strategies to prevent relapse. Overall functioning and illness management are approached through psychiatric rehabilitation techniques. Self-stigma and residual psychopathology are addressed through cognitive behavioural therapy techniques. Additional modules are available, as needed, to address SUD, traumatic experiences, and health maintenance. A training manual for IRT is available [113].

### Comprehensive FEP treatment programmes—terminable or interminable?

At 5 years, that is, 3 years after 2-year FEP programmes have ended, the large differences between patients who participated and those relegated to TAU are attenuated, and at 10 years, the differences are undetectable [114]. Three- and 5-year treatment programmes provide extended advantages for patients over TAU [115, 116].

Schizophrenia is a chronic illness for which the standard of care should be chronic comprehensive treatment to prevent progressive decline [117]. Risk for relapse continues, and relapse prevention must be sustained. Deficits endure, and accommodations to support functioning must be sustained. Traumatic life experiences and medical illnesses accrue. Family members grow old. The tasks of clinicians are long and arduous but can be rewarded by assisting patients to sustain remission and experience productive and satisfying lives.

## REFERENCES

1. noun: *treatment* the manner in which someone behaves toward or deals with someone or something. medical care given to a patient for an illness or injury. (Google Search, Google, 7 November 2017, Web, 8 November 2017).
2. Howes, O.D., McCutcheon, R., Owen, M.J., and Murray R.M. (2017). The Role of Genes, Stress, and Dopamine in the Development of Schizophrenia. *Biological Psychiatry*, **81**, 9–20.
3. Ceaser, A.E., and Barch, D.M. (2016). Striatal Activity is Associated with Deficits of Cognitive Control and Aberrant Salience for Patients with Schizophrenia. *Frontiers in Human Neuroscience*, **9**, 687.
4. Chapman, J. (1966). The early symptoms of schizophrenia. *British Journal of Psychiatry*. **112**, 225–51.
5. Valenti, O., Cifelli, P., Gill, K.M., and Grace, A.A. (2011). Antipsychotic drugs rapidly induce dopamine neuron depolarization block in a developmental rat model of schizophrenia. *Journal of Neuroscience,* **31**, 12330–8.
6. Andreasen, N.C., Carpenter, W.T. Jr., Kane, J.M., Lasser, R.A., Marder, S.R., and Weinberger, D.R. (2005). Remission in schizophrenia: proposed criteria and rationale for consensus. *American Journal of Psychiatry*, **162**, 441–9.
7. Santesteban-Echarri, O., Paino, M., Rice, S., *et al.* (2017). Predictors of functional recovery in first-episode psychosis: A systematic review and meta-analysis of longitudinal studies. *Clinical Psychology Review*, **58**, 59–75.
8. Andreasen, N.C., Liu, D., Ziebell, S., Vora, A., and Ho, B.C. (2013). Relapse duration, treatment intensity, and brain tissue loss in schizophrenia: a prospective longitudinal MRI study. *American Journal of Psychiatry,* **170**, 609–15.
9. Wunderink, L., Nieboer, R.M., Wiersma, D., Sytema, S., and Nienhuis, F.J. (2013). Recovery in remitted first-episode psychosis at 7 years of follow-up of an early dose reduction/discontinuation or maintenance treatment strategy: long-term follow-up of a 2-year randomized clinical trial. *JAMA Psychiatry*, **70**, 913–20.
10. Fusar-Poli, P., McGorry, P.D., and Kane, J.M. (2017). Improving outcomes of first-episode psychosis: an overview. *World Psychiatry*, **16**, 251–65.
11. Winton-Brown, T.T., Elanjithara, T., Power, P., Coentre, R., Blanco-Polaina, P., and McGuire, P. (2017). Five-fold increased risk of relapse following breaks in antipsychotic treatment of first episode psychosis. *Schizophrenia Research,* **170**, 50–6.
12. Alvarez-Jimenez, M., Priede, A., Hetrick, S.E., *et al.* (2012). Risk factors for relapse following treatment for first episode psychosis: a systematic review and meta-analysis of longitudinal studies. *Schizophrenia Research*, **139**, 116–28.
13. McEvoy, J.P., Johnson, J., Perkins, D., *et al.* (2006). Insight in first-episode psychosis. *Psychological Medicine*, **36**, 1385–93.
14. McEvoy, J.P., Hogarty, G.E., and Steingard, S. (1991). Optimal dose of neuroleptic in acute schizophrenia. A controlled study of the neuroleptic threshold and higher haloperidol dose. *Archive of General Psychiatry*, **48**, 739–45.
15. McEvoy, J.P. (1983). The clinical use of anticholinergic drugs as treatment for extrapyramidal side effects of neuroleptic drugs. *Journal of Clinical Pharmacology*, **3**, 288–302.
16. Lieberman, J.A., Saltz, B.L., Johns, C.A., Pollack, S., Borenstein, M., and Kane, J. (1991). The effects of clozapine on tardive dyskinesia. *British Journal of Psychiatry*, **158**, 503–10.
17. Jankovic, J. (2016). Dopamine depleters in the treatment of hyperkinetic movement disorders. *Expert Opinion on Pharmacotherapy*, **17**, 2461–70.
18. Caroff, S.N., and Mann, S.C. (1993). Neuroleptic malignant syndrome. *Medical Clinics of North America*, **77**, 185–202.
19. Grigg, J., Worsley, R., Thew, C., Gurvich, C., Thomas, N., and Kulkarni, J. (2017). Antipsychotic-induced hyperprolactinemia: synthesis of world-wide guidelines and integrated recommendations for assessment, management and future research. *Psychopharmacology (Berlin)*, **234**, 3279–97.
20. Demjaha, A., Lappin, J.M., Stahl, D., *et al.* (2017). Antipsychotic treatment resistance in first-episode psychosis: prevalence, subtypes and predictors. *Psychological Medicine*, **47**, 1981–9.
21. Gillespie, A.L., Samanaite, R., Mill, J., Egerton, A., and MacCabe, J.H. (2017). Is treatment-resistant schizophrenia categorically distinct from treatment-responsive schizophrenia? a systematic review. *BMC Psychiatry*, **17**, 12.
22. Wimberley, T., MacCabe, J.H., Laursen, T.M., *et al.* (2017). Mortality and Self-Harm in Association With Clozapine in Treatment-Resistant Schizophrenia. *American Journal of Psychiatry*, **174**, 990–8.
23. Krakowski, M.I., Czobor, P., Citrome, L., Bark, N., and Cooper, T.B. (2006). Atypical antipsychotic agents in the treatment of violent patients with schizophrenia and schizoaffective disorder. *Archive of General Psychiatry*, **63**, 622–9.
24. Meltzer, H.Y., Alphs, L., Green, A.I., *et al.*; International Suicide Prevention Trial Study Group. (2003). Clozapine treatment for suicidality in schizophrenia: International Suicide Prevention Trial (InterSePT). *Archives of General Psychiatry*, **60**, 82–91.

25. Lieberman, J.A., Stroup, T.S., McEvoy, J.P., *et al.*; Clinical Antipsychotic Trials of Intervention Effectiveness (CATIE) Investigators. (2005). Effectiveness of antipsychotic drugs in patients with chronic schizophrenia. *New England Journal of Medicine*, **353**, 1209–23.

26. Arumugham, S.S., Thirthalli, J., and Andrade, C. (2016). Efficacy and safety of combining clozapine with electrical or magnetic brain stimulation in treatment-refractory schizophrenia. *Expert Review of Clinical Pharmacology*, **9**, 1245–52.

27. Alvir, J.M., Lieberman, J.A., Safferman, A.Z., Schwimmer, J.L., and Schaaf, J.A. (1993). Clozapine-induced agranulocytosis. Incidence and risk factors in the United States. *New England Journal of Medicine*, **329**, 162–7.

28. Citrome, L., McEvoy, J.P., and Saklad, S.R. (2016). Guide to the Management of Clozapine-Related Tolerability and Safety Concerns. *Clinical Schizophrenia and Related Psychoses*, **10**, 163–77.

29. Osborne, I.J., and McIvor, R.J. (2015). Clozapine-induced myoclonus: a case report and review of the literature. *Therapeutic Advances in Psychopharmacology*, **5**, 351–6.

30. Man, W.H., Colen-de Koning, J.C., Schulte, P.F., *et al.* (2017). The Effect of Glycopyrrolate on Nocturnal Sialorrhea in Patients Using Clozapine: A Randomized, Crossover, Double-Blind, Placebo-Controlled Trial. *Journal of Clinical Pharmacology*, **37**, 155–61.

31. Every-Palmer, S., and Ellis, P.M. (2017). Clozapine-Induced Gastrointestinal Hypomotility: A 22-Year Bi-National Pharmacovigilance Study of Serious or Fatal 'Slow Gut' Reactions, and Comparison with International Drug Safety Advice. *CNS Drugs*, **31**, 699–709.

32. Paciullo, C.A. (2008). Evaluating the association between clozapine and venous thromboembolism. *American Journal of Health-System Pharmacy*, **65**, 1825–9.

33. De Hert, M., Correll, C.U., Bobes, J., *et al.* (2011). Physical illness in patients with severe mental disorders. I. Prevalence, impact of medications and disparities in health care. *World Psychiatry*, **10**, 52–77.

34. De Hert, M., Cohen, D., Bobes, J., *et al.* (2011). Physical illness in patients with severe mental disorders. II. Barriers to care, monitoring and treatment guidelines, plus recommendations at the system and individual level. *World Psychiatry*, **10**, 138–51.

35. Jensen, K.G., Correll, C.U., Rudå, D., *et al.* (2017). Pretreatment Cardiometabolic Status in Youth With Early-Onset Psychosis: Baseline Results From the TEA Trial. *Journal of Clinical Psychiatry*, **78**, e1035–46.

36. Correll, C.U., Detraux, J., De Lepeleire, J., and De Hert, M. (2015). Effects of antipsychotics, antidepressants and mood stabilizers on risk for physical diseases in people with schizophrenia, depression and bipolar disorder. *World Psychiatry*, **14**, 119–36.

37. Liu, J., Brown, J., Morton, S., *et al.* (2017). Disparities in diabetes and hypertension care for individuals with serious mental illness. *American Journal of Managed Care*, **23**, 304–8.

38. Campi, T.R. Jr., George, S., Villacís, D., Ward-Peterson, M., Barengo, N.C., and Zevallos, J.C. (2017). Effect of charted mental illness on reperfusion therapy in hospitalized patients with an acute myocardial infarction in Florida. *Medicine (Baltimore)*, **96**, e7788.

39. Irwin, K.E., Park, E.R., Shin, J.A., *et al.* (2017). Predictors of Disruptions in Breast Cancer Care for Individuals with Schizophrenia. *Oncologist*, **22**, 1374–82.

40. Bodenheimer, T., Wagner, E.H., and Grumbach, K. (2002). Improving primary care for patients with chronic illness. *JAMA*, **288**, 1775–9.

41. Torniainen, M., Mittendorfer-Rutz. E., Tanskanen. A., *et al.* (2015). Antipsychotic treatment and mortality in schizophrenia. *Schizophrenia Bulletin*, **41**, 656–63.

42. Druss, B.G., Rohrbaugh, R.M., Levinson, C.M., and Rosenheck, R.A. (2001). Integrated medical care for patients with serious psychiatric illness: a randomized trial. *Archive of General Psychiatry*, **58**, 861–8.

43. Druss, B.G., von Esenwein, S.A., Compton, M.T., Rask, K.J., Zhao, L., and Parker, R.M. (2010). A randomized trial of medical care management for community mental health settings: the Primary Care Access, Referral, and Evaluation (PCARE) study. *American Journal of Psychiatry*, **167**, 151–9.

44. Druss, B.G., Zhao, L., von Esenwein, S.A., *et al.* (2010). The Health and Recovery Peer (HARP) Program: a peer-led intervention to improve medical self-management for persons with serious mental illness. *Schizophrenia Research*, **118**, 264–70.

45. Anthenelli, R.M., Benowitz, N.L., West, R., *et al.* (2016). Neuropsychiatric safety and efficacy of varenicline, bupropion, and nicotine patch in smokers with and without psychiatric disorders (EAGLES): a double-blind, randomised, placebo-controlled clinical trial. *Lancet*, **387**, 2507–20.

46. Evins, A.E., Hoeppner, S.S., Schoenfeld, D.A., *et al.* (2017). Maintenance pharmacotherapy normalizes the relapse curve in recently abstinent tobacco smokers with schizophrenia and bipolar disorder. *Schizophrenia Research*, **183**, 124–9.

47. Hendrick, V., Dasher, R., Gitlin, M., and Parsi, M. (2017). Minimizing weight gain for patients taking antipsychotic medications: The potential role for early use of metformin. *Annals of Clinical Psychiatry*, **29**, 120–4.

48. Deutch, A.Y. (2017). Liraglutide for the Treatment of Antipsychotic Drug-Induced Weight Gain. *JAMA Psychiatry*, **74**, 1172–3.

49. Correll, C.U., Maayan, L., Kane, J., Hert, M.D., and Cohen, D. (2016). Efficacy for Psychopathology and Body Weight and Safety of Topiramate-Antipsychotic Cotreatment in Patients With Schizophrenia Spectrum Disorders: Results From a Meta-Analysis of Randomized Controlled Trials. *Journal of Clinical Psychiatry*, **77**, e745–56.

50. Miller, L.J., and Finnerty, M. (1996). Sexuality, pregnancy, and childrearing among women with schizophrenia-spectrum disorders. *Psychiatric Services*, **47**, 502–6.

51. Goodman, L.A., Dutton, M.A., and Harris, M. (1995). Episodically homeless women with serious mental illness: prevalence of physical and sexual assault. *American Journal of Orthopsychiatry*, **65**, 468–78.

52. Mehta, T.M., and Van Lieshout, R.J. (2017). A review of the safety of clozapine during pregnancy and lactation. *Archives of Women's Mental Health*, **20**, 1–9.

53. Hameed, M.A., and Lewis, A.J. (2016). Offspring of Parents with Schizophrenia: A Systematic Review of Developmental Features Across Childhood. *Harvard Review of Psychiatry*, **24**, 104–17.

54. Jones, P., Rodgers, B., Murray, R., and Marmot, M. (1994). Child development risk factors for adult schizophrenia in the British 1946 birth cohort. *Lancet*, **344**, 1398–402.

55. Puig, O., Baeza, I., de la Serna, E., *et al.* (2017). Persistent Negative Symptoms in First-Episode Psychosis: Early Cognitive and Social Functioning Correlates and Differences Between Early and Adult Onset. *Journal of Clinical Psychiatry*, **78**, 1414–22.

56. Driver, D.I., Gogtay, N., and Rapoport, J.L. (2013). Childhood onset schizophrenia and early onset schizophrenia spectrum disorders. *Child and Adolescent Psychiatric Clinics of North America*, **22**, 539–55.

57. Saykin, A.J., Gur, R.C., Gur, R.E., *et al.* (1991). Neuropsychological function in schizophrenia. Selective impairment in memory and learning. *Archives of General Psychiatry*, **48**, 618–24.

58. Keefe, R.S. (2014). The longitudinal course of cognitive impairment in schizophrenia: an examination of data from premorbid through posttreatment phases of illness. *Journal of Clinical Psychiatry*, **75 Suppl 2**, 8–13.

59. McTeague, L.M., Huemer, J., Carreon, D.M., Jiang, Y., Eickhoff, S.B., and Etkin, A. (2017). Identification of Common Neural Circuit Disruptions in Cognitive Control Across Psychiatric Disorders. *American Journal of Psychiatry*, **174**, 676–85.

60. Levitt, J.J., Nestor, P.G., Levin, L., *et al.* (2017). Reduced Structural Connectivity in Frontostriatal White Matter Tracts in the Associative Loop in Schizophrenia. *American Journal of Psychiatry*, **174**, 1102–11.

61. Yamaguchi, S., Sato, S., Horio, N., *et al.* (2017). Cost-effectiveness of cognitive remediation and supported employment for people with mental illness: a randomized controlled trial. *Psychological Medicine*, **47**, 53–65.

62. Kimhy, D., Vakhrusheva, J., Bartels, M.N., *et al.* (2015). The Impact of Aerobic Exercise on Brain-Derived Neurotrophic Factor and Neurocognition in Individuals With Schizophrenia: A Single-Blind, Randomized Clinical Trial. *Schizophrenia Bulletin*, **41**, 859–68.

63. Buchanan, R.W. (2007). Persistent negative symptoms in schizophrenia: an overview. *Schizophrenia Bulletin*, **33**, 1013–22.

64. Marder, S.R., and Galderisi, S. (2017). The current conceptualization of negative symptoms in schizophrenia. *World Psychiatry*, **16**, 14–24.

65. Barch, D.M. (2017). The Neural Correlates of Transdiagnostic Dimensions of Psychopathology. *American Journal of Psychiatry*, **174**, 613–15.

66. Veerman, S.R.T., Schulte, P.F.J., and de Haan, L. (2017). Treatment for Negative Symptoms in Schizophrenia: A Comprehensive Review. *Drugs*, **77**, 1423–59.

67. Bombin, I., Arango, C., and Buchanan, R.W. (2005). Significance and meaning of neurological signs in schizophrenia: two decades later. *Schizophrenia Bulletin*, **31**, 962–77.

68. Janssen, J., Diaz-Caneja, A., Reig, S., *et al.* (2009). Brain morphology and neurological soft signs in adolescents with first-episode psychosis. *British Journal of Psychiatry*, **195**, 227–33.

69. McEvoy, J.P., and Keefe, R.S.E. (1999). Informing subjects of risks and benefits. In: Pincus, H.A., Lieberman, J.A., and Ferris, S. (eds). *Ethics in Psychiatric Research: A Resource Manual for Human Subjects Protection*. American Psychiatric Association, Washington, DC; pp. 129–57.

70. Faden, R.R., and Beauchamp, T.L. (1986). *A History and Theory of Informed Consent*. Oxford University Press, New York, NY.

71. Killaspy, H. (2016). Supported accommodation for people with mental health problems. *World Psychiatry*, **15**, 74–5.

72. Green, M.F., Horan, W.P., Lee, J., McCleery, A., Reddy, L.F., and Wynn, J.K. (2018). Social Disconnection in Schizophrenia and the General Community. *Schizophrenia Bulletin*, 44, 242–9.

73. Falkum, E., Klungsøyr, O., Lystad, J.U., *et al.* Vocational rehabilitation for adults with psychotic disorders in a Scandinavian welfare society. *BMC Psychiatry*, **17**, 24.

74. Kuhn, W., Bellinger, J., Stevens-Manser, S., and Kaufman, L. (2015). Integration of peer specialists working in mental health service settings. *Community Mental Health Journal*, **51**, 453–8.

75. Duckworth, A.L. (2011). The significance of self-control. *Proceedings of the National Academy of Sciences of the United States of America*, **108**, 2639–40.

76. Moffitt, T.E., Arseneault, L., Belsky, D., *et al.* (2011). A gradient of childhood self-control predicts health, wealth, and public safety. *Proceedings of the National Academy of Sciences of the United States of America*, **108**, 2693–8.

77. Mischel, W., Ayduk, O., Berman, M.G., *et al.* (2011). 'Willpower' over the life span: decomposing self-regulation. *Social Cognitive and Affective Neuroscience*, **6**, 252–6.

78. Parnas, J. (1985). Mates of schizophrenic mothers. A study of assortative mating from the American-Danish high risk project. *British Journal of Psychiatry*, **146**, 490–7.

79. Kirkegaard-Sorensen, L., and Mednick, S.A. (1975). Registered criminality in families with children at high risk for schizophrenia. *Journal of Abnormal Psychology*, **84**, 197–204.

80. Thomsen, A.F., Olsbjerg, M., Andersen, P.K., and Kessing, L.V. (2013). Cohabitation patterns among patients with severe psychiatric disorders in the entire Danish population. *Psychological Medicine*, **43**, 1013–21.

81. Abdel-Baki, A., Ouellet-Plamondon, C., Salvat, É., Grar, K., and Potvin, S. (2017). Symptomatic and functional outcomes of substance use disorder persistence 2 years after admission to a first-episode psychosis program. *Psychiatry Research*, **247**, 113–19.

82. Faridi, K., Pawliuk, N., King, S., Joober, R., and Malla, A.K. (2009). Prevalence of psychotic and non-psychotic disorders in relatives of patients with a first episode psychosis. *Schizophrenia Research*, **114**, 57–63.

83. Dervaux, A., Bayle, F.J., Laqueille, X., *et al.* (2001). Is substance abuse in schizophrenia related to impulsivity, sensation seeking, anhedonia?. *American Journal of Psychiatry*, **158**, 492–4.

84. Hodgins, S., Tiihonen, J., and Ross, D. (2005). The consequences of conduct disorder for males who develop schizophrenia: associations with criminality, aggressive behavior, substance use, and psychiatric services. *Schizophrenia Research*, **78**, 323–35.

85. Volavka, J. (2014). Comorbid personality disorders and violent behavior in psychotic patients. *Psychiatric Quarterly*, **85**, 65–78.

86. Hjorthøj, C., Østergaard, M.L., and Benros, M.E., *et al.* (2015). Association between alcohol and substance use disorders and all-cause and cause-specific mortality in schizophrenia, bipolar disorder, and unipolar depression: a nationwide, prospective, register-based study. *Lancet Psychiatry*, **2**, 801–8.

87. Koola, M.M., Wehring, H.J., and Kelly, D.L. (2012). The Potential Role of Long-acting Injectable Antipsychotics in People with Schizophrenia and Comorbid Substance Use. *Journal of Dual Diagnosis*, **8**, 50–61.

88. Akerman, S.C., Brunette, M.F., Noordsy, D.L., and Green, A.I. (2014). Pharmacotherapy of Co-Occurring Schizophrenia and Substance Use Disorders. *Current Addiction Reports*, **1**, 251–60.

89. Bellack, A.S., Bennett, M.E., Gearon, J.S., Brown, C.H., and Yang, Y. (2006). A randomized clinical trial of a new behavioral treatment for drug abuse in people with severe and persistent mental illness. *Archive of General Psychiatry*, **63**, 426–32.

90. Bond, G.R., and Drake, R.E. (2015). The critical ingredients of assertive community treatment. *World Psychiatry*, **14**, 240–2.

91. van Vugt, M.D., Kroon, H., Delespaul, P.A., and Mulder, C.L. (2012). Consumer-providers in assertive community treatment programs: associations with client outcomes. *Psychiatry Services*, **63**, 477–81.

92. Felitti, V.J., Anda, R.F., Nordenberg, D., *et al.* (1998). Relationship of childhood abuse and household dysfunction to many of the leading causes of death in adults. The Adverse Childhood Experiences (ACE) Study. *American Journal of Preventative Medicine*, **14**, 245–58.

93. Mersky, J.P., Topitzes, J., and Reynolds, A.J. (2013). Impacts of adverse childhood experiences on health, mental health, and substance use in early adulthood: a cohort study of an urban, minority sample in the U.S. *Child Abuse and Neglect*, 37, 917–25.

94. Rosenberg, S.D., Lu, W., Mueser, K.T., Jankowski, M.K., and Cournos, F. (2007). Correlates of adverse childhood events among adults with schizophrenia spectrum disorders. *Psychiatric Services*, 58, 245–53.

95. Ross, R.G., Hunter, S.K., Hoffman, M.C., et al. (2016). Perinatal Phosphatidylcholine Supplementation and Early Childhood Behavior Problems: Evidence for CHRNA7 Moderation. *American Journal of Psychiatry*, 173, 509–16.

96. Raine, A., Mellingen, K., Liu, J., Venables, P., and Mednick, S.A. (2003). Effects of environmental enrichment at ages 3-5 years on schizotypal personality and antisocial behavior at ages 17 and 23 years. *American Journal of Psychiatry*, 160, 1627–35.

97. Jaffee, S.R., Bowes, L., Ouellet-Morin, I., et al. (2013). Safe, stable, nurturing relationships break the intergenerational cycle of abuse: a prospective nationally representative cohort of children in the United Kingdom. *Journal of Adolescent Health*, 53(4 Suppl), S4–10.

98. Luthar, S.S. (2006). Resilience in development: a synthesis of research across five decades. In: Cicchetti, D. and Cohen, D.J. (eds.). *Developmental Psychopathology: Risk, Disorder, and Adaptation*. Wiley, New York, NY; pp. 739–95.

99. Saltzman, W.R., Lester, P., Beardslee, W.R., Layne, C.M., Woodward, K., and Nash, W.P. (2011). Mechanisms of risk and resilience in military families: theoretical and empirical basis of a family-focused resilience enhancement program. *Clinical Child and Family Psychology Review*, 14, 213–30.

100. Oliveira, S.E., Esteves, F., and Carvalho, H. (2015). Clinical profiles of stigma experiences, self-esteem and social relationships among people with schizophrenia, depressive, and bipolar disorders. *Psychiatry Research*, 229,167–73.

101. Moritz, S., Mahlke, C., Westermann, S., et al. (2018). Embracing Psychosis: A Cognitive Insight Intervention Improves Personal Narratives and Meaning-Making in Patients With Schizophrenia. *Schizophrenia Bulletin*, 44, 307–16.

102. Lau, Y.W., Picco L., Pang, S., et al. (2017). Stigma resistance and its association with internalised stigma and psychosocial outcomes among psychiatric outpatients. *Psychiatry Research*, 257, 72–8.

103. Pernice, F.M., Biegel, D.E., Kim, J.Y., and Conrad-Garrisi, D. (2017). The Mediating Role of Mattering to Others in Recovery and Stigma. *Psychiatric Rehabilitation Journal*, 40, 395–404

104. Ong, H.C., Ibrahim, N., and Wahab, S. (2016). Psychological distress, perceived stigma, and coping among caregivers of patients with schizophrenia. *Psychology Research and Behavior Management*, 9, 211–18.

105. Magaña, S.M., Ramírez García, J.I., Hernández, M.G., and Cortez, R. (2007). Psychological distress among latino family caregivers of adults with schizophrenia: the roles of burden and stigma. *Psychiatric Services*, 58, 378–84.

106. Stuber, J.P., Rocha, A., Christian, A., and Link, B.G. (2014). Conceptions of mental illness: attitudes of mental health professionals and the general public. *Psychiatric Services*, 65, 490–7.

107. Corrigan, P.W. (2016). Lessons learned from unintended consequences about erasing the stigma of mental illness. *World Psychiatry*, 15, 67–73.

108. Subotnik, K.L., Casaus, L.R., Ventura, J., et al. (2015). Long-Acting Injectable Risperidone for Relapse Prevention and Control of Breakthrough Symptoms After a Recent First Episode of Schizophrenia. A Randomized Clinical Trial. *JAMA Psychiatry*, 72, 822–9.

109. Pillinger, T., Beck, K., Gobjila, C., Donocik, J.G., Jauhar, S., and Howes, O.D. (2017). Impaired Glucose Homeostasis in First-Episode Schizophrenia: A Systematic Review and Meta-analysis. *JAMA Psychiatry*, 74, 261–9.

110. Firth, J., Carney, R., French, P., Elliott, R., Cotter, J., and Yung, A.R. (2018). Long-term maintenance and effects of exercise in early psychosis. *Early Intervention in Psychiatry*, 12, 578–85.

111. Lal, S., Malla, A., Marandola, G., et al. (2019). "Worried about relapse": Family members' experiences and perspectives of relapse in first-episode psychosis. *Early Intervention in Psychiatry*, 13, 24–9.

112. Becker, D.R., Drake, R.E., and Bond, G.R. (2014). The IPS supported employment learning collaborative. *Psychiatric Rehabilitation Journal*, 7, 79–85.

113. Penn, D.L., Meyer, P.S., and Gottlieb, J.D. (2014). *Individual Resiliency Training (IRT). A Part of the NAVIGATE Program for First Episode Psychosis*. Clinician Manual. 1 April 2014.

114. Secher, R.G., Hjorthøj, C.R., Austin, S.F., et al. (2015). Ten-year follow-up of the OPUS specialized early intervention trial for patients with a first episode of psychosis. *Schizophrenia Bulletin*, 41, 617–26.

115. Chang, W.C., Chan, G.H., and Jim, O.T. (2015). Optimal duration of an early intervention programme for first-episode psychosis: randomised controlled trial. *British Journal of Psychiatry*, 206, 492–500.

116. Malla, A., Joober, R., Iyer, S., et al. (2017). Comparing three-year extension of early intervention service to regular care following two years of early intervention service in first-episode psychosis: a randomized single blind clinical trial. *World Psychiatry*, 16, 278–86.

117. Kotov, R., Fochtmann, L., Li, K., et al. (2017). Declining Clinical Course of Psychotic Disorders Over the Two Decades Following First Hospitalization: Evidence From the Suffolk County Mental Health Project. *American Journal of Psychiatry*, 174, 1064–74.

# SECTION 10
# Mood disorders

# 66

# Diagnosis, classification, and differential diagnosis of mood disorders

*S. Nassir Ghaemi and Sivan Mauer*

## Diagnosis

### Phenomenology

Phenomenology precedes diagnosis. Phenomenology reflects not only observed signs and symptoms, but also the subjective experience of the person with signs and symptoms. Further, phenomenology involves the interpretation of data obtained in the context of our current knowledge and prior theories. Based on phenomenology, this chapter analyses standard DSM and alternative non-DSM diagnostic approaches to mood disorders.

### DSM-based definitions

The standard DSM-based definition for a depressive episode involves the occurrence of 2 weeks or more of depressive neurovegetative criteria, defined as the following: sleep alterations (insomnia or hypersomnia), appetite alterations (increased or decreased), diminished interest or anhedonia, decreased concentration, low energy, guilt, psychomotor changes (agitation or retardation), and suicidal thoughts. Along with depressed mood, the presence of four of eight of these criteria for 2 weeks or longer represents the standard definition of a DSM-5 'major depressive episode'.

If no manic or hypomanic episodes in the past are identified, then the diagnosis of a current major depressive episode leads to a longitudinal diagnosis of 'major depressive disorder' (MDD), which will be discussed in more detail later. Subtypes in DSM-5 for MDD are atypical features (which represent mainly increased sleep and appetite, along with heightened mood reactivity), melancholic features (defined by no mood reactivity, along with marked psychomotor retardation and anhedonia), and psychotic features (the presence of delusions/hallucinations).

Manic episodes are defined as euphoric or irritable mood with three or more of seven manic criteria, as follows: decreased need for sleep with increased energy, distractibility, grandiosity or inflated self-esteem, flight of ideas or racing thoughts, increased talkativeness or pressured speech, increased goal-directed activities or psychomotor agitation, and impulsive behaviour (such as sexual impulsivity or spending sprees). If such symptoms are present for 1 week or longer with notable functional impairment, a manic episode

is diagnosed, leading to a DSM-5 diagnosis of type I bipolar disorder. If such symptoms are present for at least 4 days, but without notable functional impairment, a hypomanic episode is diagnosed. If not a single manic episode had occurred ever, but only hypomanic episodes are present, along with at least one major depressive episode, then the DSM-5 diagnosis of type II bipolar disorder is made.

If manic symptoms occur for less than 4 days, or if other specific thresholds are not met for manic or hypomanic episodes, then the DSM-5 diagnosis for such bipolar-like conditions is 'unspecified bipolar disorder'.

Manic episodes can be characterized by psychotic features (presence of delusions/hallucinations). If psychotic features are present, then hypomania cannot be diagnosed (since such features involve notable impairment by definition). Similarly, if a patient is hospitalized, irrespective of duration of manic symptoms, a manic episode is diagnosed, not a hypomanic episode, again because hospitalization involves notable functional impairment by definition.

If manic or hypomanic episodes are caused by drugs (like antidepressants), then the diagnosis of bipolar disorder is still made in DSM-5. This is an important change from DSM-IV where antidepressant related mania/hypomania was viewed as an exclusion factor, which could not be used to diagnose bipolar disorder. Extensive research in the last two decades has shown that this DSM-IV exclusion is not supported scientifically and that mania/hypomania occur with antidepressants almost exclusively in persons who have bipolar illness, rather than in unipolar depression [1, 2].

### Non-DSM-based definitions

In a non-DSM based approach to diagnosis, beginning with the phenomenology of mood disorders, an initial observation is that these conditions are not primarily disorders of mood. The term 'mood disorders' is a misnomer, if interpreted, as is commonly the case, to mean that mood is central to diagnosis. In fact, mood is variable in the phenomenology of these conditions, and the most consistent clinical features for diagnosis are psychomotor changes. One can have depression without any sad mood at all; instead anhedonia is present. One can have mania without any euphoric mood at all; instead irritability is present. Classically, depression was characterized by the slowing down of one's thoughts, feelings, and movements. In other words, depression involved psychomotor retardation. Classically, mania was characterized by the speeding up of one's thoughts, feelings, and movements. In other words, mania involved psychomotor activation. Thus, psychomotor aspects can be seen as central to these conditions [3, 4].

It might be suggested therefore that these conditions should not be called mood disorders, a term which was instituted officially by DSM-III in 1980. The older term 'affective' disorder captures some of the larger context of the phenomenology of these conditions. Some have suggested another phrase, like 'mood and movement' disorders [5], be used instead to capture the importance of the motor aspects of these conditions.

The term 'disorder' also can be questioned. It is another official term instituted by DSM-III in 1980, with the conscious intention of being 'neutral' as to aetiology. This neutrality, however, can come at the expense of clarity. The term 'disorder' is intentionally vague—some interpret it biologically to reflect a disease concept; others interpret it psychologically to reflect thought patterns or emotional experiences from the present or past; still others view it socially as reflecting medical interpretations of social conflict. The range of affective conditions is broad enough that it includes disease entities, as well as social problems and some forms of psychological developmental changes. All these varieties of affective conditions are conflated into one word with many meanings.

### Mixed states

The most common approach to the description of the phenomenology of mood conditions contrasts depression and mania. While this clinical distinction can and should be made, it is not easy to make. It also is important to acknowledge that the phenomenology of mood conditions involves the frequent, if not usual, admixture of manic and depressive symptoms at the same time—called mixed states. In this scenario, a full-blown clinical depression may be present, but some manic symptoms may also be present such as rapid thoughts, increased sexual drive, and marked anger and mood lability. Thus, one can think of mood episodes on a spectrum from pure depression to pure mania, with many mixed states in between (Fig. 66.1).

Another variety involves classic psychomotor retarded depression, lasting weeks to months, interspersed with very brief bursts of manic symptoms lasting hours to days. A third variety involves a full-blown manic episode, but with the presence of sad mood or suicidal thoughts or other potential depressive symptoms such as guilt or low self-esteem.

When defined in this manner broadly, mixed states have been reported to be the most common presentation of mood states [6]. This broad definition includes concepts such as agitated depression and dysphoric mania. If defined in this way, mania and depression would be seen as uncommon pure variants of mood states, while the most common mixed states are a mixture of two.

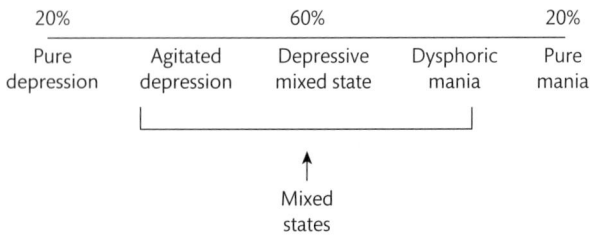

**Fig. 66.1** The mood episode spectrum.

If this phenomenology is correct, then it has important implications for the classification of diagnoses. The current diagnostic system is based completely on the distinction of depression and mania. If manic vs depressive states cannot be distinguished in most cases, then the current diagnostic system would be very difficult to implement validly. Put otherwise, the frequent presence of mixed states would invalidate the diagnostic system built on a mania vs depression dichotomy.

### Psychosis

Classically, the key controversy in the phenomenology of mood disorders involved psychotic conditions like schizophrenia. This past debate thankfully has yielded to a gradual consensus, as the conceptualization of schizophrenia has evolved to a chronic and constant disease of delusions or hallucinations. This view, which dates back to Kraepelin, still is challenged at times, though often with a misinterpretation of Kraepelin's view of manic–depressive illness (MDI). His original MDI concept involved the basic idea that psychotic symptoms, if present, were not constant. They came and went. In contrast, psychotic symptoms were present in dementia praecox all the time. Kraepelin can be misinterpreted to hold that mood conditions recover completely forever. Then contemporary critics point to the fact that long-term symptoms are present in mood disorders, as in other chronic conditions like schizophrenia. In fact, the Kraepelinian view was simply that mood episodes are episodic, which means they have a beginning and an end. This episodicity does not imply that once an episode ends, there will never be any future episodes, that is, that the patient is 'recovered' forever. It implies that acute episodes end and temporary recovery occurs, unlike schizophrenia where acute exacerbations merge into chronic psychosis. Recurrence, not permanent recovery, was the essential feature of MDI [7]. In sum, the distinction between mood vs psychotic conditions can be made well by focusing on recurrence vs chronicity of symptoms. Cross-sectionally, as Kraepelin always held, they can look the same. The clinical picture of schizoaffective illness raises the question of occasional overlap between psychotic and affective conditions, which we will discuss later in this chapter.

### Temperament

The concept of affective temperaments dates back at least 200 years and was systematized about a century ago by Emil Kraepelin and Ernst Kretschmer. In Kraepelin's texts, we read about 'manic temperaments' and 'depressive temperaments' [8]. Kretschmer developed these concepts [9], which eventually led to the concepts of hyperthymia and dysthymia, respectively. The main idea is that manic and depressive states present not only in episodes of attacks of severe symptoms, but also as mild symptoms that are present all the time, as part of the baseline personality of an individual. Thus, temperaments can be defined as mild versions of mood states, but they go beyond that initial concept to include basic differences in personality traits and in energy levels, as expressed in sleep patterns and behaviours such as sexual and social or work-related activities. Hence, the following brief descriptions apply [10]:

*Hyperthymia* involves a mild manic state as part of one's basic temperament. Such persons are high in energy, need less sleep than most people (often 4–6 hours nightly), have high sex drives, and are highly social, extroverted, often workaholics, and frequently humorous. They are described as the life of the party, as fun-loving, and can engage in risk-taking behaviours that others avoid such as skydiving or bungee-jumping or motorcycle or airplane flying. They dislike routine and are spontaneous. They can be quite anxious and inattentive.

*Dysthymia* is the reverse, a mild depressive state as part of one's basic temperament. Such persons are low in energy, need more sleep than most people (often 10–12 hours nightly), have low sex drives, and are socially anxious, introverted, low in work productivity, and not humorous. They avoid risk-taking behaviours, are devoted to routine, and can be obsessive. They can be quite anxious, but not usually inattentive.

*Cyclothymia* involves constant alternation between mild manic and depressive states on a day-to-day, or a few days at time, basis. Such persons go up and down in mood and energy and activity levels, though they can be generally mostly extroverted and productive and social. They tend to be risk-takers at times and are unpredictable and spontaneous. They can be quite anxious and inattentive.

In the original view of Kraepelin and Kretschmer, these temperaments are mild variations of MDI. They are not separate or independent diseases or disorders, as the DSM system sets them up. They are part of the same condition, just mild versions, '*formes frustes*', as in the French term. This is no different than saying that mild adrenal insufficiency is related to, but not the same as, Addison's disease or that mild hypothyroidism is related to, but not the same as, Graves' disease. Affective temperaments are different in severity, but not in kind from severe depressive or manic illness.

This perspective differs from the DSM-III-based view of dysthymia and cyclothymia as 'axis I' conditions, rather than aspects of personality. Further successive DSM revisions have ignored hyperthymia completely. A useful resource is the TEMPS (Temperament Evaluation scale from Memphis, Pisa, and San Diego) scale, which is the most validated research scale to assess affective temperaments. As an aid to clinical diagnosis, a short self-report TEMPS scale can be invaluable [11].

### Insight and the diagnostic process

A major aspect to the diagnosis of affective illness is the psychopathology of insight. In general, insight is preserved in depression, and impaired in mania [12]. Specifically, about one-half of patients with severe mania and the majority of patients with hypomanic states deny having those symptoms despite the actual presence of those symptoms observed by researchers. Further, insight appears to have a U-shaped curve in relation to severity; it is most impaired in hypomania and in severe mania but may be more present in moderate states of mania.

Since patients realize they are depressed but are often unaware that they are having hypomanic or manic states, they will present to clinicians complaining of the former and ignoring or denying the latter. Hence, clinicians may misdiagnose such patients as being depressed, rather than manic or mixed, or as having unipolar depression, as opposed to bipolar illness.

There are many reasons for the problem of lack of insight in mania. Part of the phenomenon probably is biological, with frontal or parietal function being affected in the manic state. Such lack of insight is known to occur in parietal lobe strokes and in association with frontal lobe injury, as well as other diseases such as Alzheimer's dementia and schizophrenia [13]. In addition to this biological basis, insight may be further impaired because of the cultural impact of stigma against manic states, as well as simple lack of knowledge about such states.

To address this problem of insight and misdiagnosis, it is important to include family members and/or friends in the diagnostic interviews and even in treatment sessions, so as to get information from more than one source. While patients and family members report depressive symptoms equally, family members report manic symptoms twice as frequently as patients [14].

The patient, in short, is not a sufficient source of information to make diagnoses of affective illness. Confidentiality is not relevant, since at this stage the clinician is gathering information, not divulging it. It is a common clinical error to refuse to engage with family at the outset of a treatment relationship. This mistake, which is not needed to protect confidentiality, will lead to misdiagnosis in many patients.

In addition to obtaining information from outside sources, clinicians should use interviewing methods that take into account patients' natural inclination to deny manic symptoms. Generally speaking, it is best not to ask patients about manic criteria directly, but rather to ask open-ended questions that would capture those criteria. This way, the patient would report manic symptoms spontaneously without realizing that they are doing so. An example might be: 'Other than your depressive states, have you had periods of time where you felt the opposite?' Patients tend to want to discuss their depressive states in detail. Clinicians can begin the interview by allowing such discussion and by going into detail to understand the features of the depressive states. Assessment of manic states should be left to later in the interview. Further, even if specific manic or hypomanic episodes are denied by patients, the clinician should then turn to family members present and ask them about the same symptoms. If all episodic symptoms are denied by both patient and family, then the likelihood of misdiagnosis of bipolar illness is lowered notably.

Even then, clinicians should ask patients and family about their baseline temperament, to identify possible hyperthymia or cyclothymia. Again, open-ended questions are more likely to receive accurate answers: 'Tell me what your personality is usually like, when you're not depressed? What's your usual energy and activity level?'. Since 'energy' is a vague concept, it is useful to be specific about sleep—not just whether the patient feels it is adequate or not, but the actual time one goes to bed, the time one wakes up, and the quality of sleep during that time. Whether energy is high or low should not be based on the patient's opinion alone, again, but also based on the observation of family and friends, and also compared to the norm of the patient's peers.

### Biological aspects of diagnosis

It is stated often that there are no valid biological 'markers' for psychiatric diagnosis. This statement is oversimplified. In the case of affective conditions, there are some biological testing methods that can be relevant to a more accurate diagnosis. Among these, the most important method is assessment of genetics via family history, but also in various settings, important evidence is relevant from neuroimaging, EEG testing, and neuropsychological testing.

Family history is very important in the diagnosis of mood conditions since bipolar illness is highly genetic, almost completely so based on twin studies, while DSM-defined MDD is much less genetic [15]. Further, other differential diagnostic conditions, like personality disorder, also have much lower genetic heritabilities, based on a meta-analysis [16], than bipolar illness. Thus, a positive family history for bipolar illness is diagnostically important and rather specific for that condition. The absence of such family history needs to be investigated, rather than simply being accepted as reflecting no such family history. This is the case because bipolar illness, and MDI in general, have been proven to be underdiagnosed for at least half a century or longer [17]. Thus, even if family members sought psychiatric or medical diagnosis, the statistical probability would be that bipolar or manic conditions would be diagnosed less frequently than would have been truly the case. Further, social stigma is high now, but was even greater in previous generations, and is greater in non-Western cultures, all of which may be reflected in the absence of family histories for mood conditions in prior generations or in other cultures.

Neurological evaluation can inform diagnosis, specifically EEG, neuroimaging, and neuropsychological testing. These tests tend to be informative for mood conditions in a way that is different than how they are used for neurological diagnoses. For instance, EEGs are often seen as within the normal range if there is no epileptiform activity, but spiking or slowing of EEG activity has been associated with mood conditions, depending on location and laterality [4]. In general, it has been found that right temporal abnormalities are associated with depression, and left temporal abnormalities with mania. Quantitative EEG may be more sensitive to such mild abnormalities, as compared to standard EEG [4]. On neuroimaging, depression has been associated with hippocampal atrophy, and mania with amygdala enlargement, among other changes [18]. Further, white matter infarcts, often dismissed as variants of normal, are common and specific to vascular depression [19].

Perhaps the most common, and most misused, diagnostic test is neuropsychological testing. Misuse of such testing occurs when a cognitive function is identified immediately with a diagnosis; for example, attentional impairment is quantified and then 'diagnosed' as attention deficit disorder (ADD). In fact, attentional impairment can occur because of either depression and mania [20]. Neuropsychological testing is a snapshot in time and thus reflects the current mood state, rather than the longitudinal diagnosis. It can provide corroborative evidence for mood diagnoses or other cognitive conditions though. For instance, learning disabilities or IQ abnormalities can be identified. The pattern of abnormalities can suggest right vs left hemisphere dysfunction, which, combined with quantitative EEG and/or MRI, may support a pure depressive vs a bipolar diagnosis, with a predominance of left hemispheric abnormalities for manic or bipolar states, as opposed to right hemispheric abnormalities for pure depressive states.

## Classification

### Current classification of mood disorders

The current classification of mood disorders is based on the *Diagnostic and Statistical Manual of Mental Disorders*, the fifth edition of which (DSM-5) was published recently in 2013 [21]. Changes in DSM-5, compared to DSM-IV, were minimal for mood disorders. Specifically, for the diagnosis of a manic episode, a requirement for increased energy was added to the prior criterion of decreased need

for sleep. This requirement is redundant because the entire concept of decreased *need* for sleep implies increased energy. Nonetheless, the energy criterion was made explicit. For MDD, no changes beyond minor modifiers have been made since the basic criteria were set with DSM-III in 1980.

The most important change in DSM-5 was not to the criteria for manic or depressive episodes, but rather to the modifier for 'mixed features'. The change here was that the prior mood episode definition for 'mixed episodes' was dropped, and the concept was moved to become a modifier for manic or depressive episodes. Thus, in DSM-5, mixed episodes are replaced with the terms 'Bipolar disorder, current manic episode with mixed features' or 'Bipolar disorder, current depressive episode with mixed features' and, importantly, 'MDD, current major depressive episode with mixed features'. Thus, for the first time, a DSM revision acknowledges the diagnostic relevance of manic symptoms in persons who do *not* have bipolar disorder, that is, MDD with mixed features, which will be discussed further.

The DSM-5 concept of mixed features is defined as the presence of non-overlapping mood symptoms from the opposite mood states. Thus, a depressive episode would be said to have mixed features if multiple manic symptoms were present, excluding distractibility and irritability and agitation, which are considered 'overlapping' symptoms since they are part of the definition of a major depressive episode as well. The critique has been made that these overlapping symptoms are exactly those symptoms that are most common in mixed states; thus, excluding them would be like saying that one could not use the symptom of headache to diagnose migraine, since pain in the head overlaps with other non-migraine headache syndromes [22].

### Critique of DSM-based classification

Besides specific issues related to mood conditions, as described in this chapter, DSM-based classification, in general, has been subject to criticism in recent years. The critiques that may have the most scientific merit are as follows.

DSM-based diagnosis is 'pragmatic' and is not based primarily on scientific studies. Leaders of DSM-III, IV, and 5 have been explicit that certain changes based on abundant scientific data, such as dimensions of personality traits, would not be included in official DSM diagnoses, while other definitions with very limited scientific data, like dysphoric mood dysregulation disorder, were included. These changes and failures to make change were based on judgements termed 'pragmatic', based on preferences of the psychiatric profession in the United States. This decision-making process may be utilitarian and socially needed, but it does indicate that scientific data are not the main sources of decision-making [23].

DSM-based diagnosis is overly conservative and resistant to change. The publication of DSM-5 in 2013 occurred with minor changes to DSM-IV overall (published in 1994), which also reflected little change from DSM-III (published in 1980).

As a corollary, DSM-based diagnosis impedes scientific research and hence retards progress in the profession [24]. This observation led the US National Institute of Mental Health (NIMH) in 2013 to direct that no future funded research should use DSM-based criteria. Alternative criteria—the Research Domain Criteria (RDoC)—have been instituted [25].

## Non-DSM-based classification: manic–depressive illness and neurotic depression

The critique described is a rationale for being open to non-DSM-based classifications for mood conditions. Three major non-DSM approaches involve the diagnostic groupings of MDI, neurotic depression, and affective temperaments.

### Manic–depressive illness

The central non-DSM-based classification of mood conditions is the pre-DSM III concept of MDI or the post-DSM definitions of mood spectra.

Manic depressive illness (MDI) was defined by Emil Kraepelin in 1898 and later editions of his textbooks, and used as thus defined for about century, until DSM-III in 1980. The Kraepelinian definition of MDI was that any recurrent mood episodes of any kind, depressive OR manic, constituted the diagnosis of MDI [7, 8, 26]. This is *not* the same thing as bipolar disorder, which became official with DSM-III, which meant the presence of depressive AND manic episodes, not depressive OR manic episodes. In other words, MDI meant bipolar illness *plus* unipolar depressive illness. It represented what is defined by DSM terms as bipolar disorder *and* most of MDD.

MDI was defined by *recurrence* of mood episodes as its diagnostic standard, not *polarity* of mood episodes. As long as recurrent episodes occurred, that is, they came and went and were repeated, the diagnosis was MDI. It did not matter if the diagnosis reflected 100 depressive episodes and zero manic episodes, or 100 manic episodes and zero depressive episodes. The diagnosis of MDI was the same in both cases. In other words, bipolar and unipolar courses were subtypes of the same illness, MDI, rather than two separate purported illnesses, as in the DSM system.

One reason that Kraepelin de-emphasized polarity and focused on recurrent course of illness was his observation, along with others, that most mood states were neither purely depressive nor manic, but rather mixed. Kraepelin defined six different types of mixed states, building on Weygandt [27], as opposed to the two pure depressive or manic states. Mixed states were the most common presentation of MDI, and thus it was not possible to define the illness by polarity, since most mood states were not at one pole or the other. DSM-III tried to ignore this problem away by refusing to define mixed episodes and by defining manic episodes very narrowly as being severe and lasting 1 week or longer. This definition, which conflicted with a large literature on mixed states and hypomanic episodes, was partially rectified by DSM-IV which accepted a definition of milder hypomanic episodes and introduced a definition of mixed episodes. However, hypomanic episodes were cut off at 4 days, without any scientific evidence for that cut-off duration, and mixed episodes were defined narrowly (requiring the presence of full syndromal mania and depression at the same time). DSM-5 has broadened the mixed definition somewhat, as noted, but it did not change the hypomania duration definition, despite the absence of evidence for the 4-day cut-off and the presence of some data supporting a shorter cut-off of 2 days [28]. Further, the definition of mixed states proposed by DSM-5 has been criticized as being conceptual primarily (focused on the concept of 'non-overlapping' symptoms), as opposed to extensive empirical evidence that most mixed states are broader and characterized primarily by psychomotor excitation—like rapid thoughts, marked rage/irritability, agitation, and impulsivity—added to depressive features [22]. These empirically based mixed features are not part of the DSM-5 definition but are central to the non-DSM concept of mixed depressive and dysphoric manic states [29].

These DSM debates about duration of hypomania and definitions of mixed states are only relevant if the DSM distinction between bipolar disorder and MDD is accepted. If the older concept of MDI is accepted, then DSM controversies over details of mood states would not change the MDI diagnosis in any case.

### Neurotic depression

Besides MDI, the other major non-DSM classification in mood conditions is neurotic depression [30, 31]. This diagnosis was made commonly before DSM-III in 1980, and it was targeted specifically for exclusion from DSM-III [32]. It was defined, as with MDI and unlike DSM definitions, primarily by its course, rather than cross-sectional symptoms; neurotic depression reflected a mood condition that was not severe, episodic, and recurrent—like MDI—but rather chronic, constant, but mild to moderate in severity. The mood symptoms were never manic, but rather depressed and anxious. Brief exacerbations could occur to higher severity, usually in the setting of psychosocial stress, but these periods of worsening were brief, usually days to weeks, followed by a return to a chronic baseline. In the United States, the terms 'neurotic and psychotic' were used in the mid-twentieth century loosely, based on psychoanalytic assumptions about the severity of repressed unconscious emotions. In Europe, the terms were used phenomenologically, with neurosis simply reflecting anxiety with some admixture of mild depressive symptoms, and psychosis reflecting the presence of delusions or hallucinations.

There was a robust debate about the validity of neurotic depression as a diagnosis in the 1970s, especially in the UK, but also in the United States [33]. Since the term was used differently in the two nations, the debate was not the same exactly. In the UK, neurotic depression became identified with 'exogenous' or 'reactive' depression, while psychotic depression was defined as 'endogenous'. Since MDI was always seen as a biological, and thus 'endogenous', disease, neurotic depression was seen in Europe as an entirely different kind of depressive condition than MDI. However, not all depressive episodes in MDI were psychotic, which led to the problem of how to differentiate non-psychotic depression in MDI (both bipolar and unipolar subtypes) from neurotic depression. In the UK debate, the focus was on the exogenous vs endogenous distinction, that is, on whether psychosocial stressors could be shown to differ in non-psychotic depressive states. As this factor was thrown into doubt based on research, the concept of neurotic depression was weakened accordingly. The definition of endogenous depression primarily based on the course of illness did not receive adequate attention though.

In the United States, the concept of neurotic depression fell into disfavour as being Freudian, even though it did not have psychoanalytic roots in Europe. In the course of DSM-III debates and decisions, as now documented in new historical research [32], the evolution of neurotic depression was as follows. It was replaced initially by the term 'minor' depression, as opposed to 'major' depression which was to be reserved for the more severe mood states of MDI (renamed bipolar disorder and unipolar major depressive disorder). Psychoanalytic groups in the United States objected to the term 'unipolar' as being seen as 'endogenous', and thus leading to likely drug, as opposed to psychotherapy, treatments. Those same groups objected to the term 'minor' as likely to result in minor insurance reimbursement. Thus, all the proposed terms were lumped eventually into the diagnosis of 'major depressive disorder'. There was still reluctance in the American clinical community to give up the term neurotic depression, so additional diagnoses were created or redefined—namely, generalized anxiety disorder and dysthymia—to compensate clinicians for giving up the concept of neurotic depression.

### Affective temperaments

The third major non-DSM approach is the concept of affective temperaments, namely, dysthymia (constant mild depression), hyperthymia (constant mild mania), and cyclothymia (constant mild alternation between the two), as described previously. Using validated scale measures, about one-half of persons with mood conditions have an affective temperament [34]. Affective temperaments simply are milder versions of affective illnesses, as opposed to being categorically different conditions. A patient can have both unipolar depression and cyclothymic temperament, or bipolar illness and hyperthymic temperament. Indeed, genetic studies find that affective temperaments are quite frequent diagnoses in family members of persons with affective illnesses [35].

The concept of affective temperaments provides a dimensional approach to personality, with origins in affective illness, as opposed to the DSM-based categorical approach, with origins in psychoanalytic constructs. While the DSM revisions have recognized dysthymia and cyclothymia, those conditions have not been viewed as personality constructs, but as 'axis I' disorders, equivalent to bipolar illness or unipolar depression. This approach is not how those conditions have been defined and used for over a century. Further, DSM revisions have excluded and ignored the condition of hyperthymic temperament.

Like DSM-defined personality disorders, affective temperaments are present throughout life, persisting from childhood and adolescence. Thus, patients with cyclothymia have constant mood lability and impulsive sexuality, often interpreted as borderline personality, or constant problems with attention, often interpreted as attention-deficit/hyperactivity disorder (ADHD), as discussed in this chapter.

### A post-DSM classification: spectrum concepts

After almost half a century of more research and clinical experience, one might ask how well DSM-based definitions of mood disorders have held up.

The main question relates to the radical distinction between MDI, as a single broad disease, vs two different and separate bipolar and unipolar conditions. The bipolar/unipolar dichotomy was justified in the 1970s, leading up to DSM-III, based on differences in the classic diagnostic validators of course, genetics, biological markers, and treatment response [36]. In other words, the claim that the presence or absence of manic episodes marked different diseases was supported by observations of differences in course, genetics, biology, and treatment between bipolar and unipolar groups. In particular, bipolar illness had an early age of onset (mean age of about 19 years vs about the late 20s for unipolar depression), brief depressive episodes (3 months or less, on average, in bipolar illness vs 6–12 months, on average, in unipolar depression), highly recurrent course (more frequent episodes in bipolar than unipolar illness, with rapid cycling, defined as four or more episodes yearly happening in about 25% of

bipolar illness cases, but in <1% of unipolar depression cases), genetic specificity (manic episodes were found in families of persons with manic episodes, but not in families of persons with unipolar depression), and differential treatment (antidepressants for unipolar depression vs neuroleptics and lithium for mania) [26].

In the intervening half century, all of these distinctions have been weakened and/or refuted. Regarding the course of illness, the common diagnosis of MDD in children, far below the mean onset of the late 20s, conflicts completely with the rationale that bipolar illness and MDD differ on that course criterion. Brief depressive episodes that occur multiple times yearly are diagnosed in patients with MDD commonly [37], whereas such course of illness should be rare if MDD was a different illness than bipolar disorder. Genetic studies have found high rates of depressive episodes, without mania, in persons with bipolar illness, and also frequent occurrence of bipolar illness in relatives of those with unipolar depression [35, 38, 39]. Treatment now overlaps considerably, with neuroleptic agents proven effective not only for mania, but also for depression, both in bipolar and unipolar types [40, 41]. Lithium has been well known to be effective not only for mania, but also for depression, both in bipolar and unipolar types [42, 43].

In short, the bipolar/unipolar distinction, now calcified in DSM-III through 5, has not been supported by further research in mood disorders and, in fact, research could be used to support the original MDI perspective of one broad mood illness.

Another perspective taken on this research would be to maintain the bipolar/unipolar dichotomy, but to recognize that it is not a strict distinction, but rather that there is one mood spectrum, with extremes of classic bipolar and unipolar cases, but with many cases in the middle of that spectrum. Some have called this concept a 'bipolar spectrum' [44] or a 'manic–depressive spectrum' (Fig. 66.2).

One might also refer to an 'MDD spectrum' which captures the different subtypes of depression described in this chapter, all of which were lumped together in DSM-III into one broad MDD category.

Such views would incorporate both the original MDI concept and the later observations of bipolar and unipolar variations [45] (Fig. 66.3).

The DSM approach to diagnosis generally is opposed to spectrum concepts, on a priori 'pragmatic' grounds of wanting to have a high threshold for psychiatric diagnosis to avoid 'overdiagnosis' [46]. Separate from the fact that this belief reflects stigma against psychiatric illness, it is not based on empirical evidence, but rather reflects a conceptual assumption. For that reason, the scientific evidence supporting spectrum concepts in mood disorders was rejected in the DSM-5 process.

Any future change likely will await a move away from the DSM process of diagnositic criteria towards something different, such as new research-based clinical criteria for diagnosis.

## Differential diagnosis

The differential diagnosis of mood conditions involves distinctions within the mood dichotomy (bipolar vs unipolar) and distinctions with other conditions based on overlapping symptoms such as personality changes (borderline, antisocial, narcissitic personality disorders), delusions or hallucinations (schizophrenia and/or

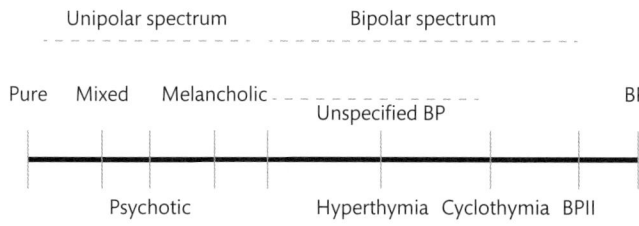

Unspecified BP is DSM terminology for bipolar aspects of a case that do not meet mania or hypomania criteria, such as recurrent depressive episodes with underlying hyperthymia, or recurrent depressive episodes with a first-degree relative with bipolar illness.

**Fig. 66.2** The manic–depressive spectrum.

schizoaffective illness), and cognition (ADD). An important aspect to approaching differential diagnosis is the concept of a diagnostic hierarchy, which has been rejected by DSM nosology. In the hierarchy approach, diagnoses with multiple symptoms should be diagnosed preferentially to diagnoses with fewer symptoms [47]. Thus, pneumonia would be the only diagnosis in a case of fever with lung infection, as opposed to 'fever disorder' comorbidity. Since mood disorders cause personality changes, delusions, and cognitive effects, they should be diagnosed, instead of assuming the presence of personality disorders, schizophrenia, and/or ADD. Further, the assumption of 'comorbidity', which is encouraged by the DSM approach, would be challenged by a hierarchy concept. Multiple diagnoses would not be made, unless other symptoms could be shown to exist, independent of the mood condition.

### Within the mood dichotomy: unipolar vs bipolar

In the DSM polarity-based nosology of mood disorder, the differential diagnosis of unipolar vs bipolar illness rests completely on the identification of manic or hypomanic episodes. Most patients present for treatment in the depressive phase; thus, the differential diagnosis rests entirely on past manic/hypomanic episodes. As noted, patients deny having manic episodes about half the time, due to lack of insight. Such impaired insight is even worse in hypomania. Thus, in most cases, patients will deny manic/hypomanic episodes, leading to underdiagnosis of bipolar illness and overdiagnosis of MDD, which has been shown empirically [17]. Interviewing should include family and friends, who report manic symptoms more accurately than patients, to correct for this diagnostic bias. Patient self-report is not sufficient to rule out past manic/hypomanic episodes.

A non-DSM-based approach would emphasize all diagnostic validators, including the course of illness and genetics, and not just symptoms, to differentiate bipolar vs unipolar depression. The depressive states themselves are somewhat different, with more melancholia, mixed states, and delusions/hallucinations in bipolar than unipolar depression [48]. Family genetics of bipolar illness would argue against the legitimacy of diagnosing MDD in a depressed person. A course of illness with early age of onset (that is, 20 years or earlier), brief depressive episodes (3–6 months or less), and high recurrence (multiple depressive episodes yearly) all would argue for the diagnosis of bipolar illness and against unipolar depression [26].

The therapeutic relevance of this distinction is that antidepressants appear to be mostly ineffective in acute bipolar depression [49] and in prophylaxis [50]. They also can cause acute manic/hypomanic episodes [51] and, more importantly, have been shown to worsen the long-term course of bipolar illness in some subjects, especially those with a rapid-cycling course [52]. In rapid-cycling cases, randomized data show that more mood episodes, including depressive states, occur over time with antidepressants than if those agents are discontinued or foregone altogether [53].

### Personality disorders

#### Borderline, narcissistic, and antisocial personality disorders

Bipolar illness and borderline personality share some features and differ in others. Shared features include rapid mood swings, unstable interpersonal relationships, impulsive sexual behaviour, and suicidality. DSM-III through 5 criteria for borderline personality are met with the four criteria described, along with one more out of nine total criteria. Thus, using DSM definitions, most persons with bipolar illness would meet borderline criteria automatically. This apparent 'comorbidity' is questionable due to overlapping diagnostic definitions. As examined in a review [54], true comorbidity would be definable with the other five borderline criteria which are less common in bipolar illness, especially dissociative states and self-mutilations. If sexual trauma is added, which is not even one of the DSM criteria for borderline personality, then it has been shown that specific differentiation of bipolar illness from borderline personality is feasible. Further, the presence of bipolar family genetics would strongly argue for bipolar illness and against borderline personality, with the former being about twice as heritable genetically than the latter.

When manic or as part of hyperthymic or cyclothymic temperament, persons with bipolar illness have high self-esteem, which can get reflected in lack of empathy towards others and a range of selfish behaviours. If seen through a Freudian and DSM-based lens, many clinicians misdiagnose such persons as having narcissistic personality disorder (NPD), characterized by a pervasive pattern of grandiosity, a need for admiration, and low empathy. This approach would ignore the diagnostic validators that would support mood illness,

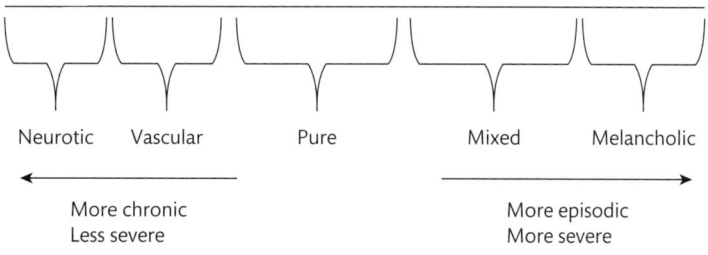

**Fig. 66.3** The major depressive disorder (MSD) spectrum.

such as family bipolar genetics, and other manic symptoms that are irrelevant to NPD such as high energy levels and decreased need for sleep. It is relevant that NPD has been invalidated by research with diagnostic validators, being unable to be distinguished from multiple other personality disorders (that is, borderline, histrionic, dependent, antisocial) [55]. The DSM-5 Personality Disorders Task Force recommended the removal of NPD, but this recommendation was rejected by the APA Board of Trustees. Thus, the scientific legitimacy of NPD as a diagnosis is questionable.

In contrast, antisocial personality has been diagnosed and validated for a century or more in psychiatry. Again, there is overlap with manic behaviours, which can be aggressive and impulsive, leading to legal troubles. If those behaviours are viewed solely from a social perspective, the antisocial diagnosis may seem relevant. Such an approach would be corrected if other diagnostic validators were taken into account, again emphasizing family bipolar genetics, but also the course of illness with different behaviours in and out of mood episodes, as well as the presence of other manic symptoms that are irrelevant to antisocial personality such as high energy levels and decreased need for sleep.

### Schizophrenia/schizoaffective illness

When delusions or hallucinations are present, the differential diagnosis of mood conditions includes schizophrenia and schizoaffective illness. Delusions or hallucinations occur in about one-half of manic states and in about 10% of depressive states, somewhat more in bipolar than unipolar illness [56]. When present, such symptoms are qualitatively similar to the delusions or hallucinations of schizophrenia and thus can be mistaken for the latter. Further, negative symptoms of schizophrenia like apathy, lack of affect, low energy, and social isolation can appear like symptoms of depression episode. In both conditions, cognitive impairment is present. This misdiagnosis was common throughout the twentieth century, when schizophrenia was diagnosed cross-sectionally by the presence of delusions/hallucinations (as Eugen Bleuler popularized), as opposed to longitudinally by a chronic declining course (as Emil Kraepelin taught). This course was key, in the Kraepelinian view—dementia praecox was chronic and MDI was episodic. The Bleulerian view was disproved by the seminal United States–U.K diagnostic project and other research, which led to the return to the Kraepelinian course criterion with DSM-III in 1980 [57].

Some recent genetics studies indicate common genetic aetiologies for schizophrenia and affective illness, which some interpret as challenging the nosological dichotomy. Other genetic studies differentiate the two basic diagnostic groupings, as do other diagnostic validators such as course and neuroimaging [58, 59].

Some patients share features of both conditions, defined in the DSM system as schizoaffective disorder. Various studies of the classic diagnostic validators suggest that schizoaffective illness does not breed true and does not appear to represent a valid third psychotic disease [60]. Instead, it likely is sometimes a more severe variant of affective illness and sometimes a less severe variant of schizophrenia. In some cases, it could represent the chance comorbidity of schizophrenia and affective illness in the same person.

### Attention deficit disorder

Depressive and manic states are characterized by impaired concentration, as well as executive function impairment, and abnormal working and short-term memory [61]. These cognitive states are also present in ADD, leading to the diagnosis of ADD in persons who have manic and depressive symptoms. This misdiagnosis would be common, especially in hyperthymia and cyclothymia, where chronic problems with attention are present due to constant manic and depressive symptoms. Using the hierarchy concept, such persons would be diagnosed preferentially as having mood conditions; using DSM definitions, the comorbidity of both diagnoses would be asserted. In contrast to bipolar illness definitions, which have remained restrictive, DSM-5 broadened the diagnosis of childhood ADD, requiring fewer criteria to be met and extending the age of onset range from a maximum of 6 years to 12 years. DSM-5 also formalized a definition of ADD in adulthood as well.

Again differential diagnosis would be assisted by attention to all diagnostic validators, not just symptoms; thus, family genetics of bipolar illness would argue against the ADD diagnosis, as would recurrent depressive episodes. Since amphetamines are used to treat ADD and they have been associated with worsening of manic states [62], as well neurotoxicity in animal studies [63], the differential diagnosis has important practical implications.

### REFERENCES

1. Perlis RH, Uher R, Ostacher M, *et al.* Association between bipolar spectrum features and treatment outcomes in outpatients with major depressive disorder. *Arch Gen Psychiatry.* 2011;68:351–60.
2. Goldberg JF, Perlis RH, Ghaemi SN, *et al.* Manic symptoms : findings from the STEP-BD. *American J Psychiatry.* 2007;164:1348–55.
3. Koukopoulos A, Sani G, Koukopoulos AE, Manfredi G, Pacchiarotti I, Girardi P. Melancholia agitata and mixed depression. *Acta Psychiatr Scand Suppl.* 2007;433:50–7.
4. Flor-Henry P. *Cerebral Basis of Psychopathology* (1st edn). Bristol: John Wright PSG Inc; 1983.
5. Joseph A, Young R. *Movement Disorders in Neurology and Neuropsychiatry* (2nd edn). Malden, MA: Blackwell Science; 1999.
6. Dilsaver SC, Benazzi F, Akiskal HS. Mixed states: the most common outpatient presentation of bipolar depressed adolescents? *Psychopathology.* 2005;38:268–72.
7. Trede K, Salvatore P, Baethge C, Gerhard A, Maggini C, Baldessarini RJ. Manic-depressive illness: evolution in Kraepelin's Textbook, 1883–1926. *Harv Rev Psychiatry.* 2005;13:155–78.
8. Kraepelin E. *Manic-Depressive Insanity and Paranoia.* In: Robertson GM (ed). Edinburgh: E & S Livingstone; 1921.
9. Kretschmer E. *Physique and Character.* New York, NY: Cooper Square Publishers.; 1925.
10. Rihmer Z, Akiskal KK, Rihmer A, Akiskal HS. Current research on affective temperaments. *Curr Opin Psychiatry.* 2010;23:12–18.
11. Akiskal HS, Mendlowicz M V., Jean-Louis G, *et al.* TEMPS-A: validation of a short version of a self-rated instrument designed to measure variations in temperament. *J Affect Disord.* 2005;85:45–52.
12. Ghaemi SN, Rosenquist KJ. Insight in mood disorders: an empirical and conceptual review. In: Amador XF, David A (eds). *Insight and Psychosis.* Oxford: Oxford University Press; 2004. pp. 101–18.
13. Shad MU, Tamminga CA, Cullum M, Haas GL, Keshavan MS. Insight and frontal cortical function in schizophrenia: a review. *Schizophr Res.* 2006;86:54–70.

14. Keitner GI, Solomon DA, Ryan CE, *et al.* Prodromal and residual symptoms in bipolar I disorder. *Compr Psychiatry.* 1996;37:362–7.

15. Bienvenu OJ, Davydow DS, Kendler KS. Psychiatric 'diseases' versus behavioral disorders and degree of genetic influence. *Psychol Med.* 2011;41:33–40.

16. Moor MHM, Costa PT, Terracciano A, *et al.* Meta-analysis of genome-wide association studies for personality. *Mol Psychiatry.* 2010;337–49.

17. Ghaemi SN, Ko JY, Goodwin FK. 'Cade's disease' and beyond: misdiagnosis, antidepressant use, and a proposed definition for bipolar spectrum disorder. *Can J Psychiatry.* 2002;47:125–34.

18. Savitz J, Drevets WC. Bipolar and major depressive disorder: neuroimaging the developmental-degenerative divide. *Neurosci Biobehav Rev.* 2009;33:699–771.

19. Taylor WD, Aizenstein HJ, Alexopoulos GS. The vascular depression hypothesis: mechanisms linking vascular disease with depression. *Mol Psychiatry.* 2013;18:963–74.

20. Camelo EVM, Velasques B, Ribeiro P, Netto T, Cheniaux E. Attention impairment in bipolar disorder: a systematic review. *Psychol Neurosci.* 2013;6:299–309.

21. American Psychiatry Association. *Diagnostic and Statistical Manual of Mental Disorders (DSM-5)* (5th edn). Washington, DC: American Psychiatric Publishing; 2013.

22. Koukopoulos A, Sani G, Ghaemi SN. Mixed features of depression: why DSM-5 is wrong (and so was DSM-IV). *Br J Psychiatry.* 2013;203:3–5.

23. Ghaemi SN. Taking disease seriously: beyond 'pragmatic' nosology. In: Kendler KS, Parnas J (eds). *Philosophical Issues in Psychiatry II: Nosology.* Oxford: Oxford University Press; 2012. pp. 42–53.

24. Ghaemi SN. Taking disease seriously in DSM. *World Psychiatry.* 2013;12:210–12.

25. Insel T, Cuthbert B, Garvey M, *et al.* Research domain criteria (RDoC): toward a new classification framework for research on mental disorders. *Am J Psychiatry.* 2010;167:748–51.

26. Goodwin FK, Jamison KR. *Manic Depressive Illness* (2nd edn). New York, NY: Oxford University Press; 2007.

27. Salvatore P, Baldessarini RJ, Centorrino F, *et al.* Weygandt's On the Mixed States of Manic-Depressive Insanity: a translation and commentary on its significance in the evolution of the concept of bipolar disorder. *Harv Rev Psychiatry.* 2002;10:255–75.

28. Ghaemi SN, Bauer M, Cassidy F, *et al.* Diagnostic guidelines for bipolar disorder: a summary of the International Society for Bipolar Disorders Diagnostic Guidelines Task Force Report. *Bipolar Disorders.* 2008;10:117–28.

29. Koukopoulos A, Sani G. DSM-5 criteria for depression with mixed features: a farewell to mixed depression. *Acta Psychiatr Scand.* 2014;129:4–16.

30. Roth SM, Kerr TA. The concept of neurotic depression: a plea for reinstatement. In: Pichot P, Rein W (eds). *The Clinical Approach in Psychiatry.* Paris: Synthelabo; 1994. pp. 339–68.

31. Ghaemi SN. Why antidepressants are not antidepressants: STEP-BD, STAR*D, and the return of neurotic depression. *Bipolar Disord.* 2008;10:957–68.

32. Decker H. *The Making of DSM-III: A Diagnostic Manual's Conquest of American Psychiatry* (1st edn). Oxford: Oxford University Press; 2013.

33. Shorter E. The doctrine of the two depressions in historical perspective. *Acta Psychiatr Scand Suppl.* 2007;433:5–13.

34. Vohringer PA, Whitham EA, Thommi SB, Holtzman NS, Khrad H, Ghaemi SN. Affective temperaments in clinical

practice: a validation study in mood disorders. *J Affect Disord.* 2012;136:577–80.

35. Kelsoe JR. Arguments for the genetic basis of the bipolar spectrum. *J Affect Disord.* 2003;73:183–97.

36. Robins E, Guze SB. Establishment of diagnostic validity in psychiatric illness: its application to schizophrenia. *Am J Psychiatry.* 1970;126:983–7.

37. Angst J, Merikangas K, Scheidegger P, Wicki W. Recurrent brief depression: a new subtype of affective disorder. *J Affect Disord.* 1990;19:87–98.

38. Lee SH, Ripke S, Neale BM, *et al.* Genetic relationship between five psychiatric disorders estimated from genome-wide SNPs. *Nat Genet.* 2013;45:984–94.

39. Wiste A, Robinson EB, Milaneschi Y, *et al.* Bipolar polygenic loading and bipolar spectrum features in major depressive disorder. *Bipolar Disord.* 2014;16:608–16.

40. Nelson JC, Papakostas GI. Atypical antipsychotic augmentation in major depressive disorder: a meta-analysis of placebo-controlled randomized trials. *Am J Psychiatry.* 2009;166:980–91.

41. De Fruyt J, Deschepper E, Audenaert K, *et al.* Second generation antipsychotics in the treatment of bipolar depression: a systematic review and meta-analysis. *J Psychopharmacol.* 2012;26:603–17.

42. Bauer M, Adli M, Ricken R, Severus E, Pilhatsch M. Role of lithium augmentation in the management of major depressive disorder. *CNS Drugs.* 2014;28:331–42.

43. Malhi GS, Tanious M, Das P, Coulston CM, Berk M. Potential mechanisms of action of lithium in bipolar disorder: current understanding. *CNS Drugs.* 2013;27:135–53.

44. Akiskal HS. The bipolar spectrum--the shaping of a new paradigm in psychiatry. *Curr Psychiatry Rep.* 2002;4:1–3.

45. Ghaemi SN, Dalley S. The bipolar spectrum: conceptions and misconceptions. *Aust N Z J Psychiatry.* 2014;48:314–24.

46. Spitzer RL, Wakefield JC. DSM-IV diagnostic criterion for clinical significance: does it help solve the false positives problem? *Am J Psychiatry.* 1999;156:1856–64.

47. Surtees PG, Kendell RE. The hierarchy model of psychiatric symptomatology: an investigation based on present state examination ratings. *Br J Psychiatry.* 1979;135:438–43.

48. Mitchell PB, Goodwin GM, Johnson GF, Hirschfeld RM. Diagnostic guidelines for bipolar depression: a probabilistic approach. *Bipolar Disord.* 2008;10(1 Pt 2):144–52.

49. Sidor MM, Macqueen GM. Antidepressants for the acute treatment of bipolar depression: a systematic review and meta-analysis. *J Clin Psychiatry.* 2011;72:156–67.

50. Ghaemi SN, Wingo AP, Filkowski MA, Baldessarini RJ. Long-term antidepressant treatment in bipolar disorder: meta-analyses of benefits and risks. *Acta Psychiatr Scand.* 2008;118:347–56.

51. Goldberg JF, Truman CJ. Antidepressant-induced mania: an overview of current controversies. *Bipolar Disord.* 2003;5:407–20.

52. Ghaemi SN, Hsu DJ, Soldani F, Goodwin FK. Antidepressants in bipolar disorder: the case for caution. *Bipolar Disord.* 2003;5:421–33.

53. Ghaemi SN, Ostacher MM, El-Mallakh RS, *et al.* Antidepressant discontinuation in bipolar depression: a Systematic Treatment Enhancement Program for Bipolar Disorder (STEP-BD) randomized clinical trial of long-term effectiveness and safety. *J Clin Psychiatry.* 2010;71:372–80.

54. Ghaemi SN, Dalley S, Catania C, Barroilhet S. Bipolar or borderline: a clinical overview. *Acta Psychiatr Scand.* 2014;130:99–108.

55. Widiger TA. The DSM-5 dimensional model of personality disorder: rationale and empirical support. *J Pers Disord.* 2011;25:222–34.

56. Dunayevich E, Keck PE. Prevalence and description of psychotic features in bipolar mania. *Curr Psych*. 2000;2: 286–90.

57. Cooper J, Kendell RE, Gurland BJ, Sharpe L, Coperland JR, Simon R. *Psychiatric Diagnosis in New York and London. A Comparative Study of Mental Hospital Admissions* (1st edn). London: Oxford University Press; 1972.

58. Craddock N, Sklar P. Genetics of bipolar disorder. *Lancet*. 2013;381:1654–62.

59. Lichtenstein P, Yip BH, Björk C, *et al*. Common genetic determinants of schizophrenia and bipolar disorder in Swedish families: a population-based study. *Lancet*. 2009;373:234–9.

60. Kendler KS, McGuire M, Gruenberg AM, Walsh D. Examining the validity of DSM-III-R schizoaffective disorder and its putative subtypes in the Roscommon Family Study. *Am J Psychiatry*. 1995;152:755–64.

61. Cullen B, Ward J, Graham NA, *et al*. Prevalence and correlates of cognitive impairment in euthymic adults with bipolar disorder: a systematic review. *J Affect Disord*. 2016;205:165–81.

62. Vergne DE, Whitham E a, Barroilhet S, Fradkin Y, Ghaemi SN. Adult ADHD and amphetamines: a new paradigm. *Neuropsychiatry*. 2011;1:591–8.

63. Urban KR, Gao WJ. Methylphenidate and the juvenile brain: Enhancement of attention at the expense of cortical plasticity? *Med Hypotheses*. 2013;81:988–94.

# 67

# Epidemiology of mood disorders

*Lars Vedel Kessing*

## Introduction

Unipolar depressive disorder and bipolar disorder are common mental diseases that impose a very high societal burden in terms of morbidity, mortality, lost productivity, and costs [1]. The Global Burden of Disease study, which is a comprehensive assessment of disability and mortality from diseases and injuries from 1990 and projected to 2020, highlights the importance of mood disorders for the world. Using the measure of disability-adjusted life years (DALYs), the World health Organization (WHO) revealed that depressive disorder was the fourth leading cause of disease burden and bipolar disorder was the sixth leading cause in the world in 1990, and it was projected that, in the year 2020, depressive disorder would be the second leading cause of disease burden. In 2010, mental and substance abuse disorders accounted for 7% all DALYs worldwide, and within mental and substance abuse disorders, depressive disorder accounted for 40% and bipolar disorder for 7% of DALYs [2]. Together, mood disorders burden society with the highest health care costs of all psychiatric and neurological disorders [3]. One DALY represents the loss of a healthy year of life and aggregates the years of life lived with disability (YLDs) with the years of life lost (YLLs) due to premature mortality. In 2010, depressive disorders were the second leading cause of YLDs due to population growth and ageing [4]. These estimations have contributed to shifting international focus towards mood disorders as a leading cause of burden in its own right and also in comparison to more recognized physical disorders.

Mood disorders have received considerable attention in psychiatric epidemiology over the last 25 years. These received particular attention in the five-site United States National Institutes of Mental Health Epidemiologic Catchment Area Study (*ECA*), as well as in epidemiological studies in other countries around the world that used the ECA methodology. Mood disorders also received particular attention in the National Comorbidity Survey (*NCS*) in the United States, in the National Psychiatric Morbidity Survey of Great Britain, and most recently in the World Mental Health Survey (*WMH*) across many countries. Thus, there are substantial data from around the world on the epidemiology of these disorders. In addition, many of the population-based case registers and twin registries have also paid particular interest in mood disorders, and

some of these registers have the additional advantage of being able to consider genetic, as well as environmental, risk factors.

Depressive disorder and bipolar disorder hold large similarities in pathogenesis, course of illness, and outcomes, and it is estimated that approximately 1% of patients convert from depressive disorder to bipolar disorder per year as patients develop hypomanic or manic episodes [5, 6], approximating 20–40% during the lifetime course.

## Bipolar disorders

### Diagnostic issues

While classical bipolar disorder, with episodes of euphoric mania interspersed with episodes of depression, is one of the clearest clinical syndromes in psychiatry, the boundaries of bipolar disorder remain contested. As case definition is central to epidemiology, all the contested boundaries of bipolar disorder could influence prevalence rates and our understanding of risk factors. Some of the major boundary issues for bipolar disorder include the overlap of bipolar disorder with psychotic features with schizoaffective disorder and schizophrenia, and the overlap of bipolar disorder with unipolar depressive disorder when patients who present primarily with depression have brief or mild episodes of hypomania. There is also an overlap of bipolar disorder with apparent personality disorder, especially Cluster B personality disorders such as borderline and narcissism, and the issue of when hyperthymic personality merges into bipolar disorder. When bipolar disorder is comorbid with alcohol or substance abuse, there are also important diagnostic issues.

Another important issue in determining caseness of bipolar disorder for epidemiological surveys is symptom pattern and duration. A number of the diagnostic instruments for assessing bipolarity in population surveys limit the questions on mania to a type of symptom profile characterized by euphoria, grandiosity, increased energy, and decreased sleep. Whether the commonly used epidemiology interviews adequately detect those individuals who have manic episodes, characterized by irritability, anger, and activation, is very debatable. The other key diagnostic issue is what criteria are used to categorize the minimum duration for hypomania; are 4 days too long? Are even 2 days too long? Furthermore, as insight is sometimes impaired in hypomania and mania, and as these are low-prevalence disorders, the accuracy of case detection of bipolar disorders in populations remains an issue for further research.

## Prevalence

Prior population studies, such as the ECA and its related cross-national studies and the NCS, reported that the lifetime prevalence of bipolar I disorder varied from 0.3% to 1.5% [7, 8]. More recent studies, such as the NCS replication study [9], reported data on both bipolar I and bipolar II disorders and found lifetime (and 12-month) prevalence estimates of 1.0% (0.6%) for bipolar I, 1.1% (0.8%) for bipolar II, and 2.4% (1.4%) for subthreshold bipolar disorder. Broader definitions of mania/hypomania have resulted in lifetime prevalence rates increasing to about 4% or even higher [10].

In bipolar I disorder, the prevalence in males and females is similar. This is in contrast to the reasonably consistent female excess found in bipolar II disorder and depressive disorder.

The incidence of bipolar I and II disorders is estimated to be 10–30 per 100,000 year (0.01–0.03% per year).

## Comorbidity

In the NCS, all identified bipolar I individuals suffered from at least one, and often up to three or more, comorbid disorder. The most common comorbid disorders included the full range of anxiety disorders, alcohol and drug dependence, and antisocial behaviours.

Alcohol and drug abuse and/or dependence are commonly comorbid with bipolar disorder. Clinical studies find that bipolar patients with comorbid substance dependence are less adherent to prescribed mood stabilizers and have more frequent hospital re-admissions. Stimulant abuse/dependence rates are especially increased in bipolar disorder.

Individuals with bipolar disorder have the full range of anxiety disorders, including phobias, panic disorder, and obsessive–compulsive disorder.

A controversial area of comorbidity with bipolar disorder is that of childhood attention deficit disorder. Early studies have suggested high comorbidity between attention deficit disorder and child and adolescent mania/bipolar disorder [11, 12], whereas longitudinal data [13–15], as well as studies with more careful diagnostic sorting of symptoms [16], have revealed lower comorbidity and supported the differentiation of child and adolescent mania/bipolar disorder from hyperkinetic disorder/attention deficit disorder. As argued by Arnold and colleagues, 'Indeed, if one automatically count such symptoms as hyperactivity and impaired attention towards both disorders without noting association with mood episodes, and especially if one does not require episodicity for bipolar disorder it may artificially inflate the comorbidity rate' [16]. In this way, longitudinal results seem to confirm the observation that even though the symptoms may not be so different between mania and attention-deficit/hyperactivity disorder (ADHD), the clinical presentation and illness course with an episodic course in bipolar disorder and a more chronic course in ADHD differ between the disorders [15, 17].

## Risk factors for bipolar disorders

In considering the risk factors for bipolar disorder, it is useful to separate risk factors into those that are risk factors for lifetime vulnerability (for example, genetic factors) and those that are risk factors for the onset of an episode of depression or mania (for example, life events). Thus, in determining the risk factors for lifetime vulnerability, genetic factors constitute the largest single risk factor. Bipolar disorder is one of the psychiatric disorders with the highest heritability at about 70–80%.

However, if one is considering who is vulnerable to an episode of mania over the next 6 months, genetic factors will play a relatively smaller part and predictions may be best based on other factors such as past history, childbirth, the presence of subsyndromal affective symptoms and cognitive deviances, being treated for depression with antidepressant medication, and the approach of spring or summer.

Although organic factors, such as some types of central nervous system damage, are unusual risk factors in young adults, in late-onset bipolar disorder (age of onset more than 50 years), organic disease of the central nervous system is an increasing factor for the development of mania.

## Age of onset and course of illness

Early-onset bipolar I disorder is more familial and is associated with a higher genetic load. Different population studies show that the mean age of onset of bipolar disorder varies from 17 to 30 years, but there seems to be differences between Europe and the United States. European data suggest a mean age in the late twenties, whereas United States data suggest a mean age in the early twenties. Reasons for these substantial differences are not known but may include greater genetic loading due to a higher risk of affective illness in those who migrated from Europe to the United States, a higher rate of assortative mating in the United States, as well as various genetic mechanisms, including anticipation and gene–environment interactions that may also differ in importance between the United States and Europe. Further, increasing overweight among children and adolescents has been suggested as a contributing factor being more prevalent in the United States.

Nevertheless, as age of onset is not normally distributed, the mean is a slightly misleading variable, while the mean age of onset may be in the twenties; for a large proportion of patients, the age of onset are the teenage years.

The majority of first episodes in bipolar I disorder are depressive; approximately 85% of patients have a depressive first episode, 10% a manic episode, and 3–5% a mixed episode. Typically, the duration of depressive episodes is between 2 and 5 months, although longer durations are often seen. The duration of manic episodes averages around 2 months.

Long-term studies suggest that the vast majority of patients with bipolar I disorder, approximating 90–100%, will develop more episodes after the first manic episode. The course of illness is heterogenous—some will develop few episodes, and some many—but, on average, the risk of recurrence increases with the number of prior affective episodes, suggesting a clinical progression of the illness [18, 19]. Long-term studies also show that despite treatment, patients with bipolar disorder type I or II suffer from affective symptoms of some severity approximately half of their lifetime. Over the course of illness, 80% of affective episodes are of the depressive type and 20% of the manic or mixed type. The presence of even milder affective symptoms is associated with decreased quality of life and functional and cognitive problems.

## Social, functional, and cognitive outcomes

Approximately 40–60% of patients with bipolar disorder present with persistent cognitive deficits in the remitted state and across several cognitive domains, including attention, verbal learning, and executive function [20, 21]. Such cognitive deficits may be prevalent even among healthy relatives of patients with bipolar disorder or early in the course of illness. There is robust evidence from several studies that patients' persistent cognitive dysfunction is a key contributor to their socio-occupational disability, independent of mood symptoms [22–24]. Functional impairment is prevalent in bipolar disorder, with unemployment rates 4- and 10-fold higher than in the general population [25, 26]. Approximately two-thirds of the patients are unable to regain premorbid levels of social and vocational functioning following a single episode [25], and verbal memory and executive function seem moderately related to employment outcome [27].

Patients with bipolar disorder have 2–3 times increased risk of developing dementia in the long run [28–32], and there are some suggestions that the risk of developing dementia may increase with the number of episodes in patients with depressive disorder and those with bipolar disorder [33]. Long-term treatment with lithium may decrease the risk of developing dementia [34–36], further supporting a link between bipolar disorder and dementia.

## Undiagnosed bipolar disorder and use of health services

There is often an interval between the onset of mood episodes and seeking help (on average 8–10 years), and it may take a decade for a bipolar patient to receive both the correct diagnosis and be prescribed mood-stabilizing medication, resulting in an extended period of untreated illness [37].

Receiving a correct bipolar diagnosis at initial assessment is complicated by few depressed patients seeking help for hypomanic/manic episodes and more seeking assistance only for their depressive episodes, while viewing any hypomanic/manic episodes as neither harmful or problematic nor particularly pathological. In combination with assessment nuances, this leads to an estimated 20–40% of bipolar patients being misdiagnosed as having a unipolar depressive disorder and administered antidepressant medication that can worsen the longitudinal course of bipolar disorder, principally by causing more switching or more mixed states [37]. Further, the proportion of undiagnosed bipolar disorder in epidemiological samples diagnosed with depressive disorder is high, quantified as up to half of identified depressive cases, depending on the sensitivity of the criteria from which bipolar disorder can be accurately recognized, as well as practice and referral nuances [37].

In the ECA study, 39% of those with bipolar I or bipolar II disorder received outpatient psychiatric treatment within 1 year and about 10% would receive inpatient treatment within a 6-month period. In the NCS study, 45% of those with bipolar disorder had received psychiatric treatment in the previous 12 months, although 93% reported lifetime treatment for their bipolar disorder. However, both of these studies suggest that more than half of individuals with bipolar disorder are not currently in psychiatric treatment.

Misdiagnosis or delayed help-seeking has been considered as a major contributor to poor outcome in bipolar disorder, with 80% of undiagnosed patients experiencing psychosocial problems impacting on their relationships, employment, finances, and health.

Further consequences of inappropriately treated bipolar disorder include an increased risk of suicide, longer hospitalizations, poorer social functioning, and general deterioration of the condition.

## Use of pharmacotherapy

Major changes have taken place since 2000 in prescription patterns for bipolar disorder in mental care in Western countries in general [38]. Nation-wide and other population-based longitudinal pharmaco-epidemiological studies on prescription patterns have shown that lithium is prescribed less and anti-epileptics and dopamine antagonists are prescribed substantially more in recent years. In particular, the prescription of lamotrigine and quetiapine has increased substantially (from 0–3% in 2000 to approximately 40% of all patients in 2011 [38]). In many areas of the world, lithium has gone from being the first drug prescribed as maintenance therapy for bipolar disorder to being replaced by dopamine antagonists or anti-epileptics. The use of drugs for depression has been constantly high in Western countries, approximating 70–80% of all patients since 2000 [38, 39]. Combination therapy of lithium, anti-epileptics, drugs for psychosis (see Chapter 140), and also antidepressants has increased substantially during the last decade.

Overall, the development in prescription patterns during the last decade has not been in accordance with the evidence and recommendations in international guidelines in relation to the use of lithium [40–44] and antidepressants [43–47] in bipolar disorder. Changes in study populations do not seem to explain the changes in prescription pattern and use [38]. The high rates of combination therapy reflect that, in real life, patient response and remission rates are low with monotherapy for acute episodes and relapse rates are high during maintenance monotherapy therapy [48].

## Adherence to treatment

Pharmaco-epidemiological studies have consistently shown that adherence to medication is a major clinical challenge in the treatment of bipolar disorder. As much as half of the patients do not take medication or take it in other durations and doses than prescribed, although randomized trials show that group-based psychoeducation can substantially add to improve adherence.

## Risk factors for affective episodes in patients with bipolar disorder

A range of other biological factors are risk factors particularly relevant to the onset of episodes of illness, but they may contribute a relatively small part to lifetime vulnerability. Many women have their first episode of depression or mania in the post-partum period. There is substantial evidence that seasonal patterns influence the onset of manic and depressive episodes. There are consistent findings of an excess of manic episodes in late spring and early summer. To date, however, the nature of the environmental factors that influence this late spring, early summer peak of manic episodes is less clear.

There is also substantial evidence that disruptions of normal biological rhythms may precipitate the onset of manic or depressive episodes. This has been documented in relation to international travel involving east–west or west–east travel with disruption of circadian rhythms. Disruption of circadian rhythms through shift work or other factors which disrupt the normal sleep cycles may also be important triggers to the onset of episodes of mania.

Adverse life events have been well documented to be precipitants of manic episodes, as well as depression. It appears that life events are more likely prior to the first or second episode of mania and are less likely later in the course of illness.

## Life expectancy, mortality, and causes of death

Standardized mortality rates (SMRs) among patients with bipolar disorder have been found consistently to be increased 2–3 times, compared to the general population [49–51], and life expectancy has been reported to be decreased 8–12 years for patients with bipolar disorder, compared to the general population [52]. The increased mortality is related to increased mortality due to suicide [51, 53], unintentional injuries [49, 51], and comorbid general medical illnesses, including cardiovascular disease [49–51, 54], diabetes [51, 55, 56], and chronic obstructive pulmonary disease [51, 57].

The SMR for completed suicide is estimated to be between 10 and 15 [58]. The lifetime risk of suicide may have been overestimated in some prior studies, due to incomplete follow-up in selected samples or rather short-term follow-up of patients with first-time treated mental disorders [59]. The absolute risk of committing suicide within 36 years after the first psychiatric contact has been estimated to be 8% for men and 5% for women [59]. Suicide is a prevalent reason for lost life years specifically during adolescence and early and mid adulthood, and that risk clearly decreases with age [60]. Among 15-year-old patients with bipolar disorder, suicide accounted for 23–24% of all lost life years, decreasing to 0–5% for patients aged 75 years [60]. However, rather surprisingly, natural causes of death is the most prevalent reason for lost life years already from adolescence and increased substantially during early and mid adulthood, that is, from age of 15 years and during the twenties, thirties, and forties [60]. For 15-year-old boys with bipolar disorder, natural causes of death have been found to account for 58% of 12 lost life years, and for 15-year-old girls, natural causes account for 67% of 9 lost life years, increasing to 74% and 80% for 45-year-old men and women, respectively [60].

Reasons for increased mortality due to comorbid general medical illness in bipolar disorder may include unhealthy lifestyle, decreased health care, adverse pharmacological effects, and biological factors [61]. In relation to biological factors, accelerated ageing has recently been proposed as a mechanism explaining the increased prevalence of comorbid medical illness due to disparate pathophysiological changes observed in bipolar disorder such as brain structural alterations, cognitive deficits, oxidative stress imbalance, amyloid metabolism, immunological deregulation, immunosenescence, neurotrophic deficiencies, and telomere shortening [62]. It is well established that, in addition to being differentially affected by chronic medical disorders, the age of onset of medical chronic disorders is much earlier, when compared to individuals in the general population [63].

## Depressive disorders

### Diagnostic issues

A key issue for the epidemiology of depressive disorders is defining the boundaries of major depression and dysthymia. Depressive symptoms in the community are common, and defining both the symptom count and the duration at which depressive symptoms

count as part of a clinical disorder is arbitrary. Provided that one accepts the arbitrary definition of major depression, then determining the rates of current depressive disorders is not especially problematic. However, there are major methodological issues involved in determining whether an individual has ever had a lifetime episode of major depression. Lifetime prevalence rates vary from 4.4% in the United States ECA study to 17.1% in the NCS and to over 30% in the Kendler's Virginia twin sample of women. In part, subjects in the community may forget or fail to report past episodes of major depression (recall bias), and the manner in which the questions are asked may importantly influence lifetime rates of depression. In the diagnostic interview schedule, which was used in the ECA, respondents were asked about lifetime symptoms, a lifetime diagnosis was made, and then recency of the lifetime diagnosis was determined. Diagnostic interview schedules, such as the Composite International Diagnostic Interview, first ask about current depressive symptoms and then, having 'primed' individuals about depressive symptoms, go on to enquire about past depressive episodes. Interviews that follow the schedule of 'priming' before asking about past episodes appear to obtain considerably higher rates of lifetime major depression. Determining lifetime rates of depression with greater precision is an important task, as the vulnerability to depression conferred by risk factors such as genetic factors and childhood experiences may be wrongly estimated if lifetime rates of major depression are imprecise.

DSM-5 allows major depression to be further sub-classified into subtypes, such as melancholia, atypical, psychotic, and by severity and recurrence. Most of the traditional epidemiology studies have tended to ignore the issue of subtyping major depression.

### Prevalence

In the ECA, the 6-month prevalence of major depression across five sites was 2.2 per 100. In the NCS, the 1-month prevalence of a major depressive episode was 6.1 per 100 [64]. In the National Psychiatric Morbidity Surveys of Great Britain, the 1-week rate of a depressive episode was 2.1 per 100 [65], and in the European Study of the Epidemiology of Mental Disorders, the 1-year prevalence of major depressive disorder was 3.9% [66]. Together, these studies would suggest that the current rate of major depression is in the realm of 2–5%.

Estimates of the lifetime rate of major depression are much more variable. The lowest rate reported is 4.4 per 100 from the ECA study, while in the study of Virginia twins, the lifetime rate of major depression is over 30%. It is reasonable to believe that the true lifetime rate of major depression is probably in the realm of 10–20 per 100, but caution should be exercised in expressing lifetime rates of depression with undue precision.

Over the past decade, one of the controversial findings in the epidemiology of major depression has been whether the rates of depression are increasing and whether it is occurring at a younger age. Despite methodological concerns about the reliability of lifetime major depression, studies across countries have reasonably consistently documented an increasing rate of major depression with an earlier age of onset [67, 68]. As mood disorders are the single largest risk factor for suicide, it is also of note that, in most Western countries, the rate of suicide, especially in young adults, increased considerably from the 1970s to the 1990s, although the suicide rate is now declining in many countries. This could, however, reflect better recognition and treatment of depression.

## Comorbidity

Comorbidity is prevalent in depressive disorder. Not surprisingly, the most common comorbid disorders are anxiety disorders and substance abuse disorders. In the NCS, the anxiety disorders with the highest odds ratios indicating comorbidity were generalized anxiety disorder, panic disorder, and post-traumatic stress disorder. It is also important to note that for most anxiety disorders, with the exception of panic disorder, the anxiety disorder usually predates the onset of the depressive disorder. This is of considerable importance, as the risk factors for pure major depression differed from the risk factors for comorbid major depression. Furthermore, the cohort effects of increasing rates of major depression were largely attributable to increasing rates of comorbid major depression, rather than to increasing rates of pure major depression. These results raise important issues for prevention, as it may well be that targeting young people with anxiety disorders could be a major step towards prevention of the development of later major depressive disorders.

The second key area of comorbidity with major depression is with alcohol dependence. Data from the Virginia Twin Register suggest that part of this comorbidity is due to shared genetic factors, although there is also a smaller common environmental risk factor to both disorders.

Another area of considerable comorbidity with depressive disorder is the personality disorders. Comorbidity between depression and these disorders is receiving considerable attention in clinical samples, but to date, there are only limited data from epidemiological samples on the importance of these patterns of comorbidity.

## Risk factors

### Genetics

There is substantial evidence that genetic factors are of major importance as risk factors for vulnerability to major depression, with a heritability at about 40%. Genes for major depression do not appear to be unique for depression but overlap with genes for anxiety and genes for neuroticism. The greater prevalence of depression in women may be due to the strong association of anxiety and neuroticism with depression and the fact that higher rates of anxiety and neuroticism in women lead to higher rates of depression.

### Stressful life events and childhood adversities

Although the experience of a stressful life event is a well-known risk factor for developing depression, the associations are complicated. Firstly, causation may be unclear, as life events may cause depression and depression may result in stressful life events. Further, the type and timing of stressful life events play a role, including the experience of acute vs more chronic stressors and the experience during childhood and the adolescent period or during different age spans in adulthood. Secondly, the impact of life events differs in relation to the onset of the first depressive episode and to subsequent depressive episodes. Approximately 60–80% of patients with a first and single depressive episode have experienced stressful life events in a 6-month period prior to the onset of depression, whereas the prevalence of life events is decreased to 20–40% or less in relation to subsequent depressive episodes. Finally, the experience of life events is highly individual and may be stressful for one person or life situation but positive for another. Overall, assessment of life events based on self-report may be influenced by recall bias and those based on interviews may be influenced by observer bias and interpretation.

### Gene–environment interaction

In 2003, Caspi et al. showed that risk for depression was related to an interaction between the serotonin transporter-linked polymorphic region (5-HTTLPR) and stressful life events, with persons carrying the short, less transcriptionally active 5-HTTLPR allele more vulnerable to depression after stressful life events [69]. The study sparked research into interactions between candidate genes and environmental exposures on risk for psychiatric disorders, but although this field of research has now persisted for more than a decade, it has been characterized by much controversy. Nevertheless, studies identifying stress using objective measures, such as specific medical conditions, or observer-based measures, such as in-person interviews, seem to have found stronger evidence for a gene–environment interaction than studies measuring stress by self-report [70].

### Gender

One of the most consistent findings in the epidemiology of major depression is that the ratio of women to men is approximately 2:1. This increased rate of major depression in women arises during puberty, as in childhood, there is a slightly higher prevalence of depression in boys than girls. The timing of this transition in rates by gender is related to biological puberty, rather than just to age. Intriguingly, a new population-based cohort study found that use of hormonal contraception among adolescent women is associated with an increased risk of subsequent development of depression, suggesting depression as a potential side effect to hormonal contraceptive use on a population level [71].

### Personality

There has been a long history of interest in the likelihood that people with certain personality traits are more vulnerable to depression than others. It is likely that those individuals who are unduly anxious, impulsive, and obsessional may have increased rates of later major depression. The best data exist for neuroticism, which emerges as a clear risk factor for the later development of depressive and anxiety disorders. However, as already mentioned, the same genes seem to contribute to the development of neuroticism and to later anxiety and depressive disorders.

### Physical illness

Having a chronic or severe physical illness is associated with an increased risk for depression. The mechanisms behind this increased risk may vary, depending upon the physical disorder. In disorders such as Parkinson's disease, it is possible that there are shared neurotransmitter abnormalities between Parkinson's disease and depression. In post-stroke depression, there is good evidence that the location of the lesion, at least in part, contributes to the rate of depression, which suggests a neuroanatomical/neurotransmitter connection between the physical illness and the likelihood of depression. For non-central nervous system disorders, such as acute myocardial infarction, diabetes, and cancers, the mechanism for this association is less clear. Further, stress associated with a serious or chronic physical illness may act by bringing out an individual's lifetime vulnerability to depression.

## An integrated aetiological model

The ultimate purpose of studying risk factors for depressive disorders is to contribute to the development of an integrated aetiological model. The most promising research in this area has been performed by Kendler and colleagues on twins from the Virginia Twin Register [72] who developed a model that predicted over 50% of the variance in the liability to develop major depression in the next 12 months. The strongest predictors to depression were as follows:

- Stressful life events.
- Genetic factors.
- Previous history of major depression.
- Neuroticism.

Approximately 60% of the effect of genetic factors on the liability to depression was direct, but the remaining 40% was indirect and largely mediated by past episodes of depression, stressful life events, and neuroticism.

## Use of health services and untreated depression

One of the major challenges for psychiatry presented by epidemiological studies of depression has been the consistent finding that the majority of cases of depression in the community are not recognized, diagnosed, or treated. In the ECA study, it was found that 65–70% of people with depression had visited a health professional in the last 6 months, but only 15–20% had had a visit for a mental health reason and only about 10% had seen a mental health specialist. Among individuals with a 12-month diagnosis of pure major depression in the European Study of the Epidemiology of Mental Disorders, only 21.2% had received any antidepressant treatment within the same period; the exclusive use of approved drugs for depression was even lower (4.6%), while more individuals took only drugs for anxiety (18.4%) [73].

Patients with depression who present with largely somatic, rather than psychological, symptoms are unlikely to be recognized by general practitioners. Even if major depression is recognized in the primary care setting, it is often not adequately treated.

The duration of untreated illness (DUI), defined as the time interval between first onset of the illness and initiation of (pharmacological) treatment, has increasingly been considered to influence the clinical course of different psychiatric disorders. Knowledge of the potential consequences of postponing medical treatment of depression is of crucial importance, when the choice stands between a drug for depression, other therapies, or watchful waiting. Unfortunately, the effects of DUI have been investigated only scarcely in first-episode depression. The largest study found that initiation of appropriate drug treatment more than 6 months after the onset of first-episode depression reduces the chance of obtaining remission to 50% [74].

## Use of pharmacotherapy

Non-adherence to medication is a major challenge concerning up to 50% of patients and is associated with an increased risk of relapse and hospitalization.

## Age of onset and course of illness

Age of onset is later for depressive disorder than for bipolar disorder, with a mean age of around 30 years—however, with a substantial proportion of patients having age at onset of below 21 years. The distribution of age of onset is bimodal, with peaks in the thirties and fifties.

Length of episodes is typically 3–12 months (median duration of 5 months), but 10–20% of patients experience depressive periods of longer than 2 years (that is, a chronic depressive episode). Results from up to 25 years of follow-up studies show that approximately 30–50% of patients remain symptom-free after a depressive episode, while the remaining 50–70% develop new episodes or chronic depression. In a recent 5-year follow-up of patients with psychiatric hospital contact for the first lifetime episode of depression, 83% obtained remission and among these, 32% experienced recurrence of depression and 9% converted to bipolar disorder [6].

Approximately 1% convert from unipolar depressive disorder to bipolar disorder per year [5, 6], approximating 20–40% during the lifetime course.

## Social and cognitive outcomes

Dysfunctions in social interactions remain persistent several years after recovery from depressive symptoms and are correlated with unemployment, disability, and decreased work performance. Within 5 years, 20% of psychiatric inpatients and outpatients with major depression and belonging to the labour force at baseline in Finland were granted a disability pension [75].

Cognitive dysfunction in attention, memory, and executive function is less prevalent in the remitted state of depressive disorder than in bipolar disorder and schizophrenia. However, self-reported attention and concentration difficulties mediate as much as 25% of the impact of depression on patients' psychosocial impairment. Long-term studies rather consistently show that depressive disorder is associated with a 2–3 times increased risk of developing dementia eventually [28–30, 32, 76].

## Life expectancy and mortality

The SMR for completed suicide is estimated to be increased 20-fold [58]. In the longest population-based follow-up study, a 36-year study after the first psychiatric hospital contact, the absolute risk of committing suicide was 7% for men and 4% for women [59].

Life expectancy is decreased approximately 12 years and 10 years in men and women, respectively [77]. SMR is highest for death due to suicide and accidents, but the absolute number of deaths is highest for natural causes.

As bipolar and depressive disorders are associated with long-term deficits in social, functional, and cognitive outcomes and a substantially decreased life expectancy, there is a need for future studies on early and lifestyle interventions. A recent randomized trial has shown that early intervention, combining optimized pharmacological treatment and psychoeducation, following the onset of bipolar disorder substantially improves the outcome of the bipolar illness [78] and specifically so among young adults below 25 years of age [79].

## Acknowledgement

The author wishes to acknowledge Professor Peter R. Joyce, the author of this chapter in the second edition of the *New Oxford Textbook of Psychiatry*.

# REFERENCES

1. Wang PS, Simon G, Kessler RC. The economic burden of depression and the cost-effectiveness of treatment. *Int J Methods Psychiatr Res* 2003;12:22–33.

2. Whiteford HA, Degenhardt L, Rehm J, *et al.* Global burden of disease attributable to mental and substance use disorders: findings from the Global Burden of Disease Study 2010. *Lancet* 2013;382:1575–86.

3. Olesen J, Gustavsson A, Svensson M, Wittchen HU, Jonsson B. The economic cost of brain disorders in Europe. *Eur J Neurol* 2012;19:155–62.

4. Ferrari AJ, Charlson FJ, Norman RE, *et al.* Burden of depressive disorders by country, sex, age, and year: findings from the global burden of disease study 2010. *PLoS Med* 2013;10:e1001547.

5. Angst J, Sellaro R, Stassen HH, Gamma A. Diagnostic conversion from depression to bipolar disorders: results of a long-term prospective study of hospital admissions. *J Affect Disord* 2005;84:149–57.

6. Bukh JD, Andersen PK, Kessing LV. Rates and predictors of remission, recurrence and conversion to bipolar disorder after the first lifetime episode of depression—a prospective 5-year follow-up study. *Psychol Med* 2016;46:1151–61.

7. Weissman MM, Bland RC, Canino GJ, *et al.* Cross-national epidemiology of major depression and bipolar disorder. *JAMA* 1996;276:293–9.

8. Kessler RC, Rubinow DR, Holmes C, Abelson JM, Zhao S. The epidemiology of DSM-III-R bipolar I disorder in a general population survey. *Psychol Med* 1997;27:1079–89.

9. Merikangas KR, Akiskal HS, Angst J, *et al.* Lifetime and 12-month prevalence of bipolar spectrum disorder in the National Comorbidity Survey replication. *Arch Gen Psychiatry* 2007;64:543–52.

10. Hoertel N, Le SY, Angst J, Dubertret C. Subthreshold bipolar disorder in a U.S. national representative sample: prevalence, correlates and perspectives for psychiatric nosography. *J Affect Disord* 2013;146:338–47.

11. Geller B, Sun K, Zimerman B, Luby J, Frazier J, Williams M. Complex and rapid-cycling in bipolar children and adolescents: a preliminary study. *J Affect Disord* 1995;34:259–68.

12. Geller B, Luby J. Child and adolescent bipolar disorder: a review of the past 10 years. *J Am Acad Child Adolesc Psychiatry* 1997;36:1168–76.

13. Craney JL, Geller B. A prepubertal and early adolescent bipolar disorder-I phenotype: review of phenomenology and longitudinal course. *Bipolar Disord* 2003;5:243–56.

14. Youngstrom EA, Birmaher B, Findling RL. Pediatric bipolar disorder: validity, phenomenology, and recommendations for diagnosis. *Bipolar Disord* 2008;10:194–214.

15. Kessing LV, Vradi E, Kragh AP. Diagnostic stability in pediatric bipolar disorder. *J Affect Disord* 2015;172:417–21.

16. Arnold LE, Demeter C, Mount K, *et al.* Pediatric bipolar spectrum disorder and ADHD: comparison and comorbidity in the LAMS clinical sample. *Bipolar Disord* 2011;13:509–21.

17. Carlson GA, Klein DN. How to understand divergent views on bipolar disorder in youth. *Annu Rev Clin Psychol* 2014; 10:529–51.

18. Kessing, L. V. Course and cognitive outcome in major affective disorder. Dissertation for Doctor of Medical Science (DMSc), 2001. *Dan Med J* 2015;62:B5160(11), 1–44.

19. Kessing LV, Andersen PK. Predictive effects of previous episodes on the risk of recurrence in depressive and bipolar disorders. *Curr Psychiatry Rep* 2005;7:413–20.

20. Burdick KE, Russo M, Frangou S, *et al.* Empirical evidence for discrete neurocognitive subgroups in bipolar disorder: clinical implications. *Psychol Med* 2014;44:3083–96.

21. Reichenberg A, Harvey PD, Bowie CR, *et al.* Neuropsychological function and dysfunction in schizophrenia and psychotic affective disorders. *Schizophr Bull* 2009;35:1022–9.

22. Depp CA, Mausbach BT, Harmell AL, *et al.* Meta-analysis of the association between cognitive abilities and everyday functioning in bipolar disorder. *Bipolar Disord* 2012;14:217–26.

23. Martinez-Aran A, Vieta E, Torrent C, *et al.* Functional outcome in bipolar disorder: the role of clinical and cognitive factors. *Bipolar Disord* 2007;9:103–13.

24. Mur M, Portella MJ, Martinez-Aran A, Pifarre J, Vieta E. Influence of clinical and neuropsychological variables on the psychosocial and occupational outcome of remitted bipolar patients. *Psychopathology* 2009;42:148–56.

25. Huxley N, Baldessarini RJ. Disability and its treatment in bipolar disorder patients. *Bipolar Disord* 2007;9:183–96.

26. Kogan JN, Otto MW, Bauer MS, *et al.* Demographic and diagnostic characteristics of the first 1000 patients enrolled in the Systematic Treatment Enhancement Program for Bipolar Disorder (STEP-BD). *Bipolar Disord* 2004;6:460–9.

27. Tse S, Chan S, Ng KL, Yatham LN. Meta-analysis of predictors of favorable employment outcomes among individuals with bipolar disorder. *Bipolar Disord* 2014;16:217–29.

28. Kessing LV, Olsen EW, Mortensen PB, Andersen PK. Dementia in affective disorder: a case-register study. *Acta Psychiatr Scand* 1999;100:176–85.

29. Kessing LV, Nilsson FM. Increased risk of developing dementia in patients with major affective disorders compared to patients with other medical illnesses. *J Affect Disord* 2003;73:261–9.

30. da SJ, Goncalves-Pereira M, Xavier M, Mukaetova-Ladinska EB. Affective disorders and risk of developing dementia: systematic review. *Br J Psychiatry* 2013;202:177–86.

31. Wu KY, Chang CM, Liang HY, *et al.* Increased risk of developing dementia in patients with bipolar disorder: a nested matched case-control study. *Bipolar Disord* 2013;15:787–94.

32. Chen MH, Li CT, Tsai CF, *et al.* Risk of subsequent dementia among patients with bipolar disorder or major depression: a nationwide longitudinal study in Taiwan. *J Am Med Dir Assoc* 2015;16:504–8.

33. Kessing LV, Andersen PK. Does the risk of developing dementia increase with the number of episodes in patients with depressive disorder and in patients with bipolar disorder? *J Neurol Neurosurg Psychiatry* 2004;75:1662–6.

34. Kessing LV, Sondergard L, Forman JL, Andersen PK. Lithium treatment and risk of dementia. *Arch Gen Psychiatry* 2008;65:1331–5.

35. Kessing LV, Forman JL, Andersen PK. Does lithium protect against dementia? *Bipolar Disord* 2010;12:87–94.

36. Gerhard T, Devanand DP, Huang C, Crystal S, Olfson M. Lithium treatment and risk for dementia in adults with bipolar disorder: population-based cohort study. *Br J Psychiatry* 2015;207:46–51.

37. McCraw S, Parker G, Graham R, Synnott H, Mitchell PB. The duration of undiagnosed bipolar disorder: effect on outcomes and treatment response. *J Affect Disord* 2014;168:422–9.

38. Kessing LV, Vradi E, Andersen PK. Nationwide and population-based prescription patterns in bipolar disorder. *Bipolar Disord* 2016;18:174–82.

39. Haeberle A, Greil W, Russmann S, Grohmann R. Mono- and combination drug therapies in hospitalized patients with bipolar depression. Data from the European drug surveillance program AMSP. *BMC Psychiatry* 2012;12:153.

40. Severus E, Taylor MJ, Sauer C, *et al.* Lithium for prevention of mood episodes in bipolar disorders: systematic review and meta-analysis. *Int J Bipolar Disord* 2014;2:15.

41. Goodwin GM. Evidence-based guidelines for treating bipolar disorder: revised second edition--recommendations from the British Association for Psychopharmacology. *J Psychopharmacol* 2009;23:346–88.

42. Grunze H, Vieta E, Goodwin GM, *et al.* The World Federation of Societies of Biological Psychiatry (WFSBP) guidelines for the biological treatment of bipolar disorders: update 2012 on the long-term treatment of bipolar disorder. *World J Biol Psychiatry* 2013;14:154–219.

43. Yatham LN, Kennedy SH, Parikh SV, *et al.* Canadian Network for Mood and Anxiety Treatments (CANMAT) and International Society for Bipolar Disorders (ISBD) collaborative update of CANMAT guidelines for the management of patients with bipolar disorder: update 2013. *Bipolar Disord* 2013; 15:1–44.

44. National Institute for Health and Care Excellence. *Bipolar disorder: the assessment and management of bipolar disorder in adults, children and young people in primary and secondary care.* NICE Clinical Guideline [CG185]. 2015.

45. Sidor MM, MacQueen GM. Antidepressants for the acute treatment of bipolar depression: a systematic review and meta-analysis. *J Clin Psychiatry* 2011;72:156–67.

46. Grunze H, Vieta E, Goodwin GM, *et al.* The World Federation of Societies of Biological Psychiatry (WFSBP) Guidelines for the Biological Treatment of Bipolar Disorders: update 2010 on the treatment of acute bipolar depression. *World J Biol Psychiatry* 2010;11:81–109.

47. Pacchiarotti I, Bond DJ, Baldessarini RJ, *et al.* The International Society for Bipolar Disorders (ISBD) task force report on antidepressant use in bipolar disorders. *Am J Psychiatry* 2013;170:1249–62.

48. Kessing LV, Hellmund G, Andersen PK. Predictors of excellent response to lithium: results from a nationwide register-based study. *Int Clin Psychopharmacol* 2011;26:323–8.

49. Osby U, Brandt L, Correia N, Ekbom A, Sparen P. Excess mortality in bipolar and unipolar disorder in Sweden. *Arch Gen Psychiatry* 2001;58:844–50.

50. Laursen TM, Munk-Olsen T, Nordentoft M, Mortensen PB. Increased mortality among patients admitted with major psychiatric disorders: a register-based study comparing mortality in unipolar depressive disorder, bipolar affective disorder, schizoaffective disorder, and schizophrenia. *J Clin Psychiatry* 2007;68:899–907.

51. Crump C, Sundquist K, Winkleby MA, Sundquist J. Comorbidities and mortality in bipolar disorder: a Swedish national cohort study. *JAMA Psychiatry* 2013;70:931–9.

52. Kessing LV, Vradi E, Andersen PK. Life expectancy in bipolar disorder. *Bipolar Disord* 2015;17:543–8.

53. Harris EC, Barraclough B. Suicide as an outcome for mental disorders. A meta-analysis. *Br J Psychiatry* 1997;170:205–28.

54. Weiner M, Warren L, Fiedorowicz JG. Cardiovascular morbidity and mortality in bipolar disorder. *Ann Clin Psychiatry* 2011;23:40–7.

55. McIntyre RS, Konarski JZ, Misener VL, Kennedy SH. Bipolar disorder and diabetes mellitus: epidemiology, etiology, and treatment implications. *Ann Clin Psychiatry* 2005;17:83–93.

56. Calkin CV, Gardner DM, Ransom T, Alda M. The relationship between bipolar disorder and type 2 diabetes: more than just co-morbid disorders. *Ann Med* 2013;45:171–81.

57. Laursen TM, Munk-Olsen T, Gasse C. Chronic somatic comorbidity and excess mortality due to natural causes in persons with schizophrenia or bipolar affective disorder. *PLoS One* 2011;6:e24597.

58. Zoltan R, Fawcett J. Suicide and bipolar disorder. In: Yatham LN, Maj M (eds). *Bipolar Disorder. Clinical and Neurobiological Foundations.* John Wiley & Sons, Chichester. 2010. pp. 62–8.

59. Nordentoft M, Mortensen PB, Pedersen CB. Absolute risk of suicide after first hospital contact in mental disorder. *Arch Gen Psychiatry* 2011;68:1058–64.

60. Kessing LV, Vradi E, McIntyre RS, Andersen PK. Causes of decreased life expectancy over the life span in bipolar disorder. *J Affect Disord* 2015;180:142–7.

61. Roshanaei-Moghaddam B, Katon W. Premature mortality from general medical illnesses among persons with bipolar disorder: a review. *Psychiatr Serv* 2009;60:147–56.

62. Rizzo LB, Costa LG, Mansur RB, *et al.* The theory of bipolar disorder as an illness of accelerated aging: Implications for clinical care and research. *Neurosci Biobehav Rev* 2014;42C:157–69.

63. McIntyre RS, Jerrell JM. Metabolic and cardiovascular adverse events associated with antipsychotic treatment in children and adolescents. *Arch Pediatr Adolesc Med* 2008;162:929–35.

64. Blazer DG, Kessler RC, McGonagle KA, Swartz MS. The prevalence and distribution of major depression in a national community sample: the National Comorbidity Survey. *Am J Psychiatry* 1994;151:979–86.

65. Jenkins R, Lewis G, Bebbington P, *et al.* The National Psychiatric Morbidity surveys of Great Britain--initial findings from the household survey. *Psychol Med* 1997;27:775–89.

66. Alonso J, Angermeyer MC, Bernert S, *et al.* Prevalence of mental disorders in Europe: results from the European Study of the Epidemiology of Mental Disorders (ESEMeD) project. *Acta Psychiatr Scand Suppl* 2004;420:21–7.

67. Cross National Collaborative Group. The changing rate of major depression. Cross national comparisons. *JAMA* 1992;268:3098–105.

68. Spiers N, Brugha TS, Bebbington P, McManus S, Jenkins R, Meltzer H. Age and birth cohort differences in depression in repeated cross-sectional surveys in England: the National Psychiatric Morbidity Surveys, 1993 to 2007. *Psychol Med* 2012;42:2047–55.

69. Caspi A, Sugden K, Moffitt TE, *et al.* Influence of life stress on depression: moderation by a polymorphism in the 5-HTT gene. *Science* 2003;301:386–9.

70. Karg K, Burmeister M, Shedden K, Sen S. The serotonin transporter promoter variant (5-HTTLPR), stress, and depression meta-analysis revisited: evidence of genetic moderation. *Arch Gen Psychiatry* 2011;68:444–54.

71. Skovlund CW, Mørch LN, Kessing SV, Lidegaard O. Association of hormonal contraception with depression. *JAMA Psychiatry* 2016;73:1154–62.

72. Kendler KS, Gardner CO, Prescott CA. Toward a comprehensive developmental model for major depression in women. *Am J Psychiatry* 2002;159:1133–45.

73. Alonso J, Angermeyer MC, Bernert S, *et al.* Psychotropic drug utilization in Europe: results from the European Study of the Epidemiology of Mental Disorders (ESEMeD) project. *Acta Psychiatr Scand Suppl* 2004;55–64.

74. Bukh JD, Bock C, Vinberg M, Kessing LV. The effect of prolonged duration of untreated depression on antidepressant treatment outcome. *J Affect Disord* 2013;145:42–8.

75. Holma IA, Holma KM, Melartin TK, Rytsala HJ, Isometsa ET. A 5-year prospective study of predictors for disability pension among patients with major depressive disorder. *Acta Psychiatr Scand* 2012;125:325–34.

76. Kessing LV. Depression and the risk for dementia. *Curr Opin Psychiatry* 2012;25:457–61.

77. Zoltan R, Fawcett J. Suicide and bipolar disorder. In: Yatham LN, Maj M (eds). *Bipolar Disorder. Clinical and Neurobiological Foundations.* John Wiley & Sons, Chichester. 2010. pp. 62–8.

77. Laursen TM, Musliner KL, Benros ME, Vestergaard M, Munk-Olsen T. Mortality and life expectancy in persons with severe unipolar depression. *J Affect Disord* 2016;193:203–7.

78. Kessing LV, Hansen HV, Hvenegaard A, *et al.* Treatment in a specialised out-patient mood disorder clinic v. standard out-patient treatment in the early course of bipolar disorder: randomised clinical trial. *Br J Psychiatry* 2013;202:212–19.

79. Kessing LV, Hansen HV, Christensen EM, Dam H, Gluud C, Wetterslev J. Do young adults with bipolar disorder benefit from early intervention? *J Affect Disord* 2014;152–4:403–8.

# 68

# Primary prevention of mood disorders: building a target for prevention strategies

*Gin S. Malhi*

## Introduction

Mood disorders, both depressive and bipolar, are seemingly ubiquitous in modern-day society and, once established, cannot be cured. Research efforts in the latter half of the last century focused largely on diagnosis and optimal treatment of mood disorders, with the implicit aim of illness containment, rather than its complete removal. But even symptomatic management of mood disorders has been less than optimal. Part of the reason for this is that there has been a widespread lack of consensus regarding whether psychiatric disorders are discrete entities or lie on a continuum defined by dimensional constructs, and though the key features that characterize the disorders have been reliably identified, the construction of a meaningful hierarchy has eluded both researchers and clinicians alike. Apart from creating difficulties in diagnosis, this has meant that defining targets for treatment, clinically and for research purposes, has proven to be challenging. It remains unclear, for example, which symptoms or clusters of symptoms are most closely coupled with functional recovery and which symptoms are most likely to herald a recurrence or re-emergence of the illness. Therefore, treatment has generally been symptom-focused and its main goal has been to limit acute episodes of illness and to return the individual to wellness. Only relatively recently has there been a shift towards longer-term prophylaxis and maintenance of well-being, with a growing emphasis on prevention. Clearly, prevention is the ultimate and ideal goal, namely, to intercept the illness before it takes hold by stopping processes that lead to the emergence of mood disorders. But to achieve this, a deeper understanding of the pathophysiology of mood disorders is necessary. Sadly, our current knowledge of how mood disorders evolve is incomplete and insufficient for this purpose. Nevertheless, attempts at prevention have begun in earnest, and emerging evidence suggests that, when such efforts are suitably targeted, reasonable benefits can be achieved, in the short term at least. Whether these outcomes can be sustained, and for how long, is the key question—the answer to which remains elusive. Therefore, this chapter briefly discusses some models of prevention, the types of interventions and treatments that are currently being trialled, and where future insights in this field might lead us.

## The burden of mood disorders

By their very nature, mood disorders distress the affected individual, but they also impact their families, friends, peers, colleagues, and the broader community. This makes mood disorders a tremendous burden to bear. Among mental disorders, the highest global burden, as explained by disability-adjusted life years (DALYs), that is, the cumulative number of years of productive life lost to disability, ill health, or early death, occurs in adolescents and the young to middle-aged and is associated with depressive and anxiety disorders, while the burden from bipolar disorders is ranked fourth overall [1, 2]. This 'quantitative' evidence underscores the need to avert or reduce the qualitatively palpable burden exerted by these disorders at an earlier stage, and it has been suggested that evidence-based interventions may be capable of doing just this [3]. But presently, and somewhat alarmingly, based on the WHO projections for 2030, this burden is not being diminished [4]. So what are the impediments to reducing this burden, and how can these barriers be overcome?

## Barriers to reducing the burden

Although gaps in the scientific knowledge base regarding prevention and treatment of mood disorders are gradually narrowing, puzzlingly, the actual burden is not diminishing at a commensurate rate. This is attributable to a number of factors, including the conflicting and disparate priorities of diverse stakeholders who collectively shoulder the burden of mood disorders. Consequently, barriers exist at all levels—from individuals and families to communities, societies, and organizations. To overcome this, an integrated approach is needed, one that targets modifiable barriers by

**Table 68.1** Modifiable barriers that hinder efforts to reduce the burden of mood disorders, and potential strategies to overcome them

| Barriers | Strategies |
|---|---|
| Delayed diagnosis* | 1. Early identification of risk and protective factors<br>2. Early detection and diagnosis |
| Delayed initiation of treatment** | Use of early intervention strategies (mainly those that have the potential to cause little harm) |
| Stigmatization (constrains uptake of services) | 1. Psychoeducation (factual information regarding the nature, causes, risks, and protective factors of mood disorders)<br>2. Awareness campaigns to enhance attitude and behaviour change<br>3. Supportive community engagement campaigns |
| Uneven distribution of funding | 1. Clarity of policies governing resource allocation<br>2. Availability of resources for training needs |
| Paucity of evidence-based interventions and treatments | Translating research from the laboratory to the real world |

* Especially likely with bipolar disorder where the illness usually manifests with depression and is therefore misdiagnosed [41].
** A tentative approach to intervention (especially the prescription of medications) is understandable where the diagnosis may be speculative.
Source: data from *Ment Health Serv Res*, 4(4), Bruce ML, Wells KB, Miranda J, *et al.*, Barriers to reducing burden of affective disorders, pp. 187–197, Copyright (2002), Plenum Publishing Corporation; *Psychiatr Serv*, 63(10), Corrigan PW, Morris SB, Michaels PJ, *et al.*, Challenging the Public Stigma of Mental Illness: A Meta-Analysis of Outcome Studies, pp. 963–973, Copyright ( 2012); American Psychiatric Association Publishing; *Biol Psychiatry*, 52(6), Wells KB, Miranda J, Bauer MS, *et al.*, Overcoming barriers to reducing the burden of affective disorders, pp. 655–675, Copyright (2002), Society of Biological Psychiatry.

taking into consideration contributions from the various stakeholders (Table 68.1) [5–7].

It is estimated that primary care interventions have the potential to reduce the burden of mood disorders by 10–30%, but because of a *delay in diagnosis* and the subsequent *initiation of treatment*, this reduction may not be sufficient [8]. Another barrier—*stigmatization*—which is largely based on fear, embarrassment, little or insufficient knowledge, and restrictive policies for those with mood disorders, further limits access to services and their uptake. Therefore, to provide sustainable and effective evidence-based interventions, it is necessary to identify changes in mental health policies and research services and to address inefficiencies in the distribution of funding and training needs [7]. At the same time, it is also important to understand the causes and underlying mechanisms involved in the development of mood disorders, to enable timely identification of the factors that contribute to their development. With early identification of risk and protective factors, it may be possible to intervene sooner to either prevent onset or delay progression to full-blown mood disorders.

## Causes of mood disorders

To be able to intervene in an effective way so as to prevent and treat mood disorders, a deeper understanding of the *risk factors* that predispose young people to developing mood disorders and the *protective factors* that may increase resilience and adequately buffer them from the development of mood disorders, or at least their consequences, is critical. Understanding these factors may reveal targets for preventative and early interventions, as well as measurable outcomes that allow assessment of their efficacy and effectiveness.

But despite extensive research in recent years, it has become increasingly evident that the causes of mood disorders are multifactorial and that numerous variables contribute to the myriad of manifestations encountered clinically. For example, mood disorders are often preceded or triggered by life events—implicating a set of interactions between environmental and intrinsic risk factors that presumably converge on any number of neural systems and pathways. Identification of such intrinsic and extrinsic risk factors that increase the probability of developing mood disorders may assist in predicting onset and serve to focus prevention endeavours. This is exciting because some of these factors may be discernible from a relatively early age [9–12], and while many are seemingly irreversible, others are modifiable and may potentially serve as targets for prevention strategies.

At the same time, enhancing protective factors may also serve to delay or prevent the deterioration of mental health. Thus, to maintain an optimal level of well-being, any imbalance between risk and protection needs to shift so as to favour resilience. However, while exposure to risks and protective factors is inherent in the course of everyone's life, critically, it is the extent of exposure and the individual's response to this that varies. Interestingly, despite individual differences, there seems to be a developmental trajectory to exposure, that is, some risks and protective factors seem to be phase (stage of life)-dependent while others are more stable and present throughout the course of life.

In the context of mood disorders, there seems to be a cumulative effect of risk and protective factors, wherein as the number of risk factors and the duration of exposure to these increases, so do the odds of developing a depressive or bipolar disorder, whereas a greater number of protective factors decreases these odds [13–16]. Specifically, emerging evidence suggests that through cumulative damage over time or disruptions during particularly sensitive developmental periods (phase-dependent), the emergence of enduring mood disorders can be traced to exposure to adversity in the early years of life, from birth and infancy throughout childhood and adolescence into young adulthood (Fig. 68.1) [11, 14, 17–24]. At the same time, throughout these periods of growth and development, protective factors (intrinsic and extrinsic) act as buffers to minimize the deleterious effects of such adversity, and from the standpoint of prevention, these may also serve as targets that can be potentially enhanced as part of preventative strategies.

For instance, from birth, there is a genetic predisposition, via parental transmission, that interacts with environmental risk factors to increase the likelihood of developing mood disorders, but there is no particular time period during which this interaction is destined to exert an effect. As such, through the interaction between the cumulative effects of, or exposure to, adversity at 'critical' time points and the individual's genetic disposition, a somewhat delayed, but chronic, expression of mood disorders may ensue years, or even decades, after the adverse event. These cumulative effects are thought to arise as a result of the 'wear and tear' or allostatic load of the body and the brain due to persistent exposure to adversity at multiple time points [16, 25, 26]. On the other hand, latent, but enduring, effects of exposure to adversity during sensitive periods

| | Box 1 | Box 2<br>Box 1-perinatal insults+ | Box 3<br>Box 2+ | Box 4<br>Box 3+ | Box 5<br>Box 4+ | Box 6<br>Box 5+ | Box 7<br>Box 6+ |
|---|---|---|---|---|---|---|---|
| **Risk factors** | Genetics<br>Maternal illness/inflammation<br>Parental depression<br>Parental substance misuse<br>Perinatal insults<br>Parental stress<br>Poverty/socio-economic status (SES) | Insecure attachment<br>Ongoing family stress<br>Difficult temperament<br>Frontal lobe hypo-activation | Parental discord conflict<br>Trauma. Abuse, maltreatment, bullying<br>Poor academic achievement performance<br>Sub-syndromal symptoms<br>Dysregulated growth hormone process<br>Hostility | Difficult interpersonal/peer relationships<br>Self-regulation difficulty<br>Poor social problem-solving skills<br>Negative cognitions/self-image<br>Anxiety<br>Stressful life events<br>Sexual identity | Early puberty<br>Parent-child conflict<br>Low self-esteem<br>Disengagement<br>Extreme need for approval and social support<br>Emotion-focused coping | Early-onset depression<br>Decrease in and need for social support<br>Need to adapt to new social contexts | Full-blown episode |
| **Developmental stage** | From conception to birth | Infancy<br>Under 2 years | Early childhood<br>3–8 years | Middle childhood<br>9–11 years | Adolescence<br>12–18 years | Early adulthood<br>19–24 years | Adulthood<br>Over 25 years |
| **Protective factors** | Successful treatments of illness/condition<br>Adequate parenting<br>Adequate stress management<br>Adequate socio-economic resources | Secure attachments<br>Frontal lobe activation | Parental harmony/conflict resolution<br>Security and safety provision/reliable support and discipline<br>Academic competence<br>Healthy physical development<br>Self-regulation<br>Ability to make friends/get along with others | Healthy peer relationships and social skills<br>Positively biased cognitions and self-image<br>Protection from harm and fear<br>Supportive environments | Adequate educational support<br>Positive physical development<br>Consistent and predictable rules/limits<br>Clear values<br>High self-esteem<br>Engagement in school/extracurricular activities and family life<br>Emotional self-regulation | Early intervention<br>Extending social networks<br>Explore self-identity in romantic relationships<br>Balance autonomy and relatedness to family | Treatment |

Scope of intervention: —— Maternal —— Family —— School —— Community ——

**Fig. 68.1** Risk and protective factors by developmental stage, reflecting the cumulative and latent effects of stressful life events, culminating in the development of mood disorders or resilience. These factors also span the affected individual's lifetime. Maternal health is important, especially during pregnancy. Similarly, early childhood milieu is critical in defining secure attachment to the 'world' and understanding interpersonal interactions. Family, peer groups, and school provide evolving and iterative environments that shape aspects of personality and lay down the foundation for later stages of development. Puberty and adolescence mark a period of rapid social, emotional, and cognitive development that culminates in a sophisticated understanding of oneself and the world, and as such, it is this phase of life during which most psychiatric disorders first appear. Throughout, the balance between risks and protective factors oscillates, eventuating, over time, in the development of vulnerabilities and resilience.

when the brain is presumed to be more responsive to positive and negative environmental triggers may become intricately embedded in underlying neurobiological processes [16, 18]. However, though it is likely that there are sensitive or 'critical' periods during which vulnerability to mood disorders is increased, the difference is probably modest, and evidence for such epochs of heightened susceptibility has thus far proven to be relatively weak and largely circumstantial [16, 18, 19].

Nevertheless, as a general rule, the earlier the intervention, the better the long-term outcomes are likely to be, and thus far, the evidence for this also seems to hold [27–30]. Most important, however, is to target the risk and protective factors that have a demonstrable causal link with mood disorders, and doing so earlier in development, as this has the greatest potential to produce the most robust, and possibly long-term positive outcomes [28, 29, 31].

## Nature of mood disorders

The major psychiatric taxonomies—the Diagnostic and Statistical Manual of Mental Disorders (DSM) and the International Classification of Diseases (ICD)—define mood disorders cross-sectionally, and they give relatively little consideration to their longitudinal course (while they acknowledge that they are chronic lifelong illnesses—often with an early age of onset) [24, 32–39]. This myopic view is, in part, pragmatic—because the trajectory of mood disorders is difficult to predict and the illnesses are intrinsically capricious. But, because the propensity for recurrence binds all mood disorders, a longitudinal and longer-term perspective is essential. In this context, recurrence refers to the repeated occurrence of episodes of depression and mania, but in reality, the underlying pathophysiology of the illness, once established, is always present; it is merely its clinical expression that ebbs and flows. This concept is not fully captured in classification systems, which instead emphasize the impact of acute exacerbations and infer that in between episodes of illness, patients recover as the illness remits. But when considering

prevention, it is the underlying processes, that is, the subsyndromal pathological activity, that need to be targeted (Fig. 68.2).

## Prevention strategies

When to intervene for maximum benefit is a crucial question that requires an understanding of the developmental trajectory of mood disorders. For instance, Howes and Falkenberg [40] have identified potential points for prevention in the developmental trajectory of bipolar disorder (BD). The earliest point in this schema is when there is fluctuation of mood that represents an underlying cyclothymia or a mental state of 'being at risk' of developing BD. The second stage is when precipitating life events accumulate to the extent they cross a threshold and transition the illness into the 'prodromal phase'—in other words, the last stage where prevention is possible. However, as BD is often initially diagnosed as MDD, and the transition from MDD to BD can take up to 5 years, and even then, only a small proportion of cases make the transition, waiting for the prodromal phase before intervening risks altogether missing the window for prevention [41–43]. One advance could be to regard the developmental trajectory of some depressive disorders as the prelude to that of BD, and in such instances, by focusing on the prevention of depression, it may be possible, in fact, to prevent the development of BD. Similarly, a step further (backwards) builds on the observation that anxiety (and anxiety disorders) often precedes major depression and is a common 'comorbidity' of both depression and BD [44–48]. Therefore, anticipating and targeting anxiety may aid the prevention of mood disorders. With this developmental and chronological perspective in mind, it is important to note that while vulnerabilities for anxiety and mood disorders may be established in adulthood, it is adolescence that seems to be the critical period for their clinical emergence and that this is set against a background of considerable neurobiological and psychosocial change that begins post-puberty [34, 49, 50]. The impact of these changes can be protective or detrimental to long-term health outcomes, and so in either case, targeting

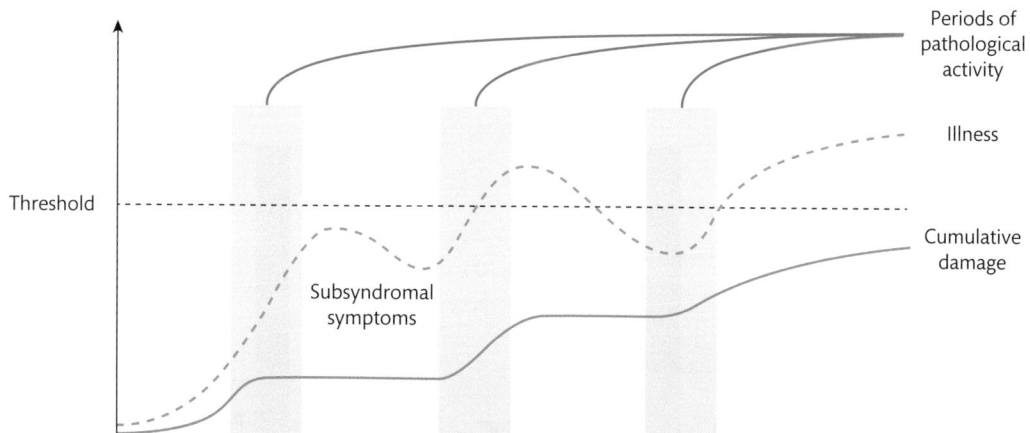

**Fig. 68.2** The clinical trajectory of mood disorders and their underlying components. The shaded blue zones represent periods of pathological activity that drive the core pathological processes underpinning the illness. This leads to damage which then accumulates. Cumulative damage is shown as a blue line, and this indicates how, as the illness progresses, it scars brain functioning—impacting reserve and resilience. The underlying pathological processes and cumulative damage lead to clinical symptoms. The dashed line depicts clinical symptomatology upon which diagnoses are dependent. This transitions from being subsyndromal to eventuating in illness. The troughs and peaks illustrate the seemingly episodic nature of the illness, as it traverses the threshold for clinical diagnosis.

this stage could hold potential to benefit long-term outcomes [50]. Therefore, targeting the developmental trajectory of anxiety and depression may be a productive prevention strategy, with a particular focus on early vulnerability markers.

## 'Prevention' vs treatment

Prevention is the reduction of risk factors and enhancement of protective factors prior to the onset of disease. Prevention interventions occur before the onset of a clinical episode and precede treatment interventions, and therefore, they lie intermediate on a continuum between health promotion and treatment [51, 52]. Effectiveness of prevention strategies appears to depend on the identification of risk factors for mood disorders and protective factors that produce resilience and defend against the development of mood disorders—even in extreme adversity. Treatment, on the other hand, is the reduction of disease-related symptoms and the enhancement of protective factors and is usually only prescribed once an illness has formed and a clinical diagnosis has been made.

However, the distinction between prevention and treatment is somewhat blurred. Some time ago, the Institute of Medicine recommended prevention should target only those with early symptoms that are not sufficiently severe to warrant a diagnosis of a mental disorder [53]. But this somewhat narrow definition overlooks a large pre-symptomatic group that may be at increased risk of mental disorders, and given our current understanding of the aetiology of mood disorders, waiting until symptoms emerge, apart from being less effective, may primarily be regarded as unethical—especially if timely interventions can be shown to have a substantial impact. An alternative perspective on the prevention of depression stipulates that for an intervention to be preventive, it has to show a post-intervention increase in depressive symptoms in the control group and either no increase or an attenuated increase in depressive symptoms in the intervention group [54]. This suggests that post-intervention, a reduction in depressive symptoms, in the absence of an increase or no change in depressive symptoms in the control group, may be indicative of a treatment effect, rather than a prevention effect (Fig. 68.3).

## Rationale for prevention

The difficulty of diagnosing mood disorders in children and adolescents is widely acknowledged, and as a consequence, diagnostic criteria originally created for adults have been modified to capture mood disorders as they evolve in young people. But a lack of specificity and the variability in presentation mean that depression is often misdiagnosed and likely overlooked. Naturally, this impacts treatment decisions. The efficacy of drugs, in combination with psychotherapy, for the treatment of unipolar depression is well established, and medications are a key component of any treatment regimen for bipolar disorders. However, the long-term consequences of pharmacotherapy are yet to be fully determined, especially if commenced early in life [55–57]. For example, in the treatment of paediatric BD, pharmacological agents and cognitive behavioural, as well as interpersonal, therapies produce some benefit [intermediate effect sizes (ES)], but these are thought to be unsustainable over time [56]. Interestingly, randomized controlled studies of psychosocial treatments suggest they may be effective in delaying the time to relapse, facilitating mood stabilization, reducing the severity of symptoms of depression, and improving psychosocial functioning [58]. Intriguingly, such evidence points to the possibility that treatments, while ameliorating indicated symptoms, do not necessarily prevent the onset of mood disorders and the recurrence of future episodes, but instead may limit negative consequences. Therefore, while treatment is often regarded as having a preventive component, in actuality, true prevention is rarely achieved with treatment alone.

Evidence suggests that in primary care patients, prevention is more cost-effective than care as usual [59]. This is because the earlier the onset of mood disorders, the poorer the long-term prognosis—as demonstrated by a poorer overall quality of life, significantly dysfunctional interpersonal relationships, a greater number of recurrences, with shorter euthymic periods in between, greater comorbidity, and an increased likelihood of suicide attempts [60, 61]. Thus, it is no surprise that the most effective strategies to reduce the health burden of mood disorders are those most likely to prevent the onset of mood disorders, particularly in vulnerable young people [14, 60, 62–64].

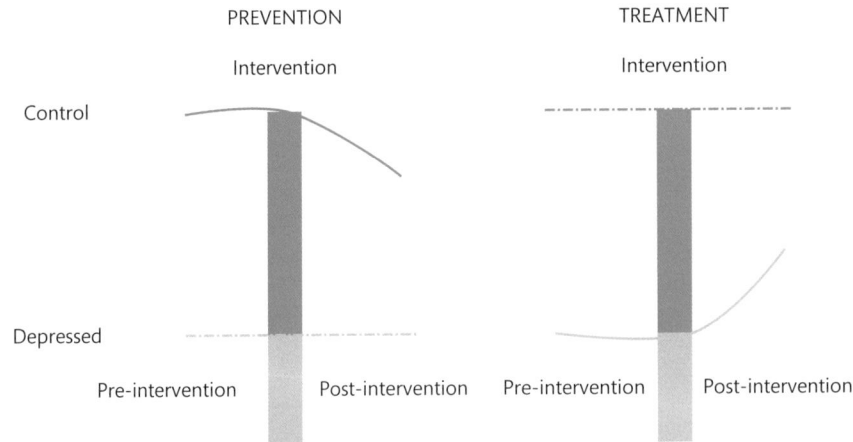

**Fig. 68.3** A comparison of the effects of prevention and treatment interventions in depressed patients vs healthy subjects. Vertical bars represent implementation of either a prevention or treatment strategy. Horizontal lines represent risk of depression during prevention, and clinical change in response to treatment. An intervention that is an effective treatment decreases depression in depressed patients but has no tangible effect on controls. An intervention that is preventive does not impact those that have already established illness (patients) but moderates the risk, and therefore reduces the likelihood, of depression in healthy controls.

## Intended target of prevention strategies

The main aim of mood disorders prevention strategies is to reduce the likelihood of developing the disorders and, as discussed, the benefits should readily outweigh any potential risks [14]. When considering prevention strategies, it is important to understand for whom they are intended and how they would be implemented, but most critical is to identify the target for which they are aiming. In this respect, according to the Institute of Medicine report [53], prevention strategies can be grouped into three categories: *universal, selective*, and *indicated* programmes (Table 68.2).

## Impact of prevention strategies

The success of a prevention strategy is determined by its outcome, but measuring this is a complex task. Gauging the efficacy or effectiveness of prevention approaches requires establishing clear outcomes, and unfortunately these are not easily defined. For instance, using a change in mood state as an outcome is not particularly useful in assessing universal and selective prevention strategies, whereas it is ideal for indicated prevention. This is because universal and selective approaches target intervention groups that may include those with low mood state levels from the outset and whose mood state changes are unlikely to be sufficiently large and clinically meaningful in comparison to other groups. This is because subthreshold depressive symptoms and syndromes seem to be prevalent (ranging from 10% to 50%) in community samples of youth who are the focus of universal and selective interventions [65–67]. On the other hand, the indicated approach will reveal clinically significant mood changes due to initial subsyndromal mood elevations in the intervention group, compared to other groups. Conversely, quality of life is an outcome measure that can be applied broadly across

different types of strategies, but because it is a very general measure that is only loosely coupled with the intervention itself, its utility, particularly in differentiating different prevention approaches, is limited. Therefore, the selection of outcome measures is critical. Furthermore, in the absence of clearly defined causal mechanisms, it is difficult to identify not only reliable and measurable outcomes, but especially the ones that have clinical salience. Another pertinent issue regarding prevention approaches is the number of people needed to show the benefits of an intervention, in other words, its ES. Across the various prevention strategies, the numbers vary, with universal strategies usually requiring much larger numbers and indicated prevention strategies generally requiring smaller numbers to demonstrate an effect [51].

## Professional responsibility

Globally, mental health services (MHS) are often multi-disciplinary, and a number of different disciplines and professionals can assume responsibility for the prevention of mood disorders and the promotion of well-being. For instance, a social worker from child services may be in a position to monitor interactions within families and identify problematic interactions that may be addressed with specific strategies to prevent the escalation of maladaptive behaviours. Indeed, ideally, the delivery of interventions has to be multi-disciplinary but integrated [68]. However, careful justification is needed when considering prevention because there are significant financial implications that affect funding policies governing the distribution of resources and training needs across disciplines. However, the prevention of mood disorders has been positioned as a global priority, and its goals extend beyond the narrow strictures of interdisciplinary MHS [69]. For instance, the Australian

**Table 68.2** Intervention programmes aimed at preventing or reducing mood disorders

| Features | Universal | Selective | Indicated |
|---|---|---|---|
| Target | Intended for the general public or community, regardless of risk status | Target a subgroup that is at higher risk, based on biological, psychological, or social/environmental risk factors, for example offspring of depressed parents, those with traumatic or life events such as divorce, bereavement, those experiencing marital or family conflict | Target people who display subthreshold signs and symptoms of a given disorder. For example: For bipolar disorder—those in the prodromal phase exhibiting mood dysregulation, fluctuation of energy levels, and anxiety symptoms. For depression—those with subclinical depressive symptoms (that do not fulfil the criteria of a diagnosis). Proximal to first onset/case identification and treatment |
| Impact | If successful, have a greater public health impact | If successful, have the potential to block the transgenerational transfer of mood disorders | If successful, can reduce the incidence of mood disorder onset and recurrences |
| Risk | Degree of individual risk is not taken into account | Risk may not always be imminent; it could be a lifetime risk | Risk is often imminent, needing swift attention |
| Risk/cost benefit | Ideal when their risk and cost are minimal | Preferred when the risk of the intervention is minimal or non-existent while the cost is not too high | Intervention would be deemed necessary, even if the risk and cost of the intervention are high |
| Examples | School-based and community/primary interventions, for example PRP [93, 94], mindfulness-based interventions [115, 116], beyondblue [123], PSL [95], PRP [143], CB and IP interventions [144] | Parenting focused and family-based interventions, for example ROSE programme [72], Preparation for Parenthood/Surviving Parenthood [145], FOCUS [76], EFFEKTE-E [77], FGCB [78], Family Options [79], KFS [80], FTI [81, 82] | ** School- and family-based CBT interventions, for example [87, 96, 113]; Effective Child and Family programme [83, 105, 106], ** STERK [142] |

** This is an ongoing intervention evaluation protocol.
PRP, Penn Resiliency Program; PSL, Problem Solving for Life; CB & IP, cognitive behavioural and Interpersonal Psychotherapy; ROSE, Reach Out, Stand Strong, Essentials; FOCUS, Families OverComing Under Stress; KFS, Keeping Families Strong; EFFEKT-E, Entwicklungsförderung in Familien: Eltern- und Kinder-Training in emotional belasteten Familien; FGCB, Family Group Cognitive-Behavioural; CBT: cognitive behavioural therapy; STERK: Screening and Training: Enhancing Resilience in Kids.

Government National Standards for Mental Health Services [70] recommended that MHS should identify individuals who are 'accountable for developing, implementing and evaluating prevention activities', while ensuring adequate training in the principles of prevention for the workforce, with appropriate support provided for the implementation of prevention activities. However, it is not clear how these individuals can be identified. Likewise, the EU Compass for Action on Mental Health and Well-being—Prevention of Depression and Promotion of Resilience, in its consensus paper, has promoted intersectorial collaborations between the health, educational, labour sector, informational technology, and economic stakeholders and the building of capacity through training in order to tackle and alleviate the burden of depression in Europe. But in practice, it is possible that any number of individuals can be identified for such roles, and those need to be determined on the basis of implementation requirements [31] (Fig. 68.4).

Lastly, prevention has to be targeting specific individuals or groups, and in that case, the contexts under which the prevention will be implemented, for the individual/parents/extended family members/peers/colleagues/schools/communities, have to be well understood. In this regard, the developmental and contextual framework that determines when and how interventions are implemented has to be taken into account. For instance, the National Research Council [14] recommended that besides multiple contexts, age-related patterns of competency and disorders and developmental tasks, as well as the interactions between biological, psychological, and social risk factors, have to be taken into consideration when designing prevention interventions.

The section on Preventative interventions, p. 706, illustrates the complexity of difficulties faced when making these considerations, with a summary of interventions implemented to date that directly or indirectly target the earliest developmental stage, that is, youth, and the setting under which they were implemented.

## Preventative interventions

### Parenting and family-based interventions

Parenting and family-based interventions target parents or the family as a unit in order to reduce risk factors and enhance protective factors in the offspring. This encourages changes in maladaptive parenting skills, attitudes to parenting, and interactions between the parent and the child. Therefore, adaptive parenting skills and functional parent–child interactions are crucial at very early stages of child development and can be commenced perhaps during pregnancy and early infancy, so that parents can be prepared emotionally and feel capable of nurturing their offspring and providing an environment that fosters secure attachment. Thus, early childhood

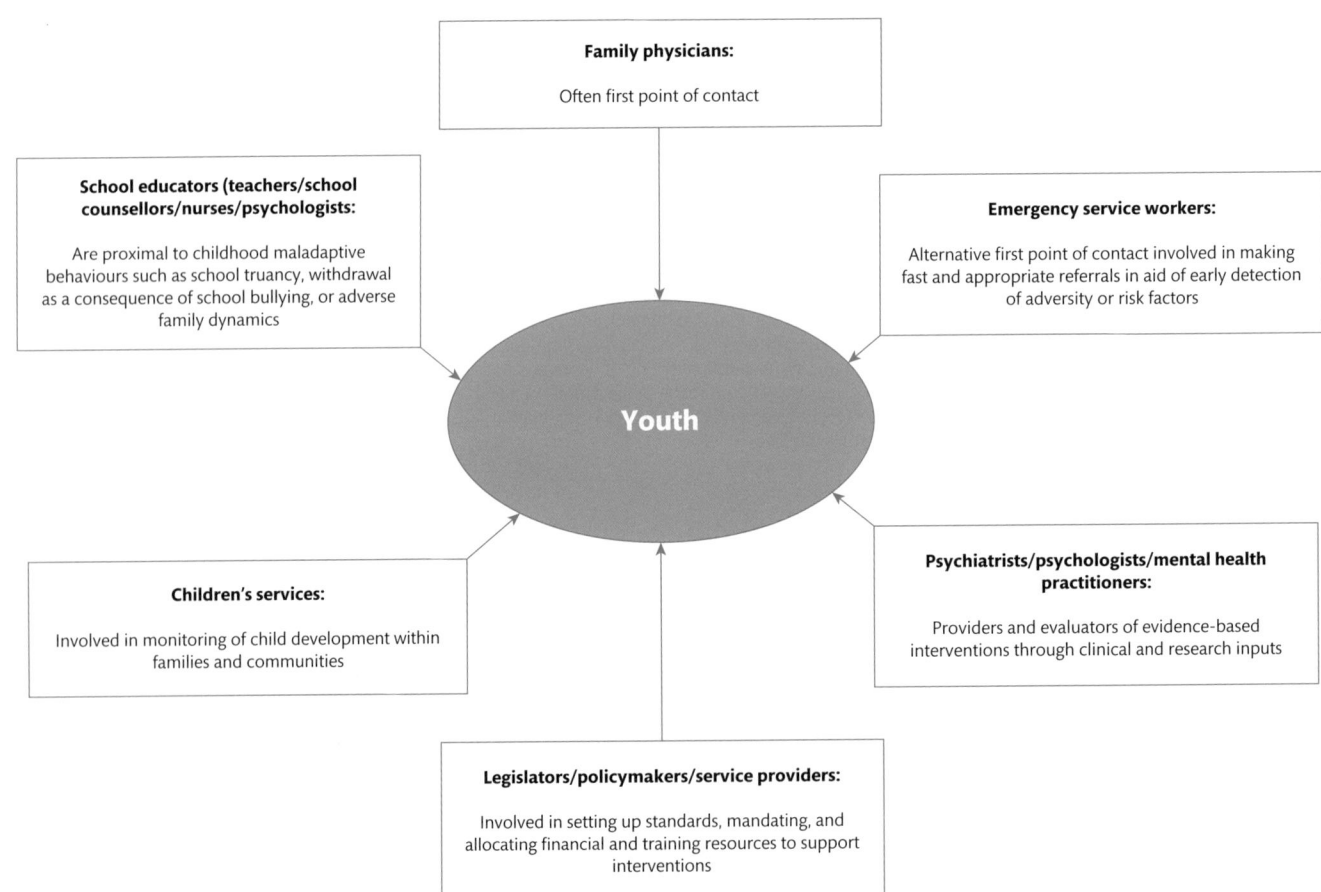

**Fig. 68.4** Professionals that have the potential to contribute to the prevention of mood disorders. Six groups of professionals, among others, have the potential to directly contribute to the prevention of mood disorders. Where possible, those involved should be working collaboratively and ideally targeting youth populations.

environments and social networks have been identified as critical in shaping emotional development because strong social supportive relationships and networks determine positive and enduring mental well-being that extends to adulthood [27]. The ultimate aim of these interventions is to limit the transgenerational transmission of mood disorders, and several interesting strategies have been developed to achieve this goal.

Core features of parenting and family-based interventions include enhancing resilience, building of interpersonal relationships and supportive networks, parental skill enhancement, and problem-solving, as well as raising awareness of the impact of mental disorders on the individual and the family, particularly the offspring. In this regard, it is encouraging to note that prevention interventions can be implemented at very early stages of development, that is, during prenatal and perinatal stages, and can restrict maladaptive or enhance adaptive parenting skills so as to modify neurocognitive development in offspring [71]. Indeed, an example of such an intervention is the Reach Out, Stand Strong, Essentials for new mothers (ROSE) programme that targets disadvantaged pregnant women deemed to be at risk of post-partum depression [72]. The ROSE programme intervention is an interpersonal therapy (IPT)-based intervention that puts emphasis on building supportive interpersonal relationships. While limited by a very small sample size, the larger reduction (20%) in parental incidence of depression in the intervention group, compared to the smaller reduction in the comparison antenatal-only group (4%), is supportive of the potential utility of such interventions. Furthermore, psychosocial and interpersonal postnatal depression prevention strategies focusing on the perinatal phase may at least reduce the incidence of postnatal depression, a promising finding for infant well-being and development. Indeed, recent evidence for a direct and sustained effect of perinatal maternal mood on the offspring's neuropsychological development is strong and has prompted for calls for in utero programming and activation of the stress–immune systems [19, 21, 73]. Although promising, the specific effects of such interventions on offspring mood states are not known, as the follow-up periods in most studies have thus far tended to be relatively brief—lasting typically no more than 6 months. Therefore, longer-term follow-up of offspring cohorts is urgently needed to initially verify and then quantify these effects.

Fostering adaptive interactions between parents and their adolescent offspring requires different parenting approaches to those employed in rearing infants and children. To identify parenting strategies that could potentially prevent depressive and anxiety symptoms in adolescent offspring, a poll of experts was undertaken using the Delphi Consensus method [74, 75]. This identified parenting strategies, such as establishing clear ground rules and consequences, establishing and maintaining a good relationship with the adolescent, and showing affection, as important. These strategies could be used in a manualized format, targeting parents as a checklist that they employ to help monitor their own behaviours in the implementation of interventions.

## Families at risk interventions

Evidence from other parenting and family-based interventions of families at risk because of the presence of parental depression seem to show short-term benefits on the functioning of the family as a unit. These interventions do not target the offspring but instead target parents with children aged 18 months to 18 years, for example the Families OverComing Under Stress (FOCUS) intervention for youth aged 3–17 years [76]; Entwicklungsförderung in Familien: Eltern- und Kinder-Training in emotional belasteten Familien (EFFEKT-E) intervention for children aged 4–6 years [77]; Family Group Cognitive-Behavioural (FGCB) for youth aged 9–15 years [78]; Family Options for children and adolescents aged 18 months to18 years [79]; and Keeping Families Strong (KFS) intervention for youth aged 9–16 years [80]. The core features of these interventions are problem-solving and skill building, mainly parenting and coping skills, as well as providing psychoeducation on various issues related to depression and its impact on the affected individual and the rest of the family, particularly the offspring. This, in turn, raises awareness and possibly tolerance, thus enhancing resilience and minimizing maladaptive stress responses.

Generally, these interventions show short-term benefits for both the children and their parents, with reductions in parental depressive symptoms and an increase in the offspring's prosocial behaviours and emotional expression that are mediated by ameliorating parental depression. However, one intervention evaluation did not have child-specific outcomes [79], and another showed improvements in child behaviour within the family that could not be transferred to the school environment where an increase in school maladjustment was seen [80]. The FGCB intervention, based on clinician ratings of mood changes, showed sustained benefits lasting 24 months, while the Youth Self-Report (YSR) measure showed intermittent and inconsistent benefits that could not be explained [78]. It could be that the sensitivity of the outcome measure might be crucial in the detection of changes.

Family therapeutic interventions (FTIs) target both mentally ill parents and their offspring aged 8–17 years [81–83]. These interventions employ CBT and psychoeducation components. Generally, these interventions have been shown to produce variable effects on mood state. For instance, FTIs produced inconsistent improvements in mood that were short term [83]. Interestingly, it is possible that these were mediated by improvements in anxiety, which often precedes depression and is thought to increase its likelihood and advance its onset to an earlier age [84]. Therefore, perhaps measures of anxiety should be routinely included when evaluating outcomes of prevention interventions [85]. However, FTIs also seem to have widespread effects in reducing risk and increasing protective factors of mood disorders through facilitation of a stronger child–parent relationship. Such improvements in family functioning have been shown to be sustained for up to 5 years, but this effect is not specific to FTIs and can also be achieved through brief parental psychoeducation [81–82].

CBT-based interventions have also been shown to have sustained reductions in the incidence of depression that is detectable for up to 75 months post-intervention and is moderated by baseline parental depression [86]. This means that, for maximum benefit, it might be prudent to treat parental depression prior to the initiation of prevention intervention programmes. Perhaps the successful treatment of parental depression fosters an environment that facilitates the preventative effects of interventions on depression. Interestingly, this series of evaluations [86–88] also seem to suggest that overall a smaller number of adolescents need to undergo an intervention to prevent the onset of depression (NNT = 9 at 9 months to NNT = 6 at 33 months). However, these findings have to be interpreted with caution because the inclusion of adolescents with a prior history of depression might, to some extent, be responsible for the observed intervention effects—obfuscating whether the intervention is truly preventative or simply therapeutic.

## School-based interventions

There have been an increasing number of school-based interventions in the last two decades, with similar overarching principles. Primarily, they are aimed at preventing the development of mood disorders, particularly depressive disorders in children and adolescents. School-based interventions offer advantages over other intervention settings because they provide ready access to large groups of young people and also remove some of the physical and economic barriers to access of services that usually limit their uptake [89]. School-based interventions, such as the CBT-based Penn Resilience Program (PRP) intervention, beyondblue, Problem Solving for Life, Resourceful Adolescent program, Positive Thoughts and Actions, and mindfulness-based programmes, have been implemented with varying degrees of success (Table 68.3). Each of these interventions has a number of core characteristic features, with some modest variations, involving mostly universal or targeted (selective and indicated) approaches. A selection of some recent interventions illustrates these similarities and differences.

### Penn Resiliency Program

The PRP [90] is the most evaluated CBT- and strength-based prevention programme designed for children and adolescents aged 10–14. It is aimed at increasing resilience, reducing depressive symptoms, and preventing the development of depressive disorders. Typically, it is a 12-week programme focused on changing cognitions, linking these to emotions, challenging negative explanations for events, handling and resolving conflict, problem-solving, and coping strategies, with weekly homework assignments between sessions. It is primarily a school-based intervention but has been evaluated in other settings such as primary care clinics. Its effectiveness seems to be independent of the expertise of the personnel leading its implementation, although the effects are slightly larger when implemented by research leaders than trained community leaders. It has been evaluated both as a targeted and as a universal intervention programme, and the former seems to be more beneficial [91–94].

### Problem Solving for Life

The Problem Solving for Life (PSFL) [95] intervention is a universal intervention that is teacher-led and incorporated into the school-term schedule. It is offered in weekly sessions over an 8-week period during a term, with each session lasting for 40–50 minutes. All sessions use various teaching methods, including interactive exercises, diary keeping, homework assignments, and the use of cartoons and class discussions. The intervention focuses on integrating cognitive restructuring and problem-solving. Targeted core skills include the identification of cognitive styles and challenging maladaptive problem-solving tendencies by teaching life problem-solving skills, enhancing the development of a positive problem-solving orientation, and optimistic thinking styles [95].

**Table 68.3** Examples of school-based programmes

| Programme | Prevention type | Age range | Programme content | Comparison programme | Number of sessions | Evaluation duration | Author |
|---|---|---|---|---|---|---|---|
| Penn Resiliency Program (PRP) | Selective (high risk based on low socio-economic status) | 10–13 years | CBT-based manualized group intervention | No intervention | 12 | Up to 12 and 24 months | [91, 92] |
| PRP | Universal (girls only and co-ed) | 11–14 years | CBT-based | Co-ed no intervention | 12 | Up to 12 months | [93] |
| PRP | Universal | 11–14 years | CBT-based | Penn Enhancement Program (identification of depression-related stressor) or no intervention | 12 | Every 6 months up to 3 years | [94] |
| Problem Solving for Life (PSFL) | Universal | 12–14 years | CBT-based | Monitoring control | 8 | Up to 1 year | [95] |
| Resourceful Adolescent Program (RAP) | Universal (RAP-Adolescent or RAP-Parent) | 12–15 years | CBT | Adolescent Watch (no intervention) | RAP-A: 11 RAP-P: 3 | Up to 10 months | [97] |
| RAP-Kiwi | Universal | 13–14 years | CBT and IPT | IPT only | 11 | Up to 18 months | [96] |
| beyondblue | Universal | 13–14 years | Multicomponent | Community focus | 10 | Annually for 3 years and up to 5 years | [122, 123] |
| | Selective (attributional styles) Indicated (subthreshold depressive symptoms) | 14–15 years | Adaptive coping skills training, enhancement of self-esteem and personal development | Assessment only conducted at beginning and end of active intervention | 14 | 6 and 12 months | [105, 106] |
| Positive Thoughts and Action (PTA) | Indicated (subthreshold depressive symptoms) | 12–14 years | CBT | Individual Support Program | 12 | 6 and 12 months | [99, 100] |

## The Resourceful Adolescent Program

The Resourceful Adolescent Program (RAP) [96–98] is a universal school-based intervention designed for adolescents (RAP-A) and their parents (RAP-P). The RAP-A component is fully manualized and implemented by school personnel at baseline during classes to groups of adolescents, aged 14–15, in Year 9. It is implemented in 11-weekly sessions per term, with each session lasting for 40–50 minutes. It is strength-based to enhance resilience through implementation of CBT and interpersonal therapy techniques. The focus is on stress management, cognitive restructuring, problem-solving, managing and resolving conflict, and building supportive networks. The RAP-P component is offered to parents of a cohort of adolescents and is usually delivered as a series of two separate 2- to 3-hour long workshops. The focus is on building parent's strengths, stress management, examination of parental roles in the development of their adolescent children while promoting positive family relationships, and conflict management and resolution.

## Positive Thoughts and Action Program

The Positive Thoughts and Action Program (PTA) [99–100] is a manualized indicated prevention programme that is developmentally sensitive, targeting early adolescents. It is a CBT-based group intervention, focusing on cognitive style, problem-solving, coping skills, and the application of learnt skills in social functioning and behaviours. It is implemented in weekly sessions lasting 50 minutes in groups of 4–6 adolescents. Parental involvement is encouraged via two home visits with the child and parents, as well as parent workshops. Parent workshops involve psychoeducation regarding adolescent development and skills training.

## Beyondblue intervention

The beyondblue intervention [101] is a flexible universal intervention established as part of the national depression initiative in Australia that fosters a stronger partnership between health and education services. It is implemented to Year 8 adolescents aged 13–14 years and follows them up for the next 3 years, in each year building on skills that have been previously taught and learnt. Each year, adolescents participate in 10-weekly classroom sessions lasting for 30–40 minutes. The intervention has four core features. It is a curriculum intervention, which is focused on building supportive environments, while building pathways for care and education and the use of community forums. As a curriculum intervention, it promotes well-being and enhances core skills and resilience. During the classroom sessions, core skills are taught in an interactive manner with the use of role plays, videos, quizzes, group exercises, and discussions. Core skills include problem-solving, conflict resolution, assertiveness, stress reduction, social skills, emotional education, self-efficacy and awareness, building of positive expectations of self in relation to the world and the future, greater understanding of mental health problems, and capacity to seek help.

## Summary

The PRP intervention effects have been variable, with some evaluations revealing short-term benefits that are not sustainable in the long term, while others have shown longer-term benefits for up to 2 years. Interestingly, the longer duration of benefits seems to depend on the presence of subthreshold symptoms at baseline and their severity. This raises the question of whether the PRP was preventative or merely a treatment of mild depressive symptoms, which, in turn, raises issues regarding conceptualization as a determining factor in prevention vs treatment. Furthermore, the strength of intervention effects seems to be dependent on symptoms at baseline, with stronger effects in those with subthreshold symptoms at baseline and only trend effects in those who are asymptomatic. It has also been suggested that the most reliable PRP effects are produced in research settings when the intervention is implemented by the developers and their expert colleagues. This means that while it is efficacious, its effectiveness is questionable. However, it does seem to have potential for those with mild to moderate depressive symptoms.

The PSFL intervention has also been shown to be superior to monitoring in the short term, with reductions in depressive symptoms that are clinically equivalent to the normative sample. The use of the Beck Depression Inventory (BDI) as an outcome measure in non-clinical populations has not been promoted due to questionable sensitivity in this population group [102, 103], but there is a possibility that booster sessions might have been helpful in maintaining benefits from the initial intervention.

Although, conceptually, the beyondblue intervention has multiple components, each of which is evidence-based, it failed to show effectiveness in reducing adolescent depressive symptoms or improving their well-being. It could be that, while the efficacy of the cognitive and IPT-based components of the intervention is somewhat established, efficacy of the building pathways for care and education and community focus components is largely unknown. Therefore, the effects of these components, separately and combined, have not been well tested and estimated. However, a meta-analytic review has suggested that the programme content does not moderate intervention effects [104]. Perhaps, with so many components to address, ten sessions per term is too conservative and does not allow for an in-depth exploration and analyses of all the issues raised by participants to their satisfaction. Another challenge brought to the fore is the need for adequate and in-depth training of teachers to implement the intervention with fidelity, which requires significant resources. This further highlights the difficulty of incorporating and integrating such complex multicomponent interventions within the school setting.

Contrary to this, a selective (based on the presence of a cognitive risk factor—attributional style) and indicated (based on the presence of subthreshold depressive symptoms) prevention programme targeting adolescents aged 14–15 years was successfully implemented in a school setting in Iceland [105, 106]. The intervention was aimed at enhancing adaptive coping, self-esteem, and personal development, while the comparison was only an assessment conducted at the beginning and at the end of the active programme, although participants in this intervention were allowed to seek treatment elsewhere at any time, if needed. It was implemented by school psychologists and regular school staff trained in its implementation and assessment procedures. This intervention showed no new episodes of depression/dysthymia in the intervention group, compared to a 2.5% increase in the usual treatment group, and at 6 and 12 months' follow-up, there was a 1.6% and 3.92% increase, respectively, in new episodes of depression/dysthymia for the intervention group, compared to a 13.3% and 20.97% increase, respectively, in the treatment as usual group. This increase was twice and three times as large in females, compared to males, at 6 and 12 months. This evidence suggests that sustained gains in the prevention of the onset of depression/dysthymia can be achieved with an intervention that enhances adaptive coping and personal development. The authors also identified the age of 14 years as potentially a good age to commence preventive intervention in those at high risk. Interestingly, this tallies with neurobiological research that shows the biggest changes occurring in 15-year-old girls with emotional symptoms—thought to be antecedents [107]. By using school personnel for the implementation of the programme, the authors point to its potential for real-world utility and effectiveness in significantly reducing the onset of depression, further bolstering the potential of targeted interventions in preventing or possibly delaying the onset of depression/dysthymia by at least a year.

The universal implementation of the RAP intervention is considered to have the potential to either shift about 13% adolescents out of depression or prevent them from developing subclinical or clinical depression, at least within 10 months of receiving the intervention. However, although well tolerated by adolescents, teachers were less optimistic about the programme, stating the manual was restrictive and inflexible for addressing the unique needs of individual classes. Furthermore, the intervention effects seem to vary, depending on the outcome measure used. For instance, although both the self-report Reynolds Adolescent Depression (RAD) scale and the Beck Depression Inventory-II (BDI-II) revealed initial intervention benefits, only the RAD revealed sustained effects to 18 months post-intervention. This again perhaps points to a lack of sensitivity of BDI measures in non-clinical populations. However, the results have to be interpreted with some caution because the analysis was performed based on the assumption that the intervention would be more beneficial than placebo. The presence of some deterioration in mood state for both interventions over time may suggest that such an assumption was premature. Statistical analysis should have taken this possibility into account but has likely compromised the detection of intervention effects.

A recent systematic review and meta-analysis of school-based interventions for depression only and depression and anxiety, respectively, have revealed very small and short-term intervention effects that are seemingly influenced by the type of prevention and the proficiency of the personnel delivering them [89]. In terms of how long the effects last for, on average, they tend not to last for more than 24 months; indeed, the effects are stronger immediately following the intervention (ES, $g = 0.23$), reducing to $g = 0.20, 0.12$, and $0.11$ in the first 6 months, 6–12 months, and over 12 months, respectively. It is not clear whether it is loss of power to detect long-term effects or a natural process of decline that explains the loss of benefit over time. If it is the latter, then perhaps booster sessions may be necessary to maintain improvements long term. However, if the issue is simply that of the studies being underpowered, then there is a need for further evaluations that are suitably powered to gauge long-term effects involving larger numbers of subjects. Alternatively, other measures that can perhaps detect more subtle changes over time with relatively smaller numbers may be trialled. Interestingly, a recent Cochrane review of CBT- and IPT-based interventions has revealed short-term benefits lasting no more than 12 months, and an estimated number to treat of 11, which is comparable to other public health interventions [108].

### Internet-based interventions

Emerging evidence from the few Internet-based interventions reveal moderate to large effects of the intervention on reducing depressive

symptoms that are sustainable for 2.5 years. For instance, the targeted Competent Adulthood Transition with Cognitive Behavioural and Interpersonal Training (CATCH-IT) intervention for adolescents and young adults aged 14–21 years was developed to establish strategies physicians could use to actively engage young people at risk of depression [109–112]. As a behaviour change and resiliency-building Internet-based intervention, it was implemented by physicians offering motivational interviewing (MI) or brief advice (BA). Both interventions elicited prevention and treatment effects, with an increasing percentage of symptom-free individuals from baseline to 12 months and reductions in clinically significant depressive symptoms over the 2.5-year follow-up. Furthermore, when comparing the CATCH-IT to reported face-to-face cognitive behavioural-based interventions, it was revealed that they produced larger effects, with a lower NNT for depressive episode (Internet NNT = 4.79 vs face-to-face NNT = 11.4) [113]. Also, CATCH-IT produced large effects (ES 0.96), compared to face-to-face interventions (ES 0.51) [113]. These ES are comparable to BDI-measured treatment effects in adults [114].

### Mindfulness-based interventions

Mindfulness interventions are based on adult mindfulness-based stress reduction (MBSR)/mindfulness-based cognitive therapy (MBCT) principles and were implemented in a cluster of 50 schools in Belgium [115] and in Australian schools [116]. During sessions, guided and unguided mindfulness practices and relaxation were taught, followed by manualized homework exercises. Practices included breath counting, stopping and being present, mindfulness of daily activities, for example walking or watching thought traffic, two guided audio (9 minutes long) of seated and lying body scans, and breath awareness. The control arm involved normal curricular activities.

Interestingly, mindfulness has significant and sustained beneficial effects on self-report depressive symptoms, at least in the short term of 6 months' duration, suggestive of preventative and treatment features in Belgium studies, whereas none of these effects were seen in Australian studies. It could be because the Belgian cohort was slightly older than the Australian cohort (14–17 years vs 12–14 years) [115, 116]. The developmental trajectory of mindfulness is not fully understood, and it could be that younger participants are at a different developmental stage and are not ready, or able, to process and use the concepts of mindfulness. Furthermore, in the Australian study, mindfulness seemed to produce anxiety [116]. The increase in anxiety in the mindfulness intervention group might be associated with, or driven by, an increase in ruminative processes where attention is perhaps drawn to issues that would normally be ignored or avoided.

### Universal vs targeted interventions

In general, universal interventions produce smaller effects ($g = 0.19$), compared to targeted interventions ($g = 0.32$), and indeed a systematic review revealed that targeted CBT-based interventions produce moderate to large ES (ranging from 0.21 to 1.40) [117]. Interestingly, these effects were achieved only when the intervention was delivered by mental health professionals, while teacher-led interventions produced significantly smaller effects, suggesting that the personnel delivering the intervention and, in particular, the extent of their training contribute to the effects. Specifically, school-based personnel achieved the smallest effects ($g = 0.17$) and their experience was variable. This is potentially problematic because it could encourage reluctance to incorporate and embed such interventions within regular school schedules where teachers and school counsellors have to invest a lot of time in class preparation, training, and supervision for relatively small gains. It has also been suggested that the magnitude of these effects may be influenced by the gender composition of participants, along with their age, and the duration of intervention. Thus far, larger effects have been seen with interventions involving more females, older adolescents, and shorter-duration programmes with homework assignments.

At the same time, it has been argued that regardless of the fact that the effects are small, they can potentially translate to meaningful improvements at a population level, with enormous implications for preventing the onset of mood disorders. Indeed, it has been shown that up to 9 months, implementing preventative interventions reduces the risk of developing depression, with RR 0.45, 0.61, and 0.79 for universal, selective, and indicated interventions, respectively, although the indicated intervention maintains reductions up to 18 months (RR = 0.23) [118]. This therefore supports the notion that, despite the smaller ES of universal interventions in reducing depressive symptoms, they may have greater utility in preventing the onset of depression. Hence, a combination of both universal and targeted interventions is needed.

### Evaluation duration

There is a growing need for long-term evaluations not only because the long-term sustained effects of prevention interventions have been variable, but because the initial effects of interventions have been shown to surface years later, during subsequent developmental phases, possibly because of having been missed earlier at times of greater 'noise' [119]. Perhaps initial intervention effects are masked by other processes or events occurring simultaneously, such that when emotional stability and maturity have been achieved, they re-emerge. Indeed, in one series of studies, intervention effects on risky behaviour seen at age 13, were no longer discernible for 4 years and then resurfaced at age 18 [28, 29]. This poses the quandary of whether initial intervention benefits need to be demonstrated before one can have some confidence in their likely downstream effects. Naturally, in the absence of initial benefits, one would assume that the intervention was not successful. The other point to consider regarding duration is the possibility that prevention interventions may not necessarily prevent the onset of mood disorders but may merely delay their onset [120]. If so, it remains to be seen how long this delay is in reality, and thus intervention evaluations may provide evidence for this alternate hypothesis. Furthermore, longer-duration evaluations may also reveal whether intervention effects decay after a while, and the potential of interim booster sessions to reignite intervention effects that may well be on their way to decay, and whether the strength of initial benefits determines the rate of decay.

### Age effects on interventions

The question of when to intervene or which age to target is a separate question that seems to be dependent on the content of the intervention. For instance, evidence from mindfulness-based interventions seems to suggest intervention efficacy in later adolescence (14–17 years), compared to early adolescence (12–14 years) [115, 116]. This is most likely because the concepts of mindfulness are too complicated for younger adolescents to comprehend and process. On the other hand, other school-based interventions that are largely based on cognitive behavioural techniques reveal stronger effects among children ($g = 0.50$), compared to early adolescents ($g = 0.23$) and older adolescents ($g = 0.22$), although the sample of interventions targeting younger children is relatively small [89]. Together, it suggests that each type of intervention is likely to be age-specific.

## Conclusions

The evidence from school-based interventions does not seem to be as strong as initially envisaged. Indeed, numerous null findings and non-significant trend effects have been reported [94, 121–123]. Factors contributing to the inconsistencies need clarification to help improve future prevention endeavours.

At the same time, while universal interventions produce the smallest short-term or intermittent effects, targeted interventions seem to produce the largest ES. Furthermore, it seems that ES are dependent on the type of intervention, and also, there may be an issue with the reliability and sensitivity of outcome measures that fail to detect significant effects but tend to reveal non-significant trend effects. Furthermore, intervention effects tend to be short term, and those showing sustained effects tend to be indicated, rather than selective and universal interventions. Only a few have revealed truly prevention vs treatment effects; only targeted interventions show small numbers needed to treat. When to intervene and the possible need for booster sessions to sustain long-term benefits need further clarification.

### Future directions

It is clear that the potential for prevention interventions is largely untapped. This is due to several reasons. Firstly, the issue of whether to intervene universally or to target specific populations remains unclear, despite superior gains from targeted interventions, as compared to universal interventions. This is because the nature of mood disorders is unpredictable. For example, although it can be predicted, with some confidence, that those who have parents with depression or have been themselves exposed to childhood adversity are more likely to develop mood disorders at some point in their lives, not everyone with these risk factors will go on to do so. On the other hand, there are many who develop mood disorders but have not been seemingly exposed to these risk factors. But prevention should aim to benefit both sets of individuals—those at high risk who go on to develop mood disorders and those at low risk who happen to develop mood disorders because of factors that are as yet unknown. Clearly, both groups should benefit from intervention, and hence the need for both targeted and universal interventions.

Specifically, in order to target only those who need the intervention, it has been suggested that a multi-level, integrated approach to prevention is needed—one that takes into account the multitude of key risk and protective factors [31, 88]. But this approach, aimed at enhancing resilience, needs to be dynamic and contextual, because each developmental stage is characterized by the emergence of new risks that may override or negate earlier protective factors, necessitating ongoing adaptation [119, 124]. Indeed, although exposure to regular and controlled stress is necessary for adaptation, the development of effective coping strategies, and maintenance of allostasis, it is when the stress is uncontrollable, irregular, and unpredictable that allostatic overload and ensuing problems arise, and are qualitatively compounded by environmental factors and individual differences such as genetic disposition and personality traits [23]. This is particularly relevant to children and adolescents who have to be taught the best ways of dealing and coping with stress in different contexts. For instance, when taught strategies that are maladaptive or that become maladaptive in a particular context, a flexible and integrated approach is needed for countering elicited stress. This is because prolonged exposure to stress potentially results in cumulative damage that is undetectable at first but causes subliminal pathological activity that eventuates in mood disorders. Therefore, neurobiological and psychosocial processes provide important substrates that underpin the integrated approach to prevention [119, 124]. Remarkably, to date, prevention approaches have focused largely on psychosocial aspects of mood disorders.

There is also an incentive to target the prodrome of mood disorders, because the benefits of intervention reductions in subclinical symptoms may be easier to measure. This reduction is presumed to reflect a slowing of any underlying process, thereby delaying the onset of the disorder or instigating the expression of a full-blown episode. However, a reduction in symptoms is perhaps more of a therapeutic than a preventive effect. Furthermore, delaying to intervene until prodromal symptoms present might also be too late to enact, 'true prevention'—that is, preventing the initiation of underlying pathological processes. Such subtle underlying pathological activity is undetectable using current tools and measures. However, recent technological advances bode well for the prevention of mood disorders, and perhaps it is time to shift towards more sensitive and specific measures that are able to target the underlying pathological activity before it escalates and leads to a mood disorder [23]. Lastly, there are ongoing protocols that address some of the limitations in previous intervention protocols such as the inclusion of quality of life and cost-effectiveness measures as outcomes. Also, the computation of a high risk index (HRI) as a measure of risk loading might be a useful tool to use for stratification.

## Contributions from genetic studies

A potential avenue that is yet to be fully understood is the genetic contribution to the risk of mood disorders. The evidence accumulated from studies of candidate genes and single-nucleotide polymorphisms (SNPs) provided no clear answers, largely because of the clinical heterogeneity of mood disorders and the large numbers of data points required for such investigations.

However, in recent times, with the use of much more powerful genome-wide association studies (GWAS), genetic risk prediction scores for individuals can be obtained that may well lead to new strategies for understanding and preventing mood disorders [125, 126]. For example, the polygenic risk score (PGRS) is a 'measure' that can be obtained by aggregating effects of SNPs (alleles) associated with disease status present in each individual, and this can be robustly applied to small samples [126–128]. Using this approach, PGRS has been applied prospectively to predict the risk of BD where the PGRS was found to be higher in high-risk young individuals (offspring and siblings of individuals with BD), compared to controls, and to provide a useful means of identifying traits linked to the genetic risk of mood disorders [20, 129–132]. The potential

to apply the PGRS as an outcome measure in prevention interventions has already been demonstrated in medical conditions. For example, in a 10-year coronary heart disease risk study, those receiving statins had a significant (3%) reduction in relevant PGRS, compared to controls. Similarly, in a 30-year risk of cancer, a lifestyle change (stopping smoking) had a significant (5.4%) reduction in PGRS. Importantly, these reductions were seen in those with a high PGRS score, compared to those with a moderate score. Furthermore, the risk threshold for screening for breast and colon cancer has been found to be reached much earlier by those with a high PGRS and family history of the disease [133]. Therefore, primary prevention strategies could potentially be facilitated by incorporating PGRS and other biological factors to identify those at different levels of risk of developing mood disorders. In other words, interventions could be tailored according to risk [133]. Furthermore, modification of the PGRS and, in turn, gene expression through psychosocial interventions serves as demonstration of the impact and importance of epigenetic processes. However, ethical, legal, and organizational considerations affecting the perception of genetic testing would have to be explored and addressed in order for polygenic predictions to be widely adopted in clinical practice.

### Filling in the gaps

The missing link in prevention programmes that may contribute to the less than robust effects of interventions on measured outcomes could also be the use of more sensitive and possibly reliable outcome measures targeting individual biology. While social processes are fluid and changing practically on a daily basis and self-reported functioning may be biased, other measures targeting biomarkers may be more subtle and stable. It has been suggested that identification of blood biomarkers for mood disorders may provide more specific and sensitive outcomes measures, while other potentially promising biomarkers of both resilience and vulnerability include measures of hypothalamic–pituitary–adrenal (HPA) axis dysregulation, oxidative stress, inflammation, autonomic responses, telomere length, and epigenetic profiles [15, 16, 23, 134]. Indeed, the course of stress exposure may not always be current or traumatic in its intensity but often can be traced to the prenatal period which seems to prime future neural and physiological responses, and these effects may persist throughout life [23]. The use of such measures in conjunction with the PGRS may eliminate the inherent problems of deciding who to target, irrespective of the risk status, whether at increased or low risk at the time of testing. Thus, in this context, the ultimate aim of prevention is not just to prevent the behavioural and clinical manifestations of mood disorders, but also to go deeper and redress or modify imbalances at cellular, neural, psychological, and behavioural levels. Indeed, there is potential utility in targeting significant mediating biomarkers for depression such as oxidative stress and inflammation, for instance with lifestyle changes and increasing the consumption of antioxidant-rich foods and omega-3 fatty acids and engaging in regular, but moderate, physical activity, along with ensuring adequate production of melatonin through sufficient sleep, but there are several problems that need to be solved to make these measures viable. Research in this area is still in its infancy and possibilities for the prevention of mood disorders are emerging; therefore, these investigations are crucial [135–137].

## When to intervene

At the same time as considering what to intervene with, the timing of any preventative measures is a key decision—for which there is no clear answer. Should preventative measures be instituted in early or middle childhood, or later still in adolescence, or are there specific critical periods that yield the most beneficial outcomes? Perhaps a standard cannot be developed and instead it is necessary to tailor interventions to individual needs based on specific risk markers. This would also mean that monitoring and follow-up adopt a personalized approach. Driving the need for prevention/early intervention is the fact that the cumulative effects of stress exposure are increasingly damaging, the longer they are present; and the earlier an intervention is instituted, the greater the potential long-term benefits [15, 16]. Prevention strategies that have been used so far, with variable success, include mindfulness- and CBT-based interventions, IPT interventions, psychoeducation, and skill training (parenting, coping, and problem-solving skills). Mindfulness prevention techniques have produced less than robust effects with respect to depression, and research thus far suggests that late adolescents may benefit more than early adolescents [115, 116]. However, understanding the mechanism of action and targeting those mechanisms may be more efficacious than self-reported mood changes. It has recently been revealed that mindfulness exerts effects on enhancing self-regulation through neuroplasticity changes in several brain regions implicated in mood disorders and their development, including the anterior cingulate cortex (ACC), the insula, the temporo-parietal junction, fronto-limbic connectivity, the default mode networks (DMNs), and grey matter volume (GMV) increases in neural structures involved in emotion regulation, learning, and memory [88, 138–140]. This burgeoning body of research provides further evidence for the need to incorporate biological consequences of interventions in the evaluation of such prevention strategies, and their potential to identify when responsiveness to interventions occurs in the developmental trajectory.

## Model generation

While our understanding remains incomplete, working models of the emotional mind are important but need to be constantly reviewed as new knowledge comes to light. It is therefore necessary to refine the models underpinning prevention interventions, so as to integrate neurobiology, neuropsychology, and social aspects of depression/mood disorders. For instance, if there are intervention gains in depression but not a significant mediator on which the intervention is based, for example cognition, or there is a change in cognition but not depression, then the accuracy of the original model and the sensitivity, reliability, and validity of the outcome measures need to be modified [104]. In this vein, it has also been posited that '*identification of genetic variants and understanding the molecular mechanisms may lead to prevention strategies aimed at correcting molecular disturbances in the pathways that lead from genes to behaviour, including the molecular pathways that underlie the effects of known risk factors for the disorder*' [14]. However, scrutiny of recent systematic reviews and meta-analyses of various approaches for the prevention of depression in children and adolescents published in the decade since this proposal was made reveal a huge gap that has not even begun to be narrowed [63, 89, 108,

117, 118]. Fundamentally, integration of our knowledge is lacking, and common and consistent approaches are yet to be developed and agreed upon. It may be that such endeavours are under way, but based on the few published protocols of ongoing evaluations, this seems unlikely [141, 142]. Therefore, renewed efforts are needed that integrate the use of biomarkers and epigenetic processes, with a view to developing a robust and testable model that traces the developmental trajectory of mood disorders within a meaningful ecological framework. Ultimately, our focus and energies to such an approach is long overdue—especially given that success in preventing mood disorders is too great an opportunity to ignore.

## REFERENCES

1. Gore, F. M., Bloem, P. J., Patton, G. C., *et al.* (2011). Global burden of disease in young people aged 10–24 years: a systematic analysis *The Lancet*, 377, 2093–102.
2. Whiteford, H. A., Degenhardt, L., Rehm, J., *et al.* (2013). Global burden of disease attributable to mental and substance use disorders: findings from the Global Burden of Disease Study 2010. *The Lancet*, 382, 1575–86.
3. Andrews, G., Issakidis, C., Sanderson, K., Corry, J., and Lapsley, H. (2004). Utilising survey data to inform public policy: comparison of the cost-effectiveness of treatment of ten mental disorders. *British Journal of Psychiatry*, 184, 526–33.
4. Mathers, C. D., and Loncar, D. (2006). Projections of global mortality and burden of disease from 2002 to 2030. *PLoS Medicine*, 3, e442.
5. Bruce, M. L., Wells, K. B., Miranda, J., Lewis, L., and Gonzalez, J. J. (2002). Barriers to reducing burden of affective disorders *Mental Health Services Research*, 4, 187–97.
6. Corrigan, P. W., Morris, S. B., Michaels, P. J., Rafacz, J. D., and Rusch, N. (2012). Challenging the public stigma of mental illness: a meta-analysis of outcome studies. *Psychiatric Services*, 63, 963–73.
7. Wells, K. B., Miranda, J., Bauer, M. S., *et al.* (2002). Overcoming barriers to reducing the burden of affective disorders. *Biological Psychiatry*, 52, 655–75.
8. Chisholm, D., Sanderson, K., Ayuso-Mateos, J. L., and Saxena, S. (2004). Reducing the global burden of depression. *British Journal of Psychiatry*, 184, 393–403.
9. Avenevoli, S. and Merikangas, K. R. (2006). Implications of high-risk family studies for prevention of depression. *American Journal of Preventive Medicine*, 31, 126–35.
10. Jaffee, S. R., Moffitt, T. E., Caspi, A., Fombonne, E., Poulton, R., and Martin, J. (2002). Differences in early childhood risk factors for juvenile-onset and adult-onset depression. *Archives of General Psychiatry*, 59, 215–22.
11. Rice, F., Sellers, R., Hammerton, G., *et al.* (2017). Antecedents of new-onset major depressive disorder in children and adolescents at high familial risk. *JAMA Psychiatry*, 74, 153–60.
12. Tandon, M., Cardeli, E., and Luby, J. (2009). Internalizing disorders in early childhood: a review of depressive and anxiety disorders. *Child and Adolescent Psychiatric Clinics of North America*, 18, 593–610.
13. McDermott, B., Baigent, M., Chanen, A., *et al.* (2010). *Clinical practice guidelines: depression in adolescents and young adults*. Melbourne: beyondblue: the national depression initiative.
14. National Research Council. (2009). *Preventing mental, emotional, and behavioral disorders among young people: progress and possibilities*. Washington, DC: National Academies Press.

15. Shonkoff, J. P. (2010). Building a new biodevelopmental framework to guide the future of early childhood policy. *Child Development*, 81, 357–67.

16. Shonkoff, J. P., Boyce, W. T., and McEwen, B. S. (2009). Neuroscience, molecular biology, and the childhood roots of health disparities: building a new framework for health promotion and disease prevention. *JAMA*, 301, 2252–9.

17. Aas, M., Henry, C., Andreassen, O. A., Bellivier, F., Melle, I., and Etain, B. (2016). The role of childhood trauma in bipolar disorders. *International Journal of Bipolar Disorders*, 4, 2.

18. Danese, A., Moffitt, T. E., Harrington, H., *et al.* (2009). Adverse childhood experiences and adult risk factors for age-related disease: depression, inflammation, and clustering of metabolic risk markers. *Archives of Pediatrics and Adolescent Medicine*, 163, 1135–43.

19. Gilman, S. E., Cherkerzian, S., Buka, S. L., *et al.* (2016). Prenatal immune programming of the sex-dependent risk for major depression. *Translational Psychiatry*, 6, e822.

20. Mullins, N., Power, R. A., Fisher, H. L., *et al.* (2016). Polygenic interactions with environmental adversity in the aetiology of major depressive disorder. *Psychological Medicine*, 46, 759–70.

21. O'Donnell, K. J., Glover, V., Barker, E. D., and O'Connor, T. G. (2014). The persisting effect of maternal mood in pregnancy on childhood psychopathology. *Development and Psychopathology*, 26, 393–403.

22. Patel, V., Flisher, A. J., Hetrick, S., McGorry, P. (2007). Mental health of young people: a global public-health challenge. *The Lancet*, 369, 1302–13.

23. Walker, A. J., Kim, Y., Price, J. B., *et al.* (2014). Stress, inflammation, and cellular vulnerability during early stages of affective disorders: biomarker strategies and opportunities for prevention and intervention. *Frontiers in Psychiatry*, 5, 34.

24. Wilson, S., Vaidyanathan, U., Miller, M. B., McGue, M., and Iacono, W. G. (2014). Premorbid risk factors for major depressive disorder: are they associated with early onset and recurrent course?. *Development and Psychopathology*, 26, 1477–93.

25. McEwen, B. S. (2003). Mood disorders and allostatic load. *Biological Psychiatry*, 54, 200–7.

26. McEwen, B. S. (2006). Protective and damaging effects of stress mediators: central role of the brain. *Dialogues in Clinical Neuroscience*, 8, 367.

27. Charles, S. T. and Carstensen, L. L. (2010). Social and emotional aging. *Annual Review of Psychology*, 61, 383–409.

28. Hawkins, J. D., Kosterman, R., Catalano, R. F., Hill, K. G., and Abbott, R. D. (2005). Promoting positive adult functioning through social development intervention in childhood: long-term effects from the Seattle Social Development Project. *Archives of Pediatrics and Adolescent Medicine*, 159, 25–31.

29. Hawkins, J. D., Kosterman, R., Catalano, R. F., Hill, K. G., and Abbott, R. D. (2008). Effects of social development intervention in childhood 15 years later. *Archives of Pediatrics and Adolescent Medicine*. 162, 1133–41.

30. Reynolds, A. J., Temple, J. A., Ou, S. R., *et al.* (2007). Effects of a school-based, early childhood intervention on adult health and well-being: a 19-year follow-up of low-income families. . *Archives of Pediatrics and Adolescent Medicine*, 161, 730–9.

31. Giesen, F., Searle, A., and Sawyer, M. (2007). Identifying and implementing prevention programmes for childhood mental health problems. *Journal of Paediatrics and Child Health*. 43, 785–9.

32. American Psychiatric Association. (2013). *Diagnostic and statistical manual of mental disorders (DSM-5®)*. Washington, D.C.: American Psychiatric Association.

33. Andrews, G., Slade, T., and Peters, L. (1999). Classification in psychiatry: ICD-10 versus DSM-IV. *British Journal of Psychiatry*, 174, 3–5.

34. Costello, E. J., Pine, D. S., Hammen, C., *et al.* (2002). Development and natural history of mood disorders. *Biological Psychiatry*, 52, 529–42.

35. De Girolamo, G., Dagani, J., Purcell, R., Cocchi, A., and McGorry, P. D. (2012). Age of onset of mental disorders and use of mental health services: needs, opportunities and obstacles. *Epidemiology and Psychiatric Sciences*, 21, 47–57.

36. Joslyn, C., Hawes, D. J., Hunt, C., and Mitchell, P. B. (2016). Is age of onset associated with severity, prognosis, and clinical features in bipolar disorder? A meta-analytic review. *Bipolar Disorders*, 218, 389–403.

37. Oquendo, M. A., Ellis, S. P., Chesin, M. S., *et al.* (2013). Familial transmission of parental mood disorders: unipolar and bipolar disorders in offspring. *Bipolar Disorders*, 15, 764–73.

38. World Health Organization. (1993). *The ICD-10 classification of mental and behavioural disorders: diagnostic criteria for research*. Geneva: World Health Organization.

39. Perlis, R. H., Miyahara, S., Marangell, L. B., *et al.* (2004). Long-term implications of early onset in bipolar disorder: data from the first 1000 participants in the systematic treatment enhancement program for bipolar disorder (STEP-BD). *Biological Psychiatry*, 55, 875–81.

40. Howes, O. D. and Falkenberg, I. (2011). Early detection and intervention in bipolar affective disorder: targeting the development of the disorder. *Current Psychiatry Reports*, 13, 493–9.

41. Fritz, K., Russell, A. M., Allwang, C., Kuiper, S., Lampe, L., and Malhi, G. S. (2017). Is a delay in the diagnosis of bipolar disorder inevitable? *Bipolar Disorders*, 19, 396–400.

42. Malhi, G. S., Morris, G., Hamilton, A., and Outhred, T. (2019). Early intervention in bipolar disorders: setting the stage from mechanisms to models. In: Chen, E. Y. H., Ventriglio, A., and Bhugra, D. (eds.). *Early intervention in psychiatric disorders across cultures*. Oxford: Oxford University Press; pp. 145–66.

43. Muneer, A. (2016). Staging models in bipolar disorder: a systematic review of the literature. *Clinical Psychopharmacology and Neuroscience*, 14, 117–30.

44. Dalrymple, K. L. and Zimmerman, M. (2011). Age of onset of social anxiety disorder in depressed outpatients. *Journal of Anxiety Disorders*, 25, 131–7.

45. Eisner, L. R., Johnson, S. L., Youngstrom, E. A., and Pearlstein, J. G. (2017). Simplifying profiles of comorbidity in bipolar disorder. *Journal of Affective Disorders*, 220, 102–7.

46. Frías, Á., Palma, C., and Farriols, N. (2015). Comorbidity in pediatric bipolar disorder: prevalence, clinical impact, etiology and treatment. *Journal of Affective Disorders*, 174, 378–89.

47. Malhi, G. S. (2002). The case for cothymia: an open verdict? *British Journal of Psychiatry*, 180, 380.

48. Perich, T., Lau, P., Hadzi-Pavlovic, D., *et al.* (2015). What clinical features precede the onset of bipolar disorder? *Journal of Psychiatric Research*, 62, 71–7.

49. Paus, T., Keshavan, M., & Giedd, J. N. (2008). Why do many psychiatric disorders emerge during adolescence? *Nature Reviews Neuroscience*, 9, 947–57.

50. Sawyer, S. M., Afifi, R. A., Bearinger, L. H., *et al.* (2012). Adolescence: a foundation for future health *The Lancet*, 379, 1630–40.

51. Muñoz, R. F., Cuijpers, P., Smit, F., Barrera, A. Z., and Leykin, Y. (2010). Prevention of major depression. *Annual Review of Clinical Psychology*, 6, 181–212.

52. Weisz, J. R., Sandler, I. N., Durlak, J. A., and Anton, B. S. (2005). Promoting and protecting youth mental health through evidence-based prevention and treatment. *American Psychologist*, 60, 628–48.

53. Mrazek, P. J. and Haggerty, R. J. (1994); Committee on Prevention of Mental Disorders, Institute of Medicine. *Reducing risks for mental disorders: frontiers for preventive intervention research.* Washington, D.C.: National Academies Press.

54. Horowitz, J. L. and Garber, J. (2006). The prevention of depressive symptoms in children and adolescents: a meta-analytic review. *Journal of Consulting and Clinical Psychology*, 74, 401–15.

55. Malhi, G. S., Bassett, D., Boyce, P., *et al.* (2015). Royal Australian and New Zealand College of Psychiatrists clinical practice guidelines for mood disorders. *Australian and New Zealand Journal of Psychiatry*, 49, 1087–206.

56. Rocha, T. B. M., Zeni, C. P., Caetano, S. C., and Kieling, C. (2013). Mood disorders in childhood and adolescence. *Revista Brasileira de Psiquiatria*, 35, S22–31.

57. Szentagotai, A. and David, D. (2010). The efficacy of cognitive-behavioral therapy in bipolar disorder: a quantitative meta-analysis. *Journal of Clinical Psychiatry*, 71, 66–72.

58. Miklowitz, D. J. and Scott, J. (2009). Psychosocial treatments for bipolar disorder: cost-effectiveness, mediating mechanisms, and future directions. *Bipolar Disorders*, 11, 110–22.

59. Smit, F., Willemse, G., Koopmanschap, M., Onrust, S., Cuijpers, P., and Beekman, A. (2006). Cost-effectiveness of preventing depression in primary care patients. *British Journal of Psychiatry*, 188, 330–6.

60. Gladstone, T. R. G. and Beardslee, W. R. (2009). The prevention of depression in children and adolescents: a review. *Canadian Journal of Psychiatry*, 54, 212–21.

61. Perlis, R. H., Miyahara, S., Marangell, L. B., *et al.* (2004). Long-term implications of early onset in bipolar disorder: data from the first 1000 participants in the systematic treatment enhancement program for bipolar disorder (STEP-BD). *Biological Psychiatry*, 55, 875–81.

62. Gladstone, T. R. G., Beardslee, W. R., and O'Connor, E. E. (2011). The prevention of adolescent depression. *Psychiatric Clinics of North America*, 34, 35–52.

63. Mendelson, T. and Tandon, S. D. (2016). Prevention of depression in childhood and adolescence. *Child and Adolescent Psychiatric Clinics of North America*, 25, 201–18.

64. Miklowitz, D. J. and Chang, K. D. (2008). Prevention of bipolar disorder in at-risk children: theoretical assumptions and empirical foundations. *Development and Psychopathology*, 20, 881–97.

65. Lewinsohn, P. M., Shankman, S. A., Gau, J. M., and Klein, D. N. (2004). The prevalence and co-morbidity of subthreshold psychiatric conditions. *Psychological Medicine*, 34, 613–22.

66. Merikangas, K. R., Nakamura, E. F., and Kessler, R. C. (2009). Epidemiology of mental disorders in children and adolescents. *Dialogues in Clinical Neuroscience*, 11, 7–20.

67. Merikangas, K. R., Nakamura, E. F., and Kessler, R. C. (2009). Epidemiology of mental disorders in children and adolescents. *Dialogues in Clinical Neuroscience*, 11, 7–20.

68. Richter, L. M., Daelmans, B., Lombardi, J., *et al.* (2017). Investing in the foundation of sustainable development: pathways to scale up for early childhood development. *The Lancet*, 389, 103–18.

69. Cuijpers, P., Beekman, A. T., and Reynolds, C. F. (2012). Preventing depression: a global priority *JAMA*, 307, 1033–4.

70. Australian Government National Standards for Mental Health Services. (2010). *National standards for mental health services 2010*. National Mental Health Strategy. Canberra: Australian Government.

71. Stafford, M., Kuh, D. L., Gale, C. R., Mishra, G., and Richards, M. (2016). Parent–child relationships and offspring's positive mental wellbeing from adolescence to early older age. *Journal of Positive Psychology*, 11, 326–37.

72. Zlotnick, C., Miller, I. W., Pearlstein, T., Howard, M., and Sweeney, P. (2006). A preventive intervention for pregnant women on public assistance at risk for postpartum depression. *American Journal of Psychiatry*, 163, 1443–5.

73. Kim, D. R., Bale, T. L., and Epperson, C. N. (2015). Prenatal programming of mental illness: current understanding of relationship and mechanisms. *Current Psychiatry Reports*, 17, 1–9.

74. Cairns, K. E., Yap, M. B., Reavley, N. J., and Jorm, A. F. (2015). Identifying prevention strategies for adolescents to reduce their risk of depression: a Delphi consensus study. *Journal of Affective Disorders*, 183, 229–38.

75. Yap, M. B. H., Fowler, M., Reavley, N. J., and Jorm, A. F. (2015). Parenting strategies for reducing the risk of childhood depression and anxiety disorders: a Delphi consensus study. *Journal of Affective Disorders*, 183, 330–8.

76. Lester, P., Liang, L. J., Milburn, N., *et al.* (2016). Evaluation of a family-centered preventive intervention for military families: parent and child longitudinal outcomes. *Journal of the American Academy of Child and Adolescent Psychiatry*, 55, 14–24.

77. Bühler, A., Kötter, C., Jaursch, S., and Lösel, F. (2011). Prevention of familial transmission of depression: EFFEKT-E, a selective program for emotionally burdened families. *Journal of Public Health*, 19, 321–7.

78. Compas, B. E., Forehand, R., Thigpen, J. C., *et al.* (2011). Family group cognitive–behavioral preventive intervention for families of depressed parents: 18-and 24-month outcomes. *Journal of Consulting and Clinical Psychology*, 79, 488–99.

79. Nicholson, J., Albert, K., Gershenson, B., Williams, V., and Biebel, K. (2009). Family options for parents with mental illnesses: a developmental, mixed methods pilot study. *Psychiatric Rehabilitation Journal*, 33, 106–14.

80. Valdez, C. R., Mills, C. L., Barrueco, S., Leis, J., and Riley, A. W. (2011). A pilot study of a family-focused intervention for children and families affected by maternal depression. *Journal of Family Therapy*, 33, 3–19.

81. Beardslee, W. R., Gladstone, T. R., Wright, E. J., and Cooper, A. B. (2003). A family-based approach to the prevention of depressive symptoms in children at risk: evidence of parental and child change. *Pediatrics*, 112, e119–31.

82. Beardslee, W. R., Wright, E. J., Gladstone, T. R., and Forbes, P. (2007). Long-term effects from a randomized trial of two public health preventive interventions for parental depression. *Journal of Family Psychology*, 21, 703–13.

83. Solantaus, T., Paavonen, E. J., Toikka, S., and Punamäki, R. L. (2010). Preventive interventions in families with parental depression: children's psychosocial symptoms and prosocial behaviour. *European Child and Adolescent Psychiatry*, 19, 883–92.

84. Malhi, G. S., Parker, G. B., Gladstone, G., Wilhelm, K., and Mitchell, P. B. (2002). Recognizing the anxious face of depression. *Journal of Nervous And Mental Disease*, 190, 366–73.

85. Knox, M., Lentini, J., Cummings, T. S., McGrady, A., Whearty, K., and Sancrant, L. (2011). Game-based biofeedback for paediatric anxiety and depression. *Mental Health in Family Medicine*, 8, 195–203.

86. Brent, D. A., Brunwasser, S. M., Hollon, S. D., *et al.* (2015). Effect of a cognitive-behavioral prevention program on depression 6 years after implementation among at-risk adolescents: a randomized clinical trial. *JAMA Psychiatry*, 72, 1110–18.

87. Beardslee, W. R., Brent, D. A., Weersing, V. R., *et al.* (2013). Prevention of depression in at-risk adolescents: longer-term effects. *JAMA Psychiatry*, 70, 1161–70.

88. Garber, J. (2006). Depression in children and adolescents: linking risk research and prevention. *American Journal of Preventive Medicine*, 31, 104–25.

89. Werner-Seidler, A., Perry, Y., Calear, A. L., Newby, J. M., and Christensen, H. (2017). School-based depression and anxiety prevention programs for young people: a systematic review and meta-analysis. *Clinical Psychology Review*, 51, 30–47.

90. Brunwasser, S. M., Gillham, J. E., and Kim, E. S. (2009). A meta-analytic review of the Penn Resiliency Program's effect on depressive symptoms. *Journal of Consulting and Clinical Psychology*, 77, 1042–54.

91. Cardemil, E. V., Reivich, K. J., Beevers, C. G., Seligman, M. E., and James, J. (2007). The prevention of depressive symptoms in low-income, minority children: two-year follow-up. *Behaviour Research and Therapy*, 45, 313–27.

92. Cardemil, E. V., Reivich, K. J., and Seligman, M. E. (2002). The prevention of depressive symptoms in low-income minority middle school students. *Prevention and Treatment*, 5, 1522–3736.

93. Chaplin, T. M., Gillham, J. E., Reivich, K., *et al.* (2006). Depression prevention for early adolescent girls: a pilot study of all girls versus co-ed groups. *Journal of Early Adolescence*, 26, 110–26.

94. Gillham, J. E., Reivich, K. J., Freres, D. R., *et al.* (2007). School-based prevention of depressive symptoms: a randomized controlled study of the effectiveness and specificity of the Penn Resiliency Program. *Journal of Consulting and Clinical Psychology*, 75, 9–19.

95. Spence, S. H., Sheffield, J. K., and Donovan, C. L. (2003). Preventing adolescent depression: an evaluation of the problem solving for life program. *Journal of Consulting and Clinical Psychology*, 71, 3–13.

96. Merry, S., McDowell, H., Wild, C. J., Bir, J., and Cunliffe, R. (2004). A randomized placebo-controlled trial of a school-based depression prevention program. *Journal of the American Academy of Child and Adolescent Psychiatry*, 43, 538–47.

97. Shochet, I. M., Dadds, M. R., Holland, D., Whitefield, K., Harnett, P. H., and Osgarby, S. M. (2001). The efficacy of a universal school-based program to prevent adolescent depression. *Journal of Clinical Child Psychology*, 30, 303–15.

98. Shochet, I. M. and Ham, D. (2004). Universal school-based approaches to preventing adolescent depression: past findings and future directions of the Resourceful Adolescent Program. *International Journal of Mental Health Promotion*, 6, 17–25.

99. Duong, M. T., Cruz, R. A., King, K. M., Violette, H. D., and McCarty, C. A. (2016). Twelve-month outcomes of a randomized trial of the Positive Thoughts and Action Program for depression among early adolescents. *Prevention Science*, 17, 295–305.

100. McCarty, C. A., Violette, H. D., Duong, M. T., Cruz, R. A., and McCauley, E. (2013). A randomized trial of the positive thoughts and action program for depression among early adolescents. *Journal of Clinical Child and Adolescent Psychology*, 42, 554–63.

101. Spence, S. H., Burns, J., Boucher, S., *et al.* (2005). The beyondblue Schools Research Initiative: conceptual framework and intervention. *Australasian Psychiatry*, 13, 159–64.

102. LeBlanc, J. C., Almudevar, A., Brooks, S. J., and Kutcher, S. (2002). Screening for adolescent depression: comparison of the Kutcher Adolescent Depression Scale with the Beck Depression Inventory. *Journal of Child and Adolescent Psychopharmacology*, 12, 113–26.

103. Roberts, R. E., Lewinsohn, P. M., and Seeley, J. R. (1991). Screening for adolescent depression: a comparison of depression scales. *Journal of the American Academy of Child and Adolescent Psychiatry*, 30, 58–66.

104. Stice, E., Shaw, H., Bohon, C., Marti, C. N., and Rohde, P. (2009). A meta-analytic review of depression prevention programs for children and adolescents: factors that predict magnitude of intervention effects. *Journal of Consulting and Clinical Psychology*, 77, 486–503.

105. Arnarson, E. O. and Craighead, W. E. (2009). Prevention of depression among Icelandic adolescents. *Behaviour Research and Therapy*, 47, 577–85.

106. Arnarson, E. O. and Craighead, W. E. (2011). Prevention of depression among Icelandic adolescents: a 12-month follow-up. *Behaviour Research and Therapy*, 49, 170–4.

107. Cyranowski, J. M., Frank, E., Young, E., and Shear, M. K. (2000). Adolescent onset of the gender difference in lifetime rates of major depression: a theoretical model. *Archives of General Psychiatry*, 57, 21–7.

108. Hetrick, S. E., Cox, G. R., Witt, K. G., Bir, J. J., and Merry, S. N. (2016). Cognitive behavioural therapy (CBT), third-wave CBT and interpersonal therapy (IPT) based interventions for preventing depression in children and adolescents. *Cochrane Database of Systematic Reviews*, 2016, 1–279.

109. Richards, K., Marko-Holguin, M., Fogel, J., Anker, L., Ronayne, J., and Van Voorhees, B. W. (2016). Randomized clinical trial of an Internet-based intervention to prevent adolescent depression in a primary care setting (CATCH-IT): 2.5-year outcomes. *Journal of Evidence-Based Psychotherapies*, 16, 113–34.

110. Saulsberry, A., Monika Marko-Holguin, M., Kelsey Blomeke, K., *et al.* (2013). Randomized clinical trial of a primary care internet-based intervention to prevent adolescent depression: one-year outcomes. *Journal of the Canadian Academy of Child and Adolescent Psychiatry*, 22, 106–17.

111. Van Voorhees, B. W., Fogel, J., Reinecke, M. A., *et al.* (2009). Randomized clinical trial of an Internet-based depression prevention program for adolescents (Project CATCH-IT) in primary care: 12-week outcomes. *Journal of Developmental and Behavioral Pediatrics*, 30, 23–37.

112. Van Voorhees, B. W., Vanderplough-Booth, K., Fogel, J., *et al.* (2008). Integrative internet-based depression prevention for adolescents: a randomized clinical trial in primary care for vulnerability and protective factors. *Journal of the Canadian Academy of Child and Adolescent Psychiatry*, 17, 184–96.

113. Garber, J., Clarke, G. N., Weersing, V. R., *et al.* (2009). Prevention of depression in at-risk adolescents: a randomized controlled trial. *JAMA*, 301, 2215–24.

114. Andersson, G., Bergström, J., Holländare, F., Carlbring, P. E. R., Kaldo, V., and Ekselius, L. (2005). Internet-based self-help for depression: randomised controlled trial. *British Journal of Psychiatry*, 187, 456–61.

115. Raes, F., Griffith, J. W., Van der Gucht, K., and Williams, J. M. G. (2014). School-based prevention and reduction of depression in adolescents: a cluster-randomized controlled trial of a mindfulness group program. *Mindfulness*, 5, 477–86.

116. Johnson, C., Burke, C., Brinkman, S., and Wade, T. (2016). Effectiveness of a school-based mindfulness program for trans diagnostic prevention in young adolescents. *Behaviour Research and Therapy*, 81, 1–11.

117. Calear, A. L., & Christensen, H. (2010). Systematic review of school-based prevention and early intervention programs for depression. *Journal of Adolescence*, 33, 429–38.

118. Stockings, E. A., Degenhardt, L., Dobbins, T., *et al.* (2016). Preventing depression and anxiety in young people: a review of the joint efficacy of universal, selective and indicated prevention. *Psychological Medicine*, 46, 11–26.

119. Masten, A. S. (2004). Regulatory processes, risk, and resilience in adolescent development. *Annals of the New York Academy of Sciences*, 1021, 310–19.

120. Cuijpers, P., van Straten, A., Smit, F., Mihalopoulos, C., and Beekman, A. (2008). Preventing the onset of depressive disorders: a meta-analytic review of psychological interventions. *American Journal of Psychiatry*, 165, 1272–80.

121. Pattison, C. and Lynd-Stevenson, R. M. (2001). The prevention of depressive symptoms in children: the immediate and long-term outcomes of a school-based program. *Behaviour Change*, 18, 92–102.

122. Sawyer, M. G., Harchak, T. F., Spence, S. H., *et al.* (2010). School-based prevention of depression: a 2-year follow-up of a randomized controlled trial of the beyondblue schools research initiative. *Journal of Adolescent Health*, 47, 297–304.

123. Sawyer, M. G., Pfeiffer, S., Spence, S. H., *et al.* (2010). School-based prevention of depression: a randomised controlled study of the beyondblue schools research initiative. *Journal of Child Psychology and Psychiatry*, 51, 199–209.

124. Silk, J. S., Vanderbilt-Adriance, E., Shaw, D. S., *et al.* (2007). Resilience among children and adolescents at risk for depression: mediation and moderation across social and neurobiological contexts. *Development and Psychopathology*, 19, 841–65.

125. Cross-Disorder Group of the Psychiatric Genomics Consortium. (2013). Identification of risk loci with shared effects on five major psychiatric disorders: a genome-wide analysis. *The Lancet*, 381, 1371–9.

126. Wray, N. R., Lee, S. H., Mehta, D., Vinkhuyzen, A. A., Dudbridge, F., and Middeldorp, C. M. (2014). Research review: polygenic methods and their application to psychiatric traits. *Journal of Child Psychology and Psychiatry*, 55, 1068–87.

127. Dima, D. and Breen, G. (2015). Polygenic risk scores in imaging genetics: usefulness and applications. *Journal of Psychopharmacology*, 29, 867–71.

128. Middeldorp, C. M., De Moor, M. H. M., McGrath, L. M., *et al.* (2011). The genetic association between personality and major depression or bipolar disorder. A polygenic score analysis using genome-wide association data. *Translational Psychiatry*, 1, e50.

129. Fullerton, J. M., Koller, D. L., Edenberg, H. J., *et al.* (2015). Assessment of first and second degree relatives of individuals with bipolar disorder shows increased genetic risk scores in both affected relatives and young at-risk individuals. *American Journal of Medical Genetics Part B: Neuropsychiatric Genetics*, 168B, 617–29.

130. Luciano, M., Huffman, J. E., Arias-Vásquez, A., *et al.* (2012). Genome-wide association uncovers shared genetic effects among personality traits and mood states. *American Journal of Medical Genetics Part B: Neuropsychiatric Genetics*, 159, 684–95.

131. Whalley, H. C., Papmeyer, M., Sprooten, E., *et al.* (2012). The influence of polygenic risk for bipolar disorder on neural activation assessed using fMRI. *Translational Psychiatry*, 2, e130.

132. Whalley, H. C., Sprooten, E., Hackett, S., *et al.* (2013). Polygenic risk and white matter integrity in individuals at high risk of mood disorder. *Biological Psychiatry*, 74, 280–6.

133. Chatterjee, N., Shi, J., and García-Closas, M. (2016). Developing and evaluating polygenic risk prediction models for stratified disease prevention. *Nature Reviews Genetics*, 17, 392–406.

134. Le-Niculescu, H., Kurian, S. M., Yehyawi, N., *et al.* (2009). Identifying blood biomarkers for mood disorders using convergent functional genomics. *Molecular Psychiatry*, 14, 156–74.

135. Lopresti, A. L., Maker, G. L., Hood, S. D., and Drummond, P. D. (2014). A review of peripheral biomarkers in major depression: the potential of inflammatory and oxidative stress biomarkers. *Progress in Neuro-Psychopharmacology and Biological Psychiatry*, 48, 102–11.

136. Parker, G., Gibson, N. A., Brotchie, H., Heruc, G., Rees, A.-M., and Hadzi-Pavlovic, D. (2006). Omega-3 fatty acids and mood disorders. *American Journal of Psychiatry*, 163, 969–78.

137. Poljsak, B. (2011). Strategies for reducing or preventing the generation of oxidative stress. *Oxidative Medicine and Cellular Longevity*, 194586.

138. Davidson, R. J., Kabat-Zinn, J., Schumacher, J., *et al.* (2003). Alterations in brain and immune function produced by mindfulness meditation. *Psychosomatic Medicine*, 65, 564–70.

139. Hölzel, B. K., Carmody, J., Vangel, M., *et al.* (2011). Mindfulness practice leads to increases in regional brain gray matter density. *Psychiatry Research: Neuroimaging*, 191, 36–43.

140. Hölzel, B. K., Lazar, S. W., Gard, T., Schuman-Olivier, Z., Vago, D. R., and Ott, U. (2011). How does mindfulness meditation work? Proposing mechanisms of action from a conceptual and neural perspective. *Perspectives on Psychological Science*, 6, 537–59.

141. Bellón, J. Á., Conejo-Cerón, S., Moreno-Peral, P., *et al.* (2013). Preventing the onset of major depression based on the level and profile of risk of primary care attendees: protocol of a cluster randomised trial (the predictD-CCRT study). *BMC Psychiatry*, 13, 171.

142. Nauta, M. H., Festen, H., Reichart, C. G., *et al.* (2012). Preventing mood and anxiety disorders in youth: a multi-centre RCT in the high risk offspring of depressed and anxious patients. *BMC Psychiatry*, 12, 31.

143. Gillham, J. E., Hamilton, J., Freres, D. R., Patton, K., and Gallop, R. (2006). Preventing depression among early adolescents in the primary care setting: A randomized controlled study of the Penn Resiliency Program. *Journal of Abnormal Child Psychology*, 34, 195–211.

144. Horowitz, J. L., Garber, J., Ciesla, J. A., Young, J. F., and Mufson, L. (2007). Prevention of depressive symptoms in adolescents: a randomized trial of cognitive-behavioral and interpersonal prevention programs. *Journal of Consulting and Clinical Psychology*, 75, 693–706.

145. Elliott, S. A., Leverton, T. J., Sanjack, M., Turner, H., Cowmeadow, P., Hopkins, J., and Bushnell, D. (2000). Promoting mental health after childbirth: A controlled trial of primary prevention of postnatal depression. *British Journal of Clinical Psychology*, 39, 223–241.

# 69

# Basic mechanisms of and treatment targets for bipolar disorder

*Grant C. Churchill, Nisha Singh, and Michael J. Berridge*

## Introduction

In our coverage of this area, we emphasize depth, rather than breadth, and focus on current leads in the basic mechanisms underlying bipolar disorder and its treatment targets, suggested by recent advances, and place these against a background of historical concepts. For more encyclopaedic accounts, we point readers in the direction of the excellent reviews available [1–3]. We take as our starting point the mechanism of action of a drug (lithium) of known efficacy and translate this information into a biologically meaningful and unifying working hypothesis, in which all molecular defects and treatment targets for bipolar disorder are directly or indirectly linked to calcium signalling. We will illustrate the utility of this conceptual framework by providing examples of how these pathways encompass current, and how they could be used to great advantage in the future for, drug discovery.

## Bipolar disorder is related to intracellular signalling pathways

Other neuropsychiatric disorders have basic mechanisms and treatment targets that directly implicate neurotransmitter systems. For example, schizophrenia has strong ties to overactive dopamine and D2 receptor activation, with D2 receptor antagonists being effective antipsychotics. Depression is also empirically linked to the serotonergic system as selective serotonin reuptake inhibitors (SSRIs) that increase the availability of serotonin in the synaptic cleft. In contrast, bipolar disorder does not implicate preferentially one neurotransmitter system, but rather is linked to several [2, 4]. Moreover, studies have demonstrated that there are changes in almost all the major neurotransmitters in studies using blood samples and post-mortem tissues [2]. Therefore, the gold standard treatment for bipolar disorder remains lithium (see Chapter 72).

## Lithium and its possible targets

Lithium arguably exerts the most specific clinical effect in psychiatry and is highly effective in reducing the risk of relapse [3]. Only lithium meets the stringent criteria of a true mood stabilizer [5]. Lithium works in acute mania and depression and as maintenance therapy, and is the only proven anti-suicidal drug [6]. However, monotherapy is rare [4], and though lithium remains the gold standard [7], it is often combined with other pharmacological agents such as the anticonvulsants valproate, carbamazepine, and lamotrigine, as well as dopamine antagonists such as olanzapine and quetiapine [4].

The treatment targets of lithium and, by extrapolation, the pathological targets of bipolar disorder have been the Holy Grail in the field ever since lithium's discovery in 1949. Despite its toxic side effects, lithium revolutionized the treatment of bipolar disorder and its success has been impossible to replicate with other drugs because we do not understand exactly how lithium works at the molecular and cellular levels. Lithium's simplicity—the third lightest element—obscures its action on multiple targets and pathways. In the past, potential drug targets for lithium have come and gone in response to scientific fashion, rather than experimental evidence. This is nicely outlined by Belmaker [8] who noted that the suggested targets varied through the decades according to the latest knowledge of brain function.

The early years of lithium research focused on neurotransmitter systems, and although lithium has definite effects on these, it is now becoming increasingly evident that the targets of all mood stabilization lie not at the receptor level, but downstream of it [2].

The most effective drugs for treating bipolar disorder share a complex pharmacology that modulates second messenger pathways. Evidence for second messenger modulation comes not only from lithium, but also from the efficacy of certain anticonvulsants. Valproate and carbamazepine both show efficacy towards bipolar disorder and affect second messenger systems; in contrast, the anticonvulsants topiramate and gabapentin do not show efficacy and do not affect second messenger systems, based on current evidence [9]. Historically, drugs used to treat bipolar disorder have been suggested to act at many intracellular targets within: the adenylyl cyclase (AC)/cyclic adenosine monophosphate (cAMP)/cAMP response element binding protein (CREB) pathway; the extracellular regulated kinase (ERK)/mitogen-activated protein kinase (MAPK) pathway; the phosphoinositide (PI)/inositol-1,4,5-triphosphate ($IP_3$)/protein kinase C (PKC)/diacylglycerol kinase (DAGK) pathway; and the Wnt/frizzled (Fz)/dishevelled (Dvl)/glycogen synthase kinase-3 beta (GSK-3β) pathway. Because of the intertwined nature of these signalling networks, with much crosstalk through feedback loops, dysfunction in unrelated gene products can give rise to similar cellular and neural network dysfunction; similarly, drugs with distinct mechanisms of action can all affect a similar cellular signalling pathway and yield the same effect on neural activity. Lithium is exceptionally promiscuous because it competes for magnesium at binding sites, due to a similar atomic radius, and can inhibit all magnesium-dependent processes, depending on its concentration. Lithium's large number of potential targets can be reduced by comparing the concentration of lithium required to inhibit a putative therapeutic target with the concentration that is therapeutically relevant (0.6–1.2 mM) [10] and by considering the likely biological relevance of a given target.

## Guanine nucleotide-binding proteins (G proteins)

Substantial evidence implicates G proteins in bipolar disorder [2, 3, 11]. G proteins are a large ubiquitous family of proteins that transduce signals from the cell surface into the cell (Fig. 69.1). The heterotrimeric class of G proteins are made up of three subunits (alpha, beta, and gamma) and couple signals from activated G protein-coupled receptors (GPCRs) to enzymes (effectors) that generate second messengers. The effector enzyme and second messenger pathway is largely dictated by the alpha subunit. The alpha subunits Gs (stimulatory) and Gi (inhibitory) control the activity of adenylyl cyclase, which makes cAMP. Conversely, the alpha subunit Gq activates phospholipase C (PLC) beta. The pathways have numerous points where they can interact to increase or decrease the

function of the other. In this manner, cAMP can amplify or inhibit calcium signals, and vice versa.

When a GPCR is activated, it causes a conformational change that results in guanosine diphosphate (GDP) being exchanged for guanosyl triphosphate (GTP), causing dissociation of the $G_\alpha$ and $G_{\beta\gamma}$ subunits, which then activate a variety of signalling pathways, depending on the location and coupling to second messengers and effectors (Fig. 69.1). Eventually, GTP is hydrolysed to GDP by the intrinsic enzymatic activity of the $G_\alpha$ subunit or the presence of other enzymes that hydrolyse GTP, and it re-joins the $G_{\beta\gamma}$ subunit to revert to the inactive trimer. This 'off-mechanism' is governed by different regulatory enzymes such as GTPase activating proteins which facilitate the $G_\alpha$ subunit's intrinsic GTPase activity. For more detailed information, see a review [12]. Additionally, there is a family of G protein receptor kinases (GRKs) which work to phosphorylate the activated receptors directly and prevent the binding of G proteins [12] (Fig. 69.1). Evidence suggests that lithium does not act directly on G proteins but, after chronic treatment, leads to the stabilization of the inactive heterotrimeric state [3, 13].

Based on the hypothesis that overactive GPCR signalling is causal in bipolar disorder, lithium could dampen overactivation by stabilizing the inactive heterotrimeric G protein, leading to a reduction in G protein–effector coupling. Neural hyperactivity in bipolar disorder is based on several lines of evidence. Post-mortem, as well as genetic, studies have shown that there exist regulatory differences in GRKs in affective disorders [14]. More specifically, a single nucleotide polymorphism of the *GRK-3* gene has been associated with bipolar disorder [2]. Other findings show hyperfunctional G protein function in leucocytes [14] and increased $G_\alpha$ subtypes in post-mortem brain tissue, platelets, and leucocytes [2]. This is suggestive of an overall amplification of signalling, as the receptors are less likely to be phosphorylated and therefore inactivated. Hence, it is feasible that lithium's therapeutic effects may be related to its ability to reduce the increased signalling as a virtue of a polymorphism in *GRK-3*. When tested *in vitro* in platelets from bipolar manic patients, valproate also showed evidence of reducing G protein coupling, and thereby attenuating signalling [15].

## AC/cAMP/CREB pathway

The initiation of the cAMP signalling pathway occurs when a hormone or neurotransmitter binds to the receptor and induces either an increase (Gαs coupled) or a decrease (Gαi coupled) in AC activity. The latter is a dimeric enzyme which catalyses the conversion of adenosine triphosphate (ATP) to cAMP, which further amplifies the signalling by acting on numerous effector proteins (Fig. 69.2), the most well characterized of which is protein kinase A (PKA). Many physiological effects of cAMP are mediated by PKA (Fig. 69.2), which phosphorylates its targets to increase or decrease cell signalling-related physiological effects. Overall, PKA activation increases cytosolic calcium via entry through L-type Cav1.1 and L-type Cav1.2 channels. Another important action of PKA is its ability to induce gene transcription via the transcription factor CREB. The catalytic subunit of PKA translocates to the nucleus and phosphorylates CREB, which, in turn, binds to the DNA promoter region and turns on or off the transcription of certain genes. Some genes regulated by CREB relevant to bipolar disorder include the ones

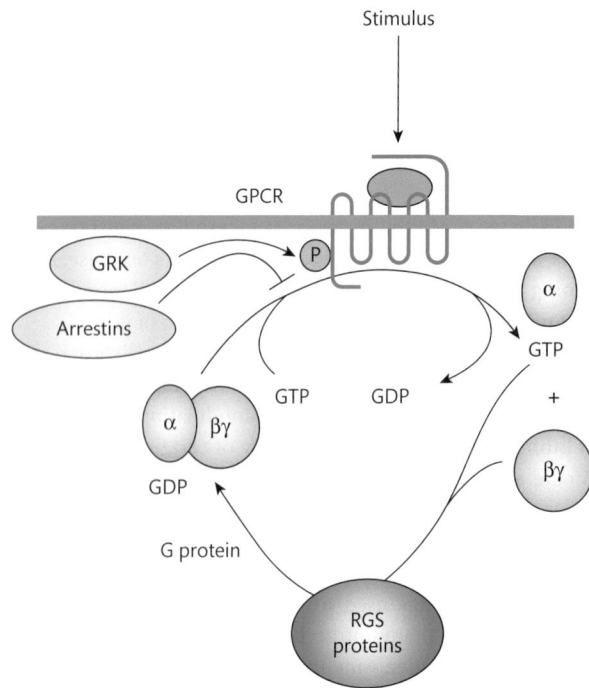

**Fig. 69.1** A simplified mechanism illustrating heterotrimeric G protein signalling.
Adapted from *Cell Signalling Biology*, 6, Berridge MJ, Module 2: Figure heterotrimeric G protein signalling, Copyright (2014), with permission from Portland Press Limited.

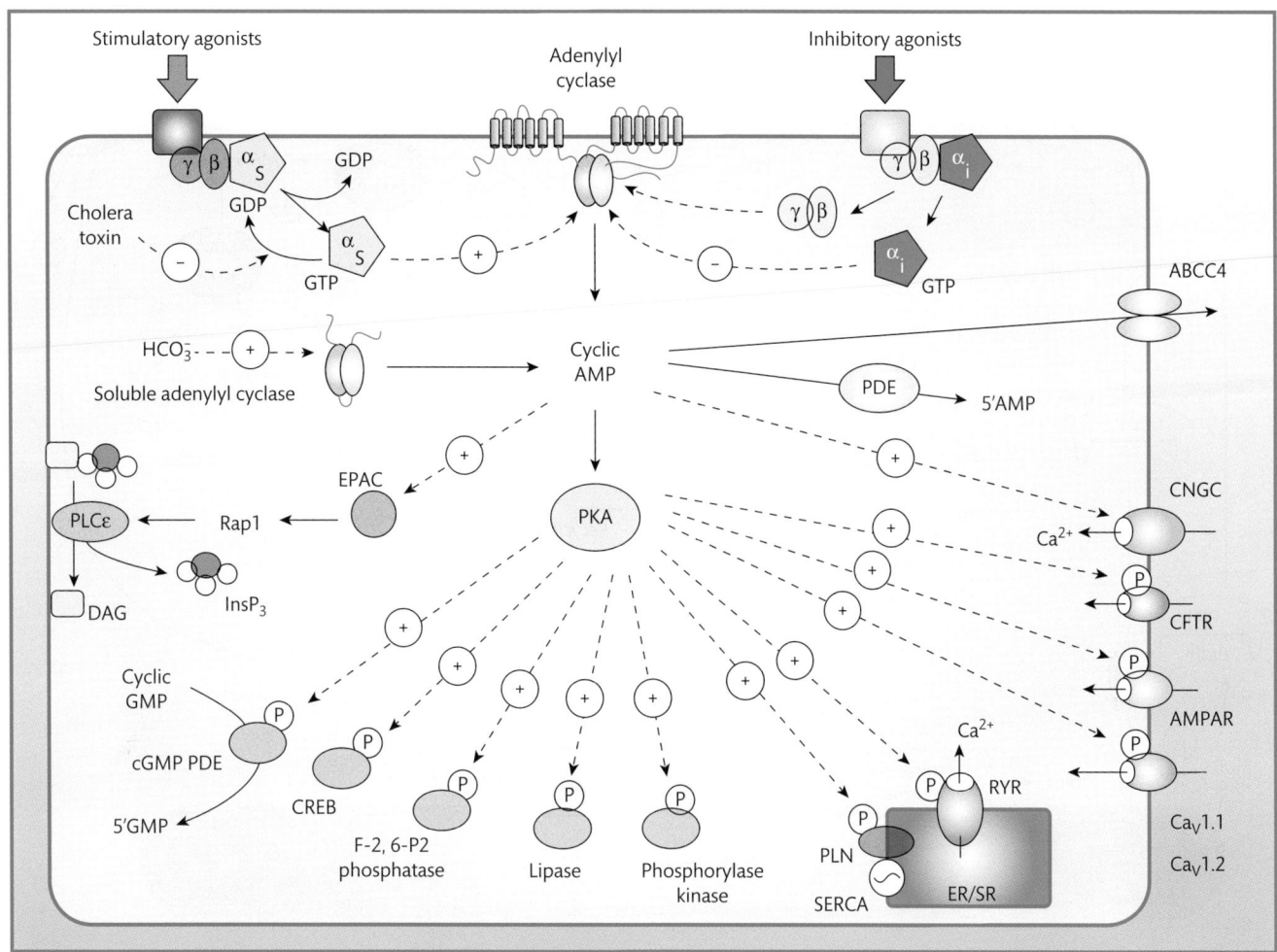

**Fig. 69.2** Summary of the control of cyclic AMP levels and its cellular targets.
Adapted from *Cell Signalling Biology*, 6, Berridge MJ, Module 2: Figure heterotrimeric G protein signalling, Copyright (2014), with permission from Portland Press Limited.

that code for brain-derived neurotrophic factor (BDNF), tyrosine hydroxylase, and circadian regulators.

Lithium produces complex effects on this cAMP signalling pathway [2, 3]. It inhibits cAMP accumulation in response to stimulation; however, paradoxically, it increases basal, and in some cases stimulated, AC activity, resulting therefore in an increase in basal cAMP [16]. Moreover, lithium's effects on cAMP and AC are tissue-specific [16, 17]. It has also been suggested that chronic lithium treatment might be producing these effects on G proteins, rather than on AC directly, as these effects were reversible *in vitro* only when increasing concentrations of GTP [18] were added, and not by increasing magnesium. If the effect of lithium were mediated by inhibition of AC, increasing magnesium would reverse the effect, as it does during acute treatment. Overall, chronic treatment with lithium showed reduced CREB phosphorylation in rat brains [2], indicative of an attenuation of this pathway, at least with respect to CREB activity. By comparison, valproate also decreased cAMP production on stimulation, but chronically it did not affect CREB.

## Phosphoinositide pathway

Much of the early work implicating phosphoinositide signalling in the pathogenesis of bipolar disorder and as providing targets for

drugs was equivocal because of the limitations of the experimental models and chemical tools available at the time. Now with new models, such as mice with genes knocked out for IMPase 1, IMPase 2, and *myo*-inositol uptake, combined with a blood–brain barrier-permeant putative lithium mimetic ebselen and with L690330 delivered directly into mouse brains [19], the phosphoinositide area is experiencing a renaissance.

Receptors that employ this pathway are coupled to Gαq, which activates phospholipase C (PLC), which catalyses the hydrolysis of phosphotidyl inositol 4,5-biphosphate (PIP$_2$) to diacylglycerol (DAG) and IP$_3$ (Fig. 69.3). Both IP$_3$ and DAG then go on to control several physiological processes, before being recycled back to PIP$_2$ via a series of intermediary phosphoinositides. As Gq is linked to nearly all of the known neurotransmitter systems (noradrenergic, serotonergic, glutamatergic, cholinergic, as well as dopaminergic through heterodimers), it is perfectly plausible that lithium might be regulating mood via its actions on phosphoinositide signalling.

Allison and Stewart first showed that inositol levels were decreased in rat brains treated with lithium and postulated that this reduction might be due to lithium interfering with active transport, synthesis, or incorporation into phosphoinositides [20]. Although *myo*-inositol levels decreased in the cerebral cortex of rats treated with lithium, levels of Ins1P increased [21], suggesting inhibition of the enzyme inositol monophosphatase (IMPase), which converts

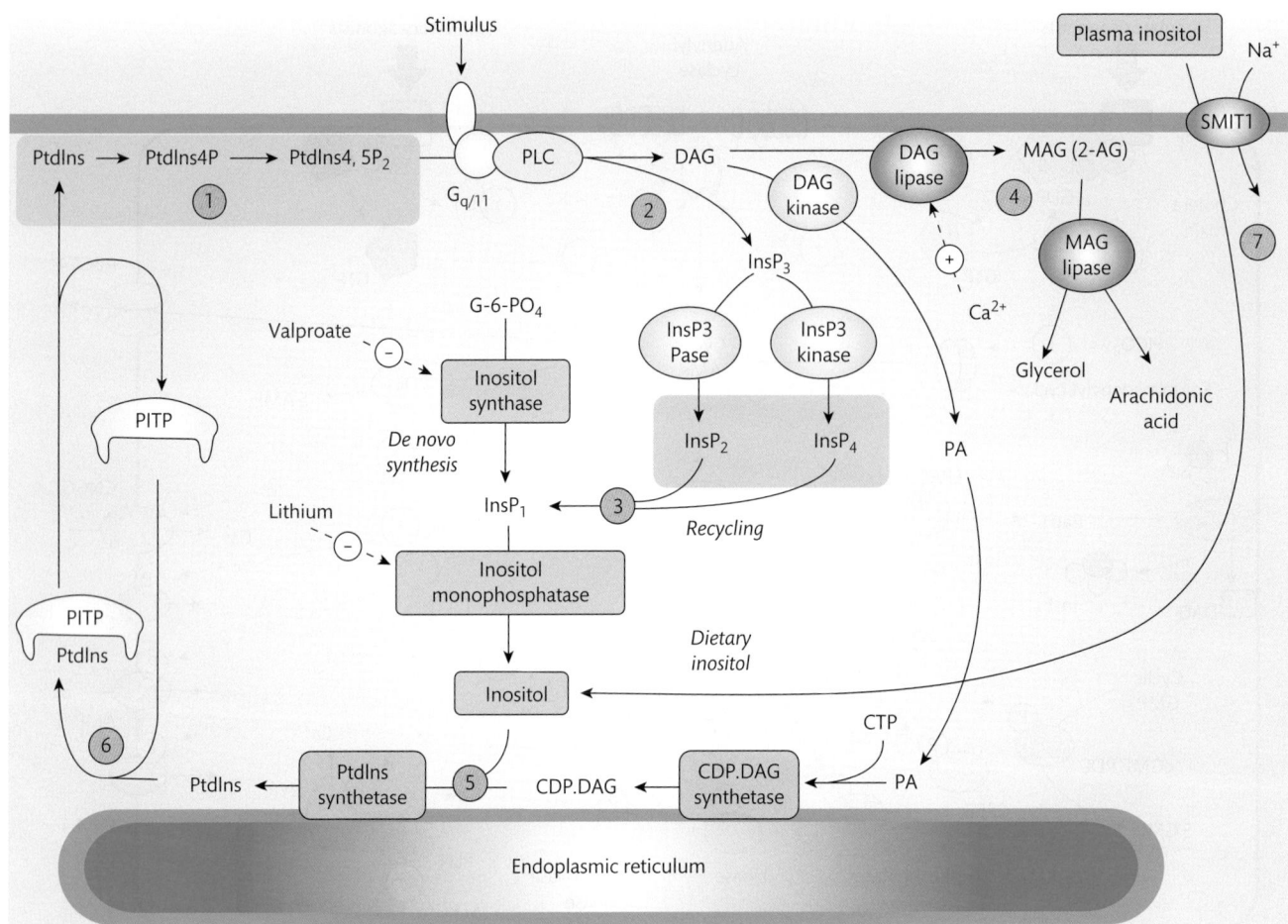

**Fig. 69.3** Summary of the phosphoinositol cycle and the possible mechanism of action of lithium and valproate.
Adapted from *Cell Signalling Biology*, 6, Berridge MJ, Module 2: Figure heterotrimeric G protein signalling, Copyright (2014), with permission from Portland Press Limited.

Ins1P into inositol. Hallcher and Sherman demonstrated that at therapeutically relevant concentrations, lithium uncompetitively inhibits IMPase [22]. This mechanism of uncompetitive inhibition is rare and was an important consideration in the development of the inositol depletion hypothesis proposed by Berridge in 1982 [23, 24].

### Inositol depletion hypothesis

The inositol depletion hypothesis proposes an elegant scheme for lithium's therapeutic efficacy in bipolar disorder [23, 24]. It is hypothesized that in bipolar patients, the phosphoinositide signalling pathway is hyperactive (Fig. 69.4). Lithium, by inhibiting IMPase, impedes this pathway by depleting the cell of inositol, which is required for the regeneration of active signalling molecules such as $IP_3$ (Figs. 69.3 and 69.4). Moreover, lithium inhibits the enzyme uncompetitively [22], that is, the level of inhibition intensifies with increasing substrate concentration. Therefore, lithium is more effective on pathways that are hyperfunctional, and not as much on those pathways that are effective at basal levels. Interestingly, IMPase is also at the juncture of another inositol recycling pathway. Glucose 6-phosphate is converted by 1-D-*myo*-inositol-3-phosphate synthase (MIPS) into Ins1P [23, 24], which is then converted to inositol

by IMPase (Fig. 69.3). Therefore, inhibition of IMPase ensures that both pathways (inositol recycling and synthesis) in the brain are inhibited.

### Inositol and the brain

The brain is uniquely sensitive to inositol depletion, because poor blood–brain barrier permeability of inositol renders it heavily dependent on recycling (Figs. 69.3 and 69.4), in contrast to tissues in the periphery which have easy access to dietary inositol. Although this depletion of inositol phosphates may be relatively small, as inositol phosphates comprise a small component of the cellular machinery, the changes they can influence may be of considerable proportion. A small change in inositol phosphatases may produce an amplification (and flux) leading to substantial cellular signalling and gene expression, which ultimately underlies lithium's therapeutic efficacy in bipolar disorder.

The premise that inositol signalling is a valid therapeutic target in the treatment of bipolar disorder is strengthened by the fact that both valproate and carbamazepine also cause a depletion of inositol phosphates, although not always by inhibiting IMPase. Valproate and carbamazepine inhibit MIPS [25] (Fig. 69.3). Furthermore, all

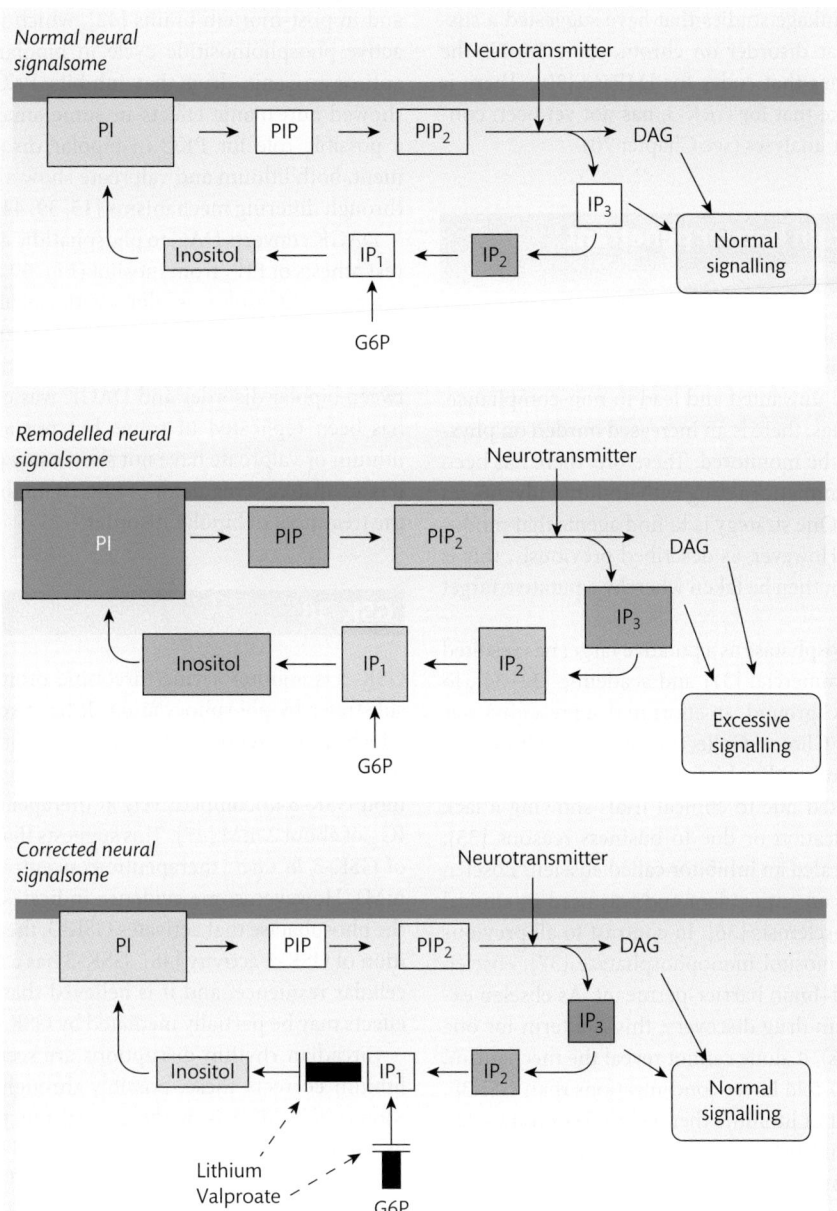

**Fig. 69.4** Diagram illustrating the inositol depletion hypothesis whereby overactive signalling in neurons can be corrected by slowing the inositol cycle.
Adapted from *Cell Signalling Biology*, 6, Berridge MJ, Module 2: Figure heterotrimeric G protein signalling, Copyright (2014), with permission from Portland Press Limited.

three mood stabilizers lithium, valproate, and carbamazepine inhibit the uptake of *myo*-inositol from blood into the brain using the sodium/*myo*-inositol transporter 1 (SMIT1) [26].

## Evidence for inositol depletion

Besides the observation that lithium, valproate, and carbamazepine all deplete inositol, the strongest evidence for the inositol depletion hypothesis comes from lithium's inhibition of IMPase at therapeutic concentrations. This inhibition causes a decrease in inositol and $PIP_2$, which can be measured. Shimon *et al.* in 1997 showed decreased levels of inositol in the prefrontal cortex in post-mortem brains

of bipolar patients using gas chromatographic techniques [27]. Magnetic resonance spectroscopy has also been extensively used, with mixed findings [28], but several studies have found decreased levels of *myo*-inositol in the frontal lobe of bipolar patients treated acutely and chronically with lithium, compared to controls [28]. Additionally, increased levels of phosphomonoesters (including Ins1P) have been shown to be increased in the frontal lobe of both bipolar manic and bipolar depressed patients treated with lithium [28]. According to the inositol depletion theory, a decrease in inositol leads to a reduction in phosphoinositides, such as $PIP_2$, a precursor for $IP_3$. This was demonstrated by showing that reduced $PIP_2$ levels were found in platelets from bipolar I patients treated with lithium, compared to control volunteers [29]. Preliminary evidence also comes from genetic linkage studies that have suggested a susceptibility locus for bipolar disorder on chromosome 18p11, the location of one of the genes that codes for IMPase [30]. There is a caveat that this locus, like that for *GRK-3*, has not yet been confirmed in subsequent meta-analyses (see Chapter 70).

## Ebselen: a blood–brain barrier penetrant IMPase inhibitor

Lithium has wanted and unwanted effects that are concentration-dependent, but the therapeutic index is small. It does not work in all patients; side effects are unwanted and lead to non-compliance, and compared to other drugs, there is an increased burden on physicians as blood levels must be monitored. Therefore, there has been an effort to find a 'lithium mimetic': a drug with lithium's advantages without its disadvantages. One strategy is to find agents that modulate the target of lithium. However, as described previously, this is unknown. An approach can then be taken whereby a putative target is explored.

Taking inositol monophosphatase as a putative target has resulted in several efforts, both commercial [31] and academic [32–34], to find inhibitors. On this background, an effort in drug rescuing was undertaken using the NIH Clinical Collection, which is a library of drugs known to be safe and with a history of use in humans but that have not been marketed due to clinical trials showing a lack of efficacy in a given indication or due to business reasons [35]. Using isolated IMPase revealed an inhibitor called ebselen. Ebselen was originally designed as an antioxidant and was used in clinical trials for stroke and atherosclerosis [36]. In contrast to all previous studies with inhibitors of inositol monophosphatase [37], ebselen was bioavailable and blood–brain barrier-permeant. As ebselen exhibits polypharmacology (in drug discovery, this is a term for one drug affecting many targets), it alone cannot reveal the mechanism, but it inhibits IMPase at 40-fold lower concentrations than GSK3β, the other most likely target of lithium's therapeutic action. Ebselen exhibited certain lithium-like behavioural effects in animal models that were reversed *in vivo* by the administration of inositol, strongly indicating IMPase inhibition as the mechanism [33, 34]. More directly, ebselen reduced *myo*-inositol in both mouse brains, as well as in the anterior cingulate cortex in healthy volunteers, consistent with the inositol depletion hypothesis [23, 24]. Ebselen also decreased impulsivity [38], which may relate to lithium's anti-suicidal effects.

## Protein kinase C and diacylglycerol kinase

PKC is a serine/threonine kinase that phosphorylates substrates to activate or inactivate them and thus modulates cell signalling pathways. PKC itself is activated by DAG and calcium ($Ca^{2+}$). Although lithium does not directly inhibit PKC, chronic administration decreases the activity of two isoforms of PKC—PKCα and PKCε—in the frontal cortex and hippocampus [39], without affecting the other PKC isoforms [40]. PKC, as a component of the calcium signalling pathway discussed previously, can modulate glutamatergic, noradrenergic, and serotonergic pathways in the CNS, indicative that it may be important for mood stabilization [39]. PKC shows increased activity in platelets from patients in the manic phase [41]

and in post-mortem brains [42], which is consistent with a hyperactive phosphoinositide cycle in bipolar disorder. Tamoxifen, an anti-oestrogenic drug that inhibits PKC at high concentrations, showed anti-manic effects in some small trials [43], highlighting a possible role for PKC in bipolar disorder. After chronic treatment, both lithium and valproate show a reduction in PKC activity, through differing mechanisms [15, 39, 44].

DAGK converts DAG to phosphatidic acid, an essential step in the resynthesis of $PIP_2$ from inositol (Fig. 69.3). Additionally, DAG also activates PKC isoforms, along with calcium. Therefore, hyperactive production or reduced removal of DAG may further result in PKC hyperactivity. In a genome-wide association study, a strong link between bipolar disorder and DAGK was observed [45]. This finding has been replicated in some, but not all, studies [46]. Although lithium or valproate have not shown any direct effects on DAGK, as it is an upstream regulator of PKC, it might be another valid target in the treatment of bipolar disorder.

## GSK-3β

GSK-3 is another serine/threonine protein kinase that modulates substrates by phosphorylation. It has two isoforms GSK-3α and β, which have essentially the same function. GSK-3 phosphorylation of glycogen synthase renders it inactive. Lithium was shown to inhibit GSK-3 uncompetitively at therapeutic concentrations with an $IC_{50}$ of about 2 mM [47]. This suggests that there is partial inhibition of GSK-3 *in vivo* (therapeutic concentration of approximately 0.8 mM). However, some evidence indicates that lithium also inhibits the phosphatase that activates GSK-3, thereby reinforcing the inhibition of GSK-3 activity [48]. GSK-3 has a role in neuroplasticity and cellular resilience, and it is believed that lithium's neuroprotective effects may be partially mediated by GSK-3 inhibition [49].

Circadian rhythm disruptions are seen in bipolar patients, and lithium corrects these, possibly through GSK-3β inhibition [49]. Moreover, GSK-3 is at the crucial juncture of neurotransmitters, like noradrenaline, dopamine, and 5-HT, and gene transcription. GSK-3 inhibition may also be involved in the teratogenic effects seen with lithium treatment [47]. Overall, GSK-3 has only recently been considered as a target for lithium and hence requires further investigation to understand lithium's effects via GSK-3β. Given that lithium must be dosed chronically to be effective, more studies are needed. Valproate does not directly inhibit GSK-3β at therapeutic concentrations [49].

Although GSK-3β has been contested vociferously as a likely target for lithium's efficacy, there are substantial caveats. For an excellent review, see [50]. Briefly, the phosphorylation patterns are inconsistent with lithium therapy. Additionally, inhibiting GSK-3β signalling causes stabilization of β-catenin and activation of the canonical Wnt signalling pathway [51]. The Wnt pathway is strongly associated with oncogenic changes, and even a moderate surge in β-catenin promotes oncogenesis [50].

## Calcium signalling as a central unifying concept

The best experimental evidence, both historical and current, from pathophysiology, genetics, and drugs is converging on calcium signalling. Calcium controls all facets of brain function, including axonal growth, memory, excitability, brain rhythms, gene transcription, neuronal firing, neurotransmitter uptake, hormone release, mitochondrial activity, neurogenesis, and apoptosis [51, 52]. Thus, calcium can control brain activity in several ways, including effects on neural circuit activity generated through interactions between excitatory and inhibitory neurons and short-term events that underlie neural excitability, as well as long-term processes such as gene transcription (Fig. 69.5). Calcium relays and integrates signals from extracellular messengers (neurotransmitters and neuromodulators) and other intracellular signalling pathways, to affect neuronal excitability over the short term and gene transcription over the longer term. Therefore, calcium is uniquely placed at a key position to influence neural activity, growth, and neural plasticity. Indeed, excessive calcium signalling has been hypothesized to drive the neuronal excitatory–inhibitory imbalance that can explain mood swings in bipolar disorder [52]. Although there is great complexity in the number and interactions of genes and molecular players in calcium signalling (Fig. 69.5), it does not mean that it will take a drug for each defect; rather, promisingly, it means that there are a great number of ways to intervene with a single drug that would affect the entire pathway.

## An overview of calcium signalling

Unlike other messengers that can be created and destroyed, calcium can only be moved around in time and space (Fig. 69.6). Cytosolic calcium concentration is at steady state and is the sum of the activity of all channels and pumps at both the plasma membrane and intracellular organelles. Extracellular calcium is approximately 1 mM and intracellular cytosolic calcium is approximately 100 nM, so there is a chemical gradient of about 10,000-fold, as well as an electrical gradient combined to drive calcium into a cell. Inside cells, many organelles also store calcium to create approximately the same concentration gradient. Maintaining low cytosolic calcium is essential, as calcium itself is inherently toxic as it precipitates phosphates and phosphate-containing molecules and induces cell death through apoptosis. The cell expends much energy maintaining low cytosolic calcium through pumps at the plasma membrane such as the plasma membrane calcium–ATPase and a sodium/calcium exchanger. The endoplasmic reticulum is the major intracellular calcium store and has the sarco(endo)plasmic reticulum calcium ATPase (SERCA) on it. Mitochondria take up calcium through an electrogenic uniporter that operates in the presence of high cytosolic calcium in microdomains close to channels.

In the cytosol, calcium is heavily bound by immobile binding proteins (buffers), which greatly limits its diffusion. This enables calcium increases to be very rapid and localized, or as calcium can stimulate its own release at certain channels, the responses can be greatly amplified in time and space. This highlights that not all calcium within a cell has the same effect—what matters is the spatial distribution, the timing, and the amplitude [51]. Indeed, different frequencies of calcium spikes can drive different transcription factors. Similarly, the amplitude of localized calcium responses in neuronal growth cones controls attractive or repulsive migration towards a chemotactic substance. There are many families and isoforms of each pump and channel to provide for fine-tuning calcium signals and their cellular

responses (Fig. 69.5). In one example, there is plasma membrane to nucleus signalling in which the calcium emanating from a Cav1.2 channel can result in changes in gene transcription, whereas calcium emanating from an NMDA receptor channel is far less effective [52]. This selectivity results from better coupling to MAPK and cAMP signalling cascades through calcium.

In neurons, calcium signalling can operate in a primary or modulatory mode [53] (Fig. 69.7). In the primary mode, calcium enters through channels in the plasma membrane, which may be amplified by ryanodine receptors through calcium-induced calcium release and often drives presynaptic vesicle fusion and neurotransmitter release. In the modulatory mode, calcium signalling is controlled through the IP$_3$/calcium pathway (Fig. 69.7). This modulatory calcium regulates membrane excitability and, in turn, neural networks and mood. Alteration in the function of components in either the primary or the modulatory pathways can contribute to the onset and treatment of bipolar disorder.

## Plasma membrane calcium channels

The plasma membrane contains many diverse families of calcium channels, all with unique activation and physiological function and classified as operating in the primary mode, as defined previously (Fig. 69.7). Voltage-operated calcium channels mediate calcium influx upon plasma membrane depolarization and are classified as L-, N-, and P/Q- types (Fig. 69.5). Calcium influx controls physiological responses such as neurotransmitter release and gene expression [51–53]. Receptor-operated types respond to neurotransmitters such as the NMDA receptor that responds to glutamate and the 5-HT$_3$ receptor that responds to serotonin. There are also second messenger-operated channels (SMOCs) that respond to calcium, cyclic nucleotides [for example, the cyclic nucleotide-gated channel (CNGC)], and arachidonic acid (AA), as well as store-operated channels (SOCs) that respond to the calcium load in the endoplasmic reticulum (Fig. 69.8). Intracellular calcium can modulate membrane excitability by acting on other channels such as inhibition of the KV7.2/KV7.3 channels responsible for the hyperpolarizing M current or stimulation of the non-selective cation channel leading to a depolarizing current.

## Intracellular calcium channels

Calcium signals that arise from intracellular channels operate in the modulatory mode and are common to all types of neurons. The regulation is also subtler in that it will influence excitability, but not actually cause firing of action potentials. There are two well-characterized families of intracellular calcium channels: the IP$_3$ receptor and the ryanodine receptor (Fig. 69.7). The IP$_3$ receptor is under control of extracellular signals, including neurotransmitters, neuromodulators, and hormones when they act through GPCRs or receptor tyrosine kinases or through the phosphoinositol pathway, as described previously (Fig. 69.5). In this pathway, a soluble messenger IP$_3$ is generated and binds to, and opens, a ligand-gated ion channel called the IP$_3$ receptor, located on the endoplasmic reticulum, to release calcium. The ryanodine receptor is primarily regulated by calcium through a process termed calcium-induced calcium release, but it is also sensitized by the second messenger

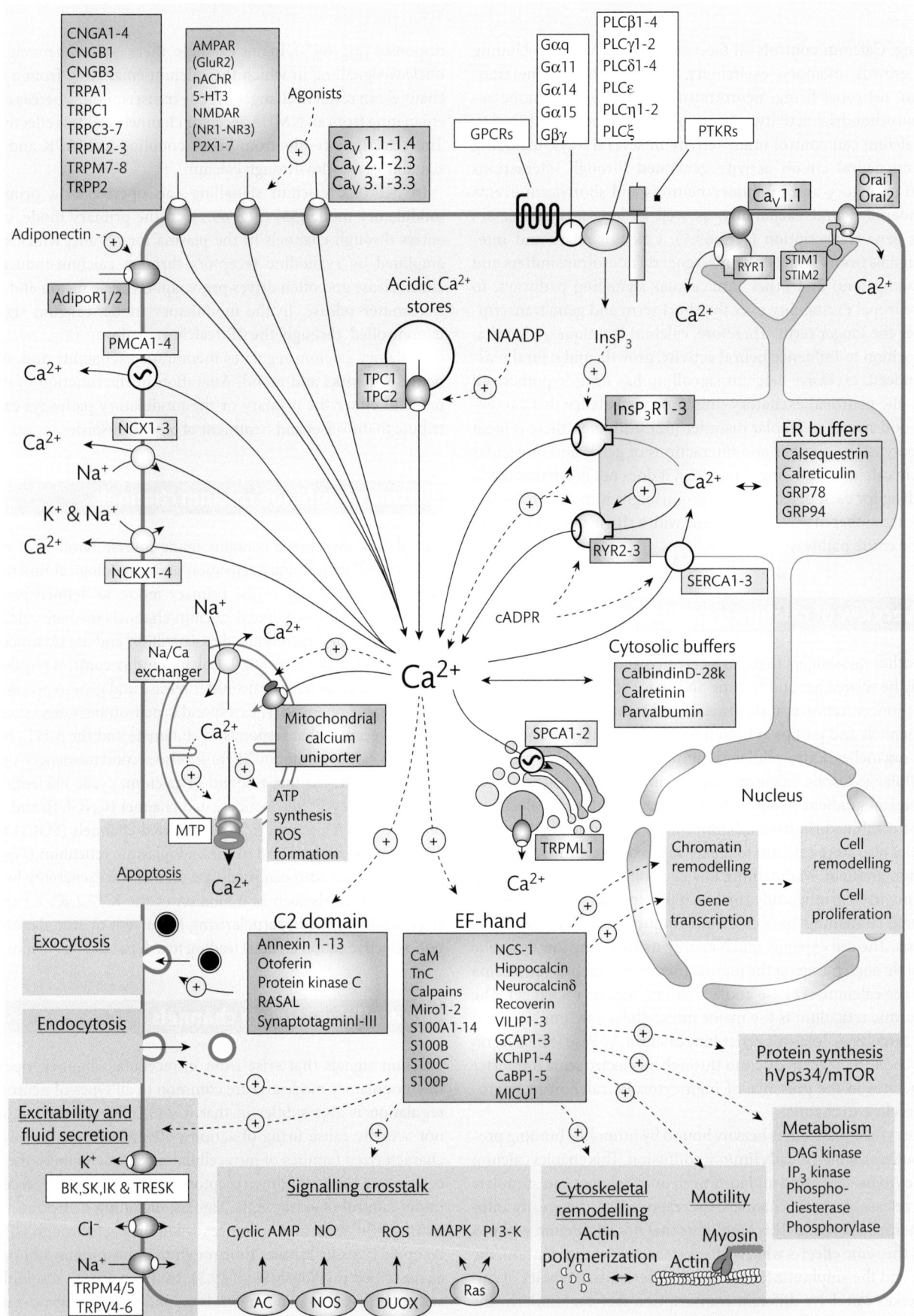

**Fig. 69.5** Calcium signalling plays a central role as a transducer of signal inputs and outputs and can be finely tuned by selecting components (channels, pumps, and effectors) from the calcium signalling toolkit. The green boxes illustrate the membrane calcium channels, whereas the red boxes are the pumps and exchangers that move calcium either out of the cell or back into the endoplasmic reticulum (ER). The purple boxes represent the buffers located in the cytoplasm or in the ER.

Adapted from *Cell Signalling Biology*, 6, Berridge MJ, Module 2: Figure heterotrimeric G protein signalling, Copyright (2014), with permission from Portland Press Limited.

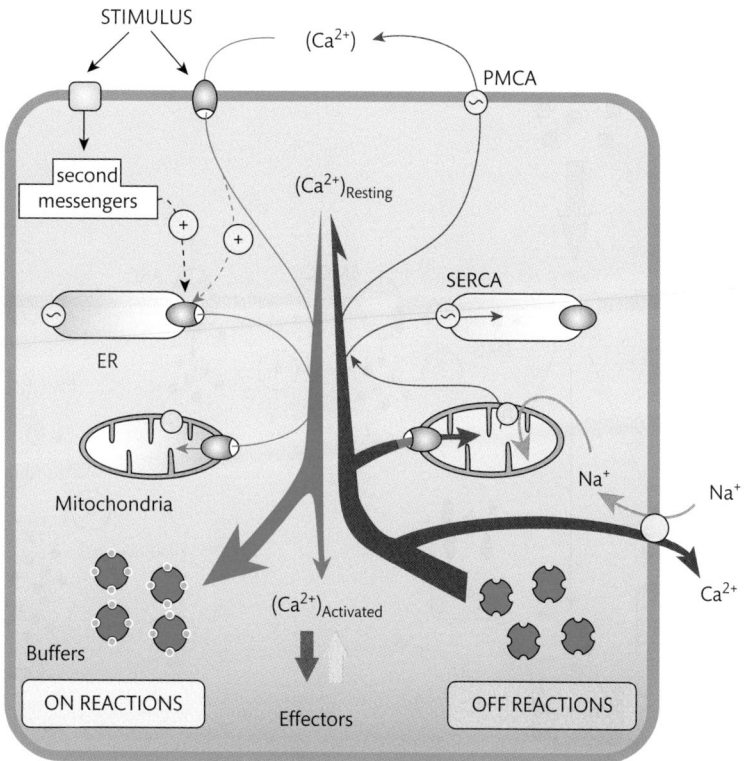

**Fig. 69.6** The 'on' and 'off' of calcium signals is controlled by channels and pumps at the plasma membrane and on organelles. PMCA, plasma membrane $Ca^{2+}$-ATPase; SERCA, sarco-/endoplasmic reticulum $Ca^{2+}$-ATPase.
Adapted from *Cell Signalling Biology*, 6, Berridge MJ, Module 2: Figure heterotrimeric G protein signalling, Copyright (2014), with permission from Portland Press Limited.

cyclic adenosine diphosphate (ADP) ribose. Calcium-induced calcium release amplifies calcium responses in amplitude, time, and space (Fig. 69.9). The $IP_3$ receptor also shows this phenomenon. Both channels have very large cytosolic heads with sites for regulation by almost all kinases, to sense calcium, ATP, redox, and other metabolites, so that they can integrate many facets of cellular status and integrate these into a calcium signal.

## Relation to treatment

In terms of drugs, most bipolar patients respond to lithium and valproate. As these are mood stabilizers and buffer swings to either pole, they are telling us something about the underlying regulation. These drugs have different chemical structures and possibly different molecular targets. They unify in their action at the level of intracellular

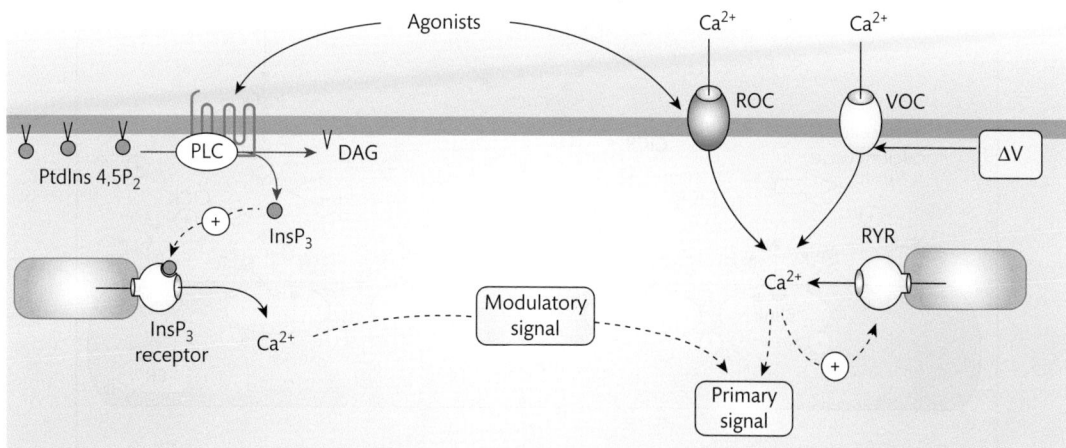

**Fig. 69.7** In neurons, calcium acts in either a primary or a modulatory mode. The primary calcium signal is generated by receptor-operated channels (ROCs) or voltage-operated channels (VOCS) that promote the entry of external calcium. This primary signal can be augmented by calcium-stimulating ryanodine receptors (RYRs) to release calcium from internal stores. The modulatory calcium signal is generated by agonists operating through InsP3 and calcium release from intracellular stores.
Adapted from *Physiol. Rev.* 96(4), Berridge MJ, The Inositol Trisphosphate/Calcium Signaling Pathway in Health and Disease, pp. 1261–96, Copyright (2016), with permission from the American Psychological Society.

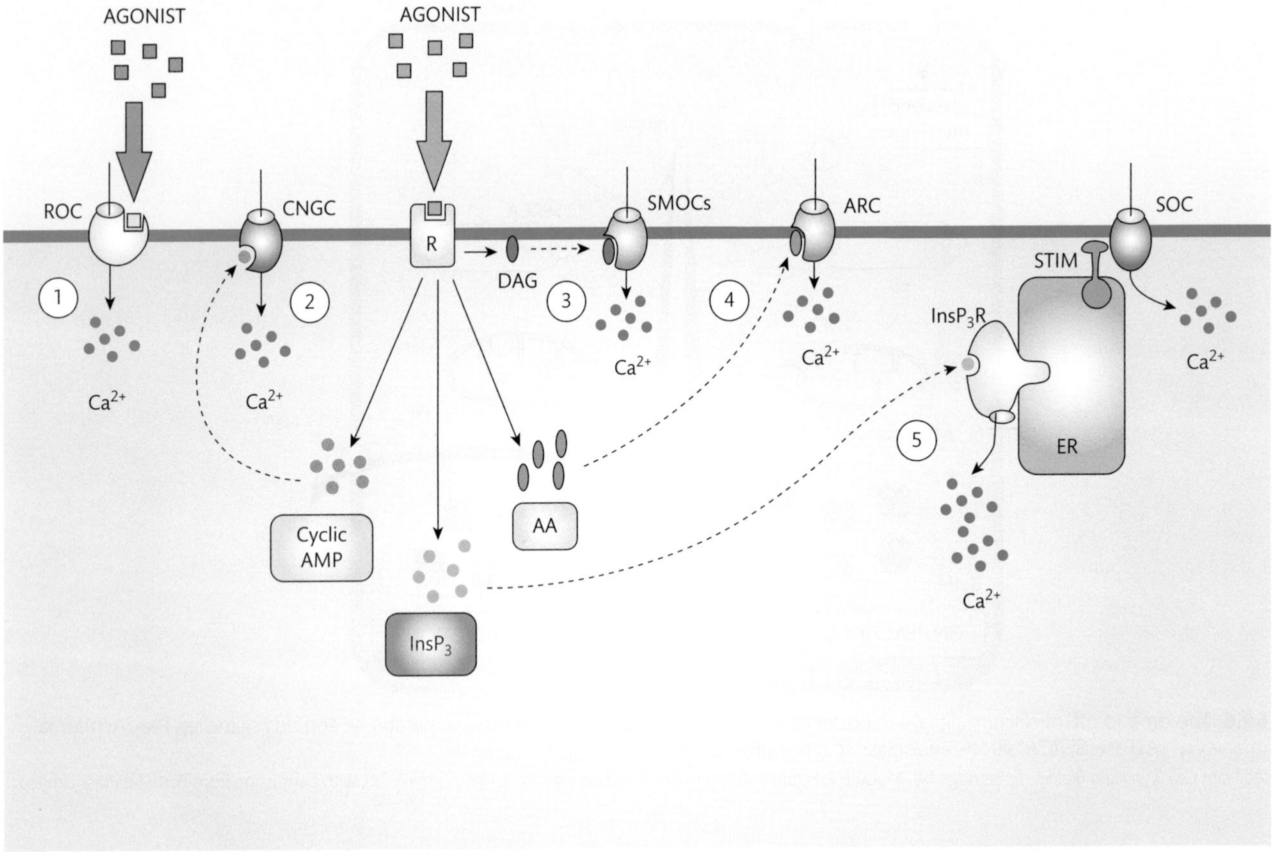

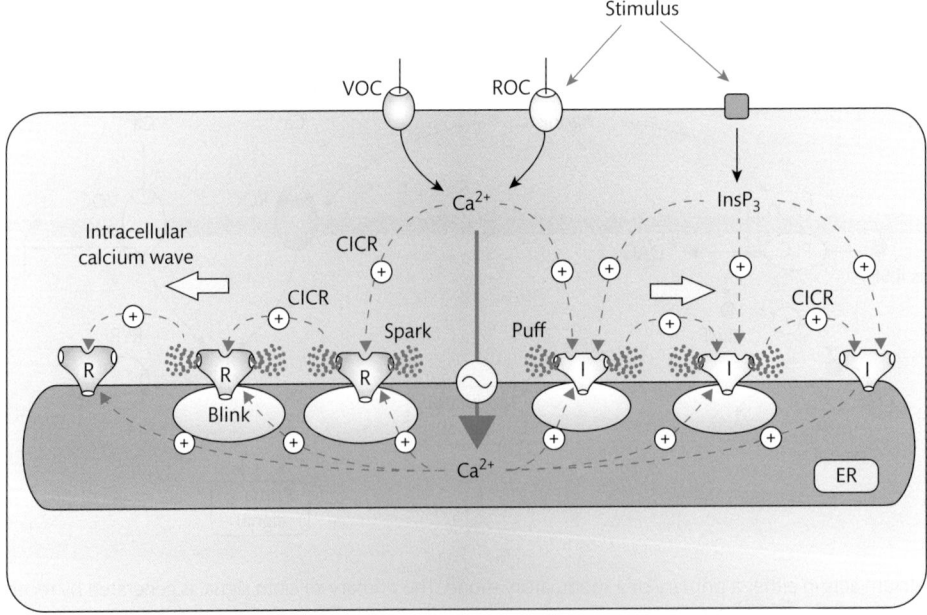

**Fig. 69.8** Mechanisms of calcium entry through agonist-operated calcium channels on the plasma membrane. The most direct mechanism occurs in the receptor-operated channels (ROCs) where the agonist binds directly to the ion channel. Agonists can also activate entry indirectly by recruiting various internal signalling pathways to activate second messenger-operated channels (SMOCs) or a store-operated channel (SOC).

Adapted from *Cell Signalling Biology*, 6, Berridge MJ, Module 2: Figure heterotrimeric G protein signalling, Copyright (2014), with permission from Portland Press Limited.

**Fig. 69.9** Calcium-induced calcium release (CICR) amplifies calcium increases in space. Calcium influx activates either ryanodine receptors or IP$_3$ receptors, which sets off a chain reaction, resulting in a calcium wave (yellow arrows). R, ryanodine receptors; I, IP$_3$ receptors; ER, endoplasmic reticulum; VOCs, voltage-operated channels.

Adapted from *Cell Signalling Biology*, 6, Berridge MJ, Module 2: Figure heterotrimeric G protein signalling, Copyright (2014), with permission from Portland Press Limited.

signal transduction, at the pathways leading to and from calcium signalling (Fig. 69.5). Efficacious drugs do not induce an all-or-none effect, but a subtle modulation of calcium release and uptake which creates an environment where variations from the mean are prohibited. The calcium signalling pathway provides for numerous unexplored potential treatment targets for new drugs.

## Evidence for calcium signalling defects in peripheral cells

Elevated intracellular $Ca^{2+}$ is recognized as a marker of bipolar disorder [54, 55]. In platelets and lymphocytes from patients with bipolar disorder, both baseline and agonist-stimulated levels of calcium were greater, consistent with overall calcium overload [55, 56]. Moreover, thapsigargin, an inhibitor of the SERCA calcium pump (Figs. 69.5 and 69.6), also showed an increase, indicating increased storage of calcium [55]. Increased cytosolic calcium occurred in both depression and mania [56]. However, elevated basal calcium concentrations have been detected in transformed B lymphoblasts from patients with bipolar I disorder, compared with those with bipolar II disorder or major depression or healthy controls [55]. Increased total serum and ionized calcium have also been reported in euthymic lithium-treated patients, compared to healthy controls [57]. Thus, calcium homeostasis appears altered across all mood states in bipolar disorder and treatment relating to bipolar disorder [2]. The mechanistic origins of these elevations in calcium are unknown, but suggestions have included dysfunction of almost all calcium pumps and channels (Fig. 69.5) [55].

## Evidence from iPSCs, genetics, and calcium antagonist drugs implicates calcium channels

An obvious limitation of studies with peripheral cells is whether calcium signalling in these cells accurately represents signalling in neurons. Recent studies with induced pluripotent stem cells (iPSCs), fibroblasts dedifferentiated and then redifferentiated into neurons, also add support to a defect in calcium signalling that can be normalized with drugs used to treat bipolar disorder. For example, iPSC neurons derived from fibroblasts taken from lithium responders showed hyperexcitability and signalling defects in both calcium and mitochondria [58]. Importantly, this hyperactivity and calcium signalling were corrected with lithium when the fibroblasts were taken from lithium responders [58]. Additionally, compared to controls, iPSC neurons derived from bipolar patients exhibited dysregulated calcium transients and wave amplitudes that were corrected with lithium [59].

One of the most promising findings is that a component of the calcium signalling pathway appears to be both involved in bipolar disorder and a therapeutic target. Specifically, the voltage-operated calcium channel Cav1.2, for which the gene *CACNA1* encodes its alpha subunit, which forms the pore, voltage sensor, and drug-binding sites (Fig. 69.10), is implicated by several distinct sources of evidence [54]. *CACNA1C* is consistently identified in genome-wide association studies (GWAS) [60, 61].

As with most findings in bipolar disorder, this hypothesis has not been fully tested but is tantalizing and theoretically straightforward.

Evidence comes from peripheral cells taken from bipolar patients, the efficacy in certain individuals with bipolar disorder of drugs that block voltage-operated calcium channels, and GWAS [54]. The voltage-operated calcium channel Cav1.2 is encoded by the gene *CACNA1*, and this has turned up reproducibly in several GWAS and has the strongest evidence of any GWAS hit [61]. Interestingly, the risk locus is within the large third intron (non-coding), and therefore, it likely affects function through the level of expression or alternative splicing. Indeed, when iPSCs were made from individuals with this variant, the cells had elevated mRNA expression and more calcium influx [62]. Results from GWAS reveal polymorphisms in the alpha 1C subunit of the L-type voltage-gated calcium channel gene (*CACNA1C*) as a risk factor for bipolar disorder. In regard to iPSCs, cells derived from bipolar patients and patients with *CACNA1* (which encodes the L-type calcium channel Cav1.2 α1) risk genotype exhibit aberrant calcium channel gene expression and functional calcium signalling. The risk variant is likely associated with increased channel expression and function.

Consistent with the involvement of Cav1.2 is that calcium channel blockers designed to treat cardiovascular disorders have been used to treat bipolar disorder. Although all three main groups of calcium channel blockers have been tested—dihydropyridines (for example, nifedipine), phenylalkylamines (for example, verapamil), and benzothiazepines (for example, diltiazem), the results are conflicting and lack definitive evidence for efficacy [54]. Problems include cohort size and low statistical power, lack of penetration of the blood–brain barrier, and lack of selectivity for isoforms found in the brain, limiting the dose to that tolerable for peripheral side effects. A recent meta-analysis concluded that the current evidence is equivocal but deserves proper study, both through design and through the development of blockers selective for the brain splice variant isoforms [54].

Theoretically, the involvement Cav1.2 will have profound effects on neural function, as it regulates both excitability and synaptic plasticity [52]. Indeed, in a model system in which a mutation in Cav1.2 in mice gives rise to Timothy syndrome, in humans, this shows effects on synaptic plasticity and spatial learning [63]. Mutations in Cav1.2 result in Timothy syndrome, dysfunction in multiple organs, and severe cognitive impairment [52].

## Future drug discovery

All drugs used in bipolar disorder were either approved before current rigorous regulatory and ethically sound clinical trials (lithium) or were repurposed from other uses as antipsychotics and antiepileptics. The community hopes to pursue rational drug design, in which our understanding of the pathophysiological or pharmacological mechanism will reveal targets for which we can develop drugs. Impeccable logic, but unfortunately there exist precious few examples where this has been achieved. The problem is that, of the many suggested therapeutic targets, none have been rigorously tested, and as the focus of biological interests in neuroscience has shifted, so has interest in possible targets. As none are validated or invalidated, we exist in a form of purgatory. Also, all mood stabilizers exhibit polypharmacology, making therapeutic target identification difficult. We need to move forward, using the best imperfect knowledge we have. For example, the putative targets of lithium have

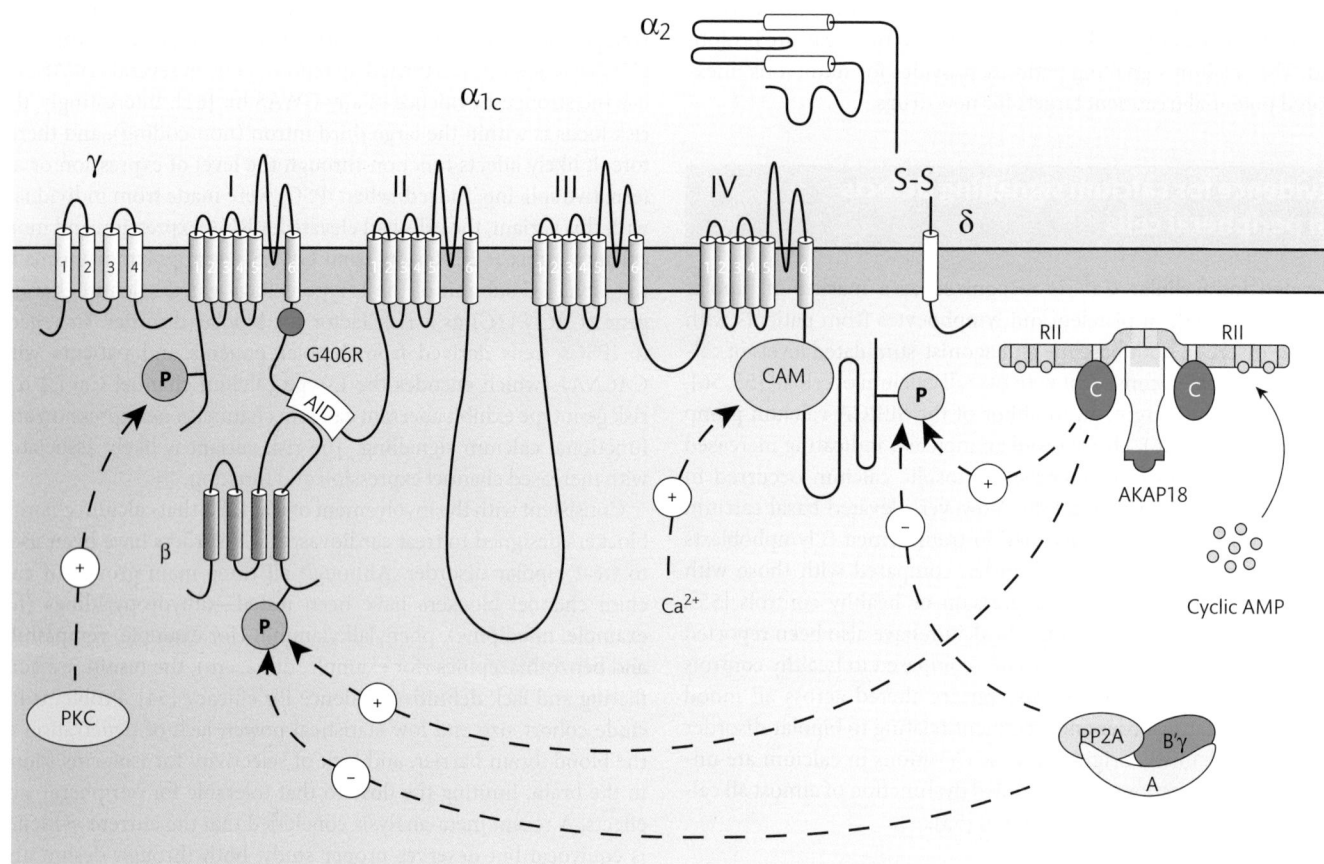

**Fig. 69.10** Structure and regulation of the Cav1.2 L-type calcium channel implicated in bipolar disorder. PKA, protein kinase A; AKAP18, A-kinase-anchoring protein; PKC, protein kinase C; CaM, calmodulin.

Adapted from *Cell Signalling Biology*, 6, Berridge MJ, Module 2: Figure heterotrimeric G protein signalling, Copyright (2014), with permission from Portland Press Limited.

not been properly explored and thus cannot conclusively be validated or invalidated. Similarly, there is much evidence from several sources that converges on the involvement of L-type calcium channels. This forms a solid working hypothesis that can be pursued. If we had drugs with good selectivity and favourable blood–brain barrier permeability, we could test these hypotheses and targets. To move on, a definitive 'no' would be more useful than a feeble 'yes'.

## REFERENCES

1. Geddes JR, Miklowitz DJ. Treatment of bipolar disorder. *Lancet*. 2013;381:1672–82.
2. Goodwin FK, Jamison KR. *Manic–Depressive Illness: Bipolar Disorders and Recurrent Depression* (2nd edn). New York, NY: Oxford University Press; 2007.
3. Manji HK, Potter WZ, Lenox RH. Signal transduction pathways. Molecular targets for lithium's actions. *Arch Gen Psychiatry*. 1995;52:531–43.
4. Goodwin GM, Haddad PM, Ferrier IN, *et al*. Evidence-based guidelines for treating bipolar disorder: revised third edition recommendations from the British Association for Psychopharmacology. *J Psychopharmacol*. 2016;30:495–553.
5. Bauer MS, Mitchner L. What is a 'mood stabilizer'? An evidence-based response. *Am J Psychiatry*. 2004;161:3–18.
6. Cipriani A, Pretty H, Hawton K, Geddes JR. Lithium in the prevention of suicidal behavior and all-cause mortality in patients with mood disorders: a systematic review of randomized trials. *Am J Psychiatry*. 2005;162:1805–19.
7. BALANCE investigators and collaborators, Geddes JR, Goodwin GM, Rendell J, *et al*. Lithium plus valproate combination therapy versus monotherapy for relapse prevention in bipolar I disorder (BALANCE): a randomised open-label trial. *Lancet*. 2010;375:385–95.
8. Belmaker RH. Bipolar Disorder. *N Engl J Med*. 2004;351:476–86.
9. Rogawski MA. Molecular targets versus models for new antiepileptic drug discovery. *Epilepsy Res*. 2006;68:22–8.
10. Gelenberg AJ, Kane JM, Keller MB, *et al*. Comparison of standard and low serum levels of lithium for maintenance treatment of bipolar disorder. *N Engl J Med*. 1989;321:1489–93.
11. Manji HK, Bowden CL, Belmaker RH. *Bipolar Medications: Mechanisms of Action*. Washington, DC: American Psychiatric Press; 2008.
12. Oldham WM, Hamm HE. Heterotrimeric G protein activation by G-protein-coupled receptors. *Nat Rev Mol Cell Biol*. 2008;9:60–71.
13. Manji HK, Bitran JA, Masana MI, *et al*. Signal transduction modulation by lithium: cell culture, cerebral microdialysis and human studies. *Psychopharmacol Bull*. 1991;27:199–208.

14. Avissar S, Schreiber G. The involvement of G proteins and regulators of receptor–G protein coupling in the pathophysiology, diagnosis and treatment of mood disorders. *Clin Chim Acta*. 2006;366:37–47.

15. Hahn C-G, Umapathy, Wang H-Y, Koneru R, Levinson DF, Friedman E. Lithium and valproic acid treatments reduce PKC activation and receptor-G protein coupling in platelets of bipolar manic patients. *J Psychiatr Res*. 2005;39:355–63.

16. Risby ED, Hsiao JK, Manji HK, *et al*. The mechanisms of action of lithium. II. Effects on adenylate cyclase activity and beta-adrenergic receptor binding in normal subjects. *Arch Gen Psychiatry*. 1991;48:513–24.

17. Mann L, Heldman E, Shaltiel G, Belmaker RH, Agam G. Lithium preferentially inhibits adenylyl cyclase V and VII isoforms. *Int J Neuropsychopharmacol*. 2008;11:533–9.

18. Mørk A, Geisler A. Effects of GTP on hormone-stimulated adenylate cyclase activity in cerebral cortex, striatum, and hippocampus from rats treated chronically with lithium. *Biol Psychiatry*. 1989;26:279–88.

19. Shtein L, Toker L, Bersudsky Y, Belmaker RH, Agam G. The inositol monophosphatase inhibitor L-690,330 affects pilocarpine-behavior and the forced swim test. *Psychopharmacology (Berl)*. 2013;227:503–8.

20. Allison JH, Stewart MA. Reduced brain inositol in lithium-treated rats. *Nature New Biol*. 1971;233:267–8.

21. Allison JH, Blisner ME, Holland WH, Hipps PP, Sherman WR. Increased brain myo-inositol 1-phosphate in lithium-treated rats. *Biochem Biophys Res Commun*. 1976;71:664–70.

22. Hallcher LM, Sherman WR. The effects of lithium ion and other agents on the activity of myo-inositol-1-phosphatase from bovine brain. *J Biol Chem*. 1980;255:10896–901.

23. Berridge MJ, Downes CP, Hanley MR. Lithium amplifies agonist-dependent phosphatidylinositol responses in brain and salivary glands. *Biochem J*. 1982;206:587–95.

24. Berridge MJ, Downes CP, Hanley MR. Neural and developmental actions of lithium: a unifying hypothesis. *Cell*. 1989;59:411–19.

25. Williams RSB, Cheng L, Mudge AW, Harwood AJ. A common mechanism of action for three mood-stabilizing drugs. *Nature*. 2002;417:292–5.

26. Harwood AJ, Agam G. Search for a common mechanism of mood stabilizers. *Biochem Pharmacol*. 2003;66:179–89.

27. Shimon H, Agam G, Belmaker RH, Hyde TM, Kleinman JE. Reduced frontal cortex inositol levels in postmortem brain of suicide victims and patients with bipolar disorder. *Am J Psychiatry*. 1997;154:1148–50.

28. Silverstone PH, McGrath BM, Kim H. Bipolar disorder and myo-inositol: a review of the magnetic resonance spectroscopy findings. *Bipolar Disord*. 2005;71–10.

29. Soares JC, Chen G, Dippold CS, *et al*. Concurrent measures of protein kinase C and phosphoinositides in lithium-treated bipolar patients and healthy individuals: a preliminary study. *Psychiatry Res*. 2000;95:109–18.

30. Sjøholt G, Gulbrandsen AK, Løvlie R, Berle JO, Molven A, Steen VM. A human myo-inositol monophosphatase gene (*IMPA2*) localized in a putative susceptibility region for bipolar disorder on chromosome 18p11.2: genomic structure and polymorphism screening in manic-depressive patients. *Mol Psychiatry*. 2000;5:172–80.

31. Atack JR. Inositol monophosphatase inhibitors--lithium mimetics? *Med Res Rev*. 1997;17:215–24.

32. Fauroux CMJ, Freeman S. Inhibitors of inositol monophosphatase. *J Enzym Inhib*. 1999;14:97–108.

33. Singh N, Halliday AC, Thomas JM, *et al*. A safe lithium mimetic for bipolar disorder. *Nat Commun*. 2013;4:1332.

34. Singh N, Sharpley AL, Emir UE, *et al*. Effect of the putative lithium mimetic ebselen on brain myo-inositol, sleep, and emotional processing in humans. *Neuropsychopharmacology*. 2016;41:1768–78.

35. Nosengo N. Can you teach old drugs new tricks? *Nature*. 2016;534:314.

36. Parnham MJ, Sies H. The early research and development of ebselen. *Biochem Pharmacol*. 2013;86:1248–53.

37. Atack JR, Prior AM, Fletcher SR, Quirk K, McKernan R, Ragan CI. Effects of L-690,488, a prodrug of the bisphosphonate inositol monophosphatase inhibitor L-690,330, on phosphatidylinositol cycle markers. *J Pharmacol Exp Ther*. 1994;270:70–6.

38. Masaki C, Sharpley AL, Cooper CM, *et al*. Effects of the potential lithium-mimetic, ebselen, on impulsivity and emotional processing. *Psychopharmacology (Berl)*. 2016;233:2655–61.

39. Manji HK, Lenox RH. Protein kinase C signaling in the brain: molecular transduction of mood stabilization in the treatment of manic-depressive illness. *Biol Psychiatry*. 1999;46:1328–51.

40. Bitran JA, Manji HK, Potter WZ, Gusovsky F. Down-regulation of PKC alpha by lithium in vitro. *Psychopharmacol Bull*. 1995;31:449–52.

41. Wang H-Y, Markowitz P, Levinson D, Undie AS, Friedman E. Increased membrane-associated protein kinase C activity and translocation in blood platelets from bipolar affective disorder patients. *J Psychiatr Res*. 1999;33:171–9.

42. Wang HY, Friedman E. Enhanced protein kinase C activity and translocation in bipolar affective disorder brains. *Biol Psychiatry*. 1996;40:568–75.

43. Amrollahi Z, Rezaei F, Salehi B, *et al*. Double-blind, randomized, placebo-controlled 6-week study on the efficacy and safety of the tamoxifen adjunctive to lithium in acute bipolar mania. *J Affect Disord*. 2011;129(1–3):327–31.

44. Manji HK, Chen G. PKC, MAP kinases and the bcl-2 family of proteins as long-term targets for mood stabilizers. *Mol Psychiatry*. 2002;7 Suppl 1:S46–56.

45. Baum AE, Akula N, Cabanero M, *et al*. A genome-wide association study implicates diacylglycerol kinase eta (*DGKH*) and several other genes in the etiology of bipolar disorder. *Mol Psychiatry*. 2008;13:197–207.

46. Sakane F, Mizuno S, Komenoi S. Diacylglycerol kinases as emerging potential drug targets for a variety of diseases: an update. *Front Cell Dev Biol*. 2016;4:82.

47. Klein PS, Melton DA. A molecular mechanism for the effect of lithium on development. *Proc Natl Acad Sci U S A*. 1996;93:8455–9.

48. Zhang F, Phiel CJ, Spece L, Gurvich N, Klein PS. Inhibitory phosphorylation of glycogen synthase kinase-3 (GSK-3) in response to lithium. Evidence for autoregulation of GSK-3. *J Biol Chem*. 2003;278:33067–77.

49. Gould TD, Quiroz JA, Singh J, Zarate CA, Manji HK. Emerging experimental therapeutics for bipolar disorder: insights from the molecular and cellular actions of current mood stabilizers. *Mol Psychiatry*. 2004;9:734–55.

50. Frame S, Cohen P. GSK3 takes centre stage more than 20 years after its discovery. *Biochem J*. 2001;359(Pt 1):1–16.

51. Berridge M. Cell Signalling Pathways. *Cell Signal Biol*. 2014;2014:1–138.

52. Berridge MJ. Calcium signalling and psychiatric disease: bipolar disorder and schizophrenia. *Cell Tissue Res*. 2014;357:477–92.

53. Berridge MJ. The inositol triphosphate/calcium signaling pathway in health and disease. *Physiol Rev*. 2016;96:1261–96.

54. Cipriani A, Saunders K, Attenburrow M-J, *et al.* A systematic review of calcium channel antagonists in bipolar disorder and some considerations for their future development. *Mol Psychiatry.* 2016;21:1324–32.

55. Warsh JJ, Andreopoulos S, Li PP. Role of intracellular calcium signaling in the pathophysiology and pharmacotherapy of bipolar disorder: current status. *Clin Neurosci Res.* 2004;4(3–4):201–13.

56. Dubovsky SL, Thomas M, Hijazi A, Murphy J. Intracellular calcium signalling in peripheral cells of patients with bipolar affective disorder. *Eur Arch Psychiatry Clin Neurosci.* 1994;243:229–34.

57. El Khoury A, Petterson U, Kallner G, Åberg-Wistedt A, Stain-Malmgren R. Calcium homeostasis in long-term lithium-treated women with bipolar affective disorder. *Prog Neuropsychopharmacol Biol Psychiatry.* 2002;26:1063–9.

58. Mertens J, Wang Q-W, Kim Y, *et al.* Differential responses to lithium in hyperexcitable neurons from patients with bipolar disorder. *Nature.* 2015;527:95–9.

59. Chen HM, DeLong CJ, Bame M, *et al.* Transcripts involved in calcium signaling and telencephalic neuronal fate are altered in induced pluripotent stem cells from bipolar disorder patients. *Transl Psychiatry.* 2014;4:e375.

60. Cross-Disorder Group of the Psychiatric Genomics Consortium, Lee SH, Ripke S, Neale BM, *et al.* Genetic relationship between five psychiatric disorders estimated from genome-wide SNPs. *Nat Genet.* 2013;45:984–94.

61. Ferreira MAR, O'Donovan MC, Meng YA, *et al.* Collaborative genome-wide association analysis supports a role for ANK3 and CACNA1C in bipolar disorder. *Nat Genet.* 2008;40:1056–8.

62. Yoshimizu T, Pan JQ, Mungenast AE, *et al.* Functional implications of a psychiatric risk variant within CACNA1C in induced human neurons. *Mol Psychiatry.* 2015;20:162–9.

63. Moosmang S, Haider N, Klugbauer N, *et al.* Role of hippocampal Cav1.2 $Ca^{2+}$ channels in NMDA receptor-independent synaptic plasticity and spatial memory. *J Neurosci.* 2005;25:9883–92.

# 70

# Genetics of bipolar disorder

*Francis J. McMahon and Sevilla Detera-Wadleigh*

## Genetic epidemiology

The earliest studies of the genetic basis of bipolar disorder (BD) were based on families, twins, and adoptees and used epidemiologic methods to draw their conclusions (Fig. 70.1). These studies provided the first systematic evidence of a genetic basis for BD, setting the stage for the molecular genetic studies of recent years.

### Family studies

The tendency of illnesses to run in families is one of the most obvious observations giving rise to genetic hypotheses. Familial transmission of BD was reported long before modern concepts of the illness [1, 2] were widely adopted. In one of the earliest systematic family studies, Slater [3] described rates of 'manic–depressive' disorder among the parents and children of diagnosed patients that were remarkably close to the estimates of modern studies using criterion-based diagnoses and family study [4] or population-based methods [5].

Family studies may reveal patterns of transmission that can give clues about the nature of genetic influences. In segregation analysis, observed patterns of transmission in families are compared to patterns that would be expected under various inheritance models such as autosomal dominant or X-linked recessive. Many such studies were carried out for BD in the 1980s and 1990s (reviewed in [6]). While some studies reported transmission patterns that were most consistent with a single major (dominant) gene, most could not confidently reject more complex, multifactorial models. Such inconsistency probably reflects what we now know to be the considerable genetic heterogeneity that underlies BD.

Family studies have also been used to explore the range of phenotypes that cluster among close relatives. Such studies can give clues to the variable expressivity of shared genetic factors. Most family studies of BD have used a proband-wise, case-control approach, comparing the rates of various illnesses among the relatives of 'cases' diagnosed with BD vs relatives of psychiatrically healthy 'controls'. Results of the largest studies are reviewed in [6]. Most studies found that 10–15% of first-degree relatives of people diagnosed with bipolar I disorder met criteria for a major mood disorder themselves when directly interviewed, although the disorder could range from major depression to schizoaffective disorder. Increased rates of other disorders were also found, including alcoholism and anxiety disorders. Some studies also reported an increased rate of schizophrenia, but this was an inconsistent observation [4, 7, 8].

Some family studies have examined clinical features of BD or its associated neurocognitive traits. These studies have found that age at onset [9], psychotic features [10], frequency of episodes [11], polarity (manic or depressive) of the initial episode [12], suicidal behaviour [13], and response to lithium treatment [14] are all familial. Studies of neurocognitive traits have also reported a number of measures that are associated with BD in families [15]. Some traits, such as resting state EEG and deficits in facial recognition, also seem to occur in unaffected relatives, suggesting that they reflect a subthreshold liability distinct from recognized clinical manifestations of the illness [16, 17]. Daily activity patterns also seem to run in families and are associated with BD in some studies [18]. So far it has proven difficult to define robust subtypes of BD based on any of these traits, but this is an area of active investigation.

Population-based family studies have only become possible in recent years, thanks to universal health registries and electronic health records. Lichtenstein and colleagues have exploited the electronic records of the Swedish health system to link related individuals who received psychiatric diagnoses at multiple time points. These studies have shown results that largely agree with the proband-wise case-control studies, but with much larger sample sizes, reduced recall bias, and more complete ascertainment [5]. The results support the finding that schizophrenia is increased among the close relatives of individuals diagnosed with bipolar I disorder, but at less than half the rate of major mood disorders [19].

While they have provided some important clues to the familiality of BD, its complex mode of transmission, and its familial clustering with other diagnoses, family studies in themselves provide only weak evidence in support of genetic aetiology. Families share environments, life experiences, and habits that could easily contribute to illness, with no necessary contribution of genes per se. Other study designs are needed to dissociate the effects of genes and family environment.

### Twin studies

Twin studies allow a more unbiased estimate of genetic influences, since they control for shared non-genetic influences that complicate the interpretation of family studies. Twin studies typically compare monozygotic (MZ or identical) twins—who inherit the same

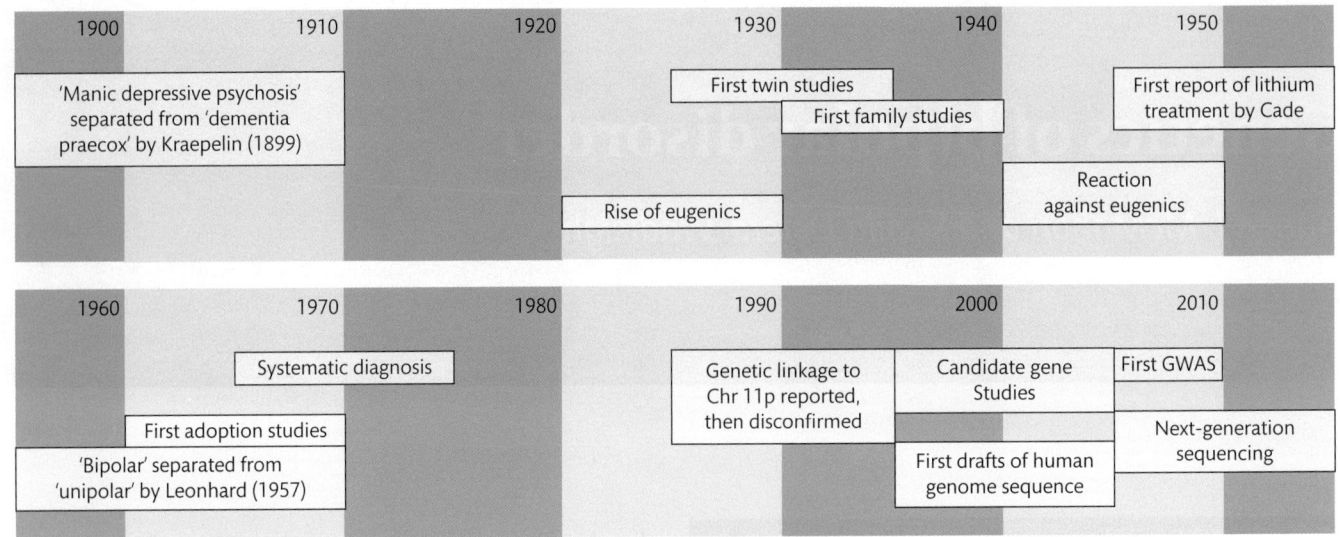

**Fig. 70.1** A timeline of bipolar disorder genetics discoveries over the past century, with a selection of key findings placed in approximate chronological order.

DNA—with dizygotic (DZ or non-identical) twins—who share, on average, half their DNA. Since both MZ and DZ twins are expected to experience the same family environment and similar early life experiences, non-genetic influences should be the same in both types of twins and traits influenced by inherited genetic factors should show more resemblance between MZ than DZ twins. Based on this principle, twin studies can estimate the fraction of trait variability that is attributable to genetic differences, a quantity known as heritability (for review, see [20]).

Twin studies have been conducted in BD since at least the 1930s. While methods of ascertainment, diagnosis, and statistics have changed substantially, heritability estimates have been remarkably consistent (reviewed in [6]). Most studies find that BD is 70–90% heritable. Such heritability estimates are among the highest of the major mental illnesses [21] and underscore the major role that inheritance plays in the aetiology of BD.

Twin studies have several limitations. Most importantly, they do not indicate which genes or how many different genes are involved. Even a highly heritable trait like BD seems to be influenced by numerous genes of small effect (see Polygenic models, p. 737). Twin studies may underestimate genetic influences when non-inherited sources of genetic variation, such as epigenetic marks and somatic mutation, play a major role. Twin studies may also overestimate heritability when the assumptions about shared environment are violated, when genetic and environmental influences are strongly correlated, or when ascertainment is biased or incomplete [22]. Despite these inherent limitations, the consistency in heritability estimates over many different studies and decades of investigation suggests any error should be modest.

### Adoption studies

Another approach to parsing the influence of genes and environment is the adoption study. Typically, adoption studies compare traits in the biological and adoptive parents of adoptees who manifest a trait of interest. This approach thus separates the effects of parental environment from those of inheritance, reducing or eliminating gene–environment correlations that can complicate the interpretation of twin studies [8]. Adoption studies cannot control for the effects of the intrauterine environment, which may play a role in some mental illnesses such as schizophrenia [23].

Three adoption studies of BD have been published [24–26]. Although they differed somewhat in methodology and had small sample sizes, all three studies found that rates of BD were increased in the biological parents of adoptees with BD, while no such increase was observed in their adoptive parents. These results support the view that inherited influences are most important in BD.

One population-based study linked electronic health records of adoptees with those of their biological and adoptive parents [19]. This study achieved a much larger sample size than the traditional adoption studies, although parents and adoptees with BD who did not seek treatment would be missed by this study design. The results again showed that rates of BD were elevated among the biological parents of adoptees diagnosed with BD.

### Assortative mating

Assortative mating describes mating patterns in a population that are non-random with regard to particular traits. For example, people tend to choose mates of similar height, education, and smoking habits. Assortative mating is important since it can concentrate genetic risk factors in certain families (while reducing them in others), increasing the risk or severity of illness in the offspring.

Assortative mating for mood disorders has long been observed in both clinical and epidemiological samples [27–29]. While such mating patterns could, in principle, reflect the influence of secondary factors associated with mood disorders (such as alcoholism), most studies have found that people often choose mates with similar (or identical) psychiatric diagnoses. A large electronic health record-based study in the Swedish population confirmed these findings and revealed strong patterns of assortative mating across a range of mental illnesses [30].

## Molecular genetics

### Genetic linkage in bipolar disorder

The ultimate goal of genetic linkage studies is to define genetic loci that underlie an inherited disorder. A considerable number of genetic linkage studies of BD were conducted between the 1980s and 1990s. To support this effort, collections of densely affected pedigrees and sib-pairs were assembled. The National Institute of Mental Health (NIMH) Genetics Initiative (https://explorer.nimhgenetics.org/subject-counts/explore/?c=bipolar-disorder), one of the largest efforts, established a resource of DNA, immortalized cell lines, and extensive clinical phenotype information from over 4000 individuals in 850 families. The DNA and associated source information are available to qualified researchers studying the genetics of mental disorders and other complex diseases at recognized biomedical research facilities.

Early linkage studies depended on phenotypic markers such as blood type or colour blindness (reviewed in [31]). Genetically mapped DNA markers, including restriction fragment length polymorphisms (RFLPs) [32] and highly informative short tandem repeat or microsatellite markers [33], were later developed.

An early study in an extended Old Order Amish pedigree reported linkage to a locus on chromosome 11 [34], but this finding was not supported in an independent set of pedigrees [35] and the original evidence for linkage was greatly diminished after a relative developed BD [36]. Linkage to chromosome 18 was also reported [37], with some support in an independent sample [38], but a causal gene was not identified.

In 1997, the NIMH Genetics Initiative published a genome-wide scan of 97 families with 540 individuals [39]. Non-parametric methods showed the strongest findings on chromosomes 1, 6, 7, 10, 16, and 22. To increase power, meta-analytic studies were performed that combined several different sets of pedigrees [40–42]. The results were stronger, but no more consistent.

Some studies sought to reduce genetic heterogeneity by focusing on clinical subtypes of BD. While most were unsuccessful, increased linkage signals were found for bipolar II disorder [43], BD with psychosis [10], age at onset [44], and polarity at onset [12]. These reports were not followed by clear replications, suggesting that the subtype strategy did not identify subsets of families that were substantially more homogenous.

### Candidate gene studies

For many years, candidate gene screening was pursued as an alternative to linkage studies. The aim was to determine whether genes postulated to serve important neuronal functions had a role in genetic predisposition to BD. The burgeoning list of potential candidate genes was presented previously [45]. So far, definitive evidence is lacking for the role of three of the most commonly investigated brain-expressed genes: brain-derived neurotrophic factor (*BDNF*), catecholamine-*O*-methyl transferase (*COMT*), and serotonin transporter (*SLC6A4*). Methodological limitations of the candidate gene strategy eventually led to its replacement by genome-wide association studies (GWAS) [46].

### Genome-wide association studies

#### Design and theory

GWAS were initially conceived as a way to overcome many of the problems inherent in candidate gene studies [47]. Initially a theoretical idea, GWAS soon became practical with the advent of microarrays. Thanks to this technology, it is now routine to genotype millions of common genetic variants (known as single nucleotide polymorphisms, or SNPs) in thousands of samples, at less than a penny per genotype. GWAS have represented a major breakthrough for BD (and hundreds of other common, complex traits), for the first time revealing robust biomarkers that point towards genes. GWAS have also revealed the hitherto underappreciated role of small chromosomal deletions and duplications (known as copy number variants, or CNVs) in risk for a range of neuropsychiatric disorders.

Since the typical GWAS assays thousands of independent SNPs, statistical testing needs to correct for the large number of hypotheses tested. This is typically accomplished by use of a Bonferroni-corrected significance threshold of $P < 5 \times 10^{-8}$. One consequence of this multiple testing problem is that GWAS need very large samples to achieve adequate statistical power. Thousands of cases and controls are typical; some studies use even more. Such sample sizes are difficult to achieve in a single collection, so many GWAS use meta-analysis methods to combine the results of different collections. This calls for sophisticated detection and correction of biases that can arise from even subtle differences in ancestry, genotyping platform, or other sample-specific sources.

GWAS are best powered for detecting association with common variants [48]. Such common variants typically confer only a slight increase in disease risk, since natural selection keeps higher-risk variants from rising to high frequencies under most circumstances [49]. The goal of GWAS is to detect genes involved in the trait of interest, but the genetic markers used in a GWAS do not unambiguously implicate particular genes and often fall within large stretches of DNA between genes. For a review of the experimental route from GWAS hit to disease gene, see [50].

### Results to date

The first GWAS of BD were published in 2007, with few genome-wide significant markers [51–53]. As samples have grown, findings have grown as well. To date, over 20 distinct genetic associations with BD have been detected at genome-wide significance (Fig. 70.2). Some of these have been replicated in at least one independent sample. This is perhaps the greatest advance of the GWAS method for psychiatry—identification of robust genetic markers for disorders that had hitherto defied genetic analysis. Given the steady pace of new findings—approximately one new genetic association for every 1000 cases of BD studied—it seems likely that GWAS will yield many additional associations as sample sizes increase [54].

As expected, all of the markers found so far are common and each confers a modest increased risk for illness (odds ratios <1.2). The associated SNPs lie near genes that encode signalling molecules, ion channels, neuronal growth factors, and other molecules [55], but as noted previously, firm experimental links between associated SNPs and particular genes remain to be established. Interestingly, many of the same genetic markers have been implicated by GWAS of schizophrenia, supporting the view that BD and schizophrenia share some genetic risk factors [5, 56].

### Polygenic models

The large number of associated markers and low risk conferred by each marker have led to intensive investigation of the ways in which markers found by GWAS may act together to influence risk in each individual case. Early expectations of multiplicative

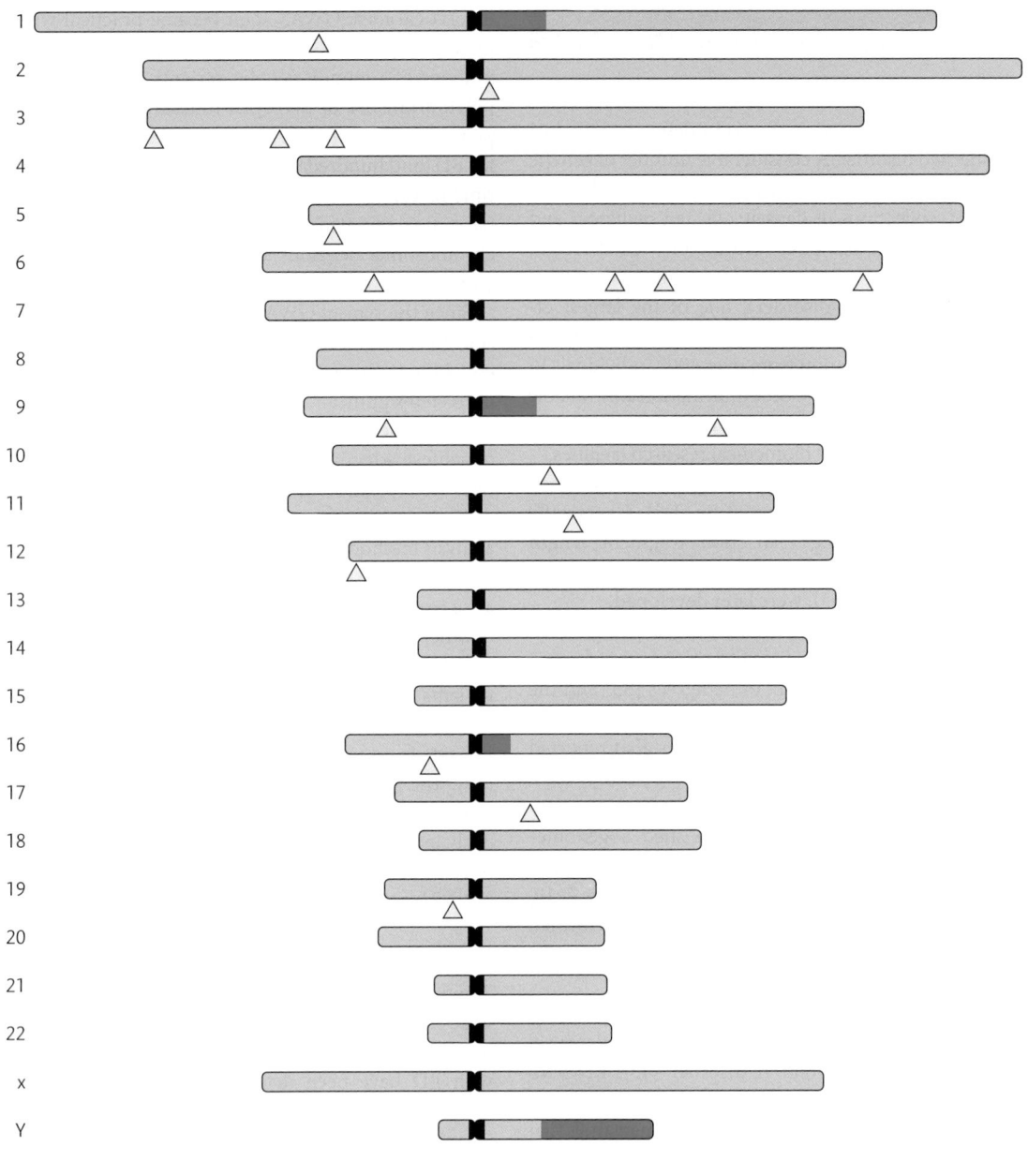

△ BP GWAS hits Dec 2016

**Fig. 70.2** Significant associations with bipolar disorder from genome-wide association studies published through December 2016.
Source: data from NHGRI-EBI GWAS Catalog; graphic generated with NCBI Genome Decoration Page.

effects—where the risk conferred by a set of distinct markers is greater than the sum of each individual marker—have been largely unfulfilled. Instead, it appears that common risk variants add together to confer risk, in much the same way as predicted by classic polygenic models [57].

A landmark study [56], published in 2009, offered one way to assess the effects of many markers of small effect. By assigning each allele a weight, based on its association odds ratio, that study showed that it is possible to estimate the total risk of illness conferred by the full set of alleles carried by each individual. Known as the polygenic risk score, this estimate has proven to be useful to gauge the impact of common risk variation across studies and traits. Since it does not seek to implicate any one particular marker, the polygenic risk score

can use information from markers that have not yet been implicated at the stringent genome-wide significance threshold.

The polygenic risk score approach shows that common variants can account for approximately 5% of the variance in risk for BD [58]. The remaining risk remains unexplained, leading to what has come to be known throughout the GWAS literature as the 'missing heritability' problem [59]. As sample sizes grow, we expect that the proportion of risk that can be explained by common variants will grow but will probably remain below the inherited genetic risk estimated by twin studies. This is one of the rationales for studies of rare variation, discussed later in this chapter.

The polygenic risk score approach has also shown that most of the common genetic risk for BD overlaps with that seen in schizophrenia and—to a lesser extent—major depression [58]. This important finding is again consistent with the idea that the major mood and psychotic disorders share many common genetic risk factors.

## SNP heritability

Since they sample genetic variation across the entire genome, SNPs can also be used to estimate distant relatedness between individuals. This fact can be harnessed to estimate heritability without some of the limitations and challenges inherent in traditional twin studies. This has come to be known as the 'SNP heritability' [60].

Several SNP heritability studies have been published. Heritability estimates have generally been far below those of twin studies. SNP heritability estimates for BD are typically in the range of 30–40%, less than half the heritability estimated from twin studies [61]. Additional research is needed to understand the sources of this large difference in heritability estimates.

## Copy number variants

As high-resolution studies of human chromosomes became feasible in recent years, it became clear that SNPs were not the only kind of variation in the human genome. Copy number variants, or CNVs, are small chromosomal segments that are deleted or duplicated across individuals in the population [62]. Individually rare, CNVs that may span several genes are, as a group, quite common in the human genome. Some of these CNVs play a role in human disease. For reasons not yet fully understood, CNVs seem to play an especially important role in diseases of the central nervous system, such as intellectual disability, autism, and schizophrenia, where they can contribute to over 5% of cases [63].

While it seems clear that CNVs do not play a major role in BD [64], several large studies have implicated particular CNVs in a range of psychiatric disorders, including BD [65, 66]. The clearest example is a duplication on chromosome 16p11.2 that spans about 650,000 base pairs of DNA and encodes a number of genes [67]. The 16p11.2 duplication is found in under 1% of people with BD but appears to confer a substantial risk of illness—about 10-fold—much higher than any other known single genetic event [65]. This same duplication also confers a high risk of schizophrenia and intellectual disability, so it cannot be considered a specific risk factor for BD. Further research is needed to understand how this CNV affects gene function and neurodevelopment and why it is such a potent risk factor for a range of neuropsychiatric disorders.

## Sequencing studies

Thanks to advances in sequencing technology, it is now possible to determine the precise nucleotide sequence of long stretches of DNA with great accuracy and relatively low cost. Sequencing can be performed at the level of individual genes, expressed sequences (known as the exome), or whole genomes, including long stretches of DNA that are coming to be understood as the major sites of gene expression regulation.

Since they do not rely on discreet genetic markers, sequencing studies can uncover the full range of genetic variation, both common and rare, that exists in the human genome. Large-scale studies have already demonstrated that each individual harbours numerous rare variants [68], including 1-3 that arose de novo as new mutations not present in either parent [69]. Variants within coding regions of genes may change amino acids, alter splice patterns, or shift the reading frame, leading to substantial differences in protein function, including complete loss of function.

Rare alleles could help explain the large portion of heritability apparently not explained by common variants [59]. This hope has fuelled a growing set of studies aimed at sequencing individuals with common neuropsychiatric disorders. Only a few large-scale sequencing studies have been performed so far in BD. Both case-control and family designs have been utilized [70–73]; one study has focused on de novo variants [74]. The results have been largely inconclusive, probably owing to the very large samples needed to establish unambiguous associations with rare variants [75]. As sample sizes grow, rare risk alleles may be found that will contribute to a more complete understanding of the full range of genetic variation underlying BD.

## Genetic modelling studies

### Animal models

Modelling psychiatric disorders in animals is challenging, since current psychiatric diagnosis is based on aspects of mood, cognition, and perception that are difficult to infer in animals. Despite this problem, certain behavioural phenotypes thought to model aspects of BD have been widely studied in rodents such as hyperactivity as a model for mania, and learned helplessness as a model for depression. Animal models offer many advantages such as rapid evaluation of therapeutic interventions, genetic engineering, and experimental control of environmental risk factors. Critical reviews on animal models for neuropsychiatric disorders [76], recurrent or bipolar depression [77], and bipolar mania [78] have been presented recently.

General approaches for creating animal models are typically based on genetics, pharmacology, environmental manipulation, or brain lesions [76]; each of these approaches has its own limitations. Evaluating the appropriateness of a model is fraught with many challenges. The latter review listed three types of validators: construct, face, and predictive validity. Criteria for construct validity could be met, for example, by knockout of a highly penetrant single gene, but such genes have not been identified in BD. Face validity depends on the extent to which the animal model displays biochemical, neuropathological, and behavioural properties analogous to those observed in human disease. Predictive validity can be claimed when the response to pharmacologic agents in the animal model predicts drug response in human patients.

Numerous attempts at modelling a specific phenotype relevant to BD have been published. Mania-like behaviour in animals has been induced through administration of psychostimulants such as amphetamine, oubain, or quinpirole [76, 78]. In these animals, hyperactivity has been shown to be diminished by mood-stabilizing agents such as lithium or valproate. A review of studies modelling mania in mice through genetic manipulations has been presented recently [78]. Expression profiling of genes changed under mania-like conditions and during subsequent behavioural rescue with drugs could reveal perturbed pathways that may have a role in pathophysiology.

Some examples illustrate the strengths and weaknesses of this strategy. GSK-3β is a well-established target of lithium via the Wnt signalling pathway. Overexpression of GSK-3β in mice induces hyperactivity, lower food intake, and other behavioural abnormalities broadly resembling mania in humans (reviewed in [78]). The *Clock*Δ19 mutant mouse, which could model some of the circadian rhythm disturbances in BD, exhibits various mania-like behaviours that can be normalized by chronic lithium treatment (reviewed in [78]). Knockdown or heterozygous disruption of exon 1b in the gene *ANK3*, which has been implicated in BD by GWAS, provokes mania-like behaviour in mice that can be reversed by lithium (reviewed in [78]). The function of genes implicated in BD is perturbed in each of these models, thus providing support for an impact of these individual genes on behaviour, as well as an experimental system in which mechanisms can be investigated. However, such models cannot capture the additive effects of multiple common variants in several genes, even though this is currently the most widely accepted genetic architecture for BD and other mental illnesses.

Animal models that might recapitulate both mania and depressive-like behaviours could meet requirements of construct, face, and predictive validity. Two such mouse models have been developed and studied—the Black Swiss mouse, which was generated by crossing outbred Swiss mice with the inbred strain C57BL6/JN, and the Madison mouse [78]. Lithium treatment reverses some of the mania-like phenotypes in both of these models, suggesting they may be exploited to screen new compounds for lithium-like effects.

Several mouse models of depression have been developed. Most are built on the learned helplessness construct [79], such as the forced swim test and the tail suspension test (reviewed in [77]). Historically, these models have played a valuable role in the discovery of antidepressants [80], which are often prescribed for people with BD, but the heuristic value of the learned helplessness construct has been questioned in recent years as the pace of discovering new antidepressants has slowed [81].

### Cellular models

Various cells, including lymphoblastoid cell lines, fibroblasts, and immortalized neuronal cells, have been used to examine diverse aspects relevant to BD. In this section, we will focus our discussion on induced pluripotent stem cells (iPSCs). The development of iPSC technology through the Nobel Prize-winning work of Yamanaka [82, 83] has provided the unprecedented power to study previously inaccessible live human tissues by reprogramming an individual's adult somatic cells to stem cells. iPSCs could then be differentiated into cells of interest, including neural progenitor cells, astrocytes, and neurons that could be targeted for various studies. iPSCs and their derivatives provide a person-specific cellular template to pursue functional, drug response, drug discovery, and toxicology studies. In contrast to animal models, studies on iPSC derivatives would deliver data on cells that carry the genetic background of the patient or that of the person under study. In addition, dish-derived stem cells could be tapped for further investigations *in vivo*, for example in mouse models, to either cause or rescue an abnormal phenotype.

To help assemble, characterize, generate, store, distribute, and promote expansion of the iPSC collection, the NIMH Repository and Genomics Resource (NIMH-RGR) (https://www.nimhgenetics.org/stem_cells/) established the NIMH Stem Cell Center to act as a repository for stem cells for neuropsychiatric disorders, assuring the research community of the availability of study samples.

Disease modelling in iPSC and iPSC derivatives in neurologic, neurodevelopmental, and neuropsychiatric disorders was recently reviewed [84]. The ability to transform stem cells into various neuronal derivatives permits the comparative analysis of transcriptome, proteome, and epigenetic patterns at each stage of differentiation of cells that originate from affected and unaffected individuals. Integration of expression patterns with GWAS findings could strengthen support for loci and signalling pathways that contribute to disease risk. Cellular phenotypes revealed in the presence or absence of various pharmacologic or environmental agents, that could distinguish patients from controls, could be harnessed to develop functional assays and lead to the discovery of candidate therapeutic compounds. Production of isogenic lines using genome-editing methods, such as CRISPR-Cas9, might reduce the requirement for large sample sizes; however, the lack of a penetrant major effect mutation in BD presents a key impediment for such an approach.

Several studies on iPSC neuronal derivatives in BD have claimed phenotype differences between cells derived from people with BD and those from healthy controls [85–87]. Each study focused on different cellular phenotypes in small samples, highlighting the need for higher-throughput, standardized measures that can be carried out and tested for replication in larger samples. If consistent cellular phenotypes can be identified, they could serve as a basis for many important studies such as screening for novel therapeutic compounds.

## Future directions

One of the important near-term tasks is to establish firm links between common variants identified by GWAS and specific genes. This task has become more tractable, as we learn more about the mechanisms of gene regulation [88]. At the same time, the task has also grown more complex. It is becoming increasingly clear that physical proximity is a poor indicator of which SNPs regulate which genes [89], that each SNP may regulate many different genes, and that the relationship between SNPs and the genes they regulate may vary by cell type and developmental stage. The identification of specific genes is important if we are to succeed in extracting insight from GWAS into the biological basis of BD.

In addition to those genes implicated by GWAS, many other genes may harbour rare variants that contribute to BD. While more difficult to achieve, firm rare variant associations may be particularly informative since they may be more easily linked to specific genes and often confer much larger risk than common variants.

The field of complex genetic disorders still lacks a unified framework that can fully encompass both common and rare genetic variants. How can both forms of variation be used to develop a more complete account of the inherited risk of BD? Are certain kinds of variants specific to BD, or are they all shared to some extent with other major mental illnesses such as schizophrenia or major depression? How can genetic variation be leveraged to improve and refine our diagnostic categories?

While it is clear that disease modelling using animal or cellular models cannot recapitulate, in its entirety, the complexity of BD, these models can illuminate certain aspects of pathophysiology. Recent developments in the generation of three-dimensional cultures and brain organoids [90] may lead to the creation of more physiologically meaningful models. Engrafting patient iPSC-derived neurons into rat brain could disclose impairments in connectivity and axonal transport that might be operative in neuropsychiatric disorders [91].

The potential role of glial cells may be revealed by tools such as chimeric mice whose native glia are replaced by human-derived cells [92, 93]. These advances and others that are being developed, such as optical electrophysiology [94], could help spur improvements in disease modelling and assay development that will form the basis for high-throughput therapeutic screening and the identification of novel drug treatments for BD.

As we move towards the identification of genetic variants that, taken together, confer substantial risk for BD, we will also have the opportunity to investigate more powerfully the role of non-genetic risk factors. By contrasting the life histories of individuals at high genetic risk who do or do not develop BD, we may finally be able to define specific non-genetic events that contribute to risk for bipolar illness. This could ultimately lead to preventive approaches, based on risk factors that are more easily modifiable than inherited genetic variants.

## Conclusions

The last century has seen enormous progress in our understanding of the genetic basis of BD. From early studies aimed at assessing the overall contribution of genes to the obvious familial clustering of BD, we have now progressed to the point where we have reliably identified dozens of common genetic markers for this common disorder. Complex inheritance patterns, substantial genetic heterogeneity, and considerable genetic overlap with other major mental illnesses remain as real barriers to a complete genetic account of individual risk. Much still needs to be done to translate the great progress in genetic research into biological insights that can inform an understanding of the causes, treatment, and prevention of BD.

## Acknowledgements

Supported by the Intramural Research Program of the National Institute of Mental Health.

We thank Christopher Song for production assistance.

## REFERENCES

1. Kraepelin E. Manic depressive insanity and paranoia. *J Nerv Ment Dis*. 1921;53:350.
2. Leonhard K. *Aufteilung der endogen Psychosen*. Akademie Verlag, Berlin; 1957.
3. Slater E. The Inheritance of manic-depressive insanity (Section of Psychiatry). *Proc R Soc Med*. 1936;29:981.
4. Gershon ES, Hamovit J, Guroff JJ, et al. A family study of schizoaffective, bipolar I, bipolar II, unipolar, and normal control probands. *Arch Gen Psychiatry*. 1982;39:1157–67.
5. Lichtenstein P, Yip BH, Björk C, et al. Common genetic determinants of schizophrenia and bipolar disorder in Swedish families: a population-based study. *Lancet*. 2009;373:234–39.
6. Tsuang MT, Faraone SV. *The Genetics of Mood Disorders*. Johns Hopkins University Press, Baltimore, MD; 1990. http://psycnet.apa.org/psycinfo/1990-97997-000
7. Helzer JE, Winokur G. A family interview study of male manic depressives. *Arch Gen Psychiatry*. 1974;31:73–7.
8. Smoller JW, Finn CT. Family, twin, and adoption studies of bipolar disorder. *Am J Med Genet C Semin Med Gen*. 2003;123C:48–58.
9. Schulze TG, Hedeker D, Zandi P, Rietschel M, McMahon FJ. What is familial about familial bipolar disorder? Resemblance among relatives across a broad spectrum of phenotypic characteristics. *Arch Gen Psychiatry*. 2006;63:1368–76.
10. Potash JB, Chiu Y-F, MacKinnon DF, et al. Familial aggregation of psychotic symptoms in a replication set of 69 bipolar disorder pedigrees. *Am J Med Genet B Neuropsychiatr Genet*. 2003;116B:90–7.
11. Fisfalen ME, Schulze TG, DePaulo JRJ, DeGroot LJ, Badner JA, McMahon FJ. Familial variation in episode frequency in bipolar affective disorder. *Am J Psychiatry*. 2005;162:1266–72.
12. Kassem L, Lopez V, Hedeker D, Steele J, Zandi P, McMahon FJ. Familiality of polarity at illness onset in bipolar affective disorder. *Am J Psychiatry*. 2006;163:1754–9.
13. Egeland JA, Sussex JN. Suicide and family loading for affective disorders. *JAMA*. 1985;254:915–18.
14. Grof P, Duffy A, Alda M, Hajek T. Lithium response across generations. *Acta Psychiatr Scand*. 2009;120:378–85.
15. Fears SC, Service SK, Kremeyer B, et al. Multisystem component phenotypes of bipolar disorder for genetic investigations of extended pedigrees. *JAMA Psychiatry*. 2014;71:375–87.
16. Flint J, Timpson N, Munafò M. Assessing the utility of intermediate phenotypes for genetic mapping of psychiatric disease. *Trends Neurosci*. 2014;37:733–41.
17. Meda SA, Ruano G, Windemuth A, et al. Multivariate analysis reveals genetic associations of the resting default mode network in psychotic bipolar disorder and schizophrenia. *Proc Natl Acad Sci U S A*. 2014;111:E2066–75.
18. Pagani L, Clair PAS, Teshiba TM, et al. Genetic contributions to circadian activity rhythm and sleep pattern phenotypes in pedigrees segregating for severe bipolar disorder. *Proc Natl Acad Sci U S A*. 2016;113:E754–61.
19. Song J, Bergen SE, Kuja-Halkola R, Larsson H, Landén M, Lichtenstein P. Bipolar disorder and its relation to major psychiatric disorders: a family-based study in the Swedish population. *Bipolar Disord*. 2015;17:184–93.
20. Visscher PM, Hill WG, Wray NR. Heritability in the genomics era—concepts and misconceptions. *Nat Rev Genet*. 2008;9:255–66.
21. Polderman TJC, Benyamin B, de Leeuw CA, et al. Meta-analysis of the heritability of human traits based on fifty years of twin studies. *Nat Genet*. 2015;47:702–9.
22. Zuk O, Hechter E, Sunyaev SR, Lander ES. The mystery of missing heritability: Genetic interactions create phantom heritability. *Proc Natl Acad Sci U S A*. 2012;109:1193–8.
23. Susser ES, Lin SP. Schizophrenia after prenatal exposure to the Dutch Hunger Winter of 1944–1945. *Arch Gen Psychiatry*. 1992;49:983–8.
24. Mendlewicz J, Rainer JD. Adoption study supporting genetic transmission in manic depressive illness. *Nature*. 1977;268:327–9.
25. Wender PH, Kety SS, Rosenthal D, Schulsinger F, Ortmann J, Lunde I. Psychiatric disorders in the biological and adoptive families of adopted individuals with affective disorders. *Arch Gen Psychiatry*. 1986;43:923–9.
26. Cadoret RJ. Evidence for genetic inheritance of primary affective disorder in adoptees. *Am J Psychiatry*. 1978;135:463–6.
27. Baron M, Mendlewicz J, Gruen R, Asnis L, Fieve RR. Assortative mating in affective disorders. *J Affect Disord*. 1981;3:167–71.

28. Dunner DL, Fleiss JL, Addonizio G, Fieve RR. Assortative mating in primary affective disorder. *Biol Psychiatry*. 1976;11:43–51.

29. Gershon ES, Dunner DL, Sturt L, Goodwin FK. Assortative mating in the affective disorders. *Biol Psychiatry*. 1973;7:63–74.

30. Nordsletten AE, Larsson H, Crowley JJ, Almqvist C, Lichtenstein P, Mataix-Cols D. Patterns of nonrandom mating within and across 11 major psychiatric disorders. *JAMA Psychiatry*. 2016;73:354–61.

31. Reich T, Clayton PJ, Winokur G. Family history studies: V. The genetics of mania. *Am J Psychiatry*. 1969;125:1358–69.

32. Botstein D, White RL, Skolnick M, Davis RW. Construction of a genetic linkage map in man using restriction fragment length polymorphisms. *Am J Hum Genet*. 1980;32:314–31.

33. Weber JL. Human DNA polymorphisms and methods of analysis. *Curr Opin Biotechnol*. 1990;1:166–71.

34. Egeland JA, Gerhard DS, Pauls DL, et al. Bipolar affective disorders linked to DNA markers on chromosome 11. *Nature*. 1987;325:783–7.

35. Detera-Wadleigh SD, Berrettini WH, Goldin LR, Boorman D, Anderson S, Gershon ES. Close linkage of c-Harvey-ras-1 and the insulin gene to affective disorder is ruled out in three North American pedigrees. *Nature*. 1987;325:806–8.

36. Kelsoe JR. Re-evaluation of the linkage relationship between chromosome 11 p loci and the gene for bipolar affective disorder in the Old Order Amish. *Nature*. 1989;342:238–43.

37. Berrettini WH, Ferraro TN, Goldin LR, et al. Chromosome 18 DNA markers and manic-depressive illness: evidence for a susceptibility gene. *Proc Natl Acad Sci U S A*. 1994;91:5918–21.

38. Stine OC, Xu J, Koskela R, et al. Evidence for linkage of bipolar disorder to chromosome 18 with a parent-of-origin effect. *Am J Hum Genet*. 1995;57:1384–94.

39. Nurnberger JI, DePaulo JR, Gershon ES, et al. Genomic survey of bipolar illness in the NIMH genetics initiative pedigrees: a preliminary report. *Am J Med Genet*. 1997;74:227–37.

40. Badner JA, Gershon ES. Meta-analysis of whole-genome linkage scans of bipolar disorder and schizophrenia. *Mol Psychiatry*. 2002;7:405–11.

41. McQueen MB, Devlin B, Faraone SV, et al. Combined analysis from eleven linkage studies of bipolar disorder provides strong evidence of susceptibility loci on chromosomes 6q and 8q. *Am J Hum Genet*. 2005;77:582–95.

42. Segurado R, Detera-Wadleigh SD, Levinson DF, et al. Genome scan meta-analysis of schizophrenia and bipolar disorder, part III: bipolar disorder. *Am J Hum Genet*. 2003;73:49–62.

43. McMahon FJ, Simpson SG, McInnis MG, Badner JA, MacKinnon DF, DePaulo JR. Linkage of bipolar disorder to chromosome 18q and the validity of bipolar II disorder. *Arch Gen Psychiatry*. 2001;58:1025–31.

44. Faraone SV, Glatt SJ, Su J, Tsuang MT. Three potential susceptibility loci shown by a genome-wide scan for regions influencing the age at onset of mania. *Am J Psychiatry*. 2004;161:625–30.

45. Serretti A, Mandelli L. The genetics of bipolar disorder: genome 'hot regions,' genes, new potential candidates and future directions. *Mol Psychiatry*. 2008;13:742–71.

46. Risch N, Merikangas K. The future of genetic studies of complex human diseases. *Science*. 1996;273:1516–17.

47. Risch N, Merikangas K, others. The future of genetic studies of complex human diseases. *Science*. 1996;273:1516–17.

48. Sham PC, Purcell SM. Statistical power and significance testing in large-scale genetic studies. *Nat Rev Genet*. 2014;15:335–46.

49. Pritchard JK. Are rare variants responsible for susceptibility to complex diseases? *Am J Hum Genet*. 2001;69:124–37.

50. Gandal MJ, Leppa V, Won H, Parikshak NN, Geschwind DH. The road to precision psychiatry: translating genetics into disease mechanisms. *Nat Neurosci*. 2016;19:1397–407.

51. Baum AE, Akula N, Cabanero M, et al. A genome-wide association study implicates diacylglycerol kinase eta (*DGKH*) and several other genes in the etiology of bipolar disorder. *Mol Psychiatry*. 2008;13:197–207.

52. Ferreira MAR, O'Donovan MC, Meng YA, et al. Collaborative genome-wide association analysis supports a role for ANK3 and CACNA1C in bipolar disorder. *Nat Genet*. 2008;40:1056–8.

53. Burton PR, Clayton DG, Cardon LR, et al. Genome-wide association study of 14,000 cases of seven common diseases and 3,000 shared controls. *Nature*. 2007;447:661–78.

54. Sullivan PF. The psychiatric GWAS consortium: big science comes to psychiatry. *Neuron*. 2010;68:182–6.

55. Craddock N, Sklar P. Genetics of bipolar disorder. *Lancet*. 2013;381:1654–62.

56. Purcell SM, Wray NR, Stone JL, et al. Common polygenic variation contributes to risk of schizophrenia and bipolar disorder. *Nature*. 2009;460:748–52.

57. Falconer DS. The inheritance of liability to certain diseases, estimated from the incidence among relatives. *Ann Hum Genet*. 1965;29:51–76.

58. Wray NR, Lee SH, Mehta D, Vinkhuyzen AAE, Dudbridge F, Middeldorp CM. Research review: Polygenic methods and their application to psychiatric traits. *J Child Psychol Psychiatry*. 2014;55:1068–87.

59. Manolio TA, Collins FS, Cox NJ, et al. Finding the missing heritability of complex diseases. *Nature*. 2009;461:747–53.

60. Lee SH, Yang J, Chen G-B, et al. Estimation of SNP heritability from dense genotype data. *Am J Hum Genet*. 2013;93:1151–5.

61. Gratten J, Wray NR, Keller MC, Visscher PM. Large-scale genomics unveils the genetic architecture of psychiatric disorders. *Nat Neurosci*. 2014;17:782–90.

62. Malhotra D, Sebat J. CNVs: harbingers of a rare variant revolution in psychiatric genetics. *Cell*. 2012;148:1223–41.

63. Lupski JR. Brain copy number variants and neuropsychiatric traits. *Biol Psychiatry*. 2012;72:617–19.

64. Grozeva D, Kirov G, Ivanov D, et al. Rare copy number variants: a point of rarity in genetic risk for bipolar disorder and schizophrenia. *Arch Gen Psychiatry*. 2010;67:318–27.

65. Green EK, Rees E, Walters JTR, et al. Copy number variation in bipolar disorder. *Mol Psychiatry*. 2016;21:89–93.

66. Malhotra D, McCarthy S, Michaelson JJ, et al. High frequencies of de novo CNVs in bipolar disorder and schizophrenia. *Neuron*. 2011;72:951–63.

67. Heinzen EL, Radtke RA, Urban TJ, et al. Rare deletions at 16p13.11 predispose to a diverse spectrum of sporadic epilepsy syndromes. *Am J Hum Genet*. 2010;86:707–18.

68. Fu W, O'Connor TD, Jun G, et al. Analysis of 6,515 exomes reveals the recent origin of most human protein-coding variants. *Nature*. 2013;493:216–20.

69. Gratten J, Visscher PM, Mowry BJ, Wray NR. Interpreting the role of de novo protein-coding mutations in neuropsychiatric disease. *Nat Genet*. 2013;45:234–8.

70. Cruceanu C, Ambalavanan A, Spiegelman D, et al. Family-based exome-sequencing approach identifies rare susceptibility variants for lithium-responsive bipolar disorder. *Genome*. 2013;56:634–40.

71. Goes FS, Pirooznia M, Parla JS, et al. Exome sequencing of familial bipolar disorder. *JAMA Psychiatry*. 2016;73:590–7.

72. Ament SA, Szelinger S, Glusman G, *et al.* Rare variants in neuronal excitability genes influence risk for bipolar disorder. *Proc Natl Acad Sci U S A.* 2015;112:3576–81.

73. Yang S, Wang K, Gregory B, *et al.* Genomic landscape of a three-generation pedigree segregating affective disorder. *PLoS One.* 2009;4:e4474.

74. Kataoka M, Matoba N, Sawada T, *et al.* Exome sequencing for bipolar disorder points to roles of de novo loss-of-function and protein-altering mutations. *Mol Psychiatry.* 2016;21:885–93.

75. Zuk O, Schaffner SF, Samocha K, *et al.* Searching for missing heritability: designing rare variant association studies. *Proc Natl Acad Sci U S A.* 2014;111:E455–64.

76. Nestler EJ, Hyman SE. Animal models of neuropsychiatric disorders. *Nat Neurosci.* 2010;13:1161–9.

77. Kato T, Kasahara T, Kubota-Sakashita M, Kato TM, Nakajima K. Animal models of recurrent or bipolar depression. *Neuroscience.* 2016;321:189–96.

78. Logan RW, McClung CA. Animal models of bipolar mania: the past, present and future. *Neuroscience.* 2016;321:163–88.

79. Abramson LY, Seligman ME, Teasdale JD. Learned helplessness in humans: critique and reformulation. *J Abnorm Psychol.* 1978;87:49–74.

80. Porsolt RD, Anton G, Blavet N, Jalfre M. Behavioural despair in rats: a new model sensitive to antidepressant treatments. *Eur J Pharmacol.* 1978;47:379–91.

81. Yin X, Guven N, Dietis N. Stress-based animal models of depression: do we actually know what we are doing? *Brain Res.* 2016;1652:30–42.

82. Takahashi K, Yamanaka S. Induction of pluripotent stem cells from mouse embryonic and adult fibroblast cultures by defined factors. *Cell.* 2006;126:663–76.

83. Takahashi K, Tanabe K, Ohnuki M, *et al.* Induction of pluripotent stem cells from adult human fibroblasts by defined factors. *Cell.* 2007;131:861–72.

84. Karmacharya R, Haggarty SJ. Stem cell models of neuropsychiatric disorders. *Mol Cell Neurosci.* 2016;73:1–2.

85. Chen HM, DeLong CJ, Bame M, *et al.* Transcripts involved in calcium signaling and telencephalic neuronal fate are altered in induced pluripotent stem cells from bipolar disorder patients. *Transl Psychiatry.* 2014;4:e375.

86. Madison JM, Zhou F, Nigam A, *et al.* Characterization of bipolar disorder patient-specific induced pluripotent stem cells from a family reveals neurodevelopmental and mRNA expression abnormalities. *Mol Psychiatry.* 2015;20:703–17.

87. Mertens J, Wang Q-W, Kim Y, *et al.* Differential responses to lithium in hyperexcitable neurons from patients with bipolar disorder. *Nature.* 2015;527:95–9.

88. Akbarian S, Liu C, Knowles JA, *et al.* The PsychENCODE project. *Nat Neurosci.* 2015;18:1707–12.

89. Stranger BE, Montgomery SB, Dimas AS, *et al.* Patterns of cis regulatory variation in diverse human populations. *PLoS Genet.* 2012;8:e1002639.

90. Lancaster MA, Renner M, Martin C-A, *et al.* Cerebral organoids model human brain development and microcephaly. *Nature.* 2013;501:373–9.

91. Korecka JA, Levy S, Isacson O. *In vivo* modeling of neuronal function, axonal impairment and connectivity in neurodegenerative and neuropsychiatric disorders using induced pluripotent stem cells. *Mol Cell Neurosci.* 2016;73:3–12.

92. Benraiss A, Wang S, Herrlinger S, *et al.* Human glia can both induce and rescue aspects of disease phenotype in Huntington disease. *Nat Commun.* 2016;7:11758.

93. Goldman SA, Nedergaard M, Windrem MS. Modeling cognition and disease using human glial chimeric mice. *Glia.* 2015;63:1483–93.

94. Zhang H, Reichert E, Cohen AE. Optical electrophysiology for probing function and pharmacology of voltage-gated ion channels. *eLife.* 2016;5.

# 71

# Neuroimaging of bipolar disorder

*Mary L. Phillips and Wayne C. Drevets*

## Functional neuroimaging studies of bipolar disorder

### Abnormal activity in emotion processing and emotion regulation neural circuitry

Emotional over-reactivity and emotion dysregulation are key clinical features of bipolar disorder [1]. Given this, it is not surprising that the majority of functional neuroimaging studies in bipolar disorder examined functioning in neural circuitries supporting emotion processing and emotional regulation when participants performed emotion processing and emotional regulation tasks. These neural circuitries centre on the amygdala, a region important for emotion processing, threat, and salience perception [2], and prefrontal cortical regions important for emotion regulation. Emotion regulation has been subdivided into voluntary and automatic (implicit) subprocesses where different prefrontal cortical regions, including the orbitofrontal cortex, ventrolateral prefrontal cortex, dorsolateral prefrontal cortex, and medial prefrontal cortex (including the anterior cingulate cortex and mediodorsal prefrontal cortex), underlie these different subprocesses [3]. Here, a predominantly lateral prefrontal cortical system, centred on the dorsolateral prefrontal cortex and ventrolateral prefrontal cortex, is thought to be important for *voluntary* emotion regulation, while a medial prefrontal cortical system, including the orbitofrontal cortex, anterior cingulate cortical subregions (subgenual, pregenual, and dorsal subregions), mediodorsal prefrontal cortex, and also the hippocampus, is thought to be important for *automatic* emotion regulation [3] (Fig. 71.1a).

Earlier studies reported abnormally elevated amygdala activity to emotional stimuli, and abnormally reduced activity in lateral and medial prefrontal cortical regions supporting emotion regulation [3] in individuals with bipolar disorder. More recent studies focused on elucidating specific fronto-subcortical functional abnormalities in adults with bipolar disorder during emotion regulation and inhibitory control [4]. Specifically, these studies showed abnormally decreased inferior frontal cortical activity, especially in the ventrolateral prefrontal cortex, during different positive and negative emotion processing and emotion regulation tasks in adults with bipolar disorder, even across different mood states. Altered (including abnormally elevated and abnormally decreased) activity in the amygdala and other emotion regulation circuitry regions was also

demonstrated in adults with bipolar disorder in these studies (Table 71.1; Fig. 71.2).

### Abnormal activity in emotion processing circuitry to positive emotional stimuli

Other findings highlight abnormally elevated amygdala and striatal and medial prefrontal cortical activity to positive emotional stimuli in individuals with bipolar disorder (Table 71.1), with more recent studies demonstrating abnormally increased amygdala and medial prefrontal cortex activity [4] to emotional, especially happy, faces in adults with bipolar disorder. These findings may reflect a dysregulated amygdala response and an underlying attentional bias to positive emotional stimuli in individuals with bipolar disorder that predisposes to hypomania and mania.

### Abnormal functional connectivity in prefrontal cortical–amygdala circuitries important for emotion processing and regulation

Several studies reported abnormally increased positive functional connectivity (that is, positive coupling of changes in magnitude of activity over time) or abnormally reduced inverse functional connectivity (that is, negative coupling of changes in magnitude of activity over time) between the amygdala and the ventrolateral prefrontal cortex in individuals with bipolar disorder, compared with healthy individuals, during performance of emotion processing and emotion regulation tasks [5] (Table 71.1). For example, studies reported weaker inverse functional connectivity or abnormal positive functional connectivity between the ventrolateral prefrontal cortex and the amygdala in individuals with bipolar disorder, compared with healthy controls, during emotion regulation tasks. Interactions between the amygdala and the ventrolateral prefrontal cortex may also be influenced by different types of emotional stimuli in individuals with bipolar disorder, but not in healthy individuals.

Other studies focused on functional connectivity between the amygdala and the medial regions of the orbitofrontal cortex. Here, reduced functional connectivity between the medial orbitofrontal cortex and the amygdala has been reported in depressed individuals with bipolar disorder, relative to healthy individuals, in both hemispheres, and on the left relative to depressed individuals with major depressive disorder. Functional connectivity between the amygdala and other medial regions of the prefrontal cortex is also altered in

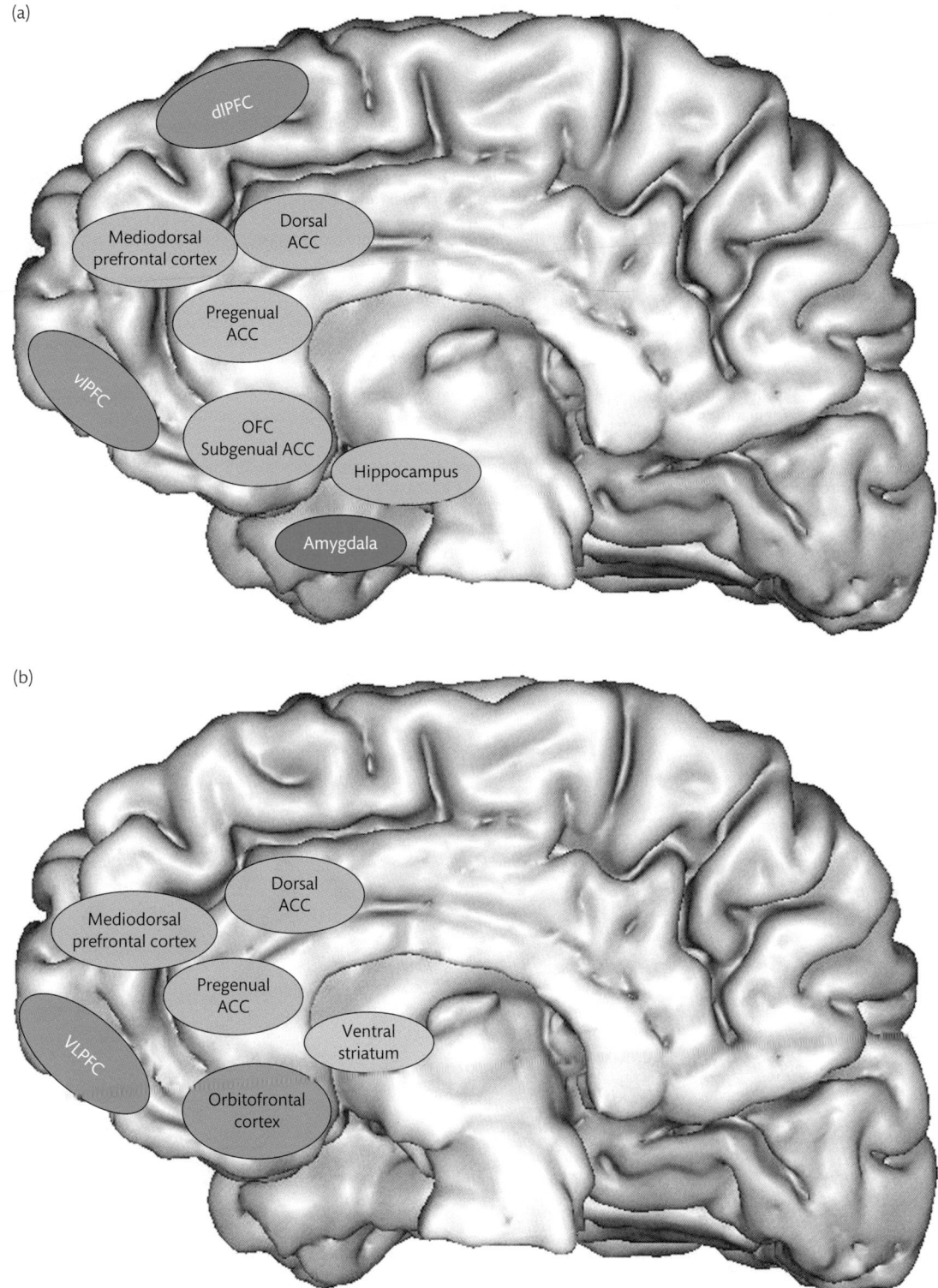

**Fig. 71.1** (a) Key nodes in emotion processing and emotion regulation and neural circuitries in healthy individuals. dlPFC, dorsolateral prefrontal cortex; vlPFC, ventrolateral prefrontal cortex; ACC, anterior cingulate cortex. Regions in blue are involved in voluntary emotion regulation processes. Regions in purple are involved in automatic emotion regulation processes. In red is the amygdala, a key node in emotion processing, threat, and salience perception.

(b) Key nodes in reward processing neural circuitry in healthy individuals. In orange is the ventral striatum, a key neural region involved in the orientation to reward cues and prediction error encoding. In red is the orbitofrontal cortex, a key neural region important for encoding the incentive value of stimuli. In purple are different medial prefrontal cortical regions, including different anterior cingulate cortical regions and mediodorsal prefrontal cortex, that are implicated in the regulation of appetitive behaviours and regulation of the ventral striatum in rewarding or potentially rewarding contexts. In blue is the ventrolateral prefrontal cortex, which, in rewarding contexts, links stimulus representations to reward outcomes and encodes the value of different decision-making options.

**Table 71.1** Main themes from functional neuroimaging studies in bipolar disorder

| | |
|---|---|
| Abnormal activity in emotion processing and emotion regulation neural circuitry | 1. Abnormally increased amygdala activity to emotional stimuli<br>2. Abnormally decreased ventrolateral prefrontal cortical activity during emotion processing, emotion regulation, and response inhibition |
| Abnormal activity in emotion processing circuitry to positive emotional stimuli | 1. Abnormally increased amygdala, striatal, and medial prefrontal cortical activity to positive emotional stimuli |
| Abnormal functional connectivity in prefrontal cortical–amygdala circuitries important for emotion processing and regulation | 1. Abnormally increased positive functional connectivity or abnormally reduced inverse functional connectivity between amygdala and ventrolateral prefrontal cortex during emotion processing and emotion regulation<br>2. Abnormally reduced or altered functional connectivity between medial orbitofrontal cortex and amygdala during emotion processing<br>3. Altered functional connectivity between ventrolateral prefrontal cortex and medial prefrontal cortex during task performance<br>4. Altered functional connectivity between dorsolateral prefrontal cortex and amygdala, and between dorsolateral prefrontal cortex, anterior cingulate cortex, and ventrolateral prefrontal cortex during emotion processing and emotion regulation |
| Abnormal activity and functional connectivity in emotion processing and emotion regulation neural circuitry during performance of non-emotional tasks | 1. Abnormally increased amygdala, medial prefrontal cortical, orbitofrontal cortical, and temporal cortical activity during non-emotional cognitive task performance |
| Abnormal activity and functional connectivity in reward processing neural circuitry | 1. Abnormally increased left ventrolateral prefrontal cortical activity and left orbitofrontal cortical activity during reward anticipation and receipt<br>2. Abnormally increased ventral striatal activity to reward anticipation and receipt in euthymic, but not in depressed, individuals with bipolar disorder<br>3. Abnormally reduced inverse functional connectivity between ventral striatum and medial prefrontal cortex |

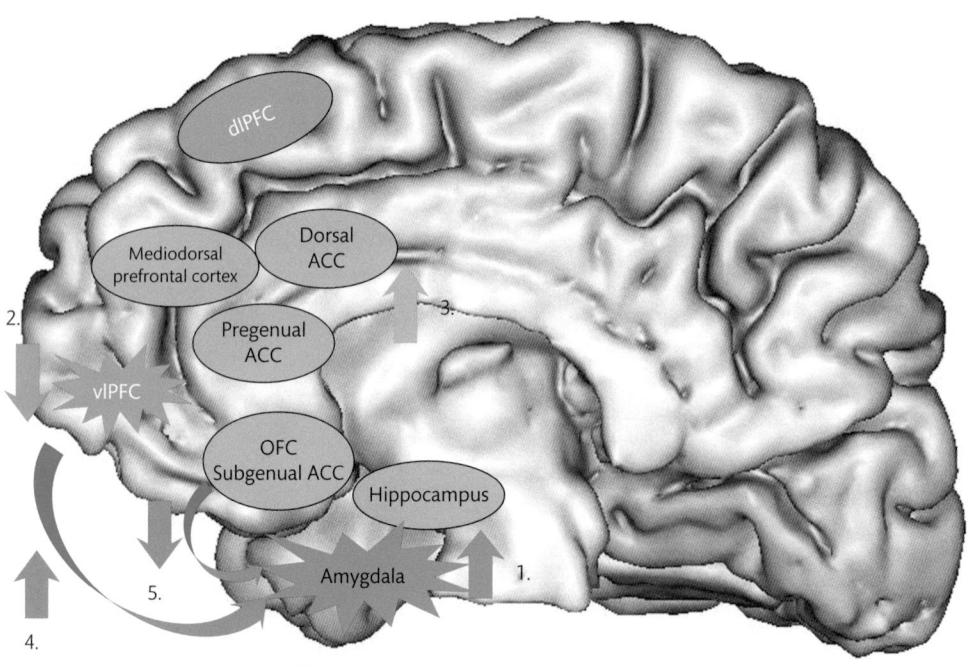

**Fig. 71.2** Key functional abnormalities in emotion regulation neural circuitry in individuals with bipolar disorder. The most consistent abnormalities include: 1. abnormally increased amygdala activity to emotional stimuli; 2. abnormally decreased ventrolateral prefrontal cortical activity during emotion processing, emotion regulation, and response inhibition; 3. abnormally increased amygdala and medial prefrontal cortical activity to positive emotional stimuli; 4. abnormally increased positive functional connectivity or abnormally reduced inverse functional connectivity between the amygdala and the ventrolateral prefrontal cortex during emotion processing and emotion regulation; and 5. abnormally reduced or altered functional connectivity between the medial orbitofrontal cortex and the amygdala during emotion processing. Star shapes refer to neural regions that are most consistently reported as being affected as described previously in bipolar disorder. In parallel, there are widespread abnormal decreases in grey matter volume and cortical thickness in prefrontal cortical regions, decreased grey matter volume in the amygdala and the hippocampus, and abnormally decreased fractional anisotropy in white matter tracts connecting the ventral prefrontal cortex and anterior temporal regions. There are also abnormalities of regional glucose metabolism and microglial activation in the same regions showing grey matter loss.

individuals with bipolar disorder during task performance, but without a clear direction of effect emerging (Table 71.1). The differential pattern of findings regarding functional connectivity between the amygdala and the ventrolateral prefrontal cortex and between the amygdala and regions of the medial prefrontal cortex may thus reflect specific functional abnormalities in lateral prefrontal cortical-based voluntary/effortful emotion regulation pathway and medial prefrontal cortical-based automatic/implicit emotion regulation pathway. Abnormally elevated positive functional connectivity in the former pathway may reflect abnormally elevated encoding of emotion in the amygdala, resulting in an inefficient, compensatory regulation of the amygdala by the ventrolateral prefrontal cortex or by abnormally elevated signalling of emotion from the amygdala to the ventrolateral prefrontal cortex. By contrast, abnormally reduced functional connectivity in the latter pathway may reflect a relative disconnectivity pattern, resulting in deficient amygdala regulation by medial prefrontal cortical regions (Fig. 71.2).

There are also observations of altered connectivity between the ventrolateral prefrontal cortex and the medial prefrontal cortex in individuals with bipolar disorder. The dorsolateral prefrontal cortex may also play a role in regulating the amygdala, with alterations in dorsolateral prefrontal cortical–amygdala and dorsolateral prefrontal cortical–anterior cingulate cortical–ventrolateral prefrontal cortical functional connectivity reported in individuals with bipolar disorder (Table 71.1).

### Abnormal activity and functional connectivity in emotion processing and emotion regulation neural circuitry during performance of non-emotional tasks

Abnormal patterns of activity in emotion processing circuitry, including the amygdala, medial prefrontal cortex, orbitofrontal cortex and temporal cortex, during non-emotional, cognitive task performance have also been reported in individuals with bipolar disorder [4] (Table 71.1). Key findings include abnormally elevated amygdala activity, abnormally reduced inverse functional connectivity between the amygdala and cortical regions, and abnormally reduced activity in prefrontal cortical regions implicated in cognitive control processes in adults with bipolar disorder during a variety of cognitive and motor tasks. These findings suggest a heightened perception of emotional salience in non-emotional contexts in bipolar disorder.

### Abnormal activity and functional connectivity in reward processing neural circuitry

A number of behavioural and event-related potential studies have highlighted heightened reward sensitivity in individuals with bipolar disorder. The key role of the ventral striatum (nucleus accumbens) in response to reward cues, reward receipt, and prediction error (the difference between expected and actual outcomes) is well established [6]. Specific prefrontal cortical regions also have specific roles in reward processing. The ventrolateral prefrontal cortex, in addition to its role in emotion regulation, is activated during arousal in the context of emotional stimuli, encodes the value of different decision-making options, and links stimulus representations to specific reward outcomes [7]. The orbitofrontal cortex encodes reward values. In humans, both of these regions may have excitatory afferent connections with the ventral striatum, given studies reporting excitatory afferent connections between the homologues of these

prefrontal cortical regions and the ventral striatum in rodents. The medial prefrontal cortex (including dorsal and pregenual anterior cingulate cortical subregions and mediodorsal prefrontal cortex) regulates the ventral striatum and appetitive behaviours in potentially rewarding contexts [8] (Fig. 71.1b).

Functional neuroimaging studies of reward processing neural circuitry in individuals with bipolar disorder indicate abnormally elevated activity in the ventral striatum and left prefrontal cortex, in particular, the left orbitofrontal cortex and the left ventrolateral prefrontal cortex, during reward processing [4]. Here, studies reported abnormally increased left ventrolateral prefrontal cortical activity to reward anticipation in adults with bipolar disorder across different mood states and abnormally increased ventral striatal activity during reward anticipation in euthymic individuals with bipolar disorder; abnormally elevated left orbitofrontal cortex and amygdala activity to reward reversal and elevated left orbitofrontal cortex activity to reward in euthymic adults with bipolar disorder; and elevated ventral striatal activity to reward cues and outcomes in individuals with subthreshold hypomania. By contrast, patterns of either no ventral striatal activity abnormality during reward anticipation or receipt or abnormally reduced ventral striatal activity to reward receipt have been demonstrated in depressed individuals with bipolar disorder. Another study reported no differential activity in the ventral striatum to reward receipt vs omission in manic adults with bipolar disorder. These findings indicate abnormally elevated activity in distributed reward circuitry, particularly in the left ventrolateral prefrontal cortex, during reward processing in individuals with bipolar disorder (Table 71.1; Fig. 71.3). Only a small number of recent studies reported altered functional connectivity in reward circuitry, including significantly reduced inverse functional connectivity between the ventral striatum and medial prefrontal cortical regions. This is an area requiring future research effort.

## Intrinsic (resting state) connectivity studies

These studies provide measures of tonic functional connectivity in neural circuitries of interest, rather than stimulus-related, phasic functional connectivity in these circuitries, and can thereby identify context-independent functional abnormalities that potentially represent core functional abnormalities in such circuitries in a given disorder. The majority of these studies in bipolar disorder employed a region of interest approach to examine functional connectivity among a priori regions and localized neural circuitries at rest, measuring, for example, correlations between time series of low-frequency fluctuations in activity among these regions. Predominant findings from these studies in individuals with bipolar disorder parallel findings from task-based fMRI studies [5] and include: (1) abnormally decreased, but also abnormally increased, positive resting connectivity between medial prefrontal cortical and amygdala and striatal regions; (2) abnormal positive and abnormally reduced inverse resting connectivity between the medial prefrontal cortex and the ventrolateral prefrontal cortex, but also abnormally reduced positive resting functional connectivity among medial and lateral prefrontal cortical regions; (3) abnormally elevated positive resting state connectivity between the ventrolateral prefrontal cortex (and the anterior cingulate cortex) and amygdala; and (4) abnormally reduced inverse resting connectivity between the amygdala

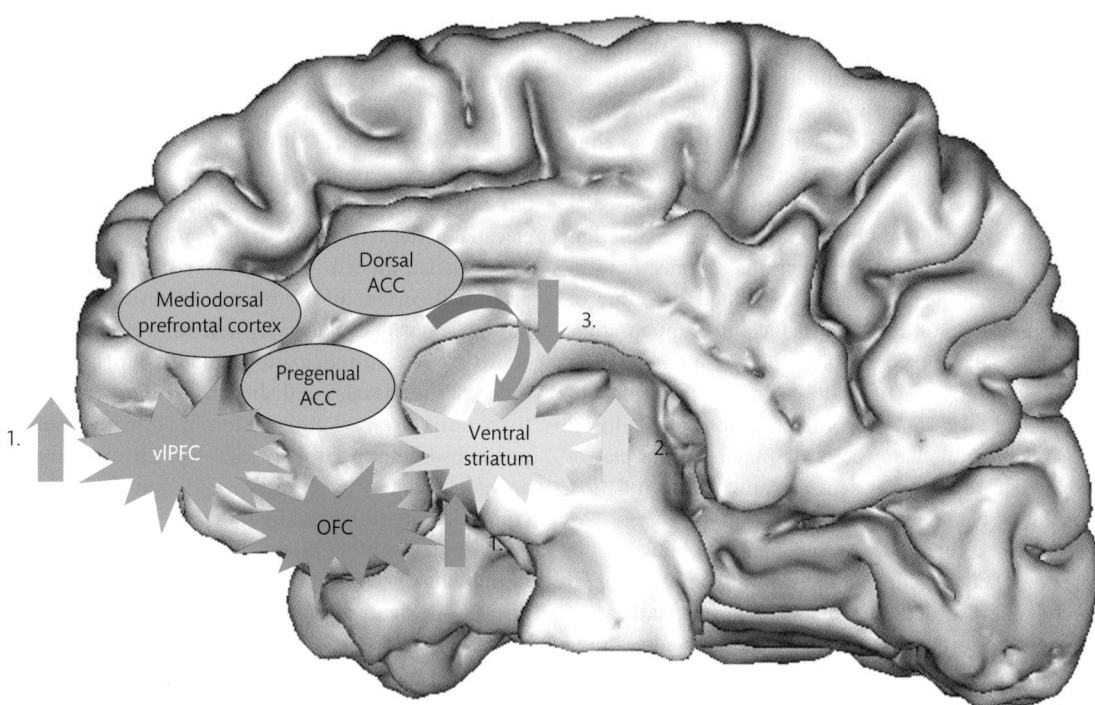

**Fig. 71.3** Key functional abnormalities in reward processing neural circuitry in individuals with bipolar disorder, including: 1. abnormally increased left ventrolateral prefrontal cortical activity and left orbitofrontal cortical activity during reward anticipation and receipt; 2. abnormally increased ventral striatal activity to reward anticipation and receipt in euthymic, but not in depressed, individuals with bipolar disorder; 3. abnormally reduced inverse functional connectivity between the ventral striatum and the medial prefrontal cortex. Star shapes refer to neural regions that are most consistently reported as being affected as described previously in bipolar disorder. In parallel, there are widespread decreases in grey matter volume and cortical thickness in prefrontal cortical regions and striatal regions in individuals with bipolar disorder.

and the dorsolateral prefrontal cortex. Other studies in individuals with bipolar disorder show more widespread patterns of abnormally reduced positive functional connectivity among different prefrontal cortical and temporal regions, and reduced positive functional connectivity among midline cortical regions. Abnormalities in amygdala–ventrolateral prefrontal cortical resting functional connectivity may be determined, at least in part, by the medial prefrontal cortex.

Other resting state functional connectivity studies focused on larger-scale networks and reported in individuals with bipolar disorder diverse patterns of abnormally increased resting connectivity in paralimbic and fronto-temporal/paralimbic networks, abnormally decreased connectivity in the medial prefrontal cortex, and abnormal positive resting connectivity between the medial prefrontal cortex and the ventrolateral prefrontal cortex, and between the medial prefrontal cortex and the insula, together with abnormal decoupling between the mediodorsal prefrontal cortex and the dorsolateral prefrontal cortex.

Fewer studies used global connectivity methods (for example, independent components analyses) to study patterns of whole brain study resting functional connectivity in individuals with bipolar disorder. Findings from these studies are somewhat mixed, showing diverse patterns of abnormally elevated or reduced resting connectivity within and among different large-scale neural networks implicated in salience processing, executive function, emotion, and 'default mode' (non-task performance).

Recent studies examined the amplitude of low-frequency fluctuations (ALFF) and the homogeneity of time series within specific neural regions, as alternative measures of resting state connectivity. These studies reported both abnormally increased and decreased ALFF in fronto-temporal–striatal regions in individuals with bipolar disorder vs healthy individuals, decreased ALFF in left post-central parahippocampal regions in individuals with bipolar disorder vs healthy individuals, and greater regional homogeneity in left fronto-parietal cortices in depressed bipolar disorder (subtype unspecified) vs healthy adults.

Together, these studies indicate intrinsic, context-independent abnormalities, both in functional connectivity between regions and in the amplitude and homogeneity of low-frequency fluctuations within neural regions, predominantly within prefrontal cortical, amygdala, and striatal circuitries implicated in emotion processing, emotion regulation, and reward processing in individuals with bipolar disorder [5]. Findings largely parallel those from task-based fMRI studies in bipolar disorder and also suggest abnormalities in resting state functional connectivity among larger-scale neural networks in the disorder (Table 71.2). The relative paucity of resting state functional connectivity studies, in comparison with task-based fMRI studies, in bipolar disorder, particularly those employing global network approaches, suggests that future studies should employ such approaches, in conjunction with task-based fMRI studies, to facilitate understanding of relationships between phasic and tonic-level functioning in neural circuitries of interest in bipolar disorder.

**Table 71.2** Main themes from intrinsic resting state connectivity studies in bipolar disorder

| Region of interest approaches | 1. Abnormal changes in resting connectivity between medial prefrontal cortical and amygdala and striatal regions (both abnormally increased and decreased resting connectivity) |
| | 2. Abnormal changes in resting connectivity between medial prefrontal cortex and ventrolateral prefrontal cortex (both abnormal positive and abnormally reduced inverse, and abnormally reduced positive, resting connectivity) |
| | 3. Abnormally elevated positive resting state connectivity between ventrolateral prefrontal cortex (and anterior cingulate cortex) and amygdala |
| | 4. Abnormally reduced inverse resting connectivity between amygdala and dorsolateral prefrontal cortex |
| | 5. Larger-scale network abnormalities across different prefrontal and temporal cortical and subcortical regions |
| Global connectivity approaches | 1. Diverse patterns of abnormally elevated or reduced resting connectivity within and among different large-scale neural networks implicated in salience processing, executive function, emotion, and 'default mode' (non-task performance) |
| Approaches using amplitude of low frequency fluctuations (ALFF) and regional homogeneity of time series | 1. Abnormally increased and decreased ALFF in fronto-temporal–striatal regions |
| | 2. Abnormally increased regional homogeneity in left fronto-parietal cortices |

## Structural neuroimaging studies

Key findings from earlier studies in bipolar disorder were an increased number of white matter hyperintensities [9] and enlarged amygdala grey matter volumes [10, 11], highlighting the potential role of abnormalities in emotion processing neural circuitry in bipolar disorder. More recent studies examined regional grey matter volumes in a wider range of cortical and subcortical regions in adults with bipolar disorder. Two main themes have emerged from these later studies that relate to emotion processing and regulation neural circuitries [4]. Firstly, findings indicate abnormally decreased grey matter volume, decreased white matter volume, and decreased thickness in cortical regions implicated in emotion processing and cognitive processes important for emotion regulation, that is, the prefrontal and anterior temporal cortices, and in cortical regions underlying salience perception, that is, the insula and the dorsal anterior cingulate cortex, in individuals with bipolar disorder, with some exceptions. One study implicated the ventrolateral prefrontal cortex, in particular, in bipolar disorder, reporting a negative association between right ventrolateral prefrontal cortex grey matter volume and illness duration, and smaller right ventrolateral prefrontal cortex grey matter volume in adults with bipolar disorder with long-term illness and minimal lifetime exposure to lithium vs healthy adults, but abnormally increased right ventrolateral prefrontal cortex grey matter volume in relatives of individuals with bipolar disorder and in younger adults in early stages of bipolar disorder [12]. Other studies replicated the finding of reduced right

ventrolateral prefrontal grey matter volume in bipolar disorder. Indeed, several findings indicate that prefrontal cortical grey matter volumes in general may decrease with illness progression, including a greater number of manic episodes, but may normalize (or even increase) with lithium. These findings of reduced grey matter volume in prefrontal cortical regions, especially in the right ventrolateral prefrontal cortex in adults with bipolar disorder, suggest a structural basis for findings from fMRI studies of decreased activity in this region during emotion processing and emotion regulation tasks.

A second key finding regarding structural findings in emotion processing and regulation neural circuitries in bipolar disorder is decreased subcortical regional volumes, especially in the amygdala, particularly during depressive episodes, which may normalize with lithium. For example, a meta-analysis reported amygdala volume decreases in youth, but not in adults, with bipolar disorder [13], suggesting a normalization of amygdala volume over development in bipolar disorder, potentially due to medication [12]. Abnormally decreased hippocampal and parahippocampal volumes have also been reported in adults with bipolar disorder; such abnormalities may also be masked by lithium.

Recent studies also provide evidence for abnormally increased gyrification of the anterior cingulate cortex in adults with bipolar disorder and have also employed newer techniques, such as high angular resolution molecular diffusion imaging, to examine the microstructure of different brain tissues in individuals with bipolar disorder. Findings confirm the presence of structural abnormalities in the hippocampus and striatum in bipolar disorder.

## Diffusion imaging studies

The main diffusion imaging measures are longitudinal/axial diffusivity (AD), the diffusivity of water molecules along the principal axis; radial diffusivity (RD), the diffusivity of water molecules along transverse directions perpendicular to the longitudinal axis; and fractional anisotropy (FA), the ratio of longitudinal vs transverse diffusivity in white matter tracts. Given the properties of white axonal membranes and myelin sheaths, FA will be high in white matter tracts with densely packed collinear axons, but low in white matter with non-collinear axons. By contrast, RD will be high in white matter with non-collinear axons, but also high in white matter with damaged axonal membranes and/or myelin sheaths.

Studies measuring FA, RD, and AD reported specific abnormalities in the microstructure of white matter tracts in neural circuitries important for emotion processing, emotion regulation, and reward processing in individuals with bipolar disorder. Initial diffusion imaging studies reported white matter abnormalities in frontally situated white matter tracts in adults with bipolar disorder [4]. Recent diffusion imaging studies of adults with bipolar disorder reported abnormally reduced FA, often paralleled by abnormally increased RD, in these tracts, especially in tracts connecting prefrontal cortical and anterior limbic structures supporting emotion regulation and in temporal white matter. White matter tracts that most consistently show these abnormalities are the anterior regions of the corpus callosum, the anterior cingulum, the uncinate fasciculus, and the superior longitudinal fasciculus, tracts that interconnect frontal regions, and connect frontal regions with more posterior regions (including occipital, parietal, and temporal regions). These abnormalities may be more apparent in a depressive episode than in remission and may be normalized by lithium. One study reported abnormal nodal networks in the left ventrolateral prefrontal cortex, left hippocampus, and bilateral mid anterior cingulate cortex in adults with bipolar disorder vs healthy adults [14], that may suggest a specific white matter structural basis for the observed pattern of abnormal left ventrolateral prefrontal cortex and orbitofrontal cortex activity during reward processing in bipolar disorder.

Together, findings from diffusion imaging studies in adults with bipolar disorder thus suggest either abnormal myelination or abnormal orientation of axons in white matter tracts connecting frontal and temporal (and also occipital and parietal) cortices, cortical regions that are in neural circuitries important for emotion regulation and reward processing. Interestingly, a recent diffusion imaging study measured magnetization transfer ratio (MTR) to assess the degree of myelin content in white matter tracts, and diffusion tensor spectroscopy (DTS) to measure metabolite diffusion specifically within axons in these tracts, in individuals with bipolar disorder [15]. This study reported specific reductions in MTR, but no abnormalities in DTS, in right prefrontal cortical white matter in individuals with bipolar disorder. These findings suggest that the major finding of reduced FA reported previously may result from reduced myelin content, rather than changes in axonal structure, in bipolar disorder.

These data appear consistent with post-mortem histopathological evidence showing a reduction in oligodendroglial cell counts and in the expression of myelin basic protein (MBP) and other oligodendroglial genes in the medial prefrontal cortical network in bipolar disorder [16]. In prefrontal cortical and hippocampal tissue of bipolar patients' studied post-mortem (predominantly from medicated subjects in the depressed or mixed phases prior to death), the genes involved in energy metabolism and mitochondrial function also are downregulated, while genes involved in immune response and inflammation are upregulated [17]. These data, taken together with the evidence reviewed in the following sections that bipolar disorder is associated with abnormal energy metabolism and neuroinflammation, may relate mechanistically to the white matter abnormalities identified using DTI, DTS, and structural MRI.

## Magnetic resonance spectroscopy studies

Data obtained using magnetic resonance spectroscopy (MRS) technologies are relevant to functional and structural neuroimaging abnormalities since they can identify alterations in the bioenergetics underlying the metabolic and haemodynamic signals assessed during functional neuroimaging. Corroborating the evidence for reduced mitochondrial gene expression in bipolar disorder, *in vivo* MRS studies have revealed an abnormal reduction in frontal lobe pH in both medicated and unmedicated individuals with bipolar disorder, and a shift from oxidative phosphorylation to glycolysis in medication-free individuals with bipolar disorder [18]. More recently, phosphorus-31 (P-31) MRS studies of bioenergetics in bipolar disorder provided additional *in vivo* evidence of mitochondrial dysfunction in bipolar disorder.

Furthermore, since cerebral blood flow, glucose metabolism, and BOLD-fMRI signals are most heavily influenced by glutamatergic transmission, the application of proton (H-1) MRS to quantitate

glutamate, glutamine, and 'Glx' (a composite measure consisting mainly of glutamate and glutamine) levels in brain tissue also holds relevance for the interpretation of functional imaging data. In general, studies applying these methods have shown a pattern of abnormally elevated Glx levels in bipolar disorder, in contrast to abnormally reduced Glx levels in major depressive disorder. Moreover, the glutamine/glutamate ratio appears abnormally decreased in depression (whether unipolar or bipolar), but elevated in mania. In contrast to functional neuroimaging measures of cerebral glucose metabolism and blood flow, which predominantly reflect glutamatergic transmission, the H-1 MRS measures of glutamate and glutamine almost entirely reflect the intracellular pools, with glutamate residing largely in neurons and glutamine in glia. The abnormal patterns found in mood disorders thus have been interpreted to indicate that the glutamate-related metabolite pool is constricted in major depressive disorder, but expanded in bipolar disorder, and that depressive and manic episodes are characterized by modulation of the glutamine/glutamate ratio in opposite directions, suggesting reduced vs elevated glutamate conversion to glutamine within glial cells, respectively. Since glutamate is converted to glutamine in glial cells, and glutamine is converted to glutamate in neurons, these data suggest an abnormality in neuronal–glial cell interactions. The MRS literature thus appears consistent with the post-mortem findings of reduced oligodendroglial cell counts, impaired astrocyte function (especially with respect to glutamate transport), and loss of GABAergic neurons in structures where the glutamine/glutamate ratio also is altered in bipolar disorder (for example, pregenual anterior cingulate cortex) [16].

## Positron emission tomography studies

PET studies of bipolar disorder have employed various radioligands to measure regional blood flow, glucose metabolism, neuroreceptor binding potential, or other parameters. Most of this literature is beyond the scope of this chapter and is reviewed elsewhere [19, 20]. A few pertinent studies are discussed here, which converge with the literature described in the preceding sections to implicate alterations in bioenergetic and neuroinflammation in the pathophysiology of bipolar disorder.

The concept that bioenergetics abnormalities exist in bipolar disorder has face validity because of the clinical observation and symptomatology indicating that psychomotor activity and subjective energy are generally elevated in mania, but reduced in depression. Consistent with this concept, glucose metabolism is increased in the unmedicated manic phase, but decreased in the unmedicated depressed phase of bipolar disorder in limbic–cortical regions such as the subgenual prefrontal cortex [21]. These data thus appear consistent with the P-31 MRS data reviewed previously, which suggested that the glutamine/glutamate ratio is modulated in opposite directions in mania vs depression.

The recent development of PET radioligands for the translocator protein (TSPO) on the outer mitochondrial membranes in microglia has enabled *in vivo* measures of microglial activation. This phenomenon is a central component of neuroinflammation and is manifest by a range of phenotypic changes in microglial cell morphology, as well as upregulation of cellular proteins, including TSPO. The first study using PET-TSPO imaging in bipolar disorder found that individuals with bipolar disorder type 1 had elevated TSPO binding, relative to healthy controls, in the hippocampus [22].

It remains unclear whether microglial activation in these regions reflects a repair response or instead constitutes a pathological process that disrupts the normal physiology and precipitates disease in bipolar disorder. One line of evidence suggests that inflammation may contribute to reductions in hippocampal volume, as pro-inflammatory drive on the kynurenine metabolic pathway reduces the concentrations of the neuroprotective metabolite kynurenic acid, relative to levels of the putatively neurotoxic metabolites 3-hydroxykynurenine and quinolinic acid. Savitz *et al.* [23] reported that this ratio was reduced in plasma in bipolar disorder individuals, relative to controls, and also correlated directly with hippocampal volume in bipolar individuals (that is, lower neuroprotective indices were associated with smaller hippocampal volumes). Similarly, within the anterior cingulate cortex, a post-mortem study of brain tissue from a combined sample of unipolar and bipolar depressed individuals who died by suicide showed that microglial activation and quinolinic acid expression were increased to the greatest extent in the subgenual anterior cingulate cortex [24], which has been associated with reduced grey matter in both mood disorder subtypes [21].

## Interim summary

Neural circuitry abnormalities in bipolar disorder thus comprise: (1) dysfunction in bilateral prefrontal cortical (especially ventrolateral prefrontal cortex and orbitofrontal cortex)–hippocampal–amygdala emotion processing and emotion regulation neural circuitries; (2) hyperactivity in predominantly left-sided ventral striatal–ventrolateral prefrontal cortex reward processing circuitry; (3) parallel resting state functional connectivity abnormalities in these, and more widespread, neural circuitries; (4) abnormalities in regional grey matter structure in these neural circuitries; (5) microstructural abnormalities in white matter tracts in these neural circuitries, with more recent findings suggesting myelin abnormalities in these tracts; (6) bioenergetic abnormalities suggestive of mitochondrial dysfunction and altered neuronal glial interactions; and (7) abnormalities of regional glucose metabolism and microglial activation in the same regions showing grey matter loss. The combination of these functional and structural abnormalities may be characteristic of the behavioural abnormalities associated with bipolar disorder, that is, emotional lability, emotional dysregulation, and reward sensitivity (Figs. 71.2 and 71.3).

## Newer neuroimaging research areas in bipolar disorder

(See Table 71.3.)

### Mood state-specific functional abnormalities in emotion processing, emotion regulation, and reward processing in neural circuitries

A small number of cross-sectional studies examined individuals with bipolar disorder in different mood states during emotion processing and emotion regulation [4, 5]. One finding is abnormally

**Table 71.3** Newer neuroimaging research areas in bipolar disorder

| | |
|---|---|
| Mood state-specific abnormalities | 1. Cross-sectional studies of emotion processing and emotion regulation neural circuitries: (1) differential patterns of activity in orbitofrontal cortex, insula, ventrolateral prefrontal cortex, amygdala, and dorsolateral prefrontal cortex across different mood states; (2) differential patterns of emotion processing task-based connectivity and resting connectivity between amygdala and medial prefrontal cortex, hippocampus, and orbitofrontal cortex<br>2. Longitudinal studies: differential patterns of prefrontal cortical and amygdala activity and amygdala connectivity across different mood states |
| Different bipolar disorder subtypes | 1. Abnormally decreased prefrontal cortical activity (especially ventrolateral prefrontal cortex) across different tasks in bipolar disorder type II<br>2. Similar patterns of abnormally elevated activity in amygdala and dorsolateral prefrontal cortex during emotion regulation and working memory, and abnormally elevated left ventrolateral prefrontal cortical and ventral striatal activity during reward anticipation, in bipolar disorder types I and II. Graded differences in magnitude of activity between bipolar disorder subtypes<br>3. More widespread reductions in grey matter across different cortical regions in bipolar disorder type I, relative to bipolar disorder type II |
| Youth with bipolar disorder | 1. Similar patterns to adult bipolar disorder of abnormally increased amygdala activity, decreased ventrolateral prefrontal cortical activity, and decreased prefrontal cortical–amygdala functional connectivity during emotion processing and emotion regulation<br>2. Abnormally decreased amygdala volumes and abnormally reduced prefrontal cortical volumes and cortical thickness<br>3. Abnormally reduced FA in white matter tracts connecting prefrontal cortical and subcortical regions |
| Adults and youth at risk of bipolar disorder | 1. Healthy at-risk adults and youth: (a) abnormally increased prefrontal cortical and amygdala activity during emotion and cognitive control tasks; (b) abnormally increased left ventrolateral prefrontal cortical activity to reward; (c) abnormally increased frontal and subcortical grey matter volumes; (d) abnormally reduced FA in white matter tracts connecting prefrontal cortical and subcortical regions<br>2. Psychiatrically affected at-risk adults and youth: (a) predominantly abnormally increased prefrontal cortical activity and prefrontal cortical–amygdala functional connectivity during emotion regulation and cognitive control tasks; (b) abnormally increased activity in *left-sided* prefrontal cortical regions and insula, regardless of task; (c) abnormally decreased grey matter volumes in prefrontal and temporal cortical regions, striatum, and insula; but increased volumes in right ventrolateral prefrontal cortex and left caudate; (d) decreased white matter volume and white matter integrity, especially in prefrontal regions |

decreased orbitofrontal cortex activity during emotion processing across different mood states. Other findings indicate differing roles of the insula and ventrolateral prefrontal cortex in adults with bipolar disorder across different mood states during emotion regulation; different mood state-specific increases in amygdala activity to negative emotional faces; abnormally decreased right dorsolateral prefrontal cortex activity during non-emotional working memory across different mood states; increased ventrolateral prefrontal cortex–thalamic activity in adults with bipolar disorder in mixed mood episode vs depression during response inhibition; and failure to deactivate ventral regions of the medial prefrontal cortex during a working memory task.

Cross-sectional studies also reported differences in amygdala–medial prefrontal cortical functional connectivity across different mood states, including differential patterns of amygdala functional connectivity with the medial prefrontal cortex between depressed and remitted individuals with bipolar disorder during emotion processing; differential patterns of resting state functional connectivity between the amygdala and the anterior cingulate cortex (pregenual subdivision) in manic and depressed mood states and between manic and euthymic states; and abnormally increased vs reduced resting state connectivity between the amygdala and the hippocampus in mania vs depression, respectively. Contrasting patterns of variability in large-scale network resting state signal amplitude in bipolar depression vs mania are also reported [25].

Longitudinal studies reported an abnormally reduced extent of activity in prefrontal cortical regions implicated in emotion regulation during an emotional face–word interference emotion regulation task in individuals with bipolar disorder, relative to healthy controls, but to a greater extent during hypomanic than depressed and euthymic mood states; differential patterns of amygdala functional connectivity in the same individuals with bipolar disorder during mania vs depression; and normalized activity in the amygdala and prefrontal cortical regions in remitted vs manic adults with bipolar disorder during reward and motor tasks.

While there are no clear patterns of mood state-specific functional neural abnormalities in bipolar disorder, findings suggest amygdala–prefrontal cortical functional abnormalities across different mood states, which normalize with remission. Clearly, more longitudinal, within-subject studies are required to identify functional abnormalities in neural circuitries that predispose to switches between different mood states in bipolar disorder.

### Bipolar disorder subtypes

A small, but increasing, number of neuroimaging studies focused on adults with bipolar disorder type II [4]. One study reported abnormally reduced amygdala and bilateral ventrolateral prefrontal cortex activity, and reduced amygdala–orbitofrontal cortex and amygdala–dorsolateral prefrontal cortex functional connectivity, during emotional face processing in depressed adults with bipolar disorder type II. Other studies reported abnormally reduced activity in different prefrontal cortical regions during working memory and response inhibition in depressed individuals with bipolar disorder type II. The finding of decreased prefrontal cortical activity, in particular in the ventrolateral prefrontal cortex, parallels that shown during similar tasks by euthymic and depressed adults with bipolar disorder type I and suggests that reduced ventrolateral prefrontal cortex activity during emotion processing and emotion regulation may be a trait marker of bipolar disorder across types I and II.

Other fMRI studies directly compared adults with bipolar disorder type I and bipolar disorder type II and healthy adults. One study compared euthymic adults with bipolar disorder type I, euthymic adults with bipolar disorder type II, and healthy controls during a working memory task and reported a graded pattern of abnormally

elevated activity in the dorsolateral prefrontal cortex during the task in individuals with bipolar disorder type I, relative to bipolar disorder type II, suggesting greater functional abnormalities in prefrontal cortical recruitment during the task in bipolar disorder type I than in type II. Another study reported similar patterns of abnormally elevated activity in the amygdala and dorsolateral prefrontal cortex during an emotion regulation task in both euthymic individuals with bipolar disorder type I and euthymic individuals with bipolar disorder type II, but abnormally increased inverse functional connectivity between the amygdala and the dorsolateral prefrontal cortex during the task only in individuals with bipolar II disorder.

Another study focused on reward circuitry and reported significantly increased ventral striatal and left ventrolateral prefrontal cortical activity in adults with bipolar disorder type II vs adults with bipolar disorder type I and healthy adults during reward anticipation, again paralleling previous studies that highlighted abnormally increased left ventrolateral prefrontal cortex and ventral striatal activity during reward anticipation in euthymic and depressed adults with bipolar disorder type I [26]. Findings from this study are the first to suggest that bipolar disorder type II may be characterized by a greater magnitude of functional abnormalities in reward neural circuitry than bipolar disorder type I, supporting findings associating bipolar disorder type II with more disabling functional impairments in daily living than bipolar disorder type I [27, 28].

Regarding other neuroimaging modalities, abnormally elevated resting state functional connectivity across several regions within a temporo-insular neural network, identified with independent components analysis, was observed in individuals with bipolar disorder type II. Other studies reported more widespread grey matter reductions in the prefrontal, temporal, and parietal cortices in euthymic/moderately depressed adults with bipolar disorder type I vs depressed adults with bipolar disorder type II, and greater magnitude of reductions in grey matter volume and cortical thickness in individuals with bipolar disorder type I relative to bipolar disorder type II. Diffusion imaging studies that compared individuals with bipolar disorder type I and those with bipolar disorder type II reported abnormalities in fronto-thalamic-temporal white matter in both disorders, although findings across studies are inconsistent, with abnormalities only in bipolar disorder type I or, by contrast, abnormalities only in bipolar disorder type II.

There is clearly a need for more neuroimaging studies comparing individuals with bipolar disorder type I with those with bipolar disorder type II and those with other bipolar disorder subtypes.

### Neuroimaging studies adopting dimensional approaches

Guided by the NIMH Research Domain Criteria initiative (see Chapter 8), neuroimaging studies are beginning to adopt a dimensional approach to the study of psychiatric disorders, including bipolar disorder. One focus has been to examine individuals across the mood disorders spectrum. One study reported a positive correlation between reward sensitivity (fun-seeking) and ventral striatal activity across adults with bipolar disorder type I, adults with bipolar disorder type II, and healthy adults [26]. This study thus associated patterns of function in reward circuitry with information processing domains that cut across diagnostic boundaries.

Another focus has been to examine the psychosis spectrum by including individuals with bipolar disorder and individuals with schizophrenia. Here, studies examined relationships between neuroimaging measures of structure and function across the whole brain and in neural circuitries of interest and psychotic symptoms, regardless of diagnosis. Recent findings include significant relationships between psychotic symptom severity and abnormally reduced local resting state functional connectivity [29] and reductions in prefrontal cortical and temporal cortical grey matter volume [30] across individuals with schizophrenia and bipolar disorder.

These findings suggest that the conceptualization of mood disorders and schizophrenia in terms of different psychiatric spectrum disorders may lead to a better understanding of neuropathophysiological processes in these illnesses [31]. Here, for example, bipolar disorder type I, bipolar disorder type II, other bipolar disorder subtypes, and major depressive disorder could perhaps be included along a mood disorders spectrum, and schizophrenia and bipolar disorder along a psychotic disorders spectrum.

## Youth with bipolar disorder

Studies reported in youth with bipolar disorder similar patterns to those in adult with bipolar disorder of abnormally increased amygdala activity, decreased ventrolateral prefrontal cortical activity, and decreased prefrontal cortical–amygdala functional connectivity during emotion processing and emotion regulation paradigms [32]. Abnormally increased amygdala activity may be more evident in youth than in adults with bipolar disorder. Studies in bipolar disorder youth also demonstrated abnormally decreased amygdala volumes; reduced orbitofrontal cortex and anterior cingulate cortex grey matter and reduced prefrontal cortical thickness; abnormally reduced FA in white matter tracts connecting prefrontal and subcortical regions, and reduced volume of the corpus callosum; and altered resting state and regional homogeneity in prefrontal cortical–amygdala–striatal circuitry and large-scale networks.

## Adults and youth at risk of bipolar disorder

These studies can be divided into those examining healthy adults and youth at future risk of bipolar disorder by virtue of having a parent or sibling with the disorder, and those examining at-risk adults and youth who are already affected with some psychiatric symptoms, but not with bipolar disorder (reviewed in [32]).

### Healthy adults and youth at risk of bipolar disorder

During emotion processing, healthy at-risk youth show abnormally elevated amygdala activity, abnormal inverse anterior cingulate–amygdala functional connectivity, and abnormally elevated left ventrolateral prefrontal cortical–amygdala functional connectivity during emotion processing. During emotion regulation and non-emotional cognitive control tasks, healthy at-risk adults and youth showed abnormally elevated, predominantly right-sided activity in frontal control regions (ventrolateral and dorsolateral prefrontal cortices) and in the amygdala, and decreased right ventrolateral prefrontal cortical–amygdala and dorsolateral prefrontal cortical–amygdala functional connectivity. Regarding reward processing, healthy at-risk youth showed abnormally elevated left ventrolateral prefrontal cortical activity to reward, and abnormally reduced functional connectivity between the ventrolateral prefrontal cortex and the anterior cingulate cortex during reward anticipation. In unaffected relatives of adults with bipolar disorder, abnormally elevated right orbitofrontal cortical activity to reward, but abnormally

elevated left orbitofrontal cortical activity to loss, was reported. Resting state findings indicate abnormally reduced resting state functional connectivity between the amygdala and the anterior cingulate cortex and between the amygdala and the ventrolateral prefrontal cortex in healthy at-risk youth.

Regarding structural findings, the main pattern is abnormally *increased* grey matter volume in several areas, including the amygdala, the bilateral ventrolateral prefrontal cortex, the left dorsolateral prefrontal cortex, the left parahippocampal gyrus, and the left caudate. Diffusion imaging studies indicate abnormal, predominantly right-sided decreases in FA and volume in white matter tracts connecting prefrontal cortical and subcortical regions.

These findings may represent two separate kinds of markers: those representing resilience and those representing risk. Resilience markers might include increased prefrontal activity and increased frontal and subcortical volumes, given that at-risk individuals who demonstrated these patterns were psychiatrically healthy at the time of study. Risk markers might include increased amygdala activity and abnormal prefrontal white matter, as these patterns are similar to findings from studies of adults with bipolar disorder.

### Psychiatrically affected adults and youth at future risk of bipolar disorder

Regarding emotion processing, findings indicate abnormally elevated amygdala activity, abnormal inverse anterior cingulate–amygdala functional connectivity and abnormally elevated left ventrolateral prefrontal cortical–amygdala functional connectivity during emotion processing, and abnormal functional connectivity among the ventrolateral prefrontal cortex, the anterior cingulate gyrus, and the dorsolateral prefrontal cortex in affected first-degree relatives of individuals with bipolar disorder. During emotion regulation and non-emotional cognitive control tasks, studies indicate abnormally increased dorsolateral prefrontal cortical activity and increased ventrolateral prefrontal cortical–bilateral amygdala functional connectivity in youth with milder-level behavioural and emotional dysregulation symptoms, and abnormally increased activity in the left frontal pole in first-degree relatives who currently have depression or substance abuse diagnoses. Such individuals also show abnormally decreased activity in cognitive control regions and abnormally decreased functional connectivity between prefrontal cortical regions implicated in emotion regulation and subcortical regions.

Regarding reward processing, one study reported increased left ventrolateral prefrontal cortical/middle prefrontal cortical activity to reward, with increasing magnitude of non-specific behavioural and mood dysregulation symptoms in youth. A meta-analysis concluded that high-risk individuals (both those with and without a current psychiatric diagnosis) showed abnormally increased activity in *left-sided* prefrontal cortical regions and the insula, regardless of task [33].

Structural findings indicate abnormally decreased volumes in a variety of regions, including the dorsolateral prefrontal cortex, orbitofrontal cortex, insula, anterior cingulate cortex, ventral striatum, and bilateral frontal and left temporo-parietal regions. Increased volumes are also observed in the right ventrolateral prefrontal cortex [12], the left insula, and the left caudate. Diffusion imaging studies report decreased white matter volume and white matter integrity, particularly in prefrontal regions.

Abnormally increased prefrontal cortical activity during emotion regulation and non-emotional cognitive control tasks may represent resilience factors in non-bipolar disorder-affected at-risk individuals. Similarly, findings of abnormally increased prefrontal cortical volume may also represent resilience factors, while findings of abnormally decreased prefrontal cortical volumes parallel findings in adults with bipolar disorder. Risk factors include left-sided subcortical volume increases that may be associated with left-sided increases in prefrontal cortical and subcortical activity during reward and other task performances observed across at-risk individuals and individuals with bipolar disorder. Diffusion imaging studies reporting decreased white matter volume in these at-risk individuals may also represent risk factors as they, too, parallel findings in adults with bipolar disorder.

Longitudinal studies are clearly needed to examine developmental trajectories of structural and functional changes in prefrontal cortical–subcortical circuitry in individuals with bipolar disorder and those youth at risk of future mood and psychotic disorders. Such studies will help identify abnormal developmental trajectories in this circuitry that are associated with having bipolar disorder or other mood disorders in youth, and biomarkers that can help identify which at-risk youth are most likely to develop these disorders in the future.

### Multimodal neuroimaging studies

A future area for neuroimaging research in bipolar disorder is the use of multimodal techniques to identify structure–function relationships in the neural circuitry. A very small number of studies examined structure–function relationships in the prefrontal cortical–amygdala circuitry in adults with bipolar disorder type I and bipolar disorder type II, but there is a need for more such studies in individuals across the mood disorders spectrum. In parallel, studies are beginning to identify relationships between genetic variants and functioning and structure within the neural circuitry in adults and youth with bipolar disorder and in individuals at risk for bipolar disorder. Ultimately, an integrated systems approach will help identify biomarkers that reflect the neuropathophysiological processes in individuals with mood, psychotic, and other psychiatric disorders that span genetic, molecular, neural circuitry, and behavioural levels of investigation [31, 34, 35].

### Neuroimaging studies using pattern recognition approaches

A key criticism of neuroimaging studies is their reliance upon group-level statistics, rather than providing data that are useful at the individual level. If neuroimaging techniques are to provide clinically relevant information, then useful individual-level measures of brain structure and function need to be obtained from these techniques. One recent advance has been to combine neuroimaging with pattern recognition approaches, which develop algorithms to automatically learn and recognize complex patterns to inform decision-making based on large data sets. Studies combining these approaches have been able to help classify individuals, case by case, into different diagnostic categories, including bipolar disorder vs major depression, based on their patterns of neural activity [36, 37] and grey and white matter structure [38]; bipolar disorder vs schizophrenia, based on grey matter structure [39]; and youth with bipolar disorder vs healthy youth, based on grey matter structure [40]; and also accurately discriminated between individual healthy youth at high genetic risk vs those at low risk for future bipolar disorder

[41]. Combining neuroimaging with pattern recognition techniques thus holds much promise for future elucidation of clinically useful, individual-level biomarkers to inform diagnosis, risk identification, and personalized treatment choice.

### Limitations of extant studies

There are many limitations of existing neuroimaging studies in bipolar disorder. Firstly, the majority of studies, especially studies employing fMRI or resting state, recruited relatively modest (for example, <30) numbers of participants per group, thereby allowing only limited conclusions about the generalizability of the findings to the wider population of individuals with bipolar disorder. Similarly, there are few studies comparing individuals with bipolar disorder across different mood states and few replication findings, especially for fMRI and resting state studies. For resting state studies, this is likely due to the different resting state methodologies used, in addition to modest sample sizes. Many studies focused solely on a priori prefrontal cortical–subcortical regions of interest, with little reporting of findings in other regions, thereby limiting inferences about potential roles of other neural circuitries in bipolar disorder. Furthermore, there is a dearth of neuroimaging studies directly comparing different bipolar disorder subtypes (for example, bipolar disorder type I vs bipolar disorder type II) or bipolar disorder vs other major psychiatric disorders (for example, schizophrenia). It is therefore difficult to determine the extent to which bipolar disorder subtypes or different psychiatric disorders share, or are distinguished by, underlying neural mechanisms. Such studies can identify neural biomarkers reflecting these neural mechanisms that can aid diagnosis and treatment choice, particularly for those disorders that are often difficult to distinguish, based on clinical assessment alone, for example, bipolar disorder type I vs bipolar disorder type II, bipolar disorder types I and II vs major depressive disorder, and bipolar disorder vs schizophrenia. There are also few multimodal neuroimaging studies examining relationships between structure and function in neural circuitries of interest in bipolar disorder, or between resting and task-related functional connectivity in these neural circuitries in bipolar disorder. These studies will facilitate more in-depth understanding of the neural mechanisms underlying bipolar disorder.

Another major criticism is the potentially confounding effects of psychotropic medication upon neuroimaging measures. An increasing number of studies in bipolar disorder suggest that psychotropic medications either have normalizing effects on neuroimaging measures or do not significantly impact these measures [42], although, as is apparent from these studies, lithium in particular may have neurotrophic effects in some neural regions in bipolar disorder, while antipsychotic medications are associated with grey matter decreases [43]. Further studies are thus needed to determine the nature of effects of specific medications on neural circuitries of interest in bipolar disorder. Longitudinal neuroimaging studies examining individuals pre- and post-medication can address this important point, as can large cross-sectional studies comparing medication-free individuals with those taking different medication types.

## Summary

The field of neuroimaging in bipolar disorder is progressing considerably, with findings from these studies making significant contributions to understanding of the neuropathophysiology of bipolar disorder [4]. To move the field forward, the next wave of bipolar disorder neuroimaging studies should aim to adopt the following strategies. Firstly, studies should examine emotion processing, emotion regulation, and reward neural circuitry functional, structural, white matter, and intrinsic connectivity abnormalities associated with dimensions of pathological behaviours that cut across conventionally defined bipolar disorder and other mood disorder diagnostic categories. These studies should also include longitudinal designs to identify the extent to which alterations in these neural circuitry abnormalities are associated with changes in affective state. This approach has potential to identify neural circuitry markers that better reflect neuropathophysiological processes in bipolar disorder and other mood disorders and the nature of neural mechanisms underlying abnormal mood switches. Secondly, studies should examine developmental trajectories of these neural circuitries in individuals with bipolar disorder across the lifespan and in at-risk youth, with longitudinal follow-up designs. This approach will identify neural circuitry markers that can help identify those individuals at highest risk of developing future affective pathology, and thereby pave the way forward for studies that utilize these markers to guide early intervention and prevention strategies. Thirdly, studies should incorporate multimodal neuroimaging techniques and biological system level approaches, to examine the impact of genetic variation and molecular-level processes upon neural circuitry development in at-risk individuals and individuals with bipolar disorder and other mood disorders. Fourthly, studies should take advantage of advances in the application of pattern recognition techniques to neuroimaging to identify individual-level neural circuitry markers that not only help classify individuals into present diagnostic groups, but also help predict individual-level future clinical course. Fifthly, collectively, these four approaches will help elucidate more complex neuropathophysiological processes underlying the dimensions of abnormal behaviours associated with affective pathology and yield individual-level biological markers reflecting these processes that have clinical utility for diagnosis, future illness development prediction, and guiding personalized treatment choice in at-risk and mood-disordered individuals.

## REFERENCES

1. Goodwin FK, Jamison KR, Ghaemi SN. *Manic-depressive Illness: Bipolar Disorders and Recurrent Depression* (2nd edn). New York, NY: Oxford University Press; 2007.
2. Davis M, Whalen PJ. The amygdala: vigilance and emotion. *Mol Psychiatry*. 2001;6:13–34.
3. Phillips ML, Ladouceur CD, Drevets WC. A neural model of voluntary and automatic emotion regulation: implications for understanding the pathophysiology and neurodevelopment of bipolar disorder. *Mol Psychiatry*. 2008;13:829, 833–57.
4. Phillips ML, Swartz HA. A critical appraisal of neuroimaging studies of bipolar disorder: toward a new conceptualization of underlying neural circuitry and a road map for future research. *Am J Psychiatry*. 2014;171:829–43.
5. Chase HW, Phillips ML. Elucidating neural network functional connectivity abnormalities in bipolar disorder: toward a harmonized methodological approach. *Biol Psychiatry Cogn Neurosci Neuroimaging*. 2016;1:288–98.
6. Wise RA. Dopamine, learning and motivation. *Nat Rev Neurosci*. 2004;5:483–94.
7. Noonan MP, Kolling N, Walton ME, Rushworth MF. Re-evaluating the role of the orbitofrontal cortex in reward and reinforcement. *Eur J Neurosci*. 2012;35:997–1010.
8. Rogers RD, Ramnani N, Mackay C, et al. Distinct portions of anterior cingulate cortex and medial prefrontal cortex are activated by reward processing in separable phases of decision-making cognition. *Biol Psychiatry*. 2004;55:594–602.
9. Soares JC, Mann JJ. The anatomy of mood disorders--review of structural neuroimaging studies. *Biol Psychiatry*. 1997;41:86–106.
10. Altshuler LL, Bartzokis G, Grieder T, Curran J, Mintz J. Amygdala enlargement in bipolar disorder and hippocampal reduction in schizophrenia: an MRI study demonstrating neuroanatomic specificity. *Arch Gen Psychiatry*. 1998;55:663–64.
11. Strakowski SM, DelBello MP, Sax KW, et al. Brain magnetic resonance imaging of structural abnormalities in bipolar disorder. *Arch Gen Psychiatry*. 1999;56:254 60.
12. Hajek T, Cullis J, Novak T, et al. Brain structural signature of familial predisposition for bipolar disorder: replicable evidence for involvement of the right inferior frontal gyrus. *Biol Psychiatry*. 2013;73:144–52.
13. Pfeifer JC, Welge J, Strakowski SM, Adler CM, DelBello MP. Meta-analysis of amygdala volumes in children and adolescents with bipolar disorder. *J Am Acad Child Adolesc Psychiatry*. 2008;47:1289–98.
14. Leow A, Ajilore O, Zhan L, et al. Impaired inter-hemispheric integration in bipolar disorder revealed with brain network analyses. *Biol Psychiatry*. 2013;73:183–93.
15. Lewandowski KE, Ongür D, Sperry SH, et al. Myelin vs axon abnormalities in white matter in bipolar disorder. *Neuropsychopharmacology*. 2015;40:1243–9.
16. Savitz JB, Price JL, Drevets WC. Neuropathological and neuromorphometric abnormalities in bipolar disorder: view from the medial prefrontal cortical network. *Neurosci Biobehav Rev*. 2014;42:132–47.
17. Konradi C, Sillivan SE, Clay HB. Mitochondria, oligodendrocytes and inflammation in bipolar disorder: evidence from transcriptome studies points to intriguing parallels with multiple sclerosis. *Neurobiol Dis*. 2012;45:37–47.
18. Dager SR, Friedman SD, Parow A, et al. Brain metabolic alterations in medication-free patients with bipolar disorder. *Arch Gen Psychiatry*. 2004;61:450–8.
19. Savitz JB, Drevets WC. Neuroreceptor imaging in depression. *Neurobiol Dis*. 2013;52:49–65.
20. Price JL, Drevets WC. Neural circuits underlying the pathophysiology of mood disorders. *Trends Cogn Sci*. 2012;16:61–71.
21. Drevets WC, Price JL, Simpson JR, et al. Subgenual prefrontal cortex abnormalities in mood disorders. *Nature*. 1997;386:824–7.
22. Haarman BCB, Riemersma-Van der Lek RF, de Groot JC, et al. Neuroinflammation in bipolar disorder–A [11 C]-(R)-PK11195 positron emission tomography study. *Brain Behav Immun*. 2014;40:219–25.
23. Savitz J, Dantzer R, Wurfel BE, et al. Neuroprotective kynurenine metabolite indices are abnormally reduced and positively associated with hippocampal and amygdalar volume in bipolar disorder. *Psychoneuroendocrinology*. 2015;52:200–11.
24. Steiner J, Walter M, Gos T, et al. Severe depression is associated with increased microglial quinolinic acid in subregions of the anterior cingulate gyrus: evidence for an immune-modulated

glutamatergic neurotransmission? *J Neuroinflammation*. 2011;8:1.

25. Martino M, Magioncalda P, Huang Z, *et al*. Contrasting variability patterns in the default mode and sensorimotor networks balance in bipolar depression and mania. *PNAS*. 2016;113:4824–9.

26. Caseras X, Lawrence NS, Murphy K, Wise RG, Phillips ML. Ventral dtriatum activity in response to reward: differences between bipolar I and II disorders. *Am J Psychiatry*. 2013;170:533–41.

27. Judd LL, Akiskal HS, Schettler PJ, *et al*. The comparative clinical phenotype and long term longitudinal episode course of bipolar I and II: a clinical spectrum or distinct disorders? *J Affect Disord*. 2003;73:19–32.

28. Maina G, Albert U, Bellodi L, *et al*. Health-related quality of life in euthymic bipolar disorder patients: differences between bipolar I and II subtypes. *J Clin Psychiatry*. 2007;68:207–12.

29. Anticevic A, Savic A, Repovs G, *et al*. Ventral anterior cingulate connectivity distinguished nonpsychotic bipolar illness from psychotic bipolar disorder and schizophrenia. *Schizophrenia Bull*. 2015;41:133–43.

30. Padmanabhan JL, Tandon N, Haller CS, *et al*. Correlations between brain structure and symptom dimensions of psychosis in schizophrenia, schizoaffective, and psychotic bipolar I disorders. *Schizophrenia Bull*. 2015;41:154–62.

31. Phillips ML, Kupfer DJ. Bipolar disorder diagnosis: challenges and future directions. *Lancet*. 2013;381:1663–71.

32. Frank E, Nimgaonkar VL, Phillips ML, Kupfer DJ. All the world's a (clinical) stage: rethinking bipolar disorder from a longitudinal perspective. *Mol Psychiatry*. 2015;20:23–31.

33. Fusar-Poli P, Howes O, Bechdolf A, Borgwardt S. Mapping vulnerability to bipolar disorder: a systematic review and meta-analysis of neuroimaging studies. *J Psychiatry Neurosci*. 2012;37:170–84.

34. McIntosh AM. Toward a systems biology of mood disorder. *Biol Psychiatry*. 2013;73:107–8.

35. Phillips ML. Brain-behavior biomarkers of illness and illness risk in bipolar disorder: present findings and next steps. *Biol Psychiatry*. 2013;74:870–1.

36. Almeida JR, Mourao-Miranda J, Aizenstein HJ, *et al*. Pattern recognition analysis of anterior cingulate cortex blood flow to classify depression polarity. *Br J Psychiatry*. 2013;203:310–11.

37. Grotegerd D, Stuhrmann A, Kugel H, *et al*. Amygdala excitability to subliminally presented emotional faces distinguishes unipolar and bipolar depression: an fMRI and pattern classification study. *Hum Brain Mapp*. 2014;35:2995–3007.

38. Redlich R, Almeida JR, Grotegerd D, *et al*. Brain morphometric biomarkers distinguishing unipolar and bipolar depression: a voxel-based morphometry–pattern classification approach. *JAMA Psychiatry*. 2014;71:1222–30.

39. Schnack HG, Nieuwenhuis M, van Haren NE, *et al*. Can structural MRI aid in clinical classification? A machine learning study in two independent samples of patients with schizophrenia, bipolar disorder and healthy subjects. *Neuroimage*. 2014;84:299–306.

40. Mwangi B, Spiker D, Zunta-Soares GB, Soares JC. Prediction of pediatric bipolar disorder using neuroanatomical signatures of the amygdala. *Bipolar Disord*. 2014;16:713–21.

41. Mourao-Miranda J, Oliveira L, Ladouceur CD, *et al*. Pattern recognition and functional neuroimaging help to discriminate healthy adolescents at risk for mood disorders from low risk adolescents. *PLoS One*. 2012;7:e29482.

42. Hafeman DM, Chang KD, Garrett AS, Sanders EM, Phillips ML. Effects of medication on neuroimaging findings in bipolar disorder: an updated review. *Bipolar Disord*. 2012;14:375–410.

43. Moncrieff J, Leo J. A systematic review of the effects of antipsychotic drugs on brain volume. *Psychol Med*. 2010;40:1409–22.

# 72

# Management and treatment of bipolar disorder

*Eduard Vieta, Isabella Pacchiarotti, and David J. Miklowitz*

## Pharmacological treatment of bipolar disorder

### Introduction

The pharmacological treatment of bipolar disorder (BD) is complex because it combines different therapeutic approaches and needs to take into account acute phases and long-term management [1, 2]. Several factors are involved in the treatment choice such as the predominant polarity [3], the risk of suicide, the treatment adherence, and the polarity index of a drug [4, 5]. Clinical guidelines have been published recently on the latest developments on pharmacological treatment of BD [6–10]. A summary of the clinical management of BD is synthesized in Table 72.1.

The challenge of treating bipolar disorder in women in the perinatal period is considered in some detail in Chapter 73.

### Mania and mixed states

The treatment of mania aims at managing the core manic symptoms and psychosis, at reducing any behavioural component typically associated with this condition, and at minimizing the risk of side effects in order to improve treatment adherence [11, 12].

A recent meta-analytic review ($N = 13{,}073$) [13] found that dopamine antagonists/partial agonists are more effective than anticonvulsants for the treatment of manic episodes, making them the most appropriate short-term choice for mania. Haloperidol, risperidone, and olanzapine (OLZ) were ranked as the most effective. Quetiapine (QTP), risperidone, and OLZ showed the best results for tolerability.

Another recent meta-analysis showed the efficacy for mania of aripiprazole (ARP), asenapine (ASN), cariprazine, haloperidol, OLZ, paliperidone (PAL), QTP, risperidone, and ziprasidone (ZIP), in comparison with placebo [14]. A network meta-analysis performed by the same author found that ARP, OLZ, QTP, risperidone, and valproate (VPA) had lower all-cause discontinuation rates than placebo. Moreover, sensitivity analysis by drug class indicated similar efficacy profiles for haloperidol, newer dopamine antagonists/partial agonists, and mood stabilizers [15].

The availability of injectable extended-release formulations (of OLZ, risperidone, ARP, PAL, and ZIP) may also represent a therapeutic option in mania, with the aim to improve treatment adherence [16].

Combined treatment with lithium or VPA and a dopamine antagonist/partial agonist should be considered when patients show breakthrough mania with the first agent [6–10].

### Bipolar depression

In contrast to the treatment of mania, enthusiasm for pharmacological strategies in BD depression is tempered by uncertainty, despite the high burden and prevalence of this phase of BD [17, 18]. Currently, none of the available antidepressants (that is, drugs licensed for the indication of major depression in a unipolar illness course) is officially recognized as monotherapy for the treatment of BD despite their common use in clinical practice. To date, only QTP (approved by the FDA and EMA), OLZ–fluoxetine combination, and lurasidone (LUR) (approved in some countries, but not by EMA) have regulatory approval for BD depression.

OLZ has been found to be effective in BD depression both in monotherapy and in association with fluoxetine [19, 20]. The efficacy of QTP monotherapy for the treatment of BD depression has been demonstrated in two placebo RCTs of similar design [21, 22]. Another two subsequent RCTs showed some superiority of QTP monotherapy over both lithium and paroxetine in BD depressive episodes [23, 24]. Two recent RCTs have demonstrated the efficacy of LUR monotherapy or in combination with lithium or VPA in BD depressed patients [25]. A more recent study of adjunctive LUR found that the significant improvement in depressive symptoms on the Montgomery-Åsberg Depression Rating Scale (MADRS) from weeks 2 to 5 disappeared at week 6 [26].

Despite preliminary evidence suggesting a possible beneficial effect of adjunctive ARP on BD depression [27], two subsequent RCTs failed to find any significant superiority of ARP over placebo [28].

With respect to lithium and anticonvulsants, use of lithium in monotherapy for an episode of BD depression seems to have no support, based on available evidence [23]. Nonetheless, for its proven effectiveness as prophylaxis of BD, as an augmentation strategy of unipolar depression, and for its effect in preventing the risk of suicide [29], lithium continues to be considered as a first-choice

**Table 72.1** Pharmacological management of bipolar disorder (BD) in mania, depression, and maintenance phases[1]

| | Clinical management[1] | | | Advantages | Disadvantages |
|---|---|---|---|---|---|
| | Mania | Depression | Maintenance | | |
| **Mood stabilizers** | | | | | |
| Valproate | +++ | + | ++ | Useful in BD episodes with mixed features<br>Prophylactic effect in BD<br>Possible effect in bipolar depression | CYP450 inhibitor, not recommended in women at childbearing age<br>Hyponatraemia |
| Lamotrigine | – – – | ++ | +++ | Predominant depressive polarity, depressive recurrences<br>Possible effect in bipolar depression | Slow titration<br>Risk of rush |
| Lithium | +++ | ++ | +++ | Anti-suicidal properties, prophylaxis in BD, manic-predominant polarity | Not recommended in renal failure |
| Carbamazepine | +++ | + | ++ | Prophylactic effect in BD, less effective than lithium and valproate, in BD with non-classical features | CYP450 inducer<br>Effects on leucocyte count |
| Oxcarbazepine | + | | + | Fewer adverse effects than carbamazepine.<br>Prophylactic effect in BD, less effective than lithium and valproate, in BD with non-classical features | Hyponatraemia |
| **Antipsychotics** | | | | | |
| Aripiprazole | +++ | – | ++ | Manic-predominant polarity, lower rates of discontinuation<br>Intramuscular long-acting formulation available | Akathisia |
| Asenapine | +++ | + | + | Manic-predominant polarity<br>Possible treatment of BD with mixed features | Moderate metabolic syndrome<br>Efficacy related to feeding |
| Lurasidone | | +++ | | Predominant depressive polarity<br>Approved by FDA for bipolar disorder | Akathisia, sedation |
| Olanzapine | +++ | +++[2] | ++ | Manic-predominant polarity, manic recurrences<br>Intramuscular long-acting formulation available<br>Olanzapine + fluoxetine approved by FDA in bipolar depression | Severe metabolic syndrome |
| Paliperidone | ++ | – | ++ | Manic-predominant polarity<br>Intramuscular formulation available<br>Minimal liver metabolism | High doses are often needed<br>Hyperprolactinaemia |
| Quetiapine | +++ | +++ | +++ | The only antipsychotic with indications for both acute episodes and maintenance in BD, for manic- and depressive-predominant polarity. Approved by FDA and EMA for bipolar depression | Sedation |
| Risperidone | ++ | – | ++ | Manic-predominant polarity, prevention of manic relapses, not depressive (risperidone long-acting injectable) | Risk of switch to depression, EPS<br>Hyperprolactinaemia |
| Ziprasidone | ++ | | ++ | Manic-predominant polarity<br>Intramuscular long-acting formulation available | Good metabolic profile |
| **Antidepressants** | | | | | |
| | – – | + | + | Controversial issue. Not in monotherapy in BDI disorder. Applicable in resistant bipolar depression combined with mood stabilizers in individual cases | Risk of switch to mania, mixed states and rapid cycling, mood destabilization |

CYP, cytochrome; EPS, extra-pyramidal symptoms.

[1] Reported clinical management reflects our interpretation of available evidence and do not necessarily imply regulatory endorsement. For further information, refer to guidelines [6–10]. The list includes some clinically significant adverse effects which can be experienced by a fraction of patients exposed. This list is by no means exhaustive and is not meant as a comparison between the different drugs.

[2] Olanzapine + fluoxetine.

+++, highly recommended; ++, very recommended; +, recommended; –, not much recommended; – –, not recommended; – – –, not at all recommended.

strategy in BDI depression by many guidelines on BD, as well as in clinical practice [9].

Use of VPA monotherapy for BD depression was supported in a recent review and meta-analysis of four small studies [30]. The effect of lamotrigine (LTG) on BD depression appeared weak in a first analysis of five double-blind RCTs [31]. However, more recent studies on LTG, mostly as adjunctive treatment to lithium or QTP, found a modest effect in BD depression [32–34]. Some clinical guidelines consider it as a first- or second-choice therapeutic strategy for the treatment of acute depressive phase [7].

One of the most controversial issue in BD is the use of ADs, since it has been associated with the risk of (hypo-) manic or mixed switch, with the risk of suicide or with a rapid cycling course [18, 35–38]. The International Society for Bipolar Disorders (ISBD) has recently assembled an international group of experts to find a clinically and evidence-based consensus on this issue [39]. They concluded that the use of ADs to treat depressive phases of BD should neither be condemned nor endorsed without carefully evaluating individual clinical cases. In general, antidepressant monotherapy should be avoided in BD. If ADs are used, they should be prescribed along with an anti-manic treatment. In BD types I and II depression, with two or more concomitant core manic symptoms and with a history of rapid cycling or mood instability, ADs should be used with caution, due to the risk of worsening of the illness course. Treatment with some ADs in BD type II appears to be otherwise relatively well tolerated. Multi-functional ADs acting on serotonergic and adrenergic systems appear to carry a particularly high risk of inducing pathologically elevated states of mood and behaviour and should be used with caution [39].

During the last years, new therapeutic strategies have been investigated for the treatment of BD depression. Limited evidence of efficacy in BD depression has been found for the dopaminergic drug modafinil and its R-enantiomer armodafinil [40, 41].

Several lines of research have suggested dysfunction of N-methyl-D-aspartate (NMDA) receptors could play an important role in the pathophysiology of BD [42], and a single intravenous dose of the NMDA receptor antagonist ketamine has been found to be effective in treating severe and resistant acute BD depression. Unfortunately, this effect is relatively short-lasting, so that finding a place in the long-term treatment is problematic [43, 44].

## Maintenance phase

The primary objectives of maintenance treatment of BD are preventing new (hypo)manic/mixed or depressive episodes and suicidal behaviour and improving residual symptoms and treatment adherence, but also optimizing functional recovery and quality of life [2].

In considering long-term treatment, the predominant polarity of the individual's illness [45] and the polarity index (PI) of any drug [4, 5] should be taken into account. The PI indicates the relative effectiveness in preventing mania against the efficacy in preventing depression of drugs commonly used for maintenance treatment of BD (Fig. 72.1); it is calculated as the ratio of the number needed to treat (NNT) for the prevention of depression and the NNT for preventing mania, based on the results of relevant RCTs for maintenance treatment of BD.

A PI >1 indicates a greater relative anti-manic prophylactic polarity; a PI <1 indicates a greater relative antidepressant prophylactic polarity, while a PI near to 1 indicates similar relative manic and antidepressant prophylaxis, so a possible ideal 'mood stabilizer'.

A predominantly anti-manic PI was found for PAL, ARP, risperidone (long-acting injectable, RLai), and ZIP, followed by OLZ, ASN, and lithium. Of all the agents tested, QTP presented a PI closest to 1. A predominantly antidepressant PI was found for LTG, oxcarbazepine (OXC), and VPA. From available recent data (not fully published), LUR would represent the first dopamine antagonist with a PI inferior to 1, so predominantly an antidepressant. The PI for VPA and OXC appears <1 but should be interpreted with caution because clinical trials for these two drugs showed no statistical superiority over placebo. In general, anticonvulsants (VPA, OXC, and LTG) appear to be slightly more effective in preventing depressive episodes, while dopamine antagonists/partial agonists (with the exception of QTP and LUR) and lithium are more effective in preventing mania. In maintenance, monotherapy is the goal, but combination treatment is often needed. Typical combinations are lithium or VPA with OLZ, QTP, LTG, or ARP, especially in patients with a depressive-predominant polarity or in the absence of a predominance of polarity. When monotherapy is preferred, in patients with a manic-predominant polarity, lithium, risperidone (RIS), ZIP, ARP, PAL, ASN, and OLZ can be used, while LTG and LUR should be used when depression prevails during the course of the illness.

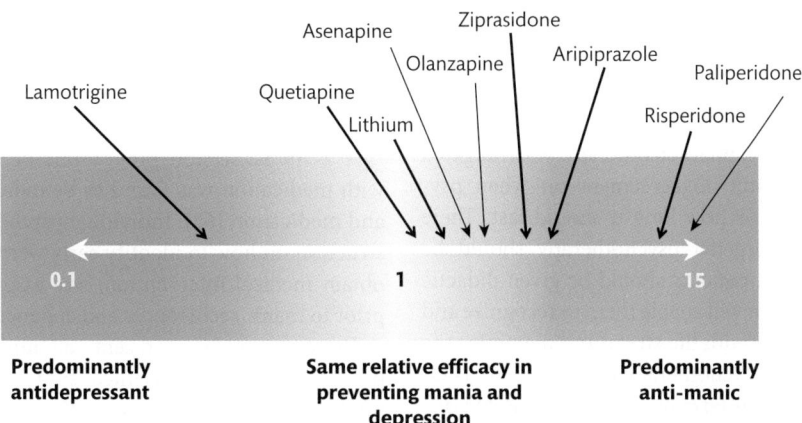

**Fig. 72.1** Long-term relative efficacy according to the polarity index.

RCT data suggest QTP monotherapy should prevent both phases of the illness (Fig. 72.1).

Regarding the efficacy of mood stabilizers and lithium during maintenance, lithium remains the most effective treatment in preventing manic relapses and, less effectively, depressive relapses and in reducing the risk of suicide and hospitalizations [29, 46].

The efficacy of LTG in preventing depression in BD patients with a predominantly depressive polarity is considered the true strength of this drug [47].

VPA monotherapy is considered less effective than lithium in the prevention of relapse and more effective in depressive relapses, and should not usually be considered for women of childbearing potential [48].

Carbamazepine (CBZ) monotherapy is less effective than lithium in preventing recurrences, and the main risk is the unsafe side effect profile and interference with the metabolism of other drugs [17]. OLZ has been studied as a comparator to depot risperidone (RLai) and showed a reduction in manic and depressive relapses [49].

The long-term use of LUR was demonstrated by a recent 28-week study of continued treatment with LUR plus lithium or VPA, with a trend in reduction in time to recurrence of any mood event, compared with placebo, and a significant reduction in time to recurrence of a depressive episode [50]. ARP in monotherapy has shown superiority over placebo for acute and continuation treatment of mania (no depression), with low rates of discontinuation [15, 51]. Similarly, ZIP and PAL have demonstrated a positive effect in preventing manic recurrences [52, 53].

The use of injectable formulations (LAIs) in long-term treatment may be considered in cases of poor adherence (that is, more than 30% of BD patients) [54]. LAIs could be used in BD patients where the treatment plan is continuation with dopamine antagonists, but adherence to oral medication is poor. The available data for LAI risperidone are positive for preventing mania, but not depression [49, 55]. PAL extended-release significantly delayed the time to recurrence of any mood symptoms vs placebo in a randomized study of maintenance treatment in patients with BD after an acute manic or mixed episode [53].

Evidence for the long-term prophylactic effect of antidepressant treatment of patients with BD type I or II remains poorly studied, despite common clinical use of antidepressants; the ideal use is always in combination with an anti-manic drug [39].

## Psychosocial management of bipolar disorder

Given the high rates of recurrence among patients with BD when maintained on standard pharmacotherapy [56], effective clinical practice recommends combining pharmacotherapy with targeted psychotherapy. There is currently no agreement on when psychotherapy should be initiated or how long it should last. There is, however, agreement that targeted psychotherapy should be *psychoeducational*, meaning that patients should be given didactic instructions and skill training that will enable them to recognize and manage their mood swings, cope with life stress, and maximize the quality of life. Several forms of psychotherapy have emerged as effective in the stabilization and long-term maintenance of BD in different age groups [57–59].

### Psychoeducational approaches

In structured group psychoeducation, between eight and 12 patients with BD meet weekly for a group session led by a mental health clinician and focusing on illness awareness, treatment compliance, early detection of prodromal symptoms and recurrences, and lifestyle regularity. Colom et al. [60] assessed the efficacy of group psychoeducation among 120 adult patients with bipolar type I who had been in remission for at least 6 months. All patients received mood-stabilizing medications. One group received 21 weekly sessions of structured group psychoeducation, and the other group 21 non-didactic group support sessions. At the end of 2 years, fewer of the group psychoeducation patients (67%) than the control patients (92%) had relapsed, and fewer had been hospitalized. The group differences remained over a 5-year post-treatment follow-up [61].

A replication study was carried out in Brazil [62]. A total of 55 bipolar type I and II outpatients in remission received 16 sessions of group psychoeducation (using the Colom et al. model) or 16 sessions of a 'matched' (that is, non-randomized) group placebo treatment. Over 1 year, there were no differential effects of group psychoeducation on recurrence or psychosocial functioning, although patients in group psychoeducation subjectively reported more clinical improvement. Non-randomized selection of the comparison participants may have attenuated treatment effects.

Two large-scale studies examined group psychoeducation within the context of larger care management programmes. Bauer et al. [63] compared 'collaborative care management' (CCM) for 306 BD patients treated at 11 U.S. Department of Veterans Affairs sites. The core of treatment—the Life Goals programme—emphasized illness management skills. CCM also included enhanced access to care through a nurse co-ordinator and support for physicians to follow medication practice guidelines. Over 3 years, patients in CCM spent fewer weeks in manic episodes and had greater improvements in social functioning and quality of life than patients who received care as usual.

In a group health network, Simon et al. [64] randomly assigned 441 patients to a similar care management intervention or to treatment as usual (TAU). Care management consisted of pharmacotherapy, group psychoeducation sessions, telephone-based monitoring, interdisciplinary care planning, and relapse prevention planning. Over 2 years, patients in care management had significantly lower mania scores and spent less time in manic or hypomanic episodes than those in TAU, but there were no effects on depressive symptoms. Both studies strongly support the beneficial effects of psychoeducation about illness management. It was not possible to determine the unique contributions of each treatment component to outcomes.

A 7- to 12-session programme of individual psychoeducation with medication was found to be more effective than routine care and medication [65]. Individual psychoeducation, consisting of instruction on how to identify early warning signs of recurrence and obtain medical intervention, was associated with longer intervals prior to manic recurrences and enhanced social functioning.

There have been recent attempts to test the effects of psychoeducationally oriented clinics on the course of BD. In a randomized trial in Denmark, Kessing et al. [66] assigned 158 patients to treatment in a specialized outpatient clinic that integrated pharmacotherapy with group psychoeducation or to a standard care outpatient clinic. There was an overall beneficial effect of psychoeducationally oriented clinics on rehospitalization, but also a statistical trend for those between the ages of 18 and 25 years to benefit more than those over the age of 25. This study may indicate that younger (or less recurrent) patients may benefit more from psychoeducation than older and more recurrent patients.

In summary, group psychoeducation and individual relapse prevention strategies are effective adjuncts to pharmacotherapy in reducing the risk of mood relapses. Studies that examine treatments at the clinic level, rather than the individual patient level, may be quite informative for community dissemination.

## Functional remediation

A multi-site study in Spain has examined the effectiveness of 21 90-minute sessions of functional remediation, in comparison with 21 sessions of structured psychoeducation groups [61] or TAU [67]. All patients received medication management. Functional remediation addresses neurocognitive issues through exercises to enhance memory, attention, problem-solving, reasoning, multitasking, and organization. In 183 euthymic patients who completed 21 weeks of treatment, functional remediation was more effective than TAU and as equally effective as structured psychoeducation in enhancing functioning.

## Family intervention approaches

Family interventions for BD first appeared in the 1970s (for example, [68]). Miklowitz and Goldstein [69, 70] developed family-focused treatment (FFT) for patients with BD who had just had an episode of mania or depression. This approach, given in 21 sessions over 9 months, consists of psychoeducation about BD for the patient and family members (parents, siblings, spouse), to assist in identifying and intervening in prodromal symptoms of relapse; communication enhancement training, and problem-solving skills training. The core assumption of FFT is that enhancing knowledge of BD, reducing high expressed emotion (critical, hostile, or overprotective attitudes in caregivers), and enhancing family interactions will promote environments that are protective against relapses.

In the Colorado Treatment/Outcome study [71], BD type I patients who were in the process of recovering from an acute episode (N = 101) were randomly assigned to 9 months of FFT with pharmacotherapy or crisis management (CM) (two sessions of family psychoeducation plus crisis intervention sessions) with pharmacotherapy. Over 2 years, patients in FFT were three times more likely to complete the study without relapsing (52% vs 17%) and had longer periods of stability without relapse (73.5 weeks vs 53.2 weeks) than those in CM. They also had greater improvements over time in depression, less severe manic symptoms, and better adherence to medications than patients in CM.

Rea and colleagues [72] compared FFT plus pharmacotherapy to an equally intensive (21 sessions), individually focused psychoeducational treatment plus pharmacotherapy for BD type I patients who had just been hospitalized for a manic episode (N = 53). Over a 1- to 2-year post-treatment follow-up, patients in FFT had much lower rates of rehospitalization (12%) and symptomatic relapse (28%) than patients in individual therapy (60% and 60%, respectively). There were no differences between the groups in medication regimens or adherence over 2 years.

## Family focused treatment for adolescents with bipolar disorder

In a two-site randomized trial, Miklowitz et al. [73] assigned 58 adolescents with BD type I, type II, or not otherwise specified to a developmentally appropriate version of FFT (FFT-A) plus pharmacotherapy or a 3-session 'enhanced care' (EC) family psychoeducational treatment plus pharmacotherapy. Over 2 years, adolescents in FFT-A had more rapid time to recovery from depressive symptoms, less time in depressive episodes, and greater stabilization of depressive symptoms over 2 years than adolescents in EC. Comparable effects were not observed on manic or mixed symptoms. A secondary analysis revealed that adolescents in high expressed emotion families showed greater reductions in both mania and depression if they received FFT-A than if they received EC [74, 75].

A second trial involving three study sites and 145 adolescents with BD type I or II did not replicate these results [76]. Adolescents in FFT-A and the 3-session EC comparator did not differ in time to recovery from their acute episode at study entry or in time to relapse over 2 years. However, the stage of treatment had a moderating effect on FFT-A; during the 1-year post-treatment phase, adolescents in FFT-A had significantly lower mania symptom scores than those in EC, and significantly higher quality of life scores. Families may need time to absorb communication, problem-solving, and relapse prevention skills that are the focus of FFT. Once skills are put into use, family environments may become more protective against mood exacerbations in bipolar illness.

## Family focused treatment for children at risk for bipolar disorder

FFT has been tested in children and adolescents who are at risk for BD—those with a family history of BD type I or II plus a current diagnosis in the child of major depressive disorder (MDD), BD not elsewhere classified (NEC: recurrent manic or hypomanic phases that do not meet the DSM-5 duration criteria), or cyclothymic disorder. In a 1-year RCT, 40 high-risk children (aged 9–17) with MDD or BD-NEC were randomly assigned to either 12 sessions of FFT high-risk version (FFT-HR) or a 1- or 2-session education control [77]. The FFT-HR focused on mood management, sleep/wake rhythm regulation, and communication/problem-solving exercises to reduce family tension. The participants in FFT-HR demonstrated more rapid recovery from their initial mood symptoms, more weeks in remission from mood symptoms, and more improvement in hypomania symptoms over 1 year than participants in the education control. Once again, the largest treatment effect sizes were among children in high expressed emotion families.

FFT is only one approach to family intervention. Reinares et al. [78] examined 12 sessions of group psychoeducation for caregivers of adult BD patients (for example, early detection of prodromes, promoting healthy sleep), stress management strategies, and encouraging self-care through expanding one's social network, exercise, and other means. Compared to usual care, caregiver psychoeducation groups were associated with longer time to manic recurrence in patients over 18 months. Caregivers also had increased knowledge of how to manage BD, decreases in subjective feelings of burden, and fewer attributions of blame towards the patients [78].

Other investigators have examined family intervention protocols that are more suited to younger bipolar patients. Multiple family groups [79] and a 12-session integrated programme of individual CBT and FFT sessions known as the 'Rainbow' programme [80] were both found to be effective in randomized trials for children with bipolar spectrum disorders (aged 12 or under).

## Cognitive behavioural therapy

CBT aims to modify maladaptive thoughts through restructuring of patients' self-defeating thoughts or beliefs and behavioural components such as scheduling pleasurable events to improve mood. Therapy usually incorporates problem-solving and interpersonal skills training as well. Several major trials of CBT have been conducted in BD. These trials have tested CBT manuals that differed to some extent (for example, whether or not patients were assumed to be in remission or not), which may, in part, explain the disparate results.

Lam and colleagues [81], compared pharmacotherapy plus 6 months of CBT (12–18 sessions) with pharmacotherapy plus TAU for 103 patients in remission from mood episodes. At 1 year, relapse rates were 44% in CBT and 75% in usual care. Patients in CBT also spent fewer days in illness episodes. One year to 30 months after treatment, CBT no longer prevented relapse, relative to usual care, but continued to show a positive influence on mood symptoms [82]. Unlike the individual psychoeducation study [65], the effects of CBT were stronger on depression than on mania.

A UK trial conducted across five sites [83] compared 22 sessions of CBT plus medication to TAU plus medication for 253 patients who began in various clinical states. No effects of CBT vs TAU were observed on time to recurrence over 18 months. A post hoc analysis revealed that patients with fewer than 12 prior episodes had fewer recurrences if treated with CBT than with TAU, whereas the opposite pattern was apparent among patients with 12 or more episodes. It is not clear whether patients with fewer than 12 episodes were less ill/episodic or younger or had been ill for fewer years than patients with 12 or more episodes.

In a four-site Canadian trial [84], 204 patients were randomly assigned to 20 weekly sessions of CBT or to six group psychoeducation sessions (using Bauer and McBride's Life Goals [63] programme) with pharmacotherapy. There were no differences in relapses or symptom severity over 72 weeks. Group treatment was clearly the more cost-effective alternative in this study.

Meyer and Hautzinger [85] examined 76 patients in a variety of clinical states who were randomly assigned to CBT plus pharmacotherapy (20 therapy sessions over 9 months) or an equally intensive individual supportive therapy plus pharmacotherapy. Over 33 months, there were no differences between the groups in relapse or time to relapse.

Thus, no RCT has shown the superiority of CBT over other forms of therapy matched on duration and the number of sessions. Meta-regression analyses of the psychosocial treatment literature may be able to specify the conditions under which CBT is effective in BD. Trials have varied in the heterogeneity of patient symptomatic states at entry, the number of prior episodes, the intensity of the comparator, or the nature of the outcome variable. It may also be that 'third-wave' approaches, such as dialectical behaviour therapy or mindfulness-based cognitive therapy, will prove effective where CBT was not [86, 87].

## Interpersonal and social rhythm therapy

The interpersonal and social rhythm therapy (IPSRT) is based on the assumptions that: (1) symptoms of BD are triggered by disruptions in daily routines and sleep/wake cycles; and (2) stabilization of these routines is essential to mood stabilization. IPSRT begins during, or shortly following, an acute period of illness and focuses on stabilizing daily and nightly rhythms and resolving interpersonal problems that preceded the acute episode. Patients learn to track their routines and sleep/wake cycles and identify events (for example, job changes) that may provoke changes in these routines.

In the Pittsburgh Maintenance Therapies study [88], 175 acutely ill patients were randomly assigned to IPSRT or active clinical management, both given weekly with medication management. Clinical management emphasized symptom control and medication adherence. Once patients were stabilized, they were randomly reassigned to IPSRT or active clinical management for a 2-year maintenance phase. The findings suggested that IPSRT in the acute phase was associated with longer time before recurrence in the maintenance phase than was clinical management, regardless of what treatment patients were assigned during maintenance care. IPSRT was most effective in delaying recurrences in the maintenance phase when patients succeeded in stabilizing their daily routines and sleep/wake cycles during acute treatment.

A study of IPSRT in New Zealand [89] examined 100 adolescent to young adult patients (aged 15–36) who were randomly assigned to 26–78 weeks of IPSRT or supportive care, both given with medications. There were no differences between groups—over the interval, both groups improved in depressive symptoms, manic symptoms, and social functioning. It is unclear whether the degree of change was attributable to non-specific elements of the two treatments (for example, duration of care or number of sessions), the effects of pharmacotherapy, or the passage of time.

Swartz *et al.* [90] compared IPSRT with placebo vs IPSRT plus QTP in 92 patients with bipolar type II depression, one of the few studies to compare psychotherapy to medications directly. Patients in the two groups had equivalent rates of treatment response over 20 weeks (60% in IPSRT plus placebo vs 74.5% in IPSRT plus QTP). Patients in the IPSRT plus QTP group had greater stabilization of Hamilton depression scores (without evidence of treatment-emergent manic symptoms) but were also more likely to gain weight during the trial. Identification of patients most likely to benefit from psychotherapy as monotherapy is an important direction for research in BD.

## The STEP-BD study

In the U.S. NIMH's multi-site study of BD, the Systematic Treatment Enhancement Program for Bipolar Disorder (STEP-BD) [91], investigators at 15 sites compared IPSRT, FFT, and CBT (30 sessions over 9 months) to a three-session individual psychoeducational intervention (collaborative care, or CC) on time to recovery from a bipolar type I or II depressive episode. Patients ($N$ = 293) received pharmacotherapy with at least one mood stabilizer with or without adjunctive ADs, atypical antipsychotics, or anxiolytics. Over 1 year, patients under intensive therapy conditions were more likely to recover from depression (64%) and recovered more rapidly (mean 169 days) than patients in CC (52%, 279 days, respectively). One-year rates of recovery, which did not statistically differ, were 77% for FFT, 65% for IPSRT, and 60% for CBT [92]. Patients in the intensive therapies were also more likely to remain well in any given month of the 12-month study than patients in CC and had better overall functioning, relationship functioning, and life satisfaction over time [93]. The STEP-BD programme suggests that intensive psychotherapy is a vital part of the effort to stabilize episodes of depression and enhance functioning in BD, although it did not show that any one of these approaches was better than the others.

## Conclusions

The broad emphasis on pharmacological management in BD has sometimes obscured the role of adjunctive psychotherapy in modulating life stressors and enhancing coping mechanisms. Bipolar patients may spend over one-third of their lives in states of depression [94], and mood-stabilizing medications are generally more effective for mania than depression [95]. Thus, integration of pharmacological and psychosocial treatments for bipolar depression seems increasingly important. The use of psychotherapy to enhance compliance with mood-stabilizing medications and to develop a relapse prevention plan may also augment the protective effects of medication maintenance.

There are three interventions with consistent empirical evidence for adults and, in some cases, adolescents: group psychoeducation (often with accompanying care management programmes), FFT, and IPSRT. The evidence for CBT is too mixed at present to list this option as evidence-based for BD. There is beginning evidence for functional remediation treatment for bipolar patients with neurocognitive impairment.

We have a considerable amount to learn about what elements of psychosocial care are most effective in stabilization or long-term treatment. Possibly, strategies like mindfulness meditation, smartphone-based mood reporting, and online psychoeducation programmes will reduce the costs of care without reducing efficacy. However, these programmes are likely to serve as supplements to major psychosocial approaches, rather than as substitutes, until randomized trial data suggest that they are just as effective as the *in vivo* intensive approaches described here.

Use of psychosocial interventions early in the illness course of BD raises the hope that we will one day be able to prevent conversions from subthreshold to threshold versions of this disorder in children. FFT has been examined in a preliminary way in pre-adolescents and adolescents at high risk for BD [77], but participants have not been followed long enough to determine the effects on conversion.

Finally, the subpopulation of patients with BD who respond most consistently to different psychosocial treatments needs to be clarified. Treatments like CBT or group psychoeducation appear to be most effective in patients with few prior episodes [78, 83, 97], although not all studies have shown this (for example, [96]). Ideally, predictive algorithms will be developed to select the type and duration of treatment that is most likely to bring about clinical improvement in patients defined by unique characteristics (personalized medicine).

## REFERENCES

1. Grande I, Berk M, Birmaher B, Vieta E. Bipolar disorder. Lancet. 2016;387:1561–72.
2. Samalin L, Murru A, Vieta E. Management of inter-episodic periods in patients with bipolar disorder. Expert Rev Neurother. 2016;16:659–70.
3. Colom F, Vieta E, Daban C, et al. Clinical and therapeutic implications of predominant polarity in bipolar disorder. J Affect Disord. 2006;93:13–17.
4. Popovic D, Reinares M, Goikolea JM, et al. Polarity index of pharmacological agents used for maintenance treatment of bipolar disorder. Eur Neuropsychopharmacol. 2012;22:339–46.
5. Popovic D, Torrent C, Goikolea JM, et al. Clinical implications of predominant polarity and the polarity index in bipolar disorder: a naturalistic study. Acta Psychiatr Scand. 2014;129:366–74.
6. Grunze H, Vieta E, Goodwin GM, et al. The WFSBP Task Force on Treatment Guidelines for Bipolar Disorders. The World Federation of Societies of Biological Psychiatry (WFSBP) guidelines for the biological treatment of bipolar disorders: update 2012 on the long-term treatment of bipolar disorder. World J Biol Psychiatry. 2013;14:154–219.
7. Yatham LN, Kennedy SH, Parikh SV, et al. Canadian Network for Mood and Anxiety Treatments (CANMAT) and International Society for Bipolar Disorders (ISBD) 2018 guidelines for the management of patients with bipolar disorder. Bipolar Disord. 2018;20(2):97–170.
8. National Institute for Health and Care Excellence (2014). *Bipolar Disorder: Assessment and Management*. Available at: https://www.nice.org.uk/guidance/cg185.
9. Malhi GS, Bassett D, Boyce P, et al. Royal Australian and New Zealand College of Psychiatrists clinical practice guidelines for mood disorders. Aust N Z J Psychiatry. 2015;49:1087–206.
10. Goodwin GM, Haddad PM, Ferrier IN, et al. Evidence-based guidelines for treating bipolar disorder: Revised third edition recommendations from the British Association for Psychopharmacology. J Psychopharmacol. 2016;30:495–553.
11. Vieta E, Langosch JM, Figueira ML, et al. Clinical management and burden of bipolar disorder: results from a multinational longitudinal study (WAVE-bd). Int J Neuropsychopharmacol. 2013;16:1719–32.
12. Garriga M, Pacchiarotti I, Kasper S, et al. Assessment and management of agitation in psychiatry: expert consensus. World J Biol Psychiatry. 2016;17:86–128.
13. Cipriani A, Barbui C, Salanti G, et al. Comparative efficacy and acceptability of antimanic drugs in acute mania: a multiple-treatments meta-analysis. Lancet. 2011;378:1306–15.
14. Yildiz A, Vieta E, Leucht S, Baldessarini RJ. Efficacy of antimanic treatments: meta-analysis of randomized, controlled trials. Neuropsychopharmacology. 2011;36:375–89.
15. Yildiz A, Nikodem M, Vieta E, Correll CU, Baldessarini RJ. A network meta-analysis on comparative efficacy and all-cause discontinuation of antimanic treatments in acute bipolar mania. Psychol Med. 2015;45:299–317.
16. Vieta E, Azorin JM, Bauer M, et al. Psychiatrists' perceptions of potential reasons for non- and partial adherence to medication: results of a survey in bipolar disorder from eight European countries. J Affect Disord. 2012;143:125–30.
17. Vieta E, Locklear J, Günther O, et al. Treatment options for bipolar depression: a systematic review of randomized, controlled trials. J Clin Psychopharmacol. 2010;30:579–90.
18. Vieta E. Antidepressants in bipolar I disorder: never as monotherapy. Am J Psychiatry. 2014;171:1023–6.
19. Tohen M, Vieta E, Calabrese J, et al. Efficacy of olanzapine and olanzapine-fluoxetine combination in the treatment of bipolar I depression. Arch Gen Psychiatry. 2003;60:1079–88.

20. Tohen M, McDonnell DP, Case M, *et al.* Randomized, double-blind, placebo-controlled study of olanzapine in patients with bipolar I depression. Br J Psychiatry. 2012;201:376–82.

21. Calabrese JR, Keck PE Jr, Macfadden W, *et al.* A randomized, double-blind, placebo-controlled trial of quetiapine in the treatment of bipolar I or II depression. Am J Psychiatry. 2005;162:1351–60.

22. Thase ME, Macfadden W, Weisler RH, *et al.*; BOLDER II Study Group. Efficacy of quetiapine monotherapy in bipolar I and II depression: a double-blind, placebo-controlled study (the BOLDER II study). J Clin Psychopharmacol. 2006;26:600–9. Erratum in: J Clin Psychopharmacol. 2007;27:51.

23. Young AH, McElroy SL, Bauer M, *et al.*; EMBOLDEN I (Trial 001) Investigators. A double-blind, placebo-controlled study of quetiapine and lithium monotherapy in adults in the acute phase of bipolar depression (EMBOLDEN I). J Clin Psychiatry. 2010;71:150–62.

24. McElroy SL, Weisler RH, Chang W, *et al.*; EMBOLDEN II (Trial D1447C00134) Investigators. A double-blind, placebo-controlled study of quetiapine and paroxetine as monotherapy in adults with bipolar depression (EMBOLDEN II). J Clin Psychiatry. 2010;71:163–74.

25. Loebel A, Cucchiaro J, Silva R, *et al.* Lurasidone monotherapy in the treatment of bipolar I depression: a randomized, double-blind, placebo-controlled study. Am J Psychiatry. 2014;171:160–8.

26. Suppes T, Kroger H, Pikalov A, Loebel A. Lurasidone adjunctive with lithium or valproate for bipolar depression: a placebo-controlled trial utilizing prospective and retrospective enrolment cohorts. J Psychiatr Res. 2016;78:86–93.

27. Dunn RT, Stan VA, Chriki LS, Filkowski MM, Ghaemi SN. A prospective, open-label study of Aripiprazole mono- and adjunctive treatment in acute bipolar depression. J Affect Disord. 2008;110:70–4.

28. Thase ME, Jonas A, Khan A, Bowden CL, *et al.* Aripiprazole monotherapy in nonpsychotic bipolar I depression: results of 2 randomized, placebo-controlled studies. J Clin Psychopharmacol. 2008;28:13–20. Erratum in: J Clin Psychopharmacol. 2009;29:38.

29. Cipriani A, Hawton K, Stockton S, *et al.* Lithium in the prevention of suicide in mood disorders: Updated systematic review and meta-analysis. BMJ. 2013;346:f3646.

30. Smith LA, Cornelius VR, Azorin JM, *et al.* Valproate for the treatment of acute bipolar depression: systematic review and metaanalysis. J Affect Disord. 2010;122:1–9.

31. Calabrese JR, Huffman RF, White RL, *et al.* Lamotrigine in the acute treatment of bipolar depression: results of five double-blind, placebo-controlled clinical trials. Bipolar Disord. 2008;10:323–33.

32. van der Loos ML, Mulder PG, Hartong EG, *et al.* Efficacy and safety of lamotrigine as add-on treatment to lithium in bipolar depression: a multicenter, double-blind, placebo-controlled trial. J Clin Psychiatry. 2009;70:223–31.

33. van der Loos ML, Mulder P, Hartong EG, *et al.* Long-term outcome of bipolar depressed patients receiving lamotrigine as add-on to lithium with the possibility of the addition of paroxetine in nonresponders: a randomized, placebo-controlled trial with a novel design. Bipolar Disord. 2011;13:111–17.

34. Geddes JR, Gardiner A, Rendell J, *et al.* Comparative evaluation of quetiapine plus lamotrigine combination versus quetiapine monotherapy (and folic acid versus placebo) in bipolar depression (CEQUEL): a 2 × 2 factorial randomised trial. Lancet Psychiatry. 2016;3:31–9.

35. Pacchiarotti I, Mazzarini L, Kotzalidis GD, *et al.* Mania and depression. Mixed, not stirred. J Affect Disord. 2011;133:105–13.

36. Pacchiarotti I, Valentí M, Colom F, *et al.* Differential outcome of bipolar patients receiving antidepressant monotherapy versus combination with an antimanic drug. J Affect Disord. 2011;129:321–6.

37. Valentí M, Pacchiarotti I, Rosa AR, *et al.* Bipolar mixed episodes and antidepressants: a cohort study of bipolar I disorder patients. Bipolar Disord. 2011;13:145–54.

38. Valentí M, Pacchiarotti I, Bonnín CM, *et al.* Risk factors for antidepressant-related switch to mania. J Clin Psychiatry. 2012;73:e271–6.

39. Pacchiarotti I, Bond DJ, Baldessarini RJ, *et al.* The International Society for Bipolar Disorders (ISBD) task force report on antidepressant use in bipolar disorders. Am J Psychiatry. 2013;170:1249–62.

40. Frye MA, Grunze H, Suppes T, *et al.* A placebo-controlled evaluation of adjunctive modafinil in the treatment of bipolar depression. Am J Psychiatry. 2007;164:1242–9.

41. Calabrese JR, Ketter TA, Youakim JM, Tiller JM, Yang R, Frye MA. Adjunctive armodafinil for major depressive episodes associated with bipolar I disorder: a randomized, multicenter, double-blind, placebo-controlled, proof-of-concept study. J Clin Psychiatry. 2010;71:1363–70.

42. León-Caballero J, Pacchiarotti I, Murru A, *et al.* Bipolar disorder and antibodies against the N-methyl-d-aspartate receptor: A gate to the involvement of autoimmunity in the pathophysiology of bipolar illness. Neurosci Biobehav Rev. 2015;55:403–12.

43. Diazgranados N, Ibrahim L, Brutsche NE, *et al.* A randomized add-on trial of an N-methyl-D-aspartate antagonist in treatment-resistant bipolar depression. Arch Gen Psychiatry. 2010;67:793–802.

44. Zarate CA Jr, Brutsche NE, Ibrahim L, *et al.* Replication of ketamines antidepressant efficacy in bipolar depression: a randomized controlled add-on trial. Biol Psychiatry. 2012;71:939–46.

45. Colom F, Vieta E, Daban C, Pacchiarotti I, Sánchez-Moreno J. Clinical and therapeutic implications of predominant polarity in bipolar disorder. J Affect Disord. 2006;93:13–17.

46. Severus E, Taylor MJ, Sauer C, *et al.* Lithium for prevention of mood episodes in bipolar disorders: systematic review and meta-analysis. Int J Bipolar Disord. 2014;2:15.

47. Vieta E, Gunther O, Locklear J, *et al.* Effectiveness of psychotropic medications in the maintenance phase of bipolar disorder: a meta-analysis of randomized con- trolled trials. Int J Neuropsychopharmacol. 2011;14:1029–49.

48. Cipriani A, Reid K, Young AH, *et al.* Valproic acid, valproate and divalproex in the maintenance treatment of bipolar disorder. Cochrane Database Syst Rev. 2013;10:CD003196.

49. Vieta E, Montgomery S, Sulaiman AH, *et al.* A randomized, double-blind, placebo-controlled trial to assess prevention of mood episodes with risperidone long-acting injectable in patients with bipolar I disorder. Eur Neuropsychopharmacol. 2012;22:825–35.

50. Calabrese J, Pikalov A, Cucchiaro J, *et al.* Lurasidone adjunctive to lithium or divalproex for prevention of recurrence in patients with bipolar i disorder: results of a 28-week, randomized, double-blind, placebo-controlled study. Neuropsychopharmacology. 2015;40:S479–80.

51. Marcus R, Khan A, Rollin L, *et al.* Efficacy of aripiprazole adjunctive to lithium or valproate in the long-term treatment of patients with bipolar I disorder with an inadequate response to

lithium or valproate monotherapy: a multicenter, double-blind, randomized study. Bipolar Disord. 2011;13:133–44.

52. Bowden CL, Vieta E, Ice KS, et al. Ziprasidone plus a mood stabilizer in subjects with bipolar I disorder: a 6-month, randomized, placebo-controlled, double-blind trial. J Clin Psychiatry. 2010;71:130–7.

53. Berwaerts J, Melkote R, Nuamah I, et al. A randomized, placebo- and active-controlled study of paliperidone extended-release as maintenance treatment in patients with bipolar I disorder after an acute manic or mixed episode. J Affect Disord. 2012;138:247–58.

54. Murru A, Pacchiarotti I, Amann BL, et al. Treatment adherence in bipolar I and schizoaffective disorder, bipolar type. J Affect Disord. 2013;151:1003–8.

55. Quiroz JA, Yatham LN, Palumbo JM, Karcher K, Kushner S, Kusumakar V. Risperidone long-acting injectable monotherapy in the maintenance treatment of bipolar I disorder. Biol Psychiatry. 2010;68:156–62.

56. Gignac A, McGirr A, Lam RW, Yatham LN. Recovery and recurrence following a first episode of mania: a systematic review and meta-analysis of prospectively characterized cohorts. J Clin Psychiatry. 2015;76:1241–8.

57. Salcedo S,., Gold AK, Sheikh S, et al. Empirically supported psychosocial interventions for bipolar disorder: current state of the research. J Affect Disord. 2016;201:203–14.

58. Swartz HA, Swanson J. Psychotherapy for bipolar disorder in adults: a review of the evidence. Focus Psychiatry. 2014;12:251–66.

59. Vallarino MA, Henry C, Etain B, et al. An evidence map of psychosocial interventions for the earliest stages of bipolar disorder. Lancet Psychiatry. 2015;2:548–63.

60. Colom F, Vieta E, Martinez-Aran A, et al. A randomized trial on the efficacy of group psychoeducation in the prophylaxis of recurrences in bipolar patients whose disease is in remission. Arch Gen Psychiatry. 2003;60:402–7.

61. Colom F, Vieta E, Martinez-Aran A, Reinares M, Goikolea JM, Martínez-Arán A. A randomized trial on the efficacy of group psychoeducation in the prophylaxis of bipolar disorder: A five year follow-up. Br J Psychiatry. 2009;194:260–5.

62. de Barros Pellegrinelli K, de O Costa LF, Silval KI, et al. Efficacy of psychoeducation on symptomatic and functional recovery in bipolar disorder. Acta Psychiatr Scand. 2013;127:153–8.

63. Bauer MS, McBride L, Williford WO, et al. Collaborative care for bipolar disorder: Part II. Impact on clinical outcome, function, and costs. Psychiatr Serv. 2006;57:937–45.

64. Simon GE, Ludman EJ, Bauer MS, Unutzer J, Operskalski B. Long-term effectiveness and cost of a systematic care program for bipolar disorder. Arch Gen Psychiatry. 2006;63:500–8.

65. Perry A, Tarrier N, Morriss R, McCarthy E, Limb K. Randomised controlled trial of efficacy of teaching patients with bipolar disorder to identify early symptoms of relapse and obtain treatment. BMJ. 1999;318:149–53.

66. Kessing LV, Hansen HV, Christensen EM, et al. Do young adults with bipolar disorder benefit from early intervention? J Affect Disord. 2014;152–4:403–8.

67. Torrent C, del Mar Bonnin C, Martinez-Aran A, et al. Efficacy of functional remediation in bipolar disorder: a multicenter randomized controlled study. Am J Psychiatry. 2013;170:852–9.

68. Fitzgerald RG. Mania as a message: treatment with family therapy and lithium carbonate. Am J Psychotherapy. 1972;26;547–55.

69. Miklowitz DJ, Goldstein MJ. Bipolar disorder: a family-focused treatment approach. New York, NY: Guildford Press; 1997.

70. Miklowitz DJ, Goldstein MJ. Behavioral family treatment for patients with bipolar affective disorder. Behav Modif. 1990;14:457–89.

71. Miklowitz DJ, George EL, Richards JA, Simoneau TL, Suddath RL. A randomized study of family-focused psychoeducation and pharmacotherapy in the outpatient management of bipolar disorder. Arch Gen Psychiatry. 2003;60:904–12.

72. Rea MM, Tompson M, Miklowitz DJ, Goldstein MJ, Hwang S, Mintz J. Family focused treatment vs. individual treatment for bipolar disorder: results of a randomized clinical trial. J Consulting Clin Psychol. 2003;71:482–92.

73. Miklowitz DJ, Axelson DA, Birmaher B, et al. Family-focused treatment for adolescents with bipolar disorder: results of a 2-year randomized trial. Arch Gen Psychiatry. 2008;65:1053–61.

74. Miklowitz DJ, Axelson DA, George EL, et al. Expressed emotion moderates the effects of family-focused treatment for bipolar adolescents. J Am Acad Child Adolesc Psychiatry. 2009;48:643–51.

75. Sullivan AE, Judd CM, Axelson DA, Miklowitz DJ. Family functioning and the course of adolescent bipolar disorder. Behav Ther. 2012;43:837–47.

76. Miklowitz DJ, Schneck CD, George EL, et al. Pharmacotherapy and family-focused treatment for adolescents with bipolar I and II disorders: a 2-year randomized trial. Am J Psychiatry. 2014;171:658–67.

77. Miklowitz DJ, Schneck CD, Singh MK, et al. Early intervention for symptomatic youth at risk for bipolar disorder: a randomized trial of family-focused therapy. J Am Acad Child Adolesc Psychiatry. 2013;52:121–31.

78. Reinares M, Sánchez-Moreno J, Fountoulakis KN. Psychosocial interventions in bipolar disorder: what, for whom, and when. J Affect Disord. 2014;156:46–55.

79. Fristad MA, Verducci JS, Walters K, Young ME. Impact of multifamily psychoeducational psychotherapy in treating children aged 8 to 12 years with mood disorders. Arch Gen Psychiatry. 2009;66:1013–21.

80. West AE, Weinstein SM, Peters AT, et al. Child- and family-focused cognitive-behavioral therapy for pediatric bipolar disorder: a randomized clinical trial. J Am Acad Child Adolesc Psychiatry. 2014;53:1168–78.

81. Lam DH, Watkins ER, Hayward P, et al. A randomized controlled study of cognitive therapy for relapse prevention for bipolar affective disorder: outcome of the first year. Arch Gen Psychiatry. 2003;60:145–52.

82. Lam DH, Hayward P, Watkins ER, Wright K, Sham P. Relapse prevention in patients with bipolar disorder: cognitive therapy outcome after 2 years. Am J Psychiatry. 2005;162:324–9.

83. Scott J. Psychotherapy for bipolar disorders-efficacy and effectiveness. J Psychopharmacology. 2006;20:46–50.

84. Parikh SV, Zaretsky A, Beaulieu S, et al. A randomized controlled trial of psychoeducation or cognitive-behavioral therapy in bipolar disorder: a Canadian Network for Mood and Anxiety treatments (CANMAT) study. J Clin Psychiatry. 2012;73:803–10.

85. Meyer TD, Hautzinger M. Cognitive behaviour therapy and supportive therapy for bipolar disorders: relapse rates for treatment period and 2-year follow-up. Psychol Med. 2012;42:1429–39.

86. Goldstein TR, Fersch-Podrat RK, Rivera M, et al. Dialectical behavior therapy (DBT) for adolescents with bipolar disorder: results from a pilot randomized trial. J Child Adolesc Psychopharmacol. 2015;25:140–9.

87. Deckersbach T, Hölzel BK, Eisner LR, et al. (2012). Mindfulness-based cognitive therapy for nonremitted patients with bipolar disorder. CNS Neurosci Ther. 2012;18:133–41.

88. Frank E, Kupfer DJ, Thase ME, *et al.* Two-year outcomes for interpersonal and social rhythm therapy in individuals with bipolar I disorder. Arch Gen Psychiatry. 2005;62:996–1004.

89. Inder ML, Crowe MT, Luty SE, *et al.* Randomized, controlled trial of Interpersonal and Social Rhythm Therapy for young people with bipolar disorder. Bipolar Disord. 2015;17:128–38.

90. Swartz HA, Rucci P, Thase ME, *et al. Interpersonal and Social Rhythm Therapy and as a Treatment for Bipolar II Depression.* International Society for Bipolar Disorders, 14 July 2016. Amsterdam: The Netherlands; 2016.

91. Sachs GS, Nierenberg AA, Calabrese JR, *et al.* Effectiveness of adjunctive antidepressant treatment for bipolar depression. N Engl J Med. 2007;356:1711–22.

92. Miklowitz DJ, Otto MW, Frank E, *et al.* Psychosocial treatments for bipolar depression: a 1-year randomized trial from the Systematic Treatment Enhancement Program. Arch Gen Psychiatry. 2007;64:419–27.

93. Miklowitz DJ, Otto MW, Frank E, *et al.* Intensive psychosocial intervention enhances functioning in patients with bipolar depression: results from a 9-month randomized controlled trial. Am J Psychiatry. 2007;164:1340–7.

94. Judd LL, Akiskal HS, Schettler PJ, *et al.* The long-term natural history of the weekly symptomatic status of bipolar I disorder. Arch Gen Psychiatry. 2002;59:530–7.

95. Keck PEJ, McElroy SL, Richtand N, Tohen M. What makes a drug a primary mood stabilizer? Mol Psychiatry. 2002;7(Suppl 1): S8–14.

96. Lam DH, Burbeck R, Wright K, Pilling S. Psychological therapies in bipolar disorder: the effect of illness history on relapse prevention—a systematic review. Bipolar Disord. 2009;11:474–82.

97. Deckersbach T, Peters AT, Sylvia LG, *et al.* A cluster analytic approach to identifying predictors and moderators of psychosocial treatment for bipolar depression: results from STEP-BD. J Affect Disord. 2016;203:152–7.

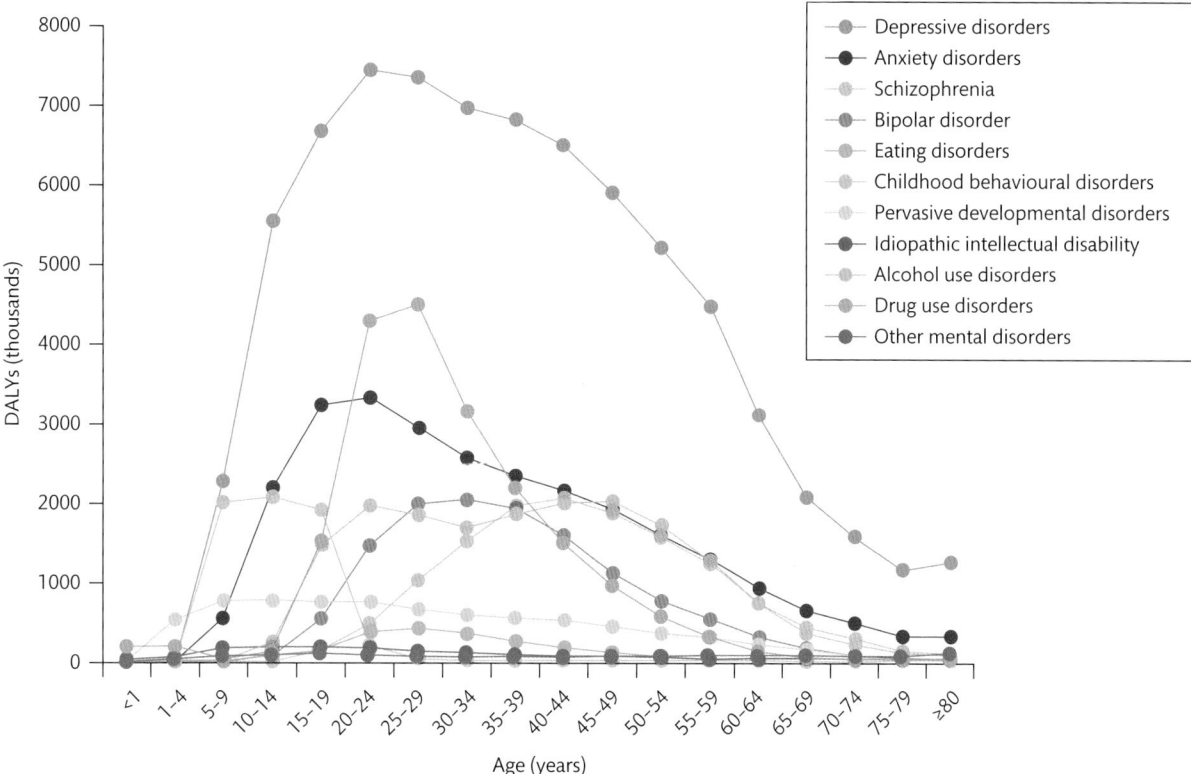

**Fig. 3.1** Disability-adjusted life years (DALYs) for each mental and substance use disorder in 2010, by age.

Reproduced from *The Lancet*, 382(9904), Whiteford HA, Degenhardt L, Rehm J, *et al.*, Global burden of disease attributable to mental and substance use disorders: findings from the Global Burden of Disease Study 2010, pp. 1575–86, Copyright (2013), with permission from Elsevier Ltd.

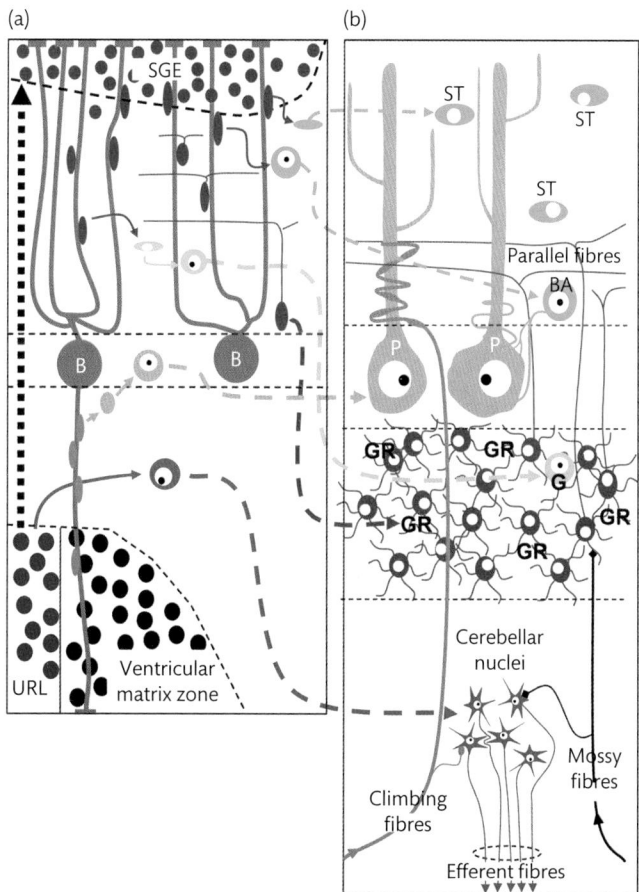

**Fig. 11.3** Development of the cerebellar cortex and nuclei. (a) Fetal development. (b) Adult stage. B, Bergmann glia; BA, basket cell; G, Golgi cell; GR, granular cell; P, Purkinje cell; SGE, stratum granulosum externum; ST, stellate cell; URL, upper rhombic lip.

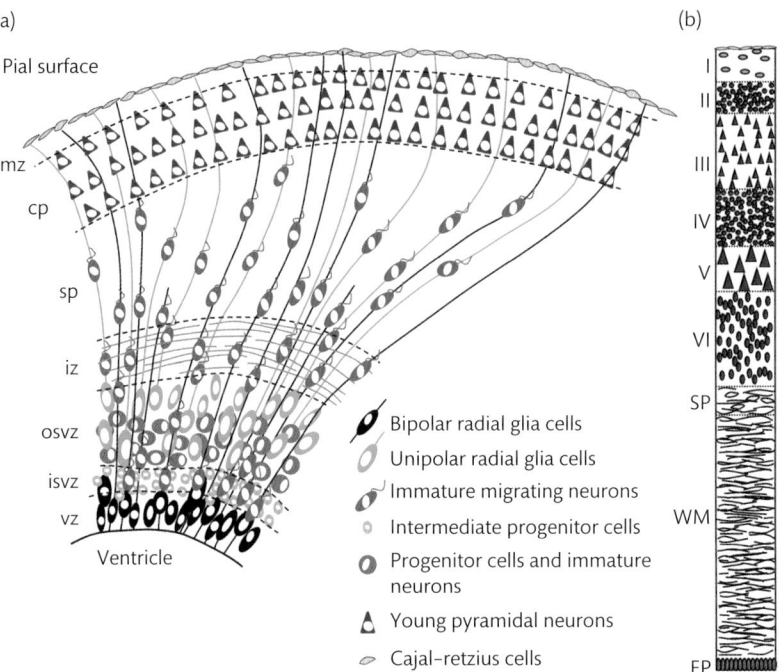

**Fig. 11.4** Histogenesis and radial migration in the cerebral cortex. (a) Development in the fetal hemispheric wall based on recent data [48, 54–56, 62, 63]. (b) Adult cortical layering in the human neopallium. I–VI, cortical layers; EP, ependymal layer; cp, cortical plate; isvz, inner subventricular zone; iz, intermediate zone with the first arriving nerve fibres establishing connection with immature neurons; mz, marginal zone; sp, subplate; osvz, outer subventricular zone; vz, ventricular zone; WM, white matter.

Legend:
- Bipolar radial glia cells
- Unipolar radial glia cells
- Immature migrating neurons
- Intermediate progenitor cells
- Progenitor cells and immature neurons
- Young pyramidal neurons
- Cajal–retzius cells

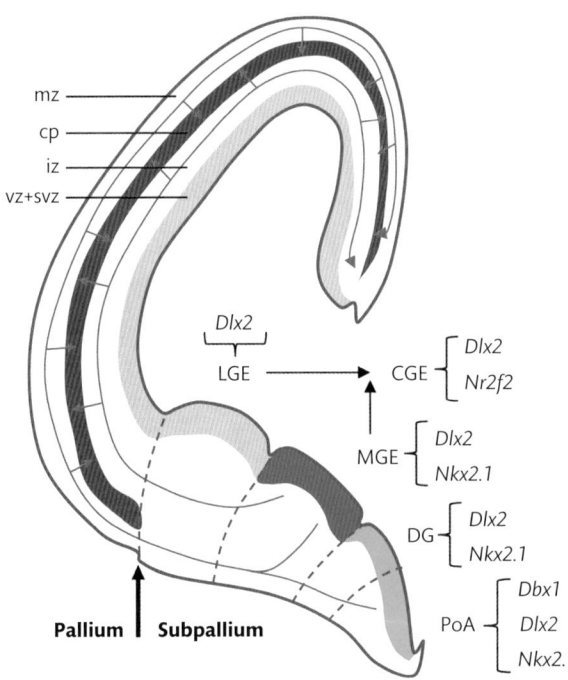

**Fig. 11.5** Schematic drawing of the precursor regions of inhibitory neurons later found in the cerebral cortex, basal ganglia, amygdala, and basal forebrain [64]. Precursor regions: CGE, caudal ganglionic eminence; DG, diagonal area; LGE, lateral ganglionic eminence; MGE, medial ganglionic eminence; PoA, preoptic area. Transcription factors: Dbx1, developing brain homeobox protein 1; Dlx2, Distal-less protein 2; Nkx2.1, thyroid transcription factor 1; Nr2f2, ligand-activated transcription factor Nr2f2. Cp, cortical plate; iz, intermediate zone; mz, mantle zone; vz + svz, ventricular + subventricular zone.

Source: data from Nieuwenhuys R, Puelles L, *Towards a new neural morphology*, Copyright (2016), Springer International Publishing Switzerland.

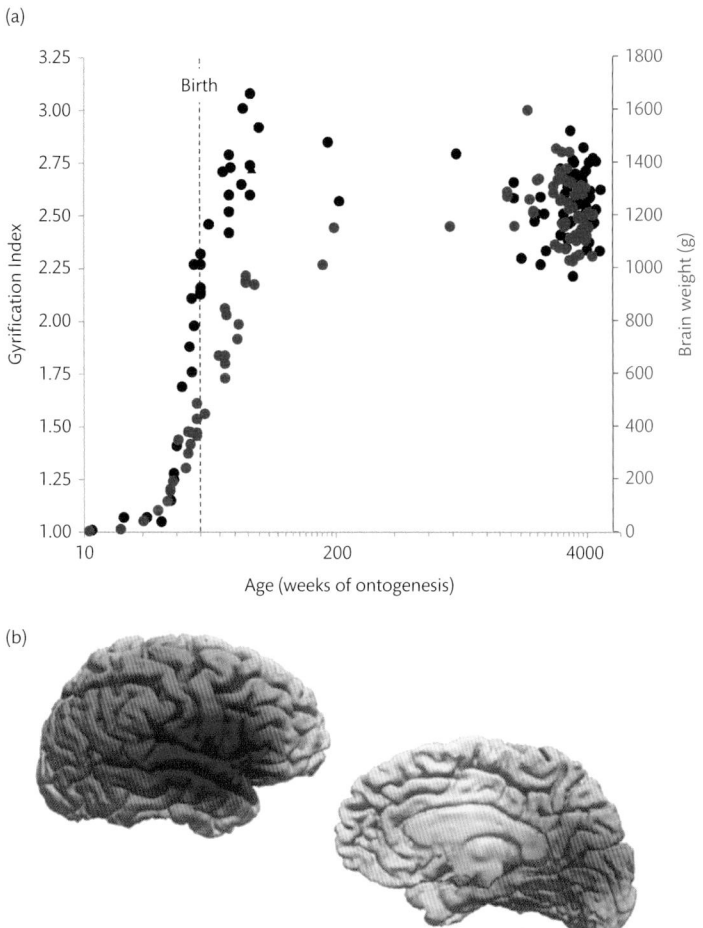

**Fig. 11.7** (a) Development of brain weight and gyrification index (GI) as a measure of the intensity of cortical folding during human lifespan. Data from Zilles *et al.* [44] and Armstrong *et al.* [45]. (b) Distribution of the local degree of cortical folding throughout the adult human brain, after Jockwitz *et al.* [46]. Red (dark grey in the printed version) indicates highest, yellow (pale grey in the printed version) lowest degrees of cortical folding.

Reproduced from *Brain Structure and Function*, 222(1), Jockwitz C, Caspers S, Heine H, *et al.*, Age- and function-related regional changes in cortical folding of the default mode network in older adults, pp. 83–99, Copyright (2017), with permission from Springer Nature.

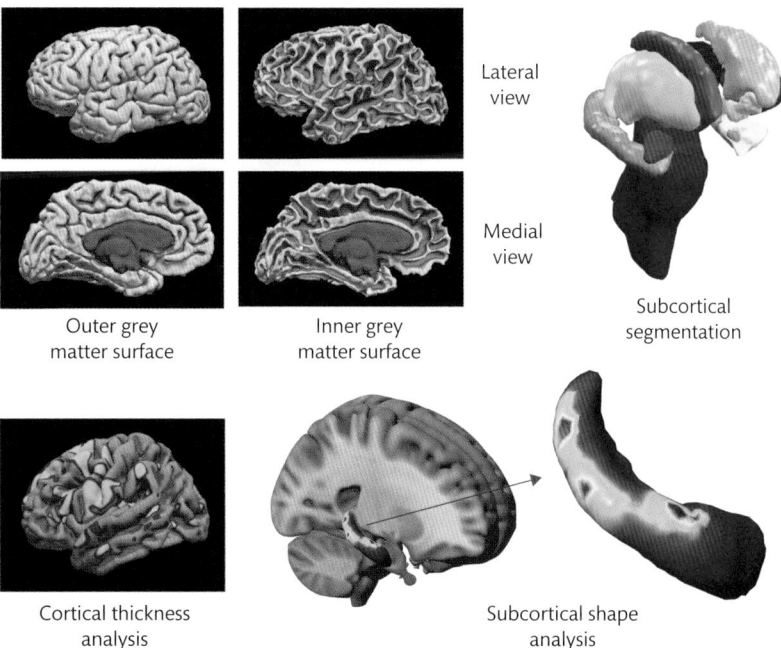

**Fig. 12.2** Examples of structural segmentation and analysis. Top left shows cortical segmentation (left hemisphere) where the inner and outer surfaces of the cortical grey matter are modelled, and from this, the cortical thickness can be calculated and analysed to show areas of differing thickness between groups (bottom left). Top right shows a set of subcortical structures (for example, caudate, hippocampus, brainstem, etc.), and bottom right shows an example of a shape analysis (hippocampus) displaying localized areas of difference in the shape between a patient and control group.

Adapted from Jenkinson M, Chappell M, *Introduction to Neuroimaging Analysis*, Copyright (2017), with permission from Oxford University Press.

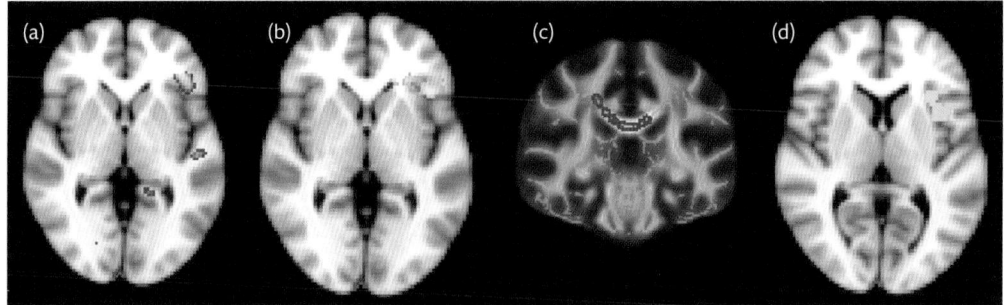

**Fig. 12.3** Example of standard analysis techniques in patients with schizophrenia (a–c) and carriers of the VAL and MET alleles of the *COMT* gene (d). (a) VBM analysis with areas of significant grey matter reduction in schizophrenia relative to controls shown in red-yellow. (b) fMRI using a letter fluency task showing significant areas of reduced activity in schizophrenia, relative to controls. (c) Diffusion MRI-based TBSS (tract-based spatial statistics) analysis of the same patients with schizophrenia, relative to controls, showing reduced fractional anisotropy in the corpus callosum and forceps major. (d) Resting fMRI analysis of healthy VAL and MET allele homozygotes of the *COMT* gene, showing greater functional connectivity in VAL carriers, relative to METs.

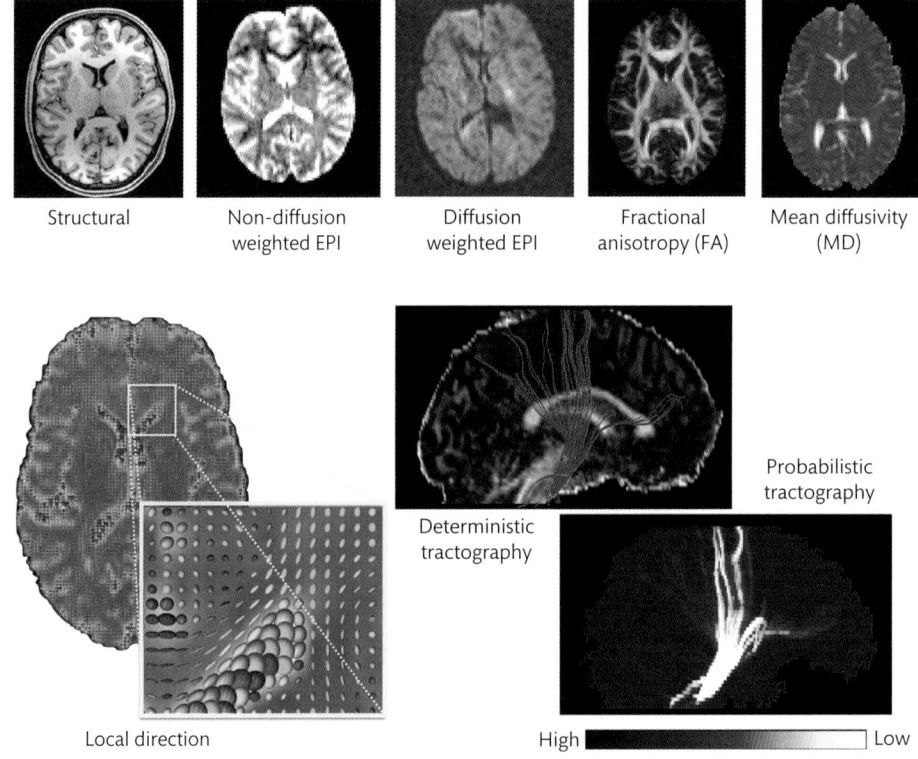

**Fig. 12.4** Examples of diffusion MRI and analysis results. Top row shows a structural image (left) for comparison, along with a non-diffusion-weighted image and a single diffusion-weighted image. Many of these EPI-based images need to be acquired in a diffusion MRI study. The two images on the right of the top row show DTI-based measures calculated from the diffusion-weighted acquisitions, which are often used as surrogate measures of white matter microstructure. The bottom row shows an example of estimated white matter tract directions on the left (colour coding based on direction: red = left–right, green = anterior–posterior, blue = inferior–superior), and the tractography results based on these (right) using either deterministic or probabilistic methods for tracing major fibre pathways.

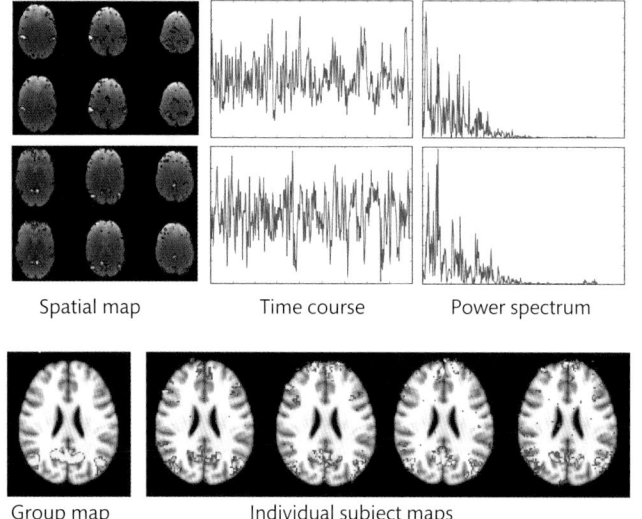

Spatial map        Time course        Power spectrum

Group map        Individual subject maps

**Fig. 12.6** Illustration of resting state networks. Top panel shows ICA components corresponding to two networks (motor and default mode in the first and second rows, respectively). These have spatial maps (left) that show the brain areas involved in each network (red-yellow), and time courses (middle) of fMRI signal fluctuations that are common across all parts of that network. The power spectra of the time courses (right) show low frequency fluctuations, characteristic of slow neuronally induced haemodynamic changes. Bottom panel shows an example of the spatial map of a resting state network (default mode network) estimated from a group of subjects (left) and from individual subjects (right). Features from these intrinsic networks can be analysed for differences across clinical populations or experimental conditions.

Adapted from Jenkinson M, Chappell M, *Introduction to Neuroimaging Analysis*, Copyright (2017), with permission from Oxford University Press; Bijsterbosch J, Smith SM, Beckmann CF, *Introduction to Resting State fMRI Functional Connectivity*, Copyright (2017), with permission from Oxford University Press.

Aβ: [$^{18}$F]AV45        Tau: [$^{18}$F]AV1451

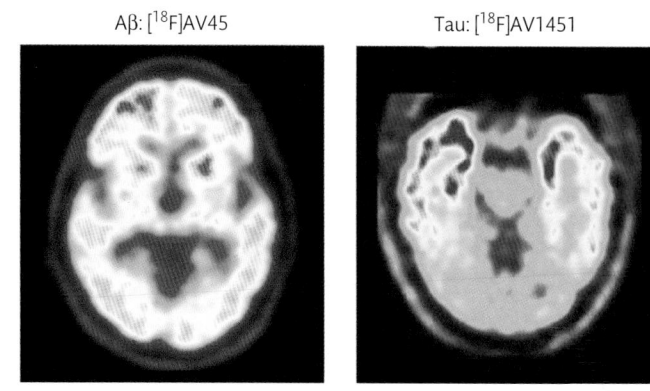

**Fig. 12.9** Examples of protein aggregate tracers for Alzheimer's disease. Reproduced courtesy of Roger Gunn and Azadeh Firouzian.

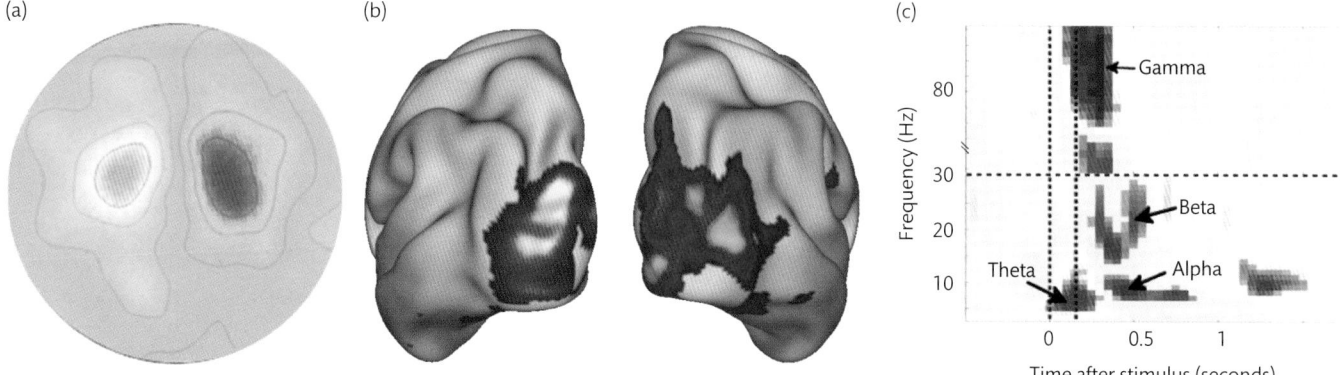

**Fig. 12.11** (a) Sensor space MEG data presented as a two-dimensional (2D) topographic sensor map of contrasted oscillatory power (between 8 and 12 Hz) in a visual attention task. Power is lower in the contralateral (attending) hemisphere. (b) The same MEG data shown reconstructed into the source (brain) space and presented on a three-dimensional cortical map. (c) Time–frequency plot of oscillatory power in MEG sensors above the visual cortex following presentation of a visual stimulus. Changes in power can be resolved at sub-second resolution, with increases (synchronization) occurring in some frequencies and reductions (desynchronization) occurring in others. Vertical lines denote stimulus onset/offset.

Reproduced from *Practical Neurology*, 14(5), Proudfoot M, Woolrich MW, Nobre AC, *et al.*, Magnetoencephalography, pp. 285–285, Copyright (2014), with permission from *British Medical Journal*.

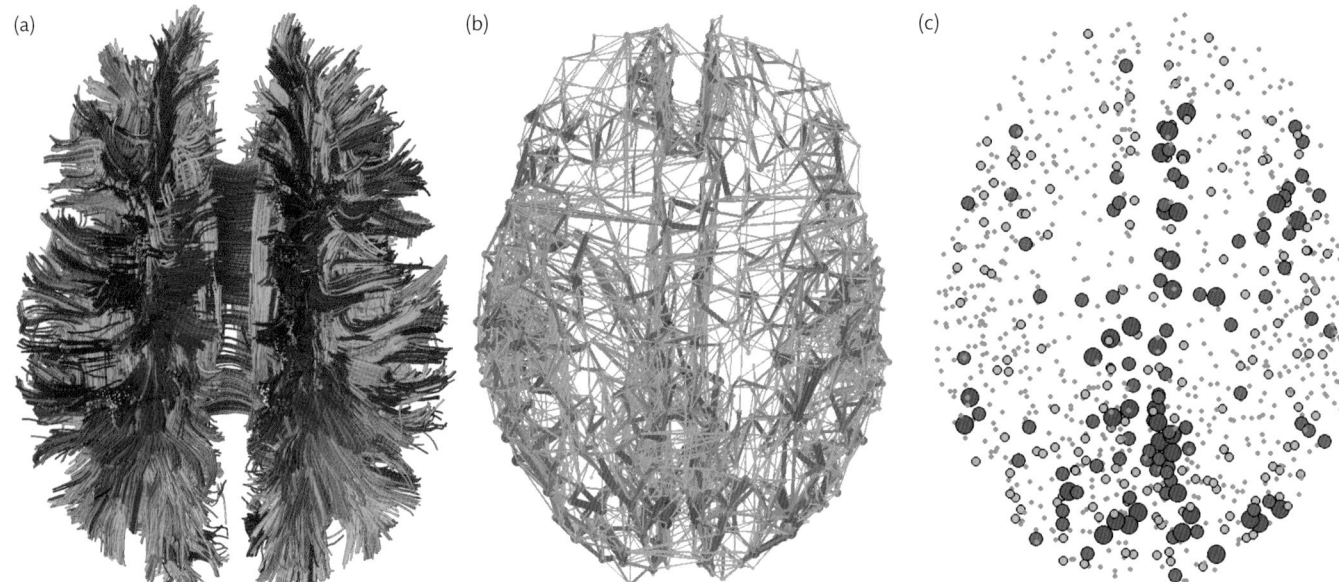

**Fig. 13.2** Different representations of the connectome. (a) A set of streamlines, derived from diffusion imaging and computational tractography. Red, green, and blue lines indicate putative white matter tracts running along the medial–lateral, anterior–posterior, and dorsal–ventral directions, respectively. (b) Nodes derived from a cortical parcellation are shown as red dots, connected by edges (blue lines) that correspond to the density of streamlines linking each pair of nodes. For clarity, the diagram shows the strongest edges only. (c) Nodes are arranged in the same anatomical positions as in panel (b), with blue-coloured nodes indicating high betweenness centrality, a measure of influence that is computed as the number of optimally short communication paths to which each node contributes. Node diameter is proportional to the number of subjects (0–5), for which a given node received high betweenness scores.

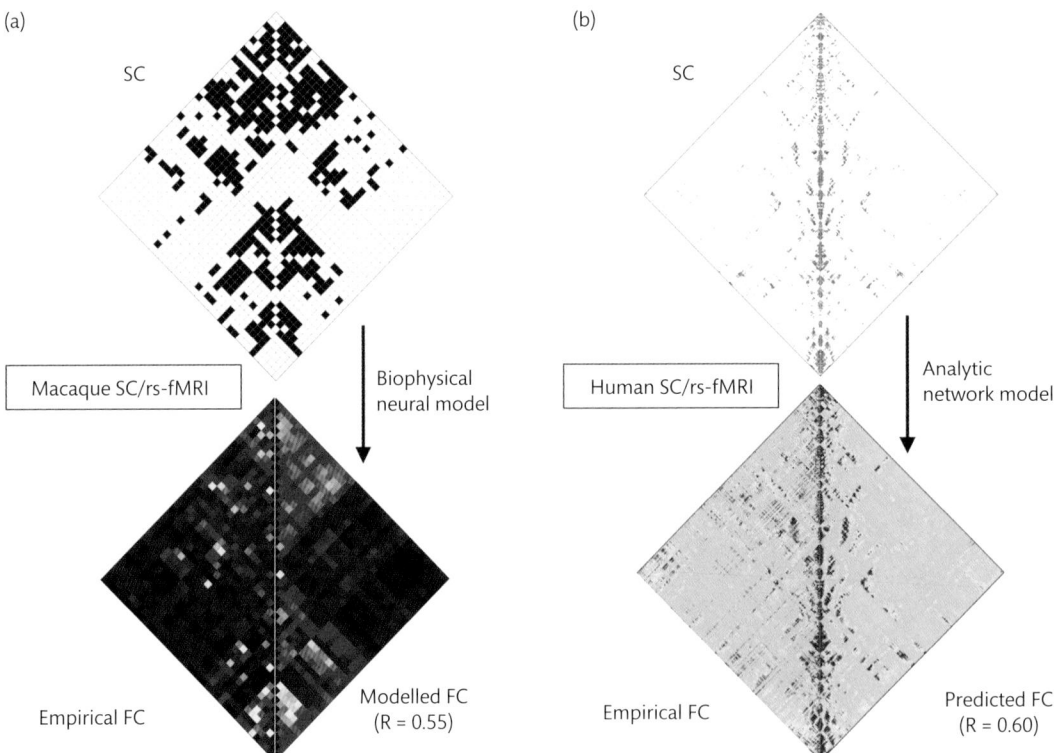

**Fig. 13.3** Connectome-based computational models of functional connectivity. (a) The matrix at the top shows structural connectivity (SC) of directed projections among a set of macaque cortical areas. This connectome formed the coupling structure for a simulation of neural mass dynamics that generated synthetic fMRI time courses and a 'modelled FC' (functional connectivity) matrix (lower plot, right half). This computational analogue of macaque FC can be compared to empirical recordings of resting-state fMRI. The correlation between the empirical and modelled FC patterns is R = 0.55 [54]. (b) Human SC matrix (from [30]) and empirical FC (from [30]), as well as predicted FC (from [61]). The predicted FC was computed from an analytic model based on measures of communication in the structural graph SC. The correlation between the empirical and predicted FC patterns is R = 0.60 [61].

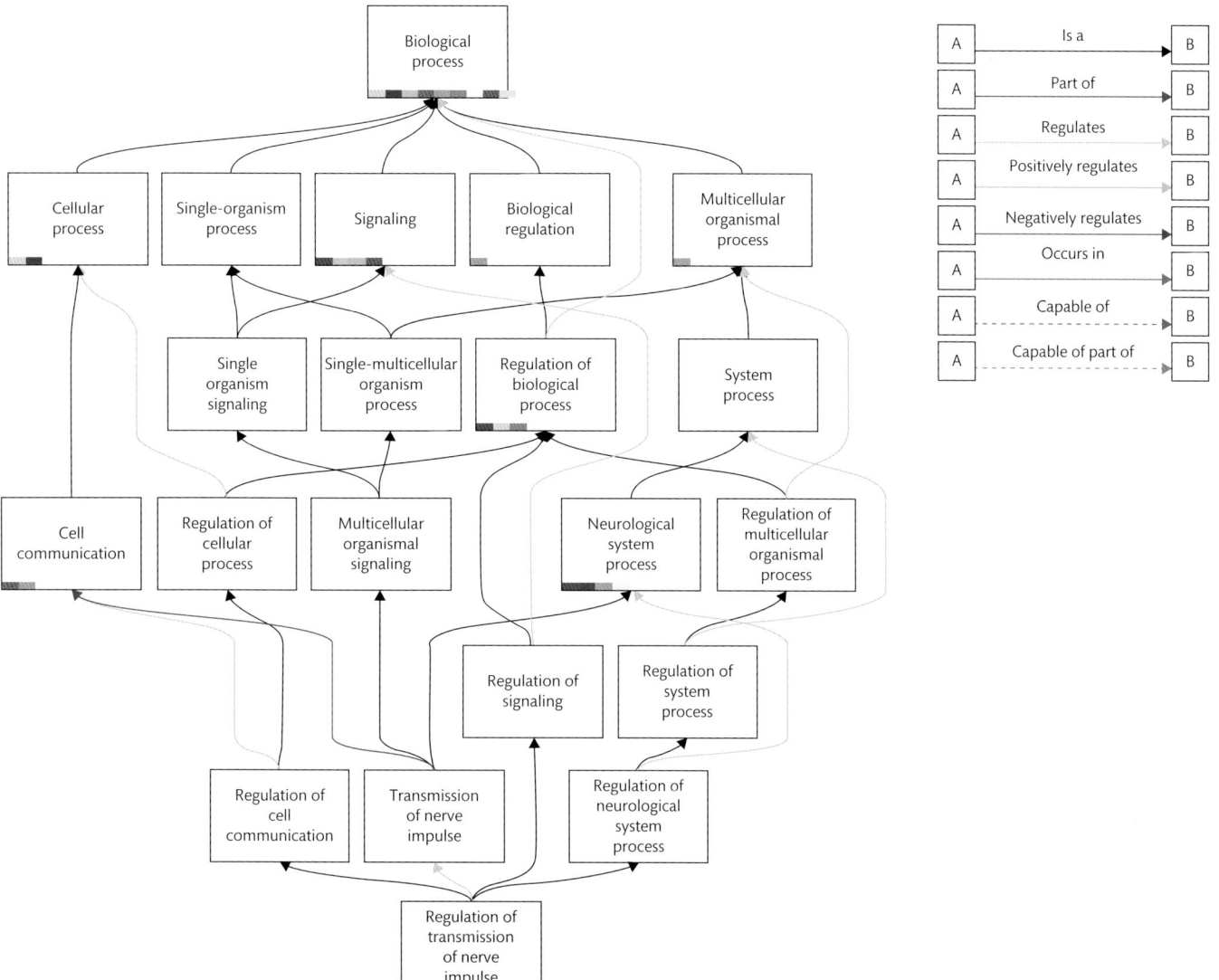

**Fig. 16.3** An example of hierarchical relationships in the Gene Ontology (GO) [58]. In this example, we show the GO annotation terms that lie above the term '*regulation of transmission of nerve impulse*'. Following this GO hierarchy, a gene that was ascribed the function of *regulation of transmission of nerve impulse* would automatically also be assigned all of the functional terms listed. As with other structured ontologies discussed in the main text, an explicit understanding of knowledge relationships between annotation terms makes it possible to identify similarities between gene functions. For example, if we were comparing a gene assigned with the term *regulation of cell communication* to another gene assigned the term *transmission of nerve impulse*, the graph identifies *cell communication* as a common role. Although many of these relationships may seem obvious to a researcher, ontologies are computable, such that we can rapidly compute the similarity between thousands of genes enabling us to statistically identify unusually common functions among sets of genes, for example those found to be dysregulated in a diseased tissue.

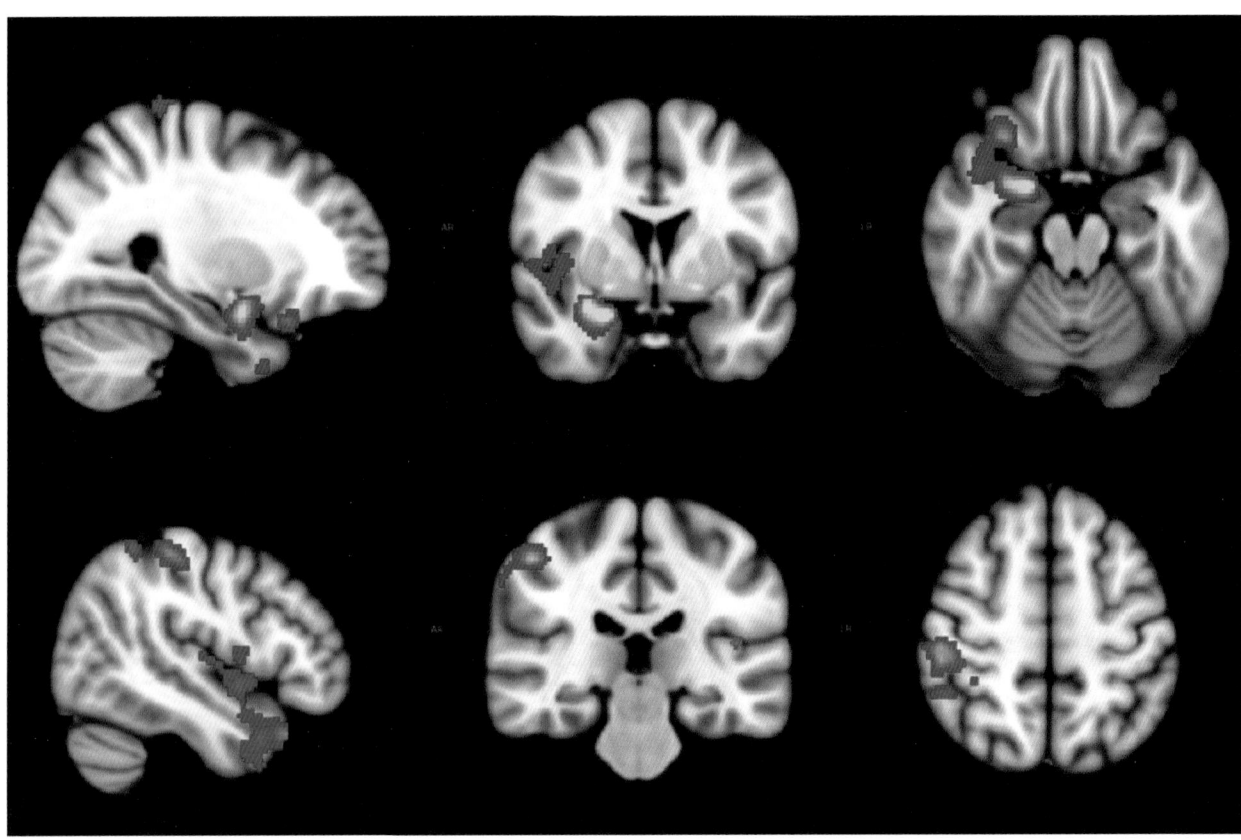

**Fig. 18.2** Negative association of vascular risk (Framingham Stroke Risk Score) averaged over 20 years from mid- to later life and grey matter density (GMD) in members of the Whitehall II cohort (N = 405). Images were analysed using FSL-VBM, an optimized voxel-based morphometry (VBM) protocol (for more details, see [140]). Using randomized and correcting for multiple comparisons, a voxel-wise general linear model (GLM) was applied between average Framingham Stroke Risk Scores and GMDs, correcting for age and sex. Significance threshold was set at $P < 0.05$, using the threshold-free cluster enhancement (TFCE) method. Significant negative association is present in the right cerebral cortex: in the medial temporal lobe, temporal pole, planum polare (a), and post-central gyrus (b). A = anterior; R = right.

Image courtesy of Dr Enikő Zsoldos.

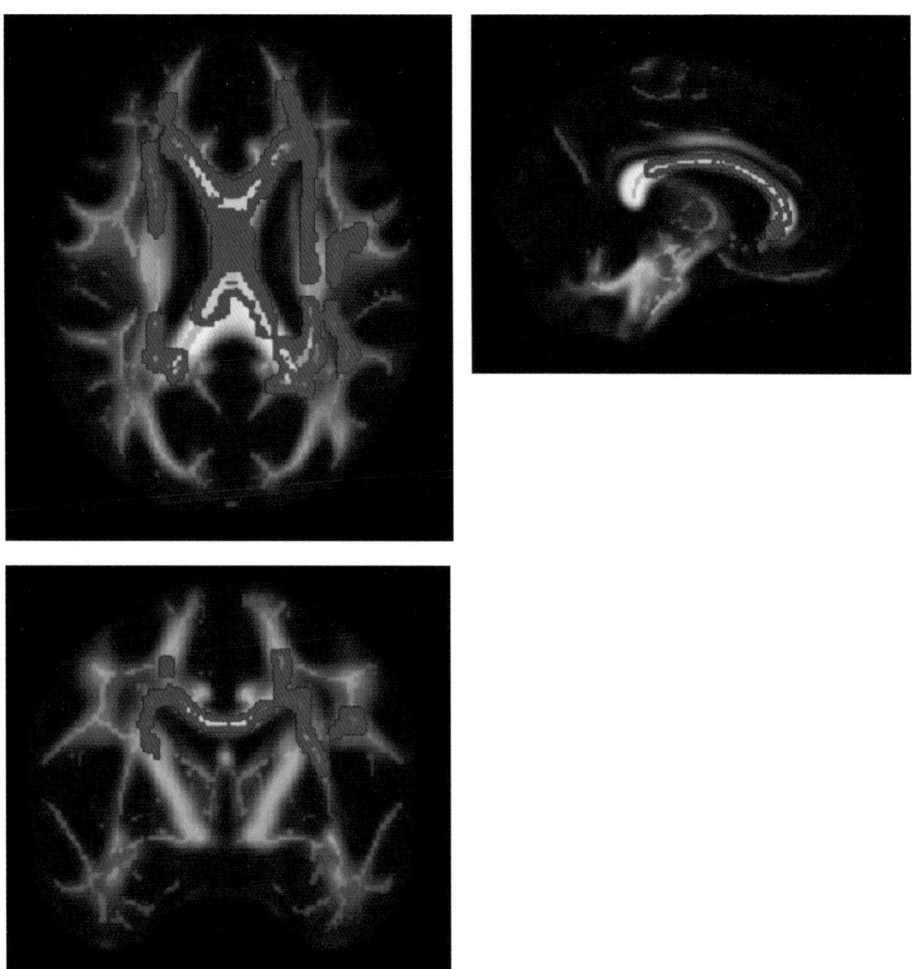

**Fig. 18.3** Associations of *large vessel elasticity* (from pulse wave velocity data supplied by Eric Brunner, University College London) with mean diffusivity in white matter (a, b, c: negative association) and grey matter density (d: positive association) (N = 444). Model: sex, education, mean arterial pressure, alcohol, antihypertensive medication, chronic illness, ethnicity, social class, and FRS (for image acquisition and analysis, see [140]).
Image courtesy of Dr Sana Suri.

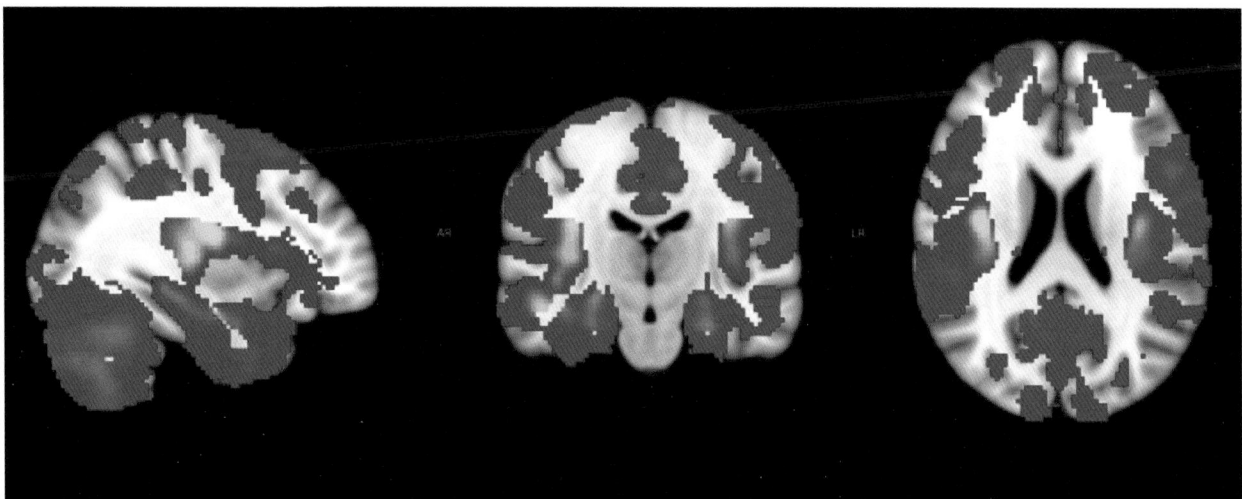

**Fig. 18.4** Widespread negative association of grey matter density (GMD) with age in members of the Whitehall II cohort (N = 405). Images were analysed using FSL-VBM, an optimized voxel-based morphometry (VBM) protocol. Using randomized and correcting for multiple comparisons, a voxel-wise general linear model (GLM) was applied between age and GMD, correcting for sex and socio-economic status defined by employment grade. Significance threshold was set at $P < 0.05$, using the threshold-free cluster enhancement (TFCE) method [140]. A = anterior; R = right.
Image courtesy of Dr Enikő Zsoldos.

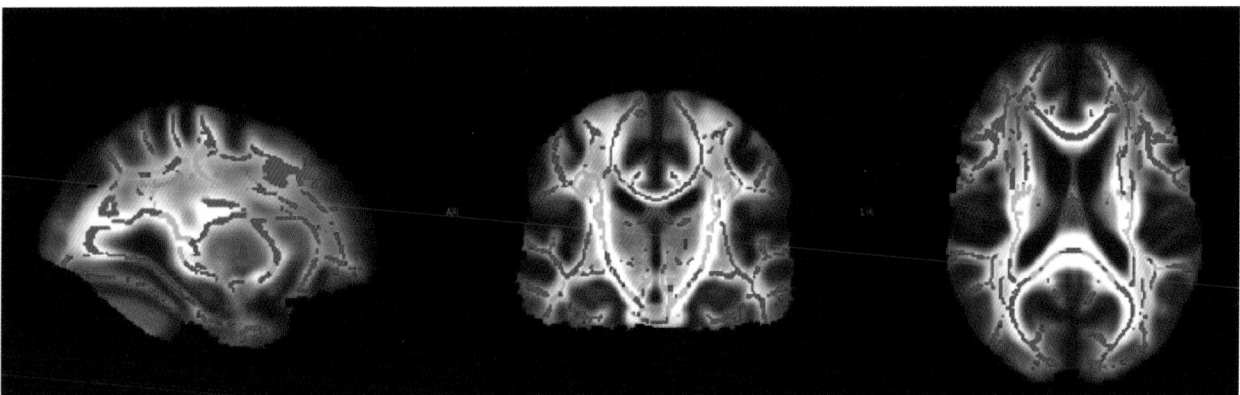

**Fig. 18.5** Widespread negative association of white matter integrity [fractional anisotropy (FA)] with age (in blue overlaid on green white matter skeleton) in members of the Whitehall II cohort (*N* = 395). Images were analysed using FSL-TBSS, an optimized tract-based spatial statistics (TBSS) protocol. Using randomized and correcting for multiple comparisons, a voxel-wise general linear model (GLM) was applied between age and FA, correcting for sex and socio-economic status defined by employment grade. Significance threshold was set at *P* <0.05, using the threshold-free cluster enhancement (TFCE) method [140]. A = anterior; R = right.
Image courtesy of Dr Enikő Zsoldos.

**Fig. 18.6** Default mode networks generated from 323 Whitehall II participant scans (MoCA >25), showing split between frontal (top) and posterior (bottom) components in older people (mean age 70 years) (for method, see [140]).
Image courtesy of Dr Sana Suri.

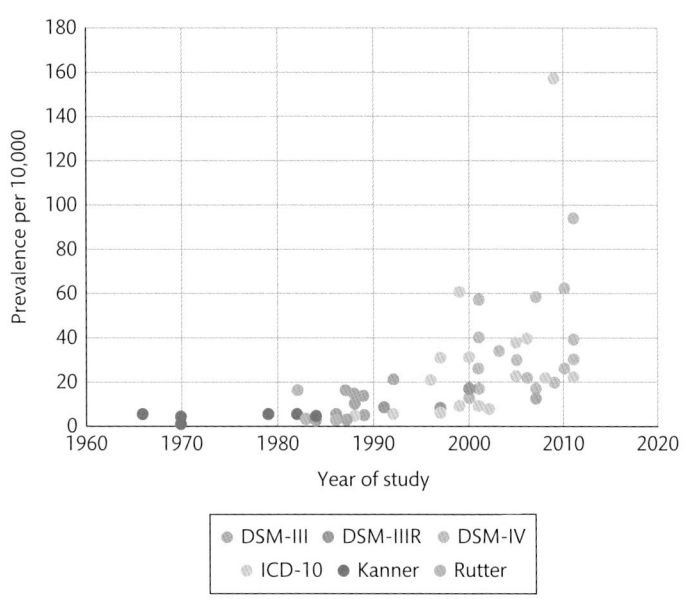

**Fig. 27.1** Prevalence of autism since the 1960s to 2015 according to the diagnostic criteria.

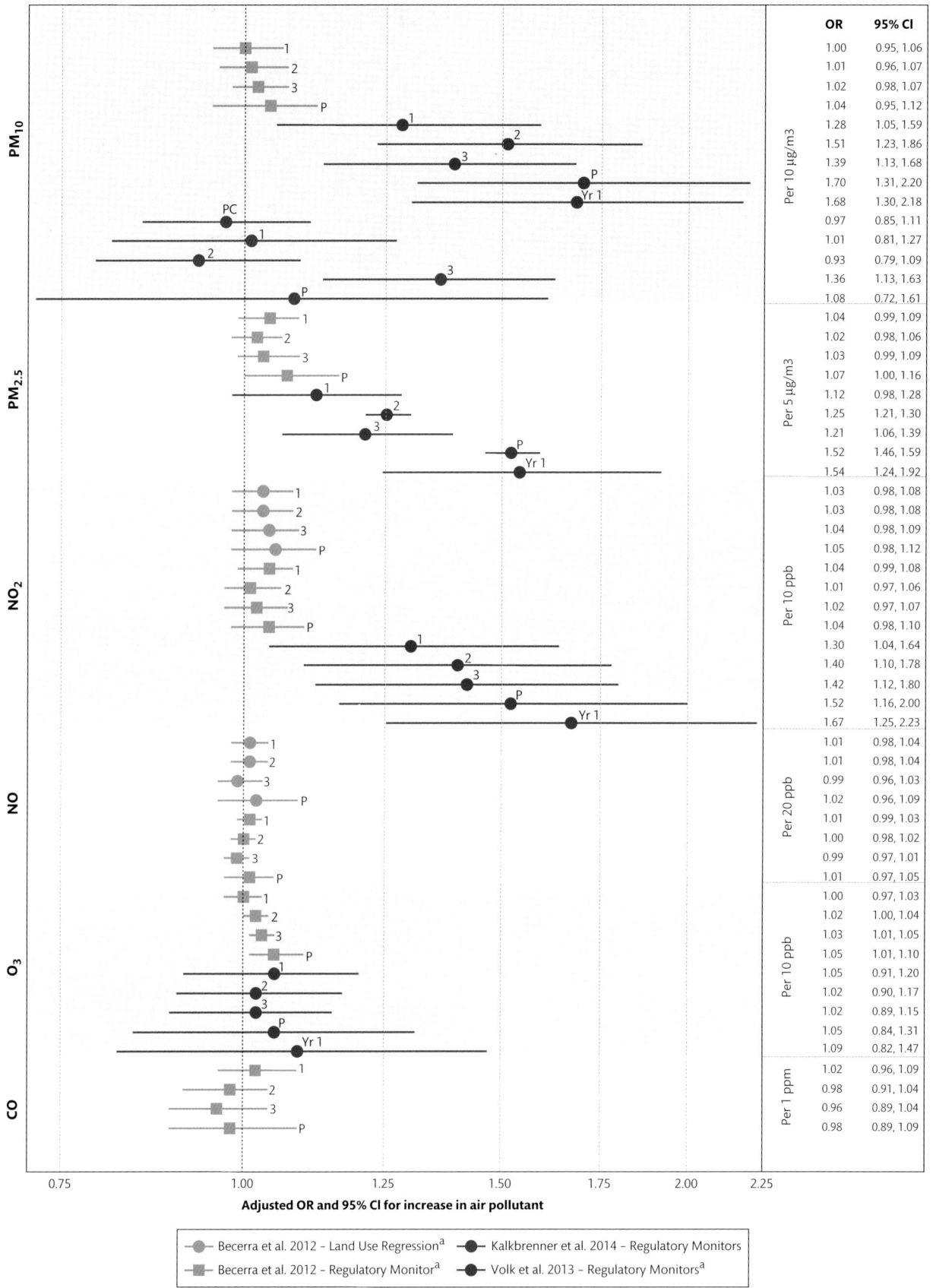

|  | OR | 95% CI |
|---|---|---|
| PM₁₀ (Per 10 µg/m3) | 1.00 | 0.95, 1.06 |
|  | 1.01 | 0.96, 1.07 |
|  | 1.02 | 0.98, 1.07 |
|  | 1.04 | 0.95, 1.12 |
|  | 1.28 | 1.05, 1.59 |
|  | 1.51 | 1.23, 1.86 |
|  | 1.39 | 1.13, 1.68 |
|  | 1.70 | 1.31, 2.20 |
|  | 1.68 | 1.30, 2.18 |
|  | 0.97 | 0.85, 1.11 |
|  | 1.01 | 0.81, 1.27 |
|  | 0.93 | 0.79, 1.09 |
|  | 1.36 | 1.13, 1.63 |
|  | 1.08 | 0.72, 1.61 |
| PM₂.₅ (Per 5 µg/m3) | 1.04 | 0.99, 1.09 |
|  | 1.02 | 0.98, 1.06 |
|  | 1.03 | 0.99, 1.09 |
|  | 1.07 | 1.00, 1.16 |
|  | 1.12 | 0.98, 1.28 |
|  | 1.25 | 1.21, 1.30 |
|  | 1.21 | 1.06, 1.39 |
|  | 1.52 | 1.46, 1.59 |
|  | 1.54 | 1.24, 1.92 |
| NO₂ (Per 10 ppb) | 1.03 | 0.98, 1.08 |
|  | 1.03 | 0.98, 1.08 |
|  | 1.04 | 0.98, 1.09 |
|  | 1.05 | 0.98, 1.12 |
|  | 1.04 | 0.99, 1.08 |
|  | 1.01 | 0.97, 1.06 |
|  | 1.02 | 0.97, 1.07 |
|  | 1.04 | 0.98, 1.10 |
|  | 1.30 | 1.04, 1.64 |
|  | 1.40 | 1.10, 1.78 |
|  | 1.42 | 1.12, 1.80 |
|  | 1.52 | 1.16, 2.00 |
|  | 1.67 | 1.25, 2.23 |
| NO (Per 20 ppb) | 1.01 | 0.98, 1.04 |
|  | 1.01 | 0.98, 1.04 |
|  | 0.99 | 0.96, 1.03 |
|  | 1.02 | 0.96, 1.09 |
|  | 1.01 | 0.99, 1.03 |
|  | 1.00 | 0.98, 1.02 |
|  | 0.99 | 0.97, 1.01 |
|  | 1.01 | 0.97, 1.05 |
| O₃ (Per 10 ppb) | 1.00 | 0.97, 1.03 |
|  | 1.02 | 1.00, 1.04 |
|  | 1.03 | 1.01, 1.05 |
|  | 1.05 | 1.01, 1.10 |
|  | 1.05 | 0.91, 1.20 |
|  | 1.02 | 0.90, 1.17 |
|  | 1.02 | 0.89, 1.15 |
|  | 1.05 | 0.84, 1.31 |
|  | 1.09 | 0.82, 1.47 |
| CO (Per 1 ppm) | 1.02 | 0.96, 1.09 |
|  | 0.98 | 0.91, 1.04 |
|  | 0.96 | 0.89, 1.04 |
|  | 0.98 | 0.89, 1.09 |

Adjusted OR and 95% CI for increase in air pollutant

Becerra et al. 2012 – Land Use Regression[a]     Kalkbrenner et al. 2014 – Regulatory Monitors
Becerra et al. 2012 – Regulatory Monitor[a]     Volk et al. 2013 – Regulatory Monitors[a]

**Fig. 27.2** Associations between autism and estimates of exposure to individual traffic-related and criteria air pollutants.
PM₁₀, particulate matter <10 µm in diameter; PM₂.₅, particulate matter <2.5 µm in diameter; NO₂, nitrogen dioxide; NO, nitrogen oxide; O₃, ozone; CO, carbon monoxide. Exposure measured during developmental windows: PC, peri-conceptual; 1, trimester 1; 2, trimester 2; 3, trimester 3; P, pregnancy; Yr 1, first postnatal year. We recalculated parameters to reflect a change in the exposure comparison, to be consistent with other comparisons in the figure, involving calculations assuming that parameters were normally distributed.

Reproduced from *Curr Probl Pediatr Adolesc Health Care*, 44(10), Kalkbrenner AE, Schmidt RJ, Penlesky AC, Environmental chemical exposures and autism spectrum disorders: a review of the epidemiological evidence, pp. 277–318, Copyright (2014), with permission from Mosby, Inc.

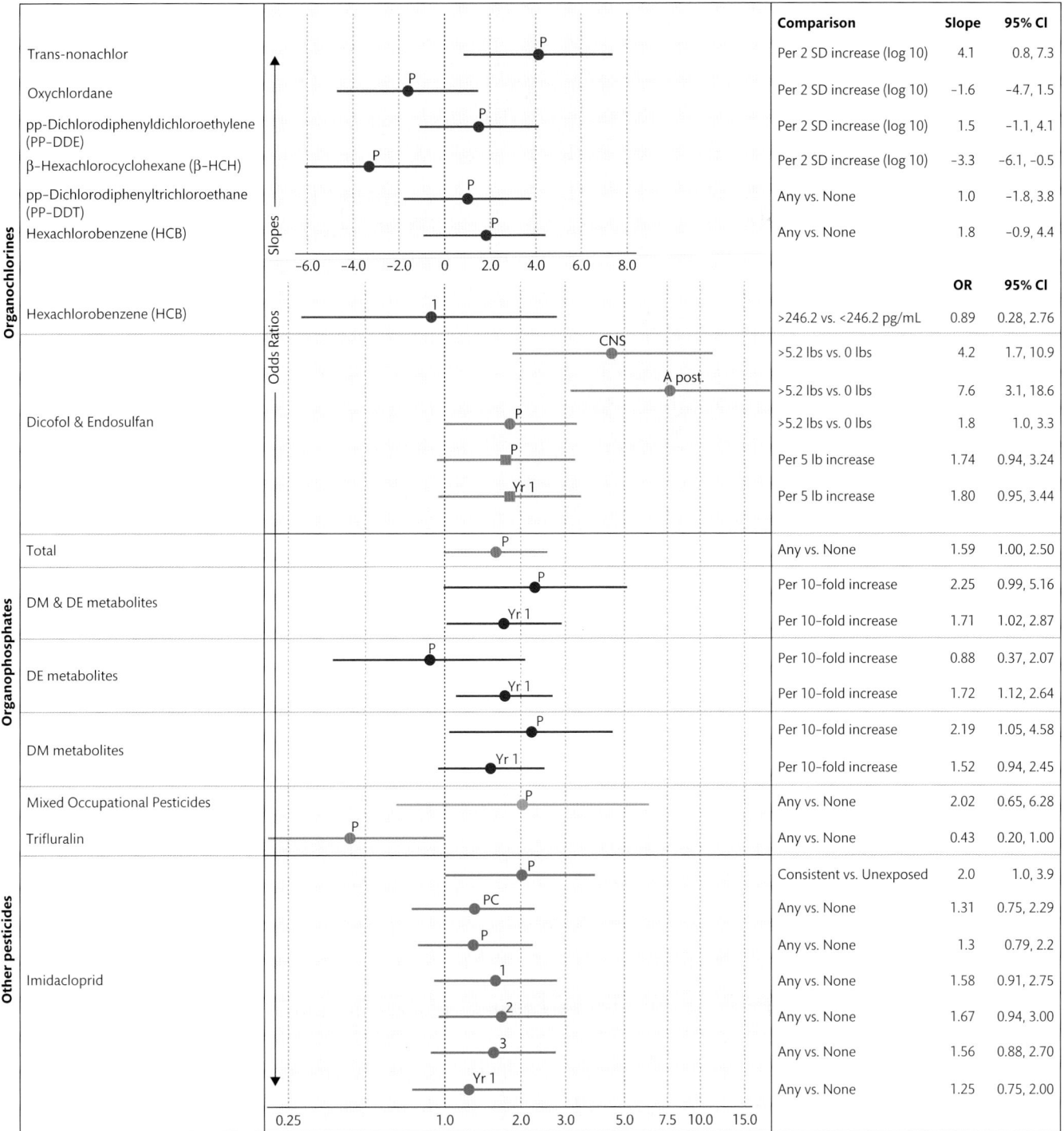

**Fig. 27.3** Associations between autism and estimates of exposure to pesticides.
DE metabolites, diethyl phosphate metabolites of organophosphate pesticides; DM metabolites, dimethyl phosphate metabolites of organophosphate pesticides. Exposure measured during developmental windows: CNS, a priori period of central nervous system development (7 days pre-fertilization to 49 days post-fertilization); a period of development (26–81 days post-fertilization); 1, trimester 1; 2, trimester 2; 3, trimester 3; P, pregnancy; Yr 1, first postnatal year. Other results not reported as measures of association with confidence intervals included pesticides that were determined not to be associated with increased autism risk and were not included in subsequent analyses from Roberts et al. 138: pesticide classes (cholinesterase inhibitors, copper-containing compounds, fumigants, avermectins, halogenated organics, N-methyl carbamates, pyrethroids, and thiocarbamates) and individual pesticide compounds (1,3-dichloropropene, chloropicrin, cypermethrin, fenarimol, methyl bromide, norflurazon, bromacil acid, chlorpyrifos, dazomet, glyphosate, molinate, oxadiazon, bifenthrin, diuron, metam-sodium, myclobutanil, and paraquat).

Reproduced from *Curr Probl Pediatr Adolesc Health Care*, 44(10), Kalkbrenner AE, Schmidt RJ, Penlesky AC, Environmental chemical exposures and autism spectrum disorders: a review of the epidemiological evidence, pp. 277–318, Copyright (2014), with permission from Mosby, Inc.

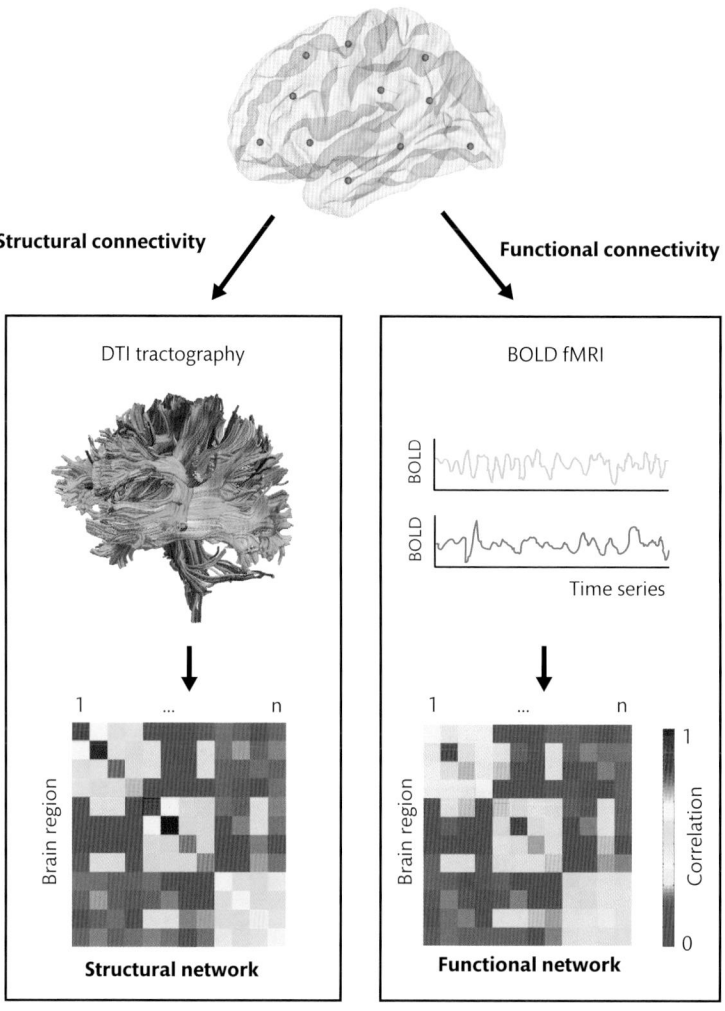

**Fig. 29.3** Schematic illustration of the underlying concepts behind atypical structural and functional brain connectivity in ASD.

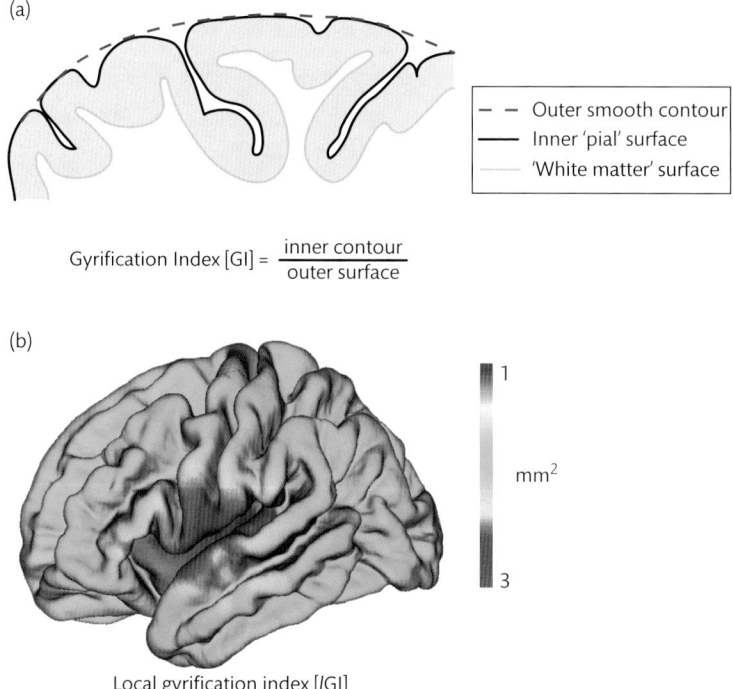

(a)

Gyrification Index [GI] = $\dfrac{\text{inner contour}}{\text{outer surface}}$

- - - Outer smooth contour
— Inner 'pial' surface
 'White matter' surface

(b)

Local gyrification index [*l*GI]

**Fig. 29.4** Computation of the gyrification index (GI) as the ratio between the inner (i.e. pial) surface of the brain and the outer smooth contour. The GI can be calculated within brain slices in 2D (a) and at each location on the cortical surface in 3D (b).

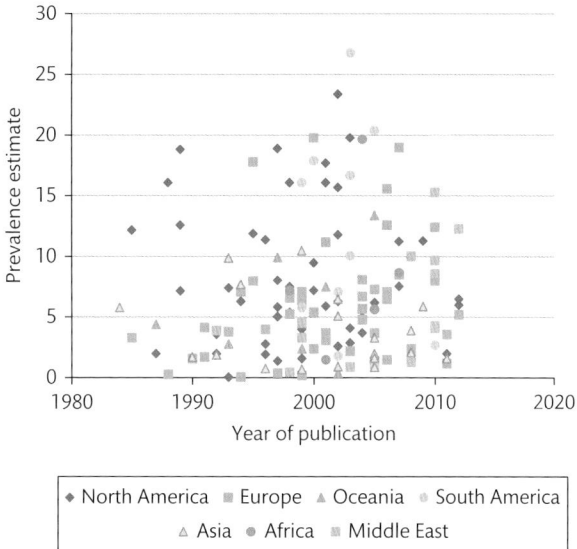

**Fig. 33.4** ADHD prevalence estimates over time as a function of geographic location of the studies.

Reproduced from *International Journal of Epidemiology*, 43(2), Polanczyk G, Guilherme V, Willcutt, EG, ADHD prevalence estimates across three decades: an updated systematic review and meta-regression analysis, pp. 434–442, Copyright (2014) with permission from Oxford University Press.

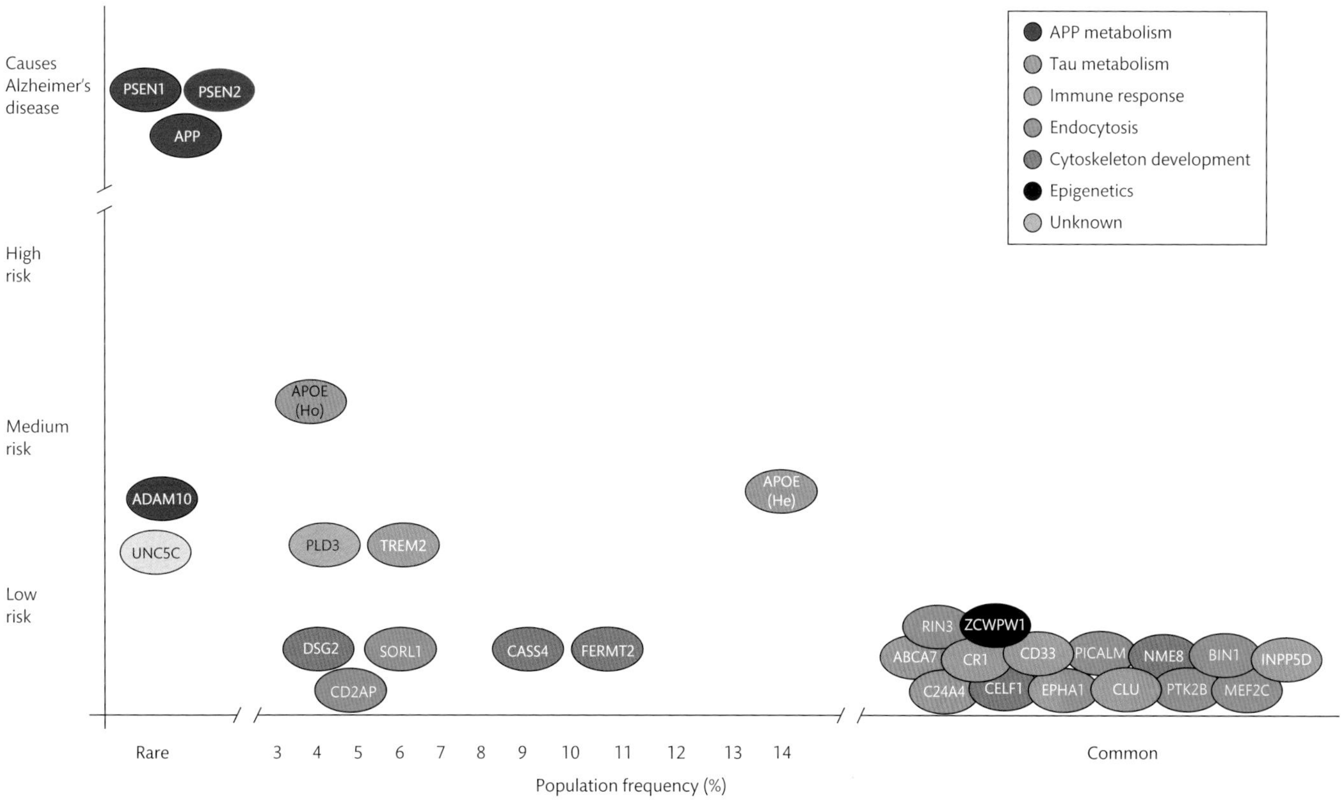

**Fig. 40.1** Risk genes for Alzheimer's disease identifying the primary mechanism, risk conferred, and population allele frequency.

Adapted from *Biol Psychiatry*, 77(1), Karch CM, Goate AM, Alzheimer's disease risk genes and mechanisms of disease pathogenesis, pp. 43–51, Copyright (2015), with permission from Society of Biological Psychiatry.

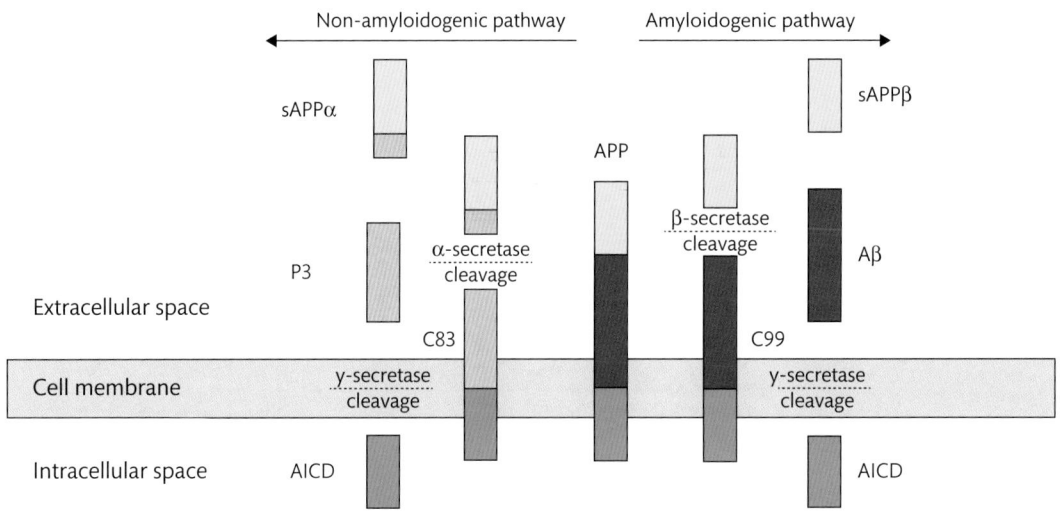

**Fig. 40.2** Schematic of amyloidogenic and non-amyloidogenic APP processing pathways.

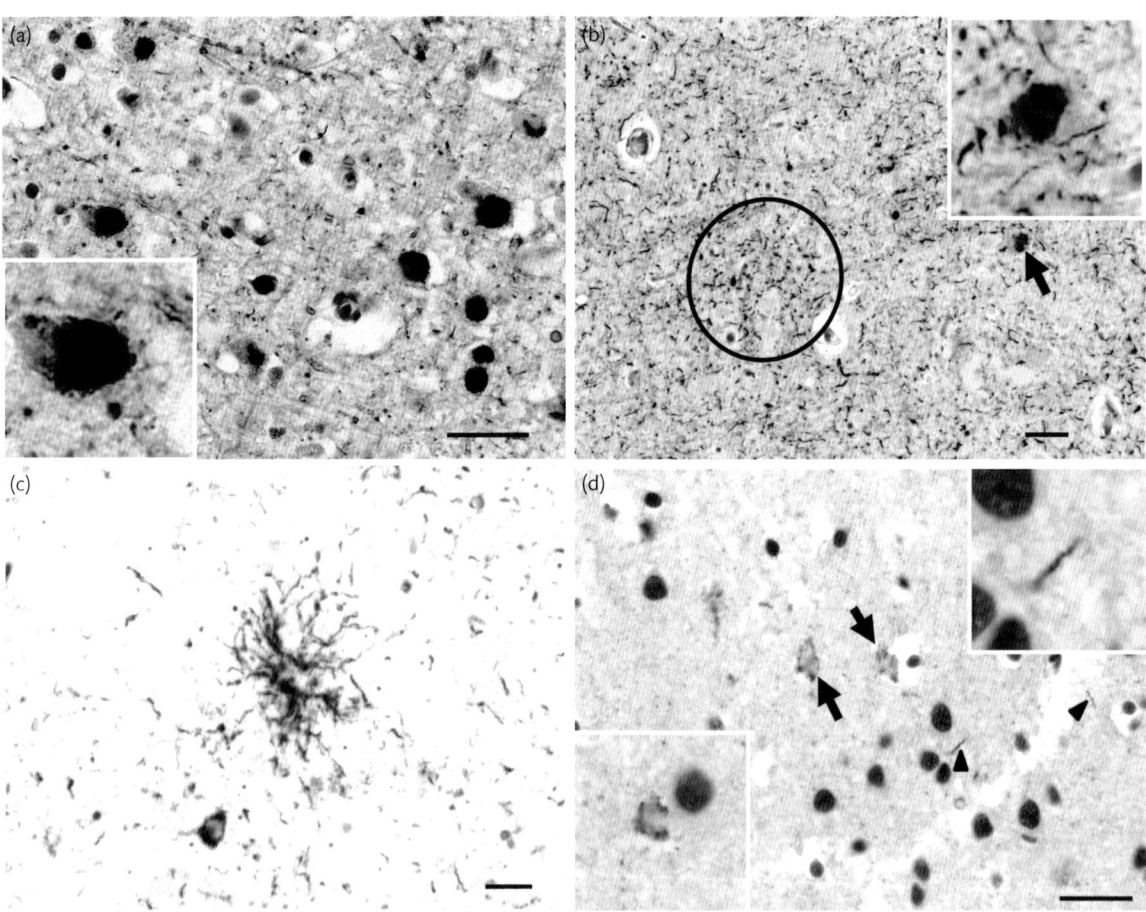

**Fig. 41.2** Histological features of FTLD-tau and FTLD-TDP. (a) Pick's disease. Pick bodies (lower inset) in the inferior temporal gyrus. (b) Cortico-basal degeneration. Astrocytic plaque (circle) and neuronal cytoplasmic inclusions (arrow and upper inset) in the precentral gyrus. (c) Progressive supranuclear palsy. Tufted astrocyte in the sensorimotor cortex. (d) FTLD-TDP type B. Neuronal cytoplasmic inclusions (arrow and lower inset) and neuropil threads (arrowheads and upper inset) in the middle frontal gyrus. Immunostains are phospho-tau (a–c) and TDP-43 (d). All scale bar represents 10 μm.

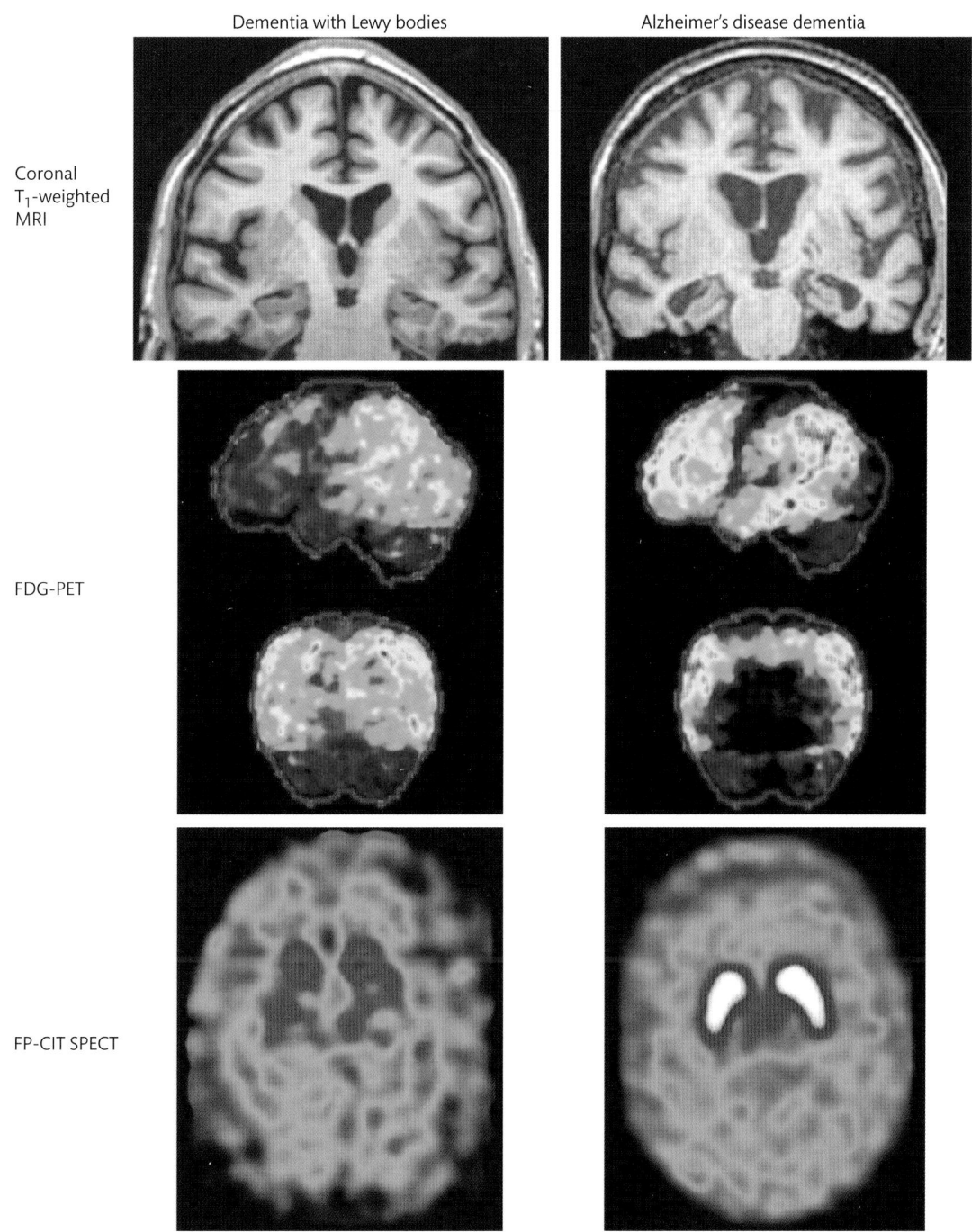

**Fig. 43.1** Representative coronal MRI, FDG-PET, and FP-CIT SPECT images in DLB and AD.

Reprinted from *The Lancet* 386(10004), Walker Z, Possin KL, Boeve BF, Aarsland D., Lewy body dementias, Pages 1683–97. Copyright 2015 with permission from Elsevier.

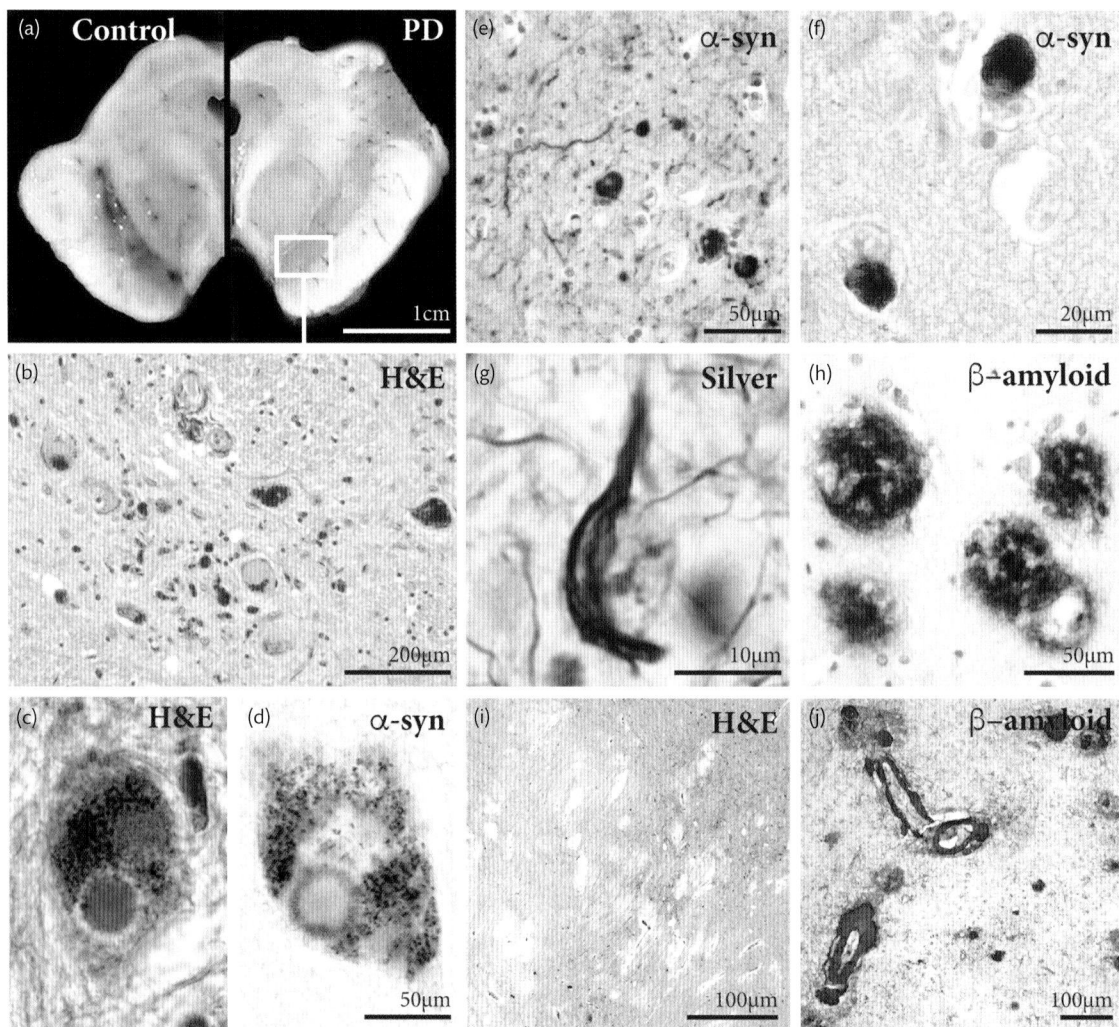

**Fig. 44.2** Tissue histopathology of PD and PDD. (a) Transverse section through the midbrain of a control (at left) showing the darkly pigmented SN in the ventral aspect of the midbrain, whereas the pigmented neurons in this structure are lost in patients with PD (at right). (b) Higher magnification (box in (a)) of a haematoxylin and eosin-stained section through the SN, showing only a few pigmented neurons remaining with many smaller phagocytic microglia. (c) and (d) Higher magnification of a haematoxylin and eosin-stained (c) and an a-Syn-immunoreactive (d) pigmented neuron in the SN of a PD patient containing an LB. (e) and (f) a-Syn-immunoreactive LBs and Lewy neurites in the amygdala (e) and anterior cingulate cortex (f) of a patient with PDD. (g) Silver-stained neurofibrillary tangle in the cortex of a patient with PDD. (h) Beta-amyloid-immunoreactive plaques in the cortex of a patient with PDD. (i) Vascular ischaemic tissue damage identified in a haematoxylin and eosin-stained section of the globus pallidus in a patient with PDD. (j) Beta-amyloid-immunoreactive congophilic angiopathy in the cortex of a patient with PDD.

Reproduced from *Mov Disord.*, 29(5), Halliday GM, Leverenz JB, Schneider JS, *et al.*, The neurobiological basis of cognitive impairment in Parkinson's disease, pp. 634–50, Copyright (2014), with permission from John Wiley and Sons.

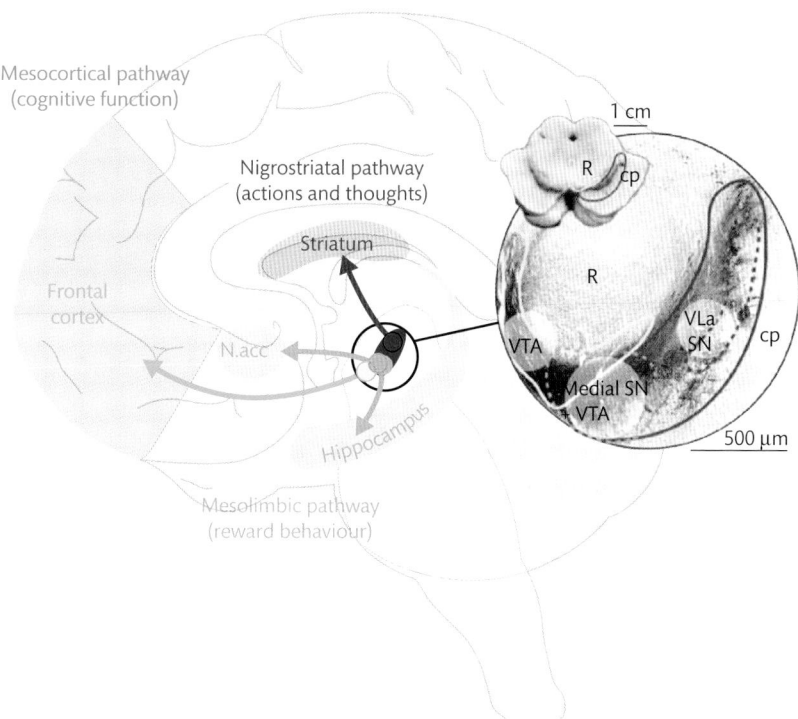

**Fig. 44.3** Dopamine pathways affected in PD and PDD. Red outline: SN, which contains both dopamine neurons in the pars compacta that give rise to the nigrostriatal projections, and GABA neurons in the pars reticulate, which innervate the thalamus. Dotted red line: ventrolateral (VLa) SN, which is selectively damaged in patients with PD. Yellow outline: ventral tegmental area (VTA), which contains both dopamine and non-dopamine neurons that project to limbic and cortical regions. Dotted orange outline: medial SN and VTA, which give rise to mesolimbic projections affected in patients with PDD. cp, cerebral peduncle; N. acc, nucleus accumbens; R, red nucleus.

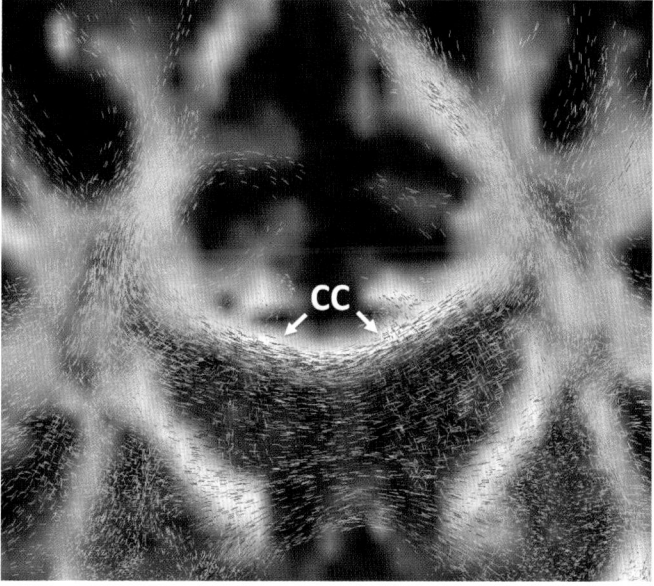

**Fig. 47.3** Diffusion tensor imaging measures the preferred direction of diffusion of water molecules. High directionality of diffusion can be observed in well-organized regions of the brain such as in the corpus callosum, as depicted here (see arrows). Diffusion tensor imaging provides information about the microstructure of brain tissue and thus may provide useful information in patients with TBI where diffuse axonal injury that involves the white matter is common.

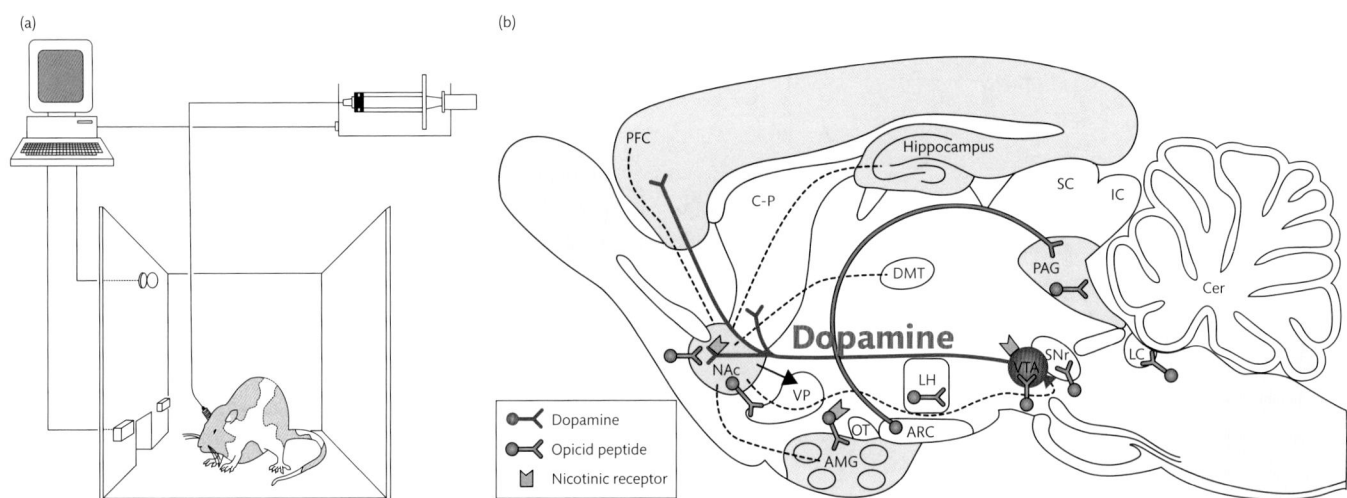

**Fig. 48.2** (a) Intracerebral drug self-administration. By pressing a lever in an operant chamber, rats can deliver microlitre and microgram quantities of drugs, such as amphetamine, directly into the brain. A major neural locus that supports such drug self-administration is the nucleus accumbens. (b) A schematic sagittal section of the rat brain showing the mesolimbic dopamine system, comprising cell bodies in the ventral tegmental area (VTA), axons that run in the medial forebrain bundle in the lateral hypothalamus, and terminals in the nucleus accumbens (NAc), medial prefrontal cortex (PFC), and amygdala (AMG), among other forebrain structures. Nicotinic and opioid receptors are shown on both dopamine neuron cell bodies and terminals in the nucleus accumbens. Some major cortical afferents to the nucleus accumbens are also shown and include the amygdala, hippocampal formation, and prefrontal cortex. Opioidergic (beta-endorphin-containing) projections are shown originating in the hypothalamic arcuate nucleus (ARC) and innervating the midbrain periaqueductal grey matter (PAG). Small encephalin-containing interneurons are represented in green. There is widespread agreement that all drugs of abuse, in addition to actions on their specific molecular targets, can increase activity in the mesolimbic dopamine system and dopamine release in the nucleus accumbens and is often therefore referred to as the common reward pathway. (See [90].)

Reproduced from *Trends Pharmacol Sci.*, 13(5), Koob G, Drugs of abuse: anatomy, pharmacology and function of reward pathways, pp. 177–84, Copyright (1992) with permission from Elsevier Ltd.

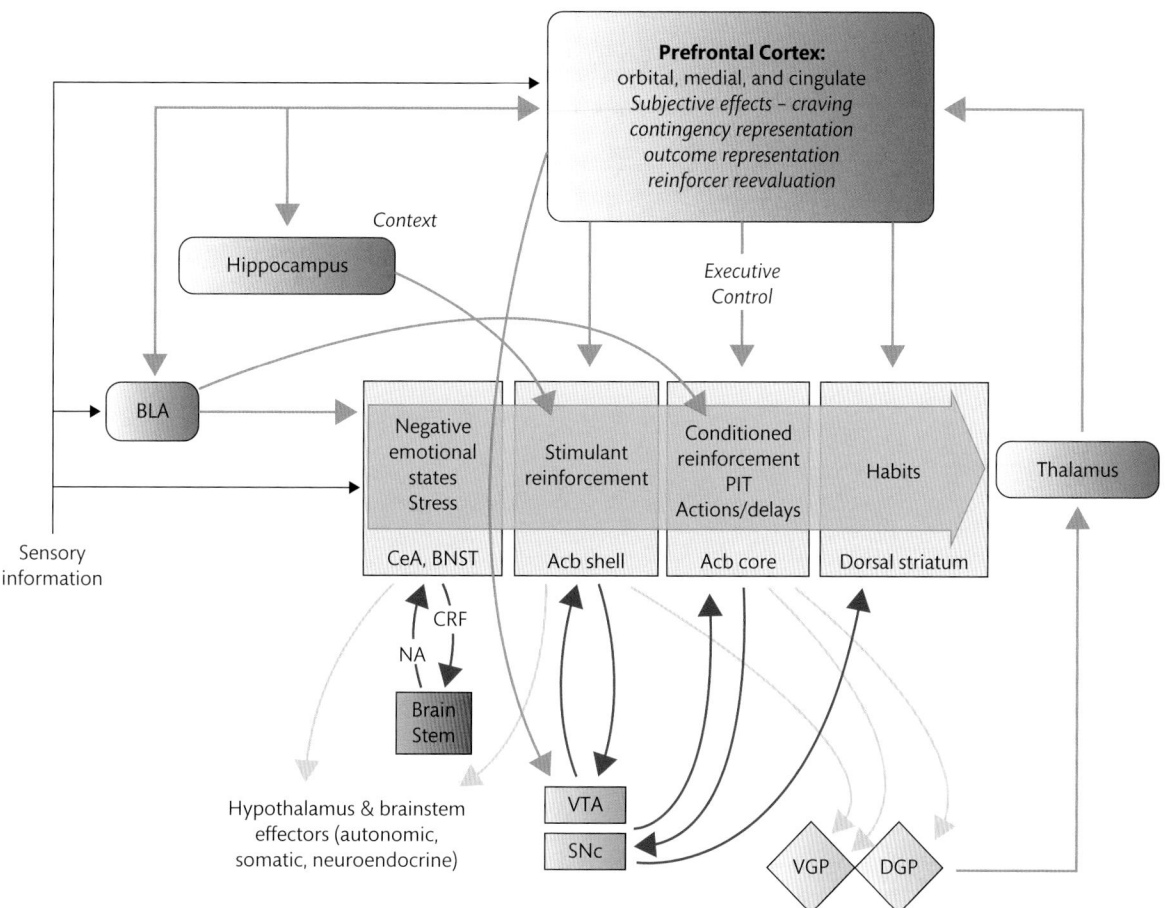

**Fig. 48.3** Representation of key components of limbic cortico- striatal circuitry in which psychological and physiological processes important in drug addiction are indicated. These include: (1) the processing of conditioned reinforcement (and Pavlovian associations between environmental stimuli and drugs in general) by the basolateral amygdala and of contextual information by the hippocampus; (2) goal- directed actions involve interactions between prefrontal cortical areas (orbitofrontal, ventromedial) and the dorsomedial striatum; (3) habits (stimulus– response associations) depend on interactions between the prefrontal cortex (sensorimotor) and dorsolateral striatum; (4) 'executive control' depends on the prefrontal cortex and includes representation of contingencies and outcomes and their value and subjective states (craving and feelings) associated with drugs; (5) in functional imaging studies, drug craving involves activation of the orbital, anterior cingulate, and insular cortices and temporal lobe structures, including the amygdala; (6) connections between dopaminergic neurons and the striatum, linking the ventral with the dorsal striatum via interactions organized in a striato- midbrain- striatal spiralling cascade of neuronal interconnections; (7) reinforcing effects of drugs may engage stimulant Pavlovian influences on behaviour such as Pavlovian- instrumental transfer, or conditioned motivation, and conditioned reinforcement processes in the nucleus accumbens shell and core and then engage stimulus– response habits that depend on the dorsal striatum; (8) the extended amygdala is composed of several basal forebrain structures, including the bed nucleus of the stria terminalis, the centromedial amygdala, and, more controversially, the medial portion (or shell) of the nucleus accumbens. A major transmitter in the extended amygdala is the corticotropin- releasing factor, which projects to the brainstem where noradrenergic neurons provide a major projection reciprocally to the extended amygdala. Activation of this system is closely associated with the negative affective state that occurs during withdrawal. Green/ blue arrows, glutamatergic projections; orange arrows, dopaminergic projections; pink arrows, GABAergic projections. Acb, nucleus accumbens; BLA, basolateral amygdala; VTA, ventral tegmental area; SNc, substantia nigra pars compacta. VGP, ventral globus pallidus; DGP, dorsal globus pallidus; BNST, bed nucleus of the stria terminalis; CeA, central nucleus of the amygdala; NA, noradrenaline; CRF, corticotropin- releasing factor; PIT, Pavlovian- instrumental transfer. (See [91].)

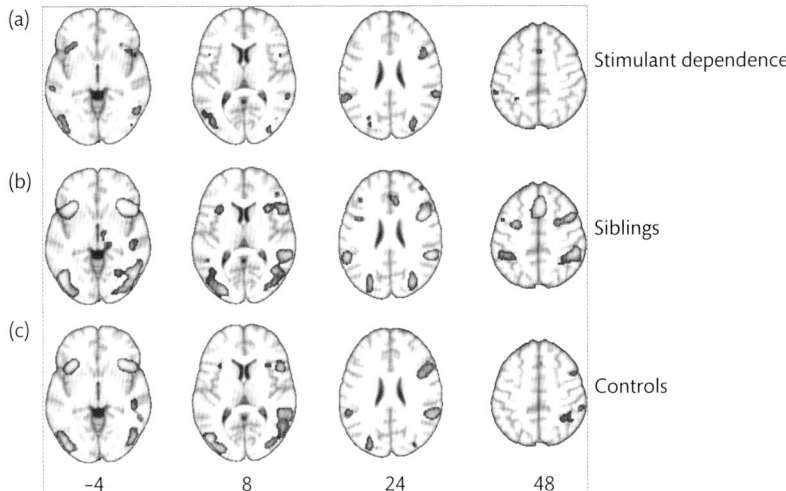

Endophenotypes for stimulant abuse: neuroimaging evidence
for resilience and compensation?

**Fig. 48.6** Evidence of hypothetical resilience factors operating in siblings of stimulant-dependent individuals (bottom row scans) in terms of BOLD response overactivation of the right inferior frontal gyrus during functional magnetic resonance imaging study of the stop-signal reaction time task, as compared with healthy control volunteers (middle row scans) and stimulant-dependent individuals (top row)—the latter showing significant reductions, compared with controls. Significant brain activation maps were associated with stopping in each group ($P$ <0.05, family-wise error). Axial brain slices demonstrate main activation clusters per group at family-wise error, $P$ <0.05. The $z$-co-ordinate slices are: −4, 8, 24, and 48. The right side of each slice corresponds to the right side of the brain.

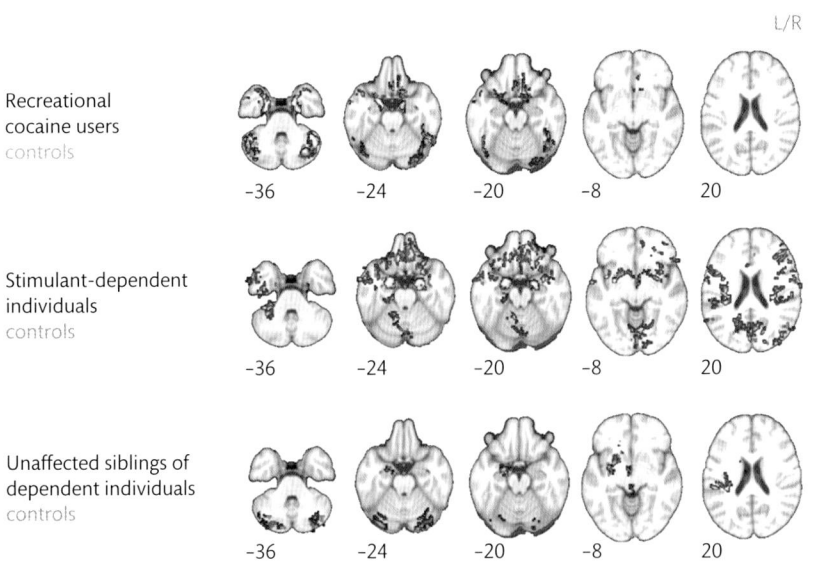

**Fig. 48.7** Structural brain abnormalities associated with stimulant exposure and familial risk. Blue voxels indicate a decrease, and red voxels indicate an increase, in grey matter volume, compared with control volunteers. Both recreational and dependent stimulant users showed significant increases in the parahippocampal gyrus, compared with healthy control volunteers, but differed with regard to abnormalities in the orbitofrontal cortex. Recreational users did not show any of the changes in brain regions associated with familial risk such as increased volume of the amygdala and putamen and decreased volume in the posterior insula. Siblings of stimulant-dependent stimulant abusers showed larger grey matter volumes in the basal ganglia, particularly the putamen. Sections and horizontal numbers below each section of the image refer to its plane position (mm) relative to the origin in MNI stereotactic space. L, left; R, right.

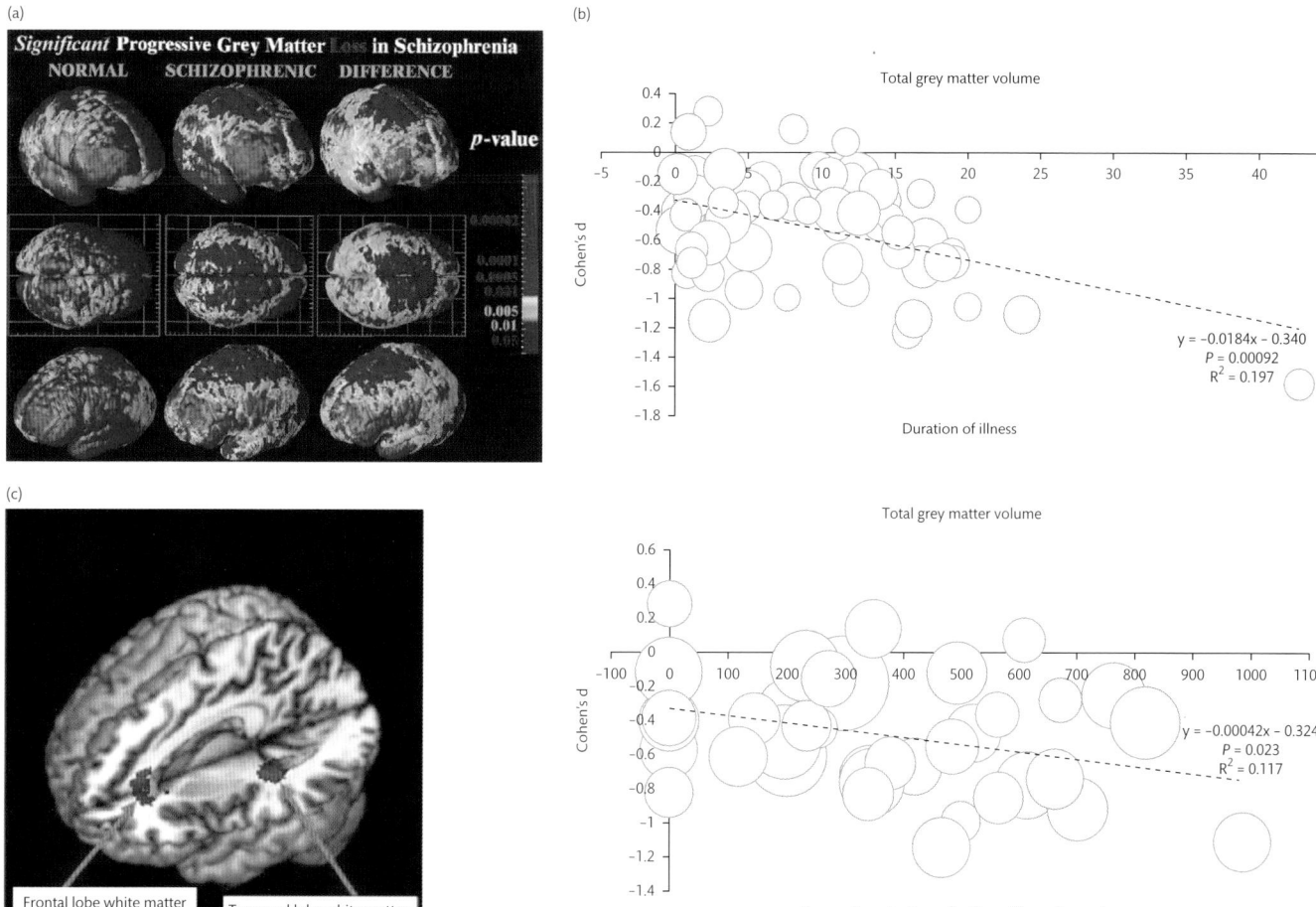

**Fig. 60.2** Progressive grey and white matter loss in schizophrenia.

(a) Significant grey matter loss in normal adolescents and schizophrenia (see Colour Plate section).

Reproduced from *Proc Natl Acad Sci U S A*, 98(20), Thompson PM, Vidal C, Giedd JN, *et al.*, Mapping adolescent brain change reveals dynamic wave of accelerated gray matter loss in very early-onset schizophrenia, pp. 11650–5, Copyright (2001), with permission from National Academy of Sciences.

(b) Upper panel: total grey matter volume reduction depends on duration of illness; lower panel: total grey matter volume reduction was more pronounced in patients using a higher dose of atypical antipsychotics.

Reproduced from *Schizophr Bull.*, 39(5), Haijma SV, Haren NV, Cahn W, *et al.*, Brain Volumes in Schizophrenia: A Meta-Analysis in Over 18 000 Subjects, pp. 1129–38, Copyright (2013), with permission from Oxford University Press.

(c) Regional fractional anisotropy reductions in the deep white matter of the left frontal and left temporal lobes in schizophrenia (see Colour Plate section).

Reproduced from *Schizophr Res*, 108(1–3), Ellison-Wright I, Bullmore E, Meta-analysis of diffusion tensor imaging studies in schizophrenia, pp. 3–10, Copyright (2009), with permission from Elsevier B.V.

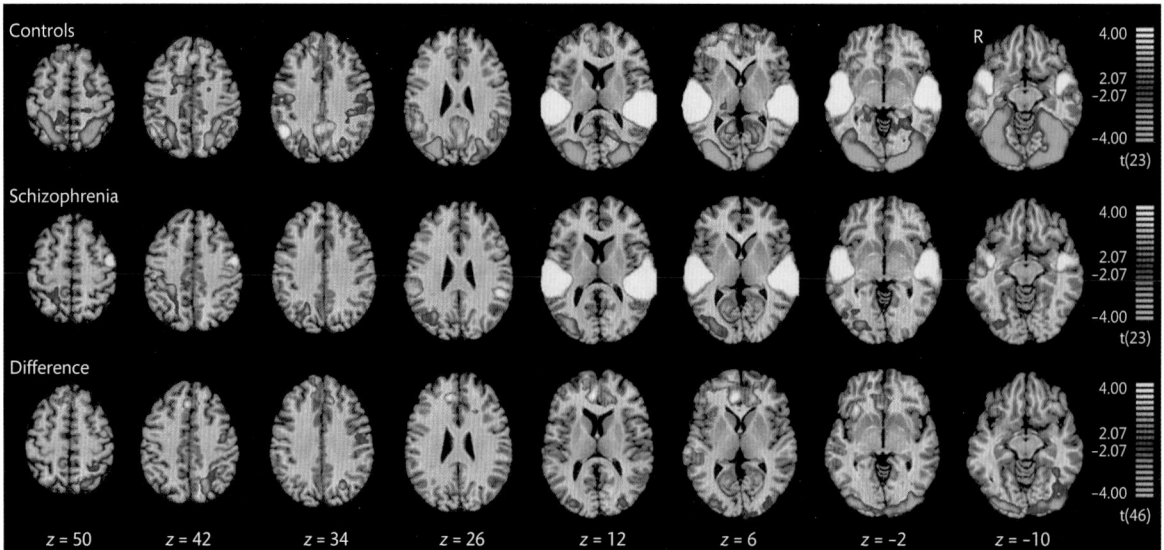

**Fig. 60.3** Haemodynamic response to mismatch blocks (*P* <0.05). A corrected cluster size threshold was based on a Monte Carlo simulation. First row: healthy controls; second row: schizophrenia patients; third row: difference between healthy controls and schizophrenia patients for the contrast mismatch > standard (baseline) condition. Schizophrenia patients exhibited less activity in the auditory cortex and prefrontal and salience network (bilateral ACC, medial frontal gyrus, and right insula). Enhanced activity was found in schizophrenia patients in the pre- and post-central gyri, compared to the control group. *z*-co-ordinates refer to the Talairach system.

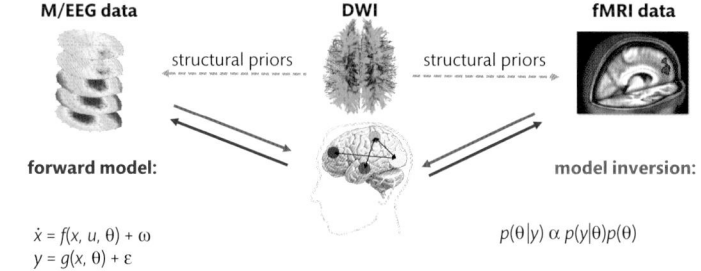

**Fig. 60.4** Generative models for neuroimaging data.
Generative models applied to neuroimaging data propose that we can infer on neural activity (for example, firing rate) from the measured signal. Constrained by priors that define neuroanatomical connectivity obtained by DWI techniques, generative models comprise neural state equations, which describe the hidden dynamics in terms of differential equations that are parameterized, and a forward model that describes a mapping from the neural state to the measured signal. To estimate how neural states translate into the measured signal, the model is inverted, that is, fitted to the neuroimaging data and the connectivity parameters that generated the observed data are estimated. DWI, diffusion-weighted imaging; M/EEG, magneto-/electroencephalography.

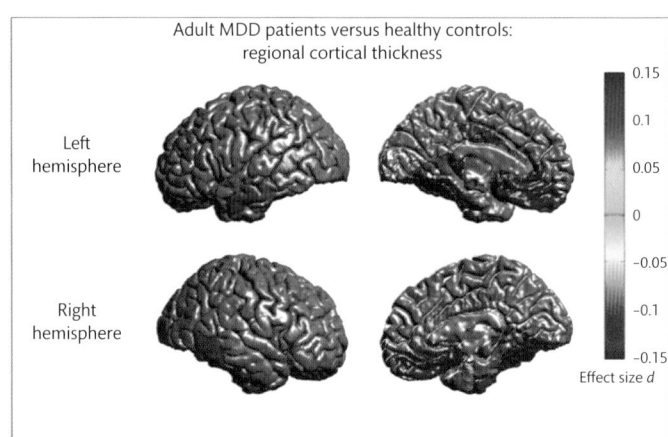

**Fig. 76.1** Meta-analysis of magnetic resonance scans from patients with major depression, compared with controls, from the ENIGMA working group [34]. Effect sizes for regions with significant (PFDR <0.05) cortical thinning are shown in red. Negative effect sizes *d* indicate cortical thinning in MDD, compared to controls.

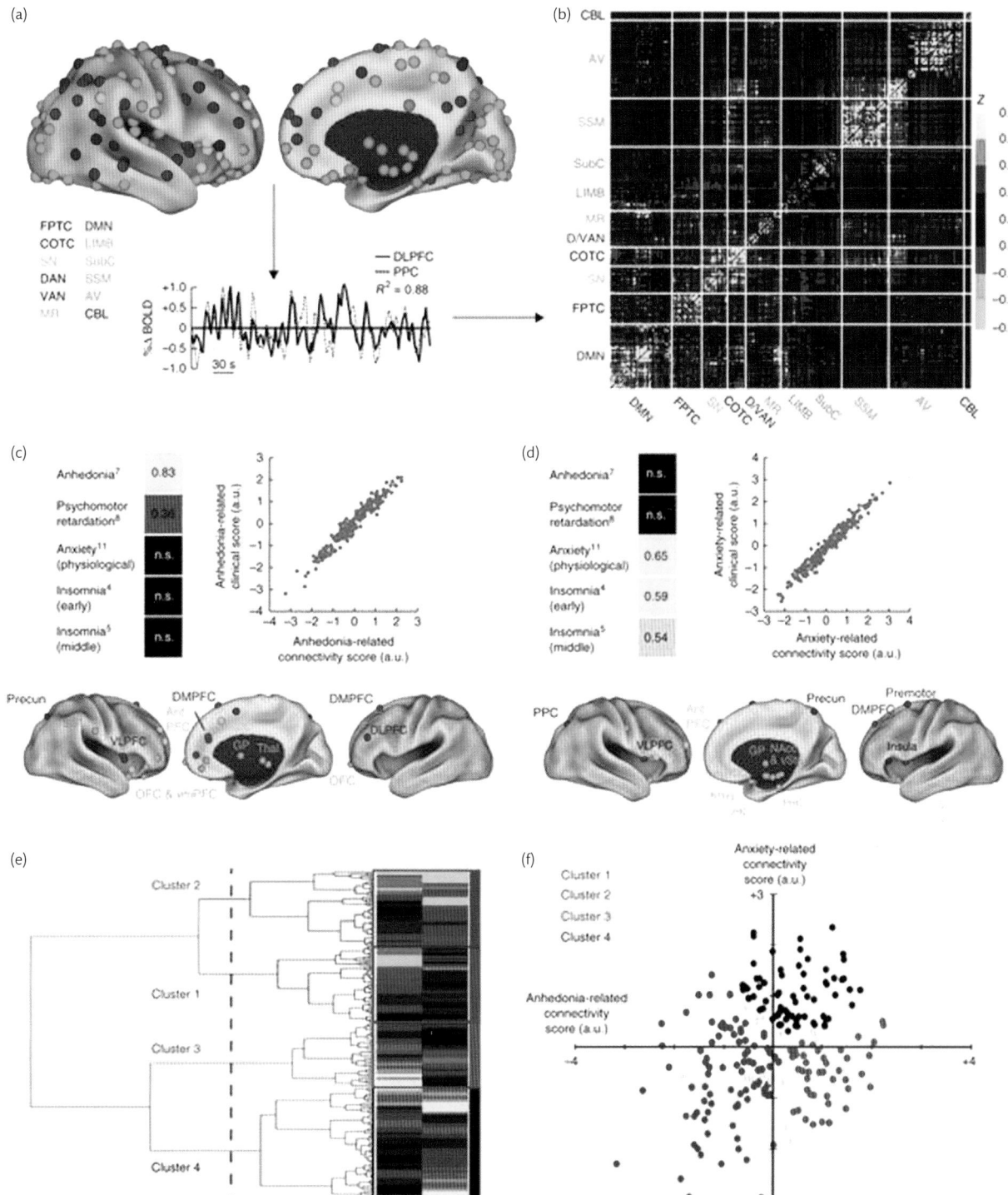

**Fig. 76.2** Definition of subtypes of depression using resting state fMRI data taken from [44]. Resting state data from depressed patients and control subjects were collected. (a) Regions of interest were defined across the brain, and the mean BOLD time series from each of these regions was extracted for each subject. (b) For each subject, the correlation between all pairs of time series was calculated as a measure of connectivity. The figure illustrates the correlation between the regions of interest which are arranged depending on the neural system of which they are a member. (c) and (d) A data reduction method (canonical correlation; CC) was then used to find simple relationships between the imaging data shown in (b) and patient depression scores measured using the Hamilton Depression Rating Scale. CC looks for common factors in the imaging and symptom score data sets; here two were found: (c) an 'anhedonia'-related scale and (d) an 'anxiety'-related scale. The brain images display the regions of interest between which resting state correlations were most closely related to the specific factor. (e) The strength of these two factors was estimated for each patient, and then an unsupervised classification procedure—hierarchical clustering—was used to try and find clusters of patients who differed on the two measures. (f) Four clusters of patients were found, with each cluster defined by a different combination of the two factors. The scatter plot shows data from patients colour-coded by the cluster to which they are assigned; grey dots represent patients who could not be confidently classified.

The authors next demonstrated that these clusters could be reliably detected in a second data set and that cluster membership could be assigned using just the neuroimaging data. Lastly, it was shown that the clusters predicted treatment response to transcranial magnetic stimulation (TMS) therapy—a greater proportion of patients in clusters 1 and 3 responded to TMS than those in clusters 2 and 4.

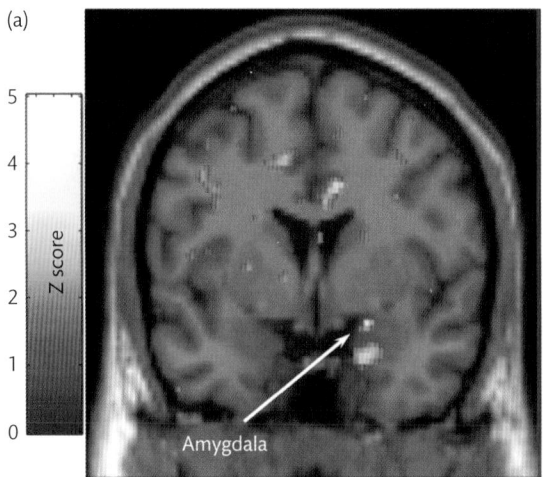

(a)

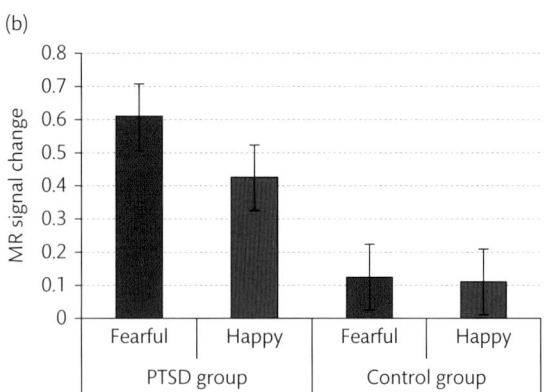

(b)

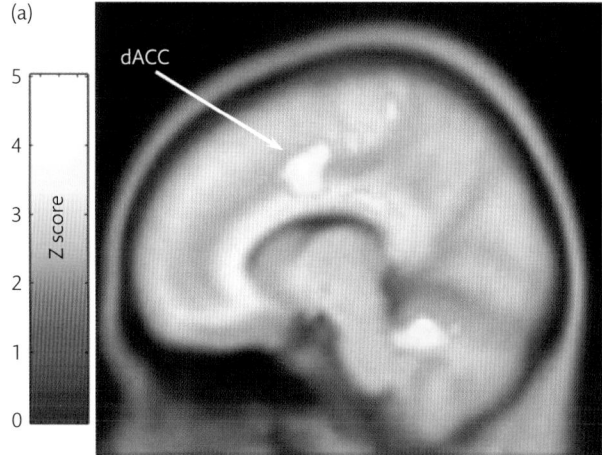

(a)

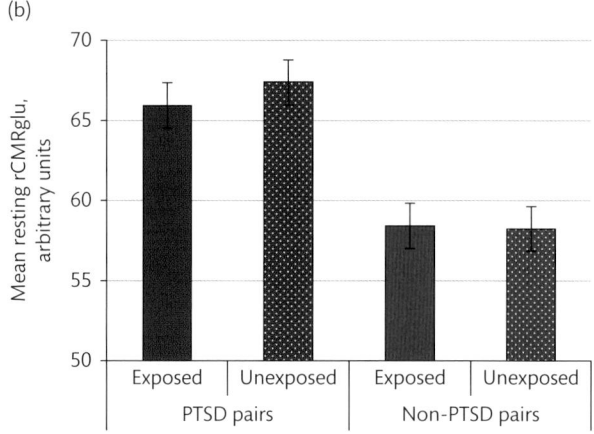

(b)

**Fig. 81.2** Example of functional magnetic resonance imaging (fMRI) data. (a) Amygdala activation to fearful vs happy facial expressions was greater in the PTSD group vs control group. (b) MR signal change in the amygdala in each condition for each group. Error bars represent the standard error of the mean.

Adapted from *Arch Gen Psychiatry*, 62(3), Shin LM, Wright CI, Cannistraro PA, *et al.*, A functional magnetic resonance imaging study of amygdala and medial prefrontal cortex responses to overtly presented fearful faces in posttraumatic stress disorder, pp. 273–81, Copyright (2005), with permission from American Medical Association.

**Fig. 81.3** Example of positron emission tomography (PET) data. (a) Greater resting regional cerebral metabolic rate for glucose (rCMRglu) in the dorsal anterior cingulate cortex (dACC)/mid cingulate cortex (arrow) in combat-exposed twins with PTSD and their identical co-twins, compared with combat-exposed twins without PTSD and their identical co-twins. (b) Group rCMRglu means. Error bars represent the standard error of the mean.

Adapted from *Arch Gen Psychiatry*, 66(10), Shin LM, Lasko NB, Macklin ML, *et al.*, Resting metabolic activity in the cingulate cortex and vulnerability to posttraumatic stress disorder, pp. 1099–107, Copyright (2009), with permission from American Medical Association.

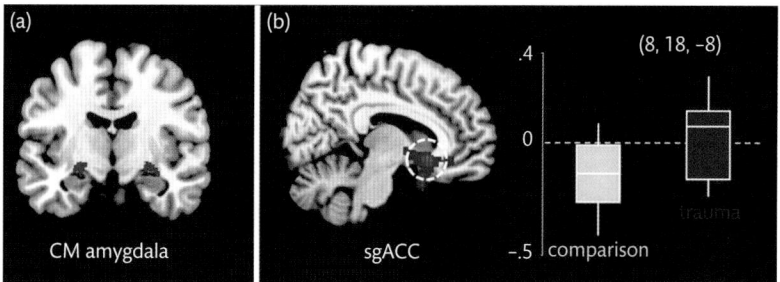

**Fig. 90.1** Absent negative connectivity between the centromedial (CM) amygdala and the subgenual anterior cingulate cortex (sgACC) in trauma-exposed youth. (a) Anatomically defined seed region of interest for the connectivity analysis within bilateral CM amygdala. (b) Tukey's boxplots depicting connectivity values by group centred on the sgACC peak. The middle line indicates the median, the vertical line the range, and the limits of the box represent the upper and lower quartiles.

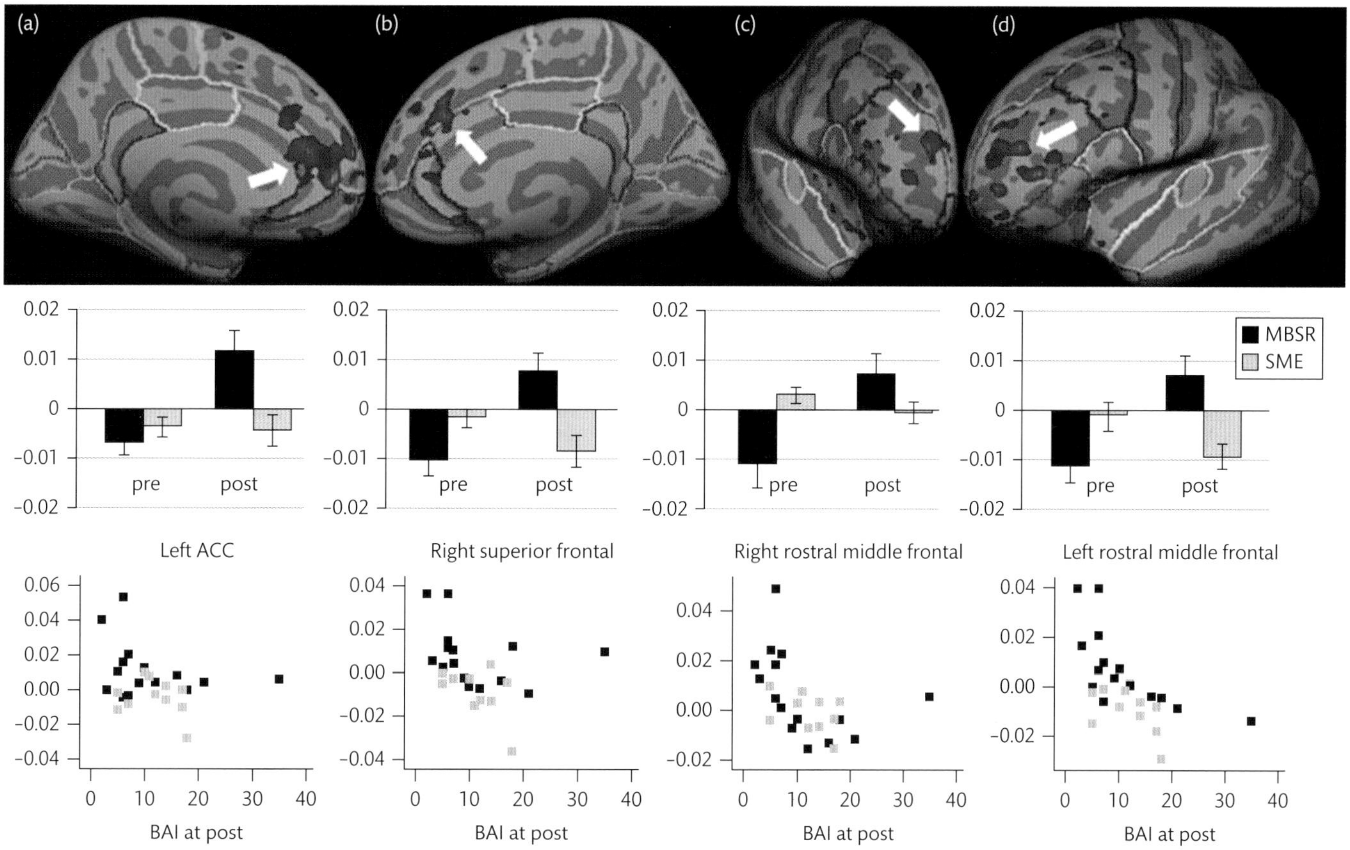

**Fig. 90.2** Functional connectivity between the seed region in the right amygdala and several regions in the frontal cortex increased from pre- to post-intervention with mindfulness-based stress reduction (MBSR) therapy in patients with generalized anxiety disorder, but not in control subjects who underwent a stress management education (SME) class. Top row: anatomical location displayed on an inflated surface. Middle row: regression coefficients extracted from the clusters from MBSR (black) and SME (blue) participants at pre- and post-interventions. Bottom row: scatter plots for correlations between pre- to post-increase in connectivity (y-axis) in the frontal cortex region and Beck Anxiety Inventory (BAI; x-axis) for MBSR and SME participants at post-intervention. ACC, anterior cingulate cortex.

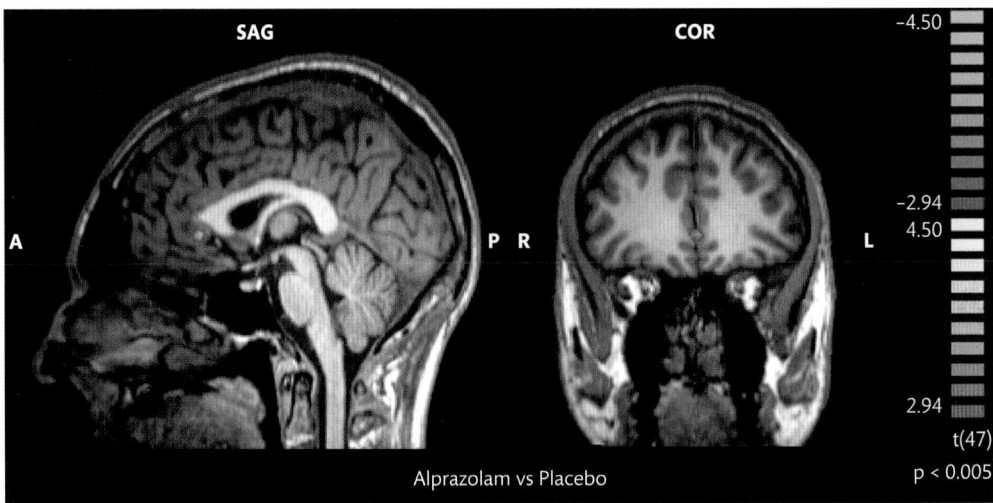

**Fig. 90.3** Contrasts of functional magnetic resonance imaging responses compared between different treatment conditions. Group analysis (*n* = 16) of the blood oxygen level-dependent response (functional magnetic resonance imaging) to challenge with cholecystokinin-tetrapeptide after alprazolam vs placebo pretreatment (Talairach co-ordinates: *x* = −1, *y* = 30). Activation of the rostral anterior cingulate cortex was reduced after pretreatment with alprazolam, but not after pretreatment with placebo. SAG, sagittal; COR, coronary; A, anterior; P, posterior; L, left; R, right.

Reproduced from *Biol Psychiatry*, 73(4), Leicht G, Mulert C, Eser D, *et al.*, Benzodiazepines Counteract Rostral Anterior Cingulate Cortex Activation Induced by Cholecystokinin-Tetrapeptide in Humans, pp. 337–344, Copyright (2013), with permission from Society of Biological Psychiatry.

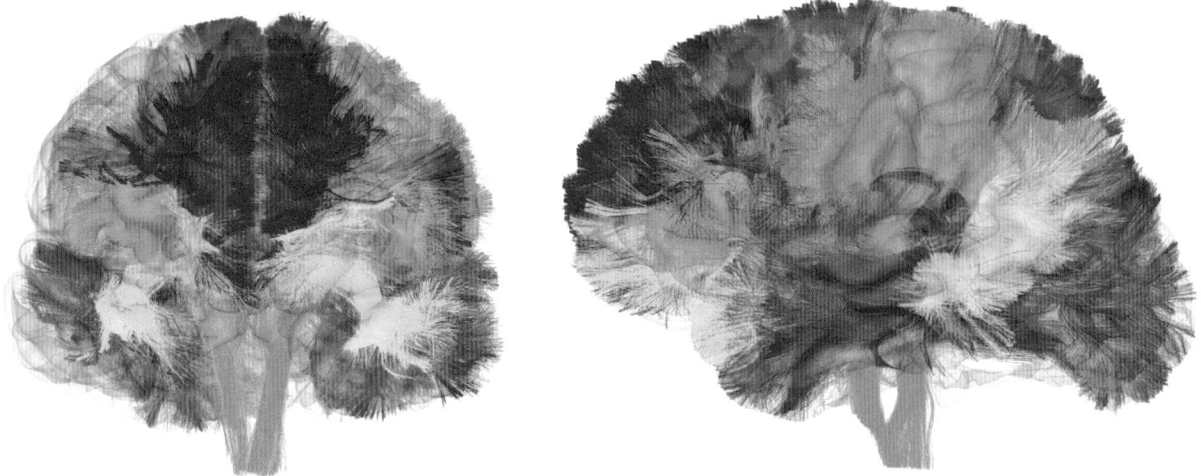

**Fig. 94.3** CONNECT/Archi atlas of the human brain white matter connectivity developed at NeuroSpin, as part of the European CONNECT FP7 project.

Reproduced courtesy of Cyril Poupon,CEA NeuroSpin.

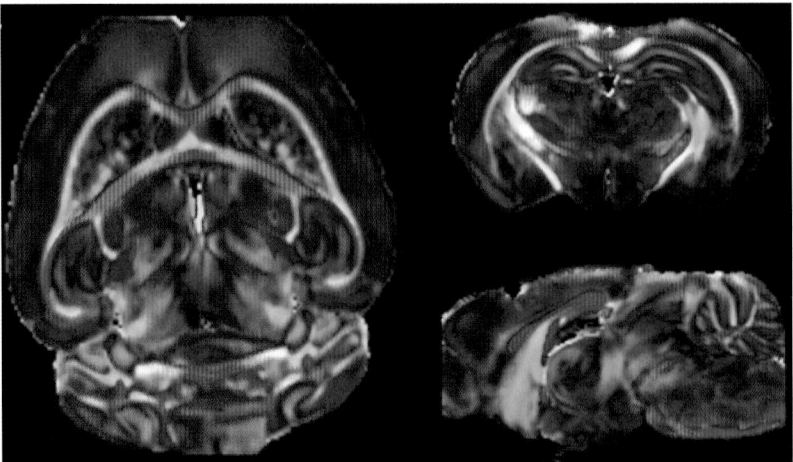

**Fig. 94.4** Representative three-dimensional image of colour-coded fractional anisotropy in a mouse brain based on diffusion MRI at 11.7 T.

Reproduced courtesy of S. B. Seébille and M. D. Santin, ICM-CENIR.

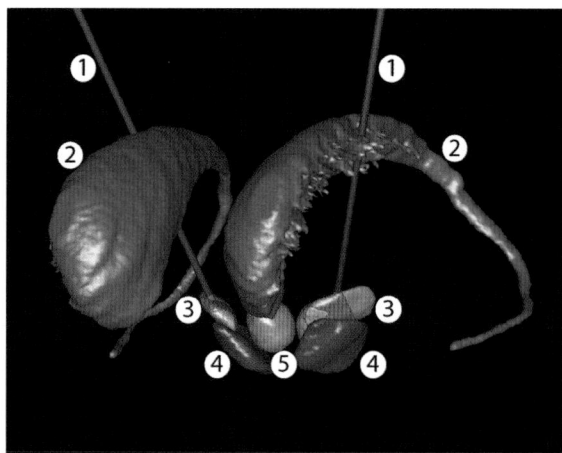

**Fig. 94.5** Three-dimensional image of electrodes implantated in a DBS procedure. Depending on the stimulating electrode (5) configuration and stereotactic co-ordinates, several anatomical sites can be targeted. Two brain targets are represented in this example: the caudate caudate nucleus (2) and the subthalamic nucleus (2). Other brain structures, such as the substantia nigra (3) and the red nucleus (4), can be used as anatomical landmarks.

Adapted courtesy of Jerome Yelnik, INSERM/ICM.

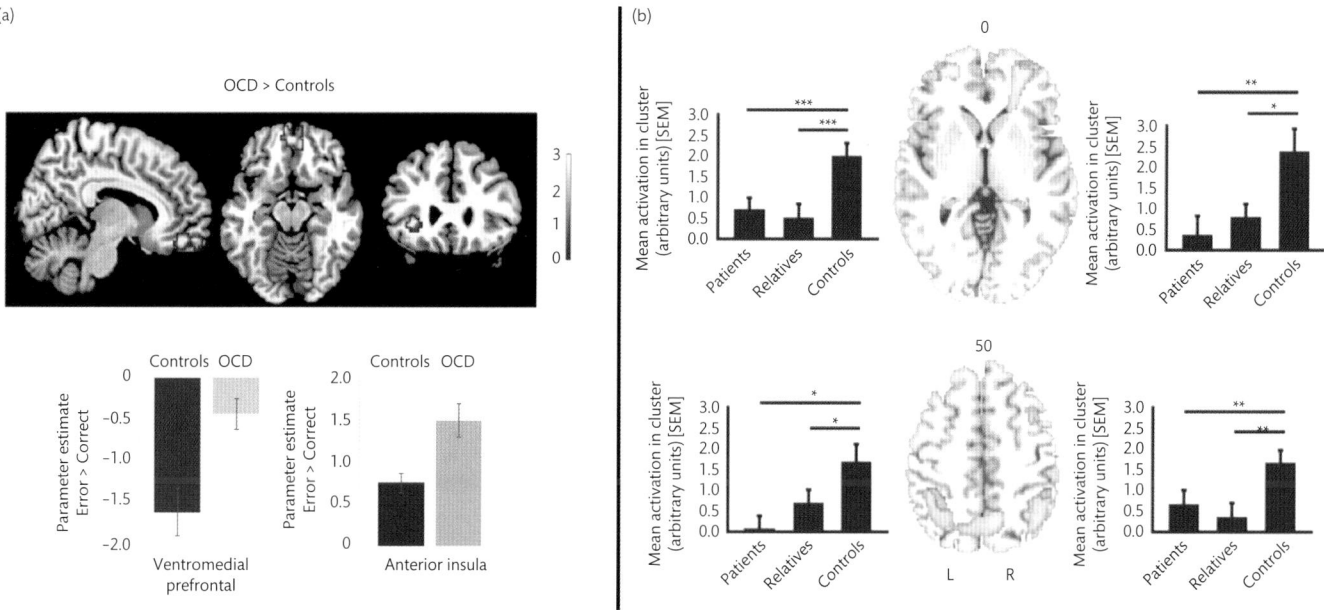

**Fig. 97.1** (a) Results from [15] showing greater error-related activity in the ventromedial prefrontal cortex and anterior insula in OCD patients, compared to controls.

Reproduced from *Biol Psychiatry*, 69(6), Stern ER, Welsh RC, Fitzgerald KD, *et al.*, Hyperactive error responses and altered connectivity in ventromedial and frontoinsular cortices in obsessive-compulsive disorder, pp. 583–91, Copyright (2011), with permission from Society of Biological Psychiatry.

(b) Results from [54] showing regions activated for (successful) reversal (areas in yellow), overlaid with orbitofrontal and parietal areas showing reduced activity during reversal, for both OCD patients and their unaffected relatives, compared to controls (areas in blue).

Reproduced from *Science*, 321(5887), Chamberlain SR, Menzies L, Hampshire A, *et al.*, Orbitofrontal Dysfunction in Patients with Obsessive-Compulsive Disorder and Their Unaffected Relatives, pp. 421–2, Copyright (2008), with permission from American Association for the Advancement of Science.

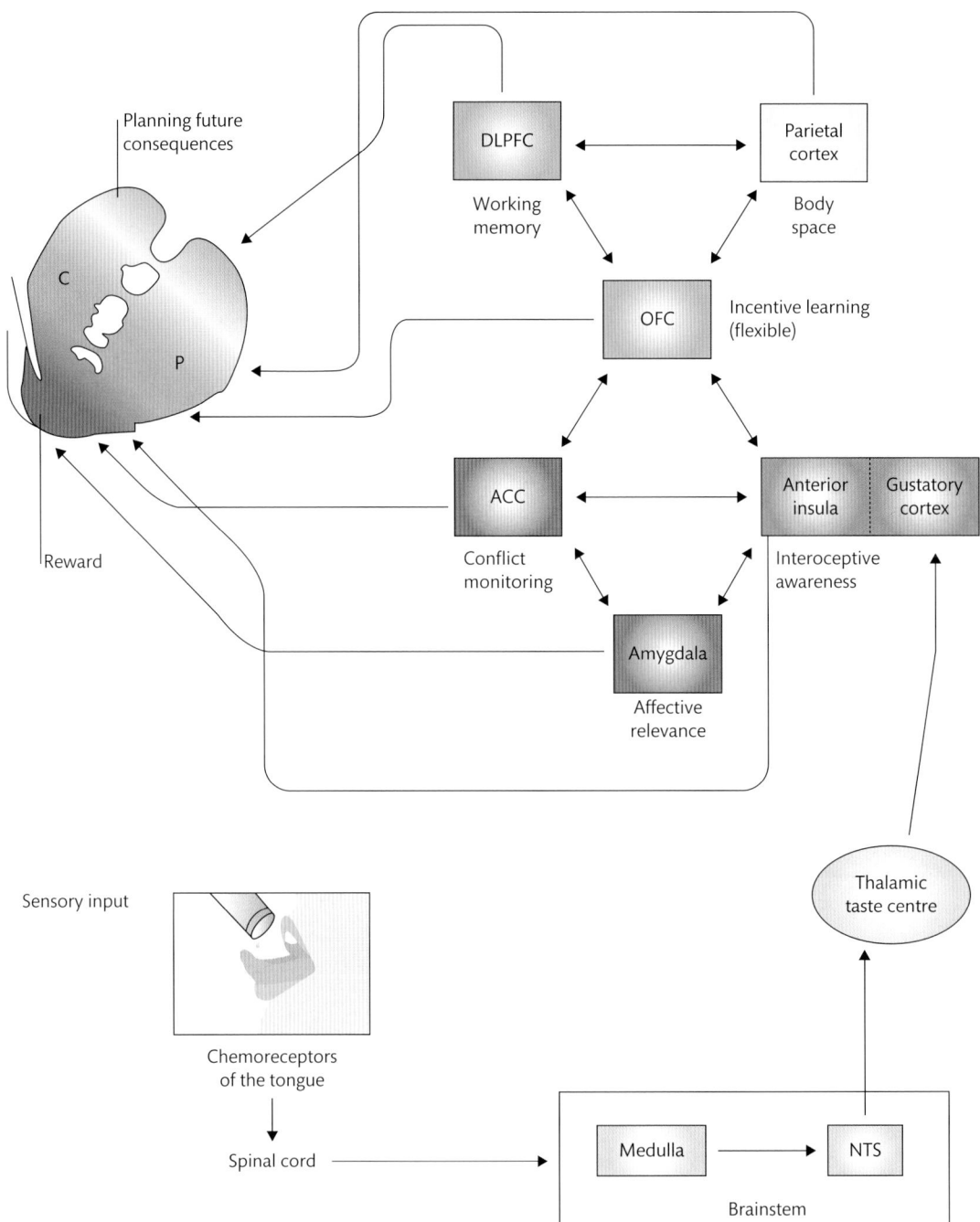

**Fig. 105.1** Cortical taste circuitry. Chemoreceptors on the tongue detect a sweet taste, which is transmitted through brainstem and thalamic centres to the primary gustatory cortex, adjacent to, and interconnected with, the insula. The anterior insula is a part of the ventral neurocircuit and is connected with the ACC and OFC. Cortical structures in the ventral neurocircuit send signals to the ventral striatum, while structures involved in cognitive strategies send input to the dorsal striatum. Taste and motivation are integrated in a decision to approach or avoid food. The figure links cortical structures with arrows, and all cortical structures project to the striatum in a topographic manner.

Reproduced from *Nat Rev Neurosci.*, 10(8), Kaye W, Fudge J, Paulus M, New insight into symptoms and neurocircuit function of anorexia nervosa, pp. 573–84, Copyright (2009), with permission from Springer Nature.

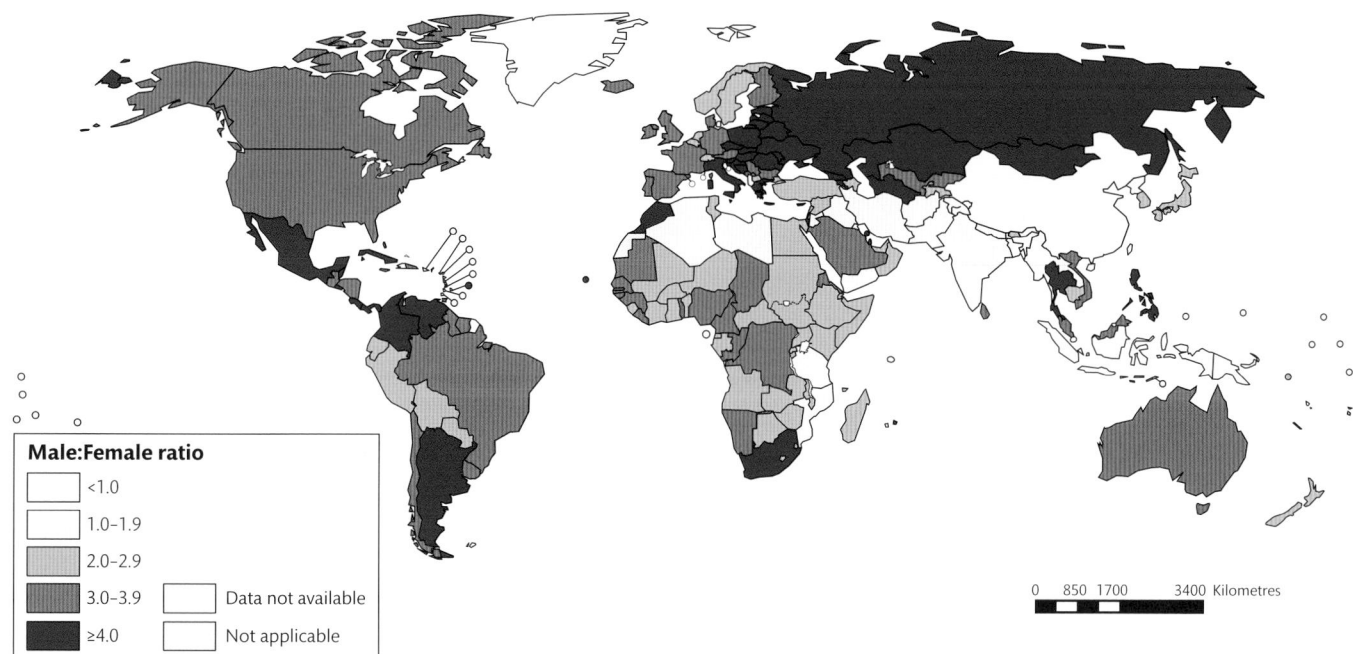

**Fig. 125.1** Age-standardized suicide rates for both genders by country (2012).

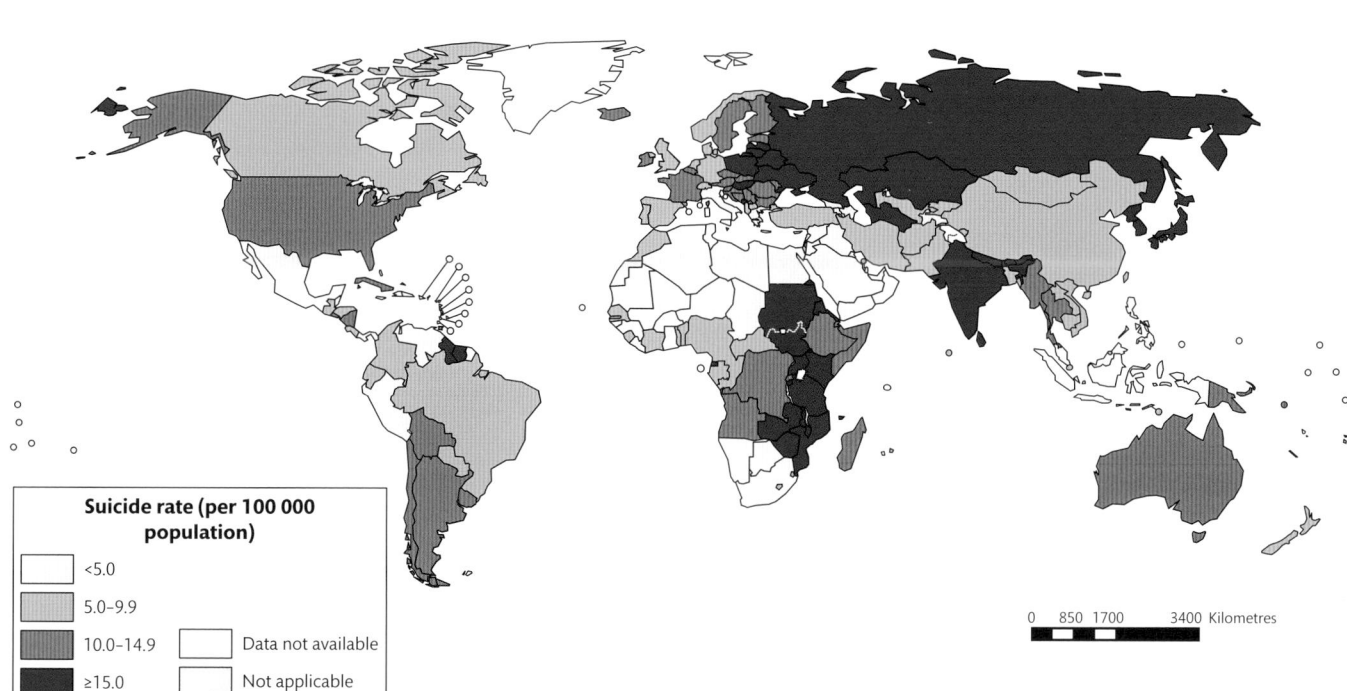

**Fig. 125.3** Sex ratio of age-standardized suicide rates by country (2012).

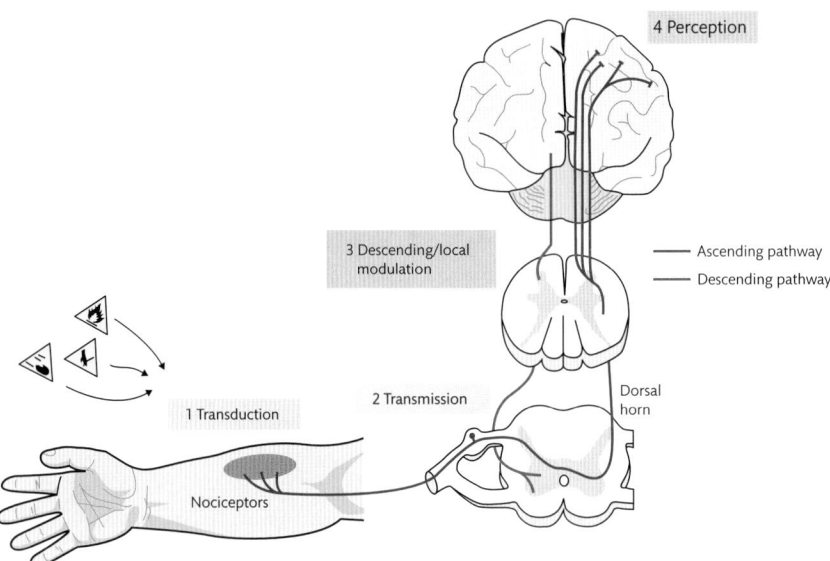

**Fig. 130.1** Acute nociception as a three-neuron order system. The peripheral nociceptor is responsible for the transduction into a neural signal (1). This is followed by transmission through neurons (2), with possible descending and local modulation (3), leading to the final perception at the cortical level (4).

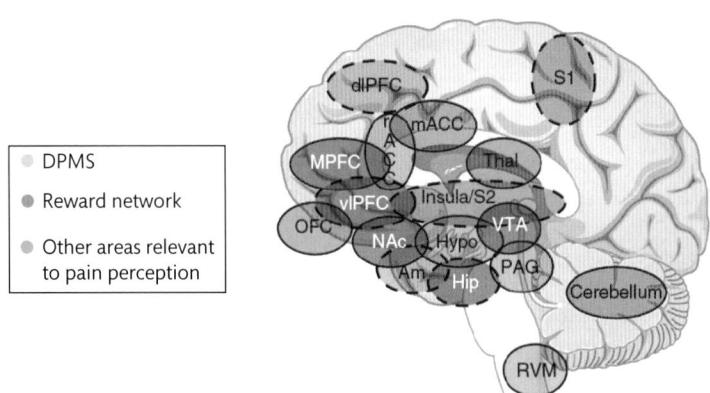

**Fig. 130.2** Cerebral areas and networks involved in pain perception and regulation, as well as reward. The key networks consist of the descending pain modulatory system (DPMS, green) and the reward network (purple). Alterations in function, connectivity, and structure have been described in these networks in chronic pain. rACC/mACC, rostral/medial anterior cingulate cortex; vlPFC, ventrolateral prefrontal cortex; dlPFC, dorsolateral prefrontal cortex; mPFC, medial prefrontal cortex; OFC, orbitofrontal cortex; insula/S2, insular and secondary somatosensory cortex; S1, primary somatosensory cortex; Am, amygdala; Hip, hippocampus; Hypo, hypothalamus; Thal, thalamus; PAG, periaqueductal grey; VTA, ventral tegmentum.

Adapted from *Nat Neurosci.*, 17(2), Denk F, McMahon SB, Tracey I, Pain vulnerability: a neurobiological perspective, pp. 192–200, Copyright (2014), with permission from Springer Nature.

# 73

# Perinatal psychiatry

*Ian Jones and Arianna Di Florio*

## Introduction

The links between childbirth and mental disorders have been described for hundreds, if not thousands, of years [1], but post-partum episodes are not merely of historical interest. Perinatal mental illness remains a great health challenge in the twenty-first century, no better illustrated than by the findings of the UK Confidential Enquiries into Maternal Deaths, which have found suicide to be a leading cause of maternal death [2]. The impact of these conditions is wider than merely maternal health, however, with the economic impact of perinatal psychiatric disorders in the UK estimated to be approximately £8.1 billion for each year's birth cohort, with the majority of costs due to consequences on the child [3]. Despite their undoubted clinical importance, perinatal mental illnesses have not received the attention, in terms of clinical practice and research, they deserve.

### Terminology and classification

#### Terminology

A range of terms are used in this area of psychiatry, including perinatal, peripartum, antenatal, prenatal, preconception, pregnancy, puerperal, postnatal, and post-partum. In other branches of medicine, the term perinatal may be used differently, but in the context of 'perinatal psychiatry', it is generally taken to refer to pregnancy and the post-partum—the period following childbirth. Although, as discussed in later sections, the common psychiatric classification systems define the post-partum as 4 or 6 weeks following delivery, in clinical practice, it is common to extend the post-partum period to at least 6 months after childbirth or even up to 1 year. Indeed, the UK National Institute for Health and Care Excellence (NICE)'s *Antenatal and Postnatal Mental Health: Clinical Management and Service Guidance* defined the post-partum period as up to 1 year following childbirth [4]. In this chapter, we will therefore take the perinatal period to be pregnancy and the first post-partum year.

#### Classification

Before a discussion of individual conditions, it is worth pausing to consider how perinatal episodes are treated by the commonly used classification systems. Unfortunately, the classification of episodes of psychiatric disorder in relationship to childbirth is an area that leads to much confusion, both clinically and in research. The *Diagnostic and Statistical Manual of Mental Disorders* (DSM) does not include separate categories for perinatal episodes. Rather, DSM-5 allows episodes of some disorders occurring in pregnancy or within 4 weeks of delivery to be given a peripartum-onset specifier [5]. Turning to the International Classification of Diseases (ICD) [6], the way perinatal disorders are dealt with in ICD-10 is also problematic. There is a category for disorders associated with the puerperium (F53), which covers those with onset within 6 weeks of delivery and includes categories for mild and severe episodes under which the terms postnatal depression and puerperal psychosis are used. However, these categories are unique in that ICD-10 states they should only be used for episodes which 'do not meet the criteria for disorders classified elsewhere'. The vast majority of perinatal episodes that would meet criteria for categories such as depression, mania, or psychosis would therefore not be diagnosed as perinatal if the instructions of the classification systems were strictly adhered to. Relying on the ICD-10 F53 diagnostic categories therefore would grossly underrepresent the true prevalence of perinatal mental health conditions.

Thus, both DSM and ICD follow the generally accepted position that conditions we will consider in this chapter, such as post-partum psychosis and postnatal depression, are not separate nosological entities but merely represent episodes of psychiatric disorder triggered by childbirth. Despite the post-partum labels not having a place in the classification systems, they remain in common use by professionals, the public, and most importantly women who experience episodes of illness at this time. One further problem with the nosology of perinatal mental health conditions is the ubiquitous use of the term 'post-partum depression' to refer to all forms of psychological distress following pregnancy—from mild and transient mood changes to some of the most severe psychotic conditions seen in psychiatry. This inappropriate usage not only can trivialize severe episodes of illness with an underestimation of risk in future pregnancies, but also supports the inappropriate labelling of a normal mood variation as a psychiatric disorder.

Women can be affected by a range of mental health problems in pregnancy and the post-partum period, including, but not limited to: depression, anxiety, eating disorders, OCD, personality disorders, bipolar disorder, schizophrenia, and other psychotic disorders. In fact, all the conditions discussed in other chapters of this textbook may present in the perinatal period. In this chapter, we will discuss both severe perinatal mental illnesses and more common mental health conditions. We will discuss disorders with first onset in the perinatal period and the course and management of women with pre-existing illness. We will first consider the presentation, epidemiology, prognosis, and management of a range of conditions presenting in relationship to pregnancy and childbirth, before finishing the chapter discussing what is known about the aetiology of these episodes. However, the most dangerous of the perinatal conditions are associated with a bipolar diagnosis, and for this reason, the chapter belongs in this section of the textbook.

## Severe perinatal mental illness

Severe episodes of mental illness occurring in the perinatal period can be a recurrence of an existing condition, such as bipolar disorder or schizophrenia, or may be the first episode of psychiatric illness a woman has experienced.

The perinatal period, as we will see, is a time of high risk for new onset of an episode of severe psychiatric illness. We will therefore also deal with the diagnosis and treatment of severe episodes of affective psychosis with onset in the immediate post-partum period—episodes that have traditionally been referred to as puerperal or post-partum psychosis. In addition, we will consider the management of women with pre-existing severe mental illness, such as bipolar disorder or schizophrenia, who become pregnant. We will examine the impact that pregnancy and childbirth may have on the condition, but also consider the implications that the mental illness may have on the pregnancy.

## Post-partum psychosis

The most severe forms of post-partum mood disorder have traditionally been labelled post-partum (or puerperal) psychosis (PP) [7]. These terms are usually used to refer to new onset, although not necessarily the first episode, of severe affective psychosis in the immediate puerperium. Although there is no consensus about what is meant by immediate, it is of note that in 90% of cases, the onset is within 2 weeks of delivery [8]. While the boundaries of this condition are not easy to define, the core concept is the acute post-partum onset of mania or affective psychosis. Accordingly, the continuation of a more chronic psychosis, such as schizophrenia, would not be appropriately labelled as post-partum psychosis. In the majority of cases, in fact, the symptomatology and prognosis of PP resemble those of an affective disorder, rather than those of schizophrenia. Symptoms are those of a severe mood disorder often accompanied by psychotic symptoms such as delusions and hallucinations. The word 'psychosis' in the context of PP can, however, be confusing as some women with severe manic episodes with early post-partum onset may receive the label but not experience actual psychotic symptoms [9]. Mixed episodes, in which manic and depressive symptoms occur simultaneously, are common, and the clinical picture often shows a constantly changing 'kaleidoscopic' picture. The latter point raises an important clinical lesson, in the assessment of women with significant psychiatric symptoms with onset in the immediate post-partum period—one evaluation is usually not enough, as the picture fluctuates over time and can escalate rapidly and severity is sometimes difficult to recognize [7, 10]. In addition,

confusion and perplexity are common symptoms and some women may present in a way typical of the so-called 'polymorphic or cycloid psychosis' [11].

In summary, although, as discussed here, puerperal/post-partum psychosis is not a prominent diagnostic category in the major classification systems, it remains an important concept. It is commonly used in clinical practice and research and, most importantly perhaps, by women who experience these episodes, as illustrated by 'Action on Postpartum Psychosis' being the major third-sector organization in the UK dedicated to helping women and their families with this condition [12]. Although the classification systems appear set on relegating the term 'puerperal psychosis' to the history books, there are advantages in the diagnosis of PP in both research and clinical practice [13].

### Differential diagnosis

In addition to other psychiatric disorders, several physical health conditions occurring in the perinatal period can be associated with, or even present with, psychosis and are therefore important in the differential diagnosis. These include: infections, pre-eclampsia and eclampsia, autoimmune, metabolic, encephalitis, and cerebral vascular diseases and syndromes associated with substance abuse and withdrawal [14]. The Confidential Enquiries into Maternal Deaths in the UK has reported a number of maternal deaths that were due to misattribution of psychotic symptoms to PP, rather than the true underlying condition, and therefore emphasize the need to consider physical conditions in the assessment of women who have sudden onset of a severe psychiatric episode in the perinatal period [2]. The Confidential Enquiries into Maternal Deaths have also found that a substantial proportion of women who committed suicide following PP were misdiagnosed as suffering from anxiety, moderate depression, or adjustment disorder and did not receive adequate treatment [2]. Untreated severe post-partum disorders are associated with an increased risk of both suicide [15] and infanticide [16].

### Epidemiology

Although, when compared to other conditions occurring in the perinatal period, PP is a less common disorder [13], as a severe and potentially fatal condition, it is important to recognize and manage appropriately. Studies based on hospital admission in the post-partum period have estimated an incidence of 1–2 in 1000 deliveries [17]. This estimate, however, does not account for women with PP who are not admitted and will, of course, also include women admitted for other reasons.

The specific link between childbirth and the triggering of mania or an affective psychosis is well established, with the post-partum a period of very high risk [17–21]. For example, data from Danish population registries have established that the risk of a first lifetime manic episode in the first 4 weeks post-partum is 23 times higher than a comparison period 1 year after childbirth [17]. Further work from Denmark has established that even if admitted for another psychiatric disorder, such as major depression, a first admission within the first month after childbirth increases four times the likelihood of developing bipolar disorder within 15 years, compared to any first psychiatric admission outside the childbearing period [20].

In more than 50% of women experiencing PP, it is their first psychiatric episode and therefore difficult to predict [22]. For women with a psychiatric history, however, there are a number of factors which identify women who are at a particularly high risk of PP. Women with a history of bipolar disorder have a 1 in 5 chance of PP for each delivery [18], and a previous episode of PP confers an even higher risk in excess of 1 in 2 [23]. A family history of PP has also been identified as doubling the risk of PP in women with a personal history of bipolar disorder [24]. For this reason, establishing a family history of perinatal episodes is clearly important in the assessment of women in pregnancy with existing mental health conditions. In contrast, for women with no personal history that puts them at high risk, the importance of a positive family history is less clear.

## Management of post-partum psychosis

PP is a psychiatric emergency, and admission is necessary in the majority of cases [7, 25]. In around 50%, the episode will be the first contact with psychiatric services and therefore could not have been predicted, emphasizing the need for prompt assessment, diagnosis, and treatment [22]. In the UK, NICE guidelines recommend admission to specialized mother and baby units (MBUs) [4], but there remains a postcode lottery in provision; MBU beds are commonly not available, necessitating admission for many women to general adult wards. Although further evidence for the efficacy of MBUs is clearly needed, there is preliminary evidence that MBUs are preferred by women [26] and also lead to better outcomes and shorter duration of admission [25].

The mainstay of the management of PP, in addition to admission, is pharmacological treatment, but there is a paucity of specific evidence to guide us, that is, no RCTs. However, response to medication is good. For example, a study from the Netherlands evaluated the efficacy of an empirical treatment algorithm for PP, consisting sequentially of: (1) a GABA-modulating drug (benzodiazepine); (2) adding a dopamine antagonist/partial agonist; and (3) adding lithium. With adherence to this stepped regime, they observed complete remission in more than 98% of cases, with 80% of women maintaining remission for 9 months [27]. Significantly higher relapse rates were seen in women maintained on a dopamine antagonist/partial agonist alone, compared to those treated with lithium [27].

Despite no RCTs for electroconvulsive therapy in PP, the evidence of its effectiveness is promising [28]. The potential side effects (anterograde amnesia in 18%, prolonged seizures in 11%, according to a recent study [29]) need to be weighed against its efficacy in those resistant to medication and the potentially very rapid response in very severe, life-threatening episodes of illness.

## Prognosis

In the modern era, the prognosis for promptly identified and treated PP is good, with over 95% of patients achieving remission within 1 year [27]. The median duration of illness is considerably shorter for women treated with pharmacotherapy (40 days) [27] than for a historical comparison with those treated prior to the era of pharmacotherapy (8 months) [30]. Having an episode of PP has a long-lasting impact beyond the acute episode. Recurrence rates are around 50% for further post-partum episodes and between 50% and 70% for bipolar recurrences not related to childbirth [31, 32]. In addition, there may be an impact on decisions about future pregnancies and on relationships. One retrospective study of 116 women, for example, found that only 58% of women went on to have a further pregnancy and that 18% of relationships ended after the severe post-partum episode [22].

## Women with existing severe mental illness

As discussed in the previous section, although an episode of severe perinatal illness may be the first psychiatric presentation, in at least 50% of cases, the episode will be in the context of a history of severe mental illness such as bipolar disorder or schizophrenia.

### Bipolar disorder

A considerable body of evidence points to the high risk of post-partum episodes in women with bipolar disorder. In a large retrospective study of 1212 parous women with bipolar disorder, over 70% had experienced at least one episode of mood disorder in the perinatal period and over 1 in 4 had experienced an episode of PP [18]. However, although the relative risk of PP was greatly increased in these women with bipolar disorder, it was non-psychotic depression that was the most commonly reported mood episode in the perinatal period [18]. Regarding the timing of episodes, although over 90% of manic or psychotic episodes occur within the first 4 weeks after childbirth, the pattern of onset is different for non-psychotic depression, with 25% having an onset after the first post-partum month [18].

### Management

For women with a history of bipolar disorder, there are difficult decisions to be made around becoming pregnant and about management in pregnancy and the post-partum period. Potential pregnancy should be considered in all women with bipolar disorder in their reproductive years, and women should have access to preconception counselling if they are considering pregnancy [4]. In counselling women about pregnancy, the known or potential risks of taking medication in pregnancy must always be weighed against the high risk of recurrence discussed previously [4, 7, 25, 33].

The evidence base to guide these decisions is admittedly sparse, and more research is clearly needed. However, there are data that can help women and clinicians. For example, it is likely that the recurrence risk in the perinatal period is higher for women who stop mood-stabilizing medication, with one study finding 2-fold higher risk of a recurrence in those who discontinued lithium due to pregnancy [34]. Further guidance on the exact period of risk comes from a naturalistic, longitudinal study which found that women with a history of PP were at high risk in the post-partum period, but not one of the 29 women with a history had a recurrence during a subsequent pregnancy. In contrast, ten of 41 women with a history of bipolar disorder outside the puerperium experienced a recurrence during pregnancy, with the risk doubled in those not taking a drug to stabilize mood (19% vs 40%, respectively) [22]. The results of this study suggest therefore that while prophylactic medication should be considered in all women at high risk in the post-partum period, in pregnancy, it should be considered in women with a history of bipolar disorder not related to childbirth.

Regarding the reproductive safety of specific medications, the evidence base is continuously developing and clinical guidelines, such as from NICE [4] or the British Association of Psychopharmacology [35], may not include the latest research. Advice in individual cases may be sought from perinatal specialist services or from websites, such as that provided by the UK Teratology Information Service (http://www.uktis.org). Although we are not able to provide a detailed consideration of all medications here, there is considerable evidence that children exposed to valproate *in utero* are at high risk of developmental disorders and congenital malformations [36]. In contrast, lithium does not appear to be as problematic in pregnancy as initial studies indicated [37].

Finally, although specific evidence for psychosocial interventions for bipolar disorder in the perinatal period may be lacking, it is vital that these approaches, particularly psychoeducation, are considered [4, 25].

Readers are referred to Chapter 75 for a more detailed account of the treatment options for bipolar disorder.

### Schizophrenia

Although a considerable body of evidence points to an aetiological overlap across the mood psychosis spectrum (see Chapter 59), the triggering of episodes by childbirth is an interesting area of distinction. We do not see the same massively increased risk of a new episode of a schizophrenia-like psychosis in the immediate post-partum, as we see for episodes of bipolar disorder [17, 19]. Women with schizophrenia may require admission in the first post-partum year, however, often to deal with issues around becoming a new mother, even in the absence of a severe symptomatic recurrence.

As for bipolar disorder, specific evidence on the management of schizophrenia in the perinatal period is lacking. A preliminary study found that collaboration between services and the women's partner in the care of the baby leads to an improvement in symptomatology [38]. Motherhood can be very challenging for women with schizophrenia, and this diagnosis, together with that of personality disorders and substance abuse or dependence, has been shown to be associated with increased involvement of social services [25]. Tragically, when it does occur, the loss of child custody is a traumatic event that can precipitate a crisis and has been associated with maternal suicide [2, 26].

## Common mental disorders

Having considered the presentation of severe perinatal mental illness, we turn now to consideration of other mental disorders that may occur in pregnancy and the post-partum.

### Depression

Depression, the leading cause of disability worldwide, is the most common medical complication of maternity [39].

#### Clinical presentation

The weight of evidence suggests that there is no difference in clinical presentation between post-partum depression and depression occurring at other times [40, 41]. There are, however, issues with some somatic depressive symptoms (that is, fatigue, loss of libido, appetite, and weight, and sleep changes), as these are commonly experienced by all women following childbirth, so they need to be assessed with care [42]. Thoughts of self-harm are common in perinatal depression; an American national survey found 30% of women who screened positive for post-partum depression endorsed thoughts of self-harm [43]. Differences between the presentation of depression in pregnancy and following childbirth have been described, with intrusive violent thoughts and psychosis more common in women with post-partum onset [44].

#### Differential diagnosis

Episodes of major post-partum depression need to be distinguished from minor mood change, the so-called baby or maternity blues, and from episodes of PP as discussed previously [45]. The blues are characterized by emotional lability in the first post-partum week. This occurs commonly and does not require treatment. Assessment of minor mood change in the post-partum period should ensure that the woman is not, and does not, become more severely depressed. Physical conditions associated with low mood in the perinatal period, such as thyroid dysfunction and anaemia, should also be assessed.

It is important to be aware that post-partum depression can be a manifestation of a bipolar disorder; for example, over 50% of cases of bipolar post-partum depression in one study were initially misdiagnosed as unipolar disorder by clinicians [46], and in another study, over 20% of women who screened positive for post-partum depression were found to have bipolar disorder [43]. Indeed, women with episodes of unipolar depression with post-partum onset have been found to be more likely to develop a future bipolar disorder than women with depression occurring at other times [20]. Episodes of psychotic depression in the immediate post-partum period should raise the possibility of an underlying bipolar diathesis, even in the absence of manic symptoms [47]. Recognition of the bipolar nature of depression is important for management. This is illustrated by a small study of 34 women with bipolar post-partum depression, initially misdiagnosed as unipolar, that showed the discontinuation of antidepressants (that is, drugs licensed for the treatment of unipolar depression) and the introduction of a mood stabilizer (drugs licensed for bipolar disorder) improved symptoms in 88% of cases [46].

#### Epidemiology

The point prevalence of major depression in the perinatal period varies widely across studies, ranging from 0% to over 30% [42, 48–50], and it is likely that methodological differences, particularly in the assessment of depression, account for this variability. A systematic review estimated the point prevalence of major depressive disorder to be between 3.1% and 4.9% during pregnancy and 4.7% in the first 3 months post-partum [49]. If minor depression is included, these rates are higher—11% in pregnancy and 13% in the post-partum [49]. There has been great debate over the question of whether depression is more common in the perinatal period and the data are not consistent. It does seem clear, however, that pregnancy is not protective against depression, with both a systematic review [49] and a large epidemiological study from the United States finding no significant difference in prevalence or incidence of depression [51]. However, there may be differences for more severe episodes with a Danish registry-based study finding the relative risk of first admission to hospital for major depression is halved during pregnancy, but more than doubled in the first 2 months after childbirth, compared to 1 year post-partum [17].

The risk factors for perinatal depression show considerable overlap with depression occurring at other times. Established risk factors for depression occurring in the post-partum include a history of mood or anxiety disorders, stressful life events, poor social support, and domestic violence [42]. The factors associated with depression in pregnancy are similar (poor social support, adverse life events, domestic violence, a history of mental illness) but include some additional factors related to the pregnancy (unplanned or unwanted pregnancy, present/past pregnancy complications) [52].

## Prognosis

Although women can be reassured that the prognosis of post-partum depression is good, with episodes lasting 3–6 months on average, 30% of women remain depressed beyond the first post-partum year [42]. It should also be discussed with women that they are at an increased risk of further episodes of depression, with recurrence rates of around 40% for both perinatal and non-perinatal episodes [53].

## Screening

It is not in doubt that many episodes of perinatal depression go undetected; some estimates suggest this may be up to 50% of cases [3]. However, there is considerable debate over the benefit of screening all women for depression in the perinatal period. The high prevalence and the potentially serious negative consequences of perinatal depression have led many to advocate for universal screening, most recently, for example, by the U.S. Preventative Services Task Force [54]. However, others have pointed to potential negative consequences of universal screening, including misdiagnosis and increasing stigma, and results from economic modelling have suggested that screening may not meet thresholds to be considered cost-effective [55]. Certainly screening tools must not be viewed as comprehensive and clinical guidelines emphasize that the clinical decision about the presence of depression should always be made on the basis of a further comprehensive assessment [4, 56]. A number of self-report measures of depression have been advocated to screen for perinatal depression; the Edinburgh Postnatal Depression scale (EPDS), which has been widely translated, is perhaps most commonly used around the globe. Despite the widespread use of the EPDS, NICE [4] recommends that health care professionals in contact with women in the perinatal period use the Whooley questions:

- During the past month, have you often been bothered by feeling down, depressed, or hopeless?
- During the past month, have you often been bothered by having little interest or pleasure in doing things?

Although formal screening programmes for maternal depression remain controversial, what is not in doubt is that all health professionals should be aware of a woman's mental health in the perinatal period, in addition to her physical well-being.

## Treatment

Perinatal depression responds to the same treatments as depression at other times. Given issues around the use of medication in pregnancy and in breastfeeding women (discussed in the following sections), psychological and psychosocial approaches are perhaps of particular relevance. A range of psychosocial interventions have been shown to be effective in a Cochrane meta-analysis, including peer support and non-directive counselling, cognitive behavioural therapy, psychodynamic psychotherapy, and interpersonal therapy [57]. In addition, for some women, further interventions directed at the mother–baby relationship may be appropriate if this remains impaired and has not responded to treatment of maternal depression [4, 56].

For many women, particularly for those with moderate to severe episodes of depression, medication will be required. It is clear that the use of drugs for depression in pregnancy has increased considerably in recent decades, with rates varying widely from around 3% in Denmark [58] to over 13% in the United States [59]. Pregnancy and breastfeeding are often exclusion criteria in drug trials, and as a result, there is little specific evidence for the pharmacologic management of post-partum or pregnancy depression [60]. Decisions must therefore be extrapolated from evidence for the efficacy of approaches accumulated in the non-perinatal context. Medication trials in women with severe post-partum depression are possible, however, and there may be scope for innovation; a 60-hour hormonal infusion appeared very promising in a small early-stage trial, for example, but obviously requires replication [61, 62].

For women already on drugs for depression, the data are inconsistent regarding the impact of medication being continued or stopped. A longitudinal study of 201 euthymic pregnant women found that 68% of those who discontinued treatment had a relapse during pregnancy, compared with 26% of those who continued medication [63]. In contrast, another study of 778 pregnant women with a history of major depression found that staying on, or stopping, drug treatment had little influence on psychiatric outcome [64]. Differences in the severity of depressive histories probably account for these conflicting findings. We would emphasize the need to take account of the specific history of each woman, the severity of her illness, and the evidence for her response to individual medications, when making these difficult decisions.

Other interventions for perinatal depression have a limited evidence base and include the use of oestrogens and progestins, N-3 fatty acids, exercise, and integrated yoga [65–67].

Just as for pregnancy, decisions regarding medication in breastfeeding women must be made following a full risk–benefit analysis that considers the options available. As new data on medication safety in pregnancy and during lactation are emerging regularly, up-to-date advice from specialist services should be sought in individual cases.

## Anxiety disorders

Despite often being overlooked [42] and mislabelled with the pervasive term 'post-partum depression', perinatal anxiety disorders are common [68, 69]. Prevalence rates for anxiety disorders range widely from 6% to 39% in pregnancy [70] and from 16% to 50% in the post-partum period [71]. In addition, both pregnant and post-partum women are at increased risk of developing OCD (risk ratios 1.45 and 2.38, respectively) [72], with 2.5% of women experiencing a clinical episode of OCD in the perinatal period [72]. In making a clinical assessment of women with OCD symptoms, it should be remembered that obsessional thinking is common in the perinatal period, but that some women are much more significantly affected with obsessional thoughts and compulsive behaviours that can often involve the child, and obsessions need to be distinguished from delusions that may pose a risk to the baby.

Perhaps to an even greater extent than for perinatal depression, there is a lack of data to guide the treatment of perinatal anxiety disorders; RCTs are lacking, and even naturalistic studies are rare [42]. Again, management decisions must be made on the basis of evidence obtained in studies of anxiety disorders not related to pregnancy and the post-partum. One group of approaches that have received interest in the perinatal period are the so-called 'mind-body' interventions that encompass a large group of therapies such as hypnosis, meditation, yoga, biofeedback, t'ai chi, and visual imagery. Although increasingly popular, there is a lack of rigorous evidence to support their effectiveness for the management of perinatal anxiety [73].

## Post-traumatic stress disorder

For many years, childbirth was not recognized as a potential trigger for PTSD, and although this has changed, perinatal PTSD still has not perhaps received the attention it deserves. Studies have examined symptoms occurring after a range of pregnancy outcomes, including miscarriage, termination, stillbirth [74], and traumatic birth [75]. The prevalence of perinatal PTSD is estimated to be between 1% and 8% [42, 76], with a higher prevalence in low-income countries and high rates of comorbidity with major depression, anxiety, and substance misuse [42, 77]. Particularly high rates of PTSD have been described in low-income pregnant women exposed to intimate partner violence, with rates as high as 40% according to one study [76]. There is not a large evidence base to guide management, but consistent with data for PTSD more generally, a Cochrane systematic review found little or no evidence to support routine psychological debriefing for women who have experienced a traumatic birth [78].

## Eating disorders

Anorexia nervosa impacts a woman's fertility [79], but eating disorders more generally do affect considerable numbers in the perinatal period. One study has reported the prevalence of eating disorders during pregnancy to be 7.5% (compared to 9.2% pre-pregnancy) [80]. For some women with a history of eating disorders, however, pregnancy is associated with symptomatic improvement. A study from Norway, for example, reported remission rates of between 29% and 78%, depending on the specific condition [81]. Eating disorder symptoms have also been reported to increase the risk of post-partum depression [82]. There is no trial evidence for the prevention of recurrence in women at risk. Management should be aimed at maintaining regular eating patterns, supporting realistic goals, and optimizing nutrition for the mother and the fetus [42].

## Personality disorders

Despite the potential for personality disorders to cause significant difficulties in pregnancy and the post-partum period, there has been little research conducted to date on their impact and management in the perinatal period. The prevalence of personality disorders in pregnancy, as assessed by self-report, was found to be around 6% in one Scandinavian study [83]. An important point is that personality disorders can occur alongside many of the other disorders discussed previously and are associated with poor prognosis [42, 83].

## Substance misuse

Substance misuse in pregnancy is common, with a study in the United States estimating 9.0% of pregnant women aged 18–25 and 3.4% of those aged 26–44 using illicit drugs or misusing prescription drugs. However, these rates were roughly half of those observed in non-pregnant women in the same age group [84]. Substance misuse is often comorbid with other psychiatric conditions and impact negatively on prognosis. In particular, the Confidential Enquiries into Maternal Deaths described a number of cases where substance abuse is a significant feature in those women who died [2]. Women with substance use disorders require intensive and multidisciplinary care in pregnancy. A harm reduction approach, aimed at periods of abstinence while recognizing the likelihood of relapse, should be adopted [84].

## Aetiology: understanding the puerperal trigger

Given the post-partum is a period of high risk for episodes of psychiatric disorder, particularly for severe illness, it has long been seen as offering potential clues to the mechanisms underlying such illness. PP affects women primarily with a bipolar disorder diathesis, acted on by a specific puerperal trigger [25]. Understanding the nature of this trigger will be of great benefit, allow for the development of novel treatments, and enable the prevention of illness in those women at high risk. There are several hypotheses of puerperal triggering that have been explored.

### Changes in medication

Perhaps the simplest explanation could be that the high-risk post-partum is a result of women stopping medication because of concerns over the safety of medication in pregnancy. The illness might be simply a result of acute withdrawal of medication. Evidence against this hypothesis comes from a study that compared the course of 42 women with previous bipolar episodes who stopped lithium due to pregnancy, compared to 59 age-matched non-pregnant lithium discontinuers [33]. Rates of recurrence were very similar for both groups up to 40 weeks, implying that drug withdrawal per se had no effect. However, following delivery, a large and highly significant difference in recurrence rates was observed (70% vs 24% recurrence, respectively). Thus, withdrawal of medication had an important impact on the vulnerability to the puerperal trigger but exerted no discernible effect on the recurrence risk in itself.

### Psychosocial factors

Becoming a mother is a complex and often difficult psychosocial transition, but psychosocial factors have not been shown to play a major role in vulnerability to psychosis in the puerperium. A number of studies have found no association between stressful life events and PP in women at high risk [85, 86].

### Genetic factors

Studies have suggested both that episodes of PP are a marker for a more familial form of bipolar disorder [87] and that a specific vulnerability to the puerperal triggering of bipolar illness is familial [24]. The relationship between genetic factors influencing puerperal triggering and those for the underlying bipolar disorder is still to be established, however, and is likely only to be clear when the genetic variation underpinning vulnerability to post-partum episodes are identified. Molecular genetic studies of PP have been conducted [88, 89], but in the age of GWAS, no genome-wide associations have been reported to date. Sample sizes available for genetic studies will have to be far bigger than those available at present to achieve the power needed to identify genes of likely small to modest effect (see Chapters 59 and 70).

### Hormones

The abrupt onset of illness during a time of major physiological change suggests hormonal factors may play an important role in aetiology. It is increasingly recognized that ovarian sex steroids have important functions in the central nervous system. Oestrogen and progesterone receptors are widespread in the brain where they modulate neurotransmission and neuroplasticity via both genomic and non-genomic mechanisms and regulate not only maternal behaviour, but also emotion processing, arousal, cognition, and motivation [90–93]. Gonadal steroids have been implicated in a number of neuropsychiatric illnesses, including migraine and neurodegenerative and premenstrual dysphoric disorders [93, 94].

The evidence pointing to reproductive hormones in the aetiology of post-partum episodes is predominantly circumstantial. The study of Bloch and colleagues [95], however, provides more direct evidence for the involvement of oestrogen and progesterone in the post-partum triggering of mood episodes. This study that simulated the supraphysiologic gonadal steroid levels of pregnancy and post-partum withdrawal found five of eight women with a history of post-partum depression and none of eight of the women with no history of post-partum depression developed significant mood symptoms during the withdrawal period. It is possible therefore that women vulnerable to post-partum episodes do not show gross abnormalities in endocrine physiology, but rather an abnormal response to the normal hormonal fluctuations of pregnancy and childbirth.

The role of gonadal steroids in the pathogenesis of perinatal mood disorders is still to be established, and its clinical implications are unclear. At present, however, there is no support for the routine use of hormonal treatments in the prevention or management of perinatal mood disorders [65].

### Sleep

It is well established that sleep and circadian rhythm disruption can trigger the onset of manic episodes very rapidly [96]. Sleep loss is also, of course, very common in pregnancy and the post-partum. It is surprising therefore that this potential trigger has not received more attention, with only a few studies addressing this very plausible hypothesis [97].

### Other potential factors

Several obstetric-related factors have been explored, but the only robust risk factor identified is primiparity [98, 99], which has held up even in analyses that take account of women with severe post-partum episodes being less likely to go on to have further pregnancies. The effect of primiparity has been hypothesized to be due to the biological differences between first and subsequent pregnancies and has raised the possibility of an aetiological link with other medical conditions showing a similar increase in first pregnancies such as pre-eclampsia [99]. Intriguingly, pre-eclampsia and PP have both been associated with immune dysregulation, for example the observation of a marked increase in the rates of post-partum autoimmune thyroiditis and immune biomarker alterations in women with PP [100]. In addition, pre-eclampsia and PP share other overlaps; for example, both have been found to be inversely correlated with tobacco smoking [101].

## REFERENCES

1. Brockington, I. F. Puerperal psychosis. In: Brockington, I. F. *Motherhood and Mental Health*. Oxford: Oxford University Press; 1996. pp. 200–84.
2. Knight, M., Nair, M., Tuffnell, D., *et al.* (eds), on behalf of MBRRACE-UK. *Saving Lives, Improving Mothers' Care—Surveillance of maternal deaths in the UK 2012–14 and lessons learned to inform maternity care from the UK and Ireland Confidential Enquiries into Maternal Deaths and Morbidity 2009–14*. Oxford: University of Oxford; 2016.
3. Bauer, A., Parsonage, M., Knapp, M., Iemmi, V., and Adelaja, B. *Costs of perinatal mental health problems*. London: London School of Economics and the Centre for Mental Health; 2014.
4. National Institute for Health and Care Excellence. *Antenatal and postnatal mental health: clinical management and service guidance*. 2014. Available at: http://www.nice.org.uk/guidance/cg192
5. American Psychiatric Association. *Diagnostic and Statistical Manual of Mental Disorders*, fifth edition. Washington, DC: American Psychiatric Association; 2013.
6. World Health Organization. *ICD-10 : The ICD-10 Classification of Mental and Behavioural Disorders : Clinical Descriptions and Diagnostic Guidelines*. Geneva: World Health Organization; 1992.
7. Di Florio, A., Smith, S., and Jones, I. Postpartum psychosis. Obstet Gynecol. 15, 145–50 (2013).
8. Heron, J., McGuinness, M., Blackmore, E. R., Craddock, N., and Jones, I. Early postpartum symptoms in puerperal psychosis. BJOG. 115, 348–53 (2008).
9. Sharma, V. and Sommerdyk, C. Postpartum psychosis: what is in a name? Aust N Z J Psychiatry, 48, 1081–2 (2014).
10. Jones, I. and Craddock, N. Bipolar disorder and childbirth: the importance of recognising risk. Br J Psychiatry. 186, 453–4 (2005).
11. Pfuhlmann, B., Stöber, G., Franzek, E., and Beckmann, H. Cycloid psychoses predominate in severe postpartum psychiatric disorders. J Affect Disord. 50, 125–34 (1998).
12. Action on Postpartum Psychosis. Available at: http://www.app-network.org
13. Di Florio, A., Munk-Olsen, T., and Bergink, V. The birth of a psychiatric Orphan disorder: postpartum psychosis. Lancet Psychiatry. 3, 502 (2016).
14. Brockington, I. F. *In Eileithyia's Mischief: the Organic Psychoses of Pregnancy, Parturition and the Puerperium*. Bredenbury: Eyry Press; 2006.
15. Khalifeh, H., Hunt, I. M., Appleby, L., and Howard, L. M. Suicide in perinatal and non-perinatal women in contact with psychiatric services: 15 year findings from a UK national inquiry. Lancet Psychiatry. 3, 233–42 (2016).
16. Spinelli, M. G. Postpartum psychosis: detection of risk and management. Am J Psychiatry. 166, 405–8 (2009).
17. Munk-Olsen, T., Laursen, T. M., Pedersen, C. B., Mors, O., and Mortensen, P. B. New parents and mental disorders. JAMA. 296, 2582–9 (2006).
18. Di Florio, A. *et al.* Perinatal episodes across the mood disorder spectrum. JAMA Psychiatry. 70, 168–75 (2013).
19. Munk-Olsen, T. *et al.* Risks and predictors of readmission for a mental disorder during the postpartum period. Arch Gen Psychiatry. 66, 189–95 (2009).
20. Munk-Olsen, T., Laursen, T. M., Meltzer-Brody, S., Mortensen, P. B., and Jones, I. Psychiatric disorders with postpartum onset: possible early manifestations of bipolar affective disorders. Arch Gen Psychiatry. 69, 428–34 (2012).
21. Di Florio, A. *et al.* Bipolar disorder, miscarriage, and termination. Bipolar Disord, 17, 102–5 (2015).
22. Blackmore, E. R. *et al.* Reproductive outcomes and risk of subsequent illness in women diagnosed with postpartum psychosis. Bipolar Disord. 15, 394–404 (2013).
23. Bergink, V. *et al.* Prevention of postpartum psychosis and mania in women at high risk. Am J Psychiatry. 169, 609–15 (2012).

24. Jones, I. and Craddock, N. Familiality of the puerperal trigger in bipolar disorder: results of a family study. Am J Psychiatry. 158, 913–17 (2001).

25. Jones, I., Chandra, P. S., Dazzan, P., and Howard, L. M. Bipolar disorder, affective psychosis, and schizophrenia in pregnancy and the post-partum period. Lancet. 384, 1789–99 (2014).

26. Dolman, C., Jones, I., and Howard, L. M. Pre-conception to parenting: a systematic review and meta-synthesis of the qualitative literature on motherhood for women with severe mental illness. Arch Womens Ment Health. 16, 173–96 (2013).

27. Bergink, V. et al. Treatment of psychosis and mania in the postpartum period. Am J Psychiatry. 172, 115–23 (2015).

28. Focht, A. and Kellner, C. H. Electroconvulsive therapy (ECT) in the treatment of postpartum psychosis. J ECT. 28, 31–3 (2012).

29. Babu, G. N., Thippeswamy, H., and Chandra, P. S. Use of electroconvulsive therapy (ECT) in postpartum psychosis—a naturalistic prospective study. Arch Womens Ment Health. 16, 247–51 (2013).

30. Protheroe, C. Puerperal psychoses: a long term study 1927–1961. Br J Psychiatry. 115, 9–30 (1969).

31. Chaudron, L. H. and Pies, R. W. The relationship between postpartum psychosis and bipolar disorder: a review. J Clin Psychiatry. 64, 1284–92 (2003).

32. Robertson, E., Jones, I., Haque, S., Holder, R., and Craddock, N. Risk of puerperal and non-puerperal recurrence of illness following bipolar affective puerperal (post-partum) psychosis. Br J Psychiatry. 186, 258–9 (2005).

33. Viguera, A. C. et al. Risk of recurrence of bipolar disorder in pregnant and nonpregnant women after discontinuing lithium maintenance. Am J Psychiatry. 157, 179–84 (2000).

34. Viguera, A. C. et al. Risk of recurrence in women with bipolar disorder during pregnancy: prospective study of mood stabilizer discontinuation. Am J Psychiatry. 164, 1817–24; quiz 1923 (2007).

35. British Association for Psychopharmacology. Available at: https://www.bap.org.uk/guidelines

36. Medicines and Healthcare products Regulatory Agency.Valproate and risk of abnormal pregnancy outcomes: new communication materials. 2016. Available at: https://www.gov.uk/drug-safety-update/valproate-and-of-risk-of-abnormal-pregnancy-outcomes-new-communication-materials

37. Wesseloo, R., Wierdsma, A.I., van Kamp, I.L., et al. Lithium dosing strategies during pregnancy and the postpartum period. Br J Psychiatry. 211, 31–6 (2017).

38. Nishizawa, O., Sakumoto, K., Hiramatsu, K.-I., and Kondo, T. Effectiveness of comprehensive supports for schizophrenic women during pregnancy and puerperium: preliminary study. Psychiatry Clin Neurosci. 61, 665–71 (2007).

39. Whiteford, H. A. et al. Global burden of disease attributable to mental and substance use disorders: findings from the Global Burden of Disease Study 2010. Lancet. 382, 1575–86 (2013).

40. Di Florio, A. and Meltzer-Brody, S. Is postpartum depression a distinct disorder? Curr Psychiatry Rep. 17, 76 (2015).

41. Cooper, C. et al. Clinical presentation of postnatal and non-postnatal depressive episodes. Psychol Med. 37, 1273–80 (2007).

42. Howard, L. M. et al. Non-psychotic mental disorders in the perinatal period. Lancet. 384, 1775–88 (2014).

43. Wisner, K. L. et al. Onset timing, thoughts of self-harm, and diagnoses in postpartum women with screen-positive depression findings. JAMA Psychiatry. 70, 490–8 (2013).

44. Altemus, M. et al. Phenotypic differences between pregnancy-onset and postpartum-onset major depressive disorder. J Clin Psychiatry. 73, e1485–91 (2012).

45. Jones, I., and Shakespeare, J. (2014). Easily missed? Postnatal depression. BMJ. 349, g4500 (2014).

46. Sharma, V. and Khan, M. Identification of bipolar disorder in women with postpartum depression. Bipolar Disord. 12, 335–40 (2010).

47. Bergink, V. and Koorengevel, K. M. Postpartum depression with psychotic features. Am J Psychiatry. 167, 476–7; author reply 477 (2010).

48. Halbreich, U. and Karkun, S. Cross-cultural and social diversity of prevalence of postpartum depression and depressive symptoms. J Affect Disord. 91, 97–111 (2006).

49. Gavin, N. I. et al. Perinatal depression: a systematic review of prevalence and incidence. Obstet Gynecol. 106, 1071–83 (2005).

50. Fisher, J. et al. Prevalence and determinants of common perinatal mental disorders in women in low- and lower-middle-income countries: a systematic review. Bull World Health Organ. 90, 139–49H (2012).

51. Vesga-López O, Blanco C, Keyes K, Olfson M, Grant BF, Hasin DS. Psychiatric disorders in pregnant and postpartum women in the United States. Arch Gen Psychiatry. 2008; 65: 805–15.

52. Biaggi, A., Conroy, S., Pawlby, S., and Pariante, C. M. Identifying the women at risk of antenatal anxiety and depression: a systematic review. J Affect Disord. 191, 62–77 (2016).

53. Cooper, P. J. and Murray, L. Course and recurrence of postnatal depression. Evidence for the specificity of the diagnostic concept. Br J Psychiatry. 166, 191–5 (1995).

54. O'Connor, E., Rossom, R. C., Henninger, M., Groom, H. C., and Burda, B. U. Primary care screening for and treatment of depression in pregnant and postpartum women: evidence report and systematic review for the us preventive services task force. JAMA. 315, 388–406 (2016).

55. Paulden M, Palmer S, Hewitt C, Gilbody S. Screening for postnatal depression in primary care: cost effectiveness analysis. BMJ. 2010, 340, b5203.

56. Scottish Intercollegiate Guidelines Network (SIGN). Available at: http://www.sign.ac.uk/

57. Dennis, C.-L. and Dowswell, T. Psychosocial and psychological interventions for preventing postpartum depression. Cochrane Database Syst Rev. 2, CD001134 (2013).

58. Munk-Olsen, T., Gasse, C., and Laursen, T. M. Prevalence of antidepressant use and contacts with psychiatrists and psychologists in pregnant and postpartum women. Acta Psychiatr Scand. 125, 318–24 (2012).

59. Cooper, W. O., Willy, M. E., Pont, S. J., and Ray, W. A. Increasing use of antidepressants in pregnancy. Am J Obstet Gynecol. 196, 544.e1–5 (2007).

60. Molyneaux, E., Howard, L. M., McGeown, H. R., Karia, A. M., and Trevillion, K. Antidepressant treatment for postnatal depression. Cochrane Database Syst Rev. 9, CD002018 (2014).

61. Kanes, S., Colquhoun, H., Gunduz-Bruce, H., et al. Brexanolone (SAGE-547 injection) in post-partum depression: a randomised controlled trial. Lancet. 390, 480–9.

62. Jones, I. Post-partum depression-a glimpse of light in the darkness? Lancet. 390, 434–5 (2017).

63. Cohen, L. S. et al. Relapse of major depression during pregnancy in women who maintain or discontinue antidepressant treatment. JAMA. 295, 499–507 (2006).

64. Yonkers, K. A. *et al.* Does antidepressant use attenuate the risk of a major depressive episode in pregnancy?: Epidemiology. 22, 848–54 (2011).

65. Dennis, C.-L., Ross, L. E., and Herxheimer, A. Oestrogens and progestins for preventing and treating postpartum depression. Cochrane Database Syst Rev. 4, CD001690 (2008).

66. Gong, H., Ni, C., Shen, X., Wu, T., and Jiang, C. Yoga for pre-natal depression: a systematic review and meta-analysis. BMC Psychiatry. 15, 14 (2015).

67. Miller, B. J., Murray, L., Beckmann, M. M., Kent, T., and Macfarlane, B. Dietary supplements for preventing postnatal depression. Cochrane Database Syst Rev. 10, CD009104 (2013).

68. Navarro, P. *et al.* Non-psychotic psychiatric disorders after childbirth: prevalence and comorbidity in a community sample. J Affect Disord. 109, 171–6 (2008).

69. Matthey, S., Barnett, B., Howie, P., and Kavanagh, D. J. Diagnosing postpartum depression in mothers and fathers: whatever happened to anxiety? J Affect Disord. 74, 139–47 (2003).

70. Goodman, J. H., Chenausky, K. L., and Freeman, M. P. Anxiety disorders during pregnancy: a systematic review. J Clin Psychiatry. 75, e1153–84 (2014).

71. Marchesi, C. *et al.* Clinical management of perinatal anxiety disorders: a systematic review. J Affect Disord. 190, 543–50 (2016).

72. Russell, E. J., Fawcett, J. M., and Mazmanian, D. Risk of obsessive-compulsive disorder in pregnant and postpartum women: a meta-analysis. J Clin Psychiatry. 74, 377–85 (2013).

73. Marc, I. *et al.* Mind-body interventions during pregnancy for preventing or treating women's anxiety. Cochrane Database Syst Rev. 7, CD007559 (2011).

74. Daugirdaitė, V., van den Akker, O., and Purewal, S. Posttraumatic stress and posttraumatic stress disorder after termination of pregnancy and reproductive loss: a systematic review. J Pregnancy. 2015, 646345 (2015).

75. James, S. Women's experiences of symptoms of posttraumatic stress disorder (PTSD) after traumatic childbirth: a review and critical appraisal. Arch Womens Ment Health. 18, 761–71 (2015).

76. Kastello, J. C. *et al.* Posttraumatic stress disorder among low-income women exposed to perinatal intimate partner violence: posttraumatic stress disorder among women exposed to partner violence. Arch Womens Ment Health. 19, 521–8 (2016).

77. Smith, M. V., Poschman, K., Cavaleri, M. A., Howell, H. B., and Yonkers, K. A. Symptoms of posttraumatic stress disorder in a community sample of low-income pregnant women. Am J Psychiatry. 163, 881–4 (2006).

78. Bastos, M. H., Furuta, M., Small, R., McKenzie-McHarg, K., and Bick, D. Debriefing interventions for the prevention of psychological trauma in women following childbirth. Cochrane Database Syst Rev. 4, CD007194 (2015).

79. Easter, A., Treasure, J., and Micali, N. Fertility and prenatal attitudes towards pregnancy in women with eating disorders: results from the Avon Longitudinal Study of Parents and Children. BJOG. 118, 1491–8 (2011).

80. Easter, A. *et al.* Recognising the symptoms: how common are eating disorders in pregnancy? Eur Eat Disord Rev. 21, 340–4 (2013).

81. Bulik, C. M. *et al.* Patterns of remission, continuation and incidence of broadly defined eating disorders during early pregnancy in the Norwegian Mother and Child Cohort Study (MoBa). Psychol Med. 37, 1109–18 (2007).

82. Micali, N., Simonoff, E., and Treasure, J. Pregnancy and post-partum depression and anxiety in a longitudinal general population cohort: the effect of eating disorders and past depression. J Affect Disord. 131, 150–7 (2011).

83. Börjesson, K., Ruppert, S., and Bågedahl-Strindlund, M. A longitudinal study of psychiatric symptoms in primiparous women: relation to personality disorders and sociodemographic factors. Arch Womens Ment Health. 8, 232–42 (2005).

84. Gopman, S. Prenatal and postpartum care of women with substance use disorders. Obstet Gynecol Clin North Am. 41, 213–28 (2014).

85. Dowlatshahi, D. and Paykel, E. S. Life events and social stress in puerperal psychoses: absence of effect. Psychol Med. 20, 655–62 (1990).

86. Brockington, I. F., Martin, C., Brown, G. W., Goldberg, D., and Margison, F. Stress and puerperal psychosis. Br J Psychiatry. 157, 331–4 (1990).

87. Jones, I. R. and Craddock, N. J. Do puerperal psychotic episodes identify a more familial subtype of bipolar disorder? Results of a family history study. Psychiatr Genet. 12, 177–80. (2002).

88. Coyle, N., Jones, I. R., Robertson, E., Lendon, C., and Craddock, N. J. Variation at the serotonin transporter gene influences susceptibility to bipolar affective puerperal psychosis. Lancet. 356, 1490–1 (2000).

89. Jones, I. R., Hamshere, M. L., Nangle, J.-M., *et al.* Bipolar affective puerperal psychosis: genome-wide significant evidence for linkage to chromosome 16. Am J Psychiatry. 164, 1099–104 (2007).

90. Arevalo, M.-A., Azcoitia, I., and Garcia-Segura, L. M. The neuroprotective actions of oestradiol and oestrogen receptors. Nat Rev Neurosci. 16, 17–29 (2015).

91. Jensik, P. J. and Arbogast, L. A. Differential and interactive effects of ligand-bound progesterone receptor A and B isoforms on tyrosine hydroxylase promoter activity. J Neuroendocrinol. 23, 915–25 (2011).

92. Zlotnik, A. *et al.* The effects of estrogen and progesterone on blood glutamate levels: evidence from changes of blood glutamate levels during the menstrual cycle in women. Biol Reprod. 84, 581–6 (2011).

93. Belelli, D. and Lambert, J. J. Neurosteroids: endogenous regulators of the GABA(A) receptor. Nat Rev Neurosci. 6, 565–75 (2005).

94. Rubinow, D. R. and Schmidt, P. J. Gonadal steroid regulation of mood: the lessons of premenstrual syndrome. Front Neuroendocrinol. 27, 210–16 (2006).

95. Bloch, M. *et al.* Effects of gonadal steroids in women with a history of postpartum depression. Am J Psychiatry. 157, 924–30 (2000).

96. Murray, G. and Harvey, A. Circadian rhythms and sleep in bipolar disorder. Bipolar Disord. 12, 459–72 (2010).

97. Lewis, K. J., Foster, R. G., and Jones, I. R. Is sleep disruption a trigger for postpartum psychosis? Br J Psychiatry. 208, 409–11 (2016).

98. Munk-Olsen, T., Jones, I., and Laursen, T. M. Birth order and postpartum psychiatric disorders. Bipolar Disord. 16, 300–7 (2014).

99. Di Florio, A. *et al.* Mood disorders and parity—a clue to the aetiology of the postpartum trigger. J Affect Disord. 152–4, 334–9 (2014).

100. Bergink, V., Gibney, S. M., and Drexhage, H. A. Autoimmunity, inflammation, and psychosis: a search for peripheral markers. Biol Psychiatry. 75, 324–31 (2014).

101. Di Florio, A. *et al.* Smoking and postpartum psychosis. Bipolar Disord. 17, 572–3 (2015).

# SECTION 12
# Depressive disorders

# 74

# Basic mechanisms of, and treatment targets for, depressive disorders

*Marcela Pereira, Roberto Andreatini, and Per Svenningsson*

## Introduction

The diagnosis of major depressive disorder (MDD) relies on the presence of a certain number of signs and symptoms, including feelings of guilt, hopelessness, dysphoria, cognitive dysfunction, persistent sleep, and appetite abnormalities. These signs and symptoms overlap with other conditions such as anxiety, bipolar, and seasonal affective disorders. In this chapter, we provide an overview of the basic neurobiological mechanisms underlying MDD and its treatment. There are several alterations in the molecular pathways and neuronal networks associated with MDD. We focus here on: gene × environment interactions, dysfunctional brain circuitries, neurotransmitter alterations, maladaptation in neurotrophins and neuroplasticity, hypothalamus–pituitary–adrenal (HPA) axis dysfunction, abnormal immune system responses, circadian arrhythmicity, and sleep disturbances (Fig. 74.1). We briefly describe the mechanisms of actions for approved antidepressant therapies and also discuss recent insights into the pathophysiology of MDD and future possible therapy targets.

## Gene × environment (G × E) interactions

There is increasing evidence that MDD is best understood in a lifelong perspective as changes in neuronal circuit function through stressful life events acting in genetically predisposed individuals. The genetic liability of MDD is 30–40% [1, 2]. It is likely that several genes, and their protein products, are involved both in the pathophysiology of the disease and in mediating antidepressant responses. Several genetic polymorphisms have been associated with depression, but in most instances, these studies have not been replicated. According to a large-scale GWAS, 15 loci and 17 independent SNPs were related to depression [3]. GWAS of both MDD and bipolar depression share 11p11.2 and 12p13.33 polymorphisms, including an SNP in *CACNA1C* encoding the α1C subunit of the voltage-gated L-type calcium channel $Ca_v1.2$ [4, 5]. A recent paper, which identified genetic determinants associated with personality traits, describes a genetic dimension which relates introversion and neuroticism to MDD [6].

A polymorphism in the 5-HT transporter results in long or short alleles, the short allele being less functional [7]. Influential G × E studies in humans [8] have reported a positive relationship between the number of self-reported early life stressors (for example, childhood maltreatment) and increased depression risk among individuals who had one or two copies of the short allele, compared with those homozygous for the long allele [8]. Similar results were observed in experimentally stressed non-human primates [9]. However, it should be noted that there have been difficulties in replicating these findings [10].

Epigenetics is an area of research intimately related to G × E interactions. It is defined as heritable cell characteristics (phenotype), which are not determined in the DNA sequence (genotype), but rather are determined by G × E interactions [11]. Environmental factors may lead to DNA methylation in cytosine bases and methylation, phosphorylation, or acetylation of histones, resulting in changes of gene expression via activation or inactivation of specific gene promoters [11]. In studies of MDD, most of the epigenetic changes have been experimentally induced by stress, especially early in life. Stressors, among other things, decrease the gene expression of both brain-derived neurotrophic factor (BDNF) and the glucocorticoid receptor [12] (Fig. 74.1). Epigenetic states might be reversible, even in adulthood. This has important implications for potential pharmacological treatment; for example, drugs that inhibit histone deacetylation (HDAC), such as valproic acid, could be used to reverse epigenetic changes [13, 14]. No human studies have been performed, but preclinical research has demonstrated that local administration of HDAC inhibitors in the nucleus accumbens can reverse depressive behaviour in rodents [13]. In addition, DNA methylation changes (for example, by acetyl-*L*-carnitine) can promote antidepressant-like behaviour in rats [15]. It is important to note, however, that drugs regulating epigenetic mechanisms have pleiotropic actions in different cell types, thus increasing the risk for side effects [12].

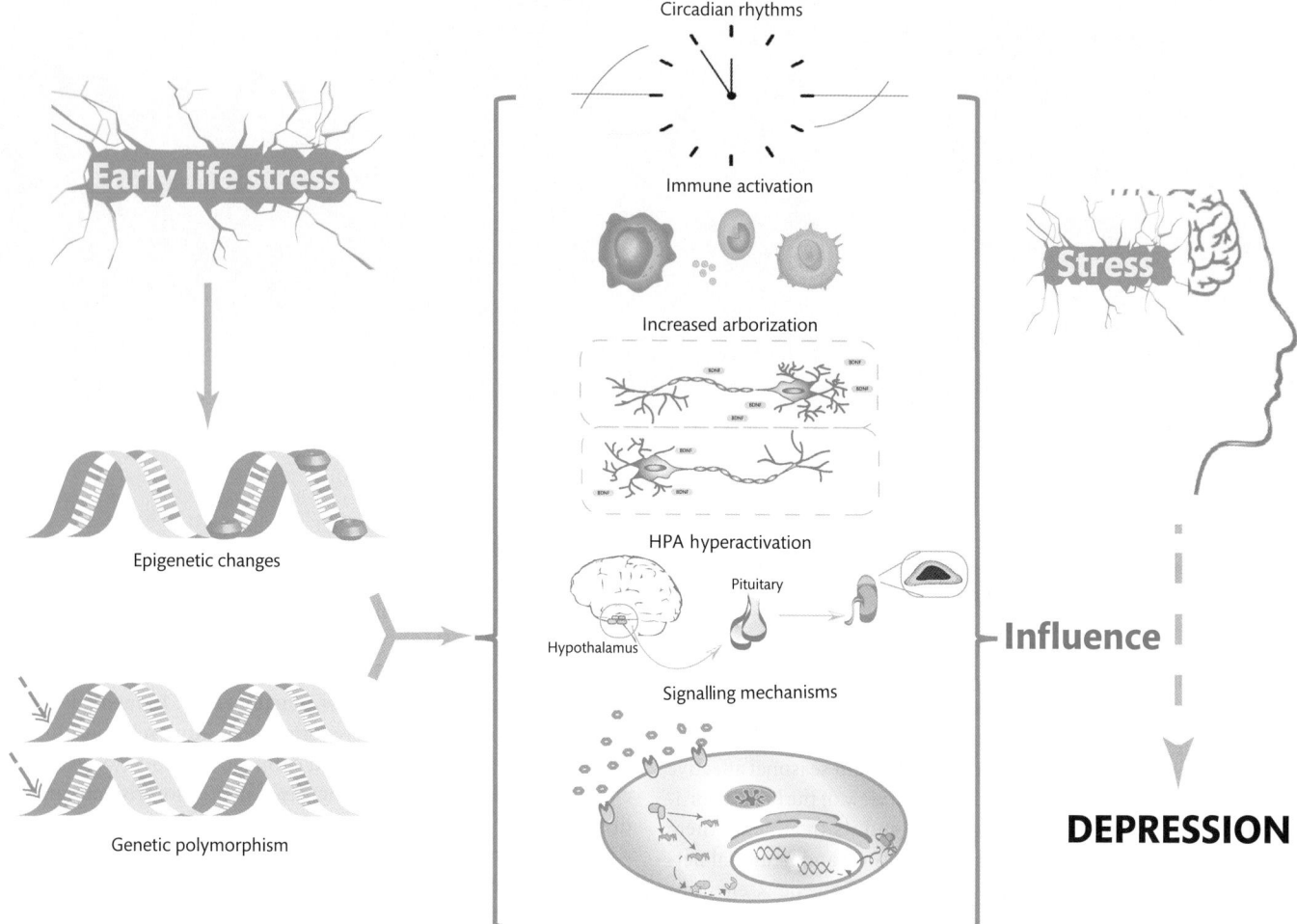

**Fig. 74.1** Neurobiological mechanisms underlying major depressive disorder. Stress, particularly in early life, causes epigenetic changes which interact with genetic vulnerability, resulting in several pathophysiological processes. Such G × E interactions affect circadian rhythms, immune activation, cellular arborization, HPA axis activity, and signalling mechanisms. Alterations in these neurobiological mechanisms contribute to the development of depression.

## Dysfunctional brain circuitries

Neuroimaging approaches, including volumetric magnetic resonance imaging (MRI), diffusion tensor imaging (DTI), functional MRI, and $^{18}$F-fluorodeoxyglucose positron emission tomography (FDG-PET), provide a versatile platform to characterize structural and functional connectomes. Imaging studies have improved neurocircuitry models of mood, emotionality, and behavioural regulation [16, 17].

Studies have reported morphological changes in MDD patients, in both neurons and glia in the hippocampus, amygdala, and prefrontal cortex (PFC) [16, 18]. The decrease in hippocampal volume is directly proportional to the number and duration of depressive episodes, especially in early-onset MDD [19]. The decrease of hippocampal volume seems to be related to prolonged increased levels of cortisol, which may relate to the fact that the hippocampus is the brain region with the highest levels of receptors for glucocorticoids [16, 20]. The hippocampus is critical for learning and memory processes. In depressive patients, memory formation is skewed towards negative events; this is known as negative bias. Negative bias is characterized by an enhanced focus on negative stimulus,

enhanced attention towards potentially threatening stimuli, and the attribution of negative emotional value to environmental stimuli that are considered to have neutral valance by healthy individuals [21]. Negative bias-related memories involve the amygdala, hippocampus, anterior cingulate cortex, PFC, and caudate–putamen [21]. In addition, the lateral habenula (LHb) may be a key subcortical structure in the generation of negative cognitive biases. LHb plays a crucial role in encoding aversive states [21, 22]. Deep brain stimulation (DBS) of the LHb can reverse depressive-like behaviours in rodents [23], reinforcing a role of the LHb in depression. DBS has also been examined in MDD patients. Based on the observation that some brain regions (including the subgenual cingulate cortex or Brodmann area 25) are metabolically overactive in treatment-resistant depression, DBS was applied to Brodmann area 25. This resulted in a striking and sustained remission of depression in some previously treatment-resistant patients in an open study [24, 25]. However, there is no published randomized controlled trial (RCT) to confirm this antidepressant effect. Another observational study showed an antidepressant effect of DBS in the ventral striatum [26], but a subsequent RCT failed to demonstrate an antidepressant effect of DBS in this region [27]. More advanced strategies for directly and focally altering neural activity, such as gene therapy, chemogenetics, and optogenetics, are successfully being developed in animals. This line of research has revealed that control of projection-specific dynamics is well suited for modulation of behavioural patterns that are relevant to a broad range of psychiatric diseases, including depression. For example, optogenetic targeting of projections from the medial PFC to the dorsal raphe nucleus will control mobility in the forced swim test, while targeting projections from the basolateral amygdala to the nucleus accumbens produces an appetitive or aversive response, depending on the type of stimulus [28].

## Neurotransmitter alterations and therapy targets

A critical role of monoamines in depression was initially supported by two independent serendipitous findings in drug discovery. Iproniazid was developed against tuberculosis but was found to exhibit antidepressant properties via monoamine oxidase (MAO) inhibition [29]. Several irreversible and non-selective MAO inhibitors were then developed, but they all have cardiovascular side effects due to the accumulation of tyramine. Accumulation of this trace amine depends upon MAO-B inhibition, and thus more recent antidepressant MAO inhibitors, such as moclobemide, target MAO-A and are reversible. Imipramine was found during efforts to develop an antipsychotic agent. Surprisingly, imipramine showed antidepressant properties and was approved as the first tricyclic drug for depression [30]. Pioneering work showed that imipramine could counteract noradrenaline uptake into presynaptic neurons [31]. It was later found that desipramine, a metabolite of imipramine, is a selective noradrenaline reuptake inhibitor (NRI). This finding, together with data showing lowered activity of noradrenergic neurons in depression, led to the catecholamine hypothesis of depression [32]. It was subsequently found that several tricyclic drugs for depression also inhibit serotonin (5-HT) reuptake, and a serotonin hypothesis of depression was conceived [33]. Currently, agents that selectively inhibit the reuptake of either noradrenaline (that is, reboxetine) or serotonin (SSRIs; for example, fluoxetine, paroxetine, sertraline, and citalopram), or both (that is, venlafaxine and duloxetine) are commonly used as drugs for depression and anxiety [34] (Fig. 74.2).

Several serotonin and noradrenaline receptors are implicated in antidepressant actions and side effects of reuptake inhibitors [34]. Many receptors are now targeted by more recently developed drugs for depression and anxiety. The 5-HT1A somatodendritic autoreceptor, which negatively controls 5-HT release, is an interesting target, since its blockade augments extracellular serotonin levels [34]. Accordingly, vilazodone is a combined 5-HT1A partial agonist and an SSRI, and is used for the treatment of depression [34]. Another compound that both inhibits serotonin reuptake and targets 5-HT receptors is vortioxetine, which binds to 5-HT1A (agonist), 5-HT1B (partial agonist), 5-HT3 (antagonist), and 5-HT7 (antagonist) receptors. In addition to these serotonin receptors, antagonism at 5-HT2C receptors plays an important role in the antidepressant actions of mirtazapine and agomelatine [34, 35]. Mirtazapine is also a noradrenergic α2A autoreceptor antagonist and enhances fronto-cortical serotonergic and noradrenergic transmission to elevate mood. Agomelatine combines 5-HT2C receptor antagonism with melatonin receptor agonism and has antidepressant

properties, along with beneficial effects on sleep, due to the restoration of circadian rhythmicity.

Antidepressant responses can also be obtained by enhancing dopaminergic transmission. Dopamine enhances motivation, reward response, and plays a crucial role in the reinforcement systems, often dysfunctional in MDD [36]. Bupropion, a dopamine and noradrenaline reuptake inhibitor, is an antidepressant drug with energizing and mood-elevating properties [34]. Several studies have also reported that D2 agonists may present antidepressant actions, some of which (for example, pramipexole) are used in the treatment of Parkinson's disease. A large proportion of patients with Parkinson's disease suffer from depression and, interestingly, depressive symptoms often precede the onset of motor symptoms and diagnosis, suggesting a largely neurochemical cause [37].

An approach to study the role of monoamine transmission in depression and antidepressant effect is monoamine depletion. Serotonin levels can be reduced by para-chlorophenylalanine (PCPA), an inhibitor of tryptophan hydroxylase, the rate-limiting step in 5-HT synthesis, or by acute depletion of tryptophan (an essential amino acid that is the precursor of 5-HT). On the other hand, inhibition of tyrosine hydroxylase by α-methyl-para-tyrosine decreases noradrenaline and dopamine synthesis. These depletion procedures induce a depressive relapse in remitted MDD patients taking drugs for depression, and there is a correlation between the target of the procedure (5-HT or noradrenaline/dopamine) and the site of action of the drug [SSRI or NRI/dopamine reuptake inhibitor (DARI)] [38]. Moreover, while depletion of monoamines lowered mood in normal volunteers with a family history of MDD, it did not affect normal volunteers without a family history of MDD. These results can be interpreted as an indication that monoamines may be related to a biological vulnerability to MDD, rather than to mood state [38, 39].

There is a delay in therapeutic onset after the start of antidepressant treatment, indicating that the antidepressant action is not strictly related to an increase in monoamine levels, but rather to molecular and cellular processes initiated by them [40]. Several molecules, including p11 (also termed S100a10), BDNF, glial cell-derived neurotrophic factor (GDNF), vascular endothelial growth factor (VEGF), insulin-like growth factor-1 (IGF-1), fibroblast growth factor-2 (FGF-2), and glutamate receptors, are induced by monoaminergic antidepressants and mediate beneficial effects on neuronal plasticity, such as increased spine density and neurogenesis, correlating with antidepressant responses [16, 40–42] (Fig. 74.2).

In contrast to monoaminergic drugs, some compounds acting via glutamate receptors possess rapid antidepressant effects. Studies using magnetic resonance spectroscopy (MRS) to measure the concentration of intra- and extracellular glutamate, glutamine, and GABA have shown changes in the glutamate system (for example, reduced levels of glutamine, the precursor of glutamate) in MDD [43–45]. It has been reported that glutamate-reducing agents, such as riluzole and lamotrigine, exert antidepressant actions by lowering extracellular levels of glutamate [46–48] (Fig. 74.2). Moreover, it has been established that blockade of NMDA receptors by a single injection of the non-competitive antagonist ketamine causes a rapid (within hours) and long (weeks) antidepressant effect [45, 49, 50]. However, the psychotomimetic, anaesthetic, amnestic, and addictive properties of ketamine preclude usage on a larger scale, and intense

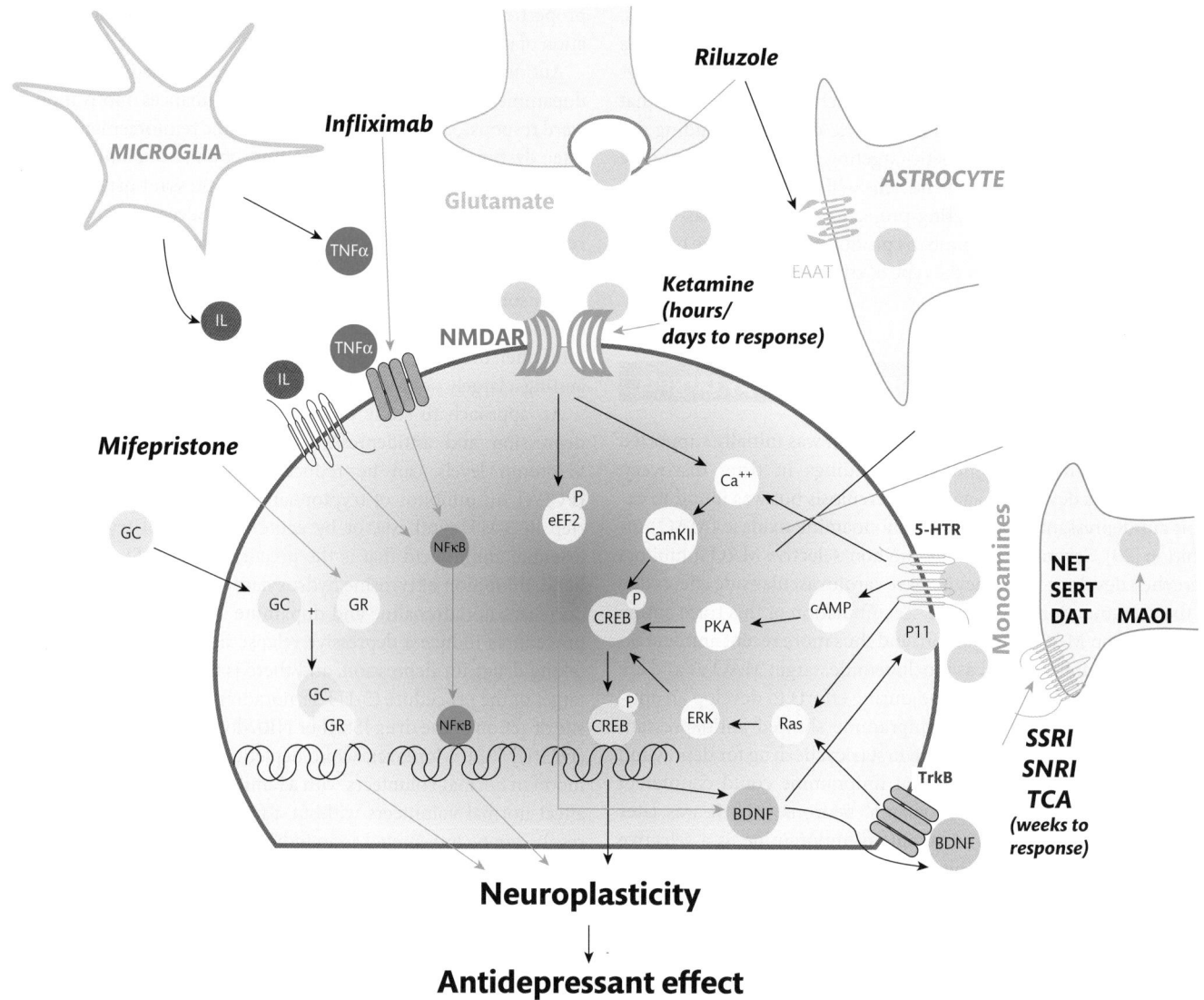

**Fig. 74.2** Cellular mediators altered in depression and by antidepressant agents. Schematic drawing showing cross-talk between neurons, microglia, and astrocytes. Selected neurotransmitters, immune mediators, and glucocorticoid hormones involved in depression are shown. Targets for antidepressant therapies are pointed out. Some intracellular signalling cascades regulating neuronal plasticity are indicated. Red indicates inhibition; black indicates stimulation.

research is focused on finding alternative ways of interfering with glutamate neurotransmission to achieve fast antidepressant actions without severe side effects. Antagonism of the NMDA/NR2B subunit presents antidepressant-like effects in animal models, but has so far failed to show antidepressant actions in clinical trials [51]. Another approach has been to develop antidepressant agents acting at the glycine modulatory site of the NMDA receptor such as the partial agonist GLYX-13 (rapastinel) [45]. Moreover, a metabolite of ketamine—(2R,6R)-hydroxynorketamine—has shown promising antidepressant-like effects in animal models [52]. The mechanism of action of (2R,6R)-hydroxynorketamine remains to be fully understood, but reported data indicate that it is not an NMDA receptor antagonist, but rather an AMPA receptor potentiator [52]. In this context, it is interesting to note that tianeptine, an atypical drug for depression, enhances 5-HT reuptake, potentiates AMPA receptor function, and promotes synaptic plasticity [53]. Moreover, it has also recently been demonstrated that tianeptine acts as a μ opioid receptor

agonist. In addition to targeting ionotropic glutamate receptors, antagonism at metabotropic glutamatergic 2, 3, or 5 receptors have shown antidepressant actions in rodent models [45] (Fig. 74.2).

There is also considerable evidence that depressed patients have reduced GABA levels in the brain and that the subunit composition of GABA(A) receptors are changed following stress and in MDD, particularly in interneurons [54].

## Maladaptation in neurotrophins and neuroplasticity

BDNF plays a central role in the neurotrophic theory of depression [20, 55]. BDNF is highly expressed and inducible in the hippocampus and PFC where it critically regulates neurotransmitter release, neurogenesis, neuronal survival, and synapse plasticity [56]. In accordance, peripheral blood markers from both unipolar and bipolar depression patients and depression-like animals have decreased levels of BDNF [20, 56, 57]. In contrast, treatment with different antidepressant drugs, for example SSRIs and ketamine, increases the levels of BDNF in the PFC and hippocampus [56, 57]. In the nucleus accumbens, low levels of BDNF seem to have antidepressant effects, being therefore the opposite from other areas, which complicates therapy development [16]. In addition to BDNF, other neurotrophins have been implicated in depression. Several studies have shown changes in GDNF and VEGF levels in depression [58]. FGF-2 level is decreased in depression, while treatment with drugs for depression increases FGF-2 levels [59]. Likewise, FGF-2 exerted an antidepressant-like effect in the chronic mild stress model, and furthermore, FGF-2 antagonists blocked the antidepressant effect of imipramine and fluoxetine [60]. Besides pharmacological treatments, cognitive behavioural therapy (CBT), electroconvulsive therapy (ECT), and exercise seem to be effective in the treatment of depression by stimulating neuroplasticity. CBT is effective both in the short and long term [61, 62], although its mechanisms of action are not yet well understood. Regarding ECT, the literature reports different procedures on how to perform it (uni- or bilateral and brief or ultrabrief pulse), and all are effective [63, 64]. The antidepressant action of ECT can be related to 5-HT, noradrenaline, and dopamine neurotransmission potentiation, hippocampal neuroplasticity, glutamate neurotransmission, and rapid eye movement (REM) sleep suppression [65, 66]. These multiple-target actions have been associated with the greater and faster effect of ECT, compared to monoaminergic drugs [63, 64]. Some data suggest that exercise can exert an antidepressant effect and may improve antidepressant drug effects [67, 68]. Exercise has been reported to affect growth hormone, inflammatory cytokines, neurotrophins, and neurogenesis [67].

## HPA axis dysfunction

Exposure to prolonged stress can lead to persistently changed responsivity of the HPA axis. Since the pre- and postnatal periods are fundamental to the development of the central nervous system, stress during these periods can promote long-term changes in the brain function, increasing the risk of depression. Accordingly, studies have shown that poor maternal care during early life can induce epigenetic changes in the neuron-specific glucocorticoid receptor NR3C1 promoter [69].

The HPA axis activity is governed by different hormones: corticotropin-releasing hormone (CRH) and vasopressin (AVP) from the hypothalamus; adrenocorticotrophic hormone (ACTH) from the pituitary; and glucocorticoids (cortisol) from the adrenal cortex. Increased levels of CRH and AVP will lead to increased ACTH that will, in turn, increase the secretion of cortisol. Cortisol has a negative feedback action on CRH, AVP, and ACTH release, thereby decreasing the activity of the HPA axis. Cortisol is fundamental to homeostatic and allostatic control of responses to the environment such as cognitive and affective coping mechanisms. Numerous studies have shown that chronic administration of glucocorticoids leads to changes in mood and cognition [70].

A significant number of depressive patients show increased levels of glucocorticoids and glucocorticoid resistance, that is, a lack of feedback suppression of the HPA axis by glucocorticoids [40,

70–72]. Glucocorticoids can activate two distinct types of receptors: mineralocorticoid (MR) and glucocorticoid (GR) receptors; MRs are related to a basal tone of activation of the HPA axis, while GRs play a more important role in the response to stress and in the negative feedback loop of HPA activation [70]. Studies have shown an imbalance in the expression of GRs and MRs in depressive patients, leading to prolonged HPA axis activation, with resistance of the negative feedback loop [70, 72].

Activity of the HPA axis is fundamental to the control of several body functions, including metabolism, the immune system, and several brain functions such as neuronal survival, neurogenesis, and memory acquisition. In rodents, repeated glucocorticoid administration has been shown to reduce hippocampal neurogenesis and volume [73]. Depressed patients with psychotic features showed high evening cortisol levels, which is associated with poor cognitive performance [74]. Moreover, Cai and co-workers [75] showed that early life stress can lead to increased mitochondrial DNA (mtDNA) dysfunction and shortening of telomeric DNA, and that these changes were tissue-specific due to glucocorticoid secretion. Drugs for depression can improve HPA axis abnormalities through modulation of GR function [73]. Several studies in depressive patients have reported increased levels of cortisol in saliva, plasma, and urine, along with hypertrophic pituitary and adrenal glands [70, 76]. Based on the HPA axis dysfunction theory of depression, mifepristone, a GR and progesterone receptor antagonist and an MR receptor agonist, has been studied in patients with bipolar depression, with mixed results (for example, [77]).

## Abnormal immune system responses

Glucocorticoids regulate not only the HPA axis, but also metabolism and immunity. There are data suggesting that increased levels of pro-inflammatory cytokines can induce glucocorticoid resistance and promote HPA axis hyperactivity in depressive patients [72, 73, 78] (see also Chapter 15). Cytokines also activate microglia, causing neuroinflammation and amplification in inflammatory signals through release of reactive oxygen and nitrogen species and chemokines [78]. This activation leads to sustained long-lasting brain inflammation that may contribute to depressive-like states and sickness behaviour.

Studies have shown changes in the regulation of both pro- and anti-inflammatory cytokines in depression, and it is proposed that such changes are due to external (for example, family loss) or internal (for example, changes in gut flora) stressors [40, 79]. Preclinical research using administration of lipopolysaccharide (LPS), a major component of the outer membrane of Gram-negative bacteria, showed increased brain levels of tumour necrosis factor alpha (TNFα) up to 10 months after exposure [80]. Moreover, LPS can induce depressive-like behaviours in rodents, which can be attenuated by anti-inflammatory drugs [81]. Increased plasma cytokines (IL-6 and TNFα) and depressed mood are also observed in normal volunteers who received a low dose of this endotoxin [82]. Although there are some discrepancies between studies regarding changes in certain cytokines in depressed patients, elevated IL-6 has been found repeatedly [83, 84]. Increased levels of IL-6 have been linked to an increase in C-reactive protein (CRP), bacterial translocation in the gut, increased oxidative and nitrosative stress, hyperactivity of the HPA axis, and a shift in the tryptophan pathway to the TRYCAT (tryptophan catabolite) pathway [85]. Due to its many pro-depressive features, antagonism of IL-6 may be a possible target to treat depression. Indeed, addition of the IL-6 receptor (IL-6R) antagonist tocilizumab to drugs for depression could be useful [86]. Recently, a proof-of-concept RCT of infliximab, a TNFα-specific monoclonal antibody, has reported improvements in patients with treatment-resistant depression characterized by high inflammation at baseline [87]. Other promising therapies include antibodies against signal transducer and activator of transcription 3 (STAT3) or soluble glycoprotein 130 (sgp130) [88].

In bipolar depression, a recent meta-analysis indicated that anti-inflammatory drugs exert antidepressant effects and can potentiate the efficacy of monoaminergic antidepressant drugs. Accordingly, N-acetylcysteine (NAC) shows an antidepressant effect; NAC also has an antioxidant effect, which may contribute to its effect on bipolar depression. On the other hand, omega-3 fatty acids and ethyl-eicosapentanoate (EPA), which are also antioxidants, have shown mixed results in adjunctive treatment studies [88]. However, not all depressed patients show cytokine changes, and positive results with drugs that target inflammation appear to be restricted to a subset of patients with increased inflammatory biomarkers [78].

Increased oxidative and nitrosative stress is associated with increased inflammation, and studies have reported that even in the absence of a depressive phenotype, long-term stress exposure, especially in early life, can lead to an increase in pro-inflammatory markers in blood [89, 90]. An increase in oxidative and nitrosative stress can also lead to decreased levels of neurotransmitters such as serotonin, noradrenaline, dopamine, and glutamate [91].

## Circadian arrhythmicity and sleep disturbances

Circadian rhythms are responsible for our adaptation to a 24-hour day schedule and to keep the homeostasis of the organism. Functions of the brain, peripheral organs (for example, heart and liver), hormone release, and the immune system all present a circadian rhythm. Several findings suggest an association between depression and circadian rhythm changes. For example, sleep change (insomnia or hypersomnia) is one of the criteria for MDD diagnosis, and it is present in 60–90% of depressive patients. Furthermore, depressive symptoms can exhibit a circadian fluctuation, generally being more prominent in the morning than in the evening [92].

Each cell in our body contains a set of circadian genes that are differently expressed along the day. The main pacemaker, responsible for keeping the whole body in synchronicity, is located in the suprachiasmatic nucleus (SCN) in the anterior hypothalamus. The main circadian genes (circadian locomotor output cycles kaput— Clock; brain and muscle ARNT-Like 1—Bmal1; Period—Per1,2,3; Cryptochrome—Cry1,2) work in transcriptional/translational feedback loops, that is, a positive and a negative loop that will stimulate and inhibit each other to keep the cycle going [93]. More specifically, increased levels of the heterodimer CLOCK–BMAL1 will increase the transcription of Per and Cry (that will heterodimerize) and REV-ERBα and RORα (retinoic acid-related orphan nuclear receptors) (another heterodimer). Once the expression of these two heterodimers increases, they will inhibit the expression of Clock and

Bmal1. However, during the day, they will be degraded, resulting in increased levels of CLOCK and BMAL1 again [93, 94].

The homeostatic functionality of the circadian system is dependent on the genes that control it, the levels of several neurotransmitters, including serotonin, noradrenaline, dopamine, and acetylcholine, and hormones [95, 96]. In homeostatic conditions, serotonin, that has its synthesis peak in the morning and presents seasonal rhythmicity fluctuations, is the precursor to the synthesis of melatonin, one of the main controllers of rhythms. Serotonergic projections go from the raphe to the SCN, and vice versa. Noradrenaline, in turn, regulates melatonin synthesis, while dopaminergic neurons from the ventral tegmental area play a role in the control of REM sleep and adaptation to light [95–98]. Acetylcholine release is highest during awake time and REM sleep, but reduced during non-REM (NREM) sleep, and consequently loss of cholinergic neurons leads to sleep disturbances [99]. Regarding hormonal regulation, growth-hormone releasing factor (GHRF) (that is predominantly expressed in the first half of the night and is secreted in the hypothalamus and arcuate nucleus) plays a role in the control of NREM sleep [100]. Increasing levels of cortisol and CRH, which build up during the night, increase the frequency of REM sleep in the second half of the night [101, 102]. In MDD, the reduction of REM latency seems to be related to decreased cholinergic and monoaminergic activity, while increased NREM duration appears to be related to low levels of CRH, and shorter sleep episodes are related to decreased cortisol [101, 102]. This could be due to crosstalk between HPA dysfunction and sleep disturbance in depressive patients.

Depressive patients seem to present arrhythmicity or lengthening of the circadian period and disruption in sleep architecture, and it is proposed that part of the effect of drugs for depression, particularly agomelatine, can be due to re-establishment of normal circadian rhythm by shortening of the circadian period [103]. Polysomnographic studies have shown changes in the electroencephalographic profile of individuals with MDD. Depressed patients presented diminished sleep efficiency, shorter sleep period, and increased REM time with shorter REM latency [102].

Regarding the use of circadian rhythm interventions to treat depression, sleep deprivation (SD) is a promising therapy. Several different procedures for SD have been proposed: total SD, partial SD, and selective REM SD [104]. A few hours of SD appear to improve mood in depressive patients. SD appears to potentiate monoaminergic transmission, influence glutamatergic neurotransmission, increase metabolism in specific brain areas (ventral/lateral cingulate cortices and medial PFC), and increase neurogenesis, while resetting the circadian rhythm of the patient [104, 105].

Another non-pharmacological therapy employed to treat depression is light therapy. Light therapy is frequently used to treat seasonal affective disorder (SAD) or MDD with seasonal patterning [106]. A defining characteristic of SAD is its seasonality, with depressive episodes commonly occurring during wintertime [106]. SAD is a complex disease and appears to be polyfactorial and polygenetic and involves circadian arrhythmicity [106]. There is a correlation between latitude and the prevalence of SAD. Indeed SAD is more prevalent in northern latitudes [106, 107]. SAD appears to respond to light therapy, although data are limited [108]. The idea behind light therapy is that exposure to a strong light pulse daily at a specific time will help to keep the circadian rhythm by synchronizing the SCN [109]. The main components of light therapy are intensity, wavelength, and duration and time of exposure. In patients with SAD, light therapy reduced 5-HT transporter binding in the PFC [110].

## Concluding remarks and future perspectives

The discovery of iproniazid and imipramine and its molecular targets resulted in the monoamine hypothesis of depression. Several improvements of monoamine-based drugs have been made, but their efficacy is still limited, with less than 50% of depressed patients remitting. It is therefore crucial to identify relevant targets for novel antidepressant treatment strategies to alleviate this serious, unmet medical need. Fundamental knowledge of the neurobiological systems and molecular targets related to the pathophysiology of depression has improved significantly over the past years. As briefly reviewed in this chapter, abnormal G × E interactions, dysfunctional brain circuitries and neurotransmitter systems resulting in maladaptive neuroplasticity, and HPA axis dysfunction, along with abnormal immune system responses and circadian arrhythmicity, all play a role in depression. The glutamatergic system, inflammatory pathways, and neuromodulation of specific brain circuitries are all promising new targets for novel therapies. In addition, several preclinical studies suggest that neuropeptides, such as galanin, neuropeptide Y (NPY), and CRH, are targets for drug development. However, there are major species differences in the expression levels and anatomical location of neuropeptides and their receptors, which complicates translation of preclinical data to the clinic.

With the advancement of genetics, epigenetics, and neuroimaging, stratification of patients with distinct diagnostic subtypes, therapy responses, dosing regimens, and likelihood for side effects will develop over the coming years. Moreover, gender is an important and largely ignored factor in depression. Indeed two-thirds of patients with unipolar depression are female, and furthermore, the hormonal status of female patients can impact depression symptomatology [111–113]. Despite the fact that some initial studies suggested that depressed female patients would respond better to SSRIs, while male patients would respond better to tricyclic drugs, the influence of gender in drug treatment response is poorly understood [112, 114, 115].

It is likely that precision medicine utilizing recent neurobiological insights and pharmacogenomic approaches will result in more personalized therapies for a large proportion of depressed patients. This development will also have a major impact on our view of depressive disorder.

## REFERENCES

1. Sullivan PF, Neale MC, Kendler KS (2000) Genetic epidemiology of major depression: review and meta-analysis. *Am J Psychiatry*. 157:1552–62.
2. Ripke S, Wray NR, Lewis CM, *et al.* (2013) A mega-analysis of genome-wide association studies for major depressive disorder. *Mol Psychiatry*. 18:497–511.
3. Hyde CL, Nagle MW, Tian C, *et al.* (2016) Identification of 15 genetic loci associated with risk of major depression in individuals of European descent. *Nat Genet*. 48:1031–6.
4. Nurnberger JI, Koller DL, Jung J, *et al.* (2014) Identification of pathways for bipolar disorder: a meta-analysis. *JAMA Psychiatry*. 71:657–64.
5. Cross-Disorder Group of the Psychiatric Genomics Consortium (2013) Identification of risk loci with shared effects on five major psychiatric disorders: a genome-wide analysis. *Lancet*. 381:1371–9.
6. Lo MT, Hinds DA, Tung JY, *et al.* (2017) Genome-wide analyses for personality traits identify six genomic loci and show correlations with psychiatric disorders. *Nat Genet*. 49:152–6.
7. Bennett AJ, Lesch KP, Heils A, *et al.* (2002) Early experience and serotonin transporter gene variation interact to influence primate CNS function. *Mol Psychiatry*. 7:118–22.
8. Caspi A, Sugden K, Moffitt TE, *et al.* (2003) Influence of life stress on depression: moderation by a polymorphism in the 5-HTT gene. *Science*. 301:386–9.
9. Lesch K-P, Bengel D, Heils A, *et al.* (1996) Association of anxiety-related traits with a polymorphism in the serotonin transporter gene regulatory region. *Science*. 274:1527–31.
10. Uher R, McGuffin P (2008) The moderation by the serotonin transporter gene of environmental adversity in the aetiology of mental illness: review and methodological analysis. *Mol Psychiatry*. 13:131–46.
11. Sun H, Kennedy PJ, Nestler EJ (2013) Epigenetics of the depressed brain: role of histone acetylation and methylation. *Neuropsychopharmacol*. 38:124–37.
12. Silberman DM, Acosta GB, Zorrilla Zubilete MA (2016) Long-term effects of early life stress exposure: role of epigenetic mechanisms. *Pharmacol Res*. 109:64–73.
13. Covington HE, Maze I, LaPlant QC, *et al.* (2009) Antidepressant actions of histone deacetylase inhibitors. *J Neurosci*. 29:11451–60.
14. Phiel CJ, Zhang F, Huang EY, *et al.* (2001) Histone deacetylase is a direct target of valproic acid, a potent anticonvulsant, mood stabilizer, and teratogen. *J Biol Chem*. 276:36734–41.
15. Bigio B, Mathé AA, Sousa VC, *et al.* (2016) Epigenetics and energetics in ventral hippocampus mediate rapid antidepressant action: implications for treatment resistance. *Proc Natl Acad Sci U S A*. 113:7906–11.
16. Krishnan V, Nestler EJ (2008) The molecular neurobiology of depression. *Nature*. 455:894–902.
17. Alhourani A, McDowell MM, Randazzo MJ, *et al.* (2015) Network effects of deep brain stimulation. *J Neurophysiol*. 114:2105–17.
18. Schmaal L, Veltman DJ, van Erp TGM, *et al.* (2016) Subcortical brain alterations in major depressive disorder: findings from the ENIGMA major depressive disorder working group. *Mol Psychiatry*. 21:806–12.
19. MacQueen G, Frodl T (2011) The hippocampus in major depression: evidence for the convergence of the bench and bedside in psychiatric research? *Mol Psychiatry*. 16:252–64.
20. Dunlop BW, Mayberg HS (2014) Neuroimaging-based biomarkers for treatment selection in major depressive disorder. *Dialogues Clin Neurosci*. 16:479–90.
21. Everaert J, Koster EHW, Derakshan N (2012) The combined cognitive bias hypothesis in depression. *Clin Psychol Rev*. 32:413–24.
22. Russo SJ, Nestler EJ (2013) The brain reward circuitry in mood disorders. *Nat Rev Neurosci*. 14:609–25.
23. Li B, Piriz J, Mirrione M, *et al.* (2011) Synaptic potentiation onto habenula neurons in the learned helplessness model of depression. *Nature*. 470:535–9.

24. Mayberg HS, Lozano AM, Voon V, *et al.* (2005) Deep brain stimulation for treatment-resistant depression. *Neuron.* 45:651–60.

25. Holtzheimer PE, Kelley ME, Gross RE, *et al.* (2012) Subcallosal cingulate deep brain stimulation for treatment-resistant unipolar and bipolar depression. *Arch Gen Psychiatry.* 69:150–8.

26. Malone DA, Dougherty DD, Rezai AR, *et al.* (2009) Deep brain stimulation of the ventral capsule/ventral striatum for treatment-resistant depression. *Biol Psychiatry.* 65:267–75.

27. Dougherty DD, Rezai AR, Carpenter LL, *et al.* (2015) A randomized sham-controlled trial of deep brain stimulation of the ventral capsule/ventral striatum for chronic treatment-resistant depression. *Biol Psychiatry.* 78:240–8.

28. Deisseroth K (2014) Circuit dynamics of adaptive and maladaptive behaviour. *Nature.* 505:309–17.

29. Loomer HP, Saunders JC, Kline NS (1957) A clinical and pharmacodynamic evaluation of iproniazid as a psychic energizer. *Psychiatr Res Rep Am Psychiatr Assoc.* 8:129–41.

30. Kuhn R (1958) The treatment of depressive states with G 22355 (imipramine hydrochloride). *Am J Psychiatry.* 115:459–64.

31. Axelrod J, Whitby LG, Hertting G (1961) Effect of psychotropic drugs on the uptake of h3-norepinephrine by tissues. *Science.* 133:383–4.

32. Schildkaut JJ (1965) The catecholamine hypothesis of affective disorders: a review of supporting evidence. *Am J Psychiatry.* 122:509–22.

33. Coppen A (1967) The biochemistry of affective disorders. *Br J Psychiatry.* 113:1237–64.

34. Millan MJ (2006) Multi-target strategies for the improved treatment of depressive states: Conceptual foundations and neuronal substrates, drug discovery and therapeutic application. *Pharmacol Ther.* 110:135–370.

35. Dale E, Bang-Andersen B, Sánchez C (2015) Emerging mechanisms and treatments for depression beyond SSRIs and SNRIs. *Biochem Pharmacol.* 95:81–97.

36. Treadway MT, Zald DH (2011) Reconsidering anhedonia in depression: Lessons from translational neuroscience. *Neurosci Biobehav Rev.* 35:537–55.

37. Aarsland D, Påhlhagen S, Ballard CG, *et al.* (2011) Depression in Parkinson disease—epidemiology, mechanisms and management. *Nat Rev Neurol.* 8:35–47.

38. Ruhé HG, Mason NS, Schene AH (2007) Mood is indirectly related to serotonin, norepinephrine and dopamine levels in humans: a meta-analysis of monoamine depletion studies. *Mol Psychiatry.* 12:331–59.

39. Goodwin G (2000) Neurobiological aetiology of mood disorders. In: Gelder MG, Ibor JJL, Andreasen NC (eds). *New Oxford Textbook of Psychiatry* (1st edn). Oxford: Oxford University Press; pp. 711–19.

40. Duman RS, Aghajanian GK, Sanacora G, *et al.* (2016) Synaptic plasticity and depression: new insights from stress and rapid-acting antidepressants. *Nat Med.* 22:238–49.

41. Miller BR, Hen R (2015) The current state of the neurogenic theory of depression and anxiety. *Curr Opin Neurobiol.* 30:51–8.

42. Covington HE, Vialou V, Nestler EJ (2010) From synapse to nucleus: novel targets for treating depression. *Neuropharmacology.* 58:683–93.

43. Yüksel C, Öngür D (2010) Magnetic resonance spectroscopy studies of glutamate-related abnormalities in mood disorders. *Biol Psychiatry.* 68:785–94.

44. Arnone D, Wise T, Cleare A, *et al.* (2014) Diagnostic and therapeutic utility of neuroimaging in depression: an overview. *Neuropsychiatry Dis Treat.* 10:1509–22.

45. Murrough JW, Abdallah CG, Mathew SJ (2017) Targeting glutamate signalling in depression: progress and prospects. *Nat Rev Drug Discov.* 16:472–86.

46. Solmi M, Veronese N, Zaninotto L, *et al.* (2017) Lamotrigine compared to placebo and other agents with antidepressant activity in patients with unipolar and bipolar depression: a comprehensive meta-analysis of efficacy and safety outcomes in short-term trials. *CNS Spectr.* 21:403–18.

47. Mathew SJ, Gueorguieva R, Brandt C, *et al.* (2017) A randomized, double-blind, placebo-controlled, sequential parallel comparison design trial of adjunctive riluzole for treatment-resistant major depressive disorder. *Neuropsychopharmacology.* 42:2567–74.

48. Pittenger C, Coric V, Banasr M, *et al.* (2008) Riluzole in the treatment of mood and anxiety disorders. *CNS Drugs.* 22:761–86.

49. Berman RM, Cappiello A, Anand A, *et al.* (2000) Antidepressant effects of ketamine in depressed patients. *Biol Psychiatry.* 47:351–4.

50. Abdallah CG, Averill LA, Krystal JH (2015) Ketamine as a promising prototype for a new generation of rapid-acting antidepressants. *Ann N Y Acad Sci.* 1344:66–77.

51. Sanacora G, Johnson MR, Khan A, *et al.* (2017) Adjunctive lanicemine (AZD6765) in patients with major depressive disorder and history of inadequate response to antidepressants: a randomized, placebo-controlled study. *Neuropsychopharmacology.* 42:844–53.

52. Zanos P, Piantadosi SC, Wu H-Q, *et al.* (2015) The prodrug 4-chlorokynurenine causes ketamine-like antidepressant effects, but not side effects, by nmda/glycineb-site inhibition. *J Pharmacol Exp Ther.* 355:76–85.

53. McEwen BS, Chattarji S, Diamond DM, *et al.* (2010) The neurobiological properties of tianeptine (Stablon): from monoamine hypothesis to glutamatergic modulation. *Mol Psychiatry.* 15:237–49.

54. Luscher B, Shen Q, Sahir N (2011) The GABAergic deficit hypothesis of major depressive disorder. *Mol Psychiatry.* 16:383–406.

55. Duman RS, Aghajanian GK, Sanacora G, Krystal JH (2016) Synaptic plasticity and depression: new insights from stress and rapid-acting antidepressants. *Nat Med.* 22:238–49.

56. Castrén E, Kojima M (2017) Brain-derived neurotrophic factor in mood disorders and antidepressant treatments. *Neurobiol Dis.* 97(Pt B):119–26.

57. Haile CN, Murrough JW, Iosifescu D V, *et al.* (2014) Plasma brain derived neurotrophic factor (BDNF) and response to ketamine in treatment-resistant depression. *Int J Neuropsychopharmacol.* 17:331–6.

58. Sharma AN, da Costa e Silva BF, Soares JC, *et al.* (2016) Role of trophic factors GDNF, IGF-1 and VEGF in major depressive disorder: a comprehensive review of human studies. *J Affect Disord.* 197:9–20.

59. Turner CA, Watson SJ, Akil H (2012) Fibroblast growth factor-2: an endogenous antidepressant and anxiolytic molecule? *Biol Psychiatry.* 72:254–5.

60. Elsayed M, Banasr M, Duric V, *et al.* (2012) Antidepressant effects of fibroblast growth factor-2 in behavioral and cellular models of depression. *Biol Psychiatry.* 72:258–65.

61. Gloaguen V, Cottraux J, Cucherat M, *et al.* (1998) A meta-analysis of the effects of cognitive therapy in depressed patients. *J Affect Disord.* 49:59–72.

62. Cuijpers P, Hollon SD, van Straten A, *et al.* (2013) Does cognitive behaviour therapy have an enduring effect that is superior to keeping patients on continuation pharmacotherapy? A meta-analysis. *BMJ Open.* 3:e002542.

63. UK ECT Review Group (2003) Efficacy and safety of electroconvulsive therapy in depressive disorders: a systematic review and meta-analysis. *Lancet*. 361:799–808.

64. Merkl A, Heuser I, Bajbouj M (2009) Antidepressant electroconvulsive therapy: mechanism of action, recent advances and limitations. *Exp Neurol*. 219:20–6.

65. McCall WV, Andrade C, Sienaert P (2014) Searching for the mechanism(s) of ECT's therapeutic effect. *J ECT*. 30:87–9.

66. Grover S, Mattoo SK, Gupta N (2005) Theories on mechanism of action of electroconvulsive therapy. *Ger J Psychiatry*. 8:70–84.

67. Schuch FB, Dunn AL, Kanitz AC, *et al.* (2016) Moderators of response in exercise treatment for depression: a systematic review. *J Affect Disord*. 195:40–9.

68. Kvam S, Kleppe CL, Nordhus IH, *et al.* (2016) Exercise as a treatment for depression: a meta-analysis. *J Affect Disord*. 202:67–86.

69. McGowan PO, Sasaki A, D'Alessio AC, *et al.* (2009) Epigenetic regulation of the glucocorticoid receptor in human brain associates with childhood abuse. *Nat Neurosci*. 12:342–8.

70. Pariante CM, Lightman SL (2008) The HPA axis in major depression: classical theories and new developments. *Trends Neurosci*. 31:464–8.

71. McEwen BS (2003) Mood disorders and allostatic load. *Biol Psychiatry*. 54:200–7.

72. Zunszain PA, Anacker C, Cattaneo A, *et al.* (2011) Glucocorticoids, cytokines and brain abnormalities in depression. *Prog Neuropsychopharmacol Biol Psychiatry*. 35:722–9.

73. Anacker C, Zunszain PA, Carvalho LA, *et al.* (2011) The glucocorticoid receptor: pivot of depression and of antidepressant treatment? *Psychoneuroendocrinology*. 36:415–25.

74. Keller J, Gomez R, Williams G, *et al.* (2017) HPA axis in major depression: cortisol, clinical symptomatology and genetic variation predict cognition. *Mol Psychiatry*. 22:527–36.

75. Cai N, Chang S, Li Y, *et al.* (2015) Molecular signatures of major depression. *Curr Biol*. 25:1146–56.

76. McKay MS, Zakzanis KK (2010) The impact of treatment on HPA axis activity in unipolar major depression. *J Psychiatr Res*. 44:183–92.

77. Watson S, Gallagher P, Porter RJ, *et al.* (2012) A randomized trial to examine the effect of mifepristone on neuropsychological performance and mood in patients with bipolar depression. *Biol Psychiatry*. 72:943–9.

78. Miller AH, Raison CL (2016) The role of inflammation in depression: from evolutionary imperative to modern treatment target. *Nat Rev Immunol*. 16.22–34.

79. Dinan TG, Cryan JF (2013) Melancholic microbes: a link between gut microbiota and depression? *Neurogastroenterol Motil*. 25:713–19.

80. Qin L, Wu X, Block ML, *et al.* (2007) Systemic LPS causes chronic neuroinflammation and progressive neurodegeneration. *Glia*. 55:453–62.

81. Remus JL, Dantzer R (2016) Inflammation models of depression in rodents: relevance to psychotropic drug discovery. *Int J Neuropsychopharmacol*. 19:pyw028.

82. Reichenberg A, Yirmiya R, Schuld A, *et al.* (2001) Cytokine-associated emotional and cognitive disturbances in humans. *Arch Gen Psychiatry*. 58:445–52.

83. Dowlati Y, Herrmann N, Swardfager W, *et al.* (2010) A meta-analysis of cytokines in major depression. *Biol Psychiatry*. 67:446–57.

84. Haapakoski R, Mathieu J, Ebmeier KP, *et al.* (2015) Cumulative meta-analysis of interleukins 6 and 1β, tumour necrosis factor α and C-reactive protein in patients with major depressive disorder. *Brain Behav Immun*. 49:206–15.

85. Leonard B, Maes M (2012) Mechanistic explanations how cell-mediated immune activation, inflammation and oxidative and nitrosative stress pathways and their sequels and concomitants play a role in the pathophysiology of unipolar depression. *Neurosci Biobehav Rev*. 36:764–85.

86. Kappelmann N, Lewis G, Dantzer R, *et al.* (2016). Antidepressant activity of anti-cytokine treatment: a systematic review and meta-analysis of clinical trials of chronic inflammatory conditions. *Mol Psychiatry*. 23:335–43.

87. Raison CL, Rutherford RE, Woolwine BJ, *et al.* (2013). A randomized controlled trial of the tumor necrosis factor antagonist infliximab for treatment-resistant depression: the role of baseline inflammatory biomarkers. *JAMA Psychiatry*. 70:31–41.

88. Rosenblat JD, Kakar R, Berk M, *et al.* (2016) Anti-inflammatory agents in the treatment of bipolar depression: a systematic review and meta-analysis. *Bipolar Disord*. 18:89–101.

89. Raison CL, Capuron L, Miller AH (2006) Cytokines sing the blues: inflammation and the pathogenesis of depression. *Trends Immunol*. 27:24–31.

90. Hughes MM, Connor TJ, Harkin A (2016). Stress-related immune markers in depression: implications for treatment. *Int J Neuropsychopharmacol*. pii:pyw001.

91. Scapagnini G, Davinelli S, Drago F, *et al.* (2012) Antioxidants as antidepressants: fact or fiction? *CNS Drugs*. 26:477–90.

92. Bunney BG, Li JZ, Walsh DM, *et al.* (2015) Circadian dysregulation of clock genes: clues to rapid treatments in major depressive disorder. *Mol Psychiatry*. 20:48–55.

93. Partch CL, Green CB, Takahashi JS (2014) Molecular architecture of the mammalian circadian clock. *Trends Cell Biol*. 24:90–9.

94. McClung CA (2007) Circadian genes, rhythms and the biology of mood disorders. *Pharmacol Ther*. 114:222–32.

95. Weber F, Dan Y (2016) Circuit-based interrogation of sleep control. *Nature*. 538:51–9.

96. Rothchild AE, Rothschild G, Giardino WJ, *et al.* (2016) VTA dopaminergic neurons regulate ethologically relevant sleep-wake behaviors. *Nat Neurosci*. 19:1356–66.

97. Foulkesa NS, Assone-Corsia P, Borjiginb J, Snyder SH (1997) Rhythmic transcription: the molecular basis of circadian melatonin synthesis. *Trends Neurosci*. 20:487–92.

98. Meyer-Bernstein EL, Blanchard JH, Morin LP (1997) The serotoninergic projection from the median raphe nucleus to the suprachiasmatic nucleus modulates activity phase onset, but not other circadian rhythm parameters. *Brain Res*. 755:112–20.

99. Vazquez J, Baghdoyan HA (2001) Basal forebrain acetylcholine release during REM sleep is significantly greater than during waking. *Am J Physiol Regul Integr Comp Physiol*. 280:R598–601.

100. Steiger A (2007) Neurochemical regulation of sleep. *J Psychiatr Res*. 41:537–52.

101. Rumble ME, White KH, Benca RM (2015) Sleep disturbances in mood disorders. *Psychiatr Clin North Am*. 38:743–59.

102. Suchecki D, Tiba PA, Machado RB (2012) REM sleep rebound as an adaptive response to stressful situations. *Front Neur*. 3:41.

103. Martynhak BJ, Pereira M, de Souza CP, *et al.* (2015) Stretch, shrink, and shatter the rhythms: the intrinsic circadian period in mania and depression. *CNS Neurol Disord Drug Targets*. 14:963–9.

104. Dallaspezia S, Benedetti F (2015) Sleep deprivation therapy for depression. *Curr Top Behav Neurosci*. 25:483–502.

105. Wolf E, Kuhn M, Normann C, *et al.* (2016) Synaptic plasticity model of therapeutic sleep deprivation in major depression. *Sleep Med Rev*. 30:53–62.

106. Basnet S, Merikanto I, Lahti T, *et al.* (2016) Seasonal variations in mood and behavior associate with common chronic diseases and symptoms in a population-based study. *Psychiatry Res.* 238:181–8.

107. Kelly J. Rohan, Kathryn A, *et al.* (2009) Biological and psychological mechanisms of seasonal affective disorder: a review and integration. *Curr Psychiatry Rev.* 5:37–47.

108. Mårtensson B, Pettersson A, Berglund L, *et al.* (2015) Bright white light therapy in depression: a critical review of the evidence. *J Affect Disord.* 182:1–7.

109. Wirz-Justice A, Benedetti F, Terman M (2013) *Chronotherapeutics for Affective Disorders* (2nd revised edn). Basel: Karger.

110. Tyrer AE, Levitan RD, Houle S, *et al.* (2016) Serotonin transporter binding is reduced in seasonal affective disorder following light therapy. *Acta Psychiatr Scand.* 134:410–19.

111. Hodes GE, Walker DM, Labonté B, *et al.* (2017) Understanding the epigenetic basis of sex differences in depression. *J Neurosci Res.* 95:692–702.

112. Keers R, Uher R (2012) Gene–environment interaction in major depression and antidepressant treatment response. *Curr Psychiatry Rep.* 14:129–37.

113. McEwen BS, Gray JD, Nasca C (2015) 60 years of neuroendocrinology: redefining neuroendocrinology: stress, sex and cognitive and emotional regulation. *J Endocrinol.* 226:T67–83.

114. Krivoy A, Balicer RD, Feldman B, *et al.* (2015) The impact of age and gender on adherence to antidepressants: a 4-year population-based cohort study. *Psychopharmacol (Berl).* 232:3385–90.

115. Kokras N, Antoniou K, Mikail HG, *et al.* (2015) Forced swim test: what about females? *Neuropharmacology.* 99:408–21.

# 75

# Genetic epidemiology of depression in the molecular era

*Alison K. Merikangas and Kathleen R. Merikangas*

## Introduction–genetic epidemiology of depression

The familial nature of major depression has been well established. The results of twin, family, and adoption studies demonstrated that both genetic and environmental factors contribute to the aetiology of depression. More recently, progress in molecular biology has led to greater insight into the specific genetic factors that may underlie depression. This chapter updates information on the genetic epidemiology of depression and reviews results of molecular genetics studies of depression. The sub-discipline of genetic epidemiology focuses on the identification of the role of genetic factors and their joint influence with environmental factors in disease aetiology. Genetic epidemiology employs traditional epidemiologic study designs, including case-control and cohort studies, to evaluate the aggregation in groups as closely related as twins or as loosely related as migrant cohorts.

Prior to the molecular genetics era, study designs in genetic epidemiology were devised to infer genetic causation by controlling for genetic background while letting the environment vary (for example, migrant cohorts, half siblings, separated twins) or, conversely, controlling for the environment while allowing variance in the genetic background (for example, siblings, twins, adoptees, non-biologic siblings). Measures of risk in genetic epidemiology include *familial relative risk* (disease risk in relatives of cases vs controls) and *genetic attributable risk* (the proportion of a particular disease that would be eliminated if a particular gene or genes were not involved in the disease). As described in the next section, sophisticated methods have been developed to compare combinations of genetic markers between cases and controls (for example, polygenic scores) and to estimate the proportion of phenotypic variance explained by genetic variants (typically SNPs) for complex traits [that is, genome-wide complex trait analysis (GCTA)] [1].

Major depressive disorder (MDD) is characterized by low mood and energy, the inability to experience enjoyment, changes to eating and sleep patterns, feelings of guilt or worthlessness, and suicidal thoughts. MDD is the second leading cause of disability worldwide [2]. Depression is highly heterogenous, and there are eight major subtypes of MDD that are associated with different levels of disability and different patterns of familiality (the tendency of a trait to occur among members of a family, usually by heredity), comorbidity, and heritability (the proportion of variability that is genetic in origin, that is, the ratio of the genetic variance of a population to its phenotypic variance).

### Genetic epidemiology of depression

There has been a substantial body of research that investigates the familial and genetic factors underlying depression. There are several reviews of family, twin, and adoption studies of depression over the past decade [3–5]. Increased recognition of the role of biologic and genetic vulnerability factors for psychiatric disorders has led to research with increasing methodological sophistication over the past two decades.

### Family studies

Familial aggregation is generally the first source of evidence that genetic factors may play a role in the aetiology of a disorder. The most common indicator of familial aggregation is the *relative risk ratio*, computed as the rate of a disorder in families of affected persons divided by the corresponding rate in families of controls. The patterns of genetic factors underlying a disorder can be inferred from the extent to which patterns of familial resemblance adhere to the expectations of Mendelian laws of inheritance. The degree of genetic relatedness among relatives is based on the proportion of shared genes between a particular relative and an index family member or proband.

The familial aggregation of major depression has been examined in numerous controlled studies. Aggregate estimates of the familial associations for major depression, based on reviews and meta-analyses of controlled family study [5] and registry [6] data, are substantially lower than those of bipolar disorder, with familial risk ratios averaging about 2.5–2.8, familial heritability of 0.32, and average twin heritability of 0.3–0.4 [7].

### Adoption studies

Adoption studies have been a major source of evidence regarding the joint contribution of genetic and environmental factors to disease aetiology. However, with recent trends towards selective adoption and the diminishing frequency of adoptions in the United States, adoption studies are becoming less feasible methods for identifying genetic and environmental sources of disease aetiology (http://www.johnstonsarchive.net/policy/adoptionstats.html).

As reviewed by Sullivan *et al.* [5], few adoption studies of depressive disorders have been completed and report conflicting findings. These studies are difficult to carry out and often involve indirect sources of diagnostic information, for example using a sick leave registry as the source of clinical information [8] or obtaining only limited data on the biological parents [9]. More recent analyses of Swedish registry data revealed that both genetic and environmental factors had influences on depression in adopted offspring [10]. The most compelling finding from adoption studies, however, is the dramatic increase in completed suicide among biological, as opposed to adoptive, relatives of mood disorder probands [11, 12].

## Twin studies

Twin studies that compare concordance rates for monozygotic twins (who share the same genotype) with those of dizygotic twins (who share an average of 50% of their genes) provide estimates of the degree to which genetic factors contribute to the aetiology of a disease phenotype. Path analytic approaches that estimate the proportion of variance attributable to additive genes and common and unique environment have been the standard method of analysis of data from large twin studies. The twin family design is one of the most powerful study designs in genetic epidemiology because it yields estimates of heritability, but also permits evaluation of multigenerational patterns of expression of genetic and environmental risk factors. Finally, twin studies may inform the spectrum of expression of diseases and disease subtypes through identification of the components of the phenotype that are the most heritable.

Twin studies of depression have been conducted on both clinical (for example, [13]) and community (for example, [14–16]) samples, or both (for example, [17]). Regardless of the method of data collection, the heritability point estimates were broadly similar, and the 95% confidence intervals were quite wide; there were no obvious gender differences, and shared environmental influences seemed to have little impact on liability to depression. Instead, the greater proportion of variance was due to individual specific environmental effects [5].

Heritability in twin studies of depression parallels the familial risks, demonstrating the contribution of genetic factors to the aetiology. During the past decade, there has been a shift from small clinical studies to studies with larger samples from registries and population samples, that has increased our ability to identify shared familial risk across these conditions, as well as patterns of familial specificity. The newer generation of family studies has also begun to expand phenotypic assessments to include dimensional measures of phenotypes and biologic measures that may be closer manifestations of the underlying genetic factors [18, 19].

## Molecular genetics

The major approaches that have successfully led to gene identification for Mendelian disorders are linkage and association studies. These approaches were highly successful for rare diseases that followed traditional modes of transmission, including autosomal dominant, recessive, or sex-linked patterns in families. With completion of the human genome project, nearly all of the genes underlying rare Mendelian disorders have been identified.

## Linkage

Genetic linkage is the tendency of DNA sequences that are located close together on a chromosome to be inherited together during the meiosis phase of sexual reproduction. This tendency is exploited in linkage analysis, a genetic mapping technique that identifies regions of chromosomes that are likely to contain a risk gene, and is measured by the percentage recombination between loci. The logarithm of the odds (LOD) score is the statistical estimate of whether two genes, or a gene and a disease gene, are likely to be located near each other on a chromosome and are therefore likely to be inherited together. A LOD score of 3 or higher is generally understood to mean that two genes are located close to each other on the chromosome and indicates a statistically significant result. After linkage is established, fine mapping must be completed to attempt to isolate which gene or genes may be driving the linkage signal. Multiple genome-wide linkage studies of depression have been completed and report variable results. Statistically significant or suggestive results have been presented for depression on chromosomes 2, 3, 7, 8, 10, 15, and 17 [20–33], with few replications.

## Association

Although there have been dozens of studies of candidate genes in case-control studies of depression, none stood the test of independent replication [34]. These studies were intuitively appealing, but the low a priori probability rate that any particular locus could have a strong association with depression led to high false-positive rates that often misled the field [35]. The lack of identification of these candidate genes in genome-wide association studies (GWAS) was also disappointing. However, few of these studies were adequately powered to identify genes of small effect. A candidate gene approach, based on replicated findings identified in GWAS, may still be a promising future tactic to dissect the genetic architecture of subgroups of depression.

## Genome-wide association studies

With advances in molecular biology, there has been a flood of information on the contribution of genetic risk factors to complex diseases. This has transformed the sub-discipline of genetic epidemiology that previously relied solely on inferences based on phenotypic disease manifestations in relatives. These advances are largely attributable to GWAS that identify common genetic variants or SNPs (common DNA variants with >1% population frequency) that are significantly more frequent in cases than in controls [36], with an a priori statistical significance threshold of $5 \times 10^{-8}$. Structural variation, such as segmental duplications and deletions, or copy number variants (CNVs) can also be identified in GWAS.

During the past decade, there has been dramatic growth in large-scale case-control studies to identify genetic markers associated with major mental disorders. To date, ten GWAS of MDD have been published [37–46], with only three loci of genome-wide significance reported [41, 46]. It is notable that many of the studies contain overlapping samples, especially since the advent of large international data-sharing initiatives such as the Psychiatric Genomics Consortium (PGC) (http://www.med.unc.edu/pgc/) (Table 75.1). The PGC has completed the largest GWAS to date of MDD and found

**Table 75.1** Genome-wide association studies of major depressive disorder published through 2016

| Author | Year | Sample | Diagnosis | Array | N (cases) | N (controls) | Results | Reference |
|---|---|---|---|---|---|---|---|---|
| Sullivan | 2009 | Netherlands Study of Depression and Anxiety (NESDA), Netherlands Twin Registry (NTR), Netherlands Mental Health Survey and Incidence Study (NEMESIS), Adolescents at Risk for Anxiety and Depression (ARIADNE) | Lifetime DSM-IV MDD | Perlegen Sciences high-density oligonucleotide arrays | 1738 | 1802 | No hits | [37] |
| Lewis | 2010 | Depression Case Control [DeCC] study, Depression Network [DeNT] study, Genome-Based Therapeutic Drugs for Depression [GENDEP] | Recurrent depression | Illumina Human610-Quad BeadChip | 1636 | 1594 | No hits | [38] |
| Muglia | 2010 | Max-Planck Institute of Psychiatry | DSM-IV or ICD-10 recurrent MDD | Illumina HumanHap550 SNP chip | 926 | 866 | No hits | [39] |
| | | CoLaus | Recurrent MDD | Affymetrix 500K SNP chip | 492 | 1052 | No hits | |
| | | Meta-analysis | | | 1359 | 1782 | No hits | |
| Rietschel | 2010 | Department of Psychiatry, University of Bonn, Germany | DSM-IV MDD | Illumina HumanHap 550v3 (controls), Illumina human 610 W quad BeadChips (cases) | 604 | 1364 | No hits | [40] |
| Kohli | 2011 | Munich Antidepressant Response Signature (MARS) | At least a moderate depressive episode | Illumina 100k, 300k Beadchips | 353 | 366 | rs1545843 | [41] |
| Shi | 2011 | Genetics of Recurrent Early-Onset Depression (GenRED) | Recurrent early-onset MDD | Affymetrix 6.0 | 1020 | 1636 | No hits | [42] |
| Shyn | 2011 | Sequenced Treatment Alternatives to Relieve Depression (STAR*D) | MDD | Affymetrix 6.0, 5.0, 500 K, and Perlegen | 1221 | 1636 | No hits | [43] |
| Wray | 2012 | Queensland Institute of Medical Research (QIMR, Australia), The Netherlands Study of Anxiety and Depression (NESDA), The Netherlands Twin Registry (NTR), The University of Edinburgh (UK), The Molecular Genetics of Schizophrenia study (controls only, USA) | MDD | Illumina and Affymetrix platforms | 2431 | 3673 | No hits | [44] |
| Ripke | 2013 | Major Depressive Disorder Working Group of the Psychiatric GWAS Consortium | DSM-IV lifetime MDD | Multiple arrays | 9240 | 9519 | No hits | [45] |
| Direk | 2017 | CHARGE consortium, PGC | Lifetime MDD | Multiple arrays | 9240 | 9519 | rs9825823, rs9323497 | [46] |
| | | CHARGE consortium, PGC | MDD | | 6718 | 13,453 | | |

no statistically significant hits [45]. More recently, however, the PGC presented the results of an analysis that stratified the sample by age at onset (AAO) and identified one replicated genome-wide significant locus associated with adult-onset (>27 years) MDD (rs7647854; odds ratio 1.16; 95% confidence interval 1.11–1.21; $P = 5.2 \times 10^{-11}$) [47]. The technique of subsetting sample cases on the basis of characteristics, such as AAO, recurrence, or episodicity of depressive episodes, and treatment response may help to disentangle the genetic heterogeneity of depression. Also, by examining a broad depression phenotype that included both MDD and depressive symptoms with data from the PGC and the Cohorts for Heart and Aging Research in Genomic Epidemiology (CHARGE) Consortium, a significant hit was found through a meta-analysis [46], whereas another study

examining depressive symptoms in African American and Latina women found no genome-wide significant hits [48]. Subsequent to the submission of this chapter in March 2016, six additional GWAS studies of depression have been completed and published; details of these are summarized by Ormel *et al.* [48a].

Despite the enthusiasm generated by the positive findings for many of these disorders, the total proportion of variance explained by even the largest international collaborative studies with hundreds of thousands of cases is still quite small (17–29% in cross-disorder analyses and much lower in others) [49]. This has led to substantial discussion regarding the so-called 'missing heritability' in GWAS. However, the findings that common genetic variants explain only a limited proportion of the variance is not surprising in light of growing evidence regarding the role of undetected rare variants, environmental factors, and sources of misclassification of cases and controls in GWAS, including aetiologic and clinical heterogeneity within cases, misclassification of controls, and other factors that might reduce the power of these studies. The clinical samples from these studies have been highly heterogenous in terms of sampling source and diagnostic characteristics, and few of the control samples would meet traditional criteria for controls in epidemiology [50]. Future studies will require large systematic samples that are either directly recruited for a cohort study or existing registries and/or biobanks that have sufficiently large and well-characterized samples of cases, as well as built-in controls without the index conditions.

### Sequencing

More recently, international collaborations have focused on genome-wide or exome (protein-coding) sequencing techniques, and this has been proposed as a tool that can be used in risk prediction and lead to a greater understanding of the aetiology, prognosis, and treatment response in psychiatric disorders [51]. Moreover, the analytic challenges will be quite complex, and novel techniques are in development [52]. Success of the sequencing approach has been shown in schizophrenia, where an exome sequencing study of 2536 schizophrenia cases and 2543 controls showed polygenic burden from rare (<1 in 10,000), disruptive mutations distributed across many genes [53]. The first major success of genome sequencing in MDD was reported by the CONVERGE (China, Oxford, and Virginia Commonwealth University Experimental Research on Genetic Epidemiology) Consortium, which used low-coverage whole-genome sequencing of 5303 Chinese women with recurrent MDD and 5337 controls, and reported two loci contributing to risk of MDD on chromosome 10: one near the *SIRT1* gene ($P = 2.53 \times 10^{-10}$), and the other in an intron of the *LHPP* gene ($P = 6.45 \times 10^{-12}$). Additional analyses of 4509 cases with melancholia yielded an increased genetic signal at the *SIRT1* locus [54].

### SNP-based polygenic approaches

Several statistical approaches that take advantage of markers identified in GWAS have also advanced our understanding of the genetic architecture of psychiatric disorders, notably genomic profile (or polygenic) risk scores and GCTA.

### *Genomic profile (or polygenic) risk scores*

Polygenic scores summarize the genetic effects in a GWAS by computing a weighted sum of associated 'risk' alleles within each subject. Initially, markers (typically SNPs) are selected based on their evidence for association, typically their *P*-values, using a 'training' or discovery sample, and the weighted score is then constructed in an independent 'testing' or replication sample. If an association is found between a trait/disorder and the polygenic score, one assumes that a genetic signal is present among the selected markers. Later, this score can then be used for prediction of individual trait values [55]. The original use of polygenic scores has now been extended to include detecting shared genetic aetiology among traits or to infer the genetic architecture of a trait, to establish the presence of a genetic signal in underpowered studies, and can act as a biomarker for a phenotype [56]. Recently, Power *et al.* [47] used polygenic score analyses to show that earlier-onset major depression is genetically

more similar to other major psychiatric disorders, e.g. schizophrenia and bipolar disorder, than later-onset depression is.

### *Genome-wide complex trait analysis*

GCTA is used to estimate the proportion of phenotypic variance explained by genetic variants (typically SNPs) for complex traits, and has been used to better understand the genetic architecture of complex traits [1]. It can be completed genome- or chromosome-wide, and using genomic-relatedness-matrix restricted maximum likelihood (GREML). It provides an estimate of narrow heritability that does not rely on the assumptions defined in standard twin studies. Instead it assumes that environmental factors are uncorrelated, with differences in the degree of genetic similarity for individuals who are not in the same extended families, and estimates genetic relatedness directly from the SNP data. This is contrary to the method used in standard behavioural genetics studies where pedigree-defined relatedness is assumed [57].

In addition to defining the genetic relationship from genome-wide SNPs, GCTA can also be used to predict the genome-wide additive genetic effects for individual subjects and for individual SNPs, to estimate the linkage disequilibrium (LD) structure encompassing a list of target SNPs and to estimate the genetic correlation between two traits or diseases using SNP data (http://www.complextraitgenomics.com/software/gcta/index.html). This method was first successfully applied to analyse the genetic contribution to human height [58], but its use has now expanded to psychiatric disorders, including depression. Using this method, Ferentinos *et al.* [59] reported an SNP-based heritability estimate of 0.17 for the presence/absence of early AAO of depression. Slightly higher estimates have been reported in a sample from China where common SNPs explained between 20% and 29% of the variance in MDD risk, and the heritability in MDD explained by each chromosome was proportional to its length ($r = 0.680$; $P = 0.0003$), supporting a common polygenic aetiology [60].

It should be noted that polygenic scoring and GCTA assume additive genetic variance, which does not take into account potential multiplicative gene–gene (G × G) interactions nor do they consider gene–environment (G × E) interactions. Furthermore, polygenic scoring and GCTA estimates are typically derived from SNPs, but other types of genetic variants (CNVs, segmental duplications, etc.) may also underlie disease aetiology.

### Pharmacogenetics

Pharmacogenetics is the study of genetic differences in drug metabolic pathways that can affect drug response. Given that treatment response with selective serotonin reuptake inhibitors (SSRIs) and other antidepressant medication varies considerably between patients but demonstrates familial aggregation [61, 62], and with only one-third of patients reaching remission [63], there has been a push to establish more rigorous biological markers of treatment response. The pharmacogenetics of depression has been reviewed by Fabbri *et al.* [64], Hamilton [65], Lin and Lane [66], and others. A number of GWAS [67–73] and meta-analyses [74, 75] have been completed to investigate the genetics of antidepressant response, as well as side effect profiles [76, 77]. Generally, these studies have not yielded positive results, and this has been attributed, in part, to the heterogenous nature of depressive disorders, the lower rates of heritability when compared to other psychiatric disorders, and poor medication adherence [78].

## Challenges in identifying genetic factors underlying depression

The heterogeneity of depression has been widely documented. The concept of unipolar depression from early therapeutic and genetic research referred to severe cases of depression that led to hospitalization. As the concept was extended to MDD that only required a 2-week episode, depression was characterized by substantially greater heterogeneity in terms of broadened symptom expression, comorbidity with anxiety and other conditions, and stronger association with environmental stressors. Both genetic epidemiologic and molecular genetic studies of depression have systematically investigated these sources of heterogeneity in order to define more homogenous subgroups that may be more likely to reflect common underlying genetic architecture.

### Subtypes

The major subtypes of depression in the *Diagnostic and Statistical Manual of Mental Disorders* (DSM) system are melancholic and atypical subtypes. There is substantial evidence from twin and family studies that the atypical subtype is more familial and may reflect inflammatory processes that lead to elevated body mass index (BMI) and other cardiovascular risk factors. Other subtypes that have been examined in genetic studies include persistent depressive disorder (dysthymia), bipolar disorder, seasonal affective disorder (SAD), psychotic depression, perinatal/peripartum/post-partum depression, and premenstrual dysphoric disorder (PMDD). The overlap across these subtypes and the lack of specificity in families, however, has not yielded greater specificity of genetic factors underlying these subtypes.

### Endophenotypes

Another widely employed approach to reduce the heterogeneity of major depression has been the exploration of endophenotypes, defined as phenotypic traits or markers that may represent intermediate forms of expression between the output of underlying genes and the broader disease phenotype [79–81]. Studies of the role of genetic factors involved in these systems may be more informative than studies of the aggregate psychiatric phenotypes because they may represent more closely the expression of underlying biologic systems. A recent meta-analysis of psychiatric endophenotypes [81] suggests that currently identified endophenotypes are not superior to conventional phenotypic disease definitions.

### Incorporation of environmental factors

To date, most of the molecular genetics studies in psychiatry have not incorporated environmental factors as a source of variance in aetiologic models. Most of the evidence for the role of the common and unique environment has been based on residuals from path analytic models employed in twin studies. Stressful life events have been consistently associated with increased risk of mood disorders, but mood disorders also elevate the risk of life events, so the directional links have been complex [82]. More recent research has identified infections [83] and inflammation or immune response [84], which may elevate the risk of depression. However, this association may be related to comorbid conditions or may actually be bi-directional,

as demonstrated in recent prospective studies of large population-based samples [84].

Although intriguing, studies that have examined candidate genes that may interact with stressful life events in the aetiology of depression have generally not been replicated. The widely cited study of Caspi *et al.* [85] has not been replicated in similar prospective studies, even in New Zealand [86], and meta-analyses have demonstrated that the original findings reflected a false-positive report [87, 88], with the most recent meta-analysis of more than 30,000 subjects concluding that there is no interaction between the *5HTTLPR* locus with life events in the aetiology of depression [89]. Duncan and Keller [90] concluded that low power, along with low prior probability that a G × E hypothesis is true, suggests that most or even all positive candidate gene G × E findings represent type I errors. Methods to combine genetic susceptibility factors with environmental exposures will be a major challenge in the next phase of psychiatric genetics, as described in the following section.

### Combining genetic and environmental factors

The next phase of research in genetic epidemiology will require integration of research on the genetic and environmental risk factors already described. Traditional study designs in genetic epidemiology that can be used to study the joint influence of genetic and environmental factors include case-only studies and cross-sectional cases-control studies, as well as cohort studies on gene–environment interaction [91–93]. These study designs can now be extended to condition upon broad or specific genotypic similarity, based on GWAS, to identify environmental exposures that influence gene expression.

There are a growing number of studies that have incorporated findings from genetic studies to identify the effect of environmental factors for diseases that have well-established genetic risk factors. The large scope of studies that will be required to detect the joint impact of genetic with environmental factors is daunting [94]. Although gene–environment interaction is generally assumed to be a key mechanism for links between genetic susceptibility and environmental exposures in complex diseases, analyses of several of these cohort studies have yielded additive, rather than interactive, influences of genetic and environmental risk factors. Likewise, studies of environmental factors among those with the APOE-$\varepsilon_4$ genotype that confers increased risk of cognitive decline and Alzheimer's disease have found additive, rather than interactive, influences of other environmental risk factors [95, 96]. Incorporation of phenotyping that taps the domains underlying broad diagnostic categories, based on knowledge of underlying biologic pathways, coupled with built-in hypothesis-based environmental exposures, will facilitate the integration of advances in molecular genetics and environmental science.

## Summary and conclusions

The results of twin, family, and adoption studies demonstrated that both genetic and environmental factors contribute to the aetiology of depression. Depression is highly familial, with familial risk ratios averaging about 2.5–2.8, a familial heritability of 0.32, an average twin heritability of 0.3–0.4, and a SNP-based heritability of 0.17 for the presence/absence of early AAO of depression. To date, no genetic markers have been associated with aggregate major depression nor its major subtypes in GWAS of tens of thousands of people; however, stratification of the sample by AAO allowed for the identification of one replicated genome-wide significant locus associated with adult-onset MDD. The first major success of genome sequencing was reported by the CONVERGE Consortium, which reported two loci contributing to risk of MDD.

Challenges to studying the genetic underpinnings of depression include its heterogeneity, multifactorial aetiology, and pervasive comorbidity with other conditions. Over time, as the concept of MDD was broadened, depression was characterized by substantially greater heterogeneity in terms of symptom expression, comorbidity with anxiety and other conditions, and stronger association with environmental stressors. Both genetic epidemiologic and molecular genetics studies of depression have systematically investigated these sources of heterogeneity in order to define more homogenous subgroups that may be more likely to reflect a common underlying genetic architecture. Incorporating environmental factors has been a challenge, and though stressful life events have been consistently associated with increased risk of mood disorders, mood disorders also elevate the risk of life events, so establishing the directional links has been complex.

The next phase of research in genetic epidemiology will require integration of research on the genetic and environmental risk factors already described. Building upon traditional study designs in genetic epidemiology that can be used to study the joint influence of genetic and environmental factors include case-only studies and cross-sectional case-control studies, as well as cohort studies on gene–environment interaction, which can now be extended to condition upon broad or specific genotypic similarity, based on GWAS, to identify environmental exposures that influence gene expression. This has led to increased recognition of the role of biologic and genetic vulnerability factors for mood disorders and to research with increasing methodological sophistication over the past two decades. This review also demonstrates the heterogeneity of depression and its multifactorial aetiology that will require future research that embraces sources of complexity, including genetic, biologic, and environmental factors.

## REFERENCES

1. Yang, J., *et al.* GCTA: a tool for genome-wide complex trait analysis. *Am J Hum Genet*, 2011. **88**:76–82.
2. Vos, T., *et al.* Years lived with disability (YLDs) for 1160 sequelae of 289 diseases and injuries 1990-2010: a systematic analysis for the Global Burden of Disease Study 2010. *Lancet*, 2012. **380**:2163–96.
3. Middeldorp, C.M., *et al.* The co-morbidity of anxiety and depression in the perspective of genetic epidemiology. A review of twin and family studies. *Psychol Med*, 2005. **35**:611–24.
4. Flint, J. and K.S. Kendler. The genetics of major depression. *Neuron*, 2014. **81**:484–503.
5. Sullivan, P.F., M.C. Neale, and K.S. Kendler. Genetic epidemiology of major depression: review and meta-analysis. *Am J Psychiatry*, 2000. **157**:1552–62.
6. Wilde, A., *et al.* A meta-analysis of the risk of major affective disorder in relatives of individuals affected by major depressive disorder or bipolar disorder. *J Affect Disord*, 2014. **158**:37–47.
7. Wray, N.R. and Gottesman, II. Using summary data from the danish national registers to estimate heritabilities for schizophrenia, bipolar disorder, and major depressive disorder. *Front Genet*, 2012. **3**:118.
8. von Knorring, A.L., et al. An adoption study of depressive disorders and substance abuse. *Arch Gen Psychiatry*, 1983. **40**:943–50.
9. Cadoret, R.J., *et al.*, Genetic and environmental factors in major depression. *J Affect Disord*, 1985. **9**:155–64.
10. McAdams, T.A., *et al.* The relationship between parental depressive symptoms and offspring psychopathology: evidence from a children-of-twins study and an adoption study. *Psychol Med*, 2015. **45**:2583–94.
11. Mendlewicz, J. and J.D. Rainer. Adoption study supporting genetic transmission in manic–depressive illness. *Nature*, 1977. **268**:327–9.
12. Wender, P.H., *et al.* Psychiatric disorders in the biological and adoptive families of adopted individuals with affective disorders. *Arch Gen Psychiatry*, 1986. **43**:923–9.
13. McGuffin, P., *et al.* A hospital-based twin register of the heritability of DSM-IV unipolar depression. *Arch Gen Psychiatry*, 1996. **53**:129–36.
14. Bierut, L.J., *et al.* Major depressive disorder in a community-based twin sample: are there different genetic and environmental contributions for men and women? *Arch Gen Psychiatry*, 1999. **56**:557–63.
15. Kendler, K.S. and C.A. Prescott. A population-based twin study of lifetime major depression in men and women. *Arch Gen Psychiatry*, 1999. **56**:39–44.
16. Lyons, M.J., *et al.* A registry-based twin study of depression in men. *Arch Gen Psychiatry*, 1998. **55**:468–72.
17. Kendler, K.S., *et al.* A pilot Swedish twin study of affective illness including hospital- and population-ascertained subsamples: results of model fitting. *Behav Genet*, 1995. **25**:217–32.
18. Gur, R.E., *et al.* The Consortium on the Genetics of Schizophrenia: neurocognitive endophenotypes. *Schizophr Bull*, 2007. **33**:49–68.
19. Glahn, D.C., *et al.* High dimensional endophenotype ranking in the search for major depression risk genes. *Biol Psychiatry*, 2012. **71**:6–14.
20. Abkevich, V., *et al.* Predisposition locus for major depression at chromosome 12q22-12q23.2. *Am J Hum Genet*, 2003. **73**:1271–81.
21. Ayub, M., *et al.* Linkage analysis in a large family from Pakistan with depression and a high incidence of consanguineous marriages. *Hum Hered*, 2008. **66**:190–8.
22. Breen, G., *et al.* A genome-wide significant linkage for severe depression on chromosome 3: the depression network study. *Am J Psychiatry*, 2011. **168**:840–7.
23. Gizer, I.R., *et al.* Genome-wide linkage scan of antisocial behavior, depression, and impulsive substance use in the UCSF family alcoholism study. *Psychiatr Genet*, 2012. **22**:235–44.
24. Hodgson, K., *et al.* The genetic basis of the comorbidity between cannabis use and major depression. *Addiction*, 2017. **112**:113–23.
25. Holmans, P., *et al.* Genetics of recurrent early-onset major depression (GenRED): final genome scan report. *Am J Psychiatry*, 2007. **164**:248–58.
26. Holmans, P., *et al.* Genomewide significant linkage to recurrent, early-onset major depressive disorder on chromosome 15q. *Am J Hum Genet*, 2004. **74**:1154–67.

27. Knowles, E.E., *et al*. Genome-wide linkage on chromosome 10q26 for a dimensional scale of major depression. *J Affect Disord*, 2016. **191**: 123–31.

28. Kuo, P.H., *et al*. Genome-wide linkage scans for major depression in individuals with alcohol dependence. *J Psychiatr Res*, 2010. **44**:616–19.

29. McGuffin, P., *et al*. Whole genome linkage scan of recurrent depressive disorder from the depression network study. *Hum Mol Genet*, 2005. **14**:3337–45.

30. Middeldorp, C.M., *et al*. Suggestive linkage on chromosome 2, 8, and 17 for lifetime major depression. *Am J Med Genet B Neuropsychiatr Genet*, 2009. **150B**:352–8.

31. Schol-Gelok, S., *et al*. A genome-wide screen for depression in two independent Dutch populations. *Biol Psychiatry*, 2010. **68**:187–96.

32. Zubenko, G.S., *et al*. Genome-wide linkage survey for genetic loci that influence the development of depressive disorders in families with recurrent, early-onset, major depression. *Am J Med Genet B Neuropsychiatr Genet*, 2003. **123B**:1–18.

33. Zubenko, G.S., *et al*. Genome-wide linkage survey for genetic loci that affect the risk of suicide attempts in families with recurrent, early-onset, major depression. *Am J Med Genet B Neuropsychiatr Genet*, 2004. **129B**:47–54.

34. Cohen-Woods, S., I.W. Craig, and P. McGuffin. The current state of play on the molecular genetics of depression. *Psychol Med*, 2013. **43**:673–87.

35. Abbott, A. Psychiatric genetics: The brains of the family. *Nature*, 2008. **454**:154–7.

36. Risch, N. and K. Merikangas. The future of genetic studies of complex human diseases. *Science*, 1996. **273**:1516–17.

37. Sullivan, P.F., *et al*. Genome-wide association for major depressive disorder: a possible role for the presynaptic protein piccolo. *Mol Psychiatry*, 2009. **14**:359–75.

38. Lewis, C.M., *et al*. Genome-wide association study of major recurrent depression in the U.K. population. *Am J Psychiatry*, 2010. **167**:949–57.

39. Muglia, P., *et al*. Genome-wide association study of recurrent major depressive disorder in two European case-control cohorts. *Mol Psychiatry*, 2010. **15**:589–601.

40. Rietschel, M., *et al*. Genome-wide association-, replication-, and neuroimaging study implicates HOMER1 in the etiology of major depression. *Biol Psychiatry*, 2010. **68**:578–85.

41. Kohli, M.A., *et al*. The neuronal transporter gene *SLC6A15* confers risk to major depression. *Neuron*, 2011. **70**:252–65.

42. Shi, J., *et al*. Genome-wide association study of recurrent early-onset major depressive disorder. *Mol Psychiatry*, 2011. **16**:193–201.

43. Shyn, S.I., *et al*. Novel loci for major depression identified by genome-wide association study of sequenced treatment alternatives to relieve depression and meta-analysis of three studies. *Mol Psychiatry*, 2011. **16**:202–15.

44. Wray, N.R., *et al*. Genome-wide association study of major depressive disorder: new results, meta-analysis, and lessons learned. *Mol Psychiatry*, 2012. **17**:36–48.

45. Ripke, S., *et al*., A mega-analysis of genome-wide association studies for major depressive disorder. *Mol Psychiatry*, 2013. **18**:497–511.

46. Direk, N., *et al*. An analysis of two genome-wide association meta-analyses identifies a new locus for broad depression phenotype. *Biol Psychiatry*, 2017. 82:322–9.

47. Power, R.A., *et al*. Genome-wide association for major depression through age at onset stratification: Major Depressive Disorder Working Group of the Psychiatric Genomics Consortium. *Biol Psychiatry*, 2017. **81**:325–35.

48. Dunn, E.C., *et al*. Genome-wide association study (GWAS) and genome-wide by environment interaction study (GWEIS) of depressive symptoms in African American and Hispanic/Latina women. *Depress Anxiety*, 2016. **33**:265–80.

48a. Ormel J, Hartman CA, Snieder H. The genetics of depression: successful genome-wide association studies introduce new challenges. *Transl Psychiatry*, 2019. **9**(1), 114.

49. Lee, S.H., *et al*. Genetic relationship between five psychiatric disorders estimated from genome-wide SNPs. *Nat Genet*, 2013. **45**:984–94.

50. Wacholder, S., M. Garcia-Closas, and N. Rothman. Study of genes and environmental factors in complex diseases. *Lancet*, 2002. **359**:1155; author reply 1157.

51. Biesecker, B.B. and H.L. Peay. Genomic sequencing for psychiatric disorders: promise and challenge. *Int J Neuropsychopharmacol*, 2013. **16**:1667–72.

52. Pabinger, S., *et al*. A survey of tools for variant analysis of next-generation genome sequencing data. *Brief Bioinform*, 2014. **15**:256–78.

53. Purcell, S.M., *et al*. A polygenic burden of rare disruptive mutations in schizophrenia. *Nature*, 2014. **506**:185–90.

54. CONVERGE consortium. Sparse whole-genome sequencing identifies two loci for major depressive disorder. *Nature*, 2015. **523**:588–91.

55. Dudbridge, F. Power and predictive accuracy of polygenic risk scores. *PLoS Genet*, 2013. **9**:e1003348.

56. Euesden, J., C.M. Lewis, and P.F. O'Reilly. PRSice: polygenic risk score software. *Bioinformatics*, 2015. **31**:1466–8.

57. Benjamin, D.J., *et al*. The genetic architecture of economic and political preferences. *Proc Natl Acad Sci U S A*, 2012. **109**:8026–31.

58. Yang, J., *et al*. Common SNPs explain a large proportion of the heritability for human height. *Nat Genet*, 2010. **42**:565–9.

59. Ferentinos, P., *et al*. Familiality and SNP heritability of age at onset and episodicity in major depressive disorder. *Psychol Med*, 2015. **45**:2215–25.

60. Peterson, R.E., *et al*. The genetic architecture of major depressive disorder in Han Chinese women. *JAMA Psychiatry*, 2017. **74**:162–8.

61. Franchini, L., *et al*. Familial concordance of fluvoxamine response as a tool for differentiating mood disorder pedigrees. *J Psychiatr Res*, 1998. **32**:255–9.

62. O'Reilly, R.L., L. Bogue, and S.M. Singh. Pharmacogenetic response to antidepressants in a multicase family with affective disorder. *Biol Psychiatry*, 1994. **36**:467–71.

63. Rush, A.J., *et al*. Acute and longer-term outcomes in depressed outpatients requiring one or several treatment steps: a STAR*D report. *Am J Psychiatry*, 2006. **163**:1905–17.

64. Fabbri, C. and A. Serretti. Pharmacogenetics of major depressive disorder: top genes and pathways toward clinical applications. *Curr Psychiatry Rep*, 2015. **17**:50.

65. Hamilton, S.P. The promise of psychiatric pharmacogenomics. *Biol Psychiatry*, 2015. **77**:29–35.

66. Lin, E. and H.Y. Lane. Genome-wide association studies in pharmacogenomics of antidepressants. *Pharmacogenomics*, 2015. **16**:555–66.

67. Garriock, H.A., *et al*. A genomewide association study of citalopram response in major depressive disorder. *Biol Psychiatry*, 2010. **67**:133–8.

68. Ising, M., *et al.* A genomewide association study points to multiple loci that predict antidepressant drug treatment outcome in depression. *Arch Gen Psychiatry*, 2009. **66**:966–75.

69. Uher, R., *et al.* Genome-wide pharmacogenetics of antidepressant response in the GENDEP project. *Am J Psychiatry*, 2010. **167**:555–64.

70. Tansey, K.E., *et al.* Genetic predictors of response to serotonergic and noradrenergic antidepressants in major depressive disorder: a genome-wide analysis of individual-level data and a meta-analysis. *PLoS Med*, 2012. **9**:e1001326.

71. Myung, W., *et al.* A genome-wide association study of antidepressant response in Koreans. *Transl Psychiatry*, 2015. **5**:e633.

72. Biernacka, J.M., *et al.* The International SSRI Pharmacogenomics Consortium (ISPC): a genome-wide association study of antidepressant treatment response. *Transl Psychiatry*, 2015. **5**: e553.

73. Adkins, D.E., *et al.* A genomewide association study of citalopram response in major depressive disorder-a psychometric approach. *Biol Psychiatry*, 2010. **68**:e25–7.

74. Niitsu, T., *et al.* Pharmacogenetics in major depression: a comprehensive meta-analysis. *Prog Neuropsychopharmacol Biol Psychiatry*, 2013. **45**: 183–94.

75. GENDEP Investigators1; MARS Investigators; STAR*D Investigators. Common genetic variation and antidepressant efficacy in major depressive disorder: a meta-analysis of three genome-wide pharmacogenetic studies. *Am J Psychiatry*, 2013. **170**:207–17.

76. Clark, S.L., *et al.* Pharmacogenomic study of side-effects for antidepressant treatment options in STAR*D. *Psychol Med*, 2012. **42**:1151–62.

77. Adkins, D.E., *et al.* Genome-wide pharmacogenomic study of citalopram-induced side effects in STAR*D. *Transl Psychiatry*, 2012. **2**:e129.

78. Malhotra, A.K. The pharmacogenetics of depression: enter the GWAS. *Am J Psychiatry*, 2010. **167**:493–5.

79. Gottesman, II and L. Erlenmeyer-Kimling. Family and twin strategies as a head start in defining prodromes and endophenotypes for hypothetical early-interventions in schizophrenia. *Schizophr Res*, 2001. **51**:93–102.

80. Gottesman, II and T.D. Gould. The endophenotype concept in psychiatry: etymology and strategic intentions. *Am J Psychiatry*, 2003. **160**:636–45.

81. Flint, J. and M.R. Munafo. The endophenotype concept in psychiatric genetics. *Psychol Med*, 2007. **37**:163–80.

82. Hammen, C. Depression and stressful environments: identifying gaps in conceptualization and measurement. *Anxiety Stress Coping*, 2016. **29**:335–51.

83. Benros, M.E., *et al.* Autoimmune diseases and severe infections as risk factors for mood disorders: a nationwide study. *JAMA Psychiatry*, 2013. **70**:812–20.

84. Glaus, J., *et al.* Associations between mood, anxiety or substance use disorders and inflammatory markers after adjustment for multiple covariates in a population-based study. *J Psychiatr Res*, 2014. **58**:36–45.

85. Caspi, A., *et al.* Influence of life stress on depression: moderation by a polymorphism in the *5-HTT* gene. *Science*, 2003. **301**:386–9.

86. Fergusson, D.M., *et al.* Impact of a major disaster on the mental health of a well-studied cohort. *JAMA Psychiatry*, 2014. **71**:1025–31.

87. Zammit, S. and M.J. Owen. Stressful life events, 5-HTT genotype and risk of depression. *Br J Psychiatry*, 2006. **188**: 199–201.

88. Risch, N., *et al.* Interaction between the serotonin transporter gene (*5-HTTLPR*), stressful life events, and risk of depression: a meta-analysis. *JAMA*, 2009. **301**:2462–71.

89. Culverhouse, R.C., *et al.* Protocol for a collaborative meta-analysis of 5-HTTLPR, stress, and depression. *BMC Psychiatry*, 2013. **13**:304.

90. Duncan, L.E. and M.C. Keller. A critical review of the first 10 years of candidate gene-by-environment interaction research in psychiatry. *Am J Psychiatry*, 2011. **168**:1041–9.

91. Ottman, R. An epidemiologic approach to gene-environment interaction. *Genet Epidemiol*, 1990. **7**:177–85.

92. Beaty, T.H. Evolving methods in genetic epidemiology. I. Analysis of genetic and environmental factors in family studies. *Epidemiol Rev*, 1997. **19**:14–23.

93. Yang, Q. and M.J. Khoury. Evolving methods in genetic epidemiology. III. Gene–environment interaction in epidemiologic research. *Epidemiol Rev*, 1997. **19**:33–43.

94. Langenberg, C., *et al.* Gene-lifestyle interaction and type 2 diabetes: the EPIC interact case-cohort study. *PLoS Med*, 2014. **11**:e1001647.

95. Andrews, S., *et al.*, Interactive effect of APOE genotype and blood pressure on cognitive decline: the PATH through life study. *J Alzheimers Dis*, 2015. **44**:1087–98.

96. Wirth, M., *et al.* Gene–environment interactions: lifetime cognitive activity, APOE genotype, and beta-amyloid burden. *J Neurosci*, 2014. **34**:8612–17.

# 76

# Imaging of depressive disorders

*Guy M. Goodwin and Michael Browning*

## Introduction

A range of neuroimaging techniques have the potential and, indeed, are contributing to the understanding of the aetiology, progression, and treatment of affective disorder. In the case of unipolar depression, they have underlined the message that depression is, in some sense, a brain disease. At the same time, they have reinforced the continuity with studies of emotion and cognition in the general population and in other disorders. However, they have also highlighted some of the weaknesses of a biological approach based on small samples and inadequate mechanistic understanding. There are important overlaps between this chapter and Chapter 71 on imaging studies in bipolar disorder (BD).

## Study designs used when imaging major depression: what they can and cannot tell us

The majority of imaging studies relevant to major depression have employed case-control designs in which a group of patients with, or at risk of, depression are compared to a control group. These studies report group-level differences in one or more neuroimaging measures, quantifying the significance of their findings using statistical approaches which estimate the probability of the group differences arising by chance. The aim of this approach is to identify features of the brain's structure or function which differ between groups from which inferences about illness mechanism may be drawn. However, as discussed in Chapter 75, it is likely that a number of distinct mechanistic processes lead to the expression of the major depressive phenotype. The ability to determine an imaging signature of a diagnosis is clearly bounded by the degree to which individuals with the diagnosis share common aetiological processes; the absence of the same [1] will make it much more difficult to identify clear neural signatures when comparing groups of depressed and non-depressed individuals. A second limitation to case-control designs is that they provide only weak evidence that the identified neuroimaging processes are causally related to pathology. Group differences in neuroimaging outcomes between patients with depression and controls may arise because: (1) changes in the identified neural system are causally related to the disorder; (2) having the disorder causes changes (for example, taking medication or leaving the house less) which then leads to the observed neuroimaging effect; or (3) a third factor causes both the expression of the illness and, separately, the observed neuroimaging finding. These limitations are widely acknowledged and can be mitigated by imaging studies using alternative designs, the most prominent of which are briefly summarized in the following sections.

### Prospective studies

Prospective cohort studies can demonstrate whether a neural process temporally precedes illness and may have a causal role in outcomes. Studies of increasing ambition have recently begun to be established, with early results relevant to depression already published [2].

### Experimental studies

Experimental studies measure the effects of interventions which manipulate neural systems potentially relevant to pathology. They are able to provide strong evidence on the causal role of the system in disease. While the capacity to target and manipulate specific neural circuits is clearly limited in human, compared to animal, models, a degree of anatomical specificity can be achieved in human subjects using electrical or magnetic stimulation, and some biochemical specificity is possible using pharmacological manipulations. For example, increased serotonergic function reduces amygdala activity in response to negative stimuli in both non-depressed control [3] and patient [4] populations, with the degree of this reduction predicting later response in patients [5].

### Classification studies

Lastly, there has been increasing recent interest in study designs in which neuroimaging techniques are used to classify patients. Broadly, two procedures have been used. Firstly, unsupervised classification attempts to find structure in the imaging data itself, for example by asking whether the data from depressed patients can be clustered into separate groups (see later in this chapter for detailed examples). A particular advantage of this approach is that it is less a hostage to heterogeneity than case-control designs. Unsupervised classification techniques could conceivably identify the neural signatures of different mechanistic processes which lead to major depression. Secondly, supervised classification uses some sort of ground truth value to determine the group to which a person belongs (for example, has a patient responded or not to their treatment?). The supervised classification procedure then attempts to uncover a rule by which the neuroimaging data may be used to arrive at this ground truth.

The statistical underpinning of these classification designs is quite different from that of case-control studies. Whereas case-control studies examine the mean differences between groups of patients and controls, asking 'what is the probability that this group difference occurred by chance?', classification studies develop a rule to separate individuals into different groups and then ask 'does my rule work when I apply it to a different set of data?'. Thus, the measure of whether a classification process is meaningful is its capacity to predict the structure of new data (sometimes called 'out-of-sample data'). The focus on predicting the properties of new data means that there is potential application in clinically relevant situations. For example, a classification rule which accurately predicts response to treatment may, in principle, be used to personalize treatment choice for individual patients.

The neuroimaging literature for major depression is split into studies which have examined genetic risk factors for major depression, those which have examined the broader risk phenotype, and finally those which have examined the phenotype itself. This literature is reviewed later in this chapter, with findings which progress beyond case-control evidence particularly highlighted. Imaging studies in psychiatry have often been too small and have reported effect sizes that are potentially inflated by post hoc statistical methods and publication bias [6]. In addition, cases and controls ought to be recruited using comparable methods, which is a challenge for clinical case series. To allow confidence in what we describe here, we will describe pooled analyses of data from many comparable studies, in preference to single studies, where possible.

## Imaging the brain at risk for major depression: 'imaging genomics'

As Chapters 70, 71, and 72 illustrate, a major depressive episode arises on a background of risk determined by genetics and early experience. The genetic basis of MDD implicates many genes of modest effect, whose identity is only now emerging from the very large samples required for statistical confidence in association studies. Such genes might be operating through anxiety proneness, since the personality trait of neuroticism is a strong predictor of the risk of MDD. Alternatively, new genes may implicate new mechanisms related to decompensation in the face of life stresses or 'events'. Imaging can identify brain structure and brain function, and both must be, in part, under genetic control and vary accordingly. Historically, there have been two distinct phases of 'imaging genomics', as it has been ambitiously named. The first focused on candidate genes that had been suggested might be contributory to genetic risk, based on contemporary understanding of neurobiology. The second, into which we are now emerging, can be described as discovery-based and relies on post hoc associations derived from GWAS.

Of the candidate gene approaches, the serotonin transporter (SERT) has long seemed a potential locus for a genetic effect. Indeed the first putative association between a polymorphism in the regulatory region of the SERT gene and anxiety trait appeared over 20 years ago. It was apparently supported by other very highly cited research [7], which suggested an interaction between the polymorphism and MDD, modulated by exposure to adverse life events. In support of these findings, both functional and structural studies of the brain in healthy volunteers suggested an association between the SERT polymorphism and brain function. The original study suggested that individuals with one or two copies of the short allele of the SERT promoter polymorphism exhibited greater amygdala neuronal activity, as assessed by BOLD, in response to fearful stimuli, compared with individuals homozygous for the long allele [8]. Further studies reported reduced grey matter volumes in the limbic system of healthy volunteers in association with the short allele [9] and that MDD was associated with the polymorphism [10]. The apparent coherence of these findings led to an increasingly optimistic view that imaging provided endophenotypes that were easier to study and more valid than 'disorders' for genetic analysis. On this view, an endophenotype could provide a target between the genotype and any disease; this could speed the development of precision medicine and would also be easier to model in animal studies [11].

The subsequent developments around this topic have been highly contested. In essence, the best known findings linking the SERT either with MDD or with abnormal brain function were shown to be at best overstated, and at worst, artefacts of enthusiasm. It has highlighted the general problem of statistical power, excess positive findings, and the problem of reproducibility in such studies. In relation to the BOLD imaging findings, a recent review concluded ' … there was considerable between-study heterogeneity, which could not be fully accounted for by the study design and sample characteristics that we investigated. In addition, there was evidence of excess statistical significance among published studies. These findings indicate that the association between the 5-HTTLPR and amygdala activation is smaller than originally thought, and that the majority of previous studies have been considerably under powered to reliably demonstrate an effect of this size'[1] [12]. Moreover, the assumption that endophenotypes will usually turn out to demonstrate larger genetic effect sizes appears to go beyond the evidence from the existing animal models as well [13]. The imaging genomics field continues to struggle with the paradox of a continuing plethora of positive findings from studies that are simply underpowered to detect reliably what is often claimed from post hoc analysis of data.

Discovery-based approaches will inform imaging in two ways. Any GWAS or CNV-based variant showing a strong association with a phenotype of interest is likely to be a better choice of candidate gene than, for example, the SERT (which does not emerge reliably from GWAS). Secondly, pooled imaging data can be directly related to GWAS data in discovery-based designs. For example, the Enhancing NeuroImaging Genetics through Meta-Analysis (ENIGMA) Consortium has identified common genetic variants associated with hippocampal volume. Their philosophy for pooling many data sets promises results for genes with clear effects on brain development [14]. However, a link through this approach to major depression has not yet been reported and the power of even very large genetic studies to detect depression-related genes suggests caution (see Chapter 75).

1. Reproduced from *Mol Psychiatry*, 18(4), Murphy SE, Norbury R, Godlewska BR, *et al.*, The effect of the serotonin transporter polymorphism (5-HTTLPR) on amygdala function: a meta-analysis, pp. 512–20, Copyright (2013), with permission from Springer Nature.

## Imaging the at-risk phenotype in major depression

Imaging young people at risk for depression is an obvious way to relate risk for depression to brain structure and function. Perhaps surprisingly, such studies have not been very numerous, but systematic reviews suggest they have been generally consistent. Being at risk may mean by virtue of familial risk or early adverse experience. The children of a proband with MDD are at risk for MDD. However, they are also at risk for anxiety disorders. Moreover, the child of a parent with BD may also be at risk for MDD and anxiety disorders (and not necessarily BD). Thus, the state of being 'at risk' may not be very specific. As a further complication, some children will prove to be resilient, so not actually at risk at all. These complexities confound all such studies designed on the basis of family history, unless there is a prolonged follow-up to determine actual outcomes. This is not always feasible. Most studies of at-risk offspring are conducted in teenagers.

Being at risk due to early abuse and neglect risks confounding by psychiatric illness in the parent. Thus, the at-risk phenotype may be at risk by virtue of both the early abuse and neglect inflicted by the parent(s) and by virtue of genes inherited from the parent. In practice, it will always be difficult, if not impossible, to control for the latter.

### Structural imaging: brain volumes and white matter integrity

Volumetric studies of the developing human brain across adolescence show early cortical grey matter volume (CGMV) increases, followed by decreases, and monotonic increases in cerebral white matter volume (CWMV) [15]. There are no consistent reports of an abnormal growth trajectory for either CGMV or CWMV in young people *at risk* for depression, but the fact that the brain is changing over the critical decades makes such studies additionally difficult. Differences in the brain of adolescent patients with MDD, compared with controls, are seen in the cortex.

Pooling of studies of subjects at risk by virtue of childhood abuse and neglect offers some preliminary findings. In such an analysis, increased exposure to childhood adversity was associated with smaller caudate volumes bilaterally, only in girls. All subcategories of childhood adversity showed the effect, independent of an MDD diagnosis [16]. The absence of the effect in boys is a striking example of sexual dimorphism, but it is not paralleled by different causal pathways to depression in men and women [17]. There was no effect of childhood adversity on hippocampal volume.

Diffusion-weighted MR (magnetic resonance) imaging (diffusion tensor imaging, or DTI) is being used increasingly to determine the integrity of white matter in MDD. DTI resolves the diffusibility of water in different directions to give a measure called fractional anisotropy (FA). If diffusion is highly constrained, as along the axons of a white matter tract, FA values are high. Unconstrained diffusion, as in saline solution or the cerebrospinal fluid, has zero FA. Reduced FA may imply white matter disorganization, either as a developmental or as an acquired property of the brain.

A small, but growing, number of studies have addressed 'at-risk' populations. Participants with a family history of depression have reduced FA in the cingulum and other white matter tracts [18].

Indeed, reduced FA has been a common finding in a range of at-risk studies—for psychosis [19], BD [20], and even antisocial personality disorder [21]. There has been usually a quite surprisingly diffuse effect across the white matter skeleton. Most studies have been individually underpowered, but a substantial overall effect is obvious.

### Functional imaging: resting states and brain activation

Functional imaging studies might be predicted to be a sensitive method to distinguish high-risk from low-risk subjects. Resting state connectivity and the patterns of activation in cognitive tasks have provided convincing methodology. However, differences in experimental design often make data pooling difficult. While still preliminary, the published studies have highlighted the insula cortex and its connections and the inferior frontal regions as key components within the networks processing emotional experience. Lesion studies had already suggested that the insula is important for integrating cognitive, affective, sensory, and autonomic information to create a conscious experience of feeling [22]. Frontal areas have been implicated as possible brain regions mediating cognitive control or feedback to brain regions with more reflexive reactions to threat such as the amygdala.

Young relatives of bipolar probands are at risk for both MDD and BD. Those who subsequently developed MDD demonstrated relatively increased activation in the insula cortex in a challenge task, compared to controls and high-risk subjects who remained well. In the latter groups, this region demonstrated reduced engagement with increasing task difficulty. The high-risk subjects who subsequently developed MDD did not demonstrate normal disengagement [23]. Insula involvement may not be specific; young unmedicated participants with BD type II had increased coherence across several brain regions at rest in a temporo-insular network, including the bilateral insula and putamen [24].

Other work has highlighted the inferior frontal cortex as a locus showing weaker connectivity at rest with other regions (including the insula and temporal gyrus in both BD and young people at risk for bipolar and other mood disorder [25]. The same group had shown reduced activation of the inferior frontal lobe when inhibiting response to fearful faces in at-risk subjects [26] and reduced cortical thickness in the left pars orbitalis of the inferior frontal gyrus (IFG), compared with controls [27]. So far, at-risk studies have not differentiated well between bipolar and unipolar risks. Indeed, at a brain systems level, they may be very similar.

The risk for future episodes of depression is increased in patients who have remitted from previous episodes. Thus, remitted patients may also be considered an 'at-risk' group. Interpretation of neuroimaging findings comparing remitted patients and never-depressed control subjects is complicated by the possibility that persistent effects between episodes of the illness may be related to trait-like risk processes or to a scarring effect of previous episodes. Resting connectivity in such patients has been reported to be reduced within cognitive control networks [28], as has default mode activity during effortful tasks [29]. Additionally, activity within reward-related circuitry has been reported to be disordered [30] and amygdala responses to faces increased [31].

There have been also a limited number of functional neuroimaging studies of children and adolescents exposed to early neglect and/or maltreatment (physical, sexual, and emotional). In reviewing these findings, there have been reports of heightened and reduced amygdala responses to threat in maltreated samples, blunted striatal response to anticipation and receipt of rewards, and increased activation in the anterior cingulate cortex during processing of emotional stimuli and executive control tasks [32].

## Imaging the MDD phenotype

### Structural imaging: brain volumes and white matter integrity

Patients with MDD are probably a highly heterogenous group, especially when studied in their maturity with an established pattern of illness. Thus, one may anticipate an impact from the current illness itself, any vulnerability factor as described in the previous paragraphs, and the uncertain effects of physical illness and lifestyle choices. All or any of these cumulative influences may produce acquired brain changes in mature patients. In addition, current or previous drug treatment may contribute to the picture either as an ongoing 'drug effect' or as a consequence of a relatively recent withdrawal. The impact of these confounding factors has been greatly increased by the use of relatively small samples drawn from individual sites. However, this problem has now been well recognized.

Systematic reviews of published data provide one solution. Judicious exclusion criteria can then identify very comparable studies that control for one or more of the obvious confounds. For example, 14 published studies of about 400 *medication-free* cases with MDD showed reduced grey matter in the prefrontal and limbic cortices (including the hippocampus bilaterally) [33]. The alternative to controlling for variables in this piecemeal way is to pool as many individual data sets as possible and allow statistical power to overcome the confounds in a single mega-analysis. This is the principle behind the ENIGMA project (http://enigma.ini.usc.edu). Thus, three-dimensional brain imaging data from 1728 MDD patients and 7199 controls (15 research projects worldwide) showed

that patients had significantly lower hippocampal volumes (Cohen's $d = -0.14$; % difference = $-1.24$). The effect was driven by patients with recurrent MDD (Cohen's $d = -0.17$; % difference = $-1.44$), so there were no differences between first-episode patients and controls. These effects are, of course, small. They may imply that loss of hippocampal volume is an acquired feature of MDD, related to the illness course. However, no cross-sectional study can prove that. Earlier age of onset was associated with a smaller hippocampus and a trend towards a smaller amygdala and larger lateral ventricles. Current symptoms, use of drugs for depression, and methodology had no effect [34]. The absence of effect in first-episode MDD patients echoes findings in individual, relatively well-powered, and controlled studies [35].

The ENIGMA group's study of cortical volumes in 2148 MDD patients and 7957 controls showed thinner cortical grey matter in the orbitofrontal cortex, anterior and posterior cingulate, insula, and temporal lobes in adults aged over 21 years (effect sizes $-0.10$ to $-0.14$) (Fig. 76.1). These effects were *more* pronounced in first-episode and early-onset cases. By contrast, effects in adolescents were larger but occurred as changes in regional brain volume, not cortical thickness. The affected brain areas included medial and superior frontal areas and somatosensory and motor areas (effect sizes $-0.26$ to $-0.57$) and were most striking in recurrent MDD [36]. This complex pattern implies different developmental trajectories for the cerebral cortex in early-onset cases, compared with controls.

It is an open question whether improved-quality multimodal imaging can refine methodology to produce more precise results in smaller samples. A pooled analysis from a selection of such studies employing peak co-ordinates for MR structural data showed reduced grey matter in the amygdala, dorsal fronto-median cortex, and right para-cingulate cortex. In the same patients, PET demonstrated increases in glucose metabolism in the right subgenual and pregenual anterior cingulate [37]. The connectivity of the subgenual region had previously been shown to suggest projections to the nucleus accumbens, amygdala, hypothalamus, and orbitofrontal cortex [38].

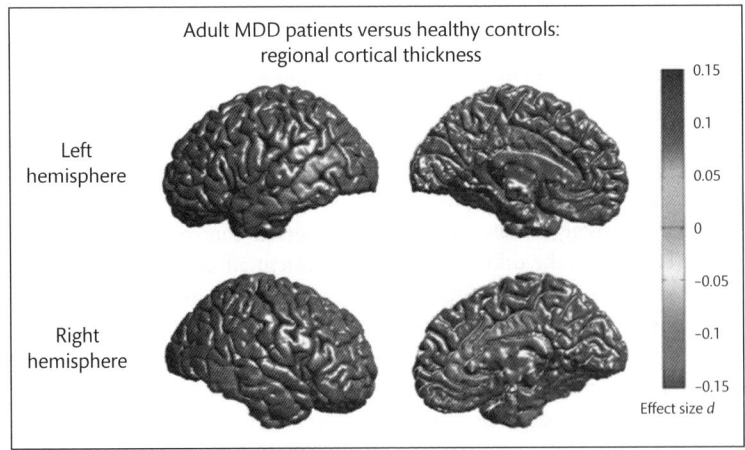

**Fig. 76.1** (see Colour Plate section) Meta-analysis of magnetic resonance scans from patients with major depression, compared with controls, from the ENIGMA working group [34]. Effect sizes for regions with significant (PFDR <0.05) cortical thinning are shown in red. Negative effect sizes *d* indicate cortical thinning in MDD, compared to controls.

## Functional imaging: resting state and task-based studies

In one sense, resting state data are well suited to aggregation in secondary analyses; the lack of any task for subjects to perform during scanning means that their experience inside the scanner should be reasonably consistent across studies. However, a large variety of statistical approaches are used in the first-level analysis of resting state data; the choice can profoundly influence the connectivity metrics generated. The two common methods for analysing resting state data involve either correlating BOLD signal against a range of seed regions (with different sets of seeds used in different laboratories) or using data-driven independent component analyses of whole brain data. It is difficult to draw firm conclusions from such variable approaches, although increased connectivity in depressed patients within the default mode network is perhaps the most consistently reported finding [39]. While it is an advantage of resting state data that the same networks can be identified with reasonable reliability across studies, it is less clear how differences in these networks relate to cognitive function or why they may be related to symptoms [40]. This explanatory gap means we do not understand what role increased connectivity within the default mode network plays in major depression.

In contrast, task-based fMRI studies in depressed patients have been influenced by dual-process, mechanistic models of emotional and cognitive control. These models suggest two neural systems to be key—firstly, a bottom–up, limbic-based system which responds relatively automatically to salient stimulus features, and secondly, a top–down frontal-based control system which responds more flexibly and is able to modify activity of the limbic system. Published studies have tended to report altered activity of frontal regions during emotional or effortful tasks, which has been interpreted as reflecting reduced or deficient function of the top–down control systems [41, 42]. This goes along with evidence of increased activity of limbic regions, particularly in response to negative affective stimuli [43]. One attraction of this proposal is that it links imaging findings not only to symptoms, but also to cognitive abnormalities observed in patients such as reduced executive function or processing biases for negative information. However, very similar 'hyperactive limbic system combined with deficient control system' models have been proposed for a range of psychiatric diagnoses such as anxiety, BD, and attention-deficit/hyperactivity disorder (ADHD). Whether this explanatory overlap between diagnoses is a result of common neural mechanisms across disorders, a reflection of the current technical limitations of neuroimaging modalities, or of a relatively under-developed imaging literature is not clear. Whatever the explanation, current imaging-based mechanistic models of major depression do not have the specificity to distinguish between different illness phenotypes.

## Classification studies in major depression

The RDoC project has exemplified the search for objective measures, such as those from neuroimaging, to inform novel categorical schemes in mental health and disease (see Chapter 8). It has led to an increased focus on studies which recruit patients with a range of difficulties and diagnoses in order to identify common processes across conventional symptom-based diagnoses. A slightly less ambitious approach attempts to identify subcategories within existing diagnoses. The common observation that patients with major depression show heterogenous illness courses, response to treatment,

and risk factors has prompted a number of early attempts to identify subgroups of depressed patients such as those with a melancholic vs a reactive illness course. Historically, it proved challenging to demonstrate that such subgroups were clinically meaningful, for example that they provide useful information on prognosis or response to treatment. A recent influential study provides a first hint that neuroimaging measures may be useful in this project. In the study illustrated in Fig. 76.2, Drysdale and colleagues amassed over 1000 resting state scans from depressed patients and controls [44]. Using an unsupervised classification approach, based on resting state connectivity measures and symptom score measures, the authors claim to have identified four distinct subgroups of patients. The groups displayed a reasonably specific pattern of resting state connectivity and associated cluster of symptoms. They then demonstrated that they were able to identify patients with these symptom clusters using just the connectivity data, in a sample of 400 new participants. However, the validity of the reported clustering of patients has been questioned in recent work (44a) and, even if the clusters do turn out to be reliable, this does not not guarantee that they will be clinically useful. The authors provided important initial reassuring evidence on this point. The four clusters of patients responded differently to repeated transcranial magnetic stimulation (rTMS). Further assessment of the utility of this clustering technique will require replication of the cluster identification process by other research groups and confirmation that cluster assignment is associated with response to more mainstream treatments or to general illness course. However, the study demonstrates a potentially exciting development beyond symptoms; this has been long anticipated, but not hitherto delivered.

Supervised learning, the second approach to classification, has most commonly been employed to classify depressed patients into responders vs non-responders to treatment. The majority of pharmacological and psychological treatments for depression take weeks to fully influence subjective symptom measures. A significant proportion of patients do not respond to the initial treatment regime. As a result, there is often a long delay before patients are started on effective therapy. A number of studies have looked at whether an individual will respond to a specific treatment, based on structural and/or functional neuroimaging data collected before treatment is initiated or over the first few days of treatment. The rationale is that such measures could pave the way to personalized therapy in which the neuroimaging outcomes would be used to select the treatment that is most likely to help an individual patient. Published studies to date have employed modest sample sizes and have been unable to test the performance of the classifiers using a fully held-out sample [45]; within-sample accuracies (that is usually estimated using 'leave-one-out' procedures) have tended to range between 60% and 70%. Response rates to antidepressants in unstratified clinical trials are often around 50%, so a 10–20% improvement appears promising for clinical settings. Ongoing projects are collecting larger sample sizes, which will allow more robust out-of-sample validation of classifier performance.

Improvements in methodology may well identify reliable subgroups of patients or classifiers which identify treatment responders vs non-responders. The next stage will be to test the use of these classifiers in RCTs. Imaging is still both unwieldy and relatively expensive, and other methods of objectifying behavioural phenotypes will be developed from self-rating and wearable devices, which may

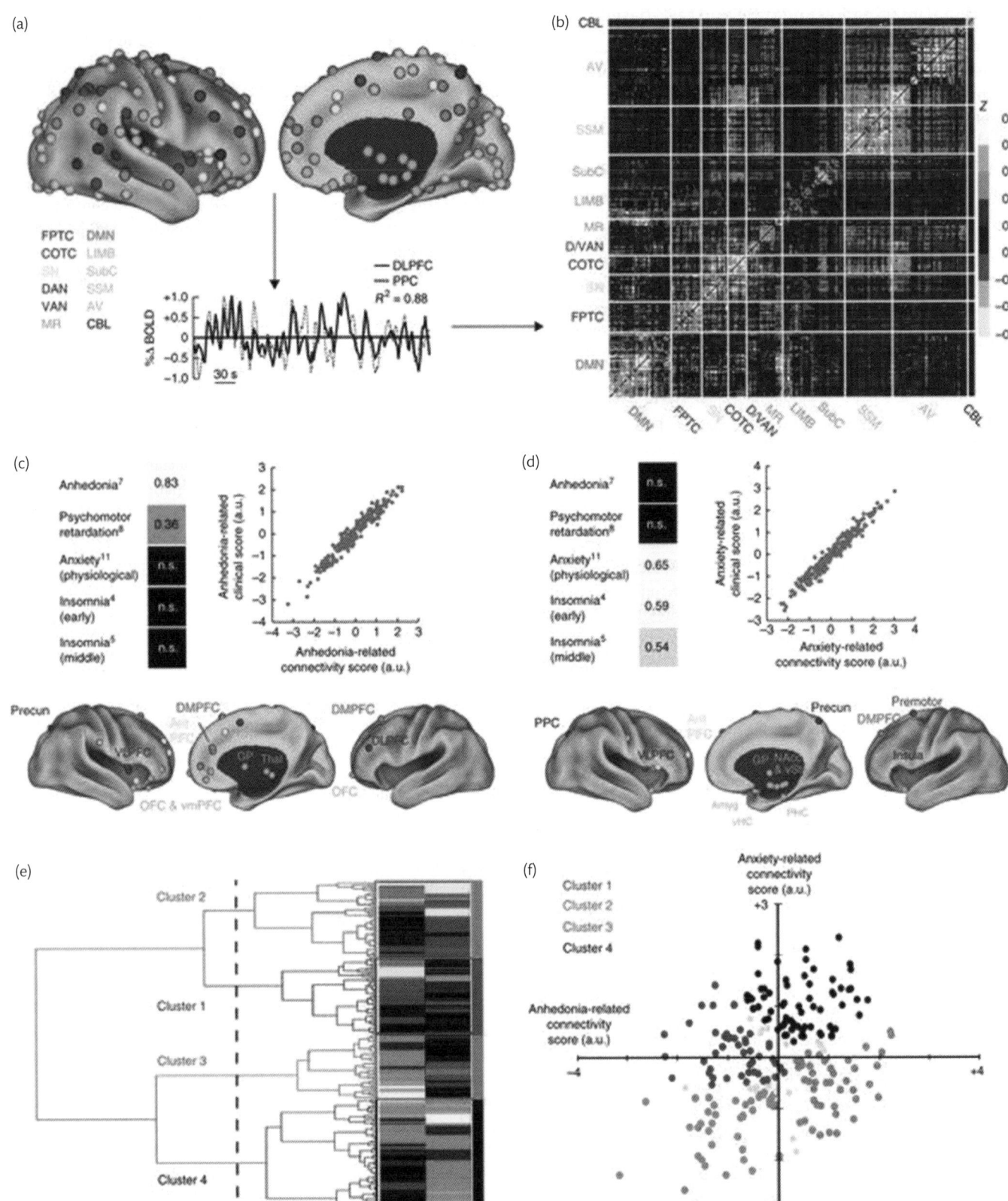

**Fig. 76.2** (see Colour Plate section) Definition of subtypes of depression using resting state fMRI data taken from [44]. Resting state data from depressed patients and control subjects were collected. (a) Regions of interest were defined across the brain, and the mean BOLD time series from each of these regions was extracted for each subject. (b) For each subject, the correlation between all pairs of time series was calculated as a measure of connectivity. The figure illustrates the correlation between the regions of interest which are arranged depending on the neural system of which they are a member. (c) and (d) A data reduction method (canonical correlation; CC) was then used to find simple relationships between the imaging data shown in (b) and patient depression scores measured using the Hamilton Depression Rating Scale. CC looks for common factors in the imaging and symptom score data sets; here two were found: (c) an 'anhedonia'-related scale and (d) an 'anxiety'-related scale. The brain images display the regions of interest

provide cheaper means of patient stratification. Whether imaging will find a role generating classifiers in clinical practice is still uncertain. Its widespread adoption will require evidence for meaningful and cost-effective improvement in outcomes.

## White matter integrity and neurodevelopment

As already noted, diffusion-weighted MR imaging (DTI) offers a sensitive way to determine the integrity of white matter. Apparent abnormalities are seen in at-risk samples. A quantitative voxel-based pooled meta-analysis of FA of almost 400 first-episode, drug-naïve MDD revealed reductions in the corpus callosum, bilateral anterior internal capsule, and right inferior temporal and right superior frontal gyri. FA reductions in some of these areas correlated with symptom scores and duration of depression [46]. In a similar large pooled analysis comparing over 500 more heterogenous MDD patients and controls, there were trends to reduced FA in the corpus callosum (CC) and inferior fronto-occipital fasciculus (effect sizes –0.19 and –0.20, respectively) [47].

These findings in people early in the illness course suggest decreased fibre coherence or glial distribution [48] to be associated with MDD. Given similar findings in at-risk populations and first-episode cases, the abnormality appears likely to be neurodevelopmental, rather than acquired, as a result of illness course or medication. FA increases monotonically during adolescence, but at different rates in different brain structures; thus, the splenium appears to stabilize by age 15, while the uncinate fasciculus appears still to be changing at age 30 [49]. Therefore, development of the splenium would be complete by age 20 and the difference in FA would then be enduring. Some prospective longitudinal data in young people with first-degree relatives with BD suggest no catch-up of the decreased FA when first seen, over the next 2 years [50]. This finding clearly complements, and must partly explain, the findings of reduced FA in mature patients. Studies of twins and siblings suggest that FA in multiple cortical regions is under genetic control [51]. Therefore, diffuse FA abnormalities in white matter appear to be a neurodevelopmental marker of vulnerability to MDD and other psychiatric disorders, including BD (see Chapter 71), ADHD (see Chapter 35), schizophrenia (see Chapter 60), and impulse control disorders (see Chapter 123). How alterations in white matter microstructure can be such a general marker of neurodevelopmental abnormality is not established. White matter investigation using more advanced MR methods will clearly be increasingly possible.

Given the findings in young people at risk of MDD or with early-onset psychiatric disorder, it is unsurprising that mature patients show the same pattern of diffuse reductions in white matter FA. It could be an enduring mark of their early vulnerability. A preliminary description of DTI data from the pooled ENIGMA MDD cohort showed the largest differences in white matter between cases

and controls in the body and genu of the CC [52]. The effect sizes for different areas varied up to a maximum of –0.34 in the body of the CC. Such effects for the white matter microstructure are stronger than those reported in their similar meta-analysis of subcortical grey matter volume in MDD described previously. The sample size is still modest, and moderating factors remain to be studied in larger samples.

In an early study of patients with *onset* of MDD over 60 years, FA reductions were marked, even when grey matter volume changes were undetectable [53]. In addition, these patients performed worse than appropriate controls in tests of executive function, processing speed, episodic memory, and language. There were meaningful correlations between FA in individual brain areas and cognitive impairments: reduced FA of the anterior thalamic radiation and uncinate fasciculus with executive function; the genu of the CC with processing speed and anterior thalamic radiation; and the genu and body of the CC and the fornix with episodic memory. While exploratory, these findings supported the internal validity of the findings in a small study. Moreover, they predicted a closer link between acquired or progressive white matter disruption and cognitive deficits than for the superficially similar reductions seen in younger patients with MDD.

For the late-onset group, acquired white matter disruption may be a particular risk factor. This is supported firstly by the observation that DTI changes are more striking in late-onset patients, compared with age-matched early-onset patients [54]. Secondly, there was an association between *subthreshold* depressive symptoms and FA reductions in an intensively studied cohort of now ex-civil servants aged almost 70 years (effect size –0.2) [55]. This group gave no history of depressive episodes. In this study, there was no association with grey matter volume, and the sample size was 350. However, only 10% of the total sample had excess depressive symptoms. The anatomy of the largest effects was diffuse, involving particularly the CC and the inferior and superior longitudinal fasciculi. Vascular risk factors are believed to contribute to the development of DTI changes in the elderly. Scores for vascular risk (Framingham Stroke Risk Profile) correlated with DTI measures in late-life MDD [56].

Reduced FA has been a highly consistent finding in studies of more heterogenous groups of older patients. In a review of nine such studies, the dorsolateral prefrontal cortex and uncinate fasciculus in patients with MDD had lower FA than controls (effect sizes 0.7 and 0.23, respectively), although heterogeneity and publication bias were evident for the dorsolateral prefrontal cortex [57].

## White matter integrity, neurodegeneration, and cerebral lesions

White matter abnormalities were originally described in mood disorder patients in the earliest studies with CT and MR imaging

**Fig. 76.2** Continued

between which resting state correlations were most closely related to the specific factor. (e) The strength of these two factors was estimated for each patient, and then an unsupervised classification procedure—hierarchical clustering—was used to try and find clusters of patients who differed on the two measures. (f) Four clusters of patients were found, with each cluster defined by a different combination of the two factors. The scatter plot shows data from patients colour-coded by the cluster to which they are assigned; grey dots represent patients who could not be confidently classified. The authors next demonstrated that these clusters could be reliably detected in a second data set and that cluster membership could be assigned using just the neuroimaging data. Lastly, it was shown that the clusters predicted treatment response to transcranial magnetic stimulation (TMS) therapy—a greater proportion of patients in clusters 1 and 3 responded to TMS than those in clusters 2 and 4.

as 'white matter hyperintensities' [58, 59] and are most often seen in older patients [60] (see Chapter 66). They are clearly correlated with vascular disease [53]. They do not, in themselves, explain any of the findings already described for older patient samples, because white matter changes appear to be so diffuse. Notwithstanding the foregoing emphasis on *neurodevelopmental* abnormality in young people and stable FA reductions in mature patients with MDD, white matter disruption appears also to be a manifestation of progressive brain changes in ageing. Correlates of microstructure abnormality with cognitive function are more evident in a healthy ageing population; progressive reduction in FA was seen with age and correlated selectively with working memory among several tests of executive function and processing speed [61].

## Brain diseases or injury and depression

Post-stroke depression (PSD) is a common complication of rehabilitation after stroke. The location of brain injury predisposing to depression is of obvious interest, although not without controversy [62, 63]. A recent systematic meta-analysis aimed to determine the mapping between PSD and lesion location. Forty-three studies involving 5507 patients suffering from stroke were included [64]. Only studies with 1–6 months post-stroke group showed a statistical association between right hemisphere stroke and risk of depression (OR 0.79, 95% CI 0.66–0.93). This contrasts with earlier claims that lesions of the *left* hemisphere were associated with an increased risk of depression after stroke [63].

Rather differently, mood and anxiety disorders may be presenting symptoms of brain tumours or other brain disease. Imaging can be highly relevant to neurological diagnosis. Depressive illness may be the only complaint in the presentation of meningioma for as many as 20% of the cases occurring in the fifth decade of life. As many as 75% of some series of patients with multiple sclerosis experience a delay in multiple sclerosis diagnosis due to symptoms of MDD. A missed or delayed diagnosis is clinically significant if it postpones effective intervention, increases the burden of disease/disability, and reduces the quality of life. Rather similarly, major depression may precede the diagnosis of Parkinson's disease in as many as 37% of younger, especially female, patients presenting with motor signs [65].

Traumatic brain injury (TBI) is receiving increasing attention because of the impact on survivors of head trauma in civilian and military life and in contact sports. In a review of almost 100 publications, 27% of cases of TBI were diagnosed with MDD/dysthymia using formal criteria and 38% reported clinically significant depression with self-report scales, which makes it a common complication of TBI [66]. Interestingly, DTI investigations of white matter integrity can effectively differentiate patients with TBI from controls [67]. There also appears to be a relationship between DTI measures and TBI outcomes. However, a specific relationship with depression in this patient group, perhaps mediated by white matter damage, has not yet been described, even if it can be anticipated from what has been foregoing in this chapter.

As with other MR measures, DTI may prove useful in patient stratification and prediction of treatment response. Lower FA has been related to treatment resistance [68] and reduced resilience to MDD after early-life adversity [69].

## Isotope-based imaging

Isotope-based imaging (PET and SPET or SPECT) has assumed marginal importance in recent years. PET and SPECT provide the initial evidence, based on cerebral blood flow, for functional abnormality in the brain in depression [70, 71]. These methods remain the only way in which specific binding to brain receptors can be measured in the living human. We do not propose to review here the literature relating to the 5-HT1 receptor [72], the D2 receptor [73], or the serotonin transporter [74], all of which are relevant to depression.

The findings in isotope imaging studies are limited by the costs of such studies (which result in small samples) and the complicated context for their interpretation (provided by genotype, development, early experience, previous exposure to medication or drug/alcohol use, data from post-mortem studies, and our understanding of animal experiments on the same receptors).

## Conclusions

MR measures have an obvious direct appeal for neuroscience, and the biology of MDD has proved no exception. To date, definitive advances that change practice have not been made. As a marker of neurodevelopmental abnormality, the white matter may prove to be an important tissue for understanding behavioural pathology; as such, it provides a candidate target for understanding gene and gene × environment interactions on the one hand and impairment of emotional control and cognition on the other.

### REFERENCES

1. Kendler KS. The dappled nature of causes of psychiatric illness: replacing the organic-functional/hardware-software dichotomy with empirically based pluralism. *Mol Psychiatry*. 2012;17:377–88.
2. Papmeyer M, Sussmann JE, Stewart T, *et al*. Prospective longitudinal study of subcortical brain volumes in individuals at high familial risk of mood disorders with or without subsequent onset of depression. *Psychiat Res*. 2016;248:119–25.
3. Murphy SE, Norbury R, O'Sullivan U, Cowen PJ, Harmer CJ. Effect of a single dose of citalopram on amygdala response to emotional faces. *Br J Psychiatry*. 2009;194:535–40.
4. Godlewska BR, Norbury R, Selvaraj S, Cowen PJ, Harmer CJ. Short-term SSRI treatment normalises amygdala hyperactivity in depressed patients. *Psychol Med*. 2012;42:2609–17.
5. Godlewska BR, Browning M, Norbury R, Cowen PJ, Harmer CJ. Early changes in emotional processing as a marker of clinical response to SSRI treatment in depression. *Transl Psychiatry*. 2016;6:e957.
6. Kempton MJ, Geddes JR, Ettinger U, Williams SC, Grasby PM. Meta-analysis, database, and meta-regression of 98 structural imaging studies in bipolar disorder. *Arch Gen Psychiatry*. 2008;65:1017–32.
7. Caspi A, Sugden K, Moffitt TE, *et al*. Influence of life stress on depression: moderation by a polymorphism in the *5-HTT* gene. *Science*. 2003;301:386–9.
8. Hariri AR, Mattay VS, Tessitore A, *et al*. Serotonin transporter genetic variation and the response of the human amygdala. *Science*. 2002;297:400–3.

9. Pezawas L, Meyer-Lindenberg A, Drabant EM, *et al.* 5-HTTLPR polymorphism impacts human cingulate–amygdala interactions: a genetic susceptibility mechanism for depression. *Nat Neurosci.* 2005;8:828–34.

10. Frodl T, Koutsouleris N, Bottlender R, *et al.* Reduced gray matter brain volumes are associated with variants of the serotonin transporter gene in major depression. *Mol Psychiatry.* 2008;13:1093–101.

11. Prathikanti S, Weinberger DR. Psychiatric genetics—the new era: genetic research and some clinical implications. *Br Med Bull.* 2005;73–4:107–22.

12. Murphy SE, Norbury R, Godlewska BR, *et al.* The effect of the serotonin transporter polymorphism (5-HTTLPR) on amygdala function: a meta-analysis. *Mol Psychiatry.* 2013;18:512–20.

13. Flint J, Munafo MR. The endophenotype concept in psychiatric genetics. *Psychol Med.* 2007;37:163–80.

14. Thompson PM, Stein JL, Medland SE, *et al.* The ENIGMA Consortium: large-scale collaborative analyses of neuroimaging and genetic data. *Brain Imaging Behav.* 2014;8:153–82.

15. Mills KL, Goddings A-L, Herting MM, *et al.* Structural brain development between childhood and adulthood: convergence across four longitudinal samples. *Neuroimage.* 2016;141:273–81.

16. Frodl T, Janowitz D, Schmaal L, *et al.* Childhood adversity impacts on brain subcortical structures relevant to depression. *J Psychiatr Res.* 2017;86:58–65.

17. Kendler KS, Gardner CO, Prescott CA. Toward a comprehensive developmental model for major depression in men. *Am J Psychiatry.* 2006;163:115–24.

18. Keedwell PA, Chapman R, Christiansen K, Richardson H, Evans J, Jones DK. Cingulum white matter in young women at risk of depression: the effect of family history and anhedonia. *Biol Psychiatry.* 2012;72:296–302.

19. Vijayakumar N, Bartholomeusz C, Whitford T, *et al.* White matter integrity in individuals at ultra-high risk for psychosis: a systematic review and discussion of the role of polyunsaturated fatty acids. *BMC Psychiatry.* 2016;16:287.

20. Miskowiak KW, Kjaerstad HL, Meluken I, *et al.* The search for neuroimaging and cognitive endophenotypes: a critical systematic review of studies involving unaffected first-degree relatives of individuals with bipolar disorder. *Neurosci Biobehav Rev.* 2017;73:1–22.

21. Waller R, Dotterer HL, Murray L, Maxwell AM, Hyde LW. White-matter tract abnormalities and antisocial behavior: a systematic review of diffusion tensor imaging studies across development. *Neuroimage Clin.* 2017;14:201–15.

22. Jones CL, Ward J, Critchley HD. The neuropsychological impact of insular cortex lesions. *J Neurol Neurosurg Psychiatry.* 2010;81:611–18.

23. Whalley HC, Sussmann JE, Romaniuk L, *et al.* Prediction of depression in individuals at high familial risk of mood disorders using functional magnetic resonance imaging. *PLoS One.* 2013;8:e57357.

24. Yip SW, Mackay CE, Goodwin GM. Increased temporo-insular engagement in unmedicated bipolar II disorder: an exploratory resting state study using independent component analysis. *Bipolar Disord.* 2014;16:748–55.

25. Roberts G, Lord A, Frankland A, *et al.* Functional dysconnection of the inferior frontal gyrus in young people with bipolar disorder or at genetic high risk. *Biol Psychiatry.* 2017;81:718–27.

26. Roberts G, Green MJ, Breakspear M, *et al.* Reduced inferior frontal gyrus activation during response inhibition to emotional

stimuli in youth at high risk of bipolar disorder. *Biol Psychiatry.* 2013;74:55–61.

27. Roberts G, Lenroot R, Frankland A, *et al.* Abnormalities in left inferior frontal gyral thickness and parahippocampal gyral volume in young people at high genetic risk for bipolar disorder. *Psychol Med.* 2016;46:2083–96.

28. Stange JP, Bessette KL, Jenkins LM, *et al.* Attenuated intrinsic connectivity within cognitive control network among individuals with remitted depression: temporal stability and association with negative cognitive styles. *Hum Brain Mapp.* 2017;38:2939–54.

29. Norbury R, Godlewska B, Cowen PJ. When less is more: a functional magnetic resonance imaging study of verbal working memory in remitted depressed patients. *Psychol Med.* 2014;44:1197–203.

30. Dichter GS, Kozink RV, McClernon FJ, Smoski MJ. Remitted major depression is characterized by reward network hyperactivation during reward anticipation and hypoactivation during reward outcomes. *J Affect Disord.* 2012;136:1126–34.

31. Jenkins LM, Kassel MT, Gabriel LB, *et al.* Amygdala and dorsomedial hyperactivity to emotional faces in youth with remitted major depression. *Soc Cogn Affect Neurosci.* 2016;11:736–45.

32. McCrory EJ, Gerin MI, Viding E. Annual research review: childhood maltreatment, latent vulnerability and the shift to preventative psychiatry—the contribution of functional brain imaging. *J Child Psychol Psychiatry.* 2017;58:338–57.

33. Zhao YJ, Du MY, Huang XQ, *et al.* Brain grey matter abnormalities in medication-free patients with major depressive disorder: a meta-analysis. *Psychol Med.* 2014;44:2927–37.

34. Schmaal L, Veltman DJ, van Erp TGM, *et al.* Subcortical brain alterations in major depressive disorder: findings from the ENIGMA Major Depressive Disorder working group. *Mol Psychiatry.* 2016;21:806–12.

35. Cheng YQ, Xu J, Chai P, *et al.* Brain volume alteration and the correlations with the clinical characteristics in drug-naive first-episode MDD patients: a voxel-based morphometry study. *Neurosci Lett.* 2010;480:30–4.

36. Schmaal L, Hibar DP, Samann PG, *et al.* Cortical abnormalities in adults and adolescents with major depression based on brain scans from 20 cohorts worldwide in the ENIGMA Major Depressive Disorder Working Group. *Mol Psychiatry.* 2017;22:900–9.

37. Sacher J, Neumann J, Funfstuck T, Soliman A, Villringer A, Schroeter ML. Mapping the depressed brain: a meta-analysis of structural and functional alterations in major depressive disorder. *J Affect Disord.* 2012;140:142–8.

38. Johansen-Berg H, Gutman DA, Behrens TEJ, *et al.* Anatomical connectivity of the subgenual cingulate region targeted with deep brain stimulation for treatment-resistant depression. *Cereb Cortex.* 2008;18:1374–83.

39. Kaiser RH, Andrews-Hanna JR, Wager TD, Pizzagalli DA. Large-scale network dysfunction in major depressive disorder: a meta-analysis of resting-state functional connectivity. *JAMA Psychiatry.* 2015;72:603–11.

40. Hamilton JP, Farmer M, Fogelman P, Gotlib IH. Depressive rumination, the default-mode network, and the dark matter of clinical neuroscience. *Biol Psychiatry.* 2015;78:224–30.

41. Price JL, Drevets WC. Neural circuits underlying the pathophysiology of mood disorders. *Trends Cogn Sci.* 2012;16:61–71.

42. Rive MM, van Rooijen G, Veltman DJ, Phillips ML, Schene AH, Ruhe HG. Neural correlates of dysfunctional emotion

regulation in major depressive disorder. A systematic review of neuroimaging studies. *Neurosci Biobehav Rev*. 2013;37:2529–53.

43. Jaworska N, Yang XR, Knott V, MacQueen G. A review of fMRI studies during visual emotive processing in major depressive disorder. *World J Biol Psychiatry*. 2015;16:448–71.

44. Drysdale AT, Grosenick L, Downar J, *et al*. Resting-state connectivity biomarkers define neurophysiological subtypes of depression. *Nat Med*. 2017;23:28–38.

44a. Dinga R, Schmaal L, Penninx BWJH, *et al*. Evaluating the evidence for biotypes of depression: Methodological replication and extension of Drysdale et al. (2017). *NeuroImage: Clinical*. 2019;22: 101796.

45. Chi KF, Korgaonkar M, Grieve SM. Imaging predictors of remission to anti-depressant medications in major depressive disorder. *J Affect Disord*. 2015;186:134–44.

46. Chen G, Guo Y, Zhu H, *et al*. Intrinsic disruption of white matter microarchitecture in first-episode, drug-naive major depressive disorder: a voxel-based meta-analysis of diffusion tensor imaging. *Prog Neuro-Psychoph*. 2017;76:179–87.

47. Kelly S, van Velzen L, Veltman D, *et al*. White matter microstructural differences in major depression: meta-analytic findings from ENIGMA-MDD DTI. *Biol Psychiatry*. 2017; 81:S381-S.

48. Walhovd KB, Johansen-Berg H, Karadottir RT. Unraveling the secrets of white matter--bridging the gap between cellular, animal and human imaging studies. *Neuroscience*. 2014;276:2–13.

49. Lebel C, Walker L, Leemans A, Phillips L, Beaulieu C. Microstructural maturation of the human brain from childhood to adulthood. *Neuroimage*. 2008;40:1044–55.

50. Ganzola R, Nickson T, Bastin ME, *et al*. Longitudinal differences in white matter integrity in youth at high familial risk for bipolar disorder. *Bipolar Disord*. 2017;19:156–67.

51. Kochunov P, Jahanshad N, Marcus D, *et al*. Heritability of fractional anisotropy in human white matter: a comparison of Human Connectome Project and ENIGMA-DTI data. *Neuroimage*. 2015;111:300–11.

52. Kelly S, van Velzen LS, Hatton S, *et al*. White matter differences in major depression: meta-analytic findings from enigma-MDD DTI. *Bipolar Disord*. 2016;18:114–15.

53. Sexton CE, Allan CL, Le Masurier M, *et al*. Magnetic resonance imaging in late-life depression: multimodal examination of network disruption. *Arch Gen Psychiatry*. 2012;69:680–9.

54. Sexton CE, Le Masurier M, Allan CL, *et al*. Magnetic resonance imaging in late-life depression: vascular and glucocorticoid cascade hypotheses. *Br J Psychiatry*. 2012;201:46–51.

55. Allan CL, Sexton CE, Filippini N, *et al*. Sub-threshold depressive symptoms and brain structure: a magnetic resonance imaging study within the Whitehall II cohort. *J Affect Disord*. 2016;204:219–25.

56. Allan CL, Sexton CE, Kalu UG, *et al*. Does the Framingham Stroke Risk Profile predict white-matter changes in late-life depression? *Int Psychogeriatr*. 2012;24:524–31.

57. Wen M-C, Steffens DC, Chen M-K, Zainal NH. Diffusion tensor imaging studies in late-life depression: systematic review and meta-analysis. *Int J Geriatr Psychiatry*. 2014;29:1173–84.

58. Brown FW, Lewine RJ, Hudgins PA, Risch SC. White matter hyperintensity signals in psychiatric and nonpsychiatric subjects. *Am J Psychiatry*. 1992;149:620–5.

59. Brown FW, Lewine RR, Hudgins PA. White matter hyperintensity signals associated with vascular risk factors in schizophrenia. *Prog Neuropsychopharmacol Biol Psychiatry*. 1995;19:39–45.

60. Dupont RM, Jernigan TL, Heindel W, *et al*. Magnetic resonance imaging and mood disorders. Localization of white matter and other subcortical abnormalities. *Arch Gen Psychiatry*. 1995;52:747–55.

61. Charlton RA, Landau S, Schiavone F, *et al*. A structural equation modeling investigation of age-related variance in executive function and DTI measured white matter damage. *Neurobiol Aging*. 2008;29:1547–55.

62. Carson AJ, MacHale S, Allen K, *et al*. Depression after stroke and lesion location: a systematic review. *Lancet*. 2000;356:122–6.

63. Narushima K, Kosier JT, Robinson RG. A reappraisal of poststroke depression, intra- and inter-hemispheric lesion location using meta-analysis. *J Neuropsychiatry Clin Neurosci*. 2003;15:422–30.

64. Wei N, Yong W, Li X, *et al*. Post-stroke depression and lesion location: a systematic review. *J Neurol*. 2015;262:81–90.

65. Cosci F, Fava GA, Sonino N. Mood and anxiety disorders as early manifestations of medical illness: a systematic review. *Psychother Psychosom*. 2015;84:22–9.

66. Osborn AJ, Mathias JL, Fairweather-Schmidt AK. Depression following adult, non-penetrating traumatic brain injury: a meta-analysis examining methodological variables and sample characteristics. *Neurosci Biobehav Rev*. 2014;47:1–15.

67. Hulkower MB, Poliak DB, Rosenbaum SB, Zimmerman ME, Lipton ML. A decade of DTI in traumatic brain injury: 10 years and 100 articles later. *AJNR Am J Neuroradiol*. 2013;34:2064–74.

68. Zhou Y, Qin LD, Chen J, *et al*. Brain microstructural abnormalities revealed by diffusion tensor images in patients with treatment-resistant depression compared with major depressive disorder before treatment. *Eur J Radiol*. 2011;80:450–4.

69. Frodl T, Carballedo A, Fagan AJ, Lisiecka D, Ferguson Y, Meaney JF. Effects of early-life adversity on white matter diffusivity changes in patients at risk for major depression. *J Psychiatry Neurosci*. 2012;37:37–45.

70. Goodwin GM. Neuropsychological and neuroimaging evidence for the involvement of the frontal lobes in depression. *J Psychopharmacol*. 1997;11:115–22.

71. Goodwin GM. Neuropsychological and neuroimaging evidence for the involvement of the frontal lobes in depression: 20 years on. *J Psychopharmacol*. 2016;30:1090–4.

72. Kaufman J, DeLorenzo C, Choudhury S, Parsey RV. The 5-HT1A receptor in major depressive disorder. *Eur Neuropsychopharmacol*. 2016;26:397–410.

73. Grace AA. Dysregulation of the dopamine system in the pathophysiology of schizophrenia and depression. *Nat Rev Neurosci*. 2016;17:524–32.

74. Kambeitz JP, Howes OD. The serotonin transporter in depression: meta-analysis of *in vivo* and post mortem findings and implications for understanding and treating depression. *J Affect Disord*. 2015;186:358–66.

# 77

# Management and treatment of depressive disorders

*Philip J. Cowen*

## Introduction

'But one need not sound the false or inspirational note to stress the truth that depression is not the soul's annihilation; men and women who have recovered from the disease—and they are countless—bear witness to probably what is probably its only saving grace: it is conquerable.' [1]. William Styron here elegantly expresses the notion that the prognosis of most depressive episodes is eventually favourable, and indeed much depression in the community resolves without specific treatment. However, depression can be persistent and disabling, and in these circumstances, the use of effective therapies is appropriate and important.

This chapter will first examine evidence for the efficacy of the wide range of treatments employed in depression. The subsequent section (see Management of depressive disorders, p. 810) will deal with the way in which these treatments are best integrated into specific clinical management plans. It should be noted that controlled trials of treatment usually involve patients with a depressive episode diagnosed according to DSM or ICD criteria and in the moderate range of clinical severity. There are less controlled data available about the treatment of milder depressions or those that are particularly severe.

## Evidence for efficacy of treatment

### Antidepressant medication

#### Treatment of acute major depression

The first widely used drugs for depression were tricyclic antidepressants (TCAs) such as imipramine and amitriptyline. Their mechanism of action in depression was eventually shown to be due to blockade of the reuptake of noradrenaline (NA) and serotonin [5-hydroxytryptamine (5-HT)] at nerve terminals, thus prolonging the action of these monoamines in the synapse. The majority of drugs developed subsequently for depression share this therapeutic mechanism [2] (Table 77.1). Despite their efficacy, TCAs have significant safety problems, particularly potential lethality in overdose through cardiotoxicity. In addition, their anticholinergic properties can

make tolerance of a therapeutic dose challenging and, for example, place older male patients at risk of urinary retention [2].

Newer drugs, in particular selective serotonin reuptake inhibitors (SSRIs), have replaced TCAs as first line [3]. SSRIs are better tolerated and much safer in overdose than TCAs, but commonly cause gastrointestinal and CNS adverse effects (Box 77.1). Serotonin and noradrenaline reuptake inhibitors (SNRIs), such as venlafaxine and duloxetine, are primarily 5-HT reuptake blockers but also have some modest effects to inhibit the reuptake of NA. Their side effect profile is similar to that of SSRIs, but venlafaxine appears less safe in overdose [2]. A number of other antidepressant drugs are available, including mirtazapine, which has antagonist properties at $5\text{-HT}_{2/3}$ and NA $\alpha_2$-adrenoceptors, and trazodone, which is a weak 5-HT reuptake inhibitor and is metabolized to a 5-HT receptor agonist. Both latter drugs have a sedating profile [2]. Agomelatine is licensed for depression in Europe; its main action is stimulation of melatonin receptors, but it may also antagonize $5\text{-HT}_{2C}$ receptors [4].

Other recent developments have led to drugs that block 5-HT reuptake, while having additional effects on a variety of 5-HT receptor subtypes. For example, vilazodone has partial agonist activity at the $5\text{-HT}_{1A}$ receptor, while vortioxetine binds to several other 5-HT receptor subtypes ($5\text{-HT}_{1A/1B/1D}$, $5\text{-HT}_3$, $5\text{-HT}_7$). Whether these agents have advantages over SSRI treatment is not fully clear, though vilazodone is claimed to produce less sexual dysfunction and vortioxetine to have particular benefits in depression-related cognitive impairment [5, 6].

All the drugs listed in Table 77.1 are efficacious in the acute treatment of major depression, with the largest effects, relative to placebo, being seen in patients with major depression whose symptoms are of at least moderate severity. Short-term response rates in controlled trials are about 50% for patients on active treatment, and about 30% for those on placebo, with the number needed to treat (NNT) being between 5 and 6 [3]. Several meta-analyses have assessed the differences in efficacy and general tolerability between the newer agents. There are suggestions that, among the SSRIs, sertraline and escitalopram are the most effective, while venlafaxine is slightly more efficacious than SSRIs, though less well tolerated [7]. Whether these differences are clinically important has been disputed [8]. In

**Box 77.1** Some side effects of SSRIs

| | |
|---|---|
| Gastrointestinal | Common: nausea, appetite loss, dry mouth, diarrhoea, constipation, dyspepsia |
| | Uncommon: vomiting, weight loss |
| Central nervous system | Common: headache, insomnia, dizziness, anxiety, agitation, fatigue, tremor, somnolence |
| | Uncommon: extra-pyramidal reaction, seizures, mania |
| Other | Common: sweating, delayed orgasm, anorgasmia |
| | Uncommon: rash, bleeding, pharyngitis, dyspnoea, serum sickness, hyponatraemia, alopecia |
| Drug interactions | NSAIDs, aspirin, anticoagulants (bleeding), lithium, triptans, MAOIs (including selegiline), tryptophan, linezolid, pethidine, St John's Wort (5-HT toxicity). Some SSRIs (fluoxetine, fluvoxamine, and paroxetine) strongly inhibit hepatic metabolizing enzymes and increase levels of other drugs; numerous examples reported, including antipsychotic drugs, anticonvulsants, and antiarrhythmics |

Adapted from Cowen P, Harrison P, Burns T, *Shorter Oxford Textbook of Psychiatry*, Sixth Edition, Copyright (2012), with permission from Oxford University Press.

some meta-analyses, the selective NA reuptake inhibitor reboxetine performs poorly in terms of tolerability and efficacy [7].

Monoamine oxidase inhibitors (MAOIs) were among the first drugs discovered that treat depression, but they are little used nowadays because of their liability to cause dangerous reactions with other drugs and tyramine-containing foods. However, controlled trials have shown that MAOIs can be effective in depressed patients who have not responded to numerous other pharmacological and non-pharmacological treatments, and for this reason, they retain some specialist use [9]. The reversible type A MAOI moclobemide has the advantage of not requiring adherence to a special diet. However, it can still produce hazardous interactions with other

drugs, and it is doubtful whether moclobemide at standard doses is as effective as conventional MAOIs for patients with resistant depression.

### Other depressive conditions

Drugs for major depression, in particular SSRIs, have been shown to be effective in dysthymia, with an NNT of 3–4 [10]. This suggests that medication can be effective in milder depressive conditions of lengthy duration. However, for milder depressions of more recent onset, antidepressant medication does not seem specifically useful [11].

### Longer-term treatment

By convention, the term 'relapse' is used to describe the worsening of depressive symptoms after an initial improvement, following the acute treatment of a depressive episode. 'Recurrence', on the other hand, refers to a new episode of depression that develops after a sustained period (of at least several months) of complete recovery. Treatment to prevent relapse is called 'continuation treatment', while that employed to prevent recurrence is known as 'prophylactic' or 'maintenance' therapy [3].

It is well established that stopping antidepressant treatment soon after an acute treatment response is associated with a high risk of relapse. Placebo-controlled studies indicated that continuing effective acute phase treatment for 6 months halves relapse rates [3]. For patients at high risk of recurrence (for example, those with three or more previous depressive episodes), extending antidepressant medication after this period is highly effective in lowering recurrence rates. A systematic review found that prescription of maintenance medication, relative to placebo, diminished the recurrence rate over the next 1–2 years from 40% to 18% (NNT = 4.5) [12]. Maintaining the dose at the level which was required to achieve acute symptomatic remission, if tolerability permits, appears the most effective strategy.

### Electroconvulsive therapy

Controlled trials indicate that electroconvulsive therapy (ECT) is more effective than simulated ECT (anaesthesia with electrode

**Table 77.1** Pharmacological properties of some antidepressants

| Drug | 5-HT reuptake | NA reuptake | Anticholinergic | Sedating | Overdose toxicity | Sexual dysfunction | Weight gain |
|---|---|---|---|---|---|---|---|
| Amitriptyline | ++ | ++ | +++ | +++ | +++ | + | +++ |
| Lofepramine | + | +++ | ++ | + | 0 | + | + |
| Fluoxetine | +++ | 0 | 0 | 0 | 0 | +++ | 0 |
| Paroxetine | +++ | 0 | + | + | 0 | +++ | ++ |
| Venlafaxine | +++ | + | 0 | 0 | ++ | +++ | + |
| Reboxetine | 0 | +++ | +[1] | 0 | 0 | + | 0 |
| Bupropion | 0 | +[2] | 0 | 0 | ++ | 0 | 0 |
| Mirtazapine | 0 | 0[3] | 0 | +++ | 0 | 0 | +++ |
| Trazodone | + | 0 | 0 | +++ | + | +[4] | + |

0, minimal effect; +, some effect; ++, moderate effect; +++, marked effect.
[1] Indirect anticholinergic effects through NA potentiation.
[2] Also blocks dopamine reuptake to some extent.
[3] Increases NA through $\alpha_2$-adrenoceptor blockade.
[4] Rarely causes priapism.

application, but no passage of current) in patients with major depression. The overall response rate is about 70% for ECT, and 40% for simulated treatment (NNT = 3.5) [13]. Randomized trials also suggest that ECT is slightly more effective and more rapid-acting than antidepressant medication, at least in the short term [13]. Generally, ECT is employed in patients who have not responded to other antidepressant therapies, and it may often prove effective in these circumstances; however, relapse rates in the months following treatment are high [14, 15].

ECT is generally a safe treatment. However, there is concern about its deleterious effects on memories for more remote personal events (autobiographical memory loss). While objective measures suggest that this loss largely resolves within 6 months, subjective reports by patients indicate that the loss can extend for longer and might sometimes be permanent [2].

## Other neurostimulatory treatments

A number of other neurostimulatory treatments have been tested in depressed patients, often where conventional therapies have not been helpful. Deep brain stimulation is discussed in Chapter 20. Other neurostimulatory approaches include vagal nerve stimulation (VNS) and transcranial magnetic stimulation (TMS), both of which have been approved for the treatment of depression in the United States. TMS has also been approved in several other countries for the management of resistant depression.

VNS has a slow onset of antidepressant action, over many months, which means that long-term follow-up studies are needed to assess its effectiveness. A meta-analysis of six outpatient multi-centre trials involving patients with refractory depression showed higher response rates in the VNS group at 96 weeks than a matched group of patients receiving standard treatment (32% vs 14%, respectively; NNT = 5.5). However, most of the studies were not randomized [16].

TMS uses a powerful magnetic field to produce a current flow in neural tissue. The use of appropriately shaped coils allows localization of stimulation to the main cortical regions. TMS has been used successfully to relieve depressive states, but there are still uncertainties about the best coil placement and stimulus parameters. The usual mode of administration is to administer stimulation to the left prefrontal cortex, with treatments being given 5 days a week for 2 weeks.

In a meta-analysis of trials involving about 1300 depressed patients randomized to either active or sham TMS, there was a greater clinical response in patients receiving active treatment (36% vs 15%, respectively; NNT = 9) [17]. However TMS appeared less effective than ECT in producing remission in severely depressed patients (34% vs 52%, respectively; NNT = 5.5) [18]. Nevertheless, TMS would be expected to be relatively free of the personal memory deficits induced in some patients by ECT.

## Bright light treatment

The use of phototherapy, or artificial bright light, as a treatment for depression was first studied systematically by Rosenthal and colleagues who used morning bright light to treat patients with the newly identified syndrome of 'seasonal affective disorder' [19]. Since then, phototherapy has become the mainstay of treatment of 'winter depression', particularly in patients whose clinical features include hyperphagia, hypersomnia, and diminished energy.

A meta-analysis of eight randomized studies found that morning bright light was significantly superior to a dim light control in reducing symptomatology in patients with winter depression, with an effect size of about 0.5 [20]. In winter depression, the therapeutic effects of bright light, fluoxetine, and cognitive behavioural therapy (CBT) appear generally equivalent, although cognitive therapy may have a better long-term outcome [3].

## Psychotherapy

### Treatment of acute depression

Individual CBT is the most studied psychological treatment in the management of acute depression, and there is strong evidence for its efficacy. Not surprisingly, the effect size of CBT is greatest in studies that compare it to a wait-list' control or 'treatment as usual' (TAU). Direct comparisons of CBT to other structured psychological treatments, such as interpersonal psychotherapy (IPT) and behavioural activation, tend not to show important differences in outcome. Similarly, most studies show similar efficacy when CBT is compared to antidepressant medication in the treatment of acute depression. However, the combination of CBT with antidepressant medication is probably better than drug treatment alone [21, 22].

Many psychiatrists do not consider that CBT is effective for patients with severe depression, but this view does not have support from randomized trials. However, defining 'severity' by means of a score on a rating scale may not capture specific factors that could compromise the efficacy of psychological treatment such as significant cognitive impairment and psychomotor retardation. Also the expertise of the therapist and their adherence to treatment protocols significantly influences outcome in CBT trials [23].

Systematic reviews indicate that other individual structured psychological treatments, such as IPT, behavioural activation, and problem-solving therapy, are effective in treating depression, in comparison to both placebo treatment and TAU [22]. However, the efficacy of short-term psychodynamic therapy is less certain [24]. The utility of behavioural activation and problem-solving therapy is important because such therapies require less therapist training and are easier to implement than CBT. Because of the high prevalence of depression in primary care and the preference of many patients for psychological treatments, there has been much interest in developing ways of increasing the availability of psychological therapies. Approaches range from group CBT formats to self-help booklets and therapy delivered via the Internet. Generally, in mild to moderate depression, all these treatments have some efficacy, relative to wait-list control, and there are no clear-cut differences between them [25].

This is also a convenient place to discuss the efficacy of exercise in treating depression. While there has been some controversy, the more recent systematic reviews suggest large effects of supervised, moderate-intensity aerobic exercise to decrease depressive symptomatology, compared to no treatment, and a moderate effect in comparison to TAU [26]. Again such treatment is likely to be most beneficial for patients with mild to moderate depression.

### Other depressive conditions

Where depression has persisted for a considerable period, and particularly in dysthymia, CBT appears less effective than antidepressant medication [27]. There are few trials of other psychological treatments in chronic depression, but psychodynamic therapy may be superior to TAU in patients with long-term resistant depression [28].

## Continuation and maintenance treatment

There is evidence that in patients randomized to CBT during the acute phase of depression, there is sustained improvement in depressive symptomatology over the next few months, even after the end of treatment. The risk of relapse after CBT is significantly less than that of patients withdrawn from pharmacotherapy (NNT = 5). There is also good evidence that CBT given in the continuation phase lowers relapse rates, compared to CBT given in the acute phase only (10% vs 31%, respectively; NNT = 5) [29].

Mindfulness-based cognitive therapy (MBCT) integrates CBT with meditation techniques designed to lower stress by facilitating acceptance and self-compassion. There is evidence that MBCT lowers the risk of recurrence in patients with a history of frequent episodes of depression and is as effective as maintenance antidepressant treatment in this respect [29, 30]. However, reliable identification of the specific elements of treatment and patient characteristics that may be linked to therapeutic response has proved difficult.

Combining IPT with medication in the treatment of acute episodes decreases relapse rates over the following 12 months [29]. In patients who achieve remission from depression, with IPT as sole treatment, maintenance therapy is also helpful in preventing recurrence. In a 3-year follow-up of elderly depressed patients, the combination of nortriptyline and IPT was more effective in preventing relapse (20% relapse rate) than nortriptyline alone (43% relapse rate), which itself was more effective than IPT alone (64% relapse rate) [31].

## Management of depressive disorders

### Assessment

The key aspects of the assessment of depression are summarized in Box 77.2. The critical factors that facilitate assessment are careful history taking and mental state examination. These also provide an invaluable opportunity to build a rapport with the patient, which is essential if constructive management plans are to be mutually agreed. The availability of a close friend or relative, able to provide collateral information, can be very helpful.

In the history, particular attention should be paid to previous episodes of mood disturbance, which can offer important clues to the likely prognosis of the present disorder. A careful search for symptoms of hypomania and mania should be made, as the presence of bipolar disorder indicates that a different kind of management of

---

**Box 77.2** Assessment of a depressive condition

- Is the diagnosis major depression (DSM-5) or depressive episode (ICD-10)?
- How severe is this episode, and what is its duration?
- What is the past history of mood disturbance?
- What is the risk of suicide?
- What are the important causal factors?
- What are the patient's social resources?
- How is the depression affecting others?

---

the depressive episode is likely to be necessary (see Chapter 72). The severity of the depressive disorder will have important implications for the kind of treatment that might be suggested first. Here, it is necessary to gauge both the intensity and the range of current symptoms, as well their duration. Identification of melancholic depression or depressive psychosis will also influence treatment selection. The risk of suicide should be assessed in every patient presenting with depression.

Coming to an understanding with the patient about the aetiology of the depressive episode is important in management. As pointed out by Aubrey Lewis [32], in most patients, the depressive episode appears to be the result of a combination of personal predisposition and current life difficulties, though, with the latter, it is important to try to establish which problems have arisen as a result of the depressive condition—often a difficult task. It is important to remember that depressive symptoms may be secondary to another psychiatric disorder or an underlying general medical condition—or its treatment.

Another important part of the assessment is learning about the patient's current social resources, for example how well they are supported in their home and work life and whether they have an understanding confidant. It is also important to consider the effects of the depressive condition on other people, both those close to the patient, such as dependent children, or others who might be affected by the patient's occupation, for example coach drivers or medical workers.

### Treatment setting

The majority of patients with depression are treated in primary care, and many continue to work and carry out family and social activities, albeit with reduced efficiency and enjoyment. Patients with more severe depressive disorders are often quite unable to function and may be in states of considerable anguish and distress, with significant suicidal ideation. An early treatment consideration therefore is how far patients need additional support and what form this should take. A few patients, perhaps because of poor self-care and worrying levels of suicidal thinking, will require inpatient admission. However, if sufficient family support is available, even very ill patients may be managed at home, in conjunction with frequent home visiting and monitoring by a community psychiatric team.

The next question is whether the patient should continue to work. If the disorder is of mild to moderate severity, work can provide a valuable distraction from depressive thoughts and be a source of companionship. If the disorder is more severe, slowness, poor concentration, and low energy are likely to impair work performance, which can increase feelings of hopelessness and may pose risks to others. If patients are not engaged in work, it is important to plan day-to-day activities because depressed patients often give up activities and withdraw from other people. As a result, they become deprived of social stimulation and potentially rewarding experiences, which increases feelings of depression. It is therefore important to make sure that the patient is occupied adequately, although they should not be pushed into activities which will be too demanding.

The appropriate kind of psychological treatment should also be decided in each case. All depressed patients require support, encouragement, and an explanation that they are suffering from an illness, and not some form of moral or other personal failure. Similar counselling of partners and other family members is often useful. It is also important to try and tackle any psychosocial problems that

1. Patients with short-lived mild depression who may recover quickly without treatment should be offered an early review ('active monitoring').
2. Antidepressants are not recommended for the treatment of mild depression.
3. Patients with persistent mild depression should be recommended a guided self-help programme, based on cognitive behavioural therapy. Group cognitive behavioural therapy is an alternative. An exercise programme can also be recommended.
4. For patients with persistent mild depressive symptoms who do not respond to these measures, consider drug treatment with an SSRI or higher-intensity psychological treatment.
5. Patients who present with moderate or severe depression should be treated with a combination of antidepressant medication and a high-intensity psychological intervention.
6. Patients who respond to antidepressant medication should continue treatment for at least 6 months. Patients at high risk of relapse should be advised to continue antidepressant treatment for 2 years.
7. Consider cognitive behavioural therapy for patients who have relapsed despite antidepressant treatment, or mindfulness-based cognitive therapy for patients who are well but who have experienced three or more previous episodes of depression.

Source: data from National Institute for Health and Care Excellence, CG90 *Depression in adults: recognition and management*, Copyright (2009; updated 2018), National Institute for Health and Care Excellence.

are making an important contribution to the depression. For example, couple therapy can be a helpful addition in depressed patients where problems with a partner are playing a role in maintaining the disorder. Other more specific psychological treatments will be indicated for some (see Box 77.3).

## The stepped-care approach

The majority of patients with depression present in primary care with mild to moderate symptoms. It is generally agreed that depressive symptomatology in the community follows a dimensional distribution, with no clear cut-off between the mild and transient depressive feelings common in everyday life and the more severe depressive states that are an indication for some form of medical intervention. In practice, the latter judgement is made on the basis of the number and severity of clinical symptoms, the subjective level of distress, the level of functional impairment, and the length of time for which the symptoms have persisted [33].

Current guidance from the National Institute for Health and Care Excellence (NICE) advises a stepped-care approach, so that depressed patients are treated with the least intrusive approaches first, with more intensive treatments being introduced where improvement does not occur [25, 34] (Box 77.2). Patients with milder symptoms can be helped by the less intensive approaches described earlier, including self-help treatment, group CBT, or exercise. It should be noted, however, that in people with a history of recurrent depressive episodes, even mild symptoms may be a sign of an impending relapse and more active treatment may be indicated.

For patients with moderate levels of depression or greater, NICE recommends a combination of high-intensity psychological treatment (which generally would be individual CBT) and antidepressant medication. This treatment is suggested because systematic reviews indicate that a combination of CBT and medication is superior to medication given alone. However, in practice, it may be difficult to access expert CBT in a timely way, in which case starting treatment with antidepressant medication is appropriate. If, however, individual CBT or IPT are available from a suitably experienced therapist, it is reasonable to use psychotherapy as sole first-line treatment in moderate depression, if the patient prefers.

### Antidepressant medication

Antidepressant medication can be considered for most patients with a major depressive syndrome of at least moderate severity, and particularly those with features of melancholic depression in DSM-5 or somatic depression in ICD-10. Dysthymia is also an indication for antidepressant medication [10, 27].

Most guidelines recommend initial treatment with an SSRI [3, 34]. Several preparations are available, and the differences between them relate largely to the pharmacokinetic profile and the risk of drug interaction (Table 77.2). There have been concerns that early in treatment, SSRI use may be associated with an increased risk of hostile and suicidal behaviour, but meta-analyses of placebo-controlled trials in adults suggest no increase in fatal suicide outcomes. SSRIs may be associated with a small increased risk of non-fatal self-harm,

**Table 77.2** SSRIs available to treat depression

| Drug (daily dose range) | Half-life (hours) | Withdrawal syndrome | CYP inhibition[1] | Cardiotoxicity |
|---|---|---|---|---|
| Citalopram (20–40mg) | 36 | + | 0 | Prolongation of QTc at higher doses |
| Escitalopram (10–20mg) | 30 | + | 0 | Prolongation of QTc at higher doses |
| Fluoxetine (20–60mg) | 90 (plus long-acting metabolite) | 0 | 2D6/2C9 | 0 |
| Fluvoxamine (100–300mg) | 20 | +++ | 1A2/2C9/2C19/3A4 | 0 |
| Paroxetine (20–50mg) | 24 | +++ | 2D6 | 0 |
| Sertraline (50–200mg) | 26 | ++ | 2D6 (modest) | 0 |

[1] Hepatic metabolizing enzymes.

but the number need to harm (759) is much greater than the NNT (about 5) [35]. However, the first few weeks in the clinical management of depression do seem to be a time of increased risk of suicidal behaviour across a range of treatment modalities [36]. Careful and frequent monitoring of patients over this period is therefore prudent.

Patients should be warned about the delayed onset of action of SSRI, as well likely side effects, including nausea and some restlessness during sleep—a forewarned patient is more likely to continue with medication. A number of patients become more anxious and agitated early during SSRI treatment; therefore, it is important to explain that such effects are sometimes experienced during treatment but do not mean that the underlying depression is worsening. If the patient persists with treatment, such anxiety and agitation usually diminish, but short-term treatment with a benzodiazapine may be helpful, particularly if sleep disturbance is a problem. Patients should be reviewed frequently during the first few weeks of treatment, when support and advice are helpful both to maintain morale and to ensure compliance with medication.

If the use of SSRI medication is not suitable or not well tolerated (Box 77.1), a number of other options are available. Mirtazapine has a sedating profile. Less sedating alternatives include the NA and dopamine reuptake inhibitor bupropion, which is licensed for treating major depression in the United States, but not in Europe. In Europe, it is possible to use lofepramine, a tricyclic drug which is predominantly an NA reuptake inhibitor and appears relatively safe in overdose [2].

### Special situations

#### Depression in pregnancy

The management of depression in pregnancy involves careful assessment, together with the provision of accurate information about the risks of depression to the mother and baby and the risks and benefits of different forms of treatment. If a woman has a history of recurrent moderate to severe depression and has been effectively maintained on antidepressant medication, it is generally better to continue this treatment during pregnancy because the risk of relapse is high if medication is withdrawn and there are risks to the fetus of untreated maternal depression. However, women with a history of less severe depression can often withdraw antidepressant medication successfully [37, 38].

Women not taking antidepressant medication who become depressed during pregnancy should be provided with psychoeducation and psychological treatment in a stepped-care manner, depending on the severity of their condition (Box 77.3). If the depression is severe, or if a moderate depressive episode fails to respond to psychological management, antidepressant medication should be offered, usually an SSRI [38]. Generally, the risks of SSRI treatment in pregnancy are low and are outweighed by those of untreated depression. However, self-limiting neonatal withdrawal syndromes have been described, although the incidence across studies varies widely. SSRI use in later pregnancy may also be associated with a small increase (1–2 per 1000 live births) in the risk of pulmonary hypertension of the newborn, a potentially fatal condition [39]. Paroxetine has been associated with cardiac defects and should therefore be avoided in pregnancy; other SSRIs appear to be safe in this respect [38]. There may also be an increased risk of autism in offspring born to mothers taking SSRIs in pregnancy, but whether this is a causal effect of SSRI treatment has yet to be determined.

Antidepressant drugs should also be prescribed cautiously to women who are breastfeeding. The amount of drug that enters breast milk varies according to the individual agent. In terms of SSRI treatment, sertraline is present in milk in only small amounts and breastfeeding may continue while the baby is observed for effects such as sedation and feeding difficulties [2].

#### Depression in childhood and adolescence

For children and young people with persistent depressive disorders that have not responded to simple supportive measures, psychological treatment is regarded as the first-line approach. A systematic review found that both CBT and IPT were superior to wait-list control, whereas psychodynamic therapy was not. IPT and CBT were also superior to problem-solving therapy, but IPT had fewer all-cause discontinuations than CBT [40].

Antidepressant medication seems less effective in child and adolescent depression than in adults, and there is greater evidence for an increased risk of self-harm with SSRIs. A network meta-analysis of several drugs, including TCAs, SSRIs, venlafaxine, and mirtazapine, found that only fluoxetine was reliably better than placebo [41]. Another meta-analysis of 27 placebo-controlled trials of SSRI therapy in young people found no completed suicides, but a small significant increase in suicidal ideation and self-harm attempts in association with SSRI treatment (number needed to harm = 143) [42].

There have been few direct comparisons of medication and psychological treatment in adolescent depression, but the Treatment for Adolescents with Depression Study (TADS), sponsored by the United States National Institute for Mental Health (NIMH), found that after 12 weeks of treatment, response rates for pill placebo (34%) and CBT (43%) were significantly less than for fluoxetine alone (61%) and the combination of CBT and fluoxetine (71%). By 18 weeks, the response to CBT was similar to that found with fluoxetine alone, while the response to combination treatment was still superior. Fluoxetine treatment alone was associated with an increased risk of suicidal ideation and self-harm relative to placebo; however, this increase was not seen in patients in whom fluoxetine was combined with CBT [43]. TADS suggests that the best current treatment for moderate to severe depression in adolescence is a combination of fluoxetine and CBT.

#### Psychotic depression

Determining when the negative thinking of a severely depressed patient has reached delusional intensity is not easy. However, recognizing patients suffering from psychotic depression is important because antidepressant medication is unlikely to be effective as sole treatment. There is a long-held clinical view that pharmacological treatment of depressive psychosis requires combination therapy with antidepressant medication and a dopamine antagonist drug—the latter given at antipsychotic doses. A meta-analysis of nine trials confirmed that such combination treatment was superior to either treatment alone (NNT = 7 vs antidepressant monotherapy; NNT = 5 vs antipsychotic monotherapy) [44]. It is also worth noting that TCAs may be more effective than the newer more pharmacologically selective drugs in the treatment of depressive psychosis [45].

## Use of electroconvulsive therapy

ECT will, very rarely, be part of the first-line treatment of depression and, in such circumstances, will usually be considered only where there is a need to bring about improvement as rapidly as possible. In practice, this applies mainly to patients who are unable to drink enough fluid to maintain an adequate output of urine, including the rare cases of depressive stupor. In depressive psychosis, ECT is considerably more effective than an antidepressant given alone, but probably about the same therapeutic effect can be achieved, albeit more slowly, if a combination of an antidepressant drug and an antipsychotic drug is used [46].

The main use of ECT is in severely depressed patients who have failed to respond to other antidepressant treatments. In these circumstances, a response rate of at least 50% can be expected, though the relapse rate over the next 6 months is high, emphasizing the importance of continuation of pharmacological and psychological treatment [9].

## Failure to respond to first-line antidepressant treatment

If a moderate to severe depressive condition does not respond within a number of weeks to psychological treatment or antidepressant medication, the diagnosis should be reviewed carefully and further assessment made as to whether continuing psychosocial difficulties are perpetuating the disorder. Substance misuse, which is commonly comorbid with depression, may also hinder the response to treatment and may need to be separately addressed (Box 77.2).

If a patient has failed to respond to appropriately delivered psychological treatment, then a trial of medication can be considered. Where there has been a lack of response to antidepressant treatment, it is important to check that the patient has been taking medication as prescribed. If not, the reasons for this should be sought. The patient may be convinced that no treatment can help or may find the side effects unpleasant. If this enquiry is unrevealing, antidepressants should be continued at an increased dose, if possible. In general, SSRIs do not have well-described dose–response relationships, although some patients respond to higher doses, particularly if a partial response has been observed at a standard dose. If psychotherapy has not been offered at this point, a structured psychological treatment, such as CBT or IPT, should be considered if it is available in a timely way.

The large pragmatic Sequenced Treatment Alternatives to Relieve Depression (STAR*D) study found similar response rates when SSRI-non-responsive patients were randomized to CBT or to pharmacological augmentation; however, the pharmacological approach worked more quickly [47]. A study of primary care patients who had failed to respond adequately to antidepressant medication found that CBT (a median of 11 sessions given over 6 months) was markedly superior to TAU in terms of response rate at 6 months (46% vs 22%, respectively; NNT = 4) [48].

If it becomes clear that the patient is not getting better, a number of further steps can be taken to improve pharmacological treatment (Box 77.4). There is not a fixed order in which treatments should be offered. Prescribing decisions should be made in collaboration with the individual patient, taking into account factors such as specific symptomatology, how far the condition may have shown a partial response, and the side effect profile of the various treatment options [46].

---

> **Box 77.4** Some pharmacological treatments for resistant depression
>
> - Increase antidepressant to the maximum dose, if tolerance permits; if the patient has depressive psychosis, add an antipsychotic drug; try a different class of antidepressant drug, including venlafaxine and tricyclic antidepressants.
> - Try an antidepressant combination (for example, an SSRI or venlafaxine with mirtazapine).
> - Add an atypical antipsychotic drug to an SSRI or venlafaxine.
> - Add lithium to antidepressant drug treatment.
> - MAOIs (can be usefully combined with lithium).
> - ECT.
>
> Reproduced from Cowen P, Harrison P, Burns T, *Shorter Oxford Textbook of Psychiatry*, Sixth Edition, Copyright (2012), with permission from Oxford University Press.

### Switching antidepressants

If a patient does not respond to one antidepressant, the first step is usually to stop the first medication and try another. If a patient has not responded to one kind of antidepressant, it would seem sensible to switch to an antidepressant that has different pharmacological properties. However, a meta-analysis showed that switching from an ineffective SSRI to a different class of antidepressant (mirtazapine, venlafaxine, or bupropion) was only marginally better in terms of remission rate than switching to a second SSRI (28% vs 23.5%, respectively; NNT = 22) [49]. Overall, however, around 30% of patients unresponsive to a first antidepressant medication will show some benefit from a switch to a second compound.

Both amitriptyline and venlafaxine appear somewhat more effective than SSRIs in patients with severe depression; these drugs are therefore worth trying at some point in the management of patients who are unresponsive to initial medication trials [9]. While MAOIs are also clearly beneficial in some patients with resistant depression, the food and drug restrictions required mean that these drugs are likely to be used as something of a last resort, unless a patient has responded well to them in the past [9].

### Combination/augmentation of antidepressants

When switching antidepressant preparations, withdrawal of the first compound may not be straightforward. For example, patients may have gained some small symptomatic benefit from the treatment and this may be lost. Also, if the first medication is stopped quickly, withdrawal symptoms can result. On the other hand, a protracted changeover in medication may be distressing for a patient who is in despair about ever feeling better.

For this reason, in patients who are unresponsive or partly responsive to first-line medication, it may be more appropriate to add a second compound to the antidepressant. This is called 'combination therapy' where the second compound is itself considered to be an antidepressant. The term 'augmentation' refers to the addition of a drug that is not by itself regarded as an effective antidepressant but is nevertheless able to produce an therapeutic response when added to ineffective antidepressant medication.

Combination therapy is widely used in patients who have failed to respond to first-line antidepressant treatments, with drugs such as mirtazapine and bupropion commonly being added to ineffective

SSRI and SNRI treatment. However, the evidence that these are efficacious strategies is not well supported by large randomized trials [9]. There is more evidence for the benefit of augmentation therapy, particularly using low-dose atypical antipsychotic drugs. A meta-analysis involving about 3500 patients found that, relative to placebo, the addition of antipsychotics such as aripiprazole and quetiapine to SSRI treatment was significantly more likely to result in clinical remission (NNT = 9) [50]. However, atypical antipsychotics are not well tolerated because of sedation and weight gain in the case of quetiapine, and restlessness and agitation with aripiprazole.

Lithium also appears effective in augmentation treatment when added to ineffective antidepressant medication. Meta-analyses of randomized studies suggest an NNT of around 5, but overall the total number of patients studied is relatively small [51]. In addition, many lithium augmentation studies involved a primary TCA treatment and the efficacy of lithium in augmentation of newer antidepressants is less firmly established. Because of the potential for serotonin toxicity, the addition of lithium to SSRIs and SNRIs should be carried out cautiously, starting at low lithium doses.

### Ketamine

Ketamine is a dissociative anaesthetic that blocks the *N*-methyl-*D*-aspartate (NMDA) subtype of the glutamate receptor. Recent controlled studies have shown that ketamine, given intravenously at a sub-anaesthetic dose, produces a striking and rapid remission of depressive symptoms in patients resistant to conventional pharmacotherapy. The improvement in depression begins about 1 hour after ketamine administration, as dissociative symptoms wane, and can last up to 7 days. A systematic review of controlled studies involving 180 patients with depression found higher rates of clinical response to ketamine than to intravenous saline or intravenous midazolam at 1, 3, and 7 days, with an NNT of 3–5 [52].

The rapid and striking antidepressant effect of ketamine in resistant depression is of great interest. However, it has not proved possible in most patients to maintain the antidepressant effect with the use of oral glutamatergic agents such as riluzole or memantine, which means that repeated administration of intravenous ketamine is often necessary to maintain the therapeutic response. A form of intranasal ketamine has been developed that appears to have acute antidepressant effects and that might be feasible to use for repeated treatment. However, there are concerns about possible ketamine toxicity after repeated use, including bladder changes, as well adverse psychological effects such as dependence [9]. Nevertheless, the antidepressant effect of ketamine has focused attention on the role of glutamate in antidepressant action and might conceivably lead to novel classes of agents for the common clinical problem of resistant depression.

## Continuation and maintenance treatment

### Continuation treatment

After symptomatic remission, follow-up for several months is usually recommended. If the improvement in depression appears to have been brought about by an antidepressant drug, that drug should usually be continued for about 6 months and then gradually withdrawn over a period of several weeks, provided longer-term maintenance treatment is not indicated. If residual depressive symptoms are still present, it is safer not to withdraw medication [3]. At follow-up interviews, a careful watch should be kept for signs of discontinuation reactions or relapse. It is helpful to discuss with the patient the possible early signs of relapse and to develop a plan of action, should any of these signs appear. Involving relatives in this plan can be helpful.

If a patient has responded to CBT or IPT, having some additional sessions during the continuation phase lessens the risk of relapse. It is known that patients with residual depressive symptoms are at greater risk of relapse, and the use of CBT, whatever the primary treatment, can have a useful prophylactic effect in this situation [29]. As noted earlier, there is a high risk of relapse in the 6 months after the use of ECT for resistant depression, and the best continuation therapy is not yet determined. Some benefit has been claimed for a continuation regime of lithium and nortriptyline [15]. The STAR*D study showed that, in general, depressed patients who required several treatment steps to achieve remission had high relapse rates over the next year [53]. In such patients, additional psychological treatment may have a useful role in improving outcome [9].

### Maintenance treatment

Major depression is often recurrent, and long-term maintenance treatment may need to be considered. It is estimated that, among patients who have had three episodes of major depression, the likelihood of another episode is 90%. The usual recommendation is that maintenance drug treatment should be considered if a patient has had two previous episodes of depression within a 5-year period, particularly if there is a family history of recurrent major depression or personal and social factors predictive of recurrence [3]. In addition, the clinician will need to take into account factors such as the likely impact of a recurrence on the patient's life and the previous response to drug treatment, as well as the patient's view of long-term drug therapy [46].

For patients taking antidepressant medication, the longer-term treatment choice is most readily based on the response to acute phase therapy. If, however, a change needs to be made because of adverse effects (for example, sexual dysfunction with SSRIs), an alternative choice can be decided on the basis of the side effect profile. Lithium is not generally employed as monotherapy in longer-maintenance treatment of depression but can be added to antidepressant treatment if the response is inadequate or there is a high risk of suicide [3].

For patients who do not do well with these measures or where a patient at high risk of relapse wishes to discontinue antidepressant medication, there is growing evidence for a role of mindfulness CBT [29, 30]. Sometimes, it appears that the depressive disorder is related to continuing life stressors such as overwork, complicated social relationships, or substance misuse. In this case, various forms of psychotherapy may help adjustment to a lifestyle that is less likely to lead to further illness.

Another important aspect of longer-term follow-up is attention to the physical health of the patient, bearing in mind that people with depression are at substantially increased risk of medical comorbidities, particularly cardiovascular disease and metabolic syndrome [54]. Regular monitoring of relevant aspects of physical health is therefore an important part of overall management.

## REFERENCES

1. Styron W (2004) *Darkness Visible: A Memoir of Madness*. Vintage Books, London.

2. Cowen P, Harrison P, Burns T (2012) Drugs and other physical treatments. In: Cowen P, Harrison P, Burns T. *Shorter Oxford Textbook of Psychiatry* (6th edn). Oxford University Press, Oxford; pp. 507–70.

3. Cleare A, Pariante CM, Young AH, *et al.* (2015) Evidence-based guidelines for treating depressive disorders with antidepressants: a revision of the 2008 British Association for Psychopharmacology guidelines. *Journal of Psychopharmacology*, 29, 459–525.

4. Whiting D and Cowen PJ (2013) Drug information update: agomelatine. *The Psychiatrist*, 37, 356–58.

5. Citrome L (2012) Vilazodone for major depressive disorder: a systematic review of the efficacy and safety profile for this newly approved antidepressant—what is the number needed to treat, number needed to harm and likelihood to be helped or harmed? *International Journal of Clinical Practice*, 66, 356–68.

6. Citrome L (2014) Vortioxetine for major depressive disorder: a systematic review of the efficacy and safety profile for this newly approved antidepressant—what is the number needed to treat, number needed to harm and likelihood to be helped or harmed? *International Journal of Clinical Practice*, 68, 60–82.

7. Cipriani A, Furukawa TA, Salanti G, *et al.* (2009) Comparative efficacy and acceptability of 12 new-generation antidepressants: a multiple-treatments meta-analysis. *The Lancet*, 373, 746–58.

8. Gartlehner G, Gaynes BN, Hansen RA, *et al.* (2008) Comparative benefits and harms of second-generation antidepressants: background paper for the American College of Physicians. *Annals of Internal Medicine*, 149, 734–50.

9. Cowen PJ and Anderson IM (2015) New approaches to treating resistant depression. *Advances in Psychiatric Treatment*, 21, 315–23.

10. Levkovitz Y, Tedeschini E, Papakostas GI (2011) Efficacy of antidepressants for dysthymia: A meta-analysis of placebo-controlled randomized trials. *Journal of Clinical Psychiatry*, 72, 509–14.

11. Barbui C, Cipriani A, Patel V, Ayuso-Mateos JL, van Ommeren M (2011) Efficacy of antidepressants and benzodiazepines in minor depression: systematic review and meta-analysis. *British Journal of Psychiatry*, 198, 11–16.

12. Geddes JR, Carney SM, Davies C, *et al.* (2003) Relapse prevention with antidepressant drug treatment in depressive disorders: a systematic review. *The Lancet*, 361, 653–61.

13. Carney S, Cowen P, Geddes J, *et al.* (2003) Efficacy and safety of electroconvulsive therapy in depressive disorders: a systematic review and meta-analysis. *The Lancet*, 361, 799–808.

14. Birkenhager TK, van den Broek WW, Moleman P, Bruijn JA (2006) Outcome of a 4-step treatment algorithm for depressed inpatients. *Journal of Clinical Psychiatry*, 67, 1266–71.

15. Kellner CH, Knapp RG, Petrides G, *et al.* (2006) Continuation electroconvulsive therapy vs pharmacotherapy for relapse prevention in major depression: a multisite study from the Consortium for Research in Electroconvulsive Therapy (CORE). *JAMA Psychiatry*, 63, 1337–44.

16. Berry SM, Broglio K, Bunker M, Jayewardene A, Olin B, Rush AJ (2013) A patient-level meta-analysis of studies evaluating vagus nerve stimulation therapy for treatment-resistant depression. *Medical Devices* 6, 17–35.

17. Allan CL, Herrmann LL, Ebmeier KP (2011) Transcranial magnetic stimulation in the management of mood disorders. *Neuropsychobiology*, 64, 163–9.

18. Berlim MT, Van den Eynde F, Daskalakis ZJ (2013) Efficacy and acceptability of high frequency repetitive transcranial magnetic stimulation (RTMS) versus electroconvulsive therapy (ECT) for major depression: a systematic review and meta-analysis of randomized trials. *Depression and Anxiety*, 30, 614–23.

19. Rosenthal NE, Sack DA, Gillin JC, *et al.* (1984) Seasonal affective disorder: a description of the syndrome and preliminary findings with light therapy. *JAMA Psychiatry*, 41, 72–80.

20. Mårtensson B, Pettersson A, Berglund L, Ekselius L (2015) Bright white light therapy in depression: a critical review of the evidence. *Journal of Affective Disorders*, 15, 182, 1–7.

21. Cuijpers P, Berking M, Andersson G, Quigley L, Kleiboer A, Dobson KS (2013) A meta-analysis of cognitive-behavioural therapy for adult depression, alone and in comparison with other treatments. *Canadian Journal of Psychiatry*, 58, 376–85.

22. Cuijpers P, van Straten A, Andersson G, van Oppen P (2008) Psychotherapy for depression in adults: a meta-analysis of comparative outcome studies. *Journal of Consulting and Clinical Psychology*, 76, 909–22.

23. Shafran R, Clark DM, Fairburn CG, *et al.* (2009) Mind the gap: Improving the dissemination of CBT. *Behaviour Research and Therapy*, 47, 902–9.

24. Fonagy P (2015) The effectiveness of psychodynamic psychotherapies: an update. *World Psychiatry*, 14, 137–50.

25. National Institute for Health and Care Excellence (2009, updated 2018) *Depression in adults: recognition and management.* Clinical guideline [CG90]. Available at: https://www.nice.org.uk/guidance/cg90/evidence

26. Kvam S, Kleppe CL, Nordhus IH, Hovland A (2016) Exercise as a treatment for depression: a meta-analysis. *Journal of Affective Disorders*, 202, 67–86.

27. Cuijpers P, van Straten A, Schuurmans J, van Oppen P, Hollon SD, Andersson G (2010) Psychotherapy for chronic major depression and dysthymia: a meta-analysis. *Clinical Psychology Review*, 28, 51–62.

28. Fonagy P, Rost F, Carlyle JA, *et al.* (2015) Pragmatic randomized controlled trial of long-term psychoanalytic psychotherapy for treatment-resistant depression: the Tavistock Adult Depression Study (TADS). *World Psychiatry*, 14, 312–21.

29. Bockting CL, Hollon SD, Jarrett RB, Kuyken W, Dobson K (2015) A lifetime approach to major depressive disorder: the contributions of psychological interventions in preventing relapse and recurrence. *Clinical Psychology Review*, 41, 16–26.

30. Kuyken W, Warren FC, Taylor RS, *et al.* (2016) Efficacy of mindfulness-based cognitive therapy in prevention of depressive relapse: an individual patient data meta-analysis from randomized trials. *JAMA Psychiatry*, 73, 565–74.

31. Reynolds III CF, Frank E, Perel JM, *et al.* (1999) Nortriptyline and interpersonal psychotherapy as maintenance therapies for recurrent major depression: a randomized controlled trial in patients older than 59 years. *JAMA Psychiatry*, 281, 39–45.

32. Lewis AJ (1934) Melancholia: a clinical study of depressive states. *British Journal of Psychiatry*, 80, 277–378.

33. Maj M (2011) When does depression become a mental disorder? *British Journal of Psychiatry*, 199, 85–6.

34. National Institute for Health and Care Excellence (2009, updated 2018) *Depression in adults: recognition and management.* Clinical guideline [CG90]. Available at: https://www.nice.org.uk/guidance/cg90/evidence

35. Gunnell D, Saperia J, Ashby D (2005) Selective serotonin reuptake inhibitors (SSRIs) and suicide in adults: meta-analysis of drug company data from placebo controlled, randomised controlled trials submitted to the MHRA's safety review. *BMJ*, 330, 385–90.

36. Simon GE, Savarino J (2007) Suicide attempts among patients starting depression treatment with medications or psychotherapy. *American Journal of Psychiatry*, 164, 1029–34.

37. Jarde A, Morais M, Kingston D, *et al.* (2016) Neonatal outcomes in women with untreated antenatal depression compared with women without depression: a systematic review and meta-analysis. *JAMA Psychiatry*, 73, 826–37.

38. Vigod SN, Wilson CA, Howard LM (2016) Depression in pregnancy. *BMJ*, 352, i1547.

39. Huybrechts KF, Bateman BT, Palmsten K, *et al.* (2015) Antidepressant use late in pregnancy and risk of persistent pulmonary hypertension of the newborn. *JAMA*, 313, 2142–51.

40. Zhou X, Hetrick SE, Cuijpers P, *et al.* (2015) Comparative efficacy and acceptability of psychotherapies for depression in children and adolescents: a systematic review and network meta-analysis. *World Psychiatry*, 14, 207–22.

41. Cipriani A, Zhou X, Del Giovane C, *et al.* (2016) Comparative efficacy and tolerability of antidepressants for major depressive disorder in children and adolescents: a network meta-analysis. *The Lancet*, 388, 881–90.

42. Bridge JA, Iyengar S, Salary CB, *et al.* (2007) Clinical response and risk for reported suicidal ideation and suicide attempts in pediatric antidepressant treatment: a meta-analysis of randomized controlled trials. *JAMA*, 297, 1683–96.

43. March JS, Vitiello B (2009) Clinical messages from the treatment for adolescents with depression study (TADS). *American Journal of Psychiatry*, 166, 1118–23.

44. Farahani A, Correll CU (2012) Are antipsychotics or antidepressants needed for psychotic depression? A systematic review and meta-analysis of trials comparing antidepressant or antipsychotic monotherapy with combination treatment. *Journal of Clinical Psychiatry*, 73, 486–96.

45. Wijkstra J, Burger H, Van den Broek WW, *et al.* (2010) Treatment of unipolar psychotic depression: a randomized, double-blind study comparing imipramine, venlafaxine, and venlafaxine plus quetiapine. *Acta Psychiatrica Scandinavica*, 121, 190–200.

46. Cowen P, Harrison P, Burns T (2012) Mood disorders. In: Cowen P, Harrison P, Burns T. *Shorter Oxford Textbook of Psychiatry* (6th edn). Oxford University Press, Oxford; pp. 205–254.

47. Thase ME, Friedman ES, Biggs MM, *et al.* (2007) Cognitive therapy versus medication in augmentation and switch strategies as second-step treatments: a STAR* D report. *American Journal of Psychiatry*, 164, 739–52.

48. Wiles N, Thomas L, Abel A, *et al.* (2013) Cognitive behavioural therapy as an adjunct to pharmacotherapy for primary care based patients with treatment resistant depression: results of the CoBalT randomised controlled trial. *The Lancet*, 381, 375–84.

49. Papakostas GI, Fava M, Thase ME (2008) Treatment of SSRI-resistant depression: a meta-analysis comparing within-versus across-class switches. *Biological Psychiatry*, 63, 699–704.

50. Spielmans GI, Berman MI, Linardatos E, *et al.* (2013) Adjunctive atypical antipsychotic treatment for major depressive disorder: a meta-analysis of depression, quality of life, and safety outcomes. *PLoS Medicine*, 10, e1001403.

51. Nelson JC, Baumann P, Delucchi K, Joffe R, Katona C (2014) A systematic review and meta-analysis of lithium augmentation of tricyclic and second generation antidepressants in major depression. *Journal of Affective Disorders*, 15, 269–75.

52. McGirr A, Berlim MT, Bond DJ, Fleck MP, Yatham LN, Lam RW (2015) A systematic review and meta-analysis of randomized, double-blind, placebo-controlled trials of ketamine in the rapid treatment of major depressive episodes. *Psychological Medicine*, 45, 693–704.

53. Rush AJ, Trivedi MH, Wisniewski SR, *et al.* (2006) Acute and longer-term outcomes in depressed outpatients requiring one or several treatment steps: a STAR* D report. *American Journal of Psychiatry*, 163, 1905–17.

54. Nemeroff CB, Goldschmidt-Clermont PJ (2012) Heartache and heartbreak—the link between depression and cardiovascular disease. *Nature Reviews Cardiology*, 9, 526–39.

# SECTION 13
# Trauma- and stress-related and adjustment disorders

# 78

# Classification and descriptive psychopathology of post-traumatic stress disorder and other stressor-related disorders

*Dean G. Kilpatrick, Matthew J. Friedman, and Amanda K. Gilmore*

## Introduction

Exposure to stressful adverse events has always been an important part of human life, and the notion that exposure to such events can have a profound impact on our emotions and behaviour was described by philosophers, writers, and artists long before it became the focus of mental health professionals and researchers. Prior to the introduction of the post-traumatic stress disorder (PTSD) diagnosis into the third edition of the *Diagnostic and Statistical Manual of Mental Disorders* (DSM-III) [1], there was widespread recognition that experiencing stressful life events could have numerous negative effects on physical and mental health [2, 3], but there was little to no focus on distinguishing between potentially traumatic vs other stressor events. The PTSD Criterion A (the stressor criterion) serves an important gatekeeping function by distinguishing between stressor events that are and are not considered to be potentially traumatic and capable of producing PTSD. Thus, it is not surprising that one of the most controversial and challenging aspects of the PTSD diagnosis has been defining potentially traumatic events (PTEs) and distinguishing PTEs from other stressor events (OSEs) [4].

PTSD was initially categorized as an anxiety disorder, whereas other disorders that are clearly precipitated by exposure to adverse stressor events [for example, adjustment disorders (ADs) and reactive attachment disorder (RAD)] were placed elsewhere in the DSM. An unintended consequence of this distinction between PTEs and OSEs and the placement of PTSD and other stressor-related disorders in different chapters of prior additions of the DSM was that it obscured the extent to which exposure to stressor events can produce a broad range of mental disorders and health problems. Perhaps the most important change regarding PTSD in DSM-5 [5] was its removal from the 'Anxiety disorders' category and reclassification within a new diagnostic category that captures problems that emerge following exposure to PTEs and OSEs. Although PTSD

may be expressed as a fear-based anxiety disorder, as defined in both DSM-III [1] and DSM-IV [6], it may be expressed also as an anhedonic/dysphoric, externalizing, or dissociative disorder [7].

Given abundant evidence that post-traumatic psychopathology is characterized by a wider range of cognitions, emotions, and behaviour than seen in an anxiety disorder, DSM-5 created a new classification for PTSD and related disorders—'Trauma- and stressor-related disorders'. All diagnoses included in this new chapter have two things in common: (1) a discrete traumatic/adverse event or experience that preceded the onset or aggravation of symptoms; and (2) a wide range of cognitions, emotions, and behaviours embedded within DSM-5 diagnostic criteria for each disorder. This new category includes five specific disorders: PTSD, ASD, AD, RAD, and disinhibited social engagement disorder (DSED). This chapter reviews each of these disorders with respect to DSM-5 diagnostic criteria, separated into adult- and child-specific disorders, describes notable changes from DSM-IV, and discusses theoretical and clinical implications of these changes.

The DSM-5 revision process adopted a very conservative approach and required very strong evidence to modify, delete, or add any symptoms to any diagnostic disorder [8]. As detailed later in this chapter and elsewhere [8, 9], major changes for PTSD were revisions of the stressor criterion (Criterion A1), deletion of Criterion A2, reconceptualizing PTSD's symptom meta-structure as a four-factor model (rather than three factors, as in DSM-IV and DSM-III), revising specific diagnostic criteria, addition of a pre-school subtype, and addition of a dissociative subtype. As with PTSD, ASD diagnostic criteria were modified to recognize the variability of post-traumatic distress responses. Further, the DSM-IV stipulation that three dissociative symptoms were required to meet diagnostic criteria was eliminated from ASD. AD, previously a residual diagnostic category in a class by itself in DSM-IV, was moved into the 'Trauma- and stress-related disorders' category because onset is preceded by an adverse event (PTE or OSE). Finally, the absence of adequate caregiving (for example, extreme insufficient care) is a prerequisite for two childhood disorders—RAD and DSED.

Recognition of the heterogeneity of post-traumatic distress in both PTSD and ASD, with consequent removal of these diagnoses from the 'Anxiety disorders' category raised a number of important theoretical issues. This is highlighted by the very different PTSD conceptualization offered by DSM-5's broad construct, in contrast to the WHO's forthcoming ICD-11 [10], which proposes a very narrow construct of PTSD. The broad DSM-5 approach seeks to 'provide clinicians with a menu of symptoms and symptom clusters that would adequately cover the most typical clinical presentations' [8, p. 550], but ICD-11's narrow approach restricts PTSD diagnostic criteria to symptoms that are unique to PTSD, and not found in other anxiety or mood disorders [10]. Therefore, symptoms, such as insomnia, irritability, cognitive impairment, dysphoria, alienation, and detachment, which occur in DSM-5's PTSD, as well as in other DSM-5 disorders, are eliminated in ICD-11's PTSD criteria. There are 20 PTSD symptoms in DSM-5, with a minimum of six symptoms needed to meet the diagnostic threshold, whereas ICD-11 only has six PTSD symptoms and requires a minimum of three symptoms to meet the diagnostic threshold. As stated elsewhere, to extend the ICD-11 approach to medical diagnoses, 'one would eliminate symptoms such as fever, pain, and edema from the diagnostic criteria of a specific disease because they are found in so many other diseases' [8, p. 550].

## Categorical vs dimensional diagnostic approaches

Both the DSM and ICD systems take categorical approaches towards PTSD and other diagnoses (for more information, see Chapter 7). That is, a person either has a diagnosis based on meeting symptoms and functional impairment thresholds or they do not have a diagnosis because they do not meet these thresholds. This categorical approach has the advantage of simplicity by making it easier to study groups of individuals with and without diagnoses and to determine eligibility for services or compensation based on diagnosis. However, categorical diagnostic approaches have disadvantages and have been criticized on theoretical, empirical, and practical grounds.

The case can be made that the latent construct of PTSD is more dimensional than categorical. Two lines of evidence support this contention. Firstly, a series of studies examined the latent structure of PTSD, using a sophisticated set of statistical procedures called taxometric analysis which used national probability samples of adult women and adolescents in the United States [11], randomly selected combat veterans in Australia [12], and United States combat veterans [13]. Taxometrics is a branch of applied mathematics that determines whether the latent structure of a phenomenon is a taxon (that is, a latent category whose members are qualitatively different from non-members of that category) or non-taxonic (that is, the latent structure is continuous in nature and the differences are quantitative, not qualitative). Analysis of the latent structure of PTSD in these three studies obtained indicators of PTSD symptomatology from individuals that were subjected to taxometric analyses to determine whether the data fit a categorical or a continuous solution. All studies found that the latent structure of PTSD is continuous in nature, not a taxon or distinct category. Secondly, studies of individuals

with PTE exposure with several PTSD symptoms, but not enough to meet diagnostic criteria, still have elevated rates of suicidal behaviours and other problems in functioning [14, 15]. This suggests that it may be more useful to think about people having degrees of PTSD, as opposed to either having PTSD or not.

Although the DSM-5 planning process recognized some of the limitations of its current categorical approach to diagnosis and conducted preliminary work investigating the feasibility of adopting a more dimensional approach, a decision was made that this was premature for DSM-5. Therefore, PTSD remained a categorical diagnosis in DSM-5 and will remain so in ICD-11.

## Post-traumatic stress disorder

### DSM-5 PTSD description and revisions from DSM-IV

The PTSD diagnostic criteria have evolved incrementally with each DSM revision. However, the core features of PTSD have remained similar throughout these evolutionary changes. The underlying assumption of this diagnosis is that exposure to PTEs has the potential to produce a characteristic set of symptoms, resulting in substantial psychological distress and/or functional impairment. Many individuals exposed to PTEs are resilient and do not develop PTSD [16], confirming that PTE exposure is a necessary, but not sufficient, condition for PTSD development and highlighting the importance of understanding factors associated with PTSD. DSM-5 contains PTSD diagnostic criteria, as well as detailed text that describes and elaborates upon these criteria and symptoms.

In DSM-5, Criterion A defines eligible PTEs as an event or events that involve exposure to: (1) death (either actual death or threats of being killed); (2) serious injury; or (3) sexual violence. Exposure to PTEs can happen in one or more of the following four ways: (1) experiencing the event directly; (2) witnessing the PTE happening to someone else in real time, in person, and not via electronic media; (3) learning that the PTE happened to a family member or close friend (note: if the PTE involved the death of a family member or close friend, the cause of death must have been violent or accidental); and (4) experiencing extreme or repeated exposure to disturbing details or aspects of PTEs experienced by other people, usually in a work-related context (for example, collecting human remains following combat, crime, or disasters; law enforcement personnel viewing photos of, or hearing, depictions of child murders or child pornography cases; military drone operators viewing death, destruction precipitated by drone attacks, and psychotherapists exposed to details of their patients' traumatic experiences). In the latter type of exposure, there is exclusion of cases in which exposure occurs through electronic media, television, movies, or pictures, unless the exposure is work-related.

The DSM-5 text gives numerous examples of the types of PTEs that are included in Criterion A. These include serious accidents and natural and man-made disasters, including terrorist attacks; combat or war zone exposure; physical or sexual assault; exposure to hazardous chemicals; torture; witnessing dead bodies or parts of dead bodies; witnessing physical or sexual assaults; threats of injury or death to family members or close friends; deaths of family members or close friends due to violence, accidents, or disasters; and the types of extreme or repeated exposure to disturbing aspects of PTEs experienced by others described previously. Medical procedures can also qualify as PTEs if they 'involve sudden, catastrophic events (for example, waking during surgery, anaphylactic shock)' [5, p. 274].

Four points are important to note about PTEs described in DSM-5. Firstly, the text indicates that the list of PTEs described in the text is not inclusive, so other events can qualify as PTEs, even if they are not specifically listed. Secondly, the Criterion A text and accompanying explanation clearly acknowledge the possibility that many individuals have experienced more than one PTE. Thirdly, the DSM-IV Criterion A (for example, A2) requirement that an event must produce fear, helplessness, or horror to qualify as a PTE was removed from DSM-5, which would likely result in an increase in the number of events qualifying as PTEs in DSM-5 vs in DSM-IV. However, DSM-5 also excluded some events that were included as PTEs in DSM-IV (for example, non-violent deaths of family members or close friends; observing violent events such as mass shootings or terrorist attacks exclusively via electronic media, unless the viewing was work-related), which would reduce the number of events qualifying as PTEs in DSM-5, as compared to DSM-IV. One study with a national sample of United States adults compared the prevalence of lifetime exposure to PTEs using DSM-5 vs DSM-IV Criterion A definition and found that lifetime prevalence was high using both definitions, but that lifetime prevalence of exposure was slightly lower using the DSM-5 Criterion A definition [16]. This suggests that the DSM-5 revisions of Criterion A had largely offsetting effects on the proportion of individuals with a qualifying PTE. However, this study did find that the biggest reason individuals had PTSD with DSM-IV, but not DSM-5, criteria, was exclusion in DSM-5 of deaths that were not violent or accidental. Finally, it is extremely important to understand that defining an event as a qualifying PTE does not mean that everyone exposed to that event will develop PTSD or that all qualifying PTEs have an equal probability of producing PTSD if they are experienced. Some PTEs have a much higher probability of increasing the risk of PTSD than others, as is described in the DSM-5 text.

Criterion B symptoms are: (1) recurrent memories of the PTE that are involuntary, intrusive, and distressing; (2) distressing dreams of the PTE or something that is closely related to the PTE; (3) flashbacks or other dissociative reactions in which the person feels as if the PTE is happening again (note: these dissociative reactions are on a continuum, ranging from feelings that are reliving the PTE all over again to experiencing fragmentary sensory or perceptual sensations that occurred during the PTE); (4) intense or prolonged psychological distress that occurs when someone encounters an internal or external cue that reminds them of the PTE or something that is closely associated with it; and (5) physiological reactions of an extreme nature that occur when a person encounters internal or external cues that remind them of the PTE or something closely associated to it. Criterion B is met if an individual has one or more of these symptoms. Criterion B in DSM-IV was revised in very minor ways, so this criterion is virtually the same as in DSM-5, with the exception of minor changes in language.

Criterion C has two symptoms that measure persistent avoidance of stimuli that are associated with a PTE: (1) avoiding, or attempts to avoid, distressing memories, thoughts, or feelings about a PTE or something that is closely associated with a PTE; and (2) avoiding or attempting to avoid external reminders of the PTE that arouse distressing memories, thoughts, or feelings about the PTE or things that are closely associated with it. Examples of such external

reminders include people, places, conversations, activities, objects, or situations. Criterion C is met if an individual has at least one of these symptoms.

One of the biggest revisions of DSM-IV criteria in DSM-5 was constructing a new Criterion C that contains only two active avoidance symptoms by pulling these symptoms out of DSM-IV Criterion C that included both avoidance and numbing symptoms. DSM-IV Criterion C had two avoidance symptoms and five numbing symptoms, and three Criterion C symptoms were required to meet the threshold. This meant that someone could meet the DSM-IV Criterion C threshold of three symptoms without having any active avoidance symptoms. Numerous factor-analytic studies found that DSM-IV Criterion C symptoms were split into an avoidance symptom factor and a numbing symptom factor. This provided ample justification for creating a separate criterion for active avoidance symptoms [7]. Some critics of DSM-5 have expressed concern that requiring the presence of at least one active avoidance symptom to obtain a PTSD diagnosis in DSM-5 will result in some people not having PTSD using DSM-5 criteria who would have PTSD using DSM-IV criteria [17]. Others argue that avoidance has always been an important part of the PTSD construct and clinical picture [16] and that the presence of active avoidance distinguishes PTSD from other disorders, including major depression [12]. The Kilpatrick et al. study [16] did find that failure to have at least one active avoidance symptom was the second biggest reason for persons meeting DSM-IV but failing to meet DSM-5 criteria for PTSD, but this occurred in a very small number of cases. Taking all of this into consideration, the DSM-5 revision requiring active avoidance is well justified because avoidance has always been a key component of the PTSD construct.

Criterion D has seven symptoms measuring negative alterations in cognition and mood. These symptoms must be associated with the PTE and must have either begun after, or been aggravated by exposure to, the PTE. Criterion D symptoms are: (D1) inability to recall important aspects of the PTE, typically due to dissociative amnesia and not due to other factors such as head injury or heavy alcohol or drug use; (D2) negative beliefs and/or expectations about others or the world that are persistent and exaggerated; (D3) distorted cognitions about the cause or consequences of the PTE that result in the person unreasonably blaming themselves or others for what happened; (D4) negative emotional states such as feelings of fear, horror, anger, guilt, or shame; (D5) diminished interest or participation in important life activities; (D6) feeling detached or estranged from other people; and (D7) inability to experience positive emotions such as happiness, satisfaction, or loving feelings. At least two of these symptoms are required to meet Criterion D.

ICD-11 proposed criteria for PTSD have no negative cognition or mood symptoms [10, 18]. However, there is substantial evidence that exposure to PTEs can produce these alterations and that exposed individuals who develop PTSD are significantly more likely to have negative alterations in cognition and mood. Two papers using data from a large national sample of United States adults addressed this issue. The first paper compared the prevalence of D2 and D3 symptoms among individuals with no PTE exposure, PTE exposure that did not result in PTSD, and PTE exposure that did result in PTSD [19]. Participants identified the type of cognitive distortion experienced if D2 or D3 was endorsed. No significant differences were found between groups with no PTE exposure or PTE exposure that did not result in PTSD. However, those with PTSD were significantly more likely to believe that they were a bad person; that they could not trust anyone; that nothing good would ever occur; that they had no chance for a career, relationship, marriage, or children; that their soul or spirit was permanently damaged; and that the world was completely dangerous. The group with PTSD was also significantly more likely to exhibit beliefs that the PTE happened because of something they did wrong; that they should have been able to prevent it; that the event happened because of something about them; and that they blamed themselves for not being able to recover and get on with their lives.

The second paper examined associations between specific negative emotions in symptom D4 and a DSM-5 PTSD diagnosis among adults who had experienced a PTE involving a physical or sexual assault [20]. Compared to individuals with assault histories who did not develop PTSD, individuals with assault-related PTSD were significantly more likely to have several negative emotions, including anger, guilt, shame, and horror, as well as fear. This study also found that the emotion of anger among those with PTSD was more prevalent than the emotion of fear.

Criterion E consists of major alterations in arousal and reactivity associated with the PTE. There are six symptoms, two or more of which are required and most of which are identical to those in DSM-IV Criterion D. However, two symptoms are new or substantially modified. Symptom E1 is irritable behaviour and angry outbursts that are expressed as verbal or physical aggression towards other people or objects. This symptom requires some behavioural manifestation of anger and aggression, not just an angry mood, and there is considerable evidence that individuals with PTSD have a substantially higher prevalence of the symptom than those without PTSD [20, 21]. Symptom E2 is reckless or self-destructive behaviour such as dangerous driving, excessive alcohol or drug abuse, or risky sexual behaviour. The behaviours described in E1 and E2 have long been a part of the clinical picture of many patients with PTSD and have also been an important focus of clinical treatment efforts. The remaining Criterion E symptoms are hypervigilance, exaggerated startle response, problems with concentration, and sleep difficulties.

As was the case with DSM-IV, PTSD in DSM-5 cannot be diagnosed unless the symptoms persist for at least 1 month (Criterion F). Likewise, PTSD cannot be diagnosed unless symptoms produce significant distress and/or functional impairment (Criterion G).

PTSD in DSM-5 has two other additions of note. Firstly, there is a new explicit set of PTSD criteria for children aged 6 years or younger. Child trauma professionals had observed that young children had extremely low rates of PTSD, using DSM-IV criteria, primarily due to adult-centric phrasing of symptoms and the requirement to have an inappropriately high number of symptoms within the DSM-IV Criteria C and D to meet the diagnostic threshold. Consequently, the DSM-5 child PTSD diagnostic criteria use a more child-centric language focus on observable behaviours, while eliminating subjective symptoms, and reduce the number of symptoms per criterion to meet the diagnosis. Secondly, there is a new dissociative subtype of PTSD, defined on the basis of repeated experiencing of either depersonalization or derealization. This addition was based on evidence of neurobiological differences among individuals with PTSD with and without these dissociative symptoms [22], as well as evidence that treatment outcome is worse among PTSD-positive patients with dissociative symptoms [7, 23].

## PTSD prevalence

Obtaining accurate estimates of PTSD prevalence requires the use of a probability sample of the population in question, comprehensive assessment of PTE exposure, and thorough assessment of PTSD symptoms and symptom-related distress/functional impairment [24, 25]. Several good studies provide information about PTSD prevalence using DSM-IV criteria. The National Comorbidity Survey-Replication (NCS-R) [26] found that the lifetime prevalence of PTSD among a national probability sample of United States adults was 6.8% overall, 7.9% among women, and 3.6% among men. The National Epidemiologic Survey on Alcohol and Related Conditions (NESARC) [27] reported that the lifetime prevalence PTSD was 7.3%. A study of PTSD among a national household probability sample of United States adolescents found that the past 6-month prevalence of PTSD was 6.3% among female adolescents and 3.7% among male adolescents [28].

Limited data are available about the impact of the DSM-5 revisions on PTSD prevalence. However, one study that compared PTSD prevalence using DSM-IV and DSM-5 criteria in a large national sample of United States adults found slightly lower prevalence using DSM-5 vs DSM-IV criteria for lifetime (8.3% vs 9.8%, respectively), the past 12 months (4.7% vs 6.3%, respectively), and the past 6 months (3.8% vs 4.7%, respectively) PTSD [16]. Another major study with a large national probability sample of United States adults reported that the lifetime and past-year prevalence of PTSD using DSM-5 criteria were, respectively, 6.1% and 4.7% [29], but this is clearly an underestimate of DSM-5 PTSD prevalence due to the use of an incorrect diagnostic algorithm requiring three symptoms each for Criteria D and E, instead of the two symptoms in each that are actually required. Another study of United States Army soldiers by Hoge and colleagues [30] confirmed that PTSD prevalence using DSM-5 vs DSM-IV criteria was slightly lower (11.5% and 12.3, respectively). In summary, the data are clear that DSM-5 PTSD is a prevalent disorder, with a prevalence that appears to be slightly lower overall than when using DSM-IV criteria.

## PTSD in ICD-11

The ICD-11 revision is scheduled for completion in 2019, so no proposed changes have been finalized. However, it is apparent from a draft of the proposed criteria and descriptions of the proposed approach that the ICD-11 version of PTSD is likely to be a radical departure from the DSM-5 version of PTSD, as well as from the DSM-IV and ICD-10 version of PTSD [10, 18]. The most radical proposed change separates PTSD into two disorders: PTSD and complex PTSD. The stated rationale is to narrow the scope of the PTSD construct, reduce the number of symptoms from 20 in DSM-5 to six in the ICD-11 proposal, increase diagnostic reliability, and eliminate a large number of symptoms that overlap with other disorders such as depression [10, 18].

The ICD-11 proposed definition of Criterion A describes exposure to an extremely threatening or horrific event or a series of events which is substantially less specific than the DSM-5 definition. The ICD-11 PTSD proposal focuses on three core elements: (1) re-experiencing of the trauma; (2) avoidance of reminders of the event; and (3) a heightened perception of threat and arousal. This ICD-11 proposal for PTSD is operationalized by requiring at least one (of two) re-experiencing symptom (that is, flashbacks or nightmares), one (of two) avoidance symptom (that is, avoidance of internal or external reminders), and one (of two) hyperarousal symptom (that is, hypervigilance or exaggerated startle response) [10, 18, 31]. The ICD-11 proposal omits the entire DSM-5 Criterion D and omits four of the DSM-5 Criterion E hyperarousal symptoms (that is, E1 irritable behaviour and angry outbursts; E2 reckless and self-destructive behaviour; E5 concentration difficulties; and E5 sleep difficulties). This PTSD proposal, like DSM-5, but unlike ICD-10, requires the symptoms to produce distress and/or functional impairment.

Complex PTSD is a controversial diagnosis which has been criticized on conceptual and empirical grounds [27, 31]. Under the ICD-11 proposal, the first requirement for complex PTSD is to have the diagnosis of PTSD. Complex PTSD, as defined by ICD-11 proposal [10, 18], requires at least one symptom in each of three complex PTSD symptom clusters: (1) affect dysregulation (that is, emotional reactivity, dissociation, anger, aggression, and emotional numbing); (2) negative self-concept (that is, negative beliefs about the core value of the self, along with feelings of guilt and shame); and (3) interpersonal disturbances (that is, avoidance of relationships, estrangement, and lack of emotional intimacy in relationships). Complex PTSD was not included in DSM-5 due to a lack of supporting evidence [7].

An obvious question is the effect these extensive revisions might have on PTSD prevalence and whether there is an impact on the percentage of those exposed to a PTE who meet diagnostic criteria for PTSD, because having a diagnosis is often required to qualify for treatment services or other benefits. The few head-to-head comparisons of ICD-11 vs DSM-5 prevalence and caseness indicate that the ICD-11 proposal may produce a dramatic reduction in PTSD prevalence and caseness. Wisco and colleagues [32] compared past-month PTSD prevalence using DSM-5 and ICD-11 criteria in a national sample of United States adults and a sample of United States military veterans. The prevalence of past-month PTSD prevalence using ICD-11 criteria was lower than when using DSM-5 criteria in both national adult and veteran samples. O'Donnell and colleagues [33] also reported the same pattern of findings in a probability sample of injury patients from four hospitals. A study from Denmark [34] also found that PTSD prevalence was lower using ICD-11, as opposed to DSM-5, criteria. An international study conducted in 13 countries [15] did not actually assess PTSD using DSM-5 and ICD-11 criteria but approximated these diagnoses using data from DSM-IV assessments. This study reported a slightly higher PTSD prevalence estimate when using the ICD-11 approximation (3.2% vs 3.0% for DSM-5), but the DSM-5 estimate was clearly lower than it should have been due to the three new symptoms not having been measured. Although more research on this topic is needed, findings suggest that the proposed ICD-11 PTSD criteria are likely to have the unintended consequence of reducing the prevalence of PTSD and the number of people with a PTSD diagnosis that could qualify them for treatment and other services.

## Acute stress disorder

Acute stress disorder (ASD) was first introduced in DSM-IV and significantly updated in DSM-5. The DSM-5 definition includes exposure to a Criterion A PTE, as described previously in the PTSD criteria. The key difference between PTSD and ASD is time and markers of distress. ASD is defined as distress occurring after 3 days, but within 1 month of a Criterion A PTE. Further, ASD requires nine or more symptoms in the five major categories of intrusion, negative mood, dissociative, avoidance, and arousal symptoms (DSM-5). Consistent with other mental health disorders, the symptoms must cause clinically significant distress or functional impairment.

DSM-III [1] did not permit a trauma-related diagnosis prior to 1-month post-traumatic event exposure, perhaps due to the normative symptoms associated with experiencing traumatic events. The introduction of ASD as a mental health disorder within DSM-IV [6] allowed for individuals who have marked distress due to a PTE within 1 month of the PTE to receive clinical services that may potentially decrease distress and the development of PTSD. However, the DSM-IV definition of ASD gave excessive weight to dissociative symptoms. Although other symptoms, including anxiety and arousal, were part of the diagnosis, individuals needed three or more dissociative symptoms in order to meet the criteria. In fact, several other acute symptoms are associated with the development of PTSD, rather than only peritraumatic dissociation [35]. When developing DSM-5, several critiques regarding DSM-IV definitions of ASD were considered, including questioning the predictive value of ASD in predicting the development of PTSD, differentiating ASD from other mental health disorders, the utility of ASD to enhance early intervention, and the general utility of the ASD diagnosis. These critiques have been described elsewhere in more detail [35–37], but recommendations for DSM-5 primarily focused on the broadening of symptoms to remove DSM-IV's unjustified emphasis on dissociative symptoms.

The DSM-5 definition of ASD differs from that of the DSM-IV definition in several ways. Firstly, the definition of a PTE was updated to be consistent with the new definition of a PTE, as described in PTSD. The most marked change in symptom presentation was the elimination of DSM-IV's requirement of three or more dissociative symptoms, while giving greater weight to a broader set of symptoms in DSM-5. Although DSM-5 does recognize that some people may experience dissociative symptoms, others may now meet ASD criteria without a single dissociative symptom. In other words, there has been a shift in our understanding of ASD from a predominantly dissociative disorder to one that includes a greater variability in symptom presentation.

Preliminary evidence suggests that both DSM-IV and DSM-5 criteria have equal predictive value related to the development of PTSD, but DSM-5 criteria have greater specificity, compared to DSM-IV criteria [35]. According to DSM-5, there are higher rates of ASD among individuals who have experienced interpersonal PTEs (20–50%), compared to non-interpersonal PTE (<20%) [5, p. 284]. Therefore, ASD is quite common and should be regularly assessed for among populations who have experienced recent PTEs. Although ASD is not always predictive of PTSD, individuals with ASD (and those without) should also be assessed for PTSD if they continue (or develop) significant symptoms of distress or impairment 1 month following a PTE.

## Adjustment disorders

Until DSM-5, ADs constituted a cluster of residual diagnoses that occupied their own space in DSM-III or DSM-IV. Divided into anxiety and depressed and disturbed conduct subtypes (or some combination of these), ADs were perhaps the most poorly characterized set of diagnoses within DSM. There were no specific symptoms needed to make the diagnoses. Indeed, all that was necessary was prior exposure to an adverse event (PTE or OSE) and a clinician's judgement that 'significant distress or functional impairment' had its onset because the exposure took place. In many cases, ADs have been considered subthreshold anxiety or mood disorders, although it has never been clear how disturbed conduct relates to better explicated DSM diagnoses.

The AD diagnosis seems to be relatively common. According to DSM-5, 'prevalence may vary widely as a function of the population studied and the assessment methods used' [5, p. 287]. In outpatient cohorts, the prevalence ranges from 5% to 20%. In hospital psychiatric consultation settings, the prevalence may reach 50% [5].

When considering ADs, the DSM-5 workgroup was faced with various definitions of AD—was it a bona fide diagnosis in its own right, a subthreshold anxiety/mood disorder (like dysthymia and cyclothymia), or something else? Given the lack of rigorous research and poor validation for the various AD subtypes, it was unclear how and whether they related to one another [38]. Some investigators formulated the diagnosis as a subthreshold PTSD syndrome [39], but again, evidence was lacking. Finally, given the DSM-5 ground rules that no diagnostic criterion could be added, deleted, or modified without strong empirical evidence and given the almost complete lack of such evidence (because of the lack of published research) when it came to ADs, it is not surprising that the DSM-5 version of ADs resembles the DSM-IV version very closely.

There were two important decisions regarding ADs that should promote research, which should usefully guide future revisions of DSM-5. Firstly, ADs were removed from their own category and moved into the 'Trauma and stressor-related disorders' chapter of DSM-5. Secondly, ADs were reconceptualized as a stress-related disorder that might share a common pathophysiology with PTSD and ASD, since failure to cope with an overwhelming stressor appears to characterize all of these disorders.

## Child-specific symptoms and disorders

In addition to the mental health disorders described, there are specific disorders for children within the trauma- and stressor-related disorders section of DSM-5. This includes PTSD, RAD, and DSED.

PTSD can be diagnosed among children; however, as discussed, DSM-5 outlines several modifications for children under the age of 6 (the preschool subtype). These child-specific symptoms were suggested after compiling 15 years of research suggesting that there may be specific developmental manifestations of symptoms [13]. Specifically, intrusive memories may manifest as re-enactment of the traumatic event; children may not be able to connect the content of nightmares to the traumatic event, and irritable behaviour may manifest as extreme temper tantrums. It is important to consider these child-specific manifestations of symptomology related to traumatic event exposure, as they differ from adults.

RAD and DSED are both diagnoses for young children older than 9 months. Both RAD and DSED are thought to be caused by social neglect, defined by DSM-5 as 'the absence of adequate caregiving during childhood' [5, p. 265]; therefore, this is a requirement for

both diagnoses. DSM-IV included only one disorder—RAD—with two subtypes (inhibited and disinhibited), but now the two subtypes are considered separate disorders in DSM-5. RAD includes predominantly internalizing symptoms, while DSED includes predominantly externalizing symptoms. Both disorders are considered to be rare, and the prevalence, even among severely neglected children, ranges from 10% for RAD to 20% for DSED [5].

Diagnostic criteria for RAD include symptoms of emotional withdrawal towards an adult caregiver and marked social and emotional disturbance, both presumably caused by social neglect. Children who meet criteria for RAD must engage in both minimal comfort-seeking and minimal responding to comfort from the caregiver when distressed. Further, children must exhibit two of the following: social withdrawal prior to the age of 2, persistent lack of positive mood, and 'episodes of unexplained irritability, sadness, or fearfulness' with their caregivers [5, p. 265]. Children are eligible for this diagnosis between the ages of 9 months and 5 years.

In contrast, DSED occurs when a child regularly interacts with unfamiliar adults in a disinhibited manner. Children who meet criteria for DSED must engage in two behaviours related to interacting with unfamiliar adults, including: (1) approaching unfamiliar adults; (2) in a disinhibited manner, including being overfamiliar with the unfamiliar adults; (3) without checking in with the caregiver; and (4) leaving with the unfamiliar adults. Similar to RAD, there must be a pattern of social neglect from the caregiver. Although both child-specific disorders are rare, they have the potential to have a significant impact on the children's lives if left untreated.

## Other specified trauma- and stressor-related disorders

In addition to the disorders described, there are several disorders that are considered to be trauma- and stressor-related but did not fit the previously referenced diagnoses. These disorders cause significant distress and functional impairment but are either not specified within the already described disorders, are culturally specific disorders, or require further study in order to determine their existence as separate disorders. These include adjustment-like disorders with delayed onset or prolonged duration, ataque de nervios and other culturally specific disorders, and unspecified trauma- and stressor-related disorders. Persistent complex bereavement disorder (PCBD) embodies symptoms otherwise categorized as complicated grief or prolonged grief disorder. Because it has not been established which symptoms best characterize pathological grief reactions, PCBD now only appears only in the DSM-5 appendix as a presumptive disorder that requires future research (for more information, see Chapter 84).

Although there is currently not a specific diagnosis for those who have PTSD symptoms but fail to meet all of the diagnostic criteria of PTSD, this 'diagnosis' is currently best captured within the 'Other trauma-related disorder' category. This is sometimes referred to as subthreshold, subsyndromal, subclinical, or partial PTSD, but the term partial PTSD has achieved the most widespread usage [15]. Partial PTSD has been operationally defined several ways, but they all require individuals to have several PTSD symptoms. Unfortunately, there is no current consensus on a case definition for partial PTSD in DSM-5, since different investigators have used different criteria in their research. Achievement of such a case definition should be a high priority for research in this field. As noted in Schnurr's recent review [15], partial PTSD is prevalent, and individuals with partial PTSD often have lower rates of functional impairment/distress than those with full PTSD, but higher rates than their counterparts who were exposed to PTEs but who had no PTSD symptoms.

Such findings are strikingly similar to what would be predicted if PTSD is continuous, as opposed to categorical. Also, many individuals with partial PTSD seek clinical services or attempt to enrol in PTSD research studies. Lacking one PTSD symptom can sometimes make the difference between having PTSD and having partial PTSD, and the former would be eligible for treatment services or research studies recruiting individuals with PTSD, whereas the latter would not.

## Co-occurring disorders

Trauma- and stressor-related disorders often have several key co-occurring disorders. Many disorders may co-occur partially due to overlapping symptomology (that is, which include both depressive and anxiety disorders). Other disorders co-occur possibly as a means to cope with the symptoms associated with experiencing stress and trauma (that is, substance use disorders). Other disorders may also be related to PTE exposure (that is, borderline personality disorder and dissociative identity disorder). When the psychological trauma is accompanied by head injury (for example, combat and motor vehicle accidents), traumatic brain injury is often a co-occurring condition. Although a thorough discussion of co-occurring disorders is beyond the scope of the current chapter, it is important to mention that co-occurring disorders can significantly complicate treatment and therefore should be thoroughly assessed. Historically, it was thought that disorders like PTSD should not be treated if there are other disorders that may complicate treatment (that is, substance use disorders or borderline personality disorder). However, recent treatment outcome research indicates that concurrent treatment of trauma-related disorders and other disorders should be strongly considered due to its efficaciousness [27, 40, 41].

## What is needed to move the science forward in understanding trauma- and stressor-related disorders?

For a better understanding of how to best classify, assess, and treat trauma- and stressor-related disorders, more research is needed in several areas. More work is needed to integrate the dimensional approach into the current categorical diagnostic criteria. With respect to PTSD, there are three major ways to accomplish this. Firstly, it is important to conduct taxometric analyses with DSM-5 PTSD symptoms to confirm the continuous nature of PTSD latent structure using the new criteria. Secondly, there is great merit to utilize continuous, as well as categorical, measures of PTSD symptoms/symptom frequency/symptom intensity in research and clinical practice. Thirdly, both research and clinical practice should make more use of the partial PTSD construct, because it is clear that individuals not meeting full diagnostic criteria still have significant problems that could benefit from increased research and clinical attention. Moreover, increased use of the partial PTSD construct might also be useful in

addressing discrepancies in PTSD caseness using DSM-5 vs DSM-IV criteria. To the best of our knowledge, no research has been done to date, in which comparisons of the overlap between PTSD cases using DSM-IV and DSM-5 criteria also included individuals with partial PTSD. Our hypothesis is that the inclusion of partial PTSD cases would substantially increase the diagnostic concordance and reduce discrepancies.

### PTSD assessment

There is a substantial literature on specific structured interview and self-report measures that have been used to assess PTSD [42, 43], so we will make three general points, rather than provide a detailed discussion of assessment measures. Firstly, an accurate assessment cannot be conducted without a thorough assessment of PTE exposure across the lifespan. In clinical, as well as research, settings, this requires asking a series of behaviourally specific questions about all types of relevant PTE exposure.

Secondly, you cannot accurately assess for PTSD or partial PTSD unless your assessment asks about all 20 DSM PTSD symptoms. It is relatively common for some PTSD assessment instruments to use screening questions or skip-outs in which individuals are not asked about all PTSD symptoms once it becomes clear that they cannot meet the full diagnostic criteria. However, these skip-outs make it impossible to determine whether someone has partial PTSD, and we believe that a strong case can be made that skip-outs should never be used in PTSD assessment.

Thirdly, the typical approach to PTSD assessment in multiple PTE exposure cases is to assess PTSD symptoms in reference to one index PTE (for example, the most recent PTE, the most serious or worse PTE, a PTE of particular interest such as rape or military combat, or a randomly selected PTE). However, exposure to multiple PTEs can result in composite PTSD, defined as meeting PTSD diagnostic criteria in which the PTSD symptoms incorporate content related to more than one PTE [16]. This requires a different assessment approach that first determines whether individuals have each PTSD symptom and then determines which PTE or PTEs caused or aggravated the symptom. Not surprisingly, composite PTSD was more prevalent than PTSD to a single event, and its prevalence increased as a function of the number of PTEs that were experienced [16]. We believe that a challenge to PTSD researchers and clinicians will be to develop assessment strategies that better address the issue of how multiple PTE exposure relates to PTSD symptomatology. Further, more research concerning the other trauma- and stressor-related disorders, specifically with respect to PCBD and ADs. Research is needed regarding the diagnostic criteria of ADs and PCBD and how these disorders may or may not overlap with other disorders within this diagnostic cluster.

It remains to be seen whether there are similar or overlapping psychobiological consequences of traumatic event exposure in PTSD and ASD, adverse experiences in ADs, and insufficient care in RAD and DSED. Research on biomarkers and underlying pathophysiological abnormalities promises to improve our understanding of how effective psychobiological mechanisms for stress and adaptation are dysregulated in the five trauma- and stressor-related disorders.

### Are there different PTSD phenotypes?

By the time DSM-6 is published, it is possible that there will be no longer a PTSD diagnosis, as we have known it since DSM-III. When first introduced in 1980, PTSD was revolutionary because it validated the notion that an overwhelming stressor can produce stable alterations in cognitions, emotions, and behaviours that result in recognizable symptom clusters. The explosion of research, since that time, has made it abundantly clear that there are a variety of post-traumatic clinical presentations that meet diagnostic criteria for PTSD. Currently, this is best exemplified in DSM-5 ASD, as discussed previously. Indeed, DSM-5 PTSD has been criticized because it has so many different symptoms, in contrast to most other psychiatric disorders such as major depressive disorder and most anxiety disorders [17, 44].

To us, the best explanation for such complexity is that we have tried to sweep all significant post-traumatic symptomatology under a single PTSD rug. Indeed, based on clinical phenomenology alone, there appear to be four different PTSD phenotypes: (1) an adrenergic fear-based anxiety disorder; (2) an anhedonic/dysphoric disorder; (3) an externalizing disorder; and (4) a dissociative disorder [45]. It is likely that the ongoing Research Domain Criteria (RDoC) approach will identify different genetic or other biomarkers that may be more strongly associated with one phenotype than another (see Chapter 8 for more on RDoC). For example, the dissociative phenotype (currently categorized as PTSD's dissociative subtype) is characterized by unique brain imagery patterns and treatment responsivity [22]. Evidence for an adrenergic subtype is indicated by selective responsivity to the adrenergic antagonist prazosin among soldiers with PTSD who recorded the highest blood pressure [46]. A specific biological marker dopamine-beta-hydroxylase (DBH), which catalyses the conversion of dopamine to noradrenaline, is uniquely associated with Criterion B intrusion symptoms; indeed, preliminary data have shown that plasma DBH levels appear to be causally related to the development of PTSD intrusion symptoms [44]. We expect that progress along these fronts may eventually result in explication of a number of more specific post-traumatic syndromes, rather than the very complex array of clinical presentations currently embodied in the solitary DSM-5 PTSD diagnosis. A list of potential phenotypes might include: post-traumatic hyperarousal/hyperadrenergic, post-traumatic anhedonic/serotonin-deficient, post-traumatic dissociative, etc. syndromes. If and when we can confidently identify different PTSD phenotypes, it is likely to have two major implications for diagnosis and treatment. Firstly, it may result in a spectrum of post-traumatic syndromes differentiated by a more concise set of diagnostic criteria that will include phenotype-specific biomarkers. Secondly, it may facilitate treatment matching, so that individuals with a certain phenotype will receive treatments best suited for their specific post-traumatic phenotype.

In short, DSM-5 has opened the way for considering PTSD as a spectrum disorder, in which research on phenotypes is the inevitable next step. We look forward to the future identification of distinct post-traumatic diagnoses with different underlying pathophysiologies that will respond best to different optimal treatments.

## Conclusions

The diagnostic criteria and classification for trauma- and stressor-related disorders have undergone significant changes with DSM-5 and are proposed to include even more drastic changes within ICD-11. The iterative changes in diagnostic criteria and classification highlights not only the extensive research that has gone into understanding these phenomena, but also the challenges that arise when examining disorders that stem from PTEs and OSEs. Given the current knowledge, there are several needed next steps to understand how to best classify trauma- and stressor-related disorders which includes, but is not limited to: (1) further clarifying partial PTSD and deciding whether classification under a dimensional vs a categorical approach would be beneficial; (2) continuing to refine assessments to ensure that PTEs and OSEs are thoroughly assessed and symptoms after these experiences are best captured; and (3) continuing to examine potential phenotypes of trauma- and stressor-related disorders.

## REFERENCES

1. American Psychiatric Association. *Diagnostic and Statistical Manual of Mental Disorders* (3rd edn). American Psychiatric Association: Washington, DC; 1980.
2. Dohrenwend BS, Dohrenwend BP. *Stressful Life Events: Their Nature and Effects*. John Wiley: New York, NY; 1974.
3. Meyer A. *Psychobiology, A Science of Man*. Thomas: Springfield, IL; 1957.
4. Cougle JR, Kilpatrick DG, Resnick H. Defining traumatic events: research findings and controversies. In: Beck JG, Sloan DM (eds). *The Oxford Handbook of Traumatic Stress Disorders*. Oxford University Press: New York, NY; 2012. pp. 11–27.
5. American Psychiatric Association. *Diagnostic and Statistical Manual of Mental Disorders* (5th edn). American Psychiatric Association: Washington, DC; 2013.
6. American Psychiatric Association. *Diagnostic and Statistical Manual of Mental Disorders* (4th edn, text revision). American Psychiatric Association: Washington, DC; 2000.
7. Friedman MJ, Resick PA, Bryant RA, Brewin CR. Considering PTSD for DSM-5. *Depress Anxiety*. 2011;28:750–69.
8. Friedman MJ. Finalizing PTSD in DSM-5: getting here from there and where to go next. *J Trauma Stress*. 2013;26:548–56.
9. Friedman MJ, Kilpatrick DG, Schnurr PP, Weathers FW. Correcting misconceptions about the diagnostic criteria for posttraumatic stress disorder in DSM-5. *JAMA Psychiatry*. 2016;73:753–54.
10. Maercker A, Brewin CR, Bryant RA, *et al*. Proposals for mental disorders specifically associated with stress in the International Classification of Diseases-11. *Lancet*. 2013;381:1683–5.
11. Broman-Fulks JJ, Ruggiero KJ, Green BA, *et al*. Taxometric investigation of PTSD: Data from two nationally representative samples. *Behav Ther*. 2006;37:364–80.
12. Forbes D, Haslam N, Williams BJ, Creamer M. Testing the latent structure of posttraumatic stress disorder: a taxometric study of combat veterans. *J Trauma Stress*. 2005;18:647–56.
13. Ruscio AM, Ruscio J, Keane TM. The latent structure of posttraumatic stress disorder: a taxometric investigation of reactions to extreme stress. *J Abnorm Psychol*. 2002;111:290–301.
14. McLaughlin KA, Koenen KC, Friedman MJ, *et al*. Subthreshold posttraumatic stress disorder in the world health organization world mental health surveys. *Biol Psychiatry*. 2015;77:375–84.
15. Schnurr PP. A guide to the literature on partial PTSD. *PTSD Research Quarterly*. 2014;25:1–8.
16. Kilpatrick DG, Resnick HS, Milanak ME, Miller MW, Keyes KM, Friedman MJ. National estimates of exposure to traumatic events and PTSD prevalence using DSM-IV and DSM-5 criteria. *J Trauma Stress*. 2013;26:537–47.

17. Hoge CW, Yehuda R, Castro CA, *et al*. Unintended consequences of changing the definition of posttraumatic stress disorder in DSM-5: critique and call for action. *JAMA Psychiatry*. 2016;73:750–2.

18. Maercker A, Brewin CR, Bryant RA, *et al*. Diagnosis and classification of disorders specifically associated with stress: proposals for ICD-11. *World Psychiatry*. 2013;12:198–206.

19. Cox KS, Resnick HS, Kilpatrick DG. Prevalence and correlates of posttrauma distorted beliefs: Evaluating DSM-5 PTSD expanded cognitive symptoms in a national sample. *J Trauma Stress*. 2014;27:299–306.

20. Badour CL, Resnick HS, Kilpatrick DG. Associations between specific negative emotions and DSM-5 PTSD among a national sample of interpersonal trauma survivors. *J Interpers Violence*. 2017;32:1620–41.

21. Koffel E, Polusny MA, Arbisi PA, Erbes CR. A preliminary investigation of the new and revised symptoms of posttraumatic stress disorder in DSM-5. *Depress Anxiety*. 2012;29:731–8.

22. Lanius RA, Vermetten E, Loewenstein RJ, *et al*. Emotion modulation in PTSD: Clinical and neurobiological evidence for a dissociative subtype. *Am J Psychiatry*. 2010;167:640–7.

23. Jaycox LH, Foa EB, Morral AR. Influence of emotional engagement and habituation on exposure therapy for PTSD. *J Consult Clin Psychol*. 1998;66:185.

24. Badour CL, Gilmore AK, Resnick HS. *Challenges and options for adding trauma items to the National Survey on Drug Use and Health (NSDUH)*. Commissioned paper for the National Academies of Sciences Standing Committee on Integrating New Behavioral Health Measures into the Substance Abuse and Mental Health Services Administration's Data Collection Programs. 2016. Available from: http://sites.nationalacademies.org/cs/groups/dbassesite/documents/webpage/dbasse_173301.pdf

25. Kilpatrick DG, Badour CL, Resnick HS. Trauma and posttraumatic stress disorder prevalence and sociodemographic characteristics. In: Gold SN (ed). *APA Handbook of Trauma Psychology: Foundations in Knowledge*. American Psychological Association: Washington, DC; 2017. pp. 63–85.

26. Kessler RC, Chiu WT, Demler O, Walters EE. Prevalence, severity, and comorbidity of 12-month DSM-IV disorders in the National Comorbidity Survey Replication. *Arch Gen Psychiatry*. 2005;62:617–27.

27. Resick PA, Bovin MJ, Calloway AL, *et al*. A critical evaluation of the complex PTSD literature: implications for DSM-5. *J Trauma Stress*. 2012;25:241–51.

28. Kilpatrick DG, Ruggiero KJ, Acierno R, Saunders BE, Resnick HS, Best CL. Violence and risk of PTSD, major depression, substance abuse/dependence, and comorbidity: results from the National Survey of Adolescents. *J Consult Clin Psychol*. 2003;71:692–700.

29. Goldstein RB, Smith SM, Chou SP, *et al*. The epidemiology of DSM-5 posttraumatic stress disorder in the United States: results from the National Epidemiologic Survey on Alcohol and Related Conditions-III. *Soc Psychiatry Psychiatr Epidemiol*. 2016;51:1137–48.

30. Hoge CW, Riviere LA, Wilk JE, Herrell RK, Weathers FW. The prevalence of post-traumatic stress disorder (PTSD) in US combat soldiers: a head-to-head comparison of DSM-5 versus DSM-IV-TR symptom criteria with the PTSD checklist. *Lancet Psychiatry*. 2014;1:269–77.

31. Wolf EJ, Miller MW, Kilpatrick D, *et al*. ICD-11 Complex PTSD in US National and veteran samples prevalence and structural associations with PTSD. *Clin Psychol Sci*. 2015;3:215–29.

32. Wisco BE, Miller MW, Wolf EJ, *et al*. The impact of proposed changes to ICD-11 on estimates of PTSD prevalence and comorbidity. *Psychiatr Res*. 2016;240:226–33.

33. O'Donnell ML, Alkemade N, Nickerson A, *et al*. Impact of the diagnostic changes to post-traumatic stress disorder for DSM-5 and the proposed changes to ICD-11. *Br J Psychiatry*. 2014;205:230–5.

34. Hansen M, Hyland P, Armour C, Shevlin M, Elklit A. Less is more? Assessing the validity of the ICD-11 model of PTSD across multiple trauma samples. *Eur J Psychotraumatol*. 2015;6:1–11.

35. Bryant RA, Creamer M, O'Donnel M., Silove D, McFarlane AC, Forbes D. A comparison of the capacity of the DSM-IV and DSM-5 acute stress disorder definitions to predict posttraumatic stress disorder and related disorders. *J Clin Psychiatry*. 2015;76:391–7.

36. Bryant RA, Friedman MJ, Spiegel D, Ursano R, Strain J. A review of acute stress disorder in DSM-5. *Depress Anxiety*. 2011;28:802–17.

37. Bryant RA, Harvey AG. Acute stress disorder: a critical review of diagnostic issues. *Clin Psychol Rev*. 1997;32:757–73.

38. Strain JJ, Friedman MJ. Considering adjustment disorders as stress response syndromes for DSM-5. *Depress Anxiety*. 2011;28:818–23.

39. Maercker A, Einsle F, Köllner V. Adjustment disorders as stress response syndromes: a new diagnostic concept and its exploration in a medical sample. *Psychopathology*. 2007;40:135–46.

40. Back SE, Foa EB, Killeen TK, *et al. Concurrent Treatment of PTSD and Substance Use Disorders Using Prolonged Exposure (COPE): Therapist Guide*. Oxford University Press, New York, NY; 2014.

41. Harned MS, Korslund KE, Foa EB, Linehan MM. Treating PTSD in suicidal and self-injuring women with borderline personality disorder: development and preliminary evaluation of a Dialectical Behavior Therapy Prolonged Exposure Protocol. *Behav Res Ther*. 2012;50:381–6.

42. Briggs EC, Nooner K, Amaya-Jackson LM. Assessment of childhood PTSD. In: Friedman MJ, Keane TM, Resick A (eds). *Handbook of PTSD: Science and Practice* (2nd edn). Guilford: New York, NY; 2014. pp. 391–405.

43. Reardon AF, Brief DJ, Miller MW, Keane TM. Assessment of PTSD and its comorbidities in adults. In: Friedman MJ, Keane TM, Resick A (eds). *Handbook of PTSD: Science and Practice* (2nd edn). Guilford: New York, NY; 2014. pp. 369–90.

44. Vermetten E, Baker DG, Jetly R, McFarlane AC. Concerns over divergent approaches in the diagnostics of posttraumatic stress disorder. *Psychiatr Ann*. 2016;46:498–509.

45. Friedman MJ. Deconstructing PTSD. In: Bromet EJ (ed). *Long-term Outcomes in Psychopathology Research: Rethinking the Scientific Agenda*. Oxford University Press: Oxford; 2016. pp. 123–39.

46. Raskind MA, Millard SP, Petrie EC, *et al*. Higher pretreatment blood pressure is associated with greater posttraumatic stress disorder symptom reduction in soldiers treated with prazosin. *Biol Psychiatry*. 2016;80:736–42.

# 79

# Basic mechanisms of, and treatment targets for, stress-related disorders

*Bruce S. McEwen*

## Introduction

'Stress' is a commonly used word that generally refers to experiences that cause feelings of anxiety and frustration, because they push us beyond our ability to successfully cope. 'Stress' has become a major focus of modern life, but what do we mean by 'stress'? Besides time pressures and daily hassles at work and home, there are stressors related to economic insecurity, loneliness, poor health, and interpersonal conflict. More rarely, there are situations that are life-threatening—accidents, natural disasters, violence—and these evoke the classical 'fight-or-flight' response and can cause traumatic memories and post-traumatic stress disorder (PTSD).

The most common stressors are the ones that operate chronically, often at a low level, and that cause us to behave in certain ways. For example, being 'stressed out' may cause us to be anxious and/or depressed, to lose sleep at night, to eat comfort foods and take in more calories than our bodies need, and to smoke or drink alcohol excessively. Being 'stressed out' may also cause us to neglect seeing friends, or to take time off from our work, or to reduce our engagement in regular physical activity as we, for example, sit at a computer and try to get out from under the burden of too much to do. Often we are tempted to take medications—anxiolytics, sleep-promoting agents—to help us cope, and, with time, our bodies may increase in weight and develop other symptoms of an unhealthy lifestyle. Thus, health-promoting and health-damaging behaviours must be included when we discuss 'stress', and this leads us to the concepts of 'allostasis' and 'allostatic load and overload' that will be discussed in this chapter.

The brain is the organ that determines what is stressful and the behavioural and physiological responses, whether health-promoting or health-damaging (Fig. 79.1). And the brain is a biological organ

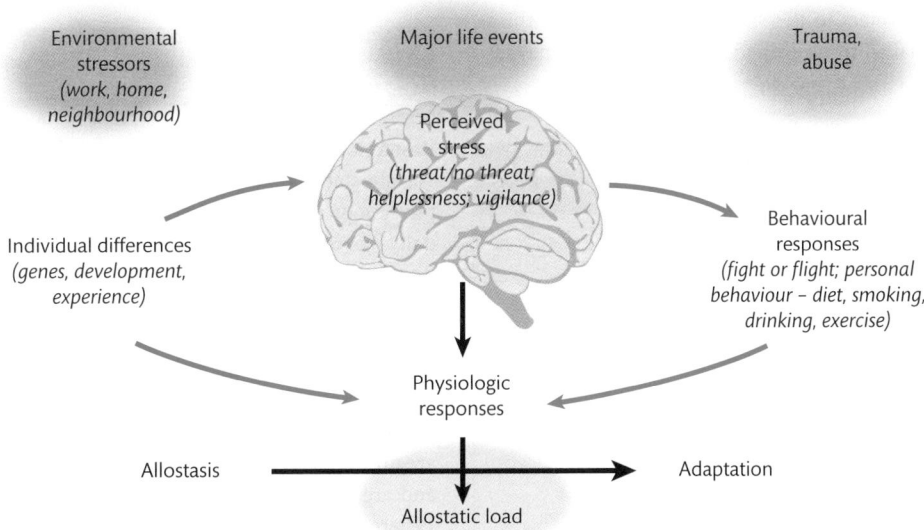

**Fig. 79.1** Central role of the brain in allostasis and the behavioural and physiological response to stressors [122].
Reproduced from *New Eng J Med*, 338(3), McEwen BS, Protective and Damaging Effects of Stress Mediators, pp. 171–9, Copyright (1998), with permission from Massachusetts Medical Society.

that changes in its architecture, molecular profile, and neurochemistry under acute and chronic stress and directs many systems of the body—metabolic, cardiovascular, immune—that are involved in the short- and long-term consequences of being 'stressed out' and the consequent health-damaging behaviours. This chapter summarizes some of the current information, placing emphasis on how the stress hormones and other hormones can play both protective and damaging roles in the brain and body, depending on how tightly their release is regulated and how harmoniously the network of stress mediators functions. The chapter discusses implications for mental, as well as physical, health and describes some of the approaches for dealing with stress in our complex world.

## Types of stress

This chapter will use the following classifications of the types of stress: good stress, tolerable stress, and toxic stress (Box 79.1). See (http://developingchild.harvard.edu/library/reports_and_working_papers/policy_framework/) for paper related to toxic stress.

Good stress is a term used in popular language to refer to the experience of rising to a challenge, taking a risk, and feeling rewarded by an often positive outcome. A related term is 'eustress'. Good self-esteem and good impulse control and decision-making capability, all functions of a healthy architecture of the brain, are important here! Even adverse outcomes can be 'growth experiences' for individuals with such positive, adaptive characteristics that promote resilience in the face of adversity.

'Tolerable stress' refers to those situations where bad things happen, but the individual with a healthy brain architecture is able to cope, often with the aid of family, friends, and other individuals who provide support. These adverse outcomes can be 'growth experiences' for individuals with such positive, adaptive characteristics and support systems that promote resilience. Here, 'distress' refers to the uncomfortable feeling related to the nature of the stressor and the degree to which the individual feels a lack of ability to influence or control the stressor [1–3].

Finally, 'toxic stress' refers to the situation in which bad things happen to an individual who has limited support and who may also

have a brain architecture that reflects the effects of adverse early life events that have impaired the development of good impulse control and judgement and adequate self esteem. Here, the degree and/or duration of 'distress' may be greater. With toxic stress, the inability to cope is likely to have adverse effects on behaviour and physiology, and this will result in a higher degree of allostatic overload, as will be explained later in this chapter.

## Definition of stress, allostasis, and allostatic load

In spite of the further definitions of the types of stress, the word 'stress' is still an ambiguous term and has connotations that make it less useful in understanding how the body handles the events that are stressful. Insight into these processes can lead to a better understanding of how best to intervene, a topic that will be discussed at the end of this article. There are two sides to this story—on the one hand, the body responds to almost any event or challenge, whether or not we call it 'stress', by releasing chemical mediators, for example catecholamines that increase the heart rate and blood pressure, that help us cope with the situation; on the other hand, chronic elevation of these same mediators, for example chronically increased heart rate and blood pressure, produces chronic wear-and-tear on the cardiovascular system that can result, over time, in disorders such as strokes and heart attacks. For this reason, the term 'allostasis' was introduced by Sterling and Eyer in 1988 to refer to the active process by which the body responds to daily events and maintains homeostasis (allostasis literally means 'achieving stability through change'). Because chronically increased allostasis can lead to disease, we introduced the term 'allostatic load or overload' to refer to the wear-and-tear that results from either too much stress or from the inefficient management of allostasis, for example not turning off the response when it is no longer needed. Other forms of allostatic load are summarized in Fig. 79.2 and involve not turning on an adequate response in the first place or not habituating to the recurrence of the same stressor and thus dampening the allostatic response.

## Protection and damage as the two sides of the response to experiences

Protection via allostasis and wear-and-tear on the body and brain via allostatic load/overload are the two contrasting sides of the physiology involved in defending the body against the challenges of daily life. Besides adrenaline and noradrenaline, there are many mediators that participate in allostasis, and they are linked together in a network of regulation that is non-linear, meaning that each mediator has the ability to regulate the activity of the other mediators, sometimes in a biphasic manner [4]. Glucocorticoids, produced by the adrenal cortex in response to ACTH from the pituitary gland, is the other major 'stress hormone'. Pro- and anti-inflammatory cytokines are produced by many cells in the body, and they regulate each other and are, in turn, regulated by glucocorticoids and catecholamines. Whereas catecholamines can increase pro-inflammatory cytokine production, glucocorticoids are known to inhibit this production. And yet, there are exceptions—pro-inflammatory effects of glucocorticoids that depend on the dose and cell or tissue type [5, 6]. The parasympathetic nervous system also plays an important regulatory

---

**Box 79.1** Levels of stressful experiences: their causes, consequences, and why we experience them!

- Result: sense of mastery and control
- HEALTHY BRAIN ARCHITECTURE
  - Good self-esteem, judgement, and impulse control

Tolerable stress
- Adverse life events buffered by supportive relationships
- Result: coping and recovery
- HEALTHY BRAIN ARCHITECTURE
  - Good self-esteem, judgement, and impulse control

Toxic stress
- Unbuffered adverse events of greater duration and magnitude
- Result: poor coping and compromised recovery
- Result: increased life-long risk for physical and mental disorders
- COMPROMISED BRAIN ARCHITECTURE
  - Dysregulated physiological systems

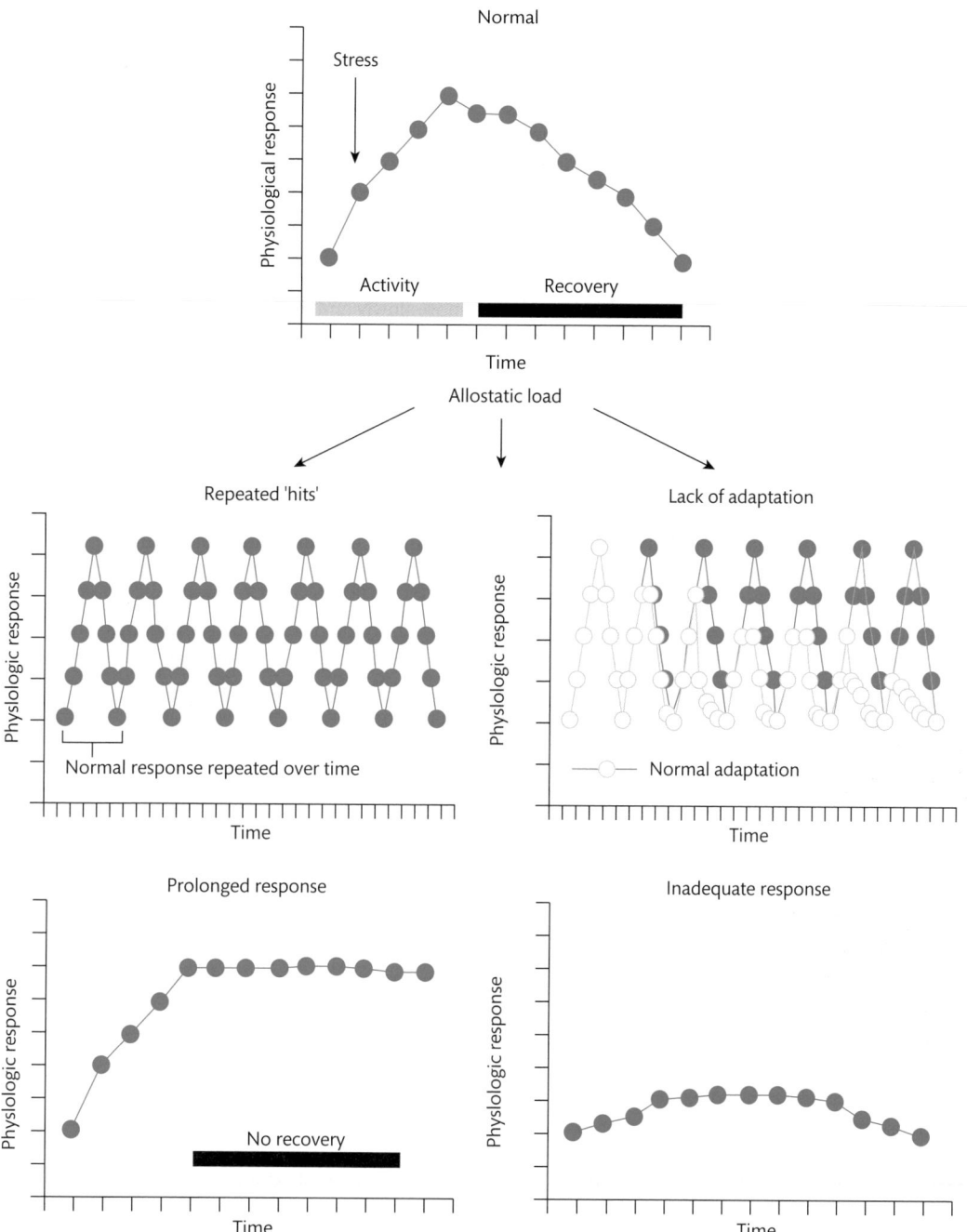

**Fig. 79.2** Four types of allostatic load. The top panel illustrates the normal allostatic response, in which a response is initiated by a stressor, sustained for an appropriate interval, and then turned off. The remaining panels illustrate four conditions that lead to allostatic load: top left, *repeated 'hits'* from multiple stressors; top right, *lack of adaptation*; bottom left, *prolonged response* due to delayed shutdown; and bottom right, *inadequate response* that leads to compensatory hyperactivity of other mediators (for example, inadequate secretion of glucocorticoid, resulting in increased levels of cytokines that are normally counter-regulated by glucocorticoids) [122].

Reproduced from *New Eng J Med*, 338(3), McEwen BS, Protective and Damaging Effects of Stress Mediators, pp. 171–9, Copyright (1998), with permission from Massachusetts Medical Society.

role in this non-linear network of allostasis, since it generally opposes the sympathetic nervous system and, for example, slows the heart and also has anti-inflammatory effects [7, 8].

What this non-linearity and interaction among mediators mean is that when any one mediator is increased or decreased, there are compensatory changes in the other mediators that depend on the time course and level of change of each of the mediators. Unfortunately,

we cannot measure all components of this system simultaneously, and we must therefore rely on measurements of only a few of them in any one study. Yet the non-linearity must be kept in mind in interpreting the results.

A good example of the biphasic actions of stress, that is, 'protection vs damage', is in the immune system, in which an acute stressor activates an acquired immune response via mediation by catecholamines and glucocorticoids and locally produced immune mediators; and yet a chronic exposure to the same stressor over several weeks has the opposite effect and results in immune suppression [9, 10]. Acute stress-induced immune enhancement is good for enhancing immunization, fighting an infection, or repairing a wound, but it is deleterious to health for autoimmune conditions such as psoriasis or Crohn's disease. On the other hand, immune suppression is good in the case of an autoimmune disorder and deleterious for fighting an infection or repairing a wound. In immune-sensitive skin cancer, acute stress is effective in inhibiting tumour progression, while chronic stress exacerbates progression [11, 12].

## Stress and disease

Cardiovascular disease and depression are recognized as consequences of 'toxic psychological stress', using the definition of toxic stress discussed earlier [13]. There are conditions that lead to allostatic load and overload and exacerbate pathophysiology, besides the well-known factors associated with diet, alcohol consumption, and smoking and other unhealthy behaviours (Box 79.2). We shall discuss physical activity and lack thereof below, in connection with interventions. In particular, the social and physical environments are huge factors. Human beings are social creatures, and loneliness is a contributor to allostatic overload. Likewise, neighbourhoods matter and living in ugly, noisy, and dangerous neighbourhoods with a lack of green space contribute to allostatic overload.

### Circadian disruption

One of the key systems in the brain and body that regulate homeostasis of these varied physiological and behavioural variables is the circadian system. Based in the suprachiasmatic nucleus (SCN) of the hypothalamus, the brain's clock controls the rhythms in the rest of the brain and body through both neural and diffusible signals. Disruption of these key homeostatic systems contributes to allostatic overload [14]. Reduced sleep duration is associated with increased body mass and obesity, and sleep restriction to 4 hours per night increases blood pressure, decreases parasympathetic tone, increases evening cortisol and insulin levels, and promotes increased appetite, possibly through the elevation of ghrelin, a pro-appetitive hormone, along with decreased levels of leptin. Moreover, pro-inflammatory cytokine levels are increased with sleep deprivation, along with decreased performance in tests of psychomotor vigilance, and this has been reported to result even from a modest sleep restriction to 6 hours per night [14, 15].

Circadian disruption has sometimes been overlooked as a separate, yet related, phenomenon to sleep deprivation. In modern industrialized societies, circadian disruption can be induced in numerous ways, the most common of which are shift work and jet lag that contribute to weight gain and obesity (reviewed in [14]). Animal models have provided additional insights; for example, normal C57Bl/6 mice housed in a disrupted 10-hour light:10-hour dark cycle showed accelerated weight gain and disruptions in metabolic hormones and also showed cognitive inflexibility and shrinkage of dendrites in the medial prefrontal cortex [16], similar to reports of long-recovery vs short-recovery flight crews where short-recovery crews had impaired performance in a psychomotor task, reacting more slowly and with more errors [17].

## Key role of the brain in response to stress

The brain is the key organ of the stress response because it determines what is threatening, and therefore stressful, and also controls the behavioural and physiological responses (Fig. 79.1). There are enormous individual differences in the response to stress, based upon the experience of the individual early in life and in adult life. Positive or negative experiences in school, at work, or in romantic and family interpersonal relationships can bias an individual towards either a positive or a negative response in a new situation.

Early life experiences carry an even greater weight in terms of how an individual reacts to new situations. Early life physical and sexual abuse carry with it a life-long burden of behavioural and pathophysiological problems [18]. Cold and uncaring families produce long-lasting emotional problems in children [19]. Some of these effects are seen on the brain structure and function and in the risk for later depression and PTSD [20]. One of the biological consequences of early life adversity is prolonged elevation of inflammatory cytokines, as well as poor dental health, obesity, and elevated blood pressure, in children and young adults [21]. Harsh language is among the components of early life adversity and has been shown to increase inflammatory markers [22].

And the physical environment makes a huge difference, with crowding, noise, and ugliness, along with physical danger, being major contributors to allostatic overload both during development and throughout adult life [2, 23, 24].

Animal models have been useful in providing insights into behavioural and physiological mechanisms. Individual differences in anxiety-like behaviours are evident [25, 26]. Early life maternal care in rodents is a powerful determinant of life-long emotional reactivity and stress hormone reactivity, and increases in both are associated with earlier cognitive decline and a shorter lifespan [27]. Effects of early maternal care are transmitted across generations by the subsequent behaviour of the female offspring as they become mothers, and methylation of DNA in key genes appears to play a role in this epigenetic transmission [28, 29]. Yet, the mother is not the sole determinant of offspring emotional and physical development, but rather modulates it by her behaviour towards the infant, particularly in the immediate aftermath of infant experiences of novelty inside or outside of the home cage [30].

Furthermore, in rodents, abuse of the young is associated with an attachment, rather than an avoidance, of the abusive mother, an effect that increases the chances that the infant can continue to obtain food and other support until weaning [31]. Moreover, other conditions that affect the rearing process can also affect emotionality

---

**Box 79.2** Causes of allostatic load/overload [122]

- Loneliness [123]
- Circadian disruption: jet lag, shift work, sleep deprivation [14, 15, 17, 82]
- Lack of physical activity [124]
- Ugly, noisy, dangerous living environment and lack of green space [2, 23, 24]
- Health behaviours: type and quantity of food, alcohol consumption, smoking

in offspring. For example, uncertainty in the food supply for rhesus monkey mothers leads to increased emotionality in offspring and possibly an earlier onset of obesity and diabetes [32, 33].

Besides the important role of the social and physical environment and experiences of individuals in health outcomes, genetic factors also play an important role. Different alleles of commonly occurring genes determine how individuals will respond to experiences. For example, the short form of the serotonin transporter is associated with a number of conditions such as alcoholism, and individuals who have this allele are more vulnerable to respond to stressful experiences by developing depressive illness [34, 35]. In childhood, individuals with an allele of the monoamine oxidase A gene are more vulnerable to abuse in childhood and more likely to themselves become abusers and to show antisocial behaviours, compared to individuals with another commonly occurring allele [36]. Nevertheless, in a positive, nurturing environment, as formulated by Suomi and by Tom Boyce and colleagues [37–39], these same alleles may lead to successful outcomes, which has led them to be called 'reactive or context-sensitive alleles', rather than 'bad genes'.

## Brain as a target of stress

### The hippocampus

One of the ways that stress hormones modulate function within the brain is by changing the structure of neurons. The hippocampus is one of the most sensitive and malleable regions of the brain and is also very important in cognitive function and mood regulation [40]. The dentate gyrus (DG)-CA3 system, which is delicately balanced anatomically, and thus vulnerable to overstimulation, as in seizures, is believed to play a role in the memory of sequences of events, although long-term storage of memory occurs in other brain regions [41]. Moreover, the anterior part of the hippocampus has strong connections to the amygdala and prefrontal cortex and is a nexus of vulnerability to depression. But, because the DG-CA3 system is so delicately balanced in its function and vulnerability to damage, there is also adaptive structural plasticity, in that new neurons continue to be produced in the dentate gyrus throughout adult life [42], and CA3 pyramidal cells undergo reversible remodelling of their dendrites in conditions such as hibernation and chronic stress [43, 44]. The role of this plasticity may be to protect against permanent damage. As a result, the hippocampus undergoes a number of adaptive changes in response to acute and chronic stress via a host of cellular and molecular mechanisms [45] and also shows positive effects of regular physical activity on hippocampal volume and memory [46].

### Prefrontal cortex and amygdala

Repeated stress also causes changes in other brain regions such as the prefrontal cortex and amygdala. Repeated stress causes dendritic shortening in the medial prefrontal cortex [47] but produces dendritic growth in neurons in the amygdala, as well as in the orbitofrontal cortex. Excitatory amino acids and BDNF are involved [47–49].

### Contrasting effects

Acute stress induces spine synapses in the CA1 region of the hippocampus, and both acute and chronic stress also increases spine synapse formation in the amygdala, but chronic stress decreases it in the hippocampus. Moreover, chronic stress for 21 days or longer impairs hippocampal-dependent cognitive function and enhances amygdala-dependent unlearnt fear and fear conditioning, which are consistent with the opposite effects of stress on hippocampal and amygdala structure [49]. Chronic stress also increases aggression between animals living in the same cage, and this is likely to reflect another aspect of hyperactivity of the amygdala [50]. Behavioural correlates of remodelling in the prefrontal cortex include impairment in attention set shifting, possibly reflecting structural remodelling in the medial prefrontal cortex [51].

### Sex differences

Animal models of stress effects on the brain show that females and males respond differently to acute and chronic stressors because of developmental factors involving both epigenetic effects of hormones along with genes in the sex chormosomes themselves [52]. Sex differences in the brain are subtle but widespread [53], and yet males and females do many things equally well; for example, in human subjects taking tests on empathy, men and women do equally well, but the brain activation patterns during the tests show different brain regions are activated [54]. This is reminiscent of an animal model study in which, despite no overall sex differences in fear conditioning freezing behaviour, the neural processes underlying successful or failed extinction maintenance are sex-specific [55]. Given other work showing sex differences in stress-induced structural plasticity in prefrontal cortex projections to the amygdala and other cortical areas [56], these findings are relevant not only to sex differences in fear conditioning and extinction, but, according to Gruene et al. 'also to exposure-based clinical therapies, which are similar in premise to fear extinction and which are primarily used to treat disorders that are more common in women than in men' [55].

## Translation to the human brain

### MRI and fMRI imaging studies of stress, depression, and Cushing's disease

Much of the impetus for studying the effects of stress on the structure of the human brain has come from the animal studies summarized thus far. Although there is very little evidence regarding the effects of ordinary life stressors on brain structure, there are indications from functional imaging of individuals undergoing ordinary stressors, such as counting backwards, that there are lasting changes in neural activity [57], and a 20-year history of chronic perceived stress has been linked to smaller hippocampal volume [58]. Moreover, the study of depressive illness and anxiety disorders has also provided some insights. Life events are known to precipitate depressive illness in individuals with certain genetic predispositions [34, 59, 60]. Moreover, brain regions such as the hippocampus, amygdala, and prefrontal cortex show altered patterns of activity in PET and fMRI and also demonstrate changes in volume of these structures with recurrent depression—decreased volume of the hippocampus and prefrontal cortices and the amygdala [61–64] (Fig. 79.3). Interestingly, amygdala volume has been reported to increase in the first episode of depression, whereas hippocampal volume is not decreased [65, 66]. It has been known

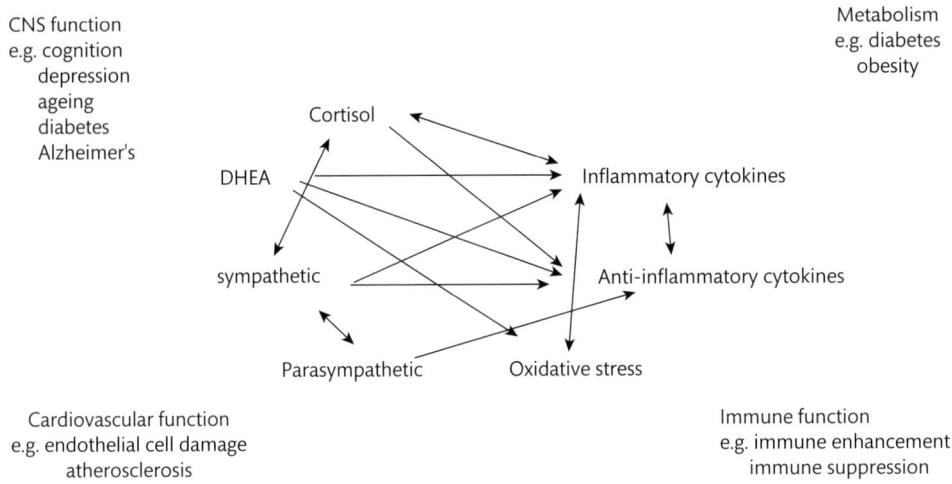

**Fig. 79.3** Non-linear network of mediators of allostasis involved in the stress response. Arrows indicate that each system regulates the others in a reciprocal manner, creating a non-linear network. Moreover, there are multiple pathways for regulation; for example, inflammatory cytokine production is negatively regulated via anti-inflammatory cytokines, as well as via parasympathetic and glucocorticoid pathways, whereas sympathetic activity increases inflammatory cytokine production. Parasympathetic activity, in turn, contains sympathetic activity.
Adapted from *Dialogues Clin Neurosci*, 8(4), McEwen BS, Protective and damaging effects of stress mediators: central role of the brain, pp. 367–81, Copyright (2006), LLS SAS. Reproduced under the Creative Commons Attribution License (CC BY-NC-ND 3.0).

for some time that stress hormones, such as cortisol, are involved in psychopathology, reflecting emotional arousal and psychic disorganization, rather than the specific disorder per se [67]. We now know that adrenocortical hormones enter the brain and produce a wide range of effects upon it.

In Cushing's disease, there are depressive symptoms that can be relieved by surgical correction of hypercortisolaemia [68, 69]. Both major depression and Cushing's disease are associated with chronic elevation of cortisol that results in gradual loss of minerals from bone and abdominal obesity. In major depressive illness, as well as in Cushing's disease, the duration of the illness, and not the age of the subjects, predicts a progressive reduction in volume of the hippocampus, determined by structural MRI [61, 70]. Moreover, there are a variety of other anxiety-related disorders, such as PTSD [71, 72] and borderline personality disorder [73], in which atrophy of the hippocampus has been reported, suggesting that this is a common process reflecting chronic imbalance in the activity of adaptive systems, such as the HPA axis, but also including endogenous neurotransmitters such as glutamate.

### Glucose regulation

Another important factor in hippocampal volume and function is glucose regulation. Poor glucose regulation is associated with smaller hippocampal volume and poorer memory function in individuals in their 60s and 70s who have 'mild cognitive impairment' (MCI) [74–76], and both MCI and type 2, as well as type 1, diabetes are recognized as risk factors for dementia [77–80]. Moreover, depression is often associated with insulin resistance (IR) and metabolic syndrome, and treatment with the peroxisome proliferator-activated receptor (PPAR) gamma agent pioglitazone showed improvement in depressive symptoms, but only in subjects with IR (81). Inflammation is also a factor related to many disorders of modern life, and elevation of IL-6 has been linked to reduced hippocampal volume [82], as well as to poor sleep (83). Regarding allostatic overload, a bifactorial model for calculating its impact on poor health

shows that mediators of inflammation, glucose level, and lipids are the most salient [84].

### Insulin resistance

The original hypothesis that IR is a missing link between mood disorders and dementia [80, 85] has recently been supported by data on all components of the model, starting with the connection between depressive disorders and IR [86, 87] and also confirming a role of depressive disorders in accelerating the onset of dementia [88–90]. As IR is a modifiable metabolic pro-inflammatory state underlying type 2 diabetes mellitus, cumulative data indicate that, in middle-aged adults, IR is associated with disrupted memory and executive function and a corresponding metabolic decline in the medial pre-frontal cortex, reductions in hippocampal volumes, and aberrant intrinsic connectivity between the hippocampus and the medial pre-frontal cortex [91–93]. These findings are supported by recent work in animal models, in which antisense inactivation of the insulin receptor in the hippocampus leads to cognitive impairment without systemic consequences [94], whereas antisense inactivation of the hypothalamic insulin receptor creates systemic insulin resistance and dyslipidaemia and also insulin resistance in the hippocampus, along with depressive-like behaviour and cognitive impairment [95]. Remarkably, these changes are reversed by dietary restriction [96, 97], indicating that the brain can be resilient.

### Progression towards dementia

Yet there is, at some point, a 'switch' that triggers irreversible changes that lead towards amyloid beta (Abeta) toxicity and dementia [89]. These authors point out that synaptic NMDA receptor activation normally has an antioxidant role by suppressing FOXO1 transcription factor in the hippocampus, but abnormal and excessive NMDA activation in the insulin-resistant state appears to enable FOXO1 translocation to the cell nucleus, leading to the generation of reactive oxygen species and possibly also activation of stress kinases, which further impairs insulin signalling. Moreover, Abeta production is accelerated and Abeta oligomers enter into a vicious cycle, leading to further damage [89]. Mitochondrial function declines under these conditions and contributes to the positive feedback cycle of toxicity [98].

## Epigenetics: two meanings that are both important for prevention and treatment

'Epigenetics' now refers to events 'above the genome' that regulate the expression of genetic information without altering the DNA sequence. Besides CpG methylation described earlier, other mechanisms include histone modifications that repress or activate chromatin unfolding [99] and the actions of non-coding RNAs [100], as well as transposons and retrotransposons [101] and RNA editing [102]. For prevention and treatment, in the spirit of integrative medicine, it is important to let the 'wisdom of the body' prevail and to focus upon strategies that centre around the use of targeted behavioural therapies, along with treatments, including pharmaceutical agents, that 'open up windows of plasticity' in the brain and facilitate the efficacy of the behavioural interventions [103]. This is because a major challenge throughout the life course is to find ways of *redirecting future behaviour and physiology in more positive and healthy directions* [104]. In keeping with the original definition of epigenetics [105] as the emergence of characteristics not previously evident or even predictable from an earlier developmental stage (for example, think about a fertilized frog or human egg which look similar and what happens as each develops!), *we do not mean 're-versibility' as in 'rolling back the developmental clock' but rather 're-direction' as well as 'resilience', which can be defined as 'achieving a successful outcome in the face of adversity'.*

## Interventions that change the brain and improve health

Can the effects of stress and adverse early life experiences on the brain be treated and compensated, even though there are no 'magic bullets' like penicillin for stress-related disorders [104]? For psychiatric illnesses such as depression and anxiety disorders, including PTSD, it is necessary to complement, and even replace, existing drugs and adopt strategies that centre around the use of targeted behavioural therapies, along with treatments, including pharmaceutical agents, that open up 'windows of plasticity' in the brain and facilitate the efficacy of the behavioural interventions [103, 106, 107]. To that extent, meeting the demands imposed by stressful experiences via various coping resources can lead to growth, adaptation, and learning to promote resilience and improved mental health [108, 109]. BDNF is a mediator of plasticity and, while it can facilitate beneficial plasticity (for example, see [48]), it should be noted that BDNF also has the ability to promote pathophysiology, as in seizures [110–112].

### How the brain gets 'stuck'

Depression and anxiety disorders are examples of a loss of resilience, in the sense that changes in brain circuitry and function, caused by stressors that precipitate the disorder, become 'locked' in

---

**Box 79.3** Reactivating and redirecting brain plasticity

- *'Releasing the brakes'* that retard structural and functional plasticity [105]. Example amblyopia first done using fluoxetine [121] and caloric restriction [125], in which reducing inhibitory neuronal activity appears to play a key role. Replicated by putting cortisol in drinking water, instead of caloric restriction [125]. NOTE: ultradian fluctuations of cortisol according to a diurnal pattern modulate turnover of some spine synapses, in relation to motor learning and possibly other forms of learning [126, 127].
- *Opening windows of plasticity with physical activity*: regular physical activity, which has actions that improve prefrontal and parietal cortex blood flow and enhance executive function [128], increases hippocampal volume in previously sedentary elderly adults [46, 129] and complements work showing that fit individuals have larger hippocampal volumes than sedentary adults of the same age range [130]. Regular physical activity is an effective antidepressant and protects against cardiovascular disease, diabetes, and dementia [131, 132]. Moreover, intensive learning has also been shown to increase the volume of the human hippocampus, based on a study on medical students [133].
- *Successful cognitive behavioural therapies*, which are tailored to individual needs, can produce volumetric changes in both the prefrontal cortex in the case of chronic fatigue [134] and in the amygdala in the case of chronic anxiety [135], and in a brainstem area associated with well-being [136]. Mindfulness-based stress reduction (MBSR) practice has been shown to increase regional brain grey matter density in the hippocampus, cerebellum, and prefrontal cortex, the brain regions involved in learning and memory processes, emotion regulation, self-referential processing, and perspective-taking [137]. Enhancing self-regulation of mood and emotion appears to be an important outcome [138, 139].
- *Meditation* is reported to enlarge the volume of the hippocampus and to do so differently in men and women, suggesting to the authors that mindfulness practices operate differently in males and females [140].

---

a particular state and thus need external intervention. Indeed, prolonged depression is associated with shrinkage of the hippocampus [62, 113] and prefrontal cortex [63]. While there appears to be no neuronal loss, there is evidence for glial cell loss and smaller neuronal cell nuclei [114, 115], which is consistent with shrinking of the dendritic tree, described earlier, after chronic stress. Indeed, a few studies indicate that pharmacological treatment may reverse the decreased hippocampal volume in unipolar [116] and bipolar [117] depression, but the possible influence of concurrent cognitive behavioural therapy in these studies is unclear.

Even in adulthood, gene expression in the brain continually changes with experience [118] and there is loss of resilience of the neural architecture with ageing [119] that can be redirected by exercise [46] and by pharmacological intervention [120, 121]. Beyond ageing, there are new approaches to 'opening windows of plasticity' and redirecting the brain towards a more health-promoting state, and these are summarized in Box 79.3.

## Conclusions: what can one do about being 'stressed out'?

If being 'stressed out' has such pervasive effects on the brain, as well as the body, what are the ways in which individuals, as well as policymakers in government and business, can act to reduce the negative effects and enhance the ability of the body and brain to deal with stress with minimal consequences? The answers are simple and obvious, but often difficult to achieve.

From the standpoint of the individual, a major goal should be to try to improve sleep quality and quantity, have good social support and a positive outlook on life, maintain a healthy diet, avoid smoking, and have regular moderate physical activity. Concerning physical activity, it is not necessary to become an extreme athlete, and moderate physical activity helps, as noted earlier, in relation to enlarging hippocampal volume.

From the standpoint of policy, the goal should be to create incentives at home and in work situations and to build community services and opportunities that encourage the development of the beneficial individual lifestyle practices.

As simple as the solutions seem to be, changing behaviour and solving problems that cause stress at work and at home are often difficult and may require professional help on a personal level, or even a change of job or profession. Yet these are important goals because the prevention of later disease is very important to increase 'healthspan' and promote full enjoyment of life and also to reduce the financial burden of disease and disability on the individual and on society.

## REFERENCES

1. Lazarus RS, Folkman S (eds). *Stress, Appraisal and Coping*. New York, NY: Springer Verlag; 1984.
2. Diez Roux AV, Mair C. Neighborhoods and health. *Ann N Y Acad Sci*. 2010;1186:125–45.
3. Theall KP, Brett ZH, Shirtcliff EA, Dunn EC, Drury SS. Neighborhood disorder and telomeres: connecting children's exposure to community level stress and cellular response. *Soc Sci Med*. 2013;85:50–8.
4. McEwen BS. Protective and damaging effects of stress mediators: central role of the brain. *Dial in Clin Neurosci: Stress*. 2006;8:367–81.
5. Dinkel K, MacPherson A, Sapolsky RM. Novel glucocorticoid effects on acute inflammation in the CNS. *J Neurochem*. 2003;84:705–16.
6. Frank MG, Thompson BM, Watkins LR, Maier SF. Glucocorticoids mediate stress-induced priming of microglial pro-inflammatory responses. *Brain Behav Immun*. 2012;26:337–45.
7. Borovikova LV, Ivanova S, Zhang M, *et al*. Vagus nerve stimulation attenuates the systemic inflammatory response to endotoxin. *Nature*. 2000;405:458–62.
8. Sloan RP, McCreath H, Tracey KJ, Sidney S, Liu K, Seeman T. RR interval variability is inversely related to inflammatory markers: The CARDIA study. *Mol Med*. 2007;13:178–84.
9. Dhabhar FS. Enhancing versus suppressive effects of stress on immune function: implications for immunoprotection and immunopathology. *Neuroimmunomodulation*. 2009;16:300–17.
10. Dhabhar FS, Malarkey WB, Neri E, McEwen BS. Stress-induced redistribution of immune cells--from barracks to boulevards to battlefields: a tale of three hormones—Curt Richter Award winner. *Psychoneuroendocrinology*. 2012;37:1345–68.
11. Dhabhar FS, Saul AN, Daugherty C, Holmes TH, Bouley DM, Oberyszyn TM. Short-term stress enhances cellular immunity and increases early resistance to squamous cell carcinoma. *Brain Behav Immun*. 2010;24:127–37.
12. Saul AN, Oberyszyn TM, Daugherty C, *et al*. Chronic stress and susceptibility to skin cancer. *J Natl Cancer Inst*. 2005;97:1760–7.
13. Cohen S, Janicki-Deverts D, Miller GE. Psychological stress and disease. *JAMA*. 2007;298:1685–8.
14. McEwen BS, Karatsoreos IN. Sleep deprivation and circadian disruption: stress, allostasis, and allostatic load. *Sleep Med Clin*. 2015;10:1–10.
15. Spiegel K, Leproult R, Van Cauter E. Impact of sleep debt on metabolic and endocrine function. *Lancet*. 1999;354:1435–9.
16. Karatsoreos IN, Bhagat S, Bloss EB, Morrison JH, McEwen BS. Disruption of circadian clocks has ramifications for metabolism, brain, and behavior. *Proc Natl Acad Sci U S A*. 2011;108:1657–62.
17. Cho K. Chronic 'jet lag' produces temporal lobe atrophy and spatial cognitive deficits. *Nature Neurosci*. 2001;4:567–8.
18. Felitti VJ, Anda RF, Nordenberg D, *et al*. Relationship of childhood abuse and household dysfunction to many of the leading causes of death in adults. The adverse childhood experiences (ACE) study. *Am J Prev Med*. 1998;14:245–58.
19. Repetti RL, Taylor SE, Seeman TE. Risky families: family social environments and the mental and physical health of offspirng. *Psychol Bull*. 2002;128:330–66.
20. Shonkoff JP, Boyce WT, McEwen BS. Neuroscience, molecular biology, and the childhood roots of health disparities. *JAMA*. 2009;301:2252–9.
21. Danese A, McEwen BS. Adverse childhood experiences, allostasis, allostatic load, and age-related disease. *Physiol Behav*. 2012;106:29–39.
22. Miller GE, Chen E. Harsh family climate in early life presages the emergence of a proinflammatory phenotype in adolescence. *Psychol Sci*. 2010;21:848–56.
23. Chang VW, Hillier AE, Mehta NK. Neighborhood racial isolation, disorder and obesity. Social forces; a scientific medium of social study and interpretation. 2009;87:2063–92.
24. Evans GW, Gonnella C, Marcynyszyn LA, Gentile L, Salpekar N. The role of chaos in poverty and children's socioemotional adjustment. *Psychol Sci*. 2005;16:560–5.
25. Cavigelli SA, McClintock MK. Fear of novelty in infant rats predicts adult corticosterone dynamics and an early death. *Proc Natl Acad Sci USA*. 2003;100:16131–6.
26. Nasca C, Bigio B, Zelli D, Nicoletti F, McEwen BS. Mind the gap: glucocorticoids modulate hippocampal glutamate tone underlying individual differences in stress susceptibility. *Mol Psychiatry*. 2015;20:755–63.
27. Meaney M, Aitken D, Bhatnagar S, Sapolsky R. Postnatal handling attenuates certain neuroendocrine, anatomical and cognitive dysfunctions associated with aging in female rats. *Neurobiol Aging*. 1991;12:31–8.
28. Meaney MJ, Szyf M. Environmental programming of stress responses through DNA methylation: life at the interface between a dynamic environment and a fixed genome. *Dialogues Clin Neurosci*. 2005;7:103–23.
29. Francis D, Diorio J, Liu D, Meaney MJ. Nongenomic transmission across generations of maternal behavior and stress responses in the rat. *Science*. 1999;286:1155–8.
30. Tang AC, Reeb-Sutherland BC, Romeo RD, McEwen BS. On the causes of early life experience effects: evaluating the role of mom. *Front Neuroendocrinol*. 2014;35:245–51.
31. Moriceau S, Sullivan R. Maternal presence serves as a switch between learning fear and attraction in infancy. *Nat Neurosci*. 2006;8:1004–6.
32. Coplan JD, Smith ELP, Altemus M, *et al*. Variable foraging demand rearing: Sustained elevations in cisternal cerebrospinal fluid corticotropin-releasing factor concentrations in adult primates. *Biol Psychiat*. 2001;50:200–4.

33. Kaufman D, Banerji MA, Shorman I, *et al.* Early-life stress and the development of obesity and insulin resistance in juvenile bonnet macaques. *Diabetes.* 2007;56:1–5.

34. Caspi A, Sugden K, Moffitt TE, *et al.* Influence of life stress on depression: Moderation by a polymorphism in the *5-HTT* gene. *Science.* 2003;301:386–9.

35. Spinelli S, Schwandt ML, Lindell SG, *et al.* The serotonin transporter gene linked polymorphic region is associated with the behavioral response to repeated stress exposure in infant rhesus macaques. *Dev Psychopathol.* 2012;24:157–65.

36. Caspi A, McClay J, Moffitt TE, *et al.* Role of genotype in the cycle of violence in maltreated children. *Science.* 2002;297:851–4.

37. Suomi SJ. Risk, resilience, and gene × environment interactions in rhesus monkeys. *Ann N Y Acad Sci.* 2006;1094:52–62.

38. Obradovic J, Bush NR, Stamperdahl J, Adler NE, Boyce WT. Biological sensitivity to context: the interactive effects of stress reactivity and family adversity on socioemotional behavior and school readiness. *Child Dev.* 2010;81:270–89.

39. Boyce WT, Ellis BJ. Biological sensitivity to context: I. An evolutionary-developmental theory of the origins and functions of stress reactivity. *Dev Psychopathol.* 2005 Spring;17:271–301.

40. McEwen BS, Nasca C, Gray JD. Stress effects on neuronal structure: hippocampus, amygdala and prefrontal cortex. *Neuropsychopharmacology.* 2016;41:3–23.

41. Lisman JE. Relating hippocampal circuitry to function: recall of memory sequences by reciprocal dentate-CA3 interactions. *Neuron.* 1999;22:233–42.

42. Cameron HA, Tanapat P, Gould E. Adrenal steroids and N-methyl-D-aspartate receptor activation regulate neurogenesis in the dentate gyrus of adult rats through a common pathway. *Neuroscience.* 1998;82:349–54.

43. McEwen BS. Stress and hippocampal plasticity. *Annu Rev Neurosci.* 1999;22:105–22.

44. Magarinos AM, McEwen BS, Saboureau M, Pevet P. Rapid and reversible changes in intrahippocampal connectivity during the course of hibernation in European hamsters. *Proc Natl Acad Sci U S A.* 2006;103:18775–80.

45. McEwen BS, Bowles NP, Gray JD, *et al.* Mechanisms of stress in the brain. *Nat Neurosci.* 2015;18:1353–63.

46. Erickson KI, Voss MW, Prakash RS, *et al.* Exercise training increases size of hippocampus and improves memory. *Proc Natl Acad Sci U S A.* 2011;108:3017–22.

47. McEwen BS, Morrison JH. The brain on stress: vulnerability and plasticity of the prefrontal cortex over the life course. *Neuron.* 2013;79:16–29.

48. Lakshminarasimhan H, Chattarji S. Stress leads to contrasting effects on the levels of brain derived neurotrophic factor in the hippocampus and amygdala. *PLoS One.* 2012;7:e30481.

49. Chattarji S, Tomar A, Suvrathan A, Ghosh S, Rahman MM. Neighborhood matters: divergent patterns of stress-induced plasticity across the brain. *Nat Neurosci.* 2015;18:1364–75.

50. Wood GE, Norris EH, Waters E, Stoldt JT, McEwen BS. Chronic immobilization stress alters aspects of emotionality and associative learning in the rat. *Behav Neurosci.* 2008;122:282–92.

51. Liston C, Miller MM, Goldwater DS, *et al.* Stress-induced alterations in prefrontal cortical dendritic morphology predict selective impairments in perceptual attentional set-shifting. *J Neurosci.* 2006;26:7870–4.

52. McCarthy MM, Arnold AP. Reframing sexual differentiation of the brain. *Nat Neurosci.* 2011;14:677–83.

53. McEwen BS, Milner TA. Understanding the broad influence of sex hormones and sex differences in the brain. *J Neurosci Res.* 2017;95:24–39.

54. Derntl B, Finkelmeyer A, Eickhoff S, *et al.* Multidimensional assessment of empathic abilities: neural correlates and gender differences. *Psychoneuroendocrinology.* 2010;35:67–82.

55. Gruene TM, Roberts E, Thomas V, Ronzio A, Shansky RM. Sex-specific neuroanatomical correlates of fear expression in prefrontal-amygdala circuits. *Biol Psychiatry.* 2015;78:186–93.

56. Shansky RM, Hamo C, Hof PR, Lou W, McEwen BS, Morrison JH. Estrogen promotes stress sensitivity in a prefrontal cortex-amygdala pathway. *Cereb Cortex.* 2010;20:2560–7.

57. Wang J, Rao H, Wetmore GS, *et al.* Perfusion functional MRI reveals cerebral blood flow pattern under psychological stress. *Proc Natl Acad Sci USA.* 2005;102:17804–9.

58. Gianaros PJ, Jennings JR, Sheu LK, Greer PJ, Kuller LH, Matthews KA. Prospective reports of chronic life stress predict decreased grey matter volume in the hippocampus. *NeuroImage.* 2007;35:795–803.

59. Kessler RC. The effects of stressful life events on depression. *Annu Rev Psychol.* 1997;48:191–214.

60. Kendler KS. Major depression and the environment: a psychiatric genetic perspective. *Pharmacopsychiatry.* 1998;31:5–9.

61. Sheline YI, Sanghavi M, Mintun MA, Gado MH. Depression duration but not age predicts hippocampal volume loss in medically healthy women with recurrent major depression. *J Neurosci.* 1999;19:5034–43.

62. Sheline YI. Neuroimaging studies of mood disorder effects on the brain. *Biol Psychiatry.* 2003;54:338–52.

63. Drevets WC, Price JL, Simpson JR Jr, *et al.* Subgenual prefrontal cortex abnormalities in mood disorders. *Nature.* 1997;386:824–7.

64. Sheline YI, Gado MH, Price JL. Amygdala core nuclei volumes are decreased in recurrent major depression. *Neuro Report.* 1998;9:2023–8.

65. Frodl T, Meisenzahl EM, Zetzsche T, *et al.* Larger amygdala volumes in first depressive episode as compared to recurrent major depression and healthy control subjects. *Biol Psychiatry.* 2003;53:338–44.

66. MacQueen GM, Yucel K, Taylor VH, Macdonald K, Joffe R. Posterior hippocampal volumes are associated with remission rates in patients with major depressive disorder. *Biol Psychiatry.* 2008;64:880–3.

67. Sachar EJ, Hellman L, Roffwarg HP, Halpern FS, Fukushima DK, Gallagher TF. Disrupted 24-hour patterns of cortisol secretion in psychotic depression. *Arch Gen Psychiatry.* 1973;28:19–24.

68. Starkman MN, Schteingart DE. Neuropsychiatric manifestations of patients with Cushing's syndrome. *Arch Intern Medicine.* 1981;141:215–19.

69. Murphy BEP. Treatment of major depression with steroid suppressive drugs. *J Steroid Biochem Molec Biol.* 1991;39:239–44.

70. Starkman MN, Gebarski SS, Berent S, Schteingart DE. Hippocampal formation volume, memory dysfunction, and cortisol levels in partiens with Cushing's syndrome. *Biol Psychiatry.* 1992;32:756–65.

71. Vythilingam M, Heim C, Newport J, *et al.* Childhood trauma associated with smaller hippocampal volume in women with major depression. *Am J Psychiatry.* 2002;159:2072–80.

72. Pitman RK. Hippocampal diminution in PTSD: More (or less?) than meets the eye. *Hippocampus.* 2001;11:73–4.

73. Driessen M, Hermann J, Stahl K, *et al.* Magnetic resonance imaging volumes of the hippocampus and the amygdala in women with borderline personality disorder and early traumatization. *Arch Gen Psychiatry.* 2000;57:1115–22.

74. Convit A, Wolf OT, Tarshish C, de Leon MJ. Reduced glucose tolerance is associated with poor memory performance and hippocampal atrophy among normal elderly. *Proc Natl Acad Sci USA.* 2003;100:2019–22.

75. Gold SM, Dziobek I, Sweat V, *et al.* Hippocampal damage and memory impairments as possible early brain complications of type 2 diabetes. *Diabetologia.* 2007;50:711–19.

76. Yau PL, Javier DC, Ryan CM, *et al.* Preliminary evidence for brain complications in obese adolescents with type 2 diabetes mellitus. *Diabetologia.* 2010;53:2298–306.

77. Ott A, Stolk RP, Hofman A, van Harskamp F, Grobbee DE, Breteler MMB. Association of diabetes mellitus and dementia: The Rotterdam study. *Diabetologia.* 1996;39:1392–7.

78. de Leon MJ, Convit A, Wolf OT, *et al.* Prediction of cognitive decline in normal elderly subjects with 2-[$^{18}$F]fluoro-2-deoxy-D-glucose/positron-emission tomography (FDG/PET). *Proc Natl Acad Sci USA.* 2001;98:10966–71.

79. Haan MN. Therapy insight: type 2 diabetes mellitus and the risk of late-onset Alzheimer's disease. *Nat Clin Pract Neurol.* 2006;2:159–66.

80. Rasgon N, Jarvik GP, Jarvik L. Affective disorders and Alzheimer disease: a missing-link hypothesis. *Am J Geriatr Psychiatry.* 2001;9:444–5.

81. Lin KW, Wroolie TE, Robakis T, Rasgon NL. Adjuvant pioglitazone for unremitted depression: clinical correlates of treatment response. *Psychiatry Res.* 2015;230:846–52.

82. Marsland AL, Gianaros PJ, Abramowitch SM, Manuck SB, Hariri AR. Interleukin-6 covaries inversely with hippocampal grey matter volume in middle-aged adults. *Biol Psychiatry.* 2008;64:484–90.

83. Friedman EM, Hayney MS, Love GD, *et al.* Social relationships, sleep quality, and interleukin-6 in aging women. *Proc Natl Acad Sci USA.* 2005;102:18757–62.

84. Wiley JF, Gruenewald TL, Karlamangla AS, Seeman TE. Modeling multisystem physiological dysregulation. *Psychosom Med.* 2016;78:290–301.

85. Rasgon N, Jarvik L. Insulin resistance, affective disorders, and Alzheimer's disease: review and hypothesis. *J Gerontology.* 2004;59A:178–83.

86. Nouwen A, Winkley K, Twisk J, *et al.* Type 2 diabetes mellitus as a risk factor for the onset of depression: a systematic review and meta-analysis. *Diabetologia.* 2010;53:2480–6.

87. van Dooren FE, Nefs G, Schram MT, Verhey FR, Denollet J, Pouwer F. Depression and risk of mortality in people with diabetes mellitus: a systematic review and meta-analysis. *PLoS One.* 2013;8:e57058.

88. Cooper C, Sommerlad A, Lyketsos CG, Livingston G. Modifiable predictors of dementia in mild cognitive impairment: a systematic review and meta-analysis. *Am J Psychiatry.* 2015;172:323–34.

89. De Felice FG, Lourenco MV, Ferreira ST. How does brain insulin resistance develop in Alzheimer's disease? *Alzheimers Dement.* 2014;10(1 Suppl):S26–32.

90. Li JQ, Tan L, Wang HF, *et al.* Risk factors for predicting progression from mild cognitive impairment to Alzheimer's disease: a systematic review and meta-analysis of cohort studies. *J Neurol Neurosurg Psychiatry.* 2016;87:476–84.

91. Rasgon NL, Kenna HA, Wroolie TE, *et al.* Insulin resistance and hippocampal volume in women at risk for Alzheimer's disease. *Neurobiol Aging.* 2011;32:1942–8.

92. Wroolie TE, Kenna HA, Williams KE, *et al.* Differences in verbal memory performance in postmenopausal women receiving hormone therapy: 17beta-estradiol versus conjugated equine estrogens. *Am J Geriatr Psychiatry.* 2011;19:792–802.

93. Kenna H, Hoeft F, Kelley R, *et al.* Fasting plasma insulin and the default mode network in women at risk for Alzheimer's disease. *Neurobiol Aging.* 2013;34:641–9.

94. Grillo CA, Piroli GG, Lawrence RC, *et al.* Hippocampal insulin resistance impairs spatial learning and synaptic plasticity. *Diabetes.* 2015;64:3927–36.

95. Grillo CA, Piroli GG, Kaigler KF, Wilson SP, Wilson MA, Reagan LP. Downregulation of hypothalamic insulin receptor expression elicits depressive-like behaviors in rats. *Behav Brain Res.* 2011;222:230–5.

96. Grillo CA, Piroli GG, Evans AN, *et al.* Obesity/hyperleptinemic phenotype adversely affects hippocampal plasticity: effects of dietary restriction. *Physiol Behav.* 2011;104:235–41.

97. Grillo CA, Mulder P, Macht VA, *et al.* Dietary restriction reverses obesity-induced anhedonia. *Physiol Behav.* 2014;128:126–32.

98. Yao J, Irwin RW, Zhao L, Nilsen J, Hamilton RT, Brinton RD. Mitochondrial bioenergetic deficit precedes Alzheimer's pathology in female mouse model of Alzheimer's disease. *Proc Natl Acad Sci U S A.* 2009;106:14670–5.

99. Allfrey VG. Changes in chromosomal proteins at times of gene activation. *Fed Proc.* 1970;29:1447–60.

100. Mehler MF. Epigenetic principles and mechanisms underlying nervous system functions in health and disease. *Prog Neurobiol.* 2008;86:305–41.

101. Griffiths BB, Hunter RG. Neuroepigenetics of stress. *Neuroscience.* 2014;275:420–35.

102. Mehler MF, Mattick JS. Noncoding RNAs and RNA editing in brain development, functional diversification, and neurological disease. *Physiol Rev.* 2007;87:799–823.

103. McEwen BS. Brain on stress: how the social environment gets under the skin. *Proc Natl Acad Sci U S A.* 2012;109 Suppl 2:17180–5.

104. Halfon N, Larson K, Lu M, Tullis E, Russ S. Lifecourse health development: past, present and future. *Matern Child Health J.* 2014;18:344–65.

105. Waddington CH. The epigenotype. *Endeavour.* 1942;1:18–20.

106. Bavelier D, Levi DM, Li RW, Dan Y, Hensch TK. Removing brakes on adult brain plasticity: from molecular to behavioral interventions. *J Neurosci.* 2010;30:14964–71.

107. Castren E, Rantamaki T. The role of BDNF and its receptors in depression and antidepressant drug action: reactivation of developmental plasticity. *Dev Neurobiol.* 2010;70:289–97.

108. McEwen BS, Gianaros PJ. Stress- and allostasis-induced brain plasticity. *Annu Rev Med.* 2011;62:431–45.

109. Russo SJ, Murrough JW, Han MH, Charney DS, Nestler EJ. Neurobiology of resilience. *Nat Neurosci.* 2012;15:1475–84.

110. Heinrich C, Lahteinen S, Suzuki F, *et al.* Increase in BDNF-mediated TrkB signaling promotes epileptogenesis in a mouse model of mesial temporal lobe epilepsy. *Neurobiol Dis.* 2011;42:35–47.

111. Kokaia M, Ernfors P, Kokaia Z, Elmer E, Jaenisch R, Lindvall O. Suppressed epileptogenesis in BDNF mutant mice. *Exp Neurol.* 1995;133:215–24.

112. Scharfman HE. Hyperexcitability in combined entorhinal/ hippocampal slices of adult rat after exposure to brain-derived neurotrophic factor. *J Neurophysiol*. 1997;78:1082–95.

113. Sheline YI. Hippocampal atrophy in major depression: a result of depression-induced neurotoxicity? *Mol Psychiatry*. 1996;1:298–9.

114. Rajkowska G. Postmortem studies in mood disorders indicate altered numbers of neurons and glial cells. *Biol Psychiatry*. 2000;48:766–77.

115. Stockmeier CA, Mahajan GJ, Konick LC, *et al*. Cellular changes in the postmortem hippocampus in major depression. *Biol Psychiatry*. 2004;56:640–50.

116. Vythilingam M, Vermetten E, Anderson GM, *et al*. Hippocampal volume, memory, and cortisol status in major depressive disorder: effects of treatment. *Biol Psychiatry*. 2004;56:101–12.

117. Moore GJ, Bebehuk JM, Wilds IB, Chen G, Manji HK. Lithium-induced increase in human brain grey matter. *Lancet*. 2000;356:1241–2.

118. Gray JD, Rubin TG, Hunter RG, McEwen BS. Hippocampal gene expression changes underlying stress sensitization and recovery. *Mol Psychiatry*. 2014;19:1171–8.

119. Bloss EB, Janssen WG, McEwen BS, Morrison JH. Interactive effects of stress and aging on structural plasticity in the prefrontal cortex. *J Neurosci*. 2010;30:6726–31.

120. Pereira AC, Lambert HK, Grossman YS, *et al*. Glutamatergic regulation prevents hippocampal-dependent age-related cognitive decline through dendritic spine clustering. *Proc Natl Acad Sci U S A*. 2014;111:18733–8.

121. Bloss EB, Hunter RG, Waters EM, Munoz C, Bernard K, McEwen BS. Behavioral and biological effects of chronic S18986, a positive AMPA receptor modulator, during aging. *Exp Neurol*. 2008;210:109–17.

122. McEwen BS. Protective and damaging effects of stress mediators. *N Engl J Med*. 1998;338:171–9.

123. Luders E, Thompson PM, Kurth F. Larger hippocampal dimensions in meditation practitioners: differential effects in women and men. *Front Psychol*. 2015;6:186.

124. Hawkley LC, Cacioppo JT. Loneliness matters: a theoretical and empirical review of consequences and mechanisms. i. 2010;40:218–27.

125. Vetencourt JFM, Sale A, Viegi A, *et al*. The antidepressant fluoxetine restores plasticity in the adult visual cortex. *Science*. 2008;320:385–8.

126. Spolidoro M, Baroncelli L, Putignano E, Maya-Vetencourt JF, Viegi A, Maffei L. Food restriction enhances visual cortex plasticity in adulthood. *Nat Commun*. 2011;2:320.

127. Liston C, Gan WB. Glucocorticoids are critical regulators of dendritic spine development and plasticity *in vivo*. *Proc Natl Acad Sci U S A*. 2011;108:16074–9.

128. Liston C, Cichon JM, Jeanneteau F, Jia Z, Chao MV, Gan WB. Circadian glucocorticoid oscillations promote learning-dependent synapse formation and maintenance. *Nat Neurosci*. 2013;16:698–705.

129. Kramer AF, Colcombe SJ, McAuley E, *et al*. Enhancing brain and cognitive function of older adults through fitness training. *J Mol Neurosci*. 2003;20:213–21.

130. Colcombe SJ, Kramer AF, Erickson KI, *et al*. Cardiovascular fitness, cortical plasticity, and aging. *Proc Natl Acad Sci U S A*. 2004;101:3316–21.

131. Erickson KI, Prakash RS, Voss MW, *et al*. Aerobic fitness is associated with hippocampal volume in elderly humans. *Hippocampus*. 2009;19:1030–9.

132. Snyder MA, Smejkalova T, Forlano PM, Woolley CS. Multiple ERbeta antisera label in ERbeta knockout and null mouse tissues. *J Neurosci Methods*. 2010;188:226–34.

133. Babyak M, Blumenthal JA, Herman S, *et al*. Exercise treatment for major depression: maintenance of therapeutic benefit at 10 months. *Psychosom Med*. 2000;62:633–8.

134. Draganski B, Gaser C, Kempermann G, *et al*. Temporal and spatial dynamics of brain structure changes during extensive learning. *J Neurosci*. 2006;26:6314–17.

135. de Lange FP, Koers A, Kalkman JS, *et al*. Increase in prefrontal cortical volume following cognitive behavioural therapy in patients with chronic fatigue syndrome. *Brain*. 2008;131: 2172–80.

136. Holzel BK, Carmody J, Evans KC, *et al*. Stress reduction correlates with structural changes in the amygdala. *Soc Cogn Affect Neurosci*. 2010;5:11–17.

137. Singleton O, Holzel BK, Vangel M, Brach N, Carmody J, Lazar SW. Change in brainstem gray matter concentration following a mindfulness-based intervention is correlated with improvement in psychological well-being. *Front Hum Neurosci*. 2014;8:33.

138. Holzel BK, Carmody J, Vangel M, *et al*. Mindfulness practice leads to increases in regional brain gray matter density. *Psychiatry Res*. 2011;191:36–43.

139. Gard T, Taquet M, Dixit R, *et al*. Fluid intelligence and brain functional organization in aging yoga and meditation practitioners. *Front Aging Neurosci*. 2014;6:76.

140. Tang YY, Holzel BK, Posner MI. The neuroscience of mindfulness meditation. *Nat Rev Neurosci*. 2015;16:213–25.

# 80

# Genetics of stress-related disorders

*Michael G. Gottschalk and Katharina Domschke*

## Introduction

This chapter will highlight the genetic architecture of trauma- and stress-related disorders, exemplified by post-traumatic stress disorder (PTSD), which itself overlaps in symptom dimensions with acute stress disorder and adjustment disorder. Within DSM-5, this nosological group shares, as part of their diagnosis, the specific call for an environmental component in the form of direct or indirect exposure to a causative traumatic incident [1]. This unique position among psychiatric disorders is particularly relevant for studying the interaction of an organism's internal biological component with external stimuli in the pathogenesis of a mental disorder.

Here, we will review the genetics of stress-related disorders, focusing on clinical genetic approaches such as family and twin studies and molecular genetic studies, that is candidate gene and hypothesis-generating genome-wide association studies (GWAS), as well as gene–environment and epigenetic approaches. Due to the close phenomenological relationship between the categories of trauma- and stress-related disorders and anxiety disorders, the genetics of cross-disorder phenotypes and cross-cutting symptom measurements will build an additional focus.

## Genetics of stress-related disorders

### Family studies and twin studies

The requirement for trauma exposure as a key factor in the diagnosis of PTSD poses a challenge to estimates of familial aggregation, since the exact degree of trauma exposure is likely to vary between otherwise comparable relatives. The task to distinguish the heritable components of PTSD is difficult. Indeed, biological factors could affect an individual's liability to PTSD in several ways, including, but not limited to an increased susceptibility to trauma exposure (gene–environment correlation), an increased susceptibility to PTSD independent of the trauma, an influence on risk factors potentially linked to PTSD (for example, the personality trait of increased risk-seeking behaviour), and/or mediation of a pleiotropic effect on several of these. For example, in one family study, PTSD lifetime symptoms of mothers were significantly associated with PTSD symptoms in

children in a dose-dependent fashion, while similarly predicting increased trauma exposure in children, which accounted for 74% of the increased PTSD incidence rate [2].

Quantitative genetic analysis of Vietnam-era veteran monozygotic and dizygotic male twin pairs overcame some of the problems of unequal trauma exposure. It revealed a substantial genetic influence on the susceptibility to all assessed PTSD symptoms; a bivariate genetic model, adjusted for combat exposure, estimated the heritability of re-experiencing symptoms to range between 0.13 and 0.30 [3]. The heritability of avoidance and arousal symptoms varied between 0.30–0.34 and 0.28–0.32, respectively, with no evidence for a shared environmental component [3]. In a study of genetic and environmental effects on exposure to assaultive and non-assaultive trauma and occurrence of PTSD symptoms in male and female twin pairs of non-veteran volunteers with trauma exposure, the variance of reported symptoms was best explained by genetic factors for assaultive trauma (overall heritability of 0.53), with genetic factors particularly contributing to symptoms of re-experiencing (0.36) and numbing (0.36), whereas no genetic component was found in non-assaultive trauma (mainly explained by non-shared environmental factors) [4] (Table 80.1).

While both genetic and non-shared environmental influences affected PTSD symptoms, and the severity of PTSD symptoms has been linked to the number of assaultive traumatic events suffered, the influence of genetic factors has been suggested to decline with increase in total trauma number [5]. In other words, there appears to be a threshold beyond which the quantitative summation of environmental factors supervenes [5]. Another population-based twin sample estimated the magnitude of additive genetic influences, based on trauma quality, and reported a greater genetic contribution in high-risk trauma (0.60; trauma reported as most disturbing), as compared to low-risk trauma (0.47), with a genetic correlation between high-risk trauma and PTSD of 0.89, whereas for low-risk trauma and additive genetic and non-shared environmental influences, a lower correlation of 0.57 was observed [6].

### Structural and rare variant studies

No systematic research efforts have been published linking PTSD to recognized neurodevelopmental disorders, structural genetic variations, or rare single-nucleotide polymorphisms (SNPs).

Table 80.1 Trauma- and symptom-focused perspectives on the heritability of stress-related disorders

| | Additive genetic factors | | Shared environment | | Unique environment | |
|---|---|---|---|---|---|---|
| | a² | 95% CI | c² | 95% CI | e² | 95% CI |
| **Trauma exposure** | | | | | | |
| Assaultive trauma[a] | 0.53 | 0.40–0.67 | – | – | 0.42 | 0.33–0.60 |
| Non-assaultive trauma[a] | – | – | 0.32 | 0.21–0.45 | 0.68 | 0.55–0.80 |
| Low-risk trauma[b] | 0.47 | 0.35–0.57 | – | – | 0.53 | 0.43–0.65 |
| High-risk trauma[b] | 0.60 | 0.49–0.71 | – | – | 0.40 | 0.29–0.51 |
| **Clinical presentation** | | | | | | |
| Re-experiencing symptoms[a] | 0.36 | 0.23–0.51 | – | – | 0.64 | 0.54–0.80 |
| Avoidance symptoms[a] | 0.28 | 0.14–0.44 | – | – | 0.72 | 0.56–0.86 |
| Numbing symptoms[a] | 0.36 | 0.22–0.50 | – | – | 0.64 | 0.50–0.78 |
| Hyperarousal symptoms[a] | 0.29 | 0.15–0.44 | – | – | 0.71 | 0.56–0.85 |
| Total PTSD symptoms[a] | 0.38 | 0.24–0.52 | – | – | 0.62 | 0.48–0.76 |
| PTSD diagnosis[b] | 0.46 | 0.31–0.62 | – | – | 0.54 | 0.38–0.69 |

Assaultive trauma comprised captivity and physical/sexual assault. Non-assaultive trauma comprised natural disasters, motor vehicle accidents, and the occurrence of a sudden death in the family. Low-risk trauma comprised combat exposure and accidents. High-risk trauma comprised rape, sexual molestation, and childhood neglect/abuse. Heritability estimates not adding up to 1.0 are derived from rounding up/down effects.

PTSD, post-traumatic stress disorder; CI, confidence interval; a², additive genetic factors; c², shared environmental factors; e², unique environmental factors.

[a] [4].
[b] [6].

## GWAS, candidate genes, gene–environment interaction, and 'therapy genetics' studies

The first GWAS of PTSD was performed in a small trauma-exposed cohort of African-American veterans and their intimate partners (295 cases, 196 controls) and yielded several SNPs with suggestive associations, with one polymorphism in the RAR (retinoic acid receptor)-related orphan receptor alpha gene (*RORA*) reaching genome-wide significance (rs8042149, C allele) [7]. The rs8042149 finding failed to replicate in two independent replication samples, but interestingly, other *RORA* SNPs were implicated as PTSD risk variants [7] . Notably, a subsample analysis of the initial GWAS cohort, screening 606 SNPs spanning the *RORA* gene, significantly associated rs8042149 with the fear sub-factor of PTSD comorbidities (outcome of a 3-factor confirmatory factor analysis, next to an internalizing and an externalizing sub-factor) [8].

A GWAS conducted in a cohort of European-Americans (300 cases, 1278 controls) yielded rs406001 on chromosome 7p12 as a genome-wide significant hit, the nearest gene being the protein cordon-bleu (*COBL*) and the second-best hit located in the first intron of the tolloid-like protein 1 (*TLL1*), barely missing genome-wide significance (rs6812849, $P = 2.99 \times 10^{-7}$) [9]. A SNP replication analysis of the top GWAS hits in another cohort and a subsequent combined cohort analysis resulted in a more favourable overall genome-wide statistical outcome for *TLL1* rs6812849 [9]. An analysis of the main effects of *COBL* SNPs in an African-American civilian population did not replicate, but a significant genotype–environment interaction with childhood trauma was found for *COBL* rs406001 [10]. The T allele mediated higher PTSD symptom intensity and was associated with significantly decreased fractional anisotropy in left hemisphere structures (inferior fronto-occipital fasciculus, uncinate fasciculus, orbitofrontal white matter tracts, and inferior longitudinal fasciculus) [10].

Screening for genome-wide significant association in a sample of trauma-exposed African-American women (94 cases, 319 controls) identified the minor G allele of rs10170218, a SNP within the long intergenic non-coding RNA sequence *AC068718.1* gene located at 2q32.1 [11]. This was replicated in a second independent cohort of European-American women [11]. A functional enrichment analysis of the nominally significant GWAS findings highlighted pathways related to the maintenance of telomere length [11].

Another GWAS (3167 cases, 4607 trauma-exposed controls) found a genome-wide significant hit in the ankyrin repeat domain-containing protein 55 gene (*ANKRD55*, rs159572) in subjects of African-American ancestry and one close to the zinc finger protein 626 gene (*ZNF626*, rs11085374) in the European-American subsamples [12].

A study analysing 3742 SNPs of over 300 genes previously reported as PTSD candidate risk genes in trauma-exposed European-American women (845 cases, 1693 controls) in a categorical and dimensional fashion found the most significant association between the intronic synaptic vesicular amine transporter (*SLC18A2*, involved in the ATP-dependent neurotransmitter storage) rs363276 A allele and a PTSD diagnosis [13]. In a similar experimental design examining the association of 3755 candidate genes and PTSD in a gene–environment interaction approach with childhood trauma in a cohort of male soldiers of European ancestry (810 samples), an association was identified between the beta-2 adrenergic receptor (*ADRB2*) rs2400707 G allele and increased childhood adversity load, resulting in heightened PTSD symptom intensity, which was subsequently replicated in an independent sample of predominantly female African-American civilians (2083 samples) [14].

A GWAS in trauma-exposed United States marines of mixed ancestry (940 cases, 2554 controls) resulted in a significant association for the phosphoribosyltransferase domain-containing protein 1

(*PRTFDC1*); the rs6482463 minor A allele was under-represented in PTSD. A replication attempt in an independent military cohort failed, and although a candidate gene screen, including *RORA, TLL1,* and *AC068718.1* SNPs, yielded nominally significant associations, no finding survived correction for the number of polymorphisms tested per gene [15]. In general, results of hypothesis-generating studies in such small samples must be viewed with caution, since it is difficult to exclude chance findings.

Finally, the largest GWAS of PTSD to date (5182 cases; 15,548 controls, 13,638 of which were trauma-exposed) suggested a genome-wide significant finding in the kelch-like protein 1 gene (*KLHL1*, rs139558732) detected in its African-American subsample (2520 cases, 7171 controls) [16]. However, recent GWAS investigations in

a cohort of mixed-ancestry Iraq–Afghanistan-era veterans [17] and of the DSM-5 dissociative subtype of PTSD in a cohort of European-American United States military veterans [18] did not report any genome-wide significant results.

In addition to GWAS, the impact of specific genetic variation in PTSD has focused on genes related to monoaminergic neurotransmission (Fig. 80.1) analogous to candidate studies performed in anxiety disorders (see Chapter 89) and neuroendocrine functioning, in particular the hypothalamic–pituitary–adrenal (HPA) axis. A recent meta-analysis of trauma-exposed samples found only a trend towards significance between PTSD and the short (s) allele of the serotonin transporter (*SLC6A4*, chromosome 17q11.2) *5-HTTLPR* (5-hydroxytryptamine transporter-linked polymorphic region;

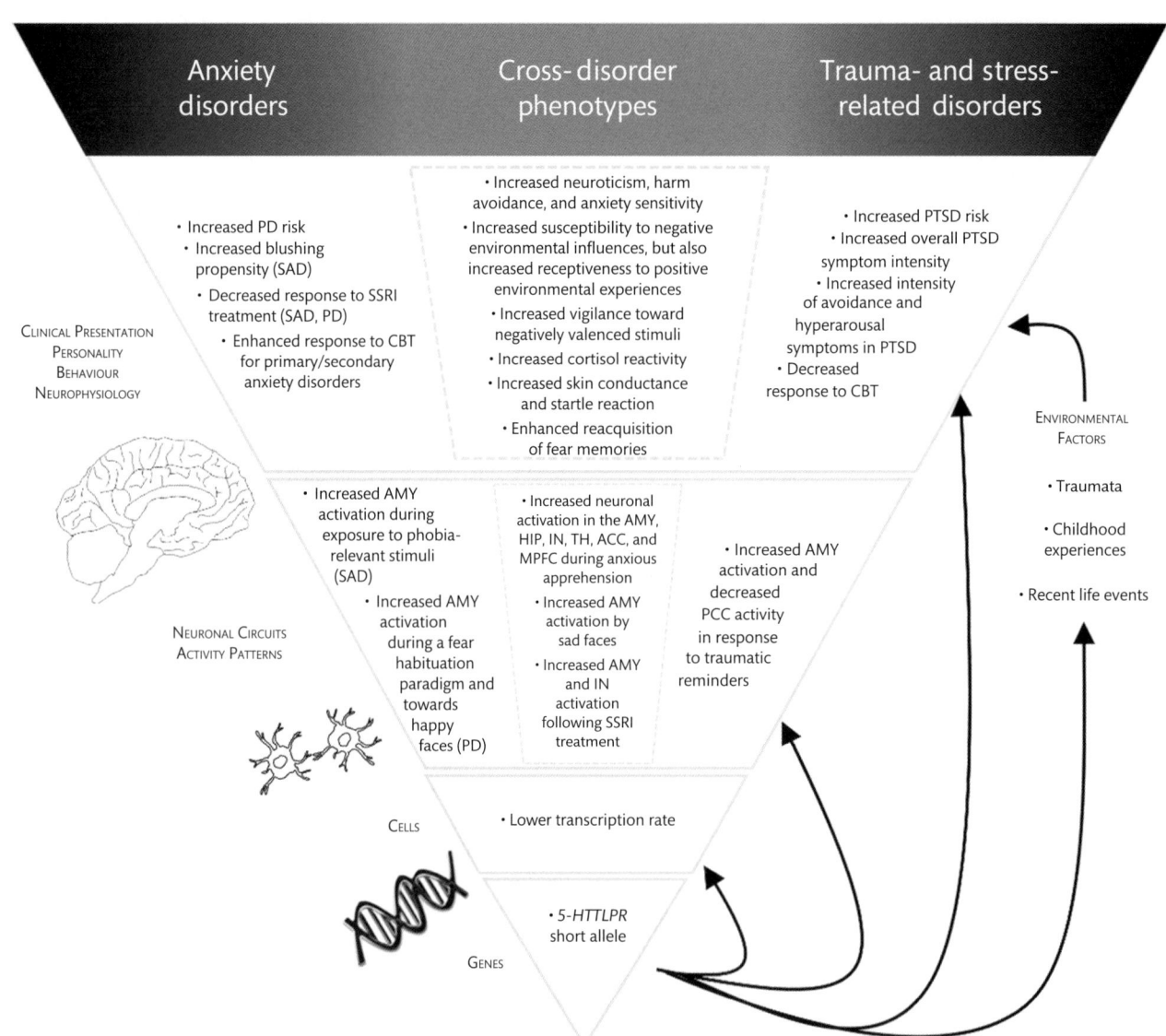

**Fig. 80.1** Multi-level evidence linking the serotonergic system to trauma- and stress-related disorders, cross-disorder phenotypes, and anxiety disorders. The short allele/low transcriptional activity variants of the *5-HTTLPR* were chosen as seed node. Arrows represent domain interrelations of systems analysis mediating interactions between genetic and environmental factors, potentially leading to observable meta-phenomena crossing classic nosological boundaries and connecting different spectra of psychopathology. Note that some authors include the *rs25531* polymorphism in their analyses, with the minor G allele rendering transporter expression levels of the long *5-HTTLPR* allele more closely to the short allele. Refer to the text for detailed supporting literature. ACC, anterior cingulate cortex; AMY, amygdala; CBT, cognitive behavioural therapy; HIP, hippocampus; IN, insula; MPFC, medial prefrontal cortex; PCC, posterior cingulate cortex; PD, panic disorder; PTSD, post-traumatic stress disorder; SAD, social anxiety disorder; SSRI, selective serotonin reuptake inhibitor; TH, thalamus.

the s allele is linked to decreased expression/transporter activity, compared to the long [l] variant) [19]. However, the s/s genotype and high trauma exposure were associated with PTSD, arguing for a further exploration of gene–environment interaction to clarify the polymorphism's role in trauma-related psychopathology [19]. Soldiers with one or two copies of the low-functioning 5-HTTLPR/rs25531 alleles (the minor rs25531 G allele reduces transporter expression levels like the s variant) reported increased symptoms of PTSD and anxiety in response to heightened exposure to war zone stressors, as compared to carriers of high-functioning alleles [20]. Accordingly, the genotype with low transcriptional efficiency was associated with PTSD diagnoses and PTSD symptom severity in veterans [21]. Interestingly, the low-functioning 5-HTTLPR/rs25531 alleles mediated an interaction effect of increased PTSD symptoms during battle deployment only in individuals with greater attentional avoidance of threats, rather than in individuals with vigilant threat appraisal [22]. Similarly, following a university campus shooting, the low-functioning 5-HTTLPR/rs25531 genotypes predicted increased acute stress symptom intensity 2–4 weeks after the event, even when correcting for shooting exposure; symptoms of avoidance and hyperarousal, but not of re-experiencing, were the most implicated [23].

Remarkably, a pharmacogenetic study examining the 4- and 12-week PTSD treatment response to sertraline linked l allele homozygosity to reduced dropout rates due to adverse effects and increased efficacy; most strikingly, there was a 48% response rate (defined as a minimum symptom reduction of 30%) by week 12, as compared to a 0% response rate in s allele carriers [24]. Correspondingly, low-expression 5-HTTLPR/rs25531 genotype carriers displayed a significantly worse 6-month treatment outcome following an 8-week exposure-based cognitive behavioural therapy (CBT) programme, controlling for pre-CBT symptom severity and the number of treatment sessions [25].

The catechol-O-methyltransferase COMT (chromosome 22q11.21) rs4680 A/A genotype has been associated with PTSD, particularly in patients who had experienced childhood adversities and possessed high neuroticism scores [26]. The minor A allele results in an exchange of amino acid 158 valine (major G allele) to methionine and significantly increased degradation of catecholamine neurotransmitters—often referred to as the val158met polymorphism. Surprisingly, it has been indicated further that, while COMT rs4680 G (val) allele carriers showed a classic dose–response relationship of lifetime trauma abundance and PTSD incidence rate, met/met genotype carriers exhibited an increased risk of PTSD, independent of trauma load [27].

The peptidyl-prolyl cis–trans isomerase FKBP5, commonly referred to as the FK506 binding protein 5 (FKBP5, chromosome 6p21.31), is probably one of the most extensively characterized candidate genes associated with PTSD. FKBP5 is an immunophilin family member with isomerase and chaperone functions; it interacts with unligated steroid receptor heterocomplexes through heat shock protein 90 (HSP90), influencing intracellular trafficking behaviour, receptor affinity, and nuclear translocation. Since FKBP5 transcription is activated by glucocorticoid receptors via steroid response elements, a direct negative feedback loop is created [28]. Several SNPs within the FKPB5 gene (rs1360780 T allele, rs3800373 C allele, rs9296158 A allele, and rs9470080 T allele) do not directly predict PTSD symptom outcome or interact with non-childhood trauma [29]. Instead, they appear to interact with the severity of child abuse to predict increased levels of adult PTSD symptom levels and a greater suppression of cortisol release during a pharmacological challenge with dexamethasone [29]. A study evaluating FKBP5 SNPs in a trauma-exposed African-American cohort (1963 samples) reported a significant association between the rs1360780 A allele (located in a functional enhancer region in intron 2 488 bp away from a glucocorticoid response element) and childhood trauma on PTSD symptoms [30]. The FKBP5 rs1360780 T allele has been independently reported to predict an increased risk of long-term PTSD symptom relapse following narrative exposure therapy [31]. In the same African-American cohort, the rs9470080 T allele increased the risk to be diagnosed with PTSD in an interaction with childhood maltreatment; yet surprisingly, T/T genotype carriers without childhood trauma had the lowest risk of PTSD [32]. In studies with diffusion tensor imaging and resting state functional magnetic resonance imaging (fMRI), rs1360780 T allele carriers with PTSD displayed a decreased structural, as well as functional, connectivity between the anterior cingulate cortex and the hippocampus, which has been suggested as a source of the pathologically increased neuronal salience observed in PTSD [33]. Moreover, in an attempt to evaluate different biologically distinct subtypes of PTSD, it has been found that rs9296158 A allele carriers display increased plasma cortisol levels [34]. These, in turn, correlated with symptom intensity and significantly influenced peripheral mRNA levels of genes carrying steroid hormone transcription factor binding sites in whole blood [34].

Other work has focused on different elements of neurohormonal stress response regulation such as the gene coding for the pituitary adenylyl cyclase-activating polypeptide type I receptor (ADCYAP1R1, chromosome 7p14.3), a G protein-coupled receptor implicated in the modulation of adrenocorticotrophic hormone (ACTH) secretion. The C allele of ADCYAP1R1 rs2267735, located in a putative oestrogen response element, has been linked to PTSD symptom intensity and PTSD diagnosis in females and reduced discrimination of danger and safety cues in a fear conditioning paradigm [35]. Subsequent gene–environment studies found significant interactions of the ADCYAP1R1 rs2267735 C allele and the total amount of suffered traumata [36], or the degree of experienced childhood maltreatment [37], in predicting increased female PTSD symptom intensity. Imaging has revealed decreased hippocampal activity during contextual, but not during cued, fear conditioning in female ADCYAP1R1 rs2267735 C allele carriers [38] and an increased reactivity of the amygdala and hippocampus to threat stimuli, as well as decreased functional connectivity between the amygdala and the hippocampus during passive viewing of threatening stimuli [39]. Moreover, with regard to HPA axis regulation, two SNPs (rs8192496 and rs2190242) in the corticotropin-releasing hormone receptor 2 (CRHR2, chromosome 7p14.3) gene have been linked to a decreased risk of suffering from PTSD in female trauma-exposed veterans, a proposed effect of an attenuated neurohormonal stress response [40]. Finally, in a prospective emergency department setting, a composite additive risk score derived off genes related to stress response and arousal, including, among others, FKBP5, ADCYAP1R1, the CRH receptor 1 gene (CRHR1, chromosome 17q21.31), and COMT, predicted increased PTSD symptoms in subjects without early post-trauma intervention classified as 'risk' carriers, as compared to 'low-risk' and 'resilience' genotypes [41]. Additionally, PTSD symptom intensity 12 weeks after trauma only correlated with the genetic risk load in the group without intervention, but not in patients with imaginal exposure therapy to trauma memory, with the overall number of risk alleles significantly associated with an increased PTSD incidence rate [41].

### Epigenetic studies

The potential relevance of maladaptive changes in chromatin structure and DNA methylation as mediators of the influence of traumatic experiences cannot be underestimated. An impact can be expected from the single cell level up to cognitive patterns and behaviour in the organism's allostatic biological load in general, and in manifestations of PTSD in particular.

A large microarray approach evaluating DNA methylation of more than 14,000 genes in 23 PTSD-affected and 77 PTSD-unaffected individuals suggested traumatic events to induce downstream alterations in immune system functions by reducing methylation levels of genes related to cytokine production and innate immunity [42].

At the candidate gene level, overall *SLC6A4* promoter region methylation influenced the risk of PTSD, independently of the *5-HTTLPR* genotype, with low methylation levels correlating with an increased PTSD incidence rate in people who experienced multiple traumata [43]. Similarly significant associations were discerned between *SLC6A4* hypomethylation and increased PTSD symptom intensity and symptom quantity [43].

A study in a trauma-exposed African-American cohort found that *FKBP5* rs1360780 influenced chromatin conformation with respect to the transcription start site—A allele carriers exposed to childhood trauma displayed decreased methylation levels close to, and within, glucocorticoid response elements in intron 7, independent of recent lifetime trauma exposure [30]. It was hypothesized that this hypomethylation in risk allele carriers would imply an increased induction of *FKBP5* by glucocorticoid receptor activation and enhancement of the ultra-short negative HPA feedback loop, leading to increased glucocorticoid receptor resistance [30]. Additionally, structural imaging data revealed a significant negative correlation between peripheral *FKBP5* intron 7 methylation and hippocampal volume [30]. Thus, epigenetic changes in these genes not only alter the sensitivity of peripheral glucocorticoid receptors, but are also associated with morphological changes in limbic areas already believed to be indicative of a higher stress hormone system reactivity [30].

Transgenerational effects of trauma exposure have been explored in a study of Holocaust survivors and their offspring; survivors showed significantly increased *FKPB5* methylation, yet decreased levels in their offspring [44]. At the same time, significant interactions of the *FKBP5* rs1360780 T allele and CpG-specific methylation levels with either parental trauma intensity or the severity of self-experienced childhood trauma were reported, providing insights into the psychophysiological epigenetic integration of trauma across age groups [44].

Finally, in a cohort of children undergoing CBT for anxiety disorders, there was a significant correlation between the change in *FKBP5* methylation and therapy response, with responders demonstrating the greatest decrease in methylation, an effect which was specific to *FKBP5* rs1360780 T allele carriers [45].

Additional epigenetic evidence links other HPA regulators to PTSD. Remarkably, while increased *ADCYAP1R1* methylation was

associated with a PTSD diagnosis, rs2267735 C allele carriers displayed reduced cerebral mRNA expression levels [35]. Furthermore, decreased glucocorticoid receptor (*NR3C1*, chromosome 5q31.3) promoter region methylation in peripheral blood mononuclear cells was detected in veterans with PTSD [46]. It was further associated with increased cortisol levels following the dexamethasone suppression test, reports of psychiatric distress, peritraumatic dissociation, and poor sleep quality [46]. In Holocaust survivors' offspring with both parents suffering from PTSD, lower *NR3C1* methylation was observed, compared to offspring with only paternal PTSD, and lower methylation levels correlated with increased post-dexamethasone cortisol suppression [47].

Interestingly, the methylation state of DNA methyltransferases themselves has been investigated following trauma exposure, with probands developing PTSD later on showing increased methylation of DNA (cytosine-5)-methyltransferase 1 (*DNMT1*), whereas low pre-trauma methylation of DNA (cytosine-5)-methyltransferase 3B (*DNMT3B*) predicted increased levels of PTSD symptom severity [48].

## Genetics of cross-disorder phenotypes of post-traumatic stress and anxiety

Heritability estimate studies suggest a shared genetic signature underlying PTSD and anxiety spectrum conditions, namely specific phobia (SP), social anxiety disorder (SAD), agoraphobia (AP), panic disorder (PD), and generalized anxiety disorder (GAD) [49]. A common diathesis of PTSD is further suggested with intermediate phenotypes, such as fear generalization, avoidance behaviour, anxiety sensitivity, state/trait anxiety, harm avoidance, and physiological hyper-responsiveness to certain stimuli, supported by their genetic correlation and joint cross-disorder familial risk [50, 51].

Unsurprisingly, in addition to an overlap in the genetic architecture of trauma- and stress-related disorders and anxiety disorders, both diagnostic categories are based upon a selection of highly connected, psychometrically assessable constructs, outlining, for example, the gradual development of normative stimulus-specific fears into functionally impairing generalized anxiety. Primarily, the study of these cross-disorder post-traumatic stress and anxiety phenotypes has focused on continuous traits, which are hypothesized to represent different forms of neuropsychiatric vulnerability for the diagnosis of the corresponding disorders during development. As outlined in later sections, various intermediate phenotype concepts have been suggested to affect the onset, therapy, or disease course of trauma-inflicted psychological stress. (Also see Chapter 89 for additional remarks on potentially relevant cross-disorder phenotypes.)

### Serotonergic system

Fig. 80.1 depicts the multi-level, cross-disorder genetic vulnerability mediated by several intermediate phenotypes and environmental factors for *SLC6A4/5-HTT* gene variation. A meta-analysis of cortisol reactivity (1686 cases) to acute psychosocial stress reported a moderating effect of the *5-HTTLPR* polymorphism, with homozygous s allele carriers demonstrating increased cortisol reactivity [52]. Increased vigilance towards negatively valenced stimuli in carriers of low-active *5-HTTLPR* alleles was further confirmed via a meta-analysis (807 cases) of studies focusing on attentional biases [53]. However, the low-expression forms of *5-HTTLPR* could rather represent a plasticity factor capable of developing stronger biases for both negative and positive affective stimuli [54]. Thus, it has been suggested that the increased amygdala response to aversive stimuli in carriers of the short *5-HTTLPR* allele is not mediated by 5-HTT availability in adults, but rather by amygdala size, with smaller amygdala volumes correlating with increased neural activation, suggesting a neurodevelopmental influence of the serotonergic polymorphism [55]. Another meta-analysis (9361 cases) of gene–environment studies in children and adolescents revealed that Caucasian carriers of the *5-HTTLPR* s allele are not only significantly more vulnerable to negative environmental influences, but also more receptive to positive input than l/l carriers [56]. In a cohort of healthy subjects, the *5-HTTLPR* l/l genotype resulted in higher anxiety sensitivity scores in an interaction with childhood trauma exposure, in particular with regard to somatic sub-dimensions of anxiety sensitivity [57]. Nevertheless, despite most studies focusing on risk factors, few have also included protective, resilience-increasing factors such as self-efficacy. When childhood trauma and self-efficacy were assessed in relation to trait anxiety, social anxiety, and agoraphobic anxiety in healthy adults genotyped for the *5-HTTLPR*/rs25531, s allele carriers showed a positive correlation of trauma and anxiety, independent of self-efficacy [58]. Conversely, $l_A/l_A$ homozygotes with low self-efficacy scored significantly higher in all available anxiety assessments when they had experienced childhood trauma but were resilient when they possessed high self-efficacy [58].

### Hormone system

In relation to the HPA axis, carriers of the *CRHR1* rs110402 A allele, which has been implicated in elevated cortisol reactivity to acute stressors, displayed blunted basolateral amygdala habituation in a fear extinction paradigm, and an increased risk to be diagnosed with any anxiety disorder [59]. The *CRHR1* rs878886 minor G variant has been associated with reduced fear-conditioned responses to a threat cue and a tendency towards anxious generalization and increased contextual anxiety in an interaction with the low-activity alleles of the *5-HTTLPR* [60]. A replication study confirmed the acquisition deficit and increased contextual anxiety in rs878886 G allele carriers and suggested a tri-allelic interaction with low-expression *5-HTTLPR*/rs25531 variants on cued fear acquisition [61]. In imaging genetic approaches, several SNPs in both HPA-relevant genes, *CRHR1* and *NR3C1*, have been linked to increased amygdala activation during the acquisition phase of a fear conditioning paradigm and decreased prefrontal activity during the extinction phase, respectively [62]. Interestingly, to note from an epigenetic viewpoint, currently healthy subjects with a lifetime anxiety disorder diagnosis have lower levels of *NR3C1* promoter region methylation, while the number of experienced childhood adversities negatively correlated with promoter region methylation only in subjects without a lifetime diagnosis [63]. A microsatellite marker [64] and several SNPs [65] within the *CRH* gene itself have also been linked to behavioural inhibition in children with a familial loading of PD. Moreover, carriers of the *FKBP5* rs1360780 T allele have been shown to display heightened levels of harm avoidance [66] and an attention bias towards threat cues and

increased hippocampal activation during threat evaluation [67], while amygdala activation was increased in risk allele carriers exposed to emotional neglect in childhood [68].

### Catecholaminergic system

Evaluation of the *COMT* val158met polymorphism in association with childhood maltreatment demonstrated that *val/val* allele carriers displayed a significantly increased startle response to aversive pictures, while *met/met* carriers showed blunted responses to unpleasant stimuli [69]. The effect in *val* carriers was discerned to be potentiated by increased amounts of maltreatment, which had no interaction effect in *met* allele carriers [69]. In a double-blind, placebo-controlled design, it has also been shown that *val* allele carriers displayed an increased startle potentiation towards aversive stimuli, independently of an acute injection of levodopa (L-dopa), whereas in *met* allele carriers, the startle response to unpleasant pictures was only enhanced under L-dopa administration, but not by placebo [70]. This would support the influence of catecholaminergic neurotransmission on the emotion-potentiated startle reflex either by increased phasic dopamine abundance, as conferred by the high-activity *val* allele, or by pharmacologically enhanced dopamine availability, eventually leading to a maladaptive predisposition of the emotional valence system.

## Clinical challenges and future perspectives

The gene–environment interactions reported in relation to PTSD highlight not only very appealing candidates, such as the serotonergic or HPA system, but also underline the importance of *individual vulnerability windows* in personal development, for example reflected by 'plasticity polymorphisms' influencing gene expression or protein activity, which interact with childhood experiences, yet are not influenced by recent life events. Due to the special position of PTSD in psychiatric nosology, genetic association and gene–environment studies pose the challenge that *causative and non-causative trauma* exposures are correlated and difficult to disentangle [71]. While trauma exposure is a diagnostic criterion of PTSD, one must distinguish that category which is sufficient to cause PTSD and that which increases the risk of a future PTSD diagnosis (but, by itself, is not enough to warrant a diagnosis) [72]. Another aspect, not to be underestimated, is the influence genetic polymorphisms may have on the exposure to trauma per se, mediated by a *gene-by-environment correlation*. Thus, a polymorphism might not only increase the susceptibility to trauma (and thereby to develop subsequent PTSD), but also rather influence the risk of a PTSD diagnosis via an increased trauma incidence rate (either of causative or risk-increasing trauma). With the ever growing feasibility and accessibility of large sample numbers in psychiatric genetics, the identification of rare variants with high penetrance could further substantiate efforts at multilocus predictions, by simultaneously integrating an array of molecular variations, next to other biological, developmental, environmental, epidemiological, or temperamental risk factors. Large-scale *machine-learning algorithms* have, for example, already been applied to identify the most significant predictors of PTSD, including demographic factors (females, married), traumatic experience (almost exclusively violence-related, including organized violence, interpersonal violence, and relationship/sexual violence), and psychiatric lifetime diagnoses (attention-deficit/hyperactivity disorder, separation anxiety disorder, SP, GAD, and prior unrelated PTSD) [73]. Moreover, genetic findings in stress-related intermediate phenotypes point towards a *bottom–up, multi-dimensional, cross-disorder taxonomy*, for example, by suggesting a considerable degree of genetic correlation between trauma-related and anxiety disorders, spanning categorical classifications, subsyndromal dimensional constructs of symptoms, temperament and environmental risk, and behavioural, neurophysiological, and neuronal circuit readouts (Fig. 80.1). This could result in specified functional domains of behaviour built upon aggregated cross-discipline evidence and grouped into higher-level processes of emotional and cognitive functioning. These may then inform major constructs, like, for example, the negative valence system within the Research Domain Criteria (RDoC) initiative [74]. Finally, future studies will have to systematically explore the potential of genetic/epigenetic tools for treatment response prediction, aiming at establishing a biomarker-driven personalized, individually tailored 'precision medicine' approach in stress-related disorders [75].

## Conclusions

Stress-related disorders display moderate heritability, as outlined by family and twin studies. Molecular genetic studies have begun to elucidate to what extent genetic and epigenetic variations shape the onset, clinical presentation, and therapy of stress-related disorders. So far, these have notably highlighted the relevance of the serotonergic and catecholaminergic systems, as well as HPA axis regulation in stress-related disorders (Table 80.2). GWAS and subsequent cross-sample meta-analyses in large cohort sizes complement the findings on candidate gene and gene–environment approaches. The potentially artificial boundaries created by a categorical diagnostic system are challenged by interdisciplinary studies gathering multi-level evidence for a common, cross-disorder genetic trunk. In light of the apparent intricacy of the implicated principal components and the heterogeneity of interaction effects and genetic pleiotropy, tools offered by systems biology could promote the synthesis of candidate genes into functional molecular processes linking environmental and psychological readouts. A central equivalent of

**Table 80.2** Overview of genetic variants implicated in PTSD and cross-disorder post-traumatic stress and anxiety phenotypes. The overall degree of confidence was ranked from '+' = 'low' to '++++' = 'high', based on the reviewed evidence (refer to the individual sections in this chapter for detailed supporting literature)

| Gene | Top risk variant | Evidence from structural, rare variant, GWAS, candidate gene, gene–environment, and epigenetic studies | Overall degree of confidence |
|---|---|---|---|
| SLC6A4 | Serotonin transporter polymorphic region (5-HTTLPR) short allele | Meta-analytical evidence for increased PTSD risk [19]<br>Meta-analytical evidence for interaction with high trauma exposure in PTSD risk [19]<br>Increased PTSD symptoms in response to increased trauma exposure [20]<br>Increased PTSD incidence rate and symptom severity [21]<br>Interaction with attentional avoidance of threats, leading to increased PTSD symptoms [22]<br>Increased acute stress symptom intensity [23]<br>Decreased response to sertraline treatment [24]<br>Decreased response to exposure-based CBT [27]<br>Decreased promoter methylation associated with increased PTSD incidence rate and symptom intensity [43]<br>Meta-analytical evidence for increased cortisol response to psychosocial stress [52]<br>Meta-analytical evidence for attentional bias to negatively valenced stimuli [53]<br>Meta-analytical evidence for increased vulnerability to negative environmental influences, but also increased receptiveness to positive influences [56] | ++++ |
| FKBP5 | rs1360780 T allele | Increased PTSD symptoms in interaction with childhood trauma [29]<br>Increased PTSD symptom relapse following narrative exposure therapy [31]<br>Decreased functional and structural connectivity between the anterior cingulate cortex and the hippocampus [33]<br>Interaction between CpG-specific methylation levels and parental or childhood trauma [44]<br>Decreased methylation associated with increased CBT therapy response for anxiety disorders [45]<br>Increased harm avoidance [67]<br>Increased attentional bias towards threat cues and increased hippocampal activation during threat evaluation [68]<br>Increased amygdala activation in interaction with emotional neglect during childhood [69] | ++++ |
| ADCYAP1R1 | rs2267735 C allele | Increased PTSD symptom intensity and PTSD incidence rate in females and reduced discriminative fear conditioning [35]<br>Increased female PTSD symptom intensity in interaction with trauma intensity [36]<br>Increased female PTSD symptom intensity in interaction with childhood maltreatment [37]<br>Increased amygdala and hippocampus activity during threat processing [39]<br>Increased methylation associated with increased PTSD incidence rate [35] | +++ |
| KLHL1 | rs139558732 C allele | Nominal genome-wide significance in the African-American subgroup of the largest PTSD GWAS to date [16] | ++ |
| ADRB2 | rs2400707 G allele | Top hit in a multi-candidate gene association study in interaction with childhood trauma exposure and replication in an independent cohort [14] | ++ |
| COMT | rs4680 G allele (val158met, val variant) | Increased PTSD incidence in interaction with lifetime trauma abundance [27]<br>Increased startle response to aversive pictures, especially in interaction with childhood maltreatment [70] | + |

PTSD, post-traumatic stress disorder; GWAS, genome-wide association study; CBT, cognitive behavioural therapy.

this integration between organism–internal molecular layout and organism–external environmental impact is emerging with psychiatric epigenetics. The potential of a dynamic gene-specific structural change in covalent DNA modifications or histone assembly could finally bridge the gap between genetics and environment. Besides its relevance for innovative and personalized treatments, the clinical potential of psychiatric genetics/epigenetics with regard to stress-related disorders lies in the prospective characterization of disease risk allowing for targeted prevention strategies, designed to counteract genetically determined at-risk states with resilience-increasing interventions and thus lower the incidence of stress-related disorders.

## Acknowledgements

This work has been supported by the German Research Foundation (DFG) (SFB-TRR-58, grant number 44541416, subprojects C02 and Z02 to K.D.) and the Federal Ministry of Education and Research (BMBF) (PROTECT-AD, grant number 14 01EE1402A, subproject P5 to K.D.).

## REFERENCES

1. American Psychiatric Association. *Diagnostic and Statistical Manual of Mental Disorders* (5th edn). Arlington, VA: American Psychiatric Publishing; 2013.
2. Roberts AL, Galea S, Austin SB, *et al.* Posttraumatic stress disorder across two generations: concordance and mechanisms in a population-based sample. *Biol Psychiatry*. 2012;72:505–11.
3. True WR, Rice J, Eisen SA, *et al.* A twin study of genetic and environmental contributions to liability for posttraumatic stress symptoms. *Arch Gen Psychiatry*. 1993;50:257–64.
4. Stein MB, Jang KL, Taylor S, Vernon PA, Livesley WJ. Genetic and environmental influences on trauma exposure and posttraumatic stress disorder symptoms: a twin study. *Am J Psychiatry*. 2002;159:1675–81.
5. Jang KL, Taylor S, Stein MB, Yamagata S. Trauma exposure and stress response: exploration of mechanisms of cause and effect. *Twin Res Hum Genet*. 2007;10:564–72.
6. Sartor CE, Grant JD, Lynskey MT, *et al.* Common heritable contributions to low-risk trauma, high-risk trauma, posttraumatic stress disorder, and major depression. *Arch Gen Psychiatry*. 2012;69:293–9.
7. Logue MW, Baldwin C, Guffanti G, *et al.* A genome-wide association study of post-traumatic stress disorder identifies the retinoid-related orphan receptor alpha (*RORA*) gene as a significant risk locus. *Mol Psychiatry*. 2013;18:937–42.
8. Miller MW, Wolf EJ, Logue MW, Baldwin CT. The retinoid-related orphan receptor alpha (*RORA*) gene and fear-related psychopathology. *J Affect Disord*. 2013;151:702–8.
9. Xie P, Kranzler HR, Yang C, Zhao H, Farrer LA, Gelernter J. Genome-wide association study identifies new susceptibility loci for posttraumatic stress disorder. *Biol Psychiatry*. 2013;74:656–63.
10. Almli LM, Srivastava A, Fani N, *et al.* Follow-up and extension of a prior genome-wide association study of posttraumatic stress disorder: gene x environment associations and structural magnetic resonance imaging in a highly traumatized African-American civilian population. *Biol Psychiatry*. 2014;76:e3–4.
11. Guffanti G, Galea S, Yan L, *et al.* Genome-wide association study implicates a novel RNA gene, the lincRNA AC068718.1, as a risk factor for post-traumatic stress disorder in women. *Psychoneuroendocrinology*. 2013;38:3029–38.
12. Stein MB, Chen CY, Ursano RJ, *et al.* Genome-wide association studies of posttraumatic stress disorder in 2 cohorts of US Army soldiers. *JAMA Psychiatry*. 2016;73:695–704.
13. Solovieff N, Roberts AL, Ratanatharathorn A, *et al.* Genetic association analysis of 300 genes identifies a risk haplotype in SLC18A2 for post-traumatic stress disorder in two independent samples. *Neuropsychopharmacology*. 2014;39:1872–9.
14. Liberzon I, King AP, Ressler KJ, *et al.* Interaction of the *ADRB2* gene polymorphism with childhood trauma in predicting adult symptoms of posttraumatic stress disorder. *JAMA Psychiatry*. 2014;71:1174–82.
15. Nievergelt CM, Maihofer AX, Mustapic M, *et al.* Genomic predictors of combat stress vulnerability and resilience in U.S. Marines: a genome-wide association study across multiple ancestries implicates *PRTFDC1* as a potential PTSD gene. *Psychoneuroendocrinology*. 2015;51:459–71.
16. Duncan LE, Ratanatharathorn A, Aiello AE, *et al.* Largest GWAS of PTSD (N=20 070) yields genetic overlap with schizophrenia and sex differences in heritability. *Mol Psychiatry*. 2018;23:666–73.
17. Ashley-Koch AE, Garrett ME, Gibson J, *et al.* Genome-wide association study of posttraumatic stress disorder in a cohort of Iraq-Afghanistan era veterans. *J Affect Disord*. 2015;184:225–34.
18. Wolf EJ, Rasmusson AM, Mitchell KS, Logue MW, Baldwin CT, Miller MW. A genome-wide association study of clinical symptoms of dissociation in a trauma-exposed sample. *Depress Anxiety*. 2014;31:352–60.
19. Gressier F, Calati R, Balestri M, *et al.* The 5-*HTTLPR* polymorphism and posttraumatic stress disorder: a meta-analysis. *J Trauma Stress*. 2013;26:645–53.
20. Telch MJ, Beevers CG, Rosenfield D, *et al.* 5-HTTLPR genotype potentiates the effects of war zone stressors on the emergence of PTSD, depressive and anxiety symptoms in soldiers deployed to iraq. *World Psychiatry*. 2015;14:198–206.
21. Wang Z, Baker DG, Harrer J, Hamner M, Price M, Amstadter A. The relationship between combat-related posttraumatic stress disorder and the 5-*HTTLPR*/rs25531 polymorphism. *Depress Anxiety*. 2011;28:1067–73.
22. Wald I, Degnan KA, Gorodetsky E, *et al.* Attention to threats and combat-related posttraumatic stress symptoms: prospective associations and moderation by the serotonin transporter gene. *JAMA Psychiatry*. 2013;70:401–8.
23. Mercer KB, Orcutt HK, Quinn JF, *et al.* Acute and posttraumatic stress symptoms in a prospective gene x environment study of a university campus shooting. *Arch Gen Psychiatry*. 2012;69:89–97.
24. Mushtaq D, Ali A, Margoob MA, Murtaza I, Andrade C. Association between serotonin transporter gene promoter-region polymorphism and 4- and 12-week treatment response to sertraline in posttraumatic stress disorder. *J Affect Disord*. 2012;136:955–62.
25. Bryant RA, Felmingham KL, Falconer EM, *et al.* Preliminary evidence of the short allele of the serotonin transporter gene predicting poor response to cognitive behavior therapy in posttraumatic stress disorder. *Biol Psychiatry*. 2010;67:1217–19.
26. Boscarino JA, Erlich PM, Hoffman SN, Rukstalis M, Stewart WF. Association of *FKBP5*, *COMT* and *CHRNA5* polymorphisms

with PTSD among outpatients at risk for PTSD. *Psychiatry Res.* 2011;188:173–4.

27. Kolassa IT, Kolassa S, Ertl V, Papassotiropoulos A, De Quervain DJ. The risk of posttraumatic stress disorder after trauma depends on traumatic load and the catechol-o-methyltransferase Val(158)Met polymorphism. *Biol Psychiatry.* 2010;67:304–8.

28. Zannas AS, Binder EB. Gene-environment interactions at the *FKBP5* locus: sensitive periods, mechanisms and pleiotropism. *Genes Brain Behav.* 2014;13:25–37.

29. Binder EB, Bradley RG, Liu W, et al. Association of FKBP5 polymorphisms and childhood abuse with risk of posttraumatic stress disorder symptoms in adults. *JAMA.* 2008;299:1291–305.

30. Klengel T, Mehta D, Anacker C, et al. Allele-specific FKBP5 DNA demethylation mediates gene-childhood trauma interactions. *Nat Neurosci.* 2013;16:33–41.

31. Wilker S, Pfeiffer A, Kolassa S, et al. The role of FKBP5 genotype in moderating long-term effectiveness of exposure-based psychotherapy for posttraumatic stress disorder. *Transl Psychiatry.* 2014;4:e403.

32. Xie P, Kranzler HR, Poling J, et al. Interaction of FKBP5 with childhood adversity on risk for post-traumatic stress disorder. *Neuropsychopharmacology.* 2010;35:1684–92.

33. Fani N, King TZ, Shin J, et al. Structural and functional connectivity in posttraumatic stress disorder: associations with *Fkbp5.* *Depress Anxiety.* 2016;33:300–7.

34. Mehta D, Gonik M, Klengel T, et al. Using polymorphisms in *FKBP5* to define biologically distinct subtypes of posttraumatic stress disorder: evidence from endocrine and gene expression studies. *Arch Gen Psychiatry.* 2011;68:901–10.

35. Ressler KJ, Mercer KB, Bradley B, et al. Post-traumatic stress disorder is associated with PACAP and the PAC1 receptor. *Nature.* 2011;470:492–7.

36. Almli LM, Mercer KB, Kerley K, et al. ADCYAP1R1 genotype associates with post-traumatic stress symptoms in highly traumatized African-American females. *Am J Med Genet B Neuropsychiatr Genet.* 2013;162B:262–72.

37. Uddin M, Chang SC, Zhang C, et al. *Adcyap1r1* genotype, posttraumatic stress disorder, and depression among women exposed to childhood maltreatment. *Depress Anxiety.* 2013;30:251–8.

38. Pohlack ST, Nees F, Ruttorf M, et al. Neural mechanism of a sex-specific risk variant for posttraumatic stress disorder in the type I receptor of the pituitary adenylate cyclase activating polypeptide. *Biol Psychiatry.* 2015;78:840–7.

39. Stevens JS, Almli LM, Fani N, et al. PACAP receptor gene polymorphism impacts fear responses in the amygdala and hippocampus. *Proc Natl Acad Sci U S A.* 2014;111:3158–63.

40. Wolf EJ, Mitchell KS, Logue MW, et al. Corticotropin releasing hormone receptor 2 (*CRHR-2*) gene is associated with decreased risk and severity of posttraumatic stress disorder in women. *Depress Anxiety.* 2013;30:1161–9.

41. Rothbaum BO, Kearns MC, Reiser E, et al. Early intervention following trauma may mitigate genetic risk for PTSD in civilians: a pilot prospective emergency department study. *J Clin Psychiatry.* 2014;75:1380–7.

42. Uddin M, Aiello AE, Wildman DE, et al. Epigenetic and immune function profiles associated with posttraumatic stress disorder. *Proc Natl Acad Sci U S A.* 2010;107:9470–5.

43. Koenen KC, Uddin M, Chang SC, et al. SLC6A4 methylation modifies the effect of the number of traumatic events on risk for posttraumatic stress disorder. *Depress Anxiety.* 2011;28:639–47.

44. Yehuda R, Daskalakis NP, Bierer LM, et al. Holocaust exposure induced intergenerational effects on *FKBP5* methylation. *Biol Psychiatry.* 2016;80:372–80.

45. Roberts S, Keers R, Lester KJ, et al. HPA axis related genes and response to psychological therapies: genetics and epigenetics. *Depress Anxiety.* 2015;32:861–70.

46. Yehuda R, Flory JD, Bierer LM, et al. Lower methylation of glucocorticoid receptor gene promoter 1F in peripheral blood of veterans with posttraumatic stress disorder. *Biol Psychiatry.* 2015;77:356–64.

47. Yehuda R, Daskalakis NP, Lehrner A, et al. Influences of maternal and paternal PTSD on epigenetic regulation of the glucocorticoid receptor gene in Holocaust survivor offspring. *Am J Psychiatry.* 2014;171:872–80.

48. Sipahi L, Wildman DE, Aiello AE, et al. Longitudinal epigenetic variation of DNA methyltransferase genes is associated with vulnerability to post-traumatic stress disorder. *Psychol Med.* 2014;44:3165–79.

49. Smoller JW. Disorders and borders: psychiatric genetics and nosology. *Am J Med Genet B Neuropsychiatr Genet.* 2013;162B:559–78.

50. Hettema JM, Prescott CA, Myers JM, Neale MC, Kendler KS. The structure of genetic and environmental risk factors for anxiety disorders in men and women. *Arch Gen Psychiatry.* 2005;62:182–9.

51. Loken EK, Hettema JM, Aggen SH, Kendler KS. The structure of genetic and environmental risk factors for fears and phobias. *Psychol Med.* 2014;44:2375–84.

52. Miller R, Wankerl M, Stalder T, Kirschbaum C, Alexander N. The serotonin transporter gene-linked polymorphic region (5-HTTLPR) and cortisol stress reactivity: a meta-analysis. *Mol Psychiatry.* 2013;18:1018–24.

53. Pergamin-Hight L, Bakermans-Kranenburg MJ, van Ijzendoorn MH, Bar-Haim Y. Variations in the promoter region of the serotonin transporter gene and biased attention for emotional information: a meta-analysis. *Biol Psychiatry.* 2012;71:373–9.

54. Fox E, Zougkou K, Ridgewell A, Garner K. The serotonin transporter gene alters sensitivity to attention bias modification: evidence for a plasticity gene. *Biol Psychiatry.* 2011;70:1049–54.

55. Kobiella A, Reimold M, Ulshofer DE, et al. How the serotonin transporter 5-HTTLPR polymorphism influences amygdala function: the roles of *in vivo* serotonin transporter expression and amygdala structure. *Transl Psychiatry.* 2011;1:e37.

56. van Ijzendoorn MH, Belsky J, Bakermans-Kranenburg MJ. Serotonin transporter genotype 5HTTLPR as a marker of differential susceptibility? A meta-analysis of child and adolescent gene-by-environment studies. *Transl Psychiatry.* 2012;2:e147.

57. Klauke B, Deckert J, Reif A, et al. Serotonin transporter gene and childhood trauma--a G x E effect on anxiety sensitivity. *Depress Anxiety.* 2011;28:1048–57.

58. Schiele MA, Ziegler C, Holitschke K, et al. Influence of 5-HTT variation, childhood trauma and self-efficacy on anxiety traits: a gene-environment-coping interaction study. *J Neural Transm (Vienna).* 2016;123:895–904.

59. Demers CH, Drabant Conley E, Bogdan R, Hariri AR. Interactions between anandamide and corticotropin-releasing factor signaling modulate human amygdala function and risk for anxiety disorders: an imaging genetics strategy for modeling molecular interactions. *Biol Psychiatry.* 2016;80:356–62.

60. Heitland I, Groenink L, Bijlsma EY, Oosting RS, Baas JM. Human fear acquisition deficits in relation to genetic variants of the

corticotropin releasing hormone receptor 1 and the serotonin transporter. *PLoS One.* 2013;8:e63772.

61. Heitland I, Groenink L, van Gool JM, Domschke K, Reif A, Baas JM. Human fear acquisition deficits in relation to genetic variants of the corticotropin-releasing hormone receptor 1 and the serotonin transporter—revisited. *Genes Brain Behav.* 2016;15:209–20.

62. Ridder S, Treutlein J, Nees F, *et al.* Brain activation during fear conditioning in humans depends on genetic variations related to functioning of the hypothalamic-pituitary-adrenal axis: first evidence from two independent subsamples. *Psychol Med.* 2012;42:2325–35.

63. Tyrka AR, Parade SH, Welch ES, *et al.* Methylation of the leukocyte glucocorticoid receptor gene promoter in adults: associations with early adversity and depressive, anxiety and substance-use disorders. *Transl Psychiatry.* 2016;6:e848.

64. Smoller JW, Rosenbaum JF, Biederman J, *et al.* Association of a genetic marker at the corticotropin-releasing hormone locus with behavioral inhibition. *Biol Psychiatry.* 2003;54: 1376–81.

65. Smoller JW, Yamaki LH, Fagerness JA, *et al.* The corticotropin-releasing hormone gene and behavioral inhibition in children at risk for panic disorder. *Biol Psychiatry.* 2005;57:1485–92.

66. Minelli A, Maffioletti E, Cloninger CR, *et al.* Role of allelic variants of FK506-binding protein 51 (*FKBP5*) gene in the development of anxiety disorders. *Depress Anxiety.* 2013;30:1170–6.

67. Fani N, Gutman D, Tone EB, *et al.* FKBP5 and attention bias for threat: associations with hippocampal function and shape. *JAMA Psychiatry.* 2013;70:392–400.

68. White MG, Bogdan R, Fisher PM, Munoz KE, Williamson DE, Hariri AR. FKBP5 and emotional neglect interact to predict individual differences in amygdala reactivity. *Genes Brain Behav.* 2012;11:869–78.

69. Klauke B, Winter B, Gajewska A, *et al.* Affect-modulated startle: interactive influence of catechol-*O*-methyltransferase Val158Met genotype and childhood trauma. *PLoS One.* 2012;7:e39709.

70. Domschke K, Winter B, Gajewska A, *et al.* Multilevel impact of the dopamine system on the emotion-potentiated startle reflex. *Psychopharmacology (Berl).* 2015;232:1983–93.

71. Koenen KC, Moffitt TE, Poulton R, Martin J, Caspi A. Early childhood factors associated with the development of posttraumatic stress disorder: results from a longitudinal birth cohort. *Psychol Med.* 2007;37:181–92.

72. Ozer EJ, Best SR, Lipsey TL, Weiss DS. Predictors of posttraumatic stress disorder and symptoms in adults: a meta-analysis. *Psychol Bull.* 2003;129:52–73.

73. Kessler RC, Rose S, Koenen KC, *et al.* How well can posttraumatic stress disorder be predicted from pre-trauma risk factors? An exploratory study in the WHO World Mental Health Surveys. *World Psychiatry.* 2014;13:265–74.

74. Cuthbert BN. The RDoC framework: facilitating transition from ICD/DSM to dimensional approaches that integrate neuroscience and psychopathology. *World Psychiatry.* 2014;13:28–35.

75. Ross DA, Arbuckle MR, Travis MJ, Dwyer JB, van Schalkwyk GI, Ressler KJ. An integrated neuroscience perspective on formulation and treatment planning for posttraumatic stress disorder: an educational review. *JAMA Psychiatry.* 2017;74:407–15.

# 81

# Imaging of stress-related disorders

*Navneet Kaur, Cecilia A. Hinojosa, Julia Russell, Michael B. VanElzakker, and Lisa M. Shin*

## Introduction

Over the past two decades, researchers have used structural and functional neuroimaging techniques and neuroscience-based paradigms to study the mediating neurocircuitry of stress-related psychiatric disorders, with a focus on post-traumatic stress disorder (PTSD). The ultimate goals of such investigations are to identify neurocircuitry abnormalities, to determine whether those abnormalities are useful in diagnosis or in predicting treatment response, and to elucidate treatments that could address the abnormalities and ameliorate symptoms. In the text that follows, we will review the imaging methods, paradigms, and findings of neuroimaging studies of PTSD and acute stress disorder (ASD). We will present the results in the context of a neurocircuitry model of PTSD that emerged from basic neuroscience studies of fear conditioning and extinction. Finally, we will identify current gaps in our knowledge regarding brain structure and function in PTSD and discuss how future studies might address those gaps.

## Imaging methods

The structure and function of the human brain have been assessed using neuroimaging techniques, including magnetic resonance imaging (MRI), functional MRI (fMRI), and positron emission tomography (PET) (for a review, see Chapter 12).

MRI generates three-dimensional images of the brain structure [1]. MRI data can be gathered and analysed in different ways, including traditional morphometry, voxel-based morphometry (VBM), and diffusion tensor imaging (DTI). In traditional morphometry, the borders of specific brain regions of interest are traced, and the volumes of these regions are calculated and compared between patients and comparison groups [2]. In VBM, grey matter density is measured at each voxel (that is, three-dimensional pixel) in the entire brain, averaged across participants, and compared between patient and control groups [3]. By measuring the linear diffusion of water molecule protons along axons, DTI can indicate the location, thickness, health, and orientation of white matter tracts [4].

fMRI measures blood oxygen level-dependent (BOLD) signal, which is the difference in magnetic susceptibility in oxygenated vs deoxygenated blood and an indicator of brain activity [1]. During emotional or cognitive tasks, brain structures become metabolically active and consume oxygen. The flow of oxygenated blood to that specific brain region is increased, creating a measurable magnetic resonance (MR) signal [5]. fMRI has good spatial and fair temporal resolution and does not use ionizing radiation, thus making it a highly desirable psychiatric neuroimaging technique.

PET is a functional neuroimaging technique that allows researchers to assess regional cerebral metabolic rate for glucose (rCMRglu), regional cerebral blood flow (rCBF), or receptor occupancy [6]. Due to its poor spatial and temporal resolution and because PET requires the injection of radioactive isotopes, it is not the preferred method for measuring the brain's responses to stimuli or tasks. However, PET is the preferred method for measuring rCMRglu and receptor occupancy.

## Paradigms

Functional neuroimaging studies of stress-related disorders commonly use behavioural or cognitive paradigms such as fear conditioning and extinction, symptom provocation, cognitive activation, and resting state methods. For example, fear conditioning and extinction paradigms elucidate the neurobiological basis of failure to extinguish fear responses to stimuli that formerly predicted threat but no longer do—a model for some PTSD symptoms. Fear conditioning involves repeated predictive pairings of a previously neutral conditioned stimulus (CS) (for example, a coloured light) with an aversive unconditioned stimulus (US) (for example, a shock), to create an association resulting in the CS alone eliciting a conditioned response (CR) (for example, increased skin conductance) [7]. Later, during extinction, the CS is repeatedly presented without the US, typically resulting in a diminished CR. Then 24 hours later, the memory of extinction training can be assessed by presenting the CS without the US. In symptom provocation paradigms, researchers present participants with audiotaped descriptions of traumatic events (known as 'scripts') or trauma-related pictures, odours, or sounds during functional neuroimaging in order to elucidate the brain regions and networks that mediate the symptomatic state [8]. In cognitive activation paradigms, researchers implement cognitive tasks that are known to activate specific brain regions or networks in order to test their function in PTSD vs comparison groups. Finally, resting state paradigms measure fMRI BOLD signal or rCMRglu in the absence of a task [9]. Resting state fMRI permits the examination of functional connectivity, that is, associations between different brain regions.

## Neurocircuitry model

Early psychophysiological and neuroimaging studies began gathering evidence for a fear conditioning model of PTSD, which posits that the principles of Pavlovian fear conditioning and extinction underlie the acquisition and maintenance of anxiety and stress-related disorders (reviewed in [7, 10]). Through the lens of the fear conditioning model, sustained symptoms of PTSD and related conditions can be conceptualized as an overexpression of fear to cues that once predicted a threat but should now be considered safe (for example, a veteran who was once injured in a loud combat explosion and who now experiences fear upon hearing loud fireworks). Neuroimaging studies of PTSD have demonstrated structural and functional abnormalities in the brain circuits that underlie fear conditioning and extinction, as well as emotion regulation and memory (Fig. 81.1).

Consistent with its role in the acquisition and expression of conditioned fear and related defensive behaviours, the amygdala is generally hyper-responsive in PTSD, and in many studies, its activation is positively correlated with symptom severity. The structures comprising the ventromedial prefrontal cortex (vmPFC) generally hold inhibitory influence over the amygdala and are key to the learning and subsequent recall of fear extinction. These vmPFC structures, such as the rostral anterior cingulate cortex (rACC), subgenual anterior cingulate cortex (sgACC), and medial frontal gyrus (MFG), are hyporesponsive in PTSD, indicating functional deficits in learning and remembering safety information and inhibiting fear responses. Conversely, the dorsal anterior cingulate cortex (dACC) is implicated in the expression of learned fear and is hyper-responsive in PTSD, and its activation often positively correlates with amygdala activation. Likewise, the insular cortex tends to be hyper-responsive in PTSD. Given its role in monitoring bodily states, insula activation in PTSD may be related to subjective experiences like anxiety and pain. Findings regarding the hippocampus in PTSD are mixed, with some studies showing hyper-responsiveness and some showing hyporesponsiveness. In PTSD, difficulty identifying safe contexts and updating contextual cues to include safety information, as well as more general deficits in declarative and episodic memory, may reflect hippocampal dysfunction.

While the fear conditioning-based neurocircuitry model of PTSD has been quite fruitful (for example, [7, 10]), it cannot directly account for several important aspects of PTSD symptomatology, including endocrine abnormalities, deficits in executive cognitive function, and ongoing anxiety, in the absence of a conditioned stimulus or context (for example, [11, 12]). However, one of the most striking aspects of the functional neurocircuitry abnormalities seen in PTSD is that they are expressed not only in studies that directly assess fear conditioning and extinction, but also in symptom provocation, cognitive activation, and resting state studies [13]. The following sections will review some of these studies.

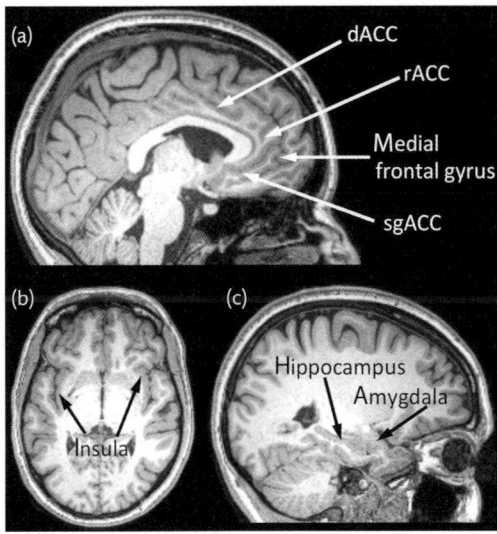

**Fig. 81.1** Structural magnetic resonance images showing brain regions of interest in PTSD. (a) A sagittal section showing the dorsal anterior cingulate cortex (dACC), as well as structures that comprise the ventromedial prefrontal cortex (vmPFC) such as the rostral anterior cingulate cortex (rACC), medial frontal gyrus, and subgenual anterior cingulate cortex (sgACC). (b) A horizontal section showing the bilateral insular cortex. (c) A sagittal section showing the hippocampus and amygdala. In PTSD, the amygdala, dACC, and insula tend to be hyper-responsive, and the vmPFC tends to be hyporesponsive. Findings regarding the hippocampus have been more mixed, as they may depend on the specific experimental paradigm.

## Amygdala

### Function

Exaggerated amygdala activation in PTSD is now a well-replicated finding that can be observed during fear conditioning paradigms, for example in response to an electric shock US [14] and to the CS during acquisition of conditioned fear (for example, [15, 16]). Furthermore, in PTSD, the amygdala continues to be hyper-responsive to the CS, even during or after extinction (for example, [16, 17]). These findings are evidence that, relative to controls, the amygdala in those with PTSD is hyper-responsive to threat and to cues that predict threat and continues to be hyper-responsive to such cues after they no longer predict threat. The amygdala also shows exaggerated responses to trauma recollection (for example, [18, 19]) and trauma-related sensory stimuli (for example, [20–22]). Interestingly, amygdala hyper-responsivity can occur in response to trauma-unrelated emotional stimuli such as emotional facial expressions (Fig. 81.2) (for example, [23–27]) and aversive images (for example, [28, 29]). Individuals with PTSD even show exaggerated amygdala activity at rest [30] or in response to tasks using neutral stimuli [31]. However, not all studies have found increased amygdala activation in PTSD (for example, [32–34]).

(a)

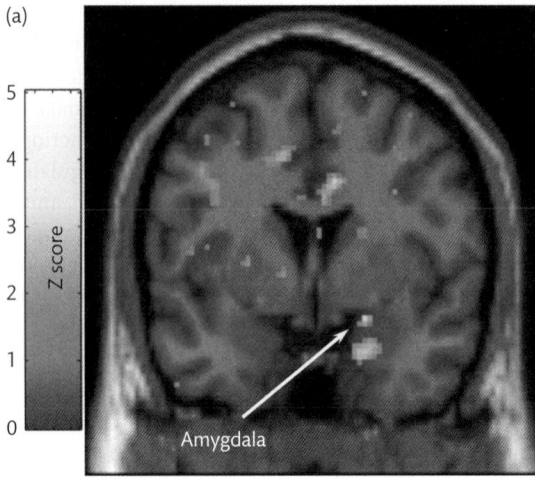

(b)

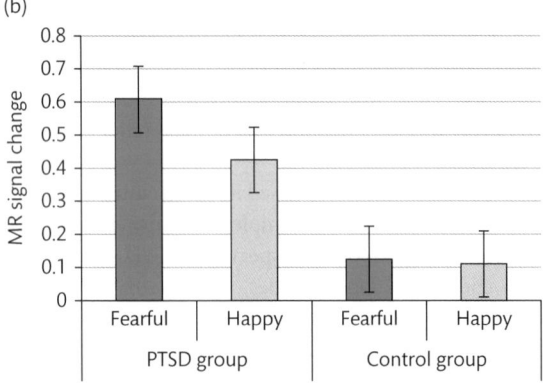

**Fig. 81.2** (see Colour Plate section) Example of functional magnetic resonance imaging (fMRI) data. (a) Amygdala activation to fearful vs happy facial expressions was greater in the PTSD group vs control group. (b) MR signal change in the amygdala in each condition for each group. Error bars represent the standard error of the mean.

Adapted from *Arch Gen Psychiatry*, 62(3), Shin LM, Wright CI, Cannistraro PA, *et al.*, A functional magnetic resonance imaging study of amygdala and medial prefrontal cortex responses to overtly presented fearful faces in posttraumatic stress disorder, pp. 273–81, Copyright (2005), with permission from American Medical Association.

Within PTSD groups, amygdala activation is positively correlated with PTSD symptom severity (for example, [18, 23, 26, 35–37]), and symptomatic improvement is associated with a decrease in amygdala activation (for example, [38–40]). Although these findings might suggest that exaggerated amygdala activation is a state-like, acquired characteristic of PTSD, other findings suggest that it may reflect a trait-like vulnerability factor—pre-trauma amygdala responses predict greater PTSD symptoms following trauma (for example, [41, 42]). Finally, pretreatment amygdala activation appears to predict a less favourable response to treatment (for example, [43, 44]).

Far less research has been conducted on amygdala function in ASD. In a small longitudinal study, Reynaud and colleagues (2015) found that firefighters who developed ASD showed a greater increase in amygdala activation post-trauma, relative to pre-trauma baseline, despite not showing differences in amygdala activation before trauma [45]. However, given the small sample in the ASD group ($n = 2$), this study requires replication.

## Structure

Findings regarding amygdala structure in PTSD are somewhat mixed. Several studies have found smaller amygdala volumes or reduced grey matter density in PTSD [46–50], with some studies reporting a negative correlation between amygdala volume and symptom severity (for example, [46, 51, 52]). However, some studies have found greater amygdala volumes in PTSD (for example, [53–55]) or no group differences (for example, [56–60]). These discrepancies could be attributed, in part, to variability in imaging methods and/or in participant samples across studies. Indeed, one meta-analysis suggested that diminished amygdala volumes are significant when PTSD groups are compared to trauma-unexposed control groups, but not trauma-exposed control groups [61]. In general, the latter is a more appropriate comparison group as it controls for exposure to trauma. Furthermore, because attempts to relate structural and functional abnormalities in the amygdala in PTSD have been lacking, it is difficult to determine whether structural abnormalities in the amygdala in PTSD are the origin of corresponding functional abnormalities. More studies examining amygdala structure and function within the same cohort are needed.

In the only study to examine amygdala structure in ASD, no abnormalities were found [62].

## Ventromedial prefrontal cortex

### Function

Individuals with PTSD show relatively diminished vmPFC activation during extinction learning and recall (for example, [15, 17, 63]), during the recollection of traumatic events (for example, [18, 33, 64–71], but see [72]), in response to other trauma-related stimuli (for example, [21, 67, 73–75]), in response to trauma-unrelated emotional stimuli such as fearful facial expressions or unpleasant scenes (for example, [22, 24, 27, 76–78]), and even in response to neutral stimuli or at rest (for example, [31, 79–85]). Finally, successful treatment with cognitive behavioural therapy (CBT), eye movement desensitization and reprocessing (EMDR), or a serotonin reuptake inhibitor (SSRI) appears to be related to increased prefrontal cortex activation (for example, [39, 40, 43, 86]).

However, not all studies have reported diminished vmPFC activation in PTSD; some have reported no group differences or greater activation in PTSD (for example, [87, 88]). The direction of the functional abnormality in the vmPFC may depend on the state of the participants and the nature of the task completed in the scanner. For example, greater vmPFC activation can be observed when PTSD groups experience a dissociative state (for example, [87, 89]) or view stimuli below the threshold of conscious awareness [90].

### Structure

Structural MRI studies of PTSD have reported abnormalities in the vmPFC in the form of reduced volumes (for example, [50, 53, 57, 91–96]), reduced white matter tract integrity (for example, [97, 98]), and reduced grey matter density (for example, [99–108]). In addition, relatively smaller pretreatment grey matter density in the pregenual ACC predicted a less favourable response to CBT [43]. Kasai and colleagues used monozygotic twin pairs discordant for combat exposure to determine whether grey matter density reductions observed in PTSD are familial vulnerability factors for developing PTSD or an acquired characteristic of PTSD. Results showed that grey matter volume density reductions in the pregenual ACC were an acquired characteristic of PTSD [102].

The only study of vmPFC structure in ASD did not find abnormalities [62].

## Dorsal anterior cingulate cortex

### Function

Neuroimaging studies have shown dACC hyperactivation in PTSD, relative to trauma-exposed control groups, during conditioning, early extinction learning, and extinction recall (for example, [17, 63, 109]). Furthermore, dACC activation is negatively correlated with extinction recall in PTSD and trauma-exposed non-PTSD controls [17], and dACC resting metabolism in PTSD is positively correlated with both activation during extinction recall and symptom severity in PTSD [109].

dACC hyper-responsivity in PTSD has also been found in studies presenting trauma scripts [18] and words [110], emotional facial expressions [81], neutral stimuli (for example, [31, 82, 111]), and in resting state studies [112]. In one study, greater dACC activation in response to negative vs neutral photographs predicted a poorer outcome following treatment [44].

The findings of two twin studies have suggested that dACC hyperactivity and hyper-responsivity are familial vulnerability factors for developing PTSD following trauma exposure. In the first, Shin and colleagues assessed rCMRglu in combat-exposed veterans with PTSD and their identical co-twins unexposed to combat, as well as combat-exposed veterans without PTSD and their identical co-twins unexposed to combat. Veterans with PTSD and their co-twins had significantly greater resting rCMRglu in the dACC/mid cingulate cortex (MCC), compared with veterans without PTSD and their co-twins (Fig. 81.3) [112]. Similarly, using fMRI and the Multi-Source Interference Task, Shin and colleagues found greater dACC activation in combat-exposed veterans with PTSD and their unexposed co-twins, as compared to combat-exposed veterans without PTSD and their co-twins [111].

Whether the dACC is hyperactivated in ASD is not clear. In one symptom provocation study, Cwik and colleagues found greater dorsal medial frontal cortex activation in participants with ASD, compared to healthy trauma-unexposed control participants [113]. However, this increased activation occurred not in dACC proper, but in a region just dorsal to that.

### Structure

Reduced grey matter volume in the dACC has been observed in trauma survivors with PTSD, compared to those without PTSD (for example, [103, 114]).

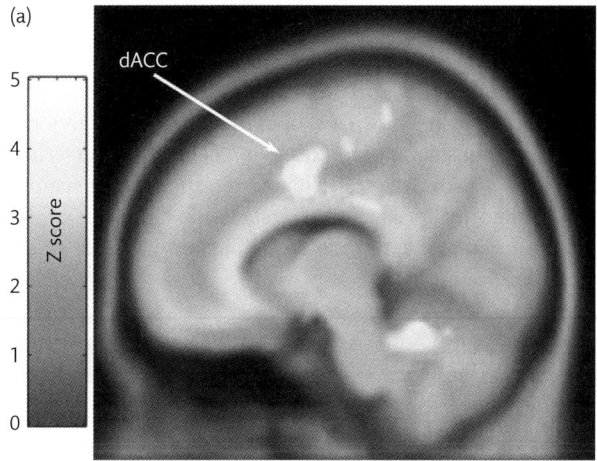

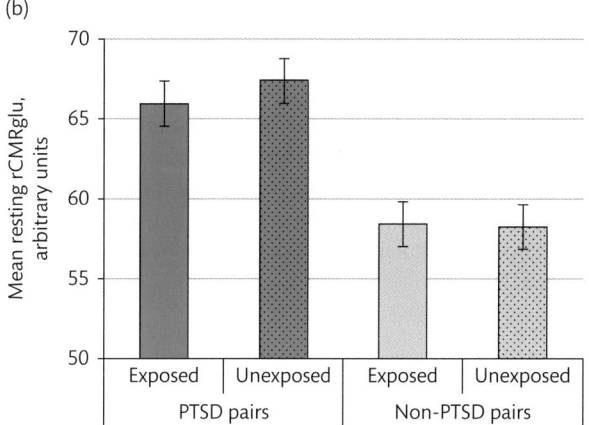

**Fig. 81.3** (see Colour Plate section) Example of positron emission tomography (PET) data. (a) Greater resting regional cerebral metabolic rate for glucose (rCMRglu) in the dorsal anterior cingulate cortex (dACC)/mid cingulate cortex (arrow) in combat-exposed twins with PTSD and their identical co-twins, compared with combat-exposed twins without PTSD and their identical co-twins. (b) Group rCMRglu means. Error bars represent the standard error of the mean.

Adapted from *Arch Gen Psychiatry*, 66(10), Shin LM, Lasko NB, Macklin ML, *et al.*, Resting metabolic activity in the cingulate cortex and vulnerability to posttraumatic stress disorder, pp. 1099–107, Copyright (2009), with permission from American Medical Association.

## Insula

### Function

The insula is hyper-responsive in PTSD during the recollection of traumatic events (for example, [64, 115, 116]), the presentation of other trauma-related stimuli (for example, [21, 110, 117, 118]), the presentation of emotional, but trauma-unrelated, stimuli such as negative words, fearful facial expressions, and aversive photographs (for example, [76, 87, 119, 120]), and at rest [85]. In addition, greater insula activation in response to negative vs neutral photographs predicted a poorer outcome following treatment [44]. However, not all studies have reported insula hyper-responsivity in PTSD (for example, [22, 29, 68]).

### Structure

Insula volume [57] and grey matter density (for example, [100, 102, 104, 121]) are reduced in PTSD, relative to comparison groups. Furthermore, a twin study has shown that diminished grey matter volume in the insula appears to be an acquired characteristic of PTSD and is negatively correlated with re-experiencing symptoms. Thus, this abnormality appears to be state-like and hence could potentially be used in diagnosis or as a biological indicator of symptomatic improvement [102].

## Hippocampus

### Function

Functional neuroimaging studies of the hippocampus in PTSD have been mixed. Some studies found that the hippocampus is hyporesponsive in PTSD, for example during extinction recall [17], script-driven imagery (for example, [40, 69]), trauma-unrelated and neutral stimuli (for example, [73, 122–124]), and at rest (for example, [125, 126]). However, other studies show that the hippocampus is hyper-responsive in PTSD during tasks with trauma-related stimuli such as words [127] and emotional and neutral stimuli (for example, [28, 79, 90, 123, 128]). These mixed findings may be accounted for by differences in task demands upon the hippocampus or imaging modality [129].

### Structure

Many studies have reported reduced overall hippocampal volume or grey matter volume in PTSD, compared to control groups (for example, [48, 57, 80, 93, 108, 130–141]). In addition, one study found that relatively smaller hippocampal volume predicted a less favourable response to treatment with prolonged exposure [142]. However, a few studies have reported larger hippocampal volume in PTSD (for example, [53, 143]) or no differences in hippocampal volume (for example, [50, 144–148]).

The results of at least one study suggest that diminished hippocampal volume is a familial vulnerability factor rather than an acquired characteristic of PTSD. In a twin design similar to those described previously (for example, [111, 113]), Gilbertson and colleagues found smaller hippocampal volumes in combat veterans with PTSD and their identical co-twins, relative to combat veterans without PTSD and their identical co-twins. Furthermore, severity of PTSD in the combat veterans was negatively correlated with hippocampal volume of their identical co-twins, consistent with a vulnerability factor [149].

## Future directions

Over the past 20 years, an enormous amount of progress has been made in our understanding of the neurocircuitry of PTSD. Despite this, many questions remain either unanswered or entirely unaddressed. For example, we do not yet know whether neurocircuitry abnormalities differ by trauma type, duration of trauma, and age of trauma onset. Part of the problem lies in the fact that single studies tend to focus on just one trauma type, duration, and age of onset. In the future, different imaging data sets, all using the same paradigm (for example, fear conditioning/extinction), might be combined to permit a proper examination of these variables.

Most studies that we reviewed have included participants with chronic PTSD, and whether the findings extend to acute PTSD is undetermined. On a related note, as shown in our literature review, very little is currently known about the neurocircuitry of ASD. Practically speaking, ASD is difficult to study because an ASD diagnosis must be made within the first month after a traumatic event. This requirement makes it challenging to find and enrol such participants for imaging studies.

Another question that is not yet fully answered relates to the origin of neurocircuitry abnormalities in PTSD. Most current studies are cross-sectional and hence cannot determine whether these abnormalities reflect pre-existing familial vulnerability factors or acquired characteristics of the disorder. If an abnormality, such as dACC hyper-responsivity, is a familial vulnerability factor and can increase the risk for developing PTSD, it could potentially be used to screen individuals who are likely to experience trauma and develop PTSD such as police officers and firefighters. In contrast, if an abnormality is an acquired characteristic of PTSD, it could potentially be used as a biological marker in diagnosis or in the assessment of treatment response. In the future, studies implementing longitudinal designs (that include a baseline assessment of participants prior to trauma exposure and follow participants over time after trauma) or twin designs will help clarify the origin of neurocircuitry abnormalities in PTSD.

In the United States, the National Institute of Mental Health (NIMH) is now requiring that all psychiatry research it funds be conducted in a new framework that focuses on symptom dimensions, rather than on categorical diagnoses. This means that future studies of PTSD will be based on correlational analyses associating symptom severity with other measures like brain activation, psychophysiology, behavioural performance, and self-report. One difficulty with this change in approach is that the results of new studies may be difficult to fully reconcile with those of existing studies that took a more categorical approach.

One of the goals of neuroimaging studies is to elucidate the brain regions or networks that function abnormally in PTSD. Such information could lead to new treatments that are focused on 'normalizing' that brain function. In the future, researchers will undoubtedly use non-invasive neuromodulation tools and techniques such as transcranial direct current stimulation (tDCS) and transcranial magnetic stimulation (TMS) to determine whether modulating brain function can ameliorate symptoms.

Another important potential clinical application of neuroimaging data in psychiatry is the prediction of response to treatment. For example, although CBT is arguably the most effective in the treatment of PTSD, not all patients respond well, and finding a good treatment fit can take months to years. Thus, patients and clinicians would benefit from having objective pretreatment measures that can be used to predict treatment response. Neuroimaging could be such a measure. Furthermore, researchers are beginning to use sophisticated machine-learning algorithms (which include multiple measures such as imaging, genetic, psychophysiological, behavioural, clinical, and demographic) to best distinguish between treatment responders and non-responders and hence improve the prediction of treatment response.

## Conclusions

Neuroimaging studies of stress disorders (predominantly PTSD) have revealed functional abnormalities consistent with a fear conditioning model. The results reviewed herein suggest that the amygdala and dACC are hyper-responsive in PTSD, consistent with their involvement in fear learning and expression. In contrast, the vmPFC is hyporesponsive, as might be predicted, given its role in inhibiting the amygdala during the successful extinction of fear. The insula is hyper-responsive in PTSD, likely reflecting the processing of interoceptive cues such as anxiety. Finally, functional abnormalities in the hippocampus have been more mixed in PTSD, and further research ought to clarify its role in memory and identifying safe contexts in this disorder.

Overall, although much progress has been made in our understanding of the neurocircuitry of PTSD, many questions remain unanswered. Future research will be needed to clarify the trauma-related factors that affect neurocircuitry abnormalities, the origin of such abnormalities, and the role of neuroimaging in assessing and predicting treatment response.

## REFERENCES

1. Buxton RB. *Introduction to Functional Magnetic Resonance Imaging: Principles and Techniques* (2nd edn). Cambridge and New York, NY: Cambridge University Press; 2009.
2. Shapleske J, Rossell SL, Chitnis XA, *et al*. A computational morphometric MRI study of schizophrenia: effects of hallucinations. *Cereb Cortex*. 2002;12:1331–41.
3. Ashburner J, Friston KJ. Voxel-based morphometry--the methods. *Neuroimage*. 2000;11(6 Pt 1):805–21.
4. Le Bihan D, Mangin JF, Poupon C, *et al*. Diffusion tensor imaging: concepts and applications. *J Magn Reson Imaging*. 2001;13:534–46.
5. Heeger DJ, Ress D. What does fMRI tell us about neuronal activity? *Nat Rev Neurosci*. 2002;3:142–51.
6. Ziegler SI. Positron emission tomography: principles, technology, and recent developments. *Nuclear Physics A*. 2005;752.
7. VanElzakker MB, Dahlgren MK, Davis FC, Dubois S, Shin LM. From Pavlov to PTSD: the extinction of conditioned fear in rodents, humans, and anxiety disorders. *Neurobiol Learn Mem*. 2014;113:3–18.
8. Hughes KC, Shin LM. Functional neuroimaging studies of post-traumatic stress disorder. *Expert Rev Neurother*. 2011;11:275–85.
9. Barkhof F, Haller S, Rombouts SA. Resting-state functional MR imaging: a new window to the brain. *Radiology*. 2014;272:29–49.
10. Rauch SL, Shin LM, Phelps EA. Neurocircuitry models of posttraumatic stress disorder and extinction: human neuroimaging research—past, present, and future. *Biol Psychiatry*. 2006;60:376–82.
11. Pitman RK, Rasmusson AM, Koenen KC, *et al*. Biological studies of post-traumatic stress disorder. *Nat Rev Neurosci*. 2012;13:769–87.
12. Zoladz PR, Diamond DM. Current status on behavioral and biological markers of PTSD: a search for clarity in a conflicting literature. *Neurosci Biobehav Rev*. 2013;37:860–95.
13. VanElzakker MB, Staples-Bradley LK, Shin LM. The neurocircuitry of fear and PTSD. In: Vermetten E, Neylan T, Pandi-Perumal SR, Kramer M (eds). *Sleep and Combat-Related Post-Traumatic Stress Disorders*. New York, NY: Springer-Verlag; 2016. pp. 111–26.
14. Linnman C, Zeffiro TA, Pitman RK, Milad MR. An fMRI study of unconditioned responses in post-traumatic stress disorder. *Biol Mood Anxiety Disord*. 2011;1:8.
15. Bremner JD, Vermetten E, Schmahl C, *et al*. Positron emission tomographic imaging of neural correlates of a fear acquisition and extinction paradigm in women with childhood sexual-abuse-related post-traumatic stress disorder. *Psychol Med*. 2005;35:791–806.
16. Garfinkel SN, Abelson JL, King AP, *et al*. Impaired contextual modulation of memories in PTSD: an fMRI and psychophysiological study of extinction retention and fear renewal. *J Neurosci*. 2014;34:13435–43.
17. Milad MR, Pitman RK, Ellis CB, *et al*. Neurobiological basis of failure to recall extinction memory in posttraumatic stress disorder. *Biol Psychiatry*. 2009;66:1075–82.
18. Shin LM, Orr SP, Carson MA, *et al*. Regional cerebral blood flow in amygdala and medial prefrontal cortex during traumatic imagery in male and female Vietnam veterans with PTSD. *Arch Gen Psychiatry*. 2004;61:168–76.
19. St Jacques PL, Botzung A, Miles A, Rubin DC. Functional neuroimaging of emotionally intense autobiographical memories in post-traumatic stress disorder. *J Psychiatr Res*. 2011;45:630–7.
20. Hendler T, Rotshtein P, Yeshurun Y, *et al*. Sensing the invisible: differential sensitivity of visual cortex and amygdala to traumatic context. *Neuroimage*. 2003;19:587–600.
21. Vermetten E, Schmahl C, Southwick SM, Bremner JD. Positron tomographic emission study of olfactory induced emotional recall in veterans with and without combat-related posttraumatic stress disorder. *Psychopharmacol Bull*. 2007;40:8–30.
22. Zhang JN, Xiong KL, Qiu MG, *et al*. Negative emotional distraction on neural circuits for working memory in patients with posttraumatic stress disorder. *Brain Res*. 2013;1531:94–101.
23. Rauch SL, Whalen PJ, Shin LM, *et al*. Exaggerated amygdala response to masked facial stimuli in posttraumatic stress disorder: a functional MRI study. *Biol Psychiatry*. 2000;47:769–76.
24. Shin LM, Wright CI, Cannistraro PA, *et al*. A functional magnetic resonance imaging study of amygdala and medial prefrontal cortex responses to overtly presented fearful faces in posttraumatic stress disorder. *Arch Gen Psychiatry*. 2005;62:273–81.
25. Simmons AN, Matthews SC, Strigo IA, *et al*. Altered amygdala activation during face processing in Iraqi and Afghanistani war veterans. *Biol Mood Anxiety Disord*. 2011;1:6.
26. Stevens JS, Jovanovic T, Fani N, *et al*. Disrupted amygdala-prefrontal functional connectivity in civilian women with posttraumatic stress disorder. *J Psychiatr Res*. 2013;47:1469–78.
27. Williams LM, Kemp AH, Felmingham K, *et al*. Trauma modulates amygdala and medial prefrontal responses to consciously attended fear. *Neuroimage*. 2006;29:347–57.
28. Brohawn KH, Offringa R, Pfaff DL, Hughes KC, Shin LM. The neural correlates of emotional memory in posttraumatic stress disorder. *Biol Psychiatry*. 2010;68:1023–30.
29. Xiong K, Zhang Y, Qiu M, *et al*. Negative emotion regulation in patients with posttraumatic stress disorder. *PLoS One*. 2013;8:e81957.
30. Chung YA, Kim SH, Chung SK, *et al*. Alterations in cerebral perfusion in posttraumatic stress disorder patients without re-exposure to accident-related stimuli. *Clin Neurophysiol*. 2006;117:637–42.

31. Bryant RA, Felmingham KL, Kemp AH, *et al*. Neural networks of information processing in posttraumatic stress disorder: a functional magnetic resonance imaging study. *Biol Psychiatry*. 2005;58:111–18.

32. Brashers-Krug T, Jorge R. Bi-directional tuning of amygdala sensitivity in combat veterans investigated with fMRI. *PLoS One*. 2015;10:e0130246.

33. Lanius RA, Williamson PC, Densmore M, *et al*. Neural correlates of traumatic memories in posttraumatic stress disorder: a functional MRI investigation. *Am J Psychiatry*. 2001;158:1920–2.

34. van Rooij SJ, Rademaker AR, Kennis M, Vink M, Kahn RS, Geuze E. Neural correlates of trauma-unrelated emotional processing in war veterans with PTSD. *Psychol Med*. 2015;45: 575–87.

35. Armony JL, Corbo V, Clement MH, Brunet A. Amygdala response in patients with acute PTSD to masked and unmasked emotional facial expressions. *Am J Psychiatry*. 2005;162:1961–3.

36. Mazza M, Catalucci A, Mariano M, *et al*. Neural correlates of automatic perceptual sensitivity to facial affect in posttraumatic stress disorder subjects who survived L'Aquila earthquake of April 6, 2009. *Brain Imaging Behav*. 2012;6:374–86.

37. White SF, Costanzo ME, Blair JR, Roy MJ. PTSD symptom severity is associated with increased recruitment of top-down attentional control in a trauma-exposed sample. *Neuroimage Clin*. 2015;7:19–27.

38. Aupperle RL, Allard CB, Simmons AN, *et al*. Neural responses during emotional processing before and after cognitive trauma therapy for battered women. *Psychiatry Res*. 2013;214:48–55.

39. Felmingham K, Kemp A, Williams L, *et al*. Changes in anterior cingulate and amygdala after cognitive behavior therapy of posttraumatic stress disorder. *Psychol Sci*. 2007;18:127–9.

40. Peres JF, Newberg AB, Mercante JP, *et al*. Cerebral blood flow changes during retrieval of traumatic memories before and after psychotherapy: a SPECT study. *Psychol Med*. 2007;37:1481–91.

41. Admon R, Lubin G, Stern O, *et al*. Human vulnerability to stress depends on amygdala's predisposition and hippocampal plasticity. *Proc Natl Acad Sci U S A*. 2009;106:14120–5.

42. McLaughlin KA, Busso DS, Duys A, *et al*. Amygdala response to negative stimuli predicts PTSD symptom onset following a terrorist attack. *Depress Anxiety*. 2014;31:834–42.

43. Bryant RA, Felmingham K, Whitford TJ, *et al*. Rostral anterior cingulate volume predicts treatment response to cognitive-behavioural therapy for posttraumatic stress disorder. *J Psychiatry Neurosci*. 2008;33:142–6.

44. van Rooij SJ, Kennis M, Vink M, Geuze E. Predicting treatment outcome in PTSD: a longitudinal functional MRI study on trauma-unrelated emotional processing. *Neuropsychopharmacology*. 2016;41:1156–65.

45. Reynaud E, Guedj E, Trousselard M, *et al*. Acute stress disorder modifies cerebral activity of amygdala and prefrontal cortex. *Cogn Neurosci*. 2015;6:39–43.

46. Depue BE, Olson-Madden JH, Smolker HR, Rajamani M, Brenner LA, Banich MT. Reduced amygdala volume is associated with deficits in inhibitory control: a voxel- and surface-based morphometric analysis of comorbid PTSD/mild TBI. *Biomed Res Int*. 2014;2014:691505.

47. Karl A, Schaefer M, Malta LS, Dorfel D, Rohleder N, Werner A. A meta-analysis of structural brain abnormalities in PTSD. *Neurosci Biobehav Rev*. 2006;30:1004–31.

48. Morey RA, Gold AL, LaBar KS, *et al*. Amygdala volume changes in posttraumatic stress disorder in a large case-controlled veterans group. *Arch Gen Psychiatry*. 2012;69:1169–78.

49. Starcevic A, Postic S, Radojicic Z, *et al*. Volumetric analysis of amygdala, hippocampus, and prefrontal cortex in therapy-naive PTSD participants. *Biomed Res Int*. 2014;2014:968495.

50. Veer IM, Oei NY, van Buchem MA, Spinhoven P, Elzinga BM, Rombouts SA. Evidence for smaller right amygdala volumes in posttraumatic stress disorder following childhood trauma. *Psychiatry Res*. 2015;233:436–42.

51. Pietrzak RH, Averill LA, Abdallah CG, *et al*. Amygdala-hippocampal volume and the phenotypic heterogeneity of posttraumatic stress disorder: a cross-sectional study. *JAMA Psychiatry*. 2015;72:396–8.

52. Shucard JL, Cox J, Shucard DW, *et al*. Symptoms of posttraumatic stress disorder and exposure to traumatic stressors are related to brain structural volumes and behavioral measures of affective stimulus processing in police officers. *Psychiatry Res*. 2012;204:25–31.

53. Baldacara L, Zugman A, Araujo C, *et al*. Reduction of anterior cingulate in adults with urban violence-related PTSD. *J Affect Disord*. 2014;168:13–20.

54. Corbo V, Salat DH, Amick MM, Leritz EC, Milberg WP, McGlinchey RE. Reduced cortical thickness in veterans exposed to early life trauma. *Psychiatry Res*. 2014;223:53–60.

55. Kuo JR, Kaloupek DG, Woodward SH. Amygdala volume in combat-exposed veterans with and without posttraumatic stress disorder: a cross-sectional study. *Arch Gen Psychiatry*. 2012;69:1080–6.

56. Chalavi S, Vissia EM, Giesen ME, *et al*. Similar cortical but not subcortical gray matter abnormalities in women with posttraumatic stress disorder with versus without dissociative identity disorder. *Psychiatry Res*. 2015;231:308–19.

57. Chao L, Weiner M, Neylan T. Regional cerebral volumes in veterans with current versus remitted posttraumatic stress disorder. *Psychiatry Res*. 2013;213:193–201.

58. Cheng B, Huang X, Li S, Hu X, Luo Y, Wang X, *et al*. Gray matter alterations in post-traumatic stress disorder, obsessive-compulsive disorder, and social anxiety disorder. *Front Behav Neurosci*. 2015;9:219.

59. Levy-Gigi E, Szabo C, Kelemen O, Keri S. Association among clinical response, hippocampal volume, and FKBP5 gene expression in individuals with posttraumatic stress disorder receiving cognitive behavioral therapy. *Biol Psychiatry*. 2013;74:793–800.

60. Meng Y, Qiu C, Zhu H, *et al*. Anatomical deficits in adult posttraumatic stress disorder: a meta-analysis of voxel-based morphometry studies. *Behav Brain Res*. 2014;270:307–15.

61. O'Doherty DC, Chitty KM, Saddiqui S, Bennett MR, Lagopoulos J. A systematic review and meta-analysis of magnetic resonance imaging measurement of structural volumes in posttraumatic stress disorder. *Psychiatry Res*. 2015;232:1–33.

62. Szabo C, Kelemen O, Levy-Gigi E, Keri S. Acute response to psychological trauma and subsequent recovery: no changes in brain structure. *Psychiatry Res*. 2015;231:269–72.

63. Rougemont-Bucking A, Linnman C, Zeffiro TA, *et al*. Altered processing of contextual information during fear extinction in PTSD: an fMRI study. *CNS Neurosci Ther*. 2011;17:227–36.

64. Liberzon I, Britton JC, Phan KL. Neural correlates of traumatic recall in posttraumatic stress disorder. *Stress*. 2003;6:151–6.

65. Lindauer RJ, Booij J, Habraken JB, *et al*. Cerebral blood flow changes during script-driven imagery in police officers with posttraumatic stress disorder. *Biol Psychiatry*. 2004;56:853–61.

66. Britton JC, Phan KL, Taylor SF, Fig LM, Liberzon I. Corticolimbic blood flow in posttraumatic stress disorder during script-driven imagery. *Biol Psychiatry*. 2005;57:832–40.

67. Hou C, Liu J, Wang K, *et al*. Brain responses to symptom provocation and trauma-related short-term memory recall in coal mining accident survivors with acute severe PTSD. *Brain Res*. 2007;1144:165–74.

68. Lanius RA, Frewen PA, Girotti M, Neufeld RW, Stevens TK, Densmore M. Neural correlates of trauma script-imagery in posttraumatic stress disorder with and without comorbid major depression: a functional MRI investigation. *Psychiatry Res*. 2007;155:45–56.

69. Bremner JD, Narayan M, Staib LH, Southwick SM, McGlashan T, Charney DS. Neural correlates of memories of childhood sexual abuse in women with and without posttraumatic stress disorder. *Am J Psychiatry*. 1999;156:1787–95.

70. Shin LM, McNally RJ, Kosslyn SM, *et al*. Regional cerebral blood flow during script-driven imagery in childhood sexual abuse-related PTSD: a PET investigation. *Am J Psychiatry*. 1999;156:575–84.

71. Gold AL, Shin LM, Orr SP, *et al*. Decreased regional cerebral blood flow in medial prefrontal cortex during trauma-unrelated stressful imagery in Vietnam veterans with post-traumatic stress disorder. *Psychol Med*. 2011:1–10.

72. Piefke M, Pestinger M, Arin T, *et al*. The neurofunctional mechanisms of traumatic and non-traumatic memory in patients with acute PTSD following accident trauma. *Neurocase*. 2007;13:342–57.

73. Bremner JD, Vythilingam M, Vermetten E, *et al*. Neural correlates of declarative memory for emotionally valenced words in women with posttraumatic stress disorder related to early childhood sexual abuse. *Biol Psychiatry*. 2003;53:879–89.

74. Bremner JD, Staib LH, Kaloupek D, Southwick SM, Soufer R, Charney DS. Neural correlates of exposure to traumatic pictures and sound in Vietnam combat veterans with and without posttraumatic stress disorder: a positron emission tomography study. *Biol Psychiatry*. 1999;45:806–16.

75. Yang P, Wu MT, Hsu CC, Ker JH. Evidence of early neurobiological alternations in adolescents with posttraumatic stress disorder: a functional MRI study. *Neurosci Lett*. 2004;370:13–18.

76. Aupperle RL, Allard CB, Grimes EM, *et al*. Dorsolateral prefrontal cortex activation during emotional anticipation and neuropsychological performance in posttraumatic stress disorder. *Arch Gen Psychiatry*. 2012;69:360–71.

77. Crozier JC, Wang L, Huettel SA, De Bellis MD. Neural correlates of cognitive and affective processing in maltreated youth with posttraumatic stress symptoms: does gender matter? *Dev Psychopathol*. 2014;26:491–513.

78. Kim MJ, Chey J, Chung A, Bae S, Khang H, Ham B, *et al*. Diminished rostral anterior cingulate activity in response to threat-related events in posttraumatic stress disorder. *J Psychiatr Res*. 2008;42:268–77.

79. Felmingham KL, Williams LM, Kemp AH, Rennie C, Gordon E, Bryant RA. Anterior cingulate activity to salient stimuli is modulated by autonomic arousal in posttraumatic stress disorder. *Psychiatry Res*. 2009;173:59–62.

80. Molina ME, Isoardi R, Prado MN, Bentolila S. Basal cerebral glucose distribution in long-term post-traumatic stress disorder. *World J Biol Psychiatry*. 2010;11(2 Pt 2):493–501.

81. Pannu Hayes J, Labar KS, Petty CM, McCarthy G, Morey RA. Alterations in the neural circuitry for emotion and attention associated with posttraumatic stress symptomatology. *Psychiatry Res*. 2009;172:7–15.

82. Shin LM, Bush G, Whalen PJ, *et al*. Dorsal anterior cingulate function in posttraumatic stress disorder. *J Trauma Stress*. 2007;20:701–12.

83. Yin Y, Li L, Jin C, *et al*. Abnormal baseline brain activity in posttraumatic stress disorder: a resting-state functional magnetic resonance imaging study. *Neurosci Lett*. 2011;498:185–9.

84. Yan X, Brown AD, Lazar M, *et al*. Spontaneous brain activity in combat related PTSD. *Neurosci Lett*. 2013;547:1–5.

85. Zhu H, Zhang J, Zhan W, *et al*. Altered spontaneous neuronal activity of visual cortex and medial anterior cingulate cortex in treatment-naive posttraumatic stress disorder. *Compr Psychiatry*. 2014;55:1688–95.

86. Lansing K, Amen DG, Hanks C, Rudy L. High-resolution brain SPECT imaging and eye movement desensitization and reprocessing in police officers with PTSD. *J Neuropsychiatry Clin Neurosci*. 2005;17:526–32.

87. Felmingham K, Kemp AH, Williams L, *et al*. Dissociative responses to conscious and non-conscious fear impact underlying brain function in post-traumatic stress disorder. *Psychol Med*. 2008;38:1771–80.

88. Mazza M, Tempesta D, Pino MC, *et al*. Neural activity related to cognitive and emotional empathy in post-traumatic stress disorder. *Behav Brain Res*. 2015;282:37–45.

89. Lanius RA, Williamson PC, Boksman K, *et al*. Brain activation during script-driven imagery induced dissociative responses in PTSD: a functional magnetic resonance imaging investigation. *Biol Psychiatry*. 2002;52:305–11.

90. Felmingham K, Williams LM, Kemp AH, *et al*. Neural responses to masked fear faces: sex differences and trauma exposure in posttraumatic stress disorder. *J Abnorm Psychol*. 2010;119:241–7.

91. Rauch SL, Shin LM, Segal E, *et al*. Selectively reduced regional cortical volumes in post-traumatic stress disorder. *Neuroreport*. 2003;14:913–16.

92. Woodward SH, Kaloupek DG, Streeter CC, Martinez C, Schaer M, Eliez S. Decreased anterior cingulate volume in combat-related PTSD. *Biol Psychiatry*. 2006;59:582–7.

93. Felmingham K, Williams LM, Whitford TJ, *et al*. Duration of posttraumatic stress disorder predicts hippocampal grey matter loss. *Neuroreport*. 2009;20:1402–6.

94. Kroes MC, Rugg MD, Whalley MG, Brewin CR. Structural brain abnormalities common to posttraumatic stress disorder and depression. *J Psychiatry Neurosci*. 2011;36:256–65.

95. Eckart C, Stoppel C, Kaufmann J, *et al*. Structural alterations in lateral prefrontal, parietal and posterior midline regions of men with chronic posttraumatic stress disorder. *J Psychiatry Neurosci*. 2011;36:176–86.

96. Schulz-Heik RJ, Schaer M, Eliez S, *et al*. Catechol-O-methyltransferase Val158Met polymorphism moderates anterior cingulate volume in posttraumatic stress disorder. *Biol Psychiatry*. 2011;70:1091–6.

97. Kim MJ, Lyoo IK, Kim SJ, *et al*. Disrupted white matter tract integrity of anterior cingulate in trauma survivors. *Neuroreport*. 2005;16:1049–53.

98. Schuff N, Zhang Y, Zhan W, *et al*. Patterns of altered cortical perfusion and diminished subcortical integrity in posttraumatic stress disorder: an MRI study. *Neuroimage*. 2011;54 Suppl 1:S62–8.

99. Corbo V, Clement MH, Armony JL, Pruessner JC, Brunet A. Size versus shape differences: contrasting voxel-based and volumetric analyses of the anterior cingulate cortex in individuals with acute posttraumatic stress disorder. *Biol Psychiatry*. 2005;58:119–24.

100. Chen S, Xia W, Li L, Liu J, He Z, Zhang Z, *et al*. Gray matter density reduction in the insula in fire survivors with

posttraumatic stress disorder: a voxel-based morphometric study. *Psychiatry Res*. 2006;146:65–72.

101. Hakamata Y, Matsuoka Y, Inagaki M, *et al*. Structure of orbitofrontal cortex and its longitudinal course in cancer-related post-traumatic stress disorder. *Neurosci Res*. 2007;59:383–9.

102. Kasai K, Yamasue H, Gilbertson MW, Shenton ME, Rauch SL, Pitman RK. Evidence for acquired pregenual anterior cingulate gray matter loss from a twin study of combat-related posttraumatic stress disorder. *Biol Psychiatry*. 2008;63:550–6.

103. Thomaes K, Dorrepaal E, Draijer N, *et al*. Reduced anterior cingulate and orbitofrontal volumes in child abuse-related complex PTSD. *J Clin Psychiatry*. 2010;71:1636–44.

104. Herringa R, Phillips M, Almeida J, Insana S, Germain A. Posttraumatic stress symptoms correlate with smaller subgenual cingulate, caudate, and insula volumes in unmedicated combat veterans. *Psychiatry Res*. 2012;203:139–45.

105. Tavanti M, Battaglini M, Borgogni F, *et al*. Evidence of diffuse damage in frontal and occipital cortex in the brain of patients with post-traumatic stress disorder. *Neurol Sci*. 2012;33:59–68.

106. Rocha-Rego V, Pereira MG, Oliveira L, *et al*. Decreased premotor cortex volume in victims of urban violence with posttraumatic stress disorder. *PLoS One*. 2012;7:e42560.

107. Bing X, Ming-Guo Q, Ye Z, *et al*. Alterations in the cortical thickness and the amplitude of low-frequency fluctuation in patients with post-traumatic stress disorder. *Brain Res*. 2013;1490:225–32.

108. Nardo D, Hogberg G, Lanius RA, *et al*. Gray matter volume alterations related to trait dissociation in PTSD and traumatized controls. *Acta Psychiatr Scand*. 2013;128:222–33.

109. Marin MF, Song H, VanElzakker MB, *et al*. Association of resting metabolism in the fear neural network with extinction recall activations and clinical measures in trauma-exposed individuals. *Am J Psychiatry*. 2016;173:930–8.

110. Shin LM, Whalen PJ, Pitman RK, *et al*. An fMRI study of anterior cingulate function in posttraumatic stress disorder. *Biol Psychiatry*. 2001;50:932–42.

111. Shin LM, Bush G, Milad MR, *et al*. Exaggerated activation of dorsal anterior cingulate cortex during cognitive interference: a monozygotic twin study of posttraumatic stress disorder. *Am J Psychiatry*. 2011;168:979–85.

112. Shin LM, Lasko NB, Macklin ML, *et al*. Resting metabolic activity in the cingulate cortex and vulnerability to posttraumatic stress disorder. *Arch Gen Psychiatry*. 2009;66:1099–107.

113. Cwik JC, Sartory G, Schurholt B, Knuppertz H, Seitz RJ. Posterior midline activation during symptom provocation in acute stress disorder: an fMRI study. *Front Psychiatry*. 2014;5:49.

114. Yamasue H, Kasai K, Iwanami A, *et al*. Voxel-based analysis of MRI reveals anterior cingulate gray-matter volume reduction in posttraumatic stress disorder due to terrorism. *Proc Natl Acad Sci U S A*. 2003;100:9039–43.

115. Lindauer RJ, Booij J, Habraken JB, *et al*. Effects of psychotherapy on regional cerebral blood flow during trauma imagery in patients with post-traumatic stress disorder: a randomized clinical trial. *Psychol Med*. 2008;38:543–54.

116. Nardo D, Hogberg G, Flumeri F, *et al*. Self-rating scales assessing subjective well-being and distress correlate with rCBF in PTSD-sensitive regions. *Psychol Med*. 2011;41:2549–61.

117. Ke J, Zhang L, Qi R, *et al*. A longitudinal fMRI investigation in acute post-traumatic stress disorder (PTSD). *Acta Radiol*. 2016;57:1387–95.

118. Simmons AN, Flagan TM, Wittmann M, *et al*. The effects of temporal unpredictability in anticipation of negative events in combat veterans with PTSD. *J Affect Disord*. 2013;146:426–32.

119. Moser DA, Aue T, Suardi F, *et al*. Violence-related PTSD and neural activation when seeing emotionally charged male-female interactions. *Soc Cogn Affect Neurosci*. 2015;10:645–53.

120. Simmons AN, Paulus MP, Thorp SR, Matthews SC, Norman SB, Stein MB. Functional activation and neural networks in women with posttraumatic stress disorder related to intimate partner violence. *Biol Psychiatry*. 2008;64:681–90.

121. Chen S, Li L, Xu B, Liu J. Insular cortex involvement in declarative memory deficits in patients with post-traumatic stress disorder. *BMC Psychiatry*. 2009;9:39.

122. Astur RS, St Germain SA, Tolin D, Ford J, Russell D, Stevens M. Hippocampus function predicts severity of post-traumatic stress disorder. *Cyberpsychol Behav*. 2006;9:234–40.

123. Geuze E, Vermetten E, Ruf M, de Kloet CS, Westenberg HG. Neural correlates of associative learning and memory in veterans with posttraumatic stress disorder. *J Psychiatr Res*. 2008;42:659–69.

124. Shin LM, Shin PS, Heckers S, Krangel TS, Macklin ML, Orr SP, *et al*. Hippocampal function in posttraumatic stress disorder. *Hippocampus*. 2004;14:292–300.

125. Sachinvala N, Kling A, Suffin S, Lake R, Cohen M. Increased regional cerebral perfusion by 99mTc hexamethyl propylene amine oxime single photon emission computed tomography in post-traumatic stress disorder. *Mil Med*. 2000;165:473–9.

126. Molina ME, Isoardi R, Prado MN, Bentolila S. Basal cerebral glucose distribution in long-term post-traumatic stress disorder. *World J Biol Psychiatry*. 2007;1–9.

127. Thomaes K, Dorrepaal E, Draijer NP, *et al*. Increased activation of the left hippocampus region in Complex PTSD during encoding and recognition of emotional words: a pilot study. *Psychiatry Res*. 2009;171:44–53.

128. Whalley MG, Rugg MD, Smith AP, Dolan RJ, Brewin CR. Incidental retrieval of emotional contexts in post-traumatic stress disorder and depression: an fMRI study. *Brain Cogn*. 2009;69:98–107.

129. Woon FL, Sood S, Hedges DW. Hippocampal volume deficits associated with exposure to psychological trauma and posttraumatic stress disorder in adults: a meta-analysis. *Prog Neuropsychopharmacol Biol Psychiatry*. 2010;34:1181–8.

130. Bremner JD, Randall P, Vermetten E, *et al*. Magnetic resonance imaging-based measurement of hippocampal volume in posttraumatic stress disorder related to childhood physical and sexual abuse—a preliminary report. *Biol Psychiatry*. 1997;41:23–32.

131. Gurvits TV, Shenton ME, Hokama H, *et al*. Magnetic resonance imaging study of hippocampal volume in chronic, combat-related posttraumatic stress disorder. *Biol Psychiatry*. 1996;40:1091–9.

132. Bremner JD, Vythilingam M, Vermetten E, *et al*. MRI and PET study of deficits in hippocampal structure and function in women with childhood sexual abuse and posttraumatic stress disorder. *Am J Psychiatry*. 2003;160:924–32.

133. Lindauer RJ, Vlieger EJ, Jalink M, *et al*. Smaller hippocampal volume in Dutch police officers with posttraumatic stress disorder. *Biol Psychiatry*. 2004;56:356–63.

134. Wignall EL, Dickson JM, Vaughan P, *et al.* Smaller hippocampal volume in patients with recent-onset posttraumatic stress disorder. *Biol Psychiatry.* 2004;56:832–6.

135. Vythilingam M, Luckenbaugh DA, Lam T, *et al.* Smaller head of the hippocampus in Gulf War-related posttraumatic stress disorder. *Psychiatry Res.* 2005;139:89–99.

136. Bossini L, Tavanti M, Calossi S, *et al.* Magnetic resonance imaging volumes of the hippocampus in drug-naive patients with post-traumatic stress disorder without comorbidity conditions. *J Psychiatr Res.* 2008;42:752–62.

137. Schmahl C, Berne K, Krause A, *et al.* Hippocampus and amygdala volumes in patients with borderline personality disorder with or without posttraumatic stress disorder. *J Psychiatry Neurosci.* 2009;34:289–95.

138. Wang Z, Neylan TC, Mueller SG, *et al.* Magnetic resonance imaging of hippocampal subfields in posttraumatic stress disorder. *Arch Gen Psychiatry.* 2010;67:296–303.

139. Shu XJ, Xue L, Liu W, Chen FY, Zhu C, Sun XH, *et al.* More vulnerability of left than right hippocampal damage in right-handed patients with post-traumatic stress disorder. *Psychiatry Res.* 2013;212:237–44.

140. Zhang Q, Zhuo C, Lang X, Li H, Qin W, Yu C. Structural impairments of hippocampus in coal mine gas explosion-related posttraumatic stress disorder. *PLoS One.* 2014;9: e102042.

141. Chalavi S, Vissia EM, Giesen ME, *et al.* Abnormal hippocampal morphology in dissociative identity disorder and post-traumatic stress disorder correlates with childhood trauma and dissociative symptoms. *Hum Brain Mapp.* 2015;36:1692–704.

142. Rubin M, Shvil E, Papini S, *et al.* Greater hippocampal volume is associated with PTSD treatment response. *Psychiatry Res.* 2016;252:36–9.

143. Tupler LA, De Bellis MD. Segmented hippocampal volume in children and adolescents with posttraumatic stress disorder. *Biol Psychiatry.* 2006;59:523–9.

144. Golier JA, Yehuda R, De Santi S, Segal S, Dolan S, de Leon MJ. Absence of hippocampal volume differences in survivors of the Nazi Holocaust with and without posttraumatic stress disorder. *Psychiatry Res.* 2005;139:53–64.

145. Freeman T, Kimbrell T, Booe L, *et al.* Evidence of resilience: Neuroimaging in former prisoners of war. *Psychiatry Res.* 2006;146:59–64.

146. Landre L, Destrieux C, Baudry M, *et al.* Preserved subcortical volumes and cortical thickness in women with sexual abuse-related PTSD. *Psychiatry Res.* 2010;183: 181–6.

147. Hall T, Galletly C, Clark CR, *et al.* The relationship between Hippocampal asymmetry and working memory processing in combat-related PTSD - a monozygotic twin study. *Biol Mood Anxiety Disord.* 2012;2:21.

148. Eckart C, Kaufmann J, Kanowski M, *et al.* Magnetic resonance volumetry and spectroscopy of hippocampus and insula in relation to severe exposure of traumatic stress. *Psychophysiology.* 2012;49:261–70.

149. Gilbertson MW, Shenton ME, Ciszewski A, *et al.* Smaller hippocampal volume predicts pathologic vulnerability to psychological trauma. *Nat Neurosci.* 2002;5:1242–7.

# 82

# Primary prevention and epidemiology of trauma- and stress-related disorders

*Maria Bragesjö, Emily A. Holmes, Filip K. Arnberg, and Erik M. Andersson*

## Introduction

In this chapter, we will focus on prevention of disorders that largely arise after single traumatic events. Such events can strike many people at once, such as disasters or terrorist attacks, or only single or few individuals such as severe motor vehicle crashes or a sexual assault. We focus on strategies to help prevent post-traumatic stress disorder (PTSD) and acute stress disorder (ASD). These are the two most well-researched disorders within the new *Diagnostic and Statistical Manual of Mental Disorders*, fifth edition (DSM-5) 'Trauma- and stressor related disorders' chapter [1]. Further, a unique aspect of both these disorders within DSM-5 is the presence of an *index traumatic event* or events. Therefore, once we know that such an event has occurred, PTSD and ASD are mental disorders for which we could, and should, seek strategies to prevent the emergence of the full-blown disorder. We first discuss what prevention means in this context. Next, we consider diagnostic features of PTSD and ASD to understand what it is that could be prevented after trauma. Then, we consider the associated epidemiology and risk indicators of developing these disorders, that is, the scale of the prevention challenge and who we might target. Given the limited prevention strategies to date, considerable further research is needed to advance the field.

## Trauma- and stressor-related disorders

In DSM-5, a new chapter 'Trauma- and stressor-related disorders' was formed that includes seven diagnoses (Box 82.1) [1]. The focus in this chapter is on PTSD and ASD as the two most well-researched disorders within this new DSM-5 chapter [1]—and the ones for which there is a clear clinical demand for prevention. Critically, a unique aspect of both these disorders within DSM-5 is the occurrence of an *index traumatic event* or events. A traumatic event here is defined as exposure to actual or threatened death, actual or threatened serious injury, or actual or threatened sexual violence [1]. Therefore, once we know that such an event

> **Box 82.1** Trauma- and stress-related disorders according to DSM-5
>
> - Acute stress disorder
> - Post-traumatic stress disorder
> - Reactive attachment disorder
> - Disinhibited social engagement disorder
> - Adjustment disorders
> - Other specified trauma- and stressor-related disorder
> - Trauma- and stress-related disorder not otherwise specified
>
> Source: data from *Diagnostic and Statistical Manual of Mental Disorders*, Fifth Edition, DSM-5, Copyright (2013), American Psychiatric Association.

has occurred, PTSD and ASD are mental disorders for which we could, and should, seek strategies to prevent the emergence of the full-blown disorder.

Regarding the other diagnoses in the 'Trauma- and stressor-related' section of this book (see Chapters 78–85), reactive attachment disorder and disinhibited social engagement disorder are viewed as general consequences of inadequate child care or maltreatment. The diagnosis of adjustment disorder reflects the case when someone is in a serious crisis and experiences very distressing reactions to, and cannot cope with, any of a great variation of stressors, often related to life events such as unemployment or divorce. The crisis is expected to resolve within a few months. The diagnoses of 'other specified' or 'not otherwise specified' trauma- and stressor-related disorder are clinically relevant when someone presents with, for example, a debilitating reaction to a sudden death in the family that is beyond a crisis or when the presenting problems do not match any other trauma-related disorder. All of the last three disorders in Box 82.1 are of clinical utility but have not been researched to any greater extent—because of their great variation in what they encompass, they are difficult targets for *prevention*. The childhood-onset disorders require preventive strategies targeted towards parents and are not described further in this text.

## Prevention strategies adapted to trauma- and stressor-related disorders

Prevention is, broadly speaking, defined as stopping 'something' from happening or arising [2]. Preventive interventions can be implemented in many different ways. A long-used medical model of prevention is the 'three-level concept of prevention' developed by Leavell and Clark [3, 4] in the late fifties. This model makes a distinction between primary, secondary, and tertiary prevention interventions from a physical health perspective. The primary prevention level refers to health promotion and protection from a disease or disorder, for example immunization from a disease through vaccination. The secondary prevention level refers both to early detection and treatment of a disease in order to avoid chronicity (for example, prostate-specific antigen screening to detect prostate cancer). Tertiary preventions are interventions that aim to reduce as much damage as possible from a disease and can be considered equivalent to physical rehabilitation.

Prevention for mental disorders also has as its aim the reduction of symptoms, and ultimately the disorder [4]; the term primary prevention can encompass a wider range of definitions, compared with this medical model [3, 5]. Primary prevention for mental disorders has been described as including interventions which are 'universal' (targeting the whole population), 'selective' (targeting population subgroups or individuals who are at higher risk than the average population), and 'indicated' (targeting high-risk people who are identified as *having minimal detectable signs or symptoms foreshadowing mental disorder or biological markers indicating a predisposition but who do not meet diagnostic criteria for the disorder at that time*' [3, 5]. Of note here is that, according to this latter aspect, primary prevention in a trauma context could include targeting those with early symptoms (such as intrusive memories of the traumatic event) which may precede the diagnosis of a full-blown disorder such as ASD and PTSD. In a mental health context, secondary prevention has been described as seeking to lower the prevalence through early detection and treatment of a diagnosable disease. Tertiary prevention interventions include those to reduce disability and prevent relapse. The World Health Organization [3, 5] uses similar terms regarding mental health and notes that given that while the traditional medical model '*works well for medical disorders with a known etiology. Mental disorders, on the other hand, often occur due to the interaction of environmental and genetic factors at specific periods of life. It becomes difficult even to agree on the exact time of onset of a mental disorder*'. However, as discussed, PTSD and ASD are unique in DSM-5 in that their aetiology is clear and forms part of the diagnosis—the presence of an index traumatic event.

In relation to aetiology, another question of importance in prevention research is *when* a preventive intervention should be administered. The definition of primary prevention requires further thought when applied to psychological trauma. Several terms are in use synonymously. Some argue that primary prevention for trauma- and stress-related disorders should only encompass interventions *before* trauma exposure, while any intervention after trauma exposure, but before the development of PTSD (for example, before 1 month of symptoms), is to be considered secondary prevention [6]. However, as described, a form of prevention focusing on early symptoms prior to a diagnosis may have utility; traumatic events

are often unpredictable, which restricts knowledge of who to target in advance in the reality of limited health care resources. Therefore, there would be benefits for the mental health field in developing 'selective' intervention strategies and tools to offer soon *after* a traumatic event where the applicability is restricted to a group with higher known risk of the disease emerging (see Epidemiology of ASD and PTSD, p. 862). Thus, another related view is that, in the mental health field, it may also be possible, by analogy, to provide a form of 'therapeutic vaccination' after an index traumatic event has occurred (that is, a *post-event* preventive intervention). For example, in physical medicine, *after* a patient is bitten by a dog, a 'therapeutic vaccine' [7] is given to protect against rabies. After a traumatic event, an equivalent 'primary' prevention approach would be the metaphor of a 'cognitive therapeutic vaccine' that could be administered soon *after* the event—whether psychological or pharmacological. We are not at the stage where there is a strong evidence base for this approach, but the analogy of preventing the worsening of symptoms soon after an index stressor is a useful one, both clinically and to guide research.

While the remainder of this chapter will focus on pragmatic and research approaches to prevention from a mental health perspective, it should be noted that many other fields have a role to play in achieving a wider prevention agenda related to trauma. For example, public health and efforts in society in general should seek to prevent potentially traumatic events such as road traffic accidents, assault with weapons, rape, and so forth. Reducing the incidence of potentially traumatic events would clearly have a major role to play in reducing the incidence of disorders such as ASD and PTSD. Examples of such intervention include implementation of blood alcohol limits for drivers, addition of separation barriers to freeways, strengthening of community-based support services, and laws limiting access to firearms.

## About post-traumatic stress disorder

We first consider the background, the definition of traumatic events, and the diagnostic features of PTSD to understand the nature of symptoms from this particular disorder that could be prevented after trauma. PTSD is defined by a set of criteria that include the event characteristics, four groups of symptoms, a duration criterion, and a distress/disability criterion [1]. The disorder is seen as the cardinal psychopathological consequence of traumatic events, although such events may also contribute to several other forms of psychopathology [8]. PTSD is often associated with high levels of distress, a high degree of chronicity, and high levels of disability [9–11].

The traumatic event that precipitates PTSD is defined as the 'index event' and means that the individual is exposed to actual or threatened death, actual or threatened serious injury, or actual or threatened sexual violence [1]. Thus, everyday stressors, like losing a job or going through a divorce, do not meet the criterion for a potentially traumatic event in DSM-5. The exposure to the event could have occurred directly or indirectly (learning that a close relative/friend has been through a trauma or being exposed to aversive material through work). It is not possible to receive a diagnosis of PTSD after being exposed indirectly through electronic media, television, or movies (that is, by watching a frightful film clip on the Internet), unless it occurred in the line of work (such as by police reviewing traumatic crime footage). It is important to note that no set of objectively discerned individual characteristics of any kind of event have been found to consistently lead to PTSD [12–14]. The subjective experience of the threatening nature of the event appears to be key factor in the 'toxicity' of an event [15]. That is, people who experience high levels of threat peritraumatically have higher risk for later PTSD [15–17].

The four symptom clusters of PTSD in DSM-5 include intrusion symptoms, avoidance, cognitive and mood changes, and arousal. The intrusion symptoms include intrusive memories of the trauma, flashbacks, nightmares, and distress in response to reminders of the trauma.

The core clinical feature of PTSD is arguably the recurrent, involuntary, and intrusive distressing memories of the traumatic event [18]. Such memories are intrusive in that they spring to mind unwanted and unbidden. They typically take the form of discrete episodes from within a trauma—so called 'hotspots' in the memory [19]. They are recurrent in that it is often the same selection of hotspot scenes that appear repeatedly (rather than, say, the whole trauma from beginning to end). Such memories are 'seen in the mind's eye' and 'heard in the mind's ear'—that is, they comprise typically visual, but multisensory, mental images [20].

The next symptom cluster of PTSD involves avoidance. PTSD patients often try to avoid stimuli that are associated with the traumatic event. They therefore often avoid thoughts and feelings or situations/persons/places that are reminders of the experienced trauma (for example, car crash survivors often avoid driving or using public transportation). Consequently, many trauma survivors live restricted lives, constantly avoiding reminders of the trauma.

The third symptom cluster involves marked changes in cognitions and mood after trauma. Some trauma survivors with PTSD report a persistent negative emotional state (e.g. shame), or that they feel numb and cannot get in touch with their emotions as they did before (e.g. happiness). They can experience persistent cognitive symptoms, with negative beliefs about themselves (for example, 'I'm a bad person'), others, and the world (for example, 'The world is unsafe'), and distorted perceptions about why the trauma occurred are also common (for example, 'It was my fault that the trauma occurred').

The fourth symptom cluster of PTSD involves arousal symptoms. PTSD patients often describe themselves as in a chronic state of alert, constantly scanning the environment for potential threats. This group of symptoms also includes insomnia, irritability, and concentration—these symptoms can follow from the hypervigilance and disrupted stress responses.

The symptoms must have been present for at least 1 month since the index event. This is called the 'duration criterion', and was originally introduced to reduce the risk of overdiagnosis of common acute responses to distressing events. The symptoms should cause clinically significant distress or impairment in social, occupational, or other important areas of functioning, and they should not be better explained by another psychiatric or somatic disorder. Hence, it is important to note that the symptoms must not be attributable to the effects of a substance (for example, medication, alcohol) or another psychiatric or medical condition, stating the importance of a good differential diagnosis.

## About acute stress disorder

ASD was introduced in DSM-IV as a way to describe a distressing response *within* the first month after the event that could identify patients at high risk for developing PTSD [21]. The diagnostic criteria of ASD are similar to those of PTSD, except that the presenting problems do not have to be as many as for PTSD and they should be present during the first month.

ASD was originally thought to be an antecedent to PTSD, and although it has some bearing on how to identify trauma survivors who are at high risk for developing PTSD, it has become evident that many patients with ASD never develop PTSD. In fact, of those diagnosed with ASD, less than half will meet criteria for PTSD after 12 months [22].

### Assessing PTSD and ASD

The assessment of ASD and PTSD is slightly different from the assessment of other mental disorders in that the clinician must assess not only the presence and severity of the symptoms, but also whether or not the individual's experience satisfies the traumatic event criterion and if the presenting symptoms started or worsened after the event. It should be evident to the reader that in order to make a diagnosis of ASD or PTSD, it requires both trained assessors and time for the assessments. The clinician should be trained and preferably use well-described methods such as the Acute Stress Disorder Interview [23] or the Clinician-Administered PTSD Scale [24]. Next, we consider the scale of occurrence of traumatic events and stress-related disorders.

## Epidemiology of ASD and PTSD

### Prevalence rates

Traumatic events are common in the population. In the large World Mental Health (WMH) surveys, where more than 70,000 respondents were interviewed between 2001 and 2012, the lifetime exposure to potentially traumatic events was estimated to be 70% across 24 countries [25].

How prevalent is PTSD? One influential study was the National Comorbidity Survey, conducted in the United States in 1995, in which the lifetime prevalence rate of PTSD in the United States was estimated to be 8% [10]. Within the UK, the best estimate of the whole population PTSD point prevalence is 3%, which is derived from the 2007 Adult Psychiatric Morbidity Study [26]. In the WMH surveys, the lifetime prevalence of PTSD was estimated to be 3.9%, with two-thirds having an adult age of onset [25]. Interestingly, in populations with a high risk of exposure, the prevalence rates vary and are not necessarily higher than the general population estimates. For example, United States military veterans seem to be at higher risk of combat-related PTSD than UK veterans [27]. Among UK veterans, the prevalence was 3–6%, which is close to the estimates of PTSD in the general population. A review of resettled refugees concluded that resettled refugees in western countries could be approximately ten times more likely to have PTSD than the general population in those countries [28], which is perhaps unsurprising, given the dose-wise effect of trauma exposure and the multiple exposure of different events, for example, war, torture, and rape, in this group. Additional studies of rescue and recovery workers suggest that the risk of PTSD decreases, the more training and familiarity the personnel in high-risk occupations have with the task [29].

Some research studies have pointed to evidence that certain types of traumatic events make it more likely to develop PTSD. Notably, high rates of occurrence are seen after rape and torture. For example, the risk of developing PTSD is approximately ten times higher in populations exposed to assault, compared to populations that survive a motor vehicle crash [30]. It should be noted that there are challenges with comparing the conditional prevalence across event types; for example, people at risk of an assault can be more likely than others to have a history of potentially traumatic events. Prevention strategies aimed towards victims of high-risk events such as interpersonal violence would therefore benefit from taking into account the influences of past stressors [31].

## The time course of trauma symptoms

As previously mentioned, it is common to experience some adverse reactions such as intrusive memories, avoidance, and hyperarousal in the immediate aftermath of trauma. For many these symptoms disappear without professional help [32]. This is thought to be the case in most trauma populations, including motor vehicle accidents [33], rape victims [34], New York City residents following the terrorist attacks of 11 September 2001 [35, 36], and for individuals who experienced the 2004 South East Asia tsunami [37].

The high proportion of exposed individuals who either are resilient or experience a natural recovery after trauma means that the timing of preventive interventions is important to consider. High natural recovery rates mean that many people that are encompassed by unselective prevention strategies shortly after an event could recover anyway, raising issues of cost and efficiency. Interventions that target high-risk groups among survivors need to consider the time frame. For example, an initial screening to select people for preventive interventions may be based on current distress levels, though more research on screening would be needed to inform evidence-based practice.

The risk of negative consequences of intervening in people who otherwise would recover anyway is also important to consider. Adverse effects of psychological interventions have only recently received greater attention, driven particularly by the discovery of adverse consequences from some early interventions for trauma survivors and bereaved individuals [38, 39]. Several reviews has shown that critical stress incident debriefing, a widely disseminated intervention after trauma, may *increase*, rather than decrease, the risk of developing PTSD [40]. In summary, to establish successful prevention strategies of trauma-related disorders in populations exposed to highly distressing events, there is a need to consider not only what the strategies should be, but also to pay careful attention to the target population and the time course of action.

## Trauma and risk indicators

There has been extensive research in the last decades on risk factors in the trauma population and identifying individuals most vulnerable following exposure to a traumatic event. A common classification of different types of indicators of risk are pre-trauma, peritraumatic, and post-trauma indicators.

### Pre-trauma risk indicators

Gender is perhaps the most well-known pre-trauma risk factor. A consistent finding has been that women have more or less twice the risk of PTSD, as compared to men overall [41–44]. For example, one large study found a lifetime prevalence of PTSD of 20.4% in female trauma survivors and 8.2% of male trauma survivors [10]. However, studies are also needed which control for exposure to the same type of event. Low socio-economic status, previous exposure to highly distressing events, previous psychiatric symptoms, and high levels of neuroticism also increase the risk of later developing PTSD [16, 45]. New research suggests that there may be genes that make certain people susceptible to PTSD. Genetic research has expanded greatly the last decade, and twin studies estimate the heritability of PTSD to up to 35%, but this varies when individual PTSD symptoms are examined [46].

### Peritraumatic risk indicators

What happens during the event plays an important role in the development of PTSD. People who thought that they would be killed or severely injured during the event have a higher risk of developing PTSD [16, 17], and very high levels of distress emotions or dissociative symptoms during, and immediately after, the trauma are strong indicators of PTSD [16, 47, 48]. In contrast, the degree of physical injuries of the trauma, sometimes thought of as an objective measure of exposure severity, does not seem to affect the probability of developing PTSD [16, 49, 50].

### Post-trauma risk indicators

Low socio-economic status plays a role post trauma as well as pre trauma in the development of PTSD [16, 51, 52]. Perceptions of a lack of social support is one of the strongest indicators of PTSD [16]. Catastrophic appraisal of the traumatic event in the long-term aftermath of trauma is also considered a risk factor [32].

Some studies have elucidated a relationship between biomarkers and the development of PTSD [53]. One recent meta-analysis showed that higher heart rate after trauma exposure predicted long-term PTSD symptoms. Neither cortisol nor blood pressure was associated with any elevations in PTSD symptoms [54]. Heart rate, cortisol, and systolic blood pressure played a significant role in developing PTSD in younger patients, but not in the older population [54]. Inflammatory responses in the aftermath of trauma has also been investigated in several studies, showing heightened concentrations of inflammatory signals, including cytokines and C-reactive protein [55].

Although there has been considerable research on the determinants of trauma and PTSD, science has not yet found decision algorithms that can reliably distinguish patients who require intervention from those who will recover on their own.

## Primary prevention of PTSD

Primary prevention strategies for PTSD have traditionally used two types of approaches—they have either targeted all individuals exposed to a trauma (for example, a disaster) or targeted those individuals who are displaying symptoms of ASD. The most effective approach remains unclear. Although several risk indicators for

PTSD have been identified, their clinical application is underdeveloped for targeting preventive interventions, and more evidence is needed.

## Screening in the aftermath of trauma

The diagnostic accuracy of screening instruments in the immediate aftermath of traumatic events is unclear at this point. Although there have been several studies investigating the usefulness of PTSD/ASD questionnaires in the immediate aftermath of trauma, results have shown overall low positive predictive values [56, 57], meaning that if we would screen all individuals who were afflicted by an event by using a cut-off value on a self-report screening measure, the number of false positives could far outnumber the true cases that would be detected. Consequently, the development of European guidelines for psychosocial services following a disaster [58] reached a consensus against screening everyone affected because of the absence of evidence for the effectiveness of screening and scarce resources could be better allocated elsewhere.

## Pharmacological prevention

Several pharmacological treatments have been proposed as possible preventive strategies of PTSD. The first trials testing pharmacological agents in a preventive context for PTSD have used benzodiazepines. However, these trials showed negative results. If anything, there were tendencies on harmful effects, that is, benzodiazepines could potentially increase the risk of developing PTSD [59, 60].

Another pharmacological preventive approach that has been tested is the β-adrenergic blocker propranolol. Propranolol is thought to block and disrupt the consolidation of newly acquired trauma memory via post-synaptic β-adrenergic receptors in the basolateral nucleus of the amygdala [61]. One double-blinded trial conducted in 2002 with 41 participants found positive results in preventing PTSD with propranolol in an emergency room setting [62]. However, a subsequent trial comparing propranolol with gabapentin and placebo ($N$ = 38) administered propranolol within 48 hours of trauma exposure and found no difference in PTSD rates in physically ill patients [63]. One study randomized 29 children to propranolol or placebo; results showed a tendency to negative effects in girls and no significant difference in PTSD rates overall, compared to placebo [64]. One double-blinded trial with 41 participants attempted to prevent PTSD by administering propranolol within 6 hours after exposure to trauma in an emergency room context. Results were overall negative, but patients randomized to propranolol showed less psychological reactivity, compared to the placebo group, when confronted with a trauma reminder 3 months later [65].

The administration of glucocorticoids is thought to result in the impairment of retrieval of declarative memory and to decrease the hyperactive fear response that is associated with the newly acquired trauma memory [66]. Schelling *et al.* performed two RCTs examining the effects of stress doses of hydrocortisone in preventing PTSD symptoms, following septic shock and cardiac surgery, in intensive care units. They found a significant reduction of PTSD symptoms in long-term survivors, as well as improvements in quality of life outcomes [67, 68]. Another RCT in an emergency room context on high-dose hydrocortisone treatment administered in the first hours after trauma exposure was associated with a lower risk of

developing PTSD [69]. Administration of low-dose hydrocortisone in another RCT was found to prevent the onset of PTSD, compared to placebo, particularly in acutely injured trauma victims without a history of significant psychopathology [70].

There have also been attempts to test other pharmacological agents such as morphine [71], SSRIs [72], and ketamine [73], but high-quality randomized trials are currently lacking. Two naturalistic studies of morphine administration following trauma exposure in civilian and combat-related injury have suggested that morphine may prevent later PTSD [71, 74]. One RCT on the effect on early administration of imipramine and fluoxetine in thermally injured children showed no effect in preventing PTSD [72]. Intranasal oxytocin has also been evaluated as a prevention strategy for PTSD, showing effect in patients with a high acute clinician-rated PTSD symptom severity [75]. Ketamine administration in naturalistic studies on moderately injured accident victims has been shown to decrease the incidence of PTSD [76, 77].

To summarize, although some important steps have been taken, more research on pharmacological agents to prevent the development of PTSD is still needed. Some studies have shown promising effects, but it is too soon to provide any definite recommendation in clinical practice yet. Importantly, one systematic review concluded that the small number of studies and their limited methodological quality cast uncertainty about the effects [78].

## Psychological prevention

A range of different early psychological interventions have been developed in order to prevent negative psychological reactions after trauma. However, as in the pharmacofield, high-quality clinical trials have been lagging considerably behind. Descriptions of the most well-researched interventions are given in the following sections.

### Critical incident stress debriefing

Critical incident stress debriefing (also commonly known as 'debriefing') takes place in the first hours following a traumatic event and typically consists of one individual or group session (1–3 hours), in which the participants describe what they experienced, their thoughts and feelings during the event, and how they think of how this event will influence them in their future [79]. Interestingly, there are several reviews of this intervention that have found that it may actually *increase*, rather than decrease, the risk of developing PTSD, that is, interfering with the natural psychological recovery after trauma [80, 81]. This is of some concern, as this is a commonly used intervention worldwide by, for example, first responders, government organizations on victims of mass disasters, and responders to traumatic incidents in the work setting. A summary of the Cochrane review even stated that 'compulsory debriefing of victims of trauma should cease' [40].

### Cognitive behavioural interventions

Trauma-focused cognitive behavioural therapy (CBT) has been tested as a secondary preventive strategy (that is, treating patients with ASD with the aim to lower the incidence of PTSD) in several trials, showing a decreased incidence of PTSD, in comparison to supportive counselling [82, 83, 84]. In this treatment, the patient usually receives 4–5 sessions covering standard CBT techniques (psychoeducation, anxiety management, exposure, and cognitive restructuring) a couple of weeks after the traumatic event.

In the case of mental health primary prevention (that is, treating individuals immediately after trauma exposure), the evidence base is more limited. Resnick et al. [85] developed a psychological intervention for rape victims that consists of a 17-minute video presentation consisting of general psychoeducation and coping strategies for anxiety. This intervention was shown to decrease both PTSD symptoms and marijuana abuse compared with standard care in a randomized trial with 140 participants with sustained long-term effects [86].

Another primary prevention strategy tested is 'prolonged exposure' (PE) which is a form of CBT. In PE treatment, PTSD symptoms are seen as signs of an incompletely processed trauma memory, making the memory associated with high levels of fear and stress. The high level of distress drives avoidance behaviours that prevent the person from facing their memories and situations that, since the trauma, are perceived as dangerous, although objectively safe, and from overcoming their problems. Thus, in this model, the patient is asked to reactivate the trauma memory repeatedly in a safe and non-stressful context (that is, visualizing the event in their mind's eye several times—the so-called imaginal exposure). The aim of this is to allow the fearful responses associated with the memory to gradually decline and afterwards to verbally process the revisiting of the traumatic memory. The patient is also asked to confront objectively safe but feared situations (the so-called exposure *in vivo*).

There is, to date, one randomized trial that has tested prolonged exposure as an early intervention after trauma [87]. In this study, 137 emergency trauma care patients received three sessions with a clinical psychologist, starting the intervention 12–24 hours after trauma exposure in the emergency department. Results showed that, compared to a control group consisting of assessment only, the modified PE intervention decreased PTSD symptoms at 12 weeks later [87]. Trials that aim to replicate and extend these promising findings are needed.

## Cognitive science-driven interventions

A new line of enquiry from experimental psychopathology studies has sought to create psychological prevention techniques '*de novo*' from cognitive science—that is, suggesting that by translating emerging neuroscientific insights and experimental research, we begin to develop new low-intensity psychiatric intervention that could prevent intrusive memories following trauma [88]. It differs from the application of PE or CBT techniques in several ways. First, this line of research focuses on targeting a core clinical feature of post-traumatic distress, rather than a whole disorder—here the recurrent intrusive visual memories of a traumatic event which are distressing and disruptive. Second, the preventive behavioural intervention is derived from various combined aspects of cognitive neuroscience (rather than being an adaptation of an existing talking therapy). The hypothesis is that engaging in a visuo-spatial task during memory consolidation competes for working memory resources with visual imagery and interferes with the formation of intrusive memories. Dual-task experiments also indicate that when similar cognitive tasks compete for shared resources, they interfere with each other and thereby impede memory processing; for example, a visuo-spatial pattern-tapping task interfered with holding a visual mental image in mind (making it become less vivid and emotional) [89]. An example of such a visuo-spatial task is the computer game Tetris [90, 91]. Critically, a competing task needs to be done within the time period of memory consolidation—within an estimated 6 hours following an event [92], during which time memory for events is still labile and vulnerable to disruption. Several laboratory experiments were done using healthy volunteers before bringing this approach to 'the real world'.

As a first proof-of-concept step towards clinical translation, Iyadurai et al. [88] compared a Tetris-based intervention (trauma memory reminder cue plus about 20 minutes of Tetris game play) vs attention-placebo control (written activity log for the same duration), both delivered in an emergency department within 6 hours of a traumatic motor vehicle accident. The primary outcome of the RCT was the number of intrusive trauma memories (core clinical feature post-trauma) measured daily in the subsequent week. Results supported the efficacy of the Tetris-based intervention, compared with the control condition; there were fewer intrusive memories overall, while time-series analyses showed that intrusion incidence declined more quickly. Convergent findings were found on a measure of clinical post-trauma intrusion symptoms at 1 week, but not on other symptom clusters or at 1 month [88]. This proof-of-concept study opens the way for a larger trial, powered to detect differences at 1 month.

A similar pattern of results has been found in a conceptual replication by Horsch et al. [93] who tested the Tetris intervention on women in hospital who had a traumatic childbirth in the previous few hours [93]. The treatment group received usual care plus the Tetris-based intervention (20 minutes of Tetris game play, but no reminder cue as mothers were in the same hospital context as where the index trauma occurred, so a reminder was not deemed necessary) vs a control group of usual care. The reduction in the number of intrusive memories was almost two-thirds in the following week in mothers who played Tetris, compared with the control group. At 1 month, there was an indication of a lower rate of PTSD in the treatment condition.

Advantages of this type of cognitive science-driven approach include the fact that it is brief (approximately one half-hour session), it does not require a highly skilled therapist or talking about the trauma—and it could be readily scalable, which is required for preventive approaches post-trauma.

## Other psychosocial interventions

Psychoeducation delivered via a self-help booklet has also been investigated in two trials but has not demonstrated any effect in preventing PTSD [94, 95]. An RCT using an early eye movement desensitization and reprocessing (EMDR) protocol delivered either 48 or 72 hours after exposure to trauma showed a decreased incidence of PTSD symptoms 3 months later in patients exposed to workplace violence [96]. However, the control group in this study consisted of debriefing, and as debriefing can potentially be harmful (see Critical incident stress debriefing, p. 864), the results should be interpreted with caution.

Psychological first aid (PFA) is a set of practices that were compiled in their current form by the National Child Traumatic Stress Network and the National Center for PTSD to reduce PTSD in adolescents, adults, and their families. The model is based on a set of principles: sense of safety, calming, sense of self, and community efficacy, connectedness, and hope [97]. Importantly, despite the widespread acclamation of PFA as an 'evidence-informed' intervention

[98], comprehensive literature reviews have not yet found evidence of its efficacy in the prevention of PTSD.

To summarize, as in the case of pharmacological agents, there are to date as yet no psychological interventions that have shown consistent, reliable results in preventing the development of PTSD, with the exception of a form of trauma-focused CBT with patients who already have ASD for which there is some evidence. Importantly, there are too few published high-quality large-scale trials to give any consistent recommendation of what psychological treatment to use for trauma survivors in the early aftermath of trauma.

## Conclusions

A considerable amount of research has looked at risk factors for PTSD, but no stable and reliable decision algorithm has been developed that can distinguish patients who require intervention from those who will recover on their own. Some early trials on primary intervention have shown promising effects, but it appears it is too soon to provide strong recommendations for clinical practice. After high-profile events such as a disaster, immediate post-trauma support can be demanded—it is as important to know the evidence on what interventions *not* to give (for example, debriefing is counterindicated). Meanwhile, active research efforts are needed to develop a range of interventions that could be used soon after trauma. Given the presence of an index traumatic event—a known aetiology—prevention efforts based on science and clinical practice should be within our reach.

## REFERENCES

1. American Psychiatric Association. *Diagnostic and Statistical Manual of Mental Disorders*, fifth edition (DSM-5). 2013. Washington, DC: American Psychiatric Association.
2. *Oxford English Dictionary*, Prevent. 2017. Oxford: Oxford University Press.
3. World Health Organization. *Prevention and Promotion in Mental Health*. Geneva: World Health Organization. 2002.
4. Leavell, H.R. and E.G. Clark. *Preventive Medicine for the Doctor in His Community: An Epidemiologic Approach*. 1965. Blakiston Division, McGraw-Hill.
5. Saxena, S., E. Jane-Llopis, and C. Hosman. Prevention of mental and behavioural disorders: implications for policy and practice. *World Psychiatry*, 2006. **5**:5–14.
6. Skeffington, P.M., C.S. Rees, and R. Kane. The primary prevention of PTSD: a systematic review. *J Trauma Dissociation*, 2013. **14**:404–22.
7. Poland, G.A., D. Murray, and R. Bonilla-Guerrero. New vaccine development. *BMJ*, 2002. **324**:1315–19.
8. Norris, F.H., *et al.* 60,000 disaster victims speak: Part I. An empirical review of the empirical literature, 1981–2001. *Psychiatry*, 2002. **65**:207–39.
9. Arnberg, F.K., K. Bergh Johannesson, and P.O. Michel. Prevalence and duration of PTSD in survivors 6 years after a natural disaster. *J Anxiety Disord*, 2013. **27**:347–52.
10. Kessler, R.C., *et al.* Posttraumatic stress disorder in the national comorbidity survey. *Arch Gen Psychiatry*, 1995. **52**:1048–60.
11. Kessler, R.C., *et al.* Prevalence, severity, and comorbidity of 12-month dsm-IV disorders in the national comorbidity survey replication. *Arch Gen Psychiatry*, 2005. **62**:617–27.
12. Rosen, G.M. and S.O. Lilienfeld. Posttraumatic stress disorder: an empirical evaluation of core assumptions. *Clin Psychol Rev*, 2008. **28**:837–68.
13. Boals, A. and D. Schuettler. PTSD symptoms in response to traumatic and non-traumatic events: the role of respondent perception and A2 criterion. *J Anxiety Disord*, 2009. **23**:458–62.
14. Bodkin, J.A., *et al.* Is PTSD caused by traumatic stress? *J Anxiety Disord*, 2007. **21**:176–82.
15. Heir, T., I. Blix, and C.K. Knatten. Thinking that one's life was in danger: perceived life threat in individuals directly or indirectly exposed to terror. *Br J Psychiatry*, 2016. **209**:306–10.
16. Ozer, E.J., *et al.* Predictors of posttraumatic stress disorder and symptoms in adults: a meta-analysis. *Psychol Bull*, 2003. **129**:52–73.
17. Resnick, H.S., *et al.* Vulnerability-stress factors in development of posttraumatic stress disorder. *J Nerv Ment Dis*, 1992. **180**:424–30.
18. Kupfer, D.J. and D.A. Regier. Neuroscience, clinical evidence, and the future of psychiatric classification in DSM-5. *Am J Psychiatry*, 2011. **168**:672–4.
19. Grey, N. and E.A. Holmes. 'Hotspots' in trauma memories in the treatment of post-traumatic stress disorder: a replication. *Memory*, 2008. **16**:788–96.
20. Pearson, J., *et al.* Mental imagery: functional mechanisms and clinical applications. *Trends Cogn Sci*, 2015. **19**:590–602.
21. American Psychiatric Association. *Diagnostic and Statistical Manual of Mental Disorders*, fourth edition, text revision. 2000. Washington, DC: American Psychiatric Association.
22. Bryant, R.A., *et al.* A comparison of the capacity of DSM-IV and DSM-5 acute stress disorder definitions to predict posttraumatic stress disorder and related disorders. *J Clin Psychiatry*, 2015. **76**:391–7.
23. Bryant, R.A., Harvey, A.G., Dang, S.T., and Sackville, T. Assessing acute stress disorder: Psychometric properties of a structured clinical interview. *Psychological Assessment*, 1998. **10**:215–20.
24. Weathers, F.W., D.D. Blake, P.P. Schnurr, D.G. Kaloupek, B.P. Marx, and T.M. Keane. *The Clinician-Administered PTSD Scale for DSM-5 (CAPS-5)*. 2013. National Center for PTSD. http://www.ptsd.va.gov.
25. Koenen, K.C., *et al.* Posttraumatic stress disorder in the World Mental Health Surveys. *Psychol Med*, 2017. **47**: 1–15.
26. McManus, S., *et al. Adult psychiatric morbidity in England, 2007: results of a household survey*. 2009. The NHS Information Centre for Health and Social Care.https://digital.nhs.uk/data-and-information/publications/statistical/adult-psychiatric-morbidity-survey/adult-psychiatric-morbidity-in-england-2007-results-of-a-household-survey
27. Richardson, L.K., B.C. Frueh, and R. Acierno. Prevalence estimates of combat-related post-traumatic stress disorder: critical review. *Aust N Z J Psychiatry*, 2010. **44**:4–19.
28. Fazel, M., J. Wheeler, and J. Danesh. Prevalence of serious mental disorder in 7000 refugees resettled in western countries: a systematic review. *Lancet*, 2005. **365**:1309–14.
29. Perrin, M.A., *et al.* Differences in PTSD prevalence and associated risk factors among World Trade Center disaster rescue and recovery workers. *Am J Psychiatry*, 2007. **164**:1385–94.
30. Breslau, N., *et al.* Trauma and posttraumatic stress disorder in the community: The 1996 detroit area survey of trauma. *Arch Gen Psychiatry*, 1998. **55**:626–32.
31. Darves-Bornoz, J.M., *et al.* Main traumatic events in Europe: PTSD in the European study of the epidemiology of mental disorders survey. *J Trauma Stress*, 2008. **21**:455–62.

32. Bryant, R.A. Early predictors of posttraumatic stress disorder. *Biol Psychiatry*, 2003. **53**:789–95.

33. Blanchard, E.B., *et al.* One-year prospective follow-up of motor vehicle accident victims. *Behav Res Ther*, 1996. **34**:775–86.

34. Rothbaum, B.O., *et al.* A prospective examination of post-traumatic stress disorder in rape victims. *J Traumatic Stress*, 1992. **5**:455–75.

35. Galea, S., *et al.* Psychological sequelae of the September 11 terrorist attacks in New York City. *N Engl J Med*, 2002. **346**:982–7.

36. Galea, S., *et al.* Trends of probable post-traumatic stress disorder in New York City after the September 11 terrorist attacks. *Am J Epidemiol*, 2003. **158**:514–24.

37. van Griensven, F., *et al.* Mental health problems among adults in tsunami-affected areas in southern thailand. *JAMA*, 2006. **296**:537–48.

38. Jonsson, U., *et al.* Reporting of harms in randomized controlled trials of psychological interventions for mental and behavioral disorders: a review of current practice. *Contemp Clin Trials*, 2014. **38**:1–8.

39. Lilienfeld, S.O. Psychological treatments that cause harm. *Perspect Psychol Sci*, 2007. **2**:53–70.

40. Rose S, Bisson J, Churchill R, Wessely S. Psychological debriefing for preventing post traumatic stress disorder (PTSD). *The Cochrane database of systematic reviews*. 2002(2):Cd000560.

41. Olff, M., *et al.* Gender differences in posttraumatic stress disorder. *Psychol Bull*, 2007. **133**:183–204.

42. McLean, C.P., *et al.* Gender differences in anxiety disorders: prevalence, course of illness, comorbidity and burden of illness. *J Psychiatr Res*, 2011. **45**:1027–35.

43. Breslau, N., *et al.* Traumatic events and posttraumatic stress disorder in an urban population of young adults. *Arch Gen Psychiatry*, 1991. **48**:216–22.

44. Breslau, N., *et al.* Sex differences in posttraumatic stress disorder. *Arch Gen Psychiatry*, 1997. **54**:1044–8.

45. Brewin, C.R., B. Andrews, and J.D. Valentine. Meta-analysis of risk factors for posttraumatic stress disorder in trauma-exposed adults. *J Consult Clin Psychol*, 2000. **68**:748–66.

46. Ryan, J., *et al.* Biological underpinnings of trauma and post-traumatic stress disorder: focusing on genetics and epigenetics. *Epigenomics*, 2016. **8**:1553–69.

47. Marmar, C.R., *et al.* Characteristics of emergency services personnel related to peritraumatic dissociation during critical incident exposure. *Am J Psychiatry*, 1996. **153**(7 Suppl):94–102.

48. Sijbrandij, M., *et al.* The structure of peritraumatic dissociation: a cross validation in clinical and nonclinical samples. *J Trauma Stress*, 2012. **25**:475–9.

49. Sijbrandij, M., *et al.* The role of injury and trauma-related variables in the onset and course of symptoms of posttraumatic stress disorder. *J Clin Psychol Med Settings*, 2013. **20**:449–55.

50. Dyster-Aas, J., *et al.* Impact of physical injury on mental health after the 2004 Southeast Asia tsunami. *Nord J Psychiatry*, 2012. **66**:203–8.

51. Bryant, R.A. and A.G. Harvey. Psychological impairment following motor vehicle accidents. *Aust J Public Health*, 1995. **19**:185–8.

52. King, L.A., *et al.* Resilience-recovery factors in post-traumatic stress disorder among female and male Vietnam veterans: hardiness, postwar social support, and additional stressful life events. *J Pers Soc Psychol*, 1998. **74**:420–34.

53. Michopoulos, V., S.D. Norrholm, and T. Jovanovic. Diagnostic biomarkers for posttraumatic stress disorder: promising horizons from translational neuroscience research. *Biol Psychiatry*, 2015. **78**:344–53.

54. Morris, M.C., *et al.* Cortisol, heart rate, and blood pressure as early markers of PTSD risk: a systematic review and meta-analysis. *Clin Psychol Rev*, 2016. **49**:79–91.

55. Michopoulos, V., *et al.* Inflammation in fear- and anxiety-based disorders: PTSD, GAD, and beyond. *Neuropsychopharmacology*, 2017. **42**:254–70.

56. Brewin, C.R. Systematic review of screening instruments for adults at risk of PTSD. *J Trauma Stress*, 2005. **18**:53–62.

57. Brewin, C.R., *et al.* Promoting mental health following the London bombings: a screen and treat approach. *J Trauma Stress*, 2008. **21**:3–8.

58. Bisson, J.I., *et al.* TENTS guidelines: development of post-disaster psychosocial care guidelines through a Delphi process. *Br J Psychiatry*, 2010. **196**:69–74.

59. Gelpin, E., *et al.* Treatment of recent trauma survivors with benzodiazepines: a prospective study. *J Clin Psychiatry*, 1996. **57**:390–4.

60. Guina, J., *et al.* Benzodiazepines for PTSD: a systematic review and meta-analysis. *J Psychiatr Pract*, 2015. **21**:281–303.

61. Cahill, L., *et al.* Beta-adrenergic activation and memory for emotional events. *Nature*, 1994. **371**:702–4.

62. Pitman, R.K., *et al.* Pilot study of secondary prevention of posttraumatic stress disorder with propranolol. *Biol Psychiatry*, 2002. **51**:189–92.

63. Stein, M.B., *et al.* Pharmacotherapy to prevent PTSD: results from a randomized controlled proof-of-concept trial in physically injured patients. *J Trauma Stress*, 2007. **20**:923–32.

64. Nugent, N.R., *et al.* The efficacy of early propranolol administration at reducing PTSD symptoms in pediatric injury patients: a pilot study. *J Trauma Stress*, 2010. **23**:282–7.

65. Hoge, E.A., *et al.* Effect of acute posttrauma propranolol on PTSD outcome and physiological responses during script-driven imagery. *CNS Neurosci Ther*, 2012. **18**:21–7.

66. Miller, M.W., *et al.* Hydrocortisone suppression of the fear-potentiated startle response and posttraumatic stress disorder. *Psychoneuroendocrinology*, 2011. **36**:970–80.

67. Schelling, G., *et al.* The effect of stress doses of hydrocortisone during septic shock on posttraumatic stress disorder in survivors. *Biol Psychiatry*, 2001. **50**:978–85.

68. Schelling, G., *et al.* Efficacy of hydrocortisone in preventing posttraumatic stress disorder following critical illness and major surgery. *Ann N Y Acad Sci*, 2006. **1071**:46–53.

69. Zohar, J., *et al.* High dose hydrocortisone immediately after trauma may alter the trajectory of PTSD: interplay between clinical and animal studies. *Eur Neuropsychopharmacol*, 2011. **21**:796–809.

70. Delahanty, D.L., *et al.* The efficacy of initial hydrocortisone administration at preventing posttraumatic distress in adult trauma patients: a randomized trial. *CNS Spectr*, 2013. **18**:103–11.

71. Holbrook, T.L., *et al.* Morphine use after combat injury in Iraq and post-traumatic stress disorder. *N Engl J Med*, 2010. **362**:110–17.

72. Robert, R., *et al.* Treating thermally injured children suffering symptoms of acute stress with imipramine and fluoxetine: a randomized, double-blind study. *Burns*, 2008. **34**:919–28.

73. McGhee, L.L., *et al.* The correlation between ketamine and posttraumatic stress disorder in burned service members. *J Trauma*, 2008. **64**(2 Suppl):S195–8; discussion S197–8.

74. Bryant, R.A., *et al.* A study of the protective function of acute morphine administration on subsequent posttraumatic stress disorder. *Biol Psychiatry*, 2009. **65**:438–40.

75. van Zuiden M, et al. Intranasal oxytocin to prevent posttraumatic stress disorder symptoms: a randomized controlled trial in emergency department patients. *Biol Psychiatry*, 2017. **81**:1030-40.

76. Schonenberg, M., *et al*. Effects of peritraumatic ketamine medication on early and sustained posttraumatic stress symptoms in moderately injured accident victims. *Psychopharmacology (Berl)*, 2005. **182**:420–5.

77. McGhee LL, et al. The correlation between ketamine and posttraumatic stress disorder in burned service members. *Journal Trauma*, 2008. **64**(2 Suppl):S195–8; Discussion S197-198.

78. Sijbrandij, M., *et al*. Pharmacological prevention of post-traumatic stress disorder and acute stress disorder: a systematic review and meta-analysis. *Lancet Psychiatry*, 2015. **2**:413–21.

79. Mitchell, J.T. When disaster strikes … the critical incident stress debriefing process. *JEMS*, 1983. **8**:36–9.

80. McNally, R.J., R.A. Bryant, and A. Ehlers. Does early psychological intervention promote recovery from posttraumatic stress? *Psychol Sci Public Interest*, 2003. **4**:45–79.

81. Rose, S., Bisson, J. and Wessely S. A systematic review of single-session psychological interventions ('debriefing') following trauma. *Psychother Psychosom*, 2003. **72**:176– 84.

82 Bryant, R.A., *et al*. Treatment of acute stress disorder: a comparison of cognitive-behavioral therapy and supportive counseling. *J Consult Clin Psychol*, 1998. **66**:862–6.

83. Bryant, R.A., et al. Treating acute stress disorder: an evaluation of cognitive behavior therapy and supportive counseling techniques. Am J Psychiatry, 1999. 156(11):1780–6.

84. Bryant, R. A., et al. The additive benefit of hypnosis and cognitive-behavioral therapy in treating acute stress disorder. J Consulting Clinical Psychology, 2005. 73(2):334.

85. Resnick, H., *et al*. Randomized controlled evaluation of an early intervention to prevent post-rape psychopathology. *Behav Res Ther*, 2007. **45**:2432–47.

86. Miller, K.E., *et al*. Psychological outcomes after a sexual assault video intervention: a randomized trial. *J Forensic Nurs*, 2015. **11**:129–36.

87. Rothbaum, B.O., *et al*. Early intervention may prevent the development of posttraumatic stress disorder: a randomized pilot civilian study with modified prolonged exposure. *Biol Psychiatry*, 2012. **72**:957–63.

88. Iyadurai, L., *et al*. Preventing intrusive memories after trauma via a brief intervention involving Tetris computer game play in the emergency department: a proof-of-concept randomized controlled trial. *Mol Psychiatry*, 2018. **23**:674–82.

89. Baddely, A. and J. Andrade. Working memory and the vividness of imagery. *J Exp Psychol Gen*, 2000. **129**:126–45.

90. Holmes, E.A., *et al*. Can playing the computer game 'Tetris' reduce the build-up of flashbacks for trauma? A proposal from cognitive science. *PLoS One*, 2009. **4**:e4153.

91. Holmes, E.A., *et al*. Key steps in developing a cognitive vaccine against traumatic flashbacks: visuospatial Tetris versus verbal Pub Quiz. *PLoS One*, 2010. **5**:e13706.

92. Nader, K., G.E. Schafe, and J.E. Le Doux. Fear memories require protein synthesis in the amygdala for reconsolidation after retrieval. *Nature*, 2000. **406**:722–6.

93. Horsch, A., *et al*. Reducing intrusive traumatic memories after emergency Caesarean section: a proof-of-principle randomized controlled study. *Behav Res Ther*, 2017. **94**:36–47.

94. Turpin, G., M. Downs, and S. Mason. Effectiveness of providing self-help information following acute traumatic injury: randomised controlled trial. *Br J Psychiatry*, 2005. **187**:76–82.

95. Scholes, C., Turpin, G., Mason, S. A randomised controlled trial to assess the effectiveness of providing self-help information to people with symptoms of acute stress disorder following a traumatic injury. *Behav Res Ther*, 2007. **45**(11):2527–36.

96. Arquinio, C., et al. Early psychological preventive intervention for workplace violence: a randomized controlled explorative and comparative study between EMDR-recent event and critical incident stress debriefing. *Issues Ment Health Nurs*, 2016. **37**(11):787–99.

96. Hobfoll, S.E., *et al*. Five essential elements of immediate and mid-term mass trauma intervention: empirical evidence. *Psychiatry*, 2007. **70**:283–315; discussion 316–69.

97. Shultz, J.M. and D. Forbes. Psychological first aid: rapid proliferation and the search for evidence. *Disaster Health*, 2014. **2**:3–12.

# 83

# Management and treatment of stress-related disorders

*Leigh van den Heuvel and Soraya Seedat*

## Introduction

Mental disorders where trauma or stress plays a central role are grouped together in 'Trauma- and stressor-related disorders' in the *Diagnostic and Statistical Manual of Mental Disorders*, fifth edition (DSM-5) [1] and in 'Disorders specifically associated with stress' in the beta version of the *International Classification of Diseases*, eleventh revision (ICD-11) [2]. This group of disorders can only be diagnosed following exposure to a stressful or traumatic event. In DSM-5 and the beta version of ICD-11, these include reactive attachment disorder, disinhibited social engagement disorder, post-traumatic stress disorder (PTSD), and adjustment disorders (ADs). DSM-5 also includes acute stress disorder (ASD), whereas the beta version of ICD-11 distinguishes between PTSD and complex PTSD and includes prolonged grief disorder. The beta version of ICD-11 specifies an acute stress reaction, but this is dissimilar from ASD as it is viewed as a normal response to trauma that subsides within a few days. Here we will focus on the management of PTSD, ASD, and ADs in adults. The management of ASD is discussed in the context of prevention of PTSD.

## Post-traumatic stress disorder

### Prevention

Both ASD and PTSD develop following exposure to a traumatic event involving actual or threatened death, serious injury, or sexual violence; ASD occurs 3 days to 1 month following the trauma, and PTSD is diagnosed when the symptoms have lasted at least 1 month [1]. Their clear relation to an instigating event(s) provides an opportunity to institute strategies to prevent the development of ASD and PTSD. Preventing the development of PTSD is of major societal significance, as the disorder is often chronic and disabling once it sets in. Although several individuals who have ASD go on to develop PTSD, there are also many who develop PTSD without a prior diagnosis of ASD [3]. In the context of PTSD, primary prevention refers to preventing exposure to traumatic events or strategies aimed at enhancing resilience (for more information on primary prevention, see Chapter 82) [4]. Secondary prevention entails interventions instituted after trauma exposure, with the intention of preventing the development of PTSD. Once PTSD symptoms are present, the aim of tertiary prevention is to treat symptoms early and try to avert the development of chronic PTSD. Prevention strategies can be universal, aimed at all individuals exposed to a traumatic event, or can be targeted towards individuals at higher risk of developing PTSD, such as individuals with ASD.

### Psychological interventions

Various psychological interventions have been investigated in the prevention of PTSD, as well as in the treatment of ASD. These include single-session interventions, such as debriefing, and multiple-session interventions such as counselling, multiple-session debriefing, cognitive behavioural therapy (CBT), memory restructuring, and psychoeducation. Debriefing is a psychological intervention usually provided in a group format, as a single session, within a few days after exposure to a traumatic event. Debriefing sessions usually involve a discussion of the traumatic event and encourage participants to recollect their experience and to express their emotional reactions to the event. The intention of debriefing is to reduce acute distress and prevent the development of psychiatric disorders—PTSD, in particular. Systematic reviews and meta-analyses have consistently found that debriefing does not reduce the incidence of PTSD nor does it lead to improvements in PTSD symptoms, depression, anxiety, or functioning [5, 6]. There is even some evidence that debriefing may worsen PTSD outcomes [6]. Similarly, a Cochrane review found that early multiple-session psychological interventions were not superior to control conditions for any PTSD-related outcomes when administered to all trauma survivors [7]. There is, however, evidence from meta-analyses that trauma-focused CBT (TF-CBT) is superior to waitlist/treatment as usual (TAU), as well as supportive counselling in the treatment of ASD (TF-CBT is described in Psychotherapy, p. 870) [5, 8]. Although various other psychosocial interventions have been investigated, there is insufficient evidence at this stage to support any of them in the prevention of PTSD.

## Pharmacotherapy

Medications that have been investigated in the prevention of PTSD include steroids (hydrocortisone), beta-blockers (propranolol), drugs for depression (fluoxetine, escitalopram, sertraline, and imipramine), benzodiazepines (BZDs) (temazepam, alprazolam, and clonazepam), anticonvulsants (gabapentin), opioids (morphine), beta-adrenergic agonists (albuterol), NMDA receptor antagonists (ketamine), and omega-3 fatty acids. The only drug that has demonstrated efficacy in preventing PTSD in meta-analyses is hydrocortisone. In two meta-analyses ($n$ = 5 studies; $n$ = 164), hydrocortisone was superior to placebo in reducing the incidence of PTSD [number needed to treat (NNT) = 7–13], as well as in improving PTSD symptom severity [9, 10]. In the studies, hydrocortisone was usually administered within 6–12 hours of trauma exposure at doses of between 20 mg and 140 mg. Glucocorticoids are hypothesized to work by facilitating extinction learning and impairing memory consolidation of the traumatic event. The known adverse effects of hydrocortisone, such as affective changes, increased susceptibility to infection, and detrimental cardiovascular outcomes, remain a concern. Another drug investigated in PTSD prevention—propranolol—showed promise in early trials but has not demonstrated efficacy in meta-analyses [9, 10]. Beta-blockers are thought to disrupt memory consolidation and to dampen sympathetic tone and, in so doing, to reduce hyperarousal and intrusive symptoms. The few studies that have evaluated drugs for depression, BZDs, anticonvulsants, and omega-3 fatty acids have largely been negative [9, 10]. Morphine administered following trauma exposure, in cohort studies, may reduce the risk of PTSD presumably by impairing amygdala fear conditioning [4, 9]. Similarly, there is limited evidence from cohort studies that ketamine and albuterol administration following trauma may moderate the incidence of PTSD [4, 9]. At this stage, there is insufficient evidence to recommend the routine clinical use of any pharmacologic intervention.

## Other interventions

Another approach examined in the prevention of PTSD involves collaborative stepped care where trauma-exposed individuals are assigned case managers and referred for evidence-based treatments (CBT and/or pharmacologic treatments), according to individual requirements. Although studies are limited, collaborative care appears to lead to improved outcomes, compared to usual care [4, 5].

## Conclusions

Overall, there is a lack of evidence to draw clear conclusions for most interventions [5]. The only intervention that can be firmly recommended is TF-CBT, but only once symptoms of ASD are present. No universal interventions aimed at all trauma-exposed individuals can currently be supported. A collaborative care approach could possibly assist in identifying individuals with PTSD symptoms earlier and increasing access to evidence-based interventions. Without clear evidence to guide interventions, clinicians should employ a pragmatic approach. This entails not interfering with spontaneous recovery, but rather providing practical assistance and support and monitoring for the emergence of symptoms of ASD or PTSD and timely referral for appropriate treatment if symptoms persist or are distressing. Providing information regarding responses to trauma and when to seek help to trauma-exposed individuals and encouraging them to engage with their available sources of social support may also be helpful. Further research is required to improve detection of individuals at increased risk of PTSD to allow for targeted interventions. Well-designed trials are required to determine the efficacy of interventions and to determine individual factors influencing treatment outcomes. Timing of preventive interventions may be of particular importance, especially if the aim is to disrupt memory consolidation of the traumatic event.

## Treatment

### Psychotherapy

#### Trauma-focused cognitive behavioural therapies

TF-CBT is the most frequently studied form of psychotherapy in PTSD. TF-CBT is a broad category of therapies where the principles of CBT have been adapted to focus on behaviours and cognitions central to the disorder. Some TF-CBTs are primarily behavioural, while others are predominantly cognitive, and others have a combined behavioural and cognitive approach. TF-CBT is usually provided in weekly sessions lasting 60–90 minutes for around 8–12 weeks and can be delivered individually or in groups. All TF-CBTs incorporate psychoeducation regarding PTSD, particularly during initial sessions, and frequently also impart anxiety management techniques. The broad aim of TF-CBT is to alter maladaptive thinking and behaviours that develop in relation to the traumatic event and thereby alleviate symptoms and improve functioning. Cognitive-based therapies focus on altering trauma-derived cognitive distortions and negative beliefs. Specific manualized variants of cognitive therapy have been developed, such as cognitive restructuring and cognitive processing therapy (CPT), which allow for a standardized approach. The behavioural-based interventions usually involve exposure therapies, which are founded on the principles of extinction learning, whereby repeated exposure to trauma-related cues in a safe environment leads to extinction of the fear response. The most frequently studied form of exposure therapy in PTSD is prolonged exposure (PE), a manualized intervention. Exposure therapy involves either imaginal or *in vivo* exposure to trauma-related stimuli, while anxiety and distress are managed with a relaxation technique such as controlled breathing. In imaginal exposure, the person recalls memories of the event, while *in vivo* exposure involves exposure to situations that the person avoids because they trigger reminders of the trauma. Recent meta-analyses have demonstrated the efficacy of individual TF-CBT in changing PTSD diagnostic status (NNT 2–4), improving PTSD symptoms, depression, anxiety, and functioning, as compared to waitlist/TAU [11–14]. The results remain similar, whether the focus is on cognitive therapy, exposure therapy, or mixed TF-CBT approaches, and effects appear to persist up to 12 months following completion. Group TF-CBT has also demonstrated efficacy for PTSD-related outcomes, although the number of studies are limited [11]. Gender appears to influence outcomes, as effects are larger in women-only studies [11]. Meta-analyses have reported higher dropout rates for TF-CBT than for waitlist/TAU, which raises concerns regarding the acceptability of TF-CBT [11].

## Non-trauma-focused cognitive behavioural therapies

Other CBT-based therapies that do not focus on the specific trauma have also been investigated in PTSD. The most frequently studied non-TF-CBT is stress inoculation training (SIT), which focuses on increasing an individual's ability to manage stress and to prevent future episodes of anxiety. It incorporates coping skills training and relaxation techniques, as well as broad CBT-based approaches. The frequency and duration of sessions are similar to those used in TF-CBT. Although fewer studies have investigated non-TF-CBT, results indicate efficacy in improving PTSD symptoms, depression, and anxiety directly following treatment [11, 14]. Other meta-analyses, however, cite insufficient evidence for the efficacy of SIT [12].

## Eye movement desensitization and reprocessing

Eye movement desensitization and reprocessing (EMDR) has features in common with other TF-CBTs and is one of the most commonly studied forms of psychotherapy in PTSD. During EMDR sessions, individuals bring to mind the traumatic experiences and negative cognitions associated with the trauma, while performing saccadic eye movements as they follow the therapist's finger from left to right for a few seconds. The process is repeated until the person becomes desensitized to the distressing content, after which the individual practises holding positive self-efficacious statements in mind, while imagining the trauma. The saccadic eye movements are thought to interfere with working memory and to reduce distress related to the trauma and thus reduce avoidance [15]. Treatment with EMDR also usually involves 8- to 12-weekly sessions, lasting around 60–90 minutes each. Meta-analyses have reported that EMDR is superior to waitlist/TAU in changing PTSD diagnostic status (NNT = 2), improving PTSD symptoms, depression, and anxiety up to 3 months following treatment [11–14].

## Other psychotherapies

Psychodynamic psychotherapy, which is usually a longer-term intervention, employs traditional psychodynamic principles of bringing unconscious content into conscious awareness where it can be processed and conflict surrounding the trauma can be resolved. Brief eclectic therapy (BET) is a manualized therapy provided over 16 sessions that combine CBT and psychodynamic approaches. Interpersonal therapy (IPT) is usually provided in 10–20 sessions and concentrates on improving interpersonal relationships to enhance the management of interpersonal distress. Narrative exposure therapy (NET) combines features of exposure therapy, as well as narrative therapy, to allow desensitization and reframing of the traumatic experience within the person's life story. Person-centred therapy and supportive counselling are non-directive and allow the person to talk about their problems and feelings, with support from an accepting therapist. Supportive therapy is often used as an active comparator in clinical trials. A Cochrane review that combined 'other therapies' reported superiority to waitlist/TAU in PTSD symptoms, depression, and anxiety directly following treatment; however, dropout rates were higher than waitlist/TAU [11]. There is some evidence of efficacy, based on a limited number of studies, for NET and BET in improving PTSD-related outcomes above waitlist/TAU [12, 13]. IPT was not superior to waitlist/TAU in one meta-analysis [14], but group IPT demonstrated efficacy in a single trial [13]. Psychodynamic psychotherapy, resilience therapy, and hypnotherapy have demonstrated efficacy only in single small trials [13].

A meta-analysis of six hypnotherapy trials found large effects in improvements of PTSD symptoms post-treatment but did not report outcomes, as compared to control conditions [16].

## Comparative effectiveness of psychotherapies

In terms of efficacy, the largest body of evidence, supported by the largest effect sizes [13], is for TF-CBT, followed by EMDR. Although there is some evidence for non-TF-CBT and other psychotherapies, these results are less clear. Effect sizes for all psychotherapeutic interventions are larger when compared against waitlist/TAU than against active comparators [13]. Fewer head-to-head comparisons for psychotherapies exist. One meta-analysis found no difference between PE and cognitive-based TF-CBTs, SIT, or EMDR [17]. Exposure therapy has demonstrated superiority to relaxation in reducing PTSD symptoms [12]. There is some evidence that TF-CBT and EMDR are superior to non-TF-CBT and 'other therapies' for certain PTSD-related outcomes [11]. One meta-analysis found that EMDR was superior to TF-CBT only in improving anxiety symptoms directly following treatment [17]. Only one study observed non-TF-CBT was superior to 'other therapies' [11].

## Pharmacotherapy

The most commonly studied medications are drugs for depression, SSRIs in particular, followed by drugs for psychosis.

### Drugs for depression (antidepressants)

Meta-analyses have demonstrated small, but significant, effects favouring these drugs overall [13], and SSRIs as a class [13, 18], above placebo. Although guidelines often combine SSRIs as a drug class in treatment recommendations, the evidence reveals that this may not be appropriate in the management of PTSD. Currently, paroxetine and sertraline are the only two SSRIs that are FDA-approved for PTSD. Of the individual SSRIs, paroxetine and fluoxetine have consistently been found superior to placebo in meta-analyses [13, 14, 18]. There are some inconsistencies in meta-analyses regarding the efficacy of sertraline, with some reporting superiority to placebo [13, 14] and others not [18]. These inconsistencies can be explained by varying inclusion criteria in clinical trials (that is, some more stringent than others) and by whether or not unpublished results were included. Citalopram and escitalopram have failed to demonstrate efficacy in a few studies [13, 14, 18]. The serotonin and noradrenaline reuptake inhibitor (SNRI) venlafaxine has demonstrated superiority over placebo in meta-analyses including two RCTs [13, 14, 18]. Meta-analyses have not shown efficacy for the monoamine oxidase inhibitor (MAOI) brofaromine, the tricyclic antidepressants (TCAs) desipramine and imipramine, and the noradrenaline/dopamine reuptake inhibitor (NDRI) bupropion [13, 14, 18]. The results for the MAOI phenelzine, the TCA amitriptyline, the noradrenergic and specific serotonergic antidepressant (NaSSA) mirtazapine, and the discontinued serotonin antagonist and reuptake inhibitor (SARI) nefazodone have been inconsistent in meta-analyses [13, 14, 18]. Even in those reporting superiority over placebo, the results were based on single trials.

### Drugs for psychosis (antipsychotics)

In two meta-analyses, dopamine antagonists were superior to placebo overall, but with a small effect [13, 14]. In two meta-analyses, olanzapine failed to demonstrate efficacy [13, 18], but in another, it was superior to placebo as monotherapy, but not when used as augmentation of an antidepressant [14]. Risperidone was superior to placebo, both as monotherapy and when used in augmentation in two meta-analyses [13, 14], but failed to demonstrate any efficacy in another [18]. Based on a single trial, aripiprazole was not superior to placebo [14]. Despite these small positive effects, their use is limited by their significant adverse effects.

### Anticonvulsants

Anticonvulsants as a class have not demonstrated efficacy [13, 14]. One meta-analysis found that topiramate was superior to placebo as monotherapy in two trials and as augmentation in a single trial [13], whereas others did not observe evidence of its efficacy [13, 18]. The other anticonvulsants valproate semisodium, tiagabine, and lamotrigine have failed to demonstrate efficacy in limited trials [13, 14, 18].

### Benzodiazepines

Systematic reviews and meta-analyses have consistently found that BZDs are ineffective in preventing or treating PTSD symptoms [13, 14, 18, 19]. Furthermore, BZDs increased the likelihood of developing PTSD and were associated with other negative sequelae such as worsened PTSD severity, psychotherapy outcomes, depression, anxiety, aggression, and substance use [19].

### Adrenergic drugs

Although there have been some negative findings [13], the alpha-1 adrenergic receptor antagonist prazosin has been found to be superior to placebo in meta-analyses in improving PTSD symptoms and sleep quality and in reducing nightmares [14, 20]. Prazosin presumably works by dampening noradrenergic activity, and thereby decreasing hyperarousal, as well as by disrupting reconsolidation of fear memories [19]. Prazosin is usually initiated at 1 mg and titrated up every 2–3 days up to mean daily doses of between 3 mg and 15 mg. It is usually well tolerated, although dizziness is the most commonly reported adverse effect. The alpha-2 agonist guanfacine has not demonstrated efficacy in PTSD thus far [13, 14].

### Other emerging drugs

Efficacy has been demonstrated for GR205171 (a neurokinin-1 antagonist) [18] and the herbal drug gingko biloba [13] in single RCTs. Due to its positive effects in depression, ketamine has received increased interest in the treatment of PTSD. Ketamine, commonly used as an anaesthetic for surgical procedures, was associated in a case series with both worsened and improved PTSD symptoms. A pilot RCT (ketamine vs midazolam) and a case study reported improvements in PTSD symptom severity [21]. A meta-analysis of 19 intranasal oxytocin trials in various mental disorders, including two PTSD trials, reported a small effect favouring oxytocin; however, of the individual disorders, significant improvements were only found for autism spectrum disorders. The two trials evaluating oxytocin in PTSD were, however, very small ($n = 18$–30), one of which showed promising results [22]. Both oxytocin and ketamine warrant further investigation in PTSD.

### Combined psychotherapy and pharmacotherapy

A Cochrane review evaluated whether combined pharmacotherapy and psychotherapy was superior to either treatment modality alone [23]. Only four trials were eligible for the review, and all of the trials utilized SSRIs and TF-CBT. Two trials compared combined treatment to pharmacotherapy alone and found no evidence that combined treatment was superior. Two trials, one in adults ($n = 25$) and one in children ($n = 24$), compared combined treatment to psychotherapy alone and found no difference between the groups. A more recent RCT ($n = 228$) similarly found that the combination of PE and paroxetine was not superior to either alone in achieving remission; PE, however, was superior to paroxetine alone in adults with PTSD secondary to a motor vehicle accident (MVA) [24]. In contrast, another RCT ($n = 37$) found combined paroxetine and PE to be superior to PE alone in improving PTSD symptom severity and in achieving remission [25]. No clear conclusions on the benefits of combination therapy can be drawn until larger well-designed RCTs are executed to address this question (Table 83.1).

**Table 83.1** Evidence-based treatments for stress-related disorders

| | First line | Second line | Third line (reserved for specialist practice and treatment resistance) | Interventions demonstrating potential |
|---|---|---|---|---|
| **PTSD** | | | | |
| **Prevention** | No evidence for any universal preventative interventions<br>*TF-CBT* for symptomatic individuals or those diagnosed with ASD | | | Collaborative care approaches<br>Hydrocortisone |
| **Treatment** | *TF-CBT*<br>*EMDR* | Other psychotherapies (group TF-CBT, non-TF-CBT, NET, BET)<br>Drugs for depression (paroxetine, fluoxetine, venlafaxine, sertraline)<br>Combined pharmacotherapy and psychotherapy | Other medications [prazosin, risperidone (monotherapy and augmentation), olanzapine (monotherapy), topiramate] | Distance-delivered TF-CBT<br>VRET<br>Mindfulness-based therapies<br>Drug-assisted psychotherapies<br>TMS<br>Exercise |
| | Problem-solving therapy | Other brief psychotherapies | Targeted pharmacotherapy | Resiliency training programmes<br>Mindfulness-based therapies<br>Exercise |

ASD, acute stress disorder; BET, brief eclectic therapy; EMDR, eye movement desensitization and reprocessing; NET, narrative exposure therapy; PTSD, post-traumatic stress disorder; TF-CBT, trauma-focused cognitive behavioural therapy; TMS, transcranial magnetic stimulation; VRET, virtual reality exposure therapy.

## Treatment selection

Effects sizes for TF-CBT and EMDR, whether compared to waitlist/TAU or comparator conditions, are significantly larger than those found in pharmacotherapy trials, which are generally small [14]. Psychotherapy benefits also persisted after therapy completion, whereas medication had to be continued to maintain efficacy [14]. The effect sizes for drugs, however, are equivalent to those observed in depression trials [18]. Based on the available evidence, TF-CBT and EMDR are first-line interventions and other psychotherapies and psychopharmacological interventions can be considered as second-line interventions. Drugs with the best evidence for efficacy are fluoxetine, paroxetine, and venlafaxine. Even though the findings of meta-analyses have been inconsistent, sertraline was equivalent to venlafaxine in one RCT [14] and can thus be considered as well. In individuals with prominent sleep difficulties, prazosin may be an option, and atypical antipsychotics, as monotherapy or augmentation, should rather be reserved for treatment-resistant cases.

Generally, dropout rates for pharmacotherapy trials have not been significantly different from placebo, suggesting that overall psychopharmacological treatment was well tolerated. Acceptability of psychotherapies is of concern, as dropout rates in studies are often high, particularly in TF-CBT, which may be related to avoidance of trauma-related reminders. A systematic review evaluating patient preferences regarding treatments for PTSD largely found that individuals preferred psychotherapy above medication; they, however, preferred medication to receiving no treatment [26]. Medication was generally preferred when there was comorbidity (depression, insomnia) and when there were practical concerns such as perceived faster effect with pharmacotherapy. Predictors of psychotherapy preference were PTSD as a primary diagnosis, perceived threat to life, previous psychiatric history, traumatic injuries, sexual assault, and female gender.

There is a lack of evidence to guide treatment selection based on trauma type or individual-level characteristics. For both psychotherapy and pharmacotherapy, studies with women only had larger effect sizes and studies with veterans smaller effect sizes [13]. Concerns regarding methodological quality and publication bias have been raised for both psychotherapeutic and pharmacologic interventions [13, 14]. Of note, individuals in psychotherapy trials are often on concomitant medications and tend to have had more prior treatments than those in pharmacotherapy trials [14]. Another factor that influences treatment choice is the availability of various treatment options. Access to psychotherapy is limited in many settings. Perceived barriers to treatment that have been identified include stigma, shame, and fear of negative social consequences, low mental health literacy, doubts regarding treatments, limited resources and time, and apprehension regarding re-experiencing the trauma [27], whereas perceived facilitators of treatment include social support and acceptance, severity of the disorder, and recognizing a need to change, positive experiences with health professionals, and avoiding negative social interactions [27]. Individual preference, along with current best evidence, should guide treatment selection.

## Special populations

### Children and adolescents

Meta-analyses have demonstrated evidence favouring psychological therapies overall in the treatment of PTSD in children and adolescents (C&A) [28, 29]. Psychological interventions studied included TF-CBT (including PE), EMDR, narrative therapy, supportive counselling, psychodynamic psychotherapy, child-centred therapy, multi-disciplinary treatment, meditation, and classroom-based interventions. Effect sizes overall were larger when compared to waitlist/TAU than to active controls. Psychological therapies were superior to control conditions in changing PTSD diagnostic status and improving PTSD symptom severity up to 1-year follow-up, as well as depression and anxiety in the short term. The only individual therapy type that was superior to both TAU/waitlist and supportive counselling was TF-CBT. A Cochrane review of psychological therapies for preventing PTSD in trauma-exposed C&A also showed a benefit for psychological treatments as a whole in preventing PTSD and in reducing PTSD symptoms, when compared to waitlist/TAU/no treatment (NNT = 6.3), for up to a month follow-up [30]. There was a small effect demonstrating superiority of TF-CBT over EMDR, play therapy, and supportive therapy in improving PTSD symptoms.

There have been very few trials evaluating pharmacotherapy in the management of PTSD in C&A. A recent systematic review of RCTs in C&A identified only two pharmacotherapy trials, both evaluating sertraline; they could not perform a meta-analysis due to the limited number of studies [28]. Another systematic review that evaluated psychopharmacology in the management of PTSD in C&A reported that in three RCTs of SSRIs (two sertraline, one fluoxetine), there was no benefit to SSRI treatment, and in one brief RCT of imipramine, the latter was superior to chloral hydrate in improving ASD symptoms in child burn victims [31]. They also found small open-label studies that demonstrated improvements in PTSD symptoms when using citalopram, quetiapine, carbamazepine, high- vs low-dose valproate semisodium, and the alpha-2 agonists clonidine and guanfacine (clonidine improved re-enactment symptoms, and guanfacine improved nightmares). However, beta-blockers did not prevent PTSD or reduce symptoms severity in an open study. In C&A with PTSD, pharmacotherapy is not routinely indicated and should be reserved for the management of treatment resistance in specialist practice.

### Psychiatric comorbidity

There is very little evidence to inform the management of PTSD with psychiatric comorbidity, although PTSD is highly comorbid with depressive, anxiety, and substance use disorders (SUDs). Many of the psychotherapies investigated in PTSD improve associated depression and anxiety symptoms as well. The same drugs with evidence in PTSD can also be utilized in the management of depressive and anxiety disorders because of their broad spectrum of action. A Cochrane review of psychological therapies for comorbid SUD and PTSD found that TF-CBT was superior to TAU in improving symptoms of PTSD and SUDs, but not when compared to active comparators [32]. Treatment completion rates were lower in TF-CBT groups. Non-TF-CBT-based therapies were not superior to TAU, whether delivered in a group/individual format. A meta-analysis evaluating integrated treatment for SUD and PTSD, which involves simultaneous treatment for both disorders by the same treatment team, found that integrated programmes improved PTSD and SUD symptoms, but integrated programmes were not superior to non-integrated programmes [33]. Thus far, there is no clear evidence of specific pharmacotherapy interventions that improve symptoms of both PTSD and SUDs in individuals with comorbidity [34].

## Emerging interventions

### Alternative psychotherapy delivery modes

Due to problems with access to evidence-based psychotherapies, efforts have been under way to examine alternative methods of delivering psychotherapies. Existing therapies have been adapted into remotely delivered interventions (Internet, telephone, email, and videoconferencing). Meta-analyses have found that Internet-delivered CBT was superior to waitlist/TAU in improving PTSD symptom severity and depressive and anxiety symptoms, but not when compared to active controls [35–37]. Virtual reality exposure therapy (VRET) follows the same principles as traditional exposure therapies, but the person is exposed to cues related to the trauma in a computer-generated virtual reality (VR). In VR, the person can interact with the environment, allowing for an immersive experience. A systematic review of VRET in PTSD identified ten studies, seven of which demonstrated that VRET was superior to waitlist, although no difference was found between VRET and traditional exposure therapies [38]. Although preliminary, these results suggest the potential utility of VRET, particularly as VR headsets have become increasingly available and affordable.

### Mindfulness-based therapies

Over the last three decades, there has been a proliferation of research into mindfulness-based interventions. Mindfulness has its origin in Buddhist contemplative teachings, and current therapies have been adapted in accordance with medical and scientific practice. The practice of mindfulness involves a non-judgemental moment-to-moment observation of internal and external experiences, with the aim of enhancing awareness. Through sustained practice, mindfulness aims to decrease distress by developing greater acceptance of things as they are and enhance self-regulation and positive qualities such as compassion and equanimity [39]. Mindfulness has been incorporated into various therapeutic approaches such as mindfulness-based stress reduction (MBSR), mindfulness-based cognitive therapy (MBCT), acceptance and commitment therapy (ACT), and dialectical behaviour therapy (DBT) [39, 40]. MBSR and MBCT are manualized programmes delivered in eight weekly group sessions, lasting around 2 hours, with one full-day session. Both MBSR and MBCT incorporate mindfulness meditation and yoga practices. MBCT also has a cognitive component where participants are instructed to change their relationship to their thoughts, rather than to challenge the content, as is commonly done in CBT. A recent systematic review of mindfulness-based interventions, mostly MBSR, in trauma-exposed adults reported that overall studies demonstrated positive effects and improvements in PTSD symptoms, particularly avoidance subscales [40]. However, the results were based on small studies with variable methodological rigour, and further studies of higher methodological quality are required before any clear conclusions can be drawn. Another meta-analysis reported that meditation-based interventions (MBSR, yoga, and mantra repetition programmes) were superior to waitlist/TAU in improving PTSD and depressive symptoms [41]. A benefit of mindfulness-based interventions is that they are often delivered in groups and thus increase accessibility.

### Drug-assisted psychotherapies

There is an increased interest in the therapeutic potential of methylenedioxymethamphetamine (MDMA), commonly known by its recreational use name 'ecstasy', in the treatment of PTSD [42]. The psychoactive properties of MDMA were first investigated in the late 1970s, and prior to it being classified as an illegal Schedule 1 drug in the mid-1980s, it was utilized by clinicians as an adjuvant to psychotherapy. For more than 20 years, research into MDMA was limited to investigations of the risks and potential neurotoxicity of MDMA, particularly with regard to its recreational use. Despite extensive research, the debate on whether MDMA is neurotoxic persists. There are, however, known potential dangers associated with recreational 'ecstasy' use such as dehydration and brain oedema [42]. MDMA-assisted psychotherapy (MDMA-AP) typically involves 1–3 drug-assisted psychotherapy sessions, lasting 8 hours each, with non-drug psychotherapy sessions provided prior to, and following, the MDMA-AP sessions. MDMA putatively assists in the treatment of PTSD by decreasing anxiety and increasing the individual's ability to trust, and thus strengthening the therapeutic alliance, by providing a sense of increased insight, and by enabling memory retrieval and reconsolidation [42]. This is partly due to its known physiological effects such as increased serotonin, dopamine, noradrenaline, oxytocin, and vasopressin release. In a preliminary meta-analysis of two RCTs ($n = 35$), the authors demonstrated large effects sizes for PTSD symptoms, favouring MDMA-AP [43]. They also compared the effect sizes and dropout rates against those reported in a meta-analysis of PE17 and found that the effect sizes were slightly larger for MDMA-AP, and that dropout rates were lower in MDMA-AP (12.7%) than in PE (27.0%).

Most of the studies evaluating cognitive enhancers of CBT have used d-cycloserine (DCS). DCS is thought to enhance extinction learning due to its partial agonism of the N-methyl-D-aspartate (NMDA) receptor complex. A recent Cochrane review evaluated the efficacy of DCS augmentation of CBT in anxiety disorders, including PTSD and included 21 RCTs, five of which were on PTSD [44]. Overall, DCS-augmented CBT was not superior to placebo-augmented CBT in both adults and C&A. The studies were heterogenous, and the quality of evidence overall was low. The subgroup analysis revealed that DCS-augmented CBT was superior to placebo in achieving remission of PTSD at 1–6 months' follow-up and in improving comorbid anxiety symptoms. In C&A, however, placebo-augmented CBT was superior to DCS-augmented CBT in improving anxiety and depressive symptoms in one study ($n = 57$).

### Transcranial magnetic stimulation

Transcranial magnetic stimulation (TMS) is a non-invasive neuromodulation modality. Electromagnetic pulses are delivered by a TMS stimulator via a coil placed over the scalp. TMS presumably works by inducing changes in the electrical field in the focal brain region being stimulated and through altering function downstream via connected neural circuits. Repetitive TMS (rTMS) is a type of TMS usually utilized in treatment protocols and can vary according to the stimulation site and the intensity, frequency, duration, and sequence of pulses. Low-frequency (LF) rTMS (≤1 Hz) is generally considered to have inhibitory effects, and high-frequency (HF) rTMS (≥5 Hz) to be excitatory. rTMS is generally considered safe when administered according to accepted safety guidelines [45]. The most frequently reported adverse effects include headaches and facial pain, and the most severe adverse effect is the induction of seizures, though the risk is very low. Since the late 1990s, rTMS has been investigated as a potential treatment for PTSD in different patient populations, utilizing varying protocols [46]. Due to its role in complex cognitive and behavioural functions, the dorsolateral prefrontal cortex (DLPFC) has been researched as a treatment target in PTSD and several other neuropsychiatric disorders. A meta-analysis and systematic review evaluating the efficacy of rTMS to the DLPFC in PTSD identified three RCTs ($n = 64$) of HF and LF rTMS to the right DLPFC, and one RCT evaluating HF rTMS to the left DLPFC [47]. All rTMS protocols were administered over ten sessions, with a mean total number of 6250 pulses. Their meta-analysis demonstrated statistically significant improvements in PTSD symptoms, anxiety, and depression, favouring active rTMS to the right DLPFC. Dropout rates did not differ between active and sham rTMS, although individuals in the active rTMS group had more severe PTSD symptoms at baseline. The RCT investigating the left DLPFC had similar results. A more recent meta-analysis pooled the results of five RCTs ($n = 108$) for HF rTMS and LF rTMS to the right and left DLPFCs, as well as HF deep TMS to the bilateral medial prefrontal cortices (mPFC) [48]. They also demonstrated an overall benefit favouring active rTMS, and a meta-regression identified no specific variables that influenced outcomes. Although preliminary, the results suggest that rTMS holds promise as a treatment option for PTSD. Further studies with larger sample sizes are required to prove efficacy for routine clinical practice, and ideal treatment protocol parameters still need to be defined.

### Exercise

Akin to many other psychiatric disorders, cardiovascular disease (CVD) risk is higher in individuals with PTSD. One meta-analysis revealed that individuals with PTSD had almost double the risk of metabolic syndrome than matched general population controls [49]. A recent systematic review and meta-analysis evaluated the efficacy of physical activity as a treatment for PTSD [50]. They included four RCTs ($n = 200$); two trials evaluated active yoga, one evaluated an aerobic intervention (stationary cycling) and one evaluated a combined resistance and aerobic intervention. The duration of the interventions varied between 6 and 12 weeks, with 1–2 supervised sessions per week. The meta-analysis found that the exercise interventions were superior to the comparator interventions in improving PTSD and depressive symptoms, with no significant adverse effects. There were insufficient data to evaluate the effect on anthropometric measurements. Although preliminary, the results suggest that exercise interventions hold potential as an adjunct in the treatment of PTSD.

### Other interventions

Biofeedback involves a process whereby an individual can gain voluntary control of a physiological process by receiving electronic monitoring feedback. When the feedback incorporates brain function, such as electroencephalography (EEG), it is called neurofeedback. A recent systematic review including three studies (one RCT) reported improvements in PTSD symptoms and associated neurobiological changes [51]. A meta-analysis of hyperbaric oxygen therapy (HOT) (100% oxygen being delivered at an increased atmospheric pressure) in traumatic brain injury (TBI) found that although HOT led to improved Glasgow coma scale (GCS) scores, there was no effect on PTSD severity [52]. Stellate ganglion block, an anaesthetic procedure where a local anaesthetic is injected next to the cervical

sympathetic ganglion, has shown promise as a treatment for PTSD in case studies and case series [53].

Deep brain stimulation (DBS) of brain regions involved in PTSD pathophysiology could be a potential treatment option for refractory PTSD. Preclinical studies have demonstrated promising results with stimulation of the basolateral amygdala (BLA), ventral striatum, hippocampus, and PFC, and one case study reported an improvement in PTSD symptoms in a veteran treated with BLA DBS [54].

Of six studies identified in a systematic review of art therapy in traumatized adults, two studies reported significant improvements in PTSD-related symptoms and two in anxiety, compared to waitlist/TAU or an art control condition [55]. A recent systematic review evaluated animal-assisted therapy in the treatment of trauma-exposed individuals; three studies were in adults, and seven in C&A. The animals most frequently utilized were dogs, followed by horses. Although very preliminary, results overall were promising, demonstrating improvements in PTSD symptoms, depression, and anxiety [56].

## Adjustment disorders

An AD involves a maladaptive response, either emotionally or behaviourally, or both, to an identifiable stressful situation or multiple stressors. ADs usually have their onset within 1 [2] to 3 [1] months after the onset of a stressful event and usually resolve within 6 months after the stressor has terminated. The types of stressful events that can lead to an AD are broad and can include severe traumas or more common events such as financial difficulties, interpersonal conflict, illness, or work-related stressors. ADs cannot be diagnosed if the person meets criteria for another mental disorder, such as major depressive disorder (MDD) or PTSD, and is distinguished from a normal response to a stressful situation by significant functional impairments or severe distress, out of proportion to what would be accepted culturally. Although ADs are frequently encountered and can be a useful clinical diagnostic classification, research specifically evaluating ADs is scant. Here we expand the discussion by including interventions in non-clinical populations or in subclinical depression and anxiety. ADs are associated with heightened suicide risk, and thus suicide risk assessment should form part of the routine management of ADs [57, 58].

### Psychological therapies

Due to the time-limited nature of ADs, brief therapies are usually preferred, unless the stressor is more chronic in nature. Interventions can be aimed at reducing or removing the stressor, facilitating adaptation, or reducing distress and functional impairment [57]. Problem-solving-based approaches can assist in directly dealing with the stressor. Adaptation to the stressor can be facilitated by approaches that reframe the stressor and with practical interventions. The specific symptoms of ADs can be addressed by similar psychological interventions used to treat depression, anxiety, and stress-related disorders such as CBT, relaxation therapies, IPT, and supportive and psychodynamic therapies [57]. Resilience-enhancing approaches can assist both with reducing the risk of developing ADs as well as with the treatment thereof. A Cochrane review evaluated CBT and problem-solving therapy (PST) to assist individuals with ADs to return to work [59]. PST involves identifying problems and then generating, implementing, and evaluating solutions to the problems. There was evidence that PST, but not CBT, had significant effects on AD-related symptoms and on the time to return to partial, but not full, work.

A meta-analysis evaluating group CBT in subclinical depression reported that group CBT was superior to waitlist, but not to comparator interventions, and did not reduce the risk of incident depression [60]. Meta-analyses of the efficacy of resiliency training programmes in diverse clinical and non-clinical populations found these programmes had a moderate effect on improving resilience overall, and trauma-focused resilience training programmes, specifically, had a moderate effect in reducing stress and depression [61, 62]. Meta-analyses of mindfulness-based interventions in diverse psychiatrically or medically ill and non-clinical populations have demonstrated improvements in anxiety, depression, stress, and quality of life [63, 64]. Meditation-based programmes were, however, not superior to active comparators. Self-help-based mindfulness interventions, such as Internet-based therapies and books, have also been demonstrated superior to control groups in improving stress, depression, anxiety, and mindfulness in meta-analyses involving non-clinical populations [65, 66]. Relaxation training, such as progressive relaxation, autogenic training, and meditation, has also demonstrated efficacy in a meta-analysis of mixed clinical and non-clinical samples [67].

### Pharmacotherapy

There are very few trials evaluating pharmacotherapy for ADs. Intervention that have been studied include BZDs, drugs for depression, and other anxiolytics. Single studies have found that etifoxine, a non-BZD anxiolytic, was superior to lorazepam, while others demonstrated no differences between drugs for depression (mianserin, tianeptine, viloxazine, trazodone) and BZDs (alprazolam, clorazepate, lormetazepam) and s-adenosyl methionine in improving anxiety [57]. Herbal medicines, such as kava-kava, valerian, gingko biloba, and plant extracts, have also demonstrated superiority in improving anxiety, compared to placebo, in one or two studies [57, 58, 68]. In practice, drugs for depression are frequently prescribed for ADs, despite the available evidence [68]. A meta-analysis of their efficacy in subthreshold depression demonstrated a small, but significant, effect favouring the SSRIs, fluoxetine, and citalopram, but not paroxetine, above placebo [69]. A Cochrane review also reported that kava was significantly superior to placebo in improving anxiety symptoms; however, concerns regarding liver toxicity limit the use of kava [70].

### Exercise

A recent meta-analysis found that physical activity improved depression and anxiety in non-clinical adults [71]. Exercise is postulated to have beneficial effects on anxiety and depressive symptoms due to neurophysiological effects such as HPA axis regulation, increased monoamine levels, and increased neurogenesis in limbic structures [72]. Yoga has also been demonstrated to improve ADs in a single study [68].

Overall, the quality of evidence for treatments in ADs is poor, and it is difficult to draw clear conclusions. In general, practical problem-focused approaches are supported by the evidence and make clinical sense (Box 83.1).

---

**Box 83.1** Practical approach to the management of PTSD

**General guidelines**
- Routinely screen for a history of trauma exposure and for symptoms of PTSD.
- Assess for ongoing trauma and ensure individual safety.
- A sensitive and empathic approach is required in dealing with trauma-exposed individuals.
- Respect autonomy, and involve the individual in treatment choices and in their management plan.
- Be aware of existing treatment options for PTSD in your community of practice, and build a referral database, including organizations that provide support to trauma-exposed individuals.
- Follow available treatment guidelines and evidence-based practices.
- Avoid potentially harmful interventions such as debriefing or prescribing benzodiazepines.

**Following trauma exposure**
- Do not interfere with spontaneous recovery.
- Provide practical support and assistance.
- Provide information regarding responses to trauma and when to seek help.
- Encourage utilization of social support structures.
- Monitor for symptom emergence.
- If ASD is diagnosed, refer for TF-CBT.

**Management of PTSD**
- Assess for suicidality and other risk behaviours.
- Confirm that PTSD is present, and exclude other differential diagnoses.
- Assess for comorbidity (medical/psychiatric/substance use), and manage comorbidity appropriately.
- Refer on to the appropriate level of care, depending on severity and complexity.
- Address potential barriers to treatment.
- Consider risks and benefits of treatment, alongside individual factors, when formulating a management plan.
- Institute first-line treatments, unless specific reasons exist for an alternative treatment option that is not first line (for example, availability, individual preference, comorbidity).
- Monitor adherence, response to treatment, and tolerability, and adjust the management plan accordingly.
- If first-line treatment has failed, confirm that the diagnosis is correct and assess for any complicating factors before instituting second-line interventions.
- Treatment-resistant individuals should ideally be managed in specialist practice.

ASD, acute stress disorder; EMDR, eye movement desensitization and reprocessing; PTSD, post-traumatic stress disorder; TF-CBT, trauma-focused cognitive behavioural therapy.

---

## REFERENCES

1. American Psychiatric Association. *Diagnostic and Statistical Manual of Mental Disorders* (5th edn). Washington, DC: American Psychiatric Association; 2013.
2. World Health Organization. *International Classification of Diseases* (11th revision). https://icd.who.int/en/
3. Bryant RA. Acute stress disorder as a predictor of posttraumatic stress disorder: a systematic review. *J Clin Psychiatry* 2011; 72: 233–9.

4. Howlett JR and Stein MB. Prevention of trauma and stressor-related disorders: a review. *Neuropsychopharmacology* 2016; 41: 357–69.

5. Forneris CA, Gartlehner G, Brownley KA, *et al*. Interventions to prevent post-traumatic stress disorder: a systematic review. *Am J Prev Med* 2013; 44: 635–50.

6. Rose SC, Bisson J, Churchill R, *et al*. Psychological debriefing for preventing post traumatic stress disorder (PTSD). *Cochrane Database Syst Rev* 2002; 2: CD000560.

7. Roberts NP, Kitchiner NJ, Kenardy J, *et al*. Multiple session early psychological interventions for the prevention of post-traumatic stress disorder. *Cochrane Database Syst Rev* 2009; 3: CD006869.

8. Roberts NP, Kitchiner NJ, Kenardy J, *et al*. Early psychological interventions to treat acute traumatic stress symptoms. *Cochrane Database Syst Rev* 2010; 3: CD007944.

9. Sijbrandij M, Kleiboer A, Bisson JI, *et al*. Pharmacological prevention of post-traumatic stress disorder and acute stress disorder: a systematic review and meta-analysis. *Lancet Psychiatry* 2015; 2: 413–21.

10. Amos T, Stein DJ, Ipser JC. Pharmacological interventions for preventing post-traumatic stress disorder (PTSD). *Cochrane Database Syst Rev* 2014; 7: CD006239.

11. Bisson JI, Roberts NP, Andrew M, et al. Psychological therapies for chronic post-traumatic stress disorder (PTSD) in adults. *Cochrane Database Syst Rev* 2013; 12: CD003388.

12. Cusack K, Jonas DE, Forneris CA, *et al*. Psychological treatments for adults with posttraumatic stress disorder: a systematic review and meta-analysis. *Clin Psychol Rev* 2016; 43: 128–41.

13. Watts BV, Schnurr PP, Mayo L, *et al*. Meta-analysis of the efficacy of treatments for posttraumatic stress disorder. *J Clin Psychiatry* 2013; 74: 541–50.

14. Lee DJ, Schnitzlein CW, Wolf JP, *et al*. Psychotherapy versus pharmacotherapy for posttraumatic stress disorder: systematic review and meta-analyses to determine first-line treatments. *Depress Anxiety* 2016; 33: 792–806.

15. Lancaster CL, Teeters JB, Gros DF, *et al*. Posttraumatic stress disorder: overview of evidence-based assessment and treatment. *J Clin Med* 2016; 5: 105.

16. O'Toole SK, Solomon SL, Bergdahl SA. A meta-analysis of hypnotherapeutic techniques in the treatment of PTSD symptoms. *J Trauma Stress* 2016; 29: 97–100.

17. Powers MB, Halpern JM, Ferenschak MP, *et al*. A meta-analytic review of prolonged exposure for posttraumatic stress disorder. *Clin Psychol Rev* 2010; 30: 635–41.

18. Hoskins M, Pearce J, Bethell A, *et al*. Pharmacotherapy for post-traumatic stress disorder: systematic review and meta-analysis. *Br J Psychiatry* 2015; 206: 93–100.

19. Guina J, Rossetter SR, DeRHODES BJ, *et al*. Benzodiazepines for PTSD: a systematic review and meta-analysis. *J Psychiatr Pract* 2015; 21: 281–303.

20. Khachatryan D, Groll D, Booij L, *et al*. Prazosin for treating sleep disturbances in adults with posttraumatic stress disorder: a systematic review and meta-analysis of randomized controlled trials. *Gen Hosp Psychiatry* 2016; 39: 46–52.

21. Averill LA, Purohit P, Averill CL, *et al*. Glutamate dysregulation and glutamatergic therapeutics for PTSD: evidence from human studies. *Neurosci Lett* 2017; 649: 147–55.

22. Bakermans-Kranenburg M and Van Ijzendoorn M. Sniffing around oxytocin: review and meta-analyses of trials in healthy and clinical groups with implications for pharmacotherapy. *Transl Psychiatry* 2013; 3: e258.

23. Hetrick SE, Purcell R, Garner B, *et al*. Combined pharmaco-therapy and psychological therapies for post traumatic stress disorder (PTSD). *Cochrane Database Syst Rev* 2010; 7: CD007316.

24. Popiel A, Zawadzki B, Pragłowska E, *et al*. Prolonged exposure, paroxetine and the combination in the treatment of PTSD following a motor vehicle accident. A randomized clinical trial—The 'TRAKT' study. *J Behav Ther Exp Psychiatry* 2015; 48: 17–26.

25. Schneier FR, Neria Y, Pavlicova M, *et al*. Combined prolonged exposure therapy and paroxetine for PTSD related to the World Trade Center attack: a randomized controlled trial. *Am J Psychiatry* 2012; 169: 80–8.

26. Simiola V, Neilson EC, Thompson R, *et al*. Preferences for trauma treatment: a systematic review of the empirical literature. *Psychol Trauma* 2015; 7: 516.

27. Kantor V, Knefel M, Lueger-Schuster B. Perceived barriers and facilitators of mental health service utilization in adult trauma survivors: a systematic review. *Clin Psychol Rev* 2017; 52: 52–68.

28. Morina N, Koerssen R, Pollet TV. Interventions for children and adolescents with posttraumatic stress disorder: a meta-analysis of comparative outcome studies. *Clin Psychol Rev* 2016; 47: 41–54.

29. Gillies D, Taylor F, Gray C, *et al*. Psychological therapies for the treatment of post-traumatic stress disorder in children and ado-lescents (review). *Evid Based Child Health* 2013; 8: 1004–116.

30. Gillies D, Maiocchi L, Bhandari AP, *et al*. Psychological ther-apies for children and adolescents exposed to trauma. *Cochrane Database Syst Rev* 2016; 10: CD012371.

31. Strawn JR, Keeshin BR, DelBello MP, *et al*. Psychopharmacologic treatment of posttraumatic stress disorder in children and ado-lescents: a review. *J Clin Psychiatry* 2010; 71: 932–41.

32. Roberts NP, Roberts PA, Jones N, *et al*. Psychological therapies for post-traumatic stress disorder and comorbid substance use disorder. *Cochrane Database Syst Rev* 2016; 38: 25–38.

33. Torchalla I, Nosen L, Rostam H, *et al*. Integrated treatment programs for individuals with concurrent substance use dis-orders and trauma experiences: a systematic review and meta-analysis. *J Subst Abuse Treat* 2012; 42: 65–77.

34. Flanagan JC, Korte KJ, Killeen TK, *et al*. Concurrent treatment of substance use and PTSD. *Curr Psychiatry Rep* 2016; 18: 1–9.

35. Kuester A, Niemeyer H and Knaevelsrud C. Internet-based inter-ventions for posttraumatic stress: a meta-analysis of randomized controlled trials. *Clin Psychol Rev* 2016; 43: 1–16.

36. Sijbrandij M, Kunovski I and Cuijpers P. Effectiveness of Internet-delivered cognitive behavioral therapy for posttraumatic stress disorder: a systematic review and meta-analysis. *Depress Anxiety* 2016; 33: 783–91.

37. Olthuis JV, Wozney L, Asmundson GJ, *et al*. Distance-delivered interventions for PTSD: A systematic review and meta-analysis. *J Anxiety Disord* 2016; 44: 9–26.

38. Gonçalves R, Pedrozo AL, Coutinho ESF, *et al*. Efficacy of virtual reality exposure therapy in the treatment of PTSD: a systematic review. *PLoS One* 2012; 7: e48469.

39. Crane R, Brewer J, Feldman C, *et al*. What defines mindfulness-based programs? The warp and the weft. *Psychol Med* 2016: 1–10.

40. Banks K, Newman E and Saleem J. An overview of the research on mindfulness-based interventions for treating symptoms of posttraumatic stress disorder: a systematic review. *J Clin Psychol* 2015; 71: 935–63.

41. Hilton L, Maher AR, Colaiaco B, *et al*. Meditation for posttraumatic stress: systematic review and meta-analysis. *Psychol Trauma* 2017; 9: 453–60.

42. Mithoefer MC, Grob CS and Brewerton TD. Novel psychopharmacological therapies for psychiatric disorders: psilocybin and MDMA. *Lancet Psychiatry* 2016; 3: 481–8.

43. Amoroso T, Workman M. Treating posttraumatic stress disorder with MDMA-assisted psychotherapy: a preliminary meta-analysis and comparison to prolonged exposure therapy. *J Psychopharmacol* 2016; 30: 595–600.

44. Ori R, Amos T, Bergman H, *et al.* Augmentation of cognitive and behavioural therapies (CBT) with d-cycloserine for anxiety and related disorders. *Cochrane Database Syst Rev* 2015; 5: CD007803.

45. Rossi S, Hallett M, Rossini PM, *et al.* Safety, ethical considerations, and application guidelines for the use of transcranial magnetic stimulation in clinical practice and research. *Clin Neurophysiol* 2009; 120: 2008–39.

46. Clark C, Cole J, Winter C, *et al.* A review of transcranial magnetic stimulation as a treatment for post-traumatic stress disorder. *Curr Psychiatry Rep* 2015; 17: 1–9.

47. Berlim MT, Van Den Eynde F. Repetitive transcranial magnetic stimulation over the dorsolateral prefrontal cortex for treating posttraumatic stress disorder: an exploratory meta-analysis of randomized, double-blind and sham-controlled trials. *Can J Psychiatry* 2014; 59: 487–96.

48. Trevizol AP, Barros MD, Silva PO, *et al.* Transcranial magnetic stimulation for posttraumatic stress disorder: an updated systematic review and meta-analysis. *Trends Psychiatry Psychother* 2016; 38: 50–5.

49. Rosenbaum S, Stubbs B, Ward PB, *et al.* The prevalence and risk of metabolic syndrome and its components among people with posttraumatic stress disorder: a systematic review and meta-analysis. *Metab Clin Exp* 2015; 64: 926–33.

50. Rosenbaum S, Vancampfort D, Steel Z, *et al.* Physical activity in the treatment of post-traumatic stress disorder: a systematic review and meta-analysis. *Psychiatry Res* 2015; 230: 130–6.

51. Reiter K, Andersen SB, Carlsson J. Neurofeedback treatment and posttraumatic stress disorder: effectiveness of neurofeedback on posttraumatic stress disorder and the optimal choice of protocol. *J Nerv Ment Dis* 2016; 204: 69–77.

52. Wang F, Wang Y, Sun T, *et al.* Hyperbaric oxygen therapy for the treatment of traumatic brain injury: a meta-analysis. *Neurol Sci* 2016; 37: 693–701.

53. Lipov E, Ritchie EC. A review of the use of stellate ganglion block in the treatment of PTSD. *Curr Psychiatry Rep* 2015; 17: 1–5.

54. Reznikov R, Hamani C. Posttraumatic stress disorder: perspectives for the use of deep brain stimulation. *Neuromodulation* 2017; 20: 7–14.

55. Schouten KA, de Niet GJ, Knipscheer JW, *et al.* The effectiveness of art therapy in the treatment of traumatized adults: a systematic review on art therapy and trauma. *Trauma Violence Abuse* 2015; 16: 220–8.

56. O'Haire ME, Guerin NA, Kirkham AC. Animal-Assisted Intervention for trauma: a systematic literature review. *Front Psychol* 2015; 6: 1121.

57. Casey P. Adjustment disorder. *CNS Drugs* 2009; 23: 927–38.

58. Carta MG, Balestrieri M, Murru A, *et al.* Adjustment disorder: epidemiology, diagnosis and treatment. *Clin Pract Epidemiol Ment Health* 2009; 5: 15.

59. Arends I, Bruinvels DJ, Rebergen DS, *et al.* Interventions to facilitate return to work in adults with adjustment disorders. *Cochrane Database Syst Rev* 2012; 12: 12.

60. Krishna M, Lepping P, Jones S, *et al.* Systematic review and meta-analysis of group cognitive behavioural psychotherapy treatment for sub-clinical depression. *Asian J Psychiatry* 2015; 16: 7–16.

61. Leppin AL, Bora PR, Tilburt JC, *et al.* The efficacy of resiliency training programs: a systematic review and meta-analysis of randomized trials. *PLoS One* 2014; 9: e111420.

62. Macedo T, Wilheim L, Gonçalves R, *et al.* Building resilience for future adversity: a systematic review of interventions in non-clinical samples of adults. *BMC Psychiatry* 2014; 14: 227.

63. Khoury B, Sharma M, Rush SE, *et al.* Mindfulness-based stress reduction for healthy individuals: a meta-analysis. *J Psychosom Res* 2015; 78: 519–28.

64. Goyal M, Singh S, Sibinga EM, *et al.* Meditation programs for psychological stress and well-being: a systematic review and meta-analysis. *JAMA Intern Med* 2014; 174: 357–68.

65. Cavanagh K, Strauss C, Forder L, *et al.* Can mindfulness and acceptance be learnt by self-help? A systematic review and meta-analysis of mindfulness and acceptance-based self-help interventions. *Clin Psychol Rev* 2014; 34: 118–29.

66. Jayewardene WP, Lohrmann DK, Erbe RG, *et al.* Effects of preventive online mindfulness interventions on stress and mindfulness: a meta-analysis of randomized controlled trials. *Prev Med Rep* 2017; 5: 150–9.

67. Manzoni GM, Pagnini F, Castelnuovo G, *et al.* Relaxation training for anxiety: a ten-years systematic review with meta-analysis. *BMC Psychiatry* 2008; 8: 41.

68. Casey P. Adjustment disorder: new developments. *Curr Psychiatry Rep* 2014; 16: 1–8.

69. Cameron IM, Reid IC, MacGillivray SA. Efficacy and tolerability of antidepressants for sub-threshold depression and for mild major depressive disorder. *J Affect Disord* 2014; 166: 48–58.

70. Pittler MH, Ernst E. Kava extract versus placebo for treating anxiety. *Cochrane Database Syst Rev* 2002; 2: CD003383.

71. Rebar AL, Stanton R, Geard D, *et al.* A meta-meta-analysis of the effect of physical activity on depression and anxiety in non-clinical adult populations. *Health Psychol Rev* 2015; 9: 366–78.

72. Wegner M, Helmich I, Machado S, *et al.* Effects of exercise on anxiety and depression disorders: review of meta-analyses and neurobiological mechanisms. *CNS Neurol Disord Drug Targets* 2014; 13: 1002–14.

# 84

# Bereavement

*Beverley Raphael[†], Sally Wooding, and Julie Dunsmore*

## Introduction

Bereavement is the complex set of reactions that occur with the death of a loved one: the emotions of grief with yearning, angry protest, and sadness; the cognitive processes of understanding and making meaning of the finality and nature of death; and the social, cultural, spiritual, and religious contexts of adaptation. Grief may also result from other losses such as health, home, country, and safe worlds. There have been investigations into potential neurobiological substrates, without, as yet, a consensus about the explanatory model. In *Mourning and Melancholia*, Freud [1] described the psychological processes of mourning which involved the gradual relinquishment of bonds with the deceased, and how mourning differed from melancholia. Lindemann [2] described the symptomatology and management of acute grief in his classic paper on his experiences assessing and treating the survivors of a nightclub fire. Engel [3] asked, 'Is grief a disease?' and concluded in the negative. Bowlby's work on attachment, separation, and loss [4–6] has been the most influential in informing research and clinical practice, with many studies of both adults and children utilizing such concepts. Early research focused chiefly on bereavement following the death of a spouse, describing normal, high-risk, and pathological patterns of grief [7–9]. There is also a number of excellent reviews of theory and research, including those of Stroebe's group [10, 11].

## Phenomenology of 'normal grief'

Common phenomena of the grief experience of adults, identified through many research studies [12–14], relate to similar domains influenced by developmental trajectories through childhood and adolescence. Adult studies indicate consistent patterns: numbness and disbelief; yearning, angry protest, and 'searching' behaviours representing separation distress; sadness with reviewing of memories of the lost relationship, with a range of associated emotions; and progressive acceptance of the death and changed circumstances, sometimes referred to as resolution. Bonanno *et al.* [14] has shown that resilient trajectories, defined by low overall distress, are common. Other transient phenomena described by clinicians working with bereaved people [15] include: identificatory symptoms, reflecting the deceased's illness; and a sense of the deceased's ongoing presence, at times as though seeing the face, hearing the voice, or feeling the touch of the dead person. 'Yearning' is considered to be the most pathognomonic of these grief phenomena, which usually settle over the first year but may continue, triggered by anniversaries or specific memories. Older people who have had a long relationship with a spouse may continue this relationship in their minds for the comfort of 'talking' with the person and a need for the ongoing closeness [16]. Recent research [17] has modelled sequential peaks of the reactive phenomena: disbelief, yearning, anger, and depression, which bereaved people more usually describe as sadness. Grief may be a precipitant of depression in those with pre-existing or bereavement-related vulnerabilities, and the differentiation of normal and more pathological forms of grief from depression is important clinically [15, 18]. Intense grief and the peaks of distress identified in this chapter do not usually continue beyond the first 4–6 months [12, 13]. Continuing 'acute' grief beyond this time suggests the possibility of a pathological response, as do other risk indicators, although some phenomena may continue intermittently for many years. Comparative studies have demonstrated that the intensity of adult grief is likely to be greatest for the death of a child, then spouse or partner, then parent [12, 19].

## Neurobiology of bereavement

Recent research has examined the neurobiology of grief through studies using functional magnetic resonance imaging of grief [20] and brain activity in women grieving the break-up of a romantic relationship [21]. Workers have attempted to develop a theoretical model, based on a wide range of relevant data, encompassing a 'neurobiopsychosocial' framework for sadness and loss [22]. Stress hormones [23] and psychoimmune function is a further area of research. A comprehensive model integrating the relevant research findings is yet to be established.

## Risk and protective factors influencing course and outcome

Pre-existing vulnerabilities that may influence the course and outcome have been reviewed, alongside other risk factors [24].

[†] It is with regret that we report that Beverley Raphael died on 21 September 2018.

These include personality vulnerabilities related to relationship styles such as avoidant and insecure attachments. Genetic factors do not appear to have been directly studied, but it is likely that the short allele of the serotonin gene promoter polymorphism of *5HTTLPR*, which influences response to adversity, may contribute through gene–environment interactions [25]. Prior loss and adverse experiences may add vulnerability, for instance multiple losses faced by indigenous peoples, with loss of culture, land, and loved ones, with multiple premature deaths and separations [26]. Separation anxiety in childhood, as well as pre-existing psychiatric disorder, family psychiatric disorder, and substance abuse, may add to vulnerability. Successful negotiation of earlier losses, mature defence styles, and optimism may be protective. The nature of the lost relationship has been identified in a number of studies as being a significant factor [15, 27]. The special relationship between parent and child is associated with greater vulnerabilities, including an increased risk of psychiatric hospitalization and even death by suicide. Patterns of distress differ by gender with stillbirth, neonatal deaths, and sudden infant death syndromes, perhaps suggesting different attachment patterns [28]. The death of an adolescent child is not infrequently by accident, suicide, or risk-taking with illicit drugs, bringing the extra complexities of adaptation for the grieving parents. A great deal of research has explored the grief associated with the death of a partner or spouse, both young and old. High levels of dependence and ambivalence have been shown to complicate grief and to be associated with more difficult bereavement [15, 27], and prolonged or complicated grief may be more likely. Family members may have different relationships with the deceased, and thus varying patterns and trajectories of grief, which may cloud the recognition of children's and others' needs. Adults' loss of an older parent appears to be the least distressing, although there is still sadness plus the recognition of one's own mortality. Here, as at any age, intense fantasies of reunion with the deceased may indicate a risk of suicide, especially for older widowed men. Circumstances of the death may influence outcome. When dying is prolonged, as in the later stages of a terminal illness, the dying person may experience grief over his or her own life and the loved ones who will be lost to him, alongside the anticipatory grieving of family members. While palliative care systems may provide bereavement programmes, families have complex dynamics and may require family-focused interventions [29]. Sudden unexpected deaths bring an extra level of emotional shock [30], especially if also untimely, as with children's death. When violent death occurs, as with homicide or the mass violence of terrorism or war, those bereaved may experience a complex mixture of traumatic stress reactions and grief reactions, sometimes called traumatic grief [31]. The specific issues facing those bereaved by violent deaths of loved ones have been reported in a recent volume by Rynearson [32], which deals with homicide, terrorism, and other violent deaths. The prolonged and difficult grief in such circumstances is highlighted by findings from September 11, Oklahoma, and Bali bombings. When people are missing, believed dead, the uncertainty and other stressors, including complex legal and evidentiary processes (for example, Disaster Victim Identification requirements), may lead to alternating hope and dread. When there are no remains, it will be more difficult for those bereaved to accept the reality of the death. Seeing and 'saying goodbye' to the dead person have been shown to help those bereaved in disasters. If remains are much disfigured, as with burns, it is important that those bereaved are supported in their choice about this. Social support, particularly the perceptions of the supportiveness of the family and social network, are likely to be protective and assist the bereaved psychologically [33], while perceptions of unhelpfulness may be associated with more negative outcomes [9]. Cultural requirements for social support may differ, as may the delineation of the period of mourning, the roles of the bereaved, and associated spiritual and religious needs [34]. Multiple other adversities may occur, either coincidentally or as a consequence of the circumstances and the loss of the person, for instance financial difficulties, loss of resources, changed status, loss of meaning and identity, or other profound stressors of illness, injury, or other bereavements. Such additional stressors may increase vulnerability [15]. In terms of prolonged grief disorder (previously known as complicated grief disorder, and initially traumatic grief), Prigerson *et al.* [35] have carried out extensive research to refine this syndrome. Bringing together the views of international researchers, they have developed consensus criteria for a distinct psychiatric disorder to be considered for inclusion in DSM-5. This definition requires that the reaction to loss encompasses one of three symptoms of separation distress (for example, yearning) and a minimum of five from a total of nine other symptoms, experienced at least daily, to a distressing or disruptive level. These include: shock; emotional numbing; avoidance of the reality of the loss; difficulty accepting the loss; feelings of meaninglessness; difficulty moving on with life; bitterness over the loss; mistrust; and a diminished sense of self. Such symptoms would need to last at least 6 months and be associated with significant levels of functional impairment. These findings fit well with earlier research identifying more chronic patterns of grief [12, 13].

## Physical and mental health consequences of bereavement

A recent valuable review [36] outlined the evidence of increased mortality for bereaved spouses, particularly males, which is most pronounced in the first 6 months and includes a range of conditions such as heart disease, leading to death from a 'broken heart'. It is also more pronounced for those younger. Death of a child is associated with an even greater mortality risk, particularly for mothers. Suicide is one of the heightened risks, especially for mothers and older males. Physical health impairments are also found [36], with a variety of physical symptoms, as well as greater use of medical services and medications. Further research is needed to clarify the nature of any increased rate of specific diseases. Changed health behaviours, the impact of loss of a health-supporting partner, functional or social changes, or shared environments of risk may contribute. With regard to mental health, there may be an increased level of anxiety and depressive symptoms. There may be a heightened risk for some bereaved individuals for exacerbations of pre-existing conditions or the precipitation of new illnesses, including post-traumatic stress disorder when there is a violent death [32]. Other anxiety disorders, major depression, substance use disorder, and bipolar disorder may be precipitated by bereavement. Complicated or prolonged grief disorder may also represent a psychiatric consequence [35].

## Assessment and management

Most bereaved people do not require counselling, so assessment must be a basis for intervention. Assessment should be simple and synchronous with need and do no harm, addressing the death and its circumstances, the relationship, and the bereaved's experience since, including social support [31]. A more structured format, potentially including grief measures [37], can clarify the presence of PTSD, depression, or prolonged grief, or other health needs, including physical health changes or problems, establishing the basis for intervention. Initial management of acutely bereaved persons requires empathic, compassionate support, and responding to any acute needs in ways that are protective of their mental health, recognizing the 'rollercoaster' of emotions that may occur, and facilitating natural resilience. Concepts of psychological first aid are also valuable in the immediate period after the death [38]. Dealing with concerns about the deceased's suffering and support to view the dead person's remains, should the bereaved choose to, are likely to be helpful. Most evidence-based interventions focus on psychotherapeutic methods, ranging from preventive counselling of those with demonstrated heightened risk [39] to self-help guided interventions [40], interpersonal psychotherapy modifications for traumatic grief [41], integrated cognitive behavioural therapy models [42], or psychodynamically informed models [43] and web-based treatments [44]. Counselling models [45] and psychoeducation have also focused on those bereaved through specific deaths such as those of infants [46]. Other models deal with grief work and tasks [47], as well as specific treatment for morbidity of complicated grief [48] and depressive or anxiety disorders, including the use of pharmacotherapy for such conditions when indicated [49]. Rynearson's [32] work with 'restorative retelling' following violent deaths emphasizes the narrative story which is central to much bereavement counselling and testimony. A practical approach to assessment and counselling may be initiated with some gentle queries such as: 'Can you tell me a little about your loss?', 'What happened with 'John's' death?', 'Can you tell me about 'John' and your relationship?', 'What's been happening since?'. If there is intense continuing distress, circumstances of death which are untimely or traumatic, a complex relationship with the deceased, disruption of family functioning which is impacting on the needs of children, inadequacies of social support, 'unresolved' earlier losses, and multiple additional stressors, the bereaved may be at heightened risk of adverse outcomes. Preventive counselling, which facilitates grieving, is attuned to the bereaved person's readiness, vulnerabilities, and strengths, and helps them to tell the story of their experiences and the person they have lost, is likely to improve outcomes [39]. If assessment indicates that psychiatric disorders have arisen, for instance depression, post-traumatic stress disorder, anxiety, or substance use disorders, these conditions should be managed appropriately, alongside counselling for the bereavement, should this be required. The use of antidepressants or other medication is not indicated for bereavement itself but may be appropriate for such complications [49]. Monitoring for suicide risk should accompany clinical management.

Prolonged or complicated grief may benefit from cognitive behavioural therapy interventions, as well as relevant rehabilitation. Those who are both traumatized and bereaved may need the traumatic stress issues to be dealt with first, and facilitation of grieving following this [43]. There is a need for more comprehensive research and evaluation of prevention, early intervention and treatment modalities, and their appropriate provision to individuals, families, or groups [50]. Culturally appropriate models of support and intervention also need to be further developed. Many bereaved people present first within primary care settings and to their general practitioners who will need the skills and knowledge to deal with their distress, assess their needs, counsel them as appropriate, and refer when necessary. Much support also comes from community and non-government agencies, including bereavement focused groups for specific losses or for grief generally, and from specialized services in public or private mental health sectors. Telling the bereaved person how to grieve, that they should 'forget about the past', and that 'time heals all' is usually perceived as unhelpful. Treating grief as a disease, for example antidepressant medication for normal sadness, is seen by many bereaved people as interfering with their capacity to grieve for their loved one. Counselling bereaved people requires hopeful, compassionate psychotherapeutic intervention, which recognizes the human suffering involved, validates the person's strengths, and respects their spiritual needs. Loss is a central issue for all of us, both our fears of it and its reality. Counselling requires those involved to recognize their own sensitivities in this regard and to assist the 'journey' of those affected in dealing with their loss. Most people grieve, remember with love those whom they have lost, and continue to love and love anew.

## FURTHER INFORMATION

Kellehear, A. (2007). *A Social History of Dying*. Cambridge University Press, Cambridge.

National Centre for Childhood Grief. http://www.childhoodgrief.org.au/

## REFERENCES

1. Freud, S. (1915). Mourning and melancholia. In: J. Strachey (ed.) *Sigmund Freud: Collected Papers*, Vol. 4. Basic Books, New York, NY.
2. Lindemann, E. (1944). Symptomatology and management of acute grief. *American Journal of Psychiatry*, 101, 141–8.
3. Engel, G.L. (1961). Is grief a disease? *Psychosomatic Medicine*, 23, 18–22.
4. Bowlby, J. (1969). *Attachment and Loss, Vol. 1. Attachment*. Hogarth, London.
5. Bowlby, J. (1973). *Attachment and Loss, Vol. 2. Separation, Anxiety and Anger*. Hogarth, London.
6. Bowlby, J. (1980). *Attachment and Loss, Vol. 3. Loss: Sadness and Depression*. Hogarth, London.
7. Parkes, C.M. (1996). *Bereavement: Studies of Grief in Adult Life* (3rd edn). Routledge, London.
8. Maddison, D.C. and Walker, W.L. (1967). Factors affecting the outcome of conjugal bereavement. *British Journal of Psychiatry*, 113, 1057–67.
9. Jacobs, S. (1993). *Pathologic Grief: Maladaptation to Loss*. American Psychiatric Press, Washington, DC.
10. Stroebe, M.S., Hansson, R.O., Stroebe, W., *et al.* (eds.) (2001). *Handbook of Bereavement Research: Consequences, Coping, and Care*. American Psychological Association, Washington, DC.

11. Stroebe, M.S., Hansson, R.O., Stroebe, W., *et al.* (eds.) (2007). *Handbook of Bereavement Research and Practice: 21st Century Perspectives.* American Psychological Association, Washington, DC.

12. Middleton, W., Raphael, B., Burnett, P., *et al.* (1998). A longitudinal study comparing bereavement phenomena in recently bereaved spouses, adult children and parents. *Australian and New Zealand Journal of Psychiatry*, 32, 235–41.

13. Byrne, G.J. and Raphael, B. (1994). A longitudinal study of bereavement phenomena in recently widowed elderly men. *Psychological Medicine*, 24, 411–21.

14. Bonanno, G.A., Wortman, C.B., Lehman, D.R., *et al.* (2002). Resilience to loss and chronic grief: a prospective study from preloss to 18-months postloss. *Journal of Personality and Social Psychology*, 83, 1150–64.

15. Raphael, B. (1983). *The Anatomy of Bereavement: A Handbook for the Caring Professions.* Basic Books, New York, NY.

16. Moss, M.S., Moss, S.Z., and Hansson, R.O. (2001). Bereavement and old age. In: M.S. Stroebe, R.O. Hansson, W. Stroebe, and H. Schut (eds.) *Handbook of Bereavement Research: Consequences, Coping, and Care.* American Psychological Association, Washington, DC. pp. 241–60.

17. Maciejewski, P.K., Zhang, B., Block, S.D., *et al.* (2007). An empirical examination of the stage theory of grief. *JAMA*, 297, 716–23.

18. Prigerson, H.G., Bierhals, A.J., Kasl, S.V., *et al.* (1996). Complicated grief as a distinct disorder from bereavement-related depression and anxiety: a replication study. *American Journal of Psychiatry*, 153, 84–6.

19. Sanders, C.M. (1980). A comparison of adult bereavement in the death of a spouse, child, and parent. *Omega*, 10, 303–22.

20. Gündel, H., O'Connor, M., Littrell, L., *et al.* (2003). Functional neuroanatomy of grief: an fMRI study. *American Journal of Psychiatry*, 160, 1946–53.

21. Najib, A., Lorberbaum, J., Kose, S., *et al.* (2004). Regional brain activity in women grieving a romantic relationship break up. *American Journal of Psychiatry*, 161, 2245–56.

22. Freed, P.J. and Mann, J.J. (2007). Sadness and loss: toward a neurobiopsychosocial model. *American Journal of Psychiatry*, 164, 28–34.

23. McCleery, J.M., Bhagwagar, Z., Smith, K.A., *et al.* (2000). Modelling a loss event: effect of imagined bereavement on the hypothalamicpituitary–adrenal axis. *Psychological Medicine*, 30, 219–23.

24. Stroebe, M., Folkman, S., Hansson, R.O., *et al.* (2006). The prediction of bereavement outcome: development of an integrative risk factor framework. *Social Science and Medicine*, 63, 2446–51.

25. Kaufman, J., Yang, B.-Z., Douglas-Palumberi, H., *et al.* (2004). Social supports and serotonin transporter gene moderate depression in maltreated children. *Proceedings of the National Academy of Sciences of the United States of America*, 101, 17316–21.

26. Raphael, B., Swan, P., and Martinek, N. (1998). Intergeneration aspects of trauma for Australian aboriginal people. In: Y. Danieli (ed.) *An International Handbook of Multigenerational Legacies of Trauma.* Plenum Press, New York, NY. pp. 327–39

27. Parkes, C.M. (2006). *Love and Loss: The Root of Grief and Its Complications.* Routledge, Hove.

28. Vance, J.C., Boyle, F.M., Najman, J.M., *et al.* (2002). Couple distress after sudden infant or perinatal death: a 30-month follow-up. *Journal of Paediatrics and Child Health*, 38, 368–72.

29. Kissane, D.W., McKenzie, M., Bloch, S., *et al.* (2006). Family focused grief therapy: a randomized controlled trial in palliative care and bereavement. *American Journal Psychiatry*, 163, 1208–18.

30. Lundin, T. (1984). Morbidity following sudden and unexpected bereavement. *British Journal of Psychiatry*, 144, 84–8.

31. Raphael, B., Martinek, N., and Wooding, S. (2004). Assessing loss, psychological trauma and traumatic bereavement. In: J. Wilson (ed.) *Assessing Psychological Trauma and PTSD* (2nd edn). Guilford Press, New York, NY. pp. 492–510.

32. Rynearson, E.K. (ed.) (2006). *Violent Death: Resilience and Intervention Beyond the Crisis.* Routledge Psychosocial Stress Series, Taylor & Francis, New York, NY.

33. Vanderwerker, L.C. and Prigerson, H.G. (2004). Social support and technological connectedness as protective factors in bereavement. *Journal of Loss and Trauma*, 9, 45–57.

34. Parkes, C.M., Laungani, P., and Young, B. (1997). *Death and Bereavement Across Cultures.* Routledge, London.

35. Prigerson, H., Horowitz, M.J., Jacobs, S.C., *et al.* (2009). Prolonged grief disorder: Psychometric validation of criteria proposed for DSM-IV and ICD-11. *PLOS Medicine*, 6(8), 1–12.

36. Stroebe, M., Schut, H., and Stroebe, W. (2007). The physical and mental health consequences of bereavement: a review. *Seminar for Lancet*, 8, 1960–73.

37. Neimeyer, R.A. and Hogan, N.S. (2001). Quantitative or qualitative? Measurement issues in the study of grief. In: M.S. Strobe, R.O. Hansson, W. Stroebe, and H. Schut (eds.) *Handbook of Bereavement Research: Consequences, Coping, and Care.* American Psychological Association, Washington, DC. pp. 89–118.

38. Wooding, S. and Raphael, B. (2012). NSW Health Disaster Mental Health Guidebook. Handbook 2: Psychological First Aid (PFA) (Level 1 Intervention following Mass Disaster) prepared by the Disaster Response, Resilience and Research Group (DRRRG), University of Western Sydney (UWS). https://www.health.nsw.gov.au/emergency_preparedness/mental/Documents/handbook-2-PFA.pdf

39. Raphael, B. (1977). Preventive intervention with the recently bereaved. *Archives of General Psychiatry*, 34, 1450–4.

40. Vachon, M.L.S., Lyall, W.A.L., Rogers, J., *et al.* (1980). A controlled study of self-help interventions for widows. *American Journal of Psychiatry*, 137, 1380–4.

41. Shear, K., Frank, E., Houck, P.R., *et al.* (2005). Treatment of complicated grief: a randomized controlled trial. *JAMA*, 293, 2601–8.

42. Shear, K. and Frank, E. (2006). Treatment of complicated grief: integrating cognitive–behavioral methods with other treatment approaches. In: V. Follette and J. Ruzek (eds.) *Cognitive Behavioural Therapies for Trauma.* pp. 290–320. Guilford Press, New York, NY.

43. Raphael, B., Dunsmore, J., and Wooding, S. (2004). Early mental health interventions for traumatic loss in adults. In: B. Litz (ed.) *Early Intervention for Trauma and Traumatic Loss.* Guilford Press, New York, NY. pp. 147–78.

44. Wagner, B., Knaevelsrud, C., and Maercker, A. (2006). Internet-based cognitive–behaviorial therapy (INTERAPY) for complicated grief: a randomized controlled trial. *Death Studies*, 30, 429–53.

45. Rando, T.A. (1993). *The Treatment of Complicated Mourning.* Research Press, Champaign, IL.

46. Murray, J.A., Terry, D.J., Vance, J.C., *et al.* (2000). Effects of a program of intervention on parental distress following infant death. *Death Studies*, 24, 275–305.

47. Worden, J.W. (1991). *Grief Counselling and Grief Therapy*. Springer Publishing Company, New York, NY.

48. Boelen, P.A. (2005). *Complicated Grief: Assessment, Theory, and Treatment*. Ipskamp, Enscede/Amsterdam.

49. Raphael, B., Dobson, M., and Minkov, C. (2001). Psychotherapeutic and pharmacological intervention for bereaved people. In: M.S. Stroebe, R.O. Hansson, W. Stroebe, and H. Schut (eds.) *Handbook of Bereavement Research: Consequences, Coping, and Care*. American Psychological Association, Washington, DC. pp. 587–612.

50. Schut, H., Stroebe, M.S., Van Den Bout, J., *et al.* (2001). The efficacy of bereavement interventions: determining who benefits. In: M.S. Stroebe, R.O. Hansson, W. Stroebe, and H. Schut(eds.) *Handbook of Bereavement Research: Consequences, Coping, and Care*. American Psychological Association, Washington, DC. pp. 705–37.

# 85

# Recovered memories and false memories

*Deborah Davis and Elizabeth F. Loftus*

## Introduction

The concept of repressed memory has been around for at least a century. It is the notion that, as a defence mechanism, horribly traumatic experiences can be involuntarily banished into the unconscious, even for decades, yet at some later point return to awareness, unchanged, vivid, and accurate—protected from the ravages of time and immune to the normal laws of memory functioning and decay.

The idea of repression is everywhere. Characters in television shows, movies, and books repress memories of their dark pasts and recover them with the help from fictional therapists—using memory recovery tools such as hypnosis, guided imagery, or age regression. Or memories return in fragments until the full story bursts into memory in time to solve a crime, to prompt a long awaited reckoning, or to allow recovery from psychological problems. And national media discuss claims involving repressed memories of satanic abuse, witnessing murder, alien abduction, and other fantastical events, some disclosed by celebrities. Psychologists are exposed to the concept of repression in introductory psychology classes and throughout their careers. Moreover, the police use memory recovery techniques with witnesses and suspects. And innocent suspects confess to crimes they did not commit and did not remember when the police convinced them they 'repressed' the memory of committing the heinous act [1, 2].

Though the idea of repression and memory recovery had been part of cultural and professional zeitgeists for decades, controversy regarding the validity of so-called 'recovered memories' broke out in force during the late 1980s and early 1990s. Cases in which a memory allegedly 'repressed' for years, even decades, was 'recovered' fully intact and in detail formed the basis of widely publicized criminal charges ranging from sexual abuse to murder. Families were destroyed; personal careers, reputations, and liberty were lost, and millions were spent on litigation of the claims.

Controversy regarding the reality of these claims was fuelled by several forces. For decades after Freud repudiated his initial view that many psychological problems were caused by child sexual abuse (CSA) by family members and theorized instead that the many accounts he heard in therapy were fantasies, CSA was widely considered to be rare and lacking in severe consequences. Changes to these assumptions began during the 1960s and 1970s among professionals and feminist writers. At the same time, there were a number of widely publicized cases of alleged sexual abuse involving multiple children in day care centres across the country. In this context, new data were emerging that suggested that CSA had been occurring more frequently than previously assumed. Together, these forces significantly increased scholarly research on the topic (for reviews of this history, see [3, 4]).

Feminists adopted the view that CSA was a violent crime of rape, not simply an inappropriate sexual act. This encouraged the trauma perspective on CSA, emphasizing the severity of short- and long-term effects of abuse that took hold during the late 1970s and 1980s. Dozens of books (many by victims), news articles, movies, and television documentaries increased public awareness of the frequency of CSA (and specifically incest) and dramatically portrayed the proposed traumatic nature of abuse and the severity of its consequences [4].

Among such reports was that of actress Roseanne Barr in 1991 [5]. She appeared on the cover of *People* magazine, claiming recent recovery of memories of abuse by her mother in infancy and later her father, who continued to abuse her until she was 17. Also in *People* magazine that year was the story of former Miss America Marilyn Van Derbur, who claimed to have recovered repressed memories of abuse by her father [6]. *Ms.* Magazine, perhaps the most prominent feminist publication of the time, published an issue with the cover 'BELIEVE IT! Cult Ritual Abuse Exists (January/February, 1993). The author described her mother as a Satanist and alleged activities such as witnessing multiple murders, cannibalization of her baby sister, and others.

A number of self-help books focusing on the link between sexual abuse and repression were published during this time frame, claiming that sexual abuse was more common than recognized, that it is traumatic and therefore memories of abuse are often repressed, that these repressed memories are the source of many psychological problems (including multiple personality disorder), and that repressed memories can be brought back into consciousness, with the result that the psychological problems will resolve. Prominent among these were *The Courage to Heal* [7], *Secret Survivors* [8], and *Repressed Memories: A Journey to Recovery From Sexual Abuse* [9].

Collectively, these influences encouraged many to self-diagnose repressed memories and/or to seek the help of therapists in recovering them, and led some therapists to focus on the possibility that repressed memories of sexual abuse were responsible for their patients' problems. Some even began to describe themselves as 'recovered memory' therapists. But the same reports and writings that, in some quarters, encouraged belief in repression and the role of sexual abuse in causing it fuelled disbelief and criticism in others. In part, disbelief stemmed from incompatibility of claims regarding trauma and repression with theoretical and empirical work on memory. And, in part, it stemmed from the very nature of many reported recovered memories. Both children's reports of day care abuse and adults' reports of their recovered memories were peppered with fantastical allegations, not all relating to sexual abuse. Children reported activities such as riding on flying cows, being forced to eat faeces, being flushed down toilets, or killing and burying large animals. Adults reported recovered memories of Satanic ritual abuse, forced impregnation by Satan, ritual human sacrifice, alien abduction, multiple past lives, or witnessing murder. Some claims were patently impossible (such as riding flying cows, being flushed down toilets). Many were regarded by most as impossible (such as alien abduction, forced sex and breeding with aliens, multiple past lives, impregnation by Satan, memory for events within the scope of infantile amnesia, and others) [10]. For critics, the question became one of how such clearly false memories had been created.

The ensuing widespread debate has left us with two clear practical problems without clear solutions. Firstly, how should therapists deal with the issue of sexual abuse and the potential existence of repressed memories underlying patients' problems? Secondly, how should claims of recovered memories be treated in legal contexts?

In sections to follow, we focus on a question informing both issues. How can false memories of such dramatic autobiographical events as sexual and/or satanic abuse be created? We explicate the repression hypothesis and point readers to excellent reviews of the positions of supporters and critics and the evidence offered in support of each position. We then turn to the false memory perspective, focusing on empirical literature demonstrating the processes and procedures through which false memories for autobiographical events are formed. We end with commentary on implications of this literature for therapeutic practices and for the legal system.

## The repression hypothesis

The repression hypothesis offers the seemingly counterintuitive proposition that the more traumatic an event at the time it occurs, the more likely the memory of the event is to be repressed, banished from consciousness, and unresponsive to attempts to retrieve it until it is psychologically 'safe' to again become aware of it (for example, [11–14]). This view is rooted in Charcot, Janet, and Freud's theories of the role of sexual abuse in prompting repression (for a review of such theories, see [15]). Central to these theories is the idea that victims may be completely unaware of the traumatic event during repression, yet it will nevertheless cause psychological problems, acting 'like a foreign body which long after its entry must continue to be regarded as an agent that is still at work' [11, p. 6].

Though Freud eventually abandoned his initial theory implicating repressed memories of CSA as the foundation of psychological problems, modern repression theorists have adopted and expanded them (for example, [13, 16]). One variant of the repression perspective—the betrayal trauma theory [14]—entails predictions that are even more counterintuitive than the basic proposition that

trauma promotes repression. For example, it asserts that sexual abuse is more likely to be forgotten if it involves greater betrayal such as when committed by an adult on whom one depends (such as a father or other close family member). The betrayal trauma theory also asserts that memory for other (particularly emotional) types of events is facilitated by repetition. But traumatic amnesia or repression is assumed to be more, rather than less, likely with repetition of traumatic events such as abuse.

The original Freudian notion of repression and variants, such as the betrayal trauma theory, have directly promoted the recovered memory movement among therapists. The assumption was that if the repressed memories could be 'recovered', processed, and integrated into the patient's life narrative, the patient's problems would improve. This led therapists to adopt suggestive techniques to uncover memories of the offending events. Principal among these was the explicit suggestion to patients that their symptoms reflect sexual abuse and that failure to remember that abuse reflects repression of the memories. Secondary to this was the use of a variety of suggestive memory recovery techniques such as hypnosis, guided imagery, dream interpretation, participation in 'survivor' support groups, and others (for reviews, see [17, 18]).

## The critics

Though the repression hypothesis has enjoyed widespread support in the therapeutic community, this has been much less true within the scientific community, particularly among memory scientists and many clinical scientists. Many criticisms address the incompatibility of the repression hypothesis with theory and research on memory. Inherent to the notion of repression is the idea that all stages of memory operate differently and through different mechanisms for traumatic material. While many on both sides of the controversy would agree that there are differences between the operation of memory for traumatic, highly emotional, and more neutral events, controversy centres on the nature of those differences.

For critics, the view is that more traumatic or emotional memories are more likely to be remembered, to be highly accessible, and to be remembered through normal processes of retrieval—though some argue for greater equivalence between traumatic and non-traumatic material. For repression theorists, the view is generally that traumatic material is more likely to be forgotten (repressed), to be inaccessible, and to be resistant to recall through normal mechanisms such as salient cues or reminders or efforts to recall (thereby necessitating the extraordinary efforts to retrieve the memories). Moreover, it is assumed that memory for traumatic material does not decay or become distorted in the normal manner, such that even when retrieved after decades of disuse, such memories will be accurate and detailed (for explication and reviews, see [19]).

Secondly, disagreement surrounds whether, and by what methods, each side's claims can be validly tested. Each has offered methodological criticisms of the efforts of the other. Though there have been some attempts to provide laboratory demonstrations of processes related to repression (such as memory suppression or blocking) (for reviews, see [20, 21]), repression theorists have largely attempted to demonstrate the reality of repression for traumatic events such as CSA or to test the conditions under which it is most likely to occur with real-life alleged victims. Critics have raised such concerns as: (1) verification of alleged abuse (that is, of the same actions entailed in the recovered memories); (2) verification of a period of inability to remember the abuse (vs failure to think about the abuse or episodes of remembering that are themselves forgotten); (3) verification of repression as the mechanism of failure to remember (vs normal mechanisms of forgetting); or (4) verification that even if an episode seemed inaccessible to memory for some period, the episode was indeed traumatic in nature. The latter concern is important, in that studies showing some report that they had been abused, but had not remembered it for long periods of time, are not relevant if the unremembered event was not traumatic. Essentially, critics argue that these concerns indicate that the hypothesis has not been adequately tested and arguably may be untestable (for reviews of these concerns, see [4, 18, 22]).

On the other hand, proponents of the repression hypothesis have argued that laboratory demonstrations of techniques and processes promoting the development of false memories are not relevant to the kinds of traumatic events that might trigger repression. Ethical constraints on laboratory research prevent either exposure to traumatic events or efforts to implant memories of such events. Moreover, though many real-life patients who have claimed to have recovered false memories of abuse through therapy have later recanted and claimed the new memories were false, repression proponents claim that these recantings are themselves subject to doubt (for example, they might be the product of social influence to recant), and not evidence of false recovered memories (for a discussion of retractor experiences, see [23]).

These debates continue. Nevertheless, we believe that the reality of false memories of highly traumatic autobiographical events has been convincingly demonstrated, if nothing else by the fantastical nature of many purportedly recovered memories, such as those for sex, childbearing, and infanticide with Satan; alien abduction and impregnation; impossible memories from beyond the veil of infantile amnesia; past lives; and others. Moreover, these false memories were developed through normal processes of memory distortion. Next, we discuss how this occurs.

## If this memory is not real, where did it come from?

Of issues relevant to the controversy, questions of whether and how false memories can be created are, in some respects, the easiest to answer. To understand this, it is important to begin with the concept of memory itself.

### The nature of memory

Many laypersons think of memory as akin to an enhanced movie consisting of sensory images replaying the event in question. Memory science has revealed that instead memory consists of at least sensory images, beliefs (the story we tell ourselves about what happened), and information relevant to the plausibility of those beliefs. A memory judgement criterion is then applied to these narrative cognitions, assessing whether the 'memory' is or is not a real memory for a real event. Some, for example, may require of themselves clear detailed sensory images to decide something is a memory. At the other extreme, a person may be convinced that a bodily sensation is an embodied memory of sexual abuse (for a review, see [24]).

Given that a real event did occur, each memory component can change over time. But each can also be fully created independent of the occurrence of a real event. We review the evidence of whether and how this happens in the sections to follow. We present evidence that false autobiographical memories can be fabricated, even for relatively extreme events and even for events that would seem rather implausible.

### Evidence that extreme false memories do occur

False autobiographical memories can develop for events ranging from the relatively mundane (for example, school performance) to the seemingly impossible (for example, having been abducted by aliens, having sex with the devil). Many find it implausible that a person could falsely remember 'extreme' experiences such as alien abduction, satanic ritual abuse, sexual abuse by one's father, or having witnessed or committed a horrific crime.

#### Real-life examples

Nevertheless, real-life examples of each of the aforementioned extreme false memories have been documented in the scientific literature: witnessing murder [25, 26], alien abduction [27], enduring the painful surgical removal of one's clitoris, sexual abuse (including satanic ritual abuse [18, 25]), witnessing dramatic fatal accidents [23, 28], and committing a crime that one did not actually commit [1, 2, 29].

#### Laboratory studies

Research demonstrating that false memories for events that never happened can be easily planted is commonplace in psychology. Many such demonstrations involve planting false memories for relatively trivial events such as hearing sounds or words, seeing various (actually unseen) objects, saying things one did not actually say, and many more [30]. False memories can be developed in people of normal cognitive function and lacking any mental illness or abnormality. Even those exceptional people who purportedly have near-perfect autobiographical memory (who can remember every day of their lives) have been led to develop false memories [31].

Though laboratory procedures for planting such false memories may seem inadequate to provoke the relatively extreme false memories of concern here, it is important to note that they involve similar processes. Countless demonstrations of schema-consistent memory intrusions illustrate the tendency to develop false memories based on what makes sense, given other relevant knowledge of similar situations, such as to falsely remember seeing books in a professor's office that had none (for example, [32]).

Plausibility and inference are also implicated in the development of dramatic false autobiographical memories. But perhaps the most relevant research has been experiments demonstrating that procedures leading to relatively mundane false memories (such as establishing plausibility, active imagination, suggestive interviewing, etc.) can also lead to the development of rich (realistic sensory detail) false autobiographical memories in a subset of study participants.

One paradigm for planting false autobiographical memories is the 'familial informant false narrative procedure' or simply the 'lost-in-the-mall' technique [33, 34]. Researchers first solicit the cooperation of a 'familial informant' (such as a parent) to ensure that a target event did not actually happen to the participant. Participants are told the family member had told researchers about several events that happened to the participant as a child. Some are true, but the target event is false. The participant may be interviewed several times about the target event, using suggestive procedures (sometimes including guided imagination). In a final session, participants report on, and describe, any memories they have developed of the target event.

Across many studies, an average of approximately 30% of subjects have developed partial or complete false memories (for reviews, see [33, 35]), varying from 0% (when an odd variation was used to attempt to plant a relatively implausible event memory) to more than 50% for more mundane events (a ride in a hot air balloon). More developed false memories either with imagination procedures included or with additional 'evidence' included (such as a doctored photo). Some develop false memories right away, whereas others begin with little memory but, after several suggestive interviews, begin to recall false events in great detail. While researchers have not attempted to plant memories of abuse, they have planted memories for highly unpleasant events such as hospitalizations, medical procedures, near drowning, or vicious animal attacks. They have also planted highly implausible memories for both mundane (for example, rubbing chalk on one's head or kissing a plastic frog) and strange or dramatic events (witnessing demonic possession as a child) (for reviews, see [17, 36]), and for personally committing specific aggressive acts [37] or crimes [38].

Notably, such false memories are consequential. Participants led to develop false beliefs or memories of being made sick by particular foods in the past avoided eating the food in follow-up assessments of a week to a month later (for example, [39, 40]).

## The path to false memory

Memory is essentially a narrative story of the event, combined with sensory images. A memory judgement criteria is applied to assess the likelihood that the 'memory' is a true memory of a real event. In part, the question of whether the 'memory' is accurate is evaluated in light of other knowledge. In part, it is evaluated in light of other criteria one may use to decide the reality of the memory, such as the clarity of the sensory images or the way it was remembered (for example, in a dream or under hypnosis). Thus, to consider how false memories might be constructed, we must consider how the narrative or images may be constructed or altered and how one's other relevant knowledge might be altered in a way favouring the validity of a new narrative, as well as how memory judgement criteria can be altered.

## Developing plausibility as the foundation for belief in the narrative

Memory is primarily semantic—the story we tell ourselves about what happened, accompanied by sensory images that become increasingly vague over time. This story is informed by other relevant knowledge suggesting that the story does or does not make sense. This knowledge can affect our interpretations of events at the time they happen and also cause them to change over time.

It is easy to see how our general knowledge and beliefs can affect the immediate interpretation of experiences. For example, shadows in one's bedroom at night might be interpreted as an alien visitation by those who believe that aliens visit the earth and make such personal visits. For those who do not possess such beliefs, the shadows are more likely to be interpreted as created by wind in the trees outside one's window.

But in a related way, they direct the development of false memories. The formation of false memories entails the construction of a narrative that is plausible in light of one's other knowledge and beliefs, including beliefs about oneself, others involved, and the way the world works. Thus, it is important to understand how a narrative involving seemingly impossible or improbable events can become plausible. Without such an element of plausibility, the person is unlikely to believe the false narrative and thus will not consider it a memory.

Regarding sexual abuse, this can happen via multiple pathways. It can begin with psychological issues leading the person to search for explanations and solutions. In the course of this search, the person may be exposed to information that increases the plausibility of: (1) repression itself; (2) sexual abuse as a cause of repression; (3) sexual abuse as a cause of symptoms such as the person is experiencing; and (4) the possibility that one could have personally experienced abuse (or that a specific person could have committed it). This can happen via exposure to media accounts of repressed and recovered memories and through exposure to self-help literature, accounts of friends or family, among many other sources.

Cultural acceptance of the trauma narrative, the idea of repression, and the link between sexual abuse and many symptoms can lend plausibility to the ideas that one may have personally been sexually abused (even in the absence of any memory of it) and that this unremembered abuse is causing most psychological/behavioural symptoms for which the person is most likely to seek psychotherapy or self-help advice. If the person sees a therapist, the therapist may further magnify the plausibility of repression and abuse narratives by actively discussing trauma and repression and/or alleged links between specific symptoms and sexual abuse or by explaining why he or she believes the patient was abused. Once beliefs linking sexual abuse, trauma, and repression are adopted, this can facilitate the formation of false memories of abuse via several mechanisms.

## Implications of fuzzy trace theory

'Fuzzy trace theory' (for example, [24]) explicates how general knowledge and beliefs can distort memories or create false memories. When one thinks about an event, both event-related images and beliefs *and* our general relevant knowledge and beliefs about such types of events and people are activated in memory. When clear verbatim sensory images (like an enhanced video) are not available to distinguish what actually happened from other information activated in memory, the person may misattribute the additional activated information from his or her general knowledge store as part of the event in question. Essentially, expectations based on our additional relevant knowledge and beliefs can result in false memories or false details, consistent with those expectations (for a review of schematic effects, see [32]).

Schemas for specific persons (oneself or others involved in the event in question) will include expectations of behaviour—how the person thinks he or she is likely to behave, as well as expectations for others' behaviour. 'Negative stereotyping' of a person suspected of CSA is commonly viewed as contributing to false memories of sexual abuse and refers to conveying information about the accused, characterizing him as the 'type of person' likely to commit abuse specifically or other damaging or aggressive acts (for example, [41]). Beliefs that sexual abuse tends to cause specific physical or psychological effects will also tend to make the belief that a person experiencing those symptoms was indeed abused more plausible.

It is easier to create false beliefs and memories if the event itself is viewed as more plausible. False memories for actions have been more easily planted in experimental subjects if the person found it plausible that he or she *would have* committed such an act (such as when a person who often behaves aggressively finds it plausible that he or she *would have* committed another aggressive act (for example, [37]). It is also easier to plant memories for things others have done if those actions are seen as plausible for the other person. Whereas it may be more difficult to plant implausible memories in many circumstances, implausibility itself is malleable [42]. For example, Mazzoni *et al.* [43] first exposed some participants to material designed to enhance the plausibility of demon possession and later attempted to plant memories of having witnessed such an event. Those exposed to the plausibility-enhancing manipulation later reported greater likelihood of having witnessed demon possession.

Many things can happen to increase the plausibility of an event. Among these is exposure to information that the type of behaviour or event in question happens relatively frequently (vs rarely) (for example, [44]) or repeatedly imagining the event in question (for example, [45]). Regarding sexual abuse, many popular books claim a high prevalence of sexual abuse and offer lists of symptoms purportedly characteristic of abuse survivors (including failure to remember the abuse) that are so inclusive as to encourage almost anyone with problems to attribute them to abuse. E. Sue Blume, in *Secret Survivors* [8], lists the most common problems for which therapy is sought: depression, addiction, phobias, sexual issues, self-destructiveness, obsessions, and countless others. It includes many opposites such as too much or too little eating, sex, sleeping, etc. It even includes failure to remember abuse as a symptom of abuse, asserting that failure to remember abuse is not evidence that one has not been abused. Such claims and lists of abuse symptoms in the survivor literature at the least make plausible that virtually any problem can be caused by sexual abuse.

Perhaps reflecting the influence of widespread depictions of abuse and repression, Rubin and Boals [46] found a relationship between self-rated likelihood of entering therapy and beliefs that one had experienced (and could not now remember) childhood trauma and abuse. Notably, such patients may influence their therapists to focus upon abuse, creating a bi-directional cycle of suggestion [17].

At some point, the person may become fully convinced that sexual abuse did occur and even develop false memories of that abuse. Kihlstrom [47] described a condition in which a person's identity, lifestyle, and interpersonal relationships are centred around an objectively false memory of traumatic experience that the person strongly believes is true. This 'false memory syndrome'—or the definition of one's identity as an abuse survivor—becomes a central aspect of relevant knowledge that serves as context for interpretation and evaluation of new information as plausible or not and as the schematic basis of memory intrusions [17].

Finally, related to the issue of plausibility, it is important to note that it is easier to convince a person that they must have done or experienced something that would otherwise seem implausible

(or to otherwise alter beliefs) if they doubt their own memories—a phenomenon Gudjonsson has dubbed 'memory distrust'. This phenomenon has been implicated in many cases of internalized false confession (that is, a confession where the person comes to believe falsely that they did commit the crime) [1, 2]. Therapeutic clients may, for various reasons, doubt the reliability of their memories and therefore be more easily convinced of things they do not initially remember.

## The role of belief: the transition from 'it could have happened' to 'it did happen'

Many false memories develop through persuasion that an event happened or happened in a particular way (for example, [17, 48, 49]). In practice, there are many pathways through which beliefs regarding sexual abuse or other seemingly implausible events can be created or altered. These include conversations with other witnesses, police, therapists, and other interviewers, exposure to media accounts, and exposure to 'evidence' that the event occurred in a particular way or was committed by a particular person. Internal processes are also important, such as attempts to reason about what must have happened or attempts to understand the 'evidence' the person is aware of. Some may interpret dreams as reflecting reality. Essentially, any source of information or argument can convince the person that a particular event, or a version of that event, is true.

Loftus and Davis [17] describe influence processes in therapy that can convince a client he or she must have been abused. This may happen at first in the absence of 'memory' of abuse. The therapist may tell clients that their symptoms suggest abuse, offer information and arguments to support the assertion, refuse to accept denials, and persist in asserting they were abused until the clients agree. These assertions can be supplemented by a variety of therapeutic procedures that appear to offer 'evidence' that clients were abused.

Evidence of many kinds can lead people to falsely believe they experienced specific autobiographical events. In the 'lost-in-the-mall' procedure, family members' assertions that an event did happen to participants as young children provided evidence crucial for the development of the many different false memories elicited through the procedure. False evidence against criminal suspects has been implicated as an important contributor to false confessions, particularly of the sort where suspects come to falsely believe (and sometimes falsely remember) that they committed the crime (for reviews, see [1, 2]). Dream interpretation suggesting that a specific type of event happened or exposure to doctored photographs depicting events that did not occur have led subjects to falsely believe and/or remember that they experienced events ranging from before the age of 3 to their recent past [36, 50].

Therapeutic techniques and persuasion can enhance belief in an event directly, by seeming to provide evidence that the event did happen. They can also do so indirectly, by making it more plausible that the event happened as believed, such as when information that a person is generally aggressive or has a criminal record can make it more plausible that he or she committed a specific aggressive act. Or information that sexual abuse is often committed by stepfathers can make it more plausible that one's own stepfather would plausibly engage in abuse.

Beliefs regarding sexual abuse can come from many sources of suggestion. These can include others who have become concerned about the possibility of abuse, others who talk to the person about the general issue of abuse or their own (or about the abuser), information acquired in sex education classes, media, etc., forensic interviewers, popular 'survivor' literature, and others.

Even the simple process of thinking about an event can make it seem more likely to have happened in the past or to happen in the future. Studies of imagination inflation have demonstrated this with a very simple procedure. Participants first rate the likelihood that specific events happened to them in the past (or will in the future). Then they imagine that event happening. Finally, they rerate the likelihood of the event's occurrence. Imagination increases the perceived likelihood that the event did (or will) happen (for example, [51]). Analogous to the process of imagination inflation, Sharman, Manning, and Garry [52] illustrated 'explanation inflation' whereby the process of explaining how or why childhood events *could have* happened leads persons to become more confident that they *did* happen. Both imagination inflation and explanation inflation have been demonstrated for a variety of past and/or future events [52].

Another laboratory procedure is analogous to situations where a therapist provides feedback to clients that their symptoms suggest abuse. Participants first rate the likelihood that certain events occurred during particular periods of their life. They then answer a series of questions (sometimes by computer) and receive false feedback that their scores indicate they experienced a particular kind of event. Sometimes this is followed by imagination procedures to picture the event in question. Finally, participants again rate the likelihood that the event actually happened and, in some studies, indicate the extent to which they recall the event. Like the imagination or explanation inflation studies, some participants in the false feedback studies develop stronger beliefs that the target event did happen and some also develop memories of the event.

Generally, procedures targeting belief that an event did occur vary in suggestiveness, with imagination/explanation procedures falling at the lower end of suggestion, false feedback studies suggesting that the person did or probably did experience the event in the middle, and those providing 'evidence' that the event did occur at the high end (such as false claims by family or doctored photos). The more suggestive procedures tend to more strongly affect belief in, and/or memories of, the suggested event (for a review, see [35]). These processes can make the event more familiar, more accessible in memory, and more fluent (easy to picture or understand), all bases upon which people judge whether or not something is or is not a memory. Moreover, the procedures can cause the person to generate images of the event that can become misinterpreted as veridical memory.

## The role of sensory images: developing what 'feels' like a memory

Most think of event memory in terms of the ability to replay sensory images of the event in one's mind. Some might not think of newly developed autobiographical beliefs as memories, until they can produce a sensory replay of the event. Sensory images are indeed one component of memory. But what is less well known is that over time, the images one associates with events can change—and even be created through a number of processes. These may consist of exposure to verbal or written accounts causing the person to generate images of the event, sensory images from other sources (such as pictures or video depictions), or internal processes such as the person's attempts to remember and picture the event or efforts to imagine how things must have happened. Some internal processes are triggered by therapeutic procedures involving active imagination/imaging (for example, guided imagery or hypnosis). Others may occur spontaneously such as dreams or sensory image associations triggered by exposure to reminders of the type of event. They may also be created through conversations with others or interviews, as described more fully in the section on suggestion.

If the person mistakenly attributes the source of such images to the experience of the original event, rather than to the real source, the images may be interpreted as a 'memory'. Indeed, a substantial body of scientific literature has shown that it is commonplace to confuse sensory images acquired independently of the original event (or any event) as 'memories' for the event in question (for reviews, see [24, 30, 51]).

With a foundation of plausibility for abuse, such misattributions become more likely. Mazzoni *et al.* [43], for example, suggested that imagination procedures can create false memories in a three-stage process by which a person first perceives the event as more plausible, then comes to believe the event actually did occur, and finally reinterprets the narrative as actual memories. Imagery is crucial to this process, in that Green and Brock [53] have shown that narratives are persuasive to the extent they evoke imagery of the event.

### Imagery in the context of suggestion

Essentially, suggestion involves any statement or action asserting or implying a particular version of an event is true or that others are not true. It may also state or imply that the speaker strongly believes what is suggested and/or the speaker strongly prefers that the listener reports a particular version of events. In effect, suggestion plants an idea in the target's mind about either what might have or probably did happen or what another person wants the target to say or do.

Suggestion can create imagery of events that did not occur and increase belief that the events did occur. Suggestion can also create expectations of more approval/reinforcement for giving specific memory reports and expectations of disapproval/punishment for continuing to give the initial report. These processes have been shown to lead to false memories and false reports of relatively trivial events in the laboratory, as well as of dramatic personal experiences among both children and adults, including false confessions to heinous crimes such as murder of one's own children, parents, siblings, and others [30, 54].

Some common therapeutic techniques are inherently suggestive or are executed in a suggestive manner. They can simultaneously encourage imagery of suggested events and increase plausibility and belief. Guided imagery, for example, may be practised alone or in the context of other suggestive techniques. It involves efforts to induce the client to picture an event through multiple sensory modalities and can involve suggestions for both focus and content. Though sufficient alone to produce false memories, false memories become more likely when guided imagery is combined with other suggestive techniques. Herndon and colleagues [55] tested combined effects of guided imagery and an analogue to survivor group therapy. Each increased false memories and participants' confidence in the memories they reported. But when exposed to both, fully 75%

of participants developed false memories for a suggested early childhood medical procedure (compared to 5% among those exposed to neither and 41–50% among those exposed to one source of suggestion) (for a demonstration of additive effects of guided imagery, peer pressure, and repeated interviewing, see [56]).

One frequently practised memory recovery technique is hypnosis, often used in conjunction with guided imagery or efforts towards age or past life regression. Though hypnosis does increase the amount recalled, even without suggestion, much new information is false. But unless carefully trained otherwise, therapists can be very suggestive with their hypnotic subjects—both through suggested focus and content and through selective reinforcement of expected reports of abuse, satanic ritual abuse, alien abduction, womb, birth, infantile, or past life experiences, etc. They may also be suggestive through directed imagery such as when therapists instruct clients to change the view of the 'camera' of memory to focus on a person, action, or location not originally noticed. This not only suggests memory content but also suggests unrealistic processes and abilities of memory. Given widespread public and professional beliefs in the ability of hypnosis to enhance recall, it is not surprising that both place greater confidence in memories recovered under hypnosis (for reviews, see [57–59]). The role of hypnosis in false memories appears to be, in part, rooted in the vulnerability of those who are hypnotized, in that hypnotizability itself is related to vulnerability to development of false memories [60].

These are only a few among many techniques that can alter the components of memory (plausibility, narrative, images, etc.). Others include survivor group participation, journaling and other 'homework', and eye movement desensitization and reprocessing (EMDR)—and even use of drugs such as sodium pentothal [3, 17, 18].

Finally, related to the adoption of a 'survivor' identity, some research has shown that when led under hypnosis to believe in characterizations of themselves that were inconsistent with their current identities, participants have shown selective attention to, and enhanced memory for, other information consistent with the new characterizations. In addition, they tended to perceive information consistent with the new characterizations as more self-relevant and personally meaningful and to more easily access autobiographical information consistent with the new characterizations. These accessed memories often entail a reinterpretation of previous experiences that seemed to verify the new characterizations (for a review, see [58]).

## The role of a memory judgement criterion

An additional step in the development of consequential false memories is that the person must apply one or more criteria to assess whether a new narrative is a memory of a real event.

Generally, the stronger the verbatim images or gist traces and the weaker the memory judgement criterion, the more likely a particular narrative is to be judged a memory. Verbatim images developed and strengthened through the many processes described thus far can be sufficiently vivid and detailed to pass even the most stringent memory judgement criterion. Gist traces (an abuse narrative) can likewise be strengthened by processes such as imagination, exposure to plausibility-enhancing information, the development of

abuse-related personal identities, and others. The more plausible the narrative in light of the person's general knowledge and beliefs, or the more information of any kind that appears consistent with the narrative in question, the more likely it will be judged an actual memory. Moreover, the sense of familiarity with an image or narrative, which grows stronger the more it is discussed or brought to mind, can be interpreted as memory.

Neither the strength of verbatim and gist traces or their plausibility nor their familiarity are necessary criteria for a person to conclude the memory is real, however. Loftus and Davis [17] described in detail the way in which the criteria one uses to assess whether or not a memory is real may be highly variable and malleable. Some people may require of themselves that they have very clear sensory images of an event in order to interpret or report it as a memory. Others may consider beliefs without images or very vague images to be memories.

These and other memory judgement criteria are malleable and can exert significant influence on reports and behaviour. Some therapists and survivor literature encourage beliefs that dreams can be verbatim replays of actual events, and therefore that a specific dream is a memory of a real event. But given that dreams are most likely to reflect daily events and what is on one's mind, a person who is exposed to content about abuse or who is thinking a great deal about abuse might dream about abuse for that reason. Beaulieu-Prevost and Zadra [61] provide a recent review of research showing that dreams are a common source of false memories and addressing the conditions under which dreams are most likely to be interpreted as memories, even in the absence of suggestion (and they further demonstrated that false memories for dreams themselves can be planted).

Other therapy-related beliefs promote very liberal memory judgement criteria that can lead clients to classify a variety of questionable experiences as true event memories. For example, Francine Shapiro's book [62] on EMDR states that any memory that emerges during EMDR is, in fact, true. A therapist may also encourage the belief, already prevalent among laypersons, that all memories that emerge during hypnosis are true. Some therapists and survivor literature have also promoted the belief that bodily sensations are 'body memories' of abuse (for example, [63]).

Bass and Davis [7] discussed body memories and promoted liberal memory judgement criteria: 'You may have forgotten large chunks of your childhood … yet there are things you do remember. When you are touched in a certain way, you feel nauseated' (p. 22). The authors suggested that although memories might be hazy, dream-like, or fragmentary, this was not evidence of inauthenticity: 'if you … have a feeling that something happened to you, it probably did' (p. 21). Though the authors recounted stories of those who doubted their new memories, or explicitly said they knew they were not real, they also suggested these feelings did not justify discounting the memories: 'It's natural that you have periodic doubts … But that's because accepting memories is painful, not because you weren't abused' (p. 86).

Beliefs that bodily sensations can be, or reflect, traumatic event memories are widespread among practising therapists, laypersons, and students. From one-third to over three-quarters of therapists in the United States and Canada report beliefs that body pains and other physical symptoms are symptoms of sexual abuse and/or that sensory impressions from early life can represent reliable memories that can be recovered (for a review, see [64]). Therapists adopting such beliefs may tell patients that a particular bodily sensation is, or reflects, a memory of abuse and thereby justify a series of suggestive therapeutic procedures to unearth a more explicit narrative or sensory 'memory'.

## Summary

Influences that can distort or fabricate memories are well established within the scientific literature. Remaining controversy concerns the nature of events for which false memories can be created. Some argue that memories for traumatic events cannot be planted and laboratory studies of less dramatic false memories are not applicable to sexual abuse. Nevertheless, many accounts of 'retractors' (those who reported recovered memories and later recanted them) have suggested that indeed false memories for horrific forms of abuse can be planted (for reviews, see [17, 18]).

While laboratory studies are limited by ethical constraints to avoid attempts to create potentially very consequential false memories, a substantial and growing literature has demonstrated that false memories for a variety of relatively dramatic, sometimes scary, autobiographical events can be planted in mentally healthy participants across the lifespan. And they can be planted by means of procedures used within therapy (such as dream interpretation, hypnosis, guided imagery, and others) or practised by the person (active imagination, reading survivor literature, exposure to abuse accounts in media, and others). Together with suggestion (that abuse may have, or must have, taken place) and loosening of memory judgement criteria, such procedures greatly increase the likelihood of the development of false memories of sexual abuse, satanic ritual abuse, or other seemingly implausible events.

## Conclusions

Although our view is that evidence for massive repression is lacking, by endorsing this conclusion, we in no way deny the reality of sexual abuse. All parties in this controversy can appreciate the widespread nature of the problem and the severity of the consequences for many victims. However, we suggest two important conclusions.

Firstly, claims of repressed and recovered memories are inherently suspect. The repression hypothesis has itself proven difficult, and some believe virtually impossible, to test. And it is fundamentally incompatible in many respects with the science of memory. Moreover, a very large and growing scientific literature has shown that common therapeutic procedures and other influences can distort memories or lead to the development of fully fabricated false memories of sexual abuse and other dramatic and/or traumatic life events.

When such claims are litigated, at the very least they should be given significantly reduced weight. There are two possible explanations for a subjectively 'recovered' memory: (1) that the memory is real, that it has indeed been repressed for as long as decades, and that it has now been recovered intact; or (2) that the memory was at best distorted—or at worst entirely fabricated—through processes shown across many scientific studies to have such effects. Even continuous memories, whether reported immediately after an event or significantly later, can be distorted. Memories can also be totally confabulated, even if no claim of repression or suspect

memory recovery procedures are involved. But when there is a claim of repression, and particularly when the claimant has been subject to influences shown to distort or fabricate memories, research suggests the claim must be given reduced weight, if not fully discounted. A plausible explanation, one that is arguably much more plausible than the reality of the memory, exists for where the memory came from (for reviews of legal issues entailed in the recovered memory debate, see [65–67]).

Secondly, research suggests that some therapeutic practices should be avoided—prominently direct suggestions and arguments to clients claiming that they have likely been sexually abused, particularly in the absence of clients' initial memories of abuse or in the face of an absolute denial. Also undesirable are focusing therapy on the issue of abuse with such clients, using memory recovery procedures within therapy focused upon retrieval of memories of abuse, and recommendations for outside activities focused on recovery of such memories (such as reading abuse centred self-help literature, participation in survivor groups, and other 'homework'). These are all procedures known to increase the risk of memory distortion and fabrication [17, 18, 68].

These recommendations may be controversial, since despite the highly publicized nature of the controversy, belief in repression remains widespread within the therapeutic community and among some clinical or memory scientists (for surveys assessing such beliefs, see [64, 69]). Many popular therapies endorse the idea of memory 'recovery' and include techniques for that purpose, for example EMDR, sensorimotor psychotherapy, somatic experiencing therapy, neurolinguistic programming, alien abduction therapy, internal family systems therapy, and others [64]. Many therapists incorporate one or more practices that increase the risks of false memory development. Beliefs supporting such practices are likely to remain widespread for some time to come.

Our hope and expectation is that researchers will continue the rapid development of new research and paradigms to inform the disputed issues and to discourage practices with known risks. While many false memories may be benign, those regarding sexual abuse are highly consequential and toxic for both the accused and the accuser.

Finally, we hope that better education of professionals and the public will improve understanding of memory and that this education will provide inoculation against many faulty claims prevalent in popular culture. Although some widely held beliefs are correct, many respondents across varied populations have endorsed beliefs diametrically opposed to the actual operation of memory (for a review, see [64]).

## REFERENCES

1. Gudjonsson, G. H., Sigurdsson, J. F., Sigurdardottir, A. S., Steinthorsson, H., and Sigurdardottir, M. (2014). The role of memory distrust in cases of internalized false confession. *Applied Cognitive Psychology*, 28, 336–48.
2. Kassin, S. M. (2007). Internalized false confessions. In: M. P. Toglia, J. D. Read, D. F. Ross, and R. C. L. Lindsay (eds). *The Handbook of Eyewitness Psychology, Vol I: Memory for events.* Mahwah, NJ: Lawrence Erlbaum Associates Publishers; pp. 175–92.
3. Beck, R. (2015). *We Believe the Children: A Moral Panic in the 80s.* New York, NY: Public Affairs Books.

4. Clancy, S. A. (2009). *The Trauma Myth: The Truth About the Sexual Abuse of Children—and its Aftermath*. New York, NY: Basic Books.

5. Barr, R. (1991). A star cries incest. *People*, 36 (13); 7 October 1991.

6. Van Derbur Atler, M. (1991). The darkest secret. *People*, 35 (22); 10 June 1991.

7. Bass, E. and Davis, L. (1988). *The Courage to Heal: A Guide for Women Survivors of Child Sexual Abuse*. New York, NY: Perennial Library/Harper and Row.

8. Blume, E. S. (1998). *Secret Survivors: Uncovering Incest and its Aftereffects in Women*. New York, NY: Ballantine Books.

9. Frederickson, R. (1992). *Repressed Memories: A Journey to Recovery From Sexual Abuse*. New York, NY: Simon and Schuster.

10. Howe, M. L. and Knott, L. M. (2015). The fallibility of memory in judicial processes: lessons from the past and their modern consequences. *Memory*, 23, 633–56.

11. Breuer, J. and Freud, S. (1893). On the psychical mechanism of hysterical phenomena: preliminary communication. In: J. Strachey (ed. and trans, 1955). *The Standard Edition of the Complete Psychological Works of Sigmund Freud*, Vol. 2. London: Hogarth Press; pp. 3–17.

12. Breuer, J. and Freud, S. (1895). Studies on hysteria. In: J. Strachey (ed. and trans, 1955). *The Standard Edition of the Complete Psychological Works of Sigmund Freud*, Vol. 2. London: Hogarth Press; pp. 1–335.

13. Brown, D., Scheflin, A. W., and Hammond, D. C. (1998). *Memory, Trauma Treatment, and the Law*. New York, NY: WW Norton.

14. Freyd, J. J. (1996). *Betrayal Trauma: The Logic of Forgetting Childhood Abuse*. Cambridge, MA: Harvard University Press.

15. Borch-Jacobsen, M. (2009). *Making Minds and Madness: From Hysteria to Depression*. Cambridge: Cambridge University Press.

16. Terr, L. (1991). Childhood traumas: an outline and overview. *American Journal of Psychiatry*, 148, 10–20.

17. Loftus, E. F. and Davis, D. (2006). Recovered memories. *Annual Review of Clinical Psychology*, 2, 469–98.

18. McNally, R. J. (2003). *Remembering Trauma*. Cambridge, MA: Harvard University Press.

19. Sotgiu, I. and Rusconi, M. L. (2014). Why autobiographical memories for traumatic and emotional events might differ: theoretical arguments and empirical evidence. *Journal of Psychology*, 148, 523–47.

20. Anderson, M. C. and Huddleston, E. (2012). Towards a cognitive and neurobiologial model of motivated forgetting. In: R. F. Belli (ed.). *True and False Recovered Memories: Toward a Reconciliation of the Debate*. New York, NY: Springer; pp. 53–120.

21. DePrince, A. P., Brown, L. S., Cheit, R. E., *et al.* (2012). Motivated forgetting and misremembering: perspectives from betrayal trauma theory. In: R. F. Belli (ed.). *True and False Recovered Memories: Toward a Reconciliation of the Debate*. New York, NY: Springer; pp. 193–242.

22. Davis, D. and Loftus, E. F. (2009). The scientific basis of testimony regarding recovered memories of sexual abuse. In: K. S. Douglas, J. L. Skeem, and S. O. Lilienfeld (eds.). *Psychological Science in the Courtroom: Controversies and Consensus*. New York, NY: Guilford Press; pp. 55–79.

23. Ost, J., Costall, A., and Bull, R. (2002). A perfect symmetry? A study of retractors' experiences of making and then repudiating claims of early sexual abuse. *Psychology, Crime, and Law*, 8, 155–81.

24. Brainerd, C. J. and Reyna, V. F. (2005). *The Science of False Memory*. New York, NY: Oxford University Press.

25. Loftus, E. F. and Ketcham, K. (1994). *The Myth of Repressed Memory: False Memories and Allegations of Sexual Abuse*. New York NY: St. Martin's Griffin.

26. Jelicic, M., Smeets, T., Peters, M. J. V., Candel, I., Horselenberg, R., and Merckelbach, H. (2006). Assassination of a controversial politician: remembering details from another non-existent film. *Applied Cognitive Psychology*, 20, 591–6.

27. Clancy, S. (2005). *Abducted: How People Come to Believe They Were Abducted by Aliens*. Cambridge, MA: Harvard University Press.

28. Crombag, H. F. M., Wagenaar, W. A., and Van Koppen, P. J. (1996). Crashing memories and the problem of source monitoring. *Applied Cognitive Psychology*, 10, 95–104.

29. Wright, L. (1994). *Remembering Satan*. New York, NY: Vintage Books.

30. Davis, D. and Loftus, E. F. (2007). Internal and external sources of misinformation in adult witness memory. In: M. P. Toglia, J. D. Read, D. F. Ross, and R. C. L. Lindsay (eds.). *Handbook of Eyewitness Psychology: Memory for Events* (Vol. l). Mahwah, NJ: Erlbaum; pp. 195–237.

31. Patihis, L., Frenda, S. J., LePort, A. K. R., *et al.* (2013). False memories in highly superior autobiographical memory individuals. *Proceedings of the National Academy of Sciences of the United States*, 110, 20947–52.

32. Wyer, R. S. (2004). *Social Comprehension and Judgment: The Role of Situation Models, Narratives, and Implicit Theories*. Mahwah, NJ: Erlbaum.

33. Lindsay, D. S., Hagen, L, Read, J. D., Wade, K. A., and Garry, M. (2004). True photographs and false memories. *Psychological Science*, 15, 149–54.

34. Loftus, E. F. and Pickrell, J. E. (1995). The formation of false memories. *Psychiatric Annals*, 25, 720–5.

35. Brewin, C. R. and Andrews, B. (2017). Creating memories for false autobiographical events in childhood: a systematic review. *Applied Cognitive Psychology*, 31, 2–23.

36. Loftus, E. F. (2003). Make-believe memories. *American Psychologist*, 58, 864–73.

37. Laney, C. and Takarangi, M. K. T. (2013). False memories for aggressive acts. *Acta Psychologica*, 143, 227–34.

38. Shaw, J. and Porter, S. (2015). Constructing rich false memories of committing crime. *Psychological Science*, 26, 291–301.

39. Geraerts, E., Bernstein, D., Merckelbach, H., Linders, C., Raymaekers, L., and Loftus, E. F. (2008). Lasting false beliefs and their behavioral consequences. *Psychological Science*, 19, 749–53.

40. Scorboria, A., Mazzoni, G., Jarry, J. L., and Bernstein, D. M. (2012). Personalized and not general suggestion produces false autobiographical memories and suggestion-consistent behavior. *Acta Psychologica*, 139, 225–32.

41. O'Donohue, W. T., Benuto, L., and Fanetti, M. (2010). Children's allegation of sexual abuse: a model for forensic assessment. *Psychological Injury and Law*, 3, 148–54.

42. Hyman, I. E. and Loftus, E. F. (2002) False childhood memories and eyewitness memory errors. In: M. L. Eisen, J. A. Quas, and G. S. Goodman (eds.). *Memory and Suggestibility in the Forensic Interview*. Mahwah, NJ: Erlbaum; pp. 63–84.

43. Mazzoni, G. A. L., Loftus, E. F., and Kirsch, I. (2001). Changing beliefs about implausible autobiographical events: a little plausibility goes along way. *Journal of Experimental Psychology: Applied*, 7, 51–9.

44. Golde, C. V., Sharman, S. J., and Candel, I. (2010). High prevalence information from different sources affects the development of false beliefs. *Applied Cognitive Psychology*, 24, 152–63.

45. Bays, B., Zabrucky, K. M., and Gagne, P. (2012). When plausibility manipulations work: an examination of their role in
the development of false beliefs and memories. *Memory*, 20,
638–44.

46. Rubin, D. C. and Boals, A. (2010). People who expect to enter
psychotherapy are prone to believing that they have forgotten
memories of childhood trauma and abuse. *Memory*, 18, 556–62.

47. Kihlstrom J. F. (1998). Exhumed memory. In: K. M. McConkey
(ed.). *Truth in Memory*. New York, NY: Guilford; pp. 3–31.

48. Leding, J. K. (2012). False memories and persuasion strategies.
*Review of General Psychology*, 16, 256–68.

49. Nash, R. A., Wheeler, R. L., and Hope, L. (2015). On the persuad-
ability of memory: is changing people's memories no more than
changing their minds? *British Journal of Psychology*, 106, 308–26.

50. Mazzoni, G. A. L., Loftus, E. F., Seitz, A, and Lynn, S. J. (1999).
Creating a new childhood: changing beliefs and memories
through dream interpretation. *Applied Cognitive Psychology*, 13,
125–44.

51. Mazzoni, G. A. L. and Memon, A. (2003). Imagination can
create false autobiographical memories. *Psychological Science*,
14, 186–8.

52. Sharman, S. J., Manning, C. G., and Garry, M. (2004). Explain
this: explaining childhood events inflates confidence for those
events. *Applied Cognitive Psychology*, 19, 67–74.

53. Green, M. C. and Brock, T. C. (2002). In the mind's
eye: transportation-imagery model of narrative persuasion. In: M. C. Green, J. J. Strange, and T. C. Brock (eds.).
*Narrative Impact: Social and Cognitive Foundations*. New York,
NY: Psychology Press; pp. 313–42.

54. Davis, D. and O'Donohue, W. T. (2004). The road to perdi-
tion: 'extreme influence' tactics in the interrogation room. In: W.
T. O'Donohue and E. Levensky (eds.). *Handbook of Forensic
Psychology*. New York, NY: Elsevier Academic Press; pp. 897–996.

55. Herndon, P, Myers, B., Mitchell, K., Kehn, A., and Henry, S.
(2014). False memories for highly aversive early childhood
events: effects of guided imagery and group influence. *Psychology
of Consciousness: Theory, Research Practice*, 1, 20–31.

56. Bruck, M., Hembrooke, H., and Ceci, S. (1997). Children's reports
of pleasant and unpleasant events. In: J. Read and D. Lindsay
(eds.). *Recollections of Trauma: Scientific Evidence and Clinical
Practice*. New York, NY: Plenum Press; pp. 199–219.

57. Mazzoni, G. A. L. and Lynn, S. J. (2007). Using hypnosis in
eyewitness memory: past and current issues. In: M. P. Toglia,

J. D. Read, D. R. Ross, and R. C. L. Lindsay (eds.). *Handbook
of Eyewitness Memory: Memory for Events* (Vol. 1). Mahwah,
NJ: Erlbaum; pp. 323–38.

58. Mazzoni, G., Laurence, J.-R., and Heap, M. (2014). Hypnosis
and memory: two hundred years of adventures and still going.
*Psychology of Consciousness: Theory, Research, and Practice*, 1,
153–67.

59. Patihis, L. and Burton, H. J. Y. (2015). False memories in therapy
and hypnosis before 1980. *Psychology of Consciousness: Theory,
Research, and Practice*, 2, 153–69.

60. Dasse, M. N., Elkins, G. R., and Weaver III, C. A. (2015).
Hypnotizability, not suggestion influences false memory de-
velopment. *International Journal of Clinical and Experimental
Hypnosis*, 63, 110–28.

61. Beaulieu-Prevost, D. and Zadra, A. (2015). When people remember dreams they never experienced: a study of the malle-
ability of dream recall over time. *Dreaming*, 25, 18–31.

62. Shapiro, F. (2001). *Eye Movement Desensitization and
Reprocessing (EMDR): Basic Principles, Protocols, and Procedures*
(2nd edn). New York, NY: Guilford Press.

63. van der Kolk, B. A. (1994). The body keeps the score: memory
and the evolving psychobiology of posttraumatic stress. *Harvard
Review of Psychiatry*, 1, 253–65.

64. Lynn, S. J., Evans, J., Laurence, J.-R., Lilienfeld, S. O. (2015).
What do people believe about memory? Implications for the sci-
ence and pseudoscience of clinical practice. *Canadian Journal of
Psychiatry*, 60, 541–7.

65. Milchman, M. S. (2012). From traumatic memory to traumatized remembering: beyond the memory wars, Part 1: agreement.
*Psychological Injury and Law*, 5, 37–50.

66. Milchman, M. S. (2012). From traumatic memory to traumatized
remembering: beyond the memory wars, Part 2: disagreement.
*Psychological Injury and Law*, 5, 51–62.

67. Milchman, M. S. (2012). From traumatic memory to traumatized
remembering: beyond the memory wars, Part 3: an integrative
schema. *Psychological Injury and Law*, 5, 63–70.

68. Follette, W. C. and Davis, D. (2008). Clinical practice and the
issue of repressed memories: avoiding an ice patch on the
slippery slope. In: W. T. O'Donohue and S. Graybar (eds.).
*Handbook of Contemporary Psychotherapy: Toward an Improved
Understanding of Effective Psychotherapy*. Thousand Oaks,
CA: Sage; pp. 47–73.

69. Patihis, L., Ho, L. Y., Tingen, I. W., Lilienfeld, S. O., and Loftus, E.
F. (2014). Are the 'memory wars' over? A scientist-practitioner
gap in beliefs about repressed memory. *Psychological Science*, 25,
519–30.

# SECTION 14
# Anxiety disorders

# 86

# Core dimensions of anxiety disorders

*Nastassja Koen and Dan J. Stein*

## Introduction

Contemporary clinical approaches to anxiety disorders are based on a categorical approach. The *Diagnostic and Statistical Manual of Mental Disorders*, third edition (DSM-III) [1] provided a key impetus to the field by providing operational diagnostic criteria for a range of different anxiety disorders and by clearly demarcating these conditions from normal anxiety responses. Subsequent decades saw progress in delineating the neurobiology of each of the anxiety disorders, as well as the introduction of specific pharmacotherapies and psychotherapies for the treatment of generalized anxiety disorder, panic disorder, specific phobia, and social anxiety disorder.

However, several factors have also suggested the value of a return to a more dimensional approach to anxiety. First, there is significant comorbidity among the anxiety disorders, and the severity of anxiety symptoms in community and clinical symptoms falls on a continuum [2]. Second, psychobiological research has emphasized that multiple genes of small effect and perhaps common environmental factors are implicated in anxiety disorders, and that overlapping neural circuits and molecular mechanisms underpin these conditions [3]. Third, there is overlap in interventions for anxiety disorders, and there is value in a transdiagnostic approach to treatment [4].

It is important to emphasize that categorical and dimensional approaches can readily complement each other [5–7]. Any dimensional variable can be split to form categories, and categorical constructs can be evaluated with dimensional measures. Categorical constructs may have significant clinical utility, facilitating decision-making and treatment, while dimensional constructs may be particularly important in research settings where fine delineation of underlying mechanisms is needed to advance diagnostic validity. Still, while categorical and dimensional approaches are complementary, it is timely to focus here on dimensions.

This chapter will provide a theoretical basis for approaching the psychobiological dimensions that underpin the anxiety disorders. We first begin with a brief description of categorical approaches. We then outline, in turn, dimensional approaches to the assessment of anxiety, the range of mechanisms underlying anxiety disorders, and transdiagnostic approaches to treatment. Subsequent chapters in this section of the volume will provide additional detail on each of these topics (for example, see Chapters 80, 87, 89, 90, and 92).

## Categorical approaches

DSM-II [8] was strongly influenced by the psychodynamic theory and described a number of categories of neuroses, including hysterical neurosis (modifiable symptoms symbolized underlying conflicts), phobic neurosis (fears are displaced from a focus unknown to the patient, to a phobic object), neurasthenic neurosis (characterized by somatic symptoms such as chronic weakness), obsessive–compulsive neurosis, and depressive neurosis. These were viewed as predominantly characterized by anxiety, which produced a range of symptoms (for example, anxious over-concern, panic, somatic manifestations) and which were experienced as subjective distress from which relief was desired [9]. The *International Classification of Diseases*, ninth revision (ICD-9) chapter on neurotic disorders similarly covers a fairly broad range of conditions [10].

DSM-III attempted to take a more atheoretical stance to classification, introducing a chapter on anxiety disorders and providing operational diagnostic criteria for each of these conditions [1]. DSM-III anxiety disorders included agoraphobia, generalized anxiety disorder, obsessive–compulsive disorder (OCD), panic disorder, post-traumatic stress disorder, simple phobia, and social phobia. DSM-IV also emphasized that panic attacks could occur in a range of different anxiety disorders and introduced the constructs of acute stress disorder, anxiety disorders due to a general medical condition, and substance-induced anxiety disorder [11]. The ICD-10 chapter on 'neurotic, stress-related, and somatoform disorders' includes these various conditions, as well as a number of additional disorders [12].

In DSM-5 [13] and ICD-11, the category of anxiety disorders has continued to evolve. The development of DSM-5 saw a strong focus on diagnostic validity and the inclusion of neuroscientific data, while the development of ICD-11 has emphasized the issue of clinical utility and considerations of public mental health [14, 15]. Both classification systems have now removed obsessive–compulsive and related disorders and trauma- and stressor-related conditions from the anxiety disorders, and placed them in separate chapters. At the same time, in both classification systems, the new chapters remain adjacent to that on anxiety disorders, and the overlap in their symptomatology is emphasized.

Fear may be described as 'an emotional response to perceived imminent threat or danger associated with urges to flee or fight' [13]. This 'fight-or-flight response' is characterized by an increased startle reaction and physiological autonomic alterations [16, 17]. In contrast, anxiety is 'the apprehensive anticipation of future danger or misfortune accompanied by a feeling of worry, distress, and/or somatic symptoms of tension. The focus of anticipated danger may be internal or external' [13]. From an evolutionary perspective, fear and anxiety appear to be adaptive responses [18]; and in the clinical setting, it is important to differentiate normal functional anxiety from pathological dysfunctional anxiety.

Since the fourth edition of the DSM, the differentiation of normal and pathological anxiety is crucially dependent on the clinical criterion; disorders are characterized by clinical distress or by significant impairment [19]. The field is unfortunately unable to rely on biomarkers for this differentiation [20]. Instead, clinical judgement is key; considerations such as duration and persistence, frequency or intensity of symptoms, disproportionality of symptoms (given the context), and pervasiveness of symptom expression across contexts all point to evidence of underlying dysfunction and so help differentiate normal and pathological anxiety [21].

## Dimensional approaches to anxiety assessment

Although current psychiatric classification systems primarily employ categorical constructs, it is notable that during the development of DSM-5, significant emphasis was placed on dimensional assessments of anxiety disorders [2]. Partly as a result, DSM-5 includes cross-cutting questions to assess anxiety symptoms, emphasizes that panic attacks may occur in a range of anxiety and other disorders, and underscores the value of assessing anxiety severity in depression [13]. In this section, we focus on a number of non-diagnostic constructs that are relevant to the dimensional assessments of anxiety: behavioural inhibition (BI), anxiety sensitivity (AS), and neuroticism.

### Behavioural inhibition

BI is a heritable temperamental trait characterized by restraint, caution, or fearfulness and withdrawal in response to unfamiliar or novel people, stimuli, or situations [22, 23]. Approximately 15–20% of young children are born with marked BI, which is usually identified early in life when children transition from the normative developmental stage of 'stranger anxiety' and begin to adapt behaviourally to threat stimuli [24, 25, 26]. The temperamental bias categorizing BI may be underpinned by varying responses to novel stimuli by the amygdala [22]. For example, adults previously categorized as behaviourally inhibited in childhood have been found to demonstrate greater amygdala response to novel (vs familiar) faces, when compared to non-behaviourally inhibited controls [27].

Behaviourally inhibited children appear to be at increased risk of developing anxiety disorders in adulthood, particularly social anxiety disorder (SAD) [23, 28]. In their recent meta-analysis, Clauss and Blackford [26] found that BI was associated with a clear increase in the risk of developing SAD (OR = 7.59). This risk remained significant after considering individual study differences in phenotype assessment, parental risk, age of anxiety diagnosis, and other potential confounders.

The conceptualization of BI as a variant of normal (i.e. a temperament) emphasizes the value of a dimensional approach to the spectrum of normal and pathological anxiety. In particular

environments, BI may have adaptive value [29], but increased BI may also increase sensitivity to the development of anxiety disorders. Further work is needed on how particular environments may intersect with BI to increase the risk for such conditions [30, 31]. Research elucidating the neurobiological underpinning of BI, as well as its role in predicting adult anxiety, may ultimately inform primary prevention tools to identify BI in children and to pre-empt the development of subsequent SAD.

### Anxiety sensitivity

AS is the fear of anxiety-related sensations, based on the belief that such sensations are harmful [32, 33]. AS may be conceptualized as an 'anxiety amplifier' [33], which increases arousal-related sensations, thus worsening anxiety in affected individuals. Individuals with AS are at increased risk of developing anxiety symptoms, particularly those pertaining to panic [34]. One meta-analysis [35] reported greater AS among patients diagnosed with an anxiety disorder vs non-clinical control participants. Further, panic disorder was found to be associated with greater AS, compared to the other anxiety disorders (with the exception of PTSD).

AS is widely believed to comprise three interrelated phenotypic concerns: physical, cognitive, and social [33, 36]. The aetiology of these dimensions may be influenced by additive genetic and/or cumulative environmental effects. Preliminary evidence suggests that AS is heritable in women [33, 37], which may be attributable to hormonally driven gene expression [38].

The Anxiety Sensitivity Index (ASI) [39] is the most widely used tool to assess AS. The ASI comprises 16 items to ascertain an individual's beliefs about the sequelae of anxiety-related sensations. Again, it is possible that AS and other markers of risk for the development of anxiety disorders could be screened for, and in those at high risk, preventive interventions could be developed and investigated.

### Neuroticism

Neuroticism—a personality trait predisposing individuals to higher negative affect—has been rigorously studied for several decades and has been strongly associated with common mental disorders (CMDs) in general and internalizing disorders, including anxiety disorders, in particular [40, 41]. This association is consistent with Clark and Watson's [42] influential tripartite model which suggested that high negative affect is common to both anxiety and depression (with physiological hyperarousal specific to anxiety, and anhedonia specific to depression). Indeed, an early proposal for DSM-5 was for an emotional cluster of disorders characterized by negative affectivity [43].

A causative model would predict that shared genetic and environmental factors lead to both neuroticism and internalizing disorders [44]. In confirmation, a large population-based twin study found that genetic factors common to neuroticism accounted for up to half of the genetic risk across internalizing disorders [45]. This genetic overlap may also help to account for the extensive comorbidity among the internalizing disorders. Indeed, in their recent meta-analysis of genome-wide linkage scans of anxiety-related phenotypes [46], Webb and colleagues reported a high global correlation between neuroticism and anxiety disorders.

A cross-cutting dimensional (rather than categorical) approach to assessing neuroticism [2] may be useful for the assessment of both anxiety and non-anxiety disorders, and there are well-validated scales for the assessment of neuroticism [44, 47].

## Mechanisms underlying anxiety disorders

### Animal models of fear

Pathological anxiety is often characterized by more rapid attentional threat engagement, elevated stress reactivity to potentially threatening stimuli, threat-based assessment of ambiguous stimuli, and impaired disengagement and avoidance of threat stimuli [48–50]. Further, increased amygdala responses to threat stimuli are often noted in pathological anxiety [50]. Fear conditioning and extinction have long been used to develop translational models of anxiety, as discussed in detail in Chapter 87. The amygdala and prefrontal areas of the brain are key components of the neurocircuitry underlying fear conditioning and extinction [51, 52] (see Chapter 90).

### Research Doman Criteria approach

The Research Domain Criteria (RDoC) approach [49, 53–55]—developed by the NIMH and described in detail in Chapter 8—is informed by a translational formulation of anxiety disorders as arising from neurobiological, cognitive–affective, and neural circuit dysfunction. This model represents anxiety disorders (and indeed all mental disorders) on a continuum, and not as discrete entities that are separate from mental health and well-being. In contrast to the categorical DSM approach (see Chapter 7), the RDoC approach presents a matrix of key behavioural dimensions or 'domains' (represented by rows), as well as a number of analytical tools, as follows (Fig. 86.1) [56]:

- Rows (domains of function): negative valence systems, positive valence systems, cognitive systems, social processes, arousal/regulatory systems, sensorimotor systems.
- Columns (modes of analyses): genes, molecules, cells, circuits, physiology, behaviour, self-report, paradigms.

Thus, psychiatric symptoms represent variation (deviation) in normal traits (ranging from normal to abnormal functioning) across one or more of the RDoC's functional domains. Currently, the RDoC model holds promise as a research framework for the dimensional assessment of anxiety disorders, rather than as a diagnostic tool. Ultimately, such models—in conjunction with categorical diagnoses that remain integral to clinical practice—may assist in incorporating advances in neurogenetics, behavioural science, and the neurosciences, thus allowing the translation of basic work into clinically useful constructs.

While quite promising as an approach to anxiety disorders, RDoC constructs are potentially no less complex than clinical disorders [57]. Further, the RDoC model has been criticized for an overly reductionist approach to psychiatric disorders, emphasizing the pathophysiological role of discrete neurocircuits and ignoring a range of other possible approaches to the conceptualization of mental illness [58].

### Transdiagnostic neural circuitry

Human functional imaging studies have built on the basic constructs of fear conditioning and extinction to address anxiety-related symptoms and behaviours (see Chapter 90). Broadly, such neuroimaging studies have suggested involvement of the insula, periaqueductal (PA) grey matter, and hypothalamus—which together are responsible for registering negative stimuli, processing resultant emotions, and autonomic regulation—in the neurocircuitry of fear and anxiety [59]. Further, amygdala hyperactivity has been found in response to disorder-specific stimuli in social phobia, specific phobia, and PTSD [60–63].

There are fewer data on the role of the amygdala in panic disorder and generalized anxiety disorder, and OCD and related syndromes are likely underpinned by dysfunctional cortico-striato-thalamo-cortical (CSTC) circuitry (see Chapters 93–100). Nonetheless, hyperactivity of the amygdala in human subjects with certain anxiety disorders is consistent with the neurocircuitry of fear conditioning proposed in animal studies.

In summary, a transdiagnostic neural circuit network, informed by classical fear conditioning paradigms, may underlie a number of the commonly occurring anxiety disorders [64, 65]. Specific functional and structural abnormalities in this large-scale neural circuit may result in biotypes which not only differ from traditional categorical DSM diagnoses, but also overlap, intersect, and interact [66]. Further delineation and validation of this network may be of value in informing novel diagnostic and therapeutic interventions for anxiety disorders, thus potentially bridging the gap between neuroscientific advances and clinical practice and perhaps even ultimately contributing towards precision medicine in psychiatry.

### Transdiagnostic neurogenetics

Genetic epidemiological studies have reported anxiety disorders to be moderately heritable, with heritability estimates ranging from 30% to 50% [67]. Further, genetic factors underlying anxiety disorders may be correlated with those underlying related phenotypes such as neuroticism [46] and may be transdiagnostic. Thus, 'overlapping genes' may account partially for the lifetime co-occurrence both of anxiety disorders and of related phenotypes. A detailed update on the genetics of anxiety and stress disorders is found in Chapters 80 and 89. However, a brief summary of the major findings will illuminate the dimensional issues described here.

Candidate gene association studies have suggested a number of genes that may be involved in increasing vulnerability both to normal anxiety traits and to pathological anxiety, including those in the serotonergic (for example, 5-HTT), noradrenergic (for example, COMT), and hypothalamic–pituitary–adrenal (HPA) axis (for example, CRHR1, FKBP5) systems [68]. These findings are endorsed and complemented by a large body of work on animal models of anxiety, including a number of mouse studies mapping several genetic loci thought to affect anxiety-like behaviour in rodents [69]. Human and animal studies have also suggested a role for both gene–gene and gene–environment interactions in contributing to the overall risk for anxiety disorders. Further, there is some evidence suggesting a role for epigenetic DNA modifications (for example, DNA methylation) and changes in gene expression in the effect of early life stress—such as poor maternal care—on anxiety-like behaviours in mice. Genetic variants may also confer risk via intermediate phenotypes (endophenotypes) such as BI, AS, and trait neuroticism [46]. Indeed, it is likely that anxiety disorders and phenotypes are polygenic with multifactorial aetiology.

| CONSTRUCT/SUB-CONSTRUCT | | GENES | MOLECULES | CELLS | CIRCUITS | PHYSIOLOGY | BEHAVIOUR | SELF-REPORT | PARADIGMS |
|---|---|---|---|---|---|---|---|---|---|
| **NEGATIVE VALENCE SYSTEMS** | | | | | | | | | |
| Acute Threat ("Fear") | | | | | | | | | |
| Potential Threat ("Anxiety") | | | | | | | | | |
| Sustained Threat | | | | | | | | | |
| Loss | | | | | | | | | |
| Frustrative Nonreward | | | | | | | | | |
| **POSTIVE VALENCE SYSTEMS** | | | | | | | | | |
| Reward Responsiveness | Reward Anticipation | | | | | | | | |
| | Initial Response to Reward | | | | | | | | |
| | Reward Satiation | | | | | | | | |
| Reward Learning | Probabilistic and Reinforcement Learning | | | | | | | | |
| | Reward Prediction Error | | | | | | | | |
| | Habit - PVS | | | | | | | | |
| Reward Valuation | Reward (probability) | | | | | | | | |
| | Delay | | | | | | | | |
| | Effort | | | | | | | | |
| **COGNITIVE SYSTEMS** | | | | | | | | | |
| Attention | | | | | | | | | |
| Perception | Visual Perception | | | | | | | | |
| | Auditory Perception | | | | | | | | |
| | Olfactory/Somatosensory/Multimodal /Perception | | | | | | | | |
| Declarative Memory | | | | | | | | | |
| Language | | | | | | | | | |
| Cognitive Control | Goal Selection; Updating, Representation, and Maintenance ⇒ Focus 1 of 2 ⇒ Goal Selection | | | | | | | | |
| | Goal Selection; Updating, Representation, and Maintenance ⇒ Focus 2 of 2 ⇒ Updating, Representation, and Maintenance | | | | | | | | |
| | Response Selection; Inhibition/Suppression ⇒ Focus 1 of 2 ⇒ Response Selection | | | | | | | | |
| | Response Selection; Inhibition/Suppression ⇒ Focus 2 of 2 ⇒ Inhibition/Suppression | | | | | | | | |
| | Performance Monitoring | | | | | | | | |

| Domain / Construct | Subconstruct | | | | | | | |
|---|---|---|---|---|---|---|---|---|
| Working Memory | Active Maintenance | | | | | | | |
| | Flexible Updating | | | | | | | |
| | Limited Capacity | | | | | | | |
| | Interference Control | | | | | | | |

**SOCIAL PROCESSES**

| Domain / Construct | Subconstruct | | | | | | | |
|---|---|---|---|---|---|---|---|---|
| Affiliation and Attachment | | | | | | | | |
| Social Communication | Reception of Facial Communication | | | | | | | |
| | Production of Facial Communication | | | | | | | |
| | Reception of Non-Facial Communication | | | | | | | |
| | Production of Non-Facial Communication | | | | | | | |
| Perception and Understanding of Self | Agency | | | | | | | |
| | Self-Knowledge | | | | | | | |
| Perception and Understanding of Others | Animacy Perception | | | | | | | |
| | Action Perception | | | | | | | |
| | Understanding Mental States | | | | | | | |

**AROUSAL AND REGULATORY SYSTEMS**

| Construct | | | | | | | | |
|---|---|---|---|---|---|---|---|---|
| Arousal | | | | | | | | |
| Circadian Rhythms | | | | | | | | |
| Sleep-Wakefulness | | | | | | | | |

**SENSORIMOTOR SYSTEMS**

| Domain / Construct | Subconstruct | | | | | | | |
|---|---|---|---|---|---|---|---|---|
| Motor Actions | Action, Planning and Selection | | | | | | | |
| | Sensorimotor Dynamics | | | | | | | |
| | Initiation | | | | | | | |
| | Execution | | | | | | | |
| | Inhibition and Termination | | | | | | | |
| Agency and Ownership | | | | | | | | |
| Habit - Sensorimotor | | | | | | | | |
| Innate Motor Patterns | | | | | | | | |

**Fig. 86.1** RDoC Matrix.

Adapted from The National Institute of Mental Health, RDoC Matrix. Retrieved September 13, 2019, from https://www.nimh.nih.gov/research/research-funded-by-nimh/rdoc/constructs/rdoc-matrix.shtml, with permission from The National Institute of Mental Health.

## Transdiagnostic approaches to treatment of anxiety disorders

The concept of 'pharmacotherapeutic dissection', with different disorders responding to different drugs, was key in delineating different categories of anxiety disorders, including panic disorder [70]. However, there is also long-standing evidence that a range of different psychotropic agents (for example, benzodiazepines, SSRIs, $D_2$ blockers) are useful across several different anxiety conditions (see also Chapter 92). Somewhat analogously, early interest in specific cognitive behavioural therapy (CBT) treatments for particular anxiety disorders has been replaced by a growing interest in transdiagnostic CBT. Indeed, transdiagnostic CBT interventions are increasingly viewed as efficacious across anxiety disorders, with a large treatment effect size and stable maintenance of improvement during follow-up [4, 71].

More recently, the Unified Protocol for Transdiagnostic Treatment of Emotional Disorders (UP) has emerged as a focus of transdiagnostic CBT studies. The UP comprises five treatment modules to target emotion processing, regulation, and extinction, as follows [72–74]: to increase present-focused emotion awareness; to increase cognitive flexibility; to identify/prevent emotion avoidance and maladaptive behaviours; to increase awareness and tolerance of emotion-related physical sensations; and interoceptive and situation-based emotion-focused exposure.

One small randomized controlled trial of clinical patients with heterogenous anxiety disorder diagnoses [72] found that immediate UP treatment resulted in significant improvement in outcome measures of general anxiety/depressive symptoms, clinical severity, and functional impairment, as compared with delayed treatment following a waitlist period. Similarly, another study of UP treatment in two consecutive trials [75] reported decreased AS from pre- to post-treatment; and the majority of this change coincided largely with the introduction of interoceptive exposure therapy.

The next step in this area is work on combined transdiagnostic pharmacotherapy and psychotherapy. One study has investigated the effect of SSRIs/SNRIs and sedatives on the efficacy of transdiagnostic 5-week group CBT [76]. These authors found that combined antidepressant/CBT resulted in greater improvement in depressive symptoms when compared to CBT monotherapy (and that the efficacy of combined therapy was less for those patients also treated with sedatives). Nevertheless, given the evident paucity of empirical data on transdiagnostic combined psychotherapy and pharmacotherapy for anxiety disorders, further work is required before such interventions are routinely advised. An even greater transdiagnostic challenge is primary prevention of anxiety disorders, described at length in Chapter 91.

## Conclusions

Categorical approaches to anxiety are currently key in the clinical diagnosis and management of DSM-5- and ICD-11-defined disorders. Dimensional approaches may hold promise for future research and clinical innovation. These approaches are informed by a growing body of evidence that dimensional assessments of anxiety and related symptoms are informative, that spectrum approaches to understanding cognitive–affective mechanisms and the underlying neurocircuitry are useful, and that transdiagnostic treatment interventions are effective. However, dimensional approaches are, for now, a complement to—rather than a substitute for—current categorical approaches to anxiety disorders.

## REFERENCES

1. American Psychiatric Association (APA). *Diagnostic and Statistical Manual of Mental Disorders*, third edition (DSM-III). Washington, D.C.: American Psychiatric Association; 1980.
2. Shear MK, Bjelland I, Beesdo K, Gloster AT, Wittchen HU. Supplementary dimensional assessment in anxiety disorders. *Int J Methods Psychiatr Res*. 2007;16 Suppl 1:S52–64.
3. Martin EI, Ressler KJ, Binder E, Nemeroff CB. The neurobiology of anxiety disorders: brain imaging, genetics, and psychoneuroendocrinology. *Clin Lab Med*. 2010;30:865–91.
4. Norton PJ, Philipp LM. Transdiagnostic approaches to the treatment of anxiety disorders: a quantitative review. *Psychotherapy (Chic)*. 2008;45:214–26.
5. Kessler RC. The categorical versus dimensional assessment controversy in the sociology of mental illness. *J Health Soc Behav*. 2002;43:171–88.
6. Borsboom D, Rhemtulla M, Cramer AO, van der Maas HL, Scheffer M, Dolan CV. Kinds versus continua: a review of psychometric approaches to uncover the structure of psychiatric constructs. *Psychol Med*. 2016;46:1567–79.
7. Ruscio J, Ruscio AM. Categories and dimensions advancing psychological science through the study of latent structure. *Curr Dir Psychol Sci*. 2008;17:203–7.
8. American Psychiatric Association (APA). *Diagnostic and Statistical Manual of Mental Disorders*, second edition (DSM-II). Washington, D.C.: American Psychiatric Association; 1968.
9. Crocq MA. A history of anxiety: from Hippocrates to DSM. *Dialogues Clin Neurosci*. 2015;17:319–25.
10. World Health Organization. *International Classification of Diseases*, ninth Revision (ICD-9). Geneva: World Health Organization; 1979.
11. American Psychiatric Association. *Diagnostic and Statistical Manual of Mental Disorders*, fourth Edition (DSM-IV). Washington, D.C.: American Psychiatric Association; 1994.
12. World Health Organization. *International Classification of Diseases*, tenth revision (ICD-9). Geneva: World Health Organization; 1992.
13. American Psychiatric Association. *Diagnostic and Statistical Manual of Mental Disorders*, fifth edition (DSM-5). Arlington, VA: American Psychiatric Association; 2013.
14. Stein DJ, Craske MG, Friedman MJ, Phillips KA. Meta-structure issues for the DSM-5: how do anxiety disorders, obsessive-compulsive and related disorders, post-traumatic disorders, and dissociative disorders fit together? *Curr Psychiatry Rep*. 2011;13:248–50.
15. Kogan CS, Stein DJ, Maj M, First MB, Emmelkamp PM, Reed GM. The classification of anxiety and fear-related disorders in the ICD-11. *Depress Anxiety*. 2016;33:1141–54.
16. Cannon WB. Bodily changes in pain, hunger, fear and rage. New York, NY: Harper & Row; 1915.
17. Rosen JB, Schulkin J. From normal fear to pathological anxiety. *Psychol Rev*. 1998;105:325–50.
18. Stein DJ, Nesse RM. Threat detection, precautionary responses, and anxiety disorders. *Neurosci Biobehav Rev*. 2011;35:1075–9.

19. Spitzer RL, Wakefield JC. DSM-IV diagnostic criterion for clinical significance: does it help solve the false positives problem? *Am J Psychiatry*. 1999;156:1856–64.

20. Bandelow B, Baldwin D, Abelli M, *et al*. Biological markers for anxiety disorders, OCD and PTSD—a consensus statement. Part I: Neuroimaging and genetics. *World J Biol Psychiatry*. 2016;17:321–65.

21. First MB, Wakefield JC. Diagnostic criteria as dysfunction indicators: bridging the chasm between the definition of mental disorder and diagnostic criteria for specific disorders. *Can J Psychiatry*. 2013;58:663–9.

22. Kagan J, Reznick JS, Snidman N. Biological bases of childhood shyness. *Science*. 1988;240:167–71.

23. Muris P, van Brakel AM, Arntz A, Schouten E. Behavioral inhibition as a risk factor for the development of childhood anxiety disorders: a longitudinal study. *J Child Fam Stud*. 2011;20:157–70.

24. Kagan J, Snidman N. Early childhood predictors of adult anxiety disorders. *Biol Psychiatry*. 1999;46:1536–41.

25. Fox AS, Kalin NH. A translational neuroscience approach to understanding the development of social anxiety disorder and its pathophysiology. *Am J Psychiatry*. 2014;171:1162–73.

26. Clauss JA, Blackford JU. Behavioral inhibition and risk for developing social anxiety disorder: a meta-analytic study. *J Am Acad Child Adolesc Psychiatry*. 2012;51:1066–75.

27. Schwartz CE, Wright CI, Shin LM, Kagan J, Rauch SL. Inhibited and uninhibited infants 'grown up': adult amygdalar response to novelty. *Science*. 2003;300:1952–3.

28. Rosenbaum JF, Biederman J, Bolduc-Murphy EA, *et al*. Behavioral inhibition in childhood: a risk factor for anxiety disorders. *Harv Rev Psychiatry*. 1993;1:2–16.

29. Marks I, Nesse R. Fear and fitness: an evolutionary analysis of anxiety disorders. *Ethol Sociobiol*. 1994;15:247–61.

30. Callaghan BL, Richardson R. The development of fear and its inhibition: knowledge gained from preclinical models. In: Ressler K, Pine D, Rothbaum B, Muskies A (eds). *Anxiety Disorders: Translational Perspectives on Diagnosis and Treatment*. Oxford: Oxford University Press, 2015; pp. 83–94.

31. McLaughlin KA, Sheridan MA, Lambert HK. Childhood adversity and neural development: deprivation and threat as distinct dimensions of early experience. *Neurosci Biobehav Rev*. 2014;47:578–91.

32. Reiss S, McNally RJ. Expectancy model of fear. In: Reiss S, Bootzin RR (eds). *Theoretical Issues in Behaviour Therapy*. San Diego, CA: Academic Press, 1985; pp. 107–21.

33. Taylor S, Jang KL, Stewart SH, Stein MB. Etiology of the dimensions of anxiety sensitivity: a behavioral-genetic analysis. *J Anxiety Disord*. 2008;22:899–914.

34. Schmidt NB, Zvolensky MJ, Maner JK. Anxiety sensitivity: prospective prediction of panic attacks and Axis I pathology. *J Psychiatr Res*. 2006;40:691–9.

35. Olatunji BO, Wolitzky-Taylor KB. Anxiety sensitivity and the anxiety disorders: a meta-analytic review and synthesis. *Psychol Bull*. 2009;135:974–99.

36. Deacon BJ, Valentiner DP. Dimensions of anxiety sensitivity and their relationship to nonclinical panic. *J Psychopathol Behav Assessment*. 2001;23:25–33.

37. Jang KL, Stein MB, Taylor S, Livesley WJ. Gender differences in the etiology of anxiety sensitivity: a twin study. *J Gend Specif Med*. 1999;2:39–44.

38. Hiroi R, McDevitt RA, Neumaier JF. Estrogen selectively increases tryptophan hydroxylase-2 mRNA expression in distinct subregions of rat midbrain raphe nucleus: association between gene expression and anxiety behavior in the open field. *Biol Psychiatry*. 2006;60:288–95.

39. Peterson RA, Reiss S. *Anxiety Sensitivity Index Revised Manual*. Worthington, OH: International Diagnostic Systems; 1992.

40. Kotov R, Gamez W, Schmidt F, Watson D. Linking 'big' personality traits to anxiety, depressive, and substance use disorders: a meta-analysis. *Psychol Bull*. 2010;136:768–821.

41. Jeronimus BF, Kotov R, Riese H, Ormel J. Neuroticism's prospective association with mental disorders halves after adjustment for baseline symptoms and psychiatric history, but the adjusted association hardly decays with time: a meta-analysis on 59 longitudinal/prospective studies with 443 313 participants. *Psychol Med*. 2016;46:2883–906.

42. Clark LA, Watson D. Tripartite model of anxiety and depression: psychometric evidence and taxonomic implications. *J Abnorm Psychol*. 1991;100:316–36.

43. Goldberg DP, Krueger RF, Andrews G, Hobbs MJ. Emotional disorders: cluster 4 of the proposed meta-structure for DSM-V and ICD-11. *Psychol Med*. 2009;39:2043–59.

44. Ormel J, Jeronimus BF, Kotov R, *et al*. Neuroticism and common mental disorders: meaning and utility of a complex relationship. *Clin Psychol Rev*. 2013;33:686–97.

45. Hettema JM, Neale MC, Myers JM, Prescott CA, Kendler KS. A population-based twin study of the relationship between neuroticism and internalizing disorders. *Am J Psychiatry*. 2006;163:857–64.

46. Webb BT, Guo AY, Maher BS, *et al*. Meta-analyses of genome-wide linkage scans of anxiety-related phenotypes. *Eur J Hum Genet*. 2012;20:1078–84.

47. Ferrando PJ. The measurement of neuroticism using MMQ, MPI, EPI and EPQ items: a psychometric analysis based on item response theory. *Personality and Individual Differences*. 2001;30:641–56.

48. Cisler JM, Koster EH. Mechanisms of attentional biases towards threat in anxiety disorders: An integrative review. *Clin Psychol Rev*. 2010;30:203–16.

49. Rosso IM, Dillon DG, Pizzagalli DA, Lauch SL. Translational perspective on anxiety disorders and the Research Domain Criteria construct of potential threat. In: Ressler K, Pine D, Rothbaum B, Muskies A (eds). *Anxiety Disorders: Translational Perspectives on Diagnosis and Treatment*. Oxford: Oxford University Press, 2015; pp. 17–29.

50. Craske MG, Rauch SL, Ursano R, Prenoveau J, Pine DS, Zinbarg RE. What is an anxiety disorder? *Depress Anxiety*. 2009;26:1066–85.

51. Likhtik E, Stujenske JM, Topiwala MA, Harris AZ, Gordon JA. Prefrontal entrainment of amygdala activity signals safety in learned fear and innate anxiety. *Nat Neurosci*. 2014;17:106–13.

52. Gore F, Schwartz EC, Brangers BC, *et al*. Neural representations of unconditioned stimuli in basolateral amygdala mediate innate and learned responses. *Cell*. 2015;162:134–45.

53. Insel T, Cuthbert B, Garvey M, *et al*. Research domain criteria (RDoC): toward a new classification framework for research on mental disorders. *Am J Psychiatry*. 2010;16:748–51.

54. Cuthbert BN. The RDoC framework: facilitating transition from ICD/DSM to dimensional approaches that integrate neuroscience and psychopathology. *World Psychiatry*. 2014;13:28–35.

55. Simpson HB. The RDoC project: a new paradigm for investigating the pathophysiology of anxiety. *Depress Anxiety*. 2012;29:251–2.

56. National Institute of Mental Health (NIMH). *RDoc Matrix*. Available at: http://www.nimh.nih.gov/research-priorities/rdoc/constructs/rdoc-matrix.shtml. [accessed 21 July 2016].

57. Zoellner LA, Foa EB. Applying Research Domain Criteria (RDoC) to the study of fear and anxiety: a critical comment. *Psychophysiology*. 2016;53:332–5.

58. Lieblich SM, Castle DJ, Everall IP. RDoC: we should look before we leap. *Aust N Z J Psychiatry*. 2015;49:770–1.

59. Etkin A. Functional neuroanatomy of anxiety: a neural circuit perspective. *Curr Top Behav Neurosci*. 2010;2:251–77.

60. Hattingh CJ, Ipser J, Tromp SA, *et al*. Functional magnetic resonance imaging during emotion recognition in social anxiety disorder: an activation likelihood meta-analysis. *Front Hum Neurosci*. 2013;6:347.

61. Ipser JC, Singh L, Stein DJ. Meta-analysis of functional brain imaging in specific phobia. *Psychiatry Clin Neurosci*. 2013;67:311–22.

62. Etkin A, Wager TD. Functional neuroimaging of anxiety: a meta-analysis of emotional processing in PTSD, social anxiety disorder, and specific phobia. *Am J Psychiatry*. 2007;164:1476–88.

63. Shin LM, Liberzon I. The neurocircuitry of fear, stress, and anxiety disorders. *Neuropsychopharmacology*. 2010;35:169–91.

64. Cannistraro PA, Rauch SL. Neural circuitry of anxiety: evidence from structural and functional neuroimaging studies. *Psychopharmacol Bull*. 2003;37:8–25.

65. Kent JM, Rauch SL. Neurocircuitry of anxiety disorders. *Cur Psychiatry Rep*. 2003;5:266–73.

66. Williams LM. Precision psychiatry: a neural circuit taxonomy for depression and anxiety. *Lancet Psychiatry*. 2016;3:472–80.

67. Shimada-Sugimoto M, Otowa T, Hettema JM. Genetics of anxiety disorders: genetic epidemiological and molecular studies in humans. *Psychiatry Clin Neurosci*. 2015;69:388–401.

68. Domschke K, Maron E. Genetic factors in anxiety disorders. *Mod Trends Pharmacopsychiatry*. 2013;29:24–46.

69. Hettema JM, Webb BT, Guo AY, *et al*. Prioritization and association analysis of murine-derived candidate genes in anxiety-spectrum disorders. *Biol Psychiatry*. 2011;70:888–96.

70. Klein DF. Delineation of two drug-responsive anxiety syndromes. *Psychopharmacologia*. 1964;5:397–408.

71. Norton PJ, Price EC. A meta-analytic review of adult cognitive-behavioral treatment outcome across the anxiety disorders. *J Nerv Ment Dis*. 2007;195:521–31.

72. Farchione TJ, Fairholme CP, Ellard KK, *et al*. Unified protocol for transdiagnostic treatment of emotional disorders: a randomized controlled trial. *Behav Ther*. 2012;43:666–78.

73. Ellard KK, Fairholme CP, Boisseau CL, Farchione TJ, Barlow DH. Unified protocol for the transdiagnostic treatment of emotional disorders: Protocol development and initial outcome data. *Cog Behav Practice*. 2010;17:88–101.

74. Wilamowska ZA, Thompson-Hollands J, Fairholme CP, Ellard KK, Farchione TJ, Barlow DH. Conceptual background, development, and preliminary data from the unified protocol for transdiagnostic treatment of emotional disorders. *Depress Anxiety*. 2010;27:882–90.

75. Boswell JF, Farchione TJ, Sauer-Zavala S, Murray HW, Fortune MR, Barlow DH. Anxiety sensitivity and interoceptive exposure: a transdiagnostic construct and change strategy. *Behav Ther*. 2013;44:417–31.

76. Eriksson EB, Kristjansdottir H, Sigurdsson JF, Agnarsdottir A, Sigurdsson E. [The effect of antidepressants and sedatives on the efficacy of transdiagnostic cognitive behavioral therapy in groups in primary care] [Article in Icelandic]. *Laeknabladid*. 2013;99:505–10.

# 87

# Basic mechanisms, genetics, targets, and animal models for anxiety disorders

*Martien J. Kas and Berend Olivier*

## Introduction

Existing anxiolytic drugs, such as benzodiazepines (BZs) and selective serotonin reuptake inhibitors (SSRIs), have been developed several decades ago, partly as a result of serendipity (BZs), partly because they were primarily targeted at major depressive disorder (SSRIs). Extensive search has occurred in the ensuing decades to find new targets for anxiolytics, based on the known and anticipated neurochemical mechanisms underlying anxiety. However, no real breakthroughs have emerged. Currently, SSRIs remain the preferred drugs for the treatment of anxiety disorders (and augmented with BZs for a limited time interval). Although efficacious, some patients are treatment-resistant, and inherent disadvantages are attached to SSRI use, including lasting side effects. Therefore, in the last decades, preclinical and clinical studies have extensively focused on other mechanisms to target anxiety processes in order to ultimately treat anxiety disorders. Since then, evidence has emerged pointing to a modulating role of corticotrophin-releasing factor 1 (CRF1) receptors, neurokinin 1 (NK-1) receptors, and glucocorticoid receptors (for a review, see [1]). Although the efficacy of such drugs during development often looked promising in the preclinical phase, therapeutic anxiolytic effects were often absent or inferior to the existing drugs. Thus, so far no 'superior' drugs have reached the market that will replace the current treatment choices.

As described in Chapter 86 in the new DSM-5, the former DSM-IV category of 'Anxiety disorders' became three separate categories: 'Anxiety disorders', 'Obsessive compulsive disorders', and 'Trauma and stress-related disorders'. This categorization does not create an easier pathway for new drugs or an easier discovery track. Thus, the creation of preclinical models for each individual anxiety disorder is not only impractical, but actually impossible. Therefore, it has been proposed that a classification based on the neurobiological mechanisms underlying anxiety and pathological anxiety (intermediate phenotypes) would enhance drug development [2]. Another classification approach would be based on dysfunctional neurotransmitter systems, for example, abnormal serotonin transporter function [3]. In the present chapter, we mainly focus on what we know on the pharmacology of GABA-ergic and serotonergic drugs, and we try to outline, focusing on genetic and genomic approaches and innovative animal models of anxiety disorder, how to find putative new targets and some new promising avenues and technologies in the anxiety field.

## GABA$_A$ receptor α subunits and anxiety

In the 1950s, BZs were serendipitously found as having therapeutically interesting activity with anxiolysis, sedation, anticonvulsive activity, and muscle relaxation. It took more than 20 years to discover the molecular target of BZs—the GABA$_A$ receptor [4]. It is now known that the GABA-ergic system has ionotropic (GABA$_A$) and metabotropic (GABA$_B$) receptors that are ubiquitously expressed and distributed in the CNS [5, 6]. The GABA$_A$ receptor (GABA$_A$R) is the target of clinically important anxiolytics, including BZs [7]. A role for GABA$_B$R in anxiety and stress has been found preclinically but has not (yet) led to clinical applications [7, 8].

GABA$_A$Rs are ligand-gated ion channels that mediate fast inhibitory effects on many post-synaptic sites and are ubiquitously present in the CNS, although there is a specific and differential subunit distribution. When the endogenous ligand gamma-aminobutyric acid (GABA) binds to its receptor, chloride ions flow into the neuron, causing hyperpolarization of the cell membrane and inhibiting cell firing. GABA$_A$Rs occur synaptically and extra-synaptically and display large molecular heterogeneity made up via a variable subunit composition. This heterogeneity in composition determines the physiological and pharmacological properties and contributes to the flexibility in signal transduction and modulation [7]. GABA$_A$Rs are always composed of five subunits, a complex that forms a heteropentamer creating a channel permeable to chloride ions. The subunits can be made up, although not randomly, from 19 subunits (α1–6; β1–3; γ1–3; δ, ε, θ, and ρ1–3). Most GABA$_A$ receptors are built from two α, two β, and one γ subunit (Fig. 87.1 from [9]). The endogenous neurotransmitter GABA binds to the GABA site, which is formed by α and β subunits, whereas the binding site for BZs is formed by one of the α subunits (α1, α2, α3, or α5) and a γ subunit (almost exclusively the γ2 subunit). GABA$_A$ receptors with α4 or α6 subunits do not bind to classic BZs. The most frequent subtype in the CNS is a pentameric complex, consisting of two α,

(a)

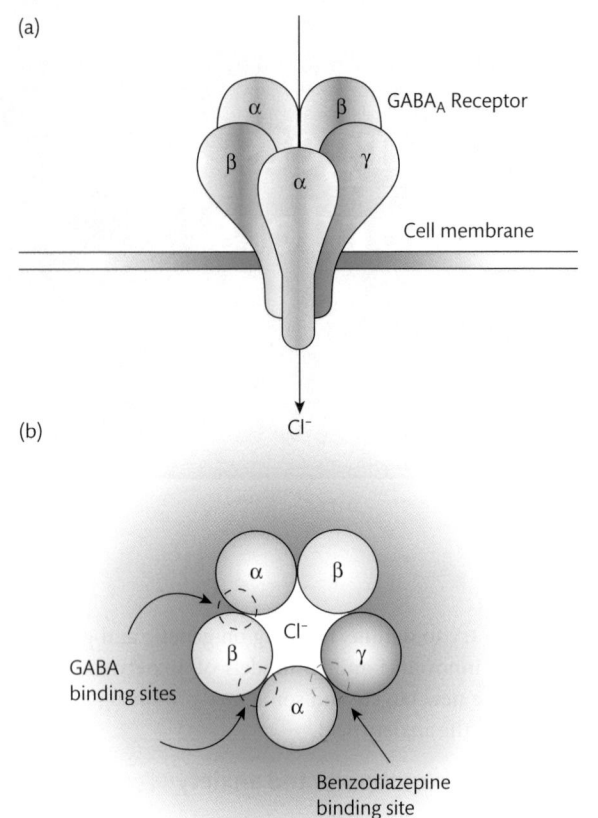

GABA$_A$ Receptor

Cell membrane

Cl$^-$

(b)

GABA binding sites

Cl$^-$

Benzodiazepine binding site

**Fig. 87.1** Schematic picture of the GABA$_A$ receptor. (a) A global picture of the two α, two β, and one γ subunits and the direction of the chloride influx. (b) A top view with the subunits arranged around a central pore—the chloride channel. The GABA and benzodiazepine binding sites are indicated.

two β, and one γ subunit. Approximately 60% of all GABA$_A$ receptors are α1β2γ2 subunits, 15–20% α2β3γ2, 10–15% α3βnγ2, and 5% α4βnγ or α4βnδ, and <5% have α6β2/3γ2 subunits [10]. GABA$_A$ receptors are the main inhibitory neurons in the CNS, and it is estimated that 20–30% of all neurons in the CNS are of the GABA$_A$ type. BZs do not open the chloride channel in the absence of GABA. Different classes of pharmacological agents act at different sites of the GABA$_A$R, including the endogenous agonist GABA and various GABA$_A$R agonists (for example, muscimol) or antagonists (for example, bicuculline). Classical BZs (for example, chlordiazepoxide, diazepam) bind to the GABA$_A$R BZ modulatory site. Other drug classes also bind to the GABA$_A$R, including alcohol, barbiturates, and neurosteroids. BZs mediate their action via the modulatory binding site that is present on most, but not all, GABA$_A$Rs. The allosteric binding site for BZs is always formed by two α subunits (α1, α2, α3, or α5), two β subunits, and the γ2 subunit. Only if the GABA receptor site is activated (by GABA or external receptor agonists) may activation of the BZ site modulate the opening of the channel (frequency and/or time). Ligands at the BZ binding site are called allosteric modulators. They modify the efficacy and/or affinity of GABA in positive allosteric modulation (PAM) or negative allosteric

modulation (NAM) or have neutral effects by stabilizing different three-dimensional conformations of the GABA$_A$R complex. Selectivity of a ligand for a specific receptor subtype can be obtained by affinity and/or efficacy changes that determine the potential potency of a ligand [11]. Benzodiazepines have anxiolytic, sedative, hypnotic, muscle relaxant, and anticonvulsive properties. The sedative–hypnotic properties are useful for, for example, insomnia treatment but are unwanted side effects if anxiolysis is the primary indication. Classic BZs (for example, diazepam) are non-selectively activating α1, α2, α3, and α5 subunits, but extensive research, mainly in genetically modified mice in which individual GABA$_A$Rα subunits (GABRA) were made insensitive to diazepam binding (by histidine-to-arginine point mutations at a conserved residue in the α1, α2, α3, or α5 subunits, whereas the actions of the endogenous ligand GABA remained intact) showed that the different subunits represent different functions. It has become clear that the broad profile of therapeutic effects of BZs is dependent on activation of selective α -subunits. Strong evidence was gathered that α1 subunits are involved in sedative and anterograde amnesia effects mediated by diazepam (α1(H101R)mice); α2 point mutations (α2(H101R) mice) led to absence of the anxiolytic and diminished muscle relaxant action, but intact anxiolytic effects, and in α3 (α3(H126R) mice) and α5 point mutations (α5(105R)mice), diazepam did not induce myorelaxation, whereas sedation and anxiolysis were intact. Such data strongly suggest a functional differentiation in the GABA$_A$ receptors, depending on the α subunit composition (for reviews, see [12, 13]).

Classic BZs, still frequently prescribed, have therapeutic activity but, inherent to the activation of all relevant α subunits, come with built-in side effects. If used as an anxiolytic tool, sedation is one of the troubling side effects. Furthermore, upon chronic use, BZs can lead to dependency and tolerance and induce abuse liability, limiting long-term use [14]. Recent efforts have tried to synthesize new drugs that have selectivity and potency for specific α subunits [13], although relatively selective drugs for the α1 subunit are already in use for sedation/hypnotic purposes (zolpidem, zopiclone, (S)-zopiclone, and zaleplone). Compounds that selectively activate the α2 subunits and have no effects on any other α subunit might constitute an ideal non-sedative anxiolytic, although activation of α3 subunits might contribute to an anxiolytic profile [15–17]. L-838417, a partial PAM at α2-, α3-, and α5-containing GABA$_A$ receptors and an antagonist at α1-containing receptors has a non-sedating anxiolytic profile in mice [18, 19] and primates [20]. Development of this compound has been stopped due to an unfavourable pharmacokinetic profile [21]. TPA023, an α2/α3 PAM, has anxiolytic and no sedative effects in rodents [22]. TPA023 was evaluated in three phase 2 studies in GAD and proved preliminary indications of anxiolytic activity without sedation [17]. However, this compound had to be withdrawn due to severe preclinical toxicity. A comparable story holds for ocinaplon, having a non-sedative, anxiolytic profile in humans but which also had to be withdrawn due to hepatotoxicity [23, 24]. Several other ligands have been synthesized and tested, mostly restricted to preclinical phases. It appears possible to make compounds with some selectivity for specific α subunits, but *in vivo* efficacy is extremely difficult to design; both PAMs and NAMs have been found, and sometimes even mixed PAM/NAM effects on different α subunits are present or no selectivity is present *in vitro*, whereas *in vivo*, some efficacy is found (for example, ocinaplon). MRK-409, an extremely low partial agonist (PAM) at α1-, α2-, and α5-containing GABA$_A$ receptors, but with higher intrinsic activity at α3 subunit GABA$_A$ receptors, appeared to be anxio-selective in animals but sedative in humans, already at low (<10%) receptor occupancy [25].

Another class of compounds—the neurosteroids (for example, allopregnanolone, alphaxolone)—have modulatory effects (PAM) on the GABA$_A$R, comparable to BZs. However, due to several differential mechanistic differences, the neurosteroids have not emerged as potent anxiolytics [26].

One of the unresolved issues around subunit selective GABAergic compounds is the issue of tolerance and abuse potential. Does activation of all α subunit-containing GABA$_A$ receptors lead to addiction or is that caused by specific α subunits [27]? This is an important issue because the development of medications with potential for misuse may not be possible. There is some evidence that activation of α1 subunits is essential in the addictive properties of BZs [14, 28]. However, the processes of tolerance development are complex and endpoint-dependent [29]. If the therapeutic effects of activation of α1-containing GABA$_A$ receptors cannot be separated from potential addictive side effects, no further development of α1 subunit-specific ligands can be expected. However, if addictive properties are not entwined in (chronic) activation of the other α2, α3, α5 subunits, new developments in the field

of anxiety (and others like cognition and analgesia) might be expected [9, 29, 30].

## The 5-HT$_{1A}$ receptor

The 5-HT$_{1A}$ receptor has been implicated in anxiety because 5-HT$_{1A}$ receptor agonists exert anxiolytic activity in rodent models of anxiety [31, 32], whereas buspirone, a partial 5-HT$_{1A}$ receptor agonist, exerts mild anxiolytic effects in human anxiety patients, particularly in GAD [33]. Although clinically the development of new 5-HT$_{1A}$ receptor agonists for anxiety disorders (for example, ipsapirone, gepirone, tandospirone, flesinoxan) failed, the 5-HT$_{1A}$ receptor has received considerable interest as a critical target implied in anxiety and depression [31–37]. 5-HT$_{1A}$ receptors are G-protein-coupled inhibitory receptors expressed in serotonergic neurons as auto-receptors and in non-serotonergic neurons as heteroreceptors (Fig. 87.2). The somatodendritic 5-HT$_{1A}$ auto-receptor controls serotonergic tone via feedback inhibition in concert with 5-HTT, the target of the most commonly used anxiolytic/antidepressant SSRIs. It has been hypothesized that desensitized 5-HT$_{1A}$ auto-receptors delay the onset of action of SSRIs that act by enhancing brain serotonin levels [38, 39]. 5-HT$_{1A}$ receptors are quite abundantly distributed and expressed, although restrictedly present in some brain areas. Auto-receptors are mainly, if not only, found in the dorsal

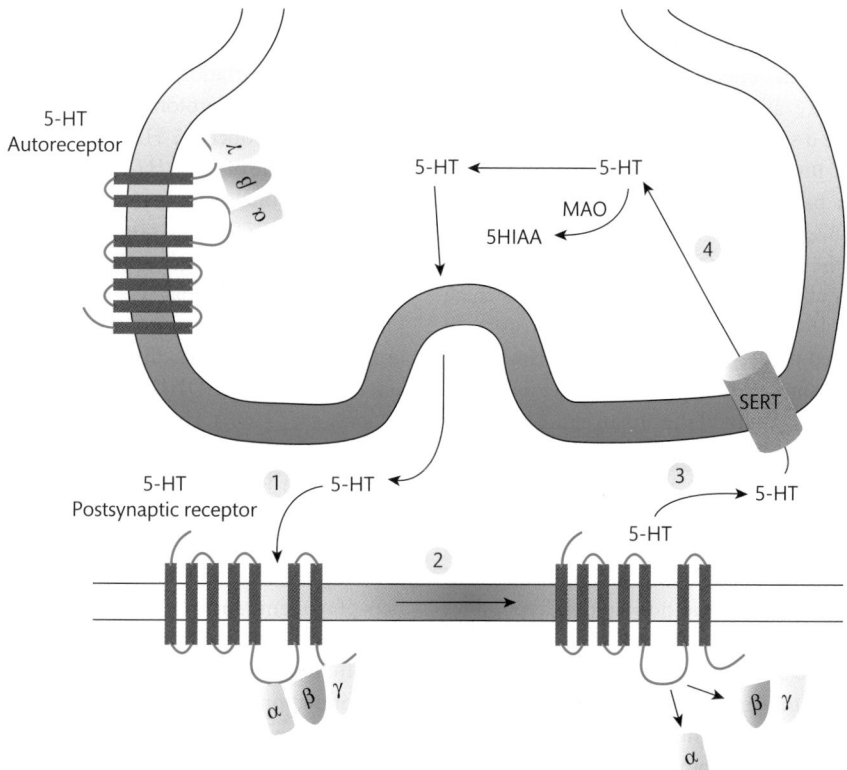

**Fig. 87.2** Schematic representation of serotonin (5-HT) in the terminal and synapse. G-protein-coupled receptors are located presynaptically [5-HT auto-receptor (5-HT$_{1A/1B}$)] or post-synaptically (5-HT$_{1/2/4/5/6/7}$ receptors). (1) 5-HT is released from the presynaptic neuron and binds to a heterotrimeric G-protein post-synaptic receptor. Heterotrimeric G-protein complexes contain an α, a β, and a γ subunit, which, in an inactive state, are bound to GDP. (2) 5-HT acts on post-synaptic receptors and induces a change in the conformation of the post-synaptic receptor. GDP is phosphorylated to GTP and binds to the α subunit, which subsequently becomes active. The β and γ subunits are freed. (3) Extracellular 5-HT is taken up by the SERT into the presynaptic neuron. (4) Back in the presynaptic neuron, 5-HT is broken down by MAO to 5-HIAA (occurs also extracellularly) or is being stored in the vesicles for future release. MAO, monoamine oxidase; 5-HIAA, 5-hydroxyindole acetic acid; SERT, serotonin transporter.

and median raphe nuclei, whereas post-synaptic heteroreceptors are found in high densities in limbic regions (including the hippocampus) and in the frontal, medial prefrontal, and entorhinal cortices.

Genetic and imaging studies in humans suggest that 5-HT$_{1A}$ receptor density or regulation are associated with depression and anxiety, but also with the response to antidepressants [40]. Recently, an association was found between a C(-1019)G polymorphism (rs6295G/C) in the promoter region of the 5-HT$_{1A}$ receptor gene (*Htr1a*) and mood-related variables, including amygdala reactivity [41] and depression [42]. Enrichment with the G-allele is associated with enhanced raphe (presynaptic) 5-HT$_{1A}$ auto-receptor expression, whereas post-synaptically, the reverse occurs with the 5-HT$_{1A}$ heteroreceptor [42]. A clear hypothesis of how such changes contribute to an anxious/depressed phenotype has, however, not emerged yet. More polymorphisms in the *Htr1a* gene are known, but no clear data on their influence on anxiety are present [43].

Studies in rodents found that 5-HT$_{1A}$ receptors modulate anxiety and depression. Three independent research groups generated 5-HT$_{1A}$ receptor knockout (KO) mice [44–46], and all KO strains displayed enhanced anxiety in standard anxiety paradigms. The unanimous finding that inactivation of the 5-HT$_{1A}$ receptor gene (both auto- and heteroreceptor) resulted in an anxious phenotype in all three lines was rather striking. The picture became even more blurred when the anxious phenotype appeared dependent on the paradigm used [47]. Moreover, in one of the strains (Swiss-Webster), the 5-HT$_{1A}$ receptor KO mouse displayed reduced sensitivity to the anxiolytic and sedative effects of diazepam, an α subunit non-selective GABA$_A$-positive allosteric modulator [48, 49], attributed to changes in some α subunits of the GABA$_A$–BZ receptor complex. However, this BZ insensitivity was not present in the KO mice in both other genetic backgrounds [49, 50]. Apparently, dysfunction of the GABA$_A$–BZ system is not a prerequisite for the 'anxiogenic' phenotype of the 5-HT$_{1A}$ KO mouse model. Along with the anxiogenic phenotype in the 5-HT$_{1A}$ receptor null mouse, which was unresponsive to SSRIs [51], it appeared that overexpression of the 5-HT$_{1A}$ receptor reduced anxiety [52]. Rescue experiments of forebrain 5-HT$_{1A}$ receptors showed that post-synaptic 5-HT$_{1A}$ receptors are critical in the development of the anxiogenic phenotype in the null mutations [53]. The latter authors showed that transgenic developmental overexpression of 5-HT$_{1A}$ receptors in the rostral brain in the early stages of life (not adulthood) was sufficient to restore normal anxiety levels. Pharmacological blockade of 5-HT$_{1A}$ receptors in early development, but not in adulthood, appeared sufficient to enhance anxious behaviour in normal (wildtype) mice [9, 54]. The complex regulation of anxiety (and depression) processes during development and adulthood illustrates the complexity of the neural substrate, including genetic regulation of anxiety and its pathology, and makes clear that straightforward and simple relationships between the function of a certain receptor and anxiety are not very likely.

By genetic modification, Richardson-Jones *et al.* [55] manipulated the level of presynaptic 5-HT$_{1A}$ auto-receptors at adult age, without changing post-synaptic 5-HT$_{1A}$ heteroreceptors. Mice with higher (1A-high) or lower (1A-low) levels of auto-receptors were tested on their vulnerability to stress and response to antidepressants. The investigators suggested that 1A-low mice showed an enhanced 5-HT tone and decreased depression-like behaviour and still responded to an SSRI, whereas 1A-high mice had a decreased 5-HT tone and more depressed-like behaviour and were unresponsive to SSRIs. In their modelling, they suggested that 1A-lows reflect human C/C, whereas 1A-highs model G/G carriers of the *Htr1a* C(-1019)G polymorphism. Such genetic mouse models are extremely useful in studying the underlying processes emerging in depression and anxiety disorders. Further molecular biological studies into the role of 5-HT$_{1A}$ receptors implicate, in particular, 5-HT$_{1A}$ post-synaptic receptors in the prefrontal cortex in the expression of anxiety [56]. In the prefrontal cortex, those heteroreceptors are expressed on two antagonistically acting neuronal populations—excitatory pyramidal neurons and inhibitory interneurons. These populations play an important role in the expression of anxiety over the lifespan and may be generating new targets for future therapeutic approaches.

### The serotonin transporter (5-HTT)

The 5-HTT has, for a long time, been implicated in the processes underlying mood and anxiety and its associate disorders mainly because the SSRI antidepressants block the serotonin uptake into the neuron thereby increasing the serotonergic output (Fig. 87.2). As outlined in the introduction, polymorphisms in the *5-HTT* gene and its associated transcriptional control region have influence on the functioning of the serotonergic system [57]. Although we restrict ourselves here to anxiety disorders, it is noteworthy to realize that several human behavioural traits and whole-body medical disorders (for example, myocardial infarction, pulmonary hypertension, irritable bowel syndrome, and sudden infant death syndrome) are associated with variations in the *5-HTT* gene (*SLC6A4*), indicating the importance of serotonin neurotransmission in all aspects of our biology [3]. Reduced 5-HTT expression and function associated with the S-allele of the *5-HTTLPR* is associated with anxiety and depression personality traits [58, 59]. In the ensuing decade, it became clear that *5-HTTPRL* and other variations in coding and non-coding regions of the *5-HTT* gene play a wide role in neuropsychiatric disorders, including bipolar disorders, depression, anxiety disorders [also obsessive–compulsive disorder (OCD)], suicide, eating disorders, substance abuse disorders, autism, attention-deficit/hyperactivity disorder (ADHD), and neurodegenerative disorders (for reviews, see [3, 60]). Human 5-HTT maps to chromosome 17q11.2, has 14 exons that span around 40 kB, and produces a 630-amino acid protein with 12 membrane domains. The expression of the gene in humans is modulated by a variation in the length of the 5-HTTLPR, together with two SNPs in this region (rs25531 and rs25332), all located upstream of the transcription start. Moreover, variable numbers of tandem repeat (VNTR) polymorphisms are known in intron 2, as well as several SNPs that influence the structure of the 5-HTT protein. In particular, the rs2551 polymorphism is quite frequent in the population and interacts with 5-HTTLPR in 5-HTT transcription [3]. This makes the modulation of serotonergic transmission via the 5-HTT mechanism highly complex and gives probably an important insight in the factors that play a role in the genetic complexity of any psychiatric disorder. The identification of specific gene variants remains a tricky avenue. It becomes increasingly clear that such variations influence intermediate biological phenotypes, in concert with other (background) genes, epigenetic variation, and environmental and developmental factors, and this complex interaction contributes to risk or resilience to develop a psychiatric condition. One avenue to pursue would be to try to find associations between specific candidate genes (for example, the *5-HTT* gene) and intermediate phenotypes mediating between a moderating allele and a more complex disease phenotype [61]. Studies on the *5-HTTLPR* gene are now under way that explicitly test gene × environment and gene × gene interaction. One study [62] found that a significant interaction between maternal anxiety during gestation and subsequent levels of infant negative emotionality at 6 months of age was modulated by 5-HTTLPR of the child. S-allele-carrying children showed high levels of negative emotionality, with mothers showing high maternal anxiety during pregnancy, whereas no such association was found in L-allele-carrying infants. In a BOLD-fMRI study, healthy women were threatened with unpredictable electric shocks of uncertain intensity, and activation was measured in several cortico-limbic networks upon threat anticipation [63]. During stress exposure, neural systems enhancing fear and arousal modulated attention towards threat and SS-individuals appeared particularly sensitive towards the stress, suggesting that such a mechanism may underlie the risk for psychopathology. In a different study, deductive reasoning appeared also dependent on the *5-HTTPRL* genotype. Apparently, differences in the functioning of the 5-HTT renders some individuals more vulnerable to emotional factors, thereby generating a deleterious effect on rational reasoning [64].

In another study, an interaction between the *5-HTTLPR* (measure in LL-variants) and an oxytocin receptor variant (TT variant of the SNP rs2268498) that influences the number of oxytocin receptors was found in individual differences in negative emotionality, indicating a gene × gene interaction [65]. Such data indicate that serotonergic and oxytocinergic neurotransmission processes are somewhere entwined and seem to play a role in affective disorders. In general, S-alleles of the *5-HTTLPR* are associated with increased risk for a variety of psychiatric disorders, including anxiety. The S-allele is considered a 'risk' or 'vulnerability' allele [66], whereas the function of the L-allele is far less clear, although this allele has been suggested as a potential risk factor for the development of psychopathic traits too [67]. Because every human has either the L or the S allele, or both, and most people do not suffer from psychiatric abnormalities, it must be assumed that the genome includes several 'protective' alleles that make many individuals resilient to stress and pathology. Such protective genes have been suggested, for example the CRF1-receptor variants that have been associated with protection from the extreme stresses of maltreatment during childhood [68] and protective emotional resilience-enhancing effects of the L-allele in students [69]. Belsky and colleagues [70] suggested that S-allele carriers are more vulnerable in general, not only negatively, but also positively. Thus, 'vulnerability genes' or 'risk alleles' seem to make individuals more susceptible to environmental influences—for better and for worse. Homberg and Lesch [71] postulated a similar picture of the functions of the allelic variants in *5-HTTLPR*. They did not portray the S-allele as a 'risk' allele and the L-allele as a 'resilient' allele but took the hypothesis that S-carriers (both in humans and in non-human primates) perform better in cognitive tasks than L-carriers. They argue for a switch from a deficit-orientated connotation of *5-HTTLPR* variants to a cognitive superiority of S-allele carriers (which have enhanced reactivity of the cortico-limbic neural circuitry) and that environmental conditions will determine whether a positive (cognitive) or negative (emotional) response will happen. Part of their support comes from studies in genetically modified mice and rats (heterozygote and homozygote) *5-HTT*

KOs. *5-HTT$^{-/-}$* rodents show brain and behavioural phenotypes rather similar to S-allele carriers such as increased emotionality, improved cognition, and increased sensitivity to psychosocial factors (reviewed in [72]). This seems present without environmental influence in the homozygote KOs, but in the heterozygotes, early or later life stress is additionally needed to show the same phenotypes [3, 72, 73].

## Genetic background of anxiety disorders

Genes certainly contribute to the risk for developing anxiety disorders. An update of the current findings is given in Chapters 80 and 89. No 'candidate' genes have emerged that play a straightforward role in the expression for vulnerability to anxiety or anxiety disorders [74]. This is probably due to the fact that several or more risk factors have individually small effects. Among those neurotransmitter systems which have provided targets to develop anxiolytic drugs are serotonin (5-HT), noradrenaline (NA), glutamate, dopamine, GABA, RGS2, and neuropeptides (corticotrophin-releasing factor, neuropeptide Y, brain-derived neurotrophic factor). Regulator of G-protein signalling proteins (RGS) are key modulators of G-protein-coupled receptor signalling. RGS2 modulates anxiety both in mice [75] and in humans [76]. In mice, a quantitative trait locus (QTL) on chromosome 1 was associated with anxiety-related phenotype [77]; the principal quantitative trait gene for this linkage signal appeared to be RGS2 [78].

In conclusion, it has proved a challenge to find loci involved in anxiety disorders, which is likely due to a complex and polygenic genetic background. Probably many genes influence the risk for developing anxiety disorders, each of them with a small effect. Moreover, epistatic processes, having the ability to mask the phenotype derived from other genes, are also very likely to be involved, whereas environmental factors induce complex gene–environment (G × E) interactions.

Another strategy has been to study endophenotypes or intermediate phenotypes in man. Such familial or heritable traits are assumed first to underlie relevant disorders and second, more controversially, to be more susceptible to genetic analysis. The amygdala shows enhanced activity in phobias and PTSD, compared to healthy individuals [79]. The function of the amygdala in processing emotion and the mechanisms underlying fear conditioning have provided important paradigms for imaging studies in man (see Chapter 90). The link with genetics has proved more challenging. There was great interest when the *5-HTTLPR* polymorphism was associated with amygdala reactivity [80, 81], implicating the S-allele in the increased amygdala reactivity towards external stimuli [82]. This kind of finding in small samples has proved difficult to replicate (see Chapters 80 and 89).

## Preclinical genetic approaches to fear and anxiety

Animal models of anxiety and fear have greatly enhanced our knowledge in the neurobiological mechanisms underlying fear and anxiety. Anxiety and fear represent the most translatable processes from animal to human. Indeed, animal pathology appears to resemble human pathology to a certain (but varying) degree [83]. Such models can be powerful in dissecting putative genes in anxiety and anxiety-associated traits [84, 85]. Apart from large-scale mouse

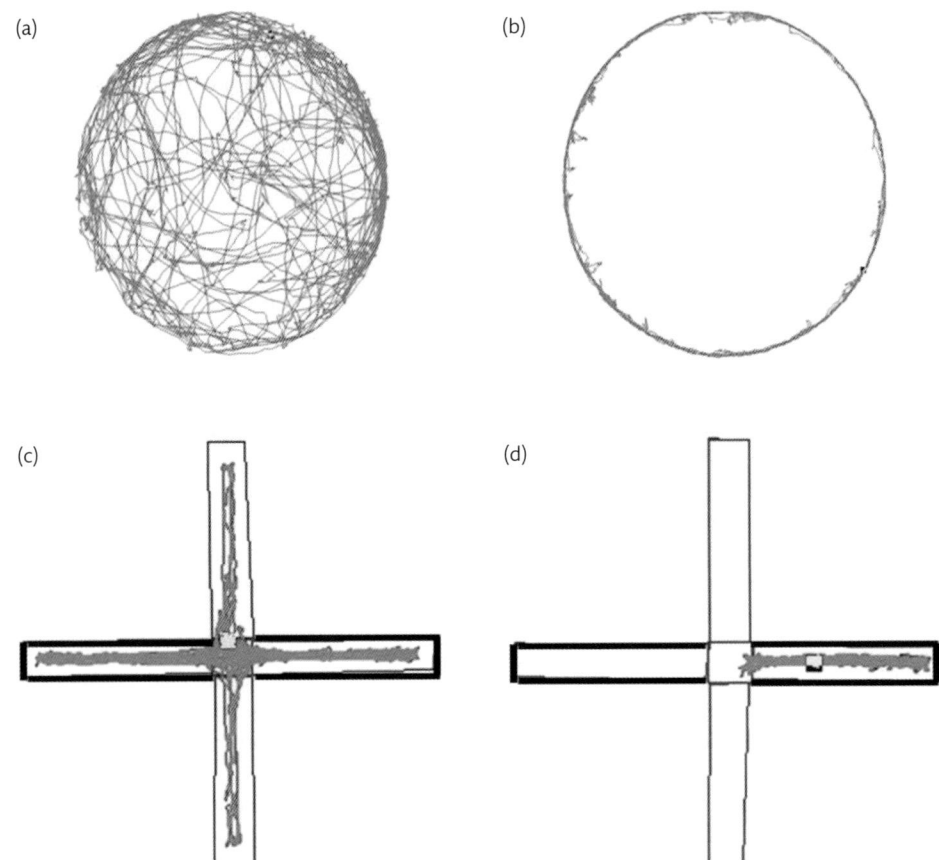

**Fig. 87.3** Traditionally, novelty-induced exploratory behaviour in the open field and the elevated plus maze are assessed to study anxiety-related behaviours in rodent species. In these representative data examples, video-tracking summary plots indicate the location of the mouse during a short session of open field exploration (a, b) or of exploration of an elevated plus maze (c, d). Different inbred strains of mice showed robust behavioural differences in these paradigms, as can be visualized in the data samples given. For example, C57BL/6J mice showed high levels of movement throughout the open field (a) and the elevated plus maze (c). In contrast, A/J mice showed lower levels of movement and stay close to the wall of the open field (b) and preferred the closed arms of the elevated plus maze (d) [closed arms are indicated by dark black lines (c, d)]. Based on the avoidance of the centre of the open field and the open arms of the elevated plus maze, A/J mice are considered to express higher levels of anxiety-related behaviour, when compared to C57BL/6J mice.

crossings for genetic mapping, leading to, for example, localization and identification of one gene *rgs2*, which influences anxious behaviours [76, 78, 86], gene-targeting approaches can be applied in rodents (Fig. 87.3).

Apart from classical searching for an animal model of anxiety, one can also try to use cross-species trait genetics in combination with an endophenotype approach [87, 88]. Using chromosome substitution strains, in which a single chromosome from one inbred strain (donor) is substituted with that of another inbred strain (host), makes it possible to locate a certain parameter or phenotype (such as avoidance behaviour) on a locus of a particular chromosome. Via further genetic crossings, the location can be refined and this may lead to candidate genes [89, 90]. By integrating genetic data from the mouse and from a large human GWAS on bipolar disorder, novel candidate genes for bipolar disorder were unravelled [91] (Fig. 87.4).

In the next section, some examples will be given of established targets involved in anxiety. A target can be defined as a neurobiological or cellular mechanism that, upon systematic manipulation, causes correlated effects on circuit function (in this case, anxiety), as well as behavioural/cognitive processes [92]. Because genomic technology advances rapidly, linkage between targets and neuronal circuitry and genetic factors involved in anxiety disorders are becoming increasingly elucidated. Fundamental research aimed at these targets may contribute to unravelling novel insights in anxiety processes and consequently engender new opportunities for drug discovery.

Although the 5-$HT_{1A}$ receptor, 5-HTT, and $GABA_A$ receptor complex belong to the most known and discussed targets in the field, human and animal research still continues to find new mechanisms around these targets that opens new possibilities to apply in animal models and human psychopathology. The future needs a strict translational approach; data found in human (anxiety) research, including genetic and environmental factors, should be used to formulate scientific approaches in animals, and vice versa. In animals, we have the opportunity to apply cell-specific inducible KOs or knock-ins. Moreover, new optogenetic technology enables selective manipulation of cellular mechanisms and circuit functions linked to the gene's suggested function [93].

### Integration

As genetic studies advance, validated animal anxiety models with translational validity are increasingly needed to study the biological role of genes found and their possible contribution to anxiety. In

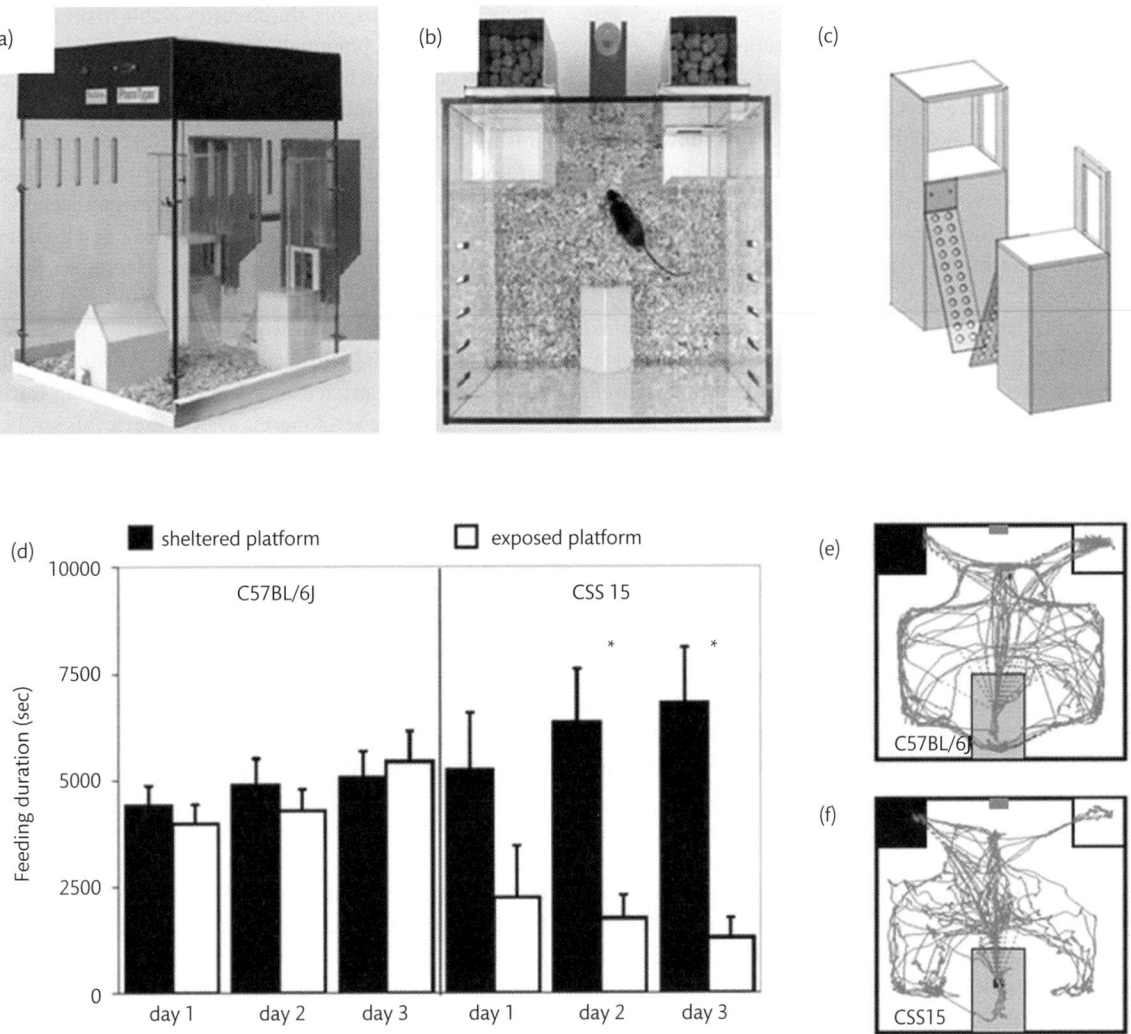

**Fig. 87.4** Behavioural screening of a chromosome substitution strain (CSS) panel revealed a locus for avoidance behaviour in an automated home cage environment on mouse chromosome 15. The automated home cage environment is equipped with a home base shelter (in which mice mainly sleep during the light phase) (a, b), a drinking spout, and two feeding platforms—one feeding platform exposed to the environment, and one allowing sheltered feeding (c). The PhenoTyper® top unit contains an infra-red camera and infra-red LED lights, allowing continuous recording, independent of lighting conditions in the test room. C57BL/6J and CSS15 females; feeding duration on the two platforms on 3 days of testing. CSS15 females showed an increasing preference for the sheltered platform over consecutive days (d). * Exposed vs sheltered feeding platform per day; P <0.05. Representative track samples during automated baseline behavioural registration, showing a reduction in visitation of the exposed feeding platform for CSS15 (f), compared to C57BL/6J (e). Further genetic fine mapping of the locus on mouse chromosome 15 revealed a homologous human locus on chromosome 8 previously associated with bipolar disorders.

Reproduced from *Biol Psychiatry*, 66(12), de Mooij-van Malsen AJ, van Lith HA, Oppelaar H, *et al.*, Inter-species Trait Genetics Reveals Association of Adcy8 with Mouse Avoidance Behavior and a Human Mood Disorder, pp. 1123–1130, Copyright (2009), with permission from Society of Biological Psychiatry.

search for animal paradigms with high translational value, we extensively explored a readout parameter of autonomic nervous system activation—stress-induced hyperthermia (SIH). SIH occurs in animals and man and depends on stress intensity, and individual differences in response to stress are dependent on genetic and environmental factors [94, 95]. In humans, autonomic stress responses correlate with perceived stress levels. Although the SIH response does not specifically model any psychiatric disease, SIH may be very useful as a readout parameter of stress or an anxiety-like response. It can be studied at preclinical and clinical levels, using different and varied stressful experimental conditions. It is highly suitable to detect genetic effects and anxiolytic properties of drugs, for example in 5-HT$_{1A}$ receptor KO mice [50, 94, 96]. The SIH response

can be reduced using GABA$_A$ receptor agonists and 5-HT$_{1A}$ receptor agonists [95, 97]. Baseline body temperature and circadian rhythmicity were comparable, but SIH was lower in 5-HTT KO than in the corresponding wildtypes. Pharmacological studies revealed that 5-HT$_{1A}$ receptors modulating SIH belong to a population of receptors that differ from those involved in hypothermia [98]. Later research found also changed sensitivity in dopamine and NA receptors in 5-HTT KO rats [99]. It might be postulated that the 5-HTT KO rat constitutes an animal model of certain psychiatric disorders, including anxiety disorders. A preliminary study [100] tried to find a genetic basis for the sensitivity of various chromosome substitution mouse strains [101] for diazepam (a non-subunit selective GABA$_A$ receptor agonist) and flesinoxan, a highly selective 5-HT$_{1A}$ receptor agonist

[102], using the SIH paradigm as experimental paradigm. Using the SIH paradigm, eight chromosomal substitution strains (CSS) on a C57BL6/J (host) × A/J (donor) background were screened to localize chromosomes involved in GABA$_A$ and 5-HT$_{1A}$ receptor sensitivity. Preliminary data indicated that some strains showed clear differences in either diazepam or flesinoxan sensitivity. Further research is ongoing to unravel underlying putative genes.

GABA-ergic and serotonergic mechanisms play an important role in SIH, and rodent and human studies into the underlying brain mechanisms indicate high translational comparability. Mouse genetic mapping studies (by using chromosomal substitution strains) indicated genetic loci involved in the pharmacological mechanisms behind the SIH processes. If such loci and genes can be localized, human counterparts have to be sought in the quest for novel candidate genes involved in anxiety and its disorders.

Besides SIH, other highly valuable translational animal paradigms also have been developed. For instance, the startle reflex methodology can translate animal research into human experimentations, and vice versa. Especially the combination of the startle reflex methodology with Pavlovian aversive conditioning makes it a powerful procedure to develop cross-species studies [103]. The startle reflex is a response to an intense and unexpected stimulus. In animals, this reflex can be measured by assessing the whole body reflex. In humans, the eyeblink reflex is used to measure the amplitude and latency of a startle reflex. Davis and colleagues [104] extensively investigated the fear-potentiated startle, which refers to the increase (potentiation) of the startle reflex during a state of fear. This state of fear is induced by the anticipation of an aversive stimulus (for example, a shock). Animals and humans display similar effects, that is, the amplitude of the startle reflex is greater in the presence of conditioned stimuli than in their absence [104–107]. The advantage of the fear-potentiated startle procedure is that the startle in animals and humans are potentiated by similar procedures. Thus, findings in humans can be replicated in animals, and vice versa, increasing the translational value of animal models of human anxiety. When a new gene is discovered by means of, for example, GWAS, an animal model can be genetically manipulated and used to study the underlying mechanisms or to investigate new potential anxiolytics.

### Translational studies into anxiety

Can data on the involvement of serotonin in anxiety and anxiety disorders (here illustrated with the 5-HTT and the 5-HT$_{1A}$ receptor) be used to design translational research that possibly will generate new hypotheses and targets for anxiolytic therapeutics? Recently, Jasinska *et al.* [108] formulated a hypothesis around the involvement of the *5-HTT* gene, stress, and raphe–raphe interactions in order to try to explain the risk of depression as a result of gene–environment interactions between the *5-HTT* gene and stress. Different populations of serotonergic neurons in the dorsal raphe (DR) nucleus exist that differentially contribute to the response to stress. Although the authors hypothesize this mechanism mainly for depression, there is no a priori reason why anxiety disorders would not be mediated by this or a similar mechanism. The authors propose that the G × E interaction of the *5-HTTPRL* and stress depends on the genetically produced variability in serotonin reuptake during stressor-induced raphe–raphe interactions and alters the balance in the amygdala–ventromedial prefrontal cortex–DR circuitry that underlie reactivity to stressors and regulation of emotion. In LL-individuals with an

efficient 5-HT transport, the circuitry is able to normalize, but not so in SS-individuals, potentially leading to abnormal activity and pathology. Whether such a mechanism also acts in human pathology is as yet unresolved but could lead to specific searches for new mechanisms causing pathological anxiety. Next to different functional serotonergic populations in the DR, serotonin transporters appear very dynamically regulated [109] and undergo regulated membrane trafficking, as well as transitions between low and high activity states, with many signalling pathways involved. Moreover, 5-HTT exhibits dynamic associations with cytoskeletal binding proteins; actually, Chang *et al.* [110] found two pools of 5-HTT proteins on the surface of serotonergic cells, with one relatively with free diffusion and the other with restricted mobility due to binding to the cytoskeleton. Whether the serotonergic system exerts this kind of extremely variability, which might lead to new and better understanding of the role of the 5-HTT complex, including its genetic variability, is still a matter of the future, but it remains fully possible that new mechanisms involved in anxiety and its disorders might emerge.

### Conclusions

The discovery and development of novel anxiolytic drugs are hampering. The existing anxiolytics have been around for decades, and no subsequent breakthrough has come through. Especially, the lack of innovative and effective novel drug targets is disappointing. The reasons for this lack of progress are not completely clear but may be due to the complex regulatory and financial regulations in the finding of new 'druggable' targets (we do not go into many other financial, outsourcing, human, and marketing reasons (see, for example, [111]).

However, central to the continued paucity of new targets for anxiolytic drugs is our limited knowledge of the mechanisms and pathology underlying the various anxiety disorders. We simply do not know what is wrong in the brain of pathologically anxious people and whether the DSM-based anxiety disorders constitute independent entities. Therefore, we have to invest in fundamental research in the neurobiological mechanisms involved in anxiety processes in healthy people and look for what is different in diseased brains. Because intrusive investigations of the human brain are often not (or never) possible, animal research is inevitable and can contribute considerably to find the neural substrates for anxiety and its pathology, although it is not realistic to think that such knowledge is 100% translatable to the human situation. Any strategy to find new targets to modulate aspects of anxiety (and hopefully its pathology) will use genetic and genomic approaches. Our initial hope was that, after elucidation of the human genome, we would be able to pinpoint certain genes as the perpetrator causing the problem. However, it soon became clear that that is an illusion. Notwithstanding a high heritability in many of the anxiety disorders, no single gene or a small number of genes have emerged from a large number of studies on large cohorts of patients thus far. It has become increasingly clear that anxiety disorders, similar probably to the fundamental mechanisms involved in anxiety processes, are caused by action at many hundreds of genes with very complex interactions, including both environmental factors and gene × gene interactions. It is difficult to expect that one single gene contributes sufficient influence to modulate anxiety processes to a large degree, and no specific drug will probably be developed for such a target. In the present contribution, three (druggable) targets have been presented, with all three somewhere involved in the (genetic) pathways of anxiety processes (5-HT$_{1A}$ receptor, 5-HTT, and GABA$_A$ receptor). Although it is not known how these three targets are involved in 'normal' or 'pathological' anxiety in the brain, we know at least that they are involved in several aspects of anxiety and may aid in our further understanding of the underlying mechanisms. Whether they represent real direct targets that are changed under pathological conditions or only as primary entrance to influence underlying mechanisms is not clear. In the case of serotonin modulation (via 5-HT$_{1A}$ receptor activation or blockade of the serotonin transporter), an indirect effect is possibly the most logical explanation, because treatment of anxiety disorders with SSRIs or buspirone takes weeks, or even months, before anxiolytic activity is seen. This points to an induction of mechanisms that slowly change and need time to become effective (plasticity changes). Anxiolytic effects after activation of GABA$_A$ receptors seem acute and might point to a primary mechanism directly involved in anxiety-regulating mechanisms. Close collaboration between fundamental academic research into anxiety mechanisms in the brain and drug discovery research and development might lead to breakthroughs in our search for new and better anxiolytics. Clearly, animal models will play an important role in future anxiolytic drug development, but only as a component of a broad and integrated multi-disciplinary approach. To be successful, preclinical researchers need to ensure that novel clinical insights into the aetiology of anxiety disorders are integrated in the design and use of animal models and tests.

## REFERENCES

1. Cryan, J.F., Sweeney, F.F. 2011. The age of anxiety: role of animal models of anxiolytic action in drug discovery. *Br. J. Pharmacol.* 164, 1129–61.

2. Ressler, K.J., Mayberg, H.S. 2007. Targeting abnormal neural circuits in mood and anxiety disorders: from the laboratory to the clinic. *Nat. Neurosci.* 10, 1116–24.

3. Murphy, D.L., Lesch, K.P. 2008. Targeting the murine serotonin transporter: insights into human neurobiology. *Nat. Rev. Neurosci.* 9, 85–96.

4. Möhler, H., Okada, T. 1977. Benzodiazepine receptor: demonstration in the central nervous system. *Science.* 198, 849–51.

5. Pirker, S., Schwarzer, C., Wieselthaler A., *et al.* 2000. GABA(A) receptors: immunocytochemical distribution of 13 subunits in the adult rat brain. *Neuroscience.* 101, 815–50.

6. Castelli M.P., Ingianni, A., Stefanini, E., Gessa, G.L. 1999. Distribution of GABA(B) receptor mRNA in the rat brain and peripheral organs. *Life Sci.* 64, 1321–8.

7. Rudolph, U., Möhler, H. 2006. GABA-based therapeutic approaches: GABA$_A$ receptor subtype functions. *Curr. Opin. Pharmacol.* 6, 18–23.

8. Jacobson L.H., Vlachou S., Slattery, D.A., *et al.* 2018. The gamma-butyric acid B receptor in depression and reward. *Biol. Psychiatry,* 83, 963–76.

9. Vinkers, C.H., Mirza, N.R., Olivier, B., Kahn, R.S. 2010. The inhibitory GABA system as a therapeutic target for cognitive symptoms in schizophrenia: investigational agents in the pipeline. *Expert Opin. Investig. Drugs.* 19, 1217–33.

10. Möhler, H., Fritschy, J.M., Rudolph, U. 2002. A new benzodiazepine pharmacology. *J. Pharmacol. Exp. Ther.* 300, 2–8.

11. Farb, D.H., Ratner, M.H. 2014. Targeting the modulation of neural cicuitry for the treatment of anxiety disorders. *Pharmacol. Rev.* 66, 1002–32.

12. Möhler, H. 2006. GABA$_A$ receptors in central nervous system disease: anxiety, epilepsy, and insomnia. *J. Recept. Signal. Transduct. Res.* 26, 731–40.

13. Rudolph, U., Knoflach, F. 2011. Beyond classical benzodiazepines: novel therapeutic potential of GABA(A) receptor subtypes. *Nat. Rev. Drug Discov.* 10, 685–97.

14. Tan, K.R., Rudolph, U., Luscher, C. 2011. Hooked on benzodiazepines: GABAA receptor subtypes and addiction. *Trends Neurosci.* 34, 188–97.

15. Dias, R., Sheppard, W.F., Fradley, R.L., *et al.* 2005. Evidence for a significant role of alpha 3-containing GABA$_A$ receptors in mediating the anxiolytic effects of benzodiazepines. *J. Neurosci.* 25, 10682–8.

16. Vinkers, C.H., Klanker, M., Groenink, L., *et al.* 2009. Dissociating anxiolytic and sedative effects of GABA$_A$ergic drugs using temperature and locomotor responses to acute stress. *Psychopharmacology (Berl).* 204, 299–311.

17. Atack, J.R. 2010. GABA$_A$ receptor alpha2/alpha3 subtype-selective modulators as potential nonsedating anxiolytics. *Curr. Top. Behav. Neurosci.* 2, 331–60.

18. McKernan, R.M., Rosahl, T.W., Reynolds, D.S. *et al.*, 2000. Sedative but not anxiolytic properties of benzodiazepines are mediated by the GABA(A) receptor alpha1 subtype. *Nat. Neurosci.* 3, 587–92.

19. Van Bogaert, M.J., Oosting, R., Toth, M., Groenink, L., van Oorschot, R., Olivier, B. 2006. Effects of genetic background and null mutation of 5-HT1A receptors on basal and stress-induced body temperature: modulation by serotonergic and GABA$_A$-ergic drugs. *Eur. J. Pharmacol.* 550, 84–90.

20. Rowlett, J.K., Platt, D.M., Lelas, S., Atack, J.R., Dawson, G.R. 2005. Different GABAA receptor subtypes mediate the anxiolytic, abuse-related, and motor effects of benzodiazepine-like drugs in primates. *Proc. Natl. Acad. Sci. U. S. A.* 102, 915–20.

21. Scott-Stevens, P., Atack, J.R., Sohal, B., Worboys, P. 2005. Rodent pharmacokinetics and receptor occupancy of the GABA$_A$ receptor subtype selective benzodiazepine site ligand L-838417. *Biopharm. Drug Dispos.* 26, 13–20.

22. Atack, J.R., Wafford, K.A., Tye, S.J., *et al.* 2006. TPA023 [7-(1,1-dimethylethyl)-6-(2-ethyl-2H-1,2,4-triazol-3-ylmethoxy)-3-(2-fluorophenyl)-1,2,4-triazolo[4,3-b]pyridazine], an agonist selective for alpha2- and alpha3-containing GABA$_A$ receptors, is a nonsedating anxiolytic in rodents and primates. *J. Pharmacol. Exp. Ther.* 316, 410–22.

23. Lippa, A., Czobor, P., Stark, J., *et al.* 2005. Selective anxiolysis produced by ocinaplon, a GABA(A) receptor modulator. *Proc. Natl. Acad. Sci. U. S. A.* 102, 7380–5.

24. Czobor, P., Skolnick, P., Beer, B., Lippa, A. 2010. A multicenter, placebo-controlled, double-blind, randomized study of efficacy and safety of ocinaplon (DOV 273,547) in generalized anxiety disorder. *CNS Neurosci. Ther.* 16, 63–75.

25. Atack, J.R., Wafford, K.A., Street, L.J., *et al.* 2011. MRK-409 (MK-0343), a GABAA receptor subtype-selective partial agonist, is a non-sedating anxiolytic in preclinical species but causes sedation in humans. *J. Psychopharmacol.* 25, 314–28.

26. Reddy, D.S., Estes, W.A. 2016. Clinical potential of neurosteroids for CNS disorders. *Trends Pharmacol. Sci.* 37, 543–61.

27. Vinkers, C.H., van Oorschot, R., Nielsen, E.Ø., *et al.* 2012. GABA(A) receptor α subunits differentially contribute to diazepam tolerance after chronic treatment. *PLoS One.* 7, e43054.

28. Tan, K.R., Brown, M., Labouebe, G., *et al.* 2010. Neural bases for addictive properties of benzodiazepines. *Nature.* 463, 769–74.

29. Vinkers, C.H., Olivier, B. 2012. Mechanisms underlying tolerance after long-term benzodiazepine use: a future for subtype-selective GABA(A) receptor modulators? *Adv. Pharmacol. Sci.* 2012, 416864.

30. Mirza, N.R., Munro, G. 2010. The role of GABA(A) receptor subtypes as analgesic targets. *Drug News Perspect.* 23, 351–60.

31. Olivier, B., Soudijn, W., van Wijngaarden, I. 1999. The 5-HT$_{1A}$ receptor and its ligands: structure and function. *Prog. Drug Res.* 52, 103–65.

32. Olivier, B. 2015. Serotonin: a never ending story. *Eur. J. Pharmacol.* 753, 2–18.

33. Goldberg, H.L., Finnerty, R.J. 1979. The comparative efficacy of buspirone and diazepam in the treatment of anxiety. *Am. J. Psychiatry.* 136, 1184–7.

34. Holmes, A. 2008. Genetic variation in cortico-amygdala serotonin function and risk for stress-related disease. *Neurosci. Biobehav. Rev.* 32, 1293–314.

35. Lanfumey, L., Mongeau, R., Cohen-Salmon, C., Hamon, M. 2008. Corticosteroid-serotonin interactions in the neurobiological mechanisms of stress-related disorders. *Neurosci. Biobehav. Rev.* 32, 1174–84.

36. Savitz, J., Lucki, I., Drevets, W.C. 2009. 5-HT(1A) receptor function in major depressive disorder. *Prog. Neurobiol.* 88, 17–31.

37. Akimova, E., Lanzenberger, R., Kasper, S., 2009. The serotonin-1A receptor in anxiety disorders. *Biol. Psychiatry.* 66, 627–35.

38. Gardier, A.M., Malagie, I., Trillat, A.C., Jacquot, C., Artigas, F. 1996. Role of 5-HT$_{1A}$ autoreceptors in the mechanism of action of serotoninergic antidepressant drugs: recent findings from *in vivo* microdialysis studies. *Fundam. Clin. Pharmacol.* 10, 16–27.

39. Blier, P., Pineyro, G., el Mansari, M., Bergeron, R., de Montigny, C. 1998. Role of somatodendritic 5-HT autoreceptors in modulating 5-HT neurotransmission. *Ann. N. Y. Acad. Sci.* 861, 204–16.

40. Lesch, K.P., Gutknecht, L. 2004. Focus on The 5-HT1A receptor: emerging role of a gene regulatory variant in psychopathology and pharmacogenetics. *Int. J. Neuropsychopharmacol.* 7, 381–5.

41. Fakra, E., Hyde, L.W., Gorka, A., *et al.* 2009. Effects of HTR1A C(-1019)G on amygdala reactivity and trait anxiety. *Arch. Gen. Psychiatry.* 66, 33–40.

42. Le François, B., Czesak, M., Steubl, D., Albert, P.R. 2008. Transcriptional regulation at a HTR1A polymorphism associated with mental illness. *Neuropharmacology.* 55, 977–85.

43. Drago, A., Ronchi, D.D., Serretti, A. 2008. *5-HT1A* gene variants and psychiatric disorders: a review of current literature and selection of SNPs for future studies. *Int. J. Neuropsychopharmacol.* 11, 701–21.

44. Ramboz, S., Oosting, R., Amara, D.A., *et al.* 1998. Serotonin receptor 1A knockout: an animal model of anxiety-related disorder. *Proc. Natl. Acad. Sci. U. S. A.* 95, 14476–81.

45. Heisler, L.K., Chu, H.M., Brennan, T.J. *et al.*, 1998. Elevated anxiety and antidepressant-like responses in serotonin 5-HT$_{1A}$ receptor mutant mice. *Proc. Natl. Acad. Sci. U. S. A.* 95, 15049–54.

46. Parks, C.L., Robinson, P.S., Sibille, E., Shenk, T., Toth, M. 1998. Increased anxiety of mice lacking the serotonin1A receptor. *Proc. Natl. Acad. Sci. U. S. A.* 95, 10734–9.

47. Pattij, T., Hijzen, T.H., Groenink, L., *et al.* 2001. Stress-induced hyperthermia in the 5-HT(1A) receptor knockout mouse is normal. *Biol. Psychiatry.* 49, 569–74.

48. Sibille, E., Pavlides, C., Benke, D., Toth, M. 2000. Genetic inactivation of the serotonin(1A) receptor in mice results in downregulation of major GABA(A) receptor alpha subunits, reduction of GABA(A) receptor binding, and benzodiazepine-resistant anxiety. *J. Neurosci.* 20, 2758–65.

49. Olivier, B., Pattij, T., Wood, S.J., Oosting, R., Sarnyai, Z., Toth, M. 2001. The 5-HT(1A) receptor knockout mouse and anxiety. *Behav. Pharmacol.* 12, 439–50.

50. Pattij, T., Groenink, L., Oosting, R.S., van der Gugten, J., Maes, R.A., Olivier, B. 2002. GABA(A)-benzodiazepine receptor complex sensitivity in 5-HT(1A) receptor knockout mice on a 129/Sv background. *Eur. J. Pharmacol.* 447, 67–74.

51. Santarelli, L., Saxe, M., Gross, C., *et al.* 2003. Requirement of hippocampal neurogenesis for the behavioral effects of antidepressants. *Science.* 301, 805–9.

52. Kusserow, H., Davies, B., Hortnagl, H., *et al.* 2004. Reduced anxiety-related behaviour in transgenic mice overexpressing serotonin 1A receptors. *Brain Res. Mol. Brain Res.* 129, 104–16.

53. Gross, C., Zhuang, X., Stark, K., *et al.* 2002. Serotonin1A receptor acts during development to establish normal anxiety-like behaviour in the adult. *Nature.* 416, 396–400.

54. Lo Iacono, L., Gross, C. 2008. Alpha-Ca$^{2+}$/calmodulin-dependent protein kinase II contributes to the developmental programming of anxiety in serotonin receptor 1A knock-out mice. *J. Neurosci.* 28, 6250–7.

55. Richardson-Jones, J.W., Craige, C.P., Guiard, B.P., *et al.* 2010. 5-HT1A autoreceptor levels determine vulnerability to stress and response to antidepressants. *Neuron.* 65, 40–52.

56. Albert, P.R., Vahid-Ansari, F., Luckhart, C. 2014. Serotonin-prefrontal cortical circuitry in anxiety and depression phenotypes: pivotal role of pre- and post-synaptic 5-HT$_{1A}$ receptor expression. *Front. Behav. Neurosci.* 8, 199.

57. Lesch, K.P. 2001. Molecular foundation of anxiety disorders. *J. Neural Transm.* 108, 717–46.

58. Lesch, K.P., Bengel, D., Heils, A., *et al.* 1996. Association of anxiety-related traits with a polymorphism in the serotonin transporter gene regulatory region. *Science.* 274, 1527–31.

59. Caspi, A., Sugden, K., Moffitt, T.E., *et al.* 2003. Influence of life stress on depression: moderation by a polymorphism in the *5-HTT* gene. *Science.* 301, 386–9.

60. Haddley, K., Bubb, V.J., Breen, G., Parades-Esquivel, U.M., Quinn, J.P. 2012. Behavioural genetics of the serotonin transporter. *Curr. Topics Behav. Neurosci.* 12, 503–35.

61. Murrough, J.W., Charney, D.S. 2011. The serotonin transporter and emotionality: risk, resilience, and new therapeutic opportunities. *Biol. Psychiatry.* 69, 510–12.

62. Pluess, M., Velders, F.P., Belsky, J., *et al.* 2011. Serotonin transporter polymorphism moderates effects of prenatal maternal anxiety on infant negative emotionality. *Biol. Psychiatry.* 69, 520–5.

63. Drabant, E.M., Ramel, W., Edge, M.D., *et al.* 2012. Neural mechanisms underlying 5-HTTLPR-related sensitivity to acute stress. *Am. J. Psychiatry.* 169, 397–405.

64. Stollstorff, M., Bean, S.E., Anderson, L.M., Devaney, J.M., Vaidya, C.J. 2013. Rationality and emotionality: serotonin transporter genotype influences reasoning bias. *Soc. Cogn. Affect. Neurosci.* 8, 404–9.

65. Montag, C., Fiebach, C.J., Kirsch, P., Reuter, M. 2011. Interaction of 5-HTTLPR and a variation on the oxytocin receptor gene influences negative emotionality. *Biol. Psychiatry.* 69, 601–3.

66. Caspi, A., Hariri, A.R., Holmes, A., Uher, R., Moffitt, T.E. 2010. Genetic sensitivity to the environment: the case of the serotonin transporter gene and its implications for studying complex diseases and traits. *Am. J. Psychiatry.* 167, 509–27.

67. Glenn, A.L. 2011. The other allele: exploring the long allele of the serotonin transporter gene as a potential risk factor for

psychopathy: a review of the parallels in findings. *Neurosci. Biobehav. Rev.* 35, 612–20.

68. Polanczyk, G., Caspi, A., Williams, B. *et al.*, 2009. Protective effect of *CRHR1* gene variants on the development of adult depression following childhood maltreatment: replication and extension. *Arch. Gen. Psychiatry.* 66, 978–85.

69. Stein, M.B., Campbell-Sills, L., Gelernter, J. 2009. Genetic variation in 5HTTLPR is associated with emotional resilience. *Am. J. Med. Genet. B. Neuropsychiatr. Genet.* 150B, 900–6.

70. Belsky, J., Jonassaint, C., Pluess, M., Stanton, M., Brummett, B., Williams, R. 2009. Vulnerability genes or plasticity genes? *Mol. Psychiatry.* 14, 746–54.

71. Homberg, J.R., Lesch, K.P. 2011. Looking on the bright side of serotonin transporter gene variation. *Biol. Psychiatry.* 69, 513–19.

72. Kalueff, A.V., Olivier, J.D., Nonkes, L.J., Homberg, J.R. 2010. Conserved role for the serotonin transporter gene in rat and mouse neurobehavioral endophenotypes. *Neurosci. Biobehav. Rev.* 34, 373–86.

73. Neumann, I.D., Wegener, G., Homberg, J.R., *et al.* 2011. Animal models of depression and anxiety: what do they tell us about human condition? *Prog. Neuropsychopharmacol. Biol. Psychiatry.* 35, 1357–75.

74. Smoller, J.W., Block, S.R., Young, M.M. 2009. Genetics of anxiety disorders: the complex road from DSM to DNA. *Depress. Anxiety.* 26, 965–75.

75. Oliveira-Dos-Santos, A.J., Matsumoto, G., Snow, B.E., *et al.*, 2000. Regulation of T cell activation, anxiety, and male aggression by RGS2. *Proc. Natl. Acad. Sci. U. S. A.* 97, 12272–7.

76. Smoller, J.W., Paulus, M.P., Fagerness, J.A., *et al.* 2008. Influence of RGS2 on anxiety-related temperament, personality, and brain function. *Arch. Gen. Psychiatry.* 65, 298–308.

77. Flint, J. 2003. Analysis of quantitative trait loci that influence animal behavior. *J. Neurobiol.* 54, 46–77.

78. Yalcin, B., Willis-Owen, S.A., Fullerton, J., *et al.* 2004. Genetic dissection of a behavioral quantitative trait locus shows that Rgs2 modulates anxiety in mice. *Nat. Genet.* 36, 1197–202.

79. Etkin, A., Wager, T.D. 2007. Functional neuroimaging of anxiety: a meta-analysis of emotional processing in PTSD, social anxiety disorder, and specific phobia. *Am. J. Psychiatry.* 164, 1476–88.

80. Hariri, A.R., Mattay, V.S., Tessitore, A., *et al.* 2002. Serotonin transporter genetic variation and the response of the human amygdala. *Science.* 297, 400–3.

81. Hariri, A.R., Holmes, A. 2006. Genetics of emotional regulation: the role of the serotonin transporter in neural function. *Trends Cogn. Sci.* 10, 182–91.

82. Hariri, A.R. 2009. The neurobiology of individual differences in complex behavioral traits. *Annu. Rev. Neurosci.* 32, 225–47.

83. Fernando, A.B., Robbins, T.W. 2011. Animal models of neuropsychiatric disorders. *Annu. Rev. Clin. Psychol.* 7, 39–61.

84. Flint, J., Shifman, S. 2008. Animal models of psychiatric disease. *Curr. Opin. Genet. Dev.* 18, 235–40.

85. Kas, M.J., Krishnan, V., Gould, T.D., *et al.* 2011. Advances in multidisciplinary and cross-species approaches to examine the neurobiology of psychiatric disorders. *Eur. Neuropsychopharmacol.* 21, 532–44.

86. Leygraf, A., Hohoff, C., Freitag, C., *et al.* 2006. *Rgs 2* gene polymorphisms as modulators of anxiety in humans? *J. Neural Transm.* 113, 1921–5.

87. Kas, M.J., Van Ree, J.M. 2004. Dissecting complex behaviours in the post-genomic era. *Trends Neurosci.* 27, 366–9.

88. Kas, M.J., Fernandes, C., Schalkwyk, L.C., Collier, D.A. 2007. Genetics of behavioural domains across the neuropsychiatric spectrum; of mice and men. *Mol. Psychiatry.* 12, 324–30.

89. Kas, M.J., de Mooij-van Malsen, A.J., Olivier, B., Spruijt, B.M., Van Ree, J.M. 2008. Differential genetic regulation of motor activity and anxiety-related behaviors in mice using an automated home cage task. *Behav. Neurosci.* 122, 769–76.

90. de Mooij-van Malsen, A.J., Olivier, B., Kas, M.J. 2008. Behavioural genetics in mood and anxiety: a next step in finding novel pharmacological targets. *Eur. J. Pharmacol.* 585, 436–40.

91. de Mooij-van Malsen, A.J., van Lith, H.A., Oppelaar, H., *et al.* 2009. Interspecies trait genetics reveals association of Adcy8 with mouse avoidance behavior and a human mood disorder. *Biol. Psychiatry.* 66, 1123–30.

92. Sarter, M., Tricklebank, M. 2012. Revitalizing psychiatric drug discovery. *Nature Rev. Drug Discov.* 11, 423–4.

93. Tye, K.M., Deisseroth, K. 2012. Optogenetic investigation of neural circuits underlying brain disease in animal models. *Nature Rev. Neurosci.* 13, 251–66.

94. Bouwknecht, J.A., Olivier, B., Paylor, R.E. 2007. The stress-induced hyperthermia paradigm as a physiological animal model for anxiety: a review of pharmacological and genetic studies in the mouse. *Neurosci. Biobehav. Rev.* 31, 41–59.

95. Vinkers, C.H., van Bogaert, M.J., Klanker, M., *et al.* 2008. Translational aspects of pharmacological research into anxiety disorders: the stress-induced hyperthermia (SIH) paradigm. *Eur. J. Pharmacol.* 585, 407–25.

96. Vinkers, C.H., Oosting, R.S., van Bogaert, M.J., Olivier, B., Groenink, L. 2010. Early-life blockade of 5-HT$_{1A}$ receptors alters adult anxiety behaviour and benzodiazepine sensitivity. *Biol. Psychiatry.* 67, 309–16.

97. Olivier, B., Zethof, T., Pattij, T., *et al.* 2003. Stress-induced hyperthermia and anxiety: pharmacological validation. *Eur. J. Pharmacol.* 463, 117–32.

98. Olivier, J.D., Cools, A.R., Olivier, B., Homberg, J.R., Cuppen, E., Ellenbroek, B.A. 2008. Stress-induced hyperthermia and basal body temperature are mediated by different 5-HT(1A) receptor populations: a study in SERT knockout rats. *Eur. J. Pharmacol.* 590, 190–7.

99. Olivier, J.D., Cools, A.R., Deen, P.M., Olivier, B., Ellenbroek, B.A. 2010. Blockade of dopamine, but not noradrenaline, transporters produces hyperthermia in rats that lack serotonin transporters. *Eur. J. Pharmacol.* 629, 7–11.

100. de Mooij-van Malsen, A.J., Vinkers, C.H., Peterse, D.P., Olivier, B., Kas, M.J. 2011. Cross-species behavioural genetics: a starting point for unravelling the neurobiology of human psychiatric disorders. *Prog. Neuropsychopharmacol. Biol. Psychiatry.* 35, 1383–90.

101. Nadeau, J.H., Singer, J.B., Matin, A., Lander, E.S. 2000. Analysing complex genetic traits with chromosome substitution strains. *Nat. Genet.* 24, 221–5.

102. Olivier, B., Tulp, M.Th.M., van der Poel, A.M. 1991. Serotonergic receptors in anxiety and aggression: evidence from animal pharmacology. *Hum. Psychopharmacol.* 6, S73–8.

103. Grillon, C. 2002. Startle reactivity and anxiety disorders: aversive conditioning, context and neurobiology. *Biol. Psychiatry.* 52, 958–75.

104. Davis, M. 1998. Are different parts of the extended amygdala involved in fear versus anxiety? *Biol. Psychiatry.* 44, 1239–47.

105. Grillon, C., Davis, M. 1997. Fear-potentiated startle conditioning in humans: explicit and contextual cue conditioning

following paired versus unpaired training. *Psychophysiology.* 34, 451–8.

106. Hamm, A.O., Greenwald, M.K., Bradley, M.M., Lang, P.J. 1993. Emotional learning, hedonic changes, and the startle probe. *J. Abnorm. Psychol.* 102, 453–65.

107. Spence, K., Norris, E. 1950. Eyelid conditioning as a function of the inter-trial interval. *J. Exp. Psychol.* 40, 716–20.

108. Jasinska, A.J., Lowry, C.A., Burmeister, M. 2012. Serotonin transporter gene, stress and raphe-raphe interactions: a molecular mechanism of depression. *Trends Neurosci.* 35, 395–402.

109. Steiner, J.A., Carneiro, A.M., Blakely, R.D. 2008. Going with the flow: trafficking-dependent and -independent regulation of serotonin transport. *Traffic.* 9, 1393–402.

110. Chang, J.C., Tomlinson, I.D., Warnement, M.R., *et al.* 2012. Single molecule analysis of serotonin transporter regulation using antagonist-conjugated quantum dots reveals restricted, p38 MAPK-dependent mobilization underlying uptake activiation. *J. Neurosci.* 32, 8919–29

111. Knutsen, L.J. 2011. Drug discovery management, small is still beautiful: why a number of companies get it wrong. *Drug Discov. Today.* 16, 476–84.

# 88

# Epidemiology of anxiety disorders

*Hans-Ulrich Wittchen and Katja Beesdo-Baum*

## Introduction

For an understanding of anxiety disorders, it is helpful to distinguish anxiety and fear as different, though overlapping and related, constructs. Anxiety is a basic emotion and is typically adaptive, and not pathological. It can be described as a future oriented mood state associated with the anticipation of future threat and possibly its avoidance. Fear is the organism's response to present/imminent real or perceived threat and is associated with autonomic arousal and escape [1]. Clinically relevant anxiety disorders differ descriptively from non-pathological forms of fear and anxiety by being considerably more persistent and excessive, causing significant distress and impairment [2]. It is assumed that various conditioned dysfunctions in the regulation of the complex neurobiological and psychological fear/anxiety circuits are responsible for pathological anxiety [3]. In childhood and adolescence, anxiety often manifests as part of typical development, which can render identification and diagnosis of pathological anxiety difficult. However, it is particularly this sensitive phase of life when initially transient and circumscribed neurobiological, cognitive, affective, and behavioural dysfunctions may generalize and escalate, leading to psychopathologic forms of anxiety associated with distress, impairment, and negative developmental outcomes [3].

Anxiety disorders represent a phenotypically heterogenous class of disorders. Although the individual anxiety disorders share several clinical diagnostic features (that is, excessive levels of fear or anxiety, physical symptoms, and avoidance behaviour resulting in distress and/or impairment [1, 2, 4]), the specific anxiety disorders (such as separation anxiety disorder, panic disorder, agoraphobia, social anxiety disorder, generalized anxiety disorder, and the specific phobia subtypes animal, natural environment, blood injection injury, situational, and 'other') also differ from each other significantly in terms of their typical focus of fear and anxiety, form, type, and severity of the psychophysiological fear response and the associated cognitions, as well their onset and patterns of course and the clinical and neurobiological correlates, as well as risk factors [1, 5–7]. Moreover, the way fear and anxiety are expressed across different developmental periods and stages may differ in the various anxiety disorders [8] and may hinder diagnosis [3]. For example, particularly in children, anxiety disorders may manifest in non-specific somatic symptoms or anxiety-related symptoms such as crying, irritability, or tantrums, often resulting in misinterpretation by adults as oppositional or disobedience [9]. However, no separate sets of criteria or classifications exist for children and adults in the most recent international diagnostic classification system DSM-5 [2] (Table 88.1). Even separation anxiety disorder and selective mutism—traditionally regarded as childhood anxiety disorders—were moved from the previous DSM-IV category of 'disorders usually first diagnosed in infancy, childhood or adolescence' to the anxiety disorder class. Yet, in order to account for differences in the symptom expression of children and adults, the individual diagnostic criteria sets in DSM-5 provide additional notes to guide the clinicians in the diagnostic process [2]. Some noteworthy differences between children and adults are: different symptom presentations (for example, clinging or tantrums in children with social anxiety disorder), duration (for example, 4 weeks in children and 6 months in adults in separation anxiety disorder), symptom type or count (for example, one physical symptom in children and at least three in adults to diagnose generalized anxiety disorder), and level of insight into the excessiveness/inadequacy of fear (children may lack insight).

This chapter summarizes current knowledge on the epidemiology of anxiety disorders across the lifespan, with a particular focus on childhood and adolescence, given the usually early onset of anxiety disorders. It describes the prevalence, onset, course, persistence, comorbidity, and outcome, as well as correlates and risk factors of separation anxiety disorder, specific phobia (and the various subtypes), social anxiety disorder, agoraphobia, panic disorder, and generalized anxiety disorder. We do not address selective mutism because of a lack of data in epidemiological studies, and post-traumatic stress disorder and obsessive–compulsive disorder—despite being closely associated with pathological anxiety—have now been moved from anxiety disorders into separate diagnostic groups in DSM-5 (see Sections 13 and 15).

**Table 88.1** Anxiety disorders in DSM-IV and DSM-5, highlighting different symptomatology in youth

| DSM-IV-TR | | DSM-5 | | Different criteria in children (vs adults) |
|---|---|---|---|---|
| Disorders usually first diagnosed in infancy, childhood, or adolescence | | Anxiety disorders | | *Information on childhood anxieties as highlighted in DSM text portion* |
| 309.21 | Separation anxiety disorder | 309.21 | Separation anxiety disorder | A5: *Children may be unable to stay in or go to a room by themselves. They may also display 'clinging' behaviour, staying near or 'shadowing' the parent around the house, or needing someone to be with them when switching to a different room in the house.* <br> A6: *Children often have difficulty during bedtime and may insist that someone stays with them till they fall asleep. In addition, they may make their way to their caretaker's bed (or that of a significant other, ex, sibling). Children may refuse or be reluctant to go to camp, attend sleepovers, or run errands.* <br> A8: *Headaches, abdominal complaints, nausea, and vomiting are common in children. Cardiovascular symptoms, such as palpitations, dizziness, and feeling faint, are less common in younger children. However, they may occur in adolescents and adults.* <br> B: *Duration is at least 4 weeks in children and adolescents and 6 months or longer in adults. Younger children are reluctant to go or may avoid going to school altogether. They may not express worries or fears about threats to their home, parents, or themselves, because the anxiety manifests only when separation takes place. As they age, they often worry about specific dangers (kidnappings, accidents, muggings, and death) or will have vague concerns about not being reunited with their attachment figures* |
| 313.23 | Selective mutism | 312.23 | Selective mutism | *In children, when encountering individuals in social interations, they do not initiate speech or reciprocally respond when spoken to by others. In addition, they will speak in their homes in the presence of immediate family, but not too often in front of extended family or even close friends. They often refuse to speak at school and sometimes use non-verbal means (grunting, pointing, writing) to communicate. They may be more willing and eager to engage in social encounters when speech is not required or necessary.* <br> C: *In children, duration of disturbance is not limited to the first month of school* |
| **Anxiety disorders** | | | | |
| 300.01 | Panic disorder without agoraphobia | 300.01 | Panic disorder | B: *Adolescents may be less worried about additional panic attacks than young adults* |
| 300.21 | Panic disorder with agoraphohia | | | |
| 300.22 | Agoraphobia without history of panic disorder | 300.22 | Agoraphobia | B: *'Other incapacitating or embarrassing symptoms' in children include a sense of disorientation and getting lost* |
| 300.23 | Social phobia | 300.23 | Social anxiety disorder | A: Social anxiety must occur in peer settings, not just in interactions with adults |
| | *(Specify if: generalized)* | | *(Specify if: performance only)* | C: In children, the anxiety may be expressed by crying, tantrums, freezing, clinging, shrinking, or failing to speak in social situations |
| | | | | F. *Duration of disturbance is at least 6 months, for that aids in distinguishing the disorder from transient social fears that are common, particularly among children. Adolescents display a broader pattern of fear and avoidance, compared to younger children. Older adults display lower levels of anxiety across a broader range of situations, whereas younger adults express high levels of social anxiety for specific situations* |
| 300.29 | Specific phobia | 300.29 | Specific phobia | A: In children, the fear or anxiety may be expressed by crying, tantrums, freezing, or clinging |
| | *(Specify type: animal, natural environment, blood injection injury, situational, other)* | | *(Specify if: animal, natural environment, blood injection injury, situational, other)* | *When a diagnosis of this disorder is being considered, it is important to evaluate the degree of impairment and the duration of fear, anxiety, or avoidance, and the typicality of such behaviour, relative to the child's particular developmental stage. Fear and anxiety are often expressed differently between children and adults. In children, the C criterion (which recognizes that fear is excessive/unreasonable) may be absent. Children are typically unable to understand the concept of avoidance* |
| 300.02 | Generalized anxiety disorder | 300.02 | Generalized anxiety disorder | C: In children, one, instead of three, out of six symptoms is required |
| | | | | *In children and adolescents, the anxieties and worries often concern the quality of their performance or competence at school or in sporting events, even when their performance is not being evaluated by others. It is possible for children with this disorder to worry about catastrophic events (such as earthquakes or nuclear war), in addition to mundane habits such as punctuality. Children may be perfectionists, redoing tasks due to dissatisfaction with their own performance. They are, more often than not, eager to seek approval and require a substantial amount of reassurance about their performance and their worries* |
| 300.00 | Anxiety disorders not otherwise specified | 300.00 | Unspecified anxiety disorder | |
| | | 300.09 | Other specfied anxiety disorder | |

**Table 88.1** Continued

| DSM-IV-TR | | DSM-5 | |
|---|---|---|---|
| **Obsessive-compulsive and related disorders** | | | |
| 300.3 | Obsessive-compulsive disorder | 300.3 | Obsessive-compulsive disorder |
| **Trauma- and stressor-related disorders** | | | |
| 308.3 | Acute stress disorder | 308.3 | Acute stress disorder |
| 309.81 | Post-traumatic stress disorder | 309.81 | Post-traumatic stress disorder |

Source: data from *DSM-IV-TR: Diagnostic and Statistical Manual of Mental Disorders*, 4th Revised edition (DSM-IV-TR), Copyright (1994), American Psychiatric Association; *Diagnostic and statistical manual of mental disorders*, 5th edition (DSM-5), Copyright (2013) American Psychiatric Association.

## Prevalence of anxiety disorders

Cross-sectional community surveys conducted in many countries around the globe [10–14] have shown the prevalence of anxiety disorders to be the highest among all classes of mental disorders (that is, mood, substance use, impulse-control, somatoform, and eating disorders) in most countries, with estimates of up to 30% for lifetime and 14% for the past 12 months. The estimated lifetime risk up to age 75 is even higher (up to 41% in the United States [15]). In addition, prospective longitudinal studies that examine mental disorders in the same study cohort at multiple points in time provide consistent evidence that the cumulative rates go beyond 30% when entering early adulthood [16–18]. Thus, anxiety disorders are already the most common class of mental disorders in childhood and adolescence [8, 19–21].

Cross-sectionally, the most frequent anxiety disorders in adulthood are specific phobias, followed in frequency by social anxiety disorder, with 12-month prevalence estimates of up to 10% and 8%, respectively [13, 15]. In children, in addition to specific phobias and social anxiety disorder, separation anxiety disorder is highly prevalent, with quite variable 12-month prevalence estimates across studies, ranging from 2.8% and 8% [8]. It is noteworthy that the National Comorbidity Survey Adolescent Supplement (NCS-A) found that separation anxiety disorder had a low current period prevalence (12 months: 1.6%; 30 days: 0.6%) [22] but displayed a high lifetime prevalence (7.6%) [19]. This might indicate that this early childhood anxiety condition rarely persists into adolescence and adulthood. Consistent with these data, adult surveys have found a relatively low 12-month prevalence of separation anxiety disorder in adulthood of 1–1.5% [23, 24].

The less prevalent anxiety conditions across all ages are generalized anxiety disorder, panic disorder, and agoraphobia. These three anxiety disorders reveal low prevalence estimates in childhood (1% or lower); somewhat higher estimates are found in adolescence (2–3% for panic disorder and 3–4% for agoraphobia and generalized anxiety disorder) (for comprehensive reviews, see [6, 8]).

## Onset of anxiety disorders

There is abundant epidemiological evidence that the developmental period of childhood, adolescence, and young adulthood constitutes the core high-risk phase for the onset of anxiety disorders [5, 25–27].

Noteworthy heterogeneity, however, exists in the specific age of onset patterns for the various types of anxiety disorders. The bars in Fig. 88.1 show the cumulative age of onset distribution for specific anxiety disorders by gender, as derived from data from the Early Developmental Stages of Psychopathology (EDSP) study [18, 28]. Separation anxiety disorder and specific phobias are the earliest forms of anxiety disorders, revealing an emergence of 50% of all onsets prior to the age of 8 years; almost all affected cases have emerged by the age of 12. Social anxiety disorder begins to develop later in childhood, showing a steep increase in incidence in early adolescence. Although agoraphobia, panic disorder, and generalized anxiety disorder reveal some onset cases in childhood, their core onset risk period is in later adolescence and early adulthood. Despite differences in prevalence estimates for females and males (the former being more commonly affected than the latter), no remarkable gender differences in the age of onset patterns are observed. Slightly earlier onsets are seen for specific phobias in males, which are due to an earlier onset of the natural environmental subtype of specific phobias in males [8], and for generalized anxiety disorder in females. Similar age of onset findings have emerged in other epidemiologic studies conducted in both adult and adolescent samples [15, 21, 26, 27].

## Natural course and outcome of anxiety disorders

Given that current 12-month period prevalence estimates are not considerably lower than the lifetime estimates for most anxiety disorders, we can assume that anxiety disorders typically have a persistent course, either in terms of chronic symptoms or in terms of a waxing and waning or frequent recurrent course [8]. For example, the 12-month/lifetime prevalence ratios in the National Comorbidity Surveys in the United States are higher for anxiety disorders (any: 0.7) than for depressive disorders (0.5), with variations across the anxiety disorders (0.5 for generalized anxiety disorder to 0.8 for specific phobia). The prevalence ratio is highest in adolescents (0.8), as compared to adults (0.6) and the elderly (0.5) [15]. However, this decrease is not uniform across the anxiety disorders, with generalized anxiety disorder (0.4–0.5) and specific phobia (0.7–0.8) showing similar ratios across all age groups [15].

Persistence estimates for anxiety disorders from cross-sectional studies may overestimate the chronicity or recurrence of anxiety

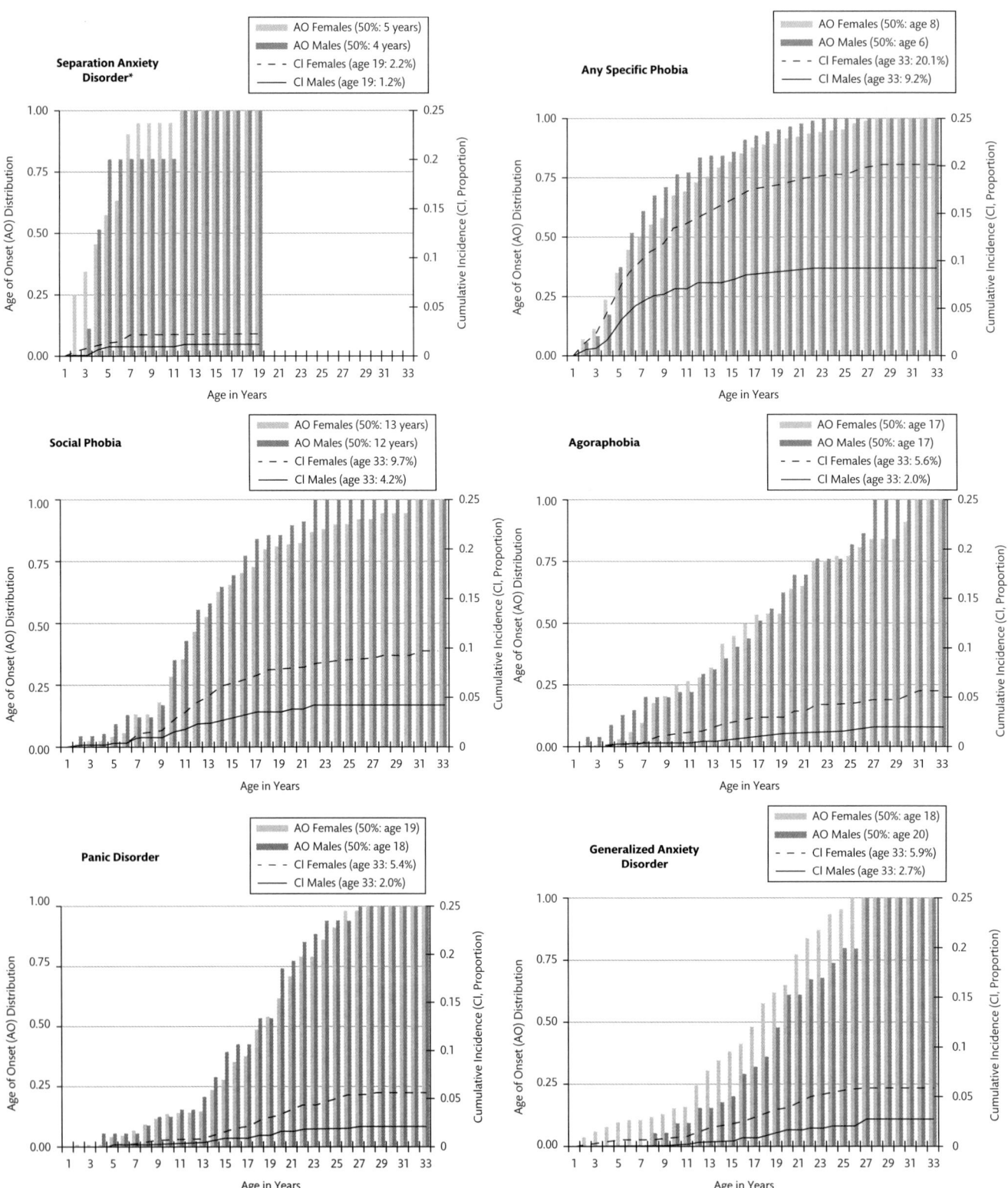

**Fig. 88.1** Cumulative incidence and age of onset distribution of anxiety disorders by gender. The EDSP study is a prospective longitudinal study in a representative sample of adolescents and young adults aged 14–24 years from the general population (Munich, Germany; N = 3021). Anxiety and other mental disorders were assessed using the standardized and computerized composite international diagnostic interview (DIA-X/M-CIDI), according to DSM-IV criteria, on a lifetime basis at baseline and for the interval period since the last assessment at 1-, 4-, and 8-year follow-up, respectively. Bars in the figure show the cumulative age of onset distribution; lines show the age-dependent cumulative lifetime incidence; in phobias, impairment was required among subjects aged 18 years or older; * Separation anxiety disorder was only assessed once at 1-year follow-up in subjects of the younger age cohort (aged 14–17 years at baseline).

problems in the general population, given the potential memory and recall bias in lifetime symptom reports and the age of onset/recency information [8]. Prospective longitudinal study approaches are able to provide a more reliable picture of the natural course and outcome of anxiety disorders (Fig. 88.2). However, given the considerable efforts and financial resources required for such studies, prospective course data are still scarce, particularly for longer time scales of 10 years or more. The data available indicate that the stability or persistence is probably less pronounced than expected, based on the estimates of cross-sectional studies, at least when focusing on

full-threshold diagnosis (*diagnostic stability*). For example, in the 15-year prospective Zurich Cohort study [29], a low stability rate of 4% was found for pure (non-comorbid) anxiety disorders (generalized anxiety or panic disorder). For children and adolescents with anxiety disorders, Last and colleagues [30, 31] reported that 80% remitted from the anxiety shown initially, over a 3- to 4-year follow-up. The prospective longitudinal EDSP study among adolescents and young adults found that 2 years after the baseline investigation, 19.7% of adolescents with baseline anxiety disorder met the threshold criteria again at follow-up, with the probability

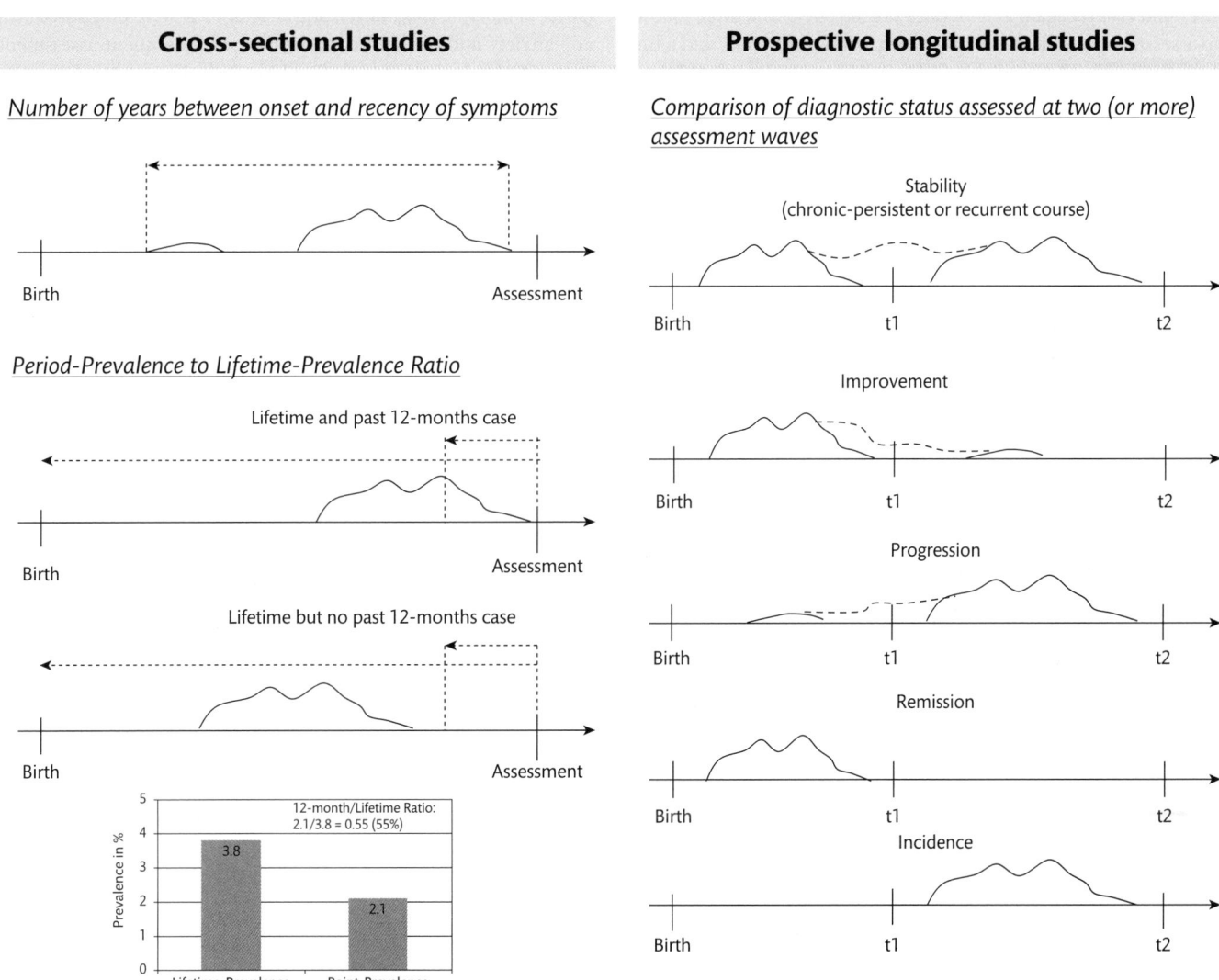

**Fig. 88.2** Approaches to the natural course assessment of anxiety disorders in cross-sectional and prospective longitudinal epidemiological community-based studies. Cross-sectional studies most frequently utilize retrospective age of onset and age of recency reports to estimate the persistence of anxiety, as indicated by the duration of a condition in years. This approach assumes the continuous presence of a disorder, neglecting waxing and waning in symptom severity, including symptom-free intervals, and may thus overestimate the stability (or persistence/chronicity). Another indirect indicator of disorder chronicity is the 12-month to lifetime prevalence ratio. The higher the proportion of 12-month cases among lifetime cases, the higher the assumed chronicity of a condition. Because only categorical diagnoses are considered here (no symptomatic improvements below the diagnostic threshold), this may lead to underestimation of chronicity. On the other hand, as lifetime occurrence prior to the past 12 months may have not been reported or remembered by study participants, this ratio may also overestimate the chronicity. Thus, cross-sectional studies only allow for crude estimations of the natural course of anxiety disorders. Longitudinal studies, in contrast, allow for a more realistic and comprehensive course description as 'true persistence', recurrence, progression, improvement, and remission can be mapped using the diagnostic information on a threshold and subthreshold level available from two (or more) assessment waves months to many years apart.

Adapted from *Psychiatr Clin of North Am.*, 32(3), Beesdo K, Knappe S, Pine DS, Anxiety and anxiety disorders in children and adolescents: Developmental issues and implications for DSM-V, pp 483–524, Copyright (2009), with permission from Elsevier Inc.

of a negative outcome increasing as a function of baseline anxiety severity [32]. Considerable variability in stability rates by type of anxiety diagnosis have been observed. For example, when taking threshold and subthreshold anxiety diagnoses from both baseline and follow-up of the EDSP study into account, panic disorder (44%) and specific phobia (30.1%) were found to be the most stable; other anxiety disorders showed lower stability rates, particularly agoraphobia (13.4%) and social phobia (15.8%) [32]. Of course, stability rates at least slightly increase when following up individuals who have been affected for longer periods of time. There is then a higher chance for recurrence to have occurred. For social anxiety disorder in the EDSP study, for example, 15.5% of baseline cases met threshold criteria again at least once during any of the three follow-up assessments conducted over a time period of 10 years, and a further 19.7% had at least subthreshold social anxiety disorder [33].

To summarize, these findings seem to indicate that anxiety disorders in the community are typically not chronic, in the sense that the symptoms are consistently stable above the diagnostic threshold. Instead, the symptoms typically wax and wane over time around the diagnostic threshold, with spontaneous complete remissions being the rare exceptions (Fig. 88.3) [32].

It is also a consistent finding from prospective studies on the course of anxiety that there is a considerable degree of homotypic continuity. This is despite the proportion of youth diagnosed again with the same anxiety disorder or symptoms thereof being numerically rather low to moderate (for comprehensive reviews of studies, see [8, 34, 35]). Individuals diagnosed with an anxiety disorder, compared to those without, are at a statistically higher risk of having the same disorder (for example, [36–38]) or symptoms of the same disorder [32, 33] at later points in time (*homotypic prediction*) [39]. Moreover, the limited *homotypic continuity* of anxiety disorders observed in prospective longitudinal community studies does not mean that anxiety disorders completely remit (Fig. 88.3). In the EDSP study, only 10% of children and adolescents with (pure or comorbid) specific phobia at baseline had no mental disorder at the 10-year follow-up (*full diagnostic remission*); 41% reported specific phobia again (*strict homotypic continuity*), and overall 73% were diagnosed with any anxiety and/or depressive disorder at subsequent assessments (*heterotypic continuity*) [40]. Similarly, only 13% of baseline social anxiety disorder cases were free of any mental disorder during the 10-year follow-up, while the remaining 87% reported having other types of anxiety disorders or depressive disorders. All of the baseline generalized anxiety disorder cases revealed either homotypic or heterotypic continuity. Other multi-wave, prospective longitudinal studies revealed similar findings [29, 31, 37, 41]. Thus, after onset of the first (that is, pure) anxiety disorder emerges in childhood or early adolescence, a pattern with continuous and frequently variable anxiety develops by later adolescence or early adulthood [6, 42].

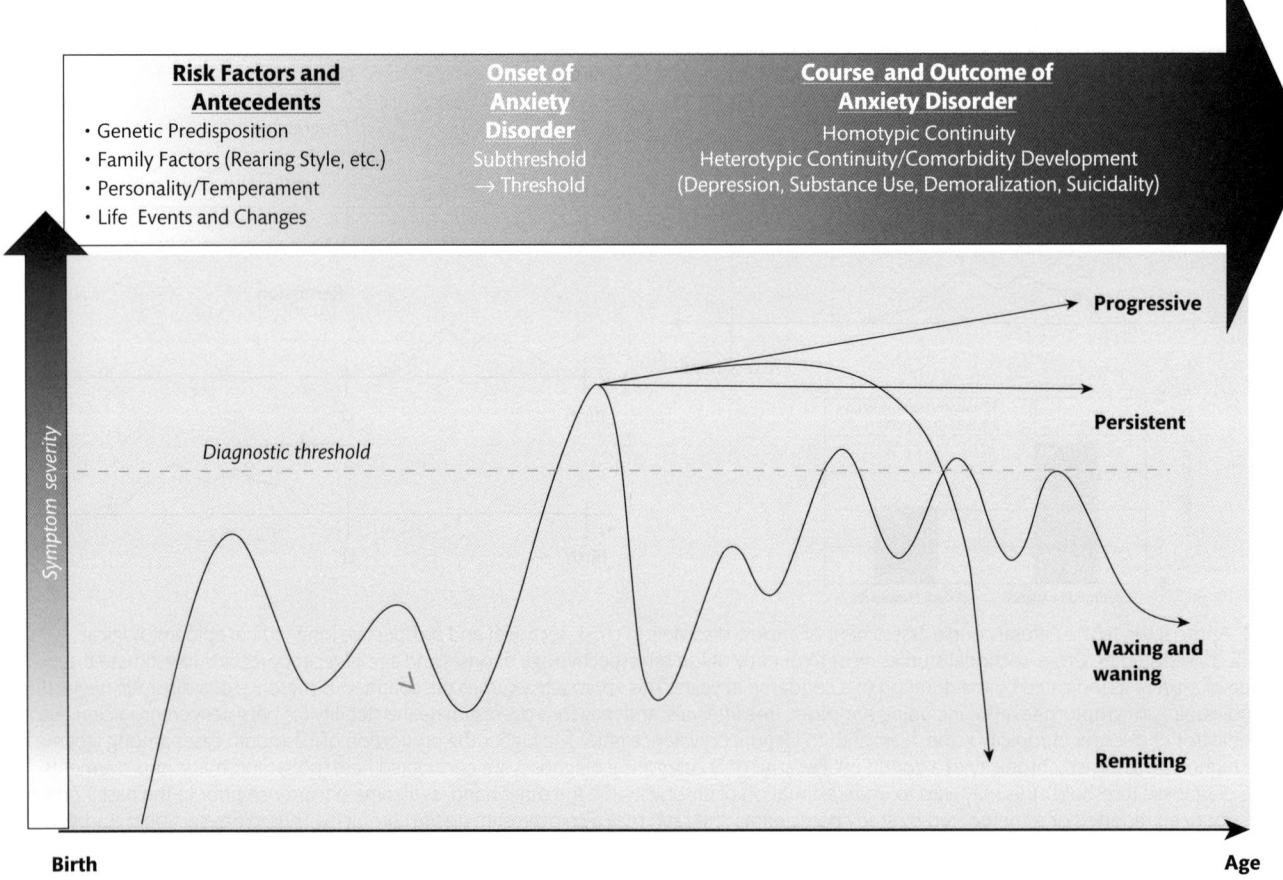

**Fig. 88.3** The evolution of anxiety disorders.

Adapted from *Compr Psychiatry*, 41(2, suppl. 1), Wittchen H-U, Lieb R, Pfister H, *et al.*, The waxing and waning of mental disorders: evaluating the stability of syndromes of mental disorders in the population, pp. 122–32, Copyright (2000), with permission from Elsevier Inc.

## Complications and development of comorbid disorders

A frequent outcome of primary anxiety disorders is the development of a cascade of other psychopathological complications [4]. Anxiety disorders have been consistently shown to contribute not only to the development of further anxiety disorders, but also to depressive disorders, substance use disorders, and suicidality, as well as to other adverse developmental outcomes (such as educational underachievement, early parenthood, and financial disadvantage [25, 43]). Thus, for anxiety cases in which *homotypic continuity* is not observed, there is a substantial degree of *heterotypic continuity* in both cross-sectional and longitudinal epidemiological studies [39]. The longitudinal associations between anxiety and subsequent depression are particularly strong [5, 21, 31, 43–47]. Prospective epidemiological studies investigating particular anxiety diagnoses found that children and adolescents with specific fears and phobias (especially fear of darkness) [48], social anxiety disorder [49–51], and other types of anxiety disorders, such as agoraphobia, panic disorder, and generalized anxiety disorder [5, 38, 51], are all at significantly increased risk for subsequent depression.

There is also consistent epidemiologic evidence that certain clinical characteristics of anxiety disorders, such as greater severity (multiple anxiety diagnoses or more severe impairment of individual anxiety disorders), greater impairment or persistence, and co-occurring panic attacks, are associated with an increased risk of depression [49, 51], suggesting that anxiety disorders may play a causal role in depression development [52].

Substance abuse or dependence is also a frequent heterotypic problem outcome of primary anxiety disorders [43, 45, 53–56], providing some evidence that alcohol or other drug use is possibly motivated by self-medication for pathological anxiety symptoms [57].

## Correlates and risk factors

A range of sociodemographic, individual, and environmental factors assessed have been found to be associated with anxiety disorders in epidemiological studies. We will describe these factors as correlates *or* risk factors, not speculating whether they should be considered as distal or proximal vulnerability factors or risk factors in a strict sense. This is because cross-sectional studies predominate and identify correlates; prospective longitudinal studies are required to evidence risk factor status [58], either for the first onset of an anxiety disorder or for an adverse course after the anxiety disorder has initially developed (chronicity/persistence/progression/recurrence vs improvement/remission) (Fig. 88.3). Course predictors have been less extensively studied, compared to risk factors for first onset; yet both appear crucial, and at least partly different factors could emerge relevant for prevention and early intervention. Moreover, while the correlates overlap, risk factors and course predictors for the individual anxiety disorders or for anxiety vs depressive or other comorbid disorders may be different. They may be implicated in the heterogeneity of the various disorder types and classes in relation to the phenomenology, onset, and course.

## Sociodemographic factors

Female gender is the most consistent risk factor for the development of each of the specific anxiety disorders (for a review, see [8]). Gender differences are usually small in childhood and grow with age, reaching a ratio of approximately 2:1 to 3:1 for females vs males in late adolescence. The recent NCS-A found a higher prevalence of anxiety disorders among non-Hispanic black, compared to non-Hispanic white, adolescents, as well as among respondents with divorced or separated parents, compared to married or cohabiting parents [19]. Anxiety disorders are frequently also found among individuals with lower, compared to higher, education (for example, [59]). In NCS-A, low parental education was also shown to be associated with adolescent anxiety disorders. Low household income or precarious financial situations have been shown to be associated with anxiety disorders (for example, [59]), and there is evidence of adverse financial outcomes in young adulthood among children and adolescents with anxiety disorders, particularly generalized anxiety disorder/overanxious disorder [25]. As sociodemographic risks co-occur, Copeland and colleagues [60] identified a moderate-risk class containing low parental education and poverty being associated with offspring anxiety disorders, as well as with depressive disorders, but not with externalizing disorders. After taking into account comorbidity and multiple other risk factors, Shanahan *et al.* [61] found that parental unemployment was associated with anxiety and behavioural disorders, but not with depressive disorders.

## Familial aggregation

Anxiety disorders consistently 'run in families', with strong associations between parental and offspring anxiety diagnoses [5, 52, 62–65]. A particularly strong risk is present for offspring with two affected parents [62, 65] and for offspring of severely affected parents as indicated by impairment, number of anxiety disorders, and early onset of anxiety disorders [66]. However, not only parental anxiety disorders increase the risk for anxiety in offspring, but parental depression was also found to be associated with offspring anxiety [67, 68]. Investigations into the specificity of the familial aggregation of anxiety and other mental disorders revealed mixed findings, with some evidence for specificity [5, 69, 70]. Furthermore, some specificity appears to exist in the familial aggregation of certain anxiety disorders [5, 71]. The exact mechanism of 'familial transmission' of anxiety from parents to offspring is complex and still far from being well understood. Biology in terms of genetic or physiological (intrauterine) factors, the family environment in terms of living with an anxious parent (for example, modelling, anxious rearing, insecure attachment), or both (additive risks or gene–environment interactions) are implicated [72–74]. Twin studies indicate that the genetic liability for specific anxiety disorders, as well as for depression and anxiety, may overlap with different environmental risks, resulting in phenotypically diverse outcomes [74–76]. For more detail on genetic factors, see Chapters 80 and 89.

## Temperament/personality

Personality traits such as neuroticism, trait anxiety, or negative affect, as well as temperamental styles often investigated in epidemiological studies in terms of behavioural inhibition are likely overlapping constructs that can be viewed as precursor conditions to anxiety disorders, with some indications of specificity between anxiety and depression outcomes [5, 77–83].

## Environmental factors

Adverse life events and conditions in childhood and adolescence, as well as unfavourable parental rearing styles, have been linked in many epidemiologic studies to the development of anxiety disorders in offspring. Indeed, loss of a parent by death, separation, or divorce, as well as physical or sexual abuse or neglect in childhood, have been associated with almost all mental disorders, including anxiety disorders (for example, [70, 84–86]). In the EDSP study data, there was nevertheless some indication that childhood separation events were specifically associated with pure anxiety, as well as with comorbid anxiety and depression, but not with pure depression [5]. Other negative life events have also not just been evidenced as risk factors for depression [87, 88], but also for anxiety disorders [89]. In particular, threat events tend to precede anxiety disorders (or comorbid anxiety and depressive disorders), whereas loss events tend to precede depression [61, 90–92].

Parenting styles have also been linked in epidemiologic studies with offspring anxiety disorders. For example, in the EDSP study, parental overprotection and parental rejection were associated with increased prevalence of social anxiety disorder in offspring [63, 71]. Overprotection was found to increase the risk for anxiety disorders, but not for pure depressive disorders, while parental rejection was linked with depressive disorder [5]. After adjusting for comorbidity and other putative risk factors, Shanahan et al. [61] found harsh discipline to be specifically associated with generalized anxiety disorder or overanxious disorder (among a range of poor emotional and behavioural outcomes); overintrusive parenting was revealed as a non-specific risk factor for anxiety and behavioural disorders.

## Course predictors

Sociodemographic, individual, and environmental factors have been less frequently examined as course predictors for anxiety disorders, particularly when based on prospective longitudinal data [35]. Contrasting to correlates and risk factors for onset, sociodemographic factors are not consistently associated with an adverse course of anxiety disorders. In a cross-sectional study among adolescents in the United States, for example, female gender was the only demographic variable found to be associated with a higher persistence of most anxiety disorders, while race/ethnicity, family income, or family composition were not consistently implicated [22]. Symptom severity and duration of illness are the best prognostic indicators for anxiety in both epidemiologic and clinical studies [8]. For example, the prospective longitudinal EDSP study revealed several clinical features, such as early age of onset, the generalized subtype, a high number of catastrophic anxiety cognitions, severe avoidance, and impairment, as predictors for higher persistence, as well as prospectively assessed diagnostic stability for social anxiety disorder [33]. Comorbidity with other disorders was not found to predict the course of social phobia, with the exception of co-occurring panic attacks that were associated with both higher persistence and diagnostic stability of social anxiety. Established vulnerability characteristics for the onset of anxiety conditions, such as parental social anxiety disorder and depression, as well as a behavioural inhibited temperament, were related to poor prognosis. Thus, besides gender and clinical diagnostic information, familial

and temperamental characteristics may inform estimates of prognosis for anxiety disorders and appear useful to target treatment interventions.

## Summary and implications

Anxiety disorders are frequent clinical conditions with an early onset in life, associated with considerable developmental, psychosocial, and psychopathological complications. Early anxiety syndromes in children may remit spontaneously, but most children and adolescents with an anxiety disorder continue to suffer from anxiety or other psychopathological problems for the major part of their subsequent life. This persistent course is causally related to a tremendous personal, economical, and societal burden (11, 93, 94]. Recent EU-wide calculations rank anxiety disorders as the third most burdensome group of disorders [3]. Although effective cognitive behavioural and pharmacological treatments exist for anxiety disorders and related conditions, the vast majority of anxiety disorders typically never receive any appropriate treatment and the majority remains undiagnosed and untreated, even in the most advantaged countries. Evidence suggests that treatment only occurs after many years when additional psychopathological complications like depression have developed. The degree of often lifelong non-recognition, underdiagnosis, and undertreatment has been related to the tremendous burden caused by anxiety in the United States, the EU, and worldwide [11]. Given that available treatments are highly effective and cost-efficient, timely and earlier treatment has the potential of substantially reducing the burden (see Chapter 92). Moreover, given the early onset of anxiety disorders, the burden of anxiety on the population level might be substantially reduced by concerted action, with targeted preventive interventions in children and adolescents, before the disorder becomes persistent and before comorbid complications arise (see Chapter 91). In order to work towards these goals, considerably more basic research is needed to identify the most powerful and specific risk factors for the first onset, as well as poor course of anxiety disorders, and to delineate the complex underlying psychological, behavioural, and biological mechanisms and interactions [3, 95–97]. Focusing on 'optimal outcomes' of anxiety problems experienced by children and adolescence is a core societal challenge [98].

## REFERENCES

1. Craske MG, Rauch SL, Ursano R, Prenoveau J, Pine DS, Zinbarg RE. What is an anxiety disorder? *Depression and Anxiety*. 2009;26:1066–85.
2. American Psychiatric Association. *Diagnostic and Statistical Manual of Mental Disorders*, fifth edition (DSM-5). Arlington, VA: American Psychiatric Association; 2013.
3. Craske MG, Stein MB, Eley TC, *et al.* Anxiety disorders. *Nature Reviews Disease Primers*. 2017;3:18.
4. Shear MK, Bjelland I, Beesdo K, Gloster AT, Wittchen H-U. Supplementary dimensional assessment in anxiety disorders. *International Journal of Methods in Psychiatric Research*. 2007;16(Suppl 1):S52–64.
5. Beesdo K, Pine DS, Lieb R, Wittchen HU. Incidence and risk patterns of anxiety and depressive disorders and categorization

of generalized anxiety disorder. *Archives of General Psychiatry.* 2010;67:47–57.

6. Beesdo-Baum K, Knappe S. Developmental epidemiology of anxiety disorders. *Child and Adolescent Psychiatric Clinics of North America.* 2012;21:457–78.

7. Lueken U, Kruschwitz JD, Muehlhan M, Siegert J, Hoyer J, Wittchen H-U. How specific is specific phobia? Different neural response patterns in two subtypes of specific phobia. *Neuroimage.* 2011;56:363–72.

8. Beesdo K, Knappe S, Pine DS. Anxiety and anxiety disorders in children and adolescents: Developmental issues and implications for DSM-V. *Psychiatric Clinics of North America.* 2009;32:483–524.

9. Wehry A, Beesdo-Baum K, Hennelly MM, Connolly SD, Strawn JR. Assessment and treatment of anxiety disorders in children and adolescents. *Current Psychiatry Reports.* 2015;17:1–11.

10. Kessler RC, Aguilar-Gaxiola S, Alonso J, et al. The burden of mental disorders worldwide: results from the World Mental Health surveys. In: Galea NCS (ed). *Population Mental Health: Evidence, Policy, and Public Health Practice.* Abingdon: Routledge; 2011. pp. 9–37.

11. Wittchen HU, Jacobi F, Rehm J, et al. The size and burden of mental disorders and other disorders of the brain in Europe 2010. *European Neuropsychopharmacology.* 2011;21:655–79.

12. Wang PS, Aguilar-Gaxiola S, Alonso J, et al. Assessing mental disorders and service use across countries: the WHO World Mental Health Survey Initiative. In: Regier DA, Narrow WE, Kuhl EA, Kupfer DJ (eds). *The Conceptual Evolution of DSM-5.* Arlington, VA: American Psychiatric Publishing; 2011. pp. 231–66.

13. Jacobi F, Hofler M, Siegert J, et al. Twelve-month prevalence, comorbidity and correlates of mental disorders in Germany: the Mental Health Module of the German Health Interview and Examination Survey for Adults (DEGS1-MH). *International Journal of Methods in Psychiatric Research.* 2014;23:304–19.

14. Remes O, Brayne C, van der Linde R, Lafortune L. A systematic review of reviews on the prevalence of anxiety disorders in adult populations. *Brain and Behavior.* 2016;6:e00497.

15. Kessler RC, Petukhova M, Sampson NA, Zaslavsky AM, Wittchen HU. Twelve-month and lifetime prevalence and lifetime morbid risk of anxiety and mood disorders in the United States. *International Journal of Methods in Psychiatric Research.* 2012;21:169–84.

16. Copeland W, Shanahan L, Costello EJ, Angold A. Cumulative prevalence of psychiatric disorders by young adulthood: a prospective cohort analysis from the Great Smoky Mountains Study. *Journal of the American Academy of Child and Adolescent Psychiatry.* 2011;50:252–61.

17. Moffitt TE, Caspi A, Taylor A, et al. How common are common mental disorders? Evidence that lifetime prevalence rates are doubled by prospective versus retrospective ascertainment. *Psychological Medicine.* 2010;40:899–909.

18. Beesdo-Baum K, Knappe S, Asselmann E, et al. The 'Early Developmental Stages of Psychopathology (EDSP) study': A 20 year review of methods and findings. *Social Psychiatry and Psychiatric Epidemiology.* 2015;50:851–66.

19. Merikangas KR, He JP, Burstein M, et al. Lifetime Prevalence of mental disorders in U.S. adolescents: results from the National Comorbidity Survey Replication-Adolescent Supplement (NCS-A). *Journal of the American Academy of Child and Adolescent Psychiatry.* 2011;49:980–9.

20. Polanczyk GV, Salum GA, Sugaya LS, Caye A, Rohde LA. Annual research review: A meta-analysis of the worldwide prevalence of mental disorders in children and adolescents. *Journal of Child Psychology and Psychiatry.* 2015;56:345–65.

21. Ormel J, Raven D, van Oort F, et al. Mental health in Dutch adolescents: a TRAILS report on prevalence, severity, age of onset, continuity and co-morbidity of DSM disorders. *Psychological Medicine.* 2015;45:345–60.

22. Kessler RC, Avenevoli S, Costello EJ, et al. Prevalence, persistence, and sociodemographic correlates of DSM-IV disorders in the National Comorbidity Survey Replication Adolescent Supplement. *Archives of General Psychiatry.* 2012;69:372–80.

23. Silove D, Alonso J, Bromet E, et al. Pediatric-onset and adult-onset separation anxiety disorder across countries in the World Mental Health Survey. *American Journal of Psychiatry.* 2015;172:647–56.

24. Shear K, Jin R, Ruscio AM, Walters EE, Kessler RC. Prevalence and correlates of estimated DSM-IV child and adult separation anxiety disorder in the national comorbidity survey replication. *American Journal of Psychiatry.* 2006;163:1074–83.

25. Copeland WE, Angold A, Shanahan L, Costello EJ. Longitudinal patterns of anxiety from childhood to adulthood: The Great Smoky Mountains Study. *Journal of the American Academy of Child and Adolescent Psychiatry.* 2014;53:21–33.

26. Kessler RC, Berglund P, Demler O, Jin R, Merikangas KR, Walters EE. Lifetime prevalence and age-of-onset distributions of DSM-IV disorders in the national comorbidity survey replication. *Archives of General Psychiatry.* 2005;62:593–602.

27. Merikangas KR, He J-P, Burstein M, et al. Lifetime prevalence of mental disorders in U.S. adolescents: results from the National Comorbidity Survey Replication-Adolescent Supplement (NCS-A). *Journal of the American Academy of Child and Adolescent Psychiatry.* 2010;49:980–9.

28. Wittchen H-U, Perkonigg A, Lachner G, Nelson CB. Early developmental stages of psychopathology study (EDSP) – objectives and design. *European Addiction Research.* 1998;4:18–27.

29. Angst J, Vollrath M. The natural history of anxiety disorders. *Acta Psychiatrica Scandinavica.* 1991;84:446–52.

30. Last CG, Hansen C, Franco N. Anxious children in adulthood: a prospective study of adjustment. *Journal of the American Academy of Child and Adolescent Psychiatry.* 1997;36:645–52.

31. Last CG, Perrin S, Hersen M, Kazdin AE. A prospective study of childhood anxiety disorders. *Journal of the American Academy of Child and Adolescent Psychiatry.* 1996;35:1502–10.

32. Wittchen H-U, Lieb R, Pfister H, Schuster P. The waxing and waning of mental disorders: evaluating the stability of syndromes of mental disorders in the population. *Comprehensive Psychiatry.* 2000;41(2, suppl 1):122–32.

33. Beesdo-Baum K, Knappe S, Fehm L, et al. The natural course of social anxiety disorder among adolescents and young adults. *Acta Psychiatrica Scandinavica.* 2012;126:411–25.

34. Pine DS, Klein RG. Anxiety disorder. In: Rutter M, Bishop D, Pine DS, et al. (eds). *Rutter's Child and Adolescent Psychiatry*, fifth edition. Oxford: Blackwell Publishing; 2008. pp. 628–46.

35. Asselmann E, Beesdo-Baum K. Predictors of the course of anxiety disorders in adolescents and young adults. *Current Psychiatry Reports.* 2015;17:1–8.

36. Bittner A, Egger HL, Erkanli A, Costello EJ, Foley DL, Angold A. What do childhood anxiety disorders predict? *Journal of Child Psychology and Psychiatry.* 2007;48:1174–83.

37. Pine DS, Cohen P, Gurley D, Brook J, Ma Y. The risk for early-adulthood anxiety and depressive disorders in adolescents with anxiety and depressive disorders. *Archives of General Psychiatry.* 1998;55:56–64.

38. Copeland WE, Shanahan L, Costello J, Angold A. Childhood and adolescent psychiatric disorders as predictors of young adult disorders. *Archives of General Psychiatry*. 2009;66:764–72.

39. Costello EJ, Copeland W, Angold A. Trends in psychopathology across the adolescent years: What changes when children become adolescents, and when adolescents become adults? *Journal of Child Psychology and Psychiatry*. 2011;52:1015–25.

40. Emmelkamp PMG, Wittchen HU. Specific phobias. In: Andrews G, Charney DS, Sirovatka PJ, Regier DA (eds). *Stress-induced and Fear Circuitry Disorders: Refining the Research Agenda for DSM-V*. Arlington, VA: American Psychiatric Association; 2009. pp. 77–101.

41. Wittchen H-U. Der Langzeitverlauf unbehandelter Angststörungen: Wie häufig sind Spontanremissionen? *Verhaltenstherapie*. 1991;1:273–82.

42. Wittchen H-U, Lecrubier Y, Beesdo K, Nocon A. Relationships among anxiety disorders: patterns and implications. In: Nutt DJ, Ballenger JC (eds). *Anxiety Disorders*. Oxford: Blackwell Science; 2003. pp. 25–37.

43. Woodward LJ, Fergusson DM. Life course outcomes of young people with anxiety disorders in adolescence. *Journal of the American Academy of Child and Adolescent Psychiatry*. 2001;40:1086–93.

44. Fergusson DM, Woodward LJ. Mental health, educational, and social role outcomes of adolescents with depression. *Archives of General Psychiatry*. 2002;59:225–31.

45. Kessler RC, Nelson CB, McGonagle KA, Liu J, Schwartz M, Blazer DG. Comorbidity of DSM-III-R major depressive disorder in the general population: results from the US National Comorbidity Survey. *British Journal of Psychiatry*. 1996;168:17–30.

46. Kessler RC, Stang P, Wittchen H-U, Stein MB, Walters EE. Lifetime comorbidities between social phobia and mood disorders in the U.S. National Comorbidity Survey. *Psychological Medicine*. 1999;29:555–67.

47. Kim-Cohen J, Caspi A, Moffitt TE, Harrington H, Milne BJ, Poulton R. Prior juvenile diagnoses in adults with mental disorder. *Archives of General Psychiatry*. 2003;60:709–17.

48. Pine DS, Cohen P, Brook J. Adolescent fears as predictors of depression. *Biological Psychiatry*. 2001;50:721–4.

49. Beesdo K, Bittner A, Pine DS, *et al*. Incidence of social anxiety disorder and the consistent risk for secondary depression in the first three decades of life. *Archives of General Psychiatry*. 2007;64:903–12.

50. Stein MB, Fuetsch M, Müller N, Höfler M, Lieb R, Wittchen H-U. Social anxiety disorder and the risk of depression. A prospective community study of adolescents and young adults. *Archives of General Psychiatry*. 2001;58:251–6.

51. Bittner A, Goodwin RD, Wittchen H-U, Beesdo K, Höfler M, Lieb R. What characteristics of primary anxiety disorders predict subsequent major depressive disorder? *Journal of Clinical Psychiatry*. 2004;65:618–26.

52 Wittchen H-U, Kessler RC, Pfister H, Lieb R. Why do people with anxiety disorders become depressed? A prospective-longitudinal community study. *Acta Psychiatrica Scandinavica*. 2000;102(Suppl 406):14–23.

53. Kessler RC, Crum RM, Warner LA, Nelson CB, Schulenberg J, Anthony JC. Lifetime co-occurrence of DSM-III-R alcohol abuse and dependence with other psychiatric disorders in the National Comorbidity Survey. *Archives of General Psychiatry*. 1997;54:313–21.

54. Merikangas KR, Mehta RL, Molnar BE, *et al*. Comorbidity of substance use disorders with mood and anxiety disorders: results of the international consortium in psychiatric epidemiology. *Addictive Behaviors*. 1998;23:893–907.

55. Kessler RC, Chiu WT, Demler O, Walters EE. Prevalence, severity, and comorbidity of 12-month DSM-IV disorders in the National Comorbidity Survey Replication. *Archives of General Psychiatry*. 2005;62:617–27.

56. Wittchen H-U, Frohlich C, Behrendt S, *et al*. Cannabis use and cannabis use disorders and their relationship to mental disorders: a 10-year prospective-longitudinal community study in adolescents. *Drug and Alcohol Dependence*. 2007;88(Suppl 1):S60–70.

57. Zimmermann P, Wittchen HU, Höfler M, Pfister H, Kessler RC, Lieb R. Primary anxiety disorders and the development of subsequent alcohol use disorders: a 4-year community study of adolescents and young adults. *Psychological Medicine*. 2003;33:1211–22.

58. Kraemer HC, Kazdin AE, Offord DR, Kessler RC, Jensen PS, Kupfer DJ. Coming to terms with the terms of risk. *Archives of General Psychiatry*. 1997;54:337–43.

59. Wittchen H-U, Nelson CB, Lachner G. Prevalence of mental disorders and psychosocial impairments in adolescents and young adults. *Psychological Medicine*. 1998;28:109–26.

60. Copeland W, Shanahan L, Costello EJ, Angold A. Configurations of common childhood psychosocial risk factors. *Journal of Child Psychology and Psychiatry*. 2009;50:451–9.

61. Shanahan L, Copeland W, Costello EJ, Angold A. Specificity of putative psychosocial risk factors for psychiatric disorders in children and adolescents. *Journal of Child Psychology and Psychiatry*. 2008;49:34–42.

62. Merikangas KR, Avenevoli S, Dierker L, Grillon C. Vulnerability factors among children at risk for anxiety disorders. *Biological Psychiatry*. 1999;46:1523–35.

63. Lieb R, Wittchen H-U, Höfler M, Fuetsch M, Stein MB, Merikangas KR. Parental psychopathology, parenting styles, and the risk for social phobia in offspring: A prospective-longitudinal community study. *Archives of General Psychiatry*. 2000;57:859–66.

64. Hettema JM, Neale MC, Kendler KS. A review and meta-analysis of the genetic epidemiology of anxiety disorders. *American Journal of Psychiatry*. 2001;158:1568–78.

65. Johnson JG, Cohen P, Kasen S, Brook JS. Parental concordance and offspring risk for anxiety, conduct, depressive, and substance use disorders. *Psychopathology*. 2008;41:124–8.

66. Schreier A, Wittchen HU, Höfler M, Lieb R. Anxiety disorders in mothers and their children: prospective longitudinal community study. *British Journal of Psychiatry*. 2008;129:308–9.

67. Lieb R, Isensee B, Höfler M, Pfister H, Wittchen H-U. Parental major depression and the risk of depressive and other mental disorders in offspring: a prospective-longitudinal community study. *Archives of General Psychiatry*. 2002;59:365–74.

68. Weissman MM, Wickramaratne P, Nomura Y, Warner V, Pilowsky D, Verdeli H. Offspring of depressed parents: 20 years later. *American Journal of Psychiatry*. 2006;163:1001–8.

69. Klein DN, Lewinsohn PM, Rohde P, Seeley JR, Shankman SA. Family study of co-morbidity between major depressive disorder and anxiety disorders. *Psychological Medicine*. 2003;33:703–14.

70. Moffitt TE, Caspi A, Harrington H, *et al*. Generalized anxiety disorder and depression: childhood risk factors in a birth cohort followed to age 32. *Psychological Medicine*. 2007;37:441–52.

71. Knappe S, Lieb R, Beesdo K, *et al*. The role of parental psychopathology and family environment for social phobia in the first three decades of life depression and anxiety. *Depression and Anxiety*. 2009;26:363–70.

72. Martini J, Knappe S, Beesdo-Baum K, Lieb R, Wittchen H-U. Anxiety disorders before birth and self-perceived distress during

pregnancy: associations with maternal depression and obstetric, neonatal and early childhood outcomes. *Early Human Development*. 2010;86:305–10.

73. Alder J, Fink N, Bitzer J, Hosli I, Holzgreve W. Depression and anxiety during pregnancy: A risk factor for obstetric, fetal and neonatal outcome? A critical review of the literature. *Journal of Maternal-Fetal and Neonatal Medicine*. 2007;20:189–209.

74. Hettema JM, Prescott CA, Myers JM, Neale MC, Kendler KS. The structure of genetic and environmental risk factors for anxiety disorders in men and women. *Archives of General Psychiatry*. 2005;62:182–9.

75. Scherrer JF, True WR, Xian H, *et al*. Evidence for genetic influences common and specific to symptoms of generalized anxiety and panic. *Journal of Affective Disorders*. 2000;57:25–35.

76. Kendler KS. Major depression and generalised anxiety disorder. same genes, (partly) different environments – revisited. *British Journal of Psychiatry*. 1996;168(suppl 30):68–75.

77. Hayward C, Killen JD, Kraemer HC, Taylor CB. Predictors of panic attacks in adolescents. *Journal of the American Academy of Child and Adolescent Psychiatry*. 2000;39:207–14.

78. de Graaf R, Bijl RV, Ravelli A, Smit F, Vollebergh WAM. Predictors of first incidence of DSM-III-R psychiatric disorders in the general population: findings from the Netherlands Mental Health Survey and incidence study. *Acta Psychiatrica Scandinavica*. 2002;106:303–13.

79. Biederman J, Hirshfeld-Becker DR, Rosenbaum JF, *et al*. Further evidence of association between behavioral inhibition and social anxiety in children. *American Journal of Psychiatry*. 2001;158:1673–9.

80. Rohrbacher H, Hoyer J, Beesdo K, *et al*. Psychometric properties of the retrospective self report of inhibition (RSRI) in a representative German sample. *International Journal of Methods in Psychiatric Research*. 2008;17:80–8.

81. Hayward C, Killen JD, Kraemer HC, Taylor CB. Linking self-reported childhood behavioral inhibition to adolescent social phobia. *Journal of the American Academy of Child and Adolescent Psychiatry*. 1998;37:1308–16.

82. Mick MA, Telch MJ. Social anxiety and history of behavioral inhibition in young adults. *Journal of Anxiety Disorders*. 1998;12:1–20.

83. Schwartz CE, Snidman N, Kagan J. Adolescent social anxiety as an outcome of inhibited temperament in childhood. *Journal of the American Academy of Child and Adolescent Psychiatry*. 1999;38:1008–15.

84. Kessler RC, Davis CG, Kendler KS. Childhood adversity and adult psychiatric disorder in the US National Comorbidity Survey. *Psychological Medicine*. 1997;27:1101–19.

85. Bijl RV, Ravelli A, Van Zessen G. Prevalence of psychiatric disorder in the general population: results of the Netherlands

Mental Health Survey and Incidence Study (NEMESIS). *Social Psychiatry and Psychiatric Epidemiology*. 1998;33:587–95.

86. Fergusson DM, Horwood J, Lynskey MT. Childhood sexual abuse and psychiatric disorder in young adulthood. II. Psychiatric outcomes of childhood sexual abuse. *Journal of the American Academy of Child and Adolescent Psychiatry*. 1996;35:1365–74.

87. Pine DS, Cohen P, Johnson J, Brook J. Adolescent life events as predictors of adult depression. *Journal of Affective Disorders*. 2002;68:49–57.

88. Friis RH, Wittchen H-U, Pfister H, Lieb R. Life events and changes in the course of depression in young adults. *European Psychiatry*. 2002;17:241–53.

89. Perkonigg A, Kessler RC, Storz S, Wittchen H-U. Traumatic events and post-traumatic stress disorder in the community: prevalence, risk factors and comorbidity. *Acta Psychiatrica Scandinavica*. 2000;101:46–59.

90. Finlay-Jones R, Brown GW. Types of stressful life event and the onset of anxiety and depressive disorders. *Psychological Medicine*. 1981;11:803–15.

91. Asselmann E, Wittchen H-U, Lieb R, Höfler M, Beesdo-Baum K. Danger and loss events and the incidence of anxiety and depressive disorders: a prospective-longitudinal community study of adolescents and young adults. *Psychological Medicine*. 2015;45:153–63.

92. Kendler KS, Hettema JM, Butera F, Gardner CO, Prescott CA. Life event dimensions of loss, humiliation, entrapment, and danger in the prediction of onsets of major depression and generalized anxiety. *Archives of General Psychiatry*. 2003;60:789–96.

93. Gustavsson A, Svensson M, Jacobi F, *et al*. Cost of disorders of the brain in Europe 2010. *European Neuropsychopharmacology*. 2011;21:718–79.

94. Trautmann S, Rehm J, Wittchen H-U. The economic costs of mental disorders. *EMBO Reports*. 2016;17:1245–9.

95. Wittchen H-U, Knappe S, Schumann G. The psychological perspective on mental health and mental disorder research: introduction to the ROAMER work package 5 consensus document. *International Journal of Methods in Psychiatric Research*. 2014;23(S1):15–27.

96. Wittchen H-U, Knappe S, Andersson G, *et al*. The need for a behavioural science focus in research on mental health and mental disorders. *International Journal of Methods in Psychiatric Research*. 2014;23(S1):28–40.

97. Verhulst FC, Tiemeier H. Epidemiology of child psychopathology: major milestones. *European Child and Adolescent Psychiatry*. 2015;24:607–17.

98. Costello EJ, Maughan B. Annual research review: optimal outcomes of child and adolescent mental illness. *Journal of Child Psychology and Psychiatry*. 2015;56:324–41.

# 89

# Genetics of anxiety disorders

*Michael G. Gottschalk and Katharina Domschke*

## Introduction

The present chapter provides a review of the current state of genetic studies across the spectrum of anxiety disorders, including specific phobias (SP), social anxiety disorder (SAD, also referred to as social phobia), agoraphobia (AP), panic disorder (PD), and generalized anxiety disorder (GAD), with a special focus on genome-wide association studies (GWAS), candidate gene studies, gene–environment studies, and recent advances in epigenetics. Given the interrelatedness of mental disorders in general and of anxiety disorders in particular, we will expand upon the genetics of intermediate phenotypes, crossing classic categorical disorder definitions, and give a critical assessment of related upcoming clinical challenges and future perspectives.

## Genetics of anxiety disorders

### Family studies and twin studies

Anxiety disorders show significant familial aggregation, with a meta-analysis of epidemiological family studies calculating substantial summary odds ratios for SP and SAD (4.1), PD (5.0), and GAD (6.1) in first-degree relatives [1]. Heritability of PD, as determined by a meta-analysis of twin studies, was 0.43 and of GAD 0.32, with mainly non-shared environmental influences contributing to the remaining variance in liability for PD [1]. GAD appeared to display a significant influence of shared environmental influences in females [1] (Table 89.1). Heritability for phobic disorders has been estimated to range between 0.43 and 0.63 [1] (Table 89.1), and factor analysis suggested one common genetic factor underlying SP and one shared factor underlying SAD and AP [2]. However, the influence of genetic factors on anxiety disorders has been suggested to decrease from childhood towards adolescence, while the influence of shared environmental factors has been reported to increase [3]. This could be explained by an increased direct environmental transmission from parents to their adolescent offspring, in line with developmental theories of fear–anxiety learning [4].

Other studies have reached similar heritability estimates, although very rarely have they corrected for the unreliability of a single lifetime assessment that is most commonly used in these investigations.

When accounting for variability in the recall of unreasonable fears and interviewer bias towards which fears constitute phobias, twin resemblance due to genetic factors of phobias was determined to be 0.46–0.59 for SP, 0.51 for SAD, and 0.67 for AP [5]. This hints at a universal underestimation of the true genetic contribution at least in phobic disorders [5]. Unsurprisingly, both family studies and twin studies in the anxiety spectrum have acknowledged that the influence of genes respects neither hierarchic diagnostic disease boundaries nor the threshold between rational and irrational pathological anxiety or fear. Comparing genetic correlations from twin studies among SAD, AG, PD, and GAD, the lowest correlation of pairwise comparisons with 0.65 was found to exist between SAD and AP, while PD and GAD reached an almost perfect correlation coefficient of 0.98 [6]. This position is further supported by the fact that when twin data of SP, SAD, PD, AP, and GAD were combined in one single analysis, the latent liability to all anxiety disorders was more heritable than for any individual disorder [7].

In summary, the classic genetic studies of anxiety disorders suggest the potential for success in identifying the genes involved. The current landscape includes interesting findings from structural and rare variant studies, genome-wide association studies (GWAS), and candidate gene studies.

### Structural and rare variant studies

A genome-wide copy number variation (CNV) association study in 535 PD cases and 1520 control subjects yielded Bonferroni-corrected significant common duplications in the pericentromeric region of 16p11.2, including genes like the immunoglobulin heavy locus (*IGH*) and solute carrier family 6 member 8 (*SLC6A8*, creatine transporter 1) [8]. Furthermore, a meta-analysis of PD linkage studies amounting to over 700 analysed subjects reported significant bins on chromosomes 1, 5, 15, 16, and 22 [9].

The follow-up with GWAS or next-generation sequencing studies appears to be a promising avenue for future rare variant research efforts. For example, the transmembrane protein 132D (*TMEM132D*) locus, a gene previously associated with PD and anxiety severity (see GWAS, candidate gene, gene–environment interaction, and 'therapy genetics' studies, p. 929), has a 40-kb region spanning all exons now fully sequenced in a cohort of 300 anxiety disorder patients, including 262 PD, compared with 300 healthy controls [10]. A total of 371 variants were identified, most of which (76%) had a minor

**Table 89.1** Heritability of anxiety disorders

| | a² | 95% CI | c² | 95% CI | e² | 95% CI |
|---|---|---|---|---|---|---|
| SP[a] | 0.46–0.59 | NA | – | – | 0.41–0.53 | NA |
| SAD[a] | 0.51 | NA | – | – | 0.48 | NA |
| AP[a] | 0.67 | NA | – | – | 0.33 | NA |
| PD[b] | 0.43 | 0.32–0.53 | – | – | 0.57 | 0.47–0.68 |
| GAD[b] | 0.32 | 0.24–0.39 | 0.17 | 0.03–0.29 | 0.51 | 0.41–0.64 |

Heritability estimates not adding up to 1.0 are derived from rounding up/down effects.
SP, specific phobias; SAD, social anxiety disorder; AP, agoraphobia; PD, panic disorder; GAD, generalized anxiety disorder; CI, confidence interval; a², additive genetic factors; c², shared environmental factors; e², unique environmental factors; NA, information not available in the respective study.
a [5].
b [1].

allele frequency of under 5%, with an overrepresentation of functional coding variants in control subjects, suggesting that putatively protective *TMEM132D* variants decreased the risk to be affected by an anxiety disorder [10].

## GWAS, candidate gene, gene–environment interaction, and 'therapy genetics' studies

Within the anxiety disorder spectrum, PD has received the most attention in GWAS. Initially, two single-nucleotide polymorphisms (SNPs) within *TMEM132D* (rs7309727 T allele, rs11060369 A allele) were discovered as top hits in independent and combined GWAS approaches in three samples of patients with PD or PD and AP diagnoses (totalling 909 cases and 915 controls) [11]. The variants were associated with the severity of anxiety symptoms in patients affected by PD or panic attacks, and post-mortem studies revealed an increased expression of *TMEM132D* mRNA in the frontal cortex [11]. Subsequently, these results were replicated in a meta-analysis combining cases with primary PD (patients without major psychiatric comorbidities, 1039 cases and 2411 controls), which confirmed the rs7309727 T risk allele and a combined T/A rs7309727–rs11060369 risk genotype [12]. An independent meta-analysis further supported the PD 'risk' allele status of the rs7309727 T allele (2630 cases, 3294 controls; and 1867 cases, 2527 controls, respectively) and the rs11060369 C allele (2609 cases, 3279 controls; and 1852 cases, 2516 controls, respectively) in samples of primary PD and European PD [13].

Based on the assumption that different diagnostic definitions reflect alternative expressions of a common underlying anxiety diathesis, a recent meta-analysis of GWAS totalling over 18,000 unrelated individuals followed a dual approach by comparing cases (SP, SAD, PD, AP, and GAD, combined into one group of subjects with any anxiety disorder) to controls and employing, as a phenotypic score, an overall latent anxiety disorder factor [14]. The case-control design revealed a so far uncharacterized non-coding RNA (ncRNA) locus on chromosome 3q12.3 (*LOC152225*), with the rs1709393 T allele as a 'protective' factor against any anxiety disorder diagnosis, while analysis of the quantitative factor score highlighted a linkage disequilibrium block on chromosome 2p21 spanning three genes coding for the neutral and basic amino acid transport protein rBAT (*SLC3A1*), the prolyl endopeptidase-like protein (*PREPL*), and the calmodulin-lysine *N*-methyltransferase (*CAMKMT*), exceeding genome-wide significance, with the *CAMKMT* rs1067327 minor G allele as the top hit 'risk' SNP [14].

Candidate gene association studies of anxiety disorders have been based on the mechanism of action of anxiolytic drugs, preclinical models, or GWAS results for categorical or dimensional anxiety disorder traits. Within anxiety spectrum conditions, studies of common genetic variation have mainly investigated the serotonergic system, including its transporter and receptors, enzymes related to the synthesis or degradation of catecholamines and other neurotransmitters, or components of neuropeptide and hormonal systems.

The implication of the serotonin transporter (*SLC6A4*, chromosome 17q11.2) polymorphic region (*5-HTTLPR*) in animal models of anxiety [15] sparked interest in the evaluation of genes related to serotonergic neurotransmission in the human anxiety spectrum. The more active (higher transcription rate) long allele (l) has been associated with lower anxiety-related personality traits and implicated as a protective factor against the development of a depressive episode due to an individual's experienced amount of lifetime stress [16]. Conversely the short (s) allele was claimed to be associated with increased anxiety-related traits (neuroticism and harm avoidance) and vulnerability for an affective disorder diagnosis [15, 16]. The less active forms of the *5-HTTLPR* have been associated with a variety of clinical phenotypes in anxiety disorders, for example increased blushing propensity in SAD patients [17], increased and more persistent activation of the amygdala during an auditory habituation paradigm [18], and increased amygdala activation during exposure to happy faces [19] (for a review of imaging genetic effects on amygdala responsiveness in anxiety disorders, see [20]).

Unfortunately, several studies have not shown a direct association between *5-HTTLPR* variation and categorical PD (see, for example, [21]), and a meta-analysis of candidate gene studies failed to find supporting evidence for a significant effect [22]. Somewhat similarly, in a therapy-genetic approach, the *5-HTTLPR* genotype was successfully included, alongside other factors like gender and comorbid mood and externalizing disorders, in a risk index predicting the response of children (384 cases) to cognitive behavioural therapy (CBT) for primary anxiety disorders [23]. However, replication of the association between the short *5-HTTLPR* variant and increased response to CBT in a cross-cohort meta-analysis (1044 cases) failed for primary anxiety disorders, albeit s/s allele carriers were more likely to be free of any anxiety disorder post-CBT treatment [24]. Positive results have been reported in pharmacogenetic studies focusing on selective serotonin reuptake inhibitors (SSRIs), with the l variant predicting an increased reduction of SAD symptoms [25] and a significant reduction of panic attacks in female PD patients [26].

A recent systematic literature review of neurobiological markers of treatment response in anxiety disorders supported the role of a functional polymorphism within the l variant of the polymorphic region (5-HTTLPR/rs25531; the minor G allele renders the l variant transporter expression levels more closely to the 'risk' s variant [27]) in the prediction of therapy outcome [28]. The ultimate status of the 5-HTTLPR gene as a successful candidate remains to be definitively established in larger studies or by meta-analysis of smaller studies with sufficiently similar designs.

The G/G genotype of the serotonin receptor 1A gene (HTR1A, chromosome 5q12.3) rs6295 polymorphism (also referred to as -1019C/G, due to its position in the transcriptional control region) has been associated with increased escape behaviour during an avoidance task prior to CBT in patients suffering from PD with AP, as well as increased amygdala activity towards threat and safety cues and reduced self-initiated exposure to aversive stimuli following CBT [29]. Correspondingly, the G allele predicted a significant persistence of panic attacks in PD patients treated with SSRIs [30]. Nonetheless, the pharmacogenetic study was relatively underpowered.

Monoamine oxidase A (MAOA) is responsible for the oxidative deamination of serotonin, noradrenaline, dopamine, and xenobiotic amines; its gene on chromosome Xp11.3 has a functional polymorphism in the promoter region. The relevant location of the variation is commonly referred to as the upstream variable number of tandem repeats (uVNTR); it can take several forms generally distinguished in short (low transcriptional activity) or long alleles (high transcriptional activity), the latter of which has already been shown to occur significantly more frequently in female PD patients than in corresponding control samples [31]. Meta-analytical evaluation (1115 cases, 1260 controls) of candidate gene studies exploring the MAOA uVNTR validated a female-specific allelic association between the long, high-expression gene variants and PD [32]. Remarkably, a controlled and randomized multi-centre analysis (283 cases) discovered that the long alleles of the MAOA uVNTR resulted in significantly worse outcome measurements on dimensional scales of anxiety, following CBT, in patients suffering from PD with AP [33]. Inferior therapy outcome among long allele PD carriers, as compared to short allele carriers, was also accompanied by increased heart rate and reported fear during a behavioural avoidance task involving agoraphobic conditions and impaired habituation to the task upon repeated exposure [33]. Also, the T allele of the T941G polymorphism in the MAOA gene sequence has been possibly linked to GAD [34].

The catechol-O-methyltransferase (COMT, chromosome 22q11.21) is essential for the degradation of catecholamine neurotransmitters via the S-adenosyl methionine-coupled methylation of a hydroxyl group. It displays a SNP at base pair position 472 replacing a G with an A (rs4680, commonly referred to as the val158met polymorphism), causing a 3- to 4-fold lower overall COMT activity [35]. Initial association analysis revealed the G allele (that is, the valine/high-activity variant) to be overrepresented in female PD patients [36]. A recent meta-analysis (1130 cases, 1783 controls), including Asian and European-Caucasian samples, confirmed the 'risk' status of the rs4680 COMT G allele in European PD samples, regardless of gender [13]. Interestingly, the 158met/met genotype has been suggested to profit less from exposure-based CBT for PD, as compared to carriers of at least one val allele, who reported higher symptom intensity prior to CBT [37]. Additionally, while the COMT val variant

has been linked to SP [38], internalizing disorders, including SAD and GAD, have been associated with other genetic variation related to the catecholaminergic system, including the sodium-dependent dopamine transporter (SLC6A3) [39].

Given the pivotal role of corticotropin-releasing hormone (CRH) in the hypothalamic–pituitary–adrenal (HPA) axis, and therefore as a regulator of cortisol release in the stress response, the CRH receptors CRHR1 and CRHR2 have been an additional focus in the exploration of anxiety disorder genetics, particularly in PD. A joint cohort approach genotyping nine CRHR1 (chromosome 17q21.31) SNPs in 531 matched PD case-control pairs delivered evidence of four SNPs (rs7209436, rs12936181, rs17689918, and rs17689966) to be associated with PD in at least one subsample, with the minor A allele of rs17689918 remaining statistically significant in PD females across all cohorts, even following conservative post hoc correction [40]. Multi-level evidence suggests the rs17689918 A allele is associated with decreased CRHR1 mRNA expression in the frontal cortex and amygdala of post-mortem brains, aberrant differential conditioning in the prefrontal cortex, and impaired safety signal processing in the amygdala in an imaging paradigm [40]. Furthermore, the risk allele caused carriers to show less escape tendencies in a behavioural avoidance task, yet increased levels of nervous apprehension and anxiety sensitivity [40]. This suggests reduced CRHR1 expression to be linked to an increased susceptibility to anxious sensations accompanied by feelings of sustained fear [40]. Additionally, an investigation of several anxiety disorder candidate gene effects on serotonin–noradrenaline reuptake inhibitor (SNRI) treatment response in GAD supported an association of CRHR1 SNPs with therapy outcome [41].

Among the neuropeptide class and their respective receptors, genetic variation of neuropeptide S (NPS) and the NPS receptor (NPSR1, chromosome 7p14.3) correlates psychopathological processes relating to stress, arousal, and fear, and to their mediation in particular, with anxiety-related behaviour and anxiety disorders (Fig. 89.1) [42]. Upon binding of NPS, the G-protein coupled NPSR1 promotes the mobilization of intracellular calcium stores and thereby affects second messenger signalling [43]. In independent, as well as joint, analyses of case-control cohorts (766 cases and 776 controls), the NPSR1 rs324981 T allele (replacing an asparagine in amino acid position 107 with an isoleucine [Asn$^{107}$Ile], leading to receptor hyper-responsiveness) has been significantly associated with PD with and without AP in females in a categorical analysis approach and, dimensionally, with increased levels of anxiety sensitivity [44]. Evaluations of the NPSR1 rs324981 T allele in PD females demonstrated increased heart rates and other symptom measures during a behavioural avoidance task and decreased activation of the anterior cingulate cortex top–down control following exposure to emotionally relevant fear stimuli [44]. The status of NPSR1 as a PD 'risk' gene has been highlighted recently by a replication of the NPSR1 rs324981 T allele association with PD in samples of European ancestry in a meta-analysis of candidate gene studies (914 cases, 1028 controls) [13]. For a review of the NPSR1 gene in mechanisms of anxiety, also see [45].

A further valuable candidate gene strategy targets mediating models of anxiety proneness, for example increased sensitivity to carbon dioxide. Hypercapnia reliably elicits a panicogenic effect in PD patients. Following linkage evidence for the chromosomal region 12q13 and PD [46], further studies expanded upon a

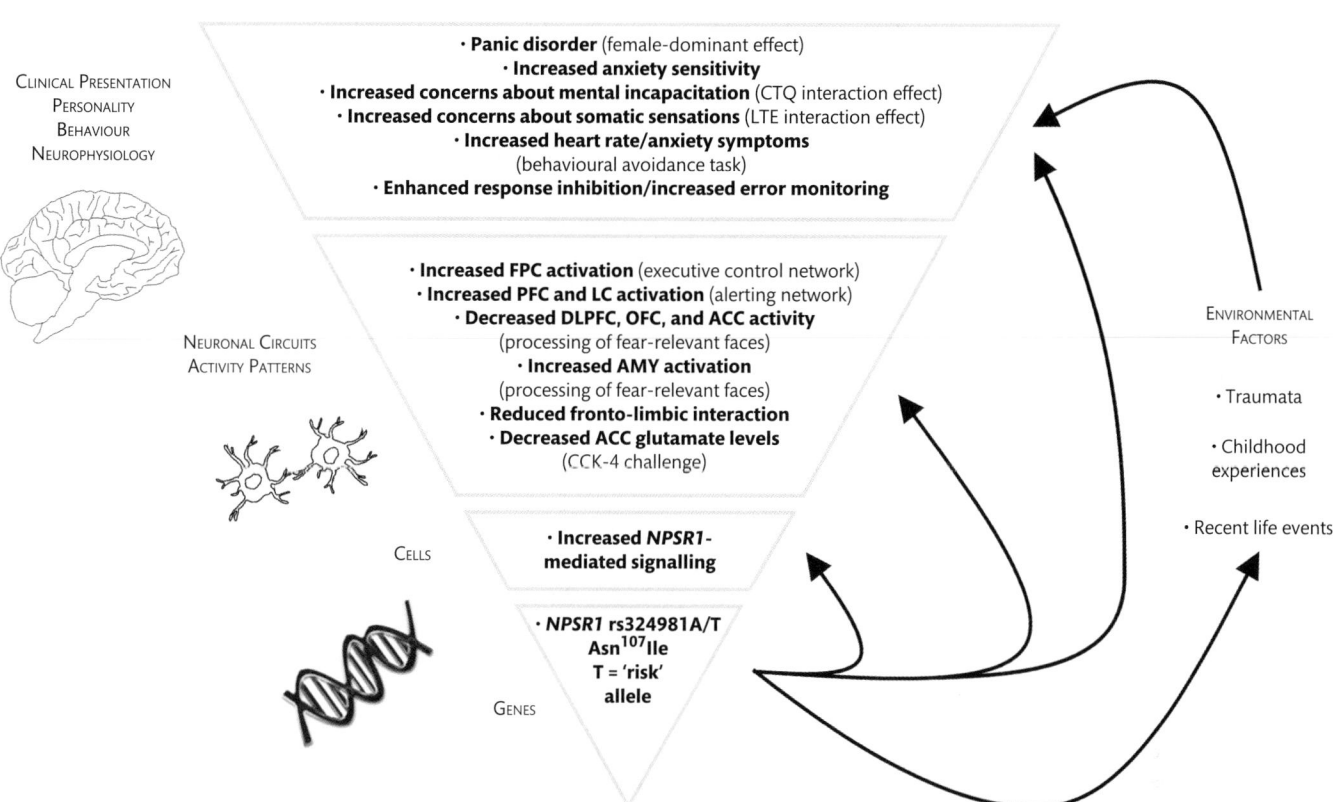

**Fig. 89.1** Multi-level evidence linking the neuropeptide S receptor 1 gene (*NPSR1*) to anxiety disorders and anxiety-related cross-disorder intermediate phenotypes. The *NPSR1* rs324981 T allele was chosen as seed node. Arrows represent domain interrelations of systems analysis mediating interactions between genetic and environmental factors, potentially leading to observable meta-phenomena crossing classic nosological boundaries and connecting different spectra of psychopathology. Refer to the individual sections in this chapter for detailed supporting literature. ACC, anterior cingulate cortex; AMY, amygdala; CCK-4, cholecystokinin tetrapeptide; CTQ, Childhood Trauma Questionnaire; DLPFC, dorsolateral prefrontal cortex; FPC, frontoparietal cortex; LC, locus coeruleus; LTE, list of threatening experiences/lifetime events; OFC, orbitofrontal cortex; PFC, prefrontal cortex.

potential role of the acid-sensing ion channel 1 (*ACCN1*, chromosome 12q13.12) in mediating the detection of brain acidosis/hypercarbia and acting as a chemosensor triggering fear-related behaviour. *ACCN1* SNPs rs685012 (C allele) and rs10875995 (C allele) have been associated with PD in a case-control analysis, with a particularly strong association in either early-onset PD or PD with primarily respiratory symptoms [47]. There was also an increased amygdala volume and reactivity to emotional stimuli in a cohort of healthy subjects [47]. Interestingly, following the recent interest in carbon dioxide-induced acidosis related to *ACCN1* in patients suffering from PD, an investigation in mice established that exposure to early-life adversity induced separation anxiety-related behaviour and hyperventilation upon carbon dioxide inhalation [48]. This phenotype was further associated with epigenetic histone modifications and a gene expression network in the medulla oblongata, not only confirming increased expression of the murine *ACCN1* orthologue, but also affecting biological processes related to neurodevelopment and emotionality, as well as actual drug targets in the form of the mammalian/mechanistic target of rapamycin (mTOR) signalling pathway [48].

## Epigenetic studies

Given the substantial impact of gene–environment interactions in the aetiology, disease course, and treatment of psychiatric disorders [49], the rising field of epigenetics has the potential to expand our

knowledge of systemic biological alterations underlying anxiety-related inter-individual differences. Given the implied intrinsic mechanistic capacity for plasticity, and therefore reversibility, the potential for treatment innovation is particularly exciting.

Assessments of epigenetic DNA methylation patterns spanning the transcription regulatory site and exon 1/intron 1 region of the *MAOA* gene in PD patients and matched controls revealed significantly reduced methylation levels in female PD patients [50]. Notably, across patients and controls, the occurrence of recent negative life events resulted in relatively decreased *MAOA* methylation levels, while positive life events were associated with increased methylation levels [50]. The potential clinical relevance of this dynamic epigenetic state of *MAOA* methylation was supported by the hypomethylation pattern in female PD patients and the correlation of decreased methylation levels with increased panic attack frequency and heightened agoraphobic avoidance in the absence or presence of a trusted person [51]. Exceptionally, following CBT, the average methylation of therapy responders increased to a level indistinguishable from that of healthy controls, while methylation of non-responders remained unchanged or even declined [51]. Further evidence for an epigenetic role in the serotonergic system was provided by a study assessing methylation levels upstream of the *SLC6A4* promoter region in children with a variety of anxiety disorders pre- and post-CBT, with one CpG site differentiating responders with increasing methylation, along with treatment success, from non-responders with decreasing methylation [52].

Oxytocin has repeatedly been implicated in social functioning and potentially SAD (for a review of oxytocin's role in anxiety disorders, see [53]). Epigenetic screening of a CpG island just downstream of the oxytocin receptor (OXTR, chromosome 3p25.3) exon 3 translation start site in a cohort of 110 medication-free SAD patients and 110 gender-matched controls revealed a decreased methylation pattern in SAD patients, with both overall and CpG3 methylation negatively correlating with SAD symptom intensity in patients, as well as dimensional social anxiety in controls [54]. OXTR methylation negatively correlated with the cortisol response to the Trier Social Stress Test (TSST) in healthy controls and amygdala activity levels upon exposure to social phobia-related words in SAD patients [54].

Finally, decreased CRHR1 promoter methylation was associated with PD in a case-control design and with heightened anxiety ratings in an independent sample of healthy volunteers [54]. A functional luciferase assay linked an unmethylated CRHR1 promoter region to increased gene expression, implicating C1 hypomethylation and a resulting CRHR1 overabundance in a dysfunctional stress response as possibly pathogenetically relevant in PD [55].

## Genetics of cross-disorder anxiety phenotypes

Family studies and twin studies support the genetic clustering and co-heritability of SP, SAD, AP, PD, and GAD, along with post-traumatic stress disorder (PTSD) [56–58]. In line with their epidemiological, as well as nosological, overlap and their shared genetic background, anxiety disorders and trauma- and stress-related disorders represent closely interrelated diagnostic constructs. They exist beyond a threshold where subsyndromal anxiety and fear responses grade into degrees of psychopathology. Accordingly, genetic investigations of cross-disorder anxiety and post-traumatic stress phenotypes have explored temperamental traits considered to mediate the susceptibility of children, adolescents, and adults to suffer from the respective disorders; these include neuroticism/negative affectivity, introversion, anxiety sensitivity, behavioural inhibition, insecure attachment styles, and harm avoidance. Further relevant cross-disorder phenotypes are expanded upon in Chapter 80.

Several GWAS have reported on genome-wide significant associations for neuroticism. One approach (106,716 samples) implicated risk genes like the glutamate ionotropic receptor kainate type subunit 3 (GRIK3, rs490647) and CRHR1 (rs111433752), as well as a 4-Mb region on chromosome 8 spanning more than 36 genes [59]. Another genome-wide analysis of 170,911 subjects identified 11 other variants associated with neuroticism; a genetic correlation based on linkage disequilibrium score regression between five different neuropsychiatric phenotypes and neuroticism was highest for anxiety disorders (0.88) [60]. Furthermore, a GWAS twin study in 730 monozygotic and dizygotic twin pairs, exploring the genetic basis of anxiety sensitivity estimated a heritability of 0.44 and identified a top hit within the coding region of the RNA binding protein fox-1 homolog 1 gene (RBFOX1, rs13334105) [61]. Notably, a genome-wide genetic linkage of neuroticism quantitative trait loci (QTLs) in extremely discordant and concordant sibling pairs established a locus on chromosome 1 spanning the regulator of the G-protein

signalling gene (RGS2) [62]. This proved to be syntenic with a QTL modulating anxiety-related behaviour in mice [63], marking a rare occasion of inter-species QTL concordance. Moreover, the RGS2 rs4606 C allele (hypothesized to lead to increased mRNA stability, and therefore higher expression levels) has been associated with increased incidence rates of PD [64] and GAD [65].

Based on a PD- and AP-related dimensional intermediate phenotype (Agoraphobia Cognition Questionnaire [ACQ]), a GWAS in healthy German probands (1370 samples) found genome-wide associations between increased agoraphobic scores and SNPs in the glycine receptor subunit beta (GLRB), one of which (rs7688285) was successfully replicated in an independent dimensional sample and a case/control sample [66]. The minor rs7688285 A allele was subsequently demonstrated to be linked to increased GLRB expression in the midbrain of post-mortem tissue, reduced startle habituation and increased startle potentiation and generalization, as well as stronger amygdala and insula activation, during the acquisition phase and thalamus, putamen/pallidum and skin conductance responses, following the acquisition phase in a fear conditioning paradigm [66]. A comparable dimensional GWAS approach in a Hispanic community sample (11,456 samples free of antidepressant or anxiolytic medication) detected a genome-wide significant association between a self-constructed GAD symptom score and the thrombospondin 2 gene (THBS2, rs78602344) [67]. Despite these encouraging advances with regard to personality dimensions and psychometric scores, so far, no genome-wide significant associations have been reported for a continuous measure of phobic anxiety [68], anxiety-related behaviour in childhood [69], or harm avoidance [70].

### Serotonergic system

Complementary to GWAS, candidate gene, and gene–environment studies outlined previously, the serotonergic system, and therein particularly the 5-HTTLPR, has been a focus of attention in the investigation of cross-disorder and dimensional anxiety-related phenotypes. Anticipation of an unpredictable shock following a long phase of expectation resulted in increased neuronal activation of the amygdala, hippocampus, anterior insula, thalamus, pulvinar nucleus, caudate nucleus, precuneus, anterior cingulate cortex, and medial prefrontal cortex and increased positive coupling between the medial prefrontal cortex and physiological anxiety experience based on insular activity in 5-HTTLPR s/s homozygotes, while in l allele carriers, a negative coupling was observed [71]. Additionally, increased activation of the dorsomedial prefrontal cortex in 5-HTTLPR short allele carriers mediated increased psychophysiological reactions in anticipation of future aversive events, explicitly by increased skin conductance and startle reaction [72]. The low-expression 5-HTTLPR risk alleles have also been implicated in an increased amygdala response to sad emotional faces [73]. Furthermore, healthy controls homozygous for the 5-HTTLPR l allele reacted with increased amygdala and insula activity towards the presentation of fearful faces, if they were treated with citalopram, as compared to placebo treatment, yielding interesting insights into the often reported 'jitteriness' phenomenon accompanying SSRI treatment during the titration phase [74].

Moreover, decreased SLC6A4 promoter methylation levels have been linked to increased cortisol secretion, following the TSST in 5-HTTLPR s allele carriers in a dose-dependent fashion, while no such association was detectable in s allele carriers with high methylation levels [75].

## Catecholaminergic system

In healthy female subjects, the *COMT* 158val allele conferred increased amygdala responses to fearful and angry facial stimuli, as well as heightened activation of the ventral visual stream and the lateral prefrontal cortex, pointing to a gender-specific effect of altered catecholaminergic activity on emotional processing [76]. Focusing on cross-generational interaction and neuronal development, it has also been shown that increased antenatal maternal anxiety was significantly positively correlated with ventrolateral prefrontal cortex thickness in neonates when carrying the *COMT* val/val genotype, suggesting a complex genetic interaction between maternal susceptibility to anxiety disorders and *in utero* development of anxiety-relevant cortical areas [77].

## Neuropeptide systems

The multi-level disease framework depicted in Fig. 89.1 reflects the converging evidence for a role of the NPS system in categorical anxiety diagnoses and cross-disorder intermediate phenotypes. Additional evidence for a key function of this system in panic-related anxiety emerges from a challenge approach, allowing for studying an unfolding panic attack by injection of the panicogenic pharmacological agent cholecystokinin tetrapeptide (CCK-4) [78]. Following CCK-4 injection, healthy *NPSR1* rs324981 T allele carriers showed lower levels of excitatory neurotransmitter abundance in the anterior cingulate cortex, as measured by magnetic resonance spectroscopy, during the course of a panic attack [79]. This suggests reduced inhibitory top–down control, allowing maladaptive behavioural responses [79]. A further pertinent link between the NPS system and phenotypes with particular relevance to anxiety-related disorders has been established by an imaging genetics approach; the *NPSR1* rs324981 T risk allele has been associated not only with increased amygdala activation in response to fear-relevant stimuli, but also with increased harm avoidance traits, potentially connecting the *NPSR1* risk allele to disorder-specific neuronal processes shaping pathological fear reactions in the limbic system [80]. Furthermore, study of event-related potentials uncovered intensified response inhibition and error monitoring to be associated with the *NPSR1* rs324981 T allele, with the latter also mediating increased levels of anxiety sensitivity [81]. Similarly, higher activation patterns in the prefrontal cortex and the locus coeruleus region during an alerting condition and increased activations in fronto-parietal regions during an executive control condition in T/T genotype carriers correlated with heightened anxiety sensitivity scores [82]. This hints at an influence of the *NPSR1* rs324981 polymorphism on neuronal processes of anxiety-relevant attentional functioning [82]. Remarkably, analysis of fronto-limbic connectivity during brain development revealed a higher connectivity between the middle frontal gyrus and the amygdala in older adolescents carrying the *NPSR1* rs324981 A allele, while T/T homozygosity was linked to a reduced connection between the medial frontal gyrus and both the amygdala and insula [83]. Hence, the *NPSR1* genotype has a potential role in dysfunctional development of cortico-limbic interaction during a crucial time window of anxiety disorder onset [83]. The effect of the *NPSR1* rs324981 genotype on anxiety sensitivity revealed that T/T homozygosity and high levels of childhood trauma resulted in increased levels of anxiety sensitivity, particularly concerns about mental incapacitation and physical sensations, while acute somatic concerns interacted with the *NPSR1* genotype and the amount of recent life events [84]. Interestingly, from the perspective of innovative future treatment strategies, intranasal NPS administration has been shown to reach the anterior olfactory area, nucleus accumbens, thalamus, hypothalamus, and particularly the hippocampus where it modulates synaptic transmission and plasticity, next to exerting anxiolytic properties in multiple behavioural tests [85].

Moreover, the influence of a less secure attachment style on increased levels of social anxiety may be partially modulated by the *OXTR* rs53576 A/G polymorphism, with the A allele exerting a significantly greater negative influence of insecure attachment on SAD-related dimensional traits, as compared to the G/G genotype [86]. The potential for a paradigm shift from 'risk' genes towards a notion of 'plasticity' genes is exemplified by a neuroimaging study assessing *OXTR* gene–environment interactions for the very same polymorphism previously linked to protective, as well as maladaptive, properties. *OXTR* rs53576 G/G homozygotes exhibited a significant reduction of bilateral ventral striatum grey matter volume interacting with the extent of childhood trauma suffered and increased amygdala reactivity towards emotional facial stimuli [87]. In turn, decreased ventral striatum grey matter volumes were also associated with the prosocial trait of lower reward dependence in G/G homozygotes [87]. Thus, the G allele may not only mediate the vulnerability of limbic structures to adverse childhood events but could also confer resilience in the form of increased limbic responsiveness to emotional interaction [87].

## Clinical challenges and future perspectives

The establishment of the genetic variation influencing anxiety disorders is an ongoing process. Recent advances converge on a cross-disorder explanation of psychopathology, pointing towards the need for a revised understanding of mental disease frameworks (Fig. 89.1), which may be translated into novel clinical tools. Specifically, the field of psychiatric genetics/epigenetics holds the promise to catalyse a paradigm shift in drug discovery, treatment response prediction, individual risk evaluation, and nosological conceptionalization, by ultimately answering questions regarding the molecular plasticity of anxiety and fear, experience and trauma, and resilience and susceptibility [45].

The inspection of a given gene, or rather a gene set, in relation to biological pathways and processes yields the potential to uncover *innovative molecular treatment targets* and pioneer alternative mechanisms of action. This is why especially the follow-up of unbiased GWAS by candidate gene studies and functional *in silico* enrichment analyses represents a pivotal step in the identification and prioritization of therapeutic objectives. The greatest present challenge is the consistent replication of findings. However, as reviewed in detail previously, several genes (for example, *NPSR1* or *ACCN1*) and systemic processes (for example, glucocorticoid or oxytocinergic signalling) have accumulated considerable evidence for their modulation of disease-relevant traits like fear generalization or perseverative thought patterns.

In addition to the provision of novel therapeutic targets, psychiatric genetics may also contribute to the discovery of clinically valid phenotypes, exploring the molecular characterization of patient subgroups that would allow for an improved pairing of patient and treatment in an *individualized precision medicine approach*. Future steps might comprise the combination of several or even many

SNPs, as well as the inclusion of environmental factors to account for the phenotypic heterogeneity observed in anxiety disorders. A polygenic risk score of environmental sensitivity based on within-pair variability in emotional problems of monozygotic twins has been found to significantly moderate the effect of parenting on emotional problems in an independent group [88]. It also predicted a better response to CBT for childhood anxiety disorders in individual, rather than in group, sessions, suggesting that, in line with the differential susceptibility hypothesis, individuals with greater environmental vulnerability are at an increased likelihood to develop emotional problems in an adverse environment but correspondingly benefit more from an intense form of treatment [88].

Finally, as summarized, a growing body of evidence suggests *dynamic epigenetic changes* in chromatin structure and methylation patterns to underlie anxiety-related phenotypes, their pathophysiological signature, their disease course, and perhaps most strikingly—in a possibly mechanistic way—their clinical response to psychotherapeutic or psychopharmacological interventions. For example, increased *MAOA* methylation levels following successful CBT might not only constitute a plastic epigenetic marker of therapy response [51] but could also pave the way for personally tailored therapy augmentation. This could be provided in the form of monoamine oxidase inhibitors (MAOIs) as an adjunct to psychotherapy in order to supplement for the degree of *MAOA* hypomethylation in patients suffering from PD. Although the particular attractiveness of epigenetic risk markers lies in their inherent capacity for reversibility, permanent (for example, SNPs), as well as transient (for example, methylation), changes to the DNA strand might not always be reducible to 'risk' and 'resilience' markers, but rather be viewed in the perspective of *differential susceptibility*. Thus, individuals most vulnerable to environmental adversity due to their genetic loading might simultaneously be most receptive to beneficial experiences, which would consequently result in their nomenclature being relabelled as *'plasticity' genes* [89]. Following their consistent validation in longitudinal studies of diagnosis and treatment, epigenetic signatures like methylation patterns could eventually meet the

**Table 89.2** Overview of genetic variants implicated in anxiety disorders and cross-disorder anxiety phenotypes. The overall degree of confidence was ranked from '+' = 'low' to '++++' = 'high', based on the reviewed evidence (refer to the individual sections in this chapter for detailed supporting literature)

| Gene | Top risk variant | Evidence from structural, rare variant, GWA, candidate gene, gene - environment, and epigenetic studies | Overall degree of confidence |
|------|------------------|-----------------------------------------------------------------------------------------------------------|------------------------------|
| *MAOA* | Upstream variable number of tandem repeats (uVNTR) Long allele | Candidate gene association with PD in females [31] <br> Meta-analytical candidate gene association with PD in females [32] <br> Association with decreased PD CBT treatment response [33] <br> Reduced methylation in the transcription-regulatory region in female PD patients [50] <br> Negative life events resulted in decreased *MAOA* methylation levels; positive life events were associated with increased methylation [50] <br> Decreased methylation correlated with increased symptom measures in female PD patients [51] <br> Response to PD CBT was linked to increased methylation [51] | ++++ |
| *NPSR1* | rs324981 T allele | Candidate gene association with PD in females [44] <br> Increased symptom measures during behavioural avoidance and decreased anterior cingulate cortex top–down control towards fear-relevant stimuli [44] <br> Gene–environment interaction with childhood trauma associated with increased anxiety sensitivity [84] <br> Meta-analytical candidate gene association with PD [13] <br> Lower anterior cingulate cortex excitatory neurotransmitter levels during a panic attack [79] <br> Increased amygdala response to fear-relevant stimuli and increased harm avoidance [80] <br> Increased frontal and locus coeruleus activation in the neuronal alerting network [82] <br> Increased fronto-parietal activation in the executive control network correlating with anxiety sensitivity [82] <br> Reduced development of neuronal fronto-limbic connectivity [83] | ++++ |
| *TMEM132D* | rs7309727 T allele | Rare functional coding variants protective of PD [10] <br> Top hit in PD/PD+AP GWAS [11] <br> Confirmed in follow-up candidate gene association [12] <br> Meta-analytical candidate gene association with PD [13] | +++ |
| *COMT* | rs4680 G allele (val158met, val variant) | Candidate gene association with PD in females [36] <br> Meta-analytical candidate gene association with PD [13] <br> Increased amygdala response to negative emotional stimuli [76] | +++ |
| *SLC6A4* | Serotonin transporter polymorphic region (5-*HTTLPR*) short allele | Increased neuroticism and harm avoidance [15] <br> Increased blushing propensity in SAD [17] <br> Increased amygdala activation during auditory habituation [18] <br> Meta-analysis of PD candidate gene studies found no association [22] <br> Contradictory findings of association with anxiety disorder CBT treatment response in children [23, 24] <br> Association with decreased SSRI treatment response [25, 26] <br> Increased coupling of insular activity and physiological anxiety [71] <br> Increased amygdala response to sad faces [73] <br> Decreased methylation levels linked to increased cortisol response to social stress [75] | ++ |
| *CRHR1* | rs17689918 A allele | Cross-cohort candidate gene association with PD in females [40] <br> Increased anxiety sensitivity and impaired safety signal processing in the amygdala [40] <br> Different SNP (rs111433752) implicated in neuroticism GWAS [59] <br> Decreased promoter methylation associated with PD [55] | ++ |

AP, agoraphobia; SAD, social anxiety disorder; PD, panic disorder; CBT, cognitive behavioural therapy; GWAS, genome-wide association study; SNP, single nucleotide polymorphism.

clinical need for an easily accessible peripheral biomarker, allowing the stratification of patients in susceptibility classes. Subsequently, regular quantitative observations could guide the development and provision of targeted, and thus the most effective, preventive, as well as interventional measures. The next generation of psychotherapeutic and psychopharmacological treatments might also be evaluated by the speed, strength, and permanence with which they alter the multilocus impact of environmental stimuli and traumata on the epigenetic architecture of anxiety disorders.

## Conclusions

Anxiety disorders display a distinct familial clustering, and heritable factors contribute significantly to their disease burden. Large-scale unbiased GWAS and meta-analyses have begun to reach the necessary sample sizes to uncover meaningful SNP associations and have been complemented and extended by candidate gene and gene–environment studies implicating the serotonergic and catecholaminergic, as well as neuropeptide and hormonal, systems (Table 89.2). The polygenic nature of anxiety disorders suggests that the still incompletely unravelled molecular signature of anxiety might transcend traditional hierarchical diagnostic boundaries. Facing the complexity of potential pleiotropic effects and their interactions with each other, systems–biological methods could facilitate the mapping of candidate genes and functional pathways onto cross-cutting symptom measures and uncover their interface with temperamental, developmental, and environmental variables. One of the emerging key mechanistic processes potentially unifying these components appears to be psychiatric epigenetics. Given the dynamic nature of chromatin structure and methylation patterns related to environmental influences, as well as psychotherapeutic and psychopharmacological interventions, epigenetics may explain part of the missing heritability of anxiety disorders, constitute a mechanistic link between stress and biological vulnerability, and finally—in synopsis with genetic and other risk factors—inform personalized treatment and indicated prevention in anxiety disorders.

## Acknowledgements

This work has been supported by the German Research Foundation (DFG) (SFB-TRR-58, grant number 44541416, subprojects C02 and Z02 to K.D.) and the Federal Ministry of Education and Research (BMBF) (PROTECT-AD, grant number 14 01EE1402A, subproject P5 to K.D.).

## REFERENCES

1. Hettema JM, Neale MC, Kendler KS. A review and meta-analysis of the genetic epidemiology of anxiety disorders. *Am J Psychiatry.* 2001;158:1568–78.
2. Czajkowski N, Kendler KS, Tambs K, Roysamb E, Reichborn-Kjennerud T. The structure of genetic and environmental risk factors for phobias in women. *Psychol Med.* 2011;41:1987–95.
3. Zheng Y, Rijsdijk F, Pingault JB, McMahon RJ, Unger JB. Developmental changes in genetic and environmental influences on Chinese child and adolescent anxiety and depression. *Psychol Med.* 2016;46:1829–38.
4. Eley TC, McAdams TA, Rijsdijk FV, et al. The intergenerational transmission of anxiety: a children-of-twins study. *Am J Psychiatry.* 2015;172:630–7.
5. Kendler KS, Karkowski LM, Prescott CA. Fears and phobias: reliability and heritability. *Psychol Med.* 1999;29:539–53.
6. Hettema JM, Neale MC, Myers JM, Prescott CA, Kendler KS. A population-based twin study of the relationship between neuroticism and internalizing disorders. *Am J Psychiatry.* 2006;163:857–64.
7. Tambs K, Czajkowsky N, Roysamb E, et al. Structure of genetic and environmental risk factors for dimensional representations of DSM-IV anxiety disorders. *Br J Psychiatry.* 2009;195:301–7.
8. Kawamura Y, Otowa T, Koike A, et al. A genome-wide CNV association study on panic disorder in a Japanese population. *J Hum Genet.* 2011;56:852–6.
9. Webb BT, Guo AY, Maher BS, et al. Meta-analyses of genome-wide linkage scans of anxiety-related phenotypes. *Eur J Hum Genet.* 2012;20:1078–84.
10. Quast C, Altmann A, Weber P, et al. Rare variants in TMEM132D in a case-control sample for panic disorder. *Am J Med Genet B Neuropsychiatr Genet.* 2012;159B:896–907.
11. Erhardt A, Czibere L, Roeske D, et al. TMEM132D, a new candidate for anxiety phenotypes: evidence from human and mouse studies. *Mol Psychiatry.* 2011;16:647–63.
12. Erhardt A, Akula N, Schumacher J, et al. Replication and meta-analysis of TMEM132D gene variants in panic disorder. *Transl Psychiatry.* 2012;2:e156.
13. Howe AS, Buttenschon HN, Bani-Fatemi A, et al. Candidate genes in panic disorder: meta-analyses of 23 common variants in major anxiogenic pathways. *Mol Psychiatry.* 2016;21:665–79.
14. Otowa T, Hek K, Lee M, et al. Meta-analysis of genome-wide association studies of anxiety disorders. *Mol Psychiatry.* 2016;21:1391–9.
15. Lesch KP, Bengel D, Heils A, et al. Association of anxiety-related traits with a polymorphism in the serotonin transporter gene regulatory region. *Science.* 1996;274:1527–31.
16. Caspi A, Sugden K, Moffitt TE, Taylor A, Craig IW, Harrington H, et al. Influence of life stress on depression: moderation by a polymorphism in the 5-HTT gene. *Science.* 2003;301:386–9.
17. Domschke K, Stevens S, Beck B, et al. Blushing propensity in social anxiety disorder: influence of serotonin transporter gene variation. *J Neural Transm (Vienna).* 2009;116:663–6.
18. Pfleiderer B, Zinkirciran S, Michael N, et al. Altered auditory processing in patients with panic disorder: a pilot study. *World J Biol Psychiatry.* 2010;11:945–55.
19. Domschke K, Braun M, Ohrmann P, et al. Association of the functional -1019C/G 5-HT1A polymorphism with prefrontal cortex and amygdala activation measured with 3 T fMRI in panic disorder. *Int J Neuropsychopharmacol.* 2006;9:349–55.
20. Domschke K, Dannlowski U. Imaging genetics of anxiety disorders. *Neuroimage.* 2010;53:822–31.
21. Deckert J, Catalano M, Heils A, et al. Functional promoter polymorphism of the human serotonin transporter: lack of association with panic disorder. *Psychiatr Genet.* 1997;7:45–7.
22. Blaya C, Salum GA, Lima MS, Leistner-Segal S, Manfro GG. Lack of association between the serotonin transporter promoter polymorphism (5-HTTLPR) and panic disorder: a systematic review and meta-analysis. *Behav Brain Funct.* 2007;3:41.
23. Hudson JL, Lester KJ, Lewis CM, et al. Predicting outcomes following cognitive behaviour therapy in child anxiety disorders: the influence of genetic, demographic and clinical information. *J Child Psychol Psychiatry.* 2013;54:1086–94.

24. Lester KJ, Roberts S, Keers R, *et al*. Non-replication of the association between 5HTTLPR and response to psychological therapy for child anxiety disorders. *Br J Psychiatry*. 2016;208:182–8.

25. Stein MB, Seedat S, Gelernter J. Serotonin transporter gene promoter polymorphism predicts SSRI response in generalized social anxiety disorder. *Psychopharmacology (Berl)*. 2006;187:68–72.

26. Perna G, Favaron E, Di Bella D, Bussi R, Bellodi L. Antipanic efficacy of paroxetine and polymorphism within the promoter of the serotonin transporter gene. *Neuropsychopharmacology*. 2005;30:2230–5.

27. Praschak-Rieder N, Kennedy J, Wilson AA, *et al*. Novel 5-*HTTLPR* allele associates with higher serotonin transporter binding in putamen: a [(11)C] DASB positron emission tomography study. *Biol Psychiatry*. 2007;62:327–31.

28. Lueken U, Zierhut KC, Hahn T, *et al*. Neurobiological markers predicting treatment response in anxiety disorders: a systematic review and implications for clinical application. *Neurosci Biobehav Rev*. 2016;66:143–62.

29. Straube B, Reif A, Richter J, *et al*. The functional-1019C/G HTR1A polymorphism and mechanisms of fear. *Transl Psychiatry*. 2014;4:e490.

30. Yevtushenko OO, Oros MM, Reynolds GP. Early response to selective serotonin reuptake inhibitors in panic disorder is associated with a functional 5-HT1A receptor gene polymorphism. *J Affect Disord*. 2010;123:308–11.

31. Deckert J, Catalano M, Syagailo YV, *et al*. Excess of high activity monoamine oxidase A gene promoter alleles in female patients with panic disorder. *Hum Mol Genet*. 1999;8:621–4.

32. Reif A, Weber H, Domschke K, *et al*. Meta-analysis argues for a female-specific role of MAOA-uVNTR in panic disorder in four European populations. *Am J Med Genet B Neuropsychiatr Genet*. 2012;159B:786–93.

33. Reif A, Richter J, Straube B, *et al*. MAOA and mechanisms of panic disorder revisited: from bench to molecular psychotherapy. *Mol Psychiatry*. 2014;19:122–8.

34. Tadic A, Rujescu D, Szegedi A, *et al*. Association of a MAOA gene variant with generalized anxiety disorder, but not with panic disorder or major depression. *Am J Med Genet B Neuropsychiatr Genet*. 2003;117B:1–6.

35. Lachman HM, Papolos DF, Saito T, Yu YM, Szumlanski CL, Weinshilboum RM. Human catechol-*O*-methyltransferase pharmacogenetics: description of a functional polymorphism and its potential application to neuropsychiatric disorders. *Pharmacogenetics*. 1996;6:243–50.

36. Domschke K, Freitag CM, Kuhlenbaumer G, *et al*. Association of the functional V158M catechol-*O*-methyl-transferase polymorphism with panic disorder in women. *Int J Neuropsychopharmacol*. 2004;7:183–8.

37. Lonsdorf TB, Ruck C, Bergstrom J, *et al*. The COMTval158met polymorphism is associated with symptom relief during exposure-based cognitive-behavioral treatment in panic disorder. *BMC Psychiatry*. 2010;10:99.

38. McGrath M, Kawachi I, Ascherio A, Colditz GA, Hunter DJ, De Vivo I. Association between catechol-*O*-methyltransferase and phobic anxiety. *Am J Psychiatry*. 2004;161:1703–5.

39. Rowe DC, Stever C, Gard JM, *et al*. The relation of the dopamine transporter gene (DAT1) to symptoms of internalizing disorders in children. *Behav Genet*. 1998;28:215–25.

40. Weber H, Richter J, Straube B, *et al*. Allelic variation in *CRHR1* predisposes to panic disorder: evidence for biased fear processing. *Mol Psychiatry*. 2016;21:813–22.

41. Perlis RH, Fijal B, Dharia S, Houston JP. Pharmacogenetic investigation of response to duloxetine treatment in generalized anxiety disorder. *Pharmacogenomics J*. 2013;13:280–5.

42. Pape HC, Jungling K, Seidenbecher T, Lesting J, Reinscheid RK. Neuropeptide S: a transmitter system in the brain regulating fear and anxiety. *Neuropharmacology*. 2010;58:29–34.

43. Bernier V, Stocco R, Bogusky MJ, *et al*. Structure-function relationships in the neuropeptide S receptor: molecular consequences of the asthma-associated mutation N107I. *J Biol Chem*. 2006;281:24704–12.

44. Domschke K, Reif A, Weber H, *et al*. Neuropeptide S receptor gene – converging evidence for a role in panic disorder. *Mol Psychiatry*. 2011;16:938–48.

45. Gottschalk MG, Domschke K. Novel developments in genetic and epigenetic mechanisms of anxiety. *Curr Opin Psychiatry*. 2016;29:32–8.

46. Smoller JW, Acierno JS, Jr., Rosenbaum JF, *et al*. Targeted genome screen of panic disorder and anxiety disorder proneness using homology to murine QTL regions. *Am J Med Genet*. 2001;105:195–206.

47. Smoller JW, Gallagher PJ, Duncan LE, *et al*. The human ortholog of acid-sensing ion channel gene ASIC1a is associated with panic disorder and amygdala structure and function. *Biol Psychiatry*. 2014;76:902–10.

48. Cittaro D, Lampis V, Luchetti A, *et al*. Histone Modifications in a mouse model of early adversities and panic disorder: role for Asic1 and neurodevelopmental genes. *Sci Rep*. 2016;6:25131.

49. Schuebel K, Gitik M, Domschke K, Goldman D. Making sense of epigenetics. *Int J Neuropsychopharmacol*. 2016;19: pii: pyw058.

50. Domschke K, Tidow N, Kuithan H, *et al*. Monoamine oxidase A gene DNA hypomethylation – a risk factor for panic disorder? *Int J Neuropsychopharmacol*. 2012;15:1217–28.

51. Ziegler C, Richter J, Mahr M, *et al*. MAOA gene hypomethylation in panic disorder-reversibility of an epigenetic risk pattern by psychotherapy. *Transl Psychiatry*. 2016;6:e773.

52. Roberts S, Lester KJ, Hudson JL, *et al*. Serotonin transporter [corrected] methylation and response to cognitive behaviour therapy in children with anxiety disorders. *Transl Psychiatry*. 2014;4:e444.

53. Gottschalk MG, Domschke K. Oxytocin and anxiety disorders. *Curr Top Behav Neurosci*. 2018;35:467–98.

54. Ziegler C, Dannlowski U, Brauer D, *et al*. Oxytocin receptor gene methylation: converging multilevel evidence for a role in social anxiety. *Neuropsychopharmacology*. 2015;40:1528–38.

55. Schartner C, Ziegler C, Schiele MA, *et al*. CRHR1 promoter hypomethylation: an epigenetic readout of panic disorder? *Eur Neuropsychopharmacol*. 2017;27:360–71.

56. Smoller JW. Disorders and borders: psychiatric genetics and nosology. *Am J Med Genet B Neuropsychiatr Genet*. 2013;162B:559–78.

57. Hettema JM, Prescott CA, Myers JM, Neale MC, Kendler KS. The structure of genetic and environmental risk factors for anxiety disorders in men and women. *Arch Gen Psychiatry*. 2005;62:182–9.

58. Loken EK, Hettema JM, Aggen SH, Kendler KS. The structure of genetic and environmental risk factors for fears and phobias. *Psychol Med*. 2014;44:2375–84.

59. Smith DJ, Escott-Price V, Davies G, *et al*. Genome-wide analysis of over 106 000 individuals identifies 9 neuroticism-associated loci. *Mol Psychiatry*. 2016;21:749–57.

60. Okbay A, Baselmans BM, De Neve JE, *et al*. Genetic variants associated with subjective well-being, depressive symptoms, and neuroticism identified through genome-wide analyses. *Nat Genet*. 2016;48:624–33.

61. Davies MN, Verdi S, Burri A, *et al*. Generalised anxiety disorder—a twin study of genetic architecture, genome-wide association and differential gene expression. *PLoS One*. 2015;10:e0134865.

62. Fullerton J, Cubin M, Tiwari H, *et al*. Linkage analysis of extremely discordant and concordant sibling pairs identifies quantitative-trait loci that influence variation in the human personality trait neuroticism. *Am J Hum Genet*. 2003;72:879–90.

63. Yalcin B, Willis-Owen SA, Fullerton J, *et al*. Genetic dissection of a behavioral quantitative trait locus shows that Rgs2 modulates anxiety in mice. *Nat Genet*. 2004;36:1197–202.

64. Hohoff C, Weber H, Richter J, *et al*. RGS2 ggenetic variation: association analysis with panic disorder and dimensional as well as intermediate phenotypes of anxiety. *Am J Med Genet B Neuropsychiatr Genet*. 2015;168B:211–22.

65. Koenen KC, Amstadter AB, Ruggiero KJ, *et al*. RGS2 and generalized anxiety disorder in an epidemiologic sample of hurricane-exposed adults. *Depress Anxiety*. 2009;26:309–15.

66. Deckert J, Weber H, Villmann C, *et al*. GLRB allelic variation associated with agoraphobic cognitions, increased startle response and fear network activation: a potential neurogenetic pathway to panic disorder. *Mol Psychiatry*. 2017;22:1431–9.

67. Dunn EC, Sofer T, Gallo LC, *et al*. Genome-wide association study of generalized anxiety symptoms in the Hispanic Community Health Study/Study of Latinos. *Am J Med Genet B Neuropsychiatr Genet*. 2017;174:132–43.

68. Walter S, Glymour MM, Koenen K, *et al*. Performance of polygenic scores for predicting phobic anxiety. *PLoS One*. 2013;8:e80326.

69. Trzaskowski M, Eley TC, Davis OS, *et al*. First genome-wide association study on anxiety-related behaviours in childhood. *PLoS One*. 2013;8:e58676.

70. Service SK, Verweij KJ, Lahti J, *et al*. A genome-wide meta-analysis of association studies of Cloninger's Temperament Scales. *Transl Psychiatry*. 2012;2:e116.

71. Drabant EM, Ramel W, Edge MD, *et al*. Neural mechanisms underlying 5-HTTLPR-related sensitivity to acute stress. *Am J Psychiatry*. 2012;169:397–405.

72. Klumpers F, Kroes MC, Heitland I, *et al*. Dorsomedial prefrontal cortex mediates the impact of serotonin transporter linked polymorphic region genotype on anticipatory threat reactions. *Biol Psychiatry*. 2015;78:582–9.

73. Dannlowski U, Konrad C, Kugel H, *et al*. Emotion specific modulation of automatic amygdala responses by 5-HTTLPR genotype. *Neuroimage*. 2010;53:893–8.

74. Ma Y, Li B, Wang C, Zhang W, Rao Y, Han S. Allelic variation in *5-HTTLPR* and the effects of citalopram on the emotional neural network. *Br J Psychiatry*. 2015;206:385–92.

75. Alexander N, Wankerl M, Hennig J, *et al*. DNA methylation profiles within the serotonin transporter gene moderate the association of 5-HTTLPR and cortisol stress reactivity. *Transl Psychiatry*. 2014;4:e443.

76. Domschke K, Baune BT, Havlik L, *et al*. Catechol-O-methyltransferase gene variation: impact on amygdala response to aversive stimuli. *Neuroimage*. 2012;60:2222–9.

77. Qiu A, Tuan TA, Ong ML, *et al*. COMT haplotypes modulate associations of antenatal maternal anxiety and neonatal cortical morphology. *Am J Psychiatry*. 2015;172:163–72.

78. Zwanzger P, Domschke K, Bradwejn J. Neuronal network of panic disorder: the role of the neuropeptide cholecystokinin. *Depress Anxiety*. 2012;29:762–74.

79. Ruland T, Domschke K, Schutte V, *et al*. Neuropeptide S receptor gene variation modulates anterior cingulate cortex Glx levels during CCK-4 induced panic. *Eur Neuropsychopharmacol*. 2015;25:1677–82.

80. Dannlowski U, Kugel H, Franke F, *et al*. Neuropeptide-S (NPS) receptor genotype modulates basolateral amygdala responsiveness to aversive stimuli. *Neuropsychopharmacology*. 2011;36:1879–85.

81. Beste C, Konrad C, Uhlmann C, Arolt V, Zwanzger P, Domschke K. Neuropeptide S receptor (*NPSR1*) gene variation modulates response inhibition and error monitoring. *Neuroimage*. 2013;71:1–9.

82. Neufang S, Geiger MJ, Homola GA, *et al*. Modulation of prefrontal functioning in attention systems by *NPSR1* gene variation. *Neuroimage*. 2015;114:199–206.

83. Domschke K, Akhrif A, Romanos M, *et al*. Neuropeptide S receptor gene variation differentially modulates fronto-limbic effective connectivity in childhood and adolescence. *Cereb Cortex*. 2017;27:554–66.

84. Klauke B, Deckert J, Zwanzger P, *et al*. Neuropeptide S receptor gene (NPSR) and life events: G x E effects on anxiety sensitivity and its subdimensions. *World J Biol Psychiatry*. 2014;15:17–25.

85. Ionescu IA, Dine J, Yen YC, *et al*. Intranasally administered neuropeptide S (NPS) exerts anxiolytic effects following internalization into NPS receptor-expressing neurons. *Neuropsychopharmacology*. 2012;37:1323–37.

86. Notzon S, Domschke K, Holitschke K, *et al*. Attachment style and oxytocin receptor gene variation interact in influencing social anxiety. *World J Biol Psychiatry*. 2016;17:76–83.

87. Dannlowski U, Kugel H, Grotegerd D, *et al*. Disadvantage of social sensitivity: interaction of oxytocin receptor genotype and child maltreatment on brain structure. *Biol Psychiatry*. 2016;80:398–405.

88. Keers R, Coleman JR, Lester KJ, *et al*. A genome-wide test of the differential susceptibility hypothesis reveals a genetic predictor of differential response to psychological treatments for child anxiety disorders. *Psychother Psychosom*. 2016;85:146–58.

89. Belsky J, Jonassaint C, Pluess M, Stanton M, Brummett B, Williams R. Vulnerability genes or plasticity genes? *Mol Psychiatry*. 2009;14:746–54.

# 90

# Neuroimaging of anxiety disorders

*Gregor Leicht and Christoph Mulert*

## Introduction

The development of neuroimaging techniques, such as functional magnetic resonance imaging (fMRI), has enabled neuroimaging researchers to identify structural and functional patterns in the brain underlying mental disorders. Thus, neuroimaging has helped to shed light on the neurobiological basis of anxiety and the pathophysiological mechanisms in anxiety disorders [1]. A large body of research has been conducted on experimentally induced anxiety in healthy individuals. Fear conditioning and fear generalization paradigms serve as models for the development and maintenance of pathological anxiety and for the maladaptive overgeneralization of fear [2, 3]. Studies investigating pharmacologically induced panic in healthy individuals tried to exemplarily resemble symptoms of patients with panic disorder (PD) [4]. Neuroimaging studies investigating patients with anxiety disorders have attempted to disentangle the neurobiological characteristics specific to each disorder [5]. Furthermore, more and more effort is focused on understanding the neural mechanisms of successful treatment of anxiety disorders [6].

The present review attempts to introduce a comprehensive overview of the current neuroimaging findings from research on anxiety disorders. In the following, we discuss evidence from neuroimaging studies on experimentally induced anxiety in healthy subjects, results of studies investigating neuronal patterns in patients with anxiety disorders, and finally findings from neuroimaging research on treatment effects in anxiety disorders.

## Neuroimaging of experimentally induced anxiety in healthy individuals

The functional neuroanatomy of anxiety in healthy humans has been investigated using experimentally induced anxiety. Such studies considerably enhanced the knowledge on pathophysiological aspects of anxiety disorders and offer the possibility to develop new treatment strategies. Mainly two different approaches of anxiety induction in healthy subjects have been applied in the recent past: fear conditioning paradigms and pharmacologically or respiratory-induced panic. In classical fear conditioning studies, a previously neutral stimulus becomes 'conditioned' after repeatedly pairing it with an aversive stimulus which elicits an autonomic fear response. After several paired presentations, the previously neutral stimulus elicits the autonomic fear response by itself [7]. For instance, this was done by conditioning neutral faces with an unpleasantly loud tone [3]. Thus, conditioned neutral faces elicited brain activity in a 'fear network' comprising the anterior cingulate cortex (ACC), the anterior insula, and the amygdala. Activity within this network evoked by aversive conditioned stimuli has repeatedly been shown in several fear conditioning studies [8, 9]. Moreover, this 'fear network' is also known to be active during symptom provocation in patients with anxiety disorders.

The idea of fear conditioning in healthy subjects has recently been used in neuroimaging studies investigating the neurobiological mechanisms involved in fear generalization. Healthy organisms tend to generalize conditioned fear responses to a certain stimulus and transfer it to perceptually close events in order to adapt behavioural responses to complex real-world situations by means of fear learning [10]. A maladaptive overgeneralization of fear is considered as a core pathophysiological mechanism of anxiety disorders [11, 12]. A first fMRI study investigating neurobehavioural mechanisms of human fear generalization revealed brain activity within regions also involved in the acquisition of conditioned fear in response to stimuli resembling an aversive conditioned stimulus. Activity within this network comprising the insula, caudate, thalamus, and ACC increased with growing similarity of the probe stimulus to the aversive conditioned stimulus, whereas the ventromedial prefrontal cortex (PFC) showed increased activity in response to a stimulus resembling a non-conditioned stimulus [13]. These results were replicated by studies presented in [2] and [14]. Additionally, Lissek *et al.* showed an increase in the involvement of the hippocampus and its connectivity to the ventromedial PFC with increasing similarity of the stimulus to a cue representing safety (in contrast to the danger-conditioned cue). The functional connectivity between the hippocampus and the amygdala, as well as the insula, increased in response to stimuli more and more resembling the danger-conditioned cue [14] . On basis of these findings, a fear generalization model has been proposed, suggesting that sensory information on stimuli resembling danger-conditioned cues is directly forwarded from the thalamus to the amygdala, bypassing the sensory cortex. Thus, conditioned fear is rapidly expressed via connections between the amygdala and, for example, the insula. Furthermore and according to this model, the hippocampus is suggested to contribute processes of pattern completion in case of presentation of stimuli resembling danger-conditioned cues, which initiates the conditioned fear response. On the other hand, in case of pattern separation processes in the hippocampus due to presentation of a cue not resembling the danger-conditioned cue, the ventromedial PFC is activated and downregulates the amygdala [15]. However, in view of the results of their recently published fMRI study, Onat et al. suggest that fear generalization is not only passively dependent from the perceptual similarity of a stimulus to a danger-conditioned cue, but also a mechanism which enables the human brain to actively transfer the threat classification to perceptually similar stimuli, using additional variables besides perceptual similarity [16].

In order to expand the understanding of neurobiological mechanisms of psychotherapeutic interventions in the treatment of anxiety disorders, fear conditioning paradigms also were used to investigate processes of fear extinction in neuroimaging studies [8]. Therefore, fear extinction has experimentally been modelled by repeatedly presenting a previously neutral, but aversive, conditioned stimulus without the aversive stimulus. Thus, the conditioned fear response can gradually be eliminated. There is evidence for activation in the ventromedial PFC and the hippocampus during fear extinction that might reflect a regulating inhibition effect on the amygdalar fear reaction [17]. Fear conditioning is differentiated from extinction learning by an anti-correlated dynamic competition between the large-scale functional networks underlying conditioning (amygdala-thalamo-cortical network) and extinction (hippocampal-prefrontal network) [18]. Moreover, a contribution of the cerebellar vermis to the extinction of conditioned fear has been shown [19]. Eckstein et al. recently found that oxytocin facilitates the extinction of conditioned fear by increasing PFC activity and inhibition of amygdalar responses during extinction [20].

An experimental model of the relapse of anxiety symptoms after successful therapeutic intervention in anxiety disorders is provided by a number of studies using return of fear experiments. For this purpose, the aversive event is re-presented after extinction [21]. Return of fear processes critically involve brain structures within the hippocampus and the ventromedial PFC [22]. The return of fear could be prevented experimentally by administration of the dopamine precursor l-3,4-dihydroxyphenylalanine (l-DOPA) [23], intake of the β-blocker propranolol [24], or REM sleep [25], which, in all cases, was accompanied by alterations of activity in return of fear-related brain regions.

The experimental induction of panic attacks with panicogenic substances in healthy subjects is another approach of modelling human anxiety. Different substances have been used to elicit panic symptoms in healthy individuals. For instance, the respiratory induction of panic symptoms has been conducted using lactate or carbon dioxide administration simulating life-threatening hypoxia. Pharmacological approaches involved noradrenergic (for example, yohimbine) and serotonergic (for example, meta-chlorophenylpiperazine) panic induction strategies. However, the most commonly used panicogenic agent is the synthetic neuropeptide cholecystokinin-tetrapeptide (CCK-4), a synthetic analogue of the endogenous neuropeptide cholecystokinin. It is considered as an ideal, safe, and valid experimental model of panic, serving as a useful approach to study the pathophysiology and neurobiology of PD [26]. CCK-4 induces symptoms closely resembling spontaneously occurring panic attacks in patients with PD [27]. Additionally, antipanic pharmacological treatment like imipramine reduces CCK-4-induced panic symptoms [28]. To this day, several neuroimaging studies have used the CCK-4 panic model in healthy participants in order to characterize brain regions which might be involved in the generation of panic attacks. The first studies investigating the functional neuroanatomy of CCK-4-induced panic in healthy participants using positron emission tomography (PET) showed an increase in cerebral blood flow (CBF) in the ACC, the claustrum-insular-amygdala region, and the cerebellar vermis [29, 30]. These results were confirmed by a first fMRI study contrasting brain activity induced by CCK-4 vs placebo administration [31]. However, the authors did not report amygdala activation elicited by CCK-4. In contrast, Eser et al. showed significantly stronger amygdala activation after CCK-4, in comparison to placebo administration, and five out of 11 healthy subjects with high amygdala activity reported more pronounced fear symptoms, in contrast to subjects with low amygdala activity. According to the authors' discussion, these findings indicate that the extent of amygdala activation might modulate the experience of CCK-4-induced fear, emphasizing the role of this structure in fear and anxiety. Moreover, CCK-4, in comparison to placebo, elicited large responses in several other brain regions, for example, the ventral ACC. In contrast, anticipatory anxiety in expectance of CCK-4 administration led to increased activity in the dorsal part of the ACC. Eser et al. interpreted this differential activation of the ACC as a correlate of a diverse functional neuroanatomy between cognitive anticipation and real autonomic and affective responses to CCK-4 in healthy subjects [32]. Using a data-driven fMRI analysis approach called tensorial probabilistic independent component analysis, Dieler et al. identified strong increases of activity in 12 different brain networks being active only after CCK-4, but not after placebo, administration or showing a significant increase in activity after CCK-4 administration, compared to placebo. The way of analysis in this study additionally allows to explore the time courses of each activated network and could enable future studies to quantify and visualize changes in CCK-4-activated neural networks, for example, elicited by pharmacological treatment of CCK-4 induced panic [33]. The CCK-4 model of PD was used not only to reveal the functional neuroanatomy of panic attacks, but also to investigate putative genomic risk factors for anxiety [34]. For instance, using magnetic resonance spectroscopy, Ruland et al. showed that the brain glutamate/glutamine levels in bilateral ACC during an acutely occurring CCK-4-induced panic attack is dependent on the neuropeptide S receptor gene variation [35]. Neuropeptide S is suggested to be involved in the pathogenesis of anxiety and PD. Accordingly, the CCK-4 panic challenge might be able to help to uncover genetic mechanisms influencing anxiety brain networks.

## Imaging neural correlates of anxiety disorders

Symptom provocation is the most commonly used procedure for the investigation of anxiety disorders in neuroimaging studies. For this purpose, anxiety-specific brain activity is induced by negative emotional stimuli such as, for example, angry faces [36], trauma-related visual or auditory stimuli [37], or pictures of phobia-related contents [38]. Most of the studies revealed increased activity of the 'fear network' comprising the amygdala, insula, ACC, and medial PFC [7] in patients with anxiety disorders, compared to healthy control groups, during symptom provocation. The appearance of anxiety symptoms seems to involve a pathologically hyperactivated amygdala under insufficient frontal top–down control [39].

The amygdala is considered to be involved in grading the biological significance of a stimulus [40]. Thus, it plays a crucial role in the processing of emotionally and socially relevant information [41]. The insula is another brain structure which is related to the processing of emotional contents [42] and interoceptive awareness [43]. Mechanisms of fear learning critically involve the medial PFC [44]. Thus, the crucial relevance of these regions for fear and anxiety may arise from its engagement in 'the processing of emotions as they relate to the self' [45].

Patients with generalized anxiety disorder (GAD) show a deficient ability of regulating their emotions. The results of the neuroimaging studies investigating this cognitive dysfunction in GAD patients suggest that the dysregulation of emotions is related to a malfunction of the medial PFC and alterations of its connectivity to the amygdala in terms of an insufficient top–down control [46]. This frontal control may be realized by means of theta oscillations, for example during emotion regulation [47]. Reduced mPFC activity was found in GAD patients during viewing emotional faces [48], suppressing worries [49], and reappraising emotional responses to negative pictures [50]. In a fear generalization experiment, the mPFC was not sufficiently recruited during fear inhibition in GAD patients [51]. Moreover, the connectivity between the mPFC and the amygdala has been shown to be altered in GAD patients [52].

The first functional neuroimaging studies investigating patients with PD have reported alterations of the blood flow in hippocampal brain regions [53, 54]. Results of fMRI studies investigating the processing of emotional stimuli suggest that hyperactivity of several different brain regions, including the amygdala, dorsolateral and medial PFC, ACC, insula, inferior frontal gyrus, orbitofrontal cortex, striatum, and hippocampus, are involved in the pathophysiology of PD [55, 56]. For instance, stronger activations were found in the bilateral ventral striatum and the left insula in PD patients during the anticipation of agoraphobia-specific pictures [57]. Increased anxiety sensitivity, which is known to be an important component of PD, has been linked to activity in regions encompassing the PFC, ACC, and insula during emotional processing [58]. A neural correlate of the altered interoceptive processing in patients with PD

might be represented by an increased functional connectivity between the somatosensory cortex and thalamus in the resting state brain [59]. The hypersensitivity of PD individuals to inhaled carbon dioxide goes along with alterations of the acid-sensing ion channel ASIC1a, and ASIC1a risk allele carriers showed increased amygdala volume, as well as task-evoked amygdala reactivity to fearful and angry faces [60]. Domschke *et al.* showed a reduction of effective connectivity between the middle frontal gyrus and both the amygdala and the insula, reflecting an impaired frontal top–down control of limbic structures in adolescent carriers of a variant in the neuropeptide S receptor gene which has been associated with PD [61]. Another imaging genetics study investigated the influence of the corticotropin-releasing hormone receptor gene *CRHR1* as a risk factor for PD on brain activity during fear conditioning. Risk allele carriers showed aberrant activity predominantly in bilateral prefrontal regions and the amygdala, implicating altered generalization of fear processes [62].

Post-traumatic stress disorder (PTSD) has been associated recurrently with amygdala hyperactivity [63, 64] and hypoactivity in the medial PFC [65] in functional neuroimaging studies. Moreover, a lack of negative connectivity between the amygdala and the subgenual ACC has been observed (Fig. 90.1) [66]. Among others, one established model of PTSD assumes that amygdala hyperactivity reflects permanently increased fear responses, whereas the observed hypoactivity in frontal regions might be a correlate of an aberrant ability of top–down regulation and fear extinction [67]. Moreover, a reduction of hippocampal activity has been observed in PTSD patients [68], which has been interpreted as a disturbed ability of the hippocampus to provide context information, especially with respect to the identification of safe contexts [69]. This exemplary conception is further strengthened by structural changes in several brain regions, including the hippocampus, amygdala, and medial PFC observed in PTSD patients [65, 70, 71]. Interestingly, some studies report increased activity in the dorsal part of the ACC and dorsolateral PFC which might be the correlate of an increased recruitment of top–down attentional control [72]. Disturbances of fear generalization processes in military veterans with PTSD have been linked to an increase of amygdala connectivity with sensory brain regions and the thalamus and a decrease of connectivity between the amygdala and the ventromedial PFC [73]. Spielberg *et al.* reported an association between PTSD re-experiencing symptoms

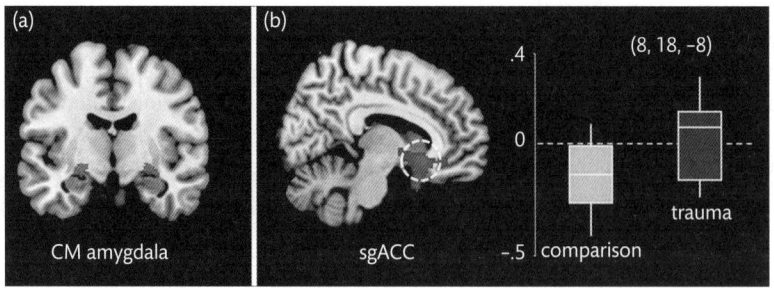

**Fig. 90.1** (see Colour Plate section) Absent negative connectivity between the centromedial (CM) amygdala and the subgenual anterior cingulate cortex (sgACC) in trauma-exposed youth. (a) Anatomically defined seed region of interest for the connectivity analysis within bilateral CM amygdala. (b) Tukey's boxplots depicting connectivity values by group centred on the sgACC peak. The middle line indicates the median, the vertical line the range, and the limits of the box represent the upper and lower quartiles.

Reproduced from *Soc Cogn Affect Neurosci.*, 10(11), Thomason ME, Marusak HA, Tocco MA, *et al.*, Altered amygdala connectivity in urban youth exposed to trauma, pp. 1460-8, Copyright (2015), with permission from Oxford University Press.

and a weakened connectivity in a hippocampus–PFC network involved in providing contextual information [74]. The fact that exposure to a traumatic event does not necessarily lead to the development of PTSD raises the question of whether the structural and functional abnormalities predispose to or follow the development of PTSD [75]. For instance, a smaller hippocampal volume has been shown to predict pathological vulnerability to psychological trauma [76]. On the other hand, hippocampal grey matter loss is predicted by the duration of PTSD [77].

Neuroimaging studies investigating the neural alterations underlying specific phobia mainly focused on the animal subtype, particularly spider phobia subjects. These studies consistently reported hyperactivation in fear-relevant structures such as the amygdala, dorsal ACC, PFC, thalamus, and insula [5]. For instance, spider-phobic subjects showed stronger responses of both amygdalae during exposure to pictures of spiders. The magnitude of amygdala responses was positively correlated with the intensity of disorder-related vigilance for threat [78]. At the same time, there are reports on reduced activity in both the dorsolateral PFC and the lateral orbitofrontal cortex during conscious perception of phobia-related pictures. Taken together, these results have been suggested to reflect an increased activation of the fear circuit, accompanied by an insufficient top–down control in response to phobia-related stimuli [79]. The exaggeration of the expectancy to be faced with the phobic threat was shown to be related to decreased activity in the lateral PFC, precuneus, and visual cortex, reflecting irrationality in encounter expectancies and deficiencies in cognitive control and contextual integration [80]. The overestimation of the relationship between fear-relevant stimuli and aversive consequences, the so-called covariation bias, was found to be predicted by connectivity between the paracentral lobule (PCL) and sensory cortices, whereas reduced covariation bias was predicted by connectivity between the PCL and the PFC [81]. In contrast to the phasic fear responses to threatening stimuli associated with increased amygdala activity, sustained anxiety in phobic patients has been related to increased activity in the bed nucleus of the stria terminalis (BNST) and the ACC, as well as to enhanced connectivity between the BNST and the amygdala [82]. Increased activity of the ACC has also been linked to anticipatory anxiety in phobia patients [83]. Moreover, structural brain abnormalities of fear-related brain regions in patients with specific phobia have also been reported [84].

## Neuroimaging of treatment effects in anxiety disorders

Neuroimaging techniques offer the opportunity to monitor structural and functional neuronal changes as a result of psychotherapy in anxiety disorders or to predict the efficacy of psychotherapeutic interventions. For example, behavioural changes in patients with social anxiety disorder after mindfulness-based stress reduction (MBSR) therapy seem to be reflected by distinct patterns of neural activity [85]. Hölzel et al. demonstrated that GAD patients with higher amygdala activity in response to neutral faces than healthy participants showed a decrease in amygdala reactivity following 8 weeks of MBSR. Moreover, the activity in the ventrolateral PFC and the functional connectivity between the amygdala and PFC regions

increased after MBSR, in comparison to a stress management education active control group (Fig. 90.2) [86].

Cognitive behavioural therapy (CBT) is known to be an effective first-line intervention in the treatment of patients with PD. Neuroimaging studies have shown that neural activation patterns predict and moderate the therapeutic success of CBT in PD [87]. For instance, CBT in patients with PD led to a significant greater reduction in bilateral amygdala activation during the processing of agoraphobia-related pictures than treatment with selective serotonin reuptake inhibitors (SSRIs) [88]. Another sample of PD patients revealed normalization of PFC hypoactivation and hyperactivation of the amygdala and hippocampus after CBT, when panic-related symptoms had improved [89]. In a fear conditioning study, patients with PD showed a CBT-induced reduction of activity in the left inferior frontal gyrus (IFG) during the conditioned response and an increase of connectivity between the IFG and regions of the 'fear network' such as the amygdalae, insulae, and ACC after CBT. The change of neuronal patterns was correlated with a reduction in agoraphobic symptoms [90]. An increase of activation of the hippocampus and a decrease of its connectivity with the IFG have also been reported as an effect of successful CBT in PD [91]. Moreover, neuroimaging data were able to predict the treatment response to CBT in PD with high accuracy on single-patient level [92]. For instance, improved response to brief CBT was predicted by increased pretreatment activation in bilateral insulae and the left dorsolateral PFC during threat processing [93]. Lueken et al. showed an association between treatment response to CBT and increased right hippocampal activation, as well as inhibitory functional coupling between the ACC and the amygdala [94].

Studies investigating the functional neuroimaging correlates of PTSD treatment have shown a correlation between improvement of PTSD symptoms after trauma therapy and alterations of activity in different brain regions such as the amygdala, insula, hippocampus, ACC, and dorsolateral PFC [95–98]. Treatment with eye movement desensitization and reprocessing (EMDR) in PTSD patient has been shown to modulate activity in limbic and prefrontal regions [99, 100] and to increase the amygdala volume [101], along with significant improvements in PTSD symptoms. The functional connectivity within the fear extinction network seems to be modified by PTSD treatment with repeated exposure to the traumatic memory, which emphasizes the relationship between human fear extinction and trauma memories [102]. Studies applying neuroimaging measures in order to predict trauma therapy responses in PTSD patients have revealed relationships between the degree of symptom reduction and the pretreatment activity of bilateral amygdalae [103], the cortical thickness in the subgenual ACC [104], or the hippocampal volume [105].

There is strong evidence for high efficacy of exposure therapy during CBT in the treatment of specific phobia patients [106]. The neural mechanisms underlying the reduction of anxiety symptoms after CBT have been extensively investigated in recent neuroimaging studies showing that processes of fear extinction and the corresponding mechanisms in the brain might play a crucial role. Different studies demonstrated a decrease in amygdala activity and normalization of insular and ACC activity after successful exposure therapy in specific phobia patients [107]. Reductions in amygdala responsiveness have been associated with self-reported symptom improvement [108]. An improvement in the effectiveness

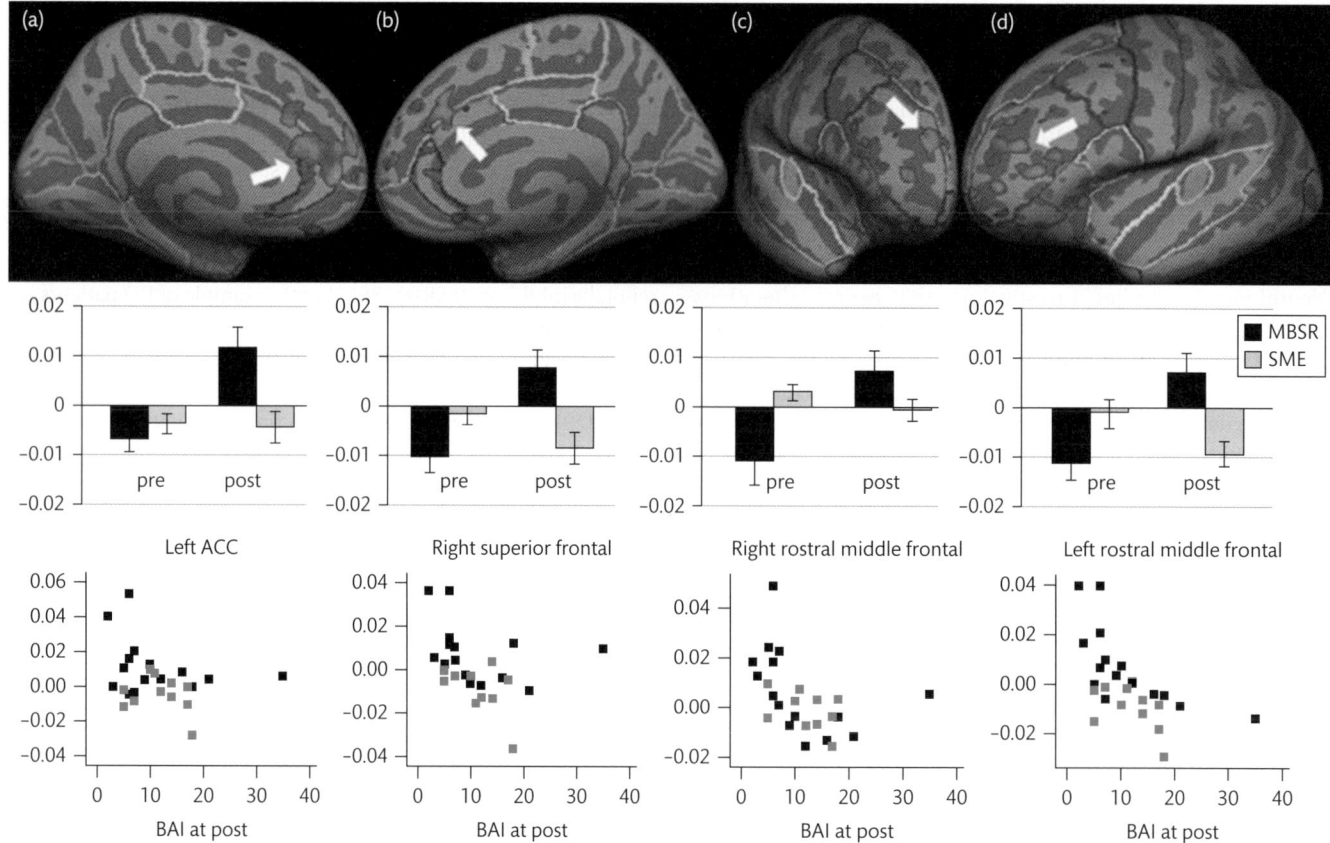

**Fig. 90.2** (see Colour Plate section) Functional connectivity between the seed region in the right amygdala and several regions in the frontal cortex increased from pre- to post-intervention with mindfulness-based stress reduction (MBSR) therapy in patients with generalized anxiety disorder, but not in control subjects who underwent a stress management education (SME) class. Top row: anatomical location displayed on an inflated surface. Middle row: regression coefficients extracted from the clusters from MBSR (black) and SME (blue) participants at pre- and post-interventions. Bottom row: scatter plots for correlations between pre- to post-increase in connectivity (y-axis) in the frontal cortex region and Beck Anxiety Inventory (BAI; x-axis) for MBSR and SME participants at post-intervention. ACC, anterior cingulate cortex.

of exposure therapy via faster fear extinction processes has been reported for the application of D-cycloserine, a partial *N*-methyl-D-aspartate (NMDA) receptor agonist, in combination with exposure-based therapy [109]. This might be due to enhancement of activation in regions involved in cognitive control and interoceptive integration, such as the PFC, ACC, and insula, during symptom provocation [110]. A novel psychotherapeutic approach is provided by applying neurofeedback techniques during training of anxiety regulation by cognitive reappraisal. fMRI neurofeedback has recently been shown to enable spider-phobic patients to downregulate insula activation levels by cognitive reappraisal strategies, accompanied by lower anxiety levels. Feedback had been provided, based on activation in the left dorsolateral PFC and the right insula. The achieved changes in insula activation levels seemed to be based on a learning mechanism and predicted long-term anxiety reduction [111].

Psychopharmacological treatments of anxiety disorders have also been shown to alter abnormal neural processes that were found to be key characteristics of fear and anxiety in neuroimaging studies. For instance, SSRI treatment attenuated activity in prefrontal regions, the striatum, the insula, and paralimbic regions during listening to worry sentences in GAD [112], reduced amygdala and enhanced ventral medial PFC reactivity to emotional faces in social phobia patients (113), and increased activation in the dorsolateral PFC during emotion regulation (114), as well as increased mean hippocampal volume in PTSD patients (115). The anxiolytic effect of benzodiazepines, such as alprazolam, seems to involve a reduction of rostral ACC activity and changes of its connectivity with the dorsolateral PFC and the amygdala, as revealed by means of CCK-4 panic challenge in healthy subjects (Fig. 90.3) [4].

The use of the neuropeptide oxytocin has been suggested as a promising approach for the facilitation of psychotherapy effects in anxiety disorders. Recent neuroimaging studies have extensively illustrated its stress-reducing, anxiolytic, and prosocial properties [116]. For instance, oxytocin attenuated the exaggerated amygdala activity [117] and enhanced the functional connectivity of the amygdala with the insula, medial PFC, and ACC [118, 119] in pathological social anxiety. Furthermore, intranasal application of oxytocin normalized the amygdala functional connectivity to the dorsal ACC and the ventromedial PFC in PTSD patients, indicating suppression of the anxiety and fear expression of the amygdala via increased top–down control of the ventromedial PFC or decreased salience processing of the dorsal ACC [120]. In summary, recent evidence from neuroimaging findings suggests that oxytocin could

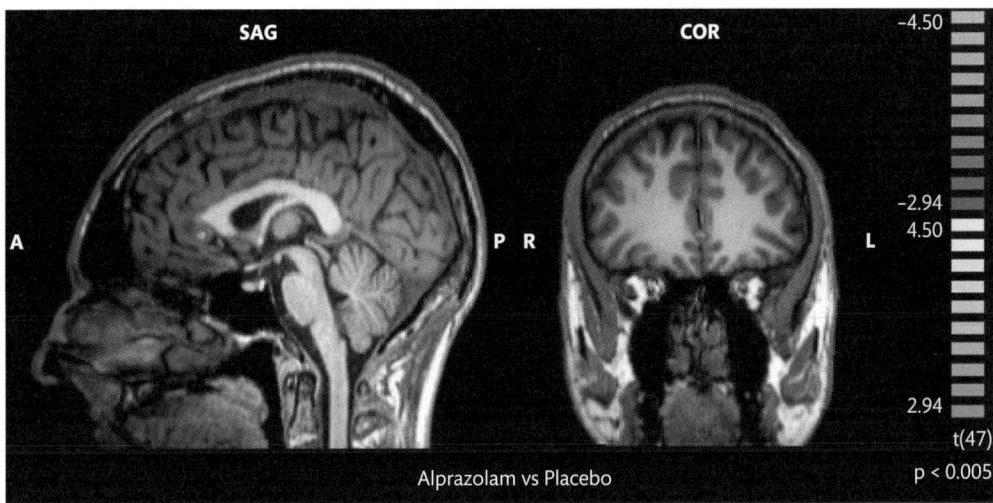

**Fig. 90.3** (see Colour Plate section) Contrasts of functional magnetic resonance imaging responses compared between different treatment conditions. Group analysis ($n$ = 16) of the blood oxygen level-dependent response (functional magnetic resonance imaging) to challenge with cholecystokinin-tetrapeptide after alprazolam vs placebo pretreatment (Talairach co-ordinates: $x$ = -1, $y$ = 30). Activation of the rostral anterior cingulate cortex was reduced after pretreatment with alprazolam, but not after pretreatment with placebo. SAG, sagittal; COR, coronary; A, anterior; P, posterior; L, left; R, right.

Reproduced from *Biol Psychiatry*, 73(4), Leicht G, Mulert C, Eser D, *et al.*, Benzodiazepines Counteract Rostral Anterior Cingulate Cortex Activation Induced by Cholecystokinin-Tetrapeptide in Humans, pp. 337–344, Copyright (2013), with permission from Society of Biological Psychiatry.

potentially enhance treatment response in PTSD by modulating the fear network.

These lines of research suggest that neuroimaging techniques could potentially identify the mode of action of anxiety treatment drugs and therefore facilitate the development of new pharmacological treatment options for anxiety disorders. Furthermore, there is evidence that pretreatment patterns of functional neuronal activity might predict the treatment response to pharmacological interventions. For instance, the treatment response to venlafaxine was predicted by greater pretreatment ACC activity and lesser reactivity in the amygdala in GAD patients [121, 122].

## Conclusions

In the present article, we have provided an overview of the results of current neuroimaging studies in fear and anxiety. Human models of anxiety in healthy individuals serve as an experimental tool for the investigation of neural processes underlying the pathophysiology of clinically relevant anxiety disorders, for example, with respect to the expression of fear during symptom provocation or fear generalization. Moreover, neurobiological aspects of therapeutic interventions have been uncovered in fear extinction studies. Studies in human models of anxiety, as well as investigations in anxiety disorder patients, consistently demonstrated the pathophysiological role of a 'fear network' comprising the amygdala, insula, medial PFC, and ACC. Symptoms of anxiety are considered to be due to a pathologically hyperactivated amygdala and insufficient top–down regulation by frontal brain regions. Moreover, a disturbed function of the hippocampus with respect to processes of pattern completion, pattern separation, and integration of contextual information seems to crucially contribute to the development and maintenance of anxiety disorders.

Effective psychotherapeutic and pharmacological treatments of anxiety occurring along with normalization in patients' perception and behaviour seem to specifically alter patterns of brain activation in these structures. Neuroimaging techniques might enable therapists and researchers to continuously monitor treatment success and thus may contribute to the refinement of existing approaches and the development of more effective therapeutic options. Furthermore, neuroimaging parameters can help to predict the success of certain treatment strategies. Thus, clinicians might prospectively be able to assign the most promising treatment option to individual patients.

## REFERENCES

1. Holzschneider K, Mulert C. Neuroimaging in anxiety disorders. *Dialogues Clin Neurosci*. 2011;13:453–61.
2. Greenberg T, Carlson JM, Cha J, Hajcak G, Mujica-Parodi LR. Neural reactivity tracks fear generalization gradients. *Biol Psychol*. 2013;92:2–8.
3. Buchel C, Morris J, Dolan RJ, Friston KJ. Brain systems mediating aversive conditioning: an event-related fMRI study. *Neuron*. 1998;20:947–57.
4. Leicht G, Mulert C, Eser D, *et al*. Benzodiazepines counteract rostral anterior cingulate cortex activation induced by cholecystokinin-tetrapeptide in humans. *Biol Psychiatry*. 2013;73:337–44.
5. Etkin A, Wager TD. Functional neuroimaging of anxiety: a meta-analysis of emotional processing in PTSD, social anxiety disorder, and specific phobia. *Am J Psychiatry*. 2007;164:1476–88.
6. Lueken U, Hahn T. Functional neuroimaging of psychotherapeutic processes in anxiety and depression: from mechanisms to predictions. *Curr Opin Psychiatry*. 2016;29:25–31.
7. Buchel C, Dolan RJ. Classical fear conditioning in functional neuroimaging. *Curr Opin Neurobiol*. 2000;10:219–23.

8. Sehlmeyer C, Schoning S, Zwitserlood P, *et al.* Human fear conditioning and extinction in neuroimaging: a systematic review. *PLoS One.* 2009;4:e5865.

9. Fullana MA, Harrison BJ, Soriano-Mas C, *et al.* Neural signatures of human fear conditioning: an updated and extended meta-analysis of fMRI studies. *Mol Psychiatry.* 2016;21:500–8.

10. Dymond S, Dunsmoor JE, Vervliet B, Roche B, Hermans D. Fear Generalization in Humans: Systematic Review and Implications for Anxiety Disorder Research. *Behav Ther.* 2015;46:561–82.

11. Lissek S, Kaczkurkin AN, Rabin S, Geraci M, Pine DS, Grillon C. Generalized anxiety disorder is associated with overgeneralization of classically conditioned fear. *Biol Psychiatry.* 2014;75:909–15.

12. Beckers T, Krypotos AM, Boddez Y, Effting M, Kindt M. What's wrong with fear conditioning? *Biol Psychol.* 2013;92:90–6.

13. Dunsmoor JE, Prince SE, Murty VP, Kragel PA, LaBar KS. Neurobehavioral mechanisms of human fear generalization. *Neuroimage.* 2011;55:1878–88.

14. Lissek S, Bradford DE, Alvarez RP, *et al.* Neural substrates of classically conditioned fear-generalization in humans: a parametric fMRI study. *Soc Cogn Affect Neurosci.* 2014;9:1134–42.

15. Lissek S. Toward an account of clinical anxiety predicated on basic, neurally mapped mechanisms of Pavlovian fear-learning: the case for conditioned overgeneralization. *Depress Anxiety.* 2012;29:257–63.

16. Onat S, Buchel C. The neuronal basis of fear generalization in humans. *Nat Neurosci.* 2015;18:1811–18.

17. Milad MR, Wright CI, Orr SP, Pitman RK, Quirk GJ, Rauch SL. Recall of fear extinction in humans activates the ventromedial prefrontal cortex and hippocampus in concert. *Biol Psychiatry.* 2007;62:446–54.

18. Marstaller L, Burianova H, Reutens DC. Dynamic competition between large-scale functional networks differentiates fear conditioning and extinction in humans. *Neuroimage.* 2016;134:314–19.

19. Utz A, Thurling M, Ernst TM, *et al.* Cerebellar vermis contributes to the extinction of conditioned fear. *Neurosci Lett.* 2015;604:173–7.

20. Eckstein M, Becker B, Scheele D, *et al.* Oxytocin facilitates the extinction of conditioned fear in humans. *Biol Psychiatry.* 2015;78:194–202.

21. Lonsdorf TB, Haaker J, Kalisch R. Long-term expression of human contextual fear and extinction memories involves amygdala, hippocampus and ventromedial prefrontal cortex: a reinstatement study in two independent samples. *Soc Cogn Affect Neurosci.* 2014;9:1973–83.

22. Scharfenort R, Lonsdorf TB. Neural correlates of and processes underlying generalized and differential return of fear. *Soc Cogn Affect Neurosci.* 2016;11:612–20.

23. Haaker J, Lonsdorf TB, Kalisch R. Effects of post-extinction l-DOPA administration on the spontaneous recovery and reinstatement of fear in a human fMRI study. *Eur Neuropsychopharmacol.* 2015;25:1544–55.

24. Kroes MC, Tona KD, den Ouden HE, Vogel S, van Wingen GA, Fernandez G. How Administration of the Beta-Blocker Propranolol Before Extinction can Prevent the Return of Fear. *Neuropsychopharmacology.* 2016;41:1569–78.

25. Menz MM, Rihm JS, Buchel C. REM Sleep Is Causal to Successful Consolidation of Dangerous and Safety Stimuli and Reduces Return of Fear after Extinction. *J Neurosci.* 2016;36:2148–60.

26. Eser D, Schule C, Baghai T, *et al.* Evaluation of the CCK-4 model as a challenge paradigm in a population of healthy volunteers within a proof-of-concept study. *Psychopharmacology (Berl).* 2007;192:479–87.

27. Bradwejn J, Koszycki D, Shriqui C. Enhanced sensitivity to cholecystokinin tetrapeptide in panic disorder. Clinical and behavioral findings. *Arch Gen Psychiatry.* 1991;48:603–10.

28. Bradwejn J, Koszycki D. Imipramine antagonism of the panicogenic effects of cholecystokinin tetrapeptide in panic disorder patients. *Am J Psychiatry.* 1994;151:261–3.

29. Benkelfat C, Bradwejn J, Meyer E, *et al.* Functional neuroanatomy of CCK4-induced anxiety in normal healthy volunteers. *Am J Psychiatry.* 1995;152:1180–4.

30. Javanmard M, Shlik J, Kennedy SH, Vaccarino FJ, Houle S, Bradwejn J. Neuroanatomic correlates of CCK-4-induced panic attacks in healthy humans: a comparison of two time points. *Biol Psychiatry.* 1999;45:872–82.

31. Schunck T, Erb G, Mathis A, *et al.* Functional magnetic resonance imaging characterization of CCK-4-induced panic attack and subsequent anticipatory anxiety. *Neuroimage.* 2006;31:1197–208.

32. Eser D, Leicht G, Lutz J, *et al.* Functional neuroanatomy of CCK-4-induced panic attacks in healthy volunteers. *Hum Brain Mapp.* 2009;30:511–22.

33. Dieler AC, Samann PG, Leicht G, *et al.* Independent component analysis applied to pharmacological magnetic resonance imaging (phMRI): new insights into the functional networks underlying panic attacks as induced by CCK-4. *Curr Pharm Des.* 2008;14:3492–507.

34. Eser D, Uhr M, Leicht G, *et al.* Glyoxalase-I mRNA expression and CCK-4 induced panic attacks. *J Psychiatr Res.* 2011;45:60–3.

35. Ruland T, Domschke K, Schutte V, *et al.* Neuropeptide S receptor gene variation modulates anterior cingulate cortex Glx levels during CCK-4 induced panic. *Eur Neuropsychopharmacol.* 2015;25:1677–82.

36. Klucken T, Kagerer S, Schweckendiek J, Tabbert K, Vaitl D, Stark R. Neural, electrodermal and behavioral response patterns in contingency aware and unaware subjects during a picture-picture conditioning paradigm. *Neuroscience.* 2009;158:721–31.

37. Bremner JD, Staib LH, Kaloupek D, Southwick SM, Soufer R, Charney DS. Neural correlates of exposure to traumatic pictures and sound in Vietnam combat veterans with and without posttraumatic stress disorder: a positron emission tomography study. *Biol Psychiatry.* 1999;45:806–16.

38. Schweckendiek J, Klucken T, Merz CJ, *et al.* Weaving the (neuronal) web: fear learning in spider phobia. *Neuroimage.* 2011;54:681–8.

39. MacNamara A, DiGangi J, Phan KL. Aberrant Spontaneous and Task-Dependent Functional Connections in the Anxious Brain. *Biol Psychiatry Cogn Neurosci Neuroimaging.* 2016;1:278–87.

40. Pessoa L, Adolphs R. Emotion processing and the amygdala: from a 'low road' to 'many roads' of evaluating biological significance. *Nat Rev Neurosci.* 2010;11:773–83.

41. Sabatinelli D, Fortune EE, Li Q, *et al.* Emotional perception: meta-analyses of face and natural scene processing. *Neuroimage.* 2011;54:2524–33.

42. Phan KL, Wager T, Taylor SF, Liberzon I. Functional neuroanatomy of emotion: a meta-analysis of emotion activation studies in PET and fMRI. *Neuroimage.* 2002;16:331–48.

43. Critchley HD, Wiens S, Rotshtein P, Ohman A, Dolan RJ. Neural systems supporting interoceptive awareness. *Nat Neurosci.* 2004;7:189–95.

44. Buchanan SL, Powell DA. Cingulate cortex: its role in Pavlovian conditioning. *J Comp Physiol Psychol.* 1982;96:755–74.

45. Paulus MP. The role of neuroimaging for the diagnosis and treatment of anxiety disorders. *Depress Anxiety.* 2008;25:348–56.

46. Mochcovitch MD, da Rocha Freire RC, Garcia RF, Nardi AE. A systematic review of fMRI studies in generalized anxiety

disorder: evaluating its neural and cognitive basis. *J Affect Disord.* 2014;167:336–42.

47. Ertl M, Hildebrandt M, Ourina K, Leicht G, Mulert C. Emotion regulation by cognitive reappraisal - the role of frontal theta oscillations. *Neuroimage.* 2013;81:412–21.

48. Palm ME, Elliott R, McKie S, Deakin JF, Anderson IM. Attenuated responses to emotional expressions in women with generalized anxiety disorder. *Psychol Med.* 2011;41:1009–18.

49. Andreescu C, Gross JJ, Lenze E, et al. Altered cerebral blood flow patterns associated with pathologic worry in the elderly. *Depress Anxiety.* 2011;28:202–9.

50. Ball TM, Ramsawh HJ, Campbell-Sills L, Paulus MP, Stein MB. Prefrontal dysfunction during emotion regulation in generalized anxiety and panic disorders. *Psychol Med.* 2013;43:1475–86.

51. Greenberg T, Carlson JM, Cha J, Hajcak G, Mujica-Parodi LR. Ventromedial prefrontal cortex reactivity is altered in generalized anxiety disorder during fear generalization. *Depress Anxiety.* 2013;30:242–50.

52. Etkin A, Prater KE, Hoeft F, Menon V, Schatzberg AF. Failure of anterior cingulate activation and connectivity with the amygdala during implicit regulation of emotional processing in generalized anxiety disorder. *Am J Psychiatry.* 2010;167:545–54.

53. Reiman EM, Raichle ME, Butler FK, Herscovitch P, Robins E. A focal brain abnormality in panic disorder, a severe form of anxiety. *Nature.* 1984;310:683–5.

54. Pannekoek JN, van der Werff SJ, Stein DJ, van der Wee NJ. Advances in the neuroimaging of panic disorder. *Hum Psychopharmacol.* 2013;28:608–11.

55. de Carvalho MR, Dias GP, Cosci F, et al. Current findings of fMRI in panic disorder: contributions for the fear neurocircuitry and CBT effects. *Expert Rev Neurother.* 2010;10:291–303.

56. Engel KR, Obst K, Bandelow B, et al. Functional MRI activation in response to panic-specific, non-panic aversive, and neutral pictures in patients with panic disorder and healthy controls. *Eur Arch Psychiatry Clin Neurosci.* 2016;266:557–66.

57. Wittmann A, Schlagenhauf F, Guhn A, et al. Anticipating agoraphobic situations: the neural correlates of panic disorder with agoraphobia. *Psychol Med.* 2014;44:2385–96.

58. Poletti S, Radaelli D, Cucchi M, et al. Neural correlates of anxiety sensitivity in panic disorder: A functional magnetic resonance imaging study. *Psychiatry Res.* 2015;233:95–101.

59. Cui H, Zhang J, Liu Y, et al. Differential alterations of resting-state functional connectivity in generalized anxiety disorder and panic disorder. *Hum Brain Mapp.* 2016;37:1459–73.

60. Smoller JW, Gallagher PJ, Duncan LE, et al. The human ortholog of acid-sensing ion channel gene ASIC1a is associated with panic disorder and amygdala structure and function. *Biol Psychiatry.* 2014;76:902–10.

61. Domschke K, Akhrif A, Romanos M, et al. Neuropeptide S Receptor Gene Variation Differentially Modulates Fronto-Limbic Effective Connectivity in Childhood and Adolescence. *Cereb Cortex.* 2017;27:554–66.

62. Weber H, Richter J, Straube B, et al. Allelic variation in CRHR1 predisposes to panic disorder: evidence for biased fear processing. *Mol Psychiatry.* 2016;21:813–22.

63. Shin LM, Orr SP, Carson MA, et al. Regional cerebral blood flow in the amygdala and medial prefrontal cortex during traumatic imagery in male and female Vietnam veterans with PTSD. *Arch Gen Psychiatry.* 2004;61:168–76.

64. Brohawn KH, Offringa R, Pfaff DL, Hughes KC, Shin LM. The neural correlates of emotional memory in posttraumatic stress disorder. *Biol Psychiatry.* 2010;68:1023–30.

65. Shin LM, Rauch SL, Pitman RK. Amygdala, medial prefrontal cortex, and hippocampal function in PTSD. *Ann N Y Acad Sci.* 2006;1071:67–79.

66. Thomason ME, Marusak HA, Tocco MA, Vila AM, McGarragle O, Rosenberg DR. Altered amygdala connectivity in urban youth exposed to trauma. *Soc Cogn Affect Neurosci.* 2015;10:1460–8.

67. Shin LM, Liberzon I. The neurocircuitry of fear, stress, and anxiety disorders. *Neuropsychopharmacology.* 2010;35:169–91.

68. Hayes JP, LaBar KS, McCarthy G, et al. Reduced hippocampal and amygdala activity predicts memory distortions for trauma reminders in combat-related PTSD. *J Psychiatr Res.* 2011;45:660–9.

69. Deckersbach T, Dougherty DD, Rauch SL. Functional imaging of mood and anxiety disorders. *J Neuroimaging.* 2006;16:1–10.

70. Wang Z, Neylan TC, Mueller SG, et al. Magnetic resonance imaging of hippocampal subfields in posttraumatic stress disorder. *Arch Gen Psychiatry.* 2010;67:296–303.

71. Pietrzak RH, Averill LA, Abdallah CG, et al. Amygdala-hippocampal volume and the phenotypic heterogeneity of posttraumatic stress disorder: a cross-sectional study. *JAMA Psychiatry.* 2015;72:396–8.

72. White SF, Costanzo ME, Blair JR, Roy MJ. PTSD symptom severity is associated with increased recruitment of top-down attentional control in a trauma-exposed sample. *Neuroimage Clin.* 2015;7:19–27.

73. Morey RA, Dunsmoor JE, Haswell CC, et al. Fear learning circuitry is biased toward generalization of fear associations in posttraumatic stress disorder. *Transl Psychiatry.* 2015;5:e700.

74. Spielberg JM, McGlinchey RE, Milberg WP, Salat DH. Brain network disturbance related to posttraumatic stress and traumatic brain injury in veterans. *Biol Psychiatry.* 2015;78:210–16.

75. Robinson BL, Shergill SS. Imaging in posttraumatic stress disorder. *Curr Opin Psychiatry.* 2011;24:29–33.

76. Gilbertson MW, Shenton ME, Ciszewski A, et al. Smaller hippocampal volume predicts pathologic vulnerability to psychological trauma. *Nat Neurosci.* 2002;5:1242–7.

77. Felmingham K, Williams LM, Whitford TJ, et al. Duration of posttraumatic stress disorder predicts hippocampal grey matter loss. *Neuroreport.* 2009;20:1402–6.

78. Lipka J, Miltner WH, Straube T. Vigilance for threat interacts with amygdala responses to subliminal threat cues in specific phobia. *Biol Psychiatry.* 2011;70:472–8.

79. Carlsson K, Petersson KM, Lundqvist D, Karlsson A, Ingvar M, Ohman A. Fear and the amygdala: manipulation of awareness generates differential cerebral responses to phobic and fear-relevant (but nonfeared) stimuli. *Emotion.* 2004;4:340–53.

80. Aue T, Hoeppli ME, Piguet C, Hofstetter C, Rieger SW, Vuilleumier P. Brain systems underlying encounter expectancy bias in spider phobia. *Cogn Affect Behav Neurosci.* 2015;15:335–48.

81. Wiemer J, Pauli P. Enhanced functional connectivity between sensorimotor and visual cortex predicts covariation bias in spider phobia. *Biol Psychol.* 2016;121:128–37.

82. Munsterkotter AL, Notzon S, Redlich R, et al. Spider or No Spider? Neural Correlates of Sustained and Phasic Fear in Spider Phobia. *Depress Anxiety.* 2015;32:656–63.

83. Straube T, Mentzel HJ, Miltner WH. Neural mechanisms of automatic and direct processing of phobogenic stimuli in specific phobia. *Biol Psychiatry.* 2006;59:162–70.

84. Hilbert K, Evens R, Maslowski NI, Wittchen HU, Lueken U. Neurostructural correlates of two subtypes of specific phobia: a voxel-based morphometry study. *Psychiatry Res.* 2015;231:168–75.

85. Goldin PR, Gross JJ. Effects of mindfulness-based stress reduction (MBSR) on emotion regulation in social anxiety disorder. *Emotion*. 2010;10:83–91.

86. Holzel BK, Hoge EA, Greve DN, *et al*. Neural mechanisms of symptom improvements in generalized anxiety disorder following mindfulness training. *Neuroimage Clin*. 2013;2:448–58.

87. Yang Y, Kircher T, Straube B. The neural correlates of cognitive behavioral therapy: recent progress in the investigation of patients with panic disorder. *Behav Res Ther*. 2014;62:88–96.

88. Liebscher C, Wittmann A, Gechter J, *et al*. Facing the fear - clinical and neural effects of cognitive behavioural and pharmacotherapy in panic disorder with agoraphobia. *Eur Neuropsychopharmacol*. 2016;26:431–44.

89. Beutel ME, Stark R, Pan H, Silbersweig D, Dietrich S. Changes of brain activation pre- post short-term psychodynamic in-patient psychotherapy: an fMRI study of panic disorder patients. *Psychiatry Res*. 2010;184:96–104.

90. Kircher T, Arolt V, Jansen A, *et al*. Effect of cognitive-behavioral therapy on neural correlates of fear conditioning in panic disorder. *Biol Psychiatry*. 2013;73:93–101.

91. Straube B, Lueken U, Jansen A, *et al*. Neural correlates of procedural variants in cognitive-behavioral therapy: a randomized, controlled multicenter FMRI study. *Psychother Psychosom*. 2014;83:222–33.

92. Hahn T, Kircher T, Straube B, *et al*. Predicting treatment response to cognitive behavioral therapy in panic disorder with agoraphobia by integrating local neural information. *JAMA Psychiatry*. 2015;72:68–74.

93. Reinecke A, Thilo K, Filippini N, Croft A, Harmer CJ. Predicting rapid response to cognitive-behavioural treatment for panic disorder: the role of hippocampus, insula, and dorsolateral prefrontal cortex. *Behav Res Ther*. 2014;62:120–8.

94. Lueken U, Straube B, Konrad C, *et al*. Neural substrates of treatment response to cognitive-behavioral therapy in panic disorder with agoraphobia. *Am J Psychiatry*. 2013;170:1345–55.

95. Aupperle RL, Allard CB, Simmons AN, *et al*. Neural responses during emotional processing before and after cognitive trauma therapy for battered women. *Psychiatry Res*. 2013;214:48–55.

96. Simmons AN, Norman SB, Spadoni AD, Strigo IA. Neurosubstrates of remission following prolonged exposure therapy in veterans with posttraumatic stress disorder. *Psychother Psychosom*. 2013;82:382–9.

97. Dickie EW, Brunet A, Akerib V, Armony JL. Neural correlates of recovery from post-traumatic stress disorder: a longitudinal fMRI investigation of memory encoding. *Neuropsychologia*. 2011;49:1771–8.

98. Thomaes K, Dorrepaal E, Draijer N, *et al*. Treatment effects on insular and anterior cingulate cortex activation during classic and emotional Stroop interference in child abuse-related complex post-traumatic stress disorder. *Psychol Med*. 2012;42:2337–49.

99. Lansing K, Amen DG, Hanks C, Rudy L. High-resolution brain SPECT imaging and eye movement desensitization and reprocessing in police officers with PTSD. *J Neuropsychiatry Clin Neurosci*. 2005 Fall;17:526–32.

100. Pagani M, Hogberg G, Salmaso D, *et al*. Effects of EMDR psychotherapy on 99mTc-HMPAO distribution in occupation-related post-traumatic stress disorder. *Nucl Med Commun*. 2007;28:757–65.

101. Laugharne J, Kullack C, Lee CW, *et al*. Amygdala Volumetric Change Following Psychotherapy for Posttraumatic Stress Disorder. *J Neuropsychiatry Clin Neurosci*. 2016 Fall;28:312–18.

102. Cisler JM, Steele JS, Lenow JK, *et al*. Functional reorganization of neural networks during repeated exposure to the traumatic memory in posttraumatic stress disorder: an exploratory fMRI study. *J Psychiatr Res*. 2014;48:47–55.

103. Cisler JM, Sigel BA, Kramer TL, *et al*. Amygdala response predicts trajectory of symptom reduction during Trauma-Focused Cognitive-Behavioral Therapy among adolescent girls with PTSD. *J Psychiatr Res*. 2015;71:33–40.

104. Dickie EW, Brunet A, Akerib V, Armony JL. Anterior cingulate cortical thickness is a stable predictor of recovery from post-traumatic stress disorder. *Psychol Med*. 2013;43:645–53.

105. Rubin M, Shvil E, Papini S, *et al*. Greater hippocampal volume is associated with PTSD treatment response. *Psychiatry Res*. 2016;252:36–39.

106. Olatunji BO, Cisler JM, Deacon BJ. Efficacy of cognitive behavioral therapy for anxiety disorders: a review of meta-analytic findings. *Psychiatr Clin North Am*. 2010;33:557–77.

107. Goossens L, Sunaert S, Peeters R, Griez EJ, Schruers KR. Amygdala hyperfunction in phobic fear normalizes after exposure. *Biol Psychiatry*. 2007;62:1119–25.

108. Lipka J, Hoffmann M, Miltner WH, Straube T. Effects of cognitive-behavioral therapy on brain responses to subliminal and supraliminal threat and their functional significance in specific phobia. *Biol Psychiatry*. 2014;76:869–77.

109. Grillon C. D-cycloserine facilitation of fear extinction and exposure-based therapy might rely on lower-level, automatic mechanisms. *Biol Psychiatry*. 2009;66:636–41.

110. Aupperle RL, Hale LR, Chambers RJ, *et al*. An fMRI study examining effects of acute D-cycloserine during symptom provocation in spider phobia. *CNS Spectr*. 2009;14:556–71.

111. Zilverstand A, Sorger B, Sarkheil P, Goebel R. fMRI neurofeedback facilitates anxiety regulation in females with spider phobia. *Front Behav Neurosci*. 2015;9:148.

112. Hoehn-Saric R, Schlund MW, Wong SH. Effects of citalopram on worry and brain activation in patients with generalized anxiety disorder. *Psychiatry Res*. 2004;131:11–21.

113. Phan KL, Coccaro EF, Angstadt M, *et al*. Corticolimbic brain reactivity to social signals of threat before and after sertraline treatment in generalized social phobia. *Biol Psychiatry*. 2013;73:329–36.

114. MacNamara A, Rabinak CA, Kennedy AE, *et al*. Emotion Regulatory Brain Function and SSRI Treatment in PTSD: Neural Correlates and Predictors of Change. *Neuropsychopharmacology*. 2016;41:611–18.

115. Vermetten E, Vythilingam M, Southwick SM, Charney DS, Bremner JD. Long-term treatment with paroxetine increases verbal declarative memory and hippocampal volume in posttraumatic stress disorder. *Biol Psychiatry*. 2003;54:693–702.

116. Wigton R, Radua J, Allen P, *et al*. Neurophysiological effects of acute oxytocin administration: systematic review and meta-analysis of placebo-controlled imaging studies. *J Psychiatry Neurosci*. 2015;40:E1–22.

117. Labuschagne I, Phan KL, Wood A, *et al*. Oxytocin attenuates amygdala reactivity to fear in generalized social anxiety disorder. *Neuropsychopharmacology*. 2010;35:2403–13.

118. Gorka SM, Fitzgerald DA, Labuschagne I, *et al*. Oxytocin modulation of amygdala functional connectivity to fearful faces in generalized social anxiety disorder. *Neuropsychopharmacology*. 2015;40:278–86.

119. Dodhia S, Hosanagar A, Fitzgerald DA, *et al.* Modulation of resting-state amygdala-frontal functional connectivity by oxytocin in generalized social anxiety disorder. *Neuropsychopharmacology.* 2014;39:2061–9.

120. Koch SB, van Zuiden M, Nawijn L, Frijling JL, Veltman DJ, Olff M. Intranasal Oxytocin Normalizes Amygdala Functional Connectivity in Posttraumatic Stress Disorder. *Neuropsychopharmacology.* 2016;41:2041–51.

121. Whalen PJ, Johnstone T, Somerville LH, *et al.* A functional magnetic resonance imaging predictor of treatment response to venlafaxine in generalized anxiety disorder. *Biol Psychiatry.* 2008;63:858–63.

122. Nitschke JB, Sarinopoulos I, Oathes DJ, *et al.* Anticipatory activation in the amygdala and anterior cingulate in generalized anxiety disorder and prediction of treatment response. *Am J Psychiatry.* 2009;166:302–10.

# 91

# The primary prevention of anxiety disorders

*Aliza Werner-Seidler, Jennifer L. Hudson, and Helen Christensen*

## Introduction

Anxiety disorders comprise the most prevalent class of psychological disorders across the lifespan. Onset frequently occurs early in life, with a median age of onset at 11 years [1]. The 12-month prevalence estimates exceed 10% [2] and affect approximately 8% of youth in a 12-month period [3]. Anxiety disorders are also highly comorbid with other mental disorders such as behavioural disorders, substance use disorder, and eating disorders [4], and frequently co-occur with depression, even in youth [5]. There has been some suggestion that anxiety in childhood acts as a precursor and risk factor for the subsequent development of depression [6, 7]. A more detailed description of the epidemiology is given in Chapter 88.

The adverse consequences of anxiety disorders are well documented and cause impairment across social, emotional, and academic domains [8, 9]. For example, young people with anxiety disorders have lower self-esteem, are more likely to be socially isolated, and perform worse academically than their non-disordered counterparts [10]. The economic impact of anxiety disorders is substantial, with current estimates of £9.8 billion per year in the United Kingdom in terms of lost productivity and direct costs to the health system [11]. This picture is mirrored in the United States, with costs reaching $42.3 billion per year during the 1990s [12]. The financial and societal burden posed by anxiety disorders has been recognized by world health authorities who have identified it as a public health priority [13].

One way to address this burden is via prevention. While effective treatments for anxiety disorders exist, the shift towards prevention has been driven by increased recognition of the shortcomings of treatment. It has become clear that the demand for mental health services far exceeds the availability of such services and that these services are costly and often inaccessible to many [8]. Additionally, more than half of individuals with mental health disorders do not receive clinical treatment [14], and of those who do, many fail to respond or they terminate treatment prematurely [8, 15]. Young people have particularly low levels of help-seeking, for reasons that include stigma, confidentiality concerns, and beliefs about the value of treatment [16]. Accordingly, there is a legitimate case for developing preventive interventions for anxiety disorders, which may avert some of the aforementioned limitations associated with treatment.

## Conceptual issues and definitions

Three levels of prevention were first described by public health researchers in the 1940s: primary, secondary, and tertiary. Primary prevention refers to a reduction in the incidence of a disorder by intervening in advance of disorder onset. Secondary prevention seeks to reduce the prevalence of psychopathology once symptoms have been identified but are not yet severe or do not meet the threshold level for the disorder, while tertiary prevention involves the treatment of disorders and relapse prevention [17, 18]. Although this classification system is pervasive in public health domains, the conceptual overlap between prevention and treatment has led to inconsistencies in how prevention is discussed and examined in the literature. As a result, the Institute of Medicine (IOM) [19] developed a definitional system specific to mental health research, which suggested that prevention should comprise programmes designed at reducing incidence rates, that is, delivered in advance of disorder onset. Three types were described: universal, selective, and indicated prevention. Universal prevention is delivered to all individuals within an identified population, regardless of risk. For example, universal prevention programmes for youth anxiety are typically delivered on a large scale in the school environment to every child in the grade [20]. Selective prevention refers to delivering interventions to individuals who have an increased risk profile for a specific disorder. Risk factors can be conceptualized as a characteristic, an experience, or an event that increases the likelihood of an adverse outcome, relative to the general population [21]. A sound knowledge of risk factors is therefore necessary to inform selective prevention efforts. Several comprehensive reviews document the risk and protective factors of anxiety disorders [8, 22], which include genetic (for example, family history), individual (for example, temperament, anxiety sensitivity), and environmental factors (for example, parental divorce, exposure to violence and crime). Finally, indicated prevention refers to approaches that are delivered to individuals who have subclinical symptoms but do not yet have a clinical disorder.

The present chapter aims to provide a systematic review of the psychological interventions that aim to prevent anxiety. This review is broader than previous reviews that either have focused individually on specific prevention settings, such as school environments [20], community settings [23], workplaces [24], or primary care settings

[25], or have examined specific age groups [26]. Although broad, with respect to setting, we restrict our focus on studies which specifically measure anxiety outcomes, rather than include studies measuring a less specific range of psychopathology, health, or well-being.

## Chapter outline

Firstly, we will review the existing research studies examining primary prevention. We believe it is important in a textbook such as this one to establish firmly the effectiveness of prevention for anxiety disorders, to consider the size of the effect, and to indicate for which population groups prevention may be of most use. Healthy scepticism about anxiety prevention is useful, but if these interventions result in a reduction of anxiety in a percentage of the population, there is an imperative to begin to systematically apply them. Secondly, we then consider the key elements common to effective prevention programmes, before thirdly considering barriers to the implementation of prevention programmes. Fourthly, we conclude with a summary of the current challenges facing the field and suggestions for future research.

## Systematic review of effectiveness

Adopting Mrazek and Haggerty's IOM conceptualization, primary prevention is defined here as interventions delivered in advance of the onset of anxiety symptoms or disorder and thus include universal and selective prevention approaches. It excludes indicated approaches targeting specific individuals with symptoms, which could be considered early intervention. By including universal approaches that target the whole population, it is assumed that approximately 8% of those included will already be experiencing an anxiety disorder [3]. Although a reduction in incidence is the gold standard for prevention studies, we have opted to include studies which focus on the total population group, including those universal studies that do not explicitly exclude individuals who may already have a diagnosis of anxiety. In large universal studies, screening for anxiety diagnosis or elevated symptoms prior to study entry is often impractical and expensive, and prevention interventions delivered in real-world situations are likely to include the full population cohort. For these practical reasons, studies that relied on continuous symptom measures, rather than diagnostic assessment tools, were included, although it is acknowledged in the case of some participants already experiencing the disorder that this could be considered early intervention.

## A systematic review of prevention of anxiety studies

### Methods

#### Search and screening procedures

PsycINFO, PubMed, and the Cochrane Library databases were electronically searched for articles with the key search terms 'prevent*' AND 'anxiety' OR 'anxious' OR 'internalising' OR 'internalizing' AND 'control*' OR 'random*' OR 'trial'. Reference lists from relevant reviews were hand-searched for additional articles.

The criteria for study inclusion were the following: (1) the clearly stated goal of the study was to prevent the incidence of anxiety or reduce symptoms; (2) the presence of anxiety disorder or symptoms was the primary outcome (or one of two or three outcomes in the absence of identified primary outcomes); (3) a universal or selective approach was employed; (4) the study was a randomized controlled trial (RCT); and (5) the study was published in a peer-reviewed English language journal. Studies were excluded if: (1) the focus was on medical or dental anxiety or trauma, post-traumatic stress disorder, or acute stress disorder; (2) the study targeted general mental health or well-being, operationalized by the inclusion of anxiety as one of more than three outcomes when no primary outcome was identified; (3) the study focused on transitory changes in state anxiety; and (4) the study conducted a diagnostic assessment or screening measure at baseline and allowed those with current or past disorder or those with high symptom levels to remain in the study (for example, indicated prevention/early intervention). Selective prevention studies that did not involve a screening procedure were permitted. There were no restrictions in terms of the setting, target group, intervention type, or control condition type. Studies were examined according to inclusion criteria using a checklist and were coded by the first author. Decisions about borderline trials (N = 4) were made by the first author and were then discussed with the final author. All decisions made by the first author were endorsed, and complete agreement reached.

### Effect size calculations

Standardized effect size estimates for continuous outcomes were calculated using Cohen's d [27] whereby d is calculated by subtracting the mean score of the intervention group from the mean score of the control group at post-test or follow-up, and dividing by the pooled standard deviation. Effect size estimates are reported for between group differences at post-test and follow-up intervals. According to Cohen, effect sizes of 0.20, 0.50, and 0.80 are considered small, medium, and large, respectively. Standardized effect size estimates for dichotomous outcomes were first transformed into ln (the natural logarithm of the odds ratio) and then converted into a standardized effect size equivalent to Cohen's d, using the method described by Chinn [28]. Where diagnostic and continuous outcomes were both included in a study, both effect size estimates are reported. In studies where follow-up occurred at very short intervals (for example, every month), data were extracted for key follow-up periods (for example, 6, 12, and 18 months).

### Results

#### Study selection

The search returned a total of 5276 articles after duplicates were removed (n = 367). The titles and abstracts of the 5276 articles were screened for relevance. Completely irrelevant articles that were unrelated to the topic were excluded at this stage, while relevant articles were retained and full texts were examined (n = 128). Of these, 42 articles describing 38 trials met inclusion criteria. The remaining 86 articles were excluded due to: not universal or selective prevention (n = 36), not anxiety-focused (n = 21), not prevention (n = 16), not an RCT (n = 12), and no full text available (n = 1). See Tables 91.1 and 91.2 for details of included universal and selective prevention studies, respectively.

**Table 91.1** Universal prevention studies

| Setting | Study | Age range | N | Programme | Content | Control group | Outcome measure | Post-test effect size | Follow-up effect size |
|---|---|---|---|---|---|---|---|---|---|
| School | Anticich et al., 2013 (Australia) | 4–7 years | 488 | FRIENDS | CBT | AC + WL | PAS | WL = 0.09 AC = 0.08 | WL = 0.33 (12M) AC = 0.27 (12M) |
| School | Aunes and Stiles, 2009 (Norway) | 11–15 years | 1439 | NUPP-SA | CBT | NI | SPAI-C | 0.34* | – |
| School | Barrett and Turner, 2001 [39] (Australia) | 10–12 years | 489 | FRIENDS | CBT | NI | SCAS | Teacher = 0.31* MHP = 0.32* | – |
| School | Bouchard et al., 2013 (Canada) | 9–12 years | 59 | DHS | CBT | WL | MASC | 0.48* | – |
| School | Calear et al., 2009 (Australia) | 12–17 years | 1477 | MG | iCBT | WL | RCMAS | 0.15* | 0.25* (6M) |
| School | Calear et al., 2016 [41] (Australia) | 12–18 years | 1767 | eCouch | iCBT | WL | GAD-7 | School = 0.58* Health = 1.74* | School = 1.78a (6M) Health = 0.32a (6M) School = 1.30a (12M) Health = 0.10a (12M) |
| School | Essau et al., 2012 (England) | 9–12 years | 638 | FRIENDS | CBT | WL | SCAS | 0.20* | 0.47* (6M) 0.69* (12M) |
| School | Kraag et al., 2009 (Netherlands) | NR | 1467 | LYLF | CBT | NI | STAI | 0.02 | 0.01 (9M) |
| School | Lock and Barrett, 2003; Barrett et al., 2006 (Australia) | 9–16 years | 737 | FRIENDS | CBT | WL | SCAS | 0.28* | 0.20* (12M) 0.42c (24M) 0.62c (36M) |
| School | Lowry-Webster et al., 2001; 2003 (Australia) | 10–13 years | 594 | FRIENDS | CBT | NI | SCAS | 0.66* | 0.69* |
| School | Miller et al., 2010 (Canada) | 7–12 years | 116 | TWD | CBT | WL | MASC | 0.32 | – |
| School | Miller et al., 2011a (Canada) | 7–13 years | 533 | FRIENDS-CE | CBT | WL | MASC | 0.12 | – |
| School | Miller et al., 2011b (Study 2; Canada) | 9–12 years | 253 | FRIENDS | CBT | AC | MASC | -0.18 | – |
| School | Roberts et al., 2010 (Australia) | 11–13 years | 496 | AOP | CBT | NI | RCMAS | -0.19 | 0.00 (6M) 0.17 (18M) |
| School | Rodgers and Dunsmuir, 2015 (Ireland) | 12–13 years | 62 | FRIENDS | CBT | WL | SCAS | 0.04a | 0.40 (4M)a |
| School | Stallard et al., 2014 [40] (England) | 9–10 years | 1448 | FRIENDS | CBT | AC + NI | RCADS | NR | School = -0.03 (12M) Health = 0.20* (12M) |
| School | Williford et al., 2012 [30] (Finland) | NR (child) | 7741 | KiVa | SD | NI | FNE + SADS | 0.13* | – |
| School | Wong et al., 2014 (Australia) | 14–16 years | 976 | TWU-S | iCBT | NI | GAD-7 | Anx program = 0.18* Dep program = 0.29* | – |
| University | Cukrowicz and Joiner, 2007 [37] (America) | 18–21 years | 152 | CBASP | CBT | AC | BAI | 0.58* | – |

| | | | | | | | | |
|---|---|---|---|---|---|---|---|---|
| University | Braithwaite and Fincham, 2007 [36] (America) | NR | ePREP & CBASP | iRFT | AC | BAI | NA[b] | – |
| University | Braithwaite and Fincham, 2009 [35] (America) | 18–25 years | ePREP | iRFT | AC | BAI | 1.51* | 1.01* (10M) |
| Community | Main et al., 2005 [38] (England) | 20–81 years | – | CBT | WL | STAI | CBT = −0.05[a] CT = 0.30[a] BT = 0.20[a] | – |

Note:

*Programs:* FRIENDS, Friends Program; NUPP-SA, Norwegian Universal Preventative Program for Social Anxiety; DHS, Dominique's Handy Tricks; MG, MoodGYM online program; eCOUCH, eCOUCH online program; LYLF, Learn Young Learn Fair; TWD, Taming Worry Dragons; FRIENDS-CE, Friends Program–Culturally Enriched Version; AOP, Aussie Optimism Program; KiVa, KiVa anti-bullying program; TWU-S, Thiswayup Schools: Combating Depression and Overcoming Anxiety; CBASP, Cognitive Behavioural Analysis System of Psychotherapy; ePREP, computer-based relationship focused preventive intervention.

*Content:* CBT, cognitive behavioural therapy; iCBT, Internet-based cognitive behavioural therapy; SD, skills development; iRFT, Internet-based relationship-focused therapy; CT, cognitive therapy; BT, behaviour therapy.

*Control group:* AC, active control; WL, wait-list control; NI, no-intervention control or usual care.

*Outcome measures:* PAS, Preschool Anxiety Scale; SPAI-C, Social Phobia and Anxiety Inventory for Children; SCAS, Spence Children's Anxiety Scale; MASC, Multidimensional Anxiety Scale for Children; RCMAS, Revised Children's Manifest Anxiety Scale; GAD-7, Generalized Anxiety Disorder Scale-7; STAI, State-Trait Anxiety Inventory; FNE, Fear of Negative Evaluation Scale; SADS, Social Avoidance and Distress Scale; BAI, Beck Anxiety Inventory.

*Effect size key:*

* Between-group difference.

[a] Between-group differences at post-test or follow-up not reported in manuscript.

[b] Insufficient data reported for effect size calculation.

M, months; MHP, mental health professional.

**Table 91.2** Selective prevention studies

| Setting | Study | Risk profile | Screened? | Age range | N | Programme | Content | Control group | Outcome measure(s) | Post-test effect size | Follow-up effect size |
|---|---|---|---|---|---|---|---|---|---|---|---|
| School | Balle and Tortella-Feliu, 2010 (Spain) | Anxiety sensitivity | Yes | 11–17 years | 145 | FRIENDS | CBT | WL | SCAS | 0.09 | 0.22 (6M) |
| School | Johnstone et al., 2014; Rooney et al., 2013a; 2013b (Australia) | Schools with low socio-economic status | No | 9–10 years | 910 | AOP-PTS | CBT | NI | SCAS | 0.08 | 0.03 (6M) 0.10 (18M) 0.01 (30M) 0.11 (42M) 0.05 (54M) |
| University | Feldner et al., 2008 (America) | Smoking and high anxiety sensitivity | Yes | NR (M = 19.8) | 96 | PIAS | CBT | AC | MASQ | – | 0.16 (6M) |
| University | Gallego et al., 2014 [31] (Spain) | Education students | Yes | 18–43 years | 125 | – | MCBT | NI + AC | DASS (Anx) | NI = 0.97* AC = 0.41 | – |
| University | Kang et al. 2009 [32] (Korea) | Nursing students undergoing clinical training | Yes | NR | 41 | – | MBSR | NI | STAI | 0.51* | – |
| University | Seligman et al., 1999 (America) | Negative attributional style | Yes | NR | 225 | – | CBT | NI | SCID-GAD BAI | BAI = 0.08 | BAI = 0.21* (12M) BAI = 0.03 (24M) BAI = 0.21 (36M) SCID-GAD = 0.22* (36M) |
| University | Sharif and Armitage, 2004 [42] (Iran) | Nursing students | NR | NR | 100 | – | CBT | NI | HARS | NA[b] | – |
| Workplace | Sheppard et al., 1997 [33] (America) | High-security government workers | No | NR (M = 50.5) | 44 | – | Meditation | AC | STAI (T) | 0.60* | 0.55* (36M) |
| Community | Ginsburg. 2009 [29] (America) | Parent with past or current anxiety disorder | Yes | 7–12 years | 40 | CAPS | CBT + PST | WL | ADIS SCARED | ADIS = 1.08* SCARED = 0.01 | ADIS = 1.08* (6M) ADIS = 1.42* (12M) SCARED = 0.08 (6M) SCARED 0.18 (12M) |
| Community | Ginsburg et al., 2015 (America) | Parent with a current anxiety disorder | Yes | 6–13 years | 136 | CAPS | CBT + PST | AC | ADIS | – | 0.79* (6M) 1.22* (12M) |
| Community | Joling et al., 2012 (Netherlands) | Primary caregiver for family member with dementia | Yes | 65+ | 192 | – | FS | NI | MINI (Anx) HADS-A | NA[b] | MINI = 0.02 (12M) |
| Hospital | Livermore et al., 2010 (Australia) | COPD patients | Yes | NR (M = 73) | 65+ | – | CBT | NI | ADIS (#PA; PD) | PA = 1.79* | PA = 1.78* (18M) PD = 0.90* (18M) |
| Hospital | Mikami et al., 2014 [34] (America) | Stroke patients | Yes | 50–90 years | 149 | – | PST or drug | AC | SCID-GAD | NA[b] | Drug = 0.81* (12M) PST = 0.58* (12M) |
| Hospital | Petersen and Quinlivan, 2002 (Australia) | Cancer patients | NR | NR (M = 61–63years) | 53 | – | Relaxation | NI | HADS | NA[b] | – |

| Hospital | Pitceathly et al., 2009 (England) | Cancer patients | Yes | 18–70 years | 188 | – | CBT | NI | SCID-Anxiety | 0.21 | – |
| Hospital | Tsai, 2003 (Taiwan) | Patients with high blood pressure or hypertension | No | 35–65 | 52 | – | T'ai chi | NI | STAI (T) | 1.10* | – |

*Note:*

*Risk profile:* COPD, chronic obstructive pulmonary disease.

*Programs:* FRIENDS, Friends Program; AOP-PTS, Aussie Optimism Program-Positive Thinking Skills Program; PIAS, psychosocial intervention targeting anxiety sensitivity and smoking.

*Content:* CBT, cognitive behavioural therapy; MBCT, mindfulness-based cognitive therapy; MBSR, mindfulness-based stress reduction; FS, family support; PST, Problem Solving Therapy.

*Control group:* WL, wait-list control; NI, no intervention control or usual care; AC, active control.

*Outcome measures:* SCAS, Spence Children's Anxiety Scale; MASC, Multidimensional Anxiety Scale for Children; DASS, Depression Anxiety Stress Scale; STAI, State-Trait Anxiety Inventory; STAI(T), State-Trait Anxiety Inventory Trait Subscale; SCID-GAD, Structured Clinical Interview for DSM Disorders; Generalised Anxiety Disorder Module; HARS, Hamilton Anxiety Rating Scale; MINI, Mini International Neuropsychiatric Interview; HADS-A, Hamilton Anxiety and Depression Rating Scale; ADIS, Anxiety Disorder Interview Schedule; PA, panic attacks; PD, panic disorder.

*Effect size key:*

* Between-group difference.

[a] Between-group differences at post-test or follow-up not reported in manuscript.

[b] Insufficient data reported for effect size calculation.

M, months.

## Study characteristics

There were 38 unique studies identified in the current review, which included a total of 23,772 participants. Sample size of the included studies varied considerably from between 40 participants [29] to 7741 participants [30], with a median of 188 participants. Included studies were published between 1997 and 2016, with 50% between 2010 and 2016 (and only two studies prior to the year 2000). A majority of studies were delivered either in Australia (11; 29%) or in America (9; 24%), with a further seven across mainland Europe (18.5%), four in Canada (10.5%), four in the United Kingdom (10.5%), two in Asia (Taiwan and Korea; 5%), and one in Iran (2.5%).

## Prevention type

Twenty-two of the studies were universal prevention trials (58%), and 16 were selective (42%). Of the 16 trials delivered to selective groups, risk was defined as: anxiety sensitivity ($n = 2$), having a negative attributional style ($n = 1$), attending a low socio-economic school ($n = 1$), having a parent with a past or current anxiety disorder ($n = 2$), being an undergraduate student for a high-risk profession (teacher, $n = 1$; nurse, $n = 2$), having a high-stress job ($n = 1$), having a physical chronic illness such as stroke, cancer, or hypertension ($n = 5$), or being the primary carer of someone with dementia ($n = 1$).

## Population and setting

Recipients of more than half ($n = 20$) of the programmes were children or adolescents (53%); two programmes were delivered to families (5%); eight were delivered to university students (21%); one was delivered to carers (3%); five were delivered to patients with a physical illness (13%), and two were delivered to the general adult population (5%). Of programmes delivered to children and adolescents, effect sizes could be calculated for 18 studies, and of these, eight (45%) reported significant reductions in symptoms of anxiety (ES = 0.15–0.66), while ten found no difference relative to the control condition. Of the trials delivered to university and college students, four of the five studies for which effect sizes could be calculated (90%) reported positive effects on anxiety prevention (ES = 0.51–1.51). The two studies delivered to families prevented the onset of an anxiety disorder over the 12-month follow-up period (ES = 1.22–1.42). The intervention delivered to carers was not effective in preventing anxiety, and of the five programmes delivered to individuals with a physical illness (including stroke, hypertension, chronic obstructive pulmonary disease, and cancer), effect sizes could be calculated for four. Of these, three (75%) were effective in preventing depression (ES = 0.58–1.79). Of the two programmes delivered to the general adult population, one study reported positive effects (ES = 0.66), while the other did not. The most common setting in which prevention was delivered was the school environment ($n = 20$; 53%), of which 90% were delivered universally. Eight trials targeted university and college students and were delivered in the university setting (22%). A single study was conducted in the workplace (3%), and three studies were conducted in general community-based settings (8%). Six trials were conducted in hospital or clinic settings (16%), and these were predominantly delivered to patients with a chronic illness.

## Content

A majority of trials ($n = 26$) delivered a prevention intervention based on cognitive behavioural therapy (CBT; 68.4%) or incorporated at least some element of CBT, blending it with problem-solving therapy ($n = 2$; 5.3%). Of the programmes based on CBT, effect sizes could be calculated for 24, and 15 of these (62.5%) were effective in preventing anxiety or reducing symptoms (ES = 0.20–1.79). The median effect size for all programmes evaluating CBT (regardless of outcome) was 0.25. The programme receiving the most attention was the FRIENDS programme (evaluated in ten studies), which is a manualized face-to-face programme for children and adolescents that can be delivered by teachers or mental health professionals. Four of these studies found FRIENDS to be an effective intervention at post-test (ES = 0.20–0.66), while six did not (ES = –0.18 to 0.20). Two studies evaluated the Aussie Optimism Programme, which is another standardized CBT school-based programme designed to teach young people about the connection between how they think, feel, and behave. Neither of these studies found significant effects (ES = –0.19 to 0.17). Other CBT prevention interventions included MoodGYM, eCouch, Dominique's Handy Tricks, Learn Young Play Young, Cool Kids, Taming Worry Dragons, and ThisWayUp Schools. Ten studies investigated approaches that were not CBT-based. Two of these tested a mindfulness intervention, one derived from mindfulness-based cognitive therapy and the other from mindfulness-based stress reduction (5.3%). Two studies ($n = 2$; 5.3%) involved relationship-focused therapy, delivering the Prevention and Relationship Enhancement Programme (ePREP). The remaining therapeutic approaches included a meditation programme, a t'ai chi programme, a relaxation programme, support and counselling, problem-solving therapy and escitalopram (an antidepressant medication), and a standardized anti-bullying programme known as KiVa based on education and skill development (each making up 2.6%). Of the ten trials that delivered therapeutic techniques that were not CBT-based, eight reported enough data for effect size calculation at post-test, of which six studies (75%) [30–35] were effective (ES = 0.41–1.10) in preventing anxiety.

## Programme format, length, and mode of delivery

More than half ($n = 23$, 60.5%) of the included programmes were delivered in a small group format (typically of groups comprising 6–10 individuals), and three programmes (7.9%) involved a group component, combined with individual sessions ($n = 2$) or combined with a self-directed computer-delivered programme ($n = 1$). Six programmes (15.8%) were delivered entirely individually face-to-face, and six programmes were delivered by computer (15.8%). Programme length ranged considerably from a single intervention session to 22 sessions, with most programmes (90%) being delivered in between 6 and 12 sessions (median = 8 sessions), usually on a weekly or a fortnightly basis. There was substantial variability in the duration over which these programmes were delivered, ranging from between a single session to 52 weeks (median = 8 weeks), although it needs to be noted that three studies delivered a single session, followed by 7 weeks of reminder emails encouraging participants to implement the skills they acquired during the session [35–37]. Sessions ranged in duration from 35 to 120 minutes, with the exception of one study where day-long workshops were delivered [38] and one study that did not report on session length [34].

In terms of personnel delivering the programme, ten studies were delivered exclusively by psychologists or mental health professionals (26%); five studies were delivered by researchers or graduate students (13%), and three programmes were delivered by either psychologists or graduate students (7.9%). One study was delivered by a t'ai chi instructor (3%), and one by a specialist physician (3%). Of these 20 studies delivered by professionals, effect sizes could be calculated for 18, and of these, 13 studies (72%) reported a significant preventive effect on anxiety (ES = 0.20–1.79). Nine of the included studies were delivered exclusively by teachers or school staff within the school environment (23.5%), of which two (22%) were effective (ES = 0.13–0.66). Two school-based studies involved both school and external staff, comparing a school-led version of the programme to a health professional-delivered version [39, 40]. In the Barrett and Turner study [39], the personnel delivering the intervention did not impact effect size, with both health- and school-led delivery producing significant reductions in anxiety (health ES = 0.32; teacher ES = 0.31). Conversely, a difference between school-led and health-led prevention was detected in the Stallard *et al.* study [40], with health-led programmes producing significant preventive effects at 12 months (ES = 0.20), while teacher-led prevention had no effect (ES = 0.03). Of the six computer-delivered programmes, two (5%) were delivered in the school environment and supported by teachers and one (3%) involved a comparison between a school-supported version to a version supported by a mental health organization [41]. The remaining three (7.9%) computer-based programmes were entirely self-directed and delivered to adults. Of the six computer-delivered programmes, four of the five (80%) for which effect sizes could be calculated were effective (ES = 0.15–1.51). One study (3%) did not report on personnel delivering the programme [42].

### Evaluation control groups

Seventeen of the included studies (45%) compared the prevention programme to either a no-intervention control group or usual care (NI), nine studies involved a wait-list control group (WL; 23.6%), seven studies used an attention control group (AC; 18.4%), and six studies involved more than one control group (15.7%). Of these six studies involving more than one comparison, three included an NI and an AC arm, and two involved a WL arm and an AC condition. Usual care typically involved regular class attendance in school-based programmes or standard care (education, check-ups) in medical settings. Attention control conditions are used to control for extraneous factors (such as attention, exposure to educational material, and non-specific prevention factors such as being in a group) that could feasibly impact preventive outcomes. Of the studies that included an attention control condition, 60% reported significant effects on anxiety (ES = 0.20–1.22), while 58% of trials employing NI or WL groups found a significant reduction in anxiety (ES = 0.15–1.78).

### Outcome measures

Anxiety symptoms were measured as outcomes on all but two of the included studies (95%). Two studies used diagnostic instruments exclusively, and five studies included both diagnostic and symptom outcomes. Of the studies using diagnostic tools, three studies (43%) used the Anxiety Disorder Interview Schedule [43], three used the Structured Clinical Interview for DSM-IV disorders [44], and the final study (14%) employed the MINI International Neuropsychiatric Interview [45]. Anxiety symptoms were measured most frequently with the Spence Children's Anxiety Scale (22%) [46], followed by the Multidimensional Anxiety Scale for Children (14%) [47] and the State-Trait Anxiety Inventory (14%)

[48], followed by the Beck Anxiety Inventory (11%) [49] and finally the Revised Children's Manifest Anxiety Scale (8%) [50].

### Overall outcomes

From the 38 studies included in this review, eight studies did not include enough information for effect sizes to be calculated or did not collect data at post-test (for example, some studies included follow-up data only). Of the 30 (79%) studies for which effect sizes could be calculated, three of these reported change score analyses only, and so group differences at post-test could not be ascertained. Out of the 27 (71%) remaining studies, 17 (63%) trials reported that the prevention programme significantly improved anxiety outcomes (ES = 0.15–1.79), while ten (37%) trials did not (ES = –0.19 to 0.21). Twenty-one studies (55%) collected follow-up data, for which effect sizes and between-group differences could be calculated for 19 (50% overall). Of these, 12 (63%) studies reported significant effects on anxiety (ES = 0.25–1.78), while seven (37%) did not (ES = 0.00–0.33). Of the studies that included follow-up periods, 15 studies (39%) did not follow up beyond 12 months, two studies included a final follow-up at 18 months (5%), and only three studies followed up individuals for longer than 2 years (8%).

### Universal programme outcomes

Effect sizes could be calculated for all but two of the 22 universal trials, but a further three did not report between-group outcomes at post-test and/or follow-up. Of the 17 (53%) trials for which effect sizes and group differences could be ascertained, 11 trials (65%) found positive outcomes on anxiety (ES = 0.15–1.51), while six did not (ES = –0.19 to 0.32). Eleven studies included follow-up data, for which group differences were reported for nine. Six studies (67%) reported an impact of anxiety prevention at follow-up (ES = 0.25–1.01), while three trials did not (ES = 0.03–0.33).

### Selective programme outcomes

Effect sizes for the 16 selective prevention programmes could be calculated for ten of the studies and ranged from 0.08 to 1.78. Of these ten studies, six (60%) found a significant preventive effect on anxiety (ES = 0.60–1.79), while four did not (ES = 0.08–0.21). Ten selective studies reported follow-up information, with six finding a positive effect of anxiety prevention (ES = 0.58–1.78) and four reporting no difference between groups on anxiety at follow-up (ES = 0.01–0.22).

## Effectiveness of the primary prevention of anxiety

Overall, this review suggests that there is legitimate value in pursuing primary prevention of anxiety disorders using both universal and selective approaches, with a median effect size for all included studies of 0.21. More than half of the trials (63%) found that the prevention programme either prevented onset of an anxiety disorder or reduced anxiety symptoms, both at post-test and at follow-up. Small (0.15) to large (1.78) effect sizes were reported for both universal and selective interventions. As might be expected, 80% of the studies included were delivered to children, adolescents, or university students, which is appropriate, given that anxiety often develops early in life. Preventive interventions delivered to young people have the greatest chance of preventing first onset, which can have implications for the trajectory of disorder across the lifespan.

Studies that involved prevention in adults and the elderly were more likely to be selective prevention programmes, delivered to those at risk for disorder development (for example, diagnosis of cancer, experience of stroke).

There has been considerable debate in the literature about whether universal or targeted prevention approaches are more effective, and to date, there does not seem to be a clear advantage of one over the other (for example, [18, 20, 51]). A common argument against universal prevention is that programmes are delivered to large samples with relatively low levels of need. However, the counter-argument is that unless prevention is universal, individuals who are on the trajectory to disorder but do not yet meet a given definition of being 'at risk' will not be captured. Furthermore, anxiety disorders can be extremely difficult to detect in children by parents and teachers, relative to other disorders [52], making universal approaches delivered in the school environment particularly attractive in terms of reaching these individuals. Another advantage of school-based universal approaches is that they minimize stigma and are usually easier for school administrators to schedule by directly integrating them into the school curriculum. Although universal programmes are associated with advantages for delivery in schools, outside of this environment, universal implementation is more difficult—we identified only a single community-based universal programme [38] and three universal programmes delivered in university settings [35–37].

Control group type did not appear to influence effectiveness outcomes. It is encouraging that approximately 32% of the studies included an active control group, which is double what has been reported previously [20]. This may reflect an increasing awareness of the importance of active control conditions to control for non-specific factors associated with the prevention programme, something which prevention researchers have been calling for [53]. There was virtually no difference in the proportion of studies reporting significant preventive effects on anxiety as a function of control group type (60% of studies with an active condition found effects, while 58% of those employing inactive control group types reported positive effects).

There was substantial variability in effect size estimates, and this likely reflects the heterogeneity in study variables (for example, setting, age, content). The fact that most selective prevention programmes screened participants for a history of anxiety or mental disorder and excluded participants on this basis, while universal prevention studies did not involve a screening process, is likely to have impacted effect sizes. Furthermore, the quality of the research methodology also varied significantly, which is very likely to have influenced effect size estimates. For example, many studies did not report attrition rates or whether fidelity measures were used (for example, independent coding of therapy tapes).

Although our results provide consistent evidence for the effectiveness of anxiety prevention programmes, findings need to be interpreted in the context of several limitations, including the fact that three studies reported only change scores, so between-group effect size estimates at post-test and follow-up could not be calculated. A further five studies did not report enough information for effect sizes to be calculated. Therefore, the effect size estimates from this review are based on 30 studies, and not the 38 that met inclusion criteria. Finally, a single rater (the first author) screened and extracted the data, without an independent coder.

## Key elements common to effective prevention programmes

A consistent finding from both the literature and the current review is that programmes can be effective in preventing anxiety. What is now needed is insight into the elements of consistently effective prevention programmes. There is not yet enough existing research to confidently address this issue, although there are some emerging patterns.

Much of the research that has been carried out in the field of anxiety prevention has tested psychological approaches and, most frequently, CBT. More than 70% of the included programmes in the current review delivered at least some component of CBT, including several trials delivering automated, computer-delivered CBT. CBT typically involves a range of different cognitive and behavioural strategies, meaning that the active ingredient and corresponding mechanisms of change cannot be identified when the overall package is examined. Dismantling studies will help to address this issue, which may inform the development of more effective prevention programmes in the future.

Drawing on the existing literature and the results from the current review, factors such as age, gender, prevention type, and setting have not consistently been associated with effect size outcomes (for example, [20, 26]). Notably, personnel delivering the programme may impact outcome. Existing evidence and data from the current review suggests that programmes delivered by mental health professionals could be more effective than those delivered by teachers [26], although this finding has not been consistently replicated [20, 51]. In our review, programmes that were delivered by mental health professionals (including psychologists, psychiatrists, doctors, graduate students, or researchers) or by computers were associated with a higher percentage of successful preventive outcomes than those delivered by teachers. However, fewer than one-third of included studies were delivered by teachers, and so a relatively low number of teacher-delivered programmes precludes strong conclusions about the effectiveness of these programmes being drawn. Of note, two studies directly compared teacher- vs mental health professional-led face-to-face prevention programmes, of which one noted superiority in the professional-delivered programme, while the other did not [39, 40]. More research is required to resolve this issue, and regardless of outcome, future studies should focus on identifying ways to improve the effects of programmes delivered by school staff, which may involve the development of teacher training and support structures to scaffold teacher competence in delivering mental health programmes.

## Barriers to the implementation of prevention programmes

### Engagement and fidelity

Engagement is a key barrier to delivering effective prevention programmes. These programmes are notoriously challenging to make appealing and relevant to the target audience, who might not perceive the need for the material or appreciate its value, particularly when there is no obvious immediate benefit. A discussion about prevention necessarily includes a focus on young people, and the emergence of programmes that use technology may have greater appeal to young people, particularly those involving gamified and interactive components (for example, [41, 54]). These programmes also lend themselves to being updated and incorporating technological innovations that may be particularly appealing to young people, such as completing mood ratings on their own digital device, rather than in a classroom setting. Systematic evaluation of engagement factors is likely to inform how prevention programmes might best be delivered at a population level.

Evidence-based anxiety prevention programmes are unlikely to be effective if they are not delivered as intended. Poor adherence to the protocol could reflect inadequate training or competence on the part of the provider or an overall lack of engagement with the programme. In the current review, most studies did not report on how fidelity to the programme was measured (if it was at all), and it is important to keep in mind that fidelity is likely to be higher in a rigorous research trial than under real-world conditions. One way this barrier might be overcome is for implementation and effectiveness–implementation hybrid trials to systematically examine factors that are associated with higher levels of engagement and fidelity to the programme and how these relate to effectiveness, uptake, and completion rates.

### Organizational priority and fit

A related issue is the compatibility of the prevention programme to the culture in which it is being delivered. In the example of school settings, the fit within the school culture and the willingness of school administrators to schedule time in the school curriculum for delivery are likely to influence outcomes. There are many demands placed on an already crowded school curriculum, and one of the key emerging barriers from our work in the field is willingness of school executives to prioritize mental health prevention programmes over other valid educational programmes. One way to overcome this is to align school prevention programmes with curriculum outcomes, such that teachers can fulfil teaching requirements by delivering mental health prevention programmes without having to find extra time in their schedule. Issues of fit and priority against competing demands are likely to apply more broadly to general workplace settings as well where it might be expected that initiatives and programmes that fit with the culture of a workplace would be prioritized. Mediating factors likely to influence implementation in a particular context include the attitude of the organization to the programme, existing stigma, and the attitude and skills of the provider. Empirical investigation into these factors as a way to promote engagement and adherence to the programme is now needed.

### Cost and sustainability

The delivery of prevention programmes is expensive. It requires investment in terms of paying professionals to deliver the programme or training non-mental health specialists to deliver the programme. Programmes delivered by lay people, including school staff, provide information about whether a programme is likely to be effective and suitable for sustainable, large-scale implementation because these programmes ultimately need to be delivered by individuals who will be available to do so over the long term. Technology-based approaches show tremendous promise in providing a low-cost and potentially sustainable avenue through which large-scale rollout might occur. Individuals with minimal training in the community can support a computer-delivered programme at much lower cost than undergoing training themselves to deliver complicated psychological therapies.

## Current challenges facing the field and suggestions for future longer research follow-up

Most of the research in the field of anxiety prevention has been conducted over the past decade. Although growing, the existing evidence base is relatively scarce, compared to the treatment literature, and even research into the prevention of depression. What this means is that we do not yet know what the longer-term impact of delivering prevention programmes is, and the field now needs studies that assess participants over longer follow-up periods. To detect a true preventive effect, a difference in the incidence of disorder or symptoms needs to be identified as differentially increasing between prevention and control groups. The use of latent growth curve modelling techniques may help to identify the impact of prevention programmes on trajectories towards disorder over time. The impact of prevention is hypothesized to be long term, and yet there are not enough data available to address this question, with only three of the included studies following participants over 2 years or longer. Researchers are encouraged to assess participants over significantly longer periods, so that genuine long-term effects can be detected. The increase in the use of digital technology may assist in the ease with which participants may be contacted and followed over longer periods.

## More rigorous research methods

Many of the studies in this review, together with previous prevention reviews, were of poor methodological quality. For example, 47% of the included studies involved less than 200 participants, suggesting inadequate power to detect preventive effects, while fewer than half of the studies in the current review did not conduct intent-to-treat analyses. These statistics are not unique to the current review and are broadly consistent with what has been reported previously (for example, [20, 51]). Given some of these methodological weaknesses, it is possible that effect size estimates are inflated, and so results need to be interpreted cautiously. The increasingly common requirement to publish protocol papers in advance of completing an RCT and to adhere to Consolidated Standards of Reporting Trials (CONSORT) guidelines [55] is likely to enhance the overall quality of RCTs moving forward.

## Cost estimates

An important next step in this line of research is to identify the cost-effectiveness of delivering anxiety prevention programmes in these environments. We know of one study that has examined the cost of delivering the FRIENDS programme universally in schools, with researchers reporting no evidence for its cost-effectiveness [56]. This is clearly an important issue from a public health perspective that future work will need to address. Again, the issue of cost may be addressed, at least in part, by the emergence of new, effective digital platforms through which prevention programmes might be delivered.

## Final comment

A common criticism of prevention programmes is that they are associated with modest effect sizes. Prevention studies require very large sample sizes to detect effects because of relatively low base rates of disorder incidence found in unselected samples [3, 57]. The picture emerging from the literature is that with enough statistical power, genuine small preventive effects may exist. Even small effect sizes are likely to be associated with meaningful and clinically important improvements at a population level. The current review found a median effect size of 0.21 at post-test, which includes all studies meeting inclusion criteria (not just those with significant between-group differences). This estimate is in line with mean weighted effect sizes reported in a previous meta-analysis of youth anxiety where Cohen's *d* at post-test was 0.18 (for example, [26]). Specifically, the median effect size for CBT programmes, the most widely studied approach, was 0.25 at post-test. Effect sizes of this magnitude may be of practical significance, as they apply to a whole population. Adopting the Kraemer approach [58] to estimate the number needed to treat, approximately 9.2 individuals would need to be delivered the prevention programme for a favourable prevention outcome in one individual. It is not possible to know exactly how many people are needed to prevent onset, as the reliance in the studies reviewed largely rely on symptom measures, for which we cannot be sure what reduction is needed to prevent incidence. However, given that comparable effect sizes in studies using diagnostic vs continuous measures (and specifically those included in this review), this suggests that 9.2 is a valid estimate. Considering that participants included universal, non-selected samples, the potential impact of prevention is substantial, particularly if prevention can be delivered to large samples at low cost, possibly using digital technologies. The successful prevention of anxiety disorders has important implications at both an individual and societal level, and investigation into the factors that promote the successful implementation of prevention programmes, together with more attention to factors which moderate outcomes and whether they are sustained, is now warranted.

## REFERENCES

1. Kessler RC, Berglund P, Demler O, Jin R, Merikangas KR, Walters EE. Lifetime prevalence and age-of-onset distributions of DSM-IV disorders in the National Comorbidity Survey Replication. *Arch Gen Psychiatry*. 2005;62:593–602.
2. Kessler RC, Aguilar-Gaxiola S, Alonso J, *et al.* The global burden of mental disorders: an update from the WHO World Mental Health (WMH) surveys. *Epidemiol Psychiatr Soc*. 2009;18:23–33.
3. Merikangas KR, Nakamura EF, Kessler RC. Epidemiology of mental disorders in children and adolescents. *Dialogues Clin Neurosci*. 2009;11:7–20.
4. Kessler RC, Chiu WT, Demler O, Merikangas KR, Walters EE. Prevalence, severity, and comorbidity of 12-month DSM-IV disorders in the National Comorbidity Survey Replication. *Arch Gen Psychiatry*. 2005;62:617–27.

5. Seligman LD, Ollendick TH. Comorbidity of anxiety and depression in children and adolescents: an integrative review. *Clin Child Fam Psychol Rev*. 1998;1:125–44.
6. Cole DA, Peeke LG, Martin JM, Truglio R, Seroczynski AD. A longitudinal look at the relation between depression and anxiety in children and adolescents. *J Consult Clin Psychol*. 1998;66:451–60.
7. Wittchen HU, Beesdo K, Bittner A, Goodwin RD. Depressive episodes – evidence for a causal role of primary anxiety disorders? *Eur Psychiatry*. 2003;18:384–93.
8. Donovan CL, Spence SH. Prevention of childhood anxiety disorders. *Clin Psychol Rev*. 2000;20:509–31.
9. Rapee RM, Schniering CA, Hudson JL. Anxiety disorders during childhood and adolescence: origins and treatment. *Annu Rev Clin Psychol*. 2009;5:311–41.
10. Strauss CC, Frame CL, Forehand R. Psychosocial impairment associated with anxiety in children. *J Clin Child Psychol*. 1987;16:235–9.
11. Fineberg NA, Haddad PM, Carpenter L, *et al.* The size, burden and cost of disorders of the brain in the UK. *J Psychopharmacol*. 2013;27:761–70.
12. Greenberg PE, Sisitsky T, Kessler RC, *et al.* The economic burden of anxiety disorders in the 1990s. *J Clin Psychiatry*. 1999;60:427–35.
13. World Health Organization. mhGAP: *Mental Health Gap Action Programme: scaling up care for mental, neurological and substance use disorders*. Geneva: World Health Organization; 2008.
14. Andrews G, Issakidis C, Carter G. Shortfall in mental health service utilisation. *Br J Psychiatry*. 2001;179:417–25.
*15. Essau CA. Frequency and patterns of mental health services utilization among adolescents with anxiety and depressive disorders. *Depress Anxiety*. 2005;22:130–7.
16. Gulliver A, Griffiths KM, Christensen H. Perceived barriers and facilitators to mental health help-seeking in young people: a systematic review. *BMC Psychiatry*. 2010;10:1–9.
17. Caplan G. *Principles of Preventive Psychiatry*. Oxford: Basic Books; 1964.
18. Feldner MT, Zvolensky MJ. Prevention of anxiety psychopathology: a critical review of the empirical literature. *Clin Psychol: Sci Prac*. 2004;11:405–24.
19. Mrazek PJ, Haggerty RJ. *Reducing Risks for Mental Disorders: Frontiers for Preventive Intervention Research*. Washington, DC: The National Academies Press; 1994.
20. Neil AL, Christensen H. Efficacy and effectiveness of school-based prevention and early intervention programs for anxiety. *Clin Psychol Rev*. 2009;29:208–15.
21. Kazdin AE, Kraemer HC, Kessler RC, Kupfer DJ, Offord DR. Contributions of risk-factor research to developmental psychopathology. *Clin Psychol Rev*. 1997;17:375–406.
22. Hudson JL, Flannery-Schroeder E, Kendall PC. Primary prevention of anxiety disorders. In: Dozois D, Dobson K (eds). *The Prevention of Anxiety and Depression: Theory, Research and Practice*. Washington, D.C.: American Psychological Association; 2004. pp. 101–30.
23. Christensen H, Pallister E, Smale S, Hickie IB, Calear AL. Community-based prevention programs for anxiety and depression in youth: a systematic review. *J Prim Prev*. 2010;31:139–70.
24. Martin A, Sanderson K, Cocker F. Meta-analysis of the effects of health promotion intervention in the workplace on depression and anxiety symptoms. *Scand J Work Environ Health*. 2009;35:7–18.
25. Garcia-Campayo J, del Hoyo YL, Valero MS, *et al.* Primary prevention of anxiety disorders in primary care: a systematic review. *Prev Med*. 2015;76 Suppl:S12–15.

26. Fisak BJ, Jr., Richard D, Mann A. The prevention of child and adolescent anxiety: a meta-analytic review. *Prev Sci.* 2011;12:255–68.

27. Cohen J. *Statistical Power Analysis for the Behavioural Sciences.* Hillsdale, NJ: Erlbaum; 1988.

28. Chinn S. A simple method for converting an odds ratio to effect size for use in meta-analysis. *Stat Med.* 2000;19:3127–31.

*29. Ginsburg GS. The child anxiety prevention study: intervention model and primary outcomes. *J Consult Clin Psychol.* 2009;77:580–7.

*30. Williford A, Boulton A, Noland B, Little TD, Karna A, Salmivalli C. Effects of the KiVa anti-bullying program on adolescents' depression, anxiety, and perception of peers. *J Abnorm Child Psychol.* 2012;40:289–300.

*31. Gallego J, Aguilar-Parra JM, Cangas AJ, Langer AI, Manas I. Effect of a mindfulness program on stress, anxiety and depression in university students. *Span J Psychol.* 2014;17:E109.

*32. Kang YS, Choi SY, Ryu E. The effectiveness of a stress coping program based on mindfulness meditation on the stress, anxiety, and depression experienced by nursing students in Korea. *Nurse Educ Today.* 2009;29:538–43.

*33. Sheppard WD, Staggers FJ, John L. The effects of a stress management program in a high security government agency. *Anxiet Stress Coping.* 1997;10:341–50.

*34. Mikami K, Jorge RE, Moser DJ, et al. Prevention of post-stroke generalized anxiety disorder, using escitalopram or problem-solving therapy. *J Neuropsychiatry Clin Neurosci.* 2014;26:323–8.

*35. Braithwaite SR, Fincham FD. A randomized clinical trial of a computer based preventive intervention: replication and extension of ePREP. *J Fam Psychol.* 2009;23:32–8.

*36. Braithwaite SR, Fincham FD. ePREP: Computer based prevention of relationship dysfunction, depression and anxiety. *J Soc Clin Psychol.* 2007;26:609–22.

*37. Cukrowicz KC, Joiner TEJ. Computer-based intervention for anxious and depressive symptoms in a non-clinical population. *Cognit Ther Res.* 2007;31:677–93.

*38. Main NA, Elliot SA, Brown JSL. Comparison of three different approaches used in large-scale stress workshops for the general public. *Behav Cogn Psychother.* 2005;33:299–309.

*39. Barrett PM, Turner C. Prevention of anxiety symptoms in primary school children: preliminary results from a universal school-based trial. *Br J Clin Psychol.* 2001;40(Pt 4):399–410.

*40. Stallard P, Skryabina E, Taylor G, et al. Classroom-based cognitive behaviour therapy (FRIENDS): A cluster randomised controlled trial to prevent anxiety in children through education in schools (PACES). *Lancet Psychiatry.* 2014;1:185–92.

*41. Calear AL, Batterham PJ, Poyser CT, Mackinnon AJ, Griffiths KM, Christensen H. Cluster randomised controlled trial of the e-couch anxiety and worry program in schools. *J Affect Disord.* 2016;196:210–17.

*42. Sharif F, Armitage P. The effect of psychological and educational counselling in reducing anxiety in nursing students. *J Psychiatr Ment Health Nurs.* 2004;11:386–92.

43. Brown TA, Barlow DH, Di Nardo PA. *Anxiety Disorders Interview Schedule for DSM-IV (ADIS-IV): Client Interview Schedule.* Graywind Publications Incorporated; 1994.

44. First MB, Spitzer RL, Gibbons M, Williams JBW. *Structured Clinical Interview for DSM-IV Axis I Disorders (SCID-IV).* Washington, D.C.: American Psychiatric Press; 1996.

45. Sheehan DV, Lecrubier Y, Sheehan KH, et al. The Mini-International Neuropsychiatric Interview (MINI): the development and validation of a structured diagnostic psychiatric interview for DSM-IV and ICD-10. *J Clin Psychiatry.* 1998;59(Suppl 20):22–33.

46. Spence SH. A measure of anxiety symptoms among children. *Behav Res Ther.* 1998;36:545–66.

47. March JS, Parker JD, Sullivan K, Stallings P, Conners CK. The Multidimensional Anxiety Scale for Children (MASC): factor structure, reliability, and validity. *J Am Acad Child Adolesc Psychiatry.* 1997;36:554–65.

48. Spielberger CD, Gorsuch RL, Lushene R, Vagg PR, Jacobs GA. *Manual for the State-Trait Anxiety Inventory.* Palo Alto, CA: Consulting Psychologists Press; 1983.

49. Steer RA, Beck AT. *Beck Anxiety Inventory.* San Antonio, TX: Harcourt Brace and Company; 1997.

50. Reynolds C, Richmond BO. What I think and feel: a revised measure of children's manifest anxiety. *J Abnorm Child Psychol.* 1978;6:271–80.

51. Stockings EA, Degenhardt L, Dobbins T, et al. Preventing depression and anxiety in young people: a review of the joint efficacy of universal, selective and indicated prevention. *Psychol Med.* 2015;46:1–16.

52. Kovacs M, Devlin B. Internalizing disorders in childhood. *J Child Psychol Psychiatry.* 1998;39:47–63.

53. Merry SN, Hetrick SE, Cox GR, Brudevold-Iversen T, Bir JJ, McDowell H. Psychological and educational interventions for preventing depression in children and adolescents. *Cochrane Database Syst Rev.* 2011;12;CD003380.

54. Perry Y, Calear AL, Mackinnon A, et al. Trial for the Prevention of Depression (TriPoD) in final-year secondary students: study protocol for a cluster randomised controlled trial. *Trials.* 2015;16:1–17.

55. Schulz KF, Altman DG, Moher D. CONSORT 2010 Statement: updated guidelines for reporting parallel group randomised trials. *BMJ.* 2010;340:c332.

*56. Stallard P, Skryabina E, Taylor G, et al. A cluster randomised controlled trial comparing the effectiveness and cost-effectiveness of a school-based cognitive-behavioural therapy programme (FRIENDS) in the reduction of anxiety and improvement in mood in children aged 9/10 years. *J Public Health Res.* 2015; 3.

57. Munoz RF, Cuijpers P, Smit F, Barrera AZ, Leykin Y. Prevention of major depression. *Annu Rev Clin Psychol.* 2010;6:181–212.

58. Kraemer HC, Kupfer DJ. Size of treatment effects and their importance to clinical research and practice. *Biol Psychiatry.* 2006;59:990–6.

* Included in systematic review.

References included in systematic review not referred to in text

Anticich SAJ, Barrett PM, Silverman W, Lacherez P, Gillies R. The prevention of childhood anxiety and promotion of resilience among preschool-aged children: a universal school based trial. *Adv Sch Ment Health Promot.* 2013;6:93–121.

Aune T, Stiles TC. Universal-based prevention of syndromal and subsyndromal social anxiety: A randomized controlled study. *J Consult Clin Psychol.* 2009;77:867–79.

Balle M, Tortella-Feliu M. Efficacy of a brief school-based program for selective prevention of childhood anxiety. *Anxiety Stress Coping.* 2010;23:71–85.

Barrett PM., Farrell LJ, Ollendick TH, Dadds M. Long-term outcomes of an Australian universal prevention trial of anxiety and depression symptoms in children and youth: an evaluation of the friends program. *J Clin Child Adolesc Psychol*. 2006;35:403–11.

Bouchard S, Gervais J, Gagnier N, Loranger C. Evaluation of a primary prevention program for anxiety disorders using story books with children aged 9-12 years. *J Prim Prev*. 2013;34:345–58.

Calear AL, Christensen H, Mackinnon A, Griffiths KM, O'Kearney R. The YouthMood Project: a cluster randomized controlled trial of an online cognitive behavioral program with adolescents. *J Consult Clin Psychol*. 2009;77:1021–32.

Essau CA, Conradt J, Sasagawa S, Ollendick TH. Prevention of anxiety symptoms in children: results from a universal school-based trial. *Behav Ther*. 2012;43:450–64.

Feldner MT, Zvolensky MJ, Babson K, Leen-Feldner EW, Schmidt NB. An integrated approach to panic prevention targeting the empirically supported risk factors of smoking and anxiety sensitivity: theoretical basis and evidence from a pilot project evaluating feasibility and short-term efficacy. *J Anxiety Disord*. 2008;22:1227–43.

Ginsburg GS, Drake KL, Tein J-Y, Teetsel R, Riddle MA. Preventing onset of anxiety disorders in offspring of anxious parents: a randomized controlled trial of a family-based intervention. *Am J Psychiatry*. 2015;172:1207–14.

Joling KJ, van Marwijk HW, Smit F, *et al*. Does a family meetings intervention prevent depression and anxiety in family caregivers of dementia patients? A randomized trial. *PLoS One*. 2012;7:e30936.

Johnstone J, Rooney RM, Hassan S, Kane RT. Prevention of depression and anxiety symptoms in adolescents: 42 and 54 months follow-up of the Aussie Optimism Program-Positive Thinking Skills. *Front Psychol*. 2014;5:364.

Kraag G, Van Breukelen GJ, Kok G, Hosman C. 'Learn Young, Learn Fair', a stress management program for fifth and sixth graders: longitudinal results from an experimental study. *J Child Psychol Psychiatry*. 2009;50:1185–95.

Livermore N, Sharpe L, McKenzie D. Prevention of panic attacks and panic disorder in COPD. *Eur Respir J*. 2010;35:557–63.

Lock S, Barrett PM. A longitudinal study of developmental differences in universal preventive intervention for child anxiety. *Behav Change*. 2003;20:183–99.

Lowry-Webster HM, Barrett PM, Dadds MR. A universal prevention trial of anxiety and depressive symptomatology in childhood: preliminary data from an Australian study. *Behav Change*. 2001; 18:36–50.

Lowry-Webster HM, Barrett PM, Lock S. A universal prevention trial of anxiety symptomology during childhood: results at 1-year follow-up. *Behav Change*. 2003;20:25–43.

Miller LD, Laye-Gindhu A, Bennett JL, *et al*. An effectiveness study of a culturally enriched school-based CBT anxiety prevention program. *J Clin Child Adolesc Psychol*. 2011a;40:618–29.

Miller LD, Laye-Gindhu A, Liu Y, March JS, Thordarson DS, Garland EJ. Evaluation of a preventive intervention for child anxiety in two randomized attention-control school trials. *Behav Res Ther*. 2011b;49:315–23.

Miller LD, Short C, Garland E, Clark S. The ABCs of CBT (cognitive behavior therapy): Evidence-based approaches to child anxiety in public school settings. *J Couns Dev*. 2010;88:432–9.

Petersen RW, Quinlivan JA. Preventing anxiety and depression in gynaecological cancer: a randomised controlled trial. *BJOG*. 2002;109:386–94.

Pitceathly C, Maguire P, Fletcher I, Parle M, Tomenson B, Creed F. Can a brief psychological intervention prevent anxiety or depressive disorders in cancer patients? A randomised controlled trial. *Ann Oncol*. 2009;20:928–34.

Roberts CM, Kane R, Bishop B, Cross D, Fenton J, Hart B. The prevention of anxiety and depression in children from disadvantaged schools. *Behav Res Ther*. 2010;48:68–73.

Rodgers A, Dunsmuir S. A controlled evaluation of the 'FRIENDS for life' emotional resiliency programme on overall anxiety levels, anxiety subtype levels and school adjustment. *Child Adol Ment Health*. 2015;20:13–19.

Rooney RM, Morrison D, Hassan S, Kane R, Roberts C, Mancini V. Prevention of internalizing disorders in 9–10 year old children: efficacy of the Aussie Optimism Positive Thinking Skills Program at 30-month follow-up. *Front Psychol*. 2013a;4:988.

Rooney R, Hassan S, Kane R, Roberts CM, Nesa M. Reducing depression in 9–10 year old children in low SES schools: a longitudinal universal randomized controlled trial. *Behav Res Ther*. 2013b;51:845–54.

Seligman MEP, Schulman P, DeRubeis RJ, Hollon SD. The prevention of depression and anxiety. *Prevention and Treatment*. 1999;2:8a.

Tsai JC, Wang WH, Chan P, *et al*. The beneficial effects of Tai Chi Chuan on blood pressure and lipid profile and anxiety status in a randomized controlled trial. *J Altern Complement Med*. 2003;9:747–54.

Wong N, Kady L, Mewton L, Sunderland M, Andrews G. Preventing anxiety and depression in adolescents: a randomised controlled trial of two school based Internet-delivered cognitive behavioural therapy programmes. *Internet Interventions*. 2014;1:90–4.

# 92

# Treatment of anxiety disorders

*David S. Baldwin and Nathan T.M. Huneke*

## Anxiety symptoms and anxiety disorders

Anxiety is an understandable response to perceived threat or experienced stress and is typically fleeting and controllable. It can be conceptualized as an 'alarm', allowing a physical and mental response to perceived danger (the 'fight-or-flight' response). Anxiety symptoms are mostly mild and transient, though many individuals experience severe and persistent symptoms that cause considerable personal distress and impair social and occupational function. A distinction is often made between physical (or 'somatic') symptoms, which mainly result from autonomic arousal or muscular tension (for example, shortness of breath, palpitations, tremor, and headache) and psychological (or 'psychic') symptoms, including apprehension, irritability, and worrying.

Anxiety symptoms are common among patients undergoing examination, investigation, and medical or surgical treatment but are also frequent in community settings in physically well individuals. If distressing and impairing anxiety exceeds specified severity thresholds and persists beyond minimum duration requirements, and providing its symptoms are not explicable by another condition, an anxiety disorder can be diagnosed. These disorders share common psychological and physical symptoms but differ in the characteristic features that aid specific diagnosis (Table 92.1), for example recurrent unexpected panic attacks in panic disorder or the fear of embarrassment and humiliation in social anxiety disorder. Accurate delineation of a suspected anxiety disorder can be challenging, but a simple algorithm can aid diagnosis (Fig. 92.1). Differential diagnosis from depression and other mental disorders is usually simple (Table 92.2).

## Treatment need and treatment choice

Some people with anxiety receive unnecessary or inappropriate treatment, as mild symptoms of recent onset and associated with stressful events will often improve spontaneously. However, the persistence and associated disability of anxiety disorders means that most patients who meet criteria for diagnosis are likely to benefit from pharmacological or psychological interventions. Unfortunately, many patients who could benefit from treatment are not recognized. The need for treatment should be determined by ascertaining the severity and persistence of symptoms, their impact on everyday life, the level of coexisting depressive symptoms, and other features such as a previous good response to medication or psychotherapy [1].

The choice of treatment is influenced by clinical characteristics, patient and doctor preferences, and the local availability of potential interventions. There is much overlap across anxiety disorders for evidence-based effective therapies—such as prescription of a selective serotonin reuptake inhibitor (SSRI) or a course of individual cognitive behavioural therapy (CBT)—but there are

**Table 92.1** Characteristic features of anxiety disorders

| | |
|---|---|
| Generalized anxiety disorder | Prolonged excessive worrying that is not restricted to particular circumstances. Worries often centre on possible physical ill health affecting themselves or family members, and patients can repeatedly present with medically unexplained physical symptoms or craving reassurance or requesting medical investigations. |
| Panic disorder | Recurrent unexpected surges of severe anxiety ('panic attacks'), which typically reach a peak within 10 minutes and last around 30–45 minutes. Patients may believe they are in imminent danger of death or collapse and seek urgent medical attention. |
| Agoraphobia | Fear and avoidance of public spaces and other situations (crowds, transportation) from which immediate escape may be difficult; in clinical samples, most patients also have expected panic attacks and some have comorbid panic disorder. |
| Social anxiety disorder (social phobia) | Marked and persistent fear of being observed or evaluated negatively by other people, in social or performance situations. Many avoid consulting doctors, but some present with physical symptoms (such as excessive perspiration) or psychological symptoms (such as fear of vomiting in public). |
| Simple phobia | Excessive or unreasonable fear of (and restricted to) single people, animals, objects, or situations (for example, dentists, spiders, lifts, flying, seeing blood), which are either avoided or are endured with significant personal distress. |
| Separation anxiety disorder | Fear or anxiety concerning separation from those to whom an individual is attached; common features include excessive distress when experiencing or anticipating separation from home and persistent excessive worries about potential harms to attachment figures or untoward events that might result in separation. |

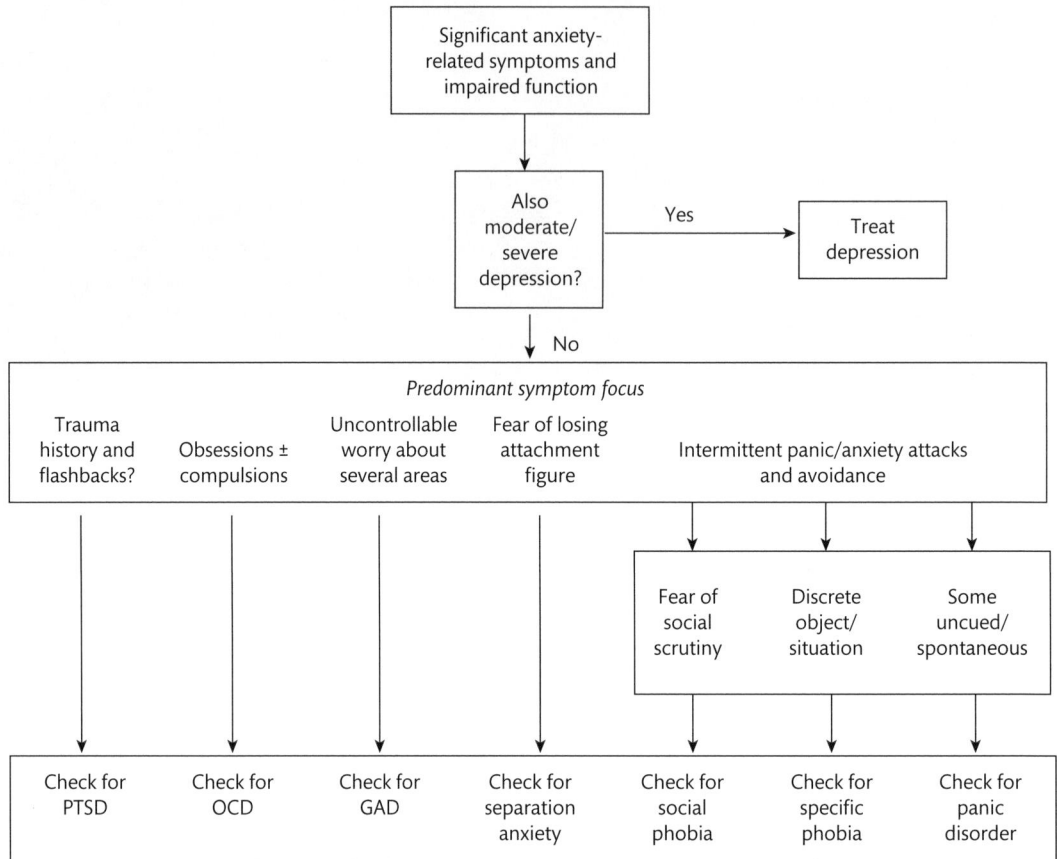

**Fig. 92.1** Suggested scheme for exploring a suspected anxiety disorder.

differences in treatment response between disorders, and it helps to be familiar with the evidence base for each condition (Table 92.3). Depressive symptoms often accompany anxiety disorders; around one-third of people with anxiety disorders also fulfil diagnostic criteria for a depressive episode. Treatment of depression will usually relieve anxiety symptoms when depression is the primary diagnosis, but if depression is comorbid or follows an anxiety disorder, each condition requires separate consideration and often specific treatment [1].

### Pharmacological and psychological treatments

The overall efficacy of psychological and pharmacological approaches in acute treatment of anxiety disorders has been regarded as broadly similar, although the findings of a recent meta-analysis have questioned this assumption [2]. The strongest evidence for acute treatment is for judicious prescription of an SSRI or undertaking manualized CBT delivered by trained and supervised staff. It is uncertain whether combining these approaches is associated with greater improvement than with either treatment given alone, at least in some disorders. Sequential steps in patient management, such as the 'stepped care' approach recommended by the National Institute for Health and Care Excellence (NICE), are recommended if a patient does not respond to first-line approaches [3]. Continuation treatment, following a satisfactory response to acute treatment (ideally resulting in remission of symptoms), is needed in all patients with anxiety disorders to consolidate the response and reduce the risk of relapse. It has been argued that psychological treatments

may be more effective than pharmacological treatments in keeping patients well, though the evidence to support this view is limited and has been questioned.

Many patients worry about starting and continuing pharmacological treatment, fearing problems such as unwanted sedation, weight gain, or the potential risk of becoming dependent on prescribed medication. By contrast, others are reluctant to engage in a psychological treatment that is often limited in availability, emotionally intrusive, and time-consuming. Regardless of the recommended treatment modality, patients should be advised that transient worsening of symptoms can occur and that prolonged efforts are needed to consolidate and maintain an initial response to treatment.

### Access to treatment and referral to psychiatric services

Stigma influences the perception of psychiatric illness and its treatment. Patients with anxiety disorders may fear being dismissed as having minor 'lifestyle' complaints and can be discouraged from seeking help and undergoing treatment. Many patients may receive conflicting messages about the benefits and risks of pharmacological treatment. Similarly, access to evidence-based psychological treatments is often prioritized for those with 'severe and enduring mental illnesses' such as schizophrenia, though this rationing reflects the widespread failure to recognize the impairment and chronicity of many anxiety disorders.

Most patients with anxiety disorders can be managed effectively within primary care, but some need the extra expertise of secondary

**Table 92.2** Important common differential diagnoses in anxiety disorders

| Condition | Differentiation from anxiety disorder |
|---|---|
| Depressive illness | Early morning waking, feeling worse in the morning, loss of capacity for pleasure, constipation, guilty thoughts, and suicidal thoughts all suggest depression, rather than anxiety. Depressive symptoms in anxiety disorders tend to develop after the psychological and somatic symptoms that characterize the anxiety disorder (for example, anticipation of embarrassment, anxiety, and avoidance in social phobia). |
| Psychotic illness | Delusions, hallucinations, and thought disorder are not seen in patients with primary anxiety disorders. |
| Psychostimulant use | Use of amphetamines, ecstasy, cocaine, and hallucinogens can all result in agitation and severe anxiety, including panic attacks. Primacy of drug-seeking behaviour and physical signs of intoxication (such as stereotypic movements with amphetamine use) support the diagnosis of drug dependency. Excess consumption of caffeine-containing drugs can result in physical and psychological symptoms of anxiety. Many novel psychoactive substances can cause anxiety, but their full effects are still not established. |
| Drug withdrawal | Abrupt withdrawal of opiates, alcohol, barbiturates, benzodiazepines, or antidepressants can result in agitation, tremor, dizziness, gastrointestinal upset, and insomnia. Anxiety disorders are not associated with acute confusional states or with marked autonomic instability. Characteristic physical signs are seen after withdrawal from certain drug classes such as pupillary dilatation when withdrawing from opiates. |
| Physical ill health | Anxiety symptoms are common in many physical health problems and can be the presenting feature (for example, in thyrotoxicosis, recurrent hypoglycaemia, complex partial seizures, paroxysmal tachycardia, and phaeochromocytoma). |

care mental health services. Referral criteria will vary, depending on service availability. It seems reasonable to expect that patients should be referred by general practitioners to secondary care services when there is uncertainty regarding a possible underlying diagnosis (such as schizophrenia), after the non-response to two evidence-based acute treatment approaches, when there has been a recurrence of symptoms despite continuing treatment, when anxiety disorders are comorbid with other disorders (for example, depression or substance use), when there is a risk of suicide, or when there is a need for specialist intervention (for example, dopamine antagonist augmentation after a partial response to an SSRI) [1].

## Generalized anxiety disorder

Generalized anxiety disorder (GAD) is characterized by excessive worrying, lasting more than 6 months and not restricted to particular circumstances (for example, only when attending a social gathering). Common features include apprehension, tension, and difficulty in concentrating, and autonomic symptoms such as dry mouth and abdominal discomfort. GAD is one of the most common mental disorders in primary care but is often not recognized, possibly because only a minority of patients present with its characteristic psychological symptoms. The most important differential diagnosis is depressive illness (although GAD and major depression often occur together), and patients should be asked about key depressive symptoms such as reduced interest, loss of weight, and suicidal thoughts, but distinction between the two conditions can be difficult.

Psychological and pharmacological treatments have broadly similar efficacy. Based on efficacy, safety, and tolerability, first-line pharmacological treatment will usually involve an SSRI, a serotonin–noradrenaline reuptake inhibitor (SNRI), or pregabalin (a calcium channel modulator). Once a drug is started, patients should be treated for a minimum of 4 weeks before deciding whether or not that treatment is working. If no response is seen after this time, increasing the dosage or switching to an alternative treatment may be advisable. The optimal duration of any drug treatment remains unclear, but a minimum of 12 months' further treatment is recommended in patients who have responded to medication [1].

A meta-analysis suggests fluoxetine may be the most likely drug for achieving response and symptomatic remission, while sertraline is the best tolerated [4]. Neither is currently licensed for treatment of GAD in the UK, though NICE recommends sertraline as initial treatment. At present, five medications are licensed for GAD in the UK: escitalopram and paroxetine (both are SSRIs), duloxetine and venlafaxine (both are SNRIs), and pregabalin. Among these drugs, the same meta-analysis found duloxetine was most likely to produce a beneficial response, escitalopram most likely to establish symptom remission, and pregabalin most likely to be best tolerated. Relative to SSRIs or SNRIs, pregabalin might have an earlier onset of effect. It also reduces the sleep disturbance commonly seen in GAD, both directly and indirectly, via the reduction of anxiety. It is generally tolerated well (although dizziness and drowsiness are common during acute treatment), is eliminated unchanged in the urine and has few drug interactions, and has a low rate of discontinuation symptoms

**Table 92.3** Summary of possible treatment options in anxiety disorders

| | Generalized anxiety disorder | Panic disorder with/without agoraphobia | Specific phobia | Social anxiety disorder |
|---|---|---|---|---|
| **First line** | | | | |
| Psychological | CBT | CBT | Exposure-based therapy | CBT |
| Pharmacological | SSRI | SSRI | SSRI | SSRI |
| **Second line** | | | | |
| Psychological | Applied relaxation | Supportive psychotherapy | CBT | Combination (CBT + SSRI) |
| Pharmacological | SSRI, SNRI, pregabalin | SSRI, SNRI | SSRI | SSRI, SNRI, SSRI plus benzodiazepine |
| **Third line** | | | | |
| Psychological | Uncertain | Combination (CBT + SSRI) | Uncertain | Uncertain |
| Pharmacological | Agomelatine, buspirone, quetiapine, TCA, benzodiazepine | Psychodynamic psychotherapy TCA, MAOI, benzodiazepine | Uncertain | MAOI, pregabalin, benzodiazepine |

No randomized controlled trials of adult separation anxiety disorder are currently published (August 2017).

[5]. However, concern has been raised about the possible risks of dependence and abuse [6].

Dopamine–serotonin antagonists, particularly quetiapine, have been investigated in GAD, both as monotherapy and as adjuncts to antidepressants. A potential benefit is an earlier onset of action, but this must be balanced against potential adverse effects such as metabolic syndrome. Use of quetiapine is therefore mainly limited to a second-line role, but it might be appropriate to use quetiapine in primary care in this way as long as the clinician feels s/he has sufficient experience and competence. Agomelatine, which acts as an agonist at melatonin MT1 and MT2 receptors and as an antagonist at $5HT_{2C}$ receptors, is generally well tolerated and has no significant discontinuation symptoms and relatively few drug interactions, when compared with SSRIs and SNRIs. Agomelatine is also efficacious in GAD, both in acute treatment and in preventing relapse [7]. Due to its mechanism of action, it may be particularly beneficial in patients with marked sleep disturbance. Preclinical studies with the novel 'multimodal' antidepressant drug vortioxetine suggested potential anxiolytic effects, and it reduces anxiety symptoms in depressed patients; however, despite its efficacy in preventing relapse, randomized placebo-controlled trials of acute treatment of GAD have produced inconsistent findings [8]. Vilazodone has both SSRI and $5\text{-HT}_{1A}$ partial agonist properties and is effective in acute treatment of GAD [9]; it may have an advantage, compared with SSRI or SNRI treatment, in having a lower incidence of treatment-emergent sexual dysfunction.

There is uncertainty about how best to proceed after a non-response to first-line treatment. A pragmatic approach suggests employing a further monotherapy before proceeding to augmentation strategies. Other efficacious drugs (usually reserved for specialist psychiatric treatment) include benzodiazepines (alprazolam, diazepam), imipramine, and the $5\text{-HT}_{1A}$ partial agonist buspirone. Clinicians and patients have concerns about the use of benzodiazepines, mainly the long-term risk of dependence, though this risk has to be weighed against the potential relief an individual with chronic, severe, distressing, and disabling symptoms might derive from intermittent use or more prolonged treatment [10]. When attempting to relieve acute exacerbations of symptoms, a short-acting benzodiazepine (for example, lorazepam) may be preferable to a longer-acting alternative due to its more rapid onset of effect and a lower risk of sedation. A prescriber should evaluate the likelihood of developing problematic use before issuing a first or subsequent prescription [11] (Box 92.1); for example, individuals who abuse drugs and/or alcohol and those with chaotic lifestyles are more likely to develop long-term problems with benzodiazepines.

Many psychological treatments have been investigated in GAD, but CBT and applied relaxation have the strongest supporting evidence.

CBT offers an effective alternative to pharmacological treatments and can help around half of patients with GAD to achieve significant symptom reduction and to improve their level of functioning. Although other psychological approaches may produce some benefit, relapse rates over the longer term are probably lower with CBT [12]. However, CBT may be less efficacious in older adults than in adults of 'working age' [13]. Augmentation of escitalopram treatment with CBT is more effective in reducing worrying than escitalopram alone, but there is at present minimal evidence for an additional benefit when combining other

> **Box 92.1** Predictors of the risk of dependence upon benzodiazepines
>
> 1 Participation in self-help group for medication dependence
> 2 Younger age
> 3 Longer duration of use
> 4 Higher dose use
> 5 Lower level of education
> 6 Non-native cultural origin
> 7 Outpatient treatment for alcohol and/or drug dependence
> 8 Short duration of elimination half-life
> 9 Higher levels of depression and anxiety
>
> Reproduced from *Compr Psychiatry*, 45(2), Kan CC, Hilberink SR, Breteler MH, Determination of the main risk factors for benzodiazepine dependence using a multivariate and multidimensional approach, pp 88–94, Copyright (2004), with permission from Elsevier Inc.

pharmacological and psychological treatments, although this is often done in practice.

## Panic disorder with or without agoraphobia

Accurate diagnosis depends on establishing the presence of recurrent unexpected panic attacks, with relative freedom from anxiety (at least initially) between these attacks, together with associated concern, worry, or change in behaviour. Coexisting depressive symptoms are common, and patients with comorbid depressive episodes are typically more impaired by symptoms, make greater use of health services, and have a worse prognosis. Panic disorder can occur with or without agoraphobia—anxiety in feared situations from which escape might prove difficult or embarrassing—and agoraphobia can either precede or follow the development of panic attacks.

Treatment is aimed at achieving complete recovery from panic attacks, resolution of anticipatory anxiety (fearful expectation of attacks), and abolition of agoraphobia [1]. Panic attacks can be shortened by rebreathing exhaled air, which corrects the abnormal blood chemistry that arises from rapid shallow breathing. In established panic disorder, psychological and pharmacological interventions are helpful. As with GAD, NICE guidance for panic disorder recommends a stepwise approach to patient management.

SSRIs are the preferred first-line drug treatments in primary care, as they cause less drowsiness and carry lower risks of tolerance and dependence than benzodiazepines. In secondary care, treatments include venlafaxine, the selective noradrenaline reuptake inhibitor reboxetine, and the tricyclic antidepressants (TCAs) imipramine and clomipramine. Certain SSRIs, venlafaxine, some TCAs, and the reversible monoamine oxidase inhibitor (MAOI) moclobemide have demonstrated long-term efficacy in clinical trials, though SSRIs tend to be better tolerated. Patients must follow a restricted diet while taking an MAOI, and these compounds are therefore reserved for second- or third-line treatment.

There are few studies to guide pharmacological management of treatment resistance, but several strategies may be beneficial. These include augmentation of fluoxetine with the beta-blocker pindolol, switching to an agent that acts via different receptors (for example, non-responders to citalopram could be switched to reboxetine, and vice versa), augmentation of a TCA with fluoxetine or augmentation of fluoxetine with a TCA, combination therapy with sodium valproate and clonazepam, or augmentation of clomipramine with lithium.

Psychological and pharmacological interventions have broadly similar efficacy and acceptability [14]. A network meta-analysis indicates that CBT is probably superior to other psychological treatments, though non-specific supportive psychotherapy also appears efficacious and psychodynamic psychotherapy may have fewer associated dropouts from treatment [15]. Routinely combining CBT with medication as a first-line approach in all patients is not recommended, but findings from a meta-analysis suggest that combining CBT with drug treatment can enhance the efficacy of CBT. CBT alone may be more cost-effective than either SSRI alone or SSRI when combined with CBT [16].

## Specific (simple) phobia

Specific fears of particular objects, animals, or situations are very common, but only a minority of affected people present for treatment, this often being at the time of changes in domestic or career responsibilities. The impairment associated with specific phobia is usually limited, but the presence of comorbid specific phobia in other anxiety disorders or depression can increase their associated disability. The effectiveness and acceptability of psychological or pharmacological treatments for specific phobia are less well researched than in other anxiety disorders.

A meta-analysis of randomized controlled trials indicated that exposure-based therapies (particularly those involving *in vivo* exposure) are more effective than other psychological interventions—effectiveness being seen regardless of the nature of the phobia, and greater with multiple, rather than single, sessions [17]. Patients with 'blood-injury phobia' can develop hypotension and bradycardia during exposure sessions, so they may require additional muscular tension exercises to benefit fully from treatment. Most patients respond to a few treatment sessions based on exposure techniques, but SSRI treatment (escitalopram, paroxetine) is helpful when patients have not responded to exposure therapy. It is unclear if concomitant benzodiazepine use enhances or reduces the efficacy of exposure therapy. Efficacy may be increased marginally by d-cycloserine administration prior to a session, though not all evidence is consistent [18].

## Social anxiety disorder (social phobia)

Social anxiety disorder is characterized by the intense, persistent fear of being scrutinized or evaluated negatively by others. Patients anticipate ridicule or humiliation and either avoid many social situations or endure them with great distress. Some experience panic attacks, but the condition can be distinguished from panic disorder, as in social phobia, the attacks occur expectedly in feared situations. Furthermore, in panic disorder, the presence of a friend typically provides some reassurance, but in social phobia, this makes little difference. Shyness is a core symptom of social phobia, though this should be distinguished from healthy individuals who are merely shy and typically experience little anxiety, functioning well at home and at work. A significant proportion of patients develop depression, and differentiating the disorders can sometimes be difficult, but in social phobia, the capacity to enjoy oneself remains and energy levels are not impaired significantly. Many patients use alcohol or other drugs in an attempt to quell anxiety symptoms prior to a social encounter.

Medications with proven efficacy in acute treatment include most SSRIs (escitalopram, fluoxetine, fluvoxamine, paroxetine, and sertraline), venlafaxine, the MAOIs phenelzine and moclobemide,

some benzodiazepines (bromazepam, clonazepam), some anticonvulsants (gabapentin, pregabalin), and olanzapine. There is little evidence of a dose–response relationship in acute treatment. Response is more likely in patients whose symptoms have reduced in intensity within 2 weeks of starting treatment. Beta-blockers can reduce physical symptoms of anxiety in some discrete performance activities (for example, acting or singing), but they do not help in patients with generalized social phobia who fear and avoid multiple social situations. As with GAD, SSRI treatment is usually regarded as being first line, based on efficacy, tolerability, and safety [1].

CBT is the most established psychological treatment. A network meta-analysis of the comparative efficacy of pharmacological and psychological treatments indicated that SSRIs and venlafaxine are superior to pill placebo, and CBT superior to 'psychological placebo' (that is, non-specific psychological intervention) [19]. In one study, the combination of phenelzine and group CBT was more effective than either treatment given alone, on measures of both response and remission, but there is inconsistent evidence regarding whether the combination of CBT with medication is associated with greater improvement than with either treatment given alone [20].

SAD is typically a long-lasting condition, and successful response to acute treatment should be followed by at least 6 months of continuation treatment, in order to consolidate recovery and prevent an early relapse of symptoms. However, relapse prevention studies demonstrating the long-term efficacy of pharmacological treatments (escitalopram, paroxetine, sertraline, pregabalin) are limited. Patients who make only a limited initial response to CBT may benefit if further CBT is combined with medication, and those who respond only partially to pharmacological treatment may benefit if further drug treatment is combined with CBT. Combination of an SSRI (sertraline) with a benzodiazepine (clonazepam) has been found superior to continuing with sertraline alone or switching to venlafaxine [21].

## Separation anxiety disorder

Differential diagnosis between separation anxiety disorder and panic disorder is difficult, but in patients with the former, the primary concern is fear of separation, rather than fear of a panic attack. Furthermore, patients with panic disorder are preoccupied with their personal health and safety, whereas individuals with separation anxiety disorder are concerned for the well-being of their attachment figures. Differential diagnosis between separation anxiety disorder and GAD can also be troublesome, as worrying that something bad might happen to loved ones is a feature common to the two conditions. Distinction largely rests on establishing that in GAD, the fear and worry of losing loved ones is just one of a wide range of worrisome themes, whereas in separation anxiety disorder, the central and often only concern is fear of, and worry about, losing a major attachment figure. Other important differential diagnoses include dependent personality disorder, emotionally unstable personality disorder, and morbid jealousy [22].

The efficacy of psychological or pharmacological treatment in adults with separation anxiety disorder has not been studied extensively, and treatment studies in children have often involved mixed diagnostic groups. The findings of randomized, placebo-controlled trials of pharmacological treatment in children with separation anxiety disorder provide no convincing evidence of benefit for any medication. However, the SSRIs fluvoxamine and sertraline have been found efficacious among the separation anxiety disorder subgroup of patients within mixed diagnostic samples. Psychological treatment studies in children find some evidence of benefit with CBT, parent–child interaction training, and 'summer camp' programmes [23].

## Room for improvement in the treatment of anxiety disorders

A wide range of options is available for the pharmacological and psychological treatment of patients with anxiety disorders. Current recommendations included within evidence-based guidelines and consensus statements are derived mainly from the findings of randomized, double-blind controlled trials, which suggested robust efficacy and generally good tolerability for many interventions, both in acute treatment and in preventing relapse. However, the patient groups that participate in randomized controlled trials may have a better prognosis than patients treated in 'real-world' clinical settings. In routine practice, response rates to initial treatment can be disappointing; many patients will experience unwanted effects during treatment; others will relapse despite adhering to treatment, and some will be affected by troublesome discontinuation symptoms. Furthermore, at present, it is not possible for doctors to predict the likelihood of a treatment response in an individual patient with great accuracy, and there are continuing uncertainties about optimal steps in the further management of patients after non-response to first-line treatment approaches.

For the time being, attempts to optimize clinical outcomes rest largely on making the best use of currently available treatments. However, there is much room for improvement in the pharmacological and psychological treatment of anxiety disorders. Improvements in clinical outcomes could result from the development and arrival of approaches with novel mechanisms of action, leading to greater efficacy and improved acceptability in all patient groups. Alternatively, novel treatments could lead to enhanced effectiveness and higher acceptability in certain specific patient subgroups, when combined with the use of reliable biomarkers for identifying which individuals are most likely to benefit.

## REFERENCES

1. Baldwin DS, Anderson IM, Nutt DJ, et al. Evidence-based pharmacological treatment of anxiety disorders, post-traumatic stress disorder and obsessive-compulsive disorder: a revision of the 2005 guidelines from the British Association for Psychopharmacology. Journal of Psychopharmacology 2014; 28: 403–39.
2. Bandelow B, Reitt M, Röver C, Michaelis S, Görlich Y, Wedekind D. Efficacy of treatments for anxiety disorders: a meta-analysis. International Clinical Psychopharmacology 2015; 30: 183–92.
3. Ho FY, Yeung WF, Ng TH, Chan CS. The efficacy and cost-effectiveness of stepped care prevention and treatment for depressive and anxiety disorders: a systematic review and meta-analysis. Scientific Reports 2016; 6: 29821.
4. Baldwin DS, Woods R, Lawson R, Taylor D. Efficacy of drug treatments for generalised anxiety disorder: systematic review and meta-analysis. BMJ 2011; 342: d1199.
5. Baldwin DS, den Boer JA, Lyndon G, Emir B, Schweizer E, Haswell H. Efficacy and safety of pregabalin in generalized anxiety disorder: a critical review of the literature. Journal of Psychopharmacology 2015; 29: 1047–60.
6. Schjerning O, Rosenzweig M, Pottegard A, Damkier P, Nielsen J. Abuse potential a pregabalin: a systematic review. CNS Drugs 2016; 30: 9–25.
7. Buoli M, Grassi S, Serati M, Altamura AC. Agomelatine for the treatment of generalized anxiety disorder. Expert Opinion on Pharmacotherapy 2017; 28: 1–7.
8. Pae CU, Wang SM, Han C, Lee SJ, Patkar AA, Masand PS, Serretti A. Vortioxetine, a multimodal antidepressant for generalized anxiety disorder: a systematic review and meta-analysis. Journal of Psychiatric Research 2015; 64: 88–98.
9. Khan A, Durgam S, Tang X, Ruth A, Mathews M, Gommoll CP. Post hoc analyses of anxiety measures in adult patients with generalized anxiety disorder treated with vilazodone. Primary Care Companion for CNS Disorders 2016; 18(2). Doi: 10.4088?PCC.15m01904.eCollection 2016.
10. Baldwin DS, Aitchison K, Bateson A, et al. Benzodiazepines: risks and benefits. A reconsideration. Journal of Psychopharmacology 2013; 27: 967–71.
11. Kan CC, Hilberink SR, Breteler MH. Determination of the main risk factors for benzodiazepine dependence using a multivariate and multidimensional approach. Comprehensive Psychiatry 2004; 45: 88–94.
12. Cuijpers P, Sijbrandij M, Koole S, Huibers M, Berking M, Andersson G. Psychological treatment of generalized anxiety disorder: a meta-analysis. Clinical Psychology Review 2014; 34: 130–40.
13. Kishita N, Laidlaw K. Cognitive behavior therapy for generalized anxiety disorder: is CBT equally efficacious in adults of working age and older adults? Clinical Psychological Review 2017; 52: 124–36.
14. Imai H, Tajika A, Chen P, Pompoli A, Furukawa TA. Psychological therapies versus pharmacological interventions for panic disorder with or without agoraphobia in adults. Cochrane Database of Systematic Reviews 2016; 10: CD011170.
15. Pompoli A, Furukawa TA, Imai H, Tajika A, Efthimiou O, Salanti G. Psychological therapies for panic disorder with or without agoraphobia in adults: a network meta-analysis. Cochrane Database of Systematic Reviews 2016; 4: CD011004.
16. van Appledoorn FJ, Stant AD, van Hout WJ, Mersch PP, den Boer JA. Cost-effectiveness of CBT, SSRI and CBT+SSRI in the treatment for panic disorder. Acta Psychiatrica Scandinavica 2014; 129: 286–95.
17. Wolitzky-Taylor KB, Horowitz JD, Poewres MB, Telch MJ. Psychological approaches in the treatment of specific phobias: a meta-analysis. Clinical Psychology Reviews 2008; 28: 1021–37.
18. Mataix-Cols D, Fernandez de la Cruz L, Monzani B, et al. D-cycloserine augmentation of exposure-based cognitive therapy for anxiety, obsessive-compulsive, and post-traumatic stress disorders: a systematic review and meta-analysis of individual participant data. JAMA Psychiatry 2017; 74: 501–10.
19. Mayo-Wilson E, Dias S, Mavranezouli I, et al. Psychological and pharmacological interventions for social anxiety disorder in adults: a systematic review and network meta-analysis. Lancet Psychiatry 2014; 1: 368–76.
20. Canton J, Scott KM, Glue P. Optimal treatment of social phobia: systematic review and meta-analysis. Neuropsychiatric Disease and Treatment 2012; 8: 203–15.
21. Pollack MH, Van Ameringen M, Simon NM, et al. A double-blind randomized controlled trial of augmentation and switch strategies for refractory social anxiety disorder. American Journal of Psychiatry 2014; 171: 44–53.
22. Baldwin DS, Gordon R, Abelli M, Pini S. The separation of separation anxiety disorder. CNS Spectrums 2016; 21: 289–94.
23. Ehrenreich J, Santucci LC, Weiner CL. Separation anxiety disorder in youth: phenomenology, assessment, and treatment. Psicologia Conductual 2008; 1: 389–412.

# SECTION 5

# Obsessive-compulsive and related disorders

# 93

# Core dimensions of obsessive–compulsive disorder

*Sophie C. Schneider, Eric A. Storch, and Wayne K. Goodman*

## Introduction

Obsessive–compulsive disorder (OCD) was once thought to be a relatively rare disorder; however, the lifetime population prevalence is now estimated at 2.3% [1]. Sustained research efforts have led to a better understanding of the aetiology, presentation, and treatment of OCD. However, debate continues regarding the conceptualization and classification of OCD in diagnostic systems. Further, there is increasing recognition that OCD is a clinically heterogenous disorder, and thus treating OCD as a unitary disorder may obscure important aetiological and clinical variables. This has led to an interest in identifying subtypes and dimensions of OCD and examining dimension-specific associations between OCD and important constructs.

## Classification of OCD

Historically, OCD was classified as an anxiety-related disorder due to similarities between OCD and anxiety disorders across core symptoms of fear and avoidance, cognitive styles, and response to pharmacological and psychological therapies [2]. However, a competing conceptualization of OCD is that it belongs to a separate group of disorders characterized by repetitive thoughts and behaviours, often referred to as the obsessive–compulsive spectrum [3]. Evidence supporting this approach has emerged from studies of genetic risk factors, comorbidity, familial transmission, neuroanatomical correlates, neuropsychological functioning, and treatment response [4, 5]. Despite initially proposing the creation of a shared anxiety and obsessive–compulsive spectrum [6], the fifth edition of the *Diagnostic and Statistical Manual of Mental Disorders* (DSM-5) [4] saw the creation of a separate 'Obsessive–Compulsive and Related Disorders' (OCRD) chapter, placed after the 'Anxiety Disorders' chapter. The DSM-5 OCRD chapter includes OCD, body dysmorphic disorder, hoarding disorder, trichotillomania (hair pulling disorder), excoriation (skin picking disorder), and other specified and unspecified OCRDs. A similar OCRD chapter is proposed for the forthcoming eleventh edition of the *International Classification of Diseases and Related Health Problems* (ICD-11), which will also include hypochondriasis and olfactory reference disorder [5].

The creation of a separate OCRD chapter is not without criticism, particularly regarding the close relationship between OCD and the anxiety disorders, the limited evidence for the association between some OCRD disorders, and the distinctive presentation of excoriation and trichotillomania (for example, see [2] for a critique of the empirical validity of the DSM-5 OCRD chapter). Further research on the classification of OCD is clearly needed, especially given that some of the OCRD diagnoses are new or have been substantially changed, for example hoarding disorder and excoriation in DSM-5 and body dysmorphic disorder in ICD-11. Despite the ongoing debate about the classification of OCD, there is a strong consensus regarding the diagnostic criteria and clinical features of OCD.

## Clinical features of OCD

### Core symptoms

Obsessions are persistent and unwanted thoughts, images, or urges that evoke distress or negative affect such as anxiety, disgust, feelings of incompleteness, or unease [5, 7]. Individuals typically attempt to counteract obsessions, either by ignoring, resisting, or controlling them, avoiding things that may trigger the obsession, or by neutralizing their obsessions with a thought or action. Compulsions are repetitive behaviours or mental acts performed in response to an obsession, to achieve a feeling of completeness or rightness, or following very specific rules. Compulsions are unrealistic or excessive and function to relieve distress or negative affect or to prevent a feared outcome from occurring. Compulsions can include observable behaviours, such as rearranging items or excessive cleaning, or mental acts such as making mental lists, neutralizing unacceptable thoughts with 'good' thoughts, or praying in response to sexual thoughts [8]. Examples of common types of obsessions and compulsions are presented in Table 93.1.

Although a diagnosis of OCD only requires the presence of obsessions or compulsions, they co-occur in 99% of cases of OCD [8]. To meet diagnostic criteria, obsessions or compulsions must be

**Table 93.1** Examples of obsessive–compulsive disorder symptom dimensions

| Symptom type | Obsession | Compulsion |
| --- | --- | --- |
| Symmetry/ordering | Uncomfortable sensation that things do not 'feel right'; for example, household objects are misaligned | Touching, tapping, or rubbing things in special ways |
| Contamination/cleaning | Concern about developing cancer from environmental pollution | Repeated and excessing cleaning such as cleaning all household surfaces with bleach every day |
| Harm/aggression | I may be responsible for a murder | Checking that nothing bad happened, asking others if they are ok, checking the news for reports of murders |
| Sexual/religious | Unwanted images of violent sexual behaviour towards others | Praying over and over to prevent the sexual behaviour from occurring |
| Hoarding | Do not throw things away as they may be important in the future | Hoarding unusual items or excessive acquisition of objects like magazines |
| Miscellaneous | Intrusive non-sensical images, songs, or words | Getting stuck performing everyday tasks such as getting dressed, eating, and work tasks |

Source: data from *Mol Psychiatr.*, 11(5), Rosario-Campos MC, Miguel EC, Quatrano S, *et al.*, The Dimensional Yale-Brown Obsessive-Compulsive Scale (DY-BOCS): an instrument for assessing obsessive-compulsive symptom dimensions, pp. 495–504, Copyright (2006), Springer Nature.

associated with significant distress or impairment and usually occur for at least 1 hour per day [4]. Obsessions and compulsions should be carefully assessed to differentiate them from symptoms of other mental disorders, for example from worries as found in generalized anxiety disorder, appearance preoccupation in body dysmorphic disorder, and ritualized eating in eating disorders.

### Clinical correlates

Lifetime comorbidity is very common, reported by 90–92% of those with OCD [1, 9]. The most common types of comorbid disorders, as defined using the fourth edition of the *Diagnostic and Statistical Manual of Mental Disorders* [10], were anxiety disorders (70–76%), mood disorders (61–63%), impulse-control disorders (36–56%), and tic disorders (28%). The most common individual disorders were major depressive disorder (41–56%), social phobia (31–44%), specific phobia (31–43%), separation anxiety disorder (28–37%), alcohol use disorders (8–39%), and generalized anxiety disorder (8–34%). Further details are given in Chapter 95.

OCD is associated with high levels of functional impairment in both community [1] and clinical populations [11]. Individuals with OCD reported poor social functioning, particularly relating to social and leisure activities and romantic relationships [12]. Their social functioning quality of life was poorer than those with schizophrenia, panic disorder, or major depressive disorder [11]. This may be due to the excessive time spent on obsessions or compulsions and the often secretive nature of their symptoms. Suicidality appears to be relatively common in OCD; thoughts that life was not worth living were reported by 60% of those with OCD, 38% reported suicidal thoughts, 22% had suicidal plans, and 11% had attempted suicide [13].

Family accommodation of OCD symptoms is also common, whereby parents or partners of the affected individual engage in OCD-related behaviours such as washing their hands excessively, changing family routines to avoid triggering or exacerbating OCD symptoms, taking on responsibilities for the individual such as a child's chores, or providing reassurance [14].

OCD is typically a chronic disorder, with a 5-year full remission rate of 17% and a partial remission rate of 22%, and a relapse rate of 59% [15]. Chronic OCD was associated with longer illness duration, higher baseline OCD severity, and greater burden of illness [15, 16].

### Insight

Insight refers to the extent to which the individual recognizes that they are experiencing obsessions and compulsions, that these symptoms are excessive, and that their concerns are unrealistic [17]. Insight occurs on a spectrum—good or fair insight indicates that the individual recognizes that their OCD-related beliefs are untrue or that they may be false; poor insight indicates that the individual believes these are likely to be true, and absent insight or delusional beliefs indicate that the individual is convinced that their beliefs are true [4]. Although OCD with absent insight is often referred to as delusional OCD, it is not considered to be a psychotic disorder [4]. This is clinically important as those with delusional OCD should receive treatment recommended for OCD, rather than treatment indicated for psychotic disorders [18].

Absent or poor insight was reported in 9–22% of clinical samples and was associated with greater OCD severity and earlier OCD onset, a lower probability of achieving remission following treatment, and a need for a higher number of medication trials during treatment [8, 19, 20]. Poor insight can complicate the process of psychotherapy; thus, therapists should adapt the therapy content to the level of OCD insight, for example, including additional psychoeducation about insight, spending extra time on symptom identification, and adding additional sessions [17].

## Subtypes of OCD

OCD is a highly heterogenous disorder. The heterogeneity of OCD has led to concerns that treating OCD as a unitary disorder may obscure differential associations between OCD subtypes and aetiological factors, clinical features, and even treatment response [21]. This has led to efforts to identify meaningful subtypes of OCD based on specific clinical features.

### Tic-related OCD

Tics are particularly common in those with OCD, with a history of tics reported by 30–55% of youth with OCD [22, 23] and by 24% of adults with OCD [8]. Simple tics involve rapid and recurrent movements or sounds with no clear purpose such as jerking limbs, blinking eyes, grunting, or squeaking [24]. In contrast, complex tics involve repetitive behaviours that appear purposeful, such as touching and rubbing in certain ways, imitating people's mannerisms, or repeating phrases, and tics which are often elicited by specific stimuli. Tic-related OCD was characterized by a higher proportion of males, an earlier onset of OCD, and possibly with greater OCD severity and higher rates of some comorbid disorders [8, 22, 23, 25]. Tic-related OCD may be associated with lower overall efficacy of SSRIs and greater response to neuroleptic augmentation of SSRIs [25], but was not associated with differences in cognitive behavioural therapy (CBT) outcome [22, 23]. Due to the evidence that tics may be associated with distinctive clinical features, tic-related OCD was added as a specifier to DSM-5, and tic disorders will be cross-referenced with OCD in ICD-11 [4, 5].

### Age of onset

The mean age of OCD onset was reported at 19–22 years [1, 26], though symptoms are often present for several years before full disorder onset. Age of onset has been proposed to delineate subtypes, with studies suggesting that early onset may be associated with male gender, greater OCD severity, more symptoms of attention-deficit/hyperactivity disorder, lower rates of employment, and a greater probability of living alone in adulthood [26–28]. Conversely, later disorder onset is relatively rare, and onset after the age of 40 was associated with female gender, greater frequency of precipitating factors and traumatic events, and lower odds of a positive family history of OCD [26, 29]. Unfortunately, interpretation of age of onset findings across studies is complicated due to the use of different criteria for onset. Further, some studies divide participants based on pre-determined developmental groups such as child, adolescent, or adult, while others use statistical methods to determine group membership. Further research is needed before robust subtypes of OCD based on age of onset can be identified; thus, age of onset was not included as a specifier in DSM-5 [25].

### Symptom presentation

Many studies have attempted to classify participants based on the focus of their OCD symptoms, for example washing or checking. The most common measure used to assess OCD is the Yale-Brown Obsessive–Compulsive Scale (Y-BOCS), which contains checklists of obsessions and compulsions grouped into similar symptom types, and items assessing the severity of obsessions and compulsions [30]. Factor analysis of the Y-BOCS typically identifies four or five factors, and a meta-analysis of 21 studies reported a four-factor solution: (1) symmetry, repeating, ordering, and counting; (2) cleaning and contamination; (3) forbidden thoughts, aggression, sexual, religious, and somatic; and (4) hoarding [31]. These factors were similar across child, adolescent, and adult samples [32] and were temporally stable [33].

Another common measure for assessing OCD dimensions is the Dimensional Yale-Brown Obsessive–Compulsive Scale (DY-BOCS), which identifies six dimensions: (1) symmetry, 'just right', counting, and arranging; (2) contamination and cleaning; (3) harm content, including aggression, injury, violence, and accidents; (4) moral, sexual, and religious content; (5) hoarding; and (6) miscellaneous, including somatic and superstition [21].

A review of studies that classified participants according to their primary OCD symptoms found differences across treatment response, neuroimaging findings, and neuropsychological deficits [34]. However, 81% of those with OCD reported symptoms across multiple symptom groups [1], challenging the validity of assigning individuals into discreet symptom-specific groups. Instead, a multi-dimensional model of OCD symptoms has been proposed [35].

## A multi-dimensional approach to OCD symptoms

In the multi-dimensional model of OCD, symptoms are conceptualized as forming several overlapping dimensions based on the content of these symptoms [35]. Although there are some differences in the factors identified in the Y-BOCS and DY-BOCS, the following factors are the most robustly identified.

### Symmetry/ordering

Symmetry/ordering symptoms may be the most frequently reported OCD symptom type [9, 36] They involve obsessions about things being symmetrical or 'just right', for example the alignment of objects or needing school work to be done perfectly. Compulsions can involve rewriting over and over, performing actions a special number of times, or touching or tapping in specific ways. A review of studies found that symmetry/ordering symptoms have been associated with perfectionism, 'not just right' sensations, magical thinking, and compulsive slowness [37]. There may also be associations between symmetry/ordering and anger, suicide, and traumatic life events.

### Contamination/cleaning

Contamination/cleaning symptoms are often considered 'classic' symptoms of OCD. Contamination obsessions often involve concerns about contracting an illness or disease, sensations of being dirty or unclean, and fears of spreading contaminants to others. A wide range of contaminants can be feared such as germs, pollution, bodily fluids, and household/environmental chemicals. Individuals often go to great length to avoid dirty or contaminated objects, people, or situations and, when exposed to these, may compulsively and excessively clean themselves or contaminated objects. Contamination/cleaning symptoms may be closely associated with feelings of disgust, which can take longer to habituate than feelings of anxiety [37].

### Forbidden thoughts

Symptoms related to forbidden thoughts are sometimes identified as a single dimension [31], but they are often divided into separate dimensions [4, 21] of harm/aggression and sexual/religious symptoms. Harm/aggression symptoms include obsessions about causing harm to self or others, or other violent or aggressive acts occurring. Associated compulsions can include checking that the feared outcome did not occur or mental rituals to neutralize or distract from the thoughts. Sexual/religious obsessions involve religious taboos and blasphemy, morality, and improper sexual thoughts, and associated compulsions can involve ritualized praying and religious behaviour, avoidance of situations that may trigger the obsessions, and checking that the feared outcome did not occur.

Forbidden thoughts may vary from other OCD dimensions in their personal significance; for example, obsessions about sexually assaulting someone may be associated with greater shame and negative self-perceptions, compared to obsessions that are morally neutral such as symmetry concerns [38]. The fear of harming others may be associated with particularly severe social withdrawal, due to the feared outcomes of the obsessions [12]. Forbidden thought obsessions may also face a greater burden of stigma; individuals in the community are least likely to recognize forbidden thoughts as a symptom of OCD, compared to other symptom types, and community members report a greater level of fear and perceived dangerousness and a greater desire for social distance in those with forbidden thought symptoms, compared to other OCD symptoms [39].

## Other symptoms

Hoarding symptoms were initially considered a subtype of OCD and thus are included in OCD measures. However, hoarding disorder has since been established as a separate diagnosis due to its distinct genetic risk factors, phenotype, comorbidity patterns, and poor response to OCD-focused treatment [2, 40]. As hoarding is discussed in depth in Chapter 99, it will not be a focus of this chapter. The Y-BOCS and DY-BOCS also contain miscellaneous symptoms such as appearance obsessions, intrusive thoughts about numbers, and excessive list-making. The miscellaneous group of symptoms are generally not considered to be a discreet OCD dimension due to the heterogeneity of the symptom content and thus are not analysed in most studies.

## Evidence supporting the multi-dimensional model of OCD symptoms

The interest in identifying OCD symptom dimensions stemmed not only from a desire to better characterize the disorder, but also from the possibility that symptom dimensions may have differential associations with important aetiological and clinical factors. Evidence supporting the multi-dimensional model of OCD has been reported across a diverse range of research areas. A summary of key findings is presented, but note that the identified symptom dimensions vary somewhat across studies, depending on the measures and methodology used.

## Genetics and family history

The familial transmission of OCD has long been recognized, with twin studies and family linkage studies indicating that OCD involves polygenic influences, likely on serotonergic, glutamatergic, and dopaminergic neural systems [41]. For a full discussion of the genetics of OCD, see Chapter 96. A small number of studies have explored dimension-specific familial and genetic associations. In sibling pairs with OCD, forbidden thought symptoms had the highest sibling concordance, whereas other symptoms were weakly or non-significantly associated [42]. Interestingly, sibling associations were strongest among female pairs, and weaker in male and cross-sex pairs. In OCD patients, those with a family history of OCD were more likely to report symptoms of contamination/cleaning and symmetry/ordering than those without a family history of OCD [43]. A population study of Brazilian children also reported familial transmission of OCD symptom dimensions, with the strongest familiality found for contamination/cleaning symptoms [36]. Another family history study found specific familial transmission of contamination/cleaning symptoms, but not of other symptom types [44].

Studies of the genetic heritability of OCD dimensions indicate both common and dimension-specific genetic influences. In one family history study, all OCD symptom dimensions were heritable, but specific genetic associations were found between forbidden thoughts and both contamination/cleaning and doubting symptoms [45]. A large twin study indicated that around 50% of the variance in OCD symptoms was due to genetic factors, that 30–35% of the genetic effect in checking, obsessing, and ordering symptoms was due to specific genetic factors, but that washing symptoms showed no specific genetic factors [40]. Another twin study found evidence of differential associations between OCD symptom dimensions and the genetic overlap with OCRD and anxiety disorders [46]. Specifically, sexual/religious and contamination/cleaning symptoms had a stronger genetic association with anxiety disorders than with OCRDs; symmetry/ordering and harm/aggression symptoms had a stronger association with OCRDs than anxiety disorders, and symmetry/ordering showed a high proportion of specific genetic factors. In most cases, common genetic factors were strongest when considering both anxiety disorders and OCRDs in the models. Single gene studies have also reported dimension-specific associations; symmetry/ordering symptoms were associated with the DRD4 dopamine receptor gene [47], and washing symptoms with the HTR3E serotonin receptor gene [48].

## Neuroanatomy and neuropsychology

Abnormalities in fronto-striatal functioning are robustly associated with OCD [41], and there appears to be dimension-specific associations with anatomical and functional differences in these brain regions [49]. In studies using whole-brain voxel-based morphometry, symmetry/ordering symptoms were associated with differences in the volume of the left lateral orbitofrontal cortex and insula, aggressive/checking symptoms with differences in insula volume, and washing symptoms with the volume of the premotor cortex [50]. Patterns of striatal functional connectivity also differ across the dimensions; aggressive symptoms were associated with decreased connectivity with the amygdala and increased connectivity with the ventromedial frontal cortex, whereas sexual/religious symptoms were associated with greater connectivity between the ventral caudate and the mid and anterobasal insular cortex [51]. Further, heightened amygdala activation to fearful faces was associated with increased severity of aggressive/checking and sexual/religious symptoms, suggesting that these types of symptoms may be particularly related to abnormal fear processes [52]. Theories of psychopathology are now increasingly informed by neuroscience (see Chapters 94 and 97).

There is also evidence of dimension-specific neuropsychological deficits. Contamination/washing symptoms were associated with deficits in visuo-spatial skills, working memory and attention, and impulsive response patterns; checking was associated with deficits in association learning, and symmetry with poorer verbal fluency; and forbidden thoughts with improved performance on attention and working memory and visuo-spatial scanning [53]. Symmetry/ordering symptoms have been associated with specific forms of neuropsychological impairment (for a review, see [54]); for example, in youth with OCD, symmetry/ordering symptoms are associated with greater deficits in non-verbal fluency, processing speed, and inhibition and switching [54].

## Clinical features

A range of clinical features have been associated with OCD symptom dimensions. In those seeking treatment for OCD, forbidden thoughts were associated with higher overall OCD severity, both before and after receiving CBT [38]. OCD-related insight also varied by dimension; higher scores for contamination symptoms predicted poorer insight, whereas higher forbidden thoughts scores predicted better insight [19]. There are also differences in the association between OCD dimensions and broader obsessive–compulsive cognitive domains; symmetry/ordering was specifically associated with perfectionism and intolerance of uncertainty cognitions, forbidden thoughts with importance and control of thoughts cognitions, and doubt/checking with cognitions related to increased responsibility and threat estimation [55]. Contamination/cleaning symptoms were not significantly associated with the examined obsessive–compulsive cognitive domains, suggesting either a lack of specific cognitive associations or associations with cognitions not assessed by the study measure.

Suicidal ideation and behaviours have been independently associated with symmetry/ordering symptoms [56] and with sexual/religious symptoms [57]. Sexual/religious symptoms were also associated with poorer social functioning [12]. Another study found specific associations between quality of life and OCD symptom dimensions; contamination/cleaning symptoms were associated with impairment in leisure, social, and health-related quality of life, symmetry/ordering symptoms with social quality of life, and forbidden thought symptoms with health-related quality of life [58].

The onset and course of OCD may also vary across symptom dimensions. In one study, early disorder onset was associated with religious and symmetry obsessions and repeating compulsions [27]. Symmetry concerns had the earliest age of onset of the dimensions, and the presence of forbidden thoughts was associated with a more fluctuating course of illness and reduced chances of reporting a deteriorating course [59]. Contamination/cleaning symptoms were associated with a chronic OCD course [16]. Primary harm obsessions have been associated with higher odds of OCD remission over time [15].

Some studies have explored the association of OCD symptom dimensions with other demographic variables. For example, those with tic-related OCD report an earlier age of onset for cleaning symptoms than those without tics [59]. Symptom dimensions may also vary by gender; females report a greater frequency and severity of harm/aggression and contamination/cleaning symptoms, whereas males report a greater frequency and severity of sexual/religious symptoms [13]. Although symmetry/ordering frequency did not differ by gender, it was reported as more severe by females.

There is also evidence that symptom dimensions may be associated with different comorbidity profiles [9]. Sexual/religious symptoms were specifically associated with mood disorders, panic/agoraphobia, social phobia, separation anxiety disorder, non-paraphilic sexual disorder, somatoform disorders, body dysmorphic disorder, and tic disorders. Harm/aggression symptoms were associated with comorbid post-traumatic stress disorder, separation anxiety, impulse control disorders, and excoriation. Contamination/cleaning was associated with hypochondriasis. Interestingly, there were no specific comorbidity associations for symmetry/ordering symptoms. In a different study of siblings with OCD, forbidden thoughts were associated with higher odds of comorbid major depressive and bipolar disorders, hypochondriasis, separation anxiety disorder, tic disorder, and body dysmorphic disorder; symmetry/ordering symptoms with higher odds of alcohol dependence, bulimia nervosa, and attention-deficit/hyperactivity disorder; and contamination/cleaning symptoms with separation anxiety disorder [42].

## Overview of findings

Studies have replicated a multi-dimensional model of OCD symptoms across individuals from different developmental stages, cultural backgrounds, and recruitment settings. Further, there is support for dimension-specific associations in genetic, neural, and clinical features of OCD. However, future research should focus on further characterizing the nature of these dimensions to resolve discrepancies across studies. Further development of assessment measures and statistical techniques is also required to better assess these dimensions. Consistency in identified dimensions will allow clearer comparisons across studies and may help to clarify associations with meaningful clinical variables. Despite these limitations, there is evidence that OCD symptoms comprise several overlapping dimensions that have differential associations to important aetiological and clinical variables.

## Summary

Important research advances have led to an improved understanding of the core features of OCD and to the reclassification of OCD in DSM-5 and ICD-11. A core focus of OCD research has been to better understand the heterogenous presentation of the disorder, with the aim of identifying meaningful disorder subtypes. Studies attempting to classify participants using features like age of onset, tic status, or primary symptom types have largely been superseded by the multi-dimensional model of OCD symptoms. This notion that OCD symptoms can be understood as a number of overlapping symptom dimensions has received support across a wide range of studies. Further, there is evidence of dimension-specific associations across studies of family history and genetics, neuroanatomy and neuropsychological functioning, clinical features, and treatment response. The multi-dimensional model of OCD thus provides a framework for an improved understanding of OCD.

## REFERENCES

1. Ruscio AM, Stein DJ, Chiu WT, Kessler RC. The epidemiology of obsessive-compulsive disorder in the National Comorbidity Survey Replication. *Mol Psychiatry*. 2010;15:53–63.

2. Abramowitz JS, Jacoby RJ. Obsessive-compulsive and related disorders: A critical review of the new diagnostic class. *Annu Rev Clin Psychol*. 2015;11:165–86.

3. Phillips KA, Stein DJ. Introduction and major changes for the obsessive-compulsive and related disorders in DSM-5. In: Phillips KA, Stein DJ, editors. *Handbook on Obsessive-Compulsive and Related Disorders*. Arlington, VA: American Psychiatric Publishing; 2015. pp. 1–24.

4. American Psychiatric Association. *Diagnostic and Statistical Manual of Mental Disorders*, 5th edn. Arlington, VA: American Psychiatric Publishing; 2013.

5. Stein DJ, Kogan CS, Atmaca M, *et al*. The classification of obsessive–compulsive and related disorders in the ICD-11. *J Affect Disord*. 2016;190:663–74.

6. Phillips KA, Stein DJ, Rauch SL, *et al*. Should an obsessive-compulsive spectrum grouping of disorders be included in DSM-V? *Depress Anxiety*. 2010;27:528–55.

7. Okuda M, Simpson HB. Obsessive-compulsive disorder. In: Phillips KA, Stein DJ, editors. *Handbook on Obsessive-Compulsive and Related Disorders*. Arlington, VA: American Psychiatric Publishing; 2015. pp. 25–56.

8. Shavitt RG, de Mathis MA, Oki F, *et al*. Phenomenology of OCD: lessons from a large multicenter study and implications for ICD-11. *J Psychiatr Res*. 2014;57:141–8.

9. Torres AR, Fontenelle LF, Shavitt RG, *et al*. Comorbidity variation in patients with obsessive–compulsive disorder according to symptom dimensions: results from a large multicentre clinical sample. *J Affect Disord*. 2016;190:508–16.

10. American Psychiatric Association. *Diagnostic and Statistical Manual of Mental Disorders*, 4th edn. Washington, DC: American Psychiatric Publishing; 1994.

11. Kugler BB, Lewin AB, Phares V, Geffken GR, Murphy TK, Storch EA. Quality of life in obsessive-compulsive disorder: the role of mediating variables. *Psychiatry Res*. 2013;206:43–9.

12. Rosa AC, Diniz JB, Fossaluza V, *et al*. Clinical correlates of social adjustment in patients with obsessive-compulsive disorder. *J Psychiatr Res*. 2012;46:1286–92.

13. Torresan RC, Ramos-Cerqueira ATA, Shavitt RG, *et al*. Symptom dimensions, clinical course and comorbidity in men and women with obsessive-compulsive disorder. *Psychiatry Res*. 2013;209:186–95.

14. Wu MS, McGuire JF, Martino C, Phares V, Selles RR, Storch EA. A meta-analysis of family accommodation and OCD symptom severity. *Clin Psychol Rev*. 2016;45:34–44.

15. Eisen JL, Sibrava NJ, Boisseau CL, *et al*. Five-year course of obsessive-compulsive disorder: Predictors of remission and relapse. *J Clin Psychiatry*. 2013;74:233–9.

16. Visser HA, van Oppen P, van Megen HJ, Eikelenboom M, van Balkom AJ. Obsessive-compulsive disorder; chronic versus non-chronic symptoms. *J Affect Disord*. 2014;152–4: 169–74.

17. Larson MJ, Whitcomb K, Hunt IJ, Bjorn D. Treatment of individuals with obsessive-compulsive disorder who have poor insight. In: Storch EA, Lewin AB, editors. *Clinical Handbook of Obsessive-Compulsive and Related Disorders: A Case-Based Approach to Treating Pediatric and Adult Populations*. Cham: Springer International Publishing; 2016. pp. 399–413.

18. Stein DJ, Phillips KA. Conclusions. In: Phillips KA, Stein DJ, editors. *Handbook on Obsessive-Compulsive and Related Disorders*. Arlington, VA: American Psychiatric Publishing; 2015. pp. 273–85.

19. Cherian AV, Narayanaswamy JC, Srinivasaraju R, *et al*. Does insight have specific correlation with symptom dimensions in OCD? *J Affect Disord*. 2012;138:352–9.

20. Catapano F, Perris F, Fabrazzo M, *et al*. Obsessive–compulsive disorder with poor insight: a three-year prospective study. *Prog Neuropsychopharmacol Biol Psychiatry*. 2010;34:323–30.

21. Rosario-Campos MC, Miguel EC, Quatrano S, *et al*. The Dimensional Yale-Brown Obsessive-Compulsive Scale (DY-BOCS): an instrument for assessing obsessive-compulsive symptom dimensions. *Mol Psychiatry*. 2006;11:495–504.

22. Højgaard DRMA, Skarphedinsson G, Nissen JB, Hybel KA, Ivarsson T, Thomsen PH. Pediatric obsessive–compulsive disorder with tic symptoms: clinical presentation and treatment outcome. *Eur Child Adolesc Psychiatry*. 2017;26:681–9.

23. Conelea CA, Walther MR, Freeman JB, *et al*. Tic-related obsessive-compulsive disorder (OCD): Phenomenology and treatment outcome in the pediatric OCD treatment study II. *J Am Acad Child Adolesc Psychiatry*. 2014;53:1308–16.

24. Ramanujam K, Himle MB. Treatment of a youngster with tourettic obsessive-compulsive disorder. In: Storch EA, Lewin AB, editors. *Clinical Handbook of Obsessive-Compulsive and Related Disorders: A Case-Based Approach to Treating Pediatric and Adult Populations*. Cham: Springer International Publishing; 2016. pp. 305–19.

25. Leckman JF, Denys D, Simpson HB, *et al*. Obsessive-compulsive disorder: a review of the diagnostic criteria and possible subtypes and dimensional specifiers for DSM-V. *Depress Anxiety*. 2010;27:507–27.

26. Sharma E, Sundar AS, Thennarasu K, Reddy YJ. Is late-onset OCD a distinct phenotype? Findings from a comparative analysis of 'age at onset' groups. *CNS Spectr*. 2015;20:508–14.

27. Albert U, Manchia M, Tortorella A, *et al*. Admixture analysis of age at symptom onset and age at disorder onset in a large sample of patients with obsessive–compulsive disorder. *J Affect Disord*. 2015;187:188–96.

28. Anholt GE, Aderka IM, van Balkom AJLM, *et al*. Age of onset in obsessive–compulsive disorder: admixture analysis with a large sample. *Psychol Med*. 2013;44:185–94.

29. Frydman I, do Brasil PE, Torres AR, *et al*. Late-onset obsessive-compulsive disorder: risk factors and correlates. *J Psychiatr Res*. 2014;49:68–74.

30. Goodman W, Price LH, Rasmussen SA, *et al*. The yale-brown obsessive compulsive scale: I. development, use, and reliability. *Arch Gen Psychiatry*. 1989;46:1006–11.

31. Bloch MH, Landeros-Weisenberger A, Rosario MC, Pittenger C, Leckman JF. Meta-analysis of the symptom structure of obsessive-compulsive disorder. *Am J Psychiatry*. 2008;165:1532–42.

32. Stewart SE, Rosario MC, Baer L, *et al*. Four-factor structure of obsessive-compulsive disorder symptoms in children, adolescents, and adults. *J Am Acad Child Adolesc Psychiatry*. 2008;47:763–72.

33. Fernández de la Cruz L, Micali N, Roberts S, *et al*. Are the symptoms of obsessive-compulsive disorder temporally stable in children/adolescents? A prospective naturalistic study. *Psychiatry Res*. 2013;209:196–201.

34. McKay D, Abramowitz JS, Calamari JE, *et al*. A critical evaluation of obsessive–compulsive disorder subtypes: symptoms versus mechanisms. *Clin Psychol Rev*. 2004;24:283–313.

35. Mataix-Cols D, Rosario-Campos MC, Leckman JF. A multidimensional model of obsessive-compulsive disorder. *Am J Psychiatry*. 2005;162:228–38.

36. Alvarenga PG, Cesar RC, Leckman JF, *et al*. Obsessive-compulsive symptom dimensions in a population-based, cross-sectional sample of school-aged children. *J Psychiatr Res*. 2015;62:108–14.

37. Williams MT, Mugno B, Franklin M, Faber S. Symptom dimensions in obsessive-compulsive disorder: phenomenology and treatment outcomes with exposure and ritual prevention. *Psychopathology*. 2013;46:365–76.

38. Chase T, Wetterneck CT, Bartsch RA, Leonard RC, Riemann BC. Investigating treatment outcomes across OCD symptom dimensions in a clinical sample of OCD patients. *Cogn Behav Ther*. 2015;44:365–76.

39. McCarty RJ, Guzick AG, Swan LK, McNamara JPH. Stigma and recognition of different types of symptoms in OCD. *J Obsessive Compuls Relat Disord*. 2017;12:64–70.

40. Iervolino AC, Rijsdijk FV, Cherkas L, Fullana MA, Mataix-Cols D. A multivariate twin study of obsessive-compulsive symptom dimensions. *Arch Gen Psychiatry*. 2011;68:637–44.

41. Pauls DL, Abramovitch A, Rauch SL, Geller DA. Obsessive-compulsive disorder: an integrative genetic and neurobiological perspective. *Nat Rev Neurosci*. 2014;15:410–24.

42. Hasler G, Pinto A, Greenberg BD, *et al*. Familiality of factor analysis-derived YBOCS dimensions in OCD-affected sibling pairs from the OCD collaborative genetics study. *Biol Psychiatry*. 2007;61:617–25.

43. Arumugham SS, Cherian AV, Baruah U, *et al*. Comparison of clinical characteristics of familial and sporadic obsessive-compulsive disorder. *Compr Psychiatry*. 2014;55:1520–5.

44. Brakoulias V, Starcevic V, Martin A, Berle D, Milicevic D, Viswasam K. The familiality of specific symptoms of obsessive-compulsive disorder. *Psychiatry Res*. 2016;239:315–19.

45. Katerberg H, Delucchi KL, Stewart SE, *et al*. Symptom dimensions in OCD: item-level factor analysis and heritability estimates. *Behav Genet*. 2010;40:505–17.

46. López-Solà C, Fontenelle LF, Verhulst B, *et al*. Distinct etiological influences on obsessive-compulsive symptom dimentions: a multivariate twin study. *Depress Anxiety*. 2016;33:179–91.

47. Taj MJ, RJ, Viswanath B, Purushottam M, Kandavel T, Janardhan Reddy YC, Jain S. *DRD4* gene and obsessive compulsive disorder: Do symptom dimensions have specific genetic correlates? *Prog Neuropsychopharmacol Biol Psychiatry*. 2013;41:18–23.

48. Lennertz L, Wagner M, Grabe HJ, *et al*. 5-HT3 receptor influences the washing phenotype and visual organization in obsessive-compulsive disorder supporting 5-HT3 receptor antagonists as novel treatment option. *Eur Neuropsychopharmacol*. 2014;24:86–94.

49. Koch K, Wagner G, Schachtzabel C, *et al*. White matter structure and symptom dimensions in obsessive–compulsive disorder. *J Psychiatr Res*. 2012;46:264–70.

50. Piras F, Piras F, Chiapponi C, Girardi P, Caltagirone C, Spalletta G. Widespread structural brain changes in OCD: a systematic review of voxel-based morphometry studies. *Cortex*. 2015;62:89–108.

51. Harrison BJ, Pujol J, Cardoner N, *et al*. Brain corticostriatal systems and the major clinical symptom dimensions of obsessive-compulsive disorder. *Biol Psychiatry*. 2013;73:321–8.

52. Via E, Cardoner N, Pujol J, *et al*. Amygdala activation and symptom dimensions in obsessive-compulsive disorder. *Br J Psychiatry*. 2014;204:61–8.

53. Kashyap H, Kumar JK, Kandavel T, Reddy YCJ. Relationships between neuropsychological variables and factor-analysed symptom dimensions in obsessive compulsive disorder. *Psychiatry Res*. 2017;249:58–64.

54. McGuire JF, Crawford EA, Park JM, *et al*. Neuropsychological performance across symptom dimensions in pediatric obsessive compulsive disorder. *Depress Anxiety*. 2014;31:988–96.

55. Brakoulias V, Starcevic V, Berle D, Milicevic D, Hannan A, Martin A. The relationships between obsessive-compulsive symptom dimensions and cognitions in obsessive-compulsive disorder. *Psychiatr Q*. 2014;85:133–42.

56. Alonso P, Segalàs C, Real E, *et al*. Suicide in patients treated for obsessive–compulsive disorder: a prospective follow-up study. *J Affect Disord*. 2010;124:300–8.

57. Torres AR, Ramos-Cerqueira A, Ferrão YA, Fontenelle LF, do Rosário MC, Miguel EC. Suicidality in obsessive-compulsive disorder: prevalence and relation to symptom dimensions and comorbid conditions. *J Clin Psychiatry*. 2011;72:17–26; quiz 119–20.

58. Schwartzman CM, Boisseau CL, Sibrava NJ, Mancebo MC, Eisen JL, Rasmussen SA. Symptom subtype and quality of life in obsessive-compulsive disorder. Psychiat Res. 2017;249:307–10.

59. Kichuk SA, Torres AR, Fontenelle LF, *et al*. Symptom dimensions are associated with age of onset and clinical course of obsessive–compulsive disorder. *Prog Neuropsychopharmacol Biol Psychiatry*. 2013;44:233–9.

# 94

# Basic mechanisms of, and treatment planning/targets for, obsessive–compulsive disorder

*Eric Burguière and Luc Mallet*

## Introduction

As described in Chapter 93, obsessive–compulsive disorder (OCD) is a condition featuring obsessions (intrusive ideas) and compulsions (repetitive behaviours such as checking, washing, or iterated thought patterns) associated with high levels of anxiety, and conservative estimates suggest it may affect 2.9 million persons across the EU (that is, 0.7% prevalence) [1]. The most severe forms lead to high costs both for the individual and society as a whole [2]. While there are currently many validated pharmacological and psychotherapeutical treatments for OCD, 20–30% of patients do not respond to them [3]. This is particularly problematic, given that 10% of these patients show severe symptoms (for example, compulsions taking >4 hours/day), resulting in high social and financial burdens to both families and society in general.

In this chapter, we describe some promising approaches that have been developed in recent decades to better understand the functional and pathophysiological basis of OCD at various different levels, including:

- Improved understanding of functional impairments and behavioural dimensions that most affect patients (*macro-scale level*).
- Characterization of dysfunctional brain activities and their related neural circuits (*meso-scale level*).
- Identification of specific cell type and neuronal assemblages implicated in obsessive and/or compulsive disorders (*micro-scale level*).

Importantly, we refer to studies carried out both on humans and animal models, providing a wider range of tools to investigate the dysfunctional neural activity associated with this condition. In particular, we consider the extracellular recording of single neurons at different brain sites during specific behaviours and also the recent development of optogenetic approaches that allow the study of neural activity with a high degree of spatial, cellular, and temporal specificity. Despite the major challenges and limitations in conducting such a translational approach across species, we believe that

it offers the best means of unravelling the neural basis of psychiatric diseases [4, 5]. Our description of studies in human is complemented and extended in Chapter 97.

We do not aim exhaustively to review all the possible therapeutic strategies to treat OCD here but will illustrate the potential of a multi-level approach using powerful, recently developed tools to develop new treatments for OCD, using some relevant examples.

## Expanding the toolbox to find relevant targets for OCD

Numerous studies on OCD patients over the past two decades have consistently identified abnormal patterns of activity in one neural circuit in particular—the cortico-basal ganglia (CBG) loop [6], which is known to serve both motor and cognitive functions. Anatomical and functional studies of the CBG provide further evidence of their role in the parallel processing of sensorimotor, associative, and limbic information arising from topographically and functionally distinct cortical areas [7]; sensorimotor, associative, and limbic information appears to be segregated along a dorsolateral to ventromedial axis within the CBG (Fig. 94.1).

These circuits are used to differing extents during the learning of a behaviour (either motor or cognitive). While the ventral loop—the 'reward circuit'—is more important during initial behaviour acquisition, it is the dorsolateral loop that is crucial once learning becomes habitual [7, 8, 9]. Recent studies have supported the view that the dorsomedial and the dorsolateral striatum complement each other in the elaboration and consolidation of learnt behavioural sequences. This associative CBG loop is essential in linking contextual information with its appropriate motor response. The associative loops can therefore modulate the action of sensorimotor loops in the control of stereotyped actions [10, 11].

This organization within distinct functional loops has been characterized in the context of the pathophysiology of OCD through

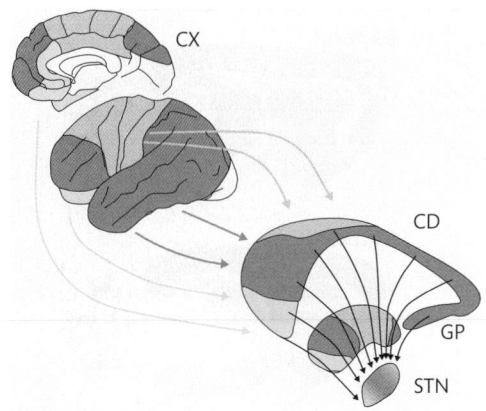

**Fig. 94.1** Schematic illustration of the convergence of projections from the cerebral cortex (CX), caudate nucleus (CD), and globus pallidus (GP) in the basal ganglia. Different colours represent the types of information processed through the CBG: limbic (light blue), associative (dark grey), and sensorimotor (light grey).
Adapted from *Proc Natl Acad Sci*, 104(25), Mallet L, Schüpbach M, N'Diaye K, *et al*, Stimulation of subterritories of the subthalamic nucleus reveals its role in the integration of the emotional and motor aspects of behaviour, pp. 10661–10666, Copyright (2007), with permission from National Academy of Sciences, U.S.A.

a number of studies on both human and animal models. In recent years, novel investigative techniques have emerged while more established methods have improved, allowing more detailed studies of dysfunctional brain circuits and the neural basis of OCD.

## Animal models

Detailed experimental evidence on the role of the different CBG loops in OCD is scarce in human subjects, mostly due to ethical issues arising from the use of invasive procedures and the time and spatial specificity constraints inherent in non-invasive imaging techniques. For these reasons, and with the development of genetically engineered mutant mice, we have witnessed the emergence of numerous animal models relevant to OCD-like behaviours within the last decade [12]. These animal models allow detailed study of the specific mechanistic processes that could be altered in OCD treatments; the results of recent studies are promising and point to investigations of specific targets in human patients. Two recent studies have shown that in a mouse model expressing compulsive-like behaviour, compulsions could be drastically reduced by targeting the lateral orbitofrontal cortex (OFC) and the medial part of the striatum (that is, the caudate in humans) [13, 14]. The combination of animal models of obsessive–compulsive spectrum symptoms with new methods available to neuroscientists should allow to better investigate the links between the genes implicated in OCD-related disorders and the neurophysiological circuits affected and behavioural phenotypes [13, 15–17].

The main characteristics of validating mutant animals as models of OCD are functional (OCD-related behaviour), neurophysiologic (the neural circuits affected by the mutation), and genetic (OCD candidate genes). The most promising mouse models developed so far share common behavioural phenotypes characterized by excessive grooming, which can be interpreted as a proxy for compulsive behaviour in mice, that is, an analogue of abnormal ritualistic and stereotyped behaviours that are overexpressed despite their negative consequences (for example, deleterious skin lesions). From a neural

circuits point of view, there is striking evidence that a mutation in all these mouse models alters the normal functioning of the CBG circuits known to be implicated in OCD (Fig. 94.2).

The introduction of gene mutations causing symptoms related to OCD had anatomical consequences such as a decrease in striatal volume [15], but also more consistently pointed towards dysfunctional synaptic transmission, particularly in the striatum compartment (for example, equivalent to caudo-putamen areas in humans) receiving cortical inputs. These features have been shown following the deletion of genes coding for SAPAP3, Slitrk5, and EAAC1—proteins located post-synaptically in striatal neurons [13, 15, 18]. These mutations had electrophysiological consequences resulting in abnormally hyperactive striatal neurons, supporting the idea that elevated striatal activity is implicated in OCD pathophysiology, as suggested by some imaging studies in human patients [14, 16].

## Imaging

### Structural connectivity MRI

Diffusion-weighted imaging (DTI) is now a well-established technique to infer brain connectivity based on magnetic resonance imaging (MRI) of the random motion of water molecules in tissues [19] (see Chapter 12). Because this motion is firmly restricted by the sheets of myelin surrounding the axons, the diffusion pattern reveals the main direction of these axons locally. The integration of information on the local directionality of white matter fibres can then be used to infer the entire network of connections within the brain using the tractography techniques now popular.

The directional dependence of molecular diffusion in white matter ('anisotropy') can be used to reconstruct tracts through the brain *in vivo* by assuming that the main direction of diffusion in a voxel indicates the local orientation of white matter fibres [20, 21]. A number of DTI tractography algorithms have been proposed to reconstruct fibre tracts [20]. Tractography enables the investigation of both tract-specific white matter lesions and the changes in connection probability between distinct brain regions (Fig. 94.3).

DTI has been used recently to study the pathophysiology of OCD and possible deficits in neural circuit connectivity in particular. Most of the studies have confirmed the implication of the CBG and its related fibres such as the cingulate bundle, the corpus callosum, and the anterior limb of the internal capsule [22].

Thanks to the increasing resolution and refinement of analytical algorithms in the field of anatomical imaging, it has been possible to discover new connections of interest. For example, the subthalamic nucleus (STN) has only recently been the subject of structural connectivity studies using diffusion MRI. Very few empirical data have yet been collected on the role of this nucleus in OCD, although its direct connectivity to the cortical areas, known as the hyperdirect pathway, has been implicated in action selection and decision-making [23]. A detailed connectivity map of the cortico-STN pathway in OCD patients, compared to healthy subjects, would therefore be of great interest in assessing its involvement in this condition.

With the advent of high magnetic field systems (>3 T) capable of producing strong gradients, diffusion methods have been extended from human to small animal imaging. With such MRI systems, high resolution can be achieved (in the order of 100 microns) and very small structures in rodent brains can be visualized to study the

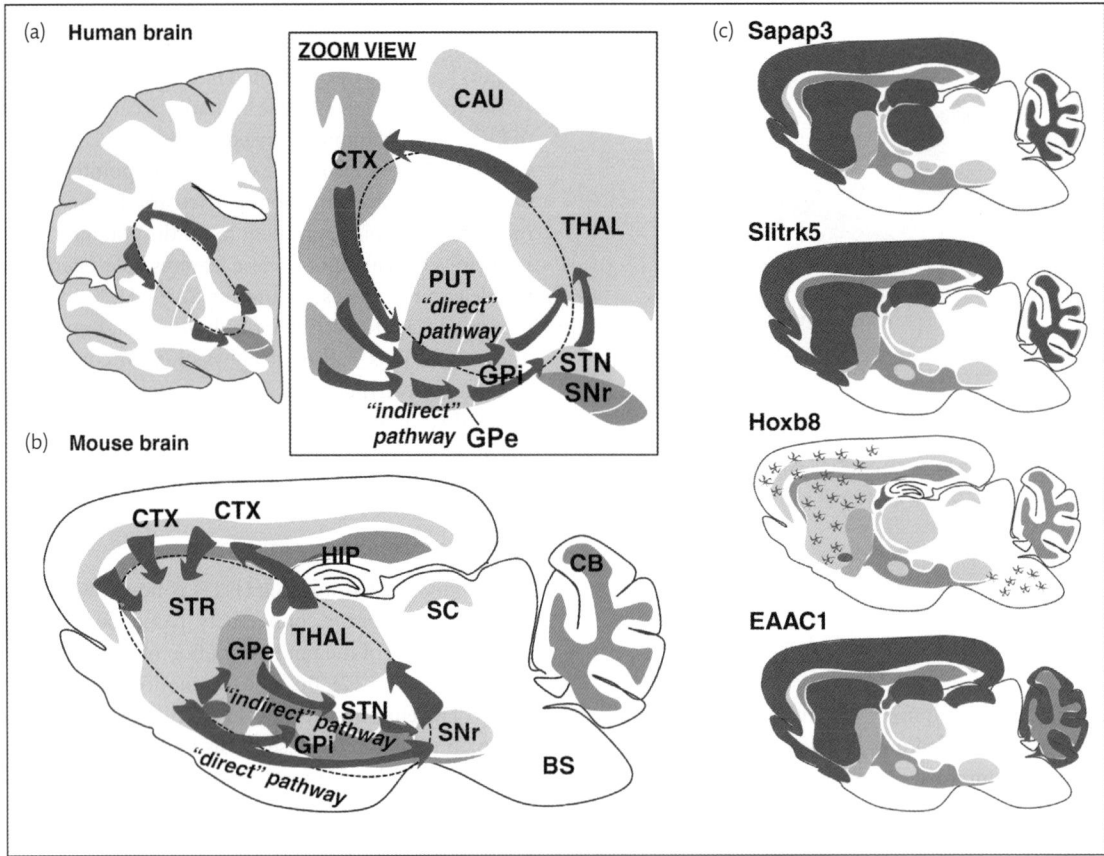

**Fig. 94.2** Central role of the CSTC circuitry in obsessive–compulsive disorder in humans and compulsive–repetitive behaviours in mice. (a) Illustration of CBG loops in the human brain. (b) Illustration of equivalent CBG loops in a mouse brain. CTX, cortex; STR, striatum; CAU, caudate; PUT, putamen; HIP, hippocampus; THAL, thalamus; STN, subthalamic nucleus; SNr, substantia nigra pars reticulata; GPe, globus pallidus externa; GPi, globus pallidus interna; SC, superior colliculus; BS, brainstem; CB, cerebellum. (c) Examples of four candidate OCD gene expression patterns that have been targeted in mutant models. Note the overlapping implication of the CBG in these different expression patterns.

Reproduced from *Curr Opin Neurobiol.*, 21(6), Ting JT, Feng G, Neurobiology of obsessive–compulsive disorder: insights into neural circuitry dysfunction through mouse genetics, pp 842–848, Copyright (2011), with permission from Elsevier Ltd.

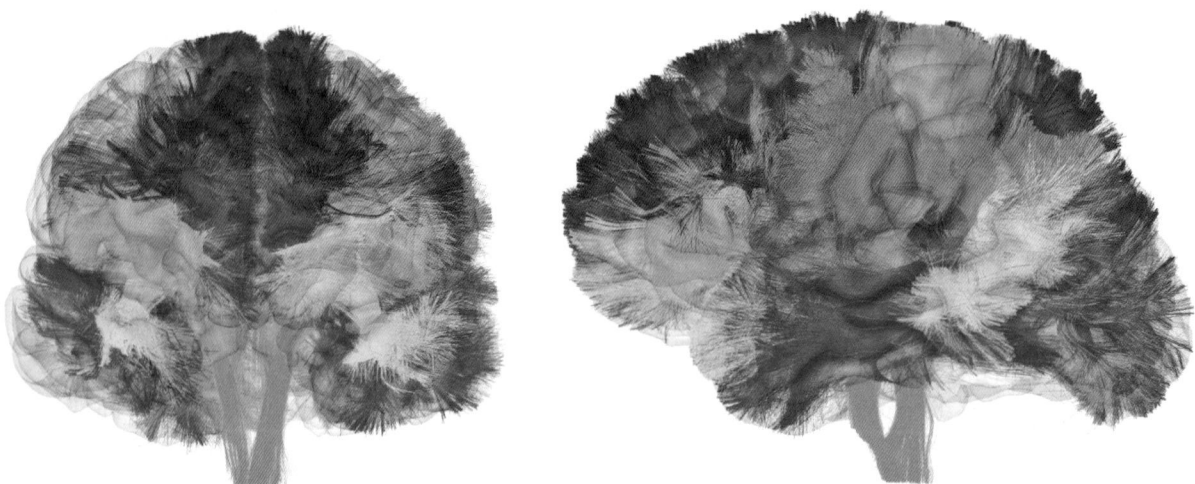

**Fig. 94.3** (see Colour Plate section) CONNECT/Archi atlas of the human brain white matter connectivity developed at NeuroSpin, as part of the European CONNECT FP7 project.

Reproduced courtesy of Cyril Poupon,CEA NeuroSpin.

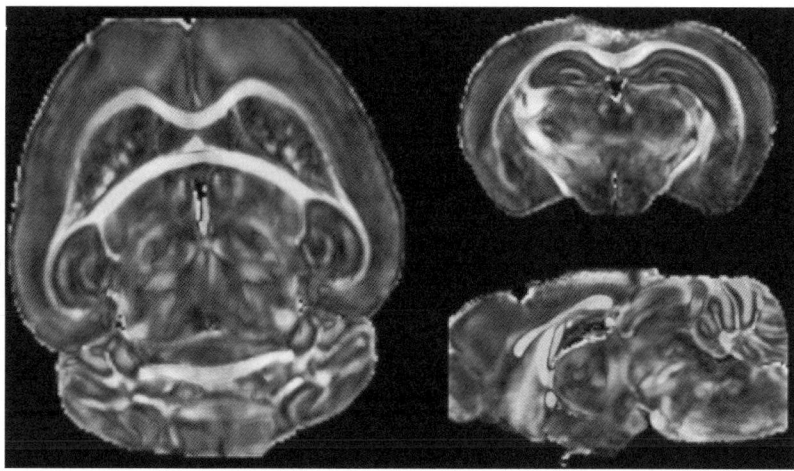

**Fig. 94.4** (see Colour Plate section) Representative three-dimensional image of colour-coded fractional anisotropy in a mouse brain based on diffusion MRI at 11.7 T.
Reproduced courtesy of S. B. Sébille and M. D. Santin, ICM-CENIR.

peripheral nervous system [24], as well as neurodegenerative diseases such as multiple sclerosis, Alzheimer's disease, and Parkinson's disease (PD) [25]. Recently, feasibility studies of DTI tractography have allowed the identification of neural networks in rodent brains in target regions relating to homologous limbic and associative regions [26] (Fig. 94.4).

With the high definition offered by recent MRI systems (up to 17 T), one could hope to detect potential structural differences in the CBG circuits between wildtype and animal models of OCD. One of the main advantages using anatomical connectivity in these models is that these data can be compared to the functional connectivities which can be finely characterized in animal models by using innovative investigative tools (for example, dense chronic single neurons recording and/or optogenetic neuromodulation).

### Functional connectivity MRI

Once the anatomical features of a given circuit are established, the next challenge is to describe its functional aspects. Such characterization may be achieved by analysing the long-distance synchronization between structures connected by the circuit.

By using fMRI [for example, echo planar imaging (EPI)] to measure the slow changes in blood oxygenation level-dependent (BOLD) signal across distant brain regions, one can identify connected networks. This technique allows the detection of spontaneous patterns of functional connectivity MRI (fcMRI). In recent years, the fcMRI approach has identified large-scale brain networks interacting, while the subject is at rest, as well as while engaged in an active task. Across neurological and psychiatric disorders, abnormal patterns of fcMRI have been interpreted as correlates of altered brain-scale network functioning, so providing a potential marker for abnormalities in information processing. For example, recent studies of fcMRI in OCD have reported changes in functional coupling between the striatum and frontal regions, compared to healthy controls. Nakame *et al.* [27] found increased functional connectivity between the ventral striatum and the OFC and ventral medial prefrontal and dorsal lateral prefrontal cortices of subjects with OCD using this method. Similarly, Harrison and colleagues

[28, 29] consistently found that this augmented functional connectivity between the OFC and the ventral striatum was positively correlated with OCD severity. However, in the particular case of the associative-limbic hyperdirect pathway, the small volume of the STN (relatively to the typical voxel size used with functional imaging, for example 2 mm isotropic) poses special difficulties.

At the whole-brain scale, functional imaging of OCD points towards hyperactivity in the limbic and associative cortical regions [anterior cingulate cortex (ACC) and OFC] and related basal ganglia areas [30]. Additionally, studies from our groups and others identified abnormalities in the CBG circuits in OCD. Indeed, in fMRI studies of OCD patients, abnormal haemodynamic responses in the OFC and ACC may decrease as patients improve either through deep brain stimulation (DBS) therapies [31] or psychotherapy [32]. These data support the involvement of limbic/associative frontal-basal ganglia loops in OCD and suggest that their dysfunction might result in pathological doubt, obsessive anxiety, and compulsive behaviours.

### Neural recording and neuromodulation

#### Electrophysiology and long-range synchronization

Unlike metabolic measures, electrophysiological recordings provide a unique source of information to assess long-distance synchronization at sub-millimetre scales with sub-millisecond resolution. Two main types of signal can be recorded—either using micro-electrodes (diameter <50 μm), which allows the identification of spike activity, and therefore single- or multi-neuron activities; or macro-electrodes (diameter >500 μm), which collect local field potentials (LFPs) that sum the relatively low-frequency (<150 Hz) electrical activity of millions of neurons and their afferences in the area surrounding the tip of the electrode. The micro-electrodes are typically used in animal studies, but they can also be used during DBS neurosurgery to confirm the targeting of the intended structure. In DBS-treated patients, LFPs may be directly recorded from the definitive stimulating electrodes, while their leads are still externalized prior to connection to the pulse generator.

To date, electrophysiological assessment of long-distance network connections has been little used in OCD patients. Most recently, simultaneous recording of the STN, LFPs, and cortical activity from scalp measurements [such as magneto- or electroencephalography (MEG/EEG)] has allowed the identification of long-distance coherence between the STN and motor cortical areas, in specific frequency bands (alpha and beta, 7–12 Hz and 13–35 Hz, respectively), suggestive of the involvement of the motor hyperdirect pathway [33, 34]. Interestingly, functional connectivity measures using electrophysiological recordings have been conducted on DBS-treated PD patients and shown increased values at higher frequencies when levodopa was concurrently administered to improve motor symptoms.

Characterizing the differences in neural activity between OCD patients and unaffected subjects would show how neural activity within elements of the CBG pathway is altered in DBS-implanted OCD patients and provide valuable data on the functional interactions between the various brain areas. By providing insight into how limbic cortical activity is co-ordinated with subcortical activity, such analyses would be crucial in understanding the pathophysiology of OCD and begin to dissect the mechanisms by which DBS functions in OCD patients. Finally, these data could lead to novel DBS technologies to target specific pathways to normalize the information transfer along the cortico-subcortical pathway that is disrupted in OCD.

### Deep brain stimulation

DBS (see Chapter 19) represents a promising type of intervention for severe, resistant forms of OCD, based principally on the serendipitous observation that DBS of the basal ganglia can reduce OCD symptoms in those patients suffering from comorbid OCD [35, 36]. Independent studies have proposed multiple targets in the CBG for DBS in OCD, such as the anterior limb of the internal capsule and the STN [37–39] (Fig. 94.5), as an alternative to stereotactic lesional neurosurgery. But progress has been limited by the lack of understanding of the pathophysiology of OCD at both the neural

and behavioural levels and how DBS operates on these brain circuits and their functions. Two meta-analyses have suggested that OCD symptoms showed a mean improvement of 45% after 3–36 months of DBS, with 60% of patients being considered responders (>35% reduction in OCD severity) and found no significant differences between the brain structures targeted [40, 41]. Yet according to Kisely et al. [40], only one study meets all four of the quality criteria, namely the first randomized double-blind study performed on 16 OCD patients which showed that 3 months of DBS of the STN is sufficient to decrease OCD severity [38]. Only a few studies report long-term efficacy (>3 years) and sustained toleration of DBS in OCD patients. Stimulation of the nucleus accumbens, the ventral caudate/ventral striatum and the anterior limb of the internal capsule, and the bed nucleus of the stria terminalis have been associated with a median reduction of 46%, 36–64%, and 45% in OCD severity, respectively, 36–171 months after surgery [42–45, 45a].

Understanding the contribution of cortico-subcortical circuits to OCD pathophysiology and therapeutic interventions therefore represents a major challenge in improving the selection of candidate patients and the optimization of treatment strategies. As recognized by various authors [46], traditional nosography—even when combined with more recent techniques such as brain imaging, has made limited progress in this direction, and novel approaches combining hypothesis-driven experimental studies of endophenotypes, animal models, and neuromodulation may be essential to open the way to translational research for innovative treatments.

As an example, therapeutic mechanisms underlying the action of STN high-frequency stimulation (HFS) involve the hyperdirect pathway. This pathway provides direct cortical inputs to the STN. It was first described in the motor/premotor domain and was considered to act through motor selection [23]. Recent evidence shows a limbic element stemming from the OFC and ACC [47]. Current proposals regarding DBS treatment in humans now incorporate the hyperdirect pathway not only for motor disorders, but also for psychiatric conditions such as OCD [48, 49]. Indeed, the effective target for OCD was the associative-limbic part of the STN-HFS [38], which is the target of hyperdirect afferents from the limbic and associative prefrontal regions (ACC and OFC).

Interestingly, per-operative recordings have revealed that populations of neurons from the associative-limbic part of the STN exhibit electrophysiological correlates of OCD symptoms (for example, repetitive checking [50]). At the cellular level, burst and oscillatory patterns of activity from the associative-limbic part of the STN correlate with OCD symptomatology (across patients) and predict the post-operative long-term response of STN-HFS [51].

However, the nature of the benefit is not clear and difficult to investigate in patients, as the amount of physiological data simultaneously available at each node of the cortico-subcortical loops is limited. Moreover, the use of DBS is today empirically driven. The exact effects of this technique are not known, especially the physiological consequences of such stimulations on the CBG loop [52]. Finally, electrical currents may trigger antidromic effects in afferent neurons, most notably in limbic cortical areas, paralleling the effects shown in cases of Parkinsonism [53].

### Optogenetics

The functional deconstruction of neuronal circuits can now be achieved in animal models using optogenetic techniques [54]. These

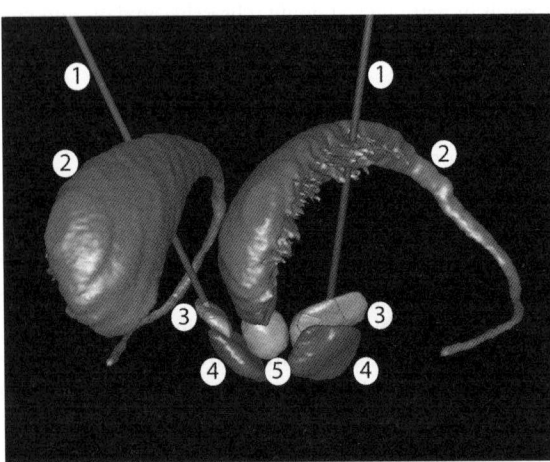

**Fig. 94.5** (see Colour Plate section) Three-dimensional image of electrodes implantated in a DBS procedure. Depending on the stimulating electrode (5) configuration and stereotactic co-ordinates, several anatomical sites can be targeted. Two brain targets are represented in this example: the caudate caudate nucleus (2) and the subthalamic nucleus (2). Other brain structures, such as the substantia nigra (3) and the red nucleus (4), can be used as anatomical landmarks.
Adapted courtesy of Jerome Yelnik, INSERM/ICM.

have already been used in rodents to decipher neural codes of basic motor, cognitive, and emotional behaviours [14, 53, 55, 56]. These techniques allow the manipulation of neuronal activity using optical stimulation by expressing, through viral vectors, specific light-sensitive membrane proteins—called opsins—in neural cells. This approach is of great interest in the selective inhibition or excitation of nodes of given targeted circuits and can be used to assess physiological and functional causal links. Using a combination of genetic and stimulation-dependent effects, optogenetics allows a high level of temporal, spatial, and cell type specificity.

It can also be used to overcome certain issues encountered in previous classical approaches. For example, the observation of electrophysiological effects of DBS in OCD patients is challenging because of the electrical artefacts it induces. DBS effects also depend on cell type, active fibres, and nearby structures. These issues could be overcome by taking advantage of the optogenetic technology, which avoids electrical artefacts and allows the stimulation of specific cell types only.

Primary applications of optogenetics have been used to better analyse and understand discrete and specific normal or abnormal behaviours in rodents. To effectively validate and translate this novel knowledge to clinical applications, the next step is to scale up these optical experiments to animal models displaying greater anatomical and physiological similarities with human beings, especially in complex behavioural abnormalities. In particular, rodents allow for a wide range of tools to be used in order to manipulate the cortex–basal ganglia circuits, yielding models of neurologic and psychiatric disorders.

Using optogenetics in rodents, some recent studies have suggested new targets that could be considered to be causally linked to OCD symptomatology. Optogenetic manipulation of specific brain circuits, such as the orbitofrontal–striatal pathway, could induce or decrease compulsive-like behaviours [14, 57]. Although these brain areas have previously been regularly identified as abnormally active in OCD patients, these studies were the first to show their manipulation could elicit/decrease compulsive-like behaviours. Thus, an optogenetic approach in animal models not only allows the testing of circuit-level hypotheses for OCD, but also challenges further the micro-circuitry within various brain areas. Indeed, genetic studies in human patients have already indicated that genes affecting the serotonergic, dopaminergic, and glutamatergic systems, and the interaction between them, may be affected in OCD and many potential therapeutic targets may arise from these biological systems [58]. Furthermore, Burguière et al. [14] focused on a new potential cellular subtype—the striatal interneurons—which may play an essential role in regulating the expression of striatal-dependent behaviours and could be implicated in OCD (Fig. 94.6).

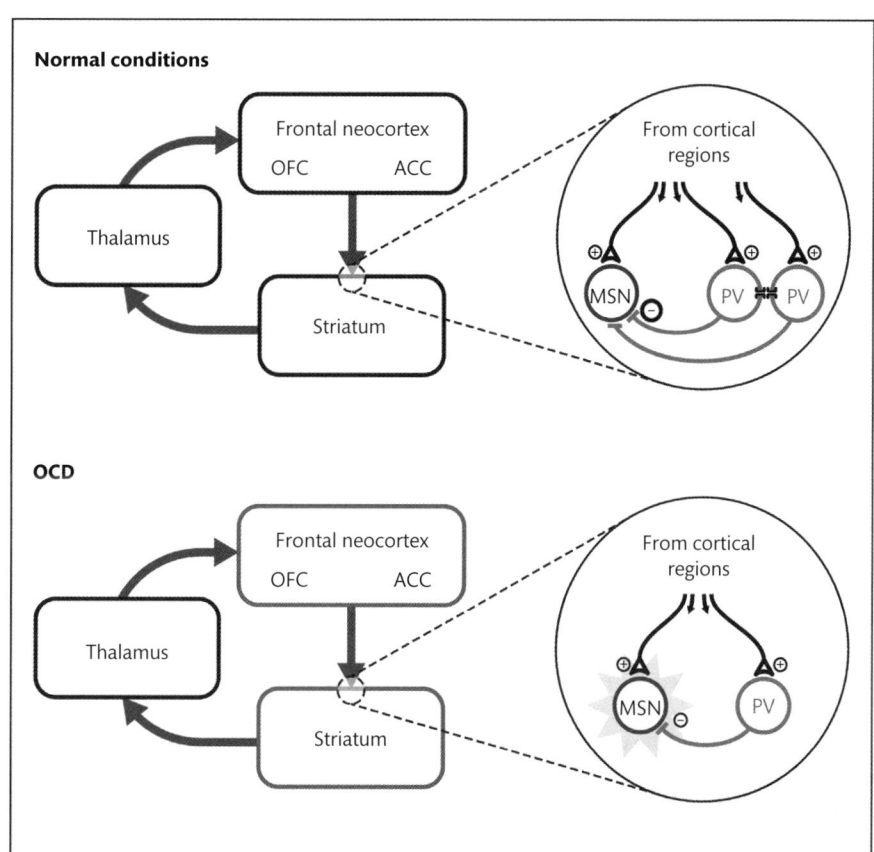

**Fig. 94.6** Hypothetical model to illustrate striatal hyperactivity as a consequence of interneuronal network deficiency. Above: in normal conditions, an extensive inhibitory network in the striatum preserves a balance of excitation and inhibition driven by the cortex. Below: in the OCD condition, there is an imbalance towards excitation in the striatal region due to a lack of interneurons. As a result, there will be hyperactivation of the entire CBG loops. ACC, anterior cingulate cortex; MSN, medium spiny neurons; OFC, orbitofrontal cortex; PV, parvalbumin-positive interneurons.

In fact, it has been shown that a powerful inhibitory network of parvalbumin (PV)-immunoreactive and cholinergic (Chat)-immunoreactive interneurons is crucial for the functional regulation of striatal networks [59]. Moreover, depending on whether either the sensorimotor or associative-limbic cortico-striatal pathways are affected by a lack of interneurons, the functional consequences can be drastically different. According to human imaging studies, it has been suggested that cortico-striatal sensorimotor pathways (including the dorsolateral part of the striatum equivalent to the putamen in humans) are more likely to be affected in Tourette's patients, while cortico-striatal associative-limbic pathways (including the medio-ventral part of the striatum or caudate nucleus in humans) are more likely to be affected in OCD patients, although some overlap can be observed in the pathophysiology of these behaviours [60–63].

## Linking behavioural and neurophysiological endophenotypes of OCD to strengthen target validity

Experimental psychologists and clinicians have performed numerous studies on OCD patients to assess their performance in the main cognitive domains (memory, attention, verbal fluency, etc.) using classical behavioural test batteries. Even if some deficits have been observed, no clear magnitudes of effects for each cognitive domain have been observed using meta-analyses [64–66]. So in order to identify the relevant behavioural dimensions that might be affected by OCD, investigators must focus on more selective cognitive processes. To illustrate this approach, we will discuss three dimensions that could prove dysfunctional in OCD, as well as the underlying brain circuits that play a role in these processes and that often overlap with those identified in the pathology.

### Uncertainty monitoring

Compulsive checking is a core symptom of OCD. It is characterized by the urge to verify repeatedly that an action, usually aimed at preventing a possible harm, has been properly completed [67]. The clinical phenomenology of compulsive checking illustrates two hypotheses regarding its psychopathological mechanisms—compulsive checking may proceed from a maladaptive goal-directed behaviour towards uncertainty reduction; or, in the context of habit-driven behaviours, it may result from a failure to control impulses to check. These two alternatives fit nicely into two lines of research on the behavioural functions of the basal ganglia in general, and the STN in particular.

A growing number of studies have expanded the role of the STN from purely motor functions to include higher-level processes such as emotion and decision-making [68, 69]. In PD patients (for whom STN-HFS treatment is most widespread), the STN has been associated with the regulation of behaviour in the face of conflicting stimuli [70], for example postponement when faced with two positively reinforced cues in reward-based motor tasks [70–72]. Conversely, lesion and stimulation studies in animals have also shown that various forms of STN intervention result in premature responses and increased attentional errors [73, 74]. Interestingly, the hyperdirect pathway, which connects the cortical frontal areas to the STN [23], as previously described, could constitute an anatomical route for such

decisional signals whereby behaviour is regulated according to the strength of the sensory evidence. Indeed, the hyperdirect pathway not only connects motor/premotor functions, but also the limbic/associative regions, such as the ACC to the anterior-medial STN, precisely the target of DBS in the context of OCD [47]. Considering the role of the ACC and other associative/limbic frontal cortices in action selection and decision-making, one could surmise that the STN receives higher-level decisional signals [69] to regulate a behaviour adaptively.

Recently, new behavioural paradigms have been developed to assess uncertainty monitoring in animals, revealing that, when given the opportunity, rats can adaptively 'opt out' and move on to the next, possibly easier, trial of the task [75, 76]. In such tasks, varying uncertainty about stimulus identity (hence decision difficulty) leads the animal to discard the trials where its response is most uncertain. Indeed, simultaneous electrophysiological recordings have shown that stimulus-related uncertainty is encoded in the spike rate of the OFC neurons. However, despite putative connectivity (via the hyperdirect pathways), it is still unknown whether these uncertainty monitoring signals reach the STN and participate in the regulation of goal-directed behaviour, either to opt out from a trial or to check back at the stimulus.

Paradoxically, empirical studies in humans have reported that repetitive checking, even in healthy subjects, instead of reducing stimulus-related uncertainty, actually decreases subjective confidence [77]. To investigate repetitive checking in the laboratory, we introduced a so-called 'verification task', based on a working memory paradigm in which, on each trial, participants could review the stimulus before proceeding to the feedback. This paradigm allowed us to provoke and assess compulsive checking in OCD patients [78, 79] and also to reproduce this pathological behaviour during the DBS surgery when the patient is awake and behaving [50]. We were therefore able to record the STN from populations of neurons, as OCD patients entered bouts of repetitive checking. The STN showed a significant increase in the population spike rate when the patient was about to perform another checking action, compared to when he/she was about to proceed to the next trial. These results suggest that uncertainty signals anticipating checking actions may be detected in STN neurons [50].

### Behavioural inhibition

A different and contrasting line of research has focused on action control [80, 81], comprising behavioural inhibition and the cessation of ongoing motor programmes before they have reached overt expression. According to the classical model of the basal ganglia-thalamo-cortical loops, the major output nuclei of the basal ganglia (the STN and the internal globus pallidus) maintain sustained inhibition at the cortical level via the thalamic relay. To explore behavioural inhibition in humans, clinical [35], functional [68], and electrophysiological studies in DBS-treated PD patients have proved critical, linking successful behavioural inhibition to frequency-specific changes of oscillatory activity within the STN [71], as well as between the STN and prefrontal cortices [82]. As a consequence, a lesion or inactivation of the STN performed in rats leads to impulsive behaviour, characterized by failed inhibition of prepotent responses initiated in the striatum–pallidum circuits [83]. In this context, compulsive behaviour may reflect a functional deficit at the STN level, causing failure to inhibit prepotent or habitual actions that are produced, irrespective of the behavioural context.

Indeed, neural representations of habitual sequences of actions triggered as encapsulated motor programmes, or 'chunks', have been observed in the striatal circuits of rodents [84–86]. Additionally, perturbation of the fronto-striatal circuitry could indeed modulate the execution of habitual actions and prevent compulsive behaviour, as has been shown using optogenetic manipulation in mice [14] and DBS in OCD patients [31]. Therefore, the fronto-striato-pallidal pathway may play an important role in the emergence of motor programmes and, if dysfunctional, provoke their overexpression, leading to compulsive behaviours. Complementary to the cortico-striatal pathway, the cortico-STN pathway (that is, the hyperdirect pathway) has been shown to stop habitual behaviours before they reach completion [82, 87]. In this context, compulsive behaviour may reflect a functional deficit which fails to inhibit prepotent or habitual actions that are produced, irrespective of the behavioural context.

## Behavioural flexibility

OCD in humans is characterized by repetitive behaviour, performed through rigid rituals. This phenomenological observation has led to exploration of the idea that OCD patients have diminished behavioural flexibility (that is, the ability to change one's behaviour according to contextual cues). Behavioural flexibility may be challenged in experimental tasks such as reversal learning paradigms. In these tasks, the participant has to respond to either of two visual stimuli. In the deterministic version, one stimulus is positively rewarded while the other is not. Unbeknown to the participant, the reward contingencies are reversed after a certain number of trials, so that the previously neutral stimulus is now rewarded while the previously rewarded stimulus is not. In this deterministic version, healthy adult humans immediately detect the change in contingencies and start responding to the other stimulus. In addition, the task may be rendered more challenging using a probabilistic version of it [88]. Here, the reward is not systematically delivered after the subject has chosen the rewarding stimulus, providing uncertainty regarding the current state of the reward contingencies. Only after having collected enough evidence that the previously reinforced stimulus has changed, will the participant shift to the newly (but still varyingly) reinforced stimulus. Performance in reversal learning is scored according to the number of persistent errors committed when participants maintain their response towards previously reinforced stimuli in spite of a negative reward. At the brain level, behavioural flexibility tasks, and reversal learning in particular, appear to engage the OFC and ACC regions. In a 2006 study, Remijnse et al. [89] showed that OCD was associated with a reduced response in the orbitofrontal–striatal network during adaptive switching to the new stimulus reinforcement regime. Using a different type of behavioural flexibility task, Chamberlain et al. [90] has demonstrated that OCD patients, as well as their relatives, show diminished OFC responses to behavioural adaptation triggered by the task, pointing towards the existence of an OCD endophenotype. Interestingly, in PD, STN stimulation has a beneficial effect on mental flexibility and working memory [91] and on cognitive flexibility, as expressed by the inhibition of habitual responses tested in a random number generation task [92]. Unsurprisingly, similar behavioural tasks have long been used with mice using various response modalities (T-maze, lever press, nose-poke), and animal studies have confirmed the role of OFC or OFC homologous regions in behavioural flexibility.

## Conclusions

Within the last decade, a multi-dimensional approach has been proposed to better link clinical observations with the increasing amount of data obtained in biological psychiatry studies [93, 94].

In fact, the integrative view of complementary research fields, including neuroimaging, genetics, experimental psychology, computational psychiatry, and animal models, has led to a redefinition of OCD nosography and its heterogenous expression. In the future, further insights may come from studies combining different fields, as illustrated by recent pioneering work with OCD patients which has combined computational and neurophysiological approaches [95] or experimental psychology with neuroimaging [96]. The identification of new targets using such complementary approaches could also be used to develop entirely novel animal models of psychiatric diseases. It would open the way to developing new ideas by manipulating brain circuits, for example using optogenetic manipulations that would reproduce relevant aspects of the OCD symptomatology.

To analyse and understand abnormal behavioural functions in OCD patients, a promising perspective comes from the recent field of computational psychiatry. It sets out to investigate the changes in elementary cognitive processes in dysfunctional patients, such as behavioural flexibility or uncertainty monitoring, as described previously. Using the computational approach, researchers try to infer the hidden variables and states associated with the computations the brain might use when performing a task. Indeed, mathematical models of how choices emerge from elementary computations can potentially bridge the gap between neural activities and the behavioural choices.

A more translational and comprehensive approach that integrates novel fields of fundamental and clinical research should therefore be used to unveil the neurobiology of OCD and possibly lead to the development of more effective treatments.

## REFERENCES

1. Wittchen HU, Jacobi F, Rehm J, et al. The size and burden of mental disorders and other disorders of the brain in Europe 2010. *Eur Neuropsychopharmacol* 2011, 21:655–79.
2. World Health Organization. *The World Health Report 2004: Changing History*. Geneva: World Health Organization; 2004.
3. Abramowitz JS, Taylor S, McKay D. Obsessive-compulsive disorder. *Lancet* 2009, 374:491–9.
4. Insel TR. From animal models to model animals. *Biol Psychiatry* 2007, 62:1337–9.
5. Nestler EJ, Hyman SE. Animal models of neuropsychiatric disorders. *Nat Neurosci* 2010, 13:1161–9.
6. Saxena S, Rauch SL. Functional neuroimaging and the neuroanatomy of obsessive-compulsive disorder. *Psychiatr Clin North Am* 2000, 23:563–86.
7. Alexander GE, DeLong MR, Strick PL. Parallel organization of functionally segregated circuits linking basal ganglia and cortex. *Annu Rev Neurosci* 1986, 9:357–81.
8. Graybiel AM. Habits, rituals, and the evaluative brain. *Annu Rev Neurosci* 2008, 31:359–87.

9. Yin HH, Knowlton BJ. The role of the basal ganglia in habit formation. *Nat Rev Neurosci* 2006, 7:464–76.

10. Thorn CA, Atallah H, Howe M, Graybiel AM. Differential dynamics of activity changes in dorsolateral and dorsomedial striatal loops during learning. *Neuron* 2010, 66:781–95.

11. Yin HH, Mulcare SP, Hilário MRF, et al. Dynamic reorganization of striatal circuits during the acquisition and consolidation of a skill. *Nat Neurosci* 2009, 12:333–41.

12. Ting JT, Feng G. Neurobiology of obsessive–compulsive disorder: insights into neural circuitry dysfunction through mouse genetics. *Curr Opin Neurobiol* 2011, 21:842–8.

13. Welch JM, Lu J, Rodriguiz RM, et al. Cortico-striatal synaptic defects and OCD-like behaviours in *Sapap3*-mutant mice. *Nature* 2007, 448:894–900.

14. Burguière E, Monteiro P, Feng G, Graybiel AM. Optogenetic stimulation of lateral orbitofronto-striatal pathway suppresses compulsive behaviours. *Science* 2013, 340:1243–6.

15. Shmelkov SV, Hormigo A, Jing D, et al. Slitrk5 deficiency impairs corticostriatal circuitry and leads to obsessive-compulsive-like behaviours in mice. *Nat Med* 2010, 16:598–602.

16. Burguière E, Monteiro P, Mallet L, Feng G, Graybiel AM. Striatal circuits, habits, and implications for obsessive–compulsive disorder. *Curr Opin Neurobiol* 2015, 30:59–65.

17. Greer JM, Capecchi MR. Hoxb8 is required for normal grooming behaviour in mice. *Neuron* 2002, 33:23–34.

18. Aoyama K, Suh SW, Hamby AM, et al. Neuronal glutathione deficiency and age-dependent neurodegeneration in the EAAC1 deficient mouse. *Nat Neurosci* 2006, 9:119–26.

19. Le Bihan D. Looking into the functional architecture of the brain with diffusion MRI. *Nat Rev Neurosci* 2003, 4:469–80.

20. Mori S, Crain BJ, Chacko VP, van Zijl PC. Three-dimensional tracking of axonal projections in the brain by magnetic resonance imaging. *Ann Neurol* 1999, 45:265–9.

21. Poupon C, Clark CA, Frouin V, et al. Regularization of diffusion-based direction maps for the tracking of brain white matter fascicles. *NeuroImage* 2000, 12:184–95.

22. Koch K, Reess TJ, Rus OG, Zimmer C, Zaudig M. Diffusion tensor imaging (DTI) studies in patients with obsessive-compulsive disorder (OCD): a review. *J Psychiatr Res* 2014, 54:26–35.

23. Nambu A, Tokuno H, Takada M. Functional significance of the cortico–subthalamo–pallidal 'hyperdirect' pathway. *Neurosci Res* 2002, 43:111–17.

24. Takagi T, Nakamura M, Yamada M, et al. Visualization of peripheral nerve degeneration and regeneration: monitoring with diffusion tensor tractography. *NeuroImage* 2009, 44:884–92.

25. Soria G, Aguilar E, Tudela R, Mullol J, Planas AM, Marin C. In vivo magnetic resonance imaging characterization of bilateral structural changes in experimental Parkinson's disease: a T2 relaxometry study combined with longitudinal diffusion tensor imaging and manganese-enhanced magnetic resonance imaging in the 6-hydroxydopamine rat model. *Eur J Neurosci* 2011, 33:1551–60.

26. Gutman DA, Keifer OP, Magnuson ME, et al. A DTI tractography analysis of infralimbic and prelimbic connectivity in the mouse using high-throughput MRI. *NeuroImage* 2012, 63:800–11.

27. Nakamae T, Sakai Y, Abe Y, et al. Altered fronto-striatal fiber topography and connectivity in obsessive-compulsive disorder. *PLoS One.* 2014, 9:e112075.

28. Harrison BJ, Soriano-Mas C, Pujol J, et al. Altered corticostriatal functional connectivity in obsessive-compulsive disorder. *Arch Gen Psychiatry* 2009, 66:1189–200.

29. Harrison BJ, Pujol J, Cardoner N, et al. Brain corticostriatal systems and the major clinical symptom dimensions of obsessive-compulsive disorder. *Biol Psychiatry* 2013, 73:321–8.

30. Menzies L, Achard S, Chamberlain SR, et al. Neurocognitive endophenotypes of obsessive-compulsive disorder. *Brain* 2007, 130:3223–36.

31. Figee M, Luigjes J, Smolders R, et al. Deep brain stimulation restores frontostriatal network activity in obsessive-compulsive disorder. *Nat Neurosci* 2013, 16:386–7.

32. Morgiève M, N'Diaye K, Haynes WIA, et al. Dynamics of psychotherapy-related cerebral haemodynamic changes in obsessive compulsive disorder using a personalized exposure task in functional magnetic resonance imaging. *Psychol Med* 2014, 44:1461–73.

33. Hirschmann J, Özkurt TE, Butz M, et al. Distinct oscillatory STN-cortical loops revealed by simultaneous MEG and local field potential recordings in patients with Parkinson's disease. *NeuroImage* 2011, 55:1159–68.

34. Williams D, Tijssen M, Van Bruggen G, et al. Dopamine-dependent changes in the functional connectivity between basal ganglia and cerebral cortex in humans. *Brain J Neurol* 2002, 125:1558–69.

35. Mallet L, Mesnage V, Houeto J-L, et al. Compulsions, Parkinson's disease, and stimulation. *Lancet* 2002, 360:1302–4.

36. Nuttin B, Cosyns P, Demeulemeester H, Gybels J, Meyerson B. Electrical stimulation in anterior limbs of internal capsules in patients with obsessive-compulsive disorder. *Lancet* 1999, 354:1526.

37. Nuttin BJ, Gabriëls LA, Cosyns PR, et al. Long-term electrical capsular stimulation in patients with obsessive-compulsive disorder. *Neurosurgery* 2008, 62:966–77.

38. Mallet L, Polosan M, Jaafari N, et al. Subthalamic nucleus stimulation in severe obsessive-compulsive disorder. *N Engl J Med* 2008, 359:2121–34.

39. Greenberg BD, Gabriels LA, Malone DA Jr, et al. Deep brain stimulation of the ventral internal capsule/ventral striatum for obsessive-compulsive disorder: worldwide experience. *Mol Psychiatry* 2010, 15:64–79.

40. Kisely S, Hall K, Siskind D, Frater J, Olson S, Crompton D. Deep brain stimulation for obsessive-compulsive disorder: a systematic review and meta-analysis. *Psychol Med* 2014, 44:3533–42.

41. Alonso P, Cuadras D, Gabriëls L, et al. Deep brain stimulation for obsessive-compulsive disorder: a meta-analysis of treatment outcome and predictors of response. *PLoS One* 2015, 10:e0133591.

42. Ooms P, Mantione M, Figee M, Schuurman PR, van den Munckhof P, Denys D. Deep brain stimulation for obsessive-compulsive disorders: long-term analysis of quality of life. *J Neurol Neurosurg Psychiatry* 2014, 85:153–8.

43. Greenberg BD, Malone DA, Friehs GM, et al. Three-year outcomes in deep brain stimulation for highly resistant obsessive-compulsive disorder. *Neuropsychopharmacol* 2006, 31:2384–93.

44. Luyten L, Hendrickx S, Raymaekers S, Gabriëls L, Nuttin B. Electrical stimulation in the bed nucleus of the stria terminalis alleviates severe obsessive-compulsive disorder. *Mol Psychiatry* 2016, 21:1272–80.

45. Fayad SM, Guzick AG, Reid AM, et al. Six-nine year follow-up of deep brain stimulation for obsessive-compulsive disorder. *PLoS One* 2016, 11:e0167875.

45a. Mallet L, Du Montcel ST, Clair AH, et al. STOC Long-term Study Group. Long-term effects of subthalamic stimulation in obsessive-compulsive disorder: Follow-up of a randomized controlled trial. *Brain Stimul* 2019, 12(4):1080–2.

46. Rasmussen SA, Eisen JL, Greenberg BD: Toward a neuroanatomy of obsessive-compulsive disorder revisited. *Biol Psychiatry* 2013, 73:298–9.

47. Haynes WIA, Haber SN. The organization of prefrontal-subthalamic inputs in primates provides an anatomical substrate for both functional specificity and integration: implications for basal ganglia models and deep brain stimulation. *J Neurosci* 2013, 33:4804–14.

48. Le Jeune F, Vérin M, N'Diaye K, et al. Decrease of prefrontal metabolism after subthalamic stimulation in obsessive-compulsive disorder: a positron emission tomography study. *Biol Psychiatry* 2010, 68:1016–22.

49. Haynes WIA, Mallet L. High-frequency stimulation of deep brain structures in obsessive-compulsive disorder: the search for a valid circuit. *Eur J Neurosci* 2010, 32:1118–27.

50. Burbaud P, Clair A-H, Langbour N, et al. Neuronal activity correlated with checking behaviour in the subthalamic nucleus of patients with obsessive-compulsive disorder. *Brain J Neurol* 2013, 136:304–17.

51. Welter M-L, Burbaud P, Fernandez-Vidal S, et al. Basal ganglia dysfunction in OCD: subthalamic neuronal activity correlates with symptoms severity and predicts high-frequency stimulation efficacy. *Transl Psychiatry* 2011, 1:e5.

52. McIntyre CC, Grill WM, Sherman DL, Thakor NV. Cellular effects of deep brain stimulation: model-based analysis of activation and inhibition. *J Neurophysiol* 2004, 91:1457–69.

53. Gradinaru V, Mogri M, Thompson KR, Henderson JM, Deisseroth K. Optical deconstruction of parkinsonian neural circuitry. *Science* 2009, 324:354–9.

54. Deisseroth K. Optogenetics. *Nat Methods* 2011, 8:26–9.

55. Tye KM, Prakash R, Kim S-Y, et al. Amygdala circuitry mediating reversible and bidirectional control of anxiety. *Nature* 2011, 471:358–62.

56. Yizhar O, Fenno LE, Prigge M, et al. Neocortical excitation/inhibition balance in information processing and social dysfunction. *Nature* 2011, 477:171–8.

57. Ahmari SE, Spellman T, Douglass NL, et al. Repeated corticostriatal stimulation generates persistent OCD-like behaviour. *Science* 2013, 340:1234–9.

58. Pauls DL, Abramovitch A, Rauch SL, Geller DA. Obsessive-compulsive disorder: an integrative genetic and neurobiological perspective. *Nat Rev Neurosci* 2014, 15:410–24.

59. Kreitzer AC. Physiology and pharmacology of striatal neurons. *Annu Rev Neurosci* 2009, 32:127–47.

60. Beucke JC, Sepulcre J, Talukdar T, et al. Abnormally high degree connectivity of the orbitofrontal cortex in obsessive-compulsive disorder. *JAMA Psychiatry* 2013, 70:619–29.

61. Lewis M, Kim S-J. The pathophysiology of restricted repetitive behaviour. *J Neurodev Disord* 2009, 1:114–32.

62. Rotge J-Y, Guehl D, Dilharreguy B, et al. Meta-analysis of brain volume changes in obsessive-compulsive disorder. *Biol Psychiatry* 2009, 65:75–83.

63. Worbe Y, Mallet L, Golmard J-L, et al. Repetitive behaviours in patients with Gilles de la Tourette syndrome: tics, compulsions, or both? *PLoS One* 2010, 5:e12959.

64. Shin NY, Lee TY, Kim E, Kwon JS. Cognitive functioning in obsessive-compulsive disorder: a meta-analysis. *Psychol Med* 2013, 44:1121–30.

65. Abramovitch A, Abramowitz JS, Mittelman A. The neuropsychology of adult obsessive-compulsive disorder: a meta-analysis. *Clin Psychol Rev* 2013, 33:1163–71.

66. Snyder HR, Kaiser RH, Warren SL, Heller W. Obsessive-compulsive disorder is associated with broad impairments in executive function: a meta-analysis. *Clin Psychol Sci* 2015, 3:301–30.

67. Rachman S. A cognitive theory of compulsive checking. *Behav Res Ther* 2002, 40:625–39.

68. Mallet L, Schüpbach M, N'Diaye K, et al. Stimulation of subterritories of the subthalamic nucleus reveals its role in the integration of the emotional and motor aspects of behaviour. *Proc Natl Acad Sci U S A* 2007, 104:10661–6.

69. Weintraub DB, Zaghloul KA. The role of the subthalamic nucleus in cognition. *Rev Neurosci* 2013, 24:125–38.

70. Frank MJ. Hold your horses: a dynamic computational role for the subthalamic nucleus in decision making. *Neural Netw* 2006, 19:1120–36.

71. Brittain J-S, Brown P. Oscillations and the basal ganglia: motor control and beyond. *NeuroImage* 2014, 85 Pt 2:637–47.

72. Zaghloul KA, Weidemann CT, Lega BC, Jaggi JL, Baltuch GH, Kahana MJ. Neuronal activity in the human subthalamic nucleus encodes decision conflict during action selection. *J Neurosci* 2012, 32:2453–60.

73. Baunez C, Lardeux S. Frontal cortex-like functions of the subthalamic nucleus. *Front Syst Neurosci* 2011, 5:83.

74. Coulthard EJ, Bogacz R, Javed S, et al. Distinct roles of dopamine and subthalamic nucleus in learning and probabilistic decision making. *Brain* 2012, 135:3721–34.

75. Foote AL, Crystal JD. Metacognition in the rat. *Curr Biol* 2007, 17:551–5.

76. Kepecs A, Uchida N, Zariwala HA, Mainen ZF. Neural correlates, computation and behavioural impact of decision confidence. *Nature* 2008, 455:227–31.

77. van den Hout M, Kindt M. Repeated checking causes memory distrust. *Behav Res Ther* 2003, 41:301–16.

78. Rotge JY, Clair AH, Jaafari N, et al. A challenging task for assessment of checking behaviours in obsessive-compulsive disorder. *Acta Psychiatr Scand* 2008, 117:465–73.

79. Clair AH, N'Diaye K, Baroukh T, et al. Excessive checking for non-anxiogenic stimuli in obsessive-compulsive disorder. *Eur Psychiatry J* 2013, 28:507–13.

80. Mink JW. The basal ganglia: focused selection and inhibition of competing motor programs. *Prog Neurobiol* 1996, 50:381–425.

81. Ridderinkhof KR, Ullsperger M, Crone EA, Nieuwenhuis S. The role of the medial frontal cortex in cognitive control. *Science* 2004, 306:443–7.

82. Alegre M, Lopez-Azcarate J, Obeso I, et al. The subthalamic nucleus is involved in successful inhibition in the stop-signal task: a local field potential study in Parkinson's disease. *Exp Neurol* 2013, 239:1–12.

83. Eagle DM, Baunez C, Hutcheson DM, Lehmann O, Shah AP, Robbins TW. Stop-signal reaction-time task performance: role of prefrontal cortex and subthalamic nucleus. *Cereb Cortex* 2008, 18:178–88.

84. Barnes TD, Kubota Y, Hu D, Jin DZ, Graybiel AM. Activity of striatal neurons reflects dynamic encoding and recoding of procedural memories. *Nature* 2005, 437:1158–61.

85. Jin X, Costa RM. Start/stop signals emerge in nigrostriatal circuits during sequence learning. *Nature* 2010, 466:457–62.

86. Cui G, Jun SB, Jin X, et al. Concurrent activation of striatal direct and indirect pathways during action initiation. *Nature* 2013, 494:238–42.

87. Anzak A, Gaynor L, Beigi M, *et al*. Subthalamic nucleus gamma oscillations mediate a switch from automatic to controlled processing: a study of random number generation in Parkinson's disease. *NeuroImage* 2013, 64:284–9.

88. Cools R, Clark L, Owen AM, Robbins TW. Defining the neural mechanisms of probabilistic reversal learning using event-related functional magnetic resonance imaging. *J Neurosci* 2002, 22:4563–7.

89. Remijnse PL, Nielen MMA, van Balkom AJLM, *et al*. Reduced orbitofrontal-striatal activity on a reversal learning task in obsessive-compulsive disorder. *Arch Gen Psychiatry* 2006, 63:1225–36.

90. Chamberlain SR, Fineberg NA, Blackwell AD, *et al*. Motor inhibition and cognitive flexibility in obsessive-compulsive disorder and trichotillomania. *Am J Psychiatry* 2006, 163:1282–4.

91. Jahanshahi M, Ardouin CMA, Brown RG, *et al*. The impact of deep brain stimulation on executive function in Parkinson's disease. *Brain* 2000, 123:1142–54.

92. Witt K, Pulkowski U, Herzog J, *et al*. Deep brain stimulation of the subthalamic nucleus improves cognitive flexibility but impairs response inhibition in parkinson disease. *Arch Neurol* 2004, 61:697–700.

93. Mataix-Cols D, Rosario-Campos MC, Leckman JF. A multi-dimensional model of obsessive-compulsive disorder. *Am J Psychiatry* 2005, 162:228–38.

94. Katerberg H, Delucchi KL, Stewart SE, *et al*. Symptom dimensions in OCD: item-level factor analysis and heritability estimates. *Behav Genet* 2010, 40:505–17.

95. Palminteri S, Clair A-H, Mallet L, Pessiglione M. Similar improvement of reward and punishment learning by serotonin reuptake inhibitors in obsessive-compulsive disorder. *Biol Psychiatry* 2012, 72:244–50.

96. Chamberlain SR, Menzies L, Hampshire A, *et al*. Orbitofrontal dysfunction in patients with obsessive-compulsive disorder and their unaffected relatives. *Science* 2008, 321:421–2.

# 95

# Obsessive–compulsive disorder

*Lior Carmi, Naomi A. Fineberg, Oded Ben Arush, and Joseph Zohar*

## Introduction

Up to the early 1980s, obsessive–compulsive disorder (OCD) was considered a rare (less than 0.5%) treatment-refractory, chronic condition of psychological origin. Dynamic psychotherapy was widely used and yet had little benefit; this was also the case for pharmacological interventions [1].

The observation that clomipramine, a tricyclic drug for depression with a serotonergic profile, is effective in treating symptoms of OCD [2, 3] has increased clinical interest in this disorder, including its epidemiology; several researchers have since reported a prevalence of OCD of about 2% in the general population [4, 5]. However, changes to the diagnostic system, especially the addition of OCD-related disorders (OCRDs) to OCD (and creating the OCRD cluster) [6], have dramatically increased the calculated prevalence of this cluster to close to 9%.

## Diagnosis

The diagnosis of OCD according to DSM-5 criteria is based on the presence of either obsessions or compulsions, which cause marked distress, are time-consuming (more than an hour daily), or significantly interfere with a person's normal routine and social and occupational activities. Notably, in DSM-5, two specifiers were added: the degree of insight (ranging from good or fair to absent) and the presence (or absence) of tics.

According to DSM-5 [6], obsessions are repetitive, intrusive, and distressing thoughts, ideas, images, or urges that are often experienced as meaningless, inappropriate, and irrelevant, and persist despite efforts to suppress, resist, or ignore them. Compulsions are repetitive, stereotyped behaviours and/or mental acts that a person feels driven to perform as a standalone urge or as a perceived reaction to an obsession. Though such intrusive thoughts and ritualistic behaviours are also frequently reported in the general population [7–9], those seen in OCD are considered psychopathological as they are time-consuming and cause marked distress and significant functional impairment [10]. OCD can express itself in various ways. The obsession component includes: dirt/germs, aggression/harm, religious/moral issues, and sexual obsessions. The compulsion component include: washing, checking, ordering, counting, reassurance seeking, and symmetry acts and various mental compulsions [11].

In accordance, a common expression of OCD is an obsession around dirt or 'germs', together with washing or avoiding presumed contaminated objects (door knobs, electrical switches, newspapers, peoples' hands, telephones, etc.). It contains 'hard-to-avoid' substances (for example, faeces, urine, dust, or germs), to the extent that individuals sometimes avoid leaving home. Another common expression of OCD involves pathological doubt, which is frequently accompanied by a compulsion to check. For example, the person may need to check whether the oven is turned off or the front and back doors are closed—the checking may involve many trips back home to recheck what was already checked. In OCD, the checking procedure, instead of resolving uncertainty, often contributes to even greater doubt, which leads to further checking. Other common expressions of OCD are related to the fear of causing harm, for example by being neglectful (for instance, an obsession of hurting someone while driving, leading to driving back towards the relevant spot repeatedly and checking no one was hurt).

The need for symmetry or precision, which may interfere with task completion and result in pathological slowness, is another presentation of OCD. For those patients, it can take hours to eat a meal or shave, in an attempt to do things 'just right'. Other common expressions include hoarding, involving the urge to accumulate and difficulty with discarding objects ('What if I will need it'?) and religious obsessions (fear of blasphemy).

At times, patients complain of intrusive thoughts without noticeable compulsions. However, such patients are often found to be engaging in mental compulsions, for example mental checking or analysing (for instance, whether the intrusive thought exists).

Several studies [12–16] have used factor-analytic methods to systematically examine the structural characteristics of OCD symptoms, revealing four main obsessive–compulsive (OC) factors:

1. Aggressive/sexual/religious/somatic obsessions accompanied by checking compulsions.

2. Symmetry obsessions accompanied by ordering and arranging/counting/repeating compulsions.
3. Contamination obsession accompanied by cleaning compulsions.
4. Hoarding obsession accompanied by hoarding and collecting compulsions.

Other theories [17–20] have suggested that the heterogeneity of OCD may be better understood with two core dimensions: harm avoidance and sense of incompleteness. They suggested that OCD is characterized either 'by anxious apprehension and exaggerated avoidance of potential harm' (for example, washing, repugnant obsessions, harm-avoidant checking) or alternatively by attempts to reduce feeling of incompleteness (for example, symmetry, counting, repeating, slowness). Interestingly, these feelings of incompleteness were first described in 1903 [21] as a central phenomenological feature of OCD, according to which OCD patients are tormented by the feeling that their actions are incompletely achieved or do not produce the expected satisfaction. Their inability to achieve 'closure' concerning actions/perceptions leads to what later was labelled as the 'not just right experience' (NJRE) [22, 23].

However, it should be noted that recent studies [24] documented that obsession may not always precede compulsion, as the traditional acronym OCD suggests. Alternatively, the pathological loop may start with the actual urge to perform the compulsion (not as a purposeful, goal-driven act, but as a habit), while the obsessional component develops later as a secondary phenomenon. The acronym OCD may be used to describe this course of illness.

Indeed, obsessions and compulsions are not necessarily rationally related; hence, a patient might perform a compulsion of clapping hands in a specific way, in order to prevent an obsession of being contaminated with germs.

Most patients present with multiple obsessions and compulsions. The symptoms may shift over time; for example, a patient who had washing rituals during childhood may present with checking rituals as an adult [19, 20].

As OCD symptoms are usually embedded within the updated culture and technology, it often assimilates with the frequent usage of the Internet and smartphones in daily life. Harnessing this technology into compulsive behaviours (for example, compulsive checking of emails/posts, taking photos as another presentation of list makings, electronic hoarding, etc.) might not always be diagnosed, since it often camouflages as proper Internet use.

### Diagnosis and differential diagnosis

As OCD has diverse expressions, the diagnosis, as well as differential diagnosis, requires careful and thorough evaluation.

The NICE guidelines include five simple questions that might help identify OCD (Box 95.1) [25]. These questions are recommended whenever a mental status examination is carried out; since patients tend to hide their symptoms (due to the ego-dystonic nature of OCD), asking direct, specific questions is often the only way to diagnose OCD.

Another clue may be past or current tics (including vocal tics) and a family history of OCD or OC spectrum disorders (OCSDs) which include: hoarding disorder; body dysmorphic disorder (BDD); and body-focused repetitive behaviours such as trichotillomania (hair pulling), onychophagia (nail biting), and excoriation (skin picking). Personal distress and functional impairment, which are required for

---

**Box 95.1** Quick screen for obsessive–compulsive disorder

- Do you wash or clean a lot?
- Do you check things a lot?
- Is there any thought that keeps bothering you that you would like to get rid of but can't?
- Do your daily activities take a long time to finish?
- Are you concerned about orderliness or symmetry?
- Do these problems trouble you?

Source: data from National Collaborating Centre for Mental Health, *Obsessive-compulsive disorder: Core interventions in the treatment of obsessive-compulsive disorder and body dysmorphic disorder*, Copyright (2006), The British Psychological Society and The Royal College of Psychiatrists.

---

diagnosis, differentiate OCD from ordinary or mildly excessive worries, thoughts, and habits.

Psychiatric diagnoses that show a presentation similar to that of OCD include schizophrenia, depressive disorder, post-traumatic stress disorder (PTSD), social anxiety, eating disorder, and phobias. The importance of an accurate diagnosis is due to the uniqueness that underlines the treatment, as well as the course, prognosis, and therapeutic goals for these disorders. Severe, bizarre, and incapacitating OCD symptoms, especially when accompanied with a lack of insight (delusions), are often misdiagnosed as schizophrenia. By introducing the lack of insight specifier and by restricting the diagnosis of schizophrenia to only those with primary symptoms, DSM-5 might help to reduce such misdiagnoses.

At times, OCD symptoms may appear as a phobia. While the classic phobic objects are avoidable (for example, tunnels, dogs, elevators) and the anxiety is reduced in the absence of the stimulus, the 'phobic' stimulus in OCD are often unavoidable (for example, germs, dirt, radioactive waves, etc.).

Major depressive disorder (MDD) is frequently associated with ruminations that are mood-congruent and, unlike OCD, usually involve beliefs of personal failure related to past events. Although MDD is common in OCD, in the majority of cases, the OCD had started first and depression developed later as a secondary response to the substantial difficulties resulting from OCD.

## Epidemiology

### Prevalence

OCD is a global phenomenon, with substantial similarity across cultures in symptom clusters, gender distribution, age of onset, and comorbidities [26]. However, regional and historical variations in symptom expression exist, and cultural factors may shape the content layer of obsessions and compulsions (for example, contamination by syphilis in the past and by AIDS nowadays; repetition of prayers by religious individuals vs personal mantras in secular persons).

Using the restricted DSM-IV definition (that is, not including OCD-related disorders), the lifetime prevalence of OCD in the general population was calculated at 2–3% in a number of seminal studies [4, 27]. Those percentages have been confirmed across cultures [5] and support the biological basis of OCD. Although the cultural, economic, and social factors play a role in the presentation of

OCD (that is, the content of obsessions and the shape of the compulsions), yet its prevalence is equally distributed across the globe.

More recent large-scale cross-sectional surveys of US and European citizens using diagnostic instruments compatible with DSM-IV produced a more conservative estimate of a 1.6% [28, 29] and 0.8% [30, 31] lifetime prevalence, respectively. In contrast, a detailed longitudinal prospective study of community respondents in the Swiss Canton of Zurich, [32], that additionally looked for subthreshold forms of OCD, reported a prevalence rate of 3.5% for OCD (males: 1.7%; females: 5.3%), 9.7% for obsessive–compulsive syndrome (males: 1.7%; females: 5.3%), and 11.2% for obsessive–compulsive symptoms (males: 13.7%; females: 8.8%). Thus, in this study, taking into account the whole spectrum of obsessive–compulsive symptomatology, over 10% of the population were affected.

In DSM-5, OCD was separated from the anxiety disorders and categorized within a new diagnostic category ('Obsessive–compulsive and related disorder'), which includes, in addition to OCD, disorders such as: hoarding disorder; BDD; and body-focused repetitive behaviours such as trichotillomania (hair pulling), onychophagia (nail biting), and excoriation (skin picking). Considering this spectrum-oriented view of OCRDs, the cumulative prevalence of OCSDs is much higher than that of OCD alone. Summing up the prevalence of the individual OCRDs (Table 95.1) and factoring in the comorbidity rates, the overall prevalence of OCRDs as a group could be as high as 9.5%.

## Gender

OCD is overrepresented in females (around 1.5:1) [32], and gender differences in the pattern of symptom dimensions have been reported. For example, females are more likely to have contamination obsessions and symptoms in the cleaning dimension and males are more likely to have symptoms in forbidden thoughts and religious and symmetry rituals [41]. Males are more prone to be associated with significant interference in life; for example, two-thirds remain single vs only one-third of women. Moreover, almost half of male patients continued to live with their original families or in assisted homes, compared with only 20% of women. These rates might be due to the relatively earlier onset of the pathology in males [41] or the different course of OCD in males vs females.

## Course of OCD

The onset of OCD is often spontaneous; however, in some cases, OCD symptoms follow a stressful or traumatic event (for example, pregnancy, labour, accident, etc.) [42, 43]. Due to the secretive nature of the disorder, there is often a delay (of up to several years [44]) before patients are adequately diagnosed. However, the delay may shorten with increased public awareness to the disorder, for example through articles, books, and movies, and if specific questions regarding OCD are included in the mental status examination (Box 95.1).

The course is usually chronic; yet some patients experience a fluctuating course [45]. In a 40-year longitudinal study (1953–1993), during which no effective and long-lasting therapies were available, the duration of illness was chronic for most patients, with half still experiencing clinically relevant symptoms and another third subclinical symptoms at 40 years' follow-up [46]. Among those followed up for half a century since onset, 37% still had OCD. Although, in the study, most patients showed some improvement along the years, complete recovery occurred in only about one-fifth of patients. A study prospectively examined 113 OCD patients (all of whom had a history of at least one other comorbid anxiety disorder) and found that the probability of OCD remission was 0.16 at year 1 and reached 0.42 by year 15 [47]. For those who remitted, the probability of recurrence of OCD remained low, approximating 0.25 from year 5 onwards. Those who were married and those without comorbid MDD were more likely to enter remission. A relatively high rate of remission at a specialist paediatric OCD clinic was also found in a 2010 study [48] where approximately 60% of 142 young people with OCD assessed at baseline did not have a full clinical syndrome of OCD after up to 9 years. However, approximately 50% of participants were still receiving treatment and about 50% expressed a need for further treatment. In the same study, the main predictor for persistent OCD was the duration of illness at assessment. Indeed, a meta-analysis of 22 studies ($n = 521$) of child/adolescent-onset OCD found that earlier age at onset and increased duration predicted persistence of illness [49].

Environmental factors like family accommodation or compliance with OCD symptoms are also important variables. Those kinds of family interactions, while understandable, can be destructive. For example, answering reassurance questions or participating in avoidance behaviours (for example, 'I will open the door for you so you will not need to wash', 'I will turn the stove off so you will not need to check', etc.) stands as a significant barrier to recovery.

## Age at onset of OCD

The mean age at onset of OCD has traditionally been reported to be late adolescence [50–52], with a range of 10–22 years [32]. However, recent studies report an even earlier mean age at onset of around 15 years [53], with onset after 30 years being uncommon

**Table 95.1** Summary of prevalence of OCRD

| Disorder | Prevalence | Comorbidity with OCD | Net prevalence (prevalence – comorbidity) |
|---|---|---|---|
| Body dysmorphic disorder | 1.9–2.2% [33] | 30–35% [34] | 1.4% |
| Hoarding disorder | 2–5% [35] | 8–35% [36] | 2.4% |
| Trichotillomania (hair pulling disorder, HPD) | 0.6–2% [37] | 13% [38] | 1% |
| Excoriation (skin picking disorder) | 1.4–5.4% [39] | 16% [40] | 3% |

Net prevalence equals prevalence (mean) minus comorbidity (mean).
Comorbidity equals comorbidity (mean) times prevalence (mean).
Sum of OCRD = 1.6% (OCD) + 1.4% (pure BDD) + 2.4% (pure hoarding) + 1% (pure trichotillomania) + 3% (pure skin picking disorder) = 9.4% (OCRD).

[54]. Females are overrepresented in late-onset OCD (around 1.5:1), while in the earlier onset of illness grouping, males are more representative [55]. Nearly 25% of males have an onset before the age of 10 years [56].

In a 40-year longitudinal study [46], early-onset OCD was associated with poorer outcome, especially in men. More recent studies have reported a negative correlation between age at onset and duration of illness [53]. Additionally, an association between early onset and greater symptom severity [57], male gender [58], genetic loading [59], [60], severity of compulsions [61], poor insight [62], co-occurring tic disorders [63], hair pulling [64], multiple anxiety disorders [61], and OC personality disorders [65] has been identified.

Late-onset OCD may include cases of OCD that have been developed after exposure to traumatic events (post-traumatic OCD) [66]. Females may develop OCD in pregnancy or after parturition or miscarriage [42].

## OCD and suicidal risk

Historically, OCD was considered a psychiatric disorder with relatively low rates of suicidal ideation (which was attributed to its compulsive domain). However, recent studies have challenged this perception and concluded that the risk of attempted and completed suicide among individuals with OCD is substantial [67]. Some authors suggested that suicide risk is more strongly predicted by psychiatric comorbidity, for example rates of comorbid depression and anxiety, rather than OCD itself [10, 11]. However, even when controlling for comorbidity, the risk of suicidality remains significant among OCD sufferers [68], and rates of suicidal ideation ranging between 20% and 46% have been reported [11–15]. Sixty-five per cent of one OCD sample had endorsed at least one of the questions about suicidal phenomena as positive. Of these, 32% had made suicidal plans and 19.4% had attempted suicide [16]. Nevertheless, it is important to note that suicidal thoughts may sometimes be a symptom of OCD (for example, 'I might commit suicide', 'what is the preferable way to commit suicide'), and not a genuine suicidal ideation.

## OCD and insight

Classically, OCD is defined as an ego-dystonic disorder, that is, a disorder in which the patient realizes that the obsessions and/or compulsions are irrational or excessive.

However, keeping in mind the diversity of the disorder, DSM-IV included the subtype of 'poor insight'.

DSM-5 extended the diagnostic boundaries of OCD by allowing to include absent insight or delusions in OCD [6]. Even if the clinician spotted a clear-cut delusion, that is, the individual is completely convinced that the OCD beliefs are true, a diagnosis of OCD may be appropriate. The diagnosis should, however, be based on careful history-taking; in OCD, the disorder usually starts as ego-dystonic and slowly moves on the continuum of insight to delusional symptomatology. Moreover, in the case of OCD diagnosis, other compulsive components (now or in the past) are present and help to differentiate OCD from delusional disorders.

## Comorbidity

If another Axis I disorder is present, the diagnosis of OCD requires that the content of the obsessions or compulsions is not restricted to that disorder (for example, a preoccupation with food or weight in eating disorders, or guilt feelings in the presence of a major depressive episode). Similarly, OCD should not be diagnosed if it is due to the direct effects of a substance (for example, a drug abuse or a medication) or a general medical condition.

In a national survey of adults in the United States [44], OCD was associated with substantial comorbidity, not only with anxiety (75.8%) and mood disorders (63.3%), but also with impulse control (55.9%) and substance use disorders (38.6%).

### Anxiety disorders

In a lifetime comorbidity community study [69], 73% of OCD patients experienced an anxiety disorder (specifically: GAD 50%, social phobia 40%, agoraphobia 30%, simple phobia 20%, and panic disorder 17%). However, a recent international study reported a more conservative prevalence of comorbidity, with 14% of patients experiencing social anxiety, 13% experiencing GAD, and 12% experiencing panic disorder with or without agoraphobia [26].

### Obsessive–compulsive spectrum disorders

An early study by Du Toit and colleagues [70] showed that 57.6% of their OCD sample currently met the criteria for at least one putative OCSD and that 67.1% had a lifetime history of at least one comorbid OCSD. In that study, the OCSDs with the highest prevalence were compulsive self-injury (22.4%), compulsive buying (10.6%), and intermittent explosive disorder (10.6%). More recently, a cluster analysis of OCSDs in a sample of 210 OCD patients identified three separate clusters that were named: (1) 'reward deficiency' [including hair pulling disorder (trichotillomania or HPD), pathological gambling, hypersexual disorder, and Tourette's disorder (TD)]; (2) 'impulsivity' (including compulsive shopping, kleptomania, eating disorders, self-injury, and intermittent explosive disorder); and (3) 'somatic' [including body dysmorphic disorder (BDD) and hypochondriasis] [9]. Along these lines, a report from the International College of Obsessive–Compulsive Spectrum Disorders (ICOCS) showed that rates of comorbid OCSDs were high, particularly given the relatively low base rate of such disorders in the general population [26]. This is consistent with earlier work [4], which has emphasized the high prevalence of tic disorders, as well as of OCSD, in OCD.

### Depression and bipolar disorder

The lifetime prevalence for a major depressive episode in individuals with OCD ranges from 40% to 80% [44]. However, depression is usually secondary (that is, the OCD started first). Depression in children and adults with OCD has been related to variables, including an early age at onset, more severe obsessive–compulsive symptoms, lower levels of perceived competence, and family history of recurrent MDD [71]. This comorbidity is often associated with greater illness severity [72] and reduced quality of life [73].

Few studies have identified a greater likelihood of bipolar (especially bipolar-II) disorder comorbidity in OCD, as compared to its prevalence in the general population [44].

## Addiction

Up to the 1980s, OCD was regarded as a disorder of 'overcontrol' and the consensus was that substance use would be incompatible with OCD [74]. This notion has been dramatically changed with later studies [75–78], which found a strong association between OCD and substance abuse/dependence (including alcohol). Earlier age at OCD onset was associated with an increased risk of alcohol use disorders, but only comorbid bipolar disorder was associated with an increased risk of drug use disorders, suggesting that patients with early-onset OCD or comorbid BPD may be especially vulnerable to substance abuse disorder [79].

## Schizophrenia

Up to 30% of patients with chronic schizophrenia experience OC symptoms, and about 12% of them may be qualified for the diagnosis of OCD [80].

As in OCD in general, the OCD symptoms in these patients do not necessarily surface, unless specific questions are asked. Moreover, compulsive behaviour may be interpreted as 'stereotypic behaviours'. Patients with schizophrenia can distinguish (if properly questioned) ego-dystonic OC symptoms (perceived as coming from within) from schizophrenic ego-syntonic delusions (perceived as introduced from the outside). Follow-up studies demonstrated that a 'schizo-obsessive' diagnosis has stability over the years and is characterized by poor prognosis, especially if appropriate (that is, symptomatic, rather than syndromatic) treatment is not administered [81].

The poor prognosis of patients with schizophrenia and OCD, along with preliminary data regarding their response to a specific combination of treatments [specific drugs for psychosis (for example, amisulpride, ziprasidone, aripiprazole) in combination with serotonin reuptake inhibitors (SRIs)], has led several researchers to suggest that a 'schizo-obsessive' category may be of value [82].

## Post-traumatic stress disorder

PTSD–OCD comorbidity and post-traumatic obsessions have been reported [83, 84]. In one study, 41% out-of-combat PTSD patients were diagnosed with OCD, while an additional 6% had subthreshold OC symptoms [66]. No difference was found between PTSD and PTSD–OCD participant characteristics (including demographics, trauma-related factors, and other psychiatric comorbidity). The surprisingly high number of OCD found in this study suggests that PTSD–OCD (post-traumatic OCD) might be underdiagnosed and signifies the importance of direct assessment of OCD in patients with PTSD.

## Tic disorder

The high comorbidity with tic disorders raises interesting pathophysiological and therapeutic implications. The rate of tic disorders approaches 40% in juvenile OCD [85, 86], and the prevalence of Tourette's syndrome is increased among the relatives of OCD patients [87]. Due to its high prevalence, tic disorder was introduced as a specifier in DSM-5. Namely, each time that OCD is diagnosed, a specific and extra question needs to be included in order to identify tics. The importance of the specific attention to tics is related to different pharmacological intervention; augmentation (of serotonergic medications) with very small doses of a D2 receptor antagonist (for example, Haldol⁺) or a D2/5-HT2 receptor antagonist (for example,

risperidone) or a partial agonist (for example, aripiprazole) in those cases was repeatedly found to be clinically effective [88].

## Prognosis

OCD is traditionally considered to be a relatively chronic disorder [46, 89, 90]. However, some studies reported a more favourable prognosis and outcome [48, 89]. In a prospective, community-based study that followed up respondents for up to 30 years [32], almost two-thirds of individuals with OCD entered a sustained period of remission. The median duration for OCD was 16 years, suggesting a better prognosis for remission for less severe illness. Individuals with a longer duration of illness (more than 14 years) and a greater number of OC-burdened years (more than 5 years) and those seeking professional help (probably due to a more severe condition) experienced significantly delayed remission. In addition, these factors, together with comorbid anxiety and—to a lesser extent—affective disorders, were associated with significantly reduced remission rates.

With adequate treatment [which includes ERP, family guidance, encouragement to return to full activity, and therapeutically appropriate (that is, medium to high) doses of SRI], a significant percentage of patients show considerable to full improvement in their symptoms [91]. Prognosis in children is even better, with up to 80% achieving partial or full remission in a 3-year prospective study [92]. Good prognosis is associated with compliance to treatment of both the family and the patient, good social and occupational adjustment, and less avoidance [45]. The obsessional content does not seem to be related to the prognosis, except for hoarding, which is usually considered to have a less favourable outcome.

## Conclusions

OCD is a chronic condition, considered by the World Health Organization as one of the ten most disabling disorders. Two main changes took place in DSM-5 in relation to OCD: the creation of the 'Obsessive–compulsive and related disorders' cluster and the addition of two specifiers to the diagnosis procedure—the degree of insight [ranging from good or fair to absent (delusional)] and the presence (or absence) of tics. OCD is a worldwide disorder, with substantial similarity across cultures in symptom clusters, gender distribution, age of onset, and comorbidities. Mood disorders and other OCRDs are among the most common comorbidities in OCD. While the life prevalence of OCD is about 2% of the population, the life prevalence of OCRD is about 9%.

The mean age at onset of OCD is late adolescence, with a range of 10–22 years. Females are overrepresented in late-onset OCD, while in the earlier onset of illness grouping, males are more representative. Early onset and long duration of illness have been reported to be associated with poor prognosis. OCD is associated with substantial comorbidities, among which anxiety, mood disorders, and other OCRDs stand with the highest prevalence.

As OCD symptoms are usually embedded within the related culture, Internet-related compulsion is becoming more and more frequent. Taking into account its diverse expressions and its ego-dystonic manner/presentation (which make it difficult for patients to come forward with their symptoms), the diagnosis, as well as differential diagnosis, requires careful and thorough evaluation.

## REFERENCES

1. Salzman, L. and F.H. Thaler. Obsessive-compulsive disorders: a review of the literature. *American Journal of Psychiatry*, 1981. **138**: 286–96.
2. Zohar, J. and T.R. Insel. Obsessive-compulsive disorder: psychobiological approaches to diagnosis, treatment, and pathophysiology. *Biological Psychiatry*, 1987. **22**: 667–87.
3. Zohar, J., *et al.* Serotonergic responsivity in obsessive-compulsive disorder: comparison of patients and healthy controls. *Archives of General Psychiatry*, 1987. **44**: 946–51.
4. Robins, L.N., *et al.* Lifetime prevalence of specific psychiatric disorders in three sites. *Archives of General Psychiatry*, 1984. **41**: 949–58.
5. Weisman, M., *et al.* The cross national epidemiology of obsessive-compulsive disorder. *Journal of Clinical Psychiatry*, 1994. **55**(3 Suppl.): 5–10.
6. American Psychiatric Association. *Diagnostic and Statistical Manual of Mental Disorders*, fifth edition (DSM-5). Washington, DC: American Psychiatric Association; 2013.
7. Rachman, S. A cognitive theory of obsessions. *Behaviour Research and Therapy*, 1997. **35**: 793–802.
8. Salkovskis, P.M. and J. Harrison. Abnormal and normal obsessions—a replication. *Behaviour Research and Therapy*, 1984. **22**:549–52.
9. Muris, P., H. Merckelbach, and M. Clavan. Abnormal and normal compulsions. *Behaviour Research and Therapy*, 1997. **35**: 249–52.
10. American Psychiatric Association. *Diagnostic and Statistical Manual of Mental Disorders*, fifth edition (DSM-5). Washington, DC: American Psychiatric Association; 2013.
11. Pinto, A., *et al.* The Brown Longitudinal Obsessive Compulsive Study: clinical features and symptoms of the sample at intake. *Journal of Clinical Psychiatry*, 2006. **67**: 703.
12. Leckman, J.F., *et al.* Symptoms of obsessive-compulsive disorder. *American Journal of Psychiatry*, 1997. **154**: 911–17.
13. Bloch, M.H., *et al.* Meta-analysis of the symptom structure of obsessive-compulsive disorder. *American Journal of Psychiatry*, 2008. **165**: 1532–42.
14. Baer, L. Factor analysis of symptom subtypes of obsessive compulsive disorder and their relation to personality and tic disorders. *Journal of Clinical Psychiatry*, 1994. **55**(Suppl): 18–23.
15. Summerfeldt, L.J., *et al.* Symptom structure in obsessive-compulsive disorder: a confirmatory factor-analytic study. *Behaviour Research and Therapy*, 1999. **37**: 297–11.
16. Zohar, J. *Obsessive Compulsive Disorder: Current Science and Clinical Practice.* Chichester: John Wiley & Sons; 2012.
17. Summerfeldt, L.J., *et al.* The relationship between miscellaneous symptoms and major symptom factors in obsessive-compulsive disorder. *Behaviour Research and Therapy*, 2004. **42**: 1453–67.
18. Summerfeldt, L.J. Treating incompleteness, ordering, and arranging concerns. In: M.M. Antony, C. Purdon, and L.J. Summerfeldt (eds.). *Psychological Treatment of Obsessive-Compulsive Disorder: Fundamentals and Beyond.* Washington, DC: American Psychological Association; 2007. pp. 187–207.
19. Calamari, J.E., *et al.* Obsessive–compulsive disorder subtypes: an attempted replication and extension of a symptom-based taxonomy. *Behaviour Research and Therapy*, 2004. **42**: 647–70.
20. McKay, D., *et al.* A critical evaluation of obsessive–compulsive disorder subtypes: symptoms versus mechanisms. *Clinical Psychology Review*, 2004. **24**: 283–313.
21. Pitman, R.K. Pierre Janet on obsessive-compulsive disorder (1903): review and commentary. *Archives of General Psychiatry*, 1987. **44**: 226–32.
22. Coles, M.E., *et al.* Not just right experiences and obsessive–compulsive features: Experimental and self-monitoring perspectives. *Behaviour Research and Therapy*, 2005. **43**: 153–67.
23. Hellriegel, J., *et al.* Is 'not just right experience'(NJRE) in obsessive-compulsive disorder part of an autistic phenotype? *CNS Spectrums*, 2017. **22**: 41–50.
24. Gillan, C.M., *et al.* Enhanced avoidance habits in obsessive-compulsive disorder. *Biological Psychiatry*, 2014. **75**: 631–8.
25. National Collaborating Centre for Mental Health (UK). *Obsessive-compulsive disorder: Core interventions in the treatment of obsessive-compulsive disorder and body dysmorphic disorder.* National Institute for Health and Clinical Excellence Clinical Guidelines, No. 31. Leicester: British Psychological Society; 2006. Available from: https://www.ncbi.nlm.nih.gov/books/NBK56458/
26. Lochner, C., *et al.* Comorbidity in obsessive–compulsive disorder (OCD): a report from the International College of Obsessive–Compulsive Spectrum Disorders (ICOCS). *Comprehensive Psychiatry*, 2014. **55**: 1513–19.
27. Karno, M., *et al.* The epidemiology of obsessive-compulsive disorder in five US communities. *Archives of General Psychiatry*, 1988. **45**: 1094–9.
28. Kessler, R.C., *et al.* Lifetime prevalence and age-of-onset distributions of DSM-IV disorders in the National Comorbidity Survey Replication. *Archives of General Psychiatry*, 2005. **62**: 593–602.
29. Kessler, R.C., *et al.* Lifetime prevalence and age-of-onset distributions of DSM-IV disorders in the National Comorbidity Survey replication: erratum. *Archives of General Psychiatry*, 2005. **62**: 768.
30. Wittchen, H.-U. and F. Jacobi. Size and burden of mental disorders in Europe—a critical review and appraisal of 27 studies. *European Neuropsychopharmacology*, 2005. **15**: 357–76.
31. Wittchen, H.-U., *et al.* The size and burden of mental disorders and other disorders of the brain in Europe 2010. *European Neuropsychopharmacology*, 2011. **21**: 655–79.
32. Fineberg, N.A., *et al.* A prospective population-based cohort study of the prevalence, incidence and impact of obsessive-compulsive symptomatology. *International Journal of Psychiatry in Clinical Practice*, 2013. **17**: 170–8.
33. Veale, D., *et al.* Body dysmorphic disorder in different settings: A systematic review and estimated weighted prevalence. *Body Image*, 2016. **18**: 168–86.
34. Gunstad, J. and K.A. Phillips. Axis I comorbidity in body dysmorphic disorder. *Comprehensive Psychiatry*, 2003. **44**: 270–6.
35. Mataix-Cols, D., *et al.* Hoarding disorder: a new diagnosis for DSM-V? *Depression and Anxiety*, 2010. **27**: 556–72.
36. Ameringen, M., B. Patterson, and W. Simpson. DSM-5 obsessive-compulsive and related disorders: clinical implications of new criteria. *Depression and Anxiety*, 2014. **31**: 487–93.
37. Grant, J.E. and S.R. Chamberlain. Trichotillomania. *American Journal of Psychiatry*, 2016. **173**: 868–74.
38. Hollander, E., A. Braun, and D. Simeon. Should OCD leave the anxiety disorders in DSM-V? The case for obsessive compulsive-related disorders. *Depression and Anxiety*, 2008. **25**: 317–29.
39. Grant, J.E., *et al.* Skin picking disorder. *American Journal of Psychiatry*, 2012. **169**: 1143–9.

40. Torres, A.R., *et al.* Comorbidity variation in patients with obsessive–compulsive disorder according to symptom dimensions: Results from a large multicentre clinical sample. *Journal of Affective Disorders*, 2016. **190**: 508–16.

41. Mathis, M.A., *et al.* Gender differences in obsessive-compulsive disorder: a literature review. *Revista Brasileira de Psiquiatria*, 2011. **33**: 390–9.

42. Williams, K.E. and L.M. Koran. Obsessive-compulsive disorder in pregnancy, the puerperium, and the premenstruum. *Journal of Clinical Psychiatry*, 1997. **58**: 330–4; quiz 335–6.

43. Sasson, Y., *et al.* Posttraumatic obsessive–compulsive disorder: a case series. *Psychiatry Research*, 2005. **135**: 145–52.

44. Ruscio, A., *et al.* The epidemiology of obsessive-compulsive disorder in the National Comorbidity Survey Replication. *Molecular Psychiatry*, 2010. **15**: 53–63.

45. Ravizza, L., G. Maina, and F. Bogetto. Episodic and chronic obsessive-compulsive disorder. *Depression and Anxiety*, 1997. **6**: 154–8.

46. Skoog, G. and I. Skoog. A 40-year follow-up of patients with obsessive-compulsive disorder. *Archives of General Psychiatry*, 1999. **56**: 121–7.

47. Marks, I., R. Hodgson, and S. Rachman. Treatment of chronic obsessive-compulsive neurosis by *in-vivo* exposure. *British Journal of Psychiatry*, 1975. **127**: 349–64.

48. Micali, N., *et al.* Long-term outcomes of obsessive–compulsive disorder: follow-up of 142 children and adolescents. *British Journal of Psychiatry*, 2010. **197**: 128–34.

49. Stewart, S., *et al.* Long-term outcome of pediatric obsessive–compulsive disorder: a meta-analysis and qualitative review of the literature. *Acta Psychiatrica Scandinavica*, 2004. **110**: 4–13.

50. Altamura, A.C., *et al.* Age at onset and latency to treatment (duration of untreated illness) in patients with mood and anxiety disorders: a naturalistic study. *International Clinical Psychopharmacology*, 2010. **25**: 172–9.

51. Angst, J., *et al.* Obsessive-compulsive severity spectrum in the community: prevalence, comorbidity, and course. *European Archives of Psychiatry and Clinical Neuroscience*, 2004. **254**: 156–64.

52. Dell'Osso, B., *et al.* Duration of untreated illness as a predictor of treatment response and remission in obsessive–compulsive disorder. *World Journal of Biological Psychiatry*, 2010. **11**: 59–65.

53. De Luca, V., *et al.* Age at onset in Canadian OCD patients: mixture analysis and systematic comparison with other studies. *Journal of Affective Disorders*, 2011. **133**: 300–4.

54. Grant, J.E., *et al.* Late-onset obsessive compulsive disorder: clinical characteristics and psychiatric comorbidity. *Psychiatry Research*, 2007. **152**: 21–7.

55. Rasmussen, S.A. and J.L. Eisen. The epidemiology and differential diagnosis of obsessive-compulsive disorder. In: I. Hand, W. Goodman, and U. Evers (eds.). *Zwangsstörungen/Obsessive-Compulsive Disorders*. Berlin Heidelberg: Springer-Verlag; 1992. pp. 1–14.

56. Dell'Osso, B., *et al.* Childhood, adolescent and adult age at onset and related clinical correlates in obsessive–compulsive disorder: a report from the International College of Obsessive–Compulsive Spectrum Disorders (ICOCS). *International Journal of Psychiatry in Clinical Practice*, 2016. **20**: 210–17.

57. Fontenelle, L.F., *et al.* Early-and late-onset obsessive–compulsive disorder in adult patients: an exploratory clinical and therapeutic study. *Journal of Psychiatric Research*, 2003. **37**: 127–33.

58. Zohar, A.H. The epidemiology of obsessive-compulsive disorder in children and adolescents. *Child and Adolescent Psychiatry Clinics of North America*, 1999. **8**: 445–60.

59. Walitza, S., *et al.* Genetics of early-onset obsessive–compulsive disorder. *European Child and Adolescent Psychiatry*, 2010. **19**: 227–35.

60. Eichstedt, J.A. and S.L. Arnold. Childhood-onset obsessive-compulsive disorder: a tic-related subtype of OCD? *Clinical Psychology Review*, 2001. **21**: 137–57.

61. Geller, D.A., *et al.* Developmental aspects of obsessive compulsive disorder: findings in children, adolescents, and adults. *Journal of Nervous and Mental Disease*, 2001. **189**: 471–7.

62. Kishore, V.R., *et al.* Clinical characteristics and treatment response in poor and good insight obsessive–compulsive disorder. *European Psychiatry*, 2004. **19**: 202–8.

63. Jaisoorya, T., *et al.* Obsessive-compulsive disorder with and without tic disorder: a comparative study from India. *CNS Spectrums*, 2008. **13**: 705–11.

64. Stewart, S.E., M.A. Jenike, and N.J. Keuthen. Severe obsessive-compulsive disorder with and without comorbid hair pulling: comparisons and clinical implications. *Journal of Clinical Psychiatry*, 2005. **66**: 864–9.

65. Maina, G., *et al.* Early-onset obsessive–compulsive disorder and personality disorders in adulthood. *Psychiatry Research*, 2008. **158**: 217–25.

66. Nacasch, N., L. Fostick, and J. Zohar. High prevalence of obsessive–compulsive disorder among posttraumatic stress disorder patients. *European Neuropsychopharmacology*, 2011. **21**: 876–9.

67. Dell'Osso, B., *et al.* Prevalence of suicide attempt and clinical characteristics of suicide attempters with obsessive-compulsive disorder: a report from the International College of Obsessive-Compulsive Spectrum Disorders (ICOCS). *CNS Spectrums*, 2018. **23**: 59–66.

68. de la Cruz, L.F., *et al.* Suicide in obsessive–compulsive disorder: a population-based study of 36 788 Swedish patients. *Molecular Psychiatry*, 2017; **22**: 1626–32.

69. Fineberg, N.A., *et al.* Lifetime comorbidity of obsessive-compulsive disorder and sub-threshold obsessive-compulsive symptomatology in the community: impact, prevalence, socio-demographic and clinical characteristics. *International Journal of Psychiatry in Clinical Practice*, 2013. **17**: 188–96.

70. Du Toit, P.L., *et al.* Comparison of obsessive-compulsive disorder patients with and without comorbid putative obsessive-compulsive spectrum disorders using a structured clinical interview. *Comprehensive Psychiatry*, 2001. **42**: 291–300.

71. Storch, E.A., *et al.* Depression in youth with obsessive-compulsive disorder: clinical phenomenology and correlates. *Psychiatry Research*, 2012. **196**: 83–9.

71. Goes, F., *et al.* Co-morbid anxiety disorders in bipolar disorder and major depression: familial aggregation and clinical characteristics of co-morbid panic disorder, social phobia, specific phobia and obsessive-compulsive disorder. *Psychological Medicine*, 2012. **42**: 1449–59.

72. Hou, S.-Y., *et al.* Quality of life and its correlates in patients with obsessive-compulsive disorder. *Kaohsiung Journal of Medical Sciences*, 2010. **26**: 397–407.

73. Zohar, J. and T.R. Insel. Obsessive-compulsive disorder and alcoholism. *Journal of Clinical Psychiatry*, 1986. **47**: 153.

74. el-Guebaly, N., *et al.* Compulsive features in behavioural addictions: the case of pathological gambling. *Addiction*, 2012. **107**: 1726–34.

75. Adam, Y., *et al.* Obsessive–compulsive disorder in the community: 12-month prevalence, comorbidity and impairment. *Social Psychiatry and Psychiatric Epidemiology*, 2012. **47**: 339–49.

76. Blom, R.M., *et al*. Co-occurrence of obsessive-compulsive dis-order and substance use disorder in the general population. *Addiction*, 2011. **106**: 2178–85.

77. De Bruijn, C., *et al*. Subthreshold symptoms and obsessive–compulsive disorder: evaluating the diagnostic threshold. *Psychological Medicine*, 2010. **40**: 989–97.

78. Mancebo, M.C., *et al*. Substance use disorders in an obsessive compulsive disorder clinical sample. *Journal of Anxiety Disorders*, 2009. **23**: 429–35.

79. Swets, M., *et al*. The obsessive compulsive spectrum in schizo-phrenia, a meta-analysis and meta-regression exploring preva-lence rates. *Schizophrenia Research*, 2014. **152**: 458–68.

80. Berman, I., *et al*. Treatment of obsessive-compulsive symptoms in schizophrenic patients with clomipramine. *Journal of Clinical Psychopharmacology*, 1995. **15**: 206–10.

81. Zohar, J. Is there room for a new diagnostic subtype—the schizo-obsessive subtype? *CNS Spectrums*, 1997. **2**: 49–50.

82. Fostick, L., N. Nacasch, and J. Zohar. Acute obsessive com-pulsive disorder (OCD) in veterans with posttraumatic stress disorder (PTSD). *World Journal of Biological Psychiatry*, 2012. **13**: 312–15.

83. Gershuny, B.S., *et al*. Comorbid posttraumatic stress dis-order: impact on treatment outcome for obsessive-compulsive disorder. *American Journal of Psychiatry*, 2002. **159**: 852–4.

84. Leonard, H.L., *et al*. Tics and Tourette's disorder: a 2- to 7-year follow-up of 54 obsessive-compulsive children. *Am J Psychiatry*, 1992. **149**: 1244–51.

85. Diniz, J.B., *et al*. Chronic tics and Tourette syndrome in pa-tients with obsessive–compulsive disorder. *Journal of Psychiatric Research*, 2006. **40**: 487–93.

86. Grados, M.A., *et al*. The familial phenotype of obsessive-compulsive disorder in relation to tic disorders: the Hopkins OCD family study. *Biological Psychiatry*, 2001. **50**: 559–65.

87. McDougle, C.J., W.K. Goodman, and L.H. Price. Dopamine ant-agonists in tic-related and psychotic spectrum obsessive compul-sive disorder. *Journal of Clinical Psychiatry*, 1994. **55** Suppl: 24–31.

88. Marcks, B.A., *et al*. Longitudinal course of obsessive-compulsive disorder in patients with anxiety disorders: a 15-year prospective follow-up study. *Comprehensive Psychiatry*, 2011. **52**: 670–7.

89. Rasmussen, S.A. and J.L. Eisen. Epidemiology of obsessive compulsive disorder. *Journal of Clinical Psychiatry*, 1990. **51** Suppl: 10–13; discussion 14.

90. Eisen, J.L., *et al*. Five-year course of obsessive-compulsive dis-order: predictors of remission and relapse. *Journal of Clinical Psychiatry*, 2013. **74**: 233.

91. Mancebo, M.C., *et al*. Long-term course of pediatric obsessive–compulsive disorder: 3years of prospective follow-up. *Comprehensive Psychiatry*, 2014. **55**: 1498–504.

# 96

# Genetics of obsessive–compulsive disorder

*Gerald Nestadt and Jack Samuels*

## Introduction

Clinicians have long observed that many of their patients with obsessive–compulsive disorder (OCD) have relatives with the disorder, and they have suspected that hereditary transmission underlies this familial aggregation. In an early report in 1936, of 50 cases of 'obsessional neurosis', Lewis reported that 37% of the parents and 21% of the siblings of these cases had pronounced obsessional traits; moreover, he noted two pairs of identical twins who were concordant for obsessive–compulsive features [1]. Additional clinical case series of OCD patients and their twins and other relatives have provided presumptive evidence of the inheritance of OCD. Based on these early studies, Slater concluded in 1964 that 'of all neurotic syndromes, the evidence relating to genetic predisposition is best in the case of obsessional neurosis' [2].

Since then, abundant evidence has been provided from genetic epidemiological (twin and family) studies to support a genetic contribution to OCD [3]. In contrast, apart from relatively rare instances of OCD associated with brain trauma, ischaemia, tumours, perinatal factors, or β-haemolytic streptococcal infections [4–6], there is limited evidence for a major contribution of environmental factors to most cases of OCD. Therefore, the discovery of specific genes and the functional relevance of proteins encoded by them hold promise for elucidating the molecular pathogenesis of OCD and for developing rational, mechanism-based approaches to its treatment.

Molecular genetic studies of OCD and other neuropsychiatric conditions have advanced rapidly and sequentially over the past 20 years, due to developments in genotyping technology and computational genetics. Initially, efforts were focused on specific candidate genes hypothesized to be functionally related to the disorder in question. Then, genetic linkage studies predominated; as more genetic markers were identified throughout the genome, genotyping became more rapid and less costly, and statistical genetic methods developed. During this scientific phase, the thought was that relatively few genes, that is, those with a 'major effect', make a major contribution to the risk of OCD. Subsequently, with recognition that neuropsychiatric conditions are genetically complex, the 'common disorder–common gene' hypothesis became predominant, which posited relatively frequent genetic variants, each with a small effect on the risk of disease, ushering in an era of genome-wide association studies (GWAS). As sample sizes increased to the tens of thousands, relevant findings emerged for several of the complex neuropsychiatric disorders; for example, with a sample of 37,000 cases, 108 genetic polymorphisms were found to be significantly associated with schizophrenia [7]. Nevertheless, these variants, although numerous, appeared to explain only a small proportion of the heritability of these diseases. With decreasing cost and speed of genotyping, and increasing sophistication of computational genetic methods, whole-genome and exon-wide sequencing studies of OCD are now in progress.

## Genetic epidemiological studies

### Family studies

At least 15 family studies of OCD have been conducted, and their findings support the familial aggregation of OCD. These include the most recent family studies, which used clear diagnostic criteria, direct assessment of family members, and inclusion of families of case as well as non-OCD control probands (that is, the index case or the first person identified in the family). For example, Black and colleagues found that the risk of 'broadly defined OCD' (that is, OCD plus subsyndromal obsessive–compulsive symptoms) was substantially greater in the parents of OCD probands (that is, index cases or the first person identified in the family) than parents of controls (16% vs 3%) [8]. Pauls and colleagues found a higher risk of OCD in first-degree relatives of OCD probands than controls (10% vs 2%) [9]. The Johns Hopkins Family Study also found a similarly higher prevalence of OCD in first-degree relatives of case than control probands (12% vs 2% [10], as did Grabe and colleagues in a European family study (10% vs 1%) [11]. Several studies have found even greater differences in the prevalence of OCD in the relatives of case vs control paediatric probands—for example, 23% vs 3% in the study by Hanna and colleagues [12]—suggesting that early-onset OCD may differentiate a strongly inherited subtype of the disorder. In addition, several family studies have found that additional disorders were more prevalent in relatives of OCD than control probands, including generalized anxiety disorder, body dysmorphic disorder, trichotillomania, pathologic skin picking, tic disorders, and obsessive–compulsive personality disorder, suggesting that these may be part of the spectrum of conditions aetiologically related to OCD in these families [13–15].

A statistical approach—complex segregation analysis—has been used to determine if the transmission of OCD in families is consistent with a Mendelian mode of inheritance. The five published studies support a Mendelian model, with transmission of a gene, or genes, of major effect. Three of the studies found that the data were most consistent with a dominant transmission model; however, the data could not reject alternative models such as codominant or recessive [16–18].

### Twin studies

Although evidence of familial aggregation is a necessary condition for a genetic contribution to OCD, it is not sufficient, since it does not rule out aggregation due to common exposures of family members to possible environmental factors related to the disease. Therefore, twin studies have been used to contrast concordance of OCD in monozygotic (identical) twins and dizygotic (fraternal) twins, under the assumptions that: (1) monozygotic twins are genetically identical; (2) dizygotic twins share only 50% of their genes, on average; and (3) both types of twins share similar environments. Thus, greater concordance of OCD symptoms in identical than nonidentical twins provides further support for a genetic influence. Using the Maudsley Twin Registry, concordance of 'obsessive symptoms or features' was found in 13 of 15 (87%) monozygotic twin pairs, but only seven of 15 (47%) of dizygotic twin pairs [19].

Moreover, twin studies have been used to estimate the 'heritability' of OCD, that is, the proportion of variation in dimensional obsessive–compulsive symptom scores that is explained by genetic effects, rather than by environmental influences. For example, in 4564 4-year-old twin pairs rated by their parents, the estimated heritability of obsessive–compulsive behaviours was 65%, with the remaining 35% of the variance attributed to unshared environmental influences [20]. Similarly, in 4246 child twin pairs, the estimated heritability of parent-rated obsessive–compulsive symptoms was 45–61%, with unique environmental influences of 42–55% [21].

Thus, twin studies provide further support for a substantial genetic contribution to OCD. However, unshared environmental factors also appear to contribute to OCD and interaction between genetic and environmental factors may be important. Adoption studies comparing twins raised together and apart would provide further evidence of the importance of genetic and environmental factors in OCD, although no such studies have been reported to date.

## Molecular genetic studies

### Linkage studies

The aim of genetic linkage studies in OCD is to identify chromosomal regions that contain genes for the disorder, by statistically testing whether specific genetic marker alleles cosegregate (that is, 'travel together') with OCD in families. Whereas parametric approaches analyse genetic recombination events and need to assume the mode of inheritance, non-parametric approaches evaluate the extent of sharing of marker alleles between affected relatives and do not require assumption about the mode of inheritance. If a linkage peak is identified, 'fine mapping' is often conducted by including additional markers to further narrow the linkage region, and family-based association analyses may be conducted to evaluate associations between specific single-nucleotide polymorphisms (SNPs) within these regions and OCD.

Hanna and colleagues were the first to report a linkage scan in OCD, which studied 56 individuals in seven families with a paediatric proband. Using parametric linkage analysis and assuming a dominant transmission model, they identified a linkage peak in the 9p24 region on chromosome 9. This region harbours the glutamate transporter gene SLC1A1, which is involved in neurotransmission and is a potential candidate gene for OCD [22]. This finding was replicated by Willour and colleagues in a linkage analysis in 50 OCD pedigrees, using the same 13 genetic markers in the region used by the Hanna group, and pedigree-based association analyses identified two markers associated with OCD in this region [23]. These linkage findings stimulated further studies of SLC1A1 as a candidate gene for OCD, as described in the next section.

A genome-wide linkage study was conducted in 219 families with multiple relatives affected with OCD, mostly affected sibling pairs, as part of the OCD Collaborative Genetics Study. Using non-parametric linkage analysis, the strongest suggestive linkage signal was found on chromosome 3, in the 3q27–28 region; other suggestive linkage signals were found in regions on chromosomes 1, 6, 7, and 15 [24]. Further analyses provided evidence for different linkage patterns in these families, depending on specific phenotypic characteristics of probands or families. For example, after stratifying families by proband gender, Wang and colleagues found suggestive linkage to the chromosome 11p15 region in families with male probands, and the linkage signal became substantially stronger after fine mapping in this region [25]. In another analysis, families were stratified into those with two or more individuals with compulsive hoarding behaviour and those with one or fewer hoarding relatives. In the hoarding-loaded families, there was significant linkage on the chromosome 14q23–32 region [26].

Findings from linkage studies have provided evidence linking specific chromosomal regions to OCD and suggest that genetic linkage may be stronger for specific phenotypic subtypes of the disorder. However, other than the findings for the hoarding phenotype, all of the regions identified so far have not met the threshold for 'statistically significant' linkage. The linkage finding in the 9p24 region was particularly intriguing, given that this region harbours a functional candidate gene for OCD. However, the 9p24 region spans over 7 million base pairs and contains dozens of potential OCD candidate genes; moreover, this region was not identified in the largest genome-wide linkage scan, which found several other regions more strongly linked to OCD. It may be that a greater number of families are required to detect and replicate statistically significant linkage findings. Furthermore, as has emerged from genetic studies of other psychiatric disorders, including schizophrenia and bipolar disorder, OCD may have a complex pattern of inheritance, with multiple genes each exerting a small effect, and genes of 'major effect' may be rare in OCD and may occur in only relatively few families.

### Candidate gene studies

Genes have been identified as potential candidate genes for OCD, based on their location within linkage peaks and/or knowledge of the pathophysiology and pharmacology of the disorder. The neuronal glutamate transporter gene SLC1A1 was hypothesized as a primary candidate gene for OCD, based on its location within a linkage peak, as described; the protein it encodes—a neuronal transporter; and its high expression in the cerebral cortex, striatum, and thalamus, which are regions connected in functional circuits are implicated in

OCD. Several research groups have reported associations between OCD and SNPs in this gene, while another found an association with SNPs about 9 kilobases 'upstream' of the gene. Moreover, the findings were specific to families with male probands or to males affected with OCD [27]. These replicated association findings implicating the *SLC1A1* gene in OCD are intriguing, and further investigations of this and possibly other interacting glutamatergic genes are warranted.

Given the therapeutic effect of serotonin reuptake inhibitors (SRIs) in the treatment of OCD, the serotonergic system also has been a major focus of candidate gene studies. Polymorphisms in the promoter region of the serotonin transporter gene (*5HTTPLR*), 5-hydroxytryptamine (serotonin) receptor 1D (*5HT1-D*), and 5-hydroxytryptamine (serotonin) receptor 1D (*5HT2C*) have been reported associated with OCD. Of these the serotonin transporter polymorphism (*5HTTPLR*), located on chromosome 17, has received the most attention. Findings from these association analyses have unfortunately been conflicting. It is interesting that the short (s) allele of this polymorphism is consistently reported associated with anxiety, depression, and neuroticism, whereas it is the long (l) allele often reported to be associated with OCD, although other studies have implicated the S-allele, rather than the L-allele, in OCD. Nevertheless, meta-analyses of polymorphisms in the *5HTTPLR* and *5HT2* genes support an association with OCD [28].

Several studies have found an association between OCD and alleles of the dopamine receptor 4 (*DRD4*) gene on chromosome 11. In some studies, the association was specific to a phenotypic subtype, for example tics or early onset of OCD. Other studies, however, have been negative, as have studies of other dopaminergic genes, including *DRD2*, *DRD3*, and the dopamine transporter *SLC6A3*. Association studies of other genes have been reported, including the catechol-*O*-methyltransferase (*COMT*) gene, the monoamine oxidase A (*MAO*) gene, the brain-derived neurotrophic factor (*BDNF*) gene, and the oligodendrocyte lineage transcription factor 2 (*OLIG2*) gene. Some of the positive findings have been gender-specific. In general, however, the positive findings have not been consistently replicated [28].

Thus, although there have been many reports of a positive association between functional candidate genes and OCD, the lack of consistent replication 'in the majority of OCD psychiatric genetic association studies may seem discouraging', as noted by Hemmings and Stein [29]. At least part of the inconsistency may be due to differences between study samples, including clinical and underlying genetic heterogeneity, as well as methodology differences, including sample size and statistical power. Taylor conducted a comprehensive meta-analysis of 230 polymorphisms that had been investigated in 113 genetic association studies of OCD. The analysis found that OCD was significantly associated with serotonin-related (5-HTTLPR and HTR2A) and, in males only, catecholamine-related (*COMT* and *MAOA*) genes; an additional 18 polymorphisms had significant odds ratios. The findings support a polygenic model of OCD, in which multiple genes each have a small, incremental effect on the risk for development of OCD [28].

### Genome-wide association studies

GWAS of OCD involve scanning hundreds of thousands, or even millions, of SNPs across the genome to detect relatively common genetic variants associated with the disorder. The studies have compared the variants in individuals with and without OCD or have focused the analysis on 'trios', affected individuals and their parents, whether affected or unaffected.

Three GWAS of OCD have been reported to date. The International OCD Foundation Genetics Collaborative (IOCDF-GC) analysed almost 1500 OCD cases, 5600 controls, and 400 trios with nearly 500,000 SNPs. In the case-control analysis, the two most significantly associated SNPs were located within the *DLGAP1* gene, although no association had 'genome-wide significance' after correcting for the large number of comparisons. In the analysis of trios, but not in the combined case-control–trio analysis, an SNP near the *BTBD3* gene was found to be significantly associated with OCD [30].

The OCD Collaborative Genetic Association Study (OCGAS) analysed over 1000 families and 500,000 SNPs. Although no association was found with genome-wide significance, the most significant finding was for an SNP on chromosome 9, near the protein tyrosine phosphate receptor D (*PTPRD*) gene. Several additional candidate genes emerged from these two studies, including Fas apoptotic inhibitory molecule 2 (*FAIM2*), glutamate ionotropic receptor NMDA type subunit 2B (*GRIN 2B*), and the cadherin genes *CDH9* and CDH10. Several of these genes appear to be involved in glutamatergic neurotransmission [31].

The third GWAS analysed almost 7000 individuals and 31,000,000 SNPs as part of the Netherland National Twin Registry, using a quantitative measure of obsessive–compulsive symptoms. A genome-wide significant finding was found for an SNP in the myocyte enhancer factor 2B neighbour (*MEF2BNB*) gene in region 19p13 on chromosome 19. Additional gene-based testing found four significantly associated genes in the same region—*MEF2BNB*, *MEF2B* and *MEF2BNB-MEF2B*, and *RFXANK* [32].

Several analytic approaches have recently been developed to estimate heritability based on genotype information collected in GWAS, that is, SNP-based heritability. Using the genome-wide complex trait analysis (GCTA) approach, the estimated heritability of quantitative obsessive–compulsive symptoms was 34%, based on the Netherlands twin genotypes. In another study, the estimated heritability of OCD was 37%, based on OCGAS genotypes. Also it was found that common alleles contribute more to the heritability of OCD than did rarer alleles and that certain chromosomes contribute more than others to OCD risk [33].

The experience with other disorders, particularly neuropsychiatric conditions, with complex patterns of inheritance, indicates that sample sizes for GWAS need to be an order of magnitude larger than those in the three studies reported here. This is because the magnitude of the association (odds ratio) between common genetic variants and these disorders is in the range of 1.0–1.4. GWAS in schizophrenia, for example, required samples in the tens of thousands before significant associations were detected. Meta-analyses of samples from several studies are currently being conducted, in order to increase the power to detect significant associations in OCD.

### In search of rare variants

Among the genetic complexity of OCD is genetic heterogeneity, that is, the pattern of genetic variation may be different in different cases of OCD. Although GWAS search for the more common genetic variants, the search continues for less common variants associated with the disorder, which may have a 'major effect' and provide insight into the pathophysiology of the disorder. Three types of these variants have been reported in OCD: chromosomal rearrangements, copy number variants (CNVs), and rare variants identified by 'deep sequencing' of the genome.

There are few reports of chromosomal rearrangements in OCD, and most are in cases with co-occurring Tourette's syndrome (TS). Bertelsen and colleagues reported a 21-year-old male patient with TS, OCD, and attention-deficit/hyperactivity disorder. The patient inherited a chromosome 3 to 9 translocation t(3;9) (q25.1;q34.3) from his mother, who had a complex motor tic. Sequencing revealed that the translocation breakpoints truncated the olfactomedin 1 (*OLFM1*) gene, which plays a role in neuronal development and is a likely candidate gene for other neuropsychiatric disorders [34]. Devor and Magee reported a balanced chromosomal translocation t(1;8) (q21.1; q22.1) in siblings multiply affected with TS, OCD, complex motor tics, and attention-deficit disorder [35].

McGrath and colleagues reported the only GWAS of large (>500 kilobases), rare (1%) CNVs in OCD. They found that the proportion of individuals with deletions in known pathogenic neurodevelopmental loci was four times greater in patients with OCD than in controls. Deletions in the 16p13.11 region, which contributed disproportionately in the OCD cases, have been implicated in other neuropsychiatric conditions [36]. Since this was a case-control study, it could not distinguish between inherited and *de novo* variants, which would require a study of families. (A *de novo* variant is a new mutation that occurs for the first time in a family member, arising from a germ cell mutation in one of the parents or in the fertilized egg during embryogenesis.) *De novo* mutations in sporadic cases provide more certainty with respect to the causal nature of the variant, and such studies are in progress in OCD.

'Deep sequencing' involves sequencing a genomic region multiple times, allowing detection of rare variants, including *de novo* variants. To date, only one study has been reported for OCD. Cappi and colleagues sequenced all genome-coding regions in 20 sporadic OCD cases and their unaffected parents in order to identify rare *de novo* single-nucleotide variants. The study found a higher than expected rate of *de novo* non-synonymous variants (that is, those that alter the amino acid sequence of a protein) in OCD cases. Analysis of the protein–protein interaction network suggested an enrichment of genes involved in immunological and central nervous system functioning and development [37]. Other genetic deep sequencing studies are in progress. As with CNVs, both inherited and *de novo* variants can be studied. It is clear that much larger sample sizes will be necessary to test the significance of rare causal variants. The identification of rare genetic variants through sequencing studies may be aetiologically relevant for smaller subgroups of cases, which may exhibit different treatment response profiles.

## Alternate phenotypes

An important consideration in investigating the genetic aetiology of OCD is the definition of the phenotype. Thus far, we have focused on the disorder OCD as the phenotype of interest in genetic studies. However, OCD is quite clinically heterogenous, with different cases exhibiting different constellations of symptoms, which could result from different underlying genetic or environmental aetiologies. In addition, OCD might share the same genetic basis with co-occurring disorders. Moreover, there may be subclinical dimensions

that are more proximal than the OCD diagnosis to the ultimate genetic causes of the disorder. The challenge is to identify more genetically homogenous clinical subtypes, genetically related disorders, and genetically relevant subclinical dimensions that maximize the elucidation of the underlying genetic aetiology.

### Clinical subtypes

In the preceding sections, we discussed several clinical features that may be useful for subtyping in genetic studies of OCD. For example, several family studies have reported that the relative odds of OCD in relatives are substantially greater in families of paediatric probands or of adult probands with onset in childhood or adolescence [9, 10, 12]. Several candidate gene studies have found stronger associations for one gender than the other; for example, some studies found an association with the *COMT* gene in women, but not men, while others found an association in men, but not women [38, 39]. Association studies of the *SLC1A1* gene have found a stronger association in men, but not women [27]. The OCGS study found significant linkage of OCD to a region of chromosome 14 in families with two or more hoarding relatives, but not in other families [26]. These and other potential phenotypes might be the focus of future genome-wide and newer-generation association studies. However, clinical subtyping increases the cost of studies, given the larger number of affected OCD cases with specific subtypes that must be identified and the increased time required for clinical examinations.

### Cross-disorder phenotypes

Several psychiatric disorders have been proposed to be related to OCD. This is an example of pleiotropy, that is, that the same genetic background can be expressed as clinically different disorders. The evidence for these relationships has typically been based upon the co-occurrence of these disorders with OCD, as well as by phenomenological similarities or treatment response profiles. A stronger case for a genetic relationship between OCD and these disorders is provided for by family studies, in which the relatives of OCD cases have greater prevalences of these other psychiatric conditions than do the relatives of controls. As discussed, several family studies have found that generalized anxiety disorder, body dysmorphic disorder, trichotillomania, pathologic skin picking, and obsessive–compulsive personality disorder and additional disorders were more prevalent in relatives of OCD than control probands [13–15].

There has been much interest in the genetic relationship between OCD and TS and other tic disorders. Tic disorders and OCD frequently co-occur, and family studies have found that the prevalence of OCD is significantly higher in TS than control relatives, whether or not the TS-affected proband had OCD, supporting the hypothesis that the disorders share genetic risk factors [40]. More recent analyses of SNPs collected in GWAS found a genetic correlation between OCD and TS of 0.41, comparable to heritability estimates based on twin and family studies [33]. However, Yu and colleagues found that although genetically related, the two disorders had distinct genetic components and OCD with co-occurring tic disorders may be genetically different from OCD alone [41].

### Endophenotypes

Like many other psychiatric disorders, OCD appears to be aetiologically complex, with suspected involvement of multiple genes, epigenetic factors, and environmental influences, which has complicated the search for specific genes and gene networks that may ultimately underlie the disorder. An endophenotype, or 'intermediate phenotype', is a biological marker that lies intermediate in the aetiologic pathway between genes and the clinical phenotype, that is, the signs and symptoms of the disorder. A psychiatric endophenotype may be biochemical, neuroanatomical, neurophysiological, neuropsychological, or behavioural. A useful candidate endophenotype is associated with the disorder, is heritable, cosegregates with the disorder within families, and occurs in non-affected, as well as affected, family members with greater frequency than in controls. It is a 'trait' marker underlying the disorder and independent of symptoms [42].

A large number of studies have found differences between OCD cases and non-cases in a variety of neurocognitive domains, including response inhibition, planning, decision-making, working memory, and visuo-spatial abilities [43]. Several of these domains involve functioning of orbitofrontal-striatal-thalamic networks in the brain, which imaging studies have implicated in OCD. In one of the first studies, Menzies and colleagues measured performance on a response inhibition task (Stop-Signal task) in 31 OCD patients, 31 of their first-degree relatives, and 31 non-OCD controls and their first-degree relatives. They found that OCD patients and their relatives had significantly longer reaction times than the controls, indicating reduced ability to inhibit their response. Using magnetic resonance imaging (MRI), they also found that the impairment in response inhibition was significantly associated with reduced grey matter in the orbitofrontal cortex in right inferior brain regions and increased grey matter in the cingulate, parietal, and striatal regions. Moreover, there were significant familial effects for reaction times and brain volumes in these regions [44]. Several later studies, using a variety of neurocognitive paradigms, as well as structural and functional imaging approaches, have supported deficits in inhibitory control, as well as structure, function, and connectivity in corticostriatal-thalamic-cortical circuits, as candidate endophenotypes for OCD [45].

Another neurocognitive domain of recent focus is performance monitoring. Many studies have found that OCD cases show a negative deflection of the event-related potential following making an error on a flanker task. Recently, error-related hyperactivity of the anterior cingulate cortex has been found in OCD cases and their relatives, compared to controls [46, 47]. More recently, higher-level executive functions have been investigated as candidate endophenotypes for OCD. For example, Zhang and colleagues found that OCD cases and their unaffected first-degree relatives had deficits in decision-making under ambiguous conditions, as well as in planning [48].

Although these findings are promising, additional family studies with greater numbers of cases and relatives are needed to determine the heritability and segregation patterns of candidate endophenotypes in OCD families. Those candidates and families with the strongest presumptive evidence for genetic transmission would then be useful for genetic association and sequencing studies to elucidate specific genetic aetiologies.

## Pharmacogenetics

A substantial proportion (40–60%) of OCD patients show poor response to SRIs, and others have significant adverse side effects that make treatment intolerable. Genetic variation appears to be an important contributor to antidepressant response in major depression, but less is known about the genetic contribution to pharmacologic treatment response to SRIs in OCD. Some studies have reported associations between treatment response and SNPs in genes known to be involved in serotonergic, dopaminergic, or glutamatergic neurotransmission (for example, *HTR1B, 5-HT2A, HTR2A, BDNF, SLC1A1, SLC6A4, COMT*). However, findings mostly have been based on small samples, have small effect sizes, and have not been replicated, and further studies are needed [49, 50].

Recently, results from a GWAS of SRI treatment response in nearly 1600 OCD-affected individuals in over 1000 families were reported. The most strongly associated SNP is located near the *DISP1* gene, and two other moderately associated SNPs are near the *PCDH10* gene; both genes are known to be involved in cell–cell adhesion. An additional 35 SNPs with signals of potential significance were in several genes expressed in the brain and implicated in neuronal development, psychiatric disorders, or drug effects, including *GRIN2B, GPC6, NTM, PARK2, PLCB1,* and *PKC* [51].

There has been important work on genes coding for liver enzymes involved in drug metabolism, specifically among the polymorphic cytochrome P450 enzymes. There is substantial genetic variation in the CYP2D6 and CYP2C19 enzymes, for instance. This can affect the metabolism of selective SRIs and lead to a range of treatment response in OCD patients with different genetic alleles [52]. Different medications, even those within the same class, could therefore have different effects, from reduced efficacy to increased liability to toxicity. The clinical utility of testing for these alleles remains controversial, but the implications need to be borne in mind by practitioners.

## Genetic studies in animals

### Canine compulsive behaviours

Ethologists have described stereotypical behaviours in non-human mammals that appear to be excessive, maladaptive variants of normal behaviours involved in grooming, predation, eating and suckling, or locomotion. Among the best studied are canine compulsive behaviours, including acral lick dermatitis, tail chasing, flank sucking, and pacing and circling. A GWAS of 92 Doberman pinschers with compulsive flank and/or blanket and sucking behaviours and 68 control dogs found a significant genome-wide association in chromosome 7, with an SNP in the *CDH2* gene, which codes for cadherin, a neuronal adhesion protein. Dogs having both blanket and sucking behaviours had the greatest frequency of the risk allele (60%), compared to 43% in dogs with only one behaviour and 22% in unaffected dogs [53]. Using a more powerful genotype-calling algorithm, 13 new OCD-associated regions were found, in addition to the *CDH2* locus; these regions included genes involved in catenin-binding and regulation of dendrite morphogenesis. Sequencing these regions found variants specific to dogs with OCD and were significantly more common in dog breeds at high risk for OCD; four genes in these regions are involved in synaptic function: neuronal cadherin (*CDH2*), catenin alpha2 (*CTNNA2*), ataxin-1 (*ATXN1*), and plasma glutamate carboxypeptidase (*PGPC*). Several of these genes appear to be functionally connected to several of the SNPs most strongly associated with OCD in a recent genome-wide OCD study in humans [30] and involved in glutamatergic signalling pathways [54].

Recently, variants in the *CDH2* gene have been reported to be associated with OCD in humans [55].

## Knockout mice models

A mouse model of compulsive grooming behaviour has been developed by genetic deletion of the *SAPAP3* gene, which codes for a scaffolding protein at excitatory synapses and is highly expressed in the striatum. Knockout mice express increased anxiety and compulsive grooming behaviour, leading to facial skin lesions and hair loss, and have reduced activity in cortico-striatal synapses, which comprise the majority of glutamatergic synapses in the striatum. When viruses containing the gene were injected into the striatum of these mice, excessive grooming behaviour, lesion severity, and anxious behaviour were reduced and cortico-striatal synaptic transmission increased [56]. In humans, a strong association between SNPs in the *SAPAP3* gene and grooming behaviours in OCD families has subsequently been reported [57], and mutations in SNPs in the *SAPAP3* gene have been found to be more frequent in individuals with OCD/ trichotillomania than controls [58]. Mice with deletions of other genes involved in cortico-striatal functioning, including *SLITRK5*, *HOX-B8*, and *SLC1A1*, have been studied as possible models of compulsive grooming behaviours and OCD [59].

## Conclusions and future directions

Evidence from epidemiological and molecular genetic studies strongly supports genetic susceptibility to OCD. The working hypothesis is that OCD, like several other neuropsychiatric disorders, has a complex pattern of inheritance that involves: many common genetic variants, each of which is expected to have a relatively small overall impact (effect size) on the risk of disease; rare genetic variants, each with potentially greater impact; and environmental factors, for which there are few, if any, supportable candidates thus far. However, to date, except for a few candidate genetic variants, such as *SLC1A1*, *DLGAP1*, and *PTPRD*, there is no established variant with unequivocal evidence for association with OCD. Many of the approaches outlined in this chapter, such as GWAS and whole-exome/ genome sequencing, are in progress and are likely to be productive as sample sizes increase.

It should be borne in mind that identifying associated genetic variants is only the initial step in elucidating the pathogenic process underlying OCD. Understanding the functional basis of these findings will rely on additional experimental approaches, several of which are currently available and others being developed, for integrating the information obtained from multiple domains, including gene sequence, gene expression, gene regulation, and gene–gene and protein–protein interaction networks [60]. Genetic expression studies in brain tissues from relevant brain regions and application of induced pluripotent stem cell (iPSC) technology will help identify relevant variants and elucidate their functional relevance. Epigenetic studies will be important for elucidating how modification of gene expression, apart from variation in the gene sequence, contributes to the risk of OCD. The Encyclopedia of DNA Elements (ENCODE) programme of the US National Institutes of Health, the goal of which is to identify all functional elements in the human genome, is one example of a programme that will facilitate this progress [61].

It is likely that this progress will result in a redefinition of the phenotype of OCD and related conditions. We anticipate a phenotype that will differentiate clinical subtypes within the existing diagnostic categories, will expand across current diagnostic boundaries, and ultimately will be based on genetic criteria. We also envision a future in which understanding of the molecular pathophysiology will catalyse the development of rational treatments and preventive measures for OCD.

## REFERENCES

1. Lewis, A. (1936). Problems of obsessional illness. *Proceedings of the Royal Society of Medicine*, 29, 325–36.
2. Slater, E. (1964). Genetical factors in neurosis. *British Journal of Psychology*, 55, 265–9.
3. Pauls, D. L. (2008). The genetics of obsessive compulsive disorder: a review of the evidence. *American Journal of Medical Genetics Part C (Seminars in Medical Genetics)*, 148C, 133–9.
4. Coetzer, B. R. (2004). Obsessive-compulsive disorder following brain injury: a review. *International Journal of Psychiatry in Medicine*, 34, 363–77.
5. Swedo, S. E., Seidlitz, J., Kovacevic, M., *et al.* (2015). Clinical presentation of pediatric autoimmune neuropsychiatry disorders associated with streptococcal infections in research and community settings. *Journal of Child and Adolescent Psychopharmacology*, 25, 26–30.
6. Geller, D. A., Wieland, N., Carey, K., *et al.* (2008). Perinatal factors affecting expression of obsessive compulsive disorder in children and adolescents. *Journal of Child and Adolescent Psychopharmacology*, 18, 373–9.
7. Schizophrenia Working Group of the Psychiatric Genomics Consortium (2014). Biological insights from 108 schizophrenia-associated genetic loci. *Nature*, 511, 421–7.
8. Black, D. W., Noyes, R., Jr., Goldstein, R. B., Blum, N. (1992). A family study of obsessive-compulsive disorder. *Archives of General Psychiatry*, 49, 362–8.
9. Pauls, D. L., Alsobrook, J. P., Goodman, W. K., Rasmussen, S. A., Leckman, J. F. (1995). A family study of obsessive compulsive disorder. *American Journal of Psychiatry*, 152, 76–84.
10. Nestadt, G., Samuels, J., Riddle, M. A., *et al.* (2000). A family study of obsessive-compulsive disorder. *Archives of General Psychiatry*, 57, 358–63.
11. Grabe, H. J., Ruhrmann, S., Ettelt, S., *et al.* (2006). Familiality of obsessive-compulsive disorder in nonclinical and clinical subjects. *American Journal of Psychiatry*, 163, 1986–92.
12. Hanna, G. L., Himle, J. A., Curtis, G. C., Gillespie, B. W. (2005). A family study of obsessive-compulsive disorder with pediatric probands. *American Journal of Medical Genetics Part B (Neuropsychiatric Genetics)*, 134B, 13–19.
13. Nestadt, G., Samuels, J., Riddle, M. A., *et al.* (2001). The relationship between obsessive-compulsive disorder and anxiety and affective disorders: results from the Johns Hopkins OCD Family Study. *Psychological Medicine*, 31, 481–7.
14. Bienvenu, O. J., Samuels, J. F., Riddle, M. A., *et al.* (2000). The relationship of obsessive-compulsive disorder to possible spectrum disorders: results from a family study. *Biological Psychiatry*, 48, 287–93.
15. Grados, M. A., Riddle, M. A., Samuels, J. F., *et al.* (2001). The familial phenotype of obsessive-compulsive disorder in relation to tic disorders: The Hopkins OCD Family Study. *Biological Psychiatry*, 50, 559–65.

16. Cavallini, M. C., Pasquale, L., Bellodi, L., Smeraldi, E. (1999). Complex segregation analysis for obsessive compulsive disorder and related disorders. *American Journal of Medical Genetics (Neuropsychiatric Genetics)*, 88, 38–43.

17. Nestadt, G., Lan, T., Samuels, J., *et al.* (2000). Complex segregation analysis provides compelling evidence for a major gene underlying obsessive-compulsive disorder and for heterogeneity by sex. *American Journal of Human Genetics*, 67, 1611–16.

18. Hanna, G. L., Fingerlin, T. E., Himle, J. A., Boehnke, M. (2005). Complex segregation analysis of obsessive-compulsive disorder in families with pediatric probands. *Human Heredity*, 60, 1–9.

19. Grootheest, D. S., Cath, D. C., Beekman, A. T., Boomsma, D. I. (2005). Twin studies on obsessive-compulsive disorder: a review. *Twin Research and Human Genetics*, 8, 450–8.

20. Eley, T. C., Bolton, D., O'Connor, T. G., Perrin, S., Smith, P., Plomin, R. (2003). A twin study of anxiety-related behaviours in pre-school children. *Journal of Child Psychology and Psychiatry*, 44, 945–60.

21. Hudziak, J. J., van Beijsterveldt, C. E. M., *et al.* (2004). Genetic and environmental contributions to the Child Behavior Checklist Obsessive-Compulsive Scale. *Archives of General Psychiatry*, 61, 608–16.

22. Hanna, G. L., Veenstra-VanderWeele, J., Cox, N. J., *et al.* (2002). Genome-wide linkage analysis of families with obsessive-compulsive disorder ascertained through pediatric probands. *American Journal of Medical Genetics (Neuropsychiatric Genetics)*, 114, 541–52.

23. Willour, V. L., Shugart, Y. Y., Samuels, J., *et al.* (2004). Replication study supports evidence for linkage to 9p24 in obsessive-compulsive disorder. *American Journal of Human Genetics*, 75, 508–13.

24. Shugart, Y. Y., Samuels, J., Willour, V. L., *et al.* (2006). Genomewide linkage scan for obsessive-compulsive disorder: evidence for susceptibility loci on chromosomes 3q, 7p, 1q, 15q, and 6q. *Molecular Psychiatry*, 11, 763–70.

25. Wang, Y., Samuels, J. F., Chang, Y. C., *et al.* (2009). Gender differences in genetic linkage and association on 11p15 in obsessive-compulsive disorder families. *American Journal of Medical Genetics Part B (Neuropsychiatric Genetics)*,150B, 33–40.

26. Samuels, J., Shugart, Y. Y., Grados, M. A., *et al.* (2007). Significant linkage to compulsive hoarding on chromosome 14 in families with obsessive-compulsive disorder: results from the OCD Collaborative Genetics Study. *American Journal of Psychiatry*, 164, 493–9.

27. Samuels, J., Wang, Y., Riddle, M. A., *et al.* (2011). Comprehensive family-based association study of the glutamate transporter gene *SLC1A1* in obsessive-compulsive disorder. *American Journal of Medical Genetics (Neuropsychiatric Genetics)*, 156, 472–7.

28. Taylor, S. (2013). Molecular genetics of obsessive-compulsive disorder: a comprehensive meta-analysis of genetic association studies. *Molecular Psychiatry*, 18, 799–805.

29. Hemmings, S. M. J., Stein, D. J. (2006). The current status of association studies in obsessive-compulsive disorder. *Psychiatric Clinics of North America*, 29, 411–44.

30. Stewart, S. E., Yu, D., Scharf, J. M., *et al.* (2013). Genome-wide association study of obsessive-compulsive disorder. *Molecular Psychiatry*, 18, 788–98.

31. Mattheisen, M., Samuels, J. F., Wang, Y., *et al.* (2015). Genome-wide association study in obsessive compulsive disorder: results from the OCGAS. *Molecular Psychiatry*, 20, 337–44.

32. den Braber, A., Zilhao, N. R., Fedko, I. O., *et al.* (2016). Obsessive-compulsive symptoms in a large population-based twin-family sample are predicted by clinically based polygenic scores and by genome-wide SNPs. *Translational Psychiatry*, 6, e731.

33. Davis, L. K., Yu, D., Keenan, C. L., *et al.* (2013). Partitioning the heritability of Tourette Syndrome and obsessive compulsive disorder reveals differences in genetic architecture. *PLoS Genetics*, 9, e1003864.

34. Bertelsen B., Melior, L., Jensen, L. R., *et al.* (2015). A t(3;9)(q25.1;q34.3) translocation leading to OLFM1 fusion transcripts in Gilles de la Tourette syndrome, OCD, and ADHD. *Psychiatry Research*, 225, 268–75.

35. Devor, E. J., Magee, H. J. (1999). Multiple childhood behavioral disorder (Tourette Syndrome, multiple tics, ADD and OCD) presenting in a family with a balanced chromosomal translocation (t1;8)(q21.1;q22.1). *Psychiatric Genetics*, 9, 149–51.

36. McGrath, L. M., Yu, D., Marshall, C., *et al.* (2014). Copy number variation in obsessive-compulsive disorder and Tourette Syndrome: a cross-disorder study. *Journal of the American Academy of Child and Adolescent Psychiatry*, 53, 910–19.

37. Cappi, C., Brentani, H., Lima, L., *et al.* (2016). Whole-exome sequencing in obsessive-compulsive disorder identifies rare mutations in immunological and neurodevelopmental pathways. *Translational Psychiatry*, 6, e764.

38. Karayiorgou, m., Altemus, M., Galke, B. L., *et al.* (1997). Genotype determining low catechol-O-methyltransferase activity as a risk factor for obsessive-compulsive disorder. *Proceedings of the National Academy of Sciences of the United States of America*, 94, 4572–5.

39. Alsobrook, J. P., Zohar, A. H., Leboyer M., *et al.* (2002). Association between the *COMT* locus and obsessive-compulsive disorder in females but not males. *American Journal of Medical Genetics*, 114, 116–20.

40. Pauls, D. L. Raymond, C. L., Stevenson, J. M., Leckman, J. F. (1991). A family study of Gilles de la Tourette Syndrome. *American Journal of Human Genetics*, 48, 154–63.

41. Yu, D., Mathews, C. A., Scharf, J. M., *et al.* (2015). Cross-disorder genome-wide analyses suggest a complex genetic relationship between Tourette Syndrome and obsessive-compulsive disorder. *American Journal of Psychiatry*, 172, 82–93.

42. Gottesman, I. I., Gould, T. D. (2003). The endophenotype concept in psychiatry: etymology and strategic intentions. *American Journal of Psychiatry*, 160, 636–45.

43. Chamberlain, S. R., Blackwell, A. D., Fineberg, N. A., Robbins, T. W., Sahakian, B.J. (2005). The neuropsychology of obsessive compulsive disorder: the importance of failures in cognitive and behavioural inhibition as candidate endophenotypic markers *Neuroscience and Biobehavioral Reviews*, 23, 399–419.

44. Menzies, L., Achard, S., Chamberlain, S. R., *et al.* (2007). Neurocognitive endophenotypes of obsessive-compulsive disorder. *Brain*, 130, 3223–36.

45. Chamberlain, S. R., Menzies, L. (2009). Endophenotypes of obsessive-compulsive disorder: rationale, evidence and future potential. *Expert Review of Neurotherapeutics*, 9, 1133–46.

46. Riesel, A., Endrass, T., Kaufmann, C., Kathmann, N. (2011). Overactive error-related brain activity as a candidate endophenotype for obsessive-compulsive disorder: evidence from unaffected first-degree relatives. *American Journal of Psychiatry*, 168, 317–24.

47. Carrasco, M., Harbin, S. M., Nienhuis, J. K., Fitzgerald, K. D., Gehring, W. J., Hanna, G.L. (2013). Increased error-related brain activity in youth with obsessive-compulsive disorder and unaffected siblings. *Depression and Anxiety*, 30, 39–46.

48. Zhang, L., Dong, Y., Ji, Y., *et al.* (2015). Dissociation of decision making under ambiguity and decision making under risk: a neurocognitive endophenotype candidate for obsessive-compulsive disorder. *Progress in Neuro-Psychopharmacology and Biological Psychiatry*, 57, 60–8.

49. Brandl, E. J., Müller, D. J., Richter, M. A. (2012). Pharmacogenetics of obsessive-compulsive disorder. *Pharmacogenomics*, 13, 71–81.

50. Zai, G., Brandl, E. J., Müller, D. J., Richter, M. A., Kennedy, J. L. (2014). Pharmacogenetics of antidepressant treatment in obsessive-compulsive disorder: an update and implications for clinicians. *Pharmacogenomics*, 15, 1147–57.

51. Qin, H., Samuels, J. F., Wang, Y., *et al.* (2016). Whole genome association analysis of treatment response in obsessive-compulsive disorder. *Molecular Psychiatry*, 21, 270–6.

52. Probst-Schendzielorz, K., Viviani, R. K., Stingl, J. C. (2015). Effect of Cytochrome P450 polymorphism on the action and metabolism of selective serotonin reuptake inhibitors. *Expert Opinion on Drug Metabolism and Toxicology*, 11, 1219–32.

53. Dodman, N. H., Karlsson, E. K., Moon-Fanelli, A., *et al.* (2010). A canine chromosome 7 locus confers OCD susceptibility. (2010). *Molecular Psychiatry*, 15, 8–10.

54. Tang, R., Noh, H. J., Wang, D., *et al.* (2014). Candidate genes and functional noncoding variants identified in a canine model of obsessive-compulsive disorder. *Genome Biology*, 15, R25.

55. McGregor, N. W., Lochner, C., Stein, D. J., Hemmings, S. M. (2016). Polymorphisms within the neuronal cadherin gene (*CDH2*) are associated with obsessive-compulsive disorder (OCD) in a South African cohort (2016). *Metabolic Brain Disease*, 31, 191–6.

56. Welch, J. M., Lu, J., Rodriguez, R. M., *et al.* (2007). Corticostriatal synaptic defects and OCD-like behaviors in *Sapap3*-mutant mice, *Nature*, 448, 894–900.

57. Bienvenu, O. J., Wang, Y., Shugart, Y. Y., *et al.* (2009). *Sapap3* and pathological grooming in humans. *American Journal of Medical Genetics Part B, Neuropsychiatric Genetics*, 50B, 710–20.

58. Zuchner, S., Wendland, J. R., Ashley-Koch, A. E., *et al.* (2009). Multiple rare SAPAP3 missense variants in trichotillomania and OCD. *Molecular Psychiatry*, 14, 6–9.

59. Ting, J. T., Feng, G. (2011). Neurobiology of obsessive-compulsive disorder: insights into neural circuitry dysfunction through mouse genetics. *Current Opinion in Neurobiology*, 21, 842–8.

60. Schadt, E. E. (2006). Novel integrative genomics strategies to identify genes for complex traits. *Animal Genetics*, 37 (Supplement 1), 18–23.

61. The ENCODE Project Consortium (2004). The ENCODE (Encyclopedia of DNA Elements) Project. *Science*, 306, 636–40.

# 97

# Imaging of obsessive–compulsive disorder

*Rebbia Shahab and Emily R. Stern*

## Introduction

For the past several decades, neuroimaging techniques, such as functional magnetic resonance imaging (fMRI) and positron emission tomography (PET), have been used to investigate neurocircuit functioning in OCD. While earlier studies examining neural responses to symptom provocation have identified altered brain activity in OCD and are clearly relevant for the disorder, they do not address whether basic cognitive–affective mechanisms are impaired in the absence of direct symptom exacerbation. In this article, we discuss findings from cognitive neuroscientific studies probing basic cognitive–affective constructs that may underlie the complex phenomenology of OCD, including conflict and error monitoring, response inhibition, task switching and reversal, decision-making, and reward processing. Although several cognitive neuroscientific studies that are not discussed here have used task paradigms that tap into theoretically driven core mechanisms of OCD (including impaired fear extinction [1] or altered habit formation [2, 3]), we focus the main part of this review on those topics where at least four studies compared adults with OCD with a healthy control group. We conclude by discussing findings in the context of OCD heterogeneity and reviewing the small literature comparing functional neuroimaging findings between OCD subtypes. Our review is complementary to the description of brain circuits in Chapter 94.

## Conflict and error monitoring

Much research into the cognitive neuroscience of OCD has taken place in the field of conflict monitoring and error detection. This approach is based on the proposal that obsessions are caused by an overactive conflict or error signal continually telling the patient that 'something is wrong' despite evidence to the contrary [4]. In this view, compulsions are behaviours that attempt to reduce this heightened conflict signal or to correct perceived errors. Cognitive conflict is typically studied in tasks where there is a mismatch between what a subject would automatically do (that is, a prepotent response) and what is required in the task. The classic example of a conflict monitoring paradigm is the Stroop task where subjects must make a response according to the font colour of a word, where the word itself is the name of a colour that is different from the font colour (that

is, the word 'blue' written in red font). In this case, the prepotent response is to read the name of the word, yet the task requires a response according to the colour of the word, which creates conflict that significantly increases response times, compared to trials where the colour and word name are the same [5]. Conflict monitoring in healthy controls fairly consistently implicates the dorsal medial frontal cortical (MFC) regions including the dorsal anterior cingulate cortex (dACC) and the supplementary motor area (SMA) and pre-SMA [6–9], yet results from the many neuroimaging studies investigating this process in OCD do not present a coherent picture. While some investigations have indeed found hyperactivity of the dorsal MFC regions during conflict in OCD [10, 11], other studies have identified reduced activity in this region [6–9, 12, 13] or no differences between patients and controls [14–16]. Many studies have reported differences between patients and controls during conflict monitoring in several other brain regions outside the dorsal MFC, including the parietal cortex [17, 18], inferior frontal gyrus/insula [19], ventral/rostral regions of the MFC [11, 20, 21], lateral [13, 17] and medial [18] temporal cortex, and striatum including the caudate nucleus and putamen [12, 13]. However, these results are often contradictory, with some studies finding activations to be greater in OCD than controls and other studies reporting the opposite effect.

Errors reflect a specific instance of conflict where the intended or correct response does not match the actual response made by the subject. Similar to conflict monitoring, errors elicit activation in the dorsal MFC regions, including the dACC and SMA. In addition, errors tend to elicit an emotional reaction related to frustration, disappointment, or fear of punishment and typically activate a broad range of brain regions, including the bilateral anterior insula, the rostral ACC (rACC), and the ventromedial prefrontal cortex (vmPFC), the dorsolateral prefrontal cortex (DLPFC), and the orbitofrontal cortex (OFC) [22]. The anterior insula, rACC/vmPFC, and OFC have been associated with valuation and emotion [23–26]; as such, activation of these brain regions to errors may reflect the neural processing of the emotional/motivational significance of mistakes [27]. Unlike the conflict processing literature, data somewhat consistently point to an enhanced error detection mechanism in OCD. The error-related negativity (ERN), a negative event-related potential (ERP) that peaks approximately 100 ms after an error and is thought to be generated in the dorsal MFC, is consistently larger in OCD than controls (for a review, see [28]). In fMRI studies, OCD

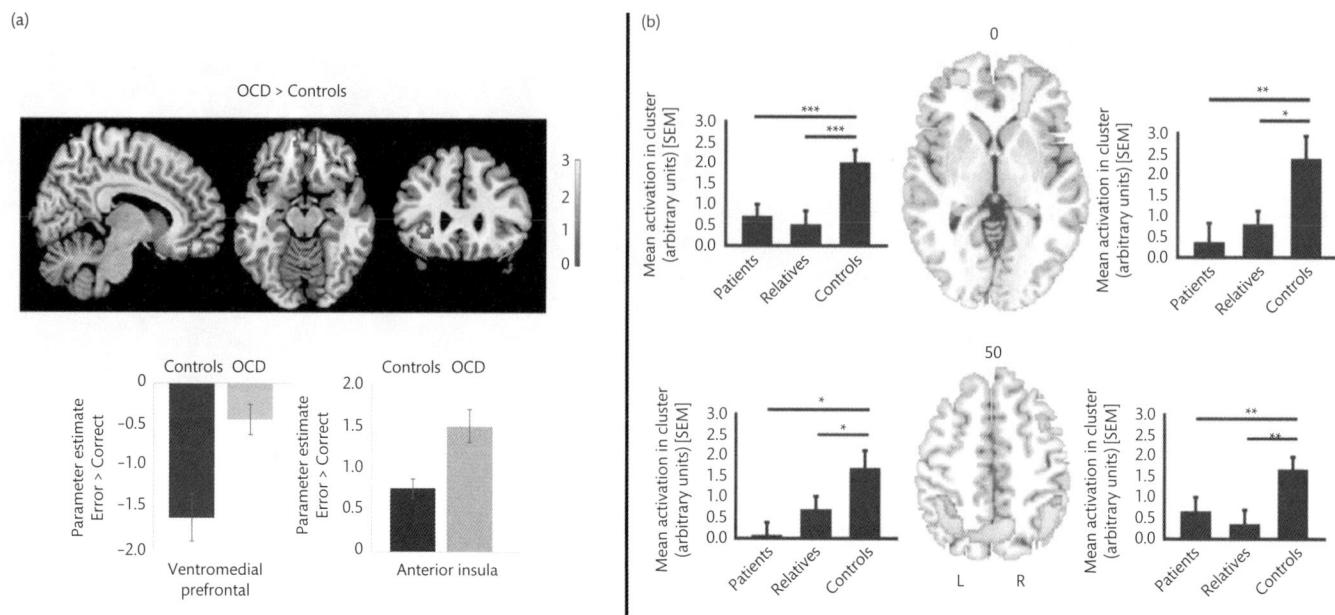

**Fig. 97.1** (see Colour Plate section) (a) Results from [15] showing greater error-related activity in the ventromedial prefrontal cortex and anterior insula in OCD patients, compared to controls.

Reproduced from *Biol Psychiatry*, 69(6), Stern ER, Welsh RC, Fitzgerald KD, *et al.*, Hyperactive error responses and altered connectivity in ventromedial and frontoinsular cortices in obsessive-compulsive disorder, pp. 583–91, Copyright (2011), with permission from Society of Biological Psychiatry.

(b) Results from [54] showing regions activated for (successful) reversal (areas in yellow), overlaid with orbitofrontal and parietal areas showing reduced activity during reversal, for both OCD patients and their unaffected relatives, compared to controls (areas in blue).

Reproduced from *Science*, 321(5887), Chamberlain SR, Menzies L, Hampshire A, *et al.*, Orbitofrontal Dysfunction in Patients with Obsessive-Compulsive Disorder and Their Unaffected Relatives, pp. 421–2, Copyright (2008), with permission from American Association for the Advancement of Science.

patients have shown an increased neural response to errors in dACC [10, 29], rACC [29], and lateral frontal cortex, including the OFC and DLPFC [14, 29]. Fitzgerald *et al.* [12] found hyperactivity in the vmPFC in a small group of patients with OCD, a finding that was replicated in a larger study [15], which also identified hyperactivity of the anterior insula (Fig. 97.1a). Despite some variation among the studies, overall these data suggest that OCD patients respond more strongly to errors than healthy individuals, particularly in ventral frontal regions potentially involved in processing the value or emotional importance of the error. However, it is important to note that these studies examine OCD patients' responses to actual errors (and conflict), whereas the phenotype of the disorder is more consistent with the detection of errors (or conflict) where there are none (or at least where their presence is uncertain). Thus, while hyperactive error responses in OCD may reflect an important characteristic of the disorder related to sensitivity to mistakes, these studies do not directly probe the neural mechanisms associated with the feeling that something is wrong, even in the absence of overt errors. ERP studies that have attempted to address this issue by examining the 'correct related negativity' (CRN)—a small negative deflection that is the analogue to the ERN on correct trials—have been somewhat inconsistent as to whether OCD patients show an enhanced CRN [28].

## Response inhibition/motor output suppression

It has been suggested that compulsions in OCD may result from an inability to engage mechanisms of response inhibition [30]. Response inhibition is commonly studied using a go/no-go task (or

a variant thereof such as the stop-signal task) where subjects make button-press responses to frequent stimuli ('go' trials) and are required to inhibit responses to infrequently presented stimuli ('no-go' trials). Even though this task inevitably involves conflict monitoring between the frequent 'go' and infrequent 'no-go' trials, these paradigms additionally involve a specific motor suppression component not present in conflict studies. Accordingly, while 'no-go' trials are associated with activation of some of the same regions as for conflict monitoring, including the dACC and SMA/pre-SMA [31–34], they also elicit activation in subcortical structures, including the thalamus and basal ganglia, as well as predominantly right hemisphere lateral frontal and inferior parietal regions [31–35]. In a meta-analysis, the right inferior frontal gyrus (IFG) has been most consistently associated with 'no-go' trials [32], which has been supported by lesion and brain stimulation studies showing impaired response inhibition after inactivation of this region [36, 37].

Studies comparing OCD patients and controls have found reduced activity in the SMA, ACC, right IFG, inferior parietal cortex, striatum, and thalamus in OCD patients during correct no-go trials (that is, successful response inhibition) [17, 38–41], which would suggest reduced recruitment of the response suppression network, even during inhibition success. However, OCD hyperactivity in the caudate nucleus and thalamus [29, 41], as well as the medial and lateral frontal regions, insula, premotor cortex, middle temporal cortex, posterior cingulate cortex, and cerebellum [17, 38–41], has also been reported for successful inhibition, which has been interpreted as compensatory activation [17]. Given the variability of findings, it is not clear whether abnormal hypoactivity or hyperactivity of a response inhibition network is a core feature of OCD. These equivocal results may stem partially from the focus on neural differences during successful inhibitions (as opposed to inhibition failures, which would be most relevant for the disorder). Further research linking brain function to behaviour will be needed to address this issue.

## Task switching and reversal

Another approach to investigating the basic mechanisms of OCD has focused on how patients switch attention between two or more different tasks, stimuli, or rewards. Rather than hypothesizing an overactive conflict or error signal or a failure to suppress motor output, these studies hypothesize that OCD patients exhibit an inflexibility that prevents them from shifting attention away from stimuli or features that are no longer relevant to the task at hand. For an in-depth discussion of behavioural measures of cognitive inflexibility in OCD, the reader is referred to a review article by Gruner and Pittenger [42].

Many studies of switching have investigated neural activity associated with shifting attention between features or dimensions of stimuli ('cognitive' switching tasks). Not surprisingly, in a meta-analysis examining brain regions involved in cognitive switching and motor suppression, overlap between these processes were found in the dACC/SMA, IFG, DLPFC, and inferior parietal cortex [32]. However, fronto-parietal activations were more widespread and bilateral for cognitive switching [32, 35], appearing very similar to a frontal-parietal network (FPN) often described as being involved in executive functions and task control [43, 44]. Studies looking at brain activity in OCD during cognitive switching have found reduced activation in patients, compared to controls, in FPN as well as in the OFC, caudate nucleus, temporal cortex, and medial parietal regions [17, 45, 46]. Two studies reported widespread reductions across the cortex and basal ganglia [45, 46], whereas two reported hypoactivations localized to only a few regions of the frontal and parietal cortices [17]. In addition to hypoactivation of the anterior prefrontal cortex extending into the lateral OFC, a recent study also found *hyper*activation of the dACC and putamen and post-central gyrus activity during task switching in OCD [47].

Another type of switching that has been of interest in OCD involves reversing stimulus–reward contingencies (sometimes referred to as 'affective' switching). In reversal tasks, the reward and punishment value of two stimuli switch, so that the currently rewarded stimulus is punished and the previously punished stimulus is rewarded. There is some evidence to suggest that reversal of reward–punishment contingencies relies primarily on the OFC, rather than the lateral prefrontal regions involved in cognitive switching [35, 48–50]. Studies of reversal in OCD have examined neural activation on trials where subjects made a reversal error that lead to a successful switch, compared with errors that did not lead to a successful switch (thereby isolating activity associated with the moment subjects learn that a switch is required) [51–53], or during the correct choice after a successful reversal [54]. For these comparisons, OCD patients exhibit reduced activation in the OFC, but similar to results from cognitive switching studies, reductions have also been found throughout the FPN, including the DLPFC, bilateral insula, lateral parietal cortex, and putamen [51–54]. In one study, unaffected relatives of OCD also showed reduced activity in

the lateral OFC, DLPFC, and lateral parietal cortex during reversal [54] (Fig. 97.1b), suggesting that impaired frontal recruitment during reversal may be an endophenotype of the disorder. With a slightly different approach using a fear conditioning reversal task, OCD patients showed reduced medial orbitofrontal activity, when compared with controls, when viewing a stimulus that was previously associated with shock but was now safe [55].

Overall, these data generally support the notion that OCD patients show hypoactivation in a variety of cortical regions, both during task switching and when reversing reward–punishment contingencies. Despite the dissociation of lateral and orbital frontal involvement in these processes, dysfunctional brain activity in OCD does not appear to be localized to one of these systems. Reduced recruitment of both the DLPFC and OFC has been found when patients switch cognitive set, as well as when they reverse reward contingencies. Similar to the concerns discussed for the other approaches, interpretation of results from switching studies is complicated by the fact that neural differences between OCD patients and controls are examined during successful switches (either at the time of the correct switch response or at the time of the error right before a correct switch), rather than for unsuccessful switches. Future work focusing on brain activity during switch failures would further elucidate the neural mechanisms of cognitive inflexibility in OCD.

## Decision-making

OCD has been characterized as a disorder associated with impaired decision-making [56, 57]. Clinically, OCD often manifests as risk aversion and intolerance of uncertainty [58, 59], and experimentally, OCD patients show reduced risk-taking [60] (but see [61]) and excessive information gathering in the face of uncertainty [62–65]. In healthy individuals, risk and uncertainty are associated with activation of the FPN [66, 67], with effects most consistently found in the anterior insula and dorsal MFC [67–72]. In a study where OCD patients played an interactive game where they could make risky or safe choices and anticipate outcomes of their choices, patients made fewer risky choices than controls and showed greater amygdala activation when anticipating outcomes of their risky choices [60]. By contrast, a recent study found that OCD patients did not show any differences from controls in risky decision-making both behaviourally and in the brain, although patients did show a stronger correlation between individual level of risk aversion and activation of the insula, DLPFC, and precentral/post-central gyri when making risky choices [61]. In an examination of uncertainty and checking, Rotge et al. [73] found that OCD patients showed reduced mid-OFC activity, compared to controls, for decisions that lead to subsequent checking behaviour. In another task investigating uncertainty, patients were required to make decisions based on evidence that was either uncertain (that is, the likelihoods for two different outcomes being similar) or certain (for example, the likelihood for one outcome being 100% and for the other being 0%) [74]. In this study, OCD patients reported more subjective uncertainty than controls, and showed increased activation of the amygdala, parahippocampus and hippocampus, temporal cortex, ventral anterior insula, lateral OFC, and vmPFC, when making decisions based on 'certain' (that is, unequivocal) evidence but showed no differences for decisions based on uncertain evidence. Interestingly, in the studies of Admon

[60] and Stern [74], hyperactivations in OCD were found in brain regions not typically linked to risk and uncertainty in healthy populations such as the amygdala, parahippocampus and hippocampus, lateral temporal cortex, and vmPFC [69]. One could speculate that recruitment of these additional limbic and paralimbic regions when processing risk and uncertainty may reflect greater emotional involvement during decision-making in OCD or an excessive internal focus associated with 'default mode network' activity [75]. This hypothesis is consistent with the finding that OCD patients hyperactivate the vmPFC and lateral temporal cortex (both areas of default mode network [75]), when making decisions about moral dilemmas [76]. Overall, these data suggest that OCD patients do engage different brain regions than controls when making decisions, although differences between paradigms and the relatively few studies investigating these behaviours in OCD suggest the need for additional study.

## Reward processing

It has been suggested that the difficulty exhibited by OCD patients in terminating inappropriate responses is related to a reduced signal of goal attainment or satiety [77]. Within this framework, OCD patients continue to engage in compulsive behaviours, such as checking, washing, or repeating/ordering, because the normal 'reward' signal associated with successfully completing these tasks is not attained. In healthy individuals, rewards elicit activation in a network of brain regions, including the ventral striatum, thalamus, putamen, hippocampus, anterior insula, MFC, and parietal cortex [78]. Prior studies in OCD have found reduced activation in patients in some of these regions during reward feedback or anticipation, including the vmPFC in a reversal paradigm [52, 53] and the putamen in a spatial reward learning task [79]. However, using a version of the monetary incentive delay (MID) task [80], Jung et al. [81] reported increased activity in cortical and subcortical regions, including the putamen and dorsal MFC, to monetary reward in OCD patients, with no regions showing reduced activity, compared to controls. In another study also using a version of the MID, OCD patients showed reduced dorsal MFC activation, compared to controls, during reward feedback, as well as reduced activation in the ventral striatum when anticipating an upcoming trial that could potentially provide reward [82]. This latter finding contrasts with three other studies showing no difference in striatal activation between OCD patients and controls during anticipation of trials where reward was possible [81, 83, 84]. Overall, it is not yet clear whether dysfunctional brain responses to reward contribute to OCD, although impaired recruitment of the striatum during reward processing has not been consistently implicated in the disorder. Future work may benefit from examining reward processing from the standpoint of goal attainment or task completion, which may be particularly relevant for the symptoms of the disorder.

## Neural correlates of OCD subtypes

As can be seen, results from fMRI studies are variable, with many revealing abnormalities of widespread fronto-parietal and fronto-striatal networks and others identifying more circumscribed differences between patients and controls. Given the heterogeneity of the disorder, it is possible that the discrepant findings may be attributed to differing neural mechanisms mediating the various symptoms of OCD. There are several ways that OCD can be segregated into symptom clusters, including by distinguishing patients with sensory phenomena from those without [85] or by focusing on severity of harm avoidance symptoms in OCD [86]. While these approaches are critical to the future understanding of how dimensional (and fundamentally trans-diagnostic) symptoms manifest in the brain not only in OCD, but also in other psychiatric disorders (that is, sensory phenomena are prevalent not only in OCD but also in tic disorders; harm avoidance is a feature not only of OCD, but also of other anxiety disorders), the majority of work to date on OCD heterogeneity has focused on investigating subtypes that have been identified through factor analyses of Yale-Brown Obsessive–Compulsive Scale (Y-BOCS) responses [87–89]. Although there are slight variations, typically these studies identify 3–5 dissociable factors of contamination/washing, aggressive/checking, symmetry/ordering, sexual/religious, and hoarding symptoms. This section will review the literature on fMRI studies that examine the neural substrates of these different symptom subtypes.

## Contamination/washing

OCD patients with contamination/washing symptoms are heavily concerned about cleanliness and disease. Washing compulsions have been associated with activation in several prefrontal regions, such as the OFC, ACC, and DLPFC, as well as the insula, during a symptom provocation [90] and continuous performance task [91]. Greater insular activation has also been associated with washers' sensitivity to disgusting stimuli in general, including pictures and facial expressions of disgust [92, 93]. A recent study [94] found increased functional connectivity between the insula and the ventral striatum also during the provocation of contamination symptoms. The findings of insula hyperactivation are particularly interesting because the insula is one of the primary regions involved in processing disgusting stimuli [90, 95, 96], potentially due to its role in interoception [97]. Of importance, one study looking at the neural substrates of washing symptoms in a medication and comorbidity-free sample of OCD patients found decreased activation in the anterior prefrontal cortex, DLPFC, OFC, ACC, insula, parietal cortex, and caudate [98]. Although the same brain regions were implicated, the activity was in the opposite direction of that in previous studies on washers. Although these results suggest that some of the prior findings of hyperactivation could be related to confounding factors, the consistency of the insula hyperactivation finding in washers and the link between disgust processing and insula activity suggest a primary role for the insula in this OCD subtype.

## Aggressive/checking, sexual/religious, and symmetry/ordering

The aggressive/checking, sexual/religious, and symmetry/ordering subtypes of OCD have not been widely studied, and the results paint an incomplete picture about the neural substrates of these subtypes. In a symptom provocation study, patients with checking compulsions showed greater activation than healthy controls in various brainstem nuclei, globus pallidus, and right thalamus, as well as in the dACC, precentral gyrus, and superior frontal gyrus [90]. In a study looking at blood flow during a continuous performance task using PET [91], there was a positive correlation between severity of aggressive/checking and sexual/religious symptoms and blood flow in bilateral striatum, including areas of the caudate nucleus, putamen, and pallidum. Many of these regions are associated with sensorimotor functions that could possibly mediate some of the motor components of checking behaviour. Greater severity of aggressive obsessions has been correlated with increased resting-state functional connectivity between the ventral caudate and the vmPFC and decreased connectivity between the ventral caudate and the amygdala [99], and amygdala activity has also been correlated with the severity of both aggressive/checking and sexual/religious symptoms in OCD patients when viewing fearful faces [100]. Given the amygdala's role in fear processing [101], these data suggest that these subtypes may be associated with altered amygdala-based fear reactivity related to concerns about causing harm and having what are deemed to be morally unacceptable thoughts related to sexual or religious themes. Interestingly, patients with more severe sexual/religious obsessions also demonstrated relatively greater connectivity between the ventral caudate and the insula [99]. The involvement of the insula in the sexual/religious subtype could reflect a type of 'moral disgust' (which also activates the insula [102]) that is characteristic of patients with these types of obsessions. Few studies have reported relationships between brain function and symmetry/ordering symptoms, although the PET study using the continuous performance task described above did find that the severity of symmetry/ordering symptoms was negatively correlated with right caudate nucleus activity [91].

## Hoarding

Hoarding is characterized by excessive collecting, or being unable to discard, items, even though they might not have objective value. Hoarders have emotional attachment to their possessions and face great difficulty in deciding what to keep or throw out. Although there is debate on whether hoarding is a subtype of OCD or is better characterized as its own distinct disorder [103], several studies have investigated hoarding symptoms within the context of OCD. One PET study found diminished glucose metabolism in the posterior cingulate cortex (PCC), occipital cortex, and ACC in hoarders, compared to non-hoarders or a control group [104]. Relatedly, anxiety evoked during the viewing of hoarding-relevant pictures was associated with reduced activity in the dACC, parieto-occipital regions, basal ganglia, and temporal cortex in a group of OCD patients including both hoarders and non-hoarders [105]. However, other work has shown that hoarding severity in OCD patients correlates positively with activation and connectivity in the vmPFC and OFC, as well as in the precentral and post-central gyri, which may point to a sensorimotor component of the hoarding phenotype [90, 99, 105]. The vmPFC has been implicated in compulsive hoarding in animal and brain lesion studies [106–108] and is also considered to be crucial for decision-making [109], suggesting that hyperactivation in this region may underlie the difficulty in making decisions regarding which objects to collect and discard.

## Conclusions

The summary provides a selective review of neuroimaging correlates of psychological processes that could potentially underlie the complex symptom presentation of patients with OCD. The most consistent findings were hyperactivation in response to errors and hypoactivation during switching tasks, with both effects occurring predominantly in the prefrontal cortex, but with findings also noted in other areas, including the striatum, parietal cortex, and temporal cortex. Given the complexity of the brain in general, and OCD in particular, no one task paradigm is likely to fully explain the disorder, and it is clear that the task chosen is absolutely critical for interpreting findings. Indeed, other approaches investigating fear extinction [1], habit formation [2, 3, 110], emotional face and picture processing [93, 100, 111–115], planning [116, 117], and working memory [118–122] have identified neural alterations in OCD that may also contribute to the phenomenology of the disorder. Some of the variability in findings may be related to the heterogeneity of symptoms in OCD, with some studies identifying distinctions in limbic and sensorimotor regions based on subtype. Taken together, the many paradigms used in cognitive neuroscientific research provide powerful probes that have already shed some light on the underlying mechanisms of OCD. Future work would benefit from combining the strengths from these many approaches by further interrogating core processes and symptom dimensions in OCD in order to design novel treatments targeting symptom-specific neural markers.

## REFERENCES

1. Milad MR, Furtak SC, Greenberg JL, et al. Deficits in conditioned fear extinction in obsessive-compulsive disorder and neurobiological changes in the fear circuit. JAMA Psychiatry. 2013;70:608–18; quiz 554.
2. Gillan CM, Apergis-Schoute AM, Morein-Zamir S, et al. Functional neuroimaging of avoidance habits in obsessive-compulsive disorder. Am J Psychiatry. 2015;172:284–93.
3. Rauch SL, Wedig MM, Wright CI, et al. Functional magnetic resonance imaging study of regional brain activation during implicit sequence learning in obsessive-compulsive disorder. Biol Psychiatry. 2007;61:330–6.
4. Pitman RK. A cybernetic model of obsessive-compulsive psychopathology. Compr Psychiatry. 1987;28:334–43.
5. MacLeod CM. Half a century of research on the Stroop effect: an integrative review. Psychol Bull. 1991;109:163–203.
6. Botvinick MM, Braver TS, Barch DM, Carter CS, Cohen JD. Conflict monitoring and cognitive control. Psychol Rev. 2001;108:624–52.
7. Garavan H, Ross TJ, Kaufman J, Stein EA. A midline dissociation between error-processing and response-conflict monitoring. Neuroimage. 2003;20:1132–9.
8. Hester R, Fassbender C, Garavan H. Individual differences in error processing: a review and reanalysis of three event-related fMRI studies using the GO/NOGO task. Cereb Cortex. 2004;14:986–94.
9. Ridderinkhof KR, Ullsperger M, Crone EA, Nieuwenhuis S. The role of the medial frontal cortex in cognitive control. Science. 2004;306:443–7.
10. Ursu S, Stenger VA, Shear MK, Jones MR, Carter CS. Overactive action monitoring in obsessive-compulsive disorder: evidence

from functional magnetic resonance imaging. *Psychol Sci.* 2003;14:347–53.

11. Yucel M, Harrison BJ, Wood SJ, *et al.* Functional and biochemical alterations of the medial frontal cortex in obsessive-compulsive disorder. *Arch Gen Psychiatry.* 2007;64:946–55.

12. Fitzgerald KD, Welsh RC, Gehring WJ, *et al.* Error-related hyperactivity of the anterior cingulate cortex in obsessive-compulsive disorder. *Biol Psychiatry.* 2005;57:287–94.

13. Nakao T, Nakagawa A, Yoshiura T, *et al.* A functional MRI comparison of patients with obsessive-compulsive disorder and normal controls during a Chinese character Stroop task. *Psychiatry Res.* 2005;139:101–14.

14. Hough CM, Luks TL, Lai K, *et al.* Comparison of brain activation patterns during executive function tasks in hoarding disorder and non-hoarding OCD. *Psychiatry Res.* 2016;255:50–9.

15. Stern ER, Welsh RC, Fitzgerald KD, *et al.* Hyperactive error responses and altered connectivity in ventromedial and frontoinsular cortices in obsessive-compulsive disorder. *Biol Psychiatry.* 2011;69:583–91.

16. Viard A, Flament MF, Artiges E, *et al.* Cognitive control in childhood-onset obsessive-compulsive disorder: a functional MRI study. *Psychol Med.* 2005;35:1007–17.

17. Page LA, Rubia K, Deeley Q, *et al.* A functional magnetic resonance imaging study of inhibitory control in obsessive-compulsive disorder. *Psychiatry Res.* 2009;174:202–9.

18. van den Heuvel OA, Veltman DJ, Groenewegen HJ, *et al.* Disorder-specific neuroanatomical correlates of attentional bias in obsessive-compulsive disorder, panic disorder, and hypochondriasis. *Arch Gen Psychiatry.* 2005;62:922–33.

19. Marsh R, Horga G, Parashar N, Wang Z, Peterson BS, Simpson HB. Altered activation in fronto-striatal circuits during sequential processing of conflict in unmedicated adults with obsessive-compulsive disorder. *Biol Psychiatry.* 2014;75:615–22.

20. Harrison BJ, Yucel M, Shaw M, *et al.* Evaluating brain activity in obsessive-compulsive disorder: preliminary insights from a multivariate analysis. *Psychiatry Res.* 2006;147:227–31.

21. Nabeyama M, Nakagawa A, Yoshiura T, *et al.* Functional MRI study of brain activation alterations in patients with obsessive-compulsive disorder after symptom improvement. *Psychiatry Res.* 2008;163:236–47.

22. Taylor SF, Stern ER, Gehring WJ. Neural systems for error monitoring: Recent findings and theoretical perspectives. *Neuroscientist.* 2007;13:160–72.

23. Harrison NA, Gray MA, Gianaros PJ, Critchley HD. The embodiment of emotional feelings in the brain. *J Neurosci.* 2010;30:12878–84.

24. Kober H, Barrett LF, Joseph J, Bliss-Moreau E, Lindquist K, Wager TD. Functional grouping and cortical-subcortical interactions in emotion: a meta-analysis of neuroimaging studies. *Neuroimage.* 2008;42:998–1031.

25. Kringelbach ML, Rolls ET. The functional neuroanatomy of the human orbitofrontal cortex: evidence from neuroimaging and neuropsychology. *Prog Neurobiol.* 2004;72:341–72.

26. Lebreton M, Jorge S, Michel V, Thirion B, Pessiglione M. An automatic valuation system in the human brain: evidence from functional neuroimaging. *Neuron.* 2009;64:431–9.

27. Taylor SF, Martis B, Fitzgerald KD, *et al.* Medial frontal cortex activity and loss-related responses to errors. *J Neurosci.* 2006;26:4063–70.

28. Endrass T, Ullsperger M. Specificity of performance monitoring changes in obsessive-compulsive disorder. *Neurosci Biobehav Rev.* 2014;46 Pt 1:124–38.

29. Maltby N, Tolin DF, Worhunsky P, O'Keefe TM, Kiehl KA. Dysfunctional action monitoring hyperactivates frontal-striatal circuits in obsessive-compulsive disorder: an event-related fMRI study. *Neuroimage.* 2005;24:495–503.

30. Chamberlain SR, Menzies L. Endophenotypes of obsessive-compulsive disorder: rationale, evidence and future potential. *Expert Rev Neurother.* 2009;9:1133–46.

31. Aron AR, Poldrack RA. Cortical and subcortical contributions to stop signal response inhibition: role of the subthalamic nucleus. *J Neurosci.* 2006;26:2424–33.

32. Buchsbaum BR, Greer S, Chang WL, Berman KF. Meta-analysis of neuroimaging studies of the Wisconsin card-sorting task and component processes. *Hum Brain Mapp.* 2005;25:35–45.

33. Garavan H, Hester R, Murphy K, Fassbender C, Kelly C. Individual differences in the functional neuroanatomy of inhibitory control. *Brain Res.* 2006;1105:130–42.

34. Garavan H, Ross TJ, Stein EA. Right hemispheric dominance of inhibitory control: An event-related functional MRI study. *Proc Natl Acad Sci U S A.* 1999;96:8301–6.

35. Robbins TW. Shifting and stopping: fronto-striatal substrates, neurochemical modulation and clinical implications. *Philos Trans R Soc Lond B Biol Sci.* 2007;362:917–32.

36. Aron AR, Fletcher PC, Bullmore ET, Sahakian BJ, Robbins TW. Stop-signal inhibition disrupted by damage to right inferior frontal gyrus in humans. *Nat Neurosci.* 2003;6:115–16.

37. Chambers CD, Bellgrove MA, Stokes MG, *et al.* Executive 'brake failure' following deactivation of human frontal lobe. *J Cognitive Neurosci.* 2006;18:444–55.

38. Berlin HA, Schulz KP, Zhang S, Turetzky R, Rosenthal D, Goodman W. Neural correlates of emotional response inhibition in obsessive-compulsive disorder: a preliminary study. *Psychiatry Res.* 2015;234:259–64.

39. de Wit SJ, de Vries FE, van der Werf YD, *et al.* Presupplementary motor area hyperactivity during response inhibition: a candidate endophenotype of obsessive-compulsive disorder. *Am J Psychiatry.* 2012;169:1100–8.

40. Kang DH, Jang JH, Han JY, *et al.* Neural correlates of altered response inhibition and dysfunctional connectivity at rest in obsessive-compulsive disorder. *Prog Neuropsychopharmacol Biol Psychiatry.* 2013;40:340–6.

41. Roth RM, Saykin AJ, Flashman LA, Pixley HS, West JD, Mamourian AC. Event-related functional magnetic resonance imaging of response inhibition in obsessive-compulsive disorder. *Biol Psychiatry.* 2007;62:901–9.

42. Gruner P, Pittenger C. Cognitive inflexibility in obsessive-compulsive disorder. *Neuroscience.* 2017;345:243–55.

43. Bressler SL, Menon V. Large-scale brain networks in cognition: emerging methods and principles. *Trends Cogn Sci.* 2010;14:277–90.

44. Power JD, Cohen AL, Nelson SM, *et al.* Functional Network Organization of the Human Brain. *Neuron.* 2011;72:665–78.

45. Gu BM, Park JY, Kang DH, *et al.* Neural correlates of cognitive inflexibility during task-switching in obsessive-compulsive disorder. *Brain.* 2008;131:155–64.

46. Han JY, Kang DH, Gu BM, *et al.* Altered Brain Activation in Ventral Frontal-Striatal Regions Following a 16-week Pharmacotherapy in Unmedicated Obsessive-Compulsive Disorder. *J Korean Med Sci.* 2011;26:665–74.

47. Remijnse PL, van den Heuvel OA, Nielen MM, *et al.* Cognitive inflexibility in obsessive-compulsive disorder and major depression is associated with distinct neural correlates. *PLoS One.* 2013;8:e59600.

48. Dias R, Robbins TW, Roberts AC. Dissociation in prefrontal cortex of affective and attentional shifts. *Nature*. 1996;380:69–72.

49. Fellows LK, Farah MJ. Ventromedial frontal cortex mediates affective shifting in humans: evidence from a reversal learning paradigm. *Brain*. 2003;126:1830–7.

50. Hampshire A, Owen AM. Fractionating attentional control using event-related fMRI. *Cereb Cortex*. 2006;16:1679–89.

51. Freyer T, Kloppel S, Tuscher O, *et al*. Frontostriatal activation in patients with obsessive-compulsive disorder before and after cognitive behavioral therapy. *Psychol Med*. 2011;41:207–16.

52. Remijnse PL, Nielen MMA, van Balkom AJLM, *et al*. Reduced orbitofrontal-striatal activity on a reversal learning task in obsessive-compulsive disorder. *Arch Gen Psychiatry*. 2006;63:1225–36.

53. Remijnse PL, Nielen MMA, van Balkom AJLM, *et al*. Differential frontal-striatal and paralimbic activity during reversal learning in major depressive disorder and obsessive-compulsive disorder. *Psychol Med*. 2009;39:1503–18.

54. Chamberlain SR, Menzies L, Hampshire A, *et al*. Orbitofrontal dysfunction in patients with obsessive-compulsive disorder and their unaffected relatives. *Science*. 2008;321:421–2.

55. Apergis-Schoute AM, Gillan CM, Fineberg NA, Fernandez-Egea E, Sahakian BJ, Robbins TW. Neural basis of impaired safety signaling in Obsessive Compulsive Disorder. *Proc Natl Acad Sci U S A*. 2017;114:3216–21.

56. Cavedini P, Gorini A, Bellodi L. Understanding obsessive-compulsive disorder: focus on decision making. *Neuropsychol Rev*. 2006;16:3–15.

57. Sachdev PS, Malhi GS. Obsessive-compulsive behaviour: a disorder of decision-making. *Aust N Z J Psychiatry*. 2005;39:757–63.

58. Steketee G, Frost RO. Measurement of Risk-Taking in Obsessive-Compulsive Disorder. *Behav Cogn Psychother*. 1994;22:287–98.

59. Tolin DF, Abramowitz JS, Brigidi BD, Foa EB. Intolerance of uncertainty in obsessive-compulsive disorder. *J Anxiety Disord*. 2003;17:233–42.

60. Admon R, Bleich-Cohen M, Weizmant R, Poyurovsky M, Faragian S, Hendler T. Functional and structural neural indices of risk aversion in obsessive-compulsive disorder (OCD). *Psychiatry Res*. 2012;203:207–13.

61. Luigjes J, Figee M, Tobler PN, *et al*. Doubt in the Insula: Risk Processing in Obsessive-Compulsive Disorder. *Front Hum Neurosci*. 2016;10:283.

62. Fear CF, Healy D. Probabilistic reasoning in obsessive-compulsive and delusional disorders. *Psychol Med*. 1997;27:199–208.

63. Volans PJ. Styles of decision-making and probability appraisal in selected obsessional and phobic patients. *Br J Soc Clin Psychol*. 1976;15:305–17.

64. Foa EB, Mathews A, Abramowitz JS, *et al*. Do patients with obsessive-compulsive disorder have deficits in decision-making? *Cogn Ther Res*. 2003;27:431–45.

65. Milner AD, Beech HR, Walker VJ. Decision processes and obsessional behavior. *Br J Soc Clin Psychol*. 1971;10:88–9.

66. Huettel SA. Behavioral, but not reward, risk modulates activation of prefrontal, parietal, and insular cortices. *Cogn Affect Behav Neurosci*. 2006;6:141–51

67. Krain AL, Hefton S, Pine DS, *et al*. An fMRI examination of developmental differences in the neural correlates of uncertainty and decision-making. *J Child Psychol Psychiatry*. 2006;47:1023–30.

68. Grinband J, Hirsch J, Ferrera VP. A neural representation of categorization uncertainty in the human brain. *Neuron*. 2006;49:757–63

69. Mohr PN, Biele G, Heekeren HR. Neural processing of risk. *J Neurosci*. 2010;30:6613–19.

70. Preuschoff K, Quartz SR, Bossaerts P. Human insula activation reflects risk prediction errors as well as risk. *J Neurosci*. 2008;28:2745–52.

71. Stern ER, Gonzalez R, Welsh RC, Taylor SF. Medial frontal cortex and anterior insula are less sensitive to outcome predictability when monetary stakes are higher. *Soc Cogn Affect Neurosci*. 2014;9:1625–31.

72. Volz KG, Schubotz RI, von Cramon DY. Predicting events of varying probability: uncertainty investigated by fMRI. *Neuroimage*. 2003;19(2 Pt 1):271–80.

73. Rotge JY, Langbour N, Dilharreguy B, *et al*. Contextual and behavioral influences on uncertainty in obsessive-compulsive disorder. *Cortex*. 2015;62:1–10.

74. Stern ER, Welsh RC, Gonzalez R, Fitzgerald KD, Abelson JL, Taylor SF. Subjective uncertainty and limbic hyperactivation in obsessive-compulsive disorder. *Hum Brain Mapp*. 2013;34:1956–70.

75. Andrews-Hanna JR. The brain's default network and its adaptive role in internal mentation. *Neuroscientist*. 2012;18:251–70.

76. Harrison BJ, Pujol J, Soriano-Mas C, *et al*. Neural correlates of moral sensitivity in obsessive-compulsive disorder. *Arch Gen Psychiatry*. 2012;69:741–9.

77. Szechtman H, Woody E. Obsessive-compulsive disorder as a disturbance of security motivation. *Psychol Rev*. 2004;111:111–27.

78. Liu X, Hairston J, Schrier M, Fan J. Common and distinct networks underlying reward valence and processing stages: A meta-analysis of functional neuroimaging studies. *Neurosci Biobehav Rev*. 2011;35:1219–36.

79. Marsh R, Tau GZ, Wang Z, *et al*. Reward-based spatial learning in unmedicated adults with obsessive-compulsive disorder. *Am J Psychiatry*. 2015;172:383–92.

80. Knutson B, Fong GW, Bennett SM, Adams CM, Hommer D. A region of mesial prefrontal cortex tracks monetarily rewarding outcomes: characterization with rapid event-related fMRI. *Neuroimage*. 2003;18:263–72.

81. Jung WH, Kang DH, Han JY, *et al*. Aberrant ventral striatal responses during incentive processing in unmedicated patients with obsessive-compulsive disorder. *Acta Psychiatr Scand*. 2011;123:376–86.

82. Figee M, Vink M, de Geus F, *et al*. Dysfunctional Reward Circuitry in Obsessive-Compulsive Disorder. *Biol Psychiatry*. 2011;69:867–74.

83. Choi JS, Shin YC, Jung WH, *et al*. Altered brain activity during reward anticipation in pathological gambling and obsessive-compulsive disorder. *PLoS One*. 2012;7:e45938.

84. Kaufmann C, Beucke JC, Preusse F, *et al*. Medial prefrontal brain activation to anticipated reward and loss in obsessive-compulsive disorder. *Neuroimage Clin*. 2013;2:212–20.

85. Subira M, Sato JR, Alonso P, *et al*. Brain structural correlates of sensory phenomena in patients with obsessive-compulsive disorder. *J Psychiatry Neurosci*. 2015;40:232–40.

86. Ecker W, Gonner S. Incompleteness and harm avoidance in OCD symptom dimensions. *Behav Res Ther*. 2008;46:895–904.

87. Baer L. Factor analysis of symptom subtypes of obsessive compulsive disorder and their relation to personality and tic disorders. *J Clin Psychiatry*. 1994;55 Suppl:18–23.

88. Leckman JF, Grice DE, Boardman J, *et al*. Symptoms of obsessive-compulsive disorder. *Am J Psychiatry*. 1997;154:911–17.

89. Mataix-Cols D, Rauch SL, Manzo PA, Jenike MA, Baer L. Use of factor-analyzed symptom dimensions to predict outcome with serotonin reuptake inhibitors and placebo in the treatment of obsessive-compulsive disorder. *Am J Psychiatry*. 1999;156:1409–16.

90. Mataix-Cols D, Wooderson S, Lawrence N, Brammer MJ, Speckens A, Phillips ML. Distinct neural correlates of washing, checking, and hoarding symptom dimensions in obsessive-compulsive disorder. *Arch Gen Psychiatry*. 2004;61:564–76.

91. Rauch SL, Dougherty D, Shin LM, et al. Neural correlates of factor-analyzed OCD symptom dimensions: a PET study. *CNS Spectrums*. 1998;1;3(:37–43.

92. Shapira NA, Liu Y, He AG, et al. Brain activation by disgust-inducing pictures in obsessive-compulsive disorder. *Biol Psychiatry*. 2003;54:751–6.

93. Lawrence NS, An SK, Mataix-Cols D, Ruths F, Speckens A, Phillips ML. Neural responses to facial expressions of disgust but not fear are modulated by washing symptoms in OCD. *Biol Psychiatry*. 2007;61:1072–80.

94. Jhung K, Ku J, Kim SJ, et al. Distinct functional connectivity of limbic network in the washing type obsessive-compulsive disorder. *Prog Neuropsychopharmacol Biol Psychiatry*. 2014;53:149–55.

95. Wicker B, Keysers C, Plailly J, Royet JP, Gallese V, Rizzolatti G. Both of us disgusted in My insula: the common neural basis of seeing and feeling disgust. *Neuron*. 2003;40:655–64.

96. Olatunji BO, Cisler J, McKay D, Phillips ML. Is disgust associated with psychopathology? Emerging research in the anxiety disorders. *Psychiatry Res*. 2010;175:1–10.

97. Craig AD. How do you feel—now? The anterior insula and human awareness. *Nat Rev Neurosci*. 2009;10:59–70.

98. Agarwal SM, Jose D, Baruah U, et al. Neurohemodynamic correlates of washing symptoms in obsessive-compulsive disorder: a pilot fMRI study using Symptom provocation paradigm. *Indian J Psychol Med*. 2013;35:67–74.

99. Harrison BJ, Pujol J, Cardoner N, et al. Brain corticostriatal systems and the major clinical symptom dimensions of obsessive-compulsive disorder. *Biol Psychiatry*. 2013;73:321–8.

100. Via E, Cardoner N, Pujol J, et al. Amygdala activation and symptom dimensions in obsessive-compulsive disorder. *Br J Psychiatry*. 2014;204:61–8.

101. Davis M. The role of the amygdala in fear and anxiety. *Annu Rev Neurosci*. 1992;15:353–75.

102. Schaich Borg J, Lieberman D, Kiehl KA. Infection, incest, and iniquity: investigating the neural correlates of disgust and morality. *J Cogn Neurosci*. 2008;20:1529–46.

103. Mataix-Cols D, Frost RO, Pertusa A, et al. Hoarding disorder: a new diagnosis for DSM-V? *Depress Anxiety*. 2010;27:556–72.

104. Saxena S, Brody AL, Maidment KM, et al. Cerebral glucose metabolism in obsessive-compulsive hoarding. *Am J Psychiatry*. 2004;161:1038–48.

105. An SK, Mataix-Cols D, Lawrence NS, et al. To discard or not to discard: the neural basis of hoarding symptoms in obsessive-compulsive disorder. *Mol Psychiatry*. 2009;14:318–31.

106. Cohen L, Angladette L, Benoit N, Pierrot-Deseilligny C. A man who borrowed cars. *Lancet*. 1999;353:34.

107. Volle E, Beato R, Levy R, Dubois B. Forced collectionism after orbitofrontal damage. *Neurology*. 2002;58:488–90.

108. Blundell JE, Herberg LJ. Effectiveness of lateral hypothalamic stimulation, arousal, and food deprivation in the initiation of hoarding behaviour in naive rats. *Physiol Behav*. 1973;10:763–7.

109. Bechara A, Tranel D, Damasio H. Characterization of the decision-making deficit of patients with ventromedial prefrontal cortex lesions. *Brain*. 2000;123 (Pt 11):2189–202.

110. Rauch SL, Savage CR, Alpert NM, et al. Probing striatal function in obsessive-compulsive disorder: a PET study of implicit sequence learning. *J Neuropsychiatry Clin Neurosci*. 1997;9:568–73.

111. Cannistraro PA, Wright CI, Wedig MM, et al. Amygdala responses to human faces in obsessive-compulsive disorder. *Biol Psychiatry*. 2004;56:916–20.

112. Cardoner N, Harrison BJ, Pujol J, et al. Enhanced brain responsiveness during active emotional face processing in obsessive compulsive disorder. *World J Biol Psychiatry*. 2011;12:349–63.

113. Goncalves OF, Soares JM, Carvalho S, et al. Brain activation of the defensive and appetitive survival systems in obsessive compulsive disorder. *Brain Imaging Behav*. 2015;9:255–63.

114. Weygandt M, Blecker CR, Schafer A, et al. fMRI pattern recognition in obsessive-compulsive disorder. *Neuroimage*. 2012;60:1186–93.

115. Simon D, Adler N, Kaufmann C, Kathmann N. Amygdala hyperactivation during symptom provocation in obsessive-compulsive disorder and its modulation by distraction. *Neuroimage Clin*. 2014;4:549–57.

116. van den Heuvel OA, Veltman DJ, Groenewegen HJ, et al. Frontal-striatal dysfunction during planning in obsessive-compulsive disorder. *Arch Gen Psychiatry*. 2005;62:301–9.

117. van den Heuvel OA, Mataix-Cols D, Zwitser G, et al. Common limbic and frontal-striatal disturbances in patients with obsessive compulsive disorder, panic disorder and hypochondriasis. *Psychol Med*. 2011;41:2399–410.

118. de Vries FE, de Wit SJ, Cath DC, et al. Compensatory frontoparietal activity during working memory: an endophenotype of obsessive-compulsive disorder. *Biol Psychiatry*. 2014;76:878–87.

119. Henseler I, Gruber O, Kraft S, Krick C, Reith W, Falkai P. Compensatory hyperactivations as markers of latent working memory dysfunctions in patients with obsessive-compulsive disorder: an fMRI study. *J Psychiatry Neurosci*. 2008;33:209–15.

120. Koch K, Wagner G, Schachtzabel C, et al. Aberrant anterior cingulate activation in obsessive-compulsive disorder is related to task complexity. *Neuropsychologia*. 2012;50:958–64.

121. Nakao T, Nakagawa A, Nakatani E, et al. Working memory dysfunction in obsessive-compulsive disorder: a neuropsychological and functional MRI study. *J Psychiatr Res*. 2009;43:784–91.

122. van der Wee NJ, Ramsey NF, van Megen HJ, Denys D, Westenberg HG, Kahn RS. Spatial working memory in obsessive-compulsive disorder improves with clinical response: a functional MRI study. *Eur Neuropsychopharmacol*. 2007;17:16–23.

# 98

# Management and treatment of obsessive–compulsive disorder

*Naomi A. Fineberg, Lynne M. Drummond, Jemma Reid, Eduardo Cinosi, Lior Carmi, and Davis N. Mpavaenda*

## Introduction

The earliest reports of the potential efficacy in obsessive–compulsive disorder (OCD) of pharmacotherapy with the tricyclic drug clomipramine and of behavioural forms of psychotherapy, initiated in the 1960s and 1970s and subsequently validated in a series of seminal studies in the 1980s, produced a dramatic change in the psychiatric management of this serious and previously treatment-refractory disorder. Since that time, treatments for OCD have been subject to considerable scientific scrutiny and treatment 'standards' have been developed and refined in succeeding evidence-based treatment guidelines [1, 2].

The disorder usually arises in childhood or early adulthood, follows a chronic course (though episodic forms do occur), and is associated with substantial psychiatric comorbidity, frequently in the form of anxiety disorders, affective disorders, and other obsessive–compulsive and related disorders. Whereas substantial improvement can be achieved in many patients following standard treatment with serotonin reuptake inhibitors (SRIs) [selective serotonin reuptake inhibitors (SSRIs), clomipramine] and cognitive behavioural therapy (CBT), for approximately 50%, the response is incomplete and new treatment paradigms are sought. Several other conventional drug treatments for depression and anxiety have been investigated and found not to be effective in OCD, though evidence has accrued that dopamine receptor antagonists may be effective for individuals with SRI-resistant OCD when prescribed as an adjunct to the SRI. In this context, a developing role for somatic treatments has also emerged, with implications for clinical service development [1].

In this chapter, we review the management and treatment of OCD, including rational options for those failing to respond to standard treatments, based, as far as possible, on randomized controlled trial (RCT) data. Where relevant, we have cited review papers of good quality to maximize efficiency.

## Defining treatment response, remission, and relapse

The introduction of methods for the standardized assessment of OCD has contributed substantially to the evidence-based treatment of the disorder. Of the several available scales, the 10-item Yale-Brown Obsessive Compulsive Scale (Y-BOCS) [3] emerged as the most widely accepted instrument for rating the magnitude of symptomatic change, based on reliability, acceptability, and sensitivity to change. Pallanti *et al.* [4] were some of the first to advocate the use of standardized operational 'responder' criteria across OCD treatment trials. They proposed that a meaningful clinical response could be conservatively represented by an improvement of 25–35% in the baseline Y-BOCS, or a score of 'much' or 'very much improved' on the Clinical Global Impression of Improvement (CGI-I) Scale [5], whereas 'remission' necessitated a total Y-BOCS score of less than 16 (out of a total score of 40). Relapse, on the other hand, was defined as a worsening by 25% of the remission Y-BOCS score. Other suggested relapse criteria include a worsening by ≥50% of post-baseline Y-BOCS scores, a 5-point worsening of the total Y-BOCS score, a total Y-BOCS score of ≥19, and CGI-I scores of 'much' or 'very much worse' [6].

A disadvantage of so much variability in these criteria is that very different claims about efficacy and relapse may ensue. Hollander *et al.* [7] attempted to validate the previously empirical responder and relapse criteria using trial data. When the treatment response was defined as at least 25% improvement in the Y-BOCS score relative to baseline, the data showed both a statistically significant and a clinically relevant differentiation in social and occupational functioning and health-related quality of life (HR-QoL) measures between responders and non-responders. This suggests that a 25% improvement in the baseline Y-BOCS does represent a *clinically relevant* change equivalent to a minimal partial response. Similarly, the analysis validated a definition of relapse represented by a 5-point worsening of the remission Y-BOCS [7].

# Evidence-based psychological therapies for OCD

## Exposure and response prevention

Prior to the mid 1960s, there were no known effective treatments for OCD. Therefore, the development of new effective psychological treatments based on the principles of exposure to the feared object or situation, combined with compulsive ritual prevention, has had a huge and lasting impact. Victor Meyer, a psychologist working at St Luke's Woodside Hospital and the Middlesex Hospital Medical School, developed a treatment for children and adults with OCD, based on earlier experimental work with animals. This treatment involved exposing the patient to situations which would normally provoke compulsive rituals and then actively preventing them from performing these rituals [8]. As OCD had previously been considered an intractable condition with no effective treatment, this was a remarkable breakthrough. Isaac Marks, a psychiatrist working with the psychologists Stanley Rachman and Ray Hodgson, took this pioneering work further by developing a treatment based on exposure but in which the patient themselves took responsibility for preventing their compulsive rituals. This treatment proved to be effective, to have results which persisted over at least 2 years, and had fewer ethical issues than previous treatments when nurses and other health care workers had actively prevented patients from performing rituals [9].

Over the years, exposure treatment has been modified so that what is practised today is prolonged graded *exposure* in real life to the feared situation, combined with self-imposed *response prevention* (ERP). In order to perform this treatment, the patient needs to be educated about OCD and how the temporary reduction in anxiety produced by performance of compulsive rituals actually serves to strengthen the association between obsessive thought and compulsive ritual, thus worsening the condition.

Compulsive rituals and other behaviours, such as repeated reassurance seeking, reduce anxiety; because high anxiety is unpleasant, this reduction acts like a reward. Thus, repeated performance of compulsions strengthens the link between obsessions and compulsions, which frequently results in increasing the amount of time spent in rituals. In order to overcome the OCD, the patient needs to face up to the feared situation without performing the compulsions. Initially, the urge to perform the ritual will rise, but if the compulsions are successfully resisted, the urge will reduce and habituation will occur.

It can be too stressful for a patient to initially face their most threatening situation. For this reason, the patient and therapist will usually construct a *hierarchy* of fear-provoking situations for exposure, ranging from those that would invoke minor fear if faced without anxiety-reducing compulsions to those that would produce panic. The patient also needs to expose themselves to the fear-provoking situation *for long enough* to enable their anxiety to habituate. Due to the complexity of compulsive rituals and the fact that patients often give themselves reassurance mentally, it will generally take up to 2 hours until the anxiety of OCD has fully subsided. This is known as 'within-session habituation'.

There are several full descriptions of the treatment given elsewhere [9]. In summary, the therapist and the patient agree a task expected to induce moderate anxiety if performed without compulsive rituals and the patient is asked to perform this task. This exposure may be performed by the patient on their own or together with a therapist or a family member or friend working with the patient. Once it has been successfully performed, then the task should be repeated in the same way approximately three times a day. This repetition of the ERP is usually referred to as 'ERP Homework'. As the task is repeated without compulsive rituals, each successive performance will generally become easier and the anxiety will last for a shorter time. This reduction in anxiety on successive repetitions is known as 'between-session habituation'. Once this task has been successfully performed, the patient tackles more difficult items on the hierarchy.

Standing the test of time, ERP treatment has been proven to be a successful treatment for patients with OCD. The theory behind it is relatively simple to apply, and it has been used effectively in a variety of self-help methods, including using computerized manuals [10]. Following on from the initial studies, evidence of the robust improvements produced with ERP has accumulated [11]. Recent studies have often assessed ERP in OCD together with other interventions, including psychopharmacological treatments [12, 13].

It is important to remember that one of the most common reasons for ERP not being successful is that it is not prescribed or performed in a regular, prolonged, predictable manner. For the best results, ERP should be practised three times a day and for sufficient time to allow the anxiety to reduce consistently by at least 50%. ERP can be applied most usefully in the patient's home where the symptoms are usually maximal [13].

## Cognitive behavioural therapies in OCD

In recent years, there has been increasing usage of cognitive and behavioural methods to treat OCD. There are, of course, a variety of different forms of cognitive therapy which work on a variety of different principles. Rational emotive therapy was developed by Albert Ellis in the 1960s for depressive and anxiety disorders and is a confrontative type of therapy where beliefs are actively challenged by the therapist [14]. A rationale for using rational emotive therapy to treat OCD rests on the observation that OCD patients do not sufficiently challenge their beliefs before acting on them by performing compulsions.

Early developers of ERP theorized that OCD patients would experience a reduction in symptoms if they felt less responsible for any feared disastrous or harmful outcome resulting from their failure to perform compulsions. In the UK, a cognitive form of treatment, based on the theory that an over-inflated sense of responsibility is key to the symptomatology of OCD, leading to increased performance of compulsions, increased sense of threat, and depressed mood, thereby establishing a vicious cycle of excessive responsibility and guilt, was developed [15].

However, it was observed by others that ideas about danger were more highly correlated with compulsive activity than were ideas of responsibility, self-efficacy, perfectionism, or anticipated anxiety. Danger ideation reduction therapy (DIRT) is another form of psychotherapy that provides information about harm in a systematized way, combined with rational emotive therapy [16]. DIRT was initially developed for OCD patients with contamination fears and washing rituals. More recently, it has been trialled with patients with compulsive-checking rituals [17].

## ERP or CBT?

Despite both the superficial attractiveness of the cognitive method of treatment, compared with ERP, and numerous studies designed to demonstrate its efficacy, there is little evidence to suggest that adding cognitive therapy to ERP offers any distinct advantage [18–20]. One of the problems with adding cognitive therapy to ERP is that it requires more training and supervision of the therapist and may thus be less cost-efficient. Some studies have found that cognitive methods can be as effective as ERP, but few have shown any clear advantage. This is true of rational emotive behaviour therapy [21]. Indeed a recent study demonstrated that in patients who initially failed to respond to ERP, there was no value in following this with a course of cognitive therapy in an attempt to improve outcome. These workers advocated using a serotonin reuptake-inhibiting drug (SRI) and demonstrated that this was a more effective second-line treatment [22].

Studies examining specific cognitive interventions aimed at an over-inflated sense of responsibility, similarly, have generally failed to demonstrate an advantage over ERP. Studies comparing ERP and cognitive therapy found that both had equal efficacy [23] or failed to demonstrate any improved efficacy of CBT, compared to ERP, on core OCD symptoms (although Cottraux et al. did find that depressive symptoms may improve more with CBT) [24]. A study examining group treatment for OCD found that ERP produced significantly better results than did CBT [25].

A major problem with most studies involving CBT or ERP is that the numbers of participants are small. Many studies also include pharmacological treatment. Inevitably, this leads to a higher chance of type 2 error and difficulty demonstrating statistical differences between treatments. It is for this reason that meta-analyses may be the most useful.

An early study [26] examining the use of ERP in severe, chronic, refractory OCD suggested that whereas ERP should be the treatment of choice, CBT may be useful for specific difficulties. A recent meta-analysis of available studies similarly concluded that 'The available research indicates that ERP is the first line evidence based psychotherapeutic treatment for OCD and that concurrent administration of cognitive therapy that targets specific symptom-related difficulties characteristic of OCD may improve tolerance of distress, symptom-related dysfunctional beliefs, adherence to treatment, and reduce drop out' [27].

## Evidence-based pharmacotherapies for OCD

### Clomipramine

#### Adults

Evidence from a series of small historical studies dating back to the 1960s [28] identified clomipramine as the first potentially effective treatment for OCD. Subsequent RCTs of clomipramine in adult OCD patient samples demonstrated efficacy in the presence of low mood or comorbid depression. A seminal placebo-referenced RCT in patients with *no coexisting depression* showed a significant advantage for clomipramine using relatively low, fixed daily dosages of 75 mg [29]. Two large multi-centre, double-blind RCTs, comprising a total of 520 patients, conclusively demonstrated significant

placebo-referenced superiority for clomipramine in non-depressed adults with OCD, using flexible daily dosages of up to 300 mg [30].

Further OCD RCTs comparing clomipramine 'head to head' with other tricyclic drugs, including imipramine, amitriptyline, nortriptyline, and desipramine [28], confirmed the superiority of clomipramine. Clomipramine has greater SRI activity than the other compounds, and this property was considered relevant in its anti-OCD effect.

#### Children and adolescents

Similar results were obtained in clomipramine studies of children and adolescents with OCD [28]. Not only was clomipramine found to be superior to desipramine, but a significant proportion of patients who had received clomipramine as their first active treatment also showed evidence of relapse when switched to desipramine, highlighting the efficacy of clomipramine, compared to desipramine.

#### Summary

These results suggest that clomipramine is an effective treatment for OCD, irrespective of the presence of comorbid depression across the young adult age range. However, there is a want of studies in the elderly population, who may be more susceptible to the adverse effects of tricyclic drugs. Moreover, the robustly successful results from these studies apply largely to patients with stable, severe, and untreated OCD. There were not many treatment-refractory cases included within the study groups.

### Selective serotonin reuptake inhibitors

Following the success of clomipramine, the SSRIs fluvoxamine, fluoxetine, sertraline, paroxetine, citalopram, and escitalopram were tested in large adult OCD samples, in a series of well-powered multi-centre placebo-referenced RCTs, and consistently found to be efficacious [31, 32]. Similarly, evidence for the efficacy of the SSRIs fluvoxamine, sertraline, fluoxetine, and paroxetine subsequently accrued from RCTs of children and adolescents with OCD [33]. Each SSRI is reviewed in the next sections. The decision to use SSRIs in children and adolescents with OCD has to be weighed against the possible risk of behavioural disinhibition, including suicidal ideation, as a recognized concomitant of SSRI treatment in young people.

#### Fluvoxamine

*Adults*

The finding from a number of small randomized placebo-controlled trials that fluvoxamine appeared efficacious in adults with OCD was substantiated in multi-centre placebo-controlled studies [34]. An earlier improvement was seen for obsessions vs compulsions, and significant improvement on the total Y-BOCS was evident by 6 weeks. Efficacy for fluvoxamine (100–300 mg) delivered in controlled-release form was also demonstrated [35].

*Children and adolescents*

Fluvoxamine was also efficacious and well tolerated in a multi-centre study of 120 young patients (8–17 years) with OCD [36]. Insomnia, asthenia, and behavioural disinhibition were reported as possible adverse events. It has been suggested that paediatric OCD patients with comorbid impulsive or tic disorders may be at increased risk of developing behavioural disinhibition after initiation of SRI treatment.

### Sertraline

#### Adults

Positive placebo-referenced RCTs, as well as a multi-centre 12-week RCT involving 324 OCD patients [37], demonstrated that sertraline, flexibly prescribed in daily dosages of 50–200 mg/day, was effective in adults with OCD.

#### Children and adolescents

Evidence from large multi-centre RCTs, demonstrated a significant advantage for sertraline (≥200 mg/day), delivered as monotherapy or in combination with CBT, compared to placebo [38]. Prospective evaluation did not reveal clinically meaningful drug-related changes in vital signs, ECG indices, or cardiovascular adverse events in any of the study subjects.

### Fluoxetine

#### Adults

The first placebo-referenced fixed-dose RCT of an SSRI in OCD, which allowed the direct comparison of different daily dosages, demonstrated placebo-referenced superiority for fluoxetine with a marginally statistically greater improvement for patients receiving the highest fluoxetine dosage (60 mg daily) and a significantly higher responder rate in patients receiving fluoxetine 40 mg or 60 mg daily, implying the existence of a dose–response relationship [39]. In a larger 13-week multi-centre RCT of 355 OCD patients [40], all fixed daily doses of fluoxetine (20 mg, 40 mg, 60 mg) were efficacious, compared to placebo, with a non-significant trend towards greater efficacy evident for the 60 mg daily dosage. Fluoxetine was adequately tolerated, even at the higher dosages. Another study [41] found fluoxetine to be superior to phenelzine, which did not differentiate from placebo.

#### Children and adolescents

The first controlled study in young OCD patients found fixed daily dosages of 80 mg fluoxetine demonstrated efficacy over placebo, with reports of discontinuation on account of suicidal ideation (resolved when fluoxetine was discontinued) and adverse events, particularly dose-related behavioural activation [42]. Thus, it was advocated that treatment should be initiated at low dosages in childhood OCD. More recent evidence confirmed fluoxetine to be significantly superior to placebo in terms of efficacy and just as well tolerated in terms of adverse event-related discontinuation. Moreover, after the first 6 weeks, the fluoxetine dose could be increased to 80 mg/day [43]. At week 16, those taking fluoxetine demonstrated a significant improvement in Children's Yale-Brown Obsessive Compulsive Scale (CY-BOCS) scores, and no patients discontinued due to adverse events. Taken together, these results suggest satisfactory efficacy and tolerability for fluoxetine in childhood OCD, imply that the treatment effect may take several weeks to develop, and draw attention to behavioural disinhibition and suicidal ideation as possible dose-related adverse effects.

### Paroxetine

#### Adults

Paroxetine (20–60 mg/day) was superior to placebo and of comparable efficacy with the active comparator clomipramine (50–250 mg/ day) in a multi-national 12-week RCT of 406 adults with OCD [44]. Of note, paroxetine showed significantly better tolerability than clomipramine. In addition, a 12-week placebo-referenced fixed-dose RCT in 348 adult OCD patients [45] also found efficacy for paroxetine, compared to placebo, at fixed daily dosages of 40 or 60 mg/day, but no demonstrable efficacy over placebo at fixed dosages of 20 mg/day.

#### Children and adolescents

A multi-centre 10-week RCT in 207 children and adolescents [46] found paroxetine (10–50 mg/day) to be superior to placebo. Adverse events with paroxetine were of mild to moderate intensity, and the authors concluded it was generally well tolerated.

### Citalopram

#### Adults

A 12-week multi-centre placebo-referenced fixed-dose RCT of 401 adults with OCD found that citalopram (20, 40, and 60 mg) was significantly superior to placebo [47]. Whereas no significant difference between the individual doses of citalopram was seen on the primary outcome, a dose vs time-to-response relationship favoured the 60 mg dose. Citalopram was well tolerated and associated with improved psychosocial functioning.

### Escitalopram

#### Adults

A multi-centre fixed-dose RCT in 466 adults with OCD compared escitalopram (10 or 20 mg) and paroxetine (40 mg) with placebo [48] over 24 weeks. Escitalopram and paroxetine were each superior to placebo from 6 weeks onwards. Those in the escitalopram 10 mg/day group also exhibited improvement, compared to placebo, on the Y-BOCS, though this effect took more than 12 weeks to become significant. The higher (20 mg/day) escitalopram dose produced additional advantages (vs escitalopram 10 mg/day) on secondary efficacy measures, including remission.

## Meta-analysis of placebo-referenced SRI studies

A meta-analysis provides an objective and quantifiable measure of effect size. However, by grouping together findings from disparate studies, the analysis is relatively removed from the originating data. Several meta-analyses in adults and in children and adolescents have supported placebo-referenced efficacy for SSRIs and clomipramine in OCD [32]. The meta-analysis by Soomro et al. [49], which included 17 adult OCD studies (3097 study participants), demonstrated that in treatment trials, SSRIs were almost twice as likely as placebo to produce a clinical response. Another recent random effects meta-analysis of SRI trials involving 789 young people with OCD [50] found a moderate effect size for treatment efficacy ($g = 0.50$), treatment response [relative risk (RR) = 1.80], and symptom/diagnostic remission (RR = 2.06).

## Which SRI is the most effective?

There is a shortage of studies directly comparing available treatments for OCD. A few head-to-head comparator studies of adequate statistical power indicated equivalent efficacy for SSRIs and clomipramine, but superior tolerability for SSRIs [28]. The UK National Institute for Health and Care Excellence (NICE) meta-analysed all the available evidence [51]. They concluded there was little difference between clomipramine and SSRIs, in terms of efficacy and adverse events. However, patients were more likely to discontinue treatment prematurely due to adverse events with clomipramine, compared to SSRIs. NICE therefore recommended SSRIs as the preferred first-line treatment for OCD, with clomipramine reserved for patients for whom SSRI treatment is inefficacious or unacceptable [51].

Although SSRIs differ in pharmacokinetics, selectivity, and potency of effect on the serotonin transporter and other neurotransmitter receptor-binding properties, there is insufficient evidence to recommend one SSRI over another. Most recently, Skapinakis *et al.* [32] performed a *network meta-analysis* that combined direct and indirect evidence to rank treatments. The analysis demonstrated efficacy for SSRIs as a whole, compared to placebo; individual SSRIs produced similar effect sizes, and there was no evidence to suggest superiority of any individual compound. Clomipramine appeared to have a larger effect size, compared to placebo, than did the SSRIs, but this difference was not statistically significant.

### Optimizing SRI dosage

Cumulative evidence suggests OCD responds preferably to a higher daily dosage of SRI, compared to depression or other anxiety disorders. Fluoxetine, sertraline, paroxetine, citalopram, and escitalopram were explored in fixed-dose studies (see Selective serotonin reuptake inhibitors, p. 1013). Of these SSRIs, a positive dose–response relationship was demonstrated for paroxetine (dose range 40–60 mg), fluoxetine (dose range 20–80 mg) [40], and escitalopram (dose range 10–20 mg) [48]. Neither clomipramine nor fluvoxamine have been subjected to multiple fixed-dose comparisons. However, a relatively low, fixed daily dose of 75 mg clomipramine was found to be effective vs placebo [29].

Another meta-analysis incorporating nine studies [52] demonstrated that the highest licensed doses of SSRI were more efficacious than low or mid-range doses. However, this advantage had to be balanced against poorer tolerability at higher dose levels. The British Association for Psychopharmacology treatment guideline [2, 53] suggested starting with the lowest efficacious daily dosage of SSRIs, which may subsequently be increased in the face of insufficient response. However, slow up-titration could be problematic for severely ill patients, for whom a speedy response is needed. The APA guidelines [54] recommend up-titration of SSRIs to the maximum FDA-approved doses within 4–6 weeks and waiting for another 6 weeks to evaluate effectiveness.

### Onset of SRI efficacy

The SRI response in OCD is comparatively slow and gradual. Thus, although some well-powered studies were able to demonstrate placebo-referenced efficacy for SRIs within 2 weeks of starting treatment, in most RCTs, the onset of efficacy was delayed by several weeks. In the meta-analysis by Soomro *et al.* [49], SSRIs as a group produced a placebo-referenced statistical difference in Y-BOCS after between 6 and 13 weeks of treatment.

### Is the efficacy of SRIs sustained long term?

The limited long-term follow-up data investigating SSRI treatment responders from acute-phase OCD studies suggest that treatment-related gains are maintained without tolerance developing. For example, in a large 24-week multi-centre study by Stein *et al.* [48],

responders continued to accrue over this extended period. Other follow-up studies suggested SSRIs remain efficacious and well-tolerated for at least 2 years [31].

### SRI and relapse prevention

It is of interest that in a recent study of a community-based sample of adults with OCD, approximately 50% achieved sustained remission by the age of 50 years, suggesting natural remission occurs commonly [55]. This contrasts with OCD as seen in the clinic, which usually follows a chronic and relapsing course. Full remission is infrequent, even in expert treatment centres.

Irrespective of treatment duration, discontinuation of pharmacotherapy is frequently, but not always, associated with relapse [31]. A number of relatively short-term studies have investigated the effect of stopping clomipramine. In the majority of cases, symptoms re-emerged within a few weeks, whereas improvement to a level near to that prior to discontinuation was achieved by reinstating clomipramine [6].

The effect of discontinuing SSRI has been subject to more robust, controlled investigation. A meta-analysis of randomized placebo-referenced RCTs of stable treatment responders demonstrated that continuing treatment with SSRIs as a class reduced relapse [6]. Interestingly, individual studies testing sertraline [56] and fluoxetine [57], which may have been underpowered, did not fully differentiate between continuation treatment or switching to placebo, although patients remaining on the highest (60 mg/day) fluoxetine doses showed significantly lower relapse rates than those given placebo [57].

Together, the results suggest that SSRIs are effective at preventing relapse. A pooled analysis by Hollander *et al.* [7] demonstrated the magnitude of the negative effect of relapse on quality of life and psychosocial functioning, emphasizing the importance of early intervention and relapse prevention, through the continuation of pharmacotherapy, as rational goals for those who have responded to an SSRI or clomipramine. Regular clinic appointments have been shown to enhance treatment adherence [58]. The APA treatment guidelines [54] recommend continuation of pharmacotherapy for a minimum of 1–2 years in treatment-responsive individuals and emphasize the importance of planning long-term treatment from the outset.

## Treatment options for patients who do not respond

The clinical management of treatment-resistant OCD has not been thoroughly investigated, although studies indicating promising treatment strategies are starting to appear. The majority of such studies have investigated SRI non-responders, and there remains a want of data relating to psychotherapy resistance. Studies have also chosen different entry criteria; some included only extremely refractory cases who had failed to respond to successive sustained treatments with more than one SRI, whereas others included those who had made a partial response to treatment with a single drug.

### Defining treatment resistance

Although most individuals with OCD respond well to first-line treatment with SRIs or ERP, for most, the treatment response is not complete. In around 40% of cases, residual symptoms remain in spite of prolonged treatment [59]. There remains controversy as to the length of an adequate treatment trial before judging its success. As OCD responds in a slow, gradual way, expert guidelines suggest waiting at least 12 weeks using optimized SRI dosages [54]. For practical purposes, patients experiencing <25% reduction of their baseline Y-BOCS score, after completing 12 weeks of SRI treatment, of which at least 6 weeks should be at the maximal tolerated dose, may be considered to have failed to respond [54].

### Extending trial of original SRIs

The APA [54] recommended continuing with an SSRI for 8–12 weeks, of which 6 should be at the maximum tolerated dose, before considering a change in treatment. However, this may result in patients enduring ineffective treatment for longer than necessary. A few studies attempted to identify likely treatment non-responders within a shorter time frame, based upon their early treatment response. For example, symptomatic improvement on SRIs at 4 weeks strongly predicted subsequent clinical response at 12 weeks [60]. This finding emphasizes the importance of looking for early treatment-related improvement and hints that changing SRIs could be considered earlier than 12 weeks into the course of treatment. However, data from another study of fluoxetine non-responders [61] suggested delayed benefit accrues with extended fluoxetine treatment. Importantly, the patients in this study were not necessarily fully SSRI-resistant at baseline. However, it may still be appropriate to persist for >12 weeks with a given SRI in patients showing at least some signs of improvement, particularly if the treatment is well tolerated.

### Increasing SRI dosage

The maximum recommended dose (250 mg/day) of clomipramine should not usually be exceeded, due to the increased risk of dose-related serious adverse events, including cardiotoxicity or seizures. In contrast, some evidence suggests SSRIs may show better efficacy and are well tolerated by OCD patients at doses exceeding the licensed maximum. A double-blind study [62] randomized 66 OCD patients who had failed to respond to standard doses to receive sertraline 200 mg/day or 250–400 mg/day. Improvement (on Y-BOCS and CGI) was significantly greater for the high dose group. Both groups displayed similar levels of adverse events, suggesting sertraline is comparatively more effective and well tolerated at doses of >200 mg/day. Similarly, open-label studies that tested a 'higher than usual' dose of escitalopram (20–50 mg/day) [63] showed a significantly greater improvement in Y-BOCS scores and response rate than doses of 20 mg/day. Interestingly, the difference disappeared when baseline depression and anxiety scores were analysed as covariates, suggesting that OCD patients with comorbid depression or anxiety may specifically benefit from a higher SSRI dosage.

The APA OCD guideline [54] provides a list of upper doses of SSRIs that are occasionally prescribed for those who have failed to respond to conventional doses or are recognized to be 'fast metabolizers'. As long as the patient is not experiencing undue adverse effects, the guideline [54] recommends 'occasionally prescribed' doses of up to 120 mg/day of fluoxetine, 450 mg/day of fluvoxamine, 100 mg/day of paroxetine, and 400 mg/day of sertraline. Such doses seem most warranted when the patient experienced a partial response to a lower dose and is tolerating the medication well. However, such

an approach is not without risk. In the case of citalopram and escitalopram, dose-dependent effects are recognized to extend the ECG QT interval. Therefore, caution is required if the maximum dose is exceeded. The elderly or those with a cardiac history may be at particular risk. However, a recent study did not show an elevated cardiac risk on higher doses of citalopram [64]. If exceeding the licensed daily dosage, it is advisable to monitor for adverse effects on cardiac conduction (for example, by ECG). The elderly may also be susceptible to SSRI-induced electrolyte disturbances and bleeding tendencies, and for those on anticoagulant therapy, the international normalized ratio (INR) may require more stringent monitoring.

### Switching SRI/SSRI to SNRI

Assuming good adherence, if response to the first SRI is inadequate after 8–12 weeks on the maximum dose or is poorly tolerated, switching to another SRI or from SSRI to clomipramine is acceptable, though limited trial data support this option. The chances of responding to a second SRI were estimated at 40%, and to a third SRI at even less [59]. Some evidence supports switching SRIs in the case of non-response and suggests that paroxetine (SSRI) is more efficacious than venlafaxine (SNRI) for non-responders to a previous SRI trial [65].

### Adjunctive dopamine antagonist (antipsychotic)

Adjunctive dopamine antagonists have arguably produced the strongest evidence of effectiveness in SRI-resistant OCD. Even so, the evidence is largely derived from small RCTs and uncontrolled case series (reviewed in [59]). There have been no dose-finding studies of dopamine antagonists in OCD. Moreover, there are limited data to inform the optimal duration of adjunctive treatment, the effect on relapse prevention, and the need for metabolic monitoring for this patient group. Apart from encouraging preliminary results for aripiprazole in young people (see Aripiprazole, p. 1017), the current limited evidence does not support the use of dopamine antagonists as monotherapy in OCD.

#### Early studies with dopamine antagonists

A case series by McDougle et al. [66] reported benefit from adding open-label pimozide in patients unresponsive to fluvoxamine. Those with comorbid chronic tic or schizotypal disorder responded best. A subsequent double-blind placebo-controlled study [67] demonstrated significant improvements when haloperidol was added to fluvoxamine. Better response was reported for patients with comorbid tic. However, dose-dependent extra-pyramidal side effects, such as akathisia, occurred to the extent that in some studies [66], up to half the patients required co-administration of β-blockers and/or anticholinergics. Therefore, these agents are usually reserved as third-line treatment after a trial of a dopamine antagonist drug with serotonergic actions. It is recommended to start treatment at low dosages and increase cautiously, subject to tolerability (for example, 0.25–0.5 mg haloperidol, titrated slowly to 2–4 mg) [67].

#### Newer dopamine antagonist drugs

##### Risperidone

Several small RCTs have demonstrated efficacy for adjunctive risperidone (0.5–4 mg/day) in SSRI-resistant OCD [68]. However, a RCT [69] that treated 100 SSRI partial or non-responders found no benefit for adjunctive risperidone (up to 4 mg) over placebo. These data suggest that the benefits of adding risperidone may be limited to patients with clear evidence of SSRI resistance.

### Paliperidone

A small 8-week double-blind, placebo-referenced RCT of adjunctive paliperidone (9-OH-risperidone) (≤9 mg/day) in 34 cases of SSRI-resistant OCD did not produce statistically significant improvement [70]. Better powered studies are needed to unequivocally demonstrate efficacy.

### Olanzapine

There has been one positive and another negative placebo-referenced RCT, which may have failed because the study population was not truly SSRI-resistant prior to entering the trial (reviewed in [31, 59]).

### Quetiapine

Studies investigating adjunctive quetiapine (≤400 mg daily) in treatment-resistant OCD have also yielded mixed results (reviewed in [31, 59]). In one double-blind, placebo-controlled study, adjunctive quetiapine was efficacious. However, another smaller RCT in more highly treatment-resistant cases found that although quetiapine (mean 215 mg/day) was numerically superior to placebo, the results did not reach statistical significance. In two further RCTs, no significant difference between adjunctive quetiapine and placebo emerged. Another study found that quetiapine successfully augmented the effect of citalopram in 76 cases of non-resistant OCD, suggesting its effects may not be limited to resistant patients.

### Aripiprazole

Two small, double-blind, placebo-controlled trials of adjunctive aripiprazole (15 mg/day, 10 mg/day) found evidence of efficacy in adults with SRI-resistant OCD [(reviewed in [31, 59]). Adjunctive aripiprazole has also been subjected to a preliminary open-label study in young people with SRI-resistant OCD, with promising results. An open-label study that investigated aripiprazole *monotherapy* (2–7.5 mg/day) in 16 children with SSRI and CBT-resistant OCD also reported positive findings [71]. These results suggest promise for aripiprazole in treatment-resistant OCD across the lifespan and support further exploration of the effect of antipsychotic monotherapy in OCD.

### Meta-analysis of adding dopamine antagonist/partial agonist drugs

While studies on the aforementioned drugs have demonstrated effectiveness as augmentation agents in OCD, the overall effect size is modest and only around one-third of patients are noted to respond. In a pooled analysis [72] of data from placebo-controlled quetiapine trials, the best results were seen when quetiapine was used in combination with clomipramine, fluoxetine, or fluvoxamine and when the SRI dose was lower, suggesting quetiapine may be of most benefit in patients unable to take maximal doses of SRIs.

A subsequent meta-analysis [73], which combined results from 14 randomized, placebo-controlled studies (incorporating 491 patients), showed that significantly more participants responded to augmentation with dopamine antagonists/partial agonists 'as a group' than placebo. Furthermore, aripiprazole, haloperidol, and risperidone significantly outperformed placebo control. Another recent meta-analysis [74] that was limited to newer drugs for psychosis

and included 14 studies and 493 patients produced a similar result. Dopamine antagonists as a class were efficacious, as were aripiprazole and risperidone, but there was insufficient evidence to suggest that quetiapine or olanzapine were superior to placebo.

A mixed-model meta-regression analysis of 13 RCTs [75] correlated the efficacy of each antagonist with its neurotransmitter receptor-binding affinities. A significant positive correlation was found between dopamine receptor (D2R, D3R) affinity and clinical efficacy (standardized mean difference in Y-BOCS score), suggesting the drugs may exert their clinical effects in OCD through this mechanism.

### Intravenous administration of SRIs

The intravenous (IV) administration of SRIs is highly dependent on the configuration of health systems and has limited practicality outside inpatient settings. In a study of 54 oral clomipramine-refractory OCD patients randomized to IV clomipramine (25 mg/day, increasing to 250 mg/day) or IV placebo [76], significant advantages were seen for clomipramine on some efficacy measures, but not on the Y-BOCS. IV clomipramine was not associated with serious adverse events. In a more recent open-label study [77] of 30 multiply SRI-resistant *inpatients* administered with IV clomipramine for 1 week, followed by oral clomipramine dosed up to 225 mg/day, 76.7% were responders and 60% were still responders at 24 weeks. No relevant persistent adverse effects were reported. The results suggest IV clomipramine could be of at least short-term benefit for severe OCD cases that have not adequately responded to several therapies, but the long-term advantages need further exploration.

Another open-label study of IV citalopram in SSRI-resistant adults, which was well tolerated even at high doses (up to 80 mg daily) [78], produced satisfactory response rates. All 21 IV citalopram responders showed significant further improvement on continuation treatment with oral citalopram, suggesting that IV citalopram may be a useful method of accelerating the response for OCD patients and for predicting response to oral citalopram.

### Combining SSRIs and clomipramine

This combination should be used with caution, as pharmacokinetic interactions on hepatic P450 cytochrome isoenzymes may occur, resulting in elevated clomipramine plasma levels and potential toxicity. One study found that the combination of fluvoxamine and clomipramine was efficacious and generally well tolerated, although high plasma levels of clomipramine associated with a higher frequency of clinically relevant adverse effects were seen [79]. Therefore, ECG, EEG, and clomipramine plasma level monitoring was recommended for co-medicated patients. Compared to other SSRIs, citalopram and escitalopram are potentially less likely to interact with clomipramine. Promising results from a small open-label trial of citalopram (40 mg daily) in combination with clomipramine (150 mg daily) contrast with the results from two more recent small studies with methodological weaknesses, which found no benefit from combining clomipramine with an SSRI and highlighted the potential for adverse effects associated with this combination [61, 80]. One patient on adjunctive clomipramine had to withdraw because of serotonergic syndrome. Another three developed ECG QTc prolongation and were withdrawn. Taken together, the results suggest limited benefits for such combinations, and if they are contemplated, ECG and plasma level monitoring are advisable.

## Novel pharmacological agents

The following compounds are under investigation for OCD and have shown some evidence of efficacy, but as so far they lack convincing validation in controlled studies, they cannot at present be judged to be effective.

The glutamatergic compound memantine has appeared helpful as an adjunct to an SSRI in a few open-label trials and two small randomized, placebo-controlled trials [31, 81]. Preliminary results from open-label studies suggesting efficacy for riluzole, another glutamate-modulating agent [31], have so far not been substantiated. In a placebo-controlled trial of riluzole in children with refractory OCD, no significant difference was noted on any of the primary or secondary outcome measures [82].

The glutamatergic hypothesis of OCD has been further explored through investigation of IV ketamine. Ketamine must be used cautiously, as it is associated with urinary tract damage. A placebo-referenced cross-over RCT in eight resistant patients produced a clinical response in 50% of those receiving ketamine [83]. However, in another 3-day open-label ketamine trial in ten subjects with refractory OCD and depression, there were no responders and, although depressive symptoms improved, the improvement in Y-BOCS scores amounted to <12% [84].

The 5-HT3 receptor antagonist ondansetron, administered in combination with fluoxetine, demonstrated a superior effect over adjunctive placebo in a randomized controlled pilot study in treatment-resistant OCD [85]. However, an as yet unpublished multi-centre trial did not demonstrate an improvement in OCD symptoms vs placebo.

Mirtazapine as monotherapy was found to significantly improve outcomes in a placebo-controlled discontinuation study of 15 open-label mirtazapine responders [86].

Clonazepam, as an adjunct to an SRI, may produce symptomatic benefit, possibly through improving associated anxiety. It is less suitable in those with a previous history of benzodiazepine or other substance abuse or dependence [87].

Anti-epileptic mood stabilizers may, in combination with an SSRI, have a role in the treatment of OCD, but the supporting evidence is not strong and further placebo-controlled trials are necessary. Positive results were obtained in a small RCT of lamotrigine and another of topiramate in which the therapeutic effect was seen on reducing compulsions only (reviewed in [31]). A second RCT of adjunctive topiramate in 38 resistant patients failed to demonstrate efficacy [88]. Adjunctive pregabalin has been investigated in an open-label case series only, with signs of possible efficacy, as has gabapentin [89].

A randomized, placebo-controlled trial of single-dose D-amphetamine produced short-lived benefits, while another RCT directly comparing D-amphetamine and caffeine noted that both compounds were associated with rapid improvement of obsessive compulsive symptoms within a week, hinting that stimulants, such as D-amphetamine, could play a role in treating OCD, possibly in the context of comorbid attention-deficit/hyperactivity disorder (ADHD) [90].

## Combined CBT and pharmacotherapy

Although many specialist centres offer combined treatment, there remains uncertainty over the degree to which combining CBT with SSRIs improves outcomes, compared to monotherapy. Some studies suggested that combining CBT with pharmacotherapy produced better results than CBT monotherapy [59]. Other studies found that patients who responded only partially to an SRI fared better if CBT with ERP was added [12, 91]. Thus, a trial of combined CBT plus an SSRI would seem appropriate for those patients failing to respond adequately to SSRI monotherapy.

The APA Practice Guidelines [54] suggest using either an SRI or CBT as first-line treatment. According to a cost-effectiveness analysis, the UK NICE guidelines [51] recommend combining CBT with an SRI only in more severe or treatment-resistant OCD cases.

The network meta-analysis by Skapinasis et al. [32] highlighted that although there are limited data regarding the efficacy of combination treatment, many trials of psychological therapies can be considered as variations of combination trials, as most allowed study participants to remain on stable doses of drugs. They concluded that the combination of SRIs with psychotherapy is likely to be more beneficial for patients with severe OCD than monotherapy. Further research is necessary to substantiate this claim.

## Somatic treatments in OCD

Failure to respond to the aforementioned treatments, including combination treatment with intensive inpatient and/or home-based or clinic-based therapist-assisted CBT, may indicate refractoriness to treatment. At this stage, if the symptoms remain severe and incapacitating, it may be necessary to liaise with specialist services offering somatic treatments such as neurostimulation or neurosurgery.

### Non-invasive neurostimulation

#### Repetitive transcranial magnetic stimulation

Repetitive transcranial magnetic stimulation (rTMS) modulates neuronal activity by inducing a magnetic field pulse. rTMS directed at the prefrontal subcortical circuits is hypothesized to be beneficial in OCD [92]. However, there is presently insufficient evidence to recommend the use of rTMS as treatment, and it remains an experimental procedure. A meta-analysis [93] of ten RCTs involving 282 subjects found a moderate effect size (0.59) and the response rates were 35% and 13% for patients receiving active and sham rTMS, respectively. The most promising target areas for stimulation included the orbitofrontal cortex (OFC) and the pre-supplementary motor area (SMA). rTMS is generally safe. However, rarely, high-frequency rTMS may induce seizures. Other reported adverse effects include localized pain, paraesthesiae, hearing change, thyroid-stimulating hormone and blood lactate level changes, and hypomania; however, these problems are usually transient [92].

#### Transcranial direct current stimulation

Research on the use of transcranial direct current stimulation (tDCS) for treating OCD is still in its infancy. There are no currently published RCTs of tDCS in OCD, but results from a small number of uncontrolled tDCS treatment trials targeting either the SMA or the OFC, in which tDCS was well tolerated in all cases, appear promising [94].

### Transcranial alternating current stimulation

A recent case series showed the successful application of transcranial alternating current stimulation (tACS) in seven SSRI- and psychotherapy-resistant OCD patients [95]. Again, further sham-controlled double-blind studies are warranted if transition of this therapy from the laboratory to the clinic is to be considered.

### Deep brain stimulation

Deep brain stimulation (DBS) involves the neurosurgical implantation of electrodes that interrupt electrical impulses linking specific locations in the brain. This approach permits focal, relatively low-risk, and relatively reversible modulation of brain circuitry. It is hypothesized that DBS brings about therapeutic effects in OCD by modulating the cortico-striatal neurocircuitry proposed to mediate OCD [96]. At present, DBS remains a highly experimental treatment for extremely severe enduring illness, with evidence largely based on case series. Studies are small with, at best, partially controlled designs. Although the procedure is reported to be 'relatively safe', with limited side effects [96], the 3-year outcomes of bilateral stimulation of ventral capsule/ventral striatum in ten adult OCD patients included surgical adverse effects, such as asymptomatic haemorrhage, seizure, and superficial infection, as well as psychiatric adverse effects, including worsening of depression and OCD when DBS was interrupted [97]. Other acute adverse effects included transient hypomania, sadness, anxiety, euphoria, and giddiness.

A meta-analysis by Alonso et al. [98], which included 116 OCD patients from 31 studies, calculated the global reduction in Y-BOCS score as 45.1% and the global number of responders as 60.0%. Older age of onset of OCD and the presence of sexual or religious obsessions or compulsions were associated with a better response. Worsening of anxiety was the most commonly reported adverse event, occurring in 21.6% of patients. However, the authors state that all side effects were generally mild and transient and that the treatment appeared to be tolerable for most patients.

### Ablative neurosurgery

Modern ablative neurosurgical procedures are stereotactically guided, resulting in small and accurately placed lesions. This is most commonly achieved using thermal stimuli, although there is ongoing research into the use of radiosurgical techniques such as the gamma knife.

Anterior cingulotomy, involving lesions placed in the dorsal anterior cingulate cortex, and anterior capsulotomy, involving lesions placed within the inferior fronto-thalamic connections within the anterior limb of the internal capsule, are the most common procedures [99]. Both are hypothesized to modulate functioning within the cortico-striatal-thalamic circuitry. The available evidence suggests that neurosurgery produces significant therapeutic benefits to 30–60% of patients with otherwise highly refractory OCD. Serious adverse effects are uncommon but have been reported with both procedures (for example, intracranial haemorrhage, recurrent seizures). Anterior cingulotomy appears to offer a superior safety profile to that of anterior capsulotomy. The quality of evidence supporting each procedure is reflective of neurosurgery as a whole. A single RCT of gamma capsulotomy has been performed in 16 highly refractory patients [100]. There was a non-significant benefit on the Y-BOCS for the actively lesioned group. The most serious adverse event was a single asymptomatic radiation-induced cyst. Surgical intervention is reserved for patients with severe, incapacitating OCD who have failed an exhaustive array of expertly delivered medication trials and intensive evidence-based CBT.

## REFERENCES

1. Fineberg, N.A., et al. Obsessive–compulsive disorder (OCD): practical strategies for pharmacological and somatic treatment in adults. *Psychiatry Research*, 2015. **227**: 114–25.
2. Baldwin, D.S., et al. Evidence-based guidelines for the pharmacological treatment of anxiety disorders: recommendations from the British Association for Psychopharmacology. *Journal of Psychopharmacology*, 2005. **19**: 567–96.
3. Goodman, W.K., et al. The Yale-Brown obsessive compulsive scale: I. Development, use, and reliability. *Archives of General Psychiatry*, 1989. **46**: 1006–11.
4. Pallanti, S., et al. Treatment non-response in OCD: methodological issues and operational definitions. *International Journal of Neuropsychopharmacology*, 2002. **5**: 181–91.
5. Guy, W. *ECDEU Assessment Manual for Psychopharmacology.* Vol. 76. US Department of Health, Education, and Welfare, Public Health Service, Alcohol, Drug Abuse, and Mental Health Administration, National Institute of Mental Health, Psychopharmacology Research Branch, Division of Extramural Research Programs; 1976.
6. Fineberg, N.A., et al. Sustained response versus relapse: the pharmacotherapeutic goal for obsessive–compulsive disorder. *International clinical psychopharmacology*, 2007. **22**: 313–22.
7. Hollander, E., et al. Quality of life outcomes in patients with obsessive-compulsive disorder: relationship to treatment response and symptom relapse. *Journal of Clinical Psychiatry*, 2010. **71**: 784–92.
8. Levy, R. and V. Meyer. *New Techniques in Behaviour Therapy: Ritual Prevention in Obsessional Patients.* SAGE Publications; 1971.
9. Marks, I., R. Hodgson, and S. Rachman. Treatment of chronic obsessive-compulsive neurosis by *in-vivo* exposure. *British Journal of Psychiatry*, 1975. **127**: 349–64.
10. Kobak, K.A., et al. Computer-assisted cognitive behavior therapy for obsessive-compulsive disorder: a randomized trial on the impact of lay vs. professional coaching. *Annals of General Psychiatry*, 2015. **14**: 10.
11. Foa, E.B., et al. Randomized, placebo-controlled trial of exposure and ritual prevention, clomipramine, and their combination in the treatment of obsessive-compulsive disorder. *American Journal of Psychiatry*, 2005. **162**: 151–61.
12. Simpson, H.B., et al. A randomized, controlled trial of cognitive-behavioral therapy for augmenting pharmacotherapy in obsessive-compulsive disorder. *American Journal of Psychiatry*, 2008. **165**: 621–30.
13. Boschen, M.J., et al. Predicting outcome of treatment for severe, treatment resistant OCD in inpatient and community settings. *Journal of Behavior Therapy and Experimental Psychiatry*, 2010. **41**: 90–5.
14. Ellis, A. *Reason and Emotion in Psychotherapy.* Oxford: Lyle Stuart; 1962.
15. Salkovskis, P.M. Obsessional-compulsive problems: A cognitive-behavioural analysis. *Behaviour Research and Therapy*, 1985. **23**: 571–83.

16. Jones, M.K. and R.G. Menzies. Danger ideation reduction therapy (DIRT) for obsessive–compulsive washers. A controlled trial. *Behaviour Research and Therapy*, 1998. **36**: 959–70.

17. Vaccaro, L.D., *et al*. Danger ideation reduction therapy for obsessive–compulsive checking: Preliminary findings. *Cognitive behaviour therapy*, 2010. **39**: 293–301.

18. Ougrin, D. Efficacy of exposure versus cognitive therapy in anxiety disorders: systematic review and meta-analysis. *BMC psychiatry*, 2011. **11**: 200.

19. Tyagi, H., L.M. Drummond, and N.A. Fineberg. Treatment for obsessive compulsive disorder. *Current Psychiatry Reviews*, 2010. **6**: 46–55.

20. Öst, L.-G., *et al*. Cognitive behavioral treatments of obsessive–compulsive disorder. A systematic review and meta-analysis of studies published 1993–2014. *Clinical Psychology Review*, 2015. **40**: 156–69.

21. Emmelkamp, P.M. and H. Beens. Cognitive therapy with obsessive-compulsive disorder: A comparative evaluation. *Behaviour Research and Therapy*, 1991. **29**: 293–300.

22. Van Balkom, A.J., *et al*. Cognitive therapy versus fluvoxamine as a second-step treatment in obsessive-compulsive disorder nonresponsive to first-step behavior therapy. *Psychotherapy and Psychosomatics*, 2012. **81**: 366–74.

23. Anholt, G.E., *et al*. Cognitive versus behavior therapy: processes of change in the treatment of obsessive-compulsive disorder. *Psychotherapy and Psychosomatics*, 2008. **77**: 38–42.

24. Cottraux, J., *et al*. A randomized controlled trial of cognitive therapy versus intensive behavior therapy in obsessive compulsive disorder. *Psychotherapy and Psychosomatics*, 2001. **70**: 288–97.

25. McLean, P.D., *et al*. Cognitive versus behavior therapy in the group treatment of obsessive-compulsive disorder. *Journal of Consulting and Clinical Psychology*, 2001. **69**: 205–14.

26. Drummond, L.M. The treatment of severe, chronic, resistant obsessive-compulsive disorder. An evaluation of an in-patient programme using behavioural psychotherapy in combination with other treatments. *British Journal of Psychiatry*, 1993. **163**: 223–9.

27. McKay, D., *et al*. Efficacy of cognitive-behavioral therapy for obsessive–compulsive disorder. *Psychiatry Research*, 2015. **225**: 236–46.

28. Fineberg, N.A. and T.M. Gale. Evidence-based pharmacotherapy of obsessive–compulsive disorder. *International Journal of Neuropsychopharmacology*, 2005. **8**: 107–29.

29. Montgomery, S., Clomipramine in obsessional neurosis: a placebo-controlled trial. *Pharm Med*, 1980. **1**: 189–92.

30. Clomipramine Collaborative Study Group. Clomipramine in the treatment of patients with obsessive-compulsive disorder. The Clomipramine Collaborative Study Group. *Archives in General Psychiatry*, 1991. **48**: 730–8.

31. Fineberg, N.A., *et al*. Pharmacotherapy of obsessive-compulsive disorder: evidence-based treatment and beyond. *Australian and New Zealand Journal of Psychiatry*, 2013. **47**: 121–41.

32. Skapinakis, P., *et al*. Pharmacological and psychotherapeutic interventions for management of obsessive-compulsive disorder in adults: a systematic review and network meta-analysis. *The Lancet Psychiatry*, 2016. **3**: 730–9.

33. Varigonda, A.L., E. Jakubovski, and M.H. Bloch, Systematic review and meta-analysis: early treatment responses of selective serotonin reuptake inhibitors and clomipramine in pediatric obsessive-compulsive disorder. *Journal of the American Academy of Child and Adolescent Psychiatry*, 2016. **55**: 851–9.

34. Goodman, W., *et al*. Treatment of obsessive-compulsive disorder with fluvoxamine: a multicentre, double-blind, placebo-controlled trial. *International Clinical Psychopharmacology*, 1996. **11**: 21–30.

35. Hollander, E., *et al*. A double-blind, placebo-controlled study of the efficacy and safety of controlled-release fluvoxamine in patients with obsessive-compulsive disorder. *Journal of Clinical Psychiatry*, 2003. **64**: 640–7.

36. Riddle, M.A., *et al*. Fluvoxamine for children and adolescents with obsessive-compulsive disorder: a randomized, controlled, multicenter trial. *Journal of the American Academy of Child and Adolescent Psychiatry*, 2001. **40**: 222–9.

37. Greist, J., *et al*. Double-blind parallel comparison of three dosages of sertraline and placebo in outpatients with obsessive-compulsive disorder. *Archives of General Psychiatry*, 1995. **52**: 289–95.

38. March, J.S., *et al*. Sertraline in children and adolescents with obsessive-compulsive disorder: a multicenter randomized controlled trial. *JAMA*, 1998. **280**: 1752–6.

39. Montgomery, S., *et al*. A double-blind, placebo-controlled study of fluoxetine in patients with DSM-III-R obsessive-compulsive disorder. *European Neuropsychopharmacology*, 1993. **3**: 143–52.

40. Tollefson, G.D., *et al*. A multicenter investigation of fixed-dose fluoxetine in the treatment of obsessive-compulsive disorder. *Archives of General Psychiatry*, 1994. **51**: 559–67.

41. Rauch, S.L. and M.L. Buttolph. Placebo-controlled trial of fluoxetine and phenelzine for obsessive-compulsive disorder. *American Journal of Psychiatry*, 1997. **154**: 1261–4.

42. Riddle, M.A. *et al*. Double-blind, crossover trial of fluoxetine and placebo in children and adolescents with obsessive-compulsive disorder. *Journal of the American Academy of Child and Adolescent Psychiatry*, 1992. **31**: 1062–9.

43. Liebowitz, M.R., *et al*. Fluoxetine in children and adolescents with OCD: a placebo-controlled trial. *Journal of the American Academy of Child and Adolescent Psychiatry*, 2002. **41**: 1431–8.

44. Zohar, J. and R. Judge. Paroxetine versus clomipramine in the treatment of obsessive-compulsive disorder. OCD Paroxetine Study Investigators. The *British Journal of Psychiatry*, 1996. **169**: 468–74.

45. Hollander, E., *et al*. Acute and long-term treatment and prevention of relapse of obsessive-compulsive disorder with paroxetine. *Journal of Clinical Psychiatry*, 2003. **64**: 1113–21.

46. Geller, D.A., *et al*. Paroxetine treatment in children and adolescents with obsessive-compulsive disorder: a randomized, multicenter, double-blind, placebo-controlled trial. *Journal of the American Academy of Child and Adolescent Psychiatry*, 2004. **43**: 1387–96.

47. Montgomery, S., *et al*. Citalopram 20 mg, 40 mg and 60 mg are all effective and well tolerated compared with placebo in obsessive-compulsive disorder. *International Clinical Psychopharmacology*, 2001. **16**: 75–86.

48. Stein, D.J., *et al*. Escitalopram in obsessive–compulsive disorder: a randomized, placebo-controlled, paroxetine-referenced, fixed-dose, 24-week study. *Current Medical Research and Opinion*, 2007. **23**: 701–11.

49. Soomro, G.M., *et al*. Selective serotonin re-uptake inhibitors (SSRIs) versus placebo for obsessive compulsive disorder (OCD). Cochrane Database of Systematic Reviews, 2008. **1**: CD001765.

50. McGuire, J.F., *et al*. A meta-analysis of cognitive behavior therapy and medicaiton for child obsessive-compulsive disorder: moderators of treatment efficacy, response, and remission. *Depression and Anxiety*, 2015. **32**: 580–93.

51. National Institute for Health and Care Excellence. *Obsessive-compulsive disorder and body dysmorphic disorder: treatment*. 2005. Available from: https://www.nice.org.uk/guidance/cg31

52. Bloch, M.H., *et al.* Meta-analysis of the dose-response relationship of SSRI in obsessive-compulsive disorder. *Molecular Psychiatry*, 2010. **15**: 850–5.

53. Baldwin, D.S., *et al.* Evidence-based pharmacological treatment of anxiety disorders, post-traumatic stress disorder and obsessive-compulsive disorder: a revision of the 2005 guidelines from the British Association for Psychopharmacology. *Journal of Psychopharmacology*, 2014. **28**: 403–39.

54. American Psychiatric Association. Practice guideline for the treatment of patients with obsessive-compulsive disorder. 2007. Available from: http://psychiatryonline.org/pb/assets/raw/sitewide/practice_guidelines/guidelines/ocd.pdf

55. Fineberg, N.A., *et al.* Remission of obsessive-compulsive disorders and syndromes; evidence from a prospective community cohort study over 30 years. *International Journal of Psychiatry in Clinical Practice*, 2013. **17**: 179–87.

56. Koran, L.M., *et al.* Efficacy of sertraline in the long-term treatment of obsessive-compulsive disorder. *American Journal of Psychiatry*, 2002. **159**: 88–95.

57. Romano, S., *et al.* Long-term treatment of obsessive-compulsive disorder after an acute response: a comparison of fluoxetine versus placebo. *Journal of Clinical Psychopharmacology*, 2001. **21**: 46–52.

58. Santana, L., *et al.* Predictors of adherence among patients with obsessive-compulsive disorder undergoing naturalistic pharmacotherapy. *Journal of Clinical Psychopharmacology*, 2010. **30**: 86–8.

59. Fineberg, N.A., *et al.* Evidence-based pharmacotherapy of obsessive-compulsive disorder. *International Journal of Neuropsychopharmacology*, 2012. **15**: 1173–91.

60. da Conceição Costa, D.L., *et al.* Can early improvement be an indicator of treatment response in obsessive-compulsive disorder? Implications for early-treatment decision-making. *Journal of Psychiatric Research*, 2013. **47**: 1700–7.

61. Diniz, J.B., *et al.* A double-blind, randomized, controlled trial of fluoxetine plus quetiapine or clomipramine versus fluoxetine plus placebo for obsessive-compulsive disorder. *Journal of Clinical Psychopharmacology*, 2011. **31**: 763–8.

62. Ninan, P.T., *et al.* High-dose sertraline strategy for nonresponders to acute treatment for obsessive-compulsive disorder: a multicenter double-blind trial. *Journal of Clinical Psychiatry*, 2006. **67**: 15–22.

63. Rabinowitz, I., *et al.* High-dose escitalopram for the treatment of obsessive-compulsive disorder. *International Clinical Psychopharmacology*. 2008. **23**: 49–53.

64. Zivin, K., *et al.* Evaluation of the FDA warning against prescribing citalopram at doses exceeding 40 mg. *American Journal of Psychiatry*, 2013. **170**: 642–50.

65. Denys, D., *et al.* A double-blind switch study of paroxetine and venlafaxine in obsessive-compulsive disorder. *Journal of Clinical Psychiatry*, 2004. **65**: 37–43.

66. McDougle, C.J., *et al.* Neuroleptic addition in fluvoxamine-refractory obsessive-compulsive disorder. *American Journal of Psychiatry*, 1990. **147**: 652.

67. McDougle, C.J., *et al.* Haloperidol addition in fluvoxamine-refractory obsessive-compulsive disorder: a double-blind, placebo-controlled study in patients with and without tics. *Archives of General Psychiatry*, 1994. **51**: 302–8.

68. McDougle, C.J., *et al.* A double-blind, placebo-controlled study of risperidone addition in serotonin reuptake inhibitor–refractory obsessive-compulsive disorder. *Archives of General Psychiatry*, 2000. **57**: 794–801.

69. Simpson, H.B., *et al.* Cognitive-behavioral therapy vs risperidone for augmenting serotonin reuptake inhibitors in obsessive-compulsive disorder: a randomized clinical trial. *JAMA Psychiatry*, 2013. **70**: 1190–9.

70. Storch, E.A. Double-blind, placebo-controlled, pilot trial of paliperidone augmentation in serotonin reuptake inhibitor-resistant obsessive-compulsive disorder. *Journal of Clinical Psychiatry*, 2013. **74**: 527–32.

71. Ercan, E.S. A Promising Preliminary Study of Aripiprazole for Treatment-Resistant Childhood Obsessive-Compulsive Disorder. *Journal of Child and Adolescent Psychopharmacology*, 2015. **25**: 580–4.

72. Denys, D., *et al.* Quetiapine addition in obsessive-compulsive disorder: is treatment outcome affected by type and dose of serotonin reuptake inhibitors? *Biological Psychiatry*, 2007. **61**: 412–14.

73. Dold, M., *et al.* Antipsychotic augmentation of serotonin reuptake inhibitors in treatment-resistant obsessive-compulsive disorder: an update meta-analysis of double-blind, randomized, placebo-controlled trials. *International Journal of Neuropsychopharmacology*, 2015. **18**: pyv047.

74. Veale, D., *et al.* Atypical antipsychotic augmentation in SSRI treatment refractory obsessive-compulsive disorder: a systematic review and meta-analysis. *BMC Psychiatry*, 2014. **14**: 317.

75. Ducasse, D., *et al.* D2 and D3 dopamine receptor affinity predicts effectiveness of antipsychotic drugs in obsessive-compulsive disorders: a metaregression analysis. *Psychopharmacology*, 2014. **231**: 3765.

76. Fallon, B.A., *et al.* Intravenous clomipramine for obsessive-compulsive disorder refractory to oral clomipramine: a placebo-controlled study. *Archives of General Psychiatry*, 1998. **55**: 918–24.

77. Karameh, W.K. and M. Khani. Intravenous clomipramine for treatment-resistant obsessive-compulsive disorder. *International Journal of Neuropsychopharmacology*, 2015. **19**: pyv084.

78. Pallanti, S., L. Quercioli, and L.M. Koran. Citalopram intravenous infusion in resistant obsessive-compulsive disorder: an open trial. *Journal of Clinical Psychiatry*, 2002. **63**: 796–801.

79. Szegedi, A., *et al.* Combination treatment with clomipramine and fluvoxamine: drug monitoring, safety, and tolerability data. *Journal of Clinical Psychiatry*, 1996. **57**: 257–64.

80. Diniz, J., *et al.* Quetiapine versus clomipramine in the augmentation of selective serotonin reuptake inhibitors for the treatment of obsessive-compulsive disorder: a randomized, open-label trial. *Journal of Psychopharmacology*, 2010. **24**: 297–307.

81. Ghaleiha, A., *et al.* Memantine add-on in moderate to severe obsessive-compulsive disorder: randomized double-blind placebo-controlled study. *Journal of Psychiatric Research*, 2013. **47**: 175–80.

82. Grant, P.J., *et al.* 12-week, placebo-controlled trial of add-on riluzole in the treatment of childhood-onset obsessive–compulsive disorder. *Neuropsychopharmacology*, 2014. **39**: 1453–9.

83. Rodriguez, C.I., *et al.* Randomized controlled crossover trial of ketamine in obsessive-compulsive disorder: proof-of-concept. *Neuropsychopharmacology*, 2013. **38**: 2475–83.

84. Bloch, M.H., *et al.* Effects of ketamine in treatment-refractory obsessive-compulsive disorder. *Biological Psychiatry*, 2012. **72**: 964–70.

85. Soltani, F., *et al.* A double-blind, placebo-controlled pilot study of ondansetron for patients with obsessive-compulsive disorder. *Human Psychopharmacology*, 2010. **25**: 509–13.

86. Koran, L.M., *et al.* Mirtazapine for obsessive-compulsive disorder: an open trial followed by double-blind discontinuation. *Journal of Clinical Psychiatry*, 2005. **66**: 515–20.

87. Hewlett, W.A., S. Vinogradov, and W.S. Agras. Clomipramine, clonazepam, and clonidine treatment of obsessive-compulsive disorder. *Journal of clinical psychopharmacology*, 1992. **12**: 420–30.

88. Afshar, H., *et al*. Topiramate augmentation in refractory obsessive-compulsive disorder: a randomized, double-blind, placebo-controlled trial. *Journal of Research in Medical Sciences*, 2014. **19**: 976.

89. Cora-Locatelli, G., *et al*. Gabapentin augmentation for fluoxetine-treated patients with obsessive-compulsive disorder. *Journal of Clinical Psychiatry*, 1998. **59**: 480.

90. Koran, L.M., E. Aboujaoude, and N.N. Gamel. Double-blind study of dextroamphetamine versus caffeine augmentation for treatment-resistant obsessive-compulsive disorder. *Journal of Clinical Psychiatry*, 2009. **70**: 1530.

91. Foa, E.B., *et al*. Six-month follow-up of a randomized controlled trial augmenting serotonin reuptake inhibitor treatment with exposure and ritual prevention for obsessive-compulsive disorder. *Journal of Clinical Psychiatry*, 2013. **74**: 464.

92. Blom, R.M., *et al*. Update on repetitive transcranial magnetic stimulation in obsessive-compulsive disorder: different targets. *Current Psychiatry Reports*, 2011. **13**: 289–94.

93. Berlim, M.T., N.H. Neufeld, and F. Van den Eynde. Repetitive transcranial magnetic stimulation (rTMS) for obsessive–compulsive disorder (OCD): an exploratory meta-analysis of randomized and sham-controlled trials. *Journal of Psychiatric Research*, 2013. **47**: 999–1006.

94. D'Urso, G., *et al*. OCD, anxiety disorders, and PTSD. In: Brunoni, A., Nitsche, M., Loo, C. (eds.). *Transcranial Direct Current Stimulation in Neuropsychiatric Disorders*. Springer; 2016. pp. 265–71.

95. Klimke, A., *et al*. Case report: successful treatment of therapy-resistant OCD with application of transcranial alternating current stimulation (tACS). *Brain Stimulation*, 2016. **9**: 463–5.

96. de Koning, P.P., *et al*. Current status of deep brain stimulation for obsessive-compulsive disorder: a clinical review of different targets. *Current Psychiatry Reports*, 2011. **13**: 274–82.

97. Greenberg, B.D., *et al*. Three-year outcomes in deep brain stimulation for highly resistant obsessive-compulsive disorder. *Neuropsychopharmacology*, 2006. **31**: 2384.

98. Alonso, P., *et al*. Deep brain stimulation for obsessive-compulsive disorder: a meta-analysis of treatment outcome and predictors of response. *PLoS One*, 2015. **10**: e0133591.

99. Rück, C., *et al*. Capsulotomy for refractory anxiety disorders: long-term follow-up of 26 patients. *American Journal of Psychiatry*, 2003. **160**: 513–21.

100. Lopes, A.C., *et al*. Gamma ventral capsulotomy for obsessive-compulsive disorder: a randomized clinical trial. *JAMA Psychiatry*, 2014. **71**: 1066–76.

# 99

# Hoarding disorder

*Lorena Fernández de la Cruz and David Mataix-Cols*

## Introduction

Hoarding disorder (HD) is a mental disorder that was newly included in the *Diagnostic and Statistical Manual of Mental Disorders*, fifth edition (DSM-5) [1]. More recently, it was also included in the eleventh revision of the *International Classification of Diseases* (ICD-11) [2]. Individuals meeting the diagnostic criteria for HD experience persistent difficulty discarding or parting with possessions due to a perceived need to save the items and distress associated with discarding them. This results in the accumulation of possessions that congest and clutter active living areas and substantially compromise their intended use, causing clinically significant distress, interfering in daily life, and sometimes posing a risk to self and others. General medical conditions and other mental disorders that are known to result in excessive accumulation of objects must be ruled out before the diagnosis of HD can be made.

Hoarding as a characterological trait has its origins in the psychoanalytical descriptions of the 'anal' character [3]. The 'inability to discard worn-out or worthless objects even when they have no sentimental value' became a core diagnostic criterion for obsessive–compulsive personality disorder (OCPD) only with the publication of DSM-III-R [4]. In 1994, DSM-IV [5] introduced the idea that 'extreme' hoarding might, in fact, warrant a diagnosis of obsessive–compulsive disorder (OCD), leading to the widespread conceptualization of hoarding as a symptom dimension of OCD. However, research accumulated over the last two decades has found that most individuals who display hoarding behaviour do not endorse other symptoms of OCD and has further delineated the differences between the two constructs. This culminated in the inclusion of the new disorder in DSM-5, separate from OCD [3].

In DSM-5, HD is included under the broad umbrella of obsessive–compulsive and related disorders, which—in addition to OCD—also includes body dysmorphic disorder, hair pulling disorder (trichotillomania), and excoriation (skin picking) disorder. The reasons for including HD in this chapter are primarily historical, given the previous conceptualization of problematic hoarding as being a criterion of OCPD and/or a symptom of OCD. While there are similarities between HD and other obsessive–compulsive and related disorders [6], it is also apparent that HD shares features with other emotional, impulse control, and neurodevelopmental disorders such as attention-deficit/hyperactivity disorder (ADHD) [7].

During the process leading to DSM-5, the OCD and Related Disorders Sub-Workgroup also proposed the removal of the hoarding criterion of OCPD, a recommendation that was initially endorsed by the DSM-5 Personality Disorders Workgroup [8], but eventually not followed. Thus, in DSM-5, OCPD retains the 'inability to discard objects' criterion, but it encourages clinicians to consider the possibility of HD, rather than OCD, when the hoarding is 'extreme'.

## Clinical features and diagnosis

The DSM-5 diagnostic criteria for HD [1] are based on an earlier operational definition of 'compulsive' hoarding [9]. The landmark feature of HD is a persistent difficulty with discarding or parting with possessions (Criterion A). The most commonly saved items include newspapers, old clothing, bags, books, and paperwork, but virtually any item can be saved. The nature of items is not limited to worthless possessions, because many individuals collect and save valuable things too. These discarding difficulties are generally motivated by the perceived utility or aesthetic value of the items, a strong sentimental attachment to the possessions, the fear of losing important information, a desire to avoid being wasteful, or—typically—a combination of these factors [9]. The prospect of discarding or parting with possessions causes substantial distress to the individual (Criterion B).

These difficulties result in the disorganized accumulation of possessions that congest and clutter active living areas and substantially compromise their intended use (Criterion C). Affected individuals may not be able to sleep in their beds, cook in the kitchen, or sit on the sofas in their living rooms. Frequently, the clutter extends beyond the person's actual home, with accumulation of possessions taking place in garages, gardens, vehicles, and even workplaces. Some individuals may pay for private storage spaces or ask family members or friends to keep items in their homes. Criterion C can still be met if the living areas are uncluttered only because of the intervention of third parties (for example, family members, cleaners, or authorities). Because children and adolescents typically do not control their living environment and have limited acquisitive power, the possible intervention of third parties (for example, parents keeping the spaces useable and thus reducing interference) should be considered when making the diagnosis. Young individuals with HD who live at their parent's home may not have unduly cluttered bedrooms but still fulfil all other diagnostic criteria.

Criterion D requires that the difficulties with discarding and/or clutter cause clinically significant distress or impairment in social, occupational, or other important areas of functioning, including maintaining a safe environment for self and others. In severe cases, hoarding can put individuals at risk for fire, falling, poor sanitation, and other health risks. Some individuals, particularly those with poor insight, may not report distress, and the impairment may only be apparent to those around the individual. However, any attempts to discard or clear the possessions by third parties result in high levels of distress. Quality of life is often severely impaired, and family relationships are frequently strained [10]. Legal proceedings ranging from forced clearings to evictions and, where relevant, the removal of dependents from the home (for example, children, elderly) are relatively common [11].

A diagnosis of HD can only be given once other general medical conditions (Criterion E) and mental disorders (Criterion F) have been ruled out (see Differential diagnosis, p. 1024).

For a diagnosis of HD, all six criteria must be met. For individuals fulfilling the diagnostic criteria for HD, clinicians may also assess the presence of two specifiers: excessive acquisition and insight.

The *excessive acquisition* specifier is endorsed when the individual engages in excessive acquisition of free items, excessive buying, or—less frequently—stealing items that are not needed or for which there is no space available. Approximately 63–90% of persons with HD engage in excessive acquisition [12–15]; these individuals typically experience distress if they are unable to acquire items or are prevented from acquiring items. Reducing excessive acquisition is one of the main goals in the treatment of HD (see Treatment, p. 1027).

The *insight* specifier has three categories (good/fair, poor, and absent/delusional) and refers to the degree to which the individual recognizes that hoarding-related beliefs and behaviours are problematic. A substantial proportion of sufferers lack insight into their difficulties and are reluctant to seek help for their problems [16].

Increasing motivation for change is an integral part of the current psychological treatment for HD (see Treatment, p. 1027).

Other common features of HD include indecisiveness, perfectionism, avoidance, procrastination, difficulty with planning and organizing tasks, and distractibility [9]. Some individuals with HD live in various degrees of unsanitary conditions (*squalor*) that may be a logical consequence of severely cluttered spaces and/or related to planning and organizing difficulties [17]. However, the majority of individuals living in severe domestic squalor do not meet the criteria for HD; rather, squalid homes are typically seen in other medical or neurocognitive conditions (see Differential diagnosis, p. 1024).

Some individuals are known to accumulate large number of animals. In *animal hoarding*, there is generally failure to provide minimal standards of nutrition, sanitation, and veterinary care for the animals and failure to act on the deteriorating condition of the animals and the environment. It is unclear if animal hoarding is a special manifestation of HD, but most individuals who hoard animals also hoard inanimate objects [18].

## Differential diagnosis

A diagnosis of HD can be made only after other medical conditions and mental disorders that can lead to excessive accumulation of possessions have been ruled out. A careful psychopathological interview is necessary to establish the differential diagnosis of HD. The presence of cluttered living spaces alone does not necessarily signal the presence of HD, because cluttered (and sometimes unhygienic) living spaces may be the consequence of multiple conditions (Fig. 99.1).

### Other medical conditions

HD is not diagnosed if the symptoms are judged to be a direct consequence of another medical condition (Criterion E), such as traumatic brain injury, surgical resection for the treatment of a tumour

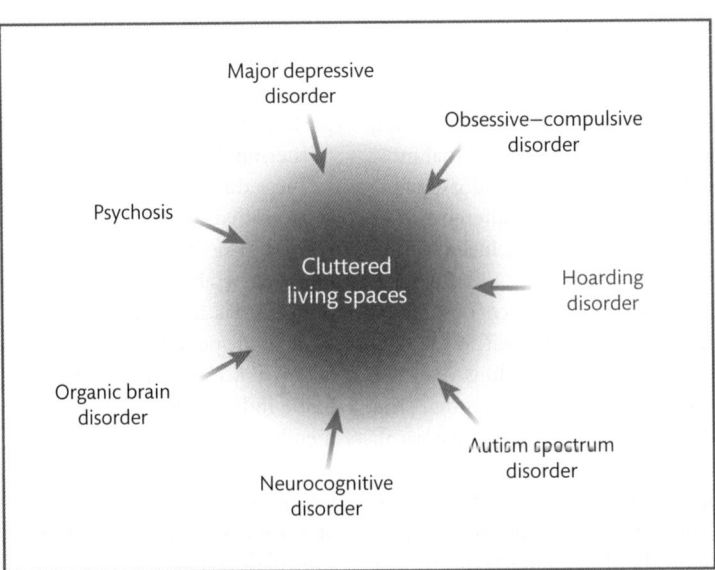

**Fig. 99.1** Differential diagnosis of hoarding disorder.

Reproduced from *N Engl J Med*, 370(21), Mataix-Cols D, Hoarding disorder, pp. 2023–2030, Copyright (2014), with permission from Massachusetts Medical Society.

or seizure control, cerebrovascular disease, infections of the central nervous system (for example, herpes simplex encephalitis), or neurogenetic conditions such as Prader–Willi syndrome [3]. Damage to the anterior ventromedial prefrontal and cingulate cortices has been particularly associated with the excessive accumulation of objects [19, 20]. In these individuals, the hoarding behaviour is not present prior to the onset of brain damage and appears shortly after brain damage occurs [19]. Some of these individuals appear to have little interest in the accumulated items and are able to discard them easily or do not care if others discard them, whereas others appear to be very reluctant to discard anything [20].

## Neurodevelopmental disorders

HD is not diagnosed if the accumulation of objects is judged to be a direct consequence of a neurodevelopmental disorder such as autism spectrum disorders (ASD) or intellectual disability. Individuals with ASD may, for example, excessively acquire or retain possessions that correspond to a particular sensory preoccupation or 'special interest'. The relevance of these behaviours should be investigated [for example, 'Do the objects you save largely share a particular physical characteristic (for example, material, texture, shape)?'].

## Schizophrenia spectrum and other psychotic disorders

HD is not diagnosed if the accumulation of objects is judged to be a direct consequence of delusions or negative symptoms in schizophrenia spectrum and other psychotic disorders [3, 21].

## Major depressive episode

HD is not diagnosed if the accumulation of objects is judged to be a direct consequence of psychomotor retardation, fatigue, or loss of energy during a major depressive episode.

## Obsessive–compulsive disorder

OCD warrants particular consideration, given the previous conceptualization of hoarding as a symptom of OCD [3]. HD is not diagnosed if the symptoms are judged to be a direct consequence of typical obsessions or compulsions such as fears of contamination, harm, or feelings of incompleteness. In such cases, OCD should be diagnosed instead [22]. Symmetry obsessions and compulsions are most commonly associated with this form of hoarding. The accumulation of objects can also be the result of persistently avoiding onerous rituals (for example, not discarding in order to avoid endless washing or checking rituals) [3, 21].

Some additional clinical features are helpful in differentiating HD from OCD. In OCD, the behaviour is generally unwanted and highly distressing, and the individual experiences no pleasure or reward from it. Excessive acquisition is usually not present; if excessive acquisition is present, items are acquired because of a specific obsession (for example, the need to buy items that have been accidentally touched in order to avoid contaminating other people), not because of a genuine desire to possess the items. These individuals are also more likely to accumulate bizarre items such as trash, faeces, urine, nails, hair, used diapers, or rotten food [23]. Accumulation of such items is very unusual in HD.

Both disorders may be diagnosed when severe hoarding appears concurrently with other typical symptoms of OCD but is judged to be independent of these symptoms [3].

## Neurocognitive disorders

HD is not diagnosed if the accumulation of objects is judged to be a direct consequence of a degenerative disorder such as neurocognitive disorder associated with fronto-temporal lobar degeneration or Alzheimer's disease. Typically, onset of the accumulating behaviour is gradual and follows the onset of the neurocognitive disorder. The accumulating behaviour may be accompanied with self-neglect and severe domestic squalor (where there is trash, rotten food, or excrement), alongside other neuropsychiatric symptoms such as disinhibition, gambling, rituals/stereotypies, tics, and self-injurious behaviours [17].

## Normal collecting

While technically not a differential diagnosis, it is worth delineating the differences between normative or healthy collecting and pathological hoarding [24]. This is particularly relevant because quite a few individuals meeting the criteria for HD define themselves as 'collectors', as they perceive this term as being somewhat less pejorative [24]. Normative collecting is a common activity that is both benign and pleasurable. Most children and up to 30% of adults collect items at some point [25]. Collectors report the acquisition of, attachment to, and reluctance to discard objects, but they do not have the disorganized clutter, distress, and impairment that is characteristic of HD. In contrast to hoarding, the process of collecting is highly structured and planned, very selective (that is, confined to a narrow range of items), pleasurable, and often a social activity. Most collectors, even those who might be considered eccentric, are unlikely to meet the diagnostic criteria for HD [24, 25].

## Comorbidities

Although approximately 5–10% of patients with OCD display hoarding symptoms, the majority of individuals (>80%) with hoarding problems do not display other OCD symptoms [12, 13, 23, 26]. In fact, hoarding symptoms may be equally prevalent in individuals with anxiety disorders other than OCD, although these symptoms often go unnoticed as clinicians do not ask about them [27].

The most common psychiatric comorbidities among hoarding cases are generalized anxiety disorder (31–37%), major depressive disorder (26–31%), OCD (15–20%), panic disorder (17%), social anxiety disorder (14%), and post-traumatic stress disorder (14%) [12, 13, 15, 21, 28]. Symptoms typical of ADHD, particularly inattention, are also commonly reported [7, 13]. These comorbidities, rather than hoarding, may often be the main reason for clinical consultation [27].

General medical conditions may also be highly frequent in patients with HD. The presence of HD has been associated with both poorer perceived physical health and higher rates of disability [15]. These limitations may be particularly evident in elderly individuals, who appear to have a disproportionally high rate of medical complications of HD, compared with age-matched control subjects [29].

## Course and prognosis

Retrospective reports indicate that hoarding difficulties begin early and span well into the late stages of life. Hoarding symptoms may first emerge around the age of 11–15 years, start interfering with the individual's everyday functioning by the mid-20s, and cause clinically significant impairment by the mid-30s [30–32]. Problems with acquisition, when they do emerge, appear to do so (or become more evident) earlier than problems with discarding [30]. Participants in clinical research studies are usually in their 50s [12, 23]. A steady worsening of symptoms is typically reported over each decade of life [33]. Once symptoms begin, the course of hoarding is often chronic, with a few individuals reporting a waxing and waning course [32]. Given the absence of treatment studies with long follow-up periods, it is currently unknown what the long-term prognosis of treated HD is.

## Epidemiology

Initial prevalence estimates, primarily from questionnaire studies conducted in Europe and the United States, estimated the point prevalence of clinically significant hoarding to be approximately 2–6% among adults [21] and 2% among adolescents [34]. However, in the only epidemiological study to date to employ the current DSM-5 criteria, conducted in England, the prevalence was estimated to be approximately 1.5% in both adult men and women [15]. This estimate, which was obtained principally through diagnostic interviews conducted face-to-face in the participant's homes, contrasts with some prior work in its suggestion that rates of HD are balanced across the genders. Help-seeking clinical samples are predominantly female, perhaps reflecting better insight and motivation for change. Epidemiological studies are more consistent in their finding that the prevalence of HD seems to increase with advancing age [15, 21].

Individuals with HD are more frequently unemployed and more often unmarried, separated, or divorced than individuals from the general community [15, 24, 35]. Additionally, they are more likely to feel that their hoarding difficulties impair their social and occupational functioning [10, 15]. The functional impairments caused by the disorder typically extend to the relatives or carers of the person who hoards [10].

## Aetiology

### Genetic and environmental factors

Although controlled family studies have not yet been carried out, patient self-report suggests that hoarding runs in families [23]. Consistently, a handful of twin studies conducted in large population-based adult twin samples suggest that this familiality is largely attributable to additive genetic factors (with heritability ranging between 36% and 50%), with the remaining variance attributable to non-shared environmental factors and measurement error [36–38]. Interestingly, a twin study in adolescents indicated possible sex-based variations regarding the role of genes and the environment in hoarding symptoms, suggesting that the aetiology of HD may be dynamic across the lifespan, with the roles of genes and the environment varying over time and between the sexes [34].

On the other hand, research in twins suggests substantial, yet incomplete, genetic overlap between core symptoms of HD (difficulties discarding and excessive acquisition), while non-shared environmental influences appear to be more specific to each of these traits [39]. Together with the fact that not all individuals with HD also excessively acquire, these twin modelling results support the current placement of excessive acquisition as a specifier in DSM-5, rather than as a core diagnostic criterion for HD.

The mechanisms by which either genetic or environmental factors, or their interaction, confer risk to the development of HD remain unknown. Specific genes implicated in HD have not yet been identified. Although research has suggested some unique environmental risk factors (for example, traumatic life events), small samples and retrospective self-report methods leave unclear the role of such exposures in the onset or exacerbation of HD [31, 36]. Anecdotal links between material deprivation (for example, childhood poverty) and hoarding have received no support in the literature [31].

Future work is warranted to understand how specific genetic and environmental risk factors interact to confer risk to individuals carefully diagnosed as having HD. It is likely that these genetic and environmental risk factors will be, at least in part, shared with related conditions such as OCD and other related disorders [40]. The potential aetiological overlaps between HD and other neuropsychiatric conditions (for example, anxiety and mood disorders, ADHD) remain to be explored.

## Neurobiology

The neural substrates of hoarding behaviour have been well studied in animals that naturally display hoarding behaviours as part of their behavioural repertoire (for example, rodents, birds), as well as primates. These studies clearly implicate subcortical limbic structures (nucleus accumbens, ventral tegmental area, amygdala, hippocampus, thalamus, hypothalamus) and the ventromedial prefrontal cortex in the mediation of hoarding behaviour [20]. Research with animals also suggests that the dopaminergic system plays a crucial role in hoarding behaviour (for a review, see [20]). Whether the known involvement of the dopaminergic system in hoarding among animals can explain the relatively poor response of hoarding individuals to serotonergic drugs [41] is an attractive hypothesis that remains to be investigated.

Much less is known about normal and abnormal hoarding behaviour in humans. Useful clues come from case studies of brain-damaged patients and of individuals with dementia, particularly of the fronto-temporal type. This research suggests that the ventromedial prefrontal/anterior cingulate cortices, as well as medial temporal regions, may be implicated in hoarding behaviour [20]. One theory is that the former cortical regions modulate or suppress subcortically driven predispositions to acquire and collect and adjust these predispositions to the environmental context [19]. Damage to these cortical regions may result in dysregulated collecting and hoarding behaviour.

The neuroimaging literature of 'non-organic' hoarding has also implicated the ventromedial prefrontal/anterior cingulate cortices and subcortical limbic structures (for example, amygdala/hippocampus) in hoarding patients [42–44]. However, the evidence is preliminary, obtained from small samples, and confounded in many cases by the presence of comorbid OCD symptoms [20].

Similarly, it is difficult to draw firm conclusions from early reports on the neurocognitive profile of HD [20]. Many of the initial neuropsychological studies recruited OCD patients with hoarding symptoms (with different degrees of severity), whereas others recruited individuals with severe hoarding, but predominantly without OCD. The neuropsychological tests employed have been heterogenous and have tapped into different domains, and few employed psychiatric control groups. Findings to date suggest possible impairments in spatial planning, visuo-spatial learning and memory, sustained attention/working memory, organization, response inhibition, set shifting, probabilistic learning, and reversal [20, 45].

Future work in this area should include carefully characterized samples of individuals meeting strict criteria for HD.

## Assessment

The diagnosis of HD is usually made on the basis of a direct interview with the person being evaluated to establish whether the diagnostic criteria are met. The Structured Interview for Hoarding Disorder (SIHD) [46] is available for this purpose.

Because hoarding may not always be the initial reason for consultation [27], clinicians often need to ask direct questions such as 'Do you find it difficult to discard or part with possessions?' or 'Do you have a large number of possessions that congest and clutter the main rooms in your home?' An affirmative answer to these questions can initiate a dialogue that may lead to diagnosis.

A home visit is recommended for the assessment of clutter, impairment, and associated risks. If a home visit is not feasible, the clinician should try to gather additional information from reliable informants such as a spouse or relative (with the patient's consent). This is particularly important for affected persons with limited insight, because they may underestimate the extent and consequences of their difficulties. Informants may also help establish whether the current presentation is long-standing or transient, whether third parties have intervened to clear away some of the clutter, and whether there are potential risks that require attention.

Photographs of the patient's home can also be very useful in helping to document the presence of clinically significant clutter and to track treatment outcomes [47, 48], particularly when home visits are not possible or are impractical. However, photographs should not be a substitute for a thorough psychopathological interview.

The diagnostic interview provides an opportunity to carry out a thorough risk assessment. Attention should be paid to potential fire hazards, the risk of a clutter avalanche, the presence of rodent or insect infestation, and unsanitary living conditions that pose a risk to health. In addition, it is important to establish whether other vulnerable persons (for example, children and elderly people) live with the person who is hoarding.

Numerous clinician and self-administered measures of hoarding severity exist and can be used to quantify the severity of various aspects of hoarding such as difficulties discarding, clutter, distress, etc. While useful, these measures do not allow a diagnosis of HD, primarily because it is not possible to rule out other disorders that may cause hoarding. Therefore, they should be restricted to quantify the severity of hoarding in already diagnosed individuals or to screen individuals in population-based studies.

Some of the most widely used clinician administered measures include the Hoarding Rating Scale-Interview (HRS-I) [49] and the Clutter Image Rating (CIR) [47]. Among the most widely used self-administered measures are the Hoarding Rating Scale-Self Report (HRS-SR) [50], the Saving Inventory-Revised (SI-R) [51],

the UCLA Hoarding Severity Scale (UHSS) [52], and the Hoarding Disorder Dimensional Scale (HD-D) [53]. Typically, these measures have empirically derived cut-offs, which give an indication of whether the person is likely to have clinically significant hoarding problems. Supplementary measures that assess saving cognitions (for example, Saving Cognitions Inventory) [54], problematic acquisition (for example, Compulsive Acquisition Scale) [55], self-reported squalor (for example, Home Environment Index) [56], and caregiver burden and accommodation (for example, Family Impact Scale for Hoarding Disorder) [57] are available and may prove useful for clarifying the clinical picture and monitoring treatment outcomes.

## Treatment

Few treatment studies have specifically included individuals fulfilling the DSM-5 criteria for HD, and therefore, the evidence to guide treatment choice is currently weak.

### Psychological treatment

Currently, the intervention that has the strongest evidence base for HD is a multicomponent psychological treatment that is based on a cognitive behavioural model [9]. The intervention includes office and in-home sessions; motivational interviewing methods to address ambivalence about therapy; education about hoarding; goal-setting; organizing, decision-making, and problem-solving skills training; exposure to sorting, discarding, and not acquiring; and cognitive strategies to facilitate this work [58].

Tolin and colleagues [59] conducted a meta-analysis of all open or randomized controlled trials (RCT) of CBT or behavioural therapy for hoarding in adults. The eligible studies used hoarding-specific outcome measures, and HD was the primary condition being studied, as opposed to hoarding measured in the context of another psychiatric disorder (for example, OCD). Ten relevant studies—comprising 12 samples—were identified, of which three were RCTs, including a total of 103 patients. Four samples used individual CBT, whereas the remaining eight used a group format. Three samples employed a peer-directed, bibliotherapy-based programme of CBT, with no professional therapist present. The number of CBT sessions ranged from 13 to 35 (mean = 20.2 sessions), and the number of visits conducted in patients' homes ranged from 0 to 33 (mean = 5.6 sessions). Overall HD symptom severity decreased significantly across studies with a large effect size (Hedges' $g = 0.82$ for the overall HD severity score). Significant effects were evident on all outcome domains. The strongest effects were seen for difficulty discarding (Hedges' $g = 0.89$). Clutter and acquiring showed effects in the moderate range (Hedges' $g = 0.70$ and 0.72, respectively). Functional impairment (which was not used in the calculation of overall HD symptom severity) showed the smallest effect in the moderate range (Hedges' $g = 0.52$) [59].

Thus, although encouraging, the clinical outcomes of CBT interventions for hoarding are relatively modest (many individuals still require additional treatment), and there is still significant room for improvement. The long-term benefit of such interventions is unclear, but data from a single trial suggest that the treatment gains of CBT for HD were largely maintained at 12-month follow-up [60]. Studies with even longer follow-up times are needed.

## Pharmacological treatment

Pharmacotherapy has also been suggested as a treatment for HD. However, data regarding the use of such treatment are limited and derived from small, uncontrolled studies. While no RCTs of medication for HD have been conducted, some data are available from studies in OCD patients with hoarding symptoms. In patients diagnosed with OCD, the presence of hoarding symptoms is associated with a worse response to serotonin reuptake inhibitors (SRIs), alone or in combination with CBT [41]. Specifically, OCD patients with hoarding symptoms are, on average, 50% less likely to respond to SRIs than non-hoarding OCD patients [41].

In an open-label study of paroxetine that included 79 OCD patients (32 patients meeting criteria for 'compulsive hoarding syndrome' [9] and 47 patients with non-hoarding OCD), hoarding symptoms improved as much as other OCD symptoms. However, paroxetine was not well tolerated (with adverse effects including sedation, fatigue, constipation, akathisia, headache, and sexual dysfunction), and the overall response was moderate in both groups.

To date, only three studies (two open-label trials and one case series) have included samples of individuals diagnosed with HD according to the DSM-5 criteria. An open study evaluated the efficacy of a 12-week trial of venlafaxine and classed 16 of 24 participants as responders (defined as at least 30% reduction in UHSS and SI-R scores, as well as a rating of at least 'much improved' on the Clinical Global Impression–Improvement) [61]. Two other studies have used ADHD treatments to treat hoarding symptoms. The first of these studies was a case series of four patients treated with methylphenidate extended-release for 4 weeks. Of the four patients, two had a modest reduction in hoarding symptoms (25% and 32% decrease in the SI-R) [62]. More recently, another uncontrolled trial reported that nine of 12 participants with HD showed some degree of reduction in their hoarding symptoms in a 12-week trial of atomoxetine [63]. Eleven patients completed the trial, and of these, six were classified as full responders based on the UHSS (mean reduction of 57%); three other patients were classified as partial responders (mean reduction of 27%).

## Future directions

Further controlled clinical trials are needed to assess the short- and longer-term efficacy of psychological and pharmacological treatments, alone and in combination, in carefully diagnosed individuals with primary HD. Additional behavioural interventions that have shown promising results and require further research include those aimed at improving cognitive functioning (for example, attention, organization) in individuals with HD [64, 65] and the development and evaluation of interventions for carers of individuals with HD [10, 66]. The development of interventions adapted for special populations (for example, hoarding symptoms in individuals ASD or intellectual disabilities) is also warranted [67, 68].

While the current psychological treatments emphasize the importance of motivational interviewing techniques, the patients included in the trials described had sufficient insight to at least seek help. It is currently unclear how to best approach individuals with absent or delusional insight and who may only come to the attention of mental health services against their will. The clinical management of these cases may require an unprecedented level of inter-agency co-ordination. Several countries have set up local or federal multi-agency task forces (often including mental health, fire, pest control, housing, legal and social services) to tackle the most severe cases of hoarding who do not voluntarily seek or want help [69].

## FURTHER INFORMATION

Frost RO, Steketee G (eds). *Oxford Handbook of Hoarding and Acquiring*. Oxford: Oxford University Press; 2014.
Mataix-Cols D. Clinical practice. Hoarding disorder. *New England Journal of Medicine*, 2014;370:2023–30.
Nordsletten AE, Mataix-Cols. Chapter 4. Hoarding disorder. In: KA Phillips, DJ Stein (eds). *Handbook on Obsessive-Compulsive and Related Disorders*. Arlington, VA: American Psychiatric Publishing; 2015. pp. 99–134.
Snowdon J, Halliday G, Banerjee S. *Severe Domestic Squalor*. Cambridge: Cambridge University Press; 2012.

## REFERENCES

1. American Psychiatric Association. *Diagnostic and Statistical Manual of Mental Disorders*, fifth edition (DSM-5). Washington, DC: American Psychiatric Association; 2013.
2. Stein DJ, Kogan CS, Atmaca M, *et al*. The classification of obsessive-compulsive and related disorders in the ICD-11. *Journal of Affective Disorders*. 2016;190:663–74.
3. Mataix-Cols D, Frost RO, Pertusa A, *et al*. Hoarding disorder: a new diagnosis for DSM-V? *Depression and Anxiety*. 2010;27:556–72.
4. American Psychiatric Association. *Diagnostic and Statistical Manual of Mental Disorders*, third edition, revised (DSM-III). Washington, DC: American Psychiatric Association; 1980.
5. American Psychiatric Association. *Diagnostic and Statistical Manual of Mental Disorders*, fourth edition (DSM-IV). Washington, DC: American Psychiatric Association; 1994.
6. Phillips KA, Stein DJ, Rauch SL, *et al*. Should an obsessive-compulsive spectrum grouping of disorders be included in DSM-V? *Depression and Anxiety*. 2010;27:528–55.
7. Tolin DF, Villavicencio A. Inattention, but not OCD, predicts the core features of hoarding disorder. *Behaviour Research and Therapy*. 2011;49:120–5.
8. Mataix-Cols D, Frost RO, Pertusa A, *et al*. Hoarding disorder: a new diagnosis for DSM-V? *Depression and Anxiety*. 2010;27:556–72.
9. Frost RO, Hartl TL. A cognitive-behavioral model of compulsive hoarding. *Behaviour Research and Therapy*. 1996;34:341–50.
10. Drury H, Ajmi S, Fernández de la Cruz L, Nordsletten AE, Mataix-Cols D. Caregiver burden, family accommodation, health, and well-being in relatives of individuals with hoarding disorder. *Journal of Affective Disorders*. 2014;159:7–14.
11. Frost RO, Steketee G, Williams L. Hoarding: a community health problem. *Health and Social Care in the Community*. 2000;8:229–34.
12. Frost RO, Steketee G, Tolin DF. Comorbidity in hoarding disorder. *Depression and Anxiety*. 2011;28:876–84.
13. Mataix-Cols D, Billotti D, Fernández de la Cruz L, Nordsletten AE. The London field trial for hoarding disorder. *Psychological Medicine*. 2013;43:837–47.
14. Frost RO, Tolin DF, Steketee G, Fitch KE, Selbo-Bruns A. Excessive acquisition in hoarding. *Journal of Anxiety Disorders*. 2009;23:632–9.

15. Nordsletten AE, Reichenberg A, Hatch SL, *et al.* Epidemiology of hoarding disorder. *British Journal of Psychiatry.* 2013;203:445–52.

16. Tolin DF, Fitch KE, Frost RO, Steketee G. Family informants' perceptions of insight in compulsive hoarding. *Cognitive Therapy and Research.* 2010;34:69–81.

17. Snowdon J, Pertusa A, Mataix-Cols D. On hoarding and squalor: a few considerations for DSM-5. *Depression and Anxiety.* 2012;29:417–24.

18. Frost RO, Patronek G, Rosenfield E. Comparison of object and animal hoarding. *Depression and Anxiety.* 2011;28:885–91.

19. Anderson SW, Damasio H, Damasio AR. A neural basis for collecting behaviour in humans. *Brain.* 2005;128:201–12.

20. Mataix-Cols D, Pertusa A, Snowdon J. Neuropsychological and neural correlates of hoarding: a practice-friendly review. *Journal of Clinical Psychology.* 2011;67:467–76.

21. Pertusa A, Frost RO, Fullana MA, *et al.* Refining the diagnostic boundaries of compulsive hoarding: a critical review. *Clinical Psychology Review.* 2010;30:371–86.

22. Pertusa A, Frost RO, Mataix-Cols D. When hoarding is a symptom of OCD: a case series and implications for DSM-V. *Behaviour Research and Therapy.* 2010;48:1012–20.

23. Pertusa A, Fullana MA, Singh S, Alonso P, Menchon JM, Mataix-Cols D. Compulsive hoarding: OCD symptom, distinct clinical syndrome, or both? *American Journal of Psychiatry.* 2008;165:1289–98.

24. Nordsletten AE, Fernández de la Cruz L, Billotti D, Mataix-Cols D. Finders keepers: the features differentiating hoarding disorder from normative collecting. *Comprehensive Psychiatry.* 2013;54:229–37.

25. Nordsletten AE, Mataix-Cols D. Hoarding versus collecting: where does pathology diverge from play? *Clinical Psychology Review.* 2012;32:165–76.

26. Samuels J, Bienvenu OJ, Grados MA, *et al.* Prevalence and correlates of hoarding behavior in a community-based sample. *Behaviour Research and Therapy.* 2008;46:836–44.

27. Tolin DF, Meunier SA, Frost RO, Steketee G. Hoarding among patients seeking treatment for anxiety disorders. *Journal of Anxiety Disorders.* 2011;25:43–8.

28. Fullana MA, Vilagut G, Rojas-Farreras S, *et al.* Obsessive-compulsive symptom dimensions in the general population: results from an epidemiological study in six European countries. *Journal of Affective Disorders.* 2010;124:291–9.

29. Ayers CR, Iqbal Y, Strickland K. Medical conditions in geriatric hoarding disorder patients. *Aging and Mental Health.* 2014;18:148–51.

30. Grisham JR, Frost RO, Steketee G, Kim HJ, Hood S. Age of onset of compulsive hoarding. *Journal of Anxiety Disorders.* 2006;20:675–86.

31. Landau D, Iervolino AC, Pertusa A, Santo S, Singh S, Mataix-Cols D. Stressful life events and material deprivation in hoarding disorder. *Journal of Anxiety Disorders.* 2011;25:192–202.

32. Tolin DF, Meunier SA, Frost RO, Steketee G. Course of compulsive hoarding and its relationship to life events. *Depression and Anxiety.* 2010;27:829–38.

33. Ayers CR, Saxena S, Golshan S, Wetherell JL. Age at onset and clinical features of late life compulsive hoarding. *International Journal of Geriatric Psychiatry.* 2010;25:142–9.

34. Ivanov VZ, Mataix-Cols D, Serlachius E, *et al.* Prevalence, comorbidity and heritability of hoarding symptoms in adolescence: a population based twin study in 15-year olds. *PLoS One.* 2013;8:e69140.

35. Timpano KR, Exner C, Glaesmer H, *et al.* The epidemiology of the proposed DSM-5 hoarding disorder: exploration of the acquisition specifier, associated features, and distress. *Journal of Clinical Psychiatry.* 2011;72:780–6; quiz 878–89.

36. Iervolino AC, Perroud N, Fullana MA, *et al.* Prevalence and heritability of compulsive hoarding: a twin study. *American Journal of Psychiatry.* 2009;166:1156–61.

37. Lopez-Sola C, Fontenelle LF, Alonso P, *et al.* Prevalence and heritability of obsessive-compulsive spectrum and anxiety disorder symptoms: a survey of the Australian Twin Registry. *American Journal of Medical Genetics. Part B, Neuropsychiatric Genetics.* 2014;165:314–25.

38. Mathews CA, Delucchi K, Cath DC, Willemsen G, Boomsma DI. Partitioning the etiology of hoarding and obsessive-compulsive symptoms. *Psychological Medicine.* 2014;44:2867–76.

39. Nordsletten AE, Monzani B, Fernández de la Cruz L, *et al.* Overlap and specificity of genetic and environmental influences on excessive acquisition and difficulties discarding possessions: implications for hoarding disorder. *American Journal of Medical Genetics. Part B, Neuropsychiatric genetics.* 2013;162B:380–7.

40. Monzani B, Rijsdijk F, Harris J, Mataix-Cols D. The structure of genetic and environmental risk factors for dimensional representations of DSM-5 obsessive-compulsive spectrum disorders. *JAMA Psychiatry.* 2014;71:182–9.

41. Bloch MH, Bartley CA, Zipperer L, *et al.* Meta-analysis: hoarding symptoms associated with poor treatment outcome in obsessive-compulsive disorder. *Molecular Psychiatry.* 2014;19:1025–30.

42. Saxena S, Brody AL, Maidment KM, *et al.* Cerebral glucose metabolism in obsessive-compulsive hoarding. *American Journal of Psychiatry.* 2004;161:1038–48.

43. An SK, Mataix-Cols D, Lawrence NS, *et al.* To discard or not to discard: the neural basis of hoarding symptoms in obsessive-compulsive disorder. *Molecular Psychiatry.* 2009;14:318–31.

44. Tolin DF, Stevens MC, Villavicencio AL, *et al.* Neural mechanisms of decision making in hoarding disorder. *Archives of General Psychiatry.* 2012;69:832–41.

45. Woody SR, Kellman-McFarlane K, Welsted A. Review of cognitive performance in hoarding disorder. *Clinical Psychology Review.* 2014;34:324–36.

46. Nordsletten AE, Fernández de la Cruz L, Pertusa A, Reichenberg A, Hatch SL, Mataix-Cols D. The Structured Interview for Hoarding Disorder (SIHD): development, usage and further validation. *Journal of Obsessive-Compulsive and Related Disorders.* 2013;2:346–50.

47. Frost RO, Steketee G, Tolin DF, Renaud S. Development and validation of the clutter image rating. *Journal of Psychopathology and Behavioral Assessment.* 2008;30:193–203.

48. Fernández de la Cruz L, Nordsletten AE, Billotti D, Mataix-Cols D. Photograph-aided assessment of clutter in hoarding disorder: is a picture worth a thousand words? *Depression and Anxiety.* 2013;30:61–6.

49. Tolin DF, Fitch KE, Frost RO, Steketee G. Family informants' perceptions of insight in compulsive hoarding. *Cognitive Therapy and Research.* 2010;34:69–81.

50. Tolin DF, Frost RO, Steketee G. A brief interview for assessing compulsive hoarding: the Hoarding Rating Scale-Interview. *Psychiatry Research.* 2010;178:147–52.

51. Frost RO, Steketee G, Grisham J. Measurement of compulsive hoarding: saving inventory-revised. *Behaviour Research and Therapy.* 2004;42:1163–82.

52. Saxena S, Ayers CR, Dozier ME, Maidment KM. The UCLA Hoarding Severity Scale: development and validation. *Journal of Affective Disorders.* 2015;175:488–93.

53. LeBeau RT, Mischel ER, Simpson HB, *et al.* Preliminary assessment of obsessive-compulsive spectrum disorder scales for DSM-5. *Journal of Obsessive-Compulsive and Related Disorders.* 2013;2:114–18.

54. Steketee G, Frost RO, Kyrios M. Cognitive aspects of compulsive hoarding. *Cognitive Therapy and Research.* 2003;27:463–79.

55. Frost RO, Steketee G, Williams L. Compulsive buying, compulsive hoarding, and obsessive-compulsive disorder. *Behavior Therapy.* 2002;33:201–14.

56. Rasmussen JL, Steketee G, Frost RO, Tolin DF, Brown TA. Assessing squalor in hoarding: The Home Environment Index. *Community Mental Health Journal.* 2014;50:591–6.

57. Nordsletten AE, Fernández de la Cruz L, Drury H, Ajmi S, Saleem S, Mataix-Cols D. The Family Impact Scale for Hoarding (FISH): measure development and initial validation. *Journal of Obsessive-Compulsive and Related Disorders.* 2014;3:29–34.

58. Steketee G, Frost RO. *Compulsive Hoarding and Acquiring: Therapist Guide (Treatments that Work).* Oxford: Oxford University Press; 2007.

59. Tolin DF, Frost RO, Steketee G, Muroff J. Cognitive behavioral therapy for hoarding disorder: a meta-analysis. *Depression and Anxiety.* 2015;32:158–66.

60. Muroff J, Steketee G, Frost RO, Tolin DF. Cognitive behavior therapy for hoarding disorder: follow-up findings and predictors of outcome. *Depression and Anxiety.* 2014;31:964–71.

61. Saxena S, Sumner J. Venlafaxine extended-release treatment of hoarding disorder. *International Clinical Psychopharmacology.* 2014;29:266–73.

62. Rodriguez CI, Bender J, Jr., Morrison S, Mehendru R, Tolin D, Simpson HB. Does extended release methylphenidate help adults with hoarding disorder? A case series. *Journal of Clinical Psychopharmacology.* 2013;33:444–7.

63. Grassi G, Micheli L, Di Cesare Mannelli L, *et al.* Atomoxetine for hoarding disorder: A pre-clinical and clinical investigation. *Journal of Psychiatric Research.* 2016;83:240–8.

64. Tolin DF, Stevens MC, Nave A, Villavicencio AL, Morrison S. Neural mechanisms of cognitive behavioral therapy response in hoarding disorder: a pilot study. *Journal of Obsessive-Compulsive and Related Disorders.* 2012;1:180–8.

65. Ayers CR, Saxena S, Espejo E, Twamley EW, Granholm E, Wetherell JL. Novel treatment for geriatric hoarding disorder: an open trial of cognitive rehabilitation paired with behavior therapy. *American Journal of Geriatric Psychiatry.* 2014;22:248–52.

66. Thompson C, Fernández de la Cruz L, Mataix-Cols D, Onwumere J. Development of a brief psychoeducational group intervention for carers of people with hoarding disorder: a proof-of-concept study. *Journal of Obsessive-Compulsive and Related Disorders.* 2016;9:66–72.

67. Kellett S, Matuozzo H, Kotecha C. Effectiveness of cognitive-behaviour therapy for hoarding disorder in people with mild intellectual disabilities. *Research in Developmental Disabilities.* 2015;47:385–92.

68. Storch EA, Nadeau JM, Johnco C, *et al.* Hoarding in youth with autism spectrum disorders and anxiety: incidence, clinical correlates, and behavioral treatment response. *Journal of Autism and Developmental Disorders.* 2016;46:1602–12.

69. Bratiotis C. Community hoarding task forces: a comparative case study of five task forces in the United States. *Health and Social Care in the Community.* 2013;21:245–53.

# 100

# Body dysmorphic disorder

*Megan M. Kelly and Katharine A. Phillips*

'The dysmorphophobic patient is really miserable; in the middle of his daily routines, talks, while reading, during meals, everywhere and at any time, he is caught by the doubt of deformity ... '

Enrico Morselli, 1891 [1]

## Introduction

Body dysmorphic disorder (BDD) (previously called 'dysmorphophobia') is a common, often severe psychiatric disorder that has been described for more than a century [1–3]. BDD is characterized by distressing or impairing preoccupations with non-existent or slight defects in physical appearance [4]. In addition, BDD consists of repetitive behaviours (that is, compulsions and rituals) that, at some point during the course of the illness, have been performed in response to the appearance concerns [4]. BDD is classified as an obsessive–compulsive and related disorder in DSM-5 [4]. In ICD-10, BDD is classified as a type of somatoform disorder, but recommendations for ICD-11 are to classify BDD in a new category of obsessive–compulsive and related disorders [5]. Psychosocial functioning is often markedly impaired in BDD [6]. In addition, BDD is characterized by high rates of suicidality and comorbid substance use [7, 8]. Despite its prevalence, severity, and negative effects on functioning, BDD is under-recognized in clinical settings [2, 3].

## Clinical features

### Demographic characteristics

BDD occurs in all age, racial, and ethnic groups [2, 3, 7, 9]. BDD appears slightly more prevalent in women than men [2, 3, 7]. Most individuals with BDD have never been in a primary relationship [10]. Occupational and academic functioning is often substantially impaired, and unemployment rates are elevated, which often appears attributable to BDD symptoms [2, 3, 6, 7].

### Bodily preoccupations

People with BDD are preoccupied with the idea that some aspect of their appearance is ugly, unattractive, deformed, flawed, or defective in some way when it actually is not [1–3, 6–7]. Concerns usually focus on the face or head but can involve any body area [1–3, 7]. Concerns with the skin (for example, perceived acne, scars, lines,

or pale skin), hair (for example, perceived thinning or excessive body or facial hair), and nose (for example, size or shape) are the most common. Concerns about perceived asymmetry of body areas occur in about a quarter of individuals (for example, concerns about perceived unevenness or asymmetry of the hair, breasts/chest, eyes, face, jawline, or lips) [11].

Most patients with BDD are preoccupied with multiple body areas; the number of body areas of concern may range from only one to virtually every aspect of one's appearance. BDD concerns may also focus on one's overall appearance. People with BDD often believe that they are unacceptable and will be rejected by others because they look abnormal [2, 3].

Muscle dysmorphia is an often more severe form of BDD and bodily preoccupation, characterized by distress over a perceived 'small' and insufficiently muscular body build, which occurs primarily in men. Individuals with muscle dysmorphia appear to have even poorer quality of life and higher rates of suicidality and substance use disorders—in particular, anabolic steroid use—than those with BDD who are preoccupied with other body areas [12]. Muscle dysmorphia may also be associated with particularly adverse psychological and medical sequelae, including an increased risk of violent behaviour, which may, in part, reflect abuse of anabolic-androgenic steroids [13].

### Insight/delusionality

BDD-related insight is typically poor but can range from good to absent insight (delusional beliefs); the latter is characterized by complete conviction that the person looks abnormal, ugly, unattractive, or deformed. Studies have found that 36–60% of individuals with BDD currently have delusional beliefs about their appearance [14, 15]. Poor insight or delusional BDD beliefs may limit patients' recognition that their appearance concerns are due to a mental illness and make them unwilling to accept mental health treatment [2, 3, 16].

In addition, a majority have ideas or delusions of reference, believing that others take special notice of the supposed appearance defects—for example, staring at them or mocking them because of how they look [16]. Referential thinking can fuel feelings of anger and rejection, as well as social isolation. These findings are consistent with evidence that individuals with BDD have an interpretive bias for threat. Compared with other groups, those with BDD more often misinterpret neutral facial expressions as contemptuous and angry, and they similarly more often misinterpret ambiguous scenarios (appearance-related, social, and general scenarios) as threatening [17, 18].

### Compulsive and safety behaviours

Compulsive behaviours, also referred to as repetitive behaviours or rituals, occur in response to preoccupations with perceived physical defects. Like the compulsive behaviours that occur in obsessive–compulsive disorder (OCD), they are usually distressing, time-consuming (occurring over an average of 3–8 hours a day), and difficult to resist or control [2, 3]. The behaviours usually aim to examine, improve, hide, or obtain reassurance about the perceived defects. These behaviours typically do not alleviate BDD-triggered distress and may even worsen it.

Common compulsive behaviours and their occurrence in those with BDD are described in the American Psychiatric Association's DSM-5 [4]. Individuals with BDD often compare their appearance to others, including people in newspapers or magazines or on television or social media. Other compulsive behaviours include repeated checking of mirrors and other reflective surfaces (for example, windows), excessive grooming (for example, hair styling, make-up application), reassurance seeking, and excessive exercise or weightlifting.

Several compulsive behaviours have potential medical risks. Compulsive skin picking, which 27–45% of BDD patients do to try to improve the appearance of their skin, can cause considerable skin damage [2, 3]. Emergency surgery is sometimes required—for example, when sharp implements are used for picking ruptured major blood vessels. Compulsive tanning to darken 'pale' skin or minimize perceived acne, scarring, or 'marks' can cause skin damage and increases cancer risk [2, 3].

Some compulsive behaviours, such as camouflaging disliked body areas (for example, hiding perceived balding with a hat or 'asymmetrical' eyes with sunglasses), may also be conceptualized as safety behaviours, as they are motivated by the desire to prevent a feared outcome. However, these behaviours may also be repetitive (for example, repeatedly reapplying and fixing make-up), and thus they may also sometimes be compulsive in nature.

### Psychosocial functioning and quality of life

BDD is associated with very poor quality of life and marked functional impairment [2, 3, 6]. Mental health-related quality of life scores in BDD are poorer than for depression, OCD, schizophrenia, and bipolar disorder [6]. Most individuals with BDD also have marked impairment in activities of daily living; many have been housebound due to their BDD symptoms [2, 3, 18]. In addition, BDD is associated with high lifetime rates of psychiatric hospitalization [19, 20]. Prospective research on the course of BDD demonstrates that functional impairment tends to be chronic over time [21], although in treatment studies, functioning usually improves when BDD symptoms do.

Social functioning is notably poor in BDD. Individuals with BDD often avoid other people because they are afraid of being rejected because of their appearance [2, 3, 10]. As a result, many people with BDD have difficulty forming and maintaining relationships with others. BDD is also associated with high rates of unemployment and often marked impairment in occupational and academic functioning [18]. In a broadly obtained sample of convenience of individuals with BDD, 38% were currently unemployed [18]. Unemployment due to BDD is associated with greater current severity of BDD and depressive symptoms, a more chronic course of BDD, and poorer current social functioning and quality of life [18]. BDD may not only negatively affect a person's ability to hold a job, but it also often impairs one's concentration, work quality, and work productivity [18]. High rates of academic impairment are also common in BDD. In one study, 18% had dropped out of elementary school or high school primarily because of BDD symptoms, and in another study, 22% of youth dropped out of school because of their BDD symptoms [22, 23].

In population-based epidemiologic studies, compared to individuals without BDD, those with BDD were more likely to be divorced and less likely to be married; they also had a lower educational level, lower household income, and greater unemployment and sick leave [24].

### Other associated features

BDD preoccupations may trigger a broad range of negative emotions. BDD is associated with an increased frequency of depression, anxiety, and social anxiety, as well as high levels of these symptoms: feelings of shame and low self-esteem; hostility and anger; rejection sensitivity; and high levels of neuroticism, introversion, perfectionism, and perceived stress [11]. Pursuit of cosmetic treatment, such as surgery and dermatologic and dental treatment, is a common feature of BDD that often leads to poor treatment outcomes.

Common core beliefs, which are addressed in cognitive behavioural therapy (CBT), include: 'I am inadequate', 'I am defective', 'I am worthless', and 'I am unlovable'. Negative core beliefs such as these are compatible with the high rates of depression and suicidality that occur in BDD.

### Suicidality

Suicidal ideation and attempts are very common in BDD. Reported lifetime rates of suicidal ideation and suicide attempts in clinical samples and broadly ascertained samples of convenience are 78–81% and 24–28%, respectively [8, 19]. In a population-based epidemiologic study, 20% of participants with BDD reported suicidal thoughts specifically because of appearance concerns, and 7% had attempted suicide because of appearance-related concerns, whereas only 1% of the non-BDD group had attempted suicide. In another epidemiologic study, 31.0% in the BDD group vs 3.5% in the non-BDD group had suicidal ideation due to appearance concerns, and 22.2% of those with BDD vs only 2.1% of those without BDD had attempted suicide specifically because of appearance concerns [24].

The rate of completed suicide, while preliminary, appears markedly high. In a prospective study, the annual suicide rate was 0.35%, which is approximately 45 times higher than for the population in the United States (adjusted for age, gender, and geographic region) and higher than for most other psychiatric disorders [25].

Preliminary evidence suggests that adolescents and Veterans with BDD, as well as those with muscle dysmorphia, appear to have significantly higher rates of suicidality than other BDD groups [25].

Variables that are independently associated with suicidal ideation and/or suicide attempts in BDD are greater BDD symptom severity; comorbid major depressive disorder, PTSD, a substance use disorder, social anxiety disorder, OCD, and three or more comorbid Axis I disorders; onset of BDD before the age of 18; being unemployed; childhood maltreatment; and BDD-related restrictive food intake [25].

BDD is associated with many risk factors that have been shown more generally to predict completed suicide. These risk factors include high rates of suicidal ideation and attempts, depression and substance use disorders, history of perceived abuse, functional impairment and social isolation, unemployment, disability, being single or divorced, and psychiatric hospitalization, as well as high levels of anxiety, depression, poor self-esteem, anger, and feelings of humiliation and shame [25]. Whether these risk factors predict completed suicide in BDD is unknown and warrants investigation.

## Comorbidity

Lifetime major depressive disorder is the most frequent comorbid disorder, occurring in about 75% of individuals with BDD [26]. The other most common co-occurring Axis I psychiatric disorders are social anxiety disorder, OCD, and substance use disorders [26]. Axis I comorbidity is associated with greater functional impairment and morbidity. In particular, the presence of comorbid major depressive disorder is associated with poorer quality of life and more functional impairment [26]. Comorbid personality disorders occur in 40–100% of individuals with BDD, with Cluster C disorders—in particular, avoidant personality disorder—occurring most frequently [26].

### Gender

BDD is slightly more common in women than in men in both clinical and non-clinical samples, with the exception of cosmetic and dermatological settings [27]. Men and women appear to have largely similar clinical features [7, 19, 28, 29]. However, there are some notable gender differences, some of which reflect gender differences in the general population. Men are more likely to be single, have a substance use disorder, and be preoccupied with thinning hair and small body build (muscle dysmorphia) [19, 29]. Women are generally more likely to be preoccupied with their weight, hips, and excessive body hair and are more likely to pick their skin and use their hands or make-up for camouflage [19, 29]. One study ($n = 58$) [28] found that women are more likely to be preoccupied with their breasts/chest and legs, check mirrors, and use camouflaging to hide disliked body areas. In addition, concerns about genitals are more common in men, and a comorbid eating disorder is more common in women [19, 28, 29].

### BDD in children and adolescents

BDD usually begins during early adolescence and can occur in childhood [30]. While data are limited, BDD's clinical features in youth appear largely similar to those in adults [30]. Youth with BDD typically have very poor psychosocial functioning and mental health-related quality of life. BDD often causes academic underachievement, social avoidance, and other types of psychosocial impairment; it may also lead to school refusal and school dropout, which can derail healthy adolescent development [30]. Suicidal ideation and attempts, physical aggression, and substance use disorders are risk behaviours that commonly occur in youth with BDD [30].

Preliminary findings suggest that BDD may be more severe in youth than in adults. Of note, children and adolescents appear to have lifetime rates of functional impairment similar to those in adults, despite having had fewer years over which to have developed these problems [30]. In addition, adolescents appear more likely than adults to have delusional BDD beliefs (as opposed to better insight), and they have a significantly higher lifetime suicide attempt rate (44% vs 24%, respectively). These findings underscore the importance of recognizing and treating BDD in this age group [30].

### Cross-cultural aspects of BDD

Case reports and case series from around the world suggest that BDD's clinical features are generally similar across cultures, but that cultural factors may produce nuances and accents on a basically invariant, or universal, expression of BDD [2, 3]. In east Asian cultures, a form of social anxiety disorder—taijin kyofusho (shubo-kyofu—'the phobia of a deformed body') [31]—has many features of BDD. Thus, in Asian cultures, BDD is considered more closely akin to social anxiety disorder; in Western countries, BDD is considered closely related to OCD due to prominent obsessive and compulsive features. Much more research has been done on BDD's relationship to OCD than to social anxiety disorder; it is likely that BDD is closely related to both of these disorders.

## Diagnosis

BDD can be diagnosed using questions at the top of Box 100.1, which are consistent with DSM-5's diagnostic criteria. Clinicians should adequately probe for examples of clinically significant distress and impairment in social, occupational, academic, and other aspects of functioning. BDD is diagnosed if the person is excessively preoccupied with one or more non-existent or slight physical flaws (for example, thinking about it for at least an hour a day) and the preoccupation causes clinically significant distress or clinically significant impairment in psychosocial functioning. In addition, at some point during the course of the illness, the appearance preoccupations must have caused repetitive behaviours such as mirror checking, excessive grooming, skin picking, reassurance seeking, or comparing one's appearance with others [4]. Finally, the appearance concerns should not be better explained by an eating disorder. However, BDD and eating disorders may co-occur, in which case both disorders should be diagnosed.

In addition, DSM-5 contains two new specifiers for BDD: muscle dysmorphia and level of BDD-related insight (good or fair, poor, or absent insight/delusional beliefs) [4]. It should be emphasized that delusional BDD beliefs should be diagnosed as BDD, not as a psychotic disorder, as this has significant implications for pharmacologic treatment. BDD-triggered panic attacks may be designated by DSM-5's panic attack specifier, which can be used for any disorder that triggers panic attacks; in BDD, common triggers are feeling scrutinized by others, looking at perceived defects in mirrors, and being under bright lights [32].

The bottom of Box 100.1 includes questions that are *not* recommended to screen for, or diagnose, BDD. The word 'imagined' is problematic, because most patients have poor or absent insight and do not think their appearance problem is imagined. Terms such as 'deformed' or 'disfigured' are too extreme for some patients to endorse. Asking if there is something wrong with one's body is too broad a question, as patients may interpret this as referring to bodily functioning.

ICD-10's description requires that patients persistently refuse to accept the advice and reassurance of doctors or healers that they do not have an abnormality. However, many people with BDD do not disclose their appearance concerns to doctors or even seek medical care because they are housebound, ashamed of their appearance concerns, believe they cannot be helped, lack health insurance, or do not have access to health care for other reasons. Using these criteria will underdiagnose BDD.

BDD usually goes undiagnosed in clinical settings [2, 3]. Sufferers often conceal their symptoms due to embarrassment and shame [2, 3]. They may volunteer only depression, anxiety, or discomfort in social situations. The compulsive and safety behaviours may be clues to BDD's presence.

BDD may also be misdiagnosed as another disorder [2, 3]. BDD may be mistaken as social anxiety disorder because of social anxiety and isolation related to appearance concerns and anxiety over being rejected by others due to the perceived appearance defects. BDD may also be misdiagnosed as OCD due to obsessional preoccupations and compulsive behaviours. Individuals with delusional BDD are sometimes misdiagnosed with schizophrenia, psychotic depression, or another psychotic disorder. People with BDD may be misdiagnosed with panic disorder because of the occurrence of panic attacks that are triggered by appearance concerns, which should instead be diagnosed as BDD with the panic attack specifier. BDD symptoms may also be misdiagnosed as trichotillomania (hair pulling disorder) when hair is repeatedly cut or plucked to improve perceived flaws in its appearance (for example, 'bushy' or uneven eyebrows). BDD may be misdiagnosed as excoriation (skin picking) disorder when skin is picked in an attempt to diminish perceived skin flaws. To diagnose BDD, patients must usually be asked directly about BDD symptoms, using questions such as those in Box 100.1.

**Box 100.1** Questions to diagnose BDD according to DSM-5 diagnostic criteria

### Questions to evaluate diagnostic criteria

*Criterion A: preoccupation with non-existent or slight appearance defects or flaws*

1 'Are you very worried about your appearance in any way?' OR 'Are you unhappy with how you look?'
2 Invite the patient to describe their concern by asking, 'What don't you like about how you look?' OR 'Can you tell me about your concern?' Listen to the patient's description; do not provide reassurance about, or comment on, their appearance.
3 Ask if there are other disliked body areas—for example, 'Are you unhappy with any other aspects of your appearance, such as your face, skin, hair, nose, or the shape or size of any other body area?'
4 Ascertain that the patient is preoccupied with these perceived flaws by asking, 'How much time would you estimate that you spend each day thinking about your appearance, if you add up all the time you spend?' OR 'Do these concerns preoccupy you?'

*Criterion B: repetitive behaviours in response to the appearance concerns*

5 Ask 'Is there anything that you do over and over again in response to your appearance concerns?' … 'For example, do you compare yourself with others, check your appearance in mirrors or other reflecting surfaces, ask other people if you look okay or what they think of your appearance, touch the disliked areas, or pick at your skin?' … 'Do you do anything else to try to check, fix, hide, or be reassured about your (fill in disliked body areas)?'

*Criterion C: clinically significant distress or impairment in functioning resulting from appearance concerns*

6 Ask 'How much distress do these concerns cause you?' Ask specifically about resulting anxiety, social anxiety, depression, panic, shame, hopelessness, guilt, and suicidal thinking.
7 Ask about effects of the appearance preoccupations on the patient's life—for example, 'Do these concerns interfere with your life or cause problems for you in any way?' Ask specifically about effects on work, school, other aspects of role functioning (for example, caring for children), relationships, intimacy, family and social activities, household tasks, and other types of interference. Examples of interference include:
   - Decreased focus and concentration.
   - Being late for, or missing, school or work.
   - Interruption of school, work, or household routines by BDD rituals (for example, leaving class to check the bathroom mirror or reapply make-up).
   - Dropping or failing grades.
   - Dropping out of school.
   - Quitting a job or being fired; being unemployed.
   - Not dating.
   - Marital conflict or divorce.
   - Sexual difficulties.
   - Not seeing friends as often or at all.
   - Missing family events.
   - Turning down or avoiding social gatherings.
   - Difficulty caring for children or managing a household, going shopping, or doing chores.
   - Avoiding activities like going to the gym.
   - Using drugs or alcohol to cope with BDD.

*Criterion D: the appearance preoccupation is not better explained by concerns with body fat or weight if these symptoms meet diagnostic criteria for an eating disorder.*

Individuals who have excessive and problematic concerns with the belief that they weigh too much or that their overall body or parts of their body are too fat should be evaluated for the presence of an eating disorder (anorexia nervosa, bulimia nervosa, and binge eating disorder). If one of these disorders explains these body image concerns, then the concerns do not count towards a diagnosis of BDD.

### Questions to evaluate specifiers

*With muscle dysmorphia*

Ask 'Are you preoccupied with the idea that your body build is too small or that you're not muscular enough?'

*Insight*

Elicit a global belief about the perceived defect(s) (rather than asking about specific body areas): 'What word would you use to describe how bad all of these areas (fill in all disliked areas) look?' If the patient has difficulty choosing a word (often because of embarrassment), ask 'Some people use words like unattractive, ugly, deformed, hideous'; do you think any of these apply to you?' Then ask 'How convinced are you that these body areas look (fill in the patient's global descriptor)?'

Source: data from *Diagnostic and Statistical Manual of Mental Disorders*, Fifth Edition, DSM-5, Copyright (2013), American Psychiatric Association.

## Epidemiology

In large population-based epidemiologic samples ($n$ = 2129 to 2891), the point prevalence of BDD ranges from 1.7% to 2.9% [24]. In military and Veteran samples, BDD's point prevalence has been much higher, ranging from 11% to 15% [33, 34]. BDD also appears fairly common in cosmetic treatment settings. A prevalence of 3–15% has been reported in cosmetic dermatology outpatient settings (weighted prevalence of 9%) [24], 11% in acne dermatology clinics, and 4–29% in general outpatient dermatology settings (weighted prevalence of 11%) [27]. In general cosmetic surgery settings, the prevalence of BDD has been found to be between 6% and 53%, with a weighted prevalence of 13% [24]; in orthognathic surgery settings, the weighted prevalence is 11%. The prevalence is higher than this in rhinoplasty samples (weighted prevalence of 20%), consistent with findings that rhinoplasty is the most common surgery received by people with BDD [24].

In samples from mental health settings, the prevalence of BDD has been reported to be 8–37% in patients with OCD, 11–13% in social phobia, 26% in trichotillomania, and 14–42% in atypical major depression [24]. In psychiatric inpatient samples, the point prevalence of BDD ranges from 6% to 13% [24].

## Pathogenesis

BDD's pathogenesis is likely complex and multifactorial, involving both 'proximal' factors, such as aberrant visual processing, as well as 'distal' factors, such as genetic predisposition, and perhaps evolutionary influences—for example, physical appearance judgements, such as those involving symmetry, are relevant to efforts to attract and secure reproductively healthy mates [35]. BDD likely involves a complex interplay of genetic and environmental risk factors [36].

BDD appears to be familial [36]. It also appears to have high familiality with OCD. For example, BDD is more common in first-degree relatives of individuals with OCD than in first-degree relatives of probands without OCD [36]. A family history study determined that 7% of BDD patients had a first-degree relative with OCD, which is elevated, compared to OCD's prevalence in the general population (about 1–2%) [36].

Twin studies, which can determine the relative contribution of genetic vs environmental factors, indicated that approximately 44% of the variance of 'dysmorphic concern' (a construct similar to BDD) is due to genetic factors [37]. BDD appears to have shared genetic liability with OCD and other obsessive–compulsive and related disorders, as well as unique disorder-specific genetic factors. Preliminary data indicate an association of the $GABA_A$-$\gamma2$ gene with BDD [38, 40].

Environmental influences for BDD and other obsessive–compulsive and related disorders appear largely disorder-specific [37]. Little is known about specific environmental risk factors in BDD, but they may include perceived childhood neglect and/or abuse, teasing, and low parental warmth [2, 3]. A role is also likely for sociocultural pressures [2, 3].

Research on BDD's neurocircuitry is still limited, but increasing, and indicates that there is likely a complex interplay of dysfunction in several neural systems [36]. Structural and functional neuroimaging studies demonstrate abnormalities within regions of the brain involved in visual processing, the limbic system (that is, the amygdala), and the orbitofrontal cortex, in addition to broadly observed changes in the white matter [36]. Findings of hyperactivity in the orbitofrontal cortex and the caudate are similar to findings in OCD [36].

Neuropsychological and neuroimaging studies indicated a tendency to focus on isolated details of visual and verbal stimuli, rather than more global, configurational attributes [39]—consistent with clinical observations that patients selectively attend to specific aspects of their appearance or minor flaws. Cognitive processing studies indicate that BDD patients tend to misinterpret ambiguous social (and other) situations as threatening and misinterpret self-referent facial expressions as contemptuous and angry [16, 17]. It can be theorized that these interpretive biases may combine with rejection sensitivity, perfectionism, and a focus on aesthetics to contribute to BDD's development [2, 3]. High neuroticism and low extroversion may also play a role [2, 3]. Many potential risk factors (for example, neuroticism) are not specific to BDD, but the overall combination of risk factors may be.

## Course and prognosis

Prospective and retrospective studies of individuals ascertained for BDD indicated that BDD is usually chronic [19, 40]. Greater severity of BDD symptoms predicts a lower likelihood of remission from BDD and a greater likelihood of relapse following remission. A longer duration of BDD also predicts a lower probability of remission [40]. However, when BDD is accurately identified and its treatment optimized, the prognosis is much more favourable.

## Treatment

BDD's treatment is described in more detail elsewhere, including in a guideline from the UK's National Institute of Health and Care Excellence (NICE) [41–43]. Serotonin reuptake inhibitors (SRIs, or SSRIs) and CBT that is specifically tailored to BDD are currently recommended as first-line treatments [41–43]. Cosmetic treatment appears ineffective for BDD [43]. Treatment studies are still limited, and more research and treatment development are needed. However, available data consistently indicate that a majority of patients improve with these treatments [41–43].

### Essential groundwork for treatment

It can be challenging to engage and retain patients with BDD in psychiatric treatment. Most have poor or absent insight, believing that they probably or certainly look abnormal. For this reason, many prefer cosmetic treatment. Depressive symptoms may cause hopelessness and decrease motivation for treatment. A number of approaches can help clinicians engage and retain patients in treatment, which are discussed in more detail elsewhere [44]:

1. First try to engage the patient and establish an alliance, so they are willing to try treatment. This can be difficult to accomplish, as many patients are delusional, prefer cosmetic treatment, are

rejection-sensitive, and do not want other people (including a clinician) to see them.

2. Empathize with the patient's suffering.

3. Take the patient's appearance concerns seriously, neither dismissing their concerns about how they look nor agreeing that there is something wrong with their appearance. Avoid debating or arguing with the patient about how they look. Trying to convince patients (especially delusional patients) that their beliefs are irrational or that they look normal is usually not helpful. It can be helpful to say that people with BDD see themselves differently than others see them and to note the findings from visual processing studies.

4. Instead, focus on the potential for psychiatric treatment to diminish their distress and preoccupation and improve their functioning and quality of life.

5. Provide psychoeducation about BDD and recommend reading.

6. For patients who wish to pursue cosmetic treatments, explain that such treatment appears ineffective for BDD.

7. Provide education about recommended treatments. It can be helpful to explain, for example, that SRIs are usually well tolerated, are not habit-forming, appear to normalize the brain (and do not cause brain damage), and often diminish suicidal thinking in people with BDD. CBT is a practical and doable 'here-and-now' treatment, in which patients actively collaborate with the therapist and learn helpful skills by attending sessions and doing homework. When patients fully adhere to, and participate in, these treatments, a majority will improve.

Treatment should be initiated with an SRI and/or CBT. SRIs are also the first-line medication for delusional BDD. All severely ill patients, especially those who are highly suicidal, should, in the authors' opinion, receive an SRI. Patients with severe comorbid depression also warrant SRI treatment. Other comorbidity may warrant additional medication.

### Surgical, dermatologic, and other cosmetic treatment

A majority of patients with BDD seek and receive often costly cosmetic treatment [3, 8, 9, 12, 26]. Some patients, including those who are turned down by physicians or cannot afford treatment, perform their own surgery [2, 3, 6]—for example, cutting open their nose with a razor blade and trying to replace their nose cartilage with chicken cartilage in the desired shape. Dermatologists and surgeons are most often consulted, but cosmetic treatment may be requested of virtually any type of physician. It appears that most BDD patients are dissatisfied with such treatment [2, 3, 26] and that cosmetic treatment is not effective for BDD. Occasional dissatisfied patients sue, or are violent towards, the physician. Thus, cosmetic treatment is not recommended for BDD.

### Pharmacotherapy and other somatic treatments

#### Serotonin reuptake inhibitors: first-line pharmacotherapy for BDD

All SRI studies to date indicate that SRIs are often efficacious for BDD [2, 3, 41] (Table 100.1). These studies include a placebo-controlled fluoxetine study ($n = 67$), a controlled and blinded crossover study comparing the SRI clomipramine to the non-SRI desipramine ($n = 29$), and open-label trials of fluvoxamine, citalopram, and escitalopram ($n = 15$–30). In these studies, 53–73% of patients responded to the SRI in intention-to-treat analyses (response rates were higher in completer analyses). The crossover trial found greater efficacy for clomipramine than desipramine, suggesting that SRIs are more efficacious than non-SRIs for BDD. This important finding is consistent with clinical series and retrospective data suggesting that SRIs are more efficacious than a broad range of non-SRI medications for BDD [2, 3, 41].

A more recent relapse prevention study treated 100 participants for 14 weeks with the SRI escitalopram (mean dose $26.2 \pm 7.2$ mg/day), with an intention-to-treat response rate of 67% and a completer response rate of 81% (Table 100.1) [45]. Escitalopram responders were randomized to continuing to take escitalopram or were switched to placebo treatment for another 6 months. Time to relapse was significantly longer among patients who continued to receive escitalopram. The proportion who relapsed while continuing escitalopram was 18%, whereas 40% relapsed after being switched to placebo. Thus, continuation of escitalopram protected against relapse.

No methodologically rigorous prospective study has compared different SRIs to one another, although they are likely all about equally efficacious. The second author often first uses escitalopram or fluoxetine; these are the best studied SRIs for BDD and are usually well tolerated, and escitalopram has the advantage of having few drug–drug interactions. Clomipramine is often reserved for use when selective SRIs (SSRIs) have not been helpful, because SSRIs are usually better tolerated. Citalopram is the least desirable choice, because the FDA dosing limit is lower than the dose typically needed to effectively treat BDD [41].

High SRI doses (higher than typically used for depression) appear to often be needed to effectively treat BDD [2, 3, 41]. Doses may sometimes need to exceed the manufacturer's maximum dose, although this is not recommended for clomipramine or citalopram. Response to an SRI usually develops gradually and may require up to 12–16 weeks of treatment (while reaching a relatively high dose) to be evident [2, 3, 41].

Response to medication usually includes a decrease in appearance preoccupations, distress, and compulsive/safety behaviours, as well as improved functioning. Suicidality, depressive symptoms, anxiety, and anger–hostility often improve [2, 3]. Of note, delusional patients often improve with SRI monotherapy, whereas limited data suggest that dopamine antagonist monotherapy is usually *ineffective* for delusional BDD [2, 3, 41]. Thus, SRIs are recommended for patients with delusional (absent insight) BDD beliefs.

If an optimal 12- to 16-week SRI trial—during which a high SRI dose is reached if needed and tolerated—improves BDD symptoms by at least 30%, it is recommended that the SRI be continued, because BDD symptoms may further improve with additional time [41].

#### Approaches if an SRI is not adequately effective

Before concluding that an SRI is ineffective, it should be tried for 12–16 weeks, reaching the highest dose recommended by the manufacturer or tolerated by the patient (if necessary) for at least 3–4 of those 12–16 weeks. Because medication adherence is often poor, the clinician should determine whether medication adherence has

**Table 100.1** Prospective controlled and open-label medication studies in adults with body dysmorphic disorder[*]

| Medication | Study design | Sample size | Trial duration and endpoint mean dose (mg/day) | Response of BDD symptoms[**] | Reference |
|---|---|---|---|---|---|
| **Serotonin reuptake inhibitor (SRI, SSRI) monotherapy** | | | | | |
| Fluoxetine (Prozac®) vs placebo | Randomized, double-blind, placebo-controlled, parallel group trial | 74 enrolled; 67 randomized | 12 weeks: 77.7 ± 8.0 | Fluoxetine significantly more effective than placebo; response rate of 53% vs 18% on BDD-YBOCS; effect size d = 0.70 | Phillips KA, et al., 2002 [60] |
| Clomipramine (Anafranil®) vs desipramine | Randomized, double-blind, controlled crossover trial | 40 enrolled; 29 randomized | 16 weeks (8 weeks on each medication) CMI: 138 ± 87 DMI: 147 ± 80 | Clomipramine significantly more effective than desipramine; response rate of 65% vs 35% on BDD-YBOCS | Hollander E, et al., 1999 [61] |
| Escitalopram (Lexapro®) vs placebo | Open-label trial with escitalopram; responders to open-label treatment were randomized to double-blind continuation treatment with escitalopram vs placebo for 6 months | 100 in open-label phase; 58 in double-blind phase | 14-week open-label phase: 26.2 ± 7.2 6-month randomized phase: 28.7 ± 4.6 | Open-label trial: BDD symptoms significantly improved; 67% of subjects (intention-to-treat) and 81% of completers responded on BDD-YBOCS Time to relapse significantly longer with escitalopram than placebo Relapse proportions: 18% for escitalopram vs 40% for placebo In continuation phase, BDD significantly improved in escitalopram-treated subjects; 36% of subjects further improved | Phillips KA, et al., 2016 [45] |
| Fluvoxamine (Luvox®) | Open-label trial | 15 | 10 weeks: 208.3 ± 63.4 | BDD symptoms significantly improved; ten subjects responded on CGI | Perugi G, et al., 1996 [62] |
| Fluvoxamine (Luvox®) | Open-label trial | 30 | 16 weeks: 238.3 ± 85.8 | BDD symptoms significantly improved; 63% of subjects responded on BDD-YBOCS | Phillips KA, et al., 1998 |
| Citalopram (Celexa®) | Open-label trial | 15 | 12 weeks: 51.3 ± 16.9 | BDD symptoms significantly improved; 73% of subjects responded on BDD-YBOCS | Phillips KA & Najjar F, 2003 [63] |
| Escitalopram (Lexapro®) | Open-label trial | 15 | 12 weeks: 28.0 ± 6.5 | BDD symptoms significantly improved; 73% of subjects responded on BDD-YBOCS | Phillips KA, 2006 [64] |
| **Serotonin–noradrenaline reuptake inhibitor (SNRI) monotherapy** | | | | | |
| Venlafaxine (Effexor®) | Open-label trial | 17 | 12–16 weeks: 163.6 ± 30.3 | BDD symptoms significantly improved; 45% responded on BDD-YBOCS | Allen A, et al., 2008 [65] |
| **Anti-epileptics** | | | | | |
| Levetiracetam (Keppra®) | Open-label trial | 17 (monotherapy in 12 cases; SRI augmentation in five cases) | 12 weeks: 2044 ± 1065 | BDD symptoms significantly improved; 53% responded on BDD-YBOCS | Phillips KA & Menard W, 2009 [66] |
| **SRI augmentation studies** | | | | | |
| Pimozide (Orap®) vs placebo augmentation of fluoxetine (Prozac®) | Randomized, double-blind, placebo-controlled, parallel-group trial | 28 | 8 weeks: 2 mg | Pimozide was not more efficacious than placebo; 18% of subjects responded to pimozide and 18% to placebo | Phillips KA, 2005 [67] |

[*] Case reports, case series, cross-sectional, and retrospective studies are not included in the table but are described in the text.

[**] Results are reported for an intention-to-treat analysis, except for the clomipramine/desipramine trial, which used a minimum treatment analysis, and the venlafaxine study, which used a completer analysis for the primary outcome. Intention-to-treat analyses are more conservative because they include study dropouts; response rates for those who completed the full trial (intention-to-treat sample) are higher than reported in this table.

Most studies defined response as 30% or greater decrease in total score on the Yale-Brown Obsessive Compulsive Scale (YBOCS).

Modified for body dysmorphic disorder (BDD-YBOCS). Other symptoms, such as depression, usually improved, as did psychosocial functioning and quality of life.

been adequate; improving adherence may convert medication non-response to response.

As a next step, the second author often raises the SRI dose even further until the following maximum doses are reached if tolerated: escitalopram 60 mg/day, fluoxetine 120 mg/day, sertraline 400 mg/day, fluvoxamine 450 mg/day, paroxetine 100 mg/day, citalopram 40 mg/day, and clomipramine 250 mg/day (with blood levels). It is recommended that an ECG be checked at a higher escitalopram dose and when using clomipramine. These doses are consistent with those in the American Psychiatric Practice Guideline for OCD [46].

If this approach does not produce the desired response, another SRI can be tried, as this may lead to a response [2, 3, 41].

Regarding SRI augmentation, a small double-blind randomized controlled trial found that the antipsychotic pimozide was not more efficacious than placebo as a fluoxetine augmenter [2, 3, 41]. However, clinical observations suggest that other dopaminergic drugs, such as aripiprazole, may be helpful as SRI augmenters and may be especially appealing for patients who are highly delusional, agitated, anxious, and/or aggressive. Clinical series suggest that augmentation of an SSRI with buspirone or clomipramine may be helpful [2, 3, 41]. (SSRIs may increase clomipramine blood levels, however, which may cause toxicity; thus, if this approach is tried, clomipramine should be started at a very low dose, with monitoring of levels.) Clinical observations suggest that SSRI augmentation with venlafaxine or bupropion may be helpful for some patients [2, 3, 41]. SRIs can also be augmented with CBT. No studies have evaluated the relative efficacy of these approaches, although clinical experience indicates that all of them may be effective.

### Monotherapy with non-SRI medications

Monotherapy with agents other than SRIs has not been well studied [2, 3, 41]. A small open-label trial ($n = 11$) suggested that the serotonin–noradrenaline reuptake inhibitor (SNRI) venlafaxine may be efficacious [2, 3]. Another small open-label trial ($n = 17$) suggested efficacy for the anti-epileptic levetiracetam [41]. For severe and treatment-refractory cases, an MAO inhibitor may be worth trying (but should never be combined with an SRI).

It appears that long-term treatment with effective medication may be needed; efficacy appears to usually be sustained over time [2, 3, 41]. For patients who appear at high risk of suicide or violence, lifelong treatment with an effective SRI is recommended, as suicides have been known to occur after SRI discontinuation.

### Other somatic treatments

Available case series and case reports, while very limited, suggested that ECT is generally ineffective for BDD and secondary depressive symptoms [2, 3, 41], although it should be considered for severely depressed and highly suicidal patients.

Improvement in BDD symptoms has been noted in case reports with a modified leucotomy, capsulotomy, bilateral anterior cingulotomy plus subcaudate tractotomy, and anterior capsulotomy, and with deep brain stimulation that targeted the ventral capsule/ventral striatum. Neurosurgery should be considered only when a patient has not responded to many adequate medication trials and to intensive CBT using an empirically based treatment manual for BDD.

## Cognitive behavioural therapy

### Research findings on CBT for BDD

In recent years, great strides have been made in understanding the cognitive behavioural processes that contribute to BDD's development and maintenance. CBT for BDD that is based on this theoretical understanding is highly effective in reducing BDD symptom severity, as well as associated symptoms [47].

In an initial small randomized controlled trial of 19 individuals with BDD who were randomized to 12 sessions of CBT or a waitlist control, the CBT group showed significantly greater improvement in BDD symptoms and depressive symptoms [48]. Another randomized controlled trial of 12 sessions of CBT, compared to an anxiety management treatment, for 46 individuals with BDD found that the CBT group showed significantly greater improvement in BDD symptoms than the anxiety management group [49]. A study of a modular 22-week CBT treatment for BDD vs a 12-week waitlist condition (followed by crossover to CBT) for 36 individuals with BDD showed that 50% of those who participated in CBT responded to CBT, compared to 12% in the control group, at week 12, a significant difference [50]. After 22 weeks of treatment, 81% of all participants (immediate treatment group plus waitlisted patients subsequently treated with CBT) who completed treatment were responders. A meta-analysis also showed that CBT is associated with more improvement in BDD symptoms than a waitlist or psychological placebo [51], resulting in a reduction in BDD symptoms, depressive symptoms, and improvement in insight and delusionality [51]. Improvement appears to be sustained over months, and even years [47, 52].

### Elements of CBT for BDD

CBT must be tailored to BDD's unique symptoms; in the authors' experience, CBT for OCD, social anxiety disorder, or other disorders will not adequately treat BDD. The authors recommend use of an empirically based CBT treatment manual, because BDD is a complex disorder that can be difficult to treat without a manual. Two such therapist manuals are available [53, 54].

Many experts recommend weekly hour-long outpatient sessions for 6 months, although some patients improve with fewer sessions and others require longer or more intensive treatment in an intensive outpatient or residential treatment setting.

CBT for BDD typically includes [53, 54]: (1) *cognitive restructuring* to identify cognitive errors and develop more accurate and helpful BDD-related thoughts and beliefs; (2) *exposure* to avoided situations (for example, leaving the house, attending social gatherings), combined with *behavioural experiments* to test the accuracy of BDD beliefs; (3) *ritual (response) prevention* to decrease or stop compulsive behaviours (for example, stopping excessive mirror checking, limiting grooming time); (4) *advanced cognitive strategies* to address maladaptive core beliefs; (5) *perceptual retraining and mindfulness*, which involves learning to see one's entire body in a non-judgemental and 'holistic' way (rather than focusing on disliked areas), while refraining from excessive mirror checking; and (6) *relapse prevention*.

One of the previously noted empirically supported treatment manuals includes the following optional modules for patients with relevant symptoms [53]: (1) *skin picking and hair pulling or plucking*; (2) *muscularity and weight/shape concerns*; (3) *cosmetic treatment*; and (4) *depression/mood management*. *Motivational interviewing* is often needed to engage and keep patients in treatment and may be used any time during treatment as needed.

Patients who are not improving with CBT may need motivational interviewing to increase engagement in treatment and homework completion, more frequent sessions, longer sessions, or a change in the current CBT focus. Maintenance/booster sessions following CBT may reduce relapse risk. It may be helpful to add an SRI to CBT if CBT alone is insufficient or the patient is too depressed to participate in CBT.

## Additional treatment considerations

### Therapy and support

Only limited research has been conducted on third-wave therapies, like acceptance and commitment therapy (ACT), although preliminary evidence from one small study is promising [55]. Clinical experience suggests that concomitant insight-oriented or supportive therapy—in addition to an SRI and/or CBT—may help some patients cope with their illness or with co-occurring problems or disorders [2, 3]. Families can be an invaluable support and facilitate treatment [2, 3]. Mental health professionals may need to interface with dermatologists, plastic surgeons, and other physicians from whom patients have requested or are receiving cosmetic treatment.

### Suicidality

Treatment approaches for more highly suicidal patients are discussed in more detail elsewhere [54]. Such patients should always receive an SRI, which has been shown to decrease suicidal thinking and protect against worsening of suicidal ideation in BDD [56]. Concomitant medication may also be helpful, depending on the patient's specific symptoms. The authors also recommend CBT for BDD if BDD appears to be the main cause of suicidal thinking. For highly suicidal patients, we recommend the use of an evidence-based CBT treatment manual that focuses on suicidal thinking [57]. Supportive therapy may be additionally helpful, depending on the patient's specific situation, and a higher level of care may be needed.

### Substance use

Substance abuse is common in individuals with BDD and often reflects attempts to self-medicate BDD-induced distress [58]. In such cases, successful treatment of BDD may reduce or eliminate problematic substance use. However, substance abuse often needs to be a major focus of treatment, using evidence-based medication (for example, naltrexone) and psychosocial treatment approaches for substance abuse, in addition to treatment for BDD.

## Conclusions

BDD is a common, but under-recognized, disorder that is often severely impairing and can lead to suicide. Research and knowledge of BDD are greatly increasing, but more research is necessary to better understand the features of this disorder and increase education, so clinicians recognize this disorder and implement recommended treatment. SRIs and CBT for BDD often improve BDD symptoms and associated symptoms such as depression, anxiety, and poor or absent insight. Clinicians should specifically screen patients for BDD in order to recognize this common disorder and provide effective treatment.

## Further information

Further information about BDD and its treatment is provided in references [2–4], [43], [53–54], and [59].

## REFERENCES

1. Morselli E. Sulla dysmorphophobia e sulla tafefobia. *Bolletinno della Raccademia di Genova.* 1891; 6: 110–19.
2. Phillips KA. *The Broken Mirror: Understanding and Treating Body Dysmorphic Disorder.* New York, NY: Oxford University Press; 2005. Revised and expanded edition, 2005.
3. Phillips KA. *Understanding Body Dysmorphic Disorder: An Essential Guide.* New York, NY: Oxford University Press; 2009.
4. American Psychiatric Association. *Diagnostic and Statistical Manual of Mental Disorders,* 5th edn. Washington, DC: American Psychiatric Association; 2013.
5. Stein DJ, Kogan CS, Atmaca M, *et al.* The classification of obsessive-compulsive and related disorders in the ICD-11. *J Affect Disord.* 2016; 190: 663–74.
6. Phillips KA, Menard W, Fay C, Pagano ME. Psychosocial functioning and quality of life in body dysmorphic disorder. *Compr Psychiatry.* 2005; 46: 254–60.
7. Phillips KA, Menard W, Fay C, Weisberg R. Demographic characteristics, phenomenology, comorbidity, and family history in 200 individuals with body dysmorphic disorder. *Psychosomatics.* 2005; 46: 317–25.
8. Phillips KA, Coles M, Menard W, *et al.* Suicidal ideation and suicide attempts in body dysmorphic disorder. *J Clin Psychiatry.* 2005; 66: 717–25.
9. Phillips KA, McElroy SL, Keck PE Jr, *et al.* Body dysmorphic disorder: 30 cases of imagined ugliness. *Am J Psychiatry.* 1993; 150: 302–8.
10. Didie ER, Tortolani C, Walters M, Menard W., Fay C., Phillips KA. Social functioning in body dysmorphic disorder: assessment considerations. *Psychiatr Q.* 2006; 77: 223–9.
11. Simmons RA, Phillips KA. Core clinical features of body dysmorphic disorder: appearance preoccupations, negative emotions, core beliefs, and repetitive and avoidance behaviors. In: Phillips KA, editor. *Body Dysmorphic Disorder: Advances in Research and Clinical Practice.* New York, NY: Oxford University Press; 2017. pp. 61–80.
12. Pope HG, Gruber AJ, Choi P, *et al.* Muscle dysmorphia: an underrecognized form of body dysmorphic disorder. *Psychosomatics.* 1997; 38: 548–57.
13. Sreshta N, Pope HG, Hudson JI, M.D, Kanayama G. Muscle dysmorphia. In: Phillips KA, editor. *Body Dysmorphic Disorder: Advances in Research and Clinical Practice.* New York, NY: Oxford University Press; 2017. pp. 81–94.
14. Eisen JL, Phillips KA, Coles ME, Rasmussen SA. Insight in obsessive-compulsive disorder and body dysmorphic disorder. *Compr Psychiatry.* 2004; 45: 10–15.
15. Phillips KA, Menard W, Pagano M, Fay C, Stout RL. Delusional versus nondelusional body dysmorphic disorder: clinical features and course of illness. *J Psychiatr Res.* 2006; 40: 95–104.
16. Buhlmann U, Etcoff NL, Wilhelm S. Emotion recognition bias for contempt and anger in body dysmorphic disorder. *J Psychiatr Res.* 2006; 40: 105–11.
17. Buhlmann U, Wilhelm S, McNally RJ, *et al.* Interpretive biases for ambiguous information in body dysmorphic disorder. *CNS Spectr.* 2002; 7: 435–6, 441–3.
18. Didie ER, Menard W, Stern AP, Phillips KA. Occupational functioning and impairment in adults with body dysmorphic disorder. *Compr Psychiatry.* 2008; 49: 561–9.
19. Phillips KA, Diaz S. Gender differences in body dysmorphic disorder. *J Nerv Ment Dis.* 1997; 185: 570–7.

20. Phillips KA, Didie ER, Menard W, *et al*. Clinical features of body dysmorphic disorder in adolescents and adults. *Psychiatry Res.* 2006; 141: 305–14.

21. Phillips KA, Quinn G, Stout RL. Functional impairment in body dysmorphic disorder: a prospective, follow-up study. *J Psychiatr Res.* 2008; 42: 701–7.

22. Albertini RS, Phillips KA. Thirty-three cases of body dysmorphic disorder in children and adolescents. *J Am Acad Child Adolesc Psychiatry.* 1999; 38: 453–9.

23. Phillips KA, Didie ER, Pagano M, Fay C, Menard W. A comparison of body dysmorphic disorder in adults versus adolescents. *Psychiatry Res.* 2006; 141: 305–14.

24. Hartmann AS, Buhlmann. Prevalence and underrecognition of Body dysmorphic disorder. In: Phillips KA, editor. *Body Dysmorphic Disorder: Advances in Research and Clinical Practice.* New York, NY: Oxford University Press; 2017. pp. 49–60.

25. Phillips KA. Suicidality and aggressive behavior in body dysmorphic disorder. In: Phillips KA, editor. *Body Dysmorphic Disorder: Advances in Research and Clinical Practice.* New York, NY: Oxford University Press; 2017. pp. 155–72.

26. Hart AS, Niemiec MA. Comorbidity and personality in body dysmorphic disorder. In: Phillips KA, editor. *Body Dysmorphic Disorder: Advances in Research and Clinical Practice.* New York, NY: Oxford University Press; 2017. pp. 125–38.

27. Veale D, Gledhill LJ, Christodoulou P, Hodsoll J. Body dysmorphic disorder in different settings: a systematic review and estimated weighted prevalence. *Body Image.* 216; 18: 168–86.

28. Perugi G, Akiskal HS, Giannotti D, *et al*. Gender-related differences in body dysmorphic disorder (dysmorphophobia). *J Nerv Ment Dis.* 1997; 185, 578–82.

29. Phillips KA, Menard W, Fay C (2006). Gender similarities and differences in 200 individuals with body dysmorphic disorder. *Compr Psychiatry* 2006; 47: 77–87.

30. Phillips KA. Body dysmorphic disorder in children and adolescents. In: Phillips KA, editor. *Body Dysmorphic Disorder: Advances in Research and Clinical Practice.* New York, NY: Oxford University Press; 2017. pp. 173–86.

31. Suzuki K, Takei N, Kawai M, *et al*. Is taijin kyofusho a culture-bound syndrome? *Am J Psychiatry.* 2003; 160: 1358.

32. Phillips KA, Menard W, Bjornsson AS. Cued panic attacks in body dysmorphic disorder. *J Psychiatr Pract.* 2013; 19: 194–203.

33. Kelly MM, Zhang J, Phillips KA. The prevalence of body dysmorphic disorder and its clinical correlates in a VA primary care behavioral health clinic. *Psychiatry Res.* 2015; 228: 162–5.

34. Campagna JD, Bowsher B. Prevalence of body dysmorphic disorder and muscle dysmorphia among entry-level military personnel. *Mil Med.* 2016; 181: 494–501.

35. Stein D. Evolutionary psychiatry and body dysmorphic disorder. In: Phillips KA, editor. *Body Dysmorphic Disorder: Advances in Research and Clinical Practice.* New York, NY: Oxford University Press; 2017. pp. 243–52.

36. McCurdy-McKinnon D, Feusner JD. Neurobiology of body dysmorphic disorder: heritability/genetics, brain circuitry, and visual processing. In: Phillips KA, editor. *Body Dysmorphic Disorder: Advances in Research and Clinical Practice.* New York, NY: Oxford University Press; 2017. pp. 253–76.

37. Monzani B, Rijsdijk F, Anson M, *et al*. A twin study of body dysmorphic concerns. *Psychol Med.* 2012; 42: 1949–55.

38. Monzani B, Rijsdijk F, Harris J, Mataix-Cols D. The structure of genetic and environmental risk factors for dimensional representations of DSM-5 obsessive-compulsive spectrum disorders. *JAMA Psychiatry.* 2014; 71: 182–9.

39. Deckersbach T, Savage CR, Phillips KA, *et al*. Characteristics of memory dysfunction in body dysmorphic disorder. *J Int Neuropsychol Soc.* 2000; 6: 673–81.

40. Phillips K, Menard W, Quinn E, Didie E, Stout R. A 4-year prospective observational follow-up study of course and predictors of course in body dysmorphic disorder. *Psychol Med.* 2013; 43: 1109–17.

41. Phillips KA. Pharmacotherapy and other somatic treatments for body dysmorphic disorder. In: Phillips KA, editor. *Body Dysmorphic Disorder: Advances in Research and Clinical Practice.* New York, NY: Oxford University Press; 2017. pp. 333–56.

42. Rasmussen J, Gomez AF, Wilhelm S. Cognitive-behavioral therapy for body dysmorphic disorder. In: Phillips KA, editor. *Body Dysmorphic Disorder: Advances in Research and Clinical Practice.* New York, NY: Oxford University Press; 2017. pp. 357–78.

43. Phillips KA. Body dysmorphic disorder: Treatment and prognosis. *UpToDate*, 2016.

44. Veale D, Phillips KA, Neziroglu F. Challenges in assessing and treating patients with body dysmorphic disorder and recommended approaches. In: Phillips KA, editor. *Body Dysmorphic Disorder: Advances in Research and Clinical Practice.* New York, NY: Oxford University Press; 2017. pp. 313–32.

45. Phillips KA, Keshaviah A, Dougherty DD, *et al*. Pharmacotherapy relapse prevention in body dysmorphic disorder: a double-blind placebo-controlled trial. *Am J Psychiatry.* 2016;173:887–95.

46. American Psychiatric Association. *Practice Guideline for the Treatment of Patients with Obsessive-compulsive Disorder.* Washington, DC: American Psychiatric Association; 2007.

47. Rasmussen J, Gomez, AF, Wilhelm S. Cognitive-behavioral therapy for body dysmorphic disorder. In: Phillips KA, editor. *Body Dysmorphic Disorder: Advances in Research and Clinical Practice.* New York, NY: Oxford University Press; 2017. pp. 357–78.

48. Veale D, Gournay K, Dryden W, *et al*. Body dysmorphic disorder: a cognitive behavioural model and pilot randomised controlled trial. *Behav Res Ther.* 1996; 34: 717–29.

49. Veale D, Anson M, Miles S, *et al*. Efficacy of cognitive behaviour therapy versus anxiety management for body dysmorphic disorder: a randomised controlled trial. *Psychother Psychosom.* 2014; 83: 341–53.

50. Wilhelm S, Phillips KA, Didie ER, *et al*. Modular cognitive-behavioral therapy for body dysmorphic disorder: a randomized controlled trial. *Behav Ther.* 2014; 45: 314–27.

51. Harrison A, Fernández de la Cruz L, Enander J, *et al*. Cognitive-behavioral therapy for body dysmorphic disorder: a systematic review and meta-analysis of randomized controlled trials. *Clin Psychol Rev.* 2016; 48: 43–51.

52. Veale D, Miles S, Anson M. Long-term outcome of cognitive behavior therapy for body dysmorphic disorder: a naturalistic case series of one to four years after a controlled trial. *Behav Ther.* 2015; 46: 775–85.

53. Wilhelm S, Phillips K, Steketee G. *A Cognitive-behavioral Treatment Manual for Body Dysmorphic Disorder.* New York, NY: Guilford; 2013.

54. Veale D, Neziroglu, F. *Body Dysmorphic Disorder: A Treatment Manual.* Chichester: Wiley-Blackwell; 2010.

55. Linde J, Rück, C, Bjureberg J, *et al.* Acceptance-based exposure therapy for body dysmorphic disorder: a pilot study. *Behav Ther.* 2015; 46: 423–31.

56. Phillips KA, Kelly MM. Suicidality in a placebo-controlled fluoxetine study of body dysmorphic disorder. *Int Clin Psychopharmacol.* 2009; 24: 26–8.

57. Wenzel A, Brown GK, Beck AT. *Cognitive Therapy for Suicidal Patients: Scientific and Clinical Applications.* Washington, DC: American Psychological Association; 2009.

58. Kelly MM, Simmons R, Wang S, *et al.* Motives to drink alcohol among individuals with body dysmorphic disorder. *J Obsessive Compuls Relat Disord.* 2017; 12: 52–7.

59. Phillips KA (editor). *Body Dysmorphic Disorder: Advances in Research and Clinical Practice.* New York, NY: Oxford University Press; 2017.

60. Phillips KA, Dwight MM, McElroy SL. Efficacy and safety of fluvoxamine in body dysmorphic disorder. *J Clin Psychiatry.* 2002; 59: 165–71.

61. Hollander E, Kwon J, Aronowitz B, et al. Clomipramine vs desipramine crossover trial in body dysmorphic disorder: selective efficacy of a serotonin reuptake inhibitor in imagined ugliness. *Arch Gen Psychiatry.* 1999; 56: 1033–9.

62. Perugi G, Giannotti D, Di Vaio S, et al. Fluvoxamine in the treatment of body dysmorphic disorder (dysmorphophobia). *Int Clin Psychopharmacol.* 1996; 11: 247–254.

63. Phillips KA, Najjar F. An open-label study of citalopram in body dysmorphic disorder. *J Clin Psychiatry.* 2003; 64: 715–720.

64. Phillips KA. An open-label study of escitalopram in body dysmorphic disorder. *Int Clin Psychopharmacol.* 2006; 21: 177–179.

65. Allen A, Hadley SJ, Kaplan A, et al. An open-label trial of venlafaxine in body dysmorphic disorder. *CNS Spectr.* 2008; 13: 138–144.

66. Phillips KA, Menard W. A prospective pilot study of levetiracetam for body dysmorphic disorder. *CNS Spect.* 2009; 14: 252–260.

67. Phillips KA. Placebo-controlled study of pimozide augmentation of fluoxetine in body dysmorphic disorder. *Am J Psychiatry.* 2005; 162: 377–379.

# SECTION 16
# Feeding , eating, and metabolic disorders

# 101

# The eating disorders

*Christopher G. Fairburn and Rebecca Murphy*

## Introduction

Eating disorders may be defined as 'a persistent disturbance of eating behaviour or behaviour intended to control weight, which significantly impairs physical health or psychosocial functioning' [1]. It is conventional to divide them into diagnostic categories, based on their clinical presentation. The three main diagnoses are anorexia nervosa, bulimia nervosa, and binge eating disorder. In addition, there are similar presentations that fall just outside these three diagnoses. We will term these the 'other eating disorders' or OEDs.

## Classification and diagnosis

The classification of eating disorders and their principal diagnostic criteria are shown in Box 101.1. Anorexia nervosa was first named and formally described in 1873 [2, 3]; the concept of bulimia nervosa was introduced in 1979 [4], and binge eating disorder was formally recognized in 2013, although the phenomenon was described in the 1950s [5]. The OEDs came to attention in the 2000s when they were encountered in large numbers with the opening of community-based eating disorder clinics [6]. The American term for OEDs used to be 'eating disorders not otherwise specified', but in DSM-5, it was changed to 'other specified feeding and eating disorders'.

Other disorders of eating are recognized. In DSM-5, these are pica, rumination disorder, and avoidant/restrictive food intake disorder. These states are quite different from the three main eating disorders and are mostly seen in children or those with intellectual disability. They are not covered in this chapter.

## General clinical features

Anorexia nervosa, bulimia nervosa, and OEDs share a common and distinctive 'core psychopathology'. This is the over-evaluation of shape and weight and their control. This psychopathology is not usually present in binge eating disorder. It is characterized by the judging of one's self-worth largely, or even exclusively, in terms of one's shape and weight and one's ability to control them. In contrast, most people judge themselves on the basis of their perceived performance in a variety domains of life, such as their performance at work, at sport, and at parenting, and the quality of their relationships.

Most features of these disorders stem from the over-evaluation and its consequences. There are repeated intense feelings of fatness, and most people either closely monitor their shape or avoid seeing it altogether. The desire to control body weight leads to persistent and strict dieting, together with other forms of extreme weight control behaviour, including self-induced vomiting, laxative misuse, and over-exercising. Strict dieting is highly impairing, as it requires a great deal of effort, often provokes anxiety, and can make socializing difficult, if not impossible. It may also lead to weight loss or binge eating, or both.

Generally, people with an eating disorder view dieting as an accomplishment, rather than a problem. It is not something that they want to change. However, in bulimia nervosa, the strict dieting is interrupted by repeated episodes of loss of control over eating, in which large amounts of food are eaten (binges). These binges are highly aversive, and as a result, they lead people to seek help. Their help-seeking is hindered, however, by the shame and secrecy that typically accompanies binge eating.

### Anorexia nervosa

In anorexia nervosa, the pursuit of weight loss is successful in that significantly low weight is achieved. In most instances, there is no true anorexia as such. The loss of weight is primarily the result of a deliberate severe and selective restriction of food intake, with foods viewed as fattening being excluded. In some people, restriction over food intake is encouraged by additional motives, including asceticism, a desire to feel 'special', and a wish to punish themselves. Self-induced vomiting and other extreme forms of weight control behaviour are practised by some. Many also engage in a driven form of over-exercising, which can also contribute to their low weight.

There is a constellation of clinical features which are a direct result of being significantly underweight and is seen in other starvation states. These features include obsessional features, low mood, irritability, impaired concentration, loss of sexual appetite, and poor sleep. Typically, these features get worse, as weight is lost, and improve with weight regain. Interest in the outside world also declines as people become underweight, with the result that most become socially withdrawn and isolated. This feature is also reversible. Some

---

**Box 101.1**  Classification and diagnosis of the eating disorders

**Definition of an eating disorder**

There is a definite disturbance of eating habits or weight control behaviour. Either this disturbance or the associated 'core psychopathology' (see text) results in clinically significant impairment of psychosocial functioning or physical health. The behavioural disturbance is not secondary to any general medical disorder or to any other psychiatric condition (for example, major depression).

**Principal diagnostic criteria**

*Anorexia nervosa*

1  Over-evaluation of shape and weight (that is, judging self-worth largely or exclusively in terms of shape and weight).

2  Active maintenance of an unduly low body weight (for example, body mass index <18·5 kg/m²).

*Bulimia nervosa*

1  Over-evaluation of shape and weight (that is, judging self-worth largely or exclusively in terms of shape and weight).

2  Recurrent binge eating (that is, recurrent episodes of uncontrolled eating in which an unusually large amount of food is eaten for the circumstances).

3  Extreme weight control behaviour (for example, strict dietary restriction, frequent self-induced vomiting, or laxative misuse).

4  The diagnostic criteria for anorexia nervosa are not met.

*Binge eating disorder*

1  Recurrent binge eating (that is, recurrent episodes of uncontrolled eating in which an unusually large amount of food is eaten for the circumstances).

2  The absence of extreme weight control behaviour (for example, strict dietary restriction, frequent self-induced vomiting, or laxative misuse).

*Other eating disorders*

Eating disorders of clinical severity that do not conform to the diagnostic criteria for anorexia nervosa, bulimia nervosa, or binge eating disorder.

---

people have times when they lose control over eating, although the amounts eaten may not be large.

### Bulimia nervosa

The main feature that distinguishes bulimia nervosa from anorexia nervosa is that attempts to restrict food intake are interrupted by repeated 'binges' (episodes of eating during which there is an accompanying sense of loss of control and an unusually large amount of food is eaten for the circumstances). The amount consumed varies greatly but is typically between 1000 and 2000 kcal. In most instances, binge eating is followed by self-induced vomiting or laxative misuse, in an attempt to avoid absorbing what has been eaten. The episodes of binge eating, together with strict dieting, result in a body weight which is generally unremarkable, providing the other obvious difference from anorexia nervosa. Depressive and anxiety features are prominent in bulimia nervosa, and as in some cases of anorexia nervosa, there is a subgroup who engage in substance misuse or self-injury, or both.

### Binge eating disorder

In binge eating disorder, there is just one primary feature. This is the occurrence of repeated episodes of binge eating. Unlike in bulimia nervosa, where the binges occur in the context of extreme attempts to diet, little or no extreme weight control behaviour is seen in binge

eating disorder. Indeed, if there is a disturbance of eating outside the binges, it is generally overeating, rather than undereating. For this reason, binge eating disorder often co-occurs with a raised body weight or frank obesity. As in bulimia nervosa, there is distress over the binge eating and accompanying shame and self-criticism.

### Other eating disorders

The OEDs are clinical states which meet the general definition of an eating disorder but do not fulfil the diagnostic criteria for any of the three specified eating disorders. They include presentations which closely resemble anorexia nervosa, bulimia nervosa, or binge eating disorder. For example, the patient's weight might be just above the diagnostic threshold for anorexia nervosa or the frequency of binge eating might not be high enough to allow a diagnosis of bulimia nervosa or binge eating disorder. Other presentations are 'mixed' in form, with features of both anorexia nervosa and bulimia nervosa being present. For instance, there may be extreme dietary restraint, pronounced over-exercising, occasional binge eating, and a low-to-normal weight. Over-evaluation of shape and weight is present in most of the OEDs, although in the early stages of the eating disorder, the focus of the over-evaluation may be primarily on maintaining strict control over eating.

## Development and course of the eating disorders

Anorexia nervosa typically starts in mid-teenage years with the onset of dietary restriction, which then proceeds to get out of control. In some instances, the disorder is short-lived and self-limiting, or only requires a brief intervention. These instances are most typical of young people. In others, the eating disorder becomes entrenched, although it is common for binge eating to develop and the weight to increase, with the result that the eating disorder evolves into bulimia nervosa. In 10–20% of people, the anorexia nervosa state persists and proves intractable [7]. This heterogeneity in the course and outcome of anorexia nervosa is often neglected in accounts of the disorder. Anorexia nervosa has been consistently found to be associated with a raised mortality rate, with the standardized mortality ratio being about 6 [8]. Most deaths are either a direct result of medical complications or due to suicide.

Bulimia nervosa has a slightly later age of onset than anorexia nervosa, although it usually starts in much the same way; indeed, in about a quarter of cases, the diagnostic criteria for anorexia nervosa are met for a time. Eventually, however, episodes of binge eating begin to interrupt the dietary self-control and, as a result, the body weight rises to normal or near-normal levels. The disorder tends to be highly self-perpetuating in the absence of effective treatment. The average length of history at presentation is about 5 years.

Little is known about the development and course of the OEDs. In many instances, they are preceded by anorexia nervosa or bulimia nervosa, in which case the current state is simply the latest expression of an enduring eating disorder.

Binge eating disorder differs from anorexia nervosa and bulimia nervosa in its course and outcome. Rather than running a persistent course, it tends to be phasic, with there being long periods free from binge eating. Indeed, there appears to be a high spontaneous remission rate, at least in the short term.

## The transdiagnostic perspective on the eating disorders

An alternative way of viewing the eating disorders is to take a 'transdiagnostic' perspective [9]. This view is based on two observations. Firstly, anorexia nervosa, bulimia nervosa, and most of the OEDs have many highly distinctive clinical features in common. These include the over-evaluation of shape and weight, a characteristic and persistent form of dieting, and a tendency to engage in extreme weight control behaviour. And secondly, patients frequently move between these diagnoses. Temporal migration between supposedly distinct mental disorders is a most unusual phenomenon outside the eating disorders, and it casts doubt over the validity of the diagnostic distinctions. However, the fact that eating disorders do not evolve into other mental disorders supports the distinctiveness of the diagnostic category as a whole.

## Acknowledgements

C.G.F. and R.M. are supported by the Wellcome Trust (grants 046386 and 094585, respectively).

## REFERENCES

1. Fairburn CG, Walsh BT. Atypical eating disorders (eating disorder not otherwise specified). In: Fairburn CG, Brownell KD (eds). *Eating Disorders and Obesity: A Comprehensive Handbook*, second edition. New York, NY: Guilford Press; 2002. pp. 171–7.
2. Gull WW. Anorexia nervosa (apepsia hysterica, anorexia hysterica). 1873. *Clin. Soc. Tr.* 1984; 7: 22.
3. Lasegue EC. On hysterical anorexia. *M. Times.* 1873; 2: 265–6.
4. Russell G. Bulimia nervosa: an ominous variant of anorexia nervosa. *Psychol. Med.* 1979; 9: 429–48.
5. Stunkard AJ. Eating patterns and obesity. *Psychiat. Quart.* 1959; 33: 284–95.
6. Fairburn CG, Bohn K. Eating disorder NOS (EDNOS): an example of the troublesome "not otherwise specified" (NOS) category in DSM-IV. *Behav. Res. Ther.* 2005; 43: 691–701.
7. Steinhausen HC. The outcome of anorexia nervosa in the 20th century. *Am. J. Psychiatry.* 2002; 159: 1284–93.
8. Arcelus J, Mitchell AJ, Wales J, Nielsen S. Mortality rates in patients with anorexia nervosa and other eating disorders. A meta-analysis of 36 studies. *Arch. Gen. Psychiatry.* 2011; 68: 724–31.
9. Fairburn CG, Cooper Z, Shafran R. Cognitive behaviour therapy for eating disorders: a "transdiagnostic" theory and treatment. *Behav. Res. Ther.* 2003; 41: 509–28.

# 102

# Basic mechanisms and potential for treatment of weight and eating disorders

*Johannes Hebebrand, Jochen Antel, and Beate Herpertz-Dahlmann*

## Introduction

In light of the current difficulties in treating feeding, eating, and weight disorders, the overall pragmatic goal is to find novel portals of entry for successful pharmacological and non-pharmacological interventions that prove superior to those currently pursued in terms of both efficacy and safety. The ongoing elucidation of the basic mechanisms underlying feeding, eating, and, in particular, weight disorders, should ideally help to develop novel treatments. However, similar to other mental disorders or complex disorders per se, the sheer number of aetiological factors, their proven and assumed small effect sizes, and their complex interactions render this a formidable task. In addition, side effects of weight loss medications have led to the withdrawal of anti-obesity drugs, which, in turn, has reduced research investment of the pharmaceutical industry.

Because of the association of specific eating disorders with different body weight categories and the obvious clinical relevance of underweight in both anorexia nervosa (AN) and avoidant restrictive food intake disorder (ARFID) and obesity in binge eating disorder (BED), one potential avenue is to focus jointly on body weight and the specific eating disorder symptomatology. Both obesity and AN have been viewed as representing behavioural addictions [1, 2]; accordingly, consideration of a treatment strategy in accordance with an addiction hypothesis is also warranted. Alterations of the microbiome have been detected in patients with AN and obesity; in animal models, evidence has accumulated that body weight can be influenced by altering the microbiome.

## The key conundrum: would patients with eating and weight disorders take a pill to restore their health?

Health care professionals are keenly aware of the hesitancy of patients with AN to readily embark on treatment schemes. In some ways, this hesitancy is similar to that observed for a substantial subgroup—if not even the majority—of patients with obesity. To gain weight or lose weight requires commitment over an extended period of time—and even then, success is by no means guaranteed; in both AN and obesity, patients have difficulties in maintaining their achieved weights. For eating and weight disorders, dropouts and lost-to-follow-ups are frequent in clinical trials [3–5], indirectly signalling that patients are unable to adhere to, or are not content with, the currently available treatment regimens.

Indeed, conventional treatment schemes do not result in quick remedies. Eating disorders, and AN in particular, run a protracted course with persistent symptoms. The mean body weight of patients remains skewed—albeit to a not as extreme extent—towards the left (underweight) side of the distribution, even after recovery from full-blown AN [6, 7]. Recent evidence now links genetic factors involved in AN to constitutional underweight [8, 9], as was already suggested over 20 years ago [10]. Obesity in adolescence or adulthood seems to be even more difficult to overcome. Thus, a meta-analysis based on behavioural intervention trials focusing on both diet and physical activity and encompassing almost 3000 adults resulted in an average difference of –1.56 kg (95% confidence interval –2.27 to –0.86 kg) at 12 months, in comparison to controls [11], which is a rather marginal effect size.

Subgroups of individuals with AN or obesity reject a patient status. Instead exceedingly low or high weight is perceived as being within the 'normal' range of the body weight distribution. Thus, the mission of the National Association to Advance Fat Acceptance [12] is 'to eliminate discrimination based on body size and provide fat people with the tools for self-empowerment though public education, advocacy, and support'. Similarly, 'it's not a diet, it's a lifestyle' is a slogan referenced in MyProAna [13]. Obviously, health care professionals are also aware of patients with eating disorders or obesity who do suffer and seek treatment. In part, this suffering is driven by comorbid somatic and/or mood disorders.

Accordingly, it is difficult to predict the extent to which patients with eating and weight disorders would indeed take a pill to overcome their disorder. Apart from ego-syntonicity, comorbidity, cultural influences, and lay beliefs, efficacy and safety represent key determinants. In addition, if the disorder, in itself, in some way has a rewarding effect, treatment-induced removal of such an effect could also influence acceptability.

## Energy homeostasis and body weight categories

A stable body weight results from a balance between energy intake and expenditure. Energy intake is a complex phenomenon which largely depends on internal (including emotional), social, time, and environmental cues to eat, feelings of appetite/hunger, food and beverage preferences, alcohol, tobacco and drug use, medication, and conscious efforts to influence eating behaviour. In sedentary individuals, total energy expenditure is determined as approximately 70% by resting energy expenditure (REE) largely accounted for by muscle and organ mass. The remaining 30% is accounted for by the thermogenic effect of food (the energy used to absorb, digest, and store nutrients) and activity subdivided into regular physical activity and non-exercise activity thermogenesis (NEAT) as in fidgeting [14].

This highly complex regulatory system has evolved to defend the individual against loss of body weight (fat and fat-free mass) and to allow adaptation to starvation [15–17]. Both intermittent experimental overfeeding and caloric restriction entail counter-regulatory adaptations of energy expenditure; upon cessation of such experiments, the body weight of participants frequently returns to the pre-intervention level. However, the recent obesity pandemic illustrates that the human organism is not well protected from the development of high body weight. In contrast, the signalling network to allow adaptation to hunger and starvation is extensive, because food supplies have repeatedly been scant during evolution.

Adult body weight categories are sub-classified according to body mass index (BMI) (Table 102.1) [18]. In healthy underweight (BMI <18.5 kg/m²) subjects, whose BMI is below the weight criterion threshold for AN, a long-standing history of underweight is the rule. Intermittent substantial weight loss is not observed, although weight loss may occur during stressful life events; furthermore, a family history of underweight and the virtual absence of obesity in first-degree relatives are common. Subjects with overweight (BMI ≥25 kg/m²) and obesity (BMI ≥30 kg/m²), including extreme obesity (BMI ≥40 kg/m²), have usually accumulated their excess adiposity over a prolonged time period; however, a more rapid weight gain leading to overweight can occur within the context of specific time periods such as, for example, puberty, pregnancy, menopause, an episode of major depression (for example, atypical depression), cessation of smoking or during treatment with drugs that induce weight gain, and even binge eating as a side effect [19].

Complex interactions of environmental factors with individual genetic factors result in normal weight, underweight, or overweight/obesity. Whereas it has proven difficult to unequivocally attribute the development of obesity to specific environmental factors entailing an increased energy intake and/or reduced energy expenditure and, as a net effect, an energy surplus, the current obesity epidemic is attributed to environmental factors (obesogenic environment). Potentially, and similar to the genetic architecture of BMI [20], the number of environmental factors is large; overall, effect sizes of single factors may well prove to be rather small; nevertheless, in a given individual genome-environment, interactions may render specific environmental factors much more important than others. Within any given society, the obesogenic environment may not differ substantially, thus enabling genetic factors to play a larger role in explaining BMI variance of the respective population. Accordingly, BMI heritability estimates based on twin studies have remained stable over the past decades [21].

Despite the assumed importance of the environment for the obesity epidemic, there is no easy way to turn the clock back; this, by itself, points to the multitude of factors involved. In industrialized countries, sedentary office workplaces, a sedentary lifestyle, and even more so overconsumption of foods are perceived as major contributors to excess weight gain. Changes in the global food system, which is producing palatable, more processed, cheap, and effectively marketed food, are thought to entail 'passive' overconsumption of energy. Overweight and obesity can thus be viewed as a predictable outcome of market economies predicated on consumption-based growth [22]. Importantly, social class is a predictor of body weight in (post-)industrial and developing countries, albeit with partially opposite effects [23, 24].

Behaviour and emotionality undoubtedly contribute to the development of eating and weight disorders. However, among laypersons, these factors frequently are perceived as the sole factors. The lay perception that behaviour is important and modifiable is, to a large extent, responsible for the stigma associated with both groups of disorders. Such lay beliefs may even have an impact on body weight; for example, subjects who believe that obesity results from a lack of exercise had a higher BMI than those who considered a poor diet at the core [25]; this effect on body weight was not explained by other factors with an influence on body weight, co-assessed in the respective study. Quite a substantial number of patients with either AN or obesity have the perception that surmounting mental problems will enable them to achieve a normal body weight; relatives, friends, and health care professionals frequently contribute to this way of thinking. This mindset can just as well be found in patients, in whom the respective condition affects multiple family members, demonstrating that the complexity of the interaction of genetic and environmental factors in the aetiologies of these disorders is frequently confusing to those most concerned. Interestingly, the lay belief that genetic factors play a major role in obesity has been associated with reports of lower levels of both physical activity and fruit and vegetable consumption [26].

**Table 102.1** Weight categories based on BMI

| Category | BMI (kg/m²) |
| --- | --- |
| Underweight | <18.5 |
| Normal weight | 18.5–24.9 |
| Overweight | ≥25 |
| Pre-obesity | 25–29.9 |
| Obesity grade I | 30–34.9 |
| Obesity grade II | 35–39.9 |
| Obesity grade III | ≥40 |

## Disordered body weight regulation

Because eating and weight disorders are associated with weight loss (AN), weight stunting (AN, ARFID), weight fluctuations (AN, bulimia nervosa, BED), and weight gain (obesity), diverse regulatory mechanisms that normally serve to defend body weight are overridden. This perturbation can stem from, *and* entail, both somatic and psychological malfunctioning, resulting in a complex intertwinement of primary and secondary factors. [27]. Neuroendocrine findings in eating disorders primarily reflect the consequences of these perturbations (Table 102.2); major causal neuroendocrine mechanisms have not been identified for eating disorders. Knowledge of the induced neuroendocrine dysregulations helps partially to understand the respective clinical symptomatology. In addition, efforts to gain weight by a patient with chronic AN may be hampered by 'physiological' counter-regulation, in addition to the primary underlying disturbances; the long-standing underweight may have led to a reduction of the body weight set-point.

## Elucidation of monogenic obesity opened the door to the neuroendocrine circuitry underlying body weight regulation and the physiological adaptation to starvation

Multifactorial obesity is the most common form of obesity in the general population [19]; this type of obesity results from the complex interaction of hundreds of polymorphisms and environmental factors. Currently, genetic variation at 941 independent loci has been detected via genome-wide association analyses; the mean allelic effects on body weight range from approximately 1.5 kg to <150 g. Approximately 6% and 22% of the BMI variance can be attributed to the currently identified polygenic loci or have been estimated to, in total, explain the polygenic contribution [20, 28].

Cloning of the leptin gene in 1994 and the identification of the rare mutations entailing the autosomal recessive phenotype of the obese mouse and the equivalent human leptin deficiency syndrome represented initial breakthroughs in our understanding of the molecular

mechanisms involved in body weight regulation and the behaviours associated with both an increased energy intake and a decreased expenditure [29]. Leptin-deficient humans for the first time revealed that extreme obesity without cognitive impairment can result from a monogenic disorder [30]; the voracious appetite and ensuing behaviours of these individuals are driven by the genetically based lack of this anorexigenic hormone.

Leptin is mainly synthesized in adipocytes and secreted into blood; circulating concentrations are correlated with BMI and fat mass in particular. Central leptin signalling is initiated via binding of leptin to its receptor at the cell surfaces of two different types of first-order neurons within the arcuate nucleus in the hypothalamus (Fig. 102.1). These neurons, in turn, convey the leptin signal to second-order neurons; brain-derived neurotrophic factor (BDNF) and its receptor are important downstream effectors of the leptin–melanocortinergic pathway, which projects to different neurotransmitter systems [15, 16, 28].

Prolonged reduced energy intake due to, for example, a famine reduces the endocrine function of adipose tissue, which is compounded by the ensuing loss of fat mass. Hence, circulating leptin drops to subnormal levels and, via this process, initiates neuroendocrine adaptation to starvation [15, 16]. Reduced leptin signalling affects the hypothalamus–pituitary axis, which down- or upregulates the functions of downstream end-organs, including the thyroid, gonads, and adrenals. In addition, growth hormone is upregulated, while others like insulin-like growth factor 1 (IGF-1), a neurotrophic polypeptide, are downregulated.

Other examples of autosomal recessive forms of monogenic obesity include those due to mutations in the genes for the leptin receptor, pro-opiomelanocortin (*POMC*) and proconvertase 1 [29]. All of the recessively inherited forms of monogenic obesity entail additional phenotypic features such as hypothalamic amenorrhoea associated with functional leptin deficiency or red hair and adreno-corticotrophic hormone (ACTH) deficiency in a subgroup of *POMC* mutation carriers; these associated phenotypes underscore the fact that the neuroendocrinology of body weight regulation is interwoven with other functions.

One of the second-order neurons expresses the melanocortin-4 receptor (*MC4R*) gene, which can harbour a vast range of functionally relevant mutations entailing dominantly inherited obesity in 1–5% of extremely obese children and adults. The anorexigenic effect of the leptin signal is diminished, if binding of the POMC cleavage product alpha-melanocyte stimulating hormone (α-MSH) to the MC4R is reduced as a consequence of such mutations. The net effects of such *MC4R* mutations result in body weight increments of approximately 15 kg and 30 kg in males and females, respectively. Obesity due to *MC4R* mutations is not associated with any readily easily recognizable associated phenotype [29].

Apart from the hypothalamus, several other subcortical and cortical brain regions, including those comprising the reward system [31], are involved in body weight regulation and adaptation to starvation. In addition to leptin, a number of peripheral hormones and peptides arising from the digestive system (gut–brain axis), muscle, and other organs provide the link between the periphery and the central nervous system via specific central receptors. Furthermore, endocrine and neurocrine pathways are assumed to be involved in gut microbiota-to-brain signalling; vice versa, the brain can alter microbial composition and behaviour via the autonomic nervous system [32].

**Table 102.2** Endocrine alterations in AN and BN[*]

| | AN | BN |
|---|---|---|
| Thyroid axis | ↓ fT3, n (↓) fT4 | n (↓) |
| Gonadal axis | ↓ FSH<br>↓ LH pulsatility<br>↓ Oestrogens<br>↓ Androgens | n (↓)<br>n (↓)<br>n (↓)<br>n (↓) |
| Adrenal axis | ↑ cortisol<br>n DHEAS | n (↑)<br>n |
| Growth hormone | GH resistance<br>(↑ GH/↓ IGF-1) | n (↑) |
| Appetite-regulating hormones | ↓ leptin<br>↑ ghrelin (fasting)<br>↑ (n) PYY (fasting) | n (↓)<br>↑<br>N |

↑, elevated; ↓, reduced; n, normal; fT3, free triiodothyronine; fT4, free thyroxine; LH, luteinizing hormone; FSH, follicle-stimulating hormone; GH, growth hormone; IGF-1, insulin-like growth factor, type 1.
[*] [90, 91].

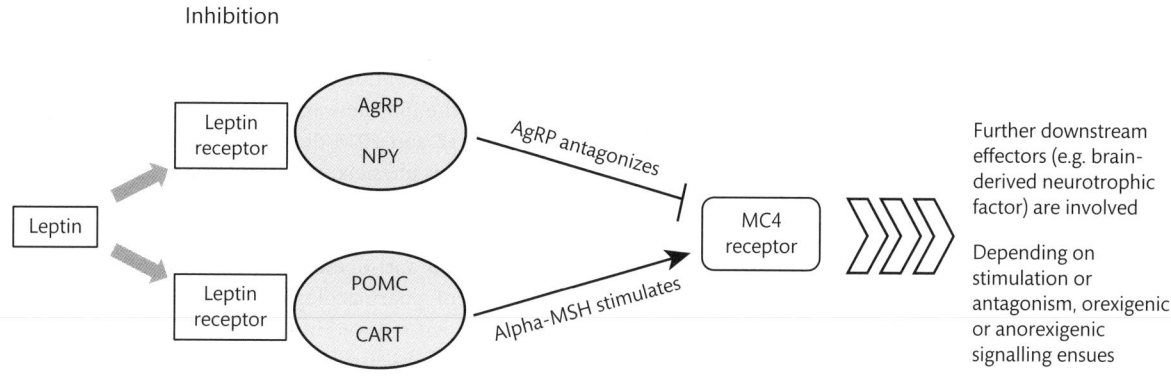

**Fig. 102.1** Leptin has central effects on feeding behaviour, appetite, motor activity, and cognitive function, but also peripheral effects on the insulin–glucose axis. In the arcuate nucleus of the hypothalamus, leptin activates two different types of first-order neurons. One co-expresses the orexigenic peptides neuropeptide Y (NPY) and agouti-related protein (AgRP), the other the anorexigenic peptides cocaine- and amphetamine-related transcript (CART) and pro-opiomelanocortin (POMC). POMC is cleaved into different peptides, including α-melanocyte-stimulating hormone (α-MSH). AgRP and α-MSH compete for the MC4 receptor (MC4R). AgRP antagonizes MC4R activity, and α-MSH stimulates MC4R activity. Decreased MC4R activity generates an orexigenic signal, whereas increased activity conveys an anorexigenic signal.

## Drug-induced weight loss and its potential for the treatment of obesity

Recent insight into the neuroendocrine regulation of body weight has led to the identification of many potential targets to influence body weight. As a consequence of the high prevalence of obesity, drug-induced weight loss has been the major focus of pharmacological research; however, AN, ARFID, sarcopenia, and cachexia due to infections, cancer, and other conditions also clearly warrant efforts to devise drugs that promote weight gain. The elucidation of polygenes in body weight regulation [20, 28] is of a too recent origin to have allowed their full exploitation with respect to a selection of drug targets. It is also questionable whether the low effect sizes of the identified genes will trigger research efforts in the pharmaceutical industry. However, the advances into treatment of different types of monogenic obesity underscore the potential of making use of the neuroendocrine mechanisms and of genetic variation underlying obesity in particular. Thus, daily treatment with subcutaneously applied recombinant leptin is able to normalize the eating behaviour of patients with inborn functional leptin deficiency within days; in the longer term, substantial weight loss ensues [30]. Two patients with a form of monogenic obesity due to *POMC* mutations benefited from treatment with the MC4R agonist setmelanotide; weight loss amounted to 51 kg and 20.5 kg after treatment for 42 and 12 weeks, respectively [33]. Functional rescue of stop mutations in *MC4R* has been demonstrated in a rodent model based on aminoglycoside-mediated read-through of stop codons [34]. MC4R agonists are currently being evaluated for the treatment of both obesity due to *MC4R* mutations and multifactorial obesity [35]. Case reports indicate that indirect sympathomimetic stimulants and atomoxetine may also induce substantial weight loss in individuals with *MC4R* mutations [36, 37].

In general terms, the known anti-obesity drugs can be classified as either centrally acting appetite suppressants and satiety enhancers (with or without additional peripheral actions) or peripherally acting agents [38]. As of today, no major clinical breakthrough has been achieved in the pharmacological treatment of multifactorial obesity or eating disorders. Whereas some drugs or drug combinations have been shown to acutely induce weight loss, clinically significant and regulatory agency-required medium-term (1 year) weight loss mostly averaged in the range of 3–5 kg in excess of placebo. Weight regain typically sets in upon discontinuation of the respective medications [38].

Apart from these disappointingly low mean weight losses, the history of anti-obesity drug development is fraught with significant cardiovascular or central nervous system side effects that have frequently led to their market removal (for example, fenfluramine, sibutramine, rimonabant [39]) or failed clinical studies prior to any new drug approval (NDA) submission; interestingly, the rare emergence of AN represents one such serious adverse event [40]. As a consequence, all large pharmaceutical companies have stopped or significantly reduced their obesity drug development programmes; in light of the regulatory requirements, the financial risks currently appear too high. Currently, only startups or some mid-sized companies pursue this challenging indication. However, paradoxically, patients with grade III (BMI ≥40 kg/m$^2$) or grade II (35 ≤ BMI < 40 kg/m$^2$) obesity and obesity-related comorbid disorders are eligible for bariatric surgery, which entails a *mortality risk* of approximately 0.5% [41]. As such, a more positive and differentiated approach to pharmacological treatment appears warranted, according to which higher risks of adverse events during pharmacological treatment of extreme obesity should not automatically entail withdrawal of the respective drug. On the other hand, regulatory agencies are justifiably concerned with off-label use of drugs to promote weight loss in less obese individuals.

Interestingly, obesity drugs have failed because of side effects due to actions in pathways overlapping with the reward and other central nervous systems. Of 25 drugs withdrawn worldwide between 1964 and 2009, 23 acted via central mechanisms, with psychiatric side effects explaining seven withdrawals; drug abuse and dependence accounted for roughly 50% of these withdrawals [39]. A centrally acting drug that leads to weight loss (or gain) frequently also affects mood, cognition, and/or behaviour. The serotonin–noradrenaline reuptake inhibitor sibutramine was originally developed as an antidepressant; due to an elevated cardiovascular risk profile and despite weight loss, which, in theory, should have reduced cardiovascular risks, the drug was taken off the market. The cannabinoid receptor-1 antagonist rimonabant (Acomplia*) was associated with depression and suicidal ideation in a small subgroup of patients, leading finally in 2009 to authorization by the European Medicines Agency (EMA) for its withdrawal from the market, 3 years after its approval in 2006; the US Food and Drug Administration (FDA) had never licensed the use of this drug in the United States due to concerns for neurologic and psychiatric side effects. The approved anticonvulsant topiramate (Topamax*), which induces weight loss in excess of both sibutramine and rimonabant, is associated with paraesthesiae, taste impairment, suicidal ideation, and psychomotor disturbances; in total, the adverse side effects again were deemed too problematic to market topiramate as a stand-alone anti-obesity drug [39]. However, low-dose combination with phentermine has received market approval.

Of the five drugs currently licensed by the FDA for the treatment of obesity, two represent combination drugs (phentermine–topiramate and naltrexone–bupropion). All five drugs are superior to placebo in inducing a weight loss of at least 5% within a clinical trial duration of 12 months. The proportions of patients meeting this threshold are shown in Table 102.3 [42].

Liraglutide and naltrexone–bupropion were associated with the highest odds of adverse event-related treatment discontinuation. Of these five drugs, the EMA has licensed the use of orlistat, naltrexone–bupropion, and liraglutide.

The ongoing elucidation of the pathways involved in energy homeostasis is continuing to turn up novel targets for anti-obesity drugs; similarly, the metabolic alterations after bariatric surgery have provided additional insight into the complex regulation of body weight [43]. Several drugs, including an MC4R agonist and an enhancer of fat oxidation, are in development for subtypes of obesity. A small number (in comparison to the era prior to 2007) of clinical trials are ongoing (see clinicaltrials.gov). Due to both the limited effect of a single drug and dose-dependent increases in side effects, combination therapies and, in particular, polypeptide hormone combinations appear promising [44].

Despite the detection of numerous targets and ongoing drug development, the four new anti-obesity drugs approved by the FDA between 2012 and 2014 did not fulfil their market expectations. Acceptance by physicians in the United States was substantially lower than for other novel drugs; furthermore, patient acceptance has only picked up slowly [45]. Obviously, the frequent market withdrawals of anti-obesity drugs have contributed to a negative perception of pharmacological treatment of elevated adiposity. This history has reduced investment in drug development for this highly relevant disease for the foreseeable future. The expectations of both patients and physicians require a realistic discussion as to the pros and cons of drug treatment of elevated adiposity; in some countries, reimbursement issues by health insurances also need to be addressed. A stand-alone drug treatment of obesity is unlikely to be successful; for the time being, lifestyle modification will remain the cornerstone of weight management [38]. Central nervous system side effects and risks for drug dependence represent serious obstacles for the development and marketing of anti-obesity drugs.

## Drug-induced weight gain and its potential for the treatment of AN and AFRID

No drugs have been specifically licensed for the treatment of AFRID or AN. As such, all medications currently used to treat these disorders symptomatically are prescribed off-label, for instance, to suppress severe eating disorder-specific cognitions. However, because starvation-associated underweight can figure prominently in both disorders, approaches for drug-induced weight gain represents a major therapeutic aim. Appetite stimulants/orexigenic drugs clearly represent an option, although drugs that reduce energy expenditure and physical activity may have potential too. Additionally, drug treatment of sarcopenia [46] and cachexia associated with cancer [47, 48], chronic kidney disease, HIV, other infectious diseases, cancer, and chronic obstructive pulmonary disease also warrants scrutiny for potential application in eating disorders. For

**Table 102.3** Obesity agents producing 5% weight loss or more (proportions of patients meeting this threshold shown as percentages)

| Drug | Mechanism of action | % meeting threshold for significant weight loss |
|---|---|---|
| Phentermine Topiramate | Phentermine: non-selective stimulator of monoamine release Topiramate acts as multifactorial: enhances GABAergic neurotransmissions, blocks voltage-dependent sodium channels, activates L-type calcium channels, enhances inhibitory activity of glutamate at AMPA (amino-3-hydroxy-5-methyl-4-isoxazole-proprionate) and kainate receptors, and inhibits several carbonic anhydrases isoenzymes [92] | 75% |
| Liraglutide | Glucagon-like peptide 1 analogue | 63% |
| Naltrexone–bupropion | Naltrexone: opiate antagonist Bupropion: previously seen as weak noradrenaline–dopamine reuptake inhibitor (NDRI), but potentially rather a noradrenaline and dopamine releasing agent (NDRA) | 55% |
| Lorcaserin | Serotonin 2C receptor agonist | 49% |
| Orlistat | Inhibitor of gastric and pancreatic lipases | 44% |
| Placebo | | 23% |

Source: data from *JAMA*, 315(22), Khera R, Murad MH, Chandar AK, *et al.*, Association of Pharmacological Treatments or Obesity With Weight Loss and Adverse Events: A systematic Review and Meta-analysis, pp 2424–34, Copyright (2016), with permission from American Medical Association.

example, given the prominent role of the MC4R as a drug target for both induction of weight loss and weight gain, it is interesting that cachexia induced by lipopolysaccharide administration and by tumour growth is ameliorated by central MC4R blockade in rodent models [49].

Several licensed drugs, particularly psychopharmacological medications, show weight gain as an unwanted side effect. Clozapine and olanzapine have the strongest effect on body weight [50]. They act via an increase of caloric intake without affecting resting energy expenditure [51] and can induce binge eating attacks [52]. Weight gains exceeding 20 kg can occur in genetically susceptible individuals [53] who are treated for psychosis or other mental disorders; the mean average weight gain after 10 weeks is between 4 kg and 4.5 kg [50]. However, use of olanzapine and related drugs in AN to promote weight gain has proven unsuccessful, as revealed by meta-analyses of randomized controlled trials [54]. It is unknown if the unresponsiveness is due to cognitive restriction or to starvation-dependent dysregulation. Interestingly, our own clinical observation is that olanzapine can induce weight gain once patients have reached their target weight.

Systematic studies of dopamine antagonists are not available for AFRID and feeding disorders associated with low body weight. The young age of the respective patients should imply a restrictive approach to treatment with off-label medications. Three case reports based on pre-adolescent patients with feeding disorders suggest that risperidone may help to increase body weight [55]. A retrospective chart review of 127 children between 7 and 80 months with feeding difficulties not exclusively fulfilling the DSM-5 criteria for ARFID suggested that cyproheptadine, an antihistaminergic and antiserotonergic agent approved for use in cold urticaria in children and adolescents, can lead to weight gain and a positive change in mealtime and feeding behaviours within the context of a complex treatment programme [56]. Mild and transient side effects, such as drowsiness, irritability, and constipation, were reported in 14% of the children.

Ghrelin represents an example of a hormone which induces food intake as an appetite stimulant; the hormone is synthesized in the enteroendocrine cells of the stomach and released upon caloric restriction—it thus signals hunger. Consistent with the neuroendocrine adaptation to starvation, serum levels are elevated in patients with AN. Based on encouraging initial findings in a small number of patients with AN, a clinical trial is currently assessing the effects of the novel ghrelin receptor agonist RM-131 for treatment of AN [57]. Apart from other functions, the hypothalamic neuropeptide oxytocin is a regulator of food intake; a clinical trial in patients with AN is looking at the effects of intranasal oxytocin on smell and food consumption. In a double-blind, single-dose, placebo-controlled crossover study, oxytocin had no effect on the 24-hour calorie intake in AN patients, whereas patients with BN consumed less calories [58]. Because testosterone increases fat-free mass, a phase 2 clinical trial is investigating the effect of transdermal testosterone on BMI of patients with AN [57]. The cannabinoid agonist dronabinol [the international non-proprietary name (INN) for delta-9-tetrahydrocannabinol (THC)] induced a small (0.73 kg in excess of placebo), but significant, weight gain after 4 weeks of treatment in the absence of severe adverse events in an add-on, prospective, randomized, double-blind, controlled crossover study, which included 25 adult patients with chronic AN [59].

## Pharmacological dissection of primary phenomena from starvation-induced symptoms in AN

Treatment of patients with AN with recombinant leptin appears to be a promising approach to ameliorate starvation-induced symptoms related to hypoleptinaemia [60]. Treatment with recombinant leptin has been shown to improve the function of the reproductive system, including resumption of menstruation in currently non-eating disordered females with hypothalamic amenorrhoea [61]. Amenorrhoea in patients with AN is induced by hypoleptinaemia [16]. The exact mechanisms linking the metabolic system with the reproductive system require further elucidation. Leptin binds to receptors on gonadotrophin-releasing hormone (GnRH) neurons. The signalling cascade for reproductive function includes gonadotrophin-inhibitory hormone (GnIH) and kisspeptin [62].

At the behavioural level, hyperactivity is encountered in a substantial subgroup of patients with AN. Hypoleptinaemia likely also plays a crucial role in the development of this phenomenon, which, if severe, substantially impedes treatment. In rats subjected to food restriction, running-wheel activity increases by 300–400%. This starvation-induced hyperactivity is assumed to facilitate food-foraging behaviour. The development of hyperactivity is completely suppressed by concomitant treatment with recombinant leptin [63]. Because removal of the adrenals also prevents the development of anorexia-based activity, it appears that leptin exerts its effects via the hypothalamic–pituitary–adrenal axis [64]. In agreement with the rat model, low serum leptin levels in patients with AN have been associated with increased activity levels [65], suggesting that the same mechanism applies. This may provide a unique example of a profound physiologically induced and hormonally determined change in activity levels. It certainly substantiates the pivotal role of leptin in the adaptation to starvation [15, 16].

Other findings supporting the role of leptin in the neuroendocrine adaptation to starvation include its suppression of growth stunting in rodent starvation models, its antidepressant effect in inborn leptin-deficient mice, and its effects on bone growth. Leptin has also been shown to have a neurotrophic effect; in leptin-deficient humans, treatment with recombinant leptin entails increments of the volume of specific brain regions [15, 16, 60]. Recombinant leptin has recently been licensed for the treatment of lipodystrophy by the FDA [66]; the EMA followed suit in 2018. Adverse effects occurred during treatment with metreleptin (Myalept®), but these seemed to be linked to the underlying disorder.

Such trials in patients with AN would enable the dissection of primary from secondary starvation-induced symptoms in AN; an amelioration of somatic, cognitive, and behavioural symptoms appears possible [66]. Patients with BN whose metabolism is in a semi-starved state might benefit as well. The risks of metreleptin treatment of patients with eating disorders might be manageable. Thus, leptin treatment of eight females with hypothalamic amenorrhoea was not associated with significant side effects [61]; in addition, long-term treatment of individuals with leptin deficiency [30] and a 24-week-long treatment of hypoleptinaemic (<5 ng/mL) adult females [67] were not associated with serious side effects. The production of antibodies neutralizing leptin has occurred after longer treatment and was countered by intermittent discontinuation and application of higher doses.

Obviously, patients with AN would have to be closely monitored during a pilot study; in particular, adequate feeding during treatment is crucial, as an elevation of leptin may reduce appetite. Preferentially, initial attempts should be directed at adult patients with hyperactivity [60, 66]. The high costs of metreleptin treatment (currently approximately half a million dollars annually for the treatment of a patient with lipodystrophy [66]) represent an important obstacle to treatment acceptance.

## Eating disorders and behavioural addictions

An addiction-like process has been suggested to explain the eating behaviour of subjects with AN [2], BED, and obesity [1]. Potentially, either overeating or caloric restriction can have a positive effect on mood, emotion regulation, and cognition in predisposed individuals. With respect to obesity, the terms 'food addiction' and 'eating addiction' illustrate the current controversy as to whether particular foods and substances (for example, sugar) can support an addictive behaviour as in substance use disorders or whether overeating is best categorized as a behavioural addiction or compulsion. The term 'paradoxical liveliness' has been coined to illustrate that some patients with AN appear more lively and become more focused and more ambitious when they initially develop their eating disorder [65]. The fact that all major religions have propagated short-term or intermittent fasting suggests that emotional and spiritual well-being may be positively influenced by the metabolic and physiological processes associated with the adaptation to starvation.

The function of leptin within the reward system warrants appreciation [1, 68]. The rewarding value of nutrients requires activation of midbrain dopamine (DA) neurons. Fasting enhances the rewarding value, whereas it is diminished by leptin. Via leptin receptors expressed on a subpopulation of midbrain DA neurons, leptin exerts an inhibitory effect on these neurons, thus potentially explaining a decreased nutrient reward and anorexia via downstream galanin-mediated inhibition of orexin neurons. Conversely, DA levels in the nucleus accumbens (NAc) are decreased in hyperphagic, leptin-deficient *obese* mice and increased by leptin injections. Food intake may thus result from DA deficiency in the NAc, entailing normalization of DA levels. Low levels of DA in the NAc have been postulated to underlie both the drive to eat in obese subjects and substance use in drug addicts [68].

Alterations of the brain reward circuitry have also been postulated to contribute to the development and maintenance of eating disorders. At the onset of AN, eating less food may be perceived as rewarding; afterwards, conditioning sets in. In the binge eating/purging type of AN, BN, and BED, patients report a strong urge to eat, together with a sense of loss of control of their energy intake and a transient reduction of negative emotional states after bingeing. Patients with eating disorders frequently present with anhedonia, meaning that they are less able to experience reward in comparison to healthy controls [69]. O'Hara and coworkers [2] hypothesized that, rather than a generalized inability to experience reward, a cognitively driven reluctance to gain weight may contribute to the aversive appraisal of food- and taste-related stimuli. Hypotheses focusing on a reduced experience of reward include inappropriate processing of visual perception of food, distinct patterns of brain activation in response to gustatory stimuli, and 'reward contamination' (normal rewarding stimuli are experienced as aversive). Patients with eating disorders may activate dopaminergic motivational circuits differently, so that normally aversive stimuli become attractive [69].

Whereas a reward-centred model of AN, and thus an overlap with addiction, appears plausible, substantial differences are also apparent. Further research is required to assess potential implications for psychotherapeutic and psychopharmacological treatment of eating disorders [2]. Prevention and treatment of obesity, based on the assumption that it (partially) results from food or eating addiction, warrants further scrutiny [1]. The 5-HT2c agonist lorcaserin, which has received FDA approval for the treatment of obesity, has further potential in substance use disorders, especially nicotine/smoking. In particular, the lorcaserin dose dependently reduces smoking rates and at the same time reduces/prevents the weight gain typically associated with cessation of smoking [70].

## Obesity, eating disorders, and the microbiome

Microbiota transplantation experiments in mouse models first indicated that the gut microbiota influences weight regulation and modulates psychopathology. Stool extracts transferred from genetically or nutritionally induced obese to germ-free (GF) mice produced a marked increase in body fat within a relatively short period of time [71]. Moreover, obesity and obesity-associated metabolic phenotypes were transmissible by uncultured microbiota of humans to GF rodents. Conversely, cohousing the microbiota-transplanted obese mouse with a mouse harbouring the microbiota from a lean individual prevented the development of obesity and the associated metabolic complications [72]. Several studies, especially those following Roux-en-Y gastric bypass, demonstrated that obesity is related to a change in the relative abundance of two bacterial strains—the *Firmicutes*-to-*Bacteroidetes* ratio is increased in obesity and reduced with weight loss. However, it is still not clear whether these changes in microbial populations directly contribute to promote weight loss or result from it [73].

The microbiome of obese individuals has an increased potential to harvest energy from nourishment, for example by nutrition absorption and polysaccharide utilization. It produces bioactive metabolites, for example short-chain fatty acids (SCFAs) (specifically acetic acid, propionic acid, and butyric acid), by fermentation of partially digestible and non-digestible carbohydrates of dietary fibres. SCFAs affect the physiology of the host organism, for example the pH level of the colon, gut transit time, and glucose metabolism, thus modifying appetite and energy metabolism [74, 75]. Obese individuals, including children and adolescents, have a higher relative abundance of microbiota able to ferment polysaccharides. The consequence is a higher amount of SCFAs providing more energy for the host, which can be stored as fat tissue or converted into glucose. In adults fed on a Western diet, the extra energy supply by producing SCFAs has been estimated to add up to 10% of the overall daily caloric intake [76]. Moreover, these metabolites are able to cross the brain–blood barrier and impact neural circuits [77].

On the other hand, the microbiome also seems to play an important role in starvation-induced weight loss. Transplantation of frozen bacterial species from children with kwashiorkor, a severe form of malnutrition often observed in developing countries, produced significant weight loss in GF mice, accompanied by severe metabolic changes. One-week application of an oral antibiotic significantly improved the nutritional status of malnourished Malawian children [78]. Significant changes of the gut microbiome were also found in the frequently used animal AN model of activity-based anorexia (ABA) [79], which stimulates weight loss by reduction of food and access to a running wheel [63, 64]. Because of the starvation- and hyperactivity-induced weight loss in the animal model, decreased thickness of the muscularis layer and significantly increased permeability of the intestine were observed [79].

Unfortunately, studies in patients with AN are still scarce. Two recent investigations found a significant difference between the abundance of certain bacterial groups in healthy controls and patients with AN, especially an increase in mucin-degraders and a decrease in butyrate producers in the latter group, which were only partly alleviated by weight gain [80, 81]. Mucin-degraders feed on mucus covering the intestinal wall and probably contribute to the increased intestinal permeability identified in the ABA model for AN mentioned previously [75].

Both in obesity and AN, there is emerging evidence for an increase in intestinal permeability, followed by low-grade inflammation, which, in turn, might contribute to the metabolic (and psychopathological) alterations found in both disorders [73]. The intestinal barrier prevents pathogenic microorganisms from spreading into the systemic circulation. However, a 'leaky gut' might facilitate the transfer of harmful microorganisms and toxins from the gut lumen to the lamina propria and mesenteric lymph nodes, from which they may reach the systemic circulation, especially if the immune system is dysfunctional. From this point, such so-called 'pathobionts' and other harmful substances could stimulate the production of pro-inflammatory peripheral and central cytokines, the latter having an impact on neuronal function (gut–brain interaction). Indeed, pro-inflammatory cytokines are known to be increased during the acute state of AN [82]. Similar processes are observed after several weeks of a high-fat diet in animals with an altered gut barrier function and elevated inflammation markers [83].

Implications for treatment of obesity and eating disorders may include changes of diet and the administration of pre- or probiotics or even of antibiotics. The composition of the human microbiome rapidly responds to a dietary change. In an informative study by David *et al.* [84], the researchers compared the effects of a shift from usual eating habits to either a vegetarian or an animal-based diet. In the group on the animal-based diet, changes in the gut microbiome occurred already 1 day after the new nourishment had reached the distal gut. The microbiome changed to an abundance of bacteria with high bile resistance (*Bilophila wadsworthia*), which is associated with the occurrence of intestinal bowel disease in mouse models. Interestingly, only this group, but not that fed on a vegetarian diet, showed significant weight loss. These findings are of potential importance for refeeding strategies in AN. After admission to hospital, the diet of the starved patient is often swiftly changed from a more plant-derived alimentation to high-calorie food rich in carbohydrates and fat to achieve weight gain. This may be doing more harm than good. Within a very short time, the microbiome of our patients is affected without considering probable consequences such as the growth of inflammation-inducing bacteria. Interestingly, an increased risk for autoimmune disorders, especially Crohn's disease, has been described in AN [85].

Prebiotics are defined as 'non-digestible food ingredients that beneficially affect the host by selectively stimulating the growth/activity of certain bacteria in the gut' [86]. Probiotics are defined as living microbial components delivered to humans or animals, with health benefits for the host. To our knowledge, there are not sufficient data to judge the effect of either prebiotics or probiotics in obesity or eating disorders. However, with further understanding of the role of the microbiome in weight and eating disorders, there is hope that modification of the gut microbes can exert a positive impact on these disorders, at least in some individuals. This could foster a more personalized treatment in these often chronic diseases [73].

Changes in the gut microbiome are also associated with symptoms of psychiatric disorders. Infections of the gastrointestinal tract are followed by anxiety-like behaviour in a rodent model (for a review, see [87]). Inflammatory bowel disease is associated with a high prevalence of anxiety and depressive disorders, which is much more pronounced than in other chronic diseases of childhood or adulthood. Further, a large case-control study in the UK demonstrated that repeated use of antibiotics was associated with an increased risk for depression and anxiety [88]. In acute AN, levels of depression, anxiety, and eating disorder psychopathology were associated with the composition and diversity of the intestinal microbiota [80].

## Conclusions

The recent years have witnessed a veritable knowledge explosion regarding the molecular mechanisms of body weight regulation [8, 9, 20, 28, 29, 89], which is currently continuing. The genetic predispositions to AN [8, 9], and possibly other eating disorders too, overlap with the molecular mechanisms involved in this complex physiology. In addition, the genetic predispositions to diverse mental and somatic disorders and quantitative somatic and mental traits overlap [89], suggesting that novel insights may have implications for the future treatment of eating disorders. Furthermore, substantial advances have been made with respect to the pathways involved in the adaptation to starvation and in considering addictive processes for both obesity and AN. Finally, microbiome-related research has come up with important findings. It appears likely that some of these novel findings will entail benefits for the treatment of patients with eating and weight disorders.

Unfortunately, pharmacological research into obesity has suffered from many setbacks that have entailed withdrawals of specific drugs. It is crucial to re-engage the pharmaceutical industry in research required to come up with novel treatments. The scientific basis for drug development in eating and weight disorders has never been as good as of today. The major challenge is to identify targets that will indeed allow the development of safe and effective drugs. The overlap of diverse functional pathways suggests that a certain degree of side effects must be taken into account in order to achieve this goal.

## REFERENCES

1. Hebebrand J, Albayrak O, Adan R, *et al.* (2014). "Eating addiction", rather than "food addiction", better captures addictive-like eating behavior. *Neurosci Biobehav Rev*, 47, 295–306.

2. O'Hara CB, Campbell IC, Schmidt U. (2015). A reward-centred model of anorexia nervosa: a focussed narrative review of the neurological and psychophysiological literature. *Neurosci Biobehav Rev*, 52, 131–52.

3. Halmi KA. (2013). Perplexities of treatment resistance in eating disorders. *BMC Psychiatry*, 13, 292.

4. Herpertz-Dahlmann, B. (2017). Treatment of eating disorders in child and adolescent psychiatry. *Curr Opin Psychiatry*, 30, 438–45.

5. Mühlig Y, Wabitsch M, Moss A, Hebebrand J. (2014). Weight loss in children and adolescents. *Dtsch Arztebl Int*, 111, 818–24.

6. Hebebrand J, Himmelmann GW, Herzog W, *et al.* (1997). Prediction of low body weight at long-term follow-up in acute anorexia nervosa by low body weight at referral. *Am J Psychiatry*, 154, 566–9.

7. Fichter MM, Quadflieg N, Crosby RD, Koch S. (2017). Long-term outcome of anorexia nervosa: Results from a large clinical longitudinal study. *Int J Eat Disord*, 50, 1018–30.

8. Hinney A, Kesselmeier M, Jall S, *et al.* (2017). Evidence for three genetic loci involved in both anorexia nervosa risk and variation of body mass index. *Mol. Psychiatry*, 22, 192–201.

9. Duncan L, Yilmaz Z, Gaspar H, *et al.* (2017). Significant locus and metabolic genetic correlations revealed in genome-wide association study of anorexia nervosa. *Am J Psychiatry*, 174, 850–8.

10. Hebebrand J, Remschmidt H. (1995). Anorexia nervosa viewed as an extreme weight condition: genetic implications. *Hum Genet*, 95, 1–11.

11. Dombrowski SU, Knittle K, Avenell A, Araújo-Soares V, Sniehotta FF. (2014). Long term maintenance of weight loss with non-surgical interventions in obese adults: systematic review and meta-analyses of randomised controlled trials. *BMJ*, 348, g2646.

12. National Association to Advance Fat Acceptance. Available from: https://www.naafaonline.com/dev2/about/

13. MyProAna. Available from: http://www.myproana.com

14. Hebebrand J. (2009). Diagnostic issues in eating disorders and obesity. *Child Adolesc Psychiatr Clin N Am*, 18, 1–16.

15. Ahima RS, Flier JS. (2000). Leptin. *Annu Rev Physiol*, 62, 413–37.

16. Hebebrand J, Muller TD, Holtkamp K, Herpertz-Dahlmann B. (2007). The role of leptin in anorexia nervosa: clinical implications. *Mol Psychiatry*, 12, 23–35.

17. Rosenbaum M, Leibel RL. (2016). Models of energy homeostasis in response to maintenance of reduced body weight. *Obesity (Silver Spring)*, 24, 1620–9.

18. World Health Organization. *Obesity: Preventing and Managing the Global Epidemic*. 2000. Available from: http://www.who.int/nutrition/publications/obesity/WHO_TRS_894/en/

19. Hebebrand J, Holm JC, Woodward E, *et al.* (2017). A proposal of the European Association for the Study of Obesity to pmprove the ICD-11 diagnostic criteria for obesity based on the three dimensions etiology, degree of adiposity and health risk. *Obes Facts*, 10, 284–307.

20. Locke AE, Kahali B, Berndt SI, *et al.* (2015). Genetic studies of body mass index yield new insights for obesity biology. *Nature*, 518, 197–206.

21. Silventoinen K, Jelenkovic A, Sund R, *et al.* (2017). Differences in genetic and environmental variation in adult body mass index by sex, age, time period, and region: an individual-based pooled analysis of 40 twin cohorts. *Am J Clin Nutr*, 106, 457–66.

22. Swinburn BA, Sacks G, Hall KD, *et al.* (2011). The global obesity pandemic: shaped by global drivers and local environments. *Lancet*, 378, 804–14.

23. Dinsa GD, Goryakin Y, Fumagalli E, Suhrcke M. (2012). Obesity and socioeconomic status in developing countries: a systematic review. *Obes Rev*, 13, 1067–79.

24. Wang Y, Lim H. (2012). The global childhood obesity epidemic and the association between socio-economic status and childhood obesity. *Int Rev Psychiatry*, 24, 176–88.

25. McFerran B, Mukhopadhyay A. (2013). Lay theories of obesity predict actual body mass. *Psychol Sci*, 24, 1428–36.

26. Wang C, Coups EJ. (2010). Causal beliefs about obesity and associated health behaviors: results from a population-based survey. *Int J Behav Nutr Phys Act*, 7, 19.

27. Hebebrand J, Bulik CM. (2011). Critical appraisal of the provisional DSM-5 criteria for anorexia nervosa and an alternative proposal. *Int J Eat Disord*, 44, 665–78.

28. Yengo L, Sidorenko J, Kemper KE, et al; GIANT Consortium (2018). Meta-analysis of genome-wide association studies for height and body mass index in ~700000 individuals of European ancestry. *Hum Mol Genet*, 27(20), 3641–9.

29. Hebebrand J, Hinney A, Knoll N, Volckmar AL, Scherag A. (2013). Molecular genetic aspects of weight regulation. *Dtsch Arztebl Int*, 110, 338–44.

30. Farooqi IS, Jebb SA, Langmack G, *et al.* (1999). Effects of recombinant leptin therapy in a child with congenital leptin deficiency. *N Engl J Med*, 341, 879–84.

31. Kenny PJ. (2011). Reward mechanisms in obesity: new insights and future directions. *Neuron*, 69, 664–79.

32. Mayer EA, Tillisch K, Gupta A. (2015). Gut/brain axis and the microbiota. *J Clin Invest*, 125, 926–38.

33. Kühnen P, Clément K, Wiegand S, *et al.* (2016). Proopiomelanocortin deficiency treated with a melanocortin-4 receptor agonist. *N Engl J Med*, 375, 240–6.

34. Brumm H, Mühlhaus J, Bolze F, *et al.* (2012). Rescue of melanocortin 4 receptor (*MC4R*) nonsense mutations by aminoglycoside-mediated read-through. *Obesity (Silver Spring)*, 20, 1074–81.

35. Bhat SP, Sharma A. (2017). Current drug targets in obesity pharmacotherapy: a review. *Curr Drug Targets*, 18, 983–93.

36. Pott W, Albayrak O, Hinney A, Hebebrand J, Pauli-Pott U. (2013). Successful treatment with atomoxetine of an adolescent boy with attention deficit/hyperactivity disorder, extreme obesity, and reduced melanocortin 4 receptor function. *Obes Facts*, 6, 109–15.

37. Albayrak O, Albrecht B, Scherag S, Barth N, Hinney A, Hebebrand J. (2011). Successful methylphenidate treatment of early onset extreme obesity in a child with a melanocortin-4 receptor gene mutation and attention deficit/hyperactivity disorder. *Eur J Pharmacol*, 660, 165–70.

38. Manning S, Pucci A, Finer N. (2014). Pharmacotherapy for obesitiy: novel agents and paradigms. *Ther Adv Chronic Dis*, 5, 135–48.

39. Onakpoya IJ, Heneghan CJ, Aronson JK. (2016). Post-marketing withdrawal of anti-obesity medicinal products because of adverse drug reactions: a systematic review. *BMC Med*, 14, 191.

40. Rosenow F, Knake S, Hebebrand J. (2002). Topiramate and anorexia nervosa. *Am J Psychiatry*, 159, 2112–13.

41. Bray GA, Frühbeck G, Ryan DH, Wilding JP. (2016). Management of obesity. *Lancet*, 387, 1947–56.

42. Khera R, Murad MH, Chandar AK, *et al.* (2016). Association of pharmacological treatments or obesity with weight loss and adverse events: a systematic review and meta-analysis. *JAMA*, 315, 2424–34.

43. Martinussen C, Bojsen-Moller KN, Svane MS, Dejgaard TF, Madsbad S. (2017). Emerging drugs for the treatment of obesity. *Expert Opin Emerg Drugs*, 22, 87–99.

44. Tschöp MH, Finan B, Clemmensen C, *et al.* (2016). Unimolecular polypharmacy for treatment of diabetes and obesity. *Cell Metab*, 24, 51–62.

45. Hendricks EJ. (2017). Off-label drugs for weight management. *Diabetes Metab Syndr Obes*, 10, 223–34.

46. Yoshimura Y, Wakabayashi H, Yamada M, Kim H, Harada A, Arai H. (2017). Interventions for treating sarcopenia: a systematic review and meta-analysis of randomized controlled studies. *J Am Med Dir Assoc*, 18, 553.e1–16.

47. Graul AI, Stringer M, Sorbera L. (2016). Cachexia. *Drugs Today (Barc)*, 52, 519–29.

48. Aversa Z, Costelli P, Muscaritoli M. (2017). Cancer-induced muscle wasting: latest findings in prevention and treatment. *Ther Adv Med Oncol*, 9, 369–82.

49. Marks DL, Ling N, Cone RD. (2001). Role of the central melanocortin system in cachexia. *Cancer Res*, 61, 1432–8.

50. Allison DB, Mentore JL, Heo M, *et al.* (1999). Antipsychotic-induced weight gain: a comprehensive research synthesis. *Am J Psychiatry*, 156, 1686–96.

51. Gothelf D, Falk B, Singer P, *et al.* (2002). Weight gain associated with increased food intake and low habitual activity levels in male adolescent schizophrenic inpatients treated with olanzapine. *Am J Psychiatry*, 159, 1055–7.

52. Theisen FM, Linden A, König IR, Martin M, Remschmidt H, Hebebrand J. (2003). Spectrum of binge eating symptomatology in patients treated with clozapine and olanzapine. *J Neural Transm (Vienna)*, 110, 111–21.

53. Gebhardt S, Theisen FM, Haberhausen M, *et al.* (2010). Body weight gain induced by atypical antipsychotics: an extension of the monozygotic twin and sib pair study. *J Clin Pharm Ther*, 35, 207–11.

54. Dold M, Aigner M, Klabunde M, Treasure J, Kasper S. (2015). Second-generation antipsychotic drugs in anorexia nervosa: a meta-analysis of randomized controlled trials. *Psychother Psychosom*, 84, 110–16.

55. Berger-Gross P, Coletti DJ, Hirschkorn K, Terranova E, Simpser EF. (2004). The effectiveness of risperidone in the treatment of three children with feeding disorders. *J Child Adolesc Psychopharmacol*, 14, 621–7.

56. Sant'Anna AM, Hammes PS, Porporino M, Martel C, Zygmuntowicz C, Ramsay M. (2014). Use of cyproheptadine in young children with feeding difficulties and poor growth in a pediatric feeding program. *J Pediatr Gastroenterol Nutr*, 59, 74–8.

57. Lutter M. (2017). Emerging treatments in eating disorders. *Neurotherapeutics*, 14, 614–22.

58. Kim YR, Eom JS, Yang JW, Kang J, Treasure J. (2015). The impact of oxytocin on food intake and emotion recognition in patients with eating disorders: a double blind single dose within-subject cross-over design. *PLoS One*, 10, e0137514.

59. Andries A, Frystyk J, Flyvbjerg A, Støving RK. (2014). Dronabinol in severe, enduring anorexia nervosa: a randomized controlled trial. *Int J Eat Disord*, 47, 18–23.

60. Hebebrand J, Albayrak O. (2012). Leptin treatment of patients with anorexia nervosa? The urgent need for initiation of clinical studies. *Eur Child Adolesc Psychiatry*, 21, 63–6.

61. Welt CK, Chan JL, Bullen J, *et al.* (2004). Recombinant human leptin in women with hypothalamic amenorrhea. *N Engl J Med*, 351, 987–97.

62. Seminara SB. (2006). Mechanisms of disease: the first kiss-a crucial role for kisspeptin-1 and its receptor, G-protein-coupled receptor 54, in puberty and reproduction. *Nat Clin Pract Endocrinol Metab*, 2, 328–34.

63. Exner C, Hebebrand J, Remschmidt H, *et al.* (2000). Leptin suppresses semi-starvation induced hyperactivity in rats: implications for anorexia nervosa. *Mol Psychiatry*, 5, 476–81.

64. Hebebrand J, Exner C, Hebebrand K, *et al.* (2003). Hyperactivity in patients with anorexia nervosa and in semistarved rats: evidence for a pivotal role of hypoleptinemia. *Physiol Behav*, 79, 25–37.

65. Holtkamp K, Herpertz-Dahlmann B, Hebebrand K, Mika C, Kratzsch J, Hebebrand J. (2006). Physical activity and restlessness correlate with leptin levels in patients with adolescent anorexia nervosa. *Biol Psychiatry*, 60, 311–13.

66. Hebebrand J, Milos G, Wabitsch M, *et al.* (2019). Clinical trials required to assess potential benefits and side effects of treatment of patients with anorexia nervosa with recombinant human leptin. *Front Psychol*, 10, 769.

67. Farr OM, Fiorenza C, Papageorgiou P, *et al.* (2014). Leptin therapy alters appetite and neural responses to food stimuli in brain areas of leptin-sensitive subjects without altering brain structure. *J Clin Endocrinol Metab*, 99, E2529–38.

68. Laque A, Yu S, Qualls-Creekmore E, *et al.* (2015). Leptin modulates nutrient reward via inhibitory galanin action on orexin neurons. *Mol Metab*, 4, 706–17.

69. Monteleone AM, Castellini G, Volpe U, *et al.* (2018). Neuroendocrinology and brain imaging of reward in eating disorders: a possible key to the treatment of anorexia nervosa and bulimia nervosa. *Prog Neuropsychopharmacol Biol Psychiatry*, 80, 132–42.

70. Shanahan WR, Rose JE, Glicklich A, Stubbe S, Sanchez-Kam M. (2017). Lorcaserin for smoking cessation and associated weight gain: a randomized 12-week clinical trial. *Nicotine Tob Res*, 19, 944–51.

71. Turnbaugh PJ, Ley RE, Mahowald MA, Magrini V, Mardis ER, Gordon JI. (2006). An obesity-associated gut microbiome with increased capacity for energy harvest. *Nature*, 444, 1027–31.

72. Ridaura VK, Faith JJ, Rey FE, *et al.* (2013). Gut microbiota from twins discordant for obesity modulate metabolism in mice. *Science*, 341, 1241214.

73. Mathur R, Barlow GM. (2015). Obesity and the microbiome. *Expert Rev Gastroenterol Hepatol*, 9, 1087–99.

74. den Besten G, van Eunen K, Groen AK, Venema K, Reijngoud DJ, Bakker BM. (2013). The role of short-chain fatty acids in the interplay between diet, gut microbiota, and host energy metabolism. *J Lipid Res*, 54, 2325–40.

75. Herpertz-Dahlmann B, Seitz J, Baines J. (2017). Food matters: how the microbiome and gut-brain interaction might impact the development and course of anorexia nervosa. *Eur Child Adolesc Psychiatry*, 26, 1031–41.

76. Brahe LK, Astrup A, Larsen LH. (2013). Is butyrate the link between diet, intestinal microbiota and obesity-related metabolic diseases? *Obes Rev*, 14, 950–9.

77. De Vadder F, Kovatcheva-Datchary P, Goncalves D, *et al.* (2014). Microbiota-generated metabolites promote metabolic benefits via gut-brain neural circuits. *Cell*, 156, 84–96.

78. Trehan I, Goldbach HS, LaGrone LN, *et al.* (2013). Antibiotics as part of the management of severe acute malnutrition. *N Engl J Med*, 368, 425–35.

79. Jesus P, Ouelaa W, Francois M, *et al.* (2014). Alteration of intestinal barrier function during activity-based anorexia in mice. *Clin Nutr*, 33, 1046–53.

80. Kleiman SC, Watson HJ, Bulik-Sullivan EC, *et al.* (2015). The intestinal microbiota in acute anorexia nervosa and during renourishment: relationship to depression, anxiety, and eating disorder psychopathology. *Psychosom Med*, 77, 969–81.

81. Mack I, Cuntz U, Gramer C, *et al.* (2016). Weight gain in anorexia nervosa does not ameliorate the faecal microbiota, branched chain fatty acid profiles, and gastrointestinal complaints. *Sci Rep*, 6, 26752.

82. Solmi M, Veronese N, Favaro A, *et al.* (2015). Inflammatory cyto-kines and anorexia nervosa: a meta-analysis of cross-sectional and longitudinal studies. *Psychoneuroendocrinol*, 51, 237–52.

83. Hamilton MK, Raybould HE. (2016). Bugs, guts and brains, and the regulation of food intake and body weight. *Int J Obes Suppl*, 6 Suppl 1, S8–14.

84. David LA, Maurice CF, Carmody RN, *et al.* (2014). Diet rapidly and reproducibly alters the human gut microbiome. *Nature*, 505, 7484, 559–63.

85. Raevuori A, Haukka J, Vaarala O, *et al.* (2014). The increased risk for autoimmune diseases in patients with eating disorders. *PLoS One*, 9, e104845.

86. Gibson GR, Roberfroid MB. (1995). Dietary modulation of the human colonic microbiota: introducing the concept of prebiotics. *J Nutr*, 125, 6, 1401–12.

87. Kelly JR, Kennedy PJ, Cryan JF, Dinan TG, Clarke G, Hyland NP. (2015). Breaking down the barriers: the gut microbiome, intestinal permeability and stress-related psychiatric disorders. *Front Cell Neurosci*, 9, 392.

88. Lurie I, Yang YX, Haynes K, Mamtani R, Boursi B. (2015). Antibiotic exposure and the risk for depression, anxiety, or psychosis: a nested case-control study. *J Clin Psychiatry*, 76, 1522–8.

89. Bulik-Sullivan B, Finucane HK, Anttila V, *et al.* (2015). An atlas of genetic correlations across human diseases and traits. *Nat Genet*, 47, 1236–41.

90. Herpertz-Dahlmann B. (2015). Adolescent eating disorders: up-date on definitions, symptomatology, epidemiology, and comorbidity. *Child Adolesc Psychiatr Clin N Am*, 24, 177–96.

91. Miller KK. (2011). Endocrine dysregulation in anorexia nervosa update. *J Clin Endocrinol Metab*. 96, 2939–49.p

92. Antel J, Hebebrand J. (2012). Weight-reducing side effects of the antiepileptic agents topiramate and zonisamide. *Handb Exp Pharmacol*, 209, 433–66.

# 103

# Epidemiology and primary prevention of feeding and eating disorders

*Katherine A. Halmi*

## Incidence and prevalence

Almost all published incidence and prevalence studies of eating disorders are based on data using DSM-IV diagnostic criteria that were obtained over at least a decade ago [1]. Most of these studies were conducted in specific population settings, such as schools, colleges, and primary care clinics, as well as from medical records. Information was collected either from standardized interviews or via self-report questionnaires. Thus, comparing the incidence and prevalence of eating disorders among various countries is more likely to be approximate than accurate. Adequate incidence studies are restricted by the need for large population samples and costs. The incidence of eating disorders, which is the number of new cases in a population over a specific period of time, is usually expressed as 100,000 persons per year. Prevalence is usually expressed either as point prevalence, which is the number of cases with a disorder at a specific point in time, or lifetime prevalence, which is the proportion of persons that had the disorder at any time in their life. There are many more published prevalence, compared to incidence, studies of eating disorders. With varying sensitivity of assessments used in these studies, comparisons are difficult to make.

The incidence of anorexia nervosa (AN) remained relatively stable between 1980 and 2000. In the United Kingdom (UK), the number of new cases from 1988 to 1993 was 4.2 per 100,000, and that from 1994 to 2000 was 4.7 per 100,000 [2]. From 1985 to 1989, the Netherlands had 7.4 new cases of AN per 100,000, and from 1995 to 1999, there were 7.7 new cases per 100,000. The incidence of eating disorders was highest among females aged 15–19 and comprised 40% of all cases—56.4 per 100,000 in 1985 and 109.2 per 100,000 in 1995–1999 [3]. The incidence of males was less than 1 per 100,000 in both countries. Incidence studies in the United States (US) are restricted to the state of Minnesota where the overall age-adjusted incidence was 15 per 100,000 in females and 1.5 per 100,000 in males from 1935 to 1989. Among 15- to 24-year-old females, the incidence rates increased from 1950 to 1984 by 1.03 per 100,000 person-years per calendar year. The increased rate was especially present in females aged 10–14 [4].

Studies on the incidence of bulimia nervosa (BN) are sparse. The incidence of BN among Finnish females aged 15–18, including those who lacked one criteria, was 438 per 100,000 person-years [5]. The incidence of BN in a nationwide primary care study in the Netherlands was 8.6 per 100,000 person-years in 1985–1989 and decreased to 6.1 per 100,000 person-years in 1995–1999 [3]. Similarly, the incidence of BN in the UK decreased from 12.2 per 100,000 person years in 1993 to 6.6 per 100,000 person years in 2000. The incidence remained stable in women aged 10–19 at 40 per 100,000 person years in 1993 and 2000 [2]. In the US, incidence rates from 1980 to 1990 in Minnesota were 26.5 per 100,000 per year in females and 0.8 per 100,000 per year in males. The mean age of onset in females was 23 years. Among 15- to 24-year-old females, it has become over twice as common as AN [6].

There are no published incidence studies for binge eating disorder (BED) or DSM-IV eating disorder not otherwise specified (EDNOS), and there are no adequate incidence studies available for rumination syndrome (RS) and pica. Avoidant/restrictive food intake disorder (ARFID), an eating disorder diagnosis created by DSM-5 [7], has only been recently defined, such that there are no published epidemiology and prevention studies as yet.

Two large-sample studies reported a lifetime prevalence of AN in the US of 0.3% among 13- to 18-year-old females and males [8], and 0.9% among adult females and 0.3% among males [9]. An 8-year prospective study of adolescent girls in the United States reported a lifetime prevalence of AN of 0.6% by age 20 and 2.0% for atypical AN using DSM-IV criteria [10]. A population-based survey in six European countries reported a lifetime prevalence of AN of 0.9% among females and 0% among males [11]. In a Dutch community sample, over 2000 children were assessed from age 11 in 2001 to age 19–20 in 2010. At age 19–20, there was a lifetime prevalence of 1.7% of DSM-5 AN among women and 0.1% among men [12].

The lifetime prevalence in the US for BN was 1.6% among 20-year-old females who were followed up for 8 years [10]. In a study across six European countries, the lifetime prevalence of BN was 0.88% among females and 0.12% among males [11]. The point prevalence of BN among university women in the US decreased from 4.2% in 1982 to 1.7% in 2002 [13]. Initially, high rates for BN found in the

1980s were based on DSM-III criteria [14]. DSM-IV criteria from 1994 for BN were more restrictive. Since the criteria for BN have become again less restrictive in DSM-5, increases in BN prevalence may be expected with DSM-5 criteria.

BED appears to be the most common of the three major eating disorders, with a lifetime prevalence in the US of 3.5% among women and 2.0% among men [9]. In US adolescents aged 13–18 years, the lifetime prevalence of BED was 2.3% among females and 0.8% among males [8]. In a study involving six European countries, the lifetime prevalence of BED was found to be 1.9% among women and 0.3% among men [11].

Prevalence data on RS are scant. One survey of 2163 children aged 10–16 years in Sri Lanka found a prevalence of RS of 5.1% among boys and 5.0% among girls. Only 8.2% had daily symptoms, and 62.7% had weekly symptoms [15]. Likewise, adequate prevalence data on pica are not available. The prevalence of pica in populations considered to be at risk was found to be up to 77% among pregnant women, 15% among persons with intellectual disabilities, 74% among sub-Saharan African children, and 61% among persons with iron deficiency [16].

## Outcome and mortality

Of psychiatric disorders, AN has one of the highest mortality rates. A meta-analysis of 36 studies showed a standardized mortality rate (SMR) of 5.86 for AN, with one in five persons dying by suicide [17]. In the US, a 20-year follow-up study reported 6.5% deaths with an SMR of 4.37 for lifetime AN. The duration of illness affected the SMR, such that those with AN for 0–15 years had an SMR of 3.25, and those with AN for 15–30 years had an SMR of 6.6 [18]. An analysis of 119 outcome studies found less than half of AN patients had full recovery, 33% improved, and 20% developed a chronic course [19]. A Dutch study found that age at the time of detection and treatment predicted recovery, with those aged 19 years and below having an odds ratio of recovery of 4.3, compared to those aged 20 years and above [20]. A US longitudinal analysis of mortality among those aged 8–25 years in 906 BN clinic outpatients found a crude mortality rate of 3.9% and an SMR of 1.57. There was a significantly elevated risk for suicide at 0.9%, which accounted for 23% of the deaths [21]. Outcome studies of BN reported recovery rates which varied from 48% [22] to 77% [23]. One large-sample, 12-year follow-up study of 68 German BED patients found a crude mortality rate of 2.9% and a non-significant SMR of 2.29 [24]. Most outcome studies of BED comprised EDNOS analyses. The overall summary is that BED remission is somewhat better than that of BN. Published outcome and mortality studies other than a few case reports are not available for RS and pica.

## Ethnicity and sociocultural demographics

Global social and cultural changes associated with industrialization and urbanization have influenced the increasing prevalence of eating disorders among minority groups in Western Europe and North America, as well as in Asian and Arab countries [25]. The prevalence of eating disorders and disturbed eating behaviours is increasing in China, Singapore, South Korea, Egypt, Pakistan, United Arab Emirates, Oman, Lebanon, Kuwait, Iran, and Jordan [25].

In the twenty-first century, the NIMH Collaborative Psychiatric Epidemiological Studies (CPES) found no significant differences in prevalence for AN and BED in the US across Latinos, Asians, African-Americans, and non-Latino whites. BN was more prevalent among Latinos and African-Americans than among non-Latino whites [26]. Utilization of mental health services was lower in all ethnic minority groups, compared to non-Latino whites [27]. Contributing factors include lack of health insurance, lack of affordable and accessible treatment services, and beliefs about seeking treatment. African-American women presenting for BED treatment had a higher BMI and binge eating frequency than whites, and lower depression than white and Hispanic groups [28]. A survey among American college students found Arab Americans reported the highest prevalence of binge eating of 10% [29].

Social factors have also been identified to be associated with the development of eating disorders. In Curacao, cases of AN were found only in mixed-ethnicity women who reported that thinness allowed them greater acceptance in the more affluent white community [30]. Higher rates of eating disorders have been reported to be associated with activities in which leanness is valued, such as dancing and gymnastics, as well as among jockeys [31].

## Primary prevention

### Risk factors

Identification of risk factors is essential for the implementation of effective intervention strategies. Risk factors for eating disorders and disordered eating behaviour diagnosed according to DSM-IV and DSM-5 increase in early adolescence, on which most studies on eating disorder risk thus focus. The majority of these studies have used self-report questionnaires to assess for disordered eating behaviour, rather than discrete eating disorder diagnoses.

For specific eating disorders, female adolescents in sixth to ninth grades reporting social pressure to be thin and body image preoccupation showed a higher risk for onset of threshold or subthreshold BN or BED over a 3-year follow-up [32]. High-school females reporting weight and shape concerns and negative affectivity had a higher risk for onset of threshold and subthreshold BN over a 4-year follow-up [33]. High dietary restraint was associated with an increased risk for onset of any eating disorder among women aged 16–23 years [34].

A study examining six risk factors at ages 13, 14, 15, and 16 found body dissatisfaction was the most consistent and robust predictor of a future eating disorder. Five of the risk factors were highly significant predictors at age 14, suggesting this age may be a key developmental time point for preventative intervention. The authors proposed a combination of physical and cognitive maturational processes such as completion of puberty, increased capacity for abstract thinking, increased peer influence, and the onset of dating and sexual experiences at this age [34].

Moderating risk factors for AN were identified in a study of children and adolescents from the Danish Psychiatric Central Research Register. Risk factors included female sex, having a sibling with AN, affective disorders in family members, and five major comorbid disorders (affective, anxiety, obsessive–compulsive, substance use, and personality disorders) present in the AN proband [35]. Eating disorders in either parent were independently associated with eating disorders in their female children in an analysis of the Stockholm Youth Cohort [36].

An analysis of obstetric records found maternal anaemia, diabetes mellitus, pre-eclampsia, placental infarction, neonatal cardiac problems, and hypoactivity were significant independent predictors of the development of AN. The risk of developing AN increased with the total number of obstetric complications. In the same study, obstetric complications significantly associated with BN were: placental infarction, neonatal hypoactivity, early eating difficulties, and low birthweight for gestational age [37]. There is some question on whether *in utero* exposure to a viral infection could increase the risk of developing AN. Exposure during the sixth month of pregnancy to the peak of chickenpox and rubella infections was significantly associated with the risk of developing AN [38]. A comparison of risk factors across AN, BN, and BED [39] showed that AN and BED were distinct from each other, with AN having greater exposure to perfectionism and BED reporting greater exposure to conduct problems, substance abuse, severe childhood obesity, and family overeating. BN shared risk factors with both AN and BED. On examining the AN subtypes, perfectionism carried a greater risk for restricting AN and family overeating while sexual abuse had a greater risk for the binge purge subtype of AN. Two-thirds of women with AN reported their eating disorder started with dieting, whereas two-thirds of women with BN and BED reported their eating disorder started with binge eating.

Risk factors have also been assessed for disordered eating and weight loss behaviours occurring without a designated eating disorder diagnosis. Depression-related symptoms and body dissatisfaction were found to be risk factors for disordered eating in overweight youths [40]. Dieting, depression, and body image distortion in adolescence predicted extreme weight loss behaviours and binge eating in young adulthood.

## Prevention programmes

### Meta-analytic reviews

Eating disorder prevention programmes that were controlled or those with systematic follow-up began in the 1980s. The outcome of these studies was determined by the decrease in related eating disorder symptoms, rather that identifying the occurrence of diagnosable eating disorders. Targeted populations have varied from at-risk individuals to all persons in specific age groups and in specific environments such as schools and colleges. A meta-analysis conducted in 2007 of 66 controlled outcome studies that targeted persons aged 15 and above with high levels of body dissatisfaction and weight concerns, using interactive paradigms administered by professionals, found small, but significant, effect sizes of these preventative interventions [41].

More recently, a study of an Internet-based prevention programme (Student Bodies) [42] and a meta-analytic review of six US and four German randomized controlled trials of 990 female high-school and college students [43] found that interventions produced moderate improvements in reduction of negative body image and the desire to be thin.

Further, a meta-analysis of 20 Internet-based programmes designed to reduce eating disorder symptoms and representing three different interventions found these programmes effective both in individuals with a clinical diagnosis of an eating disorder and in those with symptoms only [44]. Compared with control conditions, these interventions reduced body dissatisfaction, internalization of the thin ideal, shape and weight concerns, dietary restriction, drive for thinness, bulimic symptoms, purging frequency, and negative affect.

In a systematic review of interventions involving parents in the prevention of body dissatisfaction or eating disorders in children, only 20 studies were identified. Of these, only four had high-quality data, with two reporting parental involvement significantly improved children's outcome on body dissatisfaction or disordered eating. Two studies were inconclusive on the role of parental involvement [45]. However, several considerations were noted—a child's perception of their parent's behaviour is more important than the parent's perception of their own behaviour; measuring and communicating a child's at-risk status does not improve parental engagement with prevention programmes; and parents of a child with the diagnosis of an eating disorder were more likely to access prevention programmes. The benefit of involving parents in eating disorder treatment is well established. The challenge is how to motivate parents to participate in preventative research.

### Specific prevention programmes

The most frequently studied dissonance-based prevention programme is the Body Project. This paradigm is based on the proven theory that cognitive dissonance motivates participants to reduce their adherence to their original attitude. In the Body Project, participants are instructed to critique the thin ideal through verbal, written, and behavioural exercises. This is done in the context of small groups, with one or two clinicians, over four sessions. Home exercises include writing an essay about the costs of pursuing the thin ideal and standing in front of a mirror with minimal clothing while recording positive attributes about one's body. Group sessions include role plays and discussion assignments [46]. The Body Project was found to reduce caudate response to thin models in an fMRI study, providing evidence that this intervention reduces the idealization and significance attached to media images.

Another effective prevention programme tested in randomized controlled trials is the Student Bodies, which is an 8-week Internet-based programme focusing on reducing body weight and shape concerns. This programme uses cognitive behavioural therapy techniques and includes weekly exercises and journal log prompts. It is designed to create healthier behaviour patterns with eating, exercise, sleep, mood, and emotion regulation. After completion of the programme, participants are provided continued access to Student Bodies for 9 months for reviewing material as needed [47].

A mindfulness- and school-based eating disorder prevention programme of three sessions aimed to increase the capacity to refrain from automatic responses when confronted with the thin ideal and related sociocultural pressures and to reduce the impact of any experiences with a negative affective component. The sessions include common coping strategies, role play, and various guided exercises. This programme significantly reduced weight and shape concerns, dietary restraint, thin ideal internalization, eating disorder symptoms, and psychosocial impairment [48].

## Targeted populations for eating disorder prevention

Several recent controlled studies have demonstrated either efficacy or effectiveness of school-based programmes in reducing risk factors for eating disorders in adolescents. A Spanish study based on the social cognitive model, media literacy education, and cognitive dissonance found the intervention group had greater reduction in beauty ideal internalization, disordered eating attitudes, and weight-related teasing, compared to the control group, at 1 year follow-up [49]. An Australian study using a similar intervention in girls and boys in seventh and eighth grades showed similar results [50]. A US web-based intervention—Staying Fit—was effective in reducing weight/shape concerns and improving fruit and vegetable consumption in ninth-grade students at risk for eating disorders [51].

College students participating in the online programme Student Bodies in their first college year had a reduction in body image and eating concerns, continuing into their sophomore year [52]. Body dissatisfaction and shape and weight concerns decreased, whereas self-esteem increased in college students participating in a brief conditioning intervention [53].

Women with subthreshold eating disorder syndromes responded to the Internet-based prevention programme Student Bodies with a reduction or abstinence in binge eating, purging, and other disordered eating symptoms [54].

Female adolescents reporting body image dissatisfaction were recruited from two primary care clinics. They responded to a brief dissonance-based eating disorder prevention programme with reduced thin ideal internalization, pressure to be thin, dieting, and eating disorder symptoms [55].

The Parent-Based Prevention (PBP) of eating disorders targeted risk factors and facilitated behavioural change in mothers with eating disorders and their spouses to mitigate negative outcomes in their children. This uncontrolled study suggested PBP produces decreased risk of eating and mental problems in these children [56].

### Salient issues for primary prevention of eating disorders

The implementation of evidence-based eating disorder prevention programmes requires attention to issues delineated in the Consolidated Framework for Implementation Research (CFIR) model [57]. These issues, as applied to the eating disorder prevention programme Body Project, are well outlined by Shaw and Stice [58]. In summary: (1) a programme is more readily adopted if those delivering it perceive they had input into developing it; (2) there is belief among programme deliverers on the quality and validity of evidence for a desired outcome; (3) the programme has an advantage over alternative interventions; (4) the programme is accepted by participants and those delivering it and has low attrition; (5) the intervention can be adapted to meet local needs; (6) the complexity of the intervention does not inhibit its implementation; (7) design quality and packaging are appealing; and (8) costs, such as cost of manuals and related items, clinician training, and recruiting are reasonable.

For the Body Project, the most commonly reported barriers to including additional groups were limited time and high staff turnover. For participants who do not respond to the prevention programmes, revisions such as increased intensity or creative adjustments are necessary.

The problems of recruitment, screening, implementing the intervention, and influencing the community culture have been addressed in the Healthy Body Image programme [59]. This programme targets intervention across socio-environmental levels that impact students' eating and activity patterns. It aims to improve body esteem and eating attitudes and behaviours and to change cultural norms around nutrition and body image for a healthier campus community.

## Future directions

The changing demographics of eating disorders need to be continually monitored, so that all ethnic and socio-economic affected groups have access to adequate and financially feasible treatment programmes. Large population studies are needed to better ascertain the strength of the influence various moderating and mediating risk factors have on the development of eating disorders.

Specific risk factors that respond to specific treatment strategies need to be identified to create more effective preventative interventions. All interventions need to be assessed for adherence to the programme, attrition rate, and effectiveness over time.

## REFERENCES

1. American Psychiatric Association (1994). *Diagnostic and statistical manual of mental disorders*, fourth edition. Washington, DC, American Psychiatric Association.
2. Currin L, Schmidt U, Treasure J, *et al.* (2005). Time trends in the incidence of eating disorders. *Br J Psychiatry* 186: 132–5.
3. van Son GE, van Furth EF, Barteld AM, *et al.* (2006). Time trends in the incidence of eating disorders: a primary care study in the Netherlands. *Int J Eat Disord* 39: 565–9.
4. Lucas AR, Beerd CM, O'Fallon WN (1999). 50 year trend in the incidence of anorexia nervosa in Rochester Minn. A population study. *Am J Psychiatry* 148: 917–22.
5. Isomaa R, Isomaa A, Marttunen M, *et al.* (2009). The prevalence, incidence and development of eating disorders in Finnish adolescents: a two-step 3 year follow-up study. *Eur Eat Disord Rev* 17: 199–207.
6. Soundy TJ, Lucas AR, Suman VJ, *et al.* (1995). Bulimia nervosa in Rochester Minnesota, 1980–1990. *Psychol Med* 25: 1065–71.
7. American Psychiatric Association (2013). *Diagnostic and statistical manual of mental disorders*, fifth edition. Washington, DC, American Psychiatric Association.
8. Swanson SA, Crow SJ, Le Grange D, *et al.* (2011). Prevalence and correlates of eating disorders in adolescents—results from the national comorbidity survey replication adolescent supplement. *Arch Gen Psychiatry* 68: 714–23.
9. Hudson J, Hiripi E, Pope H (2007). The prevalence and correlates of eating disorders in the National Comorbidity Survey Replication. *Biol Psychiatry* 61: 348–58.
10. Stice E, Marti C, Shaw H, *et al.* (2009). An 8-year longitudinal study of the natural history of threshold, subthreshold, and partial eating disorders from a community sample of adolescents. *J Abnorm Psychol* 118: 587–97.

11. Preti A, de Girolamio G, Vilagut G, *et al.* (2009). The epidemiology of eating disorders in six European countries: results of the ESE-MED-WMH project. *J Psychiatr Res* 43: 1125–32.

12. Smink RE, Hoeken D, Oldehinkel AJ, *et al.* (2014). Prevalence and severity of DSM V eating disorders in a community cohort of adolescents. *Int J Eat Disord* 47: 610–19.

13. Keel P, Heatherton H, Dorer D, *et al.* (2006). Point prevalence of bulimia nervosa in 1982, 1992, and 2002. *Psychol Med* 36: 119–27.

14. American Psychiatric Association (1987). *Diagnostic and statistical manual of mental disorders*, third edition. Washington, DC, American Psychiatric Association.

15. Rajindrajith S, Manjuri N, Perera B (2012). Rumination syndrome in children and adolescents: a school survey assessing prevalence and symptomatology. *BMC Gastroenterol* 12: 163–8.

16. Delaney C, Eddy K, Hartmann A (2015). Pica and rumination behavior among Individuals seeking treatment for eating disorders or obesity. *Int J Eat Disord* 48: 238–48.

17. Arcelus J, Mitchell A, Wales J, *et al.* (2011). Mortality rates in patients with anorexia nervosa and other eating disorders. *Arch Gen Psychiatry* 68: 724–31.

18. Franko DL, Keskaiah A, Eddy K (2013). A longitudinal investigation of mortality in anorexia nervosa and bulimia nervosa. *Am J Psychiatry* 170: 917–25.

19. Steinhausen H (2002). The outcome of anorexia nervosa in the 20th century. *Am J Psychiatry* 159: 1284–93.

20. van Son G, Hoeken D, Furth E (2010). Course and outcome of eating disorders in a primary care based cohort. *Int J Eat Disord* 43: 130–8.

21. Crow S, Peterson C, Swanson E, *et al.* (2009). Increased mortality in bulimia nervosa and other eating disorders. *Am J Psychiatry* 166: 1342–6.

22. Fairburn C, Cooper Z, Dolt H, *et al.* (2000). The natural course of bulimia nervosa and binge eating disorder in young women. *Arch Gen Psychiatry* 57: 659–65.

23. Ben-Tovim D, Walker K, Gilchrist F, *et al.* (2001). Outcome in patients with eating disorders, a five year study. *Lancet* 357: 254–7.

24. Fichter M, Quadflieg W (2008). Twelve year course and outcome of bulimia nervosa. *Psychol Med* 43: 1396–406.

25. Pike K, Hoek H, Dunne P (2014). Cultural trends and eating disorders. *Curr Opin* 27: 436–42.

26. Heeringa SG, Berglund P (2007). *National Institutes of Mental Health (NIMH) Collaborative Psychiatric Epidemiology Survey Program (CPES) Data Set: integrated weights and sampling error codes for design-based analysis.* Ann Arbor, MI, University of Michigan, Survey Research Center.

27. Marques L, Alegria M, Becker A, *et al.* (2011). Comparative prevalence, correlates of impairment and service utilization for eating disorders across US ethnic groups. *Int J Eat Disord* 44: 412–20.

28. Lydecker J, Grilo C (2016). Different yet similar: examining race and ethnicity in treatment seeking adults with binge eating disorder. *J Consult and Clin Psychol* 84: 88–94.

29. Reslan S, Saules K (2013). Assessing the prevalence of and factors associated with overweight obesity and binge eating as a function of ethnicity. *Eat Weight Disord* 18: 209–19.

30. Katzman M, Hermans K, van Koeken D, *et al.* (2004). Not your typical island woman: anorexia nervosa is reported only in subcultures in Curacao. *Cult Med Psychiatry* 28: 463–92.

31. Thompson S, Digsby S (2004). A preliminary survey of dieting, body dissatisfaction, and eating problems among high scholl cheerleaders. *J School Health* 74: 85–90.

32. Patton GC, Selzer R, Coffey C, *et al.* (1999). Onset of adolescent eating disorders: population cohort study over 3 years. *BMJ* 318: 765–78.

33. Killen JD, Taylor CB, Hayward C, *et al.* (1996). Weight concerns influence the development of eating disorders: a 4-year prospective study. *J Consult Clin Psychol* 64: 963–740.

34. Rohde P, Stice E, Marti C (2015). Development and Predictive effects of eating disorder risk factors during adolescence; implications for preventive efforts. *Int J Eat Disord* 48: 187–98.

35. Steinhausen HC, Jacobsen H, Munk-Jorgensen P, *et al.* (2015). A nation-wide study of the family aggregation and risk factors in anorexia nervosa over three generations. *Int J Eat Disord* 48: 1–8.

36. Bould H, Sovio U, Koupil I, *et al.* (2015). Do eating disorders in parents predict eating disorders on children? Evidence from a Swedish cohort. *Acta Psychiatr Scand* 132: 51–9.

37. Favaro A, Tenconi E, Santonastaso P (2006). Perinatal factors and the risk of developing anorexia nervosa and bulimia nervosa. *Arch Gen Psychiatry* 63: 82–8.

38. Favaro A, Tenconi E, Ceschin L, *et al.* (2011). *In utero* exposure to virus infections and the risk of developing anorexia nervosa. *Psychol Med* 41: 2193–9.

39. Hilbert A, Pike K, Goldschmidt A, *et al.* (2014). Risk factors across the eating disorders. *Psychiatry Res* 220: 500–6.

40. Goldschmidt A, Wall M, Loth K (2015). Risk factors for disordered eating in overweight adolescents and young adults. *J Pediatr Psychol* 40: 1048–55.

41. Stice E, Shaw H, Marti CN (2007). A meta-analytic review of eating disorder prevention programs: encouraging findings. *Ann Rev Clin Psychol* 3: 207–31.

42. Winzelberg A, Epstein D, Eldredge E, *et al.* (2000). Effectiveness of an internet-based program for reducing risk factors for eating disorders. *J Consult Clin Psychol* 68: 346–50.

43. Beitner I, Jacobi C, Taylor CB (2012). Effects of an Internet-based prevention program for eating disorders in the US and Germany: a meta-analytic review. *Eur Eat Disord Rev* 20: 1–8.

44. Melioli, Bauer S, Moesser M, *et al.* (2016). Reducing eating disorder symptoms and risk factors using the internet: a meta-analytic review. *Int J Eat Disord* 49: 19–31.

45. Hart LM, Cornell C, Damiano SR, *et al.* (2015). Parents and prevention: a systematic review of interventions involving parents that aim to prevent body dissatisfaction or eating disorders. *Int J Eat Disord* 48: 157–69.

46. Stice E, Yocum S, Waters A (2015). Dissonance-based eating disorder prevention program reduces reward region response to thin models: how actions shape valuation. *PLoS One* 12: 1–16.

47. Kass A, Trochel M, Safer D, *et al.* (2014). Internet-based prevention intervention for reducing eating disorder risk: a randomized controlled trial comparing guided with unguided self-help. *Behav Res Ther* 63: 90–8.

48. Atkinson M, Wade T (2015). Mindfulness-based prevention for eating disorders: a school-based cluster randomized controlled study. *Int J Eat Disord* 48: 1024–37.

49. Sanchez D, Fauquet J, Lopez G, *et al.* (2016). The MABIC project: an effectiveness trial for reducing risk factors for eating disorders. *Behav Res Ther* 77: 23–33.

50. Wilksch S, Paxton S, Byrne S, *et al.* (2015). Prevention across the spectrum: a randomized controlled trial of three programs to reduce risk factors for both eating disorder and obesity. *Psychol Med* 45: 1811–23.

51. Jones M, Lynch K, Kass A, *et al.* (2014). Healthy weight regulation and eating disorder prevention in high school students: a universal and targeted web-based intervention. *J Med Internet Res* 16: 57–67.

52. Low K, Charanasomboon S, Lesser J (2006). Effectiveness of a computer-based interactive eating disorders prevention program at long-term follow-up. *Eat Disord* 14: 17–30.

53. Aspen V, Martijn C, Alleva J, *et al.* (2015). Decreasing dissatis-faction using a brief conditioning intervention. *Behav Res Ther* 69: 93–9.

54. Jacobi C, Volker U, Trockel MT, *et al.* (2012). Effects of an internet-based intervention for subthreshold eating disorders: a randomized controlled trial. *Behav Res Ther* 50: 93–9.

55. Linville D, Cobb E, Lenee T, *et al.* (2015). Effectiveness of an eating disorder preventative intervention in primary care set-tings. *Behav Res Ther* 75: 32–9.

56. Sadeh-Sharvit S, Zubery E, Mankovski E, *et al.* (2016). Parent-based prevention program for the children of mothers with eating disorders: feasibility and preliminary outcomes. *Eat Disord* 8: 1–14.

57. Damschroder L, Aron D, Keith R, *et al.* (2009). Fostering im-plementation of health services research findings into practice. *Implement Sci* 4: 50.

58. Shaw H, Stice E (2016). The implementation of evidence-based eating disorder prevention programs. *Eat Disord* 12: 71–8.

59. Jones M, Kass A, Trockel M, *et al.* (2014). A population-wide screening and tailored intervention platform for eating disorders on college campuses: the Healthy Body Image Program. *J Am Coll Health* 62: 351–7.

# 104

# Genetics of feeding and eating disorders

*Christopher Hübel, Cynthia M. Bulik, and Gerome Breen*

## Introduction

Eating disorders are serious psychiatric illnesses that are associated with a broad range of somatic and psychiatric comorbidities, high disability-adjusted life years, and premature mortality [1–4]. The *Diagnostic and Statistical Manual of Mental Disorders*, fifth edition (DSM-5) diagnostic category of feeding and eating disorders encompasses anorexia nervosa (AN), bulimia nervosa (BN), binge eating disorder (BED), avoidant and restrictive food intake disorder (ARFID), rumination disorder, pica, and other specified feeding and eating disorders (OSFED) [5]. Genetic research has primarily investigated AN, BN, and BED throughout the last 25 years, with very little research conducted into the remaining categories. This chapter therefore focuses on these three eating disorders.

## Genetic methodologies

The aetiological understanding of eating disorders is closely linked to the understanding of complex disorder genetics, which has changed fundamentally in the last two decades. Genetic research has been divided into two major fields: quantitative and molecular genetics. In quantitative genetics, twin, adoption, and family studies are used to estimate the influence and relative contribution of genetic and environmental factors on human traits. Unlike family studies, twin and adoption studies have the advantage of being able to distinguish between shared and non-shared environmental factors, while generating an estimate of the total heritable contribution to risk for developing a disorder, called heritability. Shared environmental factors are those which siblings have in common, such as their shared family home (which increase sibling similarity), while non-shared environmental factors are those which they do not have in common, such as activities or sports in which only one sibling takes part (which decrease sibling similarity) [6].

Within this framework of an integrative model of genetic and environmental factors, every individual is assumed to have a certain genetic liability to developing an eating disorder. When individuals with a genetic liability that exceeds a threshold face common environmental pressures, this may induce symptoms. If the severity or duration of symptoms exceeds a defined clinical threshold, this individual may be diagnosed as mentally or physically ill [7]. Identifying genetic and environmental risk factors could enable health care professionals to intervene at any possible stage of a disorder—before the onset, at the onset, during progression, and after remission—to guarantee the best possible prevention, diagnosis, and treatment. In practice, considerations of false positive rates mean that this is best done in high-risk populations, rather than the general population. However, the identification of genetic variants can also shed light on the underlying aetiopathology of a disorder; the identification and understanding of these biological changes may lead to the development of new medications. In molecular genetics, linkage, candidate gene, and genome-wide association studies (GWAS) have been conducted to detect genetic variants associated with some of the eating disorders. These methods differ in their underlying theoretical considerations and assumptions, particularly in how much of the genome they cover and the assumptions (or lack thereof) of what the underlying genetic architecture of a disorder is.

### Linkage studies

Linkage studies are based on the 'linkage' (that is, the co-segregation of specific genetic regions with disorders in families), using a set of a few hundred to several thousand genetic markers and testing which appear to be inherited alongside a given trait or disorder. Co-segregation is tested in large family pedigrees or in many smaller pedigrees simultaneously. Linkage studies of eating disorders have yielded inconsistent results and have not been replicated. This may be due to a number of reasons, but fundamentally the evidence is that there are no genes with large effect size mutations in families with eating disorders that are detectable by linkage studies, which are unsuitable to detect genetic risk variants that have small effects. Linkage studies are thus currently out of favour.

### Association studies

Association studies, such as candidate gene studies and GWAS, are an alternative method to investigate the genetic underpinnings of disorders by comparing frequencies of the different alleles of genetic markers between cases and healthy controls. Candidate gene studies were popular in the 1990s and 2000s and are hypothesis-driven studies that only included the analysis of one or a few genetic markers in single or several genes, with both the genes and genotyped markers selected mostly based on their biological function/impact. Single-nucleotide polymorphisms (SNPs) are used as genetic

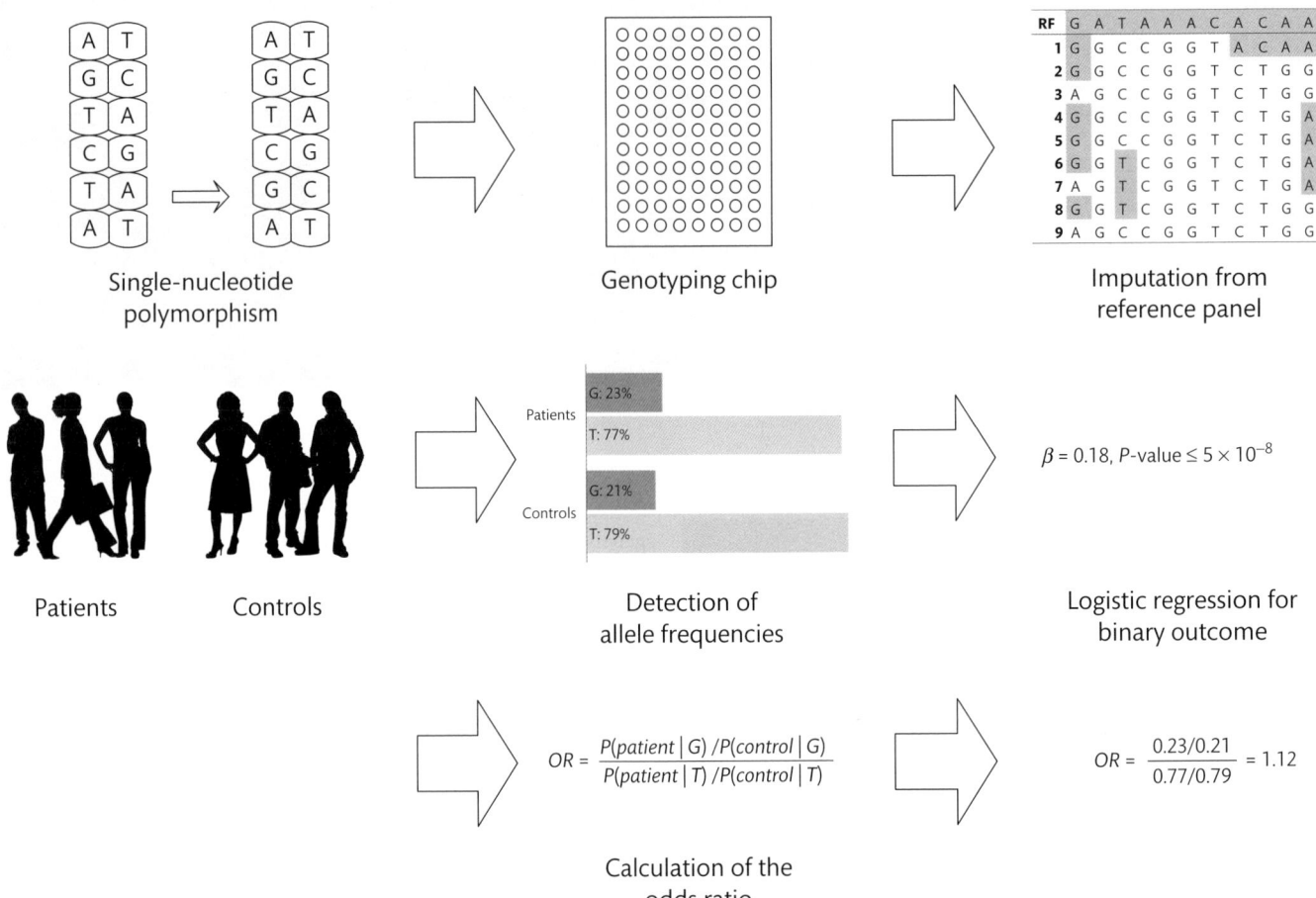

**Fig. 104.1** Genome-wide association study. Single-nucleotide polymorphisms (SNPs) are used as genetic markers for specific genetic loci. Genotyping chips can assay up to several millions of these genetic markers, and coverage of the genome can then be increased through the statistical method of imputation. Imputation predicts genotypes at unassayed locations on the basis of reference panels of the human genome. After genotyping of patients and controls, allele frequencies are compared between them and a logistic regression is performed to calculate β (the standardized regression coefficient) and odds ratios (ORs). SNPs are defined as genome-wide significant if they reach a P-value of $5 \times 10^{-8}$, which is $P = 0.05$ corrected for all the tests done in a GWAS.

markers and are the most common variants in the human genome. They are characterized by the replacement of a single nucleotide with another. For example, the base cytosine might appear at a specific base location in the majority of the population but might be replaced with guanine in an individual. Variable numbers of tandem repeats (VNTRs) and microsatellites are regions of the genome with variable numbers of a particular sequence, with a repeating unit of between two and 50 or more bases. Candidate gene studies used these VNTRs, microsatellites, or SNPs to identify which variant of a gene (that is, allele) may be associated with a symptom of disordered eating or an eating disorder, but large-scale attempts at replication of these findings have not been successful and this approach has fallen out of favour in psychiatric genetics in general [8].

### Genome-wide association studies

GWAS investigate the genetics of mental disorders using information from, and coverage of, the whole genome in a hypothesis-neutral manner (Fig. 104.1). Depending on the genotyping chip used, 500,000–1,000,000 SNPs are tested for association with a trait under study. In GWAS, SNPs are used because they are chemically easy to assay and a dense map of SNPs can 'tag' associations with a disorder

at genetic loci across the genome. GWAS are limited by the fact that they only detect chromosomal regions which can be multigenic and often do not clearly indicate the causal variants. Causal variants can be detected in further analyses such as fine mapping, exome sequencing, or whole-genome sequencing [9]. Fundamentally, GWAS are highly dependent on sample size, as shown by the results on schizophrenia [10] with, in general, >15,000 cases needed for multiple robust single genetic associations to be detected.

GWAS for eating disorders have not yet reached this sample size. However, smaller GWAS can still be used with methods such as linkage disequilibrium score regression, which uses summary statistics of GWAS to calculate the degree to which genetic variants are shared by two traits or disorders. The degree of common genetic variants shared between two traits or disorders is called a genetic correlation ($r_g$).

### Genetic architecture of mental disorders

Despite clear evidence from twin studies that eating disorders are substantially heritable, their complex genetic architecture (alongside

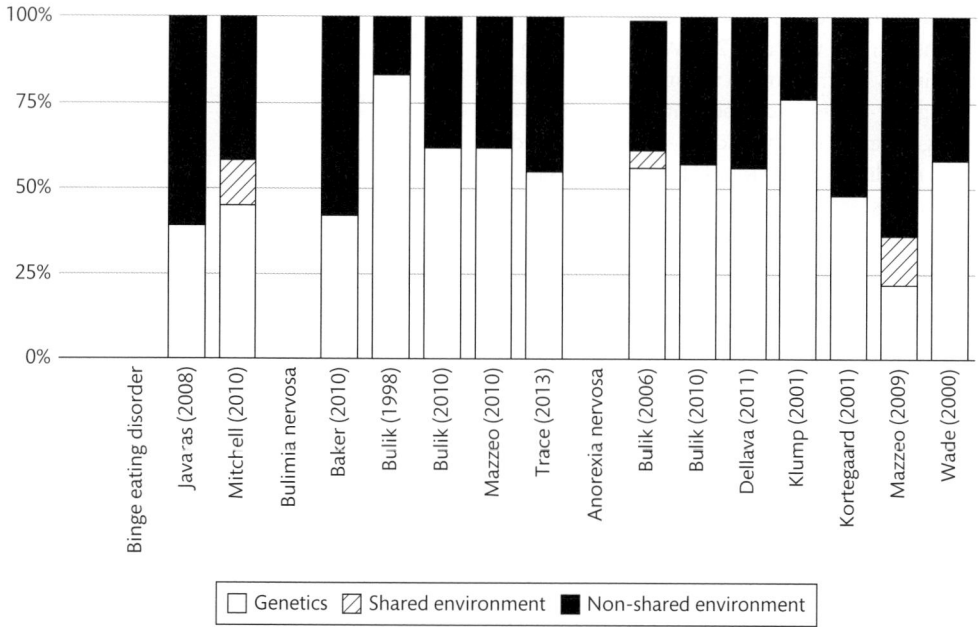

**Fig. 104.2** Heritability estimates of eating disorders derived from twin studies. Heritability estimates are expressed in percentages. Genetics (white), shared environment (striped), and non-shared (black) environment normally add up to 100%. Each bar represents one study.

a poor understanding of their neurobiology) has stymied both linkage and candidate gene studies. A large body of evidence collected over the past decade suggests that the genetic risk for psychiatric and other complex disorders is—in large part—accounted for by thousands of different genetic variations with small effect sizes [11]. For instance, GWAS on schizophrenia emphasize that this highly heritable disorder is highly polygenic, consistent with the picture in bipolar disorder and major depressive disorder (MDD) [10]. The GWAS approach also affords better estimation and control of type I errors, allowing accurate estimation of individual DNA sample quality, as well as fine-scale adjustment for ancestry differences in case-control studies—both of which can generate spurious associations and which have been considerable problems in candidate gene studies.

A complete review of a largely unsuccessful decade or more of candidate gene and linkage studies on eating disorders can be accessed elsewhere [12–15]. Our chapter focuses on the period of modern genomic approaches and the genetic overlap across the various eating disorders, as well as with common comorbid conditions. We start with the emergence of the first GWAS of AN and the formation of the Eating Disorders Working Group of the Psychiatric Genomics Consortium (PGC-ED) in 2013. We now review the quantitative and molecular (GWAS) genetic findings for AN, BN, and BED, contrasting these findings with GWAS results in food addiction, obesity, and BMI.

## Anorexia nervosa

### Family studies of anorexia nervosa

Anorexia nervosa runs in families, although sporadic cases also do occur. First-degree relatives of affected individuals are 11 times more likely to develop AN than relatives of unaffected individuals [16]. Reflecting the considerable diagnostic crossover seen during the course of eating disorders, relatives of individuals with AN are

also at increased risk for a range of eating disorders, including full and partial AN syndromes, as well as OSFED [16, 17].

### Twin studies of anorexia nervosa

A series of twin studies in European ancestry populations have suggested a fairly wide range of heritability point estimates (Fig. 104.2); the heritability of varying definitions of AN ranges from 0.28 to 0.74. Apart from genetic influence, twin studies report a significant contribution of non-shared environmental factors of 24–68%, but strikingly negligible influence of the shared environment [18–20]. As is the case with other psychiatric disorders, definitions of AN that meet the full syndrome diagnostic criteria are associated with higher heritability estimates than more loosely defined phenotypes [21]. Twin studies have also addressed the considerable diagnostic flux across eating disorder presentations, revealing that the common transition from AN to BN (and less commonly vice versa) may be due to shared genetic factors, with twin-based genetic correlations of between 0.46 and 0.79 being reported [22].

### Twin studies and comorbidity

AN is commonly comorbid in both clinical and epidemiological samples with major depression, anxiety disorders, and obsessive–compulsive disorder (OCD) [23]. Twin studies suggest that these comorbid profiles may be, at least in part, due to shared genetic factors. Bivariate twin studies of AN have revealed genetic correlations of 0.34, 0.20, and 0.52 with major depression [24], generalized anxiety disorder [21], and OCD [25], respectively. They also showed a genetic overlap between AN and suicidality [26]. The genetic overlap between AN, MDD, and suicide attempts was robustly replicated [27]. OCD is the psychiatric disorder with the strongest genetic overlap with AN.

### Developmental twin studies

Although no twin studies have been adequately powered to explore changes in heritability estimates for AN across development, this has been examined in related phenotypes. In girls, the genetic effects on eating disorder symptoms increase with age [28]. Whereas environmental factors are the primary contributors to variance in eating disorder phenotypes during pre-adolescence, the cumulative additive genetic contributions significantly increase across adolescence and remain constant through mid life. Work by Klump [28] implicates puberty and its hormonal changes (with consequent frontal temporal and other maturation of the brain), rather than a direct effect of age in this transition.

## Modern genomic approaches to anorexia nervosa

### Genome-wide association studies

The first GWAS for AN was conducted by the Children's Hospital of Philadelphia (CHOP) and the Price Foundation Collaborative Group [29]. The analysis included 1033 AN cases and 3733 paediatric controls. Given the small sample size and as predicted by experience in other psychiatric disorders, no SNPs reached genome-wide significance ($P \leq 5 \times 10^{-8}$). Also complicating the design was the fact that the control group had not yet passed through the age of risk for developing AN (mean = 12.75 years; standard deviation = 4.2 years) and so were effectively unscreened for eating disorders and other genetically related psychiatric problems, resulting in a decrease in statistical power to detect association.

The second AN GWAS was performed by the Genetic Consortium for Anorexia Nervosa (GCAN) as part of the Wellcome Trust Case-Control Consortium 3 (WTCCC3). This GWAS included 2907 AN cases of European ancestry and 14,860 ancestry-matched female controls. Although this was a larger study, it is still a modest sample size for GWAS and no genome-wide significant loci were detected, although when 72 independent markers with the lowest $P$ values were selected for replication, sign tests revealed that a highly significant 76% of these markers yielded results in the same direction in the discovery and replication samples [30]. These tests encouraged the field to continue GWAS efforts, as it suggested that the significant signal did exist in the data, but larger samples were required for detection. The controls selected for this GWAS were also not ideal as, although they were selected to be ancestrally compatible, they had been genotyped on similar (but not identical) platforms and at different times and in different laboratories (Fig. 104.3).

In an effort to unite research groups and consolidate findings, the PGC-ED was established in 2013. The first analysis of the combined CHOP and WTCCC3 data sets emerged in 2016 and has reported the first genome-wide significant locus for AN [31]. The GWAS comprised 3495 cases and 10,982 controls and now has been imputed to phase 3 of the 1000 Genomes Project to enable association statistics at millions of ungenotyped variants to be calculated [32]. A subsequent larger GWAS comprising 16,992 cases and 55,525 controls yielded eight significant loci and a pattern of genetic correlations implicating both psychiatric and metabolic origins of AN [33]. As has been seen in other mental disorders and the rest of common disorder medicine, it is reasonable to expect that the addition of samples will lead to further loci being identified, with an accelerated trajectory of significant loci.

### Low-frequency and rare variants

A GWAS focuses on common genetic variants, which occur in >1% of the population. By definition, rare variants are present in <1% of the population. During the past 3 years, some studies were performed on rare variants in the aetiology of AN. A series of sequencing and genotyping studies by Scott-Van Zeeland *et al.* [34]

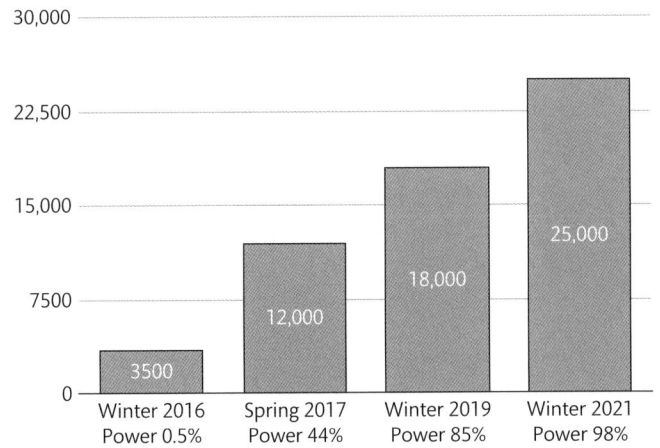

**Fig. 104.3** Expected number of cases for anorexia nervosa GWAS. Through the joint international endeavours of the Psychiatric Genetic Consortium of Eating Disorders (PGD-ED), the depicted numbers of cases are expected to have GWAS data over the new few years. The increase in cases is accompanied by a considerable increase in power, for what other disorders have suggested as plausible effect size of GWAS risk variants. The power calculation assumes an OR of 1.1 and an allele frequency of 20%.

on cases from the CHOP/Price Foundation cohort focused on the coding regions and upstream sequence of 152 candidate genes in 1205 AN cases and 1948 controls. They reported associations with variants in the oestrogen receptor β (*ESR2*) and the epoxide hydrolase 2 (*EPHX2*) genes in AN, identified via targeted gene sequencing. Case-control allele frequency differences for variants in these two genes were also observed in the CHOP/Price Foundation GWAS data set [29]. Somewhat paradoxically, hypercholesterolaemia has been reported in a subset of individuals with AN [35, 36], rendering *EPHX2* an intriguing find, as it has been implicated in cholesterol metabolism [37].

Subsequently, Cui *et al.* conducted a high-throughput sequencing study with two families who were densely affected for AN and BN [38]. They initially conducted a linkage analysis on the first pedigree (20 individuals) and identified a region on chromosome 11 from 44.1 to 64.3 cM with a significant logarithm of odds score. They then conducted whole-genome sequencing on two family members who were affected with AN and detected a missense mutation in the oestrogen-related receptor α (*ESSRA*). This pedigree was also enriched for OCD. In the second pedigree, enriched for both AN and BN cases, exome sequencing identified a rare mutation in histone deacetylase 4 (*HDAC4*). HeLa cell and mouse cortical tissue analyses demonstrated a potentially functional interaction between *ESRRA* and *HDAC4*, and using transcriptional activity assays, it was reported that *HDAC4* may act as an inhibitor of *ESRRA* activity. Given the central role of histone deacetylases in the activation and repression of gene expression genome-wide, this interaction might not be unexpected.

In order to rule in or out more common rare and functional variation in AN, an exome-array rare variant GWAS was performed in 2158 cases from nine populations of European origin and 15,327 ancestrally matched controls [39]. Cases and controls were identified from those gathered for the GCAN/WTCCC3 cohort. Sixteen independent variants were selected for *in silico* and *de novo* replication (12 common, four rare). No findings reached genome-wide significance. The authors instead highlighted two common variants—rs10791286, an intronic variant in *OPCML* ($P = 9.89 \times 10^{-6}$); and rs7700147, an intergenic variant located near *ANKRD50* ($P = 2.93 \times 10^{-5}$), reaching near suggestive significance.

## Copy number variation

Copy number variations (CNVs) are 1kb DNA segments, or larger, occurring in an altered quantity, compared with a reference genome. The most common CNVs are duplications and deletions. A genome-wide analysis of CNVs was also conducted on the CHOP/Price Foundation cohort [29]. No evidence emerged supporting enrichment of AN cases for CNVs above controls, and rare or large CNVs were not notably overrepresented in AN cases. Although a recurrent 13q12 deletion (1.5 Mb) disrupting the sacsin molecular chaperone *SACS* was seen twice in cases and CNVs disrupting the contactin 6/contactin 4 (*CNTN6/CNTN4*) region was found in multiple cases, these observations were not statistically significant. Yilmaz *et al.* [40] conducted a case-only genome-wide CNV survey in 1983 female AN cases that were part of the GCAN/WTCCC3 AN GWAS. Their case-only approach explored whether pathogenic CNVs implicated in other psychiatric and neurodevelopmental disorders were also observed in AN cases. Four of these well-established pathogenic CNVs (deletions or duplications in 1q21.1, 7q36.3, 15q13.3, or 16p11.2) were found in a small number of AN cases. One case also had a large deletion in the 13q12 region [29], and 41 cases had deletions or duplications which were 1 Mb or larger. However, at this point, it is not clear whether large-effect CNVs play a demonstrable role in AN. Larger sample sizes are required before the effect of smaller-effect CNVs can be ruled out.

## Genetic correlations with psychiatric phenotypes

A genetic correlation is an estimate of the genetic overlap between two traits. An analytic extension of linkage disequilibrium score regression [41] enables computation of cross-trait genetic correlations, and intriguing insights for AN have emerged. Bulik-Sullivan *et al.* [42] revealed a significant positive genetic correlation between AN and schizophrenia ($r_g = 0.26$), with positive, but non-significant, correlations with major depression and bipolar disorder. A second analysis replicated the positive correlation with schizophrenia ($r_g = 0.15$) and revealed a strong positive genetic correlation between AN and OCD ($r_g = 0.55$) [33, 43]. The high genetic correlation between AN and OCD parallels twin-based genetic correlations ($r_a = 0.52$) and reflects common comorbidity profiles seen clinically in AN [25, 44, 45]. The positive correlation with schizophrenia is less readily explicable, as this is not a commonly observed clinical comorbidity profile, but it should be noted that OCD also has a strong genetic correlation with schizophrenia and so could be mediating the observed correlation. However, comorbidity with schizophrenia has been documented in individuals with AN, although it has not been extensively explored [46]. The positive genetic correlation with schizophrenia thus does raise an intriguing question about whether some of the more perplexing features of AN, such as a distorted body image, as well as overvalued ideation about food and weight, may have a psychotic component.

## Genetic correlations with metabolic phenotypes

Additional intriguing genetic correlations emerged between AN and an array of anthropometric and metabolic phenotypes.

Bulik-Sullivan *et al.* first reported a significant negative correlation between AN and obesity ($r_g = -0.20$) and BMI ($r_g = -.18$), suggesting that the same genes may influence extreme dysregulation of body mass in both directions. Other genetic correlations between AN and metabolic measures were with high-density lipoprotein cholesterol, fasting insulin, fasting glucose, and type 2 diabetes. Furthermore, AN was genetically correlated with physical activity [33].

## Bulimia nervosa

### Family studies of bulimia nervosa

BN has been shown to be familial and genetically overlaps with AN; individuals with relatives who suffer from either disorder are also more likely to develop either AN or BN [16, 17]. However, relatives of cases suffering from the restrictive anorexia subtype do not show an increased liability to develop BN [47], suggesting that the overlap between the restricting type of AN and BN is, at most, modest [12].

### Twin studies of bulimia nervosa

The twin-based heritability for BN ranges between 0.55 and 0.62 [20, 22, 48, 49], suggesting that about 60% of the variance in liability can be explained by genetics (Fig. 104.2). The diagnosis of BN is somewhat unreliable in population-based samples but can be improved by including behavioural components of BN such as self-induced vomiting [50]. A twin study on specific BN symptoms showed that BN core symptoms are differentially heritable, such that specific symptoms, such as vomiting, are more heritable than, for example, the influence of weight on self-evaluation [51]. The genetic correlation reported by twin studies between the two key components of BN—binge eating and vomiting—is high, but not absolute ($r_g = 0.74$), and self-induced vomiting exhibited higher heritability of 72% vs 46% reported for binge eating alone [52]. Various twin studies have conclusively demonstrated that most of the variance in risk for BN can be explained by additive genetic effects [20, 22, 48, 49, 51]. One twin study confirmed the findings of family studies and reported the genetic correlation between AN and BN to be 0.79 [22]. This strong genetic correlation suggests that considerable overlap in the underlying biology of the two disorders may contribute to the observed diagnostic flux [12].

### Twin studies and comorbidity

BN occurs with concurrent mental illnesses. Bivariate twin studies of BN revealed a genetic overlap with major depression [53], phobia, panic disorder [54], and substance use disorder [55]. BN patients are at increased risk of suicide, which is partly influenced by common genetics [26].

### Modern genomic approaches to bulimia nervosa

#### Genome-wide association studies

Although there has been no genome-wide study testing BN per se, one major GWAS on eating behaviours investigated the bulimia subscale of the Eating Disorder Inventory-2. The study tested six eating-related traits, including drive for thinness, body dissatisfaction, bulimia, weight fluctuation symptoms, breakfast-skipping behaviour, and childhood obsessive–compulsive personality disorder traits. Furthermore, an arbitrary cut-off for case/control status determination of the bulimia scale was used, and unfortunately this was a case definition which does not fully satisfy ICD-10 or DSM-IV diagnostic criteria. The study design utilized one discovery sample and two replication samples. The study tested samples that were relatively small (approximately 2500–3000) for a GWAS, with no genetic marker reaching genome-wide significance. However, the effect sizes in the discovery sample and the replication samples were significantly in the same direction. In this study, the strongest (although non-significant) association with the bulimia scale was intergenic, lying between the cyclin L1 (*CCNL1*) and the leucine glutamate, leucine-rich 1 (*LEKR1*) genes which had previously shown multiple associations with fetal growth, birthweight, elevated insulin release, and breast cancer [56]. Effect sizes in the discovery and replication samples are concordant. GWAS of other psychiatric disorders have resulted in significant findings as sample sizes have increased. Together, these strongly suggest that increasing the sample size will enable eating disorder GWASs to reach sufficient statistical power in future.

## Binge eating disorder

Genetic research on BED is in its infancy in part due to the fact that it only became an independent diagnosis in DSM-5 in 2013. Current research focuses on neurotransmitter systems, such as dopamine and endogenous opioids, which may underlie the human central nervous reward system. Changes in the reward system are associated with addictive behaviour.

### Family studies of binge eating disorder

BED aggregates in families with a heritability of 57% [57]. Family studies [58] also showed a genetic overlap between obesity and BED. These results were replicated in additional twin studies.

### Twin studies of binge eating disorder

Twin studies of both the disorder and its cardinal symptom—binge eating—revealed consistently moderate to strong heritabilities of between 33% and 69% [57, 59–61].

#### Twin studies and comorbidities

BED is associated with obesity and the metabolic syndrome [62]. Twin studies revealed that both obesity and BED are influenced by partly shared and partly different genetic factors [63]. The direction of causality between obesity and BED is not fully elucidated and must be further investigated. Furthermore, BED exhibits a significant genetic overlap with substance use disorder [64]. Similar to the observation about other eating disorders, BED has also a significant genetic overlap with suicidality [26].

All of these observations have emerged from quantitative genetic studies, as limited molecular genetic findings and no genome-wide findings for BED exist.

### Modern genomic approaches to binge eating disorder

#### Genome-wide association studies

A GWAS on BED per se has not yet been conducted. However, the phenotypic overlap with obesity and parallel studies of phenotypes, such as food addiction, are relevant.

### Food preference patterns and food addiction

Neuroimaging studies reported altered dopamine signalling in the fronto-striatal neuronal circuitry involved in reward and self-regulatory processes [65]. From an evolutionary biology perspective, supported by epidemiological and neuroscientific evidence, certain foods, such as processed foods high in sugar, fat, and salt, may have an addictive potential similar to psychoactive substances such as cocaine or alcohol [66, 67]. This provides the foundation for the so-called construct of 'food addiction', which is assessed by self-report using the Yale Food Addiction Scale (YFAS), based on the DSM-IV diagnostic criteria for substance use disorders. Food addiction is separate from BED but is an overlapping construct that has evolved from different clinical and research areas. Genetic findings for food addiction must also be interpreted cautiously because most results are inferred from small sample sizes [68].

Food addiction is highly prevalent in patients suffering from BED [69]. A 2013 study investigated food addiction in individuals with BED. Two subgroups of BED patients with or without food addiction were equivalent in age and BMI, but BED patients also suffering from food addiction reported higher rates of emotional eating and rated themselves more responsive to rewarding food types [70].

### Twin studies of food preference patterns

Twin studies on the consumption of sugar through drinks (48%) [71], liking for sweet solutions (49%), liking for sweet foods (54%), use frequency of sweet foods (53%) [72], and food preference patterns (36–58%) [73] showed that these traits are moderately heritable.

#### Twin studies and comorbidities

One twin study showed that the association between high sugar consumption and substance use disorder is 59% genetically driven. These findings underpin the hypothesis that food addiction may be an independent entity.

### Modern genomic approaches to food addiction

#### Genome-wide association studies

A quantitative trait GWAS on the modified form of the YFAS was performed by Cornelis *et al.* [74] in 9314 women and identified genetic loci associated with food addiction but produced limited evidence for shared genetics with substance use disorder. Two genome-wide significant hits close to protein kinase C α (*PRKCA*) and neurotrimin (*NTM*) were discovered. *PRKCA* is involved in insulin signalling, inflammation, and the mitogen-activated protein kinase (MAPK) pathway. Neurotrimin was associated with opioid binding protein/cell adhesion molecule-like (*OPCML*). *OPCML* was also associated with alcohol dependence and body fat distribution [74]. However, these results require replication.

## Body mass index, obesity, and body fat genetics in relation to eating disorders

Obesity has been considered as a potential behavioural disorder, and the nature of the relation of eating disorders with BMI (body weight) and body fat is of considerable scientific and medical interest. Obesity, BMI, and body fat percentage are highly heritable, polygenic, and multifactorial human traits. Body weight is influenced by a complex interplay of genetic, environmental, and psychosocial factors. These three factors affect energy intake and energy consumption mediated by the central nervous and metabolic systems in humans [75]. BMI is commonly used as a proxy measure for both weight and body fat. However, its application has been widely criticized in healthy individuals, as well as in eating disorder patients [76, 77].

## Family and adoption studies of body mass index

Family studies generally report heritability for BMI ranging from 20% to 80%, with the observed heritability increasing with age. Data from adoption studies replicated these findings, with genetic factors accounting for 20–60% of the variation in BMI. Adoption studies showed no association between the BMI of adoptees and their adoptive parents, whereas the adoptee's BMI was associated with the biological parents' BMI [78].

## Twin studies of body mass index and body fat

### Twin studies

The (adult) twin-based heritability of BMI ranges between 59% and 64% [79, 80], with heritability estimates of about 70% for twins who were reared apart, affirming the high genetic influence [81]. Twin studies also estimated high heritability for body fat and its distribution. The heritability for total body fat is about 86%, for trunk fat about 82%, and for lower body fat about 83% [82, 83]. Parental overweight and adiposity are established risk factors for childhood obesity that are mainly genetically determined [84].

### Developmental twin studies

An extensive developmental twin study performed by Silventoinen et al. [85] shed new light on the influence of age, sex, and socio-economic background on BMI. The heritability of BMI increases from 41% after the age of 5 to 78% at the age of 19 and remains stable for the rest of the lifespan. Despite the increasing heritability, the variance of BMI also increases after the age of 5. Two possible explanations are hypothesized—either children may be able to choose their food more independently after the age of 5 or neuronal pathways involved in appetite regulation may be influenced by age-dependent gene expression. Furthermore, sex differences in BMI and its heritability are a well-known phenomenon and were replicated, which means that different genes have differential effects in both sexes. Different sets of genes seem to influence BMI before and after puberty which may be influenced by hormonal changes.

North America and Australia showed regional differences in BMI, compared with Europe and East Asia, having a higher mean and a greater variance. Including poorer socio-economic regions into the heritability analysis of BMI led to lower heritability estimates, with an increasing influence of shared environmental factors [85]. This observation may be explained by a restricted presentation of the phenotype due to limited food resources in poorer areas.

## Modern genomic approaches to weight and body fat

### Genome-wide association studies

GWAS on human obesity detected 227 independent genetic variants that are associated with BMI. These 227 SNPs were narrowed down to 97 genetic loci. These genetic loci are enriched in various biological pathways such as central nervous and peripheral appetite

regulation, adipocyte differentiation, insulin and leptin signalling, lipid metabolism, and gut microbiota. In total, common SNPs are estimated to explain about 27–30% of the phenotypic variance of BMI [86], but the identified genome-wide significant obesity SNPs only explain about approximately 3% of this variance, indicating that this is a highly polygenic trait [87]. Only two of the 97 genetic loci showed sex differences, with stronger effects in women being observed in each case.

GWAS of body fat distribution investigating the waist-to-hip ratio found 49 significant genomic loci [88, 89]. The waist-to-hip ratio was adjusted for the effect of BMI, to avoid detection of genomic loci having an effect on BMI. With 19 of the 49 loci showing a larger effect size in women, compared with men, considerable genetic sex dimorphism was uncovered. A GWAS conducted on body fat percentage revealed 12 genetic loci that were genome-wide significant. Seven of the loci showed a larger effect on body fat percentage, compared with BMI, whereas the rest showed a larger effect on BMI, suggesting an association with both fat and fat-free mass [90].

### Genetic correlations with eating disorders

As discussed earlier, Bulik-Sullivan et al. [41] achieved a major breakthrough when they developed the method of linkage disequilibrium score regression to calculate genetic correlations between different traits. They reported a significant negative correlation between AN and obesity ($r_g = -0.20$) and BMI ($r_g = -.18$), suggesting that shared genetic variants between AN and body fat may influence body mass in opposite directions. This negative genetic correlation paved the way for a more detailed exploration of AN as both a metabolic and a psychiatric disorder.

Comparing results from two genome-wide meta-analyses of AN and BMI, Hinney et al. [91] identified three independent genomic loci that were associated with both AN and a lower BMI. These three independent loci were marked by nine different SNPs. The analysis was stratified by sex and showed that the associated SNPs showed a sex-specific effect, such that the SNPs were more strongly associated with BMI in females, compared with males. The association with the region on chromosome 10 was mainly due to females. The four genes located closest to the chromosomal loci are involved in brown adipose tissue function and regulation, preadipocyte proliferation, and *BDNF* expression.

## Conclusions

A large body of evidence shows unequivocally that eating disorders are influenced by genetics. However, these findings must be interpreted cautiously. Firstly, although genetics play a significant role in the aetiology of eating disorders, it is important to bear in mind that the development of an eating disorder is also substantially influenced by environmental factors. Secondly, genetics is a highly complex, quickly developing area of research that is often difficult to comprehend and is even more so for patients and the public. Finally, it is important to communicate results correctly and in an understandable manner. It should be explained that genetics underlying eating disorders are neither deterministic nor a genetic defect and that there is no evidence that one single gene causes any of the common eating disorders.

Large numbers of eating disorder patients need to be studied more systematically to redefine the phenotypes of eating disorders. This so-called 'deep phenotyping' as part of 'phenomics' allows us to clarify diagnoses. More specific diagnoses incorporating various quantitative measures might subsequently increase the power to detect genetic variants and environmental risk factors. Increasing the sample size is a further approach to increase statistical power. Both strategies are currently being utilized by the PGC-ED on an international level. This gives hope to identify more genetic variants, environmental risk factors, and critical developmental stages involved in the aetiology of eating disorders. These identified risk factors and critical periods may ultimately be translated into more effective preventive and curative measures, but this goal can only be reached by joint efforts and expertise of clinicians, epidemiologists, neuroscientists, and geneticists.

## REFERENCES

1. Zipfel S, Giel KE, Bulik CM, Hay P, Schmidt U. Anorexia nervosa: aetiology, assessment, and treatment. *Lancet Psychiatry*. 2015;2:1099–111.
2. Herpertz-Dahlmann B. Adolescent eating disorders: update on definitions, symptomatology, epidemiology, and comorbidity. *Child Adolesc Psychiatr Clin N Am*. 2015;24:177–96.
3. Hoek HW. Incidence, prevalence and mortality of anorexia nervosa and other eating disorders. *Curr Opin Psychiatry*. 2006;19:389–94.
4. Ágh T, Kovács G, Pawaskar M, Supina D, Inotai A, Vokó Z. Epidemiology, health-related quality of life and economic burden of binge eating disorder: a systematic literature review. *Eat Weight Disord*. 2015;20:1–12.
5. American Psychiatric Association. *Diagnostic and Statistical Manual of Mental Disorders*, fifth edition. Washington, DC: American Psychiatric Association.
6. Rijsdijk FV, Sham PC. Analytic approaches to twin data using structural equation models. *Brief Bioinform*. 2002;3:119–33.
7. Wray NR, Visscher PM. Narrowing the boundaries of the genetic architecture of schizophrenia. *Schizophr Bull*. 2010;36:14–23.
8. Hodge SE. Linkage analysis versus association analysis: distinguishing between two models that explain disease-marker associations. *Am J Hum Genet*. 1993;53:367–84.
9. Corvin A, Craddock N, Sullivan PF. Genome-wide association studies: a primer. *Psychol Med*. 2010;40:1063–77.
10. Schizophrenia Working Group of the Psychiatric Genomics Consortium; Ripke S, Neale BM, Corvin A, *et al*. Biological insights from 108 schizophrenia-associated genetic loci. *Nature*. 2014;511:421–7.
11. Sullivan PF, Daly MJ, O'Donovan M. Genetic architectures of psychiatric disorders: the emerging picture and its implications. *Nat Rev Genet*. 2012;13:537–51.
12. Yilmaz Z, Hardaway JA, Bulik CM. Genetics and epigenetics of eating disorders. *Adv Genomics Genet*. 2015;5:131–50.
13. Brandys MK, de Kovel CG, Kas MJ, van Elburg AA, Adan RA. Overview of genetic research in anorexia nervosa: the past, the present and the future. *Int J Eat Disord*. 2015;48:814–25.
14. Trace SE, Baker JH, Penas-Lledo E, Bulik CM. The genetics of eating disorders. *Annu Rev Clin Psychol*. 2013;9:589–620.
15. Hinney A, Scherag S, Hebebrand J. Genetic findings in anorexia and bulimia nervosa. *Prog Mol Biol Transl Sci*. 2010;94:241–70.
16. Strober M, Freeman R, Lampert C, Diamond J, Kaye W. Controlled family study of anorexia nervosa and bulimia nervosa: evidence of shared liability and transmission of partial syndromes. *Am J Psychiatry*. 2000;157:393–401.
17. Lilenfeld LR, Kaye WH, Greeno CG, *et al*. A controlled family study of anorexia nervosa and bulimia nervosa: psychiatric disorders in first-degree relatives and effects of proband comorbidity. *Arch Gen Psychiatry*. 1998;55:603–10.
18. Bulik CM, Sullivan PF, Tozzi F, Furberg H, Lichtenstein P, Pedersen NL. Prevalence, heritability, and prospective risk factors for anorexia nervosa. *Arch Gen Psychiatry*. 2006;63:305–12.
19. Klump KL, Miller KB, Keel PK, McGue M, Iacono WG. Genetic and environmental influences on anorexia nervosa syndromes in a population-based twin sample. *Psychol Med*. 2001;31:737–40.
20. Kortegaard LS, Hoerder K, Joergensen J, Gillberg C, Kyvik KO. A preliminary population-based twin study of self-reported eating disorder. *Psychol Med*. 2001;31:361–5.
21. Dellava JE, Thornton LM, Lichtenstein P, Pedersen NL, Bulik CM. Impact of broadening definitions of anorexia nervosa on sample characteristics. *J Psychiatr Res*. 2011;45:691–8.
22. Bulik CM, Thornton LM, Root TL, Pisetsky EM, Lichtenstein P, Pedersen NL. Understanding the relation between anorexia nervosa and bulimia nervosa in a Swedish national twin sample. *Biol Psychiatry*. 2010;67:71–7.
23. Mattar L, Thiebaud MR, Huas C, Cebula C, Godart N. Depression, anxiety and obsessive-compulsive symptoms in relation to nutritional status and outcome in severe anorexia nervosa. *Psychiatry Res*. 2012;200:513–17.
24. Wade TD, Bulik CM, Neale M, Kendler KS. Anorexia nervosa and major depression: shared genetic and environmental risk factors. *Am J Psychiatry*. 2000;157:469–71.
25. Cederlöf M, Thornton LM, Baker J, *et al*. Etiological overlap between obsessive-compulsive disorder and anorexia nervosa: a longitudinal cohort, multigenerational family and twin study. *World Psychiatry*. 2015;14:333–8.
26. Wade TD, Fairweather-Schmidt AK, Zhu G, Martin NG. Does shared genetic risk contribute to the co-occurrence of eating disorders and suicidality? *Int J Eat Disord*. 2015;48:684–91.
27. Thornton LM, Welch E, Munn-Chernoff MA, Lichtenstein P, Bulik CM. Anorexia nervosa, major depression, and suicide attempts: shared genetic factors. *Suicide Life Threat Behav*. 2016;46:525–34.
28. Klump KL. Puberty as a critical risk period for eating disorders: a review of human and animal studies. *Horm Behav*. 2013;64:399–410.
29. Wang K, Zhang H, Bloss CS, *et al*. A genome-wide association study on common SNPs and rare CNVs in anorexia nervosa. *Mol Psychiatry*. 2011;16:949–59.
30. Boraska V, Franklin CS, Floyd JA, *et al*. A genome-wide association study of anorexia nervosa. *Mol Psychiatry*. 2014;19:1085–94.
31. Duncan L, Yilmaz Z, Walters R, *et al*. Eating Disorders Working Group of the Psychiatric Genomics Consortium, Thornton L, Hinney A, Daly M, *et al*. Genome-wide association study reveals first locus for anorexia nervosa and metabolic correlations. *Am J Psychiatry*. 2017;174:850–8.
32. Genomes Project Consortium; Abecasis GR, Auton A, Brooks LD, *et al*. An integrated map of genetic variation from 1,092 human genomes. *Nature*. 2012;491:56–65.
33. Watson, HJ, Yilmaz, Z, Thornton LM, *et al*. Genome-wide association study identifies either risk loci and implicated metabo-psychiatric origins for anorexia nervosa. *Nat Genet*. 2019;51:1207–14.

34. Scott-Van Zeeland AA, Bloss CS, Tewhey R, *et al*. Evidence for the role of *EPHX2* gene variants in anorexia nervosa. *Mol Psychiatry*. 2014;19:724–32.

35. Rigaud D, Tallonneau I, Verges B. Hypercholesterolaemia in anorexia nervosa: frequency and changes during refeeding. *Diabetes Metab*. 2009;35:57–63.

36. Weinbrenner T, Zuger M, Jacoby GE, *et al*. Lipoprotein metabolism in patients with anorexia nervosa: a case-control study investigating the mechanisms leading to hypercholesterolaemia. *Br J Nutr*. 2004;91:959–69.

37. Newman JW, Morisseau C, Hammock BD. Epoxide hydrolases: their roles and interactions with lipid metabolism. *Prog Lipid Res*. 2005;44:1–51.

38. Cui H, Moore J, Ashimi SS, *et al*. Eating disorder predisposition is associated with *ESRRA* and *HDAC4* mutations. *J Clin Invest*. 2013;123:4706–13.

39. Huckins L, Hatzikotoulas K, Southam L, *et al*. Investigation of common, low-frequency and rare genome-wide variation in anorexia nervosa. *Mol Psychiatry*. 2018;23:1169–80.

40. Yilmaz Z, Szatkiewicz J, Crowley JJ, *et al*. Exploration of large, rare CNVs associated with psychiatric disorders in individuals with anorexia nervosa. *Psychiatr Genet*. 2017;27:152–8.

41. Bulik-Sullivan BK, Loh PR, Finucane HK, *et al*. LD Score regression distinguishes confounding from polygenicity in genome-wide association studies. *Nat Genet*. 2015;47:291–5.

42. Bulik-Sullivan BK, Finucane HK, Anttila V, *et al*. An atlas of genetic correlations across human diseases and traits. *Nat Genet*. 2015;47:1236–41.

43. Anttila V, Bulik-Sullivan B, Finucane H, Ripke S, Malik R, Pers T. Analysis of shared heritability in common disorders of the brain. *Science*. 2018;360:pii:eaap8757.

44. Kaye WH, Bulik CM, Thornton L, Barbarich N, Masters K. Comorbidity of anxiety disorders with anorexia and bulimia nervosa. *Am J Psychiatry*. 2004;161:2215–21.

45. Godart NT, Flament MF, Curt F, *et al*. Anxiety disorders in subjects seeking treatment for eating disorders: a DSM-IV controlled study. *Psychiatry Res*. 2003;117:245–58.

46. Kouidrat Y, Amad A, Lalau JD, Loas G. Eating disorders in schizophrenia: implications for research and management. *Schizophr Res Treatment*. 2014;2014:791573.

47. Grigoroiu-Serbanescu M, Magureanu S, Milea S, Dobrescu I, Marinescu E. Modest familial aggregation of eating disorders in restrictive anorexia nervosa with adolescent onset in a Romanian sample. *Eur Child Adolesc Psychiatry*. 2003;12:i47–53.

48. Bulik CM, Sullivan PF, Kendler KS. Heritability of binge-eating and broadly defined bulimia nervosa. *Biol Psychiatry*. 1998;44:1210–18.

49. Trace SE, Thornton LM, Baker JH, *et al*. A behavioral-genetic investigation of bulimia nervosa and its relationship with alcohol use disorder. *Psychiatry Res*. 2013;208:232–7.

50. Wade TD, Bulik CM, Kendler KS. Reliability of lifetime history of bulimia nervosa. *Br J Psychiatry*. 2000;177:72.

51. Mazzeo SE, Mitchell KS, Bulik CM, Aggen SH, Kendler KS, Neale MC. A twin study of specific bulimia nervosa symptoms. *Psychol Med*. 2010;40:1203–13.

52. Sullivan PF, Bulik CM, Kendler KS. Genetic epidemiology of binging and vomiting. *Br J Psychiatry*. 1998;173:75.

53. Walters EE, Neale MC, Eaves LJ, Heath AC, Kessler RC, Kendler KS. Bulimia nervosa and major depression: a study of common genetic and environmental factors. *Psychol Med*. 1992;22:617–22.

54. Kendler KS, Walters EE, Neale MC, Kessler RC, Heath AC, Eaves LJ. The structure of the genetic and environmental risk factors for six major psychiatric disorders in women. Phobia, generalized anxiety disorder, panic disorder, bulimia, major depression, and alcoholism. *Arch Gen Psychiatry*. 1995;52:374–83.

55. Baker JH, Mitchell KS, Neale MC, Kendler KS. Eating disorder symptomatology and substance use disorders: prevalence and shared risk in a population based twin sample. *Int J Eat Disord*. 2010;43:648–58.

56. Boraska V, Davis OS, Cherkas LF, *et al*. Genome-wide association analysis of eating disorder-related symptoms, behaviors, and personality traits. *Am J Med Genet B Neuropsychiatr Genet*. 2012;159B:803–11.

57. Javaras KN, Laird NM, Reichborn-Kjennerud T, Bulik CM, Pope HG, Jr., Hudson JI. Familiality and heritability of binge eating disorder: results of a case-control family study and a twin study. *Int J Eat Disord*. 2008;41:174–9.

58. Hudson JI, Lalonde JK, Berry JM, *et al*. Binge-eating disorder as a distinct familial phenotype in obese individuals. *Arch Gen Psychiatry*. 2006;63:313–19.

59. Mitchell KS, Neale MC, Bulik CM, Aggen SH, Kendler KS, Mazzeo SE. Binge eating disorder: a symptom-level investigation of genetic and environmental influences on liability. *Psychol Med*. 2010;40:1899–906.

60. Reichborn-Kjennerud T, Bulik CM, Tambs K, Harris JR. Genetic and environmental influences on binge eating in the absence of compensatory behaviors: a population-based twin study. *Int J Eat Disord*. 2004;36:307–14.

61. Root TL, Thornton LM, Lindroos AK, *et al*. Shared and unique genetic and environmental influences on binge eating and night eating: a Swedish twin study. *Eat Behav*. 2010;11:92–8.

62. Hudson JI, Hiripi E, Pope HG, Jr., Kessler RC. The prevalence and correlates of eating disorders in the National Comorbidity Survey Replication. *Biol Psychiatry*. 2007;61:348–58.

63. Bulik CM, Sullivan PF, Kendler KS. Genetic and environmental contributions to obesity and binge eating. *Int J Eat Disord*. 2003;33:293–8.

64. Munn-Chernoff MA, Baker JH. A primer on the genetics of comorbid eating disorders and substance use disorders. *Eur Eat Disord Rev*. 2016;24:91–100.

65. Michaelides M, Thanos PK, Volkow ND, Wang GJ. Dopamine-related frontostriatal abnormalities in obesity and binge-eating disorder: emerging evidence for developmental psychopathology. *Int Rev Psychiatry*. 2012;24:211–18.

66. Davis C. Evolutionary and neuropsychological perspectives on addictive behaviors and addictive substances: relevance to the "food addiction" construct. *Subst Abuse Rehabil*. 2014;5:129–37.

67. Volkow ND, Wang GJ, Tomasi D, Baler RD. Obesity and addiction: neurobiological overlaps. *Obes Rev*. 2013;14:2–18.

68. Davis C. The epidemiology and genetics of binge eating disorder (BED). *CNS Spectr*. 2015;20:522–9.

69. Long CG, Blundell JE, Finlayson G. A systematic review of the application and correlates of YFAS-diagnosed 'food addiction' in humans: are eating-related 'addictions' a cause for concern or empty concepts? *Obes Facts*. 2015;8:386–401.

70. Davis C. Compulsive overeating as an addictive behavior: overlap between food addiction and binge eating disorder. *Curr Obesity Rep*. 2013;2:171–8.

71. Treur JL, Boomsma DI, Ligthart L, Willemsen G, Vink JM. Heritability of high sugar consumption through drinks and the genetic correlation with substance use. *Am J Clin Nutr*. 2016;104:1144–50.

72. Keskitalo K, Tuorila H, Spector TD, *et al.* Same genetic components underlie different measures of sweet taste preference. *Am J Clin Nutr.* 2007;86:1663–9.

73. Pallister T, Sharafi M, Lachance G, *et al.* Food preference patterns in a UK twin cohort. *Twin Res Hum Genet.* 2015;18:793–805.

74. Cornelis MC, Flint A, Field AE, *et al.* A genome-wide investigation of food addiction. *Obesity (Silver Spring).* 2016;24:1336–41.

75. Kopelman PG. Obesity as a medical problem. *Nature.* 2000;404:635–43.

76. Hannan WJ, Wrate RM, Cowen SJ, Freeman CPL. Body mass index as an estimate of body fat. *Int J Eat Disord.* 1995;18:91–7.

77. Trocki O, Shepherd RW. Change in body mass index does not predict change in body composition in adolescent girls with anorexia nervosa. *J Am Diet Assoc.* 2000;100:457–60.

78. Sørensen TI, Holst C, Stunkard AJ. Childhood body mass index—genetic and familial environmental influences assessed in a longitudinal adoption study. *Int J Obes Relat Metab Disord.* 1992;16:705–14.

79. Stunkard AJ, Foch TT, Hrubec Z. A twin study of human obesity. *JAMA.* 1986;256:51–4.

80. Maes HH, Neale MC, Eaves LJ. Genetic and environmental factors in relative body weight and human adiposity. *Behav Genet.* 1997;27:325–51.

81. Stunkard AJ, Harris JR, Pedersen NL, McClearn GE. The body-mass index of twins who have been reared apart. *N Engl J Med.* 1990;322:1483–7.

82. Malis C, Rasmussen EL, Poulsen P, *et al.* Total and regional fat distribution is strongly influenced by genetic factors in young and elderly twins. *Obes Res.* 2005;13:2139–45.

83. Lehtovirta M, Kaprio J, Forsblom C, Eriksson J, Tuomilehto J, Groop L. Insulin sensitivity and insulin secretion in monozygotic and dizygotic twins. *Diabetologia.* 2000;43:285–93.

84. Magnusson PKE, Rasmussen F. Familial resemblance of body mass index and familial risk of high and low body mass index. A study of young men in Sweden. *Int J Obes.* 2002;26:1225–31.

85. Silventoinen K, Jelenkovic A, Sund R, *et al.* Genetic and environmental effects on body mass index from infancy to the onset of adulthood: an individual-based pooled analysis of 45 twin cohorts participating in the COllaborative project of Development of Anthropometrical measures in Twins (CODATwins) study. *Am J Clin Nutr.* 2016;104:371–9.

86. Yang J, Bakshi A, Zhu Z, *et al.* Genetic variance estimation with imputed variants finds negligible missing heritability for human height and body mass index. *Nat Genet.* 2015;47:1114–20.

87. Locke AE, Kahali B, Berndt SI, *et al.* Genetic studies of body mass index yield new insights for obesity biology. *Nature.* 2015;518:197–206.

88. Heid IM, Jackson AU, Randall JC, *et al.* Meta-analysis identifies 13 new loci associated with waist-hip ratio and reveals sexual dimorphism in the genetic basis of fat distribution. *Nat Genet.* 2010;42:949–60.

89. Shungin D, Winkler TW, Croteau-Chonka DC, *et al.* New genetic loci link adipose and insulin biology to body fat distribution. *Nature.* 2015;518:187–96.

90. Lu Y, Day FR, Gustafsson S, *et al.* New loci for body fat percentage reveal link between adiposity and cardiometabolic disease risk. *Nat Commun.* 2016;7:10495.

91. Hinney A, Kesselmeier M, Jall S, *et al.* Evidence for three genetic loci involved in both anorexia nervosa risk and variation of body mass index. *Mol Psychiatry.* 2017;22:321–2.

# 105

# Imaging of feeding and eating disorders

*Natalie Kurniadi, Christina E. Wierenga, Laura A. Berner, and Walter H. Kaye*

## Introduction

Neuroimaging has helped refocus thinking about the aetiology and formulation of the pathophysiology of eating disorders (EDs) in the past few decades [1]. Cultural pressures to be thin were once theorized to underlie or perpetuate anorexia nervosa (AN) and bulimia nervosa (BN) almost exclusively. It is now recognized that a biological basis exists for these disorders, and neuroimaging studies provide evidence that the behavioural symptoms of EDs are associated with altered brain function and structure [2]. New insights regarding the brain pathways involved in the processing of general and taste reward, cognitive inhibition, and interoception are of particular importance. This chapter will focus primarily on functional alterations in AN, BN, and binge eating disorder (BED). The feeding disorders, including pica, avoidant restrictive food intake disorder (ARFID), and rumination disorder, will also be briefly discussed.

EDs are severe psychiatric diseases with significant physical and mental health complications. EDs occur more commonly among females than males, with the typical age of onset during early adolescence [3]. AN has the highest mortality rate of all mental illnesses and is characterized by restriction of energy intake, leading to significantly low body weight, intense fear of gaining weight, and a marked disturbance in the experience of one's weight and shape [4]. Individuals suffering from the restricting subtype of AN (AN-R) limit their caloric intake and sometimes also over-exercise, whereas those with the binge eating/purging type eat large amounts of food in a short period of time, accompanied by a sense of loss of control, and/or engage in compensatory behaviours (that is, self-induced vomiting and use of laxatives or diet pills) to prevent weight gain [4]. BN is characterized by average or above average body weight and regular binge eating and compensatory behaviours. The binge eating episodes of individuals with BN tend to include sweet, high-fat foods, and dietary restriction between binge eating episodes is common [5]. Finally, BED is associated with an increased risk of obesity and is characterized by recurrent episodes of binge eating without compensatory behaviours and marked distress about binge eating [4]. Across diagnoses, EDs are difficult to treat and have a high rate of relapse [6].

A consistent body of evidence suggests that structural and functional alterations in circuitry involved in taste and reward processing, inhibitory control, and interoception may underlie eating disorder pathology [7–12]. As such, this chapter will detail these neural circuits and associated findings in EDs. Directions for future research to better understand the aetiology of these complex disorders and implications for treatment will also be discussed.

## Structural imaging

Growing evidence suggests structural brain abnormalities among eating-disordered individuals, with the majority of research focusing on differences in brain volume. Among participants with AN, the most pronounced differences are observed during the acute stages of illness [13]. A systematic review of structural MRI studies reveals significantly lower grey matter (GM) volume and greater cerebrospinal fluid (CSF) volume among ill AN patients, relative to controls [14]. Lower GM volume was found in areas including the dorsal and rostral anterior cingulate cortex (ACC), right frontal operculum, left cerebellum, and right insula. While one study shows lower global GM volume among individuals remitted from anorexia nervosa (RAN), relative to controls, another reveals no differences in GM, white matter (WM), or CSF volume between the two groups [14]. No differences were found in WM volume between acute AN, RAN, and age-matched healthy controls (HC) [15]. Longitudinal research in AN suggests that GM volumetric differences normalize upon recovery [14], suggesting state-specific findings are likely due to malnutrition.

Inconsistent findings are also seen among patients with BN, with one study finding no differences in GM, WM, or CSF volume, compared to healthy participants [14]. However, another reveals that those with BN show greater GM volume than HC in the medial orbitofrontal cortex (OFC) and striatum. Although not significant, individuals remitted from bulimia nervosa (RBN) showed larger GM volume in the insula, relative to HC [14]. Finally, individuals with BED showed increased GM volume of the ACC and medial OFC, relative to controls [14]. Alterations in structural volume among individuals with EDs may be related to the extreme eating patterns observed among these participants.

### Structural connectivity

Only one study has examined structural connectivity among individuals with EDs. Diffusion-weighted MRI revealed that individuals with RAN showed abnormal structural connectivity in regions involving frontal, basal ganglia, and posterior cingulate nodes [16], relative to HC. RAN individuals exhibited longer normalized mean path lengths in the right caudal anterior cingulate and right posterior cingulate, which correlated to poor insight. Such findings in neural systems involved in habit formation and reward may underlie the establishment and maintenance of compulsive behaviours characteristic of AN [16].

## Functional imaging

Several studies have utilized resting-state functional magnetic resonance imaging (rsfMRI), a method that allows for making temporal correlations between brain areas using task-independent changes of blood oxygen level-dependent (BOLD) signals [17] to examine functional connectivity in EDs. A review of rsfMRI studies in AN suggests differences in functional connectivity between AN and HC in the dorsal ACC (dACC), thalamus, and right inferior frontal gyrus (IFG) [18]. AN exhibit decreased connectivity between the sensory–motor and visual networks, relative to HC [19]. Additionally, acute AN show decreased connectivity in the thalamo-insular subnetwork, relative to HC, reflecting alterations in neural systems involved in pain, body size perception, and hunger [20]. Increased functional connectivity in the default mode network (DMN), a region involved in introspective rumination, low-level arousal, and self-regulation [21], was found in AN, relative to HC [22]. Compared to HC, RAN subjects showed alterations in the DMN [23] and stronger functional connectivity between the dorsolateral prefrontal cortex (DLPFC) and medial OFC (mOFC) during a monetary incentive delay task [24]. The latter findings indicate greater cognitive control relative to motivationally salient cues among RAN. However, another study showed no differences, compared to controls [25]. Discrepant findings may be due to methodological differences, including participant characteristics and resting-state approaches [18].

Studies comparing AN, BN, and HC showed that AN individuals demonstrated stronger synchronous activity between the dACC and the retrosplenial cortex, while those with BN showed stronger synchronous activity between the dACC and the mOFC [26], relative to HC. AN and BN individuals showed stronger activity between the dACC and the precuneus, correlating to higher rates of concern with body shape on the Body Shape Questionnaire [26]. These findings indicate that greater synchrony between such regions may be associated with preoccupation with eating and body shape among individuals with EDs. Alternatively, one study using functional magnetic resonance imaging (fMRI), voxel-mirrored homotopic connectivity (VMHC), and regional interhemispheric spectral coherence (IHSC) revealed significantly reduced interhemispheric functional connectivity in patients with acute AN and BN, compared to HC [27]. Specifically, lower interhemispheric functional connectivity was shown in the precuneus, cerebellum, and posterior insula among AN patients vs HC, and in the frontal lobe of BN patients, compared to HC. Interhemispheric functional connectivity was higher in the Slow-5 band, a frequency range in which the majority of GM oscillations primarily occur [28], in all regions except the insula. There were no group differences in left–right structural asymmetries or in WM or GM volume. Functional connectivity anomalies, despite the absence of structural differences between groups, indicate that the acute phase of EDs are associated with decreased interhemispheric connectivity in regions involved in cognitive control and reward processing [27].

## General reward processing in eating disorders

Neuroimaging evidence supports a role for altered reward processing in the development and maintenance of EDs [29]. Briefly, ventral limbic neural circuitry, which includes the amygdala, rostral ACC, ventromedial prefrontal cortex (vmPFC), and anterior ventral striatum, is involved in identifying and processing rewarding or emotionally significant information and in generating affective responses to this information [30]. Through a series of non-reciprocal connections, dopamine (DA)-mediated reward and motor information travels via the limbic circuit to executive and sensorimotor areas of the striatum [31]. Together with cognitive control and sensorimotor circuits, these circuits code the rewarding value of food and non-food stimuli and evaluate and integrate reward predictions to guide behaviours [32]. The majority of research on illness-specific reward processing in EDs is based on studies examining responses to food and taste stimuli, though some studies have also examined general reward processing (for example, money) to avoid potentially eliciting symptoms caused by disorder-specific stimuli. Determining whether alterations in reward processing are specific to food or whether they generalize to secondary reinforcers (for example, money) can help elucidate neural mechanisms underlying ED pathology and identify shared and unique alterations across ED and non-ED psychiatric conditions.

### Anorexia nervosa

Individuals with AN often display anhedonia and find little pleasure outside of the pursuit of weight loss [33]. They also tend to show an enhanced capacity to delay reward, relative to their healthy peers, though only when ill [34]. Many of these characteristics typically persist to some degree following remission [35], suggesting trait-, rather than state-, related symptoms of eating disorders [36]. Individuals ill with, and remitted from, AN (RAN) show altered DA function [37] and altered brain response, particularly in striatal circuits [1, 36, 38], suggestive of abnormal reward processing. Moreover, increased DA release in the precommissural dorsal caudate has been associated with increased anxiety in RAN [39]. Since ingestion of palatable foods is associated with an increase in striatal DA [40], food restriction is thought to be an effective means of reducing the stressful experience of endogenous DA release among individuals with AN [7].

In one study, RAN adults failed to show a difference in ventral striatal response to monetary gains vs losses, suggesting an insensitivity to the distinction between positive and negative feedback that may contribute to anhedonia, difficulty with making decisions, and decreased food intake [8]. Adolescents with AN also show exaggerated neural responsivity to punishment, relative to controls, suggesting an altered ability to code for both the value and valence of potential outcomes [9]. Moreover, in contrast to healthy control women, who exhibit a greater reward response when hungry, the reward response in RAN participants does not differ significantly between hunger and satiety during a delay discounting task, suggesting reduced sensitivity to the motivational drive of metabolic state when determining the value of rewarding stimuli in AN [41]. Findings from this study suggest that hunger does not increase reward among RAN and that such individuals fail to integrate the physiological state and reward motivation into decision-making [41]. Reduced capacity to experience reward is thought to serve as a mechanism to ignore hunger and engage in prolonged periods of fasting, even in the face of physical starvation [41].

### Bulimia nervosa

Individuals who engage in binge eating and purging behaviours are typically oversensitive to reward and often engage in sensation-seeking behaviours [35]. Alterations in reward circuitry are seen in individuals with BN. For example, reduced CSF concentrations of the DA metabolite homovanillic acid (HVA) are associated with increased frequency of binge eating behaviours among individuals ill with BN [42]. Positron emission tomography (PET) studies reveal a trend towards decreased D2/D3 receptor binding potential in the posterior putamen and caudate in ill BN participants, with an inverse association between binge eating and vomiting frequencies and striatal DA response [43]. Interestingly, individuals remitted from BN (RBN) and participants with the binge eating/purging subtype of AN have normal DA D2/D3 receptor binding and CSF HVA levels [39]. Similar to RAN women, RBN women also fail to differentiate between wins and losses in ventral–striatal regions during a monetary choice task, suggesting an inability to differentiate between positive and negative feedback [11]. These findings may indicate elevated sensitivity to both reward and punishment among BN individuals, even after recovery [44].

### Binge eating disorder

Altered reward processing also has been observed among individuals with BED. Following treatment, obese individuals with BED, relative to obese individuals without BED, demonstrated diminished activation in reward circuitry during both the anticipation of rewards and actual reward processing [45]. Individuals with the greatest hypoactivation activation during reward processing engaged in more frequent binge eating [45]. In sum, research suggests that across ED diagnoses, altered reward processing, which may not be specific to food reward, likely contributes to disordered eating.

## Taste and food reward processing

Appetite is a physiological motivational drive that depends on the interaction between an individual's homeostatic needs, the rewarding aspects of food, and the cognitive ability to choose alternative behaviours to eating [36]. Cortical taste circuitry is relatively well defined. Animal studies show that sweet taste perception is mediated by tongue receptors that send signals through the brainstem and the thalamus to the primary gustatory cortex in the insula [46]. In humans, the anterior insula receives chemosensory taste information from the mid insula where it is integrated with homeostatic drives and reward value to guide motivated eating behaviour [47, 48]. Together with the amygdala, which valuates the emotional saliency of food tastes and textures [49], the anterior insula projects along the ventral aspects of the striatum to regulate palatable food intake [50]. The mOFC assesses the pleasantness of taste or smell [51] and projects to the subgenual and rostral ACC. ACC subregions

integrate reward with automatic function and motor control [52] and contribute to appetite [53]. The OFC also processes how much food an individual has eaten and guides decisions about when to stop eating one food type, while still remaining interested in other types of foods [54]. This ventral (limbic) neurocircuit thus translates taste signals into food reward and guides the approach towards, or avoidance of, food [36] (Fig. 105.1).

### Anorexia nervosa

One approach to examining food reward processing in EDs is to directly interrogate gustatory processing. Studying brain response to administration of actual tastes permits direct examination of whether individuals with EDs show alterations specific to encoding the rewarding aspects of food. Imaging studies in RAN show decreased ACC, insula, and striatal activation in response to expected sweet taste receipt, relative to controls (Fig. 105.2) [55, 56], although these studies do not directly compare responses when hungry vs satiated. Decreased brain response to palatable taste supports a role for altered reward processing of gustatory stimuli in AN. However, data from another study suggest striatal and insular activation in response to pleasant and aversive taste is increased in RAN when taste is less predictable, potentially indicating a hypersensitive salience response to unexpected food among this population [57]. Discrepant findings may relate to the predictability of the delivered taste, rather than to the tastes themselves. In addition, individuals with AN showed greater right amygdala and left medial temporal gyrus activity in response to chocolate milk than controls [58]. The amygdala is involved in the acquisition of conditioned emotional responses to neutral stimuli and is activated during fear [59]. Further research is needed to clarify the role of altered activation in response to tastes in AN.

### Bulimia nervosa

Imaging studies of BN have been somewhat inconsistent. Some research suggests reduced reward response to expected taste receipt in BN, potentially suggesting reward habituation to food [60]. It is possible that a decreased subjective sense of reward while eating may contribute to overeating in predisposed individuals [61] or that recurrent episodes of binge eating over time contribute to blunted reward responses [62]. However, other findings showed reduced reward response to unexpected taste receipt among ill BN individuals, relative to controls [10]. Exaggerated hedonic response to predictable receipt of palatable foods also has been observed among individuals with BN [5, 55]. Responsivity of reward regions during anticipation, but not receipt, of palatable food is associated with increased negative affect among women with BN [63]. This relationship has been interpreted to suggest that greater reward anticipation activation during states of negative affect in BN may make individuals with BN more likely to consume high-energy foods, and negative affect could increase the rewarding value of food if used as a temporary tool to regulate mood [63].

## Reward-based learning

### Anorexia nervosa

As learning from feedback shapes behaviour, altered feedback learning could contribute to the onset and maintenance of

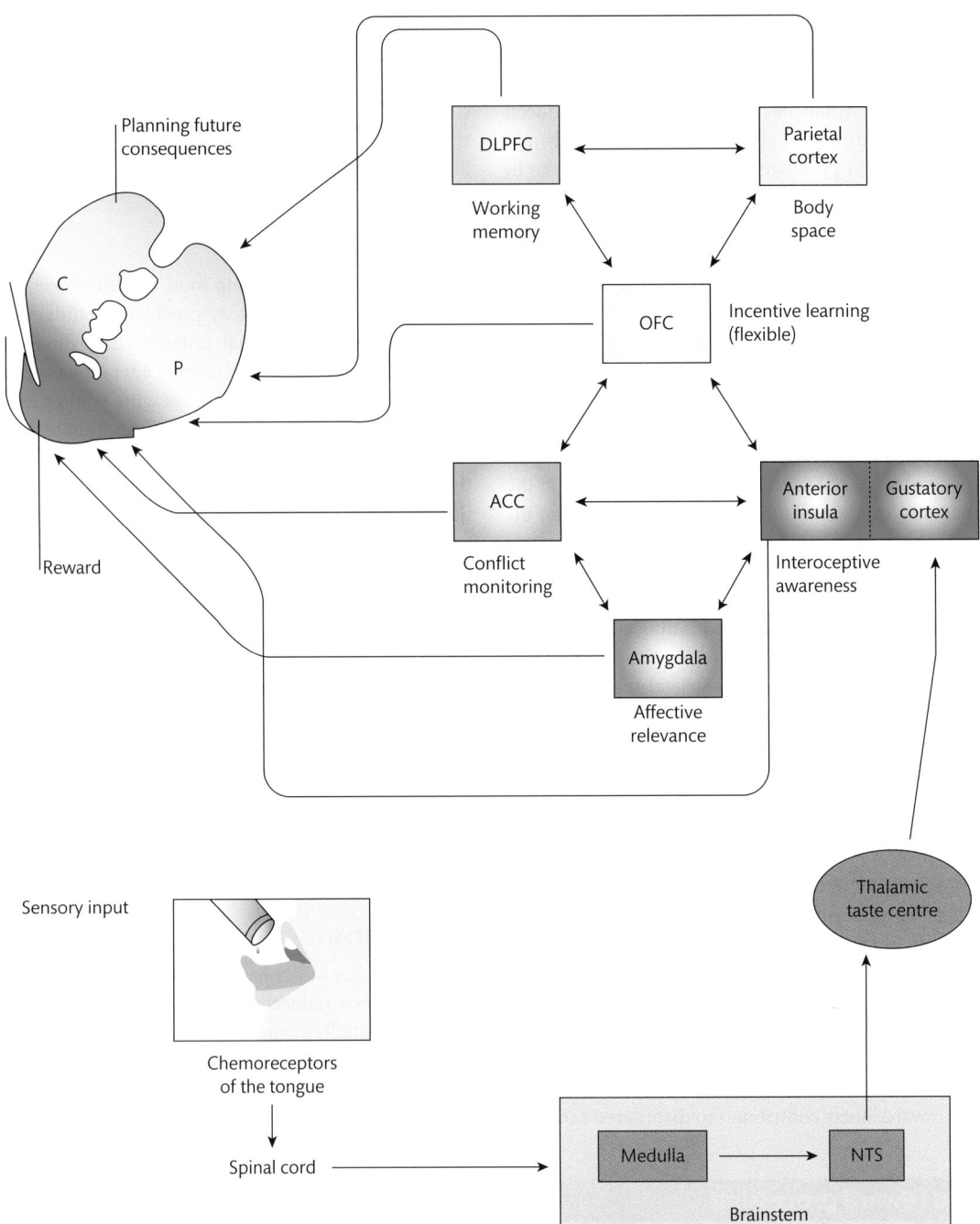

**Fig. 105.1** (see Colour Plate section) Cortical taste circuitry. Chemoreceptors on the tongue detect a sweet taste, which is transmitted through brainstem and thalamic centres to the primary gustatory cortex, adjacent to, and interconnected with, the insula. The anterior insula is a part of the ventral neurocircuit and is connected with the ACC and OFC. Cortical structures in the ventral neurocircuit send signals to the ventral striatum, while structures involved in cognitive strategies send input to the dorsal striatum. Taste and motivation are integrated in a decision to approach or avoid food. The figure links cortical structures with arrows, and all cortical structures project to the striatum in a topographic manner.

Reproduced from *Nat Rev Neurosci.*, 10(8), Kaye W, Fudge J, Paulus M, New insight into symptoms and neurocircuit function of anorexia nervosa, pp. 573–84, Copyright (2009), with permission from Springer Nature.

disordered eating. Reward-based learning can be studied by examining brain response to receipt of expected or unexpected reward stimuli [64]. DA is released during expectation of a reward, whereas omission of an expected reward is followed by a decrease in DA [65]. The difference between the value of the reward stimulus received and the stimulus predicted is known as the prediction error

(Fig. 105.3) [66] and is implicated in EDs [1, 10]. RAN participants exhibited heightened anticipatory responses to food images [67], and individuals ill with AN showed a higher brain response to unexpected taste stimuli than controls, suggesting heightened anxiety and responsivity to anticipated and unanticipated food stimuli in AN [68]. Adolescents with AN, relative to controls, showed a

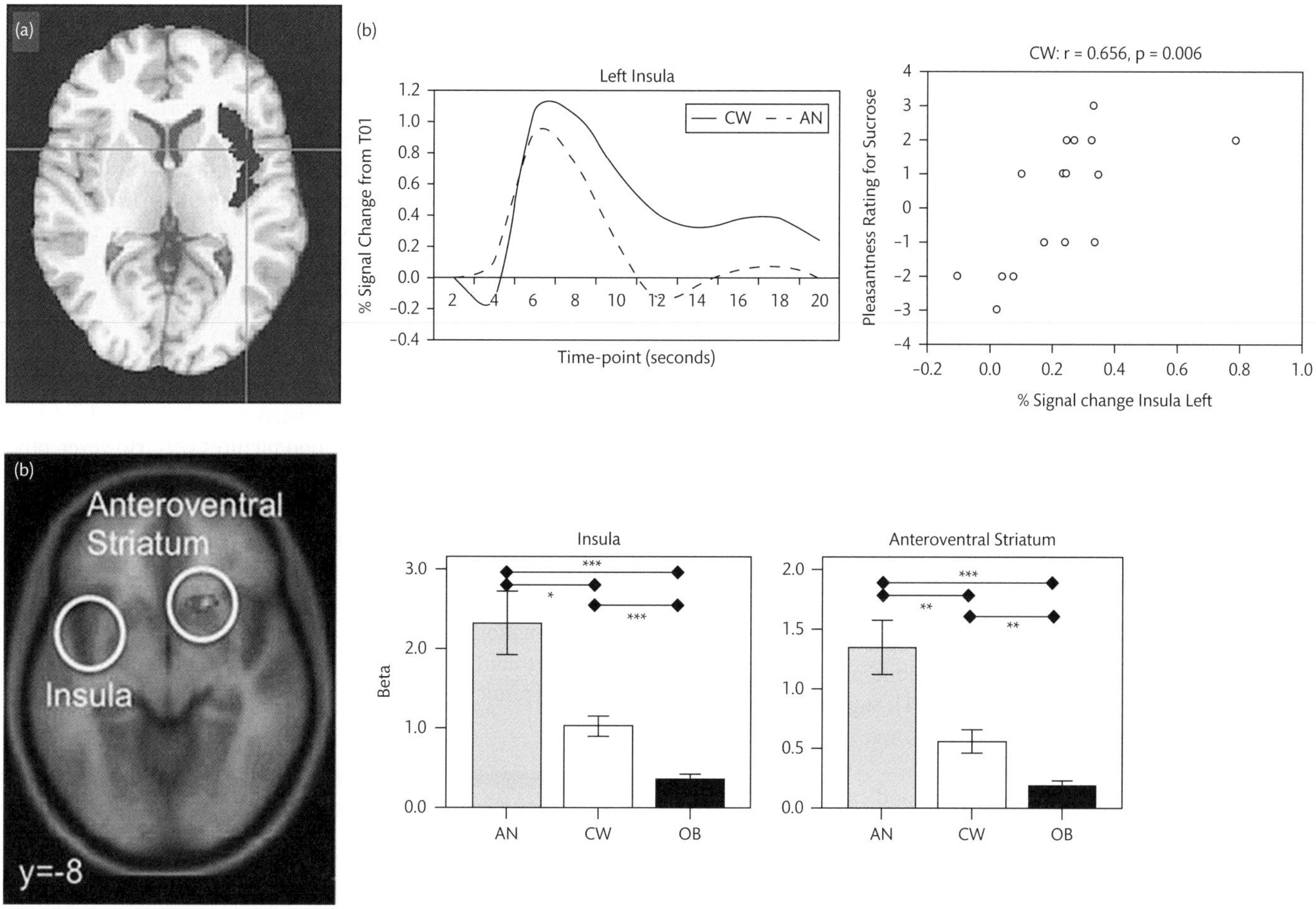

(a)

(b)

**Left Insula**

% Signal Change from T01

— CW  – – AN

Time-point (seconds)

CW: r = 0.656, p = 0.006

Pleasantness Rating for Sucrose

% Signal change Insula Left

(b)

Anteroventral
Striatum

Insula

y=-8

**Insula**

Beta

***
*
***

AN    CW    OB

**Anteroventral Striatum**

***
**
**

AN    CW    OB

**Fig. 105.2** Functional MRI studies examining taste reward processing in anorexia nervosa (AN) participants and control women (CW). (a) During taste processing of sucrose vs water, RAN, compared to CW, showed less activation of the ventral and dorsal striatum and the insula to sucrose and water. (b) Corresponding time points of the blood oxygen level-dependent (BOLD) in the left insula showed this decreased response to sucrose in RAN. BOLD response is correlated with pleasantness response for sucrose in the left and right insula in CW, but not in RAN. (c) By contrast, a taste reward conditioning tasks shows underweight AN have greater brain response in the anteroventral striatum, insula, and PF,C compared to control and obese women, during taste anticipation.

Reproduced from *Neuropsychopharmacology*, 33(3), Wagner A, Aizenstein H, Frank GK, *et al.*, Altered insula response to a taste stimuli in individuals recovered from restricting-type anorexia nervosa, pp. 513–23, Copyright (2008), with permission from Springer Nature.

greater prediction error response within the ventral caudate/nucleus accumbens, and the anterior and posterior insula during a monetary reward task [69]. They also showed an increased neural

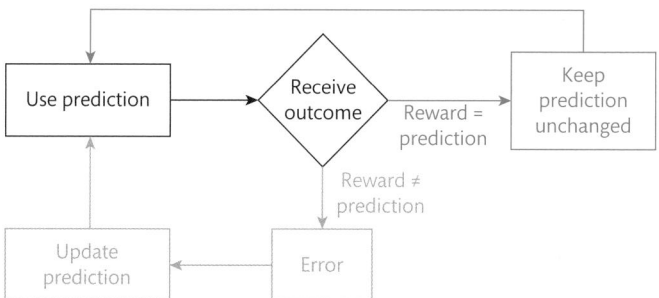

**Fig. 105.3** Learning via prediction error. Light blue lines show when reward differs from its prediction, resulting in prediction error. Dark blue lines show when outcome matches the prediction, resulting in no error and unchanged behaviour.

Reproduced from *Dialogues Clin Neurosci.*, 18(1), Schultz W, Dopamine reward prediction error coding, pp. 23–32, Copyright (2016), with permission from Institut La Conférence Hippocrate.

response to unexpected reward receipt and to unexpected reward omission. Following treatment, prediction error and response to unexpected reward omission normalized, but unexpected reward receipt remained heightened. Caudate prediction error response was negatively associated with weight gain during treatment, indicating tha a higher neural prediction error response may be a marker of illness severity or the treatment-resistant nature of adolescent AN [70]. Since depression and anxiety are significantly associated with intolerance of uncertainty and harm avoidance among AN individuals [68], an elevated prediction error in response to food could be related to higher rates of depression among AN participants, relative to controls.

## Bulimia nervosa

Opposite findings have been observed among individuals with BN. Specifically, participants with BN exhibited reduced responses to unexpected taste stimuli, relative to controls [10]. Decreased prediction error response in BN is associated with higher binge eating/purge frequency [10], potentially suggesting that repeated binge eating and purging reduce DA response in BN. Contrasting prediction error responses may play a role in the opposing patterns of food consumptions among individuals with AN and BN.

## Reward response to food cues in eating disorders

### Anorexia nervosa

The majority of research examining neural response to food among individuals with EDs uses visual food cues [2]. Functional magnetic resonance imaging (fMRI) studies investigating brain response to pictures of food revealed reduced reward brain response in AN in the inferior parietal lobe [70], OFC [71, 72], lateral PFC [72], hypothalamus [71], and insula [67, 71], but greater activation of the medial PFC and posterior cingulate [72], when viewing food images. Decreased neural responses to food images in AN may indicate innate differences in reward processing [1]. Notably, decreased reward response to food pictures in individuals with AN was significantly correlated with illness severity [70], suggesting that decreased reward sensitivity may contribute to an increased ability to restrict intake. Unlike healthy controls, both ill and weight-restored AN participants failed to demonstrate the expected associations between the levels of ghrelin, a 'hunger hormone', and brain response to visual food stimuli in limbic regions [71], suggesting a possible disconnect between brain reward response and physiological hunger signalling.

Rather than eliciting reward response, food cues may be associated with exaggerated attentional processing among ill and RAN individuals [1, 72, 73]. Early fMRI research shows that, unlike healthy controls, individuals with AN exhibited increased left amygdala response to high- vs low-calorie foods [73]. Pictures of high-calorie foods elicited high self-reported anxiety in AN individuals, along with increased left insular and ACC brain response [73], suggesting elevated fear of calorically dense foods. Elevated activation in the medial temporal gyrus when viewing high-calorie foods was also associated with self-reported anxiety [74]. More recent research showed that both ill and RAN individuals demonstrated increased activation in areas of executive function and error monitoring, relative to controls, when viewing food images [72]. Together, these findings could suggest heightened arousal, vigilance, or processing activity in response to food cues among AN individuals, possibly to predict and control the anxiety produced by food stimuli that may be experienced as unpleasant [7].

Tasks that permit examination of neural response to food images and during food-related decision-making have also been used to assess food-related processes in AN. For example, AN individuals showed greater activation of neural circuits associated with habit formation than controls when choosing low-fat vs high-fat foods [75]. Although it remains unknown whether reduced energy intake among AN individuals is a habit, these findings provide preliminary evidence that maladaptive behaviours in AN may be mediated by dorsal fronto-striatal circuits that underlie habitual behaviours [75]. Thus, alterations in these circuits may play a role in food choices in AN.

### Bulimia nervosa and binge eating disorder

Limited research examining the response to visual food cues among individuals with BN and BED has thus far yielded inconsistent findings. Participants with BN showed greater activation in the mOFC, ACC, visual cortex, and insula in response to pictures of palatable foods, relative to controls [76, 77], and heightened insular and ACC activation in response to food images, relative to participants with BED, suggesting enhanced reward processing of visual food stimuli [77]. An exaggerated response to visual food cues could increase the risk for binge eating among individuals with BN. However, other studies showed evidence of reduced reward response to food stimuli among BN, compared to controls [12, 78]. In addition, patients with BN showed decreased neural activity in the temporal lobe, inferior parietal lobule, and post-central gyrus in response to visual food stimuli [76].

Results in BED to date are similarly mixed. One study revealed increased medial PFC response, relative to controls [77], and another showed elevated response patterns of the left ventral striatum, compared to BN, in response to food pictures [79]. However, other findings revealed a negative correlation between body mass index (BMI) and neural reward response to food cues in BED, suggesting that chronic excessive caloric intake may contribute to changes in brain function or that individuals with a lower reward response are at a greater risk for weight gain [2]. It remains unclear whether functional alternations among BN individuals and those with BED are premorbid traits that contribute to binge eating behaviours or if such differences result from extreme overeating.

## Inhibitory control in eating disorders

A growing body of research suggests that EDs are marked by an imbalance between reward and inhibitory control circuitry. Homeostatic mechanisms regulating appetite interface with reward and cognitive control circuitry to guide eating behaviours [51]. Cognitive processes involved in planning, inhibitory control, and decision-making integrate interoceptive cues (for example, information about the internal physiological state) and reward signals to determine food selection, portion sizes, and frequency of eating [80]. These systems can override homeostatic signals, giving rise to extreme patterns of over- or under-consumption [81].

A network consisting of the DLPFC, ventrolateral prefrontal cortex (VLPFC), insula, dorsal caudate, and posterior parietal cortex is associated with inhibitory control [82]. The dorsal cognitive circuit modulates selective attention, planning, decision-making, and effortful regulation of affective states [83]. The ventral limbic and dorsal cognitive circuits are involved in inhibitory decision-making processes, especially involving reward-related behaviours. Through its connections with the dorsal ACC, the insula is also involved in the cognitive valuation of salient stimuli such as food [84].

### Anorexia nervosa

Individuals with AN-R often exhibit temperaments marked by behavioural inhibition, cognitive inflexibility, and emotional constraint [85]. Imaging data consistently provide evidence of alterations in dorsal inhibitory control circuits among AN and RAN individuals. Specifically, several fMRI studies revealed enhanced activity in inhibitory control regions among AN, relative to controls, during tasks requiring effortful control, cognitive inhibition, and error detection [86, 87]. RAN, relative to healthy control, participants also demonstrated enhanced activation of inhibitory control regions during both hunger and satiety [41] (Fig. 105.4). While behavioural

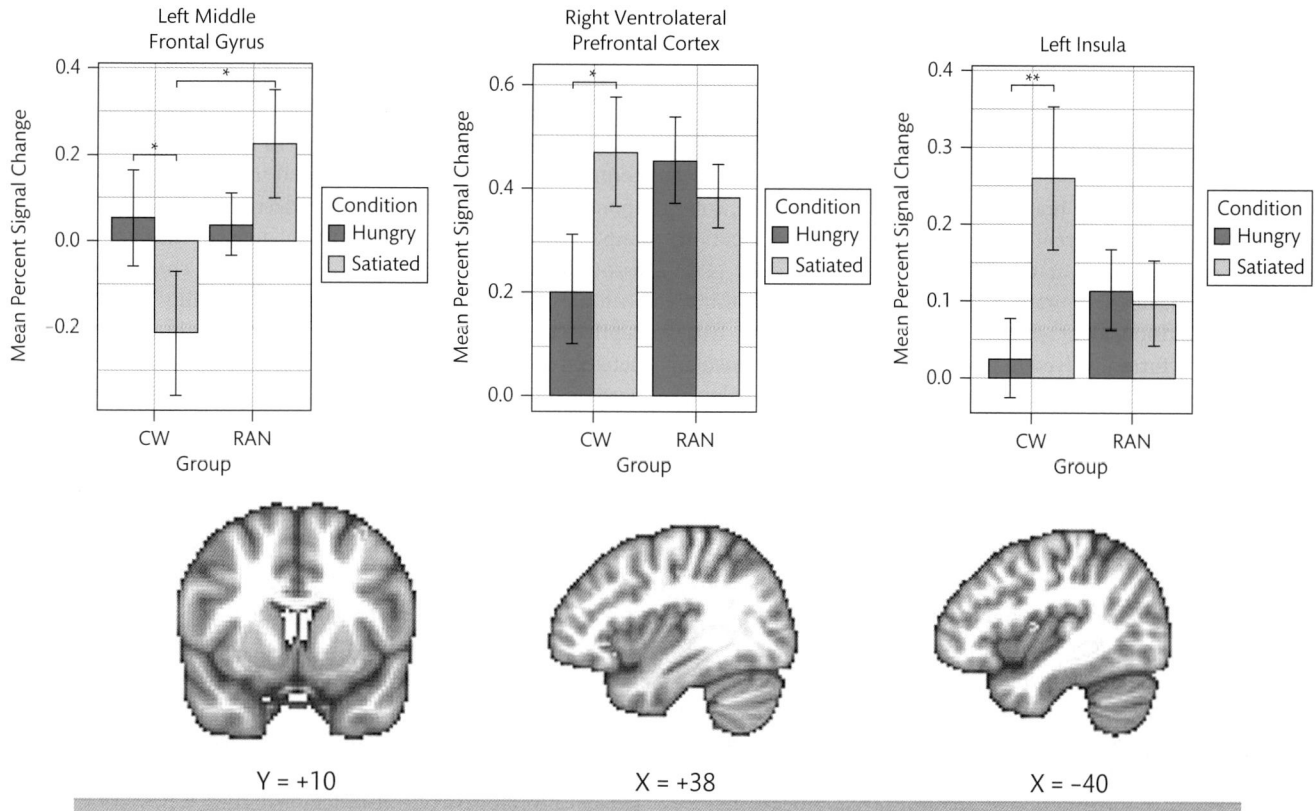

**Fig. 105.4** Functional MRI response of cognitive circuitry during a monetary decision task in RAN and CW. Left: within the left middle frontal gyrus, CW responded more strongly when hungry than when satiated ($z = 2.6$; $P = 0.04$), whereas RAN responded more than CW when satiated ($z = 2.7$; $P = 0.03$). Middle: within the right ventrolateral PFC, CW responded more when satiated than when hungry ($z = 2.0$; $P = 0.02$). Right: within the left insula, CW responded more when satiated than when hungry ($z = 3.6$; $P = 0.002$). CW, healthy comparison women; RAN, women remitted from anorexia nervosa.

findings in regard to set-shifting among adolescents with AN are mixed [88, 89], adult AN and RAN participants showed decreased neural activity in frontal regions during set-shifting [90, 91]. Such findings call into question whether cognitive inflexibility may be associated with brain development or a trait marker for AN [85]. AN participants also showed a positive association between successful inhibition and increased activation of the inferior parietal cortex [87]. Increased activation of brain regions involved in planning, control, and evaluation of negative outcomes may underlie excessive behavioural inhibition and restricted food intake characteristic of AN. Furthermore, over-control may enable AN individuals to restrict food intake in order to achieve weight loss.

### Bulimia nervosa

In addition to demonstrating high reward sensitivity, BN individuals are often emotionally dysregulated and behaviourally disinhibited [92]. They often engage in more impulsive and sensation-seeking behaviours than individuals with AN and healthy controls [93]. Inhibitory control processes are impaired in BN participants, as evidenced by poor performance on Stroop, Stop Signal, and Go/No-Go tasks [94]. Ill BN adolescents and adults, relative to controls, showed reduced fronto-striatal activation during correct responding on incongruent trials of the Simon Spatial Incompatibility Task [12, 95]. However, a study conducted by Lock *et al.* [87] revealed increased activation of the right

DLPFC among adolescents with binge eating and purging during a Go/No-Go task [87]. Reduced activation during response inhibition is associated with illness severity [12, 95]. Individuals with BN also demonstrated behavioural impairments in inhibitory control in response to food stimuli [96], indicating that altered functioning of inhibitory control circuitry may underlie eating pathology in BN.

### Binge eating disorder

Behavioural studies suggested that individuals with BED demonstrated significantly poorer performance on measures of decision-making and inhibitory control, relative to controls [97, 98]. Poor decision-making, coupled with difficulty delaying immediate rewards, may explain the tendency to binge eat despite delayed negative consequences (for example, weight gain, feelings of guilt). Imaging studies among individuals with BED showed alterations in cognitive control circuitry, namely in the prefrontal, insular, and orbitofrontal cortex in response to both food-specific and non-food stimuli [99, 100]. Obese participants with BED showed less activation in the vmPFC, IFG, and insula, compared to obese and lean controls, during a Stroop task [100]. Additionally, a negative correlation was found between activation in brain regions involved in impulse control and dietary restraint scores in the BED group, whereas no such association was found between obese non-BED and lean participants [100]. Dysregulation of these regions may contribute to the development and maintenance of binge behaviours seen among individuals with BN and BED.

## Interoception in eating disorders

Interoception refers to the brain's receipt of, and response to, continuous feedback of afferent signals that provide information about the representation of the body's physiological state [48]. Interoception includes respiration, heartbeat, pain, hunger, thirst, and intestinal tension, all of which are implicated in EDs [36, 101]. Key neural structures involved in interoception include the insula, midbrain reticular nuclei, ventromedial and ventroposterior thalami, and posterior insular cortex [48]. The insula evaluates interoceptive signals and plays a critical role in processing such sensations to guide behaviour. Evidence from neuroanatomical and functional neuroimaging indicates that the insula also plays an important role in regulating hunger, appetite, and thirst [48]. The insula receives exteroceptive signals from the spino-thalamo-cortical interoceptive pathway [48] and integrates such information with input from the hypothalamus and amygdala, creating a representation of one's internal and external environments [47]. This representation is projected to the anterior insula where it is integrated with information from cortical regions and limbic regions involved in motivation and saliency [47], evaluating how the stimulus may affect the body [102]. Ventral portions of the middle and anterior insula process social–emotional, cognitive, and sensorimotor information [48]. The mid insula also codes interoceptive prediction error, signalling a mismatch between expected and actual bodily arousal, which can elicit anxiety and approach or avoidance behaviour [47, 48, 102]. In fact, recent evidence suggests that several mood and anxiety disorders are rooted in altered interoception [103]. Altered interoception may be particularly relevant to Eds, given that individuals with AN and BN often exhibit comorbid depression and anxiety [104].

### Anorexia nervosa

Emerging evidence suggests altered interoceptive processing in ED. For example, individuals with AN demonstrate less accurate detection of interoceptive sensations (for example, cardiorespiratory changes) during meal anticipation [105]. Other studies suggested ill and RAN individuals, relative to controls, were less accurate in the perception of body signals and showed altered brain response to taste, pain, gastric interoception, and hunger [36, 105–107]. For example, despite comparable pain intensity ratings, relative to controls, RAN participants exhibited increased anterior insula response to anticipation of pain, but decreased activation to pain receipt [106]. Further, this altered right anterior insula functioning is associated with the alexithymic temperament characteristic of AN, with alexithymia possibly reflecting an inability to utilize interoceptive cues to evaluate outcomes [106]. The observed discrepancy between subjective pain experience and brain response among AN participants may indicate a disconnection between reported and actual interoceptive state [106]. Weight-restored individuals with AN showed reduced left dorsal mid-insula activity during a stomach interoceptive attention task and increased activation of the right anterior insula during heart interoceptive attention, relative to controls [107]. Altered anterior insula responsivity, as evidenced by abnormal anticipation, interpretation, and integration of internal and external stimuli, is likely to interfere with eating, social interactions, and other reward-related behaviours among individuals with AN [36].

### Bulimia nervosa

Altered interoception is also observed in BN. Patients with BN, relative to controls, reported more deficits in interoceptive awareness on the ED inventory, while also demonstrating a positive correlation between anticipatory anxiety, interoceptive awareness, and body image distortion [108]. Individuals with BN reported elevated panic and anxiety symptoms, compared to controls, following sodium lactate and isoproterenol infusions, despite exhibiting a similar sympathetic response [109]. However, RBN individuals demonstrated reduced heartbeat counting accuracy [110], and individuals with BN showed elevated thresholds for pain [111] and larger gastric capacity, in comparison to healthy controls and obese individuals [112]. Thus, findings regarding interoception among individuals with BN remain unclear, as results from these studies suggest both heightened and diminished responses to interoceptive signals among BN individuals [113]. For example, individuals with BN showed decreased baseline sympathetic tone, yet increased adrenergic sensitivity to

**Table 105.1** Summary table of neuroimaging findings of eating disorders in adults

| | | AN | RAN | BN | RBN | BED |
|---|---|---|---|---|---|---|
| Monetary reward | Expected | – | Mixed | – | – | – |
| | Unexpected | – | – | | | |
| Taste/food reward | Expected | – | – | Mixed | + | Mixed |
| | Unexpected | – | + | – | | |
| Food pictures | | – | + attentional processing | Mixed | | Mixed |
| Reward-based learning | | + anticipatory response and prediction error | + anticipatory response and prediction error | – prediction error | | |
| Inhibitory control | | Mixed | + | – | – | – |
| Interoception | | – | – | – | – | – |
| Structural findings (volume) | | Mixed | Mixed | Mixed | + | + |

(+) indicates increased neural response to stimuli, relative to controls; (–) indicates decreased neural response to stimuli, relative to controls.

**Table 105.2** Summary table of neuroimaging findings of eating disorders in adolescents

| | | AN | RAN | BN | RBN | BED |
|---|---|---|---|---|---|---|
| Monetary reward | Expected | – | | | | |
| | Unexpected | + | | | | |
| Taste/food reward | Expected | | | | | |
| | Unexpected | | | | | |
| Food pictures | | – | | Mixed | | |
| Reward-based learning | | + anticipatory response and prediction error | + anticipatory response and prediction error | | | |
| Inhibitory control | | Mixed | | Mixed | | |
| Interoception | | – | | | | |
| Structural findings (volume) | | | | | | |

(+) indicates increased neural response to stimuli, relative to controls; (–) indicates decreased neural response to stimuli, relative to controls.

isoproterenol [114]. It is hypothesized that repeated binge eating and purging may contribute to habituation or sensitization of internal body states, as evidenced by reduced salivation to food presentation among BN individuals, which normalizes after treatment [115]. Further research in individuals across all stages of illness and in recovery is needed to clarify interoceptive processes among BN individuals [113].

No studies to date have examined interoceptive awareness among individuals with BED. Research is needed to investigate the role of interoception in binge eating.

## Feeding disorders

Feeding disorders include pica, rumination disorder, and ARFID. Pica is characterized by the compulsive and persistent eating of non-nutritive substances, while the essential feature of rumination disorder is the repeated regurgitation of food occurring after feeding or eating over a period of at least 1 month [4]. Individuals with ARFID avoid or restrict food consumption, resulting in a clinically significant failure to meet nutritional requirements through the oral intake of food [4]. To date, no published neuroimaging studies of feedings disorders exist. Incidence of pica following acquired brain injury may suggest neural abnormalities among these individuals [116]. Further, some case studies suggest that selective serotonin reuptake inhibitors, in particular, are helpful in treating pica, suggesting possible serotonin dysfunction among affected individuals [117]. Although these findings support hypotheses for future investigation, imaging research is needed to better understand the neurobiological underpinnings of feeding disorders.

## Conclusions

A consistent body of research provides evidence that individuals with EDs have altered functioning in reward, control, and interoceptive circuitry (Tables 105.1 and 105.2). Reduced motivational reward response and exaggerated cognitive control, coupled with an altered ability to integrate taste, hunger, and body signals, are likely to facilitate and maintain prolonged periods of fasting in AN. By contrast, alterations in both anticipatory and actual responses to receipt of food, deficient inhibitory control circuit activation, and altered interoception are likely to underlie binge eating behaviour in BN and BED. These findings suggest potential ED phenotypes based on neural circuit abnormalities, but also provide insight for targeting behavioural and pharmacological treatment options [2].

However, many questions still remain regarding the neurobiology of EDs. For example, malnutrition, psychological comorbidities, and medication use often confound the findings of research conducted in ill individuals [1]. Many studies examine individuals in the remitted stages of illness, making it difficult to determine whether functional neural abnormalities are inherent traits or reflect scars of the illness [85]. Longitudinal studies may be one way to address this methodological question. Further research is also needed to elucidate whether neurobiological differences exist along a continuum or reflect discrete categories of eating pathology. Finally, although the hypothalamus is important in regulating food intake and body weight, evidence supporting the role of the hypothalamus in the aetiology of EDs is limited [36]. Studies combining the assessment of hypothalamic neuropeptide levels and neuroimaging may further contribute to the recent advances in understanding and treating these complex illnesses.

## REFERENCES

1. Frank G, Kaye W. Current status of functional imaging in eating disorders. *Int J Eat Disord*. 2012;45:723–36.
2. Frank G. Recent advances in neuroimaging to model eating disorder neurobiology. *Curr Psychiatry Rep*. 2015;17:559.
3. Smink F, van Hoeken D, Hoek H. Epidemiology of eating disorders: incidence, prevalence and mortality rates. *Curr Psychiatry Rep*. 2012;14:406–14.
4. American Psychiatric Association. *Diagnostic and Statistical Manual of Mental Disorders (DSM-V)*, fifth edition. Washington, DC: American Psychiatric Association; 2013.

5. Radeloff D, Willmann K, Otto L, *et al*. High-fat taste challenge reveals altered striatal response in women recovered from bulimia nervosa—a pilot study. *World J Biol Psychiatry*. 2014;15:307–16.

6. Von Hausswolff-Juhli Y, Brooks S, Larsson M. The neurobiology of eating disorders—a clinical perspective. *Acta Psychiatr Scand*. 2015;131:244–55.

7. Kaye W, Wierenga C, Bailer U, Simmons A, Bischoff-Grethe A. Nothing tastes as good as skinny feels: The neurobiology of anorexia nervosa. *Trends Neurosci*. 2013;36:110–20.

8. Wagner A, Aizenstein H, Venkatraman M, *et al*. Altered reward processing in women recovered from anorexia nervosa. *Am J Psychiatry*. 2007;164:1842–9.

9. Bischoff-Grethe A, McCurdy D, Grenesko-Stevens E, *et al*. Altered brain response to reward and punishment in adolescents with anorexia nervosa. *Psychiatry Res*. 2013;214:331–40.

10. Frank G, Reynolds J, Shott M, O'Reilly R. Altered temporal difference learning in bulimia nervosa. *Biol Psychiatry*. 2011;70:728–35.

11. Wagner A, Aizenstein H, Venkatraman V, *et al*. Altered striatal response to reward in bulimia nervosa after recovery. *Int J Eat Disord*. 2010;43:289–94.

12. Marsh R, Steinglass J, Gerber A, *et al*. Deficient activity in the neural systems that mediate self-regulatory control in bulimia nervosa. *Arch Gen Psychiatry*. 2009;66:51–63.

13. Van EF, Treasure J. Neuroimaging in eating disorders and obesity: implications for research. *Child Adolesc Psychiatr Clin N Am*. 2009;18:95–115.

14. Eynde F, Suda M, Broadbent H, *et al*. Structural magnetic resonance imaging in eating disorders: a systematic review of voxel-based morphometry studies. *Eur Eat Disord Rev*. 2012;20:94–105.

15. Pfuhl G, King J, Geisler D, *et al*. Preserved white matter microstructure in young patients with anorexia nervosa? *Hum Brain Map*. 2016;37:4069–83.

16. Zhang A, Leow A, Zhan L, *et al*. Brain connectome modularity in weight-restored anorexia nervosa and body dysmorphic disorder. *Psychol Medicine*. 2016; 46(13):2785–97.

17. Biswal BB, Mennes M, Zuo XN, et al. Toward discovery science of human brain function. *Proc Natl Acad Sci USA*. 2010;107:4734–9.

18. Gaudio S, Wiemerslage L, Brooks S J, Schiöth HB. A systematic review of resting-state functional-MRI studies in anorexia nervosa: Evidence for functional connectivity impairment in cognitive control and visuospatial and body-signal integration. *Neurosci Biobehav Rev*. 2016;71:578–89.

19. Phillipou A, Abel LA, Castle DJ, *et al*. Resting state functional connectivity in anorexia nervosa. *Psychiatry Res. Neuroimaging*. 2016;251:45–52.

20. Ehrlich S, Geisler D, Ritschel F, *et al*. Elevated cognitive control over reward processing in recovered female patients with anorexia nervosa. *J Psychiatry Neurosci*. 2015;40:307–15.

21. Smith SM, Fox PT, Miller KL, *et al*. Correspondence of the brain's functional architecture during activation and rest. *Proc Natl Acad Sci USA*. 2009;106(31):13040–5.

22. Boehm I, Geisler D, King JA, *et al*. Increased resting state functional connectivity in the fronto-parietal and default mode network in anorexia nervosa. *Front Behav Neurosci*. 2014;8:346.

23. Cowdrey FA, Filippini N, Park RJ, *et al*. Increased resting state functional connectivity in the default mode network in recovered anorexia nervosa. *Human Brain Mapp*. 2014;35:483–91.

24. Ehrlich S, Lord AR, Geisler D, *et al*. Reduced functional connectivity in the thalamo-insular subnetwork in patients with acute anorexia nervosa. *Hum Brain Mapp*. 2015;36:1772–81.

25. Boehm I, Geisler D, King JA, *et al*. Increased resting state functional connectivity in the fronto-parietal and default mode network in anorexia nervosa. *Front Behav Neurosci*. 2014;8:346.

26. Lee S, Kim KR, Ku J, *et al*. Resting-state synchrony between anterior cingulate cortex and precuneus relates to body shape concern in anorexia nervosa and bulimia nervosa. *Psychiatry Res. Neuroimaging*. 2014;221(1):43–8.

27. Canna A, Prinster A, Monteleone AM, *et al*. Interhemispheric functional connectivity in anorexia and bulimia nervosa. *Eur J Neurosci*. 2017;45(9):1129.

28. Zuo XN, Di Martino A, Kelly C, *et al*. The oscillating brain: complex and reliable. *Neuroimage*. 2010;49:1432–45.

29. O'Hara C, Schmidt U, Campberll I. A reward-centered model of anorexia nervosa: a focussed narrative review of the neurological and psychophysiological literature. *Neurosci Biobehav Rev*. 2015;52:131–52.

30. O'Doherty J. Reward representations and reward-related learning in the human brain: insights from neuroimaging. *Curr Opin Neurobiol*. 2004;14:769–76.

31. Martinez D, Slifstein M, Broft A, *et al*. Imaging human mesolimbic dopamine transmission with positron emission tomography. Part II: amphetamine-induced dopamine release in the functional subdivisions of the striatum. *J Cereb Blood Flow Metab*. 2003;23:285–300.

32. Haber S, Knutson B. The reward circuit: linking primate anatomy and human imaging. *Neuropsychopharm*. 2010;35:4–26.

33. American Psychiatric Association. *Diagnostic and Statistical Manual of Mental Disorders*, fourth edition. Washington, DC: American Psychiatric Association; 1994.

34. Steinglass JF, K, Shohamy D, Walsh B. Restrictive food choice shows neurological signature of habit. *Appetite*. 2016; 96(664).

35. Klump K, Strober M, Johnson C, *et al*. Personality characteristics of women before and after recovery from an eating disorder. *Psych Med*. 2004;34:1407–18.

36. Kaye W, Fudge J, Paulus M. New insight into symptoms and neurocircuit function of anorexia nervosa. *Nat Rev Neurosci*. 2009;10:573–84.

37. Bailer U, Frank G, Price J, *et al*. Interaction between serotonin transporter and dopamine D2/D3 receptor radioligand measures is associated with harm avoidant symptoms in anorexia and bulimia nervosa. *Psych Res Neuroimaging*. 2013;211:160–8.

38. Frank G, Collier S, Shott M, O'Reilly R. Prediction error and somatosensory insula activation in women recovered from anorexia nervosa. *J Psychiatry Neurosci*. 2016;41:150103.

39. Bailer U, Narendran R, Frankle W, *et al*. Amphetamine induced dopamine release increases anxiety in individuals recovered from anorexia nervosa. *Int J Eat Disord*. 2012;45:263–71.

40. Avena N, Bocarsly M. Dysregulation of brain reward systems in eating disorders: Neurochemical information from animal models of binge eating, bulimia nervosa, and anorexia nervosa. *Neuropharm*. 2012;63:87–96.

41. Wierenga C, Bischoff-Grethe A, Melrose A, *et al*. Hunger does not motivate reward in women remitted from anorexia nervosa. *Biol Psychiatry*. 2015;77:642–52.

42. Jimerson DC, Lesem MD, Kaye WH, Brewerton TD. Low serotonin and dopamine metabolite concentrations in cerebrospinal fluid from bulimic patients with frequent binge episodes. *Arch Gen Psychiatry*. 1992;49:132–8.

43. Broft AI, Berner LA, Martinez D, Walsh BT. Bulimia nervosa and evidence for striatal dopamine dysregulation: a conceptual review. *Physiol Behav*. 2011;104:122–7.

44. Wierenga C, Ely A, Bischoff-Grethe A, Bailer U, Simmons A, Kaye W. Are extremes of consumption in eating disorders related to an altered balance between reward and inhibition? *Front Behav Neurosci.* 2014;9:410.

45. Balodis I, Grilo C, Kober H, et al. A pilot study linking reduced fronto-Striatal recruitment during reward processing to persistent bingeing following treatment for binge-eating disorder. *Int J Eat Disord.* 2014;47:376–84.

46. Small D. Taste representation in the human insula. *Brain Struct Funct.* 2010;214:551–61.

47. Craig A. How do you feel—now? The anterior insula and human awareness. *Nat Rev Neurosci.* 2009;10:59–70.

48. Craig AD. How do you feel? Interoception: the sense of the physiological condition of the body. *Nat Rev Neurosci.* 2002;3:655–66.

49. Kadohisa M, Vernhagen J, Rolls E. The primate amygdala: neuronal representations of the viscosity, fat texture, temperature, grittiness and taste of foods. *Neuroscience.* 2005;132: 33–48.

50. Rolls E. Reward systems in the brain and nutrition. *Ann Rev Nutrition.* 2016;36:435–70.

51. Kringelbach ML, Rolls E. The functional neuroanatomy of the human orbitofrontal cortex: evidence from neuroimaging and neuropsychology. *Prog Neurobiol.* 2004;72:341–72.

52. Williams Z, Biush G, Rauch S, Cosgrove G, Eskandar E. Human anterior cingulate neurons and the integration of monetary reward with motor responses. *Nat Neurosci.* 2004;7:1370–5.

53. Appelhans B. Neurobehavioral inhibition of reward-driven feeding: implications for dieting and obesity. *Obesity (Silver Springs).* 2009;17:640–7.

54. Rolls E. Functions of the orbitofrontal and pregenual cingulate cortex in taste, olfaction, appetite and emotion. *Acta Physiol Hung.* 2008;95:131–64.

55. Oberndorfer T, Frank G, Fudge J, et al. Altered insula response to sweet taste processing after recovery from anorexia and bulimia nervosa. *Am J Psychiatry.* 2013;214:132–41.

56. Wagner A, Aizenstein H, Frank GK, et al. Altered insula response to a taste stimuli in individuals recovered from restricting-type anorexia nervosa. *Neuropsychopharmacology.* 2008;33:513–23.

57. Cowdrey F, Park R, Harmer C, McCabe C. Increased neural processing of rewarding and aversive food stimuli in recovered anorexia nervosa. *Biol Psychiatry.* 2011;70:736–43.

58. Vocks S, Herpertz S, Rosenberger C, Senf W, Gizewski E. Effects of gustatory stimulation on brain activity during hunger and satiety in females with restricting-type anorexia nervosa: an fMRI study. *J Psychiatr Res.* 2011;45:395–403.

59. Murphy FN-S, I, Lawrence A. Functional neuroanatomy of emotions: a meta-analysis. *Cogn Affect Behav Neurosci.* 2003;3:207–33.

60. Frank G, Wagner A, Brooks-Achenbach S, et al. Altered brain activity in women recovered from bulimic type eating disorders after a glucose challenge. A pilot study. *Int J Eat Disord.* 2006;39:76–9.

61. Volkow N, Wang G, Baler R. Reward, dopamine and the control of food intake: implications for obesity. *Trends Cogn Sci.* 2011;15:37–46.

62. Burger K, Stice E. Variability in reward responsivity and obesity: evidence from brain imaging studies. *Curr Drug Abuse Rev.* 2011;4:182–9.

63. Bohon C, Stice E. Negative affect and neural response to palatable food intake in bulimia nervosa. *Appetite.* 2012;58:964–70.

64. Frank G, Shott M, Hagman J, Mittal V. Alterations in brain structures related to taste reward circuitry in ill and recovered anorexia nervosa and in bulimia nervosa. *Am J Psychiatry.* 2013;170:1152–60.

65. Schultz W. Dopamine reward prediction error coding. *Dialogues Clin Neurosci.* 2016;18:23–32.

66. Rescorla R. Stimulus generalization: some predictions from a model of Pavlovian conditioning. *J Exp Psychol Anim Behav Process.* 1976;2:88–96.

67. Oberndorfer T, Simmons A, McCurdy D, et al. Greater anterior insula activation during anticipation of food images in women recovered from anorexia nervosa versus controls. *Psychiatry Res.* 2013;214:132–41.

68. Frank G, Roblek T, Shott M, et al. Heightened fear of uncertainty in anorexia and bulimia nervosa. *Int J Eat Disord.* 2012;45:227–32.

69. DeGuzman M, Shott M, Yang T, Riederer J, Frank G. Association of elevated reward prediction error response with weight gain in adolescent anorexia nervosa. *Am J Psychiatry.* 2017;174:557–65.

70. Santel S, Baving L, Krauel K, Munte T, Rotte M. Hunger and satiety in anorexia nervosa: fMRI during cognitive processing of food pictures. *Brain Res.* 2006;1114:138–48.

71. Holsen L, Lawson E, Blum K, et al. Food motivation circuitry hypoactivation related to hedonic and nonhedonic aspects of hunger and satiety in women with active anorexia nervosa and weight-restored women with anorexia nervosa. *J Psychiatry Neurosci.* 2012;37:322–32.

72. Uher R, Brammer M, Murphy T, et al. Recovery and chronicity in anorexia nervosa: brain activity associated with differential outcomes. *Biol Psychiatry.* 2003;54:934–42.

73. Ellison AR, Foong J. Neuroimaging in eating disorders. In: Hoek HW, Treasure JL, Katzman MA, editors. *Neurobiology in the Treatment of Eating Disorders.* Chichester: John Wiley & Sons; 1998. pp. 255–69.

74. Gordon CM, Dougherty DD, Fischman AJ, et al. Neural substrates of anorexia nervosa: a behavioral challenge study with positron emission tomography. *J Pediatr.* 2001;139:51–7.

75. Foerde K, Steinglass J, Shohamy D, Walsh B. Neural mechanisms supporting maladaptive food choices in anorexia nervosa. *Nat Neurosci.* 2015;18:1571–3.

76. Brooks S, O'Daly O, Uher R, et al. Differential neural responses to food images in women with bulimia versus anorexia nervosa. *PLoS One.* 2011;6:1–8.

77. Schienle A, Schafer A, Hermann A, Vaitl D. Binge-eating disorder: reward sensitivity and brain activation to images of food. *Biol Psychiatry.* 2009;65:654–61.

78. Bohon C, Stice E. Reward abnormalities in women with full and subthreshold bulimia nervosa: a functional magnetic resonance imaging study. *Int J Eat Disord.* 2010;44:585–95.

79. Weygandt M, Schaefer A, Schienle A, Haynes J. Diagnosing different binge-eating disorders based on reward-related brain activation patterns. *Hum Brain Mapp.* 2012;33:2135–46.

80. Rolls E. Taste, olfactory, and food texture processing in the brain, and the control of food intake. *Physiol Behav.* 2005;85:45–56.

81. Ely A, Berner L, Wierenga C, et al. Neurobiology of eating disorders: clinical implications. Special Report—29 April 2016. *Psychiatric Times.* 2016;33(4).

82. McClure S, Laibson D, Loewenstein G, Cohen J. Separate neural systems value immediate and delayed monetary rewards. *Science.* 2004;306:503–7.

83. Goldstein R, Volkow ND. Drug addiction and its underlying neurobiological basis: neuroimaging evidence for the involvement of the frontal cortex. *Am J Psychiatry.* 2002;159:1642–52.

84. Phillips M, Drevets WR, SL, Lane R. Neurobiology of emotion perception I: the neural basis of normal emotion perception. *Biol Psychiatry*. 2003;54:504–14.

85. Kaye W, Wierenga C, Bailer U, Simmons A, Wagner A, Bischoff-Grethe A. Does a shared neurobiology for foods and drugs of abuse contribute to extremes of food ingestion in anorexia and bulimia nervosa? *Biol Psychiatry*. 2013;73:836–42.

86. Zastrow A, Kaiser SS, C, Walthe S, et al. Neural correlates of impaired cognitive-behavioral flexibility in anorexia nervosa. *Am J Psychiatry*. 2009;166:608–16.

87. Lock J, Garrett A, Beenhakker J, Reiss A. Aberrant brain activation during a response inhibition task in adolescent eating disorder subtypes. *Am J Psychiatry*. 2011;168:55–64.

88. McAnarney E, Zarcone J, Singh P, et al. Restrictive anorexia nervosa and set-shifting in adolescents: a biobehavioral interface. *J Adolesc Health*. 2011;49:99–101.

89. Fitzpatrick K, Darcy A, Colborn D, Gudorf C, Lock J. Set-shifting among adolescents with anorexia nervosa. *Int J Eat Disord*. 2012;45:909–12.

90. Friederich H, Herzog W. Cognitive-behavioral flexibility in anorexia nervosa. *Curr Top Behav Neurosci*. 2011;6:111–23.

91. Roberts M, Tchanturia K, Treasure J. Exploring the neurocognitive signature of poor set-shifting in anorexia and bulimia nervosa. *J Psychiatr Res*. 2010;44:964–70.

92. Claes L, Nederkoorn C, Vandereycken W, Guerrieri R, Vertommen H. Impulsiveness and lack of inhibitory control in eating disorders. *Eat Behav*. 2006;7:196–203.

93. Lilenfeld L, Wonderlich S, Riso LP, Crosby R, Mitchell J. Eating disorders and personality: a methodological and empirical review. *Clin Psychol Rev*. 2006;26:299–320.

94. Wu M, Hartmann M, Skunde M, Herzog W, Friederich H. Inhibitory control in bulimic-type eating disorders: a systematic review and meta-analysis. *PLoS One*. 2013;8:e83412.

95. Marsh R, Horga G, Wang Z, et al. An fMRI study of self-regulatory control and conflict resolution in adolescents with bulimia nervosa. *Am J Psychiatry*. 2011;168:1210–20.

96. Mobbs O, Van der Linden M, d'Acremont M, Perroud A. Cognitive deficits and biases for food and body in bulimia: investigation using an affective shifting task. *Eat Behav*. 2008;9:455–61.

97. Svaldi J, Brand M, Tuschen-Caffier B. Decision-making impairments in women with binge eating disorder. *Appetite*. 2010;54:84–92.

98. Manasse S, Goldstein S, Wyckoff E, et al. Slowing down and taking a second look: inhibitory deficits associated with binge eating are not food-specific. *Appetite*. 2016;96:555–9.

99. Hege M, Stingl K, Kullmann S, et al. Attentional impulsivity in binge eating disorder modulates response inhibition performance and frontal brain networks. *Int J Obes*. 2015;39:353–60.

100. Balodis I, Molina N, Kober H, et al. Divergent neural substrates of inhibitory control in binge eating disorder relative to other manifestations of obesity. *Obesity (Silver Springs)*. 2013;21:367–77.

101. Khalsa S, Rudrauf D, Feinstein J, Tranel D. The pathways of interoceptive awareness. *Nat Neurosci*. 2009;12:1494–6.

102. Paulus M, Stein MB. An insular view of anxiety. *Biol Psychiatry*. 2006;60:383–7.

103. Paulus M, Stein M. Interoception in anxiety and depression. *Brain Struct Funct*. 2010;214:451–63.

104. Pollatos O, Gramann K, Schandry R. Neural systems connecting interoceptive awareness and feelings. *Hum Brain Mapp*. 2007;28:9–18.

105. Khalsa S, Craske M, Li W, Vangala S, Strober M, Feusner J. Altered interoceptive awareness in anorexia nervosa: Effects of meal anticipation, consumption and bodily arousal. *Int J Eat Disord*. 2015;48:889–97.

106. Strigo I, Matthews S, Simmons A, et al. Altered insula activation during pain anticipation in individuals recovered from anorexia nervosa: evidence of interocetive dysregulation. *Int J Eat Disord*. 2013;46:23–33.

107. Kerr K, Moseman S, Avery J, Bodurka J, Zucker N, Kyle Simmons W. Altered insula activity during visceral interoception in weight-restored patients with anorexia nervosa. *Neuropsychopharm*. 2016;41:521–8.

108. Zanetti T, Santonastaso P, Sgaravatti E, Degortes D, Favaro A. Clinical and temperamental correlates of body image disturbance in eating disorders. *Eur Eat Disord Rev*. 2013;21:32–7.

109. Pohl R, Yeragani V, Balon R, Lycaki H. Lactate and isoproterenol infusions in bulimic patients. *Neuropsychobiology*. 1989;22:225–30.

110. Klabunde M, Acheson DB, KN, Matthews S, Kaye W. Interoceptive sensitivity deficits in women recovered from bulimia nervosa. *Eat Behav*. 2013;14:488–92.

111. Papezova H, Yamamotova A, Uher R. Elevated pain threshold in eating disorders: physiological and psychological factors. *J Psychiatr Res*. 2005;39:431–8.

112. Geliebter A, Hashim S. Gastric capacity in normal, obese, and bulimic women. *Physiol Behav*. 2001;74:743–6.

113. Khalsa S, Lapidus R. Can interoception improve the pragmatic search for biomarkers in psychiatry? *Front Psychiatry*. 2016;7:121.

114. George DT, Kaye WH, Goldstein DS, Brewerton TD, Jimerson DC. Altered norepinephrine regulation in bulimia: effects of pharmacological challenge with isoproterenol. *Psychiatry Res*. 1990;33:1–10.

115. Bulik C, Sullivan P, Lawson R, Carter F. Salivary reactivity in women with bulimia nervosa across treatment. *Biol Psychiatry*. 1996;39:1009–12.

116. Faruqui R, El-Kadi K, Roxell A. Organic eating disorders of pica, hperphagia, and severe food restriction: presentation and prevalence after acquired brain injury. *Eur Psychiatry*. 2011;P02-119 10.1016/S0924-9338(11)72420-8.

117. Bhatia M, Gupta R. Pica responding to SSRI: an OCD spectrum disorder? *World J Biol Psychiatry*. 2009;10(4 Pt 3):936–8.

# 106

# Management and treatment of feeding and eating disorders

Susan L. McElroy, Anna I. Guerdjikova, Nicole Mori, Paul L. Houser, and Paul E. Keck, Jr.

## Introduction

Feeding and eating disorders are characterized by persistently disturbed eating behaviour that results in abnormal consumption or absorption of food that impairs health or functioning. In DSM-5, they include pica, rumination disorder, avoidant/restrictive food intake disorder (ARFID), anorexia nervosa (AN), bulimia nervosa (BN), binge eating disorder (BED), and a residual category (other specified feeding or eating disorder) that includes subthreshold AN, BN, and BED, purging disorder, and night eating syndrome (NES) [1]. The International Classification of Diseases, eleventh revision (ICD-11) will include similar disorders [2]. In this chapter, the management and treatment of these conditions are reviewed.

## Pica

Pica is the recurrent eating of non-food items or substances such as paper, paste, wood, soap, chalk, pebbles, rubber gloves, clay, paint, or faeces [1, 2]. Data on the prevalence of pica are inconclusive. Pica occurs in people of all ages but may be more common in children, those with intellectual disabilities or autism, pregnant women, and those receiving dialysis [3–5]. The presentation and medical complications of pica are highly variable and associated with the specific ingested items or substances. Pica may become a focus of clinical attention because of medical complications, such as broken teeth, choking, bowel obstruction or perforation, infection, or poisoning, some of which are potentially fatal. Pica is significantly associated with an increased risk for anaemia, low haemoglobin, low haematocrit, and low plasma zinc, although the direction of causation is unknown [6].

Management of pica starts with a thorough medical and psychological assessment to detect medical complications and any possible contributing factors. If present, medical complications of the pica must be adequately addressed. If a contributing factor (for example, iron deficiency anaemia) is identified, addressing the factor (for example, treatment with supplemental iron) may lead to resolution of pica, but this does not always occur [3].

There have been no adequately sized and designed randomized controlled treatment trials in patients with pica, and empirically derived treatment guidelines for pica do not exist. Treatment often requires a multi-disciplinary team with physicians, dieticians, and psychologists. In a review of 26 treatment studies in individuals with disabilities, it was concluded that behavioural treatments, especially those involving a combination of reinforcement response reduction procedures, were effective [7]. In another review, it was concluded that applied behaviour analysis was the most effective strategy [8].

Regarding pharmacotherapy, there are case reports of patients whose pica and attention-deficit/hyperactivity disorder (ADHD) both responded to methylphenidate, and of patients whose pica and depression or obsessive–compulsive disorder both responded to a selective serotonin reuptake inhibitor (SSRI) [9–11]. These cases suggest that treatment of comorbid psychiatric disorders might be helpful for reducing pica in some patients.

Nutritional supplements have been evaluated in pica, with negative findings. In a two-by-two factorial randomized, placebo-controlled trial of iron and multimicronutrient supplementation in 406 Zambian schoolchildren, 302 with geophagy, neither treatment was superior to placebo for decreasing geophagy prevalence [12]. Indeed, decline in geophagy prevalence was higher in children receiving placebo than those receiving iron (28.0% vs 22.3%; $P = 0.044$). There were also no interactions between iron and multimicronutrient supplementation. This trial was limited by an extremely high dropout rate. In a randomized, placebo-controlled trial of an intramuscular iron-dextran preparation in 31 African-American children with pica, improvement in pica was not significantly different at 2–3 months or at 9–10 months [13]. Patients with lower haemoglobin concentrations did not respond to iron more favourably than those with higher haemoglobin concentrations, or respond more favourably to iron than to placebo. Additionally, there was no correlation between changes in haemoglobin concentration and changes in pica severity.

## Rumination disorder

Rumination disorder is repeated regurgitation of recently ingested food (bringing previously swallowed food from the stomach back into the mouth), which may be re-chewed, re-swallowed, or spat out, that is not better explained by a gastrointestinal or other medical syndrome [1, 2, 14-17]. Of note, the Rome VI diagnostic criteria designate 'rumination syndrome' as a functional gastrointestinal disorder [18]. Though DSM-5 and the Rome criteria are silent on the relationship between rumination disorder vs rumination syndrome, the definitions are similar.

The act of regurgitation in rumination disorder is usually effortless and may be preceded by urges to regurgitate and/or a belching sensation (but not by nausea or retching). Regurgitated material contains recognizable food that may have a pleasant taste. Regurgitation tends to stop once the regurgitant becomes acidic. Although prevalence data are inconclusive, rumination disorder occurs in infancy, childhood, adolescence, and adulthood. It may be more common in certain groups such as infants and individuals with intellectual disability. Rumination can be accompanied by halitosis, chronically chapped lips, malnutrition, growth delay, or weight loss and can be life-threatening, especially in infancy. Other medical complications include tooth decay and erosion; aspiration leading to recurrent bronchitis or pneumonia, reflex laryngospasm, or asthma; and premalignant changes of the oesophageal epithelium. Patients with rumination have also been observed to have high rates of co-occurring depression and anxiety [17].

Management of rumination disorder begins with a comprehensive medical and psychological evaluation. Haematologic and chemistry tests are needed to exclude anaemia secondary to gastrointestinal bleeding and electrolyte imbalances. Rumination must be differentiated from other gastrointestinal conditions that involve gastro-oesophageal reflux or vomiting, including oesophageal stricture, achalasia, hiatal hernia, gastro-oesophageal reflux disease, Sandifer syndrome, gastroparesis, and peptic ulcer disease. Some authorities recommend studies of manometry, combined with impedance, to distinguish rumination from gastro-oesophageal reflux disease [16].

There are no randomized controlled treatment trials for rumination disorder, and it is currently thought to be best addressed with behavioural techniques across all age groups. Strategies for children include changing the child's posture during and after feeding, distracting the child when he or she starts the behaviour, and aversive conditioning (placing something bad-tasting on the child's tongue when he or she starts the behaviour). Psychotherapy for parents of children with rumination disorder may also be useful. Teaching diaphragmatic breathing to compete with the urge to ruminate may be helpful in children, adolescents, and adults [19]. In one study where 28 patients with rumination syndrome were trained to modulate abdomino-thoracic muscle activity under visual control of electromyographic recordings, the number of regurgitations decreased from 27 to eight after three sessions [20]. This improvement was maintained at 6-month follow-up. Patients with rumination associated with supragastric belching may respond well to behaviour therapy with a speech therapist [16]. There are also anecdotal reports of beneficial effects from gum chewing [16, 18].

Protein pump inhibitors may be helpful for associated oesophageal or gastric damage, but not for rumination itself. Prokinetic medications also are not effective for rumination and may worsen symptoms [17]. In an open-label trial using high-resolution manometry–impedance recordings in 12 patients with rumination or supragastric belching, treatment with the gamma-aminobutyric acid (GABA) B receptor agonist baclofen substantially reduced the number of gastrointestinal flow events, including ruminations [21]. Reduction in flow events correlated with an increase in lower oesophageal sphincter pressure and a reduction in swallowing. For treatment-resistant rumination, options include an inpatient multi-disciplinary programme [17]. Anti-reflux surgery (for example, Nissen fundoplication) has been reported to be effective, but further research is needed [16, 17].

## Avoidant restrictive food intake disorder

ARFID is characterized by avoidance or restriction of food intake accompanied by weight loss or growth delay, malnutrition, dependence on oral nutritional supplements or enteral feeding, and/or marked functional impairment that is not due to lack of food or a culturally endorsed tradition [1, 2, 22–25]. Unlike those with AN, individuals with ARFID have no disturbance in how they experience their body weight or shape and lack fear of weight gain, drive for thinness, or preoccupation with body image. Rather, they are more likely to report fear of vomiting or choking, concerns with food texture, or abdominal pain as reasons for their eating difficulties or weight loss.

ARFID most commonly develops in infancy or early childhood and may persist into adulthood. Patients with ARFID have high rates of comorbid medical and psychiatric disorders, especially low bone mineral density scores and anxiety disorders. Compared to those with AN in one study, ARFID patients were younger, more likely to be male, more likely to have a comorbid medical condition or anxiety disorder, and less likely to have a mood disorder [23].

The prevalence of ARFID is unknown. Among paediatric eating disorder inpatients, rates of ARFID have ranged from 5% [22] to 14% [23]. Initial evaluation often begins with the primary care practitioner who should address the child's prenatal, birth, and medical histories, as well as parental coping and mental health. Potential medical causes must be ruled out such as gastrointestinal disease, food allergies, or occult malignancy. Potential co-occurring medical disorders or complications and psychiatric disorders must also be determined.

No randomized controlled treatment trials have been conducted in patients with ARFID, and empirically based treatment guidelines are not available [26]. Management of ARFID usually requires a multi-disciplinary team that provides medical management, nutritional rehabilitation, and psychological treatment. Family therapy is often needed to help parents manage their child's nutritional intake. In one study, ARFID patients hospitalized for acute medical stabilization at an academic medical centre relied on more enteral nutrition and had longer hospitalizations than AN patients but had similar rates of remission and readmission 1 year after discharge [24]. In a study of 14 adolescent medicine eating disorder programmes, there were no significant differences between the types of treatments or programmes in terms of weight restoration [27]. Patients with ARFID sometimes also receive psychotropic medications, such as SSRIs for co-occurring anxiety and/or olanzapine to enhance weight gain, but the efficacy of these interventions is unknown [25].

## Anorexia nervosa

AN is characterized by persistent energy intake restriction, leading to significantly low body weight or growth failure, in combination with intense fear of gaining weight or of becoming fat or persistent behaviour that interferes with weight gain, and distorted self-perceived weight or shape [1, 2, 26, 28–30]. Physical hyperactivity, obsessive–compulsive symptoms related to eating and food, depressive and anxiety symptoms, and impaired insight are also common features. Amenorrhoea occurs in many females with AN but is no longer required for the diagnosis. DSM-5 recognizes two subtypes of AN: restrictive (where there has been no binge eating or purging behaviour in the past 3 months) and binge eating/purging (where there has been recurrent binge eating or purging in the past 3 months) [1]. Severity of AN is often determined by BMI status, with greater severity linked with lower BMI. New to DSM-5 is the diagnosis of atypical AN, in which there has been significant weight loss, but the individual's weight is within or above the normal range.

The lifetime prevalence of AN by DSM-IV criteria is around 1% in females and <0.5% in males [30]. Because amenorrhoea is no longer a defining component, AN, as defined by DSM-5 criteria, may be more common. Peak age of onset of AN is in early to mid adolescence, but the disorder may occur at any age. AN is associated with substantial medical and psychiatric comorbidity [26, 28–31]. Complications arising from the effects of starvation, binge eating, and purging occur across multiple organ systems and include: bradycardia, hypotension, and arrhythmias; reduced core body temperature; hypoglycaemia, hypercholesterolaemia, and amenorrhoea; fluid, electrolyte, and acid–base imbalances; anaemia and neutropenia; acute pancreatitis, salivary gland enlargement, Mallory–Weiss tears, elevated liver enzymes, and constipation; impaired bone quality, low bone mineral density, and increased fracture risk; depressive symptoms and cognitive impairment; and tooth decay and gum disease [26, 28–32]. Patients with AN may have an increased prevalence of autoimmune disorders, particularly type 1 diabetes, which may precede the onset of AN. More than half of adolescents and adults with AN meet criteria for another psychiatric disorder, especially mood and anxiety disorders [33, 34]. The mortality of AN is the highest of all mental disorders, with most deaths due to starvation-related medical complications and suicide [30]. Of note, AN in children and adolescents, AN in adults, and severe and enduring AN likely require different treatment approaches [26]. Early access to treatment is important, as there may be a critical window for effective intervention within the first 3 years of illness onset, beyond which full recovery becomes more difficult to achieve [30]. For younger and recently ill patients, the goal of treatment is full recovery. For patients with severe and enduring AN, treatment should focus on improving quality of life and reducing harm more than achieving full recovery.

Management of AN begins with a thorough medical and psychological evaluation, so that it can be determined where the patient should be treated—in a general medical hospital, a psychiatric hospital, or as an outpatient [26, 28–30]. There is no evidence that inpatient treatment is superior to outpatient treatment, and most patients can be treated on an outpatient basis [35]. However, a number of guidelines provide parameters for when a patient should be treated in a general medical or psychiatric hospital [26] (Table 106.1). No matter the location of care, most guidelines recommend a multi-disciplinary approach involving medical, dietetic, and psychological treatment. Whenever possible, it is crucial to involve family members or significant others in the treatment process.

Medical stabilization, refeeding, and restoration of body weight, nutritional status, and, among females, regular menses are the primary aims of initial management. There is some controversy as to how best restore body weight and nutritional status in patients with AN, as empirical data for this process are lacking and there is concern about the development of refeeding syndrome, a potentially fatal complication characterized by hypophosphataemia, hypomagnesaemia, hypokalaemia, and cardiac failure that may occur with refeeding, including with intravenous dextrose, after a sustained period of malnutrition [36–38]. The standard of care therefore is to commence refeeding at low caloric levels and increase slowly, with variable recommendations internationally as to precise caloric prescriptions. In the United States, refeeding is begun with around 1200 cal/day and increased by about 200 kcal every other day. The Royal Australian and New Zealand College of Psychiatrists (RANZP) recommends that adult AN patients should start refeeding with 6000 kJ/day, which is then increased by 2000 kJ/day every 3 days until adequate intake for weight restoration is achieved [26]. For mildly or moderately malnourished patients, there is some evidence that refeeding should start at ≥1400 kcal/day so as to avoid undernutrition.

Refeeding methods include using food, high-energy liquid supplements, nasogastric or enteral feeding, and, on rare occasions, parenteral nutrition. The least intrusive method of refeeding that can provide adequate nutrition should be used. Routine monitoring during refeeding includes regular measurement of weight, electrolytes, liver function tests, electrocardiographic findings, and other aspects of physiological functioning. In the early stages of refeeding, supplemental phosphate (500 mg twice daily) and thiamine (at least 100 mg/day) are often provided. Some guidelines argue that refeeding methods should be highly individualized. However, a study in adolescents with AN showed that a standardized caloric prescription was superior to individual prescription in facilitating early weight gain without increasing the risk of refeeding syndrome [39]. Standardized caloric prescription was also associated with a lower incidence of bed rest. Once adequate weight gain is achieved, continued dietary and psychological treatment should be provided for weight maintenance.

A wide range of psychological treatments have been evaluated in patients with AN [26, 28–30, 40–43]. For children and adolescents, the RANZP guidelines concluded that empirical evidence for efficacy was strong for family-based treatment and Maudsley family therapy; moderate for family system therapy, adolescent focused therapy, and enhanced cognitive behavioural treatment (CBT-E); and weak to moderate for cognitive behavioural therapy (CBT) [26]. The core feature of family-based treatment for adolescents with AN is that the parents are guided on how to take control of their child's eating. Of note, a recently conducted randomized controlled trial found parent-focused treatment, where the therapist meets only with the parents and a nurse monitors the patient, was superior to family-based treatment for bringing about remission in adolescents

**Table 106.1** Indicators for consideration for psychiatric and medical admission for adults with AN or BN

| | Psychiatric admission indicated | Medical admission indicated |
|---|---|---|
| Weight | Body mass index <14 kg/m² | Body mass index <12 kg/m² |
| Rapid weight loss | 1 kg per week over several weeks or grossly inadequate nutritional intake (<100 kcal daily) or continued weight loss despite community treatment | |
| Systolic BP | <90 mmHg | <80 mmHg |
| Postural BP | >10 mmHg drop with standing | >20 mmHg drop with standing |
| Heart rate | | <40 bpm or >120 bpm or postural tachycardia >20 bpm |
| Temperature | <35.5°C or cold/blue extremities | <35°C or cold/blue extremities |
| 12-lead ECG | | Any arrhythmia, including QTc prolongation or non-specific ST or T-wave changes (including inversion or biphasic waves) |
| Blood sugar | Below normal range | <2.5 mmol/L |
| Sodium | <130 mmol/L | <125 mmol/L |
| Potassium | Below normal range | <3.0 mmol/L |
| Magnesium | | Below normal range |
| Phosphate | | Below normal range |
| eGFR | | <60 mL/min/1.73m² or rapidly dropping (for example, 25% drop within a week) |
| Albumin | Below normal range | <30 g/L |
| Liver enzymes | Mildly elevated | Markedly elevated (AST or ALT >500) |
| Neutrophils | <1.5 × 10⁹/L | <1.0 × 10⁹/L |
| Psychiatric symptoms | Suicidal ideation<br>Active self-harm<br>Moderate to high agitation and distress<br>Psychosis | |

ALT, alanine aminotransferase; AST, aspartate aminotransferase; BP, blood pressure; bpm, beats per minute; ECG, electrocardiogram; eGFR, estimated glomerular filtration rate; g, gram; kg, kilogram; L, litre; mmHg, millimetres of mercury.
Adapted from *Aust N Z J Psychiatry*, 48(11), Hay P, Chinn D, Forbes D, *et al.*, Royal Australian and New Zealand College of Psychiatrists clinical practice guidelines for the treatment of eating disorders, pp. 977–1008, Copyright (2014), with permission from SAGE Publications.

with AN, though differences in remission rates were not different at 6- or 12-month follow-up [42].

For adults with AN, the RANZP guidelines concluded that there was moderately strong evidence of efficacy for CBT-E, focal dynamic therapy, Maudsley Model of Anorexia Nervosa Treatment for Adults (MANTRA), and specialist supportive clinical management (SSCM); and weak evidence for CBT, behaviour therapy, interpersonal therapy (IPT), psychodynamic therapy, and cognitive analytic therapy [26]. However, reviews of these treatments have concluded that no specific psychological therapy was consistently superior to any other specific approach [40, 41]. Thus, in a 2-year follow-up of a randomized clinical trial comparing MANTRA with SSCM in outpatient adults with AN, both treatments were comparable regarding improvement in BMI, eating disorder psychopathology, and clinical impairment [43]. In the only randomized clinical trial of psychotherapy in outpatients with severe and enduring AN, shifting focus from weight gain and recovery to improved quality of life was found to be important [44]. There is no empirical evidence that guided self-help CBT (CBT-GSH), which may be helpful in BN or BED, is an effective treatment for AN [26].

No medication has regulatory approval for the treatment of AN. The World Federation of Societies of Biological Psychiatry (WFSBP) guidelines for the pharmacological treatment of eating disorders concluded that there was weak evidence from controlled studies for zinc supplementation and olanzapine for enhancing weight gain in

AN [45]. One study found olanzapine might be helpful for promotion of weight gain in outpatients with AN when given with medication management sessions [46]. Use of both agents, however, is controversial [26, 47]. Two meta-analyses of studies of newer drugs for psychosis in AN concluded that these agents were not efficacious for weight restoration or reduction of eating disorder psychopathology in patients with AN [48, 49]. Nonetheless, certain subsets of AN patients may be responsive to dopamine antagonist drugs, including those with prominent anxiety or depression, obsessive–compulsive symptoms, hyperactivity, or antipsychotic-responsive comorbid conditions such as bipolar disorder [47].

There is no evidence of efficacy for tricyclic drugs or SSRIs for enhancing weight restoration or reducing psychopathology in the refeeding phase of AN treatment [50], while evidence for fluoxetine for relapse prevention after weight restoration is mixed [51, 52]. Drugs for depression might improve co-occurring depressive or obsessive–compulsive symptoms that persist despite successful weight restoration. Results from randomized controlled trials of alprazolam, cyproheptadine, D-cycloserine, dehydroepiandrosterone, growth hormone, lithium, naltrexone, physiologic oestrogen replacement, oxytocin, and tetrahydrocannabinol in patients with AN have been mostly negative [47]. In a small randomized controlled trial, the ghrelin agonist retamorelin improved gastric emptying (P = 0.03) and body weight (P = 0.12) more than placebo [53]. A randomized controlled trial of the synthetic cannabinoid dronabinol in patients with severe and enduring AN found small weight gain, with no side effects [54]. Different types of neuromodulation treatments (for example, deep brain stimulation, repetitive transcranial current stimulation, and transcranial direct current stimulation) have shown promise in severe and enduring AN, but systematic studies are needed before recommendations can be made [30].

Another area that has received some study is the medical treatment of AN-associated low bone mineral density. Available evidence suggests that the safest and most effective strategy for improving bone density in AN is to restore weight and, in females, menstrual function. However, even with resolution of AN, bone mineral density is not always restored. Pharmacotherapies that show promise include physiologic oestradiol replacement (that is, with a transdermal oestradiol patch) and, in adults, bisphosphonates [32].

A final important consideration is the not infrequent need for coercion in the treatment of AN [28]. Compulsory refeeding has short-term benefits, but long-term outcome is unknown [55]. More research on the potential long-term benefits and harms of compulsory refeeding in AN is needed.

## Bulimia nervosa

BN is characterized by recurrent binge eating episodes, recurrent inappropriate compensatory behaviours to prevent weight gain, and self-evaluation that is unduly influenced by body weight or shape [1, 2]. The lifetime prevalence of BN is estimated to be 1.5% in women and 0.5% in men. BN occurs in people of all ages, with the most common onset occurring in late adolescence to early adulthood. BN is associated with substantial medical and psychiatric comorbidity [31, 33, 34, 56]. Co-occurring medical conditions include complications of binge eating and inappropriate weight loss behaviours, obesity, and obesity-related disorders [26, 56]. Psychiatric comorbidity includes mood, anxiety, substance use, and impulse control disorders.

The management of BN begins with a careful medical and psychiatric evaluation, with special attention to the frequency of binge eating episodes, the types and frequencies of inappropriate compensatory behaviours, potential medical complications, and co-occurring psychiatric disorders. Physical examination and laboratory evaluation should be conducted with attention to height and weight (to determine BMI), blood pressure and pulse, electrolytes, acid–base status, and complete blood cell counts. A cardiac evaluation with an electrocardiogram may be indicated if there is hypokalaemia, postural hypertension, bradycardia, or tachycardia. If vomiting has been a prominent symptom, a dental evaluation should be done. Most patients with BN can be treated on an outpatient basis, but high frequency of binge eating and/or compensatory behaviours, medical complications, psychiatric comorbidity, such as mood disorder or suicidal ideation/behaviour, or failure to respond to outpatient treatment, may necessitate hospitalization (Table 106.1). Particularly important among medical complications of purging is pseudo-Bartter syndrome, an upregulation of aldosterone that causes hypokalaemic metabolic acidosis and, upon cessation of purging, can lead to severe oedema [31]. This syndrome may be worsened by vigorous hydration with normal saline; it can be treated by gentle rehydration with a potassium-rich fluid and with spironolactone.

Many authorities believe the first-line treatment of BN in adults is individual psychotherapy, with the strongest evidence for CBT-E [26, 28, 29, 57]. CBT-E has been found superior to both IPT (at end of treatment, but not at 1-year follow-up) and psychoanalytic psychotherapy [58–60]. A more complex form of CBT-E may be preferable for patients with affect intolerance, low self-esteem, perfectionism, or interpersonal difficulties. In a comparison trial in adolescents with BN, family-based treatment was superior to CBT at end of treatment and 6-month follow-up, but the two therapies were not statistically significantly different at 12-month follow-up [61]. Dialectical behaviour therapy (DBT) and self-help modalities, especially CBT-GSH, also hold promise in BN. Self-help modalities are probably less effective than therapist-led psychotherapies but are appropriate first-step options when such therapies are not available or affordable. This includes self-help treatments administered via the Internet.

Pharmacotherapy also has a role in the treatment of BN. The WFSBP guidelines concluded there was evidence of efficacy for tricyclics, SSRIs, and topiramate for reducing binge eating and purging in BN [45]. Indeed, fluoxetine has regulatory approval for the treatment of BN, and 60 mg/day is more efficacious than 20 mg/day [62]. Fluoxetine is also efficacious for maintenance of response, but the dropout rate is high [63]. Many other types of drugs for depression are efficacious in BN, but the weak dopamine and noradrenaline reuptake inhibitor bupropion is contraindicated due to an increased risk of seizures. There is no clear evidence that these drugs enhance the effectiveness of psychotherapy for BN. In other randomized controlled trials, ondansetron was superior to placebo for reducing binge eating and purging, methylamphetamine was superior to placebo for decreasing the amount of food eaten, lithium and the prokinetic erythromycin were not efficacious, and results for opioid antagonists were mixed [45, 64, 65].

## Binge eating disorder

BED is characterized by recurrent binge eating episodes that are accompanied by distress, but not the inappropriate compensatory weight loss behaviours of BN [1, 2]. BED is the most common eating disorder, occurring as a lifetime diagnosis in 1.9% of adults worldwide and 1.3% of adolescents in the United States [33, 34, 56]. It is associated with obesity and obesity-related medical conditions (for example, diabetes, hypertension, dyslipidaemia, and possibly metabolic syndrome) and with mood, anxiety, substance use, and impulse control disorders.

Management of BED involves a thorough psychological and medical evaluation to determine the severity of binge eating behaviour, identify comorbid medical and psychiatric disorders, and ensure that BN is ruled out (that is, that there are no surreptitious inappropriate compensatory weight loss behaviours). At a minimum, physical and laboratory examinations should include height and weight (to determine BMI), blood pressure and pulse, and fasting glucose and lipids. When surreptitious purging is a concern, serum electrolytes and amylase may be checked. Most BED patients can be treated on an outpatient basis, but psychiatric hospitalization should be considered for extremely frequent and distressing binge eating, a co-occurring mood disorder, or suicidal ideation and/or behaviour.

Psychological treatments that may be useful in patients with BED include psychoeducation, mindfulness techniques, self-help treatments (including CBT-GSH and those delivered via the Internet), behavioural weight loss therapy (BWLT), CBT, IPT, and DBT [66, 67]. The strongest evidence of efficacy is for CBT and IPT, which can work over the long term and in adolescents as well as adults [66–69]. Though CBT and IPT both reduce binge eating behaviour and associated psychopathology in BED, they are less effective for weight loss in obese patients. Patients who completely stop binge eating with these treatments, however, may lose a small amount of weight. CBT and IPT are both more effective than BWLT for reducing binge eating [69]. Though BWLT may produce greater weight loss initially, this weight loss is not maintained after 2 years.

Physical activity may also be effective for reducing binge eating behaviour and excessive body weight in BED. In a review of three randomized controlled trials of physical activity in patients with BED, aerobic and yoga exercises reduced binge eating and BMI [70]. Additionally, aerobic exercise reduced depressive symptoms; CBT with aerobic exercise, but not CBT alone, reduced BMI; and CBT with aerobic exercise was more effective for reducing depression than CBT alone.

Pharmacotherapy may be helpful for some patients with BED [45, 66, 67]. Lisdexamfetamine dimesylate (LDX), a prodrug of d-amphetamine marketed for treatment of children and adults with ADHD, is approved for the treatment of moderate to severe BED in adults in the United States. This approval was based in part on two phase 3 studies of LDX in BED, both of which found that LDX, titrated to 50 mg/day or 70 mg/day, was efficacious for reducing binge eating episodes and obsessive–compulsive features of binge eating and for inducing 4-week binge eating cessation rates [71]. An earlier phase 2 study found that LDX at 50 mg/day and 70 mg/day, but not 30 mg/day, was efficacious for reducing binge eating [72]. LDX also caused significant weight loss in these trials (most participants were obese) but is not approved for weight loss or treatment of obesity. A long-term randomized withdrawal study of LDX in BED found that LDX was superior to placebo for maintenance of response [73]. No novel safety or tolerability issues were found.

There is evidence from randomized controlled trials to support the efficacy of the anticonvulsant agents topiramate and zonisamide in BED [45, 66]. Both drugs reduce binge eating behaviour and obsessive–compulsive features of binge eating and cause clinically significant weight loss. Additionally, topiramate has been shown to augment the efficacy of CBT in obese patients with BED, enhancing weight loss and cessation of binge eating rates. However, the use of both drugs is limited by their adverse event profiles, which include cognitive dysfunction, paraesthesiae, and renal stones.

Drugs for depression are modestly effective for reducing binge eating in BED, at least over the short term. The WFSBP eating disorder pharmacotherapy guidelines concluded there was evidence of efficacy for sertraline in particular [45]. They are also effective for depressive symptoms associated with BED. In a study of patients with BED and a co-occurring depressive disorder, the serotonin/noradrenaline reuptake inhibitor duloxetine was superior to placebo in reducing binge eating behaviour, global severity of BED symptoms, global severity of depressive symptoms, and body weight [74]. In another study, bupropion (300 mg/day) was similar to placebo in reducing binge eating frequency but produced greater weight loss [75]. Also, it was well tolerated and there were no seizures. Data on

the efficacy of the combination of antidepressant drugs with CBT are mixed.

Other medications have been studied in BED. The weight loss agents orlistat (a pancreatic lipase inhibitor) and liraglutide (a glucagon-like peptide 1 analogue) may reduce body weight in obese patients with BED, but their effects on binge eating behaviour are unclear [66, 76]. Limited mixed data also exist for baclofen and chromium [66].

Treating patients with BED involves educating the patient about all treatment options, their degree of efficacy, and potential adverse effects. Determination of initial therapy often depends on patient choice and availability. As there has been virtually no research into managing treatment-resistant BED, specific recommendations cannot be made, but there is preliminary evidence that combination therapy may be helpful.

## Other eating disorders

Other eating disorders that come to clinical attention are NES and purging disorder [1]. NES is broadly defined as morning anorexia, evening hyperphagia, and insomnia. A core feature is nocturnal eating episodes, characterized by the sense that, after awakening at night, one has to eat something in order to get back to sleep. The prevalence of NES has been estimated to be 1.1–1.5% in the general population [77]. NES often co-occurs with obesity, mood disorders, and BN or BED. If possible, NES should be distinguished from the parasomnia sleep-related eating disorder, which is characterized by recurrent episodes of involuntary eating or drinking during sleep.

Study of the treatment of NES is in its infancy, and empirically based guidelines are not available. The only two randomized controlled trials were with SSRIs and had inconsistent results—sertraline was superior to placebo, but citalopram was not [77]. Preliminary data suggest CBT, progressive muscle relaxation, and topiramate may be helpful, but these treatments need study in randomized controlled trials.

Purging disorder is recurrent use of inappropriate weight loss behaviours for the purpose of influencing shape or weight, but without the binge eating episodes characteristic of BN or BED [1]. A newly recognized condition, it may be more common than realized. Though not accompanied by binge eating episodes, purging disorder may be characterized by loss of control of eating where small or normal amounts of food are ingested with a sense of loss of control.

No randomized controlled trials have yet been conducted for purging disorder, and empirically based treatment guidelines are not available. In a tertiary care treatment-seeking sample, patients with purging disorder had similar post-treatment remission or completion rates, as compared to those with AN or BN [78].

## Conclusions

Substantial advances in the management and treatment of feeding and eating disorders have been achieved, but this field lags behind that for other psychiatric disorders. The cornerstone of managing AN is refeeding, nutritional rehabilitation, and weight restoration. There is strong evidence of efficacy for family-based psychotherapy for adolescents with AN, while other forms of psychotherapy for adolescents and adults have less evidence for efficacy. No medication is approved for the treatments of AN, and the only agents with possible evidence of efficacy are zinc, olanzapine, and dronabinol. For BN, there is evidence of efficacy for CBT, IPT, drugs for depression, and topiramate. For BED, there is evidence of efficacy for CBT, IPT, LDX, topiramate, and drugs for depression. Antidepressant drugs reduce comorbid depressive symptoms, and LDX and topiramate produce clinically significant weight loss in overweight or obese patients. Less is known about the management and treatment of pica, rumination disorder, ARFID, and other specified feeding or eating disorders such as purging disorder and NES. As feeding and eating disorders often co-occur with medical and other psychiatric disorders, the management and treatment of these conditions must also be addressed.

## Acknowledgements

The authors would like to acknowledge Genie Groff for manuscript preparation.

## REFERENCES

1. American Psychiatric Association. *Diagnostic and Statistical Manual of Mental Disorders*, fifth edition. Arlington, VA: American Psychiatric Association; 2013.
2. Uher R, Rutter M. Classification of feeding and eating disorders: review of evidence and proposals for ICD-11. *World Psychiatry*. 2012;11:80–92.
3. Lanzkowsky P. Investigation into the aetiology and treatment of pica. *Arch Dis Child*. 1959;34:140–8.
4. Fawcett EJ, Fawcett JM, Mazmanian D. A meta-analysis of the worldwide prevalence of pica during pregnancy and the postpartum period. *Int J Gynaecol Obstet*. 2016;133:277–83.
5. Katsoufis CP, Kertis M, McCullough J, *et al.* Pica: an important and unrecognized problem in pediatric dialysis patients. *J Ren Nutr*. 2012;22:567–71.
6. Miao D, Young SL, Golden CD. A meta-analysis of pica and micronutrient status. *Am J Hum Biol*. 2015;27:84–93.
7. Hagopian LP, Rooker GW, Rolider NU. Identifying empirically supported treatments for pica in individuals with intellectual disabilities. *Res Dev Disabil*. 2011;32:2114–20.
8. Matson JL, Hattier MA, Belva B, Matson ML. Pica in persons with developmental disabilities: approaches to treatment. *Res Dev Disabil*. 2013;34:2564–71.
9. Herguner S, Herguner AS. Pica in a child with attention deficit hyperactivity disorder and successful treatment with methylphenidate. *Prog Neuropsychopharmacol Biol Psychiatry*. 2010;34:1155–6.
10. Stein DJ, Bouwer C, van Heerden B. Pica and the obsessive-compulsive spectrum disorders. *S Afr Med J*. 1996;86(12 Suppl):1586–8, 91–2.
11. Choure J, Quinn K, Franco K. Baking-soda pica in an adolescent patient. *Psychosomatics*. 2006;47:531–2.
12. Nchito M, Geissler PW, Mubila L, Friis H, Olsen A. Effects of iron and multimicronutrient supplementation on geophagy: a two-by-two factorial study among Zambian schoolchildren in Lusaka. *Trans R Soc Trop Med Hyg*. 2004;98:218–27.
13. Gutelius MF, Millican FK, Layman EM, Cohen GJ, Dublin CC. Nutritional studies of children with pica. I Controlled study evaluating nutritional status. *Pediatrics*. 1962;29:1012–23.

14. Chial HJ, Camilleri M, Williams DE, Litzinger K, Perrault J. Rumination syndrome in children and adolescents: diagnosis, treatment, and prognosis. *Pediatrics*. 2003;111:158–62.
15. Tack J, Blondeau K, Boecxstaens V, Rommel N. The pathophysiology, differential diagnosis and management of rumination syndrome. *Aliment Pharmacol Ther*. 2011;33:782–8.
16. Kessing BF, Smout AJ, Bredenoord AJ. Current diagnosis and management of the rumination syndrome. *J Clin Gastroenterol*. 2014;48:478–83.
17. Mousa HM, Montgomery M, Alioto A. Adolescent rumination syndrome. *Curr Gastroenterol Rep*. 2014;16:398.
18. Stanghellini V, Talley NJ, Chan F, *et al.* Rome IV—Gastroduodenal disorders. *Gastroenterology*. 2016;150:1380–92.
19. Halland M, Parthasarathy G, Bharucha AE, Katzka DA. Diaphragmatic breathing for rumination syndrome: efficacy and mechanisms of action. *Neurogastroenterol Motil*. 2016;28:384–91.
20. Barba E, Burri E, Accarino A, *et al.* Biofeedback-guided control of abdominothoracic muscular activity reduces regurgitation episodes in patients with rumination. *Clin Gastroenterol Hepatol*. 2015;13:100–6 e1.
21. Blondeau K, Boecxstaens V, Rommel N, *et al.* Baclofen improves symptoms and reduces postprandial flow events in patients with rumination and supragastric belching. *Clin Gastroenterol Hepatol*. 2012;10:379–84.
22. Norris ML, Robinson A, Obeid N, Harrison M, Spettigue W, Henderson K. Exploring avoidant/restrictive food intake disorder in eating disordered patients: a descriptive study. *Int J Eat Disord*. 2014;47:495–9.
23. Fisher MM, Rosen DS, Ornstein RM, *et al.* Characteristics of avoidant/restrictive food intake disorder in children and adolescents: a "new disorder" in DSM-5. *J Adolesc Health*. 2014;55:49–52.
24. Strandjord SE, Sieke EH, Richmond M, Rome ES. Avoidant/restrictive food intake disorder: Illness and hospital course in patients hospitalized for nutritional insufficiency. *J Adolesc Health*. 2015;57:673–8.
25. Norris ML, Spettigue WJ, Katzman DK. Update on eating disorders: current perspectives on avoidant/restrictive food intake disorder in children and youth. *Neuropsychiatr Dis Treat*. 2016;12:213–18.
26. Hay P, Chinn D, Forbes D, *et al.* Royal Australian and New Zealand College of Psychiatrists clinical practice guidelines for the treatment of eating disorders. *Aust N Z J Psychiatry*. 2014;48:977–1008.
27. Forman SF, McKenzie N, Hehn R, *et al.* Predictors of outcome at 1 year in adolescents with DSM-5 restrictive eating disorders: report of the national eating disorders quality improvement collaborative. *J Adolesc Health*. 2014;55:750–6.
28. National Institute for Health and Care Excellence. *Eating disorders. Core interventions in the treatment and managment of anorexia nervosa, bulimia nervosa and related eating disorders*. Clinical guideline [CG9]. London: National Institute for Health and Care Excellence; 2004.
29. American Psychiatric Association. Treatment of patients with eating disorders, third edition. American Psychiatric Association. *Am J Psychiatry*. 2006;163:4–54.
30. Zipfel S, Giel KE, Bulik CM, Hay P, Schmidt U. Anorexia nervosa: aetiology, assessment, and treatment. *Lancet Psychiatry*. 2015;2:1099–111.
31. Mascolo M, McBride J, Mehler PS. Effective medical treatment strategies to help cessation of purging behaviors. *Int J Eat Disord*. 2016;49:324–30.
32. Misra M, Golden NH, Katzman DK. State of the art systematic review of bone disease in anorexia nervosa. *Int J Eat Disord*. 2016;49:276–92.

33. Swanson SA, Crow SJ, Le Grange D, Swendsen J, Merikangas KR. Prevalence and correlates of eating disorders in adolescents: results from the National Comorbidity Survey Replication adolescent supplement. *Arch Gen Psychiatry*. 2011;68:714–23.

34. Hudson JI, Hiripi E, Pope HG, Jr., Kessler RC. The prevalence and correlates of eating disorders in the National Comorbidity Survey Replication. *Biol Psychiatry*. 2007;61:348–58.

35. Waller G. Recent advances in psychological therapies for eating disorders. *F1000Res*. 2016;5:F1000 Faculty Rev-702.

36. Redgrave GW, Coughlin JW, Schreyer CC, *et al*. Refeeding and weight restoration outcomes in anorexia nervosa: challenging current guidelines. *Int J Eat Disord*. 2015;48:866–73.

37. Garber AK, Sawyer SM, Golden NH, *et al*. A systematic review of approaches to refeeding in patients with anorexia nervosa. *Int J Eat Disord*. 2016;49:293–310.

38. National Institute for Health and Care Excellence. *Nutrition support for adults: oral nutrition support, enteral tube feeding and parenteral nutrition*. Clinical guideline [CG32]. London: National Institute for Health and Care Excellence; 2006.

39. Haynos AF, Snipes C, Guarda A, Mayer LE, Attia E. Comparison of standardized versus individualized caloric prescriptions in the nutritional rehabilitation of inpatients with anorexia nervosa. *Int J Eat Disord*. 2016;49:50–8.

40. Watson HJ, Bulik CM. Update on the treatment of anorexia nervosa: review of clinical trials, practice guidelines and emerging interventions. *Psychol Med*. 2013;43:2477–500.

41. Hay PJ, Claudino AM, Touyz S, Abd Elbaky G. Individual psychological therapy in the outpatient treatment of adults with anorexia nervosa. *Cochrane Database Syst Rev*. 2015;7:CD003909.

42. Le Grange D, Hughes EK, Court A, Yeo M, Crosby RD, Sawyer SM. Randomized clinical trial of parent-focused treatment and family-based treatment for adolescent anorexia nervosa. *J Am Acad Child Adolesc Psychiatry*. 2016;55:683–92.

43. Schmidt U, Ryan EG, Bartholdy S, *et al*. Two-year follow-up of the MOSAIC trial: a multicenter randomized controlled trial comparing two psychological treatments in adult outpatients with broadly defined anorexia nervosa. *Int J Eat Disord*. 2016;49:793–800.

44. Touyz S, Le Grange D, Lacey H, *et al*. Treating severe and enduring anorexia nervosa: a randomized controlled trial. *Psychol Med*. 2013;43:2501–11.

45. Aigner M, Treasure J, Kaye W, Kasper S. World Federation of Societies of Biological Psychiatry (WFSBP) guidelines for the pharmacological treatment of eating disorders. *World J Biol Psychiatry*. 2011;12:400–43.

46. Attia E, Kaplan AS, Walsh BT, *et al*. Olanzapine versus placebo for outpatients with anorexia nervosa. *Psychol Med*. 2011;41:2177–82.

47. Frank GK, Shott ME. The role of psychotropic medications in the management of anorexia nervosa: rationale, evidence and future prospects. *CNS Drugs*. 2016;30:419–42.

48. Kishi T, Kafantaris V, Sunday S, Sheridan EM, Correll CU. Are antipsychotics effective for the treatment of anorexia nervosa? Results from a systematic review and meta-analysis. *J Clin Psychiatry*. 2012;73:e757–66.

49. Lebow J, Sim LA, Erwin PJ, Murad MH. The effect of atypical antipsychotic medications in individuals with anorexia nervosa: a systematic review and meta-analysis. *Int J Eat Disord*. 2013;46:332–9.

50. Claudino AM, Hay P, Lima MS, Bacaltchuk J, Schmidt U, Treasure J. Antidepressants for anorexia nervosa. *Cochrane Database Syst Rev*. 2006;1:CD004365.

51. Kaye WH, Nagata T, Weltzin TE, *et al*. Double-blind placebo-controlled administration of fluoxetine in restricting- and restricting-purging-type anorexia nervosa. *Biol Psychiatry*. 2001;49:644–52.

52. Walsh BT, Kaplan AS, Attia E, *et al*. Fluoxetine after weight restoration in anorexia nervosa: a randomized controlled trial. *JAMA*. 2006;295:2605–12.

53. Fazeli PK, Lawson EA, Faje AT, *et al*. *Short-term treatment with a ghrelin agonist significantly improves gastric emptying in anorexia nervosa*. Presented at ENDO 2016; 1–4 April 2016; Boston, MA.

54. Andries A, Frystyk J, Flyvbjerg A, Stoving RK. Dronabinol in severe, enduring anorexia nervosa: a randomized controlled trial. *Int J Eat Disord*. 2014;47:18–23.

55. Elzakkers IF, Danner UN, Hoek HW, Schmidt U, van Elburg AA. Compulsory treatment in anorexia nervosa: a review. *Int J Eat Disord*. 2014;47:845–52.

56. Kessler RC, Berglund PA, Chiu WT, *et al*. The prevalence and correlates of binge eating disorder in the World Health Organization World Mental Health Surveys. *Biol Psychiatry*. 2013;73:904–14.

57. Hay PP, Bacaltchuk J, Stefano S, Kashyap P. Psychological treatments for bulimia nervosa and binging. *Cochrane Database Syst Rev*. 2009;4:CD000562.

58. Agras WS, Walsh T, Fairburn CG, Wilson GT, Kraemer HC. A multicenter comparison of cognitive-behavioral therapy and interpersonal psychotherapy for bulimia nervosa. *Arch Gen Psychiatry*. 2000;57:459–66.

59. Poulsen S, Lunn S, Daniel SI, *et al*. A randomized controlled trial of psychoanalytic psychotherapy or cognitive-behavioral therapy for bulimia nervosa. *Am J Psychiatry*. 2014;171:109–16.

60. Fairburn CG, Bailey-Straebler S, Basden S, *et al*. A transdiagnostic comparison of enhanced cognitive behaviour therapy (CBT-E) and interpersonal psychotherapy in the treatment of eating disorders. *Behav Res Ther*. 2015;70:64–71.

61. Le Grange D, Lock J, Agras WS, Bryson SW, Jo B. Randomized clinical trial of family-based treatment and cognitive-behavioral therapy for adolescent bulimia nervosa. *J Am Acad Child Adolesc Psychiatry*. 2015;54:886–94 e2.

62. Fluoxetine Bulimia Nervosa Collaborative Study Group. Fluoxetine in the treatment of bulimia nervosa. A multicenter, placebo-controlled, double-blind trial. *Arch Gen Psychiatry*. 1992;49:139–47.

63. Romano SJ, Halmi KA, Sarkar NP, Koke SC, Lee JS. A placebo-controlled study of fluoxetine in continued treatment of bulimia nervosa after successful acute fluoxetine treatment. *Am J Psychiatry*. 2002;159:96–102.

64. Devlin MJ, Kissileff HR, Zimmerli EJ, *et al*. Gastric emptying and symptoms of bulimia nervosa: effect of a prokinetic agent. *Physiol Behav*. 2012;106:238–42.

65. Ong YL, Checkley SA, Russell GF. Suppression of bulimic symptoms with methylamphetamine. *Br J Psychiatry*. 1983;143:288–93.

66. McElroy SL, Guerdjikova AI, Mori N, Munoz MR, Keck PE. Overview of the treatment of binge eating disorder. *CNS Spectr*. 2015;20:546–56.

67. Berkman ND, Brownley KA, Peat CM, *et al*. *Management and outcomes of binge-eating disorder*. Report No: 15(16)-EHC030-EF. AHRQ Comparative Effectiveness Reviews. Rockville, MD: Agency for Healthcare Research and Quality (US); 2015.

68. Wilfley DE, Welch RR, Stein RI, *et al*. A randomized comparison of group cognitive-behavioral therapy and group interpersonal psychotherapy for the treatment of overweight individuals with binge-eating disorder. *Arch Gen Psychiatry*. 2002;59:713–21.

69. Wilson GT, Wilfley DE, Agras WS, Bryson SW. Psychological treatments of binge eating disorder. *Arch Gen Psychiatry*. 2010;67:94–101.

70. Vancampfort D, Vanderlinden J, De Hert M, *et al.* A systematic review on physical therapy interventions for patients with binge eating disorder. *Disabil Rehabil*. 2013;35:2191–6.

71. McElroy SL, Hudson J, Ferreira-Cornwell MC, Radewonuk J, Whitaker T, Gasior M. Lisdexamfetamine dimesylate for adults with moderate to severe binge eating disorder: results of two pivotal phase 3 randomized controlled trials. *Neuropsychopharmacology*. 2016;41:1251–60.

72. McElroy SL, Hudson JI, Mitchell JE, *et al.* Efficacy and safety of lisdexamfetamine for treatment of adults with moderate to severe binge eating disorder: a randomized clinical trial. *JAMA Psychiatry*. 2015;72:235–46.

73. Hudson JI, McElroy SL, Ferreira-Cornwell C, Radewonuk J, Gaisor M. *A double-blind, placebo-controlled, randomized-withdrawal study of lisdexamfetamine dimesylate in adults with moderate to severe binge eating disorder*. 54th Annual Meeting of the ACNP; 6–10 December 2015; Hollywood, FL.

74. Guerdjikova AI, McElroy SL, Winstanley EL, *et al.* Duloxetine in the treatment of binge eating disorder with depressive disorders: a placebo-controlled trial. *Int J Eat Disord*. 2012;45:281–9.

75. White MA, Grilo CM. Bupropion for overweight women with binge-eating disorder: a randomized, double-blind, placebo-controlled trial. *J Clin Psychiatry*. 2013;74:400–6.

76. Robert SA, Rohana AG, Shah SA, Chinna K, Wan Mohamud WN, Kamaruddin NA. Improvement in binge eating in non-diabetic obese individuals after 3 months of treatment with liraglutide—a pilot study. *Obes Res Clin Pract*. 2015;9:301–4.

77. Kucukgoncu S, Midura M, Tek C. Optimal management of night eating syndrome: challenges and solutions. *Neuropsychiatr Dis Treat*. 2015;11:751–60.

78. Tasca GA, Maxwell H, Bone M, Trinneer A, Balfour L, Bissada H. Purging disorder: psychopathology and treatment outcomes. *Int J Eat Disord*. 2012;45:36–42.

# 107

# Aetiology and management of obesity

*Jamie Hartmann-Boyce, Nerys M. Astbury, and Susan A. Jebb*

## Epidemiology

The World Health Organization (WHO) estimated that in 2014, more than 1.9 billion adults (18+) had overweight, of whom 600 million had obesity, representing 39% and 13% of the world's adult population, respectively. Globally, 41 million children under the age of 5 were estimated to have overweight or obesity [1]. Obesity has more than doubled since 1980 and is projected to increase still; if current rates continue, almost half of the world's population will have overweight or obesity by 2030 [2]. Though once considered only a problem in high-income countries, recent years have seen dramatic rises in obesity rates in low- and middle-income countries, particularly in urban areas [1].

The prevalence of obesity varies by age, gender, and socioeconomic status. Globally, obesity is more prevalent in women than in men and increases with age until old age when rates again decline. In middle- and high-income countries, the socially disadvantaged appear to be more vulnerable to overweight and obesity [3, 4]. The reasons for this association are not fully explained but may include greater exposure to environmental drivers of excess weight gain (for example, limited access to healthy food and safe and affordable recreation spaces) [5], lower levels of executive functioning (a theorized control network regulating behaviours, which has been linked with poverty in childhood) [6], and a lack of cultural capital which may diminish motivation for health-related behaviour change [7].

Obesity has been formally recognized as a global epidemic by the WHO since 1997. In 2013, the American Medical Association recognized obesity as a disease.

## Definition and measurement

Overweight and obesity are defined as abnormal or excessive fat accumulation that may impair health. There are a number of ways to measure and define overweight and obesity, which are described briefly here.

Body mass index (BMI), weight in kilograms divided by the square of height in metres, is the most commonly used index for defining weight status in adults. The WHO defines adult overweight as a BMI $\geq 25$ kg/m$^2$ and adult obesity as a BMI $\geq 30$ kg/m$^2$ [1]. Some organizations use a lower BMI cut-off point for defining overweight

and obesity in Asian populations due to increased susceptibility to obesity-related illnesses at lower BMI levels than in people of other ethnicities. Typically, this cut-off is BMI $\geq 23$ kg/m$^2$ for overweight and $\geq 27.5$ kg/m$^2$ for obesity.

For children under 5 years of age, the WHO defines overweight as weight-for-height greater than two standard deviations above the WHO Child Growth Standards median, and obesity as greater than three standard deviations above the median. In children aged 5–19, the WHO defines overweight as BMI-for-age greater than one standard deviation above the WHO Growth Reference median, and obesity as greater than two standard deviations above the median [1].

Waist circumference and waist-to-hip circumference are also used as indices of excess fatness and specifically of visceral adiposity. Although some evidence points to stronger associations with metabolic health outcomes [8], the measurements are less precise than weight and height and subject to considerable inter-observer error.

Body composition measures, which aim to assess the proportion of body constituents, especially fat, are also available. Reference methods, such as whole body densitometry, dual-energy X-ray absorptiometry (DXA), and magnetic resonance imaging (MRI), are not practical in many clinical contexts. Simpler techniques, such as measurements of skinfold thickness or bioelectric impedance (measuring impedance of the body to a small electric current), are sometimes used in large surveys and cohorts, but changes in fat mass in an individual are highly correlated with changes in weight and these additional measures are unlikely to change management decisions.

Other diagnostic tools may be used to take into account obesity-related comorbidity and functional status [9].

## Aetiology

The fundamental cause of obesity is an imbalance between energy intake and expenditure (calories consumed in food and drinks vs calories expended in basal metabolism and physical activity), but the determinants of intake and expenditure are complex. Rapid increases in overweight and obesity around the world, even in places where levels were historically low, illustrate the role of environmental changes in the rise in prevalence of obesity, including readily

**Table 107.1** Drugs used to treat common mental health disorders which may predispose to weight gain

| Drug | Treatment |
| --- | --- |
| Sodium valproate | Epilepsy, bipolar disorder and mania, migraine prophylaxis |
| Lithium | Bipolar disorder and mania, recurrent depression, aggressive and self-harming behaviour |
| Clozapine | Schizophrenia and related psychoses |
| Olanzapine, risperidone, and almost all first- and second-generation antipsychotics | Schizophrenia and related psychoses, bipolar disorder, mania, agitated and disturbed behaviour |
| Amitriptyline, nortriptyline, and doxepin | Depression, neuropathic pain, migraine prophylaxis |
| Fluoxetine | Depression, bulimia nervosa, obsessive–compulsive disorder |
| Mirtazapine | Depression |

available energy-dense food and fewer imperatives for physical activity. These changes directly impact human behaviour, and urbanization serves as a clear example of this phenomenon. Numerous studies and reviews have highlighted the process by which urbanization in developing countries has led to concomitant increases in obesity prevalence [10–12]. Urbanization is characterized by marked increases in the consumption of animal fat and protein, refined grains, and added sugar—a phenomenon referred to as 'the nutrition transition' [11]. Simultaneously, the need for physical activity is reduced through decreases in active transport and increases in mechanized work where previously livelihoods were made in more manual occupations [10]. Such environmental and societal changes have been occurring worldwide and are outpacing human evolution. Humans evolved in conditions of relative food scarcity, in which high levels of physical activity were required to maintain livelihoods and lives. We evolved to conserve energy, and as a species, this leaves us genetically ill-equipped to deal with the environmental changes that have occurred over recent decades [13].

Nonetheless, within any given environment, there are marked differences in weight status between individuals, reflecting fundamental genetic differences, especially in appetite control systems (see Chapter 104) [14]. These interact with environmental drivers and behavioural differences, whether based in nature or nurture, to convey individual-level susceptibility to excess weight gain. Children are subject to the same environmental drivers as adults but are especially vulnerable. Young children lack the cognitive capacity to understand the consequences of poor dietary choices or the ability to understand the persuasive intent of food marketing, and they have limited control over their opportunities for physical activity [15]. Thus, the home environment and prevailing behaviours exert a powerful influence on a child's weight.

The systems mapping approach employed in the 2007 UK Government Foresight report on obesity concluded that energy imbalance was caused by a complex and multi-faceted system of determinants, in which no single influence dominated [16]. However, within a complex systems map, they identified primary appetite control in the brain, the force of dietary habits, physical activity levels, and ambivalence experienced by individuals in making lifestyle changes as key determinants. Psychological factors, including self-efficacy, autonomy, and the ability to cope with stress, have also been found to be associated with obesity (for more information, see Mental health, p. 1098).

Additionally, some pharmacotherapies also cause weight gain—these include sedatives and a number of medications used to treat mental health conditions (Table 107.1).

## Relationships between obesity, morbidity, and mortality

The rising prevalence of obesity presents a challenge to health care systems because elevated BMI is a major cause of morbidity and mortality [17]. The latest Global Burden of Disease study estimates that worldwide overweight and obesity caused 3.9 million deaths in 2015 and in excess of 120 million disability-adjusted life years lost in 2015, making it the fourth largest contributor to ill health [18].

### Physical health

The morbidity and premature mortality attributable to raised BMI is linearly associated with increased risk factors for a wide range of diseases, especially high blood pressure, raised low-density lipoprotein (LDL) cholesterol, insulin resistance, and non-alcoholic fatty liver disease. Together these explain much of the increased risk of coronary artery disease, stroke, and type 2 diabetes [17]. Excess weight is the most important cause of preventable cancer after smoking. Overweight and obesity are significantly associated with at least 13 types of cancer, including common (colorectal and post-menopausal breast) and hard-to-treat (pancreatic and renal) cancers [19]. The underlying mechanisms are not fully understood but include changes in hormone production, particularly oestrogen, which increases the risk of breast cancer and uterine cancer. Excess fat is also associated with over-production of insulin and other growth factors which encourage cells to divide more rapidly. Finally, as adipose tissue depots increase, macrophages within the fat secrete cytokines as part of a low-grade, chronic inflammatory response, which may increase the risk of cancer [20].

Obesity is also associated with an increased risk of musculoskeletal disorders (especially osteoarthritis and lower back pain), reproductive and urological problems (including stress incontinence, infertility, polycystic ovarian syndrome, and erectile dysfunction), and respiratory problems (including sleep apnoea and asthma) [21].

Children with overweight or obesity exhibit elevated risk factors for metabolic diseases, including raised blood pressure and insulin resistance. Moreover, they are significantly more likely to have overweight as adults, and the longer duration of excess weight further increases their risks for developing heart disease and diabetes in later life [22].

## Mental health

A high prevalence of psychological comorbidities has been reported in patients with obesity, and mood disorders, anxiety, and low self-esteem are more common in individuals with obesity than their lean counterparts [23]. However, the relationship between obesity and psychological comorbidities is complex. In some cases, the relationship may be causal (for example, obesity leads to psychological comorbidities and/or psychological comorbidities lead to obesity), and in others, the two may arise together because of common risk factors, which include lower socio-economic class, poor diet, and lower levels of physical activity [24]. A recent systematic review reported that, although obese individuals were at increased risk of developing common mental health conditions, the magnitude of the association was similar to the risk of individuals with mental health conditions developing obesity, suggesting that there is a bi-directional relationship [25].

Obesity is linked to poor self-image, low self-esteem, and social isolation, all contributors to depression [26]. People with obesity can also find themselves ostracized, stereotyped, and discriminated against, which may exacerbate the development of low mood and depressive symptoms [27]. Furthermore, individuals with obesity are more likely to develop diseases such as diabetes, osteoarthritis, and other conditions which cause disability (see Physical health, p. 1097), and many of these comorbidities independently increase the risk of depression [28, 29].

The relationship between obesity and mental health can be further complicated by the fact that some drugs used to treat mental health disorders may predispose to weight gain (Table 107.1).

## Benefits of weight loss

Many of the health risks of overweight and obesity can be mitigated by weight loss. A recent review evaluating the impact of weight loss interventions on cardiovascular risk factors found that even losses in the region of 0–2.5% of initial body weight led to statistically significant reductions in systolic and diastolic blood pressure, total cholesterol, low-density lipoprotein (LDL) cholesterol, HbA1c, and fasting plasma glucose [30].

The strongest long-term data come from the large diabetes prevention trials [31, 32]. Here, intensive lifestyle interventions, including changes to diet and physical activity to achieve weight loss, led to significant reductions in the cumulative incidence of type 2 diabetes [33]. In the 4-year diabetes prevention programme trial in the United States, the incidence of type 2 diabetes in the intensive lifestyle intervention 10 years after baseline was 4.8 cases per 100 person years (95% CI 4.1–5.7), compared to 11.0 (95% CI 9.8–12.3) in the control group [34]. Similarly, in the Finnish diabetes prevention programme trial, at 13-year follow-up, the group randomized to the intensive lifestyle intervention sustained a significantly lower incidence of diabetes, compared to a minimal control group (adjusted hazard ratio 0.61, 95% CI 0.48–0.79) [32].

Reductions in body weight are associated with a roughly linear improvement in other cardiometabolic risk factors, with every 10 kg weight loss associated with a reduction of 0.23 mmol/L in total cholesterol [35] and a decrease in blood pressure of 4.6 mmHg diastolic and 6.0 mmHg systolic [36]. In clinical practice, it may be more useful to consider the degree of weight loss which an individual needs to achieve to observe clinically measurable improvements in health. These are summarized in Table 107.2 [37].

The relationship between weight change and mental health outcomes is less well established. In cohort studies, weight loss is sometimes associated with adverse effects. However, this may be attributable to unintentional weight loss associated with disease, which adversely affects mental health, or a common antecedent such as bereavement or other life events. In contrast, randomized controlled trials of weight loss interventions tend to show improvements in mental health, in particular reductions in depression and improvements in self-esteem and general mood [38, 39]. However, it is difficult to disentangle whether these improvements are due to the weight loss or to the support provided for weight loss. Most randomized controlled trials of weight loss interventions exclude participants with serious mental illness, but those which have tested weight loss interventions in this group have not reported exacerbations of mental illness, and in some cases, there has been clinically significant weight loss and improvements to overall health [40, 41].

Evidence from randomized controlled trials largely suggests that the improvements in health outcomes are independent of the method of weight loss. However, some special considerations may apply in relation to bariatric surgery and mental health outcomes (see Bariatric surgery, p. 1100).

## Treating obesity

The rise in obesity and evidence of the health benefits of weight loss point to the need for effective interventions. Many people seeking to lose weight do so without professional support, and there is relatively limited evidence on the content or effectiveness of these efforts.

In recent years, there has been a significant expansion in the provision of weight management services within health care systems and such interventions are associated with greater weight loss than self-guided weight loss attempts. Interventions range from various forms of bariatric surgery to behavioural interventions, including individual counselling, group support, and total or partial meal replacements. There has been extensive investment by the pharmaceutical industry to develop novel anti-obesity agents, but progress has proved to be challenging.

### Behavioural interventions

Structured behavioural weight management programmes should be considered the first port of call and mainstay of treatment for people with overweight or obesity. By focusing on improvements in diet quality and increases in physical activity, these interventions can support weight loss and bring weight-independent health benefits. They can also include interventions without person-to-person contact, that is, 'self-help' interventions. A recent systematic review found that provision of self-help resources could lead to an additional 1.85 kg of weight loss at 6 months [42]. However, most behavioural weight management programmes offered in health care settings include person-to-person contact to provide support to follow a hypoenergetic diet, together with recommendations for

**Table 107.2** Therapeutic benefits of weight loss in patients with overweight or obesity

| Condition | Amount of weight loss required | Notes on possible lifestyle interventions |
|---|---|---|
| Asthma/reactive airway disease | 7–8% | No specific recommendation |
| Depression | None defined | 'Should be offered a structured lifestyle intervention' |
| Dyslipidaemia (elevated triglycerides and reduced high-density lipoprotein cholesterol) | 5–10%, as needed, to achieve therapeutic targets | Should include a physical activity programme and reduced-calorie healthy meal plan that minimizes sugars and refined carbohydrates, avoids trans fats, limits alcohol use, and emphasizes fibre |
| Female infertility | ≥10% | No specific recommendation |
| Gastro-oesophageal reflux disease | ≥10% | No specific recommendation |
| Hypertension | >5% to 15% | Should include caloric reduction and physical activity |
| Male hypogonadism | 5–10% | No specific recommendation |
| Non-alcoholic fatty liver disease | 4–10% | Caloric restriction and moderate to vigorous physical activity |
| Obstructive sleep apnoea | 7–11% | No specific recommendation |
| Osteoarthritis | ≥10% | Must include physical activity programme |
| Polycystic ovarian syndrome | 5–15% | No specific recommendation |
| Type 2 diabetes (established) | 5–15%, as needed, to lower HbA1c | Should be considered, regardless of duration or severity of disease |
| Type 2 diabetes (risk of developing) (people with 'prediabetes', metabolic syndrome, or 'high risk' based on validated paradigms) | 10% | Should include caloric reduction and physical activity |
| Urinary stress incontinence in women | 5–10% | No specific recommendation |

Source: data from *Endocr Pract.*, 22(Suppl 3), Garvey WT, Mechanick JI, Brett EM, *et al.*, American Association of Clinical Endocrinologists and American College of Endocrinology comprehensive clinical practice guidelines for medical care of patients with obesity, pp. 1–2013, Copyright (2016), American Association of Clinical Endocrinologists.

increased physical activity. A comprehensive systematic review conducted in 2014 to inform British guidelines for weight management found that, on average, participants randomized to behavioural weight management programmes, typically lasting 12–24 weeks, lost 3.7 kg after 1 year, approximately 2.8 kg more than those randomized to usual care or minimal control conditions. No adverse effects were detected. Findings from this review suggested that most, but not all, behavioural weight management programmes were effective, but the reasons behind variations in programme effectiveness remain largely unknown [43]. After many years of intense focus on the macronutrient content of the diet (for example, low fat, low carbohydrate, high protein), there is little evidence that diet composition leads to differences in weight change over a year or more and growing recognition of the importance of adherence to the programme as a predictor of weight loss [44, 45]. For example, in a 2009 trial published in *New England Journal of Medicine*, participants were randomly assigned to one of four diets which varied based on the recommended percentages of energy derived from fat, protein, and carbohydrate. Weight loss was not significantly different between treatment groups, but adherence-related measures were strongly associated with weight loss, regardless of group [45]. Accordingly, interest has grown in understanding the techniques which may help an individual change his or her behaviour, including self-monitoring, goal setting, and planning behaviours. In a 2014 systematic review to inform British guidelines, programmes which encouraged calorie counting and comparison of an individual's behaviour with that of others were associated with greater weight loss [43].

Behavioural weight management programmes may also include provision of meal replacement products to substitute for one or two usual meals or a programme involving total diet replacement with specially formulated shakes, soups, or other basic foods which are nutritionally complete with respect to micronutrients but usually contain 800 kcal per day or less, sometimes referred to as very low-energy diets. Results from a systematic review suggest a mean weight loss of 10.3 kg at 1 year after being offered a very low-energy diet with behavioural support, 3.9 kg greater weight loss than the control groups offered a behavioural programme alone [46]. Results from a recent systematic review of partial meal replacements as part of diets involving more than 800 kcal per day found weight losses midway between those reported from behavioural programmes alone and those from very low-energy diets [47]. Together, these data suggest that tight control over the type and amount of food through the use of a highly structured dietary programme can bring additional weight loss, compared to dietary advice alone, when delivered as part of behavioural weight management programmes.

## Pharmacological interventions

The physiological control systems regulating both energy intake and expenditure provide a series of logical targets for pharmacological intervention to reduce intake or increase expenditure. However, the search for safe and effective drugs to treat obesity has been difficult. Though numerous drugs have been developed which lead to successful weight loss, their side effects have frequently led to drugs being withdrawn during development or soon after coming to the market. In other cases, non-severe side effects or insufficient weight loss limit adherence and mitigate against long-term use, with weight typically regained once the medication is stopped. A new generation of treatments are now coming to market, particularly linked to the treatment of people with diabetes with overweight or obesity, though the cost is likely to be prohibitive for many health care systems.

Generally, obesity pharmacotherapies fall under three categories: those which aim to decrease energy intake; those which aim to increase energy expenditure; and those which aim to decrease energy absorption. Each of these is discussed briefly later in this chapter.

By far, the simplest are compounds that reduce absorption. The most common of these is orlistat, which is available both over-the-counter or by prescription. Orlistat prevents the absorption of a proportion of dietary fat which is instead excreted. However, unless the patient also adheres to a low-fat diet, this malabsorption will lead to oily, loose stools, which discourages patients continuing with medication. A 2011 review for the US Preventive Services Task Force found that orlistat led to an additional 3 kg weight loss at 1 year, compared to a behavioural weight management programme alone [48]. A longer-term trial in which patients were randomized to receive orlistat or placebo for 4 years found 2.8 kg greater weight loss and a 37% reduction in the incidence of diabetes [49]. For patients who are able to make the necessary dietary changes to minimize the side effects (and which also enhance weight loss), orlistat can be a useful and safe aid for weight loss.

Substances such as caffeine are known to act as metabolic stimulants and are associated with modest increases in weight loss, but are not recommended as weight loss aids [50]. Drugs which have greater metabolic effects also tend to be associated with a greater incidence and severity of adverse effects, especially increases in heart rate or blood pressure. The most well-known metabolic stimulant used to treat obesity is phentermine, today often combined with topiramate. Though clinical trials of this combination have shown greater weight loss than previously seen with orlistat, there are concerns about its long-term psychiatric and circulatory system effects, which led to its rejection by the European Medicines Agency (EMA). It is, however, available in the United States after approval by the Food and Drug Administration (FDA) in 2012 [51].

To date, the overwhelming bulk of work relating to pharmacotherapies for obesity has been focused on drugs to reduce energy intake. These include centrally acting treatments which act on neural pathways or those that work on gut mechanisms to boost gut signals and enhance appetite control. The former includes lorcaserin, which works via serotonergic mechanisms. Though phase 3 trials have demonstrated effectiveness for weight loss, use is again limited by concerns over adverse events; similar to phentermine, lorcaserin is licensed for use in the United States, but not in Europe [51]. Liraglutide, an injectable long-acting glucagon-like peptide-1 receptor agonist initially developed for the treatment of type 2 diabetes, is an example of the latter. A recent systematic review found liraglutide consistently resulted in a 4–6 kg weight loss (studies ranged from 20 weeks to 2 years), with comparative data suggesting weight loss was greater than that seen with orlistat or phentermine/topiramate [52]. Some studies also observed improvements in blood pressure and glucose. Both the FDA and EMA have licensed the use of liraglutide for weight loss, but long-term data are lacking and the high cost means this treatment is likely to be reserved for patients in whom other treatment options have failed.

## Bariatric surgery

Surgical interventions for the primary purpose of weight loss have become increasingly popular in recent years, with an estimated 10-fold increase in the number of procedures since 2000 [53]. In most countries, bariatric surgery is only recommended for people with severe obesity (BMI >35 kg/m$^2$) or for those with significant obesity-related comorbidities. Unlike behavioural interventions that rely on an individual's motivation to adhere to a hypoenergetic diet, bariatric surgery leads to weight loss either by physically restricting food intake (restriction) and/or by limiting nutrient absorption from the gastrointestinal tract (malabsorption), leading to reduced energy availability and weight loss.

There are numerous surgical procedures available, the most common being the laparoscopic adjustable gastric band (Lap-band) and Roux-En-Y gastric bypass (RYGB), the latter being associated with larger weight losses. One of the largest and longest studies of outcomes following bariatric surgery is the Swedish Obesity Study in which a cohort of 2010 patients receiving bariatric surgery were matched to a control population and followed up over 20 years [54]. The mean changes in body weight after 2, 10, 15, and 20 years were –23%, –17%, –16%, and –18% in the surgery group. Compared with control, bariatric surgery was associated with a long-term reduction in overall mortality, as well as significantly decreased incidences of diabetes, myocardial infarction, stroke, and cancer. The remission rate of type 2 diabetes was also significantly greater in the surgery group at 2 and 10 years. Though bariatric surgery clearly represents an invasive procedure, risks are low when conducted by experienced surgeons; however, patients do require long-term follow-up, especially after bypass operations where nutrient absorption is permanently impaired [55].

It is estimated that at least 40% of patients presenting for surgery have at least one psychiatric diagnosis [56], with depression, anxiety, and eating disorders being the most common conditions [57, 58]. Overall, bariatric surgery is associated with post-operative improvement in depressive symptoms, self-esteem, health-related quality of life, and body image in patients with obesity [59, 60]. However, it is of concern that there are reports that surgery may predispose to more serious psychological side effects. A systematic review reported that the rate of suicide among those who have undergone bariatric procedures is more than five times that of the general population [61]. Additionally, patients who undergo bariatric surgery may be more likely to develop alcohol and drug dependencies [62]. In light of this, careful consideration should be made as to the suitability of those presenting for surgery and ongoing provision of appropriate support to enhance physical and mental health outcomes.

### Other therapies

Though the use of other therapies for self-management of weight loss—including liposuction, food supplements, hypnotherapy, and acupuncture—is thought to be relatively common, there is very limited evidence to support their use. Where these therapies have been tested in randomized controlled trials, trials have been typically been small, short term, and limited by methodological issues, hampering the ability to draw conclusions about the effects of these therapies [63, 64].

### Treating obesity in children and adolescents

Although there has been considerable progress in developing weight management programmes for adults, there has been less success in developing effective programmes to treat obesity in children. A 2009 Cochrane review found limited quality data to recommend that one treatment programme be favoured over another but found that behavioural interventions aiming to change diet and physical activity could reduce the level of obesity in children and adolescents at 6 and 12 months after programme start. Some studies in adolescents with moderate to severe obesity found a reduction in weight with the use of medication (orlistat or sibutramine), in addition to a behavioural programme, but side effects were frequent [65].

As well as uncertainty over which types of programmes might be most effective, the provision of treatment for obesity in children and adolescents is also limited by a paucity of services in many countries. A systematic review of interventions for obesity in children and adolescents suitable for use in generalist primary care found only marginal reductions in BMI Z-score [66]. Children with severe obesity should be referred to a specialist centre able to conduct a thorough investigation of the genetic and metabolic status of the child and to offer appropriate interventions, with access to ongoing multi-disciplinary support for the child and their family [67]. On occasions, and for older children, this may include the use of pharmacotherapy or surgery; however, behavioural interventions are the mainstay of obesity treatment for children [65].

Early intervention is preferable because young children are rapidly growing and less weight change is needed to achieve a healthy weight [68]. A US task force has suggested that interventions should be of moderate to high intensity (>75 hours over 6–12 months) and include dietary, physical activity, and behavioural counselling components [69]. Some programmes focus the intervention on parents, especially for very young children, teaching an authoritative parenting style and emphasizing the importance of the family environment as a key determinant of a child's weight [70, 71]. Others, modelled on adult community weight management services, aim to equip children with practical skills relating to diet and physical activity. These interventions have shown some short-term success [72]. However, family-based programmes which take a comprehensive approach to family behaviour change appear to be more effective for older children than treating parent or child alone [73].

### Weight loss maintenance

Behavioural, pharmacological, and surgical interventions have all been shown to lead to clinically significant weight loss. However, post-intervention weight regain is very common, particularly in the case of behavioural and pharmacological treatments, as many people find it hard to maintain the cognitive control necessary to restrain their appetite and adhere to a hypoenergetic diet.

Research is ongoing into effective weight loss maintenance treatments, but to date, there is no specific intervention which has shown convincing and reproducible improvements in long-term weight control. A systematic review of non-surgical interventions for weight loss maintenance found that behavioural interventions focusing on both diet and physical activity resulted in an average difference of –1.56 kg (95% confidence interval –2.27 to –0.86 kg) in weight regain, compared with controls, at 12 months. In the same review, orlistat combined with behavioural interventions resulted in a –1.80 kg (–2.54 to –1.06) difference in regain, compared with placebo, at 12 months [74]. Data from cohort studies have identified a number of characteristics associated with long-term weight loss maintenance, including dietary restraint, frequent self-weighing, and engagement in leisure time physical activity [75]. Increases in physical activity also appear to be important in randomized controlled trials, perhaps in offsetting small excesses in energy intake;

systematic reviews have shown better long-term weight loss from interventions combining diet and physical activity than those aiming to change diet alone [76].

However, weight regain is common, and at present, many patients may need to accept the need for repeated intermittent weight loss interventions for long-term weight control. Evidence from large trials with long-term follow-up suggest some residual health benefits from initial weight loss [32, 34, 77].

## Preventing weight gain

The high and increasing prevalence of obesity makes interventions to prevent weight gain a public health priority. Such interventions offer the potential for benefit to the whole population, regardless of weight status, by preventing primary weight gain among lean individuals, reducing the risk of further weight gain among those with overweight or obesity, and reducing weight regain post-weight loss.

A 2014 systematic review found that in adults, weight gain prevention interventions such as individual counselling and exercise programmes were associated with reductions in weight and improvements in health outcomes, but it was uncertain as to whether benefits were clinically meaningful and could be maintained over time [78]. In children, a recent systematic review found moderate-quality evidence for school-based obesity prevention interventions but concluded more research was needed to evaluate programmes in other settings and of other designs [79]. Overall, progress to constrain weight gain has been limited. Though isolated areas and interventions have shown improvements, no country to date has managed to reverse the rising prevalence of obesity, suggesting that individual-level interventions or actions in specific settings may be insufficient to offset wider environmental drivers and emphasizing the need for concerted actions by the whole of society to prevent obesity across the life course [80].

## Conclusions

Obesity is a chronic, relapsing condition that is associated with significant morbidity and leads to premature death. The health risks of obesity can be offset by effective interventions, which may need to be offered on repeated occasions. As the range of effective interventions increases, attention is focusing on the personalization of care and the optimal combination of interventions to achieve weight loss and to potentially improve specific clinical conditions. Though drugs and surgery can modify an individual's internal physical environment, these treatments may be enhanced when combined with behavioural strategies to help individuals manage the external, obesogenic environment. Moreover, stronger public health interventions to prevent obesity have the potential to enhance individuals' weight loss efforts and to disproportionately benefit people with the greatest susceptibility to weight gain.

### REFERENCES

1. World Health Organization. *Obesity and Overweight: Fact Sheet.* Geneva: World Health Organization; 2016. Available from: http://www.who.int/mediacentre/factsheets/fs311/en/

2. Kelly T, Yang W, Chen C-S, Reynolds K, He J. Global burden of obesity in 2005 and projections to 2030. *Int J Obes*. 2008;32:1431–7.

3. Dinsa GD, Goryakin Y, Fumagalli E, Suhrcke M. Obesity and socioeconomic status in developing countries: a systematic review. *Obes Rev*. 2012;13:1067–79.

4. Ball K, Crawford D. Socioeconomic status and weight change in adults: a review. *Soc Sci Med*. 2005;60:1987–2010.

5. Lovasi GS, Hutson MA, Guerra M, Neckerman KM. Built environments and obesity in disadvantaged populations. *Epidemiol Rev*. 2009;31:7–20.

6. Marteau TM, Hall PA. Breadlines, brains, and behaviour. *BMJ*. 2013;347:f6750.

7. Mackenbach JP. The persistence of health inequalities in modern welfare states: the explanation of a paradox. *Soc Sci Med*. 2012;75:761–9.

8. Yusuf S, Hawken S, Ounpuu S, *et al*. Effect of potentially modifiable risk factors associated with myocardial infarction in 52 countries (the INTERHEART study): case-control study. *Lancet*. 2004;364:937–52.

9. Padwal RS, Pajewski NM, Allison DB, Sharma AM. Using the Edmonton obesity staging system to predict mortality in a population-representative cohort of people with overweight and obesity. *CMAJ*. 2011;183:E1059–66.

10. Malik VS, Willett WC, Hu FB. Global obesity: trends, risk factors and policy implications. *Nat Rev Endocrinol*. 2013;9:13–27.

11. Popkin BM. Urbanization, lifestyle changes and the nutrition transition. *World Dev*. 1999;27:1905–16.

12. Yusuf S, Reddy S, Ôunpuu S, Anand S. Global burden of cardiovascular diseases. Part I: general considerations, the epidemiologic transition, risk factors, and impact of urbanization. *Circulation*. 2001;104:2746–53.

13. Prentice AM, Hennig BJ, Fulford AJ. Evolutionary origins of the obesity epidemic: natural selection of thrifty genes or genetic drift following predation release [quest]. *Int J Obes*. 2008;32:1607–10.

14. Walley AJ, Asher JE, Froguel P. The genetic contribution to non-syndromic human obesity. *Nat Rev Genet*. 2009;10:431–42.

15. Boyland EJ, Whalen R. Food advertising to children and its effects on diet: review of recent prevalence and impact data. *Pediatr Diabetes*. 2015;16:331–7.

16. Butland B, Jebb SA, Kopelman P, *et al*. Foresight. *Tackling Obesities: Future Choices—Project Report*. London: Government Office for Science; 2007.

17. Prospective Studies Collaboration, Whitlock G, Lewington S, Sherliker P, *et al*. Body-mass index and cause-specific mortality in 900 000 adults: collaborative analyses of 57 prospective studies. *Lancet*. 2009;373:1083–96.

18. Forouzanfar MH, Afshin A, Alexander LT, *et al*. Global, regional, and national comparative risk assessment of 79 behavioural, environmental and occupational, and metabolic risks or clusters of risks, 1990–2013; 2015: a systematic analysis for the Global Burden of Disease Study 2015. *Lancet*. 2015;388:1659–724.

19. Renehan AG, Tyson M, Egger M, Heller RF, Zwahlen M. Body-mass index and incidence of cancer: a systematic review and meta-analysis of prospective observational studies. *Lancet*. 2008;371:569–78.

20. Vucenik I, Stains JP. Obesity and cancer risk: evidence, mechanisms, and recommendations. *Ann N Y Acad Sci*. 2012;1271:37–43.

21. Public Health England. *Health Risks of Adult Obesity*; 2016. Available from: http://www.noo.org.uk/NOO_about_obesity/obesity_and_health/health_risk_adult

22. Abdullah A, Wolfe R, Mannan H, Stoelwinder JU, Stevenson C, Peeters A. Epidemiologic merit of obese-years, the combination of degree and duration of obesity. *Am J Epidemiol*. 2012;176:99–107.

23. Allison DB, Newcomer JW, Dunn AL, *et al*. Obesity among those with mental disorders: a National Institute of Mental Health meeting report. *Am J Prev Med*. 2009;36:341–50.

24. Bonnet F, Irving K, Terra JL, Nony P, Berthezene F, Moulin P. Anxiety and depression are associated with unhealthy lifestyle in patients at risk of cardiovascular disease. *Atherosclerosis*. 2005;178:339–44.

25. Luppino FS, de Wit LM, Bouvy PF, *et al*. Overweight, obesity, and depression: a systematic review and meta-analysis of longitudinal studies. *Arch Gen Psychiatry*. 2010;67:220–9.

26. Minet Kinge J, Morris S. Socioeconomic variation in the impact of obesity on health-related quality of life. *Soc Sci Med*. 2010;71:1864–71.

27. Puhl RM, Heuer CA. Obesity stigma: important considerations for public health. *Am J Public Health*. 2010;100:1019–28.

28. Lustman PJ, Clouse RE. Depression in diabetic patients: the relationship between mood and glycemic control. *J Diabetes Complications*. 2005;19:113–22.

29. Bankier B, Januzzi JL, Littman AB. The high prevalence of multiple psychiatric disorders in stable outpatients with coronary heart disease. *Psychosom Med*. 2004;66:645–50.

30. Zomer E, Gurusamy K, Leach R, *et al*. Interventions that cause weight loss and the impact on cardiovascular risk factors: a systematic review and meta-analysis. *Obes Rev*. 2016;17:1001–11.

31. Diabetes Prevention Program Research Group, Knowler WC, Fowler SE, Hamman RF, *et al*. 10-year follow-up of diabetes incidence and weight loss in the Diabetes Prevention Program Outcomes Study. *Lancet*. 2009;374:1677–86.

32. Lindström J, Peltonen M, Eriksson J, *et al*. Improved lifestyle and decreased diabetes risk over 13 years: long-term follow-up of the randomised Finnish Diabetes Prevention Study (DPS). *Diabetologia*. 2013;56:284–93.

33. Merlotti C, Morabito A, Pontiroli AE. Prevention of type 2 diabetes; a systematic review and meta-analysis of different intervention strategies. *Diabetes Obes Metab*. 2014;16:719–27.

34. Diabetes Prevention Program Research Group. Long-term effects of lifestyle intervention or metformin on diabetes development and microvascular complications over 15-year follow-up: the Diabetes Prevention Program Outcomes Study. *Lancet Diabetes Endocrinol*. 2015;3:866–75.

35. Poobalan A, Aucott L, Smith WCS, *et al*. Effects of weight loss in overweight/obese individuals and long-term lipid outcomes—a systematic review. *Obes Rev*. 2004;5:43–50.

36. Aucott L, Poobalan A, Smith WC, Avenell A, Jung R, Broom J. Effects of weight loss in overweight/obese individuals and long-term hypertension outcomes: a systematic review. *Hypertension*. 2005;45:1035–41.

37. Garvey WT, Mechanick JI, Brett EM, *et al*. American Association of Clinical Endocrinologists and American College of Endocrinology comprehsive clinical practice guidelines for medical care of patients with obesity. *Endocr Pract*. 2016;22:842–84.

38. Lasikiewicz N, Myrissa K, Hoyland A, Lawton CL. Psychological benefits of weight loss following behavioural and/or dietary weight loss interventions. A systematic research review. *Appetite*. 2014;72:123–37.

39. Fabricatore AN, Wadden TA, Higginbotham AJ, *et al*. Intentional weight loss and changes in symptoms of depression: a systematic review and meta-analysis. *Int J Obes*. 2011;35:1363–76.

40. Bartels SJ, Pratt SI, Aschbrenner KA, *et al.* Pragmatic replication trial of health promotion coaching for obesity in serious mental illness and maintenance of outcomes. *Am J Psychiatry.* 2015;172:344–52.

41. Daumit GL, Dickerson FB, Wang NY, *et al.* A behavioral weight-loss intervention in persons with serious mental illness. *N Engl J Med.* 2013;368:1594–602.

42. Hartmann-Boyce J, Jebb S, Fletcher B, Aveyard P. Self-help for weight loss in overweight and obese adults: systematic review and meta-analysis. *Am J Public Health.* 2015;105:e43–57.

43. Hartmann-Boyce J, Johns D, Jebb S, Aveyard P, Behavioural Weight Management Review Group. Effect of behavioural techniques and delivery mode on effectiveness of weight management: systematic review, meta-analysis and meta-regression. *Obes Rev.* 2014;15:589–609.

44. de Souza RJ, Bray GA, Carey VJ, *et al.* Effects of 4 weight-loss diets differing in fat, protein, and carbohydrate on fat mass, lean mass, visceral adipose tissue, and hepatic fat: results from the POUNDS LOST trial. *Am J Clin Nutr.* 2012;95:614–25.

45. Sacks FM, Bray GA, Carey VJ, *et al.* Comparison of weight-loss diets with different compositions of fat, protein, and carbohydrates. *N Engl J Med.* 2009;360:859–73.

46. Parretti HM, Jebb SA, Johns DJ, Lewis AL, Christian-Brown AM, Aveyard P. Clinical effectiveness of very-low-energy diets in the management of weight loss: a systematic review and meta-analysis of randomized controlled trials. *Obes Rev.* 2016;17:225–34.

47. Astbury N, Piernas C, Hartmann-Boyce J, Lapworth S, Jebb S. A systematic review and meta-analysis on the effect of using meal replacements on weight loss in overweight and obese adults. *Obes Rev.* 2019;20:569–87.

48. Leblanc ES, O'Connor E, Whitlock EP, Patnode CD, Kapka T. Effectiveness of primary care-relevant treatments for obesity in adults: a systematic evidence review for the U.S. Preventive Services Task Force. *Ann Intern Med.* 2011;155:434–47.

49. Torgerson JS, Hauptman J, Boldrin MN, Sjostrom L. XENical in the prevention of diabetes in obese subjects (XENDOS) study: a randomized study of orlistat as an adjunct to lifestyle changes for the prevention of type 2 diabetes in obese patients. *Diabetes Care.* 2004;27:155–61.

50. Heckman MA, Weil J, Mejia D, Gonzalez E. Caffeine (1, 3, 7-trimethylxanthine) in foods: a comprehensive review on consumption, functionality, safety, and regulatory matters. *J Food Sci.* 2010;75:R77–87.

51. Dietz WH, Baur LA, Hall K, *et al.* Management of obesity: improvement of health-care training and systems for prevention and care. *Lancet.* 385:2521–33.

52. Mehta A, Marso S, Neeland I. Liraglutide for weight management: a critical review of the evidence. *Obes Sci Pract.* 2017;3:3–14.

53. Burns EM, Naseem H, Bottle A, *et al.* Introduction of laparoscopic bariatric surgery in England: observational population cohort study. *BMJ.* 2010;341:c4296.

54. Sjöström L. Review of the key results from the Swedish Obese Subjects (SOS) trial–a prospective controlled intervention study of bariatric surgery. *J Intern Med.* 2013;273:219–34.

55. Longitudinal Assessment of Bariatric Surgery (LABS) Consortium, Flum DR, Belle SH, King WC, *et al.* Perioperative safety in the longitudinal assessment of bariatric surgery. *N Engl J Med.* 2009;361:445–54.

56. Yen YC, Huang CK, Tai CM. Psychiatric aspects of bariatric surgery. *Curr Opin Psychiatry.* 2014;27:374–9.

57. Kalarchian MA, Marcus MD, Levine MD, *et al.* Psychiatric disorders among bariatric surgery candidates: relationship to obesity and functional health status. *Am J Psychiatry.* 2007;164:328–34; quiz 74.

58. Mitchell JE, Selzer F, Kalarchian MA, *et al.* Psychopathology before surgery in the longitudinal assessment of bariatric surgery-3 (LABS-3) psychosocial study. *Surg Obes Relat Dis.* 2012;8:533–41.

59. Sarwer DB, Wadden TA, Moore RH, Eisenberg MH, Raper SE, Williams NN. Changes in quality of life and body image after gastric bypass surgery. *Surg Obes Relat Dis.* 2010;6:608–14.

60. Herpertz S, Kielmann R, Wolf AM, Langkafel M, Senf W, Hebebrand J. Does obesity surgery improve psychosocial functioning? A systematic review. *Int J Obes Relat Metab Disord.* 2003;27:1300–14.

61. Peterhansel C, Petroff D, Klinitzke G, Kersting A, Wagner B. Risk of completed suicide after bariatric surgery: a systematic review. *Obes Rev.* 2013;14:369–82.

62. Conason A, Teixeira J, Hsu CH, Puma L, Knafo D, Geliebter A. Substance use following bariatric weight loss surgery. *JAMA Surg.* 2013;148:145–50.

63. Cho SH, Lee JS, Thabane L, Lee J. Acupuncture for obesity: a systematic review and meta-analysis. *Int J Obes (Lond).* 2009;33:183–96.

64. Steyer TE, Ables A. Complementary and alternative therapies for weight loss. *Primary Care.* 2009;36:395–406.

65. Oude Luttikhuis H, Baur L, Jansen H, *et al.* Interventions for treating obesity in children. The *Cochrane Database Syst Rev.* 2009;1:CD001872.

66. Sim LA, Lebow J, Wang Z, Koball A, Murad MH. Brief primary care obesity interventions: a meta-analysis. *Pediatrics.* 2016;138. pii:e20160149.

67. Coles N, Birken C, Hamilton J. Emerging treatments for severe obesity in children and adolescents. *BMJ.* 2016;354:i4116.

68. Wilfley DE, Staiano AE, Altman M, *et al.* Improving access and systems of care for evidence-based childhood obesity treatment: conference key findings and next steps. *Obesity.* 2017;25:16–29.

69. US Preventive Services Task Force, Barton M. Screening for obesity in children and adolescents: US Preventive Services Task Force recommendation statement. *Pediatrics.* 2010;125:361–7.

70. Magarey AM, Perry RA, Baur LA, *et al.* A parent-led family-focused treatment program for overweight children aged 5 to 9 years: The PEACH RCT. *Pediatrics.* 2011;127:214–22.

71. Rudolf MC, Hunt C, George J, Hajibagheri K, Blair M. HENRY: development, pilot and long-term evaluation of a programme to help practitioners work more effectively with parents of babies and pre-school children to prevent childhood obesity. *Child Care Health Dev.* 2010;36:850–7.

72. Sacher PM, Kolotourou M, Chadwick PM, *et al.* Randomized Controlled Trial of the MEND Program: a family-based community intervention for childhood obesity. *Obesity.* 2010;18(S1):S62–8.

73. Janicke DM, Steele RG, Gayes LA, *et al.* Systematic review and meta-analysis of comprehensive behavioral family lifestyle interventions addressing pediatric obesity. *J Pediatr Psychol.* 2014;39:809–25.

74. Dombrowski SU, Knittle K, Avenell A, Araujo-Soares V, Sniehotta FF. Long term maintenance of weight loss with non-surgical interventions in obese adults: systematic review and meta-analyses of randomised controlled trials. *BMJ.* 2014;348:g2646.

75. Thomas JG, Bond DS, Phelan S, Hill JO, Wing RR. Weight-loss maintenance for 10 years in the National Weight Control Registry. *Am J Prev Med.* 2014;46:17–23.

76. Johns DJ, Hartmann-Boyce J, Jebb SA, Aveyard P. Diet or exercise interventions vs combined behavioral weight management programs: a systematic review and meta-analysis of direct comparisons. *J Acad Nutr Diet.* 2014;114:1557–68.

77. Pathak RK, Middeldorp ME, Meredith M, *et al*. Long-term effect of goal-directed weight management in an atrial fibrillation cohort: a long-term follow-up study (LEGACY). *J Am Coll Cardiol*. 2015;65:2159–69.

78. Peirson L, Douketis J, Ciliska D, Fitzpatrick-Lewis D, Ali MU, Raina P. Prevention of overweight and obesity in adult populations: a systematic review. *CMAJ Open*. 2014;2:E268–72.

79. Wang Y, Cai L, Wu Y, *et al*. What childhood obesity prevention programmes work? A systematic review and meta-analysis. *Obes Rev*. 2015;16:547–65.

80. Roberto CA, Swinburn B, Hawkes C, *et al*. Patchy progress on obesity prevention: emerging examples, entrenched barriers, and new thinking. *Lancet*. 2015;385:2400–9.

# 108

# Elimination disorders in children and adolescents

*Alexander von Gontard*

## Introduction

Elimination disorders (EDs) comprise the three broad categories of faecal incontinence (FI), daytime urinary incontinence (DUI), and nocturnal enuresis (NE). They are very common and distressing disorders in children. Thus, 1–3% of typically developing 7-year-old children are affected by FI, 2–3% by DUI, and up to 10% by NE [1]. These rates are even higher in children with special needs, for example those with intellectual disability [2]. Untreated, they can persist into adolescence and even adulthood. In addition, the rate of comorbid child psychiatric disturbances is markedly increased in children with EDs—30–50% of children with FI, 20–40% of those with DUI, and 20–30% of those with NE are affected by clinically relevant behavioural or emotional disorders [3].

EDs are a heterogenous group of disorders with specific signs, symptoms, aetiologies, and treatment approaches. Although the ICD-10 [4] and DSM-5 [5] classification systems provide a general framework, they do not reflect the current state of research [6]. Most of the expanding research on EDs in the past decades has been conducted by paediatricians (especially nephrologists and gastroenterologists), as well as by paediatric urologists, epidemiologists, and basic scientists. Unfortunately, few contributions have come from the field of child psychiatry, despite the high comorbidity rate of psychiatric disorders and the preponderance and effectivity of cognitive behavioural treatment approaches. This output has resulted in two important classification systems, which have superseded those of the ICD-10 [4] and the DSM-5 [5] in clinical practice and research:

- The International Children's Continence Society (ICCS) for DUI and NE [7].
- The Rome IV classification system for FI and constipation [8].

The aim of this chapter is to provide an overview of the current state of knowledge on EDs, as well as to outline practical approaches in assessment and treatment. As EDs can coexist, the chapter will follow the treatment sequence recommended for these combined forms of incontinence—starting with FI, followed by DUI and NE.

## Faecal incontinence

FI (or encopresis) is a common disorder, which is associated with stigmatization, distress, and associated comorbid disorders despite good treatment approaches. Two main different subtypes can be differentiated: FI with and without constipation.

### Classification

According to the DSM-5 classification system, encopresis occurs either voluntarily or involuntarily and is defined by defecation in inappropriate places [5]. A duration of at least 3 months, a frequency of once per month, and a minimum age of 4 years are also required for diagnosis. This is important, because soiling is still so common in 3-year-old children that it is considered to be part of typical development. Finally, organic causes have to be ruled out. Two subtypes are differentiated, that is, encopresis 'with constipation and overflow incontinence' and 'without constipation and overflow incontinence'. As primary and secondary forms (defined by continent intervals) are identical, this differentiation is not important in encopresis.

The international Rome IV classification system avoids the term encopresis altogether and recommends the neutral term of faecal incontinence [8]. Two basic conditions are differentiated: functional constipation and non-retentive FI. The second change is that constipation is defined as the main disorder, which can coincide, but not necessarily, with soiling. Constipation is more common than FI, and the Rome IV stresses that it is aetiologically the overriding disorder. The second condition is non-retentive FI, denoting soiling without any signs of constipation. The Rome IV diagnostic criteria are listed in Box 108.1 [8]. The criteria are stricter than those of DSM-5, more specific, and based on empirical research, and the duration has been reduced to 1 month.

### Prevalence

Encopresis is a common disorder, affecting 1–3% of children from 4 years of age (the definitional age) throughout school years and can persist into adolescence and even adulthood [9, 10]. The prevalence depends on the definitions used; thus, 5.4% of 7-year-old children

I   Diagnostic criteria for functional constipation
Must include two or more of the following, occurring at least once per week for a minimum of 1 month, with insufficient criteria for a diagnosis of irritable bowel syndrome:

1   Two or fewer defecations in the toilet per week in a child of a developmental age of at least 4 years.
2   At least one episode of faecal incontinence per week.
3   History of retentive posturing or excessive volitional stool retention.
4   History of painful or hard bowel movements.
5   Presence of a large faecal mass in the rectum.
6   History of large-diameter stools that may obstruct the toilet.
After appropriate evaluation, the symptoms cannot be fully explained by another medical condition.

II  Diagnostic criteria for non-retentive faecal incontinence
At least a 1-month history of the following symptoms in a child with a developmental age older than 4 years:

1   Defecation into places inappropriate to the sociocultural context.
2   No evidence of faecal retention.
3   After appropriate medical evaluation, the faecal incontinence cannot be explained by another medical condition.

Reproduced from *Gastroenterology*, 150(6), Hyams JS, Di Lorenzo C, Saps M, *et al.*, Childhood functional gastrointestinal disorders: child/adolescent, pp. 1456–1468, Copyright (2016), with permission from the AGA Institute.

soiled in total, but only 1.4% once or more per week [11]. Boys are more commonly affected by encopresis than girls (rates: 3–4 times higher in boys). Encopresis occurs almost exclusively during the day. The rare occurrence of nocturnal encopresis is often associated with

**Table 108.1** Differences between encopresis with constipation and non-retentive faecal incontinence

| | Functional constipation | Non-retentive faecal incontinence |
|---|---|---|
| Bowel movements | Seldom | Daily |
| Large amounts of stools | Yes | No |
| Normal stools (consistency) | Half | Nearly all |
| Pain during defecation | Half | Seldom |
| Abdominal pain | Often | Seldom |
| Appetite | Reduced | Good |
| Colon transit time | Long | Normal |
| Palpable abdominal mass | Often | None |
| Palpable rectal mass | Often | Never |
| Rectal diameter (sonography) | Increased | Normal |
| Daytime urinary incontinence | Tenth | Seldom |
| Nocturnal enuresis | Third | Tenth |
| Comorbidity of behavioural and emotional disorders | 30–50% | 30–50% |
| Laxative therapy | Helpful | Not helpful, even worsening |

Source: data from *Arch Dis Child.*, 71(3), Benninga MA, Buller HA, Heymans HS, *et al.*, Is encopresis always the result of constipation?, pp. 186–193, Copyright (1994), BMJ Publishing Group Ltd and the Royal College of Paediatrics and Child Health; *Arch Dis Child*, 89(1), Benninga MA, Voskuijl WP, Akkerhuis GW, *et al.*, Colonic transit times and behaviour profiles in children with defecation disorders, pp. 13–16, Copyright (2004), BMJ Publishing Group Ltd and the Royal College of Paediatrics and Child Health.

organic causes. Constipation is more common than encopresis, with a median prevalence of 9% worldwide [12].

### Clinical signs

The two subtypes do present with different spectrum of signs and symptoms (Table 108.1) [13, 14]. Children with functional constipation have a reduced number of bowel movements with large stools of altered consistency (too soft or too hard). Defecation is often painful. Abdominal pains and reduced appetite are typical. The colon transit time is increased, and abdominal and rectal masses are palpable. The rectal diameter is increased on ultrasound (>30 mm). DUI, and even NE, can coexist. Thirty to 50% have additional emotional and behavioural disorders. Finally, laxative therapy is helpful.

Children with non-retentive FI have daily bowel movements of normal size and consistency. Pains are not typical, and appetite is good. Colon transit time is normal, and no stool masses can be palpated. Enuresis and urinary incontinence are less common, while comorbidity with psychological disturbances is also 30–50%. Finally, laxatives have no effect—and can even worsen the soiling.

### Aetiology

Genetic factors do play a role in constipation, as shown in a large twin study—less in FI [15]. Constipation often develops from acute constipation, which can be triggered by both somatic (such as painful defecation due to anal fissures) or psychological factors, including stressful life events (such as separation of parents) [16]. As a consequence, chronic stool retention can follow, characterized by painful defecation, avoidance of defecation, and contraction of the external anal sphincter. Faeces are accumulated in the colon and rectum and colon transit times increase, while peristalsis and sensation decrease. Fluid withdrawal induces large, hard faecal masses. Soiling occurs because of interference with rectal function—and by fresh stools bypassing these faecal masses.

The aetiology of non-retentive FI is not known [9]. It is not due to psychological factors alone, as the comorbidity rate of clinically relevant psychological symptoms is comparable to that of functional constipation [3, 13, 14].

Overall, 30–50% of all children with FI are affected by a comorbid emotional or behavioural disorder. In a large population-based study of children aged 7.5 years, children with encopresis had significantly increased rates of separation anxiety (4.3%), specific phobias (4.3%), generalized anxiety (3.4%), attention-deficit/hyperactivity disorder (ADHD) (9.2%), and oppositional defiant disorder (ODD) (11.9%) [11]. This means that children with FI show a heterogenous pattern of both internalizing and externalizing disorders.

### Assessment

The basic steps of assessment are shown in Table 108.2. The standard diagnostic procedures are non-invasive, are sufficient for most children, and can be performed in an outpatient setting.

The history is the most important aspect of assessment. Questionnaires can be very helpful to gain additional information. A very useful chart is the Bristol Stool Form, which depicts seven types of stool, depending on consistency and form.

A physical paediatric and neurological examination is recommended to rule out organic causes. Medical causes account for 5% in constipation and for 1% in non-retentive FI. These include anal fissures, abscesses, skin tags, dermatitis, anal stenosis, anorectal

**Table 108.2** Assessment of elimination disorders

| Faecal incontinence and constipation | Daytime urinary incontinence and nocturnal enuresis |
|---|---|
| **Standard Assessment** | |
| Sufficient for most cases | |
| History | History |
| Questionnaires and charts | 48-hour frequency/volume chart |
| Bristol Stool Form Scale | Questionnaires and charts |
| Physical examination | Physical examination |
| Sonography | Sonography |
| Screening for behavioural disorders or full child psychiatric assessment | Screening for behavioural disorders or full child psychiatric assessment |
| | Urinalysis |
| **Extended Assessment** | |
| Only if indicated | |
| | Uroflowmetry and pelvic floor EMG |
| Stool bacteriology | Urine bacteriology |
| Other diagnostic procedures: plain abdominal X-ray, colon contrast X-ray, MRI of colon, manometry, endoscopy and biopsy | Other diagnostic procedures: radiological examinations, invasive urodynamics, cystoscopy, etc. |

malformations, cystic fibrosis, Hirschsprung's disease, coeliac disease, cow milk intolerance/allergy, cerebral palsy, spina bifida, myelomeningocele, and side effects of medication.

Ultrasound is very helpful, as an enlarged rectal diameter of >30 mm is indicative of constipation [17]. Also, by sonography, a rectal examination can be avoided. Due to high comorbidity rates, a clinical child psychiatric assessment, or at least screening with validated parental behavioural questionnaires, is recommended. If many problem scores are checked, assessment and counselling or, if necessary, treatment are recommended [3]. All other examinations are not indicated routinely, but only if an organic type of FI is suspected (such as in Hirschsprung's disease).

### Treatment

The first step comprises counselling, provision of information, and psychoeducation. Unspecific measures, such as enhancing motivation and alleviating guilt feelings, are also helpful. Only if the child's food intake is restricted to low-fibre foods is a change in diet recommended. Much more important is to increase fluid intake, as many children do not drink sufficient amounts of liquids.

For both types, toilet training is the basic treatment approach. Children are asked to go to the bathroom three times a day after mealtimes and to sit on the toilet 5–10 minutes in a relaxed way. Children should be given a footstool if their feet do not reach the ground and are allowed to play or read, as they like. They do not need to pass urine or stools every time. These toilet sessions are documented in charts. The toiling training procedures have the effect of regulating defecation habits over the day, as the postprandial defecation reflexes are most active after mealtimes.

In non-retentive FI, this toilet training is the main treatment. Laxatives are not indicated. In children with constipation, toilet training is combined with laxative treatment—first disimpaction, then maintenance treatment.

Disimpaction is necessary to evacuate faecal masses at the beginning of treatment. The preferred way is orally with high doses of polyethyleneglycol (PEG—macrogol), for example up to 1.5 g/kg body weight per day, until disimpaction is successful. If not sufficient, rectal disimpaction with enemas are a good alternative—containing either phosphate or sorbite. Recommended doses are 30 mL per 10 kg body weight or half an enema for preschool children, and 3/4 to one enema in schoolchildren. Often, these have to be repeated several times. Both forms of disimpaction are effective [18].

After successful disimpaction, long-term maintenance treatment over a minimum of 6–24 months is recommended to avoid reaccumulation of stool masses. In addition to toilet training three times a day after mealtimes, oral laxatives are given. The preferred and most effective laxative is PEG (macrogol), a long, linear osmotic polymer that binds water [19, 20]. Side effects, such as abdominal pain, are rare. The initial dose is 0.4 g/kg body weight per day in two doses. If stools are too hard, the dose is increased—if too soft, reduced. The therapeutic range varies from 0.2 to 1.4 g/kg body weight per day [21]. Lactulose, a disaccharide, is less effective and has more side effects. The dosage of liquid lactulose ranges from 1 to 3 mL/kg body weight per day in 1–3 doses.

The long-term course of both types of FI is not favourable. Constipation and non-retentive FI can persist into adolescence and even young adulthood [9, 10]. Therefore, constipation and non-retentive FI needs to be treated actively, with regular follow-up visits.

In children with a combination of EDs, treatment of functional constipation and non-retentive FI should always be the first step for two reasons; on the one hand, both DUI and NE can remit by successful treatment; on the other hand, the outcomes of DUI and NE are much worse if constipation and FI are not addressed.

## Daytime urinary incontinence

DUI and NE are even more common disorders than FI. They are lumped together in the ICD-10 [4] and DSM-5 [5] classification systems under the term enuresis. DSM-5 defines enuresis as an involuntary or intentional wetting of children 5 years of age or older after organic causes have been ruled out. The wetting must have persisted for 3 months or longer and must occur at least twice per week or else must cause clinically significant distress or impairment. Only nocturnal, diurnal, or combined enuresis are differentiated—no other subtypes. As DSM-5 is not up-to-date with the current state of research, newer classification systems are needed [6].

The standard classification is provided by the ICCS [7]. It is based on international, multiprofessional consensus, including paediatricians, paediatric urologists, and child psychiatrists. The criteria have become mandatory at international meetings and for publication in journals.

According to the ICCS terminology, urinary incontinence is a general umbrella term for the symptom of any 'uncontrollable leakage of urine', which can be continuous (which is rare and usually caused by organic conditions) or intermittent (which is common and usually functional). An overview is provided in Table 108.3.

Any daytime wetting is termed daytime urinary incontinence, which can be organic (structural, neurogenic, or due to other paediatric causes) or, in most cases, functional. The term 'diurnal enuresis' is obsolete and should be avoided. If a child wets during sleep and during the day, he or she would receive two diagnoses: one for the NE and one for the DUI.

Further specifications of the ICCS criteria are shown in Table 108.3. The lower chronological age limit is 5 years, and a duration of 3 months and a frequency of once per month are required. Frequent and infrequent wetting can be differentiated. Rare wetting of less than once a month is considered to be a symptom, but not a condition. Organic causes have to be ruled out. These encompass structural causes (such as epi- and hypospadias, urethral valves and stenosis, other malformations of the urogenital tract), neurological causes (such as spina bifida, tethered cord syndrome and others), and medical causes (diabetes, urinary tract infections). Finally, many different subtypes of DUI can be differentiated.

The three main syndromes of DUI are urge incontinence, voiding postponement, and dysfunctional voiding. Each types of DUI has typical symptoms, which are summarized in Table 108.4. *Urge incontinence (or overactive bladder)* is characterized by urge symptoms, increased micturition frequency, and small voided volumes. In contrast, in *voiding postponement*, low micturition frequency and postponement of micturition are typical. In both cases, children employ holding manoeuvres to avoid wetting. *Dysfunctional voiding* is a disorder of the emptying phase; instead of relaxing the sphincter muscle, it is contracted paradoxically. Straining and an interrupted urine stream are indicative of this disorder. *Stress incontinence* is rare in children—in contrast to adults. Wetting during coughing, sneezing (that is, any increase of intra-abdominal pressure), and small volumes are typical. *Giggle incontinence* is characterized by wetting during laughing and large volumes with apparently complete emptying. *Detrusor underactivity*, a decompensation of the detrusor muscle, is marked by an interrupted stream; emptying of the bladder is possible only by straining. Wetting exclusively 5–10 minutes after normal micturition is typical of a *vaginal reflux*. *Functional obstruction* can impede urine flow, and *diurnal urinary frequency of childhood* is a benign, self-limiting condition with typical signs of frequency and urgency (often without incontinence).

## Prevalence and clinical presentation

One and a half times more girls than boys are affected by DUI. Two to 3% of 7-year olds and <1% of adolescents wet during the day. Urge incontinence and voiding postponement are the two most prevalent types. The clinical signs of the three common disorders will be presented in more detail.

Children with *urge incontinence* are characterized by a high micturition frequency of >7 times per day, with short intervals in between. Children typically have urge symptoms—sometimes with sudden, intensive (imperative) urge. They wet small volumes, especially during the afternoons, increasing with tiredness. They try to stop the urge by initiating holding manoeuvres such as contracting pelvic floor muscles, pressing the thighs together, holding the abdomen, jumping from one leg to the next, sitting on the heels, and squatting with the heels pressed against the perineum (curtsey sign). Vulvovaginitis, perigenital dermatitis, and urinary tract infections are common.

Typical signs of *voiding postponement* are a low micturition frequency (<5 times per day) and the habitual postponement of micturition in certain situations (school, play, reading, television). With increasing deferral and fullness of the bladder, holding manoeuvres are instituted (as in urge incontinence) until wetting cannot be avoided. Constipation and encopresis are common. Children have a high rate of psychological disorders such as ODD [22].

*Dysfunctional voiding* is characterized by repeated straining at the beginning and during micturition, intermittent and fractioned urine flow, incomplete bladder emptying with residual urine, urinary tract infections, stool retention, constipation, FI, and vesico-ureteral refluxes.

The comorbidity rate of psychological symptoms and disorders among children with DUI (30–40%) is higher, compared to children with enuresis (20–40%) [3]. In a population-based study of 8242 children at 7.5 years of age, externalizing disorders were prominent, with significantly increased rates of ADHD (24.8%), ODD (10.9%), and conduct disorders (11.8%) [23].

## Aetiology

Genetic factors play a role in DUI as well. In a large population-based study, the odds ratio for daytime incontinence was increased by 3.28 if the mother, and by 10.1 if the father, was affected [24]. Linkage studies demonstrated a positive linkage to chromosome 17 in urge incontinence [25]. Urge incontinence is caused by spontaneous contractions of the detrusor during the filling phase of the bladder, which are not sufficiently inhibited by the central nervous system [26]. Genetic factors also play a major role in giggle incontinence—but not in the other types of incontinence.

Psychosocial factors do, however, play a major role in the aetiology of subtypes of daytime incontinence. Voiding postponement can be due to an acquired habit—or as one of many oppositional symptoms as part of ODD [22].

## Assessment

Assessment and a detailed diagnosis is the core of successful treatment—as each subtype of DUI responds best to their specific treatment. The steps are outlined in Table 108.1 and are quite

**Table 108.3** Basic definitions of the ICCS for daytime urinary incontinence (DUI) and nocturnal enuresis (NE)

| DUI | NE (or enuresis) |
|---|---|
| Intermittent incontinence | Intermittent incontinence |
| Wetting during day (wake state) | Any wetting during sleep |
| Minimum chronological age of 5 years | Minimum chronological age of 5 years |
| Duration of 3 months | Duration of 3 months |
| Minimum frequency of once per month | Minimum frequency of once per month |
| Symptom, not disorder: less than once per month: | Symptom, not disorder: less than once per month: |
| Frequent incontinence: ≥4 times/week | Frequent incontinence: ≥4 times/week |
| Infrequent incontinence: <4 times/week | Infrequent incontinence: <4 times/week |
| Exclusion of organic causes | Exclusion of organic causes |
| Many different subtypes | Four different subtypes |

Source: data from *Neurourol Urodyn*, 35(4), Austin PF, Bauer S, Bower W, *et al.*, The Standardization of Terminology of Bladder Function in Children and Adolescents: Update Report from the Standardization Committee of the International Children's Continence Society (ICCS), pp. 471–81, Copyright (2016), John Wiley and Sons.

**Table 108.4** Classification of daytime urinary incontinence (DUI) with main distinguishing symptoms according to the ICCS

| Type of daytime wetting | Main symptoms and features |
| --- | --- |
| **Common types** | |
| Overactive bladder (OAB) and urge incontinence | Urge symptoms, increased daytime voiding frequency, and small voided volumes |
| Voiding postponement | Infrequent micturitions <5 times per day, postponement |
| Dysfunctional voiding | Straining to initiate and during micturition, interrupted stream of urine |
| **Rare types** | |
| Giggle incontinence | Wetting during laughing, large volumes with apparently complete emptying |
| Stress incontinence | Wetting during coughing and sneezing, small volumes |
| Underactive bladder | Interrupted stream, emptying of bladder possible only by straining |
| Vaginal reflux | Wetting exclusively 5–10 minutes after normal micturition due to vaginal reflux |
| Obstruction | Impediment (can be functional) to urine outflow, decreased urine flow |
| Diurnal urinary frequency of childhood | Benign, self-limiting condition with typical signs of frequency and urgency |

Source: data from *Neurourol Urodyn*, 35(4), Austin PF, Bauer S, Bower W, *et al.*, The Standardization of Terminology of Bladder Function in Children and Adolescents: Update Report from the Standardization Committee of the International Children's Continence Society (ICCS), pp. 471–81, Copyright (2016), John Wiley and Sons.

comparable to those of FI. Very important is the registration of micturition volumes and times, fluid intake, and other observations in a 48-hour micturition chart. Sonography of the bladder and kidney is a valuable instrument to detect malformations and measure the bladder wall thickness (which is often increased in DUI) and residual urine after micturition. Urinalysis is recommended, and a dipstick is usually sufficient. Uroflowmetry is also non-invasive and is performed routinely in many centres, but is mandatory only in dysfunctional voiding.

### Treatment

The basic approaches include provision of information, increasing fluid intake, counselling regarding micturition habits, and registering incontinence episodes [27]. This non-pharmacological, non-surgical treatment of incontinence has been named 'urotherapy' and contains many elements of cognitive behavioural therapy (CBT). Treatment is always symptom-oriented, with the aim of achieving complete dryness. Comorbid psychiatric disorders are addressed separately and will increase motivation and outcomes.

The main focus in the treatment of *urge incontinence* is a symptom-oriented cognitive behavioural approach aimed at conscious control of the urge without the use of the pelvic floor muscles, that is, holding manoeuvres. Children are instructed to register when they feel an urge, to go to the toilet immediately without using holding manoeuvres, and to register in a chart if their pants were dry or wet. If these simple techniques are not sufficient, pharmacotherapy with an anticholinergic medication is recommended in addition. First-line drugs are oxybutinin or propiverin. Oxybutinin is dosed

initially at 0.3 mg per kg body weight/day in three doses and can be increased to 0.6 mg per kg body weight/day (maximum of 15 mg/day). The side effects are dose-dependent and reversible. They include typical anticholinergic effects such as flushing, accommodation problems, tachycardia, hyperactivity, dryness in the mouth, residual urine, and constipation. Propiverin has fewer side effects but is not available in many countries. The dosage is a maximum of 0.8 mg per kg body weight/day in two doses (total maximum of 15 mg/day). Recently, the effects of percutaneous electrostimulation [transcutaneous electrical nerve stimulation (TENS)] have been very promising.

Timed voiding is indicated in all cases of *voiding postponement*. Children and parents are instructed to increase the micturition frequency up to seven times per day in regular intervals and to register the course in a chart. Medication is not indicated.

Treatment of *dysfunctional voiding* includes increasing motivation, cognitive behavioural elements, relaxation and general drinking, and toileting advice [28]. The most specific and effective treatment is biofeedback—either with uroflowmetry or pelvic floor electromyography (EMG). Medication is again not indicated [28].

In therapy-resistant cases, structured group therapies have been successful [29]. These combine counselling, provision of information, relaxation techniques, and cognitive behavioural, play, and group therapy approaches.

### Outlook

The outlook of DUI is quite favourable in children with DUI, provided that a specific treatment based on an exact diagnosis is provided. In children with combined EDs, the treatment of DUI should follow after that of FI and/or constipation—but before that of NE. In many children with combined DUI and NE, the NE will resolve upon successful management of the daytime problems.

## Nocturnal enuresis

NE is 2–3 times more common than DUI. As presented earlier, NE and DUI are lumped together in the ICD-10 [4] and DSM-5 [5] classification systems, although they are completely different disorders. Therefore, the ICCS classification is again important for the correct diagnosis of NE and its subtypes [7]. NE denotes any wetting during sleep (at night or daytime naps). In fact, the term enuresis can be used without the addition of the adjective nocturnal, as the term of so-called 'diurnal enuresis' is discouraged. If a child wets while sleeping and while awake, two diagnoses are given: one for the type of NE and one for the type of DUI (Table 108.5).

Many diagnostic criteria are the same in DUI as in NE (Table 108.2). The classification of NE (or enuresis for short) is simple (Table 108.1), based on the longest previous dry period and on concomitant lower urinary tract symptoms (LUTS). *Primary enuresis* means that the child has been dry for <6 months; *secondary enuresis* indicates that a relapse after a dry period of at least 6 months has occurred. Children with secondary enuresis have experienced stressful life events and have higher rates of comorbid psychiatric disorders. Otherwise, assessment and treatment of primary and secondary enuresis are exactly the same.

**Table 108.5** Subtypes of nocturnal enuresis according to ICCS terminology

| | | Maximal dry interval of <6 months | Maximal dry interval of >6 months |
|---|---|---|---|
| | | Primary nocturnal enuresis (PNE) | Secondary nocturnal enuresis (SNE) |
| No signs of bladder dysfunction* during daytime | Monosymptomatic nocturnal enuresis (MNE) | Primary monosymptomatic nocturnal enuresis (PMNE) | Secondary monosymptomatic nocturnal enuresis (SMNE) |
| Signs of bladder dysfunction* during daytime present | Non-monosymptomatic nocturnal enuresis (NMNE) | Primary non-monosymptomatic nocturnal enuresis (PNMNE) | Secondary non-monosymptomatic nocturnal enuresis (SNMNE) |

* Daytime incontinence, urgency, frequency, holding manoeuvres, interrupted flow, etc.
Source: data from *Neurourol Urodyn*, 35(4), Austin PF, Bauer S, Bower W, *et al.*, The Standardization of Terminology of Bladder Function in Children and Adolescents: Update Report from the Standardization Committee of the International Children's Continence Society (ICCS), pp. 471–81, Copyright (2016), John Wiley and Sons.

The second division is far more important—children with NE, but without daytime LUTS, have *monosymptomatic* enuresis. NE and LUTS is called *non-monosymptomatic* enuresis. In non-monosymptomatic NE, daytime symptoms have to be treated first before addressing the night-time wetting to achieve treatment success [30].

### Prevalence

One and a half to two times more boys are affected by NE than girls. The prevalence is 10% among 7-year-old children, 1–2% among adolescents, and 0.3–1.7% among adults. The mean spontaneous remission rate is 15% per year. Primary enuresis is more common than secondary enuresis, and monosymptomatic enuresis is twice as common as non-monosymptomatic enuresis.

### Signs and symptoms

Typical symptoms of *monosymptomatic NE* are deep sleep and difficult arousal and increased urine volumes at night (polyuria) with large wetted volumes. Bladder function during the day is completely normal.

Children with *non-monosymptomatic NE* have the same symptoms, but in addition, they have similar signs as those with DUI (except for wetting during the day). Also, urinary tract infections, constipation, and FI are possible.

Children with *primary* and *secondary NE* have the same symptoms, except for a higher rate of comorbid psychiatric disorders in the latter group.

Overall, 20–30% of children with enuresis, 20–40% of those with urinary incontinence, and 30–50% of those with encopresis have clinically relevant disorders [3].

Externalizing disorders predominate, but internalizing disturbances can occur as well. In a British population-based study of 8242 children at the age of 7.5 years, children with enuresis were affected by separation anxiety (8.0%), social anxiety (70%), specific phobia (14.1%), generalized anxiety (10.5%), depression (14.2%), ODD (8.8%), conduct disorders (8.5%), and ADHD (17.6%) [31]. ADHD is the most common comorbid disorder in enuresis. Enuresis in combination with ADHD is more difficult to treat due to non-compliance.

### Aetiology

Enuresis is a genetically determined maturational disorder of the central nervous system [32]. Seventy to 80% of all children with enuresis have affected relatives. The concordance rates are higher among mono- than dizygotic twins. In linkage studies, several loci on chromosomes 12, 13, and 22 could be identified—irrespective of the subtypes of enuresis [32].

Three main mechanisms are responsible for the development of enuresis. Firstly, increased urine volumes (polyuria) affects some, but not all, children. This is associated with a circadian variation (but not lack) of antidiuretic hormone (ADH). Secondly, impaired arousal is another important factor, as children do not respond to signals of their full bladder to wake up. Thirdly, children have an inhibition deficit of the brainstem and do not adequately suppress the emptying reflexes of the bladder while sleeping. The same factors are responsible for the development of non-*monosymptomatic enuresis*—in addition to local bladder dysfunction. Psychosocial factors can modulate these genetic and neurobiological risks and lead to relapses or a continuation of NE.

### Assessment and treatment

Assessment of NE is the same as that of DUI. Also, basic urotherapy, provision of information, and counselling are the first steps, combined with recording of dry and wet nights on a calendar over a baseline period of 4 weeks. Children are asked to draw a symbol for wet and dry nights (clouds and suns, stars, etc.) on a chart. Any daytime symptoms in *non-monosymptomatic* NE should be treated first [30]. These simple measures will achieve dryness in 15–20% without any further intervention.

If children continue to wet, the first-line treatment is alarm therapy, which requires active co-operation of the child and family [33]. If alarm treatment is not feasible, then it is advisable to start with desmopressin medication first.

Approximately 70% achieve dryness, with long-term cure rates of 50%. Two different types of alarms exist, the body-worn and bedside alarms, and both are equally effective. In case of wetting, the alarm is triggered and the child should wake up completely, go to the toilet, and void any remaining urine. Parents are asked to document the course of the treatment in a chart. To be successful, the alarm must be used consequently every night for a maximum of 16 weeks. After 14 consecutive dry nights, the alarm is discontinued and the child is considered to be dry. Parents are advised to restart alarm treatment if a relapse occurs. If not sufficient, alarm treatment can be combined with additional CBT components. If a child does not respond to the alarm, a switch to desmopressin, the second-line treatment, is recommended.

Indications for medication are therapy resistance towards alarm treatment, lack of motivation in the children, stress in the family, lack of co-operation, and the requirement of short-term dryness, that is, for school outings, etc. Desmopressin is the medication of choice in these cases due to positive effects and few side effects. Desmopressin (or DDAVP) is a synthetic analogue of ADH. In 70%, a reduction of wet nights or even dryness can be achieved, but after discontinuing medication, most children have a relapse, so that only

18–38% of children remain dry in the long run. It has a distinctly lower curative effect than the alarm.

Desmopressin is given 30–60 minutes before going to sleep in the evenings only. The oral dosage is 0.2–0.4 mg—or 120–240 µg as a melt tablet. It is advisable to titrate the required dose over 4 weeks, starting with the low dose first and increasing the dose only if necessary. This should be documented on a chart. If a child does not respond within 4 weeks, he or she should be considered to be a non-responder and desmopressin is discontinued. Otherwise, one can continue with the required dosage for a maximum of 12 weeks, after which desmopressin should be stopped—to check if the child can remain dry without medication. If a relapse occurs, desmopressin can be given in 3-month blocks. Adverse effects are rare and not pronounced, like headache, stomach ache, lack of appetite, etc. The most dramatic, though rare, side effect is hyponatraemia and water intoxication, which can require intensive care. Therefore, it is important not to overdose—and not to drink <8 oz (250 mL) after taking the medication.

Tricyclic drugs like imipramine have a proven antienuretic effect—and similar relapse rates as desmopressin. Due to the risk of cardiac arrhythmias and intoxication in high doses, it has become a third-line treatment in therapy-resistant cases. Also, imipramine needs close clinical and laboratory surveillance.

### Outlook

NE has the best treatment results of all EDs, again provided that an exact diagnosis is made and the recommended guidelines are followed. In children with combined EDs, NE is the last condition in the treatment sequence.

## Summary

The aim of this chapter was to provide an overview on EDs in children and adolescents. The clinical aspects of the three major groups of FI, DUI, and NE were presented. These are heterogenous disorders with divergent aetiologies, symptoms, and treatment approaches. Most EDs are functional, that is, non-organic. The guidelines for assessment and treatment are logical, and if followed, the outcome is quite promising. The treatment is symptom-oriented, with the goal of complete continence, and comorbid psychiatric disorders, which are common but do not affect most children with EDs, need to be addressed. A multi-disciplinary approach can be very helpful.

## REFERENCES

1. Franco I, Austin P, Bauer S, von Gontard A, Homsy Y (eds). *Pediatric Incontinence: Evaluation and Clinical Management*. Oxford and Hoboken, NJ: Wiley-Blackwell; 2015.
2. von Gontard A. Urinary and faecal incontinence in children with special needs. *Nat Rev Urol* 2013;10:667–74.
3. von Gontard A, Baeyens D, Van Hoecke E, Warzak W, Bachmann C. Psychological and psychiatric issues in urinary and fecal incontinence. *J Urol* 2011;185:1432–7.
4. World Health Organization. *Multiaxial Classification of Child and Adolescent Psychiatric Disorders: The ICD-10 Classification of Mental and Behavioural Disorders in Children and Adolescents*. Cambridge: Cambridge University Press; 2008.
5. American Psychiatric Association. *Diagnostic and Statistical Manual of Mental Disorders (DSM-5)*. Washington, DC: American Psychiatric Association; 2013.
6. von Gontard A. Elimination disorders—a critical comment on DSM-V proposals. *Eur Child Adolesc Psychiatry* 2011;20:83–8.
7. Austin PF, Bauer S, Bower W, *et al*. The Standardization of Terminology of Bladder Function in Children and Adolescents: Update Report from the Standardization Committee of the International Children's Continence Society (ICCS). *Neurourol Urodyn* 2016;35:471–81.
8. Hyams JS, Di Lorenzo CD, Saps M, Schulman R, Staiano A, van Tilburg M. Childhood functional gastrointestinal disorders: child/adolescent. *Gastroenterology* 2016;150:1456–68.
9. Bongers MEJ, Tabbers MM, Benninga M. Functional nonretentive fecal incontinence in children. *J Pediatric Gastroenterol Nutr* 2007;44:5–13.
10. Bongers MEJ, van Wijk MP, Reitsma JB, Benninga MA. Long-term prognosis for childhood constipation: clinical outcomes in adulthood. *Pediatrics* 2010;126:e156–62.
11. Joinson C, Heron J, Butler U, von Gontard A; Avon Longitudinal Study of Parents and Children Study Team. Psychological differences between children with and without soiling problems. *Pediatrics* 2006;117:1575–84.
12. van den Berg MM, Benninga MA, Di Lorenzo C. Epidemiology of childhood constipation: a systematic review. *Am J Gastroenterol* 2006;101:2401–9.
13. Benninga MA, Buller HA, Heymans HS, Tytgat GN, Taminiau JA. Is encopresis always the result of constipation? *Arch Disease Child* 1994;71:186–93.
14. Benninga MA, Voskuijl WP, Akkerhuis GW, Taminiau JA, Buller HA. Colonic transit times and behaviour profiles in children with defecation disorders. *Arch Dis Child* 2004;89:13–16.
15. Bakwin H, Davidson MD. Constipation in twins. *Am J Dis Child* 1971;121:179–81.
16. Cox DJ, Sutphen JL, Borrowitz SM, Korvatchev B, Ling W. Contribution of behavior therapy and biofeedback to laxative therapy in the treatment of pediatric encopresis. *Ann Behav Med* 1998;20:70–6.
17. Joensson IM, Siggard C, Rittig S, Hagstroem S, Djurhuus JC. Transabdominal ultrasound of rectum as a diagnostic tool in childhood constipation. *J Urol* 2008;179:1997–2002.
18. Bekkali N, van den Berg M, Dijkgraaf MGW *et al*. Rectal fecal impaction treatment in childhood constipation: enemas versus high doses oral PEG. *Pediatrics* 2009;124:e1108–15.
19. Candy D, Belsey J. Macrogol (polyethylene glycol) laxatives in children with functioanl constipation and faecal impaction: a systematic review. *Arch Disease Child* 2009;94:156–60.
20. Pijpers MAM, Tabbers MM, Benninga MA, Berger MY. Currently recommended treatments of childhood constipation are not evidence based: a systematic literature review on the effect of laxative treatment and dietary measures. *Arch Dis Child* 2009;94:117–31.
21. Nurko S, Youssef NN, Sabri M, *et al*. PEG3350 in the treatment of childhood constipation: a multicenter, double-blinded, placebo-controlled trial. *J Pediatr* 2008;153:254–61.
22. von Gontard A, Niemczyk J, Wagner C, Equit. Voiding postponement in children—a systematic review. *Eur Child Adolesc Psychiatry* 2016;25:809–20.
23. Joinson C, Heron J, von Gontard A. Psychological problems in children with daytime wetting. *Pediatrics* 2006;118:1985–93.

24. von Gontard A, Heron J, Joinson C. Family history of nocturnal enuresis and urinary incontinence—results from a large epidemiological study. *J Urol* 2011;185:2303–7.

25. Eiberg H, Schaumburg HL, von Gontard A, Rittig S. Linkage study in a large Danish four generation family with urge incontinence and nocturnal enuresis. *J Urol* 2001;166:2401–3.

26. Franco I. Overactive bladder in children. Part 1: pathophysiology. *J Urol* 2007;178:761–8.

27. Chang SJ, Van Laecke E, Bauer SB, *et al.* Treatment of daytime urinary incontinence: a standardization document from the International Children's Continence Society. *Neurourol Urodyn* 2017;36:43–50.

28. Chase J, Austin P, Hoebeke P, McKenna P. The management of dysfunctional voiding in children: a report from the standardisation committee of the International Children's Continence Society. *J Urol* 2010;183:1296–302.

29. Equit M, Sambach, H, Niemczyk J, von Gontard A. *Urinary and Fecal Incontinence: A Training Program for Children and Adolescents.* Boston/Göttingen: Hogrefe Publishing; 2015.

30. Franco I, von Gontard A, DeGennaro M. Evaluation and treatment of nonmonosymptomatic nocturnal enuresis: a standardization document from the International Children's Continence Society. *J Pediatr Urol* 2013;9:234–43.

31. Joinson C, Heron J, Emond A, Butler R: Psychological problems in children with bedwetting and combined (day and night) wetting: a UK population-based study. *J Ped Psychol* 2007;32:605–16.

32. von Gontard A, Schaumburg H, Hollmann E, Eiberg H, Rittig S. The genetics of enuresis—a review. *J Urol* 2001;166:2438–43.

33. Neveus T, Eggert P, Macedo A, *et al.* Evaluation of and treatment for monosymptomatic enuresis: a standardization document from the International Children's Continence Society. *J Urol* 2010;183:441–7.

# SECTION 17
# Sleep–wake disorders

# 109

# Basic mechanisms of, and possible treatment targets for, sleep–wake disorders

*David Pritchett, Angus S. Fisk, Russell G. Foster, and Stuart N. Peirson*

## Circadian rhythms

Circadian rhythms are endogenous 24-hour oscillations in physiology and behaviour that enable an organism to anticipate and adapt to the changing temporal demands of the environment [1]. The term circadian is derived from the Latin for 'around a day'. The sleep/wake cycle is the most obvious example of a circadian rhythm. Other examples include daily fluctuations in locomotor activity, core body temperature, heart rate, blood pressure, renal activity, liver metabolism, and secretion of glucocorticoids, melatonin, and testosterone [2, 3]. Circadian rhythms in physiological parameters are not unique to man; they are observed in organisms as diverse as cyanobacteria, fungi, algae, plants, *Drosophila*, and rodents [4]. Circadian rhythms confer a survival advantage to organisms that possess them, increasing their reproductive fitness. For example, ground squirrels lacking endogenous rhythms are more vulnerable to predation and show a 20% reduction in lifespan [5].

Any circadian rhythm must meet three criteria [1]. Firstly, it must persist under constant conditions (that is, in the absence of changes in temperature or light), with an endogenous (or 'free-running') period of approximately 24 hours. This distinguishes internally driven rhythms from responses to external cues. Secondly, it must be entrainable. To anticipate daily environmental events (for example, sunrise), the rhythm must be able to adjust to changes in the timing of these events. For example, the timing of sunrise varies between geographical locations and also changes across the seasons. This process of synchronization is known as entrainment, and an external stimulus that can synchronize a circadian rhythm is called a *zeitgeber*, German for 'time-giver'. Finally, a circadian rhythm must be temperature-compensated, meaning that its periodicity should remain constant over a range of physiological temperatures.

## Mechanistic basis of circadian rhythms

Mammals possess a circadian 'master clock' which resides in the suprachiasmatic nucleus (SCN), a small brain structure composed of approximately 20,000 neurons, located in the anterior hypothalamus, just above the optic chiasm [6]. The role of the SCN was first shown by rodent lesion studies; in rats, circadian rhythms in water consumption, locomotor activity, and corticosterone secretion were all abolished by SCN ablation [7, 8]. In hamsters, transplantation of neonatal hypothalamic tissue (including the SCN) can restore circadian rhythms following SCN ablation [9]. Moreover, transplanting SCN tissue from *tau* mutant hamsters, which have a 20-hour circadian period, imposes a 20-hour period on the recipient [10]. In humans, compression of the SCN by expanding pituitary tumours causes progressive circadian disintegration [11]. In the 1970s and 1980s, *in vivo* oscillations in glucose uptake and electrical activity were first reported in the rat SCN; both were upregulated in the day [12, 13]. Analogous results were subsequently reported with *in vitro* slice preparations [14]. Rhythmic firing was later observed in isolated cultured neurons, demonstrating that circadian oscillations result from subcellular mechanisms, rather than cell–cell interactions [6].

### The molecular circadian clock

Today, the molecular basis of mammalian circadian rhythms is well characterized. The basic mechanism is an autoregulatory transcriptional–translational feedback loop (TTFL), involving four core 'clock genes': Period (*Per1* and *Per2*), Cryptochrome (*Cry1* and *Cry2*), Brain and Muscle ARNT-Like (*Bmal1*), and Circadian Locomotor Output Cycles Kaput (*Clock*) [15]. These genes encode the proteins PER1-2, CRY1-2, BMAL1, and CLOCK, respectively [15]. The basic clock mechanism involves the binding of CLOCK and BMAL1 to E-box enhancers in the promoters of *Per1-2* and *Cry1-2*, driving their expression. In turn, PER and CRY form homo- and heterodimers and inhibit CLOCK/BMAL1 binding, providing a negative feedback loop. In addition, several other genes are known to regulate the mammalian TTFL. For example, casein kinase 1 (*Ck1*) plays an important role in setting the core clock speed by phosphorylating PER proteins, which targets them for ubiquitylation and proteasomal degradation [16].

The TTFL in the SCN is synchronized with the environment by light input from the retina. Light information is transmitted from the eye to the SCN via photosensitive retinal ganglion cells (pRGCs).

Although they also receive input from rod and cone photoreceptors, pRGCs are intrinsically photosensitive due to their expression of the photopigment melanopsin. Ablation of pRGCs impairs photic entrainment in mice but spares pattern-forming visual function [17]. The axons of pRGCs, which form the retinohypothalamic tract (RHT), synapse directly with the SCN [18, 19]. Glutamate and pituitary adenylyl cyclase-activating polypeptide (PACAP) are the principal neurotransmitters at these synapses [20]. Although light information is the primary *zeitgeber* for the entrainment of the circadian clock, the timing of other events such as feeding and exercise can also be considered *zeitgebers*, which affect the SCN via non-photic pathways [1].

### Clock outputs

How does the action of the TTFL translate into circadian rhythms in physiology and behaviour? The immediate output of the TTFL is the rhythmic expression of 'clock-controlled genes' within the SCN itself [11, 21]. These genes are not part of the TTFL but show rhythmic expression because they possess E-boxes. In turn, these clock-controlled genes regulate the expression of their own downstream target genes. The net result is that roughly 10% of the SCN transcriptome is rhythmically expressed. It is unclear how rhythmic patterns of electrical activity are generated in the SCN [20], but these oscillations are conveyed to other brain regions by monosynaptic or multisynaptic pathways, or via the rhythmic synthesis and secretion of peptide hormones such as vasoactive intestinal peptide (VIP) [11, 21]. The SCN's target regions are ultimately responsible for the co-ordination of circadian physiology and behaviour. Examples include the rhythmic secretion of the hormone melatonin from the pineal gland and the rhythmic secretion of corticotropin-releasing hormone (CRH) from the hypothalamus, which leads to the release of glucocorticoids from the adrenal glands [11, 21].

Multiple body tissues show self-sustained rhythmic clock gene expression *in vitro* [21, 22]. Initially observed in rodent fibroblasts [23], these peripheral rhythms are particularly well characterized in the liver [24]. As in the SCN, around 10% of the transcriptome is rhythmically expressed in most peripheral tissues [25]. In the brain, rhythmic electrical activity, hormone output, and clock gene expression has been reported in the olfactory bulb, amygdala, lateral habenula, hippocampus, motor cortex, and cerebellum, together with a variety of nuclei in the hypothalamus [21, 22]. Taken together, it appears that the brain and body are full of localized autonomous circadian clocks. The SCN synchronizes these peripheral clocks with each other and the external environment [11, 21]. Glucocorticoids may be one synchronizing signal; the administration of the glucocorticoid dexamethasone is known to synchronize 60% of the liver's circadian transcriptome [11, 21].

## Sleep

Sleep is a recurring physiological state characterized by altered consciousness, reduced perception of environmental stimuli, and inhibition of most voluntary muscles [26]. Although we spend around a third of our lives asleep, the exact functions of sleep are not well understood. Popular theories include rejuvenation of the immune system [27] and repair and regeneration of nervous tissue, bone, and muscle [26]. From a cognitive perspective, sleep may be important for memory consolidation [28], while according to the synaptic homeostasis hypothesis, sleep is required to reverse the net increase in synaptic strength which occurs in many brain circuits during wakefulness [29]. Whatever the functional roles of sleep, its importance is underscored by the myriad health problems that are associated with sleep disruption.

In humans, sleep consists of both rapid eye movement (REM) sleep and non-rapid eye movement (NREM) sleep, which has three stages [30–32]. During sleep, the body repeatedly cycles through these stages in a predictable and sequential manner, progressing through NREM stages 1, 2, and 3 and ending with REM sleep. Typically, the first cycle lasts 70–100 minutes, and subsequent cycles last 90–120 minutes. Four to five cycles are completed each night. REM sleep accounts for 20–25% of total sleep time, and the proportion of REM sleep increases across cycles. Conversely, the proportion of stage 3 NREM sleep (also known as slow-wave sleep) tends to decrease across cycles. Arousal threshold increases with each NREM stage, while muscle activity and eye movements decrease [30–32]. The three NREM stages are characterized by oscillatory brain activity of different frequencies. Sleep spindles and K-complexes occur at the onset of stage 2 NREM sleep. During REM sleep, there is vigorous eye movement, but most voluntary muscles are paralysed. Brain activity in REM sleep closely resembles that observed during wakefulness. REM sleep is also associated with dreaming, an association first noted in the early 1950s [33].

### Mechanistic basis of sleep and wakefulness

Wakefulness is a state of alertness characterized by high forebrain and cortical activity, which is promoted by the ascending arousal system (AAS) [34]. The AAS originates in the upper brainstem [35] and can be broadly divided into two separate pathways, each innervating distinct brain regions and involving different neurotransmitters [36]. The first pathway consists of cholinergic projections from the pedunculopontine (PPT) and laterodorsal tegmental (LDT) nuclei of the brainstem, which are more active during wakefulness and REM sleep and less active during NREM sleep [37]. One of their key targets is the thalamic reticular nucleus (TRN), which inhibits thalamocortical rhythms to promote wakefulness [38]. The second pathway innervates multiple targets in the hypothalamus, forebrain, and cerebral cortex [36]. It consists of noradrenergic projections from the locus caeruleus (LC), serotonergic projections from the dorsal and medial raphe nuclei (DRN and MRN), dopaminergic projections from the ventral periaqueductal grey (VPAG), and histaminergic projections from the tuberomammillary nucleus (TMN) [34]. It also includes cholinergic and GABAergic projections from basal forebrain (BF) nuclei and peptidergic projections from lateral hypothalamic (LH) nuclei [34]. These LH neurons can be subdivided into those expressing orexin (also known as hypocretin) and those expressing melatonin-concentrating hormone (MCH). Monoaminergic and orexinergic neurons are most active during wakefulness, less active during NREM sleep, and least active during REM sleep [35]. In contrast, the MCH-releasing neurons are most active during REM sleep [39], and the cholinergic neurons are most active during REM sleep and wakefulness [40].

The AAS is inhibited by the ventrolateral preoptic nucleus, or VLPO, a small cluster of neurons in the anterior hypothalamus [34]. During sleep, a subpopulation of VLPO neurons is highly active [41] and suppresses the AAS through the release of the inhibitory neurotransmitters GABA and galanin [42, 43]. Central VLPO lesions are known to reduce NREM sleep, while lesions to the extended VLPO decrease REM sleep [44]. In addition to the suppression of the AAS by the VLPO, neurons in the VLPO can be inhibited by the AAS. This inhibition is driven by noradrenergic projections to the VLPO from the LC, serotonergic projections from the MRN, and GABAergic and galinergic projections from the TMN [45]. As such, there is reciprocal inhibition between the AAS and the VLPO. The AAS inhibits the VLPO during wake, and the VLPO inhibits the AAS during sleep. It has been proposed that this reciprocal inhibition creates a bi-stable 'flip-flop' circuit—whereby sleep and wake cannot be promoted at the same time. This putative mechanism, also known as the 'sleep switch', may explain why sleep–wake transitions are swift [36, 37].

## Sleep timing: the two-process model of sleep

Sleep timing is thought to be dependent on two hypothetical mechanisms [46, 47]. The first, known as 'Process S', describes a homeostatic drive for sleep, which increases progressively during wakefulness and dissipates during sleep. The biological substrate of this mechanism is unproven, although adenosine is a likely candidate. Adenosine accumulates in the brain during wakefulness [48], while the administration of adenosine or adenosine receptor agonists promotes sleep in rats and cats [49, 50]. These pharmacological effects are likely mediated by the excitation of sleep-promoting brain regions and the inhibition of wake-promoting regions [34]. Recent evidence suggests that adenosine accumulation is also responsible for the antidepressant effect of sleep deprivation [51].

The second component of the two-process model—'Process C'—describes the contribution of the circadian clock to sleep regulation [46, 47]. More specifically, it describes a circadian drive for wakefulness, which rises during the day and falls during the evening and night. According to the two-process model, Process C counteracts Process S to keep us awake during daytime when homeostatic sleep pressure is steadily increasing. In the evening, sleep onset coincides with the opening of the 'sleep gate', the point at which the discrepancy between Processes S and C reaches a critical threshold. SCN lesions in primates result in increased sleep time, as well as arrhythmia [52]. This suggests that under normal conditions, signals from the SCN oppose the homeostatic drive for sleep, providing a plausible biological substrate for Process C. These signals may be carried by projections from the SCN to the ventral subparaventricular zone (SPZ) and the dorsomedial nucleus of the hypothalamus (DMH). In rats, lesions of both structures impair the circadian rhythmicity of the sleep/wake cycle [44, 53]. The DMH may be a critical relay between Processes C and S, as it receives inputs from the SCN and SPZ and innervates both the VLPO and the LH nuclei of the AAS [53].

## Sleep and circadian rhythm disruption in psychiatric disorders

The relationship between severe mental illness and abnormal sleep was first described in the late nineteenth century by the German psychiatrist Emil Kraepelin [54]. Today, sleep and circadian rhythm disruption (SCRD) is reported in 30–80% of patients with schizophrenia and is increasingly recognized as one of the most common features of the disorder [55]. Moreover, recent evidence suggests that the degree of SCRD is correlated with the severity of positive, negative, and cognitive symptoms [56–59]. Sleep disturbances in schizophrenia include increases in sleep latency and reductions in total sleep time, sleep efficiency, REM sleep latency, REM sleep density, and slow-wave sleep duration [54, 55, 60–62]. Schizophrenia is also associated with significant circadian disruption such as abnormal phasing, instability, and fragmentation of rest–activity rhythms [63–66]. Crucially, schizophrenia patients with SCRD score badly on many quality-of-life clinical subscales, highlighting the human cost of SCRD in schizophrenia [55, 67, 68]. Furthermore, patients often comment that an improvement in sleep is one of their highest therapeutic priorities [69].

SCRD is not limited to schizophrenia. Up to 90% of patients suffering from an acute depressive episode report simultaneous changes in their sleep profile that are usually described as difficulties initiating and maintaining sleep during the night. Significantly, persistent insomnia increases the risk of relapse into a new depressive episode [70]. Increased sleep disruption, as in mothers after childbirth, raises the risk of post-partum depression, with poorer sleep quality correlated with more severe depression [71]. Seasonal affective disorder (SAD), or 'winter depression', is clinically classified as a subtype of major depression that describes a condition of serious mood alteration associated with a change in the season towards autumn and winter. Individuals tend to show excessive daytime sleepiness, have little energy, and crave sweets and carbohydrates. SAD individuals may also feel profoundly depressed. While there is a trend suggesting an overall increase in the prevalence of SAD with increasing latitude and with the shortened daily light period during the winter season, there is considerable country-to-country variation [72, 73]. These inconsistencies in the prevalence of SAD might be because this condition is a more severe expression of the naturally occurring seasonal variation in mood experienced by a large percentage of the general population. The best evidence that there is a recurrent, seasonally influenced winter depressive condition that is a function of an interaction between light and internal circadian and/or circannual rhythms is the very high success rate of phototherapy [74]. In individuals with a diagnosis of bipolar disorder, disruption of their 24-hour sleep/wake cycle, shortened sleep, or travel across multiple time zones seems to act as an important trigger for a relapse (77% of patients) into mania [75]. By contrast, during the depressed phase, patients may become hypersomnolent, sleeping up to 12–14 hours per day [76]. Sleep in alcoholics is disturbed both on drinking nights and on nights during withdrawal. During periods of heavy drinking and up to 2 years after discontinuation of alcohol intake, sleep consists mainly of reduced NREM states, while REM sleep is suppressed and sleep duration is short, with sleep of the second half of a normal 8-hour bedtime being fragmented [77]. Rates of insomnia in this population are reported to be between 40% and 70%. Interestingly, those alcohol users who have a good prognosis for recovery are those individuals who tend to return to normal ratios of NREM/REM sleep and who overall sleep well [77]. Excessive alcohol consumption can cause depressive-like states—indeed, ethanol is classified as a depressant drug, mainly through its sedative effects via GABA facilitation and inhibition of glutamatergic NMDA function [77]. Finally, the relationship between disrupted sleep and various anxiety-related disorders is well recognized, but the cause and effect can be difficult to untangle. For example, insomnia predisposes individuals to anxiety which, in turn, precipitates sleep disruption that then increases the likelihood of panic. Conversely, studies have shown that sleep problems may actually precede conditions such as anxiety and depression [71, 78].

It is perhaps significant that behavioural abnormalities similar to those seen in psychiatric disorders can be induced in healthy individuals by sleep deprivation [79–84] or transitory circadian desynchronization [85]. For example, SCRD may exacerbate or even contribute to the cognitive impairments of schizophrenia patients. Consistent with this, associations between cognitive performance and specific sleep or circadian parameters are present in medication-naïve [86], medicated [57, 87–92], and unmedicated schizophrenia patients [93]. For example, the severity of patients' cognitive symptoms is inversely related to slow-wave sleep duration and REM sleep density [93], and the amplitude of rest–activity rhythms is strongly associated with performance in cognitive tasks that assess distractibility, reaction time, and verbal fluency [57]. A correlation is also present between attentional set-shifting performance and REM sleep latency [94]. Similar associations are evident in healthy individuals; performance in the go/no-go task (a test of response inhibition) is associated with multiple slow-wave sleep parameters [95].

Sleep makes a crucial contribution to memory consolidation [28]. Reduced overnight consolidation of procedural learning has been demonstrated in schizophrenia patients [96], and these deficits were accompanied by reduced slow-wave sleep duration [89]. Another study with schizophrenia patients showed an association between sleep spindle activity during stage 2 NREM sleep and overnight improvements in a finger-tapping, sequence-learning task [90, 91]. Sleep spindle activity is significantly reduced in schizophrenia patients [97].

In schizophrenia, where again we have the most detailed studies, positive symptoms appear to be aggravated or even triggered by SCRD. In healthy human subjects, sleep deprivation results in increased perceptual distortions [82, 98], greater paranoia [99], and reduced prepulse inhibition [82]. Clinically, sleep disturbance is a significant risk factor for the first episode of psychosis [100], as well as for relapse in recovering patients [101]. Severe sleep disturbance often precedes the onset of psychotic episodes in schizophrenia patients [59, 102, 103], while it is also predictive of the maintenance of these symptoms [103]. In addition, the severity of sleep disruption is positively correlated with the severity of psychotic symptoms [102]. Finally, the positive symptoms of schizophrenia are associated with high-frequency EEG episodes in sleep [104]. It is also interesting to note that circadian desynchronization increases negative mood, irritability, and affective volatility in healthy volunteers [85, 105]. A total of 24 hours of sleep deprivation in healthy human subjects also leads to anhedonia [82], one of the core negative symptoms of schizophrenia. Consistent with this, improvements in sleep quality are frequently correlated with amelioration of negative symptoms in schizophrenia patients [68, 106]. Moreover, the negative symptoms of schizophrenia are associated with reduced REM sleep latency and various slow-wave sleep deficits [94, 107–109]. Likewise, in adolescents at ultra-high risk for psychosis, sleep disruption is associated with greater negative symptom severity [110]. Collectively, such associations hint at causal mechanisms, and therefore possible new therapeutic targets for improved health in psychiatric disorders.

## Shared neuropathophysiology

What therefore could be the cause of SCRD in psychiatric disorders? One possibility is a shared dysfunction in common brain mechanisms (for example, specific enzymes, neuroreceptors, or neurotransmitter pathways) that contribute to the observed abnormalities [111]. According to this hypothesis, SCRD is not a consequence of the psychiatric disorder but is a core symptom intrinsically rooted in its underlying neuropathophysiology. This is plausible, given that psychiatric disorder implicates distributed brain circuits, affecting multiple neurotransmitter systems [112], many of which overlap with those involved in sleep regulation [113]. Dopamine, glutamate, and serotonin are all implicated in psychiatric disorder, while all three neurotransmitters are involved in sleep and circadian function. Moreover, multiple candidate genes for psychiatric disorder have a credible biological connection with sleep and circadian function within the brain. If these genes are the substrates of the comorbidity, their manipulation should result in both SCRD and disorder-relevant behavioural abnormalities (for example, impaired memory or reduced prepulse inhibition). Although this prediction is very difficult to address in humans, it can be tested using animal models. Indeed, there is a new, but rapidly growing, literature which speaks to this question [111].

## Studies in rodents

Just as sleep deprivation can trigger psychiatric symptoms in healthy humans, the same is true in wildtype rodents. NMDA receptor (NMDAR) antagonist-induced hyperlocomotion, a schizophrenia-relevant behaviour, is heightened by sleep deprivation in male Wistar rats [114]. Sleep deprivation is also known to cause cognitive deficits; it impairs object recognition memory [115, 116], spatial recognition memory [117, 118], long-term spatial memory in the Morris water maze [119–123] and radial arm maze [124], and attentional performance in the 5-choice serial reaction time task [125]. These findings appear to reflect genuine memory deficits, as partial sleep deprivation (by gentle handling) has little effect on exploratory locomotor activity or on indices of stress such as plasma corticosterone or adrenocorticotrophic hormone levels [116]. In rats, sleep deprivation impairs prepulse inhibition [126–128], which may be relevant to the cognitive symptoms of psychiatric disorder.

Disrupted circadian rhythms and complete arrhythmia can be induced in healthy hamsters by a single light treatment—a combination of a nocturnal light pulse and a phase delay in the light/dark (LD) cycle. Crucially, this also impairs object recognition memory performance [129, 130]. In mice, circadian rhythms can be disrupted with T7 cycles, ultradian LD cycles consisting of a 3.5-hour light phase followed by a 3.5-hour dark phase [131]. This leads to lengthening of the body temperature and rest–activity rhythms, but no change in total sleep time, REM sleep time, or the rhythmic expression of *Per2* in the SCN [132]. T7 cycles impair object recognition memory performance, although it is unclear whether this impairment reflects a genuine memory deficit or a reduction in object exploration, as locomotor activity data were not reported [131].

## Clock gene transgenic mice

Genetic manipulation of core clock genes can induce SCRD. Under 12:12 LD, circadian rhythmicity is unaffected in *Cry* single-knockout (*Cry1−/−* and *Cry2−/−*) and *Cry* double-knockout (*Cry1/*

$2^{-/-}$) mice [133, 134]. However, $Cry1^{-/-}$ mice have a shortened endogenous period and $Cry2^{-/-}$ have a lengthened endogenous period, while $Cry1/2^{-/-}$ mice become completely arrhythmic in constant darkness [133, 134]. Significantly, object recognition memory performance is impaired in $Cry1^{-/-}$, $Cry2^{-/-}$, and $Cry1/2^{-/-}$ mice. These deficits cannot be explained in terms of altered activity, since total object exploration does not differ between knockouts and wildtypes. They may be related to altered anxiety, however, as all three models exhibit heightened anxiety in the elevated plus maze [135].

## Moving from correlation to causality and new treatment targets

SCRD is rarely targeted for treatment in psychiatric patients, but when it is, individuals report improvements in both sleep quality and psychiatric symptoms. Treating insomnia with the $GABA_B$ receptor agonist sodium oxybate leads to an improvement in both the sleep quality and the negative symptoms of schizophrenia patients [136]. In another study, insomnia was treated with cognitive behavioural therapy (CBT) in 15 patients with persistent persecutory delusions and schizophrenia [58]. At least two-thirds of participants showed a substantial (>25%) improvement in insomnia, while approximately half showed a substantial (>25%) reduction in persecutory delusions. There were also reductions in hallucinations, anxiety, and depression. These studies represent an important advance, as they are the first to demonstrate that the targeted treatment of sleep disruption in schizophrenia patients can yield improvements in their 'classical' behavioural symptoms. This suggests that SCRD can make a causal contribution to the behavioural symptoms of psychiatric patients. However, both studies should be interpreted with caution, due to a number of methodological limitations; the sample sizes were small, the studies did not include control groups, and patients received medication throughout the studies. However, such issues were addressed in a very recent study where 3755 university students across the UK were randomized into two groups. One group received online CBT for insomnia; the other group did not but had access to standard treatments. The aims of the study were to explore whether sleep disruption is a driving factor in the occurrence of paranoia, hallucinatory experiences, and other mental health problems in young adults (average age of 25 years). Individuals who received the CBT intervention showed large reductions in insomnia, as well as significant reductions in paranoia and hallucinatory experiences. The treatment also led to improvements in depression, anxiety, nightmares, psychological well-being, and daytime work and home functioning [137]. These studies support the proposal that treating disrupted sleep could provide a key route for improving mental health.

SCRD in psychiatric illness such as schizophrenia has often been attributed to the side effects of medication. Although intuitively plausible, drug effects cannot be the only cause of SCRD in schizophrenia, since SCRD affects both medication-naïve [70] and medicated patients [71]. Indeed, SCRD often precedes the diagnosis of schizophrenia, prior to any medication [70, 72]. Recent and potentially exciting results have shown that dopamine antagonist drugs might actually improve sleep quality in schizophrenia [55, 71, 73], possibly due to their strong sedative effects [74]. So-called typical antipsychotics improve sleep efficiency and total sleep time [55], while atypical drugs for psychosis are even more effective at improving sleep quality in schizophrenia patients [75] (also see Chapter 64). It is also possible that antipsychotic medication might also act directly upon clock gene expression. Such actions are currently being explored by researchers at the University of Oxford.

### More evidence from rodent models

SCRD can also be targeted in rodent models that demonstrate simultaneous SCRD and psychiatric-relevant behavioural abnormalities. If SCRD makes a causal contribution to the behavioural symptoms of psychiatric disorders, then such interventions should ameliorate their behavioural impairments. Proof-of-principle for this approach is provided by the targeted 'treatment' of SCRD in the R6/2 transgenic mouse model of Huntington's disease, which displays a progressive disintegration of sleep and circadian rhythmicity across its lifespan [138]. Interventions employed include bright light therapy [139], temporally scheduled feeding [140, 141], temporally scheduled exercise [139], and pharmacological imposition of a daily sleep/wake cycle with the sedative drug alprazolam [142, 143] and/or the vigilance-promoting drug modafinil [143]. Bright light therapy and scheduled exercise delayed the disintegration of rest–activity rhythms [139], while scheduled feeding also restored behavioural rhythmicity [140, 141] but had no impact on cognitive performance [141]. Strikingly, however, alprazolam administration improved behavioural rhythmicity *and* slowed cognitive decline in the R6/2 model [140, 141]. This suggests that SCRD causally contributes to cognitive dysfunction in Huntington's disease. The same experimental approach could easily be applied to a psychiatric-relevant mouse model, or indeed any neuropsychiatrically relevant animal model. Temporally scheduled exercise has already been shown to improve behavioural rhythmicity in the schizophrenia-relevant $Vipr2^{-/-}$ mouse model [144], although cognitive performance was not assessed.

### Treatments on the horizon?

Despite our growing knowledge of the molecular mechanisms underlying the 24-hour circadian clock and its role in the development of psychiatric disease, there are very limited therapeutic options that have been developed to act on the clock directly to reduce SCRD. As light is the primary entraining agent for the SCN, bright light therapies and CBTs that strengthen natural *zeitgebers* such as scheduled outdoor exercise [145, 146] have been shown to have some success. However, potent pharmacological interventions are still lacking. Melatonin has long been characterized as an output of the circadian clock and can be used to modify the phase of the clock, presumably by acting via melatonin receptors that are expressed within the neurons of the SCN and widely across the multiple other cell populations throughout the body. Melatonin has therefore been studied as a possible chronotherapeutic drug and shows promise in certain circadian-related conditions [147, 148]. Prolonged-release melatonin (tradename Circadin) is used to treat primary insomnia [149] in the aged, and the agonist agomelatine in the treatment of major depressive disorder [150]. Most recently, tasimelteon was approved in the United States for the orphan circadian disorder non-24-hour sleep–wake disorder in the totally blind [151]. Targeting the melatonin system, however, has limited efficacy; for example, tasimelteon showed a beneficial effect on stabilizing sleep–wake in 20% of the patient population after 1 month of treatment [151]. As a consequence, recent efforts have focused on developing alternatives, mainly targeting the core clock. Solt *et al.* reported a novel

REV-ERBa receptor agonist was effective at regulating both sleep as well as metabolism in mice [152, 153], and Hirota *et al.* have developed a small-molecule cryptochrome activator [154]. An alternative strategy that is yet to be employed is the development of molecules that act on the light input pathway to the clock, providing a pharmacological replacement for light for the treatment of SCRD. Such an approach could yield an exciting alternative.

## Future perspectives

In conclusion, there are clear links between SCRD and the behavioural symptoms of psychiatric illness, although the mechanistic bases of these associations remain to be clearly defined. Rather than considering SCRD to be a by-product of medication or social isolation in psychiatric disease, it might be better conceptualized as a central feature of the condition. While SCRD is unlikely to be a primary cause of psychiatric disease, the treatment of sleep disturbances can yield improvements in the disorder's core symptoms and has the potential to significantly improve the quality of life of patients and their carers.

## REFERENCES

1. Johnson CH, Elliott JA, Foster R, Honma K, Kronauer RE. Fundamental properties of circadian rhythms. In: Dunlap JC, Loros JJ, DeCoursey PJ, editors. *Chronobiology: Biological Timekeeping*. Sunderland: Sinauer Associates; 2004. pp. 67–106.
2. Foster RG, Kreitzman L. The rhythms of life: what your body clock means to you! *Exp Physiol*. 2014;99:599–606.
3. Hastings MH. Circadian clocks. *Curr Biol*. 1997;7:R670–2.
4. Bell-Pedersen D, Cassone VM, Earnest DJ, *et al*. Circadian rhythms from multiple oscillators: lessons from diverse organisms. *Nat Rev Genet*. 2005;6:544–56.
5. DeCoursey PJ, Krulas JR, Mele G, Holley DC. Circadian performance of suprachiasmatic nuclei (SCN)-lesioned antelope ground squirrels in a desert enclosure. *Physiol Behav*. 1997;62:1099–108.
6. Welsh DK, Logothetis DE, Meister M, Reppert SM. Individual neurons dissociated from rat suprachiasmatic nucleus express independently phased circadian firing rhythms. *Neuron*. 1995;14:697–706.
7. Moore RY, Eichler VB. Loss of a circadian adrenal corticosterone rhythm following suprachiasmatic lesions in the rat. *Brain Res*. 1972;42:201–6.
8. Stephan FK, Zucker I. Circadian rhythms in drinking behavior and locomotor activity of rats are eliminated by hypothalamic lesions. *Proc Natl Acad Sci U S A*. 1972;69:1583–6.
9. DeCoursey PJ, Buggy J. Circadian rhythmicity after neural transplant to hamster third ventricle: specificity of suprachiasmatic nuclei. *Brain Res*. 1989;500:263–75.
10. Ralph MR, Foster RG, Davis FC, Menaker M. Transplanted suprachiasmatic nucleus determines circadian period. *Science*. 1990;247:975–8.
11. Hastings M. The brain, circadian rhythms, and clock genes. *BMJ*. 1998;317:1704–7.
12. Inouye ST, Kawamura H. Persistence of circadian rhythmicity in a mammalian hypothalamic "island" containing the suprachiasmatic nucleus. *Proc Natl Acad Sci U S A*. 1979;76:5962–6.
13. Schwartz WJ, Gainer H. Suprachiasmatic nucleus: use of 14C-labeled deoxyglucose uptake as a functional marker. *Science*. 1977;197:1089–91.
14. Gillette MU. The suprachiasmatic nuclei: circadian phase-shifts induced at the time of hypothalamic slice preparation are preserved *in vitro*. *Brain Res*. 1986;379:176–81.
15. Reppert SM, Weaver DR. Coordination of circadian timing in mammals. *Nature*. 2002;418:935–41.
16. Eide EJ, Woolf MF, Kang H, *et al*. Control of mammalian circadian rhythm by CKIepsilon-regulated proteasome-mediated PER2 degradation. *Mol Cell Biol*. 2005;25:2795–807.
17. Guler AD, Ecker JL, Lall GS, *et al*. Melanopsin cells are the principal conduits for rod-cone input to non-image-forming vision. *Nature*. 2008;453:102–5.
18. Hattar S, Kumar M, Park A, *et al*. Central projections of melanopsin-expressing retinal ganglion cells in the mouse. *J Comp Neurol*. 2006;497:326–49.
19. Provencio I, Cooper HM, Foster RG. Retinal projections in mice with inherited retinal degeneration: implications for circadian photoentrainment. *J Comp Neurol*. 1998;395:417–39.
20. Colwell CS. Linking neural activity and molecular oscillations in the SCN. *Nat Rev Neurosci*. 2011;12:553–69.
21. Hastings MH, Maywood ES, Reddy AB. Two decades of circadian time. *J Neuroendocrinol*. 2008;20:812–19.
22. Guilding C, Piggins HD. Challenging the omnipotence of the suprachiasmatic timekeeper: are circadian oscillators present throughout the mammalian brain? *Eur J Neurosci*. 2007;25:3195–216.
23. Balsalobre A, Damiola F, Schibler U. A serum shock induces circadian gene expression in mammalian tissue culture cells. *Cell*. 1998;93:929–37.
24. Yoo SH, Yamazaki S, Lowrey PL, *et al*. PERIOD2: LUCIFERASE real-time reporting of circadian dynamics reveals persistent circadian oscillations in mouse peripheral tissues. *Proc Natl Acad Sci U S A*. 2004;101:5339–46.
25. Duffield GE. DNA microarray analyses of circadian timing: the genomic basis of biological time. *J Neuroendocrinol*. 2003;15:991–1002.
26. Zepelin H, Siegel JM, Tobler I. Mammalian sleep. In: Kryger MH, Roth T, Dement WC, editors. *Principles and Practices of Sleep Medicine*. Philadelphia, PA: Saunders; 2005. pp. 91–100.
27. Bryant PA, Trinder J, Curtis N. Sick and tired: does sleep have a vital role in the immune system? *Nat Rev Immunol*. 2004;4:457–67.
28. Stickgold R. Sleep-dependent memory consolidation. *Nature*. 2005;437:1272–8.
29. Tononi G, Cirelli C. Sleep function and synaptic homeostasis. *Sleep Med Rev*. 2006;10:49–62.
30. Colten HR, Altevogt BM. *Sleep Physiology. Sleep Disorders and Sleep Deprivation: An Unmet Public Health Problem*. Washington, DC: National Academies Press; 2006.
31. Schulz H. Rethinking sleep analysis: comment on the AASM Manual for the Scoring of Sleep and Associated Events. *J Clin Sleep Med*. 2008;4:99–103.
32. Silber MH, Ancoli-Israel S, Bonnet MH, *et al*. The visual scoring of sleep in adults. *J Clin Sleep Med*. 2007;3:121–31.
33. Aserinsky E, Kleitman N. Regularly occurring periods of eye motility, and concomitant phenomena, during sleep. *Science*. 1953;118:273–4.
34. Schwartz JR, Roth T. Neurophysiology of sleep and wakefulness: basic science and clinical implications. *Curr Neuropharmacol*. 2008;6:367–78.
35. Fuller PM, Gooley JJ, Saper CB. Neurobiology of the sleep-wake cycle: sleep architecture, circadian regulation, and regulatory feedback. *J Biol Rhythms*. 2006;21:482–93.

36. Saper CB, Chou TC, Scammell TE. The sleep switch: hypothalamic control of sleep and wakefulness. *Trends Neurosci.* 2001;24:726–31.

37. Saper CB, Scammell TE, Lu J. Hypothalamic regulation of sleep and circadian rhythms. *Nature.* 2005;437:1257–63.

38. McCormick DA. Cholinergic and noradrenergic modulation of thalamocortical processing. *Trends Neurosci.* 1989;12:215–21.

39. Verret L, Goutagny R, Fort P, *et al.* A role of melanin-concentrating hormone producing neurons in the central regulation of paradoxical sleep. *BMC Neurosci.* 2003;4:19.

40. Lee MG, Hassani OK, Alonso A, Jones BE. Cholinergic basal forebrain neurons burst with theta during waking and paradoxical sleep. *J Neurosci.* 2005;25:4365–9.

41. Sherin JE, Shiromani PJ, McCarley RW, Saper CB. Activation of ventrolateral preoptic neurons during sleep. *Science.* 1996;271:216–19.

42. Gaus SE, Strecker RE, Tate BA, Parker RA, Saper CB. Ventrolateral preoptic nucleus contains sleep-active, galaninergic neurons in multiple mammalian species. *Neuroscience.* 2002;115:285–94.

43. Sherin JE, Elmquist JK, Torrealba F, Saper CB. Innervation of histaminergic tuberomammillary neurons by GABAergic and galaninergic neurons in the ventrolateral preoptic nucleus of the rat. *J Neurosci.* 1998;18:4705–21.

44. Lu J, Greco MA, Shiromani P, Saper CB. Effect of lesions of the ventrolateral preoptic nucleus on NREM and REM sleep. *J Neurosci.* 2000;20:3830–42.

45. Chou TC, Bjorkum AA, Gaus SE, Lu J, Scammell TE, Saper CB. Afferents to the ventrolateral preoptic nucleus. *J Neurosci.* 2002;22:977–90.

46. Achermann P, Borbely AA. Mathematical models of sleep regulation. *Front Biosci.* 2003;8:s683–93.

47. Borbely AA, Tobler I. Homeostatic and circadian principles in sleep regulation in the rat. In: McGinty D, editor. *Brain Mechanisms of Sleep.* New York, NY: Raven Press; 1985. pp. 35–44.

48. Benington JH, Kodali SK, Heller HC. Stimulation of A1 adenosine receptors mimics the electroencephalographic effects of sleep deprivation. *Brain Res.* 1995;692:79–85.

49. Scammell TE, Estabrooke IV, McCarthy MT, *et al.* Hypothalamic arousal regions are activated during modafinil-induced wakefulness. *J Neurosci.* 2000;20:8620–8.

50. Strecker RE, Morairty S, Thakkar MM, *et al.* Adenosinergic modulation of basal forebrain and preoptic/anterior hypothalamic neuronal activity in the control of behavioral state. *Behav Brain Res.* 2000;115:183–204.

51. Hines DJ, Schmitt LI, Hines RM, Moss SJ, Haydon PG. Antidepressant effects of sleep deprivation require astrocyte-dependent adenosine mediated signaling. *Transl Psychiatry.* 2013;3:e212.

52. Edgar DM, Dement WC, Fuller CA. Effect of SCN lesions on sleep in squirrel monkeys: evidence for opponent processes in sleep-wake regulation. *J Neurosci.* 1993;13:1065–79.

53. Chou TC, Scammell TE, Gooley JJ, Gaus SE, Saper CB, Lu J. Critical role of dorsomedial hypothalamic nucleus in a wide range of behavioral circadian rhythms. *J Neurosci.* 2003;23:10691–702.

54. Manoach DS, Stickgold R. Does abnormal sleep impair memory consolidation in schizophrenia? *Front Hum Neurosci.* 2009;3:21.

55. Cohrs S. Sleep disturbances in patients with schizophrenia: impact and effect of antipsychotics. *CNS Drugs.* 2008;22:939–62.

56. Afonso P, Brissos S, Figueira ML, Paiva T. Schizophrenia patients with predominantly positive symptoms have more disturbed sleep-wake cycles measured by actigraphy. *Psychiatry Res.* 2011;189:62–6.

57. Bromundt V, Koster M, Georgiev-Kill A, *et al.* Sleep-wake cycles and cognitive functioning in schizophrenia. *Br J Psychiatry.* 2011;198:269–76.

58. Myers E, Startup H, Freeman D. Cognitive behavioural treatment of insomnia in individuals with persistent persecutory delusions: a pilot trial. *J Behav Ther Exp Psychiatry.* 2011;42:330–6.

59. Waters F, Sinclair C, Rock D, Jablensky A, Foster RG, Wulff K. Daily variations in sleep-wake patterns and severity of psychopathology: a pilot study in community-dwelling individuals with chronic schizophrenia. *Psychiatry Res.* 2011;187:304–6.

60. Benca RM, Obermeyer WH, Thisted RA, Gillin J. Sleep and psychiatric disorders: a meta-analysis. *Arch Gen Psychiatry.* 1992;49:651–68.

61. Keshavan MS, Reynolds CF, Kupfer DJ. Electroencephalographic sleep in schizophrenia: a critical review. *Compr Psychiatry.* 1990;31:34–47.

62. Monti JM, BaHammam AS, Pandi-Perumal SR, *et al.* Sleep and circadian rhythm dysregulation in schizophrenia. *Prog Neuropsychopharmacol Biol Psychiatry.* 2013;43:209–16.

63. Martin J, Jeste DV, Caligiuri MP, Patterson T, Heaton R, Ancoli-Israel S. Actigraphic estimates of circadian rhythms and sleep/wake in older schizophrenia patients. *Schizophr Res.* 2001;47:77–86.

64. Martin JL, Jeste DV, Ancoli-Israel S. Older schizophrenia patients have more disrupted sleep and circadian rhythms than age-matched comparison subjects. *J Psychiatr Res.* 2005;39:251–9.

65. Wulff K, Joyce E, Middleton B, Dijk DJ, Foster RG. The suitability of actigraphy, diary data, and urinary melatonin profiles for quantitative assessment of sleep disturbances in schizophrenia: a case report. *Chronobiol Int.* 2006;23:485–95.

66. Wulff K, Porcheret K, Cussans E, Foster RG. Sleep and circadian rhythm disturbances: multiple genes and multiple phenotypes. *Curr Opin Genet Dev.* 2009;19:237–46.

67. Goldman M, Tandon R, DeQuardo JR, Taylor SF, Goodson J, McGrath M. Biological predictors of 1-year outcome in schizophrenia in males and females. *Schizophr Res.* 1996;21:65–73.

68. Hofstetter JR, Lysaker PH, Mayeda AR. Quality of sleep in patients with schizophrenia is associated with quality of life and coping. *BMC Psychiatry.* 2005;5:13.

69. Auslander LA, Jeste DV. Perceptions of problems and needs for service among middle-aged and elderly outpatients with schizophrenia and related psychotic disorders. *Community Ment Health J.* 2002;38:391–402.

70. Pigeon WR, Hegel M, Unutzer J, *et al.* Is insomnia a perpetuating factor for late-life depression in the IMPACT cohort? *Sleep.* 2008;31:481–8.

71. Posmontier B. Sleep quality in women with and without postpartum depression. *J Obstet Gynecol Neonatal Nurs.* 2008;37:722–35; quiz 35–7.

72. Levitt AJ, Boyle MH. The impact of latitude on the prevalence of seasonal depression. *Can J Psychiatry.* 2002;47:361–7.

73. Axelsson J, Ragnarsdottir S, Pind J, Sigbjornsson R. Daylight availability: a poor predictor of depression in Iceland. *Int J Circumpolar Health.* 2004;63:267–76.

74. Wirz-Justice A. Chronobiology and psychiatry. *Sleep Med Rev.* 2007;11:423–7.

75. Plante DT, Winkelman JW. Sleep disturbance in bipolar disorder: therapeutic implications. *Am J Psychiatry.* 2008;165:830–43.

76. Krystal AD. Treating the health, quality of life, and functional impairments in insomnia. *J Clin Sleep Med.* 2007;3:63–72.

77. Roehrs T, Roth T. Sleep, sleepiness, sleep disorders and alcohol use and abuse. *Sleep Med Rev.* 2001;5:287–97.

78. Monti JM, Monti D. Sleep disturbance in generalized anxiety disorder and its treatment. *Sleep Med Rev*. 2000;4:263–76.

79. Chee MW, Chuah LY. Functional neuroimaging insights into how sleep and sleep deprivation affect memory and cognition. *Curr Opin Neurol*. 2008;21:417–23.

80. Alhola P, Polo-Kantola P. Sleep deprivation: Impact on cognitive performance. *Neuropsychiatr Dis Treat*. 2007;3:553–67.

81. Horne JA. Human sleep, sleep loss and behaviour. Implications for the prefrontal cortex and psychiatric disorder. *Br J Psychiatry*. 1993;162:413–19.

82. Petrovsky N, Ettinger U, Hill A, *et al*. Sleep deprivation disrupts prepulse inhibition and induces psychosis-like symptoms in healthy humans. *J Neurosci*. 2014;34:9134–40.

83. Ratcliff R, Van Dongen HP. Sleep deprivation affects multiple distinct cognitive processes. *Psychon Bull Rev*. 2009;16:742–51.

84. Van Dongen HP, Maislin G, Mullington JM, Dinges DF. The cumulative cost of additional wakefulness: dose-response effects on neurobehavioral functions and sleep physiology from chronic sleep restriction and total sleep deprivation. *Sleep*. 2003;26:117–26.

85. Kyriacou CP, Hastings MH. Circadian clocks: genes, sleep, and cognition. *Trends Cogn Sci*. 2010;14:259–67.

86. Forest G, Poulin J, Daoust A-M, Lussier I, Stip E, Godbout R. Attention and non-REM sleep in neuroleptic-naive persons with schizophrenia and control participants. *Psychiatry Res*. 2007;149:33–40.

87. Goder R, Boigs M, Braun S, *et al*. Impairment of visuospatial memory is associated with decreased slow wave sleep in schizophrenia. *J Psychiatr Res*. 2004;38:591–9.

88. Goder R, Fritzer G, Gottwald B, *et al*. Effects of olanzapine on slow wave sleep, sleep spindles and sleep-related memory consolidation in schizophrenia. *Pharmacopsychiatry*. 2008;41:92–9.

89. Manoach DS, Thakkar KN, Stroynowski E, *et al*. Reduced overnight consolidation of procedural learning in chronic medicated schizophrenia is related to specific sleep stages. *J Psychiatr Res*. 2010;44:112–20.

90. Wamsley EJ, Shinn AK, Tucker MA, *et al*. The effects of eszopiclone on sleep spindles and memory consolidation in schizophrenia: a randomized placebo-controlled trial. *Sleep*. 2013;36:1369–76.

91. Wamsley EJ, Tucker MA, Shinn AK, *et al*. Reduced sleep spindles and spindle coherence in schizophrenia: mechanisms of impaired memory consolidation? *Biol Psychiatry*. 2012;71:154–61.

92. Wulff K, Joyce E. Circadian rhythms and cognition in schizophrenia. *Br J Psychiatry*. 2011;198:250–2.

93. Yang C, Winkelman JW. Clinical significance of sleep EEG abnormalities in chronic schizophrenia. *Schizophr Res*. 2006;82:251–60.

94. Das M, Das R, Khastgir U, Goswami U. REM sleep latency and neurocognitive dysfunction in schizophrenia. *Indian J Psychiatry*. 2005;47:133–8.

95. Mander BA, Reid KJ, Baron KG, *et al*. EEG measures index neural and cognitive recovery from sleep deprivation. *J Neurosci*. 2010;30:2686–93.

96. Manoach DS, Cain MS, Vangel MG, Khurana A, Goff DC, Stickgold R. A failure of sleep-dependent procedural learning in chronic, medicated schizophrenia. *Biol Psychiatry*. 2004;56:951–6.

97. Ferrarelli F, Huber R, Peterson MJ, *et al*. Reduced sleep spindle activity in schizophrenia patients. *Am J Psychiatry*. 2007;164:483–92.

98. Babkoff H, Sing HC, Thorne DR, Genser SG, Hegge FW. Perceptual distortions and hallucinations reported during the course of sleep deprivation. *Percept Mot Skills*. 1989;68(3 Pt 1):787–98.

99. Freeman D, Pugh K, Vorontsova N, Southgate L. Insomnia and paranoia. *Schizophr Res*. 2009;108(1-3):280–4.

100. Ruhrmann S, Schultze-Lutter F, Salokangas RK, *et al*. Prediction of psychosis in adolescents and young adults at high risk: results from the prospective European prediction of psychosis study. *Arch Gen Psychiatry*. 2010;67:241–51.

101. Birchwood M, Smith J, Macmillan F, *et al*. Predicting relapse in schizophrenia: the development and implementation of an early signs monitoring system using patients and families as observers, a preliminary investigation. *Psychol Med*. 1989;19:649–56.

102. Monti JM, Monti D. Sleep in schizophrenia patients and the effects of antipsychotic drugs. *Sleep Med Rev*. 2004;8:133–48.

103. Freeman D, Stahl D, McManus S, *et al*. Insomnia, worry, anxiety and depression as predictors of the occurrence and persistence of paranoid thinking. *Soc Psychiatry Psychiatr Epidemiol*. 2012;47:1195–203.

104. Tekell JL, Hoffmann R, Hendrickse W, Greene RW, Rush AJ, Armitage R. High frequency EEG activity during sleep: characteristics in schizophrenia and depression. *Clin EEG Neurosci*. 2005;36:25–35.

105. Murray G, Harvey A. Circadian rhythms and sleep in bipolar disorder. *Bipolar Disord*. 2010;12:459–72.

106. Yamashita H, Mori K, Nagao M, Okamoto Y, Morinobu S, Yamawaki S. Effects of changing from typical to atypical antipsychotic drugs on subjective sleep quality in patients with schizophrenia in a Japanese population. *J Clin Psychiatry*. 2004;65:1525–30.

107. Ganguli R, Reynolds CF, 3rd, Kupfer DJ. Electroencephalographic sleep in young, never-medicated schizophrenics. A comparison with delusional and nondelusional depressives and with healthy controls. *Arch Gen Psychiatry*. 1987;44:36–44.

108. Kato M, Kajimura N, Okuma T, *et al*. Association between delta waves during sleep and negative symptoms in schizophrenia. Pharmaco-eeg studies by using structurally different hypnotics. *Neuropsychobiology*. 1999;39:165–72.

109. van Kammen DP, van Kammen WB, Peters J, Goetz K, Neylan T. Decreased slow-wave sleep and enlarged lateral ventricles in schizophrenia. *Neuropsychopharmacology*. 1988;1:265–71.

110. Lunsford-Avery JR, Orr JM, Gupta T, *et al*. Sleep dysfunction and thalamic abnormalities in adolescents at ultra high-risk for psychosis. *Schizophr Res*. 2013;151:148–53.

111. Pritchett D, Wulff K, Oliver PL, *et al*. Evaluating the links between schizophrenia and sleep and circadian rhythm disruption. *J Neural Transm*. 2012;119:1061–75.

112. Weinberger DR, Harrison PJ. *Schizophrenia*, third edition. Oxford: Wiley-Blackwell; 2011.

113. Wulff K, Gatti S, Wettstein JG, Foster RG. Sleep and circadian rhythm disruption in psychiatric and neurodegenerative disease. *Nat Rev Neurosci*. 2010;11:589–99.

114. Dubiela FP, Messias MF, Moreira KD, *et al*. Reciprocal interactions between MK-801, sleep deprivation and recovery in modulating rat behaviour. *Behav Brain Res*. 2011;216:180–5.

115. Palchykova S, Crestani F, Meerlo P, Tobler I. Sleep deprivation and daily torpor impair object recognition in Djungarian hamsters. *Physiol Behav*. 2006;87:144–53.

116. Palchykova S, Winsky-Sommerer R, Meerlo P, Durr R, Tobler I. Sleep deprivation impairs object recognition in mice. *Neurobiol Learn Mem*. 2006;85:263–71.

117. Binder S, Baier PC, Molle M, Inostroza M, Born J, Marshall L. Sleep enhances memory consolidation in the hippocampus-dependent object-place recognition task in rats. *Neurobiol Learn Mem*. 2012;97:213–19.

118. Inostroza M, Binder S, Born J. Sleep-dependency of episodic-like memory consolidation in rats. *Behav Brain Res*. 2013;237:15–22.

119. Hajali V, Sheibani V, Esmaeili-Mahani S, Shabani M. Female rats are more susceptible to the deleterious effects of paradoxical sleep deprivation on cognitive performance. *Behav Brain Res.* 2012;228:311–18.

120. Smith C, Rose GM. Evidence for a paradoxical sleep window for place learning in the Morris water maze. *Physiol Behav.* 1996;59:93–7.

121. Yang RH, Hu SJ, Wang Y, Zhang WB, Luo WJ, Chen JY. Paradoxical sleep deprivation impairs spatial learning and affects membrane excitability and mitochondrial protein in the hippocampus. *Brain Res.* 2008;1230:224–32.

122. Youngblood BD, Smagin GN, Elkins PD, Ryan DH, Harris RB. The effects of paradoxical sleep deprivation and valine on spatial learning and brain 5-HT metabolism. *Physiol Behav.* 1999;67:643–9.

123. Youngblood BD, Zhou J, Smagin GN, Ryan DH, Harris RB. Sleep deprivation by the "flower pot" technique and spatial reference memory. *Physiol Behav.* 1997;61:249–56.

124. Smith CT, Conway JM, Rose GM. Brief paradoxical sleep deprivation impairs reference, but not working, memory in the radial arm maze task. *Neurobiol Learn Mem.* 1998;69:211–17.

125. Cordova CA, Said BO, McCarley RW, Baxter MG, Chiba AA, Strecker RE. Sleep deprivation in rats produces attentional impairments on a 5-choice serial reaction time task. *Sleep.* 2006;29:69–76.

126. Chang HA, Liu YP, Tung CS, Chang CC, Tzeng NS, Huang SY. Effects of REM sleep deprivation on sensorimotor gating and startle habituation in rats: role of social isolation in early development. *Neurosci Lett.* 2014;575:63–7.

127. Frau R, Orru M, Puligheddu M, *et al.* Sleep deprivation disrupts prepulse inhibition of the startle reflex: reversal by antipsychotic drugs. *Int J Neuropsychopharmacol.* 2008;11:947–55.

128. Liu YP, Tung CS, Chuang CH, Lo SM, Ku YC. Tail-pinch stress and REM sleep deprivation differentially affect sensorimotor gating function in modafinil-treated rats. *Behav Brain Res.* 2011;219:98–104.

129. Ruby NF, Fernandez F, Garrett A, *et al.* Spatial memory and long-term object recognition are impaired by circadian arrhythmia and restored by the GABAAAntagonist pentylenetetrazole. *PLoS One.* 2013;8:e72433.

130. Ruby NF, Hwang CE, Wessells C, *et al.* Hippocampal-dependent learning requires a functional circadian system. *Proc Natl Acad Sci U S A.* 2008;105:15593–8.

131. LeGates TA, Altimus CM, Wang H, *et al.* Aberrant light directly impairs mood and learning through melanopsin-expressing neurons. *Nature.* 2012;491:594–8.

132. Altimus CM, Guler AD, Villa KL, McNeill DS, Legates TA, Hattar S. Rods-cones and melanopsin detect light and dark to modulate sleep independent of image formation. *Proc Natl Acad Sci U S A.* 2008;105:19998–20003.

133. van der Horst GT, Muijtjens M, Kobayashi K, *et al.* Mammalian Cry1 and Cry2 are essential for maintenance of circadian rhythms. *Nature.* 1999;398:627–30.

134. Vitaterna MH, Selby CP, Todo T, *et al.* Differential regulation of mammalian Period genes and circadian rhythmicity by cryptochromes 1 and 2. *Proc Natl Acad Sci U S A.* 1999;96:12114–19.

135. De Bundel D, Gangarossa G, Biever A, Bonnefont X, Valjent E. Cognitive dysfunction, elevated anxiety, and reduced cocaine response in circadian clock-deficient cryptochrome knockout mice. *Front Behav Neurosci.* 2013;7:152.

136. Kantrowitz JT, Oakman E, Bickel S, *et al.* The importance of a good night's sleep: an open-label trial of the sodium salt of gamma-hydroxybyturic acid in insomnia associated with schizophrenia. *Schizophr Res.* 2010;120:225–6.

137. Freeman D, Sheaves B, Goodwin GM, *et al.* The effects of improving sleep on mental health (OASIS): a randomised controlled trial with mediation analysis. *Lancet Psychiatry.* 2017;4:749–58.

138. Morton AJ, Wood NI, Hastings MH, Hurelbrink C, Barker RA, Maywood ES. Disintegration of the sleep-wake cycle and circadian timing in Huntington's disease. *J Neurosci.* 2005;25:157–63.

139. Cuesta M, Aungier J, Morton AJ. Behavioral therapy reverses circadian deficits in a transgenic mouse model of Huntington's disease. *Neurobiol Dis.* 2014;63:85–91.

140. Maywood ES, Fraenkel E, McAllister CJ, *et al.* Disruption of peripheral circadian timekeeping in a mouse model of Huntington's disease and its restoration by temporally scheduled feeding. *J Neurosci.* 2010;30:10199–204.

141. Skillings EA, Wood NI, Morton AJ. Beneficial effects of environmental enrichment and food entrainment in the R6/2 mouse model of Huntington's disease. *Brain Behav.* 2014;4:675–86.

142. Pallier PN, Maywood ES, Zheng Z, *et al.* Pharmacological imposition of sleep slows cognitive decline and reverses dysregulation of circadian gene expression in a transgenic mouse model of Huntington's disease. *J Neurosci.* 2007;27:7869–78.

143. Pallier PN, Morton AJ. Management of sleep/wake cycles improves cognitive function in a transgenic mouse model of Huntington's disease. *Brain Res.* 2009;1279:90–8.

144. Power A, Hughes AT, Samuels RE, Piggins HD. Rhythm-promoting actions of exercise in mice with deficient neuropeptide signaling. *J Biol Rhythms.* 2010;25:235–46.

145. Atkinson G, Edwards B, Reilly T, Waterhouse J. Exercise as a synchroniser of human circadian rhythms: an update and discussion of the methodological problems. *Eur J Appl Physiol.* 2007;99:331–41.

146. Zee PC, Attarian H, Videnovic A. Circadian rhythm abnormalities. *Continuum (Minneap Min).* 2013;19(1 Sleep Disorders):132–47.

147. Dahlitz M, Alvarez B, Vignau J, English J, Arendt J, Parkes JD. Delayed sleep phase syndrome response to melatonin. *Lancet.* 1991;337:1121–4.

148. Mundey K, Benloucif S, Harsanyi K, Dubocovich ML, Zee PC. Phase-dependent treatment of delayed sleep phase syndrome with melatonin. *Sleep.* 2005;28:1271–8.

149. Lemoine P, Wade AG, Katz A, Nir T, Zisapel N. Efficacy and safety of prolonged-release melatonin for insomnia in middle-aged and elderly patients with hypertension: a combined analysis of controlled clinical trials. *Integr Blood Press Control.* 2012;5:9–17.

150. Kennedy SH, Emsley R. Placebo-controlled trial of agomelatine in the treatment of major depressive disorder. *Eur Neuropsychopharmacol.* 2006;16:93–100.

151. Lockley SW, Dressman MA, Licamele L, *et al.* Tasimelteon for non-24-hour sleep-wake disorder in totally blind people (SET and RESET): two multicentre, randomised, double-masked, placebo-controlled phase 3 trials. *Lancet.* 2015;386:1754–64.

152. Banerjee S, Wang Y, Solt LA, *et al.* Pharmacological targeting of the mammalian clock regulates sleep architecture and emotional behaviour. *Nat Commun.* 2014;5:5759.

153. Solt LA, Wang Y, Banerjee S, *et al.* Regulation of circadian behaviour and metabolism by synthetic REV-ERB agonists. *Nature.* 2012;485:62–8.

154. Hirota T, Lee JW, St John PC, *et al.* Identification of small molecule activators of cryptochrome. *Science.* 2012;337:1094–7.

# 110

# Diagnosis of sleep and circadian rhythm disorder

*Kirstie Anderson*

## Introduction

In 400 BC, Hippocrates wrote 'sleep and watchfulness, both of them when immoderate, constitute disease'. Unfortunately modern doctors in training receive little or no training in sleep medicine [1]. Disrupted sleep has immediate and long-term consequences on physical and mental health. Sleep fulfils many functions, but arguably the most important is regulation of normal affect and cognition, including a vital role in memory consolidation and new learning [2–4].

As explained at the molecular level in Chapter 109 and the systems level in Chapter 111, sleep is controlled by two neuronal circuits. The homeostat drives an increasing pressure to sleep after every hour awake and the circadian rhythm drives alertness in the day and sleep at night, with light intensity as the strongest external timekeeper [5]. Both total sleep time and the circadian rhythm change over the course of our lives [6]. As teenagers and young adults, typical sleep need is 8–9 hours for the majority, with a tendency for a delay in the sleep phase such that many comfortably fall asleep after, rather than before, midnight [7]. There is a tendency to phase-advance (that is, fall asleep earlier) with ageing. Adults fall asleep by 30 minutes earlier every decade from the third decade onwards [8]. There is greater sleep fragmentation and increased time to fall asleep in healthy older adults with and without sleep complaints [9]. At least 30% of adults in the United States regularly sleep <6 hours a night [10]. Over 7 hours of sleep at night is the adult norm, and over 9 hours is necessary for many teenagers, as well as those repaying sleep debt [11].

The physiological definition of sleep shows us to be either awake or alternating between non-rapid eye movement (NREM) or rapid eye movement (REM) sleep at approximately 90- to 120-minute cycles (Fig. 110.1).

## Current classification of sleep disorders

Sleep disorders fall into one or more of four categories: hypersomnia, insomnia, circadian rhythm disorder, and parasomnia. Common night-time disorders also include restless legs syndrome and associated periodic limb movements of sleep. The 2014 International Classification of Sleep Disorder, third edition (ICSD-3) has been used for the diagnostic criteria [13]. In addition, the most recent diagnostic criteria for restless legs syndrome (http://www.irlssg.org) improved specificity of the diagnosis and highlighted both episodic and chronic symptoms [14].

## Taking a sleep history

A sleep history should be a short, but routine, part of all psychiatry consultations. Many sleep disorders can be accurately diagnosed by clinical history alone. A limited number of things go wrong with sleep—patients complain of sleeping too much or too little, of sleeping at the wrong time of the day, and less commonly of 'things that go bump in the night' (or the complaint will come from the bed partner).

Simple screening questions are suggested in Box 110.1. A collateral history from the bed partner, where possible, is helpful to determine the presence of any snoring, periodic limb movements of sleep, sleepwalking, or other parasomnia. It is important to ask about the duration of symptoms (typically young onset for narcolepsy and NREM parasomnia) and whether they are progressive or relapse and remit. Some conditions disturb the bed partner far more than the patient, and establishing who is more concerned is important.

Discussing the patient's concerns about sleep and expectations of normal sleep is not only worthwhile, but also part of treatment in insomnia disorder. For those with significant daytime sleepiness, driving safety should be discussed when relevant. The American Academy of Sleep Medicine recommends, 'Have you had crashes, near misses, or claims on insurance in the last year?'. Those who are aware of nodding at the wheel or have modified driving are at most risk [15].

One of the most simple and cost-effective tests is a sleep diary kept for at least 2 weeks. Alongside a typical history, this may be the only diagnostic test needed for insomnia disorder, circadian rhythm disorder, or daytime sleepiness caused by sleep restriction or shift work.

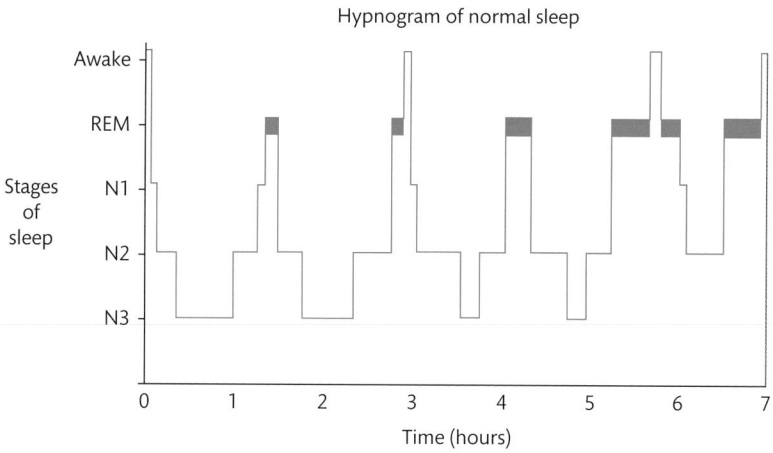

**Fig. 110.1** The sleep hypnogram. Sleep stages over a typical night as determined by polysomnography. During adult life, at night, we cycle between non-rapid eye movement (NREM) sleep and rapid eye movement (REM) sleep approximately every 90–120 minutes. REM sleep typically occurs >90 minutes into the night, and NREM sleep is divided into three stages: N1, N2, and N3. N3 is often known as slow-wave sleep (SWS). Young adults will wake 2–4 times during the night, although they may not be aware of this. Most adults will have 4–5 cycles of REM sleep, although dream recall is highly variable and few patients recall 4–5 distinct cycles of dreaming.

---

This should include: lights out, time in bed, estimated time asleep, any daytime napping, and ideally daily intake of caffeine, alcohol, meals, and exercise. There is debate about the time needed for diagnosis, but ICSD-3 highlights that certain circadian rhythm disorders will be missed with a single week of diaries. Weekends are different to weekdays, even in those who are unemployed or on work shifts. Some diaries rate satisfaction with sleep on a nightly basis, but this does not have diagnostic sensitivity and the author does not do this—generally, if they were satisfied with sleep, they would not be completing a sleep diary. Patients should complete the diary once a day, but not at night. Commercial accelerometers within smart phones and other gadgets tend to overestimate movement as wake and should not be used [16]; they can, in themselves, exacerbate insomnia. If patients awake refreshed and do not perceive a problem falling asleep, then they should largely avoid looking at movement-based data. Typical diaries are shown from normal and abnormal sleepers (Fig. 110.2).

### Screening questionnaires—which scales to use?

The Epworth Sleepiness Scale (ESS) is the most widely used questionnaire to assess daytime sleepiness as self-rated over the prior month [17] (Box 110.2). Advantages include speed and simplicity for the patient and validation within psychiatry populations. However, it correlates poorly with more objective measures of sleep in the laboratory [18]. Many typical insomniacs score 0–1; >10 is taken as daytime sleepiness, and >17 as very sleepy. Change in ESS score is often used to assess interventions for sleepiness such as stimulants [19, 20]. Added value is often obtained from asking a spouse or partner to also complete the questionnaire.

The other widely used questionnaire to separate good and bad sleepers is the Pittsburgh Sleep Quality Inventory [21]. Seven questions give a single score, with >5 indicating some form of sleep disturbance and those scoring >10 having more severe sleep disturbance. This is widely used in research but is more complex to complete.

The insomnia severity index is validated for insomnia severity and improvement after therapy, with scores ranging from 0 to 24 [22]. It is quick and easy to complete but will not distinguish between primary or secondary causes of insomnia.

---

**Box 110.1 Recommended questions for a sleep history**

**Key sleep questions**

1 Do you snore heavily? Has anyone witnessed prolonged pauses in breathing (apnoeas)?

*For typical obstructive sleep apnoea, snoring is very loud, heard outside the bedroom door; the pauses are typically 20–30 seconds, rather than brief (<5–10 seconds); and a snort or a start at the end of apnoea is characteristic.*

2 Do you have unpleasant tingling or discomfort in the legs which makes you need to kick or to move? Is it worse in the evenings? Is it helped by moving (restless in the body, rather than a racing mind)?

*Everybody needs to be asked specifically about restless legs; people can find it hard to describe the dysaesthesia—'wriggly', 'itchy', 'worms under the skin'. Bed partners can be asked about the infuriatingly regular kicks that may wake them, but not the patient—every 20–30 seconds is typical.*

3 What drugs do you take, and when do you take them, including the dose and timing of caffeine/alcohol and nicotine?

*Consider over-the-counter medication that might affect sleep, so short-acting painkillers, sedative opiates, and adrenergic drugs such as inhalers or some nasal sprays; counting the cups of coffee or tea is important.*

4 'Take me through your typical 24 hours'—describing the sleep/wake pattern over a day.

*Particularly helpful for those with sleep restriction, circadian rhythm disorder, and insomnia.*

5 Do you nap during the day—if so when and for how long? Can you get through the day without sleeping?

*Examples of when they might sleep can help to distinguish fatigue from true hypersomnia; few of us would sleep in the middle of a conversation or with food in our mouths.*

6 Do you have any history of nightmares, acting out of dreams, sleepwalking out of the bedroom? If so, what time of night do things tend to happen?

*Typically, the first cycle of REM sleep starts 90 minutes into the night, so REM parasomnias are more likely in the second half of the night. NREM parasomnias can occur within the first hour of sleep.*

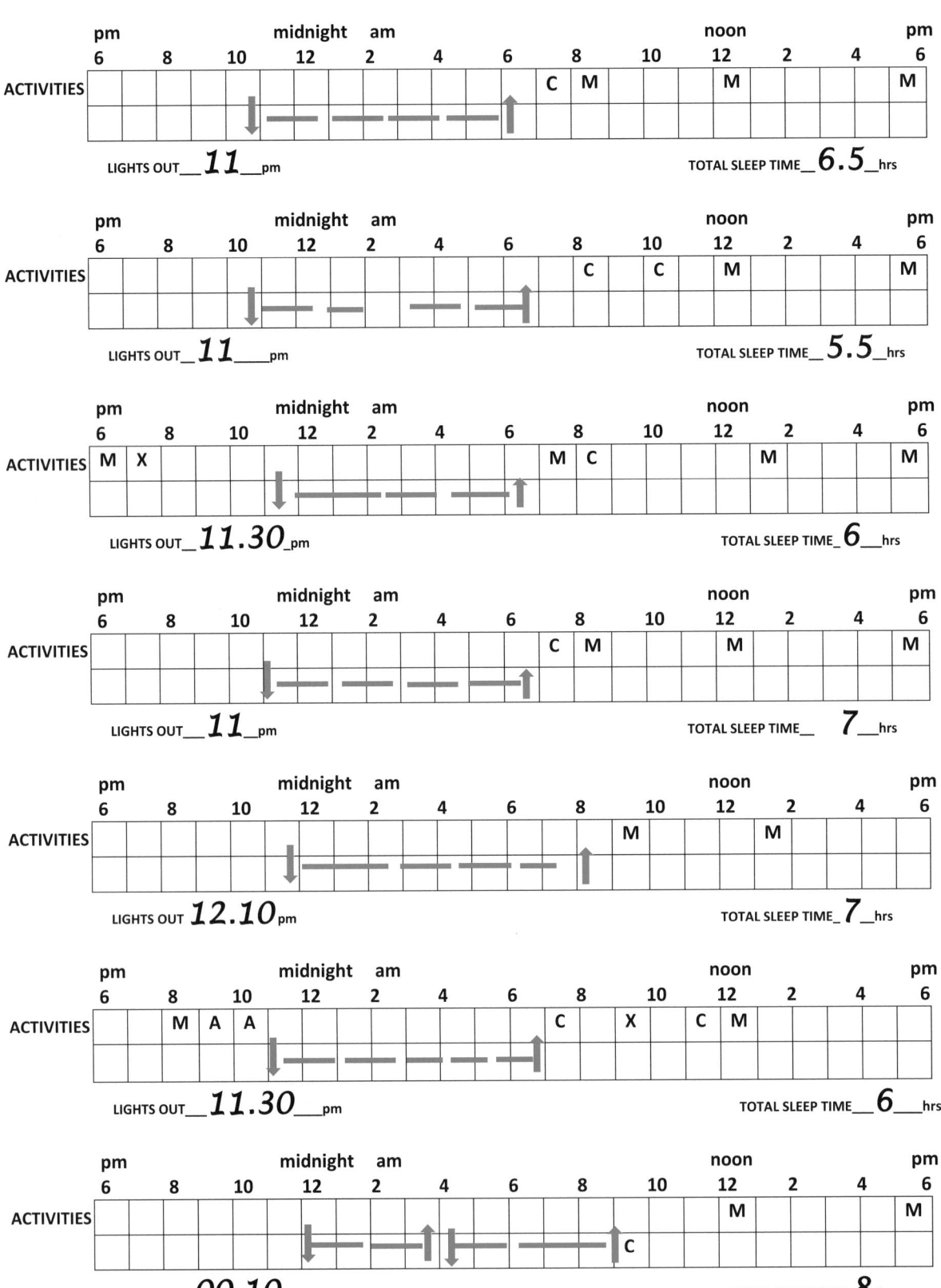

**Fig. 110.2** Sleep diaries.

(a) Diary 1. A normal (albeit slightly introspective) 45-year old with occasional brief wakenings and rapid returns to sleep. Taking up to 30 minutes to fall asleep is normal, and increased sleep time at weekends and non-work days are within current societal norms. Treatment was a clear explanation about normal sleep and advising him to avoid using his phone to record his sleep.

(b) Diary 2. Insomnia disorder where time in bed is far longer than time perceived asleep, and both difficulty initiating and maintaining sleep are seen without daytime naps. Variability among nights is seen, with occasional good nights of prolonged sleep.

(c) Diary 3. Delayed sleep phase syndrome in a 23-year-old male who has had this sleep pattern since the age of 15. The pattern is of falling asleep typically between 2.30 a.m. and 4 a.m., but waking well after 11 a.m. with a few night wakenings. The estimated total sleep time is far greater than in the patient with insomnia.

# Diary 2

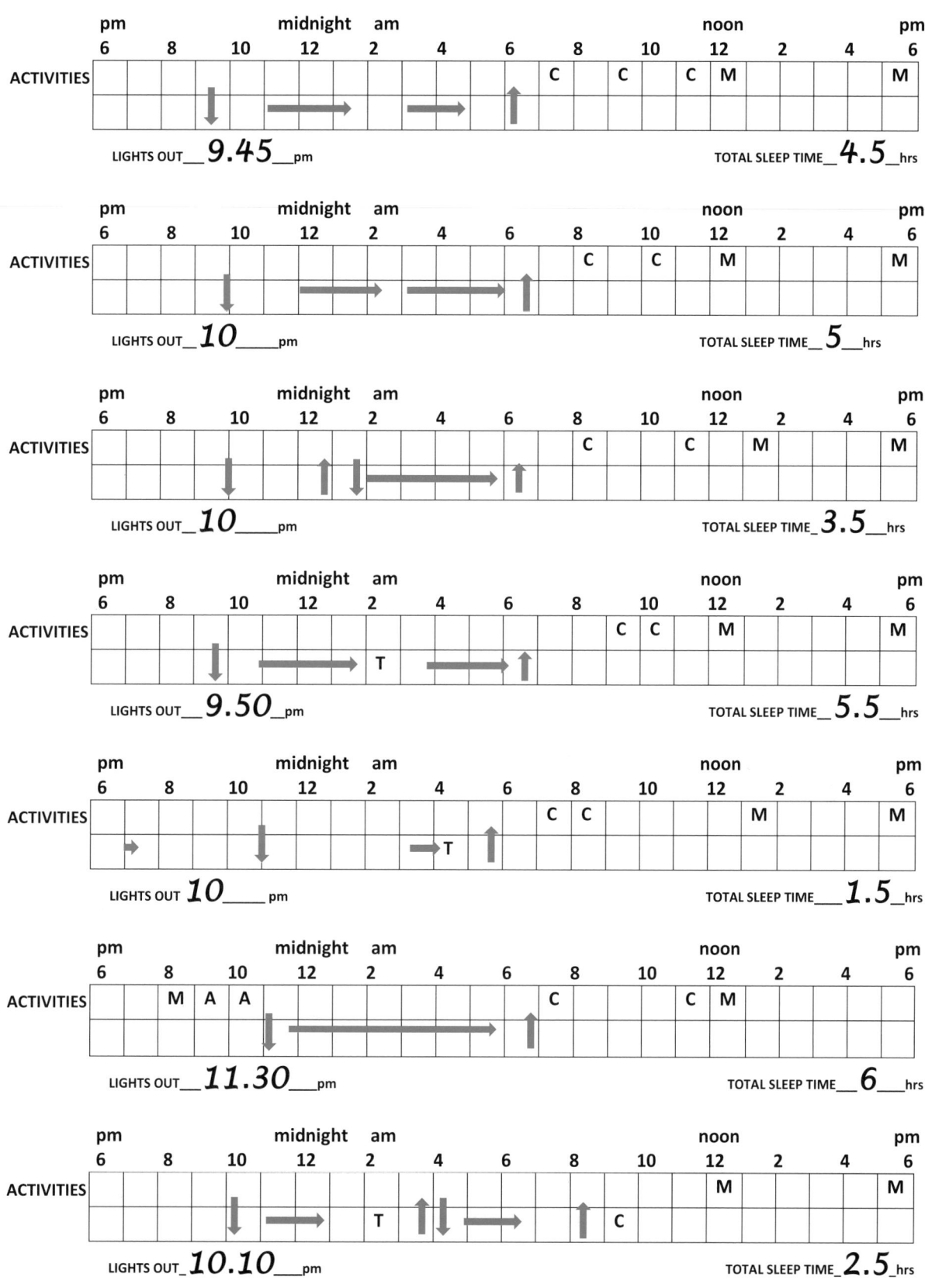

**Fig. 110.2** Continued

## Diary 3

(c)

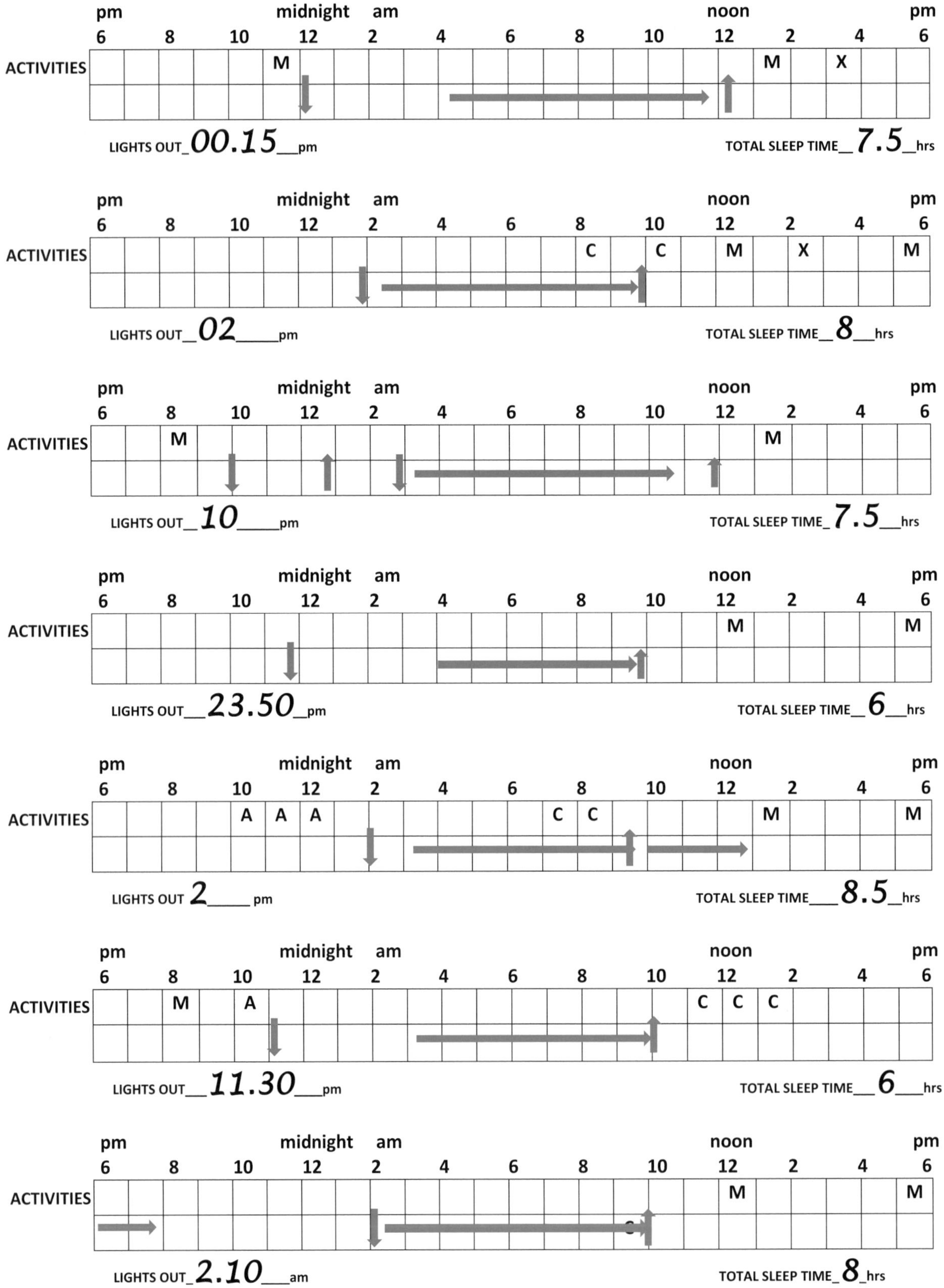

pm
midnight
am
noon
pm
6 8 10 12 2 4 6 8 10 12 2 4 6
ACTIVITIES
M
M
X
LIGHTS OUT_00.15__pm
TOTAL SLEEP TIME_7.5_hrs
ACTIVITIES
C
C
M
X
M
LIGHTS OUT__02_____pm
TOTAL SLEEP TIME__8__hrs
ACTIVITIES
M
M
LIGHTS OUT__10_____pm
TOTAL SLEEP TIME_7.5__hrs
ACTIVITIES
M
M
LIGHTS OUT__23.50_pm
TOTAL SLEEP TIME__6__hrs
ACTIVITIES
A A A
C C
M
M
LIGHTS OUT 2_____ pm
TOTAL SLEEP TIME___8.5_hrs
ACTIVITIES
M
A
C C C
LIGHTS OUT__11.30__pm
TOTAL SLEEP TIME__6___hrs
ACTIVITIES
M
M
LIGHTS OUT_2.10___am
TOTAL SLEEP TIME_8_hrs

**Fig. 110.2** Continued

## Box 110.2 Epworth Sleepiness Scale

Name: _____ Today's date: _____

Your age (Yrs): _____ Your sex (Male = M, Female = F): _____

How likely are you to doze off or fall asleep in the following situations, in contrast to feeling just tired? This refers to your usual way of life in recent times.

Even if you haven't done some of these things recently try to work out how they would have affected you.

Use the following scale to choose the most appropriate number for each situation:

0 = would never doze

1 = slight chance of dozing

2 = moderate chance of dozing

3 = high chance of dozing

It is important that you answer each question as best you can.

| Situation | Chance of dozing (0–3) |
|---|---|
| Sitting and reading | |
| Watching TV | |
| Sitting, inactive in a public place (e.g. a theatre or a meeting) | |
| As a passenger in a car for an hour without a break | |
| Lying down to rest in the afternoon when circumstances permit | |
| Sitting and talking to someone | |
| Sitting quietly after a lunch without alcohol | |
| In a car, while stopped for a few minutes in the traffic | |

THANK YOU FOR YOUR COOPERATION
© M.W. Johns 1990–1997. Used under License

Reproduced from *Sleep*, 14(6), Johns MW, A new method for measuring daytime sleepiness: the Epworth sleepiness scale, pp. 540–5, Copyright (1991), with permission from Oxford University Press.

## Hypersomnia

Hypersomnia affects up to 15% of the adult population, with 5% severely affected [23]. Differential diagnoses include obstructive sleep apnoea (OSA), sleep restriction with insufficient hours in bed for the needs of the individual, sedative medication, narcolepsy with or without associated cataplexy (transient loss of skeletal muscle tone typically triggered by strong emotion), and idiopathic hypersomnia. Excessive daytime sleepiness can be caused by head trauma (usually transient for the first 3–6 months; if it persists, other causes should be screened for) [24]. Troublesome daytime sleepiness is common in both early and more advanced neurodegenerative conditions such as Parkinson's disease where it is typically multifactorial. Louter and colleagues produced a useful diagnostic algorithm [25].

Circadian rhythm disorders can masquerade as hypersomnia, in particular in shift workers over 40 or young adults with delayed sleep phase syndrome.

## Behaviourally induced insufficient sleep syndrome (sleep restriction)

Those who are sleep-restricted for sleep will have daytime sleepiness. There are few true short sleepers, and most of the adult population sleeping <5 hours will have symptoms of poor concentration and sleepiness. 'Social jet lag' describes increased sleep over weekends to repay sleep debt. Variability over days and completion of a sleep diary, alongside a careful history, may be sufficient to make the diagnosis. Occasionally, wrist actigraphy can record sleep–wake patterns where there is diagnostic doubt.

Napoleon, Margaret Thatcher, and Thomas Edison are often acclaimed as short sleepers of only 4 hours a night. Further analysis reveals them all to be efficient power nappers. Edison, who dismissed sleep as a 'waste of time and throwback to our cave days', was once furious to be caught napping in a cupboard during the day.

## Obstructive sleep apnoea

The most common cause of significant daytime sleepiness in those over the age of 50 is OSA. It remains underdiagnosed despite having an excellent, cost-effective, symptomatic therapy—continuous positive airways pressure [26]. Risk factors include male sex, increasing age (in particular over 50), obesity, increased neck circumference (>17 inches), and retrognathic jaw. Increasing obesity means that at least 10% of men over 40 and 5% of women now have moderate or severe sleep apnoea [27]. In children, OSA is seen with adenotonsillar hypertrophy and certain dysmorphic conditions such as Down's syndrome.

Psychiatry patients have particular risk factors for sleep apnoea, and studies across a range of psychiatric disorders have reported rates of up to 66% [28, 29]. There is most evidence for increased rates in major depressive disorder and in those with elevated BMI [30]. This is a particular problem with those established on drugs for psychosis with metabolic syndrome [31, 32].

The history includes very loud snoring, progressively troublesome sleepiness, awaking unrefreshed, and often progressive over months and years. Spouses often reposition the patient onto their side, and the pauses in breathing are often long enough (>30 seconds) to cause concern. It is rare for the patient themselves to have a perception of choking, although people can wake themselves with their own snoring. Morning headache is common, often due to exacerbation of primary headache such as migraine, rather than associated respiratory failure. Clues for those who live alone include a dry, sore throat in the morning, nocturia, awaking unrefreshed, vivid dreams, and night-time sweating, alongside daytime sleepiness. Untreated OSA can cause treatment-resistant hypertension.

At least 20% of patients are not overweight, and those over 65 years of age can be slim with atypical presentations, including cognitive impairment. The STOP-Bang is a validated screening tool for OSA to assess those who may need further investigations [33] (http://www.stopbang.ca).

Those with suspected OSA should be referred for a respiratory sleep study. This detects pauses in breathing—either partial (hypopnea) or complete (apnoea)—alongside oximetry and gives an apnoea–hypopnea index (AHI). AHI of >5/hour is abnormal, but AHI of >15 (moderate) and >30 (severe) is far more likely to cause symptoms and to respond to treatment. Those with untreated OSA report more symptoms of depression and anxiety than the background population [34, 35].

Symptomatic OSA is notifiable to the driving licence authorities, but treated patients can restart driving.

It is also worth mentioning chronic fatigue syndrome. Sleep disorders must be excluded, and OSA is a common mimic. Recent polysomnography studies in those with an established diagnosis of chronic fatigue syndrome showed 21–49% had an undiagnosed sleep disorder, most commonly OSA [36, 37].

## Central sleep apnoea

Those taking sedative medication and, in particular, opiates, as well as those with heart failure, can have prolonged apnoeas without snoring as a central phenomenon. Increased opiate prescribing over the past 20 years has led to a belated recognition of their harmful effects, including sleep apnoea [38]. Those with chronic pain often complain of bad sleep, but this is mostly attributed to the pain itself. Within pain clinics, rates as high as 25–50% are reported, often with secondary respiratory failure [39, 40]. Those at highest risk are those taking >200 mg of equivalent dose of morphine, in combination with benzodiazepines. Recent changes in the Center for Disease Control prescribing guidelines in the United States have recognized the dangers and may influence prescribing in other countries [41].

## Narcolepsy

Narcolepsy, meaning 'seized by somnolence', was described by Gelineau in 1880 to include sleep attacks and falls triggered by strong emotion (cataplexy). The most recent diagnostic criteria (Box 110.3) reflect an increasing understanding of the neuropathology [42]. Narcolepsy is now characterized as type 1 or type 2, with the diagnosis made on a typical history plus supportive investigations [either polysomnography plus daytime multiple sleep latency tests or, more recently, reduced cerebrospinal fluid (CSF) hypocretin]. Its prevalence is 0.05–0.1%, but often with significant delay to diagnosis [43].

It typically develops in adolescence with excessive daytime sleepiness evolving over weeks to months and then remaining relatively fixed and unremitting over time. It is best thought of as a sleep switch problem where patients transition between sleep/ wake states more frequently than normal. The classical tetrad of excessive daytime sleepiness, hypnogogic and hypnapompic hallucinations, cataplexy, and sleep paralysis is only seen in 20% of patients at first presentation. One-third of patients will never develop cataplexy or have only very subtle symptoms. The majority will have disabling sleepiness and will not be able to get through the day without napping. Many describe naps as difficult to resist at times, but classical sleep attacks without any recollection of the event are, in fact, uncommon. The description from a relative or witness is often of a conversation stopped halfway and restarted as if no time has passed.

Key diagnostic features include the need for brief and typically refreshing naps, of sometimes just a few minutes. Adult patients will typically have a fragmented night, and some feel that this should be part of the diagnostic criteria. Certainly if an adult is very sleepy, but with a long, deep, and unbroken night, then another cause of sleepiness is more likely. Dream recall is strikingly vivid, often after even short daytime naps. The description of hypnagogic hallucinations

**Box 110.3** Diagnostic criteria for narcolepsy with and without cataplexy

**Narcolepsy type 1—narcolepsy with cataplexy**
Criteria A and B must be met:
A The patient has daily periods of an irrepressible need to sleep or daytime lapses into sleep occurring for ≥3 months.
B The presence of one or both of the following:
  1 Cataplexy and a mean sleep latency of ≤8 minutes and ≥2 sleep-onset REM periods (SOREMPs) on a multiple sleep latency test (MSLT) performed according to standard techniques. A SOREMP (within 15 minutes of sleep onset) on the preceding nocturnal polysomnogram may replace one of the SOREMPs on the MSLT.
  2 CSF hypocretin-1 concentration, measured by immunoreactivity, is either ≤110 pg/mL or <1/3 of mean values obtained in normal subjects with the same standardized assay.

**Narcolepsy type 2—narcolepsy without cataplexy**
Criteria A–E must be met:
A The patient has daily periods of an irrepressible need to sleep or daytime lapses into sleep occurring for ≥3 months.
B A mean sleep latency of ≤8 minutes and ≥2 SOREMPs are found on an MSLT performed according to standard techniques. A SOREMP (within 15 minutes of sleep onset) on the preceding nocturnal polysomnogram may replace one of the SOREMPs on the MSLT.
C Cataplexy is absent.*
D Either CSF hypocretin-1 concentration has not been measured or CSF hypocretin-1 concentration measured by immunoreactivity is either >110 pg/mL or >1/3 of mean values obtained in normal subjects with the same standardized assay.
E Hypersomnolence and/or MSLT findings are not better explained by other causes such as insufficient sleep, obstructive sleep apnoea, delayed sleep phase disorder, or the effect of medication or substances or their withdrawal.

* If cataplexy develops later, reclassify as type 1.

can vary, but unlike those with psychotic disorders, the hallucinations occur within sleep and are typically visual.

Cataplexy is typically an axial loss of posture affecting the head, face, and neck, and patients can describe their face becoming loose or their jaw dropping. Bigger attacks cause falls, but with retained consciousness; eyes close, and patients look as if they are asleep. Recovery is typically quick within a minute or so. Cataplexy is worse at times of emotional arousal. Younger children can find it harder to describe emotional triggers and may have a near permanent decrease in muscle tone, giving a tongue that lolls and a pseudomyopathic appearance with a clumsy, waddling gait [44]. Those presenting later in life have a milder phenotype, but sleepiness that is definitely new in onset over the age of 40 is rarely due to narcolepsy.

Narcolepsy is now known to be caused by a loss of hypocretin neurons within the hypothalamus [45]. Since hypocretin also has a key role in metabolism, patients typically gain weight as the condition evolves with a craving for carbohydrate-rich foods. Children, in particular, can have significant weight gain and precocious puberty as a consequence [46]. Many have parasomnia and a mild REM sleep behaviour disorder (RBD); the dream enactment rarely causes injury but can lead to diagnostic confusion and can occasionally be the presenting complaint [47].

Specific diagnostic tests include haplotyping for the commonly associated HLA-DQB1*0602 allele. This is seen in 95% of those with narcolepsy and cataplexy, but also in 25% of the background population and only in 60% of those without cataplexy, so it is of limited use.

It is strongly associated with low CSF hypocretin. The author does not use it, unless planning CSF testing. Polysomnography plus multiple sleep latency tests have for years been the gold standard objective test of both sleepiness and abnormally early-onset REM sleep (4–5 timed nap opportunities with patients given a 20-minute period and the instruction to 'try to fall asleep'). Those with a mean sleep latency of <8 minutes are said to be pathologically sleepy; many patients with narcolepsy have far shorter sleep latencies of <5 minutes [48], and the presence of REM sleep within 15 minutes on two or more occasions has 70% sensitivity and 97% specificity [49, 50]. There is no value for routine EEG to assess for the presence of sleepiness.

Differential diagnosis includes sleep restriction, and careful assessment of the average time in bed should be measured, ideally with sleep diaries. Comorbid sleep apnoea should be excluded in those with increased BMI who also snore.

## Idiopathic hypersomnia

A less well-defined condition, patients typically complain of prolonged and unrefreshing sleep, typically answering the question of 'how long do you nap?' with the answer 'until I am woken'. Naps are much more likely to last over an hour, and for these patients, there is little dream recall and no cataplexy [51, 52]. In one-third of patients, symptoms have been present since childhood. Unlike narcolepsy, there is a family history in at least a third. Typically, patients describe the phenomenon of a prolonged night sleep of often 9 or 10 hours and then marked difficulty waking (sleep drunkenness), with repeated returns to sleep. Being late into work or school is common. Diagnostic criteria again require polysomnography plus multiple sleep latency tests confirming a mean sleep latency of <8 minutes, but without sudden-onset REM sleep. Polysomnography often shows prolonged slow-wave sleep and high sleep efficiency. Unlike narcolepsy, about 10% spontaneously remit. The differential diagnosis includes hypersomnia associated with depression, but this more commonly causes more variable symptoms over weeks and months, with periods of remission [53].

## Parasomnias—'things that go bump in the night'

Described as 'undesirable physical and/or experiential phenomena accompanying sleep', parasomnias can involve complex motor acts, including walking, eating, texting, and even driving. Rarely, this can be misdiagnosed as a primary psychiatric problem or, more commonly, as possible nocturnal seizures. At least 20% of all children have some form of parasomnia, although most do not present to doctors. At least 2–3% of the adult population have some form of parasomnia, and this is increased to 4–9% in psychiatric patients [54].

Parasomnias are divided into those occurring in NREM or REM sleep.

### Non-rapid eye movement parasomnias

Confusional arousals, sleepwalking (somnambulism), sleep-related eating disorder, and sexsomnia are all NREM parasomnias. They are disorders of arousal [55], with incomplete wakening from slow-wave sleep (N3). These disorders are common in childhood,

and there is often a family history. Events can occur within the first 30–60 minutes of sleep, which is less common for REM-related events. Occasional sleep *talking* is also an NREM parasomnia, but so common as to be near universal.

Typically, there is a lack of awareness for at least some, if not all, of the events or if there is recall, it is patchy. Partners almost always describe more night-time events than the patients, and events last minutes, rather than seconds (5–15 minutes would be the average). There is variability to events, but clustering is common, with several events over a week and then periods of relative remission. Patients who are out of the bed and out of the bedroom are more likely to have NREM, rather than REM, parasomnia. Patients can be both argumentative and combative, but directed violence is rare. Hallucinatory phenomena can occur within NREM sleep.

NREM parasomnia typically decreases moving into adulthood; however, those who are predisposed can then have further symptoms with acute psychiatric illness, shift work, or irregular sleep patterns [56]. The other well-recognized trigger is another sleep disorder such as OSA or restless legs [57, 58].

Specific additional investigations include sleep diaries to look for triggers and scheduling issues and a witness history, wherever possible. The value of inpatient video polysomnography is debated, as it rarely changes the diagnosis but may detect additional sleep apnoea or restless legs [59]. If events are captured, they arise from slow-wave sleep (N3 sleep stage). If the differential diagnosis does include nocturnal seizures, then MRI brain and EEG should also be performed. However, the main value of a sleep study is to look for other sleep disorders in adults that might be triggering the event or an alternative diagnosis if no witness history is available. The current ICSD-3 criteria do not require polysomnography to make the diagnosis with a typical history.

### Rapid eye movement parasomnias

These disorders are typically brief, memorable, and dream-filled, and unlike NREM parasomnias, patients are far more likely to have recall of events. REM parasomnias include nightmare disorder, isolated sleep paralysis, and RBD.

In normal sleep, a powerful, descending glutaminergic signal inhibits the spinal motor neurons during REM sleep with reduced skeletal muscle activity or REM atonia [60]. Only the diaphragm and the extraocular muscles are active (giving the rapid, jerky eye movements on the electro-oculogram within polysomnography). In RBD, an insidious and progressive degeneration of this brainstem control causes increasingly troublesome dream enactment, alongside vivid and often violent dream content. Affected patients shout and act out dreams, and up to 70% will injure themselves or their bed partner and this is often the prompt for referral. This is typically in the second half of the night. The condition predominantly affects older men, with a reported prevalence of at least 1%. RBD was first described by Carlos Schenck in 1986 in a small series of elderly men [61]. In fact, selective brainstem lesions in animals were shown to cause dream-like behaviours many years earlier [62]. Over recent years, there has been increasing recognition of the strong association between RBD and other neurodegenerations, and in particular Parkinson's disease, dementia with Lewy bodies, and multiple system atrophy. Over 80% of those with RBD will develop one of these conditions over 15 years of follow-up [63]. Studies show subtle cognitive, olfactory, and gait disturbance in RBD patients, compared to controls

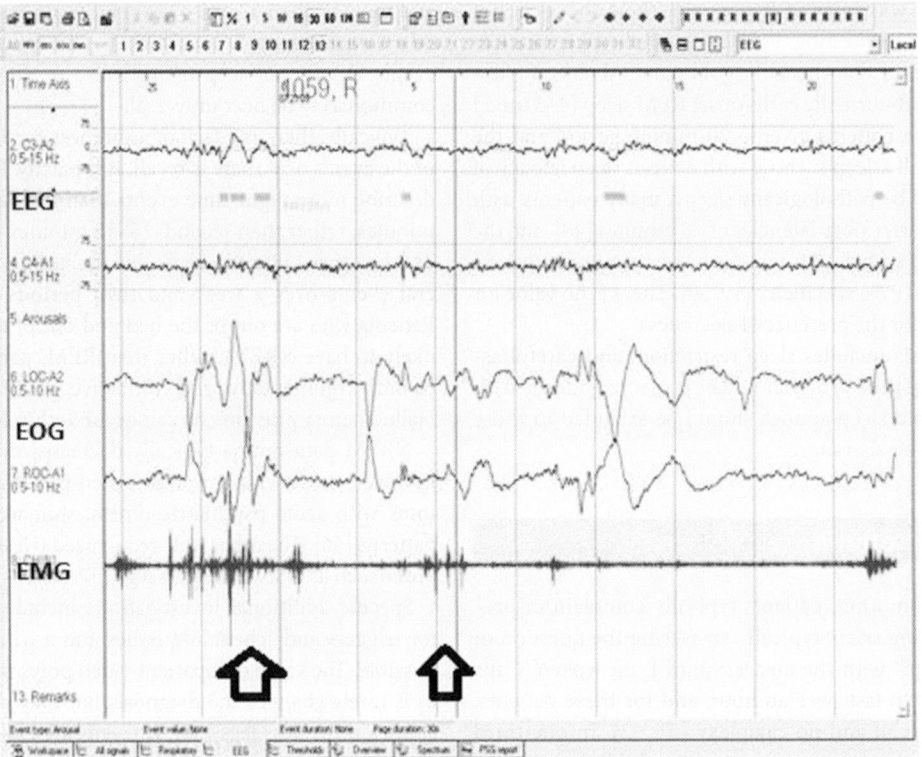

**Fig. 110.3** Inpatient video polysomnography in a patient with REM sleep behaviour disorder. A 30-second epoch of polysomnography showing EEG, EOG, and EMG, with loss of normal REM atonia (bottom line) highlighted with black arrows. This patient had a clinical history typical for REM sleep behaviour disorder (RBD).

[64]. In the Parkinson's disease clinic, at least 50% of patients will have some symptomatic RBD with a range of validated screening questionnaires primarily developed for research [65].

The ICSD-3 criteria specify the need for polysomnography in the context of a typical history, unlike other parasomnias where history alone is sufficient. This shows loss of REM atonia and occasionally abnormal behaviour on video (Fig. 110.3).

RBD is rare in children, but there is a recognized association with narcolepsy. Loss of REM atonia is seen with SSRI and SNRI antidepressants, with occasional dream enactment [66, 67].

Screening for RBD should therefore be a routine part of history taking in the memory clinic, and RBD can mimic some of the features of post-traumatic stress disorder. Key differences include a variety of different dreams, with not all of them being violent, and a lack of daytime distress. Occasionally, severe OSA can cause strikingly vivid dreams and mimics RBD. Screening for sleep apnoea should be considered in those who are sleepy or have other features to suggest OSA.

### Other REM parasomnias

Isolated sleep paralysis where someone awakes but for a minute or so cannot move. This occurs with associated dream-like imagery and occasionally with a feeling of heaviness in the chest or shortness of breath, and it is more common in the second half of the night or on waking from sleep. Touch relieves symptoms, and patients can describe trying to shout or to move. The diagnosis is made on history alone, and there are no specific tests routinely used. This is a common parasomnia experienced by at least 20% of the population

on occasion and up to 2–3% regularly [68], but it can be distressing when it first occurs. It is due to a dissociation between reactivation of skeletal muscle tone and return to wakefulness and is often seen with abrupt wakenings from REM sleep. For those with other psychopathology, the dreams can be more intrusive and involve themes of abuse. Typical triggers include irregular sleep/wake cycles for any reason. It can also be seen as a rebound phenomenon when stopping REM-suppressing antidepressants such as venlafaxine. It is seen frequently in those with narcolepsy, but alongside other features such as daytime sleepiness [69].

Nightmares are a universal phenomenon, but those with frequent and distressing nightmares have nightmare disorder. There is an association with depressive symptomatology [70]. An almost endless list of medications are said to be associated with nightmares or vivid dreams, but in practice, the common culprits are beta blockers, opiates, or cessation of REM-suppressing antidepressant medications.

### Benign hypnagogic hallucinations

There is debate about which sleep state these strikingly real, but exclusively nocturnal, and typically visual phenomena arise from. Typically occurring in the early part of the night, insects are commonly described themes, with rapid resolution of symptoms when lights come on. Insight is retained or rapidly returns with wakefulness. They seem more frequent in young women, but there are limited prevalence data.

- Advance sleep phase syndrome
- Delayed sleep phase syndrome
- Shift work disorder
- Jet lag circadian rhythm disorder
- Irregular sleep/wake syndrome
- Non-24-hour sleep/wake syndrome

## Circadian rhythm disorders

There are six distinct circadian rhythm disorders currently defined by ICSD-3 (Box 110.4) and increasing recognition of the relatively high frequency of these conditions in psychiatric patients [71]. All are caused by misalignment of the period of sleep, and many are characterized by the length of sleep time and often the quality of sleep remaining relatively normal, but simply out of sync with societal norms.

## Delayed sleep phase syndrome

This presents in teenage years with patients who typically fall asleep and wake far later than the societal norm, causing associated daytime dysfunction. The diagnosis can be made on history alone, alongside well-completed sleep diaries (Fig. 110.2). For many, the key question is 'if you were allowed to sleep when you wanted, would you sleep well?'. The quality of sleep is often good if uninterrupted, but patients simply do not feel sleepy in the first half of the night, falling asleep between 3 and 4 a.m. and then struggling to wake in the morning. Those who have sleep restriction when woken early may have daytime sleepiness; there is also evidence that the total sleep period (tau) is longer in this group. Males are more commonly affected [72].

The diagnostic criteria include either sleep diaries or actigraphy for at least 2 weeks, with a typical sleep diary shown from a teenager subsequently well treated with melatonin and light therapy (Fig. 110.2c). There are two groups: those with a lifelong tendency, often with a family history; and those that drift during teenage years. Many report symptoms persisting over years, once established. It can be misdiagnosed as insomnia or chronic fatigue syndrome.

## Shift work disorder

At least 20% of the western world do shift work, and for at least 20%, this significantly disrupts sleep. This decreases total sleep time and disrupts the circadian rhythm, with substantial evidence for increased mortality, obesity, cancer rates, and affective disorders in those who do shift work, compared to non-shift workers [73–75].

Shift work disorder occurs at greater rates in women, those over 40, and those who work rotating or back-to-back night to day shifts. Patients typically present with both insomnia when trying to sleep during the day and sleepiness during their shift, although many do not attribute either sleepiness or fatigue to their work patterns. This is often because sleep debt can accumulate over time, and shifts that may have been tolerable in the third or fourth decade become harder if there is added sleep disturbance with a young family, a longer

commute, or an additional sleep disorder such as sleep apnoea. ESS may well be increased, but the key test remains sleep diaries.

## Restless legs syndrome and periodic limb movements of sleep

This common sleep-related movement disorder is seen in at least 5% of the population at all ages [76], and diagnosis can be made on a typical clinical history for many. However, it is often missed by both patient and doctor as a cause of a disturbed night and a sleepy day. The diagnostic features, as described by the most recent International Restless Legs Syndrome Study Group (IRLSS) criteria, are an unpleasant dysaesthesia deep within the legs that causes the desire to move and is at least partially relieved by movement [14]. Twenty-five per cent of patients have daytime symptoms, but there is a clear circadian pattern, with symptoms worst in the evening and first half of the night. Patients can find it surprisingly difficult to describe the sensations; 'creeping', 'itchy', 'fidgety', and 'crawling' are all words used. Thighs and calves are affected more than the soles of the feet, and patients are restless in bed, seeking cool surfaces upon which to rest their feet. Pacing and walking during the night is seen in more severe cases. Symptoms can be asymmetric and include the low back, and less commonly the arms can be affected. Unlike arthritis pain or peripheral neuropathy, people are better or symptom-free when walking.

Symptoms can be episodic, and not all have sleep disturbance, but for those with moderate or severe symptoms, they can have considerable sleep fragmentation and subsequently a sleepy day. At least 50% will have a family history, and those with other affected family members typically present at a younger age. About 5% have had symptoms starting under the age of 16, often mislabelled as growing pains. There is an association with restless legs and high caffeine intake, smoking, and excess alcohol. Exercise close to bedtime exacerbates symptoms.

Approximately 80% of those with restless legs can describe (or a frustrated bed partner can) strikingly periodic limb movements of sleep and occasionally of wakefulness. There is a brief judder of the toe, foot, and ankle, and 20–30 seconds pass before the next. The impressive response to dopamine agonists is often both diagnostic and therapeutic.

There is an association with low ferritin levels for some and blood levels should be checked, and many psychotropic medications exacerbate symptoms, particularly those that are dopa-depleting, as well as some antidepressants and melatonin.

Polysomnography can record the periodic limb movements with both limb EMG and video. This also helps to exclude other/additional causes of sleep disturbance such as OSA. Lower limb/foot actigraphy can be used over 2–3 nights at home to measure the periodic limb movement index.

The differential diagnosis includes drug-related akathisia and hypnic jerks, but both lack the striking circadian pattern to symptoms and periodicity to night-time myoclonus.

## Insomnia disorder

Insomnia remains the most common sleep disorder in primary care, with at least 10% of the population affected [77]. Now simplified as a diagnostic entity in its own right, it is defined as difficulty initiating sleep, difficulty maintaining sleep, and associated daytime distress persisting for >3 months. It is commonly comorbid with other mental and physical health problems [78, 79]. At least 40% will have anxiety disorder. Typically, ESS will be low at 0–2, and those with high ESS should be screened for secondary causes of insomnia.

At least 10% have restless legs syndrome as the cause of their insomnia; 20% of those with sleep apnoea will perceive an unrefreshing night, although the other clues of snoring and daytime sleepiness should prompt further investigations. Gastro-oesophageal reflux can be surprisingly toxic to sleep as another secondary cause. It can be surprisingly hard to distinguish insomnia alone from insomnia with comorbid OSA in those over 65 [80].

The other common mimic is circadian rhythm disorder where patients perceive difficulty initiating sleep with delayed sleep phase, but in fact, they then stay asleep well, and sleep diaries and an accurate history should distinguish the two. There are a small number of truly short sleepers who, in fact, awake refreshed after just 5 hours but feel this is not enough. For insomnia disorder, there has to be associated daytime functional impairment.

The cornerstone of both diagnosis and therapy is sleep diaries where a typical pattern of more time in bed than being asleep is usually seen. Sleep efficiency (total sleep time/time in bed) can be calculated. Normal sleep is typically >85% sleep efficiency, and those with severe insomnia often have sleep efficiency of <50%. A typical diary is shown in Fig. 110.2. Most will have occasional nights of more normal sleep. Fatigue, rather than daytime sleepiness, is described, and documented daytime naps should be infrequent. A hypervigilant phenotype is typical, with 'My mind is racing' and 'As soon as I climb the stairs, the lights go on' as typical statements heard in clinic. Women are more affected than men, and increasing age is also a risk factor. A widely accepted model is that of predisposing factors, a precipitating trigger, and then perpetuating maladaptive behaviours that disrupt both the normal homeostatic and circadian drivers to sleep [81].

The history should include questions about the typical 24-hour pattern and the bedroom itself. Review of the prescription list for any stimulant medications is required, alongside an assessment of mood. There is often a mismatch between perceived daytime performance and more objective assessments. This is very different to the sleep apnoea or narcolepsy story where daytime function has usually been objectively affected. Use of sleeping tablets, including over-the-counter preparations, needs to be documented, as these may cause some of the daytime fatigue.

A sleep study is not indicated unless another sleep disorder is suspected, and actigraphy is rarely used outside of research. Polysomnography when performed typically shows reduced sleep efficiency, prolonged sleep latency, and early REM latency, but these changes are also seen in depressive disorder. There is often sleep misperception, with patients estimating less time asleep in the laboratory, but explaining this rarely helps the patient.

## Miscellaneous sleep disorders

### Hypnic jerks

A single shock-like jerk at sleep/wake transition is a near-universal phenomenon diagnosed by history alone, but it can be non-specifically increased by any condition that delays sleep onset or increases night wakenings.

### Exploding head syndrome

This dramatically named, but benign, phenomenon is diagnosed by history alone and is thought to be the sensory equivalent of hypnic jerks. At sleep/wake transitions, a patient will hear a single loud bang or an explosion, or occasionally there is a flash of light that can briefly seem entirely external; symptoms can cluster and be worsened by anxiety, and this tends to increase sleep latency and increase night wakenings.

### Bruxism

Those who grind their teeth at night, such that bed partners can hear, risk damage to the enamel and often disturb their partners, and some, but not all, have jaw pain. Night-time grinders tend to be daytime clenchers, with tenderness around the temporomandibular region, and there is some evidence for daytime jaw relaxation. There is some limited evidence for an association with increased anxiety and low mood [82].

## Conclusions

Unfortunately, sleep disorders remain underdiagnosed and undertreated [1, 12]. In addition, sleep disturbance in those with mental health problems is often attributed to the psychiatric diagnosis or psychotropic medication, rather than considering a distinct and treatable set of disorders. This chapter has provided the tools to identify specific sleep problems, how to take a sleep history, and how to then investigate and diagnose common sleep disorders. Their treatment is described in Chapter 114—it should assume a greater priority.

## REFERENCES

1. Stores G. Clinical diagnosis and misdiagnosis of sleep disorders. *J Neurol Neurosurg Psychiatry*. 2007;78:1293–7.
2. Diekelmann S, Born J. The memory function of sleep. *Nat Rev Neurosci*. 2010;11:114–26.
3. Stickgold R, Walker MP. Sleep-dependent memory triage: evolving generalization through selective processing. *Nat Neurosci*. 2013;16:139–45.
4. Palmer CA, Alfano CA. Sleep and emotion regulation: an organizing, integrative review. *Sleep Med Rev*. 2017;31:6–16.
5. Borbély AA, Daan S, Wirz-Justice A, Deboer T. The two-process model of sleep regulation: a reappraisal. *J Sleep Res*. 2016;25:131–43.
6. Ohayon MM, Carskadon MA, Guilleminault C, Vitiello MV. Meta-analysis of quantitative sleep parameters from childhood to old age in healthy individuals: developing normative sleep values across the human lifespan. *Sleep*. 2004;27:1255–73.
7. Crowley SJ, Acebo C, Carskadon MA. Sleep, circadian rhythms, and delayed phase in adolescence. *Sleep Med*. 2007;8:602–12.
8. Skeldon AC, Derks G, Dijk D-J. Modelling changes in sleep timing and duration across the lifespan: Changes in circadian rhythmicity or sleep homeostasis? *Sleep Med Rev*. 2016;28:96–107.
9. Gooneratne NS, Vitiello MV. Sleep in older adults: normative changes, sleep disorders, and treatment options. *Clin Geriatr Med*. 2014;30:591–627.

10. Liu Y, Wheaton AG, Chapman DP, Cunningham TJ, Lu II, Croft JB. Prevalence of healthy sleep duration among adults—United States, 2014. *MMWR Morb Mortal Wkly Rep*. 2016;65:137–41.

11. Consensus Conference Panel, Watson NF, Badr MS, Belenky G, *et al*. Joint Consensus Statement of the American Academy of Sleep Medicine and Sleep Research Society on the recommended amount of sleep for a healthy adult: methodology and discussion. *J Clin Sleep Med*. 2015;11:931–52.

12. Rosenberg RP. Clinical assessment of excessive daytime sleepiness in the diagnosis of sleep disorders. *J Clin Psychiatry*. 2015;76:e1602.

13. American Academy of Sleep Medicine. *International Classification of Sleep Disorders*, third edition. Darien, IL: American Academy of Sleep Medicine; 2014.

14. Allen RP, Picchietti DL, Garcia-Borreguero D, *et al*. Restless legs syndrome/Willis-Ekbom disease diagnostic criteria: updated International Restless Legs Syndrome Study Group (IRLSSG) consensus criteria—history, rationale, description, and significance. *Sleep Med*. 2014;15:860–73.

15. Ghosh D, Jamson SL, Baxter PD, Elliott MW. Continuous measures of driving performance on an advanced office-based driving simulator can be used to predict simulator task failure in patients with obstructive sleep apnoea syndrome. *Thorax*. 2012;67:815–21.

16. Mantua J, Gravel N, Spencer RM. Reliability of sleep measures from four personal health monitoring devices compared to research-based actigraphy and polysomnography. *Sensors (Basel)*. 2016;16:pii:E646.

17. Johns MW. A new method for measuring daytime sleepiness: the Epworth Sleepiness Scale. *Sleep*. 1991;14:540–5.

18. Fong SYY, Ho CKW, Wing YK. Comparing MSLT and ESS in the measurement of excessive daytime sleepiness in obstructive sleep apnoea syndrome. *J Psychosom Res*. 2005;58:55–60.

19. Broughton RJ, Fleming JA, George CF, *et al*. Randomized, double-blind, placebo-controlled crossover trial of modafinil in the treatment of excessive daytime sleepiness in narcolepsy. *Neurology*. 1997;49:444–51.

20. [No authors listed]. Randomized trial of modafinil for the treatment of pathological somnolence in narcolepsy. US Modafinil in Narcolepsy Multicenter Study Group. *Ann Neurol*. 1998;43:88–97.

21. Buysse DJ, Reynolds CF, Monk TH, Berman SR, Kupfer DJ. The Pittsburgh Sleep Quality Index: a new instrument for psychiatric practice and research. *Psychiatry Res*. 1989;28:193–213.

22. Bastien CH, Vallières A, Morin CM. Validation of the Insomnia Severity Index as an outcome measure for insomnia research. *Sleep Med*. 2001;2:297–307.

23. Ohayon MM, Priest RG, Zulley J, Smirne S, Paiva T. Prevalence of narcolepsy symptomatology and diagnosis in the European general population. *Neurology*. 2002;58:1826–33.

24. Gardani M, Morfiri E, Thomson A, O'Neill B, McMillan TM. Evaluation of sleep disorders in patients with severe traumatic brain injury during rehabilitation. *Arch Phys Med Rehabil*. 2015;96:1691–7.e3.

25. Louter M, Aarden WCCA, Lion J, Bloem BR, Overeem S. Recognition and diagnosis of sleep disorders in Parkinson's disease. *J Neurol*. 2012;259:2031–40.

26. McDaid C, Griffin S, Weatherly H, *et al*. Continuous positive airway pressure devices for the treatment of obstructive sleep apnoea-hypopnoea syndrome: a systematic review and economic analysis. *Health Technol Assess*. 2009;13:iii–iv, xi–xiv, 1–119, 143–274.

27. Peppard PE, Young T, Barnet JH, Palta M, Hagen EW, Hla KM. Increased prevalence of sleep-disordered breathing in adults. *Am J Epidemiol*. 2013;177:1006–14.

28. Anderson KN, Waton T, Armstrong D, Watkinson HM, Mackin P. Sleep disordered breathing in community psychiatric patients. *Eur J Psychiatry*. 26:86–95.

29. Benca RM, Obermeyer WH, Thisted RA, Gillin JC. Sleep and psychiatric disorders. A meta-analysis. *Arch Gen Psychiatry*. 1992;49:651–68; discussion 669–70.

30. Gupta MA, Simpson FC. Obstructive sleep apnea and psychiatric disorders: a systematic review. *J Clin Sleep Med*. 2015;11:165–75.

31. Henderson DC, Vincenzi B, Andrea NV, Ulloa M, Copeland PM. Pathophysiological mechanisms of increased cardiometabolic risk in people with schizophrenia and other severe mental illnesses. *Lancet Psychiatry*. 2015;2:452–64.

32. Mackin P, Waton T, Watkinson HM, Gallagher P. A four-year naturalistic prospective study of cardiometabolic disease in antipsychotic-treated patients. *Eur Psychiatry*. 2012;27:50–5.

33. Chung F, Yegneswaran B, Liao P, *et al*. STOP questionnaire: a tool to screen patients for obstructive sleep apnea. *Anesthesiology*. 2008;108:812–21.

34. Wells RD, Freedland KE, Carney RM, Duntley SP, Stepanski EJ. Adherence, reports of benefits, and depression among patients treated with continuous positive airway pressure. *Psychosom Med*. 2007;69:449–54.

35. Aloia MS, Arnedt JT, Smith L, Skrekas J, Stanchina M, Millman RP. Examining the construct of depression in obstructive sleep apnea syndrome. *Sleep Med*. 2005;6:115–21.

36. Gotts ZM, Deary V, Newton J, Van der Dussen D, De Roy P, Ellis JG. Are there sleep-specific phenotypes in patients with chronic fatigue syndrome? A cross-sectional polysomnography analysis. *BMJ Open*. 2013;3:pii:e002999.

37. Mariman A, Delesie L, Tobback E, *et al*. Undiagnosed and comorbid disorders in patients with presumed chronic fatigue syndrome. *J Psychosom Res*. 2013;75:491–6.

38. Walker JM, Farney RJ, Rhondeau SM, *et al*. Chronic opioid use is a risk factor for the development of central sleep apnea and ataxic breathing. *J Clin Sleep Med*. 2007;3:455–61.

39. Rose AR, Catcheside PG, McEvoy RD, *et al*. Sleep disordered breathing and chronic respiratory failure in patients with chronic pain on long term opioid therapy. *J Clin Sleep Med*. 2014;10:847–52.

40. Correa D, Farney RJ, Chung F, Prasad A, Lam D, Wong J. Chronic opioid use and central sleep apnea: a review of the prevalence, mechanisms, and perioperative considerations. *Anesth Analg*. 2015;120:1273–85.

41. Dowell D, Haegerich TM, Chou R. CDC guideline for prescribing opioids for chronic pain—United States, 2016. *MMWR Recomm Rep*. 2016;65(No. RR-1):1–49. Available from: https://www.cdc.gov/mmwr/volumes/65/rr/rr6501e1.htm

42. Ruoff C, Rye D. The ICSD-3 and DSM-5 guidelines for diagnosing narcolepsy: clinical relevance and practicality. *Curr Med Res Opin*. 2016;1–12.

43. Thorpy MJ, Krieger AC. Delayed diagnosis of narcolepsy: characterization and impact. *Sleep Med*. 2014;15:502–7.

44. Dauvilliers Y, Siegel JM, Lopez R, Torontali ZA, Peever JH. Cataplexy—clinical aspects, pathophysiology and management strategy. *Nat Rev Neurol*. 2014;10:386–95.

45. Mignot E, Lammers GJ, Ripley B, *et al*. The role of cerebrospinal fluid hypocretin measurement in the diagnosis of narcolepsy and other hypersomnias. *Arch Neurol*. 2002;59:1553–62.

46. Aran A, Einen M, Lin L, Plazzi G, Nishino S, Mignot E. Clinical and therapeutic aspects of childhood narcolepsy-cataplexy: a retrospective study of 51 children. *Sleep*. 2010;33:1457–64.

47. Nightingale S, Orgill JC, Ebrahim IO, de Lacy SF, Agrawal S, Williams AJ. The association between narcolepsy and REM behavior disorder (RBD). *Sleep Med*. 2005;6:253–8.

48. Aldrich MS, Chervin RD, Malow BA. Value of the multiple sleep latency test (MSLT) for the diagnosis of narcolepsy. *Sleep*. 1997;20:620–9.

49. Roehrs T, Roth T. Multiple sleep latency test: technical aspects and normal values. *J Clin Neurophysiol*. 1992;9:63–7.

50. Volk S, Dyroff J, Georgi K, Pflug B. [Quality of day time sleep in the multiple sleep latency tests in patients with narcolepsy, obstructive sleep apnea and psychogenic hypersomnia]. *EEG EMG Z Elektroenzephalogr Elektromyogr Verwandte Geb*. 1992;23:210–14.

51. Anderson KN, Pilsworth S, Sharples LD, Smith IE, Shneerson JM. Idiopathic hypersomnia: a study of 77 cases. *Sleep*. 2007;30:1274–81.

52. Billiard M, Sonka K. Idiopathic hypersomnia. *Sleep Med Rev*. 2016;29:23–33.

53. Dauvilliers Y, Lopez R, Ohayon M, Bayard S. Hypersomnia and depressive symptoms: methodological and clinical aspects. *BMC Med*. 2013;11:78.

54. Ohayon MM, Guilleminault C, Priest RG. Night terrors, sleepwalking, and confusional arousals in the general population: their frequency and relationship to other sleep and mental disorders. *J Clin Psychiatry*. 1999;60:268–76; quiz 277.

55. Guilleminault C, Kirisoglu C, da Rosa AC, Lopes C, Chan A. Sleepwalking, a disorder of NREM sleep instability. *Sleep Med*. 2006;7:163–70.

56. Pressman MR. Factors that predispose, prime and precipitate NREM parasomnias in adults: clinical and forensic implications. *Sleep Med Rev*. 2007;11:5–30; discussion 31–3.

57. Espa F, Dauvilliers Y, Ondze B, Billiard M, Besset A. Arousal reactions in sleepwalking and night terrors in adults: the role of respiratory events. *Sleep*. 2002;25:871–5.

58. Guilleminault C, Kirisoglu C, Bao G, Arias V, Chan A, Li KK. Adult chronic sleepwalking and its treatment based on polysomnography. *Brain J Neurol*. 2005;128(Pt 5):1062–9.

59. Fois C, Wright M-AS, Sechi G, Walker MC, Eriksson SH. The utility of polysomnography for the diagnosis of NREM parasomnias: an observational study over 4 years of clinical practice. *J Neurol*. 2015;262:385–93.

60. Luppi P-H, Clément O, Valencia Garcia S, Brischoux F, Fort P. New aspects in the pathophysiology of rapid eye movement sleep behavior disorder: the potential role of glutamate, gamma-aminobutyric acid, and glycine. *Sleep Med*. 2013;14:714–18.

61. Schenck CH, Bundlie SR, Ettinger MG, Mahowald MW. Chronic behavioral disorders of human REM sleep: a new category of parasomnia. *Sleep*. 1986;9:293–308.

62. Mouret J, Delorme F, Jouvet M. [Lesions of the pontine tegmentum and sleep in rats]. *C R Séances Soc Biol Fil*. 1967;161:1603–6.

63. Schenck CH, Boeve BF, Mahowald MW. Delayed emergence of a parkinsonian disorder or dementia in 81% of older men initially diagnosed with idiopathic rapid eye movement sleep behavior disorder: a 16-year update on a previously reported series. *Sleep Med*. 2013;14:744–8.

64. Postuma RB, Gagnon JF, Vendette M, Montplaisir JY. Markers of neurodegeneration in idiopathic rapid eye movement sleep behaviour disorder and Parkinson's disease. *Brain J Neurol*. 2009;132(Pt 12):3298–307.

65. Postuma RB, Pelletier A, Berg D, Gagnon J-F, Escudier F, Montplaisir J. Screening for prodromal Parkinson's disease in the general community: a sleep-based approach. *Sleep Med*. 2016;21:101–5.

66. Lee K, Baron K, Soca R, Attarian H. The prevalence and characteristics of REM sleep without atonia (RSWA) in patients taking antidepressants. *J Clin Sleep Med*. 2016;12:351–5.

67. McCarter SJ, St Louis EK, Sandness DJ, *et al*. Antidepressants increase REM sleep muscle tone in patients with and without REM sleep behavior disorder. *Sleep*. 2015;38:907–17.

68. Sharpless BA, Barber JP. Lifetime prevalence rates of sleep paralysis: a systematic review. *Sleep Med Rev*. 2011;15:311–15.

69. Sharpless BA. A clinician's guide to recurrent isolated sleep paralysis. *Neuropsychiatr Dis Treat*. 2016;12:1761–7.

70. Sandman N, Valli K, Kronholm E, Revonsuo A, Laatikainen T, Paunio T. Nightmares: risk factors among the Finnish general adult population. *Sleep*. 2015;38:507–14.

71. Abbott SM, Reid KJ, Zee PC. Circadian rhythm sleep-wake disorders. *Psychiatr Clin North Am*. 2015;38:805–23.

72. Gradisar M, Crowley SJ. Delayed sleep phase disorder in youth. *Curr Opin Psychiatry*. 2013;26:580–5.

73. Esquirol Y, Bongard V, Mabile L, Jonnier B, Soulat J-M, Perret B. Shift work and metabolic syndrome: respective impacts of job strain, physical activity, and dietary rhythms. *Chronobiol Int*. 2009;26:544–59.

74. Fekedulegn D, Burchfiel CM, Hartley TA, *et al*. Shiftwork and sickness absence among police officers: the BCOPS study. *Chronobiol Int*. 2013;30:930–41.

75. Knutsson A. Shift work and coronary heart disease. *Scand J Soc Med* (Suppl). 1989;44:1–36.

76. Ohayon MM, Roth T. Prevalence of restless legs syndrome and periodic limb movement disorder in the general population. *J Psychosom Res*. 2002;53:547–54.

77. Morin CM, LeBlanc M, Daley M, Gregoire JP, Mérette C. Epidemiology of insomnia: prevalence, self-help treatments, consultations, and determinants of help-seeking behaviors. *Sleep Med*. 2006;7:123–30.

78. Ohayon MM. Epidemiology of insomnia: what we know and what we still need to learn. *Sleep Med Rev*. 2002;6:97–111.

79. Riemann D. Insomnia and comorbid psychiatric disorders. *Sleep Med*. 2007;8 Suppl 4:S15–20.

80. Lichstein KL, Justin Thomas S, Woosley JA, Geyer JD. Co-occurring insomnia and obstructive sleep apnea. *Sleep Med*. 2013;14:824–9.

81. Spielman AJ, Caruso LS, Glovinsky PB. A behavioral perspective on insomnia treatment. *Psychiatr Clin North Am*. 1987;10:541–53.

82. Ohayon MM, Li KK, Guilleminault C. Risk factors for sleep bruxism in the general population. *Chest*. 2001;119:53–61.

# 111

# Epidemiology of sleep–wake and primary prevention of its disorders

*Lena Katharina Keller, Eva C. Winnebeck, and Till Roenneberg*

## Introduction

A recent study [1] estimated the economic costs of insufficient sleep to be roughly between 1% and 3% of the gross domestic product (GDP) in the industrialized world. To understand the mechanisms and causes behind this expensive modern sleep 'experiment', we need to strengthen sleep research both in the laboratory and in the field.

Sleep research is almost 100 years old. By studying sleep predominantly in laboratories, the physiology underlying sleep was systematically elucidated, describing, for example, the neuronal circuits and brain regions that initiate and maintain sleep [2] and how the timing of sleep and wakefulness are controlled by an internal 24-hour clock—the circadian clock [3]. Sleep research outside the laboratory in the real world, that is, the epidemiology of sleep, is even younger, looking back about only 30 years [4].

Sleep and its functions can only be understood in the context of the whole 24-hour day, which includes wake. We therefore base this review on formal considerations of the four main (albeit interrelated) aspects of sleep (and wake): duration, timing, structure, and quality (Fig. 111.1). The molecular underpinnings of the system have been described in Chapter 109.

### Duration

Wake and sleep are not identical with, but closely related to, activity and rest, which together make up the circadian day. Internal days can deviate from 24 hours, but in the long term, the duration of activity–rest (sleep–wake) averages up to 24 hours. If, on average, longer sleep was not followed by shorter wake, and vice versa, we would gradually advance or delay our sleep timing and other daily behaviours.

### Timing

The *timing* of sleep and wake, is similarly interdependent as the duration of sleep and wake. The timing is often defined by the onset and offset of the respective episodes; however, this measure is highly dependent on the episodes' durations. The timing of sleep or wake is therefore more reliably defined by the mid-points of either sleep or wake, rather than by their transitions. As will be described later, the mid-point of sleep on work-free days is used as a surrogate for chronotype. The concept of *chronotype* refers to how the circadian clock of an individual embeds itself into the 24-hour light–dark cycle—earlier or later.

Both sleep timing and duration are regulated by at least two processes [5, 6]—one homeostatic, and the other circadian. The former works like an hourglass; sleep pressure builds up during wake and dissipates during sleep (with non-linear characteristics). Sleep pressure can be estimated from the EEG, specifically the spectral power of slow-wave sleep (SWS) [7]. Yet, if sleep was solely controlled by the homeostat, sleep timing would be quite labile. Let us presume someone regularly slept 8 hours from 10 p.m. to 6 a.m. and was awake for 16 hours from 6 a.m. to 10 p.m. If this person stayed up one day until 6 a.m., he/she might sleep as long as 12 hours due to the prior sleep loss and would wake up at 6 p.m. with minimal sleep pressure. From that moment on, the homeostat would let this person sleep from 6 p.m. to 2 a.m. and be awake from 2 a.m. to 6 p.m.

But sleep—like most functions in our body—is also regulated by the circadian clock, which makes being asleep and being awake more likely to occur at certain times in the 24-hour cycle than at others. The model proposed by Borbély and Daan [5, 6] implements the circadian involvement in sleep regulation in making the thresholds that trigger falling asleep and waking up oscillate in a circadian manner. The circadian clock's influence on sleep becomes evident in jet lag situations. When we travel fast over many time zones, the resynchronization of our circadian clock lags behind (as a rule of thumb, the circadian clock adapts by no more than about 1 hour per day). As a result, we have difficulties adjusting to the new light–dark regime at our destination, cannot sleep for several days during the local night, and can hardly be awake during the local day.

Our lifestyle has drastically changed with industrialization. While we used to expose ourselves to bright natural light outdoors during the day and actual darkness during the night, we now spend most of the day inside (with light up to a 1000-fold dimmer than outside) and simply switch on artificial light from sunset to bedtime. We have thereby drastically weakened the synchronizing signals (zeitgeber) [8] that our circadian clocks use to synchronize (i.e. entrain) to the

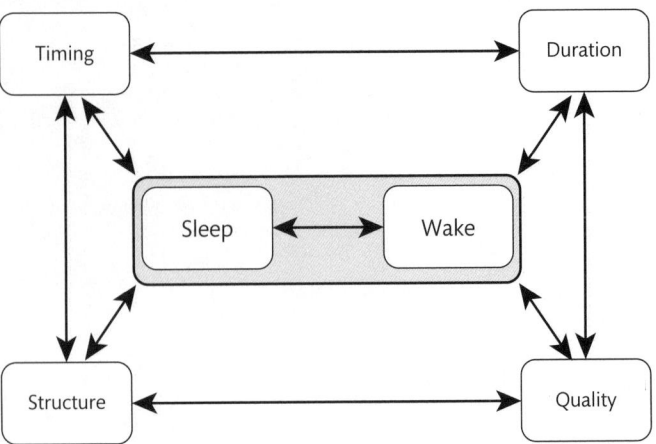

**Fig. 111.1** Key aspects of sleep–wake behaviour can be assessed separately but are highly interrelated.

24-hour cycle. In adapting to this new situation, most people's circadian clocks have become later [9]. This delayed circadian phase is quickly reversible, as Ken Wright has shown in elegant experiments where he took urban students camping for 1 week and exposed them to the strong zeitgeber of natural light and dark [10]. Especially the late chronotypes advanced, and the chronotype differences between individuals became much smaller.

### Structure

Both wake and sleep—albeit in very different ways—are also characterized by temporal structures that depend on many parameters—in our society, most importantly, on whether they occur on work-free days or workdays. This is illustrated in Fig. 111.2 where the physical activity averaged over several days rarely reaches zero in any of the subjects; this has at least two reasons: (1) sleep times can vary greatly between days (thereby 'spilling' activity into the average rest- or sleep-window); and (2) some activity can still be recorded during

sleep. Workday sleep timing is usually more regular, so that activity troughs are often more pronounced than on weekends. Although activity levels during sleep are by many factors smaller than during wake, the residual levels can still be analysed. The resulting activity structure during sleep shows a clear rhythmicity with a period of around 90–150 minutes, a property it shares with the sleep stages recorded by polysomnography (PSG) in sleep laboratories (see Activity monitoring for sleep–wake epidemiology, p. 1140).

### Quality

The fourth aspect is quality (Fig. 111.1). Although we intuitively know that sleep and wake quality are strongly interdependent, we need an objective measure for sleep quality before we can quantify the respective qualities and their interdependence scientifically. Since sleep fulfils many biological functions, which we still need to fully understand, a universal definition of sleep quality may be difficult.

Sleep science commonly distinguishes between *subjective* and *objective* sleep quality. *Subjective sleep quality* refers to how well the sleeper reports to have slept after the sleep episode or to sleep in general. This self-report is likely influenced by the sleeper's individual and cultural preconception about how sleep should be or how one should feel after waking up. It is also influenced by the sleeper's individual psychological state such as their affect [11]. *Objective sleep quality*, by contrast, compares certain objective sleep measures of an individual with normative values. These normative values may, in themselves, harbour a bias just by how they were obtained and who served as reference population—often young, healthy university students in controlled sleep laboratory environments. The most common measures for objective sleep quality are: how long people take to fall asleep (sleep latency); how often they wake and how long they are awake (wake after sleep onset); how much of their time in bed people actually sleep (sleep efficiency); the sleep architecture (shuttling between sleep stages); time in certain sleep stages; and the intensity of the slow brain waves during deep sleep (delta power).

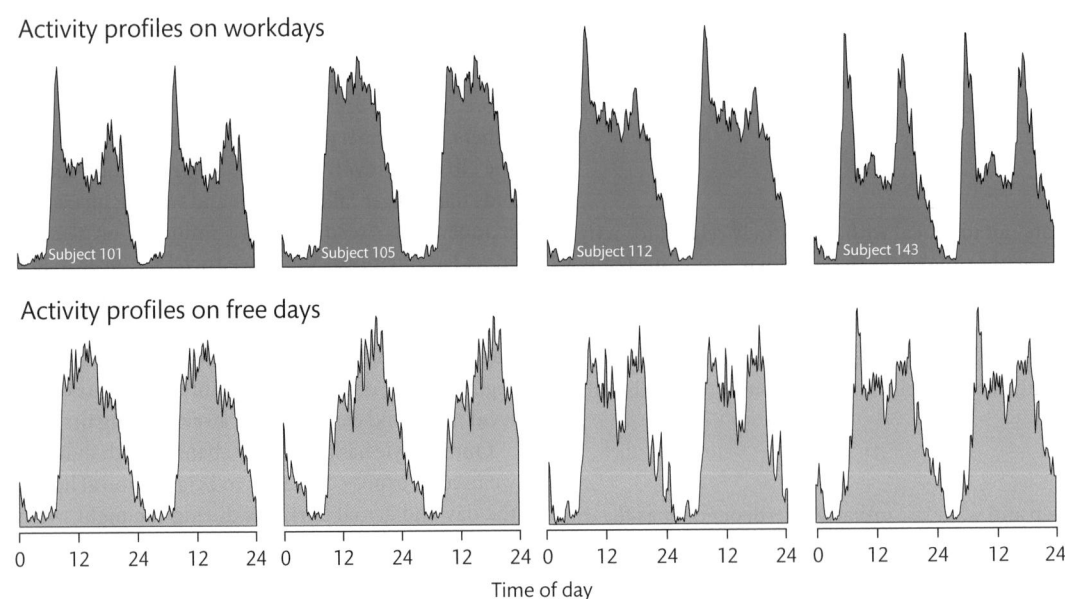

**Fig. 111.2** Activity profiles can vary in their timing, shape, and amplitude. In general, they differ greatly between workdays (top row) and work-free days (bottom row). Profiles were taken from our large actimetry database and represent averages over 23–60 days (work or work-free, respectively).

Some of these sleep measures and objective quality indicators can be subjectively assessed by questionnaires such as the Pittsburgh Sleep Quality Index (PSQI) [12], but most must be measured via PSG in the sleep laboratory.

Importantly, both objective and subjective sleep quality are biased by the modern notion of what sleep should 'look' like, namely efficient, consolidated, and, if possible, initiated 6–8 hours before one has to get up (for work). The more we find out about sleep in non-industrialized societies, that is, before the use of electrical light [13–17] or in people who have to live according to the natural photoperiod [18], the more we may have to challenge our notions and current methods of measuring sleep quality. The fact that subjective and objective sleep quality are only poorly associated with each other [11, 19, 20] indicates how difficult and highly flawed our current definition of sleep quality is.

## Epidemiology of sleep in the real world

Since 2000, we have been building a database on daily sleep behaviour using the Munich ChronoType Questionnaire (MCTQ) [21]. By now, it contains more than a quarter million entries. The MCTQ asks participants to give the times when they go to bed, prepare for sleep, fall asleep, wake up, and get up [21]. Most importantly, these questions are asked separately for workdays and work-free days. The growing database allowed us to quantify the key aspects of human sleep–wake behaviour. We assessed the amount of sleep people get and when they get it, and how different aspects of sleep change with age [22], season [23, 24], and geographical location [25], even with daylight-saving time [23]. Our results suggest that, although people sleep just as long on work-free days as they did 10 years ago, they get continuously less sleep on workdays [26]. Also, throughout their school and work life, most people alternate between under-sleeping on workdays and over-sleeping on work-free days. One factor leading to this difference in sleep duration is a change in sleep timing from workdays to work-free days. This so-called *social jetlag* [27] is quantified as the difference between the social and the biological 'time zone'. The fact that >80% of the working population in our database needs an alarm clock to wake up on workdays [26] indicates that almost the entire working population experiences a strain on their circadian clock and sleep.

### Sleep timing

Sleep times on workdays are predictably more synchronized among individuals than on work-free days, that is, they have a narrower distribution [mid-sleep on workdays (MSW); see Fig. 111.3] than on free days [mid-sleep on free day (MSF); see Fig. 111.3] (for day-specific differences in sleep timing, see also Fig. 111.5a).

The internal circadian clocks of most of us have continuously delayed during industrialization (due to decreasing zeitgeber strengths), while social times, for example work or school start times, have remained relatively stable. We fall asleep much later than our rural ancestors and use alarm clocks to wake up, thereby accumulating a sleep debt over the work week, for which we try to compensate on weekends.

For chronotype assessment, that is, how late or early one's circadian clock is embedded into the light–dark cycle, sleep timing on work-free days is a better basis than sleep timing on workdays. However,

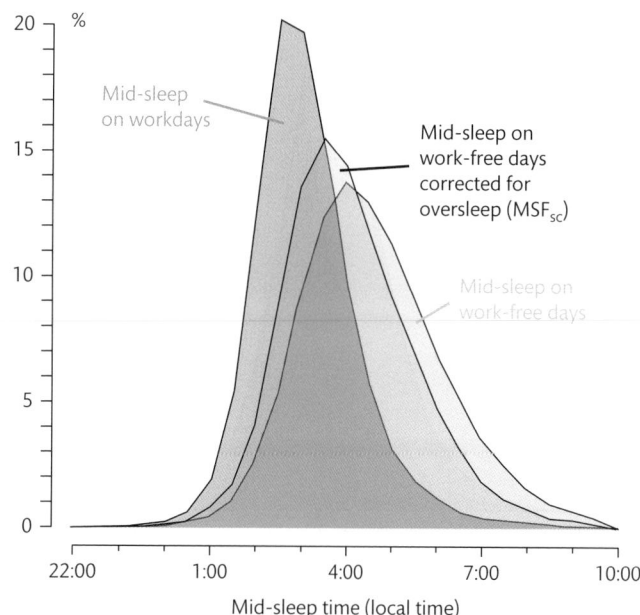

**Fig. 111.3** Distribution of mid-sleep times in the MCTQ database. The narrower distribution shows the mid-sleep times on workdays (MSW: $n$ = 197,829; mean = 3:19 $\pm$ 1.13), and the later wider distribution represents mid-sleep times on free days (MSF: $n$ = 200,260; mean = 4:47 $\pm$ 1.34; excluding people who use alarm clocks on work-free days). The assessment of chronotype involves correcting MSF for oversleep (see text for details), resulting in the distribution in the middle (MSFsc: $n$ = 181,600; mean = 4:19 $\pm$ 1.27).

since work-free days are still influenced by workdays in the form of catch-up-sleep, we correct MSF for 'over-sleep' (MSF$_{sc}$; see https://www.thewep.org/documentations/mctq for a comprehensive list of variables assessed or computed from the MCTQ). Note that MSF$_{sc}$-based chronotype should only be calculated for people who do not use alarm clocks on work-free days.

The MCTQ-assessed chronotype is not a scaled preference for doing things at specific times of day (as is the aim of the morningness–eveningness questionnaire developed in the 1970s) [28]. The MSF$_{sc}$-time should be regarded as a surrogate for the entrained phase of an individual's circadian clock. Validations with more objective measures of phase of entrainment, such as sleep-logs, actimetry, or measurements of the rise of melatonin in the evening, show good accordance [29–31] with the one-time assessment of chronotype (MSF$_{sc}$).

### Sleep duration

Most people accumulate a sleep debt on workdays. As outlined in the introduction, this is most probably due to the effects of our modern light environments on the circadian clock and fixed work schedules. Fig. 111.4 shows the distributions of sleep duration on work- and work-free days, with the former being over 1 hour shorter and just slightly narrower than its counterpart on work-free days. Fig. 111.5b shows that the day-specific sleep durations can, in some individuals, differ by >5 hours.

### Sleep quality

As discussed, we still need an objective measure for sleep quality. However, apart from pathologies that are not directly sleep-related

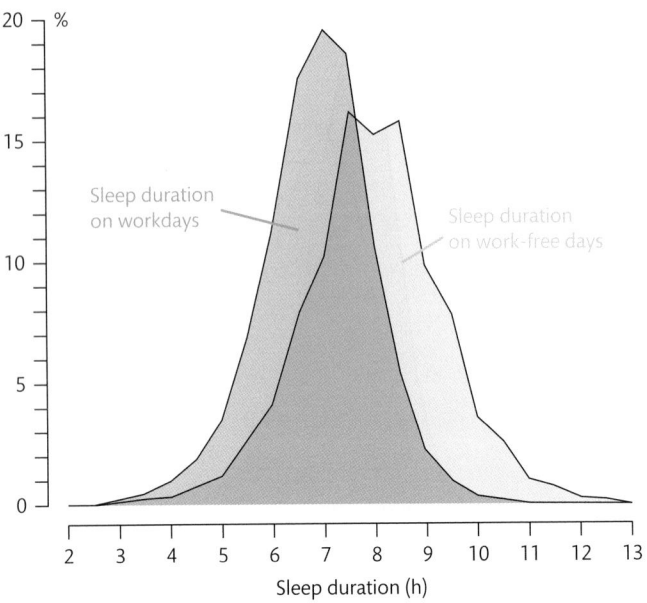

**Fig. 111.4** Distributions of sleep duration on workdays (*n* = 197,829; mean = 7.06 hours ± 1.08 hours) and on work-free days (*n* = 200,260; mean = 8.12 hours ± 1.22 hours).

sleep duration and metabolic problems [32]. Social jet lag is also associated with higher odds of being a smoker and correlates with alcohol and caffeine consumption [27], as well as with signs of depression such as appetite loss and feelings of sadness [33].

### Sleep structure

So far, there are no epidemiological data on the structure of sleep, since it is currently only accessible via measuring brain waves and other parameters in sleep laboratories using PSG. PSG recordings are subsequently analysed and 'scored' into different sleep stages. Sleep's 'architecture' cycles through these different sleep stages approximately every 90–150 minutes. This sleep-inherent 'ultradian' rhythmicity was first described by Dement and Kleitman [34]. To obtain epidemiological data on sleep structure, we recently explored how to extract this ultradian structure from activity.

(apnoea, restless legs, chronic pain, etc.), chronic accumulation of sleep debt, the habitual use of alarm clocks, and constant attempts to sleep at the wrong circadian times must greatly reduce sleep quality. All these scenarios are aspects of social jet lag (Fig. 111.5a). This modern syndrome could turn out to be the most prevalent and costly high-risk behaviour of our times. With every hour of social jet lag, the chances of being overweight or obese increase by 33% [26], substantiating an association found already much earlier between

## Activity monitoring for sleep–wake epidemiology

The methods used in sleep laboratories (for example, PSG) usually obtain detailed information on individuals in clinical settings and are less suited for large-scale studies (too costly, time-consuming, and labour-intensive). Epidemiological sleep studies require simple and cost-effective methods to assess and monitor the desired variables. They therefore often rely on self-reporting—either as one-off questionnaires (for example, the MCTQ; see Epidemiology of sleep in the real world, p. 1139) or by keeping sleep-logs.

Another method for sleep monitoring that is becoming increasingly popular is the continuous measurement of physical activity or body movement via actimetry (or 'actigraphy'). Body movements are recorded mostly with watch-like, wrist-worn devices. Since people move much more during their wake-time than during their

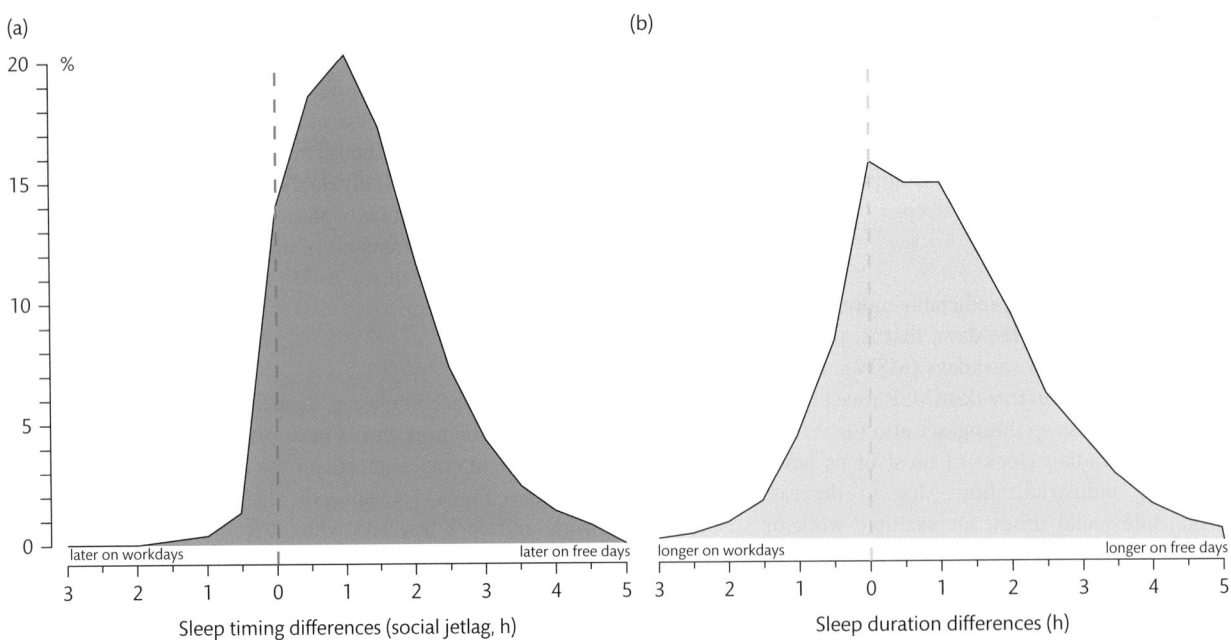

**Fig. 111.5** Differences in sleep–wake behaviour between workdays and work-free days. (a) Social jetlag is defined by the differences in sleep timing between the two day types [27]; frequencies on the right of the stippled zero line concern people who sleep later on work-free days than on workdays, while those on the left of this line sleep later on workdays. (b) Similar differences exist between sleep duration on workdays and work-free days, with the majority sleeping longer on work-free days (right of the stippled zero line).

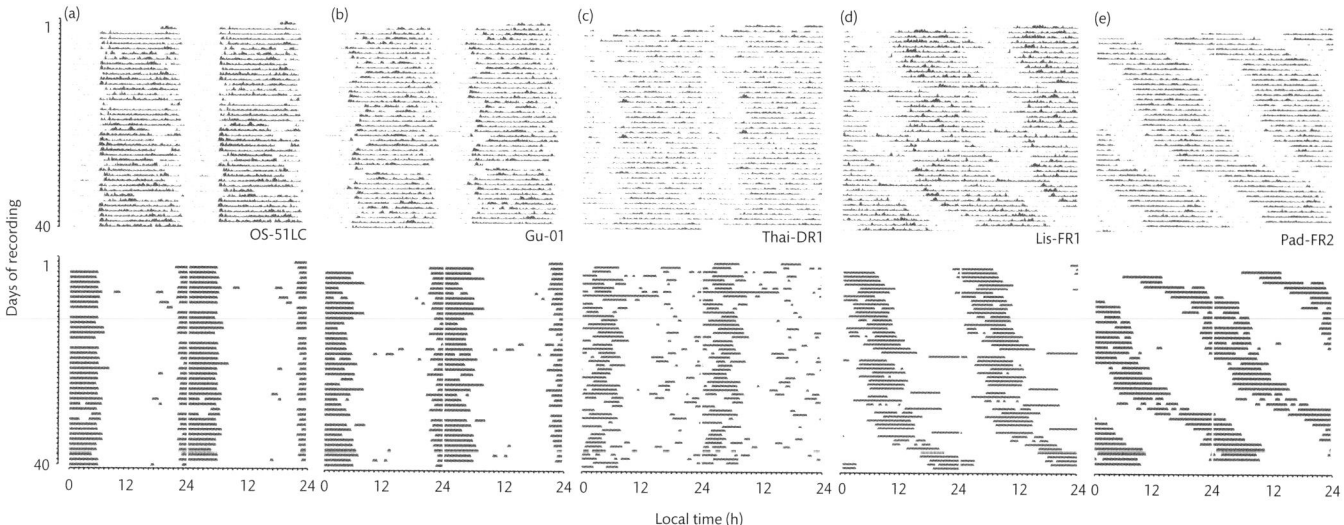

**Fig. 111.6** Activity records can be used to infer on sleep–wake times. The top row shows five 40-day activity recordings from different individuals, and the bottom row shows the respective sleep times as bars [27]. The pale backgrounds indicate photoperiods, which were calculated based on the individuals' locations (latitude and longitude) and recording dates. We selected these five examples to demonstrate how different the sleep–wake behaviour can be. The example in (a) shows a female with strict regularity in her relatively early daily sleep–wake schedules. The next pair of graphs in (b) is again a female and early chronotype whose schedules are far less regular (possibly because her partner is a late chronotype). The central pair of graphs in (c) shows a male whose nocturnal sleep episodes are late, short, and irregular and who takes naps in the early evening. The next two examples in (d) and (e) show a male and a female, respectively, whose clocks—despite being visually unimpaired individuals—have difficulties to stably synchronize to the 24-hour rhythm of the environment.

sleep (Fig. 111.2), one can estimate when and how long they sleep by the episodes of relatively low activity [35, 36], that is, rest–activity is used to assess sleep–wake (Fig. 111.6).

### Sleep timing and duration from actimetry

The many different methods to assess sleep via actimetry are either published or remain black boxes built into proprietary software. Overall, their concordance with the gold standard in sleep monitoring (PSG) is reasonably high—at least in healthy sleepers [35, 36]—but they have also been validated in sleepers suffering from common sleep pathologies such as sleep apnoea (for example, [37–39]). Most methods perform well but tend to underestimate short awakenings within a sleep episode [wake after sleep onset (WASO)]. Detection generally becomes less reliable when the difference between wake-time and sleep-time activity is low, that is, when people are bedridden or suffer from motor disorders or highly interrupted sleep.

For studies outside of laboratories and clinics, sleep detection via actimetry has many advantages despite providing much less information than PSG. Unlike self-reports, it is an objective measure of sleep timing and duration and produces—without burden—a detailed longitudinal record (over days and weeks) of an individual's rest–activity or sleep–wake behaviour. Long-term actimetry puts sleep into the context of the previous and following wake and sleep episode and thus allows, for example, teasing apart homeostatic and circadian influences on sleep (see Introduction, p. 1137). As such, long-term actimetry is superior to a single night in the sleep laboratory; it allows analysing the regularity of the sleep–wake pattern, identifying the daily phase and amplitude of general activity [for example, by a 24-hour cosine fit providing the *centre of gravity* (COG)], calculating the mid-points of sleep, or characterizing weekly patterns (for example, differences between work- and work-free days).

Long-term actimetry also allows detecting more complex sleep–wake problems, disorders or pathologies that are only apparent in long-term recordings. A good example is the N24 disorder [40] where sighted individuals cannot synchronize (i.e. entrain) to the normal light–dark cycle and therefore drift through societal time (Fig. 111.6d and e). Shift-workers have a similar problem, but the influences are inversed; societal time (for example, work schedules) make these individuals drift through their own circadian time (Fig. 111.7). Note how similar the rest–activity/sleep–wake patterns are in the individuals shown in Fig. 111.6d and e to those shown in Fig. 111.7d and e.

To make use of this strength of actimetry, its recordings need to be long enough to reveal the important patterns and be representative of an individual's sleeping habits. Since the pattern and variability in people's sleeping habits are often not known beforehand, any initial actimetry recording should cover at least 14 days (including three weekends) and ideally aim for 6 weeks. With complex disorders and sleep schedules, these initial recordings need to be complemented by even longer recordings over months.

### Sleep structure from actimetry

So far, research has usually used actimetry only to obtain information about the timing and duration of sleep episodes. However, new efforts are under way that allow extracting more information about the sleep episode itself, that is, its structure and ultradian cyclicity. This effort is based on the observation that body movements are part of sleep physiology and vary with sleep stages or sleep stage transitions (for example, [34, 41–43]). Many current commercial actimeters (notably not for use in clinical or research settings!) claim to inform consumers about their sleep depth based on their movements during sleep. Whereas these consumer products are currently not scientifically validated and their output needs to be treated with absolute

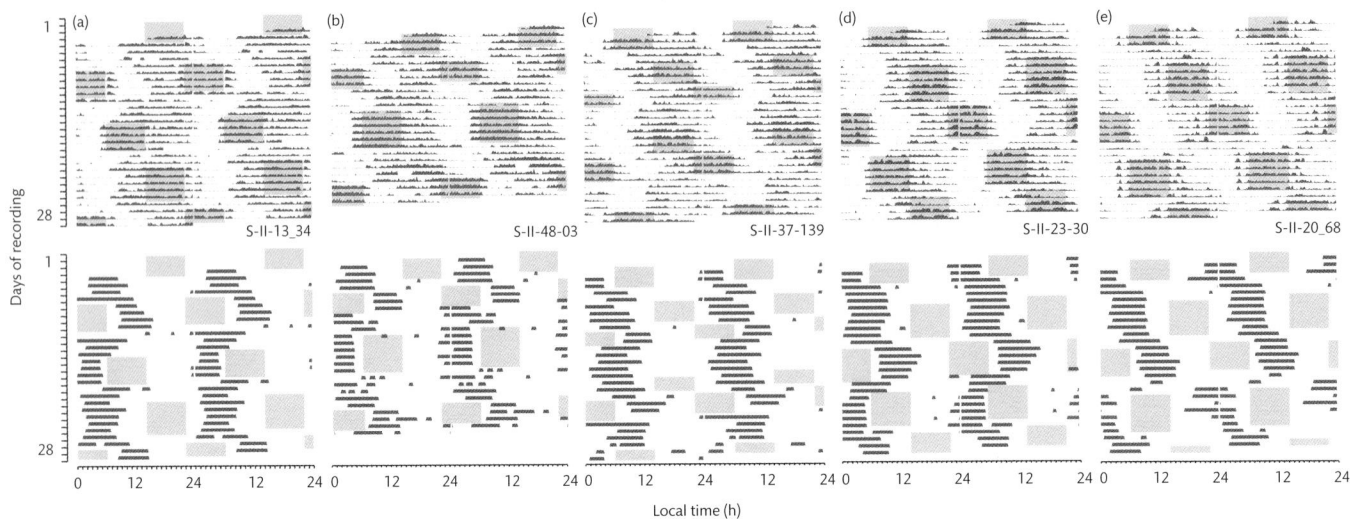

**Fig. 111.7** Actimetry and the derived sleep times in five examples of shift-workers. As in Fig. 111.6, the top row shows the activity, and the bottom row the calculated sleep times. The grey squares indicate work times.

caution [44–46], the principle on which they are based may well work. We ourselves have developed a method that reveals the rhythms in body movement during sleep in actimetry recordings—rhythms that are highly reflective of sleep cycles, as determined by clinical PSG [47]. These extended applications of actimetry in large epidemiological studies will provide valuable new insights into the structure of sleep and its relation to sleep timing, sleep duration, and sleep quality.

## Sleep–wake in psychiatric patients

The association between sleep–wake behaviour and mental disorders is apparent in the standard criteria for the diagnosis of psychiatric disorders in DSM-5 and ICD-10 [48]. Sleep problems are commonly seen as symptoms or comorbidities of the psychiatric disorder itself. For example, one of the diagnostic criteria for a depressive episode are changes in sleep (hypersomnia or insomnia); for a manic episode, a decreased need for sleep; and the criteria for post-traumatic stress disorder include nightmares and difficulty sleeping. However, the association between sleep and psychiatric pathologies is highly complex with numerous feedbacks. The causal links in this network are still not well understood but are certainly not unidirectional. While psychiatric patients frequently develop sleep problems [49], sleep problems may trigger psychiatric disorders in the general population [50]. Furthermore, psychopharmacological treatments influence sleep both by improving [51] and by creating/increasing sleep problems [51, 52]. Sleep—or rather its deprivation—is even used as therapy in major depression [53]. But again, the role of sleep deprivation in depression is complex; on the one hand, isolated sleep deprivation may acutely reduce depression [54], possibly via changing the synaptic rearrangements that occur during sleep [55]; on the other hand, chronic sleep deprivation may increase the risk for developing a variety of psychiatric (and somatic) disorders [56].

Similar to the concept of *sleep quality*, the term *sleep problems* is used for many different symptoms. Here, we try to put some order into the different aspects of sleep in the context of psychiatry by separating the individual—though interdependent—aspects of sleep, namely timing, duration, structure, and quality (see also Introduction, p. 1137 and Fig. 111.1).

### Sleep timing

Sleep timing, or chronotype, has often been associated with psychiatric syndromes (for review, see [57]). Notably, many studies ask for sleep preferences, for example for morningness (MEQ; [28]), instead of actual sleep timing (for a discussion about different chronotyping methods, see [58]). Two studies using actual sleep timing found that the later people sleep, the more depressed they are [33, 59]. In addition, Levandovski and co-workers [33] showed an association with social jet lag, indicating that the clash between chronotype and social schedules, rather than chronotype/sleep timing per se, can lead to depressive symptoms. Whether a later chronotype predisposes to depression or depression goes along with a change in chronotype still has to be worked out (for an in-depth discussion, see [60]). The fact that advancing circadian phase (chronotype) is being used as a therapeutic approach in patients suffering from depression indicates that sleep timing is being regarded as a cause—at least in part—for developing depressive symptoms [61].

Other psychiatric syndromes, such as seasonal affective disorder (SAD) [62], schizophrenia [63, 64], obsessive–compulsive disorder [65, 66], and attention-deficit/hyperactivity disorder (ADHD) [67], have also been found to be associated with delayed sleep timing. It seems that most psychiatric, as well as neurodegenerative, disorders go along with changes in sleep timing [68–71].

### Sleep duration

The most obvious example of the relationship between psychiatric syndromes and sleep duration is bipolar disorder; during depressive episodes, most patients sleep longer, whereas during manic episodes, sleep is usually shortened [49]. Notably, shortened sleep during mania is not to be confused with insomnia, the inability to initiate or maintain sleep, but is due to an apparent reduction in sleep need, that is, patients feel awake and refreshed after as little as 3 hours of sleep [49].

Other mood disorders have also been associated with changes in sleep duration; patients suffering from SAD show a prolonged sleep duration during winter [72]—as, to some extent, is also true for the general population [23]; patients with non-seasonal unipolar depression either sleep significantly longer (hypersomnia [73]) or shorter (hyposomnia [74]) than healthy controls. These changes in sleep duration are usually caused by the inability to initiate sleep and/or early morning awakenings. Another explanation for this condition is that patients adhere to habitual sleep times, even when their circadian timing changes. Some studies failed to show hypersomnia (or hyposomnia) in depressed patients in the sleep laboratory and concluded that these symptoms must be rather a subjective sleep complaint [75], but sleep measured in a one-night PSG in an artificial environment does not capture the actual sleep of patients at home.

Our own research showed that adolescent patients with remitted depressive disorder still sleep longer, compared to healthy controls [60]. Schizophrenia is also associated with hyper- [64] or hyposomnia [76]. The latter was also found in post-traumatic stress disorder [77], alcoholism [78], autism [79], and generalized anxiety disorder [80].

The relationships between psychiatric syndromes and sleep duration are all but straightforward. On the one hand, studies in the general population found sleep durations of under 5 hours increased the odds for a variety of psychiatric conditions: mood disorders such as depression [56, 81, 82]; anxiety disorders [56, 81]; obsessive–compulsive disorder [81]; and nicotine and alcohol dependence [56, 81]. On the other hand, sleep over 9 hours was associated with depression [82], anxiety disorders, social phobia, and alcohol dependence [81]. In children, both shortened and prolonged sleep increased the likelihood for ADHD [83, 84]. Although sleep duration differs significantly between workdays and work-free days [85], Park and colleagues [81] analysed the relationship of sleep duration and various psychiatric disorders only on weekdays, which predominantly reflects external (that is, social) time constraints.

## Sleep quality

Reduced subjective sleep quality can include a variety of symptoms—from trouble initiating and maintaining sleep (insomnia) to early morning awakenings, excessive daytime tiredness, and the feeling of not being refreshed despite a sufficient sleep duration. All of these symptoms have been associated with a variety of psychiatric disorders [86], both as preceding symptoms and as comorbidities. Reduced subjective sleep quality is, for example, often associated with acute depression [87, 88] and is even found in patients with remitted depression [60] either as a residual symptom or as a predictor of relapse. Sleep disturbances can be predictors for the onset of major depression [89], and subjects complaining about insomnia have a 4-fold higher chance of developing major depressive disorder [50].

## Sleep structure

The concept of sleep structure has been described (see Structure, p.1138). Due to the limited number of publications, we focus here on the main characteristics of PSG in psychiatric patients. The most obvious changes in PSG could be found in depressed patients. Many studies show a disturbed sleep consolidation, as well as changes in sleep depth and REM sleep pressure [90, 91]. Additionally, two meta-analyses found a reduced duration of SWS [90, 91], which remained

unconfirmed in another study [92], which also found none of these symptoms in SAD.

A recent meta-analysis on PSG and psychiatric disorders by Baglioni et al. [92] showed that beyond ADHD and SAD, almost every psychiatric disorder (including personality disorders, schizophrenia, and eating disorders) is associated with sleep alterations. Specific psychiatric disorders were not characterized by single PSG parameters, but rather a specific combination or profile of altered parameters.

## Primary prevention of sleep–wake disorders

Sleep disorders, according to ICD-10, refer to hyposomnia, hypersomnia, delayed or advanced sleep timing, irregular sleep, and non-24-hour sleep. The aetiology of these may be as complex as sleep itself. This complexity includes the neuronal circuits and switches that initiate, maintain, and terminate sleep [2], as well as the circadian [3] and homeostatic control [6, 93]; it also pertains to the many different functions that our brain performs during sleep such as synaptic reorganization [94], clearing of accumulated metabolites [95], consolidating memory [96], or immune functions [97]. This is a far from complete list of sleep's mechanistic gearbox that constitutes a breeding ground for sleep–wake disorders. But sleep can only be understood in context, which again constitutes a complex network of different levels. Many everyday life factors influence when, for how long, and how we sleep. Many of them are related to how we expose ourselves to light or what genetic chronotype we are: light exposure during the day—office worker vs farmer, commuting by bike or by tube; light exposure during the night—using intense, blue-rich light after sunset, sleeping in a darkened room; light exposure across the year— affected by season, longitude, timezone and 'time-meddlings' like daylight saving time; being a victim of societal time—late-chronotype teenagers learning at 8 in the morning, late chronotypes working early shifts or early chronotypes working at night. Again, this is an incomplete list of context factors, which are fertile soil for developing sleep–wake disorders. While the mechanistic complexity of sleep control does not readily lend itself to primary prevention, the contextual influences on sleep do. Here, we keep to the structure of this chapter and address this issue separately for timing, duration, structure, and quality.

### Sleep timing

Sleep timing is by far the most important and amenable toehold for preventive and therapeutic sleep medicine. Most sleep disturbances—apart from the comorbidities of psychiatric or other pathologies (pain, apnoea, etc.)—are due to living against one's internal circadian clock. This modern, highly prevalent syndrome [26] has many names: circadian disruption, circadian misalignment, circadian stress, circadian strain, or social jet lag (for details, see [98]). Its most extreme version is called shift-work. Sleeping and waking at the wrong circadian times has numerous health consequences, many of which are probably directly or indirectly related to sleep disturbances. Realigning sleep times with the temporal window provided by the circadian clock will therefore ameliorate sleep disturbances and thereby decrease health deficits. A recent epidemiological study has shown that late chronotypes have higher odds for developing type 2 diabetes if they work 'normal' day jobs, compared to working permanent night shifts [99]. Other studies have shown how sleep and health in shift-workers profit by realigning sleep and circadian time [100] or by assigning shifts according to chronotype [101].

In a majority of the population in urban/industrialized regions, circadian clocks are delayed while work schedules have hardly changed. Most people are therefore, figuratively speaking, 'permanent shift-workers'. Thus, any measure that decreases the resulting social jet lag is sleep problem-preventive. Such measures can change either the internal or the external time. The internal phase can be advanced by strengthening the zeitgeber [more light during the day and less (blue-containing) light during the night] or by ensuring an asymmetry in light exposure (more light before internal midday and less thereafter). Another point of action is delaying work and school start times or making them flexible.

### Sleep duration

Circadian misalignment and social jet lag always also affect sleep duration. Using an alarm clock and being unable to fall asleep early enough (due to the wake maintenance zone [102]) lead to chronic sleep deprivation during the work week and to over-sleep on weekends. This is also, though of a very different nature, a problem in shift-workers; shift-specific sleep problems are commonly due to forced awakenings. While late chronotypes are awoken by the external alarm clock before early shifts, early chronotypes are awoken too early by their internal (circadian) clocks when they try to get an extended sleep after night shifts [103]. Thus, changing sleep timing—as described—can, in most cases, also prevent insufficient sleep in terms of sleep duration.

### Sleep quality

Although we argued that fully consolidated sleep episodes are a modern concept, frequent interruptions are certainly a sign of poor sleep. Sleep quality and sleep interruptions change with age [104]. Alzheimer's patients often wake up during the night and are sleepy during the day. This is partly due to drastically reduced light–dark cycles in these patients, and again this syndrome is treatable with increased zeitgeber strength [105].

Low subjective sleep quality often is due to a wrong conception of what sleep should look like. For example, early chronotypes living in a predominantly late society often perceive their early tiredness and awakening as signs of a sleep disturbance, but only because they are not aware of their chronotype and the large inter-individual variability in circadian sleep timing. Once educated, society still challenges compliance with their own rhythms, but this then becomes a matter of choice, rather than a perceived illness. In other cases, simply by advising 'patients' to keep sleep diaries, which they can visualize, rectifies their misconceptions about sleep.

### Sleep structure

Abnormalities in sleep structure can be used in diagnosis and treatment of sleep disorders arising from both the mechanistic and the contextual levels. So far, sleep structure is best detected by PSG in the sleep laboratory or at home, but we are confident that actimetry can be used in future to derive the ultradian structure of sleep and thereby contribute to detection and prevention of sleep disorders. Sleep stages and structure depend on the time of day [3], so that attempts to sleep within the temporal window provided by the

circadian programme should be part of sleep hygiene and preventive sleep medicine.

## Conclusions

While we begin to understand the link between sleep timing and somatic problems (for example, metabolic syndrome), we need much more research to understand the association between sleep and psychiatric disorders. We will have to resolve several chicken-and-egg problems, and we have to look into the contexts of light, activity, food, and sleep within our weekly structures. We are optimistic that a combination of long-term activity recordings and the increasing possibilities to extrac t sleep information from activity will be a rich source for elucidating the different aetiologies of sleep pathologies, as well as the relationships between sleep and pathologies per se.

### REFERENCES

1. Hafner M, Stepanek M, Taylor J, Troxel WM. *Why sleep matters—the economic costs of insufficient sleep*. Santa Monica: CA and Cambridge, UK: RAND Corporation; 2016.
2. Saper CB, Fuller PM, Pedersen NP, Lu J, Scammell TE. Sleep state switching. *Neuron*. 2010;68:1023–42.
3. Wyatt JK, Ritz-de Cecco A, Czeisler CA, Dijk D-J. Circadian temperature and melatonin rhythms, sleep, and neurobiological function in humans living on a 20-h day. *Am J Physiol*. 1999;277:R1152–63.
4. Ferrie JE, Kumari M, Salo P, Singh-Manoux A, Kivimaki M. Sleep epidemiology—a rapidly growing field. *Int J Epidemiol*. 2011;40:1431–7.
5. Borbely AA. A two process model of sleep regulation. *Hum Neurobiol*. 1982;1:195–204.
6. Borbely AA, Daan S, Wirz-Justice A, Deboer T. The two-process model of sleep regulation: a reappraisal. *J Sleep Res*. 2016;25:131–43.
7. Dijk DJ. Regulation and functional correlates of slow wave sleep. *J Clin Sleep Med*. 2009;5(2 Suppl):S6–15.
8. Aschoff J, Klotter K, Wever R, editors. *Circadian Vocabulary*. Amsterdam: North-Holland Pulishing Company; 1965.
9. Roenneberg T, Keller LK, Fischer D, Matera JL, Vetter C, Winnebeck EC. Human activity and rest *in situ*. *Methods Enzymol*. 2015;552:257–83.
10. Wright KPJ, McHill AW, Birks BR, Griffin BR, Rusterholz T, Chinoy ED. Entrainment of the human circadian clock to the natural light-dark cycle. *Curr Biol*. 2013; 23:1554–8.
11. Jackowska M, Ronaldson A, Brown J, Steptoe A. Biological and psychological correlates of self-reported and objective sleep measures. *J Psychosom Res*. 2016;84:52–5.
12. Buysse DJ, Reynolds CF, 3rd, Monk TH, Berman SR, Kupfer DJ. The Pittsburgh Sleep Quality Index: a new instrument for psychiatric practice and research. *Psychiatry Res*. 1989;28:193–213.
13. Samson DR, Crittenden AN, Mabulla IA, Mabulla AZ, Nunn CL. Hadza sleep biology: evidence for flexible sleep-wake patterns in hunter-gatherers. *Am J Phys Anthropol*. 2017;162:573–82.
14. de la Iglesia HO, Moreno C, Lowden A, *et al*. Ancestral sleep. *Curr Biol*. 2016;26:R271–2.
15. Moreno CR, Vasconcelos S, Marqueze EC, *et al*. Sleep patterns in Amazon rubber tappers with and without electric light at home. *Sci Rep*. 2015;5:14074.

16. de la Iglesia HO, Fernandez-Duque E, Golombek DA, et al. Access to electric light is associated with shorter sleep duration in a traditionally hunter-gatherer community. J Biol Rhythms. 2015;30:342–50.

17. Yetish G, Kaplan H, Gurven M, et al. Natural sleep and its seasonal variations in three pre-industrial societies. Curr Biol. 2015;25:2862–8.

18. Wehr TA. In short photoperiods, human sleep is biphasic. J Sleep Res. 1992;1:103–7.

19. Tworoger SS, Davis S, Vitiello MV, Lentz MJ, McTiernan A. Factors associated with objective (actigraphic) and subjective sleep quality in young adult women. J Psychosom Res. 2005;59:11–19.

20. Kaplan KA, Hirshman J, Hernandez B, et al. When a gold standard isn't so golden: lack of prediction of subjective sleep quality from sleep polysomnography. Biol Psychol. 2017;123:37–46.

21. Roenneberg T, Wirz-Justice A, Merrow M. Life between clocks—daily temporal patterns of human chronotypes. J Biol Rhythms. 2003;18:80–90.

22. Roenneberg T, Kuehnle T, Pramstaller PP, Ricken J, Havel M, Guth A, et al. A marker for the end of adolescence. Curr Biol. 2004;14:R1038–9.

23. Kantermann T, Juda M, Merrow M, Roenneberg T. The human circadian clock's seasonal adjustment is disrupted by daylight saving time. Curr Biol. 2007;17:1996–2000.

24. Allebrandt KV, Teder-Laving M, Kantermann T, et al. Chronotype and sleep duration: the influence of season of assessment. Chronobiol Int. 2014;31:731–40.

25. Roenneberg T, Kumar CJ, Merrow M. The human circadian clock entrains to sun time. Curr Biol. 2007;17:R44–5.

26. Roenneberg T, Allebrandt KV, Merrow M, Vetter C. Social jetlag and obesity. Curr Biol. 2012;22:939–43.

27. Wittmann M, Dinich J, Merrow M, Roenneberg T. Social jetlag: misalignment of biological and social time. Chronobiol Int. 2006;23:497–509.

28. Horne JA, Östberg O. A self-assessment questionnaire to determine morningness-eveningness in human circadian rhythms. Int J Chronobiol. 1976;4:97–110.

29. Martin SK, Eastman CI. Sleep logs of young adults with self-selected sleep times predict the dim light melatonin onset. Chronobiol Int. 2002;19:695–707.

30. Kantermann T, Sung H, Burgess HJ. Comparing the morningness-eveningness questionnaire and Munich ChronoType Questionnaire to the dim light melatonin onset. J Biol Rhythms. 2015;30:449–53.

31. Kitamura S, Hida A, Aritake S, et al. Validity of the Japanese version of the Munich ChronoType Questionnaire. Chronobiol Int. 2014;31:845–50.

32. Spiegel K, Leproult R, Van Cauter E. Impact of sleep debt on metabolic and endocrine function. Lancet. 1999;354:1435–9.

33. Levandovski R, Dantas G, Fernandes LC, et al. Depression scores associate with chronotype and social jetlag in a rural population. Chronobiol Int. 2011;28:771–8.

34. Dement W, Kleitman N. Cyclic variations in EEG during sleep and their relation to eye movements, body motility, and dreaming. Electroencephalogr Clin Neurophysiol. 1957;9:673–90.

35. Sadeh A. The role and validity of actigraphy in sleep medicine: an update. Sleep Med Rev. 2011;15:259–67.

36. Ancoli-Israel S, Cole R, Alessi C, Chambers M, Moorcroft W, Pollak CP. The role of actigraphy in the study of sleep and circadian rhythms. Sleep. 2003;26:342–92.

37. Dick R, Penzel T, Fietze I, Partinen M, Hein H, Schulz J. AASM standards of practice compliant validation of actigraphic sleep analysis from SOMNOwatch versus polysomnographic sleep diagnostics shows high conformity also among subjects with sleep disordered breathing. Physiol Meas. 2010;31:1623–33.

38. Hyde M, O'Driscoll DM, Binette S, et al. Validation of actigraphy for determining sleep and wake in children with sleep disordered breathing. J Sleep Res. 2007;16:213–16.

39. Kushida CA, Chang A, Gadkary C, Guilleminault C, Carrillo O, Dement WC. Comparison of actigraphic, polysomnographic, and subjective assessment of sleep parameters in sleep-disordered patients. Sleep Med. 2001;2:389–96.

40. Hayakawa T, Uchiyama M, Kamei Y, et al. Clinical analyses of sighted patients with non-24-hour sleep-wake syndrome: a study of 57 consecutively diagnosed cases. Sleep. 2005;28:945–52.

41. Muzet A, Naitoh P, Townsend RE, Johnson LC. Body movements during sleep as a predictor of stage change. Psychon Sci. 1972;29:7–10.

42. Schulz H, Salzarulo P. Forerunners of REM sleep. Sleep medicine reviews. 2012;16:95–108.

43. Wilde-Frenz J, Schulz H. Rate and distribution of body movements during sleep in humans. Percept Mot Skills. 1983;56:275–83.

44. Behar J, Roebuck A, Domingos JS, Gederi E, Clifford GD. A review of current sleep screening applications for smartphones. Physiol Meas. 2013;34:R29–46.

45. Kelly JM, Strecker RE, Bianchi MT. Recent developments in home sleep-monitoring devices. ISRN Neurol. 2012;2012:768794.

46. Piwek L, Ellis DA, Andrews S, Joinson A. The rise of consumer health wearables: promises and barriers. PLoS Med. 2016;13:e1001953.

47. Winnebeck E, Fischer D, Leise T, Roenneberg T. Dynamics and ultradian structure of human sleep in real life. Curr Biol. 2018;28:49–59.

48. American Psychiatric Association. Diagnostic and Statistical Manual of Mental Disorders, fifth edition (DSM-5). Washington, DC: American Psychiatric Association; 2013.

49. Krystal AD. Psychiatric disorders and sleep. Neurol Clin. 2013;30:1389–413.

50. Breslau N, Roth T, Rosenthal L, Andreski P. Sleep disturbance and psychiatric disorders: a longitudinal epidemiological study of young adults. Biol Psychiatry. 1996;39:411–18.

51. Mayers AG, Baldwin DS. Antidepressants and their effect on sleep. Hum Psychopharmacol. 2005;20:533–59.

52. Becker SP, Froehlich TE, Epstein JN. Effects of methylphenidate on sleep functioning in children with attention-deficit/hyperactivity disorder. J Dev Behav Pediatr. 2016;37:395–404.

53. van den Burg W, van den Hoofdakker RH. Total sleep deprivation on endogenous depression. Arch Gen Psychiatry. 1975;32:1121–5.

54. Wu JC, Bunney WE. The biological basis of an antidepressant response to sleep deprivation and relapse: review and hypothesis. Am J Psychiatry. 1990;147:14–21.

55. Wolf E, Kuhn M, Normann C, et al. Synaptic plasticity model of therapeutic sleep deprivation in major depression. Sleep Med Rev. 2016;30:53–62.

56. John U, Meyer C, Rumpf HJ, Hapke U. Relationships of psychiatric disorders with sleep duration in an adult general population sample. J Psychiatr Res. 2005;39:577–83.

57. Keller LK, Zöschg S, Grünewald B, Roenneberg T, Schulte-Körne G. Chronotyp und Depression bei Jugendlichen—ein Review. Zeitschrift Für Kinder-Und Jugendpsychiatrie Und Psychotherapie. 2016;44:113–26.

58. Roenneberg T. Having trouble typing? What on Earth is chronotype? *J Biol Rhythms*. 2015;30:487–91.

59. Wittmann M, Paulus M, Roenneberg T. Decreased psychological well-being in late 'chronotypes' is mediated by smoking and alcohol consumption. *Subst Use Misuse*. 2010;45:15–30.

60. Keller LK, Grünewald B, Vetter C, Roenneberg T, Schulte-Körne G. Not later, but longer: Sleep, chronotype and light exposure in adolescents with remitted depression compared to healthy controls. *Eur Child Adolesc Psychiatry*. 2017;26:1233–44.

61. Berger M, Vollmann J, Hohagen F, *et al*. Sleep deprivation combined with consecutive sleep phase advance as a fast-acting therapy in depression: an open pilot trial in medicated and unmedicated patients. *Am J Psychiatry*. 1997;154:870–2.

62. Pandi-Perumal SR, Smits M, Spence W, *et al*. Dim light melatonin onset (DLMO): a tool for the analysis of circadian phase in human sleep and chronobiological disorders. *Progr Neuropsychopharmacol Biol Psychiatry*. 2007;31:1–11.

63. Wulff K, Joyce E, Middleton B, Dijk DJ, Foster RG. The suitability of actigraphy, diary data, and urinary melatonin profiles for quantitative assessment of sleep disturbances in schizophrenia: a case report. *Chronobiol Int*. 2006;23:485–95.

64. Wulff K, Gatti S, Wettstein JG, Foster RG. Sleep and circadian rhythm disruption in psychiatric and neurodegenerative disease. *Nat Rev Neurosci*. 2010;11:589–99.

65. Turner J, Drummond LM, Mukhopadhyay S, *et al*. A prospective study of delayed sleep phase syndrome in patients with severe resistant obsessive-compulsive disorder. *World Psychiatry*. 2007;6:108–11.

66. Mukhopadhyay S, Fineberg NA, Drummond LM, *et al*. Delayed sleep phase in severe obsessive-compulsive disorder: a systematic case-report survey. *CNS Spectr*. 2008;13:406–13.

67. Gamble KL, May RS, Besing RC, Tankersly AP, Fargason RE. Delayed sleep timing and symptoms in adults with attention-deficit/hyperactivity disorder: a controlled actigraphy study. *Chronobiol Int*. 2013;30:598–606.

68. Foster RG, Peirson SN, Wulff K, Winnebeck E, Vetter C, Roenneberg T. Sleep and circadian rhythm disruption in social jetlag and mental illness. *Progr Molecular Biol Transl Sci*. 2013;119:325–46.

69. Foster RG, Wulff K. The rhythm of rest and excess. *Nat Rev Neurosci*. 2005;6:407–14.

70. Wulff K, Dijk DJ, Middleton B, Foster RG, Joyce EM. Sleep and circadian rhythm disruption in schizophrenia. *Br J Psychiatry*. 2012;200:308–16.

71. Wulff K, Gatti S, Wettstein JG, Foster RG. Sleep and circadian rhythm disruption in psychiatric and neurodegenerative disease. *Nat Rev Neurosci*. 2010;11: 589–99.

72. Sandman N, Merikanto I, Määttänen H, *et al*. Winter is coming: nightmares and sleep problems during seasonal affective disorder. *J Sleep Res*. 2016;25:612–19.

73. Plante DT, Cook JD, Goldstein MR. Objective measures of sleep duration and continuity in major depressive disorder with comorbid hypersomnolence: a primary investigation with contiguous systematic review and meta-analysis. *J Sleep Res*. 2017;26:255–65.

74. Murray CB, Murphy LK, Palermo TM, Clarke GM. Pain and sleep–wake disturbances in adolescents with depressive disorders. *J Clin Child Adolesc Psychol*. 2012;41:482–90.

75. Dauvilliers Y, Lopez R, Ohayon M, Bayard S. Hypersomnia and depressive symptoms: methodological and clinical aspects. *BMC Med*. 2013;11:78.

76. Monti JM, Monti D. Sleep in schizophrenia patients and the effects of antipsychotic drugs. *Sleep Med Rev*. 2004;8:133–48.

77. Spoormaker VI, Montgomery P. Disturbed sleep in post-traumatic stress disorder: secondary symptom or core feature? *Sleep Med Rev*. 2008;12:169–84.

78. Brower KJ. Insomnia, alcoholism and relapse. *Sleep Med Rev*. 2003;7:523–39.

79. Johnson KP, Malow BA. Sleep in children with autism spectrum disorders. *Curr Treat Options Neurol*. 2008;10:350–9.

80. Monti JM, Monti D. Sleep disturbance in generalized anxiety disorder and its treatment. *Sleep Med Rev*. 2000;4:263–76.

81. Park S, Cho MJE, Chang SMAN, *et al*. Relationships of sleep duration with sociodemographic and health-related factors, psychiatric disorders and sleep disturbances in a community sample of Korean adults. *J Sleep Res*. 2010;19:567–77.

82. Zhai L, Zhang H, Zhang D. Sleep duration and depression among adults: a meta-analysis of prospective studies. *Depress Anxiety*. 2015;32:664–70.

83. Paavonen EJ, Räikkönen K, Lahti J, *et al*. Short sleep duration and behavioral symptoms of attention-deficit/hyperactivity disorder in healthy 7- to 8-year-old children. *Pediatrics*. 2009;123:e857–64.

84. Bogdan AR, Reeves KW. Sleep duration in relation to attention deficit hyperactivity disorder in American adults. *Behav Sleep Med*. 2018;16:235–43.

85. Roenneberg T, Kuehnle T, Juda M, *et al*. Epidemiology of the human circadian clock. *Sleep Med Rev*. 2007;11:429–38.

86. De Niet GJ, Tiemens BG, Lendemeijer HH, Hutschemaekers GJ. Perceived sleep quality of psychiatric patients. *J Psychiatr Ment Health Nurs*. 2008;15:465–70.

87. Gregory AM, Sadeh A. Annual Research Review: sleep problems in childhood psychiatric disorders—a review of the latest science. *J Child Psychol Psychiatry*. 2016;57:296–317.

88. Buysse DJ, Reynolds CF, Monk TH, Berman SR, Kupfer DJ. The Pittsburgh Sleep Quality Index: a new instrument for psychiatric practice and research. *Psychiatry Res*. 1989;28:193–213.

89. Lovato N, Gradisar M. A meta-analysis and model of the relationship between sleep and depression in adolescents: recommendations for future research and clinical practice. *Sleep Med Rev*. 2014;18:521–9.

90. Benca RM, William H, Thisted RA, Gillin JC. Sleep and psychiatric disorders. *Arch Gen Psychiatry*. 1992;49:651–68.

91. Pillai V, Kalmbach DA, Ciesla JA. A meta-analysis of electroencephalographic sleep in depression: evidence for genetic biomarkers. *Biol Psychiatry*. 2011;70:912–19.

92. Baglioni C, Nanovska S, Regen W, *et al*. Sleep and mental disorders: a meta-analysis of polysomnographic research. *Psychol Bull*. 2016;142:969–90.

93. Daan S, Beersma DG, Borbely AA. Timing of human sleep: recovery process gated by a circadian pacemaker. *Am J Physiol*. 1984;246(2 Pt 2):R161–83.

94. Tononi G, Cirelli C. Sleep and the price of plasticity: from synaptic and cellular homeostasis to memory consolidation and integration. *Neuron*. 2014;81:12–34.

95. Xie L, Kang H, Xu Q, *et al*. Sleep drives metabolite clearance from the adult brain. *Science*. 2013;342:373–7.

96. Vorster AP, Born J. Sleep and memory in mammals, birds and invertebrates. *Neurosci Biobehav Rev*. 2015;50:103–19.

97. Besedovsky L, Lange T, Born J. Sleep and immune function. *Pflugers Arch*. 2012;463:121–37.

98. Fischer D, Vetter C, Roenneberg T. A novel method to visualise and quantify circadian misalignment. *Sci Rep*. 2016;6:38601.

99. Vetter C, Devore EE, Ramin CA, Speizer FE, Willett WC, Schernhammer ES. Mismatch of sleep and work timing and risk of type 2 dabetes. *Diabetes Care*. 2015;38:1707–13.

100. Crowley SJ, Lee C, Tseng CY, Fogg LF, Eastman CI. Complete or partial circadian re-entrainment improves performance, alertness, and mood during night-shift work. *Sleep*. 2004;27:1077–87.

101. Vetter C, Fischer D, Matera JL, Roenneberg T. Aligning work and circadian time in shift workers improves sleep and reduces circadian disruption. *Curr Biol*. 2015;25:907–11.

102. Wyatt JK. Circadian rhythm sleep disorders. *Pediatr Clin North Am*. 2011;58:621–35.

103. Juda M, Vetter C, Roenneberg T. Chronotype modulates sleep duration, sleep quality and social jetlag in shift-workers. *J Biol Rhythms*. 2013;28:141–51.

104. Vitiello MV, Larsen LH, Moe KE. Age-related sleep change: gender and estrogen effects on the subjective-objective sleep quality relationships of healthy, noncomplaining older men and women. *J Psychosom Res*. 2004;56:503–10.

105. van Someren EJ, Riemersma RF, Swaab DF. Functional plasticity of the circadian timing system in old age: light exposure. *Prog Brain Res*. 2002;138:205–31.

# 112

# Genetics of sleep–wake disorders

*Diego R. Mazzotti, Allan I. Pack, and Philip R. Gehrman*

## Introduction

As with the vast majority of biological traits in humans, sleep has an important genetic component. Sleep-related traits and sleep disorders can be considered complex or multifactorial conditions, that is, the aetiology and the biological basis are a combined effect of genetic factors, environmental non-genetic components, and their interaction. Since the stimulus of the Human Genome Project, biomedical research has made real progress in characterizing the genetic architecture and molecular pathways underlying human complex diseases [1]. Establishing that a given trait is heritable implies that underlying genetic factors play a role in determining the phenotype. Despite the established genetic heritability of many sleep-related phenotypes, only a small number of validated genetic variants have been discovered so far. Thus, compared to some other fields, understanding the genetic architecture of sleep-related phenotypes through genome-wide association studies (GWAS) is in a relatively nascent stage. As methodologies for analysing these data continue to develop, research in these emerging genetic areas will improve our current knowledge. Given the known heritability of many traits of sleep and circadian rhythm in humans and also of specific sleep disorders, this is currently a major opportunity for the sleep research community.

In addition to the characterization of genetic factors underlying sleep disorders, a number of neuropsychiatric conditions have been extensively studied in regard to their genetic architecture [2]. It is also well described how sleep disorders are associated with many neuropsychiatric illnesses, and this relationship suggests that there are shared genetic components explaining this association. Only recently have advances in genomic technologies supported the development of knowledge to interpret these relationships biologically. Therefore, it is expected that a better understanding of the genetic contributions to sleep disorders and psychiatric conditions will reveal both common shared and unique molecular pathways to these traits that will help to inform the aetiology of these morbidities, thereby supporting the development of new diagnostic and therapeutic approaches.

## Genetics of sleep duration

The duration of sleep varies in individuals in the general population, and a number of studies have shown that the prevalence of self-reported short sleep duration (<6 hours per night) ranges from 14% to 35% worldwide [3]. Given the known physiological, behavioural, metabolic, and molecular consequences of lack of sleep, understanding the biological basis of short sleep duration is fundamental. Although behaviourally induced short sleep also occurs as a consequence of commitments of modern life, an important genetic contribution has been identified. Studies analysing the differences in sleep duration between monozygotic and dizygotic twins estimated the heritability of sleep duration in the order of 31–44% [4, 5].

Common and rare genetic variants have also been described as associated with this phenotype. Although an initial GWAS based on the Framingham cohort did not find any genome-wide significant single-nucleotide polymorphisms (SNPs) associated with sleep duration [6], another larger GWAS in a population with European ancestry found a significant association in an intronic variant of *ABCC9* in the discovery phase, but not on replication [7]. This gene encodes one of the 17 transmembrane domains of the pore-forming subunit of an adenosine triphosphate (ATP)-sensitive potassium channel ($K_{ATP}$) that serves as a sensor of cellular metabolism. However, the association between this variant and sleep duration was also not significant in other studies [8–10]. On the other hand, significant associations with other variants in *ABCC9* and sleep duration [11] and depressive symptoms have been found [10]. Knocking down the expression of the homologue of this gene in *Drosophila* was associated with reduced sleep amounts at night [7]. Whether variations in *ABCC9* are associated with sleep duration or with a shared mechanism between sleep duration and depression symptoms, this gene likely plays a role in the control of sleep/wake, suggesting that further investigation is needed.

In a GWAS in a Finnish cohort, no genome-wide significant associations with sleep duration were found [9]. However, some of the suggestive associations were replicated in a follow-up sample. Among the most interesting findings, the authors found an association in the *KLF6* locus. This gene encodes Kruppel-like factor 6, a transcription factor that functions as a tumour suppressor. Higher expression of *KLF6* in circulating mononuclear lymphocytes was related to shorter sleep duration, and its expression in these cells was increased with experimental sleep restriction, suggesting this gene as a modulator of the sleep/wake regulation.

A study from the CHARGE consortium used self-reported sleep duration and genotyping data from 18 community-based cohorts and found two genome-wide significant associations in European individuals. One of the significant associations was in the *PAX8* locus, which replicated in an independent African-American sample [8]. This gene encodes a thyroid-specific transcription factor involved in thyroid development and function [12], which could be potentially involved in the relationship between sleep regulation and metabolism.

Sequencing studies in individuals with extreme phenotypes in regard to sleep duration were also conducted. He *et al.* investigated two individuals who slept for 6 hours with no evidence of daytime impairments and identified a mutation in exon 5 of the *BHLEH41* (class E basic helix–loop–helix protein 41) gene, also known as *DEC2*. This mutation results in a proline-to-arginine substitution in the protein and had its sleep-affecting properties validated experimentally in *Drosophila* and mice [13]. A further study sequenced *DEC2* in two other individuals with particular sleep phenotypes and identified two new mutations in this gene [14]. In one subject, who was a member of a dizygotic twin pair, the twin with the mutation slept 2 hours less per day and had substantially less performance lapses during prolonged sleep deprivation than the other twin. The other mutation was found in three unrelated individuals, but no obvious effect of this variant on sleep duration. Interestingly, the mutations that were linked to differences in sleep showed clear functional consequences in model organisms, by affecting key mechanisms of the molecular circadian clock [14]. Based on these findings, it is expected that other variants of *DEC2* and other genes that affect the molecular circadian clock can result in short sleep.

Due to the difficulty in defining a reliable and objective phenotype that represents the habitual sleep duration, most of the studies rely only on noisy self-report measures, and conclusive studies are still not available. More objective assessment of sleep duration includes the use of actigraphy-based rest–activity patterns and GWAS, with these objective parameters only conducted recently [15], as described in more detail later in this chapter. Nevertheless, the progress so far indicates that some candidate genes deserve further functional characterization of their roles in sleep/wake regulation.

## Genetics of insomnia

Similar to sleep duration, there is a lack of comprehensive studies on the genetics of insomnia, partly because of the uncertainty in defining the appropriate phenotype. Although insomnia is a prevalent condition with defined clinical diagnostic criteria, it is difficult to establish a common biological mechanism, potentially due to the diverse underlying causes. Nevertheless, family and twin studies have been conducted, utilizing self-report measures of insomnia traits, showing that a moderate degree of the variability of these phenotypes can be explained by genetic factors.

Patients whose insomnia began in childhood reported a positive family history of sleep complaints at a higher rate than those with adult-onset insomnia [16]. In a large Australian twin study, additive genetic influences were found for sleep quality, initial insomnia, sleep latency, 'anxious insomnia', and 'depressed insomnia', with heritability ranging from 32% to 44% [4]. In a twin study from the Vietnam Era Twin Registry [17], estimates ranged from 21% to 42% for trouble falling or staying asleep, waking up several times per night, and waking up feeling tired and worn out. In a recent longitudinal

study in a representative sample of twins, there was moderate heritability in the univariate analysis (22–25%), but when accounting for the longitudinal measurement, heritability increased substantially, especially in females (59%), compared to males (38%) [18].

A GWAS for insomnia, defined using a series of questions about sleep patterns, was conducted in Korea, and an association was found with a variant in the *ROR1* locus that was not genome-wide significant [19]. This gene encodes the receptor tyrosine kinase-like orphan receptor 1, a protein that modulates synapse formation and was indicated as a potential candidate explaining genetic variability in this insomnia phenotype. Another GWAS in an Australian twin cohort did not find any genome-wide significant associations [20]. The strongest associations were between self-reported sleep latency and the *CACNA1C* locus, a gene that encodes the calcium voltage-gated channel subunit alpha 1 C and was repeatedly associated with bipolar disorder and schizophrenia [19] (see Chapters 59 and 60). This finding did not replicate in a second cohort but was then subsequently replicated in a different study [10]. More recently, genome-wide associated variants in the *RBFOX3* locus were reported with self-reported sleep latency [21]. This gene encodes the RNA-binding protein—Fox-1 homolog 3—and is believed to have a role in neuron-specific alternative splicing and to be co-expressed with genes involved with calcium channel activity and signalling of the neurotransmitter gamma-aminobutyric acid (GABA) [21]. Thus, it is of potential interest as a candidate in the aetiology of insomnia.

The fact that insomnia is mainly based on self-reported symptoms and clinical evaluation could partially explain the lack of reproducibility of studies aiming to find a strong biological basis of this disease. In this sense, objective measurements of insomnia-related traits, such as actigraphic recordings, can provide a more robust characterization of some of the phenotypes that compose the condition. Recently, the first GWAS on actigraphic sleep phenotypes found a genome-wide significant association between a variant in the *UFL1* locus and actigraphy-derived sleep efficiency on week days [15]. This gene encodes the ubiquitin-fold modifier 1 specific ligase 1, a protein that participates in the regulation of apoptosis and vesicle trafficking in the endoplasmic reticulum. Variants in other genes (*DMRT1* and *CSNK2A1*) were also associated with sleep latency and deserve further investigation. *DMRT1* encodes the double sex and Mab-3-related transcription factor 1, a protein involved in sexual differentiation and embryonic development, and *CSNK2A1* encodes the alpha subunit of casein kinase II, involved in the regulation of circadian rhythms. Even though studies can achieve more biologically meaningful phenotypes by using objective assessment, it is important to note that there is often a discrepancy between these measures and self-reports of sleep in patients with insomnia [22].

## Genetics of narcolepsy and hypersomnia

Narcolepsy is one of the most successful examples for identifying genetic factors in sleep disorders. Based on evidence from studies in mice and dogs, narcolepsy is caused by a disruption in the orexin signalling system, including selective loss of orexin-producing neurons. Although only a single patient with a mutation in the orexin receptor gene was described [23], it is established that patients with narcolepsy present with very low levels of this neuromodulator in the cerebrospinal fluid [24].

Early studies showed a 10–40 times increase in the risk of narcolepsy for someone with a first-degree relative with narcolepsy when compared to the general population [25]. In accordance with the evidence from familial aggregation, there is an established relationship between specific human leucocyte antigen (*HLA*) alleles and narcolepsy [26]. *HLA* encodes the proteins that compose the major histocompatibility complex class II expressed in immune cells, which are involved in presenting foreign peptides to receptors on T cells. In many populations, the *DQB1*0602* allele is strongly associated with narcolepsy (odds ratio approximately 250), particularly in cases that also present with cataplexy, also known as type 1 narcolepsy [27].

Regardless of its strong association with type 1 narcolepsy, the *DQB1*0602* allele is frequent in the general population, with its prevalence ranging in different ethnic groups from 12% in Japanese to 38% in African-Americans [28]. Thus, it is commonly found in many individuals without narcolepsy. In this sense, it could be that the presence of *DQB1*0602* could make individuals more susceptible to environmental insults, in a gene–environment interaction fashion. In addition, multiple gene variants other than *DQB1*0602* may be involved in narcolepsy.

In order to identify additional variants, a series of GWAS where both cases and controls were positive for the *DQB1*0602* allele were conducted. Three variants within the T cell receptor alpha (*TRCA*) locus were significantly associated with narcolepsy and were replicated in independent Caucasian and Asian samples [29], as well as in a study in Chinese patients [30]. This association within *TRCA* was also replicated in a study aimed to evaluate variants relevant to the immune system, which also identified significantly associated variants in other genes such as cathepsin H (*CTSH*) and tumour necrosis factor (ligand) super-family member 4 (*TNFSF4*) [31].

Further studies investigating *DQB1*0602*-positive individuals found additional loci associated with narcolepsy. A significant association with a variant in the promoter region of CCR1, a gene that encodes the chemokine (C-C motif) receptor 1, was reported and replicated in an independent cohort, as well as found to be associated with *CCR1* gene expression and lower migration indexes in monocytes with a CCR1 ligand [32]. Moreover, a single nucleotide variant in the purinergic receptor subtype P2Y11 (*P2RY11*) gene locus was also associated with narcolepsy and presented functional evidence of decrease in gene expression, as well as increased sensitivity of CD8+ T cells to ATP-induced cell death [33]. Interestingly, the *P2RY11* gene locus is within a region where other genes, such as *PPAN*, *EIF3G*, and *DNMT1*, are present, so the signal detected in this GWAS could be related to variants of the other genes in this region. Further studies replicated these signals and identified a strong signal in a haplotype involving *P2RY11/EIF3G* in European and Chinese cohorts [34]. Mutations in the DNA methyltransferase 1 (*DNMT1*) gene in individuals with autosomal dominant cerebellar ataxia, deafness, and narcolepsy supported the role of this region [35]. This gene encodes an enzyme responsible for maintaining methylation patterns in development and is required for the differentiation of CD4+ cells into T regulatory cells. Additionally, a genome-wide copy number variation (CNV) analysis in a Japanese cohort identified an enrichment of rare and large CNVs in different immune response-related genes, as well as duplications in the Parkinson's disease protein 2 (*PARK2*) gene in patients, compared to controls [36]. The protein encoded by this gene also participates in antigen processing and presentation, supporting the existence of an autoimmune component against orexin-producing neurons [37].

In regard to environmental influences and supporting the role of the immune system in the physiopathology of narcolepsy, a strong relationship between this sleep disorder and upper airway winter infections was described. There was a significant increase in the onset of narcolepsy after the 2009 H1N1 influenza pandemic [38], and a follow-up GWAS revealed additional loci in the *HLA* region in cases with narcolepsy with onset after the 2009 pandemic [39].

Despite efforts in the characterization of the genetic basis of type 1 narcolepsy (narcolepsy with cataplexy), a growing number of studies have been investigating the role of genetics in other forms of excessive somnolence such as essential hypersomnia syndrome (EHS). This condition differs from narcolepsy mainly because of the absence of cataplexy, but the sleep-related symptoms are indistinguishable [40]. The *DQB1*0602* allele is also associated with EHS, although not as strongly as narcolepsy with cataplexy [41]. Similarly, variants in the *TCRA* locus were described as associated with EHS in *DQB1*0602*-positive individuals [42]. A more recent GWAS in *DQB1*0602*-negative individuals with EHS reported three new loci associated with the condition (*NCKAP5*, *SPRED1*, and *CRAT*), all of which contain genes previously related to other neuropsychiatric diseases [43]. *NCKAP5* encodes NCK-associated protein 5 that still has unknown function. *SPRED1* encodes sprouty-related EVH1 domain-containing 1, a protein phosphorylated in response to growth factors. *CRAT* encodes carnitine *O*-acetyltransferase, a key enzyme in β-oxidation of fatty acids. These genes were described as candidates in EHS but still need replication and functional follow-up.

## Genetics of chronotype and circadian rhythm disorders

One of the mechanisms through with an organism responds to temporal changes in the environment as a consequence of the light–dark cycle is through regulation of the 'biological clock'. This system, also known as the molecular circadian clock, consists of autoregulatory feedback loops involving the transcription, translation, and degradation of proteins encoded by the clock genes. This set of genes includes *PER1*, *PER2*, and *PER3*, and *CRY1* and *CRY2*, as well as *CK1δ*, *CK1ε*, *CLOCK*, *NPAS1*, *NPAS2*, *DEC2*, *BMAL1*, and *BMAL2* [44]. Given the existence of a comprehensive molecular pathway regulating the generation of circadian rhythms, it is expected that variation in genes in this system could affect circadian behaviours and disorders.

Chronotype is known as the behavioural outcome that results from the generation of endogenous biological rhythms and interaction with the environment. Individuals can be classified as an evening type (that is, 'night owls'), morning type (that is, 'larks'), or intermediate. Several twin and family studies have estimated that chronotype is a moderately heritable trait, with genetic factors potentially explaining as high as 50% of the variability in this phenotype [45, 46]. This estimate can also be affected by the type of environment in which the individual lives, that is, urban or rural [47].

Linkage studies of extended families with circadian rhythm sleep disorders, primarily advanced sleep phase syndrome (ASPS), allowed the identification of specific rare variants that segregate with the disorder. A serine-to-glycine mutation in the clock gene *PER2* was reported in a family [48], and different mutations in the *CK1δ* gene were identified as the causal variant in other two studies [49, 50], supporting the role of the molecular circadian clock in ASPS. Interestingly, mouse knockouts for these genes also replicate the phenotypes seen in humans.

Common genetic variants in other genes of the molecular circadian clock, such as *CLOCK*, *PER1*, *PER2*, and *PER3*, are also associated with chronotype and other circadian rhythm disorders [51–53], but not replicated in other studies [54, 55]. One of the most studied variants is a variable number of tandem repeats polymorphism in *PER3* resulting in four or five repeats of a 54-bp motif in exon 18 [56]. This polymorphism was associated with delayed sleep phase syndrome and diurnal preference [57, 58]. The association was replicated in Brazil [59] and South Africa [60], but not in Colombia [61] or in Norway [62].

Given the evidence provided by genetic associations studies, as well as the functional nature of this polymorphism, a more in-depth characterization of sleep and circadian phenotypes was performed to evaluate the role of these variants of *PER3*. Although no significant differences were found in circadian phenotypes, differences in sleep and wake behaviour in response to sleep deprivation were found between individuals carrying *PER3*$^{4/4}$ and *PER3*$^{5/5}$ genotypes [63]. *PER3*$^{5/5}$ carriers showed increased slow-wave sleep, as well as electroencephalographic markers of slow wave activity and greater decrement in cognitive performance, in response to sleep deprivation. These findings was complemented by another study suggesting that *PER3*$^{4/5}$ is associated with greater behavioural resiliency to sleep restriction when compared to *PER3*$^{4/4}$ [64], and *PER*$^{5/5}$ carriers showed a more pronounced impact of sleep deprivation on sustained attention, with increased sleepiness, than *PER3*$^{4/4}$ carriers [65].

Genome-wide approaches were also used to potentially identify genetic loci related to circadian phenotypes. In an early family-based study in the Framingham cohort, a linkage peak close to the *CSNK2A2* gene was found with usual bedtime. This gene encodes the catalytic unit of casein kinase 2 that was described as an important component in the molecular circadian clock [6]. More recently, a large GWAS in >89,000 costumers of European ancestry of the personal genetics company 23andMe, Inc. identified 15 genome-wide significant loci associated with self-reported morningness. This study also found an enrichment of associated variants of genes in circadian and phototransduction pathways [66]. In addition, another large GWAS in the UK Biobank cohort in >100,000 individuals of European ancestry validated eight loci and reported a consistent effect of all the 15 loci reported by Hu *et al.* in 2016. A meta-analysis combining results of both studies reinforced the role of three loci: *PER3*, *VIP* and *TOX3* [67]. *VIP* encodes vasoactive intestinal peptide, a key molecule in the central nervous system. Intracerebroventricular administration of this peptide was found to increase the rapid eye movement sleep time in rabbit. *TOX3* encodes TOX high mobility group box family member 3 and was previously associated with restless legs syndrome (RLS) [68].

has been diagnosed primarily using solid symptom-based criteria [69] that allowed the identification and validation of a number of genetic risk factors, establishing it as a relevant disorder. Positive family history [70, 71], twin studies [72, 73], and complex segregation analyses [74, 75] supported the existence of an important genetic component in RLS. Most studies reported the heritability of RLS to vary between 40% and 65% [76].

Linkage analyses within large-family pedigrees were able to identify significant genetic loci linked with RLS on chromosomes 12q22–23.3, 14q13–22, 9p24–22, 2q33, 20p13, 16p12.1, 4q25–26, 17p11–13, 19p1 [76], and 13q32.3-33.2 [77]. Follow-up candidate region case-control association studies in these regions were able to find significant variants associated with RLS and potential candidate genes. Significant associations with single-nucleotide variants in *NOS1* [78] and *PTPRD* [79] were described and replicated in independent cohorts. *NOS1* encodes nitric oxide synthase 1 and has been associated with pain perception and sleep–wake control [80]. *PTPRD* encodes protein tyrosine phosphatase receptor type delta, involved in long-term potentiation in memory formation and abnormal axon targeting to motoneurons during development in mice [81, 82].

GWAS were also conducted, and the first two reports were published simultaneously and independently in Caucasian populations. One study in German and French Canadian cases, who were diagnosed by face-to-face interview with expert clinicians, identified and replicated variants associated with RLS in three different loci: *MEIS1*, *BTBD9*, and *MAP2K5/SKORK1* [83]. The other study of cases from Iceland and the United States used self-assessment questionnaires that contained the essential diagnostic criteria, as well as leg actigraphy to assess periodic limb movements during sleep, also identified variants in *BTBD9* associated with RLS. Interestingly, the association was only found in cases that also showed periodic limb movements during sleep, and this variant was also associated with ferritin levels [84]. The associations between variants in *MEIS1*, *BTBD9*, and *MAP2K5/SKORK1* have been confirmed in further independent investigations [76]. Also, an excess of loss-of-function alleles in *MEIS1* was found in RLS cases, compared to controls [85], supporting the role of these genetic loci in RLS. The functional roles of *MEIS1* (limb axis formation and neuronal differentiation), *SKOR1* (neuronal differentiation), *MAP2K5* (muscle cell differentiation), and *BTBD9* (iron and ferritin metabolism and sleep fragmentation) corroborate the associations found in variants within these genes and the pathophysiology of RLS and might suggest the role of developmental abnormality. However, better characterization of the molecular mechanisms that integrate these genes in the syndrome in humans is still warranted.

An exome sequencing study identified a rare variant in *PCDHA3* segregating in a family with multiple cases of RLS, and two additional rare missense variants in unrelated cases [86]. *PCDHA3* is expressed in neurons, and its product is present at synaptic junctions in neural cell–cell interaction [87]. This is another plausible candidate for the genetics of RLS.

## Genetics of restless legs syndrome

RLS is another successful example of how genetics has helped to identify the pathophysiology of a sleep-related condition. This disorder

## Genetics of obstructive sleep apnoea

Obstructive sleep apnoea (OSA) is a highly prevalent complex condition characterized by partial or complete blockage of the airway during sleep that leads to a repetitive reduction in blood oxygen saturation [88]. Some of the major risk factors include older age, male gender, and obesity [89], although not all cases of the disease can be explained by these factors. This suggests a high degree of heterogeneity and indicates an interesting phenotype to conduct genetic investigations.

An initial study of a single family with a high prevalence of OSA suggested for the first time the existence of an important genetic component [90]. Further investigation reported that some of the most common symptoms of OSA also aggregate in families [91], along with more refined measurements of apnoeas and hypopneas during sleep [92, 93]. Addressing the confounding effect of obesity, which is a major risk factor for OSA, the Cleveland Family Study found an increased relative risk of OSA in first-degree family members, even after controlling for body mass index [94]. This approach was supported by another investigation that identified familial aggregation of specific craniofacial features in less obese cases of OSA [95], suggesting that factors other than obesity also play an important role in the genetics of this disorder. In addition to familial aggregation, the heritability of OSA ranges between 21% and 84%, depending on the phenotype used to define the disorder and the population studied [96, 97].

There has been, however, little progress in identifying relevant and causal genetic variants accounting for the variability in OSA. Due to the heterogeneity of the phenotype, as well as technical and statistical limitations, linkage and association studies failed to report consistent results [98–100]. This led to meta-analyses of candidate genes failing to find evidence that the majority of the reported associations were replicable [98, 101], except for a polymorphism in the promoter of the *TNFA* gene. Given the participation of inflammatory response in the physiopathology of OSA [102], tumour necrosis factor alpha is an important candidate contributing to key consequences of OSA. A study in paediatric OSA patients showed higher tumour necrosis factor plasma levels, particularly in carriers of the promoter polymorphism in the *TNFA* gene [103]. In addition, these patients also presented significantly increased symptoms of excessive daytime sleepiness, suggesting that this variant might explain, in part, this particular phenotype in paediatric OSA.

A genetic association study with variants across 2000 candidate genes relevant to heart, lung, blood, and sleep disorders in the Cleveland Family Study and the Sleep Heart Health Study found a genome-wide significant association between the apnoea–hypopnea index and a variant in the *LPAR1* gene and another in the *PTGER3* gene [104]. The *LPAR1* gene encodes lysophosphatidic acid receptor I, a pro-inflammatory protein expressed in the developing cerebral cortex [105] and associated with changes in behaviour and craniofacial abnormalities in mice knockouts [106]. The product of the *PTGER3* gene—the prostaglandin E2 receptor—was described as a modulator of neurotransmitter release in central and peripheral tissues. Both genes seem to participate in important molecular pathways that could partly explain the aetiology of OSA.

Only recently has a large-scale GWAS on OSA quantitative traits been performed, in Hispanic/Latino cohorts. The authors identified two genome-wide significant candidate regions associated with the apnoea–hypopnea index and respiratory event duration in the *GPR83* and *C6ORF183/CCDC162P* loci, respectively. *GPR83* encodes a G-protein receptor expressed in different brain regions of importance to OSA, and linked to body temperature, metabolism, and

inflammatory response regulation. *C6ORF183* and *CCDC162P* are pseudogenes, and this locus was associated with red blood cell traits. Additional loci involving other plausible genes were also identified, supporting the involvement of inflammatory and hypoxia signalling pathways, as well as sleep-related gene sets [107]. However, these associations have still not been independently replicated.

Given the complexity and different proposed mechanisms and pathways contributing to OSA, the genetic study of the major risk or protective factors of this disorder can be an interesting approach and has not been explored so far. For example, there are multiple obesity and body mass index genetic loci identified by GWAS [108], but the genetic correlation between obesity and OSA is yet to be determined. Other opportunities for investigation involve the genetics of major components of OSA pathophysiology such as fat distribution [109], soft tissue volume [110], craniofacial structures [111], and hypoxic response [112], as well as other respiratory physiological parameters without genetic characterization to date. Additionally, understanding the role of ancestry and how it affects the identification of genetic risk factors of OSA has already been proposed [113], but not explored at its full potential. Although it seems a challenging task trying to dissect the complex genetic architecture of OSA, it certainly offers an exciting opportunity for future research.

## Conclusions

The genetics of sleep disorders is an emerging and rapidly evolving field in sleep medicine. Some disorders, particularly narcolepsy and RLS, present more consistent results; however, the majority of sleep-related traits still lack a robust characterization of their genetic basis. Sleep-related traits are heterogenous phenotypes, and a complex genetic architecture is expected, requiring more robust and objective ways to characterize intermediate phenotypes, as well as larger sample sizes to detect the expected low effect of variants explaining the variability in these traits. In addition, most of the identified genetic regions lack a comprehensive functional characterization of the gene and sometimes rely only on the effect of the variant on the closest gene, and not within a genomic context. Given the relationships between sleep and neuropsychiatric disorders, and the promising opportunity of more refined genetic and phenotypic characterizations, understanding the genetic basis of sleep and wake regulation could partially inform the aetiology of other relevant mental and neurological conditions for public health awareness. While understanding the genetic aspects of sleep/wake disorders imposes a challenge, it is an example of the genetic study of complex and multifactorial traits in humans.

### REFERENCES

1. Altshuler, D., Daly, M.J., and Lander, E.S. 2008. Genetic mapping in human disease. *Science*, 322, 881–8.
2. Sullivan, P.F., Daly, M.J., and O'Donovan, M. 2012. Genetic architectures of psychiatric disorders: the emerging picture and its implications. *Nature Reviews Genetics*, 13, 537–51.
3. Kronholm, E. *et al.* 2006. Self-reported sleep duration in Finnish general population. *Journal of Sleep Research*, 15, 276–90.
4. Heath, A.C. *et al.* 1990. Evidence for genetic influences on sleep disturbance and sleep pattern in twins. *Sleep*, 13, 318–35.

5. Watson, N.F. *et al.* 2010. A twin study of sleep duration and body mass index. *Journal of Clinical Sleep Medicine*, 6, 11–17.

6. Gottlieb, D.J., O'Connor, G.T., and Wilk, J.B. 2007. Genome-wide association of sleep and circadian phenotypes. *BMC Medical Genetics*, 8 Suppl 1, S9.

7. Allebrandt, K.V. *et al.* 2013. A K(ATP) channel gene effect on sleep duration: from genome-wide association studies to function in *Drosophila*. *Molecular Psychiatry*, 18, 122–32.

8. Gottlieb, D.J. *et al.* 2015. Novel loci associated with usual sleep duration: the CHARGE Consortium Genome-Wide Association Study. *Molecular Psychiatry*, 20, 1232–9.

9. Ollila, H.M. *et al.* 2014. Genome-wide association study of sleep duration in the Finnish population. *Journal of Sleep Research*, 23, 609–18.

10. Parsons, M.J. *et al.* 2013. Replication of genome-wide association studies (GWAS) loci for sleep in the British G1219 cohort. *American Journal of Medical Genetics. Part B, Neuropsychiatric Genetics*, 162B, 431–8.

11. Scheinfeldt, L.B. *et al.* 2015. Using the Coriell Personalized Medicine Collaborative Data to conduct a genome-wide association study of sleep duration. *American Journal of Medical Genetics. Part B, Neuropsychiatric Genetics*, 168, 697–705.

12. Ruiz-Llorente, S. *et al.* 2012. Genome-wide analysis of Pax8 binding provides new insights into thyroid functions. *BMC Genomics*, 13, 147.

13. He, Y. *et al.* 2009. The transcriptional repressor DEC2 regulates sleep length in mammals. *Science*, 325, 866–70.

14. Pellegrino, R. *et al.* 2014. A novel *BHLHE41* variant is associated with short sleep and resistance to sleep deprivation in humans. *Sleep*, 37, 1327–36.

15. Spada, J. *et al.* 2016. Genome-wide association analysis of actigraphic sleep phenotypes in the LIFE Adult Study. *Journal of Sleep Research*, 25, 690–701.

16. Hauri, P. and Olmstead, E. 1980. Childhood-onset insomnia. *Sleep*, 3, 59–65.

17. McCarren, M. *et al.* 1994. Insomnia in Vietnam era veteran twins: influence of genes and combat experience. *Sleep*, 17, 456–61.

18. Lind, M.J. *et al.* 2015. A longitudinal twin study of insomnia symptoms in adults. *Sleep*, 38, 1423–30.

19. Ban, H.-J. *et al.* 2011. Genetic and metabolic characterization of insomnia. *PLoS One*, 6, e18455.

20. Byrne, E.M. *et al.* 2013. A genome-wide association study of sleep habits and insomnia. *American Journal of Medical Genetics Part B-Neuropsychiatric Genetics*, 162B, 439–51.

21. Amin, N. *et al.* 2016. Genetic variants in *RBFOX3* are associated with sleep latency. *European Journal of Human Genetics*, 24, 1488–95.

22. Bianchi, M.T. *et al.* 2013. The subjective-objective mismatch in sleep perception among those with insomnia and sleep apnea. *Journal of Sleep Research*, 22, 557–68.

23. Peyron, C. *et al.* 2000. A mutation in a case of early onset narcolepsy and a generalized absence of hypocretin peptides in human narcoleptic brains. *Nature Medicine*, 6, 991–7.

24. Nishino, S. *et al.* 2000. Hypocretin (orexin) deficiency in human narcolepsy. *The Lancet*, 355, 39–40.

25. Barclay, N.L. and Gregory, A.M. 2013. Quantitative genetic research on sleep: a review of normal sleep, sleep disturbances and associated emotional, behavioural, and health-related difficulties. *Sleep Medicine Reviews*, 17, 29–40.

26. Juji, T. *et al.* 1984. HLA antigens in Japanese patients with narcolepsy. All the patients were DR2 positive. *Tissue Antigens*, 24, 316–19.

27. Tafti, M. *et al.* 2014. *DQB1* locus alone explains most of the risk and protection in narcolepsy with cataplexy in Europe. *Sleep*, 37, 19–25.

28. Faraco, J. and Mignot, E. 2012. Genetics of narcolepsy. *Sleep Medicine Clinics*, 6, 217–28.

29. Hallmayer, J. *et al.* 2009. Narcolepsy is strongly associated with the T-cell receptor alpha locus. *Nature Genetics*, 41, 708–11.

30. Han, F. *et al.* 2012. *TCRA*, *P2RY11*, and *CPT1B/CHKB* associations in Chinese narcolepsy. *Sleep Medicine*, 13, 269–72.

31. Faraco, J. *et al.* 2013. ImmunoChip study implicates antigen presentation to T cells in narcolepsy. *PLoS Genetics*, 9, e1003270.

32. Toyoda, H. *et al.* 2015. A polymorphism in *CCR1/CCR3* is associated with narcolepsy. *Brain, Behavior, and Immunity*, 49, 148–55.

33. Kornum, B.R. *et al.* 2011. Common variants in *P2RY11* are associated with narcolepsy. *Nature Genetics*, 43, 66–71.

34. Holm, A. *et al.* 2015. *EIF3G* is associated with narcolepsy across ethnicities. *European Journal of Human Genetics*, 23, 1573–80.

35. Winkelmann, J. *et al.* 2012. Mutations in *DNMT1* cause autosomal dominant cerebellar ataxia, deafness and narcolepsy. *Human Molecular Genetics*, 21, 2205–10.

36. Yamasaki, M. *et al.* 2014. Genome-wide analysis of CNV (copy number variation) and their associations with narcolepsy in a Japanese population. *Journal of Human Genetics*, 59, 235–40.

37. Mahlios, J., De la Herrán-Arita, A.K., and Mignot, E. 2013. The autoimmune basis of narcolepsy. *Current Opinion in Neurobiology*, 23, 767–73.

38. Han, F. *et al.* 2011. Narcolepsy onset is seasonal and increased following the 2009 H1N1 pandemic in China. *Annals of Neurology*, 70, 410–17.

39. Han, F. *et al.* 2013. Genome wide analysis of narcolepsy in China implicates novel immune loci and reveals changes in association prior to versus after the 2009 H1N1 influenza pandemic. *PLoS Genetics*, 9, e1003880.

40. Honda, Y. *et al.* 1986. HLA-DR2 and Dw2 in narcolepsy and in other disorders of excessive somnolence without cataplexy. *Sleep*, 9(1 Pt 2), 133–42.

41. Miyagawa, T. *et al.* 2009. Polymorphism located between *CPT1B* and *CHKB*, and *HLA-DRB1*1501-DQB1*0602* haplotype confer susceptibility to CNS hypersomnias (essential hypersomnia). *PLoS One*, 4, e5394.

42. Miyagawa, T. *et al.* 2010. Polymorphism located in *TCRA* locus confers susceptibility to essential hypersomnia with *HLA-DRB1*1501-DQB1*0602* haplotype. *Journal of Human Genetics*, 55, 63–5.

43. Khor, S.-S. *et al.* 2013. Genome-wide association study of *HLA-DQB1*06:02* negative essential hypersomnia. *Peer Journal*, 1, e66.

44. Lowrey, P.L. and Takahashi, J.S. 2011. Genetics of circadian rhythms in mammalian model organisms. *Advances in Genetics*, 74, 175–230.

45. Vink, J.M. *et al.* 2001. Genetic analysis of morningness and eveningness. *Chronobiology International*, 18, 809–22.

46. Klei, L. *et al.* 2005. Heritability of morningness-eveningness and self-report sleep measures in a family-based sample of 521 hutterites. *Chronobiology International*, 22, 1041–54.

47. von Schantz, M. *et al.* 2015. Distribution and heritability of diurnal preference (chronotype) in a rural Brazilian family-based cohort, the Baependi study. *Scientific Reports*, 5, 9214.

48. Toh, K.L. *et al.* 2001. An hPer2 phosphorylation site mutation in familial advanced sleep phase syndrome. *Science*, 291, 1040–3.

49. Xu, Y. *et al.* 2005. Functional consequences of a CKIdelta mutation causing familial advanced sleep phase syndrome. *Nature*, 434, 640–4.

50. Brennan, K.C. *et al.* 2013. Casein kinase iδ mutations in fa-milial migraine and advanced sleep phase. *Science Translational Medicine*, 5, 183ra56, 1–11.

51. Carpen, J.D. *et al.* 2006. A silent polymorphism in the *PER1* gene associates with extreme diurnal preference in humans. *Journal of Human Genetics*, 51, 1122–5.

52. Parsons, M.J. *et al.* 2014. Polymorphisms in the circadian ex-pressed genes *PER3* and *ARNTL2* are associated with diurnal preference and GNβ3 with sleep measures. *Journal of Sleep Research*, 23, 595–604.

53. Hida, A. *et al.* 2014. Screening of clock gene polymorphisms demonstrates association of a *PER3* polymorphism with morningness-eveningness preference and circadian rhythm sleep disorder. *Scientific Reports*, 4, 6309.

54. Pedrazzoli, M. *et al.* 2007. Clock polymorphisms and circadian rhythms phenotypes in a sample of the Brazilian population. *Chronobiology International*, 24, 1–8.

55. Robilliard, D.L. *et al.* 2002. The 3111 Clock gene polymorphism is not associated with sleep and circadian rhythmicity in phenotyp-ically characterized human subjects. *Journal of Sleep Research*, 11, 305–12.

56. Dijk, D.-J. and Archer, S.N. 2010. PERIOD3, circadian pheno-types, and sleep homeostasis. *Sleep Medicine Reviews*, 14, 151–60.

57. Ebisawa, T. *et al.* 2001. Association of structural polymorphisms in the human period3 gene with delayed sleep phase syndrome. *EMBO Reports*, 2, 342–6.

58. Archer, S.N. *et al.* 2003. A length polymorphism in the circadian clock gene Per3 is linked to delayed sleep phase syndrome and extreme diurnal preference. *Sleep*, 26, 413–15.

59. Pereira, D.S. *et al.* 2005. Association of the length polymorphism in the human *Per3* gene with the delayed sleep-phase syn-drome: does latitude have an influence upon it? *Sleep*, 28, 29–32.

60. Kunorozva, L. *et al.* 2012. Chronotype and *PERIOD3* variable number tandem repeat polymorphism in individual sports ath-letes. *Chronobiology International*, 29, 1004–10.

61. Perea, C.S. *et al.* 2014. Study of a functional polymorphism in the *PER3* gene and diurnal preference in a Colombian sample. *Open Neurology Journal*, 8, 7–10.

62. Osland, T.M. *et al.* 2011. Association study of a variable-number tandem repeat polymorphism in the clock gene *PERIOD3* and chronotype in Norwegian university students. *Chronobiology International*, 28, 764–70.

63. Viola, A.U. *et al.* 2007. *PER3* polymorphism predicts sleep struc-ture and waking performance. *Current Biology*, 17, 613–18.

64. Rupp, T.L. *et al.* 2013. *PER3* and *ADORA2A* polymorphisms impact neurobehavioral performance during sleep restriction. *Journal of Sleep Research*, 22, 160–5.

65. Maire, M. *et al.* 2014. Sleep ability mediates individual differences in the vulnerability to sleep loss: evidence from a *PER3* poly-morphism. *Cortex*, 52, 47–59.

66. Hu, Y. *et al.* 2016. GWAS of 89,283 individuals identifies gen-etic variants associated with self-reporting of being a morning person. *Nature Communications*, 7, 10448.

67. Lane, J.M. *et al.*, 2016. Genome-wide association analysis identi-fies novel loci for chronotype in 100,420 individuals from the UK Biobank. *Nature Communications*, 7, 10889.

68. Winkelmann, J. *et al.* 2011. Genome-wide association study iden-tifies novel restless legs syndrome susceptibility loci on 2p14 and 16q12.1. *PLoS Genetics*, 7, e1002171.

69. Allen, R.P. *et al.* 2014. Restless legs syndrome/Willis–Ekbom disease diagnostic criteria: updated International Restless Legs Syndrome Study Group (IRLSSG) consensus criteria—history, rationale, description, and significance. *Sleep Medicine*, 15, 860–73.

70. Winkelmann, J. *et al.* 2000. Clinical characteristics and frequency of the hereditary restless legs syndrome in a population of 300 patients. *Sleep*, 23, 597–602.

71. Montplaisir, J. *et al.* 1997. Clinical, polysomnographic, and gen-etic characteristics of restless legs syndrome: a study of 133 pa-tients diagnosed with new standard criteria. *Movement Disorders*, 12, 61–5.

72. Desai, A.V. *et al.* 2004. Genetic influences in self-reported symp-toms of obstructive sleep apnoea and restless legs: a twin study. *Twin Res*, 7, 589–95.

73. Xiong, L. *et al.* 2007. Canadian restless legs syndrome twin study. *Neurology*, 68, 1631–3.

74. Winkelmann, J. *et al.* 2002. Complex segregation analysis of restless legs syndrome provides evidence for an autosomal dom-inant mode of inheritance in early age at onset families. *Annals of Neurology*, 52, 297–302.

75. Mathias, R.A. *et al.* 2006. Segregation analysis of restless legs syn-drome: possible evidence for a major gene in a family study using blinded diagnoses. *Human Heredity*, 62, 157–64.

76. Schormair, B. and Winkelmann, J. 2011. Genetics of restless legs syndrome: Mendelian, complex, and everything in between. *Sleep Medicine Clinics*, 6, 203–15.

77. Balaban, H. *et al.* 2012. A novel locus for restless legs syndrome on chromosome 13q. *European Neurology*, 68, 111–16.

78. Winkelmann, J. *et al.* 2008. Variants in the neuronal nitric oxide synthase (*nNOS, NOS1*) gene are associated with restless legs syndrome. *Movement Disorders*, 23, 350–8.

79. Schormair, B. *et al.* 2008. PTPRD (protein tyrosine phosphatase receptor type delta) is associated with restless legs syndrome. *Nature Genetics*, 40, 946–8.

80. Gautier-Sauvigné, S. *et al.* 2005. Nitric oxide and sleep. *Sleep Medicine Reviews*, 9, 101–13.

81. Uetani, N. *et al.* 2006. Mammalian motoneuron axon targeting requires receptor protein tyrosine phosphatases sigma and delta. *Journal of Neuroscience*, 26, 5872–880.

82. Uetani, N. *et al.* 2000. Impaired learning with enhanced hippocampal long-term potentiation in PTP delta-deficient mice. *EMBO*, 19, 2775–85.

83. Winkelmann, J. *et al.* 2007. Genome-wide association study of restless legs syndrome identifies common variants in three gen-omic regions. *Nature Genetics*, 39, 1000–6.

84. Stefansson, H. *et al.* 2007. A genetic risk factor for periodic limb movements in sleep. *New England Journal of Medicine*, 357, 639–47.

85. Schulte, E.C. *et al.* 2014. Targeted resequencing and systematic *in vivo* functional testing identifies rare variants in *MEIS1* as signifi-cant contributors to restless legs syndrome. *American Journal of Human Genetics*, 95, 85–95.

86. Weissbach, A. *et al.* 2012. Exome sequencing in a family with restless legs syndrome. *Movement Disorders*, 27, 1686–9.

87. Wu, Q. and Maniatis, T. 2000. Large exons encoding multiple ectodomains are a characteristic feature of protocadherin genes. *Proceedings of the National Academy of Sciences of the United States of America*, 97, 3124–9.

88. Tufik, S. *et al.* 2010. Obstructive sleep apnea syndrome in the Sao Paulo Epidemiologic Sleep Study. *Sleep Medicine*, 11, 441–6.

89. Schwartz, A.R. *et al.* 2008. Obesity and obstructive sleep apnea: pathogenic mechanisms and therapeutic approaches. *Proceedings of the American Thoracic Society*, 5, 185–92.

90. Strohl, K.P. *et al.* 1978. Obstructive sleep apnea in family mem-bers. *New England Journal of Medicine*, 299, 969–73.

91. Redline, S. *et al*. 1992. Studies in the genetics of obstructive sleep apnea. Familial aggregation of symptoms associated with sleep-related breathing disturbances. *American Review of Respiratory Disease*, 145, 440–4.

92. Gislason, T. *et al*. 2002. Familial predisposition and cosegregation analysis of adult obstructive sleep apnea and the sudden infant death syndrome. *American Journal of Respiratory and Critical Care Medicine*, 166, 833–8.

93. Guilleminault, C. *et al*. 1995. Familial aggregates in obstructive sleep apnea syndrome. *Chest*, 107, 1545–51.

94. Redline, S. *et al*. 1995. The familial aggregation of obstructive sleep apnea. *American Journal of Respiratory and Critical Care Medicine*, 151, 682–7.

95. Mathur, R. and Douglas, N.J. 1995. Family studies in patients with the sleep apnea–hypopnea syndrome. *Annals of Internal Medicine*, 122, 174–8.

96. de Paula, L.K.G. *et al*. 2016. Heritability of OSA in a rural population. *Chest*, 149, 92–7.

97. Redline, S. and Tishler, P.V. 2000. The genetics of sleep apnea. *Sleep Medicine Reviews*, 4, 583–602.

98. Varvarigou, V. *et al*. 2011. A review of genetic association studies of obstructive sleep apnea: field synopsis and meta-analysis. *Sleep*, 34, 1461–8.

99. Larkin, E.K. *et al*. 2010. A candidate gene study of obstructive sleep apnea in European Americans and African Americans. *American Journal of Respiratory and Critical Care Medicine*, 182, 947–53.

100. Larkin, E.K. *et al*. 2008. Using linkage analysis to identify quantitative trait loci for sleep apnea in relationship to body mass index. *Annals of Human Genetics*, 72(Pt 6), 762–73.

101. Sun, J. *et al*. 2015. Obstructive sleep apnea susceptibility genes in Chinese population: a field synopsis and meta-analysis of genetic association studies. *PLoS One*, 10, e0135942.

102. de Lima, F.F.F. *et al*. 2016. The role inflammatory response genes in obstructive sleep apnea syndrome: a review. *Sleep and Breathing*, 20, 331–8.

103. Khalyfa, A. *et al*. 2011. TNF-α gene polymorphisms and excessive daytime sleepiness in pediatric obstructive sleep apnea. *Journal of Pediatrics*, 158, 77–82.

104. Patel, S.R. *et al*. 2012. Association of genetic loci with sleep apnea in European Americans and African-Americans: the Candidate Gene Association Resource (CARe). *PLoS One*, 7, e48836.

105. Hecht, J.H. *et al*. 1996. Ventricular zone gene-1 (*vzg-1*) encodes a lysophosphatidic acid receptor expressed in neurogenic regions of the developing cerebral cortex. *Journal of Cell Biology*, 135, 1071–83.

106. Contos, J.J. *et al*. 2000. Requirement for the lpA1 lysophosphatidic acid receptor gene in normal suckling behavior. *Proceedings of the National Academy of Sciences of the United States of America*, 97, 13384–9.

107. Cade, B.E. *et al*. 2016. Genetic associations with obstructive sleep apnea traits in Hispanic/Latino Americans. *American Journal of Respiratory and Critical Care Medicine*, 194, 886–97.

108. Locke, A.E. *et al*. 2015. Genetic studies of body mass index yield new insights for obesity biology. *Nature*, 518, 197–206.

109. Liu, C.-T. *et al*. 2013. Genome-wide association of body fat distribution in African ancestry populations suggests new loci. *PLoS Genetics*, 9, e1003681.

110. Schwab, R.J. *et al*. 2006. Family aggregation of upper airway soft tissue structures in normal subjects and patients with sleep apnea. *American Journal of Respiratory and Critical Care Medicine*, 173, 453–63.

111. Chi, L. *et al*. 2014. Heritability of craniofacial structures in normal subjects and patients with sleep apnea. *Sleep*, 37, 1689–98.

112. Collins, D.D. *et al*. 1978. Hereditary aspects of decreased hypoxic response. *Journal of Clinical Investigation*, 62, 105–10.

113. Guindalini, C. *et al*. 2010. Influence of genetic ancestry on the risk of obstructive sleep apnoea syndrome. *European Respiratory Journal*, 36, 834–41.

# 113

# Multimodal imaging of sleep–wake disorders

*Umberto Moretto, Dylan Smith, Liliana Dell'Osso, and Thien Thanh Dang-Vu*

## Introduction

The understanding of sleep and its disorders has vastly improved in recent years, aided significantly by technological and methodological advancements in neuroimaging techniques, which allowed for more precise neuroanatomical insight into the activity of the sleeping brain. Indeed, the brain does not 'turn off' during sleep and, in fact, remains active throughout the sleep cycle. While it is difficult to obtain a direct measure of neuronal activity, neuroimaging techniques have allowed sleep researchers to safely detect its correlates in human subjects during sleep and sleep/wake transitions.

The widely available research methodology include magnetic resonance imaging (MRI) and functional MRI (fMRI), magnetic resonance spectroscopy (MRS), positron emission tomography (PET), and single-photon emission computed tomography (SPET or SPECT), described in more detail in Chapter 12. When used in sleep research, these neuroimaging techniques can be powerful tools for illuminating the complex neuronal activities that shape brain function throughout the different stages of sleep.

Neuroimaging is particularly useful for studying sleep disorders. For example, insomnia has been associated with an excess of activity in brain regions responsible for processing emotion, as well as with a marked lack of activation in networks normally responsible for the inhibitory regulation of these regions, and these differences tend to be most pronounced during transitions from wakefulness to sleep. Although less consistent than functional imaging studies, neuroimaging of brain anatomy in insomnia suggests alterations in the compositional integrity of discrete brain structures such as the hippocampus and prefrontal cortex, as well as the rostral anterior cingulate cortex. Taken together, neuroimaging techniques have proven to be a powerful tool in understanding the neural mechanisms underlying sleep and pathologies leading to sleep disorders. This chapter will provide an overview of these imaging methods and discuss findings they have provided pertaining to sleep, insomnia, and other sleep–wake disorders. While this chapter focuses selectively on neurological disorders of sleep, we encourage the reader to consult dedicated works for a comprehensive overview of sleep disorders [1].

## Imaging in normal sleep

As described in detail in Chapter 109, the current predominant model of human sleep divides this physiological state into four stages, based on the characteristics of brain activity, muscle tone, and eye movements, with the main differentiation being between rapid eye movement (REM) sleep from non-REM (NREM) sleep, which is composed of stage N1, N2, and N3 sleep. Stage N3 sleep was previously further divided into stages 3 and 4 of sleep, but these were consolidated due to a lack of evidence for a neurophysiological difference between them. During a night of sleep, the brain continuously cycles through these stages in periods of approximately 90 minutes.

N1 sleep marks the transition from wakefulness to sleep. This stage of sleep, which normally constitutes 5–10% of total sleep time, shows a slower pattern of brainwave activity, compared to the awake state, when measured by electroencephalography (EEG). Stage N1 is followed by stage N2 where two distinct microarchitectural EEG patterns—K-complexes and spindles—are visible. Slow waves, also referred to as K-complexes during stage N2, are typified by a large (>75 μV), low-frequency (0.5–2 Hz) negative peak, followed immediately by a lower-frequency positive inflection. Spindles are short bursts of approximately 11–15 Hz activity lasting approximately 0.5 seconds. Spindles are thought to reflect brain processes involved in gating out of sensory stimuli that might otherwise wake the sleeper, as well as other cognitive functions such as memory consolidation. N2 sleep generally comprises 45–55% of total sleep. The next stage of NREM sleep N3 is also known as slow-wave sleep (SWS) due to an increased prevalence of slow waves on the EEG. Commonly known as 'deep sleep', N3 occurs mostly during the first half of a full night's sleep and constitutes 15–25% of total sleep time. REM sleep, characterized by rapid eye movements, is the stage of sleep most associated with dreaming. Hallmarks of REM sleep include muscle atonia, as well as an EEG profile more similar to the awake state than that of NREM sleep. For this reason, REM sleep is also known as 'paradoxical sleep'. REM sleep usually accounts for 20–25% of total sleep and occurs mostly during the second half of a normal night's sleep.

## Imaging in NREM sleep

During NREM sleep, cortical neuron activity transitions into a pattern of slow oscillations, alternating between brief bursts of neuronal firing ('up' states), followed by long intervals of hyperpolarization ('down' states). This oscillation forms the basis of cortical synchronization in NREM sleep, which is observed on EEG as spindles and slow waves. As EEG-indexed synchronization increases, down-state hyperpolarization is also associated with decreases in regional cerebral blood flow (rCBF) using PET, with gradual decreases during the transition from wakefulness to N1 and N2, reaching a minimum during N3 [2].

The induction of NREM sleep seems to be facilitated by a decreased activity in the brainstem tegmentum and its ascending pathways, as evidenced by human PET studies showing decreased activity in the pontine tegmentum during light NREM extending to the mesencephalic tegmentum during SWS [3]. Sleep spindles are thalamocortical in origin, generated by the activity of GABAergic thalamic reticular neurons and are reflected by rCBF decreases in thalamic areas during NREM sleep [3].

Moreover, the cerebral cortex also shows SWS deactivation, albeit with larger rCBF decreases in frontal and parietal cortices, with less deactivation observed in the primary cortices [3]. The observed decreases in rCBF are likely due to a larger net contribution of the down state to the overall PET signal, which is averaged across periods of several minutes. However, recent studies utilizing combined EEG and fMRI have confirmed a transient increase of brain responses in cortical and subcortical brain areas during slow waves and spindles [4, 5].

Studies of functional connectivity in NREM sleep have shown attenuated connectivity of the default mode network (DMN). The DMN, a functional neural network highly active in the absence of any stimuli or task, shows uncoupling, particularly between its anterior (medial prefrontal) and posterior (precuneus, posterior cingulate) nodes, during deep sleep [6]. In general, there is evidence that transitioning from light to deep NREM sleep is associated with uncoupling of functional neural networks in favour of an increase in local connectivity [7]. This is in line with recent consciousness theories, according to which decreasing levels of functional connectivity are the physical correlates of decreasing levels of consciousness.

## Imaging in REM sleep

In contrast with NREM sleep, REM sleep is defined by a marked desynchronization of brain waves, more closely resembling the awake state in general, with some areas showing increased activity, compared to wakefulness, and decreased activity in others.

During REM sleep, rCBF is increased specifically in limbic and paralimbic areas, the pontine tegmentum, thalamic nuclei, amygdaloid complex, anterior cingulate, orbitofrontal and insular cortices, and hippocampal formation [3, 8]. In contrast, the middle and inferior prefrontal gyri, posterior cingulate, and precuneus tend to show decreases in rCBF during REM [3, 8].

Induction of REM sleep is also believed to originate in the brainstem, as evidenced by increased activation of the mesopontine, which is thought to activate the thalamus and, in turn, the cortex [9]. Neurons in the pons generate ponto-geniculo-occipital waves, which can be recorded at different levels of this pathway: the pons, the lateral geniculate bodies, the occipital cortex, and limbic areas

[10, 11]. A time course analysis of BOLD responses during REM sleep showed activation of the pons, the thalamus, and the visual cortex, in association with REM [12]. PET-indexed rCBF analysis showed coupling of the lateral geniculate bodies, the occipital cortex, and REM during REM sleep, but not in wakefulness [13].

REM sleep has also been observed to exhibit a unique pattern of functional connectivity, exemplified by a curious dissociation between striate and extrastriate cortical areas, which is opposite to that seen in wakefulness [14]. The DMN, previously mentioned to show uncoupling in NREM sleep, demonstrates recoupling again during REM sleep between the anterior and posterior nodes of the DMN, similar to the awake state [15]. However, other changes in DMN functional connectivity occur during REM sleep such as an anti-correlation between the DMN and the thalamus, as well as sensorimotor areas [15].

Dreams, a hallmark of REM sleep, may also be related to distinct neurophysiological activity. Increased activation of the amygdala during REM is likely related to the strong emotional content experienced in dreams, and deactivation of areas associated with working memory, such as the dorsolateral prefrontal cortex, might explain the discontinuity commonly reported by dreamers [8]. The vivid visual and auditory content of dreams has been linked to hyperperfusion within occipital and temporal lobes, while the feeling of movement may be explained by increased activity within premotor and motor cortices [3, 14]. These movements are not acted out by the sleeper in normal conditions due to muscle atonia, another characteristic of REM sleep.

## Imaging in insomnia

Insomnia, defined by difficulty in sleep initiation, continuity, or quality, which leads to significant daytime impairments, has only relatively recently been considered from a neurological point of view. Current theories ascribe the aetiology of insomnia to alterations in neural control over sleep–wake regulation systems. An imbalance in these systems may be due to increased activity in networks contributing to arousal (hyperarousal), or hypofunction of those responsible for initiating or maintaining sleep [16].

A summary table of functional neuroimaging studies of insomnia can be found in Table 113.1. Compared to normal sleepers, individuals suffering from insomnia show a decrease in rCBF in the basal ganglia, medial frontal, parietal, and occipital cortices, and this decrease is most prominent in NREM sleep [17]. Interestingly, basal ganglia activity seems most sensitive to cognitive behavioural therapy for insomnia (CBTi), with one study showing a 24% increase in basal ganglia rCBF, coupled with a 43% improvement in average sleep latency, following CBTi [18]. A landmark PET imaging study in primary insomnia (that is, in the absence of major comorbidities) showed a lack of reduction in brain glucose metabolism from wakefulness to sleep, lending credence to the hyperarousal theory of insomnia where brain metabolism maintains a profile more similar to the awake state in insomnia, compared to good sleepers [19]. Specific brain areas that were affected by this failure to reduce glucose metabolism during wake–sleep transition included the ascending reticular activating system, thalamus, hypothalamus, hippocampus, amygdala, and anterior cingulate, insular, and medial prefrontal cortices. Conversely, during wakefulness, these areas—particularly the

**Table 113.1** Functional neuroimaging studies of insomnia

| Study | Neuroimaging technique | Sample size (number of females) | | Mean age in years ± SD | | PI diagnosis and assessment | PI duration | History of pharmacological treatment | Main findings in PI, compared to GS (significance level) |
|---|---|---|---|---|---|---|---|---|---|
| | | PI | GS | PI | GS | | | | |
| Smith et al. 2002 [17] | 99mTc-HMPAO SPECT | 5 (5) | 4 (4) | 37.8 ± 12.1 | 34.5 ± 11.9 | ICSD, PSG | ≥6 mo | Off-sleep aids for ≥4 weeks, off SSRIs for ≥1 year | Hypoperfusion of basal ganglia and other regions during NREM sleep (P ≤0.05 uncorr.) |
| Nofzinger et al. 2004 [19] | 18F-FDG PET | 7 (4) | 20 (13) | 34.2 ± 8.9 | 32.6 ± 8.4 | DSM-IV, PSG | ≥1 mo | PI using med. were excluded | Smaller reduction in glucose metabolism during transition to NREM sleep; prefrontal hypoactivation during wake (P ≤0.001, corr.) |
| Smith et al. 2005 [18] | 99mTc-HMPAO SPECT | 4 (4) | None | 34.5 ± 12 | None | See [17] | See [17] | See [17] | Partial re-establishment of activation in basal ganglia after BT (P ≤0.05, uncorr.) |
| Nofzinger et al. 2006 [21] | 18F-FDG PET | 15 (7) | None | 36.9 ± 10.5 | None | DSM-IV, PSG | ≥1 mo | PI using med. were excluded | Correlation between WASO and thalamocortical activation, including pontine tegmentum (P <0.05, corr.) |
| Altena et al. 2008 [22] | fMRI (1.5 T) | 21 (17) | 12 (9) | 61 ± 6.2 | 60 ± 8.2 | See [88]. PSG | ≥2.5 years | Off med. for ≥2 mo | Prefrontal hypoactivation during verbal fluency task, partially restored after CBT (P <0.05, uncorr.) |
| Huang et al. 2012 [45] | fMRI (3.0 T) | 10 (5) | 10 (5) | 37.5 ± 12.4 | 35.5 ± 8.7 | DSM-IV, PSG | n.r. | Medication-naïve | Altered connectivity between amygdala and other regions, particularly the premotor cortex; amygdala–premotor connectivity was correlated with PSQI (P <0.05, uncorr.) |
| Drummond et al. 2013 [23] | fMRI (3.0 T) | 25 (12) | 25 (12) | 32.3 ± 7.2 | 32.4 ± 7.1 | DSISD, actigraphy, PSG | ≥3 mo | PI using med. were excluded | During cognitive task, reduced activation in task-relevant areas and reduced deactivation of default mode regions (P <0.05, corr.) |
| Baglioni et al. 2014 [26] | fMRI (3.0 T) | 22 (15) | 38 (21) | 40.7 ± 12.6 | 39.6 ± 8.9 | Research diagnostic criteria for ID (not PI) [88]. PSG, ISI, PSQI | ≥1 year (10.3 ± 10.9 years) | Off psychoactive med. for ≥2 weeks | ID patients, compared to GS, have heightened amygdala responses to insomnia-related stimuli (P <0.001, uncorr.). Habituation of amygdala responses was observed only in GS, but not in patients with ID |
| Li et al. 2014 [44] | fMRI (3.0 T) | 15 (8) | 15 (8) | 39.8 ± 11.2 | 41.3 ± 8.9 | DSM-IV, PSQI | n.r. | Medication-naïve | Resting state connectivity of superior parietal lobe was decreased with superior frontal gyrus, and increased with bilateral anterior and posterior cingulate (P <0.05 uncorr.) |
| Nie et al. 2015 [43] | fMRI (3.0 T) | 42 (27) | 42 (24) | 49.24 ± 12.26 | 49.14 ± 10.20 | ICSD | >2 mo | Off psychoactive med. for ≥2 weeks | Decreased functional connectivity between medial prefrontal and right medial temporal lobes, and between left medial temporal lobe and left inferior parietal cortex (P <0.05, corr.) |
| Kay et al. 2016 [20] | 18F-FDG PET | 40 (24) | 44 (25) | 37 ± 10 | 38 ± 11 | DSM-IV, PSG | n.r. | Off psychoactive med. for ≥2 weeks | Group-by-state interactions in relative glucose metabolism showing impaired disengagement of left fronto-parietal, precuneus/ posterior cingulate and fusiform/ lingual gyri during NREM sleep, or alternatively impaired engagement of these regions during wakefulness (P <0.05, corr.) |

*Note.* corr: corrected; uncorr.: uncorrected; n.r.: not reported; SD: standard deviation; PI: primary insomnia; GS: good sleeper controls; ID: insomnia disorder; NREM: non-rapid-eye movement; BT: behaviour therapy; CBT: cognitive behavioural therapy; PSQI: Pittsburgh Sleep Quality Index; PSG: polysomnography; WASO: wake after sleep onset; med.: medication; SSRI: selective serotonin reuptake inhibitor; DSM-IV: *Diagnostic and Statistical Manual of Mental Disorders*, fourth edition; ICSD: International Classification of Sleep Disorders; DSISD: Duke Structured Interview for Sleep Disorders; mo: month.
Updated from [89].

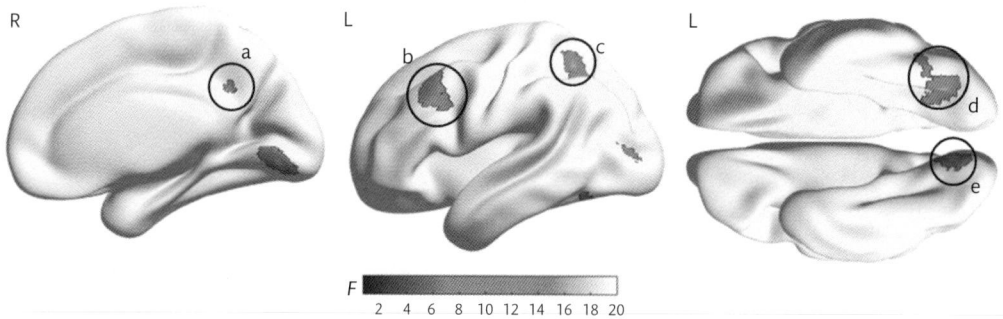

**Fig. 113.1** NREM sleep–wake differences in brain glucose metabolism—primary insomnia sufferers compared to good sleepers. Insomniacs showed smaller differences in PET-indexed glucose metabolism, compared to good sleepers, in (a) the right precuneus/posterior cingulate cortex, (b) the left middle frontal gyrus, (c) the left inferior/superior parietal lobules, (d) the left lingual/fusiform/occipital gyri, and (e) the right lingual gyrus.
Adapted from *Sleep*, 39(10), Kay DB, Karim HT, Soehner AM, *et al.*, Sleep-Wake Differences in Relative Regional Cerebral Metabolic Rate for Glucose among Patients with Insomnia Compared with Good Sleepers, pp. 1779–1794, Copyright (2016), with permission from Oxford University Press.

prefrontal cortex—showed relatively reduced glucose metabolism in insomnia sufferers, compared to good sleepers. While this initial study utilized a small sample size, a replication study comparing 44 primary insomnia sufferers with 40 good sleepers showed insomnia to exhibit smaller sleep–wake differences in glucose metabolism in brain regions involved in cognition (prefrontal), self-referential processes (precuneus/posterior cingulate), and emotion (prefrontal, fusiform/lingual gyri) during NREM sleep. These differences can be seen in Fig. 113.1. Moreover, consistent with previous findings, activation of these areas was impaired during wakefulness in insomnia, compared to good sleepers [20]. Another PET study of insomnia sufferers found that measures of WASO (wake after sleep onset) positively correlated with metabolism in the pontine tegmentum and in thalamocortical networks in a frontal, anterior temporal, and anterior cingulate distribution [21].

Neuroimaging studies investigating the waking state and cognition in insomnia have generally focused on fMRI-indexed activation of specific brain areas or networks, compared to healthy good sleepers. Insomnia was associated with lower prefrontal cortex activation during a verbal fluency task, compared to controls, and this decreased activation was partially restored after CBTi [22]. A different study showed that insomnia sufferers failed to decrease DMN activation during a working memory task, whereas controls showed attenuation of the DMN in favour of the activation of more task-specific brain areas [23]. This inability to switch neural activation patterns to those required for specific tasks may explain subjective complaints of diminished cognitive performance in insomnia. Additionally, DMN activation has also been linked to rumination in other disorders, and thus failure to attenuate this network may also provide a biological basis for cognitive rumination associated with insomnia [24, 25]. An fMRI-based investigation into amygdala activation in insomnia found heightened activation in response to insomnia-related stimuli, compared to controls, but this difference was not observed when insomnia-unrelated stimuli were tested, supporting the use of insomnia-specific cognitive restructuring that is routinely performed during CBTi [26].

MRS-based investigations in insomnia have been less consistent. Some studies have shown lower relative concentrations of brain GABA in insomnia, compared to controls, both globally [27] and localized to the occipital and anterior cingulate [28]; however, a later study showed an increase in occipital GABA concentrations [29]. A more recent study failed to replicate these results, showing no difference in GABA levels between insomnia sufferers and controls in the areas of interest (anterior cingulate cortex and dorsolateral prefrontal cortex) [30]. While the direction of effect is inconsistent, possibly due to different times of MRS data acquisition (morning vs bedtime), dysregulation of GABA neurotransmission may be a potential target for both identification and treatment of insomnia and thus warrants further study. An MRS study of phosphocreatine revealed lower levels in grey matter of insomniacs in comparison to controls. Given the fact that lower levels of this metabolite are markers of an increased energy demand, this finding provides further evidence for the hyperarousal theory of insomnia [31].

Structural MRI investigations (with volumetry and VBM analyses) in insomnia have also been inconsistent, with some observations failing replication and others not surviving statistical corrections. A summary table of structural neuroimaging studies of insomnia can be found in Table 113.2. There is some evidence for reduced hippocampal volume in insomnia, but these results are not universal [32–35]. In one study, hippocampal volume was shown to be negatively correlated with insomnia duration and arousal indices; however, no significant differences in hippocampal volume were observed between insomnia sufferers and controls [34]. A different small-sample study did report significant deficits in bilateral hippocampal volume in insomnia [32]. This was later corroborated by a different group using a larger sample size that further showed a negative correlation between CA1 volume and sleep quality [36]; the combined volume of CA3, CA4, and the dentate gyrus was also negatively correlated with cognitive performances in verbal fluency, verbal memory, and verbal information processing tasks [36]. Other areas that seem to be affected in insomniacs are the rostral anterior cingulate cortex, found to be increased in volume [37], the prefrontal (dorsolateral, orbitofrontal, medial frontal), precentral, superior, and middle temporal cortices, the precuneus, and the cerebellum, found to display decreased grey matter volume in insomniacs [38–40]. The pineal gland has also been a focus of neuroanatomical research due to its involvement in regulation of the circadian rhythm via melatonin production and release. One study revealed volume reduction of the pineal gland in insomniacs, compared to controls, with pineal gland volume also negatively correlating with age in insomnia, but not in controls [41].

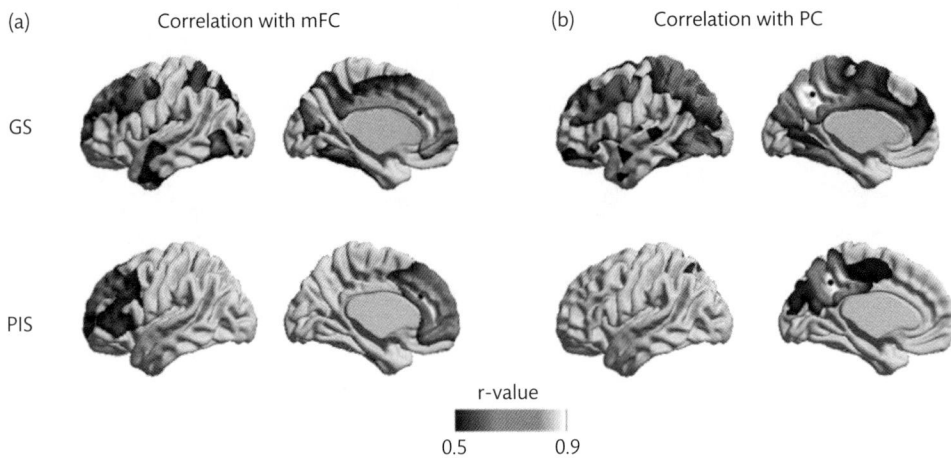

**Fig. 113.2** Structural covariance of cortical thickness—good sleepers (GS), compared to individuals with persistent insomnia symptoms (PIS). Insomnia sufferers showed a marked reduction in the spatial extent of cortical thickness correlations with regions of the default-mode network, that is, (a) the medial frontal cortex (mFC) and (b) the precuneus (PC).

Adapted from *Sleep*, 39(1), Suh S, Kim H, Dang-Vu TT, *et al.*, Cortical Thinning and Altered Cortico-Cortical Structural Covariance of the Default Mode Network in Patients with Persistent Insomnia Symptoms, pp. 161–171, Copyright (2016), with permission from Oxford University Press.

**Table 113.2** Structural neuroimaging studies of insomnia

| Study | Neuroimaging technique | Sample size (number of females) | | Mean age in years ± SD | | PI diagnosis and assessment | PI duration | History of pharmacological treatment | Main findings in PI, compared to GS (significance level) |
|---|---|---|---|---|---|---|---|---|---|
| | | PI | GS | PI | GS | | | | |
| Riemann et al. 2007 [32] | MRI (1.5 T) | 8 (5) | 8 (5) | 48.4 ± 16.3 | 46.3 ± 14.3 | DSM-IV, PSQI | 11.6 ± 8.9 years | Off medications ≥2 weeks | Reduced hippocampal volumes bilaterally (P <0.05, uncorr.) |
| Winkelman et al. 2008 [27] | 1H-MRS (4 T) | 16 (8) | 16 (7) | 37.3 ± 8.1 | 37.6 ± 4.5 | DSM-IV, PSQI, PSG | ≥6 mo | Off sleep aids ≥1 month | Average brain GABA levels were nearly 30% lower in PI. GABA levels negatively correlated with WASO (P ≤0.05) |
| Winkelman et al. 2010 [33] | MRI (3 T) | 20 (10) | 15 (6) | 39.3 (8.7) | 38.8 (5.3) | DSM-IV, ISI, PSQI, actigraphy | ≥6 months | Off psychoactive medications ≥3 months | No differences in hippocampal volume between groups |
| Altena et al. 2010 [39] | MRI (1.5 T) | 24 (17) | 13 (9) | 60.3 (6.0) | 60.2 ± 8.4 | DSM-IV | 17.7 ± 15.8 years | Off sleeping medications ≥2 months | Smaller volume of grey matter in the left orbitofrontal cortex, bilateral precuneus (P <0.05 corr.). Insomnia severity negatively correlated with left orbitofrontal cortex grey matter volume |
| Plante et al. 2012 [28] | 1H-MRS (4 T) | 20 (12) | 20 (12) | 34.3 ± 8.3 | 34.1 ± 9.9 | DSM-IV, PSQI, ISI, actigraphy | ≥1 year | Off psychoactive medications ≥2 weeks | Lower GABA levels in the occipital cortex and anterior cingulate (P ≤0.05) |
| Morgan et al. 2012 [29] | 1H-MRS (4 T) | 16 (10) | 17 (9) | 39 ± 9 | 36 ± 9 | DSM-IV, PSQI, ISI, PSG | ≥1 year | Off psychoactive medications ≥3 months | Mean occipital GABA level was 12% higher in PI. GABA levels correlated negatively with WASO (P <0.05) |
| Noh et al. 2012 [34] | MRI (1.5 T) | 20 (18) | 20 (18) | 50.8 ± 10.8 | 50.4 ± 11.7 | ICSD, PSG | 7.6 ± 6.1 years | No hypnotic med. for ≥1 month | No diff. in hippocampal volume. Hippocampal volume negatively correlated with arousal index (P <0.05 uncorr.) and insomnia duration (P <0.001 uncorr.) |

**Table 113.2** Continued

| Study | Neuroimaging technique | Sample size (number of females) | | Mean age in years ± SD | | PI diagnosis and assessment | PI duration | History of pharmacological treatment | Main findings in PI, compared to GS (significance level) |
|---|---|---|---|---|---|---|---|---|---|
| | | PI | GS | PI | GS | | | | |
| Spiegelhalder et al. 2013 [35] | MRI (3 T) | 28 (18) | 38 (21) | 43.7 ± 14.2 | 39.6 ± 8.9 | DSM-IV, PSG | 12.1 ± 11.0 years | Off psychoactive med. for ≥2 weeks | No diff. in hippocampal volume, no diff. in grey and white matter concentration (P <0.05 corr. and P <0.001 uncorr., respectively) |
| Winkelman et al. 2013 (Study 1) [37] | MRI (3 T) | 20 (10) | 15 (6) | 39.3 ± 8.7 | 38.8 ± 5.3 | DSM-IV, PSG | ≥6 months | Off psychoactive med. for ≥weeks | Increased rostral ACC volume, correlated positively with sleep onset latency and WASO, negatively with sleep efficiency (P ≤0.05 uncorr.) |
| Winkelman et al. 2013 (Study 2) [37] | MRI (3 T) | 21 (14) | 20 (12) | 35.8 ± 9.5 | 34.1 ± 9.9 | DSM-IV, PSG | ≥6 months | Off psychoactive med. for ≥2 weeks | Increased rostral ACC volume. Right ACC volume correlated with sleep onset latency (P ≤0.05 uncorr.) |
| Harper et al. 2013 [31] | [31]P-MRS (4 T) | 16 (8) | 16 (7) | 37.2 ± 8.4 | 37.6 ± 4.7 | DSM-IV, PSQI, PSG | >6 months | Off psychoactive med. for >3 months | Lower phosphocreatine in grey matter (P <0.05, corr.) |
| Joo et al. 2013 [38] | MRI (1.5 T) | 27 (25) | 27 (23) | 52.3 ± 7.8 | 51.7 ± 5.4 | ICSD-2, PSQI, ISI, PSG | 7.6 ± 6.1 years | No history of antidepressants, hypnotic agents, or anxiolytic agent use | Reduced grey matter concentrations in dorsolateral and medial prefrontal, precentral, superior and middle temporal gyri, and cerebellum (P <0.001 uncorr.) |
| Bumb et al. 2014 [41] | MRI (3 T) | 23 (11) | 27 (16) | 43 ± 7.4 | 39 ± 13.1 | DSM-IV, ICSD-2, PSG, 'Schlaffragebogen B' sleep questionnaire | 8.6 ± 7.3 years | Off psychoactive medications ≥2 weeks | Decrease in pineal gland volume (P <0.001) |
| Joo et al. 2014 [36] | MRI (1.5 T) | 27 (25) | 30 (28) | 51.2 ± 9.6 | 50.4 ± 7.1 | ICSD-2, PSQI, ISI, PSG | ≥1 year | Drug-naïve | PI showed bilateral atrophy across all hippocampal subfields (P <0.05, corr.) |
| Zhao et al. 2015 [42] | MRI (3 T) | 35 (30) | 35 (26) | 39.3 ± 8.6 | 34.9 ± 10.7 | DSM-IV, PSQI | n.r. | n.r. | Increased structural covariance between sensory and motor regions (P <0.05, corr.) |
| Suh et al. 2016 [40] | MRI (1.5 T) | 57 (22) | 40 (16) | 51.23 ± 8.07 | 47.93 ± 6.54 | Persistent insomnia symptoms, defined as difficulty to initiate or maintain sleep, early morning awakenings, and non-restorative sleep. PSQI, PSG | ≥1 month | Not on sleep or antidepressant medications at any time of the study | Cortical thinning in the anterior cingulate cortex, precentral cortex, and right lateral prefrontal cortex. Decreased structural covariance between anterior and posterior regions of the default mode network (P <0.05, corr.) |
| Spiegelhalder et al. 2016 [30] | MRS (3 T) | 20 (12) | 20 (12) | 42.7 ± 13.4 | 44.1 ± 10.6 | DSM-IV, PSQI, ISI, PSG | 9.4 ± 10.0 years | Off psychoactive medications ≥2 weeks | No difference in GABA levels in ACC and dorsolateral prefrontal cortices |

*Note.* corr.: corrected; uncorr.: uncorrected; n.r.: not reported; SD: standard deviation; PI: primary insomnia; GS: good sleeper controls; PSQI: Pittsburgh Sleep Quality Index; PSG: polysomnography; WASO: wake after sleep onset; ACC: anterior cingulate cortex; med.: medication; SSRI: selective serotonin reuptake inhibitor; DSM-IV: *Diagnostic and Statistical Manual of Mental Disorders*, fourth edition; ICSD: International Classification of Sleep Disorders.
Updated from [89].

Finally, a few studies investigated brain connectivity in insomnia. A recent structural MRI study found decreased cortical thickness correlation (that is, structural covariance) between anterior and posterior regions of the DMN in individuals with persistent insomnia symptoms (see Fig. 113.2), suggesting decreased connectivity within the DMN, and this decrease was negatively correlated with sleep quality [40]. This contrasts with other data showing increased structural covariance between sensory and motor cortices in insomnia [42]. Resting-state fMRI studies showed that insomnia was associated with disruption of medial prefrontal cortex functional connectivity with the right medial temporal cortex and left medial temporal lobe functional connectivity with the left inferior parietal cortex [43], as well as superior parietal lobe functional connectivity with the dorsolateral prefrontal cortex [44]. In line with the concept of emotional dysregulation in insomnia, resting-state fMRI data also showed increased functional connectivity between the amygdala and other regions such as sensorimotor cortices [45].

Overall, neuroimaging studies of insomnia have been mainly conducted in individuals with primary insomnia and gave further support to the hyperarousal theory—reduced deactivation during the sleep–wake transition [19], difficulty deactivating irrelevant cognitive processes [23], enhanced activity and connectivity of threat and emotional neuronal circuitry [26, 45], and reduced concentration of inhibitory neurotransmitters [28] all contribute to the incapacity to modulate levels of cortical arousal across the sleep–wake cycle. Recent data also suggest complex patterns of altered neural connectivity in insomnia. The significance of these abnormalities in structural and functional connectivity remains unclear, and further studies are warranted to confirm and clarify the relevance of these findings for the pathophysiology of insomnia.

## Imaging in other sleep disorders

### Narcolepsy

Narcolepsy is a disorder characterized by irresistible bouts of sleep throughout the day, often associated with REM-related features such as sleep paralysis, cataplexy, and hallucinations. Type 1 narcolepsy is characterized by cataplectic episodes and decreased cerebrospinal fluid levels of hypocretin. In the absence of these criteria, narcolepsy is classified as type 2. Significant DTI-indexed differences were observed between these two subtypes of narcolepsy, whereas no differences were observed between type 2 and healthy controls, suggesting the two types may result from different pathological mechanisms, with type 2 being a milder form with no apparent structural brain pathology [46]. Therefore, the bulk of neuroimaging research in narcoleptic patients focuses on type 1.

A meta-analysis of VBM in MRI studies of narcolepsy found selective grey matter loss in multiple brain areas, thought to be related to a damaged orexin/hypocretin pathway and emotional regulation system [47]. Unsurprisingly, multiple studies found alterations in the hypothalamus where orexinergic neurons are located [48], as well as the fronto-temporal cortex [47]. Further MRI analysis found a reduction in amygdalar volume, possibly serving as a mechanism for dysfunctional emotional regulation in the disorder [49].

Two fMRI studies sought to elucidate the nature of altered response to affective stimuli in narcolepsy via the presentation of humourous stimuli. Interestingly, while both studies observed increased amygdalar responses in patients, compared to healthy controls, observations in the hypothalamus were inconsistent. One study showed a decrease in hypothalamic response in response to affective stimuli [50], whereas the other study showed an increase in hypothalamic response, with the exception of one participant who experienced a cataplectic attack during the study and showed dramatic reductions in hypothalamic activity [51]. While these results seem to suggest an overdriven emotional network in narcolepsy, the role of the hypothalamus is not clear. The inconsistency in these results may be due, in part, to the relatively small sample sizes utilized in these studies.

### Restless legs syndrome

Restless legs syndrome (RLS) is characterized by an unpleasant and uncomfortable feeling in the legs, accompanied by the urge to move them in order to relieve this sensation. It occurs during the evening and at night, when sitting or lying down, and sometimes interferes with sleep onset.

The mechanism underlying RLS pathogenesis is hypothesized to involve inhibition of adrenergic, opiate, and dopaminergic descending inhibitory pathways [52]. This is supported by the observation that dopamine antagonists exacerbate RLS and dopamine agonists relieve symptoms [53].

Striatal dopamine transporter (DAT) and D2 receptor dysregulation in RLS has been extensively investigated using SPECT, but the results have been contradictory, pointing towards dysregulation, rather than a net increase or decrease of receptors [54, 55].

Similarly, PET studies using C-raclopride have found conflicting results on striatal D2 receptor binding, with differences across studies attributed to drug-naïve patients used in some studies, while others assessed patients on medication which can downregulate D2 receptors [56]. Opioid PET studies using C-diprenorphine showed no difference between RLS patients and controls; however, a relationship between RLS severity and decreased opioid binding was found, possibly due to competitive endogenous opioid release in response to pain [57].

Structural MRI studies have shown evidence of alterations in pulvinar grey matter in RLS, compared to controls, though it is unclear whether these alterations are a cause or a consequence of the syndrome [58]. A study using VBM found grey matter decreases in the primary sensorimotor cortex [59], and a DTI study revealed white matter alterations in this same area, as well as in the thalamus [60]; however, these anatomical deviations, compared to controls, were not significant when drug-naïve subjects were included [61, 62].

Functional MRI studies during resting state showed reduced thalamic connectivity with the right parahippocampal gyrus, right precuneus, right precentral gyrus, and bilateral lingual gyrus, as well as increased connectivity with the temporal and other areas. Interestingly, there was a negative correlation between RLS severity and right parahippocampal gyrus connectivity with the thalamus, suggesting dysfunction at the level of somatosensory information processing [63].

MRS studies of RLS point towards thalamic dysfunction, with one study showing decreased N-acetyl aspartate (NAA) concentrations and NAA/creatine (Cr) ratios in the medial thalamus of RLS participants, compared to controls, indicative of neuronal damage, but without showing fMRI or DTI-indexed alterations [64]. Another study found increased glutamate–glutamine/creatine ratios in the thalamic region of RLS patients, compared to controls, and interestingly, this ratio correlated with WASO [65], supporting the involvement of a glutamatergic arousal system in RLS. GABA was also investigated, with no difference in levels between RLS patients and controls. However, a positive correlation was found between thalamic GABA levels and RLS severity, as well as a negative correlation between cerebellar GABA and this same measure [66]. This suggests a role for the thalamus and the cerebellum in the modulation of RLS intensity.

## REM sleep behaviour disorder

REM sleep behaviour disorder (RBD) is a parasomnia characterized by movements or vocalizations which occur during REM sleep and are consistent with enactment of dream content. This disorder is often idiopathic but can also be comorbid with other neurological disorders or related to pharmacological effects (for example, antidepressants). The majority of idiopathic RBD patients will eventually develop neurodegenerative alpha-synucleinopathies such as Parkinson's disease (PD), multiple system atrophy, and Lewy body dementia [67].

A study attempting to elucidate the pathways involved in human RBD has employed SPECT, combined with video polysomnography, with injection of a radiotracer during an RBD episode. Increased metabolism was shown in premotor areas, the interhemispheric cleft, the periaqueductal area, the dorsal and ventral pons, and the anterior lobe of the cerebellum. Interestingly, no activation of the basal ganglia was observed, as is observed during wakeful movements. However, this study used a small sample size and no control group [68]. Other SPECT studies have reported differences in brain activation, compared to healthy controls, during resting wakefulness. A study in awake SPECT patients found decreased activity in the temporo-parietal and frontal cortices, as well as increased activity in the putamen, pons, and right hippocampus [69], and these findings have been replicated using larger populations [70, 71]. Decreased rCBF in the parietal, occipital, limbic, and cerebellar regions was observed in a group of idiopathic RBD patients, and a 2-year follow-up with the same individuals revealed further reduction of rCBF in the medial portions of the parieto-occipital lobe, with a significant decrease in rCBF in the right posterior cingulate [72]. A 3-year longitudinal SPECT study of 20 idiopathic RBD patients reported that half of these participants developed a neurodegenerative disease and hippocampal hyperperfusion was predictive of the development of neurodegeneration [71].

Due to a high degree of comorbidity with nigrostriatal dopamine pathway disorders, a number of studies have focused on unveiling a link between RBD and dopaminergic abnormalities. RBD patients showed a significant reduction in striatal DAT receptor densities, compared to controls, but not compared to PD patients [73]. Attempts to re-create these findings have been mixed, with some studies showing DAT density decrease in only a minority of RBD patients [74, 75]. Longitudinal studies of dopaminergic function have also shown a link between RBD and neurodegeneration, with presynaptic DAT densities in the substantia nigra being predictive of later onset of alpha-synucleinopathies in RBD [76]. No differences were found between RBD, PD, and healthy controls when post-synaptic D2 receptors were probed [73]. SPECT investigations

of serotonergic pathways also failed to show any involvement of these pathways in RBD [77].

Anatomical analyses using MRI confirmed that degeneration in RBD is not limited to the substantia nigra but is also observed in neighbouring pathways, as evidenced by reduced neuromelanin signal intensity in the nearby caeruleus/subcaeruleus complex; this reduction was a better predictor of alpha-synucleinopathies, compared to clinical measurements [78]. Structural studies of RBD using VBM and DTI have also revealed bilateral putamen volume decrease [79], increased hippocampal grey matter density [80], and white matter alterations in brain areas involved in REM sleep regulation [80, 81]. Decreased cortical thickness in the frontal cortex, the lingual gyrus, and the fusiform gyrus was also recently reported [82]. Using a large sample of PD patients, a recent study observed smaller volumes in the pontomesencephalic tegmentum in PD patients with probable RBD, compared to PD patients without RBD and healthy controls [83]. This area contains neurons involved in the promotion of REM sleep and muscle atonia, and it is interesting to note that animals which have lesions in this area will show RBD-like symptoms, including dream enactment and loss of REM atonia, supporting the view that the pons is a key region for RBD [84]. Furthermore, PD with probable RBD had decreased volumes extending to other subcortical and cortical regions whose loss may contribute to the dysregulation of sleep–wake states and motor activity underlying RBD in PD patients [83]. Moreover, PD patients with comorbid RBD showed reduced thalamic volume, compared to PD patients without RBD, in a VBM study [85].

MRS studies failed to reveal any differences between metabolic peaks of NAA/Cr, choline/Cr, and myoinositol/Cr ratios in the pontine tegmentum and the midbrain between idiopathic RBD patients and healthy controls [86], and between PD and RBD patients in the pontine region [87].

Taken together, these findings indicate an involvement of brain structures including (but not limited to) the pontine nuclei and the nigrostriatal dopaminergic system in the pathophysiology of RBD, although more work is required to elucidate the precise pathways involved in giving rise to this condition. The often bizarre dream enactments associated with RBD are a powerful reminder of the very active and often emotional state of the brain during REM sleep.

## Conclusions

There is still much to discover. New technological advancements in neuroimaging will allow researchers to run studies at higher and faster resolutions, which will be essential to truly elucidate the precise neural networks involved in the deceptively complex physiological state we call sleep. Furthermore, larger data sets, standardization of methodological procedures, and multimodality of imaging techniques will aid the field of sleep neuroimaging, as it expands and incorporates new results. As we further our understanding of pathologies in sleep-related neural pathways, innovative treatment interventions may emerge from better knowledge of the neural mechanisms of sleep disorders. As the physical, psychological, and cognitive costs of dysfunctional sleep become more apparent, the impetus for finding solutions to disorders of sleep will surely increase. With hope, future research in sleep neuroimaging will enable novel treatments for the many disorders of sleep.

## REFERENCES

1. Dang-Vu TT, O'Byrne J, Zhang V, et al. Neuroimaging in sleep and sleep disorders. In: Chokroverty S, editor. *Sleep Disorders Medicine*, fourth edition. Philadelphia, PA: Saunders Elsevier; 2017, 353–90.

2. Madsen PL, Schmidt JF, Wildschiødtz G, et al. Cerebral $O_2$ metabolism and cerebral blood flow in humans during deep and rapid-eye-movement sleep. *J Appl Physiol*. 1991;70:2597–601.

3. Braun AR, Balkin TJ, Wesenten NJ, et al. Regional cerebral blood flow throughout the sleep-wake cycle. An $H_2(15)O$ PET study. *Brain*. 1997:1173–97.

4. Dang-Vu TT, Schabus M, Desseilles M, Sterpenich V, Bonjean M, Maquet P. Functional neuroimaging insights into the physiology of human sleep. *Sleep*. 2010;33:1589–603.

5. Dang-Vu TT, Schabus M, Desseilles M, et al. Spontaneous neural activity during human slow wave sleep. *Proc Natl Acad Sci U S A*. 2008;105:15160–5.

6. Samann PG, Wehrle R, Hoehn D, et al. Development of the brain's default mode network from wakefulness to slow wave sleep. *Cereb Cortex*. 2011;21:2082–93.

7. Boly M, Perlbarg V, Marrelec G, et al. Hierarchical clustering of brain activity during human nonrapid eye movement sleep. *Proc Natl Acad Sci U S A*. 2012;109:5856–61.

8. Maquet P, Péters J, Aerts J, et al. Functional neuroanatomy of human rapid-eye-movement sleep and dreaming. *Nature*. 1996;383:163–6.

9. Steriade MM, McCarley RW. *Brainstem Control of Wakefulness and Sleep*. New York, NY: Plenum Press; 1990.

10. Jouvet M. Neurophysiology of the states of sleep. *Physiol Rev*. 1967;47:117–77.

11. Mikiten T NP, Hendley C. EEG desynchronization during behavioural sleep associated with spike discharges from the thalamus of the cat. *Fed Proc*. 1961;20:327.

12. Miyauchi S, Misaki M, Kan S, Fukunaga T, Koike T. Human brain activity time-locked to rapid eye movements during REM sleep. *Exp Brain Res*. 2009;192:657–67.

13. Peigneux P, Laureys S, Fuchs S, et al. Generation of rapid eye movements during paradoxical sleep in humans. *NeuroImage*. 2001;14:701–8.

14. Braun AR, Balkin TJ, Wesensten NJ, et al. Dissociated pattern of activity in visual cortices and their projections during human rapid eye movement sleep. *Science*. 1998;279:91–5.

15. Chow HM, Horovitz SG, Carr WS, et al. Rhythmic alternating patterns of brain activity distinguish rapid eye movement sleep from other states of consciousness. *Proc Natl Acad Sci U S A*. 2013;110:10300–5.

16. Santin J, Mery V, Elso MJ, et al. Sleep-related eating disorder: a descriptive study in Chilean patients. *Sleep Med*. 2014;15:163–7.

17. Smith MT, Perlis ML, Chengazi VU, et al. Neuroimaging of NREM sleep in primary insomnia: a Tc-99-HMPAO single photon emission computed tomography study. *Sleep*. 2002;25:325–35.

18. Smith MT, Perlis ML, Chengazi VU, Soeffing J, McCann U. NREM sleep cerebral blood flow before and after behavior therapy for chronic primary insomnia: preliminary single photon emission computed tomography (SPECT) data. *Sleep Med*. 2005;6:93–4.

19. Nofzinger EA, Buysse DJ, Germain A, Price JC, Miewald JM, Kupfer DJ. Functional neuroimaging evidence for hyperarousal in insomnia. *Am J Psychiatry*. 2004;161:2126–8.

20. Kay DB, Karim HT, Soehner AM, et al. Sleep-wake differences in relative regional cerebral metabolic rate for glucose among patients with insomnia compared with good sleepers. *Sleep*. 2016;39:1779–94.

21. Nofzinger EA, Nissen C, Germain A, et al. Regional cerebral metabolic correlates of WASO during NREM sleep in insomnia. *J Clin Sleep Med*. 2006;2:316–22.

22. Altena E, Van Der Werf YD, Sanz-Arigita EJ, et al. Prefrontal hypoactivation and recovery in insomnia. *Sleep*. 2008;31:1271–6.

23. Drummond SPA, Walker M, Almklov E, Campos M, Anderson DE, Straus LD. Neural correlates of working memory performance in primary insomnia. *Sleep*. 2013;36:1307–16.

24. Palagini L, Moretto U, Dell'Osso L, Carney C. Sleep-related cognitive processes, arousal, and emotion dysregulation in insomnia disorder: the role of insomnia-specific rumination. *Sleep Med*. 2017;30:97–104.

25. Kucyi A, Moayedi M, Weissman-Fogel I, et al. Enhanced medial prefrontal-default mode network functional connectivity in chronic pain and its association with pain rumination. *J Neurosci*. 2014;34:3969–75.

26. Baglioni C, Spiegelhalder K, Regen W, et al. Insomnia disorder is associated with increased amygdala reactivity to insomnia-related stimuli. *Sleep*. 2014;37:1907–17.

27. Winkelman JW, Buxton OM, Jensen JE, et al. Reduced brain GABA in primary insomnia: preliminary data from 4T proton magnetic resonance spectroscopy (1H-MRS). *Sleep*. 2008;31:1499–506.

28. Plante DT, Jensen JE, Schoerning L, Winkelman JW. Reduced γ-aminobutyric acid in occipital and anterior cingulate cortices in primary insomnia: a link to major depressive disorder? *Neuropsychopharmacology*. 2012;37:1548–57.

29. Morgan PT, Pace-Schott EF, Mason GF, et al. Cortical GABA levels in primary insomnia. *Sleep*. 2012;35:807–14.

30. Spiegelhalder K, Regen W, Nissen C, et al. Magnetic resonance spectroscopy in patients with insomnia: a repeated measurement study. *PLoS One*. 2016;11:e0156771.

31. Harper DG, Plante DT, Jensen JE, et al. Energetic and cell membrane metabolic products in patients with primary insomnia: a 31-phosphorus magnetic resonance spectroscopy study at 4 tesla. *Sleep*. 2013;36:493–500.

32. Riemann D, Voderholzer U, Spiegelhalder K, et al. Chronic insomnia and MRI-measured hippocampal volumes: a pilot study. *Sleep*. 2007;30:955–8.

33. Winkelman JW, Benson KL, Buxton OM, et al. Lack of hippocampal volume differences in primary insomnia and good sleeper controls: an MRI volumetric study at 3 Tesla. *Sleep Med*. 2010;11:576–82.

34. Noh HJ, Joo EY, Kim ST, et al. The relationship between hippocampal volume and cognition in patients with chronic primary insomnia. *J Clin Neurol*. 2012;8:130–8.

35. Spiegelhalder K, Regen W, Baglioni C, et al. Insomnia does not appear to be associated with substantial structural brain changes. *Sleep*. 2013;36:731–7.

36. Joo EY, Kim H, Suh S, Hong SB. Hippocampal substructural vulnerability to sleep disturbance and cognitive impairment in patients with chronic primary insomnia: magnetic resonance imaging morphometry. *Sleep*. 2014;37:1189–98.

37. Winkelman JW, Plante DT, Schoerning L, et al. Increased rostral anterior cingulate cortex volume in chronic primary insomnia. *Sleep*. 2013;36:991–8.

38. Joo EY, Noh HJ, Kim J-S, et al. Brain gray matter deficits in patients with chronic primary insomnia. *Sleep*. 2013;36:999–1007.

39. Altena E, Vrenken H, Van Der Werf YD, van den Heuvel OA, Van Someren EJW. Reduced orbitofrontal and parietal gray matter in chronic insomnia: a voxel-based morphometric study. *Biol Psychiatry*. 2010;67:182–5.

40. Suh S, Kim H, Dang-Vu TT, Joo E, Shin C. Cortical thinning and altered cortico-cortical structural covariance of the default mode network in patients with persistent insomnia symptoms. *Sleep*. 2016;39:161–71.

41. Bumb JM, Schilling C, Enning F, *et al.* Pineal gland volume in primary insomnia and healthy controls: a magnetic resonance imaging study. *J Sleep Res.* 2014;23:274–80.

42. Zhao L, Wang E, Zhang X, *et al.* Cortical structural connectivity alterations in primary insomnia: insights from MRI-based morphometric correlation analysis. *Biomed Res Int.* 2015;2015:817595.

43. Nie X, Shao Y, Liu S-Y, *et al.* Functional connectivity of paired default mode network subregions in primary insomnia. *Neuropsychiatr Dis Treat.* 2015;11:3085–93.

44. Li Y, Wang E, Zhang H, *et al.* Functional connectivity changes between parietal and prefrontal cortices in primary insomnia patients: evidence from resting-state fMRI. *Eur J Med Res.* 2014;19:32.

45. Huang Z, Liang P, Jia X, *et al.* Abnormal amygdala connectivity in patients with primary insomnia: evidence from resting state fMRI. *Eur J Radiol.* 2012;81:1288–95.

46. Nakamura M, Nishida S, Hayashida K, Ueki Y, Dauvilliers Y, Inoue Y. Differences in brain morphological findings between narcolepsy with and without cataplexy. *PLoS One.* 2013;8:e81059.

47. Weng H-H, Chen C-F, Tsai Y-H, *et al.* Gray matter atrophy in narcolepsy: An activation likelihood estimation meta-analysis. *Neurosci Biobehav Rev.* 2015;59:53–63.

48. Joo EY, Kim SH, Kim S-T, Hong SB. Hippocampal volume and memory in narcoleptics with cataplexy. *Sleep Med.* 2012;13:396–401.

49. Brabec J, Rulseh A, Horinek D, *et al.* Volume of the amygdala is reduced in patients with narcolepsy—a structural MRI study. *Neuro Endocrinol Lett.* 2011;32:652–6.

50. Schwartz S, Ponz A, Poryazova R, *et al.* Abnormal activity in hypothalamus and amygdala during humour processing in human narcolepsy with cataplexy. *Brain.* 2008;131(Pt 2):514–22.

51. Reiss AL, Hoeft F, Tenforde AS, Chen W, Mobbs D, Mignot EJ. Anomalous hypothalamic responses to humor in cataplexy. *PLoS One.* 2008;3:e2225.

52. Wetter TC, Pollmächer T. Restless legs and periodic leg movements in sleep syndromes. *J Neurol.* 1997;244:S37–45.

53. Trenkwalder C, Hening WA, Montagna P, *et al.* Treatment of restless legs syndrome: an evidence-based review and implications for clinical practice. *Mov Disord.* 2008;23:2267–302.

54. Eisensehr I, Wetter TC, Linke R, *et al.* Normal IPT and IBZM SPECT in drug-naive and levodopa-treated idiopathic restless legs syndrome. *Neurology.* 2001;57:1307–9.

55. Michaud M, Soucy JP, Chabli A, Lavigne G, Montplaisir J. SPECT imaging of striatal pre- and postsynaptic dopaminergic status in restless legs syndrome with periodic leg movements in sleep. *J Neurol.* 2002;249:164–70.

56. Stanwood GD, Lucki I, McGonigle P. Differential regulation of dopamine D2 and D3 receptors by chronic drug treatments. *J Pharmacol Exp Ther.* 2000;295:1232–40.

57. von Spiczak S, Whone AL, Hammers A, *et al.* The role of opioids in restless legs syndrome: an [11C]diprenorphine PET study. *Brain.* 2005;128:906–17.

58. Etgen T, Draganski B, Ilg C, *et al.* Bilateral thalamic gray matter changes in patients with restless legs syndrome. *Neuroimage.* 2005;24:1242–7.

59. Unrath A, Juengling FD, Schork M, Kassubek J. Cortical grey matter alterations in idiopathic restless legs syndrome: an optimized voxel-based morphometry study. *Mov Disord.* 2007;22:1751–6.

60. Unrath A, Müller H-P, Ludolph AC, Riecker A, Kassubek J. Cerebral white matter alterations in idiopathic restless legs syndrome, as measured by diffusion tensor imaging. *Mov Disord.* 2008;23:1250–5.

61. Comley RA, Cervenka S, Palhagen SE, *et al.* A comparison of gray matter density in restless legs syndrome patients and matched controls using voxel-based morphometry. *J Neuroimaging.* 2012;22:28–32.

62. Hornyak M, Ahrendts JC, Spiegelhalder K, *et al.* Voxel-based morphometry in unmedicated patients with restless legs syndrome. *Sleep Med.* 2007;9:22–6.

63. Ku J, Cho YW, Lee YS, *et al.* Functional connectivity alternation of the thalamus in restless legs syndrome patients during the asymptomatic period: a resting-state connectivity study using functional magnetic resonance imaging. *Sleep Med.* 2014;15:289–94.

64. Rizzo G, Tonon C, Testa C, *et al.* Abnormal medial thalamic metabolism in patients with idiopathic restless legs syndrome. *Brain.* 2012;135:3712–20.

65. Allen RP, Barker PB, Horská A, Earley CJ. Thalamic glutamate/glutamine in restless legs syndrome: increased and related to disturbed sleep. *Neurology.* 2013;80:2028–34.

66. Winkelman JW, Schoerning L, Platt S, Jensen JE. Restless legs syndrome and central nervous system gamma-aminobutyric acid: preliminary associations with periodic limb movements in sleep and restless leg syndrome symptom severity. *Sleep Med.* 2014;15:1225–30.

67. Fantini ML, Ferini-Strambi L, Montplaisir J. Idiopathic REM sleep behavior disorder: toward a better nosologic definition. *Neurology.* 2005;64:780–6.

68. Mayer G, Bitterlich M, Kuwert T, Ritt P, Stefan H. Ictal SPECT in patients with rapid eye movement sleep behaviour disorder. *Brain.* 2015;138:1263–70.

69. Mazza S, Soucy JP, Gravel P, *et al.* Assessing whole brain perfusion changes in patients with REM sleep behavior disorder. *Neurology.* 2006;67:1618–22.

70. Vendette M, Gagnon J-F, Soucy J-P, *et al.* Brain perfusion and markers of neurodegeneration in rapid eye movement sleep behavior disorder. *Mov Disord.* 2011;26:1717–24.

71. Dang-Vu TT, Gagnon J-F, Vendette M, Soucy J-P, Postuma RB, Montplaisir J. Hippocampal perfusion predicts impending neurodegeneration in REM sleep behavior disorder. *Neurology.* 2012;79:2302–6.

72. Sakurai H, Hanyu H, Inoue Y, *et al.* Longitudinal study of regional cerebral blood flow in elderly patients with idiopathic rapid eye movement sleep behavior disorder. *Geriatr Gerontol Int.* 2014;14:115–20.

73. Eisensehr I, Linke R, Noachtar S, Schwarz J, Gildehaus FJ, Tatsch K. Reduced striatal dopamine transporters in idiopathic rapid eye movement sleep behaviour disorder. Comparison with Parkinson's disease and controls. *Brain.* 2000;123:1155–60.

74. Kim YK, Yoon I-Y, Kim J-M, *et al.* The implication of nigrostriatal dopaminergic degeneration in the pathogenesis of REM sleep behavior disorder. *Eur J Neurol.* 2010;17:487–92.

75. Unger MM, Möller JC, Stiasny-Kolster K, *et al.* Assessment of idiopathic rapid-eye-movement sleep behavior disorder by transcranial sonography, olfactory function test, and FP-CIT-SPECT. *Mov Disord.* 2008;23:596–9.

76. Iranzo A, Lomeña F, Stockner H, *et al.* Decreased striatal dopamine transporter uptake and substantia nigra hyperechogenicity as risk markers of synucleinopathy in patients with idiopathic rapid-eye-movement sleep behaviour disorder: a prospective study. *Lancet Neurol.* 2010;9:1070–7.

77. Arnaldi D, Famà F, De Carli F, *et al*. The role of the serotonergic system in REM sleep behavior disorder. *Sleep*. 2015;38:1505–9.

78. Ehrminger M, Latimier A, Pyatigorskaya N, *et al*. The coeruleus/subcoeruleus complex in idiopathic rapid eye movement sleep behaviour disorder. *Brain*. 2016;139:1180–8.

79. Ellmore TM, Hood AJ, Castriotta RJ, Stimming EF, Bick RJ, Schiess MC. Reduced volume of the putamen in REM sleep behavior disorder patients. *Parkinsonism Relat Disord*. 2010;16:645–9.

80. Scherfler C, Frauscher B, Schocke M, *et al*. White and gray matter abnormalities in idiopathic rapid eye movement sleep behavior disorder: a diffusion-tensor imaging and voxel-based morphometry study. *Ann Neurol*. 2011;69:400–7.

81. Unger MM, Belke M, Menzler K, *et al*. Diffusion tensor imaging in idiopathic REM sleep behavior disorder reveals microstructural changes in the brainstem, substantia nigra, olfactory region, and other brain regions. *Sleep*. 2010;33:767–73.

82. Rahayel S, Montplaisir J, Monchi O, *et al*. Patterns of cortical thinning in idiopathic rapid eye movement sleep behavior disorder. *Mov Disord*. 2015;30:680–7.

83. Boucetta S, Salimi A, Dadar M, Jones BE, Collins DL, Dang-Vu TT. Structural brain alterations associated with rapid eye movement sleep behavior disorder in Parkinson's disease. *Sci Rep*. 2016;6:26782.

84. Sakai K, Sastre JP, Salvert D, Touret M, Tohyama M, Jouvet M. Tegmentoreticular projections with special reference to the muscular atonia during paradoxical sleep in the cat: an HRP study. *Brain Res*. 1979;176:233–54.

85. Salsone M, Cerasa A, Arabia G, *et al*. Reduced thalamic volume in Parkinson disease with REM sleep behavior disorder: volumetric study. *Parkinsonism Relat Disord*. 2014;20:1004–8.

86. Iranzo A, Santamaria J, Pujol J, Moreno A, Deus J, Tolosa E. Brainstem proton magnetic resonance spectroscopy in idopathic REM sleep behavior disorder. *Sleep*. 2002;25:867–70.

87. Hanoglu L, Ozer F, Meral H, Dincer A. Brainstem 1H-MR spectroscopy in patients with Parkinson's disease with REM sleep behavior disorder and IPD patients without dream enactment behavior. *Clin Neurol Neurosurg*. 2006;108:129–34.

88. Edinger JD, Bonnet MH, Bootzin RR, *et al*. Derivation of research diagnostic criteria for insomnia: report of an American Academy of Sleep Medicine Work Group. *Sleep*. 2004;27:1567–96.

89. O'Byrne JN, Berman Rosa M, Gouin JP, Dang-Vu TT. Neuroimaging findings in primary insomnia. *Pathol Biol (Paris)*. 2014;62:262–9.

# 114

# Management of insomnia and circadian rhythm sleep–wake disorders

*Simon D. Kyle, Alasdair L. Henry, and Colin A. Espie*

## Introduction

While sleep–wake disorders are common and impairing, they are underdiagnosed and undertreated. This notwithstanding, recent developments in the science of sleep and sleep disorders, described in Chapters 109 to 113, have given rise to the burgeoning field of sleep medicine. There has been a surge in the number of accredited sleep centres, training opportunities for health care professionals, and sleep-specific societies, all with the aim of improving sleep disorder recognition, diagnosis, and treatment.

In this chapter, we will focus on the evidence-based management of insomnia and circadian rhythm sleep–wake disorders (CRSWDs), the two classes of sleep disorder most commonly encountered in psychiatric practice. Other sleep disorders, like non-rapid eye movement (NREM) and rapid eye movement (REM)-related parasomnias, obstructive sleep apnoea (OSA), and restless legs syndrome (RLS) and periodic limb movements of sleep also co-vary with psychiatric disorder and its treatment; their recognition and diagnosis are covered in Chapter 110, but their management is beyond the scope of this chapter (for further in-depth reading, see *Oxford Textbook of Sleep Disorders* [1]).

## Insomnia disorder

Insomnia disorder (ID) is characterized by persistent problems (≥3 days per week for ≥3 months) with sleep initiation and/or maintenance, resulting in significant impairment to quality of life (QoL) [2–4]. ID is the most common sleep disorder and the second most prevalent mental health complaint in Europe, affecting 10–12% of the adult population [5, 6]. Historically viewed as a symptom of a so-called 'primary illness', ID is now recognized as: (1) a disabling, non-remitting condition in its own right [3]; and (2) a causal factor in the evolution and maintenance of physical and mental ill-health, particularly depression and cardiometabolic disease [7]. This change in understanding is reflected in the recent reclassification of primary and secondary insomnia into one overarching category ('Insomnia disorder') in both DSM-5 and the International Classification of Sleep Disorders, third edition (ICSD-3) [8]. Prospective data also suggest that persistent insomnia is a robust risk factor for all-cause mortality, after adjustment for potential confounding factors [9]. Although UK data are limited, extrapolation from per person cost data calculated in Canada [10] suggests that direct and indirect costs of insomnia are likely to exceed £14 billion per year. Associated costs reflect increased health care utilization, higher rates of workplace absenteeism, reduced productivity ('presenteeism'), and increased accident risk [11, 12].

While insomnia is a heterogenous condition, most likely comprising multiple phenotypes [7, 13], contemporary theoretical models posit that key cognitive and behavioural processes serve to disrupt sleep–wake regulation [14–18]. In Spielman's stress-diathesis conceptualization, genetic vulnerability (for example, [19]) is assumed to interact with precipitating factors (for example, stress, illness), stimulating an acute episode of insomnia. Cognitive and behavioural responses to this acute sleep loss (for example, extension of time in bed, napping, altered light exposure), driven, in part, by dysfunctional beliefs and attitudes about sleep, create sleep preoccupation and effort, conditioned arousal, sleep fragmentation, and increased night-to-night sleep variability. The end-state is persistent hyperarousal across cognitive, autonomic, and cortical domains, eroding sleep continuity and architecture and negatively affecting daytime functioning [20]. This dysfunctional arousal may also manifest in *the report of poor sleep*, despite an absence of gross sleep impairment on polysomnographic recordings [21–23].

It extends logically that treatment of insomnia should address cognitive and behavioural maintenance factors. There are two main evidence-based treatment modalities for the management of insomnia. The first comprises cognitive behavioural therapies (CBTs), reflecting a 'high-level' approach aimed at addressing sleep-related behaviours and cognitions, effectively *clearing the path* to normal sleep. The second, more 'low-level' approach involves direct pharmacological induction of sleep through, for example, the administration of hypnotics. The National Institute for Health and Care Excellence (UK) and prominent organizations in the United States (American College of Physicians) [24] endorse CBT as the *first-line treatment* for chronic insomnia, while hypnotics are recommended only for short-term use due to the risk of tolerance, withdrawal effects, and next-day side effects. We will now summarize each treatment approach.

## Cognitive behavioural therapy

CBT is a multicomponent psychological therapy, usually delivered over 4–8 sessions by a trained health care professional and after a thorough clinical history. Techniques typically have a lifestyle focus (for example, sleep hygiene), behavioural focus [for example, sleep restriction therapy (SRT), stimulus control, relaxation techniques], and cognitive focus (for example, addressing unrealistic expectations about sleep, paradoxical intention). Table 114.1 summarizes the main ingredients of CBT and proposed treatment targets. It should be noted that sleep hygiene education has no evidence as a standalone intervention in the management of insomnia but is typically incorporated to ensure that patients have basic knowledge about factors that inhibit or facilitate sleep.

Compared to CBT for other psychological disorders, insomnia-focused CBT places greater emphasis on behavioural vs cognitive modification (for an example of CBT session coverage, see Fig. 114.1). Indeed, behavioural components have the largest evidence base as standalone treatments [25, 26], and their level of implementation within multicomponent CBT is reliably associated with sleep improvement [27]. This is, in part, because sleep can be improved through attention to its fundamental biological regulation. For example, SRT, a core component of CBT, is considered to be a *psychobiological treatment* because it takes advantage of sleep homeostasis to reduce arousal and consolidate nocturnal sleep. Thus, patients are asked to keep a sleep diary for 1–2 weeks to enable calculation of the average time in bed and the average sleep duration (Table 114.2). SRT restricts time in bed to match self-reported sleep time—with the rationale that time in bed awake can maintain fragmented and poor-quality sleep. Restriction of time in bed, coupled with standardization of bed and rise-times each day, addresses both homeostatic and circadian regulation of the sleep–wake cycle, increasing the probability that patients will sleep through their allocated window each night. The successful pairing of sleepiness/sleep and the bedroom environment may also help to address conditioned (hyper)arousal that is presumed to play a role in insomnia maintenance. Titration of the sleep window each week helps to establish a robust new sleep–wake pattern for the patient and identify core sleep need. SRT has been associated with reductions in cognitive arousal, sleep effort, core body temperature, and night-to-night sleep variability [26, 28, 29].

It should be noted that any treatment that has potential to do good also has the potential to do harm—and psychological interventions are no exception [30]. SRT should be avoided or carefully adapted for populations where acute sleep loss may stimulate episodes, relapse, or symptom exacerbation (for example, epilepsy, bipolar disorder, parasomnia). Patients should also be educated about driving risks during acute implementation since vigilance is known to be compromised and daytime sleepiness enhanced [28, 31].

CBT is effective across a range of contexts, for example when delivered by different professional groups (for example, nurses, masters-level psychologists), through different delivery formats (groups, face-to-face, over the phone, Internet), and to diverse populations (for example, those with both medical and psychiatric comorbidity). The most comprehensive meta-analysis of CBT trials to date showed a large effect size (Hedges $g = 0.98$) for insomnia severity and medium to large effects for sleep continuity measures [32]. Treatment effects do not vary for patients with/without comorbid disease, by age, or whether or not patients use sleep medication. Importantly, recent studies also showed generalized benefits of CBT on other parameters of health and well-being, including inflammatory markers [33] and depressive symptoms [34]. Despite a large evidence base and endorsement in clinical guidelines, provision of CBT for insomnia within health care settings remains very limited [35]. Those in primary care are likely to receive sleep hygiene advice or be prescribed hypnotic and/or sedative antidepressant medication (off-label). Digital interventions therefore provide a unique opportunity to facilitate access at scale. Espie and colleagues [36, 37] have shown that automated CBT delivered by an animated

**Table 114.1** Principal components of cognitive behavioural therapy (CBT) for insomnia [106]

| Therapy component | Description |
|---|---|
| Cognitive therapy | Identify, challenge, and change dysfunctional beliefs and attitudes about sleep and the consequences of poor sleep that may contribute to sleep-related arousal. Use paradoxical intention techniques to reduce attempts to control sleep |
| Sleep hygiene | General recommendations that promote healthy sleep habits and practices that are conducive to healthy sleep. These can include altering the bedroom environment, scheduling a consistent pre-sleep routine, avoiding arousal-promoting activities, and limiting alcohol, caffeine, and nicotine before bed |
| Stimulus control | Behavioural instructions aimed at eliminating the association between the bedroom and arousal; instead, strengthening the bedroom environment as a stimulus for sleep and sleepiness. Examples include: only using the bedroom for sleep-related activities; only going to bed when sleepy/tired; leaving the bedroom when unable to sleep within approximately 15 minutes, and returning only when sleepy ('quarter of an hour rule') |
| Sleep restriction | A behavioural intervention which involves restricting and standardizing a patient's time in bed, with the aim of increasing homeostatic sleep pressure, overriding cognitive and physiological arousal, and strengthening circadian control of sleep. Tailored prescription of bedtime and rise-time over several weeks leads to improved sleep consolidation and quality |
| Relaxation techniques | Techniques that provide cognitive and somatic relaxation for the patient that may facilitate sleep onset/reinitiation, including progressive muscle relaxation, mindfulness, breathing meditation, and guided imagery |

Reproduced from *Br J Health Psychol.*, 22(4), Kyle S, Henry A, Sleep is a modifiable determinant of health: implications and opportunities for health psychology, pp. 661–70, Copyright (2017), with permission from John Wiley and Sons.

(a)

## Session 1   Sleep Information

**Aim**: To learn about normal sleep processes and about sleep disorders

- to understand the need for sleep and its functions
- to understand sleep pattern and how it varies during the lifetime
- to understand sleep as a process with stages and phases
- to understand factors which adversely affect sleep pattern and sleep quality
- to understand the effects of sleep loss
- to understand the concept of insomnia and how it can be measured
- to understand personal sleep histories and patterns in the above context
- to begin to correct previous misunderstandings about sleep and sleeplessness

(b)

## Session 2   Sleep Hygiene & Relaxation

**Aim**: To introduce practical steps towards developing a healthy sleep pattern without recourse to drugs

- to review progress so far and maintain treatment goals
- to create a bedroom environment that is comfortable for sleep
- to take regular exercise which promotes fitness and enhances sleep
- to develop a stable and appropriate diet
- to reduce the undesirable effects of caffeine upon sleep
- to moderate alcohol consumption and eliminate 'night-caps'
- to support people reduce and stop taking sleeping pills
- to design individualised reduction programmes
- to learn relaxation skills to apply in bed

(c)

## Session 3   Sleep Scheduling

**Aim**: To re-shape sleep patterns to correspond with individual sleep needs and to strengthen sleep rhythms

- to review progress so far and maintain treatment goals
- to develop a good pre-sleep routine
- to distance waking activities from the bedroom environment
- to establish a strong bed-sleep connection
- to eliminate wakefulness from bed
- to define restricted parameters for the individual's sleep period
- to increase sleep efficiency through scheduling sleep in relation to needs
- to eliminate daytime napping
- to establish a stable night to night sleep pattern
- to encourage and support people in changing their sleep routines

**Fig. 114.1** Session-by-session (a–e) aims for a 5-week multicomponent CBT programme.

(d)

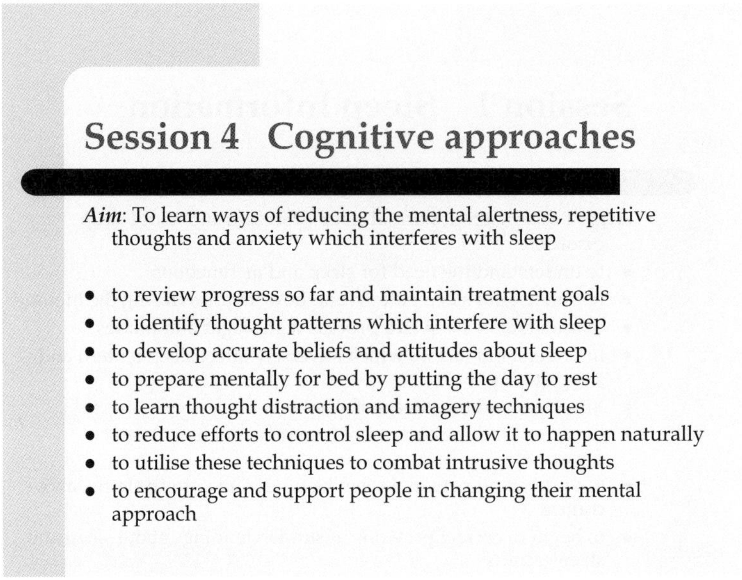

## Session 4   Cognitive approaches

*Aim*: To learn ways of reducing the mental alertness, repetitive thoughts and anxiety which interferes with sleep

- to review progress so far and maintain treatment goals
- to identify thought patterns which interfere with sleep
- to develop accurate beliefs and attitudes about sleep
- to prepare mentally for bed by putting the day to rest
- to learn thought distraction and imagery techniques
- to reduce efforts to control sleep and allow it to happen naturally
- to utilise these techniques to combat intrusive thoughts
- to encourage and support people in changing their mental approach

(e)

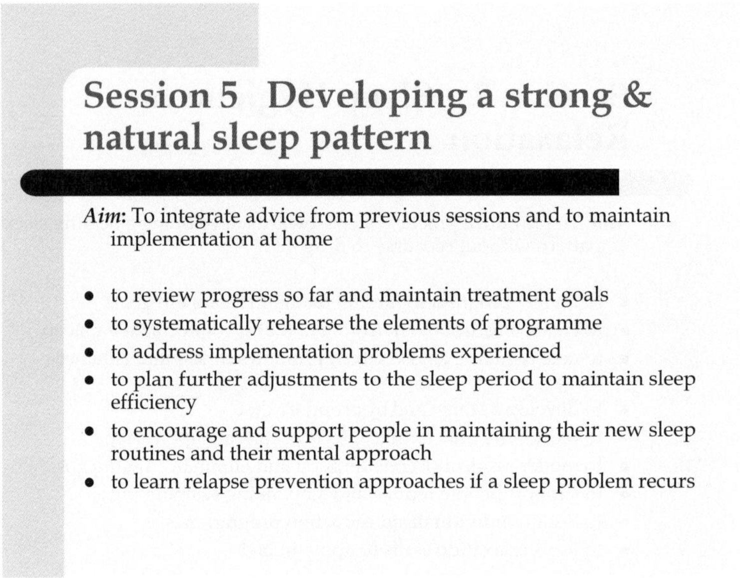

## Session 5   Developing a strong & natural sleep pattern

*Aim*: To integrate advice from previous sessions and to maintain implementation at home

- to review progress so far and maintain treatment goals
- to systematically rehearse the elements of programme
- to address implementation problems experienced
- to plan further adjustments to the sleep period to maintain sleep efficiency
- to encourage and support people in maintaining their new sleep routines and their mental approach
- to learn relapse prevention approaches if a sleep problem recurs

**Fig. 114.1** Continued

**Table 114.2** Sleep restriction therapy guidelines

| Sleep restriction therapy guidelines | Instructions |
| --- | --- |
| 1 | Patient instructed to record a sleep diary for 1–2 weeks to obtain average nightly sleep duration, for example 5 hours 30 minutes (rounded to nearest 15-minute interval). This acts as the designated sleep window |
| 2 | Therapist, in collaboration with patient, sets a morning 'rising time', for example 6.30 a.m. |
| 3 | A 'threshold time' is then calculated by subtracting the average nightly sleep duration from the specified morning rising time, for example 6.30 a.m.−5 hours 30 minutes = threshold time of 1 a.m. |
| 4 | Patient is instructed not to enter bed prior to their designated 'threshold time' and to exit bed on, or prior to, set 'rising time' |
| 5 | Patient follows this prescribed schedule every night, including weekends. Avoid driving or operating heavy machinery if experiencing excessive daytime sleepiness |
| 6 | Weekly modifications to the sleep window are based on sleep efficiency values (total time asleep/total time in bed × 100):<br>If sleep efficiency ≥90%: increase sleep window by 15 minutes<br>If sleep efficiency <85%: decrease sleep window by 15 minutes |

therapist outperformed two control conditions. This was an important trial because it incorporated an active comparator therapy (so-called imagery relief therapy, or IRT), which deliberately excluded the presumed active ingredients of CBT but was plausible because it focused on routines preparatory to sleep. Trials that so convincingly demonstrate superiority over the non-specific effects of attention and therapy involvement are rare. In addition to scale, digital technology can facilitate better matching between insomnia phenotype and specific CBT techniques [38], which may further potentiate treatment gains and reduce non-response [39].

## Pharmacotherapies

### Hypnotics

Short-term use (3–4 weeks) of sleep-prompting medication is recommended for acute insomnia (for example, insomnia caused by temporary stressor, jet lag, etc.) [40] or for chronic insomnia that fails to respond to CBT as the first-line treatment [24]. Both benzodiazepines (for example, lormetazepam) and non-benzodiazepine positive allosteric GABA-A receptor modulators (for example, zolpidem, zopiclone—the so-called 'z-drugs') are approved for the short-term management of insomnia (for dose and half-life of commonly prescribed insomnia medications, see Table 114.3). Careful consideration of pharmacological properties and risk–benefit profile, as well as any specific individual contraindications (for example, comorbidities, medications), is necessary to optimize and tailor pharmacological treatment for each patient.

These medications modify sleep and arousal via allosteric modulation of the GABA-A receptor complex, potentiating the inhibitory effects of GABA on the central nervous system. It should be noted, however, that, in general, they do not re-create normal sleep. Indeed, they may suppress power density in the low-frequency range during NREM sleep [41] and impair sleep-dependent brain plasticity [42]. Meta-analyses showed hypnotics to reliably improve insomnia symptoms, relative to placebo, when administered over a short period of time [43]. However, more recent analyses showed smaller effect size differences when

specifically investigating elderly patients [44] or when considering both published and unpublished trials of z-drugs [45]. Importantly, there is no evidence that treatment gains from hypnotics last beyond their discontinuation. Only a handful of trials have compared hypnotics directly with CBT, finding that treatment effects are comparable in the short term but that CBT outperforms medication at follow-up [46, 47].

Owing to the longer half-life of traditional benzodiazepines, physicians increasingly prefer to prescribe shorter-acting z-drugs [48]. Z-drugs are also considered more effective due to their greater selectivity for the alpha 1 subunit, thus enhancing activity in terms of sedation and limiting more generic effects involved in the interaction with other subunits [49]. Despite this assumption, meta-analyses suggested there are limited differences in efficacy or adverse effect profiles [44, 50]. Both are associated with an increased risk of adverse effects, including falls, driving accidents, and psychomotor impairment. Epidemiological studies also suggested that long-term use of hypnotics is associated with an increased risk of infection, depression, cancer, and mortality [51], although the direction of the causal relationship may be open to question.

### Melatonin receptor agonists, orexin antagonists, and off-label medication use

Melatonin receptor agonists, which act on $MT_1$ and $MT_2$ receptor sites in the suprachiasmatic nucleus (SCN) of the hypothalamus, are also licensed for the management of insomnia. Ramelteon (8 mg) is the only approved melatonin agonist for insomnia on the market (United States) and has been investigated in more than a dozen trials. Although demonstrating low potential for abuse and limited side effects, in comparison with GABA-mediated hypnotics, ramelteon appears to have only modest effects on sleep latency and little/no impact on wake-time after sleep onset or total sleep time [52]. Kuriyama et al. [53] meta-analysed 13 placebo randomized controlled trials of ramelteon, finding statistically significant, but small, effects for subjective sleep latency (mean difference = 4 minutes, compared to placebo) and self-reported sleep quality. Circadin® (2 mg), an extended-release melatonin agonist, is approved in Europe for those over 55 with insomnia. Trials have documented small to medium effects for sleep continuity parameters, sleep quality, and daytime functioning, and the safety profile appears encouraging [54, 55].

The first orexin receptor antagonist (suvorexant) has been approved by the US Food and Drug Administration (FDA) for the management of insomnia (it is not yet licensed in Europe). Orexin-producing neurons in the lateral hypothalamus innervate ascending arousal systems, helping to generate and sustain wakefulness. Hence, antagonism of orexin A and B receptors may promote sleep through blockade of the wake drive and insomnia-related hyperarousal. Prolonged treatment with suvorexant (30–40 mg) for between 3 and 12 months has been found to effectively treat insomnia symptoms, and benefits persist even after a prolonged (2-month) discontinuation phase [56, 57]. While reports of somnolence are increased, relative to placebo, the adverse effect profile appears less impairing than that of hypnotics [58]. It must be noted that the FDA recommends a maximum dose of 20 mg suvorexant—due to concerns about somnolence—but clinical trial data are less robust for this dose, relative to 30–40 mg.

Table 114.3 Benzodiazepines and non-benzodiazepine $GABA_A$ receptor positive allosteric modulators frequently used for treatment of insomnia [107]

| Drug | Usual dose (mg) | Half-life (hours) |
| --- | --- | --- |
| **Benzodiazepines** | | |
| Flunitrazepam | 0.5–2 | 16–35 |
| Flurazepam | 15–30 | 48–120 |
| Lormetazepam | 0.5–1 | 8–15 |
| Nitrazepam | 5–10 | 25–35 |
| Temazepam | 10–30 | 10–20 |
| Triazolam | 0.125–0.250 | 1.4–4.6 |
| **$GABA_A$ receptor modulators** | | |
| Zolpidem | 5–10 | 2–4 |
| Zopiclone | 3.75–7.5 | 5–6 |

A number of other drugs are also used 'off-label' to treat insomnia, including sedative antidepressants, anti-neuroleptics, and atypical (second-generation) antipsychotics. This is not evidence-based practice [24, 39]. For example, the most frequently prescribed sleep aid in the United States is the sedative antidepressant trazodone; yet there is a paucity of trials to inform efficacy or risk–benefit profile [59].

## Circadian rhythm sleep–wake disorders

CRSWDs manifest because of alterations to the endogenous circadian clock (intrinsic CRSWDs) or when there is gross misalignment between the sleep–wake cycle and the 24-hour social environment (extrinsic CRSWDs). Patients typically present with difficulty initiating sleep or maintaining sleep, or excessive sleepiness, with corresponding negative effects on daytime functioning. Because the circadian clock runs at slightly longer than 24 hours (approximately 24.2 hours), alignment between our internal rhythms and the 24-hour social environment requires daily adjustment. Light, physical activity, and melatonin are the main synchronizers of the clock and therefore form the backbone of contemporary CRSWD management. We will now provide an overview of evidence-based treatments for the following intrinsic CRSWDs: delayed sleep–wake phase disorder (DSWPD)/advanced sleep–wake phase disorder (ASWPD), irregular sleep–wake schedule disorder, and non-24-hour sleep–wake disorder. While we emphasize treatments that are endorsed by the American Academy of Sleep Medicine (AASM) task force [60], the highly specific patterning of sleep–wake timing in individual patients necessitates a tailored approach when managing CRSWDs. For the correct administration of light therapy and exogenous melatonin, it is important that the clinician is able to estimate the circadian phase. Core body temperature nadir and rise in endogenous melatonin [dim light melatonin onset (DLMO)] are the two most robust indicators of phase position. While procedures are currently being developed to reliably assess the circadian phase at home [61], clinicians will typically have to rely on questionnaire measures (sleep diary logs or psychometrics) to infer the circadian phase. In general, as a rule of thumb, the nadir of the core body temperature occurs 2 hours before habitual sleep offset, while DLMO initiates about 2–3 hours prior to habitual sleep onset (Table 114.4).

### Delayed sleep–wake phase disorder

DSWPD is one of the most common CRSWDs, affecting approximately 2% of the population [62]. It is characterized by a sleep schedule that occurs significantly later than desired or what would be considered 'normal' by society. Patients with DSWPD present with habitually delayed sleep onset and wake-times, or difficulties with sleep onset and rising when attempting to adhere to a more typical sleep schedule. When able to sleep on their preferred schedule, sleep duration and quality are normal [8]. While the aetiology of DSWPD remains unclear, longer-than-average circadian periods [63], hypersensitivity to light in the evening [64], and sleeping through the advanced period of the phase response curve in the morning [65] are all thought to play a role in perpetuating phase delay. DSWPD is overrepresented in adolescents, most likely due to puberty-related changes in sleep homeostasis and circadian timing, compounded by inflexible social schedules. Several treatments have been proposed to advance the circadian phase in DSWPD, including chronotherapy, melatonin, and phototherapy.

### Chronotherapy

Chronotherapy, or prescribed sleep scheduling, is a behavioural intervention aimed at creating a desired sleep–wake pattern by systematically delaying bedtime and rise-time by 3 hours each day [66]. Because the clock runs at >24 hours in most humans, it is easier to phase-delay than phase-advance the sleep–wake cycle. Upon achieving the desired time, individuals are instructed to rigidly adhere to strict rules around sleep and wake activity, avoiding activities that may encourage phase drift. Chronotherapy appears

**Table 114.4** Summary of clinical presentation, typical sleep–wake schedule, and evidence-based treatments for CRSWDs, based upon current AASM guidelines

| CRSWD | Clinical presentation | Typical sleep–wake pattern | Recommended treatments |
|---|---|---|---|
| DSWPD | Difficulty falling asleep and waking at times considered normal | Delayed sleep onset (2–6 a.m.) and wake-time (10 a.m.–1 p.m.) | Melatonin (0.5–3 mg) 1.5–6.5 hours prior to bedtime/DLMO |
| ASWPD | Difficulty maintaining wakefulness and sleepiness in early evening, combined with early morning awakening or sleep maintenance difficulties | Early sleep onset (6–9 p.m.) and wake (2–5 a.m.) | Bright light therapy (≥2500 lux) for 4 hours, starting at 8 p.m., or 4000 lux between 9 and 11 p.m. |
| N24SWD | Bouts of insomnia symptoms and excessive daytime sleepiness, interspersed with periods of normal alertness | Bedtime and wake-time are consistently delayed (by, for example, 1 hour) each day | Melatonin 2–3 hours before desired bedtime (0.5–5 mg) when circadian phase is approaching normal clock time, or melatonin agonist (tasimelteon) 1 hour prior to desired bedtime |
| ISWRD | Insomnia symptoms or excessive daytime sleepiness | Inconsistent and irregular patterning | Morning bright light (≥2500 lux) for 2 hours (between 8 and 11 a.m.) in elderly individuals with dementia |

ASWPD, advanced sleep–wake phase disorder; CRSWD, circadian rhythm sleep–wake disorder; DLMO, dim light melatonin onset; DSWPD, delayed sleep–wake phase disorder; ISWRD, irregular sleep–wake rhythm disorder; N24SWD, non-24-hour sleep–wake disorder.
Source: data from *J Clin Sleep Med*, 11(10), Auger RR, Burgess HJ, Emens JS, *et al.*, Clinical practice guideline for the treatment of intrinsic circadian rhythm sleep–wake disorders: advanced sleep–wake phase disorder (ASWPD), delayed sleep–wake phase disorder (DSWPD), non-24-hour sleep–wake rhythm disorder (N24SWD), and irregular sleep–wake rhythm disorder (ISWRD). An update for 2015: an American Academy of Sleep Medicine Clinical Practice Guideline, pp. 1199–236, Copyright (2015), American Academy of Sleep Medicine.

effective in laboratory demonstrations (for example, [66]), and there is some supporting evidence from observational studies (for example, [67, 68]); however, there is a dearth of robust randomized controlled trials in the home environment. Potential for creating free-running in some patients has also been observed [69]. Given the lack of controlled outcome studies, the AASM states that there is insufficient evidence to warrant recommendation of prescribed sleep scheduling for individuals with DSWPD [60].

### Morning phototherapy

Timed light therapy, also known as phototherapy, aims to take advantage of the potent role of light as a synchronizer of circadian physiology. Exposure to bright light in the morning is intended to bring about a phase advance in those with a delayed phase (while evening light can phase-delay). Phototherapy is considered more practical than chronotherapy and can harness both artificial and natural light sources. Light is typically delivered using light boxes or other specifically designed devices that emit bright broad-spectrum light (for example, re-timer glasses [70]). Light boxes usually deliver between 2500 lux and 10,000 lux, although it is important to bear in mind that these measurements are recorded at the level of the box, and not the eye [71].

A number of studies have examined the efficacy of timed light exposure in DSWPD. Rosenthal *et al.* administered 2500-lux light to patients for 2 hours between 6 a.m. and 9 a.m., in addition to light restriction in the evening. Findings revealed a phase advance in core body temperature and increased alertness in the morning [72]. Another study found that bright light (2700 lux) administered via a mask phase-advanced markers of melatonin metabolism following extended treatment for 26 days [73]. Despite these positive findings and a rich literature on the phase-shifting properties of light in healthy controls [71], there is a dearth of high-quality clinical studies. The field lacks trials with adequate sample sizes, clinical outcome measures, and appropriate control groups. Based on the low quality of evidence to date, the AASM was recently unable to recommend light therapy for the management of DSWPD, either as a monotherapy or in combination with other treatments [60]. They did, however, note that evidence is higher for the use of light therapy for children and adolescent DSWPD populations, in combination with behavioural intervention. Given the robust phase-shifting effects of light in experimental studies, there is an urgent need to develop a strong evidence base in clinical populations.

### Melatonin

Exogenous melatonin administration can shift the circadian clock to earlier or later times. Melatonin phase response curves, based on average responses from healthy participants, demonstrate phase advances when administered in late afternoon or early evening, between 5 and 7 hours before habitual bedtime [71]. Mundey *et al.* randomized DSWPD patients ($n = 13$) to one of three arms: 4 weeks of placebo, melatonin 0.3 mg or 3 mg, administered 1.5–6.5 hours prior to habitual sleep onset. Both melatonin groups displayed phase advance in DLMO, the magnitude of which was strongly correlated with the time of melatonin administration (earlier times being the most effective) [74]. A meta-analysis of nine randomized, double-blind, placebo-controlled studies confirmed that administration 1.5–6.5 hours prior to DLMO was effective at phase-advancing the clock and reducing sleep onset latency by a mean of 23 minutes [75].

At present, the AASM recommends timed melatonin for the treatment of DSWPD in adults, children, and adolescents. However, further research is required to establish optimum parameters (timing and dose), as well as long-term safety [60].

### Advanced sleep–wake phase disorder

ASWPD is characterized by persistent advancement of the major sleep period (for example, sleep onset at approximately 6–9 p.m. and sleep offset at approximately 2–5 a.m.). This advancement manifests as habitual difficulty maintaining wakefulness in early evening and wake-up times that are several hours earlier than normal. When attempting to delay sleep to a more conventional clock time—for example, to engage in social activities—patients typically experience significantly curtailed sleep duration and next-day sleepiness. The prevalence of ASWPD increases with age [76, 77], which may be a function of an age-related phase advance [78]. Possible explanatory mechanisms include a shortened endogenous circadian period and increased retinal sensitivity to light in the morning [79]. Treatment in this population relies on timed light therapy during the evening or delaying the portion of the phase response curve to bring about a phase delay of the sleep window.

### Evening phototherapy

One study in older adults showed that administration of bright light (4000 lux) between 7 and 9 p.m. for a 12-day period resulted in a 2-hour delay in core body temperature nadir and a reduction in nocturnal awakenings [80]. A more recent study by Lack and colleagues randomized 24 adults with early morning awakenings to either a bright light condition (2500 lux from 8 p.m. to 1 a.m. for two consecutive nights) or a control arm (dim red light). Participants in the bright light group evidenced a 2-hour delay in both melatonin and core body temperature rhythms and reported reductions in wake-time during the night, as well as increased total sleep duration [81].

Other studies have shown more variable results. In a study involving older adults ($n = 47$) with ASWPD, exposure to evening light (265 lux) for 2–3 hours had no effect on circadian or actigraphy outcomes. Despite this, participants reported significantly delayed sleep onset and perceived the treatment to be effective [82]. The low light intensity (just 265 lux) may have attenuated phase-shifting effects. However, a further study comparing bright light (10,000 lux) with dim light placebo similarly failed to find significant effects on sleep or circadian variables in older adults [83]. Key limitations of studies to date include gross variability in light therapy intensity and limited recruitment of well-defined ASWPD patients. This may account for the heterogeneity in trial evidence. Despite these limitations, there is some evidence to support the use of bright light therapy in early evening in those with ASWPD, which is supported by the AASM task force.

### Melatonin

Based on melatonin phase response curves, it is theoretically plausible that morning administration of melatonin will phase-delay the timing of the sleep–wake cycle. At present, however, there is little to no robust evidence regarding the effectiveness of melatonin in ASWPD [60]. Concerns about the potential for sleepiness during the day may have limited progress in this area. Morning administration of melatonin should be examined in carefully designed studies.

## Non-24-hour sleep–wake disorder

Non-24-hour sleep–wake disorder (N24SWD) is the result of the SCN failing to synchronize with the 24-hour light–dark cycle; thus, sleep–wake schedules drift progressively later each day. Patients typically experience bouts of nocturnal insomnia and daytime somnolence, the severity of which will depend on when the patient tries to sleep in relation to the current phase of the endogenous rhythm. The condition is relatively rare in sighted individuals and instead primarily affects those with total blindness due to an inability to perceive photic stimuli, impairing entrainment to the 24-hour light–dark cycle [84]. Disease mechanisms in sighted individuals may include decreased responsiveness to light entrainment or an unusually long free-running circadian period that is outside the range of entrainment [79]. Across individuals with N24SWD, treatments aim to synchronize patients' endogenous body clock with the 24-hour light–dark cycle and are initiated when the sleep–wake pattern is approaching the normal/desired clock time.

### Phototherapy

In sighted individuals, timed light exposure has been suggested as an appropriate intervention, but controlled studies are limited. Correct timing of light is important since inappropriate timing may worsen the current rhythm or induce an undesired shift in position. In a handful of case studies, administration of bright light was found to facilitate entrainment [85–88]. Nevertheless, long-term administration of this treatment appears to be difficult for patients to manage in the home environment, relative to melatonin [85]. Given the small evidence base and the absence of controlled trials, light therapy cannot yet be recommended as an effective treatment for N24SWD in sighted individuals.

### Melatonin and melatonin receptor agonists

Evidence in support of melatonin for N24SWD comes from observational studies in non-sighted individuals [89–92] and sighted individuals [85, 93, 94]. Successful entrainment depends on correct timing of melatonin since administration when the individual's free-running phase is not approaching normal can have adverse consequences and result in unwanted phase shifts. Using a placebo-controlled crossover design, Lockley and colleagues showed that administration of 5 mg of melatonin at 9 p.m. for a full circadian cycle resulted in entrainment in non-sighted individuals with N24SWD [95].

In recent years, the development of melatonin agonists has increased treatment options for those with N24SWD. Tasimelteon is an $MT_1/MT_2$ agonist which has recently been approved for treatment of N24SWD by both the FDA and the European Medicines Agency. Two consecutive placebo-controlled trials examined the effect of tasimelteon in non-sighted patients diagnosed with N24SWD. In the first of these (SET trial), participants were randomly assigned to either tasimelteon (20 mg) or placebo, 1 hour before the desired bedtime and once per day for 26 weeks. It was found that 24% of individuals receiving tasimelteon became entrained (vs 0% in the placebo arm) and patients in this group had increased night-time sleep and reduced daytime sleep [96]. The subsequent RESET trial sought to examine the effect of withdrawal from tasimelteon on entrainment. Following initial entrainment, individuals were randomized to either placebo (withdrawn group)

or continued tasimelteon. The group maintained on tasimelteon remained entrained, while those allocated to placebo withdrawal reverted back to non-24-hour rhythms [96]. Although some side effects were reported (headache, elevated liver enzymes, nightmares), tasimelteon has clear benefits for those with N24SWD. The AASM recommends melatonin for the treatment of N24SWD in blind individuals, but not in sighted individuals, given the limited evidence base for this latter population.

## Irregular sleep–wake rhythm disorder

Irregular sleep–wake rhythm disorder (ISWRD) is characterized by the absence of a clearly defined pattern in the sleep–wake cycle. While total sleep time may be normal, sleep bouts are fragmented and usually distributed in naps across a 24-hour period. There is no primary night-time sleep episode. Thus, the amplitude of the rest–activity rhythm is low and patients often report insomnia symptoms and excessive daytime sleepiness. The condition primarily affects older adults, especially those with dementia, other neurodegenerative disorders, and neurodevelopmental disorders and individuals in care home facilities.

Loss of SCN neurons, driven by dementia pathology, may be one contributor to circadian disorganization, impairing the ability to generate and sustain consolidated bouts of sleep and wakefulness [97, 98]. For patients who are institutionalized (for example, in care homes), lack of a structured schedule, reduced physical activity, and reduced exposure to light may all contribute to ISWRD [99]. The primary goal of treatment in such patients is to establish consolidated nocturnal sleep and eliminate/reduce daytime sleep episodes.

### Phototherapy

A number of studies have examined the effectiveness of timed bright light exposure in dementia patients, but findings have been inconsistent. In one study, nursing home patients with dementia were exposed to morning bright light (8–11 a.m.) for 2 hours each day for 2 weeks. Following the treatment period, patients displayed increased actigraphy-defined sleep efficiency and decreased nocturnal wake-time. Although these improvements were maintained for 4 weeks post-treatment, by 16 weeks, all improvements returned to near baseline levels [100]. Mixed effects have been shown across a number of other studies [101–103], and a recent Cochrane review found no overall effect of light therapy on cognitive function, sleep, challenging behaviour, or psychiatric symptoms in patients with dementia [104]. Taken together, there appears to be some support for the use of bright light in patients with ISWRD, but heterogeneity in design limits solid conclusions. One clear issue is the poor delineation of patient groups with ISWRD on study entry, with many studies recruiting patients with dementia and sleep difficulties (broadly defined), rather than with diagnosed ISWRD. The AASM recommends bright light as a *possible* treatment in ISWRD patients with dementia. Nevertheless, it seems clear that further research is required to optimize treatment parameters and obtain a definitive understanding of treatment benefits.

### Pharmacotherapies

Melatonin is not currently recommended for patients with ISWRD and dementia. A recent Cochrane review of four randomized controlled trials of melatonin concluded that there was no evidence of superiority, relative to placebo [105]. Similarly, current evidence and practice parameters argue against the use of sleep-promoting hypnotics in demented patients with ISWRD, owing to the potential for side effects, including falls, confusion, and physiologic dependence [60].

## Summary

Insomnia and CRSWDs are common and impairing sleep disorders. CBT is the first-line treatment for chronic insomnia, while hypnotics should only be used sparingly and for a short period of time. Digital technology is helping to disseminate evidence-based CBT to insomnia patients, while improved understanding of sleep–wake neurobiology is helping to refine pharmacological approaches beyond conventional hypnotics. Human circadian science clearly shows that melatonin and light therapy can effectively reset the clock, but these insights have only partially translated into therapeutics for patients with CRSWDs. High-quality randomized controlled trials are required to establish standardized treatment guidelines and inform on optimal timing of circadian therapeutics in the management of CRSWDs.

## REFERENCES

1. Chokroverty S, Ferini-Strambi L. *Oxford Textbook of Sleep Disorders*. Oxford: Oxford University Press; 2017.
2. Kyle SD, Espie CA, Morgan K. ' … Not just a minor thing, it is something major, which stops you from functioning daily': quality of life and daytime functioning in insomnia. *Behavioral Sleep Medicine*. 2010;8:123–40.
3. American Psychiatric Association. *Diagnostic and Statistical Manual of Mental Disorders*, fifth edition. Arlington, VA: American Psychiatric Association; 2013.
4. Kyle SD, Crawford MR, Morgan K, Spiegelhalder K, Clark AA, Espie CA. The Glasgow Sleep Impact Index (GSII): a novel patient-centred measure for assessing sleep-related quality of life impairment in insomnia disorder. *Sleep Medicine*. 2013;14:493–501.
5. Wittchen H-U, Jacobi F, Rehm J, et al. The size and burden of mental disorders and other disorders of the brain in Europe 2010. *European Neuropsychopharmacology*. 2011;21:655–79.
6. Morin CM, Benca R. Chronic insomnia. *The Lancet*. 2012;379:1129–41.
7. Vgontzas AN, Fernandez-Mendoza J, Liao D, Bixler EO. Insomnia with objective short sleep duration: the most biologically severe phenotype of the disorder. *Sleep Medicine Reviews*. 2013;17:241–54.
8. American Academy of Sleep Medicine. *International Classification of Sleep Disorders*, third edition. Darien, IL: American Academy Of Sleep Medicine; 2014.
9. Parthasarathy S, Vasquez MM, Halonen M, et al. Persistent insomnia is associated with mortality risk. *American Journal of Medicine*. 2015;128:268–75. e2.
10. Daley M, Morin CM, LeBlanc M, Grégoire J-P, Savard J. The economic burden of insomnia: direct and indirect costs for individuals with insomnia syndrome, insomnia symptoms, and good sleepers. *Sleep*. 2009;32:55–64.
11. Wickwire EM, Shaya FT, Scharf SM. Health economics of insomnia treatments: the return on investment for a good night's sleep. *Sleep Medicine Reviews*. 2016;30:72–82.
12. Léger D, Bayon V. Societal costs of insomnia. *Sleep Medicine Reviews*. 2010;14:379–89.
13. Benjamins JS, Migliorati F, Dekker K, et al. Insomnia heterogeneity: Characteristics to consider for data-driven multivariate subtyping. *Sleep Medicine Reviews*. 2017;36:71–81.
14. Spielman AJ, Caruso LS, Glovinsky PB. A behavioral perspective on insomnia treatment. *Psychiatric Clinics of North America*. 1987;10:541–53.
15. Espie CA, Broomfield NM, MacMahon KM, Macphee LM, Taylor LM. The attention–intention–effort pathway in the development of psychophysiologic insomnia: a theoretical review. *Sleep Medicine Reviews*. 2006;10:215–45.
16. Harvey AG. A cognitive model of insomnia. *Behaviour Research and Therapy*. 2002;40:869–93.
17. Perlis M, Giles D, Mendelson W, Bootzin R, Wyatt J. Psychophysiological insomnia: the behavioural model and a neurocognitive perspective. *Journal of Sleep Research*. 1997;6:179–88.
18. Espie CA. Insomnia: conceptual issues in the development, persistence, and treatment of sleep disorder in adults. *Annual Review of Psychology*. 2002;53:215–43.
19. Lane JM, Liang J, Vlasac I, et al. Genome-wide association analyses of sleep disturbance traits identify new loci and highlight shared genetics with neuropsychiatric and metabolic traits. *Nature Genetics*. 2017;49:274.
20. Kyle SD, Espie CA. Insomnias: classification, evaluation, and pathophysiology. In: Chokroverty S, Ferini-Strambi L. *Oxford Textbook of Sleep Disorders*. New York, NY: Oxford University Press; 2017. pp. 177–88.
21. Harvey AG, Tang NK. (Mis) perception of sleep in insomnia: a puzzle and a resolution. *Psychological Bulletin*. 2012;138:77.
22. Herbert V, Pratt D, Emsley R, Kyle SD. Predictors of nightly subjective-objective sleep discrepancy in poor sleepers over a seven-day period. *Brain Sciences*. 2017;7:29.
23. Buysse DJ, Germain A, Hall M, Monk TH, Nofzinger EA. A neurobiological model of insomnia. *Drug Discovery Today: Disease Models*. 2011;8:129–37.
24. Qaseem A, Kansagara D, Forciea MA, Cooke M, Denberg TD. Management of chronic insomnia disorder in adults: a clinical practice guideline from the American College of Physicians. *Annals of Internal Medicine*. 2016;165:125–33.
25. Morin CM, Bootzin RR, Buysse DJ, Edinger JD, Espie CA, Lichstein KL. Psychological and behavioral treatment of insomnia: update of the recent evidence (1998–2004). *Sleep*. 2006;29:1398–414.
26. Miller CB, Espie CA, Epstein DR, et al. The evidence base of sleep restriction therapy for treating insomnia disorder. *Sleep Medicine Reviews*. 2014;18:415–24.
27. Matthews EE, Arnedt JT, McCarthy MS, Cuddihy LJ, Aloia MS. Adherence to cognitive behavioral therapy for insomnia: a systematic review. *Sleep Medicine Reviews*. 2013;17:453–64.
28. Kyle SD, Morgan K, Spiegelhalder K, Espie CA. No pain, no gain: an exploratory within-subjects mixed-methods evaluation of the patient experience of sleep restriction therapy (SRT) for insomnia. *Sleep Medicine*. 2011;12:735–47.
29. Miller CB, Gordon CJ, Toubia L, et al. Agreement between simple questions about sleep duration and sleep diaries in a large online survey. *Sleep Health*. 2015;1:133–7.
30. Berk M, Parker G. *The Elephant on the Couch: Side-Effects of Psychotherapy*. London: Sage Publications; 2009.
31. Kyle SD, Miller CB, Rogers Z, Siriwardena AN, MacMahon KM, Espie CA. Sleep restriction therapy for insomnia is associated with

reduced objective total sleep time, increased daytime somnolence, and objectively impaired vigilance: implications for the clinical management of insomnia disorder. *Sleep*. 2014;37:229–37.

32. van Straten A, van der Zweerde T, Kleiboer A, Cuijpers P, Morin CM, Lancee J. Cognitive and behavioral therapies in the treatment of insomnia: a meta-analysis. *Sleep Medicine Reviews*. 2018;38:3–16.

33. Irwin MR, Olmstead R, Carrillo C, *et al.* Cognitive behavioral therapy vs. Tai Chi for late life insomnia and inflammatory risk: a randomized controlled comparative efficacy trial. *Sleep*. 2014;37:1543–52.

34. Christensen H, Batterham PJ, Gosling JA, *et al.* Effectiveness of an online insomnia program (SHUTi) for prevention of depressive episodes (the GoodNight Study): a randomised controlled trial. *The Lancet Psychiatry*. 2016;3:333–41.

35. Everitt H, McDermott L, Leydon G, Yules H, Baldwin D, Little P. GPs' management strategies for patients with insomnia: a survey and qualitative interview study. *British Journal of General Practice*. 2014;64:e112–19.

36. Espie CA, Kyle SD, Miller CB, Ong J, Hames P, Fleming L. Attribution, cognition and psychopathology in persistent insomnia disorder: outcome and mediation analysis from a randomized placebo-controlled trial of online cognitive behavioural therapy. *Sleep Medicine*. 2014;15:913–17.

37. Espie CA, Kyle SD, Williams C, *et al.* A randomized, placebo-controlled trial of online cognitive behavioral therapy for chronic insomnia disorder delivered via an automated media-rich web application. *Sleep*. 2012;35:769–81.

38. Luik AI, Bostock S, Chisnall L, *et al.* Treating depression and anxiety with digital cognitive behavioural therapy for insomnia: a real world NHS evaluation using standardized outcome measures. *Behavioural and Cognitive Psychotherapy*. 2017;45:91–6.

39. Espie CA, Hames P, McKinstry B. Use of the internet and mobile media for delivery of cognitive behavioral insomnia therapy. *Sleep Medicine Clinics*. 2013;8:407–19.

40. National Institute for Health and Care Excellence. *Insomnia. Clinical Knowledge Summaries*. London: National Institute for Health and Care Excellence; 2015.

41. Brunner DP, Dijk D-J, Münch M, Borbély AA. Effect of zolpidem on sleep and sleep EEG spectra in healthy young men. *Psychopharmacology*. 1991;104:1–5.

42. Seibt J, Aton SJ, Jha SK, Coleman T, Dumoulin MC, Frank MG. The non-benzodiazepine hypnotic zolpidem impairs sleep-dependent cortical plasticity. *Sleep*. 2008;31:1381–91.

43. Nowell PD, Mazumdar S, Buysse DJ, Dew MA, Reynolds CF, Kupfer DJ. Benzodiazepines and zolpidem for chronic insomnia: a meta-analysis of treatment efficacy. *JAMA*. 1997;278:2170–7.

44. Glass J, Lanctôt KL, Herrmann N, Sproule BA, Busto UE. Sedative hypnotics in older people with insomnia: meta-analysis of risks and benefits. *BMJ*. 2005;331:1169.

45. Huedo-Medina TB, Kirsch I, Middlemass J, Klonizakis M, Siriwardena AN. Effectiveness of non-benzodiazepine hypnotics in treatment of adult insomnia: meta-analysis of data submitted to the Food and Drug Administration. *BMJ*. 2012;345:e8343.

46. Morin CM, Colecchi C, Stone J, Sood R, Brink D. Behavioral and pharmacological therapies for late-life insomnia: a randomized controlled trial. *JAMA*. 1999;281:991–9.

47. Sivertsen B. Treatment of chronic insomnia with cognitive behavioral therapy vs zopiclone—reply. *JAMA*. 2006;296:2435–6.

48. Ford ES, Wheaton AG, Cunningham TJ, Giles WH, Chapman DP, Croft JB. Trends in outpatient visits for insomnia, sleep apnea, and prescriptions for sleep medications among US adults: findings from the National Ambulatory Medical Care Survey 1999–2010. *Sleep*. 2014;37:1283.

49. Nutt DJ, Stahl SM. Searching for perfect sleep: the continuing evolution of GABA$_A$ receptor modulators as hypnotics. *Journal of Psychopharmacology*. 2010;24:1601–12.

50. Dündar Y, Dodd S, Strobl J, Boland A, Dickson R, Walley T. Comparative efficacy of newer hypnotic drugs for the short-term management of insomnia: a systematic review and meta-analysis. *Human Psychopharmacology*. 2004;19:305–22.

51. Kripke DF. Mortality risk of hypnotics: strengths and limits of evidence. *Drug Safety*. 2016;39:93–107.

52. Sateia MJ, Kirby-Long P, Taylor JL. Efficacy and clinical safety of ramelteon: an evidence-based review. *Sleep Medicine Reviews*. 2008;12:319–32.

53. Kuriyama A, Honda M, Hayashino Y. Ramelteon for the treatment of insomnia in adults: a systematic review and meta-analysis. *Sleep Medicine*. 2014;15:385–92.

54. Luthringer R, Muzet M, Zisapel N, Staner L. The effect of prolonged-release melatonin on sleep measures and psychomotor performance in elderly patients with insomnia. *International Clinical Psychopharmacology*. 2009;24:239–49.

55. Wade AG, Ford I, Crawford G, *et al.* Efficacy of prolonged release melatonin in insomnia patients aged 55–80 years: quality of sleep and next-day alertness outcomes. *Current Medical Research and Opinion*. 2007;23:2597–605.

56. Michelson D, Snyder E, Paradis E, *et al.* Safety and efficacy of suvorexant during 1-year treatment of insomnia with subsequent abrupt treatment discontinuation: a phase 3 randomised, double-blind, placebo-controlled trial. *The Lancet Neurology*. 2014;13:461–71.

57. Herring WJ, Connor KM, Snyder E, *et al.* Suvorexant in elderly patients with insomnia: pooled analyses of data from Phase III randomized controlled clinical trials. *American Journal of Geriatric Psychiatry*. 2017;25:791–802.

58. Vermeeren A, Sun H, Vuurman EF, *et al.* On-the-road driving performance the morning after bedtime use of suvorexant 20 and 40 mg: a study in non-elderly healthy volunteers. *Sleep*. 2015;38:1803–13.

59. Krystal AD. A compendium of placebo-controlled trials of the risks/benefits of pharmacological treatments for insomnia: the empirical basis for US clinical practice. *Sleep Medicine Reviews*. 2009;13:265–74.

60. Auger RR, Burgess HJ, Emens JS, Deriy LV, Thomas SM, Sharkey KM. Clinical practice guideline for the treatment of intrinsic circadian rhythm sleep–wake disorders: advanced sleep–wake phase disorder (ASWPD), delayed sleep–wake phase disorder (DSWPD), non-24-hour sleep–wake rhythm disorder (N24SWD), and irregular sleep–wake rhythm disorder (ISWRD). An update for 2015: an American Academy of Sleep Medicine Clinical Practice Guideline. *Journal of Clinical Sleep Medicine*. 2015;11:1199.

61. Burgess HJ, Emens JS. Circadian-based therapies for circadian rhythm sleep–wake disorders. *Current Sleep Medicine Reports*. 2016;3:158–65.

62. Schrader H, Bovim G, Sand T. The prevalence of delayed and advanced sleep phase syndromes. *Journal of Sleep Research*. 1993;2:51–5.

63. Micic G, Bruyn A, Lovato N, *et al.* The endogenous circadian temperature period length (tau) in delayed sleep phase disorder compared to good sleepers. *Journal of Sleep Research*. 2013;22:617–24.

64. Aoki H, Ozeki Y, Yamada N. Hypersensitivity of melatonin suppression in response to light in patients with delayed sleep phase syndrome. *Chronobiology International*. 2001;18:263–71.

65. Ozaki S, Uchiyama M, Shirakawa S, Okawa M. Prolonged interval from body temperature nadir to sleep offset in patients with delayed sleep phase syndrome. *Sleep*. 1996;19:36–40.

66. Czeisler CA, Richardson GS, Coleman RM, *et al*. Chronotherapy: resetting the circadian clocks of patients with delayed sleep phase insomnia. *Sleep*. 1981;4:1–21.

67. Sharkey KM, Carskadon MA, Figueiro MG, Zhu Y, Rea MS. Effects of an advanced sleep schedule and morning short wavelength light exposure on circadian phase in young adults with late sleep schedules. *Sleep Medicine*. 2011;12:685–92.

68. de Sousa IC, Araújo JF, de Azevedo CVM. The effect of a sleep hygiene education program on the sleep–wake cycle of Brazilian adolescent students. *Sleep and Biological Rhythms*. 2007;5:251–8.

69. Oren D, Wehr T. Hypernyctohemeral syndrome after chronotherapy for delayed sleep phase syndrome. *New England Journal of Medicine*. 1992;327:1762.

70. Lovato N, Lack L. Circadian phase delay using the newly developed re-timer portable light device. *Sleep and Biological Rhythms*. 2016;14:157–64.

71. Emens JS, Burgess HJ. Effect of light and melatonin and other melatonin receptor agonists on human circadian physiology. *Sleep Medicine Clinics*. 2015;10:435–53.

72. Rosenthal NE, Joseph-Vanderpool JR, Levendosky AA, *et al*. Phase-shifting effects of bright morning light as treatment for delayed sleep phase syndrome. *Sleep*. 1990;13:354–61.

73. Cole RJ, Smith JS, Alcal YC, Elliott JA, Kripke DF. Bright-light mask treatment of delayed sleep phase syndrome. *Journal of Biological Rhythms*. 2002;17:89–101.

74. Mundey K, Benloucif S, Harsanyi K, Dubocovich ML, Zee PC. Phase-dependent treatment of delayed sleep phase syndrome with melatonin. *Sleep*. 2005;28:1271–8.

75. van Geijlswijk IM, Korzilius HP, Smits MG. The use of exogenous melatonin in delayed sleep phase disorder: a meta-analysis. *Sleep*. 2010;33:1605–14.

76. Ando K, Kripke D, Ancoli-Israel S. Estimated prevalence of delayed and advanced sleep phase syndromes. *Sleep Research*. 1995;24:509.

77. Ebisawa T. Circadian rhythms in the CNS and peripheral clock disorders: human sleep disorders and clock genes. *Journal of Pharmacological Sciences*. 2007;103:150–4.

78. Ando K, Kripke DF, Ancoli-Israel S. Delayed and advanced sleep phase symptoms. *Israel Journal of Psychiatry and Related Sciences*. 2002;39:11.

79. Lu B, Zee P. Circadian rhythm sleep disorders. *Chest*. 2006;130:1915–23.

80. Campbell SS, Dawson D, Anderson MW. Alleviation of sleep maintenance insomnia with timed exposure to bright light. *Journal of the American Geriatrics Society*. 1993;41:829–36.

81. Lack L, Wright H, Kemp K, Gibbon S. The treatment of early-morning awakening insomnia with 2 evenings of bright light. *Sleep*. 2005;28:616–23.

82. Palmer CR, Kripke DF, Savage Jr HC, Cindrich LA, Loving RT, Elliott JA. Efficacy of enhanced evening light for advanced sleep phase syndrome. *Behavioral Sleep Medicine*. 2003;1:213–26.

83. Pallesen S, Nordhus IH, Skelton SH, Bjorvatn B, Skjerve A. Bright light treatment has limited effect in subjects over 55 years with mild early morning awakening. *Perceptual and Motor Skills*. 2005;101:759–70.

84. Sack RL, Lewy AJ, Blood ML, Keith LD, Nakagawa H. Circadian rhythm abnormalities in totally blind people: incidence and clinical significance. *Journal of Clinical Endocrinology and Metabolism*. 1992;75:127–34.

85. Hayakawa T, Kamei Y, Urata J, *et al*. Trials of bright light exposure and melatonin administration in a patient with non-24 hour sleep-wake syndrome. *Psychiatry and Clinical Neurosciences*. 1998;52:261–2.

86. Watanabe T, Kajimura N, Kato M, Sekimoto M, Hori T, Takahashi K. Case of a non-24 h sleep–wake syndrome patient improved by phototherapy. *Psychiatry and Clinical Neurosciences*. 2000;54:369–70.

87. Oren DA, Giesen HA, Wehr TA. Restoration of detectable melatonin after entrainment to a 24-hour schedule in a 'free-running' man. *Psychoneuroendocrinology*. 1997;22:39–52.

88. Hoban TM, Sack RL, Lewy AJ, Miller LS, Singer CM. Entrainment of a free-running human with bright light? *Chronobiology International*. 1989;6:347–53.

89. Lewy AJ, Emens JS, Sack RL, Hasler BP, Bernert RA. Low, but not high, doses of melatonin entrained a free-running blind person with a long circadian period. *Chronobiology International*. 2002;19:649–58.

90. Hack LM, Lockley SW, Arendt J, Skene DJ. The effects of low-dose 0.5-mg melatonin on the free-running circadian rhythms of blind subjects. *Journal of Biological Rhythms*. 2003;18:420–9.

91. Lewy AJ, Emens JS, Lefler BJ, Yuhas K, Jackman AR. Melatonin entrains free-running blind people according to a physiological dose-response curve. *Chronobiology International*. 2005;22:1093–106.

92. Lewy AJ, Emens JS, Bernert RA, Lefler BJ. Eventual entrainment of the human circadian pacemaker by melatonin is independent of the circadian phase of treatment initiation: clinical implications. *Journal of Biological Rhythms*. 2004;19:68–75.

93. Siebler M, Steinmetz H, Freund H-J. Therapeutic entrainment of circadian rhythm disorder by melatonin in a non-blind patient. *Journal of Neurology*. 1998;245:327–8.

94. McArthur AJ, Lewy AJ, Sack RL. Non-24-hour sleep-wake syndrome in a sighted man: circadian rhythm studies and efficacy of melatonin treatment. *Sleep*. 1996;19:544–53.

95. Lockley S, Skene D, James K, Thapan K, Wright J, Arendt J. Melatonin administration can entrain the free-running circadian system of blind subjects. *Journal of Endocrinology*. 2000;164:R1–6.

96. Lockley SW, Dressman MA, Licamele L, *et al*. Tasimelteon for non-24-hour sleep–wake disorder in totally blind people (SET and RESET): two multicentre, randomised, double-masked, placebo-controlled phase 3 trials. *The Lancet*. 2015;386:1754–64.

97. Nakamura TJ, Takasu NN, Nakamura W. The suprachiasmatic nucleus: age-related decline in biological rhythms. *Journal of Physiological Sciences*. 2016;66:367–74.

98. Wang JL, Lim AS, Chiang WY, *et al*. Suprachiasmatic neuron numbers and rest–activity circadian rhythms in older humans. *Annals of Neurology*. 2015;78:317–22.

99. Martin JL, Ancoli-Israel S. Sleep disturbances in long-term care. *Clinics in Geriatric Medicine*. 2008;24:39–50.

100. Fetveit A, Bjorvatn B. The effects of bright-light therapy on actigraphical measured sleep last for several weeks post-treatment. A study in a nursing home population. *Journal of Sleep Research*. 2004;13:153–8.

101. Van Someren EJ, Kessler A, Mirmiran M, Swaab DF. Indirect bright light improves circadian rest-activity rhythm disturbances in demented patients. *Biological Psychiatry*. 1997;41:955–63.

102. Skjerve A, Bjorvatn B, Holsten F. Light therapy for behavioural and psychological symptoms of dementia. *International Journal of Geriatric Psychiatry*. 2004;19:516–22.

103. Dowling GA, Hubbard EM, Mastick J, Luxenberg JS, Burr RL, Van Someren EJ. Effect of morning bright light treatment for rest–activity disruption in institutionalized patients with severe Alzheimer's disease. *International Psychogeriatrics.* 2005;17:221–36.

104. Forbes D, Blake CM, Thiessen EJ, Peacock S, Hawranik P. Light therapy for improving cognition, activities of daily living, sleep, challenging behaviour, and psychiatric disturbances in dementia. *Cochrane Database of Systematic Reviews.* 2014;2:CD003946.

105. McCleery J, Cohen DA, Sharpley AL. Pharmacotherapies for sleep disturbances in dementia. *Cochrane Database of Systematic Reviews.* 2016;11:CD009178.

106. Kyle S, Henry A. Sleep is a modifiable determinant of health: implications and opportunities for health psychology. *British Journal of Health Psychology.* 2017;22:661–70.

107. Spiegelhalder K, Nissen C, Riemann D. Clinical sleep–wake disorders II: focus on insomnia and circadian rhythm sleep disorders. *Handbook of Experimental Pharmacology.* 2017 Jul 14. doi: 10.1007/164_2017_40. [Epub ahead of print].

# SECTION 18
# Gender dysphoria and sexual dysfunction

# 115

# The sexual dysfunctions and paraphilias

*Cynthia A. Graham and John Bancroft*

## Introduction

Sexual relationships are central to the lives of most of us. The sexual component of those relationships can go wrong in various ways. This may be secondary to other difficulties in the relationship, mental health problems, specific sexual vulnerabilities of the individual, or the impact of disease or medication on sexual response. This chapter will describe the more common sexual and paraphilic disorders. Evidence related to prevalence, aetiology, and treatment will be briefly reviewed. Practical guidance on how to carry out assessment and plan a treatment programme for individuals and couples with sexual dysfunction will be provided.

## Sexual dysfunctions

### Clinical features

#### Sexual problems in men

The most common sexual problems presented by men are erectile disorder (ED), premature or early ejaculation (PE), and low sexual desire. Delayed or absent ejaculation is a relatively infrequent complaint.

#### Erectile problems

Penile erection is a tangible and fundamental component of a man's experience of sexual arousal, and a lack of erection in a sexual situation often has significant negative effects on self-esteem and sexual confidence. Irrespective of whether or not there are peripheral explanations for impaired erections (for example, vascular disease), the reactions of the man and his partner have a major influence on how problematic the erectile difficulty becomes. Sexual problems in partners of men with ED have also been reported as common [1].

#### Low sexual desire

Low sexual desire is sometimes linked with erectile and/or ejaculatory concerns [2]. Men with low sexual desire often report a decline in their initiation of sexual activity and in their responses to a partner's attempts to initiate. Many men with low sexual desire also report a reduction in 'spontaneous' erections. However, a man can experience low sexual desire without having any erectile difficulties, although he may require more direct tactile stimulation to achieve erections.

#### Premature ejaculation

The key feature of PE is that ejaculation occurs prior to, or shortly after, vaginal penetration [2]. Many men also report feeling a lack of control over ejaculation and anxiety about PE occurring in future sexual encounters [3].

To meet the *Diagnostic and Statistical Manual of Mental Disorders*, fifth edition (DSM-5) diagnostic criteria for PE, ejaculation must occur within approximately 1 minute of vaginal penetration and before the man wishes it [2]. PE can be lifelong or acquired; occurring after a period of normal ejaculatory latency, acquired PE usually has a later onset.

#### Delayed ejaculation

Delayed, infrequent, or absent ejaculation occurs in men, although it is much less common than PE. A man might have difficulty ejaculating only during sexual activity with his partner and in some cases only during penetrative intercourse, or the problem may be evident even during masturbation. Delayed or absent ejaculation is a common side effect of selective serotonin reuptake inhibitor (SSRI) medications, suggesting that the primary effect of such drugs is on the triggering of orgasm [4].

#### Pain during sexual response

While there is no male sexual pain disorder listed in either the International Classification of Diseases (ICD) or DSM, pain during sexual response in men can occur [5].

### Sexual problems in women

#### Loss of sexual arousal and/or desire

Most surveys have suggested that low sexual desire is the most common sexual problem reported by women. However, low sexual desire is a heterogenous problem category, and the relationship between sexual arousal and sexual desire in women is particularly complex. Many women do not differentiate between 'arousal' and 'desire' [6], and awareness of 'desire' is usually accompanied by some degree of central arousal, whether or not any genital response is perceived [7]. There is also considerable overlap or comorbidity between problems related to sexual arousal and desire in women [8].

Although traditionally seen as the counterpart to penile erection in men, vaginal response is not central to the experience of sexual arousal in women. Vaginal dryness does not necessarily indicate lack of arousal, and conversely, a woman may experience lack of sexual arousal and yet have vaginal lubrication. An increase in vaginal blood flow has been consistently demonstrated in women reacting to sexual stimuli, whether or not they find the sexual stimulus appealing; this led Laan and Everaerd [9] to call this an 'automatic' response. The relevance of vaginal response to sexual arousal in women therefore remains unclear. Tumescence of the clitoris, on the other hand, may be more directly comparable to male genital response, but this is less easily assessed and less clearly perceived by women, compared with penile erection in men.

### Problems with genito-pelvic pain

Pain during attempted or complete vaginal entry is a common sexual problem in women with a wide range of possible causes. Fear of pain or vaginal intercourse and tension of the pelvic floor muscles are common diagnostic features [2]. Sexual pain is also frequently associated with a lack of sexual desire and/or arousal and with avoidance of sexual situations. Sometimes pain only occurs when provoked; for example, vulvar vestibulitis syndrome is a condition associated with pain on touching the labia or vaginal introitus.

### Problems with orgasm

Difficulty experiencing orgasm is not uncommon in women. Often this is situational in that orgasm is possible with masturbation, but not during sexual interaction with the partner. The capacity to experience orgasm varies considerably across women. Some women reach orgasm easily if sufficient arousal occurs; others may require more specific or more intense stimulation, and an estimated 10–15% are unable to experience orgasm throughout their lives [10]. In identifying a problem as primarily orgasmic, one needs to first establish that appropriate sexual arousal has occurred. Orgasmic difficulties can be lifelong or can be acquired, that is, problems developed after a period of normal orgasmic functioning.

### Persistent genital arousal disorder

Persistent genital arousal disorder (PGAD) is a recently recognized, but fairly uncommon, sexual problem in women. It is characterized by genital and breast vasocongestion and sensitivity which persists for hours or days and is only temporarily relieved by orgasm; genital sensations are unaccompanied by any subjective sense of sexual desire and excitement but instead are perceived as intrusive [11].

## Classification

The two major classification systems for sexual dysfunction are the American Psychiatric Association's DSM and the World Health Organization's ICD. The fifth edition of the DSM was published in 2013 [2] and ICD-11 was published in 2018 [12]. Efforts were made to harmonize the groups of disorders in ICD-11 with those included in DSM-5 [13].

DSM-5 comprises major changes in the classification of sexual disorders [14]. Specific duration and severity criteria were added to all of the sexual disorders—a requirement that the symptoms must have persisted for a minimum duration of approximately 6 months and have been experienced on all or almost all (approximately 75–100%) of sexual encounters. There is also the requirement that the symptoms cause 'clinically significant distress in the individual' [2].

Regarding female sexual disorders, there were other significant changes. Major criticisms of DSM-IV were the high comorbidity between diagnoses of sexual disorders, the 'genital' focus of the diagnostic criteria, and the neglect of psychological and relationship factors [15–17]. In response to these criticisms and to growing evidence on the overlap between arousal and desire in women, in DSM-5, 'Hypoactive sexual desire disorder' and 'Female sexual arousal disorder' were deleted and a new disorder 'Female sexual interest/arousal disorder' (FSIAD)—was added. The criteria for FSIAD include subjective, behavioural, and physical aspects of sexual interest/arousal. There were also significant changes made to female sexual pain disorders, with both vaginismus and dyspareunia deleted from DSM-5, and a new diagnosis 'Genito-pelvic pain/penetration disorder' (GPPPD) introduced (for the rationale for these changes, see [18]).

For women, the DSM-5 diagnostic categories are FSIAD, female orgasmic disorder, and GPPPD. For men, the categories are ED, PE, male hypoactive sexual desire disorder, and delayed ejaculation. Substance/medication-induced sexual dysfunction, other 'specified sexual dysfunction', and 'unspecified sexual dysfunctions' are diagnoses that can be applied to both men and women.

An important aspect of the DSM definition of sexual dysfunction is how we define a 'clinically significant disturbance', with connotations of abnormal or impaired function, and how this is distinguished from a 'sexual problem' in a more general sense. Relevant to the question of when a sexual problem becomes a 'dysfunction' is a theoretical approach called the dual control model [19, 20]. This postulates that sexual response results from an interaction between excitation and inhibition, involving relatively discrete neurophysiological systems in the brain. A central assumption of the model is that individuals vary in their propensity for both sexual excitation and sexual inhibition and that 'normal' levels of inhibition are adaptive, reducing sexual responsiveness in circumstances where sexual activity is best avoided. It is predicted that high levels of inhibition will be associated with vulnerability to sexual dysfunction, and low levels with an increased likelihood of engaging in high-risk sexual behaviour.

This faces us with the seemingly obvious, but fundamental, challenge of deciding whether a loss of sexual interest or responsiveness is an understandable, or even adaptive, reaction to current circumstances or is a result of 'malfunction' of the sexual response system, which can be appropriately called a 'sexual dysfunction'. This challenge is also central to assessment that identifies the key factors causing the sexual problem and how they should best be treated. A strategy for carrying out such assessment, which we have called the 'three-windows approach,' will be outlined further.

### Epidemiology

Many early epidemiological surveys assessed sexual problems that were relatively short term and did not ask respondents about whether they experienced any distress about symptoms. An example of this was the US National Health and Social Life survey, which asked if symptoms had occurred 'for several months or more' during the past year, but not whether the symptoms were distressing [8]. Forty-three per cent of women and 31% of men were identified as having a 'sexual dysfunction'. These figures were widely cited as evidence that sexual dysfunction is 'a significant public health problem' [8, p. 544].

More recent surveys, including the UK's third National Survey of Sexual Attitudes and Lifestyles (Natsal-3), have asked about the duration of symptoms and about associated distress [21]. These findings have demonstrated that transient sexual difficulties are very common, but more persistent problems and distress about one's sex life much less so. For example, 51.2% of women and 41.6% of men reported experience of one or more sexual problem during the previous year [21], but distress was reported by only 10.9% of women and 9.9% of men. Prevalence estimates for sexual problems also show marked reductions when duration criteria are applied; in Natsal-3, of those reporting lacking interest in sex, 35.1% of men and 55.8% of women said that the problem lasted 6 months or more [22].

Prevalence rates for specific problems vary considerably. This, in part, can be attributed to variations in how sexual problems are defined and whether distress about symptoms is assessed. Most epidemiologic research assessing sexual dysfunction was conducted in Western countries, but the limited evidence we have from other countries shows that estimated prevalence rates vary widely across cultures [23–25].

There has been more consistency across studies in the associations found between factors of possible aetiological relevance and sexual functioning. In women, sexual problems are more frequent in those with mental health problems and relationship difficulties [26, 27]. In a survey of American heterosexual women aged 20–65 years, 24.4% reported marked distress about their sexual relationship and/or their own sexuality [28]. The best predictors of distress were markers of mental health and the quality of the emotional relationship with the partner. Physical aspects of sexual response in women, such as arousal and orgasm, were relatively poor predictors.

In men, age has a predictable negative effect on erectile function [29]. Most studies have also found an association between age and loss of sexual desire [30]. There is some evidence that PE is more commonly reported by younger men than older men [21].

The association between age and sexual problems in women is more complex. Whereas the level of sexual interest typically decreases with age, older women are less likely to regard this as a problem [28]. An important predictor of sexual problems is whether a woman has a current sexual partner and, among partnered women, whether the partner has sexual difficulties [31]. Although the postmenopausal decline in oestrogens is relevant to vaginal lubrication, other factors such as mental health and the quality of the sexual relationship are more important determinants of sexual well-being than menopausal status [32].

## Aetiology

Before considering the factors that can cause sexual problems, it is worth underlining the important way that sexual function differs from most other physiological response systems. Although involving physiological mechanisms, sexual responses are most often experienced in the context of a relationship. This highlights the importance of keeping the interactive relationship components in mind when trying to assess and treat sexual problems. Sociocultural factors are also crucial to understanding how sexual problems are experienced [33]. Much of the focus in medical treatments of sexual problems has been on the individual patient, with relationship and sociocultural aspects largely ignored. The more specific aetiological factors can now be considered using the 'three-windows approach' [4].

### The first window—the current situation

Through the first window, a variety of factors in the individual's current relationship and situation may be relevant. Relationship problems, particularly resentment and insecurity within a relationship, are of particular importance. For many individuals, feeling secure and being able to 'let go' are necessary for them to enjoy sex. Other factors that may be important include: poor communication between partners about their sexual feelings and needs; misunderstandings and lack of information; unsuitable circumstances and lack of time, for example fatigue, lack of privacy; concerns about pregnancy or sexually transmitted infections; and low self-esteem and poor body image.

### The second window—vulnerability of the individual

Although a wide range of factors can impact on our sexuality, it is also clear that individuals vary substantially in the extent to which they are affected by such factors, particularly in terms of an associated inhibition of sexual response. Such vulnerabilities are likely to have been evident in earlier episodes in the current relationship or in earlier relationships.

1. Negative attitudes. Long-standing attitudes, usually stemming from childhood, that sex is inherently 'bad' or immoral are likely to interfere with an individual's ability to become involved in, and enjoy, a sexual relationship.

2. Need to maintain self-control. In some individuals, difficulty in 'letting go' sexually reflects a more general need to maintain self-control, particularly in the presence of another person.

3. Earlier experience of sexual abuse or trauma. There is now an extensive literature on the impact of sexual abuse on subsequent sexual adjustment. Whereas the mediating mechanisms are not well understood and are likely to be complex, a history of such experience should be regarded as potentially relevant to current sexual difficulties.

4. Propensity to sexual inhibition. The dual control model, discussed earlier, has led to psychometrically validated measures of propensity to sexual excitation and inhibition in men [34] and women [35]. In men, as predicted, there is a clear association between low sexual excitation and/or high sexual inhibition propensity and erectile problems, but no association with PE [36]. In women, there is a strong relationship between sexual inhibition propensity and reports of sexual problems [37, 38]. Particularly important is one inhibition subscale (labelled 'arousal contingency') that reflects susceptibility for sexual arousal to be easily affected by situational factors, for example if the circumstances are not 'just right'. Although further research is needed, these measures of sexual inhibition and excitation may prove valuable in explaining patterns of impaired sexual response and helping in the selection of appropriate treatment.

### The third window—health-related factors that alter sexual function

#### Mental health and sexuality

Psychiatric problems are commonly associated with sexual problems (for a review, see [4]). Reduction in sexual interest and, to some extent, sexual arousability is generally accepted as a common symptom of depressive illness [39]. In contrast, sexual interest tends to be increased in states of elevated mood such as hypomania [40].

With anxiety, the clinical evidence is much more limited. Higher rates of sexual dysfunction in patients with anxiety disorders have been reported [41]. Individuals with panic disorder may be particularly likely to report sexual problems. PE is a common sexual problem in men with social phobias [42].

Although most studies have focused on negative effects of mood disorders on sexual interest and response, there is evidence that a minority of individuals experience increased sexual interest during negative mood states. This paradoxical pattern has been reported in non-clinical samples of men [43] and women. [44] Although the origins of this pattern are not yet understood, it may be problematic in various ways, for example associated with sexual risk-taking or leading to sex being used as a mood regulator.

The impact of schizophrenia on sexuality is complex. Sexual thoughts and behaviours are common in schizophrenia, and there may be a relative increase in sexual activity [45].

### Physical health and sexuality

Poor physical health is associated with decreased sexual activity and reduced sexual satisfaction at all ages [46]. The impact of poor physical health on sexuality may be relatively non-specific. For example, loss of well-being and energy associated with chronic illness is likely to cause reduced sexual interest and arousability. Psychological reactions to the illness or condition (for example, the effects of breast cancer on a woman's body image, and hence her sexual enjoyment) may also be important. In addition, there are a variety of ways in which health problems can directly affect sexual interest and/or response (for a review, see [4]):

1. Damage to the neural control of genital response. This can involve peripheral mechanisms (for example, autonomic and peripheral neuropathy) or disease in the spinal cord (for example, multiple sclerosis). Injury or surgery causing nerve damage may be involved (for example, spinal cord injury, prostatectomy, or hysterectomy). The most likely consequences are ED in men and impaired vaginal response in women. Brain abnormalities, such as epilepsy or cerebral tumour, can affect central control of sexual response, the precise effect depending on the site of the abnormality or tumour. In some cases, the result is loss of sexual interest and arousability; rarely, there is disinhibition of sexual behaviour.
2. Impairment of vascular supply of the genitalia. Genital response is dependent on increased arterial inflow, as well as alteration in venous outflow.
3. Alteration of endocrine mechanisms affecting sexual interest, arousal, and response. In the male, any cause of lowered testosterone (T) levels is likely to produce loss of sexual interest and, to a varying extent, impairment of erectile response.

In women, lack of oestrogen is associated with impaired vaginal lubrication. The effects of sex steroids, either oestrogens or androgens, on sexual interest and arousability are much less predictable. The evidence is consistent with there being a proportion of women who depend on T for their normal level of sexual interest, but there are many women who can experience substantial reductions in T without obvious adverse sexual effects.

Hyperprolactinaemia, usually resulting from pituitary adenomas and hypersecretion of prolactin, may be associated with loss of sexual interest and, in men, with ED. However, this is not always the case. The precise role of prolactin in human sexuality is not understood.

Some diseases affect sexuality through more than one of the mechanisms described. Diabetes mellitus is a good example. In diabetic men, ED can result from small-vessel vascular disease and also autonomic and peripheral neuropathology. Lowered sexual interest and impairment of genital response have also been reported in diabetic women.

### Side effects of medication

We can now consider the main adverse sexual effects resulting from medication (for a review, see [47]).

#### Antidepressants

SSRIs, by inhibiting the 5-HT1A receptor, increase serotonergic transmission. The most predictable side effect, in both women and men, is inhibition of orgasm and ejaculation [48]. Other negative effects include reduced sexual interest and arousability, though they are less predictable and not always easy to distinguish from the sexual effects of the affective disorder being treated. Tricyclic antidepressants also commonly produce sexual side effects.

#### Antipsychotic medication

These drugs, used for treatment of schizophrenia and other psychotic disorders, involve a balance of dopamine antagonist and 5-HT agonist effects. The most common side effects are ED and ejaculatory difficulties in men, and orgasmic dysfunction in women.

#### Antihypertensive medication

Many drugs used to treat hypertension interfere with male sexual response. Beta-blockers (for example, propranolol), by blocking smooth muscle relaxation and leaving alpha-1-induced contraction unopposed, commonly cause ED. Centrally acting antihypertensives (for example, guanethidine) also interfere with sexual response, impairing erection and blocking ejaculation. Clonidine, an alpha-2 agonist, can also cause erectile problems. In this case, the principal effect is likely to be reduced central arousal. For a review of the effects of antihypertensive medication on male sexual response, see [49].

The effects of drugs on women's sexuality have received far less attention. Research has mostly focused on difficulties in achieving orgasm. As orgasm only occurs after sufficient sexual arousal, these effects may reflect impairment of arousal, but this has not been adequately assessed. Steroidal contraceptives, although associated with markedly reduced levels of free T, decrease sexual interest only in a minority of women [50].

## Management

In this section, we will first describe the principles of sex therapy and the main forms of psychological and pharmacological treatment, followed by an outline of the process of assessment and selection of a suitable treatment plan. There is growing recognition that integration of psychological and pharmacological methods, with emphasis on the couple, may be the most appropriate treatment model for most couples [3, 51].

## Sex therapy

Although the approach first introduced by Masters and Johnson [52] has been adapted in various ways, the core treatment techniques remain. Originally developed for helping couples, the techniques can be modified for use with individuals and with same-sex, as well as heterosexual, couples.

The key elements of the therapeutic process are:

1. Clearly defined tasks that the couple are asked to attempt before the next therapy session.
2. Those attempts, and any difficulties encountered, are examined in detail.
3. Attitudes, feelings, and conflicts that make the tasks difficult to carry out are identified.
4. These are modified or resolved, so that subsequent achievement of the tasks becomes possible.
5. The next tasks are set, and so on.

The tasks are mostly behavioural in nature. They are chosen to facilitate the identification of relevant issues but, in some cases, are sufficient in themselves to produce change. The behavioural programme is in three parts. In the first part, the couple are asked to avoid any direct genital touching or stimulation and to focus on non-genital contact, alternating who initiates and who does the touching. These first non-genital steps are effective in identifying important issues in the relationship such as lack of trust or counterproductive stereotypical attitudes (for example, once a man is aroused, he cannot be expected not to have intercourse). Once this stage can be carried out satisfactorily, and related problematic issues dealt with, the programme moves on to the second part, which allows genital touching to be combined with non-genital touching, with penile–vaginal intercourse still 'out of bounds'. In this second part, more intra-personal problems, such as long-standing negative attitudes about sex or the sequelae of earlier sexual trauma, are likely to emerge. In the third part, a gradual approach to vaginal–penile contact and insertion is undertaken. Here the most relevant issues are 'performance anxiety' and fear of pain.

As the behavioural tasks reveal key issues that need to be resolved before moving on to the next stage, a variety of psychotherapeutic approaches, including cognitive behavioural techniques, can be utilized. Although the stage at which particular issues emerge does vary from case to case, there is a tendency for problems identified through the 'first window', particularly those related to lack of trust and unresolved resentment, to appear during the first stage of the programme. Intra-personal issues (for example, as seen through the 'second window') are more likely to be recognized during the second stage.

The goals of therapy include helping the individual to accept and feel comfortable with his or her sexuality and helping the couple to establish trust and emotional security and to enhance their sexual enjoyment and intimacy. An important point is that these goals do not necessarily include reversal of specific sexual dysfunctions. There are exceptions; for example, there are specific behavioural techniques to deal with PE and orgasmic disorder (for details of these techniques, see [4]). However, the overriding principle is that, assuming there is no abnormality of the basic physiological mechanisms involved in sexual response, normal sexual function will return once these goals are achieved. In cases where impairment of physiological mechanisms does exist, the goals of sex therapy are still helpful and integrate well with the use of pharmacological treatment.

### Practical aspects

Although sex therapy varies in duration, 12 sessions over 4–5 months is typical. The therapist adjusts to the particular needs of the individual or couple. Treatment begins weekly, with the interval between sessions extended once major issues like unexpressed resentment or communication problems have been dealt with. The last two or three sessions are spaced out over a few months, so that the couple have an opportunity to consolidate their progress and cope with any setbacks before termination.

## Other psychological treatments

Apart from sex therapy, a range of other psychological treatments have been used to treat sexual dysfunction, either on their own or as a supplement to sex therapy. Two particular approaches that have generated the most interest and evaluation are cognitive behavioural therapy (CBT) and mindfulness-based intervention. There is a large literature supporting the important role for cognitive factors in the aetiology and maintenance of sexual disorders (for a review, see [53]), which suggests that CBT approaches could be effective.

## Pharmacological treatments for men

### Erectile disorders

The introduction of phosphodiesterase type 5 (PDE-5) inhibitors had a major impact on the treatment of ED. After the approval of sildenafil in 1998, other PDE-5 inhibitors, for example tadalafil and vardenafil, became available. Although these drugs were effective for approximately 75% of men, there was evidence that many men did not continue with the medication [54]. In one study done in eight countries, 2912 men identified with ED were followed up; 58% of them had sought medical help for ED, but only 16% of men maintained their use of PDE-5 inhibitors [54]. In addition, although these medications have a generally good safety and side effect profile, there are some contraindications to their use (for example, use of nitrates).

Other pharmacological treatments that were widely used before PDE-5 inhibitors became available, such as apomorphine and intracavernosal injections of phentolamine, used in combination with papaverine, are now primarily recommended for men with ED for whom PDE-5 inhibitors are either contraindicated or have been ineffective [51, 55].

Other drugs that are still in development to treat ED in men include bremelanotide, a melanocortin agonist and a synthetic peptide analogue of a naturally occurring hormone called alpha-melanocyte-stimulating hormone (MSH) [56].

### Premature ejaculation

Pharmacological treatments used for PE include SSRIs and clomipramine, a tricyclic antidepressant, and topical administration of prilocaine/lidocaine. One drug—dapoxetine, a novel, short-acting SSRI—has received approval for the treatment of PE in over 30 countries [3]. All of these medications can be taken either daily or on an as-needed basis.

### Delayed or absent orgasm/ejaculation

At the present time, there is no accepted pharmacological treatment for delayed or absent ejaculation or orgasm [57].

### Low sexual desire

The most treatable, but relatively infrequent, cause of loss of sexual desire in men is hypogonadism. Where androgen deficiency is evident, T replacement is indicated. If loss of sexual desire is associated with hyperprolactinaemia, treatment with dopamine agonists, such as bromocriptine, is recommended.

## Pharmacological treatments for women

Following the success of PDE-5 inhibitors in treating ED, there were attempts to use sildenafil to treat sexual arousal disorder in women, but the results were disappointing [58]. Attention shifted to treatment of low sexual desire in women and the use of T. Although Intrinsa, a T patch, was approved in 2006 by the European Medicines Agency, this was only for treatment of low sexual desire in women with surgically induced menopause.

The first medication to receive approval by the US Food and Drug Administration for the treatment of hypoactive sexual desire disorder in premenopausal women was flibanserin, a medication with mixed effects on serotonergic and dopaminergic transmitter systems that was originally evaluated as an antidepressant but was ineffective [59]. Flibanserin was approved amid a great deal of controversy about its safety and efficacy. Two systematic reviews on the efficacy and safety of flibanserin reached inconsistent conclusions regarding its efficacy [60, 61].

There are other drugs in development to treat women's sexual desire problems, including subcutaneously administered bremelanotide and medications that combine sildenafil and T or T and buspirone.

## Evaluation of treatments

There have been many more studies testing the effectiveness of pharmacological treatments for sexual dysfunction than of psychological or combination therapies [62]. With the exception of research on female sexual pain disorders, there has been a serious shortage of outcome research on psychological treatments. This lack of research does not reflect a lack of growth in sex therapy or of new approaches [63].

Three systematic reviews of the efficacy of psychological interventions to treat sexual dysfunction in men and women have been published [64–66]. For women, the strongest evidence exists for the use of CBT and mindfulness-based interventions in the treatment of low sexual desire [53]. For female orgasmic disorder, multimodal treatment programmes involving techniques such as directed masturbation, sexual skills training, and sex education can be effective approaches [53]. As mentioned, there have been several controlled outcome studies on psychological interventions for sexual pain disorders, and these suggest that psychological therapies are effective treatments, supporting a biopsychosocial approach [67].

For men, there have been few outcome studies on psychological treatments for ED, but the limited evidence suggests that group or couple therapy is superior to individual therapy and that combined treatments (PDE-5 inhibitors and psychological therapy) are effective [53]. For the treatment of PE, there is limited and inconsistent evidence for the effectiveness of psychological interventions. For low sexual desire and delayed ejaculation, there are very few controlled outcome studies.

## Planning a treatment programme

### Assessment

When couples present with sexual difficulties, one of them is usually regarded as having the problem, but both partners should be carefully assessed, whenever possible. There are three stages to assessment: (1) to facilitate the decision about whether sex therapy is appropriate; (2) to identify issues relevant to the sexual problem that need to be resolved; and (3) to determine whether medication or other treatments are required.

Keeping in mind the distinction between a sexual problem that is adaptive or appropriate, given an individual's current circumstances, and one that is maladaptive (and can perhaps be considered a 'dysfunction'), we can assess each individual's case through the three conceptual 'windows' described earlier. Are there problems in the couple's current relationship or situation which would make inhibition of sexual responsiveness in either partner understandable or adaptive? Does either individual give a history that suggests vulnerability to sexual problems? Are there are any mental or physical health issues or medication use in either partner that could be having a negative effect on sexual interest or response?

Although not all of the details can be obtained during the initial interview, assessment of the following topics should be carried out: the nature of the problem, including an assessment of the level of sexual interest and response in each partner; identification of other assessments that may be needed (for example, physical examination, blood tests); commitment and motivation of each partner to improving the relationship; and mental state assessment of each partner. If both partners are present, each should be interviewed separately, following a conjoint interview. As far as possible, questions should be asked about each individual's sexual history, the nature of the current relationship, contraceptive use and reproductive history, and alcohol or recreational drug use.

At the end of the initial interview, the clinician should provide a preliminary formulation of the nature of the problem and the types of intervention that may be helpful. Whatever treatment methods are used, it is important to continue to see the couple together to monitor progress and provide counselling, as needed.

If there is no evidence of causal factors of the kind viewed through the 'first' or 'second' window, then a trial of pharmacological treatment may be appropriate (although, as discussed, few pharmacological options exist for women). In such cases, a physical examination and, where relevant, laboratory investigations would normally be arranged before starting treatment. It is important to have a good 'clinical baseline' before embarking on pharmacological interventions.

If there are any indications of issues, particularly of the kind that invoke inhibition of sexual response, which need to be resolved, then pharmacological interventions should not be considered as a first step. In many such cases, more assessment is required before these factors can be adequately assessed. There are then two options: (1) further interview(s) to explore such issues; or (2) starting on a programme of sex therapy. The rationale for the second option is as follows. The initial two stages of sex therapy (that is, involving non-genital and then genital touching, with no attempts at vaginal intercourse) are particularly effective at identifying relevant issues underlying the problem. Furthermore, the process involved in those early stages is likely to benefit any sexual relationship, even those without obvious problems. After three or four sex therapy sessions, a reappraisal would be made and a decision taken about whether to continue with sex therapy alone or to combine it with an appropriate pharmacological method. For example, with a couple where the man has erectile problems, it is easier to assess the indications for the use of a PDE-5 inhibitor after the couple have gone through the first two stages of the programme where there is no 'performance pressure' and no need for an erection to occur. Similarly, it is often informative to see what impact sex therapy has on the individual who has complained of reduced sexual desire, before attempting to deal with the problem pharmacologically or hormonally.

Ideally, the use of the pharmacological method should then proceed in combination with the continuation of the sex therapy programme. In that way, a gradual transition to a satisfying sexual relationship can be achieved without renewed 'performance pressures'. If, however, progress continues to be made with sex therapy, then the addition of pharmacological interventions may not be necessary. It should be explained to the couple that, whereas pharmacological treatments often have beneficial effects on sexual response, they do not 'cure' the problem, which is likely to recur once the medication is stopped.

## Paraphilic disorders

### Clinical features

The essential feature of a paraphilia is that it involves an intense, recurrent pattern of sexual interest, manifested in sexual fantasies, urges, or behaviour, to atypical objects or activities (typically those that do not involve sexual interaction with a consenting, phenotypically normal, physically mature human partner) [2]. A paraphilia can be considered a disorder if it: (1) causes distress or other negative impact to the individual or is harmful, or potentially harmful, to other people; and (2) is manifest over at least a 6-month period. There is high comorbidity between paraphilias and mood disorders and also consistent evidence that different paraphilias often co-occur [68, 69]. Substance use disorder, neurodevelopmental conditions, and mood disorders have been reported as highly prevalent among paraphilic offenders [70].

A large number of paraphilias have been mentioned in the literature, but most of them are rare. We will focus here on the paraphilic disorders that are most common and listed in DSM-5.

### Voyeuristic disorder

The key feature is a recurring pattern of intense sexual arousal from observing an unsuspecting person or couple in the process of undressing or interacting sexually. The voyeur usually masturbates while 'peeping'.

### Exhibitionistic disorder

This involves a pattern of recurrent and intense sexual arousal from exposing one's genitalia to an unsuspecting person, experienced in fantasies, urges, or explicit behaviour. In some exhibitionists, the urge to expose themselves occurs occasionally, possibly at times of crisis or emotional distress. For others, the idea of exposing is always sexually stimulating and may feature in their masturbation fantasies.

### Frotteuristic disorder

This involves recurrent and intense sexual arousal from touching or rubbing against a non-consenting person, which is experienced in fantasies, urges, or explicit behaviour. Such individuals are also more likely to experience exhibitionist and voyeuristic disorders, and to show mood and antisocial personality disorders.

### Sexual sadism disorder

This is defined as recurrent and intense sexual arousal, as manifested by fantasies, urges, or behaviours, from the physical or psychological suffering of a non-consenting person.

### Sexual masochism disorder

This involves recurrent and intense sexual arousal from the act of being humiliated, beaten, or bound. Individuals who engage in BDSM (bondage, dominance and submission, sadism, and masochism) which is consensual and not associated with distress would not be diagnosed with either sexual sadism disorder or sexual masochism disorder.

### Paedophilic disorder

This term relates to an adult (16 years or older) being sexually attracted to a prepubertal child, engaging in sexual fantasies involving a child of either sex, and/or engaging in sexual activity with such children. In DSM-5, there is also the requirement that there must be at least a 5-year age difference between the individual and the child.

### Fetishistic disorder

This refers to recurrent and intense sexual arousal in response to a specific part of the body or to the use of non-living objects, for example rubber or leather.

### Transvestic disorder

This is a particular form of fetishism in which recurrent and intense sexual arousal arises from cross-dressing. There is evidence that some fetishistic transvestites end up transitioning to transgendered women.

### Classification

In DSM-5, there were several changes in the classification of paraphilias. Firstly, a distinction was made between paraphilias and paraphilic disorders, the latter involving behaviour that is currently either causing distress or impairment to the individual with the paraphilia or a risk of harm to others [2]. There are eight paraphilic disorders listed in DSM-5: voyeuristic disorder, exhibitionistic disorder, frotteuristic disorder, sexual masochism disorder, sexual sadism disorder, paedophilic disorder, fetishistic disorder, and transvestic disorder; there are also categories for 'other specified paraphilic disorder' and 'unspecified paraphilic disorder'. In the revision of ICD (ICD-11), several disorders listed in ICD-10 (fetishistic disorder, fetishistic transvestism, and sadomasochism) were removed from the list of paraphilic disorders [71].

Leading up to DSM-5, there were controversial proposals to introduce new disorders such as hypersexual disorder [72] and paraphilic coercive disorder [73], but these were not approved by the American Psychiatric Association. There has also been a long running and highly complex debate about whether paraphilic disorders should be removed from the DSM altogether [74].

### Epidemiology

The prevalence of paraphilic disorders is largely unknown. A consistent finding, however, has been that most paraphilias and paraphilic disorders are much less common in women than in men.

In a representative Swedish sample, 7.7% of respondents reported at least one incident of being sexually aroused by watching others having sex and 3.1% reported at least one occasion of being sexually aroused by exposing their genitals to a stranger [68].

In a representative Australian sample of 19,307 men and women aged 16–59 years, 1.8% of sexually active respondents (2.2% of men and 1.3% of women) had been involved in BDSM over the past year [75]. It is important to note that these prevalence estimates relate to paraphilic interests, and not to paraphilic disorders.

In a recent online survey of 8718 German men, 4.1% reported sexual fantasies involving prepubescent children, 3.2% reported sexual offending against prepubescent children, and 0.1% reported a paedophilic sexual preference [76]. Reviewing the literature, Seto *et al.* [69] concluded that the upper-limit prevalence of paedophilia in community settings ranged from 1% to 3% in men.

Langstrom and Zucker [77], in a representative sample of 2450 Swedish men and women, asked 'Have you ever dressed in clothes pertaining to the opposite sex and become sexually aroused by this?' Positive answers were given by 2.8% of men and 0.4% of women. However, we have no idea how many of these individuals repeated this behaviour and, in particular, how many had a transvestic disorder.

### Aetiology

There are many theories for the aetiology of paraphilias, with the most support for those involving conditioning or neurodevelopmental factors (for a review, see [78]). Because of the strong comorbidity between different paraphilic disorders, there may be common causal factors across paraphilias [69].

Although individuals with paraphilic disorders are most often seen in forensic and prison settings, they can also present in general psychiatric settings [69]. Regarding assessment, there are problems with reliance on self-report alone, and the diagnosis of a paraphilic disorder typically requires integrating many different sources of information, including a mental status examination to establish whether there are any concurrent psychiatric conditions and a careful sexual history [69]. It is important to assess whether the paraphilic interest or behaviour is stronger or weaker than normophilic interests or behaviour. Psychophysiological assessment of sexual arousal patterns, using penile plethysmography or viewing time of sexual stimuli, can be useful in this regard, particularly for individuals with a paedophilic disorder. For a review of the available self-report (through clinical interview or questionnaires) measures used in the assessment of paraphilias, see [69].

### Management

While there is no evidence that paraphilic disorders can be 'cured' [69], there is some support for pharmacological treatments such as anti-androgens and antidepressants to reduce sexual drive, in particular for men with paedophilia [78]. Cognitive behavioural approaches are often used, usually as one component in a multimodal treatment programme [78].

### Evaluation of treatments

There has been limited outcome research on treatments for the various paraphilic disorders. Although used for many years, based on a review of outcome studies, Zucker and Seto [78] concluded that there was no strong empirical evidence that pharmacological treatments to reduce sexual drive had any effect on rates of reoffending. To date, there have been very few large, controlled outcome studies of either pharmacological or psychological interventions for the treatment of paraphilic disorders.

## Conclusions

Overall, sexual dysfunctions in one or other partner of a relationship are potentially treatable in many cases. The basic sex therapy approach described in this chapter can be effective on its own or in combination with other psychological interventions such as mindfulness-based therapy or with pharmacotherapy. Paraphilias, which are of most significance when they lead to illegal behaviour, are more difficult to treat. Further research is needed on these conditions.

### REFERENCES

1. Fisher WA, Rosen RC, Eardley I, Sand M, Goldstein I. Sexual experience of female partners of men with erectile dysfunction: the Female Experience of Men's Attitudes to Life Events and Sexuality (FEMALES) study. *Journal of Sexual Medicine*. 2005;2:675–84.
2. American Psychiatric Association. *Diagnostic and Statistical Manual of Mental Disorders*, fifth edition. Arlington, VA: American Psychiatric Association; 2013.
3. Althof SE. Treatment of premature ejaculation: psychotherapy, pharmacotherapy, and combined therapy. In: Binik YM, Hall KS (editors). *Principles and Practice of Sex Therapy*, fifth edition. New York, NY: Guilford; 2014. pp. 112–37.
4. Bancroft J. *Human Sexuality and Its Problems*, third edition. Edinburgh: Elsevier; 2009.
5. Davis SN, Binik YM, Carrier S. Sexual dysfunction and pelvic pain in men: a male sexual pain disorder? *Journal of Sex and Marital Therapy*. 2009;35:182–205.
6. Graham CA, Sanders, SA, Milhausen R, McBride K. Turning on and turning off: a focus group study of the factors that affect women's sexual arousal. *Archives of Sexual Behavior*. 2004;33:527–38.
7. Laan, E, Both, S. What makes women experience desire? *Feminism and Psychology*. 2008;18:505–14.
8. Laumann EO, Paik A, Rosen RC. Sexual dysfunctions in the United States: prevalence and predictors. *JAMA*. 1999;281:537–44.
9. Laan E, Everaerd W. Determinants of sexual arousal: psychophysiological theory and data. *Annual Review of Sex Research*. 1995;6:32–76.
10. Graham CA. The DSM diagnostic criteria for female orgasmic disorder. *Archives of Sexual Behavior*. 2010; 39:256–70.

11. Goldmeier D, Sadeghi-Nejad H, Facelle TM. Persistent genital arousal disorder. In: Binik YM, Hall KS (editors). *Principles and Practice of Sex Therapy*, fifth edition. New York, NY: Guilford; 2014. pp. 263–79.

12. World Health Organization. *International Classification of Diseases*, eleventh revision. Geneva: World Health Organization. Available from https://icd.who.int/browse11/l-m/en

13. Luciano M. Proposals for ICD-11: a report for WPA membership. *World Psychiatry*. 2014;13:206–8.

14. Graham CA. Reconceptualising women's sexual desire and arousal in DSM-5. *Psychology and Sexuality*. 2015;7:34–47.

15. Brotto LA. The DSM diagnostic criteria for hypoactive sexual desire disorder in women. *Archives of Sexual Behavior*. 2010;39:221–39.

16. Graham CA. The DSM diagnostic criteria for female sexual arousal disorder. *Archives of Sexual Behavior*. 2010;39:240–55.

17. Tiefer, L. Arriving at a 'New View' of women's sexual problems: background, theory, and activism. In: Kaschak E, Tiefer L (editors). *A New View of Women's Sexual Problems*. New York, NY: Haworth Press; 2001. pp. 63–98.

18. Binik YM. The DSM diagnostic criteria for vaginismus. *Archives of Sexual Behavior*. 2010;39:278–91.

19. Bancroft J, Janssen E. The dual control model of male sexual response: a theoretical approach to centrally mediated erectile dysfunction. *Neuroscience and Biobehavioral Reviews*. 2000;24:571–9.

20. Bancroft J, Graham CA, Janssen E, Sanders SA. The dual control model: current status and future directions. *Journal of Sex Research*. 2009;46:121–42.

21. Mitchell KR, Mercer CH, Ploubidis GB, et al. Sexual function in Britain: findings from the third national survey of sexual attitudes and lifestyles (Natsal-3). *The Lancet*. 2013;382:1817–29.

22. Mitchell KR, Jones KG, Wellings K, et al. Estimating the prevalence of sexual function problems: the impact of morbidity criteria. *Journal of Sex Research*. 2016;53:955–67.

23. Gao J, Zhang X, Su P, et al. Prevalence and factors associated with the complaint of premature ejaculation and the four premature ejaculation syndromes: a large observational study in China. *Journal of Sexual Medicine*. 2013;10:1874–81.

24. Laumann EO, West S, Glasser D, et al. Prevalence and correlates of erectile dysfunction by race and ethnicity among men aged 40 or older in the United States: From the Male Attitudes Regarding Sexual Health Survey. *Journal of Sexual Medicine*. 2007;4:57–65.

25. Serefoglu EC, Yaman O, Cayan S, et al. Prevalence of the complaint of ejaculating prematurely and the four premature ejaculation syndromes: results from the Turkish Society of Andrology Sexual Health Survey. *Journal of Sexual Medicine*. 2011;8:540–8.

26. Öberg K, Sjögren Fugl-Meyer K. On Swedish women's distressing sexual dysfunctions: some concomitant conditions and life satisfaction. *Journal of Sexual Medicine*. 2005;2:169–80.

27. Witting K, Santtila P, Varjonen M, et al. Female sexual dysfunction, sexual distress, and compatibility with partner. *Journal of Sexual Medicine*. 2008;5:2587–99.

28. Bancroft J, Loftus J, Long JS. Distress about sex: a national survey of women in heterosexual relationships. *Archives of Sexual Behavior*. 2003;32:193–208.

29. Lewis RW, Fugl-Meyer KS, Corona G, et al. Definitions/epidemiology/risk factors for sexual dysfunction. *Journal of Sexual Medicine*. 2010;7:1598–607.

30. Brotto LA. The DSM diagnostic criteria for hypoactive sexual desire disorder in men. *Journal of Sexual Medicine*. 2010;7:2015–30.

31. Træen B, Hald GM, Graham CA, et al. Sexuality in older adults (65+)—an overview of the literature, part 1: sexual function and its difficulties. *International Journal of Sexual Health*. 2017;29:1–10.

32. Hayes R, Dennerstein L. The impact of aging on sexual function and sexual dysfunction in women: a review of population based studies. *Journal of Sexual Medicine*. 2005;2:317–30.

33. Hall KS, Graham CA (editors). *The Cultural Context of Sexual Pleasure and Problems: Psychotherapy With Diverse Clients*. New York, NY: Routledge; 2012.

34. Janssen E, Vorst H, Finn P, Bancroft J. The Sexual Inhibition (SIS) and Sexual Excitation (SES) Scales: I. Measuring sexual inhibition and excitation proneness in men. *Journal of Sex Research*. 2002;39:114–26.

35. Graham CA, Sanders SA, Milhausen RR. The Sexual Excitation and Sexual Inhibition Inventory for Women: psychometric properties. *Archives of Sexual Behavior*. 2006;35:397–410.

36. Bancroft J, Herbenick D, Barnes T, et al. The relevance of the Dual Control Model to male sexual dysfunction: The Kinsey Institute-BASRT Collaborative Project. *Sexual and Relationship Therapy*. 2005;20:13–30.

37. Sanders SA, Graham CA, Milhausen RR. Predicting sexual problems in women: the relevance of sexual excitation and sexual inhibition. *Archives of Sexual Behavior*. 2008;37:241–51.

38. Velten J, Scholten S, Graham CA, Margraf J. Sexual excitation and sexual inhibition as predictors of sexual function in women: a cross-sectional and longitudinal study. *Journal of Sex and Marital Therapy*. 2016; DOI: 10.1080/0092623X.2015.1115792.

39. Beck AT. *Depression: Clinical, Experimental and Theoretical Aspects*. London: Staples Press; 1967.

40. Segraves RT. Psychiatric illness and sexual function. *International Journal of Impotence Research*. 1998;10(suppl 2):S131–3.

41. Angst J. Sexual problems in healthy and depressed persons. *International Clinical Psychopharmacology*. 1998;13(suppl 6):S1–4.

42. Figueira I, Possidente E, Marques C, Hayes K. Sexual dysfunction: a neglected complication of panic disorder and social phobia. *Archives of Sexual Behavior*. 2001;30:369–77.

43. Bancroft J, Janssen E, Strong D, Vukadinovic Z, Long JS. The relation between mood and sexuality in heterosexual men. *Archives of Sexual Behavior*. 2003;32:217–30.

44. Lykins AD, Janssen E, Graham CA. The relationship between negative mood and sexuality in heterosexual college women and men. *Journal of Sex Research*. 2006;43:136–43.

45. Lilleleht E, Leiblum SR. Schizophrenia and sexuality: a critical review of the literature. *Annual Review of Sex Research*. 1993;4:247–76.

46. Field N, Mercer CH, Sonnenberg P, et al. Associations between health and sexual lifestyles in Britain: findings from the third National Survey of Sexual Attitudes and Lifestyles (Natsal-3). *The Lancet*. 2013;382:1830–44.

47. Mustanski B, Bancroft J. Sexual dysfunction. In: Gorwood P, Hamon M (editors). *Psychopharmacogenetics*. New York, NY: Kluwer Academic Plenum; 2006. pp. 479–94.

48. Baldwin DS, Foong T. Antidepressant drugs and sexual dysfunction. *British Journal of Psychiatry*. 2013;202:396–7.

49. Bochinski D, Brock GB. Medications affecting erectile function. In: Mulcahy JJ (editor). *Male Sexual Function: A Guide to Clinical Management*. Totowa, NJ: Humana; 2001. pp. 91–108.

50. Graham CA, Bancroft J, Greco T, Tanner A, Doll HA. Does oral contraceptive-induced reduction in free testosterone adversely affect the sexuality and mood of women? *Psychoneuroendocrinology*. 2007;32:246–55.

51. Rosen RC, Miner MM, Wincze JP. Erectile dysfunction: integration of medical and psychological approaches. In: Binik YM, Hall KS (editors). *Principles and Practice of Sex Therapy*, fifth edition. New York, NY: Guilford; 2014. pp. 61–85.

52. Masters WH, Johnson VE. *Human Sexual Inadequacy*. Boston, MA: Little Brown; 1970.

53. Brotto L, Atallah S, Johnson-Agbakwu C, *et al.* Psychological and interpersonal dimensions of sexual function and dysfunction. *Journal of Sexual Medicine*. 2016;13:538–71.

54. Rosen RC, Fisher WA, Eardley I, Niederberger C, Nadel A, Sand M; Men's Attitudes to Life Events and Sexuality (MALES) Study. The multinational Men's Attitudes to Life Events and Sexuality (MALES) study: I. Prevalence of erectile dysfunction and related health concerns in the general population. *Current Medical Research and Opinion*. 2004;20:607–17.

55. Hatzimouratidis K, Salonia A, Adaikan G, *et al.* Pharmacotherapy for erectile dysfunction: recommendations from the Fourth International Consultation for Sexual Medicine (ICSM 2015). *Journal of Sexual Medicine*. 2016;13:465–88.

56. Pfaus J, Giuliano F, Gelez H. Bremelanotide: an overview of pre-clinical CNS effects on female sexual function. *Journal of Sexual Medicine*. 2007;4(s4):269–79.

57. Perelman MA. Delayed ejaculation. In: Binik YM, Hall KS (editors). *Principles and Practice of Sex Therapy*, fifth edition. New York, NY: Guilford; 2014. pp. 138–55.

58. Mayor S. Pfizer will not apply for a license for sildenafil for women. *BMJ*. 2004;328:542.

59. Basson R, Driscoll M, Correia S. Flibanserin for low sexual desire in women: a molecule from bench to bed? *EBioMedicine*. 2015;2:772–3.

60. Jaspers L, Feys F, Bramer WM, Franco OH, Leusink P, Laan ET. Efficacy and safety of flibanserin for the treatment of hypoactive sexual desire disorder in women: a systematic review and meta-analysis. *JAMA Internal Medicine*. 2016;176:453–62.

61. Gao Z, Yang D, Yu L, Cui Y. Efficacy and safety of flibanserin in women with hypoactive sexual desire disorder: a systematic review and meta-analysis. *Journal of Sexual Medicine*. 2015;12:2095–104.

62. Meana M., Hall KS, Binik YM. Conclusion. Sex therapy in transition: are we there yet? In: Binik YM, Hall KS (editors). *Principles and Practice of Sex Therapy*, fifth edition. New York, NY: Guilford; 2014. pp. 541–57.

63. Binik YM, Hall KS. Introduction. The future of sex therapy. In: Binik YM, Hall KS (editors). *Principles and Practice of Sex Therapy*, fifth edition. New York, NY: Guilford; 2014. pp. 1–11.

64. Frühauf S, Gerger H, Schmidt HM, *et al.* Efficacy of psychological interventions for sexual dysfunction: a systematic review and meta-analysis. *Archives of Sexual Behavior*. 2013;42:915–33.

65. Günzler C, Berner MM. Efficacy of psychosocial interventions in men and women with sexual dysfunctions—a systematic review of controlled clinical trials: part 2—the efficacy of psychosocial interventions for female sexual dysfunction. *Journal of Sexual Medicine*. 2012;9:3108–25.

66. Berner M, Günzler C. Efficacy of psychosocial interventions in men and women with sexual dysfunctions—a systematic review of controlled clinical trials: part 1—the efficacy of psychosocial interventions for male sexual dysfunction. *Journal of Sexual Medicine*. 2012;9:3089–107.

67. Al-Abbadey M, Liossi C, Curran N, Schoth DE, Graham CA. Treatment of female sexual pain disorders: a systematic review. *Journal of Sex and Marital Therapy*. 2016;17:42:99–142.

68. Långström N, Seto MC. Exhibitionistic and voyeuristic behavior in a Swedish national population survey. *Archives of Sexual Behavior*. 2006;35:427–35.

69. Seto MC, Kingston DA, Bourget D. Assessment of the paraphilias. *Psychiatric Clinics of North America*. 2014;37:149–61.

70. Kafka M. Axis I psychiatric disorders, paraphilic sexual offending and implications for pharmacological treatment. *Israeli Journal of Psychiatry and Related Sciences*. 2012;49:255–61.

71. Giami A. Between DSM and ICD: paraphilias and the transformation of sexual norms. *Archives of Sexual Behavior*. 2015;44:1127–38.

72. Kafka MP. Hypersexual disorder: a proposed diagnosis for DSM-V. *Archives of Sexual Behavior*. 2010;39:377–400.

73. Quinsey VL. Coercive paraphilic disorder. *Archives of Sexual Behavior*. 2010;39:405–10.

74. Moser C, Kleinplatz PJ. DSM-IV-TR and the paraphilias: an argument for removal. *Journal of Psychology and Human Sexuality*. 2006;17:91–109.

75. Richters J, De Visser RO, Rissel CE, Grulich AE, Smith A. Demographic and psychosocial features of participants in bondage and discipline, 'sadomasochism' or dominance and submission (BDSM): data from a national survey. *Journal of Sexual Medicine*. 2008;5:1660–8.

76. Dombert B, Schmidt AF, Banse R, *et al.* How common is men's self-reported sexual interest in prepubescent children? *Journal of Sex Research*. 2016;53:214–23.

77. Langstrom NI, Zucker KJ. Transvestic fetishism in the general populations. *Journal of Sex and Marital Therapy*. 2005;31;87–95.

78. Zucker KJ, Seto MC. Gender dysphoria and paraphilic sexual disorders. In: Thapar A, Pine DS, Leckman JF, Scott S, Snowling MJ, Taylor E (editors). *Rutter's Child and Adolescent Psychiatry*, sixth edition. Chichester: John Wiley and Sons; 2015. pp. 983–98.

# 116

# Gender dysphoria

*Els Elaut and Gunter Heylens*

## Introduction

In the past few years, the media have covered the lives of transgenders as never before. Caitlin Jenner was on the cover of *Vanity Fair* in July 2015, and the Netflix series *Orange is the New Black* featured a trans character—Sophia Burset—embodied by a trans woman Laverne Cox. At the same time, multi-disciplinary gender clinics worldwide are reporting on rapidly growing numbers of individuals voicing a desire for gender-confirming treatment (GCT) [1–2].

## Terminology and developmental pathways

The terminology used in this chapter is summarized in Table 116.1. The term 'gender dysphoria' (GD) was first mentioned by Norman Fisk (1974) [3] to describe discomfort with the assigned gender (assignment based on biological sex), leading to a desire for sex re-assignment surgery (SRS). Until recently, gender clinics were mostly consulted by trans women (individuals who were assigned male at birth but who identify as female) and trans men (individuals who were assigned female at birth but who identify as male) requesting counselling concerning the desired social transition from one gender role to the other and requesting medical interventions (hormone treatment and genital surgery) to transition from one sex to another. Evidence shows that GCT in individuals with GD is effective [4] and leads to an improvement in psychological symptoms, improved quality of life, and diminished GD [5]. Next to the symptom, and now an official DSM-5 diagnosis, of GD today, the clinician will note a spectrum of words used to describe individuals whose gender identity, gender role behaviour, and/or gender expression do not match (or 'conform to') current local expectations and stereotypes within the binary system of male–female in society (for example, genderqueer, gender variant, genderfluid, a-gender, non-binary, transgender, trans, transsexual). Today, not all individuals with GD presenting in gender clinics desire the full range of GCTs [6]. This confronts clinicians with the challenge of providing care in the absence of evidence-based treatment for these individuals with non-binary identities [7]. This evolution of an increased awareness for a broad gender variance has led to the use of the term 'transgender', a term coined by activist Virginia Prince, referring to a diverse group of individuals who cross or transcend culturally defined categories of gender, including transsexual people, cross-dressers, drag queens and kings, non-binary people, and gender variant people [8].

Two taxonomies are dominant in describing the phenomenology of GD—based on sexual orientation [9] and on age of GD onset [10]. Blanchard proposed two possibilities in GD development (with perhaps different aetiologies), based on sexual orientation [9]: a 'homosexual' and a 'non-homosexual' (relative to birth sex) subtype (Table 116.2). Also, the non-homosexual group develops differently in trans women and men; for example, the age of first clinical contact only differed between homosexual and non-homosexual trans women, and not trans men [11]. Pioneers in transgender health care were under pressure to identify prognostic factors and select the right candidate for treatment, leading to a search for the 'true transsexual', in whom minimal post-treatment regret would be expected. In the past, clinicians have been reluctant to offer treatment to the non-homosexual group, based on (limited) evidence that regret would be more prevalent in older individuals requesting treatment [11]. This categorization based on sexual orientation hence stirs controversy until today. Individuals with GD are sometimes cautious in disclosing the history of their GD or their sexual orientation, due to fear of being denied GCT, a concern historically not unfounded.

Recently, categorization based on the age of GD onset has been used increasingly. Researchers define adults with GD who recall childhood cross-gender behaviour and identification as 'early onset', while adults in whom the indicators of GD arise during puberty, or much later, are considered 'late onset' [12]. This categorization refrains from the older terms of homosexual and non-homosexual but uses the terms 'androphilic' (sexually attracted to men) and 'gynephilic' (sexual attracted to women) to refer to sexual attraction without making assumptions about sex or gender. A recent review shows that categorization based on the anticipated post-treatment heterosexual behaviour of trans women and men (as proposed by Blanchard's typology) might not be very predictive of a good outcome after GCT [10]. Contrary to early treatment protocols, sexual orientation is currently no longer a decisive factor in treatment decisions. Considering the potential psychosocial consequences of becoming part of not one minority group (the transgender community), but two (the gay and lesbian and bisexual communities), and the need to assess the individual's skills in dealing with minority distress, sexual orientation might still be a topic in need of clinical attention.

**Table 116.1** Summary of the terminology used in this chapter

| | |
|---|---|
| Sex | The biological aspect of gender, mostly based on primary and secondary sex characteristics |
| Gender | The psychosocial aspect of sex, subjective experience |
| Assigned gender | Apart from assigning a legal sex (in most countries, male or female, based on a newborn's primary sex characteristics), children are also assigned a certain gender (role and identity), for example expectations on crying behaviour, having a calm or more aggressive temper, showing an interest in stereotypical clothing, toys, hairstyle, etc. |
| Experienced gender | Or gender identity; the subjective experience of being male, female, genderqueer, or otherwise |
| Gender role | Behaviours that are—within a certain culture and time—associated with being male or female and hence are expected from men and women |
| Transgender | An umbrella term referring to a group of individuals who cross or transcend culturally defined categories of gender, including transsexual people, cross-dressers, drag queens and kings, non-binary people, and gender variant people |
| Cisgender | Opposite of transgender; people whose gender identity matches the sex and gender assigned at birth |
| Trans woman | An individual assigned the male gender at birth who identifies as a woman |
| Trans man | An individual assigned the female gender at birth who identifies as a man |
| Non-binary | An umbrella term for all not exclusively male or female gender identities; also genderqueer, genderfluid, etc. |
| Cross-dressing | The act of assuming a gender expression commonly associated with another gender; does not necessarily imply a direct correlation with gender dysphoria, a transgender identity, or fetishist arousal |
| Androphilia and gynephilia | Terms used to describe sexual orientation without attributing a sex or gender assignment (in contrast to the terms gay, lesbian, or bisexual); androphilia describes sexual attraction to men or masculinity; gynephilia refers to sexual attraction to women or femininity |

## Diagnostics

During the past decades, gender identity and gender role diagnoses underwent category migration and renaming, both in the American Psychiatric Association's (APA) *Diagnostic and Statistical Manual of Mental Disorders* (DSM) and in the World Health Organization's (WHO) *International Classification of Diseases* (ICD) [13]. Transsexualism appeared for the first time in the DSM in 1980 ('Gender identity disorder of childhood (GIDC) and transsexualism') and was listed among the psychosexual disorders. In 1994, GIDC and transsexualism were merged into one diagnosis—'Gender identity disorder' (GID)—and clustered with paraphilias and sexual dysfunctions. In the preparation phase of DSM-5, a fundamental question was raised by some transgender activists and clinicians of whether the diagnosis of GID should be retained at all. Their main argument was that GID was not a mental disorder, a similar argument that led to the removal of homosexuality from DSM-II in 1973. The decision to keep the diagnosis within the DSM was based on two considerations: access to care (health care reimbursement) and reconceptualization of the diagnosis. The new concept of GD was introduced to emphasize the fact that incongruence between one's felt gender and assigned sex/gender (usually at birth) leading to distress and/or impairment was the core feature of the diagnosis [14].

Also in the eleventh revision of the ICD, GID will be replaced with the label of 'Gender incongruence' (GI) to a new section provisionally entitled 'Conditions related to sexual health' [15]. The main argument for shifting and renaming diagnoses is further destigmatization of trans people who are already at risk for discrimination and associated mental health problems.

## Prevalence

While studies on the prevalence of both childhood GD and GD in adults are severely hampered by the uncertain methodology and diagnostic classification, a recent review calculated a meta-analytical general prevalence for GD in adults of 4.6 in 100,000 individuals, 6.8 for trans women and 2.6 for trans men. The review also found an increase in reported prevalence over the last 50 years [1]. This might still represent an underestimation of the true prevalence, as most studies are based on the number of adult individuals seen at specialized gender clinics or on the number of legal sex changes. Recently, population-based data have become increasingly available [16–18]. Conron *et al.* estimated 0.5% of adults consider themselves as 'transgender' (for example, 'a person born into a male body but who feels female or lives as a woman'), based on a probability sample in the United States of 28,176 adults aged between 18 and 64 years

**Table 116.2** Differences between homosexual and non-homosexual subtype

| Homosexual | Non-homosexual |
|---|---|
| Stronger cross-gender identity in childhood | Less cross-gender identity in childhood |
| Younger age at first clinical contact | Older age at first clinical contact |
| Lower prevalence of being (or having been) married | Higher prevalence of being (or having been) married |
| Less sexual arousal while cross-dressing in adolescence | Greater sexual arousal when cross-dressing in adolescence |

Reproduced from *Psychiatry Res.*, 137(3), Smith Y, van Goozen S, Kuiper A, *et al.*, Transsexual subtypes: clinical and theoretical significance, pp. 151–160, Copyright (2005), with permission from Elsevier Ireland Ltd.

[16]. Kuyper and Wijsen reported on a prevalence of 'gender incongruence' ('stronger identification with other sex as with sex assigned at birth') of 1.1% in men and 0.8% in women. When also assessing a dislike of the body and a wish to obtain hormones/surgery, the percentages drop to 0.6% and 0.2%, respectively [17]. Obtaining a psychiatric diagnosis and the level of distress in population-based surveys and self-report instruments remains difficult, and hence, these numbers cannot unequivocally be interpreted as a true epidemiological estimate of GD. These numbers of GI might well consist of a theoretical potential of individuals situated in the transgender spectrum that might eventually seek medical treatment.

Valid information on the prevalence of childhood GD is currently lacking entirely. An estimate of gender non-conforming/gender variant behaviour can be made, based on Child Behavior Checklist (CBCL) studies, pointing at 2.6% of boys and 5.0% of girls who 'behave like the opposite sex' and 1.4% of boys and 2.0% of girls who 'wish to be of the other sex' [19]. Therefore, gender non-conformity/gender variance appears to be more prevalent in girls than in boys. Interestingly, based on referral rates to gender clinics, the sex ratios for prepubescent children, adolescents, and adults have always been in favour of trans women. This might be a reflection of a historically lower societal acceptance of femininity in boys, compared to tolerance for masculinity in girls. In fact, gender clinics are currently reporting a change in both prepubescent children and adolescents with GD, such that more trans boys are presenting for care [20–21].

## Associated psychopathology

The association between GD and psychopathology has been changing ever since the first publications on transsexualism in the middle of the twentieth century. Transsexualism was previously considered as a severe symptom of a psychiatric disorder (for example, schizophrenia), and it was assumed that both axis 1 and axis 2 disorders were highly prevalent in transsexualism. The viewpoint now is that transsexualism/transgenderism should no longer be included in psychiatric manuals (see Diagnostics, p. 1192) [22]. Previous attitudes were based on anecdotal, rather than systematic, evidence. Gender non-conformity is no longer judged as inherently pathological or negative. Nevertheless, more recently, methodologically sound research has shown a high prevalence of depression and anxiety symptoms in individuals with GD who are referred to gender clinics [23]. A review on the co-occurrence of mental health problems and GD clearly showed that severe psychiatric problems, such as schizophrenia and bipolar disorder, are not more prevalent in individuals with GD, compared to the general population. The prevalence of affective disorders, on the other hand, is considered to be 2–3 times as high as in the general population. Trans women are found to be more comparable to cisgender women, then to cisgender men, with regard to the prevalence and nature of associated psychopathology [24]. With regard to suicidality and self-harm, Zucker et al. reported on the results of 13 studies, showing that one in three adults with GD has experienced suicidal ideation or attempted suicide or engaged in suicidal or non-suicidal self-harm [14]. Results on the co-occurrence of axis 2 disorders and GD have been inconsistent with regard to prevalence and the nature of the personality disorder [24]. Recently, there has been increasing interest in the link between GD and autism spectrum disorder (ASD). Van Der Miesen

et al. concluded that there is evidence for an overrepresentation of co-occurring GD and ASD, compared to the general population, and that possible aetiological factors that could account for this co-occurrence are speculative [25].

Still, there are some limitations with regard to research in this field. Firstly, the sample size is still limited and only individuals attending a gender clinic and who are willing to participate are included. Secondly, no randomized controlled trials are available, mainly due to ethical reasons.

Several possible explanations for the overrepresentation of mental health problems in GD are formulated—experiencing an incongruence between one's assigned gender at birth and perceived gender leads to dysphoria, the negative psychological effects of belonging to a minority group, with the risk for prejudice, discrimination, and victimization [14].

## Aetiology

As for studies on other psychological characteristics in humans, the role of nature (biological factors) vs nurture (psychosocial factors) in the development of GD has been a subject of debate. GD should be considered as an extreme variant of a gender-atypical development. This development starts from early childhood and is characterized by cross-gender behaviour and/or the stated wish to be of the other gender. Only a small proportion of children showing gender-atypical development fulfil the criteria for childhood GD, and with the onset of puberty (with the inherent physical changes, changing social interactions, and first romantic feelings), gender dysphoric feelings desist in the majority of children with GD [26]. Historically, psychosocial factors have accounted for the development of a cross-gender identity or GD. However, there is a lack of methodologically sound studies on the causal status of these factors in the development of GD. Furthermore, causal factors for the development of GD should already be present at a very early stage of development, that is, in the prenatal and/or early postnatal period [27]. Therefore, psychosocial processes are conceptualized as having a perpetuating role, rather than a causal role [14].

With regard to biological factors, most information is gained from genetic and brain imaging studies. Twin studies suggested a heritability of GD that varied between 62% [28] and 77% [29]. Heylens et al. found a significant difference between monozygotic twins and dizygotic twins with GD, suggesting a role for genetic factors [30]. In this study, almost 40% of the 23 monozygotic twins included were concordant for GD, in contrast to none of the 21 dizygotic twins. At present, no candidate genes have been found that can account for the development of GD. Studies have focused on genes involved in sex steroid biosynthesis, but results have been inconsistent. Genome-wide studies on GD patients could give more insight into the genetic basis for GD but are presently lacking.

The effects of (prenatal) hormones on the brain can be visualized using brain imaging techniques such as magnetic resonance imaging (MRI) and diffusion tensor imaging (DTI). An overview of neuroimaging studies in patients with GD is given by Kreukels et al. [31] and Guillamon et al. [32]. Both groups concluded that the brain phenotypes of trans women and trans men differed in various ways from those of control men and women with feminine, masculine, demasculinized, and defeminized features. Evidence for these phenotypes is strongest for early-onset gynephilic trans men and androphilic trans women, and absent for androphilic trans men and gynephilic trans women, suggesting that there are different developmental pathways for different subgroups (based on sexual orientation and age of GD onset). Guillamon *et al.* concluded that the origin of these phenotypes might be caused by atypical effects of sex hormones in specific cortical regions of trans men and trans women [32]. They hypothesized that these differences are due to differently timed cortical thinning in different regions. Functional alterations in the brain of individuals with GD have also been described, using task-related imaging studies (for example, visuo-spatial tasks, verbal fluency tasks) [31].

Finally, post-mortem studies have found that in trans women, specific brain structures (the interstitial nucleus, the bed nucleus of the stria terminalis, and the intermediate nucleus of the hypothalamus) have some sex-specific characteristics that are more similar to cisgender females than males [33–35].

In summary, gender identity development in general, and GD in particular, is the result of a complex interaction between multiple genetic and environmental factors. Genes encode hormones that exert an effect on sex-dimorphic neural structures during the prenatal period. Environmental factors then could have a pivotal effect on gender-atypical development during childhood or adolescence. Since time windows for the prenatal development of the genitals and the brain are believed to differ, individuals with GD experience an incongruence between their perceived gender identity and their body.

## Clinical management of gender-dysphoric adults

### Diagnostic assessment

Most individuals attending a gender clinic arrive with a self-diagnosis. During the diagnostic phase, a detailed clinical interview is most useful to confirm the diagnosis of GD. Standardized measures can be helpful to capture multiple indicators of gender identity and GD. These measures include the Utrecht Gender Dysphoria Scale (UGDS), and the Gender Identity/Gender Dysphoria Questionnaire for Adolescents and Adults (GIDYQ-AA) [48–49]. The latter uses a specific time frame and has similar items for males and females, in contrast to the UGDS. When associated psychopathology (see Role of the mental health professional, p. 1195) is likely, further diagnostic investigations can be important, in order to initiate appropriate treatment. This can be crucial since (severe) psychiatric comorbidity is a predictor of regret and a worse outcome after GCT [5, 22]. In recent years, the diagnostic phase has shortened and the approach to gender-dysphoric patients has become more individualized. Living in the preferred/experienced gender [the so-called real life experience (RLE)] is no longer a requirement for hormonal treatment. A study by Lawrence *et al.* showed no association between the duration of preoperative RLE and any outcome measure after GCT, except for happiness with the result [50].

GD should be distinguished from simple non-conformity to stereotypical gender role behaviour. Given the increased openness of atypical gender expressions by individuals, it is important that the clinical diagnosis is limited to those whose distress and impairment meet the DSM-5 criteria. Another diagnosis that should be accounted for is transvestic disorder (characterized by the association between cross-dressing and sexual excitement, leading to distress and/or impairment). Occasionally, transvestic disorder is accompanied by GD, and in many

cases of late-onset GD in gynephilic assigned males, transvestic behaviour is a precursor. Individuals suffering from body dysmorphic disorder, obsessive–compulsive disorder, and psychotic disorders can also present with symptoms that are similar to those typical for GD. Most often, these conditions can be differentiated from GD by the presence of other symptoms that are not related to the diagnosis of GD [22].

### Role of the mental health professional

Recently, there has been a debate with regard to the role of the mental health professional (MHP) in diagnosing GD and associated psychopathology. With the introduction of the Standards of Care for the Health of Transsexual, Transgender, and Gender-Non-conforming People, Version 7 (SOC-7), any health professional who is appropriately trained in behavioural health and competent in the assessment of GD is authorized to make diagnoses and treatment recommendations [51]. This more liberalized approach is in contrast with the traditional position of MHPs as gatekeepers for adults with GD. It is too early to estimate which approach leads to the best outcome after GCT with regard to satisfaction with treatment and quality of life (for prognostic factors associated with outcome after GCT, see [8]). The SOC-7 states that GCT can be initiated if physical and/or mental health problems that co-occur with GD are sufficiently stabilized.

The use of psychotherapy merely to change a person's gender identity has been considered unethical (SOC-7). Still, psychotherapy or counselling could be useful to treat concomitant mental health problems and to deal with other issues such as grief and loss, sexual concerns, or problems related to partner relationship. If a specific treatment is needed, for example more specific psychotherapy for persons with personality disorders or pharmacotherapy for mood disorders, patients can be referred to a specialized MHP [52].

### Endocrinological interventions

Based on a thorough assessment, a qualified MHP can write a referral letter to start hormone replacement therapy (HRT). The SOC-7 outlines several criteria for commencing HRT: persistent, well-documented GD; the capacity to make a fully informed decision and to consent for treatment, having reached the age of majority in a given country; and if significant medical or mental health problems are present, they should be reasonably controlled [51]. The administration of exogenous endocrine agents to induce feminizing or masculinizing changes is a medically necessary intervention, for which the Endocrine Society has issued very specific guidelines [53]. A safe and effective hormone regimen should: (1) suppress endogenous hormone secretion as determined by the person's genetic/biological sex; and (2) maintain sex hormone levels within the normal range for the person's desired gender [53]. HRT in trans women may consist of blocking androgen action (with anti-androgens, for example GnRHa, cyproterone acetate, spironolactone, finasteride) to decrease masculinization (diminishing body hair, frequency and firmness of erections, and muscle volume and strength) and oestrogens to achieve a more feminine presentation (breast development, softer skin, female fat distribution). Unfortunately, elimination of the hormonally induced natal sex characteristics is rarely complete—HRT does not alter voice, hand, feet, or shoulder dimensions [54]. In trans men, HRT may consist of synthetic progestins (for example, lynestrenol, medroxyprogesterone acetate) to interrupt menstrual bleeding, and testosterone to obtain more masculine features (deepening of the voice, increasing muscle mass and strength, beard and body hair growth, decreased fat mass, male pattern baldness, etc.). Although generally, a good aesthetic result is achieved in trans men, the short stature and often broader hip configuration do not change with HRT.

## Surgical interventions

Gender-confirming surgeries in trans women may include breast/chest surgery (augmentation mammoplasty), genital surgery (penectomy, orchidectomy, vaginoplasty, clitoroplasty, vulvoplasty), and/or other interventions such as facial feminization surgery, liposuction, lipofilling, voice surgery, thyroid cartilage reduction, gluteal augmentation, hair reconstruction, and various aesthetic procedures. It is recommended that trans women undergo HRT (minimum of 12 months) prior to breast augmentation, to maximize breast growth and surgical results. For genital surgery, two MHP referrals are recommended. Specifically for orchidectomy, the SOC-7 recommends 12 continuous months of HRT to introduce reversible testosterone suppression before undergoing irreversible surgery. For vaginoplasty, it is additionally recommended that the GD individual lives for 12 months in the congruent gender role. Typically, it is advised to stop all HRT at least 2 weeks prior to any surgical procedure, as oestrogens in particular cause an increased risk of thromboembolic complications [51, 55].

In trans men, gender-confirming surgeries may include subcutaneous mastectomy, hysterectomy/ovariectomy, vaginectomy, reconstruction of the fixed part of the urethra (if isolated, metoidioplasty), scrotoplasty, phalloplasty, and implantation of erection and/or testicular prostheses. It is recommended that trans men undergo HRT (minimum of 12 months) prior to 'internal' genital surgery (hysterectomy/ovariectomy), to introduce a period of reversible oestrogen suppression before irreversible surgery is performed. For 'external' genital surgery (metoidioplasty), it is additionally recommended that the GD individual lives for 12 months in the congruent gender role [51, 56].

## Fertility

Although neglected for a long time, fertility issues have become an important topic in the care of transgender persons. The SOC-7 clearly emphasizes the need to discuss fertility options prior to any treatment or medical intervention, since GCT (especially genital reconstructive surgery) often has irreversible effects with regard to fertility. The development of new reproductive medicine techniques creates opportunities for preserving fertility in transgender persons. Before, losing fertility was accepted as the price to pay for transitioning [57]. For trans women, sperm cryopreservation is the simplest and most reliable method. Success rates regarding pregnancy are similar to preservation in cisgender patients. Fertility options in trans men include embryo cryopreservation, oocyte cryopreservation, and ovarian tissue cryopreservation. Each option requires the use of partner sperm or donor sperm and a recipient uterus. Success rates are lower, compared to trans women, and depend, besides specific expertise of a specialized fertility centre, also on the age of the patient at the moment of cryopreservation. An interruption of cross-sex hormones for 3 months is necessary to restore fertility, both in trans women and trans men [58].

## Sexual health

Sexuality and relationships are vital parts of almost everyone's quality of life, including GD individuals. In the past, GD was often considered to be a 'hyposexual' state. Most individuals consulting a gender clinic (80%) have had sexual experiences with a partner. About half also involved their genitals in partnered contact, although only a minority (10–15%) indicated pleasurable genital sensations. Also, most have experience with masturbation [59]. Thus, the idea of GD individuals as not being sexual creatures is an oversimplification. Sexual activity is there before, during, and after GCT. Hence, both health care providers and individuals considering whether to undergo GCT should have clear information on the potential sexual effects of treatment (for a more extensive review, see [60–61]).

While one might reduce the potential sexual effects of GCT to the effects of sex steroids (oestrogens in trans women inhibiting sexuality; testosterone in trans men stimulating sexuality), other factors such as better self-esteem, feeling more comfortable with the new genitalia, and being able to allow more sexual exploration should not be disregarded. With regard to sexual desire, when trans women and men are asked—in retrospect—whether treatment has decreased, increased, or not affected their sexual desire, remarkable results emerge. The majority of trans women (70%) report decreased sexual desire after treatment (hormones and surgery), while a minority report an increase (10%) or no effect (20%). For trans men, the picture is reversed; the majority report an increase (70%), and a minority a decrease (10%) or no effect (20%) [60]. Most trans women and men welcome these changes, as they value sexual functioning more closely resembling the 'typical' functioning of their identified gender [62]. A subgroup of trans women (one in five) experience distress from decreased sexual desire. It is unclear to what extent this subgroup struggle with developing sexual desire which is now less testosterone-driven and more driven by mental processes. In any case, GCT always demands sexual (re)development by the individual and within a partnership. Distress about both decreased (5%) and too much sexual desire (3%) is much less of a concern in trans men. Sexual arousal is found to increase after GCT [63], although it should be noted that trans women with a skin-lined vagina always need a lubricant for penetration. Trans men also cannot obtain an erection spontaneously, even with an erection prosthesis. Percentages for 'orgasm capacity' in trans women, the best studied aspect of sexuality in GD individuals, ranges from 27% to 100% and differs between countries and used techniques [61]. It should, of course, be noted that obtaining an orgasm is not only about functional nerves and adequate hormone therapy, but as much about knowledge, skill, and experience. Most trans men are able to reach orgasm after having a phalloplasty [63–64]. So both trans men and women appear to experience increased orgasmic functioning after GCT.

## Post-treatment adjustment and prognostic factors

As GCT is, at least partially, an irreversible process, it is of major importance to look at outcome with regard to feelings of GD, quality of life, and psychological functioning post-treatment. A systematic review by Murad et al. showed that, after GCT, 80% of individuals diagnosed with GD reported significant improvement in gender-dysphoric feelings and 78% reported significant improvement in psychological symptoms [5]. Also with regard to quality of life and sexual function, 80% and 72%, respectively, reported an improvement. Djehne *et al.* reported on 11 longitudinal studies investigating outcome of psychiatric disorders and psychopathology post-treatment and found that in the majority of the studies, scores on questionnaires measuring psychopathology and GD were similar to normative data [24]. In general, however, longitudinal studies on the effects of GCT are methodologically weak, and follow-up duration is limited. Only one study has a duration time of >10 years, showing an overall positive evaluation [65]. More discouragingly, a Swedish cohort study (average follow-up duration of 10.4–11.4 years) showed that overall mortality for sex-reassigned persons was higher during follow-up than for cisgender controls, particularly death from suicide. Sex-reassigned persons also had an increased risk for suicide attempts and psychiatric inpatient care [66]. The majority of the patients included in this study were diagnosed in the 70s and 80s and, along with altered societal attitudes towards persons with different gender expressions, received less qualitative care both for their GD and for co-occurring mental health problems.

Positive prognostic factors are early-onset GD and a homosexual subtype [5], being a trans man [5, 67], and a younger age at assessment [68], although results are inconsistent. Pre-existing psychopathology [5] and poor results of SRS [4] tend to have worse prognosis. Furthermore, inadequate social functioning, indicated by periodical or full dependence on social assistance, and poor support from the individual's family are considered to be negative predictive factors [69].

Regret after GCT, defined as GD in the new gender role and after GCT, and the explicit wish to revert to his/her original gender role is estimated to occur in <1% in trans men and <1–1.5% in trans women [70]. Risk factors for regret are: inadequate diagnosis of GD and/or major psychiatric comorbidity, absent or disappointing RLE, and disappointing surgical results [22, 70]. De Cuypere and Vercruysse concluded that inadequate diagnosis of GD and major psychiatric comorbidity are the predominant indicators for regret [69].

The question remains as to which part of GCT is essential with regard to improvement of psychological functioning: RLE in the preferred gender role, hormonal therapy, or SRS. Heylens *et al.* showed that after initiation of hormonal treatment, the level of psychological stress, as measured by Symptom Checklist-90 (SCL-90), became comparable to a general population control. SRS did not further change the level of psychological distress [71].

In general, GCT has proven to be the best method for treating GD. Clinicians should stay mindful of actual or potential psychiatric problems before the start of GCT and after its completion.

## REFERENCES

1. Arcelus J, Bouman WP, Van Den Noortgate W, Claes L, Witcomb G, Fernandez-Aranda F. Systematic review and meta-analysis of prevalence studies in transsexualism. *Eur Psychiatry* 2015;30: 807–15.
2. Reed B, Rhodes S, Schofield P, Wylie K. *Gender variance in the UK: prevalence, incidence, growth and geographic distribution.* Gender Identity Research and Education Society (GIRES), June 2009.
3. Fisk N. Gender dysphoria syndrome (the how, what and why of a disease). In: Lauband D, Gandy P (eds). *Proceedings of the Second Interdisciplinary symposium on Gender Dysphoria Syndrome.* Palo Alto, CA: Stanford University Press; 1974. pp. 7–14.
4. Phäfflin F, Junge A. *Sex reassignment. Thirty years of international follow-up studies after sex reassignment surgery: a comprehensive review, 1961–1991* (English edition). 1998. Available from: https://web.archive.org/web/20070503090247/http://www.symposion.com/ijt/pfacfflin/1000.htm
5. Murad MH, Elamin MB, Garcia MZ, *et al.* Hormonal therapy and sex reassignment: a systematic review and meta-analysis of quality of life and psychosocial outcomes. *Clin Endocrinol* 2010;72:214–31.
6. Beek T, Kreukels BPC, Cohen-Kettenis PT, Steensma TD. Partial treatment requests and underlying motives of applicants for gender affirming interventions. *J Sex Med* 2015;12:2201–5.
7. Richards C, Bouman WP, Leighton S, John BM, Nieder TO, T'Sjoen G. Non-binary or genderqueer genders. *Int Rev Psychiatry* 2016;28:95–102.
8. King D, Ekins R. *Pioneers of transgendering: the life and work of Virginia Prince.* 2000. Available from: http://www.gender.org.uk/conf/2000/king20.htm
9. Blanchard R. The classification and labeling of nonhomosexual gender dysphoria. *Arch Sex Behav* 1989;18:315–34.
10. Nieder TO, Elaut E, Richards C, Dekker A. Sexual orientation of trans adults is not linked to outcome of transition-related health care, but worth asking. *Int Rev Psychiatry* 2016;28:103–11.
11. Smith Y, van Goozen S, Kuiper A, Cohen-Kettenis PT. Transsexual subtypes: clinical and theoretical significance. *Psychiatry Res* 2005;137:151–60.
12. Nieder T, Herff M, Cerwenka S, *et al.* Age of onset and sexual orientation in transsexual males and females. *J Sex Med* 2011;8:783–91.
13. Drescher, J. Gender identity diagnoses: history and controversies. In: Kreukels BPC, Steensma TD, de Vries ALC (eds). *Gender Dysphoria and Disorders of Sex Development: Progress in Care and Knowledge.* New York, NY: Springer; 2013. pp. 137–50.
14. Zucker K, Lawrence A, Kreukels, BK. Gender dysphoria in adults. *Annu Rev Clin Psychol* 2016;12:217–247.
15. Drescher, J. Queer diagnoses revisited: the past and future of homosexuality and gender diagnoses in DSM and ICD. *Int Rev Psychiatry* 2015;27:386–95.
16. Conron KJ, Scot G, Stowell GS, Landers SJ. Transgender health in Massachusetts: results from a household probability sample of adults. *Am J Public Health* 2012;102:118–22.
17. Kuyper L, Wijsen C. Gender identities and gender dysphoria in the Netherlands. *Arch Sex Behav* 2014;43:377–85.
18. Van Caenegem E, Wierckx W, Elaut E, *et al.* Prevalence of gender nonconformity in Flanders, Belgium. *Arch Sex Behav* 2015;44:1281–7.
19. Verhulst F, van der Ende J, Koot H. *Handleiding voor de CBCL/4-18* (in Dutch, *Manual for the CBCL/4-18*). Rotterdam: Erasmus University; 1996.
20. Aitken M, Steensma TD, Blanchard R, *et al.* Evidence for an altered sex ratio in clinic-referred adolescents with gender dysphoria. *J Sex Med* 2015;12:756–63.
21. Wood H, Sasaki S, Bradley SJ, *et al.* Patterns of referral to a gender identity service for children and adolescence (1976–2011): age, sex ration, and sexual orientation. *J Sex Mar Ther* 2013;39:1–6.
22. Gijs L, van der Putten-Bierman E, De Cuypere G. Psychiatric comorbidity in adults with gender identity problems. In: Kreukels BPC, Steensma TD, de Vries ALC (eds). *Gender Dysphoria and Disorders of Sex Development: Progress in Care and Knowledge.* New York, NY: Springer; 2013. pp. 255–76.

23. Heylens G, Elaut E, Kreukels BPC, *et al*. Psychiatric charac-teristics in transsexual individuals: multicentre study in four European countries. *Br J Psychiatry* 2014;204:151–6.
24. Dhejne C, Van Vlerken R, Heylens G, Arcelus J. Mental health and gender dysphoria: a review of the literature. *Int Rev Psychiatry* 2016;28:44–57.
25. Van Der Miesen, A, Hurley, H, De Vries A. Gender dysphoria and autism spectrum disorder: a narrative review. *Int Rev Psychiatry* 2016;28:70–80.
26. Steensma TD, McGuire JK, Kreukels BPC, Beekman AJ, Cohen-Kettenis PT. Factors associated with desistence and persistence of childhood gender dysphoria: a quantitative follow-up study. *J Am Acad Child Adolesc Psychiatry* 2013;52:582–90.
27. Swaab DF, Garcia-Falgueras A. Sexual differentiation of the human brain in relation to gender identity and sexual orienta-tion. *Funct Neurol* 2009;24:17–28.
28. Coolidge FL, Thede LL, Young SE. The heritability of gender identity disorder in a child and adolescent twin sample. *Behav Genet* 2002;32:251–7.
29. Van Beijsterveld C, Hudziak J, Boomsma D. Genetic and en-vironmental influences on cross-gender behavior and relation to behavioral problems: a study of Dutch twins at ages of 7 and 10 years. *Arch Sex Behav* 2006;35:647–58.
30. Heylens G, De Cuypere G, Zucker KJ, *et al*. Gender identity dis-order in twins: a review of the case report literature. *J Sex Med* 2012;9:751–7.
31. Kreukels BPC, Guillamon A. Neuroimaging studies in people with gender incongruence. *Int Rev Psychiatry* 2016;28:120–8.
32. Guillamon A, Junque C, Gomez-Gil E. A review of the status of brain structure research in transsexualism. *Arch Sex Behav* 2016;45:1615–48.
33. Garcia-Falgueras A, Swaab DF. A sex difference in the hypothal-amic uncinate nucleus: relationship to gender identity. *Brain* 2008;131:3132–46.
34. Kruijver FP, Zhou JN, Pool CW, Hofman MA, Gooren LJ, Swaab DF. Male-to-female transsexuals have female neuron numbers in a limbic nucleus. *J Clin Endocrinol Metab* 2000;85:2034–41.
35. Zhou JN, Hofman MA, Gooren LJ, Swaab DF. A sex difference in the human brain and its relation to transsexuality. *Nature* 1995;378:68–70.
36. Bartlett NH, Vasey PL, Bukowski WM. Is gender identity dis-order in children a mental disorder? *Sex Roles* 2000;43:753–85.
37. Cohen-Kettenis PT. Gender identity disorder in DSM? *J Am Acad Child Adolesc Psychiatry* 2011;40:391.
38. Drummond KD, Bradley SJ, Peterson-Badali M, Zucker KJ. A follow-up study of girls with gender identity disorder. *Dev Psychol* 2008;44:34–45.
39. Wallien, MSC, Cohen-Kettenis PT. Psychosexual outcome of gender-dysphoric children. *J Am Acad Child Adolesc Psychiatry* 2008;47:1413–23.
40. Steensma TD, van der Ende J, Verhulst FC, Cohen-Kettenis PT. Gender variance in childhood and sexual orientation in adult-hood: a prospective study. *J Sex Med* 2013;10:2723–33.
41. Steensma TD, Biemond T, de Boer T, Cohen-Kettenis PT. Desisting and persisting gender dysphoria after childhood: a qualitative follow-up study. *Clin Child Psychol Psychiatry* 2011;16:499–516.
42. Cohen-Kettenis PT, Pfäfflin F. *Transgenderism and Intersexuality in Childhood and Adolescence* (Volume 46). Thousand Oaks, CA: Sage; 2003.
43. Zucker KJ. Gender identity disorder. In: Wolfe DA, Mash EJ (eds). *Behavioral and Emotional Disorder in Adolescents: Nature,*

44. de Vries ALC, Steensma TD, Doreleijers TAH, Cohen-Kettenis PT. Puberty suppression in adolescents with gender identity dis-order: a prospective follow-up study. *J Sex Med* 2011;8:2276–83.
45. de Vries ALC, Cohen-Kettenis PT. Clinical managment of gender dysphoria in children and adolescents: the Dutch approach. *J Homosex* 2012;59:301–20.
46. Delemarre-van de Waal HA. Early medical intervention in ado-lescents with gender dysphoria. In: Kreukels BPC, Steensma TD, de Vries ALC (eds). *Gender Dysphoria and Disorders of Sex Development: Progress in Care and Knowledge.* New York, NY: Springer; 2014. pp. 193–203.
47. Cohen-Kettenis PT, Delemarre-van de Waal HA, Gooren LJ. The treatment of adolescent transsexuals: changing insights. *J Sex Med* 2008;5:1892–7.
48. Schneider C, Cerwenka S, Nieder TO, *et al*. Measuring gender dysphoria: a multicenter examination and comparison of the Utrecht Gender Dysphoria Scale and the Gender Identity/Gender Dysphoria Questionnaire for Adolescents and Adults. *Arch Sex Behav* 2016;45:551–8.
49. Deogracias JJ, Johnson LL, Meyer-Bahlburg HFL, Kessler SJ, Schober JM, Zucker KJ. The gender identity/gender dysphoria questionnaire for adolescents and adults. *J Sex Res* 2007;44:370–9.
50. Lawrence A. Factors associated with satisfaction or regret fol-lowing male-to-female sex reassignment surgery. *Arch Sex Behav* 2003;32:299–315.
51. Coleman E, Bockting W, Botzer M, *et al*. Standards of Care for the Health of Transsexual, Transgender, and Gender-Nonconforming People, Version 7. *Int J Transgend* 2011;13:165–232.
52. Bockting W, Knudson G, Goldberg J. Counseling and mental health care for transgender adulst and loved ones. *Int J Transgend* 2006;9:35–82.
53. Hembree WC, Cohen-Kettenis PT, Delemarre-van de Waal HA, *et al*. Endocrine treatment of transsexual persons: an Endocrine Society clinical practice guideline. *J Clin Endocrinol Metab* 2009;94:3132–54.
54. Gooren LJ. Hormone treatment of adult transgender people. In: Ettner R, Monstrey S, Coleman E (eds). *Principles of Transgender Medicine and Surgery*. New York, NY: Routledge; 2016. pp. 165–76.
55. Colebunders B, Verhaeghe W, Bonte K, D'Arpa S, Monstrey S. Male-to-female gender reassignment surgery. In: Ettner R, Monstrey S, Coleman E (eds). *Principles of Transgender Medicine and Surgery*. New York, NY: Routledge; 2016. pp. 248–76.
56. Colebunders B, D'Arpa S, Weyers S, Lumen N, Hoebeke P, Monstrey S. Female-to-male gender reassignment surgery. In: Ettner R, Monstrey S, Coleman E (eds). *Principles of Transgender Medicine and Surgery*. New York, NY: Routledge; 2016. pp. 277–315.
57. T'Sjoen G, Van Caenegem E, Wierckx K. Transgenderism and re-production. *Curr Opin Endocrinol Diabetes Obes* 2013;20:575–9.
58. De Roo C, Tilleman K, T'Sjoen G, De Sutter P. Fertility options in transgender people. *Int Rev Psychiatry* 2016;28:112–19.
59. Cerwenka S, Nieder TO, Cohen-Kettenis PT, *et al*. Sexual behavior of gender-dysphoric individuals before gender-confirming interven-tions: a European multicenter study. *J Sex Mar Ther* 2014;40:1–15.
60. Elaut E, Weyers S, Hoebeke P, Stockman S, Monstrey S. Sexuality and relationships of transgender people. In: Arcelus J, Bouman W (eds). *Gender Dysphoria and Gender Incongruence—A Guide for Patients, Families and Professionals*. New York, NY: Nova Science Publishers Inc; 2017. pp. 117–32.

61. Klein, Gorzalka BB. Sexual functioning in transsexuals following hormone therapy and genital surgery: a review. *J Sex Med* 2009;6:2911–39.

62. Doornduin T, van Berlo W. Trans people's experience of sexuality in the Netherlands: a pilot study. *J Homosex* 2014;61:654–72.

63. De Cuypere G, T'Sjoen G, Beerten R, *et al.* Sexual and physical health after sex reassignment surgery. *Arch Sex Behav* 2005;34:679–90.

64. Wierckx W, Van Caenegem E, Elaut E, *et al.* Quality of life and sexual health after sex reassignment surgery in transsexual men. *J Sex Med* 2011;8:3378–88.

65. Ruppin U, Pfafflin F. Long-term follow-up of adults with gender identity disorder. *Arch Sex Behav* 2015;44:1321–9.

66. Dhejne C, Lichtenstein P, Boman M, Johansson A, Langstrom N, Landen M. Long-term follow-up of transsexual persons undergoing sex reassignment surgery: Cohort study Sweden. *PLoS One* 2011;6:e16885.

67. Smith YLS, van Goozen SHM, Kuiper AJ, Cohen-Kettenis PT. Sex reassignment: outcomes and predictors of treatment for adolescent and adult transsexuals. *Psychol Med* 2005; 35:89–99.

68. De Cuypere G, Elaut E, Heylens G, *et al.* Long-term follow-up: psychosocial outcomes of Belgian transsexuals after sex reassignment surgery. *Sexologies.* 2006;15:126–33.

69. De Cuypere G, Vercruysse H Jr. Eligibility and readiness criteria for sex reassignment surgery: recommendations for Revision of the WPATH Standards of Care. *Int J Transgend* 2009;11:194–205.

70. Pfäfflin F. Regrets after sex reassignment surgery. *J Psychol Hum Sex* 1993;5:69–85.

71. Heylens G, Verroken C, De Cock S, T'Sjoen G, De Cuypere G. Effects of different steps in genderreassignment therapy on psychopathology: a prospective study of persons with a gender identity disorder. *J Sex Med* 2014;11:119–26.

# SECTION 19
# Personality disorders

# 117

# Core dimensions of personality pathology

*Andrew E. Skodol and Leslie C. Morey*

## Introduction

For no realm of psychopathology has a categorical approach to classification and diagnosis proved more wanting than for personality pathology. A meta-analytic review of 177 studies with a combined sample of over 500,000 participants on the latent structure of various types of psychopathology [1] found little persuasive evidence for the existence of taxa (categories) for any of the personality disorders (PDs) classified by the DSM, with the possible exception of schizotypal personality disorder (STPD). Further, in a 2007 survey of PD experts, 87% believed that personality pathology was dimensional in nature [2]. Although the definition of PD categories by explicit diagnostic criteria since DSM-III has had beneficial effects in documenting substantial prevalence in community and clinical populations, high rates of associated social and occupational impairment, and a more chronic course for other mental disorders co-occurring with PDs, the approach embodied by the DSMs has also been fraught with problems. These include extensive co-occurrence of PDs, considerable heterogeneity within PD categories, arbitrary diagnostic thresholds without empirical bases, temporal instability, limited validity and clinical utility, and incomplete coverage of the full range of personality pathology [3]. Dimensional models of personality pathology have been proposed since the publication of DSM-III as alternative representations of PDs [4], with the goal of rectifying some of these problems. Debate and controversy over the best dimensional representations of personality pathology have played out over the past three or more decades, but considerable consensus exists now about fundamental core dimensions.

In this chapter, we will review the core *personality trait* domains underlying psychopathology in general, and personality pathology specifically. We will describe the core dimensions of *personality functioning* that can distinguish between personality styles and PDs and between PDs and other types of psychopathology. We will then review the development and longitudinal course, the impact on health and psychosocial functioning, and the clinical utility of core personality dimensions. Finally, we will illustrate how traditional PD subtypes can be rendered in terms of domains and facets of personality functioning and of personality traits in a 'hybrid' dimensional–categorical model.

## Personality domains and the meta-structure of psychopathology

Co-occurrence of categorical mental disorders is very common in clinical populations and in the community, because certain types of signs, symptoms, and personality traits tend to vary together. This co-variation has led to attempts to understand the organization of psychopathology by identifying fundamental dimensions of psychopathology that undergird groups of disorders using factor analyses of disorders and their manifestations. Two broad dimensions, or 'spectra', of psychopathology, called *internalizing* and *externalizing*, have been identified that encompass a large number of non-psychotic mental disorders [5]. The process of internalizing involves the expression of mental problems by negative feelings and behaviours directed at oneself and includes symptoms of depression and anxiety, for example; externalizing involves the expression of such problems by negative feelings and behaviours directed at other people or things in one's environment and includes symptoms of aggression, defiance, and violence. A third broad spectrum of psychopathology has been identified that includes schizophrenia and other psychotic disorders and bipolar I disorder, and has been referred to as a *thought disorder* spectrum [6]. These spectra are fundamentally dimensional in nature, because a person can exhibit more or less internalizing, externalizing, or disordered thinking, rather than an 'all or nothing', 'present or absent' (that is, categorical) expression. Spectra also represent general, consistent tendencies or proclivities to think, feel, and act in certain ways, and thus reflect personality dispositions, that is, 'enduring patterns of perceiving, relating to, and thinking about the environment and oneself that are exhibited in a wide range of social and personal contexts' [7, p. 647].

Disorders within these three broad domains have been shown to not only co-occur, but also to share genetic, environmental, and temperamental risk factors, exhibit common cognitive and emotional processing abnormalities, and respond to similar treatments, even though they are assigned to different diagnostic classes in DSM-5. A classification of mental problems based on empirical associations can include both symptoms—relatively transient forms of psychopathology—and maladaptive personality traits that are thought to form the stable core of many mental disorders. Thus, personality trait domains can be viewed as the dimensional underpinnings of the meta-structure of psychopathology in general.

An extensive literature shows that personality constructs are organized empirically into 3–5 broad domains [8]. According to the most widely studied five-factor model (FFM) of personality, these domains are labelled as neuroticism (a tendency to be depressed, anxious, and stress-reactive), agreeableness (oriented towards empathy and getting along with other people), extraversion (a disposition to be outgoing, friendly, and emotionally positive), openness (a tendency to be curious and imaginative and to try new things), and conscientiousness (a tendency to be orderly and achievement-oriented). These domains organize both normal and abnormal personality [9], because normal- and abnormal-range personality variations are continuous with each other and there is no compelling evidence that they differ in kind, as opposed to degree [10]. In working to systematically introduce an empirically based trait assessment into DSM-5, the DSM-5 Personality and Personality Disorders (P&PD) Work Group developed a model that was consistent with the well-established FFM but was an extension that specifically delineated and encompassed the more extreme and maladaptive personality variants necessary to capture the maladaptive personality dispositions of people with PDs [11]. Although the Work Group's model was not placed in Section II 'Diagnostic criteria and codes' of DSM-5, it appears as an 'alternative' dimensional–categorical model of PDs in Section III 'Emerging measures and models'.

The alternative DSM-5 model of personality disorders (AMPD) describes personality pathology in terms of five broad trait domains, within the internalizing, externalizing, and thought disorder spectra. The domains and their definitions are as follows [7, pp. 779–81]:

1. *Negative affectivity*: frequent and intense experiences of high levels of a wide range of negative emotions (for example, anxiety, depression, guilt/shame, worry, anger, etc.) and their behavioural (for example, self-harm) and interpersonal (for example, dependency) manifestations.
2. *Detachment*: avoidance of socio-emotional experience, including both withdrawal from interpersonal interactions (ranging from casual, daily interactions to friendships to intimate relationships) and restricted affective experience and expression, particularly limited hedonic capacity.
3. *Antagonism*: behaviours that put the individual at odds with other people, including an exaggerated sense of self-importance and a concomitant expectation of special treatment, as well as a callous antipathy towards others, encompassing both unawareness of others' needs and feelings and a readiness to use others in the service of self-enhancement.
4. *Disinhibition*: orientation towards immediate gratification, leading to impulsive behaviour driven by current thoughts, feelings, and external stimuli, without regard for past learning or consideration of future consequences.
5. *Psychoticism*: exhibiting a wide range of culturally incongruent, odd, eccentric, or unusual behaviours and cognitions, including both thought process (for example, perception, dissociation) and content (for example, beliefs).

The personality trait domain of negative affectivity is the personality component of the internalizing spectrum of psychopathology. The trait domains of disinhibition and antagonism are the components of the externalizing spectrum. The trait domain of psychoticism is the component of the thought disorder spectrum. A trait domain of detachment corresponding to a spectrum of pathological introversion has been found in many studies of the structure of mental disorders that have included PDs and/or pathological personality traits [12–14].

The most recent description of the PD proposal for ICD-11 also incorporates a personality trait domain schema for describing the variation in PD presentations [15]. The five trait domains included are negative affectivity, detachment, dissocial, disinhibition, and anankastic. Three of these domains are identical to the AMPD model, and dissocial corresponds closely with the AMPD antagonism domain, leaving the only difference between AMPD psychoticism and ICD-11 anankastic trait domains. The AMPD includes psychoticism to represent STPD traits in the model, and other structural studies have found that DSM-IV cluster A PDs load positively onto the thought disorder spectrum. Since STPD is not classified as a PD in ICD-11, psychoticism may be less necessary to capture the full range of PD in the ICD. Unlike the ICD-11 proposal, the AMPD conceptualizes anankastic (obsessive–compulsive) personality traits as the opposite pole of disinhibition (that is, low levels), although some empirical studies of the AMPD have suggested that it might potentially be better characterized as an independent dimension as in the ICD proposal [16]. Nonetheless, the clear similarity in these two independently developed approaches to the classification of PD speaks further to the consensus around the dimensional structure of pathological personality.

A number of researchers (for example, [8, 17]) have suggested that PD traits might be best represented as an integrative hierarchy, with broad dimensions of personality situated at the top of this hierarchy and specific trait constructs described at lower levels—with these lower-level constructs providing important bridges between personality pathology and syndromal disorders. Thus, each of the five broad trait domains of the AMPD includes from three to six more specific component trait facets. The trait facets and their definitions, used for the formulation of specific PDs according to the AMPD, can be found in DSM-5 [7, pp. 779–81].

PDs vary in their manifestations and complexity. Some PDs are related to internalizing mental disorders, such as depressive or anxiety disorders, because they are characterized primarily by traits of negative affectivity, for example depressivity or anxiousness. Dependent personality disorder (DPD) is an example of a PD within the internalizing spectrum of psychopathology. Some PDs are related to externalizing disorders, such as disruptive, impulse control, and conduct disorders or substance use disorders, because they are characterized by traits of disinhibition, for example impulsivity or risk-taking, and/or of antagonism, for example callousness, deceitfulness, or grandiosity. Antisocial personality disorder (ASPD) is an example of a PD within the externalizing spectrum of psychopathology. Some PDs are related to psychotic disorders and are characterized by traits of psychoticism, for example cognitive/perceptual dysregulation or unusual beliefs and experiences, with STPD as an example. Finally, some PDs represent constellations of broad domains; borderline personality disorder (BPD) has both internalizing and externalizing characteristics, and avoidant personality disorder (AVPD) is characterized by a combination of internalizing and detachment.

Appreciation of the relationship of pathological personality trait domains with the meta-structure of psychopathology in general makes the ubiquitous phenomenon of mental disorder comorbidity understandable. Because symptom disorders and PDs share underlying predispositions, certain patterns of co-occurrence of categorical disorders can be expected to be observed more often than others. To represent psychopathology as co-occurring disorders when some more fundamental process is operative, however, obscures the search for aetiology and pathophysiology and complicates treatment selection [18].

## Core dimensions of personality functioning

Since the same personality trait domains underlie both symptom disorders—such as depressive, anxiety, disruptive behaviour, and psychotic disorders—and PDs, core aspects of personality pathology that would distinguish PDs from other types of pathology, as well as from non-pathological personality 'styles', need to be identified. A PD is defined by general criteria in Section II of DSM-5 as an 'enduring pattern of inner experience and behaviour that deviates markedly from the expectations of the individual's culture, is pervasive and inflexible, has an onset in adolescence or early adulthood, is stable over time, and leads to distress or impairment' [7, p. 645]. The patterns are said to manifest in two or more of the following areas: *cognition, affectivity, interpersonal functioning*, and *impulse control*. Because these features are not specific to PDs and may characterize other chronic mental disorders, the DSM-5 Section III AMPD includes a more specific set of general criteria with which to define and identify PDs. According to this empirically derived model, PDs are characterized by *impairments in personality functioning*, including core functions of identity, self-direction, empathy, and intimacy, in combination with the presence of pathological personality traits [7, p. 761]. Impairment in personality functioning occurs on a continuum of severity, and greater severity of impairment in these core functions is proposed to both distinguish PDs from other types of psychopathology and from normal personality functioning. Given the presence of such impairment, various configurations of pathological personality traits can describe the myriad manifestations in the presentations of personality pathology.

The history of the study of personality is replete with classification models that are unitary, dimensional severity models [19]. From Sir Francis Galton's model of 'good and bad temper', through James Cowles Prichard's concept of 'moral insanity' and theorists such as Piaget, Erikson, and Loevinger, many personality-oriented writers emphasized a single developmental continuum over which individuals could vary, based on a principle of maturation that reflected greater (or lesser) degrees of self-control and prosocial behaviour. Along similar lines, Kernberg's construct of 'personality organization' represents a classification of character pathology arrayed along a severity continuum, with a realistic and stable sense of identity and of the experience of others reflecting the healthy end of this continuum. In fact, the significance of a severity gradient in evaluating personality problems has been described for far longer than PD categories themselves. Even according to the FFM, which posits that these personality factors are largely independent of each other, different DSM PDs consistently have been shown to exhibit quite similar profiles, consisting of high neuroticism, low agreeableness, and low conscientiousness [20].

In a literature review of clinician-administered measures for assessing personality functioning performed for the DSM-5 P&PD

Work Group, Bender *et al.* [21] found that global measures of personality pathology all referenced fundamental impairments in self and interpersonal functioning—impairments that exist on a continuum of severity, can be measured reliably, and have considerable clinical utility in determining the type and degree of personality pathology, planning treatment interventions, and anticipating treatment course and outcome. To capture this severity continuum, a 5-point scale of impairment in personality functioning, ranging from little or none (0) to some (1), moderate (2), severe (3), and extreme (4) impairment and consisting of a global rating of self (identity and self-direction) and interpersonal (empathy and intimacy) functioning—the Level of Personality Functioning Scale (LPFS)—was developed. It was tested in secondary data analyses in over 2000 patients and community members, and the construct was found to relate to the probability of receiving any PD diagnosis and the total number of DSM-IV PD features manifested, as well as the probability of receiving two or more PD diagnoses as determined by semi-structured diagnostic interviews [22]. A subsequent study [23] determined that a clinician rating of '2 (moderate)' impairment in personality functioning on the LPFS identified clinician-diagnosed DSM-IV PDs with solid sensitivity (0.846) and specificity (0.727), a cut-point which was incorporated into the DSM-5 AMPD's general criteria for a PD. This severity continuum is designed to capture the variation between PDs (which may, on average, vary in the degree of impairment typically present), but also the heterogeneity within PD categories (where some manifestations of a specific PD may be more severe than others), and to be sensitive to change. The DSM-5 AMPD definitions of the core self and interpersonal functions are as follows [7, p. 762].

### Self

1. *Identity*: experience of oneself as unique, with clear boundaries between self and others; stability of self-esteem and accuracy of self-appraisal; capacity for, and ability to regulate, a range of emotional experience.
2. *Self-direction*: pursuit of coherent and meaningful short-term and life goals; utilization of constructive and prosocial internal standards of behaviour; ability to self-reflect productively.

### Interpersonal

3. *Empathy*: comprehension and appreciation of others' experiences and motivations; tolerance of differing perspectives; understanding the effects of own behaviour on others.
4. *Intimacy*: depth and duration of connection with others; desire and capacity for closeness; mutuality of regard reflected in interpersonal behaviour.

The ICD-11 PD proposal also includes a dimensional personality pathology severity measure as its centrepiece. The scale would distinguish personality difficulty (not a disorder) from mild, moderate, and severe PD. The ICD-11 scale is to be based on interpersonal functioning only, without a self functioning component. However, recent research has demonstrated that self pathology adds incremental validity over interpersonal pathology in predicting overall severity of personality pathology [24], suggesting that the AMPD approach to characterizing severity may ultimately prove to be more valid.

In addition to clinician-rated measures (reviewed in [21]), self-report instruments to assess personality functioning also emphasize a self–other perspective. For example, the Severity Indices of Personality Problems (SIPP) [25] measures five domains of personality functioning: identity integration, self-control, relational functioning, social concordance, and responsibility. The General Assessment of Personality Disorder (GAPD) [24] measures self pathology linked to failures in the development of an integrated self system or structure, and interpersonal pathology linked to failures in the capacity for intimacy, attachment, and co-operative behaviour.

## Development and longitudinal course

Temperament can be viewed as personality traits that are present very early in life and appear to have biological origins. One widely studied model of childhood temperament is a three-factor model that includes negative affectivity, extraversion/surgency, and effortful control [26]. These personality trait domains are structurally, hierarchically, and developmentally related to the FFM domains described previously, in that neuroticism and negative affectivity and extraversion and extraversion/surgency are analogous constructs, conscientiousness and agreeableness develop from effortful control, and openness develops from extraversion [5]. So some continuity between basic temperament and personality trait domains seems likely, though relationships remain to be established through more longitudinal research.

Traditionally, personality pathology has not been assessed or diagnosed in children or young adolescents for a variety of reasons—personality was considered to be in flux; some immature attitudes and behaviours are developmentally appropriate, and diagnosis could be stigmatizing. DSM-5 Section II describes the onset of PDs as 'traced back to at least adolescence or early adulthood' and the course to be 'stable and of long duration' [7, p. 647]. However, other than ASPD, which has a minimum age of 18 years, PDs according to DSM-5 can be diagnosed in children or adolescents if an 'individual's particular maladaptive personality *traits* [italics added] appear to be pervasive, persistent, and unlikely to be limited to a particular developmental stage' [7, p. 647]. Most mental disorders have an onset in some form in childhood or adolescence, and homotypic and heterotypic continuity characterize the course of psychopathology across the lifespan [27].

Dimensional approaches to conceptualization and measurement of pathological personality in children are being developed. A model including emotional instability, introversion, compulsivity, and disagreeableness has been proposed [28]. Child clinical researchers often advocate for assessing adolescents for personality pathology, and some have specifically endorsed the DSM-5 AMPD as an approach preferable to the standard categorical approach [29, 30]. The structure of four of the five AMPD trait domains—negative affectivity, detachment, antagonism, and disinhibition—has been replicated many times in adolescents. In addition to a trait dimensional approach, incorporation of a self–other dimension to distinguish personality from PD has been endorsed, in order to better understand the processes involved in the development of personality pathology [30]. Social adaptation and emotional regulation depend on the presence of a realistic and stable sense of self, and gratifying, supportive, and maturation-promoting interpersonal relationships depend on accurate perceptions of others.

The context in which a young person's personality develops is critical. Children and young adults are at increased risk for developing personality pathology if they have experienced physical, sexual, or verbal abuse or neglect in childhood. The personality profiles of mistreated children are characterized by high neuroticism, low agreeableness, low conscientiousness, and low openness to experience—a profile of maladaptive personality very similar to that reflecting PD in adulthood—which tend to persist [31]. Child and adolescent psychopathology of other types, such as depressive, anxiety, and disruptive behaviour disorders, have been shown in longitudinal studies to predispose to the development of personality pathology in adolescents and young adults. Even according to the categorical approach to the diagnosis of personality pathology in children, research has shown that although rates of PD features decrease over time, children who report higher rates are more likely to have PDs in young adulthood and to suffer from a host of other mental disorders and psychosocial problems. Thus, the identification of personality pathology in children and adolescents presents an opportunity for early intervention to prevent future adverse consequences.

Certain critical developmental periods are implicated in the genesis of personality pathology. Abnormal attachment to a primary caregiver, due to either separation or poor parenting, has been observed. Disrupted attachment early in life is likely to lead to impairments in emotional regulation and self-control [32]. Temperamentally high stress-reactivity in a child may itself contribute to problematic attachment. In adolescence, the development of a stable identity or sense of self is a major task and, when delayed or impeded, may lead to the development of personality pathology. In early adulthood, transitions such as leaving home, becoming economically self-sufficient, and being intimately involved with people outside of the family of origin are important developmental tasks. As a consequence, personality pathology often becomes evident when young people attempt these transitions.

Traditional PD diagnostic criteria have poor face validity in later life, because they often refer to occupational or interpersonal activities that may no longer be relevant to older adults. The few longitudinal studies of PDs over the lifespan suggest a drop in PD prevalence in older adults, but it is not known how much this finding is dependent on inapplicable criteria. Some argue that personality traits are generally stable across age, with slight decreases in (FFM) neuroticism, extraversion, and openness, and slight increases in agreeableness and conscientiousness. Trait expression in later life might, however, be a function not only of underlying neurobiology, but also of different (from youth) contextual factors varying over the lifespan. Thus, the degree of social, physical, occupational, or economic stress experienced by an individual over time may determine how stable or unstable personality appears [30].

Dimensional approaches to the conceptualization of personality pathology are appropriate for the study of development and longitudinal course, since change is a matter of degree and behaviours, such as excessive dependency or obstinacy, that are developmentally appropriate at certain ages but become inappropriate at other ages. Viewed developmentally, personality pathology may be considered a manifestation of delayed or obstructed development [33]. Recent rigorous prospective longitudinal studies have shown that PDs are much less stable over time than are implied in the traditional DSM conceptualization [34, 35]. However, certain features of PD are more stable than others [36], perhaps because the severity of core personality pathology can fluctuate over time, related to situational or contextual factors, while the basic personality trait structure for any given individual may be more stable. Most studies of personality traits have shown that they change gradually over the lifespan until individuals reach the age of 50 [37]. In a clinical population, the stability of personality traits, as measured by the FFM (normal) or Schedule for Nonadaptive and Adaptive Personality (SNAP) (normal and pathological) models, was significantly higher than the stability of DSM-IV PD symptoms (that is, criteria) over 10 years of follow-up, suggesting that, from a longitudinal perspective, 'traits reflect basic tendencies that are stable and pervasive across situations, whereas ... [PD] symptoms reflect characteristic maladaptations that are a function of both basic tendencies and environmental dynamics' [38]. DSM-5 AMPD personality traits have been shown to be highly stable, to be prospectively predictive of psychosocial functioning, and to be dynamically associated with functioning over time [39]. In the Collaborative Longitudinal Personality Study (CLPS) sample, general PD features representing 'disorder' severity exhibited less stability than specific features representing 'style', consistent with the notion that personality functioning is the more dynamic and changeable aspect of personality pathology, while personality traits are stable [40].

## Impact on health and psychosocial functioning

### Physical health

PDs are known to have associations with a wide range of physical health disorders. In the National Epidemiological Survey on Alcohol and Related Conditions (NESARC), PDs within clusters A, B, and C were associated with multiple physical conditions, including cardiovascular disease, arthritis, diabetes, and gastrointestinal conditions [41]. The occurrence of physical disorders with a wide range of PDs suggests common underlying factors (that is, core dimensions) at work. From a review of population-based studies in England, Wales, Scotland, Western Europe, Norway, Australia, and the United States, Quirk and colleagues [42] concluded that the bulk of evidence supports associations between PDs from clusters A and B and cardiovascular disease and arthritis. As a result, PDs increase health care utilization, particularly in primary care. Individuals with PD have reduced life expectancy [43], with all-cause mortality predicted by alcohol and drug abuse, physical illness, and functional impairment [44].

Considerable evidence indicates that broad personality trait domains, such as neuroticism (that is, negative affectivity), adversely affect physical health and the quality and longevity of life [45]. In recent years, neuroticism has been found to be associated with asthma [46], obesity [47], Alzheimer's disease [48], and coronary heart disease [49]. Low conscientiousness (that is, disinhibition) has been found to increase the risk of diabetes [50] and risk of death [51].

The trait domain of conscientiousness appears to be protective against a number of physical conditions, possibly related to a more favourable inflammatory profile [52]. A meta-personality factor of 'stability', consisting of high conscientiousness, high agreeableness, and low neuroticism is associated with reduced cardiometabolic risk, an association that was mediated by inflammation, autonomic function, and physical activity [53]. Lower-order FFM personality trait facets of straightforwardness, self-discipline, altruism, compliance, tender-mindedness, and openness to fantasy are associated with increases in life survival time [54].

### Psychosocial functioning

All PDs, by definition, are maladaptive and accompanied by functional problems in school or at work, in social relationships, or at leisure. The requirement for impairment in psychosocial functioning is codified in DSM-5 Section II in its criterion C of the general diagnostic criteria for a PD, which states that 'the enduring pattern [of inner experience and behaviour, that is, personality] leads to clinically significant distress or impairment in social, occupational, or other important areas of functioning' [7, p. 646].

A number of studies have compared patients with PDs to those with no PD or with DSM-IV axis I disorders and have found that patients with PDs were more likely to be functionally impaired [55]. Specifically, they are more likely to be separated, divorced, or never married and to have had more unemployment, frequent job changes, or periods of disability. Fewer studies have examined quality of functioning, but in those that have, poorer social functioning or interpersonal relationships and poorer work functioning or occupational achievement and satisfaction have been found among patients with PDs than with other disorders. When patients with different PDs were compared with each other on levels of functional impairment, those with severe PDs, such as STPD and BPD, were found to have significantly more impairment at work, in social relationships, and at leisure than patients with less severe PDs, such as obsessive–compulsive personality disorder (OCPD), or with an impairing other mental disorder such as major depressive disorder (MDD) without PD. Patients with AVPD had intermediate levels of impairment.

Another important aspect of the impairment in functioning in patients with PDs is that it tends to be persistent, even beyond apparent improvement in PD psychopathology itself [34, 56]. The persistence of impairment is understandable if one considers that PD psychopathology has usually been long-standing and therefore has disrupted a person's work and social development over a period of time [57]. The 'scars' or residua of personality pathology take time to heal or be overcome. With time (and treatment), however, improvements in functioning can occur [35].

DSM-5 Section III criteria for PDs in the AMPD do not include a requirement for impairment in psychosocial functioning. This change is in keeping with some other disorders in DSM-5, which attempted to separate the manifestations of a disorder (that is, signs, symptoms, traits) from their consequences (that is, impact on occupational, social, and leisure functioning). Furthermore, Section III PDs all include specific impairments in *personality functioning* at a moderate level or greater. This change is consistent with the distinction between mental *functions* (for example, emotional regulation, reward dependence, reality testing) that lead to *symptoms* and the *disabilities* that accompany disturbances in these functions [58].

Interpersonal problems are probably most characteristic of people with PDs [59, 60], which, coupled with problems in the sense of self, are captured by the Section III LPFS and the A criteria for the six specific PDs and personality disorder–trait specified (PD-TS). Each of the six PDs has characteristic problems with empathy and intimacy, reflecting fundamental abnormalities in social cognition [61].

People with ASPD deceive and intimidate others for personal gain. Lacking in 'emotional empathy', they have no concern for the feelings of others and fail to express remorse if they hurt someone. In the area of intimacy, they are incapable of having mutually intimate relationships, as they exploit others or control them. Patients with histrionic personality disorder (HPD) and narcissistic personality disorder (NPD) need to be the centre of attention and require excessive admiration. Intimate relationships are generally shallow, and people are sought out primarily to bolster self-esteem. Empathic concerns centre on issues that have direct implications for the person with the PD.

Patients with OCPD have difficulties appreciating others' perspectives and need to control them and to have them submit to their ways of doing things. Intimacy is circumscribed by stubbornness and rigidity and a preference for engaging in tasks, rather than pursuing close relationships.

The interpersonal relationships of patients with AVPD and DPD are impoverished as a result of fear and submissiveness, respectively. Patients with AVPD are inhibited in interpersonal relationships because they are afraid of being shamed or ridiculed. Empathy is impaired because of a distorted sense of others' appraisal and an acute sensitivity to rejection. Patients with DPD will not disagree with important others for fear of losing their support or approval and will actually do things that are unpleasant, demeaning, or self-defeating in order to receive nurturance from them. With the self-sacrificing approach to relationships, real intimacy and empathy are elusive.

The empathy of patients with BPD is distorted and typically biased towards the negative tendencies and vulnerabilities of others. Intimate relationships are extremely challenging, with a pattern of becoming 'deeply' involved and dependent only to turn manipulative and demanding when their needs are not met. They have interpersonal relationships that are unstable and conflicted, and they alternate between over-involvement with others and withdrawal from them.

The degree of detachment associated with patients with paranoid PD, schizoid PD, and STPD serves as a pronounced impediment to empathy and intimacy in interpersonal relationships. Patients with schizoid PD manifest an apparent lack of need for closeness with others; people with paranoid PD do not trust others enough to become deeply involved; and patients with STPD have few friends or confidants, in part due to a lack of trust and in part as a result of poor communication and inadequate relatedness.

In addition to these core personality functions, personality traits have been found to predict concurrent and prospective function in psychiatric patients [62], with some specificity across different traits. Within the FFM traits, neuroticism was broadly related to impairment across the domains of social, occupational, and recreational functioning. Extraversion (low) was primarily related to social and recreational dysfunction, openness (low) to recreational dysfunction, agreeableness (low) to social dysfunction, and conscientiousness (low) to work dysfunction. Ro and Clark [63] compared adaptive-range traits to non-adaptive range traits in patient and non-patient samples and found that psychosocial functioning and personality traits were closely linked, particularly in patients. General well-being was negatively associated with neuroticism/ negative affectivity and positively associated with extraversion/ positive affectivity; social/interpersonal functioning was associated with dis(agreeableness) and with conscientiousness/disinhibition, and basic functioning was associated with conscientiousness/ disinhibition.

Simms and Calabrese [64] found that Section III pathological personality traits incrementally predicted psychosocial impairment over normal-range personality traits, PD criteria counts, and common psychiatric symptoms. In contrast, the incremental effects of normal traits, PD criteria counts, and common symptoms were substantially smaller than for pathological personality traits. In the CLPS follow-along [65], PD criteria counts were strongly associated with impairment in psychosocial functioning at intake (more strongly than categorical PD diagnoses), but this relationship diminished over time. The best predictors longitudinally of impairment were models that combined normative traits and maladaptive variables (that is, the SNAP model or a model composed of a DSM-IV PD criteria count and FFM domains). At 6-, 8-, and 10-year follow-ups, the SNAP continued to be the most predictive and DSM PD criteria and FFM domains tended to provide substantial incremental validity to one another, supporting a hybrid model [66]. Also, in the CLPS sample, general PD features representing 'disorder' severity were more strongly related to psychosocial functioning concurrently and prospectively than specific features representing personality 'style' [40].

## Clinical utility

In the official DSM-5 Field Trials, clinicians were asked to rate the usefulness of tested diagnostic criteria for all disorders. In both the Academic Centers and the Routine Clinical Practice Field Trials [67], the Section III PD model was rated as 'moderately', 'very', or 'extremely' useful by over 80% of clinicians. In the Academic Centers trial, more clinicians rated the Section III model as 'very' or 'extremely' useful, compared to DSM-IV than all disorders, except somatic symptom disorders and feeding and eating disorders. In the Routine Clinical Practice trial, the Section III model was more often rated as 'very' or 'extremely' useful, compared to DSM-IV than all disorders, except neurocognitive disorders and substance use and addictive disorders. In a separate investigation, Morey and colleagues [68] asked clinicians to rate the perceived utility of the proposed DSM-5 rendering of personality pathology, compared to DSM-IV. Questions addressed ease of use and usefulness for communication, patient description, and treatment planning. Although the clinicians were much more familiar with DSM-IV PDs, they rated all DSM-5 components generally as 'useful' or 'more useful' than DSM-IV for clinical description and treatment planning. Other than in ease of use and communication with other professionals, the LPFS was rated by clinicians as more useful than DSM-IV for patient description, communicating with patients about their problems, and treatment planning. Furthermore, the DSM-5 pathological trait system was rated by both psychiatrists and psychologists as easier to use and more useful for communication with other clinicians and with patients, for patient description, and for planning treatment than the DSM-IV conceptualization.

In addition to perceived utility, self interpersonal problems, such as insecure attachment and maladaptive schemas, have been shown to be associated significantly with PD psychopathology and impairments in psychosocial functioning, as well as to affect clinical outcome [3]. Self–other dimensions have discriminated different types of PD pathology, predicted various areas of psychosocial functioning, and have shown to be moderators of treatment alliance and outcome. In the Morey and colleagues' survey [23], the single-item LPFS rating predicted variance in clinician ratings of psychosocial functioning, prognosis, and treatment needs over and above that predicted by all ten DSM-IV PD diagnoses combined (that is, diagnoses based on 79 total criteria).

In addition to the independent utility of pathological personality traits and of personality functioning in identifying and describing personality pathology and in planning and predicting the outcome of treatment, a number of recent studies support a model of personality psychopathology that specifically combines ratings of disorder and trait constructs. Each has been shown to add incremental value to the other in predicting important antecedent (for example, family history, history of child abuse), concurrent (for example, functional impairment, medication use), and predictive (for example, functioning, hospitalization, suicide attempts) variables [65, 66, 69, 70].

## Dimensions and personality disorder subtypes

Each of the 'official' DSM-5 PDs can be characterized by specific impairments in personality functioning and by pathological personality traits in one or more of the DSM-5 trait domains of negative affectivity, detachment, antagonism, disinhibition, and psychoticism. Some of the simpler PDs have traits in only one domain. DPD can be described by three traits in the negative affectivity domain: submissiveness, separation insecurity, and anxiousness. Schizoid PD can be described by four traits in the detachment domain: withdrawal, intimacy avoidance, anhedonia, and restricted affectivity. Some of the more complex PDs have traits in more than one domain. Complexity in clinical presentation is also reflected by the common co-occurrence of categorical PDs with each other and with other mental disorders. Co-occurring disorders frequently, though not always, come from the same psychopathological spectrum or trait domain.

The DSM-5 alternative model includes six specific PDs—ASPD, AVPD, BPD, NPD, OCPD, and STPD—selected because of their empirical bases or their utility for clinicians [71, 72]. All PDs are required to have at least moderate impairment in personality functioning, according to the DSM-5 AMPD, because a moderate level of impairment has been empirically shown to identify PDs with maximal combined sensitivity and specificity.

PD trait domain and facet assignments were made on the basis of existing meta-analyses of FFM/PD relationships [73–75], with corroboration from data provided by clinicians that were gathered to inform the process [76]. In analyses of 33 data sets, O'Connor [73] found that DPD, AVPD, and BPD had high loadings on a factor resembling FFM neuroticism; antisocial, NPD, paranoid PD, and HPD loaded on a factor of low agreeableness; schizoid PD, STPD, AVPD, paranoid PD, and HPD (a negative loading) loaded on low extraversion, and OCPD loaded on conscientiousness. In terms of the DSM-5 trait model, these four factors would be represented by negative affectivity, antagonism, detachment, and low disinhibition, respectively.

In Morey and colleagues' study [76], ASPD was associated with traits from the antagonism and disinhibition domains. All seven traits assigned for the diagnosis of ASPD (four from the antagonism

domain and three from the disinhibition domain) had higher correlations with ASPD than any of the remaining traits in the AMPD model. STPD was associated with traits almost exclusively in the psychoticism and detachment domains, and again all six assigned traits had higher correlations with STPD than any of the other traits. BPD showed generally elevated trait associations across the negative affectivity domain, with the highest correlation being with emotional lability. Significant correlations were also found for risk-taking and impulsivity from the disinhibition domain. The two traits assigned to NPD—grandiosity and attention seeking—both had high correlations with the diagnosis. In addition, there were significant correlations with other traits from the antagonism domain such as callousness, manipulativeness, and deceitfulness. These traits of so-called 'malignant narcissism' were not assigned to NPD because to do so resulted in extensive overlap between the diagnoses of NPD and ASPD. Since reducing PD comorbidity was a goal of the AMPD, these traits were included as diagnostic 'specifiers' to be listed when warranted. OCPD had significant correlations with traits from different domains. The four highest correlated traits were assigned. AVPD had significant correlations with anxiousness from negative affectivity and several traits from the detachment domain, which were assigned. For each AMPD-specific disorder, except for STPD, it was shown that clinician ratings on the criterion A impairments in personality functioning significantly incremented the assigned traits in predicting a DSM-IV PD diagnosis, supporting the validity of the AMPD personality functioning and personality trait hybrid dimensional–categorical model.

Each PD also had a diagnostic algorithm for the trait ('B' criterion) developed from the Morey survey [77], consisting of a minimum number of assigned traits and, in some cases, a particular configuration of traits. The algorithm was developed to simultaneously maximize correspondence with DSM-IV PD diagnoses (to be minimally disruptive to clinical practice and research), to minimize overlap with other PD diagnoses (to reduce comorbidity), and to maximize relationships with functional impairment (to increase validity). The algorithms were successful in rendering DSM-IV PD diagnoses according to personality functioning impairments and pathological personality traits, with very good fidelity (correlations between DSM-IV and AMPD dimensional criteria counts for ASPD = 0.80; BPD = 0.80; AVPD = 0.77; NPD = 0.74; STPD = 0.60; OCPD = 0.57). The algorithm for the A criterion for specific PDs according to the alternative model of 'characteristic difficulties in any two of four areas' (that is, identity, self-direction, empathy, or intimacy) was found to be associated with the greatest combined sensitivity and specificity across the six specific PDs in the AMPD [77].

According to the AMPD, the other four official PDs in DSM-5, as well as any other PD presentations that would be diagnosed as 'other specified personality disorder' in DSM-5 Section II, may be diagnosed as PD-TS. Both the specific level of impairment (that is, moderate, severe, or extreme) and the specific pathological personality traits that describe the person would be noted.

## Conclusions

The classification and diagnosis of personality pathology has been slowly, but inexorably, moving from a categorical to a dimensional model. A dimensional model better reflects the phenomena of personality pathology, which are continuous in nature, and better describes the degrees of difference from normal personality and the degrees of severity. Core personality dimensions can represent the features that distinguish PDs both from normal personality functioning and from other forms of psychopathology, as well as the myriad manifestations of PD. A general consensus is that the personality trait structure of PD converges on a five-factor model of broad trait domains, with each factor composed of more narrow trait facets. The DSM-5 alternative model for PDs comprises an LPFS to identify PD and its severity and five trait domains of negative affectivity, detachment, antagonism, disinhibition, and psychoticism—the first four of which represent the pathological poles of the five factors of the five-factor model of normal personality—and their component trait facets. Personality traits and personality functioning variables will undoubtedly be more closely related than traditional categories to basic physiological and psychological processes underlying personality pathology. Personality traits and personality functioning have been shown to be associated with physical health problems and impaired psychosocial functioning, to guide treatment planning, and to predict a host of important outcomes. Clinicians find dimensional models more clinically useful than categorical models, despite their newness and unfamiliarity. The future for research and treatment of personality pathology lies in its dimensional conceptualization.

## REFERENCES

1. Haslam N, Holland E, and Kuppens P. Categories versus dimensions in personality and psychopathology: a quantitative review of taxometric research. *Psychol Med* 2012;42:903–20.

2. Bernstein DP, Iscan C, Maser J, *et al.* Opinions of personality disorder experts regarding the DSM-IV personality disorders classification system. *J Pers Disord* 2007;21:536–51.

3. Skodol AE, Bender DS, Oldham JM. An alternative model for personality disorders: DSM-5 section III and beyond. In: Oldham JM, Skodol AE, Bender DS, eds. *The American Psychiatric Publishing Textbook of Personality Disorders*, second edition. Washington DC: American Psychiatric Publishing; 2014. pp. 511–44.

4. Frances A. The DSM-III personality disorders section: a commentary. *Am J Psychiatry* 1980;137:1050–4.

5. Markon KE, Krueger RF, Watson D. Delineating the structure of normal and abnormal personality: An integrative hierarchical approach. *J Pers Soc Psychol* 2005;88:139–57.

6. Keyes KM, Eaton NR, Krueger RF, *et al.* Thought disorder in the meta-structure of psychopathology. *Psychol Med* 2013;43:1673–83.

7. American Psychiatric Association. *Diagnostic and Statistical Manual of Mental Disorders*, fifth edition. Arlington, VA: American Psychiatric Association; 2013.

8. Widiger TA, Simonsen E. Alternative dimensional models of personality disorder: finding a common ground. *J Pers Disord* 2005;19:110–30.

9. Krueger RF, Markon KE. The role of the DSM-5 personality trait model in moving toward a quantitative and empirically based approach to classifying personality and psychopathology. *Annu Rev Clin Psychol* 2014;10:477–501.

10. Eaton NR, Krueger RF, South SC, *et al.* Contrasting prototypes and dimensions in the classification of personality pathology: evidence that dimensions, but not prototypes, are robust. *Psychol Med* 2011;41:1151–63.

11. Krueger RF, Eaton NR, Derringer J, *et al.* Personality in DSM-5: helping delineate personality disorder content and framing the meta-structure. *J Pers Assess* 2011;42:325–31.

12. Markon KE. Modeling psychopathology structure: a symptom-level analysis of axis I and II disorders. *Psychol Med* 2010;40:273–88.

13. Roysamb E, Kendler KS, Tambs, K, *et al.* The joint structure of DSM-IV axis I and axis II disorders. *J Abnorm Psychol* 2011;120:198–209.

14. Wright AGC, Simms LJ. A metastructural model of mental disorders and pathological personality traits. *Psychol Med* 2015;45:2309–19.

15. Tyrer P, Crawford M, Sanatinia R, *et al.* Preliminary studies of the ICD-11 classification of personality disorder in practice. *Personal Ment Health* 2014;8:254–63.

16. Morey LC, Krueger RF, Skodol AE. The hierarchical structure of clinician ratings of DSM-5 pathological personality traits. *J Abnorm Psychol* 2013;122:836–41.

17. Wright AG, Thomas KM, Hopwood CJ, et al. The hierarchical structure of DSM-5 pathological personality traits. *J Abnorm Psychol* 2012;121:951–7.

18. Hyman SE. The diagnosis of mental disorders: the problem of reification. *Ann Rev Clin Psychol* 2010;6:155–79.

19. Morey LC, Bender DS. Articulating a core dimension of personality pathology. In: Oldham JM, Skodol AE, Bender DS, eds. *The American Psychiatric Publishing Textbook of Personality Disorders*, second edition. Washington DC: American Psychiatric Publishing; 2014. pp. 39–54.

20. Morey LC, Gunderson JG, Quigley BD, *et al.* The representation of borderline, avoidant, obsessive-compulsive, and schizotypal personality disorders by the five-factor model. *J Pers Disord* 2002;16:215–34.

21. Bender DS, Morey LC, Skodol AE. Toward a model for assessing level of personality functioning in DSM-5, part I: a review of theory and methods. *J Pers Assess* 2011;93:332–46.

22. Morey LC, Berghuis H, Bender DS, *et al.* Toward a model for assessing level of personality functioning in DSM-5, part II: empirical articulation of a core dimension of personality pathology. *J Pers Assess* 2011;93:347–53.

23. Morey LC, Bender DS, Skodol AE. Validating the proposed DSM-5 severity indicator for personality disorder. *J Nerv Ment Dis* 2013;201:729–35.

24. Hentschel AN, Livesley WJ. The General Assessment of Personality Disorder (GAPD): factor structure, incremental validity of self pathology, and relations to DSM-IV personality disorders. *J Pers Assess* 2013;95:479–85.

25. Verheul R, Andrea H, Berghout CC, *et al.* Severity Indices of Personality Problems (SIPP-118): development, factor structure, reliability, and validity. *Psychol Assess* 2008;20:23–34.

26. Rothbart MK, Ahadi SA, Hershey K, *et al.* Investigations of temperament at three to seven years: the Children's Behavior Questionnaire. *Child Dev* 2001;72:1394–408.

27. Skodol AE, Bender DS. Psychopathology across the life span. In: Tasman A, Kay J, Lieberman JA, *et al.*, eds. *Psychiatry*, third edition. Chichester: John Wiley and Sons; 2008. pp. 487–524.

28. De Clerq B, De Fruyt F, Widiger TA. Integrating a developmental perspective in dimensional models of personality disorder. *Clin Psychol Rev* 2009;29:154–62.

29. Shiner RL, Allen TA. Seven guiding principles for assessing personality disorders in adolescents. *Clin Psychol Sci Prac* 2013;20:361–77.

30. Tackett JL, Balsis S, Oltmanns TF, *et al.* A unifying perspective on personality pathology across the lifespan: developmental considerations for the fifth edition of the Diagnostic and Statistical Manual of Mental Disorders. *Dev Psychopathology* 2009;21:687–713.

31. Rogosch FA, Cicchetti D. Childhood maltreatment and emergent personality organization: perspective from the five-factor model. *J Abnorm Child Psychol* 2004;32:123–45.

32. Fonagy P, Bateman A. The development of borderline personality disorder—a mentalizing model. *J Pers Disord* 2008;22:4–21.

33. Cohen P, Crawford T. Developmental issues. In: Oldham JM, Skodol AE, Bender DS, eds. *The American Psychiatric Publishing Textbook of Personality Disorders*. Washington, DC: American Psychiatric Publishing; 2005. pp. 171–85.

34. Gunderson JG, Stout RL, McGlashan TH, et al. Ten-year course of borderline personality disorder: psychopathology and functioning from the Collaborative Longitudinal Personality Disorders Study. *Arch Gen Psychiatry* 2011;68:827–37.

35. Zanarini MC, Frankenburg FR, Reich DB, et al. Attainment and stability of sustained symptomatic remission and recovery among patients with borderline personality disorder and axis II comparison subjects: a 16-year prospective follow-up study. *Am J Psychiatry* 2012;169:476–83.

36. Morey LC, Hopwood CJ. Stability and change in personality disorders. *Annu Rev Clin Psychol* 2013;9:499–528.

37. Roberts BW, DelVecchio WF. The rank-order consistency of personality traits from childhood to old age: a quantitative review of longitudinal studies. *Psychol Bull* 2000;126:3–25.

38. Hopwood CJ, Morey LC, Donnellan MB, et al. Ten year rank-order stability of personality traits and disorders in a clinical sample. *J Pers* 2013;81:335–44.

39. Wright AGC, Calabrese WR, Rudnick MM, et al. Stability of the DSM-5 section III pathological personality traits and their longitudinal associations with psychosocial functioning in personality disordered individuals. *J Abnorm Psychol* 2015;124:199–207.

40. Wright AGC, Hopwood CJ, Skodol AE, et al. Longitudinal validation of general and specific structural features of personality pathology. *J Abnorm Psychol* 2016;125:1120–34.

41. Quirk SE, El-Gabalawy R, Brennan SL, et al. Personality disorders and physical comorbidities in adults in the United States: data from the National Epidemiologic Survey on Alcohol and Related Conditions. *Soc Psychiatry Psychiatr Epidemiol* 2015;50:807–20.

42. Quirk SE, Berk M, Chanen AM, et al. Population prevalence of personality disorder and associations with physical health comorbidities and health care utilization: a review. *Personal Disord* 2016;7:136–46.

43. Fok ML, Hayes RD, Chang CK, et al. Life expectancy at birth and all-cause mortality among people with personality disorder. *J Psychosom Res* 2012;73:104–7.

44. Fok ML, Stewart R, Hayes RD, et al. Predictors of natural and unnatural mortality among patients with personality disorder: evidence from a large UK case register. *PLoS One* 2014;9:e100979.

45. Lahey BB. Public health significance of neuroticism. *Am Psychol* 2009;64:241–56.

46. Loerbroks A, Li J, Bosch JA, et al. Personality and risk of adult asthma in a prospective cohort study. *J Psychosom Res* 2015;79:13–17.

47. Gerlach G, Herpertz S, Loeber S. Personality traits and obesity: a systematic review. *Obes Rev* 2015;16:32–63.

48. Johansson L, Guo X, Duberstein PR, et al. Midlife personality and risk of Alzheimer disease and distress: a 38-year follow-up. *Neurology* 2014;83:1538–44.

49. Jokela M, Pulkki-Raback L, Elovainio M, et al. Personality traits as risk factors for stroke and coronary heart disease mortality: pooled analysis of three cohort studies. *J Behav Med* 2014;37:881–9.

50. Jokela M, Elovainio M, Nyberg ST, et al. Personality traits and risk of diabetes in adults: a pooled analysis of 5 cohort studies. *Health Psychol* 2014;33:1618–21.

51. Jokela M, Batty GD, Nyberg ST, et al. Personality and all-cause mortality: individual-participant meta-analysis of 3,947 deaths in 76,150 adults. *Am J Epidemiol* 2013;178:667–75.

52. Luchetti M, Barkley JM, Stephan Y, et al. Five-factor model personality traits and inflammatory markers: new data and a meta-analysis. *Psychoneuroendocrinology* 2014;50:181–93.

53. Dermody SS, Wright AG, Cheong J, et al. Personality correlates of midlife cardiometabolic risk: the explanatory role of higher-order factors of the five-factor model. *J Pers* 2016;84:765–76.

54. Costa PT Jr, Weiss A, Duberstein PR, et al. Personality facets and all-cause mortality among Medicare patients aged 66–102 years: a follow-along study of Weiss and Costa (2005). *Psychosom Med* 2014;76:370–8.

55. Skodol AE, Bender DS, Gunderson JG, et al. Personality disorders. In: Hales RE, Yudofsky SC, Roberts LW, eds. *American Psychiatric Publishing Textbook of Psychiatry*, sixth edition. Arlington, VA: American Psychiatric Publishing; 2014. pp. 851–94.

56. Skodol AE, Pagano ME, Bender DS, et al. Stability of functional impairment in patients with schizotypal, borderline, avoidant, or obsessive-compulsive personality disorder over two years. *Psychol Med* 2005;35:443–51.

57. Roberts BW, Caspi A, Moffitt TE. Work experiences and personality development in young adulthood. *J Pers Soc Psychol* 2003;84:582–93.

58. Sartorius N. Disability and mental illness are different entities and should be assessed separately. *World Psychiatry* 2009;8:86.

59. Gunderson JG. Disturbed relationships as a phenotype for borderline personality disorder. *Am J Psychiatry* 2007;164:1637–40.

60. Hill J, Pilkonis P, Morse J, et al. Social domain dysfunction and disorganization in borderline personality disorder. *Psychol Med* 2008;38:135–46.

61. Herpertz SC, Bertsch K. The social-cognitive basis of personality disorders. *Curr Opin Psychiatry* 2014;27:73–7.

62. Hopwood CJ, Morey LC, Ansell EB, et al. The convergent and discriminant validity of five-factor traits: current and prospective social, work, and recreational dysfunction. *J Pers Disord* 2009;23:466–76.

63. Ro E, Clark LA. Interrelations between psychosocial functioning and adaptive- and maladaptive-range personality traits. *J Abnorm Psychol* 2013;122:822–35.

64. Simms LJ, Calabrese WR. Incremental validity of the DSM-5 section III personality disorder traits with respect to psychosocial impairment. *J Pers Disord* 2016;30:95–111.

65. Morey LC, Hopwood CJ, Gunderson JG, et al. Comparison of alternative models for personality disorders. *Psychol Med* 2007;37:983–94.

66. Morey LC, Hopwood CJ, Markowitz JC, et al. Comparison of alternative models for personality disorders, II: 6-, 8- and 10-year follow-up. *Psychol Med* 2012;42:1705–13.

67. Kraemer HC, Kupfer DJ, Narrow WE, et al. Moving toward DSM-5: the field trials. *Am J Psychiatry* 2010;167:1058–60.

68. Morey LC, Skodol AE, Oldham JM. Clinicians' judgments of clinical utility: a comparison of DSM-IV-TR personality disorders and the alternative model for DSM-5 personality disorders. *J Abnorm Psychol* 2014;123:398–405.

69. Hopwood CJ, Zanarini MC. Borderline personality traits and disorder: predicting prospective patient functioning. *J Consult Clin Psychol* 2010;78:585–9.

70. Morey LC, Zanarini MC. Borderline personality: traits and disorder. *J Abnorm Psychol* 2000;109:733–7.

71. Skodol AE, Bender DS, Morey LC, et al. Personality disorder types proposed for DSM-5. *J Pers Disord* 2011;25:136–69.

72. Skodol AE, Bender DS, Morey LC. Narcissistic personality disorder in DSM-5. *Pers Disord* 2014;5:422–7.

73. O'Connor BP. A search for consensus on the dimensional structure of personality disorders. *J Clin Psychol* 2005;61:323–45.

74. Saulsman LM, Page AC. The five-factor model and personality disorder empirical literature: a meta-analytic review. *Clin Psychol Rev* 2004;23:1055–85.

75. Samuel DB, Widiger TA. A meta-analytic review of the relationship between the five-factor model and DSM-IV-TR

personality disorders: a facet level analysis. *Clin Psychol Rev* 2008;28:1326–42.

76. Morey LC, Benson KT, Skodol AE. Relating DSM-5 section III personality traits to section II personality disorder diagnoses. *Psychol Med* 2016;46:647–55.

77. Morey LC, Skodol AE. Convergence between DSM-IV and DSM-5 diagnostic models for personality disorder: evaluation of strategies for establishing diagnostic thresholds. *J Psychiatr Pract* 2013;19:179–93.

# 118

# Basic mechanisms of, and treatment planning/targets for, personality disorders

*Kate E. A. Saunders and Steve Pearce*

## Introduction

Personality disorders are a group of disorders characterized by a pervasive set of feelings and behaviours that impair an individual's ability to function. Even when standardized approaches are employed by highly trained clinicians, the consistency of diagnosis between different clinicians is highly variable [1]. Many commentators argue that this is inevitable because current diagnostic classifications are fundamentally flawed; their explanation is that personality dysfunction is a continuum and comorbidity between the different classes is ubiquitous [2]. This debate is not unique to personality disorder, and there is increasingly a move away from observational approaches to a more integrated approach where multiple sources of information are assimilated to better understand the basic dimensions of functioning underlying the full range of human behaviour, from normal to abnormal [3]. For personality disorder, this tension between dimensional and categorical approaches to diagnosis, in combination with the dominant role of psychoanalytic and behavioural models in treatment development, has resulted in a relative paucity of research into underlying neurobiology, cognitive psychology, or physiology. As a result, evidence-based treatment targets are few and based upon a small number of studies. The interpretation of the existing literature is limited by the internal heterogeneity of each specific personality disorder, a lack of consistency in the approach to diagnosis, axis I and II comorbidity, female gender bias, small sample sizes, and cross-sectional approaches. Borderline personality disorder (BPD) has been the focus of the majority of research in personality disorder, although there is some literature on antisocial personality disorder (ASPD) and schizotypal personality disorder (SPD). Studies of other personality disorders are too few in number to draw any firm conclusions about the mechanisms or treatment targets. In this chapter, we will review the current evidence for the basic mechanisms for personality disorder, relevant to treatment development, as well as review what current treatments reveal about potential treatment targets.

## Neurobiologic targets

The neurobiology of personality disorder is poorly understood, and it seems unlikely that any of the disorders relate to the impairment of a single neurotransmitter system. This may, in part, relate to the inherent heterogeneity of personality disorder diagnoses, but also to the fact that the disorders emerge as a result of biological vulnerability in combination with environmental influences. However, the underlying neurobiology does provide useful insights into how/why personality disorders develop, and targeting specific neurotransmitter systems may lead to symptomatic relief and enhance the efficacy of existing psychological treatments. Biological approaches are widely used in the treatment of personality disorder, and there is evidence to support the role of a number of neurotransmitter systems.

### Serotonergic system

There is considerable evidence implicating serotonin in personality disorder. Serotonin regulates amygdala hyperreactivity in BPD, thought to be a central neurobiological correlate of affective instability [4]. It has been proposed that the imbalance between prefrontal and limbic responsivity may relate to impaired serotonergic facilitation of top–down control [5]. Polymorphisms in the genes for the 5-HT2 receptor, tryptophan hydroxylase, and the serotonin transport promoter are all found to be associated with BPD [6, 7], although these findings have not been replicated. However, there is more convincing evidence that gene–environment interactions are of greater relevance, with some studies suggesting that these genes mediate the impact of exposure to childhood trauma in BPD [8, 9]. The serotonin transporter gene is also associated with ASPD [10], and methylation of this gene has been shown to mediate the impact of childhood sexual abuse in ASPD [11]. Variants of monoamine oxidase (MAO), which metabolizes dopamine and serotonin, are also thought to have a role in the development of antisocial traits and again are implicated in outcomes following adverse events in childhood [12]. Positron emission tomography (PET) studies indicate that there is reduced serotonin transporter availability in the prefrontal cortex in BPD, compared with healthy controls [13]. Blunted hormonal responses to serotonergic agonists, such as fenfluramine and meta-chlorpiperazine, have been observed in BPD [14, 15], and this blunting is associated with impulsivity, anger, and self-harm, but not the social or affective components of the disorder. Increased impulse aggression has also been shown to be associated with reduced prolactin release in response to fenfluramine in obsessive–compulsive personality disorder (OCPD) [16]. These findings are consistent with preclinical studies where reductions in serotonergic activity are found to be associated with aggression [17]. Fluoxetine (a selective serotonin reuptake inhibitor) has been shown to increase the metabolic rate in the orbitofrontal cortex and to significantly improve symptoms in individuals with aggressive–impulsive personalities [18].

Despite there being considerable evidence for a role of the serotonergic system in personality disorder, there is no convincing evidence that treatment with serotonergic drugs is associated with significant or sustained improvement in symptom profiles in clinical trials [19]. This may relate to a lack of serotonin receptor specificity (impulsivity is associated with 5-HT2a, not 5-HT2c, antagonism), the complexity of the interactions between different receptor systems associated with behavioural outcomes, and the need for targeting specific brain regions [20].

### Dopaminergic system

The dopamine system has been a target of interest in SPD because of its similarity to psychotic disorders. SPD has been found to be associated with the catechol-O-methyltransferase enzyme (COMT), the D4 receptor, and dopamine beta-hydroxylase genes. Decreased dopaminergic activity in the prefrontal cortex has been observed, but there appears to be evidence of compensatory activation in other regions, such as the striatum, suggesting that individuals with SPD may have greater buffering of subcortical dopaminergic activity than that found in those with schizophrenia [21, 22]. Homovanillic acid, a proxy for dopamine levels in the brain, has been found to be elevated in both plasma [23] and the cerebrospinal fluid (CSF) [24] in SPD. SPD is associated with enhanced dopamine release in response to amphetamine [25], and both amphetamine and pergolide have been shown to improve cognitive performance [26, 27].

Use of drugs for psychosis in personality disorder is widespread [28, 29]. In a recent systematic review of their use in SPD, there was little evidence found to support it [30]. In BPD, one meta-analysis concluded that dopamine antagonists were associated with worsening of symptom severity [19]. However, there is some evidence supporting reductions in symptom severity in BPD associated with olanzapine [31, 32], quetiapine [33], and aripiprazole [34]. Ziprasidone has not proved to be efficacious in BPD, despite having a similar pharmacological profile to aripiprazole [35].

### Oxytocin

Given the centrality of interpersonal dysfunction to all personality disorders, and particularly BPD, there has been an increasing focus on oxytocin, a prosocial neuropeptide. The precise mechanism by which oxytocin exerts this effect is unknown, but there is substantial evidence in non-clinical groups that it promotes empathy, trust, and social reward [36]. There is some evidence to support the moderating role of alleles of the oxytocin receptor (OXTR) coding gene in the development of BPD symptoms, following childhood adversity [37]. There is also evidence that methylation of OXTR genes occurs rapidly after exposure to stress [38], suggesting that oxytocin may play a role in enhanced stress sensitivity found in BPD. Reduced CSF and serum oxytocin levels have been found to be associated with BPD symptoms [39]; however, these findings are not specific to BPD. It may therefore be oversimplistic to consider BPD as a disorder uniquely characterized by low oxytocin levels. Studies of the impact of oxytocin in BPD indicate that while it downregulates stress responses to social threat [40], it is not associated with increased no-verbal affiliative behaviour observed in healthy controls [41]. In another study, BPD subjects given intranasal oxytocin were found to show less co-operative behaviour while playing the assurance game (a variant of the classic prisoner's dilemma) and described higher levels of attachment anxiety [42]. Striepens et al. have proposed a paradoxical effect of oxytocin in BPD; while oxytocin may downregulate amygdala reactivity to aversive stimuli [43], it may also increase insular responses to negative stimuli, enhancing the defensive impact of negative social cues [44]. It could be that individuals with BPD experience the prosocial effects of oxytocin as aversive, given the association of the insula with the processing of complex negative emotions.

Given the conflicting evidence about the effects of oxytocin in BPD, its role in treatment remains unclear. However, all studies to date have used single doses of oxytocin and explored the possibility that BPD may be associated with dysfunctional oxytocin regulation or that the prosocial effects of oxytocin may heighten entrenched anxieties and fears about trust and attachment. Despite these uncertainties, oxytocin represents a potential treatment for the core dysfunction in BPD. Some authors have suggested that oxytocin may facilitate the learning of new relational strategies in combination with psychological interventions [42], while others have proposed that it may allow the intergenerational cycle of dysfunction to be broken [36].

### Opioids

Brain opioids play an important role in mediating the social impact of isolation and exclusion [45]. There is evidence to support the dysfunction of the endogenous opioid system (EOS) in both BPD [46] and ASPD [47], and it has been proposed that reduced EOS activity may underpin the chronic dysphoria associated with BPD [48]. It has also been suggested that self-harm represents an unconscious drive to increase EOS activity [48]. PET studies showed evidence of mu-opioid receptor binding dysfunction [46], and lower levels of endogenous opioids have been reported in the CSF of individuals with BPD [49]. To date, there have been no randomized controlled trials of opioid antagonists, but a small number of open-label studies [50, 51] in BPD suggested that targeting the EOS may be a potential treatment strategy.

The glutamatergic system has been proposed as a potential treatment target, given the role of N-methyl-D-aspartate (NMDA) in mediating a range of psychiatric symptoms and on the basis that excessive glutamatergic activity contributes to hypersensitivity of the limbic system associated with BPD [52]. There is little direct evidence directly linking personality disorders with glutamatergic dysfunction, but a randomized trial of an NMDA receptor antagonist in BPD is ongoing [53].

## Symptom-based targets

Factor analysis of the diagnostic criteria for borderline personality disorder has consistently revealed three factors: affective dysregulation, behavioural dysregulation, and interpersonal disturbances.

### Mood instability

Affective dysregulation has long been viewed as the core source of dysfunction in BPD. Recent technological developments enabling prospective real-time monitoring have confirmed this observation [54]. Although mood instability is common in other mental disorders, the high temporal frequency and characteristics observed in BPD appear to be distinct and specific to the disorder [54, 55]. Some of the most consistent neuroanatomical findings in BPD are those of reduced volumes in the amygdala, hippocampus, orbitofrontal cortex, and anterior cingulate cortex [56, 57]. These are all areas of the brain involved in emotional regulation. Multiple studies revealed decreased activation in prefrontal areas in response to emotional stimuli, suggesting that top–down emotional control may be impaired [58]. Psychophysiological studies also indicate abnormal emotional regulation in BPD [59]. Mood regulation forms one of the central components of a number of psychotherapies, and there is some limited evidence that existing treatments may reduce mood instability, although this is limited to single-study estimates of effect [60]. Specific emotion regulation training has not been found to be effective, although this may relate to short study duration [61]. While mood instability is often used as an outcome measure in trials of treatments for BPD, few studies have employed objective longitudinal measurement of mood; rather mood instability has been assessed using one-off questionnaires and items from the Structured Clinical Interview for DSM-IV Axis II personality disorders (SCID-II). Mood instability remains an important treatment target, and there is a need for large, high-quality studies using objective longitudinal measures of mood.

### Interpersonal disturbance

Social dysfunction is a prominent and pervasive feature in BPD. Impairments in social functioning are well documented in BPD and persist despite remission of other symptoms, both in children who meet criteria for borderline pathology [62] and in adults [63].

Interpersonal difficulties have been linked to impairments in decoding social signals, such as facial expressions [64], and deeper problems with trusting the motives and behaviours of others [65, 66]. Individuals with BPD appeared to lack the capacity to sustain mutually beneficial interactions with playing partners in an investment-trust game [67] and showed patterns of reduced co-operation when compared to those with bipolar disorder or healthy controls in an iterated prisoner's dilemma game [68]. In this latter study, trait aggression, hostility, and impulsivity were not found to account for the failure to co-operate; instead it was proposed that in BPD, the experience of co-operation may not be coded or experienced as rewarding and consequently cannot provide a basis for sustained future co-operation. However, in real life, decisions rarely involve interactions with one individual. To date, no one has systematically studied the responses of individuals with BPD in a group context or which factors are most influential. Given that almost all

current treatment modalities involve group treatments, enhancing our understanding of group behaviour may assist in identifying potential specific treatment targets relating to social function.

### Behavioural disturbance

Behavioural disturbance is common to all personality disorders but has been most widely studied in BPD and ASPD. Reactive aggression has been consistently described in ASPD and is associated with dysfunctional representation of the cost of aggressive behaviour and the failure of inhibitory mechanisms in response to the distress of the victim [69]. In BPD, prefrontal activation is diminished, when compared to non-aggressive healthy controls, and there is evidence of decoupling of orbitofrontal–amygdala responses in BPD, suggesting a failure of top–down control leading to more rapid escalation of angry responses to angry faces [70]. However, these findings are not specific to personality disorders, and to date, interventions specifically directly targeting aggression have been unsuccessful.

### What can we learn from effective treatments?

While there is evidence for pharmacological targets in personality disorders, the rationale for the use of medications is largely based on observed symptom control, although this is not supported by any randomized controlled trials of adequate size, observational data are poor, and studies have generally been limited by short treatment duration and inadequate follow-up time. The one independent randomized trial of a reasonable size found no beneficial effect in the use of lamotrigine in BPD [71].

In contrast, there are a wide range of psychosocial interventions that appear to be effective, in particular in BPD. The majority of randomized studies have follow-up periods of <2 years, a drawback in the treatment of trait-based disorders. Of the three studies with longer follow-ups, only mentalization-based treatment (MBT) has demonstrated a robust effect [72]. This is a small study and the nature of the intervention is unclear [73], consisting of 5-days-per-week day hospital treatment and employing a range of interventions [74]. This result may mirror Antonsen et al's [75] finding at 6-year follow-up of a superior outcome for patients with BPD who participated in day hospital treatment, when compared to a group receiving individual therapy. A 6-year follow-up of cognitive behavioural therapy (CBT) for BPD gave mixed results [76].

Authors of the psychosocial treatments that appeared to have a beneficial effect in BPD proposed a variety of mechanisms which underpin their efficacy (Table 118.1).

The wide range of therapeutic targets is likely to be a result of the complex nature of BPD, involving a wide range of high-level functions, but may also reflect the lack of current knowledge of the active elements in effective therapies and the heterogenous nature of the population.

In ASPD, the evidence is too weak to support any specific treatment targets [95]. In cluster C conditions, exposure and behavioural experimentation have been proposed as the mechanism of action of CBT and the development of emotional insight in short-term psychodynamic psychotherapy (STPP) [96].

In addition to authors' assumption/models, other themes are emerging from the existing evidence base. The majority of successful treatments involve groups (all except individual schema-focused therapy (SFT), transference-focused psychotherapy (TFP), STPP, and cognitive analytic therapy) [97]. Group membership promotes

**Table 118.1** Treatment targets/mechanisms of successful psychological treatments for BPD

| Treatment target/ mechanism | Therapy |
|---|---|
| Addressing underlying schema/cognitive distortions | SFT and CBT-PD address unhelpful cognitive schema explicitly, and 'loving kindness/self compassion' techniques are also likely to challenge putative schema [77] |
| Mentalizing capacity deficits/reflective function | MBT and DTC encourage mentalizing/reflective function explicitly, while SCM incorporates elements of the MBT theory, and TFP has been found to have a beneficial impact on reflective function [78] |
| Emotional regulation skills deficits | DBT and STEPPS incorporate group-based emotional skills sessions, which, in DBT, are then practised and reinforced in one-to-one sessions and telephone support. Mindfulness comprises an additional emotional regulation skill taught in DBT, although its applicability as a stand-alone intervention in personality disorder is not established [79] |
| Psychoeducation | Psychoeducation overlaps with emotional skills training, but in addition, STEPPS explicitly incorporates education on the nature of BPD, an approach that is also showing promise using the Internet [80] |
| Identifying recurring behavioural and emotional themes and patterns | STPP, DBT, and DTC all target problematic and recurrent behavioural and emotional patterns in order to explore their meaning (STPP and DTC) and encourage the development of alternative strategies (DTC and DBT) |
| Case management | Nidotherapy [81] and SCM both provide this as a core part of the intervention, but it is probably active in most of the approaches discussed here |
| Encouraging emotional expression and addressing emotional avoidance | A number of the models recognize the tendency of individuals with personality disorder to avoid strong emotions. STPP, DTC, MBT, and DDP all explicitly encourage the idea that this is an unhelpful coping strategy and encourage alternative ways of dealing with distress |
| Resolution of past trauma/construction of coherent narrative, development of emotional insight | Individuals with personality disorder have often experienced adverse events in childhood, and narrative reconstruction is a part of all exploratory approaches to personality disorder, including DTC, STPP, CAT, DDP, TFP, and SFT [82] |
| Social function and belongingness | Improvement in social function is probably targeted in all group-based approaches but has been specifically addressed in PEPS (although with disappointing results [83]) and interpersonal group psychotherapy [84]. Belongingness arises from frequent and positive contact with others and has a range of benefits [85], and is also likely to be active, to an extent, in group approaches but has been specifically identified in DTC |
| Deficiencies in responsible agency | Agency is the main therapeutic target in MI, and it is also targeted in DTC and MBT |

SFT, schema-focused therapy [86]; MBT, mentalization-based therapy [72]; SCM, structured clinical management [87]; DTC, democratic therapeutic community [88]; DBT, dialectical behaviour therapy [89]; STEPPS, systems training for emotional predictability and problem solving [90]; STPP, short-term psychodynamic psychotherapy [91]; PEPS, psychoeducation with problem-solving [83]; MI, motivational interviewing [92]; DDP, dynamic deconstructive psychotherapy [93]; TFP, transference-focused psychotherapy [78]; CAT, cognitive analytic therapy [94].

social learning and a sense of belongingness, and there is evidence that this is associated with more prosocial behaviour in experimental settings [98]. Many interventions improve self-efficacy and responsible agency (the concept that individuals are motivated to change, feel that they have the power to do so, and wish to exert this power to effect change). This is likely to be related to empowerment—an internal locus of control, knowledge of how to respond, and a sense of having something to offer to others. This is a particularly prominent element of democratic therapeutic communities (DTCs) where it is facilitated by support systems and member–member mentoring. All interventions probably improve social function when clinicians are empathic and reasonably skilled, but attempts to teach social problem-solving have proved disappointing [83]. Clinician attitude and faith in the model is likely to be an important ingredient in the success of any treatment [87].

Treatment strategies can also be derived from ineffective interventions. Crisis planning and motivational interviewing are too brief to be effective [99]. Failure of emotional regulation training to have any impact in adolescents with BPD may also relate to the brevity of the intervention [61]. Similarly, brief CBT seems not to help in people with personality dysfunction after self-harm [100].

The apparent effectiveness of a range of complex interventions illustrates the need for dismantling studies. The only approach in which this has been attempted to date is dialectical behaviour therapy (DBT) where Linehan *et al.* [89] found that skills training plus case management (DBT-S) showed significant advantages over DBT individual therapy plus activities group, whereas the full DBT programme was not clearly superior to DBT-S, indicating that group-based skills training constitutes an essential part of the DBT intervention and may represent the active element. Similarly, Soler *et al.* [101] found DBT skills training superior to standard group therapy. The apparent effectiveness of Systems Training for Emotional Predictability and Problem Solving (STEPPS) [90], a 20-week CBT programme that bears similarities to DBT skills training groups, provides further evidence to support this conclusion.

It has been proposed that the effectiveness of therapies for personality disorder relates to non-specific factors that all therapies share. While there are considerable overlaps between therapies, it is unlikely that this is a valid explanation, given the heterogeneity of approach and the fact that some studies have been able to differentiate between psychotherapies (for example, [102]). Nevertheless, the use of control conditions that incorporate non-specific factors such as case management and skills groups produces improvements in the control arm of trials, thus narrowing the gap with the active conditions both in trials that were still able to demonstrate some superiority for the active condition (in MBT [103] and TFP [104]) and in those that were not (in DBT [105] and cognitive analytic therapy [106]).

## Future directions

Current neuroscientific evidence supported by the theoretical underpinnings of successful psychotherapeutic interventions converge on social functioning and mood regulation as key treatment targets in personality disorder, and specifically in BPD. Current treatments may be more efficacious than they appear, but the heterogeneity of the recruited samples and poor choices of outcome measures have created too much noise for much signal to be detected. Trans-diagnostic approaches may prove more informative, given the heterogeneity of presentations within each specific personality disorder and the extent of comorbidity.

Treatment outcome trials have suffered from a number of methodological flaws which limit their usefulness, and further research is required to address these. In trials of medication, most studies have suffered from being small and funded by drug companies and having short follow-ups. Although follow-up periods have, on the whole, been longer for psychosocial interventions, long-term follow-up over 5 years remains the exception; to date, there have been no published multi-centre trials, and randomized studies have not yet been carried out for cluster A disorders and are rare for cluster C disorders (although some studies have looked at all three clusters [88, 107]). The current uncertainty over the effectiveness of psychosocial interventions for personality disorders stems also from the small numbers enrolled in studies to date for all interventions other than DBT. Finally, the active elements of effective complex interventions will need to be investigated through dismantling and component studies [108].

To date, there are no animal models of personality disorder or an experimental medicine model against which to test new treatments, and there is no consensus on outcome measures in personality disorder research [109]. Developments in mobile and wearable technologies should be exploited in the development of new treatments and objective markers of treatment success.

## REFERENCES

1. Regier, D.A., *et al.* DSM-5 field trials in the United States and Canada, Part II: test-retest reliability of selected categorical diagnoses. *Am J Psychiatry*, 2013;170:59–70.

2. Tyrer, P., *et al.* Reclassifying personality disorders. *Lancet*, 2011;377:1814–15.

3. Insel, T., *et al.* Research domain criteria (RDoC): toward a new classification framework for research on mental disorders. *Am J Psychiatry*, 2010;167:748–51.

4. New, A.S., *et al.* Recent advances in the biological study of personality disorders. *Psychiatr Clin North Am*, 2008;31:441–61, vii.

5. Siever, L.J. and L.N. Weinstein. The neurobiology of personality disorders: implications for psychoanalysis. *J Am Psychoanal Assoc*, 2009;57:361–98.

6. Siever, L.J. Neurobiology of aggression and violence. *Am J Psychiatry*, 2008;165:429–42.

7. Siever, L.J., *et al. The serotonin transporter binding and genotypes in impulsive personality disorders.* Society of Biological Psychiatry, 61st Annual Scientific Convention and Program. 2006.

8. Wilson, S.T., *et al.* Interaction between tryptophan hydroxylase I polymorphisms and childhood abuse is associated with increased risk for borderline personality disorder in adulthood. *Psychiatr Genet*, 2012;22:15–24.

9. Distel, M.A., *et al.* Life events and borderline personality features: the influence of gene-environment interaction and gene-environment correlation. *Psychol Med*, 2011;41:849–60.

10. Gunter, T.D., M.G. Vaughn, and R.A. Philibert. Behavioral genetics in antisocial spectrum disorders and psychopathy: a review of the recent literature. *Behav Sci Law*, 2010;28:148–73.

11. Beach, S.R., *et al.* Methylation at 5HTT mediates the impact of child sex abuse on women's antisocial behavior: an examination of the Iowa adoptee sample. *Psychosom Med*, 2011;73:83–7.

12. Caspi, A., *et al.* Role of genotype in the cycle of violence in maltreated children. *Science*, 2002;297:851–4.

13. Soloff, P.H., *et al.* A fenfluramine-activated FDG-PET study of borderline personality disorder. *Biol Psychiatry*, 2000;47:540–7.

14. Coccaro, E.F., *et al.* Serotonergic studies in patients with affective and personality disorders. *Arch Gen Psychiatry*, 1989;46:587–99.

15. Coccaro, E.F., R.J. Kavoussi, and R.L. Hauger. Serotonin function and antiaggressive response to fluoxetine: a pilot study. *Biol Psychiatry*, 1997;42:546–52.

16. Stein, D.J., *et al.* Impulsivity and serotonergic function in compulsive personality disorder. *J Neuropsychiatry Clin Neurosci*, 1996;8:393–8.

17. Olivier, B. Serotonin and aggression. *Ann N Y Acad Sci*, 2004;1036: 382–92.

18. New, A.S., *et al.* Fluoxetine increases relative metabolic rate in prefrontal cortex in impulsive aggression. *Psychopharmacology (Berl)*, 2004;176:451–8.

19. Lieb, K., *et al.* Pharmacotherapy for borderline personality disorder: Cochrane systematic review of randomised trials. *Br J Psychiatry*, 2010;196: 4–12.

20. Ripoll, L.H. Psychopharmacologic treatment of borderline personality disorder. *Dialogues Clin Neurosci*, 2013;15:213–24.

21. Siever, L.J. and K.L. Davis. The pathophysiology of schizophrenia disorders: perspectives from the spectrum. *Am J Psychiatry*, 2004;161:398–413.

22. Mitropoulou, V., *et al.* Effects of acute metabolic stress on the dopaminergic and pituitary-adrenal axis activity in patients with schizotypal personality disorder. *Schizophr Res*, 2004;70:27–31.

23. Siever, L.J., *et al.* Plasma homovanillic acid in schizotypal personality disorder. *Am J Psychiatry*, 1991;148:1246–8.

24. Siever, L.J., *et al.* CSF homovanillic acid in schizotypal personality disorder. *Am J Psychiatry*, 1993;150:149–51.

25. Abi-Dargham, A., *et al.* Striatal amphetamine-induced dopamine release in patients with schizotypal personality disorder studied with single photon emission computed tomography and [123I] iodobenzamide. *Biol Psychiatry*, 2004;55:1001–6.

26. McClure, M.M., *et al.* Pergolide treatment of cognitive deficits associated with schizotypal personality disorder: continued evidence of the importance of the dopamine system in the schizophrenia spectrum. *Neuropsychopharmacology*, 2010;35:1356–62.

27. Siegel, B.V., Jr., *et al.* D-amphetamine challenge effects on Wisconsin Card Sort Test. Performance in schizotypal personality disorder. *Schizophr Res*, 1996;20:29–32.

28. Crawford, M.J., *et al.* Medication prescribed to people with personality disorder: the influence of patient factors and treatment setting. *Acta Psychiatr Scand*, 2011;124:396–402.

29. Pateon, C., *et al.* The use of psychotropic medication in patients with emotionally unstable personality disorder under the care of UK mental health services. *J Clin Psychiatry*, 2015;76:512–18.

30. Jakobsen, K.D., *et al.* Antipsychotic treatment of schizotypy and schizotypal personality disorder: a systematic review. *J Psychopharmacol*, 2017;31:397–405.

31. Schulz, S.C., *et al.* Olanzapine for the treatment of borderline personality disorder: variable dose 12-week randomised double-blind placebo-controlled study. *Br J Psychiatry*, 2008;193:485–92.

32. Zanarini, M.C., *et al.* Open-label treatment with olanzapine for patients with borderline personality disorder. *J Clin Psychopharmacol*, 2012;32:398–402.

33. Black, D.W., *et al.* Comparison of low and moderate dosages of extended-release quetiapine in borderline personality disorder: a randomized, double-blind, placebo-controlled trial. *Am J Psychiatry*, 2014;171:1174–82.

34. Canadian Agency for Drugs and Technologies in Health. *Aripiprazole for Borderline Personality Disorder: A Review of the Clinical Effectiveness.* Ottawa: Canadian Agency for Drugs and Technologies in Health; 2017.

35. Pascual, J.C., et al. Ziprasidone in the treatment of borderline personality disorder: a double-blind, placebo-controlled, randomized study. J Clin Psychiatry, 2008;69:603–8.

36. Brune, M. On the role of oxytocin in borderline personality disorder. Br J Clin Psychol, 2016;55:287–304.

37. Hammen, C., J.E. Bower, and S.W. Cole. Oxytocin receptor gene variation and differential susceptibility to family environment in predicting youth borderline symptoms. J Pers Disord, 2015;29:177–92.

38. Unternaehrer, E., et al. Dynamic changes in DNA methylation of stress-associated genes (OXTR, BDNF) after acute psychosocial stress. Transl Psychiatry, 2012;2:e150.

39. Bertsch, K., et al. Reduced plasma oxytocin levels in female patients with borderline personality disorder. Horm Behav, 2013;63:424–9.

40. Bertsch, K., et al. Oxytocin and reduction of social threat hypersensitivity in women with borderline personality disorder. Am J Psychiatry, 2013;170:1169–77.

41. Brune, M., et al. Nonverbal communication of patients with borderline personality disorder during clinical interviews: a double-blind placebo-controlled study using intranasal oxytocin. J Nerv Ment Dis, 2015;203:107–11.

42. Bartz, J., et al. Oxytocin can hinder trust and cooperation in borderline personality disorder. Soc Cogn Affect Neurosci, 2011;6:556–63.

43. Evans, S., S.S. Shergill, and B.B. Averbeck. Oxytocin decreases aversion to angry faces in an associative learning task. Neuropsychopharmacology, 2010;35:2502–9.

44. Striepens, N., et al. Oxytocin facilitates protective responses to aversive social stimuli in males. Proc Natl Acad Sci U S A, 2012;109:18144–9.

45. Bodnar, R.J. Endogenous opiates and behavior: 2008. Peptides, 2009;30:2432–79.

46. Prossin, A.R., et al. Dysregulation of regional endogenous opioid function in borderline personality disorder. Am J Psychiatry, 2010;167:925–33.

47. Bandelow, B. and D. Wedekind. Possible role of a dysregulation of the endogenous opioid system in antisocial personality disorder. Hum Psychopharmacol, 2015;30:393–415.

48. Stanley, B. and L.J. Siever. The interpersonal dimension of borderline personality disorder: toward a neuropeptide model. Am J Psychiatry, 2010;167:24–39.

49. Stanley, B., et al. Non-suicidal self-injurious behavior, endogenous opioids and monoamine neurotransmitters. J Affect Disord, 2010;124:134–40.

50. Schmahl, C., et al. Evaluation of naltrexone for dissociative symptoms in borderline personality disorder. Int Clin Psychopharmacol, 2012;27:61–8.

51. Meiser, M., et al. Improvement of borderline personality disorder with naltrexone: results of a retrospective evaluation. Eur Psychiatry, 2015;30:28–31.

52. Grosjean, B. and G.E. Tsai. NMDA neurotransmission as a critical mediator of borderline personality disorder. J Psychiatry Neurosci, 2007;32:103–15.

53. Kulkarni, J., et al. A novel drug for borderline personality disorder. 2014. Available from: https://clinicaltrials.gov/ct2/show/NCT02097706

54. Tsanas, A., et al. Daily longitudinal self-monitoring of mood variability in bipolar disorder and borderline personality disorder. J Affect Disord, 2016;205:225–33.

55. Reich, D.B., M.C. Zanarini, and G. Fitzmaurice. Affective lability in bipolar disorder and borderline personality disorder. Compr Psychiatry, 2012;53:230–7.

56. Chanen, A.M., et al. Orbitofrontal, amygdala and hippocampal volumes in teenagers with first-presentation borderline personality disorder. Psychiatry Res, 2008;163:116–25.

57. Soloff, P., et al. Structural brain abnormalities in borderline personality disorder: a voxel-based morphometry study. Psychiatry Res, 2008;164:223–36.

58. Ruocco, A.C. The neuropsychology of borderline personality disorder: a meta-analysis and review. Psychiatry Res, 2005;137:191–202.

59. Hazlett, E.A., et al. Exaggerated affect-modulated startle during unpleasant stimuli in borderline personality disorder. Biol Psychiatry, 2007;62:250–5.

60. Stoffers, J.M., et al. Psychological therapies for people with borderline personality disorder. Cochrane Database Syst Rev, 2012;8:CD005652.

61. Schuppert, H.M., et al. Emotion regulation training for adolescents with borderline personality disorder traits: a randomized controlled trial. J Am Acad Child Adolesc Psychiatry, 2012;51:1314–23 e2.

62. Zelkowitz, P., et al. A five-year follow-up of patients with borderline pathology of childhood. J Pers Disord, 2007;21:664–74.

63. Gunderson, J.G., et al. Ten-year course of borderline personality disorder: psychopathology and function from the Collaborative Longitudinal Personality Disorders study. Arch Gen Psychiatry, 2011;68:827–37.

64. Minzenberg, M.J., J.H. Poole, and S. Vinogradov. Social-emotion recognition in borderline personality disorder. Compr Psychiatry, 2006;47:468–74.

65. Lieb, K., et al. Borderline personality disorder. Lancet, 2004;364:453–61.

66. Fonagy, P. and A.W. Bateman. Mechanisms of change in mentalization-based treatment of BPD. J Clin Psychol, 2006;62:411–30.

67. King-Casas, B., et al. The rupture and repair of cooperation in borderline personality disorder. Science, 2008;321:806–10.

68. Saunders, K.E., G.M. Goodwin, and R.D. Rogers. Borderline personality disorder, but not euthymic bipolar disorder, is associated with a failure to sustain reciprocal cooperative behaviour: implications for spectrum models of mood disorders. Psychol Med, 2015;45:1591–600.

69. Blair, R.J. Neuroimaging of psychopathy and antisocial behavior: a targeted review. Curr Psychiatry Rep, 2010;12:76–82.

70. Coccaro, E.F., et al. Amygdala and orbitofrontal reactivity to social threat in individuals with impulsive aggression. Biol Psychiatry, 2007;62:168–78.

71. Crawford, M.J., et al. Lamotrigine versus inert placebo in the treatment of borderline personality disorder: study protocol for a randomized controlled trial and economic evaluation. Trials, 2015;16:308.

72. Bateman, A. and P. Fonagy. 8-year follow-up of patients treated for borderline personality disorder: mentalization-based treatment versus treatment as usual. Am J Psychiatry, 2008;165:631–8.

73. Bateman, A. and P. Fonagy. Effectiveness of partial hospitalization in the treatment of borderline personality disorder: a randomized controlled trial. Am J Psychiatry, 1999;156:1563–9.

74. Mishan, J. and A. Bateman, Group-Analytic Therapy of Borderline Patients in a Day Hospital Setting. Group Analysis, 1994;27:483–95.

75. Antonsen, B.T., et al. Favourable outcome of long-term combined psychotherapy for patients with borderline personality disorder: Six-year follow-up of a randomized study. Psychother Res, 2017;27:51–63.

76. Davidson, K.M., *et al.* Cognitive therapy v. usual treatment for borderline personality disorder: prospective 6-year follow-up. *Br J Psychiatry*, 2010;197:456–62.

77. Feliu-Soler, A., *et al.* Fostering Self-Compassion and Loving-Kindness in Patients With Borderline Personality Disorder: A Randomized Pilot Study. *Clin Psychol Psychother*, 2017;24:278–86.

78. Levy, K.N., *et al.* Change in attachment patterns and reflective function in a randomized control trial of transference-focused psychotherapy for borderline personality disorder. *J Consult Clin Psychol*, 2006;74:1027–40.

79. Elices, M., *et al.* Impact of Mindfulness Training on Borderline Personality Disorder: A Randomized Trial. *Mindfulness*, 2016;7:584–95.

80. Zanarini, M.C., *et al.* Randomized Controlled Trial of Web-Based Psychoeducation for Women With Borderline Personality Disorder. *J Clin Psychiatry*, 2018;79:pii:16m11153.

81. Tyrer, P., *et al.* Nidotherapy in the treatment of substance misuse, psychosis and personality disorder: secondary analysis of a controlled trial. *The Psychiatrist*, 2011;35:9–14.

82. Young, J.E. *Cognitive therapy for personality disorders: A schema-focused approach*. Rev Professional Resource Press/Professional Resource Exchange; 1994.

83. McMurran, M., *et al.* Psychoeducation with problem-solving (PEPS) therapy for adults with personality disorder: a pragmatic randomised controlled trial to determine the clinical effectiveness and cost-effectiveness of a manualised intervention to improve social functioning. *Health Technol Assess*, 2016;20:1–250.

84. Marziali, E., H. Munroe-Blum, and L. McCleary. The effects of the therapeutic alliance on the outcomes of individual and group psychotherapy with borderline personality disorder. *Psychother Res*, 1999;9:424–36.

85. Pearce, S. and H. Pickard. How therapeutic communities work: Specific factors related to postive outcome. *Int J Soc Psychiatry*, 2013;59:636–45.

86. Farrell, J.M., I.A. Shaw, and M.A. Webber. A schema-focused approach to group psychotherapy for outpatients with borderline personality disorder: a randomized controlled trial. *J Behav Ther Exp Psychiatry*, 2009;40:317–28.

87. Bateman, A. and R. Krawitz. *Borderline Personality Disorder: An Evidence-based Guide for Generalist Mental Health Professionals*. Oxford: Oxford University Press; 2013.

88. Pearce, S., *et al.* Democratic therapeutic community treatment for personality disorder: randomised controlled trial. *Br J Psychiatry*, 2017;210:149–56.

89. Linehan, M.M., *et al.* Dialectical behavior therapy for high suicide risk in individuals with borderline personality disorder: a randomized clinical trial and component analysis. *JAMA Psychiatry*, 2015;72:475–82.

90. Blum, N., *et al.* Systems Training for Emotional Predictability and Problem Solving (STEPPS) for outpatients with borderline personality disorder: a randomized controlled trial and 1-year follow-up. *Am J Psychiatry*, 2008;165:468–78.

91. Leichsenring, F. and E. Leibing. The effectiveness of psychodynamic therapy and cognitive behavior therapy in the treatment of personality disorders: a meta-analysis. *Am J Psychiatry*, 2003;160:1223–32.

92. McMurran, M., *et al.* The addition of a goal-based motivational interview to treatment as usual to enhance engagement and reduce dropouts in a personality disorder treatment service: results of a feasibility study for a randomized controlled trial. *Trials*, 2013;14:50.

93. Monroe-Blum, H. and E. Marziali. A controlled trial of short-term group treatment for borderline personality disorder. *J Pers Disord*, 1995;9:190–8.

94. Clarke, S., P. Thomas, and K. James. Cognitive analytic therapy for personality disorder: randomised controlled trial. *Br J Psychiatry*, 2013;202:129–34.

95. Bateman, A., *et al.* A randomised controlled trial of mentalization-based treatment versus structured clinical management for patients with comorbid borderline personality disorder and antisocial personality disorder. *BMC Psychiatry*, 2016;16:304.

96. Svartberg, M., T.C. Stiles, and M.H. Seltzer. Randomized, controlled trial of the effectiveness of short-term dynamic psychotherapy and cognitive therapy for cluster C personality disorders. *Am J Psychiatry*, 2004;161:810–17.

97. Omar, H., M. Tejerina-Arreal, and M.J. Crawford. Are recommendations for psychological treatment of borderline personality disorder in current U.K. guidelines justified? Systematic review and subgroup analysis. *Pers Ment Health*, 2014;8:228–37.

98. Saunders, K.E.A., *et al. Social behaviour following group therapy*. Unpublished; 2017.

99. Borschmann, R., *et al.* Joint crisis plans for people with borderline personality disorder: feasibility and outcomes in a randomised controlled trial. *Br J Psychiatry*, 2013;202:357–64.

100. Tyrer, P., *et al.* Differential effects of manual assisted cognitive behavior therapy in the treatment of recurrent deliberate self-harm and personality disturbance: the POPMACT study. *J Pers Disord*, 2004;18:102–16.

101. Soler, J., *et al.* Dialectical behaviour therapy skills training compared to standard group therapy in borderline personality disorder: a 3-month randomised controlled clinical trial. *Behav Res Ther*, 2009;47:353–8.

102. Linehan, M.M., *et al.* Two-Year Randomized Controlled Trial and Follow-up of Dialectical Behavior Therapy vs Therapy by Experts for Suicidal Behaviors and Borderline Personality Disorder. *Arch Gen Psychiatry*, 2006;63:757–66.

103. Bateman, A. and P. Fonagy. Randomized controlled trial of outpatient mentalization-based treatment versus structured clinical management for borderline personality disorder. *Am J Psychiatry*, 2009;166:1355–64.

104. Clarkin, J.F., *et al.* Evaluating three treatments for borderline personality disorder: a multiwave study. *Am J Psychiatry*, 2007;164:922–8.

105. McMain, S.F., *et al.* Dialectical behavior therapy compared with general psychiatric management for borderline personality disorder: clinical outcomes and functioning over a 2-year follow-up. *Am J Psychiatry*, 2012;169:650–61.

106. Chanen, A.M., *et al.* Early intervention for adolescents with borderline personality disorder using cognitive analytic therapy: randomised controlled trial. *Br J Psychiatry*, 2008;193:477–84.

107. Abbass, A., *et al.* Intensive short-term dynamic psychotherapy for DSM-IV personality disorders: a randomized controlled trial. *J Nerv Ment Dis*, 2008;196:211–16.

108. Ahn, H. and B. Wampold. Where oh where are the specific ingredients? A meta-analysis of component studies in counseling in psychotherapy. *J Couns Psychol*, 2001;48:251–7.

109. COMET Initiative. Available from: www.comet-initiative.org

# 119

# Personality disorders
## Epidemiology and clinical course

*Renato D. Alarcón and Brian A. Palmer*

## Introduction

The conceptual, clinical, and nosological debates about personality disorders (PDs) as psychiatric entities reflect both the complexity of the diagnoses and the fragility of the agreements arrived at in different classification systems [1, 2]. Among the reasons, the absence of common or homogenous phenomenological and psychopathological bases for the different PD types, the multiple clinical variations or subtypes among the individual conditions, profuse comorbidity levels, and uncertain outcomes are frequently mentioned [3, 4]. Additionally, a relatively reduced prevalence of PDs in the general population, when compared with 'major' psychiatric disorders, leads to relatively scarce (and, at times, questionable) epidemiological data and to a colourful, but heterogenous, clinical course. On the other hand, the same debates and their many implications represent the growing relevance of PDs, not only as more or less permanent distortions of individual identities, but also as repositories of genetic, epigenetic, environmental, and socio-cultural factors in the construction of such identities [3–5]. Thanks to the rapidly developing field of molecular genetics, PD phenotypes may assist in better aetio-pathogenic, and therefore diagnostic, and epidemiological estimates [6]. Furthermore, in many modern approaches to the delineation of PDs, basic personality features or traits and personality functioning levels are the departure point of thorough and comprehensive clinical evaluations [7]. Different statistical methods and procedures (from multi-dimensional scaling to factor analysis through correlational analyses, to cite a few) assist in the structuring of PDs and the controversial acceptance of their three superordinate clusters in the *Diagnostic and Statistical Manual of Mental Disorders*, fifth edition (DSM-5).

Historically, the maladaptive variants of normal personality traits, grouped in the well-known Five-Factor Model [8], provide a particularly compelling tool for the identification and assessment of the 11 DSM-IV's axis II PDs, still present in DSM-5 [1]; in spite of the unevenness of studies about these factors (many more on neuroticism and extraversion than on openness, agreeableness, and conscientiousness related to former axis I disorders) [9], it is clear that personality can decisively influence much broader psychopathologies and, secondarily, epidemiological, follow-up, and outcome inquiries. Intrapersonal and interpersonal manifestations of PDs differ, and informant reports may be more valid than self-reports in both clinical evaluations and prevalence surveys, adding another important methodological layer to research in both areas. Higher-order internalizing and externalizing structural factors in different psychopathologies were correlated with 30 latent personality facets in a study by Uliaszek and Zinbarg [10]. An elevation of the neuroticism facets, along with low positive emotions, low actions, and low competence, was found for the higher-order internalizing factor entities (that is, major depression), whereas the higher-order externalizing ones were negatively associated with most conscientiousness and agreeableness factors and with an elevation of excitement-seeking impulsivity and angry hostility. These findings constitute a call for active search of PDs in different types of studies, epidemiological surveys included. In turn, environmental characteristics (including interpersonal transactions such as perceived discrimination) must be assessed in every type of study, as they have shown to be a main social pathway which, in addition to biological and developmental routes, is crucial for the establishment of the adult personality type and its detection and prognosis [11–12].

This section will examine, first, general epidemiological data on PDs through studies from different regions of the world, following immediately with studies on the prevalence and incidence of each of the PD types identified in the main world nomenclatures. Emphasis on the role and significance of socio-demographic variables, family history, and relevant comorbidities will precede the clinical course subsection, similarly focused on each PD type, with and without treatment, on pertinent risk and protective factors, and on their short- and long-term prognostic implications. Topics such as relapses and chronicity patterns will also be examined.

## Methodological issues

The considerable heterogeneity and poor discriminant validity of DSM's PDs impede accurate diagnoses and therefore can make epidemiological findings questionable. Yun *et al.* [13] proposed alternative assessment tools such as Kernberg's object relational model [14], on the basis of which develops a finite mixture modelling that harboured three components: Group 1, characterized by low levels of antisocial, paranoid, and aggressive features; Group 2, by elevated paranoid features; and Group 3, with the highest levels across the three variables. Various external measures supported the validity of this grouping structure, thus offering a substantive aid in refining PD classification and conferring additional solidity to prevalence, incidence, and clinical course studies.

Different clinical populations have been used in attempts to delineate more precisely normal personality types and actual PDs. This helps to consider pathogenic circumstances, that is, situations that contribute to the evolvement of actual psychopathologies. For instance, coping styles (relevant personality-based features) and treatment preferences were evaluated by Contractor et al. [15] in 1266 trauma-exposed military veterans (89.6% male). The results were revealing: (1) post-traumatic stress disorder (PTSD)-free and emotionally stable probands were less likely to use self-distraction, denial, and substance consumption, and more likely to use active coping; (2) those less emotionally stable and with more re-experiencing and avoidance symptoms were less likely to use denial and active coping, but more likely to use behavioural disengagement; (3) those with subsyndromal PTSD were more likely to use self-distraction, active coping, and substance use, but less likely denial, instrumental coping, positive reframing, and acceptance; and (4) those with severe PTSD and combined internalizing–externalizing traits responded similarly to (3), but also used more substances, more denial, more emotional support, and less active coping. Interestingly, emotional stability was the most distinguishing feature, and all classes were more likely to seek mental health treatment.

Similarly, the assessment of personality traits becomes an important parameter for psychological evaluations among persons seeking cosmetic surgery. In a study from Iran, Golshani et al. [16], using three well-validated instruments, evaluated 274 randomly selected individuals seeking rhinoplasty, blepharoplasty, face/jaw implant, mammoplasty, and liposuction; a prevalence of 51% of psychiatric problems was found, with interpersonal sensitivity as the highest syndrome-like endorsed (the lowest, psychosis), and agreeableness and extroversion as the highest scored features (the lowest, openness).

Sexual problems (hypersexuality, excitation, and inhibition) constitute another area of discussions and studies of this kind. Rettenberger et al. [17] investigated the impact of different personality traits on data provided by two instruments in a sample of 1749 participants in an Internet-based survey. Six per cent of the probands were categorized as hypersexual, irrespective of gender and sexual orientation. Among male recidivist offenders, Barbosa et al. [18], based on the signal detection theory, evaluated sensitivity to emotional arousal and valence induced by pictures; offenders reported higher arousal than controls and showed lower sensitivity to changes in levels of arousal, but no differences vis-à-vis controls for valence. This modality of research broadens the narrow typological taxonomy and allows indirect, but valid, assessment of PDs in special populations.

Finally, issues such as reality-testing, developmental phases of the life cycle, and traumatic experiences make prevalence and incidence studies of PDs a difficult enterprise. The associations between PDs and other conditions have shown different degrees of consistency when epidemiologically assessed by established nomenclature classifications. It can be said that the pervasive and relatively inflexible pattern of behaviours that reflect the individual's predominant mode of being is, in itself, a formidable challenge for epidemiological, field, and clinical studies.

## General epidemiology

The instruments used in epidemiological studies of personality and other disorders are a critical component of this area of knowledge. In addition to the questionnaires used in the first historical studies, a multitude of instruments reflecting different modalities of conceptualization (categorical and dimensional, and among the latter, interpersonal, clinical, bio-psychological, etc.) have been developed. Names of authors such as Goldberg, Fonagy, Widiger, Costa and McCrae, Cloninger, Millon, Gunderson, Livesley, Silver and Davies, Oldham and Skodol, Krueger, and Clark provide a sound historical background for this field of inquiry [3].

There is some variability in the estimation of general prevalence of PDs in the general population. Torgersen et al. [19] examined the issue in depth, identifying different components of any epidemiological search (that is, sample selection) that impact the final estimates. In eight prevalence studies including all PDs and covering a total of 5081 persons, with >500 as the average sample size, the findings ranked between 3.9% and 22.7%, but in small samples, the variation was smaller between 10.0% and 14.3%. The median prevalence of all studies was 11.55%, and the pooled prevalence 12.26% [20]. These data are consistent with the major large, representative national epidemiological studies, including those from Great Britain [21], which estimated an overall prevalence of 10.1%, and the US National Comorbidity Survey Replication [22] with a rate of 9.1%.

### Prevalence data

Grant et al.'s analysis of the National Epidemiological Survey on Alcohol and Related Conditions (NESARC) [23] presented nationally representative data (from a sample of 43,093 subjects) on the prevalence, socio-demographic correlates, and disability of seven of the ten DSM-IV PDs; overall, 14.8% of adult Americans (or 30.8 million) had at least one personality disorder. Another report of the same study found rates of PDs at the high end of previously published ranges (21.5% overall) [24]. Test–retest reliabilities between wave 1 (2001–2002) and wave 2 data (2004–2005), using the Alcohol Use Disorder and Associated Disabilities Interview Schedule-IV (AUDADIS-IV), were, however, low for some types [that is, 0.40 for histrionic PD (HPD)] [25]. Some have criticized the diagnostic approach, as the study required only one of the identified PD symptoms to have an association with distress or impairment. A re-analysis of the data that required an association with distress or impairment for each of the symptoms used to make the PD diagnosis [for example, five of nine borderline personality disorder (BPD) symptoms] yielded rates more in keeping with other samples (9.1%) [26].

As expected, prevalence figures increased up to 50% in studies conducted within specific clinical settings [20]. Widiger and Rojas [27] pointed out that the prevalence of PDs is generally underestimated in clinical practice due, in part, to the previously mentioned deficiencies in a comprehensive clinical assessment of the corresponding symptomatology. Moreover, Beckwith *et al.* [28] conducted a systematic literature review of studies measuring the prevalence of PDs in community secondary care settings and identified only nine out of 269 papers deserving critical appraisal; they showed a high level of heterogeneity with regard to methods, inclusion criteria, source of information, times of assessment, instruments used, and overall quality of research. Prevalence estimates in Europe varied between 40% and 92%, showed a closer range (45–51%) in the United States, and differed significantly in two Asian studies (1.07% in India and 60% in Pakistan). The low prevalence in India confirmed a previous finding by Gupta and Mattoo [29], but once again, weak methodology (case records study) may have generated questionable results.

### Socio-demographic variables

It is generally accepted that the prevalence rates are higher in urban populations and in lower socio-economic groups. Gender is probably the most controversial topic in this area. Some studies concluded that the prevalence levels of PDs in men and women are roughly equivalent, with some disorders more frequently present in each gender, whereas others seemed to indicate that only one type (borderline) is more prevalent among women. A variety of recommendations to reduce and avoid sampling, assessment, and criteria biases have been made. The differential socialization and life experiences of males and females have been used to explain the differences in personality and PDs between males' and females' innate behavioural tendencies, without excluding neurobiological (particularly physiological and endocrinological) factors. Nevertheless, the general agreement is that more than one in ten adult individuals has a PD. The average prevalence of specific PDs is a little above 1%, with variations per type. It is also important to remark that these correlations neither display one-directional causal relationships nor account for the total nature and characteristics of the individual's interpersonal experiences [30].

According to DSM-5 [1], features of a PD must have been present for at least 1 year if the diagnosis is to be made before age 18. Apparently, individuals with odd/eccentric PDs are older, and the dramatic/emotional trait dimensions decrease with age [19]. Subjects with PDs have more often been separated, unmarried, or divorced, even though there is agreement in that the real effect of marital status on PD occurrence is difficult to determine. Similarly, the trend of a negative correlation between PD prevalence and educational and income status is not uniformly agreed upon. Urban location seems more often linked to PDs, with subsequent lower quality of life and higher dysfunctional level [31]. Last, but not least, the few studies on PDs and ethnicity show methodological weaknesses, as analysed by McGilloway *et al.* [32]. Meta-analyses revealed significant differences in prevalence of PDs between black and white groups, but no differences between Asian or Hispanic groups compared with white groups; these heterogenous results may be accounted for by methodological characteristics, ranging from a true lower prevalence among black patients to a clear neglect of PD diagnoses among other ethnic groups.

### Risk and protective factors

We have touched also on risk and protective factors as important variables in the clinical evolvement of PDs and their epidemiological correlates. While the genetic load seems to be unquestionable,

particularly, for example, in the DSM-5's Cluster A types [33], epigenetic variations and environmental factors, such as child-rearing issues, intra-family relationships, parental styles, educational milieus, and opportunities or cultural and religious concerns, can play either a risk or a protective role, depending on the kind, orientation, and weight of each in everyday life [4]. Childhood and adolescence are considered critical periods in the developmental cycle of every individual. A balanced use of modelling, independence fostering, decision-making, and social/relational skills will do a lot to favour a normal personality development. Contrariwise, gender-based violence is associated with at least 38% of all PD cases, and women who have experienced it have 8.5 times the odds of PDs, compared to non-victims [34]. Needless to say, the assessment of these factors is decisive in the epidemiological and clinical evaluation of the disorders.

### Comorbidities

Another heatedly debated topic is that of the correlation (or coexistence, although some may call it comorbidity) between PDs and other psychiatric conditions—the main point of contention is the cause–effect equation, which is first, and how one can lead into the other. It must be clear that this type of studies does not refer to the clinical setting in which they take place; actually, most of them are community-based projects. A third phase of the NESARC study [23], conducted in 36,309 adults, found significant associations of 12-month and lifetime prevalence of drug use disorders (DUD) with a variety of PDs, including antisocial, avoidant, and borderline. In Denmark, Toftdahl *et al.* [35] found that 46% of 463,003 substance use disorder (SUD) patients had diagnoses of PDs.

A study in France [36] found PDs (independent of clusters) as significant risk factors for generalized anxiety disorder, and Cluster C types for major depressive disorder (MDD), in non-metastatic breast cancer patients. In a population-based 37-year follow-up cohort study of >29,000 Swedish Twin Registry members, Sieurin *et al.* [37] found neuroticism and introversion strongly associated with a risk of Parkinson's disease; smoking was a significant mediator in the relationship between personality traits and Parkinson's disease, partly accounting for the effect of introversion, while being a suppressor for the effect of neuroticism. Higher-than-normal body weight was associated with paranoid, antisocial, and avoidant PDs among women, whereas overweight men had lower rates of paranoid PD (PPD) and underweight women had higher odds of schizoid PD (SPD) [38]. An intriguing finding—among college men with purging-type eating disorders, symptoms were associated with constellations of personality traits that are typically reported among women [39]. The obvious conclusion is that, in general, PDs are highly associated with a variety of disabilities in different periods of the life cycle.

Thus, it is evident that personality and its temperamental and characterological components are always in the background of normal and ill people; among the latter, early and precise identification of such features is crucial as they can contribute, in many cases, to increased levels of severity and to a complicated clinical course of the comorbid condition. Of interest, the trait model of personality pathology in DSM-5 Section III [1] has been successfully applied to problematic alcohol use cases, with antagonism and disinhibition as the most relevant domains. It has been suggested that throughout life, higher coercion experiences are associated with lower understanding and lower reasoning which, in turn, decrease the social engagement of individuals with severe PDs [40]. On the other hand, the course of PDs themselves will depend on the timing and scope of the professional intervention. In general, an early diagnosis and appropriate therapeutic interventions can certainly be effective, improve the patient's quality of life, and disrupt the chronicity pathway characteristic of untreated conditions; the pattern is similar in the case of comorbid medical or psychiatric pictures.

## Special epidemiology, comorbidities, and clinical course

Primarily referred to data about each of the more or less established PDs in modern psychiatry, special epidemiology integrates concomitant issues such as comorbidities and risk and protective factors. At the same time, it offers much needed information for the formulation and understanding of the clinical course, prognosis, and outcomes of each of the disorders [41, 42]. Tables 119.1 and 119.2 summarize the information from this and the previous section.

### Paranoid personality disorder

#### Prevalence

Although distrust and suspiciousness, with subsequent misinterpretation of others' behaviours, may be present in 13% of adult males and 6% of females [8], the actual DSM-5 criteria for PPD seem to be met only by a population range of between 0.4% and 4.4%, according to a variety of prevalence studies [1], with a median rate of 1.6% [27]. In inpatient clinical settings, the range may increase to 10–30%, while in ambulatory services, it may oscillate between 2% and 10%. It may be worth mentioning that some studies show a 0% prevalence of PPD, which raises several of the questions examined in previous pages.

Table 119.1 Main epidemiological data about personality disorders

| PD type | Prevalence range (%) | Avg community (%) | Clinical settings (%) |
|---|---|---|---|
| All | 3.9–22.7 | 11.6 | 40.0–51.0 |
| Paranoid | 0.4–4.4 | 1.6 | Inpt 10–30; outpt 2–10 |
| Schizoid | 0.4–4.9 | 0.6 | Inpt 16 |
| Schizotypal | 0.1–5.6 | 0.8 | Inpt 2–20 |
| Antisocial | 0.2–4.5 | 1.3 | Outpt 3–30 |
| Borderline | 0.2–5.9 | 1.7 | Inpt 20; Outpt 6.0 |
| Histrionic | 0.3–3.9 | 1.6 | Outpt 10–15 |
| Narcissistic | 0.1–1.5 | 0.5 | Outpt 6.2 |
| Avoidant | 1.0–6.0 | 1.7 | Outpt 6.0 |
| Dependent | 0.1–11.0 | 0.9 | |
| Obsessive–compulsive | 2.1–7.9 | 2.1 | General 10.0–20.0 |

Inpt, inpatient; outpt, outpatient.
Main sources: [41, 42].

### Comorbidities

It has been demonstrated that the phenomenological structure of PPD can share some of its features with the other Cluster A types, all of Cluster B's, and Cluster C's avoidant PD (AvPD). The clinician must have a clear perspective about the global nature of the trait combinations, that is, the distinction between the affective distance and eccentricity of the schizoid or avoidant PD's fear of being ashamed or overwhelmed vs the hypervigilance or suspiciousness of PPD. Conversely, a careful evaluation must be pursued to rule out predictable 'paranoid-like' behaviours in members of immigrant, ethnic, or political groups.

Other forms of psychopathology may occur simultaneously (or more frequently) in individuals with PPD: psychotic conditions such as delusional disorder, schizophrenia, depressive and manic episodes, alcohol and substance dependence and abuse, criminal behaviours, and obsessive–compulsive, agoraphobic, and depressive disorders [43, 44].

### Clinical course

During childhood and early adolescence, PPD features such as hypersensitivity, social anxiety, low school performance, and poor peer relationships can elicit bullying from other children, thus accentuating paranoid attitudes. Brief psychotic episodes have been reported in connection with stressful situations throughout the life of PPD patients. A consistent employment history is relatively infrequent, mostly due to hyperdefensiveness, litigiousness, and antagonistic, or even violent, behaviour. Last, but not least, clinicians must not forget the premonitory nature of PPD features in patients that later may develop psychoses such as schizophrenia.

### Schizoid personality disorder

#### Prevalence

With two studies showing a 0% prevalence, the range in all the others goes from 0.4% to 4.9% and one study showed 7%, but the median in several tables is around 0.65%. Additional contradictions emerge from the statement that SPD is considered 'uncommon' in clinical settings, at the time that the same source (DSM-5) included prevalence levels of 4.9 and 3.1%, from Part II of the Comorbidity Survey-Replication (CMS-R) and NESARC samples, respectively [1]; in other clinical samples, the prevalence reaches 16%. Similar disagreements exist about the prevalence of SPD by gender [45, 46].

### Comorbidities

There is limited documentation of comorbidity between SPD and major psychotic conditions, probably due to difficulties in differentiating the clinical presentations of both kinds of disorders. Actually, some authors have found little or no relationship between SPD and schizophrenia when family history or clinical course were compared. The same occurs in cases of mild autism spectrum disorder that may co-occur with SPD, even though in the majority of cases, the former may be installed earlier than SPD could be detected. These problems multiply when a trait distinction is attempted between SPD and schizotypal and avoidant PDs.

### Clinical course

Usually long-lasting, but not necessarily life-long, SPD courses in a more or less 'stable' fashion, seldom exhibiting rapid or profound

Table 119.2 Comorbidities and clinical course of personality disorders

| PD types | Main comorbidities | Clinical course |
|---|---|---|
| All | Other PDs; alcohol and SUDs; mood and anxiety disorders; eating disorders; medical illnesses | Strong tendency to chronicity |
| Paranoid | Clusters A and B and AvPD; schizophrenia and other psychoses; bipolar disorder; SUDs; OCD | Bullying victims, pre-psychotic states, unstable employment |
| Schizoid | Cluster A PDs; mood and phobic disorders; autism spectrum disorder | Marital and relational difficulties; reasonable adaptation |
| Schizotypal | Cluster A PDs; AvPD and BPD; brief psychotic episode; MDD, OCD, generalized anxiety disorder | More among men; social isolation; 10% suicidal behaviour; marginal employment; no frequent psychoses |
| Antisocial | Cluster B PDs; PPD; alcohol and SUDs; hypochondriasis; gambling; ADHD | More among men; family dysfunction; unemployment; conduct disorder and law/forensic problems; criminal behaviour; frequent use of medical services; some improvement with ageing |
| Borderline | MDD, bipolar disorder, PTSD, SUDs, generalized anxiety disorder, and panic disorder | Self-mutilation episodes and suicidal behaviour; 80% remission by 10 years, 40% with high functioning; infrequent relapses, but persistent social and occupational issues |
| Histrionic | Cluster B PDs and DPD; somatization, conversion and dissociative disorders; brief reactive psychosis | More among women; problems since adolescence; suicidal attempts; occupational fragility; frequent use of medical services; improves with age |
| Narcissistic | SUDs; anxiety disorders; bipolar disorder; BPD and AsPD | 60% improve in 3 years; connection with evolution of comorbidities; prognosis worsens with AsPD |
| Avoidant | SAD, DPD | Variations in early periods; diagnostic 'stability'; many patients remain single |
| Dependent | AvPD; anxiety disorders; depressive mood | Few studies; limited reduction of symptoms |
| Obsessive-compulsive | Anxiety, mood and obsessive–compulsive disorders; Cluster C PDs | More among men; small long-term improvement of core symptoms |

changes. This does not mean that patients will not have difficulties in different settings—their more or less severe social ostracism makes them have few close relationships, including sexual partners, and occasionally become homeless. If married and having children, they have limited capacity to provide warm, supportive, or endearing affection. Clinical complications, in addition to possible psychotic occurrences, include mood, phobic, and behavioural disorders. On the other hand, and differing from the other Cluster A PDs, a relatively good number of SPD patients, particularly those with mild manifestations, may reach reasonable levels of social adaptation, work, and quality of life [45].

### Schizotypal personality disorder (StPD)

#### Prevalence

Studies that have found prevalent schizotypal personality disorder (StPD) showed a lowest level of 0.1% and a highest of 5.6% in community populations, with a median of 0.7–0.9%. In clinical populations, prevalence levels of between 2% and 20% have been found, and 14.6% among relatives of schizophrenic patients [46, 47], particularly those with a history of childhood onset and among monozygotic twins. According to Kendler et al. [33], StPD most closely reflects the genetic and environmental liability common to all three Cluster A disorders. No gender distinction appears to be unequivocal, but there seems to be more male than female StPD patients.

#### Comorbidities

About 30% of StPD patients present a comorbid pattern with SPD (with introversion as the common dominant feature), and 60% with PPD (with suspiciousness as the most shared trait). AvPD and BPD

are also frequently encountered in patients with StPD. The joint presence of paranoid, schizotypal, schizoid, and avoidant personalities among first-degree relatives of schizophrenic patients has led to the notion of schizophrenia-spectrum disorder and the identification of such PDs as psychometric high-risk groups [48]. In cases, these patients may be 'in and out' of brief psychotic episodes or present premorbid schizophreniform disorder or schizophrenia. As relevant as this, DSM-5 [1] points out that approximately half of StPD patients experience comorbid MDD and may also show evidence of obsessive–compulsive and generalized anxiety disorders [27].

#### Clinical course

Like the other Cluster A PDs, StPD patients show their main symptoms (social isolation, esoteric fantasies, peculiar thought, and language and school underachievement) early in childhood or adolescence. As adults, they may join in marginal groups with extreme socio-political or religious views which may increase their sense of alienation and interpersonal deterioration, a factor that can make them reach, according to some studies, up to 10% of suicidal behaviour. They do not seek treatment for their PD, but rather for associated depression, dysphoria, and/or anxiety. Nevertheless, only a minority falls into schizophrenia or other psychotic disorders, and a good number of patients remain marginally employed throughout their active life period [42].

### Antisocial personality disorder

#### Prevalence

One of the two most studied PDs, the prevalence figures of antisocial personality disorder (AsPD) do not escape the levels of debate or disagreement seen in other types, in spite of large-size studies and more sophisticated evaluation instruments. The highest incidence figures are seen in late adolescence and early adulthood. The range in community samples goes from 0.2% to 4.5%, with a median of between 0.9% and 1.7%, while figures in clinical populations (including prisons or other forensic settings) vary from 3% to 30%. High levels of sensation-seeking and low anxiety sensitivity indicate an increased risk for substance misuse in incarcerated male offenders [49]. In most studies, the role of socio-environmental factors has been elucidated: more often seen in men than in women (rates of 3:1) and among people of younger ages; living in urban, but deprived, areas [ergo, low socio-economic status (SES)]; members of dysfunctional families; and history of trauma, victimization, and neglect during childhood. AsPD patients also have been found to be frequent users of medical services [47]. All-cause mortality is twice as high among those imprisoned [50]. A genetic component is strongly considered by the majority of researchers [6, 33, 42, 51].

## Comorbidities

In addition to a relatively frequent co-occurrence of other Cluster B PDs like borderline, narcissistic, and histrionic, AsPD patients show frequent comorbidity with PPD, alcoholism, hypochondriac behaviour, problem-gambling, and depression [42, 52], the latter exhibiting predominantly atypical features. Substance abuse may coexist with AsPD since childhood, and antisocial behaviour may be secondary to premorbid alcoholism; this association relies on underlying dimensions of impulsivity or externalization [53, 54]. Men with attention-deficit/hyperactivity disorder (ADHD) and patterns of use of nicotine, cannabis, and other illicit drugs since early age also show high presence of AsPD [49], and almost 15% of patients on methadone maintenance therapy fulfil the diagnostic criteria [55].

## Clinical course

AsPD is probably one of the most complicated and clinically fascinating conditions, even when looking back at the childhood life period of the patients—conduct disorder diagnoses frequently precede AsPD detection by the second decade of life. Children with a history of severe conduct problems and callous-unemotional traits (that is, with limited prosocial emotions) can be identified by their peers as early as their preschool years [56] and are high on fearlessness but, like those on the other extreme of the same scales, may have the same antisocial phenotypic outcome. AsPD cannot be diagnosed before age 18, as its typical behavioural manifestations are most pronounced in early adult years [57]. In addition to serious problems with the law, other sequelae, such as unemployment, poverty, homelessness, risky driving, weapon-carrying, and increasingly brutal actions in and out of numerous and fragile marital relationships [56–58], may end up in a shorter life course. Non-domestic homicide offenders are four times more frequent users of firearms, and twice more likely than spontaneous domestic homicide's to be diagnosed as AsPD [58].

It is possible that AsPD behaviours may either gradually decrease with age in some patients, or a subgroup of them may be able to conduct seemingly acceptable social and occupational lives; thus, reduction or remission of criminal behaviour and decrease of the full spectrum of antisocial postures may occur around the fourth decade of life. On average, 20 years after the diagnosis is made, 12% of the patients are symptom-free, 27% show a notable improvement, but

60% remain unchanged [46]. Interestingly, the appearance of other conditions such as depression or hypochondriasis correlates with abandonment of rage and aggression as interpersonal life strategies, reflecting and fostering personality maturation.

## Borderline personality disorder

### Prevalence

According to DSM-5, the median population prevalence of BPD is estimated to be 1.6%, but other sources cite a range of 0.2–5.9%. The high end of this range is from the NESARC study [59], which may be inflated by oversampling young adults (prevalence decreases with age), thus requiring less robust associations with impairment. The samples have been more numerous than with any other PDs, and the clinical correlates with a variety of other conditions are abundant. The disorder is significantly more common among females, particularly widowed and unmarried women (though less clearly so in community samples), and its frequency increases in younger, nonwhite, urban, and poorer respondents. The presence of BPD patients in primary care settings seems to be about 6%, about 10% in outpatient mental health clinics, and 20% in inpatient psychiatric units [60]. A substantial genetic basis, 18–35 years as age of onset, and decreased incidence among older individuals are additional findings.

### Comorbidities

BPD is highly comorbid with a number of other disorders. Up to 75% of patients have comorbid major depression [61], and patients with BPD report MDD symptoms that are subjectively more severe and more interpersonally driven [62]. Even though the presence of MDD does not impact the accuracy of the BPD diagnosis, the latter's symptoms are less responsive to treatment with drugs for depression and electroconvulsive therapy (ECT). On the other hand, bipolar disorder is overrepresented in BPD. In two large prospective studies of BPD, bipolar disorder co-occurred in 15–20% of patients [12% bipolar disorder type I (BPI) and 8% bipolar type II (BPII) in one study [61]; 1% BPI and 14% BPII in the other [63], though BPI was initially excluded from this second cohort).

PTSD co-occurs with BPD at rates of between 17% and 50%, depending on sample and methodology, whereas BPD is found in 7–25% of people with PTSD [22, 26, 59, 64, 65]. Substance use and anxiety disorders (including panic disorder) are also quite common in BPD (upwards of 50%) and tend to remit when BPD symptoms do [60].

### Clinical course

Two large prospective, longitudinal studies inform most of what is known about the course and outcome of BPD. The McLean Study of Adult Development (MSAD), led by Zanarini [63, 66], followed 290 former inpatients for about 20 years; all met rigorous diagnostic criteria for study entry. The second study—the Collaborative Longitudinal Personality Disorders Study (CLPDS)—led by Gunderson [65] was a multi-site, more socio-economically representative inquiry and followed 175 patients with BPD (as well as patients with MDD and other PDs). Both studies demonstrated surprising levels of symptom remission. In fact, by the end of 10 years of follow-up, >80% of each sample no longer met diagnostic criteria. Moreover, when symptomatic remission was achieved, relapse was rare—cumulatively 12% in CLPDS and 15% in the MSAD study. Nonetheless, severe and persistent impairment in social and occupational functioning remained, with only a third of patients obtaining full-time employment by the end of 10 years and only 40% of previously high-functioning patients regaining that performance level.

### Histrionic personality disorder

#### Prevalence

Within ranges of 0.3–3.9% in general populations (median between 1.5% and 1.8%) and 10–15% in clinical settings, HPD is seen more frequently among women, particularly separated and divorced, but without other socio-demographic differences. This disorder seems to respond more to cultural aetio-pathogenic factors (that is, sex role stereotypes, emotional expressiveness, etc.), while some authors suggest that HPD in women is genotypically linked to AsPD in men [42, 45].

#### Comorbidities

Overlapping HPD cases and those of other clusters is a relatively frequent occurrence; borderline, narcissistic, and antisocial from Cluster B, and dependent from Cluster C are the most prevalent. As the features of the different disorders can be combined, once again, a clinically sound differential diagnosis must converge with a thorough assessment of authentic comorbidity. The most difficult comparison is with narcissistic personality disorder (NPD) and AsPD. In the former, the main distinction has to do with the narcissist's attention- and superiority-seeking vs the histrionic's inconsistent and dependency-seeking interpersonal transactions; about the latter, although both types show impulsive, manipulative, and seductive behaviours, the histrionic manipulates to capture others' attention and does not necessarily break the law to reach it, whereas the antisocial individual seduces others in search of absolute authoritarian power frequently nourished by illegal manoeuvres.

The evidence in favour of HPD's comorbidity with other psychiatric disorders is greater for somatization, conversion, and dissociative disorders, besides brief reactive psychosis and a few cases of hypomanic and manic states; the episodic nature of these, though, leads to a differential diagnosis more than to a real comorbidity process [45].

#### Clinical course

Blashfield *et al.* [67] characterized the HPD patient's adolescent period as playful, flamboyant, flirtatious, and attention-seeking. During their early adult life, superficiality, rapidly changing and inconsistent interpersonal patterns, poor sense of responsibility, competitiveness, emotional instability, and suggestibility lead them to, at times, risky or dangerous connections, theatrical and melodramatic explosions, and occupational fragility. Obviously, concomitant borderline and antisocial disorders generate severe levels of personal dysfunctionality. In these and other contexts, depressive symptoms, suicide attempts, and frequent use of medical services are common. Ageing may become a factor of sobering changes in the clinical course of a number of HPD cases.

### Narcissistic personality disorder

#### Prevalence

Perhaps the most debatable and debated PD, with serious considerations of its elimination from DSM-5 due to reasons such as limited credible research, excessive theoretical/ideological considerations, very low prevalence figures, and more dimensional or trait-related coverage and pertinence [68], NPD is, at best, a rich source of dialectics or a window into the relationship between self-esteem and emotional regulation [69] and, at worst, a questionable clinical disorder. It is the PD with the most 0% prevalence figures in the epidemiological literature (eight of 16), and with levels as low as 0.1% among general populations. It is commonly cited as having a rate of 0.5% [19–21], with a range of up to 4.4% [70] or a surprisingly high 6.2% in the NESARC study [71]. More frequently diagnosed in some female clinical populations, this gender difference becomes irrelevant, however, in most epidemiological inquiries.

#### Comorbidities

In the NESARC data, NPD was strongly associated with SUD (40% 12-month prevalence, 64% lifetime) and anxiety disorders (40% 12-month prevalence, 55% lifetime) [71]. Rates of NPD in BPI (24% lifetime) and BPI in BPD (20% lifetime) were surprisingly high, perhaps owing to the overlaps in constructs of grandiosity. Given the prevalence data being out of step with most other studies, interpretation or application of these results warrant caution. Finally, NPD can co-occur with other PDs, most commonly BPD. Estimates are that 15% of patients with BPD have NPD, and 25% of patients with NPD have BPD [60].

#### Clinical course

There are strikingly limited data about the course of NPD. One 3-year prospective study found that 60% of a sample of 20 patients improved over 3 years and that the remaining 40% showed no change; improvement was associated with achievements and new relationships, whereas disillusionments and remaining symptomatology were predicted by high narcissism in interpersonal relationships [72]. Furthermore, NPD worsens the course of comorbid BPD but will improve when BPD symptoms do, and comorbidity with AsPD worsens the prognosis of NPD [60].

### Avoidant personality disorder

#### Prevalence

The clinical expression of an intense sensitivity to rejection and criticism with resulting social isolation, AvPD was first introduced as an independent entity in DSM-III. It is considered the most prevalent PD type in clinical populations, with figures of up to 5.7% in at least one epidemiological study [70], but still above 5% in two other surveys, a rate of 1.7% in general populations [20] and much higher in psychiatric outpatients. Forty-five per cent of people with AvPD are single (never married) [19, 20], but no strong gender differences have been found [73].

#### Comorbidities

Social anxiety disorder (SAD) is both the most common comorbid condition with AvPD and the most common diagnostic confounder. Co-occurrence with SAD is seen in 40% of patients with AvPD, and in patients with SAD, AvPD can be diagnosed in 46% [74]. Social fears are more associated with self-concept AvPD and therefore are more pervasive and interfere with more life domains [75]. High comorbidity with DPD is noted, and a connection with schizoid PD has also been postulated [76].

## Clinical course

While carefully designed long-term studies of AvPD are rare, data do support the relative stability of the symptoms over time. An analysis of the CLPDS data showed that in a 10-year follow-up of AvPD patients, diagnostic stability was reasonably robust from years 6 through 10 (standardized effect 0.79 in men and 0.81 in women), with more variability earlier in the course [77]. It also seems that genetic factors contribute most robustly to AvPD's phenotypic stability [78].

## Dependent personality disorder

### Prevalence

In spite of relatively small numbers, prevalence data of DPD in different studies report significant oscillations (0.1–11%), with a median of between 0.5% and 1.4% and some predominance among women [21, 23, 78, 79]. This PD may be one of the most affected by cultural factors, as pointed out by Carrasco and Lecic-Tosevski [80], due to patterns of passivity, politeness, and submissiveness normally dominant and accepted in some societies.

### Comorbidities

DPD has reasonably high comorbidity with AvPD, as outlined [75]. It is also commonly thought to have high comorbidity with anxiety disorders, but meta-analytic data have questioned this assumption by reporting a modest association ($r = 0.11$) [81]. The submissive nature of the disorder may contribute to an ambiguous presence of a comorbid anxiety, whereas reports of depressed mood are more common.

### Clinical course

The clinical course of DPD is very poorly studied, a major gap in the epidemiological literature on PDs. Indirect evidence for diagnostic stability (vs its emergence in older age) comes from the fact that it only shows a 23.8% reduction in symptoms between ages 20 and 50 [82].

## Obsessive–compulsive personality disorder

### Prevalence

There seems to be agreement in that OCPD is, side by side with AvPD, one of the most prevalent PDs in the general population, with a range of 2.1–7.9% [1], depending in some cases on the preciseness and specificity of the instruments utilized. In clinical populations, prevalence may be as high as 10%. The most accepted median figure is 2.1%. Males may show five times higher rates than females, and the same happens among white, highly educated, married, older age, and employed subjects [83]. Clinical setting may be another differentiating factor, as the highest number of OCPD is seen in outpatient clinics and the lowest in inpatient units and private practice offices [27]. The issue of 'adaptive' (with a subtle or evident cultural input), not necessarily pathological, obsessive–compulsive personality traits has also been raised since the publication of the Epidemiologic Catchment Area (ECA) findings [41, 43, 68].

### Comorbidities

OCPD is commonly comorbid with anxiety and mood disorders, occurring at rates of over 20% in both groups of patients [84]. Among the PDs, OCPD co-occurs with the other Cluster C disorders (particularly AvPD), as well as PPD and StPD. While obsessive–compulsive disorder (OCD) is clearly a separate disorder, symmetry and hoarding symptoms can certainly co-occur, and the capacity to delay rewards contributes to this distinction [85].

### Clinical course

Data from the CLPDS documented no change in OCPD functional improvement over 2 years. Small treatment studies have shown improvement in core PD symptoms, as well as anxiety and depression measures, but data are limited regarding long-term changes in OCPD.

## Other personality disorders

### Passive–aggressive (negativistic) personality disorder

Initially considered in DSM-I as a 'personality trait disturbance', this label was taken out of DSM-IV, and in DSM-5, it could be eventually ascribed to the so-called 'Personality disorder-trait specified' (PD-TS) category included in Section III as a resource for clinicians to describe and identify types different from the generally accepted ones [86]. In European psychiatry, the label is more used and recognized than in North America. According to studies, the general population prevalence ranges from 0.9 to 3.1, but in clinical settings, it moves up to 10% [80].

### Additional PD types

There are several additional labels scattered around the existing literature. For example, some pre-DSM-5 classification instruments listed a *depressive personality disorder*, later incorporated to either 'Dysthymia', 'Major/moderate depressive disorder', or other clinical entities. In a recent study, it was found mostly associated with inattentive ADHD [87]. Similarly, *self-defeating (masochistic)* and *sadistic PDs*, with low prevalence levels (0.8% and 0.2%, respectively), have been studied primarily by Scandinavian researchers [19] and in forensic populations. Finally, a *mixed PD* could not be absent from attempts at a comprehensive clinical assessment [1].

DSM-5 [1] groups a series of personality-related conditions under the rubric of '*Personality change due to another medical condition*' (in the past also called 'Organic PD'), with specifiers that identify different types (labile, disinhibited, aggressive, apathetic, paranoid, other, combined, and unspecified) causing significant distress or impairment in social, occupational, and other areas of functioning. In this context, the issue and actual existence of defined *comorbidities* make the distinction between a pre-existing PD and personality changes secondary to medical conditions a delicate and complex clinical exercise. Furthermore, a growing variety of medical diagnoses can cause this disruption: neurological (that is, Huntington's, Parkinson's, Alzheimer's, and Pick's diseases, epilepsy and interictal status, frontal lobe syndrome, head or central nervous system trauma), neoplastic, infectious (that is, HIV), endocrinological (that is, hypo- and hyperthyroidism, hypo- and hyperadrenalism), and autoimmune conditions (that is, systemic lupus erythematosus). Thus, the *clinical course* of these variants is determined by the underlying cause and a subsequent tendency to chronicity and gradual clinical worsening.

## REFERENCES

1. American Psychiatric Association. *Diagnostic and Statistical Manual of Mental Disorders*, fifth edition. Washington, DC: American Psychiatric Publishing; 2013.

2. World Health Organization. *The ICD-10 Classification of Mental and Behavioural Disorders. Clinical descriptions and Diagnostic Guidelines*. Geneva: World Health Organization; 1992.

3. Millon T. *Disorders of Personality. Introducing a DSM/ICD Spectrum from Normal to Abnormal*, third edition. Hoboken, NJ: John Wiley and Sons; 2011.

4. Millon T, Krueger R, Simonsen E (editors). *Contemporary Directions in Psychopathology. Scientific Foundations of the DSM-5 and ICD-11*. New York, NY: Guilford; 2010.

5. Oldham JM. Personality disorders: recent history and future directions. In: Oldham JM, Skodol AE, Bender DS, editors. *The American Psychiatric Publishing Textbook of Personality Disorders*. Washington, DC: American Psychiatric Publishing; 2005. pp. 3–16.

6. Reichborn-Kjennerud T. Genetics of personality disorders. *Psychiatr Clin North Am* 2008;31:421–40.

7. Bender DS, Morey LC, Skodol AE. Toward a model for assessing level of personality functioning in DSM-5. Part I: A review of theory and methods. *J Pers Assess* 2011;93:332–46.

8. McCrae RR, Costa PT. A five-factor theory of personality. In: Pervin LA, John OP, editors. *Handbook of Personality: Theory and Research*, second edition. New York, NY: Guilford; 1999. pp. 139–53.

9. Pinto J, Carvalho J, Nobre PJ. The relationship between the FFM personality traits, state psychopathology, and sexual compulsivity in a sample of male college students. *J Sex Med* 2013;10:1773–82.

10. Uliaszek AA, Zinbarg RE. An examination of the higher-order structure of psychopathology and its relationship to personality. *J Pers Disord* 2016;30:157–76.

11. Sutin AR, Stephan Y, Terracciano A. Perceived discrimination and personality development in adulthood. *Dev Psychol* 2016;52:155–63.

12. Kantojärvi L, Hakko H, Riipinen P, Riala K. Who is becoming personality disordered? A register-based follow-up study of 508 inpatient adolescents. *Eur Psychiatry* 2016;31:52–9.

13. Yun RJ, Stern BL, Lenzenweger MF, Tiersky LA. Refining personality disorders subtypes and classification using finite mixture modeling. *Personal Disord* 2013;4:121–8.

14. Kernberg OF. *Severe Personality Disorders*. New Haven, CT: Yale University Press; 1984.

15. Contractor AA, Armour C, Shea MT, Mota N, Pietrzak RH. Latent profiles of DSM-5 PTSD symptoms and the 'big Five' personality traits. *J Anxiety Disord* 2016;37:10–20.

16. Golshani S, Mani A, Toubaei S, Farnia V, Sepehry AA, Alikhani M. Personality and psychological aspect of cosmetic surgery. *Aesthetic Plast Surg* 2016;40:38–47.

17. Rettenberger M, Klein V, Briken P. The relationship between hypersexual behavior, sexual excitation, sexual inhibition, and personality traits. *Arch Sex Behav* 2016;45:219–33.

18. Barbosa F, Almeida PR, Ferreira-Santos F, Marques-Teixeira J. Using signal detection theory in the analysis of emotional sensitivity of male recidivist offenders. *Crim Behav Ment Health* 2016;26:18–29.

19. Torgersen S, Kringlen E, Cramer V. The prevalence of personality disorders in a community sampler. *Arch Gen Psychiatry* 2001;46:590–6.

20. Torgersen S. Epidemiology. In: Widiger TA, editor. *Oxford Handbook of Personality Disorders*. New York, NY: Oxford University Press; 2012. pp. 186–205.

21. Coid JW, Yang M, Tyrer P, *et al*. Prevalence and correlates of personality disorders in Great Britain. *Br J Psychiatry* 2006;188:423–31.

22. Lenzenweger MF, Lane M, Loranger AW, Kessler RC. DSM-IV personality disorders in the National Comorbidity Survey Replication (NCSR). *Biol Psychiatry* 2007;62:553–64.

23. Grant BF, Hasin DS, Stinson FS, *et al*. Prevalence, correlates, and disability of personality disorders in the United States: results from the National Epidemiologic Survey on Alcohol and Related Conditions. *J Clin Psychiatry* 2004;65:948–58.

24. Grant BF, Saha TD, Ruan WJ, *et al*. Epidemiology of DSM-5 Drug Use Disorder: Results from the National Epidemiologic Survey on Alcohol and Related Conditions-III. *JAMA Psychiatry* 2016;73:39047.

25. Grant BF, Stinson FS, Dawson DA, Chou SP, Ruan WJ, Pickering RP. Co-occurrence of 12-month alcohol and drug use disorders and personality disorders in the United States. *Arch Gen Psychiatry* 2004;61:361–8.

26. Pietrzak RH, Goldstein RB, Southwick SM, Grant BF. Personality disorders associated with full and partial posttraumatic stress disorder in the U.S. population: results from Wave 2 of the National Epidemiologic Survey on Alcohol and Related Conditions. *J Psychiatr Res* 2011;25:456–65.

27. Widiger TA, Rojas SL. Personality disorders. In: Tasman A, Kay J, Lieberman JA, First MB, Riba MB, editors. *Psychiatry*, fourth edition, Vol. 2. Chichester: John Wiley and Sons; 2015. pp. 1706–48.

28. Beckwith H, Moran PF, Reilly J. Personality disorder prevalence in psychiatric outpatients: a systematic literature review. *Pers Ment Health* 2014;8:91–101.

29. Gupta S, Mattoo SK. Personality disorders: prevalence and demography at a psychiatric outpatient in North India. *Int J Soc Psychiatry* 2012;58:146–52.

30. Morey LC, Hopwood CJ, Gunderson JG, *et al*. Comparison of alternative models for personality disorders. *Psychol Med* 2007;37:983–94.

31. Cramer V, Torgersen S, Kringlen E. Socio-demographic conditions, subjective somatic health, Axis I disorders and personality disorders in common population: the relationship to quality of life. *J Pers Disord* 2007;21:552–67.

32. McGilloway A, Hall RE, Lee T, Bhui KS. A systematic review of personality disorder, race and ethnicity: prevalence, aetiology and treatment. *BMC Psychiatry* 2010;10:33.

33. Kendler KS, Myers J, Torgersen S, Neale MC, Reichborn-Kjennerud T. The heritability of Cluster A personality disorders assessed by both personal interview and questionnaire. *Psychol Med* 2007;37:655–65.

34. Walsh K, Hasin D, Keyes KM, Koenen KC. Association between gender-based violence and personality disorders in U.S. women. *Pers Disord* 2016;7:205–10.

35. Toftdahl NG, Nordentoft M, Hjorthøj C. Prevalence of substance use disorders in psychiatric patients: a natiowide Danish population-based study. *Soc Psychiatry Psychiatr Epidemiol* 2016;51:1290140.

36. Champagne AL, Brunault P, Huguet G, *et al*. Personality disorders but not cancer severity or treatment type, are risk factors for later generalized anxiety disorder and major depressive disorder in nonmetastatic breast cancer patients. *Psychiatry Res* 2016;236:64–70.

37. Sieurin J, Gustavsson P, Weibull CE, *et al*. Personality traits and the risk for Parkinson disease: a prospective study. *Eur J Epidemiol* 2016;31:1690175.

38. Gerlach G, Loeber S, Herpertz S. Personality Disorders and obesity: a systematic review. *Obes Rev* 2016;17:691–723.

39. Dubovi AS, Li Y, Martin JL. Breaking the silence: disordered eating and big five traits in college men. *Am J Mens Health* 2016;10:NP118–26.

40. Zlodre J, Yiend J, Burns T, Fazel S. Coercion, competence, and consent in offenders with personality disorder. *Psychol Crime Law* 2016;22:315–30.

41. Oldham J, Skodol A, Bender D (editors). *Textbook of Personality Disorders*. Washington, DC: American Psychiatric Publishing; 2005.

42. Gelder M, Andreasen N, Lopez-Ibor J, Geddes J (editors). *New Oxford Textbook of Psychiatry*, second edition. New York, NY: Oxford University Press; 2009.

43. Donadon MF, Osorio FL. Personality traits and psychiatric comorbidities in alcohol dependence. *Braz J Med Biol Res* 2016;49:e5036.

44. Lozano ÓM, Rojas AJ, Fernández Calderón F. Psychiatric comorbidity and severity of dependence on substance users: how it impacts on their health-related quality of life? *J Ment Health* 2016;25:1–8.

45. Roca-Bennasar M, Arnillas-Gómez H, Bauzá-Siddons N. Clínica. In: Vallejo-Ruiloba J, Leal-Cercós C, editors. *Tratado de Psiquiatria*, Vol. II. Madrid: Ars Medica; 2005. pp. 1421–34.

46. Koldobsky NMS, Alarcón RD. Trastornos de personalidad: clasificación y aspectos clínicos. In: Alarcón RD, Mazzotti G, Nicolini H, editors. *Psiquiatria*, third edition. Mexico, DF: Manual Moderno; 2008. pp. 529–71.

47. Guzzetta F, de Girolamo G. Epidemiology of personality disorders. In: Andreasen N, Geddes J, Goodwin G, editors. *The New Oxford Textbook of Psychiatry*, second edition. New York, NY: Oxford University Press; 2009. pp. 881–5.

48. Gooding DC, Tallent KA, Matts CW. Rates of avoidant, schizotypal, schizoid and paranoid personality disorders in psychometric high-risk groups at 5-year follow-up. *Schizophr Res* 2007;94:373–4.

49. Anthony ABH, Brunelle C. Substance use in incarcerated male offenders: Predictive validity of a personality typology of substance misusers. *Addict Behav* 2016;53:86–93.

50. Steingrimsson S, Sigurdsson MI, Gudmundsdottir H, Aspelund T, Magnusson A. Mental disorder, imprisonment and reduced life expectancy. A nationwide psychiatric inpatient cohort study. *Crim Behav Ment Health* 2016;26:6–17.

51. Tuvblad C, Wang P, Bezdjian S, Raine A, Baker LA. Psychopathic personality development from ages 9 to 18: genes and environment. *Dev Psychopathol*, 2016;28:27–44.

52. Kong G, Smith PH, Pilver C, Hoff R, Potenza MN. Problem-gambling severity and psychiatric disorders among American-Indian/Alaska native adults. *J Psychiatr Res* 2016;74:55–62.

53. Krueger RF, Hicks BM, Patrick CJ, *et al.* Etiologic connections among substance dependence, antisocial behavior, and personality: modeling the externalizing spectrum. *J Abnorm Psychol* 2002;111:411–24.

54. Ruiz MA, Pincus AL, Schinka JA. Externalizing pathology and the five-factor model: a meta-analysis of personality traits associated with antisocial personality disorder, substance use disorder, and their co-occurrence. *J Pers Disord*. 2008;44:365–88.

55. Teoh Bing Fei J, Yee A, Habil MH. Psychiatric comorbidity among patients on methadone maintenance therapy and its influence on quality of life. *Am J Addict* 2016;25:49–55.

56. Graziano PA, Ros R, Haas S, *et al.* Assessing callous-unemotional traits in preschool children with disruptive behavior problems using peer reports. *J Clin Child Adolesc Psychol* 2016;45:201–14.

57. Vasallo S, Lahausse J, Edwards B. Factors affecting stability and change in risky driving from late adolescence to the late twenties. *Accid Anal Prev* 2016;88:77–87.

58. Saukkonen S, Laajasalo T, Jokela M, Kivivuori J, Salmi V, Aronen ET. Weapon carrying and psychopathic-like features in a population-based sample of Finnish adolescents. *Eur Child Adolesc Psychiatry* 2016;25:183–91.

59. Grant BF, Chou SP, Goldstein RB, *et al.* Prevalence, correlates, disability, and comorbidity of DSM-IV borderline personality disorder: results from the Wave 2 National Epidemiological Survey on Alcohol and Related Conditions. *J Clin Psychiatry* 2008;69:533–45.

60. Gunderson JG, Links P. *Handbook of Good Psychiatric Management for Borderline Personality Disorder*. Washington, DC: American Psychiatric Publishing; 2014.

61. Gunderson JG, Weinberg I, Daversa MT, *et al.* Descriptive and longitudinal observations on the relationship of borderline personality disorder and bipolar disorder. *Am J Psychiatry* 2006;163:1173–8.

62. Yoshimatsu K, Palmer B. Depression in patients with borderline personality disorder. *Harv Rev Psychiatry* 2014;22:266–73.

63. Zanarini MC, Frankenberg FR, Hennen J, Reich DB, Silk KR. Axis I comorbidities in patients with borderline personality disorder: 6-year follow-up and prediction of time to remission. *Am J Psychiatry* 2004;161:2108–14.

64. Pagura J, Stein MB, Bolton JM, Cox BJ, Grant B, Sareen J. Comorbidity of borderline personality disorder and posttraumatic stress disorder in the U.S. population. *J Psychiatry Res* 2010;44:1190–8.

65. Gunderson JG, Stout RL, McGlashan TH, *et al.* Ten-year course of borderline personality disorder: psychopathology and function from the Collaborative Longitudinal Personality Disorders Study. *Arch Gen Psychiatry* 2011;68:827–37.

66. Zanarini MC, Frankenburg FR, Reich DB, Fitzmaurice G. Time to attainment of recovery from borderline personality disorder and stability of recovery: a 10-year prospective follow-up study. *Am J Psychiatry* 2010;167:663–7.

67. Blashfield RK, Reynolds SM, Stennett B. The death of histrionic personality disorder. In: Widiger TA, editor. *The Oxford Handbook of Personality Disorders*. New York, NY: Oxford University Press; 2012. pp. 603–27.

68. Alarcón RD, Sarabia S. Debates on the narcissism conundrum: trait, domain, dimension, type or disorder? *J Nerv Ment Dis* 2013;200:16–25.

69. Ronningstam E, Baskin-Sommers AR. Fear and decision-making in narcissistic personality disorder—a link between psychoanalysis and neuroscience. *Dialog Clin Neurosci* 2013;15:191–201.

70. Klein DN, Riso LP, Donaldson SK, *et al.* Family study of early-onset dysthymia: mood and personality disorders in relatives of outpatients with dysthymia and episodic major depression and normal controls. *Arch Gen Psychiatry* 1995;52:487–96.

71. Stinson FS, Dawson DA, Goldstein RB, *et al.* Prevalence, correlates, disability, and comorbidity of DSM-IV narcissistic personality disorder: results from the Wave 2 National Epidemiologic Survey on Alcohol and Related Conditions. *J Clin Psychiatry* 2008;69:1033–45.

72. Ronningstam E, Gunderson JG, and Lyons M. Changes in pathological narcissism. *Am J Psychiatry* 1995;152:253–7.

73. Oltmanns TF, Powers AD. Gender and personality disorders. In: Widiger TA, editor. *The Oxford Handbook of Personality Disorders*. New York, NY: Oxford University Press; 2012. pp. 206–18.

74. Friborg O, Martinussen M, Kaiser S, Overgard KT, Rosenvinge JH. Comorbidity of personality disorders in anxiety

disorders: a metaanalysis of 30 years of research. *J Affect Disord* 2013;145:143–55.

75. Weinbrecht A, Schulze L, Boettcher J, Renneberg B. Avoidant personality disorder: a current review. *Curr Psychiatry Rep* 2016;18:29–32.

76. Asarnow RF, Nuechterlein KH, Fogelson D, *et al*. Schizophrenia and schizophrenia-spectrum personality disorders in the first-degree relatives of children with schizophrenia: The UCLA Family Study. *Arch Gen Psychiatry* 2001;58:581–8.

77. Sanislow CA, Little TD, Ansell EB, *et al*. Ten-year stability and latent structure of the DSM-IV schizotypal, borderline, avoidant, and obsessive-compulsive personality disorders. *J Abnorm Psychol* 2009;118:507–19.

78. Gjerde LC, Czajkowski N, Roysamb E, *et al*. A longitudinal, population-based twin study of avoidant and obsessive-compulsive personality disorder traits from early to middle adulthood. *Psychol Med* 2015;45:1–10.

79. Brewer K. *Dependent Personality Disorder and other Personality Disorders: A Critical Introduction*. Orsett Academic Monographs, No. 6. Grays: Orsett Psychological Services; 2003.

80. Carrasco JL, Lecic-Tosevski D. Specific types of personality disorder. In: Andreasen N, Geddes J, Goodwin G, editors. *The New Oxford Textbook of Psychiatry*, second edition. New York, NY: Oxford University Press; 2009. pp. 861–81.

81. Ng HM, Bronstein RF. Comorbidity of dependent personality disorder and anxiety disorders: a meta-analytic review. *Clin Psychol Sci Pract* 2005;12:395–406.

82. Gutiérrez F, Vall G, Maria Peri J, *et al*. Personality disorder features through the life course. *J Pers Disord* 2012;26: 763–74.

83. Samuels J, Costa PT. Obsessive-compulsive personality disorder. In: Widiger TA, editor. *The Oxford Handbook of Personality Disorders*. New York, NY: Oxford University Press; 2012. pp. 566–81.

84. Grant JE, Mooney ME, Kushner MG. Prevalence, correlates, and comorbidity of DMS-IV obsessive-compulsive personality disorder: results from the National Epidemiologic Survey on Alcohol and Related Conditions. *J Psychiatr Res* 2012;46:469–75.

85. Pinto A, Steinglass JE, Greene AL, Weber EU, Simpson HB. Capacity to delay reward differentiates obsessive–compulsive disorder and obsessive–compulsive personality disorder. *Biol Psychiatry* 2014;75:653–9.

86. Krueger RF, Derringer J, Markon KE, *et al*. Initial construction of a maladaptive personality trait model and inventory for DSM-5. *Psychol Med* 2012;42:2879–90.

87. Irastorza-Eguskiza LJ, Bellón JM, Mora M. Comorbidity of personality disorders and attention-deficit hyperactivity disorder in adults. *Rev Psiquiatr Salud Ment* 2018; 11:151–5.

# 120

# Genetics of personality disorders

*C. Robert Cloninger*

## Introduction

Substantial contributions have been made to understanding personality disorders through work in psychiatric genetics in a progressive way that can be summarized in five major steps. Initially twin, family, and adoption studies were conducted in order to test whether personality disorders were familial and heritable [1, 2], and also whether there was concordance for specific categorical diagnoses in families [3]. Personality disorders were found to be familial, but patterns of comorbidity within individuals and resemblance among relatives were found to be complex [4]. Personality disorders are not inherited as discrete entities, so there was a need to quantify the descriptive features of the disorders [5].

Secondly, reliable interviews were developed with checklists of features that quantified diagnosis, and the inheritance patterns of such descriptive features were studied. The number of features of disorders was found to be moderately heritable, and some progress was made to identify which features were common to all personality disorders and which to particular subtypes [6, 7]. However, there was still much overlap within individuals and within families, calling into serious doubt the reliance on categorical diagnosis [8]. Nevertheless, categorical diagnoses communicate much information concisely, so they continue to be popular with clinicians.

Thirdly, the relationship between normal and abnormal personality traits were thoroughly studied using quantitative interviews and/or self-report inventories with many scales and subscales [9]. The structure of personality was found to be the same whether people came from the general population or from clinical samples [10, 11], indicating that people with personality disorders or prominent abnormal personality traits were simple unusual configurations of traits that vary widely in the general population [12]. Extremes of individual traits or particular combinations of traits led to problems adapting in a healthy manner. In other words, what appeared to be fuzzy categories of disorder without discrete boundaries could well be specified as specific combinations of extreme (high or low) scorers on multiple dimensions of personality [13]. At least seven dimensions of personality, as measured by various alternative models, had some genes that were unique to each dimension, even though some systems used only 3–5 dimensions [14].

Fourthly, with the ability to measure personality and its disorders as multi-dimensional configurations or profiles of traits, it quickly became clear that the inheritance of the dimensions of personality was highly complex, with resemblance in families influenced by genetics, socio-cultural learning, and environmental experiences throughout the lifespan, even though such complexity had been well described much earlier [15, 16]. Personality is a person's characteristic way of learning about, and adapting to, his or her life experiences. Human beings have multiple systems of learning and memory—procedural (behavioural conditioning for temperament traits), semantic (learning facts and propositions), and autonoetic (self-aware learning or autobiographical memory of a life narrative). Such observations facilitated the integration of genetic, biological, social, and cultural contributions to understanding personality and its disorders. Although twin studies often seemed to suggest that heritability of personality was about 50%, in fact, most of the heritability is due to complex interactions among many gene loci acting in concert, which is called epistasis [17, 18]. The average effects of individual genes on personality are weak and inconsistent until their interactions with other genetic variants and environmental events are taken into account [19, 20]. There is much gene–gene and gene–environment interaction involved in the development of healthy and unhealthy personalities [21–23]. As a result, the field was stuck for more than two decades with what was called the 'missing' or 'hidden' heritability problem—despite resemblance for personality in monozygotic (MZ) twins being very much greater than in dizygotic (DZ) twins and other relatives, most of the genetic variability could not be explained by the average effects of genetic variants despite surveying dense maps of the entire genome [24, 25]. Less than 1% of variability in personality was explained by the average effects of individual genes, even in huge samples of over 60,000 subjects collected by the Genetics of Personality Consortium [19, 26].

Fifthly, it has recently become possible to identify systematically sets of many genetic variants that influence the risk of personality disorders [24]. Using genome-wide association studies (GWAS) in moderate-sized samples with detailed genotyping of the whole genome, the hidden heritability was found distributed in networks of many genes acting in concert, rather than individually. We now have well-validated clustering methods that allow a thorough description of both the genetic and phenotypic architecture of personality [24, 27, 28]. Most of the genome is expressed in the brain, and there is much regional variability in brain gene expression, as well as much individual variability in gene expression between individuals. The genetic variants that influence personality are widespread across the genome, as illustrated later, and are found to regulate gene expression that contributes, in particular, to variability in neural development and neuroplasticity. These recent discoveries open a rich and promising field for understanding the complex genotypic networks and pathways by which personality develops and is self-regulated in human beings. Its applicability to even small and moderate samples means that the pathway from genotype to phenotype can be characterized with depth and precision in ways that are impractical in very large samples [24].

In this chapter, the basic observations along this progression in understanding the genetics of personality disorders will be described and discussed to provide an overview of the contributions of genetics to the diagnosis and treatment of personality disorders.

## Genetic variation in risk of personality disorder is quantitative, not discrete

Antisocial personality is the most consistently recognized and most extensively studied personality disorder. Family, twin, and adoption studies have all shown that liability to antisocial personality disorders varies quantitatively and is moderately heritable, regardless of methods of assessment and diagnosis. Adoption studies of psychopathy [29], antisocial personality [2, 30], and criminality [31, 32] all moderate heritability of the quantitative risk of illness. The childhood experience of an unstable, hostile, or neglectful home acted synergistically to increase the risk of adult petty criminality or antisocial personality [30, 31]. MZ twins were much more often concordant for criminality than were DZ twins, with differences in prevalence according to gender and severity of impairment explaining the degree of familial loading or concordance in relatives in population-based samples for all of Denmark and its islands [33]. A meta-analysis of 51 twin and adoption studies estimated that there were moderate proportions of variance due to additive genetic influences (0.32), non-additive genetic influences (0.09), shared environmental influences (0.16), and non-shared environmental influences (0.43) [34], but the additive genetic influences may have been inflated by the neglect of cultural inheritance and assortative mating [15].

Sex differences in prevalence in the general population have a substantial impact on the degree of familial concordance [1, 33, 35]. For example, antisocial personality disorder is more rare in women than in men, and antisocial women carry a greater genetic loading (measured by more antisocial relatives) than do antisocial men [36].

Such findings show that liability to personality and its disorders varies quantitatively, not as a discrete disease or a set of diseases. Nevertheless, categorical classifications have remained popular for use in clinical practice, even when clinicians are warned that the clinical syndromes used for classification should be reified into discrete diseases, as was done in DSM-IV. The quantitative nature of variation in personality traits suggested the possibility that the number of diagnostic symptoms would be a good index of genetic risk.

## Resemblance for personality disorder categories and symptoms in twins

Svenn Torgersen and his colleagues carried out a twin study of personality disorders using categorical diagnoses [3]. They ascertained 92 MZ and 129 DZ twin pairs, in which at least one proband had a diagnosis of personality disorder, and then classified subjects according to DSM clusters and categories. The concordances for any personality disorder were 58% for MZ pairs and 36% for DZ pairs, indicating moderate heritability (44%) (Table 120.1). When the diagnosis of personality disorder was definite, concordances for any personality disorder were 40% for MZ pairs and 29% for DZ pairs, which was highly significant ($P <0.01$). However, the results could not be explained by a single heritable factor for personality disorder in general; there were heritable influences that further differentiated personality disorder clusters (Table 120.1). Torgersen's estimates of heritability for the clusters and specific categories were moderate (that is, between 40% and 60%), just as was found for quantitative measures of normal [16, 37] and abnormal personality traits [38]. The correlations between DZ pairs were usually less than half of those of MZ pairs, which suggests that gene–gene and gene–environment interactions are important for categorical diagnoses, as they are for personality dimensions in twins reared apart [17, 39–41].

Even stronger evidence for the moderate heritability of personality disorders has been provided by more recent studies of the inheritance of the number of symptoms in each of the ten categories of personality disorders in DSM-IV, which is conserved officially in DSM-5. The sample included 1386 pairs of twins aged 19–35, as assessed by Structured Interview for DSM-IV Personality Disorders (SIDP-IV) interviews. The data were compiled from separate reports about the heritability of the number of symptoms of disorders in personality Cluster A [6], Cluster B [42], and Cluster C [7] (Table 120.2). The total heritability of liability to the number of symptoms in each category varied from weak to moderate, ranging from 28% for paranoid personality symptoms to 38% for antisocial personality symptoms (Table 120.2).

The unique heritability in Table 120.2 indicates the specificity of the genetic determinants of each disorder. Low specificity means that the genetic determinants are non-specific for various diagnoses, so that there is much overlap of diagnostic features in the same individuals and in their relatives, as is true for most personality disorders. In contrast, obsessive–compulsive personality disorder has 85% unique heritability, indicating that its genetic determinants are largely distinct from those of avoidant and dependent personality disorders. This supports the proposal that obsessional traits constitute a fourth cluster with high persistence or anankastic traits [43]. Likewise, unique genetic determinants predominate for dependent personality disorder (52%) in Cluster C, and for schizoid personality disorder (74%) and paranoid personality disorder (54%) in Cluster A. Likewise in Cluster B, antisocial and borderline personality

**Table 120.1** A study of categorical personality disorders (PDs) assessed by SCID-II interviews in 92 MZ twin pairs and 129 DZ twin pairs in Norway

| Diagnoses | MZ correlation 100($r \pm$ SE) | DZ correlation 100($r \pm$ SE) | Broad heritability (% $\pm$ SE) |
|---|---|---|---|
| Any PD | 58 ± 10 | 36 ± 10 | 44 ± 20 |
| Any Cluster A | 37 ± 14 | 9 ± 11 | 37 ± 25 |
| Any Cluster B | 60 ± 11 | 31 ± 12 | 59 ± 23 |
| Any Cluster C | 61 ± 9 | 23 ± 11 | 59 ± 20 |

Source: data from *Compr Psychiatry*, 41(6), Torgersen S, Lygren S, Oien PA, *et al.*, A twin study of personality disorders, pp. 416–25, Copyright (2000), Elsevier Inc.

**Table 120.2** Heritability of the number of symptoms in personality categories in a sample of 1386 Norwegian twin pairs aged 19–35, as assessed by SIDP-IV interviews (total heritability and the heritability unique to each disorder within the three clusters are shown)

| Clusters of PD symptoms | Total heritability (%) | Unique heritability (%) |
|---|---|---|
| **Cluster A ('odd')** | | |
| Schizotypal | 26 | 0 |
| Paranoid | 21 | 57 |
| Schizoid | 28 | 74 |
| **Cluster B ('dramatic')** | | |
| Antisocial | 38 | 15 |
| Histrionic | 31 | 0 |
| Narcissistic | 24 | 10 |
| Borderline | 35 | 0 |
| **Cluster C ('anxious')** | | |
| Avoidant | 35 | 17 |
| Dependent | 31 | 52 |
| Obsessive–compulsive | 27 | 85 |

Source: data from *Psychol Med*, 36(11), Kendler KS, Czajkowski N, Tambs K, *et al.*, Dimensional representations of DSM-IV Cluster A personality disorders in a population-based sample of Norwegian twins: a multivariate study, pp. 1583–91, Copyright (2006), Cambridge University Press [Cluster A]; *Psychol Med*, 38(11), Torgersen S, Czajkowski N, Jacobson K, *et al.*, Dimensional representations of DSM-IV cluster B personality disorders in a population-based sample of Norwegian twins: a multivariate study, pp. 1617–25, Copyright (2008), Cambridge University Press [Cluster B]; *Psychol Med*, 37(5), Reichborn-Kjennerud T, Czajkowski N, Neale MC, *et al.*, Genetic and enviromental influences on dimensional representations of DSM-IV cluster C personality disorders: a population-based multivariate twin study, pp. 645–53, Copyright (2007), Cambridge University Press [Cluster C].

disorders are more closely related genetically to each other than to histrionic and narcissistic personality disorders.

The genetic and environmental architecture of all ten DSM-IV personality disorders has been evaluated using path analysis to estimate the number of common factors and unique determinants of all ten DSM-IV personality disorders [44]. Three latent genetic factors were uncovered (Table 120.3). The first factor is a common determinant of all personality disorders. This common personality factor corresponds to what is measured as low self-directedness (that is, irresponsible, blaming) using the Temperament and Character Inventory (TCI) [10, 43]. The second genetic determinant contributes most strongly to antisocial and borderline personality disorders and most likely corresponds to low TCI Cooperativeness (that is, hostile, revengeful). The third genetic determinant contributes most strongly to schizoid and avoidant personality disorders and most likely corresponds to social detachment as a result of high TCI Harm Avoidance (that is, anxious, shy) and/or low TCI Reward Dependence (that is, aloof, detached).

The first two general factors provide support for proposals to use low Self-directedness and low Cooperativeness as indices of personality in general, as is done in the alternative criteria in DSM-5 [45] and elsewhere [46]. However, most of the disorders have additional genetic influences that are not accounted for by such character variables that define personality disorders in general. Subtypes of personality disorder are largely explained by variation in four temperament dimensions [5, 46], as proposed by Peter Tyrer for the eleventh edition of the *International Classification of Diseases* (ICD-11) [47]. Therefore, genetic evidence strongly supports classifying personality disorders on the basis of multi-dimensional inventories that distinguish character traits for identifying personality disorder in general or not, and temperament traits that distinguish subtypes in terms of their profile of emotional style [10, 43].

## Same genes influence normal and abnormal personality

Multi-dimensional inventories for assessing components of personality disorders have been developed to measure both normal and abnormal traits. One of the most robust findings about personality, but

**Table 120.3** Path coefficients (× 100) for contributions to heritability of numbers of PD symptom groupings measured by the SIDP from three latent genetic factors (GFs) and unique contributions for each grouping of symptoms in 2794 Norwegian twins

| Clusters of PD symptoms | Path from GF1 (? low Self-directedness) | Path from GF2 (? high Novelty Seeking/ low Cooperativeness) | Path from GF3 (? high Harm Avoidance/low Reward Dependence) | Path from Unique or Unexplained GF |
|---|---|---|---|---|
| **Cluster A** | | | | |
| Schizotypal | 11 | 22 | 22 | 31 |
| Paranoid | 30 | 13 | 22 | 28 |
| Schizoid | 2 | 7 | 37 | 34 |
| **Cluster B** | | | | |
| Antisocial | 6 | 63 | 9 | 0 |
| Histrionic | 49 | 23 | 14 | 0 |
| Narcissistic | 35 | 12 | 7 | 33 |
| Borderline | 32 | 43 | 16 | 24 |
| **Cluster C** | | | | |
| Avoidant | 14 | 7 | 59 | 0 |
| Dependent | 29 | 15 | 23 | 37 |
| Obsessive | 29 | 6 | 13 | 41 |

Source: data from *Arch Gen Psychiatry*, 65(12), Kendler KS, Aggen SH, Czajkowski N, *et al.*, The structure of genetic and environmental risk factors for DSM-IV personality disorders, pp. 1438–46, Copyright (2008), American Medical Association.

one that is surprising to many psychiatrists, is that the same dimensions of personality are observed whether one begins with normal personality variation in the general community, with abnormal personality traits, or with symptoms of personality disorders in treatment samples.

There are three main lines of evidence indicating that the same genes and environmental variables account for variation in both normal and abnormal personality traits. Firstly, people with personality disorders or other forms of psychopathology have extreme values on one or more personality dimensions, but the correlational structure is the same in samples from the general community and from psychiatric treatment facilities [43, 48, 49]. If personality disorders were discrete diseases unrelated to normal personality variation, then the correlational structures of personality would differ in clinical and non-clinical samples (but they do not!). Secondly, the genetic–environmental architecture of normal personality traits is indistinguishable from that of abnormal personality traits. The finding that the genes and environmental influences for normal and abnormal personality are the same is found whether twins are reared together [49] or apart [50]. Thirdly, variability in normal personality traits that are descriptive of the general population are diagnostic of personality disorders [43, 51]. Therefore, normal personality traits share a common functional foundation with abnormal personality traits and most, if not all, mental disorders. Essentially, the same genetic and bio-psychosocial systems influence individual differences in normal personality and in its disorders.

In order to understand how personality disorders arise from particular configurations of traits that characterize normal variation in the general population, it is helpful to consider information from genetic studies of both normal and abnormal personality. Twin studies of personality dimensions in the general population demonstrated moderate heritability of normal personality traits. For example, the TCI was developed based on specific neurobiological and psychosocial data [5, 10, 52–54]. It measures four dimensions of temperament (that is, behavioural biases in response to basic emotional stimuli) and three dimensions of character (that is, higher cognitive processes influencing the maturity of a person's goals and values). Initial twin studies were carried out using only measures of temperament [55, 56]. More recent twin studies have used the TCI and showed that each of the seven TCI dimensions has a unique genetic variance that is not explained by the other dimensions [14].

The TCI is descriptive of normal variation in the general population and is also highly effective in distinguishing people with and without personality disorder and in doing differential diagnosis of all personality disorder subtypes [43, 46]. The distinction between character and temperament in the TCI allows its character dimensions to be a highly effective model in distinguishing healthy from unhealthy personality traits [51]. The three character dimensions of the TCI are Self-directedness (that is, resourceful, purposeful, and responsible), Cooperativeness (that is, tolerant, helpful, and principled), and Self-transcendence (that is, idealistic, selfless, and contemplative) [57]. These dimensions correspond to variability in the intrapersonal, interpersonal, and transpersonal aspects of the self. The distinction between character (what we make of ourselves intentionally) and temperament (emotional drives) is well supported by studies of unique genetic determinants [14], phylogenesis [58, 59], brain imaging [60, 61], self-awareness and mental time-travel [62], effects of parental child rearing and early home environment [63],

and generativity (that is, fertile and/or stable marriage, sperm donation) [64–67].

The heritability of each of the seven TCI dimensions in a sample of 2517 Australian twins is summarized in Table 120.4. Total heritability varied from 27% to 45%, without correcting for the reduced reliability of the short form of the TCI used in this study. Both temperament and character traits were roughly equally heritable, and each dimension had genetic determinants unique to it (that is, not overlapping with the genetics of other dimensions).

Likewise, John Livesley and his colleagues developed the Differential Assessment of Personality Pathology (DAPP) to measure the self-report of abnormal personality traits as a hierarchy of dimensions. The questionnaire is composed of 560 items measuring 18 factorially derived dimensions, each with at least three specific facet scales [11, 38]. The heritability and concordances in 236 MZ twin pairs and 247 DZ twin pairs have been estimated for all 18 DAPP traits (Table 120.5). The heritability ranged from 35% for rejection sensitivity to 56% for conduct problems and callousness, once again showing that personality traits are moderately heritable.

Four higher-order traits have been identified that account for most of the variability in the 18 DAPP dimensions. These are described as: (1) 'emotional lability or dysregulation'; (2) 'antagonism or dissocial behavio[u]r'; (3) 'interpersonal responsiveness or inhibition'; and (4) 'compulsivity' [49]. These higher-order dimensions of abnormal personality resemble the unhealthy extreme of the dimensions of normal personality. The first three also correspond to the three factors identified in path analysis of personality disorders, as summarized previously in Table 120.3. For example, emotional dysregulation is similar to high neuroticism in the five-factor model (measured by the NEO) [68] or low Self-directedness in the seven-factor model of temperament and character (measured by TCI) [10]. Antagonism or dissocial behaviour is similar to low agreeability in the five-factor model and low Cooperativeness in the seven-factor model. Hence, these dimensions define healthy personality at one extreme (namely, high TCI Self-directedness and Cooperativeness, or low DAPP emotional dysregulation and dissocial behaviour, or low NEO Neuroticism and Agreeableness) and personality disorder at the other extreme (for example, low TCI Self-directedness and Cooperativeness, etc.) [43, 49, 68].

**Table 120.4** Total heritability of each of the seven Temperament and Character Inventory (TCI) personality dimensions estimated in 2517 twins in Australia (unique effects exclude genetic contributions shared with other TCI personality dimensions)

| Personality dimension | Total heritability (%) | Unique heritability (%) |
|---|---|---|
| Harm Avoidance | 42 | 29 |
| Novelty Seeking | 39 | 32 |
| Reward Dependence | 35 | 20 |
| Persistence | 30 | 23 |
| Self-directedness | 34 | 25 |
| Cooperativeness | 27 | 16 |
| Self-transcendence | 45 | 26 |

Source: data from *Pers Individ Dif.*, 35(8), Gillespie NA, Cloninger CR, Heath AC, *et al.*, The genetic and environmental relationship between Cloninger's dimensions of temperament and character, pp. 1931–46, Copyright (2003), Elsevier Ltd.

**Table 120.5** Heritability and concordances in 236 MZ twin pairs and 247 DZ twin pairs for 18 basic scales of the Differential Assessment of Personality Pathology in Canada

| Scale label | MZ correlation (r × 100) | DZ correlation (r × 100) | Heritability (%) |
|---|---|---|---|
| Affective lability | 49 | 12 | 45 |
| Anxiousness | 42 | 25 | 44 |
| Callousness | 56 | 32 | 56 |
| Cognitive distortion | 48 | 31 | 49 |
| Compulsivity | 40 | 19 | 37 |
| Conduct problems | 53 | 36 | 56 |
| Identity problems | 51 | 28 | 53 |
| Insecure attachment | 45 | 27 | 48 |
| Intimacy problems | 47 | 24 | 48 |
| Narcissism | 51 | 22 | 53 |
| Oppositionality | 41 | 29 | 46 |
| Rejection | 33 | 19 | 35 |
| Restricted expression | 48 | 26 | 41 |
| Self-harm | 39 | 26 | 41 |
| Social avoidance | 52 | 27 | 53 |
| Stimulus-seeking | 38 | 21 | 40 |
| Submissiveness | 41 | 29 | 45 |
| Suspiciousness | 42 | 29 | 45 |

Source: data from *Acta Psychiatr Scand.*, 94(6), Jang KL, Livesley WJ, Vernon PA, *et al.*, Heritability of personality disorder traits: a twin study, pp. 438–44, Copyright (1996), John Wiley and Sons.

Overall, twin studies showed that personality is moderately heritable whether measured as normal traits, abnormal traits, number of symptoms, or categorical diagnoses. Alternative measurement methods are highly convergent with one another.

## The complexity of personality genetics

Twin studies indicated that between 30% and 60% of the phenotypic variance in personality and its disorders, as assessed by a variety of instruments, is genetic in origin [14, 18, 39, 69, 70]. However, adoption studies, studies of twins plus other family members, and GWAS have shown that common additive genetic variants account for little of the heritability of personality traits; most of the heritability of personality and its disorders, as assessed by a variety of instruments, depends on complex interactions among multiple gene loci (that is, epistasis) and possibly multiple alleles at a locus (that is, dominance), rather than the average effects of individual genes [17, 18, 20, 39, 70–72]. As a result, little (that is, <7.2% on average) of the expected genetic effects on personality can be attributed to the average effects of individual single-nucleotide polymorphisms (SNPs) [20].

The importance of gene–gene and gene–environment interactions can be illustrated by studies of association of TCI Novelty Seeking with polymorphisms for dopamine receptor type 4 (DRD4), first reported by Jonathan Benjamin. Initially, they observed the simple association between DRD4 and Novelty Seeking, and then extended their findings to show the association depends on the three-way interaction of DRD4 with catechol-O-methyltransferase (COMT)

and the serotonin transporter locus promoter's regulatory region (5-HTTLPR). Consequently, the association of Novelty Seeking with the average effects of DRD4 is weak and inconsistent. In the absence of the short 5-HTTLPR allele (5HTLPR L/L genotype) and in the presence of the high-activity COMT Val/Val genotype, Novelty Seeking scores are higher in the presence of the DRD4 7-repeat allele than in its absence [73]. Furthermore, within families, siblings who shared identical genotype groups for all three polymorphisms (COMT, DRD4, and 5-HTTLPR) had significantly correlated TCI Novelty Seeking scores (r = 0.4 in 49 subjects; P <0.01). In contrast, sibs with dissimilar genotypes in at least one polymorphism showed no significant correlation for Novelty Seeking. Similar interactions were observed between these polymorphisms and Novelty Seeking in an independent sample of unrelated subjects [73] and have been replicated by independent investigators [74]. Likewise, there is also substantial evidence for specific gene–environment interactions on personality development [21, 75–83]. For example, TCI Novelty Seeking scores in adulthood are associated with particular DRD4 polymorphisms only if the children were reared in a hostile childhood environment with measures during childhood of maternal reports of emotional distance and punitive discipline [21]. Such complex non-linear interactions present great challenges for the identification and replication of relationships in GWAS. As a result of such complexity, despite extensive past effort, for the past decade, GWAS of personality had found few significant associations between specific SNPs and personality traits despite using a variety of well-validated personality instruments [19, 26, 84]. This is not surprising because the GWAS methods failed to account for the complexity of personality. Such failure to account for most of the heritability of complex traits has been called the 'missing' [25] or 'hidden' [85] heritability problem.

Until recently [24], the missing heritability problem had been approached in GWAS by analysing the explained variance in individual personality traits in large individual samples or by using meta-analysis to combine data sets, such as the Genetics of Personality Consortium, with more than 60,000 subjects in 30 or more demographically diverse samples assessed with a variety of personality inventories [19, 20, 26, 86–89]. Efforts have also been made to harmonize measures from moderately correlated inventories using item-response theory and to consider the impact of demographic variables or allele frequencies on variation in individual traits. Nevertheless, most of the heritability of the traits has remained unexplained because even in large samples, the methods used are effective for detecting only the average effects of individual genes, but not the non-additive interactions among multiple genes and environmental events that are actually expected [24, 28, 90] (Table 120.6).

## Genomic approaches to understanding temperament and character

Fortunately, the integration of well-validated clustering methods with GWAS has made it possible to address the complexity of personality systematically [24]. Different profiles of temperament and of character were associated with different sets of functionally interacting genes detected through SNPs. The broad heritability of the various traits of personality varies from 30% to 60%, but this

**Table 120.6** Greater importance of non-additive than additive components of heritability for Cloninger's and Eysenck's personality traits in a study of 9672 MZ and DZ twins and 3241 of their siblings (twin plus sibling design)

| Personality trait | Additive heritability (women) | Non-additive heritability (women) | Additive heritability (men) | Non-additive heritability (men) |
|---|---|---|---|---|
| TCI Harm Avoidance | 0.15* | 0.27* | – | 0.29* |
| TCI Novelty Seeking | 0.05 | 0.35* | 0.05 | 0.35* |
| TCI Reward Dependence | 0.07 | 0.31* | – | 0.11* |
| TCi Persistence | 0.00 | 0.35* | 0.00 | 0.35* |
| EPQ-R Extraversion | 0.23* | 0.24* | 0.23* | 0.24* |
| EPQ-R Neuroticism | 0.19* | 0.23* | 0.09* | 0.12* |

* Denotes components that are significant in best-fitting model

Source: data from *Behav Genet.*, 35(6), Keller MC, Coventry WL, Heath AC, *et al.*, Widespread evidence for non-additive genetic variation in Cloninger's and Eysenck's Personality Dimensions using a Twin Plus Sibling Design, pp. 707–21, Copyright (2005), Springer Science Business Media, Inc.

depends on substantial interactions among multiple genes and environmental variables. The average effects of individual genes explains <7.2% of the variability in personality, but allowing for gene–gene and gene–environment interactions accounted well for the broad heritability of temperament and character. The whole genome was screened for specific genes using about one million SNPs in >4000 people representative of the general populations of Finland, Germany, and Korea. Personality was found to be highly polygenic, with the associated genes distributed across all the human chromosomes in the Young Finns Heart Study [91], followed by replication in the other two independent samples. Fig. 120.1 shows the number of genes per chromosome that are strongly associated with clusters of people with particular temperament profiles (that is, temperament only), clusters of people with particular character profiles

(that is, character only), and clusters of people with profiles of both temperament and character traits (that is, temperament and character). Sets of multiple genes were identified, independently of information about the personality traits, and the clusters of people were identified without information about the genetic profiles. The gene sets therefore represent naturally occurring combinations of genes with distinct functional interactions [24]. The sets of genes and personality profiles were very strongly associated, but the relationships were complex in the sense that the same gene set could be expressed in multiple ways (that is, multifinality, pleiotropy) and different sets of genes could be expressed in the same way (that is, equifinality, heterogenetiy).

The complex development of personality profiles from interacting sets of multiple genes and environmental variables will be described in more detail later. Now it is fundamentally important to recognize that most of the genes that influence personality have regulatory functions, rather than being protein-coding genes (Fig. 120.2). In older genetic studies of personality, nearly all attention has been focused on protein-coding genes related to neurotransmitter functions. However, it is the regulatory genes that help us to understand change and development of human personality.

Most of the regulatory genes are long non-coding ribonucleic acids (lncRNAs), other shorter non-coding RNAs (ncRNAs), and pseudogenes. These ncRNAs (long or short) are functional RNA molecules that are transcribed from deoxyribonucleic acid (DNA) but are not translated into proteins [92]. They can regulate gene expression at both the transcriptional and post-transcriptional levels. They are involved in epigenetic processes that can be divided into two main groups: the short ncRNAs of <30 nucleotides and the lncRNAs of >200 nucleotides. The major classes of short ncRNAs are microRNAs (miRNAs), short interfering RNAs (siRNAs), and piwi-interacting RNAs (piRNAs). Both long and short RNAs are known to play a role in heterochromatin formation, histone modification, DNA methylation targeting, and gene silencing. However, lncRNAs and the shorter ncRNAs act differently.

Nearly 30% of the genes associated with character only involve lncRNAs, whereas the percentage is only 20% in the other two

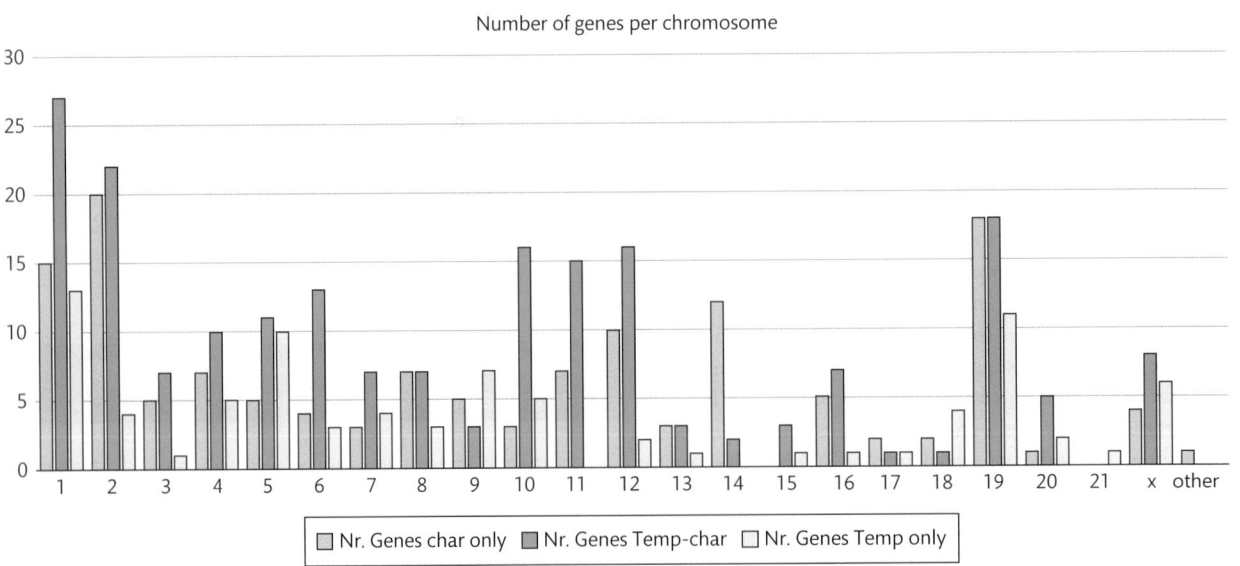

Number of genes per chromosome

**Fig. 120.1** Number of genes per chromosome for temperament and character identified and replicated in person-centred GWAS of Temperament and Character Inventory in the Young Finns Study.

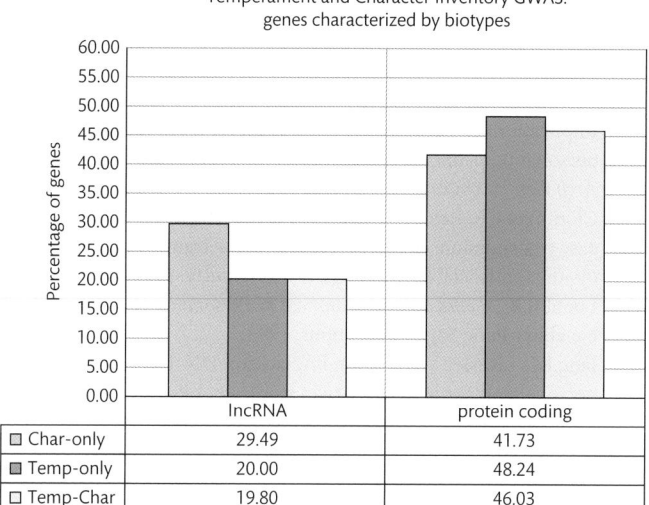

Temperament and Character Inventory GWAS: genes characterized by biotypes

| | lncRNA | protein coding |
|---|---|---|
| ☐ Char-only | 29.49 | 41.73 |
| ▣ Temp-only | 20.00 | 48.24 |
| ☐ Temp-Char | 19.80 | 46.03 |

**Fig. 120.2** Genes distinguished by biotype for temperament only, character only, and both in person-centred GWAS of Temperament and Character Inventory in the Young Finns Study.

groups, as shown in Fig. 120.2. In contrast, protein-coding genes are more often associated with temperament only than with the groups involving character. The more prominent role of lncRNAs in character is consistent with the hypothesis that epigenetic change is more important for the development of character than for temperament [63, 91].

lncRNAs form extensive networks of ribonucleoprotein (RNP) complexes with numerous chromatin regulators. These chromatin regulators target these enzymatic activities to the appropriate locations in the genome. Apparently, lncRNAs can function as modular scaffolds to specify higher-order organization in RNP complexes and in chromatin states. lncRNAs have several functions in the regulation of gene transcription, including the regulation of specific gene transcription (either activation or repression), post-transcriptional regulation, differential spicing, and regulation of epigenetic modifications, including histone and DNA methylation, histone acetylation and sumoylation, and remodelling of chromatin domains. These findings suggest the hypothesis that character development involves epigenetic processes involving regulation of gene expression and chromatin modification, which, in turn, influence neural development and neuroplasticity. lncRNA dysfunction is also often observed in common chronic diseases related to stress and lifestyle regulation, including cancer, cardiovascular diseases, neurological diseases, and immune-mediated diseases.

In contrast, the shorter ncRNAs are mostly involved in distinct temporal expression patterns during embryogenesis, acting in specific tissues to regulate expression at a post-transcriptional level. miRNAs usually bind to a specific target messenger RNA with a complementary sequence to induce cleavage and degradation or to block translation, and they have crucial roles in epigenesis. Silent-interfering RNAs function in ways similar to miRNAs to mediate post-transcriptional gene silencing as a result of messenger RNA degradation and to induce heterochromatin formation. piRNAs are so named due to their interaction with the piwi family of proteins. They are involved in chromatin regulation and suppression of transposon activity during embryogenesis. The percentage of ncRNA

genes associated with personality is only 5% and do not distinguish the temperament clusters from the character clusters.

As shown in Fig. 120.2, the distribution of the types of genes associated with character differs from that of other groups. These findings suggest that the ability of the human character to self-regulate emotion may be related to the human capacity to self-regulate gene expression, which can be cultivated by enhanced self-awareness [93]. The prominence of regulatory functions associated with personality traits that influence neural development and neuroplasticity provides a mechanism for understanding the way learning and memory processes influence personality development as a complex adaptive process.

## REFERENCES

1. Cloninger RC, Reich T, Guze SB. The multifactorial model of disease transmission: II. Sex differences in the familial transmission of sociopathy (antisocial personality). *Br J Psychiatry*. 1975;127:11–22.
2. Crowe RR. The adopted offspring of women criminal offenders: a study of their arrest records. *Arch Gen Psychiatry*. 1972;27:600–3.
3. Torgersen S, Lygren S, Oien PA, *et al.* A twin study of personality disorders. *Compr Psychiatry*. 2000;41:416–25.
4. Cloninger CR. Implications of comorbidity for the classification of mental disorders: the need for a psychobiology of coherence. In: Maj M, Gaebel W, Lopez-Ibor JJ, Sartorius N, editors. *Psychiatric Diagnosis and Classification*. New York, NY: Wiley; 2002. pp. 79–105.
5. Cloninger CR. A systematic method for clinical description and classification of personality variants. A proposal. *Arch Gen Psychiatry*. 1987;44:573–88.
6. Kendler KS, Czajkowski N, Tambs K, *et al.* Dimensional representations of DSM-IV Cluster A personality disorders in a population-based sample of Norwegian twins: a multivariate study. *Psychol Med*. 2006;36:1583–91.
7. Reichborn-Kjennerud T, Czajkowski N, Neale MC, *et al.* Genetic and enviromental influences on dimensional representations of DSM-IV cluster C personality disorders: a population-based multivariate twin study. *Psychol Med*. 2007;37:645–53.
8. Cloninger CR. Validation of psychiatric classification: the psychobiological model of personality as an exemplar. In: Zachar P, Stoyanov D, Aragona M, Jablensky A, editors. *Alternative Perspectives on Psychiatric Validation: DSM, ICD, RDoC, and Beyond*. Oxford: Oxford University Press; 2015. pp. 201–23.
9. Strack S, editor. *Differentiating Normal and Abnormal Personality*, second edition. New York, NY: Springer Publishing; 2006.
10. Cloninger CR, Svrakic DM, Przybeck TR. A psychobiological model of temperament and character. *Arch Gen Psychiatry*. 1993;50:975–90.
11. Livesley WJ, Jang KL, Vernon PA. Phenotypic and genetic structure of traits delineating personality disorder. *Arch Gen Psychiatry*. 1998;55:941–8.
12. Cloninger CR. A new conceptual paradigm from genetics and psychobiology for the science of mental health. *Aust N Z J Psychiatry*. 1999;33:174–86.
13. Cloninger CR, editor. *Personality and Psychopathology*, first edition. Washington, DC: American Psychiatric Press; 1999.
14. Gillespie NA, Cloninger CR, Heath AC, Martin NG. The genetic and environmental relationship between Cloninger's dimensions of temperament and character. *Pers Individ Diff*. 2003;35:1931–46.
15. Cloninger CR, Rice J, Reich T. Multifactorial inheritance with cultural transmission and assortative mating. II. a general model

of combined polygenic and cultural inheritance. *Am J Hum Genet*. 1979;31:176–98.

16. Eaves LJ, Eysenck HJ, Martin NG. *Genes, Culture and Personality: An Empirical Approach*. London: Academic Press; 1989.

17. Plomin R, Corley R, Caspi A, Fulker DW, DeFries J. Adoption results for self-reported personality: evidence for nonadditive genetic effects? *J Pers Soc Psychol*. 1998;75:211–18.

18. Keller MC, Coventry WL, Heath AC, Martin NG. Widespread evidence for non-additive genetic variation in Cloninger's and Eysenck's Personality Dimensions using a Twin Plus Sibling Design. *Behav Genet*. 2005;35:707–21.

19. Verweij KJH, Zietsch BP, Medland SE, et al. A genome-wide association study of Cloninger's temperament scales: implications for the evolutionary genetics of personality. *Biol Psychol*. 2010;85:306–17.

20. Verweij KJ, Yang J, Lahti J, et al. Maintenance of genetic variation in human personality: testing evolutionary models by estimating heritability due to common causal variants and investigating the effect of distant inbreeding. *Evolution*. 2012;66:3238–51.

21. Keltikangas-Jarvinen L, Raikkonen K, Ekelund J, Peltonen L. Nature and nurture in novelty seeking. *Mol Psychiatry*. 2004;9:308–11.

22. Keltikangas-Jarvinen L, Jokela M. Nature and nurture in personality. *Focus*. 2010;8:180–6.

23. Lahti J, Raikkonen K, Ekelund J, Peltonen L, Raitakari OT, Keltikangas-Jarvinen L. Novelty seeking: interaction between parental alcohol use and dopamine D4 receptor gene exon III polymorphism over 17 years. *Psychiatr Genet*. 2005;15:133–9.

24. Arnedo J, Svrakic DM, Del Val C, et al. Uncovering the hidden risk architecture of the schizophrenias: confirmation in three independent genome-wide association studies. *Am J Psychiatry*. 2015;172:139–53.

25. Eichler EE, Flint J, Gibson G, et al. Missing heritability and strategies for finding the underlying causes of complex disease. *Nat Rev Genet*. 2010;11:446–50.

26. Service SK, Verweij KJ, Lahti J, et al. A genome-wide meta-analysis of association studies of Cloninger's Temperament Scales. *Transl Psychiatry*. 2012;2:e116.

27. Arnedo J, del Val C, de Erausquin GA, et al. PGMRA: a web server for (phenotype × genotype) many-to-many relation analysis in GWAS. *Nucleic Acids Res*. 2013;41(Web Server issue):W142–9.

28. Arnedo J, Mamah D, Baranger DA, et al. Decomposition of brain diffusion imaging data uncovers latent schizophrenias with distinct patterns of white matter anisotropy. *Neuroimage*. 2015;120:43–54.

29. Schulsinger F. Psychopathy, heredity and environment. *Int J Ment Health*. 1972;1:190–206.

30. Crowe RR. An adoption study of antisocial personality. *Arch Gen Psychiatry*. 1974;31:785–91.

31. Cloninger CR, Sigvardsson S, Bohman M, von Knorring AL. Predisposition to petty criminality in Swedish adoptees. II. Cross-fostering analysis of gene-environment interaction. *Arch Gen Psychiatry*. 1982;39:1242–7.

32. Mednick SA, Gabrielli WFJ, Hutchings B. Genetic influences in criminal convictions: evidence from an adoption cohort. *Science*. 1984;22:891–4.

33. Cloninger CR, Gottesman II. Genetic and environmental factors in antisocial behavior disorders. In: Mednick SA, Moffitt TE, Stack S, editors. *The Causes of Crime: New Biological Approaches*. Cambridge: Cambridge University Press; 1987. pp. 92–109.

34. Rhee SH, Waldman ID. Genetic and environmental influences on antisocial behavior: a meta-analysis of twin and adoption studies. *Psychol Bull*. 2002;128:490–529.

35. Cloninger CR, Christiansen KO, Reich T, Gottesman, II. Implications of sex differences in the prevalences of antisocial personality, alcoholism, and criminality for familial transmission. *Arch Gen Psychiatry*. 1978;35:941–51.

36. Cloninger CR, Reich T, Guze SB. The multifactorial model of disease transmission: II. Sex differences in the transmission of sociopathy (antisocial personality). *Br J Psychiatry*. 1975;127:11–22.

37. Loehlin JC. *Genes and Environment in Personality Development*. Newbury Park: Sage Publications; 1992.

38. Jang KL, Livesley WJ, Vernon PA, Jackson DN. Heritability of personality disorder traits: a twin study. *Acta Psychiatr Scand*. 1996;94:438–44.

39. Tellegen A, Lykken TD, Bouchard TJ, Wilcox KJ, Segal NL, Rich S. Personality similarity in twins reared apart and together. *J Pers Soc Psychol*. 1988;54:1031–9.

40. Pedersen NL, Plomin R, McClearn GE, Friberg L. Neuroticism, extraversion, and related traits in adult twins reared apart and reared together. *J Pers Soc Psychol*. 1099;55:950–7.

41. Bergeman CS, Chipur HM, Plomin R, et al. Genetic and environmental effects on openness to experience, agreeableness, and conscientiousness: an adoption/twin study. *J Pers*. 1993;61:159–79.

42. Torgersen S, Czajkowski N, Jacobson K, et al. Dimensional representations of DSM-IV cluster B personality disorders in a population-based sample of Norwegian twins: a multivariate study. *Psychol Med*. 2008;38:1617–25.

43. Svrakic DM, Whitehead C, Przybeck TR, Cloninger CR. Differential diagnosis of personality disorders by the seven-factor model of temperament and character. *Arch Gen Psychiatry*. 1993;50:991–9.

44. Kendler KS, Aggen SH, Czajkowski N, et al. The structure of genetic and environmental risk factors for DSM-IV personality disorders. *Arch Gen Psychiatry*. 2008;65:1438–46.

45. Cloninger CR. Personality and temperament: new and alternative perspectives. *Focus*. 2010;8:161–3.

46. Cloninger CR. A practical way to diagnose personality disorder: a proposal. *J Pers Disord*. 2000;14:99–108.

47. Tyrer P, Crawford M, Sanatinia R, et al. Preliminary studies of the ICD-11 classification of personality disorder in practice. *Personal Ment Health*. 2014;8:254–63.

48. Krueger RF. The structure of common mental disorders. *Arch Gen Psychiatry*. 1999;56:921–6.

49. Livesley WJ, Jang KL, Vernon PA. Phenotypic and genetic structure of traits delineating personality disorder. *Arch Gen Psychiatry*. 1998;55:941–8.

50. Markon KE, Krueger RF, Bouchard TJ, Jr., Gottesman, II. Normal and abnormal personality traits: evidence for genetic and environmental relationships in the Minnesota Study of Twins Reared Apart. *J Pers*. 2002;70:661–93.

51. Grucza RA, Goldberg LR. The comparative validity of 11 modern personality inventories: predictions of behavioral acts, informant reports, and clinical indicators. *J Pers Assess*. 2007;89:167–87.

52. Cloninger CR. A unified biosocial theory of personality and its role in the development of anxiety states. *Psychiatr Dev*. 1986;4:167–226.

53. Bohman M, Cloninger R, Sigvardsson S, von Knorring AL. The genetics of alcoholisms and related disorders. *J Psychiatr Res*. 1987;21:447–52.

54. Cloninger CR. The psychobiological theory of temperament and character: comment on Farmer and Goldberg (2008). *Psychol Assess*. 2008;20:292–9; discussion 300–4.

55. Heath AC, Cloninger CR, Martin NG. Testing a model for the genetic structure of personality: a comparison of the personality systems of Cloninger and Eysenck. *J Pers Soc Psychol*. 1994;66:762–75.

56. Stallings MC, Hewitt JK, Cloninger CR, Heath AC, Eaves LJ. Genetic and environmental structure of the Tridimensional Personality Questionnaire: three or four temperament dimensions? *J Pers Soc Psychol*. 1996;70:127–40.

57. Cloninger CR. What makes people healthy, happy, and fulfilled in the face of current world challenges? *Mens Sana Monogr*. 2013;11:16–24.

58. Cloninger CR, Kedia S. The phylogenesis of human personality: identifying the precursors of cooperation, altruism, and well-being. In: Sussman RW, Cloninger CR, editors. *The Origins of Cooperation and Altruism. Developments in Primatology: Progress and Prospects*, first edition. New York, NY: Springer; 2011. pp. 63–110.

59. Cloninger CR. The evolution of human brain functions: the functional structure of human consciousness. *Austr N Z J Psychiatry*. 2009;43:994–1006.

60. Van Schuerbeek P, Baeken C, De Raedt R, De Mey J, Luypaert R. Individual differences in local gray and white matter volumes reflect differences in temperament and character: a voxel-based morphometry study in healthy young females. *Brain Res*. 2011;1371:32–42.

61. Gardini S, Cloninger CR, Venneri A. Individual differences in personality traits reflect structural variance in specific brain regions. *Brain Res Bull*. 2009;79:265–70.

62. Quoidbach J, Hansenne M, Mottet C. Personality and mental time travel: a differential approach to autonoetic consciousness. *Conscious Cogn*. 2008;17:1082–92.

63. Josefsson K, Jokela M, Hintsanen M, et al. Parental care-giving and home environment predicting offspring temperament and character traits after 18 years. *Psychiatry Res*. 2013;209:643–51.

64. Brandstrom S, Przybeck TR, Sigvardsson S. Reliability of informant ratings and spouse similarity based on the Temperament and Character Inventory. *Psychol Rep*. 2011;109:231–42.

65. Fassino S, Garzaro L, Peris C, Amianto F, Piero A, Abbate Daga G. Temperament and character in couples with fertility disorders: a double-blind, controlled study. *Fertil Steril*. 2002;77:1233–40.

66. Sydsjo G, Lampic C, Brandstrom S. Who becomes a sperm donor: personality characteristics in a national sample of identifiable donors. *BJOG*. 2012;119:33–9.

67. Rizzo A. Temperament and generativity during the life span. *Mediterranean Journal of Clinical Psychology*. 2013;1:1–31.

68. Costa PTJ, McCrae RR. Personality disorders and the five-factor model of personality. *J Pers Disord*. 1990;4:362–71.

69. Yamagata S, Suzuki A, Ando J, et al. Is the genetic structure of human personality universal? A cross-cultural twin study from North America, Europe, and Asia. *J Pers Soc Psychol*. 2006;90:987–98.

70. Finkel D, McGue M. Sex differences and nonadditivity in heritability of the Multidimensional Personality Questionnaire Scales. *J Pers Soc Psychol*. 1997;72:929–38.

71. Eaves LJ, Heath AC, Neale MC, Hewitt JK, Martin NG. Sex differences and non-additivity in the effects of genes on personality. *Twin Res*. 1998;1:131–7.

72. Eaves LJ, Heath AC, Martin NG, et al. Comparing the biological and cultural inheritance of personality and social attitudes in the Virginia 30,000 study of twins and their relatives. *Twin Res*. 1999;2:62–80.

73. Benjamin J, Osher Y, Kotler M, et al. Association between tri-dimensional personality questionnaire (TPQ) traits and three functional polymorphisms: dopamine receptor D4 (DRD4), serotonin transporter promoter region (5-HTTLPR) and catechol O-methyltransferase (COMT). *Mol Psychiatry*. 2000;5:96–100.

74. Strobel A, Lesch KP, Jatzke S, Paetzold F, Brocke B. Further evidence for a modulation of Novelty Seeking by DRD4 exon III, 5-HTTLPR, and COMT val/met variants. *Mol Psychiatry*. 2003;8:371–2.

75. Caspi A, Moffitt TE. Gene-environment interactions in psychiatry: joining forces with neuroscience. *Nat Rev Neurosci*. 2006;7:583–90.

76. Caspi A, Sugden K, Moffitt TE, et al. Influence of life stress on depression: moderation by a polymorphism in the *5-HTT* gene. *Science*. 2003;301:386–9.

77. Kim-Cohen J, Caspi A, Taylor A, et al. MAOA, maltreatment, and gene-environment interaction predicting children's mental health: new evidence and a meta-analysis. *Mol Psychiatry*. 2006;11:903–13.

78. Hintsanen M, Pulkki-Raback L, Juonala M, Viikari JS, Raitakari OT, Keltikangas-Jarvinen L. Cloninger's temperament traits and preclinical atherosclerosis: the Cardiovascular Risk in Young Finns Study. *J Psychosom Res*. 2009;67:77–84.

79. Jokela M, Raikkonen K, Lehtimaki T, Rontu R, Keltikangas-Jarvinen L. Tryptophan hydroxylase 1 gene (*TPH1*) moderates the influence of social support on depressive symptoms in adults. *J Affect Disord*. 2007;100:191–7.

80. Keltikangas-Jarvinen L, Pulkki-Raback L, Elovainio M, Raitakari OT, Viikari J, Lehtimaki T. DRD2 C32806T modifies the effect of child-rearing environment on adulthood novelty seeking. *Am J Med Genet B Neuropsychiatr Genet*. 2009;150B:389–94.

81. Keltikangas-Jarvinen L, Puttonen S, Kivimaki M, Elovainio M, Rontu R, Lehtimaki T. Tryptophan hydroxylase 1 gene haplotypes modify the effect of a hostile childhood environment on adulthood harm avoidance. *Genes Brain Behav*. 2007;6:305–13.

82. Keltikangas-Jarvinen L, Puttonen S, Kivimaki M, Rontu R, Lehtimaki T. Cloninger's temperament dimensions and epidermal growth factor A61G polymorphism in Finnish adults. *Genes Brain Behav*. 2006;5:11–18.

83. Keltikangas-Jarvinen L, Salo J. Dopamine and serotonin systems modify environmental effects on human behavior: a review. *Scand J Psychol*. 2009;50:574–82.

84. de Moor MH, Costa PT, Terracciano A, et al. Meta-analysis of genome-wide association studies for personality. *Mol Psychiatry*. 2012;17:337–49.

85. Williams SM, Haines JL. Correcting away the hidden heritability. *Ann Hum Genet*. 2011;75:348–50.

86. Verweij KJ, Burri AV, Zietsch BP. Evidence for genetic variation in human mate preferences for sexually dimorphic physical traits. *PLoS One*. 2012;7:e49294.

87. van den Berg SM, de Moor MH, McGue M, et al. Harmonization of neuroticism and extraversion phenotypes across inventories and cohorts in the Genetics of Personality Consortium: an application of Item Response Theory. *Behav Genet*. 2014;44:295–313.

88. van den Berg SM, de Moor MH, Verweij KJ, et al. Meta-analysis of genome-wide association studies for extraversion: findings from the Genetics of Personality Consortium. *Behav Genet*. 2016;46:170–82.

89. Genetics of Personality Consortium, de Moor MH, van den Berg SM, Verweij KJ, et al. Meta-analysis of genome-wide association

studies for neuroticism, and the polygenic association with major depressive disorder. *JAMA Psychiatry.* 2015;72:642–50.

90. Manolio TA. Genomewide association studies and assessment of the risk of disease. *N Engl J Med.* 2010;363:166–76.

91. Josefsson K, Jokela M, Cloninger CR, *et al.* Maturity and change in personality: developmental trends of temperament and character in adulthood. *Dev Psychopathol.* 2013;25:713–27.

92. Qureshi IA, Mehler MF. Emerging roles of non-coding RNAs in brain evolution, development, plasticity and disease. *Nat Rev Neurosci.* 2012;13:528–41.

93. Campanella F, Crescentini C, Urgesi C, Fabbro F. Mindfulness-oriented meditation improves self-related character scales in healthy individuals. *Compr Psychiatry.* 2014;55: 1269–78.

# 121

# Imaging of personality disorders

*Christian Paret and Christian Schmahl*

## Introduction

In this chapter, we will review the neuroimaging literature in personality disorders. Given its clinical importance and the rapidly grown literature on borderline personality disorder (BPD), we will focus on this condition, with some additional findings from studies on avoidant (AvPD), narcissistic (NPD), and obsessive–compulsive personality disorder (OCPD), where appropriate. Due to consistency and readability, we abstained from reviewing the large body of imaging literature on suspicious personality disorder types (paranoid, schizoid, schizotypal, antisocial), which has been covered elsewhere [1, 2].

## Emotion processing and regulation

### Emotion processing

Emotion dysregulation is a hallmark of BPD psychopathology [3]. A growing number of studies have used functional magnetic resonance imaging (fMRI) during emotional challenge (for example, presentation of emotionally arousing pictures or facial expressions) to investigate the neural correlates of emotional responding in individuals with BPD, compared to healthy individuals; the majority of fMRI studies have observed hyperreactivity of the amygdala in response to negative emotional stimuli in BPD patients, compared to healthy controls (for a meta-analysis, see [4]). In addition to an exaggerated amygdala response to emotional pictures, several studies in BPD patients found increased amygdala activation in response to pictures which have been rated as neutral in the general population (for example, [5, 6]). Both BPD and AvPD patients showed a lack of habituation to repeated presentations of emotional stimuli [7]. Increased dorsal anterior cingulate cortex (ACC) activity and amygdala–insula connectivity was observed in healthy controls, but not in BPD and AvPD [7]. This is in line with other studies revealing a lack of habituation in BPD [8–10] which may contribute to affective instability [7]. Findings of increased and prolonged amygdala activation are in line with the well-documented clinical feature of high sensitivity to emotional stimuli with intense and long-lasting reactions in patients with BPD [10–12]. Most interestingly, medication-free samples were characterized by limbic hyperactivity, whereas no such group differences were found in patients currently taking psychotropic medication [4].

In addition to amygdala hyperreactivity, increased activation in the insula has been observed in emotional challenge studies in BPD patients, compared to healthy controls, emphasizing the role of this brain area in disturbed emotion processing in BPD [5, 6, 13, 14]. In numerous studies in healthy individuals, the insula has been associated with the encoding of unpleasant feelings, interoceptive awareness (awareness of one's own bodily experiences), perceived social exclusion, and pain perception [15, 16].

Several neuroimaging studies have revealed frontal hypoactivation [17–19], especially blunted responses of the bilateral dorsolateral prefrontal cortex (dlPFC) [4], in response to emotionally arousing stimuli. Schmahl and colleagues [20] presented individualized auditory scripts of abandonment situations to their participants and found increased activation in the dlPFC and decreased activation in the medial prefrontal cortex (mPFC). Furthermore, when patients were confronted with their self-reported traumatic memories, they did not exhibit increased activity in the ACC or orbitofrontal cortex (OFC) and dlPFC, as did healthy controls. Instead, they showed unaltered or diminished activity [21]. The OFC and dlPFC are thought to be implicated in a top–down appraisal system that modulates activation in limbic and subcortical brain areas [22]. Hence, it is conceivable that the pattern of hypoactivation observed in frontal brain regions during emotional challenge in BPD might represent a neural correlate of altered processing of negative autobiographical memories and negative emotions.

Turning to studies of brain structures (for example, brain volume) in patients with BPD, compared to healthy controls, several studies have shown a reduced volume in limbic and paralimbic brain regions. A meta-analysis [23] even proposed that reduced volumes of the amygdala and hippocampus may be regarded as 'biological markers' or endophenotypes of BPD. In a recent meta-analysis on studies using voxel-based morphometry (VBM), most prominent volumetric changes in BPD were observed in the amygdala and dlPFC [4]. It is nonetheless controversial whether the observed alterations rather stem from experience of abuse in childhood [24] or might even be a substrate of comorbid post-traumatic stress disorder (PTSD), both of which are highly prevalent conditions in BPD [25, 26]. Kuhlmann and colleagues [27] further detected a reduced volume of the hypothalamus, which extends previous findings of alterations in the hypothalamic–pituitary–adrenal axis in BPD [28, 29]. The first multimodal imaging study in BPD published by Salvador and colleagues [30] complements earlier work [31–33] showing converging abnormalities in subgenual and perigenual ACC.

While no differences were found between BPD and AvPD in brain structure, both patient groups showed reduced mPFC and ACC volumes, compared to healthy controls [34]. Further, both patient groups showed a positive correlation between amygdala volume and anxiety [34].

The research depicted here has led to the current conceptualization of BPD suggesting that emotion dysregulation results from deficient 'top–down' frontal control mechanisms involved in regulating activation in hyperactive 'bottom–up' emotion-generating limbic structures. Imbalance of control such that the lower brain regions generating emotion are untethered from prefrontal control areas is also observed in anxiety disorders [35] and is probably not specific to BPD. The white and grey matter abnormality, accompanied with altered resting-state brain connectivity [36], emphasizes alterations in fronto-limbic networks as a candidate neural substrate of symptoms concerning several functions, such as emotion processing, emotion regulation, and decision-making, that are impaired in BPD and other mental disorders.

## Cognitive emotion regulation

Three studies investigated the cognitive regulation of emotions in BPD by presenting negative pictures with the instruction to regulate emotions in the MRI scanner [37–39]. The results converged to a reduced response of the dorsal mPFC and dlPFC in BPD patients when regulating emotions. More specifically, the study by Koenigsberg and colleagues [37] found diminished activity in the dlPFC and ventrolateral prefrontal cortices when patients with BPD tried to cognitively distance themselves from negative stimuli. Similarly, cognitive reappraisal yielded decreased recruitment of the OFC and increased activation of the insula in patients with BPD, relative to healthy participants [39]. In an attempt to clarify the role of trauma history on downregulation of emotional responses in BPD patients, Lang et al. [38] compared trauma-exposed BPD patients to trauma-exposed healthy subjects without BPD and non-traumatized healthy subjects. In this study, BPD patients, as well as healthy individuals with a trauma history, recruited brain regions associated with up- and downregulation of negative emotions (for example, ACC) to a lesser extent, which might reflect compensatory changes associated with trauma exposure.

Initial fMRI findings suggested changes in neural responding with psychotherapy. Goodman and colleagues [40] demonstrated a reduction of amygdala activity in a passive viewing paradigm after dialectical behaviour therapy (DBT) treatment. Testing patients receiving DBT vs patients receiving treatment as usual (TAU) and healthy controls, Winter et al. [41] found the inferior parietal lobe/supramarginal gyrus (IPL/SMG) to alter responding during emotion regulation. Decreased IPL/SMG responding predicted an improvement of symptom severity. Furthermore, DBT responders reduced perigenual ACC activation when viewing negative vs neutral pictures. Schmitt et al. [42] found decreased insula and ACC activity during reappraisal in patients with BPD. ACC connectivity to the medial and superior frontal gyri, superior temporal gyrus, and inferior parietal cortices increased after DBT. Treatment responders exhibited reduced activation in the amygdala, ACC, OFC, and dlPFC, together with increased connectivity within a limbic–prefrontal network, during reappraisal of negative stimuli after psychotherapy.

One fMRI study testing neural responses of cognitive emotion regulation in AvPD revealed amygdala hyperreactivity in anticipation of regulation and in response to negative, compared to neutral, pictures [43]. Furthermore, amygdala reactivity was correlated with anxiety ratings [43] and may be interpreted as a neural correlate of exaggerated anticipatory anxiety of social situations.

## Self-injury and altered pain processing

A very common dysfunctional behaviour, closely linked to emotion dysregulation in BPD, is non-suicidal self-injury (NSSI) [44]. Pain appears to have an important emotion-regulating effect in BPD [45]. A large body of experimental research investigating pain perception in individuals with BPD points to reduced sensitivity in BPD patients (for example, [46–49]). Schmahl and colleagues [48] showed that self-reported pain ratings were *lower* in BPD patients and that pain thresholds were altered. Interestingly, no differences were observed in discrimination task performance of laser-evoked brain potentials, which showed that the analgesic state in BPD is not explained by an impairment of the sensory-discriminative component of pain [48]. In a first neuroimaging study by Schmahl et al. [47], patients with BPD and NSSI underwent fMRI while heat stimuli were applied to their hands. BPD patients showed increased dlPFC activation, along with decreased activation of the posterior parietal cortex. Moreover, painful heat stimulation evoked neural deactivation in the amygdala and perigenual ACC in participants with BPD [47]. The observed interaction between increased pain-induced response in the dlPFC, coupled with deactivations in the ACC and amygdala, could be interpreted as an anti-nociceptive mechanism in BPD [47]. While sensory discrimination processes remain intact, this mechanism may modulate pain circuits primarily by an increased top–down regulation of emotional components of pain or an altered affective appraisal of pain [47].

Examining the neural mechanisms underlying the role of self-inflicted pain as a means of affect regulation in BPD more directly, Niedtfeld and colleagues [6] conducted an fMRI study using pictures to elicit negative affect and thermal stimuli to induce heat pain. Although the authors found an attenuation of activation in limbic areas (amygdala, insula) in response to sensory stimulation, it was specific neither to patients with BPD nor to painful stimulation. In order to identify brain mechanisms underlying the limbic deactivation observed [6], the authors measured functional connectivity between those regions that had been identified to be involved in emotional processing, namely the amygdala, insula, and ACC [50]. Results of their analyses indicated that painful sensory stimuli, as opposed to warmth perception, resulted in enhanced negative coupling between (para-) limbic and prefrontal structures in BPD, thus indicating inhibition of limbic arousal. Increased coupling between the amygdala and medial frontal gyrus (BA8 and BA9) may point to attentional distraction processes [51]. Additionally, in the patient group, the dlPFC showed enhanced coupling to the posterior insula, a brain region known to play a critical role in pain processing [52] and affective appraisal of pain perception [53].

To test the direct effect of tissue damage, two recent studies induced stress with the Montreal Imaging Stress Task, followed by either an incision into the forearm (tissue damage) or a sham condition [54, 55]. The incision resulted in a decrease in tension and heart rate in the BPD group, in contrast to a short-term increase in aversive tension in the healthy control group [55]. A resting-state fMRI scan after the incision pointed to a decrease in amygdala activity, together with normalized functional connectivity of the amygdala and superior frontal gyrus, in the BPD group [54]. These results may point to a stress-reducing effect of tissue damage that affects subjective experience, psychophysiological reactions, and brain function in BPD.

In sum, the overall reported results on pain processing in BPD suggest that NSSI may be interpreted as an attempt to compensate for a deficient emotion regulation mechanism. More specifically, the reported findings implicate that the soothing effect of pain in BPD seems to be mediated by different emotion regulation processes (attentional shift and altered appraisal of pain).

## Social interaction

### Processing of social stimuli

Izurieta Hidalgo and colleagues [56] found a decreased late centroparietal P300 response in BPD patients that may reflect diminished categorical processing of happy faces. Several fMRI studies found increased amygdala responses to emotional facial expressions [57–60], and decreased subgenual and dorsal ACC responses were reported [60]. Further, increased functional connectivity of the amygdala with the dorsal and rostral ACC was observed in overt face processing [61]. Covert face processing increased the amygdala–thalamus connectivity in BPD patients [61], and an early enhancement in electroencephalogram (EEG) responses (P100, N170) was observed [56]. Although BPD patients tended to make more and faster initial eye fixations to the eyes of angry faces [58] and to misclassify predominantly happy faces as angry faces [56], amygdala hyperactivation was not enhanced comparing angry faces to other emotions [57, 60].

### Empathy

Both increased interpersonal resonance and pervasive interpersonal disturbances are ubiquitous in BPD, possibly rooted in reduced mirroring of emotional reactions in parent–child dyads and childhood traumatic experiences [62]. Frick et al. [63] found that BPD patients were better and faster than healthy controls in infering emotional states from eye gaze pictures. This was accompanied by increased amygdala, temporal cortex, and OFC responses to emotional eye gazes and ventromedial PFC (vmPFC), ACC, and parietal activations specifically to eye gazes in faces with negative emotional expression in BPD. Increased amygdala activation was also observed in BPD patients attributing intentions to emotional face expressions [59]. Similar to posterior insula hyperactivity in BPD patients who empathized with people on violence and threat photographs [64], amygdala hyperactivity may reflect increased emotional resonance and arousal. In contrast, reduced anterior insula activations [63] may reflect divergent social expectations in BPD [65]. Moreover, empathic mindsets increased superior temporal cortex activity in healthy subjects, but not in BPD patients [59, 63, 64]. Low superior temporal cortex activity was suggested to reflect reduced meta-cognitive processes [66], which may entail inadequate emotion regulation in social situations. Paired with enhanced emotional sensitivity and affective reverberation, this may promote interpersonal disturbances [62].

Reduced grey matter volume in patients with NPD was found in the anterior insula, rostral ACC, mPFC, and medial cingulate [67]. Another study found reduced grey matter volume in the mPFC/

ACC and fusiform, temporal, and occipital cortices [68]. Higher anterior insula volume predicted higher emotional empathy [67]. These findings were further supported by diffusion tensor imaging findings, showing altered structural connectivity involving frontal lobe and thalamic regions [68]. Neural alterations were discussed to underlie decreased empathy, which is characteristic for NPD [67]. Somatosensory gating (SG) during the anticipation and observation of pain, measured with EEG, was found increased in NPD subjects [69]. According to the authors, this finding may reflect an increased somatic representation of observed pain. A positive correlation of SG with impulsivity–egocentricity ratings suggests an increased somatic representation of observed pain despite lower empathy [69]. The NPD sample consisted of patients with high psychopathic traits, limiting the generalization of results. Though the database is sparse, imaging data so far support malfunction in the frontolimbic and paralimbic systems to underlie NPD psychopathology.

### Co-operation and social exclusion

Perceived exclusion in a virtual ball-tossing game was associated with hyperactivation of the dlPFC and precuneus in patients with BPD [70]. Furthermore and independent of actual exclusion by the co-players, hyperactivation of the dorsal mPFC/ACC, parietal cortex, occipital cortex, and insula was found [70]. Unlike healthy controls, BPD patients felt excluded, even when they were actually included. Furthermore, they also felt excluded and showed neural hyperactivation when players followed predefined rules [70]. The observed pattern was discussed to possibly reflect 'hypermentalizing', that is, the tendency to attribute intentions to co-players when behaviour is actually not guided by intentions. Abnormal anterior insula activation may reflect decreased expectations of co-operative behaviour in BPD [65], a potential precursor of break-ups in interpersonal co-operation. Additionally, increased anterior PFC activation during exclusion [71] may relate to altered emotion regulation in social interactions [72]. In summary, divergent social expectations appear to promote feelings of exclusion and impede the maintenance of relationships. This is reflected by divergent neural responding to social interaction in BPD.

With regard to interpersonal aggression, patients increased both OFC and amygdala activation in an experimental manipulation provoking aggressive tendencies, while controls decreased amygdala activation [73]. As the latter study assessed patients with comorbid intermittent explosive disorder (IED), results may not generalize to BPD without IED. Mancke, Herpertz, and Bertsch [74] suggested a multi-dimensional model linking neuropsychology and neurochemistry data to the bio-behavioural dimensions of affective dysregulation, threat hypersensitivity, reduced cognitive empathy, reduced self–other differentiation, and impulsivity. The authors assumed a prefrontal–limbic imbalance to underlie impulsivity, affective dysregulation, and hypersensitivity to social threat cues, mediating aggressive tendencies often observed in BPD [74].

## Behavioural regulation

### Decision-making

Decisions are ubiquitous in daily life and 'commit the organism to one out of several possible behaviors' [75]. It is assumed that decisions are guided by the processing of subjective value that critically involves the vmPFC and OFC (reviewed, for example, in [76]). Brain volumetry analyses revealed differences in mPFC/OFC grey matter volume in BPD patients vs healthy controls [77–83] and in BPD patients vs other clinical populations [77, 84]. A meta-analysis found reduced grey matter volume in the ventral mPFC/OFC of patients with BPD [4].

fMRI studies demonstrated that BPD patients' vmPFC response did not differentiate between reward and no-reward expectations; in contrast, this pattern was observed in healthy controls [85, 86]. Notably, effects were most pronounced for reward anticipation in face of emotional pictures [85]; in the presence of emotional pictures, BPD patients did not discriminate between anticipated reward and no-reward conditions. Group differences were also observed in upstream brain regions of the reward system such as the ventral striatum, ventral tegmental area, and amygdala. Generally, healthy participants, compared to BPD patients, showed stronger deactivations in these regions if no reward was expected [85]. In line with this, reduced neural discrimination between reward and punishment in BPD was found in a simple gambling task [87, 88]. Andreou et al. [87] localized this group interaction effect to the mPFC/ACC. In addition, they observed group differences in mPFC and OFC responses to high vs low magnitudes of monetary reward and punishment. In concert with the findings reviewed in this chapter, Schuermann and colleagues [89] demonstrated reduced frontal EEG discrimination between reward and punishment in a more complex decision-making task. In addition, they observed an increased P300 response to punishments in BPD patients that may relate to delayed processing of feedback [89]. Alternatively, an increased P300 response may indicate differences in BPD patients' expectations about receiving punishment [89]. In accordance with these findings, BPD patients did not adjust their choices and kept drawing from disadvantageous card decks [89].

In summary, neuroimaging studies document a lack of discrimination between reward and punishments in the neural reward system of BPD patients.

### Learning

Classical conditioning is used as a paradigmatic task for fear learning. In turn, the unlearning of fear is studied by investigating how well subjects extinguish an established conditioned response. BPD patients reported stronger affective responses in fear extinction [9]. However, on the neural level, no significant group differences emerged comparing BPD patients and healthy controls [9].

Fear can also be learnt by verbal instruction. In research, this phenomenon is investigated in 'instructed fear' studies where investigators inform subjects about a possible negative stimulus (for example, an electrodermal pain stimulus) that might be delivered upon a certain cue but is actually never given during the experiment. BPD patients showed a prolonged amygdala response to instructed fear, while healthy controls decreased amygdala activation over time [10]. In addition, BPD patients showed altered connectivity patterns in the prefrontal–limbic regions in this paradigm [10]. While patients' amygdala activation failed to habituate, this was not represented in skin conductance responses [10].

Turning to another learning process, Soloff et al. [90] investigated episodic memory encoding and retrieval. BPD patients observed affective and neutral pictures a first and later a second time where they should identify those already known pictures among unfamiliar

pictures. Comparing with healthy control patients, differential activations in the hippocampus, ACC, dorsal PFC, and parietal cortex were seen for negative vs positive pictures. This suggests less differential recruitment of brain areas associated with episodic memory formation in BPD. Despite neural differences, patients recognized items equally well as healthy controls during retrieval.

To our knowledge, imaging studies in other personality disorders (excluding antisocial personality disorder, which are not addressed in this chapter) focusing on memory functions are not existent. Coutinho and colleagues demonstrated altered precuneus network connectivity in OCPD [91]. The authors speculated that altered precuneus connectivity may reflect over-involvement in anticipatory processes, leading to rumination in future-oriented planning at the cost of present moment experience and an attentional bias to minor details [91].

### Cognitive conflict management

Winter et al. [92] did not find a group difference comparing BPD patients to healthy controls in an fMRI study with the 'emotional Stroop' task. However, when dissociation was evoked by personalized autobiographical memory scripts, significant emotional interference was observed comparing these patients to non-dissociated BPD patients and controls [92]. Moderate activation differences in the inferior parietal cortex and inferior temporal gyrus may reflect impaired inhibition of task-irrelevant information caused by dissociation [92]. Dissociation involves disruptions of usually integrated functions such as consciousness, memory, attention, pain perception, and perception of the self and environment, and is frequently reported by patients with BPD [93–95]. Compared to healthy controls, non-dissociated patients were found to increase responses to positive words in temporal, frontal, and cingulate regions, but no differences were observed with regard to negative words [92]. In contrast, Malhi et al. [96] found increased ventrolateral PFC and decreased dlPFC and amygdala activation in BPD patients in the 'emotional Stroop' task, although lacking behavioural group differences. In their analyses, both PFC regions showed correlations with self-assessments of emotion dysregulation, which is supportive of increased involvement of the PFC in emotional interference resolution. In contrast, another study found decreased dlPFC activation [97]. Wingenfeld and colleagues [98] reported activations of a more posterior lateral PFC area when comparing the responses to negative vs neutral words in healthy controls to responses in BPD patients, in addition to temporal cortex and ACC activations.

Beyond word identification, emotional conflict can also be introduced to other cognitive processes. Krause-Utz et al. [5] found BPD patients to be more distracted by negative emotional pictures that were presented during a working memory task, evidenced by slowing of reaction times. Neurally, this was complemented by increased amygdala and anterior insula, as well as decreased dlPFC, activation [5]. Furthermore, stronger functional connectivity of the amygdala with the dorsomedial prefrontal cortex (dmPFC) was found, and stronger coupling of these regions was related to increased reaction times [99]. In addition, amygdala connectivity with the dorsal ACC was increased and amygdala activation decreased when patients reported higher dissociation [99]. These findings suggest that BPD is associated with an increased demand of cognitive resources to counteract intense emotional interference.

Presenting emotional face distractors in a flanker-task, Holtmann *et al.* [100] found stronger dorsal ACC responses to fearful vs neutral faces in BPD patients, compared to healthy controls. A negative correlation of dorsal ACC response to incongruent vs congruent trials with anxiety ratings suggests involvement of this region in conflict resolution, modulated by anxiety. Behaviourally, no effect of distraction on reaction times or accuracy was detected by the authors. As reviewed previously, emotional content is also suggested to interfere with neural representations of reward processing [85].

In contrast to emotional conflict, semantic conflict is provoked, for example in the colour-word Stroop or the face-word Stroop task [101], where semantically relevant distractors (that is, colour words or emotion words) compete with target stimuli (that is, print colour or faces with emotional expressions, respectively). To the best of our knowledge, there is currently no published study on the neural correlates of semantic conflict resolution in BPD. Though there is limited evidence for significant slowing in the colour-word Stroop task [102], we are not aware of a study testing interference with task-relevant emotional stimuli in BPD patients (utilizing the face-word Stroop task).

In summary, though several studies found neural differences in emotional conflict processing in BPD, no consistent picture can be derived from the literature. Behaviourally, though significant interference of emotional material with working memory was found, BPD patients did not show distraction effects in the majority of tasks. Negative findings may also relate to low robustness of the 'emotional Stroop' effect [89].

### Response control

The ability to inhibit a prepotent response can shed light on impulse control. Impulsivity is not assumed to be a unitary construct; thus, different facets of impulsivity have been investigated, using both behavioural experiments and self-assessment instruments, in BPD (for a review, see [103]). Subjects are required to withhold a prepotent behavioural response (usually a button press) to perform a correct action, while neural responses are measured. Jacob *et al.* [104] reported lower inferior frontal cortex (IFC) and higher subthalamic nucleus activation in BPD patients, compared to controls, after anger induction. The authors discussed this in terms of increased neural inhibitory activity of the IFC and compensatory subthalamic activity in BPD. However, behavioural data did not reveal group differences. When BPD patients were confronted with face stimuli showing affective expressions, increased brain activations were observed in task-related (parietal, basal ganglia, middle inferior OFC, hippocampus) and emotion-related (amygdala) brain areas [90]. This reflects task-dependent differences in the recruitment of neural circuits, perhaps due to increased proneness to cognitive interference from emotional distraction. In face of affective vs neutral words, which were used as distracting stimuli while subjects performed a response control task, BPD patients decreased responses in the subgenual ACC, posterior medial OFC, and posterior ACC, relative to healthy controls [97]. Conversely, patients increased responses in the lateral OFC and dlPFC, among others. There are major differences in methods and stimulus material in the latter two studies, limiting comparability. Nonetheless, they both support altered brain activations in response control in BPD patients when confronted with emotional material. With a stress induction procedure, which might more potently affect information processing

systems in BPD, Cackowski and colleagues [105] found patients to make more response errors relative to a no-stress condition.

With EEG, Ruchsow *et al.* [106] observed a reduced late positivity (P300) in BPD patients to events when subjects had to withhold a prepotent response. Conversely, no differences, compared to healthy controls, were found in the earlier N200 component. In addition, a negative correlation of the P300 component was found with cognitive impulsiveness and depressiveness in patients. The authors concluded that P300 findings point to altered response inhibition in BPD related to impulsivity and depression. On the other hand, unchanged N200 responses are in favour of intact conflict resolution. Behaviourally, no differences between patients and controls were observed. The most recent neuroimaging work found neither neural nor behavioural differences between unmedicated BPD patients and matched healthy controls in tasks probing action withholding, response interference resolution, and stop signal reactions [107]. Further, no correlations with self-assessments of impulsivity and task data were found.

In conclusion, the literature does not reflect a general impairment in the ability to control or stop actions in BPD (for reviews, see [103,107]). Cumulative evidence demonstrates that emotional provocation can deteriorate response withholding on the behavioural and neural levels in BPD.

### Closing remarks

Neuroimaging work has contributed to a better understanding of the psychophysiological correlates of personality disorders. Existing research has resulted in a comprehensive picture of the neurobiology of altered emotion processing and emotion regulation. This is fundamental for understanding BPD psychopathology, although the neural mechanisms are probably not unique to this disorder.

Hyper-responsiveness to social cues in BPD is underscored by neuroimaging studies, providing support for altered activations in the brain's attention and salience systems. Research has started to illuminate the neural basis of empathy, cooperation, and aggression in BPD. Current findings are congruent with socio-psychological models; however, neuroimaging studies in social interaction research in BPD are still sparse. As discussed previously, integration of these findings into bio-behavioural models of dysfunctioning may result in a more complete picture to guide future research.

Diverse areas of executive functioning have been explored by BPD researchers such as decision-making, learning, cognitive conflict management, and response control. Taken together, many studies using tasks that are thought to tap into aspects of BPD psychopathology (for example, impulsivity, disinhibition, risky choice behaviour, emotional learning) lack positive behavioural findings, although they produce neural effects. In addition, the latter sometimes seem inconsistent in the aggregate. Furthermore, neuroimaging research in many areas of executive functioning in BPD is rare. In light of this, we currently do not have a clear picture on how neuroimaging findings relate to behavioural dysregulation in general in BPD.

### REFERENCES

1. Raine A, Lencz T, Yaralian P, *et al.* Prefrontal structural and functional deficits in schizotypal personality disorder. *Schizophr Bull.* 2002;28:501–13.

2. Cummings MA. The neurobiology of psychopathy: recent developments and new directions in research and treatment. *CNS Spectr*. 2015;20:200–6.

3. Sanislow CA, Grilo CM, Morey LC, *et al*. Confirmatory factor analysis of DSM-IV criteria for borderline personality disorder: findings from the collaborative longitudinal personality disorders study. *Am J Psychiatry*. 2002;159:284–90.

4. Schulze L, Schmahl C, Niedtfeld I. Neural correlates of disturbed emotion processing in borderline personality disorder: a multimodal meta-analysis. *Biol Psychiatry*. 2016;79:97–106.

5. Krause-Utz A, Oei NYL, Niedtfeld I, *et al*. Influence of emotional distraction on working memory performance in borderline personality disorder. *Psychol Med*. 2012;42:2181–92.

6. Niedtfeld I, Schulze L, Kirsch P, Herpertz SC, Bohus M, Schmahl C. Affect regulation and pain in borderline personality disorder: a possible link to the understanding of self-injury. *Biol Psychiatry*. 2010;68:383–91.

7. Koenigsberg HW, Denny BT, Fan J, *et al*. The neural correlates of anomalous habituation to negative emotional pictures in borderline and avoidant personality disorder patients. *Am J Psychiatry*. 2014;171:82–90.

8. Hazlett EA, Zhang J, New AS, *et al*. Potentiated amygdala response to repeated emotional pictures in borderline personality disorder. *Biol Psychiatry*. 2012;72:448–56.

9. Krause-Utz A, Keibel-Mauchnik J, Ebner-Priemer U, Bohus M, Schmahl C. Classical conditioning in borderline personality disorder: an fMRI study. *Eur Arch Psychiatry Clin Neurosci*. 2016;266:291–305.

10. Kamphausen S, Schröder P, Maier S, *et al*. Medial prefrontal dysfunction and prolonged amygdala response during instructed fear processing in borderline personality disorder. *World J Biol Psychiatry*. 2013;14:307–18, S1–4.

11. Crowell SE, Beauchaine TP, Linehan MM. A biosocial developmental model of borderline personality: elaborating and extending Linehan's theory. *Psychol Bull*. 2009;135:495–510.

12. Gilbert R, Widom CS, Browne K, Fergusson D, Webb E, Janson S. Burden and consequences of child maltreatment in high-income countries. *Lancet*. 2009;373:68–81.

13. Beblo T, Driessen M, Mertens M, *et al*. Functional MRI correlates of the recall of unresolved life events in borderline personality disorder. *Psychol Med*. 2006;36:845–56.

14. Ruocco AC, Amirthavasagam S, Choi-Kain LW, McMain SF. Neural correlates of negative emotionality in borderline personality disorder: an activation-likelihood-estimation meta-analysis. *Biol Psychiatry*. 2013;73:153–60.

15. Damasio AR, Grabowski TJ, Bechara A, *et al*. Subcortical and cortical brain activity during the feeling of self-generated emotions. *Nat Neurosci*. 2000;3:1049–56.

16. Menon V, Uddin LQ. Saliency, switching, attention and control: a network model of insula function. *Brain Struct Funct*. 2010;214:655–67.

17. Leichsenring F, Leibing E, Kruse J, New AS, Leweke F. Borderline personality disorder. *Lancet*. 2011;377:74–84.

18. Lis E, Greenfield B, Henry M, Guilé JM, Dougherty G. Neuroimaging and genetics of borderline personality disorder: a review. *J Psychiatry Neurosci*. 2007;32:162–73.

19. O'Neill A, Frodl T. Brain structure and function in borderline personality disorder. *Brain Struct Funct*. 2012;217:767–82.

20. Schmahl CG, Elzinga BM, Vermetten E, Sanislow C, McGlashan TH, Bremner JD. Neural correlates of memories of abandonment in women with and without borderline personality disorder. *Biol Psychiatry*. 2003;54:142–51.

21. Schmahl CG, Vermetten E, Elzinga BM, Bremner JD. A positron emission tomography study of memories of childhood abuse in borderline personality disorder. *Biol Psychiatry*. 2004;55:759–65.

22. Ochsner KN, Silvers JA, Buhle JT. Functional imaging studies of emotion regulation: a synthetic review and evolving model of the cognitive control of emotion. *Ann N Y Acad Sci*. 2012;1251:E1–24.

23. Nunes PM, Wenzel A, Borges KT, Porto CR, Caminha RM, de Oliveira IR. Volumes of the hippocampus and amygdala in patients with borderline personality disorder: a meta-analysis. *J Pers Disord*. 2009;23:333–45.

24. Stein MB, Koverola C, Hanna C, Torchia MG, McClarty B. Hippocampal volume in women victimized by childhood sexual abuse. *Psychol Med*. 1997;27:951–9.

25. Krause-Utz A, Schmahl C. Neurobiological differentiation between borderline patients with and without post-traumatic stress disorder. *Eur Psychiatr Rev*. 2010;3:63–8.

26. Lieb K, Rexhausen JE, Kahl KG, *et al*. Increased diurnal salivary cortisol in women with borderline personality disorder. *J Psychiatr Res*. 2004;38:559–65.

27. Kuhlmann A, Bertsch K, Schmidinger I, Thomann PA, Herpertz SC. Morphometric differences in central stress-regulating structures between women with and without borderline personality disorder. *J Psychiatry Neurosci*. 2013;38:129–37.

28. Wingenfeld K, Wolf OT. Effects of cortisol on cognition in major depressive disorder, posttraumatic stress disorder and borderline personality disorder—2014 Curt Richter Award Winner. *Psychoneuroendocrinology*. 2015;51:282–95.

29. Wingenfeld K, Spitzer C, Rullkötter N, Löwe B. Borderline personality disorder: hypothalamus pituitary adrenal axis and findings from neuroimaging studies. *Psychoneuroendocrinology*. 2010;35:154–70.

30. Salvador R, Vega D, Pascual JC, *et al*. Converging medial frontal resting state and diffusion-based abnormalities in borderline personality disorder. *Biol Psychiatry*. 2016;79:107–16.

31. New AS, Carpenter DM, Perez-Rodriguez MM, *et al*. Developmental differences in diffusion tensor imaging parameters in borderline personality disorder. *J Psychiatr Res*. 2013;47:1101–9.

32. Maier-Hein KH, Brunner R, Lutz K, *et al*. Disorder-specific white matter alterations in adolescent borderline personality disorder. *Biol Psychiatry*. 2014;75:81–8.

33. Carrasco JL, Tajima-Pozo K, Díaz-Marsá M, *et al*. Microstructural white matter damage at orbitofrontal areas in borderline personality disorder. *J Affect Disord*. 2012;139:149–53.

34. Denny BT, Fan J, Liu X, *et al*. Brain structural anomalies in borderline and avoidant personality disorder patients and their associations with disorder-specific symptoms. *J Affect Disord*. 2016;200:266–74.

35. Killgore WDS, Britton JC, Schwab ZJ, *et al*. Cortico-limbic responses to masked affective faces across ptsd, panic disorder, and specific phobia. *Depress Anxiety*. 2014;31:150–9.

36. Doll A, Sorg C, Manoliu A, *et al*. Shifted intrinsic connectivity of central executive and salience network in borderline personality disorder. *Front Hum Neurosci*. 2013;7:727.

37. Koenigsberg HW, Fan J, Ochsner KN, *et al*. Neural correlates of the use of psychological distancing to regulate responses to negative social cues: a study of patients with borderline personality disorder. *Biol Psychiatry*. 2009;66:854–63.

38. Lang S, Kotchoubey B, Frick C, Spitzer C, Grabe HJ, Barnow S. Cognitive reappraisal in trauma-exposed women with borderline personality disorder. *Neuroimage*. 2012;59:1727–34.

39. Schulze L, Domes G, Krüger A, et al. Neuronal correlates of cognitive reappraisal in borderline patients with affective instability. *Biol Psychiatry*. 2011;69:564–73.

40. Goodman M, Carpenter D, Tang CY, et al. Dialectical behavior therapy alters emotion regulation and amygdala activity in patients with borderline personality disorder. *J Psychiatr Res*. 2014;57:108–16.

41. Winter D, Niedtfeld I, Schmitt R, Bohus M, Schmahl C, Herpertz SC. Neural correlates of distraction in borderline personality disorder before and after dialectical behavior therapy. *Eur Arch Psychiatry Clin Neurosci*. 2017;267:51–62.

42. Schmitt R, Winter D, Niedtfeld I, Herpertz SC, Schmahl C. Effects of psychotherapy on neuronal correlates of reappraisal in female patients with borderline personality disorder. *Biol Psychiatry Cogn Neurosci Neuroimaging*. 2016;1:548–57.

43. Denny BT, Fan J, Liu X, et al. Elevated amygdala activity during reappraisal anticipation predicts anxiety in avoidant personality disorder. *J Affect Disord*. 2015;172:1–7.

44. Welch SS, Linehan MM, Sylvers P, Chittams J, Rizvi SL. Emotional responses to self-injury imagery among adults with borderline personality disorder. *J Consult Clin Psychol*. 2008;76:45–51.

45. Klonsky ED. The functions of deliberate self-injury: a review of the evidence. *Clin Psychol Rev*. 2007;27:226–39.

46. Ludäscher P, Bohus M, Lieb K, Philipsen A, Jochims A, Schmahl C. Elevated pain thresholds correlate with dissociation and aversive arousal in patients with borderline personality disorder. *Psychiatry Res*. 2007;149:291–6.

47. Schmahl C, Bohus M, Esposito F, et al. Neural correlates of antinociception in borderline personality disorder. *Arch Gen Psychiatry*. 2006;63:659–67.

48. Schmahl C, Greffrath W, Baumgärtner U, al. Differential nociceptive deficits in patients with borderline personality disorder and self-injurious behavior: laser-evoked potentials, spatial discrimination of noxious stimuli, and pain ratings. *Pain*. 2004;110:470–9.

49. Schmahl C, Meinzer M, Zeuch A, et al. Pain sensitivity is reduced in borderline personality disorder, but not in posttraumatic stress disorder and bulimia nervosa. *World J Biol Psychiatry*. 2010;11(2 Pt 2):364–71.

50. Niedtfeld I, Kirsch P, Schulze L, Herpertz SC, Bohus M, Schmahl C. Functional connectivity of pain-mediated affect regulation in borderline personality disorder. *PLoS One*. 2012;7:e33293.

51. McRae K, Hughes B, Chopra S, Gabrieli JDE, Gross JJ, Ochsner KN. The neural bases of distraction and reappraisal. *J Cogn Neurosci*. 2010;22:248–62.

52. Rainville P. Brain mechanisms of pain affect and pain modulation. *Curr Opin Neurobiol*. 2002;12:195–204.

53. Treede RD, Apkarian AV, Bromm B, Greenspan JD, Lenz FA. Cortical representation of pain: functional characterization of nociceptive areas near the lateral sulcus. *Pain*. 2000;87:113–19.

54. Reitz S, Kluetsch R, Niedtfeld I, et al. Incision and stress regulation in borderline personality disorder: neurobiological mechanisms of self-injurious behaviour. *Br J Psychiatry J Ment Sci*. 2015;207:165–72.

55. Reitz S, Krause-Utz A, Pogatzki-Zahn EM, Ebner-Priemer U, Bohus M, Schmahl C. Stress regulation and incision in borderline personality disorder—a pilot study modeling cutting behavior. *J Pers Disord*. 2012;26:605–15.

56. Izurieta Hidalgo NA, Oelkers-Ax R, Nagy K, et al. Time course of facial emotion processing in women with borderline personality disorder: an ERP study. *J Psychiatry Neurosci*. 2016;41:16–26.

57. Donegan NH, Sanislow CA, Blumberg HP, et al. Amygdala hyperreactivity in borderline personality disorder: implications for emotional dysregulation. *Biol Psychiatry*. 2003;54: 1284–93.

58. Bertsch K, Gamer M, Schmidt B, al. Oxytocin and reduction of social threat hypersensitivity in women with borderline personality disorder. *Am J Psychiatry*. 2013;170:1169–77.

59. Mier D, Lis S, Esslinger C, et al. Neuronal correlates of social cognition in borderline personality disorder. *Soc Cogn Affect Neurosci*. 2013;8:531–7.

60. Minzenberg MJ, Fan J, New AS, Tang CY, Siever LJ. Fronto-limbic dysfunction in response to facial emotion in borderline personality disorder: an event-related fMRI study. *Psychiatry Res*. 2007;155:231–43.

61. Cullen KR, Vizueta N, Thomas KM, et al. Amygdala functional connectivity in young women with borderline personality disorder. *Brain Connect*. 2011;1:61–71.

62. Fonagy P, Luyten P. A developmental, mentalization-based approach to the understanding and treatment of borderline personality disorder. *Dev Psychopathol*. 2009;21:1355–81.

63. Frick C, Lang S, Kotchoubey B, et al. Hypersensitivity in borderline personality disorder during mindreading. *PLoS One*. 2012;7:e41650.

64. Dziobek I, Preissler S, Grozdanovic Z, Heuser I, Heekeren HR, Roepke S. Neuronal correlates of altered empathy and social cognition in borderline personality disorder. *Neuroimage*. 2011;57:539–48.

65. King-Casas B, Sharp C, Lomax-Bream L, Lohrenz T, Fonagy P, Montague PR. The rupture and repair of cooperation in borderline personality disorder. *Science*. 2008;321:806–10.

66. Herpertz SC, Jeung H, Mancke F, Bertsch K. Social dysfunctioning and brain in borderline personality disorder. *Psychopathology*. 2014;47:417–24.

67. Schulze L, Dziobek I, Vater A, et al. Gray matter abnormalities in patients with narcissistic personality disorder. *J Psychiatr Res*. 2013;47:1363–9.

68. Nenadic I, Güllmar D, Dietzek M, Langbein K, Steinke J, Gaser C. Brain structure in narcissistic personality disorder: a VBM and DTI pilot study. *Psychiatry Res*. 2015;231:184–6.

69. Marcoux L-A, Michon P-E, Lemelin S, Voisin JA, Vachon-Presseau E, Jackson PL. Feeling but not caring: empathic alteration in narcissistic men with high psychopathic traits. *Psychiatry Res*. 2014;224:341–8.

70. Domsalla M, Koppe G, Niedtfeld I, et al. Cerebral processing of social rejection in patients with borderline personality disorder. *Soc Cogn Affect Neurosci*. 2014;9:1789–97.

71. Ruocco AC, Medaglia JD, Tinker JR, et al. Medial prefrontal cortex hyperactivation during social exclusion in borderline personality disorder. *Psychiatry Res*. 2010;181:233–6.

72. Volman I, Roelofs K, Koch S, Verhagen L, Toni I. Anterior prefrontal cortex inhibition impairs control over social emotional actions. *Curr Biol*. 2011;21:1766–70.

73. New AS, Hazlett EA, Newmark RE, et al. Laboratory induced aggression: a positron emission tomography study of aggressive individuals with borderline personality disorder. *Biol Psychiatry*. 2009;66:1107–14.

74. Mancke F, Herpertz SC, Bertsch K. Aggression in borderline personality disorder: a multidimensional model. *Personal Disord*. 2015;6:278–91.

75. Pearson JM, Watson KK, Platt ML. Decision making: the neuroethological turn. *Neuron*. 2014;82:950–65.

76. Bartra O, McGuire JT, Kable JW. The valuation system: a coordinate-based meta-analysis of BOLD fMRI experiments examining neural correlates of subjective value. *Neuroimage.* 2013;76:412–27.

77. Bertsch K, Grothe M, Prehn K, et al. Brain volumes differ between diagnostic groups of violent criminal offenders. *Eur Arch Psychiatry Clin Neurosci.* 2013;263:593–606.

78. Brunner R, Henze R, Parzer P, et al. Reduced prefrontal and orbitofrontal gray matter in female adolescents with borderline personality disorder: is it disorder specific? *Neuroimage.* 2010;49:114–20.

79. Chanen AM, Velakoulis D, Carison K, et al. Orbitofrontal, amygdala and hippocampal volumes in teenagers with first-presentation borderline personality disorder. *Psychiatry Res.* 2008;163:116–25.

80. de Araujo Filho GM, Abdallah C, Sato JR, et al. Morphometric hemispheric asymmetry of orbitofrontal cortex in women with borderline personality disorder: a multi-parameter approach. *Psychiatry Res.* 2014;223:61–6.

81. Rossi R, Pievani M, Lorenzi M, et al. Structural brain features of borderline personality and bipolar disorders. *Psychiatry Res.* 2013;213:83–91.

82. Sato JR, de Araujo Filho GM, de Araujo TB, Bressan RA, de Oliveira PP, Jackowski AP. Can neuroimaging be used as a support to diagnosis of borderline personality disorder? An approach based on computational neuroanatomy and machine learning. *J Psychiatr Res.* 2012;46:1126–32.

83. Tebartz van Elst L, Hesslinger B, Thiel T, et al. Frontolimbic brain abnormalities in patients with borderline personality disorder: a volumetric magnetic resonance imaging study. *Biol Psychiatry.* 2003;54:163–71.

84. Richter J, Brunner R, Parzer P, Resch F, Stieltjes B, Henze R. Reduced cortical and subcortical volumes in female adolescents with borderline personality disorder. *Psychiatry Res.* 2014;221:179–86.

85. Enzi B, Doering S, Faber C, Hinrichs J, Bahmer J, Northoff G. Reduced deactivation in reward circuitry and midline structures during emotion processing in borderline personality disorder. *World J Biol Psychiatry.* 2013;14:45–56.

86. Völlm B, Richardson P, McKie S, Elliott R, Dolan M, Deakin B. Neuronal correlates of reward and loss in Cluster B personality disorders: a functional magnetic resonance imaging study. *Psychiatry Res.* 2007;156:151–67.

87. Andreou C, Kleinert J, Steinmann S, Fuger U, Leicht G, Mulert C. Oscillatory responses to reward processing in borderline personality disorder. *World J Biol Psychiatry.* 2015;16:575–86.

88. Vega D, Soto À, Amengual JL, et al. Negative reward expectations in borderline personality disorder patients: neurophysiological evidence. *Biol Psychol.* 2013;94:388–96.

89. Schuermann B, Kathmann N, Stiglmayr C, Renneberg B, Endrass T. Impaired decision making and feedback evaluation in borderline personality disorder. *Psychol Med.* 2011;41:1917–27.

90. Soloff PH, White R, Omari A, Ramaseshan K, Diwadkar VA. Affective context interferes with brain responses during cognitive processing in borderline personality disorder: fMRI evidence. *Psychiatry Res.* 2015;233:23–35.

91. Coutinho J, Goncalves OF, Soares JM, Marques P, Sampaio A. Alterations of the default mode network connectivity in obsessive-compulsive personality disorder: a pilot study. *Psychiatry Res.* 2016;256:1–7.

92. Winter D, Krause-Utz A, Lis S, et al. Dissociation in borderline personality disorder: disturbed cognitive and emotional inhibition and its neural correlates. *Psychiatry Res.* 2015;233:339–51.

93. Korzekwa MI, Dell PF, Links PS, Thabane L, Fougere P. Dissociation in borderline personality disorder: a detailed look. *J Trauma Dissociation.* 2009;10:346–67.

94. Stiglmayr CE, Ebner-Priemer UW, Bretz J, et al. Dissociative symptoms are positively related to stress in borderline personality disorder. *Acta Psychiatr Scand.* 2008;117:139–47.

95. Stiglmayr CE, Grathwol T, Linehan MM, Ihorst G, Fahrenberg J, Bohus M. Aversive tension in patients with borderline personality disorder: a computer-based controlled field study. *Acta Psychiatr Scand.* 2005;111:372–9.

96. Malhi GS, Tanious M, Fritz K, et al. Differential engagement of the fronto-limbic network during emotion processing distinguishes bipolar and borderline personality disorder. *Mol Psychiatry.* 2013;18:1247–8.

97. Silbersweig D, Clarkin JF, Goldstein M, et al. Failure of frontolimbic inhibitory function in the context of negative emotion in borderline personality disorder. *Am J Psychiatry.* 2007;164:1832–41.

98. Wingenfeld K, Rullkoetter N, Mensebach C, et al. Neural correlates of the individual emotional Stroop in borderline personality disorder. *Psychoneuroendocrinology.* 2009;34:571–86.

99. Krause-Utz A, Elzinga BM, Oei NYL, et al. Amygdala and dorsal anterior cingulate connectivity during an emotional working memory task in borderline personality disorder patients with interpersonal trauma history. *Front Hum Neurosci.* 2014;8:848.

100. Holtmann J, Herbort MC, Wüstenberg T, et al. Trait anxiety modulates fronto-limbic processing of emotional interference in borderline personality disorder. *Front Hum Neurosci.* 2013;7:54.

101. Etkin A, Egner T, Peraza DM, Kandel ER, Hirsch J. Resolving emotional conflict: a role for the rostral anterior cingulate cortex in modulating activity in the amygdala. *Neuron.* 2006;51:871–82.

102. Legris J, Links PS, van Reekum R, Tannock R, Toplak M. Executive function and suicidal risk in women with borderline personality disorder. *Psychiatry Res.* 2012;196:101–8.

103. Sebastian A, Jung P, Krause-Utz A, Lieb K, Schmahl C, Tüscher O. Frontal dysfunctions of impulse control—a systematic review in borderline personality disorder and attention-deficit/hyperactivity disorder. *Front Hum Neurosci.* 2014;8:698.

104. Jacob GA, Zvonik K, Kamphausen S, et al. Emotional modulation of motor response inhibition in women with borderline personality disorder: an fMRI study. *J Psychiatry Neurosci.* 2013;38:164–72.

105. Cackowski S, Reitz A-C, Ende G, et al. Impact of stress on different components of impulsivity in borderline personality disorder. *Psychol Med.* 2014;44:3329–40.

106. Ruchsow M, Groen G, Kiefer M, et al. Response inhibition in borderline personality disorder: event-related potentials in a Go/Nogo task. *J Neural Transm.* 2008;115:127–33.

107. van Eijk J, Sebastian A, Krause-Utz A, et al. Women with borderline personality disorder do not show altered BOLD responses during response inhibition. *Psychiatry Res.* 2015;234:378–89.

# 122

# Treatment and management of personality disorder

*Giles Newton-Howes and Roger Mulder*

## Introduction

The management of personality disorder remains a complex and challenging, but increasingly recognized and potentially rewarding, area of psychiatric practice. Our understanding of personality, personality disorder, and its interactions with mental state disorders continues to develop, and alongside this, understanding of mechanisms of management has also developed. Personality disorder is discussed in multiple places in this textbook, and some of the interventions described here are developed in greater detail elsewhere, being general interventions for a wide array of presentations, as opposed to personality disorder itself. Nonetheless, collating these into one chapter provides an overview of the current state of the evidence in the management of personality disorder and the influence of personality pathology in those with comorbidities. Before we examine the current state of the literature, it is important to consider its potential shortcomings. This allows for a balanced understanding of the evidence base and its applicability to day-to-day clinical practice.

## Difficulties with clinical interpretation of the literature

All medical evidence is open to criticism. However, as the complexity of problems being addressed increases, the need to understand the limitations of the evidence without discarding it increases. The difficulties in interpreting the evidence base for the treatment of personality disorders is considered under four headings: population studied, treatment duration, comorbidity, and outcome measures used.

## Population studied

Ideally, to allow translation of clinical trials to standard clinical practice, it is important for the study population to mirror the clinical population to which it is to be applied. This presents difficulties in the interpretation of personality disorder trials for numerous

reasons. Importantly, there are no long-term, robust studies of the epidemiology of personality disorder in a general population. This makes the interpretation of trials difficult. We do not know what the natural progression of personality disorder is in the community. This is not to say there are no data to act as a guide, but simply the data that exist require interpretation with caution. The Children in the Community study [1], based in New York state and initiated in 1975, has tracked the course of around 800 children over longer than a 20-year period. However, the inclusion of personality considerations occurred late with a 'constructed' measurement of uncertain validity, and no data were published from this study in relation to personality disorder for 18 years after its initiation [2]. The McLean Study of Adult Development (MSAD) [3] provides valuable information on the trajectory of borderline personality disorder (BPD). The Collaborative Longitudinal Personality Disorders Study (CLiPS) [4] follows the course of avoidant, obsessive–compulsive, borderline, and schizotypal personality disorders, but again broader issues as to the value of categorical diagnoses and the capacity to translate these data into other cultural settings provide at best a coarse backdrop from which to compare intervention studies.

## Treatment duration

For most mental state disorders, it is relatively clear about the duration over which to demonstrate the efficacy of a particular intervention, largely due to an understanding of the natural development of the disorder. In the case of personality disorder, since chronicity is a core feature of the condition, much longer time frames are needed than in many other disorders. Previously, periods of 2–3 years have been suggested. However, it is not clear how long is really needed. This problem is made more difficult by the relative instability of the categorical personality disorder diagnoses over time [5]. It is also clear that, in following those with categorical diagnoses longitudinally, there is a natural progression of the disorder, with many no longer reaching diagnostic criteria without targeted interventions [6]. It is not clear whether this translates into problem resolution [7]. This evidence suggests that larger numbers will be required for trials to show an effect (taking into account the potential natural resolution of some participants) conducted over a time frame that takes this natural variation into account. It also suggests studies should examine treatment effect over variable time frames, to assess the duration of treatment needed to accelerate symptom remission. Therapy studies of one [8] or more [9] years have been conducted; however, few brief interventions have been considered. For those that have, they have not reported benefit, although understanding the reasons for this is complex. What is clear is that for a treatment to be considered useful, it needs to show improvement greater than would be expected from the natural history of the disorder; the improvement needs to be sustained, and follow-up should be able to find evidence of continued effectiveness in a real-world clinical setting.

Consideration also needs to be given to the natural history of personality development and the place of extremes of personality that cause distress, namely personality disorder. It is clear that personality develops and continues to do so throughout the life course, and this needs to be considered when the outcomes of trials on management are considered. This is most clearly highlighted by work that identifies personality disorder in adolescence and its specific treatment [10]. The personality disorders that garner the most clinical (and research) attention are externalizing, and these disorders tend to peak in mid life where the bulk of the literature into interventions is focused, improving from the fourth decade onwards. Later in life, paranoid, schizoid, and schizotypal presentations become increasingly apparent. The literature is starting to recognize this better [11], as well as the problems associated with it [12], although there has been little work on the management and treatment of later-life personality disorder.

## Comorbidity

Comorbidity is 'the presence of any distinct clinical entity that has existed or that may occur during the clinical course of a patient who has the index disease under study' [13]. The key word here is 'distinct', identifying two separate disorders that are distinct and not causally related in any way. Co-occurrence ranges from comorbidity to the presence of the same disorder in two or more differing forms [14]. Historically, personality disorder itself has been questioned as a diagnostic entity, with some suggesting it is 'an adjective in search of a noun' [15]. Frustratingly, comorbidity (or consanguinity) is the norm in personality disorders, both with other personality disorders [16] and with mental state disorder [17]. This may relate to the categorical constructs used to artificially separate normal from abnormal personality. In deciding the efficacy of a treatment for personality pathology, it would be useful to examine the intervention in a population without comorbidity. However, this is difficult, with a rate of BPD without comorbidity of as low as 5% [18] and no clear indication of the rates of comorbidity for other personality disorders. This comorbidity implies undertaking efficacy studies for the management of personality disorder is difficult to impossible, and the trials described in the following sections are, in effect, effectiveness trials. While this has the advantage of clinical applicability, it leaves open the question as to whether the intervention is impacting primarily on the personality disorder or the comorbid condition. It may be more sensible to consider personality function in this

regard—an intervention may not lead to a change in personality per se; however, the functioning of the individual may markedly change on the basis of changes in the environment, mental state changes, or cognitive consideration of the person's internal world [19].

## Outcome measures

Understanding the most appropriate outcome measure in personality disorder trials is also problematic. Personality disorders that come to the attention of psychiatric services cause problems for an individual in their internal world, in their relationships with others and society in general. These are all potentially outcome targets to measure. Forensic clinicians generally consider social measures of the most importance (for example, reoffending), and this measure is often considered the most important by the general public. Although such measures offer a clear outcome target, there are so many potential confounders that it may well not reflect personal or personality change at all. Change in psychopathology is the most common measure in most psychiatric trials but may be inappropriate due to the likely presence of comorbid mental state disorder, as well as the reorientation of psychiatric services towards a recovery focus of care that minimizes the importance of symptoms over improvement in psychosocial functioning [20]. Direct use of repeated measures using personality assessment tools is also beset by problems related to the instability of these tools over time and the natural development of personality through the life course [21]. Currently, there is no agreed outcome measure in personality disorder trials, requiring careful consideration of each trial on its own. This problem needs to be kept in mind when considering meta-analyses or overviews that combine multiple trials in an effort to overcome the power problems described previously. It is probably best to have a range of outcome measures, being mindful of their shortcomings and examining for areas of convergence that may reflect more closely actual change.

## Taxonomic issues

Overarching all of the issues described previously when considering the literature related to the treatment of personality disorder is the issue of diagnosis and the use of the term 'personality disorder'. The *Diagnostic and Statistical Manual of Mental Disorders*, fifth edition (DSM-5) and the *International Classification of Diseases*, tenth revision (ICD-10) take a categorical approach to the definition of personality disorder. This is not based on in a single theoretical construct, the empirical literature, or clear divisions in the epidemiological data to suggest a set number of discrete entities. These problems may go some way to explaining the difficulties in the utility of categories that experts agree neither are helpful nor reflect empirical understandings of personality [22]. Trials of interventions are heavily skewed towards BPD and antisocial personality disorder, and care is needed not to assume the heuristic that the weight of evidence (of varying strength and quality) implies these categories are more biologically based or amenable to intervention than other conceptualizations of personality. Rather these categories cause the most social distress and the greatest economic burden for society, focusing research on them for these reasons. The recently published ICD-11 has moved away from traditional personality disorder categories [23]. Clinicians can now describe the severity of core personality dysfunction (mild, moderate, or severe) when describing personality disorders. The ICD-10 specific personality disorders are abandoned entirely in favour of five broad trait domains based on the scientific literature on personality: negative affectivity, disinhibition, dissociality, detachment, and anankastia. A borderline specifier was also added to enhance clinical utility and continuity. The utility of assessing core personality functioning is supported by research showing that severity is more predictive of clinical outcomes than specific personality disorder categories [23a]. The range of behaviours described by the domains may encourage treatment studies to venture beyond BPD into patients with detachment or anankastic symptoms.

## Psychotherapies

Psychological treatment is now clearly recognized as the most appropriate primary intervention for the treatment of BPD, and this is identified in national guidelines [25]. The evidence discussed later in this chapter is related to BPD unless stated otherwise. Although the evidence is much weaker, a similar approach is recommended for other personality pathologies. A broad spectrum of psychotherapeutic approaches have been tried, from strict behavioural approaches, through psychoeducation and supportive therapy, to analytic therapy. A recent Cochrane review identified more than 15 modalities of therapy trialled in BPD alone [26]. These have been trialled in inpatient, outpatient, and partial hospitalization settings. Length of therapy and therapy mix (individual, group, and mixed individual and group) are also variable and often based on therapist choice or model adherence, as opposed to robust clinical evidence. The UK's National Institute for Health and Care Excellence (NICE) recommends a mixed-therapy approach for patients with BPD, but little other guidance is available. Often the key determinant is resource provision, heavily working against high cost services, such as traditional therapeutic communities, and significantly advantaging treatments that reduce hospital presentations or admissions, as opposed to functional recovery. It is worth noting that the overall evidence for the effectiveness of psychotherapies is low, with the likelihood that well-designed randomized controlled trials (RCTs) in the future may lead to significant changes in clinical practice. A recent systematic review and meta-analysis concluded that psychotherapies are effective for BPD. However, effect sizes were small, inflated by risk of bias, and unstable at follow-up [26a].

## Cognitive therapies

Cognitive behavioural therapy for personality disorder (CBT-PD) [27, 28], dialectical behaviour therapy (DBT) [29], and schema-focused therapy (SFT) [30] are the three largely cognitively based psychological interventions that are most researched. They have in common an attempt to integrate biological and social factors, linking past experience and relationships with current difficulty and testing out mechanisms in the 'here and now' to normalize dysfunctional behaviours and emotional responses.

Cognitive behavioural therapy (CBT) was originally developed for the treatment of depressive disorder, designed to help the patient identify and modify dysfunctional thoughts and beliefs through the use of specific techniques such as Socratic questioning. Although therapy relies on an understanding of development, the focus of therapy is 'here and now', with symptomatic relief of central importance. CBT-PD expands this narrow window regarding problems as originating in the temperament of the child, development, and early experience. These experiences, particularly early attachment experiences, shape the style of interpersonal relatedness in adulthood and ongoing emotional and behavioural responses. With this in mind, one of the primary tasks of CBT-PD is to gain a solid understanding of childhood experience and the development of a shared formulation to link past difficulties with present problems. This understanding is then used to identify core beliefs and consequent behavioural patterns and emotional responses that are maladaptive. The meaning and content of these beliefs are explored, as well as their basis in negative early experience, possible neglect, and abuse. These experiences are likely to have led to difficulties in self-esteem, hypersensitivity to criticism, and difficult interpersonal relationships. Once these patterns are identified, the therapist and patient develop strategies to test them out in the present and learn new, more adaptive patterns of response. The emphasis may be cognitive (for example, 'How can I think about myself in positive terms and collect evidence that supports this perspective?') or behavioural ('When I feel criticized, I will not retreat and cut but ask the question, "Can you explain that to me?" to gain a better understanding of the other person's perspective') [31]. Compared to CBT for mental state disorders, CBT-PD generally takes longer, places significantly greater importance on the maintenance of the therapeutic relationship, and uses experiences occurring in the therapeutic relationship as 'microcosmic' examples of experiences occurring in the real world. The logic behind this is the more ingrained and pervasive cognitive and behavioural patterns found in personality pathology would be expected to take longer to work through and are pervasive enough to be expected to occur in the therapeutic relationship. There is evidence of effectiveness in this approach [32].

DBT is a form of CBT linked to skills training and detached (or radical) acceptance conceptualized as mindfulness. DBT was one of the first therapies formally tested for its benefits in patients with BPD [33] and has been the subject of more RCTs than any other treatment for BPD. Working from a basis of assuming BPD is primarily a dysfunction of emotion regulation based on biology and early environment, patients become emotionally vulnerable, struggling to regulate patterns of responses associated with emotional states. This leads to maladaptive behaviours and maladaptive problem-solving strategies. As the name implies, DBT has an implicit embracing of opposites, for example an acceptance of how things are and a drive to change, directed through therapy. From a working perspective, the essentials of DBT include: (1) manualized weekly individual therapy sessions; (2) group psychoeducational behavioural skills training; and (3) telephone coaching. The focus is on problem-solving skills, emotion regulation techniques, distress tolerance, validation, and mindfulness. Therapists also meet weekly to discuss therapy progress, share problems, and ensure therapy adherence [29]. Nine RCTs have examined the effectiveness of DBT and summarized in a Cochrane review [26]. These showed DBT is beneficial in reducing anger and self-harm and generally improving overall functioning for patients with BPD.

SFT has been trialled in two RCTs, one of which importantly is a head-to-head trial against transference-focused therapy (TFT) [30]. Building on CBT, SFT expands the basic notions of cognitions affecting behaviours and affects to include considerations from object–relations theory, in particular. There are assumptions of maladaptive schemas developed early in life that lead to maladaptive interpersonal relatedness in adulthood. This leads to individual therapy sessions, with a focus on understanding and redressing maladaptive schemas and elements of CBT (and gestalt) to adapt or replace maladaptive coping styles. Techniques focus on the patient–therapist relationship with SFT, describing a 'limited reparenting' role for the therapist. Some describe SFT as an integrative psychotherapy, as opposed to a predominantly cognitively based therapy. The study of Giesen-Bloo and colleagues showed advantages of SFT over TFT in most domains related to BPD.

## Dynamic therapies

Transference-focused therapy [34] and mentalization-based therapy (MBT) [35] are the two dynamically oriented therapies that have been trialled for the management of BPD. Although very different in approach, both are based on an understanding of the influence of the unconscious on the presentation of patients in their theory. They utilize this understanding of the unconscious to enable the patient to develop insight into their difficulties, enabling change.

MBT [35] was specifically designed as therapy for patients with BPD, conceptualized as a problem of disorganized attachment and subsequent failure to mentalize. Mentalization is the capacity to interpret action and derive an internal meaning for it. This is the basis of relationships (and understanding of self), and developing this enables normalization of the emotional difficulties (neither too intense nor too detached) and behaviours of those with BPD. Having stabilized emotional expression in the initial stages of therapy, the primary aim of all therapy is to increase mentalization, this being more important than the 'task' orientation of cognitively based therapies (be they cognitive or behavioural tasks). This requires a 'not knowing' stance that accepts the various positions of the patient and focuses on description ('What is going on for you now?'), as opposed to understanding ('Why are you doing that?'). It is important for the therapist to be mindful of their own mentalizing stance throughout therapy. MBT has been trialled in both partial hospitalization [36] and outpatient [37] settings and shown to be effective in BPD.

TFT is also designed to manage the problems of BPD and developed from the object–relations model of borderline personality organization [38]. It assumes internal and unconscious conflict exists between internal representations of both self and others, and this leads to emotionally unstable relationships. These distorted internal representations emerge in the process of therapy in a classic transference style of understanding and interpretation. This is a major intervention designed to lead to internal change and also (ultimately) behavioural change. The end-goal of TFT, like all psychotherapy for BPD, is amelioration of symptoms, reduction of non-suicidal self-harm, and improved relationships. TFT is a long-term individual therapy, as long as twice-weekly sessions for 3 years, and works at containing dangerous behaviours, managing behaviour that impairs therapy, and synthesizing the 'split-off' part of self into an integrated whole. Although there is evidence of effectiveness, this is a time-intensive treatment and has been shown to be inferior to SFT in a head-to-head trial.

## Other structured therapies

Interpersonal therapy (IPT) has been modified for application in patients with BPD on the basis of efficacy of IPT in patient with depression and comorbid BPD. A small trial has suggested this may be of benefit [39] but needs replication. Systems Training for Emotional Predictability and Problem Solving (STEPPS) is aligned with cognitive therapies, but largely psychoeducational. It is a structured programme of 20 2-hour weekly group sessions, with a learning goal to be derived from each session. Evidence of effectiveness exists [40]. Cognitive analytic therapy has also shown weak evidence of effectiveness in adolescents with personality disorder and traits [41], and this well-constructed trial is important not only for its evidence of effectiveness, but also for clearly displaying the utility of a BPD diagnosis in adolescence.

## Social therapies

Social therapies were the traditional mainstay for the management of personality disorders, bridging the time of development of pharmacotherapies and implementation of modern psychotherapies. Personality disorders do, by definition, cause significant distress to the community, and it is perhaps not surprising that efforts to consider alternative community settings were thought to be the best approach. In general, they recognize the influential elements of natural communities and aim to use these communities and the environment into the tolls for change. Although these approaches are used considerably less today, they remain an important element of the overall bio-psychosocial management armory and should be considered for the most severe and disruptive patients with personality disorder. Notably, the therapeutic communities described in the following paragraphs are not those utilized by correctional services in the United States, although they have at times been considered in this light.

Therapeutic communities have been described variously, although their modern context was defined and described by Maxwell Jones [42], who created a structure that ran counter to the traditional mental hospital. This can be defined as a socially cohesive structure, depending on intensive group treatments carried out by the residents who are involved in treatment in a democratic way. These communities have a strong historical basis for their effectiveness but are complex, long-term interventions and, as such, are expensive to run and difficult to assess, particularly compared to manualized psychotherapy or pharmacotherapy. Nonetheless, there is some evidence for their effectiveness in personality disorder, although there are no RCTs that have been completed.

Nidotherapy is a novel social therapy described as 'the collaborative systematic assessment and modification of the environment to minimise the impact of any form of mental disorder on the individual in society' [43]. It was developed and trialled with personality disorder as a central focus, in association with other comorbid mental state disorders [44]. Interestingly, this 'add-on therapy' does not aim to directly change psychopathology; rather it focuses on developing a better 'fit' between an individual and their environment. It is normally carried out by a nidotherapist working independently from other clinical services, while liaising with them. There is some RCT evidence this form of therapy may lead to cost savings and improvements in social functioning, the therapy's natural target endpoints [45].

## Pharmacotherapies

The rationale for using drugs in the treatment of personality disorders is that some of the behaviours associated with personality disorders may reflect disordered neurochemistry [46]. The poor empirical basis for the creation of the individual personality disorders in DSM-III, their heterogeneity, and the absence of evidence to support drug treatment of specific personality disorders have led researchers to largely ignore the DSM categories and to focus on dimensions of psychopathology. The algorithm generally used to study drug effects was proposed by Siever and Davis [47] and further developed by Soloff [48]. It suggests that four dimensions—affective instability, anxiety inhibition, cognitive-perceptual disturbances, and impulsivity aggression—cut across all personality disorder categories and that drug treatment effects on these dimensions should be studied, rather than on individual personality disorders. Although heuristically appealing, little evidence exists to support their validity. The dimensions have never been tested in hypothesis-driven studies [49]. In addition, although the algorithm was designed to study behaviours across all personality disorder categories, most clinical trials have used participants with BPD. A systematic review reported that over 70% of all drug trials used subjects with BPD [50]. The review also noted that most trials were underpowered, with a mean of 22.4 participants in the treatment group and 19.3 in the control group, were of short duration, averaging 13.2 weeks, and had a wide range of outcome measures [50]. Finally, we should note that many studies were sponsored by the pharmaceutical industry.

## Cluster A personality disorders

Studies have focused on the drug effect on cognitive perceptual disturbances in this population. Patients with schizotypal personality disorder have been studied in a few small, usually open-label studies using dopamine antagonists [51]. Patients showed some improvement in overall symptom severity, but the risk-to-benefit ratio appears poor. No RCTs for patients with schizoid or paranoid personality disorders have been undertaken, and therefore, no robust evidence about the efficacy of drugs in these patients is available at present.

## Cluster B personality disorders

As previously noted, most evidence for the use of drugs in patients with Cluster B personality disorders have been derived from studies on subjects with BPD, using the Siever and Davis algorithm [47]. This has led to a number of recommendations which are confusing and, at times, contradictory. Some guidelines advocate symptom-targeted pharmacotherapy, based on Siever and Davis' dimensions, while others state drug treatment should be avoided generally in patients with BPD.

The American Psychiatric Association (APA) guideline [52] states that symptom-targeted pharmacotherapy is an important adjunct treatment. It suggests that affective instability is treated with selective serotonin reuptake inhibitors (SSRIs) or monoamine oxidase inhibitors (MAOIs), impulsive aggression with SSRIs or mood stabilizers, and cognitive–perceptual disturbances with low-dose dopamine antagonists. The World Federation of Societies of Biological Psychiatry guidelines [53] state that moderate evidence exists for dopamine antagonist drugs being effective for cognitive–perceptual and impulsive–aggressive symptoms, some evidence exists for SSRIs being effective for emotional dysregulation, and there is some evidence for mood stabilizers being effective for emotional dysregulation and impulsive–aggressive symptoms. The most recent Cochrane review [54] partially contradicted these guidelines, reporting no evidence for the efficacy of SSRIs, but did report that mood stabilizers could diminish affective dysregulation and impulsive–aggressive symptoms in patients with BPD and antipsychotics could improve cognitive–perceptual symptoms and affective dysregulation.

In contrast, the UK NICE guidelines [55] state that drug treatment should generally be avoided, except in a crisis, and then given for no longer than 1 week. More recent guidelines for the treatment of BPD from the Australian National Health and Medical Research Council (NHMRC) [56] again reviewed the literature, including conducting a series of meta-analyses. It concluded that pharmacotherapy did not appear to be effective in altering the nature and course of BPD.

These apparently contradictory recommendations may reflect the weight given to risks, as well as benefits, of drug treatment. Both NICE and NMHRC Committees acknowledged evidence existed that some dopaminergic drugs (notably aripiprazole and olanzapine) and mood stabilizers (notably topiramate, lamotrigine, and valproate) may reduce BPD symptoms over the short term. They concluded that substantial long-term risks did not justify recommending these drugs when alternative psychosocial interventions do not carry such risks.

A pragmatic compromise may be to acknowledge the real concerns about using drugs in this population and be guided towards using drugs with at least some evidence of efficacy, using them sparingly and for short periods. The current evidence [57] would suggest using dopamine antagonists/partial agonists and mood stabilizers, rather than SSRIs, tricyclic antidepressants, and benzodiazepines. However, a recent large, well-conducted RCT testing lamotrigine for BPD reported no evidence for its efficacy or cost-effectiveness [57a]. A more radical view, articulated in the NICE guidelines [55], is that if patients have no comorbid illness, efforts should be made to reduce or stop pharmacotherapy.

Drug treatment of antisocial personality disorder has almost no evidence base [50]. The NICE guidelines for antisocial personality disorder concluded that pharmacological interventions should not be used routinely for the treatment of antisocial personality disorder or its associated behaviours. However, NICE states that drugs can be used for comorbid mental disorders. A recent meta-analysis by Khalifa and colleagues [58] reached similar conclusions.

## Cluster C personality disorders

No RCTs have been published of drug treatment for patients with Cluster C personality disorders. However, the World Federation of Societies of Biological Psychiatry guidelines [53] suggests that studies in patients with social phobia, which reported that drugs for depression are superior to placebo, might be evidence that these drugs are effective in patients with avoidant personality disorder.

In summary, the evidence base for psychopharmacology in patients with personality disorders is poor. Drug treatment should be used sparingly for short periods, with careful consideration of risks and benefits. Hopefully, more useful drugs may become available. For example, targeting $N$-methyl-$D$-aspartate signalling pathways, which have effects on disinhibition, social cognition, and dissociative symptoms, has potential [59]. There is a suggestion that opioid modulation is a possible mechanism for treatment [60, 61] and oxytocin is associated with prosocial behaviour [62]. However, small open trial results have been mixed [62, 63]. We still have a long way to go.

## Managing risk or managing needs?

In addition to interventions designed to alter the trajectory of personality disorder, a service orientation towards recognizing this problem and ensuring a seamless service is considered important. This needs to take into account the risks presented, while recognizing the limitations in the evidence for effective interventions, and not inadvertently positively reinforcing unhelpful or dangerous behaviours. For example, if hospitalization is the default response to non-suicidal self-injury and a patient with severe personality disorder is struggling in the community, there is a risk that they will self-harm in order to gain access to an inpatient ward. Developing a plan with the patient, which recognizes these difficulties, is important to ensure the patient, services, and the wider community that may be involved (for example, police and paramedical staff) are clear as to the best approach in difficult situations. Providing a consistency of response allows for a patient with personality disorder to develop an understanding of boundaries and balances long- and short-term risks. Constancy in personnel further allows for an understanding of behaviour driven by long-term traits and the more acute psychopathologically driven behaviours. This sort of conceptualization and understanding of the purpose of behaviour reflects what is known of personality disorder in regard to its structure [3, 64].

## Conclusions

Although the management of personality disorder remains in flux, much progress has been made over the last decade. Increased clarity associated with an improved understanding of taxonomy has opened the door to the development of novel trait-based psychotherapeutic interventions. The importance of psychotherapy as the primary intervention of value, particularly in BPD, has been strengthened and the relatively limited place of pharmacotherapy is clearer. The potential for 'add-on' therapy, such as STEPPS or nidotherapy, is also clearer. Having said this, there remains little evidence to guide any but BPD treatment. The evidence for antisocial personality disorder treatment suggests little leads to long-term change. Almost nothing is known as to the effectiveness of interventions for other categorical diagnoses. Added to this, it is likely that ICD-11 will take a radically different approach to diagnosis from that of DSM-5, and this

opens the door to both confusion and improved study of personality problems. In the future, well-designed large randomized or complex trials with novel findings are likely to lead to significant changes in clinical practice, suggesting the current evidence is at best weak. Despite the significant steps forward, clarity about the limits of the evidence and the need for $n = 1$ trials with our patients remain important. Acknowledging the changes in personality through the life course [21] and the need to be cognizant of our limits and expertise ensures we will be able to help patients with personality disorder, without overstating the current state of the evidence.

## REFERENCES

1. Cohen P, Crawford TN, Johnson JG, Kasen S. The children in the community study of developmental course of personality disorder. *Journal of Personality Disorders* 2005;**19**:466–86.
2. Bezirganian S, Cohen P, Brook JS. The impact of mother-child interaction on the development of borderline personality disorder. *American Journal of Psychiatry* 1993;**150**:1836.
3. Zanarini MC, Frankenburg FR, Hennen J, Reich DB, Silk KR. The McLean Study of Adult Development (MSAD): overview and implications of the first six years of prospective follow-up. *Journal of Personality Disorders* 2005;**19**:505–23.
4. Gunderson JG, Shea MT, Skodol AE, *et al*. The Collaborative Longitudinal Personality Disorders Study: development, aims, design, and sample characteristics. *Journal of Personality Disorders* 2000;**14**:300–15.
5. Zimmerman M. Diagnosing personality disorders: a review of issues and research methods. *Archives of General Psychiatry* 1994;**51**:225.
6. Zanarini MC. Diagnostic specificity and long-term prospective course of borderline personality disorder. *Psychiatric Annals* 2012;**42**:53–8.
7. Zanarini MC, Frankenburg FR, Reich DB, Fitzmaurice G. Attainment and stability of sustained symptomatic remission and recovery among patients with borderline personality disorder and axis II comparison subjects: a 16-year prospective follow-up study. *American Journal of Psychiatry* 2012;169:476–83.
8. Verheul R, van den Bosch LM, Koeter MW, De Ridder MA, Stijnen T, Van Den Brink W. Dialectical behaviour therapy for women with borderline personality disorder. *British Journal of Psychiatry* 2003;**182**:135–40.
9. Linehan MM, Comtois KA, Murray AM, *et al*. Two-year randomized controlled trial and follow-up of dialectical behavior therapy vs therapy by experts for suicidal behaviors and borderline personality disorder. *Archives of General Psychiatry* 2006;**63**:757–66.
10. Chanen AM, McCutcheon L. Prevention and early intervention for borderline personality disorder: current status and recent evidence. *British Journal of Psychiatry* 2013;**202**:s24–9.
11. Eaton NR, Krueger RF, Oltmanns TF. Aging and the structure and long-term stability of the internalizing spectrum of personality and psychopathology. *Psychology and Aging* 2011;**26**:987.
12. Oltmanns TF, Balsis S. Personality disorders in later life: Questions about the measurement, course, and impact of disorders. *Annual Review of Clinical Psychology* 2011;7:321.
13. Feinstein AR. The pre-therapeutic classification of co-morbidity in chronic disease. *Journal of Chronic Diseases* 1970;**23**:455–68.
14. Tyrer P. Comorbidity or consanguinity. *British Journal of Psychiatry* 1996;**168**:669–71.

15. Akiskal HS, Chen SE, Davis GC, Puzantian V, Kashgarian M, Bolinger J. Borderline: an adjective in search of a noun. *Journal of Clinical Psychiatry* 1985;46:41–8.

16. Trull TJ, Durrett CA. Categorical and dimensional models of personality disorder. *Annual Review of Clinical Psychology* 2005;**1**:355–80.

17. Clark LA. Assessment and diagnosis of personality disorder: Perennial issues and an emerging reconceptualization. *Annual Review of Clinical Psychology* 2007;**58**:227–57.

18. Fyer MR, Frances AJ, Sullivan T, Hurt SW, Clarkin J. Comorbidity of borderline personality disorder. *Archives of General Psychiatry* 1988;**45**:348–52.

19. Tyrer P. Personality diatheses: a superior explanation than disorder. *Psychological Medicine* 2007;**37**:1521–6.

20. Barber ME. Recovery as the new medical model for psychiatry. *Psychiatric Services* 2012;**63**:277–9.

21. Newton-Howes G, Clark LA, Chanen A. Personality disorder across the life course. *The Lancet* 2015;**385**:727–34.

22. Bernstein DP, Iscan C, Maser J. Opinions of personality disorder experts regarding the DSM-IV personality disorders classification system. *Journal of Personality Disorders* 2007;**21**:536–51.

23. Tyrer P, Mulder R, Kim YR, Crawford MJ. The development of the ICD-11 classification of personality disorders: An amalgam of science, pragmatism, and politics. *Annual Review of Clinical Psychology* 2019;**15**:481–502.

23a. Bach, B. Treating comorbid depression and personality disorders in DSM-5 and ICD-11. (Correspondence). *Lancet Psychiatry*, 2018;**5**(11):874–5.

24. Clark LA, Livesley WJ, Morey L. Special feature: Personality disorder assessment: The challenge of construct validity. *Journal of Personality Disorders* 1997;**11**:205–31.

25. National Institute for Health and Care Excellence. *Borderline Personality Disorder: Treatment and Management*. NICE Clinical Guideline No. 78. National Collaborating Centre for Mental Health, British Psychological Society; 2009.

26. Stoffers JM, Völlm BA, Rücker G, Timmer A, Huband N, Lieb K. Psychological therapies for people with borderline personality disorder. *Cochrane Database of Systematic Reviews* 2012;**8**:CD005652.

26a. Cristea IA, Gentili C, Cotet CD, Palomba D, Barbui C, Cuijpers P. Efficacy of psychotherapies for borderline personality disorder: A systematic review and meta-analysis. *JAMA Psychiatry* 2017;**74**(4):319–28.

27. Davidson K, Halford J, Kirkwood L, Newton-Howes G, Sharp M, Tata P. CBT for violent men with antisocial personality disorder. Reflections on the experience of carrying out therapy in MASCOT, a pilot randomized controlled trial. *Personality and Mental Health* 2010;**4**:86–95.

28. Tyrer P, Davidson K. Cognitive therapy for personality disorders. *Psychotherapy for Personality Disorders* 2000;**19**:131–49.

29. Linehan M. *Cognitive-behavioral Treatment of Borderline Personality Disorder*. New York, NY: Guilford Press; 1993.

30. Giesen-Bloo J, Van Dyck R, Spinhoven P, *et al.* Outpatient psychotherapy for borderline personality disorder: randomized trial of schema-focused therapy vs transference-focused psychotherapy. *Archives of General Psychiatry* 2006;**63**:649–58.

31. Davidson K. *Cognitive Therapy for Personality Disorders: A Guide for Clinicians*. New York, NY: Routledge; 2007.

32. Davidson K, Norrie J, Tyrer P, *et al.* The effectiveness of cognitive behavior therapy for borderline personality disorder: results from the borderline personality disorder study of cognitive therapy (BOSCOT) trial. *Journal of Personality Disorders* 2006;**20**:450.

33. Linehan MM, Armstrong HE, Suarez A, Allmon D, Heard HL. Cognitive-behavioral treatment of chronically parasuicidal borderline patients. *Archives of General Psychiatry* 1991;**48**:1060–4.

34. Doering S, Hörz S, Rentrop M, *et al.* Transference-focused psychotherapy v. treatment by community psychotherapists for borderline personality disorder: randomised controlled trial. *British Journal of Psychiatry* 2010;**196**:389–95.

35. Bateman A, Fonagy P. Mentalization based treatment for borderline personality disorder. *World Psychiatry* 2010;**9**:11–15.

36. Bateman A, Fonagy P. Effectiveness of partial hospitalization in the treatment of borderline personality disorder: a randomized controlled trial. *American Journal of Psychiatry* 1999;**156**:1563–9.

37. Bateman A, Fonagy P. Randomized controlled trial of outpatient mentalization-based treatment versus structured clinical management for borderline personality disorder. *American Journal of Psychiatry* 2009;**166**:1355–64.

38. Kernberg O. The treatment of patients with borderline personality organization. *International Journal of Psycho-Analysis* 1968;**49**:600.

39. Bellino S, Rinaldi C, Bogetto F. Adaptation of interpersonal psychotherapy to borderline personality disorder: a comparison of combined therapy and single pharmacotherapy. *Canadian Journal of Psychiatry* 2010;**55**:74.

40. Blum N, John DS, Pfohl B, *et al.* Systems Training for Emotional Predictability and Problem Solving (STEPPS) for outpatients with borderline personality disorder: a randomized controlled trial and 1-year follow-up. *American Journal of Psychiatry* 2008;**165**:468–78.

41. Chanen AM, Jackson HJ, McCutcheon LK, *et al.* Early intervention for adolescents with borderline personality disorder using cognitive analytic therapy: randomised controlled trial. *British Journal of Psychiatry* 2008;**193**:477–84.

42. Jones M. *The Therapeutic Community: A New Treatment Method in Psychiatry*. Oxford: Basic Books; 1953.

43. Tyrer P. Nidotherapy: a new approach to the treatment of personality disorder. *Acta Psychiatrica Scandinavica* 2008;**105**:469–71.

44. Tyrer P, Bajaj P. Nidotherapy: making the environment do the therapeutic work. *Advances in Psychiatric Treatment* 2005;**11**:232–8.

45. Ranger M, Tyrer P, Miloseska K, *et al.* Cost-effectiveness of nidotherapy for comorbid personality disorder and severe mental illness: randomized controlled trial. *Epidemiologia e Psichiatria Sociale* 2009;**18**:128–36.

46. Mulder R. The biology of personality. *Australian and New Zealand Journal of Psychiatry* 1992;**26**:364–76.

47. Siever LJ, Davis KL. A psychobiological perspective on the personality disorders. *American Journal of Psychiatry* 1991;**148**:1647–58.

48. Soloff PH. Algorithms for pharmacological treatment of personality dimensions: symptom-specific treatments for cognitive-perceptual, affective, and impulsive-behavioral dysregulation. *Bulletin of the Menninger Clinic* 1998;**62**:195–214.

49. Kendall T, Burbeck R, Bateman A. Pharmacotherapy for borderline personality disorder: NICE guideline. *British Journal of Psychiatry* 2010;**196**:158–9.

50. Duggan C, Huband N, Smailagic N, Ferriter M, Adams C. The use of pharmacological treatments for people with personality disorder: a systematic review of randomized controlled trials. *Personality and Mental Health* 2008;**2**:119–70.

51. Silk KR, Feurino L, III. Psychopharmacology of personality disorders. In: Widiger TA, ed. *Oxford Handbook of Personality Disorders*. New York, NY: Oxford University Press; 2012. pp. 713–26.

52. American Psychiatric Association Practice Guidelines. Practice guideline for the treatment of patients with borderline personality disorder. American Psychiatric Association. *American Journal of Psychiatry* 2001;**158**(10 Suppl): 1–52.

53. Herpertz SC, Zanarini M, Schulz CS, Siever L, Lieb K, Moller HJ. World Federation of Societies of Biological Psychiatry (WFSBP) guidelines for biological treatment of personality disorders. *World Journal of Biological Psychiatry* 2007;**8**:212–44.

54. Lieb K, Vollm B, Rucker G, Timmer A, Stoffers JM. Pharmacotherapy for borderline personality disorder: Cochrane systematic review of randomised trials. *British Journal of Psychiatry* 2010;**196**:4–12.

55. National Institute for Health and Care Excellence. *Borderline Personality Disorder: Recognition and Management.* Clinical guideline [CG78]. 2009. https://www.nice.org.uk/guidance/cg78

56. National Health and Medical Research Council. *Clinical Practice Guideline for the Management of Borderline Personality Disorder.* Melbourne: National Health and Medical Research Council; 2012.

57. Abraham PF, Calabrese JR. Evidenced-based pharmacologic treatment of borderline personality disorder: a shift from SSRIs to anticonvulsants and atypical antipsychotics? *Journal of Affective Disorders* 2008;**111**:21–30.

57a. Crawford MJ, Sanatinia R, Barrett B, *et al.* on behalf of the Labile Study Team. The clinical effectiveness and cost-effectiveness of lamotrigine in borderline personality disorder: A randomized placebo-controlled trial. *American Journal of Psychiatry* 2018;**175**(8):756–64.

58. Khalifa N, Duggan C, Stoffers J, *et al.* Pharmacological interventions for antisocial personality disorder. *Cochrane Database of Systematic Reviews* 2010;**8**:CD007667.

59. Ripoll LH. Clinical psychopharmacology of borderline personality disorder: an update on the available evidence in light of the Diagnostic and Statistical Manual of Mental Disorders—5. *Current Opinion in Psychiatry* 2012;**25**:52–8.

60. Bandelow B, Schmahl C, Falkai P, Wedekind D. Borderline personality disorder: a dysregulation of the endogenous opioid system? *Psychological Review* 2010;**117**:623–36.

61. Stanley B, Siever LJ. The interpersonal dimension of borderline personality disorder: toward a neuropeptide model. *American Journal of Psychiatry* 2010;**167**:24–39.

62. Bartz J, Simeon D, Hamilton H, *et al.* Oxytocin can hinder trust and cooperation in borderline personality disorder. *Social Cognitive and Affective Neuroscience* 2011;**6**:556–63.

63. Bertsch K, Gamer M, Schmidt B, *et al.* Oxytocin and reduction of social threat hypersensitivity in women with borderline personality disorder. *American Journal of Psychiatry* 2013;**170**:1169–77.

64. Skodol AE, Gunderson JG, Shea MT, *et al.* The collaborative longitudinal personality disorders study (CLPS): overview and implications. *Journal of Personality Disorders* 2005;**19**:487–504.

# SECTION 20
# Impulse-control and conduct disorders

SECTION 20

Impulse-control and conduct disorders

# 123

# Impulse-control and its disorders, including pathological gambling

*Donald W. Black*

## Introduction

The hallmark of impulse-control disorders (ICDs) is difficulty with emotional and behavioural self-regulation, as manifested by difficult, disruptive, or aggressive behaviour. Recognized in *Diagnostic and Statistical Manual of Mental Disorders*, third edition (DSM-III) [1] as 'disorders of impulse control not elsewhere classified', the category included pathological gambling, kleptomania, pyromania, and both intermittent and isolated explosive disorders. All were unified by the failure to resist an impulse to perform an act harmful to the individual or others, increasing tension before the act, and the experience of pleasure, gratification, or release at the time of the act. They were believed ego-syntonic at the 'moment of discharge', but accompanied by guilt or regret afterwards [2]. The chapter continued in DSM-III-R, DSM-IV, and DSM-IV-TR [3]. Trichotillomania was added in DSM-III-R, while isolated explosive disorder was dropped after DSM-III.

The chapter was reorganized in DSM-5 [4], with intermittent explosive disorder (IED), kleptomania, and pyromania continuing in a new chapter called 'Disruptive, impulse-control, and conduct disorders'. Pathological gambling was moved to the chapter on 'Substance-related and addictive disorders' and renamed *gambling disorder*, while trichotillomania was moved to the chapter on 'Obsessive–compulsive and related disorders'. Oppositional defiant disorder (ODD) and conduct disorder, previously included in the chapter on childhood disorders, were brought into the new chapter, reflecting the view that they too are disorders of self-regulation.

ICDs received limited recognition in *International Classification of Diseases*, ninth revision (ICD-9) [5]. The category 'Disturbances of conduct not elsewhere classified' included conditions characterized by aggressive and destructive behaviour. Kleptomania was given as an example of a 'compulsive conduct disorder'. In ICD-10 [6], the renamed category ('Habit and impulse disorders') was expanded to include gambling disorder, pyromania, pathological stealing (kleptomania), and trichotillomania (with IED listed under 'Other habit and impulse disorders'). These disorders were characterized by repeated acts having no clear rationale.

Despite their historical roots, ICDs were not officially recognized until DSM-III. In the nineteenth century, the French psychiatrist Jean Étienne Esquirol used the term monomania to describe a group of conditions in which people had irresistible urges without apparent motivation [7]. Pyromania was recognized by the nineteenth-century German psychiatrist Griesinger as a 'morbid impulse', which drives the person to commit destructive acts. In the early twentieth century, Bleuler wrote about *reactive impulses* that borrowed from Kraepelin's *impulsive insanity* [8, 9]. Included were pyromania, kleptomania, and compulsive shopping (*oniomania*). More recently, many of these conditions have been described as *behavioural addictions*, characterized by the presence of unrestrained or poorly controlled behaviours arising in the absence of alcohol or drugs of abuse [10].

This chapter discusses the following DSM-5 disorders: ODD, IED, pyromania, kleptomania, and gambling disorder. Trichotillomania is discussed in Chapter 93 on obsessive–compulsive and related disorders. For completeness, the chapter will include a discussion of three non-DSM conditions that involve poorly regulated behaviours: compulsive shopping (CS), Internet addiction, and compulsive sexual behaviour (CSB). Despite its reclassification in DSM-5, conduct disorder is discussed in Chapter 124.

## Oppositional defiant disorder

ODD is a diagnosis for persons who exhibit negativistic, hostile, defiant, and disobedient behaviours towards others. ODD is mostly a diagnosis for children and adolescents but may also be used in adults. The diagnosis is made on the basis of angry or irritable, defiant, or vindictive behaviour of at least 6 months' duration, with a minimum of four of eight symptoms in three categories: angry/irritable mood, argumentative/defiant behaviour, and vindictiveness. DSM-5 [4] considers ODD to be a developmental antecedent for some youth with conduct disorder, thereby suggesting that they may reflect different stages of a spectrum of disruptive behaviours.

ODD was introduced in DSM-III [1] as 'oppositional disorder' to characterize those with a negative and disobedient opposition to authority. The diagnosis received its current name with DSM-III-R. The diagnosis had many commonalities with DSM-II's [11] unsocialized aggressive reaction, a diagnosis used to describe loners with a pattern of hostile disobedience, aggressiveness, stealing, and lying, behaviours thought to result from inconsistent discipline and parental rejection.

The prevalence of ODD has ranged in studies from 1% to 11%, with an average of 3.3% [4]. The disorder is more common in boys than girls prior to adolescence [12]. ODD has a mean age of onset of 6 years and may precede the onset of conduct disorder. Youth with ODD are also at risk for developing mood and anxiety disorders [12, 13]. The defiant, argumentative, and vindictive symptoms carry most of the risk for conduct disorder. Angry/irritable mood symptoms carry most of the risk for internalizing disorders. While all children show oppositional behaviour from time to time, the diagnosis is given to those with frequent, recurrent, and problematic behaviours, for example temper outbursts, arguments with parents or other authority figures, and a refusal to obey orders.

The disorder tends to be stable over time [12]. Boys who develop conduct disorder have higher numbers of ODD symptoms that those who do not. There appears to be a genetic overlap of ODD with other disruptive disorders, including conduct disorder and attention-deficit/hyperactivity disorder.

Other disorders need to be ruled out. Unlike conduct disorder which specifies that the child must have violated personal rights and social rules, ODD is defined on the basis of difficult and disruptive behaviour. Attention-deficit/hyperactivity disorder may be comorbid with ODD but is a diagnosis used in those with problems of sustained effort and attention. ODD shares many features with disruptive mood dysregulation disorder, such as negative mood and temper outbursts, but the severity, frequency, and chronicity of temper outbursts are more severe in children with disruptive mood dysregulation disorder than in those with ODD. (In DSM-5, the diagnosis of disruptive mood dysregulation disorder takes precedence over ODD, if the criteria for both disorders are met.) IED also involves high rates of anger, but people with this disorder show serious aggression towards others that is not part of the definition of ODD.

There has been little neurobiologic research with regard to ODD. One study showed elevated levels of dehydroepiandrosterone sulfate in children with ODD, in contrast to children with attention-deficit/hyperactivity disorder and controls, suggesting to the authors that stress or genetic factors have led to a shift in adrenocorticotrophic hormone (ACTH)–β-endorphin functioning in the hypothalamic–pituitary–adrenal axis. Another study found a specific pattern of single-nucleotide polymorphisms associated with attention-deficit/hyperactivity disorder comorbid with ODD, compared with attention-deficit/hyperactivity disorder alone, especially for measures of argumentative and defiant behaviours.

There is no standard treatment for ODD, but common sense suggests that because most patients with ODD are children, clinical management should emphasize individual and family therapy, with treatment of co-occurring attention-deficit/hyperactivity disorder or other disorders with medications, as needed, such as stimulants, guanfacine, or clonidine [12]. Family-based interventions include parental management training and child problem skills training. The former aims to teach parents to better manage their child's behaviour, as well as to promote desired behaviours. The latter is cognitively based and aims to help children learn to manage anger, improve problem-solving ability, delay impulsive responses, and improve social interactions. School-based programmes, such as those aimed at resisting negative peer influences and reducing bullying and antisocial behaviour, may also be helpful.

## Intermittent explosive disorder

IED was new to DSM-III [1] and included as a diagnosis for those with episodes of verbal or physical aggression grossly out of proportion to the stressor. IED was considered roughly equivalent to DSM-II's [11] explosive personality. A related diagnosis—isolated explosive disorder—was also included in DSM-III and was meant to be used in persons with a single, discrete episode of uncharacteristic aggression. It was dropped from later editions.

In DSM-5 [4], IED is defined by the presence of recurrent behavioural outbursts that are grossly out of proportion to the provocation or stressors, are not premeditated, occur in an individual aged 6 or older, cause distress or functional impairment, and are not better explained by another mental disorder, medical condition, or the effects of a substance. ICD-10 [6] lists IED under 'Other habit and impulse disorders' but does not provide criteria.

People with IED describe their aggressive episodes as brief, explosive, uncontrollable, and unpremeditated, and typically provoked by minor events [14]. They may experience changes in mood, awareness, and autonomic arousal before the outburst. The frequency of episodes depends, in part, on how the disorder is defined. In the National Comorbidity Survey-Replication (NCS-R) [15], whereby DSM-IV criterion A was operationalized as ≥3 lifetime attacks, persons with IED had a mean of 43 lifetime attacks. Many people with IED have a history of chronic anger or irritability accompanied by frequent minor episodes. Subthreshold episodes are similar to the anger attacks (sudden episodes of intense anger with autonomic arousal) often described in patients with mood disorders.

Before making the diagnosis, IED needs to be distinguished from Cluster B personality disorders associated with anger outbursts (antisocial and borderline personality disorders), neurocognitive disorders characterized by verbal or physical outbursts, substance abuse and intoxication causing behavioural disinhibition, and the childhood-onset disorders disruptive mood dysregulation disorder, autism spectrum disorder, attention-deficit/hyperactivity disorder, ODD, and conduct disorder. In the case of the childhood-onset disorders, the additional diagnosis of IED may be warranted when outbursts are deemed in excess of those usually seen in the disorders and warrant independent clinical attention.

IED is common in clinical and general population samples, with an estimated lifetime prevalence in the general population of 7.3% [14]. IED is more common in men than women. IED begins in childhood or adolescence and rarely occurs after age 40. The disorder follows a chronic or episodic course and is associated with distress, morbidity (for example, accidents), and social and occupational impairment. In the NCS-R [15], IED had a mean age at onset of 14 years, was persistent over the life course (with averages of 6.2–11.8 years with attacks), and was associated with substantial role impairment. The prevalence of the disorder was much lower in persons aged 60 years and older.

Psychiatric comorbidity is common in persons with IED. In the NCS-R [15], 82% of respondents with IED met criteria for at least one other lifetime disorder, in particular depressive, anxiety, and substance use disorders. It was also significantly comorbid with ODD, conduct disorder, and attention-deficit/hyperactivity disorder.

Family studies suggested that first-degree relatives of people with IED have high rates of impulsive violence, substance misuse, and possibly mood and other ICDs [14]. A blinded, controlled family history study using broadly defined IED criteria found a significantly increased morbid risk of the condition in relatives of affected probands (26%), compared with relatives of control probands (8%).

In terms of neurobiology, people with emotion dysregulation and aggression have been shown to have disturbed serotonergic function [14] and functional abnormalities in both the limbic system and the orbitofrontal cortex. In a functional magnetic resonance imaging (MRI) study of response to social threat [16], ten subjects with IED showed exaggerated amygdala reactivity and diminished orbitofrontal cortex activation to faces expressing anger, compared with controls. The authors noted these findings were similar to other disorders characterized by impulsive aggression, including borderline personality disorder and bipolar disorder, and that they supported a link between a dysfunctional frontal–limbic network and aggression.

There are no standard treatments for IED. Cognitive behavioural therapy has been used, with a focus on anger management [17]. Patients learn to recognize when they are becoming angry and to identify and defuse the triggers that lead to outbursts. One study showed that cognitive behavioural therapy was superior to a wait list in reducing anger and hostility in persons with IED. The programme employed relaxation training, imagery, rebreathing, use of time-outs, and cognitive restructuring.

Medication has been used to reduce or eliminate aggressive impulses [17] in persons with impulsive aggression. The strongest evidence supports the use of selective serotonin reuptake inhibitors (SSRIs) in the treatment of IED. There is some evidence that mood stabilizers and drugs for psychosis may also play a role in reducing anger outbursts in persons with behavioural dyscontrol. Benzodiazepines should be avoided because of their tendency to cause behavioural disinhibition.

## Pyromania

Pyromania was first recognized in the nineteenth century, its name coined in 1833 by Marc, a French psychiatrist [3]. He described the disorder as a form of instinctive and impulsive monomania. Griesinger, Bleuler, and Kraepelin, all active at the turn of the twentieth century, considered pyromania a 'morbid impulse' [8, 9, 18]. The disorder was briefly mentioned in DSM-I [19] as a supplementary term but was not mentioned in DSM-II. Pyromania was included in DSM-III [1] and has continued to the present.

DSM-5 [4] defines pyromania as the deliberate and purposeful fire-setting on more than one occasion; tension or affective arousal before the act; fascination with, interest in, curiosity about, or attraction to fire and its contents and characteristics; and pleasure, gratification, or relief when setting fires or when witnessing or participating in their aftermath. Importantly, those who set fires for political motives, out of anger or to seek vengeance, to conceal

crimes, or to improve one's living situation (for example, by claiming insurance benefits) do not have pyromania. Likewise, the fire-setting cannot be in response to a psychosis or to impaired judgement from a neurocognitive disorder or drug of abuse. Thus, an arsonist who sets fires for monetary gain or for political or criminal purposes would not merit the diagnosis. In ICD-10 [6], pyromania is defined as multiple acts of, or attempts at, setting fire to property or other objects, without apparent motive and by a persistent preoccupation with subjects related to fire and burning.

Data show that around 1% of the general population report a lifetime history of fire-setting, though this is only one component of pyromania [20]. A study of psychiatric inpatients found that about 6% had a lifetime history of pyromania [21]. Pyromania is probably more common in men than women and usually begins in adolescence or early adulthood. Mood, substance use, and other ICDs are common in people with pyromania. Fire-setting is considered a poor prognostic sign for children with conduct disorders and is associated with adult aggression [20]. The course of pyromania is unknown, but clinical descriptions suggest that the course of pyromania is episodic and tends to wax and wane.

Before making the diagnosis, the clinician should rule out other causes of intentional fire-setting, including normal developmental experimentation (for example, playing with matches), antisocial personality disorder, and adult antisocial behaviour. Accidental fire-setting, as might occur in a person with a neurocognitive disorder, substance abuse or intoxication, and psychosis, should be ruled out.

There are no standard treatments for pyromania [22]. Much of the literature on the use of psychological treatments has focused on children and includes behavioural therapies, family therapy, and fire education. Case reports have suggested benefit from SSRIs, lithium, topiramate, olanzapine, and valproate.

## Kleptomania

Kleptomania has been recognized for nearly 200 years [3]. Bleuler provided one of the first clinical descriptions: 'The kleptomaniacs in the old sense cannot even otherwise resist the impulse of appropriating things … ' ([8], p. 539). The disorder was listed as a supplementary term in DSM-I and was formally included in DSM-III. The disorder has continued to the present.

In DSM-5 [4], kleptomania is defined as the 'recurrent failure to resist impulses to steal objects that are not needed for personal use or for their monetary value'. In addition, there is an increasing sense of tension immediately before committing the theft, followed by pleasure, gratification, or relief at the time of the theft. Importantly, individuals do not steal to express anger or vengeance, or steal in response to hallucinations or delusions. In ICD-10 [6], kleptomania (or pathological stealing) is defined as the repeated failure to resist impulses to steal objects that are not acquired for personal use or monetary gain.

Kleptomania prevalence is unknown, perhaps because individuals rarely report their symptoms. A survey of the adult general population in the United States found shoplifting to have a lifetime prevalence of 11% [23], though stealing is only one component of kleptomania. A survey of nearly 800 college students reported a 0.4% current prevalence for kleptomania [24]. Grant et al. [21] reported a 9% lifetime prevalence rate in psychiatric inpatients.

People with kleptomania describe irresistible impulses or urges to steal that build until satisfied [25]. They understand their impulses are senseless and intrusive and that their behaviour is wrong. Many try to resist the impulses with varying degrees of success. Stealing itself is accompanied by a 'rush' or 'high', although that feeling dissipates as the potential consequences of the act become apparent. While most stealing is impulsive, some is premeditated. People with kleptomania tend to steal items that they otherwise could afford such as toiletries, make-up, or jewellery. Triggers include feelings of depression, anxiety, or boredom, or sometimes the particular sights, sounds, and objects found within a store. Lying to conceal the stealing is common. Some stop stealing temporarily following an arrest for shoplifting, but the behaviour resumes unfettered for most. A small number of individuals report that they have no memory of the stealing or that it occurs in a dream-like (or dissociative) state. For these individuals, stealing may become automatic.

Clinicians should rule out other causes of stealing before making the diagnosis of kleptomania. Other possible diagnoses include antisocial personality disorder, crime occurring in the context of adult antisocial behaviour, and stealing that may occur in the course of a neurocognitive disorder, mania, or psychosis.

Kleptomania appears more common in women than in men [25]. Many cases begin in the late teens to early 20s and often follow an episodic or a chronic course. By the time patients seek treatment, women are typically in their mid- to late 30s, while men are in their 50s. Clinical studies show that kleptomania often co-occurs with other mental psychiatric disorders, including mood, anxiety, substance use, and eating disorders (particularly bulimia). Kleptomania may also be associated with compulsive shopping.

Family study data are limited, but studies suggested that people with kleptomania have first-degree relatives with high rates of mood disorders, obsessive–compulsive disorder, and substance use disorders [25].

Kleptomania may be associated with serotonergic and frontal lobe dysfunction, as evidenced by reduced [3H] paroxetine binding (a peripheral marker of serotonin function) found in a mixed group of 20 people with obsessive–compulsive-related disorders, including five with kleptomania [26]. In another study, ten women with kleptomania were more likely than controls to have decreased white matter microstructural integrity in the inferior frontal brain regions when evaluated with diffusion tensor imaging [27].

While there are no standard treatments for kleptomania [25], various forms of cognitive behavioural therapy have been recommended. Case reports and open-label studies have reported on the use of SSRIs, topiramate, and naltrexone. Interestingly, there are also case reports of persons treated for depression with SSRIs who subsequently *developed* kleptomania [28]. In a randomized controlled trial (RCT) [29], naltrexone produced significant reductions in stealing urges and behaviours, compared with placebo. Common wisdom suggests that a self-imposed ban on shopping in an attempt to head off potential thefts may help curb stealing, but this may not be sustainable.

## Gambling disorder

Recognized by both Kraepelin [10] and Bleuler [8], uncontrolled gambling was included in DSM-III [1] as pathological gambling within the chapter 'Impulse-control disorders not elsewhere classified'. In DSM-5 [4], the disorder was moved to the chapter on 'Substance related and other addictive disorders', a change made because of growing evidence of its relationship with alcohol and drug use disorders. The name was changed to *gambling disorder* (GD), in part, because of the stigma from the word 'pathological' [3]. ICD-10 [6] includes pathological gambling, which is defined as frequent and repeated episodes of gambling that dominate the person's life to the detriment of their functioning.

GD prevalence is estimated at 1.6% of the general population, but the prevalence of subclinical GD ('at-risk' gambling) is much higher at nearly 4% [30]. Gambling behaviour typically has an onset in adolescence, with GD developing by the late 20s for men and early 40s for women [31]. GD affects more men than women and progresses more rapidly in the latter, a phenomenon also observed in alcoholic persons [32]. Risk factors include a history of mental illness or substance misuse, lower levels of education, and ethnic and racial minority populations. Family and twin data show that GD is familial and has a heritable component shared with substance addictions. In a large family study involving over 1200 subjects, rates of lifetime pathological gambling were significantly greater among the first-degree relatives of people with pathological gambling (11%) than among control relatives (1%) [33].

Substance use, mood, and anxiety disorders are common in persons with GD [31]. Personality disorders are frequent, particularly the antisocial and borderline types. Compulsive shopping commonly occurs in women with GD, and the disorders run in the same families [34].

The most widely discussed clinical distinction among gamblers is that of 'escape-seekers' and 'sensation-seekers' [35]. Escape-seekers are often older persons who gamble out of boredom, to alleviate depression, or to fill time. They tend to choose passive forms of gambling such as slot machines. Sensation-seekers are younger and prefer the excitement of card games or table games that involve active input. Another model posits the existence of three subgroups of GDs: (1) behaviourally conditioned gamblers without predisposing psychopathology but who make bad judgements regarding gambling; (2) emotionally vulnerable gamblers with premorbid depression or anxiety, and a history of poor coping; and (3) impulsive gamblers who are highly disturbed with features of antisocial personality disorder [36].

GD is described in DSM-5 as chronic and progressive, though recent data have challenged the notion that GD is intractable. Instead, most GD subjects improve during follow-up, as evidenced by fewer gambling behaviours and less preoccupation [37].

Functional MRI and other technologies showed that the neurocircuitry mediating GD is similar to those seen in substance addictions [38]. The involvement of reward circuitry has also been strongly suggested by research showing that dopamine agonist medications for Parkinson's disease have led to the development or exacerbation of GD in some persons [39]. Dopamine is widely considered the neurotransmitter most involved in reward-based neurocircuitry.

While few persons with GD seek treatment, cognitive behavioural therapy and motivational interviewing are effective [40]. Gamblers Anonymous (GA), a 12-step programme patterned after Alcoholics Anonymous, is often helpful and chapters are widely available. Self-exclusion programmes in which gamblers agree not to enter a casino can be helpful. RCTs have shown naltrexone and nalmefene (not available in the United States) to be effective in reducing gambling behaviours and urges. SSRIs have also been studied, but RCTs have shown little effect [41].

## Compulsive shopping

Compulsive shopping (CS) has been recognized for over 100 years, including descriptions from Kraepelin [10] and Bleuler [8]. Despite this rich history, CS attracted little attention until interest was revived in the late 1980s and early 1990s by consumer behaviour researchers and clinicians interested in compulsive behaviours [42–44]. CS is not included in DSM-5 or ICD-10.

McElroy et al. [43] have published diagnostic criteria that have become standard in the research community. They require the presence of cognitive and behavioural aspects of CS and impairment from both subjective distress and interference in social or occupational functioning or from financial or legal problems. The criteria require that the disorder does not co-occur with mania or hypomania.

The prevalence of CS has been estimated at nearly 6% [45]. The disorder has shown a female preponderance in nearly all clinical and epidemiologic studies. CS has an onset in the late teens or early twenties that appears to correspond with emancipation from the nuclear family and establishing credit [46]. CS occurs mainly in developed countries, probably due to the availability of consumer goods and disposable income. Interestingly, after Germany reunified in 1989, the prevalence rate of CS increased, presumably due to the influx of goods into the former East Germany, combined with increased income [47].

Psychiatric comorbidity with substance use, mood, anxiety, personality, and eating disorders and other ICDs is common. Research suggests that CS is familial and co-aggregates with mood, anxiety, and substance use disorders [46]. CS has been considered chronic or episodic, but a recent study showed that CS behaviours diminished during a 5-year follow-up [48].

The hallmark of CS is a preoccupation with shopping and spending [46]. People with CS spend many hours each week engaged in shopping and spending behaviours, often preceded by increasing tension or anxiety relieved with a purchase. Compulsive shoppers are mainly interested in consumer goods such as clothing, shoes, crafts, jewellery, and make-up. The impact of the Internet on CS behaviour is unclear but could be considerable.

Neurobiologic theories of CS have focused on disturbed serotonin neurotransmission, because of hypothetical similarities between CS and obsessive–compulsive disorder, a disorder treated with SSRIs. Dopamine has been theorized to play a role in 'reward dependence', which has been linked to behavioural addictions, including CS. Functional abnormalities in limbic regions and the prefrontal cortex have been hypothesized to account for the impulsivity and poor decision-making that characterize CS. Using fMRI, Raab et al. [49] reported on differences between 23 women with CS and 26 controls. They found greater nucleus accumbens activity during product presentation in women with CS, compared to those without, and lower insula activation during the presentation of prices for the products the CS women decided to purchase. These investigators concluded that the expected loss of money led to a stronger negative emotional response in healthy controls than in women with CS.

There are no standard treatments for CS, but various forms of cognitive behavioural therapy have been shown to be effective [50]. Benson et al. [51] have developed a comprehensive programme combining cognitive behavioural therapy and elements of dialectical behaviour therapy. In an RCT, 11 subjects randomized to the group treatment had significantly greater improvement than wait list controls and the benefit was maintained at 6-month follow-up. Medication studies have had mixed success, with open-label trials showing positive results not confirmed in RCTs. SSRIs have been the most frequently used drugs in these trials. Other treatments are 12-step programmes, financial counselling, and self-help books. Common sense suggests that people with CS should avoid carrying credit cards or shopping alone.

## Internet addiction

Internet addiction is characterized by excessive and/or inappropriate use of personal computers and other electronic devices, combined with personal distress or impairment in important life domains. Young [52] has proposed criteria patterned after those used to diagnose GD. She only counts non-essential computer/Internet usage (for example, non-business or non-academic use), and Internet addiction is present when five or more symptom criteria are present during the past 6 months and mania has been ruled out. The concept of Internet addiction has been criticized because, unlike other behavioural addictions, the focus is on the medium, and not the behaviour, so that if an addiction exists, it likely pertains to the activity engaged in (for example, gaming, gambling, viewing pornography) [53]. The condition is not listed in DSM-5 or ICD-10.

The prevalence of Internet addiction is unknown, in part because surveys have produced figures that range from 0.9% to 38% [54]. In a random telephone survey of adult Americans, Aboujaoude et al. [55] reported prevalence rates ranging from 0.3% to 0.7%. The widely varying figures suggest that more work is needed to develop uniform definitions of Internet addiction. Cases of Internet addiction have been reported in many countries, showing its universality.

Data suggest that Internet addiction is more prevalent in males than females, perhaps because males are more likely to use the Internet for activities that may fuel addiction such as games, pornography, and gambling [54]. Age of onset is unknown, but Internet addiction has been reported in children as young as age 6 [55].

Psychiatric comorbidity is common, particularly for mood, anxiety, and substance use disorders and other ICDs [54]. Using a dimensional approach to assess the psychological status, increased use of the Internet was associated with higher ratings on measures of depression, loneliness, and social isolation.

Neurobiological theories of Internet addiction focus on disturbed neurotransmission, particularly serotonin and dopamine [55], but there is no direct evidence to support the role of these or other neurotransmitter systems in Internet addiction. Pallanti et al. [56] hypothesized that immaturity of the frontal cortical and subcortical monoaminergic system during normal neurodevelopment underlies adolescent impulsivity and perhaps Internet addiction. One study employing diffusion tensor imaging concluded that Internet addiction was associated with widespread reductions in fractional anisotropy in major white matter pathways that the authors believed may be linked to the abnormal behaviours exhibited by their subjects [57].

There are no standard treatments for Internet addiction [55, 58]. Young [58] has developed a guide for therapists working with Internet addicts, employing cognitive behavioural methods. SSRIs have been used to treat Internet addiction [58], but there have been no RCTs. Because Internet affects many youth, family therapy has been recommended. Support groups are available in some areas and are available online as well.

## Compulsive sexual behaviour

CSB involves excessive preoccupation and/or behaviour that causes distress or impairs one's functioning. The concept of a hypersexual disorder dates back to the work of the German psychiatrist Krafft-Ebing [59]; yet the concept of a *sexual addiction* was first recognized by Orford [60]. Diagnostic criteria have been proposed that incorporate the concepts of inappropriate or excessive sexual cognitions or behaviours, subjective distress, and impaired functioning [61]. CSB is not listed in DSM-5 or ICD-10.

CSB encompasses various problematic sexual behaviours that can roughly be divided into paraphilic and non-paraphilic subtypes [61]. The former involves pathological sexual behaviours (for example, exhibitionism, voyeurism), while the latter involves conventional sexual behaviours taken to extremes (for example, compulsive masturbation, promiscuity, pornography dependence). While hypersexual behaviour is the hallmark of CSB, it can be found in mania, substance use disorders, and neurocognitive disorders, all of which need ruling out.

The prevalence of CSB is estimated to range from 3% to 6% of the general adult population in the United States [61]. Kafka [62] has suggested that data on total sexual outlet (TSO) (or total number of orgasms achieved through any means during a designated week) may more accurately reflect CSB prevalence, at least in men. He concluded that ≥7 weekly orgasms over 6 consecutive months could be used to define hypersexual behaviour, a figure that corresponds to 3–15% of the adult male population in the United States. Grant *et al.* [21] reported a 4.9% lifetime prevalence for CSB in adult psychiatric inpatients. Whether high-frequency sexual behaviour is inherently pathological has been questioned. In one study, high-frequency sexual behaviour with a stable partner indicated *better* psychological functioning [63].

CSB is primarily a disorder of men, and there may be gender-specific differences in the way CSB manifests [61]. Men are more likely to report compulsive masturbation, to engage in paraphilias, to pay for sex, or to engage in anonymous sex. Women are more likely to engage in fantasy sex (for example, seductive behaviour leading to multiple affairs/relationships) or sadomasochism, to use sex as a business, or to see themselves as 'love addicts'. CSB has an onset in adolescence, with paraphilic behaviours frequently occurring earlier than non-paraphilic behaviours [61]. CSB appears to be chronic, though waxing and waning in frequency and severity. Psychiatric comorbidity is common in persons with CSB, particularly mood, anxiety, and substance use disorders. Some experts have suggested that CSB begins with childhood sexual abuse, but not all persons with CSB have experienced maltreatment [64].

Typical symptoms include preoccupation with one's sexual urges and fantasies and/or being overly sexually active, often spending considerable time in pursuit of sexual experiences [64]. Many will report feeling out control and being subjectively distressed by their sexual thoughts or urges. The behaviour eventually causes impairment in important life domains such as affecting their marriage or significant relationships or one's work or school life (for example, through intrusive thoughts or from frequent lateness). Persons with CBS often try unsuccessfully to resist sexual thoughts and urges.

In terms of neurobiology, Kafka [65] has focused on the possible contribution of disturbed neurotransmission, noting that noradrenaline, serotonin, and dopamine all serve to modulate sexual behaviour and other dimensions of human and animal pathophysiology. In a functional MRI study [66], sexual-cue reactivity led to greater activation in brain regions linked to drug craving and emotion processing (ventral striatum, amygdala, and dorsal anterior cingulate cortex) in 19 persons with CSB, compared to 19 controls. The authors suggested that CBS shares neural mechanisms with addictive disorders.

There are no standard treatments for CSB. Many forms of psychotherapy have been recommended, including imaginal desensitization, aversion therapy, group therapy, and psychodynamic and cognitive behavioural therapies [67]. Twelve-step programmes are available in some areas and can be helpful. SSRIs have been used in one controlled study and several open studies, leading to a reduction in sexual preoccupations and behaviours [67]. Case reports and small case series have also suggested that nefazodone, naltrexone, and anti-androgens may be effective in treating CSB. A placebo-controlled trial of the gonadotrophin-releasing hormone analogue triptorelin in men with severe paraphilias suggested that it is effective [68]. A meta-analysis of 118 patients suggested that luteinizing hormone-releasing agonists were effective in treating patients with severe paraphilias [69]. Anti-androgens should probably be reserved for men with aggressive and/or dangerous forms of CSB.

## REFERENCES

1. American Psychiatric Association (1980). *Diagnostic and Statistical Manual of Mental Disorders*, third edition. American Psychiatric Association, Washington, DC.
2. Spitzer, R.L., Williams, J.B., and Skodol, A. (1980). DSM-III: the major achievements and an overview. *American Journal of Psychiatry* 137, 151–64.
3. Black, D.W. and Grant, J.E. (2013). *DSM-5 Guidebook: The Essential Companion to the Diagnostic and Statistical Manual of Mental Disorders*, fifth edition. American Psychiatric Association, Washington, DC.
4. American Psychiatric Association. (2013). *Diagnostic and Statistical Manual of Mental Disorders*, fifth edition. American Psychiatric Association, Arlington, VA.
5. World Health Organization. (1978). *International Statistical Classification of Diseases and Related Health Problems*, ninth revision. World Health Organization, Geneva.
6. World Health Organization. (1992). *International Statistical Classification of Diseases and Related Health Problems*, tenth revision. World Health Organization, Geneva.
7. Moeller, G. (2012). Historical perspectives on impulsivity and impulse control disorders. In: J.E. Grant and M.N. Potenza, editors.

*Oxford Handbook of Impulse Control Disorders*, pp. 11–21. Oxford University Press, New York, NY.

8. Bleuler, E. (1911/1930). *Textbook of Psychiatry*. (Trans. A.A. Brill), Macmillan, New York, NY.

9. Kraepelin, E. (1915). *Psychiatrie*, eighth edition. Verlag Von Johann Ambrosius Barth, Leipzig.

10. Holden, C. (2001). Behavioral addictions; do they exist? *Science*, 294, 980–2.

11. American Psychiatric Association. (1968). *Diagnostic and Statistical Manual of Mental Disorders*, second edition. American Psychiatric Association, Washington, DC.

12. Thomas, C.R. (2016). Oppositional defiant disorder. In: M.K. Dulcan, editor. *Dulcan's Textbook of Child and Adolescent Psychiatry*, second edition, pp. 195–218. American Psychiatric Association, Arlington, VA.

13. Serra-Pinheiro, M.A., Schmitx, M., Mattos, P., and Souza, I. (2004). Oppositional defiant disorder: a review of neurobiological and environmental correlates, comorbidities, treatment, and prognosis. *Revista Brasileira de Psiquiatria*, 26, 272–5.

14. Coccaro, E.F. and Danehy, M. (2006). Intermittent explosive disorder. In: E. Hollander and D.J. Stein, editors. *Clinical Manual of Impulse Control Disorders*, pp. 19–37. American Psychiatric Association, Arlington, VA.

15. Kessler, R.C., Coccaro, E.F., Fava, M., *et al.* (2006). The prevalence and correlates of DSM-IV intermittent explosive disorder in the National Comorbidity Survey Replication. *Archives of General Psychiatry*, 63, 669–78.

16. Coccaro, E.F., McCloskey, M.S., Fitzgerald, D.A., *et al.* (2007). Amygdala and orbitofrontal reactivity to social threat in individuals with impulsive aggression. *Biological Psychiatry*, 62, 168–71

17. McCloskey, M.S., Berman, M., and Noblett, K. (2012). Assessment and treatment of intermittent explosive disorder. In: J.E. Grant and M.N. Potenza, editors. *Oxford Handbook of Impulse Control Disorders*, pp. 344–52. Oxford University Press, New York, NY.

18. Griesinger, W. (1882). *Mental Pathology and Therapeutics*, second edition. (Trans. C.L. Robertson), William Wood and Co., New York, NY.

19. American Psychiatric Association. (1952). Diagnostic *and Statistical Manual of Mental Disorders*. American Psychiatric Association, Washington, DC.

20. Lejoyeaux, M. and Germain, C. (2012). Pyromania: phenomenology and epidemiology. In: J.E. Grant and M.N. Potenza, editors. *Oxford Handbook of Impulse Control Disorders*, pp. 135–48. Oxford University Press, New York, NY.

21. Grant, J.E., Levine, L., Kim, D., and Potenza, M.N. (2005). Impulse control disorders in adult psychiatric inpatients. *American Journal of Psychiatry*. 162, 2184–8.

22. Grant, J.E., Odlaug, B.L. (2012). Assessment and treatment of pyromania. In: J.E. Grant and M.N. Potenza, editors. *Oxford Handbook of Impulse Control Disorders*, pp. 353–9. Oxford University Press, New York, NY.

23. Blanco, C., Grant, J., Petry, N.M., *et al.* (2008). Prevalence and correlates of shoplifting in the United States: results from the National Epidemiologic Survey on Alcohol and Related Conditions (NESARC). *American Journal of Psychiatry*, 165, 905–13.

24. Odlaug, B.L. and Grant, J.E. (2010). Impulse control disorders in a college sample. *Primary Care Companion Journal of Clinical Psychiatry*, 12, e1–5.

25. Grant, J.E. (2006). Kleptomania. In: E. Hollander and D.J. Stein, editors. *Clinical Manual of Impulse Control Disorders*, pp. 175–202. American Psychiatric Association, Arlington, VA.

26. Marazziti D, Dell'Osso L, Presta S, *et al.* (1999). Platelet [3H] paroxetine binding in patients with OCD-related disorders. *Psychiatry Research*, 89, 223–8.

27. Grant, J.E., Correia, S., and Brennan-Krohn, T. (2006). White matter integrity in kleptomania: a pilot study. *Psychiatry Research*, 147, 233–7.

28. Kindler, S., Dannon, P.N., Iancu, I., Sasson, Y., and Zohar, J. (1997). Emergence of kleptomania during treatment for depression with serotonin selective reuptake inhibitors. *Clinical Neuropharmacology*, 20, 126–9.

29. Grant, J.E., Kim, S.W., and Odlaug, B.L. (2009). A double-blind, placebo-controlled study of the opiate antagonist, naltrexone, in the treatment of kleptomania. *Biological Psychiatry*, 65, 600–6.

30. Grant, J.E. and Odlaug, B.L. (2010). Pathological gambling clinical aspects. In: E. Aboujaoude and L. Koran, editors. *Impulse Control Disorders*, pp. 51–74. Cambridge University Press, New York, NY.

31. Black, D.W., Coryell, W.H., Crowe, R.R., Shaw, M., McCormick, B., and Allen, J. (2015). Age at onset of DSM-IV pathological gambling in a non-treatment sample: early- versus later-onset. *Comprehensive Psychiatry*, 60, 40–6.

32. Tavares, H., Martins, S.S., Lobo, D.S.S., Silviera, C.M., Gentil, V., and Hodgins, D.C. (2003). Factors at play in faster progression for female pathological gamblers: an exploratory analysis. *Journal of Clinical Psychiatry*, 64, 433–8.

33. Black, D.W., Coryell, W.C., Crowe, R.R., McCormick, B., Shaw, M., and Allen, J. (2014). A direct, controlled, blind family study of pathological gambling. *Journal of Clinical Psychiatry*, 75, 215–21.

34. Black, D.W., Coryell, W.H., Crowe, R.R., Shaw, M., McCormick, B., and Allen J. (2015). The relationship of DSM-IV pathological gambling to compulsive buying and other possible spectrum disorders: results from the Iowa PG family study. *Psychiatry Research*, 226, 273–6.

35. Blaszczynski, A. and McConaghy, N. (1989). Anxiety and/or depression in the pathogenesis of addictive gambling. *International Journal of Addictions*, 24, 337–50.

36. Blaszczynski, A. and Nower, L. (2002). Pathways model of problem and pathological gambling. *Addiction*, 97, 487–99.

37. LaPlante, D.A., Nelson, S.E., LaBrie, R.A., and Shaffer, H.J. (2008). Stability and progression of disordered gambling: lessons from longitudinal studies. *Canadian Journal of Psychiatry*, 53, 52–60.

38. Leeman, R.F. and Potenza, M.N. (2013). A targeted review of the neurobiology and genetics of behavioral addictions: an emerging area of research. *Canadian Journal of Psychiatry*, 58, 260–78.

39. Lader, M. (2008). Antiparkinsonian medication and pathological gambling. *CNS Drugs*, 22, 407–16.

40. Tavares, H. (2012). Assessment and treatment of pathological gambling. In: J.E. Grant and M.N. Potenza, editors. *Oxford Handbook of Impulse Control Disorders*, pp. 279–312. Oxford University Press, New York, NY.

41. Bartley, C.A. and Bloch, M. (2013). Meta-analysis: pharmacological treatment of pathological gambling. *Expert Review of Neurotherapeutics*, 13, 887–94.

42. Christenson, G.A., Faber, J.R., de Zwann, M., *et al.* (1994). Compulsive buying: descriptive characteristics and psychiatric comorbidity. *Journal of Clinical Psychiatry*, 55, 5–11.

43. McElroy, S.L., Keck, P.E. Jr., Pope, H.G. Jr., *et al.* (1994). Compulsive buying: a report of 20 cases. *Journal of Clinical Psychiatry*, 55, 242–8.

44. O'Guinn, T.C. and Faber, R.J. (1989). Compulsive buying: a phenomenological exploration. *Journal of Consumer Research*, 16, 147–57.

45. Koran, L.M., Faber, R.J., Aboujaoude, E., Large, M.D., and Serpe, R.T. (2006). Estimated prevalence of compulsive buying in the United States. *American Journal of Psychiatry*, 163, 1806–12.

46. Black, D.W. (2012). Epidemiology and phenomenology of compulsive buying disorder. In: J.E. Grant and M.N. Potenza, editors. *Oxford Handbook of Impulse Control Disorders*, pp. 196–208. Oxford University Press, New York, NY.

47. Scherhorn, G., Reisch, L.A., and Raab, G. (1990). Addictive buying in West Germany: an empirical study. *Journal of Consumer Policy*, 13, 355–87.

48. Black, D.W., Shaw, M., and Allen, J. (2016). Five-year follow-up of persons reporting compulsive shopping behavior. *Comprehensive Psychiatry*, 68, 97–102.

49. Raab, G., Elger, C.E., Neuner, M., and Weber, B. (2011). The neural basis of compulsive buying. In: A. Müller and J.E. Mitchell, editors. *Compulsive Buying: Clinical Foundations and Treatment*, pp. 63–86. Routledge, New York, NY.

50. Mitchell, J.E., Burgard, M., Faber, R., and Crosby, R.D. (2006). Cognitive behavioral therapy for compulsive buying disorder. *Behavioral Research and Therapy*, 44, 1859–65.

51. Benson, A., Eisenach, D.A., Abrams, L., and Stolk-Cooke, L. (2014). Stopping overshopping: a preliminary randomized controlled trial opf group therapy for compulsive buying. *Journal of Groups in Addiction and Recovery*, 9, 97–125.

52. Young, K.S. (1996). Internet addiction: the emergence of a new clinical disorder. *Cyberpsychology and Behavior*, 1, 237–44.

53. Starcevic, V. Is Internet addiction a useful concept? (2012). *Australia and New Zealand Journal of Psychiatry*, 47, 16–19.

54. Liu, T. (2012). Epidemiology and phenomenology of problematic internet use. In: J.E. Grant and M.N. Potenza, editors. *Oxford Handbook of Impulse Control Disorders*, pp. 176–85. Oxford University Press, New York, NY.

55. Liu, T. and Potenza, M.N. (2010). Problematic Internet use: clinical aspects. In: E. Aboujaoude and L. Koran, editors. *Impulse Control Disorders*, pp. 167–81, Cambridge University Press, New York, NY.

56. Pallanti, S., Bernardi, S., and Quercioli, L. (2006). The Shorter PROMIS Questionnaire and the Internet Addiction Scale in the assessment of multiple addictions in a high-school population: prevalence and related disability. *CNS Spectrums*, 11, 966–74.

57. Lin, F., Shou, Y., Du, Y., *et al.* (2012). Abnormal white matter integrity in adolescents with Internet addiction disorder: a tract-based spatial statistics study. *PLoS One*, 7, e30253.

58. Young, K. (2012). Assessment and treatment of problematic internet use. In: J.E. Grant and M.N. Potenza, editors. *Oxford Handbook of Impulse Control Disorders*, pp. 389–97. Oxford University Press, New York, NY.

59. Krafft-Ebbing, R. (1886/1927). *Psychopathia Sexualis*. (Trans. F.J. Rebman). Physicians and Surgeons Book Company, New York, NY.

60. Orford, J. (1978). Hypersexuality: implications for a theory of dependence. *British Journal of Addictions*, 73, 299–310.

61. Schreiber, L.R.N., Grant, J.E., and Odlaug, B. (2012). Compulsive sexual behavior: phenomenology and epidemiology. In: J.E. Grant and M.N. Potenza, editors. *Oxford Handbook of Impulse Control Disorders*, pp. 165–75. Oxford University Press, New York, NY.

62. Kafka, M.P. (1997). Hypersexual desire in males: an operational definition and clinical implications for males with paraphilias and paraphilia-related disorders. *Archives of Sexual Behavior*, 26, 505–26.

63. Langstrom, N. and Hanson, R.K. (2006). High rates of sexual behavior in the general population: correlates and predictors. *Archives of Sexual Behavior*, 35, 37–52.

64. Kuzma, J. and Black, D.W. (2008). The epidemiology of compulsive sexual behavior. *Psychiatric Clinics of North America*, 31, 603–11.

65. Kafka, M.P. (2000). Psychopharmacologic treatments for nonparaphilic compulsive sexual behaviors. *CNS Spectrums*, 5, 49–59.

66. Voon, V., Mole, T.B., Banca, P., *et al.* (2014). Neural correlates of sexual cue reactivity in individuals with and without compulsive sexual behaviours. *PLoS One*, 9, e102419.

67. Coleman, E. (2012). Impulsive/compulsive sexual behavior: assessment and treatment. In: J.E. Grant and M.N. Potenza, editors. *Oxford Handbook of Impulse Control Disorders*, pp. 375–88. Oxford University Press, New York, NY.

68. Rosler, A. and Witztum, E. (1998). Treatment of men with paraphilia with a long acting analog of gonadotropin releasing hormone. *New England Journal of Medicine*, 338, 416–22.

69. Bricken, P., Hill, A., and Berner, W. (2003). Pharmacology of paraphilia with long-acting agonists of luteinizing hormone-releasing hormone: a systematic review. *Journal of Clinical Psychiatry*, 64, 890–7.

# 124

# Conduct disorders and antisocial personality disorder in childhood and adolescence

*Stephen Scott and Melanie Palmer*

## Introduction

The term conduct disorder refers to a persistent pattern of anti-social behaviour in which the individual repeatedly breaks social rules and carries out aggressive acts. It is the most common psychiatric disorder of childhood across the world. Antisocial behaviour has the highest continuity into adulthood of all measured human traits, except intelligence. A high proportion of affected children and adolescents grow up to be antisocial adults with impoverished and destructive lifestyles; some will develop antisocial personality disorder. The disorder places a large personal and economic burden on individuals and society. Juvenile delinquency is a legal term, referring to an act by a young person that breaks the law. Most recurrent juvenile offenders have conduct disorder. In this chapter, the term ODD/CD is used to denote oppositional defiant disorder (ODD) and conduct disorder (CD) together, since although they are essentially the same underlying condition of persistent antisocial behaviour expressed at different ages, in the *Diagnostic and Statistical Manual of Mental Disorders*, fifth edition (DSM 5), unlike in the *International Classification of Diseases*, tenth revision (ICD-10), they are separated. The term conduct problems will be used for less severe antisocial behaviour; when the term child is used, it refers to both children and adolescents, for brevity.

## Clinical features

Aggressive and defiant behaviour is an important part of normal child and adolescent development which ensures physical and social survival. Indeed, parents may express concern if a child is too acquiescent and unassertive. The level varies considerably among children, and it is a continuously distributed trait. Picking a particular level of antisocial behaviour to call ODD/CD is therefore necessarily arbitrary. For all children, the expression of any particular behaviour also varies according to child age; for example, physical hitting is at a maximum at around 2 years of age but declines over the next few years. Therefore, any judgement about the significance of the level of antisocial behaviour has to be made in the context of the child's age. Before deciding that the behaviour is abnormal, other clinical features have to be considered:

- Level: severity and frequency of antisocial acts, compared with children of the same age and gender.
- Pattern: the variety of antisocial acts and the setting in which they are carried out.
- Persistence: duration over time.
- Impact: distress and social impairment of the child; disruption and damage caused to others.

### Change in clinical features with age

The type of behaviour seen will depend on the age and gender of the individual.

*Younger children*, from 3 to 7 years of age, usually present with general defiance of adults' wishes, disobedience of instructions, angry outbursts with temper tantrums, physical aggression to people, especially siblings and peers, destruction of property, arguing, blaming others for things that have gone wrong, and a tendency to annoy and provoke others.

In *middle childhood*, from 8 to 11 years, these features are often present, but as the child grows older and stronger and spends more time out of the home, other behaviours are seen. They include: swearing, lying, stealing of others' belongings outside the home, persistent breaking of rules, physical fights, and bullying of other children.

In *adolescence*, from 12 to 17 years, more antisocial behaviours are often added: cruelty and hurting of other people, assault, robbery using force, vandalism, breaking and entering houses, stealing from cars, driving and taking away cars without permission, running away from home, truanting from school, and misuse of drugs.

### Girls

Severe antisocial behaviour is less common in girls who are less likely to be physically aggressive and engage in criminal behaviour, but more likely to show spitefulness, emotional bullying (such as excluding children from groups, spreading rumours so others are rejected by their peers), frequent unprotected sex leading to sexually transmitted diseases and pregnancy, drug abuse, and running away from home.

## Classification

The ICD-10 classification has a category for CDs—F91. The *ICD-10 Classification of Mental and Behavioural Disorders: Clinical Descriptions and Diagnostic Guidelines* [1] states that any one of the behaviours on which a diagnosis is based (for example, excessive levels of fighting or bullying, cruelty to animals), if marked, is sufficient for diagnosis, but isolated acts are not. An enduring pattern of behaviour should be present, but no time frame is given and there is no impairment or impact criterion stated.

ICD-10 has conduct disorder as an overarching term, which can be divided into two subtypes—ODD and CD, thus making it closely compatible with DSM-5 [2] which treats ODD and CD as completely separate conditions. There is considerable debate about the validity of this division, with many authorities considering it to be a unitary disorder, with different phenomena chiefly due to different ages of presentation. In contrast to the clinical guidelines, the *ICD-10 Classification of Mental and Behavioural Disorders: Diagnostic Criteria for Research* [3] takes a menu-driven approach that is virtually identical to DSM-5. In line with the underlying philosophy of DSM-5, ODD and CD could theoretically be used at any age, but in practice, ODD is usually used for younger children and CD for adolescents up to the age of 18. Neither term tends to be used in adults.

To diagnose *ODD* (313.81/F91.3), there should be four of the following eight symptoms over at least 6 months:

*Angry/irritable mood*

1. Has unusually frequent or severe temper tantrums for his or her developmental level.
2. Is often touchy or easily annoyed by others.
3. Is often angry or resentful.

*Argumentative/defiant behaviour*

4. Often argues with adults.
5. Often actively refuses adults' requests or defies rules.
6. Often deliberately does things that annoy other people.
7. Often blames others for their own mistakes or misbehaviour.

*Vindictiveness*

8. Has been spiteful or vindictive at least twice in the last 6 months.

The behavioural problems should be associated with distress in the individual or others around them, or affect social, educational, or other areas of function.

For the diagnosis of *CD*, three of the following 15 behaviours should have occurred in the last 6 months:
*Aggression to people and animals*

1. Often bullies, threatens, or intimidate others.
2. Frequently initiates physical fights.
3. Has used a weapon that can cause serious physical harm to others (for example, knife, gun).

4. Exhibits physical cruelty to people.
5. Exhibits physical cruelty to animals.
6. Has stolen with confrontation of victim (including purse-snatching, extortion, mugging).
7. Has forced someone into sexual activity.

*Destruction of property*

8. Deliberately sets fires with a risk or intention of causing serious damage.
9. Deliberately destroys the property of others.

*Deceitfulness or theft*

10. Has broken into someone else's house, building, or car.
11. Often lies to obtain goods or favours to avoid obligations (that is, 'cons' others).
12. Has stolen objects of significant value without confronting the victim (for example, shoplifting, burglary).

*Serious violations of rules*

13. Often stays out after dark despite parenting prohibition, beginning before age 13 years.
14. Has run away from home at least twice overnight.
15. Is frequently truant from school, beginning before age 13 years.

In DSM-5, there should be significant impairment in social, academic, or occupational functioning, whereas in ICD-10, there is no impairment criterion. Age of onset should be specified, with *childhood-onset type* (312.81) manifesting before age 10 and *adolescent-onset type* (312.89) after. Severity should be categorized as *mild, moderate,* or *severe,* according to the number of symptoms or impact on others.

New in DSM-5 is recognition of the subtype characterized by callous-unemotional traits (discussed further under 'Aetiology' p. 1268) called *with limited prosocial emotions,* which is effectively a personality trait. Two of the following four features should be persistently and pervasively present:

• *Lack of remorse or guilt*: does not feel bad or guilty when they do something wrong; unconcerned about the negative consequences of their actions, for example no remorse after hurting someone or harmful effect of breaking rules.
• *Callous—lack of empathy*: disregards, and is unconcerned about, the feelings of others; cold and uncaring. The person appears more concerned about themselves, even when their actions result in substantial harm to others.
• *Unconcerned about performance*: does not show concern about poor/problematic performance at school, work, or other important activities. Puts in insufficient effort needed to perform well, typically blames others for poor performance.
• *Shallow or deficient affect*: does not express feelings or show emotions to others, except in ways that seem shallow, insincere, or superficial or are used for gain (for example, emotions displayed to manipulate or intimidate others).

Where there are sufficient symptoms of a comorbid disorder to meet diagnostic criteria, the ICD-10 system discourages the application of a second diagnosis and instead offers two combined categories: mixed disorders of conduct and emotions where

*Depressive Conduct Disorder* (F92.0) is the best researched; and *Hyperkinetic Conduct Disorder* (F90.1). There is good evidence to suggest these combined conditions differ in the longitudinal course from the pure form, in a manner that would be expected. Comorbidity in DSM-5 is handled by giving as many separate diagnoses as necessary.

## Differential diagnosis

Making a diagnosis of CD is usually straightforward, but comorbid conditions are often missed. The differential diagnosis may include:

1. *Hyperkinetic syndrome/attention-deficit/hyperactivity disorder (ADHD).* These are the names given by ICD-10 and DSM-5, respectively, for similar conditions, except that the former is more severe. For convenience, the term *ADHD* will be used here. It is characterized by impulsivity, inattention, and motor overactivity. Any of these three sets of symptoms can be misconstrued as antisocial, particularly impulsivity which is also present in ODD/CD. However, none of the antisocial symptoms of ODD/CD are a part of ADHD, so excluding CD should not be difficult. A frequently made error, however, is to miss comorbid ADHD. Standardized questionnaires are very helpful here, such as the Conners or the Strengths and Difficulties Questionnaire, which is brief and just as effective at detecting hyperactivity as much longer alternatives [4].

2. *Adjustment reaction to an external stressor.* This can be diagnosed when onset occurs soon after exposure to an identifiable psychosocial stressor such as parental divorce or bereavement, trauma, abuse, or adoption. The onset should be within 1 month for ICD-10, and 3 months for DSM-5, and symptoms should not persist for >6 months.

3. *Mood disorders.* Depression can present with irritability and oppositional symptoms, but unlike typical ODD/CD, mood is usually clearly low and there are vegetative features; more severe conduct problems are absent. It is common—around a third of adolescents with ODD/CD have depressive or other emotional symptoms, severe enough to warrant a diagnosis. Low self-esteem is the norm in ODD/CD, as is a lack of friends or constructive pastimes, so it is easy to overlook more pronounced depressive symptoms. Early manic/bipolar depressive disorder can be harder to distinguish, as there is often considerable defiance and irritability, combined with disregard for rules and behaviour that violates the rights of others, but there should be clear evidence of elevated mood, racing thoughts, etc. [5].

A new disorder appeared in DSM-5, called *Disruptive Mood Dysregulation Disorder* (296.99). This condition does not have a solid research underpinning and has a comorbidity rate approaching 90% with ODD, so its validity as a separate entity is questionable. The motivation for introducing the new condition was to stop some psychiatrists misdiagnosing ODD with prominent temper tantrums in young children as juvenile bipolar disorder and using potentially harmful medications.

4. *Autistic spectrum disorders.* These are often accompanied by marked tantrums or destructiveness, which may be the reason for seeking a referral. Enquiring about other symptoms of autistic spectrum disorders should reveal their presence.

5. *Subcultural deviance.* Some youths are antisocial and commit crimes but are not particularly aggressive or defiant. They are well adjusted within a deviant peer culture that approves of recreational drug use, shoplifting, etc. In some localities, a quarter or more of teenage males fit this description and would meet ICD-10 diagnostic guidelines for socialized CD. Some clinicians are unhappy to label such a large proportion of the population with a psychiatric disorder. Using DSM-5 criteria would preclude the diagnosis for most youths like this, due to the requirement for significant impairment.

## Multi-axial assessment

ICD-10 recommends that multi-axial assessment be carried out for children and adolescents. A benefit of having a multi-axial system is that at least it forces the clinician to consider aspects beyond the presenting symptoms. In ICD-10, Axis I is used for psychiatric disorders; Axis II and Axis III cover specific and general intellectual disabilities, respectively; and Axis IV, Axis V, and Axis VI cover general medical conditions, psychosocial problems, and the level of social functioning, respectively. DSM-5 has abolished the first three axes as separate entities but keeps psychosocial problems and level of social functioning.

Both specific and general learning disabilities need to be assessed in individuals with conduct problems. Over a quarter of children with ODD/CD also have specific reading impairment/dyslexia [6], defined as a reading level two standard deviations below that predicted by the person's intelligence quotient (IQ). This is not just due to a lack of adequate schooling; there is good evidence that the cognitive deficits often precede the behavioural problems. The rate of ODD/CD rises several-fold as the IQ gets below 70, and general intellectual disability is often missed in children, so if school performance is markedly behind, IQ and attainment testing should be carried out.

## Epidemiology

Most surveys find ODD + CD to have a prevalence of around 5–7% when an impairment criterion is applied [7, 8]; a meta-analysis of epidemiological studies estimated that the worldwide prevalence of CD alone among children and adolescents aged 6–18 years is 3.2%, with little variation across countries or continents [9]. A modest rise in diagnosable ODD/CD over the second half of the twentieth century has also been observed, comparing assessments of three successive birth cohorts in Britain [10]. There is a very marked social class gradient, greater than for almost any other disorder, with five times the prevalence in the lowest, compared to the highest, socioeconomic group [8]. With respect to ethnicity, youth self-reports of symptoms of CD and crime victim survey reports of perpetrators' ethnicity (both of which are less likely to be influenced by racial prejudice than parent or teacher reports of CD symptoms or police arrests) show an excess of offenders of black African ancestry, whereas Hispanic Americans in the United States and British Asians in the UK do not show an excess of offending, compared to their white counterparts. The sex ratio is approximately equal with respect to ODD in younger children but then rises to 2- to 3-fold more in males than females after around 7 years. The causes of conduct problems appear to be the same, but males have more ODD/CD because they experience a greater number and intensity of individual-level risk factors (for example, hyperactivity, neurodevelopmental delays).

## Developmental subtypes

### Life course persistent versus adolescence onset

DSM-5 distinguishes between conduct problems that are first seen in early childhood versus those that start in adolescence. Early onset is a strong predictor of persistence through childhood and into adult life (Fig. 124.1) [11]. Those with early onset differ from those with later onset in that they have lower IQ, more attention and impulsivity problems, poorer scores on neuropsychological tests, greater peer difficulties, and they are more likely to come from adverse family circumstances [12]. Those with later onset become delinquent predominantly as a result of social influences such as association with other delinquent youths; they have fewer neurodevelopmental risk factors, but they are not absent [12]. Longitudinal studies support poorer adult outcomes for the early-onset group, but the doom-laden prognosis of 20 years ago has been moderated by the discovery of an early-onset group that subsequently desist, called childhood limited. Distinguishing between this group and the life course-persistent group has proved difficult, although a family history of criminal behaviour predicts persistence [13]. While many of the adolescence-onset group still engage in offending as adults and often have problems with alcohol and drugs, the level is lower than in the early-onset group.

### Progression to antisocial/dissocial personality disorder

In both ICD-10 and DSM-5, a person should be aged 18 or older before a personality disorder can be diagnosed, but it is a requirement that they should have a history of CD from before age 15. The diagnostic criterion is generous, since only one of the following seven symptoms is needed:

1. Failure to obey laws and norms by engaging in behaviour warranting criminal arrest.
2. Lying, deception, and manipulation for profit or self-amusement.
3. Impulsive behaviour.
4. Irritability and aggression, manifested as frequent assaults or fighting.
5. Blatantly disregards safety of self and others.
6. A pattern of irresponsibility.
7. Lack of remorse for actions.

Perhaps not surprisingly, given these wide criteria, prevalence rates vary from 0.2% to 3.3%; using clinical impairment criteria, the prevalence is around 1% [2]. Antisocial personality disorder is a natural progression over time in children with CD who display the subtype with limited prosocial emotions. They have difficulty learning from mistakes, are rigid in decision-making, and are typically unresponsive to punishment [14].

## Aetiology

The causes of ODD/CD vary considerably according to subtype and are multifactorial. After consideration of implicated factors, a synthesis model will be offered.

### Individual-level characteristics

#### Genetic contribution

While in former times, ODD/CD was reckoned to arise from bad socialization and a lack of self-control, it is now evident that overall, genetic factors account for around 60% of the variance [15]. Within this overall figure, for some subtypes, the genetic contribution is even stronger. Twin studies showed both substantial genetic influences and also a substantial shared environmental component [16]. The genetic contribution is higher when inattention and hyperactivity are present [17], and extremely high when there are callous-unemotional traits, when the heritability typically reaches 80% [18]. Conversely, where these factors are absent, the genetic contribution can be as low as 30% [18].

#### Identified genotypes

Genome-wide approaches looking for main effects have been disappointing so far for ODD/CD, typically accounting for at most 2% of the variance; no consistent linkage regions have been identified [19, 20]. The most studied candidate gene in relation to conduct problems is the *MAOA* promoter polymorphism. The gene encodes the MAOA enzyme, which metabolizes neurotransmitters linked to aggressive behaviour. Replicated studies showed that maltreatment history and genotype interact to predict antisocial outcome [21]. Recently, the impact of environmental influences on epigenetic processes has become prominent whereby identifiable chemical changes, such as acetylation and methylation of genes, are affected. For example, a study has shown differentially increased methylation in adolescents whose parents reported they were exposed to stress as infants [22].

#### Perinatal complications and temperament

Recent large-scale general population studies have found associations between life course-persistent type conduct problems and perinatal complications, minor physical anomalies, and

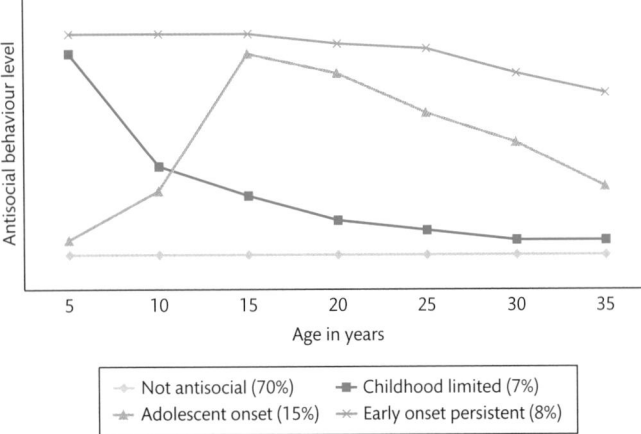

**Fig. 124.1** Subtypes of antisocial behaviour by longitudinal course (data synthesis from several longitudinal studies).

Reproduced from Scott S, Gardner F, Parenting programs. In: Thapar A, Pine D, Leckman J, *et al.* [Eds.], *Rutter's Child and Adolescent Psychiatry*, 6th ed., pp. 483–495, Copyright (2015), with permission from John Wiley and Sons.

low birthweight. Most studies support a biopsychosocial model in which obstetric complications might confer vulnerability to other co-occurring risks such as hostile or inconsistent parenting. Smoking in pregnancy is a statistical risk predictor of offspring conduct problems. Several prospective studies have shown associations between irritable temperament and conduct problems.

### Brain structure and function

Whereas ADHD has been recognized as having specific brain differences for over 20 years, it is only in the last decade that it has become clear that ODD/CD has its own and different set of brain anomalies. These are in terms of both structure, with reduced white matter connectivity with default mode regions that subsume cognitive functions about understanding self [23], and function where a recent meta-analysis of 24 studies found consistent differences in the rostro-dorsomedial, fronto-cingulate, and ventral–striatal regions that mediate reward-based decision-making, which is typically compromised in ODD/CD. Youths with callous-unemotional traits, on the other hand, had dysfunctions associated with the ventromedial prefrontal cortex and limbic system, together with dorsal and fronto-striatal hyperfunctioning, which may reflect poor affect reactivity and empathy in the presence of hyperactive executive control. In particular, these youths have a hypofunctioning amygdala, which is consistent with their fearlessness [24].

### Autonomic reactivity and intellectual and information processing deficits

A slow heart rate has been consistently associated with ODD/CD [25]. Indicators of heart rate variability and skin conductance confirm that the callous-unemotional subtype tend to be hypo-aroused, whereas the subtype with mood/internalizing problems is hyperaroused [25].

Children with ODD/CD have increased rates of deficits in language-based verbal skills. The association holds after controlling for potential confounders such as race, socio-economic status, academic attainment, and test motivation. Children who cannot reason or assert themselves verbally may attempt to gain control of social exchanges using aggression; there are likely also to be indirect effects in which low verbal IQ contributes to academic difficulties, which, in turn, mean that the child's experience of school becomes unrewarding. Children with ODD/CD also have poor executive functions such as skills in learning and applying contingency rules, abstract reasoning, problem-solving, self-monitoring, sustained attention and concentration, relating previous actions to future goals, and inhibiting inappropriate responses. These functions are largely, although not exclusively, associated with frontal lobe function. A meta-analysis with nearly 15,000 participants found that individuals with conduct problems had poorer executive functioning by an effect size of 0.54 standard deviations [26].

Dodge [27] proposed the leading information-processing model for the genesis of aggressive behaviours within social interactions. The model has good evidence that children prone to aggression focus on threatening aspects of others' actions, interpret neutral actions as hostile, and are more likely to favour aggressive solutions.

## Risks outside the family

### Risks in the neighbourhood

It has long been assumed that bad neighbourhoods promote youth antisocial behaviour. It is difficult to make direct links between neighbourhood characteristics and child behaviour, since several risk factors often coexist such as demographic factors like percentage of ethnic minority residents or single-parent households, unemployment levels, and parental mental illness. Many neighbourhood influences are mediated by supportive parenting, notably high warmth and close monitoring [28].

### Peer influences

Children with conduct problems have poorer peer relationships than non-disordered children. It often starts off with failure to have the social skills to befriend more socially successful children, so that they then tend to associate with other antisocial children and, in turn, take pleasure in being defiant and breaking rules. In adolescence, a high proportion of delinquent acts are committed in the company of other antisocial youths [29].

## Risks within the family

### Concentration of crime in families

Fewer than 10% of families in any community account for >50% of its criminal offences, reflecting the co-occurrence of genetic and environmental risks. However, knowing that conduct problems are under some genetic influence is less useful clinically than knowing that this genetic influence appears to be reduced or enhanced, depending on the quality of the child's environment. Several genetically sensitive studies have allowed interactions between family genetic liability and rearing environment to be examined. Thus, for example, genetic risk, indexed by having a criminal or an alcoholic parent, leads to tripling or so of ODD/CD in their children, compared to controls. However, if the upbringing is benign, this is reduced, whereas if it is harsh, the rate can be 8- or 10-fold greater. In short, genetic vulnerability provides a form of susceptibility to adverse child-rearing conditions [30].

### Family poverty

There is an association between severe poverty and early childhood conduct problems. Early theories proposed direct effects of poverty. Subsequent research has indicated that the association between low income and childhood conduct problems is indirect, mediated via family processes such as marital discord and parenting deficits.

### Parent–child attachment

Parent–child relationships provide the setting for the development of later social functioning, and disruption of these attachment relationships, for example through institutional care, is associated with subsequent difficulties in relating. One study found that ambivalent and controlling attachment predicted externalizing behaviours after controlling for baseline externalizing problems [31]; disorganized child attachment patterns seem to be especially associated with conduct problems. Although it seems obvious that poor parent–child relationships in general predict conduct problems, it has yet to be established whether attachment difficulties have an independent causal role in the development of behaviour problems or if classifications are markers for poor parenting.

### Discipline and parenting

Patterns of parenting associated with conduct problems were delineated by Patterson [32] in his seminal work *Coercive Family Process*. Parents of antisocial children were found to be more inconsistent in their use of rules, to issue less clear and more commands, to be more likely to respond to their children on the basis of their own mood, rather than the characteristics of the child's behaviour, to be less likely to monitor their children's whereabouts, and to fail to acknowledge or reward their children's prosocial behaviour. Patterson provided observational evidence for negative coercive cycles worsening antisocial behaviour as follows. A parent responds to mild child oppositional behaviour with a prohibition; the child responds by escalating his or her behaviour; the parent, in turn, gets angry and mutual escalation continues until exasperated and tired, the parent backs off. This has the inadvertent effect of teaching the child that if they argue and swear and are defiant, they get their way, thus reinforcing the child's behaviour and making it more likely that the child will be antisocial next time. There is ample evidence that conduct problems are associated with hostile, critical, punitive, and coercive parenting [33].

In considering the role of coercive processes in the origins or maintenance of conduct problems, we need to consider possible alternative explanations: (1) that the associations reflect familial genetic liability towards children's psychopathology and parents' coercive discipline, so they would happen whether or not they lived together; (2) that they represent evocative effects of children's behaviours on parents; and (3) that coercive parenting may be a correlate of other features of the relationship that influence children's behaviours, for example noisy living conditions that make them both more irritable. There is considerable evidence that children's difficult behaviours do indeed evoke parental negativity. The fact that children's behaviours can evoke negative parenting does not, however, mean that negative parenting has no impact on children's behaviour. The E-Risk longitudinal twin study of British families examined the effects of fathers' parenting on young children's aggression [34]. As expected, a prosocial father's *absence* predicted more aggression by his children, but the presence of an antisocial father predicted even greater aggression and his harmful effect was exacerbated the more times each week he spent taking care of the children.

### Exposure to adult marital conflict and domestic violence

Family processes other than parenting skills and the quality of parent–child attachment relationships have a role. Many studies have shown that children exposed to domestic violence between adults are subsequently more likely to themselves become aggressive. Marital conflict influences children's behaviour because of its effect on their regulation of emotion. For example, a child may respond to frightening emotion arising from marital conflict by downregulating his or her own emotion through denial of the situation. This, in turn, may lead to inaccurate appraisal of other social situations and ineffective problem-solving. Repeated exposure to family conflict is thought to lower childrens' thresholds for psychological dysregulation, resulting in greater behavioural reactivity to

stress. Children's aggression may also be increased by marital discord because children are likely to imitate aggressive behaviour modelled by their parents [35].

### Maltreatment

In the Christchurch longitudinal study, child sexual abuse predicted conduct problems, after controlling for other childhood adversities [36]. Overall, associations between physical punishment and conduct problems are well established; however, links are not straightforward. The risk for conduct problems does not apply equally to all forms of physical punishment. The E-Risk longitudinal twin study was able to compare the effects of corporal punishment (smacking, spanking) versus injurious physical maltreatment, using twin-specific reports of both experiences [37]. Results showed that children's genetic endowment accounted for virtually all of the association between their corporal punishment and their conduct problems. This indicated a 'child effect', in which children's bad conduct provokes their parents to use more corporal punishment, rather than the reverse. Findings for injurious physical maltreatment were the opposite; significant effects of maltreatment on child aggression remained after controlling for any genetic transmission of liability to aggression from antisocial parents.

## From risk predictor to causation

Associations have been documented between conduct problems and a wide range of risk factors. A variable is called a 'risk factor' if it has a documented predictive relation with antisocial outcomes, whether or not the association is causal. The causal status of most of these risk factors is unknown; we know what statistically predicts conduct problem outcomes, but not how or why. Establishing a causal role for a risk factor is by no means straightforward, particularly as it is unethical to experimentally expose healthy children to risk factors. The use of genetically sensitive designs and the study of within-individual change in natural experiments and treatment studies have considerable methodological advantages for suggesting causal influences.

## Prognosis

Many of the risk factors which predict poor outcome are associated with early onset (Table 124.1).

**Table 124.1** Factors predicting poor outcome

| | |
|---|---|
| Onset | Early onset of severe problems, before age 8 |
| Phenomenology | Antisocial acts which are severe, frequent, and varied |
| Comorbidity | Hyperactivity and attention problems |
| Intelligence | Lower IQ |
| Family history | Parental criminality, parental alcoholism |
| Parenting | Harsh and inconsistent parenting, with high criticism, low warmth, low involvement, and low supervision |
| Wider environment | Low-income family in poor neighbourhood with ineffective schools |

## Protective factors

To detect protective factors, children who do well, despite adverse risk factors, have been studied.

These so-called 'resilient' children, however, have been shown to have lower levels of risk factors, for example a boy with antisocial behaviour and low IQ living in a rough neighbourhood, but living with supportive, concerned parents. Protective factors are mostly the opposite end of the spectrum of the same risk factor. Nonetheless, there are factors which are associated with resilience, independent of known adverse influences. These include a good relationship with at least one adult who does not necessarily have to be the parent, a sense of pride and self-esteem, and skills or competencies.

## Adult outcome

Studies of groups of children with early-onset CD indicated a wide range of problems not only confined to antisocial acts, as shown in Table 124.2.

What is clear is that not only are there substantially increased rates of antisocial acts, but also the general psychosocial functioning of children with CD when they have grown up is strikingly poor. For most of the characteristics shown in Table 124.2, the increase, compared to controls, is at least double for community cases who were never referred, and 3–4 times for referred children [27].

## Pathways

The path from childhood CD to poor adult outcome is neither inevitable nor linear.

Different sets of influences impinge and shape the life course as the individual grows up. Many of these can accentuate problems. Thus, a toddler with an irritable temperament and short attention span may not learn good social skills if he or she is raised in a family lacking them and where he or she can only get his or her way by behaving antisocially and grasping for what he or she needs. At school, he or she may fall in with a deviant crowd of peers where violence and other antisocial acts are talked up and give him a sense of esteem. His or her generally poor academic ability and difficult behaviour in class may lead him to truancy increasingly, which, in turn, makes him fall further behind. He or she may then leave school with no qualifications and fail to find a job, and resort to drugs. To fund his or her drug habit, he or she may resort to crime and, once convicted, find it even harder to get a job. From this example, it can be seen that adverse experiences do not only arise passively and independently of the young person's behaviour; rather, the behaviour predisposes them to end up in risky and damaging environments. Consequently, the number of adverse life events experienced is greatly increased [38]. The path from early hyperactivity into later CD is also not inevitable. In the presence of a warm, supportive family atmosphere, it is far less likely than if the parents are highly critical and hostile.

Other influences can, however, steer the individual away from an antisocial path. For example, the fascinating follow-up of delinquent boys to age 70 by Laub and Sampson [39] showed that the following led to desistence: being separated from a deviant peer group; marrying to a non-deviant partner; moving away from a poor neighbourhood; and military service which imparted skills.

## Treatment

### Evidence-based treatments

Proven treatments include those which singly or in combination address: (1) parenting skills; (2) family functioning; (3) child interpersonal skills; (4) difficulties at school; (5) peer group influences; and (6) medication for coexisting hyperactivity.

1. Parenting skills.

*Parent management training* aims to improve parenting skills. There are scores of randomized controlled trials showing that it is effective for children aged up to about 10 years. They address the parenting practices identified in research as contributing to conduct problems. A more detailed account is given by Scott and Gardner [11]. Typically, they include five elements:

i. *Promoting play and a positive relationship.* In order to cut into the cycle of defiant behaviour and recriminations, it is important to instil some positive experiences for both sides and begin to mend the relationship. Teaching parents the techniques of how to play helps them recognize their child's needs and respond sensitively. The child, in turn, begins to like and respect their parents more and becomes more secure in the relationship.

ii. *Praise and rewards for prosocial behaviour.* Parents are helped to reformulate difficult behaviour in terms of the positive behaviour they wish to see, so that they encourage wanted behaviour, rather than criticize unwanted behaviour. For example, instead of shouting at the child not to run, they would praise him whenever he or she walks quietly; then he or she will do it more often. Through hundreds of such prosaic daily interactions, child behaviour can be substantially modified. Yet some parents find it hard to praise and fail to recognize positive behaviour when it happens, with the result that it become less frequent.

**Table 124.2** Adult outcome

| | |
|---|---|
| Antisocial behaviour | More violent and non-violent crimes, for example mugging, grievous bodily harm, theft, car crimes, fraud |
| Psychiatric problems | Increased rates of antisocial personality, alcohol and drug abuse, anxiety, depression and somatic complaints, episodes of deliberate self-harm and completed suicide, time in psychiatric hospitals |
| Education and training | Poorer examination results, more truancy and early school leaving, fewer vocational qualifications |
| Work | More unemployment, jobs held for shorter time, jobs lower in status and income, increased claiming of benefits and welfare |
| Social network | Few, if any, significant friends, low involvement with relatives, neighbours, clubs, and organizations |
| Intimate relationships | Increased rate of short-lived, violent cohabiting relationships, partners often also antisocial |
| Children | Increased rates of child abuse, conduct problems in offspring, children taken into care |
| Health | More medical problems, earlier death |

iii. *Clear rules and clear commands.* Rules need to be explicit and constant; commands need to be firm and brief. Thus, shouting at a child to stop being naughty does not tell him what he or she *should* do, whereas, for example, telling him to play quietly gives a clear instruction, which makes compliance easier.

iv. *Consistent and calm consequences for unwanted behaviour.* Disobedience and aggression need to be responded to firmly and calmly by, for example, putting the child in a room for a few minutes. This method of 'time-out from positive reinforcement' sounds simple but requires considerable skill to administer effectively. More minor annoying behaviours, such as whining and shouting, often respond to being ignored, but again parents often find this hard to achieve in practice.

v. *Reorganizing the child's day to prevent trouble.* There are often trouble spots in the day which will respond to fairly simple measures. For example, putting siblings in different rooms to prevent fights on getting home from school and banning electronic devices in the morning until the child is dressed.

Treatment can be given individually to the parent and child, which enables live feedback in light of the parent's progress and the child's response. Alternatively, group treatments with parents alone have been shown to be equally effective [40]. Trials showed that parent management training is effective in reducing child antisocial behaviour in the short term, with moderate to large effect sizes of 0.5–0.8 standard deviations, and there is little loss of effect at 1- or 3-year follow-up [41].

2. Family functioning.

*Functional family therapy, multi-systemic therapy, and treatment foster care* aim to change a range of difficulties which impede effective functioning of teenagers with CD. Functional family therapy addresses family processes which need to be present such as improved communication between parent and young person, reducing interparental inconsistency, tightening up on supervision and monitoring, and negotiating rules and sanctions to be applied for breaking them. Functional family therapy has been shown to reduce reoffending rates by around 50% [42]. Other varieties of family therapy have not been subjected to controlled trials for young people with CD or delinquency, so they cannot be evaluated for their efficacy.

In multi-systemic therapy [43], the young person's and family's needs are assessed in their own context at home and in their relations with other systems such as school and peers. Following the assessment, proven methods of intervention are used to address difficulties and promote strengths. Multi-systemic therapy differs from most types of family therapy such as the Milan or systemic approach as usually practised in a number of regards. Firstly, treatment is delivered in the situation where the young person lives, for example at home. Secondly, the therapist has a low caseload (4–6 families) and the team is available 24 hours a day. Thirdly, the therapist is responsible for ensuring appointments are kept and for making change happen—families cannot be blamed for failing to attend or 'not being ready' to change. Fourthly, regular written feedback on progress towards goals from multiple sources is gathered by the therapist and acted upon. Fifthly, there is a manual for the therapeutic approach and adherence is checked weekly by the supervisor.

Several randomized controlled trials have attested to the effectiveness, with reoffending rates typically cut by half and time spent in psychiatric hospitalization reduced further [43].

Treatment Foster Care is an approach developed in Oregon in the United States as a way to improve the quality of encouragement and supervision that teenagers with CD receive. The young person lives with a foster family specially trained in effective techniques; sometimes it is ordered as an alternative to jail. Outcome studies have shown useful reductions in reoffending [44].

3. Anger management and child interpersonal skills.

Most of the programmes to improve child interpersonal skills derive from cognitive behavioural therapy. A typical example is the *Coping Power Programme* [45]. This, and other programmes have in common, involves training the young person to:

i. Slow down impulsive responses to challenging situations by stopping and thinking.

ii. Recognize their own level of physiological arousal and their own emotional state.

iii. Recognize and define problems.

iv. Develop several alternative responses.

v. Choose the best alternative, based on anticipation of consequences.

vi. Reinforce himself or herself for use of this approach.

Over the longer term, they aim to increase positive social behaviour by teaching the young person skills to make and sustain friendships, turn taking and sharing, and express viewpoints in appropriate ways and listen to others.

Typically, given alone, treatment gains with interpersonal skills training are good within the treatment setting but only generalize slightly to 'real-life' situations such as the school playground. However, when they are part of a more comprehensive programme which has those outside the young person reinforcing the approach, they add to outcome gains [46].

4. Difficulties at school.

These can be divided into learning problems and disruptive behaviour. There are proven programmes to deal with specific learning problems such as Reading Recovery; however, few of the programmes have been specifically evaluated for their ability to improve outcomes in children with CD, although trials are in progress.

There are several schemes for improving classroom behaviour, which vary from those which stress on improved communication such as 'circle time' and those which work on behavioural principles or are part of a multimodal package. Many of these schemes have been shown to improve classroom behaviour, and some specifically target children with CD [47].

5. Peer group influences.

A few interventions have aimed to reduce the bad influence of deviant peers. However, a number attempted this through group work with other conduct-disordered youths, but outcome studies showed a *worsening* of antisocial behaviour due to forming more ties with antisocial peers. Current treatments therefore either see youths individually or work in small groups (say 3–5 youths) where the therapist can control the content of the sessions. Some interventions place youths with CD in groups with well-functioning youths, and this has led to favourable outcomes [48].

6. Medication for coexisting hyperactivity.

Where there is comorbid hyperactivity, in addition to CD, several studies attested to a large (effect size of 0.8 standard deviations or greater) reduction in both overt and covert antisocial behaviour, both at home and at school [49]. However, the impact on long-term outcome is unstudied.

## Management

Engagement of the family is particularly important for this group of children and families, as dropout from treatment is high at around 30–40%. Practical measures, such as assisting with transport, providing childcare, and holding sessions in the evening or at other times to suit the family, will all help. Many of the parents of children with CD may themselves have difficulty with authority and officialdom and be very sensitive to criticism. Therefore, the approach is more likely to succeed if it is respectful of their point of view, does not offer overly prescriptive solutions, and does not directly criticize parenting style. Practical homework tasks increase changes, as do problem-solving telephone calls from the therapist between sessions.

Parenting interventions may need to go beyond skills development to address more distal factors which prevent change. For example, drug or alcohol abuse in either parent, maternal depression, and a violent relationship with the partner are all common. Assistance in claiming welfare and benefits and help with financial planning may reduce stress from debts.

A multimodal approach is likely to get larger changes. Therefore, involving the school in treatment by visiting and offering strategies for managing the child in class is usually helpful, as is advocating for extra tuition where necessary. Avoiding antisocial peers and building self-esteem may be helped by getting the child to attend after-school clubs and holiday activities.

Where parents are not coping or an abusive relationship is detected, it may be necessary to liaise with social services to arrange respite for the parents or a spell of foster care. It is important during this time to work with the family to increase their skills, so the child can return to the family. Where there is permanent breakdown, long-term fostering or adoption may be recommended.

## Opportunities for prevention

CD should offer good opportunities for prevention since:

1. It can be detected early reasonably well.
2. Early intervention is more effective than later intervention.
3. There are a number of effective interventions.

In the United States, a number of comprehensive interventions based on up-to-date empirical findings are being carried out. Perhaps the best known is Families and Schools Together [50]. Here the most antisocial 10% of 5- to 6-year olds in schools in disadvantaged areas were selected, as judged by teacher and parent reports.

They were then offered intervention which was given for a whole year in the first instance and comprised:

1. Weekly parent training in groups with videotapes.
2. An interpersonal skills training programme for the whole class.
3. Academic tutoring twice a week.
4. Home visits from the parent trainer.
5. A pairing programme with sociable peers from the class.

Almost 1000 children were randomized to receive this condition or controls, and the project has cost over $100 million. By age 25, children in the treatment group had less antisocial behaviour and criminality and psychopathology, but only if they were in the more severe part of the sample to begin with.

In the United States, preschool education programmes for disadvantaged children have shown good outcomes in small demonstration projects, but replication on a larger scale has generally proved rather disappointing. In the UK, the government stressed the importance of helping parents of children in the first 3 years of life and put substantial resources (£540 million) into *SureStart* centres in specifically targeted high-risk neighbourhoods to support parenting. Early evaluation of outcome showed no change on 24 of 25 variables; maternal acceptance of the child was the only measured outcome to change, and child antisocial behaviour did not change [51]. However, more intensive high-quality parenting programmes started when children are young (aged 4–7 years) do have some evidence of longer-term effects, including prevention of antisocial personality traits in adolescence [52].

## Conclusions

Much is known about the risk factors leading to CD, and effective interventions exist. The challenge is to make these available on a wide scale and to develop approaches to prevention which are effective and can be put into practice at a community level.

### REFERENCES

1. World Health Organization. *The ICD-10 Classification of Mental and Behavioural Disorders: Clinical Descriptions and Diagnostic Guidelines.* Geneva: World Health Organization, 1992.
2. American Psychiatric Association. *Diagnostic and Statistical Manual of Mental Disorders*, fifth edition (DSM-5). Washington, DC: American Psychiatric Association; 2013.
3. World Health Organization. *The ICD-10 Classification of Mental and Behavioural Disorders: Diagnostic Criteria for Research.* Geneva: World Health Organisation; 1993.
4. Goodman R, Scott S. Comparing the Strengths and Difficulties Questionnaire and the Child Behaviour Checklist: is small beautiful? *Journal of Abnormal Child Psychology.* 1999;27:17–24.
5. Towbin K, Leibenluft E. Differential diagnosis of bipolar disorder in children and youth. In: Strakowski S, DelBello M, editors. *Bipolar Disorder in Youth: Presentation, Treatment and Neurobiology.* New York, NY: Oxford University Press; 2014. pp. 34–55.
6. Trzesniewski K, Moffitt T, Caspi A, Taylor A, Maughan B. Revisiting the association between reading achievement and antisocial behaviour: new evidence of an environmental explanation from a twin study. *Child Development.* 2006;77:72–88.

7. Angold A, Costello EJ. The epidemiology of disorders of conduct: nosological issues and comorbidity. In: Hill J, Maughan B, editors. *Conduct Disorders in Childhood and Adolescence.* Cambridge: Cambridge University Press; 2001. pp. 126–68.

8. Green H, McGinnity A, Meltzer H, Ford T, Goodman R. *Mental Health of Children and Young People in Great Britain.* London: The Stationery Office; 2005.

9. Canino G, Polanczyk G, Bauermeister JJ, Rohde LA, Frick PJ. Does the prevalence of CD and ODD vary across cultures? *Social Psychiatry and Psychiatric Epidemiology.* 2010;45:695–704.

10. Collishaw S, Maughan B, Goodman R, Pickles, A. Time trends in adolescent mental health. *Journal of Child Psychology and Psychiatry.* 2004;45:1350–62.

11. Scott S, Gardner F. Parenting programs. In: Thapar A, Pine D, Leckman J, Scott S, Snowling M, Taylor E, editors. *Rutter's Child and Adolescent Psychiatry*, third edition. Oxford: Wiley Blackwell; 2015. pp. 483–95.

12. Jolliffe D, Farrington DP, Piquero AR, Loeber R., Hill KG. Systematic review of early risk factors for life-course-persistent, adolescence-limited, and late-onset offenders in prospective longitudinal studies. *Aggression and Violent Behavior.* 2017;33:15–23.

13. Odgers CL, Milne BJ, Caspi A, Crump R, Poulton R, Moffitt TE. Predicting prognosis for the conduct-problem boy: can family history help? *Journal of the American Academy of Child and Adolescent Psychiatry.* 2007;46:1240–9.

14. De Brito S, Viding E, Kumari V, Blackwood N, Hodgins S. Cool and hot executive function impairments in violent offenders with antisocial personality disorder with and without psychopathy. *PLoS One.* 2013;8:e65566.

15. Porsch R, Middeldorp M, Cherny S, *et al.* (2016) Longitudinal heritability of childhood aggression. *American Journal of Medical Genetics Part B: Neuropsychiatric Genetics.* 2016;171;697–707.

16. Bornovalova MA, Hicks BM, Iacono WG, McGue M. Familial transmission and heritability of childhood disruptive disorders. *American Journal of Psychiatry.* 2010;167:1066–74.

17. Thapar A, Cooper M, Eyre O, Langley K. Practitioner review: what have we learnt about the causes of ADHD? *Journal of Child Psychology and Psychiatry.* 2013;54:3–16.

18. Viding E, Jones AP, Frick PJ, Moffitt TE, Plomin R. Heritability of antisocial behaviour at 9: do callous-unemotional traits matter? *Developmental Science.* 2008;11:17–22.

19. Plomin R, DeFries JC, Knopik VS, Neiderhiser JM. *Behavioral Genetics*, sixth edition. New York, NY: Worth; 2013.

20. Salvatore J, Dick D. Genetic influences on conduct disorder. *Neuroscience and Biobehavioral Reviews.* 2018;91:91–101.

21. Kim-Cohen J, Caspi A, Taylor A, Williams B, Newcombe R, Craig IW, Moffitt TE. MAOA, maltreatment, and gene-environment interaction predicting children's mental health: new evidence and a meta-analysis. *Molecular Psychiatry.* 2006;11: 903–13.

22. Essex MJ, Boyce WT, Hertzman C, *et al.* (2013). Epigenetic vestiges of early developmental adversity: childhood stress exposure and DNA methylation in adolescence. *Child Development.* 2013;84:58–75.

23. Broulidakis MJ, Fairchild G, Sully K, Blumensath T, Darekar A, Sonuga-Barke EJ. Reduced default mode connectivity in adolescents with conduct disorder. *Journal of American Academy of Child and Adolescent Psychiatry.* 2016;55:800–8.

24. Alegria AA, Radua J, Rubia K. Meta-analysis of fMRI studies of disruptive behavior disorders. *American Journal of Psychiatry.* 2016;173:1119–30.

25. Fanti K. Understanding heterogeneity in conduct disorder: a review of psychophysiological studies. *Neuroscience and Biobehavioural Review.* 2018;91:4–20.

26. Ogilvie JM, Stewart AL, Chan RCK, Shum DHK. Neuropsychological measures of executive function and antisocial behavior: a meta-analysis. *Criminology.* 2011;49:1063–107.

27. Dodge K. Translational science in action: hostile attributional style and the development of aggressive behaviour problems. *Development and Psychopathology.* 2006;18:791–814.

28. Odgers C, Caspi A, Russell MA, Moffitt TE. Supportive parenting mediates neighborhood socioeconomic disparities in children's antisocial behavior from ages 5–12. *Development and Psychopathology.* 2012;24:705–21.

29. Vitaro F, Brendgen M, Lacourse E. Peers and delinquency: a genetically informed, developmentally sensitive perspective. In: Morizot J, Kazemian L, editors. *The Development of Criminal and Antisocial Behaviour.* New York, NY: Springer; 2014. pp. 221–36.

30. Harold GT, Leve LD, Elam KK, *et al.* The nature of nurture: disentangling passive genotype–environment correlation from family relationship influences on children's externalizing problems. *Journal of Family Psychology.* 2013;27:12–21.

31. Moss E, Smolla N, Cyr C, Dubois-Comtois K, Mazzarello T, Berthiaume C. Attachment and behaviour problems in middle childhood as reported by adult and child informants. *Development and Psychopathology.* 2006;18:425–44.

32. Patterson GR. *Coercive Family Process.* Eugene, OR: Castalia Publishing Company; 1982.

33. Rutter M, Giller H, Hagell A. *Antisocial Behaviour by Young People.* Cambridge: Cambridge University Press; 1998.

34. Jaffee SR, Moffitt TE, Caspi A, Taylor A. Life with (or without) father: the benefits of living with two biological parents depend on the father's antisocial behavior. *Child Development.* 2003;74:109–26.

35. Harold G, Leve L, Sellers R. How can genetically informed research help inform the next generation of interparental and parenting interventions? *Child Development.* 2017;88:446–58.

36. Fergusson DM, Horwood LJ, Lynskey MT. Childhood sexual abuse and psychiatric disorder in young adulthood: II psychiatric outcomes of childhood sexual abuse. *Journal of the American Academy of Child and Adolescent Psychiatry.* 1996;35:1365–74.

37. Jaffee SR, Caspi A, Moffitt TE, Polo-Tomas M, Price TS, Taylor A. The limits of child effects: evidence for genetically mediated child effects on corporal punishment, but not on physical maltreatment. *Developmental Psychology.* 2004;40:1047–58.

38. Champion L, Goodall G, Rutter M. Behavioural problems in childhood and stressors in early adult life: a 20 year follow-up of London school children. *Psychological Medicine.* 1995;25:231–46.

39. Laub J, Sampson R. *Shared Beginnings, Divergent Lives: Delinquent Boys to Age 70.* Cambridge, MA: Harvard University Press; 2003.

40. Scott S, Spender Q, Doolan M, Jacobs B, Aspland H. Multicentre controlled trial of parenting groups for child antisocial behaviour in clinical practice. *BMJ.* 2001;323:194–7.

41. Scott S. Do parenting programmes for severe child antisocial behaviour work over the longer term, and for whom? 1 year follow up of a multi-centre controlled trial. *Behavioural and Cognitive Psychotherapy.* 2005;33:403–21.

42. Alexander JF, Holtzworth-Munroe A, Jameson PB. The process and outcome of marital and family therapy research: review

and evaluation. In: Bergin AE, Garfield S, editors. *Handbook of Psychotherapy and Behaviour Change*. New York, NY: Wiley;1994. pp. 595–630.

43. Curtis NM, Ronan KR, Borduin CM. Multisystemic therapy: a meta-analysis of outcome studies. *Journal of Family Psychology*. 2004;18:411–19.

44. Eddy JM, Whaley RB, Chamberlain P. The prevention of violent behavior by chronic and serious male juvenile offenders: a 2-year follow-up of a randomized clinical trial. *Journal of Emotional and Behavioral Disorders*. 2004;12:2–8.

45. Lochman JE, Wells KC. The coping power program for preadolescent aggressive boys and their parents: outcome effects at the 1-year follow-up. *Journal of Consulting and Clinical Psychology*. 2004;72:571–8.

46. Lochman JE, Wells KC, Qu L, Chen L. Three year follow-up of Coping Power intervention effects: evidence of neighborhood moderation? *Prevention Science*. 2013;14: 364–76.

47. Durlak J. *School-based Prevention Programs for Children and Adolescents*. Thousand Oaks, CA: Sage; 1995.

48. Feldman R. The St. Louis experiment: effective treatment of antisocial youths in prosocial peer groups. In: McCord J, Tremblay R, editors. *Preventing Antisocial Behaviour*. New York, NY: Guilford: 1992. pp. 233–52.

49. Connor DF, Glatt SJ, Lopez ID, Jackson D, Melloni RH. Psychopharmacology and aggression. I: a meta-analysis of stimulant effects on overt/covert aggression-related behaviors in ADHD. *Journal of American Academy of Child and Adolescent Psychiatry*. 2002;41:253–61.

50. Dodge KA, Bierman KL, Coie JD, *et al*. Impact of early intervention on psychopathology, crime, and well-being at age 25. *American Journal of Psychiatry*. 2015;172:59–70.

51. Belsky J, Melhuish E, Barnes J, Leyland A, Romaniuk H. Effects of Sure Start local programmes on children and families: early findings from a quasi-experimental, cross sectional study. *BMJ*. 2006;332:1476.

52. Scott S, Briskman J, O'Connor T. Early prevention of antisocial personality: long-term follow-up of two randomized controlled trials comparing indicated and selective approaches. *American Journal of Psychiatry*. 2014;171:649–57.

# SECTION 21
# Suicide

# 125

# Epidemiology and causes of suicide

*Merete Nordentoft, Trine Madsen, and Annette Erlangsen*

## Understanding suicide

Ever since the work of Charles Darwin established that the struggle for existence plays a major role as scientific explanation of diversification in nature [1], the striving to live has been considered fundamental for all living creatures, also among human beings. Therefore, suicidal impulses and suicidal behaviour must be understood as disturbances of this fundamental condition. But suicide statistics clearly demonstrate that the will to live can be broken. While the strength of the force threatening to break the will to live is crucial, individual resilience play an important role too. When suicidal behaviour occurs, it must be considered as an indication that the strain on the individual is exceeding his or her capability to cope with the situation. The diathesis–stress model can be used as a framework for understanding suicidal impulses and suicidal behaviour. In 2003, van Heeringen presented a slightly modified version of the diathesis–stress model related to suicidal behaviour [2]. The model suggests that suicidal behaviour might be explained through factors related to trait (determined by genetics, personality, intellect, and other factors) and factors related to state (which can be influenced by, for instance, depression or substance use disorder). Stressors and protective factors, as well as threshold factors (for instance, access to lethal means, alcohol intoxication, crisis, and access to help), might further act as facilitators or barriers for suicidal behaviour. Destructive forces, that is, stressors, can be manifold and diverse and modified by protective factors hosted by the individual. Humans react differently to the same condition; thus, a situation perceived stressful for one individual may not be distressing for another individual. Different individuals have different levels of resilience. This may depend upon individual trait factors, genetics, or being grounded during childhood, but it can also be influenced by more recent factors such as the support to which he or she has access. Similarly, the perception of options for help is likely to vary from one individual to another, as well as by cultural factors. Protective factors and stressors either from early life experiences or from the current context may impact traits or the state of the individual, while genetic factors are mainly thought to influence traits. Threshold factors, such as alcohol intoxication, crisis, or access to help, can act either as drivers or as barriers for suicidal behaviour.

## Prevention strategies

Suicide cannot be understood as a disease or an accident; suicidal acts should be considered as severe and preventable complications to a range of diseases and conditions in which social aspects play an important role. The understanding of suicidal acts as complications emphasizes that, like other complications, suicidal acts can be prevented.

The most frequently used model for suicide prevention is the Universal, Selected and Indicated preventive model (USI-model), which was suggested by Gordon [3] and later accepted by the Institute of Medicine [4]. This model provides a relevant and applicable framework for suicide prevention. Universal prevention strategies aim to address an entire population and is designed to influence everyone. *Universal* interventions include programmes such as: public education campaigns, restricting access to suicide means, and education programmes for the media on reporting practices related to suicide. There are several examples of universal interventions that could be considered suicide-preventive but were not launched as such, mainly because the primary focus of the intervention is not suicide—for instance, school-based programmes aiming at reducing bullying and campaigns to reduce mental health stigma. An example of successful universal suicide prevention is the restriction of pack sizes on paracetamol, which has been linked to less severe suicide poisoning [5]. *Selective* prevention strategies aim to prevent the onset of suicidal behaviours among specific subpopulations. Important high-risk groups are the mentally ill, alcohol and drug misusers, those with a newly diagnosed severe physical disorder, prisoners, and the homeless, as well as other socially marginalized groups. Crisis plans for patients with mental illness is an example of application of selective prevention strategies [6]. Another example is better education of general physicians for recognition and treatment of depression, which has been shown to reduce suicide rates [7]. *Indicated* prevention strategies are focused on high-risk groups, that is, persons who have attempted suicide or have presented themselves to health services because of suicidal ideation. An example of a promising indicated strategy is the psychosocial therapy provided to people after suicide attempt [8]. In addition, help lines, psychiatric emergency rooms, psychiatric emergency outreach, and other crisis interventions can play a role in preventing suicide attempts among persons in a suicidal crisis.

National action plans for suicide prevention generally include all three types of strategies.

## Definitions

The World Health Organization (WHO) defines *suicide* as the act of deliberately killing oneself [9]. This definition underlines that the death is caused by a deliberate act, thereby separating suicide from accidents. The definition does not mention suicidal intent, which, in some cases, can be difficult to determine after death. The number of suicides is recorded and suicidal rates are available for most high-income countries.

The WHO [9] defines *suicide attempt* as any non-fatal suicidal behaviour, such as intentional self-inflicted poisoning, injury, or self-harm, which may or may not have a fatal intent or outcome. This definition implies that non-fatal self-harm without suicidal intent is included under this term, which is problematic due to the possible variations in related interventions. However, the WHO chooses this definition because suicide intent can be difficult to determine as it may be surrounded by ambivalence or even concealment. Some countries record hospital-treated suicide attempts, but underreporting is common and suicide attempts outside hospital settings are not included in statistics. Other terms, such as deliberate self-harm, are also used for suicide attempt.

*Suicidal ideations* or thoughts may vary in terms of intensity, from being sporadic and transient to being frequent and persistent. Suicidal thoughts can be active, such as considering killing oneself, or passive such as wishing to catch an incurable disease or not waking up tomorrow. Some people might express their suicidal thoughts overtly without being prompted; others present them only after questioning or conceal them. Suicidal thoughts include suicidal plans where a distinction can be made between plans for not being alive anymore (writing a testimony, preparing economy, and writing suicidal notes) and plans for carrying out a suicidal act (selecting the method, time, and place).

## Epidemiological trends and registration of suicides

The WHO estimates that the number of suicides worldwide was 803,900 in 2012 [9].

The absolute number, that is, the actual number of people dying by suicide, in a country is dependent on the number of people living in the country. Thus, when comparing suicide figures across borders, a yearly suicide rate per 100,000 inhabitants is usually used. National suicide rates based on those countries that report data on causes of death are presented in Fig. 125.1. Specific regions are noted for high suicide rates: Eastern Europe (Russia, Ukraine, Lithuania, Latvia, Poland, Hungary, Belarus, and Kazakhstan) and Eastern sub-Saharan countries (Sudan, Uganda, Kenya, Tanzania, Zambia, Malawi, and Zimbabwe). In addition, particularly countries such as India and Japan, as well as Guyana and Suriname in South America, list high rates of suicide.

The quality of death and population statistics varies substantially across the world, and one has to bear this in mind when comparing rates. For instance, low- and middle-income countries with low infrastructure might have limited resources to dedicate to recording suicide statistics. The fact that more than 75% of all suicide takes place in low- and middle-income countries (Fig. 125.2) complicates the process of estimation. Suicide has, throughout the ages, been subjected to taboo and stigmatization. Religious and cultural norms

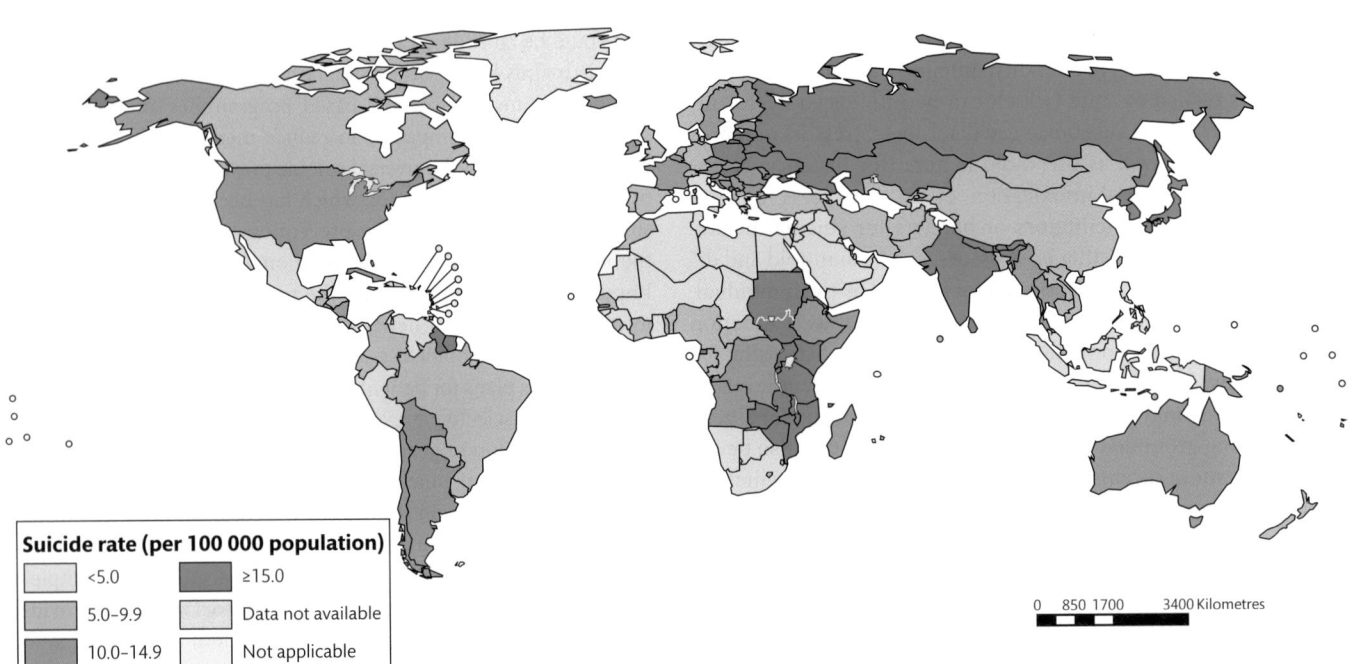

**Fig. 125.1** (see Colour Plate section)  Age-standardized suicide rates for both genders by country (2012).
Reproduced from World Health Organization, *Preventing suicide: A global imperative*, Copyright (2014), with permission from the World Health Organization.

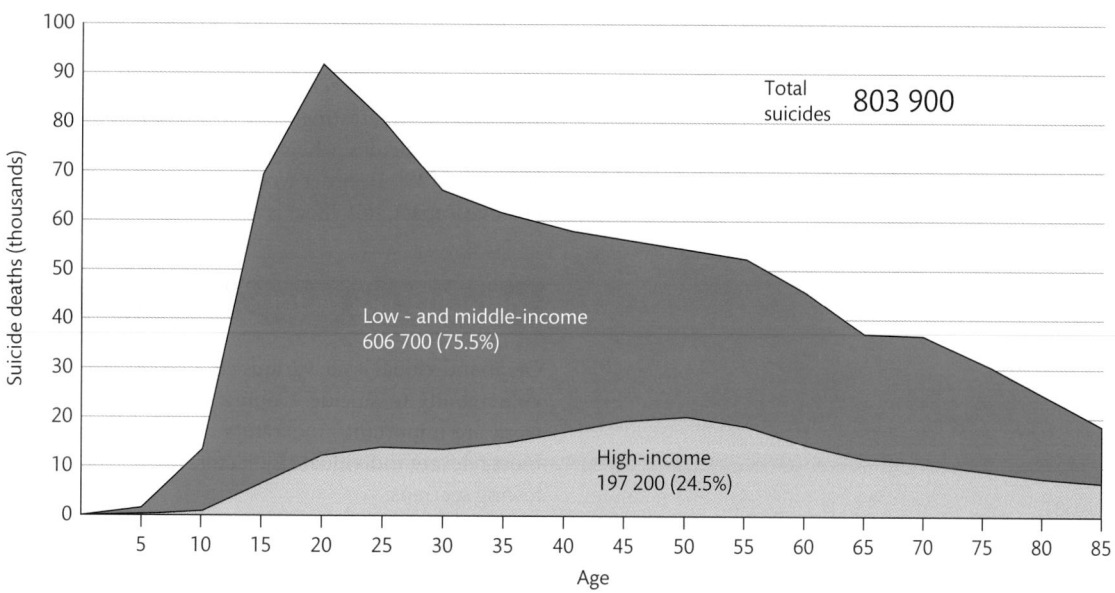

**Fig. 125.2** Absolute numbers of suicide in the world by age and income level (2012).
Reproduced from World Health Organization, *Preventing suicide: A global imperative*, Copyright (2014), with permission from the World Health Organization.

might imply that a suicide death is unacceptable or shameful, and social or legal sanctions are possible consequences. Several religions, such as Catholicism and Islam, consider suicide a sin and the burial of a deceased by suicide might not be granted the same rituals as other deceased, and relatives might experience sanctions [10]. For such reasons, it is plausible that suicide deaths in some countries might, to a larger extent, be recorded as accidents or other causes of death, partially out of concern for the relative.

The administrative procedure of recording causes of death varies substantially across the world. In the UK, for instance, a jurisdictional coroner system determines whether a death is a suicide, an accident, or undetermined, that is, an 'open verdict' [11]. In this setting, supportive evidence, such as a 'suicide note', documenting intent of suicide, might be required before a cause of death is determined to be a suicide. In other high-income countries, the presence of suicidal intent is generally determined by medical or forensic staff. For the reasons listed previously, caution has to be applied when comparing suicide rates of different countries.

## Risk factors

In the following sections, societal and individual risk factors for suicide are presented. There is no clear distinction between societal and individual risk factors; yet both groups of factors have an interdependent impact on the risk of suicide. For example, an economic crisis affects the entire society, while specific individuals will be distressed by unemployment or bankruptcy. Likewise, free-of-charge access to high-quality health care can be considered as a societal factor, while the influence by treated or untreated mental disorders on the risk of suicide is an individual factor. Still, there are clear links between the two dimensions. The relative risk associated with individual risk factors are listed in Table 125.1.

## Societal factors

On the societal level, there are factors which can be associated with high or low risk of suicide. Rather than focusing on individual risk factors, the French sociologist Durkheim attributed variations in suicidal behaviour between different countries to societal factors such as sense of connectedness and social cohesion. Durkheim used the term 'anomic' to describe suicides in societies with poor connectedness between people and where the individual behaviour was not regulated by a strong social cohesion [12]. He hypothesized that anomic suicides were likely to increase in periods when social norms and roles underwent rapid changes. As such, the steep increase in suicide rates seen in indigenous societies, for example among New Zealand's Maori population, Australia's aborigines, the United States' native Indians, and Canadian and Greenland's indigenous peoples, could be seen as examples of increasing numbers of anomic suicides [13, 14].

Societal factors influence the number of suicides occurring in a country. In the 1980s, the 'Perestroika' policy introduced by the Soviet leader Mikhail Gorbachev included restrictions on alcohol sales. Alcohol misuse is linked to suicide in some populations, and the implementation of the policy consequently resulted in a marked drop in the suicide rate [15]. After the dissolved Soviet Republic, structural changes and increasing unemployment, as well as rising alcohol sales, contributed to an increase in suicide rates in many post-Soviet countries. The global financial crisis of 2007–2008 was linked to an increase in the numbers of suicide, particularly in European countries and the United States [16]. While the financial crisis had an impact on a societal level, for instance, through cutbacks in state budgets, rising unemployment rates might act as an individual stressor, as suggested previously. Significant increases in suicide rates of age groups belonging to the working forces were noted in the years following. Interestingly, countries with social

Table 125.1 Relative risks denoting the risk of suicide with respect to select risk factors of suicide in relation to the general population

| Risk factor | Men | Women |
| --- | --- | --- |
| Schizophrenia [57] | 9 | 19 |
| Bipolar depression disorder [57] | 11 | 18 |
| Unipolar depression disorder [57] | 9 | 15 |
| Substance abuse[1] [57] | 7 | 13 |
| Any mental disorder [57] | 6 | 8 |
| Previous self-harm [73, 92–94][4] | >30 | >30 |
| Prisoner [95][3] | >3 | >6 |
| Divorced [96][2] | 3 | 3 |
| Widow/widower [97] | 2.3 | 1.7 |
| Homeless [34] | 7 | 15 |
| Same-sex married [37][6] | 4.1 | 6.4 |
| Somatic illness [98][5] | 1.8 | 2.4 |
| Transgender [99][7] | 5.7 | 2.2 |

[1] Based on a psychiatric substance abuse diagnosis.

[2] Higher in Asian countries.

[3] Inmate suicide rates in women varied widely in different countries and was based on small numbers of suicide.

[4] Based on a number of longitudinal follow-up studies of people presenting with self-harm.

[5] Based on somatic illness requiring inpatient hospitalization (adjusted analysis).

[6] Measured as persons living in a same-sex marriage, when compared to persons living in an opposite-sex marriage. Figures are adjusted for persons never married.

[7] Persons who have received hormone therapy or transgender surgery or diagnosed with transgender orientation.

welfare systems, such as Finland and Sweden, seemingly were less affected by the crisis [17].

Durkheim predicted that when a country is in war, this would increase the social cohesion and strengthen the societal influence of individual's behaviour. Some support for this hypothesis has been found, for instance among the countries participating in the First World War where a decline in suicide rate was noted over the same period [18]. Decreasing suicide rates were, among others, noted in Norway and Sweden during the Second World War [19]. Newer findings indicated that civil wars might not have this effect on suicide rate, potentially explained through the lack of social cohesion when national, oppositional groups are in conflict [20].

## Role models and media portrayal

Goethe's book *The Sorrows of Young Werther* depicts a tragic love story from the Romantic period where the main character ends up taking his own life. Legends from contemporary Germany report how young men would identify with the story and copy the behaviour of Werther—sometimes even dressed in similar ropes and found with the book next to their body [21]. The main character gave name to the phenomenon 'the Werther effect', which denotes famous suicide deaths (by fictive or actual persons) that are being copied. A more recent case of this was observed in Germany in 2009 where a former national soccer player R. Enke died by suicide. In subsequent years, a 31% increase in suicides by the same method was observed among men [22]. Fictive portrayals, as a suicide of a main character in a soap opera, have been linked to an increase in self-poisonings

admitted to hospital by women [23]. Media guidelines installing that reports of suicide should not list details regarding the method and avoid depicting the event as a heroic act have subsequently been developed [24]. Interestingly, the media might also have a preventive impact on suicides when reports are made according to media guidelines [25]. In order to emphasize that media may also have a positive impact, this effect is now called 'the Papageno effect'.

## Individual risk factors

On an individual level, various circumstances are linked to elevated vulnerability to suicide. Coping strategies and support from network are important moderators of these risk factors. Some of the most relevant individual risk factors for suicide are listed in the following sections.

### Gender and age

In most countries, suicides by men outnumber those by women at a ratio of 1:2 to 1:4. However, as can be seen in Fig. 125.3, there is great variation in the sex ratio between countries. One explanation for this is gender-specific preferences for methods; men tend to use more lethal means of suicide, while women outnumber men when it comes to suicide attempts as a result of predominantly using poisoning [26]. China is an exception to this, as Chinese women have a 25% higher suicide rate than men [27]. This is largely attributed to suicides in rural areas where young women have a very high rate of suicide and might be explained through their low social status and the availability of highly lethal means (pesticides), as well as limited options for social support.

As shown in Fig. 125.4, suicide rates increase with increasing age in those countries that report their data to the WHO. While older adults aged 75 years and older have the highest rate, more detailed studies of the suicide rates among the oldest age groups reveal even higher rates for men until age 90 years, while the rate for women peaks at age 85–94 [28, 29]. In terms of absolute numbers, most suicides in high-income countries occur among persons in mid life at around age 50. In low- and middle-income countries, most suicides take place among the very young aged 15–24 (Fig. 125.2). In all countries, suicides among children below age 15 years are very rare.

### Family and close relations

Familial conditions, such as separation, divorce, and widowhood, are linked to a higher risk of suicide, while marriage is often found to be protective against suicide [30]. Having a child, particularly a young child, protects parents against suicide [31].

Stressful life events, such as the death of a child or loss of a relative to suicide, are linked to increased risks of suicide [31, 32]. Studies showed that the recent loss of a partner constitutes a stressor that is associated with higher risks of suicide, for instance in older adults [33]. Moreover, it is plausible that humiliation, bullying, financial ruin, fear of not passing exams, or losing one's job are all factors that might be associated with an increased risk of suicide.

### Minority groups

An increased suicide mortality is found among homeless people; this is particularly dominant in younger age groups [34]. Imprisonment, but also being charged with a criminal offence, although not found

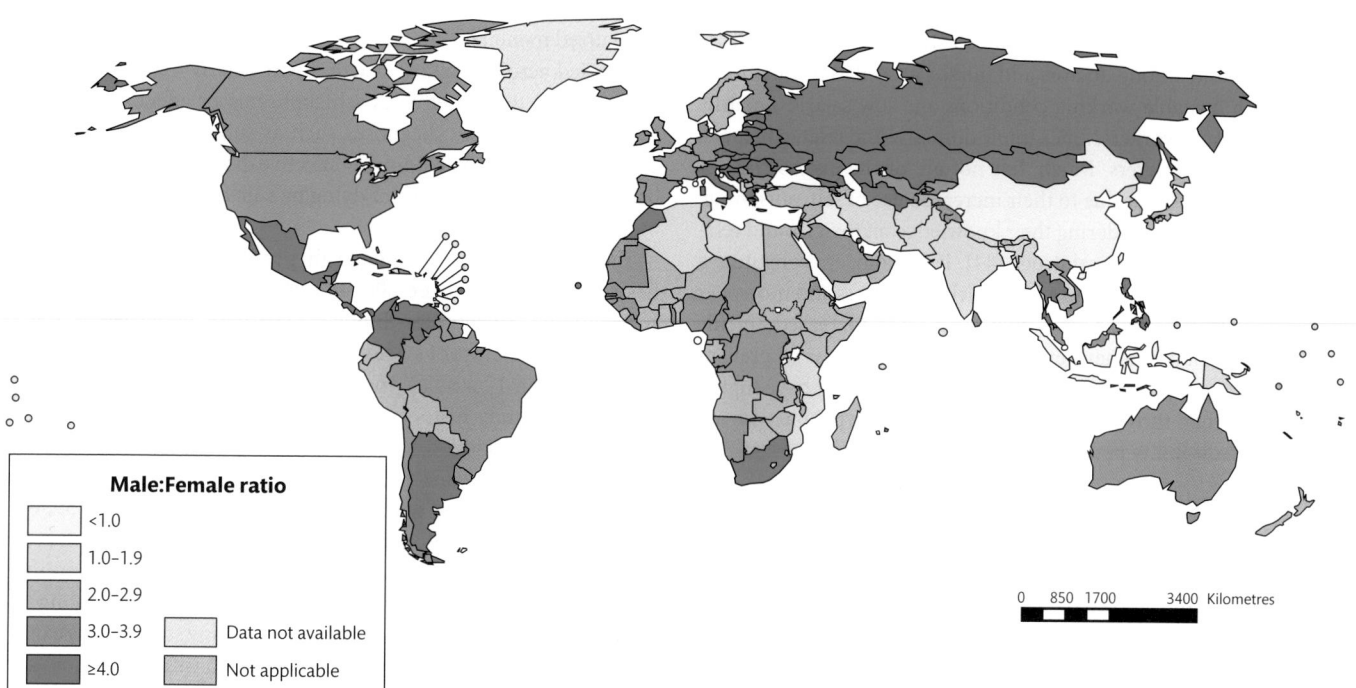

**Fig. 125.3** (see Colour Plate section)  Sex ratio of age-standardized suicide rates by country (2012).
Reproduced from World Health Organization, *Preventing suicide: A global imperative*, Copyright (2014), with permission from the World Health Organization.

guilty, are linked to increased risks of suicide [35]. The period immediately after imprisonment is associated with the highest risk of suicide [35]. For marginalized groups, such as the homeless or people with a criminal history, the elevated risk of suicide might be mediated through untreated mental disorders.

Sexual minority groups are generally thought to have a higher suicide rate, although limited evidence has been produced [36]. Based on Danish register data, persons living in same-sex partnership had higher suicide rates than those living in opposite-sex partnerships [37]. A study on transgendered persons in treatment found that these have a higher suicide rate than the general population [38].

Until recently, the rate of suicide in the military has been lower than the rate among civilians [39]. However, large cohort studies based on active US army soldiers (deployed or not) and veteran populations (that is, those who are no longer employed in the army) have shown a rise in the suicide risk in the period spanning from 2004 to 2009—even higher than in the general background population [40, 41]. In the UK, a similar trend was found in a large cohort study; however, an excess risk, when compared with a background population, applied only to veterans younger than 24 years [42]. Regarding leaving the armed forces, both US and UK studies found that the suicide risk was highest in the first years after leaving the military [42, 43].

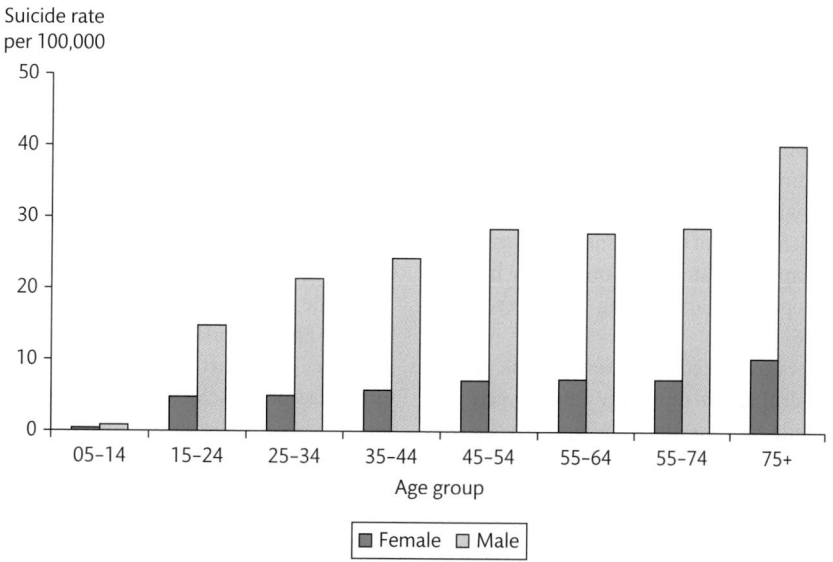

**Fig. 125.4**  Suicide rate age group for 62 countries reporting to WHO Mortality Data Bank (2004–2009).
Reproduced from World Health Organization, *Preventing suicide: A global imperative*, Copyright (2014), with permission from the World Health Organization.

Suicide rates in different occupational groups have been examined in several studies. In a large Danish study, the highest suicide rates were found among doctors and nurses, as well as occupational groups with unstable working conditions and low salaries, mainly unskilled manual workers, for example domestic and related helpers, cleaners, and launderers. Much, but not all, of the excess risk for doctors and nurses was due to their increased use of self-poisoning, a feasible method, considering their knowledge on toxicity and relatively easy access to medical drugs [44]. Police officers constitute a professional group exposed to a high level of job stress and moreover with access to firearms. Some studies reported increased suicide rates of this group and have examined the effectiveness of prevention programmes [45, 46]. People who are unemployed have higher suicide risks than those in work. The same goes for people who are retired or on disability pensions [47].

## Mental disorders

The strongest individual risk factors are mental disorders and previous suicidal behaviour. In fact, the increased risk of suicide is one of the main explanations for why people with mental disorders have a 15–20 years shorter life expectancy, compared with the general population [48]. Psychological autopsy studies where available post-mortem information on the suicide victim is collected from, for instance, family members and general practitioner found that up to 90% of people who died by suicide met the criteria for a mental disorder [49, 50]. While acknowledging that not all people with mental disorders receive treatment, a recent study found that the risk of suicide varies according to the level of mental health care received; people admitted to inpatient care had a 44-fold higher risk of suicide than the general population, whereas those receiving outpatient care or psychiatric medication had an 8- or 6-fold higher risk, respectively [51].

While suicide among psychiatric inpatients is a rare event, this population still has a high rate of suicide—147 per 100,000 patient-years [52], which is almost 13 times higher than the annual global age-standardized suicide rate of 11.4 per 100,000 provided by the WHO [9]. Two phases are linked to particularly high risks: patients who are currently admitted and those who are recently discharged from psychiatric hospital [53]. Most inpatient suicides take place within the first week of admission [54, 55]. The first days and months after discharge comprise a suicidal high-risk period, especially in the first week where the risk has been reported to be up to 102-fold (for men) and 246-fold (for women) higher, when compared to a background population with no admission history. The following clinical factors have been associated with an increased risk: history of suicide attempt, depressed mood, feelings of hopelessness or worthlessness and suicidal ideations expressed at admission, family history of suicide, diagnosis of schizophrenia, and having been prescribed antidepressant medication [56].

Virtually all mental disorders are linked to an elevated risk of suicide. A register-based long-term follow-up study investigated the cumulative incidence of suicide by time since the first psychiatric inpatient or outpatient contact for each disorder in men and women, respectively [57]. The incidences were based on a 36-year observational follow-up study of the Danish population and showed that the suicide risk is highest in the first years after first contact and that all psychiatric diagnoses had an elevated suicide risk throughout the study period. The overall cumulative risk of dying by suicide in people who had inpatient or outpatient clinical contact with specialized mental health services was 4% in men and 2% in women and varied across diagnoses, with a particularly higher risk of suicide in those diagnosed with schizophrenia or affective disorders, compared with other diagnoses such as substance abuse. Women diagnosed with bipolar/unipolar affective disorder or schizophrenia had a 4–5% long-term risk of dying by suicide, whereas this risk in men was 6–7%.

The increased risk of suicide in people with bipolar disorder has been estimated to be 200–400 per 100,000 person-years. The International Society for Bipolar Disorders published a meta-analysis of predictors of suicide death in relation to bipolar disorder [58]. Based on 12 studies, the variables being a man and having a first-degree family history of suicide were identified as significant risk factors of suicide.

Unipolar depressions occur with a prevalence of 2–3% among men and 3–5% among women in the general population [59, 60], and the general practitioner is often the first treatment contact for people with depression. It is difficult to identify who are at eminent risk of suicide, but addressing suicidal issues is important among patients who experience depressive episodes. Many studies have examined risk factors of suicide in people diagnosed with depression, and a meta-analysis based on 19 studies found that male gender, family history of psychiatric disorder, previous attempted suicide, severe depression, hopelessness, and comorbid disorders, such as anxiety and substance misuse, were significant predictors [61]. Treatment of depression is very important to reduce suicide risk. Antidepressants are commonly used in the treatment of people with depression. New generations of antidepressants, such as selective serotonin reuptake inhibitors (SSRIs) and serotonin/noradrenaline reuptake inhibitors (SNRIs), have been linked to suicidal ideation and preparative acts and behaviour in children and young people [62, 63], but protective for those older than 64 years [62]. When prescribing antidepressants, it is important to carefully monitor patients, especially when young people are treated.

In a meta-analysis, the lifetime suicide risk in schizophrenia was estimated to be 5.6% [57, 64]. In a long-term follow-up study from the UK of a large cohort of individuals, the absolute risk of suicide was 3.23% for patients 20 years after the initial diagnosis of a psychotic disorder [65]. Based on the standardized mortality ratio, this study also reported that the risk of suicide was 12-fold higher in patients with psychosis, when compared with the general population. A meta-analysis of risk factors for suicide in schizophrenia based on 29 eligible studies found robust evidence of increased risk being conferred by depressive disorders, previous suicide attempts, drug misuse, agitation and motor restlessness, fear of mental disintegration, poor adherence to treatment, and recent loss [66].

Suicide is also increased in those suffering from substance abuse [67–69] and personality disorders, especially borderline personality disorders [70]. Further, these disorders often exist as comorbidity to depression or schizophrenia. Thus, in addition to adding to the suicide risk, it also complicates the treatment and recovery of these patients [71, 72].

## History of suicide attempt

Having a history of suicide attempt is possibly the most significant risk factor of completed suicide. A meta-analysis showed that as many as 1.6% persons died of suicide within 1 year after re-presenting to hospital with a non-fatal suicide attempt and that one in 25 had died after 5 years [73]. In these studies, the suicide risk associated with the different mental disorders almost doubled if a patient had also been admitted to hospital with a suicide attempt [57].

A Swedish register-based study examined the association between the method of attempted suicide and the risk of subsequent suicide and found that individuals who had attempted suicide by hanging, strangulation, or suffocation had higher risks of dying by suicide [74]. In particular, this study highlighted that among patients who were admitted to hospital due to suicide attempt by method of hanging, strangulation, or suffocation and who had a coexisting diagnosis of a non-organic psychosis, 68.8% of women and 69.6% of men had completed suicide within a year.

### Physical disorders

Severe somatic disorders have been associated with an increased risk of suicidal behaviour. Studies of specific disorders identified that peptic ulcers [75], renal disease [75], arthritis [76], acquired immune deficiency syndrome (AIDS) [77], cancer [78, 79], cerebral stroke [80–82], myocardial infarction [83], diabetes [84], multiple sclerosis [85, 86], and epilepsy [84, 87] were linked to an elevated suicide risk. Also relatively rare diseases, such as fibromyalgia and Crohn's disease [88, 89], have been linked to increased risks of suicidal behaviour. Danish findings showed that the time immediately after discharge from treatment of somatic diseases is linked to an excess risk [90].

## Population-attributable risk

Population-attributable risk (PAR) is a useful measure when thinking in terms of suicide prevention. It estimates the potential for prevention if addressing effectively specific individual risk factors, although it does not include a measure for estimating the potential for prevention of societal risk factors. The PAR denotes the proportion of all suicides prevented if one were to avoid all suicides associated with a specific risk factor. For example, if the excess risk of suicide among single men would be reduced to the level of the general population, then the total number of suicides would be reduced with 26.2% (Table 125.2). The usefulness is apparent when comparing the PAR of different risk factors, as this provides information on which risk factors are linked to larger potentials of prevention. An important consideration is the population size affected by a risk factor. As the epidemiologist Rose noted, an intervention aimed at a large population at a low risk might result in prevention of more suicides than an intervention aimed at a small, but high-risk, group [91]. The size of the exposed population for each risk factor is also included in the PAR. As seen in Table 125.2, an intervention aimed at preventing suicides in a large population, such as single men, that has a relatively small excess suicide risk has the potential to prevent one in four of all male suicides. An intervention aimed at a proportionally smaller group, such as women who have been diagnosed with schizophrenia who have a 19-fold higher risk of suicide than the general population, would prevent 3.4% of all female suicides. The factors with the highest PAR are mental disorders, recent suicide attempt, and single marital status.

**Table 125.2** Population-attributable risk (%) associated with specific risk factors [100–101]

| Risk factor | Men | Women |
|---|---|---|
| Co-habiting marital status | 1.9 | 1.0 |
| Single | 26.2 | 20.6 |
| Unemployed | 3.0 | 2.1 |
| Age pensioner | 7.0 | 18.8 |
| Disability pensioner | 1.7 | 6.7 |
| Imprisoned | 1.0 | – |
| Lowest-income quartile | 9.3 | 7.2 |
| Sickness-related absence from work | 6.6 | 6.2 |
| Recent suicide attempt* | 11.8 | 24.4 |
| All psychiatric diagnoses | 32.5 | 53.9 |
| Any affective disorder | 8.6 | 19.2 |
| – Bipolar disorders | 1.0 | 2.2 |
| – Recurrent depression | 3.9 | 9.8 |
| – Other affective disorders | 3.7 | 7.2 |
| Schizophrenia | 3.2 | 3.4 |
| Other schizophrenic disorders | 2.3 | 3.7 |
| Borderline personality disorders | 0.1 | 1.7 |
| Other personality disorders | 3.5 | 7.7 |
| Reaction to stress/adjustment disorders | 4.0 | 5.3 |
| Other anxiety disorders | 0.4 | 1.3 |
| Substance use disorders | 7.6 | 6.0 |
| – Alcohol use disorders | 6.0 | 3.7 |
| – Drug use disorders | 1.6 | 2.3 |
| Dementia | 0.5 | 0.7 |
| Other psychiatric disorders | 2.3 | 4.9 |

* Estimated on Danish citizens in year 2010, based on numbers from the Centre for Suicide Research in DK (prevalence of suicide attempt), Statistics Denmark (population size), and Carroll et al, 2014 (73) (percentage of fatal repitition within a year).

## REFERENCES

1. Darwin C. *The Origin of Species—by Means of Natural Selection, or the Preservation of Favoured Races in the Struggle for Life.* London: John Murray; 1859.
2. Van Heeringen K. The neurobiology of suicide and suicidality. *Can J Psychiatry.* 2003;48:292–300.
3. Gordon RS. *An Operational Classification of Disease Prevention.* Geneva: World Health Organization; 1983.
4. Mrazek PJ, Haggerty RJ. *Reducing Risk for Mental Disorders: Frontiers for Preventive Intervention Research.* Washington, DC: National Academy Press; 1994.
5. Hawton K, Bergen H, Simkin S, et al. Reduced pack sizes of paracetamol: time-series analysis of long-term impacts on poisoning deaths and liver transplant long-term impacts on poisoning deaths and liver transplant activity in England and Wales. *BMJ.* 2013;346:f403.
6. Stanley B, Brown GK. Safety planning intervention: a brief intervention to mitigate suicide risk. *Cogn Behav Pract.* 2012;19:256–64.
7. Rutz W, von Knorring L, Wålinder J. Long-term effects of an educational program for general practitioners given by the Swedish

Committee for the Prevention and Treatment of Depression. *Acta Psychiatr Scand*. 1992;85:83–8.

8. Erlangsen A, Lind BD, Stuart EA, *et al*. Short-term and long-term effects of psychosocial therapy for people after deliberate self-harm: a register-based, nationwide multicentre study using propensity score matching. *Lancet Psychiatry*. 2015;2:49–58.

9. World Health Organization. *Preventing Suicide—A Global Imperative*. Geneva: World Health Organization; 2014.

10. Gearing RE, Lizardi D. Religion and suicide. *J Relig Health*. 2009;48:332–41.

11. Cooper PN. The coroner's system and under-reporting of suicide. *Med Sci Law*. 1995;35:319–26.

12. Durkheim E. *Le Suicide*. Paris: Felix Alcan; 1897.

13. Hunter E, Harvey D. Indigenous suicide in Australia, New Zealand, Canada and the United States. *Emerg Med*. 2002;14:14–23.

14. Bjerregaard P, Lynge I. Archives of suicide research: Suicide—a challenge in modern Greenland. *Suicide*. 2006;1118:37–41.

15. Värnik A, Wasserman D, Dankowicz M, Eklund G. Age-specific suicide rates in the Slavic and Baltic regions of the former USSR during perestroika, in comparison with 22 European countries. *Acta Psychiatr Scand* (Suppl). 1998;394:20–5.

16. Chang S-SS-S, Stuckler D, Yip P, Gunnell D. Impact of 2008 global economic crisis on suicide: time trend study in 54 countries. *BMJ*. 2013;347:f5239.

17. Stuckler D, Basu S, Suhrcke M, Coutts A, McKee M. The public health effect of economic crises and alternative policy responses in Europe: an empirical analysis. *Lancet*. 2009;374:315–23.

18. Stack S. Suicide: a 15-year review of the sociological literature. Part II: Modernization and social integration perpectives. *Suicide Life Threat Behav*. 2000;30:163–76.

19. Thorvik AA. [Under krigen holdt vi sammen]. *Norske og svenske suicidrater* 1940–5 (in Norwegian). 2016;1:24–33.

20. Gunnell DJ, Fernando R, Priyangika WDD, Eddleston M. The impact of pesticide regulations on suicide in Sri Lanka. *Int J Epidemiol*. 2007;36:1235–42.

21. Ziegler W, Hegerl U. Der Werther-Effekt—Bedeutung, Mechanismen, Konsequensen. *Nervenarzt*. 2002;73:41–9.

22. Hegerl U, Koburger N, Rummel-Kluge C, Gravert C, Walden M, Mergl R. One followed by many? Long-term effects of a celebrity suicide on the number of suicidal acts on the German railway. *J Affect Disord*. 2013;146:39–44.

23. Hawton K, Simkin S, Deeks JJ, *et al*. Effects of a drug overdose in a television drama on presentations to hospital for self poisoning: time series and questionnaire study. *BMJ*. 1999;318:972–7.

24. International Association for Suicide Prevention. *Media guidelines*. 2016. Available from: https://www.iasp.info/media_guide-lines.php

25. Niederkrotenthaler T, Voracek M, Herberth A, *et al*. Role of media reports in completed and prevented suicide: Werther v. Papageno effects. *Br J Psychiatry*. 2010;197:234–43.

26. O'Connor R, Nock M. The psychology of suicidal behaviour. *Lancet Psychiatry*. 2014;1:73–85.

27. Phillips MR, Li X, Zhang Y. Suicide rates in China, 1995–99. *Lancet*. 2002;359:835–40.

28. Shah A, Bhat R, Zarate-Escudero S, DeLeo D, Erlangsen A. Suicide rates in five-year age-bands after the age of 60 years: the international landscape. *Aging Ment Health*. 2016;20:131–8.

29. Shah A, Zarate-Escudero S, Bhat R, De Leo D, Erlangsen A; International Research Group on Suicide in Older Adults. Suicide in centenarians: the international landscape. *Int Psychogeriatr*. 2014;26:1703–8.

30. Agerbo E. Midlife suicide risk, partner's psychiatric illness, spouse and child bereavement by suicide or other modes of death: a gender specific study. *J Epidemiol Community Health*. 2005;59:407–12.

31. Qin P, Mortensen PB. The impact of parental status on the risk of completed suicide. *Arch Gen Psychiatry*. 2003;60:797–802.

32. Tidemalm D, Runeson B, Waern M, *et al*. Familial clustering of suicide risk: a total population study of 11.4 million individuals. *Psychol Med*. 2011;41:2527–34.

33. Erlangsen A, Jeune B, Bille-Brahe U, Vaupel JW. Loss of partner and suicide risks among oldest old: a population-based register study. *Age Ageing*. 2004;33:378–83.

34. Nielsen SF, Hjorthoj CR, Erlangsen A, Nordentoft M. Psychiatric disorders and mortality among people in homeless shelters in Denmark: a nationwide register-based cohort study. *Lancet*. 2011;377:2205–14.

35. Webb RT, Qin P, Stevens H, Mortensen PB, Appleby L, Shaw J. National study of suicide in all people with a criminal justice history. *Arch Gen Psychiatry*. 2011;68:591–9.

36. Haas AP, Eliason M, Mays VM, *et al*. Suicide and suicide risk in lesbian, gay, bisexual, and transgender populations: review and recommendations. *J Homosex*. 2011;58:10–51.

37. Frisch M, Simonsen J. Marriage, cohabitation and mortality in Denmark: national cohort study of 6.5 million persons followed for up to three decades (1982–2011). *Int J Epidemiol*. 2013;42:559–78.

38. van Kesteren PJ, Asscheman H, Megens JA, Gooren LJ. Mortality and morbidity in transsexual subjects treated with cross-sex hormones. *Clin Endocrinol (Oxf)*. 1997;47:337–42.

39. Nock MK, Deming CA, Fullerton CS, *et al*. Suicide among soldiers: a review of psychosocial risk and protectice factors. *Psychiatry*. 2014;27:380–92.

40. Schoenbaum M, Kessler RC, Gilman SE, *et al*. Predictors of suicide and accident death in the Army Study to Assess Risk and Resilience in Servicemembers (Army STARRS): results from the Army Study to Assess Risk and Resilience in Service members (Army STARRS). *JAMA Psychiatry*. 2014;71:493–503.

41. Kang HK, Bullman TA, Smolenski DJ, Skopp NA, Gahm GA, Reger MA. Suicide risk among 1.3 million veterans who were on active duty during the Iraq and Afghanistan wars. *Ann Epidemiol*. 2015;25:96–100.

42. Kapur N, While D, Blatchley N, Bray I, Harrison K. Suicide after leaving the UK armed forces—a cohort study. *PLoS Med*. 2009;6:e26.

43. Reger MA, Smolenski DJ, Skopp NA, *et al*. Risk of suicide among US military service members following operation enduring freedom or operation Iraqi freedom deployment and separation from the US military. *JAMA Psychiatry*. 2015;72:561–9.

44. Agerbo E, Gunnell D, Bonde JP, Mortensen PB, Nordentoft M. Suicide and occupation: the impact of socio-economic, demographic and psychiatric differences. *Psychol Med*. 2007;37:1131–40.

45. O'Hara AF, Violanti JM, Levenson RL Jr, Clark RG Sr. National police suicide estimates: web surveillance study III. *Int J Emerg Ment Health*. 2013;15:31–8.

46. Mishara BL, Martin N. Effects of a comprehensive police suicide prevention program. *Crisis*. 2012;33:162–8.

47. Mortensen PB, Agerbo E, Erikson T, Qin P, Westergaard-Nielsen N. Psychiatric illness and risk factors for suicide in Denmark. *Lancet*. 2000;355:9–12.

48. Wahlbeck K, Westman J, Nordentoft M, Gissler M, Laursen TM. Outcomes of Nordic mental health systems: life expectancy of patients with mental disorders. *Br J Psychiatry*. 2011;199:453–8.

49. Cavanagh JTO, Carson AJ, Sharpe M, Lawrie SM. Psychological autopsy studies of suicide: a systematic review. *Psychol Med.* 2003;33:395–405.

50. Isometsa ET. Psychological autopsy studies—a review. *Eur Psychiatry.* 2001;16:379–85.

51. Hjorthøj CR, Madsen T, Agerbo E, Nordentoft M. Risk of suicide according to level of psychiatric treatment: a nationwide nested case-control study. *Soc Psychiatry Psychiatr Epidemiol.* 2014;49:1357–65.

52. Walsh G, Sara G, Ryan CJ, Large M. Meta-analysis of suicide rates among psychiatric in-patients. *Acta Psychiatr Scand.* 2015;131:174–84.

53. Qin P, Nordentoft M. Suicide risk in relation to psychiatric hospitalization: evidence based on longitudinal registers. *Arch Gen Psychiatry.* 2005;62:427–32.

54. Madsen T, Agerbo E, Mortensen PB, Nordentoft M. Predictors of psychiatric inpatient suicide—a national prospective register-based study. *J Clin Psychiatry.* 2012;73:144–51.

55. Hunt IM, Bickley H, Windfuhr K, Shaw J, Appleby L, Kapur N. Suicide in recently admitted psychiatric in-patients: a case-control study. *J Affect Disord.* 2013;144:123–8.

56. Large M, Smith G, Sharma S, Nielssen O, Singh SP. Systematic review and meta-analysis of the clinical factors associated with the suicide of psychiatric in-patients. *Acta Psychiatr Scand.* 2011;124:18–19.

57. Nordentoft M, Mortensen PB, Pedersen CB. Absolute risk of suicide following first hospital contact with mental disorder. *Arch Gen Psychiatry.* 2011;68:1058–64.

58. Schaffer A, Isometsä ET, Tondo L, et al. International Society for Bipolar Disorders Task Force on Suicide: meta-analyses and meta-regression of correlates of suicide attempts and suicide deaths in bipolar disorder. *Bipolar Disord.* 2015;17:1–16.

59. Kessler RC, Aguilar-Gaxiola S, Alonso J, et al. The global burden of mental disorders: an update from the WHO World Mental Health (WMH) surveys. *Epidemiol Psichiatr Soc.* 2009;18:23–33.

60. Pedersen CB, Mors O, Bertelsen A, et al. A comprehensive nationwide study of the incidence rate and lifetime risk for treated mental disorders. *JAMA Psychiatry.* 2014;71:573–81.

61. Hawton K, Casañas I, Comabella C, Haw C, Saunders K. Risk factors for suicide in individuals with depression: a systematic review. *J Affect Disord.* 2013;147:17–28.

62. Stone M, Laughren T, Jones ML, et al. Risk of suicidality in clinical trials of antidepressants in adults: analysis of proprietary data submitted to US Food and Drug Administration. *BMJ.* 2009;339:b2880.

63. Sharma T, Guski LS, Freund N, Gøtzsche PC. Suicidality and aggression during antidepressant treatment: systematic review and meta-analyses based on clinical study reports. *BMJ.* 2016;352:i65.

64. Palmer BA, Pankratz VS, Bostwick JM. The lifetime risk of suicide in schizophrenia: a re-examination. *Arch Gen Psychiatry.* 2005;62:247–53.

65. Dutta R, Murray RM, Hotopf M, Allardyce J, Jones PB, Boydell J. Reassessing the long-term risk of suicide after a first episode of psychosis. *Arch Gen Psychiatry.* 2010;67:1230–7.

66. Hawton K, Sutton L, Haw C, Sinclair J, Deeks JJ. Schizophrenia and suicide: systematic review of risk factors. *Br J Psychiatry.* 2005;187:9–20.

67. Wilcox HC, Conner KR, Caine ED. Association of alcohol and drug use disorders and completed suicide: an empirical review of cohort studies. *Drug Alcohol Depend.* 2004;76(Suppl):11–19.

68. Darvishi N, Farhadi M, Haghtalab T, Poorolajal J. Alcohol-related risk of suicidal ideation, suicide attempt, and completed suicide: a meta-analysis. *PLoS One.* 2015;10:1–14.

69. Poorolajal J, Haghtalab T, Farhadi M, Darvishi N. Substance use disorder and risk of suicidal ideation, suicide attempt and suicide death: a meta-analysis. *J Public Health (Oxf).* 2016;38:e282–91.

70. Pompili M, Girardi P, Ruberto A, Tatarelli R. Suicide in borderline personality disorder: a meta-analysis. *Nord J Psychiatry.* 2005;59:319–24.

71. Yuodelis-Flores C, Ries RK. Addiction and suicide: a review. *Am J Addict.* 2015;24:98–104.

72. Kolla NJ, Eisenberg H, Links PS. Epidemiology, risk factors, and psychopharmacological management of suicidal behavior in borderline personality disorder. *Arch Suicide Res.* 2008;12:1–19.

73. Carroll R, Metcalfe C, Gunnell D. Hospital presenting self-harm and risk of fatal and non-fatal repetition: systematic review and meta-analysis. *PLoS One.* 2014;9:e89944.

74. Runeson B, Tidemalm D, Dahlin M, Lichtenstein P, Langstrom N. Method of attempted suicide as predictor of subsequent successful suicide: national long term cohort study. *BMJ.* 2010;341:c3222.

75. Stenager EN, Stenager E. *Disease, Pain and Suicidal Behavior.* New York, NY: Haworth Medical Press; 1997.

76. Treharne GJ, Lyons AC, Kitas GD. Suicidal ideation in patients with rheumatoid arthritis. *BMJ.* 2000;321:1290–1.

77. Keiser O, Spoerri A, Brinkhof MW, et al. Suicide in HIV-infected individuals and the general population in Switzerland, 1988–2008. *Am J Psychiatry.* 2010;167:143–50.

78. Schairer C, Brown LM, Chen BE, et al. Suicide after breast cancer: an international population-based study of 723810 women. *J Natl Cancer Inst.* 2006;98:1416–19.

79. Yousaf U, Christensen MLM, Engholm G, Storm HH. Suicides among Danish cancer patients 1971–1999. *Br J Cancer.* 2005;92:995–1000.

80. Forsstrom E, Hakko H, Nordstrom T, Rasanen P, Mainio A. Suicide in patients with stroke: a population-based study of suicide victims during the years 1988–2007 in northern Finland. *J Neuropsychiatry Clin Neurosci.* 2010;22:182–7.

81. Teasdale TW, Engberg AW. Suicide after stroke: a population study. *J Epidemiol Community Health.* 2001;55:863–6.

82. Stenager EN, Madsen C, Stenager E, Boldsen J. Suicide in patients with stroke: epidemiological study. *BMJ.* 1998;316:1206.

83. Larsen KK, Agerbo E, Christensen B, Sondergaard J, Vestergaard M. Myocardial infarction and risk of suicide: a population-based case-control study. *Circulation.* 2010;122:2388–93.

84. Christiansen E, Stenager E. Risk for attempted suicide in children and youths after contact with somatic hospitals: a Danish register based nested case-control study. *J Epidemiol Community Health.* 2012;66:247–53

85. Brønnum-Hansen H, Stenager E, Nylev Stenager E, Koch-Henriksen N. Suicide among Danes with multiple sclerosis. *J Neurol Neurosurg Psychiatry.* 2005;76:1457–9.

86. Pompili M, Forte A, Palermo M, et al. Suicide risk in multiple sclerosis: a systematic review of current literature. *J Psychosom Res.* 2012;73:411–17.

87. Christensen J, Vestergaard M, Mortensen PB, Sidenius P, Agerbo E. Epilepsy and risk of suicide: a population-based case-control study. *Lancet Neurol.* 2007;6:693–8.

88. Duricova D, Pedersen N, Elkjaer M, Gamborg M, Munkholm P, Jess T. Overall and cause-specific mortality in Crohn's disease: a meta-analysis of population-based studies. *Inflamm Bowel Dis.* 2010;16:347–53.

89. Dreyer L, Kendall S, Danneskiold-Samsøe B, Bartels EM, Bliddal H. Mortality in a cohort of Danish patients with fibromyalgia: increased frequency of suicide. *Arthritis Rheum.* 2010;62:3101–8.

90. Qin P, Webb R, Kapur N, Sorensen HT. Hospitalization for physical illness and risk of subsequent suicide: a population study. *J Intern Med.* 2013;273:48–58.

91. Rose G. *The Strategy of Preventive Medicine.* Oxford: Oxford University Press; 1992.

92. Cooper J, Kapur N, Webb R, *et al.* Suicide after deliberate self-harm: a 4-year cohort study. *Am J Psychiatry.* 2005;162:297–303.

93. Hawton K, Bergen H, Cooper J, *et al.* Suicide following self-harm: findings from the multicentre study of self-harm in England, 2000–2012. *J Affect Disord.* 2015;175:147–51.

94. Jenkins GR, Hale R, Papanastassiou M, Crawford MJ, Tyrer P. Suicide rate 22 years after parasuicide: cohort study. *BMJ.* 2002;325:1155.

95. Fazel S, Grann M, Kling B, Hawton K. Prison suicide in 12 countries: an ecological study of 861 suicides during 2003–2007. *Soc Psychiatry Psychiatr Epidemiol.* 2011;46:191–5.

96. Yip PSF, Yousuf S, Chan CH, Yung T, Wu KCC. The roles of culture and gender in the relationship between divorce and suicide risk: a meta-analysis. *Soc Sci Med.* 2015;128:87–94.

97. Martikainen P, Valkonen T. Mortality after the death of a spouse: rates and causes of death in a large Finnish cohort. *Am J Public Health.* 1996;86:1087–93.

98. Qin P, Hawton K, Mortensen PB, Webb R. Combined effects of physical illness and comorbid psychiatric disorder on risk of suicide in a national population study. *Br J Psychiatry.* 2014;204:430–5.

99. Asscheman H, Giltay EJ, Megens JAJ, De Ronde W, Van Trotsenburg MAA, Gooren LJG. A long-term follow-up study of mortality in transsexuals receiving treatment with cross-sex hormones. *Eur J Endocrinol.* 2011;164:635–42.

100. Qin P. The impact of psychiatric illness on suicide: differences by diagnosis of disorders and by sex and age of subjects. *J Psychiatr Res.* 2011;45:1445–52.

101. Qin P, Agerbo E, Mortensen PB. Suicide risk in relation to socioeconomic, demographic, psychiatric, and familial factors: a national register-based study of all suicides in Denmark, 1981–1997. *Am J Psychiatry.* 2003;160:765–72.

# 126

# Self-harm

## Epidemiology and risk factors

*Nav Kapur, Sarah Steeg, and Adam Moreton*

## Introduction

Self-harm is a behaviour, not a diagnosis, so why should it appear in a textbook of psychiatry? People commonly present to emergency departments or mental health services having poisoned or injured themselves and in a state of distress. Self-harm is probably the strongest risk factor for suicide, and yet services to help people are patchy or non-existent. Although the evidence base to inform management is growing, it remains thin. In this chapter, we will discuss what we know about the epidemiology and risk factors for self-harm.

## Terminology

Characterizing non-fatal suicidal behaviour is challenging, and the terminology in this area has developed over time. 'Attempted suicide' is problematic because many patients who self-harm do not wish to die or are too distressed to have formed a clear intent at the time of the episode. 'Parasuicide' describes an act of deliberate self-injury or poisoning which mimics the act of suicide but does not result in a fatal outcome [1]. However, this still contains a reference to suicide. 'Deliberate self-harm' became the preferred term in the UK, but in recent years, the prefix 'deliberate' has been dropped in response to concerns that it was judgemental and in recognition of the heterogenous nature of the phenomenon [2]. Self-harm refers to an intentional act of self-poisoning or self-injury, irrespective of motivation [3]. This is the term that will generally be used throughout this chapter, except when we describe individual studies. People can hurt themselves in a variety of ways—by poisoning, self-cutting, burning, and scratching, as well as by other forms of potentially more lethal self-injury such as hanging, stabbing, and jumping.

## Categorizing self-harm

Should people who self-harm be categorized into those who have clear suicidal intent and those who do not? Proponents have argued that a diagnosis of 'non-suicidal self-injury disorder' (NSSID) would increase precision and lead to improved communication between health professionals, as well as stimulate research into causes and prevention and the development of specific treatments. Others have argued that the term is not useful because suicidal and non-suicidal motivations often coexist, methods of self-harm change, there is no clear dichotomy of intent in self-harm populations (it is continuously distributed), and even people with low-intent episodes are at increased risk of subsequent suicide [4]. It has been suggested that there are potential problems with creating a new diagnosis of NSSID for which there are few proven treatments and which could stigmatize large numbers of young people unnecessarily. Given the uncertainty, we will use the broad and inclusive definition of self-harm, as highlighted in UK national guidance [5]. However, it should be noted that NSSID and attempted suicide disorder are included in DSM-5 as conditions requiring further study.

## Understanding the epidemiology of self-harm: the iceberg model of suicidal behaviour

It has been suggested that the epidemiology of suicidal behaviour might be best conceptualized as an iceberg (Fig. 126.1). Behaviours become more common, but less severe and less visible as one descends the iceberg. The most serious episodes are at the top—deaths by suicide. Self-harm which comes to medical attention is the next level of the iceberg. Even when people present to hospitals, some episodes may go unrecognized and are hence 'under the surface'. Self-harm in the community may be hidden and never come to the attention of health or helping services. Below this, there may be an even larger group of people who experience thoughts of self-injury without acting on them. The important point to note is that the vast majority of epidemiological research in self-harm has been carried out in hospital settings.

We know far less about self-harm in the community. It is difficult to put definitive numbers to the various levels of the iceberg, but McMahon and colleagues attempted to do just this in a recent Irish study of suicidal behaviour in young people where they estimated just 6% of self-harm episodes resulted in hospital presentation. This proportion might be higher in adults—data from a UK household survey suggested that around half of people who attempted suicide or self-harm received some form of help from clinical services [6].

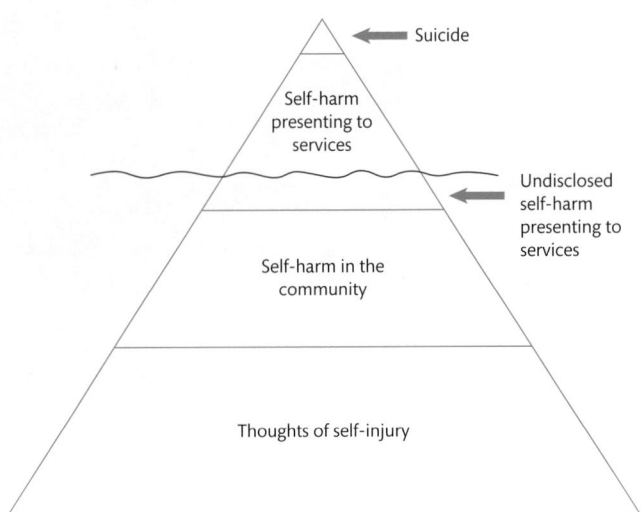

**Fig. 126.1** The iceberg of suicidal behaviour.

In the following sections, we will examine data on the community prevalence of self-harm from international and school surveys before moving on to the hospital-based epidemiology of self-harm.

## International surveys of suicidal behaviour

One of the challenges of international survey data is ensuring consistent methodology across settings. Findings need to be interpreted cautiously, as survey data tend to be self-reported. Response rates may also vary between centres.

Nock and colleagues [7] assessed the prevalence of suicidal ideation, plans, and attempts using the Composite International Diagnostic Interview, as part of the World Health Organization (WHO) World Mental Health Survey initiative. Across 17 high-, middle-, and low-income countries, the lifetime prevalence of suicide attempts was 2.7%, with a lifetime prevalence of 9.2% for ideation and 3.1% for suicide planning. There was substantial cross-national variability, with the lifetime prevalence of suicide attempts ranging from 0.7% in Nigeria to 5% in the United States.

More recently, the WHO has estimated that the global annual rate of suicide attempts is around 4 per 1000 adults on the basis of the same survey methodology [8]. Interestingly, the 12-month prevalence rates for suicidal behaviour were found to be similar for males and females in high- and low-income countries (0.3–0.4%), but higher for females (0.6%) than males (0.3%) in middle-income countries [8].

In a UK household survey, 5.6% of adults reported a lifetime history of suicide attempts and 4.9% a history of self-harm (without suicidal intent), with a 50% overlap between the groups. The prevalence of suicide attempts during the previous year was 0.7% (these previous-year data were not available for self-harm) [6].

## School surveys of self-harm

School-based surveys are a useful source of information. In an international study of self-harm in adolescents (Child and Adolescent Self-harm in Europe study), Madge and colleagues [9] reported rates for self-harm in the previous year of 8.9% for females and 2.6% for males, and lifetime rates of 13.5% and 4.3%, respectively. In terms of methods of self-harm, over half of episodes involved self-cutting and around a fifth poisoning. Many countries have shown similar rates of self-harm in their adolescent populations, (for example, [10, 11]), although some recent research reported considerable variation. A study, using self-report data on over 45,000 15- to 16-year olds from 17 countries participating in the European School Survey Project on Alcohol and Other Drugs, found the proportion reporting a lifetime suicide attempt varied from 4% in Armenia to 24% in Hungary, with a median of around 11% [12]. Female rates were consistently almost twice as high as male rates. Regardless of the precise incidence, it is clear that self-harm is a commonly reported issue in adolescence and often a major concern for young people themselves, their parents, and their teachers.

## The hospital-based epidemiology of self-harm

Register-based studies of self-harm are another valuable source of information but generally only identify people presenting to hospital. However, this is an important and relatively severe subgroup of those who self-harm.

As part of the WHO/EURO multi-centre study of suicidal behaviour, Schmidtke and colleagues [13] investigated treated episodes and found that self-harm was more common among females than males and higher rates were found among younger adults. In particular, young women aged 15–24 years and young men aged 25–29 years had the highest rates of self-harm. There was also substantial variation, with a 6- to 9-fold difference in self-harm rates, even among countries in Europe.

Ireland has a national registry of self-harm, which has been running since 2002 and collects data from hospital emergency departments [14]. In 2014, the annual rate of self-harm was 185 per 100,000 for men and 216 per 100,000 for women. The peak ages were 15–19 years for females and 20–24 years for males. In contrast to community settings, the majority of episodes (70%) involved overdoses of medication or other substances and 26% involved cutting. In interpreting these data, it should be noted that emergency department visits incur a personal cost to the patient in Ireland.

In England, self-harm data are available from 2000 for the three sites that make up the Multicentre Study of Self-harm in England (Oxford, Manchester, and Derby) [15]. In 2013, the rates of self-harm were 322 per 100,000 per year for men and 468 per 100,000 per year for women. The peak age of presentation during the study period (2000–2012) was 15–24 years for women (41% of female episodes). Men had a more even age distribution, with approximately one-third of men who self-harmed aged 15–24 years and one-third aged 35–54 years. Self-poisoning featured in 75% of episodes, and self-injury (mostly cutting) in 21% of episodes. In terms of medication ingested in overdose, despite legislation to reduce pack sizes, paracetamol was the most common substance (ingested in 35% of episodes). This was followed by selective serotonin reuptake inhibitor (SSRI) or serotonin/noradrenaline reuptake inhibitor (SNRI) antidepressants (17%), benzodiazepines (14%), and paracetamol-containing compounds (11%).

## Trends in self-harm

There was a substantial increase in the rates of self-harm during the 1960s and 1970s in the UK [16], but accurate long-term data are sparse. Data from the Oxford Monitoring system suggests hospital presentations for self-harm have increased by 60% since the 1970s, but annual rates based on individuals are not dissimilar to earlier years. It seems likely that rates of hospital-based repetition have increased, but the reasons for this are unclear.

International data suggest that the prevalence of suicidal behaviour may have remained relatively stable between 1997 and 2007 [7]. With respect to adolescent self-injury, a systematic review concluded that although rates were high, relative to other age groups, they did not seem to have increased internationally between 2007 and 2011 [17].

It seems likely that rates of self-harm in adults increased in response to the 2008 recession, especially in centres which experienced increased joblessness in the UK [18]. Research from Ireland suggests a greater impact on men [19]. There has been much recent concern about a possible epidemic of self-harm among adolescents. This has not been substantiated in the research literature but is a focus of much ongoing work.

## Risk and protective factors for self-harm

The causes of self-harm are multiple and complex. Some researchers conceptualize self-harm as part of a 'suicidal process' that ranges from thoughts through to self-injurious behaviour and ultimately suicide for a minority of people [20]. Self-harm may share many risk factors with suicide, but some are also distinct. One striking difference is the gender ratio—self-harm tends to be more common in women, and suicide much more common in men. It has been suggested that the reasons for this disparity may include methods (men may choose more lethal methods when they hurt themselves) or help-seeking behaviour (men may be less likely to seek help if they become physically or psychologically unwell). Table 126.1 summarizes some of the most important risk and protective factors for self-harm, and these will be discussed in more detail in the next section. Protective factors have been subject to much less research than risk factors.

**Table 126.1** Risk and protective factors for self-harm

| Sociodemographic factors | Gender |
| | Age |
| | Ethnicity |
| | Sexual orientation |
| | Deprivation |
| | Social support (p) |
| | Religious affiliation (p) |
| Biological factors | Genes |
| | Neurochemistry |
| Clinical factors | Psychiatric disorder |
| | Physical disorder |
| | Alcohol misuse |
| Psychological factors | Impulsivity |
| | Poor problem-solving skills |
| | Hopelessness |
| Environmental factors | Early adversity |
| | Later life events |
| | Education (p) |
| | Media |

(p) indicates a possible protective factor.

### Sociodemographic factors

Self-harm is more common in young people, particularly girls in mid to late adolescence. The increase in the incidence of self-harm in the early teenage years is striking and may be linked to the pubertal stage. Underlying mechanisms could be biological or social (for example, sensitivity to social cues or propensity to imitative self-harm). Self-harm in older adults tends to be associated with a greater suicidal intent [21] than in younger age groups, and its incidence may be increasing [21].

Socio-economic disadvantage is associated with self-harm in both high- [22] and low- and middle-income countries [23]. There is evidence that rates of self-harm may increase at times of economic adversity [18]. Social isolation is also an important factor [22], but good communication and family functioning may be protective [24]. A 2013 review by Beghi et al. reported a weak association between unmarried marital status and repetition of self-harm [25]. Although previous studies suggested that young South Asian females were at increased risk of self-harm, this has not been borne out by more recent studies and reviews [26, 27], which suggested the highest risks are in young black females. In older age groups, self-harm is most common among the white population. People from all minority ethnic groups were less likely to repeat self-harm in a large English study [26]. A review of adolescent suicidal behaviour in the United States found the highest rates among white youths [28]. Religious affiliation is likely to be protective [29], although this may be context-dependent—religious minorities may feel socially isolated and so may be at greater risk. Sexual orientation is also a risk factor for suicide attempt, with the highest risks possibly in gay and bisexual men [30].

### Genetic and biological factors

A family history of suicide increases the individual's risk of suicide, a finding that may be explained by observational learning or genetic predisposition. A genetic explanation is supported by twin studies and adoption studies which suggested a heritability of between 30% and 50% (or 17% once other psychiatric disorders have been taken into account). What is inherited is unknown. No specific genes coding for suicidal behaviour have been identified. Instead much of the research interest has shifted to the link between early life experience and epigenetic mechanisms that could explain some of the link between childhood exposures, suicide risk, brain circuitry, and neurochemistry. Studies suggested that changes in the polyamine and serotonergic systems and the hypothalamic–pituitary–adrenal axis might be implicated. These could make certain individuals more vulnerable to suicidal behaviour (for a comprehensive recent review, see [31]).

### Clinical and psychological factors

The prevalence of psychiatric disorders in people who self-harm varies according to the setting and method of assessment. Using diagnostic interviews and research criteria, as many as 90% of those who present to hospital may have an Axis I psychiatric disorder, with the most common single diagnosis being affective disorder (70%) [32]. However, it is possible that psychiatric symptoms at the time of an episode are relatively transient and may remit spontaneously in a substantial proportion of cases. A history of psychiatric disorder is also important. In a cross-national community study, a prior mental disorder was associated with significantly increased risk of developing suicidal behaviours, even after adjusting for sociodemographic factors and country of residence. Mood disorders had the strongest association [33].

Alcohol consumption is also an important contributory factor to self-harm—both acute ingestion (which may increase the risk of impulsive behaviour) and longer-term misuse [34]. Physical illness is a risk factor for self-harm, perhaps more so for women than men [35]. At least for some illnesses (asthma, back pain, diabetes, epilepsy, hypertension), the association persists after adjustment for depression [35].

A number of psychological characteristics are more common among those who self-harm; these include impulsivity, poor problem-solving, perfectionism, and hopelessness [36]. It is possible to apply diagnostic labels to some of these characteristics (for example, personality disorder), but this may have the unfortunate consequence of causing stigma, diverting attention from enabling the person to overcome their problems or even leading to them being denied help [2].

### Environmental factors

Childhood adversity, including early abusive experiences, can predispose to self-harm. A recent review suggested that sexual abuse was the most important of these antecedents, but that physical abuse and domestic violence were also associated with self-harm [37]. A classic review found strong cross-sectional associations between childhood sexual abuse and self-harm, but the lack of longitudinal prospective studies led the authors to conclude that these exposures could not be classified as true risk factors [38]. A meta-analysis, which only considered non-suicidal self-injury as an outcome, found a weak association with sexual abuse, which largely disappeared after adjustment for psychiatric factors [39]. On balance, it seems likely that adverse childhood experiences can lead to later self-harm, but this effect may be mediated through an association with clinical factors.

As well as individual exposures, there may also be an association between self-harm and the number and type of adverse events that an individual reports having experienced during their lifetime [22]. Early studies established that life events, particularly interpersonal ones, were important immediate precipitants of self-harm [40], and this has been confirmed more recently [41].

The role of the media in propagating suicidal behaviour, possibly by increasing the cognitive availability of self-harm methods or normalizing it as a coping strategy, is an additional environmental factor and the subject of much published work [42]. Social media is a further development, of course, and the subject of considerable ongoing research.

## Outcomes

Repetition, suicide, and death from all causes are outcomes of particular interest following self-harm. Each will be explored in more detail in the rest of this chapter.

### Non-fatal repetition

A recent meta-analysis of 170 cohort studies and randomized trials in people who had presented to health care services with self-harm suggested that the pooled incidence of repeat self-harm was 16.3%

at 1 year and 22.4% at 5 years [43]. Repetition rates based on patient self-report, as opposed to hospital databases, were around 5% higher at 1 year. There was also some evidence that repetition rates were lower in Asian vs non-Asian countries, perhaps due to differences in ascertainment or the method of self-harm. Poisoning in South Asia has a higher case fatality during the index episode than in the West due to the lethality of the substances ingested—for example, pesticides.

The timing of repetition is striking and has important clinical implications. Most people who repeat self-harm do so soon after they present to hospital. Data from the Manchester Self-harm Project (Fig. 126.2) suggest that 30% of people who repeat within a year will do so within 1 month of presentation and one in ten will repeat within 5 days. This means that any aftercare needs to be provided without delay.

### Suicide

The Carroll *et al.* systematic review [43] found that 1.6% of people died by suicide in year after presentation with self-harm, with a pooled suicide incidence of 3.9% at 5 years and a persistent risk of suicide in the longer term. The risk of suicide was twice as high in men than in women, and higher in studies which focused on older age groups. Self-poisoning was associated with a lower risk of subsequent suicide than other methods. Gender and age together explained nearly 70% of the between-study variation. In a UK single-centre study, suicide rates were highest within the first 6 months after the index self-harm episode [44].

### All causes of death

In an English study of over 30,000 individuals presenting with self-harm to three centres and followed up for an average of 6 years, approximately 6% of the cohort died—about four times the number of deaths that would be expected according to general population mortality rates [45]. The risk of death increased with levels of socio-economic deprivation. Diseases of the circulatory and digestive systems made a major contribution to natural mortality. This study also expressed the risk of death as mean years of life lost—25–26 years for natural-cause deaths, and 40 years for external-cause deaths (for example, accidents, suicide, and undetermined deaths).

### Outcome of self-harm in young and older people

The prognosis of self-harm is of great concern to young people and their parents. A cohort study of 1800 adolescents in Victoria, Australia provided a valuable insight into the natural history of self-harm in young people [46]. The researchers found that 4% of the sample reported self-harm within the previous 12 months at the start of the adolescent phase of data collection (mean age of cohort 15.9 years). This fell steadily through subsequent waves of data collection, so that by the end of the study (mean age of cohort at this stage 29.0 years), just 0.8% reported self-harm. Of the young people who self-harmed in adolescence, only one in ten continued to do so as young adults.

Some authors have argued that fatal and non-fatal self-harm are more closely related in the elderly than in younger age groups [47]. In a large English study of older adults (>60 years), the suicide rate was 1.5% within 12 months of self-harm, 67 times higher than in the general population of similar age and three times higher than in younger self-harm patients in the same cohort. Suicide was most common in those aged 75 years and over [48].

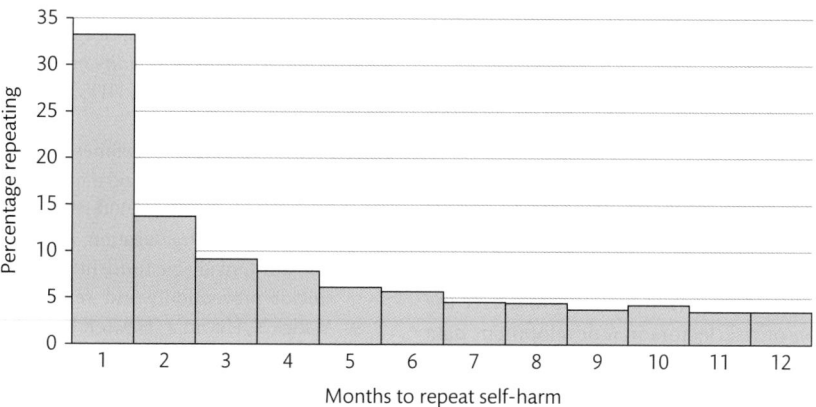

**Fig. 126.2** Timing of repeat self-harm for people repeating within a year (*N* = 3078).
Source: data from the Manchester Self-harm project.

## Risk factors for repetition

Many studies have examined the factors which might make repeat self-harm more likely. In a recent systematic review of 129 prospective studies, a number of factors were identified as consistent predictors of self-harm repetition [49]. Many of these were similar to the risk factors for incident self-harm. They included previous self-harm, personality difficulties, hopelessness, a history of psychiatric treatment, schizophrenia, and alcohol and drug misuse. However, the sensitivity of individual variables (ability to correctly identify those who went on to repeat) varied greatly between studies. Other factors were less consistently reported, but it was suggested they too were linked to increased repetition, for example impulsivity, comorbidity, poor problem-solving ability, sexual abuse, staff attitudes to self-harm, and stressful life events. Self-cutting was associated with a higher risk of repetition than self-poisoning. Area-based variables, such as deprivation, may also be important determinants of suicidal behaviour, but an English study suggested an individual's own characteristics were much more powerful predictors of repetition than the characteristics of the area in which they lived [50].

In a separate review of risk factors for suicide following self-harm, updating work carried out as part of the National Institute for Health and Care Excellence (NICE) guidelines [51], four risk factors emerged from a meta-analysis with robust effect sizes that showed little change, even after adjustment for potential confounders. These included: previous episodes of self-harm, suicidal intent, physical health problems, and male gender. However, the authors suggested that the factors might be of limited practical use because these were common in clinical populations. In a large, Manchester (UK)-based study [52], independent risk factors for suicide after hospital presentation for self-harm were: avoiding discovery at the time of self-harm, not living with a close relative, previous psychiatric treatment, self-cutting (vs self-poisoning), alcohol misuse, and physical health problems. The overall adjusted population-attributable fraction for the statistical model in the study (a measure of the overall proportion of self-harm repetition in a population that might be accounted for by the variables) was 65%.

## Drawing risk factors together—models of self-harm

Although risk factors may provide some clues to the aetiology, they are unable to explain why self-harm occurs. Explanatory models may help us to understand the phenomena better, help to formulate testable hypotheses, and ultimately facilitate the development of appropriate treatments. One of the most influential models of suicidal behaviour is a clinical model—the stress–diathesis or stress–vulnerability model [53]. This suggests that certain individuals carry with them a predisposition to suicidal behaviour (which may be related to sex, religion, familial and genetic factors, childhood experiences, psychosocial support systems, access to lethal methods, or biological factors). The vulnerability only leads to suicidal behaviour when the individual encounters a stressor (which could be a mental disorder, alcohol or drug misuse, a medical illness, or a psychosocial crisis). Other influential models of suicidal behaviour include the 'cry of pain' model (which emphasizes the role of defeat and entrapment—the sense there is nowhere else to go, following the experience of a major stressor), the interpersonal–psychological model (which suggests perceived burdensomeness and thwarted belongingness are central to suicidal ideation), and the integrated motivational–volitional model, a stress–diathesis model which highlights the pre-motivational, motivational (ideation and intent formation), and volitional (behavioural, enaction) phases of suicidality. A full review is provided in [36].

## Risk scales

Combinations of risk factors considered together in 'risk assessment scales' are in widespread use. A study from 32 hospitals in England found that the vast majority of services used risk assessment tools, and in 22 of 32 hospitals, the tools were locally developed and unvalidated [54]. A number of recent reviews [51, 55, 56] have suggested that scales are of limited usefulness in terms of predicting future outcomes such as repetition and suicide. Positive predictive values for suicide ranged from 1% to 17%, with the most relevant UK study suggesting a value of 4%. This means that of 100 people identified as being at high risk, four will die by suicide. However, a greater number of suicide deaths occur in the large low- and middle-risk groups—the so-called population paradox. These may be missed if services are organized according to high-risk paradigms. This has important implications for management, with some authorities going as far as to suggest that viewing risk assessment as risk prediction is a fallacy. Management decisions should be based on more generic models of assessment which emphasize the need to engage with patients, rather than tick-box assessments [51].

The development of novel risk measures is the subject of ongoing research. One approach is to use data-driven methods to derive the most important combination of risk factors in a development data set and then test the instrument in a separate validation data set [56]. Examples of these empirically derived tools include the Manchester Self-Harm and ReACT rules and the Repeated Episodes of Self-Harm (RESH) score. Although robustly developed, there is no good evidence that these tools are any more useful than older scales [55]. A different approach is to use neurocognitive or psychological functioning as a marker of risk. The advantage of some of these measures is that they can be used when people are unaware of their intent or not articulating it. Traits that may be predictive include deficits in attentional shifting, deficits in verbal fluency, and poor decision-making [56]. Another novel method—the Implicit Association Test—measures the reaction time for people to respond to images (related to suicidal behaviour or neutral images) [57]. Shorter reaction times are thought to be associated with a greater propensity to suicidal behaviour. The predictive ability of the test may be improved when used in conjunction with other traditional risk factors [56].

## Which risk factors are the most important clinically?

Although some risk factors are common in clinical populations and the predictive value of risk scales is dubious, clinicians clearly need to assess and treat patients. Which risk factors are the most clinically important? One practice-based review suggested that mental illness, alcohol and drug use, current thoughts and plans, gender, and previous self-harm, along with possible protective characteristics (such as dependent children, supportive family, religious beliefs) were the most important factors to take into account in a real-world clinical assessment [58].

## REFERENCES

1. Kreitman N. *Parasuicide*. Chichester: Wiley; 1977.
2. National Collaborating Centre for Mental Health. *Self-harm: the short-term physical and psychological management and secondary prevention of self-harm in primary and secondary care*. London: British Psychological Society and Royal College of Psychiatrists; 2004.
3. Hawton K, Harriss L, Hall S, Simkin S, Bale E, Bond A. Deliberate self-harm in Oxford, 1990–2000: a time of change in patient characteristics. *Psychological Medicine*. 2003;33:987–95.
4. Kapur N, Cooper J, O'Connor RC, Hawton K. Non-suicidal self-injury v. attempted suicide: new diagnosis or false dichotomy? *British Journal of Psychiatry*. 2013;202:326–8.
5. National Institute for Health and Care Excellence. *Self-harm in over 8s: long-term management*. Clinical guideline [CG133]. London: National Institute of Health and Care Excellence; 2011.
6. McManus S, Meltzer H, Brugha T, Bebbington P, Jenkins R. *Adult psychiatric morbidity in England, 2007: results of a household survey*. Leeds: The NHS Information Centre for Health and Social Care; 2009.
7. Nock MK, Borges G, Bromet EJ, et al. Cross-national prevalence and risk factors for suicidal ideation, plans and attempts. *British Journal of Psychiatry*. 2008;192:98–105.
8. World Health Organization. *Preventing suicide: a global imperative*. 2014. Available from: http://www.who.int/mental_health/suicide-prevention/world_report_2014/en/
9. Madge N, Hewitt A, Hawton K, et al. Deliberate self-harm within an international community sample of young people: comparative findings from the Child & Adolescent Self-harm in Europe (CASE) Study. *Journal of Child Psychology and Psychiatry*. 2008;49:667–77.
10. Hawton K, Rodham K, Evans E, Weatherall R. Deliberate self harm in adolescents: self report survey in schools in England. *BMJ*. 2002;325:1207–11.
11. O'Connor RC, Rasmussen S, Miles J, Hawton K. Self-harm in adolescents: self-report survey in schools in Scotland. *British Journal of Psychiatry*. 2009;194:68–72.
12. Kokkevi A, Rotsika V, Arapaki A, Richardson C. Adolescents' self-reported suicide attempts, self-harm thoughts and their correlates across 17 European countries. *Journal of Child Psychology and Psychiatry*. 2012;53:381–9.
13. Michel K, Schmidtke A. The WHO/EURO multicentre study on suicidal behaviour. *European Psychiatry*. 2004;19:7S.
14. Griffin E, Corcoran P, Cassidy L, O'Carroll A, Perry IJ, Bonner B. Characteristics of hospital-treated intentional drug overdose in Ireland and Northern Ireland. *BMJ Open*. 2014;4:e005557.
15. Geulayov G, Kapur N, Turnbull P, et al. Epidemiology and trends in non-fatal self-harm in three centres in England, 2000–2012: findings from the Multicentre Study of Self-harm in England. *BMJ Open*. 2016;6:e010538.
16. Kapur N, Gask L. Introduction to suicide and self-harm. *Psychiatry*. 2009;8:233–6.
17. Muehlenkamp JJ, Claes L, Havertape L, Plener PL. International prevalence of adolescent non-suicidal self-injury and deliberate self-harm. *Child and Adolescent Psychiatry and Mental Health*. 2012;6:10.
18. Hawton K, Bergen H, Geulayov G, et al. Impact of the recent recession on self-harm: Longitudinal ecological and patient-level investigation from the Multicentre Study of Self-harm in England. *Journal of Affective Disorders*. 2016;191:132–8.
19. Corcoran P, Griffin E, Arensman E, Fitzgerald AP, Perry IJ. Impact of the economic recession and subsequent austerity on suicide and self-harm in Ireland: an interrupted time series analysis. *International Journal of Epidemiology*. 2015;44:969–77.
20. Van Heeringen C. *Understanding Suicidal Behaviour: The Suicidal Process Approach to Research, Treatment and Prevention*. Chichester: Wiley; 2001.
21. Haw C, Casey D, Holmes J, Hawton K. Suicidal intent and method of self-harm: a large-scale study of self-harm patients presenting to a general hospital. *Suicide and Life-Threatening Behavior*. 2015;45:732–46.
22. Meltzer H, Lader D, Corbin T, Singleton N, Jenkins R, Brugha T. Non-fatal suicidal behaviour among adults aged 16 to 74 in Great Britain. Office for National Statistics, 2002.
23. Knipe DW, Carroll R, Thomas KH, Pease A, Gunnell D, Metcalfe C. Association of socio-economic position and suicide/attempted suicide in low and middle income countries in South and South-East Asia—a systematic review. *BMC Public Health*. 2015;15:1055.

24. Evans E, Hawton K, Rodham K. Factors associated with suicidal phenomena in adolescents: A systematic review of population-based studies. *Clinical Psychology Review*. 2004;24:957–79.

25. Beghi M, Rosenbaum JF, Cerri C, Cornaggia CM. Risk factors for fatal and nonfatal repetition of suicide attempts: a literature review. *Neuropsychiatric Disease and Treatment*. 2013;9:1725–35.

26. Cooper J, Steeg S, Webb R, *et al.* Risk factors associated with repetition of self-harm in black and minority ethnic (BME) groups: a multi-centre cohort study. *Journal of Affective Disorders*. 2013;148:435–9.

27. Al-Sharifi A, Krynicki CR, Upthegrove R. Self-harm and ethnicity: a systematic review. *International Journal of Social Psychiatry*. 2015;61:600–12.

28. Balis T, Postolache TT. Ethnic differences in adolescent suicide in the United States. *International Journal of Child Health and Human Development*. 2008;1:281–96.

29. Lawrence RE, Oquendo MA, Stanley B. Religion and suicide risk: a systematic review. *Archives of Suicide Research*. 2016;20:1–21.

30. King M, Semlyen J, Tai SS, *et al.* A systematic review of mental disorder, suicide, and deliberate self harm in lesbian, gay and bisexual people. *BMC Psychiatry*. 2008;8:70.

31. van Heeringen K, Mann JJ. The neurobiology of suicide. *The Lancet Psychiatry*. 2014;1:63–72.

32. Haw C, Houston K, Townsend E, Hawton K. Deliberate self-harm patients with alcohol disorders: characteristics, treatment, and outcome. *Crisis*. 2001;22:93–101.

33. Nock MK, Hwang I, Sampson N, *et al.* Cross-national analysis of the associations among mental disorders and suicidal behavior: findings from the WHO World Mental Health Surveys. *PLoS Medicine*. 2009;6:e1000123.

34. Ness J, Hawton K, Bergen H, *et al.* Alcohol use and misuse, self-harm and subsequent mortality: an epidemiological and longitudinal study from the multicentre study of self-harm in England. *Emergency Medicine Journal*. 2015;32:793–9.

35. Webb RT, Kontopantelis E, Doran T, Qin P, Creed F, Kapur N. Risk of self-harm in physically ill patients in UK primary care. *Journal of Psychosomatic Research*. 2012;73:92–7.

36. O'Connor RC, Nock MK. The psychology of suicidal behaviour. *The Lancet Psychiatry*. 2014;1:73–85.

37. Ford JD, Gomez JM. The relationship of psychological trauma and dissociative and posttraumatic stress disorders to nonsuicidal self-injury and suicidality: a review. *Journal of Trauma and Dissociation*. 2015;16:232–71.

38. Fliege H, Lee J-R, Grimm A, Klapp BF. Risk factors and correlates of deliberate self-harm behavior: a systematic review. *Journal of Psychosomatic Research*. 2009;66:477–93.

39. Klonsky DE, Moyer A. Childhood sexual abuse and non-suicidal self-injury: meta-analysis. *British Journal of Psychiatry*. 2008;192:166–70.

40. Bancroft J, Skrimshire A, Casson J, Harvardwatts O, Reynolds F. People who deliberately poison or injure themselves—their problems and their contacts with helping agencies. *Psychological Medicine*. 1977;7:289–303.

41. Johnson JG, Cohen P, Gould MS, Kasen S, Brown J, Brook JS. Childhood adversities, interpersonal difficulties, and risk for suicide attempts during late adolescence and early adulthood. *Archives of General Psychiatry*. 2002;59:741–9.

42. Gould MS. Suicide and the media. *Clinical Science of Suicide Prevention*. 2001;932:200–24.

43. Carroll R, Metcalfe C, Gunnell D. Hospital presenting self-harm and risk of fatal and non-fatal repetition: systematic review and meta-analysis. *PLoS One*. 2014 28;9:e89944.

44. Cooper J, Kapur N, Webb R, *et al.* Suicide after deliberate self-harm: a 4-year cohort study. *American Journal of Psychiatry*. 2005;162:297–303.

45. Bergen H, Hawton K, Waters K, *et al.* Premature death after self-harm: a multicentre cohort study. *The Lancet*. 2012;380:1568–74.

46. Moran P, Coffey C, Romaniuk H, *et al.* The natural history of self-harm from adolescence to young adulthood: a population-based cohort study. *The Lancet*. 2012;379:236–43.

47. Dennis MS, Owens DW. Self-harm in older people: a clear need for specialist assessment and care. *British Journal of Psychiatry*. 2012;200:356–8.

48. Murphy E, Kapur N, Webb R, *et al.* Risk factors for repetition and suicide following self-harm in older adults: multicentre cohort study. *British Journal of Psychiatry*. 2012;200:399–404.

49. Larkin C, Di Blasi Z, Arensman E. Risk factors for repetition of self-harm: a systematic review of prospective hospital-based studies. *PLoS One*. 2014;9:e84282.

50. Johnston A, Cooper J, Webb R, Kapur N. Individual- and area-level predictors of self-harm repetition. *British Journal of Psychiatry*. 2006;189:416–21.

51. Chan KY, Bhatti H, Meader N, *et al.* Predicting suicide following self-harm: systematic review of risk factors and risk scales. *British Journal of Psychiatry*. 2016;209:277–83.

52. Kapur N, Cooper J, King-Hele S, *et al.* The repetition of suicidal behavior: a multicenter cohort study. *Journal of Clinical Psychiatry*. 2006;67:1599–609.

53. Mann JJ. A current perspective of suicide and attempted suicide. *Annals of Internal Medicine*. 2002;136:302–11.

54. Quinlivan L, Cooper J, Steeg S, *et al.* Scales for predicting risk following self-harm: an observational study in 32 hospitals in England. *BMJ Open*. 2014;4:e004732.

55. Quinlivan L, Cooper J, Davies L, Hawton K, Gunnell D, Kapur N. Which are the most useful scales for predicting repeat self-harm? A systematic review evaluating risk scales using measures of diagnostic accuracy. *BMJ Open*. 2016;6:e009297.

56. Bolton JM, Gunnell D, Turecki G. Suicide risk assessment and intervention in people with mental illness. *BMJ*. 2015;351:h4978.

57. Nock MK, Park JM, Finn CT, Deliberto TL, Dour HJ, Banaji MR. Measuring the suicidal mind: implicit cognition predicts suicidal behavior. *Psychological Science*. 2010;21:511–17.

58. Morriss R, Kapur N, Byng R. Assessing risk of suicide or self harm in adults. *BMJ*. 2013;347:f4572.

# 127

# Biological aspects of suicidal behaviour

*J. John Mann and Dianne Currier*

## Modelling suicidal behaviours

To understand the biological underpinnings of multi-determined behaviours such as suicide and attempted suicide, it is best to conceptualize them within an explanatory model that describes the potential causal pathways and interrelations between biological, clinical, genetic, and environmental factors that all play a role in suicidal behaviour. Where possible, such a model should be clinically explanatory, incorporate biological correlates, be testable in both clinical and biological studies, and have some utility in identifying high-risk individuals.

One such model is the stress–diathesis model of suicidal behaviour wherein exposure to a stressor precipitates a suicidal act in those with the diathesis, or a propensity for suicidal behaviour [1]. Stressors are generally state-dependent factors such as an episode of major depression or the occurrence of an adverse life event. The diathesis comprises trait characteristics of reactive aggression, deficits in executive function, negative or rigid cognitive processes, impaired problem-solving, social distortions, and recurrent mood disorders [2]. Uncovering the biological mechanisms relevant to the stress and the diathesis dimensions of suicidal behaviour will facilitate the identification of both enduring and proximal markers of risk, and thus potential targets for prevention interventions.

This chapter gives an overview of the major neurobiological findings in suicide and attempted suicide, as well as emerging findings from studies of genes related to those neurobiological and stress response systems.

## Serotonergic system

A key biological correlate of the diathesis for suicidal behaviour appears to be low serotonergic activity. Abnormal serotonergic function may be the result of numerous factors, including genetics, early life experience, chronic medical illness, alcohol use disorders, or substance use disorder, many of which have been correlated with an increased risk for suicidal behaviour. Moreover, serotonergic dysfunction may underlie recurrent mood disorders, as well as behavioural traits that characterize the diathesis such as aggression, pessimism and dysfunctional attitudes, hopelessness, and deficits in decision-making.

Serotonin is involved in brain development, behavioural regulation, sleep, mood, anxiety, cognition, and memory and is shown to be disturbed in various psychiatric disorders. Serotonergic function is under genetic control, and moreover deficits in functioning have been shown to be enduring, marking it as a biological trait. The serotonergic system became a target for investigation in relation to suicide when, more than 40 years ago, Asberg and colleagues observed that depressed individuals who had either attempted suicide by violent means or subsequently died by suicide in the study follow-up period were more likely to have lower 5-hydroxyindoleacetic acid (5-HIAA) levels in the cerebrospinal fluid (CSF) [3]. Since that time, the function of the serotonergic system in suicide and attempted suicide has been examined in many paradigms, and while not all studies agree, there is substantial consensus that individuals who die by suicide, or make serious non-fatal suicide attempts, exhibit a deficiency in CNS serotonin neurotransmission.

Evidence of hypofunction comes from CSF and post-mortem studies. 5-HIAA is the major metabolite of serotonin, and the level of CSF 5-HIAA is a guide to serotonin activity in parts of the brain, including the prefrontal cortex. There have been over 20 studies of CSF 5-HIAA and suicidal behaviour in mood disorders, and a meta-analysis of prospective studies of 5-HIAA found that in mood disorders, lower CSF 5-HIAA levels increased the chance of death by suicide by over 4-fold over follow-up periods of 1–14 years [4].

Several post-mortem studies of suicide have reported lower brainstem levels of 5-HIAA and/or serotonin [5-hydroxytryptamine (5-HT)] (for a review, see [5]). These deficits in 5-HT or 5-HIAA are observable across diagnostic groups [6] and, despite early reports to the contrary, appear to be independent of the suicide method. A limitation of these studies is that they did not use toxicological sensitive assays of brain tissue or psychological autopsy interviews to rule out recent antemortem antidepressant exposure which would potentially lower 5-HIAA levels. A more recent study that carefully ruled out such medication exposure found higher levels of 5-HT and 5-HIAA in the brainstem of depressed suicides [7]. This observation appears to be largely specific to the brainstem, because no differences are generally found between suicides and controls in 5-HT level in other brain regions, including the hippocampus, occipital cortex, frontal cortex, temporal cortex, caudate, striatum, or hypothalamus [5]. Serotonin neuron cell bodies are in the brainstem raphe nuclei, while their axons innervate most of the brain, including the ventral prefrontal cortex. Morphological analysis of stained serotonin neurons in the brainstem of depressed suicides and non-suicides observed greater cell density in the dorsal raphe nucleus in suicides [8] and greater expression of the rate-limiting biosynthetic enzyme for serotonin—tryptophan hydroxylase—per neuron [9], suggesting that reduction in serotonin activity is associated with dysfunctional cells, and not with fewer neurons. That observation is consistent with the report of more 5-HT in the brainstem of suicides [7].

Neuroendocrine challenge studies using fenfluramine provide further evidence of anomalous serotonergic function associated with suicidal behaviour. Fenfluramine is a serotonin-releasing agent and a reuptake inhibitor that may also directly stimulate post-synaptic 5-HT receptors. The release of serotonin by fenfluramine causes an increase in serum prolactin levels that is an indirect index of central serotonergic responsiveness. In depressed patients, those with a history of suicide attempts have a more blunted prolactin response to fenfluramine challenge than non-attempters, with evidence that the effect is more related to lethality of past suicide attempts [10].

Lower serotonergic transmission in the central nervous system (CNS) may be accompanied by a compensatory upregulation of some serotonergic post-synaptic receptors, such as 5-$HT_{1A}$ and 5-$HT_{2A}$ receptors, and a decrease in the number of serotonin transporters [5]. There is a reported increase in the concentration of post-synaptic 5-$HT_{2A}$ receptors in the prefrontal cortex of suicides, compared with non-suicides [11]. This increased binding is reflected in more protein and may be due to elevated gene expression in young suicides [12]. Elevated 5-$HT_{2A}$ binding has also been reported in the amygdala in depressed suicides [13]. In depressed and non-depressed suicides, there is evidence that 5-$HT_{2A}$ receptors are upregulated in the dorsal prefrontal cortex, but not the rostral prefrontal cortex [11].

Platelet studies examine 5-$HT_{2A}$ in living subjects with respect to non-fatal suicide attempt. 5-$HT_{2A}$ receptors, serotonin reuptake sites, and serotonin second messenger systems are present in blood platelets, and changes in these platelet measurements may reflect similar changes in the CNS. Multiple studies have reported higher platelet 5-$HT_{2A}$ receptor numbers in suicide attempters, compared with non-attempters and healthy controls [14].

Studies of second messengers indicated impaired 5-$HT_{2A}$ receptor-mediated signal transduction in the prefrontal cortex of suicides [15], and in platelets, 5-$HT_{2A}$ receptor responsivity is significantly blunted in patients with major depression who have made high-lethality suicide attempts, compared to depressed patients who have made low-lethality suicide attempts [16]. The implications of such a defect in signal transduction, if present in the brain, would be that although there may be greater density of 5-$HT_{2A}$ receptors, the signal transduced by 5-$HT_{2A}$ receptor activation may be blunted.

Some post-mortem studies of the post-synaptic 5-$HT_{1A}$ receptor have reported higher binding in the prefrontal cortex and more rostral segments of the raphe nuclei, and lower binding in the more caudal raphe nuclei, hippocampus, prefrontal cortex, and temporal cortex [17]. Less 5-$HT_{1A}$ auto-receptor gene expression has also been reported in the dorsal raphe [18] and would favour higher serotonin neuron firing rates.

Post-mortem studies of depressed suicides reported fewer 5-HT transporters in the prefrontal cortex, hypothalamus, occipital cortex, and brainstem [19]. Moreover, in suicides, this deficit appears localized to the ventromedial prefrontal cortex and anterior cingulate, whereas depressed individuals who died of other causes had lower binding throughout the prefrontal cortex [20].

The emerging picture from post-mortem studies of greater 5-$HT_{2A}$ receptor binding in the frontal cortex of depressed individuals who die by suicide, fewer brainstem 5-$HT_{1A}$ auto-receptors, and fewer serotonin transporters in the cortex, as well as findings of greater tryptophan hydroxylase (the rate-limiting step in serotonin synthesis) immunoreactivity in serotonin nuclei in the brainstem [9], all point to homeostatic changes designed to increase deficient serotonergic transmission, evidenced by low 5-HIAA in the CSF and brain, and blunted prolactin response to fenfluramine challenge.

### Serotonergic dysfunction and suicide endophenotypes

Reactive aggressive traits are potentially part of the diathesis for suicidal behaviour [1]. Increased aggression has been associated with suicide and more highly lethal suicide attempts, and impulsivity has shown a stronger relationship to non-fatal suicide attempts [21]. Reduced activity of the serotonergic system has been implicated in impulsive violence and aggression in studies in a variety of paradigms, including: low CSF 5-HIAA levels in individuals with a lifetime history of aggressive behaviour with personality and other psychiatric disorders [22, 23]; a blunted prolactin response to the serotonin-releasing agent fenfluramine in personality disorder patients [24, 25]; and greater platelet 5-$HT_{2A}$ binding correlated with aggressive behaviour in personality and other psychiatric disorder patients [26, 27]. In a post-mortem study of aggression, suicidal behaviour, and serotonergic function, a positive relationship was found between lifetime history of aggression scores and 5-$HT_{2A}$ binding in several regions of the prefrontal cortex of individuals who had died by suicide [28].

Positron emission tomography (PET) studies have shown a deficient response to serotonergic challenge in the orbitofrontal cortex and medial frontal and cingulate regions in individuals with impulsive aggression, compared to controls [29, 30], and lower serotonin transporter binding in the anterior cingulate cortex in impulsive and aggressive individuals, compared to healthy controls [31]. The prefrontal cortex is important in the inhibitory control of behaviour, including impulsive and aggressive behaviour [32]. Thus, aggressive/impulsive traits, related to serotonergic dysfunction, are potentially an aspect of the diathesis for suicidal behaviour, whereby aggressive/suicidal behaviour is manifested in response to stressful circumstances or powerful emotions. This tendency might be conceived of as a diminution in brain inhibitory circuits or as a volatile cognitive decision-making trait.

## Noradrenergic system

According to the stress–diathesis model of suicidal behaviour, it is the confluence of stressful events with the diathesis that is thought to precipitate a suicidal act. Thus, investigating the functioning of stress response systems in suicidal individuals is important for elucidating neurobiological concomitants of suicidal behaviour and identifying targets for preventative intervention. The noradrenergic system and the hypothalamus–pituitary–adrenal (HPA) axis are two key stress response systems.

The majority of noradrenaline neurons in the brain are located in the brainstem's locus caeruleus. Post-mortem studies of suicides have documented fewer noradrenergic neurons in the rostral locus caeruleus, the part that projects to the brain [33]. There are also indications of cortical noradrenergic overactivity, including lower α- and high-affinity $β_1$-adrenergic receptor binding [34], and lower β-adrenoceptor density and $α_2$-adrenergic binding in the prefrontal cortex in individuals who died by suicide [35]. There is some, but not unanimous, evidence from prospective studies of lower CSF levels of 3-methoxy-4-hydroxyphenylglycol (MHPG), a metabolite of noradrenaline, in future suicides [36], although not in those making non-fatal suicide attempts [37]. Low CSF MHPG levels predict both the probability of a suicide attempt and the lethality of the attempt.

Fewer noradrenergic neurons observed in depressed suicides may indicate a lower functional reserve of the noradrenergic system, which, if accompanied by an exaggerated stress response with a greater release of noradrenaline, may result in noradrenaline depletion, leading to depression and hopelessness, both of which are contributory factors to suicidal behaviour.

Noradrenergic response to stress in adulthood appears to be greater in those reporting an abusive experience in childhood [38]. Such individuals are potentially at greater risk in adulthood for major depression and suicidal behaviour. Childhood abuse may be associated with an increased risk for depression and suicidal behaviour because of a dysfunctional stress response both via the noradrenergic system and via the HPA axis, and secondary effects of noradrenaline depletion and elevated cortisol levels. There is interaction between the noradrenergic system and the stress response activity of the HPA axis, with reciprocal neural connections between corticotropin-releasing hormone (CRH) neurons in the hypothalamic paraventricular nucleus and noradrenergic neurons in the human brainstem and locus caeruleus [39].

## The hypothalamic–pituitary–adrenal axis

The HPA axis is a major stress response system. Major depression is associated with hyperactivity of the HPA axis [40], and suicidal patients in diagnostically heterogenous populations exhibit HPA axis abnormalities, most commonly failure to suppress cortisol normally after dexamethasone [36]. We found most future suicides were dexamethasone suppression test (DST) non-suppressors [4]. In mood disorders, DST non-suppressors had a 4.5-fold greater risk of dying by suicide, compared with suppressors [4]. Moreover, non-suppression may be characteristic of more serious attempts that result in greater medical damage [41, 42] or the use of violent methods in the suicide attempt [43]. In other indices of HPA axis function, suicide attempters had attenuated plasma cortisol responses to fenfluramine, although that may indicate less serotonin release, and not an HPA abnormality [44, 45], and lower CSF CRH levels, compared to non-attempters [46], though not all studies agree.

Larger pituitary and adrenal gland volumes have been reported in depressed suicides [47, 48] and fewer CRH binding sites in the prefrontal cortex of depressed suicide victims, which may mean receptor downregulation due to elevated corticotropin-releasing factor (CRF) release [49].

As with the noradrenergic system, early life adversity appears to have lasting effects on stress response in the HPA axis in adulthood. Abnormalities in HPA axis function have been implicated in poor response to drug treatment and a greater likelihood of relapse in major depression, both of which increase the risk for suicidal acts [36]. Increased anxiety and agitation reflect another potential pathway whereby an abnormal stress response, in both the noradrenergic and the HPA axis, contributes to risk for suicidal behaviour.

## Other biologic systems

Abnormality in the dopaminergic system has been reported in depressive disorders [50]. However, studies of dopaminergic function and suicidal behaviour are relatively few and inconclusive [5]. Low dihydroxyphenylacetic acid levels, indicative of reduced dopamine turnover, in the caudate, putamen, and nucleus accumbens have been reported in depressed suicides [51], although the same group of investigators found no difference in number or affinity of the dopamine transporters [52]. Accordingly, it is unlikely that the reduced dopamine turnover initially observed in depressed suicides is a result of decreased dopaminergic innervation of those regions. Prospective studies disagree as to whether CSF homovanillic acid (HVA) levels predict suicidal behaviour [53–55]. Low CSF HVA levels may be related to higher lethality suicide attempts in males.

There is a well-documented relationship between thyroid dysfunction and depression [56], and some studies have linked thyroid function and suicide. Abnormal thyroid-stimulating hormone (TSH) response to thyrotropin-releasing hormone (TRH) has been observed in individuals who died by suicide in a follow-up study [57]. Abnormal TSH response to challenge tests has also been associated with poor response to antidepressant treatment and a higher relapse rate which may increase the risk for suicidal behaviour [58].

Neurotrophins are involved in brain development and growth, neuronal functioning, and synaptic plasticity. Lower protein levels and gene expression of brain-derived neurotrophic factor (BDNF) in the prefrontal cortex and hippocampus [59, 60] and less mRNA of nerve growth factor, neurotrophin 3, and neurotrophin 4/5 in the hippocampus [61] have been reported post-mortem in suicides. Lower plasma BDNF levels have been reported in major depressive disorder (MDD) suicide attempters, compared to MDD non-attempters and healthy controls [62].

Suicide is more common in groups with very low cholesterol levels or after cholesterol lowering by diet (for a review, see [63]). This relationship between cholesterol levels and suicide may be mediated by serotonergic function, as studies of non-human primates on a low-fat diet found lower serotonergic activity and increased aggressive behaviours [64]. Long-chain polyunsaturated fatty acids, particularly omega-3 [docosahexaenoic acid (DHA)], may also be a mediating factor in the relationship between low cholesterol levels and increased risk for depression and suicide [65]. A decrease in DHA concentration was associated with a 14% increased risk for suicide death for every standard deviation decrease in DHA level in a large study of military suicides in the United States [66]. However, other post-mortem studies did not find any association [5]. Lower DHA percentage of total plasma polyunsaturated fatty acids and a higher omega-6:omega-3 ratio predicted depressed individuals who made a suicide attempt during a 2-year follow-up [67], and lower eicosapentaenoic acid is found in red blood cells of suicide attempters, compared to controls [68].

Other potential candidate neurobiological systems for investigation with respect to suicidal behaviour come from genetic studies. One novel approach examined the correlations between candidate genes and gene expression in the prefrontal cortex of suicides, with the aim to identify correlations that were independent of mood disorder diagnosis [69]. That study identified genes related to suicidal behaviour which had not been previously identified in candidate gene studies of suicide, but which did overlap with the broad biologic domains identified in earlier expression studies in suicide, including CNS development, homophilic cell adhesion, regulation of cell proliferation, and transmission of nerve impulse [69–71]. Other recent work points to potential involvement of the immune system, for example *CD44*, a gene connected with the immune system that has been identified in three studies of suicides, and Galfalvy *et al.* additionally found its expression in both BA9 and BA24 was significantly low [69]. Immune system dysregulation has been reported in major depression [72, 73], but there has been little investigation of its role in suicide. The inflammatory and neurodegenerative hypothesis of depression hypothesizes that neurodegeneration and reduced neurogenesis are caused by inflammation, cell-mediated immune activation, and their long-term sequelae [74]. Disordered neuroimmune function may be present in suicide, and its pathogenesis related to genes identified in these studies. Finally, another area of emerging interest is a possible link between suicide and allergic reactions that may alter the function of the orbital prefrontal cortex [75, 76].

## Neurobiology, genetics, and suicidal behaviour

Family, twin, and adoption studies support a genetic contribution to suicidal behaviour, independent of psychiatric disorder (for a review, see [77]), and genetic studies have sought to determine the responsible genes for suicide and suicide attempt though linkage and single-nucleotide polymorphism (SNP) association studies. Candidate genes for most studies were selected based on evidence from neurobiological studies in suicide, as a result of which the serotonergic system has been the most extensively investigated. A tri-allelic polymorphism in the serotonin transporter promoter has two alleles with lower transcriptional activity and fewer transporters. In varied psychiatric populations, despite some negative findings, the S, or the more common lower-expressing allele, has been associated with suicide and suicide attempts, particularly violent or high-lethality attempts [78]. Functional MRI studies have found greater amygdala activation in individuals with the SS genotype when they were exposed to negative stimuli such as angry or fearful faces, negative words, or aversive pictures (for a review, see [79]). The amygdala is densely innervated by serotonergic neurons and 5-HT receptors are abundant, and the amygdala plays a central role in emotional regulation and memory. Excessive responses to emotionally negative events, such as abuse, may be over-encoded and contribute to stress sensitivity in adulthood, and thereby to major depression after stress and even suicidal behaviour.

Other genetic studies of the serotonergic system, including 5-$HT_{1A}$, 5-$HT_{2A}$, 5-$HT_{1B}$, and other serotonin receptors, have largely reported negative results, although there have been some positive findings for the 5-$HT_{2A}$ 102C allele and attempted suicide or suicidal ideation [78]. For tryptophan hydroxylase (TPH1 and TPH2 are the two forms of tryptophan hydroxylase, with TPH1 only expressed in the brain during development), associations have

been reported with suicide and suicide attempt and TPH1 SNPs; however, multiple negative findings have also been reported. Haplotype and SNP studies have suggested the involvement of the *TPH2* gene in suicide and suicide attempt; however, again not all studies agree [78]. Monoamine oxidase A (MAO-A) plays a key role in the metabolism of amines. Low MAO activity results in elevated levels of serotonin, noradrenaline, and dopamine in the brain. The *MAO-A* gene has functional variable number of tandem repeats; however, no association has been found between this upstream variable number of tandem repeats (uVNTR) and suicidal behaviour, although there is some indication that it may be related to aggression [78], and it is linked to the impact of adversity in childhood on adult antisocial behaviour and trait impulsiveness [80, 81].

Genetic studies on the dopaminergic system, noradrenergic system, and BDNF are few and generally negative [78], although there are reports of a positive association of the catechol-*O*-methyltransferase (*COMT*), a major catecholamine-catabolic enzyme, gene in Finnish and Caucasian suicide attempters [82] and Japanese suicides [83]. A recent study implicates gamma aminobutyric acid (GABA)- and glutamate-related genes and suicidal behaviour [84]. Inconsistent findings in genetic studies of suicidal behaviour may be due to the complexity of the suicide phenotype, gene–gene interactions, the presence of multiple psychiatric disorders, population racial differences, possible epigenetic effects, and the influence of gene/environment interactions. Nonetheless, new microarray technologies that test the expression of thousands of genes simultaneously, allowing better gene coverage, and haplotype mapping approaches offer promise for future investigation. Other options include examining more basic endophenotypes such as mood regulation and decision-making.

## Genes and environment

Early life stress, in conjunction with genetic vulnerability, can have enduring effects into adulthood and affect psychopathology and the functioning of biologic systems, including the serotonergic and stress response systems [85]. For example, monkeys exposed to maternal deprivation in infancy and having the 5-HTTLPR lower-expressing S allele in the serotonin transporter gene manifested a lowering of CSF 5-HIAA levels that persisted into adulthood [86]. In 6-month-old macaque monkeys exposed to social stress, those with the S allele had a higher adrenocorticotrophic hormone (ACTH) response, an HPA axis hormone related to stress response, compared with those without that allele and S allele animals who were maternally reared [87]. Thus, the low-expressing S allele not only increased vulnerability to stress in development, but early life stress may also further interact with the genotype to lower the serotonergic function and increase the sensitivity to stressful events later in life, both of which are risk factors for suicidal behaviour.

In human studies, among individuals who had experienced childhood maltreatment, those with the low-expressing S allele were at risk for suicidal ideation and suicide attempt [88], and those with a lower-expressing variant of the *MAO-A* gene were more likely to manifest antisocial behaviour and more impulsivity as adults [80, 81].

## Future directions

There is much still to be learnt about the biologic aetiology of suicidal behaviour and the pathways and mechanisms through which biologic dysfunction is involved in suicidal acts. New techniques for imaging the brain, identification of basic intermediate phenotypes, and denser gene markers will contribute to elucidating the biologic factors and mechanisms involved in suicide and attempted suicide and identifying potential targets for prevention.

## REFERENCES

1. Mann JJ, Waternaux C, Haas GL, Malone KM. Toward a clinical model of suicidal behavior in psychiatric patients. *Am J Psychiatry*. 1999;156:181–9.
2. van Heeringen K, Mann JJ. The neurobiology of suicide. *Lancet Psychiatry*. 2014;1:63–72.
3. Asberg M, Thoren P, Traskman L, Bertilsson L, Ringberger V. 'Serotonin depression'—a biochemical subgroup within the affective disorders? *Science*. 1976;191:478–80.
4. Mann JJ, Currier D, Stanley B, Oquendo MA, Amsel LV, Ellis SP. Can biological tests assist prediction of suicide in mood disorders? *Int J Neuropsychopharmacol*. 2006;9:465–74.
5. Oquendo MA, Sullivan GM, Sudol K, *et al.* Toward a biosignature for suicide. *Am J Psychiatry*. 2014;171:1259–77.
6. Mann JJ, Brent DA, Arango V. The neurobiology and genetics of suicide and attempted suicide: a focus on the serotonergic system. *Neuropsychopharmacology*. 2001;24:467–77.
7. Bach H, Huang YY, Underwood MD, Dwork AJ, Mann JJ, Arango V. Elevated serotonin and 5-HIAA in the brainstem and lower serotonin turnover in the prefrontal cortex of suicides. *Synapse*. 2014;68:127–30.
8. Arango V, Underwood MD, Gubbi AV, Mann JJ. Localized alterations in pre- and postsynaptic serotonin binding sites in the ventrolateral prefrontal cortex of suicide victims. *Brain Res*. 1995;688:121–33.
9. Boldrini M, Underwood MD, Mann JJ, Arango V. More tryptophan hydroxylase in the brainstem dorsal raphe nucleus in depressed suicides. *Brain Res*. 2005;1041:19–28.
10. Kamali M, Oquendo MA, Mann JJ. Understanding the neurobiology of suicidal behavior. *Depress Anxiety*. 2001;14:164–76.
11. Stockmeier CA. Involvement of serotonin in depression: evidence from postmortem and imaging studies of serotonin receptors and the serotonin transporter. *J Psychiatr Res*. 2003;37:357–73.
12. Pandey GN, Dwivedi Y, Rizavi HS, *et al.* Higher expression of serotonin 5-HT(2A) receptors in the postmortem brains of teenage suicide victims. *Am J Psychiatry*. 2002;159:419–29.
13. Hrdina PD, Demeter E, Vu TB, S¢t¢nyi P, Palkovits M. 5-HT uptake sites and 5-HT 2 receptors in brain of antidepressant- free suicide victims/depressives: increase in 5- HT2 sites in cortex and amygdala. *Brain Res*. 1993;614:37–44.
14. Pandey GN. Altered serotonin function in suicide. Evidence from platelet and neuroendocrine studies. *Ann N Y Acad Sci*. 1997;836:182–200.
15. Pandey GN, Dwivedi Y, Pandey SC, *et al.* Low phosphoinositide-specific phospholipase C activity and expression of phospholipase C beta1 protein in the prefrontal cortex of teenage suicide subjects. *Am J Psychiatry*. 1999;156:1895–901.
16. Malone KM, Ellis SP, Currier D, John Mann J. Platelet 5-HT2A receptor subresponsivity and lethality of attempted suicide in depressed in-patients. *Int J Neuropsychopharmacol*. 2007;10:335–43.
17. Furczyk K, Schutova B, Michel TM, Thome J, Buttner A. The neurobiology of suicide—a review of post-mortem studies. *J Mol Psychiatry*. 2013;1:2.
18. Arango V, Underwood MD, Boldrini M, *et al.* Serotonin 1A receptors, serotonin transporter binding and serotonin transporter mRNA expression in the brainstem of depressed suicide victims. *Neuropsychopharmacology*. 2001;25:892–903.
19. Purselle DC, Nemeroff CB. Serotonin transporter: a potential substrate in the biology of suicide. *Neuropsychopharmacology*. 2003;28:613–19.
20. Mann JJ, Huang YY, Underwood MD, *et al.* A serotonin transporter gene promoter polymorphism (5-HTTLPR) and prefrontal cortical binding in major depression and suicide. *Arch Gen Psychiatry*. 2000;57:729–38.
21. Oquendo MA, Galfalvy H, Russo S, *et al.* Prospective study of clinical predictors of suicidal acts after a major depressive episode in patients with major depressive disorder or bipolar disorder. *Am J Psychiatry*. 2004;161:1433–41.
22. Brown GL, Goodwin FK. Cerebrospinal fluid correlates of suicide attempts and aggression. *Ann N Y Acad Sci*. 1986;487:175–88.
23. Stanley B, Molcho A, Stanley M, *et al.* Association of aggressive behavior with altered serotonergic function in patients who are not suicidal. *Am J Psychiatry*. 2000;157:609–14.
24. Coccaro EF, Siever LJ, Klar HM, *et al.* Serotonergic studies in patients with affective and personality disorders. Correlates with suicidal and impulsive aggressive behavior. *Arch Gen Psychiatry*. 1989;46:587–99.
25. New AS, Trestman RF, Mitropoulou V, *et al.* Low prolactin response to fenfluramine in impulsive aggression. *J Psychiatr Res*. 2004;38:223–30.
26. Coccaro EF, Kavoussi RJ, Sheline YI, Berman ME, Csernansky JG. Impulsive aggression in personality disorder correlates with platelet 5-HT 2A receptor binding. *Neuropsychopharmacology*. 1997;16:211–16.
27. McBride PA, Brown RP, DeMeo M, Keilp JG, Mieczkowski T, Mann JJ. The relationship of platelet 5-HT 2 receptor indices to major depressive disorder, personality traits, and suicidal behavior. *Biol Psychiatry*. 1994;35:295–308.
28. Oquendo MA, Russo SA, Underwood MD, *et al.* Higher postmortem prefrontal 5-HT2A receptor binding correlates with lifetime aggression in suicide. *Biol Psychiatry*. 2006;59:235–43.
29. Siever LJ, Buchsbaum MS, New AS, *et al.* d,1-fenfluramine response in impulsive personality disorder assessed with [18 F]fluorodeoxyglucose positron emission tomography. *Neuropsychopharmacology*. 1999;20:413–23.
30. New AS, Hazlett EA, Buchsbaum MS, *et al.* Blunted prefrontal cortical 18fluorodeoxyglucose positron emission tomography response to meta-chlorophenylpiperazine in impulsive aggression. *Arch Gen Psychiatry*. 2002;59:621–9.
31. Frankle WG, Lombardo I, New AS, *et al.* Brain serotonin transporter distribution in subjects with impulsive aggressivity: a positron emission study with [11C]McN 5652. *Am J Psychiatry*. 2005;162:915–23.
32. de Almeida RM, Rosa MM, Santos DM, Saft DM, Benini Q, Miczek KA. 5-HT(1B) receptors, ventral orbitofrontal cortex, and aggressive behavior in mice. *Psychopharmacology (Berl)*. 2006;185:441–50.
33. Arango V, Underwood MD, Mann JJ. Fewer pigmented locus coeruleus neurons in suicide victims: preliminary results. *Biol Psychiatry*. 1996;39:112–20.

34. Arango V, Ernsberger P, Sved AF, Mann JJ. Quantitative auto-radiography of alpha 1- and alpha 2-adrenergic receptors in the cerebral cortex of controls and suicide victims. *Brain Res.* 1993;630:271–82.

35. De Paermentier F, Cheetham SC, Crompton MR, Katona CL, Horton RW. Brain beta-adrenoceptor binding sites in antidepressant-free depressed suicide victims *Brain Res.* 1990;525:71–7.

36. Mann JJ, Currier D. A review of prospective studies of biologic predictors of suicidal behavior in mood disorders. *Arch Suicide Res.* 2007;11:3–16.

37. Lester D. The concentration of neurotransmitter metabolites in the cerebrospinal fluid of suicidal individuals: a meta-analysis. *Pharmacopsychiatry.* 1995;28:77–9.

38. Heim C, Nemeroff CB. The role of childhood trauma in the neurobiology of mood and anxiety disorders: preclinical and clinical studies. *Biol Psychiatry.* 2001;49:1023–39.

39. Austin MC, Rice PM, Mann JJ, Arango V. Localization of corticotropin-releasing hormone in the human locus coeruleus and pedunculopontine tegmental nucleus: an immunocytochemical and *in situ* hybridization study. *Neuroscience.* 1995;64:713–27.

40. Carroll BJ, Feinberg M, Greden JF, et al. A specific laboratory test for the diagnosis of melancholia. Standardization, validation, and clinical utility. *Arch Gen Psychiatry.* 1981;38:15–22.

41. Norman WH, Brown WA, Miller IW, Keitner GI, Overholser JC. The dexamethasone suppression test and completed suicide. *Acta Psychiatr Scand.* 1990;81:120–5.

42. Coryell W. DST abnormality as a predictor of course in major depression. *J Affect Disord.* 1990;19:163–9.

43. Roy A. Hypothalamic-pituitary-adrenal axis function and suicidal behavior in depression. *Biol Psychiatry.* 1992;32:812–16.

44. Duval F, Mokrani MC, Correa H, et al. Lack of effect of HPA axis hyperactivity on hormonal responses to d-fenfluramine in major depressed patients: implications for pathogenesis of suicidal behaviour. *Psychoneuroendocrinology.* 2001;26:521–37.

45. Malone KM, Corbitt EM, Li S, Mann JJ. Prolactin response to fenfluramine and suicide attempt lethality in major depression. *Br J Psychiatry.* 1996;168:324–9.

46. Brunner J, Stalla GK, Stalla J, et al. Decreased corticotropin-releasing hormone (CRH) concentrations in the cerebrospinal fluid of eucortisolemic suicide attempters. *J Psychiatr Res.* 2001;35:1–9.

47. Szigethy E, Conwell Y, Forbes NT, Cox C, Caine ED. Adrenal weight and morphology in victims of completed suicide. *Biol Psychiatry.* 1994;36:374–80.

48. Dumser T, Barocka A, Schubert E. Weight of adrenal glands may be increased in persons who commit suicide. *Am J Forensic Med Pathol.* 1998;19:72–6.

49. Nemeroff CB, Owens MJ, Bissette G, Andorn AC, Stanley M. Reduced corticotropin releasing factor binding sites in the frontal cortex of suicide victims. *Arch Gen Psychiatry.* 1988;45:577–9.

50. Dailly E, Chenu F, Renard CE, Bourin M. Dopamine, depression and antidepressants. *Fundam Clin Pharmacol.* 2004;18:601–7.

51. Bowden C, Cheetham SC, Lowther S, Katona CL, Crompton MR, Horton RW. Reduced dopamine turnover in the basal ganglia of depressed suicides. *Brain Res.* 1997;769:135–40.

52. Bowden C, Theodorou AE, Cheetham SC, et al. Dopamine D1 and D2 receptor binding sites in brain samples from depressed suicides and controls. *Brain Res.* 1997;752:227–33.

53. Roy A, De Jong J, Linnoila M. Cerebrospinal fluid monoamine metabolites and suicidal behavior in depressed patients. A 5-year follow-up study. *Arch Gen Psychiatry.* 1989;46:609–12.

54. Engstrom G, Alling C, Blennow K, Regnell G, Traskman-Bendz L. Reduced cerebrospinal HVA concentrations and HVA/5-HIAA ratios in suicide attempters. Monoamine metabolites in 120 suicide attempters and 47 controls. *Eur Neuropsychopharmacology.* 1999;9:399–405.

55. Placidi GP, Oquendo MA, Malone KM, Huang YY, Ellis SP, Mann JJ. Aggressivity, suicide attempts, and depression: relationship to cerebrospinal fluid monoamine metabolite levels. *Biol Psychiatry.* 2001;50:783–91.

56. Jackson IM. The thyroid axis and depression. *Thyroid.* 1998;8:951–6.

57. Linkowski P, Van Wettere JP, Kerkhofs M, Gregoire F, Brauman H, Mendlewicz J. Violent suicidal behavior and the thyrotropin-releasing hormone-thyroid-stimulating hormone test: a clinical outcome study. *Neuropsychobiology.* 1984;12:19–22.

58. Targum SD. Persistent neuroendocrine dysregulation in major depressive disorder: a marker for early relapse. *Biol Psychiatry.* 1984;19:305–18.

59. Dwivedi Y, Rizavi HS, Conley RR, Roberts RC, Tamminga CA, Pandey GN. Altered gene expression of brain-derived neuro-trophic factor and receptor tyrosine kinase B in postmortem brain of suicide subjects. *Arch Gen Psychiatry.* 2003;60:804–15.

60. Karege F, Vaudan G, Schwald M, Perroud N, La Harpe R. Neurotrophin levels in postmortem brains of suicide victims and the effects of antemortem diagnosis and psychotropic drugs. *Brain Res Mol Brain Res.* 2005;136:29–37.

61. Dwivedi Y, Mondal AC, Rizavi HS, Conley RR. Suicide brain is associated with decreased expression of neurotrophins. *Biol Psychiatry.* 2005;58:315–24.

62. Kim YK, Lee HP, Won SD, Park EY, Lee HY, Lee BH, et al. Low plasma BDNF is associated with suicidal behavior in major depression. *Prog Neuropsychopharmacol Biol Psychiatry.* 2007;31:78–85.

63. Golomb BA. Cholesterol and violence: is there a connection? *Ann Intern Med.* 1998;128:478–87.

64. Muldoon MF, Rossouw JE, Manuck SB, Glueck CJ, Kaplan JR, Kaufmann PG. Low or lowered cholesterol and risk of death from suicide and trauma. *Metabolism.* 1993;42 Suppl. 1:45–56.

65. Brunner J, Parhofer KG, Schwandt P, Bronisch T. Cholesterol, essential fatty acids, and suicide. *Pharmacopsychiatry.* 2002;35:1–5.

66. Lewis MD, Hibbeln JR, Johnson JE, Lin YH, Hyun DY, Loewke JD. Suicide deaths of active-duty US military and omega-3 fatty-acid status: a case-control comparison. *J Clin Psychiatry.* 2011;72:1585–90.

67. Sublette ME, Hibbeln JR, Galfalvy H, Oquendo MA, Mann JJ. Omega-3 polyunsaturated essential Fatty Acid status as a predictor of future suicide risk. *Am J Psychiatry.* 2006;163:1100–2.

68. Huan M, Hamazaki K, Sun Y, et al. Suicide attempt and n-3 fatty acid levels in red blood cells: a case control study in China. *Biol Psychiatry.* 2004;56:490–6.

69. Galfalvy H, Zalsman G, Huang YY, et al. A pilot genome wide association and gene expression array study of suicide with and without major depression. *World J Biol Psychiatry.* 2013;14:574–82.

70. Sequeira A, Klempan T, Canetti L, et al. Patterns of gene expression in the limbic system of suicides with and without major depression. *Mol Psychiatry.* 2007;12:640–55.

71. Thalmeier A, Dickmann M, Giegling I, et al. Gene expression profiling of post-mortem orbitofrontal cortex in violent suicide victims. *Int J Neuropsychopharmacol.* 2008;11:217–28.

72. Mendlovic S, Doron A, Eilat E. Short note: can depressive patients exploit the immune system for suicide? *Med Hypotheses.* 1997;49:445–6.

73. Mendlovic S, Mozes E, Eilat E, *et al*. Immune activation in non-treated suicidal major depression. *Immunol Lett*. 1999;67:105–8.

74. Maes M. Inflammatory and oxidative and nitrosative stress pathways underpinning chronic fatigue, somatization and psychosomatic symptoms. *Curr Opin Psychiatry*. 2009;22:75–83.

75. Postolache TT, Lapidus M, Sander ER, *et al*. Changes in allergy symptoms and depression scores are positively correlated in patients with recurrent mood disorders exposed to seasonal peaks in aeroallergens. *Sci World J*. 2007;7:1968–77.

76. Postolache TT, Mortensen PB, Tonelli LH, *et al*. Seasonal spring peaks of suicide in victims with and without prior history of hospitalization for mood disorders. *J Affect Disord*. 2010;121:88–93.

77. Brent DA, Mann JJ. Family genetic studies, suicide, and suicidal behavior. *Am J Med Genet C Semin Med Genet*. 2005;133:13–24.

78. Bondy B, Buettner A, Zill P. Genetics of suicide. *Mol Psychiatry*. 2006;11:336–51.

79. Brown SM, Hariri AR. Neuroimaging studies of serotonin gene polymorphisms: exploring the interplay of genes, brain, and behavior. *Cogn Affect Behav Neurosci*. 2006;6:44–52.

80. Caspi A, McClay J, Moffitt TE, *et al*. Role of genotype in the cycle of violence in maltreated children. *Science*. 2002;297:851–4.

81. Huang YY, Cate SP, Battistuzzi C, Oquendo MA, Brent D, Mann JJ. An association between a functional polymorphism in the monoamine oxidase a gene promoter, impulsive traits and early abuse experiences. *Neuropsychopharmacology*. 2004;29:1498–505.

82. Nolan KA, Volavka J, Czobor P, *et al*. Suicidal behavior in patients with schizophrenia is related to COMT polymorphism. *Psychiatr Genet*. 2000;10:117–24.

83. Ono H, Shirakawa O, Nushida H, Ueno Y, Maeda K. Association between catechol-O-methyltransferase functional polymorphism and male suicide completers *Neuropsychopharmacology*. 2004;29:1374–7.

84. Olivier B, Pattij T, Wood SJ, Oosting R, Sarnyai Z, Toth M. The 5-HT(1A) receptor knockout mouse and anxiety. *Behav Pharmacol*. 2001;12:439–50.

85. Mann JJ, Currier D. Effects of genes and stress on the neurobiology of depression. *Int Rev Neurobiol*. 2006;73:153–89.

86. Bennett AJ, Lesch KP, Heils A, *et al*. Early experience and serotonin transporter gene variation interact to influence primate CNS function. *Mol Psychiatry*. 2002;7:118–22.

87. Barr CS, Newman TK, Shannon C, *et al*. Rearing condition and rh5-HTTLPR interact to influence limbic-hypothalamic-pituitary-adrenal axis response to stress in infant macaques. *Biol Psychiatry*. 2004;55:733–8.

88. Caspi A, Sugden K, Moffitt TE, *et al*. Influence of life stress on depression: moderation by a polymorphism in the *5-HTT* gene. *Science*. 2003;301:386–9.

# 128

# Prevention of suicide and treatment following self-harm

*Keith Hawton, Kate E. A. Saunders, and Alexandra Pitman*

## Introduction

The World Health Organization (WHO) estimates that approximately 800,000 people die by suicide worldwide every year and regards suicide prevention as a major public health priority [1]. However, unlike other major causes of death such as cancer or heart disease, suicide is a behaviour, not a diagnosis, with a myriad of contributory factors. Although 87–91% of people who die by suicide are thought to have had a diagnosable mental disorder [2, 3], an understanding of the suicidal mind requires consideration of other key factors underlying a person's decision to take their life. Access to methods of suicide, cognitive style, social problems, and social modelling, for example, are all targets for interventions that interrupt the pathway from suicidal ideation to suicide attempt [4]. Therefore, a number of population and high-risk approaches have been employed, with varying degrees of success, and these are summarized in this chapter.

The design of interventions to prevent suicide and respond to those who self-harm is founded on an understanding of recent international trends in suicide and self-harm. These have been described in Chapters 125–127 in this section. The changing nature of the epidemiology of suicide, both at a national and an international level, means that interventions can become outdated and may fail to target groups that have become at risk. This requires ongoing surveillance of patterns of suicide, translated into appropriate and effective new intervention approaches. Most notably, emerging methods of suicide require a rapid response in terms of restricting access to means.

It is important to note that conventions regarding suicide and self-harm nomenclature differ both temporally and internationally. For simplicity, in this chapter, the term 'self-harm' is used to include any act of intentional non-fatal self-poisoning or self-injury, irrespective of the motive or degree of suicidal intent [5]. The term 'suicide' is used in the place of completed suicide or fatal suicide attempt. Given the relationship of suicide to self-harm, this chapter should be read in conjunction with Chapter 126 describing the epidemiology and management of self-harm.

## Prevention of suicidal behaviour

The WHO recommends that for national responses to suicide to be effective, a comprehensive multi-sectoral suicide prevention strategy is needed [1]. Their emphasis is on: restricting access to means of suicide, including pesticides, firearms, and certain medications; early identification and effective management of psychiatric disorders and harmful alcohol use; and social support for vulnerable individuals in communities. High-income countries have developed suicide prevention strategies that combine broad population or universal approaches with complementary high-risk or targeted prevention interventions, discussed further later in this chapter, with evidence favouring population strategies [6]. Relatively rapid changes in the epidemiology of suicide require suicide prevention strategies to be able to respond to emergent high-risk groups [6]. They must also be able to meet the needs of the diverse groups at risk of suicidal behaviour, ranging from those with experiences of early trauma in childhood, people in specific occupational groups, those facing acute life events, to those with debilitating mental illness, including those with prior self-harm. Interventions intended to reduce the risk of suicide in these groups are likely to have their effects mediated via improvements in wider mental health and social functioning. Because the risk of suicide varies by ethnic group [7], the effectiveness and cultural acceptability of specific suicide prevention interventions are likely to vary in different cultural settings. It is therefore important that tailored suicide prevention programmes are developed both nationally and for specific cultures sub-nationally. For example, among younger age groups, the male excess of suicides observed internationally is reversed in India and China [8], identifying young women in rural areas as requiring tailored suicide prevention interventions.

While ethical issues in relation to suicide prevention are not covered in detail in this chapter, it is important that they are recognized. The concept of rational suicide and whether suicide should always be prevented is particularly contentious. For example, in the Netherlands, where euthanasia or assisted suicide (EAS) is legal, EAS of psychiatric patients tends to occur in patients with complex and chronic psychiatric, medical, and psychosocial histories, predominantly women, and usually after discussion with multiple physicians, however often with disagreement between them [9].

## Principles of prevention

Broadly there are two approaches to suicide prevention (Box 128.1). One can distinguish between population approaches, which aim to decrease risk in the population as a whole, and high-risk group strategies, in which specific groups that are at increased risk are targeted. High-risk group strategies often appear more attractive and realistic. However, risk factors for many disorders are widely spread in the population and so the high-risk strategy tends to exclude a large number of people at moderate risk and is often ineffective in reducing the burden of a disease at the population level. Conversely, population strategies may appear more difficult to achieve but are more likely to be effective in reducing population levels of disease (see also Chapter 125).

It is unclear to what extent national suicide prevention programmes are effective, although evidence of effectiveness for specific components of such strategies is emerging [11]. An impressive programme, developed in Finland, was based on information from a detailed national study of all suicides in 1 year and included a wide range of elements [12]. The programme was evaluated as relatively successful [13]. In England, a national suicide prevention strategy with a suicide target was introduced in 2002 [14], followed by a revised strategy in 2012, although this time without a target [15]. Strategies have now been introduced in a large number of countries [1]. While prevention strategies are difficult to evaluate [16], there are indications that programmes for prevention of suicide on a national scale may be effective.

It is also important to note that suicide prevention is age-specific, and preventive interventions in different age groups are likely to differ.

---

**Box 128.1** Examples of strategies for prevention of suicide and attempted suicide

**Population strategies**
- Reducing the availability of means for suicide*
- Educating primary care physicians*
- Influencing media portrayal of suicide
- Educating the public about mental illness and its treatment
- Educational approaches in schools*
- Befriending agencies and telephone helplines

**High-risk strategies**
Prevention of suicide in:
- Patients with psychiatric disorders*
- Specific age groups
- Suicide attempters
- High-risk occupational groups
- Prisoners
- People bereaved by suicide

* Denotes those with established evidence supporting effectiveness [9, 10]

---

## Population strategies

### Reducing availability of means for suicide

This is the most widely discussed population strategy [17]. It is based on evidence that if the availability and/or danger of a popular method for suicide changes, then this tends to have an impact on suicide rates. The general principles of prevention through reducing the availability of means are firstly that if a dangerous means is available, then acts of self-harm are more likely to result in death, especially when they occur impulsively, and secondly that the eventual suicide rate in survivors of serious attempts is remarkably low. Also the common adage that if people are intent on dying by suicide they will find a means is not borne out by the evidence on the effectiveness of means restriction. The success of policies to restrict access to specific means will depend on what other means are available, their relative lethality, and the extent to which substitution of a method occurs. The following are some examples of impacts of means restriction policies.

### Gas

Perhaps the clearest example of the potential effectiveness of restricting access to a common method of suicide was the reduction in suicides in the UK which occurred in the 1960s and early 1970s when toxic coal gas supplies were gradually replaced with non-toxic North Sea gas [18]. Prior to this time, coal gas poisoning through people placing their head in a gas oven was the most common method of suicide in the UK. As North Sea gas was gradually introduced, the suicide rate dropped steadily, eventually being reduced by approximately a third [18]. It is estimated that as many as 6000 deaths may have been prevented by this change [18]. The effect also illustrates the point that when one method of suicide is no longer available, people do not automatically turn to another, or if they do, it may be to one that is less likely to cause death. Thus, it was some years before the suicide rate rose again, this being related to an increase in deaths from poisoning with carbon monoxide from car exhausts. Another factor that may have been relevant to the decline in suicides was the reduction in prescribing of barbiturates, these being replaced by far less toxic benzodiazepines.

Suicide by carbon monoxide poisoning from car exhausts used to be a common method. However, this became less common as cars were fitted with catalytic converters, which detoxify the exhaust gas. This resulted in a decline in suicide rates in countries where this method of suicide had become more common, particularly in young males [19].

### Firearms

The widespread availability of guns in certain countries, particularly the United States, has been proposed as an important reason for their relatively high suicide rates. Guns are used in more than half of all suicides in the United States, and their use for suicide correlates with the holding of gun licences in households [20]. Some controversy surrounds the question of whether restricting the availability of firearms through, for example, making gun purchase more difficult and improving firearm storage in households leads to a reduction in suicide rates, but the weight of evidence seems to indicate that it does [11].

## Analgesics

In the UK and some other countries, there has been particular concern about deaths from self-poisoning with paracetamol (acetaminophen). Due to evidence that countries which have fewer tablets per pack seem to have a lower rate of mortality from paracetamol self-poisoning and because overdoses of paracetamol are often taken impulsively and involve household supplies, legislation was introduced in the UK in 1998 to reduce the number of tablets of paracetamol (and aspirin) available per pack. This resulted in fewer overdoses, decreased cases of hepatotoxicity due to paracetamol toxicity, and a reduced number of deaths from both paracetamol and aspirin [21, 22].

Also in the UK, withdrawal of the analgesic co-proxamol (paracetamol combined with the highly toxic opiate dextropropoxyphene) in 2005–2007 resulted in virtual elimination of deaths due to self-poisoning with this drug and no evidence of an increase in deaths involving other analgesics, at least until the end of 2010 [23].

## Popular sites for suicide

Much attention has been paid to improving safety at popular sites for suicide. This includes, for example, erecting suicide barriers on bridges, multi-storey car parks, and other sites. For example, erection of barriers on the Clifton Suspension Bridge in Bristol in the UK, a popular site for suicide, has resulted in far fewer deaths by jumping [24]. It has been estimated that safety measures at such sites may reduce suicide considerably [25].

## Pesticides

Ingestion of pesticides is common in several low- and middle-income countries in which there are large numbers of small rural farming communities. It is thought to be responsible for a large proportion of suicides globally [1]. Banning sales of more toxic pesticides is one approach that has been shown to have a profound effect on national suicide rates. Safer storage of pesticides in domestic settings and improved emergency access to medical treatment are other approaches.

## Hanging

Hanging is an extremely common method of suicide in many countries. This may reflect the decreased availability of other methods, together with the frequency with which it is portrayed in the media. Prevention in terms of restricting access to means is difficult, except in institutional settings. Making psychiatric hospital wards safer through removing ligature points and introducing collapsible curtain rails may reduce hanging deaths in this setting [26]. Similar safety measures in prisons may also be helpful.

Clinicians involved in the development of suicide prevention strategies should look very carefully at local patterns of suicide which might provide clues about potentially effective measures for reducing access to methods. This includes prescribing less toxic medication where feasible, especially to patients at risk of self-harm.

## Attempts to limit contagion effects

Exposure to suicidal behaviour of other people can increase the risk of suicide and self-harm. This can result in suicide clusters where a greater than expected number of suicides occur in a locality or setting in a particular time period (so-called 'point clusters'). Clusters may be temporal where, for example, there is a spike in the number of suicides that are geographically unrelated, but similar in terms of methods and characteristics of individuals involved. Clusters of suicides and of self-harm are not infrequent in young people and in institutional settings such as psychiatric hospitals, schools, and prisons [27]. In planning local suicide prevention strategies, it is important to prepare policies to address such clusters, with, for example, identification of the agency that will co-ordinate the local response, a plan for addressing media responses to the cluster, and a policy for identifying people at risk and providing help [28].

## Influencing media portrayal of suicidal behaviour

A growing, if mixed, evidence base demonstrates that irresponsible reporting and portrayal of suicide in fictional or non-fictional contexts can give rise to imitative suicidal behaviour [29, 30], through a process of social modelling [31]. Practices such as featuring a suicide on the front page of a newspaper, repeated coverage, speculation about the triggers, and publishing details of the method, location, or suicide note are thought to increase the risk of suicidal behaviour in vulnerable people.

This effect appears to be particularly powerful in relation to the death by suicide of entertainment and political celebrities [32] and in young people [29]. Conversely, reporting that highlights the ability of suicidal individuals to cope positively in adverse circumstances may be negatively associated with suicide rates [33] and is to be encouraged.

In view of these concerns, prevention agencies in several countries have attempted to work with the media to reduce sensationalism and inappropriate language when reporting or portraying suicide or self-harm to minimize possible negative influences. There is mixed evidence for the effectiveness of such media activity and of guidelines [34], and little in the way of sanctions for those who do not adhere to them [35]. Experiences of working with media agencies in Europe, Australia, and New Zealand suggest that reactive and punitive approaches, such as enforcing regulatory agencies' relatively weak penalties for breaching guidelines, are unlikely to be as effective as collaborative approaches [35]. Mental health professionals are encouraged to work with the media, where opportunities arise, to promote responsible reporting of suicide and mental ill-health and to challenge stigma.

With the growth of new media, the sheer volume of online and print content overwhelms most systems of surveillance, and it often falls on the general public to take a 'name and shame' approach to promote journalistic change. The Internet also offers multiple fora for people to describe or encourage specific suicide methods. If not moderated appropriately, there is a risk of unchecked encouragement of suicide in vulnerable individuals. Attempts to build alert systems into sites such as Facebook and Twitter have not always been successful. However, use of search engine optimization and advert targeting has the potential to promote supportive organizations such as the Samaritans.

## Education of the public about mental illness, its treatment, stigma, and help-seeking

Given estimates that 87–91% of people who die by suicide have a diagnosable mental disorder [2, 3] and that the distress caused by mental illness is a key mediator of suicidality, optimizing treatment of underlying mental health problems may contribute to decreasing suicide mortality rates. The same might be said for self-harm, given that up to 84% of patients who present to hospital having self-harmed are thought to have an underlying psychiatric diagnosis [36]. Optimal treatment for mental disorder starts with detection and referral by general practitioners (GPs)—described later in this chapter—but also the willingness of patients in distress to consult a health professional. The stigma of mental illness is a major barrier to help-seeking, as is ignorance about mental illness and the potential to treat it. The contribution of this to the reluctance of men and young people to seek formal help is a particular concern in the UK, given high rates of suicide in young and middle-aged men [8]. It has also been suggested that the stigma of mental illness contributes to suicidality, although this may be mediated by correlates of stigma such as social isolation, unemployment, hopelessness, or stress [37].

Public education about the recognition and treatment of mental illness is one approach intended to reduce stigma and increase self-presentation to health services among people suffering from mental distress. The intended effects of such programmes are to reduce stigma stress, increase detection and treatment of mental disorder, and reduce suicidal behaviour. Again, such programmes are hard to evaluate, given that mortality outcomes are so distal and subject to intercurrent socio-economic influences. Any effect on suicide rates is likely to be mediated by more proximal outcomes such as rates of depression, anxiety, and social functioning. A review of international evidence describing the impact of anti-stigma campaigns found modest evidence for their effectiveness in increasing knowledge and reducing stigmatizing attitudes, limited to short-term effects [38]. Harnessing the Internet to extend the reach of anti-stigma messages has the potential to penetrate specific groups and to reset social norms that have tended to stigmatize those who struggle with mental ill-health.

### Education of primary care physicians

Primary care physician education in the recognition and treatment of depression had previously been regarded as one of the suicide prevention interventions for which there was relatively strong evidence for effectiveness [10]. This was based on the experiences of the Swedish island of Gotland [39–41]. However, despite short-term benefits in terms of proactive treatment of depression and a reduction in suicides [39], these effects are now understood to be short-lived [40] and more marked in women [41]. An updated systematic review noted the lack of trial data published since the Gotland initiative, with weak evidence from ecological studies that primary care physician education might reduce suicide rates in Hungary, Slovenia, and Sweden [11].

Primary care is regarded as the setting in which there is great potential to identify mental illness and prevent suicide, given that in up to 75% of suicide cases in the United States [42] and up to 63% of cases in the UK [43], a primary care presentation occurred in the year before death. However, this relies on primary care practitioners making a diagnosis of depression (or other mental disorder) and initiating acceptable evidence-based treatment. Additionally, psychological autopsy studies indicate that the population attributable fraction for a mental disorder in suicide ranges from 47% to 74% [2]. Predicting which patients are most likely to attempt suicide goes beyond what can be expected from any clinician, given our current understanding of the poor predictive value of risk prediction tools [44, 45].

Given the wider benefits demonstrated in the Gotland study, GP educational interventions might be regarded as beneficial to public mental health, even if the impact on suicide rates is less marked.

### Educational approaches in schools

School or college interventions are usually universal in nature, as opposed to targeting those most at risk of youth suicide.

There have been three broad approaches in trying to prevent suicide through school-based programmes. The first of these has tended to focus on increasing pupils' knowledge and awareness of suicide. Some evidence from the United States showed that such a programme appeared to lead to a small increase in pupils' ratings of the acceptability of suicide, although it is not known if this was associated with any change in the rates of self-harm or suicide.

Suicidal behaviour in young people often appears to be related to depression, anxiety, low self-esteem, difficulties during upbringing (for example, abuse, deprivation), life events (especially break-up of relationships, family problems, and bullying), and poor problem-solving skills [46]. Troubled and suicidal young people often seek help from their peers. A second school-based strategy has been the development of educational programmes in schools about recognition of psychological distress in individuals and their peers, problem-solving, and peer support. A trial of a Youth Aware of Mental Health Programme intervention significantly reduced (by more than 50%) the incidence of suicide attempts and suicidal ideation at 12 months' follow-up, compared with the control group. Similar reductions were not associated with a manualized gatekeeper programme or screening for high-risk individuals by professionals [47]. This suggests that changes in suicidal behaviour are more likely to occur when pupils are personally engaged in the intervention.

A third approach is to screen adolescents with questionnaires to detect children and adolescents at risk of psychiatric disorder and possible suicidal behaviour. Pupils that are so detected will then need referral to an appropriate agency for further assessment and possible treatment. While this approach was not found to be associated with any reduction in suicidal behaviour, when compared to no intervention, it is likely to be important in the early detection and treatment of pupils with emerging psychopathology. (Suicide in children and adolescents is considered further in Chapter 125.)

For psychiatrists and others involved in developing local prevention strategies, it is important to recognize that school-based approaches to prevention constitute a highly sensitive area and one where the most effective (and least risky) approach is at present unclear. Another important aspect of suicidal behaviour in school pupils is management of the aftermath of suicides and its impact on other pupils (see postvention in People bereaved by suicide, p. 1309) and how to tackle outbreaks of self-harm [46].

### Telephone helplines and Internet-based support

Some individuals who attempt suicide will find the anonymity of a telephone helpline or an Internet forum more acceptable than consulting health professionals about their problems. Others prefer to use leaflets or the Internet to access information on self-management of suicidal thoughts. The voluntary sector plays a key role in the provision of Internet-based information and non-judgemental support for those who feel suicidal. This might be in the context of social isolation, mental health problems, relationship problems, or other social issues. The model used by Samaritans is one of the best known and, over the years, has evolved from a drop-in service to include a service accessible via telephone, letter, or email. Other telephone helplines offering support to suicidal people are now widely available in Australia, Canada, the United States, and northern Europe. Freephones may be installed at sites frequently used as a location for suicide [48], and helplines may be advertised on websites in a targeted fashion where suicidal language is detected on web posts.

Survey methods have demonstrated a high level of satisfaction with suicide helplines, with users tending to discuss suicidal thoughts and mental health problems and to use the service as part of a range of support sources [49]. However, methodological problems make it difficult to trial the effect of telephone helplines and other Internet resources on suicide rates. Until randomized controlled studies are conducted of callers to suicide helplines, with sufficient follow-up, it remains uncertain whether suicide helplines are effective. Their effects on the mediators of suicide risk, such as social isolation, severity of depression, and impaired problem-solving, may be easier to evaluate.

### Gatekeepers

The term gatekeepers refers to 'individuals in a community who have face-to-face contact with large numbers of community members as part of their usual routine' [50]. They are usually trained in the identification of those at risk of suicide and then in referring them for support and treatment. This approach has been used in schools and the military, as well as in primary care and emergency department settings. The use of gatekeeper programmes is popular in many countries. Observational data suggest there is only limited evidence that such approaches serve to reduce suicides or suicide attempts [11], and there have been no randomized controlled trials.

### Strategies for high-risk groups

A wide range of prevention strategies can be targeted at high-risk groups.

### Patients with psychiatric disorders

#### Risk identification and reduction

All psychiatric disorders carry an increased risk for suicidal behaviour. Those with the highest suicide risk are those with borderline personality disorder, anorexia nervosa, depression, and bipolar disorder [51]. Risk of suicide appears to be highest in the first few months following a diagnosis across all mental disorders. Other risk factors for suicide include previous attempts, family history of suicidal behaviour, and living alone. Comorbidity of alcohol abuse, personality disorder, and other psychiatric disorders also increases the risk. There is a robust association between mood instability and suicidal ideation, irrespective of the diagnosis, and this association persists even when accounting for mood, anxiety, and substance abuse [52].

One difficulty in using a risk identification approach is that the risk factors identified from studies of groups of people who have died from suicide are often misleading when applied to individual patients. Many of the identified risk factors apply to a relatively large number of individuals (for example, those living alone), the majority of whom will not be at risk. In clinical practice, it is important to be aware of patients who, due to their individual characteristics, are at long-term high risk, as well as the dynamic factors which may serve to increase risk (for example, drugs and alcohol).

#### Risk scales

There is increasing evidence that scales for predicting the risk of suicide and non-fatal suicidal behaviour are ineffective at the individual patient level [44] and that they should not be relied on to guide patient management [53]. The most pragmatic approach is to ensure that proven effective treatments for patients with psychiatric conditions are available, to focus on risk reduction in all patients, and to be particularly cautious at times of apparent high risk. The first few weeks after psychiatric hospital discharge are a key risk period [54]. In a UK study, a third of suicides among psychiatric patients occurred within 3 months of discharge from hospital, almost half of whom died within the first month [55]. Other risk periods follow a relationship break-up or other significant loss, shortly after discharge from hospital, and following recent suicidal behaviour by another patient or someone else close to the individual.

#### Preventative strategies

Prevention of suicide in patients with psychiatric disorders should be a major element of suicide prevention strategies [56]. Important strategies in preventing suicide in patients with psychiatric disorders include active treatment of individual episodes of illness, psychological therapy to improve compliance with treatment, review of access to means, and encouraging self-management.

### Pharmacological treatments

#### Antidepressants

The role of drugs licensed for depression in the treatment of suicidal behaviour is debated. In a non-systematic review, reductions in suicide attempts of between 40% and 80% have been reported in depressed patients treated with antidepressants [57]. The antidepressant response may also relate to clinical presentation. A trial in the Netherlands in which paroxetine was compared with placebo in patients who had all repeated self-harm but who did not suffer from current depressive disorder showed apparent benefits for a subgroup of patients who received paroxetine, namely those who had a history of 1–4 episodes of self-harm. Patients with a history of five or more episodes did not seem to benefit [58]. A meta-analysis of all data submitted to the US Food and Drug Administration (FDA) revealed a reduction in suicidal thoughts and behaviour in those aged 25 years and over, but an increase on those measures for participants below the age of 25 [59]. The risk of attempting suicide is 2.5 times higher in the month preceding antidepressant treatment than in the month following treatment [60].

These findings have highlighted the need to be cautious in the use of antidepressants, to provide early follow-up after initiating therapy, and to consider combining antidepressant treatment with other therapies, especially for adolescents (in whom only fluoxetine is currently recommended for the treatment of depression).

#### Lithium

The protective effect of lithium in people with affective disorders is well established. A systematic review of trials of lithium therapy vs a range of other drugs and placebo in patients with affective disorders has shown convincing evidence that lithium may prevent suicide [61]. Lithium reduced the risk of death and suicide by 60%, compared to placebo. The anti-suicidal effect was found to be greater than the effect on mood episodes, suggesting that it may be a specific effect perhaps related to changes in aggression or impulsivity. It is not known if lithium has anti-suicidal properties in other groups of patients.

### Neuroleptics

Suicidal acts are common in those suffering from psychotic illnesses. Clozapine has been identified in some studies as having a protective effect. In the Intersept (International Suicide Prevention Trial) trial, clozapine was compared to olanzapine in a multi-centre randomized, open-label study in individuals with schizophrenia or schizoaffective disorder who were deemed to be at high risk of suicide [62]. Clozapine was associated with a significant reduction in suicidal ideation and suicide attempts and fewer interventions to prevent suicide. There were also fewer deaths from suicide, but this was not a statistically significant finding. Data from the Clozaril National Register also suggest that current users of clozapine have a lower mortality rate than recent or past users [63]. However, this analysis used no control group and discontinuation of clozapine was associated with a worse clinical outcome.

### Ketamine

Ketamine can have rapid antidepressant effects and may be a useful treatment option for acute suicidality. A case series involving 14 subjects who presented to an emergency department showed rapid and significant decreases in suicidality, which were sustained over 10 days [64]. In one randomized controlled trial, total absence of suicidal ideation was observed in over half of patients treated with ketamine, compared with 24% of those given midazolam [65]. Two systematic reviews of the effectiveness of ketamine in unipolar depression have shown that it may reduce suicidality in patients being treated for depression [66]. Ketamine is also reported to be effective in reducing suicidal ideation in people with bipolar disorder [67]. These findings are promising, but little is known about the effects of ketamine on self-harm or how long the anti-suicidal effects might persist.

### Service provision and continuity of care

Aspects of the provision of mental health services can affect the rates of suicide in clinical populations. In the UK, lower suicide rates were observed in areas which implemented the recommendations of the National Confidential Inquiry into suicide and homicide by people with mental illness [68]. Recommendations included removal of ligature points, provision of 24-hour crisis teams, 7-day follow-up following discharge, and training for frontline staff. Continuity of care is likely to be a particularly important factor in preventing suicide in patients at risk, involving care being continued during periods of remission. Unlike affective disorders where risk is greatest during depressive episodes, the risk in schizophrenia tends to be highest between episodes of acute psychotic illness when patients may have insight and feel hopeless about their circumstances and prospects. Risk is related more to affective symptoms than to core features of the disorders [69]. In the UK, specific concerns have been raised about the use of out-of-area inpatient beds, given a significant increase in suicides after discharge from a non-local unit [55]. This is likely to relate to social isolation and disruption in communication and care planning associated with out-of-area admissions. Frequent reorganizations of psychiatric services have also been linked to increased suicidal behaviour [70].

## Specific at-risk groups

### Those who misuse drug and alcohol

Programmes for suicide prevention must reinforce healthy behaviours with respect to alcohol and substance misuse, irrespective of whether an individual has a formal diagnosis. Treatment of those who abuse substances is likely to be the best approach to prevention for patients, in parallel with social measures such as restricting access to alcohol or minimum pricing. The introduction of policies to restrict access to alcohol has been associated with a reduction in suicide in Slovenia and Russia, although the effect was limited to men [71–73]. The elevated risk in the weeks following the break-up of a relationship for patients with severe alcohol abuse [74] again points to the need for continuity of support in the community.

Prevention of suicide in patients with comorbid disorders, especially the combination of depression with alcohol abuse and/or personality disorder, is challenging, as compliance with treatment is often less than in patients with single disorders. Effective prevention is likely to depend on close integration of care between different statutory care agencies.

### Chronic physical illness and pain

Chronic illnesses, particularly cancer and respiratory diseases, are associated with an increased risk of suicide [75, 76]. The relationship between pain and suicidal behaviour is also highly significant [77, 78]. Risk is particularly associated with severe and recurrent headache, psychogenic pain, chronic abdominal pain, and medicolegal issues related to pain. Suicide prevention in this group is complicated by the bi-directional relationship between pain and psychopathology. All patients with chronic illness should be screened for depressive disorder and asked about suicidal ideation if screening positive. Proactive treatment should be instigated if a mood disorder is identified.

### People who self-harm

In view of the clear association between non-fatal self-harm and suicide, establishment of adequate services for people who self-harm, including the provision of careful assessments of patients in the general hospital, and offering treatments for which at least some indicators of benefit are available, are important elements in any national suicide prevention strategy. There is good evidence that well-trained non-medical psychiatric staff can effectively carry out assessments and arrange aftercare. Furthermore, psychosocial assessment following self-harm may be associated with a reduction in repeat episodes [79]. Models for ideal services exist such as those published by the National Institute for Health and Care Excellence [53, 80] in the UK.

### High-risk occupational groups

Certain occupational groups are known to be at relatively high risk of suicide. In England, recent evidence indicated that these include men in the construction industry and in media and cultural occupations and women in primary school teaching, nursing, and cultural and media occupations, together with people of both genders in caring occupations.

## Prisoners

There are relatively high suicide rates in prisoners [81], especially young males held on remand. While one aspect of prevention is through ensuring that prisons and police cells are safe in terms of absence of ligature points, there are a range of other potentially useful and humane strategies [82]. These include careful assessments of new inmates using risk assessment procedures, training of staff with regard to both assessment skills and attitudes towards mental health problems and suicide prevention, in-reach programmes by befriending organizations such as Samaritans, court diversion of individuals with major mental health treatment needs, and prompt access to psychiatric and psychological services.

## People bereaved by suicide

People bereaved by suicide have an increased risk of depression, psychiatric admission, suicide attempt, and suicide, when compared with those bereaved by other types of death [83, 84]. Risk of suicide attempt after a close contact's death is elevated, regardless of whether they were related to the deceased or not [85], suggesting that wider social networks are vulnerable to adverse mental health outcomes. The term postvention is used to describe support offered to someone after the suicide of a close contact. Such post-bereavement interventions are intended to prevent the emergence of mental health problems and include national helplines, online support, individual counselling, group work, school and college in-reach after suicide, and support from professionals. Countries such as the United States and Australia lead the way in terms of the range of services and public health resources devoted to postvention. In most countries, the majority of provision lies within the voluntary sector. Much of the momentum for this has been provided by people bereaved by suicide who, in the United States, are also known as suicide survivors.

There is weak evidence supporting the effectiveness of postvention offered in school-based, family-focused, and community-based settings to reduce the risk of suicide-related outcomes [86]. Trials of interventions to reduce other adverse outcomes of suicide bereavement have found little evidence for effectiveness [87]. Evaluations of any such interventions will need to be conducted on a country-by-country basis, given cultural dimensions of grief, bereavement, and suicide and of stigmatizing attitudes to those bereaved by suicide.

## Treatment of people who self-harm

Self-harm occurs for a wide range of reasons. In many cases, the primary aim is not death, but some other outcome such as processing distress, temporary escape, or communicating distress to other people. The needs of individual patients vary widely, meaning that a broad range of potential treatments are required. Treatments include both psychosocial and pharmacological approaches, which might be combined, for example, if a patient suffers from moderate or severe depression in the setting of employment and financial difficulties, when treatment with an effective drug might be combined with problem-solving therapy.

Factors relevant to treatment needs in people who self-harm are discussed in the following sections.

## Repetition of attempts and risk of suicide

Repetition of attempts is common, with 15–25% of those who present to hospital engaging in further self-harm within a year [88, 89]. Self-harm is also associated with an elevated risk of suicide, although the frequency of suicide following attempted suicide varies internationally [90], depending partly on the overall characteristics of the patient population and the general population suicide rates. Repetition of self-harm increases the risk of suicide [88]. Prevention of repetition of self-harm and suicide is understandably a major aim in treating people who intentionally harm themselves.

## Psychiatric disorders and psychopathology

In a systematic review of studies worldwide, an estimated 87% of adults who presented to hospital having self-harmed had at least one psychiatric disorder, with depression, anxiety, and substance misuse being particularly common [36]. In adolescents, a pooled average of 81% had psychiatric disorders, with depression, anxiety, and attention-deficit/hyperactivity disorder (ADHD) being the most frequent. In addition, some four out of ten patients may have personality disorders [91]. While treatment directed at the underlying causes of such disorders, where possible, will be important in managing patients who self-harm, often the disorders themselves will require specific treatment.

## Negative life events

Social problems are particularly common in people who self-harm [92], including difficulties in interpersonal relationships, especially with partners and other family members, employment problems, particularly in males, and financial difficulties. Physical and sexual abuse, neglect, and domestic violence are relatively common. Life events, especially loss of a relationship, a job, or housing, frequently precede self-harm [93].

## Poor problem-solving skills

Difficulties in problem-solving, particularly in relation to interpersonal relationships, are characteristic of people who self-harm [94]. This distinguishes them from patients with psychiatric disorders who have not carried out a suicidal act.

## Impulsivity and aggression

There are strong links between suicidal behaviour and impulsivity and aggression. There is also accumulating evidence that hypofunction of brain serotonergic systems is linked to aggression (and possibly impulsivity) and also to suicidal behaviour [95] (see Chapter 127). It is unclear whether this represents a state phenomenon associated with psychiatric disturbance or a trait phenomenon, but current evidence favours the latter.

## Hopelessness and low self-esteem

Hopelessness, or pessimism about the future, is an important predictor of repetition of suicidal behaviour and a risk factor for eventual suicide [93]. Low self-esteem is another important characteristic associated with suicidal behaviour [4]. There is likely to be a link between low self-esteem and a tendency to experience hopelessness when facing adverse circumstances.

## Motivational problems and poor compliance with treatment

Some people who attempt suicide may be poorly motivated to engage in aftercare, which affects treatment adherence. Organizational factors in general hospital psychiatric services (including continuity of care) and the attitudes of clinical staff may be important factors influencing whether patients engage in aftercare. In adolescents, family group interventions appear to improve adherence with aftercare, as do brief interventions in the emergency department [96].

## Psychosocial assessment

While conducting the assessment, the clinician should try to assess the imminent risk of suicide or further self-harm (Box 128.2). However, suicide risk assessment scales perform badly [44, 45] and reliance on them to determine aftercare is discouraged. Several factors associated with an increased risk of suicide following attempted suicide relate to the nature of the act (for example, violent method, leaving a suicide note, high suicidal intent), but even these have low predictive power, especially in the longer term. The best predictor of repeat self-harm is a previous episode. Rather than focusing primarily on risk assessment, it is recommended that clinicians direct their attention to risk reduction in *all* patients. This includes safety and crisis plans such as restricting access to means and collaborative crisis planning with the patient. Safety planning may be enhanced by involvement of family members and other key individuals. Another key component is clear communication between agencies, with the patient and with family members and other key individuals (as appropriate).

## Planning aftercare

Aftercare following self-harm should be planned according to each patient's specific needs. An individual with moderate to severe depression and difficulties with employment or finances might best be helped through a combination of pharmacotherapy and psychological therapy such as problem-solving and support. Someone with relationship and substance misuse difficulties might best be helped with a combination of specific substance misuse treatment and couple or family therapy. Someone with difficulties in impulse-control and attachment problems might be offered longer-term psychotherapy such as dialectical behaviour therapy (DBT). Whichever therapy is offered, risk reduction measures and careful monitoring of mood and suicidal ideation are recommended (Box 128.3).

## Psychosocial treatments

A range of psychosocial therapies for patients who self-harm have been evaluated in randomized controlled clinical trials [97, 98]. The findings from these reviews and some individual studies are summarized here.

### Brief cognitive behavioural therapy-based interventions

A meta-analysis of the results of trials of cognitive behavioural therapy (CBT)-based psychotherapy, compared with treatment as usual (TAU), indicated that CBT-based psychotherapy (including either problem-solving therapy or CBT) is associated with fewer individuals repeating self-harm [97]. There is also evidence of other positive outcomes, including greater reductions in depression, hopelessness, and suicidal ideation. This approach is useful, either used alone or in the context of other treatments.

### Dialectical behaviour therapy

DBT is a relatively intensive form of therapy, combining individual therapy sessions focused on addressing an individual's life problems, group therapy focused on acceptance of emotions, reducing emotional responsivity and development of interpersonal skills, and access to therapist support.

DBT is thought to be appropriate for patients with a history of multiple episodes of self-harm, especially those with features associated with borderline personality disorder. Treatment in adults

---

**Box 128.2** Assessment of patients who self-harm

**Factors to cover in history-taking**
- Life events preceding the attempt
- Motives for the act, including suicidal intent (Box 128.1)
- Problems facing the patient
- Psychiatric disorders
- Psychiatric history
- Previous suicide attempts
- Personality traits/disorders
- Alcohol and drug misuse
- Family and personal history
- Current circumstances
- Social (for example, nature of social relationships)
- Domestic (for example, living alone)
- Occupation (for example, whether employed)
- Exposure to suicide/self-harm in friends or family members
- Accessing Internet sites relevant to suicidal behaviour
- Online social networking or similar activities related to suicidal behaviour

**Additional suggested assessments**
- Risk of further self-harm and of suicide
- Coping resources and supports
- What treatments are appropriate to the patient's needs?
- Motivation of the patient (and significant others where appropriate) to engage in treatment

---

**Box 128.3** Factors that suggest high suicidal intent

- Act carried out in isolation
- Act timed so that intervention unlikely
- Precautions taken to avoid discovery
- Preparations made in anticipation of death (for example, making a will, organizing insurance)
- Preparations made for the act (for example, purchasing means, saving up tablets)
- Communicating intent to others beforehand
- Extensive premeditation
- Leaving a note
- Note alerting potential responders after the act
- Subsequent admission of suicidal intent

usually lasts a year. While few trials have been conducted in patients who self-harm, a meta-analysis of trials comparing DBT to TAU indicated that individuals receiving DBT had fewer subsequent episodes of self-harm. DBT has also been developed for adolescents, but in a briefer format. Early evidence suggests that, compared with TAU, DBT may reduce repetition of self-harm and benefit mood and self-esteem in adolescents with a history of repeated self-harm.

### Contact interventions

Contact interventions are those in which contact is maintained remotely with patients who have self-harmed, for example through regular mail contacts with patients, usually via postcards. Typically these include expression of concern for the patient's welfare and details of emergency contact information and are sent monthly for a few months and then bi-monthly for the remainder of the first year after a self-harm episode. A meta-analysis of trials comparing this approach combined with TAU with TAU alone suggested equivocal results in terms of self-harm repetition. However, a trial in Iran, where community psychiatric service provision (that is, TAU) is limited, suggested a significant benefit in terms of reduced repetition of self-harm [99]. There is little evidence for benefits of other contact interventions such as those via telephone.

### Other psychosocial treatment innovations

As treatment adherence is often an issue in individuals who self-harm, efforts have been made to improve attendance at treatment sessions. Continuity of care, through having the assessing clinician provide aftercare, has been shown to increase the proportion of patients who attend for treatment [100]. Among patients who failed to attend an outpatient appointment, those who had a home visit from a nurse were more likely to attend subsequent follow-up than those where no such visit occurred [101]. For adolescents, 'therapeutic assessment' has been developed, in which, in addition to a routine assessment, there is a focus on understanding the meaning of their self-harm, on formulation of their problem, and linking this to benefits of aftercare, together with family involvement in the process. In trials, this was associated with more adolescents attending treatment sessions than where a routine assessment was provided [102]. However, it should be noted that none of these service-orientated innovations was associated with reduced subsequent frequency of repeated suicide attempts, although existing trials had limited power to evaluate this outcome.

A rapidly growing recent development is the provision of therapy through mobile health applications (apps) on remote electronic devices such as smartphones [103]. This is clearly a growth area with the major advantage that it might be helpful for people who do not access clinical services. However, trials are so far lacking.

## Pharmacological treatments

In spite of the high prevalence of psychiatric disorder, particularly depression [36], in people who self-harm, there have been relatively few trials evaluating the effectiveness of pharmacological agents in this population [104]. This perhaps reflects the problems of treatment adherence and risk of overdose. The likely most effective pharmacological approach is treatment of any underlying psychiatric disorder.

Care should be taken to prescribe the safest appropriate treatment. Tricyclic antidepressants should be avoided in view of their high toxicity. Selective serotonin reuptake inhibitors (SSRIs) are generally deemed to be the safest, although citalopram is significantly more toxic than other SSRIs [105]. Prescriptions should be limited to small quantities of medications where necessary. Lithium has the strongest evidence for prevention of suicidal behaviour [61].

In adolescents, there are concerns about the use of SSRIs in particular, because of an association with suicidal ideation. However, reduced prescribing of SSRIs in response to warnings from regulatory bodies was actually associated with increased rates of suicide in young people [106]. There is also evidence that a combination of fluoxetine and CBT may have greater benefit in terms of suicidal ideation than either alone in the treatment of adolescents with depression [107]. Where a drug is prescribed for either adults or young people with depression, early follow-up (within a few days) is indicated because this is when agitation and possible suicidal ideation are most likely to occur.

## Conclusions

In this chapter, we have focused on a wide range of specific initiatives that may help prevent suicide, especially in people with psychiatric disorders. We have emphasized the need for a comprehensive multisectoral approach to suicide prevention. This should be tailored to specific local patterns of suicide. For people in contact with psychiatric services, prevention may be achieved through specific aspects of service provision, as well as through indicated therapies. Evidence of effectiveness of specific initiatives is gradually emerging. We have focused in some detail on people who have self-harmed. This is justified both because of the strength of the association between self-harm and suicide and also because of the impact that self-harm has on the individuals involved and the family and friends. Again, potentially effective therapies are being identified. In considering prevention of self-harm and suicide in people with psychiatric disorders, an essential complement is a population-based strategy that ensures easy access to well-designed and supportive services, staffed by those with an awareness of the needs after self-harm and training in suicide prevention.

### FURTHER INFORMATION

Hawton, K. *Prevention and Treatment of Suicidal Behaviour: From Science to Practice*. Oxford University Press: Oxford; 2005.

National Collaborating Centre for Mental Health. *Self-harm: the short-term physical and psychological management and secondary prevention of self-harm in primary and secondary care*. Clinical guideline [CG16]. National Institute for Health and Care Excellence: London; 2004.

National Institute for Health and Care Excellence. *Self-harm in over 8s: long term management*. Clinical guideline [CG133]. National Institute for Health and Care Excellence: London; 2011.

O'Connor, R. and J. Pirkis. *The International Handbook of Suicide and Attempted Suicide*. Wiley: Chichester; 2016.

World Health Organization. *Suicide prevention*. 2014. Available from: http://www.who.int/mental_health/prevention/suicide/suicideprevent/en/

## REFERENCES

1. World Health Organization. *Suicide prevention*. 2014. Available from: http://www.who.int/mental_health/prevention/suicide/suicideprevent/en/

2. Cavanagh, J.T.O., *et al*. Psychological autopsy studies of suicide: a systematic review. *Psychol Med*, 2003. **33**: 395–405.

3. Arsenault-Lapierre, G., C. Kim, and G. Turecki. Psychiatric diagnoses in 3275 suicides: a meta-analysis. *BMC Psychiatry*, 2004. **4**: 37.

4. O'Connor, R.C. and M.K. Nock. The psychology of suicidal behaviour. *Lancet Psychiatry*, 2014. **1**: 73–85.

5. Hawton, K., *et al*. Deliberate self-harm in Oxford, 1990–2000: a time of change in patient characteristics. *Psychol Med*, 2003. **33**: 987–95.

6. Pitman, A. and E. Caine. The role of the high-risk approach in suicide prevention. *Br J Psychiatry*, 2012. **201**: 175–7.

7. Fortune, S.A. and K. Hawton. Culture and mental disorders: suicidal behaviour. In: D. Bhugra and K. Bhui, editors. *Textbook of Cultural Psychiatry*. Cambridge University Press: Cambridge; 2007. pp. 255–71.

8. Pitman, A., *et al*. Suicide in young men. *Lancet*, 2012. **379**: 2383–92.

9. Kim, S.Y., R.G. De Vries, and J.R. Peteet. Euthanasia and assisted suicide of patients with psychiatric disorders in the Netherlands 2011 to 2014. *JAMA Psychiatry*, 2016. **73**: 362–8.

10. Mann, J.J., *et al*. Suicide prevention strategies. A systematic review. *JAMA*, 2005. **294**: 2064–74.

11. Zalsman, G., *et al*. Suicide prevention strategies revisited: 10-year systematic review. *Lancet Psychiatry*, 2016. **3**: 646–59.

12. Lonnqvist, J. National suicide prevention project in Finland: a research phase of the project. *Psychiatria Fennica*, 1988. **19**: 125–32.

13. Kerkhof, A. The Finnish national suicide prevention program evaluated. *Crisis*, 1999. **20**: 50–63.

14. Department of Health. *National Suicide Prevention Strategy for England*. Department of Health: London; 2002.

15. Department of Health. *Preventing Suicide in England: A Cross-Government Outcomes Strategy to Save Lives*. Department of Health: London; 2012.

16. Goldney, R.D. Suicide prevention is possible: a review of recent studies. *Arch Suicide Res*, 1998. **4**: 329–39.

17. Hawton, K. Restriction of access to methods of suicide as a means of suicide prevention. In: K. Hawton, editor. *Prevention and Treatment of Suicidal Behaviour: From Science to Practice*. Oxford University Press: Oxford; 2005. pp. 279–91.

18. Kreitman, N. The coal gas story: United Kingdom suicide rates 1960–1971. *Br J Prev Soc Med*, 1976. **30**: 86–93.

19. Amos, T., L. Appleby, and K. Kiernan. Changes in rates of suicide by car exhaust asphyxiation in England and Wales. *Psychol Med*, 2001. **31**: 935–9.

20. Kellermann, A.L., *et al*. Suicide in the home in relation to gun ownership. *N Engl J Med*, 1992. **327**: 467–72.

21. Hawton, K., *et al*. UK legislation on analgesic packs: before and after study of long term effect on poisonings. *BMJ*, 2004. **329**: 1076–9.

22. Hawton, K., *et al*. Long term effect of reduced pack sizes of paracetamol on poisoning deaths and liver transplant activity in England and Wales: interrupted time series analyses. *BMJ*, 2013. **346**: f403.

23. Hawton, K., *et al*. Six-year follow-up of impact of co-proxamol withdrawal in England and Wales on prescribing and deaths: time-series study. *PLoS Med*, 2012. **9**: e1001213.

24. Bennewith, O., M. Nowers, and D. Gunnell. Effect of barriers on the Clifton suspension bridge, England, on local patterns of suicide: implications for prevention. *Br J Psychiatry*, 2007. **190**: 266–7.

25. Pirkis, J., *et al*. Interventions to reduce suicides at suicide hotspots: a systematic review and meta-analysis. *Lancet Psychiatry*, 2015. **2**: 994–1001.

26. Kapur, N., *et al*. Suicide in psychiatric in-patients in England, 1997 to 2003. *Psychol Med*, 2006. **36**: 1485–92.

27. Niedzwiedz, C., *et al*. The definition and epidemiology of clusters of suicidal behavior: a systematic review. *Suicide Life Threat Behav*, 2014. **44**: 569–81.

28. Public Health England. *Identifying and Responding to Suicide Clusters and Contagion*. Public Health England: London; 2014.

29. Pirkis, J. and R.W. Blood. *Suicide and the News and Information Media: A Critical Review*. Commonwealth of Australia: Canberra; 2010.

30. Sisask, M. and A. Värnik. Media roles in suicide prevention: a systematic review. *Int J Environ Res Public Health*, 2012. **9**: 123–38.

31. Zahl, D. and K. Hawton. Media influences on suicidal behaviour: an interview study of young people. *Behav Cogn Psychother*, 2004. **32**: 189–98.

32. Stack, S. Suicide in the media: a quantitative review of studies based on non-fictional stories. *Suicide Life Threat Behav*, 2005. **35**: 121–33.

33. Niederkrotenthaler, T., *et al*. Role of media reports in completed and prevented suicide: Werther v. Papageno effects. *Br J Psychiatry*, 2010. **197**: 234–43.

34. Bohanna, I. and X. Wang Media guidelines for the responsible reporting of suicide: a review of effectiveness. *Crisis*, 2012. **33**: 190–8.

35. Pitman, A. and F. Stevenson. Suicide reporting within British newspapers' arts coverage. *Crisis*, 2015. **36**: 13–20.

36. Hawton, K., *et al*. Psychiatric disorders in patients presenting to hospital following self-harm: a systematic review. *J Affect Disord*, 2013. **151**: 821–30.

37. Rusch, N., *et al*. Does the stigma of mental illness contribute to suicidality? *Br J Psychiatry*, 2014. **205**:257–9.

38. Mehta, N., *et al*. Evidence for effective interventions to reduce mental health-related stigma and discrimination in the medium and long term: systematic review. *Br J Psychiatry*, 2015. **207**: 377–84.

39. Rutz, W., L. von Knorring, and J. Walinder. Frequency of suicide on Gotland after systematic postgraduate education of general practitioners. *Acta Psychiatr Scand*, 1989. **80**: 151–4.

40. Rutz, W., L. von Knorring, and J. Walinder. Long-term effects of an educational program for general practitioners given by the Swedish Committee for the Prevention and Treatment of Depression. *Acta Psychiatr Scand*, 1992. **85**: 83–8.

41. Rutz, W., *et al*. *An Update of the Gotland Study*. Martin Dunitz Publishers: London; 1997.

42. Luoma, J.B., C.E. Martin, and J.L. Pearson. Contact with mental health and primary care providers before suicide: a review of the evidence. *Am J Psychiatry*, 2002. **159**: 909–16.

43. National Confidential Inquiry into Suicide and Homicide by People with Mental Illness (NCISH). *Suicide in Primary Care in England: 2002–2011*. University of Manchester: Manchester; 2014.

44. Quinlivan, L., *et al*. Which are the most useful scales for predicting repeat self-harm? A systematic review evaluating risk scales using measures of diagnostic accuracy. *BMJ Open*, 2016. **6**: e009297.

45. Chan, M.K., *et al*. Predicting suicide following self-harm: systematic review of risk factors and risk scales. *Br J Psychiatry*, 2016. **209**: 277–83.

46. Hawton, K. and K. Rodham. *By Their Own Young Hand: Deliberate Self-Harm and Suicidal Ideas in Adolescents*. Jessica Kingsley Publishers: London; 2006.

47. Wasserman, D., *et al*. School-based suicide prevention programmes: the SEYLE cluster-randomised, controlled trial. *Lancet*, 2015. **385**: 1536–44.

48. Cox, G.R., *et al*. Interventions to reduce suicides at suicide hotspots: a systematic review. *BMC Public Health*, 2013. **13**: 214.

49. Coveney, C.M., *et al*. Callers' experiences of contacting a national suicide prevention helpline: report of an online survey. *Crisis*, 2012. **33**: 313–24.

50. Office of the Surgeon General (US); National Action Alliance for Suicide Prevention (US). *2012 National Strategy for Suicide Prevention: Goals and Objectives for Action: A Report of the U.S. Surgeon General and of the National Action Alliance for Suicide Prevention*. US Department of Health and Human Services: Washington, DC; 2012.

51. Chesney, E., G.M. Goodwin, and S. Fazel. Risks of all-cause and suicide mortality in mental disorders: a meta-review. *World Psychiatry*, 2014. **13**: 153–60.

52. Bowen, R., *et al*. The relationship between mood instability and suicidal thoughts. *Arch Suicide Res*, 2015. **19**: 161–71.

53. National Institute for Health and Care Excellence. *Self-Harm: Longer-Term Management*. Clinical guideline [CG133]. National Institute for Health and Care Excellence: London; 2012.

54. Goldacre, M., V. Seagroatt, and K. Hawton. Suicide after discharge from psychiatric inpatient care. *Lancet*, 1993. **342**: 283–6.

55. The National Confidential Inquiry into Suicide and Homicide by People with Mental Illness. *Making Mental Health Care Safer: Annual Report and 20-year Review*. University of Manchester: Manchester; 2016.

56. National Confidential Inquiry into Suicide and Homicide by People with Mental Illness. *Avoidable deaths. Five year report of the National Confidential Inquiry into suicide and homicide by people with mental illness*. University of Manchester: Manchester; 2006.

57. Rihmer, Z. [Antidepressants, depression and suicide]. *Neuropsychopharmacol Hung*, 2013. **15**: 157–64.

58. Verkes, R.J., *et al*. Reduction by paroxetine of suicidal behavior in patients with repeated suicide attempts but not major depression. *Am J Psychiatry*, 1998. **155**: 543–7.

59. Stone, M., *et al*. Risk of suicidality in clinical trials of antidepressants in adults: analysis of proprietary data submitted to US Food and Drug Administration. *BMJ*, 2009. **339**: 431–4.

60. Simon, G.E. and J. Savarino. Suicide attempts among patients starting depression treatment with medications or psychotherapy. *Am J Psychiatry*, 2007. **164**: 1029–34.

61. Cipriani, A., *et al*. Lithium in the prevention of suicide in mood disorders: updated systematic review and meta-analysis. *BMJ*, 2013. **346**: f3646.

62. Meltzer, H.Y., *et al*. Clozapine treatment for suicdality in schizophrenia. International Suicide Prevention Trial (InterSePT). *Arch Gen Psychiatry*, 2003. **60**: 82–91.

63. Walker, A.M., *et al*. Mortality in current and former users of clozapine. *Epidemiology*, 1997. **8**: 671–7.

64. Larkin, G.L. and A.L. Beautrais. A preliminary naturalistic study of low-dose ketamine for depression and suicide ideation in the emergency department. *Int J Neuropsychopharmacol*, 2011. **14**: 1127–31.

65. Price, R.B., *et al*. Effects of ketamine on explicit and implicit suicidal cognition: a randomized controlled trial in treatment-resistant depression. *Depress Anxiety*, 2014. **31**: 335–43.

66. Caddy, C., *et al*. Ketamine and other glutamate receptor modulators for depression in adults. *Cochrane Database Syst Rev*, 2015. **9**: CD011612.

67. Zarate, C.A., *et al*. Replication of ketamine's antidepressant efficacy in bipolar depression: a randomized controlled add-on trial. *Biol Psychiatry*, 2012. **71**: 939–46.

68. While, D., *et al*. Implementation of mental health service recommendations in England and Wales and suicide rates, 1997–2006: a cross-sectional and before-and-after observational study. *Lancet*, 2012. **379**: 1005–12.

69. Haw, C., *et al*. Schizophrenia and deliberate self-harm: a systematic review of risk factors. *Suicide Life Threat Behav*, 2005. **35**: 50–62.

70. Pirkola, S., *et al*. Community mental-health services and suicide rate in Finland: a nationwide small-area analysis. *Lancet*, 2009. **373**: 147–53.

71. Pridemore, W.A. and A.J. Snowden. Reduction in suicide mortality following a new national alcohol policy in Slovenia: an interrupted time-series analysis. *Am J Public Health*, 2009. **99**: 915–20.

72. Pridemore, W.A. and M.B. Chamlin. A time-series analysis of the impact of heavy drinking on homicide and suicide mortality in Russia, 1956–2002. *Addiction*, 2006. **101**: 1719–29.

73. Pridemore, W.A., M.B. Chamlin, and E. Andreev. Reduction in male suicide mortality following the 2006 Russian alcohol policy: an interrupted time series analysis. *Am J Public Health*, 2013. **103**: 2021–6.

74. Murphy, G.E., *et al*. Suicide and alcoholism: Interpersonal loss confirmed as a predictor. *Arch Gen Psychiatry*, 1979. **36**: 65–9.

75. Qin, P., *et al*. Combined effects of physical illness and comorbid psychiatric disorder on risk of suicide in a national population study. *Br J Psychiatry*, 2014. **204**: 430–5.

76. Singhal, A., *et al*. Risk of self-harm and suicide in people with specific psychiatric and physical disorders: comparisons between disorders using English national record linkage. *J R Soc Med*, 2014. **107**: 194–204.

77. Tang, N.K. and C. Crane. Suicidality in chronic pain: a review of the prevalence, risk factors and psychological links. *Psychol Med*, 2006. **36**: 575–86.

78. Calati, R., *et al*. The impact of physical pain on suicidal thoughts and behaviors: meta-analyses. *J Psychiatr Res*, 2015. **71**: 16–32.

79. Kapur, N., *et al*. Does clinical management improve outcomes following self-harm? Results from the Multicentre Study of Self-harm in England. *PLoS One*, 2013. **8**: e70434.

80. National Collaborating Centre for Mental Health. *Self-Harm: The Short-Term Physical and Psychological Management and Secondary Prevention of Self-Harm in Primary and Secondary Care*. Clinical guideline [CG16]. National Institute for Health and Care Excellence: London; 2004.

81. Fazel, S., *et al*. Prison suicide in 12 countries: an ecological study of 861 suicides during 2003–2007. *Soc Psychiatry Psychiatr Epidemiol*, 2011. **46**: 191–5.

82. Marzano, L., *et al*. Prevention of suicidal behavior in prisons. *Crisis*, 2016. **37**: 323–34.

83. Pitman, A. *et al*. The impact of suicide bereavement on mental health and suicide mortality. *Lancet Psychiatry*, 2014. **1**: 86–94.

84. Pitman, A.L., *et al*. Support for relatives bereaved by psychiatric patient suicide: National Confidential Inquiry Into Suicide and Homicide Findings. *Psychiatr Serv*, 2017. **68**: 337–44.

85. Pitman, A.L., *et al*. Bereavement by suicide as a risk factor for suicide attempt: a cross-sectional national UK-wide study of 3432 young bereaved adults. *BMJ Open*, 2016. **6**: e009948.

86. Szumilas, M., and Kutcher, S. Post-suicide intervention programs: a systematic review. *Can J Public Health*, 2011. **102**(1): 18–29.

87. McDaid, C., *et al*. Interventions for people bereaved through suicide: a systematic review. *Br J Psychiatry*, 2008. **193**: 438–43.

88. Zahl, D. and K. Hawton. Repetition of deliberate self-harm and subsequent suicide risk: long-term follow-up study in 11,583 patients. *Br J Psychiatry*, 2004. **185**: 70–5.

89. Corcoran, P., *et al*. Hospital-treated deliberate self-harm in the Western area of Northern Ireland. *Crisis*, 2016. **36**: 83–90.

90. Carroll, R., C. Metcalfe, and D. Gunnell. Hospital presenting self-harm and risk of fatal and non-fatal repetition: systematic review and meta-analysis. *PLoS One*, 2014. **9**: e89944.

91. Hawton, K., *et al*. Comorbidity of axis1 and axis2 disorders in patients who attempted suicide. *Am J Psychiatry*, 2003. **160**: 1494–500.

92. Townsend, E., *et al*. Self-harm and life problems: findings from the Multicentre Study of Self-harm in England. *Soc Psychiatry Psychiatr Epidemiol*, 2016. **51**: 183–92.

93. Beck, A.T., *et al*. Hopelessness and eventual suicide: a 10 year prospective study of patients hospitalised with suicidal ideation. *Am J Psychiatry*, 1985. **145**: 559–63.

94. Williams, J.M.G., *et al*. Psychology and suicidal behaviour: elaborating the entrapment model. In: K. Hawton, editor. *Prevention and Treatment of Suicidal Behaviour: From Science to Practice*. Oxford University Press: Oxford; 2005. pp. 71–90.

95. Mann, J.J. Neurobiology of suicidal behaviour. *Nat Rev Neurosci*, 2003. **4**: 819–28.

96. Lizardi, D. and B. Stanley. Treatment engagement: a neglected aspect in the psychiatric care of suicidal patients. *Psychiatr Serv*, 2010. **61**: 1183–91.

97. Hawton, K., *et al*. Psychosocial interventions following self-harm in adults: a systematic review and meta-analysis. *Lancet Psychiatry*, 2016. **3**: 740–50.

98. Hawton, K., *et al*. Psychosocial interventions for self-harm in adults. *Cochrane Database Syst Rev*, 2016. **5**: CD012189.

99. Hassanian-Moghaddam, H., *et al*. Postcards in Persia: randomised controlled trial to reduce suicidal behaviours 12 months after hospital-treated self-poisoning. *Br J Psychiatry*, 2011. **198**: 309–16.

100. Rossow, I., *et al*. Chain of care for patients with intentional self-harm: an effective strategy to reduce suicide rates? *Suicide Life Threat Behav*, 2009. **39**: 614–22.

101. Van Heeringen, C., *et al*. The management of non-compliance with referral to out-patient after-care among attempted suicide patients: a controlled intervention study. *Psychol Med*, 1995. **25**: 963–70.

102. Ougrin, D., *et al*. Adolescents with suicidal and nonsuicidal self-harm: clinical characteristics and response to therapeutic assessment. *Psychol Assess*, 2012. **24**: 11–20.

103. Marzano, L., *et al*. The application of mHealth to mental health: opportunities and challenges. *Lancet Psychiatry*, 2015. **2**: 942–8.

104. Hawton, K., *et al*. Pharmacological interventions for self-harm in adults. *Cochrane Database Syst Rev*, 2015. **7**: CD011777.

105. Hawton, K., *et al*. Toxicity of antidepressants: rates of suicide relative to prescribing and non-fatal overdose. *Br J Psychiatry*, 2010. **196**: 354–8.

106. Gibbons, R.D., *et al*. Early evidence on the effects of regulators' suicidality warnings on SSRI prescriptions and suicide in children and adolescents. *Am J Psychiatry*, 2007. **164**: 1356–63.

107. March, J.S., *et al*. The Treatment for Adolescents with Depression Study (TADS): long-term effectiveness and safety outcomes. *Arch Gen Psychiatry*, 2007. **64**: 1132–44.

# SECTION 22

# Somatic symptoms and related disorders

# 129

# Deconstructing dualism
## The interface between physical and mental illness

*Michael Sharpe and Jane Walker*

## Introduction

Patients usually attend doctors because they are concerned about symptoms. When these symptoms are associated with persistent distress and/or disability, we refer to the patient as having an illness. When assessing the patient's illness, the doctor aims to make a diagnosis, on the basis of which management can be planned. The diagnoses available to doctors are conventionally categorized into either 'medical' or 'psychiatric'. This division of illnesses into two distinct types is such an accepted feature of current medical practice that we take it for granted. But is it really the best way to think about patients' illnesses and to plan their care? In order to answer this question, we examine below what is meant by 'medical' and 'psychiatric' diagnoses. The disadvantages of this dichotomous approach will then be considered, and potential solutions outlined.

## Diagnosis

### Medical diagnosis

A medical diagnosis is a label for a type of illness that is: (1) conventionally treated by medical (non-psychiatric) doctors; and (2) listed in classifications of medical conditions such as the *International Classification of Diseases*, tenth revision (ICD-10). Most medical diagnoses are based on identifiable bodily pathology (abnormal structure and/or function). Therefore, to make a medical diagnosis (such as cancer), doctors enquire about specific bodily symptoms, before confirming the presence of bodily pathology by seeking physical signs and doing biological investigations (such as X-rays).

### Psychiatric diagnosis

A psychiatric diagnosis is a label for a condition that is: (1) conventionally treated by psychiatrists; and (2) listed in the psychiatric diagnostic classifications of ICD and the *Diagnostic and Statistical Manual of Mental Disorders* (DSM). Psychiatric diagnoses are not based on bodily pathology (with the possible exception of the so-called 'organic disorders'). They are instead associated with the idea of 'psychopathology', that is, proposed abnormalities of the mind. Unlike bodily pathology, these abnormalities of the mind cannot be objectively identified. Rather they are inferred from the patient's reported mental symptoms and their behaviour.

### What makes an illness psychiatric, rather than medical?

Why are some illnesses regarded as 'mental' or 'psychiatric', as opposed to 'medical'? Examination of the criteria for those diagnoses reveals that factors common to most 'psychiatric' illnesses are:

- An absence of identifiable bodily pathology.
- An abnormal mental state implying psychopathology.
- A presentation with abnormal behaviour.

## Mind–body dualism

The fundamental assumption underpinning this dichotomous view of illness as either medical or psychiatric is that it is both conceptually valid and clinically useful. The idea that the mind is fundamentally distinct from the body (or the brain) is referred to as mind–body dualism. Mind–body dualism is commonly attributed to the writings of the philosopher Descartes. This so-called Cartesian dualism has exerted a profound influence on Western medical thought and still shapes our thinking, training, and service provision today [1].

However, it is increasingly clear that dualism is at best an oversimplification and at worst a cause of serious theoretical and clinical problems. Theoretically, it can be argued that there is no such thing as a purely 'bodily' illness or a purely 'mental' illness and that all illnesses have both mental and bodily aspects [2]. Clinically, the associated assumption that bodily symptoms always indicate bodily pathology and that mental symptoms always indicate psychopathology is not consistent with clinical experience. Two important examples are: (1) when bodily symptoms occur without bodily pathology; and (2) when mental symptoms occur with bodily pathology (Table 129.1).

**Table 129.1** Diagnoses, symptoms, and bodily pathology

| Symptoms | Bodily pathology | Diagnosis |
|---|---|---|
| Bodily symptoms | Present | Medical diagnosis |
| | Absent | *Somatization* |
| Mental symptoms | Present | *Comorbidity* |
| | Absent | Psychiatric diagnosis |

### 'Medically unexplained symptoms'

When patients present with bodily symptoms, but *no* evidence of bodily pathology, it is unclear whether their illness should be best regarded as 'psychiatric' or as 'medical' because they do not clearly fulfil the criteria for either. But the imperative to classify every illness as either medical or psychiatric in order to determine the type of treatment requires that an allocation is made.

One solution is to allocate these illnesses to psychiatry. This is done by assuming that the patient's somatic symptoms are, in fact, explained by psychopathology. The relative absence of mental symptoms, from which psychopathology is usually inferred, is explained by the idea that the psychopathology has been 'somatized'. This means that an abnormal mental state is not apparent because it has been 'converted' into bodily symptoms. The process of somatization (literally making the mental physical) is poorly specified. However, the concept can be seen in a variety of diagnostic labels, including 'somatization', 'somatoform disorder', 'conversion disorder', and 'bodily distress disorder'.

Another solution is to allocate the illness to medicine. This is made possible by assuming that the patients really do have bodily pathology (even though it is as yet unidentifiable). The absence of identifiable bodily pathology may be explained on the basis that it is present but simply not detectable using currently available diagnostic technology. A medical diagnosis that implies disease, such as 'fibromyalgia' in rheumatology or 'syndrome X' in cardiology, is then made.

A third, and all too common solution, is for the patient to be rejected as 'not really ill' by both psychiatry and medicine, leaving them in a no-man's-land between these specialties.

The problems with all three of these solutions has been particularly well illustrated by the controversy and conflict surrounding the condition called chronic fatigue syndrome (CFS), or myalgic encephalomyelitis (ME), in which there has been often fraught controversy about the nature of the illness and an associated lack of care [3].

### Comorbidity

When a patient has both bodily pathology *and* mental symptoms, they may be given *both* a medical diagnosis (based on the bodily pathology) and a psychiatric diagnosis (based on presumed psychopathology). The resulting mental–physical 'comorbidity' or 'multimorbidity' gives rise to both theoretical and practical problems, however.

The theoretical problem concerns the psychiatric diagnosis. To make this diagnosis, the doctor must identify symptoms which are considered to be evidence of the underlying psychopathology. However, some symptoms may be considered as resulting from either psychopathology or bodily pathology. For example, if a patient

has mental symptoms of weight loss and a lack of energy and a medical diagnosis of cancer, based on bodily pathology, should the weight loss and lack of energy be counted towards a psychiatric diagnosis of depression or be regarded as a symptom of the cancer? There is no generally agreed answer to this conundrum (although a variety of ways of addressing it have been proposed [4]), probably because it is a manifestation of the fundamentally flawed dualistic assumption.

The main practical clinical problem that results from making two diagnoses, one medical and one psychiatric, is a failure to adequately treat the patient. This is because the patient is considered to have two illnesses, each of which requires diagnosis and treatment by a different specialty, often based in different hospitals. As treatment of the medical condition usually takes precedence, the patient's psychiatric diagnosis often goes untreated [5].

## Solutions to dualism

### Theoretical solutions

New scientific knowledge, such as the demonstration of a bodily (neural) basis to many 'mental' symptoms, is increasingly rendering crude dualistic thinking theoretically untenable [2]. Mind and brain are increasingly regarded as two sides of the same coin—the 'mind/brain'. If this paradigm shift is adopted, it will imply that 'psychiatric' illnesses are no more distinct from 'medical conditions' than the nervous system is separate from the rest of the body. According to this new way of thinking, it would make no sense to dichotomize illnesses into 'medical' and 'psychiatric' types. Illness is just illness [6].

### Practical solutions

However the theoretical arguments play out, for the present, we must accept that dualism continues to shape our everyday thinking, practice, and service organization. But we can surely agree already that there is a need for psychiatry to become less 'brain-less' and for medicine to become less 'mind-less' [7]. In this regard, the psychiatrist is especially well placed to make a major contribution to the care of all patients by ensuring that biological, psychological, and social aspects of illness are considered in every case. This so-called 'bio-psychosocial' approach, first proposed by George Engel, provides a framework for considering multiple causes of illness [8]. A further enhancement of this approach is to divide the relevant biological, psychological, and social aetiological factors into those that predisposed the patient to the illness, those that precipitated or triggered it, and those that are perpetuating it or impeding recovery. The last group of causes is a target for treatment, and the first two for prevention. A way of tabulating factors to consider in a bio-psychosocial formulation is shown in Table 129.2.

### Service solutions

Finally, the consequence of the long-standing professional and organizational separation of medicine and psychiatry must be addressed. One service solution has been the establishment of so-called liaison (linking) psychiatry services to general hospital inpatient units. Another recent and welcome development has been the increasing integration of psychological management into general medical care [9].

**Table 129.2** A bio-psychosocial formulation

| Main factors | Sub-factors | Predisposing | Precipitating | Perpetuating |
|---|---|---|---|---|
| Biological | Disease | | | |
| | Physiology | | | |
| Psychological | Cognition | | | |
| | Mood | | | |
| | Behaviour | | | |
| Social | Interpersonal | | | |
| | Social and occupational | | | |
| | Health care system | | | |

Such developments are likely to be important for psychiatry's future status as a medical discipline [10].

## Conclusions

Hitherto we have taken it for granted that it is both appropriate and desirable to dichotomize illnesses into medical and psychiatric types, based on identifiable bodily pathology and inferred psychopathology, respectively. Such an approach has, however, created obstacles to integrated and effective patient care. A better understanding of neuroscience is challenging the theory of dualism and may lead to a more unified conceptualization of illness. The growing need to address the epidemic of patients with multi-morbidity is already making dualistic management redundant and favouring more integrated models of care. The influence of dualism is finally on the wane. The question is, 'will it be missed?'.

## FURTHER READING

Damasio AR. *Descartes' Error*. GP Putnam's Sons, New York, NY; 1994.

Naylor K, Das P, Ross S, Honeyman M, Thompson J, Gilburt H. *Bringing Together Mental and Physical Health: A New Frontier for Integrated Care*. The Kings Fund, London; 2016.

White PD. *Biopsychosocial Medicine*. Oxford University Press, Oxford; 2005.

## REFERENCES

1. Miresco MJ, Kirmayer LJ. The persistence of mind-brain dualism in psychiatric reasoning about clinical scenarios. *Am J Psychiatry*. 2006;163:913–18.
2. Kendler KS. The dappled nature of causes of psychiatric illness: replacing the organic-functional/hardware-software dichotomy with empirically based pluralism. *Mol Psychiatry*. 2012;17:377–88.
3. Sharpe M. Chronic fatigue syndrome: neurological, mental or both. *J Psychosom Res*. 2011;70:498–9.
4. Endicott J. Measurement of depression in patients with cancer. *Cancer*. 1984;53(10:Suppl):2243–9.
5. Walker J, Hansen CH, Martin P, *et al*. Prevalence, associations, and adequacy of treatment of major depression in patients with cancer: a cross-sectional analysis of routinely collected clinical data. *Lancet Psychiatry*. 2014;1:343–50.
6. Sharpe M, Mayou R, Walker J. Bodily symptoms: new approaches to classification. *J Psychosom Res*. 2006;60:353–6.
7. Eisenberg L. Mindless and brainless in psychiatry. *Br J Psychiatry*. 1986;148:497–508.
8. Engel GL. The need for a new medical model: a challenge for biomedicine. *Science*. 1977;196:129–96.
9. Sharpe M, Naylor C. Integration of mental and physical health care: from aspiration to practice. *Lancet Psychiatry*. 2016;3:312–13.
10. Sharpe M. Psychological medicine and the future of psychiatry. *Br J Psychiatry*. 2014;204:91–2.

# 130

# Neural mechanisms in chronic pain relevant for psychiatric interventions

*Chantal Berna and Irene Tracey*

## Introduction

Pain is defined as 'an unpleasant sensory and emotional experience associated with actual or potential tissue damage, or described in terms of such damage' [1]. Acute pain is a warning system alerting the subject of possible harm and leading to corrective or preventive action, both immediate (flight or fight) and delayed (learning, avoidance). However, inherent to this definition, it is clear that pain can exist as an emotional experience also without actual 'tissue damage' or physical harm. This broad definition is important as it encapsulates what can occur in chronic pain, that is, persistent pain outliving the usual time for tissue healing (>3–6 months). Chronic pain is one of the largest medical health problems in the developed world, affecting 19% of adults in Europe, with a considerable impact on quality of life, productivity, and costs for the society [2]. A recent report by the American Institute of Medicine assessing the significance and impact of chronic pain in America presented similar figures, with an estimated cost to society of about 600 billion dollars per annum, due to both medical care and lost productivity [3].

## Pain as the transduction, transmission, and perception of a nociceptive signal

Nociception, that is, the neural and molecular processes involved in acute pain perception, has been progressively elucidated. This includes the *transduction* of the nociceptive input through different peripheral sensory neurons (nociceptors) into a neural signal, followed by the multisynaptic *transmission* to the central relays and *perception* in the sensory cortices (Fig. 130.1).

Most nociceptors are myelinated A fibres or unmyelinated small-diameter axons (C fibres). They project to the superficial laminae I and V (Aδ) and I and II (C fibre) of the dorsal horn of the spinal cord [4]. Local spinal circuits— excitatory and inhibitory—allow for bi-directional changes in spinal outputs. Excitatory transmitters, such as glutamate and substance P, can facilitate and 'wind up' neuronal responses, whereas inhibitory interneurons releasing endogenous opioids and gamma aminobutyric acid (GABA) can modulate spinal activity. From the dorsal horn, three major projection pathways lead the signal to the brain: the spinomesencephalic [to the periaqueductal grey (PAG)], the spinothalamic (to the thalamus as a relay to the cortex), and the spinoreticular pathway (to the reticular formation of the medulla and pons as a relay to the thalamus and cortex) [5]. Molecular biology and the study of patients suffering from congenital insensitivity to pain have contributed significantly over the past decades to form a more complete understanding of these mechanisms of transduction and transmission, providing new opportunities for possible pharmacological targets such as the sodium channel NAv.1.7, the transient receptor potential (TRP) family, and acid-sensing ion channels (ASICs) [6]. In parallel, improved knowledge of the molecular and cellular changes that occur post-injury and in the chronic pain state is providing novel options for therapeutic interventions such as nerve growth factor (NGF) antagonism [7]. These advances, among others, have contributed to chronic pain being classified as a disease in its own right [8, 9], with specific underlying mechanisms distinct from the ones involved in acute pain.

## Neural networks of sensory perception

Neuroimaging has helped to develop knowledge about the neural networks of sensory perception. The current concept for the central aspects of pain perception is mostly based on acute induced pain studies and considers a large bilateral network available for variable activation, including the thalamus, the posterior and anterior insulae, the secondary somatosensory cortex, the anterior cingulate cortex, and the PAG matter, among other regions (Fig. 130.2) [10, 11].

The principle is that different brain regions and networks can be recruited variably and dynamically for activation (or not), depending on the nociceptive drive, context, attention, emotions, and cognitions, allowing for rapidly adaptive behavioural responses to each individual specific situation [5]. It should be obvious that most of the brain regions active in this dynamic network are not pain-specific (that is, the 'hurt' of pain) but subserve many features

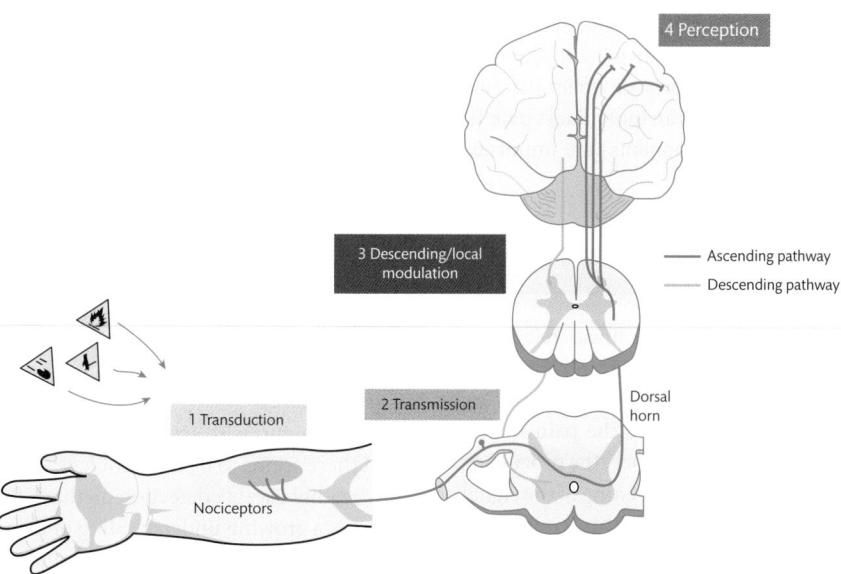

**Fig. 130.1** (see Colour Plate section) Acute nociception as a three-neuron order system. The peripheral nociceptor is responsible for the transduction into a neural signal (1). This is followed by transmission through neurons (2), with possible descending and local modulation (3), leading to the final perception at the cortical level (4).

relevant to this multifactorial experience in matters of anticipation, anxiety, attention, sensory discrimination, motor preparation, etc. (for example, [12]). Some regions of this brain network also likely encode the saliency of pain within a particular context [13]. Overlap of activity in regions like the anterior cingulate and divisions of the insula, as well as distinctions in the activated networks when comparing physical pain, empathy (that is, feeling for others in pain), and moral suffering (such as studied through social rejection), highlight that while *many cortical areas* are recruited by multiple processes, *specific networks* and *patterns of activation* can be characteristic of a certain perception or function. Such distinctions are being increasingly disambiguated with more advanced imaging analysis methods and paradigms [14–16]. We should remember that

experiencing emotional pain is what makes us human, as underlined by William James and other philosophers. Distinguishing between pain that has a peripheral maintaining drive (sometimes wrongly labelled 'physical') and centrally generated or maintained pain (oftentimes labelled 'emotional') has been a preoccupation for scientists, the medical profession, lawyers, and insurance brokers, with frequent misunderstandings and confusion—leading to downgrading the relevance of 'emotional' pain because it does not have a 'physical' origin. Newer research, taking into account the complexities of the neural pathways that integrate emotional and physical experiences, can allow distinctions at more subtle levels. Hence, an emotional response to social exclusion should not be confused or amalgamated with centrally amplified pain following a nerve injury with resulting

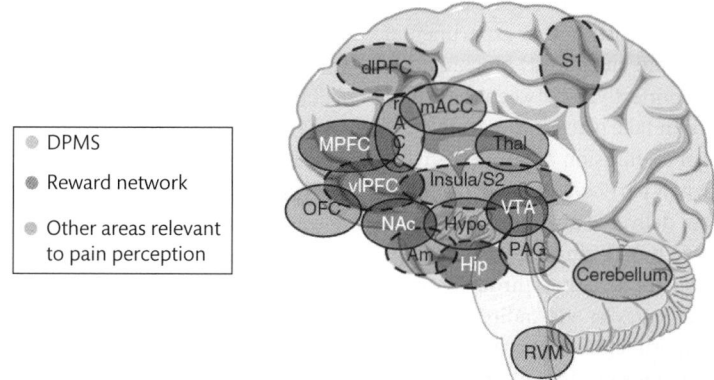

**Fig. 130.2** (see Colour Plate section) Cerebral areas and networks involved in pain perception and regulation, as well as reward. The key networks consist of the descending pain modulatory system (DPMS, green) and the reward network (purple). Alterations in function, connectivity, and structure have been described in these networks in chronic pain. rACC/mACC, rostral/medial anterior cingulate cortex; vlPFC, ventrolateral prefrontal cortex; dlPFC, dorsolateral prefrontal cortex; mPFC, medial prefrontal cortex; OFC, orbitofrontal cortex; insula/S2, insular and secondary somatosensory cortex; S1, primary somatosensory cortex; Am, amygdala; Hip, hippocampus; Hypo, hypothalamus; Thal, thalamus; PAG, periaqueductal grey; VTA, ventral tegmentum.

Adapted from *Nat Neurosci.*, 17(2), Denk F, McMahon SB, Tracey I, Pain vulnerability: a neurobiological perspective, pp. 192–200, Copyright (2014), with permission from Springer Nature.

central sensitization. We are not making judgements about which pain (or suffering) is more important—for the patient, the experience is paramount, whatever the cause. However, better discrimination and identification of what constitutes an individual's pain (that is, balance of peripheral and central components) are important if we are to target treatments more effectively.

## Modulation of pain perception

Nociception and pain can have a highly non-linear relationship; there is frequently a mismatch between the nociceptive input and the resultant pain perception. In fact, the bottom–up input can be modulated by a number of mechanisms along the pain neuraxis, leading to different final experiences. For instance, the processing of the signal can be modified through either dampening of the signal or the recruitment of supplementary cortical areas. This is important as it allows for a person's pain experience and subsequent behavioural response to adapt to the situation in which they are—enabling an improved decision and outcome. A major regulatory pathway is the descending pain modulatory system (DPMS), which has central relays in the dorsolateral prefrontal cortex (DLPFC), rostral anterior cingulate cortex (rACC), amygdala, hypothalamus, rostral ventromedial medulla (RVM), and PAG matter and releases endogenous opioids in the dorsal horn of the spinal cord, as well as noradrenaline and serotonin [10, 17] (Fig. 130.2). In the RVM, serotonin (5-HT) can inhibit (via 5-HT1 receptors) or facilitate (via 5-HT2 or 5-HT3 receptors) spinal neuronal activity; endorphins also have bi-directional effects, while noradrenaline has inhibitory activity through the α2 adrenoceptor. The DPMS is a powerful system that is recruited for its inhibitory (pain-inhibiting) features when subjects are distracted from pain or during placebo analgesia. The opposite facilitatory arm is recruited in response to injury. It is now known from animal and human studies that an imbalance in this system (too much facilitation and not enough inhibition) is a major factor explaining the chronic pain phenotype.

Many studies in healthy participants have demonstrated the potential for modulation of acute pain through cognitive processes such as distraction, expectations, or context [18–20]. The involvement of the central relays of the DPMS was demonstrated in experimental placebo analgesia, with naloxone (opioid antagonist) blocking this effect and inhibiting the functional connectivity between the rACC and the PAG [21]. Opposite effects can take place with negative expectations. For example, the effect of an infusion of remifentanil, a powerful opioid, can be annulled when participants are deceptively led to believe the medication was not delivered anymore [22].

Furthermore, anxiety and negative mood can heighten the pain experience to the same nociceptive input either through direct modulation of core pain-processing areas or via indirect means. These affective modulations in the experimental context seem to rely on recruiting other pathways, involving the prefrontal cortex (PFC), hippocampus, and amygdala, among other structures [23–27].

These concepts become more complex in the clinical situation, as the three levels (transduction, transmission, perception) can all be modified in chronic pain—as further discussed in the section on acute and chronic pain [28, 29]. For instance, the bi-directional control means that the DPMS has also been involved in facilitating nociceptive processing. Indeed, it has now been shown that an imbalance

between facilitation and inhibition (too much facilitation and too little inhibition) contributes to the development, maintenance, and exacerbation of chronic pain states in both animal (for example, [30, 31]) and human studies [32–35]. Therefore, an intervention in chronic pain only targeting the periphery (trying to dampen the volume of the transduction) is most often bound to fail, as it omits central processes, such as anxiety, depression, or central sensitization, which can upregulate the experience.

## Transition from acute to chronic pain—a process with possible predisposing factors

Not all patients with acute pain go on to develop a chronic condition, and there seems to be different levels of risk. While there are not yet any readily useable detection methods for individuals at higher risk, there is a growing understanding of the vulnerability and protective factors that might lead to implement early preventive interventions or to develop better-targeted treatments. Vulnerability factors for developing chronic pain can be present at birth, such as female gender or genetic make-up; brought on by the environment such as adverse life events; or, in many circumstances, be the result of a combination of both (Fig. 130.3) [36]. On the other hand, inherent features of resilience are progressively being investigated and demonstrated to be different from vulnerability factors (or the absence thereof) [37]. For example, a novel line of research is focusing on the value of positive affect [38]—an important area for further research and development.

### Genetic factors involved in pain perception

The genetic make-up of certain enzymes and receptors is of importance for pain perception. Catechol-*O*-methyltransferase (COMT) is an enzyme degrading catecholamine neurotransmitters (that is, adrenaline, dopamine, and noradrenaline) in the synaptic cleft, thereby regulating different neurophysiological functions. Certain frequent polymorphisms of *COMT* seem to affect experimental pain processing, endogenous opioid transmission, and perhaps the response to opioids [39]. While COMT variants do not appear to be predisposing factors for developing chronic pain, they have been shown to impact a number of affective and cognitive tasks in which the PFC plays a key role [40]. For example, COMT variations can affect the response to placebo modulations in patients [41] and could also be involved in the response to psychological approaches to pain management [40].

Preclinical models have shown that serotonin is involved in chronic pain, although it is a complex system with serotonergic receptors demonstrating pro- or anti-nociceptive function, depending on a number of factors (type of animal model, anatomical site, subtype of receptor). Polymorphisms in serotonin receptors could be involved in the regulation of pain affect and perhaps response to opioids [40].

### Priming processes

Animal studies of early-life exposures to pain are striking examples of how life events can mark future pain perception; it can result in heightened pain sensitivity in fully developed individuals [42]. In addition to prior pain, early-life stress, such as maternal separation, can also be sufficient to induce hypersensitivity in later life [43]. Increased axonal

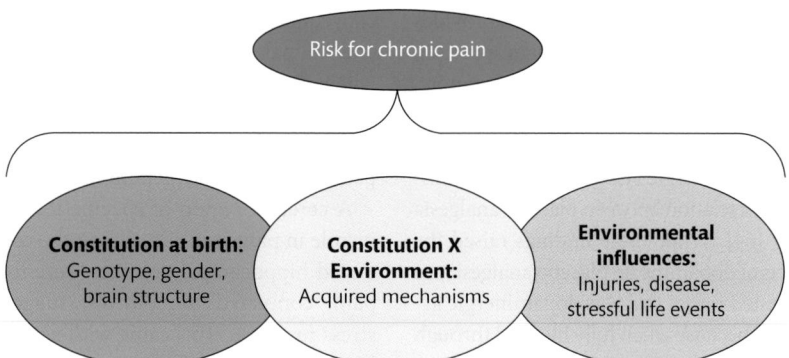

**Fig. 130.3** Factors of vulnerability for a chronic pain state. These factors emerge at different levels, whether endogenous (genetic predispositions and cerebral structures) or environmental or through a combination of the two.
Adapted from *Nat Neurosci.*, 17(2), Denk F, McMahon SB, Tracey I, Pain vulnerability: a neurobiological perspective, pp. 192–200, Copyright (2014), with permission from Springer Nature.

sprouting, NGF-induced neuronal plasticity, changes to the opioid system, or alterations in the hypothalamic–pituitary–adrenal axis and in the spinal microglia could possibly explain these processes [42, 44]. Parallel human work was done through neuroimaging in school-age children who were born preterm; central functional alterations have been demonstrated, with an impact on cognitive outcomes and pain processing [45, 46]. A similar mechanism, known as priming, has been demonstrated in adult animals; for example, repeated nerve injury or stress before an experimental nerve lesion can result in prolonged hypersensitivity, when compared to a single lesion [47]. The main pathways examined to explain this phenomenon are the peripheral afferents and the spinal microglia [36].

Hypothetically, early-life stressors that are known to relate to neuroticism and anxiety could have developmental influences on the DPMS via alterations in the coupling of the amygdala–PFC network to the brainstem nuclei, leading to an unfavourable imbalance in inhibitory and facilitatory drive, which could predispose individuals towards developing chronic pain. Based on this hypothesis, personal specificities such as variants in personality, psychological traits, response to opioids, or reactivity to standard pain testing could rely on changes in central networks and represent risk factors for increased pain perception [32, 48–51]. While differences were found at the central level between these groups and controls, it is unclear if the central correlates of these behavioural and psychological variants in healthy people translate to any clinically meaningful impact regarding the risk for chronic pain. Nevertheless, testing the DPMS function in patients could classify them for the risk in response to surgery; two pain modulatory processes thought to be mediated through the DPMS—temporal summation (that is, an individual's level of pain in response to a rapid succession of similar noxious inputs) and diffuse noxious inhibitory control (DNIC) (that is, the level of pain reduction when the stimulus of interest is associated to a second noxious stimulus)—were shown to be predictive of post-surgical pain levels [52, 53].

## Importance of the reward–motivation–learning system

While studies in patients have shown clear functional and structural differences, compared to healthy controls, this does not provide

evidence of a causal link. It also leaves open the question of whether these changes in central networks are causal or consequential to chronic pain. Yet, recent longitudinal studies have underlined the particular wiring of the central reward–motivation–learning network as a potential key factor of vulnerability (Fig. 130.2). This is especially interesting, when one considers relief as an integrated reward process in pain [54]. An impressive and large prospective observational neuroimaging study followed 159 patients with subacute low back pain over the course of a year (N = 69 completed follow-up) as they recovered (N = 30) or developed chronic pain (N = 39, prolonged follow-up to 3 years) [55–59], providing important data and insight into the evolution of chronic pain. Results from the first neuroimaging session during the subacute pain phase demonstrated that greater functional connectivity or 'coupling' of the nucleus accumbens (NAC) with the PFC was strongly predictive of pain persistence. Hence, cortico-striatal circuitry could be causally involved in the transition from acute to chronic pain. Interestingly, this stronger coupling remained present throughout the transition to chronic pain, despite grey matter density decreases in the NAC. Furthermore, in the group that went on to develop chronic pain, white matter fractional anisotropy differences in the PFC were identified at an early time point, possibly representing structural vulnerabilities. These results suggest a role for the brain's reward–motivation–learning circuitry during the transition from acute to chronic pain. Finally, stronger white matter and functional connections within the dorsal medial PFC–amygdala–accumbens circuit, as well as smaller amygdala volume, represented independent risk factors, accounting together for 60% of the variance of pain persistence at 3 years' follow-up [59].

Separate work has underlined differences in NAC activity in response to relief from acute experimental pain between controls and patients with chronic low back pain [60], as well as patients with fibromyalgia [61].

Healthy volunteer studies have also shown that baseline activity in the ventral tegmental area and the NAC was predictive of subsequent opioid-induced analgesia and central activity in the DPMS [51]. Animal studies supported also the need for a functioning reward system to experience analgesia [62].

Provided the appropriate relative context, the hedonic value of pain can be 'flipped' from threat to reward, with increased activity in reward regions, working in concert with the DPMS [18]. Such work provides further evidence for the importance of these networks in pain appraisal, which is a key feature of ongoing chronic pain states. Furthermore, dispositional optimism and pessimism influence the central processing of unexpected relief outcomes, with diametrically opposite NAC activity [63]. Finally, the dopaminergic system has also been involved in placebo effects, with a correlation between placebo analgesia and levels of dopamine release [64]. While these findings raised the question of possible direct effects of dopamine on placebo analgesia, an interesting separate study suggested rather that this dopaminergic activity is related to the relief of pain because when fully blocked through a dopamine antagonist, the placebo effect still took place [65].

It seems likely that the transition to chronic pain is dependent on the state of the mesolimbic–prefrontal connectivity and function, that is, of the motivation–learning and reward circuitry. Yet it remains ambiguous what this means. While it has been interpreted as a predictor for a *transition* from acute to chronic pain, an alternative explanation could be that these patients suffer from *an inability to experience relief and hence analgesia from treatment*, that is, they have a 'broken analgesic system' and so, by definition, remain in pain as they get no relief [66].

## Other cognitive factors of risk

Other cognitive factors have been investigated as predisposing to chronic pain. Most notably, catastrophizing, a cognitive–emotional process involving magnification, helplessness, and rumination when facing pain, has been shown to be tied to negative outcomes [67] and to be an independent predictor of ill adaptation to pain and pain-related affective dysregulation [38].

Another proposed vulnerability factor could consist of the chosen attentional focus when confronted with concomitant nociceptive stimuli and cognitive tasks. In fact, two different profiles were identified, with participants demonstrating either a 'pain focus' or being able to remain focused on a parallel cognitive task, with resulting faster reaction times [68]. Participants focusing on pain demonstrated more grey matter in regions implicated in pain and salience, greater functional connectivity in sensorimotor and salience resting-state networks, less white matter integrity in the internal and external capsules, and anterior thalamic radiation and corticospinal tract, while well matched for sex, neuroticism, pain sensitivity, and catastrophizing. Interesting parallels can be drawn with the literature on anxiety where cognitive biases towards threat, as well as inefficient attentional regulation of emotionally and non-emotionally salient stimuli, have been demonstrated [69, 70].

## Chronic pain as a brain disease: maladaptive plasticity and psychological maintaining processes

Once pain is chronic, the central circuitry involved in processing further nociceptive stimuli might be quite different from what is studied in acute pain, both at a structural and at a functional level. In fact, meta-analytic studies have shown decreases in grey matter volumes in different cortical and brainstem areas, as well as increases in the thalamus, and this has been found across different chronic pain conditions [71]. Whether these differences are causal or

consequential to chronic pain is still up for debate, although human and animal studies are suggestive of pain causing the changes, as when pain is relieved, the structural changes normalize [72–75]. Such reversal is important, as it calls into question the early interpretations of what these volume changes represent (that is, incompatible with neurodegeneration) [76].

A cerebral region of specific interest is the hippocampus, given its role in pain amplification in the context of anxiety and stress; reduced hippocampal volumes were found in patients with chronic pain, compared to controls, suggesting a sustained endocrine stress response. This came with associated increased activity in the hippocampal complex in response to acute pain [77]. These elements together could, in turn, contribute to the persistent pain state.

At a functional level, pain perception in patients with chronic low back pain involves less somatosensory and more limbic networks, compared to acute pain models [56]. As mentioned, there is also an imbalance in the DPMS, with too little descending inhibition and too much descending facilitation. In fact, central sensitization is a normal adaptive response post-injury; yet failure to resolve this beyond the acute stage is a maintaining factor of chronic pain states. The signs of central sensitization have been demonstrated by increased PAG activity in certain patients with osteoarthritis [32], replicating experimental human models of brainstem amplification mechanisms [34, 35, 78]. This factor could also be involved in functional pain syndromes or fibromyalgia [79, 80]. Importantly, central aberrant mechanisms are the target of duloxetine, a serotonin and noradrenaline reuptake inhibitor that supposedly 'rebalances' the inhibitory/facilitatory drive, as well as of tricyclic antidepressants [81]. In fact, a study in painful diabetic neuropathy found that poor DNIC efficiency predicts the efficacy of duloxetine and that this treatment allowed to re-establish normal DNIC [82].

Of course, the poster-child for maladaptive plasticity is phantom limb pain where original theories suggested that altered brain representation of body parts into the 'vacated' deprived cortex (from the missing limb) causally produced pain in patients [83]. However, recent work now suggests different interpretations might better explain the pain of phantom limb, with lively debate and discussion ensuing [84–87]. This is not only an academic question; the maladaptive model has also been used to support treatments, which might be misdirected in this newer light [88, 89].

Psychiatric comorbidity is extremely frequent, with most patients suffering from chronic pain declaring symptoms of anxiety or depression [90–92]. Post-traumatic stress disorder is also a frequent co-occurrence with possible reciprocal maintenance [93, 94]. As in the experimental context described, depressed mood can have a negative impact on pain control and perception [95]. Furthermore, catastrophic thinking has been shown to affect pain perception through altered PFC activity [96]. Anxiety, fear of pain, avoidance, and related cognitive behavioural mechanisms have been extensively described as relevant to pain suffering and loss of function [97, 98]. These factors need to be addressed through psychological or mind–body approaches in chronic pain [99–101].

## Therapeutic implications

Clarifying the maintaining factor, whether peripheral or central, and diagnosing emotional, cognitive, and neurogenic (autonomous

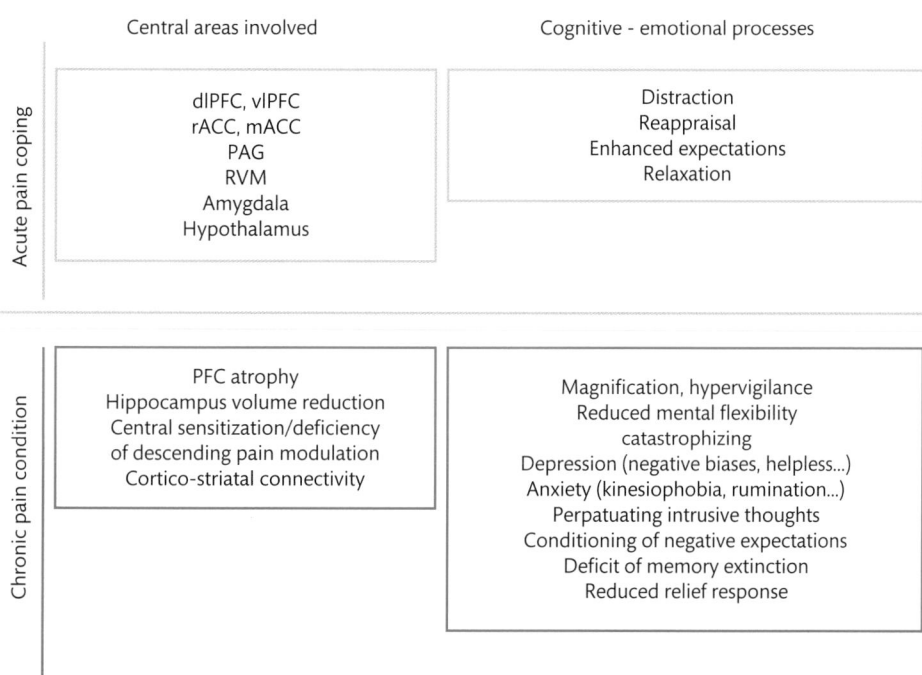

**Fig. 130.4** Contrasting acute pain coping to the chronic pain condition. This non-exhaustive graphical representation highlights some of the commonalities and differences in neural processing areas and cognitive–emotional processes between acute pain in the healthy state and chronic pain pathology. The alterations in chronic pain shown here cannot be addressed by acute pain medication and require psychiatric or rehabilitative approaches to achieve improved function.

nervous system, DPMS, etc.) processes allow for appropriate treatment targeting. When there is evidence for central maintaining factors, it appears illusory to expect that medications, which act peripherally, such as non-steroidal anti-inflammatory drugs, could address the full depth of the problem. Molecules acting centrally and psychotherapy, as well as rehabilitation, may be needed (Fig. 130.4). Hence, there is an indication for medications such as duloxetine, tricyclic antidepressants, gabapentin, and pregabalin [81]. Opioidergic agents present somewhat a special case worth discussing. Opioids act centrally, at the very core of the DPMS, and there is even evidence for acute relief of emotional suffering [102]. Yet the clinical literature suggests long-term opioid therapy has a rather poor outcome in chronic pain [103], and there is a concerning association between opioid dose and the risk of activity interference, depression, and suicide [104, 105]. Mechanisms underlying the adverse outcomes of long-term opioid therapy for chronic pain are not yet well understood, but tolerance and induced hyperalgesia (a form of central sensitization due to opioids) could be involved.

Psychological and mind–body approaches, such as cognitive behavioural therapy, meditation, hypnosis, or yoga, are supported by clinical research [101, 106–108]. Increasingly, there is also brain imaging evidence for such therapies, with hints at the mechanisms involved in their benefits, mostly from healthy volunteers [109–112]. In patients, it has been demonstrated that a course of cognitive behavioural therapy can increase PFC activation of patients with fibromyalgia in response to pain or change resting-state connectivity that seems tied to catastrophizing [113, 114].

In sum, treating the psychiatric comorbidity and adverse psychological adaptation mechanisms needs to be taken as seriously as addressing the physical injury [115, 116]. This understanding is key

to the involvement of psychiatrists in the treatment of chronic pain [117], a field where multi-disciplinary care has shown to be very important [118] and in which exclusive opioid pharmacological treatment has been recently strongly warned against [103, 119].

## Considerations on somatic symptom disorder

In certain circumstances, chronic pain is associated with somatic symptom disorders, which can be diagnosed in the presence of at least one of three psychological criteria: health anxiety, disproportionate and persistent concerns about the medical seriousness of the symptoms, and excessive time and energy devoted to the symptoms or health concerns. However, this new DSM-5 diagnostic category is under debate [120]. Beyond the syndromes including pain, the neural mechanisms involved in somatic symptom disorders are not yet well qualified [121]. Our understanding of certain functional pain syndromes, as well as somatic symptom disorders, might benefit from new theories and research regarding the nature of perception [122]. This line of research has also offered explanatory models for placebo effects [123]. Bayesian models of perception suggest that prior information can alter the *interpretation* of new stimuli, with prior beliefs and sensory information biasing new perceptions by overriding the current input [124].

## Conclusions

Finally, whatever the cause, the underlying risk factors, or the specific pathophysiological path of a chronic pain sufferer, 'terminal' chronic pain can be seen as failure of an individual's coping abilities and of their adaptation resources. If the condition has been ongoing for long enough, patients are likely to present with depression or anxiety, social isolation, functional impairment, and possibly opioid reliance. They are at a dead-end, which requires a fundamental change of course to get back to a life worth living and to experience well-being and happiness. When medications, surgeries, and procedures are not helpful, psychological techniques fostering change are required. In any case, the comorbid psychiatric or psychological conditions, which can act as maintaining factors, must be addressed.

## REFERENCES

1. International Association for Suicide Prevention (IASP) Task Force on Taxonomy (1994). Part III: pain terms, a current list with definitions and notes on usage. In: Merskey, H., Bogduk, N (editors). *Classification of Chronic Pain*, second edition. Seattle, WA: IASP Press; pp. 209–14.
2. Breivik, H., Collett, B., Ventafridda, V., Cohen, R., Gallacher, D. (2006). Survey of chronic pain in Europe: prevalence, impact on daily life, and treatment. *Eur J Pain*, 10, 287–333.
3. Institute of Medicine Committee on Advancing Pain Research, Care, and Education (2011). *Relieving Pain in America: A Blueprint for Transforming Prevention, Care, Education, and Research*. Washington, DC: National Academies Press.
4. Todd, A. J. (2010). Neuronal circuitry for pain processing in the dorsal horn. *Nat Rev Neurosci*, 11, 823–36.
5. Tracey, I., Dickenson, A. (2012). SnapShot: pain perception. *Cell*, 148, 1308–8.e2.
6. McMahon, S., Koltzenburg, M., Tracey, I., Turk, D. C. (2013). *Wall & Melzack's Textbook of Pain*. Philadelphia, PA: Elsevier/ Saunders.
7. Denk, F., Bennett, D. L., McMahon, S. B. (2017). Nerve growth factor and pain mechanisms. *Annu Rev Neurosci*, 40, 307–25.
8. Tracey, I., Bushnell, M. C. (2009). How neuroimaging studies have challenged us to rethink: is chronic pain a disease? *J Pain*, 10, 1113–20.
9. Treede, R.-D., Rief, W., Barke, A., *et al.* (2015). A classification of chronic pain for ICD-11. *Pain*, 156, 1003–7.
10. Tracey, I., Mantyh, P. W. (2007). The cerebral signature for pain perception and its modulation. *Neuron*, 55, 377–91.
11. Wager, T. D., Atlas, L. Y., Lindquist, M. A., Roy, M., Woo, C. W., Kross, E. (2013). An fMRI-based neurologic signature of physical pain. *N Engl J Med*, 368, 1388–97.
12. Ploghaus, A., Tracey, I., Gati, J. S., *et al.* (1999). Dissociating pain from its anticipation in the human brain. *Science*, 284, 1979–81.
13. Legrain, V., Iannetti, G. D., Plaghki, L., Mouraux, A. (2011). The pain matrix reloaded: a salience detection system for the body. *Progr Neurobiol*, 93, 111–24.
14. Krishnan, A., Woo, C. W., Chang, L. J., *et al.* (2016). Somatic and vicarious pain are represented by dissociable multivariate brain patterns. *eLife*, 5, e.15166.
15. Kross, E., Berman, M. G., Mischel, W., Smith, E. E., Wager, T. D. (2011). Social rejection shares somatosensory representations with physical pain. *Proc Natl Acad Sci U S A*, 108, 6270–5.
16. Woo, C. W., Koban, L., Kross, E., *et al.* (2014). Separate neural representations for physical pain and social rejection. *Nat Commun*, 5, 5380.
17. Heinricher, M. M., Tavares, I., Leith, J. L., Lumb, B. M. (2009). Descending control of nociception: Specificity, recruitment and plasticity. *Brain Res Rev*, 60, 214–25.

18. Leknes, S., Berna, C., Lee, M. C., Snyder, G. D., Biele, G., Tracey, I. (2013). The importance of context: when relative relief renders pain pleasant. *Pain*, 154, 402–10.
19. Tracey, I., Ploghaus, A., Gati, J. S., *et al.* (2002). Imaging attentional modulation of pain in the periaqueductal gray in humans. *J Neurosci*, 22, 2748–52.
20. Wiech, K., Ploner, M., Tracey, I. (2008). Neurocognitive aspects of pain perception. *Trends Cogn Sci*, 12, 306–13.
21. Eippert, F., Bingel, U., Schoell, E. D., *et al.* (2009). Activation of the opioidergic descending pain control system underlies placebo analgesia. *Neuron*, 63, 533–43.
22. Bingel, U., Wanigasekera, V., Wiech, K., *et al.* (2011). The effect of treatment expectation on drug efficacy: imaging the analgesic benefit of the opioid remifentanil. *Sci Transl Med*, 3, 70ra14.
23. Berna, C., Leknes, S., Holmes, E. A., Edwards, R. R., Goodwin, G. M., Tracey, I. (2010). Induction of depressed mood disrupts emotion regulation neurocircuitry and enhances pain unpleasantness. *Biol Psychiatry*, 67, 1083–90.
24. Fairhurst, M., Wiech, K., Dunckley, P., Tracey, I. (2007). Anticipatory brainstem activity predicts neural processing of pain in humans. *Pain*, 128, 101–10.
25. Ploghaus, A., Narain, C., Beckmann, C. F., *et al.* (2001). Exacerbation of pain by anxiety is associated with activity in a hippocampal network. *J Neurosci*, 21, 9896–903.
26. Wiech, K., Edwards, R., Moseley, G. L., Berna, C., Ploner, M., Tracey, I. (2014). Dissociable neural mechanisms underlying the modulation of pain and anxiety? An FMRI pilot study. *PLoS One*, 9, e110654.
27. Wiech, K., Kalisch, R., Weiskopf, N., Pleger, B., Stephan, K. E., Dolan, R. J. (2006). Anterolateral prefrontal cortex mediates the analgesic effect of expected and perceived control over pain. *J Neurosci*, 26, 11501–9.
28. Bushnell, M. C., Ceko, M., Low, L. A. (2013). Cognitive and emotional control of pain and its disruption in chronic pain. *Nat Rev Neurosci*, 14, 502–11.
29. Tracey, I., Bushnell, M. C. (2009). How neuroimaging studies have challenged us to rethink: is chronic pain a disease? *J Pain*, 10, 1113–20.
30. De Felice, M., Sanoja, R., Wang, R., *et al.* (2011). Engagement of descending inhibition from the rostral ventromedial medulla protects against chronic neuropathic pain. *Pain*, 152, 2701–9.
31. Wang, R., King, T., De Felice, M., Guo, W., Ossipov, M. H., Porreca, F. (2013). Descending facilitation maintains long-term spontaneous neuropathic pain. *J Pain*, 14, 845–53.
32. Gwilym, S. E., Keltner, J. R., Warnaby, C. E., *et al.* (2009). Psychophysical and functional imaging evidence supporting the presence of central sensitization in a cohort of osteoarthritis patients. *Arthritis Rheum*, 61, 1226–34.
33. Iannetti, G. D., Zambreanu, L., Wise, R. G., *et al.* (2005). Pharmacological modulation of pain-related brain activity during normal and central sensitization states in humans. *Proc Natl Acad Sci U S A*, 102, 18195–200.
34. Lee, M. C., Zambreanu, L., Menon, D. K., Tracey, I. (2008). Identifying brain activity specifically related to the maintenance and perceptual consequence of central sensitization in humans. *J Neurosci*, 28, 11642–9.
35. Wanigasekera, V., Lee, M. C., Rogers, R., Hu, P., Tracey, I. (2011). Neural correlates of an injury-free model of central sensitization induced by opioid withdrawal in humans. *J Neurosci*, 31, 2835–42.
36. Denk, F., McMahon, S. B., Tracey, I. (2014). Pain vulnerability: a neurobiological perspective. *Nat Neurosci*, 17, 192–200.

37. Sturgeon, J. A., Zautra, A. J. (2010). Resilience: a new paradigm for adaptation to chronic pain. *Curr Pain Headache Rep*, 14, 105–12.

38. Sturgeon, J. A., Zautra, A. J., Arewasikporn, A. (2014). A multi-level structural equation modeling analysis of vulnerabilities and resilience resources influencing affective adaptation to chronic pain. *Pain*, 155, 292–8.

39. Zubieta, J. K., Heitzeg, M. M., Smith, Y. R., *et al.* (2003). COMT val158met genotype affects mu-opioid neurotransmitter responses to a pain stressor. *Science*, 299, 1240–3.

40. Lee, M. C., Tracey, I. (2013). Neuro-genetics of persistent pain. *Curr Opin Neurobiol*, 23, 127–32.

41. Hall, K. T., Lembo, A. J., Kirsch, I., *et al.* (2012). Catechol-O-methyltransferase val158met polymorphism predicts placebo effect in irritable bowel syndrome. *PLoS One*, 7, e48135.

42. Low, L. A., Fitzgerald, M. (2012). Acute pain and a motivational pathway in adult rats: influence of early life pain experience. *PLoS One*, 7, e34316.

43. Moloney, R. D., O'Leary, O. F., Felice, D., Bettler, B., Dinan, T. G., Cryan, J. F. (2012). Early-life stress induces visceral hypersensitivity in mice. *Neurosci Lett*, 512, 99–102.

44. Beggs, S., Currie, G., Salter, M. W., Fitzgerald, M., Walker, S. M. (2012). Priming of adult pain responses by neonatal pain experience: maintenance by central neuroimmune activity. *Brain*, 135, 404–17.

45. Doesburg, S. M., Chau, C. M., Cheung, T. P., *et al.* (2013). Neonatal pain-related stress, functional cortical activity and visual-perceptual abilities in school-age children born at extremely low gestational age. *Pain*, 154, 1946–52.

46. Hohmeister, J., Kroll, A., Wollgarten-Hadamek, I., *et al.* (2010). Cerebral processing of pain in school-aged children with neonatal nociceptive input: an exploratory fMRI study. *Pain*, 150, 257–67.

47. Loram, L. C., Taylor, F. R., Strand, K. A., *et al.* (2011). Prior exposure to glucocorticoids potentiates lipopolysaccharide induced mechanical allodynia and spinal neuroinflammation. *Brain Behav Immunity*, 25, 1408–15.

48. Coghill, R. C., McHaffie, J. G., Yen, Y. F. (2003). Neural correlates of interindividual differences in the subjective experience of pain. *Proc Natl Acad Sci U S A*, 100, 8538–42.

49. Erpelding, N., Moayedi, M., Davis, K. D. (2012). Cortical thickness correlates of pain and temperature sensitivity. *Pain*, 153, 1602–9.

50. Ploner, M., Lee, M. C., Wiech, K., Bingel, U., Tracey, I. (2010). Prestimulus functional connectivity determines pain perception in humans. *Proc Natl Acad Sci U S A*, 107, 355–60.

51. Wanigasekera, V., Lee, M. C., Rogers, R., *et al.* (2012). Baseline reward circuitry activity and trait reward responsiveness predict expression of opioid analgesia in healthy subjects. *Proc Natl Acad Sci U S A*, 109, 17705–10.

52. Weissman-Fogel, I., Granovsky, Y., Crispel, Y., *et al.* (2009). Enhanced presurgical pain temporal summation response predicts post-thoracotomy pain intensity during the acute postoperative phase. *J Pain*, 10, 628–36.

53. Yarnitsky, D., Crispel, Y., Eisenberg, E., *et al.* (2008). Prediction of chronic post-operative pain: pre-operative DNIC testing identifies patients at risk. *Pain*, 138, 22–8.

54. Leknes, S., Tracey, I. (2008). A common neurobiology for pain and pleasure. *Nat Rev Neurosci*, 9, 314–20.

55. Baliki, M. N., Petre, B., Torbey, S., *et al.* (2012). Corticostriatal functional connectivity predicts transition to chronic back pain. *Nat Neurosci*, 15, 1117–19.

56. Hashmi, J. A., Baliki, M. N., Huang, L., *et al.* (2013). Shape shifting pain: chronification of back pain shifts brain representation from nociceptive to emotional circuits. *Brain*, 136, 2751–68.

57. Mansour, A. R., Baliki, M. N., Huang, L., *et al.* (2013). Brain white matter structural properties predict transition to chronic pain. *Pain*, 154, 2160–8.

58. Mutso, A. A., Petre, B., Huang, L., *et al.* (2014). Reorganization of hippocampal functional connectivity with transition to chronic back pain. *J Neurophysiol*, 111, 1065–76.

59. Vachon-Presseau, E., Tetreault, P., Petre, B., *et al.* (2016). Corticolimbic anatomical characteristics predetermine risk for chronic pain. *Brain*, 139, 1958–70.

60. Baliki, M. N., Geha, P. Y., Fields, H. L., Apkarian, A. V. (2010). Predicting value of pain and analgesia: nucleus accumbens response to noxious stimuli changes in the presence of chronic pain. *Neuron*, 66, 149–60.

61. Loggia, M. L., Berna, C., Kim, J., *et al.* (2014). Disrupted brain circuitry for pain-related reward/punishment in fibromyalgia. *Arthritis Rheumatol*, 66, 203–12.

62. Navratilova, E., Xie, J. Y., Meske, D., *et al.* (2015). Endogenous opioid activity in the anterior cingulate cortex is required for relief of pain. *J Neurosci*, 35, 7264–71.

63. Leknes, S., Lee, M. C., Berna, C., Andersson, J., Tracey, I. (2011). Relief as a reward: hedonic and neural responses to safety from pain. *PLoS One*, 6, e17870.

64. Scott, D. J., Stohler, C. S., Egnatuk, C. M., Wang, H., Koeppe, R. A., Zubieta, J. K. (2008). Placebo and nocebo effects are defined by opposite opioid and dopaminergic responses. *Arch Gen Psychiatry*, 65, 220–31.

65. Wrobel, N., Wiech, K., Forkmann, K., Ritter, C., Bingel, U. (2014). Haloperidol blocks dorsal striatum activity but not analgesia in a placebo paradigm. *Cortex*, 57, 60–73.

66. Tracey, I. (2016). A vulnerability to chronic pain and its interrelationship with resistance to analgesia. *Brain*, 139, 1869–72.

67. Sullivan, M. J., Thorn, B., Haythornthwaite, J. A., *et al.* (2001). Theoretical perspectives on the relation between catastrophizing and pain. *Clin J Pain*, 17, 52–64.

68. Erpelding, N., Davis, K. D. (2013). Neural underpinnings of behavioural strategies that prioritize either cognitive task performance or pain. *Pain*, 154, 2060–71.

69. Bishop, S. J. (2008). Neural mechanisms underlying selective attention to threat. *Ann N Y Acad Sci*, 1129, 141–52.

70. Ochsner, K. N., Gross, J. J. (2005). The cognitive control of emotion. *Trends Cogn Sci*, 9, 242–9.

71. Cauda, F., Palermo, S., Costa, T., *et al.* (2014). Gray matter alterations in chronic pain: A network-oriented meta-analytic approach. *Neuroimage Clin*, 4, 676–86.

72. Gwilym, S. E., Filippini, N., Douaud, G., Carr, A. J., Tracey, I. (2010). Thalamic atrophy associated with painful osteoarthritis of the hip is reversible after arthroplasty: a longitudinal voxel-based morphometric study. *Arthritis Rheum*, 62, 2930–40.

73. Rodriguez-Raecke, R., Niemeier, A., Ihle, K., Ruether, W., May, A. (2009). Brain gray matter decrease in chronic pain is the consequence and not the cause of pain. *J Neurosci*, 29, 13746–50.

74. Seminowicz, D. A., Laferriere, A. L., Millecamps, M., Yu, J. S., Coderre, T. J., Bushnell, M. C. (2009). MRI structural brain changes associated with sensory and emotional function in a rat model of long-term neuropathic pain. *Neuroimage*, 47, 1007–14.

75. Seminowicz, D. A., Wideman, T. H., Naso, L., *et al.* (2011). Effective treatment of chronic low back pain in humans reverses abnormal brain anatomy and function. *J Neurosci*, 31, 7540–50.

76. Apkarian, A. V., Sosa, Y., Sonty, S., *et al.* (2004). Chronic back pain is associated with decreased prefrontal and thalamic gray matter density. *J Neurosci*, 24, 10410–15.

77. Vachon-Presseau, E., Roy, M., Martel, M. O., *et al.* (2013). The stress model of chronic pain: evidence from basal cortisol and hippocampal structure and function in humans. *Brain*, 136, 815–27.

78. Zambreanu, L., Wise, R. G., Brooks, J. C. W., Iannetti, G. D., Tracey, I. (2005). A role for the brainstem in central sensitisation in humans. Evidence from functional magnetic resonance imaging. *Pain*, 114, 397–407.

79. Berman, S. M., Naliboff, B. D., Suyenobu, B., *et al.* (2008). Reduced brainstem inhibition during anticipated pelvic visceral pain correlates with enhanced brain response to the visceral stimulus in women with irritable bowel syndrome. *J Neurosci*, 28, 349–59.

80. Bosma, R. L., Mojarad, E. A., Leung, L., Pukall, C., Staud, R., Stroman, P. W. (2016). FMRI of spinal and supra-spinal correlates of temporal pain summation in fibromyalgia patients. *Hum Brain Mapp*, 37, 1349–60.

81. Kremer, M., Salvat, E., Muller, A., Yalcin, I., Barrot, M. (2016). Antidepressants and gabapentinoids in neuropathic pain: Mechanistic insights. *Neuroscience*, 338, 183–206.

82. Yarnitsky, D., Granot, M., Nahman-Averbuch, H., Khamaisi, M., Granovsky, Y. (2012). Conditioned pain modulation predicts duloxetine efficacy in painful diabetic neuropathy. *Pain*, 153, 1193–8.

83. Flor, H., Elbert, T., Knecht, S., *et al.* (1995). Phantom-limb pain as a perceptual correlate of cortical reorganization following arm amputation. *Nature*, 375, 482–4.

84. Devor, M., Vaso, A., Adahan, H. M., Vyshka, G. (2014). PNS origin of phantom limb sensation and pain: reply to letter to the editor regarding Foell *et al.*, peripheral origin of phantom limb pain: is it all resolved? *Pain*, 155, 2207–8.

85. Makin, T. R., Scholz, J., Filippini, N., Henderson Slater, D., Tracey, I., Johansen-Berg, H. (2013). Phantom pain is associated with preserved structure and function in the former hand area. *Nat Commun*, 4, 1570.

86. Makin, T. R., Scholz, J., Henderson Slater, D., Johansen-Berg, H., Tracey, I. (2015). Reassessing cortical reorganization in the primary sensorimotor cortex following arm amputation. *Brain*, 138, 2140–6.

87. Vaso, A., Adahan, H. M., Gjika, A., *et al.* (2014). Peripheral nervous system origin of phantom limb pain. *Pain*, 155, 1384–91.

88. Moseley, G. L., Flor, H. (2012). Targeting cortical representations in the treatment of chronic pain: a review. *Neurorehabil Neural Repair*, 26, 646–52.

89. Yanagisawa, T., Fukuma, R., Seymour, B., *et al.* (2016). Induced sensorimotor brain plasticity controls pain in phantom limb patients. *Nat Commun*, 7, 13209.

90. Bair, M. J., Robinson, R. L., Katon, W., Kroenke, K. (2003). Depression and pain comorbidity: a literature review. *Arch Intern Med*, 163, 2433–45.

91. Gureje, O., Von Korff, M., Kola, L., *et al.* (2008). The relation between multiple pains and mental disorders: results from the World Mental Health Surveys. *Pain*, 135, 82–91.

92. Knaster, P., Karlsson, H., Estlander, A.-M., Kalso, E. (2012). Psychiatric disorders as assessed with SCID in chronic pain patients: the anxiety disorders precede the onset of pain. *Gen Hosp Psychiatry*, 34, 46–52.

93. Asmundson, G. J. G., Hadjistavropolous, H. D. (2006). Addressing shared vulnerability for comorbid PTSD and chronic pain: a cognitive-behavioral perspective. *Cogn Behav Pract*, 13, 8–16.

94. Sharp, T. J., Harvey, A. G. (2001). Chronic pain and posttraumatic stress disorder: mutual maintenance? *Clin Psychol Rev*, 21, 857–77.

95. Strigo, I. A., Simmons, A. N., Matthews, S. C., Craig, A. D., Paulus, M. P. (2008). Association of major depressive disorder with altered functional brain response during anticipation and processing of heat pain. *Arch Gen Psychiatry*, 65, 1275–84.

96. Loggia, M. L., Berna, C., Kim, J., *et al.* (2015). The lateral pre-frontal cortex mediates the hyperalgesic effects of negative cognitions in chronic pain patients. *J Pain*, 16, 692–9.

97. Flink, I., Boersma, K., Linton, S. J. (2013). Pain catastrophizing as repetitive negative thinking: a development of the conceptualization. *Cogn Behav Ther*, 42, 215–23.

98. Flink, I., Boersma, K., Linton, S. J. (2014). Changes in catastrophizing and depressed mood during and after early cognitive behaviorally oriented interventions for pain. *Cogn Behav Ther*, 43, 332–41.

99. Eccleston, C., Hearn, L., Williams, A. C. (2015). Psychological therapies for the management of chronic neuropathic pain in adults. *Cochrane Database Syst Rev*, 10, CD011259.

100. Simons, L. E., Elman, I., Borsook, D. (2014). Psychological processing in chronic pain: a neural systems approach. *Neurosci Biobehav Rev*, 39, 61–78.

101. Williams, A. C., Eccleston, C., Morley, S. (2012). Psychological therapies for the management of chronic pain (excluding headache) in adults. *Cochrane Database Syst Rev*, 11, CD007407.

102. Yovell, Y., Bar, G., Mashiah, M., *et al.* (2016). Ultra-low-dose buprenorphine as a time-limited treatment for severe suicidal ideation: a randomized controlled trial. *Am J Psychiatry*, 173, 491–8.

103. Dowell, D., Haegerich, T. M., Chou, R. (2016). CDC guideline for prescribing opioids for chronic pain—United States, 2016. *JAMA*, 315, 1624–45.

104. Ilgen, M. A., Bohnert, A. S. B., Ganoczy, D., Bair, M. J., McCarthy, J. F., Blow, F. C. (2016). Opioid dose and risk of suicide. *Pain*, 157, 1079–84.

105. Turner, J. A., Shortreed, S. M., Saunders, K. W., LeResche, L., Von Korff, M. (2016). Association of levels of opioid use with pain and activity interference among patients initiating chronic opioid therapy: a longitudinal study. *Pain*, 157, 849–57.

106. Holtzman, S., Beggs, R. T. (2013). Yoga for chronic low back pain: a meta-analysis of randomized controlled trials. *Pain Res Manag*, 18, 267–72.

107. Jensen, M. P. (2009). Hypnosis for chronic pain management: a new hope. *Pain*, 146, 235–7.

108. Veehof, M. M., Trompetter, H. R., Bohlmeijer, E. T., Schreurs, K. M. (2016). Acceptance- and mindfulness-based interventions for the treatment of chronic pain: a meta-analytic review. *Cogn Behav Ther*, 45, 5–31.

109. Jensen, K. B., Berna, C., Loggia, M. L., Wasan, A. D., Edwards, R. R., Gollub, R. L. (2012). The use of functional neuroimaging to evaluate psychological and other non-pharmacological treatments for clinical pain. *Neurosci Lett*, 520, 156–64.

110. Villemure, C., Ceko, M., Cotton, V. A., Bushnell, M. C. (2014). Insular cortex mediates increased pain tolerance in yoga practitioners. *Cereb Cortex*, 24, 2732–40.

111. Zeidan, F., Adler-Neal, A. L., Wells, R. E., *et al.* (2016). Mindfulness-meditation-based pain relief is not mediated by endogenous opioids. *J Neurosci*, 36, 3391–7.

112. Zeidan, F., Emerson, N. M., Farris, S. R., *et al.* (2015). Mindfulness meditation-based pain relief employs different neural mechanisms than placebo and sham mindfulness meditation-induced analgesia. *J Neurosci*, 35, 15307–25.

113. Jensen, K. B., Kosek, E., Wicksell, R., *et al.* (2012). Cognitive behavioral therapy increases pain-evoked activation of the

prefrontal cortex in patients with fibromyalgia. *Pain*, 153, 1495–503.

114. Lazaridou, A., Kim, J., Cahalan, C. M., *et al.* (2017). Effects of cognitive-behavioral therapy (CBT) on brain connectivity supporting catastrophizing in fibromyalgia. *Clin J Pain*, 33, 215–21.

115. Gureje, O. (2007). Psychiatric aspects of pain. *Curr Opin Psychiatry*, 20, 42–6.

116. Kerns, R. D., Sellinger, J., Goodin, B. R. (2011). Psychological treatment of chronic pain. *Annu Rev Clin Psychology*, 7, 411–34.

117. Elman, I., Zubieta, J. K., Borsook, D. (2011). The missing p in psychiatric training: why it is important to teach pain to psychiatrists. *Arch Gen Psychiatry*, 68, 12–20.

118. Ebert, M., Kerns, R. D. (2011). *Behavioral and Psychopharmacologic Pain Management*. New York, NY: Cambridge University Press.

119. Volkow, N. D., McLellan, A. T. (2016). Opioid abuse in chronic pain—misconceptions and mitigation strategies. *N Engl J Med*, 374, 1253–63.

120. Rief, W., Martin, A. (2014). How to use the new DSM-5 somatic symptom disorder diagnosis in research and practice: a critical evaluation and a proposal for modifications. *Annu Rev Clin Psychol*, 10, 339–67.

121. Browning, M., Fletcher, P., Sharpe, M. (2011). Can neuroimaging help us to understand and classify somatoform disorders? A systematic and critical review. *Psychosom Med*, 73, 173–84.

122. Edwards, M. J., Adams, R. A., Brown, H., Pareés, I., Friston, K. J. (2012). A Bayesian account of 'hysteria'. *Brain*, 135, 3495.

123. Buchel, C., Geuter, S., Sprenger, C., Eippert, F. (2014). Placebo analgesia: a predictive coding perspective. *Neuron*, 81, 1223–39.

124. Wiech, K., Vandekerckhove, J., Zaman, J., Tuerlinckx, F., Vlaeyen, J. W., Tracey, I. (2014). Influence of prior information on pain involves biased perceptual decision-making. *Curr Biol*, 24, R679–81.

# 131

# Treatment of fibromyalgia (chronic widespread pain) and chronic fatigue syndrome

*Jonathan Price*

## Fibromyalgia (chronic widespread pain)

### Clinical presentation and epidemiology

Fibromyalgia (FM) is the second most common musculoskeletal presentation, after osteoarthritis. It is a complex presentation (Box 131.1) [1], combining the core symptom (chronic widespread pain) with other very commonly associated symptoms (for example, fatigue, sleep disturbance, cognitive difficulties, non-pain somatic symptoms, low mood, anxiety). In addition, coexisting somatic syndromes [for example, irritable bowel syndrome (IBS), chronic headache, temporomandibular disorder, chronic fatigue] are common. Its complex nature, spanning traditional medical specialty boundaries, presents considerable challenges to health care professionals. FM is best conceptualized as a *centralized* disease state, in which symptoms and sensations from any part of the body are centrally amplified, rather than as a peripheral disorder of fibrous tissue and muscle.

The point prevalence of FM is estimated at 2.7% globally [2]. It is higher among women, with a female:male ratio of perhaps 2:1, a ratio which has shifted to much closer to parity since the requirement for multiple tender points was dropped from the diagnostic criteria. Prevalence is higher in middle-aged and older adults and in lower socio-economic status groups, especially the unemployed.

### Diagnostic issues

FM was known by other terms until 1990 when diagnostic criteria were published that included both symptoms and, on examination, 'tender points' [3]. Recently, updated criteria have emphasized the importance of *chronic* (>3 months) pain that is *widespread* across the body [4]. Importantly, an FM diagnosis does not now exclude the diagnosis of any other disorder, and additional diagnoses are likely in order to fully describe the clinical condition of a typical patient. It is likely that the diagnosis and classification will start to consider FM and similar, often overlapping, disorders in a more integrated way, emphasizing their considerable similarities, rather than their differences [5, 6].

FM has some unique features but shares some symptoms, epidemiological features, and underlying mechanisms with other 'chronic overlapping pain conditions' (COPCs) (for example, tension-type headache, temporomandibular disorder) [5] and chronic non-pain conditions [for example, chronic fatigue syndrome CFS)]. Indeed, FM is commonly comorbid with COPCs with non-pain somatic symptom syndromes (for example, CFS and IBS) and with mental disorders (especially anxiety disorder and depressive disorder). Furthermore, the population of patients with rigorously diagnosed FM is not discrete—there is a population penumbra, with patients on either side of the cutpoints of diagnosis being similar, rather than different. In other words, we are not 'carving nature at the joints'. Finally, clinical diagnoses of FM are not confirmed by objective diagnostic tests, because such tests do not exist. These issues present major challenges for clinicians, and especially for researchers, and may also contribute to diagnostic delay; in a typical FM patient, there has often been more than 2 years of symptoms, and several medical consultations, before diagnostic confirmation [7]. A positive early diagnosis is likely to improve outcome, and FM should be suspected in any patient with chronic widespread pain not straightforwardly explained by injury or inflammation.

### Aetiology

This chapter focuses on the role of three key factors which form the focus of successful treatment: central sensitization, fear avoidance, and physical deconditioning. Interested readers are referred elsewhere [8] for a broader review of psychosocial factors in chronic pain. A broader range of relevant factors are listed in Table 131.1.

### Central sensitization

In the last two decades, the focus for understanding FM has shifted from peripheral nerves and muscles towards the role of the central nervous system (CNS). This shift is reflected in the range of recommended treatments, all of which act directly (for example,

**Box 131.1** The 'FFIBRO' mnemonic for the core symptoms of fibromyalgia

| Fatigue | Fatigue and tiredness |
|---|---|
| Fog | Cognitive dysfunction, memory and concentration impairment |
| Insomnia | Poor sleep initiation, sleep maintenance, poor sleep refreshment |
| Blues | Depression, anxiety |
| Rigidity | Stiff muscles, stiff joints |
| Ow! | Pain, which is widespread across the body and long-standing |

Source: data from *Nat Rev Rheumatol.*, 5(4), Boomershine C, Crofford L, A symptom-based approach to pharmacologic management of fibromyalgia, pp. 191–199, Copyright (2009), Springer Nature.

antidepressants) or indirectly (for example, physical exercise) on the CNS. CNS sensitization appears to play a central role, such that the brain amplifies signals arriving from the peripheries by facilitating spinal transmission and by modifying cortical processing [9]. The person therefore feels more pain than is expected from the nociceptive stimulus (hyperalgesia) or feels pain from a stimulus that does not usually cause pain (allodynia). Central sensitization therefore contributes to the development of FM, other centralized pain states, and non-pain somatic symptom syndromes and allows us to attribute and manage a single cause in complex patients presenting with multiple symptoms spanning body systems.

### Fear-avoidance (or 'kinesiophobia')

The person's fear of pain leads to avoidance of activities believed to cause or worsen the pain, that is, avoidance of movement and physical exertion. This leads to physical deconditioning and adverse psychological consequences, and thereby to exacerbation of the pain experience [10]. Importantly, the fear-avoidance model incorporates

**Table 131.1** Aetiological factors in FM (key treatment targets in italics)

| Physical | *Central sensitization*<br>*Reduced physical activity and consequent physical deconditioning*<br>Genetic/familial factors<br>Maladaptive posture/gait<br>Non-restorative sleep |
|---|---|
| Psychological | *Fear-avoidance*<br>*Cognitive factors*, including catastrophizing, reduced self-efficacy<br>*Patient behaviours*, including hypervigilance, reduction of activities<br>*Abnormal mood states*, including depression and anxiety |
| Social | *Reactions and responses of others*, including:<br>• Health care professionals, including over-investigation, medicalization, and undertreatment by psychological means<br>• Relatives and other carers<br>*Unemployment or underemployment*<br>Reinforcement of illness behaviour by, for example, financial benefits/provision of physical aids |

both cognitive elements (beliefs about the consequences of movement and about the meaning of pain) and behavioural elements (avoidance of movement and exercise). Fear-avoidance is common in FM patients and correlates well with symptom severity and physical disability [11]. It provides a target model for treatment development with wide applicability in chronic musculoskeletal pain, and emerging evidence suggests that reduced fear-avoidance mediates the physical benefits of structured exercise interventions in FM.

### Physical deconditioning

This plays a key role in the development and maintenance of central sensitivity. A vicious cycle is set up (Fig. 131.1).

These three factors—central sensitization, fear-avoidance, and physical deconditioning—usually enable a coherent explanation of causation to be provided to patients and carers. They also provide a firm basis for a management plan that is fundamentally patient-centred, incorporating: a *phenotype* that it predisposed to be pain-prone; *fears* about the impact of physical activity and *beliefs* about the need to rest and protect the body from the adverse effects of disease; and consequent and inherently reasonable *behavioural responses*, including symptom monitoring and excessive rest. These maladaptive beliefs and behaviours can be reinforced by the responses of relatives and other carers, and also by the responses of health care practitioners; both groups may encourage rest, in the hope that this may enable the body to recover from an as yet undiscovered disease process.

### Assessment

In primary care, the assessment of FM will necessarily be pragmatic. In secondary care, clinicians should aim for a thorough understanding [12]. In both settings, assessment is a key part of treatment, not only by guiding it, but also by providing the trust and reassurance that chronic pain patients need to be able to move forward with potentially counter-intuitive approaches such as exercising despite increased pain. The interested reader is referred to Lotze and Moseley [13], who eloquently integrate compassion and modern pain science in the clinical assessment.

Assessment should include:

• *Pain behaviours*, for example, complaints of pain to others, including health care professionals, requests for medicines, avoidance of feared activities, reduced mobility, use of aids, protective postures.
• *Pain cognitions*, including dysfunctional beliefs, such that pain signals an underlying disease or that pain should respond to avoidance of usual activities; a tendency to catastrophize, that is, to assume the worst possible outcome; and low self-efficacy, that is, a lack of confidence in the person's own ability to influence their pain, now and in the future.
• *Pain impacts*, including on mood (low or anxious), on sleep, and on physical, social, and occupational functioning,
• *History from corroborants*, to confirm the patient's beliefs and behaviours, and allow the assessment of carers' beliefs and behaviours.

An appropriate physical examination should be carried out to: (1) rule out the presence of the inflammatory arthritides or, if one is present, to assess its contribution to overall morbidity; (2) assess the

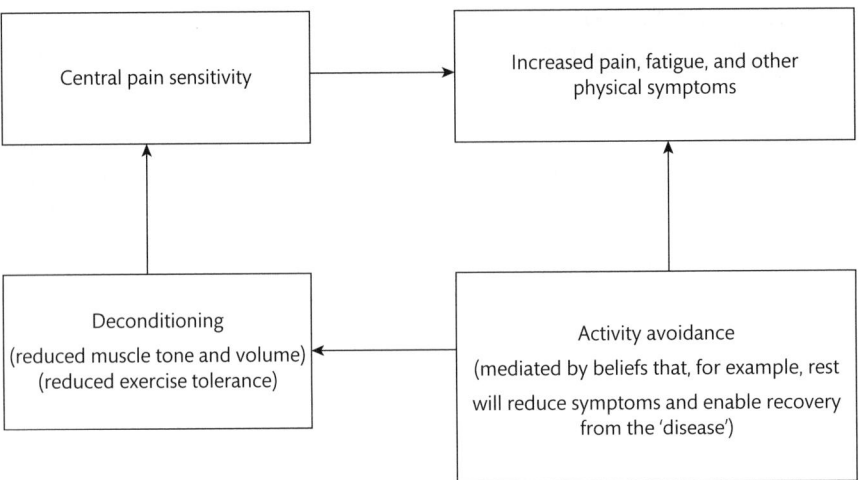

**Fig. 131.1** Vicious cycle of deconditioning.

extent of physical deconditioning; and (3) provide appropriate reassurance to the patient that important physical diagnoses have been appropriately considered and excluded. A small number of appropriately targeted investigations are likely to be appropriate, but each should be clearly justified [14]. Clinicians should carefully balance the need for physical investigation with the prudent avoidance of over-investigation and over-medicalization of FM.

### Management

FM can be challenging to manage, but clinicians should be encouraged that a reasonable evidence base exists and that this has helpfully been summarized and interpreted in recent clinical guidelines and reviews [14–18]. The guidelines differ in their details, partly due to recent changes in regulatory approvals for specific pharmacological approaches. However, there is broad agreement on principles (Box 131.2). In addition to these clinical guidelines, a recent review has documented the important academic and leadership challenges [19]. Finally, there is scope for a note of caution; for most of the evidence-based treatments described in this chapter, there remains a dearth of randomized controlled trials (RCTs) of high quality. An inevitable side effect is that robust evidence for comparative effectiveness of individual treatments is very limited. The interested reader is referred to a recent network meta-analysis [20].

### Overall approach

RCTs have demonstrated the effectiveness of several treatments, both non-pharmacological and pharmacological, in FM. Initially, non-pharmacological approaches should be pursued [18]. They may be used in combination in an integrated, multi-disciplinary way (for example, patient education plus exercise programme supervised by a physiotherapist). Failure of this approach should lead to the considered introduction of a pharmacological agent, alongside continued non-pharmacological management and with ongoing monitoring of key symptoms and function. The approach throughout is individualized for the particular needs and preferences of a particular FM patient.

Self-management plays a fundamental role in the management of FM throughout the spectrum of severity. Patients must understand the nature of the illness, its likely causes, the role of health care practitioners, and, importantly, their own role in active day-to-day management. This statement applies equally to key carers. Table 131.2 outlines the characteristics of an optimal management approach to be promoted by the health care professional to the FM patient.

The European League Against Rheumatism (EULAR) guideline [18] provides a flowchart incorporating a stepped-care approach (Table 131.3), which facilitates prompt treatment. It is important to intervene promptly when patients present with FM, because longer pain duration is associated with the development and embedding of maladaptive illness behaviours, kindling of maladaptive pain pathways, more challenging management, and poorer prognosis. Referral to secondary care is appropriate when the illness does not respond to initial treatments, when there is uncertainty over the diagnosis, perhaps in the presence of significant comorbidity, and when there is significant psychiatric comorbidity that does not respond to initial treatments.

### Empirically supported treatments

The specific treatments for FM for which there is reasonable or good evidence are now addressed in turn. Each treatment will be outlined, key clinical issues described, and the available evidence summarized.

#### Patient education

Effective patient education is pivotal to the effective care of FM. Multi-faceted, patient-focused education is likely to provide much needed coherence and reassurance that there is hope. Whenever possible, close family members/key carers should also be involved in discussion (see Table 131.4 for the key messages for patients).

---

**Box 131.2** Key aspects of management of fibromyalgia, derived from current clinical guidelines

1 Deliver initial care for FM in primary care;
2 Incorporate both pharmacological and non-pharmacological approaches, but with an initial focus on the non-pharmacological; and
3 Encourage active patient participation in treatment, facilitated by
4 High-quality patient education.

**Table 131.2** Characteristics of an optimal management plan in FM

| | |
|---|---|
| Internally consistent | That is, with a clear conceptualization of treatment that is based on an explanation of causes, especially maintaining factors |
| Externally consistent | That is, deliberately target and reduce or eliminate ambiguity between involved health care professionals concerning the causes of the illness, and the methods and goals of treatment |
| Incorporating the reduction or stopping of inappropriate medication | That is, those that are inconsistent with the aetiological understanding being promoted, and that are not required for the management of comorbidities |
| Multimodal | That is, involving both physical and educational/psychological components, in every case |
| Promoting a graded increase in physical activity | Aiming to reduce disability and improve morale and well-being, rather than to reduce pain |
| Promoting an increase in patient responsibility and independence | Rather than maintaining dependence on health services |
| Individualized | To the needs and preferences of the specific patient, and to their response or non-response to specific treatments |
| Structured | With a beginning (assessment, education, first step), a middle (empirical, stepwise approach to selecting successful treatment(s)), and an end (relapse prevention) |
| Addressing the information needs of carers | Who need to share a common understanding of causes and cures, and the chosen approach |
| Adopting the principles of stepped care | So that the maximum number of patients can benefit from appropriate management, in a resource-constrained health care system |

The first, and fundamental, part of patient education is giving the diagnosis. Most FM patients will have tolerated incoherent and inconsistent explanations, without a clear way forward, for months or years. There is reassuring evidence that an FM diagnosis does

**Table 131.3** Stepped care according to the revised EULAR guidelines

| | |
|---|---|
| Step one | Patient education and information sheet; leading to, if insufficient response … |
| Step two | Physical therapy, with individualized graded physical exercise, which may be combined with other recommended non-pharmacological therapies such as hydrotherapy/acupuncture, if necessary; leading to, if insufficient response … |
| Step three | Reassess the patient to target individualized treatment, focused as follows:<br>• If pain-related depression, anxiety, catastrophizing, overly passive—psychological therapies—mainly CBT—for more severe depression or anxiety, consider psychopharmacological treatment<br>• If severe pain or sleep disturbance, then pharmacotherapy: for severe pain—duloxetine, pregabalin, tramadol; for severe sleep problems—low-dose amitriptyline, cyclobenzaprine (tricyclic-related), or pregabalin at night<br>• If severe disability or sick leave, multimodal rehabilitation programmes |

Source: data from Ann Rheum Dis., 76(2), Macfarlane G, Kronisch C, Dean L, et al., EULAR revised recommendations for the management of fibromyalgia, pp. 318–328, Copyright (2017), BMJ Publishing Group Ltd and the European League Against Rheumatism.

not reinforce the sick role, and most patients should respond positively to a clear diagnosis, supported by a coherent and rational explanation.

Crucially, however, a diagnosis is not simply about delivering a name for the disorder. It is about explaining the nature of the illness, explaining that it is common and affects many people, and providing a coherent explanation of the cause which maps onto the proposed management plan. A high degree of fit between patient understanding of the cause (and especially maintaining factors) and the management plan is likely to predict treatment engagement and clinical response. 'Explaining pain' (EP) treatments or 'pain biology education' are of increasing interest [13, 21]. In these, the focus is on helping the pain patient understand that pain is a creation of the brain, designed to indicate the possibility of harm, rather than an accurate measure of tissue damage. The focus is on using education about pain biology to change the *meaning* of pain which then alters the experience of pain. Clearly, there is significant overlap here with more explicitly cognitive interventions.

The core of patient education should be about effective management, as patient behaviours are pivotal. The patient needs to understand what is needed to improve outcomes, and needs to feel enabled to start to act (self-efficacy). A *graded increase in physical activity* is the critical intervention, and patients must understand the rationale for this somewhat counter-intuitive approach in order to make a material and persistent change in their lifestyle. Some brief cognitive work may be needed to tackle unhelpful beliefs impeding engagement with a graded exercise programme. This emphasizes that education should be individualized to the needs of the specific patient. For example, patients who fear the adverse consequences of physical activity (fear-avoidance) need a targeted cognitive intervention, perhaps assisted by behavioural experiments. Such an intervention need not take place within the feasibility constraints of a formal psychological treatment but rather should usually be delivered by non-specialist staff in the clinic setting.

Evidence for the effectiveness of patient education in FM is extensive but is skewed towards highly time- and resource-intensive educational interventions. There are clearly important questions about the feasibility of such interventions in primary care. However, the fundamental importance of effective patient education is not doubted. The clinical challenge is to maximize its effect within the usual significant resource constraints. Undoubtedly, *good-quality written information* can help to leverage benefit, with minimal additional cost. *Careful selection of the recommendations for a particular patient* and *active endorsement of the treatment approach by a trusted clinician* are also critical.

### Graded exercise

A graded, but persistent, increase in physical activity is the critical recommendation for patients with FM. EULAR guidance [18] concludes that there is 'strong evidence for' exercise and that exercise may benefit pain, function, sleep, and morale.

The relevant evidence comprises many RCTs, which have been summarized in three key Cochrane Collaboration reviews [22–24]. The best evidence is for supervised aerobic exercise training, which improves aerobic fitness, pain, physical function, and well-being. Strength (resistance) training also has a range of benefits and appears to be more effective than flexibility training, but possibly less effective than aerobic exercise. Aquatic (that is, water-based)

**Table 131.4** Key messages for patient education

| | |
|---|---|
| *You have a real illness* | We see many patients with problems like yours. We know that you are not imagining it or making it up. We want to help. |
| *The illness is called FM* | It is common—about one in 40 people have this illness. |
| *FM is problematic, but benign* | It is an illness that causes symptoms and disability. But it is not an illness which causes a long-term decline. |
| *FM is an illness of the nervous system, not an illness of the muscles and joints* | In FM, the body is especially good at generating pain signals, even when there is no cause for the pain. This is why medicines usually used for other illnesses, such as epilepsy and depression, can help; they change the way that the nerves in the brain and spine transmit pain signals from the muscles. |
| *FM is not caused by persistent infection* | An illness, such as a flu infection, may be a trigger for the illness, but ongoing infection is very unlikely. (Note: many patients, especially those who also satisfy the criteria for CFS, believe that they are harbouring an occult infection which explains their symptoms.) |
| *Exercise is the most effective treatment that we have for FM* | Exercise helps to build up the body and make it more resistant to challenges. Exercise improves blood flow to the muscles by causing blood vessels to grow more thickly through the muscle. Exercise may help to 'reset' the nervous system, so that it deals better with pain signals. |
| *Exercise causes temporary muscle discomfort, which is a sign of the muscle reorganizing to become stronger* | Exercise breaks the body down before it builds it back up, and so muscle pain and muscle tenderness are entirely normal after exercise, and not a sign of illness or abnormality. Competitive and recreational athletes know this very well. (Use a simple model to explain this, describing, for example, how muscle fibres disaggregate after acute exercise and then reorganize over a period of 24–72 hours.) |
| *FM symptoms are worsened by stress and low mood* | Learning self-help approaches to anxiety (relaxation, cognitive approaches, behavioural approaches) and depression is important. Antidepressants and other formal treatments, including CBT, also have a role to play. |
| *FM is helped by active involvement of the patient* | I can't cure this illness for you. I need you to work hard with the treatment plan, and I will do my best to support you. |
| *With treatment, FM can have a much smaller impact on your lifestyle* | Together, we can work at enabling you to manage and control your illness, so that it has much less of an impact on your life. I want to work with you on your rehabilitation, focused on what you can do, and on what you would like to do in the future. |

exercise training appears to be as effective as land exercise training. The choice of exercise modality (aerobic vs strength/resistance; land vs water) therefore depends on patient preference and on feasibility, determined by both the availability and the impact of medical comorbidities. Fast walking, cycling, and swimming are good initial recommendations, as they have lower musculoskeletal impact than running.

FM patients have often been through a lengthy period of reduction in physical activity, frequency, duration, and intensity, due to their pain and related symptoms, and the majority would be classified as sedentary (<5000 steps per day). A sudden and significant step change in activity level is unlikely to be successful. Graded increments in activity, clearly prescribed or described by a health care professional or sports professional, are needed. Although small increases in activity (2000–3000 steps per day) may help, the greater the increase in activity, the greater the improvement in function, mood, and physical health-related quality of life, but not pain intensity [25]. Increased physical activity is, of course, also likely to have associated benefits for physical health (for example, body mass index, blood pressure, and glucose tolerance) and mental health.

Early worsening of pain and fatigue is common, and patients need encouragement to persist and to attribute such symptoms to the body's rebuilding in response to increased activity, rather than attributing them to worsening of a disease process. Many patients are concerned about pain, soreness, and tenderness arising in muscles in the hours and days following exercise, especially in the early stages of exercise training. This phenomenon is well known to athletes and others who undertake physical exercise for training purposes and is known as 'delayed onset of muscular soreness' (DOMS). This is an inevitable consequence of physical activity beyond the person's norm, in which muscular breakdown following exercise is accompanied by soreness and muscular fatigue, before the muscles rebuild

more strongly over a period of 2–3 days. In other words, increased muscle pain in this context is a sign of *adaptation* and improving physical fitness, rather than of disease. This is an important message for FM patients—physical sensations of pain and fatigue during and after exercise do not mean that the body is being damaged, but rather they are signs that the body is responding normally to the challenge and becoming stronger. It may therefore be better to use the word 'training', rather than exercise, with FM patients.

Understandably, motivation to exercise, and to exercise in a planned and strategic way over a period of weeks and months, is crucial to success. A minority of patients will find this straightforward, but a majority will struggle and need assistance at the outset and in an ongoing way. Tips for success are listed in Box 131.3.

So-called 'activity cycling' is common and unhelpful. In this situation, patients are overactive on 'good days' and then underactive on the inevitable painful and tired subsequent 'bad days'. The aim should be that the patient gradually, but steadily, increases their physical activity level, independent of how they feel on the day—in other words, on good days, they may do less than what they feel capable of, but on bad days, they aim to do more than what they feel capable of.

### Cognitive behavioural therapy

It makes intuitive good sense to incorporate *cognitive* elements into a purely *behavioural* intervention (exercise) for FM. Many patients will be reluctant to engage in a graded exercise programme, due to concerns about feasibility (for example, access to means or time), effectiveness (why should this help?), and toxicity (won't this make me worse?). Personalized assistance with overcoming practical concerns, and with the identification and challenge of maladaptive beliefs about the effectiveness and adverse effects of exercise, is highly appropriate. There are several key cognitions in FM that deserve targeting. These include that pain or other symptoms indicate actual bodily harm, that exercise will

**Box 131.3** Tips for success with exercise for FM

- Involve key carers/relatives when explaining the rationale and the detail.
- Explain the muscular deconditioning cycle, and check understanding (**Fig. 131.1**).
- Be specific about what graded exercise is, and personalize the discussion.
- Help the patient to set clear treatment goals.
- Interpret 'exercise' very broadly and sensibly, especially when there are problems starting.
- Emphasize the importance of persistent engagement with the exercise programme—stopping and starting is unlikely to be helpful.
- Consider using a mechanical pedometer or a smartphone app to provide a daily record of activity levels.
- Be aware of the potency of fear-avoidance of physical activity.
- Be aware of 'activity cycling'.

cause pain or other symptoms, and that the increased symptoms following exercise are a sign of increased activity in the disease process, which then leads logically to resumed avoidance of exercise.

EULAR guidance [18] concludes that there is 'weak evidence for' cognitive behavioural therapy (CBT), based upon a Cochrane review [26] of 23 RCTs, in which there was a statistically significant difference in pain and mood at end of CBT and in which improvement was sustained at 6 months. Unfortunately, the RCTs have substantial heterogeneity. It is therefore difficult to extrapolate directly to clinical practice in FM. Furthermore, there are several difficulties associated with the practical use of CBT, including highly varied cognitive behavioural interventions, the availability of therapists and their varied skill level, and varied treatment fidelity. Limited availability may, in part, be addressed by innovative delivery via groups or the Internet [27].

### Multicomponent treatments

EULAR guidance [18] concludes that there is 'weak evidence for' the combination of treatments, and especially psychological or educational therapies combined with graded exercise. A systematic review [28] defined multicomponent therapy as 'at least 1 educational or other psychological therapy, and at least 1 exercise therapy' and concluded that it was effective in reducing pain post-treatment, compared to control interventions. However, there is considerable complexity in the nature of 'multicomponent' interventions, especially regarding their level of integration [29]. 'Multi-disciplinary' and 'interdisciplinary' interventions lie along a continuum where the latter implies that the various disciplines have a common, coherent approach, rather than continuing to work within their own silo.

### Antidepressants and anticonvulsants (as 'neuromodulators')

Most guidance, including EULAR [18], recommends pharmacological approaches, including antidepressants, as second line, that is, following failed intervention with education and exercise. An optimal therapeutic approach may be described as 'cautious pharmacological input' [30]. A recent summary of medicines for which there is evidence of effectiveness in FM, including specific contraindications and cautions, is helpful [31].

Importantly, in treating the core syndrome of FM, antidepressants and anticonvulsants are not functioning via their impact on mood

but are functioning as *neuromodulators* influencing central sensitivity; the analgesic effect of antidepressants occurs in FM patients who are not depressed and is independent of any antidepressant effect. It is important to emphasize this to FM patients for whom these medicines are being prescribed, to avoid their objection that either their illness is 'real', and not 'mental', or that they are not depressed. Most patients will accept the explanation that antidepressants change the functioning of 'nerves in the brain', to improve the outcome of depression, and that they can also therefore change the functioning of nerves in the spine and muscles, and so can alter the experience of pain in FM.

Hauser suggested three main reasons for why antidepressants should be used second line: (1) modest evidence of effectiveness; (2) high individual variability in response; and (3) problematic adverse effects [32]. While she concludes, somewhat implausibly, that amitriptyline, duloxetine, and milnacipran 'are first-line options for the treatment of FM', she goes on, thoughtfully, to state:

> 'Physicians and patients should be realistic about the potential benefits of antidepressants in FM … A small number of patients experience a substantial symptom relief with no or minor adverse effects … However, a remarkable number of patients drop out of therapy because of intolerable adverse effects or experience only a small relief of symptoms, which does not outweigh the adverse effects.'[1]

The usual recommendation is to start with a low or very low dose of amitriptyline (25 or 10 mg, or even 5 mg, at night) and to titrate up, according to tolerance, to 75 mg. However, many patients will not be able to tolerate this modest dose and, even if they do, many will take the medicine for less than a year [33]. The usual cautions apply in older patients, and especially those with cardiac disease.

If amitriptyline is ineffective or poorly tolerated, then the serotonin/noradrenaline reuptake inhibitors (SNRIs) duloxetine or milnacipran should be considered [34]. The use of the tricyclic amitriptyline and these SNRIs is firmly rooted in the relevant biology—both serotonin and noradrenaline influence the descending modulatory pain pathways. There is little randomized evidence to support the use of the SNRI venlafaxine in FM. Cyclobenzaprine, a tricyclic-like muscle relaxant, is another alternative to amitriptyline ('weak evidence for') [18]. Finally, other alternatives include the anticonvulsants pregabalin ('weak evidence for') and gabapentin ('research only') [18]. Both of these medicines affect voltage-gated calcium channels, which are modulators of afferent pain signals.

The choice of an appropriate medicine should consider the symptom profile, likely side effects profile, likely patient tolerance of side effects, and patient preferences, which may be influenced by other FM patients' experiences. Clinical practice tends to favour amitriptyline or an SNRI with prominent depression, an anticonvulsant with prominent sleep disturbance, and an SNRI with prominent fatigue. Intolerance of medicines, even at low or very low doses, is a frequent problem [35], probably due to increased somatic sensitivity in FM, although other mechanisms are also likely to contribute to this nocebo effect.

---

[1] Reproduced from *CNS Drugs*, 26(4), Hauser W, Wolfe F, Tolle T, *et al.*, The role of antidepressants in the management of fibromyalgia syndrome: a systematic review and meta-analysis, pp. 297–307, Copyright (2012), with permission from Adis Data Information BV.

The prescription of strong opioid analgesics is inappropriate, as is long-standing prescription of any opioid. This reflects the lack of evidence for their effectiveness, with consequent lack of support from guidelines, alongside an increasing concern about their excessive use in some countries, with a high prevalence of use (10–60%) among FM opioid users [36]. Some evidence supports the use of tramadol, an opioid with some SNRI activity, and EULAR [18] concludes 'weak evidence for', but adverse effects and misuse are frequent issues.

Rather than 'prescribe and forget', an integrated approach to pharmacological treatment should be adopted. This should include:

- Careful patient and carer education;
- Continued exercise/activity intervention;
- Careful selection and targeting of medicines;
- An empirical approach, based on simple trials of one medicine at a time, with patient monitoring of key symptoms and function;
- Stepwise increase in dosing, to a dose likely to be therapeutic;
- Monitoring of adherence;
- Prompt discontinuation of ineffective medicines; and
- Pruning of medicines lists to reduce iatrogenic harm.

The last issue is crucial—FM patients are typically taking 8–10 medicines, for a variety of reasons [33], and such a number is unlikely to represent optimal management, even where there are multiple comorbidities. Application of simple $n$ of 1 trials in this patient group may advance the rigour of decision-making and improve individual patient outcomes from pharmacotherapy [37].

Emerging randomized evidence suggests that combinations of CNS-acting medicines may increase response rates. For example, in a recent randomized crossover trial, patients received placebo, pregabalin, duloxetine, and pregabalin–duloxetine combination [38], with pain response of 18%, 39%, 42%, and 68%, respectively. Unsurprisingly, adverse effects, including drowsiness, were more common with combination treatment, and it seems prudent to reserve this approach for patients who have failed both first-line non-pharmacological treatment and second-line single-agent pharmacological treatment.

### Failure to respond

Continued symptoms and disability are common, despite education, graded exercise, and a single pharmacological agent at the maximum tolerated dose. In this situation, a number of pragmatic approaches may be adopted, chosen according to the patient's particular clinical situation and preferences. These include:

- *Combinations of drugs, rather than monotherapy.* One approach is to combine a morning SNRI with an evening anticonvulsant. Another is to combine a morning selective serotonin reuptake inhibitor (SSRI) with a low dose of amitriptyline in the evening. There is some limited evidence that SSRIs alone may provide some benefit. Adjunctive medicines, such as paracetamol, tramadol, and non-steroidal anti-inflammatory drugs (NSAIDs), may give additional benefit.
- *Supervised exercise or comprehensive rehabilitation programmes.* Patients who do not respond adequately to an exercise programme, often due to either poor motivation or poor exercise tolerance, may benefit from structured exercise in a more supervised setting, perhaps following referral to a physiotherapist, or in an exercise group supervised by a health care professional.
- *Psychiatric referral.* This may be appropriate when a patient with depression has not responded to first- and second-stage antidepressant treatment, when suicidal ideation is significant or worsening, and when psychiatric problems may benefit from the input of the multi-disciplinary psychiatry team.
- *Pain management programme referral.* For more complex patients, perhaps with multiple comorbidities, consider referral to a pain management programme, which delivers more intensive support for self-management, with a mixed group of chronic pain patients, but using core principles of education, graded activity, and cognitive behavioural approaches [39].
- *Other approaches for which there is more limited evidence* such as complementary or alternative therapies. If the patient is enthusiastic about an empirically unsupported treatment, it should be considered in a non-judgemental way if the clinician does not view it as actively detrimental or unsafe—the placebo effect is a powerful tool in FM.

### Empirically unsupported treatments

EULAR guidance [18] does not recommend a variety of treatments, including biofeedback, capsaicin gel, hypnotherapy, massage, and S-adenosyl-methionine (all 'weak evidence against'); other complementary and alternative therapies ('strong evidence against'); and chiropractic ('strong against', due to safety concerns). It also does not recommend many other treatments due to inadequate evidence, including electrothermal therapy, phytothermotherapy, music therapy, storytelling, magnet therapy, transcranial magnetic therapy, and direct current stimulation.

Many FM patients use complementary and alternative therapies. Clinicians should routinely ask patients about their attitudes to such therapies and about their use of them but should be clear that there is currently insufficient evidence to recommend them. Indeed, the use of such therapies alongside treatments with an established evidence base may be counterproductive, due to concomitant engagement with an alternative aetiological model.

### Management of comorbidities

Comorbid diagnoses impact significantly on an FM patient's clinical presentation, prognosis, and treatment. It is therefore desirable to fully diagnose comorbid disorders, in order to characterize the patient's situation, understand their likely illness trajectory, and plan appropriate and comprehensive management. While targeting multiple problems simultaneously is unrealistic, and unlikely to be effective, if one or two symptoms are especially problematic, they may benefit from targeted treatment. A syndrome such as IBS, for example, may benefit from dietary advice, increased physical activity, and an antispasmodic.

Low mood sufficient to constitute a depressive episode deserves prioritization, as it reduces engagement with treatment, is associated with a worsened prognosis, and increases suicide risk, which is a significant concern in FM. In the presence of pain, mental disorders, such as depression, tend to be missed and, even when recognized, tend to be treated inadequately. This is despite their undoubted contribution to disability and chronicity.

## Prognosis

In secondary and tertiary care, continued pain, fatigue, and sleep and mood disturbance are the norm over a period of several years [40]. This reinforces the need for early identification and energetic evidence-based treatment in primary care, based upon the rehabilitative model described in the previous section. The focus of many patients is on symptoms, including pain and fatigue; while these are unlikely to resolve, the impact on them and on health services can be significantly reduced. The aims of FM treatment should therefore be broad and include increased activity/reduced disability, improved mood and self-efficacy, increased employment, reduced sickness/benefit payments, and reduced use and cost of health care services.

The prediction of outcome in an individual patient at treatment outset is challenging. Psychosocial factors may help to predict prognosis, such as: (1) beliefs that the pain is harmful or severely disabling; (2) low mood and social isolation; (3) fear-avoidance; (4) an expectation that the patient will be a passive recipient of care, rather than an active participant in treatment; and (5) comorbid depression.

Overall, FM is not associated with increased mortality, but it has been associated with a 10-fold increased risk of suicide in a secondary care population [standardized mortality ratio (SMR) 10.5, 95% confidence interval (CI) 4.5–20.7] [41]. This emphasizes the need for:

- Therapeutic optimism, facilitated by and facilitating a pain rehabilitative approach;
- The identification and management of comorbid depression; and
- Routine or urgent referral for psychiatric assessment when needed.

## Relapse prevention

Perhaps surprisingly, despite the chronicity of symptoms in most patients with FM, little attention has been paid to long-term management and prevention of relapse from treatment response. There is some evidence that the benefits of exercise may persist [42]. However, predisposing factors, such as genetic vulnerability, imply that FM responders remain vulnerable to setbacks and that continued improvement should not be taken for granted.

A common-sense approach suggests that, prior to discharge from health care, responders should be reminded that:

- They have a lifetime vulnerability to central sensitivity and FM.
- They should maintain non-sedentary levels of physical activity.
- They should identify early warning signs of a return of FM and share those signs with key relatives/carers.
- If the early warning signs emerge, they should redouble their self-care strategy.
- If their self-care fails to deliver early improvement, they should seek additional help from their health care provider.

It may be helpful to provide these key messages in written form for the patient's and carer's records.

## Chronic fatigue syndrome

CFS is a complex disorder, in which severe fatigue, combined with several other symptoms, causes impairment across a wide spectrum, from mild restriction to severe and bedbound. Clinical management and advances in understanding are impeded by entrenched and diametrically opposed positions on the roles of rest and physical activity, which are each seen variously as either cause or cure. The following text reviews in brief some of the issues and ends with a plea for a meeting of minds.

### Clinical presentation and epidemiology

Fatigue is a common, almost universal, sensation and a normal bodily response to sustained effort. The challenge for clinicians and researchers has been to determine when 'normal' fatigue ends and when an important and problematic clinical disorder begins. In essence, this relates to chronicity and severity, although, as an indicator of the extent of difficulty, no less than nine sets of diagnostic criteria have been developed in the last 30 years. These have helpfully been summarized in a recent systematic review [43]. The 'Oxford criteria' [44], used in the largest and most controversial treatment trial to date [45], are summarized in Box 131.4, and the most recent criteria [46] for 'systemic exertion intolerance disease' (SEID) in Box 131.5. This new term is intended to convey the undoubted impact of the disorder and to reduce what the authors called the 'stigmatization and trivialization' resulting from the existing terminology.

While the diagnostic criteria for CFS/SEID are relatively straightforward, it is clear that the population of patients with CFS is a complex and heterogenous one, with multiple comorbidities. Muscle pain and joint pain are common, and there is considerable overlap between FM and CFS populations, with FM co-diagnosis indicating a more burdened CFS population. Other functional somatic syndromes are common, and diagnostic overlap has contributed to an energetic debate regarding the advantages of 'lumping' such syndromes together to emphasize commonalities in features and aetiology vs 'splitting' to emphasize differences [47]. Depression and anxiety are more common in CFS than in FM or IBS, but far from universal [48].

### Epidemiology

The prevalence of CFS is uncertain, in part due to significant discrepancy between point prevalence in the community determined by self-reporting of symptoms (3.5%) and clinical assessment (0.9%) [49]. An added complication is the decline in prevalence of CFS through time. Between 1990 and 2001, combined fatigue diagnoses

---

**Box 131.4** The Oxford criteria for chronic fatigue syndrome (CFS)

- Fatigue is the main symptom.
- Fatigue is severe and disabling, and affects physical and mental function.
- Fatigue present at least 50% of the time for a period of at least 6 months.
- Other symptoms may occur, including muscle pain, mood problems (including depressive and anxiety disorder), and sleep problems.
- Not explained by a medical condition, for example severe anaemia.
- Not in a person with schizophrenia, bipolar disorder, substance misuse, eating disorder, or organic brain disease.

Source: data from *J R Soc Med.*, 84(2), Sharpe MC, Archard LC, Banatvala JE, *et al.*, A report – chronic fatigue syndrome: guidelines for research, pp. 118–121, Copyright (1991), SAGE Publications.

[CFS, post-viral fatigue syndrome (PVFS), asthenia] fell by 44% [50]. Recent findings confirmed a continued fall between 2001 and 2013 [51], with a modest decline in CFS incidence (3% annually), a more rapid decline in PVFS (8%), and a precipitate decline in asthenia (30%). Alongside this shift, there has been a rise in FM diagnosis, such that FM in the UK is now about three times more frequent than CFS [51]. This is confirmed by evidence from high-quality community surveys (0.8% CFS vs 2.7% FM) [2, 49]. The reasons for these trends are unclear; there is no good evidence for changes in diagnostic labelling. Recent data from Norway indicated two age peaks for incident CFS (10–19 and 30–39 years) and a female:male ratio of >3:1 [52].

### Aetiology

There is no clearly established, widely agreed aetiological understanding for CFS. This undoubtedly reflects the clinical heterogeneity and aetiological complexity but also reflects the fundamental disagreements about the nature and causes of the illness. The aim here is to encourage the reader to engage with the relatively rapid advance in evidence relating to relevant aetiological factors and to form balanced opinions that are supported by evidence.

There is no doubt that physical disorder, such as common viral illnesses, often acts as a trigger/precipitating factor for severe fatigue and, in some individuals, the development of CFS. What are in dispute are: (1) the extent to which psychological or social factors predict the development of CFS after such illness (that is, are predisposing factors); and (2) the extent to which ongoing physical illness (such as chronic viral infection) contributes to persistent symptomatology (that is, is a maintaining factor). In a study of patients with glandular fever, chronic fatigue was not predicted by the severity of the glandular fever, as measured by symptom count [53]. Predictors included personality factors, such as perfectionism, and also cognitive factors such as ascribing symptoms to their glandular fever, believing that the illness would last a long time and impact detrimentally on their life, and not believing that they could control their illness. Emerging evidence suggests that CFS patients have specific cognitive biases which reinforce and maintain maladaptive cognitions and associated behaviours. These include an attentional bias for fatigue-related information and a tendency to

interpret ambiguous information as implying bodily dysfunction [54]. As in FM, fear of movement and avoidance of physical activity are common in CFS and related to symptom severity and physical disability [11]. Fear-avoidance lies at the core of the cognitive behavioural model of CFS, in which catastrophic interpretations of physical symptoms (and an unhelpful focus on symptoms) motivate behaviours, including activity avoidance and activity cycling.

A fundamental divide in thinking about CFS is the role of rest. On one side, rest (or relative rest) is viewed as an essential component of *treatment* of CFS, to allow the body to recover from the illness and gain in strength to fight putative infection or other ongoing physical challenge to wellness. On the other side, rest is viewed as an essential part of the *cause* of CFS [55], by leading to deconditioning. The adverse effects of excessive rest on multiple physiological systems are well established in healthy humans [56] and in patients with chronic physical illness such as renal failure [57].

There has been an ongoing search for physical causes of chronic fatigue. There is no doubt that, in some patients, a clear physical cause can be found. Prudent history-taking, physical examination, and investigation are therefore needed in possible cases of CFS to rule out significant physical pathology. Specific red flag features have been identified such as: difficulty in focusing the eyes, inflammatory arthritis or connective tissue disease, cardiorespiratory disease, weight loss, sleep apnoea, and lymphadenopathy [58]. However, little appears to be gained by an aggressive search for a physical disorder in the presence of normal physical examination and unremarkable screening investigations. In recent years, there was much early excitement when the retrovirus xenotropic murine leukaemia virus-related virus (XMRV) was found in the blood of most CFS patients, only for new evidence to dash hopes of a cure based on this finding [59]. The meaning of abnormalities in brain regional connectivity in CFS patients, the extent of which appears correlated with fatigue severity [60], is uncertain. Demonstrable effects of exercise [61] and psychological treatment [62] on neuroinflammation offer encouragement that a more integrated understanding of the causes of CFS can be developed.

### Management

The UK's National Institute for Health and Care Excellence (NICE) guidance [58] recommends referral to specialist care within 3–4 months for adults with moderate symptoms, and immediately for patients with severe symptoms. Specialist care includes patient-centred rehabilitation programmes, which aim to improve physical and cognitive function and to manage symptoms. *Patient education* plays a key role and contributes to genuinely collaborative care, including shared decision-making. There is robust empirical support for two treatments: *graded exercise therapy* (GET) and *cognitive behavioural therapy* (CBT), and this is considered in the following sections. The evidence for *pacing* is disputed. There is little evidence for the effectiveness of *neuromodulators*, including antidepressants, unless a depressive illness is present. The evidence for pharmacological interventions has recently been reviewed, with no promising solutions evident [63].

Systematic reviews of RCTs support the use of GET [64] and CBT [65], but trials are small and there is a lack of comparative evidence with pacing. There is debate about the optimal specification of pacing in CFS, but in essence, it is an approach in which the patient functions within their perceived energy levels, rather than aiming to systematically increase their level of functioning, as in GET or CBT. It is popular with patients, often advocated by patient groups, and it is unfortunate that better evidence does not exist. The PACE trial [66] was intended to provide a definitive answer to the important question about the relative merits of specialist medical care alone vs additional pacing, GET, or CBT. The main conclusions were that CBT and GET improved outcomes when added to specialist medical care, pacing did not, and adverse events seemed similar across the trial treatments. Overall, however, outcomes were modest and the proportion of recovered patients was low, perhaps reflecting clinical heterogeneity. Unfortunately, following the publication of short-term [45], adverse events [67], and long-term [68] results, fundamental and apparently bitter disagreements between the researchers and their critics have emerged, and their positions appear entrenched to a degree that is unique in medicine. The respective positions are well summarized in recent papers [69, 70]. The differences are clearly mirrored in the divergent recommendations of patient support organizations and medical organizations [71]. Those who are interested in uncertainty and the nature of scientific evidence, facts, and beliefs are strongly encouraged to read the cited documents. As the then deputy editor of the *BMJ* stated in 2011 [72]:

'Why can't CFS/ME be like other common chronic conditions where patients, carers, doctors, and researchers work together to pose research questions, gain understanding, and—in the absence of clear explanations and cures—at least find ways to respond to patients' needs, help them live with and manage symptoms, and get more out of life?'[2]

## REFERENCES

1. Boomershine C, Crofford L. A symptom-based approach to pharmacologic management of fibromyalgia. *Nat Rev Rheumatol* 2009; 5: 191–9.
2. Queiroz L. Worldwide epidemiology of fibromyalgia. *Curr Pain Headache Rep* 2013; 17: 356.
3. Wolfe F, Smythe H, Yunus M, *et al.* Report of the Multicenter Criteria Committee. The American College of Rheumatology 1990 criteria for the classification of fibromyalgia. *Arthritis Rheumatol* 1990; 33: 160–72.
4. Wolfe F, Clauw DJ, Fitzcharles MA, *et al.* 2016 revisions to the 2010/2011 Fibromyalgia Diagnostic Criteria: 2016 Revised Fibromyalgia Criteria. *Semin Arthritis Rheum* 2016; 46: 319–29.
5. Maixner W, Finnigim R, Williams D, Smith S, Slade G. Overlapping chronic pain conditions: Implications for diagnosis and classification. *J Pain* 2016; 17 Suppl. 2: T93–107.
6. Fink P, Schroder A. One single diagnosis, bodily distress syndrome, succeeded to capture 10 diagnostic categories of functional somatic syndromes and somatoform disorders. *J Psychosom Res* 2010; 68: 415–26.
7. Choy E, Perrot S, Leon T, *et al.* A patient survey of the impact of fibromyalgia and the journey to diagnosis. *BMC Health Serv Res* 2010; 10: 102.
8. Edwards R, Dworkin R, Sullivan M, Turk D, Wasan A. The role of psychosocial processes in the development and maintenance of chronic pain. *J Pain* 2016; 17 Suppl. 2: T70–92.
9. Bourke JH, Langford RM, White PD. The common link between functional somatic syndromes may be central sensitisation. *J Psychosom Res* 2015; 78, 228–36.
10. Lethem J, Slade P, Troup J, Bentley G. Outline of a fear-avoidance model of exaggerated pain perception. *J Behav Res Ther* 1983; 21, 401–8.
11. Nijs J, Roussel N, Van Oosterwijck J, *et al.* Fear of movement and avoidance behaviour toward physical activity in chronic-fatigue syndrome and fibromyalgia: state of the art and implications for clinical practice. *Clin Rheumatol* 2013; 32: 1121–9.
12. Turk D, Fillingim R, Ohrbach R, Patel K. Assessment of psychosocial and functional impact of chronic pain. *J Pain* 2016; 17 Suppl. 2: T21–49.
13. Lotze M, Moseley G. Theoretical considerations for chronic pain rehabilitation. *Phys Ther* 2015; 95: 1316–20.
14. Rahman A, Underwood M, Carnes D. Clinical review: fibromyalgia. *BMJ* 2014; 348: 1224.
15. Fitzcharles M, Ste-Maria P, Goldenberg D, *et al.* Canadian Pain Society and Canadian Rheumatology Association recommendations for rational care of persons with fibromyalgia: a summary report. *J Rheumatol* 2013; 40:1388–93.
16. Clauw D. Fibromyalgia: a clinical review. *JAMA* 2014; 311: 1547–55.
17. Goldenberg D. *Initial Treatment of Fibromyalgia in Adults.* UpToDate, 2018. Available from: https://www.uptodate.com/contents/initial-treatment-of-fibromyalgia-in-adults
18. Macfarlane G, Kronisch C, Dean L, *et al.* EULAR revised recommendations for the management of fibromyalgia. *Ann Rheum Dis* 2017; 76: 318–28.
19. Arnold L, Choy E, Clauw D, *et al.* Fibromyalgia and chronic pain syndromes: a white paper detailing current challenges in the field. *Clin J Pain* 2016; 32: 737–46.
20. Nuesch E, Hauser W, Bernardy K, Barth J, Juni P. Comparative efficacy of pharmacological and non-pharmacological interventions in fibromyalgia syndrome: network meta-analysis. *Ann Rheum Dis* 2013; 72: 955–62.
21. Van Oosterwijck J, Meeus M, Paul L, *et al.* Pain physiology education improves health status and endogenous pain inhibition in fibromyalgia: a double-blind randomized controlled trial. *Clin J Pain* 2013; 29: 873–82.
22. Busch A, Barber K, Overend T, Peloso P, Schacter C. Exercise for treating fibromyalgia syndrome. *Cochrane Database Syst Rev* 2007; 4: CD003786.
23. Busch A, Webber S, Richards R, *et al.* Resistance exercise training for fibromyalgia. *Cochrane Database Syst Rev* 2013; 12: CD010884.
24. Bidonde J, Busch A, Webber S, *et al.* Aquatic exercise training for fibromyalgia. *Cochrane Database Syst Rev* 2014; 10: CD011336.
25. Kaleth A, Slaven J, Ang D. Does increasing steps per day predict improvement in physical function and pain interference in adults with fibromyalgia? *Arthritis Care Res* 2014; 66: 1887–94.
26. Bernardy K, Klose P, Busch A, Choy E, Hauser W. Cognitive behavioural therapies for fibromyalgia. *Cochrane Database Syst Rev* 2013; 9: CD009796.
27. Friesen L, Hadjistavropoulos H, Schneider L, Alberts N, Titov N, Dear B. Examination of an internet-delivered cognitive behavioural pain management course for adults with fibromyalgia: a randomized controlled trial. *Pain* 2017; 158: 593–604.
28. Hauser W, Bernardy K, Arnold B, Offenbacher M, Schiltenwolf M. Efficacy of multicomponent treatment in fibromyalgia syndrome: a meta-analysis of randomized controlled trials. *Arthritis Care Res* 2009; 61: 216–24.

29. Giusti E, Castelnuovo G, Molinari E. Differences in multidisciplinary and interdisciplinary treatment programs for fibromyalgia: a mapping review. *Pain Res Manage* 2017; 2017: 7261468.

30. Cohen H. Controversies and challenges in fibromyalgia: a review and a proposal. *Ther Adv Musculoskel Dis* 2017; 9: 115–127.

31. Kia S, Choy E. Update on treatment guideline in fibromyalgia syndrome with focus on pharmacology. *Biomedicines* 2017; 5: 20.

32. Hauser W, Wolfe F, Tolle T, Uceyler N, Sommer C. The role of antidepressants in the management of fibromyalgia syndrome: a systematic review and meta-analysis. *CNS Drugs* 2012; 26: 297–307.

33. Kim S, Landon J, Solomon D. Clinical characteristics and medication uses among fibromyalgia patients newly prescribed amitriptyline, duloxetine, gabapentin, or pregabalin. *Arthritis Care Res* 2013; 65: 1813–19.

34. Hauser W, Petzke F, Uceyler N, Sommer C. Comparative efficacy and acceptability of amitriptyline, duloxetine and milnacipran in FM syndrome: a systematic review with meta-analysis. *Rheumatology* 2011; 50: 532–43.

35. Mitsikostas D, Chalarakis N, Mantonakis L, Delicha E, Sfikakis P. Nocebo in fibromyalgia: metaanalysis of placebo controlled clinical trials and implications for practice. *Eur J Neurol* 2012; 19: 672–80.

36. Goldenberg D, Clauw D, Palmer R, Clair A. Opioid use in fibromyalgia: a cautionary tale. *Mayo Clin Proc* 2016; 91: 640–8.

37. Schork N. Personalized medicine: time for one-person trials. *Nature* 2015; 520: 609–11.

38. Gilron I, Chaparro L, Tu D, *et al*. Combination of pregabalin with duloxetine for fibromyalgia: a randomized controlled trial. *Pain* 2016; 157: 1532–40.

39. British Pain Society. *Guidelines for Pain Management Programmes for Adults: An Evidence-based Review Prepared on Behalf of the British Pain Society*. London: British Pain Society; 2013.

40. Wolfe F, Anderson J, Harkness D, *et al*. A prospective, longitudinal, multicenter study of service utilization and costs in fibromyalgia. *Arthritis Rheumatol* 1997; 40: 1560–70.

41. Dreyer L, Kendall S, Danneskiold-Samsoe B, Bartels E, Bliddal H. Mortality in a cohort of Danish patients with fibromyalgia: increased frequency of suicide. *Arthritis Rheum* 2010; 62: 3101–8.

42. Sanudo B, Carrasco L, de Hoyo M, McVeigh J. Effects of exercise training and detraining in patients with fibromyalgia syndrome: a 3-yr longitudinal study. *Am J Phys Med Rehab* 2012; 91: 561–73.

43. Haney E, Smith ME, McDonagh M, *et al*. Diagnostic methods for myalgic encephalomyelitis/chronic fatigue syndrome: a systematic review for a National Institutes of Health pathways to prevention workshop. *Ann Intern Med* 2015; 162: 834–40.

44. Sharpe MC, Archard LC, Banatvala JE, *et al*. A report—chronic fatigue syndrome: guidelines for research. *J R Soc Med* 1991; 84: 118–21.

45. White PD, Goldsmith KA, Johnson AL, *et al*. Comparison of adaptive pacing therapy, cognitive behaviour therapy, graded exercise therapy, and specialist medical care for chronic fatigue syndrome (PACE): a randomised trial. *Lancet* 2011; 377: 823–36.

46. Institute of Medicine. *Beyond Myalgic Encephalomyelitis/Chronic Fatigue Syndrome: Redefining an Illness*. Washington, DC: National Academies Press; 2015.

47. Chalder T, Willis C. 'Lumping' and 'splitting' medically unexplained symptoms: is there a role for a transdiagnostic approach? *J Ment Health* 2017; 26: 187–91.

48. Janssens KA, Zijlema WL, Joustra ML, Rosmalen JG. Mood and anxiety disorders in chronic fatigue syndrome, fibromyalgia, and irritable bowel syndrome: results from the LifeLines cohort study. *Psychosom Med* 2015; 77: 449–57.

49. Johnston S, Brenu EW, Staines D, Marshall-Gradisnik S. The prevalence of chronic fatigue syndrome/myalgic encephalomyelitis: a meta-analysis. *Clin Epidemiol* 2013; 5: 105.

50. Gallagher AM, Thomas JM, Hamilton WT, White PD. Incidence of fatigue symptoms and diagnoses presenting in UK primary care from 1990 to 2001. *J R Soc Med* 2004; 97: 571–5.

51. Collin SM, Bakken IJ, Nazareth I, Crawley E, White PD. Trends in the incidence of chronic fatigue syndrome and fibromyalgia in the UK, 2001–2013: a Clinical Practice Research Datalink study. *J R Soc Med* 2017; 110: 231–44.

52. Bakken IJ, Tveito K, Gunnes N, *et al*. Two age peaks in the incidence of chronic fatigue syndrome/myalgic encephalomyelitis: a population-based registry study from Norway 2008–2012. *BMC Med* 2014; 12: 167.

53. Moss-Morris R, Spence MJ, Hou R. The pathway from glandular fever to chronic fatigue syndrome: can the cognitive behavioural model provide the map? *Psychol Med* 2011; 41: 1099–107.

54. Hughes AM, Chalder T, Hirsch CR, Moss-Morris R. An attention and interpretation bias for illness-specific information in chronic fatigue syndrome. *Psychol Med* 2017; 47: 853–65.

55. Sharpe M, Wessely S. Putting the rest cure to rest—again: Rest has no place in treating chronic fatigue. *BMJ* 1998; 316: 796.

56. Greenleaf JE. *Clinical Physiology of Bed Rest*. NASA Technical Memorandum 104010. 1993. Available from: https://ntrs.nasa.gov/search.jsp?R=19940008974

57. Krasnoff J, Painter P. The physiological consequences of bed rest and inactivity. *Adv Ren Replace Ther* 1999; 6: 124–32.

58. National Institute for Health and Care Excellence. *Chronic Fatigue Syndrome/Myalgic Encephalomyelitis (or Encephalopathy): Diagnosis and Management*. Clinical guideline [CG53]. London: National Institute for Health and Care Excellence; 2007.

59. Van Kuppeveld FJ, van der Meer JW. XMRV and CFS—the sad end of a story. *Lancet* 2012; 379: e27–8.

60. Gay CW, Robinson ME, Lai S, *et al*. Abnormal resting-state functional connectivity in patients with chronic fatigue syndrome: results of seed and data-driven analysis. *Brain Connect* 2016; 6: 48–56.

61. Moylan S, Eyre HA, Maes M, Baune BT, Jacka FN, Berk M. Exercising the worry away: how inflammation, oxidative and nitrogen stress mediates the beneficial effect of physical activity on anxiety disorder symptoms and behaviours. *Neurosci Biobehav Rev* 2013; 37: 573–84.

62. Irwin MR, Olmstead R, Breen EC, *et al*. Cognitive behavioral therapy and tai chi reverse cellular and genomic markers of inflammation in late-life insomnia: a randomized controlled trial. *Biol Psychiatry* 2015; 78: 721–9.

63. Collatz A, Johnston SC, Staines DR, Marshall-Gradisnik SM. A systematic review of drug therapies for chronic fatigue syndrome/myalgic encephalomyelitis. *Clin Ther* 2016; 38: 1263–71.

64. Larun L, Brurberg KG, Odgaard-Jensen J, Price JR. Exercise therapy for chronic fatigue syndrome. *Cochrane Database Syst Rev* 2016; 6: CD003200.

65. Price JR, Mitchell E, Tidy E, Hunot V. Chronic behaviour therapy for chronic fatigue syndrome in adults. *Cochrane Database Syst Rev* 2008; 3: CD001027.

66. White PD, Sharpe MC, Chalder T, DeCesare JC, Walwyn R. Protocol for the PACE trial: a randomised controlled trial of adaptive pacing, cognitive behaviour therapy, and graded exercise as supplements to standardised specialist medical care versus standardised specialist medical care alone for patients with the chronic fatigue syndrome/myalgic encephalomyelitis or encephalopathy. *BMC Neurol* 2007; 7: 6.

67. Dougall D, Johnson A, Goldsmith K, *et al.* Adverse events and deterioration reported by participants in the PACE trial of therapies for chronic fatigue syndrome. *J Psychosom Res* 2014; 77: 20–6.
68. Sharpe M, Goldsmith KA, Johnson AL, Chalder T, Walker J, White PD. Rehabilitative treatments for chronic fatigue syndrome: long-term follow-up from the PACE trial. *Lancet Psychiatry* 2015; 2: 1067–74.
69. Wilshire C, Kindlon T, Matthees A, McGrath S. Can patients with chronic fatigue syndrome really recover after graded exercise or cognitive behavioural therapy? A critical commentary and preliminary re-analysis of the PACE trial. *Fatigue* 2017; 5:43–56.
70. Sharpe M, Chalder T, Johnson AL, Goldsmith KA, White PD. Do more people recover from chronic fatigue syndrome with cognitive behaviour therapy or graded exercise therapy than with other treatments? *Fatigue* 2017; 5: 57–61.
71. Mallet M, King E, White PD. A UK based review of recommendations regarding the management of chronic fatigue syndrome. *J Psychosom Res* 2016; 88: 33–5.
72. Groves T. Commentary: Heading for a therapeutic stalemate. *BMJ* 2011; 342: d3774.

# 132

# Factitious disorder and malingering

*Thomas Merten and Harald Merckelbach*

## Factitious disorder and malingering: two forms of feigned symptom presentation

Patients do not always present their symptoms in an honest manner. Their symptom reports may be affected by goals and motives that lie outside the realm of proper diagnosis and treatment of existing health problems. Distorted symptom presentations may occur in the forensic context where substantial incentives or secondary gain (for example, injury claims for compensation) are immanent, but also in clinical, as well as rehabilitative, settings.

Patients sometimes strive for certain benefits without their therapists being aware of this (that is, patients follow a 'hidden agenda'). Van Egmond, Kummeling, and van Balkom [1] asked psychiatric outpatients whether or not they expected to gain something from being a patient. A substantial minority (42%) said that this was indeed the case. They admitted that their patient status may help them to get a new home, sickness benefits, or a resident permit. A hidden agenda may fuel feigning and treatment stagnation [2]. The link between feigning and poor therapeutic success—including lack of co-operation, high dropout, and increased health care utilization—has now been well documented [3, 4] and should in itself be sufficient reason to consider feigning as a diagnostic option.

Exaggerated symptom reports may be motivated by a need to protect self-esteem. For example, Smith, Snyder, and Perkins [5] found that some individuals reported more symptoms in an evaluative vs non-evaluative situation, suggesting a self-protecting motive, according to the authors' interpretation. Mild symptom exaggeration or denial will not substantially hamper diagnostic decision-making. More blatant forms of distortions, however, may compromise clinical decisions. Such illness deception is commonly labelled factitious disorder or malingering. Both are commonly used categorical denominators to describe forms of significantly distorted illness behaviour, but phenomenologically they might not be distinguishable from each other at all. Indeed, some authors have argued that factitious disorder and malingering constitute one diagnostic entity [6]. We will return to this issue.

According to widely accepted definitions, malingering is the deliberate invention or gross exaggeration of health problems (symptoms), motivated by external incentives (secondary gain). The *Diagnostic and Statistical Manual of Mental Disorders*, fourth (DSM-IV) and fifth editions (DSM-5) [7, 8] described this deliberate invention as 'intentional production' of false symptoms. However, Young [9] argued that the DSM definition should be modified by substituting *production* by *presentation*, highlighting different forms of how false or exaggerated symptoms can be demonstrated. Thus, Young defines malingering as 'the intentional *presentation with* false or grossly exaggerated symptoms [physical, mental health, or both; full or partial; mild, moderate, or severe], for purposes of obtaining an external incentive . . . ' (p. 180; italics in the original).

The extant literature on malingering includes different manifestations, ranging from pure fabrications of symptomatology over grossly exaggerated symptoms and perseverations (continued assertion of symptoms that have been present in the past) to false imputations (that is, intentionally attributing genuine symptoms to a false source) [10]. The wide range of distorted symptom reports that are brought under the definition of *malingering* partly explains largely different views on its prevalence. There is no consensus on where to draw the line between mild and gross exaggeration, and how to treat the intermediate zone.

In and of itself, malingering is not a mental disorder, but rather a behavioural strategy that healthy or sick people might use in certain situations (for example, after a motor vehicle accident, in a situation of social misery). This strategy may be appropriate or not in a specific situation; it may be judged morally wrong or right (and differently so by different people or from different angles), and it may be highly adaptive or severely maladaptive.

In contrast, factitious behaviour is commonly perceived to be a mental disorder and described as such by the International Classification of Diseases (ICD) [11] and the DSM [7, 8]. Exactly like malingering, it describes the deliberate false presentation (invention, production, gross exaggeration) of health problems. Yet, the underlying motive for factitious symptom presentation is thought to be internal (that is, primary gain), rather than external, as is the case with malingering. This internal motivation is commonly assumed to be unconscious and related to the sick role (patient care, medical procedures, diagnosis and treatment of claimed health problems). The Munchausen's syndrome (named after the German Freiherr von Münchhausen, dubbed the Baron of Lies), in which patients actively try to mimic symptoms (for example, by hurting themselves), was first described by Asher [12] and continues to be considered as the most prototypical form of factitious behaviour. Factitious behaviour is closely tied to self-harm [13] (but for a discussion, see [14]). Thus,

**Table 132.1** The differential diagnosis between three forms of non-authentic symptom presentation largely rests on subjective judgment about the intention and the motivation for symptom distortion

| Diagnostic category | Distorted symptom presentation | Incentives for distorted symptom presentation | Examples of incentives |
|---|---|---|---|
| Malingering | Intentional, deliberate, controlled (conscious) | Cognizant, self-reflected (conscious); external incentive, secondary gain | Sick leave, financial compensation, escape from legal responsibility |
| Factitious disorder | Intentional, deliberate, controlled (conscious) | Non-reflective, unaware (unconscious); internal incentive, primary gain | Medical treatment, including surgery, sick role |
| Somatoform, dissociative, and conversion disorders | Unintentional, involuntary, uncontrolled (unconscious) | Non-reflective, unaware (unconscious); internal incentive, primary gain; secondary gain may also be present | Conflict management, stress reduction |

Reproduced from Merten T, False symptom claims and symptom validity assessment. In: Otgaar H, Howe M [eds]., *Finding the truth in the courtroom? Problems with deception, lies, and memories*, Copyright (2018), Oxford University Press.

unlike malingering, factitious behaviour is maladaptive, which may be the reason why it is included in subsequent versions of the DSM as a disorder.

However, motivational aspects are crucial for distinguishing between malingering and factitious disorder. The presence of external rewards per se does not exclude factitious disorder, given that the potential for some form of secondary gain is usually considerable for patients in Western welfare states (such as sick leave, sick pay). The fact that secondary gain can be identified does not automatically mean that it plays a reinforcing role in patients' symptom presentation [15]. In many cases, it will be difficult to clarify the true and complete motivational background of false or grossly distorted illness presentations. This may become completely impossible when both external and internal factors are apparently present and interact in a complex way (for case examples, see [16]). All that might be said with some confidence about such complex cases is that symptoms are *feigned*.

Feigning comprises both malingering and factitious disorder. It is defined as 'the deliberate fabrication or gross exaggeration of psychological or physical symptoms without any assumptions about its goals' ([17], p. 6). However, before an expert can ascertain feigning in a given case, he or she has to take another decision that is conceptually as complex and problematic as the clarification of the underlying motivation—whether or not false symptoms are presented intentionally, voluntarily, consciously.

## Feigning and genuine mental disorder

Striking discrepancies between subjective symptom report and objective signs are not limited to feigned health problems. In fact, they constitute the key feature of what historically has been called hysteria. In 1917, Jones and Llewellyn [18] wrote: 'Nothing, it may be said, *resembles malingering more than hysteria; nothing hysteria more than malingering*. In both alike we are confronted with the same discrepancy—between fact and statement, between objective sign and subjective symptom … ' (p. 117, *italics* in the original). Phenomenologically, patient behaviour in the context of factitious disorder, malingering, and somatoform or dissociative disorders may be completely indistinguishable. To address this problem, DSM-IV [7] stipulated as a necessary criterion for diagnosing both somatization disorders and conversion disorder: 'The symptoms are not intentionally produced or feigned (as in Factitious Disorder or

Malingering)' (p. 462). This requirement was given up in DSM-5 for *Somatic symptom and related disorders*. Still, the dimension of intentionality delineates a distinction between self-deceit (in genuine mental disorder) and other-deceit (in feigning), as described by Turner [19].

Intentionality (or not) and the nature of incentives are the two dimensions with which various forms of discrepant symptom presentations can be differentiated. The distinction between the three diagnostic entities listed in Table 132.1 critically hinges on the assumption that both intentionality and true motivation can be reliably and, much more importantly, validly ascertained by a third party (that is, the clinician or forensic expert) [20]. Many authors have criticized this assumption [21]. Moreover, in many cases, it appears doubtful whether intentionality and motivation can be reliably dichotomized at all. Diagnostic options such as *Feigning, unspecified* or *Feigning, not otherwise specified* [22], as well as previous attempts to rename somatoform disorders into *medically unexplained symptoms* [23], are reflective of this nosological inconclusiveness. However, the traditional approaches of DSM and ICD stick to the categorical system and have largely ignored attempts to introduce a multi-faceted and dimensional approach [24–26].

Incidentally, Brown's [27] definition of *medically unexplained symptoms* as 'a heterogeneous group of conditions characterized by persistent physical symptoms that cannot be explained by medical illness or injury' (p. 769) would encompass somatoform, dissociative, factitious, and malingered symptom presentations, plus symptoms in the context of a yet unknown physical disease. A more detailed discussion of the conceptual problems of distinguishing between somatoform and feigned disorders and its practical consequences can be found in Merten and Merckelbach [28].

In the descriptions below, we largely ignore the conceptual conundrum surrounding factitious disorder and malingering and depict their ideal-typical manifestations as they are treated in the literature.

## Malingering

### Definition

Malingering is the intentional false presentation (invention, gross exaggeration, or otherwise gross misrepresentation) of symptoms or health problems with the primary goal of attaining an external reward. External gain may be a financial incentive (for example, compensation), but it may also relate to obtaining drugs, escaping from formal duty (for example, sick leave, military service, sitting an exam), legal responsibility, or punishment, or obtaining other material or non-material advantage. The specifier *external* indicates that the motivation for false illness presentation does not primarily relate to stress management, internal (interpersonal) conflict, or the sick role. Malingering is not a mental illness and should not be pathologized. Still, pathologization of people who, in a certain context, engage in malingering is not uncommon [29], as indicated by phrases such as *healthy people don't do this; cry for help; you need to be mad in order to fake madness.*

In DSM-5, the term malingering has been deleted from the index and is difficult to find in the text. It is treated under the headline *Nonadherence to medical treatment,* with the code V65.2 (pp. 726–7). DSM-5 lists four criteria that were adapted from DSM-III [30], even though these criteria have repeatedly been shown to be completely inadequate [24, 31, 32]. According to DSM-5, any combination of the following four criteria would be strongly suggestive of malingering: (1) medicolegal context of presentation; (2) marked discrepancy between symptom presentation and objective findings; (3) low degree of co-operation in diagnosis and treatment; and (4) presence of an antisocial personality disorder.

To illustrate the inappropriateness of these criteria, it may suffice to note that any person with a diagnosed antisocial personality disorder who is examined in a medicolegal context should be 'strongly suspected' of malingering according to these criteria (when, in fact, the link between antisocial features and malingering is, at best, weak [33]). Also, any patient with a somatic symptom disorder or a conversion disorder should be 'strongly suspected' of malingering in any medicolegal context, given the fact that both disorders are characterized by a marked discrepancy between subjective symptom presentation and objective findings and observations.

The DSM criteria for malingering have virtually not changed since 1980. They are based on an outdated (criminological) conception of malingering prevalent in the 1970s (with antisocial personality considered to be a key issue in feigned health problems [34]), and they ignore the vast empirical and conceptual work with several thousands of publications written during the last three decades [24].

In ICD-10, malingering is coded as Z76.5, without further elaboration. Interestingly enough, ICD-10 contains another category of exaggerated or excessively prolonged symptoms that was conceptualized as *Elaboration of physical symptoms for psychological reasons* (F68.0). It corresponds roughly to the older concept of *compensation neurosis* (for a more recent appraisal, see [35]). However, for unknown reasons, it is explicitly limited to physical symptoms and is poorly defined. Cooper's pocket guide [11] stressed the psychological causation of it (including the aspiration of obtaining financial compensation). Contrary to malingering, F68.0 is conceived to be a mental disorder.

### Assessment

Different medical disciplines have developed their own strategies and lists of criteria for the detection of malingered symptomatology. Among traditional medical disciplines, ophthalmology has shown a particularly strong interest in differentiating true visual deficits from feigned impairment [36]. The determination of malingering is usually based on an analysis of plausibility and consistency within the available information or data on a case, with general criteria focusing on discrepancies, such as the following [31, 37]:

- Excessive, overgeneralized symptom report.
- Bizarre symptom presentation.
- Inconsistency in symptom presentation.
- Absence of functional impairment outside the diagnostic setting, unimpaired functional level in the private sphere.
- Disproportionate claimed disability, as compared to the objective severity of illness or injury.
- Implausibility of symptoms and complaints with regard to current medical/psychological knowledge (symptoms *do not make sense*), symptom presentation contradicts the functional–anatomic principles.
- Contradictions between claimed history and documented facts.
- No improvement under treatment with known efficiency.
- Evasiveness.

For different disciplines (for example, neurology, ophthalmology, neuropsychology), lists of special malingering markers have been developed, related to the functional system in question. In psychiatry, such lists are currently *en vogue* with regard to judging the authenticity of claimed symptoms of post-traumatic stress disorder PTSD). Such red flags may include early and spontaneous patient's symptom report, the quality of reported flashbacks, the presence or not of observable emotional arousal in the patient, the quality and extent of reported amnesia for aspects of the traumatic event, contents and the frequency of reported nightmares, temporal stability or instability of claimed symptoms, the presence or not of survivor guilt, or blame of others instead of self-blame [38, 39].

The use of checklists for malingering is hampered by a number of difficulties. Firstly, they ignore the conceptual problems. Often, the criteria used for determining malingering equally apply to factitious disorder, making them criteria for feigning, rather than malingering. Also, similar or identical criteria are used for identifying somatoform, conversion, and dissociative disorders [40]. As a consequence, they may rather be called criteria for nongenuine symptom presentation.

Secondly, the criteria on checklists often have been established intuitively, on the basis of what may be called clinical lore, but nobody knows about their reliability and validity or their accuracy of classification (sensitivity, specificity). Usually, they are poorly described and handled in an intuitive, individualized way. They have not been operationalized (that is, there are no rules that describe how to apply and score them). Inter-rater reliability must be expected to be a major problem.

Thirdly, there is no systematic knowledge about decision rules (which and how many criteria should be checked in which context, how many of them must be positive for a positive classification, etc.). A strict application of such criteria may result in an inappropriately low threshold for malingering [41].

For the last two decades, the bulk of research in the domain of malingering has been done by neuropsychologists and published in neuropsychological journals [42]. The reason for neuropsychologists' prominence is their reliance on test data. Psychological test results are highly dependent upon the individual's willingness to co-operate. With the development of what was then called symptom validity tests (SVTs), malingering assessment entered a new stage and became a primarily data-driven and evidence-based methodology. A vast number of instruments for practical use were developed, comprising cognitive SVTs (today mostly called performance validity tests), self-report validity measures (questionnaire approaches), and clinical interviews and ratings. It is beyond the scope of this chapter to give an overview over these psychological test measures; the reader can easily find summary reports in about a dozen of books available in English language [9, 43, 44]. In the past, SVTs were often referred to as malingering tests, but this is misleading because malingering is just one possible reason why individuals may fail on such tests.

Under certain circumstances, some SVTs (those that operate on a forced-choice format) are able to identify response patterns that are indicative of *intentional, voluntary* response distortions [45]. In such cases, test results are paramount to the confession of feigning. Accordingly, they occupy a special place in the most noteworthy attempt to formalize diagnostic reasoning about malingering—the criteria proposed by Slick, Sherman, and Iverson [46]. While their original criteria were related to malingered neurocognitive dysfunctions, they were later extended to other conditions, in particular to pain disorder [47].

## Prevalence

Available base rate estimates of malingering differ immensely. In clinical contexts, the base rate of malingered symptom presentations is usually expected to be very low. Consequently, the possibility of intentional response distortions is often dismissed at the outset, conforming to the traditional role concept of mental health providers. To illustrate this point, Reuber *et al.* [48] went as far as maintaining that: '*Fortunately*, it is rarely necessary for a clinician to determine whether symptoms are intentional' (p. 308, *emphasis added*). In other settings, malingering appears to be rather common. For the United States military, Morel [49] maintained that: 'No clinical opinion is more problematic, more weighty, or more pressing for a solution in military psychiatric medicine than differentiating malingering from post-traumatic stress disorder (PTSD)' (preface).

Potential factors responsible for the wide range of base rate estimates of malingering are the following:

- The exact definition or underlying concept of the phenomenon that is being evaluated (for example, feigning, malingering, symptom exaggeration, negative response bias, suboptimal effort, effort test failure, overreporting, underperformance, symptom invalidity).
- The referral context of the examination (for example, forensic, clinical, rehabilitative).
- Within forensic contexts, the legal issue at stake (for example, diminished criminal responsibility, liability, workers' compensation, disability, custody).
- The diagnostic group (diagnosed or claimed condition, for example mild traumatic brain injury, moderate or severe traumatic brain injury, PTSD, whiplash injury, chronic toxic encephalopathy, attention-deficit disorder).
- The method used for detecting feigning (for example, unspecified clinical impression, expert rating using specified criteria, rating or questionnaire methods, performance validity tests, application of the Slick criteria [46]).
- The standardized measures or SVTs if any were employed (for example, for questionnaire methods, MMPI-2 Fake Bad Scale, F scale, Response Bias Scale, combination of different scales,

Structured Inventory of Malingered Symptomatology, Assessment of Depression Inventory).

- When SVTs were used, the diagnostic decision rule (for example, based on a score in a single instrument or scores on a whole set of instruments; the number of SVTs administered and the number of positive single indicators necessary to classify the response pattern as feigned).
- The classification accuracy (sensitivity, specificity) of the specific methods used for diagnostic decision-making.
- Which cut scores were used for the single instruments (for a number of SVTs, different cut scores are available and some cut scores underwent modification or refinement in the course of time, after first publication).

Some estimates resort to the criterion of below-chance response patterns in performance validity tests [45, 46]. This is a very conservative criterion with a very high specificity, but low sensitivity in most real-world referral contexts. Consequently, such estimates necessarily result in a considerable underestimation of the true prevalence. In a similar vein, reliance on obsolete screening instruments (for example, the Fifteen-Item Test [50]) or embedded measures with known low sensitivity will yield grossly deflated estimates. Conversely, the employment of larger batteries of validity measures, and particularly of so-called embedded performance validity indicators, with a low threshold of diagnosing negative response bias will yield gross overestimations. Rogers *et al.* [41] pointed out that the influential model of Malingered Neurocognitive Dysfunction (MND) [46] defines a low threshold, in particular for the determination of possible malingering. As a consequence, prevalence estimates based on criteria suggestive of possible MND (and, to a much lower degree, probable MND) will inevitably produce grossly overestimated base rates.

With all these factors in mind, existing prevalence estimates must be understood as very rough approximations for the true base rates to be expected in different contexts. The most frequently cited prevalence data stem from a survey by Mittenberg *et al.* [51]. Probable malingering or symptom exaggeration was judged by 131 participating neuropsychologists to be present in almost a third of all litigating patients (in personal injury, disability, and workers' compensation contexts). Larrabee [52] identified mild traumatic brain injury as one of the most delicate conditions when it comes to malingering, with a prevalence of about 40% of false or grossly distorted symptom presentations (see a more recent study by Peck *et al.* [53] also reporting a 40% base rate in their sample). For some referral contexts and/or claimed conditions, base rate estimates reaching or exceeding the 50% mark have been published such as: litigating patients after whiplash injury [54]; patients with reported hearing loss, in independent medical examinations [55]; criminal defendants [56]; Social Security disability claimants in the United States [57, 58]; students with claimed attention-deficit disorders, but without learning disability [59]; British personal injury litigation patients claiming memory impairment [60]; or United States veterans claiming mild traumatic brain injury [61]. Adding to these studies, Spanish researchers [62] performed a survey among 161 Spanish medical doctors who were asked to estimate the percentage of malingering patients with different health conditions. Mean estimates of 50% or higher were reported for patients with claimed whiplash injury, fibromyalgia, chronic cervicalgia, depression, and anxiety disorders.

Young [63] performed an extensive literature search on recently published prevalence estimates and also came to the conclusion that 'it is difficult to arrive at one percentage or range of percentages that are definite about the proportion of malingering found in forensic disability and related examinations' (p. 196). He argued that 15% is the most appropriate estimate at the time being, with a large variation of another 15% in both directions, depending on the referral background, the condition in question, and other factors.

## Factitious disorder

### Definition

Factitious disorder is considered to be a mental disorder characterized by a non-authentic, feigned symptom presentation, either in the form of a voluntary production of symptoms (for example, self-inflicted injury, artificial fever, self-induced wound healing disturbance) or false, misleading, or grossly exaggerated symptom report. DSM-5 [8] describes this condition in the chapter on *Somatic symptom and related disorders*. The key criterion of factitious disorder (300.19) is described as a *falsification* of physical or mental signs or symptoms (instead of false presentation), and it extends to the induction of injury or disease. This behaviour must be deceptive and deception has to be identified. Furthermore, deceptive illness presentation is assumed to be evident, 'even in the absence of obvious external rewards' (p. 324). As with malingering, these diagnostic criteria are judged to be of little clinical validity [64]. Neither do they foster diagnostic reasoning nor do they help to arrive at a reliable diagnosis or assist in differential diagnosis.

In ICD-10, factitious disorder is coded as F68.1 under *Intentional production or feigning of symptoms or disabilities, either physical or psychological*, despite the fact that this description comprises both malingering and factitious disorder. Cooper's pocket guide [11] gives a very short description stressing that false symptom presentation which may include self-harm occurs 'for no obvious reason', with an assumed internal motivation of adopting the sick role. Included are the older concepts of the hospital hopper syndrome, Munchausen's syndrome, and the peregrinating patient. Asher [12], who originated the concept of Munchausen's syndrome, commented: 'These patients often seem to gain nothing except the discomfiture of unnecessary investigations or operations' (p. 339). Munchausen's syndrome is estimated to represent about 5–10% of all factitious cases [65].

Different types of factitious disorder have been described, first the abdominal, the haemorrhagic, and the neurological type by Asher [12] (laparatomophilia migrans, haemorrhagica histrionica, neurologica diabolica), later types like dermatitis autogenica, hyperpyrexia figmentatica, or cardiopathia phantastica. Also, pathological lying (pseudologia phantastica) is being discussed in the context of Munchausen's syndrome [66]. More recently, manifestations of factitious illness behaviour in Internet communities, such as cancer support groups, have been described [67].

### Prevalence and assessment

The incidence of factitious disorder in patient groups is estimated to be well below 1%, but using a more liberal criterion, Catalina *et al.* [68] found in their sample of psychiatric inpatients that 8% exhibited factitious symptoms. These authors further noted that in this group, women were overrepresented, the mean age was below 40, and symptoms became more intense when patients faced discharge. Fliege *et al.* [69] surveyed senior hospital consultants and physicians in private practices. They estimated the 1-year prevalence of factitious disorder at 1.3%. Relatively higher rates were reported by dermatologists and neurologists. Another study reported a prevalence of 1.8% [70]. In contrast, Wallach [71] estimated the base rate of factitious disorders at 5% of all physician encounters. With these estimates in mind, factitious disorder should not be considered a rare condition, having in mind that in any large general hospital in the Western world, several patients with factitious disorder should be expected to be present at any time—mostly going undiagnosed for this very condition.

The diversity of prevalence estimates is partly due to a lack of diagnostic guidelines or assessment procedures. With a few exceptions [72], researchers have employed little effort to develop screening methods for factitious behaviour. In most cases, factitious disorder must be expected to be left undetected. Suspicion is raised in patients with an atypical illness course and marked inconsistencies. Behavioural manifestations may include gratuitous, self-aggrandizing lying, non-compliance with medical prescriptions, disruptive actions, or excessive request for invasive medical procedures [64].

The ample literature on factitious behaviour consists, to a large extent, of case studies. One recent exception is a study by Lawlor and Kirakowski [73] who analysed text communications of two online communities of people who said they engaged in factitious behaviour. One remarkable result was that a large majority reflected upon their motives for playing the sick role, which suggests that factitious behaviour is more consciously motivated than assumed by some workers in the field.

## Feigning by proxy

Factitious disorder by proxy has long been discussed as a major problem in childcare, but it may also be present where caregivers exert pressure on persons with intellectual disability, dementia, or mental disease or directly impose symptoms on them. It includes such extreme forms as non-accidental poisoning or non-accidental suffocation [74]. Typical Munchausen presentations would then be called Munchausen by proxy (or Munchausen's syndrome by proxy). Moreover, factitious illness behaviour is sometimes related to animals, in particular pets [75].

In DSM-5, such behaviour is coded as *Factitious disorder imposed on another*, with the code 300.19. The diagnosis is given to the perpetrator, not to the victim.

Little attention has so far been paid to cases in which external gain (such as monetary benefit) is clearly sought by parents or caregivers who exert pressure on the patient (a child or a cared person) to invent or exaggerate symptoms. With a clearly identified secondary gain as the central motive for exerting this pressure, such behaviour is called malingering by proxy [76]. In cases where motivational analysis can favour neither primary nor secondary gain as being central for the grossly distorted symptom presentation, this abnormal illness behaviour may be called feigning by proxy.

## Summary and conclusions

Factitious disorder and malingering are two forms of abnormal health care-seeking behaviour [64]. Their common denominator is deception, a conscious intention to deceive medical personnel (or other people), or what Kozlowska [77] called a 'strategic use of illness behaviours in relationships with other individuals' (p. 1368). In the case of malingering, external incentives (such as monetary compensation or sick leave) prevail and health care can be considered to be only the means through which these external goals are expected to be reached. In factitious disorder, health care and the patient role are thought to central. However, both forms of deceptive behaviour can often not be reliably differentiated from each other and from what has previously been called hysteria. The core feature of all three categories—malingering, factitious disorder, and hysteria (or unexplained medical symptoms)—is the presence of marked inconsistencies, implausibilities, and contradictions within and between different sources of information. While the clinical manifestation may be indistinguishable between these forms of distorted symptom presentation, differential diagnosis requires determinations about both the motivation and the degree of consciousness about the falseness or gross exaggeration of symptoms. However, both dimensions are, in fact, neither categorical nor stable in time nor can they reliably be rated by a third party. This imposes significant limits to the validity of the clinical entities used for the description of non-genuine, feigned symptom presentations. Consequently, the utility of maintaining the distinction between malingering and factitious disorder has been questioned, and the apprehension of factious disorder as a mental disorder in its own right has likewise been questioned. Both malingering and factitious disorder can be comprehended as expressions of interpersonal behaviour; ' … they have no strategic or communicative function except when someone else can observe and respond to the behaviour' [77] (p. 1368).

In a historical perspective, factitious disorder may be conceived of as an attempt of the medical profession 'to acknowledge the deception while pathologizing it. The doctor could make a medical, not legal, 'diagnosis', keeping their medical hat on, and allowing the doctor–patient relationship to remain a therapeutic one' [78] (p. 76).

While factitious disorder is mostly discussed in the context of patient care, most studies on malingering centre on forensic or medicolegal contexts. There may be a bias in this dichotomy. Be that as it may, the bottomline of most prevalence studies is that significant response distortions, substantial symptom exaggeration, and feigning are to be expected *in a sizable proportion* of patients in medicolegal contexts. Whatever the exact numbers are, the problem of feigning is prevalent enough to proactively test it in any patient with a medicolegal background. Ruling out feigning should also be mandatory practice in clinical patients with a current or foreseeable litigation background, instead of automatically assuming that symptom presentation is genuine under all circumstances (which seems to be the common clinical stance today).

## REFERENCES

1. van Egmond J, Kummeling I, Balkom T. Secondary gain as hidden motive for getting psychiatric treatment. *Eur Psychiatry.* 2005; 20: 416–21.

2. van Egmond JJ, Kummeling I. A blind spot for secondary gain affecting treatment outcome. *Eur Psychiatry.* 2002; 17: 46–54.

3. Horner MD, VanKirk KK, Dismuke CE, Turner TH, Muzzy W. Inadequate effort on neuropsychological evaluation is associated with increased healthcare utilization. *Clin Neuropsychol.* 2014; 28: 703–13.

4. Anestis JC, Finn JA, Gottfried E, Arbisi PA, Joiner TE. Reading the road signs: the utility of the MMPI-2 Restructured Form Validity Scales in prediction of premature termination. *Assessment.* 2014; 8: 1–10.

5. Smith TW, Snyder CR, Perkins SC. The self-serving function of hypochondriacal complaints: physical symptoms as self-handicapping strategies. *J Pers Soc Psychol.* 1983; 44: 787–97.

6. Jonas JM, Pope HG. The dissimulating disorders: a single diagnostic entity? *Compr Psychiatry.* 1985; 26: 58–62.

7. American Psychiatric Association. *Diagnostic and Statistical Manual of Mental Disorders,* fourth edition (DSM-IV). International version with ICD-10 codes. Washington, DC: American Psychiatric Association; 1995.

8. American Psychiatric Association. *Diagnostic and Statistical Manual of Mental Disorders,* fifth edition (DSM-5). Washington, DC: American Psychiatric Association; 2013.

9. Young G. *Malingering, Feigning, and Response Bias in Psychiatric/Psychological Injury: Implications for Practice and Court.* Dordrecht: Springer; 2014.

10. Lipman FD. Malingering in personal injury cases. *Temple Law Q.* 1962; 35: 141–62.

11. World Health Organization. *Pocket Guide to the ICD-10 Classification of Mental and Behavioral Disorders, with Glossary and Diagnostic Criteria for Research (ICD-10: DCR-10).* Compilation and editorial arrangements by JE Cooper. Washington DC: American Psychiatric Press; 1994.

12. Asher R. Munchausen's syndrome. *Lancet.* 1951; 1: 339–41.

13. Turner MA. Factitious disorders: reformulating the DSM–IV criteria. *Psychosomatics.* 2006; 47: 23–32.

14. Krahn LE, Bostwick JM, Stonnington CM. Looking toward DSM–V: should factitious disorder become a subtype of somatoform disorder? *Psychosomatics.* 2008; 49: 277–82.

15. Fishbain DA. Secondary gain concept: Definition problems and its abuse in medical practice. *Am Pain Soc J.* 1994; 3: 264–73.

16. Eisendrath SJ. When Munchausen becomes malingering: factitious disorders that penetrate the legal system. *J Am Acad Psychiatry.* 1996; 4: 471–81.

17. Rogers R. An introduction to response styles. In: Rogers R, ed. *Clinical Assessment of Malingering and Deception,* third edition. New York, NY: Guilford; 2008. pp. 3–13.

18. Jones AB, Llewellyn LJ. *Malingering or the Simulation of Disease.* London: Heinemann; 1917.

19. Turner M. Malingering. *Brit J Psychiat.* 1997; 171: 409–11.

20. Merten T. False symptom claims and symptom validity assessment. In: Otgaar H, Howe M, eds. *Fnding the Truth in the Courtroom? Problems with Deception, Lies, and Memories.* New York, NY: Oxford University Press; 2018.

21. Bass C, Halligan PW. Illness related deception: social or psychiatric problem? *J R Soc Med.* 2007; 100: 81–4.

22. Merten T, Rogers R. An international perspective on feigned mental disabilities: conceptual issues and continuing controversies. *Behav Sci Law.* 2017; 35: 97–112.

23. Rief W, Broadbent E. Explaining medically unexplained symptoms-models and mechanisms. *Clin Psychol Rev.* 2007; 27: 821–41.

24. Berry DTR, Nelson NW. DSM-5 and malingering: a modest proposal. *Psychol Inj Law.* 2010; 3: 295–303.

25. Travin S, Protter B. Malingering and malingering-like behavior. Some clinical and conceptual issues. *Psychiat Q.* 1984; 56: 189–97.

26. Walters GD, Berry DTR, Rogers R, Payne JW, Granacher RP. Feigned neurocognitive deficit: taxon or dimension? *J Clin Exp Neuropsychol.* 2009; 31: 584–93.

27. Brown RJ. Introduction to a special issue on medically unexplained symptoms: background and future directions. *Clin Psychol Rev.* 2007; 27: 769–80.

28. Merten T, Merckelbach H. Symptom validity testing in somatoform and dissociative disorders: a critical review. *Psychol Inj Law.* 2013; 6: 122–37.

29. Green P, Merten T. Noncredible explanations of noncredible performance on symptom validity tests. In: Carone DA, Bush SS, eds. *Mild Traumatic Brain Injury: Symptom Validity Assessment and Malingering.* New York, NY: Springer; 2013. pp. 73–100.

30. American Psychiatric Association. *Diagnostic and Statistical Manual of Mental Disorders*, third edition (DSM-III). Washington, DC: American Psychiatric Association; 1980.

31. Hall HV, Pritchard DA. *Detecting Malingering and Deception. Forensic Distortion Analysis (FDA).* Delray Beach, FL: St. Lucie Press; 1996.

32. Rogers R, Harrell EH, Liff CD. Feigning neuropsychological impairment: a critical review of methodological and clinical considerations. *Clin Psychol Rev.* 1993; 13: 255–75.

33. Niesten IJ, Nentjes L, Merckelbach H, Bernstein DP. Antisocial features and 'faking bad': a critical note. *Int J Law Psychiat.* 2015; 41: 34–42.

34. Rogers R. Models of feigned mental illness. *Prof Psychol.* 1990; 21: 182–8.

35. Hall RC, Hall RC. Compensation neurosis: a too quickly forgotten concept? *J Am Acad Psychiatry Law,* 2012; 40: 390–8.

36. Incesu AI. Tests for malingering in ophthalmology. *Int J Ophthalmol.* 2013; 6: 708–17.

37. Spreen O, Strauss E. *A Compendium of Neuropsychological Tests: Administration, Norms, and Commentary*, second edition. New York, NY: Oxford University Press; 1998.

38. Resnick PJ. Malingering of posttraumatic disorders. In: Rogers R, ed. *Clinical Assessment of Malingering and Deception*, second edition. New York, NY: Guilford Press; 1997. pp. 130–52.

39. Dressing H, Foerster K. Begutachtung der posttraumatischen Belastungsstörung [Expert opinion on post-traumatic stress disorder]. *Fortschr Neurol Psychiat.* 2010; 78: 475–8.

40. Wilbourn AJ. The electrodiagnostic examination with hysteria-conversion reaction and malingering. *Neurol Clin.* 1995; 13: 385–404.

41. Rogers R, Bender SD, Johnson SF. A critical analysis of the MND criteria for feigned cognitive impairment: implications for forensic practice and research. *Psycho Inj Law.* 2011; 4: 147–56.

42. Sweet JJ, Guidotti Breting LM. Symptom validity test research: status and clinical implications. *J Exp Psychopathol.* 2013; 4: 6–19.

43. Carone D, Bush SS, eds. *Mild Traumatic Brain Injury: Symptom Validity Assessment and Malingering.* New York, NY: Springer; 2013.

44. Morgan JE, Sweet JJ, eds. *Neuropsychology of Malingering Casebook.* New York, NY: Psychology Press; 2009.

45. Merten T, Merckelbach H. Forced-choice tests as single-case experiments in the differential diagnosis of intentional symptom distortion. *J Exp Psychopathol.* 2013; 4: 20–37.

46. Slick DJ, Sherman EM, Iverson GL. Diagnostic criteria for malingered neurocognitive dysfunction: proposed standards for clinical practice and research. *Clin Neuropsychol.* 1999; 13: 545–61.

47. Bianchini KJ, Greve KW, Glynn G. On the diagnosis of malingered pain-related disability: lessons from cognitive malingering research. *Spine J.* 2005; 5: 404–17.

48. Reuber M, Mitchell AJ, Howlett SJ, Crimlisk HL, Grünewald RA. Functional symptoms in neurology: questions and answers. *J Neurol Neurosurg Psychiatry.* 2005; 76: 307–14.

49. Morel KR. *Differential Diagnosis of Malingering Versus Posttraumatic Stress Disorder: Scientific Rationale and Objective Scientific Methods.* New York, NY: Nova Science Publ; 2010.

50. Rey A. *L'Examen Clinique en Psychologie* [*The Clinical Examination in Psychology*]. Paris: Presses Universitaires de France; 1958.

51. Mittenberg W, Patton C, Canyock EM, Condit DC. Base rates of malingering and symptom exaggeration. *J Clin Exp Neuropsychol.* 2002; 24: 1094–102.

52. Larrabee GJ. Detection of malingering using atypical performance patterns on standard neuropsychological tests. *Clin Neuropsychol.* 2003; 17: 410–25.

53. Peck CP, Schroeder RW, Heinrichs RJ, *et al.* Differences in MMPI-2 FBS and RBS scores in brain injury, probable malingering, and conversion disorder groups: a preliminary study. *Clin Neuropsychol.* 2013; 27: 693–707.

54. Schmand B, Lindeboom J, Schagen S, Heijt R, Koene T, Hamburger HL. Cognitive complaints in patients after whiplash injury: the impact of malingering. *J Neurol Neurosurg Psychiatry.* 1998; 64: 339–43.

55. Streppel M, Brusis T. Zur Problematik der Simulation und Aggravation in der HNO-ärztlichen Begutachtung [Problematic medical expertise concerning malingering in audiology]. *HNO.* 2010; 58: 126–31.

56. Ardolf BR, Denney RL, Houston CM. Base rates of negative response bias and malingered neurocognitive dysfunction among criminal defendants referred for neuropsychological evaluation. *Clin Neuropsychol.* 2007; 21: 899–916.

57. Chafetz, MD, Abrahams JP, Kohlmaier J. Malingering on the Social Security Disability Consultative Exam: a new rating scale. *Arch Clin Neuropsychol.* 2007; 22: 1–14.

58. Miller LS, Boyd M, Cohn A. Prevalence of sub-optimal effort in disability applicants. *J Int Neuropsychol Soc.* 2006; 12(S1): 159.

59. Sullivan BK, May K, Galbally L. Symptom exaggeration by college adults in attention-deficit hyperactivity disorder and learning disorder assessments. *Appl Neuropsychol.* 2007; 14: 189–207.

60. Gill D, Green P, Flaro L, Pucci T. The role of effort testing in independent medical examinations. *Medico-Legal J.* 2007; 75: 64–72.

61. Armistead-Jehle, P. Symptom validity test performance in U.S. veterans referred for evaluation of mild TBI. *Appl Neuropsychol.* 2010; 17: 52–9.

62. Santamaría P, Capilla Ramírez P, González Ordi H. Prevalencia de simulación en incapacided temporal: percepción de los profesionales de la salud [Health professionals' perception of prevalence of malingering in temporary disability in Spain]. *Clínica y Salud.* 2013; 24: 139–51.

63. Young G. Malingering in forensic disability-related assessments: prevalence 15 ± 15%. *Psychol Inj Law.* 2015; 8: 188–99.

64. Bass C, Halligan P. Factitious disorders and malingering: challenges for clinical assessment and management. *Lancet.* 2014; 383: 1422–32.

65. Feldman MD, Eisendrath SJ, eds. *The Spectrum of Factitious Disorders.* Washington DC: American Psychiatric Press; 1996.

66. Feldman MD. *Playing Sick? Untangling the Web of Munchausen Syndrome, Munchausen by Proxy, Malingering & Factitious Disorder*. New York, NY: Routledge; 2004.

67. Witney C, Hendricks J, Cope V. Munchausen by Internet and nursing practice: an ethnonetnographic case study. *Int J Nurs Clin Pract*. 2015; 2: 131.

68. Catalina ML, Gómez MV, De Cos A. Prevalence of factitious disorder with psychological symptoms in hospitalized patients. *Actas Esp Psiquiatri*. 2007; 36: 345–9.

69. Fliege H, Grimm A, Eckhardt-Henn A, Gieler U. Martin K, Klapp BF. Frequency of ICD-10 factitious disorder: survey of senior hospital consultants and physicians in private practice. *Psychosomatics*. 2007; 54: 142–8.

70. Ferrara P, Vitelli O, Bottaro G, *et al*. Factitious disorders and Munchausen syndrome: the tip of the iceberg. *J Child Health Care*. 2013; 17: 366–74.

71. Wallach J. Laboratory diagnosis of factitious disorders. *Arch Intern Med*. 1994; 154: 1690–6.

72. Rogers R, Jackson RL, Kaminski PL. Factitious psychological disorders: the overlooked response style in forensic evaluations. *J Forensic Psychol Pract*. 2005; 5: 21–41.

73. Lawlor A, Kirakowski J. When the lie is the truth: grounded theory analysis of an online support group for factitious disorder. *Psychiatry Res*. 2014; 218: 209–18.

74. McClure RJ, Davis PM, Meadow SR, Sibert JR. Epidemiology of Munchausen syndrome by proxy, non-accidental poisoning, and non-accidental suffocation. *Arch Dis Child*. 1996; 75: 57–61.

75. Oxley JA, Feldman MD. Complexities of maltreatment: Munchausen by proxy and animals. *Companion Animal*. 2016; 21: 586–9.

76. Chafetz M, Prentkowski E. A case of malingering by proxy in a social security disability psychological consultative examination. *Appl Neuropsychol*. 2011; 18: 143–9.

77. Kozlowska K. Abnormal illness behaviours: a developmental perspective. *Lancet*. 2014; 383: 1368–9.

78. Kanaan RAA, Wessely SC. The origins of factitious disorder. *Hist Human Sci*. 2010; 23: 68–85.

# 133

# Functional neurological symptom disorder (conversion disorder)

*Jon Stone and Michael Sharpe*

## Introduction

Functional neurological symptom disorder, also called conversion disorder, refers to symptoms of motor and sensory dysfunction which can be positively identified as incompatible or incongruent with neurological disease. Common symptoms include blackouts (that may look like epileptic seizures or syncope), limb weakness, movement disorder such as tremor, dystonia, or jerks, and sensory disturbance, including visual loss. In this chapter, we trace the history of the disorder, especially as it relates to psychiatry, and describe the terminology, classification, epidemiology, clinical features, and treatment.

## Historical background

The term 'hysteria' has been used since the time of Hippocrates (around 400 BC) to describe symptoms that were considered to occur only in women, such as choking, and to be caused by a 'wandering womb' exerting its influence throughout the body.

From the early seventeenth century onwards, physicians, such as Lepois (1618), Willis (1667), and Sydenham (1682), located the origin of these 'hysterical' symptoms in the brain and nervous system, rather than the uterus, not only because of changes in neuroanatomical thinking, but also because of a recognition that the same symptoms also occurred in men [1].

In the nineteenth century, Briquet (1859), Charcot (1880s), and Janet (1890–1920s) pursued a more systematic approach and focused on symptoms that we would now regard as neurological such as paralysis, numbness, seizures, and blindness. Pierre Janet used the clinical study of hysteria to advance his views on 'dissociation' as a way of understanding how a person could lack the ability to control their own voluntary movements.

In 1895, Breuer and Freud's book *Studies on Hysteria* described five case studies in which hypnosis was used to find 'reminiscences' thought to be relevant to the onset of hysterical symptoms. These initial cases formed the basis not only of psychoanalytic theory, but also of the conversion hypothesis. The conversion hypothesis proposed that symptoms, such as paralysis, were created unconsciously by conversion of intrapsychic conflict. The main benefit or 'primary gain' was considered to be the reduction in the psychological conflict the person experienced. Additional benefits of 'secondary gain' were considered to occur if the symptom provided an escape from the external sources of the conflict, for example by leading to the inability to carry out an act.

Freud's ideas, despite being largely unfalsifiable, had a profound effect on clinical practice over the subsequent century, not least in the adoption of the term conversion disorder in the *Diagnostic and Statistical Manual of Mental Disorders* (DSM) of the American Psychiatric Association—the only psychoanalytic diagnosis to remain in the manual to the present day. The effect on practice was that neurologists were able to confidently dismiss the problem as psychiatric and psychiatrists felt an obligation to attempt therapy to make the proposed conflict conscious [2].

Consequently, patients have often ended up falling between neurology and psychiatry, often with neither being sure of what the correct treatment is. To add to the uncertainty, Eliot Slater's influential, but flawed, study on 'hysteria', published in 1965, suggested incorrectly that many such patients had misdiagnosed neurological disease [3].

There has been progress and in the last 20 years, it has been established that patients with neurological symptoms unexplained by an identifiable pathophysiological process are, in fact, common (the second most common reason to see a neurologist). It has also become clear that they can be reliably diagnosed using positive clinical features identified predominantly on physical assessment (and not only as a diagnosis of exclusion). Studies have also suggested that the symptoms have an inconsistent relationship to trauma and stress (that is, some have it, but some do not). In summary, after a long period of confusion and ignorance, we are starting to see progress. We are hopefully now entering a more optimistic era of clinical science which builds on the notion that a brain-and-mind approach is required to understand its aetiology and to deliver effective treatment.

## Terminology and classification

Terminology can be difficult for both doctors and patients. Broadly, the current terms can be categorized as follows:

- Psychogenic/somatization/somatoform/conversion—implying that the symptoms are essentially physical manifestation of a psychological problem.
- Non-organic/non-epileptic/medically unexplained—defining the problem as not being due to disease.
- Functional—suggesting a disorder of bodily or nervous system functioning without aetiological presumption.
- Dissociative—suggesting a disconnection between nervous system component functions.

These terms each have advantages and disadvantages. We will use the term 'functional neurological disorder' here for the scientific and pragmatic reasons outlined in this chapter.

The classification of functional neurological disorder has been through several iterations in DSM. In DSM-I, it was Conversion Reaction (DSM-I), in DSM-II Hysterical Neurosis—Conversion Type, and in DSM-III and IV Conversion Disorder [4]. In DSM-IV, conversion symptoms were also listed under somatization disorder, a relatively tightly defined long-standing vulnerability to 'somatoform' symptoms starting before the age of 30, involving symptoms which were neurological (≥1 symptoms), pain (≥4 symptoms), gastrointestinal (≥2 symptoms), and sexual (≥1 symptoms). In the latest iteration of DSM (DSM-5), the disorder is now called Conversion Disorder (Functional Neurological Symptom Disorder) (300.11).

It should be noted that wilfully manufactured or grossly exaggerated symptoms which are deliberately feigned to obtain medical care (factitious disorder, which is considered a mental disorder) or material gain (malingering, which is simply a behaviour, not a mental disorder) are classified separately.

There have also been important changes in the diagnostic criteria in DSM-5 [5] (Table 133.1).

Firstly, it has been recognized that it is not simply a diagnosis of exclusion—patients with this diagnosis should have specific findings on neurological examination such as Hoover's sign of leg weakness or a positive tremor entrainment test (see Examination, p. 1352). Importantly, this allows the diagnosis to be made even in patients with a coexisting neurological disease, as long as that condition is not a better explanation for the symptom. For example, a patient may have both epilepsy and dissociative (non-epileptic) attacks/seizures, or multiple sclerosis and functional limb weakness.

Secondly, there is a recognition that stressors are not always identifiable [6]. Sometimes this is because they only emerge later, but sometimes this may simply be because they are not present.

Lastly, the specific requirement to positively exclude feigning has been removed. While it is rarely possible to obtain positive evidence of feigning, it is arguably impossible to positively exclude it.

The World Health Organization (WHO)'s International Classification of Diseases, tenth revision (ICD-10) has, to date, preferred the term 'Dissociative Disorder', 'Dissociative (Conversion) Seizures/Paralysis', etc. Moreover, as with all ICD diagnoses, there are no operationalized diagnostic criteria.

## Epidemiology

Most of the data on functional neurological symptom disorder (FNSD) are from clinical settings, rather than the general population. It has been diagnosed from early childhood to the ninth decade but is rare before the age of 10. Patients with dissociative (non-epileptic) seizures have an average age of onset in the twenties, with a second late onset group, often in relation to the development of physical disease. Patients with functional movement disorders have a mean age of presentation in the late thirties. Most presentations of FNSD occur more commonly in females, with a ratio of 2–3:1.

Patients with FNSD are commonly encountered in neurological or general medical settings. In a study of 3781 new neurology outpatients in Scotland, 16% had a primary diagnosis of a functional disorder and 6% a primary diagnosis compatible with FNSD. Patients with functional limb weakness are probably as common as patients with multiple sclerosis, with an incidence of around 5/100,000 [7]. Patients with dissociative (non-epileptic) seizures have a similar incidence of around 5/100,000 [8]. Up to 50% of patients presenting to accident and emergency with apparent epileptic status may have dissociative (non-epileptic) seizures.

Studies of FNSD have consistently found severity of disability similar to that of patients with equivalent disease [7, 9, 10], and usually a higher rate of psychiatric disorder [11]. Health care costs are also high, especially with respect to repeated investigations and referral [12].

Epidemiological factors related to aetiology and mechanisms are discussed further later in this chapter.

**Table 133.1** A summary of the main changes in DSM-5 in relation to functional neurological symptom disorder (conversion disorder)

|  | DSM-IV | DSM-5 | Comments |
|---|---|---|---|
| Motor or sensory symptom … | ✓ | ✓ | Includes limb weakness, movement disorder, gait, blackouts, vision, speech, and hearing symptoms. Not pain, fatigue, dizziness, or memory symptoms |
| … causing distress or difficulty for the patient | ✓ | ✓ | |
| Positive physical signs of internal inconsistency or incongruity with recognized disease | ✗ | ✓ | Not a diagnosis of exclusion. Emphasizes how these disorders should be diagnosed |
| Patient must have an identifiable psychological stressor | ✓ | ✗ | Often not present. Therefore, many patients without stressors were previously rejected by psychiatrists |
| Intentional feigning must be excluded | ✓ | ✗ | This applies to all psychiatric disorders. It is impossible to exclude feigning |

## Clinical features

### History

Patients with FNSD commonly have many symptoms, in addition to motor and sensory symptoms. These may include fatigue, pain, poor memory and concentration, sleep disturbance, and symptoms of other functional disorders such as irritable bowel syndrome or chronic widespread pain/fibromyalgia. It is therapeutically and diagnostically helpful to make a list of all the patient's symptoms at the beginning of the consultation.

Dissociative symptoms, such as derealization ('feeling disconnected/unreal/cut off/floating') and depersonalization ('my leg doesn't feel part of me'), are also common in FNSD. Patients with acute-onset functional symptoms (both motor symptoms and blackouts) often describe dissociation at the moment the symptoms began. Establishing this sequence can be particularly helpful when explaining the mechanism of symptom production to the patient or, in the case of dissociative (non-epileptic) seizures, targeting the prodromal symptoms during therapy (as for panic disorder).

Enquiry about the patient's beliefs about their illness is important. A patient sent from a neurologist with a very firm belief they have 'chronic Lyme disease' or 'multiple sclerosis' is going to require a different consultation to someone who believes they have a functional disorder. When asking about beliefs, however, it is generally best to avoid getting into an unproductive debate about whether the symptoms are neurological or psychological (since they are best considered as both). It can be more helpful to establish whether the patient sees their symptoms as potentially reversible or as a result of irreversible damage (the analogy here is software vs hardware fault), as the former is less of an obstacle to rehabilitation. It can also be helpful to ask the patient's views about what treatments they think would help them and which would not, before discussing options.

Patients with FNSD may be reticent about reporting psychological symptoms. This may be, in part, because they fear being told that all their symptoms are imagined. Therefore, rather than ask direct questions about depression or anxiety, it can be more helpful to begin the enquiry by asking about the emotional and psychological consequences of having disabling physical symptoms. Panic disorder is also common, but often not recognized as such by the patient experiencing sudden chest pain or shortness of breath with dizziness. Equally, the psychiatrist must bear in mind that the patient may have no obvious psychological symptoms. This does not necessarily mean that there is 'no psychiatric disorder' and that the patient cannot be helped; FNSD remains classified as a psychiatric disorder at the interface with neurological practice and the psychiatrist has an important role, as described in this chapter.

One psychological symptom, so-called 'belle indifference', requires a particular comment. This refers to a cheerful indifference to disability and has historically been viewed as a typical clinical feature of FNSD. However, modern studies suggest that while this symptom does occur, it has no discriminating diagnostic value, as it also occurs in patients with organic brain disease, especially those with frontal lobe involvement [13]. When apparently present, in our experience, it most commonly reflects an attempt to 'put on a brave face'. Persistent 'belle indifference' may, in fact, suggest factitious disorder, a condition that can only really be diagnosed in a neurological context by finding evidence of marked discrepancy between reported and observed function (for example, walking normally when they said that would be impossible) or significant deception.

### Examination

The assessment must address the wide range of possible neurological diagnoses that may present with the observed neurological symptoms. FNSD is not a diagnosis of exclusion; rather it depends on finding positive evidence of clinical signs, which are strongly suggestive of functional disorder (Table 133.2). The diagnosis can therefore also be made in the presence of neurological disease.

The physical signs are: (1) either to aim to find out if the symptom briefly resolves when attention is directed to another body part (for example, Hoover's sign of functional leg weakness or tremor entrainment test) (Fig. 133.1); or (2) are characteristic of a functional disorder in the correct context (for example, the new onset of a clenched fist or an inverted ankle in an adult, or a sudden episode of motionless unresponsiveness and amnesia with the eyes closed for longer than 2 minutes). Awareness of how these physical signs work puts the psychiatrist in a much better position to explain the illness to the patient. Like all physical signs, none is completely reliable on its own, although published studies have suggested they have good sensitivity and specificity.

Cognitive symptoms are common in association with other presentations of FNSD, although they are not included in the DSM-5 definition [14]. Typical positive features of functional cognitive symptoms include inconsistency between reported symptoms and ability to follow dramas on television or perform a job, difficulty with easy cognitive tasks, compared to difficult ones, ability to answer multiple-component questions, and offering of elaboration and detail regarding memory lapses. Someone with more severe functional or feigned cognition difficulties may perform badly on tests of effort in which patients should score by chance or at least above patients with severe dementia. Rarely, questions such as 'how many legs has a horse got?' may be met with an 'approximate' answer such as 'five'—the so-called Ganser syndrome that often suggests factitious disorder or malingering.

Another distinct type of cognitive presentation is a pure retrograde or dissociative amnesia. This presents as a 'soap opera style' memory loss in which a portion of retrograde memory is missing, sometimes for years, but with normal anterograde memory. It can sometimes be associated with wandering geographical location when it is called fugue. Typically, there is loss of information about personal identity, which is rare in other amnestic disorders, although other causes such as encephalitis or epileptic amnesia should be considered.

Dizziness can also be a common functional symptom but again is not listed in the DSM5 criteria. Typically, the patient with chronic functional dizziness, now called 'persistent perceptual postural dizziness', reports a continuous sense of movement, often a 'swaying' sensation, worse on standing and walking, which can be mixed with dissociative symptoms. This usually arises after a vestibular trigger, such as labyrinthitis or benign paroxysmal positional vertigo, and becomes persistent through a complex process of abnormally focused attention and alteration of normal postural control [15]. Health anxiety and a daily routine dominated by the experience of dizziness can respond well to treatment with cognitive behavioural therapy and/or treatment with antidepressant medication.

**Table 133.2** Examples of positive signs in functional neurological symptom disorder

| Symptom | Positive finding of FNSD |
|---|---|
| **Functional limb weakness** | |
| Hoover's sign [44] (Fig. 133.1) | Hip extension weakness that returns to normal, with contralateral hip flexion against resistance |
| Hip abductor sign [44] | Hip abduction weakness that returns to normal, with contralateral hip abduction against resistance |
| Other clear evidence of inconsistency | For example, weakness of ankle–plantar flexion on the bed, but patient able to walk on tiptoes |
| Global pattern of weakness | Weakness that is global, affecting extensors and flexors equally |
| Dragging gait | A gait in which the forefoot remains in contact with the ground, typically with the hip externally or internally rotated |
| **Functional movement disorder/gait** | |
| Tremor entrainment test [45] | Patient with a unilateral tremor is asked to copy a rhythmical movement with their unaffected limb. The tremor in the affected hand 'entrains' to the rhythm of the unaffected hand, stops completely, or the patient is unable to copy the simple rhythmical movement |
| Typical 'functional' hemifacial overactivity [46] (Fig. 133.2) | Orbicularis oculis or oris over-contraction, especially when accompanied by jaw deviation and/or ipsilateral functional hemiparesis |
| Fixed dystonic posture [47] (Fig. 133.3) | A typical fixed dystonic posture, characteristically of the hand (with flexion of the fingers, wrist, and/or elbow) or ankle (with plantar flexion and dorsiflexion) |
| Distraction during standing [48] | Patient with an apparently positive Romberg's test is asked either to guess numbers written on their back or to carry out a complex motor task (for example, with a phone). In a functional gait problem, their balance will improve significantly |
| **Dissociative (non-epileptic) attacks [49]** | |
| Prolonged attack of motionless unresponsiveness | Paroxysmal motionlessness and unresponsiveness, with amnesia lasting longer than 2 minutes |
| Long duration | Attacks lasting longer than 2 minutes (but be careful of misleading witness histories) |
| Closed eyes | Closed eyes during an attack, especially if there is resistance to eye opening |
| Ictal weeping | Crying either during or immediately after the attack |
| Memory of being in a generalized seizure | Ability to recall the experience of being in a generalized shaking attack |
| Ictal hyperventilation | During a generalized epileptic seizure, respiration ceases, but it commonly speeds up during a non-epileptic attack |
| Presence of an attack resembling epilepsy with a normal EEG | Normal EEG does not exclude frontal lobe epilepsy or deep foci of epilepsy but does provide supportive evidence |
| **Visual symptoms [50]** | |
| Fogging test | Vision in the unaffected eye is progressively 'fogged' using lenses of increasing dioptres, while reading an acuity chart. A patient who still has good acuity at the end of the test must be seeing out of their affected eye |
| Tubular visual field (Fig. 133.4) | A patient is found to have a field defect which has the same width at 1 m as it does at 2 m |
| **Speech** | |
| Highly inconsistent speech, new-onset stuttering in an adult or telegraphic speech [51] | Patients with neurological diseases also can develop stuttering. Persistent foreign accent syndrome is often functional |

Adapted from *Neurophysiol Clin.*, 44(4), Stone J, Functional neurological disorders: The neurological assessment as treatment, pp. 363–73, Copyright (2014), with permission from Elsevier Masson SAS.

## Investigations

In the presence of typical clinical features, the role of investigation is primarily to seek comorbid neurological disease, rather than to refute the diagnosis. Patients with arm or leg weakness will typically require structural imaging with magnetic resonance imaging (MRI) or computed tomography (CT). The diagnosis of dissociative seizures can be greatly aided by recording a normal electrocardiogram (ECG) and electroencephalogram (EEG) during an attack (but note that some forms of epilepsy cannot be seen on surface EEG). It is the positive recording of an event with typical features of dissociative (non-epileptic) seizures that matters, rather than merely normal investigations. Smartphone footage from family and friends can be especially helpful. It should be remembered that investigations commonly reveal incidental abnormalities in the brain and spine. Such

abnormalities are found in around one in six on MRI brain scans. Disc prolapses occur in asymptomatic individuals at a frequency similar to the 'age of the patient plus 10' (for example, around 50% of 40-year olds have some disc prolapse) [16].

### Psychiatric examination

A skilled neurologist should be able to make a positive diagnosis of FNSD. A psychiatric assessment has an important role in ensuring a complete history has been taken and addressing the psychiatric differential diagnosis.

It may reveal important life stressors and factors inhibiting recovery (such as an insurance claim). But it should be remembered that it is not necessary to make such a finding (or to hypothesize it) to make the diagnosis.

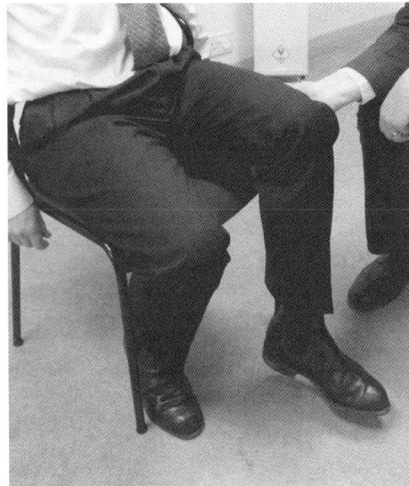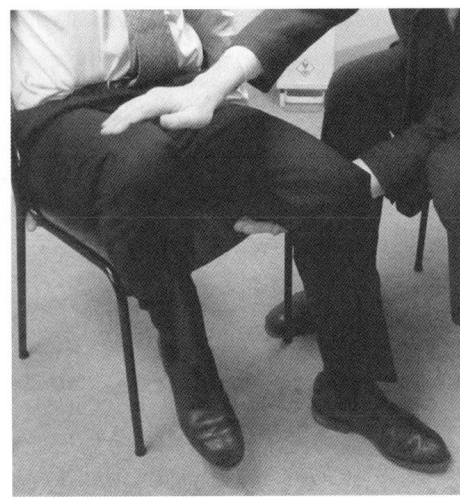

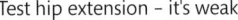

Test hip extension – it's weak

Test contralateral hip flexion against resistance–hip extension has become strong

**Fig. 133.1** Hoover's sign of functional leg weakness.

Reproduced from *Pract Neurol.*, 9(3), Stone J, Functional symptoms in neurology, pp. 179–89, Copyright (2009), with permission from *British Medical Journal*.

The assessment also provides the foundation for treatment and is an opportunity to further develop a shared and positive understanding of the disorder with the patient and carer.

## Differential diagnosis

The differential diagnosis of FNSD encompasses many neurological conditions and several psychiatric ones. It should usually be diagnosed by a neurologist or a specialist familiar with neurological diagnosis and a psychiatrist, working either together or sequentially.

A common pitfall in diagnosis is failure to consider the presence of a comorbid neurological disease, especially symptoms in the prodrome of a degenerative disease such as Parkinson's disease.

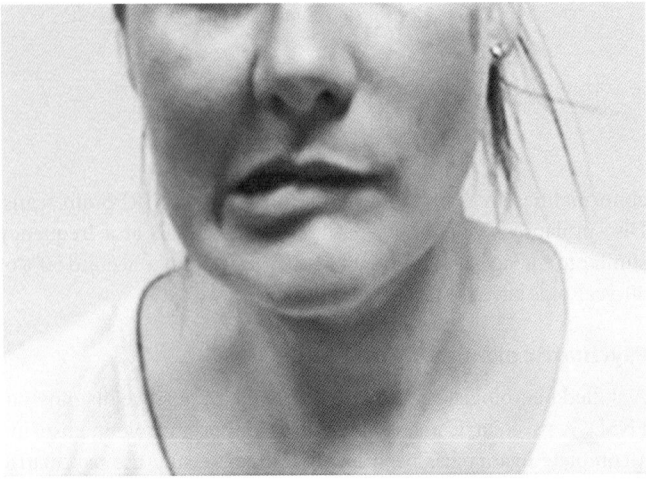

**Fig. 133.2** Functional facial overactivity can look like facial weakness—typically with platysma overactivity, jaw deviation, and/or contraction of the orbicularis oculis.

Reproduced from *Pract Neurol.*, 13(2), Stone J, Reuber M, Carson A, Functional symptoms in neurology: mimics and chameleons, pp. 104–13, Copyright (2013), with permission from *British Medical Journal*.

Misdiagnoses of neurological disease as FNSD appears especially likely in relation to an isolated gait disorder with normal examination on the bed (for example, stiff person syndrome and spastic gait from cervical myelopathy can present like this); frontal lobe epilepsy (which can look odd and present sometimes with a normal EEG); autoimmune encephalitis and other neurological disorders where there may be prominent psychiatric symptoms [17].

The psychiatric differential is anxiety and especially panic disorder, depression, obsessive–compulsive disorder, and post-traumatic stress disorder (PTSD). Symptoms of dissociation occur as part of both panic and PTSD. These disorders may be the primary diagnosis and the patient may recover with treatment for them; more often, they are comorbidities that may still require treatment in their own right.

Finally, it is important to consider the possibility that the patient is wilfully manufacturing or exaggerating their symptoms. When this is done for medical care only, it is factitious disorder, classified as a psychiatric disorder which often coexists with a personality disorder. When symptoms are manufactured for material gain only, then it is malingering, and not a psychiatric disorder. Wilful exaggeration can only be detected reliably by the presence of a marked discrepancy between reported and observed function (note that this is not the same as variability in symptoms) or by evidence of lying. Most experts seeing patients with FNSD agree that clinically significant wilful exaggeration is relatively rare outside legal scenarios. These disorders are discussed further in Chapter 132.

## Aetiology and mechanism

The 'conversion' hypothesis in which symptoms of FNSD are always presumed to be a physical manifestation of the psychological effect of a recent stressor has been superseded by a more complex model. This explains the considerable heterogeneity between patients and suggests a mechanism of symptom production (Table 133.3). Many biological, psychological, and social factors appear to be relevant,

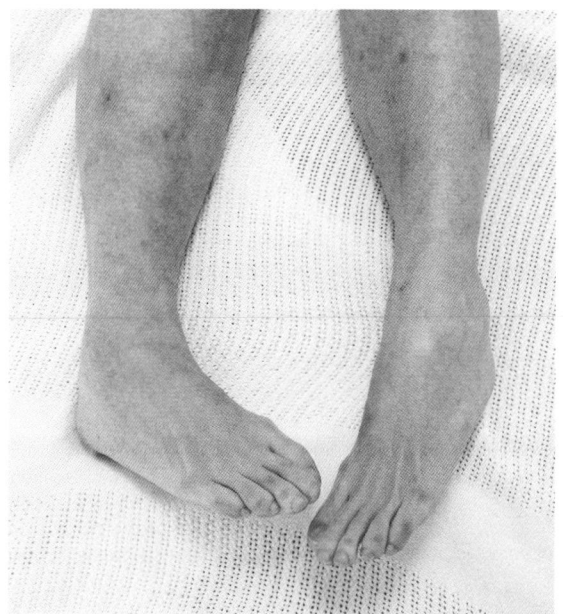

**Fig. 133.3** Functional dystonia with characteristic ankle inversion and plantar flexion.

Reproduced from *Continuum (Minneap Minn)*., 21(3), Stone J, Carson A, Functional Neurologic Disorders, pp. 818–37, Copyright (2015), with permission from American Academy of Neurology.

including childhood sexual, physical, and emotional abuse and neglect as predisposing factors and life events as precipitating factors. Adverse experiences like this can promote a vulnerability to dissociation and heighten the experience of threat produced by minor pathophysiological or physiological stimuli. Reviews of the relative magnitude of these factors in individual patients have demonstrated that although more frequent than in those with neurological disease and in healthy controls, they are not universal [6]. For example,

while a detailed study of life events in FNSD suggested an increase in frequency of events just prior to symptom onset, especially of the 'escape' type that Freud suggested, not all patients were found to have experienced severe or adverse events of any type [18].

The 'conversion model' of aetiology has also been unsatisfactory in explaining why someone should develop a weak arm or blackouts in relation to stress. The solution proposed was that the symptom was 'symbolic of the difficulty' or represented an inability to function. Systematic studies of patients with FNSD have suggested a more prosaic explanation for particular symptoms—that they are simply continuations of acute symptoms that arose for many reasons. For example, patients with dissociative (non-epileptic) seizures commonly experience transient dissociative or panic symptoms just before their blackouts [19]. Studies have supported a model in which the 'blackout' occurs as a response to this arousal which then becomes habitual, perhaps through classical conditioning [11]. More recently, evidence has accumulated to support the idea that physical injury or physiological states, such as migraine, commonly occur at the onset of these symptoms, which then become perpetuated via persistent abnormal attention [20, 21]. Cognitive neuropsychological models with their basis in a concept of the brain as a 'predictive' organ help bridge the gap between neuroscience and psychological models of this disorder and support new ways of delivering treatment [22].

Functional brain imaging of patients with FNSD has found differences between patients and volunteers pretending to have similar symptoms. In addition, functional imaging of patients in experimental hypnotic states has revealed changes similar to those seen in patients with FNSD, with hypoactivation of cortical and subcortical motor areas, without activation of prefrontal areas often involved in motor inhibition. Limbic areas, such as the amygdala, are also commonly overactive in comparison with controls [23]. In addition, some studies have suggested hypoactivation of a network identified with self-agency, including the temporo-parietal junction, in keeping with the notion that the movements do involve the

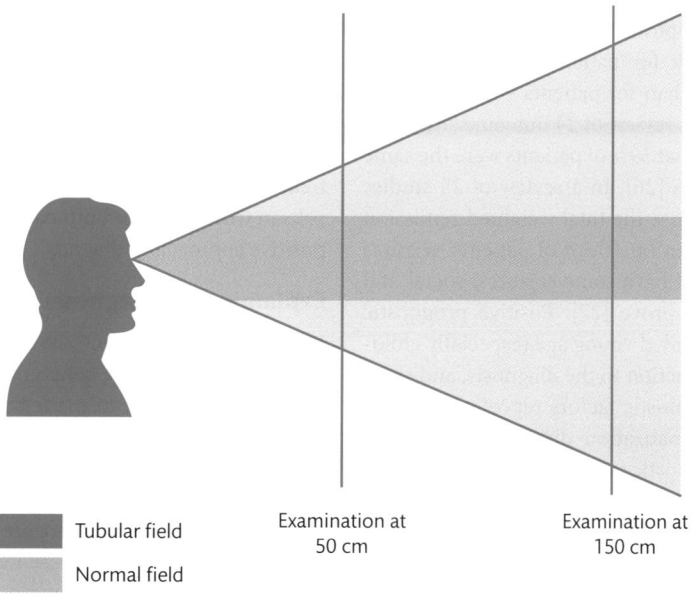

Tubular field

Normal field

Examination at 50 cm

Examination at 150 cm

**Fig. 133.4** In patients with functional visual loss, bedside testing may reveal a tubular field defect, which disobeys the laws of physics.

Reproduced from *J Neurol Neurosurg Psychiatry*, 76(Suppl 1), Stone J, Carson A, Sharpe M, Functional symptoms and signs in neurology: assessment and diagnosis, i2-12, Copyright (2005), with permission from *British Medical Journal*.

**Table 133.3** A range of potential aetiological factors in patients with functional neurological symptom disorder

| Factors | Biological | Psychological | Social |
|---|---|---|---|
| Factors acting at all stages | • Pathophysiological disease<br><br>• History of previous functional symptoms | • Emotional disorder<br>• Personality disorder | • Socio-economic deprivation<br>• Life events and difficulties |
| Predisposing | • Genetic factors affecting personality<br>• Biological vulnerabilities in nervous system? | • Perception of childhood experience as adverse<br>• Personality traits<br>• Poor attachment/coping style | • Childhood neglect/abuse<br>• Poor family functioning<br>• Symptom modelling |
| Precipitating | • Abnormal physiological event or state (for example, hyperventilation, sleep deprivation, sleep paralysis)<br>• Physical illness/injury/pain | • Perception of life event as negative, unexpected<br>• Acute dissociative episode/panic attack | |
| Perpetuating | • Plasticity in central nervous system motor and sensory (including pain) pathways<br>• Deconditioning/'habit'<br>• Neuroendocrine and immunological abnormalities similar to those seen in depression and anxiety | • Illness beliefs (patient and family)<br>• Perception of symptoms as being due to disease/damage/outwith the scope of self-help<br>• Not feeling believed<br>• Avoidance of symptom provocation | • Presence of a welfare system<br>• Social benefits of being ill<br>• Availability of legal compensation<br>• Stigma of 'mental illness' in society and from the medical profession<br>• Ongoing medical investigations and uncertainty |

Adapted from *Pract Neurol.*, 9(3), Stone J, Functional symptoms in neurology, pp. 179–89, Copyright (2009), with permission from *British Medical Journal.*

voluntary motor system, but the person genuinely does not have the sense that they are 'doing it' [24].

Neurophysiological studies have also revealed potentially intriguing differences in evoked responses between patients with FNSD and controls and also in a parameter known as sensory attenuation, which measures the person's ability to predict their own actions [25]. Interestingly, FNSD may be a paradigmatic disorder of willed action which has escaped scrutiny because of its clinical similarities to 'willed action of pretending'.

## Prognosis and misdiagnosis

The prognosis is highly variable. Symptom duration may be as brief as hours or as long as years. Symptoms may be mild or severely disabling. In general, the outlook for patients with dissociative (non-epileptic) seizures is better than for patients with functional movement disorders. A systematic review of 24 outcome studies of functional motor disorder found that 39% of patients were the same or worse after a mean of 7.5 years [26]. In a review of 25 studies of patients with dissociative seizures, the total weighted remission rate was around 33% (that is, about one-third of patients' seizures stopped). While patients may still have some seizures, social and occupational functioning may improve [27]. Positive prognostic factors noted in these studies included young age (especially childhood), early diagnosis, positive reaction to the diagnosis, and short duration of illness. Negative prognostic factors reported are presence of personality disorder, somatization disorder, or ongoing litigation. Patients with poor prognostic factors can, however, sometimes respond well to treatment, and vice versa [26].

We referred earlier to the well-known follow-up study of Slater in 1965 which suggested that as many as two-thirds of patients with a diagnosis of hysteria actually had misdiagnosed neurological disease. Although methodologically flawed, mainly by selection bias, this study convinced at least two generations of psychiatrists that they

need not worry about this disorder; it was just an example of neurologists getting it wrong. However, a systematic review of 27 studies published since Slater's found a misdiagnosis rate of <5% since 1970 (interestingly, this was long before MRI scans and videotelemetry were in routine use) (Fig. 133.5). This rate of misdiagnosis is similar to that for other neurological and psychiatric disorders. Subsequent large prospective studies have also been reassuring [28], as have follow-up studies of other somatoform disorders [29].

## Treatment

The treatment of FNSD should usually be multi-disciplinary. Its foundation is a plausible and agreed explanation of the diagnosis, followed by effective triage to the correct therapy (and in some cases recognizing that the patient is unlikely to benefit from therapy).

The traditional sequence of events has been for a neurologist to tell a patient there is 'nothing wrong' and then to refer to a psychiatrist who is expected to detect the psychological stressor and then treat the patient. It is hardly surprising that this process usually results in frustration for both patients and clinicians. A combined and positive approach to diagnosis is preferable.

### Explaining the diagnosis

It is crucial that someone, and preferably every member of the clinical team, can deliver a coherent and consistent explanation of how the diagnosis has been made and how the symptoms can be improved with therapy.

Although there is much debate about whether the patient should be told that their illness is 'psychogenic' or 'functional' or 'conversion', it seems likely that there are other more important ingredients of a useful explanation. These include: (1) taking the problem seriously; (2) giving the problem a positive diagnostic label (rather than just telling the patient what they do not have); (3) demonstrating to the patient the rationale for the diagnosis (showing the patient their

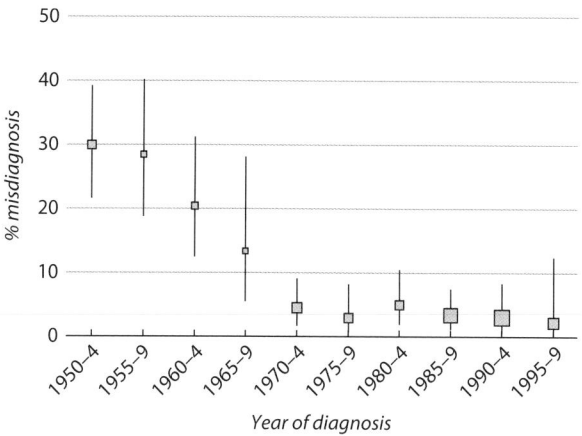

**Fig. 133.5** Frequency of misdiagnosis of functional neurological symptoms disorder/conversion disorder/hysteria in 27 studies and 1466 patients, with a mean duration of 5 years.
Reproduced from *J Neurol Neurosurg Psychiatry*, 76(Suppl 1), Stone J, Carson A, Sharpe M, Functional symptoms and signs in neurology: assessment and diagnosis, i2–12, Copyright (2005), with permission from *British Medical Journal*.

positive Hoover's sign or how their tremor stops briefly during the entrainment test, or going through the typical features of a dissociative seizure); (4) emphasizing the potential for reversibility, for example using metaphors such as software vs hardware; (5) providing written information, for example, such as that found at https://www.neurosymptoms.org or http://www.nonepilepticattacks.info; and (6) triaging to an appropriate treatment.

Our personal preference for a diagnostic label is to use the terms 'functional' or 'dissociative'. For us, these are terms most consistent with the current state of our knowledge in that they allow for a bio-psychosocial model in which there can be a discussion of abnormal brain function, as well as a discussion of how symptoms may persist because of psychological 'patterns' or habits. In addition, there is the critical implication that brain function (as opposed to structural damage) can be improved by many interventions, including medication, activity, and psychological treatment.

### Physiotherapy

Current evidence suggests that physiotherapy should be a first-line treatment for patients with functional movement disorders and limb weakness, as long as the patient has some confidence in the diagnosis and is motivated to change. In recent years, the nature of physiotherapy for functional motor disorders has become more clearly defined and is being tested in randomized trials. Physiotherapy techniques are based on an understanding of how symptoms in FNSD can be dependent on abnormally focused attention and tend to improve with distraction. There has been a realization that generic physiotherapy, as one would use for stroke, may, in fact, be counterproductive. Consensus recommendations have been published for the various motor symptoms with which patients present [30]. A case series and randomized controlled trial found evidence of efficacy for this approach in patients selected for their understanding and motivation. Despite a symptom duration of 5.8 years, 72% had a good outcome with specific therapy, compared to only 18% who had physiotherapy of a non-specific nature [31]. Another trial found sustained benefit from 3 weeks of inpatient rehabilitation [32]. Further studies of inpatient treatment are also encouraging [33, 34].

### Psychological and psychotropic drug treatment

Psychiatric assessment and formulation have a key role to play in the management of many patients with FNSD. A bio-psychosocial formulation can put together the factors seen in Table 133.3 and present them back to the patient as an explanation of what may have led to the development of their symptoms and what may now need to be addressed to achieve recovery.

Comorbid and psychiatric disorders, such as panic, anxiety, and depression, often contribute to FNSD and may need to be targeted in treatment, whether pharmacological or psychological.

A tailored cognitive behavioural therapy (CBT)—an informed guided self-help programme—was found to be better than treatment as usual for patients with a range of functional neurological symptoms in a randomized trial [35]. Another specific form of cognitive behavioural psychological therapy has been developed specifically for dissociative (non-epileptic) seizures [36, 37]. In a pilot trial of this CBT-based approach, developed from therapy for panic disorder, the number needed to treat for seizure remission was 5 [36]. This therapy involves: education about the disorder and setting of goals, teaching specific distraction techniques for episodes, learning to make connections between emotions and seizures, using graded exposure to change behaviour restricted by the events, and looking more widely, if necessary, at psychological antecedents or perpetuating factors. A large multi-centre trial is currently under way [38]. There is some evidence for a role of psychodynamic psychotherapy in other functional somatic disorders [39], but little specifically for FNSD [40].

### Other treatments

Other treatments used since the nineteenth century may still have a place. Hypnosis may have some efficacy, especially in those keen to have it [41]. Electrical stimulation of the arms and legs has been used for centuries to treat patients with functional disorders but lost popularity after the First World War. More recent studies of transcranial magnetic stimulation have suggested it may have a role, especially in demonstrating reversibility of symptoms, but trial evidence is lacking [42]. Finally, abreaction and therapeutic sedation, which were used as long ago as the First World War, may still have a role for patients with fixed dystonia, mutism, or deficits, where transient improvement cannot be demonstrated using bedside manoeuvres [43]. There is, however, no specific evidence for the use of psychotropic drugs in FNSD, although they may be required to treat comorbid anxiety or depression.

### Stopping treatment

While the prognosis for established FNSD is poor without treatment, we may have been too pessimistic about the response to treatment. However, not all patients can be successfully treated and it is at times useful to share this conclusion with the patient, where appropriate, emphasizing that this is something that can be revisited.

## Conclusions

Functional disorders are common in neurological practice and are one of the most common reasons for referral to psychiatrists working in that setting. Significant advances over recent years have improved our understanding of both aetiology and treatment. The modern clinical assessment emphasizes the primacy of diagnosis based on typical characteristics of the physical symptoms themselves. Joint neurological, psychiatric, and multi-disciplinary teamworking is the cornerstone of management for most patients.

## REFERENCES

1. Trimble M, Reynolds EH. A brief history of hysteria. In: Hallett M, Stone J, Carson A, editors. *Handbook of Clinical Neurology*, volume 139. Amsterdam: Elsevier; 2016. pp. 3–10.
2. Stone J, Hewett R, Carson A, *et al*. The 'disappearance' of hysteria: historical mystery or illusion? *J R Soc Med* 2008;**101**:12–18.
3. Stone J, Warlow C, Carson A, *et al*. Eliot Slater's myth of the non-existence of hysteria. *J R Soc Med* 2005;**98**:547–8.
4. Levenson JL, Sharpe M. Chapter 16—The classification of conversion disorder (functional neurologic symptom disorder) in ICD and DSM. In: Hallett M, Stone J, Carson A, editors. *Handbook of Clinical Neurology*, volume 139. Amsterdam: Elsevier; 2016. pp. 189–92.
5. Stone J, LaFrance WC, Brown R, *et al*. Conversion disorder: current problems and potential solutions for DSM-5. *J Psychosom Res* 2011;**71**:369–76.
6. Ludwig L, Pasman JA, Nicholson T, *et al*. Stressful life events and maltreatment in conversion (functional neurological) disorder: systematic review and meta-analysis of case-control studies. *Lancet Psychiatry* 2018;**5**:307–20.
7. Stone J, Warlow C, Sharpe M. The symptom of functional weakness: a controlled study of 107 patients. *Brain* 2010;**133**:1537–51.
8. Duncan R, Razvi S, Mulhern S. Newly presenting psychogenic nonepileptic seizures: incidence, population characteristics, and early outcome from a prospective audit of a first seizure clinic. *Epilepsy Behav* 2011;**20**:308–11.
9. Anderson KE, Gruber-Baldini AL, Vaughan CG, *et al*. Impact of psychogenic movement disorders versus Parkinson's on disability, quality of life, and psychopathology. *Mov Disord* 2007;**22**:2204–9.
10. Carson A, Stone J, Hibberd C, *et al*. Disability, distress and unemployment in neurology outpatients with symptoms 'unexplained by organic disease'. *J Neurol Neurosurg Psychiatry* 2011;**82**:810–13.
11. Brown RJ, Reuber M. Psychological and psychiatric aspects of psychogenic non-epileptic seizures (PNES): a systematic review. *Clin Psychol Rev* 2016;**45**:157–82.
12. Ahmedani BK, Osborne J, Nerenz DR, *et al*. Diagnosis, costs, and utilization for psychogenic non-epileptic seizures in a US health care setting. *Psychosomatics* 2013;**54**:28–34.
13. Stone J, Smyth R, Carson A, *et al*. La belle indifférence in conversion symptoms and hysteria: systematic review. *Br J Psychiatry* 2006;**188**:204–9.
14. Stone J, Pal S, Blackburn D, *et al*. Functional (psychogenic) cognitive disorders: a perspective from the neurology clinic. *J Alzheimer's Dis* 2015;**48**:S5–17.
15. Dieterich M, Staab JP. Functional dizziness. *Curr Opin Neurol* 2017;**30**:107–13.
16. Brinjikji W, Luetmer PH, Comstock B, *et al*. Systematic literature review of imaging features of spinal degeneration in asymptomatic populations. *Am J Neuroradiol* 2015;**36**:811–16.
17. Stone J, Reuber M, Carson A. Functional symptoms in neurology: mimics and chameleons. *Pract Neurol* 2013;**13**:104–13.
18. Nicholson TR, Aybek S, Craig T, *et al*. Life events and escape in conversion disorder. *Psychol Med* 2016;**46**:2617–26.
19. Hendrickson R, Popescu A, Dixit R, *et al*. Panic attack symptoms differentiate patients with epilepsy from those with psychogenic nonepileptic spells (PNES). *Epilepsy Behav* 2014;**37**:210–14.
20. Stone J, Warlow C, Sharpe M. Functional weakness: clues to mechanism from the nature of onset. *J Neurol Neurosurg Psychiatry* 2012;**83**:67–9.
21. Pareés I, Kojovic M, Pires C, *et al*. Physical precipitating factors in functional movement disorders. *J Neurol Sci* 2014;**338**:174–7.
22. Edwards MJ, Adams RA, Brown H, *et al*. A Bayesian account of 'hysteria'. *Brain* 2012;**135**:3495–512.
23. Aybek S, Vuilleumier P. Chapter 7—Imaging studies of functional neurologic disorders. In: Hallett M, Stone J, Carson A, editors. *Handbook of Clinical Neurology*, volume 139. Amsterdam: Elsevier; 2016. pp. 73–84.
24. Voon V, Gallea C, Hattori N, *et al*. The involuntary nature of conversion disorder. *Neurology* 2010;**74**:223–8.
25. Pareés I, Brown H, Nuruki A, *et al*. Loss of sensory attenuation in patients with functional (psychogenic) movement disorders. *Brain* 2014;**137**:2916–21.
26. Gelauff J, Stone J. Chapter 43—Prognosis of functional neurologic disorders. In: Hallett M, Stone J, Carson A, editors. *Handbook of Clinical Neurology*, volume 139. Amsterdam: Elsevier; 2016. pp. 523–41.
27. Reuber M, Mitchell AJ, Howlett S, *et al*. Measuring outcome in psychogenic nonepileptic seizures: how relevant is seizure remission? *Epilepsia* 2005;**46**:1788–95.
28. Stone J, Carson A, Duncan R, *et al*. Symptoms 'unexplained by organic disease' in 1144 new neurology out-patients: how often does the diagnosis change at follow-up? *Brain* 2009;**132**:2878–88.
29. Eikelboom EM, Tak LM, Roest AM, *et al*. A systematic review and meta-analysis of the percentage of revised diagnoses in functional somatic symptoms. *J Psychosom Res* 2016;**88**:60–7.
30. Nielsen G, Stone J, Matthews A, *et al*. Physiotherapy for functional motor disorders: a consensus recommendation. *J Neurol Neurosurg Psychiatry* 2015;**86**:1113–19.
31. Nielsen G, Buszewicz M, Stevenson F, *et al*. Randomised feasibility study of physiotherapy for patients with functional motor symptoms. *J Neurol Neurosurg Psychiatry* 2017;**88**:484–90.
32. Jordbru AA, Smedstad LM, Klungsøyr O, *et al*. Psychogenic gait disorder: a randomized controlled trial of physical rehabilitation with one-year follow-up. *J Rehabil Med* 2014;**46**:181–7.
33. Demartini B, Batla A, Petrochilos P, *et al*. Multidisciplinary treatment for functional neurological symptoms: a prospective study. *J Neurol* 2014;**261**:2370–7.
34. McCormack R, Moriarty J, Mellers JD, *et al*. Specialist in-patient treatment for severe motor conversion disorder: a retrospective comparative study. *J Neurol Neurosurg Psychiatry* 2014;**85**:895–900.
35. Sharpe M, Walker J, Williams C, *et al*. Guided self-help for functional (psychogenic) symptoms: a randomized controlled efficacy trial. *Neurology* 2011;**77**:564–72.
36. Goldstein LH, Chalder T, Chigwedere C, *et al*. Cognitive-behavioral therapy for psychogenic nonepileptic seizures: a pilot RCT. *Neurology* 2010;**74**:1986–94.
37. LaFrance WC, Baird GL, Barry JJ, *et al*. Multicenter pilot treatment trial for psychogenic nonepileptic seizures: a randomized clinical trial. *JAMA Psychiatry* 2014;**71**:997–1005.
38. Goldstein LH, Mellers JDC, Landau S, *et al*. Cognitive behavioural therapy vs standardised medical care for adults with dissociative non-epileptic seizures (CODES): a multicentre randomised controlled trial protocol. *BMC Neurol* 2015;**15**:98.

39. Abbass A, Kisely S, Kroenke K. Short-term psychodynamic psychotherapy for somatic disorders. Systematic review and meta-analysis of clinical trials. *Psychother Psychosom* 2009;**78**:265–74.

40. Reuber M, Burness C, Howlett S, *et al.* Tailored psychotherapy for patients with functional neurological symptoms: a pilot study. *J Psychosom Res* 2007;**63**:625–32.

41. Koch T, Lang E V, Hatsiopoulou O, *et al.* A randomized controlled clinical trial of a hypnosis-based treatment for patients with conversion disorder, motor type. *Int J Clin Exp Hypn* 2003;**51**:357–68.

42. Pollak T, Nicholson T. A systematic review of transcranial magnetic stimulation in the treatment of functional (conversion) neurological symptoms. *J Neurol Neurosurg Psychiatry* 2014;**85**:191–7.

43. Stone J, Hoeritzauer I, Brown K, *et al.* Therapeutic sedation for functional (psychogenic) neurological symptoms. *J Psychosom Res* 2014;**76**:165–8.

44. Daum C, Hubschmid M, Aybek S. The value of 'positive' clinical signs for weakness, sensory and gait disorders in conversion disorder: a systematic and narrative review. *J Neurol Neurosurg Psychiatry* 2014;**85**:180–90.

45. Zeuner K, Shoge R, Goldstein S, *et al.* Accelerometry to distinguish psychogenic from essential or parkinsonian tremor. *Neurology* 2003;**61**:548–50.

46. Fasano A, Valadas A, Bhatia KP, *et al.* Psychogenic facial movement disorders: clinical features and associated conditions. *Mov Disord* 2012;**27**:1544–51.

47. Schrag A, Trimble M, Quinn N, *et al.* The syndrome of fixed dystonia: an evaluation of 103 patients. *Brain* 2004;**127**:2360–72.

48. Wolfsegger T, Pischinger B, Topakian R. Objectification of psychogenic postural instability by trunk sway analysis. *J Neurol Sci* 2013;**334**:14–17.

49. Avbersek A, Sisodiya S. Does the primary literature provide support for clinical signs used to distinguish psychogenic nonepileptic seizures from epileptic seizures? *J Neurol Neurosurg Psychiatry* 2010;**81**:719–25.

50. Chen CS, Lee AW, Karagiannis A, *et al.* Practical clinical approaches to functional visual loss. *J Clin Neurosci* 2007;**14**:1–7.

51. Duffy JR. Chapter 33—Functional speech disorders: clinical manifestations, diagnosis, and management. In: Hallett M, Stone J, Carson A, editors. *Handbook of Clinical Neurology*, volume 139. Amsterdam: Elsevier; 2016. pp. 379–88.

# SECTION 23
# Service provision

# 134

# Public policy and service needs in mental health

*Martin Knapp*

## Introduction

In policy terms, mental health problems are among the most complex of all health issues, characterized by a number of pervasive challenges. Seen as a group, prevalence rates are high and onset is often relatively early in life. Most mental health problems are chronic, often with life-long negative impacts. Aetiology represents a melange of genetic and environmental influences. People who have mental health problems will often experience stigma, discrimination, and victimization—opportunities available to other people are often closed off. Psychological well-being—to be separated from psychiatric symptoms—is often very poor for people experiencing mental illness.

There are close links between mental illness, self-harm, and suicide. There are also strong links between some mental health problems, antisocial behaviour, and crime. Consequently, most countries have legal powers of compulsory detention and treatment to protect individuals from themselves or to protect other people. Mental health problems may have other negative collateral effects, including on siblings, parents, peers in schools, and work colleagues, and perhaps also in local communities.

Responses to mental health problems are many and various, and often lead to high public sector and privately borne costs that may extend over many years. Young people with mental health problems are at above-average risk of failing to achieve their educational potential. In adulthood, there are often considerable employment-related difficulties—long spells of unemployment, high rates of absenteeism, and under-par performance when at work—which can lead to substantial productivity losses for the economy and income losses for the individual and family.

It is the combination of these often very challenging characteristics and experiences—for individuals, families, and communities—which require careful, multi-dimensional, far-sighted policy responses. Mental health policy-making that concertedly aims to address these challenges will necessarily be complex. The focus of this chapter is such policy-making. I will briefly consider the main drivers of mental health problems (in Section 2) as a platform for identifying the domains where policy action might be needed to prevent or ameliorate illness and the distress associated with it. I will then turn to the main consequences of mental health problems, emphasizing how widely spread those consequences will often be (Section 3). Societal responses to those consequences will be discussed. The focus of Section 4 is on the main dimensions of a good mental health policy, providing some illustrations. A brief concluding section pulls together the main arguments.

## Drivers of mental health problems

There are many factors that can precipitate, prolong, or reignite mental health problems, representing a set of complex interactions between genes and the environment; although some mental illnesses have high rates of heritability, there are very strong environmental effects. Age and gender are relevant factors in understanding the incidence and prevalence, and demographic trends over time can affect the patterns of mental illness and the nature of the policy challenge. Traumatic experiences, lifestyle choices, and other health problems (acute or chronic) are important, and economic conditions can play a major part. Other chapters in this book have discussed many of these 'drivers' in more detail, and here I briefly summarize some of them as a way to identify individual, family, and societal consequences, which, if recognized, will then often be prompts for policy action.

Three-quarters of mental health problems (except dementia) have emerged before age 24, and perhaps as many as half by age 14 [1]. Psychoses most commonly emerge in late adolescence and early adulthood, which is precisely the age when most individuals would be making key decisions that will shape the rest of their lives: finishing their education, moving away from the parental home, taking their first steps into the world of work, and having their first serious relationships. A mental health problem that is not adequately treated can have life-long personal and economic consequences. Later in life, Alzheimer's disease and other dementias are highly prevalent; as populations age—as they are doing rapidly across the world—overall numbers of people with these disorders will grow too and will clearly need concerted policy attention, especially given that there is currently no cure.

The influences of traumatic experiences on mental health are often pernicious and persistent—experiencing war, military combat, terrorism, rape, or sexual abuse can bring on a range of mental health problems, including post-traumatic stress and depression. Bullying victimization in childhood is known to be still affecting someone's mental and physical health many decades later [2, 3], with sizeable impacts on mental health care systems.

Numerous lifestyle choices are known to affect mental health. For example, excessive cannabis use in young people is a recognized risk factor for developing schizophrenia [4]. Being breast-fed, on the other hand, can be a protective factor—not being breast-fed for very long independently predicts poor mental health during childhood and early adolescence, even after adjusting for other factors [5].

There are well-known links between other health problems and mental illness. People with long-term conditions, such as diabetes, cancer, and coronary heart disease, have above-average risks of psychiatric morbidity, which often affect how their physical health develops and is managed, with consequences for quality of life and costs [6, 7]. For example, it has been shown that the health care costs of treating 11 different chronic health problems are significantly higher when a patient has comorbid depression, while there can also be considerable impacts on workplace performance and absenteeism from work [8]. Individuals with neurodevelopmental conditions can also be at high risk; the prevalence of anxiety is as high as 42% among autistic children [9].

Economic conditions in a country and the economic status of an individual can affect mental health, and in fact, there are multiple and two-way links between economic factors and mental illness. 'Social causation' arguments suggest that core aspects of economic disadvantage, such as poverty and long-term unemployment, increase the risk of mental illness by initiating or exacerbating financial stress (particularly unmanageable debt), social exclusion, stigma, and poor diet, and also by undermining protective factors such as social capital, education, and personal resilience. An alternative explanation is the 'social selection' or 'drift' argument that people with mental health problems have higher risks of remaining or falling into poverty because of the (privately borne) costs of their treatment, disrupted employment, and reduced earnings [10]. A general economic recession, such as the recent global financial crisis, can have profound effects on employment, job security, productivity, earnings, and social cohesion, with knock-on effects on mental illness, as shown most immediately by suicide rates [11].

## Consequences and societal responses

Most mental health problems are complicated and distressing. They can cause temporary incapacity, abject misery, self-loathing, and personal shame, and lead to public stigma and discrimination in many different settings. They can prompt violent behaviour, self-harm, and suicidal ideation, causing societies to impose restrictions on individual liberty because of assumed or confirmed incapacity or dangerousness. They are associated with poor health behaviours and premature mortality. But there may occasionally also be some positive aspects; a mental illness may give an individual new insights, help them to embrace change, or energize their creativity. Overwhelmingly, however, the negatives outweigh any positives.

This wide-ranging mix of (largely negative) consequences also makes mental illness look 'economically expensive' in the sense that scarce resources must be devoted to respond to them, often over long periods of time. As a result, decision-makers in health and other systems must think carefully about how they use the resources under their control in order to meet needs and preferences associated with mental illness or—better still—how these illnesses can be prevented in the first place.

### Economic and social exclusion

As already noted, people with mental health problems have above-average rates of economic difficulties, particularly linked to employment (especially finding and keeping a job, and chronic unemployment), rent and mortgage arrears, other unsecured debt, low earnings, low household income, poor social networks, loneliness, and social isolation [12].

An authoritative commentary on some of these issues from the Organisation for Economic Co-operation and Development (OECD) drew on national statistics and robust studies [13]. It illustrated the multifarious links between mental health problems and work; people who have experienced mental health problems find it harder to acquire and retain paid employment, have higher rates of absenteeism and presenteeism (reduced productivity when at work because of symptoms), earn lower salaries, and are more likely to take early retirement [14]. The typical age of onset of serious mental health problems often prevents individuals from completing their education. For most people, employment is their primary source of income, and so long-term employment difficulties can propel people into unmanageable personal debt and poverty, which, in turn, can worsen mental health [15]. Employment is, of course, more than just a source of income—it influences social position and community roles, fosters social participation, and, for many people, is a key source of self-concept.

At a national level, these employment difficulties damage productivity and economic growth. For example, a study in eight very different countries found that the extent and costs of depression-related absenteeism and presenteeism in the workplace were considerable, both in absolute monetary terms and in relation to the proportion of the country's gross domestic product (GDP). Absenteeism had a large impact across all countries, but the costs associated with presenteeism were 5–10 times higher [16].

Employment issues mean that many individuals with mental health problems are reliant on social security (welfare) payments. The OECD report cited earlier found that between one-third and one-half of new disability benefit claims in the countries they studied were made for reasons connected to mental illness. Benefits systems need to be designed so as to provide appropriate compensation, but not to make people feel trapped—anxious, perhaps, about losing their benefit entitlements if they 'take the risk' of moving into a paid job that might prove stressful and reignite an otherwise stable condition. But benefits systems that leave people at risk of poverty could create a different kind of downward spiral—their economic circumstances could exacerbate their symptoms, which then make it harder to secure employment and lead to further social and economic exclusion. If an individual struggles to keep up their rent or mortgage payments, then homelessness might even be the result [17].

## Crime

If not treated effectively, some mental health problems can result in either antisocial or violent crime [18–20]. Drug and alcohol misuse might prompt acquisitive crime, as individuals seek to find the resources to purchase their substance of choice, and there are also associations between such misuse and violent crime. Conduct disorder—the most common childhood psychiatric disorder, with a UK prevalence of 4.9% for children aged 5–10 years [21]—is associated with antisocial behaviour (and substance misuse) in adolescence and criminal activity in young adulthood, with high costs for both criminal justice bodies and victims. Indeed, an 18-year follow-up study in London found that these crime-related costs dominated all other economic consequences of conduct disorder [22]. However, people with mental health problems are also at above-average risk of being *victims* of crime, particularly violent crime [23].

## Self-harm and suicide

According to the World Health Organization (WHO) [24], globally there are more than 800,000 suicides each year, each of them potentially preventable. Suicide and self-harm are major public health issues, and because there are links with mental health problems (especially depression, eating disorders, and alcohol misuse), some governments have included suicide prevention strategies within their mental health policy frameworks. Generally, however, WHO argues that insufficient strategic attention is paid to suicide prevention. Another obstacle is the taboo surrounding suicide. Suicide is one of the priorities in the WHO Mental Health Gap Action Programme (mhGAP) launched in 2008 in low- and middle-income countries. In high-income countries, there is strong evidence that economic difficulties are associated with higher suicide risks. For example, the global financial crisis led to significantly higher suicide rates, particularly for men [25], and an earlier recession in South Korea widened income-related inequalities in depression and suicidal behaviour, especially in lower-income groups [26]. Some authors have further argued that government 'austerity' measures have exacerbated the situation [11].

## Premature mortality

It is not only suicide rates that are higher for people with mental health problems; premature mortality for other reasons is another major challenge [24]. This is particularly so for people with more severe (schizophrenia, bipolar disorder, and moderate to severe depression). Life expectancy for people with schizophrenia is 20 years lower than for the general population [27], while for people with depression, the risk of death is 1.8 times higher than for the general population. Cardiovascular disease and type 2 diabetes are quite prevalent among people with schizophrenia, and other physical health problems commonly experienced by people with mental health problems that can shorten their lives include respiratory diseases, hypertension, and infectious diseases such as HIV, hepatitis, and tuberculosis.

Many of the reasons for poor physical health and premature morbidity are not hard to identify, linked to lifestyle, poor health behaviours, and, to some extent, the side effects of treatment. Tobacco use is high [28]. Obesity is also an issue, linked to poor diet [29], physical inactivity, and weight gain brought on by some medications (particularly some antipsychotics) [30]. Infectious diseases, such as

HIV and hepatitis, are more common among people with mental health problems, linked to socio-economic disadvantage and behaviours such as intravenous substance abuse. The symptoms of mental illness might make it hard for individuals to seek medical treatment, and social isolation and homelessness will add to the barriers. Stigma and discrimination associated with severe mental illness might also result in poorer physical health care. Every one of these risk factors is, in principle, preventable and ought to be part of any mental health policy strategy.

## Transmitted impacts on the family and others

The negative effects of mental health problems can be experienced by people other than the person with the illness. One obvious transmitted effect is the 'burden' of being a family carer; for example, supporting someone with moderate to severe dementia can be stressful, with a high risk of anxiety or depression [31], as well as requiring out-of-pocket payments for services and transport costs and missing opportunities for paid employment or social activities [32]. On the other hand, good family care for someone with dementia can greatly improve their well-being and delay nursing home admission [33]. Supporting someone with schizophrenia can be distressing and costly, and the effects on parents of a child with externalizing behavioural problems, such as conduct disorder, can be considerable [34]. Postnatal depression can affect the birth-child's emotional, behavioural, and intellectual development, with attendant long-term economic consequences [35]. Attention-deficit/hyperactivity disorder can affect classmates at school, work colleagues, and members of the local community [36].

## Stigma and discrimination

Stigma and discrimination are deep-rooted, pervasive challenges. The consequences for individuals include social isolation, bullying in schools, discrimination in the workplace, active hostility or neglectful indifference in communities, and a consequent reluctance on the part of mentally ill individuals to seek the help they need [37]. Evidence from a seven-country European study in workplaces showed that managers' attitudes, employers' policies on flexible working arrangements, and national benefits systems can have significant effects on individuals with lived experience of mental illness [38]. Negative attitudes can have serious knock-on effects on health, especially mental health, quality of life, access to opportunities, services, and welfare entitlements [12]. Stigma may stem from lack of awareness but often reflects a more insidious suspicion and hostility. A mature mental health policy framework will include concerted anti-stigma efforts, as well as intervention to tackle discrimination and victimization.

## High and wide-ranging costs

As is already clear, mental health problems generate high and wide-ranging costs, not only for the health care system, but also for public and other agencies responsible for welfare benefits, social care, education, employment, criminal justice, and other systems. There can be substantial productivity losses associated with mental illness; indeed, the costs of unemployment, absenteeism, and presenteeism tend to dominate any service-related costs. For some disorders, such as dementia, the costs directly or indirectly borne by the family and other carers are, in aggregate, larger than the costs of health and social care services that people with dementia will use [39]. Many childhood disorders will continue to generate substantial private and public costs many decades later, in terms of employment disruption [40] and earnings, criminal behaviour, and high use of health services [41].

## Policy dimensions

### What is a mental health policy?

According to the WHO, 'A mental health policy is an organized set of values, principles and objectives for improving the mental health and reducing the burden of mental disorders in a population. It defines a vision for the future and helps to establish a model of how action should be taken' [42]. Typically, a policy document will range over a number of key domains, responding to the kinds of challenge and negative consequences described in the previous section. These could include: human rights and advocacy; financing (such as taxation or insurance); payment mechanisms for providers (such as fee-for-service or capitation); organization and co-ordination of services within the health care sector and across other sectors; prevention of illness and promotion of well-being; treatment and rehabilitation interventions, including access to medicines and other services in different country contexts; quality of services and performance monitoring; information systems; recruitment, training, and retention of skilled human resources; and commitment to research and evaluation.

A recent example can be given from England—a comprehensive policy framework from the 2010–2015 Coalition government (Box 134.1) [43]. More recently, an independent Taskforce was commissioned by NHS England. Its report summarized developments in mental health treatment in England over recent decades and set out a number of 'priority actions' for the National Health Service (NHS) for the next 5 years [44].

### Financing

There are numerous reasons why a formal mental health policy is needed. There are too many distressing, damaging, and durable consequences for any civilized society to ignore. There are collateral damages for communities and the national economy. Another reason is that families cannot be left to address the issues alone, and there is only so much that relatively informal, locally initiated, and sustained community action can go. There is often market failure, which manifests itself in policy terms in an emphasis on *collective* responsibility for managing, delivering, and/or financing mechanisms.

Most high- and middle-income countries—and gradually a number of low-income countries—rely on prepayment systems of revenue collection as the basis for financing health care. In those countries, the most common methods of financing are tax-based (37% in OECD countries), mandatory (social) insurance (36%), out-of-pocket payments (19%), and voluntary (or private) insurance (6%) [45]. Prepayment through social health insurance, private health insurance, or taxation is preferable to out-of-pocket payments because each individual's need for health care is uncertain, but when that need arises, it can generate enormous (perhaps 'catastrophic') economic impacts in terms of treatment costs and lost earnings.

**Box 134.1** Closing the Gap: Priorities for Essential Change in Mental Health (UK Government, January 2014)

This policy document set out 25 priorities for change in how children and adults with mental health problems should be supported and cared for:

1. High-quality mental health services with an emphasis on recovery should be commissioned in all areas, reflecting local need.
2. We will lead an information revolution around mental health and well-being.
3. We will, for the first time, establish clear waiting time limits for mental health services.
4. We will tackle inequalities around access to mental health services.
5. Over 900,000 people with benefit from psychological therapies every year.
6. There will be improved access to psychological therapies for children and young people across the whole of England.
7. The most effective services will get the most funding.
8. Adults will be given the right to make choices about the mental health care they receive.
9. We will radically reduce the use of all restrictive practices and take action to end the use of high-risk restraint, including face-down restraint and holding people on the floor.
10. We will use the Friends and Family Test to allow all patients to comment on their experience of mental health services—including children's mental health services.
11. Poor-quality services will be identified sooner and action taken to improve care and where necessary protect patients.
12. Carers will be better supported and more closely involved in decisions about mental health service provision.
13. Mental health care and physical health care will be better integrated at every level.
14. We will change the way frontline health services respond to self-harm.
15. No-one experiencing a mental health crisis should ever be turned away from services.
16. We will offer better support to new mothers to minimize the risks and impacts of postnatal depression.
17. Schools will be supported to identify mental health problems sooner.
18. We will end the cliff edge of lost support as children and young people with mental health needs reach the age of 18.
19. People with mental health problems will live healthier lives and longer lives.
20. More people with mental health problems will live in homes that support recovery.
21. We will introduce a national liaison and diversion service so that mental health needs of offenders will be identified sooner and appropriate support provided.
22. Anyone with a mental health problem who is a victim of crime will be offered enhanced support.
23. We will support employers to help more people with mental health problems to remain in or move into work.
24. We will develop new approaches to help people with mental health problems who are unemployed to move into work and seek to support them during periods when they are unable to work.
25. We will stamp out discrimination across mental health.

Prepayment systems pool risks, thereby potentially redistributing benefits towards people with greater health needs, and can also be made progressive, so that poorer individuals pay less than wealthier people for equivalent access to health care. Obstacles to the use of prepayment mechanisms in low-income countries include the state of the economy, unstable governance structures, and the informality of much employment, making revenue collection impracticable.

Financing arrangements for *mental health* services vary considerably from country to country, with out-of-pocket payments (which are both inefficient and unfair) still dominating in most low-income countries [46], but actually still fairly common in some other countries [47]. As far as mental health systems are concerned, almost every country has a mix of public and private funding. Mental and physical health care needs are generally not treated with parity [48]; some insurance or managed care arrangements exclude mental health coverage in an attempt to cap expenditure, but this will then have predictably undesirable consequences for access, knock-on costs, societal inefficiencies, and inequity [49]. The so-called Obamacare in the United States (centred around the Affordable Care Act 2010) made important breakthroughs in expanding access to health insurance, including mental health coverage [50], and illustrates well the need for strategic policy efforts to be made to address financing issues.

The revenue collected from taxes or insurance premiums reaches service providers via various *commissioning or purchasing* routes. Provider reimbursement can be retrospective (such as fee-for-service) or prospective (capitation and fixed budgets). Fee-for-service arrangements encourage productivity but also perversely encourage resource consumption through unnecessary visits, diagnostic investigations, and hospitalization ('supplier-induced demand') and so can push up overall costs. Prospective payments are therefore increasingly being used to encourage cost-consciousness among providers. Capitation is a fixed payment for a defined set of benefits (treatments or health gains). It encourages efficiency but has some risks, including adverse selection and cream-skimming (where providers have no incentive to treat 'complicated or expensive' patients), which could shift costs onto other providers or sectors or lead to undertreatment [51]. A commonly used mode of prospective payment is by case-mix, for example using diagnosis-related groups (DRGs)—patients are categorized by clinical diagnosis and treatment process and a standard payment is made to the provider. DRG-based pricing is not always straightforward to implement in mental health contexts.

## Prevention and risk reduction

Reducing the number of people who develop mental health problems and delaying or avoiding relapse and symptom exacerbation must surely be high policy priorities—to head off or reduce distress and suffering for individuals and families, and potentially avoid substantial future streams of expenditure and productivity losses. Prevention and early intervention therefore figure prominently in many policy frameworks and may require action outside the health sector. Such actions can be highly effective and cost-effective, as the following examples illustrate.

Postnatal depression (PND) has high prevalence but is often undiagnosed and untreated. The effects for women and their children can be considerable. A recent systematic review looked at a range of interventions developed to prevent PND [52], finding a number of beneficial interventions, including midwifery-redesigned postnatal care, person-centred approaches, and cognitive behavioural therapy—which are intended to be universal—as well as some interventions targeted on high-risk women such as interpersonal psychotherapy (IPT). The study also compared interventions in terms of cost-effectiveness, compared to usual care, and although there was uncertainty about what might be the 'best buy', the accumulated international evidence clearly shows how prevention can have considerable benefits for mother and child and make economic sense.

School-based interventions can also be effective at preventing some mental health problems and also cost-effective such as those that aim to develop social and emotional development [53], build resilience and thereby reduce the risk of later depression [54], or instil positive behaviours to reduce tobacco use and improve well-being [55].

Suicide prevention is possible, but complex. The WHO recommends reducing access to the means of suicide (pesticides, guns, certain medications), more responsible media reporting, policies to reduce alcohol misuse, early identification and treatment of people with mental or substance use disorders who could be high risk, training of health workers to recognize, assess, and manage suicidal ideation, and follow-up support for people who have attempted suicide [56].

Another area where there is good evidence of the potential for risk reduction is in relation to dementia. Mid-life risk factors for developing Alzheimer's disease and other dementias in late life are physical inactivity, smoking, diabetes, hypertension, obesity, depression, and lower educational attainment [57]. These risk factors are clearly interconnected, but even after adjusting for correlations, almost a third of Alzheimer's disease cases might be 'attributable' to risk factors that are potentially modifiable [58].

## Effective treatments

An obvious element within any policy framework would be to ensure that effective treatments are available to people who are ill. There is not a bottomless pit of resources, however, and so a policy framework will also need to be clear about how to prioritize needs and target treatments and ensure that resources (public and private) are not wasted on treatments that are ineffective or expensive, relative to their outcomes. The extent to which a mental health policy engages in the details of prioritization, targeting, evidence generation, or cost-effectiveness recommendation depends heavily on a country's overall political approach to health policy. In England, with its central 'command-and-control' NHS, policy documents in mental health and other areas have often been quite prescriptive about the treatments to be delivered and the people who should receive them. In contrast, the health system in the United States is dominated by the private decisions of citizens (for example, in relation to the insurance plan they purchase), the independent case-level decisions of clinicians, and state-level decisions about priorities and funding generosity.

In England and Wales, much of the responsibility for evidence appraisal and prioritization has been devolved by the government to the National Institute for Health and Care Excellence (NICE). With its thorough technology appraisals and its transparently developed clinical guidelines, NICE aims to help individual clinicians and other professionals to choose the best treatments, defined as those of proven effectiveness and also cost-effectiveness in the context of NHS structures and resources. Some other countries also have health technology appraisal (HTA) mechanisms, varying in structure from country to country and leading to variation in decisions too [59].

One of the most impressive policy initiatives of recent years in *some* countries has been the closure of the old psychiatric asylums. In most European countries, and for many decades, large mental institutions dominated the landscape. Although originally built with some good intentions (to group people together to make best use of scarce skilled professionals, achieve economies of scale, and protect vulnerable individuals), these asylums were also convenient ways to allow families to hide away their 'disturbed' or socially embarrassing relatives and, in some countries, were instruments of political oppression. Many institutions provided appalling, abusive care, breaching internationally accepted human rights [60]. Where evaluations have been conducted, they demonstrated clearly the *potential* to replace institutional care with good-quality community-based care, so long as it is adequately funded [61].

There are areas where effective treatments are simply not reaching people who need them and where mental health policy has failed. Youth mental health is one area where there is an enormous treatment gap in many countries, with people aged 16–25 with mental health problems having low contact rates with services. Another failure is the frequent neglect of the physical health needs of people with mental health problems, leading to significantly truncated life expectancy. A third example of common policy failure is in relation to dementia where evidence on interventions is now accumulating rapidly [62], but where few countries have yet pulled together a coherent overall strategy, although with some notable exceptions [63]. But even these failings pale into insignificance when compared to the huge mental health treatment gap in most low-income countries of the world [64]. The WHO's mhGAP initiative mentioned earlier seeks to scale up services for mental, neurological, and substance use disorders for all countries.

Because mental health problems often affect families and other community members, a policy framework should include attention to the needs of family members, especially if they are regular (but unpaid) carers. Some countries have already developed formal carer strategies.

Treatments are not necessarily delivered only through the health care system, as conventionally defined, but could be delivered in schools and colleges, workplaces, prisons, and community services.

### Tackling inequity

There will always be inequalities, but not necessarily all of them are unfair. Inequality and inequity are not the same; the latter refers to an allocation of resources or responsibilities that is deemed to be unfair by reference to some external criteria, such as a decision-maker's preferences or society's agreed priorities, while inequality simply describes the difference between two or more things. According to the WHO, 'Equity is the absence of avoidable or remediable differences among groups of people, whether those groups are defined socially, economically, demographically, or geographically' [65].

What is meant by 'fair' is a value judgement, and hence likely to be reflected (though perhaps implicitly) in political statements or positions. Most people would probably agree that it would be equitable to allocate more treatment resources to people with greater needs, and fewer resources to people with less needs. But there might not

be such ready agreement that it is equitable for poorer individuals to pay less for their treatment than wealthier individuals; not everyone supports redistributive policies of this kind.

It is abundantly clear from many studies that the risk of mental illness is not equally or fairly distributed across the population, and neither is access to effective treatment. Socio-economic status plays a big part in these unequal distributions. Both absolute and relative poverty affect the development of emotional, behavioural, and psychiatric problems [10, 66]. It is not only socio-economic status that can influence incidence, prevalence, and treatment, but also race, ethnicity, gender, age, language, religion, sexual preference, and place of residence [67].

As noted earlier, there is a vicious cycle linking mental illness with social and economic disadvantage. For any mental health policy to be successful, it must surely find ways to break into that cycle. It needs to ensure that effective treatment and support are accessible to everyone, regardless of individual characteristics, social position, or the ability to pay. It should support efforts to build resilience and invest in mental health literacy. It needs to support wider efforts to tackle poor housing, unequal access to education and employment, and basic material poverty. It must protect and promote human rights [68]. In countries without prepayment financing mechanisms (tax- or insurance-based) or where such arrangements are only affordable by the wealthy, introducing funding reform would make an enormous difference to access and better mental health [46].

### Opportunities, choice, and control

When people with mental health problems were contained in large, remote asylums, they were denied the most basic of liberties and rights, often for many decades. A prominent feature of most mental health policies today is to broaden the range of opportunities that are available, tackling the endemic inequities that damage so many people's lives. Indeed, there are a number of different, but connected, themes that feature in policy discussions today, including opportunities, choice, control, personalization, and recovery.

One important area is employment; creating better opportunities and breaking down attitudinal barriers can help to socially integrate someone with a history of mental health problems, make them economically independent, and potentially head off exacerbation of their illness. Widening choice is seen as intrinsically desirable; it leads to greater autonomy and arguably better well-being. Giving people more choice and control over their lives, including the support services they use, can benefit both health and well-being and also prove cost-effective. Experiments in England in devolved funding through personal budgets for social care and continuing health care achieved encouraging results [69, 70].

The concept of recovery—not in the clinical sense of symptom alleviation or cure, but in a broader, personal sense—is attracting growing attention. It is associated particularly with arguments propounded by Bill Anthony some years ago:

'[Recovery is] a deeply personal, unique process of changing one's attitudes, values, feelings, goals, skills, and/or roles. It is a way of living a satisfying, hopeful, and contributing life even with limitations caused by illness. Recovery involves the development of new meaning and purpose in one's life as one grows beyond the catastrophic effects of mental illness.' [71]

The top priority in the English government's 2014 mental health policy statement was 'High quality mental health services with an emphasis on recovery should be commissioned in all areas' (Box 134.1). Specific recovery-focused initiatives might include peer support arrangements, opportunities for self-managing treatment, supported employment, advice on welfare entitlements and how to manage debt, advance treatment directives, health promotion, personal budgets, and recovery colleges [72].

## Attitudes and discrimination

At a strategic or societal level, policies are needed to raise awareness of mental illness, improve knowledge about prevention and treatment, tackle prejudice and stigma, and directly combat discrimination. In terms of individual experience, policies are needed to stamp out bullying and victimization. In these ways, it is hoped that there will be a number of gains—more supportive attitudes will lead to less treatment avoidance by people experiencing poor mental health, and so fewer delays in their taking up appropriate treatment, and hence better health and well-being. National anti-stigma programmes have been successful [73] and can be cost-effective [74]. More targeted anti-bullying interventions can certainly help too.

## Co-ordinated action

Policy intentions and actions must be co-ordinated, given that people with mental health problems, especially if severe or enduring, often have needs that span a number of different service systems. Their needs could require action and support from health, social care, education, housing, employment, welfare benefits, criminal justice, and other systems, and these will need co-ordination to ensure that vulnerable people do not 'fall through the cracks'. A mental health policy therefore needs to include a strategy for bringing together the various local, regional, and national bodies and processes that are involved, directly or tangentially, in supporting individuals and families. It needs to resolve funding issues (especially given the propensity for silo-budgeting), co-ordinate assessment procedures, and agree on both short-term and longer-term objectives. Co-ordination is needed not just across the public sector, but also with non-public entities such as employers, schools, and community groups.

## Concluding comments

As noted at the outset, mental health problems represent or combine a number of complex issues and characteristics. Incidence is commonly early in life, and prevalence of many conditions is enduring over much of the life-course. The distress associated with mental illness can be immense, and there can be adverse consequences for family members and friends. People with severe and enduring problems may face enormous difficulties in securing and retaining paid employment. Many will face discrimination in employment and other areas of everyday life: education, participation, citizenship, and access to community resources. It is still common in many countries today for people with mental health problems to be locked away in large institutions that deny basic human rights and offer little active treatment. People with mental health problems have shorter lives because of their poor physical health, due in large part to their lifestyle, and they are at much higher risk of self-harm and suicide. The symptoms of illness or needs for material resources may lead a

minority of people to commit violent or acquisitive crimes. All societies have the legal powers to compulsorily detain and treat people.

The policy challenges of mental illness therefore are many and huge. A policy framework needs to recognize the complex aetiology of illness and respond to the wide range of individual, social, and economic impacts that often follow. It also needs to tackle some wide inequalities, many of them representing gross inequities in individual experiences and opportunities. Commitment to social justice should be a core part of any mental health policy.

A good mental health policy would invest significant resources in prevention and risk reduction and ensure timely diagnosis and early intervention. It would include a strategy for developing, delivering, and ensuring access to effective and cost-effective treatments. Parity with physical health treatment is essential. Barriers to treatment and services need to be removed, whether due to ignorance, inability to pay, funder prejudice, or provider discrimination. The symptoms of an illness may themselves contribute to access difficulties.

A good mental health policy would adopt a life-course perspective, intervening early enough to prevent more serious symptoms and their consequences. It would promote co-ordinated multisector efforts to identify, assess, respond, and fund appropriate actions. Families and communities may need to be involved in some decisions and may themselves have needs that should be addressed. But through it all, the individual with a mental illness should be at the centre and should be given as many opportunities and as much choice and control as is possible and appropriate, given their circumstances and state of health. Finally, a good mental health policy should include ongoing commitment to change societal attitudes to mental illness, promoting recovery in its modern interpretation.

## REFERENCES

1. Kessler, Ronald C., Patricia Berglund, Olga Demler, *et al.* (2005). Lifetime prevalence and age-of-onset distributions of DSM-IV disorders in the National Comorbidity Survey Replication. *Archives of General Psychiatry*, 62: 593–602.
2. Takizawa, Ryu, Barbara Maughan, and Louise Arseneault. (2014). Adult Health Outcomes of Childhood Bullying Victimization: Evidence From a Five-Decade Longitudinal British Birth Cohort. *American Journal of Psychiatry*, 171: 777–84.
3. Evans-Lacko, Sara, Ryu Takizawa, Nicola Brimblecombe, *et al.* (2017). Childhood bullying victimisation is associated with use of mental health services over 5 decades: a longitudinal nationally-representative cohort study. *Psychological Medicine*, 47: 127–35.
4. Henquet, Cécile, Robin Murray, Don Linszen, and Jim van Os. (2005). The environment and schizophrenia: the role of cannabis use. *Schizophrenia Bulletin*, 31: 608–12.
5. Oddy, Wendy H., Garth E. Kendall, Jianghong Li, *et al.* (2010). The long-term effects of breastfeeding on child and adolescent mental health: a pregnancy cohort study followed for 14 years'. *Journal of Pediatrics*, 156: 568–74.
6. Naylor, Chris, Michael Parsonage, David McDaid, Martin Knapp, Matt Fossey, and Amy Galea. *Long-term Conditions and Mental Health: The Cost of Co-morbidities.* London: The King's Fund; 2012.
7. Welch, Charles, A., David Czerwinski, Bijay Ghimire, and Dimitris Bertsimas. (2009). Depression and costs of health care. *Psychosomatics*, 50: 392–401.
8. Das Munshi, Jayati, Rob Stewart, Khalida Ismail, Paul E. Bebbington, Rachel Jenkins and Martin J. Prince. (2007).

Diabetes, common mental disorders, and disability: findings from the UK National Psychiatric Morbidity Survey. *Psychosomatic Medicine*, 69: 543–50.

9. Simonoff, Emily, Andrew Pickles, Tony Charman, Susie Chandler, Tom Loucas, and Gillian Baird. (2008). Psychiatric disorders in children with autism spectrum disorders: prevalence, comorbidity, and associated factors in a population-derived sample. *Journal of the American Academy of Child and Adolescent Psychiatry*, 47: 921–9.

10. Murali, Vijaya and Femi Oyebode. (2004). Poverty, social inequality and mental health. *Advances in Psychiatric Treatment*, 10: 216–24.

11. Stuckler, David and Sanjay Basu. *The Body Economic: Why Austerity Kills*. London: Basic Books; 2013.

12. Evans-Lacko, Sara, Emilie Courtin, Andrea Fiorillo, *et al*. (2014). The state of the art in European research on reducing social exclusion and stigma related to mental health: a systematic mapping of the literature. *European Psychiatry*, 29: 381–9.

13. Organisation for Economic Co-operation and Development. *Sick on the Job? Myths and Realities About Mental Health and Work*. Paris: OECD Publishing; 2012.

14. Kessler, Ronald, C., Steven Heeringa, Matthew D. Lakoma, *et al*. (2008). Individual and societal effects of mental disorders on earnings in the United States: results from the national comorbidity survey replication. *American Journal of Psychiatry*, 165: 703–11.

15. Fitch, Chris, Sarah Hamilton, Paul Bassett, and Ryan Davey. (2011). The relationship between personal debt and mental health: a systematic review. *Mental Health Review Journal*, 16: 153–66.

16. Evans-Lacko, Sara and Martin Knapp. (2016). Global patterns of workplace productivity for people with depression: absenteeism and presenteeism costs across eight diverse countries. *Social Psychiatry and Psychiatric Epidemiology*, 51: 1525–37.

17. Fleischhacker, Wolfgang, Celso Arango, Paul Arteel, *et al*. (2014). Schizophrenia: time to commit to policy change', *Schizophrenia Bulletin*, vol. 40, supplement 3: 165–94.

18. Flynn, Sandra, Cathryn Rodway, Louis Appleby, and Jenny Shaw. (2014). Serious Violence by People With Mental Illness: National Clinical Survey. *Journal of Interpersonal Violence*, 29: 1438–58.

19. McCrone, Paul, Paulo Menezes, Sonia Johnson, *et al*. Service use and costs of people with dual diagnosis in South London. *Acta Psychiatrica Scandinavica*, 101: 464–72.

20. Swartz, Marvin S., Jeffrey W. Swanson, Virginia Aldigé Hiday, Randy Borum, H. Ryan Wagner, Barbara J. Burns. (1998). Violence and severe mental illness: the effects of substance abuse and nonadherence to medication. *American Journal of Psychiatry*, 155: 226–31.

21. Green, Hazel, Áine McGinnity, Howard Meltzer, Tamsin Ford, and Robert Goodman. *Mental Health of Children and Young People in Great Britain, 2004*. Basingstoke: Palgrave Macmillan; 2005.

22. Scott, Stephen, Martin Knapp, Juliet Henderson, and Barbara Maughan. (2001). Financial cost of social exclusion: follow up study of antisocial children into adulthood. *BMJ*, 323: 191–4.

23. Hughes, Karen, Mark A. Bellis, Lisa Jones, *et al*. (2012). Prevalence and risk of violence against adults with disabilities: a systematic review and meta-analysis of observational studies. *Lancet*, 379: 1621–9.

24. World Health Organization. *Information Sheet: Premature Death Among People with Severe Mental Disorder*. Geneva: World Health Organization. Available from: http://www.who.int/mental_health/management/info_sheet.pdf

25. Chang, Shu-Sen, David Stuckler, Paul Yip, and David Gunnell. (2013). Impact of 2008 global economic crisis on suicide: time trend study in 54 countries. *BMJ*, 347: f5239.

26. Hong, Jihyung, Martin Knapp and Alistair McGuire. (2011). Income-related inequalities in the prevalence of depression and suicidal behaviour: a 10-year trend following economic crisis. *World Psychiatry*, 10: 40–4.

27. Chang, Chin-Kuo, Richard D. Hayes, Gayan Perera, *et al*. (2011). Life expectancy at birth for people with serious mental illness and other major disorders from a secondary mental health care case register in London. *PLoS One*, 6: e19590.

28. McManus, Sally, Howard Meltzer, and Jonathan Campion. *Cigarette Smoking and Mental Health in England. Data from the Adult Psychiatric Morbidity Survey*. London: National Centre for Social Research; 2010.

29. McCreadie, Robin G. and Scottish Schizophrenia Lifestyle Group. (2003). Diet, smoking and cardiovascular risk in people with schizophrenia: descriptive study. *British Journal of Psychiatry*, 183: 534–9.

30. Rummel-Kluge, Christine, Katja Komossa, Sandra Schwarz, *et al*. (2010). Head-to-head comparisons of metabolic side effects of second-generation antipsychotics in the treatment of schizophrenia: a systematic review and meta-analysis. *Schizophrenia Research*, 123: 225–33.

31. Mahoney, Rachel, Ciaran Regan, Cornelius Katona, and Gill Livingston. (2005). Anxiety and depression in family caregivers of people with Alzheimer disease: the LASER-AD study. *American Journal of Geriatric Psychiatry*, 13: 795–801.

32. Martín, Josune, Angel Padierna, Bob van Wijngaarden, *et al*. (2015). Caregivers consequences of care among patients with eating disorders, depression or schizophrenia. *BMC Psychiatry*, 15: 124.

33. Yaffe, Kristine, Patrick Fox, Robert Newcomer, *et al*. (2002). Patient and caregiver characteristics and nursing home placement in patients with dementia. *JAMA*, 287: 2090–7.

34. Romeo, Renee, Martin Knapp, and Stephen Scott. (2006). Economic cost of severe antisocial behaviour in children—and who pays it. *British Journal of Psychiatry*, 188: 547–53.

35. Bauer, Annette, Martin Knapp, and Michael Parsonage. (2016). Lifetime costs of perinatal anxiety and depression. *Journal of Affective Disorders*, 192: 83–90.

36. Harpin, Val. (2005). The effect of ADHD on the life of an individual, their family, and community from preschool to adult life. *Archives of Disease in Childhood*, 90: i2–7.

37. Clement, Sarah, Oliver Schauman, Tanya Graham, *et al*. What is the impact of mental health-related stigma on help-seeking? A systematic review of quantitative and qualitative studies. *Psychological Medicine*, 45: 11–27.

38. Evans-Lacko, Sara and Martin Knapp. (2014). Importance of social and cultural factors for attitudes, disclosure and time off work for depression: findings from a seven country European study on depression in the workplace. *PLoS One*, 9: e91053.

39. Prince, Martin, Martin Knapp, Maelenn Guerchet, *et al*. *Dementia UK*, second edition. London: Alzheimer's Society; 2014.

40. Knapp, Martin, Derek King, Andrew Healey, and Cicely Thomas. (2011). Economic outcomes in adulthood and their associations with antisocial conduct, attention deficit and anxiety problems in childhood. *Journal of Mental Health Policy and Economics*, 14: 122–32.

41. D'Amico, Francesco, Martin Knapp, Jennifer Beecham, Eric Taylor, and Kapil Sayal. (2014). Use of services and associated costs for young adults with childhood hyperactivity/conduct

problems: 20-year follow-up. *British Journal of Psychiatry*, 204: 441–7.

42. World Health Organization. *The Mental Health Context*. Geneva: World Health Organization; 2003.

43. Department of Health. *Closing the Gap: Priorities for Essential Change in Mental Health*. Social Care, Local Government and Care Partnership Directorate. 2014. Available from: https://www.gov.uk/government/uploads/system/uploads/attachment_data/file/281250/Closing_the_gap_V2_-_17_Feb_2014.pdf

44. Independent Mental Health Taskforce to the NHS in England. *The Five-Year Forward View for Mental Health*. 2016. Available from: https://www.england.nhs.uk/wp-content/uploads/2016/02/Mental-Health-Taskforce-FYFV-final.pdf

45. Organisation for Economic Co-operation and Development. *Financing of health care. In Health at a Glance 2015: OECD Indicators*. Paris: OECD Publishing; 2015. Available from: http://dx.doi.org/10.1787/health_glance-2015-62-en

46. Dixon, Anna, David McDaid, Martin Knapp, and Claire Curran. (2006). Financing mental health services in low- and middle-income countries. *Health Policy and Planning*, 21: 171–82.

47. Sevilla-Dedieu, Christine, Viviane Kovess-Masféty, Fabien Gilbert, *et al.* (2011). Mental health care and out-of-pocket expenditures in Europe: results from the ESEMeD project. *Journal of Mental Health Policy and Economics*, 14: 95–105.

48. Barry, Colleen L. and Haiden A. Huskamp. (2011). Moving beyond parity—mental health and addiction care under the ACA. *New England Journal of Medicine*, 365: 973–5.

49. Knapp, Martin and David McDaid. Economic realities: financing, resourcing, challenging, resolving. In: Martin Knapp, David McDaid, Elias Mossialos, Graham Thornicroft, editors. *Mental Health Policy and Practice Across Europe*. Buckingham: Open University Press; 2007.

50. Burns, Marguerite E. and Barbara L. Wolfe. (2016). The effects of the Affordable Care Act adult dependent coverage expansion on mental health. *Journal of Mental Health Policy and Economics*, 19: 3–20.

51. Glied, Sherry and Allison Evans Cuellar. (2003). Trends and issues in child and adolescent mental health. *Health Affairs*, 22: 39–50.

52. Morrell, C. Jane, Paul Sutcliffe, Andrew Booth, *et al.* (2016). A systematic review, evidence synthesis and meta-analysis of quantitative and qualitative studies evaluating the clinical effectiveness, the cost-effectiveness, safety and acceptability of interventions to prevent postnatal depression. *Health Technology Assessment*, 20: 1–414.

53. Durlak, Joseph. A., Roger P. Weissberg, Allison B. Dymnicki, Rebecca D. Taylor, and Kriston B. Schellinger. (2011). The impact of enhancing students' social and emotional learning: a meta-analysis of school-based universal interventions. *Child Development*, 82: 405–32.

54. Stockings, Emily, Louisa Degenhardt, Timothy Dobbins, *et al.* (2016). Preventing depression and anxiety in young people: a review of the joint efficacy of universal, selective and indicated prevention. *Psychological Medicine*, 46: 11–26.

55. Aos, Steve, Roxanne Lieb, Jim Mayfield, Marna Miller, and Annie Pennucci. *Benefits and Costs of Prevention and Early Intervention Programs for Youth*. Olympia, WA: Institute for Public Policy; 2004.

56. World Health Organization. *Suicide Fact Sheet*. Geneva: World Health Organization. 2016. Available from: https://www.who.int/news-room/fact-sheets/detail/suicide

57. Barnes, Deborah and Kristine Yaffe. (2013). The projected impact of risk factor reduction on Alzheimer's Disease prevalence. *Lancet Neurology*, 10: 819–28.

58. Norton, Sam, Fiona E. Matthews, Deborah E. Barnes, Kristine Yaffe, and Carol Brayne. (2014). Potential for primary prevention of Alzheimer's disease: an analysis of population-based data. *Lancet Neurology*, 13: 788–94.

59. Cerri, Karin, Martin Knapp, and Jose-Luis Fernandez. (2015). Untangling the complexity of funding recommendations: a comparative analysis of health technology assessment outcomes in four European countries. *Pharmaceutical Medicine*, 29: 341–59.

60. Mansell, Jim, Martin Knapp, Julie Beadle-Brown, and Jennifer Beecham. *Deinstitutionalisation and Community Living: Outcomes and Costs*. Vol 1–3. Canterbury: Tizard Centre, University of Kent.

61. Knapp, Martin, Jennifer Beecham, David McDaid, Tihana Matosevic, and Monique Smith. (2011). The economic consequences of deinstitutionalisation of mental health services: lessons from European experience. *Health and Social Care in the Community*, 19: 113–25.

62. Winblad, Bengt, Philippe Amouyel, Sandrine Andrieu, *et al.* Defeating Alzheimer's disease and other dementias: a priority for European science and society. *Lancet Neurology*, 15: 455–532.

63. Department of Health. *Prime Minister's Challenge on Dementia 2020*. 2015. Available from: https://www.gov.uk/government/publications/prime-ministers-challenge-on-dementia-2020

64. World Health Organization. *WHO Mental Health Gap Action Programme (mhGAP)*. 2016. Available from: http://www.who.int/mental_health/mhgap/en/

65. World Health Organization. *Health Systems: Equity*. Available from: http://www.who.int/healthsystems/topics/equity/en/

66. Pickett, Kate E., Oliver W. James, and Richard G. Wilkinson. (2006). Income inequality and the prevalence of mental illness: a preliminary international analysis. *Journal of Epidemiology and Community Health*, 60: 646–7.

67. Alegria, Margarita, Melissa Vallas, and Andres Pumariega. (2010). Racial and ethnic disparities in pediatric mental health. *Child and Adolescent Psychiatric Clinics of North America*, 19: 759–74.

68. Lund, Crick, Mary De Silva, Sophie Plagerson, *et al.* (2011). Poverty and mental disorders: breaking the cycle in low-income and middle-income countries. *Lancet*, 378: 1502–14.

69. Netten, Ann, Karen Jones, Martin Knapp, *et al.* (2012). Personalisation through Individual Budgets: does it work and for whom. *British Journal of Social Work*, 42: 1556–73.

70. Forder, Julien, Karen Jones, Caroline Glendinning, *et al.* *Evaluation of the Personal Health Budget Pilot Programme*. London: Department of Health; 2012.

71. Anthony, William A. (1993). Recovery from mental illness: the guiding vision of the mental health system in the 1990s. *Psychosocial Rehabilitation Journal*, 16: 11–23.

72. Knapp, Martin, Alison Andrew, and David McDaid, *et al.* *Investing in Recovery*. London: Rethink Mental Illness; 2014.

73. Jorm, Anthony F., Helen Christensen, and Kathleen M. Griffiths. (2009). The impact of Beyondblue: the national depression initiative on the Australian public's recognition of depression and beliefs about treatments. *Australian and New Zealand Journal of Psychiatry*, 39: 248–54.

74. Evans-Lacko, Sara, Claire Henderson, Graham Thornicroft, and Paul McCrone. (2013). Economic evaluation of the anti-stigma social marketing campaign in England 2009–2011. *British Journal of Psychiatry* Supplement, 55: 95–101.

# 135

# Planning and providing mental health services for a community

*Tom Burns and Tony Kendrick*

## Introduction

The aim of this chapter is to assist clinicians and managers review and plan services effectively for their local population. Severe psychiatric disorders manifest themselves in social relations and often disrupt social structures; they have wide-ranging consequences, so services need to be comprehensive, providing both health and social care. Neither can be ignored in the wider context of their management.

Planning mental health services rarely starts with a clean sheet. Where there is one, Tansella and Thornicroft's 'matrix' model [1] is a particularly thorough and structured guide. It outlines service principles and needs assessment (at national, regional, and local levels) through to monitoring the cycle of planning and provision. Their hierarchical approach reflects the level of spend [2]. Case identification and outpatient treatments in primary care are the priority for low-income countries, and only with increased resources the establishment of a secondary care mental health service [usually a form of generic community mental health team (CMHT)]. Not until these are well established are specialist and inpatient services indicated. This process must, however, take account of what is already in place.

The range of spend and local cultures in mental health services is enormous, and attempting to address all of these would result in a series of unhelpful generalized statements. In this chapter, we will focus on the UK because it is an example of a relatively coherent, developed system with a culture of research. The specificity of many of the descriptions should not be interpreted as a prescription, but as a platform for local consideration and decisions.

## Mental health services research

The last 40 years have seen an explosion of mental health services research, alongside the shrinking and closure of mental hospitals (see Chapter 134). The research agenda is disproportionately anglophone, testing innovative alternatives to institutional care. More routine practices, crucial for safe and effective care, have been relatively neglected.

## Scope of chapter

This chapter will describe the essential components of a mental health service. It will cover how they relate to one another, how they are linked into other essential services, and how their evolution should be monitored. Services for adults of working age (18–65 years) will be used as template. In many settings, these may be the only services. In better-resourced systems, a range of specialized services have evolved which are described elsewhere (see Chapter 138).

## Prevalence of mental illness within the community

Mental illnesses are common, and it is estimated that around 25% of people will suffer from a mental disorder at some point in their lives. However, most of these people will not see a psychiatrist. A useful starting point in service planning is to use any available prevalence figures to estimate the number of people with particular conditions in the community. In the UK, the periodic national Psychiatric Morbidity Survey [3], run by the UK Office of National Statistics (ONS), revealed the following prevalence of disorders among adults in England in 2007 [according to the criteria of the World Health Organization's *International Classification of Diseases*, tenth revision (ICD-10)] [4]:

- Mixed anxiety and depression, 9.7%.
- Generalized anxiety disorder (GAD), 4.7%.
- Depressive episode, 2.6%.
- Phobia, 2.6%.
- Obsessive–compulsive disorder (OCD), 1.3%.
- Panic disorder, 1.2%.
- Psychotic disorders (including schizophrenia and bipolar disorder), 0.5%.

In the UK, the first six of these disorders are termed common mental health disorders (CMHDs), and the last severe (or serious) mental illness (SMI). The overall prevalence of CMHDs, which are not mutually exclusive, was found to be 17.6% [3], while the prevalence of SMI was likely to have been underestimated by the community survey, and other estimates range between 0.5% and 2%, with higher rates found in the inner city [5].

## Treatment in primary care

In the UK, around 70–80% of people with CMHDs are treated only in primary care by general practitioners (GPs), usually with SSRI antidepressants [6], while 10–15% are referred, or refer themselves, for psychological therapies offered by the Improving Access to Psychological Therapies (IAPT) programme [7]. That means only the remaining 5–10% of people with CMHDs receive care from multidisciplinary mental health services, although they will be the most severely affected people. GPs may also be involved in the mental health care of people with SMI in the UK, although the majority, at least two-thirds, will be receiving care from mental health services [8].

This means at any one time, around 15–20 adults per 1000 will be in contact with mental health services in the UK, of whom the large majority will be suffering from SMI. It also means that a relatively small increase, of say 5%, in the proportion of people with CMHDs referred from primary care to mental health services would increase the workload of those services by around a third to a half!

## Referral from primary to secondary care

Ideally, there should be a clear understanding between psychiatrists and their local GPs, to ensure that only the more needy patients who really require a specialist opinion are referred. Box 135.1 lists suggested referral criteria for patients with depression.

Agreeing referral criteria like these, however, does require the psychiatrist to accept referrals which meet them. The psychiatric team needs to offer treatments which are not usually provided by the GP, including intensive support with or without hospital admission, electroconvulsive therapy (ECT), prophylactic lithium or other mood stabilizers, etc. Simply prescribing another antidepressant and returning the person to their GP's care is not an adequate response to a GP who has already tried three courses of antidepressants combined with psychological therapy.

## Building blocks of secondary mental health services: care and treatment

Most mental health treatments (whether psychological, pharmacological, or social) involve face-to-face interviews and require no

### Box 135.1 Indications for referral of patients with depression

- Poor response to antidepressants (three different drugs sequentially) and psychological therapy (if available).
- Recurrent episode within 1 year of last episode.
- Self-neglect.
- Postnatal depression.
- Assessment for possible bipolar disorder.
- Suicidal ideas and plans (urgent referral).
- Psychotic symptoms (urgent referral).

sophisticated equipment. Asylums provided social care, protecting disabled individuals while they recovered and, sometimes, protecting society from them. Patients needing long-term institutional care are now very few, but psychiatry is still judged on how they are cared for and services must pay them due attention.

## Inpatient beds

No comprehensive service can survive without access to 24-hour nursing supervision for acute episodes of severe illness. They are needed for patients at risk from neglect or suicide, usually lacking sufficient insight to co-operate with treatment. Wards usually accommodate 10–20 patients. It is rarely possible to effectively staff and run stand-alone units of fewer than 3–4 such wards (30–60 beds). Ward size is a trade-off between privacy and domesticity against safety and effective supervision. Single rooms afford privacy and, while initially expensive, improve flexibility and reduce conflict.

Smaller, more flexible units, such as 'crisis houses', offering 24-hour care are a useful complement to inpatient wards, but not an effective replacement. Ward design and management are increasingly crucial as improved community care means that inpatients are mostly involuntary and highly disturbed.

## How many acute beds?

'How many beds do we need for our local population?' is often the first question asked by planners or managers. Unfortunately, there is no reliable or precise answer to this. Supply will drive use (perceived as need) and beds are rarely left empty despite enormous variation in their availability. International comparisons are complicated by differences in methods of reporting and a profusion of overlapping ill-defined local terms (for example, night hospitals, crisis homes, step-down wards). Levels of hostels and day care also impact the need for acute beds, which reduces as community services become more comprehensive.

European provision of general acute mental health beds in the public sector in the early 2000s ranged from 64 beds per 100,000 in Germanic settings to 6 per 100,000 in Italy and Spain [9]. However, these figures tell us relatively little unless we know the levels of private and social services care provision. In the UK, with little parallel private care, overall provision has shrunk by 62% between 1988 and 2008 [10].

Current low bed usage in the UK reflects recently established home treatment and crisis resolution teams and the expansion of forensic care, but also a shift in practice. The duration for admissions has steadily reduced over the last four decades. Mean durations are heavily skewed by short (1- to 2-day) crisis admissions, but patients with uncomplicated psychotic relapses usually stay between 3 and 6 weeks.

## Longer inpatient care

Acute inpatient wards are designed to admit patients for weeks or, at most, a couple of months, with rapid discharge anticipated, but some patients require longer or more secure care because of either illness severity or legal restrictions. Modern long-stay and rehabilitation wards are essentially restricted to patients with behaviour that is persistently unacceptable to local communities. Forensic and secure services are usually a regional or national, rather than local, responsibility.

## Diagnosis-specific wards

Alcohol and substance abuse wards are common in much of Europe, and diagnosis- or disorder-specific wards in academic services. Specialized wards for patients with anorexia nervosa or resistant schizophrenia provide highly specific regimes, but usually alongside acute admission wards, rather than as an alternative. Some services now organize wards by care pathway clusters (for example, a psychosis unit, an affective disorders ward), instead of general wards. Such specialization is still experimental and not particularly feasible in comprehensive services for smaller populations, as they reduce flexibility and absorb energy in 'boundary disputes'.

## Day care

Day care is provided either in day hospitals or in day centres. The two terms and their practices overlap and vary enormously. Attendance generally ranges from half a day to 5 days a week, and many now remain open in the evenings and at weekends.

Day hospitals are provided by the health service, include medical and nursing staff, and provide treatments such as medication and psychotherapies. They figured prominently in the plans to move to district general hospital psychiatry. However, their role shrank as CMHTs expanded, taking over much of their anticipated role. Day hospitals were scaled down or even closed, shifting ongoing support to social services day centres. However, they have recently been reinvigorated as a key ingredient in home treatment teams.

Day centres, provided by social care organizations, do not usually provide complex treatments or employ clinical staff. However, their practice is highly specific to local context. A drop-in day centre may provide psychiatric assessment and treatment in deprived areas with high levels of homelessness. Generally, day centres provide long-term social support, and day hospitals focused interventions and treatments [11]. The 'Club House' is a specialized rehabilitation day centre, popularized in the United States, where members run the centre with minimal supervision.

Acute day hospitals in Europe and partial hospitalization in the United States have been trialled as alternatives to inpatient care [12] but did not catch on, although they have been recently revitalized as bases for crisis resolution teams. Specialized therapeutic day hospitals serve specific groups such as personality disorders [13] or eating disorders. Day care is problematic in rural settings, but adaptations such as travelling day centres or open days run by CMHTs have all been tried successfully.

## Supported accommodation and residential care

Many patients can only survive outside hospital with support and supervision to ensure self-care and continued medication and to anticipate and defuse crises. This can be provided by voluntary agencies, social services, or health services. Voluntary agencies tend to be more efficient at providing long-term residential care [14], but they may be reluctant to accept high-risk patients with a history of violence or substance abuse. A mixed economy works best, and the need for health services provision will depend on the vigour of local voluntary and social services. Purpose-built units do exist, but shared adapted houses are more common and promote integration and reduce stigma.

Supported or sheltered accommodation can be classified by levels of increasing need:

1. *Group homes* have no regular staff and are reserved for relatively independent patients, with visits by CMHT staff.
2. *Day-staffed hostels* have one or two day staff to support and monitor patients (encouraging cooking and cleaning, etc.). Specific treatments are provided by the CMHT.
3. *Night-staffed hostels* have non-clinical staff sleeping over, providing safety and support.
4. *24-hour staffed/nursed hostels* have on-site clinical staff overnight either sleeping in or, sometimes, awake. They are expensive, generally for patients with long-term severe illnesses, sometimes including involuntary patients ('hospital hostels'). They tend to be larger, usually with 10–20 residents.

Most comprehensive local services provide levels 1 and 2, and most social services undertake to provide level 3. Level 4 hostels are relatively rare.

## Office-based care and outpatient clinics

In insurance-based systems (the United States and much of Europe), psychiatrists may run individual office practices and manage patients on their own. In directly state-funded systems, this is rare and most psychiatrists work in outpatient clinics or CMHTs. Financial considerations can inhibit integration and service developments if they pose a threat to practitioners' livelihoods. Office-based practice is neglected in academic and policy publications. It is usually focused on either psychotherapy or pharmacotherapy and is poorly equipped for managing severe disorders.

Outpatient clinics are increasingly replacing office practice. Psychiatrists and psychologists may still operate independently within them, but with access to enhanced resources and second opinions. In the public sector, outpatient clinics may operate either alongside CMHTs or as part of them (which works better for severe illness) [15]. They provide for efficient assessment, treatment, and monitoring.

## Community mental health centres

Mental hospitals, for all their faults, had no problems co-ordinating care; what little was available was all in the same place. Community mental health centres (CMHCs) were established in the late 1960s, initially in the United States, to provide a wide range of services located in shared buildings (for example, depot clinics, a day hospital, psychotherapy services). Early CMHCs in the United States failed to engage psychosis patients because they lacked any outreach, and this, with an ideological down-playing of the 'medical model', made it impossible to recruit psychiatrists.

Now CMHCs provide accommodation for CMHTs and other services such as day care. This shared accommodation helps sustain clinical standards by reducing professional isolation with dispersed community services otherwise risking becoming idiosyncratic and rigid in their practice.

## Multi-disciplinary community mental health teams

Most community mental health services consist of one form or another of multi-disciplinary CMHT. This comprises psychiatrists, nurses, and social workers plus other specialist staff such as psychologists, occupational therapists, employment specialists, etc. Regular meetings to assess and review the management of patients incorporate a wide range of professional perspectives and allocate tasks based on skills and needs.

## The sector CMHT ('the CMHT')

### Who it is for

The CMHT is the fundamental building block of most modern community mental health services. Mental hospital catchment areas, which often covered a whole city or county, were divided into sectors of 50,000–100,000 inhabitants to facilitate continuity of care. The team could gain familiarity with most of its long-term patients and also some personal knowledge of the referring doctors and community resources. Western European sectors now range from 20,000–50,000 population, determined both by resources (shrinking as investment and specialization increase) and by local characteristics. With more specialized teams, CMHT responsibilities shrink and sector size may increase, but keeping its caseload fairly constant. Two hundred or so patients is about the maximum manageable to exploit multi-disciplinary working effectively.

CMHTs offer assessment and care for patients who cannot be adequately treated in primary care, so they prioritize severe mental illnesses. A trial of community mental health nurse care for people with CMHDs [16] showed no benefit over usual GP care, even when the nurses were trained in problem-solving therapy (a brief CBT-based therapy for CMHDs). Diversion of mental health staff away from a focus on people with SMI does not appear to be a cost-effective strategy. However, diagnosis is not all—social adversity, personality difficulties, or substance abuse can make secondary mental health care necessary, even for apparently 'minor' disorders. Instruments to clarify this threshold have been tried and, indeed, introduced in some countries [17] but are of questionable value. Refusal to assess a patient, not surprisingly, irritates referring GPs and most teams rely on clinical assessments.

CMHTs can be remarkably inefficient if little thought is given to their structure and procedures. Agreement is needed on their purpose, clientele, and systems of management, and they have often suffered from a lack of clarity and leadership.

## Staffing and management

CMHT staffing varies enormously and there is no uniform model, although the general trend is towards bigger, better-staffed teams.

Small teams of less than six can rarely provide comprehensive care or cross-cover, while teams of more than 15 or so, or with many part-time workers, become unwieldy, overwhelmed with management and information transfer. CMHTs emphasize skill-sharing and a degree of generic working and have evolved an informal, democratic style [18]. This often generates confusion about clinical leadership (originally provided by senior medical staff). With increased staff numbers and treatment complexity, 'team managers' now co-ordinate procedures, varying from being purely administrative to setting clinical priorities and supervising staff. Establishing a clear understanding of clinical leadership in CMHTs (without inhibiting initiative and creativity) is essential for effective functioning. If leadership and management are separated, the roles need to be well defined and the relationships good.

## Assessments

The key to good care is accurate assessment (see Chapter 137). Traditionally, psychiatrists conducted all initial assessments (usually in an outpatient clinic) and involved team members in treatment. Increasingly, other disciplines have taken a role in assessments, either individually or jointly with the psychiatrist. This issue generates strong feelings, but there is surprisingly little research into it. With highly developed primary care, non-medical assessments may be effective, but otherwise medical staff should prioritize time for assessments. With severely ill patients, home-based assessments pay considerable dividends [19].

## Case management

Most CMHT staff act as clinical case managers [20, 21] with responsibility for the co-ordination, delivery, and review of care for their patients. Caseloads should be explicitly limited (usually 15–25), and reviews systematic and recorded. In the UK, this has been formalized as the Care Programme Approach (CPA) [22]. Fig. 135.1 shows a care plan indicating a patient's needs or problems, the interventions proposed to meet them, who is responsible and who is informed, plus an agreed date for review. Such concise structured paperwork (as with the risk assessment and contingency plan) (Fig. 135.2) can be adapted to any team. It co-ordinates complex care and serves as a natural focus for clinical reviews. The level of detail needs to be clinically (not managerially) determined.

## Team meetings

Many of the newer, specialized teams meet daily. For generic CMHTs, it would be an inefficient use of time. They generally have 1–2 regular meetings of 1.5–2 hours each per week to cover clinical and administrative business. The degree of structure depends on team style and remit.

## Allocation of referrals

Referrals can be allocated by who is first available or by matching the clinical problem against available skill and training. Time discussing

---

## CPA REVIEW

| | |
|---|---|
| **Patient's name: Jenny T** | **CMHT:** West Central |
| | **Phone:** |
| **Address: 56 Acacia Avenue** | **New patient:** ~~YES~~/NO |
| | **If NO, date of review: 20.10.07** |
| **Phone:** | |
| | **Diagnosis:** |
| **Date of birth: 09.06.61** | **1...Major depressive disorder..... F 32 .0** |
| **GP: Dr Findlay** | |
| **Phone:** | **2............................................**      **F __ __.__** |

**You must consider the following:** 1) Mental health, including indicators of relapse; 2) Physical health; 3) Medication; 4) Daytime activity; 5) Personal care / living skills; 6) Carers, family, children and social network; 7) Forensic history; 8) Alcohol or substance misuse

9) Cultural factors; 10) Housing/finances/legal issues.

Complete a **risk assessment** and include: **i) a crisis plan; ii) a contingency plan**

| Assessed needs or problem | Intervention | Res p.of |
|---|---|---|
| 1. Depressed mood, apathetic and self critical | • Regular home visits, assess mental state<br>• Encourage compliance with antidepressants<br>• Encourage activity – take to shops etc | BJ |
| 2. Suicidal thoughts | • Explore severity (+/- plans) at each visit<br>• Support mother and husband who are scared of suicidal thoughts | BJ/ Cons |
| 3. Daughter's school problems | • Maintain links with class teacher<br>• Keep family informed of her progress | BJ |
| 4. Plan for recovery | • Link with support group when mood lightens<br>• Help reapply for part-time cleaning job | BJ |

| | | | | | | | | |
|---|---|---|---|---|---|---|---|---|
| **Professionals involved in care:** | ✔ Dr | Psychologist | ✔CPN | OT | ~~S~~W | Ward Nurse | ACT | Other |
| **Present at planning meeting:** | ✔ Dr | ✔ Psychologist | ✔CPN | OT | ~~S~~W | Ward Nurse | ACT | Other |

Copy given to patient?    YES/ ~~NO~~        Copy sent to GP?    YES/ ~~NO~~

| | | |
|---|---|---|
| **Care co-ordinator(print):** | **Billie Jarvis (BJ)** | **Phone** |
| **Care co-ordinator (signature):** | .......................................... | **Date of next review: 20.04.08.** |
| **Job title:** | **CPN** | **Patient's signature:................................** |

| | | | | | |
|---|---|---|---|---|---|
| On Supervision Register? | ~~YES~~/ NO | Care management?  YES/ ~~NO~~ | Risk history completed?  YES/ ~~NO~~ |
| On Supervised Discharge? | ~~YES~~/ NO | Relapse + risk plan required?  YES/ ~~NO~~ |

**Fig. 135.1** Care programme review document.

allocations before assessment is wasteful, and most well-established teams delegate the task to the manager or a senior clinician.

## Patient reviews

Reviews should be held for: (1) new patients; (2) routine monitoring; and (3) discharge. Reviews can range from simply reporting the problem and proposed treatment in uncomplicated cases through to detailed, structured, multi-disciplinary case conferences, including other services (for example, GP, housing, child protection). New patient reviews are an excellent opportunity for providing a broad, experienced overview and ensuring rational and fair allocation to caseloads. Routine monitoring is often overlooked yet is probably the most important for team efficiency. It should be systematic, and not only responsive to crises and problems. It shapes and redirects

---

### CONFIDENTIAL: RELAPSE AND RISK MANAGEMENT PLAN

Name: Alastair W

**Categories of Risk Identified:**

| | | | |
|---|---|---|---|
| Aggression and violence | ~~YES~~/NO | Severe self-neglect | YES/~~NO~~ |
| Exploitation (self or others) | YES/~~NO~~ | Risk to children & young adults | YES/~~NO~~ |
| Suicide and self-harm | YES/~~NO~~ | | |
| Other (please specify} ...................... | | | |

**Current factors which suggest there is significant apparent risk:**
(For example: alcohol or substance misuse; specific threats; suicidal ideation; violent fantasies; anger; suspiciousness; persecutory beliefs; paranoid feelings or ideas about particular people)

Continued excessive drinking—especially when depressed. Makes him more suspicious and hostile.

**Clear statement of anticipated risk(s):**
(Who is at risk; how immediate is that risk; how severe; how ongoing)

Clear risk to strangers (not family or staff), usually in bars. Often when poor medication compliance.

**Action Plan:**
(Including names of people responsible for each action and steps to be taken if plan breaks down)

Relapse plan discussed and agreed—to increase antipsychotics and contact when concerned with people plotting ('to help you cope with them').
If he feels seriously threatened to seek admission through the emergency room

**Date Completed:** xx/xx/xx     **Review date:** xx/xx/xx

**Fig. 135.2** Risk assessment and contingency plan.

treatment and identifies patients ready for discharge, and monitors the burden on individual staff members. Routine monitoring is a requirement of the CPA. Discharge reviews are an excellent opportunity for audit and learning within the team.

### Managing waiting lists and caseloads

Effective CMHTs need to guarantee prompt access. Routine assessments should be within 2–4 weeks. Sooner is rarely productive, and delays above 3 weeks result in a rapidly rising rate of failed appointments [23]. Urgent assessments (most psychotic episodes) need to be seen within a week, usually within a couple of days. Emergency assessments for those at immediate risk (for example, hostile behaviour or suicidal intent) need to be seen on the same day. These pragmatic guidelines may soon be superseded by imposed targets.

A practical approach to waiting lists is to count the assessments in the preceding year and allocate routine appointments for 20% more. Thus, for a team with 400 assessments in the preceding year, allocating nine slots a week will have one slot available weekly for emergencies. Rapid routine assessment reduces pressure for urgent and emergency referrals much more efficiently than emergency rotas.

### Communication and liaison

Team meetings ensure internal communication, but CMHTs need good links with a wide network of professional colleagues. Structured liaison is advisable with primary care and general hospitals. Hospital links may be between specific CMHTs and wards,

or CMHTs may provide input to patients from their sectors in the absence of dedicated liaison psychiatry services.

### General practice liaison

As so much mental health care is delivered in primary care, effective co-ordination is essential. 'Consultation-liaison' also represents efficient use of a specialist team's time if it increases the capacity of primary care through improving GPs' skills and knowledge. However, there has been little systematic research evaluating consultation liaison interventions and this model would apply only in those countries with more developed primary and secondary care services [24]. GP liaison systems range from informal contact through to shared care and co-location of CMHTs in GP health centres [25]. An effective system need not be time-consuming but requires regular, timetabled meetings between the two teams or a 'link' CMHT member. Monthly meetings where shared and complex patients are discussed facilitate prompt problem-solving and crisis anticipation. However, it is important to be clear about responsibilities; fudging boundaries is risky.

### Liaison with other agencies

The same principles apply to liaison with other agencies (social services, housing, etc.). Whether regular meetings are feasible and cost-effective will depend on the volume of shared work, but showing up and meeting people (even just once) pays enormous dividends.

## Assertive outreach teams

The most replicated and researched specialist CMHT is the assertive outreach (AO) team. The original US model [26] substantially reduced hospitalization without increased cost. AO teams (Box 135.2) are staff-intensive and reserved for the most difficult ('hard-to-engage' or 'revolving-door') psychotic patients. These have frequent, often dangerous, relapses and poor medication compliance, complicated by alcohol or drug abuse.

AO emphasizes proactive outreach—visiting patients at home, even when they are reluctant. It exploits enhanced teamworking with daily meetings and several staff involved with most patients both for safety considerations and to meet patients' extensive needs. The culture is very practical (taking patients shopping, sorting out accommodation, delivering medicines daily if need be), often well beyond traditional professional boundaries.

AO brought much needed clear thinking and research to CMHT practice. However, they failed to deliver the same expected benefits in the UK as in the United States [27]. Similar results were found without slavishly following the original model [28, 29]. Detailed examination of AO studies [29] showed that CMHTs delivered equivalent outcomes at much less cost. Consequently, the UK requirement for these teams has been abandoned, with intensive care provided within the CMHT. A more structured approach to identifying and monitoring patients in CMHTs needing intensive care has been proposed as FACT (functional assertive community treatment) [30].

## Crisis teams

Crisis teams play a crucial role where local services are poorly developed (they may be the only community services). They prioritize rapid response and accessibility. Early crisis services often had a short lifespan as they either evolved into more durable CMHT services or became overwhelmed by inappropriate referrals.

## Crisis resolution/home treatment (CR/HT) teams

The CR/HT team model implemented in the UK and Europe reflects increased public demand for access in crises plus a drive to reduce inpatient care costs. It draws heavily on AO practice with limited shared caseloads, flexible working, extended access, and an emphasis on outreach. Reduction in hospitalization is believed

to offset much of their cost [31]. How they integrate with generic CMHTs varies markedly, but they work with patients who would otherwise be in hospital—either by supporting them in early discharge or seeking alternatives to admission. They offer intensive visiting (usually daily for a limited period) and considerable practical support and work with patients' social networks. Many are based in a crisis day hospital, and input is limited to a few weeks. Such intensive teamworking requires highly effective communication and the teams meet daily (often twice at shift handovers). Information transfer can be burdensome and liaison with CMHTs complex, requiring absolute clarity on local arrangements for clinical responsibility.

## Variations in practice and sustainability

The CR/HT teams may reduce the need for hospital care [31, 32]. The UK model is precisely specified (including who it should and should not care for) (Box 135.3), but practice varies considerably. A full 24-hour service is rarely provided; most rely on established on-call services. Strict observance of the prescribed patient group 'otherwise in hospital' is difficult to achieve, and engagement may be longer. The main criticism is of multiple repetitive visits from endlessly changing staff members. Good medical staffing is needed, and CMHT responsibilities need to be carefully negotiated, mutually agreed, and crystal clear if confusion is to be avoided.

## Crisis houses and respite care

Crisis house admissions involve a minimum of formality with less intense supervision than hospitals. They are usually small (4–8 beds) in a relatively domestic setting and admit for days, occasionally a week or two. They are favoured for vulnerable women and early intervention services. Most have one staff member overnight and a couple during the day, with input from patients' case managers. They improve acceptability and access but do not replace inpatient

---

**Box 135.2** ACT core components

- Assertive follow-up.
- Small caseloads (1:10–1:15).
- Regular (daily) team meetings.
- Frequent contact (weekly to daily).
- *In vivo* practice (treatment in home and neighbourhood).
- Emphasis on engagement and medication.
- Support for family and carers.
- Provision of services using all team members.
- Crisis stabilization 24 hours a day, 7 days a week.

---

**Box 135.3** Remit of UK crisis resolution/home treatment teams

'Commonly adults (16 to 65 years old) with severe mental illness (schizophrenia, manic depressive disorders, severe depressive disorder) with an acute psychiatric crisis of such severity that, without the involvement of the CR/HT team hospitalisation would be necessary.'

'The service is not usually appropriate for individuals with:

- Mild anxiety disorders.
- Primary diagnosis of alcohol or other substance abuse.
- Brain damage or other organic disorders including dementia.
- Learning disabilities.
- Exclusive diagnosis of personality disorder.
- Recent history of self harm but not suffering from a psychotic or serious depressive illness.
- Crisis related solely to relationship issues.'

Reproduced from Department of Health, *The mental health policy implementation guide*, Copyright (2001), Crown Copyright. Reproduced under the terms of the Open Government Licence v3.0. Available at https://webarchive.nationalarchives.gov.uk/20120514200638/http://www.dh.gov.uk/prod_consum_dh/groups/dh_digitalassets/@dh/@en/documents/digitalasset/dh_4058960.pdf

care and need careful management to avoid becoming chaotic or blocked.

## Early intervention service

Concern that a long duration of untreated psychosis (DUP) confers poorer prognosis [34] spurred the development of early intervention service (EIS) teams which have now become standard in the UK. Developed mainly from Australian and UK models [35, 36], they vary remarkably. Some down-play diagnosis in favour of easy access; others restrict to schizophrenia; some emphasize a 'youth service', while others take all first-episode patients, irrespective of age [18]. Even more confusing, there are three quite different activities which may, or may not, be part of the service (Box 135.4).

The core of EIS is a specialized CMHT based closely on AO team practice which case-manages first-episode psychosis patients. EIS emphasizes protecting social networks and functioning, aiming to keeping patients at college or work, and assuming a return to premorbid functioning. Crisis and respite houses are preferred to hospital. Some EIS teams go beyond this basic model and conduct public awareness campaigns, lecturing in schools and colleges [37]. A minority of research teams attempt to identify and treat 'ultra-high-risk' patients to prevent progression to psychosis [38]. EIS teams are highly popular with families, staff, and commissioners. They are generally better staffed and funded than other CMHTs, and inevitably problems arise with 'step-down' to routine services.

## Adjunct or replacement for CMHTs?

The four teams outlined comprise the fundamental building blocks of most community services. AO EIS and CR/HT teams were originally proposed as replacements for CMHTs. However, both experience and research evidence [39] suggest that they are better considered as additions to improve the quality of care from otherwise well-functioning CMHTs, rather than as cost-saving alternatives.

## Highly specialized and diagnosis-specific teams

Several specialized teams are generally organized at a regional level. They impact on local services, removing some of the CMHT's clinical load, but need clear and negotiable thresholds if confusion is to be avoided.

## Forensic and rehabilitation teams

Community-focused services face particular difficulties with treatment-resistant patients, particularly those with socially unacceptable or offending behaviour who fit poorly into open wards. Specialized forensic teams provide secure care. Increasingly, they also run community teams to provide intensive case management of dangerous patients. Integrating them with general services can be problematical, and boundaries are invariably controversial.

## Rehabilitation

A significant number of patients remain disabled and require long-term management of disability, rather than episode-based care, despite optimal treatment. Rehabilitation teams generally serve patients who cannot survive without supervised accommodation, even when at their best. They comprise a disturbed 'new long-stay' population, characterized by comorbid substance abuse and behavioural disturbances.

## Diagnosis-specific teams

Highly specialized teams for individual disorders (for example, eating disorders, personality disorders, bipolar patients) concentrate on specific skills and provide specialized treatments and are usually provided at a regional level. They provide settings for intensive academic research and treatment refinement, but their opportunity costs need careful thought.

## Compulsion and ethics in community mental health care

Balancing patients' welfare with their autonomy and balancing their individual rights with those of their families and the wider community have both become more complex as CMHTs have developed. The introduction of community treatment orders (CTOs) [40] highlights these dilemmas. Compulsion and coercion (either explicitly in the form of legal requirements or informally through professional or social pressure [41–43]) are now a pervasive feature of practice. Improved clinical provision and legal scrutiny make compulsory treatment possible in the community.

Most developed countries have enacted forms of CTO ('mandated community treatment', 'outpatient committal'). Their introduction has generally been controversial, and this is heightened by mounting evidence of their ineffectiveness [44]. CTOs have the advantage of legal scrutiny, unlike most of the ethical dilemmas facing CMHT staff in their day-to-day work which require case-by-case discussion. How proper is it to inform neighbours if a patient may pose a risk to them but will not give consent? Is it right for a patient to deny information on his or her treatment to parents on whom he or she is heavily dependent? Guidelines exist only for extreme circumstances, and teams need regular discussions of these issues.

## Stepwise planning and adaptation

### Local population needs assessment

Psychiatric morbidity varies considerably with social deprivation and is much higher in cities than in stable rural or suburban settings

---

**Box 135.4** Components of early intervention teams

- Case management—ongoing care of identified patients.
- Early identification—awareness-raising campaigns for psychoses.
- High-risk and prodromal patient identification and treatment.

(see Chapters 134–136). At regional and national levels, comparative need can be predicted fairly well from established indexes incorporating age profiles, number of migrants, overcrowding, poverty, etc. [45]. Catchment areas should broadly reflect these differences. At the local level, however, these figures are of limited value. How can one factor in travelling time or differences in the quality of primary care? A process of negotiation is best to agree on local allocation following these general guidelines. However, a concentration of hostels for the mentally ill or homeless or the presence of a railway station or an international airport may swamp these differences. Such local factors should be provisionally estimated in the planning process, but regularly reviewed.

## Opportunity costs and unintended consequences

Planning mental health services is driven by political and policy considerations, at least as much as on international evidence, often including cost-effectiveness analyses. However, these analyses rarely address the opportunity costs across a whole system. A study may demonstrate that one acute day hospital is more cost-effective than another, but does the whole system gain when considering diverting the inpatient nurses redeployed to staff it? Rigorous intervention studies of large systems are formidably difficult to conduct and even more so to interpret.

The impact of enthusiasm and the migration of the best staff to such research services can be especially misleading [46]. Successful new services are always reported, but not when they lose their edge or are abandoned [15, 47]. It is best to visit examples of services that you are considering, and not to assume automatically that what works for them will necessarily work for you [28].

Skilled manpower is as significant a resource limitation as funding is, hence the need for a system-wide appraisal. Although costs are usually cited, planning decisions reflect wider values and expectations, rather than simply outcomes [2].

## Cultures and funding

Health care cultures, their structures and their funding systems vary enormously. Services must be congruent with them otherwise they will not survive. The current emphasis on the 'recovery' model [48], while it may not make any major differences in practice, has to be incorporated into service planning proposals if they are to be funded. Occasionally, service planners can influence the culture but more often have to adapt to it. Obtaining relatively small changes in funding arrangements (or external governance) can deliver quite major improvements. However, caution is needed as the risks of unintended consequences and perverse incentives are ever present. Enthusiastic clinicians are often blind to the risks of overprescription which can lock in outmoded practices (for example, a highly specific form of day hospital or crisis facility) that may not meet local needs but are too rigidly prescribed to then be adapted.

How 'integrated' mental health care should be is a highly local decision. Well-established systems often strive for integration with general medicine or with social services to reduce both discrimination and administrative barriers to integrated care. The current emphasis on 'parity of esteem' for mental health is sometimes taken to imply such integration. For many services, the value of a distinct, separate identity can be considerable—not least the ability to protect its resources.

The task of integration is easily underestimated, particularly the energies required to accommodate contrasting health and social care cultures. Compromises need to be agreed before such integration and the negotiations can be exhausting, but they are infinitely preferable to fudges and misunderstandings. The costs and benefits will depend very much on the local situation, relationships, and history.

## Relationships with the voluntary sector and patients movement

Current policies emphasize outsourcing, where practical, any welfare provision for which there is a 'suitably qualified provider'. Relations with local non-health statutory services (housing, education, police) and with the voluntary sector will determine much of the success of mental health services, and their strengths need to be exploited. Non-statutory services are usually well adapted to local needs, but less comprehensive or reliable long term. Patient and carer advocacy and support organizations are now a major force; effective working with them will significantly enhance both the design and the delivery of services.

## Monitoring and review

Careful monitoring and review are as important as careful planning, probably more so. Services can easily drift to those who demand them from those who most need them; delivery of treatments (particularly psychological and psychotherapeutic treatments) may become mechanical, losing their effectiveness. The most needy patients are rarely the most demanding or well informed, and engaging them in long-term treatments is often difficult.

A consistent effort to deliver even the most basic proven interventions will make a substantial difference to patient welfare. The PORT study in the United States demonstrated how schizophrenia care was strikingly inconsistent and fell below accepted standards [49]. Regular audit, particularly of national guidelines such as those produced by the National Institute for Health and Care Excellence (NICE), ensures that services remain targeted and quality is maintained. Monitoring can vary in sophistication—from a simple head count of who is getting what (for example, clozapine treatment) through to careful evaluation of care pathways. The audit review process feeds back into the development process. Audit invariably rewards its investment.

## Routine outcome measures (ROMs)

Audit and measurement bring rigour and reflection, which are often lost in the immediacy of the therapeutic relationship. Measurement also serves a training purpose by benchmarking interdisciplinary understandings of symptoms and outcomes. Systematic, periodic recording of patients' clinical or social status is increasingly used in both planning and research. Structured outcomes can be generic [for example, Health of the Nation Outcome Scales (HoNOS) [50]] or for specific disorders (for example, the Brief Psychiatric Rating Scale [51]) or even locally developed. Their value lies in their consistency of use.

## Physical health care of people with SMI

In the UK, GPs take responsibility for health promotion and care of the physical health of people with SMI. They are incentivized through the GP contract quality and outcomes framework (QOF) to review the needs of their SMI patients annually and ensure a care plan is in place [52]. This proactive care is crucial, as mortality rates for people with SMI are 2–3 times higher than for the general population. While this is partly due to suicide, two-thirds of the excess mortality is a result of physical disorders, especially smoking- and obesity-related cardiovascular and respiratory diseases [53–55].

The annual review of physical health for people with SMI includes:

- Use of alcohol and drugs and smoking behaviour.
- Blood pressure.
- Body mass index.
- HbA1c blood test for diabetes.
- Cholesterol.
- Cervical screening, if appropriate.
- Medication review.

In addition, GPs in the UK check blood lithium levels and monitor thyroid and kidney function of people with SMI taking lithium.

Mental health service planning should take into account the physical health care needs of people with SMI. It will have to provide that care in countries with less well-developed primary care systems or residential mental health care settings. Even in the UK, the primary care of people with SMI varies widely in quality, and one cannot assume their physical health needs will automatically be met through registration with a GP. An audit of the care of schizophrenia in mental health services in England and Wales revealed only 29% received a fully comprehensive assessment of important cardiometabolic risk factors. Among those with high blood pressure and high cholesterol levels, there was frequently no evidence of appropriate investigation or treatment [56]. The authors recommended all health professionals working with such patients should have training in physical health problems and interventions for treating them, including access to the correct monitoring equipment. They also stressed that mental health services and primary care services need to work together to agree who will monitor and treat these physical health problems [56].

## Conclusions

Planning and providing mental health services require flexibility and compromise. Epidemiological and service statistics provide a framework for local planning, but it is still primarily a practical and 'political' activity. The scientific evidence is dominated by anglophone alternatives to hospital care studies, but local history, culture, mental health law, and political imperatives cannot be ignored.

---

**Box 135.5** Developing local community mental health services

- Make a careful inventory of what services exist and any special local needs.
- Consult locally and invest heavily in building coalitions with policy-makers, statutory services, and voluntary groups.
- Test research evidence for durability and relevance. If possible, visit established services and ask 'around the service'.
- Monitor and review regularly. Improved consistency of current practice often delivers more than introducing new treatments.
- Consider carefully opportunity costs. Include both the impact of a specific improvement across the whole service and the costs of system change itself.
- Avoid excessive reorganization—not all change is innovation.

---

A high-profile patient homicide, or a strong public endorsement of services by a politician or celebrity, can derail months of careful planning.

This chapter has attempted to draw out some principles (Box 135.5) for the process, but these can only be guidelines. Inevitably, the decision will be based on what is possible locally. Most solutions rely on the tried and tested structures described here, but their configuration will depend on what is available and local values. Above all, the mentally ill and their families deserve reliable and predictable services. Not all change is innovation. Research findings should be judged in terms of their sustainability and translation from research efficacy to clinical effectiveness more than on the *P*-values in individual trials.

## FURTHER INFORMATION

Burns, T. (2004). *Community Mental Health Teams*. Oxford: Oxford University Press.

Pilling, S., Whittington, C, Taylor, C., Kendrick, T. (2011). Identification and care pathways for common mental health disorders: summary of NICE guidance. *BMJ*, **342**, d2868.

Thornicroft, G., Tansella, M. (2004). Components of a modern mental health service: a pragmatic balance of community and hospital care: overview of systematic evidence. *British Journal of Psychiatry*, **185**, 283–90.

## REFERENCES

1. Tansella, M., Thornicroft, G. (1998). A conceptual framework for mental health services: the matrix model. *Psychological Medicine*, **28**, 503–8.
2. Thornicroft, G., Tansella, M. (2004). Components of a modern mental health service: a pragmatic balance of community and hospital care: overview of systematic evidence. *British Journal of Psychiatry*, **185**, 283–90.
3. McManus, S., Meltzer, H., Brugha, T. *et al.* (2009). *Adult psychiatric morbidity in England, 2007. Results of a household survey*. Leicester: National Centre for Social Research and Department of Health Sciences, University of Leicester.
4. World Health Organization (1992). *The ICD-10 classification of mental and behavioural disorders*. Geneva: World Health Organization.
5. Kai, J., Crosland, A., Drinkwater, C. (2000). Prevalence of enduring and disabling mental illness in the inner city. *British Journal of General Practice*, **50**, 992–4.

6. Kendrick, T., Dowrick, C., McBride, A. *et al*. (2009). Management of depression in UK general practice in relation to scores on depression severity questionnaires: analysis of medical record data. *BMJ*, **338**, b750.

7. Health and Social Care Information Centre (2014). *Psychological therapies, annual report on the use of IAPT services: England—2013–14*. Leeds: Health and Social Care Information Centre.

8. Reilly, S., Planner, C., Hann, M. *et al*. (2012). The role of primary care in service provision for people with severe mental illness in the United Kingdom. *PLoS One*, **7**, e36468.

9. Kallert, T.W., Glöckner, M., Onchev, G. *et al*. (2005). The EUNOMIA project on coercion in psychiatry: study design and preliminary data. *World Psychiatry*, **4**, 168–72.

10. Keown, P. (2011). Association between provision of mental illness beds and rate of involuntary admissions in the NHS in England 1988–2008: ecological study. *BMJ*, **343**, d3736.

11. Catty, J., Goddard, K., Burns, T. (2005). Social services day care and health services day care in mental health: do they differ? *International Journal of Psychoanalysis*, **51**, 151–61.

12. Marshall, M. (2003). Acute psychiatric day hospitals. *BMJ*, **327**, 116–17.

13. Bateman, A., Fonagy, P. (2008). Eight-year follow-up of patients treated for borderline personality disorder: mentalization-based treatment versus treatment as usual. *American Journal of Psychiatry*, **165**, 631–8.

14. Knapp, M., Hallam, A., Beecham, J. *et al*. (1999). Private, voluntary or public? Comparative cost-effectiveness in community mental health care. *Policy and Politics*, **27**, 25–41.

15. Wright, C., Catty, J., Watt, H. *et al*. (2004). A systematic review of home treatment services. Classification and sustainability. *Social Psychiatry and Psychiatric Epidemiology*, **39**, 789–96.

16. Kendrick, T., Simons, L., Mynors-Wallis, L. *et al*. (2006). Cost-effectiveness of referral for generic care or problem-solving treatment from community mental health nurses, compared with usual general practitioner care for common mental disorders: randomised control trial. *British Journal of Psychiatry*, **189**, 50–9.

17. Slade, M., Powell, R., Rosen, A. *et al*. (2000). Threshold assessment grid (TAG): the development of a valid and brief scale to assess the severity of mental illness. *Social Psychiatry and Psychiatric Epidemiology*, **35**, 78–85.

18. Burns, T. (2004). *Community Mental Health Teams*. Oxford: Oxford University Press.

19. Burns, T., Beadsmoore, A., Bhat, A.V., *et al*. (1993). A controlled trial of home-based acute psychiatric services. I: clinical and social outcome. *British Journal of Psychiatry*, **163**, 49–54.

20. Intagliata, J. (1982). Improving the quality of community care for the chronically mentally disabled: the role of case management. *Schizophrenia Bulletin*, **8**, 655–74.

21. Holloway, F., Oliver, N., Collins, E., *et al*. (1995). Case management: a critical review of the outcome literature. *European Psychiatry*, **10**, 113–28.

22. Department of Health (1990). *The care programme approach for people with a mental illness referred to the special psychiatric services*. Report No.: Joint Health/Social Services Circular HC (90) 23/LASS (90) 11. London: Department of Health.

23. Burns, T., Raftery, J., Beadsmoore, A., *et al*. (1993). A controlled trial of home-based acute psychiatric services. II: treatment patterns and costs. *British Journal of Psychiatry*, **163**, 55–61.

24. Gask, L., Sibbald, B., Creed, F. (1997). Evaluating models of working at the interface between mental health services and primary care. *British Journal of Psychiatry*, **170**, 6–11.

25. Burns, T., Bale, R. (1997). Establishing a mental health liaison attachment with primary care. *Advances in Psychiatric Treatment*, **3**, 219–24.

26. Stein, L.I., Test, M.A. (1980). Alternative to mental hospital treatment. I: conceptual model, treatment program, and clinical evaluation. *Archives of General Psychiatry*, **37**, 392–7.

27. Burns, T.; for the UK700 Group (2002). The UK700 trial of Intensive Case Management: an overview and discussion. *World Psychiatry*, **1**, 175–8.

28. Fiander, M., Burns, T., McHugo, G.J., *et al*. (2003). Assertive community treatment across the Atlantic: comparison of model fidelity in the UK and USA. *British Journal of Psychiatry*, **182**, 248–54.

29. Burns, T., Marshall, M., Catty, J., *et al*. (2005). *Variable outcomes in case management trials—an exploration of current theories using meta-regression and meta-analysis: final report*. London: Department of Health.

30. Firn, M., Hindhaugh, K., Hubbeling, D. *et al*. (2012). A dismantling study of assertive outreach services: comparing activity and outcomes following replacement with the FACT model. *Social Psychiatry and Psychiatric Epidemiology*, **48**, 998–1003.

31. Smyth, M.G., Hoult, J. (2000). The home treatment enigma. *BMJ*, **320**, 305–9.

32. Johnson, S., Nolan, F., Pilling, S., *et al*. (2005). Randomised controlled trial of acute mental health care by a crisis resolution team: the north Islington crisis study. *BMJ*, **331**, 599.

33. Department of Health (2001). *The mental health policy implementation guide*. London: Department of Health.

34. Marshall, M., Lewis, S., Lockwood, A., *et al*. (2005). Association between duration of untreated psychosis and outcome in cohorts of first-episode patients: a systematic review. *Archives of General Psychiatry*, **62**, 975–83.

35. Edwards, J., McGorry, P.D., Pennell, K. (2002). Models of early intervention in psychosis: an analysis of service approaches. In: Birchwood, M., Fowler, D, Jackson, C., editors. *Early Intervention in Psychosis: A Guide to Concepts, Evidence and Interventions*. New York, NY: John Wiley and Sons. pp. 281–314.

36. Birchwood, M., Todd, P., Jackson, C. (1998). Early intervention in psychosis. The critical period hypothesis. *British Journal of Psychiatry* (Supplement), **172**, 53–9.

37. McGorry, P., Jackson, H. (1999). *Recognition and Management of Early Psychosis. A Preventative Approach*. Cambridge: Cambridge University Press.

38. McGorry, P.D., Yung, A.R., Phillips, L.J., *et al*. (2002). Randomized controlled trial of interventions designed to reduce the risk of progression to first-episode psychosis in a clinical sample with subthreshold symptoms. *Archives of General Psychiatry*, **59**, 921–8.

39. Burns, T., Catty, J., Watt, H., *et al*. (2002). International differences in home treatment for mental health problems. Results of a systematic review. *British Journal of Psychiatry*, **181**, 375–82.

40. Canvin, K., Rugkasa, J., Sinclair, J. *et al*. (2014). Patient, psychiatrist and family carer experiences of community treatment orders: qualitative study. *Social Psychiatry and Psychiatric Epidemiology*, **49**, 1873–82.

41. Monahan, J., Redlich, A.D., Swanson, J., *et al*. (2005). Use of leverage to improve adherence to psychiatric treatment in the community. *Psychiatric Services*, **56**, 37–44.

42. Burns, T., Yeeles, K., Molodynski, A. *et al*. (2011). Pressures to adhere to treatment ('leverage') in English mental healthcare. *British Journal of Psychiatry*, **199**, 145–50.

43. Szmukler, G., Applebaum, P.S. (2008). Treatment pressures, leverage, coercion, and compulsion in mental health care. *Journal of Mental Health*, **17**, 233–44.

44. Kisely, S., Hall, K. (2014). An updated meta-analysis of randomized controlled evidence for the effectiveness of community treatment orders. *Can J Psychiatry*, **59**, 561–4.

45. Keown, P., McBride, O., Twigg, L., *et al.* (2016). Rates of voluntary and compulsory psychiatric in-patient treatment in England: An ecological study investigating associations with deprivation and demographics. *British Journal of Psychiatry*. **209**, 157–61.

46. Coid, J. (1994). Failure in community care: psychiatry's dilemma. *BMJ*, **308**, 805–6.

47. Cooper, J.E. Crisis admission units and emergency psychiatric services. In: Cooper, J.E. *Public Health in Europe*, No. 11. Copenhagen: Regional Office for Europe, World Health Organization; 1979. pp. iv.

48. Slade M. *Personal Recovery and Mental Illness: A Guide for Mental Health Professionals (Values-Based Practice)*. Cambridge: Cambridge University Press; 2009.

49. Lehman, A.F., Steinwachs, D.M. (1998). Translating research into practice: the Schizophrenia Patient Outcomes Research Team (PORT) treatment recommendations. *Schizophrenia Bulletin*, **24**, 1–10.

50. Orrell, M., Yard, P., Handysides, J., *et al.* (1999). Validity and reliability of the health of the nation outcome scales in psychiatric patients in the community. *British Journal of Psychiatry*, **174**, 409–12.

51. Overall, J.E., Gorham, D.L. (1962). The brief psychiatric rating scale. *Psychological Reports*, **10**, 799–812.

52. British Medical Association, NHS Employers (2006). *Revisions to the GMS contract 2006/07. Delivering investment in general practice*. London: NHS Confederation (Employers) Company Ltd.

53. McManus, S., Meltzer, H., Campion, J. (2010). *Cigarette smoking and mental health in England: data from the Adult Psychiatric Morbidity Survey 2007*. London: National Centre for Social Research.

54. McElroy, S.L. (2009). Obesity in patients with severe mental illness: overview and management. *Journal of Clinical Psychiatry*, **70**(Suppl. 3),12–21.

55. Osborn, D.P.J., Levy, G., Nazareth, I., *et al.* (2007). Relative risk of cardiovascular and cancer mortality in people with severe mental illness from the UK General Practice Research Database. *Archives of General Psychiatry*, **64**, 242–9.

56. Royal College of Psychiatrists (2012). *Report of the National Audit of Schizophrenia (NAS) 2012*. London: Healthcare Quality Improvement Partnership.

# 136

# Health economic analysis of service provision

*Judit Simon*

## Introduction

Resources available in the health care system are limited and are exceeded by needs. Public health and long-term care expenditures have been rising steadily, relative to national income, for several decades. Among the Organisation for Economic Co-operation and Development (OECD) countries, they increased by more than a fifth to approximately 6% of the annual national income or gross domestic product (GDP) between 2000 and 2010, and are predicted to more than double, increasing to almost 14% of the GDP by 2060 unless active cost containment efforts are put in place [1]. Currently, the costs of mental ill-health account for up to 14% of health spending in OECD countries and this proportion is also expected to rise further [2]. Worldwide, costs due to psychiatric diseases are expected to double by 2030 [3]. Decisions on how best to allocate scarce resources are therefore becoming increasingly prominent among health policy-makers.

This chapter summarizes the health economic methods used to inform the key questions of decision-makers in health care related to efficiency and equity, which are '*Who gets what, where, and how?*'. It provides an explanation of the underlying economic and analytical frameworks and gives a summary of the different techniques of health economic analyses, supported by a selection of recent relevant published examples from the mental health field.

## Health economic analyses

Health economic analyses are concerned with the efficient (and equitable) allocation of limited resources for the promotion of health and the prevention, treatment, and care of diseases to maximize the health of the population. *Cost descriptions* [for example, cost-of-illness studies (COIs)] assess the cost of interventions, services, or illnesses with no comparison in place. When information on outcomes is also described, but no comparison to status quo or other alternative is given, the analysis is called *cost–outcome description*. *Cost analyses* compare two or more alternatives, based only on their costs. To assess the overall value of a health intervention, however,

decision-makers need information on the effect, the resources used to generate the effect, and the cost of these resources incremental to the next best alternative action. The value of the next best alternative forgone is known as the opportunity cost. *Economic evaluations* are the comparative assessment of both costs and outcomes of alternative health care interventions. They provide an explicit economic framework for the systematic identification, measurement, and valuation of the resource inputs and outcomes of alternative activities, and the subsequent comparative analysis of these based on the evidence available [4] (Table 136.1).

### Cost descriptions

Mental health disorders are common, often recurrent or chronic, have major impacts on individual and social well-being, cause excess premature mortality, and therefore pose great disease burden. Worldwide, the burden of mental and substance use disorders increased by 38% between 1990 and 2010, driven mostly by population growth and ageing [5]. In 2010, they were among the ten leading causes of total disease burden in terms of disability-adjusted life years (DALYs) (7.4% of the total) and were the leading cause of years lived with disability (YLDs) worldwide (23% of the total) [5]. Depression particularly is considered the third leading cause of disability due to morbidity and mortality in Europe, causing 3.8% of all DALYs [6]. By 2020, depression is predicted to become the leading cause of disease burden, alongside cardiovascular diseases, worldwide [7]. *COIs* estimate the economic burden of an illness in terms of its costs either for a year based on its prevalence or for a lifetime based on its incidence. They may use top–down methods by disaggregating health (and possibly other intersectoral) expenditure data according to disease, or a bottom–up approach by projecting population-level cost of an illness from patient-level data. They are useful in providing information on resource allocation in health systems, analyse time trends, make projections of future health expenditure, and help make international comparisons. Comparability of top–down calculations between countries has improved substantially since the introduction of the System of Health Accounts (SHA) method by OECD in 2000, which provides a framework for a family of interrelated tables for standard reporting of expenditure on health [8].

**Table 136.1** Health economic analyses

| | | Is there a comparison? | |
|---|---|---|---|
| | | NO | YES |
| Is evidence only available on costs? | YES | Cost description | Cost analysis |
| | NO | Cost-outcome description | Economic evaluation |

COIs can also greatly contribute to the identification of discrepancy between epidemiological and health service use data and identify unmet needs. For example, a pan-European cost of brain disorders study from 2010 concluded that less than one-third of all cases received treatment and suggested a considerable level of unmet needs [9]. There are several potential reasons for this, besides the general underfunding of mental health services. Issues such as availability of trained personnel, poor geographical distribution of services, and other access and utilization issues (language, socio-economic status, stigma, low weight of individual needs and preferences), lack of long-term thinking at decision-making level, provision of cost-ineffective services, bureaucracy, and, last but not least, fragmented funding and provision all play a role.

## Cost categories

The *direct medical costs* of mental ill-health include medical expenditure of all goods and services related to the prevention, diagnosis, and treatment of an illness (for example, physician visits, hospitalizations, medication) due to an increased need for health care. Poor mental health also drives up the cost of treating other health problems. It is more expensive to treat physical ill-health conditions when the patient is suffering from a mental illness (for example, depression), and people with mental ill-health are more likely to suffer from physical comorbidities (for example, cardiovascular diseases) (Box 136.1).

*Direct non-medical costs* refer to the cost of other goods and services related to the disorder, including social services, long-term care, special accommodation, and costs to the patients and their families (for example, travel costs, out-of-pocket payments). Mental illnesses also have broader societal impacts that lead to significant *indirect costs*. People with mental ill-health experience higher rates of unemployment. According to OECD estimates, people with severe mental health disorders are 6–7 times more likely, while people with mild to moderate disorders are 2–3 times more likely, to be unemployed than people with no mental health disorders [2]. In addition, people with mental ill-health retire earlier, have more absences from work (absenteeism), and also suffer more from presenteeism, meaning reduced productivity at work. In the case of depression, for example, lost productivity costs due to presenteeism are five times as high as those incurred due to absenteeism [13]. Indirect costs also include economic costs attributable to lost resources, but not involving direct payments such as informal care provided by family members and friends. A full accounting of the costs of poor mental health should include relevant *intersectoral costs* of lower educational achievements, increased homelessness, and crime. The *intangible costs* of mental ill-health are considerable and include the monetary value of reduced well-being, emotional distress, pain, and other forms of suffering (for example, stigma). Due to difficulties in quantifying the latter costs, however, they are often neglected in COIs, resulting in an underestimation of the true disease costs (Box 136.2).

COIs, however, are limited regarding their interpretation and policy use in resource allocation. Bias towards already costly disease areas is likely to occur without further consideration of whether the current allocation is optimal and what kind of trade-offs may be done that represent good value for money and may contribute to the reduction of both the disease and the economic burdens effectively. As mental health services are usually complex with multiple impacts, it is difficult to estimate their real cost-saving potentials without relevant considerations in a full economic evaluation framework.

## Cost analyses

Comparative cost analyses are seen as partial economic evaluations [4]. Although, without information on outcomes, they are not useful in determining the cost-effectiveness of alternative options, cost analyses may be used to highlight the difference in costs between two alternative interventions or services and are useful tools in health services research and planning. The perspective of the analysis depends on the included cost categories. *Budget impact analyses (BIAs)* are specific cost analyses that address the expected changes in the expenditure of a health care system after the adoption of a new intervention or service in comparison to status quo. They present information on the relevant monetary impact and its diffusion, depending on the time horizon of the analysis and the included cost categories. BIAs are used for budget or resource planning by those who manage and plan health care budgets (for example, administrators of national or regional health care programmes, private health

---

**Box 136.1** Costs of medications

Often direct medical costs that are easy to estimate, for example medication costs, are in the focus of resource allocation debates. Antidepressant consumption has at least doubled in the OECD countries between 2000 and 2013 [10]. Globally, antidepressant medications were ranked ninth among all prescription drugs, with sales of over US$20 billion in 2011 [11]. Despite the general trend of increasing consumption, drug costs only have limited effect on the total direct costs (between 6% and 29% of the total), with hospitalization remaining the main cost driver (between 30% and 79%) in terms of the economic burden of depression and other mental illnesses internationally [12].

---

**Box 136.2** Costs of mental health in Europe

The total European cost of brain disorders in 2010 was estimated at €798 billion, of which direct health care costs accounted for 37%, direct non-medical costs for 23%, and indirect costs for 40%. The average cost per inhabitant was €5550. From these, the aggregated economic costs of depression were calculated at €92 billion, attributing to one-third of the total cost of brain disorders, and therefore being the most costly brain disease in Europe. The average total cost per patient for depression was estimated at €3034, of which direct health care costs amounted to €797 (26%) and direct non-medical costs at €454 (15%). With €1782 (59%), indirect costs were responsible for the highest proportion of costs per patient, making lost productivity the greatest contributor to the overall economic burden of depression and emphasizing its large societal cost [14, 15].

**Box 136.3** Costs of mental health in the UK

A recent UK cost analysis estimated the mental health service use and cost impacts of remote mood monitoring of patients with bipolar disorder introduced in a specialist mood disorders clinic via the *True Colours* system over 1 year before and after engagement with monitoring. Average compliance with monitoring was over 80%. No significant changes in the annual use and costs of mental health services were found, except for patients who were newly referred to the clinic during the pre-monitoring period. Annual psychiatric medication costs increased, however, on average by £235 across all patients due to more frequent changes to psychiatric medications and higher levels of multi-drug use as a possible consequence of a tighter medication regime [17].

insurance companies, health care providers). A BIA can be an independent analysis or part of a comprehensive economic assessment of a health care intervention, alongside an economic evaluation of its cost-effectiveness [16] (Box 136.3).

## Economic evaluations

### Techniques of economic evaluations

The main question an economic evaluation tries to answer is: 'Is an intervention or service cost-effective, that is, meaning 'good value for money', in comparison to an alternative use of resources, based on the available evidence?' For this, both costs and outcomes of competing alternatives have to be compared and an *appropriate comparator* should be chosen. For example, when the cost-effectiveness of a new antidepressant medication is investigated, it is not sufficient to compare its outcomes and costs to that of a placebo, but rather to the current gold standard active antidepressant treatment options.

Depending on the resource allocation question at hand, different *types of economic evaluations* applying different types of outcome measures are appropriate [4] (Table 136.2). When there is good evidence that the compared alternatives are equally safe and effective, and therefore have identical outcomes, the question of finding the least costly option can be answered within a so-called *cost-minimization analysis (CMA)*. Because of the inherent uncertainty around both the cost and outcome estimates, however, it has been questioned whether CMA can be seen as the correct approach in any decision situation [18]. When competing alternatives within the same disease area are compared, it is appropriate to use

**Table 136.2** Types of economic evaluations

|  | Costs | Outcomes |
|---|---|---|
| Cost-minimization analysis (CMA) | Monetary unit | (Preliminary evidence of equal outcomes) |
| Cost-effectiveness analysis (CEA) | Monetary unit | Natural units (for example, relapse prevented, life years gained) |
| Cost-utility analysis (CUA) | Monetary unit | QALY, DALY |
| Cost-benefit analysis (CBA) | Monetary unit | Monetary unit |
| Cost-consequences analysis (CCA) | Monetary unit | Multiple outcomes tabulated |

outcome measures that are common natural units meaningful for the given disease within a *cost-effectiveness analysis (CEA)*. For example, for people with depression, meaningful outcomes could be expressed as relapse prevented or depression-free days. The preferred outcome measure for economic evaluations that allows comparison across disease areas is the generic quality-adjusted life year (QALY) used in a *cost-utility analysis (CUA)*. QALYs combine both quantity of life and quality of life outcomes into a single metric. For this purpose, quality of life is measured in terms of the utility value of a given health state. The length of time an individual spends in a given health state is weighed by its utility value to calculate the QALY. Utility values of 1 indicate full health, and 0 indicate a health state value equivalent to being dead. Health states considered worse than being dead can be represented by negative values. Whether patients, experts, or the general public are best suited to perform utility valuations is an ongoing debate. From a social perspective, the general public is considered as the most appropriate group due to the dominantly public financing of health care systems and the need for unbiased valuations across a wide range of different disease areas and health states. Other generic outcome measures predominantly used in international CUAs are disability-adjusted life years (DALYs) and healthy year equivalents (HYEs) [19]. When the relevant resource allocation question crosses the boundaries of public policy sectors (for example, investment in better health care vs investment in better education), outcomes necessarily need to be measured in a metric that is common to all sectors, that is, in monetary terms within a *cost-benefit analysis (CBA)*. It is also possible to report costs and outcomes of an economic evaluation in a disaggregated way in a tabulated format within a *cost-consequences analysis (CCA)* framework. In these cases, while information on the relevant ranking of alternatives is possible alongside different criteria, no single cost-effectiveness ratio is presented, leaving the overall synthesis and trade-off between different outcome attributes for the decision-maker thereby less explicit. More recent attempts for eliciting weights by analysts for different criteria are emerging within a *multi-criteria decision analysis (MCDA)* framework [20].

The resource allocation question at hand also determines the appropriate *perspective of an economic evaluation*, which, in return, defines the categories of costs (and types of outcomes) that need to be included in the assessment. Many stakeholders require an economic evaluation to be conducted from their relevant perspective (for example, provider perspective, payer perspective). In the evaluation of mental health services (particularly with their typically fragmented financing arrangements), such an approach is usually considered insufficient as large proportions of the relevant costs and consequences fall outside the health care sector, with impacts on social care, patients and their families, and other sectors of the economy (for example, employment, justice, education). The broadest possible perspective of an economic evaluation is the societal perspective, which includes all possible costs (and outcomes). Alternative perspectives can result in different conclusions concerning the cost-effectiveness of interventions and services. Therefore, it is not uncommon for an economic evaluation to present results from several perspectives (Box 136.4).

Randomized clinical studies are a great source of collecting relevant cost and outcome data at individual patient level. Often, however, data for all relevant comparisons are not available directly. Furthermore, unless an economic evaluation is prospectively planned *alongside a clinical trial*, information on important outcomes or costs is frequently not collected. It is also important that the analytical time horizon of an economic evaluation is long enough to capture all important cost and outcome impacts of the compared alternatives. This aspect becomes extremely influential when costs and outcomes occur at different time points, for example, when assessing the value for money of preventative programmes. The time frame of clinical studies is often too short to provide all the necessary evidence. A fourth potential limitation of clinical studies as data sources is the representativeness of their investigated patient populations to real life. Due to these limitations, evidence synthesis of cost and outcome data from multiple sources, including literature, routine administrative databases, and expert opinions, within a *decision analytic modelling* framework often becomes necessary for economic evaluations [23].

### Identifying, measuring, and valuing costs

Costing in economic evaluations include the identification of the resources used as inputs in the provision of an intervention or service (for example, medications taken, days spent in hospital, GP visits), measurement of the actual *resource use* for each relevant category, and the valuation of these amounts by their respective *unit costs* (for example, cost per usual defined daily dose of an SSRI, cost of 1 day in hospital, cost of a GP visit).

Information on individual-level resource use can be derived from routinely collected data (for example, hospital records). In addition, linkage of different routine databases across multiple providers may become necessary. Alternatively, patients, caregivers, or professionals may be asked via specifically designed resource use questionnaires and diaries. A comprehensive collection of such resource use measurement instruments is publicly accessible via the DIRUM (Database of Instruments for Resource Use Measurement) database (http://www.dirum.org/). When patient-level variability of resource use is of lesser importance, relevant estimates may be taken from the literature or expert estimates are used.

Unit cost information for the valuation of health and social care resources may come from specific unit cost libraries, if available (for example, http://www.pssru.ac.uk/project-pages/unit-costs/), or be estimated anew using top–down or bottom–up (also called

micro-costing) approaches, depending on data availability and perspective. Unit cost estimates usually include relevant cost categories for staff costs, capital costs, and overhead costs [24].

### Identifying, measuring, and valuing outcomes

In clinical practice, *disease-specific and symptom-specific outcome measures* [for example, Beck Depression Inventory (BDI), Brief Psychiatric Rating Scale (BPRS)] are routinely used to monitor and evaluate outcomes focusing on a particular disease or symptom area. For the purposes of economic evaluations where often outcomes have to be measured and compared across different disease areas or patient populations or within the general population, there has been a growing interest in more *generic outcome measures* that are able to capture health or broader social functioning and well-being [for example, Short Form Health Survey 36 (SF-36), EuroQoL (EQ-5D)].

Both disease-specific and generic instruments can be further classified as *patient-reported outcome measures (PROMs)* when values for health state descriptions are directly reported by individuals who experience them, vs *assessor-reported outcome measures* when someone else, often a doctor, nurse or carer, reports the values. PROMs do not include biomedical measures or are used as specific diagnostic instruments in clinical practice. A great compilation of different PROM instruments can be found at http://phi.uhce.ox.ac.uk/home.php.

Outcome measures can also be classified as non-preference-based or preference-based instruments. *Non-preference-based instruments* measure symptoms, disease progression, or health-related quality of life, alongside a predefined profile, and yield profile scores on the relevant domains without assessing the value individuals place on the different domains. Their applicability in economic evaluations is restricted, as their comparability is frequently limited, they are not linked to any underlying valuation of health states, the trade-off across different domains in the profile is difficult to interpret, and they do not provide a single score usable for the development of a single cost-effectiveness ratio. In contrast, *preference-based instruments* combine different dimensions of health to generate quality of life estimates for multiple health states, which are then valued to yield a single summary utility score [25]. When utility values from generic preference-based outcome measures are not directly available for economic evaluations, statistical methods, known as 'mapping', can be applied to predict health state utilities from disease-specific scales, given there is an overlap in content between the measures of interest [26].

There are several instruments and elicitation methods to estimate health state utilities. Among these, the EuroQoL EQ-5D is the most widely recommended tool for quantifying utilities and conducting economic evaluations [27]. There is, however, growing concern whether generic preference-based measures, including the EQ-5D, capture all important aspects of health-related quality of life for specific mental disorders [28]. Although there are studies that have reported that the EQ-5D demonstrates construct validity and responsiveness for common mental illnesses, such as depression, the results for severe mental illnesses, including schizophrenia and bipolar disorders, are less convincing [29, 30].

In the light of the ongoing discussion on the appropriateness of the existing outcome measures for certain disease areas, including people with mental health problems, new approaches of measuring well-being based on the capability approach have emerged and been increasingly applied in general outcome measurement in health economics. Instruments, including the ICECAP (ICEpop CAPability) and ASCOT (Adult Social Care Outcome Toolkit) questionnaires, have been developed to use in the health and social care sectors [31]. The OxCAP-MH (Oxford CAPabilities questionnaire-Mental Health), a 16-item PROM, has been specifically designed for outcome measurement in mental health [32]. The validation of the instrument with patients suffering from severe mental health problems showed good feasibility, acceptability, content, and construct validities, including significant correlations with psychiatric symptoms, social functioning, and other quality of life measures [33].

### Cost-effectiveness decision framework

Economic evaluations compare the difference in costs to the difference in outcomes (effects) between two competing alternatives (alternative A vs alternative B) in the form of an *incremental cost-effectiveness ratio (ICER)*.

$$ICER = (CA - CB)/(EA - EB)$$

Depending on the type of economic evaluation, the ICER may be expressed as the 'incremental cost per case prevented' (CEA) or as the 'incremental cost per QALY' (CUA). Including the inherent uncertainty in estimating the difference in costs and outcomes, there are nine possible decision scenarios that can emerge. These scenarios are listed and depicted on the cost-effectiveness plane in Fig. 136.1.

- Scenario 1: The new intervention/service is more effective and less costly than the control one; the new intervention/service dominates and should be accepted.
- Scenario 2: The new intervention/service is less effective and more costly than the control; the new intervention/service is dominated and should be rejected.

- Scenario 3: The new intervention/service is more effective and costs the same as the control; the new intervention/service dominates and should be accepted.
- Scenario 4: The new intervention/service is less effective and costs the same as the control; the new intervention/service is dominated and should be rejected.
- Scenario 5: The new intervention/service is equally effective and less costly than the control; the new intervention/service dominates and should be accepted.
- Scenario 6: The new intervention/service is equally effective and more costly than the control; the new intervention/service is dominated and should be rejected.
- Scenario 7: The new intervention/service is more effective and more costly than the control; no clear decision.
- Scenario 8: The new intervention/service is less effective and less costly than the control; no clear decision.
- Scenario 9: The new intervention/service is equally effective and equally costly as the control; no clear decision.

In case of scenarios 7 and 8, the cost-effectiveness decision depends on the *threshold value* (T) society is willing to pay or can afford for a unit of outcome. In England, the National Institute for Health and Care Excellence (NICE) established a range between £20,000–30,000 as the relevant cost-effectiveness threshold for one QALY gained [27]. According to this, interventions/services with a cost per QALY of below £20,000 would be funded; between £20,000–30,000, the funding decision would depend mostly on other decision factors (for example, availability of alternative treatment options, burden of disease); and above £30,000, it would be funded only in rare cases. Similar affordability criteria have been set

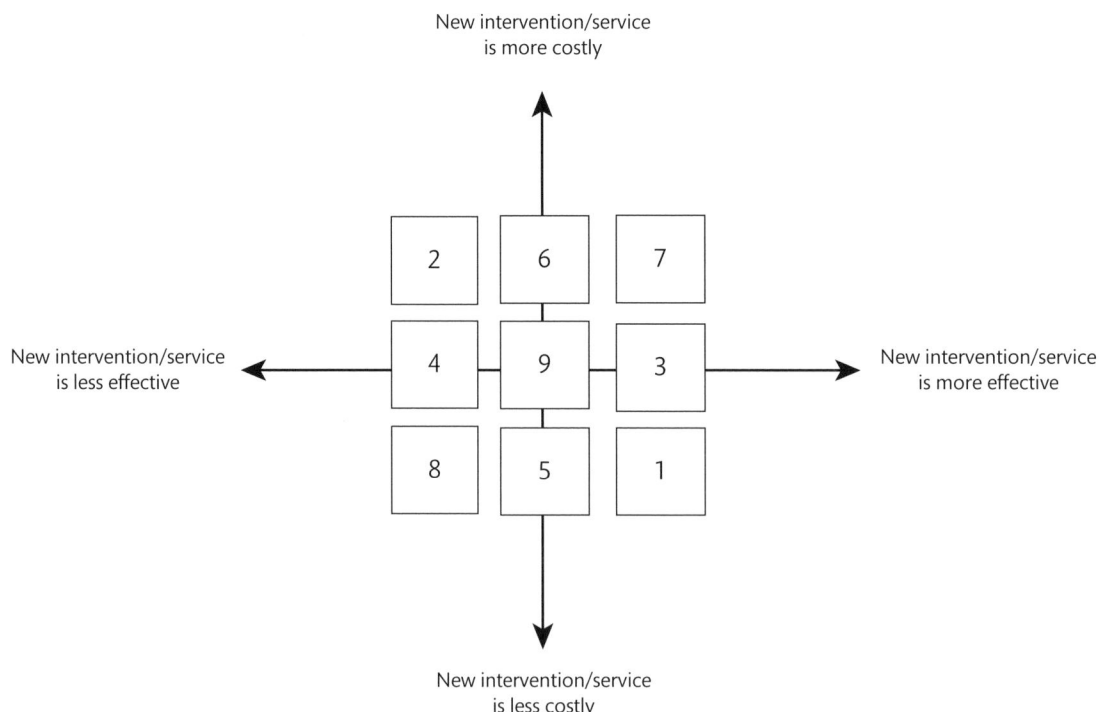

**Fig. 136.1** Cost-effectiveness plane with possible cost-effectiveness decision scenarios.

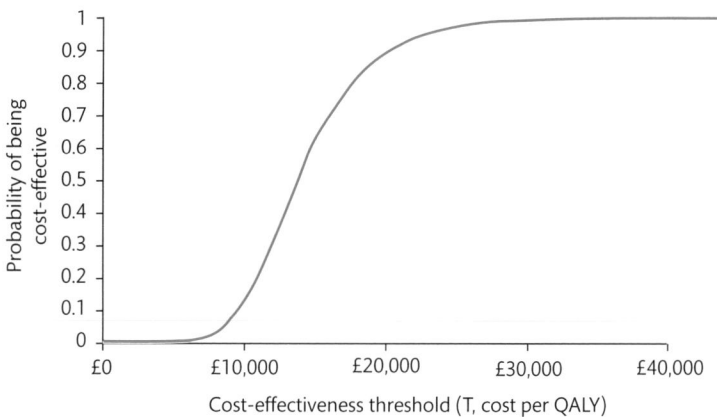

**Fig. 136.2** Cost-effectiveness acceptability curve.

up for developing countries by the WHO [34]. Here, interventions are considered very cost-effective if a DALY averted costs less than the GDP per capita, and cost-effective if a DALY averted costs less than three times the GDP per capita. *Cost-effectiveness acceptability curves* show the probability that an intervention is cost-effective, dependent on the threshold value (Fig. 136.2). These curves are based on the *net benefit (NB)*, an alternative summary measure of the value for money of interventions/services derived at by the following cost-effectiveness decision rule:

$$NB = T \times (EA - EB) - (CA - CB)$$

If NB >0, the new intervention/service is cost-effective. If NB <0, the new intervention/service is not cost-effective. If NB = 0, there is an indifference between the alternatives. A similar decision rule applies to the results of CBAs.

## Applications

Economic evaluations are seen by decision-makers as useful tools with growing importance due to the increasing need for resource allocation decisions. Many countries have now established organizations to develop economic evaluations to inform policy-making either within or outside a health technology assessment (HTA) framework (for example, NICE for England, CADTH for Canada, IQWIG for Germany, CVZ for the Netherlands). A comprehensive list of relevant HTA organizations can be found under the umbrella organizations of the International Network of Agencies for Health Technology Assessment (INAHTA) (www.inahta.org), Health Technology Assessment international (HTAi) (https://htai.org/about-htai/), and European Network for Health Technology Assessment (EUnetHTA) (https://www.eunethta.eu/about-eunethta/). Furthermore, the requirement to demonstrate cost-effectiveness evidence, in addition to quality, safety, and efficacy, for the reimbursement of pharmaceutical, medical technology, or biotech products has been introduced as a 'fourth hurdle' in many health care systems [35].

It is therefore not accidental that a rapid review of evidence on the costs and benefits of interventions in the area of mental health from Australia found that among the included 50 studies, pharmacological treatments were the most commonly studied interventions, followed by psychosocial interventions [36]. Only a few studies investigated the cost-effectiveness of employment programmes, art programmes, internet strategies, electroconvulsive therapy, discharge models, and

joint crisis plans. Most studies were from the UK and adopted a health sector perspective, with only a small number considering other sectors (for example, housing, education, employment, or (criminal) justice sectors) and relevant intersectoral aspects. In terms of disease area, depression was the most frequently studied, followed by schizophrenia, anxiety disorder, conduct disorder, attention-deficit/hyperactivity disorder (ADHD), and panic disorder [36].

Another systematic review of published economic evaluations that compared antidepressant treatments in depression, based on database analyses and prospective clinical studies, identified 40 papers that met the inclusion criteria [37]. Among these, a relatively large number of industry-sponsored evaluations of escitalopram were identified, which found escitalopram to be potentially cost-effective in depression treatment. Evidence of cost-effectiveness differences between other individual SSRIs was not unequivocally established. Inconsistent findings further emerged concerning the cost-effectiveness of SSRIs vs tricyclic antidepressants between retrospective database analyses and prospective studies [37].

Incorporation of economic analyses in evidence-based clinical guidelines is also becoming common practice. One of the first decision analytic models developed for this purpose relates to the 2004 NICE depression guideline [38, 39]. This evaluated the outcomes and likely costs of the first-line use of combination therapy of antidepressant medication with psychological therapy for moderate and severe depression in the UK. The study found that combination therapy is likely to be cost-effective for severe depression, with an average cost per QALY gained of £5777 (95% CI: £1900–33,800), while its cost-effectiveness is much more uncertain for moderate depression (average cost per QALY gained: £14,540; 95% CI: £4800–79,400).

Economic evaluations may also be used to evaluate mental health programmes for whole populations and show how much of the burden may be averted by selecting cost-effective interventions. A comparative cost-effectiveness analysis of interventions for reducing the burden of major neuropsychiatric disorders formed part of the WHO CHOICE project (CHOosing Interventions that are Cost-Effective) [40]. The project assembled databases on cost-effectiveness of key health interventions in 14 epidemiological subregions of the world, using a generalized cost-effectiveness framework in which costs and outcomes of current and new interventions were compared to 'doing nothing'. The costs and effectiveness of pharmacological and psychosocial interventions in primary care or outpatient settings for psychiatric disorders were compared in a population model. Effects were measured as DALYs averted and costs in international dollars. Compared to no treatment, the most cost-effective strategy for averting the burden of psychosis and severe affective disorders in developing regions of the world is a combined intervention of first-generation antipsychotic or mood-stabilizing drugs with adjuvant psychosocial treatment delivered by community-based outpatient services. For more common mental disorders treated in primary care settings (depressive and anxiety disorders), the single most cost-effective strategy was the scaled-up use of older antidepressants due to their lower cost, but broadly similar efficacy to newer antidepressants. However, as the price difference between older and generic newer antidepressants continued to narrow over time, generic SSRIs may represent the current treatment of choice. Proactive disease management, including long-term maintenance treatment with antidepressant drugs, also represents a cost-effective way of significantly reducing the enormous burden of depression in developing regions. As the authors point out, these findings provide relevant information regarding the relative value of investing in neuropsychiatric treatment and prevention, and so may help to remove one of many remaining barriers to a more appropriate public health response to mental health needs [40].

In addition, economic evaluations can highlight the potential economic benefits of improved service and care provision at the population level. A global return on investment analysis for scaling up depression and anxiety treatment focusing on the benefits of increased productivity found a benefit-to-cost ratio of 2.3–3.0 when only economic costs and benefits were considered, and a ratio of 3.3–5.7 when the intrinsic value of health gains were also included across the different country income groups [41].

Due to the growing number of published economic evaluations to guide resource allocation decisions, it is of utmost importance that the methods used and the standards of reporting are harmonized. International checklists to support the *critical appraisal* of the robustness of methods and results have now been developed and are used to guide publications standards as well [42, 43].

## Conclusions

Health economic analyses of mental health services are aimed to support needs assessment, service development, budget planning, and resource allocation decisions. Among these, economic evaluations provide information on the cost-effectiveness of competing alternative interventions and services. They are seen as useful decision-making tools with increasing importance worldwide.

The rising disease and economic burden of mental health problems, together with the growing economic evidence on simple cost-effective interventions with great return on investment potentials, put the scaling up of some mental health services high on the political agenda. Availability of current cost-effectiveness information reflects the increased submission requirements for the reimbursement of new technologies. As a consequence, evidence on the cost-effectiveness of preventative measures for mental health disorders remains limited, potentially shifting away the attention from such options.

Although the rigour of the methods and reporting standards of economic evaluations have considerably increased since the introduction of relevant checklists, several methodological questions persist. Outcome measurement for the evaluation of mental health services remains a major challenge. Recently growing concerns about the validity and responsiveness of common, generic quality of life measures for people with severe mental disorders point towards the need for alternative, broader well-being measures to be implemented in this context. Novel instruments using the capability approach as their underlying framework have now emerged as promising new concepts. Due to the important broader societal consequences of mental health problems, including their negative impacts on families, it is also imperative to shift standard outcome evaluation from individual patients towards family units and progress relevant methods. For the same reason, economic evaluations of mental health services require broad costing perspectives. Although the methodology of costing in economic evaluations may seem more straightforward than that of outcome measurement, internationally harmonized methods and tools for the identification, definition, measurement, and valuation of costs have received considerably less attention, and comparability among economic evaluations is often lacking in this respect. Not only is there a need for increased availability of harmonized national unit cost compendiums for health and social care services internationally, the lack of similar comprehensive intersectoral unit cost information also remains a major challenge.

## REFERENCES

1. Organisation for Economic Co-operation and Development (OECD). *What Future for Health Spending?* OECD Economics Department Policy Notes; No. 19. Paris: OECD; 2013.

2. Organisation for Economic Co-operation and Development (OECD). *Making Mental Health Count. The Social and Economic Costs of Neglecting Mental Healthcare*. OECD Health Policy Studies. Paris: OECD; 2014.

3. Bloom DE, Cafiero ET, Janeì-Llopis E, *et al. The Global Economic Burden of Noncommunicable Diseases*. Geneva: World Economic Forum; 2011

4. Drummond M, Sculpher M, Torrance G, O'Brien B, Stoddart G. *Methods for the Economic Evaluation of Healthcare Programmes*, fourth edition. New York, NY: Oxford University Press; 2015.

5. Whiteford HA, Degenhardt L, Rehm J, *et al.* Global burden of disease attributable to mental and substance use disorders: findings from the Global Burden of Disease Study 2010. *Lancet*. 2013; 382: 1575–86.

6. World Health Organization (2012). *Depression Factsheet*. Available from: http://www.euro.who.int/en/health-topics/ noncommunicable-diseases/mental-health

7. Murray CJ, Lopez AD. Global mortality, disability, and the contribution of risk factors: Global Burden of Disease Study. *Lancet*. 1997; 349: 1436–42.

8. Organisation for Economic Co-operation and Development (OECD). *Estimating Expenditure by Disease, Age and Gender Under the System of Health Accounts (SHA) Framework*. Paris: OECD Publishing; 2008.

9. Wittchen HU, Jacobi FR, Rehm J, *et al.* The size and burden of mental disorders and other disorders of the brain in Europe 2010. *Eur Neuropsychopharmacol*. 2011; 21: 655–79.

10. Organisation for Economic Co-operation and Development (OECD). *Health at a Glance: Europe 2015*. Paris: OECD Publishing; 2015.

11. IMS Health. *Health Top 20 Global Therapeutic Classes, Total Audited Markets*. Danbury, CT: IMS Health; 2011.

12. Luppa M, Heinrich S, Angermeyer MC, Konig HH, Riedel-Heller SG. Cost-of-illness studies of depression: a systematic review. *J Affect Disord*. 2007; 98:29–43.

13. Evans-Lacko S, Knapp M. Importance of social and cultural factors for attitudes, disclosure and time off work for depression: findings from a seven country European study on depression in the workplace. *PLoS One*. 2014; 9:e91053.

14. Gustavsson A, Svensson M, Jacobi F, *et al*. Cost of disorders of the brain in Europe 2010. *Eur Neuropsychopharmacol*. 2011; 21:718–79.

15. Olesen J, Gustavsson A, Svensson M, Wittchen HU, Jönsson B. The economic cost of brain disorders in Europe. *Eur J Neurol*. 2012; 19:155–62.

16. Sullivan SD, Mauskopf JA, Augustovski F, *et al*. Budget Impact Analysis—Principles of Good Practice: Report of the ISPOR 2012 Budget Impact Analysis Good Practice II Task Force. *Value Health*. 2014; 17:5–14.

17. Simon J, Budge KV, Goodwin G, Geddes J. Health economic preparatory work for OXTEXT: The development and evaluation of cost-effective systems of collaborative disease management for people with bipolar disorder. *J Ment Health Policy Econ*. 2011; 14(Suppl.1): S32.

18. Briggs AH, O'Brien BJ. The death of the cost-minimisation analysis? *Health Econ*. 2001; 10:179–84.

19. Brazier J, Ratcliffe J, Salomon JA, Tsuchiya A. *Measuring and Valuing Health Benefits for Economic Evaluation*, second edition. New York, NY: Oxford University Press; 2017.

20. Thokala P, Duenas A. Multiple criteria decision analysis for health technology assessment. *Value Health*. 2012; 15: 1172–81.

21. Burns T, Rugkåsa J, Molodynski A, *et al*. Community treatment orders for patients with psychosis (OCTET): a randomised controlled trial. *Lancet*. 2013; 381: 1627–33.

22. Simon J, Gray A, Mayer S, *et al*. Cost-effectiveness of Community Treatment Orders (CTOs): Economic Evaluation of the OCTET Study. *J Ment Health Policy Econ*. 2015; 18(S1): S36.

23. Briggs AH, Claxton K, Sculpher MJ. *Decision Modelling for Health Economic Evaluation*. New York, NY: Oxford University Press; 2006.

24. Beecham JKJ, Knapp MRJ. Costing psychiatric interventions. In: Thornicroft G, Brewin C, Wing JK (eds.). *Measuring Mental Health Needs*, second edition. London: Gaskell; 2000. pp. 200–24.

25. Gray AM, Clarke PM, Wolstenholme JL, Wordsworth S. *Applied Methods of Cost-Effectiveness Analysis in Healthcare*. New York, NY: Oxford University Press; 2010.

26. Petrou S, Rivero-Arias O, Dakin H, *et al*. The MAPS reporting statement for studies mapping onto generic preference-based outcome measures: explanation and elaboration. *Pharmacoeconom*. 2015; 33: 993–1011.

27. National Institute for Health and Care Excellence. *Guide to the Methods of Technology Appraisal*. London: National Institute for Health and Care Excellence; 2013.

28. Brazier JJ. Is the EQ–5D fit for purpose in mental health? *Br J Psychiatry*. 2010; 197: 348–9.

29. Brazier J, Connell J, Papaioannou D, *et al*. A systematic review, psychometric analysis and qualitative assessment of generic preference-based measures of health in mental health populations and the estimation of mapping functions from widely used specific measures. *Health Technol Assess*. 2014; 18:vii–viii, xiii–xxv, 1–188.

30. Payakachat N, Ali MM, Tilford JM. Can the EQ-5D detect meaningful change? A systematic review. *Pharmacoeconom*. 2015; 33: 1137–54.

31. Coast J, Kinghorn P, Mitchell P. The development of capability measures in health economics: opportunities, challenges and progress. *Patient*. 2015; 8: 119–26.

32. Simon J, Anand P, Gray A, Rugkasa J, Yeeles K, Burns T. Operationalising the capability approach for outcome measurement in mental health research. *Soc Sci Med*. 2013; 98: 187–96.

33. Vergunst F, Jenkinson C, Burns T, Anand P. Gray A, Rugkåsa J, Simon J (2017). Psychometric validation of a multi-dimensional capability instrument for outcome measurement in mental health research (OxCAP-MH). *Health and Quality of Life Outcomes*. 15: 250.

34. Commission on Macroeconomics and Health. *Macroeconomics and Health: Investing in Health for Economic Development*. Geneva: World Health Organization; 2001.

35. Rawlins MD. Crossing the fourth hurdle. *Br J Clin Pharm*. 2012; 73: 855–60.

36. Doran CM. *The Costs and Benefits in the Area of Mental Health*. An evidence check review brokered by the Sax Institute (www.saxinstitute.org.au) for the Mental Health Commission of NSW; 2013.

37. Pan YJ, Knapp M, McCrone P. Cost-effectiveness comparisons between antidepressant treatments in depression: Evidence from database analyses and prospective studies. *J Affect Disord*. 2012; 139: 113–25.

38. National Institute for Health and Care Excellence. *Depression: Management of Depression in Primary and Secondary Care*. Clinical guideline [CG23]. London: National Institute for Health and Care Excellence; 2004.

39. Simon J, Pilling S, Burbeck R, Goldberg D. Treatment options in moderate and severe depression: decision analysis supporting a clinical guideline. *Br J Psychiatry*. 2006; 189: 494–501.

40. Chisholm D. Choosing cost-effective interventions in psychiatry. *World Psychiatry*. 2005; 4: 37–44.

41. Chisholm D, Sweeny K, Sheehan P, *et al*. Scaling-up treatment of depression and anxiety: a global return on investment analysis. *Lancet Psychiatry*. 2016; 3: 415–24.

42. Drummond MF, Jefferson T. Guidelines for authors and peer reviewers of economic submissions to the BMJ. *BMJ*. 1996; 313: 275–83.

43. Husereau D, Drummond M, Petrou S, *et al*. Consolidated health economic evaluation reporting standards (CHEERS) statement. *BMC Med*. 2013; 11: 80.

# 137

# Organization of psychiatric services for general hospital departments
## Proactive and preventive interventions in psychiatry

*William H. Sledge and Julianne Dorset*

## Introduction

There are many proactive health care interventions that have proven to be effective with acceptable risk–reward ratios. Organized Western medicine, however, continues to focus on administering health care resources, particularly in hospital-based psychiatry, to those patients with advanced illnesses despite knowing about early manifestations of mental illness and associated disorders of personality and addiction. Consultation-liaison psychiatric services, where treatment may be considered reactive and minimalist, relative to what consult services within other disciplines believe is adequate care, are particularly vulnerable to glossing over early signs of illness due to the lack of mental health professionals in general hospitals and the gulf of understanding between hospital staff and psychiatric service providers. A variety of problems flow from this type of practice. Practitioners from other medical disciplines and specialties are rarely well versed in accurately recognizing subtle and/or early signs of mental illness and emotional suffering. This is a matter of training and skill, but also a product of the way that many mental illnesses are conceptualized as a continuum of traits and qualities. As such, there is no clear line of demarcation between illnesses and normality. Consequently, medical practitioners may not understand or have adequate experience utilizing psychiatric treatments that may be appropriate for their patients. This may result in 'psychiatric treatment nihilism' or a phenomenon in which the non-psychiatric practitioner feels that there is little that can be done to help the patient, partly because treatments are limited, but also because of a lack of skills and knowledge to deal with the clinical presentation accurately [1]. A sense of futility may ensue so that the practitioner calls for a psychiatric consult late in the hospitalization or does not call a mental health specialist at all.

The appropriateness of the consultation request does not always match the putative patient. Some requests for services are inappropriate such as in the case of a normal reaction to bad news or physical suffering that does not require the specialized skills and knowledge of a mental health professional. This may happen while the undetected mentally ill patient suffers in silence in the absence of appropriate care. Nursing staff members are left to use 'common sense' to manage these patients, which may suffice when distress, and not mental illness, is the cause of a patient's symptoms. Common sense in the face of mental illness, however, is often uncommon among non-psychiatric hospital clinical workers. Therefore, it is inappropriate for practitioners in disciplines other than mental health to decide whether mental health services should intervene during an episode of care for a somatic ailment. Non-psychiatric physicians do not always understand mentally ill patients nor do they have knowledge of the resources that might be available to both patients and practitioners. It is thus understandable, but not entirely forgivable, why psychiatric patients often do not get maximal care for their psychiatric troubles when they are in a non-psychiatric setting in the hospital.

Part of the responsibility for this lack of awareness about mental health issues redounds to the mental health practitioners who do not educate non-mental health providers and/or lack the ability to deal professionally with their skepticism about psychiatry. In that regard, mental health practitioners may need to be more assertive and proactive in advocating for these services. Chen, Evans, and Larkin [1] reviewed the literature from 1965 to 2015, on the reasons that hospital-based physicians are reluctant to refer to psychiatry. They noted that physicians frequently did not call for psychiatric consultations due to feeling uncomfortable with consultation-liaison psychiatry (CLP). Operant factors that favoured psychiatric referrals were a dedicated CLP service, an active consultant, and physicians who were comfortable with psychiatric patients, as well as with medically ill patients.

In this chapter, we address psychiatric consultation services for early intervention, review conceptual and practical challenges, and present where to find more detail about efforts of early intervention. We distinguish the difference between proactive and preventative services by the following—'proactive' refers to activity on the part of the practitioner that is designed to eliminate or arrest the progression of an already recognized condition and/or illness, whereas 'prevention' entails activities that keep an illness or a disability from being established. Common examples of preventative measures are vaccination programmes against infectious diseases, protective gear in athletic endeavours, or mandatory seat belts in automobiles to prevent traumatic injury. We review successful non-psychiatric proactive health care interventions to establish universal structural factors that need to be considered in any kind of proactive or preventative intervention. For ease of presentation, we will use the term 'early intervention' to describe preventative and/or proactive efforts together. While we propose a clear-line distinction between proactive and preventive, in practice, this distinction may not always be discernable.

Prevention as a concept in medicine has been modernized by an Institute of Medicine work group [2], which divides it into three subcategories: *universal* preventive interventions, *selective* preventive interventions, and *indicated* preventive interventions. Universal preventive interventions are targeted to the public or to whole population groups that have not been identified as having the illness in question but perhaps have associated increased risks for the disorder(s) being considered. In this instance, there would be no discernable, definitive evidence of the presence of the condition(s) in question, but there would be a perceived risk or vulnerability. Universal interventions are typically characterized by low risk and low cost. The annual flu shot and other vaccinations urged upon populations would be examples of universal interventions. Psychiatry does not have a disorder that clearly fits into this category.

Selective preventive interventions refer to operations and interventions for subgroups of the population whose risk for developing a disorder is higher due to present known individual traits and characteristics or social risk factors. Such a group might be the non-symptomatic carriers of a recessive gene for the development of a severe disorder such as Huntington's disease or coal miners who, due to their line of work, are at higher risk for developing black lung disease. The risk–reward ratio of the intervention and the likelihood of developing the condition dictate whether an intervention may be worth implementing.

Indicated preventive interventions are for high-risk individuals who are identified as having minimal, but detectable, signs or symptoms which foreshadow the expression of a disorder. Biological markers or symptoms that signal a predisposition for a mental disorder in the carrier, but do not meet diagnostic criteria for the disorder at the current time, would also fall into this group [2]. Indicated preventive interventions may be worthwhile, even if intervention costs are high and the intervention entails some considerable expense or risk to the patient, relative to the possible consequences of not providing the intervention. Interventions for conditions that demonstrate that a disorder is present should be considered treatment, rather than prevention.

Proactive interventions in psychiatry, and perhaps for many medical conditions, fall somewhere between treatment and indicative preventive interventions. However, psychiatric conditions present conceptual, as well as practical, challenges to this cartography of intervention in that the present diagnostic system in psychiatry is largely based on descriptive accounts, rather than precise aetiological, biologically based characteristics. Furthermore, as noted, psychiatric conditions are frequently expressed along a spectrum of the illness in question, so that there may be several conditions that create suffering and disability but do not rise to diagnosable disease proportions. There may be ambiguity as to whether a person is diagnosable as mentally ill or not. Additionally, some conditions have similar characteristics, which may result in different providers diagnosing a person differently over time. Finally, some normal symptomatic conditions are difficult to discern from mental illness, such as in the case of grief which may, in some cases, be indistinguishable from depression. These conditions can be easily confused with pathological states if the historical data are not clear or understood.

Psychiatric conditions are often chronic, beginning slowly and eventually manifesting as peaks and valleys of symptoms and morbidity, interspersed with periods of relatively normal functioning. Experienced psychiatric clinicians can usually identify prodromal symptoms and recognize deterioration in clinical status and capacity. Yet it may be difficult to differentiate between illness and normal variation in many circumstances, particularly when a clinician is without a longitudinal view of the patient or significant training for recognizing mental illness.

Diagnostic uncertainty in psychiatry has, in part, added to the lack of preventive prescriptions that are feasible in effectiveness, cost, or secondary risk, to which the interventions may expose the patient and/or others. In most of medicine, with the exception of trauma, serious diseases may present with minor symptoms or findings that are frequently ambiguous in terms of their implications. Physicians and patients are left to opt for a wait-and-see approach, to push aggressively for a definitive diagnosis immediately despite economic cost and/or personal risks, or to pursue a course of assessment and treatment somewhere in between these two polar positions. To illuminate the possibility of proactive and/or preventive measures in mental health, we review some of the literature on early interventions in other fields. In doing so, some of the conceptual considerations for proactive and preventive approaches in psychiatry will be brought to light. Desan *et al.* [3] similarly described a new vision of liaison psychiatry for the future, in which psychosomatic medicine will be proactive and increasingly integrated into specialty and general medical care.

## Structural examples of 'early recognition' interventions in clinical care

A review of the literature on early intervention revealed some common structural features of successful programmes (including assessment). Certainly, an important feature is a clear concept of the illness/disease in question, both in its treatment as well as in its morbidity and mortality. Of particular importance is its manner of early expression. In other words, detectable features (signs and/or symptoms) must be present for early detection and subsequent treatment to be applied effectively and appropriately. There must also be a means of detecting and recognizing the early signs in the form of a screening process that has acceptable accuracy and ease of use and that poses no threat to the safety of the patient. For some diseases, this may be screening for biological markers, but in psychiatry, markers will inevitably be historical facts, present symptoms, and/or behaviour (which includes thoughts, intentions, emotions, etc.). Standardization of these data is important to understand, as it is through standardization that we can compare outcomes and course, as well as risk and results. Ideally, screening is standardized across a variety of barriers such as time, place, condition, and user.

## Review of proactive treatments

One form of proactive treatment that has gained traction is the rapid response team (RRT). Most of these teams are used to counteract extreme illnesses such as cardiovascular events and other medical emergencies that respond to highly specialized technical care. Garretson et al. [4] offered that the use of rapid assessment breaks traditional hospital hierarchies or silos that delay care, noting that the role of the team is to assess the patient, assist the bedside nurse in providing the most appropriate care for the patient, and determine whether the patient needs a higher level of care and where that care can be provided. The effectiveness of RRTs has been measured by reduced unplanned intensive care unit (ICU) admissions [5, 6], reduced incidence of cardiac arrest and mortality [7], and increased patient, family, and staff satisfaction [8, 9]. These teams adopt a proactive approach, which contrasts with the reactive nature of conventional care such as traditional cardiac arrest teams [10].

One modification of the RRT is a 'rover team' which identifies at-risk patients and facilitates the prompt administration of time-sensitive therapies [11]. This proactive approach provides a critical care resource and improves clinically important outcomes, at a lower level of cost than a reactive approach. One randomized controlled study measured the efficacy of a proactive infection control team [12]. The team visited patients on the study wards daily and identified risk factors for developing health care-associated infections (HAIs). If risk factors were identified, the team worked with the treating clinicians to eliminate those risk factors, which resulted in a significant decrease in the incidence of HAIs. Another quasi-experimental study [13] found that a proactive response system identified subtle signs of deterioration faster than a control unit without a system of proactivity. This experimental unit used the physiological measures of patients to generate an alert for early warning signs of patient deterioration. These measures were updated regularly throughout the day, and if a patient generated a score above a set threshold, an RRT was activated. This is an example of delivering expedient and appropriate expertise to patients in need. On the back end of hospitalization, when cost and oversubscription become a problem, a proactive palliative care nurse consultation was shown to reduce the length of stay (LOS) in a medical ICU by almost half (8.96 vs 16.28 days; $P = 0.0001$) without any impact on mortality or other salient clinical measures [14]. In yet another study, proactive consultations for geriatric patients undergoing repair of hip fractures resulted in an 18% reduction of post-operative delirium [15]. Additionally, proactivity has been found to affect patient and staff experience, with one proactive approach to hourly rounding by nursing staff resulting in improved patient satisfaction and staff morale [16].

In several studies of medical rounding, researchers pursued a proactive approach through the inclusion of non-conventional professionals. These professionals were sought for their expertise and skills which were employed to help detect signs of problems that might cause complications in patients' hospital stays and to offer solutions. In an innovative proactive approach, investigators found that the inclusion of a clinical medical librarian as a part of the medical team during daily rounds helped to improve the performance of the team, as measured by lower LOS and lower readmission rate [17]. The librarian helped to clarify clinicians' questions immediately during rounds or after through prompt email responses. Shortened LOS and lower readmission rates were also the outcomes of a multicentre quasi-randomized controlled clinical trial that included a pharmacist on a medical team in two internal medicine and two family medicine services [18]. The pharmacist helped to resolve drug-related issues and make suggestions for improvement by reviewing patients' medication histories and participating in rounds and discharge counselling. Another example is the development of a new system of multi-disciplinary rounds [19]. A team of clinicians from medical wards, as well as other specialty services, designed a new process for performing rounds that targeted care inefficiency, poor communication, and redundant documentation. The new standardized method of rounding increased the frequency to daily, included all disciplines involved in patients' care in the interaction, and made workloads more predictable by requiring orders to be written during the rounds. The new method of rounding resulted in both decreased cost and decreased LOS in the treatment groups, as compared to controls.

This review of proactive services for disciplines outside psychiatry illuminates the critical design features that a proactive service might contain. Fig. 137.1 outlines the eight proposed critical design features. Perhaps the most important design feature for a psychiatric proactive approach is that it must comprise clinicians from various disciplines (at least nurses, physicians, and social workers). Additionally, these clinicians should be flexible and devoted, enquiring practitioners who are looking for the right clinical answers to the patients' troubles. Having multiple practitioners who overlap in tasks and skill sets offers more flexibility and depth in personnel, and knowledge. A second design feature is the availability and clear definition of discoverable facts within the patients' narratives and behaviours that may be harbingers of mental illness. Screening algorithms serve this purpose well. Furthermore, practitioners must have the skills to detect and interpret these signs and symptoms. The third necessity for a successful team is for the clinicians to be well trained, so that they can interview patients efficiently and quickly develop an accurate idea of what may be wrong. The fourth feature is to have a standardized and thorough assessment which helps to ensure accuracy of diagnosis. The fifth feature is the availability and prescription of an effective treatment. The sixth is the follow-up, monitoring, and assessment of treatment delivery and effectiveness and assisting in post-hospitalization care. A seventh feature is that the practitioners should be fluent with each other's disciplines and aware of each other's strengths and weaknesses. This allows for timely and unambiguous communications, as well as on-site education. And finally, there should always be an educational function and goal with non-specialty staff.

## Programme descriptions

Desan et al. [20] reviewed the literature on the impact of consultation services on LOS and discussed the impact of a proactive approach. In the review, ten studies were identified that demonstrated increased consultation rates, four of which demonstrated improved LOS. Twelve studies examined the salience of consultation to geriatric patients, four of which demonstrated significant improvement in LOS. This review did not include the proactive psychiatric studies from Yale, Columbia, or Birmingham City Hospital. The review

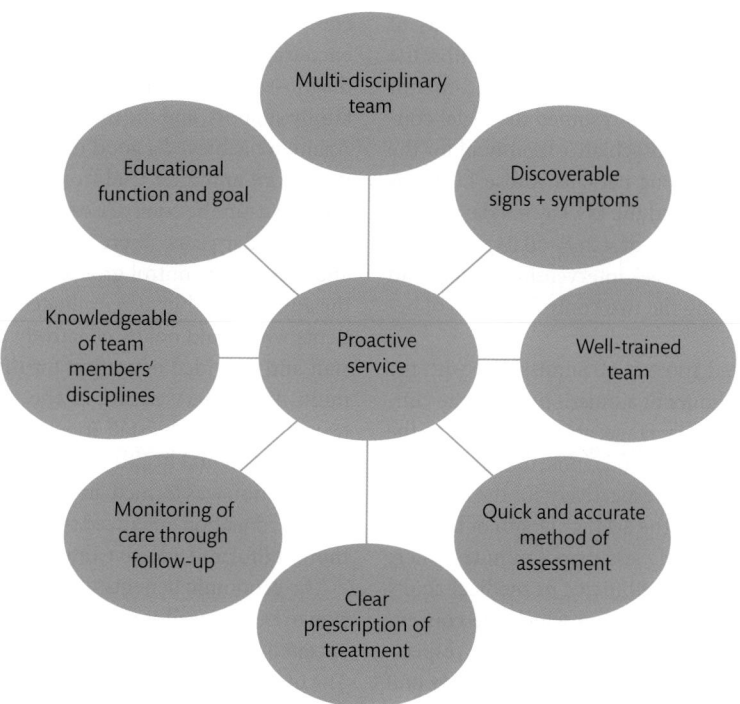

**Fig. 137.1** Design features of a proactive intervention programme.

did include the proactive geriatric service described by Sennour *et al.* [21].

Three comprehensive models of proactive psychiatric services have been developed and reported in the literature in the last 7 years. All three models are general hospital-based and would qualify as 'indicative prevention/treatment approaches', as all patients within the total inpatient population on or within an organization (service, floor, unit, etc.) are screened for the presence of mental illness, substance abuse, severe character disorders, or situational stressors. One is from the United Kingdom, and two are from the United States. All interventions came into being within a year of one another, though none were aware of the others.

The innovative proactive Rapid Assessment, Interface, and Discharge (RAID) model in the United Kingdom was developed to serve the 600-bed City Hospital of Birmingham [22]. RAID is a rapid-response, 'age-inclusive', comprehensive mental health intervention. During the study period, the team responded to 91% of accident and emergency (A&E) service cases within an hour (average of 24 minutes), and 89% of general and specialty ward cases within 24 hours (average of 16 hours). It also provided periodic training to the staff in these settings about the care of patients. The presence of RAID increased the detection of mental illness and reduced readmissions.

The assessment of the effectiveness of RAID entailed a novel approach of comparing populations in a before-and-after trial, in which patients were matched by risk factors and drawn to create three different analytic groups. The first group consisted of patients treated prior to the implementation of the RAID intervention and who had only received standard consultation services. The second group were the RAID recipients, and the third were those who were contemporaneous to the RAID recipients but had not received the intervention and were referred to as RAID-influenced. The clinical outcome variables were LOS, readmission rate, cost savings, and quality of care, as measured by the percentage of mental health diagnoses detected. The authors noted that they reduced the LOS, which equated to savings of 21–42 beds per day and reduced readmissions, saving 22 beds per day. The economic assessment carried out by the London School of Economics used the estimate of at least 44 beds per day, resulting in an estimated savings of £3.5 million. The authors believed this was a conservative estimate and that the actual savings would have been more like £4–6 million. During the intervention, the City Hospital was able to close 60 beds without cutting down on services.

From the United States, Muskin *et al.* [23] reported on a 'quality improvement program' in which psychiatrists and internists co-managed patients with comorbid psychiatric and medical conditions. In a before-and-after trial on a single unit, they found that the intervention resulted in a statistically significant reduction in LOS of 1.19 days among patients, with an LOS of less than 10 days. When annualized, the total number of saved days was 2889. The estimated cost per day was $600, resulting in an expected annual savings of over $1.7 million per year. The intervention paid for itself, as the estimated savings were more than three times the cost of the intervention teamworkers' salaries (2.5 full-time equivalent psychiatrists, in addition to a social worker).

Aspects of the Yale proactive approach have been reported in three different publications from two different, but related, interventions. The first, a pilot and feasibility study [24] demonstrated the value and effectiveness of a psychiatric proactive approach, revealing potential clinical and financial advantages, as well as areas for improvement. This initial study was conducted in a 30-bed general internal medicine inpatient unit at Yale New Haven Hospital. In an A-B-A single case study design, the patients' average LOS and consultation rates were examined in three different time frames. These were, in order, the pre-intervention period in which there was an initial study of the LOS in the usual treatment phase of the study for 6 months, the proactive intervention period for roughly 5 weeks, and the 6-month post-intervention period in which the unit resumed the usual conventional consultations as the mode of psychiatric treatment for the patients. On this general service, among patients whose LOS was 30 days or less, the intervention reduced the LOS by 0.9 days (from an average of 3.8 days, chi square = 6.38, df = 2; $P = 0.04$). The consultation rate was 22.6% during the 5-week intervention period, and 9.3% and 12.0%, respectively, during the two control periods of before and after the intervention.

The intervention team screened 100% of all admissions, with the initial contact being within 34.6 hours of admission, while the conventional consultations occurred, on average, at 72.5 hours into the admission during the two control time periods (note that the average LOS for the unit which was 3.8 and 3.7, respectively, for the two control times in the A-B-A comparison). The average length of the proactive screening assessment was slightly less than 3 minutes. There were no discernable differences in age, ethnicity, or medical acuity among the three different patient groups upon which the conventional and proactive services consulted ($N = 257, 62, 274$, respectively). The screenings revealed that 51% of patients on the study unit had a psychiatric condition that required treatment or consultation. Substance abuse disorders accounted for 43%, the largest portion of the detected difficulties. Mood and anxiety disorders (30%), psychotic disorders (13%), suicide attempts (7%), and delirium and dementia (6%) accounted for the rest.

After the initial pilot study was completed, and the service was terminated due to a shortage of staff, we used the results and experiences of the staff and patients to create a proposal for an enhanced proactive service. In addition to the reduction in LOS, responses of the nursing staff on a satisfaction measure administered after the initial study described high praise, with 80% of staff giving the service the highest rating possible. The medical team also expressed their pleasure with the increased presence of a psychiatrist [roughly 0.25 full-time equivalent (FTE)] on the unit. The estimated financial benefit was roughly $828,722 ($237,286 for cost avoidance by reduction of LOS, and $591,436 for revenue enhancement from backfilling the saved days). The only added cost was $56,550 (annualized) for the psychiatrist's extra time during the 5 weeks that the intervention was in place. The annualized net financial benefit was estimated to be $772,172, with a cost-to-revenue ratio of 4.2 (cost-effectiveness is calculated by adding the expenses of the intervention to usual costs and dividing that into the total dollars received).

Given the promising LOS reduction, high staff morale, and good contribution to the bottomline of expenses and revenues, a case was successfully made for the implementation of another version of a proactive psychiatric consultation service. This version was a team approach that was given the name behavioural intervention team (BIT). This second iteration was implemented on three internal medicine inpatient units (92 total patient bed capacity), with a team of a part-time psychiatrist (0.5 FTE), a full-time nurse practitioner (APRN), and a full-time social worker. We worked with a bio-psychosocial understanding of the patient's hospitalization, and hence the skills and perspectives of the aforementioned various medical professional groups were essential [25–28]. We decided on a team approach, as there were multiple tasks and domains that required different skills and knowledge for a maximally

effective hospital experience. Examples of such tasks are support, encouragement, reassurance, medication when needed, accurate diagnoses and formulation of their problems, education, social and family support, and the mental health practitioners' support of staff. Again, we achieved a good reduction in LOS (0.65 days; $P <0.02$) in the before-and-after trial from the three general internal medicine units. We ran the comparison for the same 11 months in two successive calendar years. There were 509 patients in the treatment group and 535 in the control group. The team not only screened 100% of the admissions, but also evaluated and cared for the psychiatric patients who could not be effectively managed by the regular medical staff and provided education for the staff about these patients. The multi-disciplinary nature of the team also allowed the treatment team to educate the staff in a practical and individualized manner about the mental health and social issues of each patient. This type of education was termed 'just-in-time education'. The added dimension of education enhanced the satisfaction of the staff and provided more skilful and effective interventions for patients.

The economic benefits of the BIT were characterized by a reduction in LOS, as well as the provision of added services and features associated with caring for patients who were behaviourally challenged. The incremental costs of the team were compared to the incremental economic benefits to the hospital as a result of the team's work. We conceptualized the economic benefit of the team's work in terms of the overall cost of the patient's hospitalization, as measured by the LOS and extra services such as sitters or other types of increased staffing. It was hypothesized that the intervention would have the greatest impact on LOS, readmission rate, and sitter use. There was an additional economic benefit of more filled beds which were made available by the increased efficiency of bed use (0.65 days of reduced LOS) without increased expense. Furthermore, when these patients with mental illness or psychological distress were given the care they needed in a timely, effective manner, both their medical and psychological outcomes improved. At the time of this study, the hospital was reimbursed for medical services almost exclusively by a case rate methodology, as opposed to a per diem rate. We compared the experience of the three medical units in a before-and-after implementation evaluation design of the intervention over successive and same 11-month calendar periods.

The average LOS for patients in the two intervention periods are presented in Table 137.1 [27]. The before-period consisted of treatment as usual with reactive conventional consultation liaison (CCL). The after-period was when the proactive BIT was employed. For the LOS expense calculations, the comparison was based on a blended rate. Included in the expenses were sitter costs, as well as room and medication costs, and associated overhead allocations. For income, a blended rate that reflected the proportion of different payers was utilized. The details of this economic relationship are presented in detail in another publication [27]. In the pilot study of proactive consultation with only a psychiatrist providing the services for one internal medicine unit, the economic benefit or cost-effectiveness ratio was estimated, conservatively to be 4.2. The same ratio in this before-and-after implementation was 1.7, meaning that for every dollar spent over and above usual care, $2.70 were received.

Table 137.2 [27] shows the direct cost metrics and comparison of the second study. The total saved cost for the intervention (not annualized) was $107,027 or a case rate of $210 saved on average per patient. There is also the opportunity for enhanced revenue by the

**Table 137.1** Length of stay metrics for the second study

| Population | CCL period N Mean (SD) | BIT period N Mean (SD) | Period effect Test statistic (df) P-value |
|---|---|---|---|
| Patients with psychiatric intervention and LOS <31 days | **535** **7.29** **(5.76)** | **509** **6.65** **(5.75)** | **T = 2.86** **(1042)** **0.004** |
| All patients with LOS <31 days | 5158 4.98 (4.62) | 5391 4.68 (4.38) | F = 8.39 (215, 457) 0.0002 |
| All patients | 5251 5.87 (8.9) | 5490 5.58 (9.12) | F = 6.90 (215, 755) 0.001 |

creation of empty beds. The value of enhanced revenue will vary by institution and setting. For instance, the freed-up bed space due to reduced occupancy from the shortened LOS allows for more revenue. Table 137.3 [27] summarizes the calculations for increased revenue realized due to the increased capacity created by the LOS reduction over 11 months.

The actual realized income will vary, depending on the mechanism of payment and the amount. For example, a case rate will be potentially more lucrative than a per diem rate, as the case rate incentivizes efficiency and reduced LOS. Furthermore, the magnitude of benefit realized by increasing capacity will vary per rate of backfill. Table 137.4 [27] illustrates the change of revenue, depending on the percentage of occupancy rate.

It should be clear there will likely be a substantial economic benefit from a proactive psychiatric consultation service, regardless of the payer, unless the utilization of beds is lower than the break-even point which, in our institution, is at 50% occupancy. The same will hold for revenue per case. Table 137.5 [27] summarizes the expected consequences of various scenarios for revenue per case.

Table 137.6 [27] summarizes the annualized costs of the programme in terms of salary expenses, incorporates the credits of reduced costs and enhanced revenue, and provides an integrated financial return on the BIT.

**Table 137.2** Direct cost comparisons

| Population | Cases | Direct cost/case |
|---|---|---|
| BIT, LOS <31 only | 509 | $6550 |
| CC, LOS <31 only | 535 | $6760 |
| Total cost per case difference | | |
| BIT minus CL ($210) times 509 cases | ($107,027) | |

**Table 137.3** Incremental net revenue (over 11 months)

| Population | Patient days | ALOS | Number of cases |
|---|---|---|---|
| BIT or CL period 3, LOS <31 only | 3383 | 6.65 | 509 |
| CL period 2, LOS <31 only | 3902 | 7.29 | 535 |
| Not BIT nor CL, LOS <31 only | 67,240 | 4.66 | 14,416 |
| LOS >31 (that is, LOS outliers) | 16,476 | 55.29 | 298 |
| Total | 91,001 | 5.77 | 15,758 |
| ALOS difference (7.29 – 6.65) | | 0.65 | |
| Patient days difference (0.65 ALOS ´ 509 cases) | 329.4 | | |
| Potential new cases (329.37 days/5.77 ALOS), assuming 100% backfill | 57.08 | | |
| Net revenue per case | $12,682 | | |
| Potential incremental revenue | $723,889 | | |

## Clinical process and considerations for the future

Clinically, in the 11-month trial, there were 5641 admissions to the three units. While we screened almost all patients on admission for the BIT trial, 945 patients, or 17%, were noted likely to be in need of psychiatric services. The incidence of the major diagnostic groups that required the attention of psychiatric services because their psychiatric condition was requiring psychiatric care was 63% (of the 945 screened); 52% required specialized (in mental health) discharge planning; 34% were seen for addiction; 18% were seen for delirium/dementia; and 17% had a behavioural issue that interfered with medical care [28].

The outcome of this study allowed us to implement the BIT on all medical units at Yale New Haven Hospital, York Street Campus, and on half of the medical units at our recently acquired nearby campus of the former Hospital of Saint Raphael. The multi-disciplinary teams perform the various clinical tasks noted in Fig. 137.1. Through screening 100% of the admitted patients, BIT staff quickly identify those who will require and/or benefit from a psychiatric consultation. This is accomplished by reviewing the medical and social histories provided in the patients' electronic medical records within 36 hours

**Table 137.4** Incremental revenue based on bed demand: alternate estimates of incremental net revenue

| Revenue | Backfill (%) | New cases | Annualized |
|---|---|---|---|
| $723,889 | 100 | 57.08 | $789,697 |
| $651,500 | 90 | 51.37 | $710,727 |
| $579,111 | 80 | 45.66 | $631,757 |
| $506,722 | 70 | 39.96 | $552,787 |
| $434,333 | 60 | 34.25 | $473,818 |
| $361,944 | 50 | 28.54 | $394,848 |

**Table 137.5** Alternative estimates of average net revenue per case

| Alternate estimates of incremental net revenue | Change to net revenue per case | Net revenue per case | |
|---|---|---|---|
| $868,667 | 110% | $13,950 | |
| $829,182 | 105% | $13,316 | |
| **$789,697** | **100%** | **$12,682** | **Our institution** |
| $750,212 | 95% | $12,048 | |
| $675,191 | 90% | $11,414 | |
| $573,912 | 85% | $10,780 | |

of their admission and discussing the patients with the admitting nurses and/or attending physicians. Those patients who screen positive for the likelihood of being able to benefit from a mental health consult are evaluated by the end of the second day of their stay. The 'treatment' that they receive may be extra support and attention to their mental illness by either the APRN or the doctor, depending on the problem and/or disposition assessment by the social worker who evaluates the various requirements related to different social elements such as family, living arrangements, and work. Those who will be at risk for difficulty at discharge due to their mental health or social issues are evaluated early on in their hospital stay, so that any serious psychiatric issues can be resolved early enough to accept an appropriate transfer to a psychiatric facility or discharge. They are evaluated by the psychiatric social worker on the team who works with the medical-floor social worker to fashion a suitable disposition. The unit's general medical nurses and the medical social workers are encouraged to support the patient in their capacity and look out for problems at disposition. If this is not enough to manage and treat the patient effectively, BIT members provide the mental health services and use that intervention as a teaching exercise for the staff on the units.

The doctors on the BIT oversee the treatment plans and spearhead the resolution of medically related problems for disposition. The doctor is also the leader of the team. However, the team is intensely nurse-oriented, and the medical-floor nurses can ask for

**Table 137.6** Summary of net financial return on BIT

| Estimated financial benefit | 11 months | 12 months |
|---|---|---|
| Incremental net revenue from backfill (filled at 100%) | $723,889 | $789,697 |
| Overall reduction in cost/case for BIT cases, including | $107,027 | $116,757 |
| Reduction in use of sitters | | |
| Subtotal, estimated financial benefit | $830,916 | $906,454 |
| Estimated additional expenses | $306,230 | $334,069 |
| Estimated benefit minus expenses | $524,686 | $572,384 |

consultations and support from any one of the team members. In terms of our cartography of the interventions for prevention and treatment noted, this is universal in that all patients get screened and may be categorized into a group that needs treatment (at least 25% of the patients have a history of mental illness). This includes our educational efforts with the nursing and medical staff at recognition, diagnosis, and treatment. The next level of preventive intervention that makes this an 'early' or proactive intervention is that those who may have a pre-existing psychiatric condition or who demonstrate some likelihood of disruptive behaviour or suffer from mental illness, such as confusion, irritability, fear, or depression, are treated immediately with no lapse in their care, before their behavioural or mental health condition can become a disruptive factor. For those who are clearly manifesting psychiatric problems, their care is taken on immediately by the mental health professionals and their condition elaborated and explained to the nursing staff as the characterization of the intervention moves from selective to indicated.

The team functions both as practitioners of psychiatric care for patients, but also as educators and assistants for the regular unit staff. BIT team members and floor staff co-monitor patients who are in the selective category of prevention and treat or supervise the care of those who are in the indicated category, while they monitor and teach the treatment given by the medical/nursing team with primary responsibility. The education can take many forms such as: formal and informal supervision, tutorials, case conferences, case reports, and orientation. One common form is the 'just-in-time' education previously mentioned. This is education in which staff observe the experts in action and may informally seek their advice. Tadros *et al.* described a similar interactive education provided by RAID and noted that the instruction of the RAID team members helped junior doctors and nurses to better manage difficult patients and more accurately identify those patients who should be referred to psychiatric services [22]. Typically, the 'just-in-time' intervention will be triggered by a request from a medical or nursing staff member for advice on the care of a patient.

The interventions employed are: (1) the assessment of risks and whether risk categories have reached the level of indicated treatment; (2) the prescription of care in the development of a behaviourally oriented treatment plan, at all times supporting the patient; (3) the provision of just-in-time education that increases the effectiveness of the floor staff in their interactions with patients and encourages them to try out the perspective and skills themselves; (4) the assessment of the family and subsequent discharge; and (5) the actual care itself for those difficult patients. The goal is to produce outstanding clinical care in the most cost-effective manner possible.

At present, we have implemented the BIT only for internal medicine services on two of the hospital campuses. The programme is especially popular with nursing staff, as nurses are the hospital professionals most directly affected by the presence of the BIT. There are plans eventually to expand to cardiology, cancer, and appropriate surgical specialties. In each of these instances, we will take into consideration the dynamics of admission, treatment, and discharge, so that we can design a programme that functions well at the decisional points in the patients' hospital career.

Common sense tells us that proactivity and early intervention are clearly strategies that are effective in the face of the cascade effect [29]. In health care, the cascade effect is the process of deterioration of health when the resources available to the patient do not match the needs of the patient's environment, so that a feed-forward state ensues, in which unmet demands in one sector (that is, attending to medical appointments) result in an ever more serious and numerous unmet demands in other sectors as the person sacrifices resources from one sector (for example, saving money previously used for transportation) in order to correct unmet other demands (buying groceries). This cycle continues until the patient's health becomes unstable to the point where hospitalization or acute care is warranted. Effective holistic programmes are those that have a clear understanding of the costs and benefits of the intervention programme in its totality, so that the system in which the patient lives can be stabilized and recovery becomes an option for more people sooner in the cycle of their illnesses than would otherwise pertain.

## The future

Other features that we intend to investigate and possibly develop are the integration of inpatient and outpatient experiences through the maintenance of continuity of care. We believe that integrating care should make the continuity of care between inpatient and outpatient more effective, which will further reduce the need for, and length of, hospital stays. In addition, we plan to document and better understand the role and value of informal consultations, or 'curbside consultations' which are not typically noted in the medical records and have no income associated with them. Nevertheless, they appear to be effective and valuable to the recipients. We believe that the RAID programme's educational effect is similar to what we call 'just-in-time' education.

And finally, our ambition for the future is to create a consortium comprising a regionally based group of hospitals or other health care entities capable of serving large populations of patients and that can develop this model and share experiences, so that information, data, ideas, and experiences can be shared and a more substantial research programme can be developed to refine and pilot innovation.

## REFERENCES

1. Chen KY, Evans R, Larkins S. Why are hospital doctors not referring to Consultation-Liaison Psychiatry?–a systemic review. *BMC Psychiatry*. 2016;16:390.
2. Muñoz RF, Mrazek PJ, Haggerty RJ. Institute of Medicine report on prevention of mental disorders: summary and commentary. *Am Psychol*. 1996;51:1116.
3. Desan, PH, Lee, HB, Zimbrean, P, Sledge, W. New models of psychiatric consultation in the general medical hospital: liaison psychiatry is back. *Psychiatr Ann*. 2017;47(7):355–61.
4. Garretson S, Rauzi MB, Meister J, Schuster J. Rapid response teams: a proactive strategy for improving patient care. *Nurs Stand*. 2006;21:35–40.
5. Szalados JE. Critical care teams managing floor patients: the continuing evolution of hospitals into intensive care units. *Crit Care Med*. 2004;32:1071–2.
6. Dacey MJ, Mirza ER, Wilcox V, *et al*. The effect of a rapid response team on major clinical outcome measures in a community hospital. *Crit Care Med*. 2007;35:2076–82.
7. Bellomo R, Goldsmith D, Uchino S, *et al*. A prospective before-and-after trial of a medical emergency team. *Med J Austr*. 2003; 179:283–8.
8. Salamonson Y, van Heere B, Everett B, Davidson P. Voices from the floor: nurses' perceptions of the medical emergency team. *Intensive Crit Care Nurs*. 2006;22:138–43.
9. Grissinger M. Rapid response teams in hospitals increase patient safety. *Pharm Ther*. 2010;35:191.
10. Daly FF, Sidney KL, Fatovich DM. The Medical Emergency Team (MET): a model for the district general hospital. *Intern Med J*. 1998;28:795–8.
11. Hueckel RM, Turi JL, Cheifetz IM, *et al*. Beyond rapid response teams: instituting a 'rover team' improves the management of at-risk patients, facilitates proactive interventions, and improves outcomes. In: Henriksen K, Battles J, Keyes M, Grady M, editors. *Advances in Patient Safety: New Directions and Alternative Approaches* (volume 3: performance and tools). Rockville, MD: Agency for Healthcare Research and Quality; 2008.
12. Korbkitjaroen M, Vaithayapichet S, Kachintorn K, Jintanothaitavorn D, Wiruchkul N, Thamlikitkul V. Effectiveness of comprehensive implementation of individualized bundling infection control measures for prevention of health care–associated infections in general medical wards. *Am J Infect control*. 2011;39:471–6.
13. Heal M, Silvest-Guerrero S, Kohtz C. Design and development of a proactive rapid response system. *Comput Inform Nurs*. 2017;35:77–83.
14. Norton SA, Hogan LA, Holloway RG, Temkin-Greener H, Buckley MJ, Quill TE. Proactive palliative care in the medical intensive care unit: effects on length of stay for selected high-risk patients. *Crit Care Med*. 2007;35:1530–5.
15. Marcantonio ER, Flacker JM, Wright RJ, Resnick NM. Reducing delirium after hip fracture: a randomized trial. *J Am Geriatr Soc*. 2001;49:516–22.
16. Tea C, Ellison M, Feghali F. Proactive patient rounding to increase customer service and satisfaction on an orthopaedic unit. *Orthop Nurs*. 2008;27:233–40.
17. Esparza JM, Shi R, McLarty J, Comegys M, Banks DE. The effect of a clinical medical librarian on in-patient care outcomes. *J Med Libr Assoc*. 2013;101:185.
18. Makowsky MJ, Koshman SL, Midodzi WK, Tsuyuki RT. Capturing outcomes of clinical activities performed by a rounding pharmacist practicing in a team environment: the COLLABORATE study. *Med Care*. 2009;47:642–50.
19. Curley C, McEachern JE, Speroff T. A firm trial of interdisciplinary rounds on the inpatient medical wards: an intervention designed using continuous quality improvement. *Med Care*. 1998;36:AS4–12.
20. Desan PH, Zimbrean PC, Lee HB, Sledge WH. Proactive psychiatric consultation services for the general hospital of the future. In: Summergrad P, Kathol R, editors. *Integrated Care in Psychiatry*. New York, NY: Springer; 2014. pp. 157–81.
21. Sennour Y, Counsell SR, Jones J, Weiner M. Development and implementation of a proactive geriatrics consultation model in collaboration with hospitalists. *J Am Geriatr Soc*. 2009;57:2139–45.
22. Tadros G, Salama RA, Kingston P, *et al*. Impact of an integrated rapid response psychiatric liaison team on quality improvement and cost savings: the Birmingham RAID model. *Psychiatrist Online*. 2013;37:4–10.
23. Muskin PR, Skomorowsky A, Shah RN. Co-managed care for medical inpatients, CL vs C/L psychiatry. *Psychosomatics*. 2016;57:258–63.
24. Desan PH, Zimbrean PC, Weinstein AJ, Bozzo JE, Sledge WH. Proactive psychiatric consultation services reduce length of stay

for admissions to an inpatient medical team. *Psychosomatics.* 2011;52:513–20.

25. Engel GL. The clinical application of the biopsychosocial model. *Am J Psychiatry.* 1980;137:535–44.

26. Engel GL. The need for a new medical model: a challenge for bio-medicine. *Holistic Medicine.* 1989;4:37–53.

27. Sledge WH, Bozzo J, White-McCullum B, Lee, H. The cost-benefit from the perspective of the hospital of proactive

psychiatric consultation service on inpatient general medicine services. *Health Econ Outcome Res.* 2016;2:122.

28. Sledge WH, Gueorguieva R, Desan P, Bozzo JE, Dorset J, Lee HB. Multidisciplinary proactive psychiatric consultation service: impact on length of stay for medical inpatients. *Psychother Psychosom.* 2015;84:208–16.

29. Mold JW, Stein HF. The cascade effect in the clinical care of patients. *N Engl J Med.* 1986;314:512–14.

# 138

# Refugees and populations exposed to mass conflict

*Mina Fazel, Susan Rees, and Derrick Silove*

## Introduction

This chapter will consider the mental health needs of refugees and other populations forcibly displaced because of exposure to mass conflict. Migration has been a hallmark of humanity over millennia, the reasons leading individuals or groups to move being numerous and often multi-faceted. Migration can be forced or by choice or a combination of these factors; for example, poverty or natural disasters might lead a person or group to leave their home out of choice, but elements of compulsion can play a role such as severe food insecurity. This chapter will consider those obliged to leave their homelands for reasons of persecution and exposure to mass conflict, populations broadly referred to as refugees. The terms utilized to describe these populations are summarized in Box 138.1 [1], highlighting the different groups to consider; however, for the purposes of this chapter, *refugees* will be used to describe this population, unless reference is made to specifically defined groups.

The mental health of refugees continues to be an important area of clinical work and research, and one that highlights the complex interplay among biological, psychological, social, and cultural processes in determining how individuals vary on a spectrum of adaptation to frank mental illness. The psychological impact on a person, family, and groups forced to migrate because of conflict can be considerable, the effects generally being negative, but, in some aspects, potentially positive. To leave an environment of extreme insecurity in order to reach a new country of safety is likely to enhance the mental health and well-being for many; the focus of this chapter, however, will be on the varied mental health risks associated with forced migration and the factors preceding and following that major event. We will describe the mental health impacts of forced displacement and the essential role that both previous and ongoing exposures to traumatic events, ongoing stresses, and broader psychosocial influences play in generating or maintaining the psychopathology and the appropriate interventions that may assist in overcoming these adverse outcomes. Selective high-risk subpopulations will be described in more detail, including unaccompanied refugee minors, persons living in states of protracted insecurity, such as in refugee camps, women and their children, and those caught in cycles of violence, for example in situations where post-traumatic anger presents a risk to the individual, those close to them, and the wider community.

The global pressures causing forced displacement show no signs of abating, including the Syrian civil unrest which has caused a substantial movement of forcibly displaced populations. In 2015, the estimated number of people displaced by mass conflict reached 65 million worldwide [2]. A total of 12 million were displaced in 2015, with at least 40 million believed to be internally displaced. The majority of refugees live in protracted insecure situations, often in makeshift settlements in countries neighbouring the site of the conflict, almost all in low-income countries. Only a small portion are able to travel to high-income countries. Table 138.1 lists refugees and asylum seeker populations by country of origin and destination [2], and Fig. 138.1 is a graph showing the changes over the last 15 years in the numbers being displaced across the globe.

## Mental health needs

Refugee populations are exposed to a number of stressors that may impact on mental health, many of these factors operating simultaneously or in sequence. Refugees commonly experience personal grief often complicated by the nature of the multiple losses they experience, including murders, disappearances, kidnapping, atrocities, and sex slavery, and more general potentially traumatic events such as violence, torture, sexual abuse, and arbitrary incarceration. As a group, refugees experience major psychosocial and cultural upheavals of having to leave their families, homes, communities, and work to seek personal security. Evidence suggests that two sets of factors are of key importance in impacting on the mental health of refugees: exposure to past and ongoing potentially traumatic events, and the complexities of navigating the post-migration environment as both individuals and groups [3–5]. These inter-relationships have been best described by Miller and Rasmussen (2016), from which Fig. 138.2 has been adapted [3].

The actual rates of mental illness identified among refugees vary by population, their exposures to potentially traumatic events, their current living arrangements (where and with whom they are currently

**Migrant:** A person who has moved across an international border or within a state away from their habitual place of residence, regardless of their legal status, whether the movement is voluntary or involuntary, what the causes for the movement are, or what the length of the stay is.

**Refugee:** A person who, owing to a well-founded fear of persecution for reasons of race, religion, nationality, membership of a particular social group, or political opinions, is outside the country of his or her nationality and unable or, owing to such fear, is unwilling to avail themselves of the protection of that country; often strictly defined according to the 1951 UNHCR Refugee Convention.

**Internally displaced person:** A person who has been forced to leave their place of habitual residence as a result of armed conflict, generalized violence, violations of human rights, or natural or human-made disasters, and who has not crossed an internationally recognized state border.

**Asylum seeker:** A person who seeks safety from persecution or serious harm in a country other than their own and awaits a decision on the application for refugee status under relevant international and national instruments.

**Stateless person:** A person who is not considered as a national by any State under the operation of its law. As such, a stateless person lacks those rights attributable to protection of a State, no inherent right of sojourn in the State of residence, and no right of return in case he or she travels.

**Irregular migrant:** A person whose movement takes place outside the regulatory norms of the sending, transit, and receiving countries and increasingly used for a person who has been smuggled or trafficked.

**Trafficked:** A person who has been recruited, transported, transferred, harboured, by force or other forms of coercion, abduction, and deception, to achieve one person having control over another person, for the purpose of exploitation. Trafficking in persons can take place within the borders of one State or may have a transnational character.

Reproduced from Institute of Migration, *Glossary on Migration, International Migration Law Series No. 25,* Copyright (2011), with permission from International Organization for Migration. Available from https://www.iom.int/key-migration-terms

**Table 138.1** Refugee data (2015) by country of origin and destination

| Top ten source countries of refugees | Top ten refugee host countries | Highest number of refugees per 100 inhabitants in host country |
|---|---|---|
| Syria | Turkey (2.5 million) | Lebanon |
| Afghanistan | Pakistan (1.6 million) | Jordan |
| Somalia | Lebanon (1.1 million) | Nauru |
| Sudan | Iran (979,400) | Chad |
| South Sudan | Ethiopia (736,100) | Djibouti |
| Democratic Republic of Congo | Jordan | South Sudan |
| Myanmar | Kenya | Turkey |
| Central African Republic | Chad | Mauritania |
| Iraq | Uganda | Sweden |
| Eritrea | China | Malta |

Reproduced from UNHCR, *Global Trends: Forced displacement in 2015,* Copyright (2016), United Nations High Commissioner for Refugees. Available from http://www.unhcr.org/576408cd7.pdf

residing), and the long-term security of their place of residence. In general, rates of depression, post-traumatic stress disorder (PTSD), and anxiety disorders are high, compared to non-displaced populations, with some suggestion that the prevalence of psychotic disorders is also increased [4, 6, 7]. Nevertheless, there is considerable heterogeneity in reported rates of mental disorder across studies, most likely because of variation in sampling, measurement, and the characteristics of the groups under inquiry. The sociodemographic profile of the population alone may influence the overall mental health status of individual groups. In a meta-analysis published in 2005 on pre- and post-displacement influences on mental health, refugees who were older, more educated, and female, those who had higher pre-displacement socio-economic status, and persons from a rural background had worse mental health outcomes [4]. Some studies have identified higher rates of somatization [5], and others have suggested an elevated suicide risk among refugees, especially when there are significant post-migration stressors [8]. Several factors have been shown to be associated with suicidal risk among refugees, including lack of employment, access to resettlement services and social support, distress related to separation from families, past trauma exposure, and integration difficulties in the resettlement country. Discrimination against ethnic minorities is also associated with poor mental health among refugees, a society-wide problem that is of particular relevance to contemporary resettlement environments. These factors, along with the stigma that often accompanies mental illness, can complicate efforts to seek treatment after resettlement [8] (Box 138.2).

## Long-term outcomes

The complexities of studying refugee populations are most evident when considering the array of long-term mental health implications associated with their experiences; although studies are limited, there is evidence that mental disorders, especially PTSD, tend to be highly prevalent in these populations, even years after resettlement [15]. As identified in a systematic review on studies of populations resettled for more than 5 years, this increased risk seems to be a consequence of exposure to both conflict-related trauma, post-migration socio-economic factors, and more general living difficulties [16]. The systematic review identified 29 studies, of which only 13 were deemed of high quality. Consistent with past findings, there was substantial heterogeneity across studies in the prevalence rates of depression (range 2.3–80%), PTSD (4.4–86%), and anxiety disorder (20.3–88%). Nevertheless, prevalence estimates were typically in the range of 20% and above for any disorder, the lowest rates being found in the higher-quality studies. Descriptive synthesis suggested that greater exposure to pre-migration traumatic experiences and post-migration stressors, the higher the rates of all three categories of mental disturbance (PTSD, depression, anxiety), while a poor post-migration socio-economic status was particularly associated with depression.

## Impact of exposure to previous and ongoing traumatic events

### Impact of other post-migration stressors

Specific post-migration displacement stressors that have been shown to influence mental health include social isolation resulting

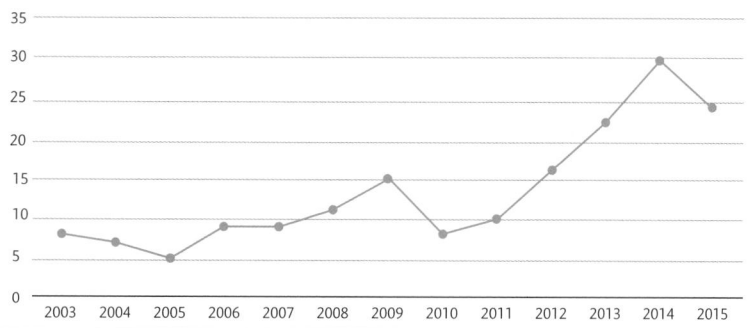

**Fig. 138.1** Graph to show rates of newly displaced persons from 2003 to 2015.

from the loss of social networks [17], unemployment (either due to limited rights to work or because of local employment demands [17, 18]), poverty [19, 20], perceived discrimination [21], increased violence against women [22–26], and a lack of safety when living in refugee camps [20, 27]. These post-migration living difficulties prolong pre-existing feelings of insecurity and deplete the capacity of displaced persons to manage ongoing challenges, a compounding of prior conflict-related experiences and ongoing stressors, a combination of factors that increase the vulnerability to disorders such as PTSD [28].

## A conceptual model for understanding the refugee experience

When attempting to understand the full range of experiences of refugees, it is important to consider a number of interacting domains: early developmental experiences; the context and culture of origin; and the sequence of changes that have occurred through the phases of mass conflict, displacement, transition, and final resettlement [29]. There are multiple levels of influences (political, social, cultural, familial, and physical/biological) that impact at each phase on the adaptive capacity of refugees, their families, and the wider community; the outcome of these attempts to adapt may be positive

or, in conditions of overwhelming stress, may result in severe distress and ultimately mental disorder. The Adaption and Development After Persecution and Trauma (ADAPT) model identifies five core psychosocial pillars challenged by the sequence of experiences that refugees encounter [30]. These pillars, which form the foundations of stable societies, maintain social cohesion, as well as individual mental health. Specifically, the pillar of *safety* and its maintenance are vital to the person's sense of security and protection, with conditions of pervasive or recurrent threat generating anxiety and fear, the extreme outcome being disorders such as PTSD. Maintaining *interpersonal bonds* (nuclear and extended family, networks) is essential to mental well-being. Multiple threats to attachments and repeated traumatic losses can lead to severe distress, including symptoms of complicated grief and separation anxiety. The maintenance of *roles and identities* (cultural, social, family, personal, work-related) is vital to prevent alienation, isolation, and marginalization, a state referred to in sociology as anomie. Finally, the sense of *meaning and coherence* in life is critical to forming a positive view of the present and future, the existential domain which may be expressed in political values, religious beliefs, social and cultural affiliations, and/or spirituality. All five domains, and the institutions and social rules that support them, tend to be undermined by the refugee experience,

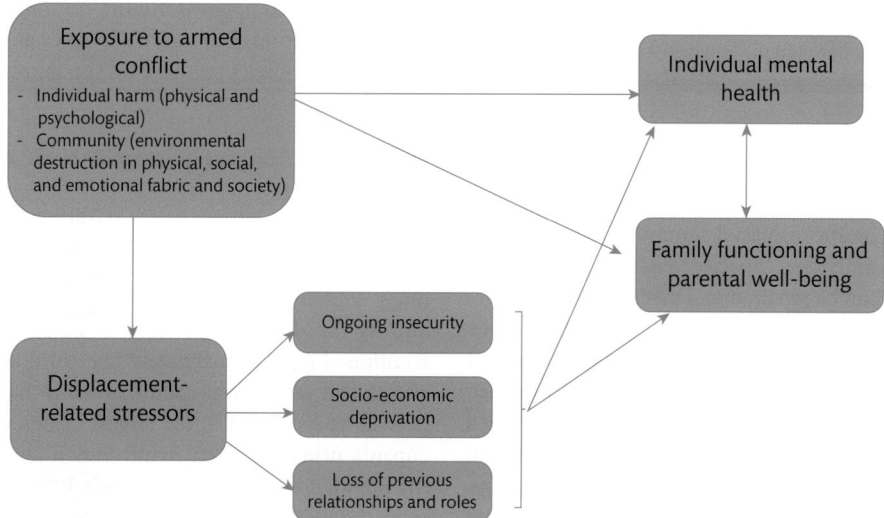

**Fig. 138.2** Relationship of armed conflict, displacement, and mental health.
Adapted from *Epidemiol Psychiatr Sci.*, 26(20), Miller K, Rasmussen A, The mental health of civilians displaced by armed conflict: an ecological model of refugee distress, pp. 129–138, Copyright (2017), with permission from Cambridge University Press.

**Box 138.2** Assessment of refugees in mental health services

In addition to the usual assessment required of any person referred to mental health services, there are a number of areas that it might be of additional importance to question. These include those identified in the ADAPT formulation described in the text, but the core elements of assessment are detailed here.

**Background history**

- Description of previous life before difficulties that led to displacement.
- Sensitive enquiry of reasons as to why they had become displaced: any experience of incarceration, torture, abuse directed to themselves or family members and other close associates, including sexual abuse. Significant losses experienced of family members, friends, and colleagues.
- Enquiry as to how they arrived in their current place of residence: how did they travel, were they placed in hands of strangers or traffickers, did they spend time in a refugee camp, experiences and exposure to abuses in these environments.
- Their perceived roles in their families, previous occupation, and communities.

**Physical health**

- Review of physical health needs is important, as this can be overlooked. It should include chronic health conditions, oral health, and skin. The screening would need to include questions about previous health and exposure to any infectious diseases endemic in the countries of origin and transit, as well as previous injuries [9–11].
- Previous head injury, especially if associated with loss of consciousness, is an important question to ascertain, as studies have demonstrated that this is highly prevalent in torture survivors and can have significant long-term psychological effects, including depression and PTSD [12–14].

**Current situation**

- Living circumstances: where are they living; with whom; how many house moves have they had since arrival; are they able to afford food, clothing, other necessities; how do they spend their time (as those awaiting more permanent legal status are often not permitted to work); any new family stressors; any family members they are trying to find.
- Immigration status and understanding of the process: these processes can often be complex and hard to understand, as information might not be available in the desired languages; legal representation can be hard to access without financial assistance, and there might be the constant threat of immigration detention and deportation back to either a country of transit or the country of origin.
- Linguistic ability and access to interpreters: this is likely to be apparent in the interview. Mental illness can impact on a person's ability to learn the host language.

impacting at every level on the displaced community and exerting reciprocal effects on the individual capacity to adapt. The extent to which these disruptions can be repaired or accommodated will determine where individuals and their collectives are located on the continuum of adaptation and functional impairment, a failure of adaptation expressing itself in the individual as mental disorder. The ADAPT system can be used as a framework for undertaking a comprehensive assessment of the experiences and psychosocial responses of individual refugees in clinical and other service settings. The model can also provide a framework for assessing the overall needs of refugee families and communities as a first step in formulating effective programmes of psychosocial and mental health interventions.

## Specific populations of note

There are a number of subpopulations requiring special attention among the heterogenous population of refugees.

### Unaccompanied minors

An unprecedented number of children and adolescents worldwide are forced to migrate on their own to escape war and persecution [31]. As minors, these individuals face extreme risks to their physical and psychological well-being at an important developmental period [27, 32]. The trauma and hardships that accompany these experiences have potential to create prolonged mental health difficulties [33].

War exposures and ongoing social hardships can be complex and severe in nature for unaccompanied refugee minors. In contrast to single-incident trauma, war-affected youth can experience chronic exposure to traumatic events for weeks, months, or even years, often representing a significant proportion of their life [34]. Among the range of traumatic incidents common in war, children may witness violence, lose family members and friends, experience physical, sexual, and psychological harm, be exploited in various ways (involvement in criminality, prostitution, sex slavery), deprived of food, water, or shelter, or be compelled to inflict harm on others. These exposures have varying impacts for each child, but some experiences are particularly harmful [35]. For example, it is not uncommon for long-term shame and guilt to be experienced by some of these children, responses that are intensified by being forced to serve as 'child soldiers' and either witnessing or participating in breaking cultural taboos such as injuring family members. Managing the social stigmatization and isolation that can follow these experiences adds to the complexities of rehabilitation of these populations.

Studies support the high-risk status of unaccompanied minors. For example, the prevalence of PTSD was increased among unaccompanied minors resettled in Belgium, Norway, and the Netherlands [33, 36–38]. War exposure was positively associated with depression among unaccompanied minors on arrival in Belgium [37] and 6 months post-arrival in Norway [36]. In a follow-up study, unaccompanied minors continued to exhibit high scores on anxiety, depression, and PTSD over an 18-month period, with negative outcomes predicted by the number of traumatic experiences and daily stressors experienced [33].

### Living in prolonged insecurity such as refugee camp settings

Refugee camps are settlements, usually built with the intention of being temporary, to receive forcibly displaced populations. However, many settlements have grown and become semi-permanent, requiring the development of systems of governance and civic institutions [39]. Approximately one-third of refugees in protracted situations live in camps, some of which have been in existence for over 20 years. In 2015, the largest camps were in Kenya, with occupants primarily from South Sudan and Somalia (for example, the population of Kakuma exceeds 180,000 and that of Hagaderaa more than 100,000); other large camps have also been established in Jordan for Syrian occupants [40].

Studies have highlighted the mental health risks of living in refugee camps [41, 42]. For example, among Rwandan and Burundese refugees in a Tanzanian refugee camp, the prevalence of serious mental health problems was estimated to be 50% [43]. Children and young people living in camps (for example, in Central America, the Middle East, and the Former Yugoslavia) have higher rates of mental illness, compared to young people living in other transitional settings [27]. Refugee camps are often unsafe situations, placing children at risk of violence and abuse and consequent negative mental health outcomes. Neglect of basic needs, such as sanitation, parental distress, high levels of poverty, and lack of access to education increase the risk of mental disorder—even though humanitarian organizations and international bodies, such as UNICEF, provide substantial assistance in these settings [44]. Not surprisingly, therefore, a systematic review of 20 mental health studies of refugee/displaced youth residing in camps highlighted high rates of maladjustment, a large number of these young persons experiencing anxiety, somatic symptoms, depression, and aggression [45].

## Women and families

Violence against women is a global public health problem. There is a clear association between exposure to gender-based violence, including intimate partner violence, rape, and sexual assault, and mental disorders including PTSD, depression, and anxiety, as well as adverse psychosocial outcomes such as increased suicidal ideation [46]. Social and cultural factors influence the risk of violence against women. In particular, violence is higher in societies that are patriarchal, that is where authority in the household is reserved for men, and many contemporary settings of mass conflict involve populations with these traditional customs. In these contexts, women are at risk because of the prevailing culture of patriarchy and the disruptive and traumatic effects of mass violence [47]. The sequence of factors that increase the risk of intimate partner violence is complex, commencing with the increased risk among those exposed to early childhood abuse and violence (involving both sexes), experiences of war-related trauma, and conditions of extreme deprivation and poverty in the post-conflict environment, stressors that are common among displaced populations in low-income countries [48, 49]. Laws and customs that promote and protect women's rights and entitlements may also be regressive or undermined by war and conflict. The society as a whole may have lost its regulatory capacity, for example to intervene in situations of family conflict, and the exigencies of survival and the stresses arising from these pressures may reinforce traditional roles, including gender-inequitable practices.

War-specific factors can directly endanger women. The militaristic culture associated with war, for example, can intensify women's subordination and increase the risk of gender-based violence [50]. Rape is commonly used as a weapon of war and intimidation, leading to demoralization, humiliation, and isolation of women survivors and impacting more widely on men, families, and communities [25]. A recent meta-analysis of studies found that one in five refugee or displaced women in complex humanitarian settings have experienced sexual violence [51]. This is likely to be an underestimate, given the multiple barriers associated with disclosure, particularly in such unsafe settings. As indicated, gender-based violence is associated with a range of mental disorders, including PTSD, outcomes that further undermine women's functioning and capacity to manage the immediate demands of the post-displacement environment [46].

Women are critically important to ensuring social stability and recovery after conflict, both in the roles they play within the family and in guiding societies towards a return to peace and security [26]. Yet, qualitative studies confirm that women are often under-represented in decision-making in situations where they could provide a significant contribution to recovery and development. For example, women's voices concerning the violent episodes in refugee camps are often muted and left unheard [50]. It is crucially important therefore to raise awareness of aid personnel and camp authorities to ensure that priority is given to promoting gender equality and to recognizing and addressing factors that may undermine women's participation such as the presence of mental health-related disabilities as a consequence of gender-based violence. Gender equity promotion programmes and an explicit social and legal infrastructure that promotes gender equality should be prioritized to reduce violence against women and promote gender equality [47].

## Cycles of violence and human rights abuses that can be perpetuated in peri- and post-migration settings

There is emerging evidence indicating that under certain circumstances, a post-conflict cycle of violence can occur within families and communities in displaced societies. The proposed cycle of violence, partly supported by a growing body of research, proposes that there is a sequence of events in which adults exposed to trauma related to human rights violations are prone to outbursts of excessive anger in the post-conflict period, a sense of enduring injustice playing an important role in engendering this tendency. As a consequence, there can be inappropriate acts of anger and aggression within the family, triggered by relatively minor frustrations and conflict. Post-migration conditions of poverty and insecurity can exacerbate this tendency (see Fig. 138.3) for a conceptual model to describe these cycles of violence. In affected families, aggression may manifest as family conflict or in the form of intimate partner violence targeting women, and/or in harsh parenting in the upbringing of children. The long-term outcome may be the initiation of pathways in which the effects of trauma are transmitted to the next generation, impacting on their mental health and their tendency towards aggression and violence. A recent study identified a key pathway in this sequence in which male and female partners of survivors of trauma were more likely to exhibit high levels of grief and anger symptoms. Only women partners of men with high levels of trauma, however, showed an increase in PTSD, an important reason appearing to be that women tended to identify with the injustices experienced by their husbands [52].

## Societal factors

### Detention

In over 60 countries worldwide, including high-, middle-, and low-income nations, immigration detention is used in inconsistent ways to incarcerate some of the persons who have been forcibly displaced. In high-income countries, these practices are applied to selective groups of refugees such as those who arrive without an entry visa and others who are deemed not to have proved their claim for protection. Existing studies suggested that immigration detention is associated with poor mental health outcomes that can last for many years after release, the overall body of evidence indicating that the relationship is likely to be causal [53–56]. Several studies from the UK and Australia showed that the majority (if not all) children surveyed in detention centres meet criteria for at least one psychiatric illness

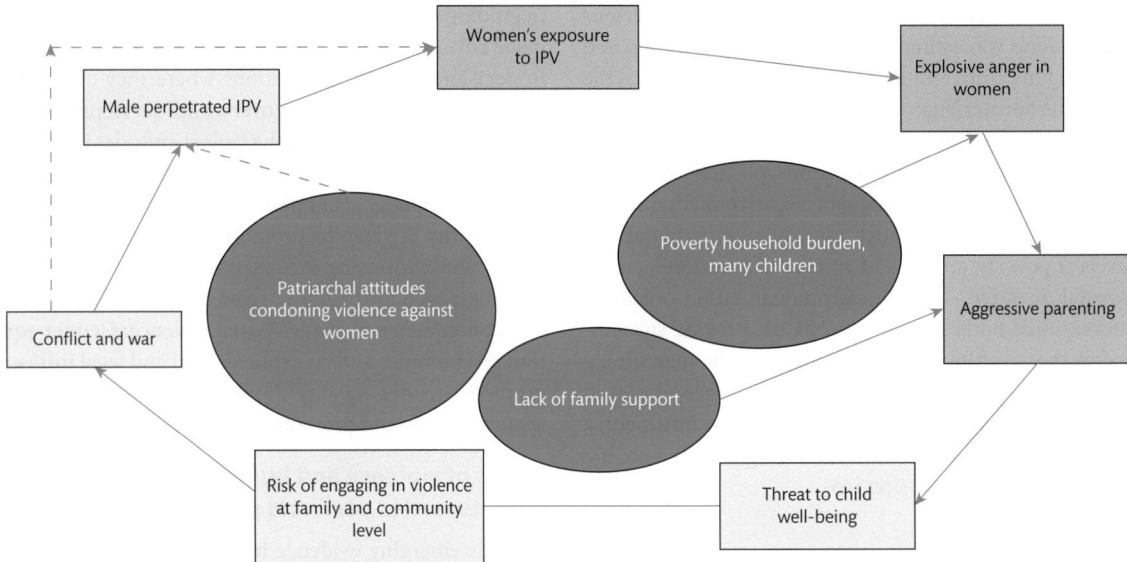

**Fig. 138.3** The conflict-related cycle of violence model.

Reproduced from *Soc Sci Med*, 132, Tay AK, Rees S, Chan J, *et al.*, Examining the broader psychosocial effects of mass conflict on PTSD symptoms and functional impairment amongst West Papuan refugees resettled in Papua New Guinea (PNG), pp. 70–8, Copyright (2015), with permission from Elsevier Ltd.

[54, 57]. The prevalence of disorder in these settings is remarkably high, with some studies showing a 10-fold increase in PTSD, anxiety disorders, depression, and sleep disturbances following detention [54, 58]. Factors such as ongoing uncertainty and stress associated with prolonged and indefinite detention, parental psychological distress, disrupted peer and family relationships, exposure to further traumatic events, human rights abuses, and witnessing attempts at self-harm all increase the risk of mental disorder in detained children and adolescents [53]. In a study of adults who had been detained, both previous detention and ongoing temporary protection after release contributed to the risk of ongoing PTSD, depression, and mental health-related disability [55].

Providing mental health care in immigration detention facilities is associated with major challenges, with the compromise of human rights in these facilities serving as an 'invalidating environment' that potentially undermines the therapist's attempts to provide psychological assistance [59, 60].

### Trafficking

Human trafficking represents a further risk for refugees, with the lack of protection many experience making them prey to both forced labour and sexual exploitation [61, 62]. Studies indicate that trafficked women, men, and children experience high levels of violence and consequent physical health symptoms, including headaches, stomach pain, and back pain. The most commonly reported mental health problems include depression, anxiety, and PTSD [62, 63]. Self-harm among these populations is prevalent. There is a greater need therefore for professionals working with refugees to focus on these high-risk groups [64, 65].

### Parenting difficulties and second-generation psychopathology

The culture of the refugee parenting experience may be characterized by disruption and alterations to family structure and organization; cultural values and norms; and gender roles [66]. Trauma-exposed parents and children may also have problems with attachment and

related parenting dysfunction [67]. Difficulties can arise in communication because of language barriers which can place children with greater access to learning the new language in a premature adult role in the family. Further, differing beliefs and behaviours concerning child-rearing practices can lead to claims of child maltreatment, as well as inter-familial conflict [68]. The situation can become more complex when older children and parents adjust to differing degrees to western cultural mores and norms regarding freedoms and rights [69]. It is important to affirm the positive parenting practices of families in post-migration environments and ensure child safeguarding needs are addressed using culturally sensitive and engaging methods. Therefore, there needs to be specific attention to promoting the welfare of children within pre- and post-resettlement contexts [32, 66, 70].

### Interventions

The study of interventions for refugee and forcibly displaced populations has grown substantially over the last decade, although only a few have been rigorously evaluated in randomized controlled trials [71–73]. This reflects many of the difficulties inherent in studying forcibly displaced populations where cultural, linguistic, financial, and practical problems abound [27, 74–76].

Refugees have diverse mental health needs, and in the ideal setting, there should be a range of networked services and agencies providing assessments and interventions for common mental disorders (depression, PTSD, anxiety), severe mental disorders (psychosis, schizophrenia, bipolar disorder) which are often neglected, 'complex cases' who may not respond to brief therapies, drug and alcohol problems, and organic disorders (often, by default, including epilepsy in low-income settings). The heterogeneity of needs makes it difficult to draw general conclusions about the effects of various interventions on a range of symptomatic and functional outcomes. The difficulty is to combine specific therapeutic components, for example, derived from cognitive behavioural therapy, in a broader and multi-level approach to psychosocial interventions, for example based on the principles of the ADAPT model [77, 78]. Specific clinical interventions at the individual level include treatments for PTSD following multiple traumatic events, commonly applied approaches being narrative exposure therapy (NET), eye movement desensitization and reprocessing (EMDR), and trauma-focused cognitive behavioural therapy (TF-CBT) [79–82]. At a more general psychosocial level, several approaches are used focusing on groups, the community as a whole, the school, and the family [83–86] (Table 138.2).

Studies of specific interventions usually targeting culturally homogenous client samples tend to demonstrate moderate to large outcome effects in relation to traumatic stress and anxiety reduction [72]. Further work is needed to ensure that these interventions can be embedded and sustained within primary health care facilities, that workers receive adequate supervision to maintain skills and prevent burnout, and that the long-term effects of treatment are maintained.

In designing intervention programmes, beliefs held by refugees about health care—its role, how to access it, and whether it can help—need to be a primary consideration. For example, a study among Somali women demonstrated how their beliefs focused on situational factors as determinants of mental health, in contrast to biological models that tend to drive interventions in Western medicine [92, 93]. These discordant health beliefs resulted in divergent expectations regarding the process and outcomes of treatment and health care interactions. Experiencing unmet and varying expectations, Somali women and their health care providers reported multiple frustrations, which often diminished the perceived quality of health care. Moreover, during the process, previously silent worries about mental health and reproductive decision-making surfaced. To provide high-quality, transcultural health care, providers must encourage patients to voice their own health explanations, expectations, and worries.

There is a consensus that in the resettlement environment, positive psychosocial outcomes for youth and adults depend to a great extent on the integrity and functioning of families. Yet few intervention programmes in mental health focus specifically on families in the refugee field. There is a pressing need therefore to devise and test mental health interventions that aim to prevent or lessen the effects of family dysfunction on individual mental health. Weine (2011) described eight characteristics that preventive mental health interventions should address to meet the needs of refugee families, including: feasibility, acceptability, culturally tailored, multi-level, time-focused, prosaicness, effectiveness, and adaptability [94]. To address these eight characteristics in the complex environment of refugee resettlement programmes requires modifying the process of research to introduce innovative strategies that build these principles into mental health services. Important principles are adopting a resilience (rather than an illness) framework; promoting community collaboration, participation, and leadership; and utilization of mixed-methods approaches, including focused ethnography. At a wider systems level, promoting preventive mental health programmes for refugee families requires appropriate supporting policy directives, multi-systemic partnerships, and training in flexible implementation research designs that ensure that innovative programmes are rigorously evaluated and the positive findings are captured and disseminated.

In general, controlled studies among refugees and asylum seekers have reported positive intervention outcomes in reducing trauma-related symptoms [84]. For example, there is evidence to support TF-CBT and NET in certain refugee populations. Findings from other intervention studies are limited by methodological constraints such as lack of randomization, absence of control groups, and small samples. Further evaluations of the array of psychotherapeutic, psychosocial, pharmacological, and other therapeutic approaches, including psychoeducational and community-based interventions that facilitate personal and community growth and change, are needed [72]. In addition, there is a need to test the effectiveness of rehabilitation strategies for more complex cases and interventions for refugees with severe mental disorders such as psychosis. There is a need for increased awareness, training, and funding to implement and assess broader psychosocial programmes (working in

**Table 138.2** Examples of mental health interventions for refugee populations

| Intervention | How delivered | Study example | Findings |
|---|---|---|---|
| Narrative exposure therapy (NET) | Individual sessions provided by lay counsellors (6–10 sessions) | Rwandan and Somali refugees in a Ugandan camp [79, 87] | Significant reduction in PTSD symptoms for NET and trauma counselling groups. Remission of 70% following NET |
| Common elements treatment approach | Individual sessions provided by lay counsellors | Burmese refugees in Thailand [85] | Significant reduction in depression, post-traumatic stress, anxiety, and aggression scores |
| Cognitive behavioural therapy (CBT) | Individual sessions (with or without interpreter) | Mixed refugee group receiving CBT in a London outpatient service [88] | Positive PTSD outcomes in both groups (interpreter or not) |
| Multiple-family group access intervention for PTSD | Multiple-family group (nine sessions) | Families from Bosnia-Herzegovina in Chicago [89] | Improved access to mental health services |
| Parenting intervention | Parenting programme (eight sessions) | African migrants and refugee families in Australia [90] | Positive change in all parenting domains tested |
| School-based theatre intervention to improve mental health and academic outcomes | Classroom-based drama workshop | Multi-ethnic high schools [91] | Significant decrease in impairment score for first-generation migrants and increase for second-generation |
| Classroom-based intervention (CBI) | CBI for aftermath of exposure to potentially traumatic events (15 sessions) | Trials in conflict-affected settings (Burundi, Sri Lanka, Indonesia, Nepal) [44] | Positive change in coping, hope, pro-social behaviour, and functional impairment |

synchrony with clinical services) that collaborate with refugee communities in promoting adaptation during the stages of resettlement, programmes that require an innovative approach to ensuring that both the host and refugee communities actively contribute in reciprocal ways to ensure successful integration.

Notwithstanding the documented risks to mental health that the refugee experience generates, these adverse outcomes must be balanced against the potential positive adaptive outcomes among many displaced populations [95]. There is growing interest in issues of youth resilience and post-traumatic growth in the face of adversity; for example, many war-affected adolescents from Uganda did not display psychosocial distress 4 years after the war had ended, despite witnessing various atrocities [96, 97]. Nevertheless, although the relevance of a resilience-oriented approach is broadly recognized, there is little consensus about the definition of resilience and substantial variation in the operationalization and measurement of that construct, a challenge that is increased in relation to ensuring the cross-cultural equivalence of relevant concepts [95]. A study of 26 qualitative studies exploring resilience in young refugees identified six sources of resilience: (1) social support; (2) acculturation strategies; (3) education; (4) religion; (5) avoidance; and (6) hope [95]. These sources indicated that both social as well as personal factors confer resilience in young refugees. Nevertheless, several fundamental issues need to be clarified, including whether resilience is a latent capacity of the individual or is invested in the social sphere in which the person is embedded; and whether resilience is a unique positive characteristic of active adaptation and maximizing the person's potential, independent of mental disorder or simply the absence of the latter.

## Conclusions

Refugee communities and people displaced by mass conflict have been increasing in numbers over the last few decades. They can experience a potent mix of biological, psychological, and social stressors that can lead to increased rates of mental health problems, especially depression, anxiety, and PTSD. Furthermore, these populations have increased exposures to a sequence of experiences of violence and abuse, both in their countries of origin, situations of transition such as refugee camps and even when reaching host countries, within their own families and self-induced, in the form of suicidal acts. Refining a suite of broad psychosocial and more specific clinical interventions to address the varied needs of this population requires much further work, the focus being both on mitigating specific mental health problems and preventing adverse society-wide outcomes, including potential cycles of violence in the family and the community.

## REFERENCES

1. International Organization for Migration. *Glossary on Migration*, second edition. International Migration Law No. 25. Geneva: International Organization for Migration; 2011.
2. United Nations High Commissioner for Refugees. *UNHCR Global Trends: Forced Displcement in 2015*. Geneva: United Nations High Commissioner for Refugees; 2016.
3. Miller K, Rasmussen A. The mental health of civilians displaced by armed conflict: an ecological model of refugee distress. *Epidemiology and Psychiatric Sciences* 2017;**26**:129–38.
4. Porter M, Haslam N. Predisplacement and postdisplacement factors associated with mental health of refugees and internally displaced persons: a meta-analysis. *JAMA* 2005;**294**:602–12.
5. Schweitzer RD, Brough M, Vromans L, Asic-Kobe M. Mental health of newly arrived Burmese refugees in Australia: contributions of pre-migration and post-migration experience. *Australian and New Zealand Journal of Psychiatry* 2011;**45**:299–307.
6. Fazel M, Wheeler J, Danesh J. Prevalence of serious mental disorder in 7000 refugees resettled in western countries: a systematic review. *Lancet* 2005;**365**:1309–14.
7. Hollander A-C, Dal H, Lewis G, Magnusson C, Kirkbride JB, Dalman C. Refugee migration and risk of schizophrenia and other non-affective psychoses: cohort study of 1.3 million people in Sweden. *BMJ* 2016;**352**:i1030.
8. Hagaman AK, Sivilli TI, Ao T, et al. An investigation into suicides among Bhutanese refugees resettled in the United States between 2008 and 2011. *Journal of Immigrant and Minority Health* 2016;**18**:819–27.
9. Davidson N, Skull S, Chaney G, et al. Comprehensive health assessment for newly arrived refugee children in Australia. *Journal of Paediatrics and Child Health* 2004;**40**:562–8.
10. Benson J, Smith M. Early health assessment of refugees. *Australian Family Physician* 2007;**36**:41–3.
11. Gerritsen AAM, Bramsen I, Devillé W, van Willigen LHM, Hovens JE, van der Ploeg HM. Physical and mental health of Afghan, Iranian and Somali asylum seekers and refugees living in the Netherlands. *Social Psychiatry and Psychiatric Epidemiology* 2006;**41**:18–26.
12. Mollica RF, Henderson DC, Tor S. Psychiatric effects of traumatic brain injury events in Cambodian survivors of mass violence. *British Journal of Psychiatry* 2002;**181**:339–47.
13. Mollica RF, Lyoo IK, Chernoff MC, et al. Brain structural abnormalities and mental health sequelae in South Vietnamese ex-political detainees who survived traumatic head injury and torture. *Archives of General Psychiatry* 2009;**66**:1221–32.
14. Keatley E, Ashman T, Im B, Rasmussen A. Self-reported head injury among refugee survivors of torture. *Journal of Head Trauma Rehabilitation* 2013;**28**:E8–13.
15. Marshall GN, Schell TL, Elliott MN, Berthold SM, Chun CA. Mental health of Cambodian refugees 2 decades after resettlement in the United States. *JAMA* 2005;**294**:571–9.
16. Bogic M, Njoku A, Priebe S. Long-term mental health of war-refugees: a systematic literature review. *BMC International Health and Human Rights* 2015;**15**:29.
17. Priebe S, Jankovic Gavrilovic J, Bremner S, et al. Psychological symptoms as long-term consequences of war experiences. *Psychopathology* 2012;**46**:45–54.
18. Silove D, Steel Z, Bauman A, Chey T, McFarlane A. Trauma, PTSD and the longer-term mental health burden amongst Vietnamese refugees: a comparison with the Australian-born population. *Social Psychiatry and Psychiatric Epidemiology* 2007;**42**:467–76.
19. Tay AK, Rees S, Chan J, Kareth M, Silove D. Examining the broader psychosocial effects of mass conflict on PTSD symptoms and functional impairment amongst West Papuan refugees resettled in Papua New Guinea (PNG). *Social Science and Medicine* 2015;**132**:70–8.
20. Rasmussen A, Nguyen L, Wilkinson J, et al. Rates and impact of trauma and current stressors among Darfuri refugees in Eastern Chad. *American Journal of Orthopsychiatry* 2010;**80**:227–36.

21. Ellis BH. New directions in refugee youth mental health services: overcoming barriers to engagement. *Journal of Child and Adolescent Trauma* 2011;**4**:69–85.

22. Betancourt TS, Newnham EA, Layne CM, *et al.* Trauma history and psychopathology in war-affected refugee children referred for trauma-related mental health services in the United States. *Journal of Traumatic Stress* 2012;**25**:682–90.

23. Panter-Brick C, Grimon MP, Eggerman M. Caregiver—child mental health: a prospective study in conflict and refugee settings. *Journal of Child Psychology and Psychiatry* 2014;**55**:313–27.

24. Rees S, Pease B. Domestic violence in refugee families in Australia. *Journal of Immigrant and Refugee Studies* 2007;**5**:1–19.

25. Stark L, Wessells M. Sexual violence as a weapon of war. *JAMA* 2012;**308**:677–8.

26. Hossain M, Zimmerman C, Watts C. Preventing violence against women and girls in conflict. *Lancet* 2014;**383**:2021.

27. Reed RV, Fazel M, Jones L, Panter-Brick C, Stein A. Mental health of displaced and refugee children resettled in low-income and middle-income countries: risk and protective factors. *Lancet* 2012;**379**:250–65.

28. Nickerson A, Steel Z, Bryant R, Brooks R, Silove D. Change in visa status amongst Mandaean refugees: relationship to psychological symptoms and living difficulties. *Psychiatry Research* 2011;**187**:267–74.

29. Silove D. The psychosocial effects of torture, mass human rights violations, and refugee trauma: toward an integrated conceptual framework. *Journal of Nervous and Mental Disease* 1999;**187**:200–7.

30. Silove D. The ADAPT model: a conceptual framework for mental health and psychosocial programming in post conflict settings. *Intervention* 2013;**11**:237–48.

31. United Nations High Commissioner for Refugees (UNHCR). *No More Excuses: Provide Education to all Forcibly Displaced People.* Geneva: UNHCR and Global Education Monitoring Report; 2016.

32. Fazel M, Reed RV, Panter-Brick C, Stein A. Mental health of displaced and refugee children resettled in high-income countries: risk and protective factors. *Lancet* 2012; **379**:266–82.

33. Vervliet M, Lammertyn J, Broekaert E, Derluyn I. Longitudinal follow-up of the mental health of unaccompanied refugee minors. *European Child and Adolescent Psychiatry* 2014;**23**:337–46.

34. Betancourt TS, Newnham EA, McBain R, Brennan RT. Post-traumatic stress symptoms among former child soldiers in Sierra Leone: follow-up study. *British Journal of Psychiatry* 2013;**203**:196–202.

35. Betancourt TS, McBain R, Newnham EA, Brennan RT. Trajectories of internalizing problems in war-affected Sierra Leonean youth: examining conflict and postconflict factors. *Child Development* 2013;**84**:455–70.

36. Jensen TK, Fjermestad KW, Granly L, Wilhelmsen NH. Stressful life experiences and mental health problems among unaccompanied asylum-seeking children. *Clinical Child Psychology and Psychiatry* 2015;**20**:106–16.

37. Vervliet M, Meyer Demott MA, Jakobsen M, Broekaert E, Heir T, Derluyn I. The mental health of unaccompanied refugee minors on arrival in the host country. *Scandinavian Journal of Psychology* 2014;**55**:33–7.

38. Smid GE, Lensvelt-Mulders GJ, Knipscheer JW, Gersons BP, Kleber RJ. Late-onset PTSD in unaccompanied refugee minors: exploring the predictive utility of depression and anxiety symptoms. *Journal of Clinical Child and Adolescent Psychology* 2011;**40**:742–55.

39. Bulley D. Inside the tent: community and government in refugee camps. *Security Dialogue* 2014;**45**:63–80.

40. United Nations High Commissioner for Refugees. *Life in Limbo: Inside the World's 10 Largest Refugee Camps.* 2016. Available from: http://storymaps.esri.com/stories/2016/refugee-camps/

41. Kane JC, Ventevogel P, Spiegel P, Bass JK, Van Ommeren M, Tol WA. Mental, neurological, and substance use problems among refugees in primary health care: analysis of the Health Information System in 90 refugee camps. *BMC Medicine* 2014;**12**:228.

42. Adaku A, Okello J, Lowry B, *et al.* Mental health and psychosocial support for South Sudanese refugees in northern Uganda: a needs and resource assessment. *Conflict and Health* 2016;**10**:18.

43. de Jong JP, Scholte WF, Koeter MW, Hart AA. The prevalence of mental health problems in Rwandan and Burundese refugee camps. *Acta Psychiatrica Scandinavica* 2000;**102**:171–7.

44. Fazel M, Patel V, Thomas S, Tol WA. Mental health interventions in schools in low-income and middle-income countries. *Lancet Psychiatry* 2014;**1**:388–98.

45. Vossoughi N, Jackson Y, Gusler S, Stone K. Mental health outcomes for youth living in refugee camps: a review. *Trauma, Violence, and Abuse* 2018;**19**:528–42.

46. Rees S, Silove D, Chey T, *et al.* Lifetime prevalence of gender-based violence in women and the relationship with mental disorders and psychosocial function. *JAMA* 2011;**306**:513–21.

47. World Health Organization. *Global and Regional Estimates of Violence Against Women: Prevalence and Health Effects of Intimate Partner Violence and Non-Partner Sexual Violence.* Geneva: World Health Organization; 2013.

48. Catani C. War at home–a review of the relationship between war trauma and family violence. *Verhaltenstherapie* 2010;**20**:1.

49. Catani C, Jacob N, Schauer E, Kohila M, Neuner F. Family violence, war, and natural disasters: A study of the effect of extreme stress on children's mental health in Sri Lanka. *BMC Psychiatry* 2008;**8**:33.

50. Beswick S. ' If you leave your country you have no life!' Rape, suicide, and violence: the voices of Ethiopian, Somali, and Sudanese female refugees in Kenyan refugee camps. *Northeast African Studies* 2001;**8**:69–98.

51. Vu A, Adam A, Wirtz A, *et al.* The prevalence of sexual violence among female refugees in complex humanitarian emergencies: a systematic review and meta-analysis. *PLoS Currents Disasters* 2014, edition 1. doi: 10.1371/currents.dis.835f10778fd80ae031aac12d3b533ca7.

52. Silove D, Tay A, Steel Z, *et al.* Symptoms of post-traumatic stress disorder, severe psychological distress, explosive anger and grief amongst partners of survivors of high levels of trauma in post-conflict Timor-Leste. *Psychological Medicine* 2017;**47**:149–59.

53. Fazel M, Karunakara U, Newnham EA. Detention, denial, and death: migration hazards for refugee children. *The Lancet Global Health* 2014;**2**:e313–14.

54. Steel Z, Momartin S, Bateman C, *et al.* Psychiatric status of asylum seeker families held for a protracted period in a remote detention centre in Australia. *Australian and New Zealand Journal of Public Health* 2004;**28**:527–36.

55. Steel Z, Silove D, Brooks R, Momartin S, Alzuhairi B, Susljik I. Impact of immigration detention and temporary protection on the mental health of refugees. *British Journal of Psychiatry* 2006;**188**:58–64.

56. Robjant K, Hassan R, Katona C. Mental health implications of detaining asylum seekers: systematic review. *British Journal of Psychiatry* 2009;**194**:306–12.

57. Lorek A, Ehntholt K, Nesbitt A, *et al*. The mental and physical health difficulties of children held within a British immigration detention center: a pilot study. *Child Abuse and Neglect* 2009;**33**:573–85.

58. Dudley M, Steel Z, Mares S, Newman L. Children and young people in immigration detention. *Current Opinion in Psychiatry* 2012;**25**:285–92.

59. Brooker S, Albert S, Young P, Steel Z. *Challenges to Providing Mental Health Care in Immigration Detention*. Global Detention Project Working Paper No. 19, Geneva: Global Detention Project; 2016.

60. Grant-Peterkin H, Schleicher T, Fazel M, *et al*. Inadequate mental healthcare in immigration removal centres. *BMJ* 2014;**349**:g6627.

61. Hebebrand J, Anagnostopoulos D, Eliez S, Linse H, Pejovic-Milovancevic M, Klasen H. A first assessment of the needs of young refugees arriving in Europe: what mental health professionals need to know. *European Child and Adolescent Psychiatry* 2016;**25**:1–6 .

62. Ottisova L, Hemmings S, Howard L, Zimmerman C, Oram S. Prevalence and risk of violence and the mental, physical and sexual health problems associated with human trafficking: an updated systematic review. *Epidemiology and Psychiatric Sciences* 2016;**25**:317–41.

63. Tsutsumi A, Izutsu T, Poudyal AK, Kato S, Marui E. Mental health of female survivors of human trafficking in Nepal. *Social Science and Medicine* 2008;**66**:1841–7.

64. Westwood J, Howard LM, Stanley N, Zimmerman C, Gerada C, Oram S. Access to, and experiences of, healthcare services by trafficked people: findings from a mixed-methods study in England. *British Journal of General Practice* 2016;**66**:e794–801.

65. Stanley N, Oram S, Jakobowitz S, *et al*. The health needs and healthcare experiences of young people trafficked into the UK. *Child Abuse and Neglect* 2016;**59**:100–10.

66. Williams N. Establishing the boundaries and building bridges. A literature review on ecological theory: implications for research into the refugee parenting experience. *Journal of Child Health Care* 2009;**14**:35–51.

67. Orlans M, Levy TM. *Attachment, Trauma, and Healing: Understanding and Treating Attachment Disorder in Children, Families and Adults*. London and Philadelphia, PA: Jessica Kingsley Publishers; 2014.

68. Pinquart M, Kauser R. Do the associations of parenting styles with behavior problems and academic achievement vary by culture? Results from a meta-analysis. *Cultural Diversity and Ethnic Minority Psychology* 2018;**24**:75–100.

69. Berry JW, Vedder P. Adaptation of immigrant children, adolescents, and their families. In: Gielen UP, Roopnarine JL, editors. *Childhood and Adolescence: Crosscultural Perspectives and Applications*, second edition. Santa Barbara, CA: Praeger; 2016. pp. 321–47.

70. Deng SA, Marlowe JM. Refugee resettlement and parenting in a different context. *Journal of Immigrant and Refugee Studies* 2013;**11**:416–30.

71. Nickerson A, Bryant RA, Silove D, Steel Z. A critical review of psychological treatments of posttraumatic stress disorder in refugees. *Clinical Psychology Review* 2011;**31**:399–417.

72. Murray KE, Davidson GR, Schweitzer RD. Review of refugee mental health interventions following resettlement: best practices and recommendations. *American Journal of Orthopsychiatry* 2010;**80**:576–85.

73. McFarlane CA, Kaplan I. Evidence-based psychological interventions for adult survivors of torture and trauma: a 30-year review. *Transcultural Psychiatry* 2012;**49**:539–67.

74. Slobodin O, de Jong JT. Family interventions in traumatized immigrants and refugees: a systematic review. *Transcultural Psychiatry* 2015;**52**:723–42.

75. Drożdek B. Challenges in treatment of posttraumatic stress disorder in refugees: towards integration of evidence-based treatments with contextual and culture-sensitive perspectives. *European Journal of Psychotraumatology* 2015;**6**:10.3402/ejpt. v6.24750.

76. Carlsson J, Sonne C, Silove D. From pioneers to scientists: challenges in establishing evidence-gathering models in torture and trauma mental health services for refugees. *Journal of Nervous and Mental Disease* 2014;**202**:630–7.

77. Betancourt TS, Gilman SE, Brennan RT, Zahn I, VanderWeele TJ. Identifying priorities for mental health interventions in war-affected youth: a longitudinal study. *Pediatrics* 2015;**136**:e344–50.

78. Lambert JE, Alhassoon OM. Trauma-focused therapy for refugees: meta-analytic findings. *Journal of Counseling Psychology* 2015;**62**:28–37.

79. Robjant K, Fazel M. The emerging evidence for narrative exposure therapy: a review. *Clinical Psychology Review* 2010;**30**:1030–9.

80. ter Heide FJJ, Mooren TM, van de Schoot R, de Jongh A, Kleber RJ. Eye movement desensitisation and reprocessing therapy v. stabilisation as usual for refugees: randomised controlled trial. *British Journal of Psychiatry* 2016;**209**:311–18.

81. Hinton DE, Jalal B. Guidelines for the implementation of culturally sensitive cognitive behavioural therapy among refugees and in global contexts. *Intervention* 2014;**12**:78–93.

82. Palic S, Elklit A. Psychosocial treatment of posttraumatic stress disorder in adult refugees: a systematic review of prospective treatment outcome studies and a critique. *Journal of Affective Disorders* 2011;**131**:8–23.

83. Tyrer RA, Fazel M. School and community-based interventions for refugee and asylum seeking children: a systematic review. *PLoS One* 2014;**9**:e89359.

84. Slobodin O, de Jong JT. Mental health interventions for traumatized asylum seekers and refugees: What do we know about their efficacy? *International Journal of Social Psychiatry* 2015;**61**:17–26.

85. Bolton P, Lee C, Haroz EE, *et al*. A transdiagnostic community-based mental health treatment for comorbid disorders: development and outcomes of a randomized controlled trial among Burmese refugees in Thailand. *PLoS Medicine* 2014;**11**:e1001757.

86. Drożdek B, Kamperman AM, Tol WA, Knipscheer JW, Kleber RJ. Seven-year follow-up study of symptoms in asylum seekers and refugees with PTSD treated with trauma-focused groups. *Journal of Clinical Psychology* 2014;**70**:376–87.

87. Neuner F, Onyut PL, Ertl V, Odenwald M, Schauer E, Elbert T. Treatment of posttraumatic stress disorder by trained lay counselors in an African refugee settlement: a randomized controlled trial. *Journal of Consulting and Clinical Psychology* 2008;**76**:686–94.

88. d'Ardenne P, Ruaro L, Cestari L, Fakhoury W, Priebe S. Does interpreter-mediated CBT with traumatized refugee people work? A comparison of patient outcomes in East London. *Behavioural and Cognitive Psychotherapy* 2007;**35**:293–301.

89. Weine S, Kulauzovic Y, Klebic A, *et al*. Evaluating a multiple-family group access intervention for refugees with PTSD. *Journal of Marital and Family Therapy* 2008;**34**:149–64.

90. Renzaho AM, Vignjevic S. The impact of a parenting intervention in Australia among migrants and refugees from Liberia, Sierra Leone, Congo, and Burundi: Results from the African Migrant Parenting Program. *Journal of Family Studies* 2011;**17**:71–9.

91. Rousseau C, Beauregard C, Daignault K, *et al*. A cluster randomized-controlled trial of a classroom-based drama workshop program to improve mental health outcomes among immigrant and refugee youth in special classes. *PLoS One* 2014;**9**:e104704.
92. Pavlish CL, Noor S, Brandt J. Somali immigrant women and the American health care system: Discordant beliefs, divergent expectations, and silent worries. *Social Science and Medicine* 2010;**71**:353–61.
93. May S, Rapee RM, Coello M, Momartin S, Aroche J. Mental health literacy among refugee communities: differences between the Australian lay public and the Iraqi and Sudanese refugee communities. *Social Psychiatry and Psychiatric Epidemiology* 2014;**49**:757–69.
94. Weine SM. Developing preventive mental health interventions for refugee families in resettlement. *Family Process* 2011;**50**:410–30.
95. Sleijpen M, Boeije HR, Kleber RJ, Mooren T. Between power and powerlessness: a meta-ethnography of sources of resilience in young refugees. *Ethnicity and Health* 2016;**21**:158–80.
96. McMullen JD, O'Callaghan PS, Richards JA, Eakin JG, Rafferty H. Screening for traumatic exposure and psychological distress among war-affected adolescents in post-conflict northern Uganda. *Social Psychiatry and Psychiatric Epidemiology* 2012;**47**:1489–98.
97. Sutton V, Robbins I, Senior V, Gordon S. A qualitative study exploring refugee minors personal accounts of post-traumatic growth and positive change processes in adapting to life in the UK. *Diversity and Equality in Health and Care* 2006;**3**:77–88.

# SECTION 24

# Forensic psychiatry

# 139

# Associations between psychiatric disorder and offending

*Seena Fazel and Mark Toynbee*

## Introduction

The perception of an association between mental illness and anti-social behaviour has been widespread historically and influenced changes in mental health services and policy, including the development of secure hospitals and specific laws for mentally disordered individuals in the criminal justice system. Over the last few decades, research evidence has clarified the nature of this association and investigated mechanisms. Most of the high-quality evidence for associations between psychiatric disorders and offending has come from epidemiology. Translating the epidemiological evidence into individual clinical assessment and decision-making remains a challenge for the field.

## Historical perspectives

Historically, many cultures have assumed a link between mental illness and criminality [1]. In the 1980s, this view was questioned by some research that suggested that schizophrenia and other psychoses did not, in fact, increase the risk of violence [2]. However, from the 1990s, longitudinal population-based studies showed clear evidence of associations between most investigated psychiatric disorders and offending, and also violent behaviour [3]. The magnitude of this association varied from study to study. The influential MacArthur Risk Assessment study that followed up discharged psychiatric patients from three inner cities in the United States reported no such association for a heterogenous group of diagnoses without substance misuse comorbidity [4]. However, the MacArthur study did find increased risks of violence for some specific mental illnesses, and in particular severe mental illness, and strong links were reported between comorbidity and violent outcomes [5]. In a 2009 systematic review of 20 studies examining the association between psychosis and violence, all included studies found an increased risk of violence when individuals with psychosis were compared with general population controls, links that were substantially increased by comorbid substance misuse [6]. Additional research using population-based sibling-control studies in Sweden [7] and Israel [8] has further

strengthened the evidence of an association. However, any such reviews of association studies need to be viewed in the context of the risks of violent victimization to individuals with schizophrenia [9, 10], the population impact of a particular diagnosis such as schizophrenia on all violent crime, and how this population impact compares with other more common diagnoses.

In addition, the robustness of the research evidence needs to be considered. Typically in this field, exposures and outcomes have been heterogenous. For exposures, different psychiatric disorders have been investigated, with varying approaches to determining diagnosis. In relation to outcomes, self-report, informant report, arrest, conviction, and imprisonment have been variously reported. Although the relative risks for self-reported and conviction data do not appear to differ in mental illness [11], absolute risks do. As any association between mental illness and offending is subject to a range of confounders and liable to reverse causality, longitudinal studies are key.

## Violent offending

Violent crime is particularly important from a public health and policy perspective, as it is less prone to measurement error than other violence outcomes, is associated with more morbidity and economic costs, and may be more generalizable than other outcomes. A consistent finding from population-based studies is that a significant proportion of violent offending is perpetrated by a relatively small number of individuals [12, 13]. Among the mental disorders, violent offending is strongly associated with substance misuse [14, 15] and personality disorder [16], and less strongly with schizophrenia and related psychoses [6], bipolar disorder [17], and depression [18].

Mechanisms linking these disorders to violence have been proposed [19, 20] that has drawn on research examining damage to certain areas of the brain (especially the orbitofrontal region) [21], genetic research [22], neurochemical investigations [23], and imaging studies [24]. There is consistent evidence from animal models that decreased serotonin transmission is associated with aggressive behaviour [25]. In humans, higher levels of serotonin in the blood of males (but not females) who have committed violent crimes have been demonstrated [26]. Serotonin is metabolized by monoamine oxidase, and it has been hypothesized that decreased expression of the gene for monoamine oxidase A is associated with an increased risk of violence [27], with a gene–environment interaction [28]. Other genes involved with serotonin metabolism have also been investigated such as the *COMT* gene (involved in the metabolism of catecholamines) [29]. However, this research has been influenced by small studies and has not been replicated. Although violence is heritable [30], genetic association studies have reported no consistent associations [31] and genome-wide association studies are now required. Statistical genetic approaches have found shared genetic liability for schizophrenia, substance misuse, and violent crime [32].

## Psychoses

Schizophrenia and other psychoses have been shown to be associated with an increased risk for a number of different crimes, including arson, drug, property, and violence [7, 33, 34]. For arson and homicide [6, 35–37], the relative risks are more than 10, compared with population controls. However, absolute risks are low, and, for example, the annual risk for a stranger homicide in schizophrenia is not higher than one in 11 million annually in Western Europe [37]. For violence, the increased odds of violent crime range between 2 and 6 in men, and slightly higher in women, and remains increased when compared with siblings who do not have schizophrenia and related psychoses [38]. The impact of environmental influences may vary with gender [39]. Overall, around one in 20 violent crimes is committed by individuals with psychosis [40].

### Risk factors

The strongest predictor of future violence in individuals with schizophrenia is a history of previous violence, especially convictions for violent crime [41]. Clinical factors include persecutory delusions [42], particular if accompanied with anger [43] (consistent with earlier work [19, 44]). This was attenuated after treatment—a finding consistent with other work using novel within-individual designs that has found a reduced rate of violence in patients on antipsychotic medication [45]. Other possible mechanisms include impulsivity, hostility, and lack of insight [41]. Poor adherence to medication and psychological treatments is another risk factor. A reliable finding is the effect of substance misuse [41], which acts as both a mediator and a moderator of the association and in homicide in individuals with psychosis [46]. Comorbidity with substance misuse increases the risk of violent outcomes 8–10 times, compared with the general population [7, 47]. Substance misuse may directly contribute to the risk of violent offending by decreasing adherence to medication, increasing impulsivity and hostility, and worsening certain psychotic symptoms, and indirectly through social networks and antisocial peers. Consistent with the importance of genetics and early environment, a review of risk factors for violence in psychosis found that a history of childhood abuse (OR 2.2, 95% CI 1.5–3.1), parental criminal history (OR 1.8, 95% CI 1.5–2.2), and parental alcohol misuse (OR 1.6, 95% CI 1.4–1.8) were all significantly associated with an increased risk [41]. No significant association has been found with many neuropsychological factors [41], including intelligence quotient (IQ) [47] (Table 139.1).

**Table 139.1** Strongest associations between risk factors and violence in individuals diagnosed with psychosis

| Risk factor | | Odds ratio (95% CI)[*] |
|---|---|---|
| Criminal history | History of assault | 21.4 (5.2–86.6) |
| | History of imprisonment for any offence | 4.5 (2.7–7.7) |
| | Recent arrest for any offence | 4.3 (2.7–6.7) |
| | History of conviction for violent offence | 4.2 (2.2–9.1) |
| | History of arrest for any offence | 3.5 (2.1–5.8) |
| | History of violent behaviour | 3.1 (2.2–4.4) |
| Substance misuse | Comorbid substance misuse disorder diagnosis | 3.1 (1.9–5.0) |
| | History of alcohol misuse | 2.3 (1.7–3.3) |
| | History of substance misuse (alcohol and/or drugs) | 2.2 (1.6–2.9) |
| | Recent drug misuse | 2.2 (1.6–3.1) |
| Treatment | Non-adherence to psychological therapies | 6.7 (2.4–19.2) |

[*] All significant to the *P* <0.001 level.
Adapted from *PloS One*, 8(2), Witt K, Van Dorn R, Fazel S, Risk factors for violence in psychosis: systematic review and meta-regression analysis of 110 studies, e55942, Copyright (2013), PloS. Reproduced under the Creative Commons Attribution License CC BY 4.0.

### First episode

Around a third of offending in schizophrenia occurs before any contact with mental health services [36], and approximately one in three individuals with first-episode psychosis exhibit some violent behaviour [48]. Hence, early diagnosis and treatment are likely to reduce violence repetition. In addition, a longer period of untreated psychosis is associated with increased risk [48]. Risk factors for violence in first-episode psychosis include hostility [odds ratio (OR) 3.5, 95% confidence interval (CI) 2.1–5.9], past violence or criminality (OR 3.3, 95% CI 1.8–6.1), and manic symptoms (OR 2.9, 95% CI 1.9–4.4) [48].

### Repeat offending

A systematic review [49] and a recent longitudinal study [50] reported a clear increased risk of recidivism in individuals with psychosis. The latter study confirmed this association using sibling pairs released from prison who were discordant for mental disorders. This is in contrast to a previous review that included studies with heterogenous comparison groups, including some with personality disorders and substance misuse, and therefore was potentially misleading [51]. Further evidence for mental illness as a risk factor for repeat offending was found in a large study of Texan prisoners [52].

## Affective disorders

Studies investigating associations between affective disorders and violence are less frequent than those investigating psychosis [53]. Depression has a high prevalence in forensic populations, with up to one in ten prison inmates clinically depressed [54]. Early studies reported an association between depression and violence, but this relationship was mostly attenuated after adjustment for confounders

[11, 55, 56]. This was not a consistent finding, however—and the MacArthur study [4] and some case register studies [57] found links. New work has more clearly demonstrated an association between depression and violence, utilizing longitudinal designs and siblings and twins as genetically informative controls [18]. The latter research reported the odds of committing a violent crime in individuals with depression, compared with the general population, was around three times higher [18]. When depressed individuals were compared to their non-depressed siblings, the increased risk was 2-fold. The absolute rate of violence in men diagnosed with depression was 3.7% over 3.2 years, higher than the rates of suicide (0.6%) and self-harm (3.3%). Rates in women were significantly lower, with 0.5% of women convicted of a violent crime after a depression diagnosis.

Bipolar disorder is clearly associated with a range of adverse outcomes. A longitudinal analysis and systematic review in 2010 investigated the risk of violent crime and bipolar disorder [17]. The 30-year prevalence of violent crime convictions for people with a diagnosis of bipolar disorder was 8.4%, compared to the general population where it was 3.5%. When meta-analysed with eight other investigations, the increased odds of violent outcomes was 4.6 (95% CI 3.9–5.4). The impact of early environment and genetic factors is important in patients with bipolar disorder, and the rate of violence in unaffected male siblings has been reported to be 6.2% [17]. In terms of risk factors, no difference in violent crime risk was found in bipolar patients if their last episode was psychotic or non-psychotic, nor according to crude markers of disease phases. More sensitive markers of clinical presentation will be required, and some work has shown that links between mania and offending may be mediated by disinhibition, irritability, and impulsivity [58].

## Substance misuse

Goldstein proposed three mechanisms through which substance misuse may cause violent behaviour—directly or 'psychopharmacological violence', or more indirectly via 'systemic' or 'economic compulsive' paths where situational and environmental factors 'impact on behaviour' [59]. Clinical studies focusing on just the 'psychopharmacological' pathways are complicated by confounding, comorbidities, and clarifying temporal and spatiotemporal relationships [20, 60, 61]. Risk factors for substance misuse and psychiatric illness overlap and have varying impacts at different points along the life course, and many studies rely on self-report. Polysubstance misuse is common, especially in individuals with serious mental illness—the odds of having another drug use disorder if also suffering from alcohol use disorder is around 4- to 5-fold, compared to those not using alcohol [62]. Despite all these difficulties, associations between violent offending and a history of substance misuse has been clearly established [20, 63].

The evidence for an association between alcohol use and violence is relatively strong. Studies have shown that the greater the number of symptoms of alcohol dependence, the higher the risk of violent offending [64]. The Dunedin birth cohort study found that 11% of the violence risk was attributable to alcohol dependence, with an adjusted OR of 3.4 (95% CI 2.0–5.9) for violence in those with significant alcohol use, compared to non-drinkers [11]. Other studies suggest a dose–response relationship, with weekly binge drinking associated with an increased risk of crime,

compared to monthly binge drinking [65]. In a case-crossover study, alcohol consumption in the previous 24 hours was associated with a relative risk of violence of 13.2 (95% CI 8.2–21.2) [66]. Individuals with a history of alcohol misuse were responsible for 16% of violent crime in Sweden [67].

Studies looking at individual substances are fewer in number and poorer in quality [68]. A 2016 review of studies of controlled substances and violence identified 22 relevant prospective studies, all of which had a moderate to serious risk of bias [68]. Eight studies investigated marijuana and showed either an increased risk or no change in risk of violence [68]. Studies of other illegal drugs have typically reported similar mixed results, with some with increased risk and others with no association. Data on barbiturates and tranquillizers, however, showed negative associations with some self-reported violence outcomes [69]. In an investigation based on an American inner-city population [69], other illegal drugs (including amphetamine, crack cocaine, opiates, and tranquillizers) were also associated with mixed results, based on self-reported violence outcomes.

There are few studies that have looked carefully at temporal relationships between substance misuse and violence. One report examined the odds of committing an act of serious violence the day after substance or alcohol misuse [70]. Consistent with other studies, it found that violence on day 1 was the largest risk factor for violence on the following day. It also found that alcohol use increased the odds of serious violence on the following day (OR 2.4, 95% CI 1.8–3.2). A possible effect of drug use alone (other than marijuana) could not be excluded (OR 1.5, 95% CI 0.8–2.8). Similar to many studies in this area, information on drug use relied on self-report.

## Personality disorders

A number of studies have investigated links between personality disorder and offending [71, 72]. Birth cohorts and population-based studies have shown associations, which tend to be stronger for Cluster B disorders (antisocial, borderline, narcissistic, and histrionic). In a meta-analysis, Yu et al. [16] found that 10.7% of individuals with a personality disorder diagnosis were violent over a median follow-up period of 4.5 years, compared to 1.2% of general population controls. This corresponded to an increase in risk (OR 3.0, 95% CI 2.6–3.5) of violent outcomes in individuals with a personality disorder diagnosis. Antisocial personality disorder was associated with the greatest increase in risk, with elevated odds of violence of more than 10, although the individual estimates contributing to this pooled estimate were mostly unadjusted. When studies that excluded patients with antisocial personality disorder were compared, the risk of violence remained significantly raised. There was no significant difference between genders in studies with samples that included all personality disorders. No explanation was found for variations between studies when age band, comparison group, or diagnostic criteria were considered. Overall, it was estimated that around a fifth of all violence could be attributed to individuals with personality disorder if causality was assumed, and the prevalence of personality disorder in the general population is typically between 5% and 10% [16].

Personality disorder is also a risk factor for repeat offending. The odds of any criminal recidivism is doubled in individuals with a personality disorder diagnosis [16], with little difference in risk if the comparison group comprised individuals with other psychiatric diagnoses or the general population. Studies have found that around two-thirds of individuals with a personality disorder diagnosis will reoffend, with no difference between different personality disorders. As individuals with personality disorder often have comorbid disorders, future research should account more carefully for this.

## Neurodegenerative disorders

There are few high-quality studies that estimate the risk of offending and violence in neurodegenerative disorders. One of the most common behavioural manifestations of dementia is aggression, with estimates of over 90% in some patient surveys [73], with plausible mechanisms such as misinterpretation of the environment [74]. Rarely, this aggression can result in a criminal offence, especially prior to a formal clinical diagnosis, and offences committed by patients with dementia are not limited to violence and range from theft [75] to homicide [76]. A case series of first-time offenders aged 65 and over have found higher rates of dementia than would be expected by age alone [77].

Fronto-temporal dementia and Huntington's disease are two disorders where illness onset is earlier than that in other neurodegenerative disorders. A recent review of offending and neurodegenerative diseases found associations with fronto-temporal dementia [behavioural variant (bvFTD)], primary progressive aphasia, and Huntington's disease, all of which have clinical conditions affecting the frontal circuits [78]. In a cohort of 2397 patients seen at a memory clinic in California, 8% presented with criminal behaviour, patients with bvFTD had the highest rates of offending (37%) and those with mild cognitive impairment the lowest (3%), and estimates for vascular dementia and Alzheimer's disease were 15% and 8%, respectively. In 4% of bvFTD patients, violence was their presenting complaint, which compares with 0.7% of Alzheimer's disease patients. Thus, degenerative processes that predominantly affect non-frontal areas, such as Alzheimer's disease, do not appear to be as strongly associated with offending [78].

## Neurological disorders

Traumatic brain injury (TBI) can lead to personality change and incident psychiatric and substance use disorders. The odds of a juvenile offender having a history of TBI, compared to a control, is 3.4 (95% CI 1.5–7.5) [79], and a 2010 meta-analysis estimated the prevalence of TBI in offender populations at 60% (95% CI 48–72) [80]. Prisoners appear to have a higher lifetime prevalence at 68% (95% CI 50–86), with more than half of these injuries including loss of consciousness (the diagnostic threshold for mild TBI or concussion). Absolute rates of violent crime in TBI patients are about 6% [81], reflected in an increased odds of 2.3 (95% CI 2.2–2.5) when adjusted for socio-economic confounders and substance misuse. When compared with unaffected siblings, the odds of violent crime remain raised at 2.0 (95% CI 1.8–2.3) [81].

Although epilepsy has been historically linked with crime and higher-than-expected rates in prisoners [82], both of these conventions have been questioned. In a population-based study, the absolute risk associated with epilepsy was slightly higher than in age-matched population controls, but not different to unaffected siblings (OR 1.1, 95% CI 0.9–1.2) [81]. Further, a systematic review found no support for the increased rates in prisoners, and previous findings of increased rates were partly based on using the wrong denominator [83]. The finding that epilepsy itself is not associated with an increased risk of violence is important, given the stigma associated with this condition.

## Neurodevelopmental disorders

Up to 10% of the child and adolescent population worldwide have neurodevelopmental disorders [84], and these disorders are overrepresented in the criminal justice system [85]. Of these disorders, attention-deficit/hyperactivity disorder (ADHD) has been consistently associated with an increased risk of offending (OR 4.6, 95% CI 2.2–10.3 in a large epidemiological study) [86]. In some studies, ADHD is a stronger predictor of violence than substance misuse [87], although comorbidity is common. Individuals with ADHD appear to be overrepresented in the criminal justice system, with an estimated prevalence of around 12% in boys in detention [88]. Among those diagnosed with ADHD, earlier onset of ADHD symptoms is associated with a higher rate of recidivism. Individuals with ADHD often have other comorbid psychiatric disorders, most often conduct disorder (17%) [89]. A longitudinal study in Sweden examined four childhood neurodevelopmental disorders and their association with future violent offending, compared to age-matched controls [90]. After adjustment for confounding, a diagnosis of ADHD was associated with an increased risk of violent offending (OR 2.7, 95% CI 2.0–3.8) [90]. When comparing full-siblings of individuals with ADHD with matched controls and adjusting for confounders, an increased risk of violent offending remained (OR 1.3, 95% CI 0.9–2.0), suggesting familial confounding.

It has been hypothesized that autism spectrum disorders (ASD) may be associated variously with higher and lower risks of offending than the general population. Studies based on offender cohorts have suggested a small increased risk of criminality in individuals with ASD [85]. More recently, no association was found between ASD and violent offending in a Swedish sibling control study (OR 1.1, 95% CI 0.6–1.9) [90]. The authors suggested that associations seen in previous studies were possibly due to other comorbid psychiatric diagnoses [90]. A study of individuals with ASD reviewed by the forensic psychiatric service in Norway found comorbidities included intellectual disability (33%), ADHD (15%) and substance misuse (19%) [91]. Risk factors for violence in individuals with ASD included comorbid psychiatric disorder (OR 4.2, 95% CI 1.8–9.8) [92]. A diagnosis of Asperger's syndrome has also been associated with a higher risk of violence than ASD [92]. Other neurodevelopmental disorders associated with offending include tic disorder [90].

## Eating disorders

There have been very few studies researching associations between eating disorders and offending. One investigation compared individuals with eating disorders to matched controls and found no difference in aggressiveness [93]. There have been case reports of an association with shoplifting; however, epidemiological data are lacking [94] (Table 139.2).

Table 139.2 Associations between psychiatric disorder and offending (comparison groups used unaffected siblings where possible; if not, systematic reviews were identified, followed by large observational studies)

| Psychiatric disorder | Odds of offending/violence (95% CI) | Comparator | Source |
|---|---|---|---|
| Schizophrenia-spectrum disorders | 4.2 (3.8–4.5) | Siblings | [47] |
| Bipolar disorder | 3.4 (risk ratio) | Siblings | [100] |
| Depression | 2.1 (1.8–2.4) | Siblings | [18] |
| Personality disorder | 3.0 (2.6–3.5) | General population | [16] |
| Substance misuse | 7.4 (4.3–12.7) | General population | [6] |
| Substance misuse (SMI + alcohol + drugs—general) | 9.8 (5.2–18.7) | General population | [6] |
| Neurodevelopmental disorder (ADHD) | 1.4 (0.9–2.1) | Siblings | [90] |
| Neurodegenerative disorder (bv-FTD) | 7.2 (P <0.001) | Alzheimer's disease | [78] |
| Neurological (TBI) | 2.0 (1.8–2.3) | Siblings | [81] |
| Neurological (epilepsy) | 1.1 (0.9–1.2) | Siblings | [81] |

SMI, severe mental illness.

## Risk assessment

There has been a proliferation of structured risk assessment tools in recent years, which rely on research on risk factors to create a checklist of items that can be scored in an unweighted or weighted manner. Current tools identify low-risk individuals with reasonable accuracy but are less accurate at identifying high-risk individuals who will actually go on to offend [95]. The rates of violence in individuals classified as high risk by these tools vary substantially [96], and trial evidence does not demonstrate improved outcomes using structured clinical judgement instruments [97]. In addition, some of these tools are subject to the prevention paradox—that most individuals with adverse outcomes are categorized in low- or medium-risk categories [17, 49], especially for rare outcomes such as homicide. Furthermore, scalability and simplicity need to be prioritized, as current instruments are time-consuming, suffer from authorship and publication biases [98], and are expensive to use (often requiring training and costs to administer). Recent work has addressed some of the limitations of previous work by using large data sets, pre-specifying risk factors and thresholds in a protocol, publishing a range of performance measures in a validation cohort, and developing a brief, scalable, and free-to-use risk assessment tool (OxMIV) for clinical decision-making in individuals with schizophrenia-spectrum and bipolar disorders [99]. The validation C-index [equivalent to area under the curve (AUC)] for this tool was 0.87, higher than comparative tools that take considerably longer and rely on interviews. Such a scalable tool can be used to screen out low-risk persons with psychosis and act as an adjunct to clinical decision-making.

## Conclusions and implications

Offending is a complex human behaviour and has many different causes, often acting at the same time. The links between psychiatric disorder and offending can be further clarified by using clear outcomes that allow for comparability, longitudinal studies to account for temporal relationships between exposure and outcome, and methods that adjust for sociodemographic and familial confounders. Overall, the data suggest that substance misuse and antisocial personality disorder are most strongly associated with an increased risk of offending, particularly violent offending, in relative and absolute terms. Schizophrenia-spectrum disorders, bipolar disorder, and clinical depression are also associated with offending, but relative and absolute risks are lower, unless there is comorbidity with substance misuse (Table 139.2). Pharmacological treatment of schizophrenia-spectrum and bipolar disorders is associated with a reduction in reoffending in observational studies and with broader violent outcomes in randomized controlled trials, which underscores the importance of early diagnosis and treatment. Violence risk assessment should consider using scalable tools, particularly to screen out low-risk persons and as an adjunct to clinical decision-making.

## REFERENCES

1. Monahan J. Mental disorder and violent behavior: perceptions and evidence. *American Psychologist.* 1992;47:511.
2. Monahan J, Steadman HJ. Crime and mental disorder: an epidemiological approach. *Crime and Justice.* 1983;145–89.
3. Swanson JW, Holzer III CE, Ganju VK, Jono RT. Violence and psychiatric disorder in the community: evidence from the Epidemiologic Catchment Area surveys. *Psychiatric Services.* 1990;41:761–70.
4. Steadman HJ, Mulvey EP, Monahan J, *et al.* Violence by people discharged from acute psychiatric inpatient facilities and by others in the same neighborhoods. *Archives of General Psychiatry.* 1998;55:393–401.
5. Grisso T, Davis J, Vesselinov R, Appelbaum PS, Monahan J. Violent thoughts and violent behavior following hospitalization for mental disorder. *Journal of Consulting and Clinical Psychology.* 2000;68:388.
6. Fazel S, Gulati G, Linsell L, Geddes JR, Grann M. Schizophrenia and violence: systematic review and meta-analysis. *PLoS Medicine.* 2009;6:e1000120.
7. Fazel S, Långström N, Hjern A, Grann M, Lichtenstein P. Schizophrenia, substance abuse, and violent crime. *JAMA.* 2009;301:2016–23.
8. Fleischman A, Werbeloff N, Yoffe R, Davidson M, Weiser M. Schizophrenia and violent crime: a population-based study. *Psychological Medicine.* 2014;44:3051–7.

9. Silver E, Arseneault L, Langley J, Caspi A, Moffitt TE. Mental disorder and violent victimization in a total birth cohort. *American Journal of Public Health*. 2005;95:2015–21.

10. Trotta A, Di Forti M, Mondelli V, *et al*. Prevalence of bullying victimisation amongst first-episode psychosis patients and unaffected controls. *Schizophrenia Research*. 2013;150:169–75.

11. Arseneault L, Moffitt TE, Caspi A, Taylor PJ, Silva PA. Mental disorders and violence in a total birth cohort: results from the Dunedin Study. *Archives of General Psychiatry*. 2000;57:979–86.

12. Moffitt TE, Caspi A. Childhood predictors differentiate life-course persistent and adolescence-limited antisocial pathways among males and females. *Development and Psychopathology*. 2001;13:355–75.

13. Farrington D, Piquero AR, Jennings WG. *Offending from Childhood to Late Middle Age: Recent Results from the Cambridge Study in Delinquent Development*. New York, NY: Springer; 2013.

14. Coid J, Yang M, Roberts A, *et al*. Violence and psychiatric morbidity in a national household population—a report from the British Household Survey. *American Journal of Epidemiology*. 2006;164:1199–208.

15. Grann M, Danesh J, Fazel S. The association between psychiatric diagnosis and violent re-offending in adult offenders in the community. *BMC Psychiatry*. 2008;8:92.

16. Yu R, Geddes JR, Fazel S. Personality disorders, violence, and antisocial behavior: a systematic review and meta-regression analysis. *Journal of Personality Disorders*. 2012;26:775.

17. Fazel S, Lichtenstein P, Grann M, Goodwin GM, Långström N. Bipolar disorder and violent crime: new evidence from population-based longitudinal studies and systematic review. *Archives of General Psychiatry*. 2010;67:931–8.

18 Fazel S, Wolf A, Chang Z, Larsson H, Goodwin GM, Lichtenstein P. Depression and violence: a Swedish population study. *The Lancet Psychiatry*. 2015;2:224–32.

19. Appelbaum PS, Robbins PC, Monahan J. Violence and delusions: data from the MacArthur violence risk assessment study. *American Journal of Psychiatry*. 2000;157:566–72.

20. Van Dorn R, Volavka J, Johnson N. Mental disorder and violence: is there a relationship beyond substance use? *Social Psychiatry and Psychiatric Epidemiology*. 2012;47:487–503.

21. Yang Y, Raine A. Prefrontal structural and functional brain imaging findings in antisocial, violent, and psychopathic individuals: a meta-analysis. *Psychiatry Research*. 2009;174:81–8.

22. Kim-Cohen J, Caspi A, Taylor A, *et al*. MAOA, maltreatment, and gene–environment interaction predicting children's mental health: new evidence and a meta-analysis. *Molecular Psychiatry*. 2006;11:903–13.

23. Retz W, Retz-Junginger P, Supprian T, Thome J, Rösler M. Association of serotonin transporter promoter gene polymorphism with violence: relation with personality disorders, impulsivity, and childhood ADHD psychopathology. *Behavioral Sciences and The Law*. 2004;22:415–25.

24. Pardini DA, Raine A, Erickson K, Loeber R. Lower amygdala volume in men is associated with childhood aggression, early psychopathic traits, and future violence. *Biological Psychiatry*. 2014;75:73–80.

25. Carrillo M, Ricci LA, Coppersmith GA, Melloni Jr RH. The effect of increased serotonergic neurotransmission on aggression: a critical meta-analytical review of preclinical studies. *Psychopharmacology*. 2009;205:349–68.

26. Moffitt TE, Brammer GL, Caspi A, *et al*. Whole blood serotonin relates to violence in an epidemiological study. *Biological Psychiatry*. 1998;43:446–57.

27. Brunner HG, Nelen M, Breakefield XO, Ropers HH, Van Oost BA. Abnormal behavior associated with a point mutation in the structural gene for monoamine oxidase A. *Science*. 1993;262:578–80

28. Caspi A, McClay J, Moffitt TE, *et al*. Role of genotype in the cycle of violence in maltreated children. *Science*. 2002;297:851–4.

29. Rujescu D, Giegling I, Gietl A, Hartmann AM, Möller HJ. A functional single nucleotide polymorphism (V158M) in the *COMT* gene is associated with aggressive personality traits. *Biological Psychiatry*. 2003;54:34–9.

30. Frisell T, Lichtenstein P, Långström N. Violent crime runs in families: a total population study of 12.5 million individuals. *Psychological Medicine*. 2011;41:97–105.

31. Vassos E, Collier DA, Fazel S. Systematic meta-analyses and field synopsis of genetic association studies of violence and aggression. *Molecular Psychiatry*. 2014;19:471–7.

32. Sariaslan A, Larsson H, Fazel S. Genetic and environmental determinants of violence risk in psychotic disorders: a multivariate quantitative genetic study of 1.8 million Swedish twins and siblings. *Molecular Psychiatry*. 2016;21:1251–6.

33. Modestin J, Ammann R. Mental disorder and criminality: male schizophrenia. *Schizophrenia Bulletin*. 1996;22:69–82.

34. Anwar S, Långström N, Grann M, Fazel S. Is arson the crime most strongly associated with psychosis?—A national case-control study of arson risk in schizophrenia and other psychoses. *Schizophrenia Bulletin*. 2011;37:580–6.

35. Fazel S, Grann M. Psychiatric morbidity among homicide offenders: a Swedish population study. *American Journal of Psychiatry*. 2004;161:2129–31.

36. Nielssen O, Large M. Rates of homicide during the first episode of psychosis and after treatment: a systematic review and meta-analysis. *Schizophrenia Bulletin*. 2010;36:702–12.

37. Nielssen O, Bourget D, Laajasalo T, *et al*. Homicide of strangers by people with a psychotic illness. *Schizophrenia Bulletin*. 2011;37:572–9.

38. Fazel S, Wolf A, Palm C, Lichtenstein P. Violent crime, suicide, and premature mortality in patients with schizophrenia and related disorders: a 38-year total population study in Sweden. *The Lancet Psychiatry*. 2014;1:44–54.

39. Frisell T, Pawitan Y, Långström N, Lichtenstein P. Heritability, assortative mating and gender differences in violent crime: results from a total population sample using twin, adoption, and sibling models. *Behavior Genetics*. 2012;42:3–18.

40. Fazel S, Grann M. The population impact of severe mental illness on violent crime. *American Journal of Psychiatry*. 2006;163:1397–403.

41. Witt K, Van Dorn R, Fazel S. Risk factors for violence in psychosis: systematic review and meta-regression analysis of 110 studies. *PLoS One*. 2013;8:e55942.

42. Keers R, Ullrich S, DeStavola BL, Coid JW. Association of violence with emergence of persecutory delusions in untreated schizophrenia. *American Journal of Psychiatry*. 2014;171:332–9.

43. Coid JW, Ullrich S, Bebbington P, Fazel S, Keers R. Paranoid ideation and violence: meta-analysis of individual subject data of 7 population surveys. *Schizophrenia Bulletin*. 2016;42:907–15.

44. Coid JW, Ullrich S, Kallis C, *et al*. The relationship between delusions and violence: findings from the East London first episode psychosis study. *JAMA Psychiatry*. 2013;70:465–71.

45. Fazel S, Zetterqvist J, Larsson H, Långström N, Lichtenstein P. Antipsychotics, mood stabilisers, and risk of violent crime. *The Lancet*. 2014;384:1206–14.

46. Short T, Thomas S, Mullen P, Ogloff JR. Comparing violence in schizophrenia patients with and without comorbid substance-use disorders to community controls. *Acta Psychiatrica Scandinavica*. 2013;128:306–13.

47. Fazel S, Wolf A, Palm C, Lichtenstein P. Violent crime, suicide, and premature mortality in patients with schizophrenia and related disorders: a 38-year total population study in Sweden. *The Lancet Psychiatry*. 2014;1:44–54.

48. Large MM, Nielssen O. Violence in first-episode psychosis: a systematic review and meta-analysis. *Schizophrenia Research*. 2011;125:209–20.

49. Fazel S, Yu R. Psychotic disorders and repeat offending: systematic review and meta-analysis. *Schizophrenia Bulletin*. 2011;37:800–10.

50. Chang Z, Larsson H, Lichtenstein P, Fazel S. Psychiatric disorders and violent reoffending: a national cohort study of convicted prisoners in Sweden. *The Lancet Psychiatry*. 2015;2:891–900.

51. Bonta J, Law M, Hanson K. The prediction of criminal and violent recidivism among mentally disordered offenders: a meta-analysis. *Psychological Bulletin*. 1998;123:123.

52. Baillargeon J, Binswanger IA, Penn JV, Williams BA, Murray OJ. Psychiatric disorders and repeat incarcerations: the revolving prison door. *American Journal of Psychiatry*. 2009;166:103–9.

53. Oakley C, Hynes F, Clark T. Mood disorders and violence: a new focus. *Advances in Psychiatric Treatment*. 2009;15:263–70.

54. Fazel S, Seewald K. Severe mental illness in 33 588 prisoners worldwide: systematic review and meta-regression analysis. *British Journal of Psychiatry*. 2012;200:364–73.

55. Brennan PA, Mednick SA, Hodgins S. Major mental disorders and criminal violence in a Danish birth cohort. *Archives of General Psychiatry*. 2000;57:494–500.

56. Elbogen EB, Johnson SC. The intricate link between violence and mental disorder: results from the National Epidemiologic Survey on Alcohol and Related Conditions. *Archives of General Psychiatry*. 2009;66:152–61.

57. Wallace C, Mullen P, Burgess P, Palmer S, Ruschena D, Browne C. Serious criminal offending and mental disorder. Case linkage study. *British Journal of Psychiatry*. 1998;172:477–84.

58. Swann AC, Lijffijt M, Lane SD, Kjome KL, Steinberg JL, Moeller FG. Criminal conviction, impulsivity, and course of illness in bipolar disorder. *Bipolar Disorders*. 2011;13:173–81.

59. Goldstein PJ. The drugs/violence nexus: a tripartite conceptual framework. *Journal of Drug Issues*. 1985;15:493–506.

60. Friedman AS. Substance use/abuse as a predictor to illegal and violent behavior: a review of the relevant literature. *Aggression and Violent Behavior*. 1999;3:339–55.

61. Boles SM, Miotto K. Substance abuse and violence: a review of the literature. *Aggression and Violent Behavior*. 2003;8:155–74.

62. Grant BF, Goldstein RB, Saha TD, et al. Epidemiology of DSM-5 alcohol use disorder: results from the National Epidemiologic Survey on Alcohol and Related Conditions III. *JAMA Psychiatry*. 2015;72:757–66.

63. Soyka M. Substance misuse, psychiatric disorder and violent and disturbed behaviour. *British Journal of Psychiatry*. 2000;176:345–50.

64. Boden JM, Fergusson DM, Horwood LJ. Alcohol misuse and violent behavior: findings from a 30-year longitudinal study. *Drug and Alcohol Dependence*. 2012;122:135–41.

65. Popovici I, Homer JF, Fang H, French MT. Alcohol use and crime: findings from a longitudinal sample of US adolescents and young adults. *Alcoholism: Clinical and Experimental Research*. 2012;36:532–43.

66. Haggård-Grann U, Hallqvist J, Långström N, Möller J. The role of alcohol and drugs in triggering criminal violence: a case-cross-over study. *Addiction*. 2006;101:100–8.

67. Grann M, Fazel S. Substance misuse and violent crime: Swedish population study. *BMJ*. 2004;328:1233–4.

68. McGinty EE, Choksy S, Wintemute GJ. The relationship between controlled substances and violence. *Epidemiologic Reviews*. 2016;38:5–31.

69. Friedman AS, Glassman K, Terras A. Violent behavior as related to use of marijuana and other drugs. *Journal of Addictive Diseases*. 2001;20:49–72.

70. Mulvey EP, Odgers C, Skeem J, Gardner W, Schubert C, Lidz C. Substance use and community violence: a test of the relation at the daily level. *Journal of Consulting and Clinical Psychology*. 2006;74:743.

71. Duggan C, Howard R. The 'functional link' between personality disorder and violence: a critical appraisal. In: McMurran M, Howard R, editors. *Personality, Personality Disorder and Violence: An Evidence-Based Approach*. Chichester: Wiley-Blackwell; 2009. pp. 19–37.

72. Fountoulakis KN, Leucht S, Kaprinis GS. Personality disorders and violence. *Current Opinion in Psychiatry*. 2008;21:84–92.

73. Keene J, Hope T, Fairburn CG, Jacoby R, Gedling K, Ware CJ. Natural history of aggressive behaviour in dementia. *International Journal of Geriatric Psychiatry*. 1999;14:541–8.

74. Patel V, Hope T. Aggressive behaviour in elderly people with dementia: a review. *International Journal of Geriatric Psychiatry*. 1993;8:457–72.

75. Kim JM, Chu K, Jung KH, Lee ST, Choi SS, Lee SK. Criminal manifestations of dementia patients: report from the national forensic hospital. *Dementia and Geriatric Cognitive Disorders Extra*. 2011;1:433–8.

76. Putkonen H, Weizmann-Henelius G, Repo-Tiihonen E, et al. Homicide, psychopathy, and aging—a nationwide register-based case-comparison study of homicide offenders aged 60 years or older. *Journal of Forensic Sciences*. 2010;55:1552–6.

77. Barak Y, Perry T, Elizur A. Elderly criminals: a study of the first criminal offence in old age. *International Journal of Geriatric Psychiatry*. 1995;10:511–16.

78. Liljegren M, Naasan G, Temlett J, et al. Criminal behavior in frontotemporal dementia and Alzheimer disease. *JAMA Neurology*. 2015;72:295–300.

79. Farrer TJ, Frost RB, Hedges DW. Prevalence of traumatic brain injury in juvenile offenders: a meta-analysis. *Child Neuropsychology*. 2013;19:225–34.

80. Shiroma EJ, Ferguson PL, Pickelsimer EE. Prevalence of traumatic brain injury in an offender population: a meta-analysis. *Journal of Correctional Health Care*. 2010;16:147–59.

81. Fazel S, Lichtenstein P, Grann M, Långström N. Risk of violent crime in individuals with epilepsy and traumatic brain injury: a 35-year Swedish population study. *PLoS Medicine*. 2011;8:e1001150.

82. Amoroso C, Zwi A, Somerville E, Grove N. Epilepsy and stigma. *The Lancet*. 2006;367:1143–4.

83. Fazel S, Vassos E, Danesh J. Prevalence of epilepsy in prisoners: systematic review. *BMJ*. 2002;324:1495.

84. Polanczyk GV, Salum GA, Sugaya LS, Caye A, Rohde LA. Annual Research Review: A meta-analysis of the worldwide prevalence of mental disorders in children and adolescents. *Journal of Child Psychology and Psychiatry*. 2015;56:345–65.

85. Ståhlberg O, Anckarsäter H, Nilsson T. Mental health problems in youths committed to juvenile institutions: prevalences and

treatment needs. *European Child and Adolescent Psychiatry*. 2010;19:893–903.

86. Satterfield JH, Faller KJ, Crinella FM, Schell AM, Swanson JM, Homer LD. A 30-year prospective follow-up study of hyperactive boys with conduct problems: adult criminality. *Journal of the American Academy of Child and Adolescent Psychiatry*. 2007;46:601–10.

87. Young S, Thome J. ADHD and offenders. *World Journal of Biological Psychiatry*. 2011;12(sup1):124–8.

88. Fazel S, Doll H, Långström N. Mental disorders among adolescents in juvenile detention and correctional facilities: a systematic review and meta-regression analysis of 25 surveys. *Journal of the American Academy of Child and Adolescent Psychiatry*. 2008;47:1010–19.

89. Jensen CM, Steinhausen HC. Comorbid mental disorders in children and adolescents with attention-deficit/hyperactivity disorder in a large nationwide study. *ADHD Attention Deficit and Hyperactivity Disorders*. 2015;7:27–38.

90. Lundström S, Forsman M, Larsson H, et al. Childhood neurodevelopmental disorders and violent criminality: a sibling control study. *Journal of Autism and Developmental Disorders*. 2014;44:2707–16.

91. Helverschou SB, Rasmussen K, Steindal K, Søndanaa E, Nilsson B, Nøttestad JA. Offending profiles of individuals with autism spectrum disorder: a study of all individuals with autism spectrum disorder examined by the forensic psychiatric service in Norway between 2000 and 2010. *Autism*. 2015;19:850–8.

92. Långström N, Grann M, Ruchkin V, Sjöstedt G, Fazel S. Risk factors for violent offending in autism spectrum disorder: a national study of hospitalized individuals. *Journal of Interpersonal Violence*. 2009;24:1358–70.

93. Miotto P, Pollini B, Restaneo A, Favaretto G, Preti A. Aggressiveness, anger, and hostility in eating disorders. *Comprehensive Psychiatry*. 2008;49:364–73.

94. Baum A, Goldner EM. The relationship between stealing and eating disorders: a review. *Harvard Review of Psychiatry*. 1995;3:210–21.

95. Fazel S, Singh JP, Doll H, Grann M. Use of risk assessment instruments to predict violence and antisocial behaviour in 73 samples involving 24 827 people: systematic review and meta-analysis. *BMJ*. 2012; 345:e4692.

96. Singh JP, Fazel S, Gueorguieva R, Buchanan A. Rates of violence in patients classified as high risk by structured risk assessment instruments. *British Journal of Psychiatry*. 2014;204:180–7.

97. Troquete NA, van den Brink RH, Beintema H, *et al*. Risk assessment and shared care planning in out-patient forensic psychiatry: cluster randomised controlled trial. *British Journal of Psychiatry*. 2013;202:365–71.

98. Singh JP, Grann M, Fazel S. Authorship bias in violence risk assessment? A systematic review and meta-analysis. *PLoS One*. 2013;8:e72484.

99. Fazel S, Wolf S, Larsson H, Lichtenstein P, Mallett S, Fanshawe T. Identification of low risk of violent crime in severe mental illness with a clinical prediction tool (Oxford Mental Illness and Violence tool [OxMIV]): a derivation and validation study. *The Lancet Psychiatry*. 2017;4:461–8.

100. Webb R, Lichtenstein P, Larsson H, Geddes JR, Fazel S. Suicide, hospital-presenting suicide attempts, and criminality in bipolar disorder: examination of risk for multiple adverse outcomes. Journal of Clinical Psychiatry. 2014;75(8):e809-e816.

# 140

# Developmental approach to understanding the needs of young people in contact with the criminal justice system

*Sue Bailey and Prathiba Chitsabesan*

## Introduction

Over the last decade, studies have highlighted that young people with disproportionately high and multiple needs have clustered in the juvenile justice system. These young people experience higher levels of diagnosable mental health problems and neurodisability than the general population.

Delinquency, conduct problems, and aggression all refer to antisocial behaviours that reflect a failure of the individual to conform his or her behaviour to the expectations of some authority figure or to societal norms, or to respect the rights of other people. The 'behaviours' can range from mild conflicts with authority figures, to major violation of societal norms, to serious violations of the rights of others. The term 'delinquency' implies that the acts could result in conviction, although most do not do so. The term 'juvenile' usually applies to the age range, extending from a lower age set by the age of criminal responsibility to an upper age when a young person can be dealt with in courts for adult crimes. These ages vary between, and indeed within, countries and are not the same for all offences.

This chapter provides a developmental approach to understanding the needs of young people in contact with the criminal justice system. It reviews the prevalence of a range of mental health and neurodevelopmental disorders in young offenders and describes the key principles of assessment and intervention approaches. The policy and legal framework have been illustrated by reference to the system in England but will have relevance to readers from further afield.

## Developmental pathways to antisocial behaviour

Adolescence is a transitional stage of development between childhood and adulthood; the developmental tasks of adolescence centre on autonomy and connection with others, rebellion and the development of independence, the development of identity, and the distinction from, and continuity with, others. Many theories of development are stage theories, in which we pass from stage to stage, completing the developmental tasks appropriate to each stage prior to moving on. However, in reality, progression across domains is not equal and frequently non-linear. Additionally, neuroscience suggests that there is a lack of synchrony in late childhood and adolescence in the development of two of the critical brain systems that enable the development of adaptive behaviour [1]. The mesolimbic system develops more quickly than the frontal system, resulting in the adolescent brain having a heightened need for basic reward, but a lower capacity to manage short-term rewards for greater long-term gains. This discrepancy may be greater for young people at risk of antisocial behaviour where reward-driven behaviour is increased and neurocognitive deficits in executive functioning more common.

Epidemiological studies suggest that the development of antisocial behaviour involves a complex interaction of intrinsic and psychosocial risk and protective factors [2]. Links between early adverse events in the prenatal period and the impact of parenting, family, and peer relationships on behaviour in early childhood have been found [2]. Heritable influences contribute towards a gene–environment interaction, suggesting pathways are complex and some vulnerabilities become increasingly evident in the context of other risk factors. Intrinsic risk factors include socio-cognitive deficits (hostile attribution bias), temperamental factors (callous-unemotional traits), and low autonomic nervous system arousal [2, 3]. The neurocognitive profiles of young offenders include deficits in language skills, attention, and impulse control, as well as low intelligence quotient (IQ) scores. Deficits in executive function can affect the young person's ability to regulate their behaviours and plan and generate alternative strategies. However, antisocial behaviour also shows strong associations with psychosocial adversity. Parental mental illness, family breakdown, parenting style, and association with other antisocial peers influence outcomes [2]. Detachment from school through truancy and exclusion may increase the risk of offending through reduced supervision and loss of any positive socialization effects of school and by creating delinquent groups of young people [4].

Distinctive pathways are described for those with early and late onset of offending behaviour, with some gender differences suggested. Girls have historically been found to have a later onset to their antisocial behaviour, compared with boys [2, 5]. Moffitt [5] proposed a developmental taxonomy whereby early-onset conduct problems were more likely to be associated with individually based risk factors that increase vulnerability to the development of behaviour problems in the context of adverse family and parenting conditions. In adolescent-onset conduct problems, by contrast, individual vulnerabilities may be less marked, and the impact of environmental risk factors, including the influence of antisocial peers, more evident. There is evidence that early-onset, life course-persistent antisocial behaviour is more likely to be associated with a greater risk of neurodevelopmental impairment [6].

However, it is important to bear in mind that protective or resilience factors for the young person or within the system around them can also modify outcomes (Fig. 140.1).This is particularly relevant for interventions and an important underpinning principle of the risk and resilience approach which focuses on building important 'assets' in the child's health and emotional well-being. Activity can include strengthening children's internal resources, as well as resilience in their families, their communities, and their broader environment.

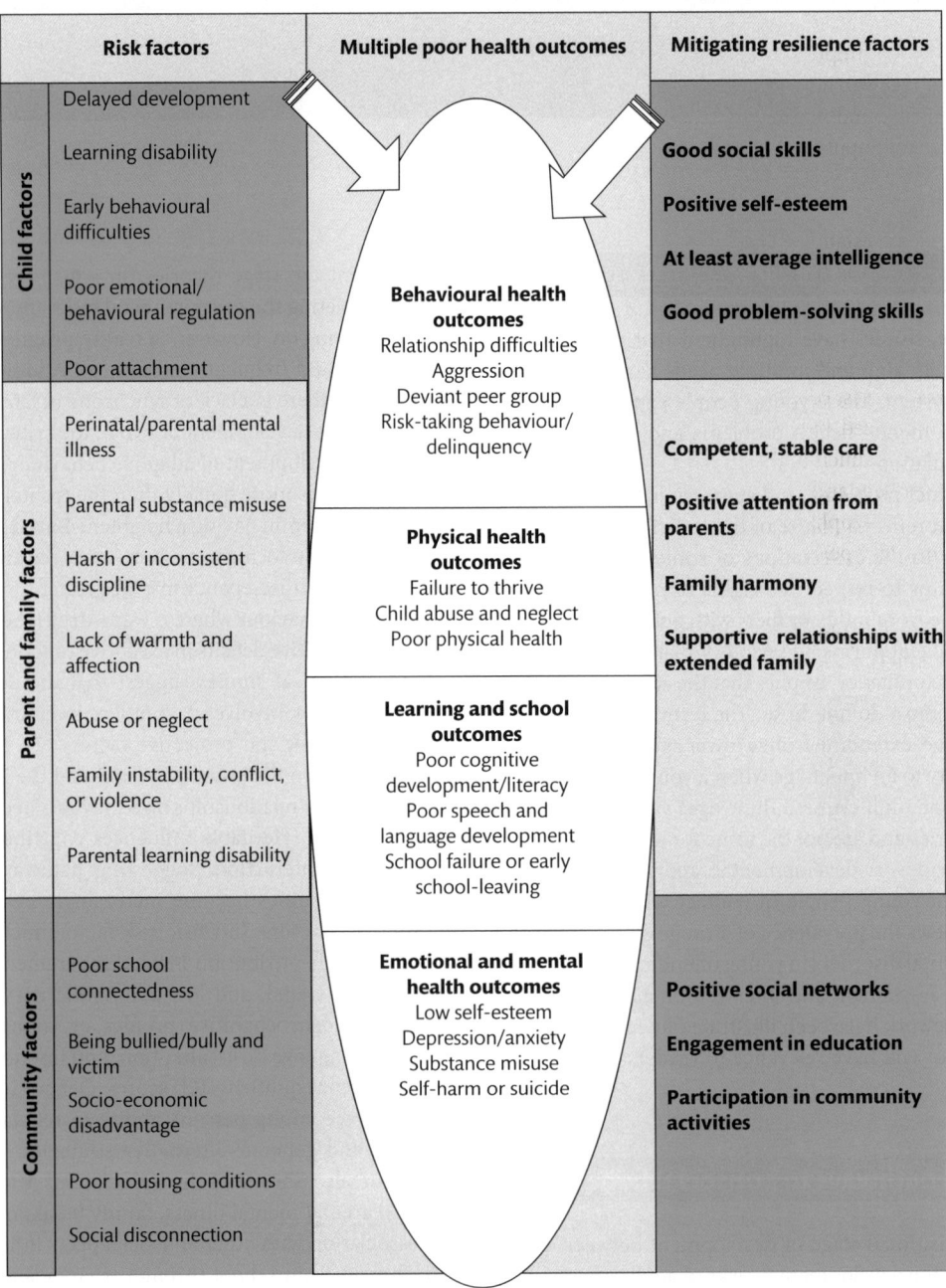

**Fig. 140.1** Risk and resilience factors affecting multiple health outcomes.

Reproduced from Chitsabesan P, Khan L, Assessment of young offenders; mental health, physical, educational and social needs. In: *Forensic Child and Adolescent Mental Health: Meeting the Needs of Young Offenders*, Bailey S, Chitsabesan P, Tarbuck P [Eds.], pp 41–54, Copyright (2017), with permission from Cambridge University Press.

## Prevalence of mental health needs and neurodevelopmental disorders

### Mental health needs

Studies have reported the prevalence of psychiatric disorders among young males in custody in the United States (US) to be between 60% and 70%, and between 60% and 80% for young females in custody [8], in contrast to rates of between 7% and 12% in the general population [9]. The high rate of psychopathology in juvenile offenders may be the consequence of shared risk factors in the development of both antisocial behaviour and psychiatric disorders.

Table 140.1 summarizes a range of studies that identify rates of specific mental health needs and neurodevelopmental disorders among young people within the youth justice system and the general population [10]. While it is important to highlight that comparing such rates is problematic due to differences in methodology between studies, prevalence rates found in young offenders are consistently higher than in the general population.

### Psychotic disorders

Young people in the secure estate are approximately ten times more likely to suffer from psychosis than the general adolescent population [11]. Fazel *et al.* [11] found that 3.3% of males and 2.7% of females in youth custody were diagnosed with a psychotic illness. A first psychotic episode may have multiple causes, including drugs, brain injury, physical illnesses, or schizophrenia. Schizophrenia is a mental illness characterized by cognitive disruption, delusions (fixed, false beliefs), and hallucinations. Sufferers frequently have comorbid depression, anxiety, and substance misuse. Mortality rates for young offenders with schizophrenia was found to be significantly higher than in non-offending peers [12].

**Table 140.1** Prevalence of psychiatric and neurodevelopmental disorders in young offenders

| Type of disorder | Reported prevalence rates among young people in the general population (%) | Reported prevalence rates among young offenders (%) |
| --- | --- | --- |
| Psychotic disorder | 0.4 | 1–3.3 |
| Depressive disorder | 0.2–3 | 8–29 |
| Anxiety disorder | 3.3 | 9–21 |
| Post-traumatic stress disorder | 0.4 | 11–25 |
| Substance misuse disorder | 7 | 37–55 |
| Learning disabilities | 2–4 | 23–32 |
| Dyslexia | 10 | 21–43 |
| Communication disorders | 5–7 | 60–65 |
| Attention-deficit/hyperactive disorder | 3–9 | 11.7–18.5 |
| Autistic spectrum disorder | 0.6–1.2 | 15 |
| Traumatic brain injury | 24–31.6 | 65 |

### Anxiety disorders and post-traumatic stress disorder

Anxiety disorders include a range of different disorders, from generalized anxiety disorder to phobias and post-traumatic stress disorder (PTSD). In their UK-based study of young offenders, Chitsabesan *et al.* [13] diagnosed anxiety disorder in 16% of cases, consistent with findings from a systematic review [14].

The NWJP study found that the vast majority of offenders had experienced at least one trauma in their lifetime (93%), while 11% met the criteria for PTSD [15]. In the UK, the Annual Report of the Chief Medical Officer stated that 9% of 13- to 18-year-old young offenders in secure care have a diagnosis of PTSD [16].

Many young people within the criminal justice system who present with pervasive and complex presentations often have an extensive history of repeated interpersonal traumatic experiences. Disruption to the early attachment process through interpersonal trauma has a direct impact on the development of a child's brain, attachment style, and emotional regulation systems [17]. Over time, the brain is more likely to develop connections between the parts of the brain based on recognizing and interpreting threat.

### Depression

A number of studies in adolescents within the criminal justice systems, both in the UK and internationally, have reported disproportionally higher prevalence rates of depressive disorders in young offenders. Fazel *et al.* [11] conducted a meta-analysis of 25 studies of psychiatric morbidity among children and young people in custody, including studies from the UK, as well as other international contexts. Their findings suggested that around 11% of boys and 29% of girls had a major depressive disorder [11]. Adolescents within the youth justice system experience high levels of psychosocial adversity and are significantly more at risk of developing depression due to both genetic and environmental factors. Additionally, these young people are at greater risk of continued depression, as they have fewer protective influences to compensate for the many adversities they face.

### Self-harm and suicidal behaviour

An association between antisocial behaviour and suicidal behaviour has also been demonstrated in research studies. A study of 200 young people sentenced to custody found that 20% were reported to have harmed themselves and 11% to have attempted suicide [18]. Self-harm is more prevalent among offenders, as certain risk factors for self-harm are more common among this group. Predictors of an increased risk include previous attempts, prolonged low mood, attention-deficit/hyperactivity disorder, impulsivity, and substance misuse [19].

Rates of suicide are similarly much higher in the offender population, compared with non-antisocial peers, possibly as a consequence of greater impulsive behaviour and substance misuse, which are more common in this group of young people [19].

### Substance misuse

Substance misuse disorders are defined by sustained maladaptive behaviours related to, or caused by, substance misuse. Young people's substance misuse differs from that of adult substance misusing offenders. Cannabis and alcohol are the main substances of choice reported by adolescents, and polydrug use is common. The mesolimbic dopaminergic system, or 'reward system in the brain', has an important role as adolescent brains appear particularly sensitized to dopamine.

Prevalence rates of substance misuse disorder in young offenders in custody have ranged from 41% to 55% [20]. Childhood exposure to violence and abuse was found to increase the likelihood of violence and problematic substance misuse in adulthood [20, 21]. Reduced parental supervision and the influence of peer relationships play a key role in both experimentation with, and ongoing use of, substances [20]. Mulvey *et al.* [21] reported that the disinhibiting effects of drugs, such as alcohol, can increase the risk of violent or risk-taking behaviour. Positive associations have also been shown between substance misuse and other disorders, including depression and attention-deficit/hyperactivity disorder (ADHD). Longitudinal studies also showed an association with persistent offending and both depressive symptoms and drug use into adulthood [22].

### Psychopathy

Psychopathy is characterized by a unique cluster of traits, including shallow affect; lack of empathy, and guilt; irresponsibility; impulsivity; and poor decision-making. A closely related construct to psychopathy is antisocial personality disorder (APD). APD is defined in the *Diagnostic and Statistical Manual of Mental Disorders*, fifth edition (DSM-V) as having a pervasive disregard for, and a willingness to, violate the rights of others [23]. While most individuals with APD do not meet the diagnostic criteria for psychopathy, psychopaths are almost invariably diagnosed with APD.

The Psychopathy Checklist Revised (PCL-R) is a well-known measure of adult psychopathic traits, although criticized for its strong focus on criminality. The Psychopathy Checklist: Youth Version (PCL:YV) was developed from the PCL-R to provide a standardized approach to assessing psychopathic-like traits in youth males and females aged 12–17 years and has demonstrated predictive validity for reoffending and violent offending [24]. An alternative approach which is still in its early stage of validation is the Comprehensive Assessment of Psychopathic Personality Disorder (CAPP) which has six dimensions: attachment, behavioural, cognitive, dominance, emotional, and self-styles of functioning [25]. The new measure attempts to encapsulate the 'clinical' construct, as well as capture change [26].

The presence of callous-unemotional (CU) traits has been shown to identify a discrete group of conduct-disordered children with more severe conduct problems and aggression. A biological theory has been proposed that children who develop CU traits have unique neural mechanisms characterized by low cortisol and underarousal, contributing to a temperamental style which has low emotional reactivity and fearfulness to threatening stimuli, poor responsiveness to cues to punishment, and reward-dominant orientation [27]. However, Johnstone [26] argues that there are developmental challenges associated with extending the construct of psychopathy to youth and that environmental factors, such as disrupted parent–child attachments and trauma, are also important risk and mediating factors which can influence neural brain processes and outcomes.

## Neurodevelopmental disorders

Neurodevelopmental impairments are expressed through a wide range of symptoms, including deficits in cognitive functions (reasoning, thinking, and perception) and social–affective functions (the expression of emotion and formation of relationships). Specifically, problems with executive functioning, cognitive empathy, and emotional regulation associated with particular neurodevelopmental disorders can directly influence propensity towards aggressive and antisocial behaviour [6].

### Attention-deficit/hyperactivity disorder

A meta-analysis reviewing 25 international studies found a rate of 11.7% for young male offenders [11], in contrast to 3–7% within the general population. Longitudinal studies have suggested that childhood ADHD predicts later antisocial behaviour, although more recent evidence suggests that this association is indirect and mediated through the development of conduct disorder, illicit drug use, and peer delinquency [28]. Young people with conduct disorder and ADHD have been shown to have greater severity and persistence of antisocial behaviour. Co-occurrence with substance misuse is also high, with evidence of increased frequency and severity of institutional behavioural disturbances while in custody [29].

### Autism spectrum disorders

Autism is a neurodevelopmental disorder characterized by a triad of impairment in social communication that affects about 1% of children and young people [30]. Certain features of autism may predispose young people to offend, including social naïvety, misinterpretation of social cues, and poor empathy [30]. While the National Autistic Society [31] suggests that young people with Asperger's syndrome are seven times more likely to come into contact with the criminal justice system than their peers, many studies demonstrating an increased prevalence rate in the criminal justice system have been conducted on a forensic psychiatry sample of offenders, suggesting further research is required. There is concern, however, about the possible links between autism and particular types of offending. Certain types of offences may raise the suspicion of autism spectrum disorder (ASD), including stalking, arson, sexual offences, inexplicable violence, computer crime, and offences arising out of misjudgement of social relationships [30].

### Learning disability

A learning disability is defined as an IQ score of less than 70, together with significant difficulties with adaptive or social functioning and onset prior to adulthood. High prevalence rates (23–32%) have been found in studies of young offenders [32]. The majority of young offenders with a learning disability frequently have an IQ in the 'mild range' (between 50 and 69) and may therefore be less likely to have had their learning needs identified in mainstream schools where those needs are often overshadowed by their challenging behaviour [33].

### Communication disorders

Communication disorders relate to problems with speech, language, and communication that significantly impact day-to-day functioning. A study of 72 young offenders attending a youth offending service found that 65% of those screened had profiles indicating that they had communication difficulties, including expressive language difficulties (28%), receptive language difficulties (45%), and articulation difficulties such as a stammer (8%) [34]. Particular deficits in verbal skills may also be highlighted through a discrepancy in verbal and performance IQ scores.

## Traumatic brain injury

A traumatic brain injury (TBI) is any injury to the brain caused by an impact, and the severity is typically measured by the depth of loss of consciousness (LOC). The majority of TBIs appear to be mild, although long-term effects on academic performance, behaviour, emotional control, and social interactions can be reported. This is reflected in a range of studies which have demonstrated an association between TBI and antisocial behaviour, including an earlier onset of offending history and more violent offending [35]. Greater severity of TBI was also found to be associated with greater impairment of cognition, earlier onset of criminal behaviour, and increased rates of mental illness and substance use. Identified prevalence rates of TBI among young offenders are variable, however, ranging from 4.5% to 72% [36].

## Gender and ethnicity

While studies of mental health needs have predominantly focused on male offenders, gender differences have been reported. The NWJP study found that female offenders were 14 times as likely as male offenders to meet the criteria for at least one mental disorder, including depression and anxiety disorders [8]. Rates of PTSD and self-harm have also been found to be significantly more prevalent in females [13]. Explanatory mechanisms may include greater genetic vulnerability, as well as increased exposure to trauma and chaotic family lifestyles. Female offenders have been shown to experience more abuse, neglect, and a family history of mental illness than male offenders. There are concerns that there is an overrepresentation of some ethnic minority groups within the criminal justice system and that these groups of young people have poorer access to services. However, studies exploring differences in the prevalence of mental disorders among young offenders by ethnicity have been sparse and findings inconsistent. A national study within the United States using the Massachusetts Youth Screening Instrument-Version 2 (MAYSI-2) found that differences in prevalence rates varied across sites and were generally small [37].

## Screening and assessment

Studies to date suggest that one of the most common reasons for unmet need is lack of appropriate and timely assessment [38]. Lack of identification hampers opportunities for early intervention and promotion of healthy development and resilience in young people.

Initial assessment is a key factor in the successful treatment of mental health needs for young offenders. Early identification of mental health needs may also reduce the later risk of mental disorders and their related health costs. However, assessment can be complicated by a number of factors, including the non-clear nature of emerging mental health symptoms in children and young people, in comparison to presentations in adults, the minimization of symptoms by young offenders, and the disinclination of young people to engage with mental health services due to fear of stigma.

Historically, screening and assessment tools have been developed focusing on single-problem areas, for example the MAYSI-2, a widely used screening tool for mental health needs within the US youth justice system [39]. However, young people who offend often have multiple areas of need. In recognition of these difficulties, the Comprehensive Health Assessment Tool (CHAT) was introduced for young offenders in custody across England and Wales [40], supported by the development of Healthcare Standards for Children and Young People in Secure Settings [41]. The CHAT is a semi-structured assessment developed to provide a standardized approach to health screening for all young offenders admitted to the secure estate and includes assessment of mental health needs, physical health, substance misuse, and neurodevelopmental impairment. Assessing and managing unmet health needs can inform individual care plans, help to address offending behaviour, and provide a valuable opportunity to re-engage young people with health and educational services to address unmet needs.

## Principles of risk assessment

Risk assessment combines statistical data with clinical information in a way that integrates historical variables, current crucial variables, and contextual or environmental factors. Structured risk assessment instruments have been developed that aim to increase the validity of clinical prediction. These scales typically contain a number of risk items selected from reviews of research, crime theories, and clinical considerations. Items are summed to form a total risk score and may also reveal specific risk patterns (for example, mainly family or child factors). The Structured Assessment of Violence Risk in Youth (SAVRY) [42] is a popular risk assessment tool which assesses 24 risk factors (ten historical risk factors, six social/contextual risk factors, eight individual/clinical risk factors) and six protective factors. The SAVRY has a good evidence base to support its predictive accuracy and clinical applicability in a range of settings.

Risk assessments can vary in the type of risk they assess, for example the Youth Level of Service/Case Management Inventory [43] assesses general offending, while the SAVRY assesses interpersonal violence.

The following five-step approach should be considered when undertaking risk assessments [44]:

- Step 1: collecting case information via interviews and collateral information from informants.
- Step 2: identifying the presence and relevance of risk factors using the structured risk assessment tool.
- Step 3: identifying the presence and relevance of protective factors using the structured risk assessment tool.
- Step 4: risk formulation.
- Step 5: management plan.

For risk and protective factors, consideration needs to be given to the presence and relevance of the factor in relation to a specific risk, as well as its severity and frequency. A rating (low, moderate, or high for risk factors, and either absent or present for protective factors) does not fully inform the subsequent risk formulation or management plans. The aim of a risk formulation is to provide a better understanding of the origins of violence and how it has developed, is maintained, and changes [44]. There are a number of frameworks which can be used to help explain and communicate risk, including the '5Ps' model (problem, predisposing factors, precipitating factors, perpetuating factors, and protective factors) and the '3Ds' model (which represents drivers, destabilizers, and disinhibitors) [44].

## Interventions

A large number of different treatments have been developed to reduce antisocial behaviour. These include psychotherapy, pharmacotherapy, school-based interventions, residential programmes, and social treatments. Meta-analyses of treatment approaches to juvenile delinquency have produced reasonably consistent findings [45]. The best results were obtained from cognitive behavioural, skills-orientated, and multimodal methods. Specifically, treatment approaches that were participatory, collaborative, and problem-solving were particularly likely to be beneficial. Family and parenting interventions also seem to reduce the risk of subsequent delinquency among older children and adolescents.

Cognitive behavioural therapy (CBT) is an effective psychological intervention for a number of mental health difficulties in childhood and adolescence, including depression, social anxiety disorder, and PTSD. Studies that have been conducted with young people engaging in high-risk behaviours indicated that CBT may be useful for young offenders with a range of mental health needs [46]. However, the format and delivery of CBT may require adaptation, taking into account the young person's level of cognitive, social, and emotional development, including neurodevelopmental impairment. Adaptations include use of visual cues, encouraging verbal learning through games, reducing distractions, and using simplified language [47].

More recently, therapies include mindfulness-based cognitive therapy, dialectical behaviour therapy (DBT), and mentalization-based therapies. Overall, the current research base provides support for the feasibility of mindfulness-based interventions with children and adolescents, and there is an emerging evidence base in relation to adolescence with behavioural problems and those in custodial settings; however, there is no generalized empirical evidence of the efficacy of these interventions at present. DBT was developed as a treatment for suicidal adults by developing specific skills in mindfulness, emotional regulation, distress tolerance, and interpersonal effectiveness through individual and group sessions. Over recent years, DBT has been modified and adapted to meet the needs of adolescents within forensic settings. Mentalization-based treatment for adolescents (MBT-A) is a psychodynamic psychotherapy programme with roots in attachment theory, aimed at enhancing the young person's capacity to represent their own and other's feelings accurately in emotionally challenging situations. MBT-A has been influential in the development of a more systemic approach called adolescent mentalization-based integrative therapy (AMBIT), specifically designed for 'hard-to-reach' adolescents with mental health problems who may be or are at risk of offending [48].

The National Institute for Health and Care Excellence (NICE) [49] recommends multimodal interventions for the treatment of conduct disorder in children and young people aged between 11 and 17 years. A meta-analysis of eight family-based treatment studies of adolescent conduct disorder found better outcomes for three family-based treatments: functional family therapy (FFT), multi-systemic therapy (MST), and multi-dimensional treatment foster care (MTFC), compared to routine treatment [50]. The most well-evaluated is MST.

MST is a multimodal intervention where interventions are targeted at not only the young person, but also their family, school, and peers. Evaluation studies of MST have been promising [51]. In particular, it has also been shown to be effective for young people with substance misuse disorders. However, criticisms of MST include the requirement for a high level of therapeutic expertise, as well as the cost of implementation.

McGuire [52] identified six principles for effective programmes:

1. The intensity should match the extent of the risk posed by the offender.
2. A focus on active collaboration, which is not too didactic or unstructured.
3. Close integration with the community.
4. Emphasis on behavioural or cognitive approaches.
5. Delivered with high quality with training and monitoring of staff.
6. Focus on the proximal causes of offending behaviour (peer groups, promoting current family communication, and enhancing self-management and problem-solving skills), rather than the distal causes (early childhood).

## Serious crimes

### Homicide

Longitudinal studies are invaluable in mapping out the range of factors and processes that contribute to the development of aggressive behaviour and in showing how they are causally related [2]. Research suggests that risk factors that increase violent offending overlap with those increasing the risk for homicides as well, for example repeat offending, substance abuse problems, and exposure to early risk factors such as family dysfunction and educational difficulties [53, 54]. The Pittsburgh study found that the strongest predictors of becoming a homicide offender were environmental, rather than individual, factors [54]. The study found that there was no single factor explaining homicide offending, but instead a cumulative effect, with the greater the number of risk factors, the more likely it was that the individual would become involved in a homicidal incident.

Murder and manslaughter are more often committed alone, and on average, the perpetrators start their criminal activities at a later age and are much less likely to have previous convictions than other minors taken into judicial youth institutions. However, there is a great variety in terms of motives and victims, etc. Studies show that children and adolescents who murder share a constellation of psychological, educational, and family system disturbance [53]. The majority of young persons who have killed initially dissociate themselves from the reality of their act but gradually experience a progression of reactions and feelings akin to a grief reaction. The young person, while facing a still adversarial and public pre-trial and trial process, has to move safely through the process of disbelief, denial, loss, grief, and anger/blame. PTSD arising from the participation in the sadistic act (either directly or observing the actions of co-defendants) has to be treated, as does trauma arising from their own past personal emotional, physical, and/or sexual abuse. A combination of verbal and non-verbal therapies are effective, but factors such as a history of severe aggression, low intelligence, and a poor capacity for insight are associated with poorer outcomes [53].

In understanding the role of violence and sadism in a young person's life, one has to understand their reaction to perceived threat and their past maladaptive behaviours aimed at allowing them to feel in control of their lives.

## Harmful sexual behaviour

Harmful sexual behaviours by children and young people is a considerable problem that impacts on victims and their perpetrators, as well as their families. The sexual behaviours of children and young people are on a continuum, which ranges, on the one hand, from normal and developmentally appropriate to highly abnormal and violent on the other. It is important to place any assessment of a child's sexual behaviour within a developmental context, as such behaviours may have substantially different motivations and different developmental significance across these two developmental stages. Models have been developed to describe children and young people's sexual behaviours at various levels of seriousness or concern, including age-appropriate and inappropriate [55].

Most, but not all, abusers are male, often come from disadvantaged backgrounds, with a history of victimization and sexual and physical abuse, and show high rates of psychopathology [55]. Females with harmful sexual behaviour were found to have higher rates of PTSD and a history of family dysfunction and have been victims of sexual abuse, in comparison to male offenders [56]. People with learning disability (LD) and ASD are overrepresented in services for sexual offenders, which may relate to a number of factors, including a lack of socio-sexual knowledge, difficulties understanding the nature of relationships and the feelings of others, and more limited opportunities for intimate relationships [30, 55].

A core part of any assessment of an adolescent sex offender should include a holistic assessment of needs and risks, including an assessment of mental health [55]. These young people often have a history of other offending behaviours, experienced trauma and loss, and are likely to suffer from a range of mental health disorders. Assessment and treatment of these disorders should be an integral part of the process, including the awareness that addressing harmful sexual behaviours may have an adverse impact on the young person's emotional well-being and behaviour.

The AIM assessment model [57] identifies mental health concerns as risk factors, distinguishing between those with strong empirical support (high levels of trauma, for example own victimization and witnessing domestic violence; a formal diagnosis of conduct disorder; poor social and intimacy skills; and highly compulsive/impulsive behaviours) and others based on practice consensus (diagnoses of ADHD, depression, or other significant mental health problems).

New approaches to CBT with sexually abusing youths have recently been described within the context of relapse prevention, and a more complex CBT intervention—mode deactivation therapy (MDT)—has been suggested for disturbed, sexually abusive young people with reactive conduct disorders or personality disorders [58]. CBT group work with sexually abusing children and young people is widely practised in the UK [59].

More recently, there has been an increased emphasis on strength-based models of intervention for young people with harmful sexual behaviours. Treatment is therefore seen as an activity that should add to the young person's skills and personal functioning [55].

For some young people with significantly risky sexually harmful behaviour, treatment needs to be undertaken within a close supervised, intensive, community-based foster placement with specially trained foster carers. Approaches include MTFC and forensic foster care. However, there continues to be a lack of longitudinal studies to measure the effectiveness of existing programmes.

## Fire-setting and arson

Arson can have a devastating impact on the victim and the wider society. Juvenile arsonists are not a homogenous group, with a wide range of familial, social, and developmental needs [60]. High-frequency fire-setters (three or more episodes in the past year) were more likely to have started their fire involvement before the age of 10 years and had cumulative risk factors and other problem behaviours, including antisocial behaviour, aggression, impulsivity, and alcohol and drug misuse [61]. Other factors identified include lower IQ, poor social judgement, lack of empathy, and poor super-ego development. Environmental factors such as parenting practices (low monitoring or absence of a parent) and experiences of physical and sexual abuse have also been reported. Epidemiological studies showed that males are more common perpetrators than females and more likely to fire-set on multiple occasions [61].

Kolko and Kazdin [62] used a bio-psychosocial framework to specify the individual, social, and environmental risk factors related to the onset, severity, and maintenance of fire-setting behaviour and highlighted the importance of attraction to fire, heightened arousal, impulsivity, and limited social competence. A review of different fire-specific assessment tools is available [60]. Assessing factors, such as caregiver supervision, behavioural modelling, and access to fire-setting materials, are included in fire risk assessment protocols [62] and as treatment targets in intervention programmes [60].

The first component of a multi-disciplinary intervention should include a home safety visit, as most fatal fires occur in the home. Other interventions include fire safety educational sessions (to promote the understanding of cause and effect), motivational interviewing (to assess capacity for change), and CBT (to increase the understanding of the behaviour, including antecedents and establishing the behavioural reinforcers) [60]. Parent management training for caregivers has been shown to be effective for young people with a range of antisocial behaviour. Caregivers working with young people provide opportunities to address environmental risk factors, including parenting approaches.

## Gangs and violence

The definition of a gang includes a relatively durable group of young people who seem themselves as a group, engage in criminal activity, and have some form of structure. Longitudinal studies have identified many risk factors for poor outcomes in later life such as poverty, a lack of positive parenting, family conflict, maltreatment, and school failure, as well as individual factors [2]. There is an association between the number of risk factors experienced by young people and gang membership [63]. Qualitative research also highlights a range of other drivers for gang involvement, including the need to feel protected and feel safe, the need to build and maintain status or to boost young people's reputation, and using gangs as a substitute family unit [63]. The literature on young women in gangs includes family histories characterized by exposure to violence, maltreatment, and abuse [64]. The gang offers an opportunity to feel safe and protected within a substitute family unit.

There is evidence that young people in gangs, and particularly young women, have higher levels of mental health needs [63, 64]. Many of these needs are long-standing and unmet, with few young people accessing early support [64].

The evidence base for interventions to reduce gang involvement is still evolving, with many interventions focusing on multiple risk factors affecting the young person or on the systems around the young person. Primarily developed in the US for males, rather than females, few of these interventions help to address young people's mental health problems. MAC-UK's Integrate approach is delivered as an adaptive, flexible intervention for young people who do not otherwise easily access support from professionals [65]. Integrate projects are intensive and use a multi-agency approach, reconfiguring staff from other agencies to work in partnership with excluded young people within their local community.

## Legal framework

A 'child' is defined by the Children Act [66] and the United Nations Convention on the Rights of the Child [67] as 'any person under the age of 18'. In England, Wales, and Northern Ireland, criminal responsibility is set at the age of 10. However, there is evidence that brain development continues into the early 20s, with the frontal lobes developing later [1]. These areas are involved in consequential thinking, inhibition of impulses, empathy, and planning. These normal developmental stages are important to consider when assessing and passing comment on a child's criminal responsibility [68]. Developmental level is important in the context of criminal liability (so-called 'mens rea', the ability to form a guilty mind).

### Fitness to plead and effective participation

Mental health professionals are frequently asked to assess a young person in relation to their 'fitness to plead', which is a standard set in caselaw (Pritchard criteria). 'Fitness to plead' in this context requires that the individual (whether adult or child):

1. Has the ability to understand the charge(s).
2. Has the ability to decide whether to plead guilty or not guilty.
3. Has the ability to follow the course of proceedings.
4. Has the ability to instruct a solicitor.
5. Has the ability to challenge a juror.
6. Has the ability to give evidence in his/her own defence.

Important for children and young people is the principle of 'effective participation'—which examines the ability of the young person to engage with the trial. A child's age, level of maturity, and intellectual and emotional capacities must be taken into account when they are charged with a criminal offence, and appropriate steps should be taken in order to promote their ability to understand and participate in the court proceedings. The responsibility therefore falls on the defence lawyer to be aware of the possibility that a young person may not be able to participate effectively in the trial process, particularly if they are under 14 years old or have learning problems or a history of absence from school.

### Capacity

One fundamental distinction in criminal law is between conditions that negate criminal liability and those that might mitigate the punishment deserved under particular circumstances. Very young children and the profoundly mentally ill may lack the minimum capacity necessary to justify punishment [68]. Those exhibiting less profound impairments of the same kind may qualify for a lesser level of deserved punishment, even though they may meet the minimum conditions for some punishment. Immaturity, like mental disorder, can serve both as an excuse and as mitigation in the determination of just punishment. Capacity is a feature that is both situation-specific and open to influence.

Capacity is multi-faceted, with four key elements:

1. The capacity to understand information relevant to the specific decision at issue (understanding).
2. The capacity to appreciate one's situation as the defendant is confronted with a specific legal decision (appreciation).
3. The capacity to think rationally about an alternative course of action (reasoning).
4. The capacity to express a choice among alternatives.

Any evaluation of competence should include an assessment of psychopathology and emotional understanding, as well the cognitive level, the child's experiences, and appreciation of situations comparable to the one relevant to the crime and to the trial, and any particular features that may be pertinent in this individual and this set of circumstances [68].

## Conclusions

Politicians and professionals have begun to acknowledge the importance of meeting the needs of offenders, as long-term costs to society become increasingly apparent. The major challenge of altering the trajectories of persistent young offenders has to be met in the context of satisfying public demands for retribution, together with welfare and civil liberties considerations. Over the last 30 years, there has been increasing research studies evidencing the risk factors and developmental pathways to antisocial behaviour.

This chapter has evidenced the high prevalence of mental health needs and neurodisability in young people who offend and outlined the implications for policy and practice, including recent developments. It demonstrates the increasing importance of providing a standardized and evidence-based approach to screening and intervention for a variety of health needs. Provision of appropriately designed programmes can reduce recidivism among persistent offenders. Initiatives within the community include the development of liaison and diversion teams within police and court interfaces to screen and divert young people away from the criminal justice system where possible. Opportunities also exist through multi-agency partnerships. Early co-ordinated care is essential in meeting the complex needs of this group of young people, highlighting the important role of a multi-agency public health strategy.

### REFERENCES

1. Steinberg, L. (2008). A social neuroscience perspective on adolescent risk-taking. *Developmental Review*, **28**, 78–106.
2. Murray, J. and Farrington, D.P. (2010). Risk factors for conduct disorder and delinquency: key findings from longitudinal studies. *Canadan Journal of Psychiatry*, **55**, 633–42.

3. Hawes, D.J., Brennan, J., and Dadds, M.R. (2009). Cortisol, callous-unemotional traits, and pathways to antisocial behaviour. *Current Opinion in Psychiatry*, **22**, 357–62.

4. Stevenson, M. (2006). *Young People and Offending: Education, Youth Justice and Social Care Inclusion*. Williams, London.

5. Moffitt, T., Caspi, A., Rutter, M., and Silva, P. (2001). *Sex Differences in Antisocial Behaviour: Conduct Disorder and Delinquency and Violence in the Dunedin Longitudinal Study*. Cambridge University Press, Cambridge.

6. Hughes, N., Williams, H., and Chitsabesan, P. (2017). The influence of neurodevelopmental impairment on youth crime. In: S. Bailey, P. Chitsabesan, and P. Tarbuck, editors. *Forensic Child and Adolescent Mental Health: Meeting the Needs of Young Offenders*. Cambridge University Press, Cambridge; pp. 68–81.

7. Chitsabesan, P. and Khan, L. (2017). Assessment of young offenders; mental health, physical, educational and social needs. In: S. Bailey, P. Chitsabesan, and P. Tarbuck, editors. *Forensic Child and Adolescent Mental Health: Meeting the Needs of Young Offenders*. Cambridge University Press, Cambridge; pp. 41–54.

8. Golzari, M., Hunt, S.J., and Anushiravani, A. (2006). The health status of youth in juvenile detention facilities. *Journal of Adolescent Health*, **38**, 776–82.

9. Roberts, R.E., Atkinson, C.C., and Rosenblatt, A. (1998). Prevalence of psychopathology among children and adolescents. *American Journal of Psychiatry*, **155**, 715–25.

10. Chitsabesan, P. and Hughes, N. (2015). Mental health and neurodevelopmental disorders amongst young offenders: implications for policy and practice. In: J. Winstone, editor. *Mental Health, Crime and Criminal Justice, Responses and Reforms*. Palgrave, Basingstoke; pp. 109–30.

11. Fazel, S., Doll, H., and Langstrom N. (2008). Mental disorders among adolescents in juvenile detention and correctional facilities: a systematic review and metaregression analysis of 25 surveys. *Journal of the American Academy of Child and Adolescent Psychiatry*, **47**, 1010–19.

12. Coffey, C., Veit, F., Wolfe, R., *et al.* (2003). Mortality in young offenders: retrospective cohort study. *BMJ*, **326**, 1064–7.

13. Chitsabesan, P., Kroll, L., Bailey, S., *et al.* (2006). National study of mental health provision for young offenders. Part 1: Mental health needs of young offenders in custody and in the community. *British Journal of Psychiatry*, **188**, 534–40.

14. Colins, O., Vermeiren, R., Vreugdenhil, C., *et al.* (2010). Psychiatric disorders in detained male adolescents in custody: a systematic literature review. *Canadian Journal of Psychiatry*, **55**, 255–63.

15. Teplin., L.A. Abram., K.M., McClelland, G.M., *et al.* (2002). Psychiatric disorders in youth in juvenile detention. *Archives of General Psychiatry*, **59**, 1133–43.

16. Lennox, C. and Khan, L. (2013). Youth justice. In: *Our Children Deserve Better: Prevention Pays. Annual Report of the Chief Medical Officer 2012*. Department of Health and Social Care, London.

17. Schore, A.N. (2001). Effects of a secure attachment relationship on right brain development, affect regulation, and infant mental health. *Infant Mental Health Journal*, **22**, 7–66.

18. Jacobson, J., Bhardiva, B., Gyateng, T., *et al.* (2010). *Punishing Disadvantage: A Profile of Children in Custody*. Prison Reform Trust, London.

19. Putnins, A.L. (2005). Correlates and predictors of self-reported suicide attempts among incarcerated youths. *International Journal of Offender Therapy and Comparative Criminology*, **49**, 143–57.

20. Theodosiou, L. (2017). Substance misuse in young people with antisocial behaviour. In: S. Bailey, P. Chitsabesan, and P. Tarbuck, editors. *Forensic Child and Adolescent Mental Health: Meeting the Needs of Young Offenders*. Cambridge University Press, Cambridge; pp. 177–89.

21. Mulvey, E., Schubert, C., and Chassin, L. (2010). Substance use and delinquent behaviour among serious adolescent offenders. *Juvenile Justice Bulletin*. Available from: https://www.ncjrs.gov/pdffiles1/ojjdp/232790.pdf

22. Chitsabesan, P., Rothwell, J., Kenning, C., *et al.* (2012). Six years on: a prospective cohort study of male juvenile offenders in secure care. *European Child and Adolescent Psychiatry*, **21**, 339–47.

23. American Psychiatric Association. (2013). *Diagnostic and Statistical Manual of Mental Disorders*, fifth edition. American Psychiatric Publishing, Arlington, VA.

24. Edens, J.F., Campbell, J.S., and Weir, J.M. (2007). Youth psychopathy and criminal recidivism: a meta-analysis of the Psychopathy Checklist Measures. *Law and Human Behavior*, **31**, 53–75.

25. Cooke, D. J., Hart, S. D., Logan, C., and Michie, C. (2012). Explicating the construct of psychopathy: Development and validation of a conceptual model, the Comprehensive Assessment of Psychopathic Personality (CAPP). *International Journal of Forensic Mental Health*, **11**, 242–52.

26. Johnston, L. (2017). Youth psychopathy: a developmental perspective. In: S. Bailey, P. Chitsabesan, and P. Tarbuck, editors. *Forensic Child and Adolescent Mental Health: Meeting the Needs of Young Offenders*. Cambridge University Press, Cambridge; pp. 217–37.

27. Frick, P.J., Ray, J.V., Thornton, L.C., and Kahn, R.E. (2014). Annual Research Review: A developmental psychopathology approach to understanding callous-unemotional traits in children and adolescents with serious conduct problems. *Journal of Child Psychology and Psychiatry*, **55**, 532–48.

28. Gudjonsson, G., Sigurdsson, J.F., Sigfusdottir, I.D., and Young, S. (2012). A national epidemiological study of offending and its relationship with ADHD symptoms and associated risk factors. *Journal of Attention Disorders*, **18**, 3–13.

29. Young, S., Greer, B., and White, O. (2017). Attention deficit hyperactivity disorder and antisocial behaviour. In: S. Bailey, P. Chitsabesan, and P. Tarbuck, editors. *Forensic Child and Adolescent Mental Health: Meeting the Needs of Young Offenders*. Cambridge University Press, Cambridge; pp. 190–200.

30. Gralton, E. and Baird, G. (2017). Autism spectrum disorders in young people in the criminal justice system. In: S. Bailey, P. Chitsabesan, and P. Tarbuck, editors. *Forensic Child and Adolescent Mental Health: Meeting the Needs of Young Offenders*. Cambridge University Press, Cambridge; pp. 201–16.

31. The National Autistic Society. (2008). *Autism: A Guide for Criminal Justice Professionals*. The National Autistic Society, London.

32. Hughes, N., Williams, H.W., Chitsabesan, P., *et al.* (2012). *Nobody Made the Connection: The Prevalence of Neurodisability in Young People Who Offend*. Office for the Children's Commissioner, London.

33. Chitsabesan, P., Bailey, S., Williams, R., *et al.* (2007). Learning disabilities and educational needs of juvenile offenders. *Journal of Children's Services*, **2**, 4–14.

34. Gregory, J. and Bryan, K. (2011). Speech and language therapy intervention with a group of persistent and prolific young offenders in a non-custodial setting with previously undiagnosed speech, language and communication difficulties. *International Journal of Language and Communication Disorders*, **46**, 202–15.

35. Williams, H.W. (2013). *Repairing Shattered Lives: Brain Injury and Its Implications for Criminal Justice*. Transition to Adulthood Alliance, London.

36. Hughes, N., Williams, H., Chitsabesan, P., *et al.* (2015). The prevalence of traumatic brain injury among young offenders in custody: a systematic review. *Journal of Head Trauma Rehabilitation*, **30**, 94–105.

37. Vincent, G.M., Grisso, T., Terry, A., *et al.* (2008). Sex and race differences in mental health symptoms in juvenile justice: the MAYSI-2 national meta-analysis. *Journal of the American Academy of Child and Adolescent Psychiatry*, **47**, 282–90.

38. Centre for Mental Health. (2010). *You Just Get on and Do it: Healthcare Provision in Youth Offending Teams*. Centre for Mental Health, London.

39. Grisso, T. and Barnum, R. (2006). *Massachusetts Youth Screening Instrument- Version 2: User Manual and Technical Report*. Professional Resource Press, Sarasota, FL.

40. Chitsabesan, P., Lennox, C., Theodosiou, L., *et al.* (2014). The development of the comprehensive health assessment tool for young offenders within the secure estate. *Journal of Forensic Psychiatry and Psychology*, **25**, 1–25.

41. Royal College of Paediatrics and Child Health. (2013). *Healthcare Standards for Children and Young People in Secure Settings*. Royal College of Paediatrics and Child Health, London.

42. Borum, R. Bartel, P., and Forth, A. (2003). *Manual for the Structured Assessment for Violence Risk in Youth (SAVRY) Version 1.1*. Florida Mental Health Institute, University of South Florida, Tampa, FL.

43. Schmidt, F., Hoge, R., and Gomes, L. (2005). Reliability and validity analyses of the Youth Level of Service/Case Management Inventory. *Criminal Justice and Behavior*, **32**, 329–44.

44. Millington, J. and Lennox, C. Risk assessment and management approaches with young offenders. In: S. Bailey, P. Chitsabesan, and P. Tarbuck, editors. *Forensic Child and Adolescent Mental Health: Meeting the Needs of Young Offenders*. Cambridge University Press, Cambridge; pp. 55–67.

45. Kazdin, A. (2007). Psychosocial treatments for conduct disorder in children and adolescents. In: P. Nathan and J. Gorman, editors. *A Guide to Treatments that Work*, third edition. Oxford University Press, New York, NY; pp. 71–104.

46. Townsend, E., Walker, D., Sargeant, S., *et al.* (2010). Systematic review and meta-analysis of interventions relevant for young offenders with mood disorders, anxiety disorders, or self-harm. *Journal of Adolescence*, **33**, 9–20.

47. Mitchell, P. and Staniforth, C. (2017). Cognitive, behavioural and related approaches in young offenders. In: S. Bailey, P. Chitsabesan, and P. Tarbuck, editors. *Forensic Child and Adolescent Mental Health: Meeting the Needs of Young Offenders*. Cambridge University Press, Cambridge; pp. 254–65.

48. Bevington, D., Fuggle, P., Fonagy, P., Target, M., and Asen, E. (2013). Innovations in Practice: Adolescent Mentalization-Based Integrative Therapy (AMBIT)—a new integrated approach to working with the most hard to reach adolescents with severe complex mental health needs. *Child and Adolescent Mental Health*, **18**, 46–51.

49. National Institute for Health and Care Excellence. (2013). *Antisocial Behaviour and Conduct Disorder in Children and Young People: Recognition, Intervention and Management*. National Institute for Health and Care Excellence, London.

50. Woolfenden, S., Williams, K., and Peat, J. (2002). Family and parenting interventions for conduct disorder and delinquency: a meta-analysis of randomised controlled trials. *Archives of Diseases in Childhood*, **86**, 251–6.

51. Henggeler, S. W. and Schaeffer, C. (2010). Treating serious anti-social behavior using multisystemic therapy. In: J.R. Weisz and A.E. Kazdin, editors. *Evidence-based psychotherapies for children and adolescents*, second edition. Guilford Press, New York, NY; pp. 259–76.

52. McGuire, J. (2013). 'What works' to reduce re-offending: 18 years on. In: L. Craig, j. Dixon, and T.A. Gannon, editors. *What Works in Offender Rehabilitation: An Evidence Based Approach to Assessment and Treatment*. Wiley-Blackwell, Chichester; pp. 20–49.

53. Bailey, S. (2000). Juvenile homicide. *Criminal Behaviour and Mental Health*, **10**, 149–54.

54. Loeber, R. and Farrington, D.P. (2011). *Young Homicide Offenders and Victims: Risk Factors, Prediction and Prevention from Childhood*. Springer, New York, NY.

55. Murphy, M., Ross, K., and Hackett, S. (2017). Sexually harmful behaviour in young people. In: S. Bailey, P. Chitsabesan, and P. Tarbuck, editors. *Forensic Child and Adolescent Mental Health: Meeting the Needs of Young Offenders*. Cambridge University Press, Cambridge; pp. 121–33.

56. Matthews, R., Hunter, J.A., and Vuz, J. (1997). Juvenile female sexual offenders: clinical characteristics and treatment issues. *Sexual Abuse*, **9**, 187–99.

57. AIM. (2001). *Working with Children and Young People Who Sexually Abuse: Procedures and Assessment*. The AIM Project, Manchester.

58. Apsche, J.A. and Ward, S.R. (2003). Mode deactivation therapy and cognitive behavioral therapy: a description of treatment results for adolescents with personality beliefs, sexual offending, and aggressive behaviors. *The Behavior Analyst Today*, **3**, 460–70.

59. Seabloom, W., Seabloom, M., Seabloom, E., *et al.* (2003). A 14- to 24-year longitudinal study of a comprehensive sexual health model treatment program for adolescent sex offenders: predictors of successful completion and subsequent criminal recidivism. *International Journal of Offender Therapy and Comparative Criminology*, **47**, 468–81.

60. Mackay, S., Feldberg, A., Ward A., and Marton, P. (2012). Research and practice in adolescent fire-setting. *Criminal Justice and Behaviour*, **39**, 842–64.

61. MacKay, S., Paglia-Boak, A., Henderson, J., Marton, P., and Adlaf, E. (2009). Epidemiology of fire-setting in adolescents: mental health and substance use correlates. *Journal of Child Psychology and Psychiatry*, **50**, 1282–90.

62. Kolko, D.J. and Kazdin, A.E. (1989). Assessment of dimensions of childhood firesetting among child psychaitric patients and non patients. *Journal of Abnormal Child Psychology*, **17**, 609–24.

63. Law, H., Khan, L., and Zlotowitz, S. (2017). Group violence and youth gangs. In: S. Bailey, P. Chitsabesan, and P. Tarbuck, editors. *Forensic Child and Adolescent Mental Health: Meeting the Needs of Young Offenders*. Cambridge University Press, Cambridge; pp. 107–20.

64. Khan, L., Saunders, A., and Plumtree, A. (2013). *A Need to Belong: What Leads Girls to Join Gangs*. Centre for Mental Health, London.

65. Zlotowitz, S., Barker, C., Moloney, O., and Howard, C. (2015). Service users as the key to service change? The development of an innovative intervention for excluded young people. *Child and Adolescent Mental Health*, **21**, 102–8.

66. The Children Act Section 105(1).

67. The United Nations Convention on the Rights of the Child (1989) (Article 1).

68. Delmage, E. (2017). Children and the law. In: S. Bailey, P. Chitsabesan, and P. Tarbuck, editors. *Forensic Child and Adolescent Mental Health: Meeting the Needs of Young Offenders*. Cambridge University Press, Cambridge; pp. 289–99.

# 141

# Child molesters and other sexual offenders

*Stephen J. Hucker*

## Introduction

Though widely condemned, and often severely punished, throughout the world, only a relatively small proportion of all reported offences involve sexual behaviour. Nonetheless, research has repeatedly shown that, even if taken only as minimal figures, large numbers of people, both children and adults, report having been subject to some form of sexually unwelcome behaviour [1]. The legal term 'sexual assault' is now widely used in most Western countries to embrace any type of non-voluntary sexual act in which the victim is coerced or physically forced to engage against their will, or any non-consensual sexual touching of another person [2]. It includes forced vaginal, anal, or oral penetration (rape), drug-facilitated sexual assault, groping, forced kissing, child sexual abuse, or sexual torture.

The long-term effects of victimization have been extensively studied, and individuals with a history of childhood sexual abuse, for example, report a wide range of long-term psychological consequences [3]. And those who have been sexually assaulted as adults similarly and uniformly report extensive psychological, if not physical, repercussions [4].

Although often perceived as the purview of specialized forensic services, nearly all psychiatrists will at some time meet victims of sex offenders, if not offenders themselves. The general psychiatrist, for example, is almost certain on occasions to encounter a 'flasher' (exhibitionist) or a 'peeping Tom' (voyeur), as these are usually viewed by authorities as minor sex offenders not needing specialist attention. It is therefore important for the generalist to have at least some knowledge of sex offenders and their treatment, as they may be called upon to provide a report for court purposes, especially in places where availability of expert forensic services is limited.

## Some definitions

A 'sex offender' is simply an individual whose sexual behaviour contravenes the law in a particular jurisdiction. However, criminological preoccupations with particular kinds of sexual offences have often varied considerably over time. The types of activities that may be proscribed will also vary considerably. Thus, in the last century, incest, homosexuality, and bigamy seem to have been the main concerns, and child molestation and sexual assault much less so. Though some are more tolerant than others, most societies provide sanctions for sexual activity involving children below the age of consent, non-consensual sexual acts, sexual relations with close family members, and sexual interference with animals or corpses. Typically also there are legal and other interventions available in cases where a person fears sexual harassment or assault, where abuse of a child is suspected, and where there has been abuse, or likelihood of abuse, in certain professional relationships. As well there is commonly regulation of pornography and other obscene material.

'Sexual deviance' refers to those sexual behaviours that go beyond societal norms. They may be subject to legal sanctions as well, though in many cases not. It involves consistent, rather than occasional, sexual interests and behaviours. Common perceptions of what is 'normal' will also be influenced by whether the acts are committed in public or private. As with sex offending, the concept of sexual deviance will vary greatly across jurisdictions and at differing times.

Finally, 'paraphilia' is a diagnostic term popularized by Money [5] and currently used in official classification systems such as the World Health Organization's *International Classification of Diseases* (ICD) and the American Psychiatric Association's *Diagnostic and Statistical Manual* (DSM) to identify the experience of intense sexual arousal to atypical objects, situations, or individuals. The current edition DSM-5 introduced the term 'paraphilic disorder' which causes the individual distress or interferes with their personal functioning, whereas a 'paraphilia' in itself does not. The ICD prefers the term 'disorders of sexual preference', but both systems require the characteristic sexual behaviours or preferences to be persistent or recurrent and to cause subjective distress or interference with their social, occupational, or other important areas of their lives.

Although Money and others list numerous unconventional sexual interests and behaviours [6], in the two dominant classifications, worldwide only a few of the most common are listed individually and others relegated to a miscellaneous category such as 'unspecified paraphilia' [7]. Not all sex offenders are paraphilic or have a paraphilic disorder, and not all those diagnosed with a paraphilia or paraphilic disorder are sexual offenders. The psychiatric categories of paraphilia and paraphilic disorders and their characteristics are outlined in Chapter 115 of this textbook.

## Types of sex offender

General psychiatrists will be concerned with sexual behaviours such as indecent exposure, obscene telephone calling, voyeurism, bestiality, incest, child molestation, and pornography collecting. Specialists will also be interested in sexually motivated homicide, the more serious forms of sexual assault, and necrophilia. Most sexual offenders are male, though a small number of women may commit similar crimes [8].

### Child molesters

Sexual abuse of children has been reported and generally condemned throughout history [9], and the reportedly more permissive attitude in ancient Greece seems more or less an exception [10].

Thus, for example, a recent meta-analysis of 217 studies based on self-report data [11] estimated a global prevalence of 12.7–18% for girls and 7.6% for boys. A World Health Organization study [12] earlier reviewed estimates of childhood sexual abuse from 39 countries and found that the prevalence of non-contact, contact, and intercourse in female children was approximately 6%, 11%, and 4%, respectively; corresponding figures for males was about 2% for all categories. It is well known that many victims do not report such experiences, and when guaranteed confidentiality, individual sex offenders admit to many more offences than they were charged with or convicted of [13]. Similarly, sex offending against adults has also been underreported, though it is estimated that about 13% of women and 3% of men have been sexually assaulted at some time during their lives [14].

An early typology [15] for this group was based on the degree of apparent paraphilic attraction (sexual deviancy). The 'fixated' subtype identifies those paedophiles with an enduring attraction to children, typically dating from adolescence, and thereby conforming to the definitions of paedophilia in DSM-5 and ICD-10. Paedophiles attracted to male children are more likely to repeat their offences with recidivism at least twice as high as those attracted to girls. Homosexual paedophiles tend to victimize boys aged 11–15 years of age, whereas heterosexual paedophiles prefer girls of 8–10 years. 'Fixated' paedophiles tend to commit premeditated offences that often involve considerable planning, manipulation, and 'grooming' behaviour to lure, and even abduct, children into sexual activity, and they may gain the trust of the parents or other caregivers. Often they appear to have an excellent rapport with the child victims and treat them kindly, but the motive is primarily for the child to meet their sexual needs, rather than the reverse. It is for this reason that 'needy' children are often selected as victims. Such offenders will typically profess their 'love' for children and convince themselves that their behaviour is not harmful. Other rationalizations, such as that they were educating the child or introducing the child to sexual love in a caring way, are also common.

'Regressed' or 'situational' child molesters are, according to this typology, attracted primarily to adult females and may be in a marital relationship at the time of their offence. They will often report feelings of personal inadequacy or low self-esteem, and their offences are typically spontaneous and occur in the context of a stressful life circumstance.

In contrast to the 'fixated' type, the 'regressed' child molester is less inclined to 'groom' victims and their caregivers. Victims of this type may be older than those involved with the 'fixated' type of molester. However, molestations may begin before and continue beyond puberty.

Critical of earlier typologies such as this, as well as of the definition in DSM, in their attempts to delineate paedophiles from other types of child molester, Knight et al. [16] developed a different model incorporating two axes that assess psychological issues, abuse behaviours, and the degree of sexual fixation. Though empirically validated, others have doubted its clinical usefulness because of its complexity [17]. It is worth noting that, in the literature, the terms 'child molester' and 'paedophile' are often used interchangeably, tacitly acknowledging that it is often difficult to differentiate the two. Moreover, the treatment may be determined by actuarial estimates and are also very similar.

Despite dire parental warnings to their children to be aware of strangers as potential sexual predators, the majority of individuals who molest children are either already acquainted or are related to them. The term 'incest' is used to identify situations in which a close blood relative is subjected to sexual abuse. Some researchers, based on statistical reoffence data, have suggested that the phenomenon is primarily a symptom of family dysfunction distinct from paedophilia, and that the perpetrator represents a low risk of extending their behaviour outside the family [18]. However, other authorities have found that as many as half of self-reported father or stepfather incest offenders had also abused children outside their families and 18% had raped adult women [13]. Some men pursue and subsequently marry or cohabit with single mothers with the intent to gain access to their children.

At one time, it was believed that paedophiles were inadequate, unaggressive men unable to form relationships with adult women. It is now well recognized that gratuitous violence is used by a substantial minority of paedophiles [19].

A further aspect of paedophilia that needs to be mentioned because of its increasing identification in the age of the Internet is the use of computers to view, manufacture, and distribute pornographic images of children [20]. Such imagery is widely used by such men to generate sexual fantasies, and the behaviour will then be reinforced by masturbation. Some have argued that this sequence essentially normalizes the fantasy and further disinhibits the user. This combination of disinhibition and cognitive distortions regarding the impact of the behaviour may stimulate the urge to seek more intense experiences from 'hands-on' experiences, rather than simply on a computer screen. However, the risk of this progression is likely exaggerated, as only a minority of Internet child pornography offenders, in fact, progress to molest a child [20]. Those with previous or concurrent contact sexual offences are more likely to have more than one reconviction, whether general or sexual, than those with child pornography offences who are only rarely reconvicted [21]. Nevertheless, research has shown that there are psychological and other similarities between men who use child pornography and those who actually do commit such offences. Child pornography offenders more often show evidence of arousal to children on phallometric laboratory testing than those who committed 'hands-on' offences against children.

### Sexual assault of adult women

As with those who molest children, men who perpetrate sexual assault on adult women (rapists) do not necessarily justify a diagnosis of a paraphilia [22]. Indeed attempts by some sexologists to have individuals who appear to prefer sexual relations with non-consenting partners identified by a paraphilia label (terms such as biastophilia, rape preference, or paraphilia-not otherwise specified—non-consenting) have been repeatedly rejected, often based on feminist arguments that to do so would thereby 'medicalize' inappropriately a predisposition in males generally to dominate women [23].

The typology proposed by Knight [24], though not extensively used and rather complicated for routine clinical use, does have the merit of highlighting the fact that several different motivations appear to underlie sexual assault of adult women. Thus, 'anger-motivated' rapists act out deviant fantasies of retaliation towards the victim, using violence as a means of expressing generalized anger, typically towards women specifically, but sometimes towards people in general. The motive of the attack is to humiliate and debase the victim who will typically have been picked randomly. The 'power-motivated' rapist is further divided into the 'power-reassurance' and 'power-assertive' subtypes. The former is afflicted by doubts and insecurities about their own masculinity and sexual adequacy, often uses minimal force, and may apologize to the victim or even seek a relationship afterwards. However, the victims may have been stalked and the attacks on them premeditated. The 'power-assertive' subtype is motivated by the desire to dominate women, and such men have no doubts about their masculinity. However, unlike the previous subtype, they typically do not use gratuitous violence to subdue the victim. On the other hand, 'sadistic' rapists, the least common but, in many ways, most worrisome subtype, derive sexual pleasure from inflicting pain and suffering on the victim. However, this is often difficult to differentiate from other rapist types where pain, suffering, and humiliation are also the consequences, but not the primary motivation for the attack [25].

Other types of sexual assault may not involve any kind of penetration but represent related behaviours, including toucheurism and frotteurism. These involve, respectively, touching or grabbing strangers, typically females, in a way that provides the perpetrator with sexual gratification. The former, in particular, may pass unnoticed by the victim, as attackers will typically touch or grab sexual areas such as breasts, buttocks, or crotch, in crowds and similar situations and the incident may be discounted as 'accidental'.

### Non-contact sexual offences

There are several common types of sexual offence that do not involve any physical contact with the victim [26]. The group includes 'peeping Toms', 'flashers', and indecent phone callers, with their corresponding psychiatric diagnoses of the paraphilias voyeurism, exhibitionism, and telephone scatalogia, respectively.

'Peepers' or voyeurs like to observe an unsuspecting female stranger undressing, or couples in the act of copulation. They may masturbate at the scene or later in private, while recalling what they saw. Most voyeurs, like most sex offenders generally who are paraphilic, are aware of their deviant impulses while still adolescent, but the behaviour may become chronic. Many men will admit to enjoying watching adult women in this situation or attend striptease shows, making these difficult to differentiate from those who prefer this activity.

'Flashers' or indecent exposers will often justify a psychiatric diagnosis of exhibitionism. These men become sexually excited while exposing their genitals, sometimes erect and sometimes not, to unsuspecting female strangers. The preferred reaction is one of shock or outrage. Complete indifference is a useful response if the victim has the presence of mind. The perpetrator may masturbate at the time or later in private. It is unusual to see an exhibitionist still active past the age of 40, but many are nevertheless for a time quite intractable and will expose themselves in situations where they may well be apprehended or reported. This suggests a degree of risk-taking that enhances the excitement.

Obscene telephone callers, corresponding to the paraphilic diagnosis of telephone scatalogia, call unsuspecting female victims and proceed to bombard them with explicit and sometimes frightening sexual comments, such that the victim may be very distressed by them. However, they often do not report them unless they are particularly persistent or if their voice or something they say reveals their identity. Often the individual masturbates while doing this. If apprehended, which is uncommon, it may be difficult to distinguish them from a simple prankster. However, a repetitive pattern will usually point to the appropriate diagnosis.

Though typically seen as 'nuisance offences', they are, in fact, much more common and more psychologically disturbing than is generally appreciated, and recent research [27] has indicated that large numbers of young women have directly experienced the behaviour of frotteurs and exhibitionists and experience considerable subsequent emotional distress.

As well, these non-contact offences are not generally regarded as a danger. However, in some cases, estimates place them somewhere around 10%, and the individual may engage in related paraphilic behaviours or progress to more serious sexual assault [28]. Attempts to approach or speak to the victim may well be warning signs of this. The behaviour therefore should not be taken lightly, and all available information about the perpetrators' actual behaviour in the index offence, as well as previous incidents, needs to be scrutinized with this possibility in mind.

## Assessment of sex offenders

As was noted at the beginning of this chapter, more serious sex offences are likely to require the expertise of specialized forensic services. The less serious or less intrusive offences may well fall into the hands of a general psychiatrist, and it is useful therefore to have a sense of what is involved if the matter requires a report or even an actual testimony in court.

Pre-trial situations usually require assessment of fitness (competence) to stand trial, though sometimes criminal responsibility will also need to be addressed. Only a small number of sex offenders show symptoms of a psychotic mental disorder such as schizophrenia or depression [29]. However, when such disorders are present, it will be necessary to explore whether and how the symptoms bear specifically on the sexual behaviour [30]. For example, the patient may report that they were acting in response to auditory hallucinations or specific delusional ideas about the victim or type of victim.

It is more likely, however, that other psychiatric disorders will be found among sex offenders. A diagnosis of mental retardation or personality disorder or, more particularly, paraphilia will be more relevant with respect to the offending behaviour [31].

Especially in more serious cases, the court may be interested in sentencing considerations, specifically the risk the offender presents to others and whether and what medical and/or other professional treatment or interventions might be ordered or recommended by the court to reduce that risk.

Few sex offenders will have presented to a psychiatrist or psychologist voluntarily. It is therefore helpful for the interviewer to assume that the subject will be at best guarded or possibly frankly hostile in their response to the assessment. It may be difficult to achieve the level of rapport more commonly experienced with non-psychotic general psychiatric patients. A non-judgemental approach is therefore desirable, regardless of the examiner's personal emotional reaction to the offences that are alleged. For example, an offender who has molested a child, or exposed to a group of children, will often arouse very strong feelings in the examiner, particularly when they have children of their own, and it is necessary to hold such reactions in check. Judging the alleged offender, especially when his guilt has not been determined by the court, is not an appropriate professional attitude.

Denials, rationalizations, distortions, and minimization are the kinds of cognitive distortions that are the norm with sex offenders. There is a frequent tendency to prevaricate or frankly lie. It is therefore essential for the examiner to have detailed information from police reports and elsewhere about the act or acts that are alleged to have occurred. Direct, interrogation-style confrontation is usually not particularly productive, and an oblique approach may obtain more information that will be useful in identifying a diagnosis and determining rational treatment possibilities.

Particularly unhelpful in gaining rapport or obtaining information is to accuse the individual of dishonesty or dissembling. A sympathetic approach, suggesting that sometimes people have difficulty accepting unpleasant aspects of themselves, may be more helpful. Alternatively, one can invite the subject to explore why the victim might have made the accusations if they are untrue and whether they can accept, if not the whole, then some parts of the accusations against them. Also important to remember is that while the individual may have been accused of one type of deviant sexual behaviour, other types of paraphilic behaviour may also have occurred and been undetected. Paraphilic disorders tend not to occur alone, but rather in association with other paraphilias [32], typically at least two or three. Thus, for example, an exhibitionist may have been reported for exposing specifically to children, rather than adults, and this will suggest an additional diagnosis of paedophilia. Similarly, an individual who is being convicted of rubbing himself against women in public places may also have made obscene phone calls and harbour fantasies of rape.

In the case of child molesters, it is important to consider how the perpetrator gained access to his victims. Exploration of the methods of 'grooming' is important in understanding ways to assist the offender to avoid risky situations in the future.

In terms of the overall assessment, identification of psychopathology outside the domain of sexual deviation is important. The presence of psychotic illness will have implications for the type of treatment to be recommended, even if it is not common among sex offenders [30]. It seems likely that, in some such offenders, the sexual behaviour is dismissed as a function of their mental illness and the underlying paraphilic disorder may easily be discounted

or not be considered at all. More commonly, it will be personality disorders or traits, alcohol or substance abuse, mild to moderate depression, and anxiety disorders [31, 33], rather than major mental illness that will be noted. Attention to these will nevertheless be an important part of any subsequent treatment or management recommendations [33].

Psychometric testing may contribute additional information to the overall assessment of a sex offender, in particular where the subject is not forthcoming in a personal interview. There are a number of general personality assessment instruments available. These include the well-known and widely used *Minnesota Multiphasic Personality Inventory* (MMPI) , the *Millon Clinical Multiaxial Inventory-III* (MCMI-III), and the *Personality Assessment Inventory* (PAI). All have been, and are being, extensively used in offender populations, including sex offenders, and common profiles have been identified. Although none can specifically identify a sex offender, the information gained concerning impulsivity, denial, judgement, and general psychopathology may be very useful.

In addition, there are a number of psychological tests that have been developed specifically for the assessment of sex offenders. These include the *Multiphasic Sex Inventory-2* (MSI-2) [34] and the revised version of the Clarke Sex History Questionnaire (SHQ) for Males [35]. The MSI-2 is designed to measure the sexual characteristics of an adult male (there is a female version as well) alleged to have committed a sexual offence or sexual misconduct, including those who deny the allegations. Though standardized in the United States on a large sample of sex offenders, it is used very widely. It consists of 560 true/false questions, and the completed questionnaire must be sent to the developers for computerized scoring and interpretation. The SHQ consists of 508 questions, and the completed questionnaire may again be sent away for scoring and an interpretive report returned.

## Phallometric testing (penile plethysmography)

Because sex offenders commonly lie and distort their self-report of deviant interests and behaviours, a more objective method of assessment has long been sought. One of the earliest to be developed was penile plethysmography (PPG)—phallometry—to measure changes in response to erotic stimulation [36]. This method involves measuring changes in the size of the penis, either in circumference or volume, while presenting the subject with carefully selected images, both still and moving, of both sexes and different age groups, and audiotaped descriptions of various sexual activities. There are certainly problems with PPG testing [37, 38], including the standardization of stimulus materials used [39, 40]. Some offenders are able to either learn to suppress their physiological response or masturbate before the testing in order to render themselves unresponsive. Nonetheless, PPG, most commonly using a circumferential device or the volumetric method, is extensively used in the assessment of sex offenders.

In the United States in particular, PPG has come under attack [41, 42] as, in addition to standardization and reliability issues, it has used pictures of children whose consent or that of their parents had never been obtained. Computer-generated images have been developed in an attempt to obviate this concern [43].

Other less intrusive methods of assessment are also widely adopted, including the Abel screen [44, 45] which measures time the subject spends viewing non-nude images.

Mention must also be made of the polygraph, or 'lie detector', with sex offenders which is being used extensively in many parts of the United States and in the United Kingdom [46, 47]. The subject is asked questions relating to the sexual interests and activities, while their pulse, respiration, and skin conductance are measured. Research in the area is generally weak, and despite its widespread use and perception of usefulness, particularly for monitoring sex offenders in the community, the method is controversial [48, 49].

## Assessment of risk in sex offenders

An assessment of the future risk of sex offending is often requested by the court, so it is important for any psychiatrist being asked to provide this to have an understanding of the factors that contribute to this (Boxes 141.1 and 141.2).

> **Box 141.1** Established risk factors for sexual recidivism
>
> - Sexual criminal history:
>   - Prior sexual offence
>   - Victim characteristics (unrelated, strangers, males)
>   - Early onset of sex offending
>   - Diverse sexual crimes
>   - Non-contact sexual offences.
> - Sexual deviance:
>   - Any deviant sexual preference:
>     - Sexual preference for children
>     - Sexualized violence
>     - Multiple paraphilias
>   - Sexual preoccupation.
> - Attitudes tolerant of sexual assault.
> - Lifestyle instability/criminality:
>   - Childhood behaviour problems (for example, running away, grade failure)
>   - Juvenile delinquency
>   - Any prior offences
>   - Lifestyle instability (reckless behaviour, employments instability)
>   - Personality disorder (especially psychopathy)
>   - Grievance/hostility.
> - Social problems/intimacy deficits:
>   - Single (never married)
>   - Conflicts with intimate partners
>   - Hostility towards women
>   - Emotional congruence with children
>   - Negative social influences.
> - Response to treatment/supervision:
>   - Treatment dropout
>   - Non-compliance with supervision
>   - Violation of conditional release.
> - Poor cognitive problem-solving.
> - Age (young).
>
> Source: data from *J Consult Clin Psychol.*, 66(2), Hanson RK, Bussiere MT, Predicting relapse: a meta-analysis of sexual offender recidivism studies, pp. 348–62, Copyright (1998), American Psychological Association; *Sex Abuse*, 22(2), Mann RE, Hanson RK, Thornton D, Assessing risk for sexual recidivism: Some proposals on the nature of psychologically meaningful risk factors, pp. 191–217, Copyright (2010), SAGE Publications.

> **Box 141.2** Characteristics with little or no relationship with sexual recidivism
>
> - Victim empathy.
> - Denial/minimization of sexual offence.
> - Lack of motivation for treatment.
> - Clinical impressions of 'benefit' from treatment.
> - Internalizing psychological problems (anxiety, depression, low self-esteem).
> - History of being sexually abused as a child.
> - Sexual intrusiveness of sexual offences (for example, intercourse).
> - Low social class.
>
> Source: data from *J Consult Clin Psychol.*, 66(2), Hanson RK, Bussiere MT, Predicting relapse: a meta-analysis of sexual offender recidivism studies, pp. 348–62, Copyright (1998), American Psychological Association; Hanson RK, Morton-Bourgon K, Predictors of sexual recidivism: An updated meta-analysis 2004-02, Copyright (2004), Public Works and Government Services Canada; *J Consult Clin Psychol.*, 73(6), Hanson RK, Morton-Bourgon KE, The characteristics of persistent sexual offenders: a meta-analysis of recidivism studies, pp. 1154–63, Copyright (2005), American Psychological Association.

Risk factors have been divided into:

1. Static risk, that is, involving those factors which cannot change, such as the offender's age, sex, or number of previous criminal convictions; and
2. Dynamic risk, that is, involving those factors which potentially could change, either as a result of treatment or some other intervention or simply the passage of time. This can be further subdivided into: relatively stable, but nonetheless potentially changeable; factors such as sexual preferences or negative attitudes; and acute factors such as access to victims, reversion to substance use, and active mental illness.

Static factors have received the most scientific study, and it is chiefly these that have been incorporated into various actuarial or statistical instruments that have been developed, based on follow-up studies of samples of sex offenders [50]. Among these instruments, the Static-99 and its recent modifications [51] and the Sex Offender Risk Appraisal Guide (SORAG), now replaced by the Violence Risk Appraisal Guide-Revised (VRAG-R) [52], are the most widely used. Though the assessment instruments have been published or are available online, a professional intending to use any of these instruments needs to be thoroughly familiar with the literature on the topic of risk assessment and to have participated in training workshops that are given at conferences and elsewhere from time to time [53]. Useful though these tools can be, too heavy reliance upon them is no substitute for a full understanding of how they were constructed and their limitations [54].

## Treatment issues

It is rare for a paraphilic individual to present for treatment in order to prevent themselves from becoming a sex offender (though see [55]). While some paraphilias are usually not associated with criminal behaviour (for example, transvestic disorder or fetishistic disorder), others, such as paedophilia or sexual sadism, are much more likely to be referred from the court or subsequently by probation and parole services.

It is important to realize that, though some dissent from this view [56], sexual preferences are highly resistant, if not impossible, to change (see [57]). The most that can usually be expected with sex offenders who have deviant sexual preferences (paraphilic disorders) is to help them learn to control their behaviour and to recognize that their propensity will always remain in the background, much as alcoholics are advised to consider themselves always vulnerable to relapse.

Psychological treatments have often been attempted with sex offenders [58]. Psychodynamically based individual and group treatments have been the most commonly used in the past. It has become clear more recently, however, that cognitive-based therapies are the preferable strategy to employ, although techniques involving classical behaviour therapy, for example covert sensitization, are also sometimes used for specific purposes such as creating aversion to deviant arousing images and replacement of these with non-deviant ones. Cognitive-based therapy itself involves helping the subject to develop strategies to alter their thought processes in order to avert their deviant behaviour, to improve their social skills, and to remedy their distorted beliefs and attitudes.

There is little or no evidence for the efficacy of psychological treatments prior to the introduction of cognitive-based therapy. Based on a meta-analysis of 43 published studies, it has been shown that treatment programmes using this approach are associated with a reduction in overall recidivism rate from about 17% to 10% [59]. Similar findings have been reported by others [60], though, as Hanson and Yates pointed out, there have been very few high-quality treatment studies [55]. The most effective programmes are those that adhere to risk/need/responsivity principles (see [61]). Thus, the highest intensity of treatment should be given to those of highest risk; treatment must address factors known to be associated with a risk of recidivism, and the therapy needs to be presented in a language and format such that the culture and learning styles of the offenders are addressed adequately.

Psychological treatments of all types have, until recently, focused on offenders' deficits and difficulties, rather than their strengths and other assets. The development of the 'Good Lives Model' [62] marked a turning point, and this approach has been integrated in to many of the programmes currently in use. The aim of this treatment is to help the sex offender meet his needs more appropriately and achieve pro-social life goals, thereby reducing the attractiveness of his offending behaviour [63].

Another approach that has yielded some very positive results has been the Circles of Support and Accountability (CoSA) [64]. Originating with leaders of the Mennonite Church in Canada, it has been adopted in a way that does not require religious affiliation. It is designed to provide intensive support for offenders upon release from prison and develop realistic risk management strategies to achieve successful community reintegration.

Despite some apparent progress, there is still controversy over the effectiveness of sex offender treatment programmes, and there remains a continuing need for better designed research.

## Medications

A number of different medications have been used to treat sex offenders [65–70]. Based on empirical observations of animals, which

become less sexually active following neutering, hormonal treatments that reduce testosterone levels have been extensively employed. All require careful discussion with the potential patient concerning side effects, and it is important to obtain written, informed consent [71].

Oestrogens proved to be problematic because of the serious risk of thromboembolic complications, and a safer alternative was found in cyproterone acetate (Androcur*) [72], an anti-androgen which is available in Europe, including the United Kingdom, and in Canada, but not in the United States. Medroxyprogesterone acetate (Provera*) [73, 74] was introduced as an alternative. Both drugs may be responsible for minor side effects such as weight gain, tiredness, and gynaecomastia (especially with cyproterone), as well as more serious problems, including thromboembolism and increased blood sugar.

More recently, luteinizing hormone-releasing hormone (LHRH) agonists [75–77], such leuprolide acetate (Lupron*), goserelin (Zoladex*), and others, have been found useful as they produce almost total suppression of testosterone production, such as would be seen following surgical castration [78]. However, they tend to be used mainly in very high-risk offenders or those who have failed with other drugs [79].

Reduction of oestrogen or androgen removes restraining effects on osteoblastogenesis and osteoclastogenesis, and causes an imbalance between resorption and formation of bone by prolonging the lifespan of osteoclasts and shortening the lifespan of osteoblasts. Thus, all of these hormone-reducing substances, though especially the LHRH agonists, have a tendency to increase the rate of bone remodelling and weaken its structure; it is necessary to monitor carefully for this side effect through annual bone density scanning and to administer antidotes, including calcium supplements, vitamin D, and possibly bisphosphonates [80].

However, the main problem with hormonal treatments is their lack of acceptance by those who might potentially benefit. An alternative approach using serotonin reuptake inhibitors has therefore been better received, though the necessary double-blind trials are still lacking [81]. They depress libido in only about 50–60% of cases. Higher doses, such as those used in obsessive–compulsive disorder, are sometimes necessary. The risk of prolonging the QT interval on the electrocardiogram is then one of the few reasons for which to choose one selective serotonin reuptake inhibitor (SSRI) over another, besides patient tolerance of different subjective side effects like nausea and sleep disturbance.

## Ethical problems

Several ethical issues have so far been mentioned in passing. However, it is worth re-emphasizing in conclusion that a disinterested professional demeanour is important when assessing sex offenders. No matter what his or her own private views, it is not the place of the clinician to decide on guilt or innocence or in any other way to pass judgement on the offender or alleged offender. Moreover, alienating the offender will present a further impediment to gaining information and to providing treatment when indicated and necessary.

It is important, at the assessment stage, to identify for the subject the nature of the evaluation, the role of the assessor, and the person or agency for whom they are acting, for example a child protection service, a defence lawyer, or a crown prosecutor. This may limit the degree of co-operation. However, when the purpose of the evaluation is solely to provide a risk assessment, not to explain this fully (and simply to present oneself as a 'doctor' in a helping role) would be unethical.

Certain assessment procedures, such as PPG or polygraphy (when used in a clinical setting), are particularly contentious. Though both may provide useful information, written and fully informed consent should always be obtained beforehand.

Finally, when the drugs that have been developed and marketed for other purposes are used to suppress sexual drive (so-called 'off-label' use), the patient needs to be fully informed of the potential benefits, as well as the risks involved, and should not be denied complementary or alternative treatments should they decide not to expose themselves to potential side effects. They also need to be aware that, though the clinician is not in a position to insist on such treatment, their refusal to participate may well have repercussions with probation and parole officers or the court itself, and these issues need to be fully discussed with the patient to avoid misunderstandings.

## REFERENCES

1. Barth J, Bermetz L, Heim E, Trelle S, Tonia T. The current prevalence of child sexual abuse worldwide: a systematic review and meta-analysis. *International Journal of Public Health.* 2013;58:469–83.
2. Ullman SE, Bhat M. Sexual assault/sexual violence. In: Naples N, Hoogland RC, Wickramasinghe M, Wong WCA, editors. *The Wiley Blackwell Encyclopedia of Gender and Sexuality Studies.* Chichester: Wiley-Blackwell; 2016. pp. 1–3.
3. Norman RE, Byambaa M, De R, Butchart A, Scott J, Vos T. The long-term health consequences of child physical abuse, emotional abuse, and neglect: a systematic review and meta-analysis. *PLoS Medicine.* 2012;9:e1001349.
4. Moor A, Ben-Meir E, Golan-Shapira D, Farchi M. Rape: a trauma of paralyzing dehumanization. *Journal of Aggression, Maltreatment and Trauma.* 2013;22:1051–69.
5. Money J. *Lovemaps.* New York, NY: Irvington; 1986.
6. Aggrawal A. *Forensic and Medico-legal Aspects of Sexual Crimes and Unusual Sexual Practices.* Boca Raton, FL: CRC Press; 2008.
7. American Psychiatric Association. *Diagnostic and Statistical Manual of Mental Disorders,* fifth edition (DSM-5). Washington, DC: American Psychiatric Association; 2013.
8. Colson M-H, Boyer L, Baumstarck K, Loundou A. Female sex offenders: a challenge to certain paradigmes. Meta-analysis. *Sexologies.* 2013;22:e109–17.
9. Seto MC. *Pedophilia and Sexual Offending Against Children: Theory, Assessment, and Intervention.* Washington, DC: American Psychological Association; 2008.
10. Ayonrinde O, Bhugra D. Paraphilias and culture. In: Bhugra D, Malhi GS, editors. *Troublesome Disguises: Managing Challenging Disorders in Psychiatry.* Chichester: John Wiley and Sons; 2014. pp. 199–217.
11. Stoltenborgh M, van IJzendoorn MH, Euser EM, Bakermans-Kranenburg MJ. A global perspective on child sexual abuse: meta-analysis of prevalence around the world. *Child Maltreatment.* 2011;16:79–101.
12. World Health Organization. *Global Health Risks: Mortality and Burden of Disease Attributable to Selected Major Risks.* Geneva: World Health Organization; 2009.
13. Abel GG, Becker JV, Mittelman M, Cunningham-Rathner J, Rouleau JL, Murphy WD. Self-reported sex crimes of nonincarcerated paraphiliacs. *Journal of Interpersonal Violence.* 1987;2:3–25.
14. Spitzberg BH. An analysis of empirical estimates of sexual aggression victimization and perpetration. *Violence and Victims.* 1999;14:241–60.
15. Groth AN, Birnbaum HJ. Adult sexual orientation and attraction to underage persons. *Archives of Sexual Behavior.* 1978;7:175–81.
16. Knight RA, Carter DL, Prentky RA. A system for the classification of child molesters reliability and application. *Journal of Interpersonal Violence.* 1989;4:3–23.
17. Robertiello G, Terry KJ. Can we profile sex offenders? A review of sex offender typologies. *Aggression and Violent Behavior.* 2007;12:508–18.
18. Hanson RK, Bussiere MT. Predicting relapse: a meta-analysis of sexual offender recidivism studies. *Journal of Consulting and Clinical Psychology.* 1998;66:348.
19. Marshall W, Christie MM. Pedophilia and aggression. *Criminal Justice and Behavior.* 1981;8:145–58.
20. Seto MC. *Internet Sex Offenders.* Washington, DC: American Psychological Association; 2013.
21. Babchishin KM, Hanson RK, VanZuylen H. Online child pornography offenders are different: A meta-analysis of the characteristics of online and offline sex offenders against children. *Archives of Sexual Behavior.* 2015;44:45–66.
22. Sheridan PM, Hucker S. Rape and sadomasochistic paraphilias. In: Kricacska JJ, Money J, editors. *The Handbook of Forensic Sexology: Biomedical and Criminological Perspectives.* Buffalo, NY: Prometheus Books; 1994. pp. 104–25.
23. Kaplan HI. Paraphilias—rape as a paraphilia? In: Kaplan HI, Sadock BJ, editors. *Comprehensive Textbook of Psychiatry,* Volume 1, fifth edition. Baltimore, MA: Williams and Wilkins; 1989. pp. 1079–80.
24. Knight RA. Validation of a typology for rapists. *Journal of Interpersonal Violence.* 1999;14:303–30.
25. Polaschek DL, Ward T, Gannon TA. Violent sex offenders. In: Hilarski C, Wodarski J, editors. *Comprehensive Mental Health Practice with Sex Offenders and Their Families.* Binghamton, NY: The Haworth Press; 2006. pp. 167–92.
26. Krueger RB, Kaplan MS. *Noncontact Paraphilic Sexual Offenses. Sexual Offending.* Springer; 2016. pp. 79–102.
27. Clark SK, Jeglic EL, Calkins C, Tatar JR. More than a nuisance: the prevalence and consequences of frotteurism and exhibitionism. *Sexual Abuse.* 2016;28:3–19.
28. McNally MR, Fremouw WJ. Examining risk of escalation: a critical review of the exhibitionistic behavior literature. *Aggression and Violent Behavior.* 2014;19:474–85.
29. Sahota K, Chesterman P. Sexual offending in the context of mental illness. *Journal of Forensic Psychiatry.* 1998;9:267–80.
30. Gordon H, Grubin D. Psychiatric aspects of the assessment and treatment of sex offenders. *Advances in Psychiatric Treatment.* 2004;10:73–80.
31. Kafka M. Axis I psychiatric disorders, paraphilic sexual offending and implications for pharmacological treatment. *Israel Journal of Psychiatry and Related Sciences.* 2012;49:255–61.
32. Abel GG, Becker JV, Cunningham-Rathner J, Mittelman M, Rouleau J-L. Multiple paraphilic diagnoses among sex offenders. *Journal of the American Academy of Psychiatry and the Law.* 1988;16:153–68.
33. Grossman LS, Martis B, Fichtner CG. Are sex offenders treatable? A research overview. *Psychiatric Services.* 1999;50:349–61.

34. Nichols H, Molinder I. *Manual for the Multiphasic Sex Inventory.* Tacoma, WA: Crime and Victim Psychology Specialists; 1984.

35. Paitich D, Langevin R, Freeman R, Mann K, Handy L. The Clarke SHQ: a clinical sex history questionnaire for males. *Archives of Sexual Behavior.* 1977;6:421–36.

36. Laws DR, Marshall WL. A brief history of behavioral and cognitive behavioral approaches to sexual offenders: Part 1. Early developments. *Sexual Abuse.* 2003;15:75–92.

37. Marshall WL. Phallometric assessments of sexual interests: an update. *Current Psychiatry Reports.* 2014;16:1–7.

38. Marshall WL, Fernandez YM. Phallometric testing with sexual offenders: limits to its value. *Clinical Psychology Review.* 2000;20:807–22.

39. Murphy L, Ranger R, Fedoroff JP, Stewart H, Dwyer RG, Burke W. Standardization of penile plethysmography testing in assessment of problematic sexual interests. *Journal of Sexual Medicine.* 2015;12:1853–61.

40. Murphy L, Ranger R, Stewart H, Dwyer G, Fedoroff JP. Assessment of problematic sexual interests with the penile plethysmograph: an overview of assessment laboratories. *Current Psychiatry Reports.* 2015;17:1–5.

41. O'Shaughnessy R. Commentary: phallometry in court—problems outweigh benefits. *Journal of the American Academy of Psychiatry and the Law.* 2015;43:154–8.

42. Purcell MS, Chandler JA, Fedoroff JP. The use of phallometric evidence in Canadian criminal law. *Journal of the American Academy of Psychiatry and the Law.* 2015;43:141–53.

43. Dombert B, Mokros A, Brückner E, *et al.* The virtual people set: developing computer-generated stimuli for the assessment of pedophilic sexual interest. *Sexual Abuse.* 2013;25:557–82.

44. Letourneau EJ. A comparison of objective measures of sexual arousal and interest: Visual reaction time and penile plethysmography. *Sexual Abuse.* 2002;14:203–19.

45. Laws DR, Gress CL. Seeing things differently: the viewing time alternative to penile plethysmography. *Legal and Criminological Psychology.* 2004;9:183–96.

46. Grubin D. The case for polygraph testing of sex offenders. *Legal and Criminological Psychology.* 2008;13:177–89.

47. Grubin D. A trial of voluntary polygraphy testing in 10 English probation areas. *Sexual Abuse.* 2010;22:266–78.

48. Cross TP, Saxe L. A critique of the validity of polygraph testing in child sexual abuse cases. *Journal of Child Sexual Abuse.* 1993;1:19–34.

49. Beech A, Friendship C, Erikson M, Hanson RK. The relationship between static and dynamic risk factors and reconviction in a sample of UK child abusers. *Sexual Abuse.* 2002;14:155–67.

50. Hanson RK, Thornton D. Improving risk assessments for sex offenders: a comparison of three actuarial scales. *Law and Human Behavior.* 2000;24:119.

51. Storey JE, Watt KA, Jackson KJ, Hart SD. Utilization and implications of the Static 99 in practice. *Sexual Abuse.* 2012;24:289–302.

52. Rice ME, Harris GT, Lang C. Validation of and revision to the VRAG and SORAG: The Violence Risk Appraisal Guide—Revised (VRAG-R). *Psychological Assessment.* 2013;25:951.

53. Brown J, Singh JP. Forensic risk assessment: a beginner's guide. *Archives of Forensic Psychology.* 2014;1:49–59.

54. Mossman D. Evaluating risk assessments using receiver operating characteristic analysis: Rationale, advantages, insights, and limitations. *Behavioral Sciences and the Law.* 2013;31:23–39.

55. Hanson RK, Yates PM. Psychological treatment of sex offenders. *Current Psychiatry Reports.* 2013;15:1–8.

56. Müller K, Curry S, Ranger R, Briken P, Bradford J, Fedoroff JP. Changes in sexual arousal as measured by penile plethysmography in men with pedophilic sexual interest. *Journal of Sexual Medicine.* 2014;11:1221–9.

57. Seto MC. Is pedophilia a sexual orientation? *Archives of Sexual Behavior.* 2012;41:231–6.

58. Kim B, Benekos PJ, Merlo AV. Sex offender recidivism revisited: review of recent meta-analyses on the effects of sex offender treatment. *Trauma, Violence, and Abuse.* 2016;17:105–17.

59. Hanson RK, Gordon A, Harris AJ, *et al.* First report of the collaborative outcome data project on the effectiveness of psychological treatment for sex offenders. *Sexual Abuse.* 2002;14:169–94.

60. Lösel F, Schmucker M. The effectiveness of treatment for sexual offenders: a comprehensive meta-analysis. *Journal of Experimental Criminology.* 2005;1:117–46.

61. Karl Hanson R. Sex offenders. In: Webster C, Haque Q, Hucker S, editors. *Violence Risk: Assessment and Management: Advances Through Structured Professional Judgement and Sequential Redirections,* second edition. Chichester: Wiley-Blackwell; 2014. pp. 148–58.

62. Ward T, Mann RE, Gannon TA. The good lives model of offender rehabilitation: clinical implications. *Aggression and Violent Behavior.* 2007;12:87–107.

63. Ward T, Gannon TA. Rehabilitation, etiology, and self-regulation: the comprehensive good lives model of treatment for sexual offenders. *Aggression and Violent Behavior.* 2006;11:77–94.

64. Clarke M, Brown S, Völlm B. Circles of Support and Accountability for Sex Offenders: a systematic review of outcomes. *Sexual Abuse.* 2017;29:446–78.

65. Garcia FD, Delavenne HG, Assumpção AdFA, Thibaut F. Pharmacologic treatment of sex offenders with paraphilic disorder. *Current Psychiatry Reports.* 2013;15:1–6.

66. Holoyda BJ, Kellaher DC. The biological treatment of paraphilic disorders: an updated review. *Current Psychiatry Reports.* 2016;18:1–7.

67. Khan O, Ferriter M, Huband N, Powney MJ, Dennis JA, Duggan C. Pharmacological interventions for those who have sexually offended or are at risk of offending. *Cochrane Database of Systematic Reviews.* 2015;2:CD007989.

68. Lehne G, Thomas K, Berlin F. Treatment of sexual paraphilias: a review of the 1999–2000 literature. *Current Opinion in Psychiatry.* 2000;13:569–73.

69. Nair M. Pharmacotherapy for sexual offenders. In: Phenix A, Hoberman HM, editors. *Sexual Offending: Predisposing Antecedents, Assessments, and Management.* New York, NY: Springer; 2016. pp. 755–67.

70. Thibaut F. Pharmacological treatment of sex offenders. *European Psychiatry.* 2016;33:S43.

71. Khan O, Mashru A. The efficacy, safety and ethics of the use of testosterone-suppressing agents in the management of sex offending. *Current Opinion in Endocrinology, Diabetes and Obesity.* 2016;23:271–8.

72. Railly DR, Delva NJ, Hudson RW. Protocols for the use of cyproterone, medroxyprogesterone, and leuprolide in the treatment of paraphilia. *Canadian Journal of Psychiatry.* 2000;45:559–63.

73. Kiersch TA. Treatment of sex offenders with Depo-Provera. *Bulletin of the American Academy of Psychiatry and the Law.* 1990;18:179–87.

74. Kravitz HM, Haywood TW, Kelly J, Wahlstrom C, Liles S, Cavanaugh JLJ. Medroxyprogesterone treatment for paraphiliacs. *Bulletin of the American Academy of Psychiatry and the Law.* 1995;23:19–33.

75. Rosler A, Witztum E. Treatment of men with paraphilia with a long-acting analogue of gonadotrophin-releasing hormone. *New England Journal of Medicine*. 1998;338:416–22.

76. Rousseau L, Couture M, Dupont A, Labrie F, Couture N. Effect of combined androgen blockade with an LHRH agonist and flutamide in one severe case of male exhibitionism. *Canadian Journal of Psychiatry*. 1990;35:338–41.

77. Schober JM, Kuhn PJ, Kovacs PG, *et al*. Leuprolide acetate suppresses pedophilic urges and arousability. *Archives of Sexual Behavior*. 2005;34:691–705.

78. Heim N. Sexual behavior of castrated sex offenders. *Archives of Sexual Behavior*. 1981;10:11–19.

79. Thibaut F, Cordier B, Kuhn J-M. Gonadotrophin hormone releasing hormone agonist in cases of severe paraphilia: a lifetime treatment? *Psychoneuroendocrinology*. 1996;21:411–19.

80. Grasswick LJ, Bradford JMW. Osteoporosis associated with the treatment of paraphilias: a clinical review of seven case reports. *Journal of Forensic Science*. 2003;48:849–55.

81. Baratta A, Javelot H, Morali A, Halleguen O, Weiner L. The role of antidepressants in treating sex offenders. *Sexologies*. 2012;21:106–8.

82. Mann RE, Hanson RK, Thornton D. Assessing risk for sexual recidivism: some proposals on the nature of psychologically meaningful risk factors. *Sexual Abuse*. 2010;22:191–217.

83. Hanson RK, Morton-Bourgon K. *Predictors of Sexual Recidivism: An Updated Meta-analysis 2004-02*. Ottawa: Public Safety and Emergency Preparedness Canada; 2004.

84. Hanson RK, Morton-Bourgon KE. The characteristics of persistent sexual offenders: a meta-analysis of recidivism studies. *Journal of Consulting and Clinical Psychology*. 2005;73:1154.

# 142

# Stalking and querulous behaviour

*Rosemary Purcell and Paul E. Mullen*

## Stalking

Stalking occurs when a person repeatedly intrudes upon another in such a manner that the recipient fears for his or her safety or experiences significant distress [1]. The intrusions can involve following, loitering nearby, maintaining surveillance, approaching the victim, and communicating via telephone, letters, email, social media, or notes attached to property. Associated behaviours include ordering or cancelling goods and services on the victim's behalf (for example, pizzas or taxis in the former, and utilities such as gas or electricity in the latter), spreading malicious rumours, vexatious complaints, threats, property damage, and assault.

Stalking is motivated by a range of intentions. Some stalk in hope, some in anger, some in lust, some in ignorance, and some in mixtures of these motives [1]. Research suggests that the overarching term 'stalking' encompasses two basic patterns [3]. The first involves incursions that are largely confined to following or unwanted approaches perpetrated usually by a stranger, which last only a day or so before ending, usually without the need for intervention. The second is characterized by a broader range of intrusions, perpetrated most commonly by someone known to the victim (for example, an ex-partner, acquaintance, colleague, or neighbour), that lasts for months or even years. The first type of stalking is often distressing but rarely culminates in threats or physical violence or inflicts psychosocial damage. The second type is far more likely to be associated with longer-term psychological disturbance and lifestyle alterations, as well as threats and assault. The watershed between these two forms of stalking is the continuation of the behaviours for more than 2 weeks [3], which is important to recognize from an early intervention perspective.

Stalking is proscribed as a criminal offence in most English-speaking countries, as well as a number of European countries (Austria, Belgium, Denmark, Germany, Italy, Malta, and the Netherlands), although to date only Japan and India have enacted laws in the Asian region. The drafting of stalking legislation has not been without controversy [4, 5], particularly since stalking behaviours can overlap with interactions that, however unwelcome or inappropriate, are nonetheless part of many people's everyday experience (such as being pursued for a relationship) or regarded as culturally acceptable.

## Epidemiology of stalking

Estimates of the prevalence of stalking, as with any other phenomenon, will vary according to definition, sampling, method of enquiry, and the willingness of subjects to respond and disclose their experience. Reported lifetime rates of victimization suggest that stalking is a prevalent social problem, affecting an estimated 10–15% of adults [6–10]. Stalking also occurs among juveniles [11, 12], with an estimated 12-month incidence of 16.5% for victimization and 5.3% for perpetration [13]. Irrespective of age, the majority of victims are female (70–80%), while stalkers are male (80–85%). Victims are typically pursued by someone known to them (80%), though strangers account for a significant minority.

Cyberstalking has attracted considerable media interest, but few systematic studies. Broadly defined as repeated, unwanted contacts via the Internet, social media, and other communication technologies, 'pure' cyberstalking is relatively uncommon, affecting an estimated 6% of Internet users [14] or 7% of stalking victims [15]. Cyberstalking appears to be one more technique in a perpetrator's arsenal, rather than a distinct type of activity. The level of concern about cyberstalking appears to be driven more so by the *potential*, rather than the actual, size of the problem. Well over half a billion people share personal information every day on Facebook alone, let alone other platforms such as Twitter or Instagram. The scope for cyberstalking, particularly gathering information about a victim, is undoubtedly immense.

## The impacts of stalking

Stalking is an act of violence in itself that causes psychological distress and social disruption (and, in many cases, occupational impairment), as well as a harbinger of assault. Being stalked can produce a corrosive state of fear, arousal, and helplessness. As with intimate partner violence, for most victims, it is not the blows which are the most destructive, but living in a chronic state of intimidation or looming vulnerability. Clinical and epidemiological studies have indicated that the majority of stalking victims report psychiatric morbidity, most commonly disruptive levels of anxiety (including hyperarousal), sleep disturbance, and lowered mood [16–18]. A significant minority also report considering suicide to escape the situation [16] and/or admit to homicidal fantasies toward the stalker [1].

Psychiatric morbidity appears to be mediated not only by stalking-related factors, particularly threats and ongoing harassment, but also by individual vulnerability factors, especially the use of avoidance as a coping strategy [19], the latter being amenable to treatment.

## Stalkers: classifications and typologies

Stalking, like most forms of complex human behaviour, can emerge from a wide range of psychological, social, and cultural influences. In the absence of any comprehensive explanatory theory of stalking, over 20 typologies have flourished [20], most of which categorize according to the stalker's prior relationship with the victim, an underlying mental disorder, and/or the primary motivation for the stalking.

Classifying stalkers by the nature of their prior relationship with the victim has the advantages of simplicity and utility. Mohandic and colleagues [21] used this approach in their classification, which divides stalkers into those with a prior relationship and those without. This classification's greatest utility is in predicting the risks of assault, with those targeting ex-intimate partners constituting the highest-risk group and those targeting public figures/strangers the lowest. The nature of the prior relationship is recognized as a critical aspect of any classification but, in isolation, is insufficient, as it is unlikely to adequately guide clinical or legal interventions.

The typology developed by Mullen and colleagues [1, 2] is multiaxial, depending primarily on the context in which the stalking emerges and the motivations which initiated and sustain the behaviour, along with the nature of the prior relationship and any underlying mental disorder in the perpetrator. Its appeal has been primarily to clinicians managing stalkers and stalking victims [22]. The typology enables predictions to be made about the duration of the stalking, the nature of the stalking behaviours, the risks of threatening and violent behaviour, and, to some extent, the response to management strategies [1, 23]. There are five main stalker types:

1. *The rejected* whose stalking begins in the context of the breakdown of a close (usually sexually intimate) relationship. The stalking is initially motivated either by the desire for reconciliation or to express rage at rejection, with a mixture of both being common. The stalking is often sustained by the pursuit becoming a substitute for the lost relationship, with the satisfactions from intrusion and control replacing those of intimacy.

2. *The intimacy seeker* who is pursuing love. The stalking begins in the context of a life lacking intimacy and is motivated by the hope, or firm expectation, of obtaining a loving relationship with a person on whom they have fixed their amorous attentions. The pursuit is sustained in the face of indifference or outright rejection, because better a love based on fantasy or delusion than no love at all.

3. *The incompetent suitor* who is pursuing a sexual encounter or friendship. This usually begins in the context of loneliness and is motivated by a desire to start some form of relationship with someone who has attracted their interest. This group often pursues intensely but rarely persists for prolonged periods, presumably because multiple rebuffs bring few rewards.

4. *The resentful*, whose stalking starts in the context of a grievance at being unjustly treated or humiliated. The initial motivation is revenge, but this gives way to the satisfactions obtained from the sense of power over someone who has previously been experienced as an oppressor.

5. *The predatory*, which begins in the context of the desire to act out violent or sexual fantasies often of a sadistic or paedophilic nature. The initial motivation is to gain information about the movements of a potential victim (usually a stranger or acquaintance). The stalking continues because of the satisfactions accruing not just from voyeurism, but from the excitement and sense of power which comes from rehearsing the planned attack in fantasy while watching the future victim.

Each of the stalker types (hopefully with the exception of the predatory) has correlates in normal behaviour [24]. When relationships break down, one partner is often confused or distressed by the separation and seeks to understand, reconcile, or express anger. The incompetent suitor is akin to the awkward adolescent or socially inept adult who fails to traverse the social minefields of dating or simply making acquaintance. The intimacy seeker is the adolescent crush and the enthusiastic fan writ large. Even the resentful is not far removed from some seekers after justice and those asserting their rights. In theory, the boundary between persistent approaches as part of socially acceptable behaviour and the crime of stalking is difficult to isolate. In practice, the distinction is rarely a problem. Stalkers are those who repeatedly impose themselves on another person in a manner that creates obvious distress. It is the disregard of, or blindness to, the disturbance that their behaviour creates that distinguishes the stalker from their more normal counterparts.

## Psychopathology of stalkers

Stalkers are rarely drawn from the psychologically adequate or socially able of the world. The proportion of stalkers whose behaviour is directly related to mental illness varies according to where the researchers derived their sample (for example, clinical settings vs law enforcement) and the proportion of strangers or acquaintances in the sample, with the rates of mental illness, particularly psychosis, highest in these groups [25, 26].

In broad terms, psychotic disorders are relatively frequent in the intimacy-seeking group. In the resentful type, paranoid disorders unsurprisingly predominate, though most are not associated with frank delusion. The rejected most often have problems around dependency, entitlement, rigidity, and control, with substance abuse and depressive states occasionally complicating the picture. The incompetent suitors are socially disabled by shyness, narcissism, intellectual limitations, or autism spectrum disorders, but always with interpersonal insensitivity or indifference. The predatory are sexually perverse and not infrequently have marked psychopathic traits, but they are rarely psychotic [1].

Attachment theory has unsurprisingly been evoked to explain stalking [27]. That stalkers as a group do not manage interpersonal relationships very well is obvious. Attachment style has been shown to differ according to stalker type [28], which may be useful in the formulation process, but what connection it may have with any theory of early development is speculative. A deficit in verbal, relative to performance, intelligence quotient (IQ) has also been found [29], which should be considered in relation to an individual's ability to engage in particular psychological treatments.

## Stalking of health professionals

Health professionals have a heightened vulnerability to being stalked by their clients [30–32]. The risk stems both from resentful, disappointed, or disgruntled patients, and lonely and disordered people who misconstrue empathy and attention for romantic interest [33, 34]. While some stalking behaviours constitute little more than minor irritations, they may also ruin a clinician's career.

Rates differ according to the setting and professional groups surveyed. For example, 53% of clinical staff in an inpatient psychiatric service reported being stalked by a patient [35], compared to 21% of psychiatrists in a large mental health organization [36]. General practitioners report high rates of intrusiveness by patients (70%), with 20% having been stalked and a further 20% subjected to a short burst of harassment [37]. Almost one in five psychologists report stalking by a client [38], 30% of whom were subjected to vexatious complaints to professional boards, which left many considering whether they wanted to continue with their profession.

Clinicians who fall victim to stalking by patients may bear the additional burden of implied or overt criticism from colleagues to the effect that, had they more adroitly managed the therapeutic encounter, they would not now find themselves in this predicament. There should be no tolerance with blaming the victim, even if it comes in the guise of collegial advice or supervision. Being stalked is an occupational hazard for the health professions. Affected colleagues should be accorded support and help, if for no other reason than we do not know when it may be our turn to face the pursuit of the vengeful or lustful patient.

## Risk assessment and risk management

Assessing and managing the stalker requires a primary focus on the risks they present to the victim, in terms of physical violence, as well as psychosocial damage. The risk that stalkers incur from their *own* behaviour also needs to be considered. The conflict between the stalker's desires and the victim's interests is obvious, but they are at one in being at risk of damage from the stalking situation. There can be a tragic symmetry between the victim becoming preoccupied with the stalking and forced to live an increasingly restricted life in a state of apprehension and the stalker devoting all his/her time and resources to a damaging and ultimately self-defeating pursuit. The victim's and the perpetrator's lives can be laid waste. This is not to argue for equivalence between victim and perpetrator, but merely to note that they share the chance of disaster. A perspective which encompasses the risks to stalkers and victims has the advantage for health professionals of reducing the ethical dilemma when treating stalkers around whose interests one is serving, the patient's or their victim's. Both are assisted to the extent that treatment stops the stalking or reduces its damaging impacts.

### The empirical basis for evaluating risk in the stalking situation

Risk assessment in stalking situations is hampered by a paucity of retrospective or prospective studies of representative samples. Clinicians do not have the luxury of deferring action until such evidence emerges, and so must instead depend on integrating knowledge from stalking research or systematic studies of risk in other areas and drawing on clinical experience [1].

## The risk of continued or recurrent stalking

Once stalking has continued for more than 2 weeks, the chances are high that it will continue for months [3]. The duration is longest for intimacy seekers and rejected stalkers pursuing ex-intimates, with the incompetents usually pursuing only briefly [1, 2]. Stalking recidivism (of the same victim) is associated with mental status, personality disorder, and prior criminal offending [39, 40].

## The risks of psychosocial damage to victims

There is some indication that female stalking victims report a greater psychological impact than males [6, 16]. Male victims are less inclined, however, to report fear (a requirement in most legal definitions) when they are stalked by a female; this likely explains the preponderance of same-gender stalking among men in community samples [6, 8]. Psychological distress is higher among victims subjected to prolonged and repeated following and the experience of property theft or destruction [17, 41, 42]. The relationship between psychological impact and the experience of physical violence is less clear, despite its intuitive appeal [42, 43].

## The risks of physical violence

### Prior relationship

Victims who have shared a prior intimate relationship with their stalker are at high risk of assault [44–47]. In a random community sample, ex-intimates were the most likely to be attacked (56%), followed by estranged relatives or friends (36%), casual acquaintances (16%), work-related contacts (9%), and strangers (8%) [8]. Such findings should not be interpreted as suggesting that victims of stalkers who are not ex-intimates are in little danger of physical violence. A chance of between 8% and 36% of being assaulted is no small risk.

### Threats

Between 30% and 60% of stalking victims are threatened [2, 26, 44]. In a community-based study, 44% of those threatened were subsequently assaulted and 73% of victims assaulted by their stalker had previously been threatened [8]. In short, threats are highly associated with violence and should be taken seriously.

### Mental disorder

Research has generally concluded that psychotic stalkers are less likely to be physically violent than their non-psychotic counterparts, but the relationship to personality disorder remains unclear [46, 48, 49].

### Substance abuse

Substance abuse is associated with violence in the stalking situation [2, 50–52].

### Prior offending and antisocial behaviour

Empirical data on the association between past criminal or violent behaviour and stalking violence are inconsistent [43]. However, the balance of the evidence favours such a relationship [44, 50].

### Demographic variables

The gender of stalkers has no impact on the rates of threats or assault [53–55]. Preliminary research indicates that the prevalence of threats and assault is higher among juvenile stalkers, compared to their adult counterparts [12], suggesting that younger perpetrators prefer more direct forms of harassment, as opposed to some of the more surreptitious pursuit employed by adults.

### The nature of the stalking

Violence is predicted by escalating intrusiveness and the intensity of the stalking behaviour [56]. The strongest association is with physical intrusions into the victim's house or place of work [49].

## Assessment and management

Initial assessments of stalkers often occur in the context of pre-sentence or parole board evaluations. Victims may be encountered in a wider range of contexts, many seeking help from general, rather than forensic, mental health professionals. Stalkers usually lack insight into their behaviour and tend to deny, minimize, and rationalize their actions. Victims often minimize the experience of stalking and over-emphasize their own responsibility for the harassment, which should be of no surprise to anybody experienced in working with victims in other contexts. Conversely, the problem of false claims of stalking victimization cannot be entirely ignored [57] and indeed can be guaranteed to be encountered among practitioners who specialize in the treatment of stalking victims. This group, particularly if delusional, are often obvious, given implausible and exuberant accounts of victimization. Care should be taken in dismissing claims of being stalked, however, as there are some calculating stalkers who leave few, if any, objective signs. False victims require help and treatment, not rejection, but they require quite different treatment from actual victims [57].

In all cases, it is essential to assess collateral information from such sources as witness statements, victim impact reports, judges' sentencing remarks, and professional-to-professional contacts, confidentiality allowing. Attempts to contact the victim when assessing the stalker, or the stalker when assessing the victim, are not advised. However, skilfully managed, such contacts tend to be experienced by the victim as the professional acting as an agent of the stalker, and by the stalker as support for their beliefs that this is a misunderstanding within a mutual relationship.

A comprehensive assessment of the stalker should answer at least the following questions, to enable a preliminary formulation:

1. What motivated the stalking, what sustains it, and what is the nature of the prior relationship with the victim (if any)?
2. What, if any, is the nature of the stalker's current mental disorder (including salient personality characteristics)? How has this been managed previously?
3. What is the nature and extent of the stalker's substance use/misuse?
4. Into which stalking type does the stalker best fit, based on these previous questions?
5. What are the stalker's current social circumstances/supports?
6. What role could treatment have in ameliorating the stalking?
7. What is the probability of continued stalking and/or physical violence?

The management of stalkers remains very much the province of forensic mental health professionals, and even among them, it is a specialist area. Basic approaches to identifying potentially remediable risks and their management, along with more specific interventions for particular stalker types, have been explored by Mullen and colleagues [1].

Stalking victims rarely present for mental health care after the fact; most will be exposed to ongoing intrusions, such that their safety needs have to be prioritized, along with their mental health. Some victims of prolonged, intense stalking can manifest symptoms of complex post-traumatic stress disorder (PTSD) [58] and may have a poorer response due to the sense of having been permanently changed or damaged by their victimization. Like many victims of crime, stalking victims may be reluctant to disclose the details or even the existence of traumatic experiences. As noted earlier, self-blame (or indeed explicit blame by those around them) is not infrequently part of the picture.

Stalking victims need good psychiatric care. Strategies to manage stress reactions are required, along with methods to ameliorate hyperarousal and/or depressed mood. The following is a brief account of key interventions to combat stalking that should be canvassed in the treatment of victims:

1. *Inform others.* It is essential that victims inform those they love or with whom they work or socialize. This performs three functions:
   i. It enables others to support the victim and to avoid inadvertently assisting the stalker.
   ii. It prevents those around the victim from being put at risk by ignorance or by provoking the stalker and exacerbating the situation.
   iii. It allows victims a 'reality check' on their fears that the stalking is occurring or about the seriousness of their situation.
2. *Avoid contact and/or confrontation.* All contacts or direct communications with a stalker risks reinforcing their behaviour and must be actively avoided. Once stalking is established, it is usually too late to resolve matters by meeting 'one last time'. Threats of suicide if the victim refuses to meet or otherwise engage with the stalker should not be rewarded or reinforced, despite an elevated risk of suicide among perpetrators [59].
3. *Documentation.* The best protection for stalking victims often lies in criminal law. The police are more likely to respond appropriately if victims can demonstrate that the behaviour is repeatedly occurring and make it relatively easy for them to pursue the allegations. Retain phone or text messages, emails, letters, and unwanted 'gifts', and keep a diary noting approaches, threats, or property damage, and, where possible, witnesses to (or photographic evidence of) such events. This will be invaluable for any prosecution and further assist the victim to take back control over their lives.
4. *Restraining/intervention/apprehended violence (and other such) orders.* The effectiveness of these orders to combat stalking is debatable, with 35–80% breached in stalking situations [60–62]. Nonetheless, these civil orders can be used to demonstrate for subsequent criminal proceedings that the stalker's behaviour was intentional, which may often be a legislative requirement. Reservations have to be expressed, however, not only about their utility (being totally ineffective, for example, for delusional intimacy seekers), but also about the level of insecurity and distress consequent on their breach. These orders are also often

*provocative*, particularly for the rejected, and victims should be advised about the potential for an escalation in violence after obtaining an order against a former intimate (particularly if the relationship was characterized by violence).

5. *Increased security.* Inexpensive measures, such as good locks, movement-triggered outdoor lighting, secure mailboxes (or post office boxes), and ensuring high-privacy settings on social media accounts, may provide a degree of reassurance and a modicum of security.

## Querulous behaviour: abnormally persistent complaining and vexatious litigation

In response to a perceived or real personal grievance, querulous individuals relentlessly pursue their notion of justice in a manner that is seriously damaging to the person's economic, social, and personal interests and disruptive to the functioning of courts and/or other agencies involved in attempts to resolve the claims [63]. A minority may engage in stalking as part of their campaign, but most pursue their quest via relentless complaining and litigation.

Psychiatry's interest in the querulous (from Latin, to mutter and to mumble) thrived in the late nineteenth and early twentieth centuries. Classical psychiatry viewed querulousness as a form of paranoia, with the term *Querulantenwahn* ('litigants' delusion') coined in 1857 by Johann Ludwig Casper to describe:

> 'A form of so called paranoia in which there exists in a patient an insuppressible and fanatic craving for going to law in order to get redress for some wrong which he believes done to him. Individuals who fall victim to this disorder are always strongly predisposed … extremely egotistical … know everything better … differs from other forms of paranoia in so far as the wrong may not be quite imaginary … the more he fails the more he becomes convinced that enormous wrong is being done to him … neglects his family and his business … going down the road to ruin' [64].

The accuracy of this description aside, the classical view of querulousness as a form of paranoia was problematic, given that the behaviour was usually based on a genuine grievance and frequently regarded as developing on the basis of vulnerabilities in the individual's personality [65–67]. The diagnosis of querulous paranoia was appealed to less and less, and by the latter half of the twentieth century, the literature largely fell silent [68]. Unreasonable complainants ultimately came to be considered as a purely legal, rather than a medical, issue [69]. The disappearance of querulousness from the realms of psychiatry paralleled the decline of paranoia as a diagnostic entity, but also reflected psychiatry's increasing reluctance to play the role of social regulator. Perhaps most significant in the diminishing interest in the querulous was the coinciding emergence of the culture of blame [70], which drew more and more vulnerable people into the systems of complaint management [1].

Cultural factors have been little explored in the querulous, but individuals who have migrated from Eastern bloc countries appear overrepresented in our clinical experience, likely reflecting the historical absence of avenues to complaint or redress from injustice under oppressive regimes. We speculate that these individuals are susceptible to becoming overwhelmed with the myriad of opportunities afforded to them with a Western 'culture of complaint' and blame.

Agencies of accountability, including courts and tribunals, Ombudsmen's offices, registration boards, and complaints departments, are those now primarily charged with navigating the problems created by a tiny fraction of people pursuing grievances with a persistence and insistence disproportionate to the substantive nature of their claim. In the civil, administrative, and family courts, the number of intractable cases being pursued—usually by self-represented litigants—increases each year. By pursuing what they regard as their rights through repeated petitions and intrusive approaches to politicians and heads of state, querulants are also distracting protection services from more substantial threats [63, 71–74].

The querulous pursue their vision of justice through litigation in courts and tribunals, through petitions to the powerful, and through the various agencies of accountability. In practice, all three avenues are exploited simultaneously. Courts and agencies of accountability are designed to deliver conciliation, mediation, reparation, and compensation, but rarely retribution, except in the exceptional case of punitive damages, and never personal vindication. As the querulous seek, above all, personal vindication and retribution, from the outset, they are doomed to fail.

### Clinical features

It is not easy to distinguish the querulant from the difficult complainant, or even from social reformers and victims of gross injustice. The following simple typology may assist [63]:

1. *Normal complainants* are aggrieved and seek reasonable compensation, reparation, or simply an apology. They can engage in, and will accept, mediation and conciliation, though they may become persistent and insistent if provoked by inefficiency or injustice.

2. *Difficult complainants* also seek compensation and reparation for their grievance but, in addition, can pursue retribution. They tend from the outset to manifest victimization and anger, and resist all solutions but their own. Eventually, they will settle for the best deal they can obtain, albeit still complaining of injustice.

3. *Altruistic reformers* pursue goals of social progress via the courts, petitions, and complaints. They sacrifice their personal interests in pursuit of better outcomes for others. Though they may have a political agenda that is sectarian (for example, genetically modified foods, fathers' rights), they do not have idiosyncratic and personalized objectives.

4. *Fraudsters* who knowingly pursue false or grossly exaggerated claims.

5. *The mentally ill* whose claims are driven by delusional preoccupations that are frequently bizarre in nature, which reflect underlying disorders often of a psychotic type.

6. *The querulous* who seek personal vindication, in addition to compensation, reparation, and retribution. They are on a quest for justice that becomes their preoccupation (and often substitutes any occupation). Unlike reformers, and most of the difficult complainants, there is an obvious discrepancy between the provoking event and the salience attached to it by the querulous. They appear to seek not resolution, but continuation of the

conflict. Their loss of perspective lays waste to their social and economic functioning.

The querulous are predominantly males, who first become embroiled in complaining and claiming later in life, usually in their fourth or fifth decade [69, 75]. Premorbidly, most function reasonably well [69] and may well be above average in intelligence or functioning. They rarely have criminal records or prior psychiatric contact, and substance abuse is not prominent. Many have close relationships, but by the time they reach mental health professionals, they have usually alienated their family and friends. Querulants are often disappointed people who feel their effort (indeed striving) and qualities have been ignored and left unrewarded. Their pursuit of justice offers an opportunity to vindicate their lives and obtain the public recognition so long denied. Their personalities tend to have the traits of self-absorption, suspiciousness, and obsessionality, combined with an enviable capacity for persistence.

Clinically, querulants typically present as energized individuals eager to convince of the merits of their case. There is an enthusiasm that can seem almost manic, but unlike the manic, they are totally focused and almost impossible to distract from their narrative of injustice. They may attend appointments with reams of documents testifying to their misplaced scholarship. If challenged, they usually become patronizing as they pedantically refute all objections, to their complete satisfaction. Alternatively, they may become menacing and overtly threatening.

Communications from querulants [75] and vexatious litigants have been observed to be often characterized by:

- Multiple methods of emphasis, including underlining, highlighting, capitalization, or italics.
- The generous use of exclamation marks and question marks.
- Numerous footnotes and marginal notes.
- The use of attachments, some potentially pertinent (for example, letters received, copies of legislation), others of less obvious relevance (for example, Magna Carta, United Nations Declaration of Human Rights).
- And many, many pages.

The content of communications may also be unusual [75], sometimes containing:

- Legal, medical, and other terms used frequently, but often incorrectly;
- Repeated rhetorical questions;
- Reference to the self in the third person;
- Veiled threats to harm themselves or others if their wishes are not granted; or
- Exaggerated politeness and attempts to ingratiate.

## Clinical assessment

The querulous can only be adequately assessed by considering the development over time of their behaviour, as well as their state of mind. In an interview, they may present as merely overenthusiastic or overly hopeful, pursuing their legitimate rights with, at worst, a degree of fanaticism. It is the unfolding of their story which reveals the damage they are suffering and that they have inflicted on those around them.

### Case example

*An academic in her mid forties, whose fixed-term contract was not renewed, complained to the University that this was a result of bullying by her supervisor, who she claimed was seeking to appropriate her intellectual property for his own career advancement. The University investigated but ultimately rejected her complaint, noting that the contract non-renewal was due to a lack of ongoing funding and role redundancy. She initiated civil action in the state administrative tribunal and submitted dozens of Freedom of Information (FoI) applications pertaining to the University, her former supervisor, and numerous other departmental colleagues. Only a handful of the FoI applications were granted, and the civil action was dismissed. She unsuccessfully appealed the latter over the next 12 years (as a self-represented litigant), including eventually to the full bench of the national administrative court. She repeatedly sought stays and postponements of court hearings that had been scheduled to determine (that is, finalize) her case, the delays causing tremendous inconvenience both to the University staff named as respondents in the claims and the court staff. A frequent tactic was to 'reserve the right' to terminate proceedings due to 'health issues', which she typically employed at the end of lengthy proceedings when an adverse decision (in her opinion) was about to be adjudicated. Her administrative court claims were joined by complaints to the privacy commissioner, the human rights commissioner, and numerous members of parliament. She also contacted the registries of each state administrative tribunal, inundating staff with emails and phone calls and revelling in any inconsistent advice provided (which she regarded as confirmation of the tribunals' gross incompetence, rather than regional procedural differences). She was ultimately instructed by the Principal Registrar to deal only with the registry manager of the tribunal in which her original claim was lodged, whom she came to believe was responsible for the failure of her various claims. She finally made death threats against the registry manager, for which she was charged and subsequently convicted. On the day of sentencing, she abused and threatened the Magistrate ('No one has the right to stop me! ... Just try and you'll pay, bitch!') and assaulted a court attendant who intervened. She was imprisoned for a brief period, after which she resumed her complaining and litigation with a vengeance. She continues to pursue various actions in the courts, with her identity (obvious to all who encounter her) inexorably linked to her dogged self-righteousness.*

Traditionally, psychiatry has attempted to distinguish between deluded querulants, who are in the business of mental health services, and the non-deluded who are not. Unfortunately, the querulous present a formidable phenomenological challenge in this regard. They advance their ideas plausibly, making apparently rational connections between the underlying grievance (which is almost always based on some actual event or injustice) and their current claims and complaints. The querulous offer a detailed and apparently logical account of the emergence of their grievances and the progress of their quest for justice—logical that is, if taken in cross-section, but not when considered over time, when gross discrepancies between the supposed initiating cause and subsequent behaviour become apparent. Their persuasive presentation can obscure the essential futility of the quest and distract attention from the chaos they have created for themselves and those around them. The temptation is to normalize the clinical presentation, but this is to ignore both the peculiarity of their behaviour and beliefs, as well as the devastation they have wrought on their own lives. Sometimes the querulous are obviously deluded, and sometimes they appear to inhibit the borderline between overvalued ideas and delusion-like ideas. Debates over the phenomenological niceties should not, however, distract from recognizing the pathological nature of such querulousness.

### Management

Psychiatrists currently only tend to be involved in the management of querulants after the situation has reached the stage of the person either becoming seriously depressed or being charged with threats, violence, or contempt. The literature on the therapeutic management of the querulous is meagre. Ungvari [76] reported successful treatment using pimozide, which is consistent with our clinical experience that relatively low doses of a dopamine antagonist are helpful, though the response is slow in coming. The critical hurdle in treatment, however, is attaining some semblance of a therapeutic alliance with the patient. This requires avoiding being caught up in discussions of the rights and wrongs of their quest. The focus should be on the price they and their loved ones are paying for the pursuit [63]. Interestingly, some of those who come on orders from the court that mandate treatment will accept medication and other therapeutic interventions, as they wish to make clear they abide by the law. Paradoxically, a number have continued voluntarily in treatment after the end of the order, though they never acknowledge either that they were in error or in need of treatment because of their querulousness. What change are the involvement in the querulous ideas, the degree of preoccupations, and the behaviour, but the core belief that they were right never wavers. Querulous behaviour appears to be sustained by a range of cognitive distortions, including:

- Those who do not fully support their cause are enemies.
- Any lack of progress is the product of malevolent interference from someone.
- Any compromise is humiliating defeat.
- The grievance is the defining moment of their lives.
- That because they are in the right, the outcomes they seek must be not only possible, but also necessary.

These distortions are open to challenge and amelioration, and the cognitive therapy approaches advocated for delusions [77, 78] should, in theory, also be of value. The problem with the therapeutic management of querulous behaviour is that there are no adequate clinical trials of treatment, or indeed much beyond case reports. This reflects the prevailing zeitgeist that the querulous are not the concern of mental health, and even if they are, they are largely untreatable. Hopefully, if this neglect is overcome and querulous behaviour is once more recognized as a legitimate concern for mental health professionals, then systematic studies of therapy will follow.

## Conclusions

Not a few psychiatrists have difficulties with the notion of problem behaviours like stalking and querulousness being a proper subject for mental health concern. Psychiatry has traditionally been wary of concerning itself directly with criminal and antisocial behaviours [79, 80]. The approach taken in this chapter was to define patterns of behaviour destructive to the interests of the perpetrator and the victim, and then to examine the origins, effects, and potential therapeutic management. By recognizing that psychiatry can have a role in assessing and managing problem behaviours, without first performing obfuscating transformations into supposed mental disorders (such as impulse-control disorders), allows a more clear-sighted and effective approach to areas of human activity where our intervention can benefit both the actor and the wider community.

## FURTHER INFORMATION

Douglas, M. (1992). *Risk and Blame: Essays in Cultural Theory*. Routledge, London.

Mullen, P.E., Lester, G. (2006). Vexatious litigants and unusually persistent complainants and petitioners: from querulous paranoia to querulous behaviour. *Behavioural Sciences and the Law*, 24, 333–49.

Mullen, P.E., Pathé, M., Purcell, R. (2009). *Stalkers and Their Victims*, second edition. Cambridge University Press, Cambridge.

Pinals, D.A., editor. (2007). *Stalking Psychiatric Perspectives and Practical Approaches*. Oxford University Press, New York, NY.

## REFERENCES

1. Mullen, P.E., Pathé, M., Purcell, R. (2009). *Stalkers and Their Victims*, second edition. Cambridge University Press, Cambridge.
2. Mullen, P.E., Pathé, M., Purcell, R., Stuart, G.W. (1999). A study of stalkers. *American Journal of Psychiatry*, 156, 1244–9.
3. Purcell, R., Pathé, M., Mullen, P.E. (2004). When do repeated intrusions become stalking? *Journal of Forensic Psychiatry and Psychology*, 15, 571–83.
4. De Fazio, L. (2011). Criminalization of stalking in Italy: one of the last among the current European member states' anti-stalking laws. *Behavioral Sciences and the Law*, 29, 317–23.
5. Purcell, R., Pathé, M., Mullen, P.E. (2004). Stalking: defining and prosecuting a new category of offending. *International Journal of Law and Psychiatry*; 27, 157–69.
6. Tjaden, P., Thoennes, N. (1998). *Stalking in America: Findings From the National Violence Against Women Survey*. National Institute of Justice and Centers for Disease Control and Prevention, Washington, DC.
7. Budd, T., Mattinson, J. (2000). *Stalking: Findings From the 1998 British Crime Survey*. Research Findings No. 129. Home Office Research Development and Statistics Directorate.
8. Purcell, R., Pathé, M., Mullen, P.E. (2002). The prevalence and nature of stalking in the Australian community. *Australian and New Zealand Journal of Psychiatry*, 36, 114–20.
9. Breiding, M.J., Smith, S.G., Basile, K.C., et al. (2014). Prevalence and characteristics of sexual violence, stalking, and intimate partner violence victimization—National Intimate Partner and Sexual Violence Survey, United States, 2011. *MMWR Surveillance Summaries*, 63, 1–18.
10. Hellmann, D.F., Kliem, S. (2015). The prevalence of stalking: current data from a German victim survey. *European Journal of Criminology*, 12, 700–18.
11. McCann, J.T. (2000). A descriptive study of child and adolescent obsessional followers. *Journal of Forensic Sciences*, 45, 195–9.
12. Purcell, R., Moller, B., Flower, T., Mullen, P.E. (2009). Stalking among juveniles. *British Journal of Psychiatry*, 194, 451–5.
13. Fisher, B.S., Coker, A.L., Garcia, L.S., Williams, C.M., Clear, E.R., Cook-Craig, P. G. (2014). Statewide estimates of stalking among

high school students in Kentucky: demographic profile and sex differences. *Violence against Women*, **20**, 1258–79.

14. Dressing, H., Anders, A., Gallas, C., *et al.* (2011). Cyberstalking: prevalence and impact on victims. *Psychiatrishe Praxis*, **38**, 336–4.

15. Sheridan, L.P, Grant, T. (2007). Is cyberstalking different? *Psychology, Crime and Law*, **13**, 627–40.

16. Pathé, M., Mullen, P.E. (1997). The impact of stalkers on their victims. *British Journal of Psychiatry*, **170**, 12–17.

17. Purcell, R., Pathé, M., Mullen, P.E. (2005). Association between stalking victimization and psychiatric morbidity in a random community sample. *British Journal of Psychiatry*, **187**, 416–20.

18. Dressing, H., Kuehner, C., Gass, P. (2005). Lifetime prevalence and impact of stalking in a European population: epidemiological data from a middle-sized German city. *British Journal of Psychiatry*, **187**, 168–72.

19. Purcell, R., Pathé, M., Baksheev, G.N., MacKinnon, A., Mullen, P.E. (2012). What mediates psychopathology in stalking victims? The role of individual-vulnerability and stalking-related factors. *Journal of Forensic Psychiatry and Psychology*, **23**, 361–70.

20. Spitzberg, B.H., Cupach, W.R. (2007). The state of the art of stalking: taking stock of the emerging literature. *Aggression and Violent Behavior*, **12**, 64–86.

21. Mohandie, K., Meloy, J.R., McGowan, M., Williams. J. (2006). The RECON typology of stalking: reliability and validity based upon a large sample of North American stalkers. *Journal of Forensic Science*, **51**, 147–55.

22. Pinals, D.A. (2007). *Stalking: Psychiatric Perspectives and Practical Applications*. American Psychiatric Association, Washington, DC.

23. Mullen, P.E., MacKenzie, R., Ogloff, J.R.P., Pathé, M., McEwan, T., Purcell, R. (2006). Assessing and managing the risks in the stalking situation. *Journal of the American Academy of Law and Psychiatry*, **34**, 439–50.

24. Mullen, P.E., Pathé, M., Purcell, R. (2001). Stalking: new constructions of human behaviour. *Australian and New Zealand Journal of Psychiatry*, **35**, 9–16.

25. McEwan, T.E., Strand, S. (2013). The role of psychopathology in stalking by adult strangers and acquaintances. *Australian and New Zealand Journal of Psychiatry*, **47**, 546–55.

26. Zona, M.A., Sharma, K.K., Lane, J. (1993). A comparative study of erotomanic and obsessional subjects in a forensic sample. *Journal of Forensic Sciences*, **38**, 894–903.

27. Patton, C.L., Nobles, M.R., Fox, K.A. (2010). Look who's stalking: obsessive pursuit and attachment theory. *Journal of Criminal Justice*, **38**, 282–90.

28. MacKenzie, R.D., Mullen, P.E., Ogloff, J.R.P., *et al.* (2008). Parental bonding and adult attachment styles in different types of stalker. *Journal of Forensic Sciences*, **53**, 1443–9.

29. MacKenzie, R.D., James, D.V., McEwan, T.E., *et al.* (2010). Stalkers and intelligence: implications for treatment. *Journal of Forensic Psychiatry and Psychology*, **21**, 852–72.

30. Mullen, P.E., Purcell, R. (2007). Stalking of therapists. In: B. van Luyn, S. Akhtar, J. Livesley, editors. *Severe Personality Disorders: Major Issues in Everyday Practice*. Cambridge University Press, Cambridge; pp. 196–210.

31. Nelsen, A.J., Johnson, R.S., Ostermeyer, B., *et al.* (2015). The prevalence of physicians who have been stalked: a systematic review. *Journal of the American Academy of Psychiatry and the Law*, **43**, 177–82.

32. Clarke, M., Yanson, I., Saleem, Y., *et al.* (2016). Staff experience of harassment and stalking behavior by patients. *International Journal of Forensic Mental Health*, **15**, 247–55.

33. Pathé, M., Mullen, P.E., Purcell, R. (2002). Patients who stalk doctors: their motives and management. *Medical Journal of Australia*, **176**, 335–8.

34. Wooster, L., Farnham, F., James, D. (2016). Stalking, harassment and aggressive/intrusive behaviours towards general practitioners: (2) associated factors, motivation, mental illness and effects on GPs. *Journal of Forensic Psychiatry and Psychology*, **27**, 1–20.

35. Sandberg, D.A., McNiel, D.E., Binder, R.L. (2002). Stalking, threatening and harassing behavior by psychiatric patients toward clinicians. *Journal of the American Academy of Psychiatry and the Law*, **30**, 221–9.

36. McIvor, R.J., Potter, L., Davies, L. (2008). Stalking behaviour by patients towards psychiatrists in a large mental health organization. *International Journal of Social Psychiatry*, **54**, 350–7.

37. Wooster, L., Farnham, F., James, D. (2013). The prevalence of stalking, harassment and aggressive/intrusive behaviours towards general practitioners. *Journal of Forensic Psychiatry and Psychology*, **24**, 514–31.

38. Purcell, R., Powell, M.B., Mullen, P.E. (2005). Clients who stalk psychologists: prevalence, methods and motives, *Professional Psychology: Research and Practice*, **36**, 527–43.

39. Rosenfeld, B. (2003). Recidivism in stalking and obsessional harassment. *Law and Human Behavior*, **27**, 251–65.

40. Eke, A.W., Hilton, N.Z., Meloy, J.R., *et al.* (2011). Predictors of recidivism by stalkers: a nine-year follow-up of police contacts. *Behavioral Sciences and the Law*, **29**, 271–83.

41. Blaauw, E., Winkel, F.W., Arensman, E., *et al.* (2002). The toll of stalking: the relationship between features of stalking and psychopathology of victims. *Journal of Interpersonal Violence*, **17**, 50–63.

42. Kamphuis, J.H., Emmelkamp, P.M.G., Bartak, A. (2003). Individual differences in post-traumatic stress following post-intimate stalking: stalking severity and psychosocial variables. *British Journal of Clinical Psychology*, **42**, 145–56.

43. McEwan, T., Mullen, P.E., Purcell, R. (2007). Identifying risk factors in stalking: a review of current research. *International Journal of Law and Psychiatry*, **30**, 1–9.

44. Harmon, R.B., Rosner, R., Owens, H. (1998). Sex and violence in forensic population of obsessional harassers. *Psychology, Public Policy and Law*, **4**, 236–49.

45. Palarea, R.E., Zona, M.A., Lane, J.C., *et al.* (1999). The dangerous nature of intimate relationship stalking: threats, violence, and associated risk factors. *Behavioral Sciences and the Law*, **17**, 269–83.

46. Meloy, J.R., Davis, B., Lovette, J. (2001). Risk factors for violence among stalkers. *Journal of Threat Assessment*, **1**, 3–16.

47. Thomas, S., Purcell, R., Pathé, M., Mullen, P.E. (2008). Harm associated with stalking victimization. *Australian and New Zealand Journal of Psychiatry*, **48**, 800–6.

48. Kienlen, K.K., Birmingham, D.L., Solberg, K.B., *et al.* (1997). A comparative study of psychotic and nonpsychotic stalking. *Journal of the American Academy of Psychiatry and the Law*, **25**, 317–34.

49. Farnham, F.R., James, D.V., Cantrell, P. (2000). Association between violence, psychosis, and relationship to victim in stalkers. *The Lancet*, **355**, 199.

50. Brewster, M.P. (2000). Stalking by former intimates: verbal threats and other predictors of physical violence. *Violence and Victims*, **15**, 41–54.

51. Roberts, K.A. (2005). Women's experience of violence during stalking by former romantic partners: factors predictive of stalking violence. *Violence Against Women*, **11**, 89–114.

52. Rosenfeld, B., Harmon, R. (2002). Factors associated with violence in stalking and obsessional harassment cases. *Criminal Justice and Behavior*, **29**, 671–91.

53. Purcell, R., Pathé, M., Mullen, P.E. (2001). A study of women who stalk. *American Journal of Psychiatry*, **158**, 2056–60.

54. Meloy, J.R., Boyd, C. (2003). Female stalkers and their victims. *Journal of the American Academy of Psychiatry and the Law*, **31**, 211–19.

55. Strand, S., McEwan, T.E. (2012). Violence among female stalkers. *Psychological Medicine*, **42** , 545–55.

56. McEwan, T. E., MacKenzie, R.D., Mullen, P.E., *et al.* (2012). Approach and escalation in stalking. *Journal of Forensic Psychiatry and Psychology*, **23**, 392–409.

57. Pathé, M., Mullen, P.E., Purcell, R. (1999). Stalking: false claims of victimisation. *British Journal of Psychiatry*, **174**, 170–2.

58. Herman J.L. (1997). *Trauma and Recovery: The Aftermath of Violence—From Domestic Abuse to Political Terror*. Basic Books, New York, NY.

59. McEwan, T., Mullen, P., MacKenzie, R. (2010). Suicide among stalkers. *Journal of Forensic Psychiatry and Psychology*, **21**, 514–20.

60. Hakkanen, H., Hagelstam, C., Santtila, P. (2003). Stalking actions, prior offender-victim relationships and issuing of restraining orders in a Finnish sample of stalkers. *Legal and Criminological Psychology*, **8**, 189–206.

61. Purcell, R., Flower, T., Mullen P.E. (2009). Adolescent stalking: offence characteristics and effectiveness of intervention orders. *Trends and Issues in Crime and Criminal Justice*, **369**, 1–6.

62. MacKenzie, R.D. (2006). *The Systematic Assessment of Stalkers*. Doctorate of Psychology Thesis. Monash University, Melbourne.

63. Mullen, P.E., Lester, G. (2006). Vexatious litigants and unusually persistent complainants and petitioners: from querulous paranoia to querulous behaviour. *Behavioural Sciences and the Law*, **24**, 333–49.

64. Hack Tuke, D. (1892). *A Dictionary of Psychological Medicine*, pp. 1060–1. Churchill, London.

65. Jaspers, K. (1923). *General Psychopathology* (trans. J. Hoenig and M.W. Hamilton, 1963). Manchester University Press, Manchester.

66. Krafft Ebing, R. (1905). *Textbook of Insanity* (trans. C.G. Chaddock), pp. 397–9. Davies Company, Philadelphia, PA.

67. Kraepelin, E. (1904). *Lectures in Clinical Psychiatry* (trans. and ed. T. Johnstone). Bailliere, Tindall, and Cox, London.

68. Caduff, F. (1995). Compulsive querulousness: a decreasing behaviour syndrome? *Fortschritte Der Neurologie Psychiatrie*, **63**, 504–10.

69. Levy, B. (2015). From paranoia querulans to vexatious litigants: a short study on madness between psychiatry and the law. Part 2. *History of Psychiatry*, **26**, 36–49.

70. Douglas, M. (1992). *Risk and Blame, Essays in Cultural Theory*. Routledge, London.

71. James, D.V., Mullen, P.E., Meloy, J.R., *et al.* (2007). The role of mental disorder in attacks on European politicians 1990–2004. *Acta Psychiatrica Scandinavica*, **116**, 334–44.

72. Mullen, P.E., James, D.V., Meloy, J.R., *et al.* (2009). The fixated and the pursuit of public figures. *Journal of Forensic Psychiatry and Psychology*, **20**, 33–47.

73. Poole, S. (2000). *The Politics of Regicide in England, 1760–1850: Troublesome Subjects*. Manchester University Press, Manchester and New York, NY.

74. James, D.V., Mullen, P.E., Meloy, J.R. (2011). Stalkers and harassers of British royalty: an exploration of proxy behaviours for violence. *Behavioral Sciences and the Law*, **29**, 64–80.

75. Lester, G., Wilson, B., Griffin, L., *et al.* (2004). Unusually persistent complainants. *British Journal of Psychiatry*, **184**, 352–6.

76. Ungvari, G.S. (1993). Successful treatment of litigious paranoia with pimozide. *Canadian Journal of Psychiatry*, **38**, 4–8.

77. Chadwick, P., Birchwood, M., Trower, P. (1996). *Cognitive Therapy for Delusions, Voices and Paranoia*. John Wiley and Sons, Chichester.

78. Bentall, R., Kinderman, P. (1994). Cognitive processes and delusional beliefs: attributions and the self behaviour. *Research and Therapy*, **32**, 331–41.

79. Lewis, A. (1955). Health as a social concept. *British Journal of Sociology*, **4**, 109–24.

80. Clare, A. (1997). The disease concept in psychiatry. In: R. Murray, P. Hill, P. McGuffin, editors. *Essentials of Postgraduate Psychiatry*. Cambridge University Press, Cambridge; pp. 41–52.

# 143

# Domestic violence and abuse and mental health

*Louise M. Howard and Deirdre MacManus*

## Introduction

Violence and abuse is a pervasive problem in our society. It includes physical, sexual, and psychological abuse, coercive behaviour, and deprivation. Violence can be perpetrated by family members, intimate partners, and ex-partners (domestic violence) or by strangers and acquaintances (non-domestic or community violence, including violence by care providers) [1] (Fig. 143.1). Domestic violence, the focus of this chapter, is a global public health problem [2]. Worldwide, intimate partner violence (IPV) (one form of domestic violence) has been estimated to account for up to 7% of the overall burden of disease among women, mostly due to its impact on mental ill health [3, 4]. Annual direct and indirect costs of domestic violence and abuse (DVA) in the UK have been estimated to amount to £16 billion per annum [5]. In the UK, DVA is defined as: '*controlling, coercive or threatening behaviour, violence or abuse between people aged 16 or over, who are or have been intimate partners or family members, regardless of gender or sexuality. It includes psychological, physical, sexual, financial and emotional abuse*' [6]. This definition applies to adult family members (>15 years of age). Emotional and psychological abuse, including coercive control, are therefore recognized as part of DVA [7, 8]. (DVA also encompasses traditional practices, including forced marriage, so-called 'honour crimes', and female genital mutilation, in addition to partner violence, but these are beyond the scope of this chapter.) The World Health Organization (WHO) focuses on IPV, defining it as: '*behaviour by an intimate partner or ex-partner that causes physical, sexual, or psychological harm, including physical aggression, sexual coercion, psychological abuse or controlling behaviours*'. In this chapter, we will use the term DVA, unless a study refers specifically to IPV only, and will specify where studies are referring to non-partner violence. It is important to note that victims of DVA are rarely subjected to just one form of abuse—around half of women suffering from DVA experience more than one type of partner violence [9, 10].

DVA is sometimes classified into typologies, for example 'situational couple violence' and 'intimate terrorism' [11–13], and there is some preliminary evidence for the existence of IPV typologies, though further research empirically validating typologies is needed [14]. Situational couple violence is generally considered much more common than intimate terrorism and includes abuse, but without a context of control. Individuals who engage in situational couple violence are characterized as poor communicators who respond to frustrations with verbal or physical aggression. Although situational couple violence is harmful, intimate terrorism is the type of DVA that accounts for most serious injury and death. It is also more gendered than situational couple violence, with women more likely to be the victims of repeated and severe DVA by men, although intimate terrorism also occurs in same-sex relationships. Perpetrators may display emotionally unstable personality traits, develop strong disordered attachment to their victims, and engage in violence in order to prevent abandonment. Other intimate terrorists may have sociopathic traits and seek to dominate and control many aspects of their lives, including their relationships [14].

## Prevalence of domestic violence and abuse

DVA is common. A systematic review of international studies of physical violence in intimate relationships found that more than one in four women (28.3%) and one in five men (21.6%) reported perpetrating physical violence in an intimate relationship [15]. The British Crime Survey estimates of DVA (using the broad definition given) showed that some 8.2% of women and 4% of men were estimated to have experienced domestic abuse in 2014/15 [16], while 27.1% of women and 13.2% of men, between the ages of 16 and 59, had experienced any domestic abuse since the age of 16. In the United States, the National Intimate Partner and Sexual Violence Survey (2011) found that severe physical violence by an intimate partner (including acts such as being hit with something hard, being kicked or beaten, or being burnt on purpose) was experienced by an estimated 22.3% of women and 14.0% of men during their lifetime and by an estimated 2.3% of women and 2.1% of men in the 12 months before taking the survey [17]. DVA has the highest rate of repeated victimization of any violent crime [18–20]. There is substantial variation globally; the WHO multi-country study of female DVA victims reported that the lifetime prevalence of physical or

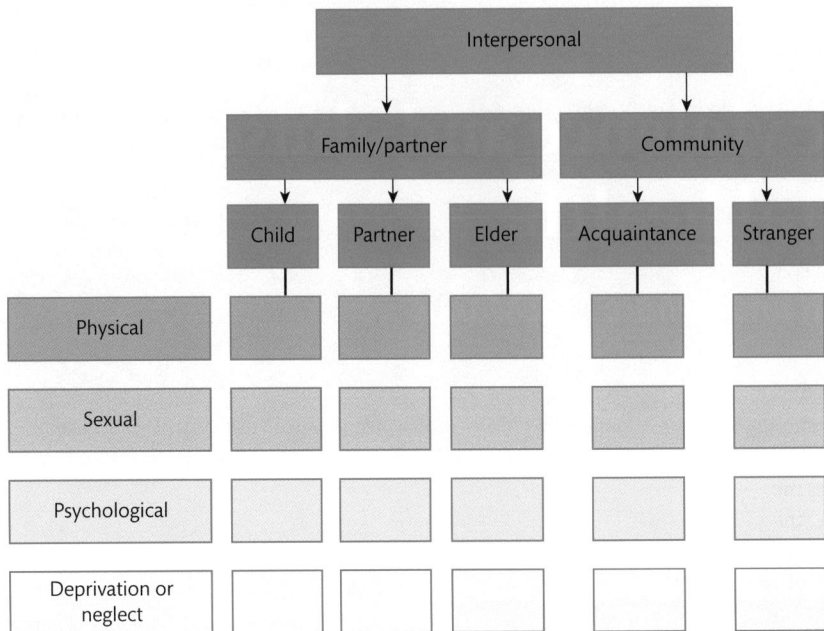

**Fig. 143.1** World Health Organization's typology of violence.
Adapted from Krug EG, Dahlberg LL, Mercy JA, *et al.* [Eds.], *World Report on Violence and Health,* Copyright (2002), with permission from World Health Organization. Available at http://www.who.int/violence_injury_prevention/violence/world_report/en/

sexual partner violence, or both, varied from 15% to 71%, and past-year violence between 4% and 54%, among the countries studied [21, 22]. Prevalence is higher in some clinical populations; for example, a systematic review found the highest prevalences of physical violence (30–50%) and sexual violence (30–35%) in studies conducted in psychiatric clinics and obstetrics and gynaecology clinics, and the highest mean lifetime prevalence of psychological violence in psychiatric clinics and emergency departments (65–87%) [23]. Adolescent and young women face a substantially higher risk of experiencing IPV than older women [24]. Lower rates of physical and sexual IPV are reported in older women, but the prevalence of emotional and economic abuse and controlling behaviours are similar to those experienced by younger women [25].

### Gender differences

While studies that have investigated the prevalence of DVA in both men and women have often found that the prevalence of victimization is similar in both genders, this masks the frequent finding that women are at greatest risk of serious and sexual assaults. A study in the United States using a representative general population sample found the lifetime prevalence of isolated domestic violence incidents to be comparable for men and women, but that nearly 25% of surveyed women, compared to 7.6% of surveyed men, reported that they were raped and/or physically assaulted by a current or former partner at some time in their lifetime [26]. Gender differences in the type of violence experienced were also found in the National Violence Against Women Survey (NVAWS), a telephone survey of over 6000 women and 7000 men across the United States. While they also found similar proportions of women and men reporting that they had experienced physical, sexual, or psychological IPV during their lifetime (28.9% and 22.9%, respectively), it was found that women were significantly more likely than men to experience physical or sexual IPV and abuse of power and control, but less likely

than men to report verbal abuse alone [27]. A systematic review of international studies of homicide revealed that one in seven of global homicides were committed by an intimate partner, and this proportion was six times higher for female homicides than for male homicides (38·6% vs 6·3%) [28]. Sexual violence against men by women partners has been found to be rare; in contrast, at least one in four women report sexual violence by a male intimate partner [29, 30].

Reports of comparable lifetime occurrence of 'all-type' DVA among men and women also mask the gender differences with regard to the number and type of specific assaults. For example, Tjaden and Thoennes [26] found that women in the United States were at greater risk of repeated coercive, sexual, or severe physical violence. British Crime Survey for England and Wales findings also suggested differences in repeat victimization; male victims may experience, on average, up to seven instances of repeat victimization, and women an average of 20 incidents [31]. Women are also more likely to report more severe injuries and to be more likely to be frightened as a result of domestic violence [29, 31].

However, there may also be gender differences in reporting. Brown [32] noted gender discrepancies in the rates of arrest and prosecution for IPV. Male victims were reluctant to report the incident, and the police were unwilling to arrest women accused of perpetrating violence, resulting in only 2% of suspected female perpetrators being arrested, which raises the concern that national prevalence rates based on surveys may not accurately reflect prevalence rates, particularly for men. A number of researchers also have challenged the assumption that IPV has a greater impact on women than men [33, 34], with studies increasingly examining the psychological impact of IPV on men [35] (see also later discussion of DVA and mental disorder).

Less is known about gender differences in male, compared with female, homosexual relationships, but a survey from the United States found that rates of emotional and physical violence victimization among urban men who have sex with men were substantially higher than previously reported among heterosexual men—34% reported psychological violence, 22% physical violence, and 5% sexual violence [36]. Studies from the United States increasingly suggest that the prevalence of DVA may be similar across same-sex and heterosexual relationships and what differs are help-seeking behaviours [37]. In a UK survey of 800 homosexual men and women, Hester (2009) reported that more than a third of respondents (38%) said that they had experienced DVA at some time in a same-sex relationship, with similar proportions in women (40%) and men (35%) [38]. However, the main prevalence data on DVA worldwide are derived from surveys that do not identify individuals in same-sex relationships, so current knowledge on violence occurring in homosexual relationships in epidemiologically representative populations is limited.

While this chapter includes more studies of women as victims and men as perpetrators of DVA, the authors acknowledge that this reflects the smaller research literature on women as perpetrators and men as victims (irrespective of whether in heterosexual or homosexual relationships).

## Risk factors for domestic violence and abuse: an ecological model

The WHO uses an ecological model when considering risk factors for DVA to provide a theoretical framework to help explain the multi-faceted nature of violence (Fig. 143.2) [1]. Risk factors operating at the level of the individual include being female, young age [39, 40], disability [41], poverty [40, 42], witnessing DVA as a child, childhood abuse [40, 43], and substance abuse [44]. Many of these factors are also risk factors for mental disorders, which emphasizes the social determinants of both mental disorders and DVA and the complex pathways involved in being a victim of violence through the lifespan. Aetiological factors also occur at the level of the relationship (for example, partner with substance misuse), community characteristics (for example, high population density, unemployment, and social isolation), and larger societal factors, including health, educational, economic, and social policies, cultural norms, gender disadvantage, and social inequalities [1, 45].

## Victimization

Being a victim of DVA is associated with mental disorders across the diagnostic spectrum, including anxiety, depression, post-traumatic stress disorder (PTSD), eating disorders, and psychosis, though there are limited data on this relationship for men [46–52]. Prospective studies have shown that psychiatric disorder can increase domestic violence perpetration and victimization, and that domestic violence is associated with both risk and chronicity of mental disorder [53, 54].

The prevalence of DVA victimization is particularly high among people in contact with secondary mental health services; a recent survey of mental health care service users in London reported that 70% of women and 50% of men had been DVA victims as adults, with many (27% of women, 10% of men) experiencing recent and current DVA, that is, significantly higher than the general population [odds ratio (OR) adjusted for sociodemographics (aOR) 2.7, 95% confidence interval (CI) 1.7–4.0 for women; aOR 1.6, 95% CI 1.0–2.8 for men] [55]. In addition, of note, family (non-partner) violence comprised a greater proportion of overall DVA among SMI than control victims (63% vs 35%; P <0.01), and adulthood serious sexual assault led to attempted suicide significantly more often among SMI than control female victims. Witnessing DVA also impacts on the health and mental health of children of adults who engage in IPV [56–58]. Mental health problems and violence can thus be transmitted through the generations [59].

The association between DVA and mental disorder is likely to be complex. Pre-existing mental health problems influence vulnerability to domestic violence. Indeed, there is evidence that a bi-directional causal relationship exists between some mental disorders and DVA. Prospective studies have shown that DVA contributes to both the emergence and the exacerbation of mental health symptoms [54, 60]. A systematic review of longitudinal studies of IPV and depressive symptoms reported both an association between depression and subsequent DVA and that DVA increases the risk of depression among women with no previous history of symptoms [61]. Moreover, data from an earlier systematic review [48] found that rates of depression declined over time once the abuse had ceased and that the severity or duration of violence was associated with the prevalence or severity of depression. Serious mental illness increases the likelihood of being in unsafe environments and relationships, and vulnerability to violent victimization [62]. There has,

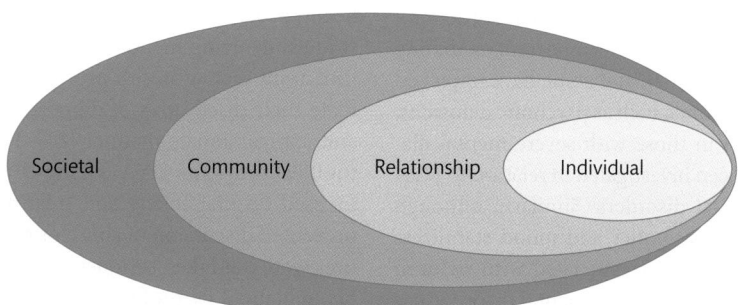

**Fig. 143.2** The ecological model for understanding violence.

Adapted from Krug EG, Dahlberg LL, Mercy JA, *et al.* [Eds.], *World Report on Violence and Health*, Copyright (2002), with permission from World Health Organization. Available at http://www.who.int/violence_injury_prevention/violence/world_report/en/

however, been limited longitudinal research into the relationship between DVA and other mental disorders, and more work is needed to disentangle the role of childhood abuse, which is associated with both mental disorder and DVA [63].

It has been suggested that DVA is more psychologically damaging than stranger violence or other forms of trauma [64]. The psychological effects of domestic violence can be conceptualized within a trauma framework, but the complex presentation of victims who have often been exposed to extensive control and repeated assaults, particularly if abuse was also experienced in childhood and escape was not possible due to physical, psychological, family, or societal factors, may be more adequately captured with the concept of 'complex PTSD' [65]. Although not a category in DSM-5 (but will be included in ICD-11), complex PTSD is considered a useful concept by many working with chronically traumatized victims [66]. Complex PTSD extends beyond the classic cluster of intrusive, avoidance, and arousal symptoms to incorporate changes in victims' attitudes about self, the perpetrator, relationships, and beliefs. Symptoms include those of PTSD, with additional disturbance in affect regulation and interpersonal relationships (see associated features of post-traumatic stress disorder in DSM-5 [67], including: feelings of ineffectiveness, shame, despair, or hopelessness; feeling permanently damaged; loss of previously sustained beliefs; hostility; social withdrawal; feeling constantly threatened; impaired relationships with others; or a change from the individual's previous personality characteristics).

### Perpetration

Although there is a wealth of research literature supporting the link between mental disorder and increased risk of perpetrating violence in general [68–70], fewer studies have examined DVA perpetration specifically. A recent systematic review found only 17 studies reporting the risk of DVA perpetration among men and women with mental disorders [71]—three reported on past-year violence, and these three studies did not consistently report increased risk for any diagnosis. Most studies examined lifetime risk of physical violence towards a partner and reported increased risk among samples with mental disorder of any diagnosis. However, most studies were cross-sectional, and importantly, alcohol and substance misuse were not examined as potential confounding or mediating factors. Further research is needed to investigate whether psychiatric disorders are associated with a current risk of violence to partners.

Recent studies of general violence and mental disorder have advanced our understanding of the link between mental disorder and violence perpetration. Some have identified the important mediating role of alcohol and substance misuse [72], and some have unpicked the mediating role of certain symptoms, such as psychotic delusions, negative affect, or anger [73, 74] in those with severe mental disorder. These pathways have not been investigated in relation to DVA perpetrated by people with mental disorders. Similarly, although treatment (for example, with antipsychotics and mood stabilizers for those with severe mental disorder) is associated with reduced violent crime [75], the impact of treatment for mental disorder has not been investigated in relation to DVA. It seems possible, however, that similar mechanisms may be important in any relationship between DVA perpetration and mental disorders.

The general premise in the literature, historically, was that even if women and men engage in equivalent rates of IPV in heterosexual relationships, male-perpetrated violence has more negative consequences for its victims than does female-perpetrated violence. Supportive evidence for this view comes from studies suggesting that women are more likely than men to sustain serious physical injury and negative psychological consequences [27, 76, 77]. However, recent cultural shifts have led to the acknowledgement that men can also be victimized in their relationships and research has shown that men can sustain similar levels of psychological injury. The NVAWS of women and men aged 18–65 found that, for both men and women, physical IPV victimization was associated with an increased risk of current poor health, depressive symptoms, substance use, and developing a chronic disease, chronic mental illness, and injury [27]. In general, psychological IPV was more strongly associated with these health outcomes than physical IPV. The proportion of IPV survivors meeting criteria for moderate to severe PTSD did not differ by gender (20% male, 24% female) [78], and psychological abuse was just as strongly associated with PTSD as physical abuse. This raises questions about the assumed lesser impact of IPV by women towards men, given findings that women are more likely to perpetrate psychological than physical aggression towards male partners. However, it is also clear that at the population level, being a victim of DVA is more prevalent in women and the psychiatric burden (estimated as population-attributable fractions, assuming causality) of DVA is higher in women [79].

## Identification of domestic violence and abuse by mental health services

### Identification of victims

Women are more likely to disclose domestic violence to a health care professional than to the police [80]. However, despite the high prevalence of DVA among mental health service users, a review in 2010 found that only 10–30% of DVA victims were identified by mental health professionals internationally [19]. Qualitative research in primary and secondary care has found that women may not disclose unless they are asked [81–83]. Barriers to disclosure for psychiatric patients include fear of consequences such as social services involvement and consequent child protection proceedings, fear that disclosure would not be believed, and fear that disclosure would lead to further violence. Other barriers included the actions of the perpetrator (such as always being present when the victim is seen by health professionals) and feelings of shame. A review of qualitative studies involving mental health service users found that DVA victims want mental health professionals to acknowledge and/or validate their disclosures of domestic violence in a non-judgemental and compassionate manner [81]. Patients reported limited opportunities to discuss DVA during clinical consultations, which were focused on diagnosing and treating psychiatric symptoms which prevented discussion of abuse or the extent of abuse. When disclosures were not taken seriously or minimized or there is the sense of being blamed by professionals, this was considered unhelpful and was associated with persistent symptoms. Concerns for future safety were prominent, with some responders expressing fear that mental health professionals' responses to the violence could place (and had placed) them at risk of further harm (for example, if the perpetrator hears about the DVA disclosure). There can be an expectation that they leave their partner, but mental health professionals may fail to understand that choosing to remain in an abusive relationship may be based on a strategic risk—benefit analysis which balances the risk of ongoing harm with the potential negative consequences of leaving their partner (financial concerns, social stigma, custody of children) and the hope that their partner may change [82, 84]. Some women fear more severe violence if they leave their partner. Indeed, it has been identified that women are at greatest risk of homicide in the months immediately following separation [85, 86].

There is some evidence that when routine enquiry about DVA is introduced across mental health services, detection rates improve. But even then, formulations and management plans rarely include issues around domestic violence and often do not include safety planning or trauma-focused therapy [87]. Therefore, it is now health policy in England, and in some parts of the United States, Australia, and New Zealand, to routinely enquire about DVA in all mental health assessments in psychiatric care [88]. Routine enquiry refers to 'asking all people within certain parameters about the experience of DVA, regardless of whether or not there are signs of abuse, or whether DVA is suspected'. Enquiry and disclosure in mental health settings have been found to be facilitated by a supportive and trusting relationship between patient and professional [82], with similar findings in other health care settings [83]. However, barriers to routine enquiry by professionals have also been identified, such as a lack of understanding of different types of DVA and a lack of confidence in facilitating and managing disclosures [82, 89]. Mental health professionals may be unsure of their role in the identification and management of DVA, and surveys have identified knowledge gaps [90]. International guidelines, including from the WHO and the National Institute for Health and Care Excellence (NICE), recommend that appropriately trained mental health professionals should facilitate DVA disclosure as part of comprehensive clinical assessments [30, 91].

Trials of systemic interventions to improve identification and response to DVA victims [92] in primary care (that is, integrated training, support, and advice from DVA advocates) have been shown to significantly improve health professionals' facilitation of disclosure and their subsequent response [92, 93]. As yet, there have been no trials in mental health settings, but a pilot has suggested that there are similar increases in identification rates of DVA victim with improvements in health and quality of life outcomes [94].

All mental health professionals need comprehensive training in how to enquire safely, with clarity on subsequent referral and care pathways [30]. The World Psychiatric Association (WPA) has just published an international competency-based curriculum for mental health care providers on IPV and sexual violence against women [95]. In England, the Department of Health has recommended that a question about any past or current violence and abuse should be asked during assessments and care programme approach meetings [96]. However, disclosure is more likely if more than one specific behaviour-based questions are used. Open questions can be asked initially about relationships, and normalization of the area of enquiry can also be helpful, but more specific questions about each type of abuse should also be asked (Boxes 143.1–143.4). Such questions can only be asked if a patient is alone or with a professional interpreter (rather than a family member).

However, there is evidence internationally that guideline dissemination and training in isolation do not necessarily create consistent,

---

**Box 143.1** Introductory open questions

- Are you having any problems with your husband/partner?
- We know that one in four women (and one in five men) experience domestic violence at some time in their life, so I ask everyone if that has ever happened to them. Has that happened to you?
- Some women have these symptoms when they are experiencing abuse. Are you afraid of anyone at home?
- Sometimes partners use physical force. Is this happening to you?
- Have you felt humiliated or emotionally abused by your partner (or ex-partner)?
- Has your partner ever physically threatened or hurt you? Or have you been kicked, hit, slapped, or otherwise physically hurt by your partner (or ex-partner)?
- In the past year, have you been forced to have any kind of sexual activity by your partner (or ex-partner)?

Reproduced from *Adv Psychiatr. Treat.*, 18(2), Howard LM, Domestic violence: its relevance to psychiatry, pp. 129–136, Copyright (2012), with permission from The Royal College of Psychiatrists.

---

sustainable improvements in identification and response to DVA [92, 97], and research into strategies to improve the integration of DVA into the scope of mental health services is needed. Integration of DVA advocates within mental health teams, with additional dedicated time for training, may improve rates of identification of DVA and outcomes for individuals [89], but training in identification may not lead to improved patient outcomes if they do not lead to increased engagement in interventions [98].

## Identification of perpetrators

A recent UK qualitative study with mental health professionals revealed that while they routinely ask about violence in general, they often fail to ask about current or ex-partner DVA (even though it has been shown that the risk of lethal violence increases after separation [99] due to inadequacy of current risk assessments, which often do not specifically refer to different types of DVA; and lack of clarity on information sharing when DVA was also a concern is disclosed [100]. In England, the National Confidential Inquiry into Homicides and the Home Office reported a failure of mental health

---

**Box 143.2** Questions about psychological abuse

- Does anyone insult you, call you names, or swear at you?
- Does anyone make it difficult for you to see friends/family or leave the house?
- Does anyone act in a jealous way or keep track of where you go?
- Does anyone put you down, embarrass you, or criticize you?
- Does anyone undermine your independence or try to make you feel small?
- Does anyone make you feel as if you have to walk on eggshells or as if you do nothing right?
- Does anyone order you around like a servant?
- Does anyone blame you for things that are not your fault?
- Does anyone control the money, make you ask for it, or stop you earning?

Reproduced from *Adv Psychiatr. Treat.*, 18(2), Howard LM, Domestic violence: its relevance to psychiatry, pp. 129–136, Copyright (2012), with permission from The Royal College of Psychiatrists.

- Do you ever feel that you have to have sex, even though you don't want to?
- Have you felt forced into sex because of what your partner might do?
- Has your partner made you have sex or carried on when it was painful?
- Has your partner made you have oral or anal sex when you didn't want to?
- Has your partner used an object in a sexual way that you didn't like?
- Has your partner made you do things or perform sexual acts that you didn't like?
- Has your partner refused safe sex or to use birth control?
- Has your partner made you have sex with another person?
- Has your partner talked about sex or done things in a way you didn't like?

Reproduced from *Adv Psychiatr. Treat.*, 18(2), Howard LM, Domestic violence: its relevance to psychiatry, pp. 129–136, Copyright (2012), with permission from The Royal College of Psychiatrists.

professionals to assess for DVA perpetration risk [101], despite a clear responsibility of mental health services to identify potential perpetrators of all forms of violence within current risk assessment frameworks. Recent studies using data from statutory domestic homicide reviews in England and confidential enquiries into homicides by people with mental illness have highlighted that a significant proportion of domestic homicides are perpetrated by male mental health service users; 14% of intimate partner homicides and 23% of adult family homicides were perpetrated by men who had been in contact with mental health services in the preceding year (men made up 80% of both types of homicide perpetrators) [72]. A study of homicide–suicides in England and Wales similarly found that current or former partners were the victims in two-thirds of cases and that 12% of perpetrators had been in contact with mental health services in the year before the offence [102].

Although there has been less research on how to respond to mental health service users who disclose DVA perpetration, there is extensive guidance on how to manage risk of violence, which includes consideration of the safety of the victim and appropriate

- Has your partner shaken you or grabbed you roughly?
- Has your partner shoved you or made you fall?
- Has your partner slapped you or smacked you?
- Has your partner tried to hit you with something or used an object as a weapon?
- Has your partner punched you?
- Has your partner tried to choke you or put his hands round your throat?
- Has your partner pushed you against the wall or thrown you down?
- Has your partner pulled your hair?
- Has your partner burnt you or scalded you with something?
- Has your partner threatened you with a knife or gun?
- Has your partner hurt you while you were pregnant?

Reproduced from *Adv Psychiatr. Treat.*, 18(2), Howard LM, Domestic violence: its relevance to psychiatry, pp. 129–136, Copyright (2012), with permission from The Royal College of Psychiatrists.

disclosure, if necessary, even if in breach of patient confidentiality. Homicide–suicides, 88% of which are perpetrated by men, with 77% of victims being female, are commonly preceded by relationship breakdown and separation [102]. With such a high proportion identified as having mental health problems, more research and guidance are needed on management risk of DVA perpetration among mental health professionals.

## How should mental health professionals respond to domestic violence and abuse experienced by psychiatric patients?

International guidelines, including from the WHO and NICE, recommend that, following the facilitation of DVA disclosure during a comprehensive clinical assessment, mental health professionals should provide support, ensure safety, and treat physical and mental disorders arising in the context of any DVA [30, 88]. There is debate about the role of universal screening for DVA in the health care system in generic services such as primary care or emergency departments [83]. However, the prevalence of violent victimization is so high in mental health service users [55, 103], and clinical guidelines recommend that mental health professionals routinely ask about DVA experienced in childhood and adulthood as part of clinical assessment and ongoing care [30, 88, 104].

As highlighted, however, routine enquiry may not improve outcomes if the enquirer is not appropriately trained in how to respond [88]. Guidelines recommend appropriate training, in combination with the establishment of protocols for inter-agency communication and information sharing, referrals to specialist DVA services, and referrals for interventions, including to specialist trauma services, if necessary. In some jurisdictions, there are specific multi-agency risk assessment conferences (MARACs) [105] which enable all services, including the DVA sector, to share information and reduce risk, and there is evidence to suggest that these can reduce risk of subsequent DVA.

Although there is limited research evidence in this area, good clinical practice includes making accurate notes, carrying out a risk assessment (particularly regarding immediate safety and considering the need for emergency action and/or child protection procedures), prioritizing safety planning, avoiding victim-blaming, and discussing available options [106]. Information about domestic violence services should be given, but professionals need to check whether it is safe for the patient to take information home with them—there may be an escalation of violence if such information is seen by the perpetrator. Potential interventions are discussed later in this chapter, but local health care trust policies (on domestic violence and on safeguarding of children and vulnerable adults), care pathways, and training should include information on what to do after disclosure [96].

When working with survivors of DVA, mental health professionals should ensure women have opportunities to be seen without partners, family members, or acquaintances present; provide access to independent interpreters; respond sensitively, compassionately, and non-judgementally to disclosure; reassure women that they are believed and not to blame for their experiences; and offer information and practical support that responds to women's concerns and respects their autonomy [30, 107]. It is also crucial for health professionals to recognize children as direct victims of domestic violence and abuse through witnessing or being aware of DVA in the family. Such experiences are associated with an increased risk of health problems and DVA in adulthood. There is also an increased risk of them being abused directly themselves by the abusive parent [91]. Professionals should recognize children's experience of the impact of DVA and strengthen professional responses to them as direct victims, not as passive witnesses to violence [108].

There is a need for greater focus on the interaction of the wider health infrastructure, including mental health services, in order to improve the management and reduction of DVA. This interdisciplinary and inter-agency approach was highlighted in the 2014 *Lancet* series on violence against women [109] and can be extrapolated beyond violence against women to DVA in general. Although additional research is needed, strengthening of health systems can enable providers to address DVA, including protocols, capacity building, effective co-ordination between agencies, and referral networks.

## What interventions are effective for psychiatric patients experiencing domestic violence?

### Interventions for victims

There is now a wealth of evidence for the effectiveness of a variety of pharmacological and psychological interventions for victims of trauma. NICE recommends cognitive behavioural therapy (CBT) and eye movement desensitization and reprocessing (EMDR) for PTSD [110], but until recently, there was a lack of research into the efficacy of these treatments for survivors of DVA who often present with more comorbidity or complex PTSD (as described). There is a growing evidence base for the treatment of complex PTSD, though this is currently under critical review [111]. However, while evidence-based interventions are already well established for victims of trauma, without identification and an understanding of the interpersonal dynamics of coercive, controlling DVA, it is likely that treatment may be less effective; indeed, some have hypothesized that DVA may be a moderator of treatment response if not identified or addressed [112].

Systematic reviews of treatment for DVA-related trauma have reported that CBT-based interventions may be associated with improved PTSD and depressive symptoms in survivors no longer in abusive relationships [84, 85]. Advocacy and CBT interventions may also be effective in reducing physical and psychological DVA [113]. However, these findings cannot be extrapolated to women with more severe psychiatric illnesses. Studies are emerging which have shown the effectiveness of NICE-recommended trauma-focused therapies in treating PTSD comorbid with psychosis [114, 115], but none have specifically focused on trauma in the context of domestic violence. Few studies have examined whether interventions are helpful in reducing psychological symptoms among women still subject to abuse.

### Interventions for perpetrators

Evidence is lacking on the effectiveness and appropriateness of DVA perpetrator programmes for people with mental disorders, and these programmes receive few referrals from mental health services [116].

However, interventions for modifiable risk factors (such as medication for persecutory delusions, psychological interventions, and treatment of comorbid alcohol and substance misuse), while ensuring the safety of the potential victim, may be expected to improve health and reduce violence for DVA perpetrators in contact with mental health services whose DVA perpetration appears linked to these factors.

## Future research

As this chapter has highlighted, there is still limited understanding of pathways to DVA and mental disorders, particularly in relation to DVA perpetration. It is also not clear how treatments need to be modified for DVA victims and perpetrators, nor how to prevent recurrent DVA. Future research needs to investigate the underlying mechanisms between DVA and mental disorders in both victims and perpetrators, develop and evaluate interventions to address these potential targets, and examine systemic interventions to improve responses of mental health services as a whole.

## Conclusions

DVA is an endemic problem in our society, but even more of an issue in psychiatric patients. Traditional training of psychiatrists has not included knowledge about DVA, and in view of the high rates of both DVA perpetrators and victims in psychiatric patients and the potential impact, this clearly needs to change. Current guidance is based on limited evidence, and further research is needed to improve the evidence base on identification and treatment of both victims and perpetrators.

### REFERENCES

1. Krug EG, Mercy JA, Dahlberg LL, Zwi AB. The world report on violence and health. *The Lancet*. 2002;360:1083–138.
2. World Health Organization and London School of Hygiene and Tropical Medicine. *Preventing Intimate Partner and Sexual Violence Against Women: Taking Action and Generating Evidence*. Geneva: World Health Organization; 2010.
3. Devries KM, Mak JY, Garcia-Moreno C, *et al*. Global health. The global prevalence of intimate partner violence against women. *Science*. 2013;340:1527–8.
4. Vos T, Astbury J, Piers L, *al*. Measuring the impact of intimate partner violence on the health of women in Victoria, Australia. *Bulletin of the World Health Organization*. 2006;84:739–44.
5. Walby S. *The Cost of Domestic Violence: Update 2009*. Lancaster: Lancaster University; 2009.
6. Home Office. *Information for Local Areas on the Change to the Definition of Domestic Violence*. London: Home Office; 2013.
7. Dutton MA, Goodman LA. Coercion in intimate partner violence: toward a new conceptualization. *Sex Roles*. 2005;52:743–56.
8. Johnson MP. Violence and abuse in personal relationships: conflict, terror, and resistance in intimate partnerships. In: Perlman ALVD, editor. *The Cambridge Handbook of Personal Relationships*. New York, NY: Cambridge University Press; 2006. pp. 557–76.
9. Coleman K, Jansson K, Kaiza P, Reed E. *Homicides, Firearms Offences and Intimate Violence 2005/6*. Home Office Statistical Bulletin. London: Home Office; 2007.

10. Donaldson A, Marshall L. *Domestic Abuse Prevalence: Argyll and Clyde DAP Study*. Glasgow: West Dunbartonshire Domestic Abuse Partnership; 2005.

11. Graham-Kevan N, Archer J. Intimate terrorism and common couple violence: a test of Johnson's predictions in four British samples. *Journal of Interpersonal Violence*. 2003;18:1247–70.

12. Johnson MP. Patriarchal terrorism and common couple violence: two forms of violence against women. *Journal of Marriage and Family*. 1995;57:283–94.

13. Kelly JB, Johnson MP. Differentiation among types of intimate partner violence: research update and implications for interventions. *Family Court Review*. 2008;46:476–99.

14. Ali PA, Dhingra K, McGarry J. A literature review of intimate partner violence and its classifications. *Aggression and Violent Behavior*. 2016;31:16–25.

15. Desmarais SL, Reeves KA, Nicholls TL, Telford RP, Fiebert MS. Prevalence of physical violence in intimate relationships, Part 2: Rates of male and female perpetration. *Partner Abuse*. 2012;3:170–98.

16. Office for National Statistics. *Focus on: Violent Crime and Sexual Offences, 2014/15*. London: Office for National Statistics; 2016.

17. Centers for Disease Control and Prevention. *Prevalence and Characteristics of Sexual Violence, Stalking, and Intimate Partner Violence Victimization—National Intimate Partner and Sexual Violence Survey, United States, 2011*. Atlanta, GA: Centers for Disease Control and Prevention; 2014.

18. Dodd T, Nicholas S, Povey D, Walker A. *Crime in England and Wales 2003/2004*. Statistical Bulletin, Home Office Research Development and Statistics Directorate. London: Home Office; 2004.

19. Howard LM, Trevillion K, Agnew-Davies R. Domestic violence and mental health. *International Review of Psychiatry*. 2010;22:525–34.

20. Walby S, Towers J, Francis B. Is violent crime increasing or decreasing? A new methodology to measure repeat attacks making visible the significance of gender and domestic relations. *British Journal of Criminology*. 2015;56:1203–34.

21. Ellsberg M, Jansen HAFM, Heise L, Watts CH, Garcia-Moreno C. Intimate partner violence and women's physical and mental health in the WHO multi-country study on women's health and domestic violence: an observational study. *The Lancet*. 2008;371:1165–72.

22. Garcia-Moreno C, Jansen HAFM, Ellsberg M, Heise L, Watts CH. Prevalence of intimate partner violence: findings from the WHO multi-country study on women's health and domestic violence. *The Lancet*. 2006;368:1260–9.

23. Alhabib S, Nur U, Jones R. Domestic violence against women: systematic review of prevalence studies. *Journal of Family Violence*. 2010;25:369–82.

24. Stöckl H, March L, Pallitto C, Garcia-Moreno C. Intimate partner violence among adolescents and young women: prevalence and associated factors in nine countries: a cross-sectional study. *BMC Public Health*. 2014;14:1–14.

25. Stöckl H, Penhale B. Intimate partner violence and its association with physical and mental health symptoms among older women in Germany. *Journal of Interpersonal Violence*. 2015;30:3089–111.

26. Tjaden P, Thoennes N. Prevalence and consequences of male-to-female and female-to-male intimate partner violence as measured by the National Violence Against Women Survey. *Violence Against Women*. 2000;6(2):142–61.

27. Coker AL, Davis KE, Arias I, *et al*. Physical and mental health effects of intimate partner violence for men and women. *American Journal of Preventive Medicine*. 2002;23:260–8.

28. Stöckl H, Devries K, Rotstein A, *et al*. The global prevalence of intimate partner homicide: a systematic review. *The Lancet*. 2013;382:859–65.

29. Barnish M. *Domestic Violence: A Literature Review*. London: HM Inspectorate of Probation; 2004.

30. World Health Organization. *Responding to Intimate Partner Violence and Sexual Violence Against Women: WHO Clinical and Policy Guidelines*. Geneva: World Health Organization; 2013.

31. Walby S, Allen J, Simmons J. *Domestic Violence, Sexual Assault and Stalking: Findings from the British Crime Survey*. London: Home Office Research, Development and Statistics Directorate; 2004.

32. Shorey RC, Ninnemann A, Elmquist J, *et al*. Arrest history and intimate partner violence perpetration in a sample of men and women arrested for domestic violence. *International Journal of Criminology and Sociology*. 2012;1:132.

33. Hines DA. Posttraumatic stress symptoms among men who sustain partner violence: an international multisite study of university students. *Psychology of Men and Masculinity*. 2007;8:225.

34. Holzworth-Munroe A. Male versus female partner violence: putting controversial findings in context. *Journal of Marriage and Family*. 2005;67:1120–5.

35. Randle AA, Graham CA. A review of the evidence on the effects of intimate partner violence on men. *Psychology of Men and Masculinity*. 2011;12:97–111.

36. Greenwood GL, Relf MV, Huang B, Pollack LM, Canchola JA, Catania JA. Battering victimization among a probability-based sample of men who have sex with men. *American Journal of Public Health*. 2002;92:1964–9.

37. Calton JM, Cattaneo LB, Gebhard KT. Barriers to help seeking for lesbian, gay, bisexual, transgender, and queer survivors of intimate partner violence. *Trauma, Violence, and Abuse*. 2016; 17(5):585–600.

38. Hester M, Donovan C. Researching domestic violence in same-sex relationships—a feminist epistemological approach to survey development. *Journal of Lesbian Studies*. 2009;13:161–73.

39. Kessler RC, Molnar BE, Feurer ID, Appelbaum M. Patterns and mental health predictors of domestic violence in the United States: results from the National Comorbidity Survey. *International Journal of Law and Psychiatry*. 2001;24:487–508.

40. Abramsky T, Watts CH, Garcia-Moreno C, *et al*. What factors are associated with recent intimate partner violence? Findings from the WHO multi-country study on women's health and domestic violence. *BMC Public Health*. 2011;11:1.

41. Khalifeh H, Howard LM, Osborn D, Moran P, Johnson S. Violence against people with disability in England and Wales: findings from a national cross-sectional survey. *PLoS One*. 2013;8:e55952.

42. Gass JD, Stein DJ, Williams DR, Seedat S. Gender differences in risk for intimate partner violence among South African adults. *Journal of Interpersonal Violence*. 2011;26:2764–89.

43. Ehrensaft MK, Cohen P, Brown J, Smailes E, Chen H, Johnson JG. Intergenerational transmission of partner violence: a 20-year prospective study. *Journal of Consulting and Clinical Psychology*. 2003;71:741.

44. Devries KM, Child JC, Bacchus LJ, *et al*. Intimate partner violence victimization and alcohol consumption in women: a systematic review and meta-analysis. *Addiction*. 2014;109:379–91.

45. Heise L, Garcia-Moreni C. Violence by intimate partners. In: Krug EG, Dahlberg LL, Mercy JA, Zwi AB, Lozano R, editors. *World Report on Violence and Health*. Geneva: World Health Organization; 2002. pp. 87–122.

46. Campbell JC. Health consequences of intimate partner violence. *The Lancet*. 2002;359:1331–6.

47. Flach C, Leese M, Heron J, et al. Antenatal domestic violence, maternal mental health and subsequent child behaviour: a cohort study. *BJOG*. 2011;118:1383–91.

48. Golding JM. Intimate partner violence as a risk factor for mental disorders: a meta-analysis. *Journal of Family Violence*. 1999;14:99–132.

49. Oram S, Trevillion K, Feder G, Howard LM. Prevalence of experiences of domestic violence among psychiatric patients: systematic review. *British Journal of Psychiatry*. 2013;202:94–9.

50. Bundock L, Howard LM, Trevillion K, Malcolm E, Feder G, Oram S. Prevalence and risk of experiences of intimate partner violence among people with eating disorders: a systematic review. *Journal of Psychiatric Research*. 2013;47:1134–42.

51. Howard LM, Oram S, Galley H, Trevillion K, Feder G. Domestic violence and perinatal mental disorders: a systematic review and meta-analysis. *PLoS Medicine*. 2013;10:e1001452.

52. Trevillion K, Oram S, Feder G, Howard LM. Experiences of domestic violence and mental disorders: a systematic review and meta-analysis. *PLoS One*. 2012;7:e51740.

53. Brown GW, Harris TO, Hepworth C, Robinson R. Clinical and psychosocial origins of chronic depressive episodes. II. A patient enquiry. *British Journal of Psychiatry*. 1994;165:457–65.

54. Ehrensaft MK, Moffitt TE, Caspi A. Is domestic violence followed by an increased risk of psychiatric disorders among women but not among men? A longitudinal cohort study. *American Journal of Psychiatry*. 2006;163:885–92.

55. Khalifeh H, Moran P, Borschmann R, et al. Domestic and sexual violence against patients with severe mental illness. *Psychological Medicine*. 2015;45:875–86.

56. Levendosky AA, Bogat GA, Martinez-Torteya C. PTSD symptoms in young children exposed to intimate partner violence. *Violence Against Women*. 2013;19:187–201.

57. Alisic E, Krishna RN, Groot A, Frederick JW. Children's mental health and well-being after parental intimate partner homicide: a systematic review. *Clinical Child and Family Psychology Review*. 2015;18:328–45.

58. Blair F, McFarlane J, Nava A, Gilroy H, Maddoux J. Child witness to domestic abuse: baseline data analysis for a seven-year prospective study. *Pediatric Nursing*. 2015;41:23.

59. Widom CS, Wilson HW. Intergenerational transmission of violence. In: Lindert J, Levav I, editors. *Violence and Mental Health: Its Manifold Faces*. New York, NY: Springer; 2015. pp. 27–45.

60. Zlotnick C, Johnson DM, Kohn R. Intimate partner violence and long-term psychosocial functioning in a national sample of American women. *Journal of Interpersonal Violence*. 2006;21:262–75.

61. Devries KM, Mak JY, Bacchus LJ, et al. Intimate partner violence and incident depressive symptoms and suicide attempts: a systematic review of longitudinal studies. *PLoS Medicine*. 2013;10:e1001439.

62. Khalifeh H, Dean K. Gender and violence against people with severe mental illness. *International Review of Psychiatry*. 2010;22:535–46.

63. Anderson F, Howard L, Dean K, Moran P, Khalifeh H. Childhood maltreatment and adulthood domestic and sexual violence victimisation among people with severe mental illness. *Social Psychiatry and Psychiatric Epidemiology*. 2016;51:961–70.

64. Sharhabani-Arzy R, Amir M, Kotler M, Liran R. The toll of domestic violence PTSD among battered women in an Israeli sample. *Journal of Interpersonal Violence*. 2003;18:1335–46.

65. Herman JL. Complex PTSD: a syndrome in survivors of prolonged and repeated trauma. *Journal of Traumatic Stress*. 1992;5:377–91.

66. Greenberg N, Brooks S, Dunn R. Latest developments in post-traumatic stress disorder: diagnosis and treatment. *British Medical Bulletin*. 2015;114:147–55.

67. American Psychiatric Association. *Diagnostic and Statistical Manual of Mental Disorders*, fifth edition. Arlington, VA: American Psychiatric Publishing; 2013.

68. Fazel S, Lichtenstein P, Grann M, Goodwin GM, Langstrom N. Bipolar disorder and violent crime: new evidence from population-based longitudinal studies and systematic review. *Archives of General Psychiatry*. 2010;67:931–8.

69. Fazel S, Wolf A, Chang Z, Larsson H, Goodwin GM, Lichtenstein P. Depression and violence: a Swedish population study. *The Lancet Psychiatry*. 2015;2:224–32.

70. Chang Z, Larsson H, Lichtenstein P, Fazel S. Psychiatric disorders and violent reoffending: a national cohort study of convicted prisoners in Sweden. *The Lancet Psychiatry*. 2015;2:891–900.

71. Oram S, Trevillion K, Khalifeh H, Feder G, Howard LM. Systematic review and meta-analysis of psychiatric disorder and the perpetration of partner violence. *Epidemiology and Psychiatric Sciences*. 2014;23:361–76.

72. Oram S, Flynn SM, Shaw J, Appleby L, Howard LM. Mental illness and domestic homicide: a population-based descriptive study. *Psychiatric Services*. 2013;64:1006–11.

73. Ullrich S, Keers R, Coid JW. Delusions, anger, and serious violence: new findings from the MacArthur Violence Risk Assessment Study. *Schizophrenia Bulletin*. 2014;40:1174–81.

74. Keers R, Ullrich S, DeStavola BL, Coid JW. Association of violence with emergence of persecutory delusions in untreated schizophrenia. *American Journal of Psychiatry*. 2014;171:332–9.

75. Fazel S, Zetterqvist J, Larsson H, Långström N, Lichtenstein P. Antipsychotics, mood stabilisers, and risk of violent crime. *The Lancet*. 2014;384:1206–14.

76. Moffitt TE, Robins RW, Caspi A. A couples analysis of partner abuse with implications for abuse-prevention policy. *Criminology and Public Policy*. 2001;1:5–36.

77. Ehrensaft MK, Moffitt TE, Caspi A. Clinically abusive relationships in an unselected birth cohort: men's and women's participation and developmental antecedents. *Journal of Abnormal Psychology*. 2004;113:258–70.

78. Coker AL, Weston R, Creson DL, Justice B, Blakeney P. PTSD symptoms among men and women survivors of intimate partner violence: the role of risk and protective factors. *Violence and Victims*. 2005;20:625–43.

79. Jonas S, Khalifeh H, Bebbington PE, et al. Gender differences in intimate partner violence and psychiatric disorders in England: results from the 2007 adult psychiatric morbidity survey. *Epidemiology and Psychiatric Sciences*. 2014;23:189–99.

80. Yearnshire S. *Analysis of Cohort. Violence Against Women*. London: Royal College of Obstetricians and Gynaecologists; 1997.

81. Trevillion K, Hughes B, Feder G, Borschmann R, Oram S, Howard LM. Disclosure of domestic violence in mental health settings: a qualitative meta-synthesis. *International Review of Psychiatry*. 2014;26:430–44.

82. Rose D, Trevillion K, Woodall A, Morgan C, Feder G, Howard L. Barriers and facilitators of disclosures of domestic violence by mental health service users: qualitative study. *British Journal of Psychiatry*. 2011;198:189–94.

83. Feder G, Ramsay J, Dunne D, et al. How far does screening women for domestic (partner) violence in different

health-care settings meet criteria for a screening programme? Systematic reviews of nine UK National Screening Committee criteria. *Health Technology Assessment*. 2009;13:iii–iv, xi–xiii, 1–113, 137–347.

84. Warshaw C, Sullivan CM, Rivera EA. *A Systematic Review of Trauma-Focused Interventions for Domestic Violence Survivors*. Chicago, IL: National Center on Domestic Violence, Trauma and Mental Health; 2013.

85. Wilson M, Daly M. Spousal homicide risk and estrangement. *Violence and Victims*. 1993;8:3.

86. Campbell JC, Webster D, Koziol-McLain J, et al. Risk factors for femicide in abusive relationships: results from a multisite case control study. *American Journal of Public Health*. 2003;93:1089–97.

87. Howard L, Trevillion K, Khalifeh H, Woodall A, Agnew-Davies R, Feder G. Domestic violence and severe psychiatric disorders: prevalence and interventions. *Psychological Medicine*. 2010;40:881–93.

88. National Institute for Health and Care Excellence. *Domestic Violence and Abuse: How Health Services, Social Care and the Organisations They Work With Can Respond Effectively*. London: National Institute of Health and Care Excellence; 2014.

89. Trevillion K, Byford S, Cary M, et al. Linking abuse and recovery through advocacy: an observational study. *Epidemiology and Psychiatric Sciences*. 2014;23:99–113.

90. Nyame S, Howard LM, Feder G, Trevillion K. A survey of mental health professionals' knowledge, attitudes and preparedness to respond to domestic violence. *Journal of Mental Health*. 2013;22:536–43.

91. National Institute for Health and Care Excellence. *Domestic Violence and Abuse: Multi-Agency Working*. London: National Institute for Health and Care Excellence; 2014.

92. Zaher E, Keogh K, Ratnapalan S. Effect of domestic violence training: systematic review of randomized controlled trials. *Canadian Family Physician*. 2014;60:618–24.

93. Feder G, Davies RA, Baird K, et al. Identification and Referral to Improve Safety (IRIS) of women experiencing domestic violence with a primary care training and support programme: a cluster randomised controlled trial. *The Lancet*. 2011;378:1788–95.

94. Trevillion K, Byford S, Cary M, et al. Linking abuse and recovery through advocacy: an observational study. *Epidemiology and Psychiatric Sciences*. 2014;23(1):99–113.

95. Stewart DE, Chabra PS. WPA international competency-based curriculum for mental health care providers on intimate partner violence and sexual violence against women. *World Psychiatry*. 2016;16:223–4.

96. Department of Health. *Domestic Violence and Abuse: Guidance for Health Professionals*. London: Department of Health; 2013.

97. Choi YJ, An S. Interventions to improve responses of helping professionals to intimate partner violence: a quick scoping review. *Research on Social Work Practice*. 2016;26:101–27.

98. Read J, Sampson M, Critchley C. Are mental health services getting better at responding to abuse, assault and neglect? *Acta Psychiatrica Scandinavica*. 2016;134:287–94.

99. Campbell JC, Glass N, Sharps PW, Laughon K, Bloom T. Intimate partner homicide review and implications of research and policy. *Trauma, Violence, and Abuse*. 2007;8:246–69.

100. Oram S, Carpon, S., Trevillion, K. *Promoting Recovery in Mental Health: Evaluation Report*. London: King's College London; 2016.

101. The National Confidential Inquiry. *The National Confidential Inquiry into Homicide and Suicide by People with Mental Illness. Annual Report 2014: England, Northen Ireland, Scotland, Wales*. Manchester: University of Manchester; 2014.

102. Flynn S, Gask L, Appleby L, Shaw J. Homicide–suicide and the role of mental disorder: a national consecutive case series. *Social Psychiatry and Psychiatric Epidemiology*. 2016;51:877–84.

103. Desmarais SL, Van Dorn RA, Johnson KL, Grimm KJ, Douglas KS, Swartz MS. Community violence perpetration and victimization among adults with mental illnesses. *American Journal of Public Health*. 2014;104:2342–9.

104. Stewart DE, Harriet MacMillan M. Intimate partner violence/ La violence entre partenaires intimes. *Canadian Journal of Psychiatry*. 2013;58:S1.

105. McCoy E, Butler N, Quigg Z. *Evaluation of the Liverpool Multi-Agency Risk Assessment Conference (MARAC)*. Liverpool: Centre for Public Health, Liverpool John Moores University; 2016.

106. Hegarty K, Taft A, Feder G. Violence between intimate partners: working with the whole family. *BMJ*. 2008;337:346.

107. HM Government. *Multi-Agency Statutory Guidance on Female Genital Mutilation*. London: Home Office; 2016.

108. Callaghan JE, Alexander JH, Sixsmith J, Fellin LC. Beyond 'Witnessing' children's experiences of coercive control in domestic violence and abuse. *Journal of Interpersonal Violence*. 2015. pii: 0886260515618946. [Epub ahead of print].

109. García-Moreno C, Hegarty K, d'Oliveira AF, Koziol-McLain J, Colombini M, Feder G. The health-systems response to violence against women. *The Lancet*. 2015;385:1567–79.

110. National Institute for Health and Care Excellence (NICE). (2018). *Post-traumatic stress disorder*. NICE guideline [NG116]. https://www.nice.org.uk/guidance/ng116

111. Jongh A, Resick PA, Zoellner LA, et al. Critical analysis of the current treatment guidelines for complex PTSD in adults. *Depression and Anxiety*. 2016;33:359–69.

112. Oram S, Khalifeh H, Howard LM. Violence against women and mental health. *The Lancet Psychiatry*. 2017;4(2):159–70.

113. Tirado-Muñoz J, Gilchrist G, Farré M, Hegarty K, Torrens M. The efficacy of cognitive behavioural therapy and advocacy interventions for women who have experienced intimate partner violence: a systematic review and meta-analysis. *Annals of Medicine*. 2014;46:567–86.

114. van den Berg DP, de Bont PA, van der Vleugel BM, et al. Trauma-focused treatment in PTSD patients with psychosis: symptom exacerbation, adverse events, and revictimization. *Schizophrenia Bulletin*. 2016;42:693–702.

115. van den Berg DP, de Bont PA, van der Vleugel BM, et al. Prolonged exposure vs eye movement desensitization and reprocessing vs waiting list for posttraumatic stress disorder in patients with a psychotic disorder: a randomized clinical trial. *JAMA Psychiatry*. 2015;72:259–67.

116. Kelly L, Westmarland N. *Domestic Violence Perpetrator Programmes: Steps Towards Change. Project Mirabel Final Report*. London and Durham: London Metropolitan University and Durham University; 2015.

# 144

# Assessing and managing the risk of violence to others

## Alec Buchanan

## Introduction

Assessing the risk of patient violence has always been integral to the practice of psychiatry. There are several reasons. Violence risk assessment is a necessary part of providing safe and effective outpatient psychiatric care. It is an essential element of proper decision-making around hospital admission and discharge and of providing a safe environment to patients and those who care for them. Finally, like many other aspects of psychiatric practice, when things go wrong, an inadequate assessment of violence risk is a potential source of legal liability for clinicians and mental health services.

While its importance is long-standing, the prominence of violence risk assessment has risen over the past 40 years. The most commonly identified causes for this increased prominence include the closure of many large psychiatric hospitals and discharge of patients to community settings, although empirical evidence linking this to an increase in violence is lacking. On both sides of the Atlantic, community care is widely regarded as inadequately resourced to manage the challenge of increased caseloads and challenging patient behaviour. Individuals and groups seeking to improve community care sometimes highlight violence rates in an attempt to highlight the need for increased resources.

These public, press, and political pressures are external. It is also the case, however, that over the past 40 years the focus of medicine itself has shifted. Public health indices, of which violence is one, have replaced the relationship between patient and doctor as the primary object of medical attention [1]. The value of screening clinics, vaccination, and antenatal care is now commonly assessed by reference to the health of the general population, not to the health of patients in care. Prevention of all types is now more than ever the province of medicine. As a recognized, if unusual, consequence of mental disorder, patient violence has become a recognized 'outcome measure'.

In some respects, psychiatry has been unprepared for this increased focus on the infrequent, but sometimes serious, violence of its clients. Throughout the developed world, bed closures have reduced the availability of psychiatry's principal tool in managing violence risk—admission to hospital. In the UK, proposals aimed at detaining people with personality disorders were justified by reference to doctors using 'loopholes' in existing legislation to discharge dangerous patients. In the United States, psychiatry has struggled to find a single path through the conflicting demands that patient confidentiality be respected and that potential victims and others be warned about risk. The primacy of the doctor–patient relationship, once unchallenged, is now seen as out of place in a world where a shrinking proportion of those in care see a doctor at each visit.

This chapter reviews the principles governing the assessment of violence risk in psychiatry. It discusses the practice of conducting such assessments and examines the limits of psychiatric violence risk assessment. In doing so, it draws on material published in previous reviews of risk assessment and management [2–4]. While not all psychiatric patient violence can be prevented, good practice in assessing violence risk is both a necessary element in ensuring the safety of patients and others and a vital aspect in the care of people with mental disorders.

## The principles of violence risk assessment

### Overview

Much violence risk assessment in psychiatry is invisible, carried out routinely by clinicians in the course of their work. Violence risk is one of many considerations that inform decisions that range from admitting a patient to hospital to deciding on the most appropriate form of outpatient care. Even when risk of harm to others becomes the principal focus of the doctor's interaction with his or her patient, the principles underlying its assessment are the same as those underlying psychiatric practice more generally. A good evaluation will usually be based on the results of obtaining a history and examining a patient's mental state.

Accurate assessment depends on the availability of accurate information. In violence risk assessment, this will usually include information obtained from collateral sources including medical records, informants, and, where the police have been involved, police reports. Assessments carried out at the point of admission to hospital are often brief and unresolved issues of risk require continued

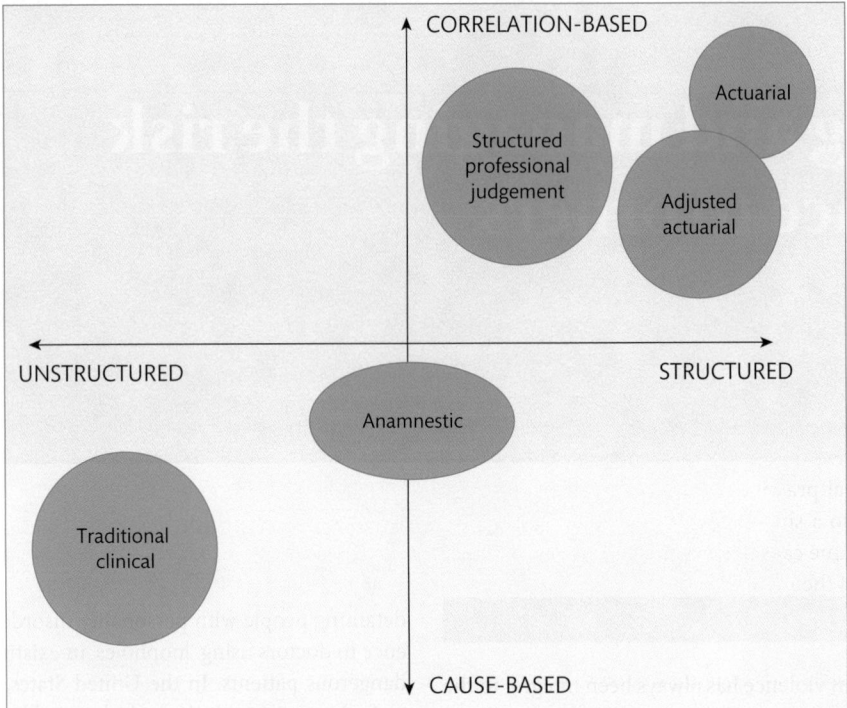

**Fig. 144.1** Approaches to violence risk assessment in psychiatry.
Reproduced from Buchanan A, Norko M, Violence risk in community settings. In: Buchanan A, Wootton L [Eds]., *Care of the Mentally Disordered Offender in the Community*, Second Edition, Copyright (2017), with permission from Oxford University Press.

attention in the course of an admission. Additional investigation, including psychological testing, may be required. Particularly with regard to specialist areas of practice, such as assessing the risk of sexual offending, it may be appropriate to ask specialist services, such as forensic psychiatry, to become involved.

The literature contains descriptions of numerous approaches to risk assessment. These approaches can usefully be described by virtue of where they fall on two dimensions. These dimensions are presented as the axes in Fig. 144.1.

The first dimension reflects whether a risk assessment method helps clinicians to assess risk by attending to known statistical correlations (sometimes referred to as a 'nomothetic' approach) or through a cause-based analysis of a client's behaviour (also known as an 'ideographic' method). The second dimension reflects the degree to which the approach provides a structure for the assessor to follow. Some risk assessment methods, including actuarial schemes, require the scoring of a prescribed list of items and the combining of a subject's scores on those items in a particular way. Other methods, particularly traditional clinical ones, permit the assessor greater discretion and, to this extent, provide less structure.

## Correlation and cause in risk assessment

Research findings from the past several decades have identified numerous factors associated with psychiatric patient violence. Psychiatric patients are, in some ways, like the general population in terms of what increases the risk for violent offending, and in other ways different. Among the psychiatric population, being male is less strongly associated with violence, first offences tend to occur later, risk reduces less with advancing age [5], and stable relationships

are not as protective, especially when individuals experience poor overall function [6–8].

There are also many similarities, in terms of risk factors, between psychiatric patients and the general population. Substance abuse is a significant risk factor, as are unemployment, living in a high-crime neighbourhood, and having antisocial peers. Violent crimes tend to be committed by young males. Recidivism is lower for violent and more serious crime than for non-violent crime. Criminal history is a particularly strong predictor [9–12].

A second way in which psychiatrists assess risk, in addition to looking for risk factors, is by comparing their understanding of the patient's personality, symptoms, and environment with their understanding of the likely causes of violence. Where someone suffers from persecutory delusions that concern their spouse, for instance, there will usually be available no empirical data from research conducted on samples of similar patients demonstrating a correlation between continued cohabitation and violence. Yet the clinician's understanding of the likely causes of violence may still allow him or her to conclude that continued cohabitation presents a risk [13].

Pollock described the processes involved:

'The skillful clinician assessing dangerous behavior formulates and tests a series of clinical hypotheses to define patterns of violence in the individual's history. Once defined, these patterns can be applied to the explanation and prediction of violence in that individual.' [14, p. 105]

Approaches to risk assessment based on explanations of this type seem to rely heavily on induction. They require the clinician to draw conclusions about the future from past observations. Future conditions will never exactly mimic the conditions in which behaviour has occurred in the past, yet the circumstances of other episodes of violence, whether in the patient's case or more generally, will usually be relevant and sometimes critical. Notwithstanding the uncertainty inherent in this process, one task of risk assessment is to determine the relevance of past patterns.

Clinicians trying to work out what might cause future violence are guided also by the understanding of patterns of behaviour that they develop in their training and through clinical practice [15, 16]. Claims that 'causal' ways of thinking are better than correlation-based ones at predicting rare events [17] have not been confirmed by empirical research. Instead, the persistence of causal approaches when clinicians think about risk may relate to the fact that many of the other judgements required in medicine are causation-based also—establishing why someone has symptoms, for instance, or deciding which further investigations are needed to complete an evaluation. Because clinical practice requires each of these judgements to be integrated into a single plan, it may be that clinicians find it helpful to use the same causal heuristic in assessing risk that they use in other aspects of their work.

### Structure in risk assessment

Although not frequently discussed in the literature on risk assessment, it is important to recognize that the cause-based analyses of many clinicians are structured. The structures are derived from their professional training. They include accepted practices and guidelines concerning taking a clinical history and examining the patient. Structure offers the same advantages to risk assessment that it offers to other areas of clinical practice. It is a means of integrating and communicating information [18]. It can be a useful aide-memoire, particularly when the clinical question being addressed is unusual (some risk factors apply particularly to sex offences, for instance). Learning how to structure the clinical approach is a key aspect of clinical training.

The correlation-based approach is most commonly structured using structured risk assessment instruments (SRAIs). Actuarial instruments, such as the Violence Risk Appraisal Guide (VRAG), formalize the process by which the simultaneous presence of more than one correlate of violence increases the perception of risk. They do this by rating variables, such as poor school adjustment and alcohol problems, and combining these mathematically to generate an overall score or category. A different type of instrument relies on 'structured professional judgement'. The Historical, Clinical Risk Management-20 (HCR-20), for instance, encourages the clinician to assess the relevance of a list of pre-identified variables, but also to take into account other information, including factors he or she considers unique to the case, before allocating a case to a risk category.

There are now a large number of such instruments [19]. Some of the most widely used are listed in Table 144.1. Using some of these instruments requires specialist training and experience, which are described in the references in Table 144.1.

Structured approaches to violence risk assessment have been shown to have greater predictive validity than unstructured ones when the follow-up period is measured in years [20, 21]. In the shorter term, unstructured predictions made by emergency room clinicians have been shown to have levels of accuracy comparable to that of structured instruments [22, 23].

The proven predictive validity of structured correlational approaches has not led to their unqualified clinical acceptance [24]. One person's structure is another's straitjacket. Clinicians complain

**Table 144.1** Structured risk assessment instruments

| Type, name, and reference | Target population |
| --- | --- |
| **Actuarial** | |
| VRAG [53] | General psychiatry, forensic |
| SORAG [53] | Sexual offenders |
| Static 99 [57] | Sexual offenders |
| COVR [58] | General psychiatry |
| PCL-R [59] | General psychiatry, forensic |
| PCL-SV [60] | General psychiatry, forensic |
| **Structured professional judgement** | |
| HCR-20 [61] | General and forensic |
| SARA [62] | Spousal assault |
| SVR-20 [63] | Sexual offenders |
| RSVP [64] | Sexual offenders |

Source: data from Buchanan A, Norko M, Violence risk assessment. In: Buchanan A, Norko M [Eds]., *The Psychiatric Report*, pp.224–239, Copyright (2011), Cambridge University Press; Buchanan A, Norko M, Violence risk in community settings. In: Buchanan A, Wootton L [Eds]., *Care of the Mentally Disordered Offender in the Community*, Second Edition, Copyright (2017), with permission from Oxford University Press.

that they have to respond both to risky circumstances not listed in an instrument and to mitigating factors such as the incapacitation through hospitalization or imprisonment of someone with a high actuarial score [25, 26]. One alternative would be to outline permissible exceptions, when the results of using a scale could be ignored, but this course has been opposed by the authors of some of the most accurate instruments [27]. A related clinicians' complaint is that it is difficult to use the score on a rating scale to guide treatment when research has yet to show whether treatment will change the score or whether the risk will then be less.

On the other hand, unstructured approaches to risk assessment may not integrate straightforwardly with other aspects of treatment, either. In addition, unstructured approaches are more vulnerable to cognitive biases, such as attending disproportionately to recent events, that afflict many of the judgements that people make [28], risk assessment included [29]. Finally, if the central task of risk assessment lies in establishing and quantifying statistical correlations, the arithmetic techniques contained in some structured approaches may be best suited to this task [30].

Criteria have been developed in other areas of medicine to establish whether a validated rating scale will be useful in an individual case [31]. Three are statistical: whether the confidence limits are acceptable; whether the scale works for all subgroups of subjects ('goodness of fit'); and whether its predictions are accurate. While the predictive accuracy of many instruments is uncontroversial, confidence intervals remain contentious [32, 33]. Non-statistical criteria are the degree to which the patient resembles patients in the validation study, the similarity between the outcome in the study and the outcome of interest to the clinician, and the availability to the clinician of data similar to those that were used in the study.

### Integration

Correlation-based approaches can indicate whether someone shares some characteristics with a high-risk group, but not whether they can properly be seen as representative of the group and what intervention is the most appropriate. Causation-based approaches can incorporate more kinds of information but offer no obvious mechanism whereby the psychiatrist can use data to compare the risk to that posed by other people. Because they offer different things, a risk assessment that makes use of both approaches is, at least in principle, in a better position to be helpful than one that chooses between them [34].

There is little agreement, however, as to how such integration might be achieved. One possibility is that the psychiatrist should proceed sequentially, first reviewing the established correlates of violence that are present and then using this review as a starting point for a cause-based analysis that makes use of the psychiatrist's understanding of the subject and his or her circumstances. Correlation-based approaches, after all, generate information that courts and others can usually obtain by other means, for instance from pre-sentence reports prepared by the probation service. In theory at least, causation-based approaches have the potential to provide something extra.

Three factors are likely to govern the extent to which they can do this in practice. The first is the degree to which the psychiatrist has had access to the patient's mental state. Only if someone is willing to discuss their feelings, intentions, and beliefs, can a clinician incorporate this information.

The second is whether circumstances may change. Where consideration is being given to treating in the community a patient who has recently acted violently, for instance, an evaluation that concentrates on identifying the population correlates of violence, such as past violence and age, is unlikely to be helpful. A more useful assessment may employ data concerning past behaviour and include a cause-based conclusion that focuses on the origins of recent violence and examines what has, and what has not, changed. Where the circumstances are dynamic, for instance when it is not known whether the subject of the evaluation will return to live with the partner he has abused, a cause-based approach that incorporates different plausible scenarios may be particularly helpful.

The third factor affecting the usefulness of a causation-based approach is the period over which the risk assessment will apply. In emergency settings, where an assessment is often required to cover days or weeks, there are few correlates to guide clinicians [35], although anger [36] and substance use [37] both seem to be important. Instead, a sound risk assessment is more likely to be based on an understanding of the likely effect on a patient of the circumstances to which they are being discharged. Assessments designed to apply over longer periods, on the other hand, are less able to rely on this kind of understanding because mental states, circumstances, and the sources of risk change. Unless they know what these changes will be, clinicians who wish to offer an estimate of risk designed to cover months or years have little choice but to concentrate on recognized risk factors, using either an unstructured approach or a recognized instrument.

## The practice of violence risk assessment

### Obtaining the background information

A number of factors that are identified in the course of taking a psychiatric history have been shown to be associated with future violence [38–42].

Table 144.2 lists those variables identified most frequently in psychiatric reviews. Because past violence is the strongest correlate of future violence, and because the risk of future violence increases with each subsequent offence [43], risk assessments should include details of the client's history of acting violently. The dates and types of violent act are important, because criminological variables, such as age of onset of violent behaviour and the number of violent convictions, are themselves correlates of future violence.

A cause-based analysis, however, will usually require more information. The circumstances of each act should be described in sufficient detail to allow the identification of patterns, if these exist. These circumstances include the individual's living situation, their relationship to the victim, what they intended to achieve, their mental state (and whether they were in treatment), and their use of drugs and alcohol. The nature of the victim's injury should be described; hospital treatment is often an indicator of severity. Collateral sources that can be of assistance in gathering this information include arrest records, police reports, trial transcripts, pre-sentence reports, and treatment records.

The association between substance use and violence is one of the most widely reported empirical findings in risk assessment. Moving beyond the statistical correlation to include a cause-based analysis requires that the assessor addresses the details of an individual's behaviour in relation to substances. Violence may be the result of intoxication, and past instances of violence when using substances should be noted. It may follow an exacerbation of mental illness precipitated by drug use, in which case the history may indicate previous instances of drug-induced relapse. Finally, violence may be a consequence of involvement in a drug market where territorial conflicts are common and where weapons are carried, although this is less of an issue for alcohol. The response of the subject to treatment for substance abuse problems will usually be important, especially in criminal sentencing.

The description of the past psychiatric history should make clear the relationship, if any, between an individual's history of violence and his mental disorder. The nature of any treatment, the individual's compliance with treatment, and his or her response to treatment will usually be important. The psychiatric history may also suggest what psychiatric measures have been helpful previously in reducing risk. The subject's social circumstances should be described for past episodes of violence (see earlier), for the present, and with reference to the period over which the risk assessment is required. Attention should be paid to the presence or absence of potentially protective factors such as stable relationships, employment, and housing. The availability of likely victims, including the victims of past violence, should be noted.

### Examining the mental state

The implications for violence risk of mental state abnormalities depend on the context. Where someone harbours delusions regarding an individual, for instance, the likelihood of their coming into contact with that individual and the likely nature of that contact are important. Pathological jealousy is likely to be managed differently if the jealous man plans to live with the wife he believes is being unfaithful. The mental state findings and circumstances most commonly listed by reviewers as associated with risk of harm to others [44–48] are listed in Table 144.3.

The weight that can be appropriately attached to mental state abnormalities depends also on the period over which the risk assessment is intended to apply. Some features listed in Table 144.3, such

**Table 144.2** Correlates I. Background factors and social circumstances linked to violence

| | Substantial correlate | Correlate | Protective |
|---|---|---|---|
| Sociodemographics | | Youth | |
| | | Male sex | |
| Past behaviour | History of violence if no change in person or circumstance | | |
| | Recent violence | | |
| | | History of threats not acted upon | |
| Psychiatric and substance abuse | Substance use, especially if rising | | |
| | | Conduct disorder | |
| Social circumstances | Availability of weapons, familiarity with their use | | |
| | | | Good social networks |
| | | Domestic conflict, especially if escalating | |
| | Future circumstances likely to resemble those in which violence has previously occurred | | |
| Traits | Hare psychopathy (Table 144.3) | | |
| | | Impulsiveness | |
| | | Feckless disregard for consequences in schizophrenia | |
| | | | Fear of own potential for violence |
| | | | Has demonstrated internal resources to cope with conflict |

Source: data from Buchanan A, Norko M, Violence risk assessment. In: Buchanan A, Norko M [Eds]., *The Psychiatric Report*, pp.224–239, Copyright (2011), Cambridge University Press; Buchanan A, Norko M, Violence risk in community settings. In: Buchanan A, Wootton L [Eds]., *Care of the Mentally Disordered Offender in the Community*, Second Edition, Copyright (2017), with permission from Oxford University Press.

**Table 144.3** Correlates II. Mental state features and interactions associated with risk of harm to others

| | Substantial correlate | Correlate | Protective |
|---|---|---|---|
| Mental state features (including recent behaviours) | Steps taken in preparation (obtaining weapons, surveillance, putting affairs in order) | | |
| | Threats creating fear and concern in people who know the person threatening | | |
| | | | Compliant with treatment |
| | | | Responding to treatment |
| | | | Perceives treatment as effective |
| | Violent thoughts or intentions | | |
| | Morbid jealousy where object of jealousy available | | |
| | Delusional systems focused on individuals seen as a threat or as obstructing an important goal | Delusions, particularly misidentification syndromes | |
| | | Clouding of consciousness and confusion | |
| | | | Insight into illness and need for treatment |
| Interactions | Depressed suicidal mothers of young children | | |
| | Suicidal seeking revenge | | |
| | Stalking with past violence | Stalking without past violence | |
| | Angry and threatening with a plan to cause harm | | |
| | Fearful with a plan to cause harm (may be pre-emptive) | | |

Source: data from Buchanan A, Norko M, Violence risk assessment. In: Buchanan A, Norko M [Eds]., *The Psychiatric Report*, pp.224–239, Copyright (2011), Cambridge University Press; Buchanan A, Norko M, Violence risk in community settings. In: Buchanan A, Wootton L [Eds]., *Care of the Mentally Disordered Offender in the Community*, Second Edition, Copyright (2017), with permission from Oxford University Press.

as threats, carry particular short-term significance. Others, such as those related to personality, will usually be more relevant when the assessment is intended to cover months or years.

The description of thought content should include reference to thoughts of violence and their quality. Obsessional thoughts concerning violence in the absence of psychotic symptoms are not unusual, and empirical research has not linked them to future violence. Command hallucinations have been described in association with violence, but the association is inconsistent, the empirical base limited and conflicting, and the implications at the population level uncertain [49]. As with other symptoms, a detailed analysis of past violence may nevertheless reveal their importance in an individual case. Violent thoughts that are pleasurable warrant particular concern and, when the pleasure has a sexual component, particular attention to the sexual history.

In describing a subject's insight into his or her past behaviour, a detailed description or verbatim account will usually be more helpful than a summary statement. 'Lack of remorse', in particular, can cover a range of phenomena, of which a general unwillingness to take responsibility probably carries fewer implications for future dangerousness than a sense of self-justification, the persistence of a grudge, or a reference to unfinished business [50]. A subject's willingness to address the causes of violence should be assessed in the light of their response to previous interventions. Ambivalence may not always have prevented successful treatment.

### Psychological testing

Psychological testing contributes to the assessment of violence risk in community settings in several respects. Firstly, the testing of personality and cognitive function can contribute to an understanding of the reasons behind an act of violence, for instance when neuropsychological testing demonstrates impaired executive function secondary to a head injury.

Secondly, some tests of personality and general psychological functioning serve as risk assessments in their own right. Of these, the best known is the Hare Psychopathy Checklist [51], which has been shown consistently to predict acts of physical violence with a level of accuracy comparable with that of the other structured instruments listed in Table 144.1 [52]. The personality traits identified include a number of negative markers encompassing inflated senses of self-worth, devious and manipulative attitudes towards others, behavioural problems, and lifestyle characteristics.

Thirdly, the understanding of someone's personality structure that testing can sometimes offer can be a valuable aid to community management, particularly when it helps the clinician to understand what aspects of their family and social environment people find most threatening, and why. Fourthly, a patient's history may indicate a need for specialized assessments such as assessments of sex-offending risk. These may need to be repeated at regular intervals, either for clinical reasons or because a court imposes such evaluations as a condition of someone remaining in the community.

Finally, a range of other investigations may be made necessary by particular aspects of a patient's case. Occupational assessments offer particular insights into the stresses that may affect a patient moving from institutional care to the community, and into possible ways of addressing these. Neurological investigation and treatment will be an enduring component of the care of some patients. One of

the tasks of the team providing care, whether they carry the label of forensic or general psychiatry, is to ensure that physical health needs are adequately met. Some of those health needs are generated by the same medications that allow some patients to remain in the community.

## The limits to risk assessment

In conducting any assessment of violence risk, it is important to bear in mind the levels of accuracy that can be expected. Those levels of accuracy are not simple to describe. One approach is to ask: if a particular structured instrument was used as a screening test and those identified as likely to be violent were not discharged, over any given period, how many patients would need to be detained to prevent one unwanted act? This statistic—the number needed to detain (NND) [51]—is the inverse of the positive predictive value (PPV) and analogous to the 'number needed to treat'. Used as a screening test where the base rate of violence is 10% and where, as a result, an unselective approach would lead to the detention of ten people in order to prevent one from acting violently, the VRAG (Table 144.1) would require the detention of five people to achieve the same end [52].

Other structured instruments could be expected to perform similarly. Unstructured approaches have been less studied, but what research does exist does not suggest that they fare better. More importantly, for risk assessments conducted in everyday clinical settings the NND rises as the prevalence falls [53]. One consequence is that the number of mistakes rises when unusual acts, such as serious acts of violence, are sought to be prevented. At the base rate recorded in the Epidemiologic Catchment Area (ECA) study, where 17% of the sample self-reported violence in the previous 12 months, the NND to prevent an act of violence is 3.5 [54]. The outcome measure in the ECA study did not require injury. When injury is required, the base rate falls. In the Clinical Antipsychotic Trials of Intervention Effectiveness (CATIE) study, the 6-month prevalence of assault with a weapon or causing serious injury was 3.6% [55]. Here, the NND at a sensitivity of 0.73 and a specificity of 0.63 is 15.

Data such as these have been used in the past to support statements to the effect that psychiatrists 'can' or 'cannot' distinguish which of their patients will act violently. This is to miss the point. There is no threshold of accuracy at which psychiatric risk assessment becomes possible or not possible. Instead, assessments of violence risk are just some of the numerous pieces of information that clinicians use to manage a case. Good assessments are more helpful in this regard than poor ones, and good assessments do not simply seek to be accurate, but also seek to inform clinical management.

## Conclusions

The limits to the accuracy of what can be achieved represent one reason why violence risk assessment will usually be one factor, among many, that clinicians consider in the course of managing a case. Particularly where a patient has a history of violence or has stated a desire to harm, however, violence risk assessments will remain an essential part of clinical practice. Specialist advice will sometimes be necessary.

It is likely that the most helpful psychiatric violence risk assessments make use of both known statistical correlations and causal explanations. As one author put it:

'By supplementing a knowledge of relevant risk factors with a detailed examination of an individual's mental state, it may be possible to build up some picture of the calculus of reasons on which that individual's future actions may be based and in this way to give a more precise prediction . . . ' [56, p. 70].

The author went on to point out that the more an action is dominated by some overriding preoccupation or delusion, the more precise will be a prediction. He also pointed out, however, that however detailed our understanding of someone's calculus of reasons, we usually cannot predict with any certainty what they will do, or when.

While the ability to inform clinical decisions is not the same as predictive accuracy, the accuracy of violence predictions is important in helping clinicians decide which approach to risk assessment they should use. Research over the past 40 years has demonstrated a modest improvement in the level of accuracy that can be achieved using structured risk assessment instruments. As those instruments are further refined and developed, further research may show that they are capable of levels of accuracy beyond those that can currently be achieved. This work should be complemented by research on the cause-based approaches to risk assessment that remain widespread in clinical practice. Finally, research should examine the ways in which correlational and causal approaches can most helpfully be combined.

## Acknowledgements

The author acknowledges the assistance of collaborators in the empirical and theoretical work cited here: Renee Binder, Morven Leese, Michael Norko, and Marvin Swartz.

## REFERENCES

1. Le Fanu J (2012). *The Rise and Fall of Modern Medicine*. Basic Books: New York, NY.
2. Buchanan A, Norko M (2011). Violence risk assessment. In: A Buchanan, M Norko, editors. *The Psychiatric Report*, pp. 224–39. Cambridge University Press: Cambridge.
3. Buchanan A, Binder R, Norko M, Swartz M (2012). *Resource Document on Psychiatric Violence Risk Assessment*. American Psychiatric Association: Washington, DC.
4. Buchanan A, Norko M (2017). Violence risk in community settings. In: A Buchanan, L Wootton, editors. *Care of the Mentally Disordered Offender in the Community*, second edition. Oxford University Press: Oxford.
5. Häfner H, Boker W (1973). *Crimes of Violence by Mentally Disordered Offenders*. Cambridge University Press: Cambridge.
6. McNiel D, Binder R, Greenfield T (1988). Predictors of violence in civilly committed acute psychiatric patients. *American Journal of Psychiatry* 145: 965–70.
7. Mullen P (1997). Assessing risk of interpersonal violence in the mentally ill. *Advances in Psychiatric Treatment* 3: 166–73.
8. Swanson J, Swartz M, Estroff S, Borum R, Wagner R, Hiday V (1998). Psychiatric impairment, social contact, and violent behavior: evidence from a study of outpatient-committed persons with severe mental disorder. *Social Psychiatry and Psychiatric Epidemiology* 33: S86–94.
9. Bonta J, Law M, Hanson K (1998). The prediction of criminal and violent recidivism among mentally disordered offenders: a meta-analysis. *Psychological Bulletin* 123: 123–42.
10. Fisher W, Silver E, Wolff N (2006). Beyond criminalization: toward a cirminologically informed framework for mental health policy and services research. *Administration and Policy in Mental Health and Mental Health Services Research* 33: 544–57.
11. Skeem J, Manchak S, Peterson J (2011). Correctional policy for offenders with mental illness; creating a new paradigm for recidivism reduction. *Law and Human Behaviour* 35: 110–26.
12. Peterson J, Skeem J, Kennealy P, Bray B, Zvonkovic A (2014). How often and how consistently do symptoms directly precede criminal behaviour among offenders with mental illness? *Law and Human Behaviour* 38: 439–49.
13. Marra H, Konzelman G, Giles P (1987). A clinical strategy to the assessment of dangerousness. *International Journal of Offender Therapy and Comparative Criminology* 31: 291–9.
14. Pollock N, McBain I, Webster C (1989). Clinical decision making and the assessment of dangerousness. In: K Howells, C Hollin, editors. *Clinical Approaches to Violence*, pp. 89–115. John Wiley: Chichester.
15. Garb H (1998). *Studying the Clinician: Judgment Research and Psychological Assessment*. American Psychological Association: Washington, DC.
16. Skeem J, Mulvey E, Lidz C (2000). Building mental health professionals' decisional models into tests of predictive validity: the accuracy of contextualized predictions of violence. *Law and Human Behavior* 24: 607–28.
17. Sreenivasan S, Korkish P, Garrick T, Weinberger L, Phenix A (2000). Actuarial risk assessment models: a review of critical issues related to violence and sex-offender recidivism assessments. *Journal of the American Academy of Psychiatry and the Law* 28: 438–48.
18. Skeem J, Golding S, Cohn N, Berge G (1998). Logic and reliability of evaluations of competence to stand trial. *Law and Human Behavior* 22: 519–47.
19. Singh J, Fazel S (2010) Forensic risk assessment. A metareview. *Criminal Justice and Behavior* 37: 965–88.
20. Grove W, Meehl P (1996). Comparative efficiency of informal (subjective, impressionistic) and formal (mechanical, algorithmic) prediction procedures: the clinical-statistical controversy. *Psychology, Public Policy and Law* 12: 293–323.
21. Grove W, Zald D, Lebow B, Snitz B, Nelson C (2000). Clinical versus mechanical prediction: a meta-analysis. *Psychological Assessment* 12: 19–30.
22. Lidz C, Mulvey E, Gardner W (1993). The accuracy of predictions of violence to others. *JAMA* 269: 1007–11.
23. Mossman D (1994). Assessing predictions of violence: being accurate about accuracy. *Journal of Consulting and Clinical Psychology* 62: 783–92.
24. Litwack T (2001). Actuarial versus clinical assessments of dangerousness. *Psychology, Public Policy and Law* 7: 409–43.
25. Rogers R (2000). The uncritical acceptance of risk assessment in forensic practice. *Law and Human Behavior* 24: 595–605.
26. Glancy G (2006). Caveat usare: actuarial schemes in real life. *Journal of the American Academy of Psychiatry and the Law* 34: 272–5.
27. Quinsey V, Harris G, Rive M, Cormier C (2006). *Violent Offenders. Appraising and Managing Risk*, second edition. American Psychiatric Association: Washington, DC.

28. Kahneman D, Slovic P, Tversky A, editors (1982). *Judgment Under Uncertainty: Heuristics and Biases*. Cambridge University Press: New York, NY.

29. Shah S (1978). Dangerousness. A paradigm foe exploring some issues in law and psychology. *American Psychologist* 33, 224–38.

30. Sarbin T (1943). A contribution to the study of actuarial and individual methods of prediction. *American Journal of Sociology* 48, 593–602.

31. Braitman L, Davidoff F (1996). Predicting clinical states in individual patients. *Annals of Internal Medicine* 125, 406–12.

32. Hart S, Michie C, Cooke D (2007). Precision of actuarial risk assessment instruments. Evaluating the 'margins of error' of group v. individual predictions of violence. *British Journal of Psychiatry* 190: s60–5.

33. Mossman D, Sellke T (2007). Avoiding errors about 'margins of error'. *British Journal of Psychiatry* 191: 561.

34. Skeem J, Mulvey E (2002). Assessing the risk of harm posed by mentally disordered offenders being treated in the community. In: A Buchanan, editor. *Care of the Mentally Disordered Offender in the Community*, pp. 111–42. Oxford University Press: Oxford.

35. Douglas K, Skeem J (2005). Violence risk assessment: getting specific about being dynamic. *Psychology, Public Policy and Law* 11: 347–83.

36. Skeem J, Schubert C, Odgers C, Mulvey E, Gardner W, Lidz C (2006). Psychiatric symptoms and community violence among high-risk patients: a test of the relationship at the weekly level. *Journal of Consulting and Clinical Psychology* 74: 967–79.

37. Mulvey E, Odgers C, Skeem J, Gardner W, Schubert C, Lidz C (2006). Substance use and community violence: a test of the relation at the daily level. *Journal of Consulting and Clinical Psychology* 74: 743–54.

38. Monahan J (1985). Evaluating potentially violent persons. In: C Ewing, editor. *Psychology, Psychiatry and the Law: A Clinical and Forensic Handbook*, pp. 9–39. Professional Resource Exchange: Sarasota, FL.

39. Otto R (2000). Assessing and managing violence risk in outpatient settings. *Journal of Clinical Psychology* 56: 1239–62.

40. Mullen P (1997). Assessing risk of interpersonal violence in the mentally ill. *Advances in Psychiatric Treatment* 3: 166–73.

41. Bonta J, Law M, Hanson K (1998). The prediction of criminal and violent recidivism among mentally disordered offenders: a meta-analysis. *Psychological Bulletin* 123: 123–42.

42. Skeem J, Mulvey E (2002). Assessing the risk of harm posed by mentally disordered offenders being treated in the community. In: A Buchanan, editor. *Care of the Mentally Disordered Offender in the Community*, pp. 111–42. Oxford University Press: Oxford.

43. Walker N, Hammond W, Steer D (1967). Repeated violence. *Criminal Law Review* 465–73.

44. Monahan J (1985). Evaluating potentially violent persons. In: C Ewing, editor. *Psychology, Psychiatry and the Law: A Clinical and Forensic Handbook*, pp. 9–39. Professional Resource Exchange: Sarasota, FL.

45. Otto R (2000). Assessing and managing violence risk in outpatient settings. *Journal of Clinical Psychology* 56: 1239–62.

46. Mullen P (1997). Assessing risk of interpersonal violence in the mentally ill. *Advances in Psychiatric Treatment* 3: 166–73.

47. Bonta J, Law M, Hanson K (1998). The prediction of criminal and violent recidivism among mentally disordered offenders: a meta-analysis. *Psychological Bulletin* 123: 123–42.

48. Skeem J, Mulvey E (2002). Assessing the risk of harm posed by mentally disordered offenders being treated in the community. In: A Buchanan, editor. *Care of the Mentally Disordered Offender in the Community*, pp. 111–42. Oxford University Press: Oxford.

49. Junginger J, McGuire L (2004). Psychotic motivation and the paradox of current research on serious mental illness and rates of violence. *Schizophrenia Bulletin* 30: 21–30.

50. Grounds A (1995). Risk assessment and management in clinical context. In: J Crichton, editor. *Psychiatric Patient Violence. Risk and Response*, pp. 43–59. Duckworth: London.

51. Buchanan A, Leese M (2001). Detention of people with dangerous severe personality disorders. *The Lancet* 358: 1955–9.

52. Buchanan A (2008). Risk of violence by psychiatric patients: beyond the 'actuarial versus clinical' assessment debate. *Psychiatric Services* 59: 184–90.

53. Quinsey V, Harris G, Rice M, Cormier C (2006). *Violent Offenders: Appraising and Managing Risk*, second edition. American Psychological Association: Washington, DC.

54. Swanson J, Holzer C, Ganju V, *et al.* (1990). Violence and psychiatric disorder in the community: evidence from the Epidemiologic Catchment Area surveys. *Hospital and Community Psychiatry* 41: 761–70.

55. Swanson J, Swartz M, Van Dorn R, *et al.* (2006). A national study of violent behavior in persons with schizophrenia. *Archives of General Psychiatry* 63: 490–9.

56. Howard C (1991). The individual's calculus of reasons: forensic psychiatry and science. *Psychiatric Bulletin Supplement* 4: 70.

57. Hanson R, Thornton D (1999). *Static 99: Improving Actuarial Risk Assessments for Sex Offenders*. Department of the Solicitor General of Canada: Ottawa.

58. Monahan J, Steadman H, Appelbaum P, *et al.* (2006). The classification of violence risk. *Behavioral Sciences and the Law* 24: 721–30.

59. Hare E (1991). *The Revised Psychopathy Checklist*. Multi-Health Systems: Toronto.

60. Hart S, Cox D, Hare R (1995). *The Hare Psychopathy Checklist: Screening Version (PCL:SV)*. Multi-Health Systems: Toronto.

61. Webster C, Douglas K, Eaves D, Hart S (1997). *HCR-20: Assessing Risk for Violence (Version 2)*. Mental Health, Law, and Policy Institute, Simon Fraser University: Vancouver.

62. Kropp P, Hart S, Webster C, Eaves D (1999). *Manual for the Spousal Assault Risk Assessment Guide*, third edition. Multi-Health Systems: Toronto.

63. Boer D, Hart S, Kropp P, Webster C (1997). *Manual for the Sexual Violence Risk—20: Professional Guidelines for Assessing Risk of Sexual Violence*. British Columbia Institute Against Family Violence: Vancouver.

64. Hart S, Kropp P, Laws R (2004). *The Risk for Sexual Violence Protocol (RSVP)*. Mental Health, Law, and Policy Institute, Simon Fraser University: Burnaby.

# 145

# The expert witness in the criminal and civil courts

*John O'Grady*

## Introduction

As an expert witness in court, the psychiatrist ceases to be simply a doctor, as a psychiatrist's report and testimony address issues on the boundary between law and psychiatry. The law is not primarily concerned with the welfare of the defendant. Criminal law is concerned with justice, fact-finding, and the attribution of guilt, while psychiatry concerns itself with the welfare of the individual, their mental disorder, and its treatment. This chapter will explore the legal framework for expert reports and testimony, expert witness standards, and an ethical framework for practice and will provide practical guidance on the preparation of reports and testimony.

Expert witness reports and testimony can only be usefully discussed within the legal framework of a particular jurisdiction. This chapter will discuss expert witness evidence in the context of jurisdictions based on common law (UK, Ireland, United States, Canada, and New Zealand). The legal framework for expert witness evidence in England and Wales is used as the primary jurisdiction, but the discussion will be applicable to other common law areas. While civil law jurisdictions (most of Europe) manage expert evidence differently from common law jurisdictions, both share concerns about admissibility, reliability, and impartiality of expert witness evidence. The focus of this chapter is on expert testimony in criminal courts, but the chapter will also discuss how expert evidence is handled in civil courts.

## Expert psychiatric evidence

Witnesses in court can only give evidence of facts they personally perceived, and not evidence of their opinion. The opinion of an expert witness is an exclusion to this general rule, because the court needs the assistance of experts to consider issues beyond their knowledge. The judge, whether sitting alone or in a jury trial, acts as gatekeeper on whether expert evidence is admissible. In criminal courts, it is for the jury to draw inferences from, and adduce weight to, the evidence. In the absence of a jury, the judge decides both on admissibility of, and weight accorded to, expert evidence [1–4].

## Miscarriages of justice and development of rules governing expert evidence

All jurisdictions have had miscarriages of justice attributed, at least in part, to poor-quality expert evidence. Two cases in the English jurisdiction—*R v Clark* and *R v Cannings*—concerned miscarriages of justice where medical evidence influenced the court's decision. Both cases concerned two infant deaths in the same family due to sudden infant death syndrome. An expert paediatrician gave evidence that there was only a 1:73 million chance of such deaths in the same family in the absence of a genetic or an environmental cause, thereby implying that the alternative proposition, that of deliberate killing, was more likely (see The prosecutor's fallacy, p. 1472). Both the statistical methodology and assumptions proved faulty, and both mothers were acquitted on appeal. The appeal court was critical of the expert medical evidence. The expert was not a trained statistician and had not consulted a trained statistical colleague before giving his opinion, thereby straying beyond his area of expertise. The opinion was dogmatic, that is, was a view based on a hypothesis not sufficiently scrutinized or supported by empirical evidence and did not give sufficient weight to conflicting views. The appeal court was concerned that the criminal court had been swayed by the aura of expertise and infallibility of the expert and had not critically appraised the reliability of the expert's evidence. These themes will be picked up in the rest of this section.

### Case law and expert witnesses

Two landmark cases from the United States—*Frye* and *Daubert*—have become highly influential in developing case law on expert testimony across jurisdictions. The English courts have cited and amended a judgement in the Australian courts (in turn, citing Frye and Daubert) *Bonython* and decided upon four criteria to be considered by the court in deciding the admissibility and reliability of expert evidence:

1. Whether the subject matter of expert evidence is beyond the 'common knowledge' of judge and jury, making such evidence necessary to the court to be able to form a sound judgement on that subject matter.

2. Whether the expert's evidence forms 'part of a body of knowledge that is sufficiently organized or recognized to be acceptable as a reliable body of knowledge or experience', thereby making the expert evidence of special assistance to the court.

3. Whether the expert has 'acquired by study or experience sufficient knowledge of the subject' to render his or her opinion of value to the court.

4. Whether the expert can demonstrate that they provide an impartial opinion, recognizing the expert's duty is to the court.

By rigorously applying these four criteria to expert evidence, courts strive to ensure scientific evidence does not contribute to miscarriages of justice.

### Common knowledge

Lawton L. J. in *R v Turner* established a 'common knowledge' rule governing expert evidence, specifically psychiatric evidence in this case, as follows:

> 'An expert opinion is admissible to furnish the Courts with scientific information which is likely to be outside the experience and knowledge of a Judge or a jury. If on the proven fact, a Judge or jury can form their own conclusions without help, then the opinion of an expert is unnecessary. In such a case if it given dressed up in scientific jargon it may make judgement more difficult. The facts that an expert witness has impressive scientific qualifications does not by that fact alone make his opinion on matters of human nature and behaviour within the limits of normality any more helpful than that of the jurors themselves; but there is a danger that they may think it does … jurors do not need psychiatrists to tell them how ordinary folk who are not suffering from any mental illness are likely to react to the stresses and strains of life.'

This seems to limit psychiatric evidence to recognized mental disorder [as in the *Diagnostic and Statistical Manual of Mental Disorders*, fifth edition (DSM-5) and the *International Classification of Diseases*, tenth revision (ICD-10)]. However, expert advice is allowed which is 'outside the experience and knowledge of a judge or jury'. The abnormal/normal dichotomy is not a rule of law, but guidance. Courts have allowed evidence on a variety of conditions which would not normally be thought of as an established mental disorder, for example 'battered women's syndrome'.

Particular problems arise for the court in respect of borderline conditions falling short of a recognized mental disorder. Here admissibility will be determined by the court's judgement as to whether the expert evidence addresses matters outside the experience or knowledge of a judge or jury. The psychiatrist will have other knowledge of assistance to the court such as assessing the risk associated with a mental disorder or providing an opinion on professional standards to be applied in cases of medical negligence. Such evidence will be deemed admissible.

Even if the evidence meets this test, the court has discretion to render it inadmissible, for example if the court deems it prejudicial or misleading.

### Body of knowledge

The second limb concerns itself with the reliability of expert testimony. Given that the court will have decided that the evidence is 'outside the experience and knowledge', it faces an inevitable dilemma in reaching a judgement as to its reliability when, by definition, it lacks the scientific knowledge to do so. Recognizing this dilemma, courts have sought tests that can be applied to determine this issue.

The most stringent is the test arrived at by the court in the United States in *Daubert v Merrell Dow Pharmaceuticals*, namely that '*the technique, body of knowledge, or theory can be tested; has been subjected to peer review and publication; has a known rate of error; is subject to maintenance of standards and controls and is generally accepted by the scientific community*'. English courts have been reluctant to adopt this test, as its stringent criteria could rule out consideration of expert evidence, based on novel or developing science for which there may be no definitive peer review and which may not be accepted fully by the wider scientific community. Psychiatric evidence derives from scientific evidence, but also from expert consensus and experience—based on knowledge, and thereby not likely to meet the Daubert test. The Law Commission [5] considers expert evidence to be a continuum between experience-based evidence and narrowly scientific evidence and recommended that the criteria applied to expert evidence be flexible enough to be able to encompass this continuum. A phrase that recurs often in addressing reliability is that the evidence should be 'soundly based', such that simply stating 'in my clinical experience…' would not be sufficient to be classed as soundly based, and courts should be mindful of the trap of accepting dubious scientific evidence on the basis of prestige and professional standing of the witness.

The Law Commission [5] considered the problem, concluded that the common law approach to the admissibility of expert witness evidence is one of laissez-faire, and recommended instead that a test of reliability be placed on a statutory basis. The Commission [5] was particularly concerned that without such a statutory test, there would be a 'danger that juries will abdicate their duty to ascertain and weigh the facts and simply accept the expert's own opinion evidence, particularly if the evidence is complex and difficult for a non-specialist to understand and evaluate'. The government was reluctant to limit the discretion of the court in admitting evidence and instead issued a practice direction [6] to the courts, with detailed guidance on criteria to be applied to expert scientific evidence to decide upon its reliability. This practice direction is reproduced in Box 145.1. Rule 702 of Federal Rules of Evidence (United States) [7] likewise provides judges with guidance.

The leading textbook on expert evidence in the UK [1] concludes 'English judges now have the benefit of the most comprehensive guidance in the common law world as to how the reliability of expert evidence should be assessed'. This guidance (Box 145.1) should be understood and applied by psychiatric experts to their reports and could form the structured criteria by which reports are subjected to peer review case conferencing.

### Acquired by study or experience

In English law, there is no statutory definition of what constitutes an expert. In *R v Bunnis*, the court stated that an expert is 'one who has by dint of training or practice acquired a good knowledge of the science concerning which his opinion is sought'. Rule 702 of the Federal Rules of Evidence (United States) [7] defines an expert as 'a witness qualified as an expert by knowledge, skill, expertise or training'. As psychiatry is a recognized specialty within medicine, which, in

## Box 145.1 Criminal Practice Directions 2015 [6]

19A Factors which the court may take into account when determining the reliability of expert opinion, and especially of expert scientific opinion, include:

1. Extent and quality of the data on which the expert's opinion is based and the validity of the methods by which they were obtained.
2. If the expert opinion relies on an inference from any findings, whether the opinion properly explains how safe or unsafe the inference is (whether by reference to statistical significance or other appropriate terms).
3. If the expert's opinion relies on the results of any method (for instance, a test, measurement, or survey), whether the opinion takes proper account of matters such as the degree of precision or margin of uncertainty affecting the accuracy or reliability of those results.
4. The extent to which any material upon which the expert opinion is based has been reviewed by others with relevant expertise (for instance, in peer-reviewed publications) and the views of those others on that material.
5. The extent to which the expert opinion is based on material falling outside the expert's own field of expertise.
6. The completeness of the information which was available to the expert and whether the expert took account of all relevant information in arriving at the opinion (including information as to the context of any facts to which the opinion relates).
7. If there is a range of expert opinion on the matter in question, where in the range the expert's opinion lies and whether the expert's preference has been properly explained.
8. Whether the expert's methods followed established practice in the field and, if they did not, whether the reason for the divergence has been properly explained.

In addition, the court should be astute to identify potential flaws in such opinion which detract from its reliability such as:

1. Being based on a hypothesis which has not been subjected to sufficient scrutiny or which has failed to stand up to scrutiny;
2. Being based on an unjustifiable assumption;
3. Being based on flawed data;
4. Relying on an examination, technique, method, or process which has not been properly carried out or applied, or was not appropriate for use in the particular case; or
5. Relying on an inference or conclusion which has not been properly reached.

turn, is accepted as a scientific discipline, psychiatrists who have completed recognized training, are members of their professional body, adhere to standards of professional practice laid down by their regulatory body, and hold registration in the area of psychiatry they practise should have no difficulty in being accepted as an expert by the court.

When giving evidence based on novel or developing science or practice or where the opinion is experience-based, the expert should be in a position to demonstrate practical knowledge or have conducted research in the relevant science or practice and be careful not to give evidence outside their professional knowledge or practice. The UK regulatory body the General Medical Council (GMC) provides the following guidance: '*You must only give expert testimony and opinions about issues that are within your professional competence or about which you have relevant knowledge including, for example, knowledge of the standards and nature of practice at the time of the incident or events that are the subject of the proceedings. If a particular question or issue falls outside your area of expertise, you should* either refuse to answer or answer to the best of your ability but make it clear that you consider the matter to be outside your competence' [8].

### Impartial evidence

Courts have, over time, defined what is expected of an expert witness. The landmark case is that of the *Ikarian Reefer*. In *Field v Leeds City Council*, the judge stated that the expert witness 'should provide independent assessment to the court by way of objective unbiased opinion'. These and other judgements have led to the overriding principle governing expert evidence being that the expert's obligation is to the court, and not to whoever has instructed them. All other standards flow from that overriding obligation.

Case law judgements on expert evidence have been drawn together into sets of Rules governing expert witnesses in court. In England and Wales, three sets of Rules have emerged:

1. Civil Procedure Rules (CPR), Rule 35 [9].
2. Criminal Procedure Rules (CrPR), Part 19 [10].
3. Family Procedure Rules (FPR) [11].

In the United States, expert evidence is governed by Federal Rules of Evidence [7] and in Australia by the Australian Evidence Act [12].

Psychiatrists are, in addition, subject to standards set out by their professional and licensing bodies [8, 13, 14].

Box 145.2 draws together common standards from court rules and professional standards.

### Bias

Bias is a shadow to impartiality [15].

#### Cognitive bias

Psychiatric experts come to the court with their own particular way of looking at the world underpinned by their values, cultural and ethnic background, professional experience, and theoretical framework and training. Experts should, through supervision and peer review, recognize their own preconceptions with resultant due weight given to contrary views. The psychiatric expert may have particular views within their field, for example particular views on the biological vs familial/interpersonal understanding of attention-deficit/hyperactivity disorder (ADHD). Particular training, for example in psychoanalysis, may shape the expert's opinion. To counter this, regulatory frameworks emphasize the expert's obligation to give due weight to the range of opinion on particular issues (see listed item 7 in Box 145.1 and listed item 4 in Box 145.2). Rix [3] recommends, as a framework, addressing the range of opinion that might be expressed in a peer review case conference by respected consultant colleagues who may hold legitimate contrary views on psychiatric issues to the expert's own. He adds that there may be times when the expert has to address unreasonable opinions by colleagues lacking respect.

#### Adversarial bias

Adversarial bias can arise through selection bias and unconscious or deliberate partisanship. Legal firms may choose particular experts because they are known to support their client's particular viewpoint (Hired Guns). Experts are human and do not like to disappoint their instructing party. Deliberate partisanship can arise from the expert subtly or otherwise moulds their opinion to whoever hires them.

*Overarching duty*: the paramount duty of the expert is to assist the court on matters within his or her own expertise, and this overrides any obligation to the person from whom the expert has received instructions or receives payment.

*Expert reports must contain:*

1. Details of academic and professional qualifications, together with experience and accreditation relevant to the opinions expressed in the report (usually as a summary in the introduction, with more detail within an appendix);
2. A statement of the range and extent of expertise, together with limitations upon that expertise, particularly declaring when a particular issue is outside his/her expertise;
3. A statement setting out the substance of all instructions received, together with a listing of all materials provided and considered, upon which the opinion is based;
4. Where there is a range of opinion on matters dealt with in the report, a summary range of opinion, together with reasons for the expert's preferred opinion;
5. A declaration of any facts, materials, or investigations which might bear upon, or be made against, the expert opinion;
6. Extracts of the literature or any other material upon which the scientific evidence is based;
7. A statement of which facts are within the expert's own knowledge and which are assumed;*
8. Where an opinion is qualified, a statement to that effect;
9. A statement that the expert will inform all parties, including the court, in the event that his or her opinion changes on any material issue; and
10. A declaration of truth.

* Courts distinguish true and assumed facts. The only facts the psychiatric expert will routinely know to be true are the results of examination and results of tests or investigations. All other facts will be assumed to be true.

## Confirmation bias

Confirmation bias can arise where the expert starts with a particular preconception on issues to be addressed to the report. Evidence is then sought and funnelled through that preconception (opinion-based evidence).

## The prosecutor's fallacy

In the cases of *R v Clark* and *R v Cannings*, two conflicting propositions to explain two unexplained infant deaths in the same family were proposed: (1) the two deaths occurred due to sudden infant death syndrome; and (2) the two deaths were due to double murder by the parent. The first was presented in court where the likelihood was judged to be one in 73 million, with the inference being that the second proposition was therefore more likely. The fact that two sudden infant deaths are unlikely by itself is misleading, as the other proposition may be even more unlikely, that is, two deaths by murder by the same parent. The presentation of only one of the competing hypotheses in these cases has been dubbed the prosecutor's fallacy, as it usually favours the prosecution case. Rules on expert evidence therefore stipulate that the expert must consider and assign due weight to alternate views on any scientific issue before expressing their own opinion (see listed item 7 in Box 145.1 and listed item 4 in Box 145.2).

Strict adherence to Court Rules (Box 145.2) and ensuring reports meet tests of reliability (Box 145.1) mitigate against bias.

Other forms of bias are recognized, which are more applicable to forensic science practice (for a full review, see [15]).

### Legal governance

Should any party in court proceedings have reason for concern regarding an expert witness's adherence to standards of practice, there are a range of remedies available (UK case law, but similar remedies apply in other jurisdictions):

1. A judge in court can refer an expert to their regulatory body (the GMC for psychiatrists) to consider their fitness to practise.
2. The court can make an expert witness subject to a wasted costs penalty if they have seriously delayed or obstructed the progress of the case through poor adherence to the standards expected of an expert witness.
3. An expert witness can be held in contempt of court through wilful disregard or disrespect for the authority of the court.
4. In *Jones v Kaney*, the Supreme Court overturned a 400-year-old convention that an expert in court should enjoy immunity from suit. This means that the expert psychiatric witness can be sued for damages, but that is limited to parties to whom the expert owes a duty of care, as when the expert is instructed by one party in a civil dispute. The implications of this judgement continue to be worked out, but it appears a professional witness to fact, court-appointed experts, or experts instructed by the presiding judge do not owe a duty of care to a particular party in an adversarial system and therefore retain immunity from suit.
5. The expert witness can be charged with perjury where they are held to be wilfully telling an untruth or making a misrepresentation in their evidence.

The practical implication for the psychiatric expert witness is that they must have their own personal indemnity insurance for court work.

## Ethical practice (with special reference to risk assessment)

Stone [16] used the term 'dual role' to describe the psychiatrist in the legal context. In Stone's view, the roles of the clinician and expert are ethically irreconcilable. The dual role arises from the conflicting expectations and responsibilities between their duty to the evaluee to maximize their welfare (medical ethics) and the duty to put their clinical knowledge and experience at the disposal of the court (justice ethics).

Evidence on the risk associated with mental disorder is an exemplar for the dual role dilemma. Judges when considering an indeterminate (life) sentence or a longer-than-usual sentence, will, for offenders who may be mentally disordered, routinely require a psychiatric opinion on mental disorder, risk, and treatability. That assessment may result in welfare disposal in the form of a hospital order for treatment, instead of a custodial sentence, or where a mental disorder (for example, personality disorder) is identified and linked to future risk, but no treatment disposal recommended, the judge may justifiably conclude that the protection of the public would be best protected by imposing an indeterminate or longer-than-usual sentence.

One solution is to separate the clinical and legal roles [16], such that the expert does not have a clinical role to play in respect of the evaluee. Adshead [17] argues that this is not viable in the UK. For any one offender, the psychiatrist may have multiple roles. In a public health system, the psychiatrist will have obligations to the state to fairly distribute health resources and thereby act as gatekeeper to psychiatric health care. At trial, the psychiatrist may give evidence on legal matters (for example, diminished responsibility) and, at the point of sentencing, provide an opinion impacting upon disposal (welfare or custodial). The psychiatrist's opinion may, at a later time, for the same offender, be central to legal decisions—the Mental Health Review Tribunal or parole hearing on release. Considering these overlapping and contradictory roles, Martinez and Candilis (United States perspective) [18] and Adshead (UK perspective) [17] reject the strict view of experts as being answerable to either the law (justice ethics) or their profession (medical ethics). Professional responsibilities cannot be divided along any absolute or clear lines.

The narrow domain of medical ethics does not remove from doctors the duty to consider the interests and the rights of other people and to consider the distribution of benefits and risks [19]. To work ethically within this framework presupposes a just state. Adshead [17] argues that the psychiatrist has duties as a citizen to participate in processes that could protect others from risk arising from individuals with mental disorder. The psychiatrist must, if acting as an expert witness, continuously negotiate a struggle between the welfare of the individual defendant, the legitimate need to the court for expert testimony, and duties to the wider society to address the risk to others associated with mental disorder. Very high standards are required of the expert in presenting findings on risk and their reliability. While probabilistic risk assessments may be accurate at a group level, at an individual level, the confidence intervals for any risk instrument are so wide as to make individual predictions highly problematic [20]. This has led Mullen [21] to conclude that 'the margin of error in every actual or conceivable risk assessment instrument is so wide at the individual level that their use for sentencing or any formal detention, is unethical'. While the court will recognize the limitations of risk assessment, nevertheless, risk assessment for the mentally disordered will fall outside the 'common knowledge' of the judge and jury. If the state has a legitimate claim on the psychiatrist's expertise in passing sentence or when considering parole, the psychiatrist would appear to have little option but to report their assessment of risk despite its clear limitations. This places grave responsibility on the psychiatric expert to report the findings on risk in a way that informs the court on the limitations of the risk assessment, particularly the problem of extracting an individual risk assessment from probabilistic group risk. Furthermore, when obtaining informed consent for reports, the psychiatrist should provide information to the evaluee on the use the court or tribunal may make of the psychiatrist's risk assessment.

Common to approaches to developing an ethical framework for the psychiatric expert witness is the necessity to draw upon multiple ethical perspectives and values when undertaking evaluations and recognizing that there may be conflict between those ethical perspectives. These approaches combine ethics derived from traditional medical ethics, but also incorporate ethics derived from the perspective of justice (for a full theoretical account of this approach,

see [19]). Martinez and Candilis [18] proposed the following principles to guide practice:

- *Respect for persons*: everyone subject to a psychiatric evaluation for the court should be regarded with respect and professional fairness.
- *Respect for privacy and confidentiality*: while acknowledging that there are inherent limitations to this value in the legal context, nevertheless, care must be exercised in dealing with sensitive information. Balance and perspective are critical to the presentation of clinical findings, avoiding the provision of gratuitous information and avoiding bias through selective use of information.
- *Respect for consent*: psychiatric experts must ensure that those they evaluate understand the purpose of the evaluation, the limitations of confidentiality, and the potential use of the expert's opinion by the court (dual-role obligations).
- *Commitment to honesty and striving for objectivity*: this is reflected in the formulation of procedure rules across jurisdictions (Box 145.2), which must be adhered to by the psychiatric expert witness. The expert must resist the hired gun bias and exhibit thoroughness and transparency in respect of their personal values.

To this list, the author would add:

- *Respect for the human rights of others*: balancing the distribution of benefits and risks for the person being evaluated and society, including fair distribution of health resources [17, 19].

Individual psychiatrists and their professional bodies have a duty to ensure that psychiatric experts are properly trained and understand their dual obligations as a doctor and as a witness in court. This can be achieved through professional development, appraisal, and revalidation. The psychiatric expert must be willing to submit their medicolegal work to peer scrutiny and, through peer review and training, gain knowledge of the values and prejudices they bring to evaluations. Professional obligations include a willingness to tackle poor practice by colleagues, including referral to professional regulatory bodies.

## The psychiatric report

Rix [22] and Buchanan and Norko [23] provide detailed guidance on the preparation of reports for courts and tribunals. The main points are summarized in Box 145.3. The court or tribunal has little time to read lengthy reports and are primarily concerned with the expert's findings and opinion. However, if detailed facts or narrative are necessary for whatever purpose, then the details can be confined to appendices. The aspiring expert should seek out formal training in medicolegal report writing and be thoroughly familiar with the subtle, but important, differences between reports for criminal, civil, and family courts (see [3]).

If there is no evidence of mental disorder, then the privileged exception accorded to psychiatric experts may no longer apply (see Common knowledge, p. 1470). However, the court may use psychiatric evidence where the boundary between disorder and normality is blurred. As in all aspects of interaction with the court, transparency is key to acting as a responsible expert. Psychiatric expertise derives from established scientific evidence, but also from expert consensus

**Box 145.3** Report structure

The report should be typed using numbered paragraphs and headings and subheadings, and should make use of short sentences and paragraphs.

The psychiatric report should contain the following sections:

**(a) Instructions, documentation, and methodology**

The report should include details of instructions received, the methodology, documents received, assumptions adopted, and interviews conducted. The overriding principle is transparency. Full disclosure of all documents and information upon which the opinion is based is essential, along with disclosure of limitations and assumptions employed. In a psychiatric report, assumptions might include that the subject has been truthful and that medical records are accurate.

**(b) The facts**

The report should record briefly the facts upon which the opinion is based and should avoid interpretation which is the proper function of the opinion section. In psychiatric reports, the only facts that are within the psychiatrist's own knowledge are likely to be those based on findings of the mental state examination. All other facts are assumed. If structured tests are utilized, they may also constitute facts within the psychiatrist's own knowledge. Sufficient detail, recognizing that the court will have full knowledge of the case, for the court or another expert to understand the basis for opinion is what is required of the report. Further detail can be relegated to appendices.

**(c) Opinion**

The role of the psychiatric expert in the criminal court is to provide an opinion on mental disorder and its implications for the matters before the court. The features that lead to a diagnosis of mental disorder should be described, avoiding jargon and including mental state findings, so that others can understand how the opinion is reached. The diagnosis or differential diagnosis should be clearly stated, using a recognized classification (ICD-10, DSM-5). Where a condition is described which is not part of such recognized classification systems or where 'leading-edge' scientific findings or opinion based on experience or special knowledge are used to support the opinion, that should be justified by disclosure (as an appendix to the report) of the relevant literature to support the expert's opinion, together with, if applicable, the expert's own experience and knowledge of the field. In the civil court, opinion in clinical negligence should be anchored to established codes of practice, clinical practice guidelines, or service protocols and should be backed by providing relevant citations (which may form the basis for cross-examination).

The second stage of the opinion is to apply the psychiatric findings to the issues to be addressed in the report. Each issue should have its own section. The content should show how the opinion derives from the facts. The opinion should highlight the strength of the opinion, giving due weight to matters that might undermine the opinion or could fairly be made against it. The opinion should highlight any unusual or contradictory findings, must be balanced, and must give due weight to the range of reasonable opinion on the issue to be addressed (the psychiatric case conference model).

**(d) Declarations and statement of truth**

Court rules require the report writer to provide a declaration that the expert understands and has complied with their duty to the court (Box 145.2). Court Rules require a statement of truth to the effect that the content of the report is true and that the report writer is aware of their liability to be prosecuted for untruth in court.

**(e) Qualifications and experience**

Usually as an appendix.

**(f) Appendices**

Included here are recorded lists of documents, publications cited, and definitions of any technical terms.

Source: data from Rix K, The structure, organisation and content of the generic report, In: Rix K, Expert *Psychiatric Evidence*, pp 35–51, Copyright (2011), The Royal College of Psychiatrists.

and experience-based knowledge. In broad terms, the court needs to be informed of the level of evidence underpinning opinion.

Particularly in the civil court, the expert may be given reports of other experts in the case and due weight should be accorded to their opinion before commenting on their opinion and setting out the basis for agreement or disagreement (see listed item 7 in Box 145.1 and listed item 4 in Box 145.2).

There may be conflict in the factual evidence, and the report should avoid preference for one side or the other but instead give alternative opinion, based on differing judgements on the evidence.

Terms such as 'diminished responsibility', 'insanity', or 'automatism' have precise legal definitions, and the report should address how the psychiatric findings translate to the legal definitions employed by the court.

Where recommendations for a mental health disposal under specific Acts are included, the precise wording of the relevant section of those Acts should be employed.

## Opinion on the ultimate issue

There is long-standing prohibition in common law jurisdictions against the expert providing an opinion on the ultimate issue before the court. The judge will decide if a hospital is negligent in a civil negligence claim. The jury will decide in a criminal court whether a defendant is guilty. In deciding upon the ultimate issue, the court may require knowledge outside their common knowledge, for example interpreting the McNaughton rules for insanity or applying the criteria for a finding of diminished responsibility. In such cases, the court has allowed opinion on the ultimate issue. The court in the United States generally allows opinion that embraces the ultimate issue, but this is limited by Rule 704 of the Federal Rules of Evidence [7], which states that the expert 'must not state an opinion about whether the defendant did or did not have a mental state or condition that constitutes an element of the crime charged or of a defence. Those matters are for the trier of fact alone'. The psychiatric expert should be careful when expressing an opinion on the ultimate issue that their opinion is necessary to assist the court on matters outside the common knowledge of the court.

## Confidentiality

Medicolegal work undertaken by psychiatrists is governed by the same rule of confidentiality as applied to other clinical work. Reports cannot be disclosed to a third party without the consent of the body commissioning the report. Psychiatric reports do not form part of a person's medical record, except by the express consent of the individual or their legal representative. Defence solicitors can exercise a right not to disclose a report to court. Failure to comply with the rules of confidentiality can lead to civil action or reporting to a professional regulatory body. Breaching confidentiality may be justified in particular cases.

While the psychiatric expert owes an overriding obligation to the court, nevertheless, the expert remains a doctor with consequent medical responsibilities. If the report writer concludes that the evaluee requires treatment, then the expert must consider whether their medical practitioner should be alerted to that treatment need.

This is usually done with the agreement of the evaluee or their legal representative. Where, for whatever reason, that recommendation is not passed on to the evaluee's medical practitioner, consideration must be given to disclosure in the person's best interests.

A psychiatrist who believes that the evaluee is not co-operating with the preparation of a report because of mental illness has a duty to consider whether the evaluee's mental illness could interfere with a fair trial (for example, fitness to plead or lack of consideration of a mental health disposal). The psychiatrist must then make a judgement whether it is in the best interests of the evaluee for sufficient information to be provided to the court to alert them of the doctor's concerns. Such disclosure will almost certainly be justified in the interests of a fair trial and justice.

The other situation where a breach of confidentiality may be justified is where a report is not disclosed, but the report writer believes that the court ought to consider the report findings on potential risk to the public or where the court is unaware of information that might have a crucial bearing on outcome. In *BW v Edgell*, the court held that the doctor's duty of confidence did not prevent a psychiatrist from taking steps to communicate the grounds of concern to the court. The strong public interest in disclosure to prevent a court from making decisions based upon inadequate information was held to override the psychiatrist's duty of confidentiality. Where a doctor is considering disclosure in these circumstances, advice should be sought from an experienced colleague and the case law consulted, and the psychiatrist should thoroughly understand their regulatory bodies' guidance on disclosure, as well as consult their indemnity insurer.

In all cases, disclosure should be limited to providing sufficient information to the receiving body (court or medical practitioner) to make a decision. In *Cornelius v DeTaranto*, a psychiatrist who wished to arrange treatment for a claimant in a civil case disclosed the full report to the claimant's medical practitioner without the claimant's consent and was held to be negligent in doing so. Limited disclosure would have been sufficient to alert the medical practitioner to the treatment need, rather than full disclosure of the report.

It is the responsibility of the expert to ensure the security of clinical records and court documents, and the expert must adhere to relevant data protection legislation. The three Rs should be followed:

- *Retain*: all documentation until the statutory time limits for retention of documents has passed and to at least the time of any potential appeal, civil suit, or referral to regulatory bodies.
- *Record*: keep structured, clear, legible, and comprehensive records in a format suitable for other instructed experts to consult.
- *Reveal*: all sources of information in the report.

## The interview

At the beginning of the interview, the examining psychiatrist should explain carefully to the defendant the nature of the doctor's dual role, the limits of confidentiality in producing a medicolegal report, and that the court will have full disclosure of all material known to the report writer (no off-record material). It is prudent to obtain a signed record of this discussion and to include it as part of the introduction to the report. Whenever possible, an informant should be interviewed—by telephone, if necessary.

## Appearing in court

Experts are allowed, unlike witnesses of fact, to sit in court and hear the evidence of other witnesses before they, themselves, give evidence. An expert can be called by any interested party in proceedings. The cardinal rule when giving oral evidence in court is that, although called by one party, the expert witness is not giving evidence for that party's side but is under duty to provide fair and impartial evidence to the court, even where this conflicts with the interests of the party calling them [1, 3].

In the criminal court, the report will have been pre-read by the judge, and it is usual for the examiner to refer to relevant sections of the report. A report with numbered paragraphs is easier for the court to follow. The jury will not have read the report and will not usually be given sight of the report. Their knowledge of the expert's report will come from submissions made by either side and through the judge's questioning and summing up.

When calling an expert witness, the advocate must elicit the following:

1. The expert's qualifications: the report should have been prepared according to court procedure rules and therefore contain a biography setting out the qualifications and experience of the witness. It will then be usual for the advocate to lead this part of the evidence by reference to the biography supplied in the report. It will be perfectly permissible for the other side to call into question the expert's qualifications. This should be met politely by outlining the reasons why the expert believes they have the requisite qualifications and experience to answer the questions posed in instructions and have not strayed beyond their area of expertise.

2. Advocates are under duty to challenge disputed evidence. Thus, where more than one expert opinion is provided and they differ, the expert must expect their opinion to be disputed. The expert must resist pressure from one party to deviate from, or express greater certainty about, an opinion they have reached in the written report. The use of joint expert statements helps this process.

3. An expert witness may be cross-examined as a hostile witness if there is good reason to suppose that they are not telling the truth. Thankfully, this is extremely rare. The possibility of deliberate or inadvertent bias must, however, always be considered.

## Civil courts

(See [1, 3, 24, 25]). This chapter has concentrated upon practice in the criminal court, and the discussion applies equally to the civil court. However, there are important differences. The civil court is far more complex than its criminal counterpart. Each jurisdiction will have its own CPR. Psychiatric experts familiar with work in the criminal court will, when undertaking occasional expert reports in the civil court, be relative novices and need to thoroughly familiarize themselves with court processes and the stringent requirements of civil proceedings. If coming to the civil court for the first time, it may be prudent to prepare reports under supervision from an experienced colleague. Adversarial bias is a particular hazard in civil proceedings.

Important differences in England and Wales include:

- The burden of proof is at the level of balance of probabilities, rather than the more stringent test—beyond reasonable doubt—in the criminal court.
- Civil actions have multiple stages governed by different rules (preliminary reports, pre-action stage, claim). Preliminary reports are for the sole use of the legal team, and not subject to CPR, while reports at the claim stage are subject to the specific and stringent CPR.
- The CPR encourage the appointment of single experts.
- Where more than one expert is involved, exchange of reports is mandatory, and case conferencing between experts with joint reports on areas of agreement/disagreements routine. While not covered specifically by CrPR, this is becoming common practice in the criminal court.

The psychiatric expert will need to take particular care to understand the questions asked of them and understand the case law applicable to the questions asked. The reliability of the expert's evidence, including evidence on standards of care in medical negligence, will be central to the court's assessment of the expert's evidence. In medical negligence cases, the opinion should be anchored to established codes of practice, clinical practice guidelines, and practice protocols applicable at the time of the medical event under scrutiny. Though the civil court does not have formal guidance on reliability in England and Wales, the guidance for the criminal court is equally applicable to the civil court (Box 145.1).

## Civil jurisdictions

It is beyond the scope of this chapter to examine the expert's role in civil jurisdictions, which includes most of Europe, but some differences and common concerns can be recognized. Inquisitorial systems typically employ two stages: an investigative stage and a trial stage. The judge is an active protagonist in adducing the truth. The divide between both systems is not clear-cut; for example, in Scotland, the Procurator Fiscal directs an investigative stage in the most serious crimes, followed by a trial employing the adversarial approach.

In contrast to common law jurisdictions, the courtroom is not the setting for examining the scientific reliability of expert evidence and the expert's evidence is not subject to cross-examination at the trial stage. Issues of admissibility or reliability are not subject to formal criteria, but there is equal concern about these matters within the European Union [26]. The examining magistrate has wide discretion in what evidence is admitted at the trial stage.

### FURTHER READING: CASE LAW

*R v Clark* [2003] EWCA Crim 1020. [2003] 2 FCR 447 (2nd appeal)
*R v Canings* [2004] EWCA Crim. [2004] 1 WLR 25707
*Frye v United States* 293F 1013 (DC Cir 1923)
*Daubert v Merrill Dow Pharmaceuticals Inc* 509 US 579 113 S Ct 2786 1993
*Bonython* [1984] 38 S A S R 45
*R v Turner* [1975] Q.B. 834 and 841

*R v Bunnis* [1964] 50 WWR ,422
*Ikarian Reefer* [1993] 2 Lloyds Rep 68 at 81
*Jones v Kaney* [2011] UKSC 13
*Daubert v Merrell Dow Pharmaceuticals Inc* [1993] 509 US 575
*Field v Leeds City Council* [2001] 2 CPLR 129
*BW v Edgell* [1990] Cr App ch 359
*Cornelius v de Taranto* [2000] EWCA Civ 1511

### REFERENCES

1. Hodgkinson T, James M. *Expert Evidence: Law and Practice*, fourth edition. London: Sweet and Maxwell; 2014.
2. Adam C. *Forensic Evidence in Court: Evaluation and Scientific Opinion*. Chichester: Wiley; 2016.
3. Rix K. *Expert Psychiatric Evidence*. London: Royal College of Psychiatrists; 2011.
4. Watson C. Expert testimony: legal principles. In: Weiss KJ, Watson C, editors. *Psychiatric Expert Testimony: Emerging Applications*. New York, NY: Oxford University Press; 2015. pp. 1–13.
5. The Law Commission. *Expert Evidence in Criminal Proceedings in England and Wales*. Law Com No. 325. 2011. Available from: https://assets.publishing.service.gov.uk/government/uploads/system/uploads/attachment_data/file/229043/0829.pdf
6. Courts and Tribunals Judiciary: UK. *Criminal Practice Directions 2015* (Expert Evidence: subsection 19 A.5 and 19 A.6). Available from: https://www.justice.gov.uk/courts/procedure-rules/criminal/rulesmenu-2015
7. United States Court. *Federal Rules of Evidence, December 1, 2017* (Opinions and Expert Testimony: Rules 701–706). Available from: https://www.rulesofevidence.org/article-vii
8. General Medical Council (UK). *Giving Evidence As An Expert Witness*. Available from: https://www.gmc-uk.org/ethical-guidance/ethical-guidance-for-doctors/acting-as-a-witness/acting-as-a-witness-in-legal-proceedings
9. Ministry of Justice (UK). *The Civil Procedure Rules. Part 35: Experts and Assessors*. Available from: www.justice.gov.uk/courts/procedure-rules/civil/rules/part35
10. Ministry of Justice (UK). *The Criminal Procedure Rules. Part 19: Expert Evidence*. Available from: https://www.justice.gov.uk/courts/procedure-rules/criminal/docs/2015/crim-proc-rules-2015-part-19.pdf
11. Ministry of Justice (UK). *The Family Procedure Rules. Practice Direction* (Part 25: Expert and Assessors: Practice Directions 25A–25E). Available from: https://www.justice.gov.uk/courts/procedure-rules/family/rules_pd_menu
12. Australian Government. *Evidence Act 1995* (Part 79: Exception: Opinions Based on Specialised Knowledge). Available from: https://www.legislation.gov.au/Details/C2012C00518
13. Royal College of Psychiatrists. *Responsibilities of Psychiatrists who Provide Expert Opinion to Courts and Tribunals*. Report Number: CR193. 2015. Available from: https://www.rcpsych.ac.uk/docs/default-source/improving-care/better-mh-policy/college-reports/college-report-cr193.pdf?sfvrsn=c0381b24_2
14. American Academy of Psychiatry and the Law. *Ethics Guidelines for the Practice of Forensic Psychiatry*. 2005. Available from: http://www.aapl.org/ethics-guidelines
15. Adam C. Cognitive bias and expert opinion. In: Adam C. *Forensic Evidence in Court: Evaluation and Scientific Opinion*. Chichester: Wiley; 2016. pp. 117–26.

16. Stone AA. The ethical boundaries of forensic psychiatry—a view from the Ivory tower. *Bulletin of the American Academy of Psychiatry and the Law*. 1984;12:209–19.

17. Adshead G. Three faces of justice: competing ethical paradigms in forensic psychiatry. *Legal and Criminological Psychology*. 2014;19:1–12.

18. Martinez R, Candilis PJ. Ethics. In: Buchanan A, Norko MA, editors. *The Psychiatric Report*. New York, NY: Cambridge University Press; 2011. pp. 56–67.

19. Beauchamp TF, Childress JF. *Principles of Biomedical Practice*, seventh edition. New York, NY: Oxford University Press; 2013

20. Hart S, Michie C, Cooke D. Precision of actuarial risk assessment instruments. Evaluating the margins of error of group versus individual predictions of violence. *British Journal of Psychiatry*. 2007;190(Supp 49):s60–5.

21. Mullen P. Dangerous and severe personality disorder and in need of treatment. *British Journal of Psychiatry*. 2007;190:s3–7.

22. Rix K. The structure, organisation and content of the generic report. In: Rix K. *Expert Psychiatric Evidence*. London: Royal College of Psychiatrists; 2011. pp. 35–51.

23. Buchanan A, Norko MA, editors. *The Psychiatric Report*. New York, NY: Cambridge University Press; 2011.

24. UK Register of Expert Witnesses. *Factsheet 01: Civil Litigation and the Expert Witness*. 2018. Available from: https://www.jspubs.com/experts/fs/01.pdf

25. Recupero PR, Price M. Civil litigation. In: Buchanan A, Norko MA, editors. *The Psychiatric Report*. New York, NY: Cambridge University Press; 2011. pp. 112–27.

26. European Parliament. *Civil-Law Expert Reports in the EU: National Rules and Practices*. Available from: http://www.europarl.europa.eu/RegData/etudes/IDAN/2015/519211/IPOL_IDA(2015)519211_EN.pdf

# 146

# Homicide

*Matthew Large and Olav Nielssen*

## Introduction

Homicide is the killing of one person by another. This simple definition unites a wide range of motives, methods, and characteristics of both the offenders and the victims. Murder has been defined as the unlawful and intentional killing of one person by another, and psychological aspects of the motive for killing are central to the legal verdict of murder. All societies with recorded history have forbidden homicide, and an enduring fascination with homicide is reflected in our myths, plays, and fiction and the continued public appetite for stories about homicide.

Most homicides are committed by people with no identifiable mental disorder, and few people with a mental disorder will ever commit a homicide. However, homicide is an important topic in psychiatry, because people with mental disorders, especially schizophrenia, commit a disproportionate number of homicides. Psychiatrists have a role in assisting the court in determining the degree of criminal responsibility of mentally disordered homicide offenders and in providing long-term care and advice regarding the release of offenders to the community. Moreover, several notorious homicides involving people with mental illness have influenced the development of mental health law, policy, and services.

## Definitions

Homicide is a type of unnatural death, along with fatal accidents and suicides [1]. Deaths from military conflicts are not usually considered to be homicides, although those resulting from civil unrest, mass killings of civilians by governments, and deaths from terrorism are included in the definition. This chapter is mainly concerned with intentional homicides, defined as 'unlawful death purposefully inflicted on a person by another person' [1]. Non-intentional homicide (such as in motor vehicle accidents) and lawful killings (in self-defence or during law enforcement) are not considered. Intentional homicides can be divided into primary, or interpersonal homicide, when the death or injury of a particular victim was the aim of the offender, and secondary homicide which is the result of other criminal activities [1].

Without wishing to understate the importance of deaths due to military conflict, civil unrest, terrorism, negligence, and lawful killings, or any overlap between primary and secondary homicide, the focus of this chapter is on primary or interpersonal homicide, particularly homicide committed by people with a mental disorder.

An equivalent to the commandment 'Thou shalt not kill' can be found in the lore of all ancient societies [2]. Most legal classifications of homicide have developed around the offender's motive and the degree of mental responsibility for their behaviour. For example, in Anglo-Saxon law, at the time of the Norman Conquest, 'slaying by stealth' was distinguished from 'slaying openly'; the former was punishable by death, and the latter could be remedied with compensation to the victim's family [3]. More modern definitions of criminal homicide emerged in twelfth-century England when 'slaying with malice aforethought' was distinguished from justified homicides, such as the killing of a thief caught in the act, and excusable homicides such as accidental homicide and homicide in self-defence [3, 4]. The perceived intent and the capacity to form the requisite intent to kill have become central to modern legal determinations. A clear-minded intention to harm or kill is what distinguishes murder from deaths resulting from dangerous acts committed without the specific intention of causing death. In most jurisdictions, there are provisions that recognize the effect of mental disorder on the ability to form the rational intention to kill, together with mechanisms for diversion for treatment and supervision of mentally ill offenders.

## Epidemiology of homicide

In 2012, almost half a million people died by homicide [1]. Most homicides are single homicides committed by one person, and therefore the rates of death by homicide and homicide offending are generally similar. The global homicide rate is about six per 100,000 people, but there is marked variation in homicide rates between regions, countries, and communities (Table 146.1). In the Americas, the rate of death by homicide was over 16 per 100,000 in 2012; in Africa, it was over 12 per 100,000, while rates of homicide in Europe, Oceania, and Asia were about three per 100,000. The homicide rate in Russia in 2012 was over nine per 100,000, whereas in England and Wales, as in most other countries in Western Europe, it was about one per 100,000. In Canada, the rate of homicide was 1.6 per 100,000; in the United States, it was 4.7 per 100,000, and in Honduras, it was over 90 per 100,000 per annum.

**Table 146.1** Homicide rate and proportion of male homicide victims in the ten most populous countries, England and Wales, Canada, Australia, and New Zealand

| Country | Homicides per 100,000 per annum | Proportion of male victims |
|---|---|---|
| China | 1.0 | 78.1 |
| India | 3.5 | 59.2 |
| United States | 4.7 | 77.8 |
| Indonesia | 0.6 | 80.3 |
| Brazil | 25.2 | 89.8 |
| Pakistan | 7.7 | 76.7 |
| Bangladesh | 2.7 | 63.3 |
| Russian Federation | 9.2 | 75.5 |
| Japan | 0.3 | 47.1 |
| England and Wales | 1.0 | 70.3 |
| Canada | 1.6 | 69.8 |
| Australia | 1.1 | 67.3 |
| New Zealand | 0.9 | 48.8 |

Source: data from UNODC, *Global Study on Homicide 2013*, Copyright (2012), United Nations Office on Drugs and Crime.

Being male is one of the most stable and well-established risk factors for homicide, and about 95% of homicide offenders are male, a proportion that does not vary much between countries or according to the rate of homicide. About 80% of homicide victims are also male, although the ratio of male-to-female victims varies more than that of offenders, and in a small number of countries, including Germany, Japan, several Nordic states, and New Zealand, the number of female victims exceeds the number of male victims [1].

Homicide offending by children is rare, and the rate of offending is highest between the ages of 15 and 29 and declines steadily with age. The age distribution of homicide victims varies between regions. In the Americas, 15- to 29-year-old men and women are most at risk, whereas in Europe, males aged 30–59 are more likely to be the victims of homicide than younger men.

Rates of homicide have declined in most economically developed countries in the last 20 years, for reasons that may include ageing of the population, better policing, changes in patterns of substance use, and a decline in the number of domestic homicides [5]. Improvement in emergency treatment of trauma victims might also have influenced the measured rates of homicide, especially in the United States [6]. Changes in homicide rates in low- and middle-income countries have been less uniform but appear to be related to economic development. For example, the greatest decline in the rate of homicide in South America has been in Chile, a country that has enjoyed consistent economic progress [7].

There is no complete explanation for the wide variation in homicide rates. Differing patterns of weapon availability and substance use are two of the most frequently cited reasons. Worldwide, more than 40% of homicides are committed using a firearm; higher rates of firearm ownership are associated with higher rates of homicide [1, 8], and being a gun owner is associated with an increased probability of committing homicide, compared to non-gun owners from the same community [9, 10]. There is clear evidence that measures to regulate gun ownership can have an impact on homicide rates. For

example, in the wake of a mass killing in Australia in 1996, stricter licensing and storage requirements and compulsory government buy-back of automatic and semi-automatic weapons was followed by an accelerated decline in firearm homicides and a marked reduction in the number of mass killings [11].

High homicide rates can be found in some areas with low levels of gun ownership, mainly in places with high-per-capita alcohol consumption. There is a well-established association between alcohol intoxication and homicide at the level of the offender [12], and there is an association between changes in national alcohol consumption and fluctuations in homicide rates [13]. There is also an association between more broadly defined rates of substance use and homicide [14], an association that might be explained by the criminal activity associated with illegal drug use and possibly even the mental effects of abuse of illegal drugs, especially stimulants. In regions with very high homicide rates, such as South Africa and some Central and South American countries, there is often a combination of ready availability of weapons, hazardous patterns of substance use, drug crime, economic deprivation, and weak law enforcement.

## Homicide and mental disorder

The two main methods of examining the association between crime and mental disorder are by psychiatric evaluation of offenders and by linking criminal and health registers. Both methods have advantages and disadvantages. The examination of offenders is liable to sampling bias, as not all offenders are the subject of a detailed examination and because those evaluations are retrospective. To date, only a few countries have had the benefit of centralized health information in order to perform large-scale data linkage studies. This method relies on the reliability of primary health diagnoses and overlooks the presence of mental illness in offenders in the first episode of an illness and those who avoided contact with health services. However, both types of study provide strong evidence for an association between schizophrenia and homicide [15]. The association between homicide and mental disorders other than schizophrenia is less clear and might well be explained by other factors such as comorbid substance use [16, 17].

### Homicide and schizophrenia

People with schizophrenia are overrepresented among samples of homicide offenders. Meta-analyses suggest that those with schizophrenia are about 20 times more likely to commit a homicide than other members of the community [18] and make up about 6.5% of all homicide offenders [15]. The population rate of homicide by people with an established diagnosis of schizophrenia appears to be about ten per 100,000 annum [19], although there is some variation, and the rate of homicide by people with schizophrenia is higher in regions with high total rates of homicides [15]. A meta-analysis found that about 40% of those homicides occur in the first episode of psychosis and the absolute risk of homicide by people during the period of their first episode of psychosis, regardless of how long the illness had been untreated, is more than ten times the annual risk of homicide after treatment [19].

Homicides by people with schizophrenia are often committed in response to frightening delusional beliefs [20]. The importance of delusional beliefs and positive symptoms of schizophrenia is supported by the association between delusions and non-lethal violence [21], the apparent fall in the homicide rates after initial treatment [19], and the decline in homicide by people with schizophrenia following the development of community mental health services in England and Wales in the 1970s [22]. However, other factors contribute to the association between schizophrenia and homicide, especially after initial treatment of the illness, including the high rates of substance use among people with schizophrenia, the emergence of schizophrenia among young males, a group already at greater risk of violence, and the association between social disadvantage and both violence and schizophrenia. The importance of factors other than delusional beliefs in homicide is evident in the finding that rates of homicide by people with schizophrenia are strongly correlated with rates of other homicides, rather than with the epidemiology of schizophrenia. One interpretation of this finding is that people with schizophrenia are vulnerable to the social factors that determine the overall rate of homicide [15].

### Homicide and other mental disorders

The proportion of homicide offenders with mental illness varies widely between studies. A nation-wide study from New Zealand found that fewer than 10% of all homicide perpetrators were determined to be 'mentally abnormal' by the courts [23]. In contrast, a national study of Swedish homicide offenders found that only 10% had no mental health diagnosis [14]. The association between homicide and mental disorders other than schizophrenia has also been studied by the psychiatric evaluation of offenders and by linking health and criminological data. Any study of the homicide rates among people with mental disorders is likely to have been affected by the proportion of homicide offences that result in the identification of an offender, whether the study was conducted by clinical interview, co-registration of criminological and health data, or research interviews. Studies that include substance use disorders and personality disorders in the definition of mental disorder are also likely to report a higher proportion of mentally disordered offenders than studies that exclude those diagnoses. It has been suggested that places with a higher homicide rate have a smaller proportion of mentally ill offenders because of a dilution effect [24], although this is disputed [25].

There is evidence for an association between substance use disorders and homicide. A case linkage study from Sweden found that 20% of homicide offenders had been identified to have a substance use disorder prior to the homicide [14], whereas a study conducted in Australia using similar methods found that 5% of homicide offenders had a previous substance use disorder [26]. Studies based on the psychiatric evaluations of homicide offenders after the offence also vary in the proportion of offenders with a substance use disorder, with studies from the United States [27], Finland [28], Austria [16], and New Zealand [23] reporting rates of substance use disorder of 47%, 12%, 1.4%, and 0.7%, respectively.

There is marked variation in the proportion of homicide offenders considered to have a mood disorder. Case linkage studies from Australia [26] and Sweden [14] both reported that about 2% of homicide offenders had been treated for depression prior to the offence, whereas studies relying on the clinical examination of offenders have reported varying proportions of offenders with mood disorders. Studies from Singapore [29] and the United States [27] both reported that 9% of homicide offenders had a diagnosis of depression. Studies from other regions have reported lower rates of depression, including 5% in Finland [28], 4% in England and Wales [30], 1.4% in Austria [16], and 1% in New Zealand [23].

There is an obvious association between antisocial personality disorder and violent crime, in part because a pattern of impulsive behaviour and criminal conduct is part of the definition of the condition, but few population-based studies of the psychiatric diagnoses of homicide offenders have specifically reported the proportion of offenders with the diagnosis of personality disorder. A Swedish case linkage study found that almost 30% of homicide offenders had been diagnosed with personality disorder prior to the homicide [14], and a recent study from the United States found that 23% of homicide offenders met the criteria for at least one personality disorder [27]. The reported rates of organic mental disorders, epilepsy, or brain damage among homicide offenders also vary. A Swedish case linkage study reported no cases of organic mental disorder [14], whereas a case linkage study from Australia reported that 7% of homicide offenders had a pre-existing organic mental disorder, most commonly a history of traumatic brain injury [26]. The reported rates of intellectual disability among homicide offenders range from 2% in Finland [28] and the United States [27] to under 1% in New Zealand [23] and Sweden [14].

## Types of primary homicide

### Domestic homicide

Domestic homicide includes the killing of an intimate partner, the killing of one's own children (filicide), the killing of parents (matricide and patricide), and the killing of siblings (fratricide). In England and Wales, about 20% of all homicides are classified as domestic homicides, 80% of which involve the killing of current or former partners [31]. Like other homicides, the offenders are mostly male and have a mean age in the late thirties. Unlike other forms of homicide, the victims are overwhelmingly female. In the United States, the pattern of male perpetrators and female victims in domestic homicide is similar, although a higher proportion of deaths involve a firearm [32]. In regions where firearm ownership is less common and total homicide rates are low, kitchen knives are the most common method [33]. Domestic homicides are often a form of fatal domestic violence, in which there has been an escalating pattern of violence in the relationship before the killing. Less common forms of domestic homicide include homicide by a mentally ill family member and homicide–suicide.

### Homicide of strangers

Stranger homicide can be defined as the killing of a person who is not known to the perpetrator until shortly before the offence. In the United Kingdom, as many as one in five homicides are stranger homicides, usually involving young men who become involved in a fight in a public place while affected by alcohol [34]. Stranger homicides by people with mental illness are very rare. A meta-analysis of data from England, Germany, Denmark, Finland, and Australia estimated the population rate of stranger homicide by people with schizophrenia to be about one in 14 million people per annum [35]. Stranger homicide offenders with psychosis are often homeless, have a history of violence, and are acutely psychotic at the time of the offence, often without any previous psychiatric treatment [35].

## Neonaticide, infant homicide, and infanticide

About half of child homicide victims are under one year of age [36]. Neonaticide is the killing of a child in the first 24 hours of life and is typically committed by disadvantaged and psychologically distressed single women who concealed their pregnancy and kill their children by abandonment or neglect [37]. Infant homicide is the killing of a child below the age of one and includes neonatacide. The most common cause of infant homicide is fatal child abuse, usually by male partners [36, 38]. Rates of infant homicide are correlated with rates of both homicide and other violent offending [39, 40].

In some jurisdictions, infanticide is a separate category of homicide offence and refers to the killing of a child less than one year of age by the mother during a post-partum mental illness. Mothers with mental illness commit a small proportion of infant homicides [36, 38]. In jurisdictions without specific infanticide laws, the role of maternal mental illness on criminal responsibility is determined in the same way as that of other forms of mental illness. Societal attitudes to the killing of infants influence the types of verdicts and the penalties imposed [41].

## Child homicide

Over 5% of homicide victims are under 15 years of age. About half are killed as a result of fatal physical abuse, and about 20% are due to parental mental illness, usually involving the child's mother [38]. Other causes are fights between teenagers, and children being caught up in criminal homicides or homicide–suicide by parents [42]. Despite the publicity that follows the offences, sexually motivated homicides of children are rare.

## Homicides by older people

People over 60 commit a small proportion of all homicides, although this proportion is likely to increase with ageing of populations around the world. Homicide by people in advanced old age is extremely rare [43–45]. Studies of older offenders emphasize the role of cognitive impairment and morbid jealousy associated with long-term alcohol use [46].

Many older homicide victims are intimate partners of a similar age to the perpetrators. Homicide of the elderly also includes homicides committed in the course of a robbery, intentional neglect, and physical abuse of a frail elderly people, and altruistic homicide of chronically ill and terminally ill partners, for example those with dementia [47].

## Homicide–suicide

Homicide that is closely followed by the suicide of the perpetrator is known as homicide–suicide or murder–suicide. Worldwide, almost one in ten homicides are followed by the suicide of the offender [48]. Most homicide–suicides are by men who kill their partners, and sometimes their children, and familial ties between the offender and the victim make suicide after homicide more likely [49]. Establishing the motives for homicide–suicide is difficult because of the death of both parties. A quantitative review of 49 international studies of homicide–suicide found that rates of homicide–suicide are strongly associated with rates of homicide, which is understandable, given that the initial event is a homicide [48]. There is less evidence for an association between rates of suicide and those of homicide–suicide, suggesting that, in most cases, homicide–suicide

should be considered to be a form of homicide, rather than 'extended suicide'. However, altruistic homicide of a sick or infirm partner, followed by the suicide of older offenders is a well-established pattern of homicide–suicide.

## Medical killings and euthanasia

A full discussion of euthanasia is beyond the scope of this chapter. However, two points are worth noting. The first is that deaths classified as euthanasia occur on a spectrum from legal and ethical decisions not to resuscitate or continue medical care of a terminally ill person to the use of terminal sedation, assisted suicide of people with varying degrees of competence, to premeditated killings by health practitioners. An increasing number of jurisdictions permit physician-assisted suicide for terminally ill people, and the responsibility for determining capacity to give consent often falls to psychiatrists. At the other end of the spectrum, physicians played a role in the state-sponsored killing of disabled patients in Nazi Germany, and England's most prolific serial killer was a trusted local doctor Harold Shipman [50].

## Homicide in institutions

Suicides and deaths from natural causes in institutional care far outnumber homicides, and state-sanctioned execution is probably more common than homicide as a cause of death among prisoners worldwide. Homicides do occur among inmates of prisons and include cases of mentally ill inmates killing their cellmates. Homicides in secure hospitals and other psychiatric hospitals are rare events. A study of homicides in Australian and New Zealand psychiatric hospitals found that all of the 11 homicides were by people with schizophrenia, and ten of the victims were fellow patients. The rate of homicides per bed day was estimated to be similar to that of the wider community, although the victims would not have been placed in danger had they not been detained in hospital [51].

## Mass killings, spree killings, and serial killings

Mass killing is variously defined as the killing of more than three or, in some studies, four people at one time. Mass killing is distinguished from spree killings, which are random killings of more than one person in a short time, sometimes in company, and from serial killings, in which a series of homicides are committed, usually by one person, over a longer period.

Mass killings have been described as a relatively modern phenomena, although there are historical accounts of random mass killings [52]. Mass killings include multiple homicides of a family by a family member, often followed by the suicide of the perpetrator, and mass killings of strangers or colleagues and acquaintances by disturbed men, often with an automatic or semi-automatic weapon. A proportion of mass killings are committed by people with mental illness, often with emerging or untreated psychosis [53].

## Homicidal ideation

The incidence of thoughts or plans to commit homicide among members of the general community has never been reported. Further, the extent of any association between homicidal ideas and actual homicide is not known. Two studies of psychiatric patients have reported the rates of homicidal ideation. One study found 22%

of 517 unselected psychiatric outpatients reported previous homicidal ideation, that 7% had persisting homicidal thoughts or a homicide plan, and about 4% had made an attempt to kill another person [54]. Gender, race, marital status, and the diagnosis of schizophrenia were not associated with homicidal ideation, but those with schizophrenia and homicidal ideation were more likely to have been violent. Another study of 223 adult patients with chronic schizophrenia found that 15% had 'severe or extreme homicidality' and that homicidal ideation was associated with the presence of mania, psychotic symptoms, and impaired social function [55]. Another study followed up 613 people who had been convicted of threatening to kill another person found that 44% were convicted of a violent offence in the next 10 years, including 3% who were charged with homicide [56]. Although this study suggested a possible link between homicidal ideation and homicide, it should not be forgotten that homicidal ideas must be several orders of magnitude more common than homicide in most patient groups.

The relationship between homicidal ideas and homicide was the subject of one of the best known legal cases in psychiatric history. In 1967, Prosenjit Poddar met Tatiana Tarasoff while they were both university students in California. Poddar was rebuffed by Tarasoff who subsequently sought psychiatric treatment. In the course of counselling, Poddar disclosed homicidal ideas towards Tarasoff, and some time later stabbed her to death. The court later held that treating doctors owed duties not only to the patient, but also to warn and protect members of the public who might be endangered by the actions of their patients [57]. Although the duty to warn after Tarasoff only applies in some states in America, it has influenced the laws and claims for negligence internationally.

## Attempted homicide

The two elements of murder are death and the intent of the offender to kill. However, even when there is a clear intention to kill, injuries inflicted are not always fatal, and the victim fighting back, the intervention of bystanders or medical care, might prevent death. Hafner and Boker's landmark study of homicide and mental disorder in West Germany between 1955 and 1965 included cases of both homicide and attempted homicide [58]. Their study found similar numbers of attempted and actual homicides, and few differences between the offenders in each group. A recent Australian study suggested there were few differences between mentally ill homicide offenders and mentally ill people who committed serious non-lethal violence [59]. Assaults by mentally ill people that result in a serious injury are rare, compared to other less serious types of assault. For example, in a recent meta-analysis, pooled estimates of the proportion of patients with first-episode psychosis committing any violence, serious violence, and violence resulting in serious injury were 34.5%, 16.6%, and 0.6%, respectively [60].

## Legal proceedings and inquiries after a homicide

Several notorious homicides by people with mental illness have resulted in changes in the way in which people with mental illness are regarded and treated. An early example was a trial following the attempted shooting of George III by James Hadfield in 1800, which led to the emergence of both the verdict of 'not guilty by reason of insanity' and of legislation to regulate the treatment and control of mentally ill offenders [61].

Homicides are usually followed by police investigations to determine the cause of death and who might be responsible. The 'clearance rate' is the proportion of homicides in which either the killer is identified or a conviction is obtained. About 60% of homicides worldwide result in an arrest, a proportion that varies markedly between jurisdictions, mainly according to the number of homicides to be investigated [1]. For example, in countries where the homicide rate is less than one per 100,000, the clearance rates are mostly above 90%. Clearance rates fall to below 80% in countries with homicide rates of between one and ten per 100,000 and below 50% when the homicide rate is above ten per 100,000 [1]. Clearance rates can affect the results of studies of the epidemiology of homicide by the mentally ill, because it may be that homicides by the mentally ill are more likely to be detected.

Criminal proceedings after homicide offences initially involve establishing that the accused person committed the homicide. However, if the facts of the offence are clear, a conviction for the most serious form of intentional homicide can depend on the motive and state of mind of the accused person. When the accused has a mental illness, the question before the court is the extent to which the mental illness reduced the defendant's degree of responsibility. Defences on the basis of mental infirmity have been described since Roman times [61]. In common law tradition, the defence of mental illness depends either on the person being aware that the killing was legally wrong or, in some places, morally wrong, from the perspective of the mentally ill offender. The most influential precedent in assessing criminal responsibility in the presence of mental illness were made by the House of Lords after the acquittal of Daniel M'Naghten for the 1843 killing of Edward Drummond, who M'Naghten had mistaken for the then British Prime Minister Robert Peel. In the M'Naghten Rules, as they came to be known, a verdict of not guilty by reason of insanity required that it be 'clearly proved that at the time of committing the act the party accused was labouring under such a defect of reason, from disease of the mind, as not to know the nature and quality of the act he was doing, or as not to know that what he or she was doing was wrong' [62].

Many jurisdictions have partial defences to murder on the basis that a psychiatric disorder may cause an offender to have reduced ability to form the required intent to commit murder or to control their actions (Box 146.1). A finding of diminished responsibility in the UK [63] reduces the verdict from murder to manslaughter, with a lower range of sentences and often an order for secure hospital treatment.

In addition to criminal proceedings, homicides are often the subject of civil inquests and proceedings on the basis of alleged negligence. In the UK, homicides by known patients are routinely examined in a process of confidential inquiry [64]. Coroners sometimes conduct inquiries to determine the cause of homicides that did not result in immediate criminal charges. Several well-publicized homicides by patients have resulted in more wide-ranging public inquiries, for example, the enquiry into the care and treatment of Christopher Clunis who killed a young man standing with his family on a London railway station [65], which produced recommendations for wide-ranging changes in clinical practice.

Homicides by patients with mental illness deserve close scrutiny to establish whether future tragedies might be prevented. However,

Box 146.1 Approximate legal definitions of homicide in English law

**Homicide:** a broad term for the killing of one human by another, sometimes restricted to unlawful killings.

**Murder:** an unlawful death inflicted with the intent to kill or seriously injure, and in the case of felony murder, a killing that takes place in the course of committing a serious crime, even if the killing was not intended.

**Manslaughter:** an unlawful death inflicted without the intent to kill or injure, including killings where the offender's criminal responsibility is reduced because of the effect of a mental disorder.

**Not guilty by reason of insanity:** at the time of committing the offence, the offender was unable to appreciate the nature and quality or the wrongfulness of his or her acts because of the effect of a mental illness or condition.

**Diminished responsibility:** where a person kills or is party to the killing of another, he or she shall not be convicted of murder if he or she was suffering from such an abnormality of the mind (whether arising from a condition of arrested or retarded development of the mind or from any inherent causes or induced by disease or injury) as substantially impairing his or her mental responsibility for his or her acts and omission in doing or being party to the killing.

**Infanticide:** when a woman or girl who unlawfully kills her child (under 12 months) under circumstances which, but for this section, would constitute wilful murder or murder, does the act which causes death when the balance of her mind is disturbed because she is not fully recovered from the effect of giving birth to the child or because of the effect of lactation consequent upon the birth of the child, she is guilty of infanticide only.

**Homicide–suicide:** when the homicide offender commits suicide shortly after the homicide, sometimes defined as within a week of the homicide.

homicide is a very rare event that is not possible to meaningfully predict [66, 67]. Decisions regarding the release of mentally ill homicide offenders should take into account the cognitive biases that influence the interpretation of catastrophic events, including the tendency to hindsight bias in apportioning blame. The rarity of homicides by the mentally ill, and the absence of identified factors associated with a greatly increased probability of homicide, means that it is not possible to predict which patients might go on to commit homicide or when a homicide might occur.

## Homicide recidivism

Homicides committed by people after the conclusion of proceedings for an earlier homicide offence are known as recidivist homicides. Schizophrenia has been reported to be a risk factor in recidivist homicide [68], but in most advanced countries, recidivist homicide by people with schizophrenia is rare or unknown, probably because of long-term secure hospitalization and effective systems for ensuring long-term care after release [69].

## The role of mental health professionals in homicide prevention

People with mental illness commit a minority of homicides, and only a small proportion of homicide offenders are in contact with

mental health services at the time of the homicide. Hence, treatment of mental illness can only ever have a small effect on the overall rate of homicide. However, mental health professionals do have a role in the prevention of some homicides, particularly domestic homicide, homicide by people seeking treatment for substance use, and homicide by people with emerging or established psychotic illness. Because domestic homicides are a common form of homicide, the most important role health professionals can play is in the detection of domestic violence and in interventions to protect the victim and treat the perpetrator. Domestic violence victims present with a range of emotional disorders and seek help from a range of services, often without disclosing their situation [70]. Health professionals can assist domestic violence victims by notifying the authorities and referral to respite and support. In many jurisdictions, there is now mandatory notification of violence involving children. Mental health professionals may also have a role in notifying licensing authorities about the emergence of mental illness or the presence of domestic violence among gun owners.

Improvements in the overall management of substance use disorders, in particular alcohol use disorders, and of comorbid substance use among people with mental illness could be expected to reduce the incidence of violence, including homicide, among those seeking care.

Health services can also play a part in reducing the incidence of violence by the mentally ill, by developing systems to ensure early treatment of psychotic illness and by ensuring the continuity and standards of ongoing care.

Threats of homicide warrant careful evaluation. Warning of potential victims and notifying authorities can be an acceptable breach of patient confidentiality, if the information that has become available to the clinician indicates the presence of a real threat to another person's safety.

While it is likely that good clinical care can prevent some homicides, the benefit of interventions is not apparent or easy to demonstrate. Most clinicians will never have a patient who commits a homicide. Psychiatrists do have a more tangible role in providing care to both mentally ill homicide offenders and a much larger number of people who have experienced the trauma and grief of the loss of a relative by homicide.

## REFERENCES

1. United Nations Office on Drugs and Crime. *Global Study on Homicide 2013: Trends, Context, Data.* Vienna: United Nations Office on Drugs and Crime; 2013.
2. Daly M, Wilson M. *Homicide.* New Brunswick, NJ: Transaction Publishers; 1988.
3. Green TA. The jury and the English Law of Homicide, 1200–1600. *Michigan Law Review.* 1976;74:413–99.
4. Stephen JF. *A History of the Criminal Law of England.* Cambridge: Cambridge University Press; 1883.
5. Blumstein A, Rosenfeld R. Explaining recent trends in U.S. homicide rates. *Journal of Criminal Law and Criminology.* 1998;88:1175–216.
6. Jena AB, Sun EC, Prasad V. Does the declining lethality of gunshot injuries mask a rising epidemic of gun violence in the United States? *Journal of General Internal Medicine.* 2014;29:1065–9.
7. Otzen T, Sanhueza A, Manterola C, Hetz M, Melnik T. Homicide in Chile: trends 2000–2012. *BMC Psychiatry.* 2015;15:312.
8. Monuteaux MC, Lee LK, Hemenway D, Mannix R, Fleegler EW. Firearm ownership and violent crime in the U.S.: an ecologic study. *American Journal of Preventive Medicine.* 2015;49:207–14.

9. Kellermann AL, Rivara FP, Rushforth NB, *et al*. Gun ownership as a risk factor for homicide in the home. *New England Journal of Medicine*. 1993;329:1084–91.

10. Wiebe DJ. Homicide and suicide risks associated with firearms in the home: a national case-control study. *Annals of Emergency Medicine*. 2003;41:771–82.

11. Chapman S, Alpers P, Agho K, Jones M. Australia's 1996 gun law reforms: faster falls in firearm deaths, firearm suicides, and a decade without mass shootings. *Injury Prevention*. 2006;12:365–72.

12. Gillies H. Murder in the west of Scotland. *British Journal of Psychiatry*. 1965;111:1087–94.

13. Pridemore WA. Vodka and violence: alcohol consumption and homicide rates in Russia. *American Journal of Public Health*. 2002;92:1921–30.

14. Fazel S, Grann M. Psychiatric morbidity among homicide offenders: a Swedish population study. *American Journal of Psychiatry*. 2004;161:2129–31.

15. Large M, Smith G, Nielssen O. The relationship between the rate of homicide by those with schizophrenia and the overall homicide rate: a systematic review and meta-analysis. *Schizophrenia Research*. 2009;112:123–9.

16. Schanda H, Knecht G, Schreinzer D, Stompe T, Ortwein-Swoboda G, Waldhoer T. Homicide and major mental disorders: a 25-year study. *Acta Psychiatrica Scandinavica*. 2004;110:98–107.

17. Bennett DJ, Ogloff JR, Mullen PE, Thomas SD, Wallace C, Short T. Schizophrenia disorders, substance abuse and prior offending in a sequential series of 435 homicides. *Acta Psychiatrica Scandinavica*. 2011;124:226–33.

18. Fazel S, Gulati G, Linsell L, Geddes JR, Grann M. Schizophrenia and violence: systematic review and meta-analysis. *PLoS Medicine*. 2009;6:e1000120.

19. Nielssen O, Large M. Rates of homicide during the first episode of psychosis and after treatment: a systematic review and meta-analysis. *Schizophrenia Bulletin*. 2010;36:702–12.

20. Nielssen OB, Westmore BD, Large MM, Hayes RA. Homicide during psychotic illness in New South Wales between 1993 and 2002. *Medical Journal of Australia*. 2007;186:301–4.

21. Keers R, Ullrich S, Destavola BL, Coid JW. Association of violence with emergence of persecutory delusions in untreated schizophrenia. *American Journal of Psychiatry*. 2014;171:332–9.

22. Large M, Smith G, Swinson N, Shaw J, Nielssen O. Homicide due to mental disorder in England and Wales over 50 years. *British Journal of Psychiatry*. 2008;193:130–3.

23. Simpson AI, McKenna B, Moskowitz A, Skipworth J, Barry-Walsh J. Homicide and mental illness in New Zealand, 1970–2000. *British Journal of Psychiatry*. 2004;185:394–8.

24. Coid J. The epidemiology of abnormal homicide and murder followed by suicide. *Psychological Medicine*. 1983;13:855–60.

25. Large M, Smith G, Nielssen O. Correspondence: the epidemiology of abnormal homicide and murder followed by suicide. *Psychological Medicine*. 2009;39:699; author reply 700–1, discussion 701.

26. Wallace C, Mullen P, Burgess P, Palmer S, Ruschena D, Browne C. Serious criminal offending and mental disorder. Case linkage study. *British Journal of Psychiatry*. 1998;172:477–84.

27. Martone CA, Mulvey EP, Yang S, Nemoianu A, Shugarman R, Soliman L. Psychiatric characteristics of homicide defendants. *American Journal of Psychiatry*. 2013;170:994–1002.

28. Eronen M, Hakola P, Tiihonen J. Mental disorders and homicidal behavior in Finland. *Archives of General Psychiatry*. 1996;53:497–501.

29. Koh KG, Gwee KP, Chan YH. Psychiatric aspects of homicide in Singapore: a five-year review (1997–2001). *Singapore Medical Journal*. 2006;47:297–304.

30. Appleby L, Shaw J. *Avoidable Deaths. Five-Year Report of the National Confidential Inquiry into Suicide and Homicide by People with Mental Illness*. Manchester: University of Manchester; 2006.

31. Oram S, Flynn SM, Shaw J, Appleby L, Howard LM. Mental illness and domestic homicide: a population-based descriptive study. *Psychiatric Services*. 2013;64:1006–11.

32. Shaw HA, Shaw JA. Domestic violence homicide in Oklahoma: 1998–1999. *Journal of the Oklahoma State Medical Association*. 2007;100:115–19.

33. Kidd S, Hughes N, Crichton J. Kitchen knives and homicide: a systematic study of people charged with murder in the Lothian and Borders region of Scotland. *Medicine, Science, and The Law*. 2013;54:167–73.

34. Shaw J, Amos T, Hunt IM, *et al*. Mental illness in people who kill strangers: longitudinal study and national clinical survey. *BMJ*. 2004;328:734–7.

35. Nielssen O, Bourget D, Laajasalo T, *et al*. Homicide of strangers by people with a psychotic illness. *Schizophrenia Bulletin*. 2011;37:572–9.

36. Makhlouf F, Rambaud C. Child homicide and neglect in France: 1991–2008. *Child Abuse and Neglect*. 2014;38:37–41.

37. Putkonen H, Weizmann-Henelius G, Collander J, Santtila P, Eronen M. Neonaticides may be more preventable and heterogeneous than previously thought—neonaticides in Finland 1980–2000. *Archives of Women's Mental Health*. 2007;10:15–23.

38. Nielssen OB, Large MM, Westmore BD, Lackersteen SM. Child homicide in New South Wales from 1991 to 2005. *Medical Journal of Australia*. 2009;190:7–11.

39. Large MM, Nielssen OB. Infant homicide in the USA between 1940 and 2005. *Journal of Epidemiology and Community Health*. 2012;66:662–3.

40. Large M, Nielssen O, Lackersteen S, Smith G. The associations between infant homicide, homicide, and suicide rates: an analysis of World Health Organization and Centers for Disease Control statistics. *Suicide and Life-Threatening Behavior*. 2010;40:87–97.

41. Spinelli MG. Infanticide: contrasting views. *Archives of Women's Mental Health*. 2005;8:15–24.

42. Logan JE, Hall J, McDaniel D, Stevens MR, National Center for Injury Prevention and Control, Centers for Disease Control and Prevention. Homicides—United States, 2007 and 2009. *Morbidity and Mortality Weekly Report Surveillance Summaries*. 2013;62 Suppl 3:164–70.

43. Overshott R, Rodway C, Roscoe A, *et al*. Homicide perpetrated by older people. *International Journal of Geriatric Psychiatry*. 2012;27:1099–105.

44. Fazel S, Bond M, Gulati G, O'Donnell I. Elderly homicide in Chicago: a research note. *Behavioral Sciences and the Law*. 2007;25:629–39.

45. Putkonen H, Weizmann-Henelius G, Repo-Tiihonen E, *et al*. Homicide, psychopathy, and aging—a nationwide register-based case-comparison study of homicide offenders aged 60 years or older. *Journal of Forensic Sciences*. 2010;55:1552–6.

46. Reutens S, Nielssen O, Large M. Homicides by older offenders in New South Wales between 1993 and 2010. *Australasian Psychiatry*. 2015;23:493–5.

47. Karch D, Nunn KC. Characteristics of elderly and other vulnerable adult victims of homicide by a caregiver: national violent death reporting system—17 U.S. states, 2003–2007. *Journal of Interpersonal Violence*. 2011;26:137–57.

48. Large M, Smith G, Nielssen O. The epidemiology of homicide followed by suicide: a systematic and quantitative review. *Suicide and Life-Threatening Behavior*. 2009;39:294–306.

49. Stack S. Homicide followed by suicide: an analysis of Chicago data. *Criminology*. 1997;35:435–53.

50. Kaplan R. The clinicide phenomenon: an exploration of medical murder. *Australasian Psychiatry*. 2007;15:299–304.

51. Nielssen O, Large MM. Homicide in psychiatric hospitals in Australia and New Zealand. *Psychiatric Services*. 2012;63:500–3.

52. Cantor CH, Mullen PE, Alpers PA. Mass homicide: the civil massacre. *Journal of the American Academy of Psychiatry and the Law*. 2000;28:55–63.

53. Lester D, Stack S, Schmidtke A, Schaller S, Muller I. Mass homicide and suicide deadliness and outcome. *Crisis*. 2005;26:184–7.

54. Asnis GM, Kaplan ML, van Praag HM, Sanderson WC. Homicidal behaviors among psychiatric outpatients. *Hospital and Community Psychiatry*. 1994;45:127–32.

55. Schwartz RC, Petersen S, Skaggs JL. Predictors of homicidal ideation and intent in schizophrenia: an empirical study. *American Journal of Orthopsychiatry*. 2001;71:379–84.

56. Warren LJ, Mullen PE, Thomas SD, Ogloff JR, Burgess PM. Threats to kill: a follow-up study. *Psychological Medicine*. 2008;38:599–605.

57. Anfang SA, Appelbaum PS. Twenty years after Tarasoff: reviewing the duty to protect. *Harvard Review of Psychiatry*. 1996;4:67–76.

58. Hafner H, Boker W. *Crimes of Violence by Mentally Abnormal Offenders: A Psychiatric and Epidemiological Study in the Federal German Republic*. New York, NY: Cambridge University Press; 1982.

59. Nielssen OB, Yee NL, Millard MM, Large MM. Comparison of first-episode and previously treated persons with psychosis found NGMI for a violent offense. *Psychiatric Services*. 2011;62:759–64.

60. Large MM, Nielssen O. Violence in first-episode psychosis: a systematic review and meta-analysis. *Schizophrenia Research*. 2011;125:209–20.

61. Moran R. The origin of insanity as a special verdict: the trial for treason of James Hadfield (1800). *Law and Society Review*. 1985;19:487–519.

62. M'Naghten's case; 8 ER 718, [1843] UKHL J16, (1843).

63. Samuels A, O'Driscoll C, Allnutt S. When killing isn't murder: psychiatric and psychological defences to murder when the insanity defence is not applicable. *Australasian Psychiatry*. 2007;15:474–9.

64. Appleby L. New confidential inquiry established into homicides and suicides by mentally ill people. *BMJ*. 1996;313:234.

65. Coid J. The Christopher Clunis enquiry. *Psychiatric Bulletin*. 1994;18:449–52.

66. Fazel S, Buxrud P, Ruchkin V, Grann M. Homicide in discharged patients with schizophrenia and other psychoses: a national case-control study. *Schizophrenia Research*. 2010;123:263–9.

67. Large MM, Ryan CJ, Singh SP, Paton MB, Nielssen OB. The predictive value of risk categorization in schizophrenia. *Harvard Review of Psychiatry*. 2011;19:25–33.

68. Eronen M, Hakola P, Tiihonen J. Factors associated with homicide recidivism in a 13-year sample of homicide offenders in Finland. *Psychiatric Services*. 1996;47:403–6.

69. Golenkov A, Nielssen O, Large M. Systematic review and meta-analysis of homicide recidivism and schizophrenia. *BMC Psychiatry*. 2014;14:46.

70. Ormon K, Sunnqvist C, Bahtsevani C, Levander MT. Disclosure of abuse among female patients within general psychiatric care a cross sectional study. *BMC Psychiatry*. 2016;16:79.

# Index

*Note:* Tables are indicated by an italic *t* following the page number.